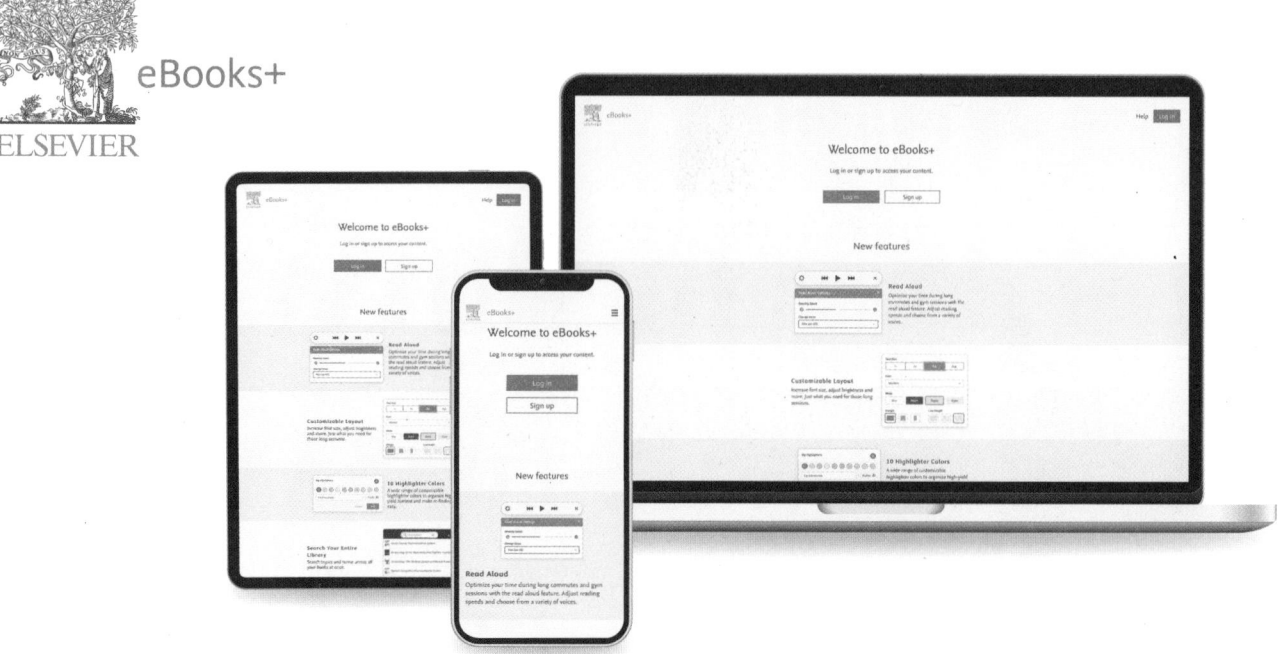

Activate your eBook today!

Elsevier eBooks+ allows you to search, browse, make notes, highlight, and have content read aloud.

1. To sign up, visit http://ebooks.health.elsevier.com/
2. Scratch to reveal your code below, and enter in **Redeem Access Code** box
3. Click **Redeem**

Contact Customer Support via
https://service.elsevier.com/app/home/supporthub/elsevierebooksplus/

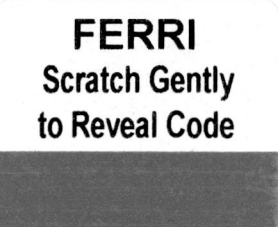

FERRI
**Scratch Gently
to Reveal Code**

2025

Ferri's CLINICAL ADVISOR

5 books in 1

FRED F. FERRI, MD, FACP

Clinical Professor
Department of Medicine
The Warren Alpert Medical School of Brown University
Providence, Rhode Island

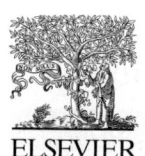

ELSEVIER

Elsevier
1600 John F. Kennedy Blvd.
Ste 1800
Philadelphia, PA 19103-2899

Notice

Practitioners and researchers must always rely on their own experience and knowledge in evaluating and using any information, methods, compounds or experiments described herein. Because of rapid advances in the medical sciences, in particular, independent verification of diagnoses and drug dosages should be made. To the fullest extent of the law, no responsibility is assumed by Elsevier, authors, editors or contributors for any injury and/or damage to persons or property as a matter of products liability, negligence or otherwise, or from any use or operation of any methods, products, instructions, or ideas contained in the material herein.

International Standard Book Number: 978-0-443-11724-4

Publisher: Sarah Barth
Senior Content Development Manager: Meghan Andress
Publishing Services Manager: Catherine Jackson
Senior Project Manager: Douglas Turner
Design Direction: Renee Duenow

Printed in Canada

Last digit is the print number: 9   8   7   6   5   4   3   2   1

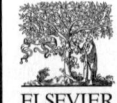
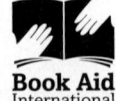

Working together
to grow libraries in
developing countries

www.elsevier.com • www.bookaid.org

Contributors

Dori Abel, MD
Division of Rheumatology
The Children's Hospital of Philadelphia
Philadelphia, PA

Rebecca A. Abelman, MD
Department of Medicine
Division of HIV, Infectious Diseases & Global Medicine
University of California, San Francisco
San Francisco, CA

Sarah Abu Kar, MD
Department of Nephrology
Vanderbilt University Medical Center
Nashville, TN

Saeed Abughazaleh, MD
Department of Internal Medicine
St. Elizabeth's Medical Center—Tufts University School of Medicine
Brighton, MA

Husam Abu-Nejim, MD
Kent Hospital Program
The Warren Alpert Medical School of Brown University
Warwick, RI

Maxwell Eyram Afari, MD
Advanced Heart Failure Attending
Cardiac Service Line
Maine Medical
Portland, ME

Hammood Ahmed, MD
Internal Medicine ABIM
Niagara Health System
St. Catharines, Ontario
Canada

Shanice Akoto, MD, MPH
Department of OB/GYN
ChristianaCare Health Services
Newark, DE

Kenneth Alabre, MD
Department of Anesthesiology
The Warren Alpert Medical School of Brown University
Providence, RI

Fahad Ali, MD
Emergency Medicine
The Warren Alpert Medical School of Brown University
Providence, RI

Tanya Ali, MD
Clinical Assistant Professor of Medicine
Department of Medicine
The Warren Alpert Medical School of Brown University
Brown University
Providence, RI

Narges Alipanah-Lechner, MD
Division of Pulmonary, Critical Care, Allergy & Sleep Medicine
University of California, San Francisco
San Francisco, CA

Erdem Altunel, MD
Division of Hematology & Oncology
Department of Medicine
UMass Chan Medical School
Worcester, MA

Lama Alzoebie, MBBS
Division of Endocrinology & Diabetes
Children's Hospital of Philadelphia
Philadelphia, PA

Chelsie Anderson, MD, MS
Department of Surgery
University of California, San Francisco
San Francisco, CA

Christine B. Andrews, MD, MPH
Department of Pediatric Gastroenterology, Hepatology & Nutrition
Hasbro Children's Hospital
Providence, RI

AnnGene Anthony, MD, MPH, FAAFP
Teaching Faculty
HMH Mountainside Family Medicine Residency Program
Assistant Professor of Family Medicine
Associate Clerkship Director/Site Director—Family Medicine Clerkship
Hackensack Meridian School of Medicine
Nutley, NJ

Paul-Hugo Arcand, BA
Department of Engineering
McGill University
Montréal, Quebec
Canada

Sohrab Arora, MD, MS, MCh
Vattikuti Urology Institute
Henry Ford Hospital
Detroit, MI

Joseph A. Asaro, DO
Attending Neonatologist
AtlantiCare Regional Medical Center
Children's Hospital of Philadelphia Newborn Care Network
Galloway, NJ

Anna Astashchanka, MD
Division of Pulmonary, Critical Care, Sleep Medicine & Physiology
UC San Diego Health
San Diego, CA

Douglas Atchison, MD, PhD
Department of Internal Medicine
Division of Nephrology
Henry Ford Health
Detroit, MI

Contributors

Sudeep K. Aulakh, MD, FACP, FRCPC
Director Ambulatory Education
Internal Medicine Residency
Department of Medicine
UMass Chan Medical School-Baystate
Springfield, MA

Taruna Aurora, MD
Hematology & Oncology
UMass Chan Medical School
Worcester, MA

Rupali Avasare, MD
Associate Professor of Medicine
Glomerular Disease Program
Division of Nephrology & Hypertension
Oregon Health & Science University
Portland, OR

Baktash Babadi, MD, PhD
Department of Psychiatry
Harvard Medical School
Massachusetts General Hospital
Harvard Medical School
Boston, MA

Tania B. Babar, MD
Department of Electrophysiology
Charleston Area Medical Center
Charleston, WV

Emelia Argyropoulos Bachman, MD, FACOG
Delaware Institute for Reproductive Medicine
Department of OB/GYN
ChristianaCare Health Services
Newark, DE

Ashika Bains, MD, MS
Department of Psychiatry
Massachusetts General Hospital
Boston, MA

Roumen Balabanov, MD
Fellowship Program Director
Division of Multiple Sclerosis & Neuroimmunology
Department of Neurology
Northwestern University Feinberg School of Medicine
Chicago, IL

Pedro Balaguera, MD
Assistant Professor of Neurology
University of Texas Health Science Center at Houston
McGovern Medical School
Houston, TX

Javier Balda, MD
Division of Cardiology
St. Elizabeth's Medical Center
Boston, MA

T. Caroline Bank, MD
Department of OB/GYN
ChristianaCare Health Services
Newark, DE

Brenda Banwell, MD
Chief of the Division of Neurology
Neurology & Pediatrics
Children's Hospital of Philadelphia
Perelman School of Medicine
University of Pennsylvania
Philadelphia, PA

Francisco J. Barrera, MD, SM
Department of Psychiatry
Massachusetts General Hospital, McLean Hospital
Harvard Medical School
Boston, MA

Samantha Barta, DO
Department of OB/GYN
ChristianaCare Health Services
Newark, DE

Craig L. Basman, MD, FACC, FSCAI
Interventional Cardiology
Cardiology/Center for Structural Heart Disease
Hackensack University Medical Center
Hackensack, NJ

Crystal T. Bass, MD
Attending Neonatologist
AtlantiCare Regional Medical Center
Children's Hospital of Philadelphia Newborn Care Network
Galloway, NJ

Scott R. Beach, MD
Psychiatrist Massachusetts General Hospital
Associate Professor of Psychiatry
Harvard Medical School
Boston, MA

Persey Bediako, MD
Cardiovascular Disease
Cardiac Service Line
Maine Medical Center
Portland, ME

Ren Belcher, MD
Lecturer in Psychiatry
Harvard Medical School
Clinical Associate
McLean Hospital
Boston, MA

Jennifer Bell, MD
Advanced Heart Failure & Transplant Specialist
Department of Cardiology
The Hartford Health Care Heart and Vascular Institute
Hartford, CT

Amy L. Bellinghausen, MD
Assistant Clinical Professor
Pulmonary, Critical Care & Sleep Medicine
University of California, San Diego
San Diego, CA

Colleen E. Bennett, MD, MSHP
Medical Director of CARE Clinics
Children's Hospital of Philadelphia
Assistant Professor, Clinical Pediatrics
Perelman School of Medicine at the University of Pennsylvania
Philadelphia, PA

Carol D. Berkowitz, MD
Division of General Pediatrics
Harbor-UCLA Medical Center
Torrance, CA

Omkar Betageri, MD
Cardiology Department
Maine Medical Center
Portland, ME

Murtaza Bharmal, MD
Interventional Cardiology
Division of Cardiology
Department of Medicine
University of California, Irvine
Orange, CA

Harikrashna B. Bhatt, MD
Assistant Professor, Clinician Educator
Division of Endocrinology
Department of Medicine
The Warren Alpert Medical School of Brown University
Providence, RI

Prachi H. Bhuptani, PhD
Rhode Island Hospital
Brown University
Providence, RI

Richard O. Bido-Medina, MD, PhD
Associate Director Hispanic Psychiatry Clinic
Director of Education & Training, Division of Public & Community
    Psychiatry
Department of Psychiatry
Massachusetts General Hospital
Harvard Medical School
Boston, MA

Kendall Bielak, MD
OB/GYN
ChristianaCare Health Services
Newark, DE

Courtney Clark Bilodeau, MD, FACP
Assistant Professor
Department of Obstetric Medicine
The Warren Alpert Medical School of Brown University
Attending Physician
Internal Medicine
Women's Medicine Collaborative
Miriam Hospital
Providence, RI

Lisa Bird, MD
Department of OB/GYN
TriHealth
Cincinnati, OH

Erin Bishop, MD
Department of OB/GYN
ChristianaCare Health Services
Newark, DE

Ghamar Bitar, MD
Maternal Fetal Medicine
The University of Texas Health Science Center at Houston (UTHealth)
Houston, TX

Craig Blakeney, MD
Emergency Medicine
University of Tennessee Health Science Center
Memphis, TN

Allison M. Blatz, MD
Division of Pediatric Critical Care
Department of Pediatrics
Nemours Children's Health
Wilmington, DE

Brian Block, MD
Assistant Professor
Associate Director Medical ICU
Pulmonary & Critical Care Medicine
University of California, San Francisco
San Francisco, CA

Christina M. Bortz, MD, FACP
Assistant Professor of Medicine
The Warren Alpert Medical School of Brown University
Attending Physician, Internal Medicine
Women's Medicine Collaborative
Providence, RI

Kristopher R. Bosse, MD
Assistant Professor of Pediatrics
Perelman School of Medicine at the University of Pennsylvania
Division of Oncology
The Children's Hospital of Philadelphia
Philadelphia, PA

Tara C. Bouton, MD, MPH, TM
Assistant Professor of Medicine
Section of Infectious Disease
Boston Medical Center
Boston University School of Medicine
Boston, MA

Mary E. Bove, MD
CHOP Care Network
Broomall, Drexell Hill, Media, PA

Lynn A. Bowlby, MD, FACP
Assistant Medical Director
Center for Primary Care
Division of General Internal Medicine
The Warren Alpert Medical School of Brown University
Providence, RI

Sean Boyden, MD
Department of Psychiatry
Massachusetts General Hospital, McLean Hospital
Boston, MA

Mark F. Brady, MD, MPH, MMSc
Assistant Professor
Department of Emergency Medicine
The Warren Alpert Medical School of Brown University
Providence, RI

Biobele Braide, MD
Department of Psychiatry
Massachusetts General Hospital, McLean Hospital
Boston, MA

Contributors

Jessica K. Brar, MD
Department of Medicine
Brown University
Providence, RI

Russell E. Bratman, MD
Assistant Professor, Clinician Educator
Division of Endocrinology
Department of Medicine
The Warren Alpert Medical School of Brown University
Providence, RI

Emily Chan Brodowsky, MD
Department of Urology – Vattikuti Urology Institute
Henry Ford Hospital
Detroit, MI

Austin K. Brown, MD
Emergency Medicine
University of Tennessee Health Science Center
Memphis, TN

Emily C. B. Brown, MD, MS
Assistant Professor of Pediatrics
Department of Pediatrics, Division of General Pediatrics
University of Washington School of Medicine
Seattle, WA

Jessalyn Brugnoni, DO
Department of Emergency Medicine
Henry Ford Hospital
Detroit, MI

Eric Bui, MD, PhD
Department of Psychiatry
University of Caen Normandy & Caen University Hospital
Caen, France

Christine Burke, MD
OB/GYN
ChristianaCare Health Services
Newark, DE

Lauren Burton, MD
Department of OB/GYN
Division of Female Pelvic Medicine & Reconstructive Surgery
Cooper University Hospital
Camden, NJ

Blythe Butler, MD
Department of Medicine
University of California, San Francisco
San Francisco, CA

William Butler, MD
Department of Psychiatry
Massachusetts General Hospital, McLean Hospital
Harvard Medical School
Boston, MA

Katerina L. Byanova, MD, MS
Department of Medicine
Division of Pulmonary, Critical Care, Allergy & Sleep Medicine
University of California, San Francisco
San Francisco, CA

Blaire Byg, MA
The Warren Alpert Medical School of Brown University
Providence, RI

Tucker C. Callanan, MD
Department of Orthopaedic Surgery
The Warren Alpert Medical School of Brown University
Providence, RI

Adriana Cantos, MD
Department of Psychiatry
Massachusetts General Hospital, McLean Hospital
Boston, MA

Katherine W. Canty, MD
Child Protection Program, Division of General Pediatrics
Boston Children's Hospital
Boston, MA

Eugene Carragee, MD
Assistant Professor
Department of Anesthesia & Perioperative Care
University of California, San Francisco
San Francisco, CA

Meredith Carrel-Lammert, MD
Department of Urogynecology
TriHealth
Cincinnati, OH

Jorge J. Castillo, MD
Associate Professor
Bing Center for Waldenström Macroglobulinemia
Dana-Farber Cancer Institute
Harvard Medical School
Boston, MA

Daniel Chait, MD, MEd
Massachusetts General Hospital, McLean Hospital
Clinical Fellow & Research Fellow
Harvard Medical School
Boston, MA

Philip A. Chan, MD, MS
Associate Professor
Department of Medicine
Brown University
Providence, RI

Arlene Chapman, MD
Professor of Medicine
Chief, Section of Nephrology
Department of Medicine
University of Chicago
Chicago, IL

Sudeshna Chatterjee-Paer, MD
Department of Gynecologic Oncology
Helen Graham Cancer Center
ChristianaCare Health Services
Newark, DE

Vicky Cheng, MD
Assistant Professor of Medicine, Clinician Educator
Division of Endocrinology
The Warren Alpert Medical School of Brown University
Providence, RI

Michael Chien, MD
Department of Urology
Henry Ford Health
Detroit, MI

Jeffrey Chilcote II, MD
Cardiovascular Medicine
St. Elizabeth's Medical Center
Brighton, MA

Candicee Childs, MD, MHA
Department of Psychiatry
Massachusetts General Hospital, McLean Hospital –
   Psychiatry Residency Program
Boston, MA

Amit Chopra, MBBS, DFAPA
Department of Psychiatry
Massachusetts General Hospital
Harvard Medical School
Boston, MA

Stella T. Chou, MD
Chief of the Division of Transfusion Medicine, Associate Professor
   of Pediatrics
Department of Pediatrics, Division of Hematology
Department of Pathology, Division of Transfusion Medicine
Children's Hospital of Philadelphia
Philadelphia, PA

Natasha Choudhury, MD
Division of Multiple Sclerosis & Neuroimmunology
Department of Neurology
Northwestern University Feinberg School of Medicine
Chicago, IL

Cindy W. Christian, MD
Professor of Pediatrics
Department of Pediatrics, Division of General Pediatrics
The Children's Hospital of Philadelphia
The Perelman School of Medicine at the University of Pennsylvania
Philadelphia, PA

Winona Chua, MD
Clinical Associate Professor of Pediatrics
Perelman School of Medicine
University of Pennsylvania
Attending Physician
Department of Pediatrics
Children's Hospital of Philadelphia
Philadelphia, PA

Andrew S. Chun, MD, MPH
Department of Psychiatry
Massachusetts General Hospital, McLean Hospital
Boston, MA

David Claman, MD
Professor of Medicine & Medical Director of Sleep Disorders Center
Division of Pulmonary, Critical Care, Allergy & Sleep Medicine
University of California, San Francisco
San Francisco, CA

Grace V. Clark, MD, BA
OB/GYN
ChristianaCare Health Services
Newark, DE

Seth Clark, MD, MPH, FASAM
Assistant Professor
Department of Medicine
Department of Psychiatry & Human Behavior
The Warren Alpert Medical School of Brown University
Providence, RI

Ross Clarke, ScM, BA
Brown University
Providence, RI

Alexandra Clay, MD
Department of Psychiatry
Massachusetts General Hospital, McLean Hospital – Psychiatry Residency
   Program
Boston, MA

Karl T. Clebak, MD, MHA, FAAFP
Associate Professor, Program Director
Department of Family & Community Medicine Residency Program
Penn State Health Milton S. Hershey Medical Center
Hershey, PA

Derrick Cleland, DO, MPH
Riverside University Health
Department of Medicine
Loma Linda University Health
Loma Linda, CA

Debbie L. Cohen, MD
Professor of Medicine
Division of Renal-Electrolyte & Hypertension
Department of Internal Medicine
Hospital of the University of Pennsylvania
Philadelphia, PA

Lisa Cohen, PharmD
Professor of Pharmacy
Department of Pharmacy Practice
University of Rhode Island, College of Pharmacy
Kingston, RI

Morgan Congdon, MD, MPH, MSEd
Clinical Assistant Professor of Pediatrics
Children's Hospital of Philadelphia
Philadelphia, PA

Maria Constantinou, MD
Medical Oncologist
Lifespan Cancer Institute
Providence, RI

James Elliott Cooper, MD
Emergency Medicine
University of Tennessee Health Science Center
Memphis, TN

James Earl Corley, MD
Assistant Professor of Emergency Medicine & Internal Medicine
Emergency Medicine & Internal Medicine
University of Tennessee Health Sciences Center
Memphis, TN

Abigail Cosgrove, MD
Assistant Professor
Emergency Medicine
University of Tennessee Health Science Center
Memphis, TN

Oscar Covarrubias, BS
Department of Orthopaedics
Division of Shoulder & Elbow
The Warren Alpert Medical School of Brown University
Providence, RI

Rebecca Craine, MSEd, CCC-SLP
Speech Language Pathologist, Rehabilitation
Bradley Hospital
East Providence, RI

Sarah Criddle, MD
Department of Orthopaedics
Brown University
Providence, RI

Patricia Cristofaro, MD
Assistant Professor
Department of Infectious Diseases
The Warren Alpert Medical School of Brown University
Providence, RI

Joanne Szczygiel Cunha, MD
Director, Rheumatology Fellowship Program
Assistant Professor of Medicine
Division of Rheumatology
The Warren Alpert Medical School of Brown University
Brown Medicine
Providence Veterans Affairs Medical Center
Providence, RI

Karlene Cunningham, PhD
Clinical Associate Professor
Department of Psychiatry & Behavioral Medicine
Brody School of Medicine at East Carolina University
Greenville, NC

Joseph Cusano, MD
Department of Orthopaedic Surgery
Rhode Island Hospital
Brown University
Providence, RI

Frank B. D'Alessandro, MD
Endocrinologist
Providence, RI

Lynn Dado, MD
Primary Care Physician
Internal Medicine
Henry Ford Health System
Bloomfield Hills, MI

Shanaz Daneshdoost, MD
Department of Pediatrics
Children's Hospital of Philadelphia
Philadelphia, PA

Nicholas Omid Daneshvari, MD
Department of Psychiatry
Massachusetts General Hospital, McLean Hospital
Boston, MA

Sabrina Darwiche, MD, MPH
Division of General Pediatrics
Children's Hospital of Philadelphia
Philadelphia, PA

Abhijit Das, MD
Child Neurology
Department of Pediatrics
Baylor College of Medicine
Houston, TX

Manuel F. DaSilva, MD
Associate Professor
Department of Orthopaedics
The Warren Alpert Medical School of Brown University
Providence, RI

Carlos De La Garza, MD
Adult Neurology
Baylor College of Medicine
Houston, TX

Alison DeDent, MD
Assistant Professor
Division of Pulmonary & Critical Care Medicine
University of California, San Francisco
San Francisco, CA

Mery Deeb, MD
Internal Medicine
The Warren Alpert Medical School of Brown University
Providence, RI

John W. Denninger, MD, PhD
Director of Research & Clinical Training
Benson-Henry Institute for Mind Body Medicine
Department of Psychiatry
Massachusetts General Hospital
Harvard Medical School
Boston, MA

Colette Desrochers, MD
Children's Hospital of Philadelphia Primary Care Attending Physician
Clinical Associate Professor of Pediatrics
Perelman School of Medicine at the University of Pennsylvania
Philadelphia, PA

Erin Pete Devon, MD, MSEd
Pediatric Hospital Medicine Physician
Division of General Pediatrics
Children's Hospital of Philadelphia
Philadelphia, PA

Joseph A. Diaz, MD, MPH
Associate Dean for Diversity & Multicultural Affairs
Associate Professor of Medicine & Medical Science
The Warren Alpert Medical School of Brown University
Providence, RI

Kyle DiGrande, MD
Department of Medicine
University of California, Irvine Medical Center
Orange, CA

Ayodeji Dina, MD, FRACP
Electrophysiology
Division of Cardiology
St. Elizabeth's Medical Center
Boston, MA

Kathleen Doo, MD, MHPE
Associate Program Director, Pulmonary & Critical Care Medicine
  Fellowship
Department of Pulmonary
Kaiser Permanente Northern California
Oakland, CA

Brian Drury, MD
Department of Emergency Medicine
The Warren Alpert Medical School of Brown University
Providence, RI

Bethany Dus, MD, MSc
OB/GYN
ChristianaCare Health Services
Newark, DE

Roop Dutta, MD
Clinical Electrophysiology
Division of Cardiology
St. Elizabeth's Medical Center
Boston, MA

Myles Dworkin, MD, MPH
Department of Orthopaedics
Brown University
Providence, RI

Timothy G. Dyster, MD
Division of Pulmonary, Critical Care & Sleep Medicine
University of California, San Francisco
San Francisco, CA

Eric Ebert, MD
Department of Emergency Medicine
Brown Emergency Medicine
Providence, RI

Joseph Edmund, MD
Hematologist Oncologist
Department of Internal Medicine, Division of Hematology & Oncology
Marshfield Clinic
Marshfield, WI

Heather L. Edward, MD
Child Abuse Pediatrics
Department of Pediatrics
The Warren Alpert Medical School of Brown University
Providence, RI

Erica Eggers, MD
Female Pelvic Medicine & Reconstructive Surgery
Department of OB/GYN
Cooper University Hospital
Camden, NJ

Christine Eisenhower, PharmD
Clinical Associate Professor
Pharmacy Practice
University of Rhode Island
Kingston, RI

Pamela Ellsworth, MD
Division of Pediatric Urology
Nemours Children's Hospital Orlando
Orlando, FL

Radowan Elnair, MD
Consultant, Bone Marrow Transplant & Cellular therapy
Department of Internal Medicine
Division of Hematology & Oncology
Roger Williams Medical Center
Providence, RI

César E. Escamilla-Ocañas, MD
Education Chief Resident
Department of Neurology
Baylor College of Medicine
Houston, TX

Patricio Sebastian Espinosa, MD, MPH, FAAN
Chief of Neurology & Institute Director
Neurology
The Espinosa Neuroscience Institute
Boca Raton, FL

Mark D. Faber, MD, MACM
Division of Nephrology & Hypertension
Henry Ford Hospital
Associate Professor
Internal Medicine
Wayne State University School of Medicine
Detroit, MI

Evan Facer, DO
Assistant Professor of Pediatrics
Division of Infectious Diseases
Washington University School of Medicine
St. Louis, MO

Paul D. Fadale, MD
Chief of Sports Medicine
Department of Orthopaedic Surgery
Brown University, University Orthopaedics
Providence, RI

Ryan T. Fallon, MD
Department of Orthopaedics
Brown University/Lifespan
Providence, RI

Michael J. Farias, BS
Orthopedic Surgery
The Warren Alpert Medical School of Brown University
Providence, RI

Jon Farkas, MD
Pediatric Hospital Medicine Attending
Pediatrics
NYU School of Medicine
New York, NY

Erica Farrand, MD
Assistant Professor
Division of Pulmonary & Critical Care Medicine
University of California, San Francisco
San Francisco, CA

Ronan Farrell, MD
Division of Gastroenterology
Brown University
Providence, RI

Kevin S. Fay, MD
Assistant Professor of Clinical Medicine
Division of Renal-Electrolyte & Hypertension
Department of Internal Medicine
Penn Presbyterian Medical Center
Philadelphia, PA

Robert Zachary Fender, MD, MSCI
OB/GYN
ChristianaCare Health Services
Newark, DE

Samantha Fernandez Hernandez, MD
Baylor College of Medicine
Houston, TX

Contributors

Carlos Fernandez-Robles, MD, MBA
Chief of Psychiatry
Brigham & Women's Faulkner Hospital
Vice-Chair of BWFH
Brigham & Women's Hospital
Boston, MA

Jason D. Ferreira, MD
Clinical Assistant Professor of Medicine
Brown University
Gastroenterology
University Gastroenterology
LLC/Miriam Hospital
Providence, RI

Fred F. Ferri, MD, FACP
Clinical Professor
Department of Medicine
The Warren Alpert Medical School of Brown University
Providence, RI

Heather Ferri, DO
Department of Medicine
Rhode Island Hospital
The Warren Alpert Medical School of Brown University
Providence, RI

Jessica C. Fields, MD
Maternal-Fetal Medicine Physician
Delaware Center for Maternal-Fetal Medicine
ChristianaCare Health Services
Newark, DE

Lauren Fields, MD
Psychiatry
Massachusetts General Hospital, McLean Hospital
Boston, MA

Staci A. Fischer, MD
Accreditation Council for Graduate Medical Education
Chicago, IL

Hannah Fiske, MD
Internal Medicine
Brown University
Providence, RI

Maria Camila Velez Florez, MD
Massachusetts General Hospital, McLean Hospital
Clinical Fellow & Research Fellow
Harvard Medical School
Boston, MA

Kellie C. Forbes, MD
Department of OB/GYN
ChristianaCare Health Services
Newark, DE

Michelle Forcier, MD, MPH
Professor Pediatrics
Assistant Dean of Admissions
The Warren Alpert Medical School of Brown University
Providence, RI

Sydney Ford, MD, MPH
Department of OB/GYN
ChristianaCare Health Services
Newark, DE

Frank G. Fort, MD, FACS, RPHS
Medical Director
Capital Region Vein Centre
Schenectady, NY

Glenn G. Fort, MD, MPH
Clinical Associate Professor of Medicine
Division of Infectious Diseases
The Warren Alpert Medical School of Brown University
Providence, RI

Eitan S. Frankel, MD
Cardiac Electrophysiology, Division of Cardiology
Thomas Jefferson University Hospital
Philadelphia, PA

Nancy Freeman, MD
Chief, Hematology & Oncology
Department of Medicine
Providence VA Medical Center
Providence, RI

Ryan Friedman, MD
Department of Medicine
Oregon Health & Science University
Portland, OR

Daniel R. Frisch, MD
Associate Professor
Division of Cardiology
Thomas Jefferson University
Philadelphia, PA

Relindis Azenwi Fru, MD
Hematology & Oncology
Doctors Hospital at Renaissance
Edinburg, TX

Lynn C. Fullenkamp, MD, JD
Assistant Professor
Pediatric Hospital Medicine & Child Advocacy Team
Children's Hospital & Medical Center
University of Nebraska Medical Center
Omaha, NE

Michael Gaffney, MD
Developmental & Behavioral Pediatrics
Boston Children's Hospital
Boston, MA

Jose P. Garcia, MD
Division of Rheumatology
Rhode Island Hospital
Brown University
Providence, RI

Paloma Jolin Garcia, MD
Division of Human Genetics
The Children's Hospital of Philadelphia & Perelman School
   of Medicine of the University of Pennsylvania
Philadelphia, PA

Jonathan S. Ge, ScB
Brown University
Providence, RI

Yaron B. Gesthalter, MD
Associate Professor of Medicine
Division of Pulmonary & Critical Care Medicine
University of California, San Francisco
San Francisco, CA

Anil Ghimire, MD
Interim Division Chief
Pulmonary, Critical Care & Sleep Medicine
Assistant Director, Faculty Development
Director, Adult CF Program
Associate Clinical Professor of Medicine
University of California, San Francisco – Fresno
Fresno, CA

Christopher Gibson, MD
Pediatric Endocrinologist
Division of Endocrinology & Diabetes
Children's Hospital of Philadelphia
Philadelphia, PA

Nisha H. Gidwani, MD
Associate Professor of Clinical Medicine
Department of Medicine
Division of Pulmonary, Critical Care, Allergy & Sleep Medicine
University of California, San Francisco
San Francisco, CA

Katarzyna Gilek-Seibert, MD
Program Director
Division of Rheumatology
Roger Williams Medical Center
Providence, RI

Vinit J. Gilvaz, MD
The Warren Alpert Medical School of Brown University
Providence, RI

Jacob Glueck, BA
Department of Orthopaedics
The Warren Alpert Medical School of Brown University
Providence, RI

Jennifer Leah Goetz, MD
Psychiatry/Child & Adolescent Psychiatry
Massachusetts General Hospital, McLean Hospital
Harvard Medical School
Boston & Belmont, MA

Alla Goldburt, MD
Assistant Clinical Professor
Family Medicine
The Warren Alpert Medical School of Brown University
Providence, RI

Corey Elam Goldsmith, MD, FAAN
Associate Professor of Neurology
Baylor College of Medicine
Houston, TX

Maheswara Satya Gangadhara Rao Golla, MD
Interventional Cardiology
Parkersburg Cardiology Associates
Camden Clark Medical Center
Parkersburg, WV

Alexander Gomez, MD
Assistant Clinical Professor
Division of Pulmonary, Critical Care, Allergy & Sleep Medicine
University of California, San Francisco
San Francisco, CA

Helen B. Gomez Slagle, MD
Maternal-Fetal Medicine
Columbia Irving Medical Center
New York, NY

H. Karl Greenblatt, MD
Division of Rheumatology
Roger Williams Medical Center
Providence, RI

Morgan Greenfield, MD
General Pediatrics
Children's Hospital of Philadelphia
Assistant Professor of Pediatrics
Perelman School of Medicine
University of Pennsylvania
Philadelphia, PA

Lindsay Gugerty, DO
Department of OB/GYN
ChristianaCare Health Services
Newark, DE

Patan Gultawatvichai, MD
Assistant Professor of Medicine
UMass Chan Medical School
Worcester, MA

Samantha Gunning, MD
Assistant Professor of Medicine
Department of Nephrology
The University of Chicago Medicine
Chicago, IL

David Guo, MD
Affiliate Clinical Assistant Professor
Department of Urology
Stanford Medical School
Kaiser Santa Clara Medical Center
Santa Clara, CA

Simran Gupta, MD
Department of Internal Medicine
Brown University
Providence, RI

Brittany Guttadauria, MD
Department of Emergency Medicine, Division of Pediatrics
Children's Hospital of Philadelphia
Philadelphia, PA

Meghan Gwinn, MD
Department of Nephrology
University of Chicago Medical Center
Chicago, IL

Mohanad Hadi, MD
Department of Rheumatology
Roger Williams Medical Center
Providence, RI

Contributors

Muhammad Ubaid Hafeez, MD
Assistant Professor of Neurology
University of Texas Medical Branch
Galveston, TX

Hayden Hall, DO
Department of Neurology
Baylor College of Medicine
Houston, TX

Sarah Hall, MD
Department of OB/GYN
ChristianaCare Health Services
Newark, DE

Sajeev Handa, MD, SFHM
Chief, Hospital Medicine
Lifespan Physician Group
Rhode Island Hospital
Clinical Assistant Professor of Medicine
Clinical Assistant Professor of Neurology
The Warren Alpert Medical School of Brown University
Providence, RI

John R. Hanna, MD
Department of Orthopaedics
Rhode Island Hospital
Brown University
Providence, RI

Nikolas Harbord, MD
Nephrologist/Internist
Private Practice
Ormond Beach, FL

Kyle Hardacker, MD
Orthopedic Surgery
Brown University
Providence, RI

Anna Hardesty, MD
Department of Infectious Diseases
University of California, Los Angeles
Los Angeles, CA

Nirav Haribhakti, MD, PharmD
Department of Internal Medicine
Rhode Island Hospital
The Warren Alpert Medical School of Brown University
Providence, RI

Daniel J. Harris, MD
Department of Psychiatry
Massachusetts General Hospital
Boston, MA

Abigail Hartmann, MD
OB/GYN
ChristianaCare Health Services
Newark, DE

Davis A. Hartnett, MD
Department of Internal Medicine
Brigham & Women's Hospital
Boston, MA

Nathan Hartvigsen, MD
Harvard Medical School Instructor in Psychiatry
Massachusetts General Hospital
Boston, MA

Brian Hawkins, MD
Assistant Professor
Emergency Medicine
University of Tennessee Health Science Center
Memphis, TN

Elaine He, BA
Brown University
Providence, RI

Rachel Wright Heinle, MD, FACOG
Department of OB/GYN
ChristianaCare Health Services
Newark, DE

Leesha A. Helm, MD, MPH
Assistant Professor of Family & Community Medicine
Penn State Hershey Medical Center
Hershey, PA

Matthew F. Helm, MD
Assistant Professor of Dermatology
Penn State Hershey Medical Center
Hershey, PA

Thomas Herlevich, MD
Emergency Medicine
University of Tennessee Health Science Center
Memphis, TN

Klodia M. Hermez, DO
Division of Nephrology & Hypertension
Henry Ford Hospital
Detroit, MI

Ross W. Hilliard, MD, FACP
Internal Medicine Residency Director
Maine Medical Center
Tufts University School of Medicine
Portland, ME

Nathaniel Hocker, MD
Nephrology
Oregon Health & Science University
Portland, OR

R. Scott Hoffman, MD
Assistant Clinical Professor
University of Louisville School of Medicine
Doctors Eye Institute & U of L Ophthalmology
Louisville, KY

Siri M. Holton, MD
Department of OB/GYN
ChristianaCare Health Services
Newark, DE

Alexander S. Homer, AB
Department of Emergency Medicine
The Warren Alpert Medical School of Brown University
Providence, RI

Benjamin E. Hook, MD
Department of Emergency Medicine
University of Tennessee Health Science Center
Memphis, TN

Raymond Hsu, MD
Department of Orthopaedic Surgery
Brown University
Providence, RI

Laurence Huang, MD, FCCP, ATSF
Professor of Medicine
Chief, HIV/AIDS Chest Clinic, Zuckerberg San Francisco General Hospital
 & Trauma Center
Division of HIV, Infectious Diseases & Global Medicine
Division of Pulmonary, Critical Care, Allergy & Sleep Medicine
University of California, San Francisco
San Francisco, CA

Mariam Hull, MD
Assistant Professor
Pediatric Movement Disorders Clinic
Section of Child Neurology & Neurodevelopmental Disabilities
Texas Children's Hospital – Baylor College of Medicine
Houston, TX

Anne L. Hume, PharmD
Professor of Pharmacy
Department of Pharmacy Practice
University of Rhode Island
Kingston, RI

Zilla Hussain, MD
Gastroenterology
Greater Baltimore Medical Center
Baltimore, MD

Donny V. Huynh, MD
Hematologist & Oncologist
McLeod Oncology & Hematology Associates
McLeod Regional Medical Center
Little River, SC

Sarah Hyder, MD, MBA
Director of Endoscopy
U Mass Memorial Medical Center
Worcester, MA

Caitlin Ingraham, MD
Department of OB/GYN
ChristianaCare Health Services
Newark, DE

Louis F. Insalaco, MD
Department of Otolaryngology
Mass Eye & Ear, Stoneham
Harvard Medical School
Stoneham, MA

James Jackson, MD
Emergency Medicine
University of Tennessee, Memphis
Memphis, TN

Shadi Jafari-Esfahani, MD
Division of Rheumatology
Roger Williams Medical Center
Providence, RI

Rishubh Jain, BA
Department of Orthopaedics
The Warren Alpert Medical School of Brown University
Providence, RI

Vanita B. D. Jain, MD
Clinical Faculty
Division of Maternal Fetal Medicine
ChristianaCare Health Services
Newark, DE

Vipul V. Jain, MD, MS
Interim Chief, UCSF Fresno Department of Medicine
Vice Chair, UCSF Department of Medicine
Professor of Clinical Medicine
University of California, San Francisco – Fresno
Fresno, CA

Fariha Jamal, MD
Assistant Professor of Neurology
Baylor College of Medicine
Michael E. DeBakey VA Medical Center
Houston, TX

Robert H. Janigian Jr., MD
Clinical Associate Professor of Surgery
The Warren Alpert Medical School of Brown University
Providence, RI

Sonia Jasuja, MD
Assistant Clinical Professor
Division of Pulmonary, Critical Care & Sleep Medicine
University of California, Los Angeles
Los Angeles, CA

Noelle Marie Javier, MD
Associate Professor
Brookdale Department of Geriatrics & Palliative Medicine
Icahn School of Medicine at Mount Sinai
New York, NY

Nishant Jayachandran, BA
Department of Orthopaedic Surgery
Brown University
Providence, RI

Vybhav Jetty, MD, MHA
Electrophysiology
Department of Cardiovascular Medicine
Saint Elizabeth's Medical Center
Boston, MA

Michael P. Johnson, MD
MDVIP-Affiliated Physician
Providence, RI

Steven D. Johnson, MD
Department of OB/GYN
TriHealth
Cincinnati, OH

Amanda Jones, MD
Department of OB/GYN
ChristianaCare Health Services
Newark, DE

Tatiana Joseph, MD
Department of Cardiology
St. Elizabeth Medical Center
Brighton, MA

Ganaelle Joseph-Senatus, MD
Department of Psychiatry
Massachusetts General Hospital
Boston, MA

Shyam Joshi, MD
Associate Professor of Medicine
Section of Allergy & Immunology
Oregon Health & Science University
Portland, OR

Joshua Justice, MD
Assistant Professor
Department of Emergency Medicine
University of Tennessee Health Science Center
Memphis, TN

Sohaip Kabashneh, MD
Hematology & Oncology
UMass Chan Medical School
Worcester, MA

Vishnu Kadiyala, MD
Division of Cardiology
The Warren Alpert Medical School of Brown University
Providence, RI

Markos Kalligeros, MD
Department of Internal Medicine
The Warren Alpert Medical School of Brown University
Providence, RI

Vanji Karthikeyan, MD
Division of Nephrology
Henry Ford Hospital
Detroit, MI

Erika Kaske, MD
Department of Psychiatry
Massachusetts General Hospital, McLean Hospital
Harvard Medical School
Boston, MA

Vania Kasper, MD
Associate Professor
Department of Pediatric Gastroenterology, Hepatology & Nutrition
Hasbro Children's Hospital
Providence, RI

Joseph S. Kass, MD, JD, FAAN
Associate Dean of Student Affairs
Professor of Neurology, Psychiatry & Medical Ethics
Director, Alzheimer's Disease & Memory Disorders Center
Baylor College of Medicine
Chief of Neurology
Director of Comprehensive Stroke Program
Ben Taub General Hospital
Houston, TX

Naomi R. Kass, BA
Baylor College of Medicine
Houston, TX

Viknesh S. Kasthuri, AB
The Warren Alpert Medical School of Brown University
Providence, RI

Luca Katz, BA
The Warren Alpert Medical School of Brown University
Providence, RI

Vera Kazakova, MD
Division of Hematology & Medical Oncology
UMass Chan Medical School
Worcester, MA

Jennifer L. Keim, MD, MPH
Clinical Assistant Professor of Pediatrics
CHOP Karabots Pediatric Care Center
Perelman School of Medicine, University of Pennsylvania
Philadelphia, PA

Nicholas Kensey, DO
The Warren Alpert Medical School of Brown University
Providence, RI

Victoria Kent, BS
The Warren Alpert Medical School of Brown University
Providence, RI

Danielle Kerrigan, MD
Department of Emergency Medicine
The Warren Alpert Medical School of Brown University
Providence, RI

Dennis Keselman, MD
Neurology
Children's Hospital of Philadelphia
Philadelphia, PA

Sarthak Khare, MD
Division of Cardiology
St. Elizabeth's Medical Center
Boston, MA

Surya Khatri, BA
Department of Orthopaedic Surgery
Brown University
Providence, RI

Hussain R. Khawaja, MD, FACP
Associate Professor of Medicine
Clinician Educator
The Warren Alpert Medical School of Brown University
Division of General Internal Medicine
Department of Medicine
Rhode Island Hospital
Providence, RI

Saranya S. Khurana, MD, MPH
Department of Psychiatry
Massachusetts General Hospital
Boston, MA

Betelhem Kifle, MD
San Francisco VA Medical Center
University of California, San Francisco
San Francisco, CA

Chan Woo Kim, MD
Internal Medicine
Rhode Island Hospital Program
Brown University
Providence, RI

Jinseong Kim, MD
Department of Orthopaedics
The Warren Alpert Medical School of Brown University
Providence, RI

Samantha Kisare, MD
Department of Pediatrics
The Children's Hospital of Philadelphia
Philadelphia, PA

Samuel I. Kohrman, MD
Department of Psychiatry
Massachusetts General Hospital
Boston, MA

Aravind Rao Kokkirala, MD, FACC
Division of Cardiology
Department of Medicine
The Warren Alpert Medical School of Brown University
Providence Veterans Affairs Medical Center
Providence, RI

Yuval Konstantino, MD
Cardiac Electrophysiology & Pacing Unit
Department of Cardiology
Soroka University Medical Center
Beersheba, Israel

Nicholas Kontos, MD
Director, Fellowship in Consultation-Liaison Psychiatry
Department of Psychiatry
Massachusetts General Hospital
Boston, MA

Nelson Kopyt, DO
Clinical Professor of Medicine
Nephrology
Lehigh Valley Hospital
Morsani College of Medicine
Allentown, PA

Savan Kothadia, MD
Gastroenterology Department
Rhode Island Hospital
Providence, RI

Ajay S. Koti, MD
Department of Pediatrics, Division of General Pediatrics
University of Washington School of Medicine
Seattle, WA

Ioannis Koulouridis, MD, MSc
Consultant in Cardiology & Cardiac Electrophysiology
Department of Medicine
Division of Cardiology
King Faisal Specialist Hospital & Research Center
Jeddah, Makkah
Saudi Arabia

Timothy R. Kreider, MD, PhD
Assistant Professor & Director of Undergraduate Medical Education in
    Psychiatry
Department of Psychiatry
Donald and Barbara Zucker School of Medicine at Hofstra/Northwell
Hempstead, NY

Kevin Kron, MD
Department of Pediatrics
Oregon Health & Science University
Portland, OR

Ilana Krumm, MD
Division of Pulmonary, Critical Care, Allergy & Sleep Medicine
Department of Medicine
University of California, San Francisco
San Francisco, CA

Elizabeth Kuhn, MD
General Pediatrics
Children's Hospital of Philadelphia
Philadelphia, PA

Lalathaksha Kumbar, MD
Division of Nephrology & Hypertension
Henry Ford Hospital
Detroit, MI

Sheng-Han Kuo, MD
H. Houston Merritt Associate Professor
Department of Neurology
Columbia University
New York, NY

Eren O. Kuris, MD
Assistant Professor
Department of Orthopaedic Surgery
The Warren Alpert Medical School of Brown University
Providence, RI

David I. Kurss, MD, FACOG, NCMP
Women's Wellness Center of Western New York
Invision Health
Amherst, NY;
Clinical Assistant Professor
School of Medicine
Department of OB/GYN
State University of New York at Buffalo
Buffalo, NY

Michael J. Kutschke, MD
Department of Orthopaedic Surgery
Brown University
Providence, RI

William F. Laband, MBBS, BSc (Hons)
Department of Medicine
St. Elizabeth's Medical Center
Boston, MA

Philip LaCombe, MD
Cardiac Service Line
Maine Medical Center
Portland, ME

Uyen T. Lam, MD
Division of Cardiology
St. Elizabeth's Medical Center
Boston, MA

Wilson Lam, MD
Associate Professor, Departments of Internal Medicine & Pediatrics
Baylor College of Medicine
Combined Adult-Pediatric Cardiology/Clinical Cardiac Electrophysiology
Texas Children's Hospital–Texas Adult Congenital Heart Center
Houston, TX

Jonathan Laredo, BS
Research Associate
Department of Trauma & Critical Care Surgery
University of Tennessee Medical Center
Knoxville, TN

Contributors

Mary Larijani, MD
Assistant Professor of Pediatrics
Attending Physician
Dermatology Section
Department of Pediatrics
Perelman School of Medicine
Children's Hospital of Philadelphia
Philadelphia, PA

Peter Le, MD
Pulmonary & Critical Care
Kaiser Permanente Oakland Medical Center
Department of Pulmonary Medicine
The Permanente Medical Group
Oakland, CA

Caroline Leahy, MD
General Pediatrics
The Children's Hospital of Philadelphia
Philadelphia, PA

Lorriana E. Leard, MD
Professor of Clinical Medicine
Associate Dean, Continuing Medical Education, UCSF School of Medicine
Vice Chief, Clinical Operations
Division of Pulmonary, Critical Care, Allergy & Sleep Medicine
University of California, San Francisco
San Francisco, CA

David A. Leavitt, MD
Vattikuti Urology Institute
Henry Ford Hospital
Detroit, MI

Christopher T. Leba, MD, MPH
Pulmonary & Critical Care Medicine Physician
Department of Pulmonary, Critical Care & Sleep Medicine
Kaiser Permanente North Valley
Sacramento, CA

Hyung Jin Lee, MS4
The Warren Alpert Medical School of Brown University
Providence, RI

Kachiu C. Lee, MD, MPH
Cosmetic Dermatologist & Laser Specialist
Main Line Center for Laser Surgery
Ardmore, PA

Tracy Leigh LeGros, MD, PhD
Emergency Medicine
University of Tennessee, Memphis
Memphis, TN

Nicholas J. Lemme, MD
Department of Orthopaedic Surgery
The Warren Alpert Medical School of Brown University
Providence, RI

Nathan L'Etoile, MD
Division of Pediatric Infectious Diseases
Children's Hospital of Philadelphia
Philadelphia, PA

Jian Li, MD, PhD
Internal Medicine
Division of Hypertension & Nephrology
Henry Ford Hospital
Detroit, MI

Carol Lim, MD, MPH
Department of Psychiatry
Massachusetts General Hospital
Harvard Medical School
Boston, MA

Chi-Ying (Roy) Lin, MD, MPH
Assistant Professor of Neurology
Director, CurePSP Center of Care for PSP, CBD, & MSA
Department of Neurology
Baylor College of Medicine
Houston, TX

Jordan Lippincott, MD
Department of Emergency Medicine
University of Tennessee Health Science Center
Memphis, TN

Jonathan Liu, MD
Department of Orthopaedic Surgery
Brown University
Providence, RI

Teresa C. Logue, MD, MPH
Department of OB/GYN
ChristianaCare Health Services
Newark, DE

Riley Longtain, MD
Department of Psychiatry
Massachusetts General Hospital, McLean Hospital
Harvard Medical School
Boston, MA

Gabriela López, PhD
Department of Behavioral & Social Sciences
Brown University School of Public Health
Providence, RI

Kito Akin Lord, MD, MBA
Assistant Professor
Department of Emergency Medicine
University of Tennessee Health Science Center
Memphis, TN

Kirsten Loscalzo, MD
Division of Internal Medicine
The Warren Alpert Medical School of Brown University
Providence, RI

Mathew J. Lucas, MD
Department of General Pediatrics
The Children's Hospital of Philadelphia
Philadelphia, PA

David J. Lucier Jr., MD, MBA, MPH
Director of Quality & Patient Safety, Hospital Medicine
Division of General Internal Medicine
Massachusetts General Hospital
Boston, MA

Marwan Ma'ayeh, MD
Maternal-Fetal Medicine
ChristianaCare Health Services
Newark, DE

Rachel L. MacLean, MD
Department of Psychiatry
Massachusetts General Hospital
Boston, MA

Maeve G. MacMurdo, MBChB, MPH
Respiratory Institute
Cleveland Clinic
Cleveland, OH

Elizabeth N. Madva, MD
Associate Program Director
Massachusetts General Hospital, McLean Hospital
Psychiatry Residency
Department of Psychiatry
Massachusetts General Hospital
Boston, MA

Lewena Maher, MD
Assistant Professor of Rheumatology
The Warren Alpert Medical School of Brown University
Providence, RI

Gretchen Makai, MD
Director, Division of Minimally Invasive Gynecologic Surgery
Department of OB/GYN
ChristianaCare Health Services
Newark, DE

Luis Malpica, MD
Assistant Professor
Department of Lymphoma & Myeloma, Division of Cancer Medicine
The University of Texas MD Anderson Cancer Center
Houston, TX

Jonathan Marks, MD
Department of Emergency Medicine
The University of Tennessee Health Science Center
Memphis, TN

Ana Paula Marques Pinheiro, MD
Department of Psychiatry
Massachusetts General Hospital, McLean Hospital
Clinical Fellow
Harvard Medical School
Boston, MA

Mollie C. Marr, MD, PhD
Department of Psychiatry
Massachusetts General Hospital
Boston, MA;
Department of Psychiatry
McLean Hospital
Belmont, MA

Adali Martinez, MD, MPH
Division of Pulmonary, Critical Care, Allergy & Sleep Medicine
University of California, San Francisco
San Francisco, CA

Adiba Matin, MD
Emergency Medicine
Mayo Clinic
Rochester, MN

Peter J. Mazzaglia, MD
Associate Professor of Surgery
The Warren Alpert Medical School of Brown University
Providence, RI

Nadine N. Mbuyi, MD
Assistant Professor of Medicine
Department of Medicine
Washington, DC

Russell J. McCulloh, MD
Professor
Pediatrics
University of Nebraska Medical Center
Omaha, NE

Donna M. McDonald-McGinn, MS, LCGC
Professor of Clinical Pediatrics
Director, 22q and You Center
Chief, Section of Genetic Counseling
Associate Director, Clinical Genetics Center
Research Scientist
The Children's Hospital of Philadelphia
Perelman School of Medicine of the University of Pennsylvania
Philadelphia, PA

Alexandra McGowen, MD
Clinical Faculty
Emergency Medicine
University of Tennessee
Memphis, TN

Katherine Elizabeth McGraw, MD
Pediatrician
Children's Hospital & Medical Center
Omaha, NE

Jaclyn McKenna, MD
Assistant Attending Physician
Primary Care Sports Medicine
Hospital for Special Surgery
White Plains, NY

Kelly McNamara, MD
Attending Physician & Associate Program Director
OB/GYN
ChristianaCare Health Services
Newark, DE

Kapil S. Meleveedu, MD
Director, Blood & Marrow, Transplant & Head, Malignant Hematology
Carole & Ray Neag Comprehensive Cancer Center University of
  Connecticut
Farmington, CT

Megan Mendez-Miller, DO
Associate Professor
Medical Director–Family & Community Medicine Inpatient Service
Department of Family & Community Medicine
Penn State Health Milton S. Hershey Medical Center
Hershey, PA

Jorge Mercado, MD
Associate Professor of Medicine
NYU School of Medicine
Director of Pulmonary Medicine
Director of Bronchoscopy
Associate Chief of Pulmonary & Critical Care Medicine
NYU Langone Brooklyn
Brooklyn, NY

Osvaldo Mercado, MD
Fellow, Department of Biomedical Health & Informatics, Division of
  Neonatology
Hospital of the University of Pennsylvania
Children's Hospital of Philadelphia
Philadelphia, PA

Rory Merritt, MD, MEHP
Assistant Dean of Medicine—PLME Advising
Assistant Professor of Emergency Medicine
The Warren Alpert Medical School of Brown University
Providence, RI

Marian G. Michaels, MD, MPH
Professor of Pediatrics & Surgery
Division of Infectious Diseases
Children's Hospital of Pittsburgh of UPMC
Pittsburgh, PA

Jeremy Michel, MD, MHS
Assistant Professor of Pediatrics
The Perelman School of Medicine
University of Pennsylvania
Philadelphia, PA

Brian D. Mikolasko, MD
Assistant Professor
Department of Medicine
The Warren Alpert Medical School of Brown University
Providence, RI

John D. Milner, MD
Department of Orthopaedic Surgery
The Warren Alpert Medical School of Brown University
Providence, RI

May Min, MD
Department of Gastroenterology
Brown University
Providence, RI

Taro Minami, MD
Director, Intensive Care Unit
Kent Hospital;
Director of Medical Simulation & Point-of-Care Ultrasound (POCUS)
    Training
Division of Pulmonary, Critical Care & Sleep Medicine
Department of Medicine at Kent Hospital & Care New England;
Associate Professor of Medicine and Medical Science, Clinician Educator
The Warren Alpert Medical School of Brown University
Providence, RI

Mouhand F. Mohamed, MD, MSc
Department of Medicine
Brown University
Providence, RI

Javad Najjar-Mojarrab, MD, MBA
Division of Nephrology & Hypertension
Henry Ford Hospital
Detroit, MI

John Molinari, MD
Department of Internal Medicine
Henry Ford Health
Detroit, MI

Philippe Montgrain, MD
Professor of Medicine
Division of Pulmonary, Critical Care & Sleep Medicine
University of California, San Diego
La Jolla, CA

Heesung Moon, MD
Department of Internal Medicine
St. Elizabeth's Medical Center
Boston, MA

Michael Z. Moore, MD
Assistant Professor of Neurology
Baylor College of Medicine
Houston, TX

Shawn D. Moore, MD
Adult Neurology
Baylor College of Medicine
Houston, TX

Leah Morelli, MD
Department of Child Psychiatry
Massachusetts General Hospital
Boston, MA

Patrick J. Morrissey, MD
Department of Orthopaedic Surgery
Brown University
Providence, RI

Aleem I. Mughal, MD, FHRS
Cardiac Electrophysiologist
Heart Center of North Texas
Fort Worth, TX

Shiva Kumar R. Mukkamalla, MD, MPH
Hematology & Oncology
Presbyterian Healthcare Services
Albuquerque, NM

Marguerite A. Mullen, BA
The Warren Alpert Medical School of Brown University
Providence, RI

Alexandra Mulliken, MD
OB/GYN
ChristianaCare Health Services
Newark, DE

Tayebah Mumtaz, MD
Cardiovascular Medicine
St. Elizabeth Medical Center
Boston, MA

Fadeke Muraina, MD
Adult Psychiatry
Massachusetts General Hospital, McLean Hospital
Boston, MA

Ahmad Mustafa, MD
Cardiovascular Disease
Staten Island University Hospital – Northwell Health
New York, NY

Ellen Myers, MD
OB/GYN
ChristianaCare Health Services
Newark, DE

Emily Mylhousen, MD
Emergency Medicine
University of Tennessee Health Sciences Center
Memphis, TN

Jack Nadaud, BS
University of Tennessee Health Science Center
Memphis, TN

Akash Nadella, BS
The Warren Alpert Medical School of Brown University
Providence, RI

Mohnish Nadella, BS
The Warren Alpert Medical School of Brown University
Providence, RI

Albert Nadjarian, MD, MPH
Department of Pulmonary Medicine & Critical Care
Kaiser Permanente Northern California
Oakland, CA

Nikita Nagpal, MD
Assistant Professor of Pediatrics
NYU Grossman School of Medicine
New York, NY

Miriam Nathan, MD
Clinical Instructor Trainee of Infectious Diseases Program, Infectious
    Diseases
Boston University Chobanian & Avedisian School of Medicine
Boston, MA

Asim Naveed, MD
Department of Neurology
Willis-Knighton Hospital
Shreveport, LA

Ahmad Al Nawaiseh, MD
Department of Internal Medicine
St. Elizabeth's Medical Center
Boston, MA

Robert Neff, MD
TriHealth Cancer Institute
Division of Gynecologic Oncology
Cincinnati, OH

Adrienne B. Neithardt, MD
Reproductive Endocrinology & Infertility
Boston IVF
Waltham, MA

Christina Nestlerode, DO
Department of OB/GYN
TriHealth
Cincinnati, OH

Azfar K. Niazi, MD
Internal Medicine
Greater Baltimore Medical Center
Baltimore, MD

Mladen Nisavic, MD
Director, Burns & Trauma Psychiatry Service
Consultation-Liaison Service, Psychiatry
Massachusetts General Hospital
Boston, MA

Natalie Nokoff, MD, MSCS
Pediatric Endocrinology
TRUE Center for Gender Diversity
SOAR Clinic
Children's Hospital Colorado
Aurora, CO

Ibrahim Z. D. Noorbhai, MD
Baylor College of Medicine
Houston, TX

James E. Novak, MD, PhD
Program Director
Division of Nephrology & Hypertension
Henry Ford Hospital
Nephrology Professor
Michigan State University
Detroit, MI

Austin Novarra, MD
Department of Psychiatry
Massachusetts General Hospital
Boston, MA

Audrey R. Odom John, MD, PhD
Stanley Plotkin Endowed Chair & Professor of Pediatrics & of Microbiology
Chief of the Division of Infectious Diseases
Department of Pediatrics
Children's Hospital of Philadelphia
Perelman School of Medicine
University of Pennsylvania
Philadelphia, PA

Jeffrey Okewunmi, MD
Department of Orthopaedic Surgery
Brown University
Providence, RI

Rebecca Oliver, DO
Department of OB/GYN
TriHealth OB/GYN
Cincinnati, OH

Adam J. Olszewski, MD
Associate Professor of Medicine
The Warren Alpert Medical School of Brown University
Providence, RI

Henry K. Onyeaka, MBChB, MPH
Department of Psychiatry
Massachusetts General Hospital
Boston, MA

Lindsay M. Orchowski, PhD
Associate Professor (Research)
Department of Psychiatry & Human Behavior
The Warren Alpert Medical School of Brown University
Rhode Island Hospital
Providence, RI

Marcela Osorio, BA
The Warren Alpert Medical School of Brown University
Providence, RI

Luis Osorio, DO
Department of Nephrology & Hypertension
Henry Ford Hospital
Detroit, MI

Cassidy O'Sullivan, MD
OB/GYN
ChristianaCare Health Services
Newark, DE

Jasmine Outlaw, MD
Department of Psychiatry
Massachusetts General Hospital
Boston, MA

Ayotomide Oyelakin, MD, MPH
Assistant Professor of Psychiatry & Behavioral Sciences McGovern
    Medical School
Director, LMHA Telehealth Program
University of Texas Health Science Center at Houston
Houston, TX

Paolo G. Pace, MASc, MD
Resident Physician
Internal Medicine
Roger Williams Medical Center
Providence, RI

John E. Paddock, MD
Assistant Professor of Ophthalmology
Department of Ophthalmology
Division of Neuro-Ophthalmology
Weill Cornell Medicine
New York, NY

David F. Painter, BS
The Warren Alpert Medical School of Brown University
Providence, RI

Alicia Palmieri, DO
Department of Urogynecology
Cooper University Hospital
Camden, NJ

Lisa Pappas-Taffer, MD
Associate Professor
Department of Dermatology
University of Pennsylvania
Philadelphia, PA

Sneha Paranandi, MD
Department of OB/GYN
ChristianaCare Health Services
Newark, DE

Mihir Parikh, MD
Assistant Professor of Medicine
Division of Thoracic Surgery & Interventional Pulmonology
Beth Israel Deaconess Medical Center
Harvard Medical School
Boston, MA

Michael T. Partin, MD
Assistant Professor
Department of Family & Community Medicine
Penn State Health Milton S. Hershey Medical Center
Hershey, PA

Birju B. Patel, MD
Assistant Professor of Medicine
Department of Medicine
Division of Geriatrics & Gerontology
Emory University School of Medicine
Atlanta Veterans Affairs Medical Center
Atlanta, GA

Melissa D. Patel, MD, MPH
Hospital Medicine
The Children's Hospital of Philadelphia
Philadelphia, PA

Minta Patel, MD
Internal Medicine
Cambridge Memorial Hospital
Cambridge, ON
Canada

Nima R. Patel, MD, MS
Minimally Invasive Gynecologic Surgeon & Residency Program Director
Department of OB/GYN
Division of MIGS
TriHealth
Cincinnati, OH

Pranav M. Patel, MD, FACC, FAHA, FSCAI
Professor, Medicine & Biomedical Engineering
Chief of the Division of Cardiology
Department of Medicine
University of California, Irvine Medical Center
Orange, CA

Vishal I. Patel, MD
Division of Cardiology
Department of Medicine
University of California, Irvine School of Medicine
Orange, CA

Brett Patrick, MD
Core Faculty
Memphis Emergency Medicine Residency
University of Tennessee Health Science Center
Memphis, TN

Shreedhar Paudel, MD, MPH
Massachusetts General Hospital
Assistant Professor of Psychiatry
Harvard Medical School
Boston, MA

Ari Pelcovits, MD
Assistant Professor of Medicine
Department of Medicine
The Warren Alpert Medical School of Brown University
Providence, RI

David L. Perez, MD, MMSc
Associate Professor of Neurology & Psychiatry
Departments of Neurology & Psychiatry
Massachusetts General Hospital
Harvard Medical School
Boston, MA

Jose J. Hermina Perez, MD
Department of Psychiatry
Massachusetts General Hospital, McLean Hospital
Harvard Medical School
Boston, MA

Clément Pétron, MD
Department of Psychiatry
University of Caen Normandy & Caen University Hospital
Caen, France

Courtney Pfeuti, MD
Department of OB/GYN
ChristianaCare Health Services
Newark, DE

Lily C. Pham, MD
Assistant Professor of Neurology & Neurosurgery
Department of Neurology
Division of Neuro-Oncology
University of Maryland
Baltimore, MD

Katharine A. Phillips, MD
Professor of Psychiatry & DeWitt Wallace Senior Scholar
Weill Cornell Medical College
Attending Psychiatrist
New York-Presbyterian Hospital, Psychiatry
New York, NY

Oliver W. Phillips, MD
Assistant Professor of Neurology
Department of Neurology
Geisel School of Medicine at Dartmouth
Hanover, NH

Tara M. Phillips, CRNP
Division of Urology
Children's Hospital of Philadelphia
Philadelphia, PA

Lauren E. Piana, MD
Department of Orthopaedics
Brown University/Lifespan
Providence, RI

Brandon S. Portnoff, BS
Department of Orthopaedic Surgery
Brown University
Providence, RI

Sovijja Pou, MD
Department of Medicine
The Warren Alpert Medical School of Brown University
Providence, RI

Rohini Prashar, MD
Division of Nephrology
Henry Ford Hospital
Detroit, MI

Christine Pulice, DO
Clinical Professor of Pediatrics
General Pediatrics
The Children's Hospital of Philadelphia
Philadelphia, PA

Diana Punko, MD, MS
Department of Psychiatry
Massachusetts General Hospital
Instructor
Harvard Medical School
Boston, MA

Ayan Purkayastha, MD
Department of Internal Medicine
The Warren Alpert Medical School of Brown University
Providence, RI

Imrana Qawi, MD
Assistant Professor of Medicine
Director Pulmonary Ambulatory Clinic
Director Critical Care Ultrasound
Division of Pulmonary, Critical Care & Sleep
Tufts Medical Center
Boston, MA

David Qu, MD
Emergency Medicine
University of Tennessee Health Sciences Center
Memphis, TN

Adrian Quesada, MD
Department of OB/GYN
ChristianaCare Health Services
Newark, DE

Matthew S. Quinn, MD
Department of Orthopaedic Surgery
Brown University
Providence, RI

Nicholas Racchi, MD
OB/GYN
TriHealth
Cincinnati, OH

Gregory S. Rachu, MD, MPH
Assistant Professor of Medicine
Division of Geriatrics and Palliative Medicine
The Warren Alpert Medical School of Brown University
Providence, RI

Suvithan Rajadurai, MD
Internal Medicine
Rhode Island Hospital
Providence, RI

Lintu Ramachandran, MD
Baylor College of Medicine
Department of Neurology
Houston, TX

Tanvi Rana, MD
Department of OB/GYN
TriHealth
Cincinnati, OH

Bharti Rathore, MD
Assistant Professor
Boston University School of Medicine
Program Director, Hematology & Oncology Fellowship
Roger Williams Medical Center
Providence, RI

Ritesh Rathore, MD
Associate Professor
Boston University School of Medicine
Director, Hematology & Oncology
Roger Williams Medical Center
Providence, RI

Neha P. Raukar, MD, MS
Emergency Medicine
Mayo Clinic
Rochester, MN

Lakshmi Ravindra, MD
Division of Endocrinology
Rhode Island Hospital
Brown University
Providence, RI

John L. Reagan, MD
Associate Professor of Medicine
Department of Medicine
The Warren Alpert Medical School of Brown University
Providence, RI

P. K. Reardon, MD, DPhil
Department of Psychiatry
Massachusetts General Hospital, McLean Hospital
Clinical Fellow
Harvard Medical School
Boston, MA

Bharathi V. Reddy, MD
Associate Professor of Medicine
Section of Nephrology
Department of Medicine
University of Chicago
Chicago, IL

Snigdha T. Reddy, MD
Associate Program Director
Division of Nephrology & Hypertension
Henry Ford Hospital
Detroit, MI

Anne Reed-Weston, MD
OB/GYN
ChristianaCare Health System
Newark, DE

Anthony M. Reginato, MD, PhD
Director, Division of Rheumatology
Associate Professor of Medicine
The Warren Alpert Medical School of Brown University
Director of Rheumatology Research & Musculoskeletal Ultrasound
Rhode Island Hospital;
Chief, Division of Rheumatology, Providence Veteran
Affairs Medical Center
Providence, RI

James P. Reichart, MD
Department of Medicine
Lehigh Valley Health Network
Allentown, PA

Victor I. Reus, MD
Emeritus Distinguished Professor
Department of Psychiatry & Behavioral Sciences
Weill Institute for Neurosciences
University of California, San Francisco – School of Medicine
San Francisco, CA

Matthew Reuter, MD, FAAPMR
Department of Physical Medicine & Rehabilitation
Lifespan Physician Group
Providence, RI

Sana Riaz, MBBS
Department of Cardiology
The Hartford Health Care Heart & Vascular Institute
University of Connecticut Medical School
Hartford, CT

Brittany Ricci, MD
Division of Endocrinology
The Warren Alpert Medical School of Brown University
Providence, RI

Harlan G. Rich, MD, FACP, AGAF
Associate Professor of Medicine
Division of Gastroenterology
Brown University
Providence, RI

Savanah Richter, MD
OB/GYN
ChristianaCare Health Services
Newark, DE

Lauren Davis Rivera, MD, MSEd
OB/GYN
ChristianaCare Health Services
Newark, DE

Melena J. Robertson, DO
Division of Infectious Diseases
Inova Children's Specialists
Fairfax, VA

Lauren C. Roby, MD
OB/GYN
ChristianaCare Health Services
Newark, DE

Meaghan Roche, MD
Clinical Assistant Professor of Medicine
Michigan State University College of Human Medicine
Department of Nephrology & Hypertension
Henry Ford Health
Detroit, MI

Alejandra E. Morfin Rodriguez, MD
Adult Psychiatry
Massachusetts General Hospital, Mclean Hospital
Harvard Medical School
Boston, MA

Perla M. Romero Gómez, MD
Department of Psychiatry
University of New Mexico
Albuquerque, NM

Hayley A. Ron, MD
Medical Geneticist
The Children's Hospital of Philadelphia
Philadelphia, PA

Michael Rossi, MD
Rhode Island Hospital, The Miriam Hospital
The Warren Alpert Medical School of Brown University
Providence, RI

David Rubin, MD
Assistant Professor
Harvard Medical School
Director, Child & Adolescent Psychiatry Residency Training
Massachusetts General Hospital, McLean Hospital
Executive Director
Massachusetts General Hospital Psychiatry Academy
Boston, MA

Lila Rubin, MD
Department of Internal Medicine
Rhode Island Hospital
Brown University
Providence, RI

Parker Rushworth, MD
Division of Cardiology
Department of Medicine
University of California, Irvine Medical Center
Orange, CA

Beth H. Rutstein, MD, MSCE
Division of Rheumatology
The Children's Hospital of Philadelphia
Assistant Professor of Clinical Pediatrics
Department of Pediatrics
University of Pennsylvania Perelman School of Medicine
Philadelphia, PA

Noushine Sadeghi, MD
OB/GYN
ChristianaCare Health Services
Newark, DE

Ruchi Jalota Sahota, MD
Mayo Clinic
Department of Pulmonary Critical Care
Rochester, MN

Emily Saks, MD, MSCE
ChristianaCare Center for Urogynecology & Pelvic Reconstructive Surgery
ChristianaCare Health Services
Newark, DE

Jeffrey W. Sall, PhD, MD
Professor
Department of Anesthesia & Perioperative Care
University of California, San Francisco
San Francisco, CA

Joshua D. Salvi, MD, PhD
Department of Psychiatry
Assistant Medical Director
Center for OCD & Related Disorders
Massachusetts General Hospital
Boston, MA

Frank A. Sanchez, MD, MBA
Division of Internal Medicine, Division of Infectious Diseases and Immunology
UMass Chan Medical School
Worcester, MA

Martha C. Sanchez, MD
Assistant Professor of Medicine
Division of Infectious Diseases
The Warren Alpert Medical School of Brown University
Providence, RI

Pranavi Sanka, MD
Department of Medicine
The Warren Alpert Medical School of Brown University
Providence, RI

Lekshmi Santhosh, MD, MAEd
Associate Professor of Clinical Medicine
Associate Program Director, Pulmonary & Critical Care Fellowship
Associate Program Director, Internal Medicine Residency
Medical Director, UCSF Post-COVID OPTIMAL Clinic
University of California, San Francisco
San Francisco, CA

Linda Herrera Santos, MD, PhD
Instructor in Psychiatry
Harvard Medical School
Attending Psychiatrist
Massachusetts General Hospital
Boston, MA

Emily Sauck, DO, MBA
OB/GYN
ChristianaCare Health Services
Newark, DE

Leah Saylor, DO
Department of OB/GYN
TriHealth
Cincinnati, OH

William J. Scheuing, MD
Department of Rheumatology
Rhode Island Hospital
The Warren Alpert Medical School of Brown University
Providence, RI

Anthony Sciscione, DO
Director of Maternal-Fetal Medicine
Director of OB/GYN Residency Program
ChristianaCare Health Services
Newark, DE

Matthew Thomas Scott, BS
University of Tennessee Health Science Center
Memphis, TN

Bethany K. Sederdahl, MPH, MD
OB/GYN
ChristianaCare Health Services
Newark, DE

Richard E. Seeber II, MD
Department of Psychiatry
Massachusetts General Hospital, McLean Hospital;
Clinical Fellow
Harvard Medical School
Boston, MA

Kyle Sellers, MD
Department of Psychiatry
Massachusetts General Hospital, McLean Hospital
Boston, MA

Aritra Sen, MD
Pulmonary/Critical Care
Tufts Medical Center
Boston, MA

Rachel Sewell, MD
Department of Pediatric Endocrinology
University of Colorado School of Medicine
Aurora, CO

Hesham Shaban, MD
Division of Nephrology & Hypertension
Henry Ford Hospital
Detroit, MI

Ankur Shah, MD
Division of Kidney Disease & Hypertension
Rhode Island Hospital
The Warren Alpert Medical School of Brown University
Providence, RI

Isha Shah, MD
Division of Rheumatology
Kent Hospital
Providence, RI

Omair Shakil, MD, MPH
Department of Neurology
Baylor College of Medicine
Houston, TX

Animesh Sharma, MD
Assistant Professor of Pediatrics
Pediatric Endocrinology
Children's Hospital of Colorado
Aurora, CO

Yuvraj Sharma, MD
Division of Nephrology & Hypertension
Henry Ford Hospital
Detroit, MI

Lydia Sharp, MD
Assistant Professor
Department of Neurology
Baylor College of Medicine
Houston, TX

Alexander Sherman, MD
Assistant Clinical Professor
Division of Pulmonary, Critical Care & Sleep Medicine
University of California, Los Angeles
Los Angeles, CA

Jessica E. Shill, MD
Division of Endocrinology, Diabetes & Bone & Mineral Disorders
Henry Ford Health System
Clinical Associate Professor of Medicine
Wayne State University School of Medicine
Detroit, MI

Alexei Shimanovsky, MD
Clinical Assistant Professor of Medicine
Hematology & Oncology
The Warren Alpert Medical School of Brown University
Lifespan Cancer Institute
The Miriam Hospital & Rhode Island Hospital
Providence, RI

Michael M. Shipp, MD
Department of Orthopaedics
Brown University/Lifespan
Providence, RI

Philip A. Shlossman, MD
Delaware Center for Maternal Fetal Medicine
Newark, DE

Khawja A. Siddiqui, MD
Assistant Professor of Neurology
Baylor College of Medicine
Houston, TX

Alyssa Siegel, MD
Clinical Associate Professor
Perelman School of Medicine at the University of Pennsylvania
Philadelphia, PA

Mark Sigman, MD
Professor of Urology
Brown University
Rhode Island & The Miriam Hospitals
Providence, RI

Harinder P. Singh, MD
Assistant Professor
Department of Pulmonary & Critical Care Medicine
Carney Hospital, Tufts University
Boston, MA

Jasneet Singh, MD
Department of Internal Medicine
The Warren Alpert Medical School of Brown University
Providence, RI

Manjot Singh, BS
Department of Orthopaedics
The Warren Alpert Medical School of Brown University
Providence, RI

Brett Slingsby, MD
Associate Professor of Pediatrics, Clinician Educator
The Warren Alpert Medical School of Brown University
Providence, RI

Amy J. Sloane, MD
Attending Neonatologist & Assistant Professor of Pediatrics
Nemours Neonatology
Thomas Jefferson University Hospital – Sidney Kimmel Medical College
Philadelphia, PA

Alexandra H. Smick, MD
Department of OB/GYN
TriHealth
Cincinnati, OH

Jeanette G. Smith, MD
Division of Gastroenterology
Brown Medicine
Providence, RI

Matthew J. Smith, MD
Physical Medicine and Rehabilitation
The Warren Alpert Medical School of Brown University
Rhode Island Hospital
Providence, RI

Ryann Sohaney, DO, MS
Division of Nephrology
Henry Ford Hospital
Detroit, MI

Vivek Soi, MD
Clinical Associate Professor Wayne State University & Michigan State University
Division of Nephrology Henry Ford Hospital
Detroit, MI

Rebecca Soinski, MD
Rheumatologist
Women's Medicine Collaborative
Providence, RI

Maria E. Soler, MD, MPH, MBA
Director, Education Division & OB Triage
Department of OB/GYN
ChristianaCare Health Services
Newark, DE

Sandeep Soman, MD, FNKF, FAMIA
Division Head
Division of Nephrology & Hypertension
Henry Ford Hospital
Chief Medical Officer
Greenfield Health Systems
Detroit, MI

Emily Sorg, MD
Massachusetts General Hospital
Harvard Medical School
Boston, MA

Olivia Sosnoski, MS
University of Tennessee Health Science Center, College of Medicine,
  % 2026
Memphis, TN

C. John Sperati, MD, MHS
Associate Professor of Medicine
Division of Nephrology
Johns Hopkins University School of Medicine
Baltimore, MD

Nathan Stanford, MD
Professor
Emergency Medicine
University of Tennessee Health Science Center
Memphis, TN

Emery Steele, MD
Department of Neurology
Baylor College of Medicine
Houston, TX

Jacqueline Steele, MD
Department of Pediatrics
Children's Hospital of Philadelphia
Philadelphia, PA

Ella Stern, MD
Division of OB/GYN
ChristianaCare Health Services
Newark, DE

James Stier, MD
Division of Medicine
Willamette Valley Medical Center
McMinnville, OR

Philip Stockwell, MD
Associate Professor of Medicine (Clinician Educator)
The Warren Alpert Medical School of Brown University
Providence, RI

Lakshmi Subramanian, MD
Department of Internal Medicine
Greenville, NC

Angela Suen, MD
Division of Pulmonary & Critical Care Medicine
University of California, San Francisco
San Francisco, CA

Edward Suh, MD, MPH
Assistant Professor of Anesthesiology
Department of Anesthesiology
The Warren Alpert Medical School of Brown University
Providence, RI

Anjali Sundaramoorthy, DO
Baylor Scott & White Headache Medicine Specialists of North Texas
Texas A&M College of Medicine
Dallas, TX

Naveena Sunkara, MD
Department of Internal Medicine
The Warren Alpert Medical School of Brown University
Providence, RI

Varut Supanakorn, MD
Head & Neck Surgeon
Department of Otolaryngology
King Chulalongkorn Memorial Hospital
Bangkok, Thailand

Priyasha Suri, MD
Department of Critical Care, Division of Critical Care
Max Healthcare
Dehradun, Uttarakhand
India

Hannah Sweeney, MD
OB/GYN
ChristianaCare Health Services
Newark, DE

Kaoru Takasaki, MD
Division of Hematology
Department of Pediatrics
Children's Hospital of Philadelphia
Philadelphia, PA

Ryosuke Takei, MD
Department of Pediatrics
Division of General Pediatrics
Children's Hospital of Philadelphia
Philadelphia, PA

Laren Tan, MD, MBA
Associate Professor of Medicine
Chair
Department of Medicine, Division of Pulmonary, Critical Care, Hyperbaric,
  Allergy & Sleep Medicine
Department of Medicine
Loma Linda University Health
Loma Linda, CA

Mohammad Tarawneh, MD
Department of Medicine
St. Elizabeth's Medical Center
Brighton, MA

Alan Taylor, MD
Program Director
Emergency Medicine
University of Tennessee Health Science Center
Memphis, TN

Kathryn Marie Taylor, PT, DPT, CLT-LANA
LANA Certified Lymphedema Therapist
Senior Instructor, Norton School of Lymphatic Therapy
Saratoga Springs, NY

Matthew A. Taylor, MD
Department of Medicine
Brown University
Providence, RI

S. Trevor Taylor, MD, MPH
Harvard Medical School;
McLean Hospital
Boston, MA

Rebecca Tenney-Soeiro, MD, MSEd
Associate Division Chief of Education & Innovation
Division of General Pediatrics
Program Director
Pediatric Hospital Medicine Fellowship
General Pediatrics
Children's Hospital of Philadelphia
Philadelphia, PA

Anthony G. Thomas, DO, FACP
Clinical Assistant Professor of Medicine
Hematology & Oncology
The Warren Alpert Medical School of Brown University;
Lifespan Cancer Institute
Providence, RI

Stefani Thompson, MD
Division of Nephrology & Hypertension, Division of Critical Care
Henry Ford Hospital
Detroit, MI

Alexandra Meyer Tien, MD
Clinical Assistant Professor
Department of Family Medicine
The Warren Alpert Medical School of Brown University
Providence, RI

David Robbins Tien, MD
Clinical Associate Professor
Department of Surgery (Ophthalmology)
The Warren Alpert Medical School of Brown University
Providence, RI

Anna-Marie Tierney, MD
The Children's Hospital of Philadelphia Care Network, South Philadelphia;
Associate Clinical Professor, Pediatrics
Perelman School of Medicine, University of Pennsylvania
Philadelphia, PA

Helen Toma, MD, MSPH
OB/GYN
ChristianaCare Health Services
Newark, DE

Kim Tran Lopez, DO
General Pediatrics
Children's Hospital of Philadelphia
Philadelphia, PA

Margaret Tryforos, MD
Assistant Professor of Family Medicine (Clinical)
Department of Family Medicine
The Warren Alpert Medical School of Brown University
Pawtucket, RI

Gal Tsaban, MD, MPH
Department of Cardiovascular Medicine
Mayo Clinic
Rochester, MN

Christine Tschoe, MD
Department of Neurology
Baylor College of Medicine
Houston, TX

Robert Tungate, MD
Department of Medicine
University of California, Irvine Medical Center
Orange, CA

Christina S. Turn, MD
Instructor of Pediatrics
Perelman School of Medicine at the University of Pennsylvania;
Division of Oncology
The Children's Hospital of Philadelphia
Philadelphia, PA

Junior Uduman, MD, MS
Division of Nephrology & Hypertension
Henry Ford Hospital
Detroit, MI

Kausik Umanath, MD, MS, FACP, FASN
Associate Program Director, Internal Medicine Residency
Internal Medicine Residency Research Director
Section Head Clinical Research
Division of Nephrology & Hypertension
Henry Ford Health
Detroit, MI

Stephanie P. Ungar, MD
Clinical Assistant Professor
Department of Pediatrics, Division of Pediatric Infectious Diseases
NYU Grossman School of Medicine
New York, NY

Babak Vakili, MD
Urogynecology
Department of OB/GYN
ChristianaCare Health Services
Newark, DE

Ella van Deventer, BA
The Warren Alpert Medical School of Brown University
Providence, RI

Ridhima Vemula, MD
TriHealth
Cincinnati, OH

Aida Venado, MD, MAS
Assistant Professor
Division of Pulmonary, Critical Care, Allergy & Sleep Medicine
University of California, San Francisco
San Francisco, CA

Kathryn G. Vollum, MD
OB/GYN
ChristianaCare Health Services
Newark, DE

Ethan Vorel, MD
Pediatric Emergency Medicine Fellow
Johns Hopkins Children's Center
Baltimore, MD

Ifeanyi Walson, DO
Perinatal & Women's Mental Health Fellow
Northwestern Medicine
Chicago, IL

Angela Wang, MD
Clinical Professor
University of California, San Diego
San Diego, CA

Emily Wang, BA
The Warren Alpert Medical School of Brown University
Providence, RI

Li Wang, MD, MHA
Assistant Professor
Division of Gastroenterology
Brown University
Providence, RI

Linsey Wehner, MPH
Research Assistant
Herbert Wertheim School of Public Health & Human Longevity Science
University of California, San Diego
San Diego, CA

Roi Westreich, MD, PhD
Department of Cardiology
Soroka University Medical Center & Faculty of Health Sciences
Ben-Gurion University of the Negev
Beer-Sheva, Israel

Ericka Wheeler, MD, MPhil
Department of Psychiatry
Massachusetts General Hospital, McLean Hospital
Boston, MA

Nakia Wighton, MD
OB/GYN
ChristianaCare Health Services
Newark, DE

Alexis Wildman, MD
Emergency Medicine
University of Tennessee Health Science Center
Memphis, TN

Annise Wilson, MD
Assistant Professor of Neurology & Medicine (Pulmonary, Critical Care & Sleep Medicine)
Baylor College of Medicine
Houston, TX

Jared M. Winikor, MD
Department of Pediatrics
Children's Hospital of Philadelphia
Philadelphia, PA

Bryce Wininger, MD
Department of Psychiatry
Massachusetts General Hospital, Harvard Medical School
Boston, MA

Julia M. Winschel, MPH
The Warren Alpert Medical School of Brown University
Providence, RI

Jaclyn Wold, MD
Pediatrics
NYU School of Medicine
New York, NY

Adam J. Wolpaw, MD, PhD
Assistant Professor of Pediatrics
Perelman School of Medicine at the University of Pennsylvania;
Division of Oncology
The Children's Hospital of Philadelphia
Philadelphia, PA

Marlene Fishman Wolpert, MPH, CIC, FAPIC
Consultant in Infection Prevention & Control
Long-Term Care Infection Preventionist
Infection Control & Epidemiology
Lifespan Health System
Providence, RI

Elisabeth A. Wong, MD
Division of Cardiology
The Warren Alpert Medical School of Brown University
Providence, RI

John Wylie, MD, FACC
Director, Cardiac Electrophysiology
Steward Health Care System
Associate Professor of Medicine
Tufts University School of Medicine;
Adjunct Associate Professor of Medicine
Boston University School of Medicine
Boston, MA

Anna Yang, MD
Assistant Professor
Emergency Medicine
University of Tennessee Health Science Center
Memphis, TN

Xuan Yao, MD
Division of Cardiology
St. Elizabeth's Medical Center
Boston, MA

Gemini Yesodharan, MD
Interventional Cardiologist
Central Maine Heart & Vascular Institute
Lewiston, ME

Jennifer Yeung, DO
Urogynecology Program Director
Department of Urogynecology
TriHealth
Cincinnati, OH

Chun H. Yin, MD
General Pediatrics, Primary Care
Children's Hospital of Philadelphia
Philadelphia, PA

Agustin G. Yip, MD, PhD
Associate Director of Clinical Operations (Inpatient)
Division of Depression & Anxiety Disorders
McLean Hospital
Belmont, MA

Diana H. Yu, MD
Assistant Professor of Medicine
Director, Interventional Pulmonology Fellowship
Division of Pulmonary, Critical Care, Allergy & Sleep Medicine
University of California, San Francisco
San Francisco, CA

Elizabeth An Yu, MD, PhD
Interventional Pulmonologist
Pulmonary & Critical Care Medicine
Palo Alto Medical Foundation
Mountain View, CA

Jeffrey Yung, MD
Internal Medicine
Oregon Health & Science University
Portland, OR

Sarah Zainelabdin, MD
Department of Medicine
Brown University
Providence, RI

Juliana Zambrano, MD, MPH
Department of Psychiatry
Massachusetts General Hospital, McLean Hospital
Harvard Medical School
Boston, MA

Emin Zargarian, MD
Division of Cardiology
Department of Medicine
University of California, Irvine Medical Center
Orange, CA

B. Shoshana Zha, MD, PhD
Assistant Professor
Division of Pulmonary, Critical Care, Allergy & Sleep Medicine
University of California, San Francisco
San Francisco, CA

Helen Zhang, BS
The Warren Alpert Medical School of Brown University
Providence, RI

Leon Zhao, BS
Department of Orthopaedics
The Warren Alpert Medical School of Brown University
Providence, RI

Diana X. Zhou, MD
Emergency Medicine
University of Tennessee Health Science Center
Memphis, TN

Navid Ziaie, MD
Oregon Health & Science University
Division of Internal Medicine
Portland, OR

Danylo Zorin, MD
Department of Cardiology
St. Elizabeth's Medical Center
Boston, MA

Section Editors

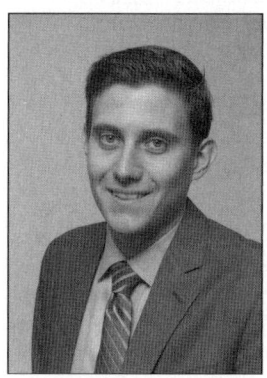

Scott R. Beach, MD
Psychiatrist
Massachusetts General Hospital
Associate Professor of Psychiatry
Harvard Medical School
Boston, Massachusetts

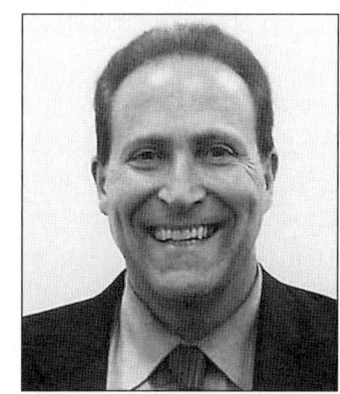

Fred F. Ferri, MD, FACP
Clinical Professor
Department of Medicine
The Warren Alpert Medical School
 of Brown University
Providence, Rhode Island

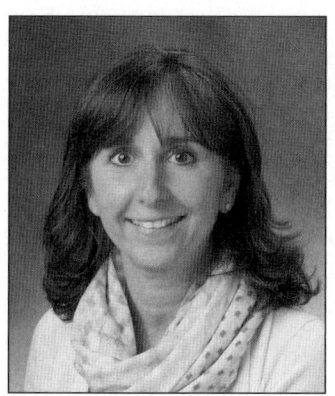

Cindy W. Christian, MD
Professor of Pediatrics
Department of Pediatrics, Division
 of General Pediatrics
The Children's Hospital of
 Philadelphia
The Perelman School of Medicine
 at the University of
 Pennsylvania
Philadelphia, Pennsylvania

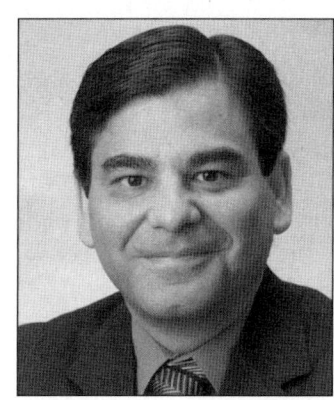

Glenn G. Fort, MD, MPH
Clinical Associate Professor of
 Medicine
Division of Infectious Diseases
The Warren Alpert Medical School
 of Brown University
Providence, Rhode Island

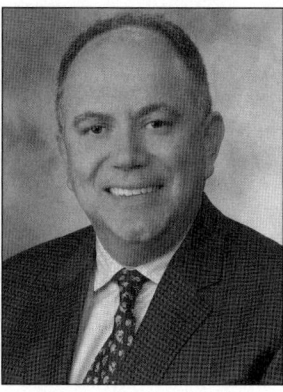

Manuel F. DaSilva, MD
Associate Professor
Department of Orthopaedics
The Warren Alpert Medical School
 of Brown University
Providence, Rhode Island

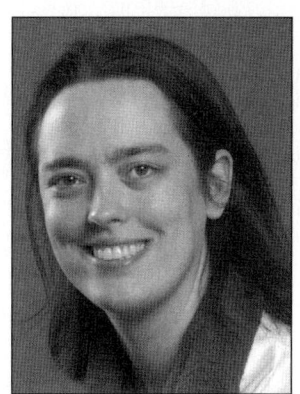

Corey Elam Goldsmith, MD, FAAN
Associate Professor of Neurology
Baylor College of Medicine
Houston, Texas

Section Editors

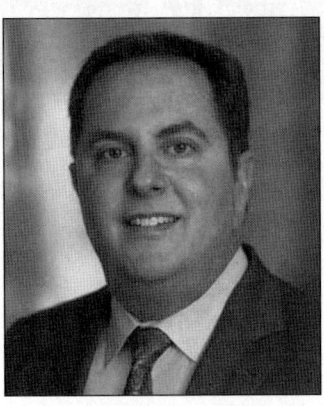

Joseph S. Kass, MD, JD, FAAN
Associate Dean of Student Affairs
Professor of Neurology, Psychiatry
 & Medical Ethics
Director, Alzheimer's Disease &
 Memory Disorders Center
Baylor College of Medicine
Chief of Neurology
Director of Comprehensive Stroke
 Program
Ben Taub General Hospital
Houston, Texas

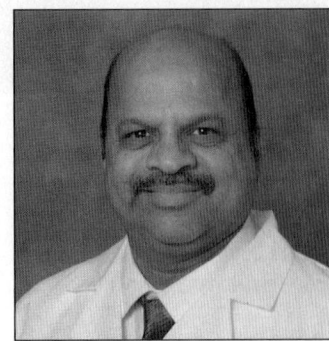

Sandeep Soman, MD, FNKF, FAMIA
Division Head
Division of Nephrology &
 Hypertension
Henry Ford Hospital
Chief Medical Officer
Greenfield Health Systems
Detroit, Michigan

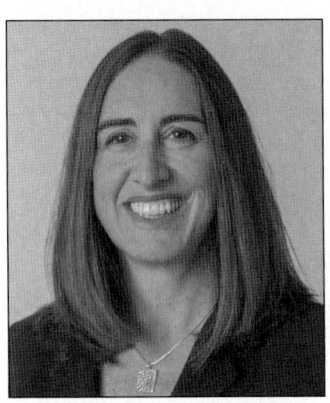

Lorriana E. Leard, MD
Professor of Clinical Medicine
Associate Dean, Continuing
 Medical Education, UCSF
 School of Medicine
Vice Chief, Clinical Operations
Division of Pulmonary, Critical
 Care, Allergy & Sleep Medicine
University of California, San
 Francisco
San Francisco, California

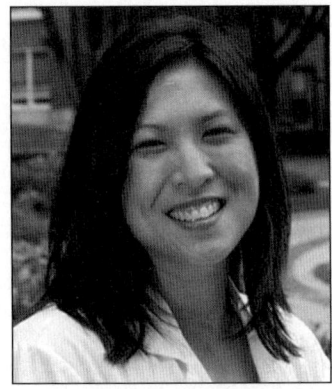

Iris L. Tong, MD
Associate Professor
Department of Medicine
The Warren Alpert Medical School
 of Brown University;
Women's Primary Care
Women's Medicine Collaborative
Providence, Rhode Island

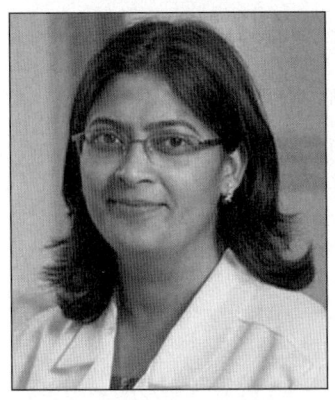

Bharti Rathore, MD
Assistant Professor
Boston University School of
 Medicine
Program Director, Hematology &
 Oncology Fellowship
Roger Williams Medical Center
Providence, Rhode Island

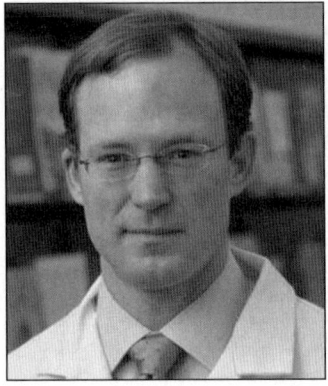

John Wylie, MD, FACC
Director, Cardiac Electrophysiology
Steward Health Care System
Associate Professor of Medicine
Tufts University School of
 Medicine;
Adjunct Associate Professor of
 Medicine
Boston University School of
 Medicine
Boston, Massachusetts

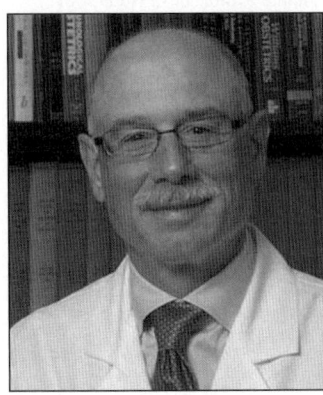

Anthony Sciscione, DO
Director of Maternal-Fetal
 Medicine
Director of OB/GYN Residency
 Program
ChristianaCare Health Services
Newark, Delaware

To my sons, Dr. Vito F. Ferri and Dr. Christopher A. Ferri,
and my daughter-in-law, Dr. Heather A. Ferri,
for their help and constant support,
and to my wife, Christina, for her patience during manuscript preparation.
A special thanks to all the readers
who have personally commented on the merits of this book
and through their suggestions have helped make this product
a bestseller in the medical field.

Fred F. Ferri, MD, FACP
Clinical Professor
Department of Medicine
Warren Alpert Medical School of Brown University
Providence, Rhode Island

Preface

This book is intended to be a clear and concise reference for physicians and allied health professionals. Its user-friendly format is designed to provide a fast and efficient way to identify important clinical information and to offer practical guidance in patient management. The book is divided into five sections and an appendix, each with emphasis on clinical information.

The tremendous success of the previous editions and the enthusiastic comments from numerous colleagues have brought about several positive changes over time. This is the 27th edition of *Ferri's Clinical Advisor*, a best-seller nationally and internationally and now available in multiple languages. Each section has been significantly expanded from prior editions, bringing the total number of medical topics covered in this book to more than 1200. New illustrations, tables, and boxes have been added to this edition to enhance recollection of clinically important facts. The expedited claims submission and reimbursement ICD-10CM codes are included in all topics.

Section I describes in detail over 1000 medical disorders and diseases—including 30 new topics this edition—arranged alphabetically and presented in outline format for ease of retrieval. Topics with an accompanying algorithm are identified with an ALG icon; similarly, those topics with an accompanying online Patient Teaching Guide (PTG) are identified with a PTG symbol. Throughout the text, key quick-access information is consistently highlighted, with clinical photographs to further illustrate selected medical conditions, and relevant ICD-10CM codes listed. Most references focus on current peer-reviewed journal articles rather than outdated textbooks and old review articles.

Topics in **Section I** use the following structured approach:
1. Basic Information (Definition, Synonyms, ICD-10CM Codes, Epidemiology & Demographics, Physical Findings & Clinical Presentation, Etiology)
2. Diagnosis (Differential Diagnosis, Workup, Laboratory Tests, Imaging Studies)
3. Treatment (Nonpharmacologic Therapy, Acute General Rx, Chronic Rx, Disposition, Referral)
4. Pearls & Considerations (Comments, Suggested Readings)

Section II includes the differential diagnosis, etiology, and classification of signs and symptoms. This practical section allows the user investigating a physical complaint or abnormal laboratory value to follow a "workup" leading to a diagnosis. The physician can then easily look up the presumptive diagnosis in Section I for information specific to that illness. Several new signs and symptoms have been added to this section for the 2025 edition.

Section III includes more than 150 clinical algorithms to guide and expedite the patient's workup and therapy. For the 2025 edition, we have continued to update algorithms and colorize online versions for improved readability. Physicians describe this section as particularly valuable in today's managed-care environment.

Section IV includes normal laboratory values and interpretation of results of commonly ordered laboratory tests. By providing interpretation of abnormal results, this section facilitates the diagnosis of medical disorders and further adds to the comprehensive "one-stop" nature of our text. New illustrations and tables have been added for this edition.

Section V focuses on preventive medicine. Information here includes screening recommendations for major diseases and disorders, patient counseling, and immunization and chemoprophylaxis recommendations.

The **Appendix** is divided into nine major sections. Appendix I contains extensive information on complementary and alternative medicine (CAM), including Common Herbs in Integrated Medicine as well as Herbal Activities Against Pain and Chronic Diseases. With this material, we aim to lessen the current scarcity of exposure of allopathic and osteopathic physicians to the diversity of CAM therapies. Appendix II focuses on nutrition, with an emphasis on dietary supplements, vitamins, and minerals. Appendix III deals with diagnosis and treatment of acute poisoning. Appendix IV is a guide on impairment and disability evaluation. Appendix V focuses on the protection of travelers. Appendix VI addresses care of the transgender patient. Appendix VII is a repository of practical patient instruction sheets, organized alphabetically, and covers the majority of topics in this book. These guides can be easily customized and printed and serve as valuable tools for improving physician-patient communication, patient satisfaction, and ultimately quality of care. Appendices VIII and IX offer guidance related to palliative care and preoperative evaluation, respectively.

I believe that we have produced a state-of-the-art information system with significant differences from existing texts. The information offered in all five sections and patient education guides could be sold separately based on their content, yet are available under a single cover, offering the reader tremendous value. I hope that the *Clinical Advisor's* user-friendly approach, numerous unique features, and yearly updates will make this book a valuable medical reference, not only to primary care physicians but also to physicians in other specialties, medical students, and allied health professionals.

Fred F. Ferri, MD, FACP
Clinical Professor
Department of Medicine
The Warren Alpert Medical School of Brown University
Providence, Rhode Island

Note: Comments from readers are always appreciated and can be forwarded directly to Dr. Ferri at fred_ferri@brown.edu.

Mouse icon: Indicates content with additional references, figures, or tables available at eBooks.Health.Elsevier.com.

PTG icon: Indicates an accompanying Patient Teaching Guide available at eBooks.Health.Elsevier.com. Many additional PTGs are available online that are not connected to topics in Section I.

ALG icon: Indicates a topic with an accompanying algorithm.

Contents

Detailed Contents

SECTION I Diseases and Disorders*

*Italic topics are available online only.

SECTION II **Differential Diagnosis**

Detailed Contents

SECTION III Clinical Algorithms*

*Italic topics are available online only.

SECTION IV Laboratory Tests and Interpretation of Results*

*Italic topics are available online only.

SECTION V Clinical Practice Guidelines*

*Italic topics are available online only.

APPENDIX I   **Complementary and Alternative Medicine Terms (available online)**

APPENDIX II   **Nutrition (available online)**

SECTION I

Diseases and Disorders
Fred F. Ferri, MD

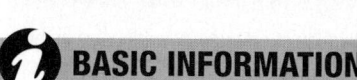
BASIC INFORMATION

DEFINITION

An abdominal aortic aneurysm (AAA) is a segmental full-thickness dilation of 1.5 times or greater than expected normal diameter of the abdominal aorta, defined as the fifth part of the aorta between the diaphragm and the aortic bifurcation. The average diameter of a human infrarenal aorta is approximately 2 cm, thus a threshold of 3 cm is commonly considered aneurysmal.[1,2] Due to a lack of definition uniformity, the term "ectasia" has fallen out of favor and is not commonly used to describe the imaging interpretation of aortic enlargement.

ICD 10-CM CODES
I71.4	Abdominal aortic aneurysm, without rupture
I71.3	Abdominal aortic aneurysm, ruptured

EPIDEMIOLOGY & DEMOGRAPHICS

- Lifetime risk for AAA is 8.2% in men and 10.5% in current smokers.[1]
- Approximately 13,000 deaths/yr in the U.S. are attributed to AAA.[2]
- AAA is predominantly a disease of older adults and affects males four times more than females.[3]
- The prevalence of AAA ranges 1.2% to 3.3% in males older than 60 yr, which is lower than had been previously reported, likely due to overall reductions in smoking. The prevalence in the U.S. specifically is unclear given that screening is rare in nonsmokers.[4]
- More than half of males with subaneurysmal aorta (2.6 to 2.9 cm) develop an AAA >3.0 cm within 5 yr of their original ultrasound. 28% of male patients with a subaneurysmal aorta will develop a large AAA >5.5 cm within 15 yr.[5]

NATURAL HISTORY

- AAAs tend to develop in the infrarenal aorta and expand at a faster rate the larger the diameter of the AAA, with each 0.5 cm increase in baseline AAA diameter increasing the rate of expansion by 0.59 mm/yr.[6]
- Larger aneurysms are associated with increased rate of expansion, and thus current guidelines recommend more frequent surveillance for larger aneurysms. Frequency of surveillance for aneurysms is as follows: 3.0 to 3.9 cm every 3 yr, 4.0 to 4.9 cm every yr, 5.0 to 5.4 cm every 6 mo.[6] Aneurysmal size is the greatest predictor of rupture.[2]
- Out of hospital AAA rupture is often lethal with mortality ranging from 80% to 90%.[2,4] Female sex, current smoking, and older age are associated with an increased risk of AAA rupture. Current smokers are two times more likely than former smokers to suffer from AAA rupture.[4]
- Annual risk for rupture of the AAA depends on the size of the AAA[2]:
  1. <1% for AAA 5.4 cm or under
  2. 9.4% for AAA between 5.5 cm and 5.9 cm
  3. 10.2% for AAA between 6.0 cm to 6.9 cm
  4. 32.5% for AAA 7.0 cm or greater
- Heavily calcified AAAs expand at a slower rate than less calcified AAAs.[7] The presumed mechanism may be stabilization of the aortic wall by calcification.

SCREENING & MONITORING

Major societal guidelines share similar screening recommendations. These include the U.S. Preventive Services Task Force (USPSTF), the Society for Vascular Surgery (SVS), the American Heart Association (AHA), and the American College of Cardiology (ACC).

- The USPSTF recommends one-time screening for AAA by ultrasonography in males ages 65 to 75 who have a history of smoking, and selectively offer screening to males 65 yr of age or older who have never smoked but have certain risk factors, including family history of AAA in a parent or sibling. This latter population has been shown to have a higher prevalence of AAA, and selectively screening this group has been shown to decrease AAA-specific mortality.[4]
- The USPSTF and AHA/ACC have found little benefit in repeat screening in males with a negative ultrasound and has determined that males over the age of 75 are unlikely to benefit from screening. It was also concluded that the current evidence is insufficient to assess the balance of the harms and benefits of screening for AAA in females ages 65 to 75 who have ever smoked or with family history of AAA, thus screening may be reasonable in certain cases.[1,4]
- The SVS recommends one-time ultrasonography screening for AAAs in males and females ages 65 to 75 yr with a history of tobacco use; in males and females 65 to 75 yr with a first-degree relative with an AAA; and in patients 75 yr or older in good health who have either a history of smoking or a first-degree relative with an AAA.[8]
- The SVS also recommends monitoring by ultrasound or CT scan should be performed every 6 mo for patients with AAAs measuring 5.0 to 5.4 cm in diameter, every 12 mo for AAAs measuring 4.0 to 4.9 cm in diameter, and every 3 yr for AAAs 3.0 to 3.9 cm in diameter.[8]

PHYSICAL FINDINGS & CLINICAL PRESENTATION

- Most aneurysms are asymptomatic and incidentally discovered on imaging studies.[9,10]
- Physical examination has moderate sensitivity for detection of AAA. Abdominal palpation may reveal a pulsatile mass and is less than 50% sensitive in detection of AAA. Detection is further limited in individuals with abdominal girth >100 cm. Palpation of the aneurysm does not increase the risk of rupture.[10]
- Symptomatic patients may present with pain of the abdomen, back, flank, or groin or sequelae secondary to compression or mass effect of adjacent organs. Early satiety, nausea, and vomiting may be caused by compression of adjacent bowel. Venous thrombosis or insufficiency may occur from iliocaval venous compression. Thromboembolization can cause lower extremity pain and discoloration. Abdominal bruits can be present in case of renal or visceral arterial stenosis. Ureteral obstruction and hydronephrosis can cause flank and groin pain and lead to obstructive renal failure.[10] Additionally, aneurysmal formation can lead to development of arteriovenous fistulas and aortoenteric fistulas, which may present as high-output heart failure and gastrointestinal blood loss, respectively.[10]
- Approximately half of patients with AAA rupture will classically present as a triad of abdominal or back pain, hypotension, and a pulsatile abdominal mass. Ruptured aneurysms (Fig. E1) lead to rapid progression to hemorrhagic shock and require emergent surgery within hours to increase chances of survival.[2,9]

ETIOLOGY

- AAA development is characterized by medial degeneration of the aortic wall via various pathophysiologic mechanisms including smooth muscle cell apoptosis and media layer thinning, vascular inflammation from lymphocyte and macrophage infiltration, and extracellular matrix degradation.[2,11] These degenerative processes deplete the normal lamellar elastin matrix leading to vascular remodeling and aneurysmal formation, expansion, and eventual rupture.[11] Matrix metalloproteinases have been implicated in the development of aneurysms as well and have been tested with variable success as a therapeutic target for prevention of AAA.[12]
- Most AAAs develop an intraluminal thrombus that contributes to wall degradation through oxidative stress, cell apoptosis, and inflammation.[1]
- Advanced age is significantly associated with AAA. Individuals over the age of 65, compared to under age 55, are 9.4 times as likely to develop AAA.[3]
- Smoking is considered one of the strongest modifiable risk factors for AAA development. A history of smoking was associated with an odds ratio of 5.07 for formation of AAA over 4 cm. Smoking was considered to be responsible for 75% of the excess prevalence of AAAs greater than 4 cm.[13]
- The association of family history of AAA suggests a role of inherited connective tissue diseases such as Marfans and Ehlers-Danlos in the pathogenesis of AAA formation.[3]
- Additional risk factors include hypertension, hyperlipidemia, obesity, prexisting peripheral arterial disease, cerebrovascular disease, coronary artery disease, and other aneurysmal vessels.[1-3]
- Regular consumption of fruits, vegetables, and nuts along with regular moderate intensity exercise were associated with reduced risk of AAA formation.[3]
- Ethnically, Caucasian race is associated with increased risk of AAA development compared to African American, Hispanic, and Asian origins.[3]

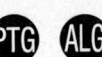
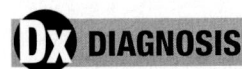 **DIAGNOSIS**

DIFFERENTIAL DIAGNOSIS

Most patients with AAA are asymptomatic, and the condition is discovered on routine examination or incidentally diagnosed when ordering studies for other symptoms.[9] Diagnosis of AAA should be considered in the differential with the following symptoms: Abdominal, back, or flank pain and/or a pulsatile abdominal mass. The differential diagnosis of these symptoms can include aortic dissection, ulcerated aortic plaque, renal colic, mesenteric ischemia, pancreatitis, diverticulitis, peptic ulcer disease, biliary tract disease, and others.

LABORATORY TESTS

In general, laboratory studies are not routinely indicated. For suspected infected or inflammatory aneurysms, white blood cell (WBC), erythrocyte sedimentation rate (ESR), C-reactive protein (CRP), and blood cultures can be considered. An elevated d-dimer may indicate a thrombus within the aneurysm. Fig. 2 describes an algorithm for the diagnosis and treatment of abdominal aortic aneurysms.

IMAGING STUDIES

- Abdominal ultrasound (Fig. 3) is 94% to 100% sensitive and 98% to 100% specific in identifying an aneurysm. Ultrasound is readily available, noninvasive, and accurate. Increasing application in emergency settings as point-of-care imaging has led to a significant reduction in time to diagnosis and treatment of AAA.[4,8]
- Computed tomography (CT) (Fig. 4) scan is recommended for preoperative aneurysm imaging due to reliability of size estimation of AAA within 0.2 mm.[3] CT scan can identify extension to renal vessels with more precision than ultrasound. It is the imaging modality of choice for symptomatic AAA and can also detect the integrity of the wall (Fig. 5) and exclude rupture.[10]
- Magnetic resonance angiography (MRA) may also be used and is more accurate than CT; however, it has a longer study acquisition time and may not be readily available.[3]

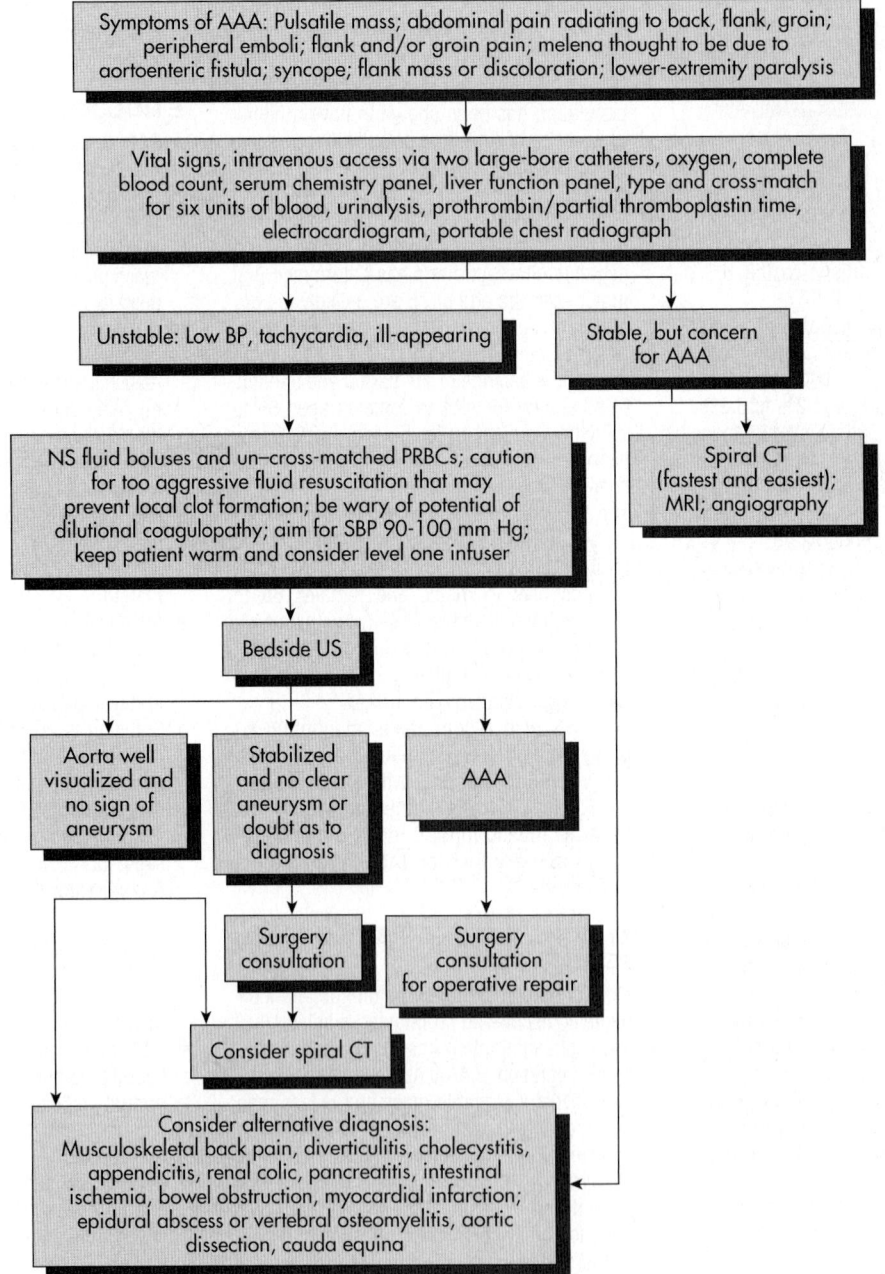

FIG. 2 Algorithm for the diagnosis and treatment of abdominal aortic aneurysms (AAAs). *BP*, Blood pressure; *CT*, computed tomography; *MRI*, magnetic resonance imaging; *NS*, normal saline; *PRBCs*, packed red blood cells; *SBP*, systolic blood pressure; *US*, ultrasonography. (From Adams JG et al: *Emergency medicine, clinical essentials*, ed 2, Philadelphia, 2013, Elsevier.)

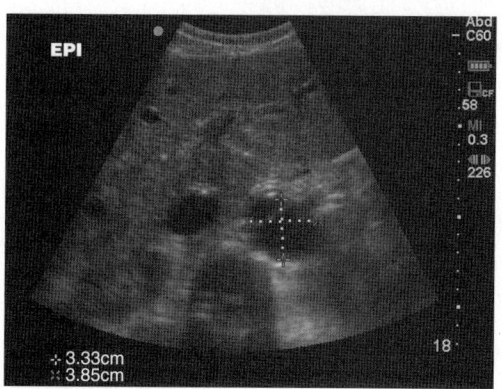

FIG. 3 Transverse image of an abdominal aortic aneurysm. Note the measurements of 3.33 × 3.85 cm. The inferior vena cava is seen to the patient's right of the aorta, and the vertebral body is seen below the two vessels. Note also that there appears to be an echogenic flap within the aorta, possibly representing an aortic dissection. (From Adams JG et al: *Emergency medicine, clinical essentials,* ed 2, Philadelphia, 2013, Elsevier.)

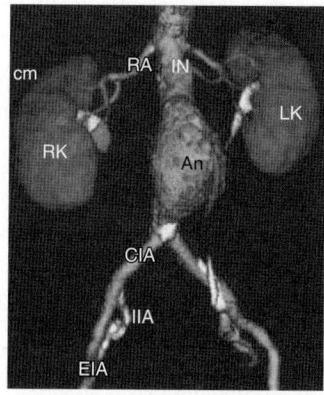

FIG. 4 Three-dimensional computed tomography image illustrates the presence of an infrarenal abdominal aortic aneurysm. *An,* Aneurysm; *CIA,* common iliac artery; *EIA,* external iliac artery; *IIA,* internal iliac artery; *IN,* infrarenal neck; *LK,* left kidney; *RA,* renal artery; *RK,* right kidney. (From Townsend CM et al [eds]: *Sabiston textbook of surgery,* ed 17, Philadelphia, 2004, Saunders.)

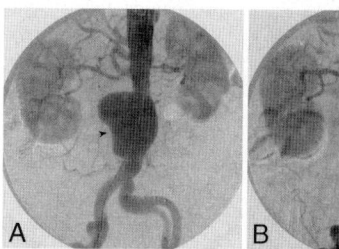

FIG. 6 A, Conventional catheter angiography with bilateral marked catheters in place demonstrates a large, lobulated, infrarenal aortic aneurysm *(arrowhead)* with a 4-cm proximal neck suitable for endovascular repair. **B,** An image after endovascular repair demonstrates complete exclusion of the aneurysm *(arrowhead)* with no endoleak and preservation of the renal and hypogastric arteries. (From Soto JA, Lucey BC: *Emergency radiology, the requisites,* ed 2, Philadelphia, 2017, Elsevier.)

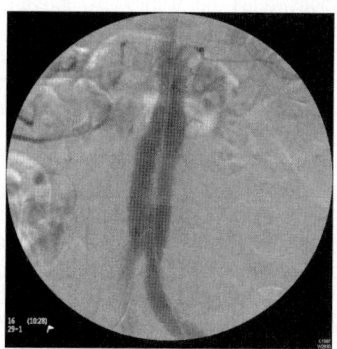

FIG. 7 Digital subtraction angiogram following endovascular aneurysm repair. (From Fillit HM: *Brocklehurst's textbook of geriatric medicine and gerontology,* ed 8, Philadelphia, 2017, Elsevier.)

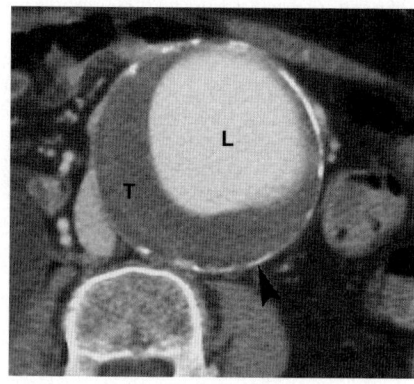

FIG. 5 Aneurysm of the abdominal aorta. A large aortic aneurysm is evident. The aorta exceeds 5 cm in diameter. A large amount of thrombus *(T)* partially surrounds the contrast-enhanced patent lumen *(L).* Note the atherosclerotic calcification *(arrowhead)* in the wall of the aneurysm.

- Plain radiographs may show the outline of an aneurysm in calcified aortas. This is an insensitive test for diagnosing AAA and is not routinely a first-line test.
- Diagnostic aortography has essentially been replaced by other noninvasive imaging modalities such as CT or MRA. Intraoperative angiography is still used for determining treatment options and postprocedure efficacy (Fig. 6).
- Endovascular aneurysm repair (EVAR) needs close and lifelong imaging surveillance of the aneurysm site for the timely detection of possible complications, including endoleaks, graft migration, fractures, graft infection, and enlargement of aneurysmal sac size with eventual rupture.[8] Contrast-enhanced computed tomography (CTA) is considered the gold standard in EVAR follow-up (Fig. 7); however, routine use is limited given cumulative radiation exposure and risk of contrast-induced renal injury. Guidelines suggest serial ultrasound surveillance if neither enoleak nor AAA enlargement is seen on CTA at 1 yr after EVAR.[8]

(Rx) TREATMENT

MEDICAL MANAGEMENT

- The primary goal of medical therapy is to reduce growth rates, subsequently reducing the need for aortic repair and aortic-related mortality. The secondary goal is to decrease risk of nonaortic cardiovascular events given shared risk factors between aortopathy and atherosclerotic disease.[1]
- Smoking cessation is critical for treatment of patients with AAAs and can decrease rate of expansion. Patients with known AAA or a family history of aneurysms should be advised to stop smoking and be offered smoking cessation interventions.[13]
- Maintaining healthy blood pressure with beta-blockers or angiotensin-receptor blockers

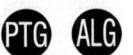

mitigates proteolysis pathways and reduces shear stress on the aortic wall.[1]

- Use of lipid-lowering therapies such as HMG-CoA reductase inhibitors (statins) helps to target inflammatory pathways, reducing medial degeneration.[1]
- Healthy diet and exercise have been observed to be associated with reduced risk of AAA via shared multifactorial mechanisms. Of note, moderate exercise does not increase the rate of aneurysm expansion or the risk of rupture.[3]
- Definitive treatment depends on the size of the aneurysm (see "Chronic Therapy").

ACUTE THERAPY

- AAA can be treated with open surgical repair (OSR) or EVAR (Fig. E8). EVAR is recommended in patients with suitable anatomy given reduced short-term morbidity compared to OSR.[8,14,15] Elective, symptomatic, or ruptured AAA repair can be performed via endovascular or open techniques.[8,10] Ruptured AAA requires emergent repair, and symptomatic AAA requires urgent repair.[8]
- Historically, emergent open repair had been the standard of care; however, trials now show no significant difference in 30-day mortality compared to EVAR.[14] There was a higher incidence of reintervention for patients undergoing EVAR, although interventions to deal with procedural complications were generally less invasive and involved catheter-based approaches.[15-17]
- The major limitations for EVAR include anatomic issues such as tortuosity or small caliber iliac arteries prohibiting graft deployment, end-organ ischemia from endograft limb occlusion, endoleak from inadequate fixation or sealing of the graft to the vessel wall, and inability to follow up patients to exclude late failure of stent-grafts and development of endoleaks.[8-10]

CHRONIC THERAPY

- Optimizing blood pressure and lipid profile is recommended for patients with hypertensive and atherosclerotic disease. AAA formation has often been recognized as a distinct degenerative process from atherosclerosis, but emerging data suggest some shared pathophysiology. Outcomes data from clinical trials of medical therapy are limited, thus conflicting guidelines regarding medical therapy still persist.[1,2,8]
- Data are also sparse as to the protective effects of antibiotics such as doxycycline and roxithromycin to limit the expansion of small AAAs.[8,18]

- AAA repair to eliminate the risk for rupture should be performed for patients with infrarenal or juxtarenal AAA of approximately 5.5 cm or larger in diameter. Repair in females can be considered at diameters larger than 5 cm per Society of Vascular Surgery guidelines. Additionally, AAAs with a rate of enlargement greater than 0.5 cm over 6 mo should be considered for repair. All patients who are symptomatic should undergo repair, regardless of size.[8]
- Smoking cessation is recommended for at least 2 wk before surgery.[8] It is reasonable to delay elective AAA repair in an effort to optimize comorbid medical conditions. Preoperative nutritional status should be optimized prior to undergoing repair. Intravenous antibiotics with a first-generation cephalosporin should be administered 30 min to 1 h prior to either OSR or EVAR.[8]
- There is no clear advantage to early repair (open or endovascular) for small asymptomatic AAAs. Meta-analysis has demonstrated no significant difference in all-cause mortality or AAA-related mortality with early treatment (EVAR vs. OSR) compared with surveillance for small AAAs.[19]
- Historically, EVAR was thought to be associated with better short-term outcomes than OSR (lower 30-day mortality and myocardial infarction [MI] rates, shorter hospital stays, and better health-related quality of life up to 12 mo postoperatively) but increased rates of graft-related complications and long-term all-cause mortality. However, there is conflicting evidence about the long-term relative benefits of OSR, with some recent trials demonstrating no significant difference in long-term mortality.[8,10,15-17]
- In patients who have undergone EVAR, long-term surveillance is required to assess for an endoleak, stent migration, change in aneurysm size, and need for reintervention.[8] Surveillance for endovascular AAA repair has typically involved use of periodic CT scans, but abdominal ultrasound is gaining widespread adoption for postprocedure monitoring. Surveillance is recommended to occur at least 1 mo and 12 mo postoperatively, followed by annually thereafter.[8]
- EVAR with proximally fenestrated grafts (FEVAR) is an alternative to open repair in the management of juxtarenal aortic aneurysms and short-neck abdominal aortic aneurysms, with the "neck" defined as the distance from the lowest main renal artery to the beginning of the aneurysm. Contemporary literature shows it is a safe and efficacious treatment, particularly for those deemed surgically high risk.[15]

- For patients with limited life expectancy, elective AAA repair is not recommended.[6]

REFERRAL

- Vascular surgical referral is recommended at the time of diagnosis of AAA.[8]
- It is important to optimize any comorbid conditions along with surgical referral, including cardiology and endocrinology referrals as indicated.[8]

PEARLS & CONSIDERATIONS

- Smoking is the strongest modifiable risk factor for AAA formation, expansion, and rupture, and cessation should strongly be encouraged through utilization of behavioral support techniques and pharmacologic therapy.
- Guidelines suggest elective repair for patients with AAA ≥5.5 cm at low or acceptable surgical risk.
- The results from multiple trials to date demonstrate no advantage to immediate repair for small AAA (4.0 to 5.5 cm).
- 5-yr all-cause mortality remains poor after elective AAA repair despite advances in short-term outcomes.

COMMENTS

- Most AAAs are infrarenal. This is thought to be due in part to decreased lamellar structural proteins in the vascular wall below the renal arteries leading to decreased vascular wall strength.[2,11]
- Surgical risk is increased in patients with coexisting coronary artery disease, pulmonary disease, or chronic renal failure. Evaluation for ischemia and aggressive perioperative hemodynamic monitoring can help identify high-risk patients to help decrease postoperative complications.[8]
- AAAs expand at a faster rate the larger the diameter of the AAA, with each 0.5 cm increase in baseline AAA diameter increasing the rate of expansion by 0.59 mm/yr.[6]

RELATED CONTENT

Abdominal Aortic Aneurysm (Patient Information)

REFERENCES

Available at eBooks.Health.Elsevier.com.

AUTHORS: **VISHAL I. PATEL, MD** and **PRANAV M. PATEL, MD, FACC, FAHA, FSCAI**

BASIC INFORMATION

DEFINITION

Abruptio placentae is the premature separation of placenta from the uterine wall before delivery of the fetus. The condition occurs in approximately 1% of pregnancies. There are three classes of abruption (Fig. 1) based on maternal and fetal status, including an assessment of uterine contractions, quantity of bleeding, fetal heart rate monitoring, and abnormal coagulation studies (fibrinogen, prothrombin time, partial thromboplastin time).

- Grade I: Mild vaginal bleeding, uterine irritability, stable vital signs, reassuring fetal heart rate, normal coagulation profile (fibrinogen 450 mg/dl). Approximately half of abruptions are grade I.
- Grade II: Moderate vaginal bleeding, hypertonic uterine contractions, orthostatic blood pressure measurements, unfavorable fetal status, fibrinogen 150 to 250 mg. Approximately a quarter of abruptions are grade II.
- Grade III: Severe bleeding (may be concealed), hypertonic uterine contractions, overt signs of hypovolemic shock, fetal death, thrombocytopenia, fibrinogen <150 mg/dl. Approximately a quarter of abruptions are grade III.

SYNONYMS

Premature separation of placenta
Placental abruption

ICD-10CM CODES
O45.8X1	Other premature separation of placenta, first trimester
O45.8X2	Other premature separation of placenta, second trimester
O45.8X3	Other premature separation of placenta, third trimester
O45.8X9	Other premature separation of placenta, unspecified trimester
O45.91	Premature separation of placenta, unspecified, first trimester
O45.92	Premature separation of placenta, unspecified, second trimester
O45.93	Premature separation of placenta, unspecified, third trimester

EPIDEMIOLOGY & DEMOGRAPHICS

INCIDENCE (IN U.S.):

- 1% of deliveries according to epidemiologic cohort studies
- Implicated in up to 10% of preterm births

PREVALENCE: 5% to 17%, some studies showing a 5- to 10-fold increase in risk; with two prior episodes, 25%.

RISK FACTORS: Abruption in a prior pregnancy (greatest association), hypertension, trauma, polyhydramnios, multifetal gestation, smoking, use of cocaine, chorioamnionitis, preterm premature rupture of membranes. Table 1 summarizes placental abruption risk factors.

PHYSICAL FINDINGS & CLINICAL PRESENTATION

- The presentation is variable; however, the classic presentation is the triad of uterine bleeding (concealed or per vagina), hypertonic uterine contractions or signs of preterm labor, and evidence of fetal compromise.
- More than 80% of cases have external bleeding; 20% of cases have no bleeding but have indirect evidence of abruption, such as failed tocolysis for preterm labor.
- Tetanic uterine contractions are found in only 17%.

ETIOLOGY

- Primary etiology: Unknown
- Hypertension: Found in 40% to 50% of grade III abruptions
- Rapid decompression of uterine cavity, as can occur in polyhydramnios or multifetal gestation
- Blunt external trauma (motor vehicle accident, spousal abuse)

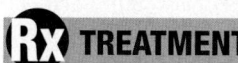 DIAGNOSIS

DIFFERENTIAL DIAGNOSIS

- Placenta previa
- Cervical or vaginal trauma
- Labor
- Cervical cancer
- Rupture of membranes

WORKUP

- Placental abruption is primarily a clinical diagnosis that is supported by laboratory, radiographic (Fig. 2), and pathologic studies.
- Initial assessment should evaluate for the source of bleeding, ruling out placenta previa that may contraindicate any type of vaginal examination (e.g., pelvic speculum examination).
- Continuous fetal heart monitoring is indicated for all viable gestations (60% incidence of

fetal distress in labor); may show early signs of maternal hypovolemia (late decelerations or fetal tachycardia) before overt maternal vital sign changes.

- Actual amount of blood loss is often greater than initially perceived because of the possibility of concealed retroplacental bleeding and apparent "normal" vital signs. The relative hypervolemia of pregnancy initially protects the patient until late in the course of bleeding, when abrupt and sudden cardiovascular collapse can occur.

LABORATORY TESTS

- Baseline serum hemoglobin helps quantify blood loss and establish baseline values for serial comparisons during expectant management.
- Coagulation profile: Platelets, fibrinogen, prothrombin, and partial thromboplastin time. Diffuse intravascular coagulation can develop with severe abruption. If fibrinogen is <150 mg/dl, estimated blood loss is approximately 2000 ml; if fibrinogen is <100 mg/dl, consider fresh frozen plasma to prevent further bleeding.
- Type and antibody screen is important to identify Rh-negative patients who need Rh immune globulin.

IMAGING STUDIES

Ultrasound should include fetal presentation and status, amniotic fluid volume, placental location, as well as any evidence of hematoma (retroplacental, subchorionic, or preplacental) (Fig. 3).

TREATMENT

ACUTE GENERAL Rx

- Stabilization of the mother is the first priority
- Treatment depends on gestational age of the fetus, severity of the abruption, and maternal status
- Initial assessment for signs of maternal hemodynamic compromise or hemorrhagic shock; large-bore intravenous access, with crystalloid fluid resuscitation using a replacement of 3 ml lactated Ringer solution for every 1 ml estimated blood loss
- Indwelling Foley catheter to monitor urine output and maternal volume status, with a goal of 0.5 cc/kg/h of urine output

TABLE 1 Placental Abruption Risk Factors

Increasing parity or maternal age
Cigarette smoking
Cocaine abuse
Trauma
Maternal hypertension
Preterm premature rupture of membranes
Rapid uterine decompression associated with multiple gestation and polyhydramnios
Inherited or acquired thrombophilia
Uterine malformations or fibroids
Placental abnormalities or ischemia
Prior abruption

From Gabbe SG: *Obstetrics,* ed 6, Philadelphia, 2012, Saunders.

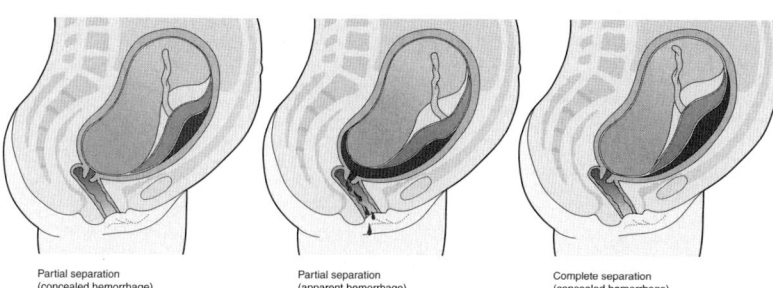

Partial separation (concealed hemorrhage)   Partial separation (apparent hemorrhage)   Complete separation (concealed hemorrhage)

FIG. 1 Classification of placental abruption. (From Magowan BA: *Clinical obstetrics & gynecology,* ed 4, 2019, Elsevier.)

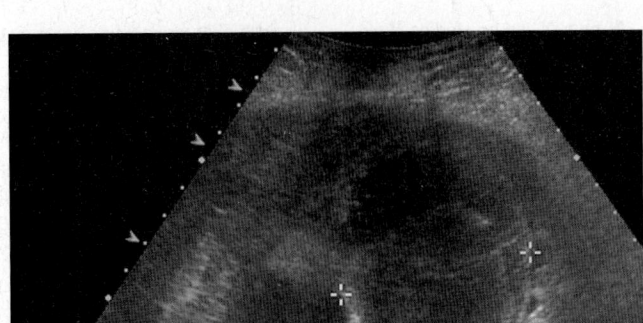

FIG. 2 Placental abruption. Transabdominal sonogram of the placenta *(PL)* with a hematoma *(calipers)* lifting the placenta away from the uterine wall. (From Rumack CM et al [eds]: *Diagnostic ultrasound,* ed 4, Philadelphia, 2011, Mosby.)

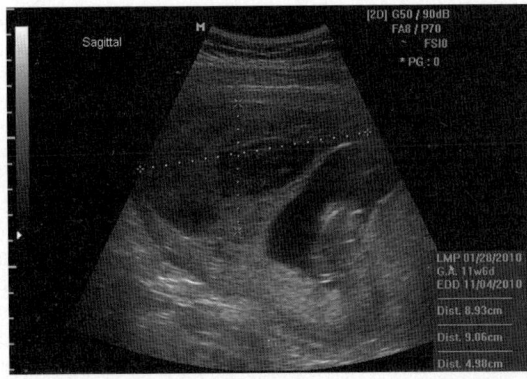

FIG. 3 Ultrasonic image of a subchorionic abruption. (Courtesy K. Francois; from Gabbe SG: *Obstetrics,* ed 6, Philadelphia, 2012, Saunders.)

- Assess fetal status and gestational age by sonogram and continuous fetal heart rate monitoring
- Because of the unpredictable nature of abruptions, cross-matched blood should be made available during the initial resuscitation period

CHRONIC Rx

- In the term fetus, delivery is indicated.
- In the preterm fetus, consider betamethasone 12.5 mg IM q24h for two doses and then delivery, depending on the severity of the abruption and the likelihood of fetal complications from preterm birth. Expectant management may be appropriate in some cases depending on maternal and fetal stability.
- Cesarean delivery should be reserved for cases of fetal distress or for standard obstetric indications. While cesarean delivery may be needed to stabilize the fetal and/or maternal status, the mother's coagulation status may complicate the procedure and availability of blood products may be critical.
- In cases of maternal stability and fetal prematurity, expectant management can occur in the setting of close follow-up, including regular evaluation of fetal growth and reassuring antenatal testing.

DISPOSITION

Because of the unpredictable nature of abruptions, expectant management should occur only under controlled circumstances.

REFERRAL

Abruptio placentae places mother and fetus in a high-risk situation and should be managed by a qualified obstetrician in a facility with capability for neonatal and maternal resuscitation, for supporting a preterm infant if delivery is indicated at an early gestational age, and for performing emergency cesarean deliveries.

RELATED CONTENT

Abruptio Placentae (Patient Information)
Premature Labor (Related Key Topic)
Vaginal Bleeding During Pregnancy (Related Key Topic)

AUTHOR: **ANNE REED-WESTON, MD**

BASIC INFORMATION

DEFINITION

Absence seizures are a type of generalized seizure characterized by brief episodes of staring with impairment of consciousness (absence). They usually last no more than 20 to 30 sec. The onset and the end of the seizures are sudden. Patients are typically unaware of the seizure and resume the activity they were performing before the seizure. The electroencephalogram signature of absence seizures consists of a generalized 3-Hz spike and slow wave discharges.

SYNONYMS

Childhood absence epilepsy
Seizures, absence

> **ICD-10CM CODE**
> G40.309 Generalized idiopathic epilepsy and epileptic syndromes, not intractable, without status epilepticus

EPIDEMIOLOGY & DEMOGRAPHICS

INCIDENCE: 1 to 10 cases per 100,000 population
PREVALENCE: Represents up to 12% to 18% of all pediatric epilepsy syndromes
PREDOMINANT SEX & AGE: More common in girls than in boys, absences typically begin between 4 and 10 yr and remit by age 20 yr.[1]
PEAK INCIDENCE: 6 to 7 yr

PHYSICAL FINDINGS & CLINICAL PRESENTATION

- Patients with absence seizures usually have normal physical and neurologic examinations. However, attention deficit hyperactivity disorder (ADHD), anxiety, mood disorders, and learning disorders are common comorbidities in children with absence seizures.
- During the seizures, the patients are unresponsive and can have motor phenomena (automatisms, eye blinks, mouth and hand movements).
- Typical seizure duration is 4 to 20 sec.
- Absence seizures are not associated with post-ictal confusion.
- They may be triggered by hyperventilation associated with activity.
- Tonic clonic seizures are not usually a feature of this syndrome. If the patient also experiences tonic clonic seizures, other etiologies should be investigated, such as juvenile absence epilepsy, juvenile myoclonic epilepsy, complex partial seizures, etc.

ETIOLOGY

Genetic

DIAGNOSIS

DIFFERENTIAL DIAGNOSIS

It is important to distinguish between focal onset impaired awareness seizures (previously called complex partial seizures) and absence seizures (Tables E1 and E2).

- Juvenile absence epilepsy
- Juvenile myoclonic epilepsy
- Complex partial seizures
- Focal seizures with altered consciousness
- Nonepileptic spells comprised of staring
- GLUT1 deficiency syndrome
- Epilepsy with eyelid myoclonia
- Epilepsy with myoclonic absences
- Atypical absence seizures

WORKUP

- Electroencephalogram (EEG) with hyperventilation and photic stimulation is crucial in the diagnosis (Fig. E1).
- Ambulatory EEG and video EEG are recommended for patients with diagnostic uncertainty.

LABORATORY TESTS

No specific studies needed

IMAGING STUDIES

- MRI of the brain with and without contrast should be performed in all epilepsy patients, especially if the EEG does not show the typical characteristic of absence seizures (3-Hz spike and slow wave discharges).
- Computed tomography scans of the head should be avoided in children due to unnecessary exposure to radiation and low yield of the test except when MRI cannot be obtained.

TREATMENT

The medication of choice based on the best current evidence available is ethosuximide, followed by valproic acid and lamotrigine.[2]

NONPHARMACOLOGIC THERAPY

Not applicable

ACUTE GENERAL Rx

- Ethosuximide: Initial dose: 5 to 10 mg/kg/day divided into two doses for children <6 yr and 250 mg/kg twice daily for children 6 yr and older; then after 7 days, the usual maintenance dose is 15 to 40 mg/kg/day in divided doses; goal therapeutic concentration is 40 to 100 micrograms/ml.
- Divalproex sodium (Depakote): Initial dose: 15 mg/kg/day (divided od, bid, or tid); dose is increased by 5 to 10 mg/kg per day at weekly intervals until seizures controlled or side effects prevent further increases; maximum/maintenance dose: 30 to 60 mg/kg/day (divided bid or tid); therapeutic concentration is 50 to 125 micrograms/ml.
- Lamotrigine (Lamictal): Dose for patients age 2.5 to 13 yr on no other antiepileptic drugs. Wk 1 and 2: 0.3 mg/kg/day. Wk 3 and 4: 0.6 mg/kg/day. Wk 5 onward: Increase every 1 to 2 wk by 0.6 mg/kg/day. Maintenance: 4.5 to 7.5 mg/kg/day. Warning: Should be used with caution due to the potential for toxicity and Stevens-Johnson syndrome. Patients on other antiepileptic drugs can also have severe adverse reactions (e.g., valproate can cause increased levels of lamotrigine, and lamotrigine must be titrated much more slowly in patients on valproate therapy).

CHRONIC Rx

- Children with recurrent seizures require chronic treatment.
- If children are seizure-free for a period of 1 to 2 yr, a trial on no medications should be considered; children typically outgrow childhood absence seizures.

DISPOSITION

- Response to treatment is excellent.
- Absence seizures tend to remit in teenage years.
- Epilepsy can be considered as resolved once 10 yr have elapsed since the last event, including 5 yr free from medications.

COMPLEMENTARY & ALTERNATIVE MEDICINE

Not applicable

REFERRAL

Patients with epilepsy should be referred for a consultation by a child neurologist, preferably one specializing in epilepsy.

PEARLS & CONSIDERATIONS

COMMENTS

- Absence seizures can be present in other epilepsy syndromes.
- Valproate should be avoided in girls and women with childbearing potential due to the risk of teratogenicity.
- Carbamazepine and phenytoin should be avoided in the treatment of absence seizures since these medications may worsen seizures and provoke absence status epilepticus.
- All women of childbearing age taking antiepileptic drugs should take folic acid supplementation (1 to 4 mg/day) for the prevention of neural tube defects.

PREVENTION

Sleep deprivation and alcohol consumption should be avoided.

PATIENT & FAMILY EDUCATION

Patients with ongoing seizures are forbidden to drive; check state regulations and laws regarding driving and epilepsy.

RELATED CONTENT

Absence Seizures (Patient Information)

> **REFERENCES**
> Available at eBooks.Health.Elsevier.com.

AUTHORS: **NAOMI R. KASS, BA** and
JOSEPH S. KASS, MD, JD, FAAN

BASIC INFORMATION

DEFINITION

Acquired immunodeficiency syndrome (AIDS) is a disorder caused by infection with the human immunodeficiency virus (HIV) and marked by progressive deterioration of the cellular immune system, leading to secondary (opportunistic) infections and/or malignancies.

SYNONYM

AIDS

ICD-10CM CODE
B20   Human immunodeficiency virus
        [HIV] disease

EPIDEMIOLOGY & DEMOGRAPHICS

INCIDENCE (IN U.S.):
- A significant number of persons are diagnosed with AIDS in the U.S. each year.
- There is a disproportionate number of new HIV/AIDS cases among Black/African Americans and Latino/Hispanic Americans compared with white Americans.
- The majority of all new HIV/AIDS diagnoses are among gay, bisexual, or other men who have sex with men (MSM).

PREVALENCE (IN U.S.): Approximately 1.2 million people in the U.S. have HIV. A subset of these have been diagnosed with AIDS.

PREDOMINANT SEX: Men constitute the majority of HIV/AIDS diagnoses in the U.S. with a disproportionate number among MSM.

PREDOMINANT AGE: The predominant age group diagnosed with HIV/AIDS is 25 to 59 yr of age.

PEAK INCIDENCE: Ages 25 to 59 yr

GENETICS:
- Familial disposition: Although there is no proven genetic predisposition, individuals with deletions in the *CCR5* gene are less susceptible to HIV infection with macrophage tropic virus (the predominant virus in sexual transmission) and may progress to AIDS more slowly.
- Congenital infection:
  1. HIV is transmittable from an infected mother to the fetus in utero in as many as 30% of pregnancies if untreated.
  2. No specific congenital malformations associated with infection; low birth weight and spontaneous abortion are possible.

PHYSICAL FINDINGS & CLINICAL PRESENTATION

- Nonspecific findings: Fever, weight loss, anorexia
- Specific syndromes:
  1. Seen in association with specific opportunistic infections and malignancies. These include:
     a. Opportunistic infections:
        (1) Disseminated strongyloidiasis
        (2) Disseminated toxoplasmosis, cryptococcosis, histoplasmosis,

cytomegalovirus (CMV), herpes simplex virus (HSV), or mycobacterial disease (most common is *Mycobacterium avium* complex)
        (3) *Candida* esophagitis or bronchopulmonary disease
        (4) Chronic cryptosporidiosis diarrhea
        (5) *Pneumocystis jiroveci* pneumonia (PJP)
        (6) Extensive pulmonary and extrapulmonary tuberculosis (TB)
        (7) Recurrent pneumonia or other bacterial infections
        (8) Progressive multifocal leukoencephalopathy (PML)
     b. AIDS-related neoplasms:
        (1) Kaposi sarcoma
        (2) Primary brain lymphoma
        (3) Invasive cervical carcinoma
        (4) High-grade B-cell non-Hodgkin lymphoma, Burkitt lymphoma, undifferentiated non-Hodgkin lymphoma, or immunoblastic lymphoma
  2. Most common:
     a. Respiratory infections (Pneumocystis jiroveci [formerly known as Pneumocystis carinii] pneumonia, TB, bacterial pneumonia, fungal infection)
     b. CNS infections (toxoplasmosis, TB)
     c. GI (cryptosporidiosis, isosporiasis, CMV); Sections II and III describe organisms associated with diarrhea in patients with AIDS
     d. Eye infections (CMV, toxoplasmosis)
     e. Kaposi sarcoma (cutaneous or visceral) or lymphoma (nodal or extranodal)
- Possibly asymptomatic
- Diagnosis of AIDS if the CD4 cell count is <200 or <14% of total lymphocyte in the presence of proven HIV infection, even in the absence of other infections
- The various manifestations of HIV infection are described in Section II

ETIOLOGY

- Caused by infection with HIV-1 or HIV-2 (less common).
- HIV is transmitted by sexual contact, needle-sharing (during injection drug use), transfusion of contaminated blood or blood products, and from infected mother to fetus or neonate.

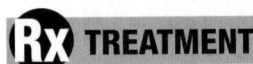 **DIAGNOSIS**

DIFFERENTIAL DIAGNOSIS

- Other wasting illnesses mimicking the nonspecific features of AIDS:
  1. TB
  2. Malignancy
  3. Disseminated fungal infection
  4. Malabsorption syndromes
  5. Depression
- Other disorders associated with dementia or demyelination producing encephalopathy, myelopathy, or neuropathy

WORKUP

Prompt evaluation of respiratory, CNS, and GI complaints. Fig. 1 illustrates a syndromic approach to suspected opportunistic infection in HIV.

LABORATORY TESTS

- HIV antibody testing. See "Human Immunodeficiency Virus" topic for the updated surveillance case definition for HIV infection
- CD4 cell count: Performed to determine the degree of immunodeficiency
- Viral load assay: To plan long-term antiviral therapy and to follow progression and success of treatment (i.e., HIV RNA PCR)
- CSF examination: For meningitis or neurologic disease (if indicated)
- Serologic tests for syphilis, hepatitis A, hepatitis B, hepatitis C, and toxoplasmosis
- Testing for other sexually transmitted infections (STIs) such as syphilis, gonorrhea, and chlamydia
- Genotypic resistance testing: Used to assess for primary resistance in naïve patients and secondary resistance in patients failing a regimen
- Eye exam: To evaluate for CMV retinitis in patients with CD4 counts <50 cells/mm^3
- Cryptococcal antigen: Part of the evaluation in AIDS patients with CD4 counts <100 cells/mm^3 who have fever, diffuse pneumonia, or evidence of meningitis
- Evaluation for infection with mycobacterium (TB or MAI) including a tuberculin skin test (TST) or interferon-gamma release assay (IGRA), sputum cultures, chest radiograph, and blood cultures for acid-fast bacteria, depending on clinical presentation

IMAGING STUDIES

- MRI or CT of head for encephalopathy or focal CNS complications (e.g., toxoplasmosis [Fig. E2], lymphoma)
- Chest radiography or CT to aid in the diagnosis of *Pneumocystis jiroveci* pneumonia (PJP), TB, or bacterial pneumonia

Rx **TREATMENT**

The most important aspect in management of AIDS due to HIV infection is the timely initiation of antiretroviral therapy. Antiretroviral therapy should be initiated regardless of CD4 cell count.

NONPHARMACOLOGIC THERAPY

- Maintain adequate caloric intake.
- Encourage good oral hygiene and regular dental care.
- Avoid high-risk behaviors that increase the risk of other potential pathogens—use condoms, avoid sharing needles, etc.
- Update vaccines—particularly Tdap (tetanus, diphtheria, and pertussis), pneumococcal, meningococcal, and hepatitis A/B vaccines along with annual influenza vaccines. COVID-19 vaccination is recommended.

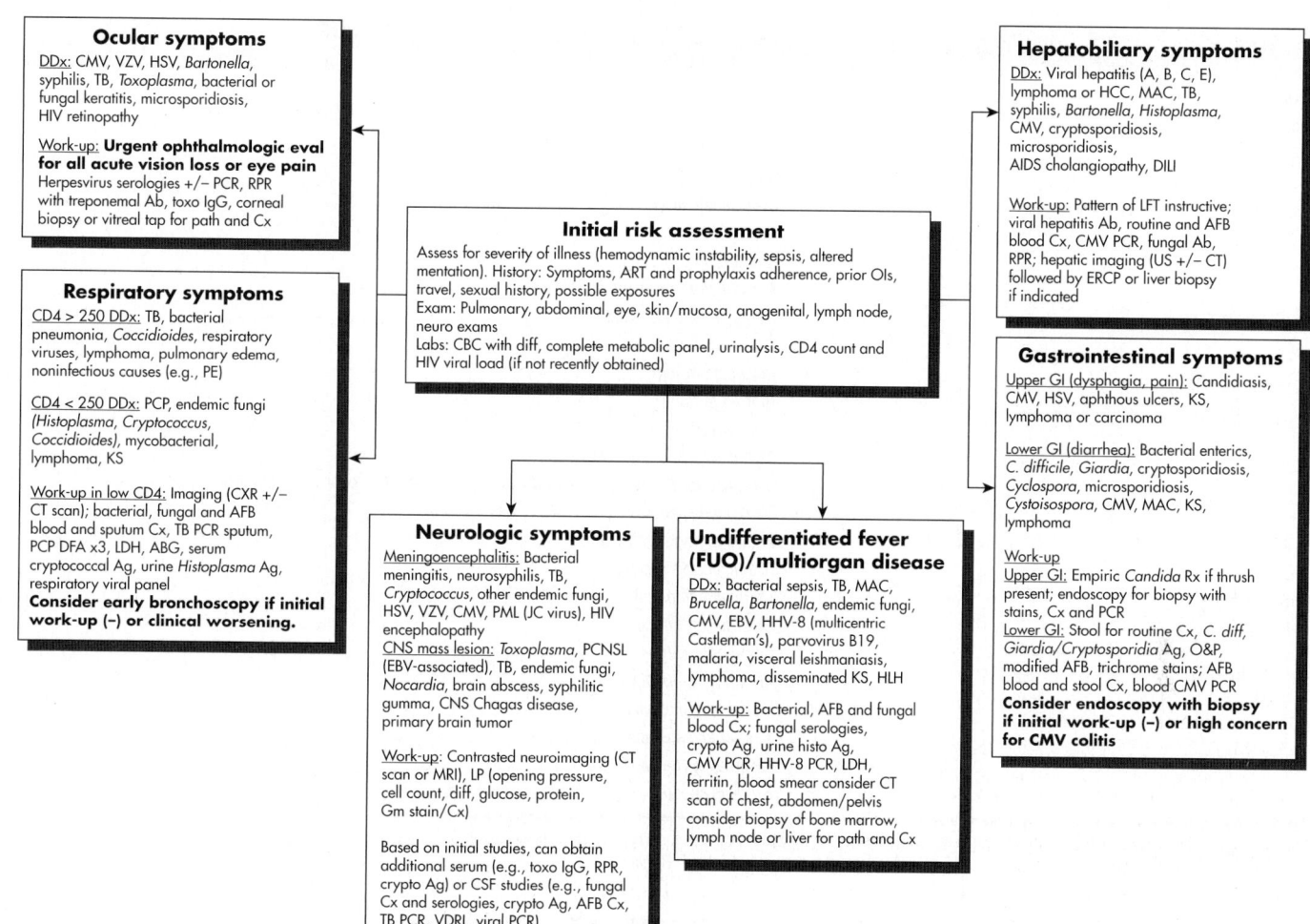

FIG. 1 Syndromic approach to suspected opportunistic infection in HIV. *ABG,* Arterial blood gas; *AFB,* acid-fast bacilli; *ART,* antiretroviral therapy; *CBC,* complete blood count; *CMV,* cytomegalovirus; *DFA,* direct fluorescent antibody; *DILI,* drug-induced liver injury; *EBV,* Epstein–Barr virus; *ERCP,* endoscopic retrograde cholangiopancreatography; *FUO,* fever of unknown origin; *HCC,* hepatocellular carcinoma; *HHV-8,* human herpes virus 8; *HLH,* hemophagocytic lymphohistiocytosis; *HSV,* herpes simplex virus; *KS,* Kaposi sarcoma; *LDH,* lactate dehydrogenase; *LP,* lumbar puncture; *MAC, Mycobacterium avium* complex; *O&P,* ova and parasite; *PCNSL,* primary CNS lymphoma; *PCP, Pneumocystis* pneumonia; *PCR,* polymerase chain reaction; *PE,* pulmonary embolism; *PML,* progressive multifocal leukoencephalopathy; *RPR,* rapid plasma reagin; *TB,* tuberculosis; *US,* ultrasound; *VDRL,* Venereal Disease Research Laboratory test; *VZV,* varicella-zoster virus. (From Spec A et al: *Comprehensive review of infectious diseases,* 2020, Elsevier.)

- Avoid administration of any live attenuated vaccines that may be a risk to these immunocompromised patients (e.g., MMR, varicella). (See "Section V" for immunization schedules for HIV-infected children.)
- When feasible, avoid activities that might increase risk of exposure to opportunistic infections (e.g., cleaning out a cat litter box [toxoplasmosis], getting scratched by a cat [*Bartonella* infections], exposure to pet reptiles [salmonellosis], traveling to developing countries [cryptosporidiosis, tuberculosis], eating undercooked foods and drinking from unsafe water supplies, etc.). A description of enteropathogens causing infections in HIV-infected patients is provided in Table 1.

ACUTE GENERAL Rx

Acute management of opportunistic infections is summarized in Table 2 and reviewed elsewhere in this text under specific AIDS-related

disorders. For management of AIDS-related malignancies, please refer to the specific malignancy elsewhere in this text.

CHRONIC Rx

For all HIV-infected patients, particularly those meeting the case definition of AIDS:

- Preventive therapy for *Pneumocystis jiroveci* pneumonia and *Mycobacterium avium* (see specific chapters elsewhere in this text). With appropriate antiretroviral therapy, many patients experience substantial restoration of cellular immune function. Preventive therapy for *Pneumocystis jiroveci* can be safely stopped if the CD4 cell count rises above 200 for at least 3 mo.
- Based on the Department of Health and Human Services (DHHS) Guidelines, active antiretroviral therapy (ART) should be started regardless of CD4 cell count. Individuals with CD4 cell counts <350 and especially CD4

cell counts <200 should be strongly encouraged to start ART in a timely fashion.
- ART usually includes three-drug combinations of:
  1. Nucleoside reverse transcriptase inhibitors (NRTI): Tenofovir disoproxil fumarate (TDF), tenofovir alafenamide fumarate (TAF), lamivudine (3TC), emtricitabine (FTC), and abacavir (ABC). Older drugs such as zidovudine (AZT), didanosine (ddI), and stavudine (d4T) are generally not recommended.
  2. Protease inhibitors (PI): Darunavir (preferred) or atazanavir.
  3. Nonnucleoside reverse transcriptase inhibitors (NNRTI): Nevirapine, efavirenz (EFV), etravirine, doravirine, and rilpivirine.
  4. Integrase inhibitors: Raltegravir, elvitegravir, bictegravir, dolutegravir, and cabotegravir.
  5. Others: Maraviroc, enfuvirtide, ibalizumab, and fostemsavir.

TABLE 1 Organisms That Cause Gastrointestinal Tract Infections in Patients With HIV/AIDS

Organisms

Esophagus	*Candida albicans*[a]
	Cytomegalovirus[a]
	Herpes simplex virus[a]
Hepatobiliary	Cytomegalovirus
	Cryptosporidium[a]
	Hepatotropic viruses
	Mycobacterium avium complex[a]
Small intestine	*Campylobacter* species
	Cytomegalovirus[a]
	Cryptosporidium[a]
	Giardia lamblia[a]
	Isospora belli[a]
	Mycobacterium avium complex[a]
	Microsporidia[a] (*Enterocytozoon bieneusi* and *Encephalitozoon intestinalis*)
	Salmonella species[a]
	Enteroaggregative *E. coli*
	Strongyloides stercoralis
Large intestine	*Campylobacter* species
	Clostridium difficile
	Cytomegalovirus[a]
	Entamoeba histolytica
	Herpes simplex virus[a]
	Salmonella species[a]
	Enteroaggregative *E. coli*
	Shigella species

[a]Diseases of the gastrointestinal tract that fulfill the Centers for Disease Control and Prevention surveillance case definition of AIDS.
From Cherry JD et al: *Feigin and Cherry's pediatric infectious diseases,* ed 8, Philadelphia, 2019, Elsevier.

TABLE 2 Treatment of AIDS-Associated Opportunistic Infections

Opportunistic Infection	Preferred Therapy	Alternative Therapy	Other Comments
PJP	• Patients who develop PJP despite TMP-SMX prophylaxis can usually be treated with standard doses of TMP-SMX. • Duration of PJP treatment: 21 days. *For Moderate to Severe PJP:* • TMP-SMX: (TMP 15-20 mg and SMX 75-100 mg/kg/day) IV given q6h or q8h, may switch to PO after clinical improvement. *For Mild to Moderate PJP:* • TMP-SMX: (TMP 15-20 mg and SMX 75-100 mg/kg/day), given PO in 3 divided doses, *or* • TMP-SMX: (160 mg/800 mg or DS) 2 tablets PO tid. *Secondary Prophylaxis, after completion of PJP treatment:* • TMP-SMX DS: 1 tablet PO daily *or* • TMP-SMX (80 mg/400 mg or SS): 1 tablet PO daily.	*For Moderate to Severe PJP:* • Pentamidine 4 mg/kg IV daily infused over ≥60 min; can reduce dose to 3 mg/kg IV daily because of toxicities, *or* • Primaquine 30 mg (base) PO daily + (clindamycin 600 mg q6h IV or 900 mg IV q8h) or (clindamycin 300 mg PO q6h or 450 mg PO q8h). *For Mild to Moderate PJP:* • Dapsone 100 mg PO daily + TMP 5 mg/kg PO tid, *or* • Primaquine 30 mg (base) PO daily + (clindamycin 300 mg PO q6h or 450 mg PO q8h), *or* • Atovaquone 750 mg PO bid with food. *Secondary Prophylaxis, after completion of PJP treatment:* • TMP-SMX DS: 1 tablet PO tiw, *or* • Dapsone 100 mg PO daily, *or* • Dapsone 50 mg PO daily + (pyrimethamine 50 mg + leucovorin 25 mg) PO weekly, *or* • (Dapsone 200 mg + pyrimethamine 75 mg + leucovorin 25 mg) PO weekly, *or*	*Indications for Adjunctive Corticosteroids:* • Pao$_2$ <70 mm Hg at room air, *or* • Alveolar-arterial O$_2$ gradient >35 mm Hg. *Prednisone Doses (beginning as early as possible and within 72 h of PJP therapy):* • Days 1-5: 40 mg PO bid. • Days 6-10: 40 mg PO daily. • Days 11-21: 20 mg PO daily. • IV methylprednisolone can be administered as 75% of prednisone dose. • Benefit of corticosteroid if started after 72 h of treatment is unknown, but some clinicians will use it for moderate-to-severe PJP. • Whenever possible, patients should be tested for G6PD before use of dapsone or primaquine. Alternative therapy should be used in patients found to have G6PD deficiency. • Patients who are receiving pyrimethamine/sulfadiazine for treatment or suppression of toxoplasmosis do not require additional PJP prophylaxis.

TABLE 2   Treatment of AIDS-Associated Opportunistic Infections—cont'd

Opportunistic Infection	Preferred Therapy	Alternative Therapy	Other Comments
		• Aerosolized pentamidine 300 mg monthly via Respirgard II nebulizer, *or* • Atovaquone 1500 mg PO daily, *or* • (Atovaquone 1500 mg + pyrimethamine 25 mg + leucovorin 10 mg) PO daily.	• If TMP-SMX is discontinued because of a mild adverse reaction, reinstitution should be considered after the reaction resolves. The dose can be increased gradually (desensitization) or be reduced, or the frequency can be modified. • TMP-SMX should be permanently discontinued in patients with possible or definite Stevens–Johnson syndrome or toxic epidermal necrosis.
Toxoplasma gondii encephalitis	*Treatment of Acute Infection:* • Pyrimethamine 200 mg PO 1 time, followed by weight-based therapy: • If <60 kg, pyrimethamine 50 mg PO once daily + sulfadiazine 1000 mg PO q6h + leucovorin 10-25 mg PO once daily. • If ≥60 kg, pyrimethamine 75 mg PO once daily + sulfadiazine 1500 mg PO q6h + leucovorin 10-25 mg PO once daily. • Leucovorin dose can be increased to 50 mg daily or bid. *Duration for Acute Therapy:* • At least 6 wk; longer duration if clinical or radiologic disease is extensive or response is incomplete at 6 wk. *Chronic Maintenance Therapy:* • Pyrimethamine 25-50 mg PO daily + sulfadiazine 2000-4000 mg PO daily (in 2-4 divided doses) + leucovorin 10-25 mg PO daily (AI).	*Treatment of Acute Infection:* • Pyrimethamine (leucovorin)* + clindamycin 600 mg IV or PO q6h *or* • TMP-SMX (TMP 5 mg/kg and SMX 25 mg/kg) IV or PO bid, *or* • Atovaquone 1500 mg PO bid with food + pyrimethamine (leucovorin), *or* • Atovaquone 1500 mg PO bid with food + sulfadiazine 1000-1500 mg PO q6h (weight-based dosing, as in preferred therapy) *or* • Atovaquone 1500 mg PO bid with food, *or* • Pyrimethamine (leucovorin)* + azithromycin 900-1200 mg PO daily. *Chronic Maintenance Therapy:* • Clindamycin 600 mg PO q8h + (pyrimethamine 25-50 mg + leucovorin 10-25 mg) PO daily *or* • TMP-SMX DS 1 tablet bid, *or* • Atovaquone 750-1500 mg PO bid + (pyrimethamine 25 mg + leucovorin 10 mg) PO daily, *or* • Atovaquone 750-1500 mg PO bid + sulfadiazine 2000-4000 mg PO daily (in 2-4 divided doses), *or* • Atovaquone 750-1500 mg PO bid with food.	• Adjunctive corticosteroids (e.g., dexamethasone) should only be administered when clinically indicated to treat mass effect associated with focal lesions or associated edema; discontinue as soon as clinically feasible. • Anticonvulsants should be administered to patients with a history of seizures and continued through acute treatment but should not be used as seizure prophylaxis. • If clindamycin is used in place of sulfadiazine, additional therapy must be added to prevent PCP.
Mycobacterium tuberculosis disease (TB)	• After collecting specimen for culture and molecular diagnostic tests, empiric TB treatment should be started in individuals with clinical and radiographic presentation suggestive of TB. *Initial Phase (2 mo, given daily):* • INH + [RIF or RFB] + PZA + EMB. *Continuation Phase:* • INH + (RIF or RFB) daily. *Total Duration of Therapy (for drug-susceptible TB):* • Pulmonary TB: 6 mo. • Pulmonary TB and culture-positive after 2 mo of TB treatment: 9 mo. • Extrapulmonary TB with CNS infection: 9-12 mo. • Extrapulmonary TB with bone or joint involvement: 6-9 mo. • Extrapulmonary TB in other sites: 6 mo. • Total duration of therapy should be based on number of doses received, not on calendar time.	*Treatment for Drug-Resistant TB* • Resistant to INH: • (RIF or RFB) + EMB + PZA + (moxifloxacin or levofloxacin) for 2 mo; followed by (RIF or RFB) + EMB + (moxifloxacin or levofloxacin) for 7 mo. *Treatment for Drug-Resistant TB* • Resistant to INH: • (RIF or RFB) + EMB + PZA + (moxifloxacin or levofloxacin) for 2 mo; followed by (RIF or RFB) + EMB + (moxifloxacin or levofloxacin) for 7 mo. *Resistant to Rifamycins ± Other Drugs:* • Regimen and duration of treatment should be individualized based on resistance pattern, clinical and microbiologic responses, and in close consultation with experienced specialists.	• Adjunctive corticosteroid improves survival for TB meningitis and pericarditis. See text for drug, dose, and duration recommendations. • RIF *is not recommended* for patients receiving HIV PI because of its induction of PI metabolism. • RFB is a less potent CYP3A4 inducer than RIF and is preferred in patients receiving PIs. • Once-weekly rifapentine can result in development of rifamycin resistance in HIV-infected patients and *is not recommended.* • Therapeutic drug monitoring should be considered in patients receiving rifamycin and interacting ART. • Paradoxical IRIS that is not severe can be treated with NSAIDs without a change in TB or HIV therapy. • For severe IRIS reaction, consider prednisone and taper over 4 wk based on clinical symptoms. For example: • *If receiving RIF:* Prednisone 1.5 mg/kg/day for 2 wk, then 0.75 mg/kg/day for 2 wk.

TABLE 2 Treatment of AIDS-Associated Opportunistic Infections—cont'd

Opportunistic Infection	Preferred Therapy	Alternative Therapy	Other Comments
			• *If receiving RFB:* Prednisone 1.0 mg/kg/day for 2 wk, then 0.5 mg/kg/day for 2 wk. • A more gradual tapering schedule over a few mo may be necessary for some patients.
Disseminated MAC disease	*At Least Two Drugs as Initial Therapy With:* • Clarithromycin 500 mg PO bid + ethambutol 15 mg/kg PO daily, *or* Azithromycin 500-600 mg + ethambutol 15 mg/kg PO daily if drug interaction or intolerance precludes the use of clarithromycin. *Duration:* • At least 12 mo of therapy, can discontinue if no signs and symptoms of MAC disease and sustained (>6 mo) CD4 count >100 cells/µl in response to ART.	• Addition of a third or fourth drug should be considered for patients with advanced immunosuppression (CD4 counts <50 cells/µl), high mycobacterial loads (>2 log CFU/ml of blood), or in the absence of effective ART. *Third or Fourth Drug Options May Include:* • RFB 300 mg PO daily (dosage adjustment may be necessary based on drug interactions), *or* • Amikacin 10-15 mg/kg IV daily, *or* • Streptomycin 1 g IV or IM daily, *or* • Moxifloxacin 400 mg PO daily, *or* levofloxacin 500 mg PO daily.	• Testing of susceptibility to clarithromycin and azithromycin is recommended. • NSAIDs can be used for patients who experience moderate to severe symptoms attributed to IRIS. • If IRIS symptoms persist, short-term (4-8 wk) systemic corticosteroids (equivalent to 20-40 mg prednisone) can be used.
Bacterial respiratory diseases *(with focus on pneumonia)*	Empiric antibiotic therapy should be initiated promptly for patients presenting with clinical and radiographic evidence consistent with bacterial pneumonia. The recommendations listed are suggested empiric therapy. The regimen should be modified as needed once microbiologic results are available. *Empiric Outpatient Therapy:* • A PO β-lactam + a PO macrolide (azithromycin or clarithromycin). • *Preferred β-lactams:* Amoxicillin/clavulanate. • *Alternative β-lactams:* Cefpodoxime or cefuroxime, *or* • *For penicillin-allergic patients:* Levofloxacin 750 mg PO once daily, *or* moxifloxacin 400 mg PO once daily. • *Duration:* 7-10 days (a minimum of 5 days). Patients should be afebrile for 48-72 h and clinically stable before stopping antibiotics. *Empiric Therapy for Non-ICU Hospitalized Patients:* • An IV β-lactam + a macrolide (azithromycin or clarithromycin). • *Preferred β-lactams:* Ceftriaxone, cefotaxime, ceftaroline, or ampicillin-sulbactam. • *For penicillin-allergic patients:* Levofloxacin, 750 mg IV once daily, *or* moxifloxacin, 400 mg IV once daily. *Empiric Therapy for ICU Patients:* • An IV β-lactam + IV azithromycin, *or* • An IV β-lactam + (levofloxacin 750 mg IV once daily or moxifloxacin 400 mg IV once daily). • *Preferred β-lactams:* Ceftriaxone, cefotaxime, ceftaroline *or* ampicillin-sulbactam. *Empiric Therapy for Patients at Risk of Pseudomonas Pneumonia:* • An IV antipneumococcal, antipseudomonal β-lactam + ciprofloxacin 400 mg IV q8-12h or levofloxacin 750 mg IV once daily.	*Empiric Outpatient Therapy:* • A PO β-lactam + PO doxycycline. • Preferred β-lactams: Amoxicillin/clavulanate. • Alternative β-lactams: Cefpodoxime or cefuroxime. *Empiric Therapy for Non-ICU Hospitalized Patients:* • An IV β-lactam + doxycycline. *Empiric Therapy for ICU Patients:* • *For penicillin-allergic patients:* Aztreonam IV + (levofloxacin 750 mg IV once daily or moxifloxacin 400 mg IV once daily). May add other agents depending on concern for MRSA. *Empiric Therapy for Patients at Risk of Pseudomonas Pneumonia:* • Above β-lactam + an aminoglycoside + (levofloxacin 750 mg IV once daily or moxifloxacin 400 mg IV once daily), *or* • *For penicillin-allergic patients:* Replace the β-lactam with aztreonam. • An IV antipneumococcal, antipseudomonal β-lactam + an aminoglycoside + azithromycin.	• Fluoroquinolones should be used with caution in patients in whom TB is suspected but is not being treated. • Empiric therapy with a macrolide alone should be used with caution in areas with high (>25%) pneumococcal resistance. • Patients receiving a macrolide for MAC prophylaxis should not receive macrolide monotherapy for empiric treatment of bacterial pneumonia. • For patients begun on IV antibiotic therapy, switching to PO should be considered when they are clinically improved and able to tolerate oral medications. • Chemoprophylaxis can be considered for patients with frequent recurrences of serious bacterial pneumonia. • Clinicians should be cautious about using antibiotics to prevent recurrences because of the potential for developing drug resistance and drug toxicities.

TABLE 2 Treatment of AIDS-Associated Opportunistic Infections—cont'd

Opportunistic Infection	Preferred Therapy	Alternative Therapy	Other Comments
	• *Preferred β-lactams:* Piperacillin-tazobactam, cefepime, imipenem, or meropenem. *Empiric Therapy for Patients at Risk for Methicillin-Resistant Staphylococcus aureus Pneumonia:* • Add vancomycin IV or linezolid (IV or PO) to the baseline regimen. • Addition of clindamycin to vancomycin (but not to linezolid) can be considered for severe necrotizing pneumonia to minimize bacterial toxin production.		
Bacterial enteric infections	• Diagnostic fecal specimens should be obtained before initiation of empiric antibiotic therapy. • Empiric antibiotic therapy is indicated for patients with advanced HIV (CD4 count <200 cells/μl or concomitant AIDS-defining illnesses), with clinically severe diarrhea (>6 stools/day), and/or accompanying fever or chills. *Empiric Therapy:* • Ciprofloxacin 500-750 mg PO (or 400 mg IV) q12h. • Therapy should be adjusted based on the results of diagnostic workup. • For patients with chronic diarrhea (>14 days) without severe clinical signs, empiric antibiotic therapy is not necessary; can withhold treatment until a diagnosis is made.	*Empiric Therapy:* • Ceftriaxone 1 g IV q24h, *or* Cefotaxime 1 g IV q8h.	• Hospitalization with IV antibiotics should be considered in patients with marked nausea, vomiting, diarrhea, electrolyte abnormalities, acidosis, and blood pressure instability. • Oral or IV rehydration if indicated. • Antimotility agents should be avoided if there is concern about inflammatory diarrhea, including *Clostridium difficile*–associated diarrhea. • If no clinical response after 5-7 days, consider follow-up stool culture with antibiotic susceptibility testing or alternative diagnostic tests (e.g., toxin assays, molecular testing), alternative diagnosis, or antibiotic resistance.
Salmonellosis	All HIV-infected patients with salmonellosis should be treated because of high risk of bacteremia.		
	• Ciprofloxacin 500-750 mg PO (or 400 mg IV) q12h, if susceptible. *Duration of Therapy:* For gastroenteritis without bacteremia: • If CD4 count ≥200 cells/μl: 7-14 days. • If CD4 count <200 cells/μl: 2-6 wk. For gastroenteritis with bacteremia: • If CD4 count ≥200/μl: 14 days; longer duration if bacteremia persists or if the infection is complicated (e.g., if metastatic foci of infection are present). • If CD4 count <200 cells/μl: 2-6 wk. *Secondary Prophylaxis Should Be Considered for:* • Patients with recurrent *Salmonella* gastroenteritis ± bacteremia, *or* • Patients with CD4 <200 cells/μl with severe diarrhea.	• Levofloxacin 750 mg (PO or IV) q24h, *or* • Moxifloxacin 400 mg (PO or IV) q24h, *or* • TMP, 160 mg-SMX 800 mg (PO or IV) q12h, *or* • Ceftriaxone 1 g IV q24h, *or* • Cefotaxime 1 g IV q8h.	• Oral or IV rehydration if indicated. • Antimotility agents should be avoided. • The role of long-term secondary prophylaxis in patients with recurrent *Salmonella* bacteremia is not well established. Must weigh benefit against risks of long-term antibiotic exposure. • Effective ART may reduce the frequency, severity, and recurrence of *Salmonella* infections.
Mucocutaneous candidiasis	*For Oropharyngeal Candidiasis; Initial Episodes (for 7-14 days):* Oral Therapy • Fluconazole 100 mg PO daily, *or* Topical Therapy • Clotrimazole troches, 10 mg PO 5 times daily, *or* • Miconazole mucoadhesive buccal 50-mg tablet—apply to mucosal surface over the canine fossa once daily (do not swallow, chew, or crush).	*For Oropharyngeal Candidiasis; Initial Episodes (for 7-14 days):* Oral Therapy • Itraconazole oral solution 200 mg PO daily, *or* • Posaconazole oral solution 400 mg PO bid for 1 day, then 400 mg daily. Topical Therapy • Nystatin suspension 4-6 ml qid or 1-2 flavored pastilles 4-5 times daily.	• Chronic or prolonged use of azoles may promote development of resistance. • Higher relapse rate for esophageal candidiasis is seen with echinocandins than with fluconazole use. • Suppressive therapy is usually not recommended unless patients have frequent or severe recurrences.

Continued

TABLE 2	Treatment of AIDS-Associated Opportunistic Infections—cont'd		
Opportunistic Infection	**Preferred Therapy**	**Alternative Therapy**	**Other Comments**
	For Esophageal Candidiasis (for 14-21 days): • Fluconazole 100 mg (up to 400 mg) PO or IV daily, *or* • Itraconazole oral solution 200 mg PO daily. *For Uncomplicated Vulvovaginal Candidiasis:* • Oral fluconazole 150 mg for 1 dose, *or* • Topical azoles (clotrimazole, butoconazole, miconazole, tioconazole, or terconazole) for 3-7 days. *For Severe or Recurrent Vulvovaginal Candidiasis:* • Fluconazole 100-200 mg PO daily for ≥7 days, *or* • Topical antifungal ≥7 days.	*For Esophageal Candidiasis (for 14-21 days):* • Voriconazole 200 mg PO or IV bid, *or* • Posaconazole 400 mg PO bid, *or* • Anidulafungin 100 mg IV 1 time, then 50 mg IV daily, *or* • Caspofungin 50 mg IV daily, *or* • Micafungin 150 mg IV daily, *or* • Amphotericin B deoxycholate 0.6 mg/kg IV daily, *or* • Lipid formulation of amphotericin B 3-4 mg/kg IV daily. *For Uncomplicated Vulvovaginal Candidiasis:* • Itraconazole oral solution 200 mg PO daily for 3-7 days.	*If Decision Is to Use Suppressive Therapy: Oropharyngeal Candidiasis:* • Fluconazole 100 mg PO daily or tiw. • Itraconazole oral solution 200 mg PO daily. *Esophageal Candidiasis:* • Fluconazole 100-200 mg PO daily. • Posaconazole 400 mg PO bid. *Vulvovaginal Candidiasis:* • Fluconazole 150 mg PO once weekly.
Cryptococcosis	*Cryptococcal Meningitis* • Induction Therapy (for at least 2 wk, followed by consolidation therapy): • Liposomal amphotericin B 3-4 mg/kg IV daily + flucytosine 25 mg/kg PO qid. (NOTE: Flucytosine dose should be adjusted in patients with renal dysfunction.) *Consolidation Therapy (for at least 8 wk followed by maintenance therapy):* • Fluconazole 800 mg PO (or IV) daily. *Maintenance Therapy:* • Fluconazole 200 mg PO daily for at least 12 mo. *For Non-CNS, Extrapulmonary Cryptococcosis and Diffuse Pulmonary Disease:* • Treatment same as for cryptococcal meningitis. *Non-CNS Cryptococcosis With Mild to Moderate Symptoms and Focal Pulmonary Infiltrates:* • Fluconazole, 400-800 mg PO daily for 12 mo.	*Cryptococcal Meningitis* • Induction Therapy (for at least 2 wk, followed by consolidation therapy): • Amphotericin B deoxycholate 0.7 mg/kg IV daily + flucytosine 25 mg/kg PO qid, *or* • Amphotericin B lipid complex 5 mg/kg IV daily + flucytosine 25 mg/kg PO qid, *or* • Liposomal amphotericin B 3-4 mg/kg IV daily + fluconazole 800 mg PO or IV daily, *or* • Amphotericin B deoxycholate 0.7 mg/kg IV daily + fluconazole 800 mg PO or IV daily, *or* • Fluconazole 800-1200 mg PO or IV daily + flucytosine 25 mg/kg PO qid, *or* • Fluconazole 1200 mg PO or IV daily. *Consolidation Therapy (for at least 8 wk followed by maintenance therapy):* • Itraconazole 200 mg PO bid for 8 wk—less effective than fluconazole. *Maintenance Therapy:* • No alternative therapy recommendation.	• Addition of flucytosine to amphotericin B has been associated with more rapid sterilization of CSF and decreased risk for subsequent relapse. • Patients receiving flucytosine should have either blood levels monitored (peak level 2 h after dose should be 30-80 μg/ml) or close monitoring of blood counts for development of cytopenia. Dosage should be adjusted in patients with renal insufficiency. • Opening pressure should always be measured when an LP is performed. Repeated LPs or CSF shunting are essential to effectively manage increased intracranial pressure. • Corticosteroids and mannitol are ineffective in reducing intracranial pressure and are not recommended. • Some specialists recommend a brief course of corticosteroid for management of severe IRIS symptoms.
Histoplasmosis	*Moderately Severe to Severe Disseminated Disease Induction Therapy (for at least 2 wk or until clinically improved):* • Liposomal amphotericin B 3 mg/kg IV daily. *Maintenance Therapy:* • Itraconazole 200 mg PO tid for 3 days, then 200 mg PO bid. *Less Severe Disseminated Disease:* Induction and Maintenance Therapy: • Itraconazole 200 mg PO tid for 3 days, then 200 mg PO bid. *Duration of Therapy:* • At least 12 mo. *Meningitis* Induction Therapy (4-6 wk): • Liposomal amphotericin B 5 mg/kg/day. *Maintenance Therapy:* • Itraconazole 200 mg PO bid to tid for ≥1 yr and until resolution of abnormal CSF findings. *Long-Term Suppression Therapy:* • For patients with severe disseminated or CNS infection after completion of at least 12 mo of therapy; and those who relapse despite appropriate therapy. • Itraconazole 200 mg PO daily.	*Moderately Severe to Severe Disseminated Disease Induction Therapy (for at least 2 wk or until clinically improved):* • Amphotericin B lipid complex 3 mg/kg IV daily, *or* • Amphotericin B cholesteryl sulfate complete 3 mg/kg IV daily. *Alternatives to Itraconazole for Maintenance Therapy or Treatment of Less Severe Disease:* • Voriconazole 400 mg PO bid for 1 day, then 200 mg bid, *or* • Posaconazole 400 mg PO bid. • Fluconazole 800 mg PO daily. *Meningitis* • No alternative therapy recommendation. Long-Term Suppression Therapy: • Fluconazole 400 mg PO daily.	• Itraconazole, posaconazole, and voriconazole may have significant interactions with certain ARV agents. These interactions are complex and can be bidirectional. • Therapeutic drug monitoring and dosage adjustment may be necessary to ensure triazole antifungal and ARV efficacy and to reduce concentration-related toxicities. • Random serum concentration of itraconazole + hydroxyitraconazole should be >1 μg/ml. • Clinical experience with voriconazole or posaconazole in the treatment of histoplasmosis is limited. • Acute pulmonary histoplasmosis in HIV-infected patients with CD4 counts >300 cells/μl should be managed as nonimmunocompromised host.

TABLE 2   Treatment of AIDS-Associated Opportunistic Infections—cont'd

Opportunistic Infection	Preferred Therapy	Alternative Therapy	Other Comments
Coccidioidomycosis	*Clinically Mild Infections (e.g., focal pneumonia):* • Fluconazole 400 mg PO daily *or* • Itraconazole 200 mg PO bid. *Severe, Nonmeningeal Infection (diffuse pulmonary infection or severely ill patients with extrathoracic, disseminated disease):* • Amphotericin B deoxycholate 0.7-1.0 mg/kg IV daily. • Lipid formulation amphotericin B 4-6 mg/kg IV daily. • Duration of therapy: Continue until clinical improvement, then switch to an azole. *Meningeal Infections:* • Fluconazole 400-800 mg IV or PO daily. *Chronic Suppressive Therapy:* • Fluconazole 400 mg PO daily, *or* • Itraconazole 200 mg PO bid.	*Mild Infections (focal pneumonia) for patients who failed to respond to fluconazole or itraconazole:* • Posaconazole 200 mg PO bid, *or* • Voriconazole 200 mg PO bid. *Severe, Nonmeningeal Infection (diffuse pulmonary infection or severely ill patients with extrathoracic, disseminated disease):* • Some specialists will add a triazole (fluconazole or itraconazole, with itraconazole preferred for bone disease) 400 mg per day to amphotericin B therapy and continue triazole once amphotericin B is stopped. *Meningeal Infections:* • Itraconazole 200 mg PO tid for 3 days, then 200 mg PO bid, *or* • Posaconazole 200 mg PO bid, *or* • Voriconazole 200-400 mg PO bid, *or* • Intrathecal amphotericin B deoxycholate, when triazole antifungals are ineffective. *Chronic Suppressive Therapy:* • Posaconazole 200 mg PO bid, *or* • Voriconazole 200 mg PO bid.	• Some patients with meningitis may develop hydrocephalus and require CSF shunting. • Therapy should be continued indefinitely in patients with diffuse pulmonary or disseminated diseases because relapse can occur in 25%-33% of HIV-negative patients. It can also occur in HIV-infected patients with CD4 counts >250 cells/μL. • Therapy should be lifelong in patients with meningeal infections because relapse occurs in 80% of HIV-infected patients after discontinuation of triazole therapy. • Itraconazole, posaconazole, and voriconazole may have significant interactions with certain ARV agents. These interactions are complex and can be bidirectional. Therapeutic drug monitoring and dosage adjustment may be necessary to ensure triazole antifungal and antiretroviral efficacy and to reduce concentration-related toxicities. • Intrathecal amphotericin B should be given only in consultation with a specialist and should be administered by an individual with experience with the technique.
Aspergillosis, invasive	*Preferred Therapy:* • Voriconazole 6 mg/kg IV q12h for 1 day, then 4 mg/kg IV q12h, followed by voriconazole 200 mg PO q12h after clinical improvement. *Duration of Therapy:* • Until CD4 cell count >200 cells/μl and the infection appears to be resolved.	*Alternative Therapy:* • Lipid formulation of amphotericin B 5 mg/kg IV daily, *or* • Amphotericin B deoxycholate 1 mg/kg IV daily, *or* • Caspofungin 70 mg IV 1 time, then 50 mg IV daily, *or* • Micafungin 100-150 mg IV daily, *or* • Anidulafungin 200 mg IV 1 time, then 100 mg IV daily, *or* • Posaconazole 200 mg PO qid, then, after condition improved, 400 mg PO bid.	• Potential for significant pharmacokinetic interactions between certain ARV agents and voriconazole; they should be used cautiously in these situations. Consider therapeutic drug monitoring and dosage adjustment if necessary.
CMV disease	*CMV Retinitis Induction Therapy for Immediate Sight-Threatening Lesions (adjacent to the optic nerve or fovea):* • Consult ophthalmologist; ganciclovir implant no longer available: • Ganciclovir 5 mg/kg IV q12h for 14-21 days followed by Valganciclovir 900 mg PO bid. *For Small Peripheral Lesions:* • Valganciclovir 900 mg PO bid for 14-21 days. • One dose of intravitreal ganciclovir can be administered immediately after diagnosis until steady-state plasma ganciclovir concentration is achieved with oral valganciclovir. *Chronic Maintenance (secondary prophylaxis):* • Valganciclovir 900 mg PO daily (for small peripheral lesion). *CMV Esophagitis or Colitis:* • Ganciclovir 5 mg/kg IV q12h; may switch to valganciclovir 900 mg PO q12h once patient can tolerate oral therapy.	*CMV Retinitis Induction Therapy:* • Ganciclovir 5 mg/kg IV q12h for 14-21 days, *or* • Foscarnet 90 mg/kg IV q12h or 60 mg q8h for 14-21 days, *or* • Cidofovir 5 mg/kg/wk IV for 2 wk; saline hydration before and after therapy and probenecid, 2 g PO 3 hours before dose, followed by 1 g PO 2 h and 8 h after the dose (total of 4 g). (Note: This regimen should be avoided in patients with sulfa allergy because of cross-hypersensitivity with probenecid.) *Chronic Maintenance (secondary prophylaxis):* • Ganciclovir 5 mg/kg IV 5-7 times weekly, *or*	• The choice of therapy for CMV retinitis should be individualized, based on location and severity of the lesions, level of immunosuppression, and other factors (e.g., concomitant medications and ability to adhere to treatment). • The choice of chronic maintenance therapy (route of administration and drug choices) should be made in consultation with an ophthalmologist. Considerations should include the anatomic location of the retinal lesion, vision in the contralateral eye, the patients' immunologic and virologic status, and response to ART.

Continued

TABLE 2 Treatment of AIDS-Associated Opportunistic Infections—cont'd

Opportunistic Infection	Preferred Therapy	Alternative Therapy	Other Comments
	• Duration: 21-42 days or until symptoms have resolved. • Maintenance therapy is usually not necessary but should be considered after relapses. *Well-Documented, Histologically Confirmed CMV Pneumonia:* • Experience for treating CMV pneumonitis in HIV patients is limited. Use of IV ganciclovir or IV foscarnet is reasonable (doses same as for CMV retinitis). • The optimal duration of therapy and the role of oral valganciclovir have not been established. *CMV Neurologic Disease:* • Note: Treatment should be initiated promptly. • Ganciclovir 5 mg/kg IV q12h + (foscarnet 90 mg/kg IV q12h or 60 mg/kg IV q8h) to stabilize disease and maximize response; continue until symptomatic improvement and resolution of neurologic symptoms. • The optimal duration of therapy and the role of oral valganciclovir have not been established.	• Foscarnet 90-120 mg/kg IV once daily, *or* • Cidofovir 5 mg/kg IV every other week with saline hydration and probenecid as above. *CMV Esophagitis or Colitis:* • Foscarnet 90 mg/kg IV q12h or 60 mg/kg q8h for patients with treatment-limiting toxicities to ganciclovir or with ganciclovir resistance, *or* • Valganciclovir 900 mg PO q12h in milder disease and if able to tolerate PO therapy, *or* • For mild cases, if ART can be initiated without delay, consider withholding CMV therapy. • Duration: 21-42 days or until symptoms have resolved.	• Patients with CMV retinitis who discontinue maintenance therapy should undergo regular eye examinations for early detection of relapse IRU—optimally every 3 mo and then annually after immune reconstitution. • IRU may develop in the setting of immune reconstitution. *Treatment of IRU:* • Periocular corticosteroid or short courses of systemic steroid. • Initial therapy in patients with CMV retinitis, esophagitis, colitis, and pneumonitis should include initiation or optimization of ART.
HSV disease	*Orolabial Lesions (for 5-10 days):* • Valacyclovir 1 g PO bid *or* • Famciclovir 500 mg PO bid *or* • Acyclovir 400 mg PO tid. *Initial or Recurrent Genital HSV (for 5-14 days):* • Valacyclovir 1 g PO bid, *or* • Famciclovir 500 mg PO bid, *or* • Acyclovir 400 mg PO tid. *Severe Mucocutaneous HSV:* • Initial therapy acyclovir 5 mg/kg IV q8h. • After lesions begin to regress, change to PO therapy as previously. Continue until lesions are completely healed. *Chronic Suppressive Therapy for Patients With Severe Recurrences of Genital Herpes or for Patients Who Want to Minimize Frequency of Recurrences:* • Valacyclovir 500 mg PO bid. • Famciclovir 500 mg PO bid. • Acyclovir 400 mg PO bid. • Continue indefinitely regardless of CD4 cell count.	*For Acyclovir-Resistant HSV:* Preferred Therapy: • Foscarnet 80-120 mg/kg/day IV in 2-3 divided doses until clinical response. *Alternative Therapy:* • IV cidofovir (dosage as in CMV retinitis), *or* • Topical trifluridine, *or* • Topical cidofovir, *or* • Topical imiquimod. *Duration of Therapy:* • 21-28 days or longer.	• Patients with HSV infections can be treated with episodic therapy when symptomatic lesions occur, or with daily suppressive therapy to prevent recurrences. • Topical formulations of trifluridine and cidofovir are not commercially available. • Extemporaneous compounding of topical products can be prepared using trifluridine ophthalmic solution and the IV formulation of cidofovir.
VZV disease	*Primary Varicella Infection (Chickenpox):* Uncomplicated Cases (for 5-7 days): • Valacyclovir 1 g PO tid *or* • Famciclovir 500 mg PO tid. *Severe or Complicated Cases:* • Acyclovir 10-15 mg/kg IV q8h for 7-10 days. • May switch to oral valacyclovir, famciclovir, or acyclovir after defervescence if no evidence of visceral involvement. *Herpes Zoster (Shingles) Acute Localized Dermatomal:* • For 7-10 days; consider longer duration if lesions are slow to resolve. • Valacyclovir 1 g PO tid *or* • Famciclovir 500 mg tid.	*Primary Varicella Infection (Chickenpox):* • Uncomplicated Cases (for 5-7 days): • Acyclovir 800 mg PO 5 times/day. *Herpes Zoster (Shingles)* *Acute Localized Dermatomal:* • For 7-10 days; consider longer duration if lesions are slow to resolve. • Acyclovir 800 mg PO 5 times/day.	• In managing VZV retinitis: Consultation with an ophthalmologist experienced in management of VZV retinitis is strongly recommended. • Duration of therapy for VZV retinitis is not well defined and should be determined based on clinical, virologic, immunologic, and ophthalmologic responses. • Optimization of ART is recommended for serious and difficult-to-treat VZV infections (e.g., retinitis, encephalitis).

Diseases and Disorders

I

TABLE 2 Treatment of AIDS-Associated Opportunistic Infections—cont'd

Opportunistic Infection	Preferred Therapy	Alternative Therapy	Other Comments
	Extensive Cutaneous Lesion or Visceral Involvement: • Acyclovir 10-15 mg/kg IV q8h until clinical improvement is evident. • May switch to PO therapy (valacyclovir, famciclovir, or acyclovir) after clinical improvement (i.e., when no new vesicle formation or improvement of signs and symptoms of visceral VZV), to complete a 10- to 14-day course. *Progressive Outer Retinal Necrosis:* • Ganciclovir 5 mg/kg + foscarnet 90 mg/kg IV q12h + ganciclovir 2 mg/0.05 ml ± foscarnet 1.2 mg/0.05 ml intravitreal injection twice weekly *or* • Initiate or optimize ART. *Acute Retinal Necrosis:* • Acyclovir 10 mg/kg IV q8h for 10-14 days, followed by valacyclovir 1 g PO tid for 6 wk.		
Progressive multifocal leukoencephalopathy (JC virus infections)	• There is no specific antiviral therapy for JC virus infection. The main treatment approach is to reverse the immunosuppression caused by HIV. • Initiate ART immediately in ART-naïve patients. • Optimize ART in patients who develop PML in phase of HIV viremia on ART.	None.	• Corticosteroids may be used for PML-IRIS characterized by contrast enhancement, edema, or mass effect and with clinical deterioration.

AIDS, Acquired immunodeficiency syndrome; *ART*, antiretroviral therapy; *ARV*, antiretroviral; *bid*, twice a day; *CD4*, CD4 T lymphocyte cell; *CFU*, colony-forming unit; *CMV*, cytomegalovirus; *CNS*, central nervous system; *CSF*, cerebrospinal fluid; *CYP3A4*, cytochrome P-450 3A4; *DS*, double strength; *EMB*, ethambutol; *G6PD*, glucose-6-phosphate dehydrogenase; *HIV*, human immunodeficiency virus; *HSV*, herpes simplex virus; *ICU*, intensive care unit; *IM*, intramuscular; *INH*, isoniazid; *IRIS*, immune reconstitution inflammatory syndrome; *IRU*, immune recovery uveitis; *IV*, intravenous; *JC*, John Cunningham (virus); *LP*, lumbar puncture; *MAC*, *Mycobacterium avium* complex; *NSAID*, nonsteroidal antiinflammatory drug; *PCP*, *Pneumocystis* pneumonia; *PI*, protease inhibitor; *PJP*, *Pneumocystis jiroveci* pneumonia; *PML*, progressive multifocal leukoencephalopathy; *PO*, oral; *PZA*, pyrazinamide; *qid*, four times a day; *RFB*, rifabutin; *RIF*, rifampin; *SS*, single strength; *TB*, tuberculosis; *tid*, three times daily; *tiw*, three times weekly; *TMP-SMX*, trimethoprim-sulfamethoxazole; *VZV*, varicella zoster virus. *Quality of Evidence for the Recommendation:* I: One or more randomized trials with clinical outcomes and/or validated laboratory endpoints. II: One or more well-designed, nonrandomized trials or observational cohort studies with long-term clinical outcomes. III: Expert opinion.
*Pyrimethamine and leucovorin doses are the same as for preferred therapy.

The medications ritonavir or cobicistat are usually used in combination with other protease inhibitors or integrase inhibitors to obtain more sustained drug levels. Usual initial dosing regimens include two NRTIs and an NNRTI or PI or integrase inhibitor. Two-drug regimens with dolutegravir and lamivudine can be considered in certain clinical situations. Currently, integrase inhibitors are recommended as first-line drugs because of tolerability. Examples of initial regimens recommended by the guidelines:
• Bictegravir/tenofovir alafenamide/emtricitabine
• Dolutegravir/abacavir/lamivudine (in patients who are HLA-B5701 NEGATIVE)
• Dolutegravir plus tenofovir/emtricitabine (tenofovir-based formulations can include tenofovir disoproxil fumarate [TDF] or tenofovir alafenamide [TAF])
• Dolutegravir and lamivudine (two-drug regimen). This regimen should not be used in individuals with HIV RNA >500,000 copies/ml, HBV coinfection, or in whom ART is to be started before the results of HIV genotypic

resistance testing for reverse transcriptase or HBV testing are available.
All these drugs have unique and class-specific side effects and require careful and expert follow-up to achieve optimal antiviral effects, ensure compliance, and maintain efficacy. Antiviral response should be monitored by baseline HIV viral load and CD4 count and repeat measurement at 2 wk and 4 wk into treatment and then periodically (3 to 6 mo) to ensure viral suppression.
• The approach to a patient with CNS signs and symptoms is described in Fig. 3, and Fig. 4 describes the management of CNS mass lesions.
• Genotypic resistance testing is strongly encouraged for all patients initiating treatment and for any patient failing antiretroviral therapy. Poor adherence to therapy, however, often underlies virologic failure.

DISPOSITION
The outlook for HIV has changed radically since the advent of ART from an essentially fatal disease to a chronic medical illness compatible

with long-term survival and remarkably good quality of life. Patients should be aggressively treated for severe illnesses as outcomes following ICU admissions remain good. This is accomplished through expert and continuous follow-up, use of ART, and careful detail to compliance to medications and lifestyle modification.

REFERRAL
All patients with HIV should be referred to a physician knowledgeable and experienced in the management of the disease and its complications.

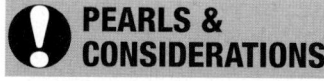 **PEARLS & CONSIDERATIONS**

• Newer agents effective against HIV have recently been approved:
1. Ibalizumab-Uiyk (Trogarzo): injectable monoclonal antibody that binds to the surface proteins of CD4 and thus prevents fusion entry of HIV virus into cells.

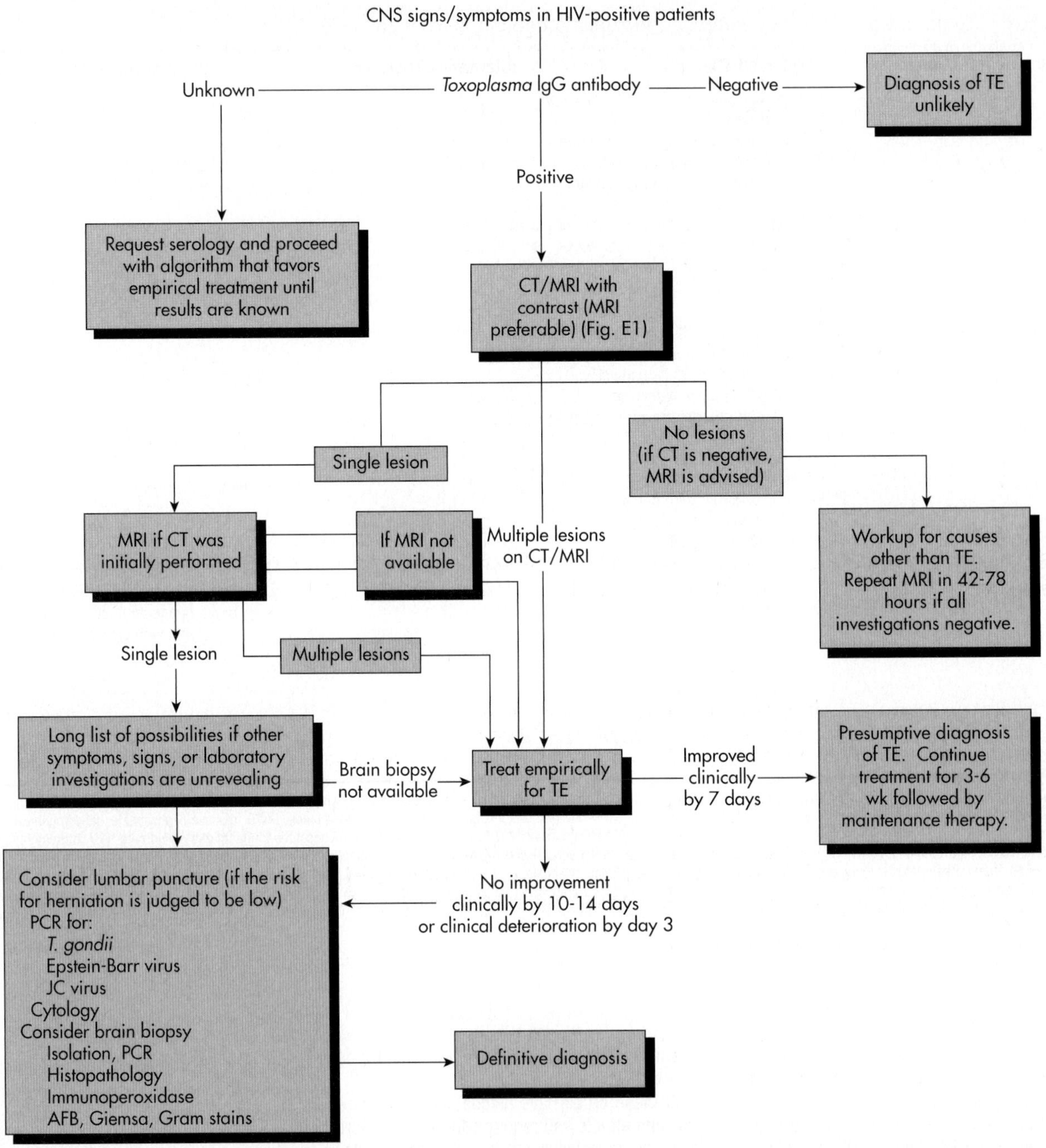

CNS signs/symptoms in HIV-positive patients

Unknown ———————— *Toxoplasma* IgG antibody ———— Negative ————→ Diagnosis of TE unlikely

Positive

Request serology and proceed with algorithm that favors empirical treatment until results are known

CT/MRI with contrast (MRI preferable) (Fig. E1)

Single lesion

No lesions (if CT is negative, MRI is advised)

MRI if CT was initially performed

If MRI not available

Multiple lesions on CT/MRI

Workup for causes other than TE. Repeat MRI in 42-78 hours if all investigations negative.

Single lesion

Multiple lesions

Long list of possibilities if other symptoms, signs, or laboratory investigations are unrevealing

Brain biopsy not available

Treat empirically for TE

Improved clinically by 7 days

Presumptive diagnosis of TE. Continue treatment for 3-6 wk followed by maintenance therapy.

No improvement clinically by 10-14 days or clinical deterioration by day 3

Consider lumbar puncture (if the risk for herniation is judged to be low)
PCR for:
   T. gondii
   Epstein-Barr virus
   JC virus
   Cytology
Consider brain biopsy
   Isolation, PCR
   Histopathology
   Immunoperoxidase
   AFB, Giemsa, Gram stains

Definitive diagnosis

FIG. 3 Diagnostic approach and management algorithm for human immunodeficiency virus *(HIV)*–infected patients with central nervous system *(CNS)* symptoms or signs that might potentially be toxoplasmic encephalitis *(TE)*. *AFB,* Acid-fast bacilli; *CT,* computed tomography; *IgG,* immunoglobulin G; *MRI,* magnetic resonance imaging; *PCR,* polymerase chain reaction. (From Bennett JE et al: *Mandell, Douglas, and Bennett's principles and practice of infectious diseases,* ed 9, Philadelphia, 2020, Elsevier.)

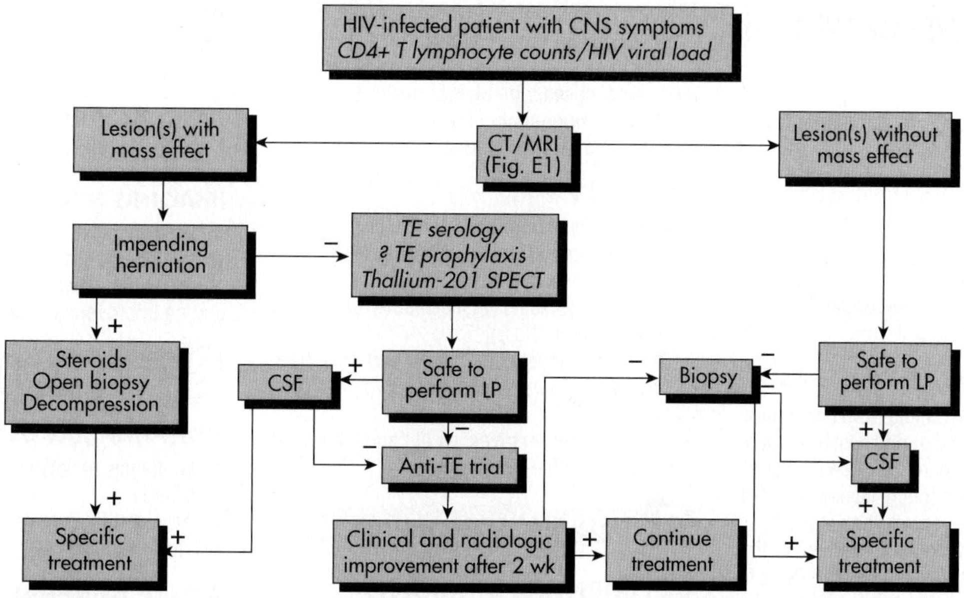

FIG. 4 Management of the human immunodeficiency virus *(HIV)* type 1–infected patient with central nervous system *(CNS)* mass lesions. The elements in *italics* represent data that contribute to the decision-making process (see text for details). *CSF,* Cerebrospinal fluid; *CT,* computed tomography; *LP,* lumbar puncture; *MRI,* magnetic resonance imaging; *SPECT,* single-photon emission computed tomography; *TE, Toxoplasma* encephalitis. (From Bennett JE et al: *Mandell, Douglas, and Bennett's principles and practice of infectious diseases,* ed 9, Philadelphia, 2020, Elsevier.)

2. Fostemsavir (Rukobia): is an attachment inhibitor that prevents viral entry into cells used in combination with other agents in patients with multidrug resistant HIV-1.
- Four patients have been cleared of their HIV after stem cell transplant for blood cancer; the most recent case was announced in July 2022: stem cell transplant for AML.

RELATED CONTENT

Acquired Immunodeficiency Syndrome (AIDS) (Patient Information)

Candidiasis, Cutaneous (Related Key Topic)
Candidiasis, Invasive (Related Key Topic)
Cryptosporidium Infection (Related Key Topic)
Cytomegalovirus Infection (Related Key Topic)
Herpes Simplex (Related Key Topic)
Histoplasmosis (Related Key Topic)
HIV-Associated Cognitive Dysfunction (Related Key Topic)
Human Immunodeficiency Virus (Related Key Topic)
Kaposi Sarcoma (Related Key Topic)

Pneumonia, *Pneumocystis jiroveci (carinii)* (Related Key Topic)
Progressive Multifocal Leukoencephalopathy (Related Key Topic)
Toxoplasmosis (Related Key Topic)
Tuberculosis, Pulmonary (Related Key Topic)

SUGGESTED READINGS

Available at eBooks.Health.Elsevier.com.

AUTHOR: **PHILIP A. CHAN, MD, MS**

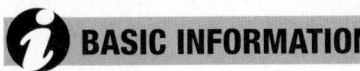 BASIC INFORMATION

DEFINITION
Acute bronchitis is a self-limited inflammation of trachea and bronchi.

SYNONYM
Chest cold

ICD-10CM CODE
J20.9   Acute bronchitis, unspecified

EPIDEMIOLOGY & DEMOGRAPHICS
- Highest incidence in smokers, older adults, and young children and during winter months.
- In the U.S. there are nearly 30 million ambulatory visits annually for cough, leading to more than 12 million diagnoses of "bronchitis."
- Acute lower respiratory tract infection is the most common condition treated in primary care.

PHYSICAL FINDINGS & CLINICAL PRESENTATIONS
- In most cases, acute bronchitis begins with signs and symptoms typical of the common cold syndrome (nasal congestion, sore throat), followed shortly by the onset of cough
- Cough, usually worse in the morning, often productive; mainly caused by transient bronchial hyperresponsiveness
- Low-grade fever
- Substernal discomfort worsened by coughing
- Postnasal drip, pharyngeal injection
- Rhonchi that may clear after cough, occasional wheezing

- Various host factors (age, immune status, smoking, underlying medical conditions) can influence illness severity and clinical presentation
- In mild cases, the illness lasts only 7 to 10 days, whereas in others, cough may persist for up to 3 wk or longer

ETIOLOGY
- Viral infections are the leading cause of bronchitis (rhinovirus, influenza virus, adenovirus, respiratory syncytial virus)
- Atypical organisms (*Mycoplasma, Chlamydia pneumoniae*)
- Bacterial infections (*Bordetella pertussis, Haemophilus influenzae, Moraxella, Streptococcus pneumoniae*)
- Table 1 summarizes viral and bacterial causes of acute bronchitis

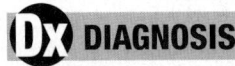 DIAGNOSIS

DIFFERENTIAL DIAGNOSIS
- Pneumonia
- Asthma
- Sinusitis
- Bronchiolitis
- Aspiration
- Cystic fibrosis
- Pharyngitis
- Cough secondary to medications
- Neoplasm (elderly patients)
- Influenza
- Allergic aspergillosis
- Gastroesophageal reflux disease
- Congestive heart failure (in elderly patients)
- Bronchogenic neoplasm

WORKUP
Seldom necessary (e.g., to rule out pneumonia, neoplasm)

LABORATORY TESTS
Laboratory tests are generally not necessary.

IMAGING STUDIES
Chest x-ray is usually reserved for patients with suspected pneumonia, influenza, or underlying chronic obstructive pulmonary disease (COPD) and no improvement with therapy.

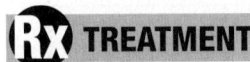 TREATMENT

NONPHARMACOLOGIC THERAPY
- Avoidance of tobacco and other pulmonary irritants
- Increased fluid intake
- Use of vaporizer to increase room humidity

ACUTE GENERAL Rx
- Therapy is generally symptomatic and directed at relief of cough and wheezing.
- Inhaled bronchodilators (e.g., albuterol, metaproterenol) as needed for 1 to 2 wk in patients with wheezing or troublesome cough. Inhaled albuterol has been proven effective in reducing the duration of cough in adults with uncomplicated acute bronchitis.
- Cough suppression with dextromethorphan and guaifenesin is commonly recommended; addition of codeine for cough suppression if cough is severe and is significantly interrupting patient's sleep pattern.

TABLE 1   Viral and Bacterial Causes of Acute Bronchitis

.	Seasonality	Comments
Influenza viruses	Winter	Local epidemics last 6-8 wk during which clinical illness of cough and fever has high predictive value; laboratory diagnosis readily available; early neuraminidase inhibitor therapy effective
Rhinoviruses	Fall and spring	Most frequent cause of common cold syndrome; immunity is serotype specific
Coronaviruses	Winter to spring	Cause common cold syndrome; newer strains are difficult to culture and require RT-PCR for diagnosis
Adenoviruses	Year round, winter epidemics	High attack rates in closed populations such as persons living in military barracks or college dormitories; serotype-specific immunity
Respiratory syncytial virus (RSV)	Late fall to early spring	Attack rates approach 75% in neonates, 3%-5% in adults; associated with wheezing in all age groups; rapid antigen test accurate in children but requires culture or RT-PCR to diagnose in adults
Human metapneumovirus (hMPV)	Winter to early spring	Associated with wheezing in adults and in infants; difficult to isolate in tissue culture and often requires RT-PCR
Parainfluenza viruses	Fall to winter	Similar to RSV and hMPV, parainfluenza viruses are primarily pediatric pathogens but can cause severe acute disease in some adults
Measles virus	Year round	Can cause respiratory disease in malnourished children; illness causes transient immune suppression
Mycoplasma pneumoniae	Year round, fall outbreaks	Long incubation period (10-21 days) results in staggered epidemic pattern in families; nonproductive persistent cough typical; diagnosed by IgM serology; treated with macrolide, quinolone, or tetracycline antibiotics
Chlamydia pneumoniae	Year round	Associated with sinusitis; diagnosis by RT-PCR not readily available
Bordetella pertussis	Year round	Severe illness in nonimmunized children; illness milder in partially immune adults; can be associated with prolonged cough; adults are often reservoirs for epidemics; early therapy with antibiotics can reduce spread

IgM, Immunoglobulin M; *RT-PCR*, reverse-transcriptase polymerase chain reaction.
From Bennett JE et al: *Mandell, Douglas, and Bennett's principles and practice of infectious diseases*, ed 8, Philadelphia, 2015, Saunders.

- Use of antibiotics (trimethoprim-sulfamethoxazole, amoxicillin, doxycycline, cefuroxime) for acute bronchitis is generally not indicated; should be considered only in patients with concomitant COPD, increased dyspnea, and purulent sputum or in patients with suspected pertussis. In the few cases of acute bronchitis caused by *B. pertussis* or atypical bacteria such as *C. pneumoniae* or *Mycoplasma pneumoniae,* early use of macrolide antibiotics is reasonable. Clinicians should limit antibiotic treatment duration to 5 days when managing patients with COPD exacerbations and acute uncomplicated bronchitis who have clinical signs of a bacteria infection.
- Antibiotics are overused in patients with acute bronchitis (70% to 90% of office visits for acute bronchitis result in treatment with antibiotics); this practice pattern is contributing to increases in resistant organisms.
- Trials have shown that there are no significant differences in patients receiving antibiotics compared with those receiving placebo in overall clinical improvements or limitations in work or other activities. There was a significant increase in adverse effects in the antibiotic group, particularly GI symptoms.

CHRONIC Rx

Avoidance of tobacco and other pulmonary irritants

DISPOSITION

- Complete recovery within 7 to 10 days in most patients.
- Patients should be informed to expect to have a cough for 10 to 14 days after the visit.

REFERRAL

For pulmonary function testing only in patients with recurrent bronchitis and suspected underlying pulmonary disease

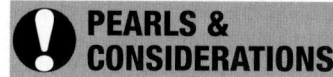

COMMENTS

- Patients are more likely to receive prescriptions for antibiotics from mid- or late-career physicians with high patient volumes and from physicians who were trained outside of Canada or the U.S. Intervention studies reveal that patient and physician education are effective in reducing the use of antibiotic therapy. No offer or delayed offer of antibiotics for acute uncomplicated lower respiratory tract infection is acceptable, is associated with little difference in symptom resolution, and is likely to reduce antibiotic use and beliefs in the effectiveness of antibiotics.
- It is helpful to refer to acute bronchitis as a "chest cold." Patients should be informed that antibiotics are probably not going to be beneficial and may result in significant side effects.

RELATED CONTENT

Acute Bronchitis (Patient Information)

AUTHOR: **FRED F. FERRI, MD**

SUGGESTED READINGS

Available at eBooks.Health.Elsevier.com

A

Diseases and Disorders

I

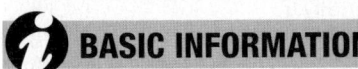

BASIC INFORMATION

Acute coronary syndrome (ACS) represents a spectrum of clinical disorders that results from a sudden decrease in blood flow to the myocardium. ACS can be a life-threatening condition that incurs high, and in some cases immediate, mortality. The most common mechanism for this disruption in blood flow is an interaction of vulnerable atherosclerotic plaque in the coronary arteries with activated clotting factors and platelets in the systemic circulation. In the modern era, management of ACS involves highly protocolized and systematic care of both procedural and medical therapies guided toward restoring blood flow to the heart. When ACS is suspected due to symptoms suggestive of cardiac ischemia (i.e., chest discomfort), it is divided into two important categories that dictate the urgency of evaluation and treatment: ST-elevation myocardial infarction (STEMI) and non-ST-elevation ACS (NSTE-ACS). STEMI, defined by the presence of ST-segment elevations on ECG, is considered to be the most severe form of ACS, and emergent evaluation for reperfusion therapy is indicated.[1] NSTE-ACS is characterized by similar presenting symptoms but without ST-segment elevations, and is further subcategorized into non-ST-elevation myocardial infarction (NSTEMI) and unstable angina (UA) based on the presence of serum cardiac biomarkers.[2] While UA has historically been defined by the absence of elevated serum cardiac biomarkers, the identification and widespread use of more sensitive biomarkers has decreased the incidence of this diagnosis. With implementation of the high-sensitivity troponin, most patients who would previously have been diagnosed with UA now fall within the diagnosis of NSTEMI.[3] ACS can be conceptualized as a continuum representing the degree to which perfusion has been impaired, with the potential to progress if left untreated (Table 1).

SYNONYMS

ACS
UA
NSTEMI
STEMI
Acute MI

ICD-10CM CODES

I20.0	Unstable angina
I21.0-I21.3	ST elevation (STEMI)
I21.4	Non-ST elevation (NSTEMI) myocardial infarction
I24.9	Acute ischemic heart disease, unspecified

EPIDEMIOLOGY & DEMOGRAPHICS

INCIDENCE: In the U.S., heart disease accounts for approximately 695,000 deaths each year based on the most recent data.[4] The estimated annual incidence of heart attacks in the U.S. is 605,000 new attacks and 200,000 recurrent attacks.[4] Approximately 70% of MIs are listed as NSTEMI, with the remainder being listed as STEMI.[5] Patients presenting with NSTE-ACS have a better short-term prognosis but worse long-term prognosis than patients presenting with STEMI, although this difference in long-term mortality is attributed to the higher comorbidity profile of patients presenting with NSTE-ACS (i.e., significantly older population, higher burden of comorbidities, and frequent history of coronary artery disease [CAD]). The underlying etiology, atherosclerotic CAD, remains the number one cause of mortality.[4]

PREDOMINANT SEX & AGE: In the U.S., the average age at first MI is 65 yr for males and 72 yr for females, and MI has a prevalence of 4.5% in males and 2.1% in females.[4] In a 2005 to 2014 study sponsored by National Heart, Lung, and Blood Institute, the incidence of MI across all age groups was higher in black men, followed by black women, white men, and then white women.[4] As evidenced by this study, heart disease affects African Americans disproportionately. Heart disease is also the leading cause of death in women, surpassing all forms of cancer.[4]

RISK FACTORS: Hypertension, diabetes mellitus, dyslipidemia, tobacco use, and family history of premature CAD (CAD in a male first-degree relative younger than 55 yr or a female younger than 65 yr of age) are all associated risk factors for CAD. There are also female-specific risk factors for CAD, including disorders of pregnancy and early onset of menopause. Refer to the topic "Angina Pectoris" for an extensive list of risk factors. Presence of these risk factors cause damage to the vascular endothelium and progression of atherosclerotic coronary artery plaques.

PHYSICAL FINDINGS & CLINICAL PRESENTATION

- Symptoms of ACS most commonly include chest discomfort described as a pressure that may radiate to the shoulders, neck, jaw, or back. Angina, or ischemic chest pain, is substernal in location, brought on by emotional or physical stress, and relieved with rest and/or nitroglycerin. The discomfort associated with an ACS event is often diffuse rather than localized and accompanied by diaphoresis.
- Women, diabetics, the elderly (>75 yr old), and postoperative patients can have nonclassic symptoms when presenting for ACS.
- UA has three typical presentations:

1. Rest angina: Angina occurring at rest and usually prolonged for longer than 20 min.
2. New-onset angina: New-onset angina of at least Canadian Cardiovascular Society (CCS) class III symptoms (Table 2).
3. Progressive angina: Previously diagnosed angina that has become distinctly more frequent, longer in duration, or lower in threshold (i.e., increased by ≥1 CCS class to at least CCS class III severity).

- "Anginal equivalents" may include dyspnea, nausea, vomiting, and fatigue.
- ECG for NSTE-ACS may reveal transient ST-segment elevation, ST-segment depression, and/or new T-wave inversion. ECG for definition of STEMI will reveal ≥1-mm ST-segment elevation at the J-point in two contiguous leads other than leads V_2-V_3 in which cut-points are ≥2 mm in men ≥40 yr, ≥2.5 mm in men <40 yr, or ≥1.5 mm in women regardless of age.[1]
- Physical examination findings alone are insufficient for the diagnosis of ACS. The physical examination may provide clues as to alternative diagnoses, such as aortic dissection (differences in pulse and blood pressure between the arms, murmur of aortic regurgitation), aortic stenosis, pericarditis (friction rub), cardiac tamponade (pulsus paradoxus), and pneumothorax (absent breath sounds). In ACS, it is important to assess the patient's hemodynamic stability, as signs of heart failure may be present. These signs include elevated jugular venous pressure (JVP), presence of an S3 gallop, rales, and to a lesser extent, peripheral edema. The degree of heart failure with MI can be represented by the Killip classification, with the greater the Killip classification, the greater the mortality noted[6]:

1. Killip Class 1 is no heart failure.
2. Killip Class 2 includes individuals with rales, elevated JVP, and S3 on examination.
3. Killip Class 3 includes individuals with frank pulmonary edema.
4. Killip Class 4 describes individuals in cardiogenic shock or hypotension with evidence of vasoconstriction noted.

ETIOLOGY

The hallmark of ACS is vulnerable atherosclerotic plaque, which typically has a thin fibrous cap

---

TABLE 1 Acute Coronary Syndromes

	SPECTRUM OF ACUTE CORONARY SYNDROME		
	Unstable Angina	**NSTEMI**	**STEMI**
Chest discomfort	1	1	1
Cardiac biomarkers	2	1	1
ECG changes	TWI and/or ST depression	TWI and/or ST depression	ST elevation or presumed new left bundle branch block
Pathophysiology	Partial/transient thrombotic occlusion	Partial/transient thrombotic occlusion	Complete thrombotic occlusion

ECG, Electrocardiogram; *NSTEMI,* non–ST-segment elevation myocardial infarction; *STEMI,* ST-segment myocardial infarction; *TWI,* T-wave inversion.

TABLE 2 Grading of Angina Pectoris According to CCS Classification

Class	Description of Stage
I	"Ordinary physical activity does not cause angina," such as walking or climbing stairs. Angina occurs with strenuous, rapid, or prolonged exertion at work or recreation.
II	"Slight limitation of ordinary activity." Angina occurs on walking or climbing stairs rapidly; walking uphill; walking or stair climbing after meals; in cold, in wind, or under emotional stress; or only during the few hours after awakening. Angina occurs on walking 0.2 blocks on the level and climbing 0.1 flight of ordinary stairs at a normal pace and under normal conditions.
III	"Marked limitations of ordinary physical activity." Angina occurs on walking 1-2 blocks on the level and climbing one flight of stairs under normal conditions and at a normal pace.
IV	"Inability to carry on any physical activity without discomfort—anginal symptoms may be present at rest."

Adapted with permission from Campeau L: Grading of angina pectoris (letter), *Circulation* 54:522-523, 1976. © 1976, American Heart Association, Inc. From Braunwald E et al: ACC/AHA guidelines for the management of patients with unstable angina and non–ST-segment elevation myocardial infarction: a report of the American College of Cardiology/American Heart Association Task Force on Practice Guidelines (Committee on the Management of Patients With Unstable Angina), *J Am Coll Cardiol* 36:970-1062, 2000.

and a large lipid core. This vulnerable plaque can spontaneously rupture, which leads to platelet activation and aggregation and a systemic inflammatory cascade, leading to thrombus formation. STEMI typically results from complete thrombotic occlusion of a coronary artery, whereas NSTE-ACS often has partial occlusion. Angiographically, it is often the intermediate coronary artery lesions (30% to 50% diameter vessel stenosis) that lead to subtotal or total vessel occlusion in two thirds of STEMI cases.

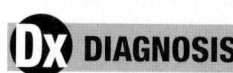 **DIAGNOSIS**

DIFFERENTIAL DIAGNOSIS

Chest pain mimicking ACS may be the result of various underlying disorders, some of which are also accompanied by ECG changes and/or cardiac biomarker release. Examples include acute pulmonary embolism, acute aortic dissection, pericarditis, myocarditis, costochondritis, pneumonia, tension pneumothorax, perforating ulcer, or esophageal perforation (i.e., Boerhaave syndrome). Refer to topics "Angina Pectoris," "Coronary Artery Syndrome," and "Myocardial Infarction" for extensive differential diagnoses of chest pain.

WORKUP

Focused history and physical examination, 12-lead ECG, serum cardiac biomarkers, and chest radiograph (CXR) are the cornerstone of the initial chest pain workup. Initial biomarkers may not be positive early in the disease process. Conventional troponin levels are often drawn every 6 to 8 h for a total of three sets for the purposes of ruling out MI or until peak to determine the severity of an established MI, but with the advent of the high-sensitivity troponin, the time to rule in MI can be done in as little as 3 h from initial presentation.[1] Echocardiogram may reveal new regional wall motion abnormalities, newly depressed left ventricular (LV) function or aneurysm formation. Fig. 1 summarizes the evaluation of patients for ACS.

LABORATORY TESTS

- Biomarkers and their trends play an important role in the early detection and diagnosis of ACS. Although troponin is essential to the diagnosis of acute MI, other markers have demonstrated utility in the setting of acute chest pain and ACS. Creatinine kinase-myocardial band (CK-MB) and myoglobin are two traditional markers that are frequently used in combination with troponin and will be elevated in the setting of NSTEMI or STEMI. See Fig. E2, *A*, for timing of release of each biomarker. Given that troponin is the most sensitive biomarker for cardiac myocyte damage and also predicts 42-day mortality in ACS, it is considered the gold standard for diagnosis of MI (Fig. E2, *B*). Newer troponin assays, referred to as high-sensitivity troponins, have the ability to detect troponin levels at thresholds approximately 100 times lower than older assays. These assays allow for improved sensitivity in diagnosis or exclusion of acute MI.[1]
- CK-MB is the cardiac specific isoform of creatinine kinase (CK) and is found in high concentrations in the myocardium. After an acute myocardial injury, CK-MB levels peak within 4 to 6 h. Its shorter half-life leads to normal values within 24 to 48 h after an event. As such, CK-MB is especially useful when assessing a patient for possible reinfarction given troponin levels can remain elevated up to 14 days or more after an acute MI.[1]
- MI is not always the cause of elevated troponin levels. Any form of myocardial injury can cause elevation in troponin. Cardiac conditions that cause supply-demand mismatch without acute coronary obstruction, such as arrhythmias, hypotension/hypertension, heart failure, and myocarditis, can lead to elevated troponin levels. Noncardiac conditions, including renal failure, sepsis, respiratory failure, and neurologic diseases, may similarly lead to elevations in troponin.
- Meanwhile, other biomarkers also have significant prognostic value. Testing for B-type natriuretic peptide (BNP) can help risk-stratify mortality in patients presenting with ACS. Notably, a BNP >80 portends a high risk of death at initial presentation of a STEMI.[1]

RISK MODELS & RISK SCORES

Risk models and scores such as TIMI (see "Risk Assessment" in "Myocardial Infarction" topic), PURSUIT, HEART, and GRACE combine clinical history, ECG findings, risk factors, and laboratory data at presentation to assess a patient's risk for short- and intermediate-term adverse outcomes (Fig. E2, *C*).[7] These risk stratification models are helpful in determining the timing and strategy of treatment.

IMAGING STUDIES

- A CXR should be obtained to assist in evaluating for volume overload and possible widened mediastinum, which could be indicative of an aortic dissection. It can be useful in assessing for pneumonia, pneumothorax, intraperitoneal free air, and other noncardiac causes of chest pain.
- In patients for whom ECG and cardiac biomarkers are nondiagnostic but the clinical suspicion for ACS remains high, an echocardiogram may be helpful to assess LV function and regional wall motion abnormalities.
- Coronary CT angiography is recommended in patients with suspected ACS who have no history of CAD, have an inconclusive initial workup, and are considered to be at intermediate risk for adverse outcome (Class I); it can also be useful in intermediate-risk patients with suspected ACS who have had a previous mildly abnormal or inconclusive stress test (Class IIa).[8]
- Cardiac stress testing (treadmill ECG, imaging stress studies using echocardiography or nuclear modalities) is helpful in further risk stratification of intermediate-risk patients. (See "Coronary Artery Syndrome" in Section I.)
- Coronary angiogram/cardiac catheterization will reveal coronary artery luminal irregularities/stenotic lesions. In patients with ACS who undergo coronary angiography, radial artery access is preferred over femoral artery access to minimize risk of bleeding complications.[5]

Rx TREATMENT

The overall goal for patients with ACS is to relieve myocardial ischemia and to prevent recurrent cardiovascular events. This is achieved by targeting both vulnerable coronary plaque and activated clotting factors and platelets in the blood. Revascularization, whether it is chemical (i.e., thrombolysis) or mechanical (i.e., percutaneous coronary intervention [PCI]), is needed to prevent further events and improve flow within the coronary artery lumen. In the modern era, PCI has improved outcomes for patients presenting with ACS.[5] For patients with STEMI, time from onset of ischemia to revascularization guides the reperfusion strategy. STEMI patients presenting to a hospital with PCI capability should be treated with primary PCI within 90 min of first medical contact (Figs. E3 and E4). At non–PCI-capable hospitals where the first medical contact to PCI is more than 120 min, thrombolytic therapy should be given to eligible patients within the first 12 h after symptom onset; thrombolytics should not be administered 24 h after initial diagnosis of STEMI (Table 3).[5]

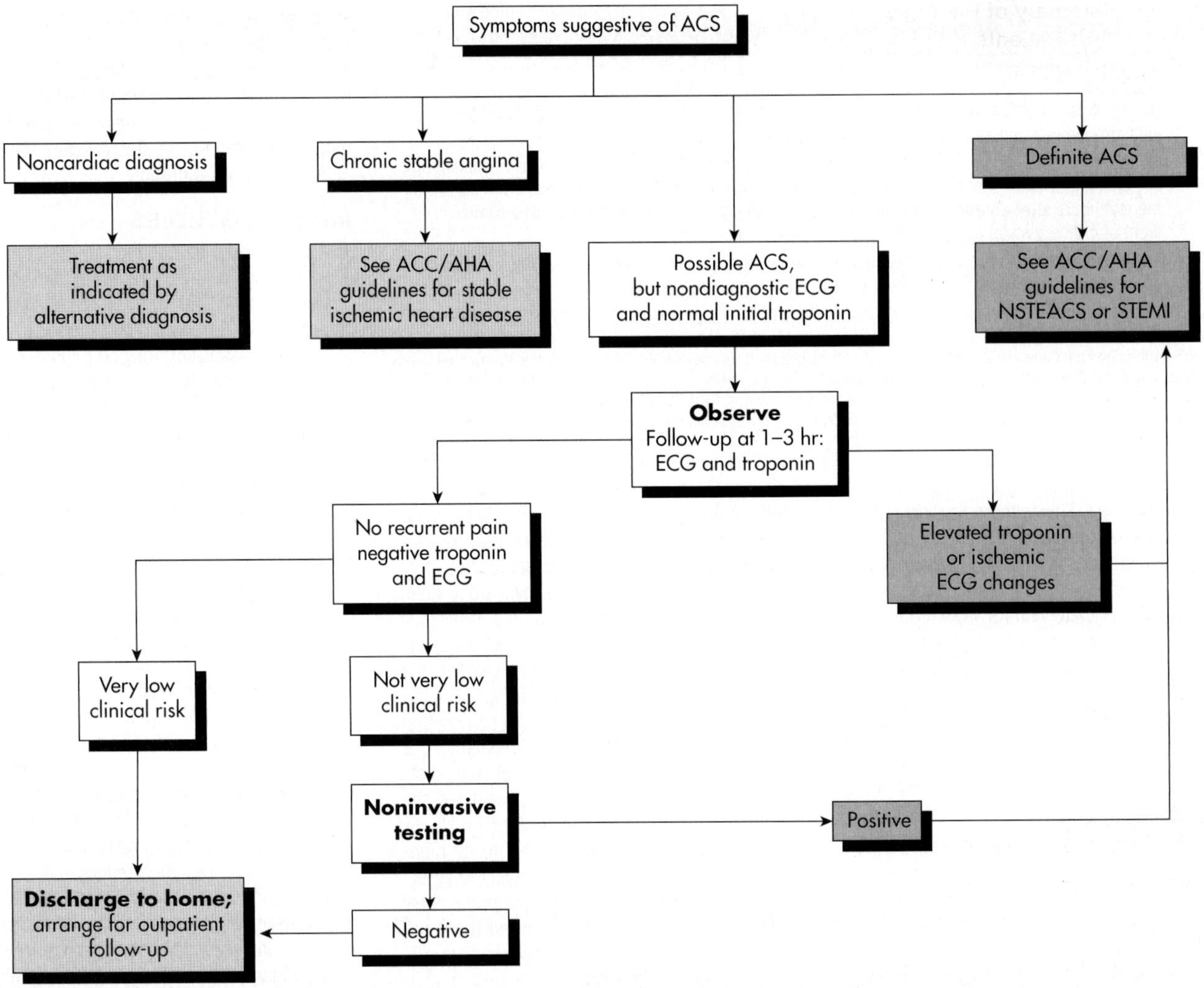

```
┌─────────────────────────────┐
│   Symptoms suggestive of ACS │
└─────────────────────────────┘
```

FIG. 1 Algorithm for the evaluation and management of patients suspected of having ACS. (Data from Amsterdam EA et al: 2014 AHA/ACC guideline for the management of patients with non-ST-elevation acute coronary syndromes: a report of the American College of Cardiology/American Heart Association Task Force on Practice Guidelines, *J Am Coll Cardiol* 64[24]:e139-e228, 2014.)

TABLE 3 Reperfusion Strategies

Anticipated time from FMC to PCI	>120 min	<120 min
	and	or
Symptom duration?	<12 h	<24 h
	and	or
Thrombolytic eligible?	YES	NO
Reperfusion strategy	Thrombolytics and transfer	Primary PCI

FMC, First medical contact; *PCI,* percutaneous coronary intervention.

In patients who receive thrombolytic agents, coronary angiography can be done at a receiving hospital as soon as possible but not within the first 2 to 3 h after administration of a fibrinolytic agent. Thrombolytic agents come in two forms, fibrin specific (alteplase, reteplase, tenecteplase) and nonfibrin specific (streptokinase).[9] Absolute contraindications to thrombolytic therapy include the following: History of intracranial hemorrhage, known structural cerebral vascular lesion, known intracranial neoplasm, ischemic stroke within 3 mo, suspected aortic dissection, active bleeding, head trauma within 3 mo, intracranial surgery within 2 mo, or severe uncontrolled hypertension. Relative contraindications include ischemic stroke more than 3 mo prior, dementia, major surgery within 3 wk, current oral anticoagulant therapy, and traumatic or prolonged CPR.[9] Antithrombotic therapy is needed to reduce thrombus burden, prevent further thrombosis, and improve coronary artery flow.

NONPHARMACOLOGIC THERAPY

- STEMI is a medical emergency and requires immediate reperfusion therapy; the best outcomes are seen with cardiac catheterization and primary PCI. Guidelines call for a goal door-to-balloon time of ≤90 min.[9]

- Patients with NSTE-ACS should be risk stratified in conjunction with the cardiology consult service. Risk scores such as the TIMI and GRACE scores can be used to decide between an early invasive strategy and an ischemia-guided strategy. Overall, an early invasive strategy is associated with better outcomes in patients with higher risk (i.e., TIMI score >3 or GRACE >140) and involves cardiac catheterization followed by revascularization with PCI or coronary artery bypass grafting (CABG) within 4 to 24 h of presentation. An ischemia-guided strategy involves aggressive medical management and revascularization only if ischemia recurs or is documented on noninvasive testing.[2] This should be reserved only for patients with low-risk scores (TIMI score 0 or 1, GRACE <109). The early invasive strategy can be further stratified by timing:

1. Immediate (within 2 h): Patients with refractory or recurrent angina despite optimal initial treatment, signs or symptoms of heart failure, new or worsening mitral regurgitation, hemodynamic instability, sustained ventricular tachycardia or ventricular fibrillation

TABLE 4 Summary of Recommendations for Standard Medical Therapy in the Early Hospital Care Phase of Management of Patients with Non–ST-Elevation Acute Coronary Syndrome (NSTE-ACS)

Recommendations	COR	LOE
Oxygen		
Administer supplemental oxygen only with oxygen saturation <90%, respiratory distress, or other high-risk features for hypoxemia.	I	C
Nitrates		
Administer sublingual NTG every 5 min ×3 for continuing ischemic pain and then assess need for IV NTG.	I	C
Administer IV NTG for persistent ischemia, HF, or hypertension.	I	B
Nitrates are contraindicated with recent use of a phosphodiesterase inhibitor.	III: Harm	B
Analgesic Therapy		
IV morphine sulfate may be reasonable for continued ischemic chest pain despite maximally tolerated antiischemic medications.	IIb	B
NSAIDs (except aspirin) should not be initiated and should be discontinued during hospitalization for NSTE-ACS because of the increased risk of MACE associated with their use.	III: Harm	B
Beta-Adrenergic Blockers		
Initiate oral beta blockers within the first 24 h in the absence of HF, low-output state, risk for cardiogenic shock, or other contraindications to beta blockade.	I	A
Use of sustained-release metoprolol succinate, carvedilol, or bisoprolol is recommended for beta-blocker therapy with concomitant NSTE-ACS, *stabilized* HF, and reduced systolic function.	I	C
Reevaluate to determine subsequent eligibility in patients with initial contraindications to beta blockers.	I	C
It is reasonable to continue beta-blocker therapy in patients with normal LV function with NSTE-ACS.	IIa	C
IV beta blockers are potentially harmful when risk factors for shock are present.	III: Harm	B
Calcium Channel Blockers (CCBs)		
Administer initial therapy with nondihydropyridine CCBs with recurrent ischemia and contraindications to beta blockers in the absence of LV dysfunction, increased risk for cardiogenic shock, PR interval >0.24 sec, or second- or third-degree atrioventricular block without a cardiac pacemaker.	I	B
Administer oral nondihydropyridine calcium antagonists with recurrent ischemia after use of beta blocker and nitrates in the absence of contraindications.	I	C
CCBs are recommended for ischemic symptoms when beta blockers are not successful, are contraindicated, or cause unacceptable side effects.*	I	C
Long-acting CCBs and nitrates are recommended for patients with coronary artery spasm.	I	C
Immediate-release nifedipine is contraindicated in the absence of a beta-blocker.	III: Harm	B
Cholesterol Management		
Initiate or continue high-intensity statin therapy in patients with no contraindications.	I	A
Obtain a fasting lipid profile, preferably within 24 h.	IIa	C

COR, Class of recommendation; *HF,* heart failure; *IV,* intravenous; *LOE,* level of evidence; *LV,* left ventricular; *MACE,* major adverse cardiovascular events; *N/A,* not available; *NSAIDs,* nonsteroidal antiinflammatory drugs; *NTG,* nitroglycerin.
*Short-acting dihydropyridine calcium channel antagonists should be avoided.
From Amsterdam EA et al: 2014 AHA/ACC guideline for the management of patients with non–ST-elevation acute coronary syndromes: a report of the American College of Cardiology/American Heart Association task force on practice guidelines, *J Am Coll Cardiol* 64:e139-228, 2014; in Libby P et al: *Braunwald's heart disease, a textbook of cardiovascular medicine,* ed 12, Philadelphia, 2022, Elsevier.

2. Early (within 24 h): No characteristics from the immediate category but new ST-segment depression, a GRACE risk score >140 or temporal change in troponin
3. Delayed invasive (25 to 72 h): None of the immediate or early characteristics but renal insufficiency, LV ejection fraction (EF) of <40%, early post-infarct angina, history of PCI within the past 6 mo, prior CABG, GRACE risk score of 109 to 140, or TIMI score of ≥2
- Continuous ECG monitoring is recommended for all ACS patients. Supplemental oxygen should be administered only to patients with arterial oxygen saturation of <90%, respiratory distress, or other high-risk features of hypoxemia. Finger pulse oximetry should be used to assess arterial oxygen saturation.[5]

ACUTE GENERAL Rx
- Table 4 is a summary of recommendations for standard medical therapy in the early hospital care phase of management of patients with NSTE-ACS.[2]
- Antithrombotic therapy (Table 5) is critical in treating the underlying pathophysiology of ACS. This consists of administering antiplatelet and anticoagulant agents (Table 6).

- Antiplatelet agents (Table 7) inhibit platelet activation and aggregation. Aspirin is an irreversible cyclooxygenase inhibitor that blocks platelet aggregation and should be administered to all ACS patients without contraindications.
- All patients with ACS should receive full-dose non–enteric-coated chewable aspirin of 162 to 325 mg to establish a high blood level for its antiplatelet effects to occur. Thereafter, daily dose of 81 mg should be continued indefinitely.[2]
- Clopidogrel is a thienopyridine agent that inhibits platelet activation and aggregation. It should be administered in all ACS patients, with the timing dependent on the clinical scenario and management strategy. It requires a loading dose of 300 to 600 mg followed by 75 mg/day. It should be discontinued at least 5 days before CABG to avoid excessive bleeding related to surgery. If a patient is unable to take aspirin in the setting of hypersensitivity or major gastrointestinal intolerance, a loading dose of clopidogrel followed by daily maintenance should be started.[2]
- Other antiplatelet agents that can be substituted instead of clopidogrel include prasugrel

and ticagrelor. Ticagrelor has a half-life of 12 h with a more rapid onset and more consistent onset of action. In the PLATO trial, there was a reduction in death from vascular causes, MI, and stroke in patients with NSTE-ACS who received ticagrelor compared to those who received clopidogrel, without an increase in the rate of overall major bleeding.[10] This benefit is limited to patients taking aspirin 75 to 100 mg/day. Prasugrel is not recommended as the initial antiplatelet agent in patients with NSTE-ACS. Multiple studies have demonstrated an increase in bleeding in patients taking prasugrel; in particular, those who are >75 yr old, with low body weight (<60 kg), or with a history of cerebrovascular events.[11] Cangrelor is an IV ADP-P2Y12 receptor antagonist that may be used initially as a load in the emergency department before an invasive strategy, given its initial action and quick platelet recovery time. As a rule, all ACS patients should have two antiplatelet agents initiated and should be continued up to 12 mo regardless of treatment strategy.[2]
- GP IIb/IIIa inhibitors (Table 8) may be considered as an intravenous antiplatelet therapy in

TABLE 5 Summary of Recommendations for Antithrombotic Therapy

Recommendations	Dosing, Special Considerations	COR	LOE
Aspirin			
Non–enteric-coated aspirin to all patients promptly after presentation	162-325 mg	I	A
Aspirin maintenance dose continued indefinitely	81-325 mg/day*	I	A
P2Y12 Inhibitors			
Clopidogrel loading dose followed by daily maintenance dose in patients unable to take aspirin	75 mg	I	B
P2Y12 inhibitor, in addition to aspirin, for up to 12 mo for patients treated initially with either an early invasive or initial ischemia-guided strategy:		I	B
• Clopidogrel	300- or 600-mg loading dose, then 75 mg/day		
• Ticagrelor	180-mg loading dose, then 90 mg twice daily		
P2Y12 inhibitor therapy (clopidogrel, prasugrel, or ticagrelor) continued for at least 12 mo in post-PCI patients treated with coronary stents	N/A	I	B
Ticagrelor in preference to clopidogrel for patients treated with an early invasive or ischemia-guided strategy	N/A	IIa	B
Glycoprotein (GP) IIb/IIIa Inhibitors			
GP IIb/IIIa inhibitor in patients treated with an early invasive strategy and DAPT with intermediate/high-risk features (e.g., positive troponin)	Preferred options are eptifibatide or tirofiban	IIb	B
Parenteral Anticoagulant and Fibrinolytic Therapy			
SC enoxaparin for duration of hospitalization or until PCI is performed	1 mg/kg SC every 12 h (reduce dose to 1 mg/kg/day SC in patients with CrCl <30 ml/min) Initial 30-mg IV loading dose in select patients	I	A
Bivalirudin until diagnostic angiography or PCI is performed in patients with early invasive strategy only	Loading dose 0.10 mg/kg, followed by 0.25 mg/kg/h Only provisional use of GP IIb/IIIa inhibitor in patients also treated with DAPT	I	B
SC fondaparinux for the duration of hospitalization or until PCI is performed	2.5 mg/day SC	I	B
Administer additional anticoagulant with antilla activity if PCI is performed while patient is on fondaparinux	N/A	I	B
IV UFH for 48 hr or until PCI is performed	Initial loading dose 60 IU/kg (max 4000 IU) with initial infusion 12 IU/kg/h (max 1000 IU/h) Adjusted to therapeutic APTT range	I	B
IV fibrinolytic treatment not recommended in patients with NSTE-ACS	N/A	III: Harm	A

APTT, Activated partial thromboplastin time; *COR*, class of recommendation; *CrCl*, creatinine clearance; *DAPT*, dual antiplatelet therapy; *IV*, intravenous; *LOE*, level of evidence; *max*, maximum; *N/A*, not available; *NSTE-ACS*, non–ST-elevation acute coronary syndromes; *PCI*, percutaneous coronary intervention; *SC*, subcutaneous; *UFH*, unfractionated heparin.
*The recommended maintenance dose of aspirin to be used with ticagrelor is 81 mg/day.
From Amsterdam EA, et al. 2014 AHA/ACC guideline for the management of patients with non-ST-elevation acute coronary syndromes: A report of the American College of Cardiology/American Heart Association task force on practice guidelines. *J Am Coll Cardiol* 2014;64:e139-e228.

TABLE 6 2014 Guideline Recommendations for Antithrombotic Agents in Patients With Non–ST-Elevation Acute Coronary Syndrome

Antiplatelet Therapy

Non–enteric-coated, chewable aspirin (162-325 mg) should be given to all patients without contraindications on presentation, and a maintenance dose of aspirin (81-325 mg/day) continued indefinitely.
In patients who are unable to take aspirin because of hypersensitivity or major gastrointestinal intolerance, a loading dose of clopidogrel (300 or 600 mg) followed by a daily maintenance dose of 75 mg should be substituted.
Either clopidogrel or ticagrelor can be used initially with either an early invasive or ischemic guided strategy (COR I, LOE: B).
Ticagrelor may be preferred over clopidogrel as the initial treatment (COR IIa, LOE: B).
In patients treated with ticagrelor, the preferred aspirin maintenance dose is 81 mg/day.
Use prasugrel only in patients receiving coronary stents (COR I, LOE: B).
The use of glycoprotein IIb/IIIa receptor inhibitors is reserved mainly to the time of PCI in high-risk patients who were not adequately pretreated with P2Y12 inhibitors (COR I, LOE: A) or in those patients who were adequately pretreated with P2Y12 inhibitors but have a high-risk profile (COR IIa, LOE: B).
Clopidogrel and ticagrelor should be discontinued at least 5 days (COR I, LOE: B) and prasugrel at least 7 days (COR I, LOE: C) before major surgery.

Anticoagulant Therapy

Enoxaparin is recommended at presentation (COR I, LOE: A); other options include unfractionated heparin (UFH) (COR I, B) and fondaparinux (COR I, LOE: B). If an early invasive strategy is planned, bivalirudin (COR I, LOE: B) is also an option.
If fondaparinux is used initially, add UFH or bivalirudin just before or during PCI to prevent catheter-related thrombosis (COR I, LOE: B).
Bivalirudin is preferred over UFH plus GP IIb/IIIa inhibitor in patients undergoing PCI who are at high risk of bleeding (COR IIa, LOE: B).
It is reasonable to use enoxaparin during PCI if it was used as the initial anticoagulant (COR IIb, LOE: B).

COR, Class of recommendation; *LOE*, level of evidence; *PCI*, percutaneous coronary intervention.
Modified from Eisen A, Giugliano RP: Antiplatelet and anticoagulation treatment in patients with non–ST-segment elevation acute coronary syndrome: comparison of the updated North American and European guidelines, *Cardiol Rev* 24:170-176, 2016; and Amsterdam EA et al: 2014 AHA/ACC guideline for the management of patients with non–ST-elevation acute coronary syndromes: a report of the American College of Cardiology/American Heart Association Task Force on Practice Guidelines, *J Am Coll Cardiol* 64: e139-228, 2014; in Zipes DP: *Braunwald's heart disease, a textbook of cardiovascular medicine*, ed 11, Philadelphia, 2019, Elsevier.

TABLE 7 Pharmacologic Characteristics of Oral Antiplatelet Drugs Commonly Used in the Management of Acute Coronary Syndrome

		ADP RECEPTOR ANTAGONISTS		
Characteristic	Aspirin	Clopidogrel	Prasugrel	Ticagrelor
Class	COX inhibitor	Thienopyridine (second generation)	Thienopyridine (third generation)	Cyclopentyl triazolopyrimidine
Target	COX-1	P2Y12	P2Y12	P2Y12
Dose	162- to 325-mg loading dose; 75-325 mg/day maintenance dose	300- to 600-mg loading dose; 75 mg/day maintenance dose	60-mg loading dose; 10 mg/day maintenance dose	180-mg loading dose; 90 mg bid maintenance dose
Prodrug	No	Yes	Yes	No
Time to effect[a]	<1 h	4-6 h[b]	<1 h	<1 h
Drug half-life	20 min	Min	Min	12 hr
Reversible	No	No	No	Yes

ADP, Adenosine diphosphate; *bid*, twice daily; *COX*, cyclooxygenase.
[a]After loading dose.
[b]Increased antithrombotic benefit was seen after the first hour in patients enrolled in the COMMIT trial who did not receive a loading dose, but maximum effect is not seen until after 4-6 h.
From Hoffman R et al: *Hematology, basic principles and practice*, ed 8, Philadelphia, 2023, Elsevier.

TABLE 8 Features of GPIIb/IIIa Antagonists

Feature	GPIIb/IIIa Antagonists		
Generic name	Abciximab	Eptifibatide	Tirofiban
Trade name	ReoPro	Integrilin	Aggrastat
Description	Fab fragment of humanized mouse monoclonal antibody	Cyclical KGD-containing heptapeptide	Nonpeptidic RGD mimetic
Specific for GPIIb/IIIa	No	Yes	Yes
Plasma half-life	Short (min)	Long (2.5 h)	Long (2.0 h)
Platelet-bound half-life	Long (days)	Short	Short
Renal clearance	No	Yes	Yes
Dosing	0.25 mg/kg bolus followed by a 12-h infusion of 10 μg/min	Two 180 μg/kg boluses given 10 min apart	25 μg/kg boluses followed by an 18-h infusion of 0.15 μg/kg/min
Adjustment for renal impairment	No	Yes	Yes

KGD, Lys-Gly-Asp; *RGD*, Arg-Gly-Asp.
From Hoffman R et al: *Hematology, basic principles and practice*, ed 8, Philadelphia, 2023, Elsevier.

addition to aspirin for medium- or high-risk patients with NSTE-ACS in whom an invasive strategy is planned (Class IIb). Eptifibatide and tirofiban are preferred agents over abciximab for NSTE-ACS patients; however, for STEMI patients undergoing primary PCI, IV abciximab has the same Class IIa indication as tirofiban and ptifibatide.[9]
- Anticoagulant agents should be administered to all ACS patients, irrespective of initial treatment strategy. Options include either unfractionated heparin (UFH), or low-molecular-weight heparin (LMWH; enoxaparin), or factor Xa inhibitors such as fondaparinux, or direct thrombin inhibitors such as bivalirudin (Table 9).[9]
- For STEMI, fondaparinux can be used for anticoagulation. It has been shown to decrease bleeding complications as compared with either UFH or LMWH. However, it should not be used as the sole anticoagulant in PCI because of the risk of catheter thrombosis.[9]
- Bivalirudin is a reversible direct thrombin inhibitor and may be considered as an alternative to UFH and GP IIb/IIIa inhibitors in patients with STEMI who are undergoing primary PCI. In a large study comparing bivalirudin to UFH in patients with STEMI and PCI, less major bleeding and a reduction in

30-day mortality in the patients who received bivalirudin was observed.[12] With bivalirudin, there is no risk of heparin-induced thrombocytopenia, less bleeding is observed, and the anticoagulant effect can be monitored during intervention by the activated clotting time. Similar results were reported in the use of bivalirudin alone in patients with UA/NSTEMI in the ACUITY trial when compared to enoxaparin/UFH with GP IIb/IIIa arms.[13]
- Beta-blocker therapy reduces ischemia by decreasing myocardial oxygen demand and has a proven long-term mortality benefit. Oral therapy should be initiated within 24 hours of onset of ACS unless signs or symptoms of heart failure and shock are present or bradycardia precludes its use. Oral administration, titrated to a heart rate of 50 to 60 beats/min, is preferred.[9] Intravenous beta-blockers can be administered to STEMI patients who are hypertensive or have ongoing ischemia; they should be avoided if the patients have any of the following:
  1. Signs of heart failure
  2. Evidence of a low output state
  3. Increased risk for cardiogenic shock
  4. Other relative contraindications to beta-blockade (PR interval >0.24 sec, second- or

third-degree heart block, active asthma, or reactive airway disease)
- Nitroglycerin is a vasodilator that should be administered to relieve chest discomfort in all ACS patients. It can be administered sublingually at first, up to 3 doses, followed by intravenous administration if symptoms persist. In the setting of an inferior STEMI, it is necessary to rule out a right ventricular (RV) infarct with a right-sided ECG before the administration of nitroglycerin.[9] This is because RV infarcts are preload dependent and nitroglycerin decreases preload through venodilation, which leads to hypotension in this setting. This can be corrected by discontinuing nitroglycerin and starting bolus intravenous fluids. Nitrates should not be administered in patients who recently received a phosphodiesterase inhibitor. Of note, nitroglycerin provides no mortality benefit in ACS patients.
- Oxygen should be administered to ACS patients with signs of respiratory distress or an arterial oxyhemoglobin saturation of <90%. The 2014 ACC/AHA guidelines report no demonstrated benefit for routine use of supplemental oxygen in normoxic patients with NSTE-ACS; rather, emerging data suggest that routine use of oxygen can lead to

TABLE 9 Pharmacologic Characteristics of Parenteral Anticoagulants Commonly Used in the Management of Patients with Acute Coronary Syndrome

	Unfractionated Heparin	Enoxaparin	Bivalirudin	Fondaparinux
Route of administration	IV	SC (first dose IV[a])	IV	SC (first dose IV[a])
Frequency of dosing	Continuous IV infusion	Twice daily; once daily if CrCl <30 ml/min	Continuous IV infusion	Once-daily injection
Clearance	Primarily nonrenal	Renal	Renal, proteolytic cleavage	Renal
Use in ACS patients with moderate renal impairment	Yes	Yes (dose reduction)	Yes (dose reduction)	Yes[b]
Use in ACS patients undergoing dialysis	Yes	No experience	Yes (dose reduction)	No experience[c]
Routine laboratory monitoring	Yes	No	No[d]	No
Dose	Adjust dose according to the results of the aPTT	Fixed weight adjusted	Fixed weight adjusted	Fixed
Accumulation in renal failure	No	Yes	Yes	Yes
Nonanticoagulant side effects	Allergy, HIT	HIT (rare)	—	—
Nonbleeding contraindications	Allergy, immune HIT	Allergy, immune HIT	Allergy	Allergy
Antidote	Protamine sulfate	Protamine sulfate partially reverses	No	No

ACS, Acute coronary syndromes; *aPTT,* activated partial thromboplastin time; *CrCl,* creatinine clearance; *HIT,* heparin-induced thrombocytopenia; *IV,* intravenous; *SC,* subcutaneous.
[a]The first dose of enoxaparin was given by the intravenous route in the TIMI-11B (Thrombolysis In Myocardial Infarction 11B) and EXTRACT-TIMI 25 (Enoxaparin and Thrombolysis Reperfusion for Acute Myocardial Infarction Treatment, Thrombolysis in Myocardial Infarction 25) studies. The first dose of fondaparinux was given by the intravenous route in the OASIS-6 (Optimal Antiplatelet Strategy for Interventions 6) trial.
[b]Acute coronary syndrome patients with creatinine up to 265 μmol/L were eligible for inclusion in the OASIS-5 and -6 trials (equivalent to an estimated creatinine clearance of 15-20 ml/min in a 70-kg patient who is 70 yr of age).
[c]Fondaparinux is contraindicated in patients with venous thromboembolism who have severe renal impairment.
[d]Monitoring and dose adjustment required in patients with creatinine clearance below 30 ml/min.
From Hoffman R et al: *Hematology, basic principles and practice,* ed 8, Philadelphia, 2023, Elsevier.

adverse effects such as increased coronary vascular resistance, reduced coronary blood flow, and increased mortality rate.[2]

- Morphine can be used intravenously in patients with NSTE-ACS if there is continued ischemic chest pain despite treatment with maximally tolerated antiischemic medications (Class IIb).[8]
- Calcium channel blockers (nondihydropyridine) may be used in patients with persisting or recurrent symptoms, despite treatment with beta-blockers and nitroglycerin. They work by having negative inotropic and chronotropic effects and causing coronary vasodilation. They are especially useful when beta-blockers are contraindicated and in patients with coronary artery spasm. Calcium channel blockers should not be used in cases of severe LV dysfunction, pulmonary edema, increased risk for cardiogenic shock or advanced heart blocks.[9]
- Patients routinely taking NSAIDs (except for aspirin), both nonselective as well as COX-2–selective agents, before ACS should discontinue those agents at the time of presentation because of the increased risks of mortality, reinfarction, hypertension, heart failure, myocardial rupture, along with overall cardiovascular and bleeding events. However, there is evolving evidence for the role of colchicine to reduce recurrent event risk in the acute post-MI period, with the COLCOT trial showing a reduction in death from cardiovascular causes, resuscitated cardiac arrest, recurrent MI, stroke or urgent hospitalization for angina leading to coronary revascularization.[14] No guidelines have been published that reflect the results of this trial.

- ACE inhibitors may be added and should be used within 24 h of onset of ACS in all patients with depressed LV function (EF <40%) and those with a history of hypertension, diabetes mellitus, or stable chronic kidney disease. Angiotensin receptor blockers (ARBs) should be used in patients who are ACE inhibitor intolerant.[2]
- Table 10 summarizes indications and cautions for adjunctive medical therapies for patients with STEMI.
- Refer to topic "Cocaine Overdose" for treatment of cocaine-related ACS.

CHRONIC Rx
- Post-ACS medical therapy involves aspirin, statin, beta-blocker, and a second antiplatelet agent such as clopidogrel, ticagrelor, or prasugrel.
- In patients already on an oral anticoagulant for another diagnosis such as atrial fibrillation, the duration of triple therapy should be minimized. Strategies aimed at minimizing the risk of bleeding in patients treated with triple therapy (dual antiplatelet therapy and an oral anticoagulant) are summarized in Table 11. Studies have shown that taking a P2Y12 inhibitor such as clopidogrel along with an oral anticoagulant results in a significant reduction in bleeding complications with no significant difference in thrombotic protection when compared with taking triple therapy of oral anticoagulant, aspirin, and clopidogrel.[5] It is a class IIB recommendation in those patients with atrial fibrillation and a CHADS-VASC score of ≥2 after coronary revascularization to consider using clopi-

dogrel concurrently with oral anticoagulant (Table 12) but without aspirin.
- Lipid lowering with high-intensity statins has been shown to reduce death, MI, and cardiac events at 16 wk when administered early (within 24 to 96 h after ACS). Additional data demonstrated the benefit of early high-intensity statin therapy with low density lipoprotein (LDL) targets <70 mg/dl in ACS.[2]
- ACE inhibitors may be added to treat hypertension and should be used in all patients with depressed LV function (EF <40%) or pulmonary vascular congestion. ARBs should be used in patients who are ACE inhibitor intolerant.[2]
- An aldosterone blocker should be used in post-MI patients without significant renal dysfunction (creatinine >2.5 mg/dl in men or creatinine >2.0 mg/dl in women) or hyperkalemia (K >5.0 mEq/L) who have an EF of <40% and are already on therapeutic doses of an ACE inhibitor and a beta-blocker.[2]
- Cardiac rehabilitation and a monitored exercise program should be recommended at the time of discharge.[2]
- Aggressive risk factor management, including smoking cessation, weight loss, diet and exercise, diabetes control, and so on, for secondary prevention of future events is crucial.[2]

REFERRAL
- All ACS patients should be cared for in conjunction with the cardiology consult service.
- When appropriate, referral to a cardiac surgeon may be necessary for CABG and comprehensive heart team approach.
- At the time of discharge, patients should be referred for cardiac rehabilitation.

A

TABLE 10 Indications and Cautions for Adjunctive Medical Therapies for Patients with ST-Elevation Myocardial Infarction

Therapy	Indications	Cautions
Beta-adrenergic receptor–blocking agents	Oral: All patients without contraindication IV: Patients with refractory hypertension or ongoing ischemia without contraindication	Signs of congestive heart failure Low-output state Increased risk for cardiogenic shock Prolonged first-degree or high-grade atrioventricular block Reactive airways disease
Angiotensin-converting enzyme (ACE) inhibitors	Anterior myocardial infarction and LVEF ≤0.40 or congestive heart failure All patients without contraindication	Hypotension Renal failure Hyperkalemia
Angiotensin receptor–blocking agents (ARBs)	Intolerant of ACE inhibitors	Hypotension Renal failure Hyperkalemia
Statins	All patients without contraindications	With drugs metabolized via CYP3A4, fibrates Monitor for myopathy, hepatotoxicity Adjust dose for lipid targets
Nitroglycerin	Ongoing chest pain Hypertension and congestive heart failure	Suspected right ventricular infarction SBP <90 (or 30 mm Hg below baseline) Recent use of a type 5 PDE inhibitor
Oxygen	Clinically significant hypoxemia (SpO_2 <90) Congestive heart failure Dyspnea	Chronic obstructive pulmonary disease and CO_2 retention
Morphine	Pain Anxiety Pulmonary edema	Lethargic or moribund patient Hypotension Bradycardia Known hypersensitivity

IV, Intravenous; *LVEF,* left ventricular ejection fraction; *PDE,* phosphodiesterase; *SBP,* systolic blood pressure.
From Zipes DP: *Braunwald's heart disease, a textbook of cardiovascular medicine,* ed 11, Philadelphia, 2019, Elsevier.

TABLE 11 Strategies Aimed at Minimizing the Risk of Bleeding in Patients Treated with Triple Therapy (Dual Antiplatelet Therapy and an Oral Anticoagulant)

Proposed Approach	Rationale
Aspirin maintenance dose ≤100 mg/day	Higher aspirin maintenance doses increase bleeding, and there is no evidence that they improve efficacy.
PPI with a preference for agents that interfere less with CYP 2C19 (e.g., pantoprazole)	Much of the excess bleeding is from the GI tract. The use of acid-suppressive agents that interfere less with CYP 2C19 minimizes the potential for a negative interaction with clopidogrel.
Preference for a nonvitamin K antagonist oral anticoagulant	Dabigatran 110 mg twice daily and apixaban 2.5 or 5.0 mg twice daily are associated with lower rates of bleeding than warfarin.
For warfarin, use a target INR of 2-2.5	Some evidence that a restricted target INR range reduces the risk of bleeding.
Manage warfarin in a specialized anticoagulation clinic	Compared with usual care, specialist clinics achieve a higher TTR of the INR.
Minimize duration of triple therapy	The risk of bleeding is highest during the first 30 days but remains elevated with long-term treatment.
Avoid NSAIDs	NSAIDs are a common cause of upper GI bleeding.
Avoid prasugrel and ticagrelor	Prasugrel and ticagrelor cannot be recommended because they are more potent than clopidogrel and cause more bleeding.

CYP, Cytochrome P-450; *GI,* gastrointestinal; *INR,* international normalized ratio; *NSAID,* nonsteroidal antiinflammatory drug; *PPI,* proton pump inhibitor; *TTR,* time in therapeutic range.
From Hoffman R et al: *Hematology, basic principles and practice,* ed 8, Philadelphia, 2023, Elsevier.

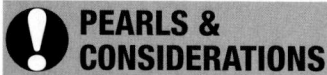

PEARLS & CONSIDERATIONS

COMMENTS
- ACS is a common life-threatening disorder and a leading cause of mortality in the U.S.
- The diagnosis hinges on the basics—history and physical, ECG, biomarkers, and CXR.
- Remember the potentially fatal non-ACS causes of chest discomfort, which include acute pulmonary embolism, acute ascending aortic dissection, pneumothorax, and esophageal rupture (Boerhaave syndrome).

- STEMI patients presenting to a hospital with PCI capability should be treated with primary PCI within 90 min of first medical contact.
- STEMI patients presenting to a hospital without PCI capability and who cannot be transferred to a PCI center and undergo PCI within 120 min of first medical contact should be treated with fibrinolytic therapy within 30 min of hospital presentation unless fibrinolytic therapy is contraindicated.
- Refer to topics "Angina Pectoris" and "Myocardial Infarction" for additional discussion of this subject matter.

RELATED CONTENT

Acute Coronary Syndrome (Patient Information)
Angina Pectoris (Related Key Topic)
Coronary Artery Disease (Related Key Topic)
Myocardial Infarction (Related Key Topic)
Hypertension (Related Key Topic)

AUTHORS: **KYLE DIGRANDE, MD,** and **PRANAV M. PATEL, MD, FACC, FAHA, FSCAI**

REFERENCES

Available at eBooks.Health.Elsevier.com.

TABLE 12 Pharmacologic Characteristics of Warfarin and New Oral Anticoagulants Evaluated in Phase III Trials for the Long-Term Management of Acute Coronary Syndrome

Characteristic	Warfarin	Rivaroxaban	Apixaban
Target	VKORC1	Factor Xa	Factor Xa
Prodrug	No	No	No
Bioavailability (%)	100	80	60
Dosing	Variable, once daily	Fixed, 2.5 or 5 mg twice daily[a]	Fixed, 5 mg twice daily (2.5 mg twice daily in selected patients)
Half-life	Mean: 40 h (range: 20-60 h)	7-11 h	12 h
Renal clearance (%)	Nil	66[b]	25
Routine coagulation monitoring	Yes (INR)	No	No
Drug interactions	Multiple	Potent inhibitors of CYP3A4 and P-gp[c]	Potent inhibitors of CYP3A4 and P-gp[c]
Antidote	Yes (vitamin K, PCC, FFP)	Yes (Andexanet alfa)	Yes (Andexanet alfa)
Approved for ACS management	Yes	Yes, in Europe	No

ACS, Acute coronary syndromes; *CYP3A4,* cytochrome P-450 3A4; *FFP,* fresh frozen plasma; *fXa,* activated factor X; *INR,* international normalized ratio; *PCC,* prothrombin complex concentrates; *P-gp,* P-glycoprotein; *VKORC1,* C1 subunit of vitamin K epoxide reductase. Strategies Aimed at Minimizing the Risk of Bleeding in Patients Treated With Triple Therapy (Dual Antiplatelet Therapy and an Oral Anticoagulant).

[a]A once-daily regimen was tested in atrial fibrillation.

[b]Half of renally cleared rivaroxaban is cleared as unchanged drug and half as inactive metabolites.

[c]Potent inhibitors of both CYP3A4 and P-glycoprotein include azole antifungals (e.g., ketoconazole, itraconazole, voriconazole, posaconazole) and protease inhibitors, such as ritonavir. Potent inhibitors of CYP3A4 include azole antifungals, macrolide antibiotics (e.g., clarithromycin), and protease inhibitors (e.g., atazanavir).

From Hoffman R et al: *Hematology, basic principles and practice,* ed 8, Philadelphia, 2023, Elsevier.

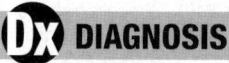
BASIC INFORMATION

DEFINITION

Acute glomerulonephritis (GN) is inflammation of the glomerulus, an intricate mesh of blood vessels that acts as the filtration system of the kidney, usually caused by an autoimmune reaction resulting in deposition of immunoreactants and recruitment of inflammatory cells. Clinically, patients present with blood and protein in the urine, acute kidney injury, and high blood pressure. If untreated, chronic glomerular inflammation leads to progressive chronic kidney disease. Rapidly progressive glomerulonephritis (RPGN) is said to be present when there is a loss in GFR of 50% or more within weeks due to acute glomerulonephritis. Kidney biopsy in patients with RPGN shows inflammatory glomerular lesions that may be associated with crescents.

SYNONYMS

Acute nephritic syndrome
Glomerulonephritis, acute GN

ICD-10CM CODES
N00.0	Acute nephritic syndrome with minor glomerular abnormality
N00.1	Acute nephritic syndrome with focal and segmental glomerular lesions
N00.2	Acute nephritic syndrome with diffuse membranous glomerulonephritis
N00.3	Acute nephritic syndrome with diffuse mesangial proliferative glomerulonephritis
N00.4	Acute nephritic syndrome with diffuse endocapillary proliferative glomerulonephritis
N00.5	Acute nephritic syndrome with diffuse mesangiocapillary glomerulonephritis
N00.6	Acute nephritic syndrome with dense deposit disease
N00.7	Acute nephritic syndrome with diffuse crescentic glomerulonephritis
N00.8	Acute nephritic syndrome with other morphologic changes
N00.9	Acute nephritic syndrome with unspecified morphologic changes

EPIDEMIOLOGY & DEMOGRAPHICS

- Incidence of primary GN varies between 0.2/100,000 (membranoproliferative GN) and 2.5/100,000 (immunoglobulin A [IgA] nephropathy) cases per patient-year.[1]
- Immunoglobulin A (IgA) nephropathy is the most common form of GN worldwide, and true incidence is likely underestimated as cases exist subclinically.
- GN accounts for 23% of end-stage kidney disease cases worldwide.
- GN affects adults and children.
- IgA nephropathy is more common in males while lupus nephritis is more common in females.[2]

PHYSICAL FINDINGS & CLINICAL PRESENTATION

- Acute onset of hypertension.
- Dark, "tea-colored" urine.
- Edema (peripheral, periorbital, or pulmonary).
- Fatigue.
- Concurrent pulmonary hemorrhage and rapidly progressive decline in kidney function is often associated with "crescentic GN," such as that seen with antineutrophil cytoplasmic antibody (ANCA) vasculitis or antiglomerular basement membrane (anti-GBM) disease (formerly Goodpasture syndrome).[3]
- Joint pains, oral ulcers, and malar rash are frequently seen with systemic lupus erythematosus (SLE).[4]
- Palpable purpura may be seen in patients with systemic vasculitides, such as IgA vasculitis (formerly Henoch-Schönlein purpura), ANCA-associated vasculitis, SLE, or cryoglobulinemia.[3]
- A recent history of endocarditis, cellulitis/impetigo, or pharyngitis preceding or occurring along with urinary abnormalities may indicate infection-related GN.
- Hepatitis C virus infection may cause membranoproliferative GN (MPGN) with or without cryoglobulinemia.[5]
- Concurrent upper respiratory tract infection (synpharyngitic infection) and gross hematuria may indicate IgA nephropathy.
- Table 1 summarizes the clinical and laboratory features of the different causes of rapidly progressive GN.

ETIOLOGY

- Acute GN may occur as a renal-limited disease or part of a systemic disorder. A description of target antigens is included in Table 2.
- In the past decade, the knowledge of the pathogenesis of several acute GNs has greatly expanded.
- IgA nephropathy is considered a multi-hit process that involves insufficiently *O*-galactosylated IgA1 forming aggregates, development of *O*-glycan-specific antibodies, and deposition of IgA1-containing immune complexes in the kidney.[6]
- Hepatitis C causes chronic immune stimulation and production of cryoglobulins that deposit in the kidney.[6]
- Poststreptococcal GN is now part of the broader category termed infection-related GN which includes IgA-dominant *Staphylococcus*-associated GN.
- ANCA-associated (pauci-immune) vasculitis is associated with antibodies to myeloperoxidase, proteinase 3, and less commonly lysosomal-associated membrane protein 2, although not all studies have supported direct disease causation.[7,8]
- Paraproteins, which are immunoglobulin components or whole immunoglobulins, may deposit in the kidney and cause a variety of glomerular lesions. When these paraproteins are not associated with a hematologic malignant condition, the kidney condition is termed monoclonal gammopathy of renal significance.[9]
- C3 glomerulopathy, composed of C3 GN and dense deposit disease, is caused by dysregulation of the alternative complement pathway. The alternative complement path-way is now implicated in several different GNs,

including IgA nephropathy and ANCA-associated vasculitis. Identification of complement activation in these disorders portends future treatment implications.[10]
- Thrombotic microangiopathy (thrombotic thrombocytopenic purpura, hemolytic uremic syndrome) in the native kidney is caused by endothelial damage that can be triggered by drugs, pregnancy, autoimmune diseases (e.g., atypical hemolytic uremic syndrome, antiphospholipid antibody disease, lupus), infection, and primary genetic disorders.[11]
- Pathologic features of immune glomerular diseases are summarized in Table 3.

DIAGNOSIS

DIFFERENTIAL DIAGNOSIS FOR HEMATURIA AND/OR PROTEINURIA IN ADDITION TO ACUTE GN

- Urinary tract infection
- Nephrolithiasis
- Urothelial malignancy
- Polycystic kidney disease
- Acute interstitial nephritis
- Acute tubular necrosis
- Nephrotic syndrome
- Hereditary nephritis (Alport syndrome and thin basement membrane nephropathy)
- Diabetic nephropathy

WORKUP

Initial evaluation of suspected GN consists of laboratory testing.

LABORATORY TESTS[13]

- Urinalysis with albuminuria (majority of proteinuria in GN is albuminuria) and hematuria (dysmorphic erythrocytes and red cell casts).
- Blood urea nitrogen and serum creatinine.
- 24-h urine collection for total protein excretion (includes albumin plus tubular proteins) and creatinine clearance to document degree of renal dysfunction and accuracy of urine collection. Random urine (spot) specimen for evaluation of the protein-to-creatinine ratio instead of a 24-h collection is also acceptable. Proteinuria in acute GN typically ranges from 500 mg/day to 3 g/day, but nephrotic-range proteinuria (>3.5 g/day) may be present.
- Streptococcal tests (Streptozyme) and antistreptolysin O (ASO) quantitative titer (highest in 3 to 5 wk). The ASO titer is not related to severity of kidney disease, duration, or prognosis.
- Additional serologic testing, including antinuclear antibody (ANA), antibody directed against double-stranded DNA (anti-dsDNA), C3, C4, hepatitis B and C viral serologies, HIV, ANCA (myeloperoxidase and proteinase-3 antigens), anti-GBM antibodies, cryoglobulins, rheumatoid factor, serum and urine protein electrophoresis with immunofixation, and serum free light chain analysis.
- Thrombotic microangiopathies present with microangiopathic hemolytic anemia—decreased hemoglobin and platelets, decreased haptoglobin, and elevated LDH, along with

TABLE 1   Clinical and Laboratory Features in the Different Causes of Rapidly Progressive Glomerulonephritis

Disease	Typical Clinical Features	Serologic Findings	Complement Levels	Immune Deposits in Glomerulus on Renal Biopsy
Vasculitis				Few/pauci-immune
Granulomatosis with polyangiitis (formerly, Wegener granulomatosis)	Prodrome of nasal stuffiness, blocked ears, arthralgia; then onset of hemoptysis, purpura, peripheral neuropathy	C-ANCA	Normal or increased	
Microscopic polyangiitis	Similar to granulomatosis with polyangiitis (Wegener granulomatosis) or affecting the kidneys only (renal-limited) or overlap with polyarteritis nodosa	P-ANCA	Normal or increased	
Anti-GBM disease	Macroscopic hematuria and hemoptysis	Anti-GBM antibodies	Normal or increased	Linear staining for IgG and C3
SLE (diffuse proliferative, WHO Class IV)	Previous history of SLE, marked hematuria and proteinuria, hypertension "telescoping" urinary sediment	ANA, anti-dsDNA antibodies	Low C3, low C4	Granular immune deposits
IgA disease	Persistent microscopic hematuria with episodes of synpharyngitic macroscopic hematuria, with proteinuria, hypertension	IgA (increased in about half of cases)	Normal or increased	
Poststreptococcal glomerulonephritis	At 1-3 wk after streptococcal pharyngitis or impetigo, macroscopic hematuria, edema, hypertension, oliguria	ASO, anti-DNase B antibodies	Low C3, normal C4	

ANA, Antinuclear antibody; *anti-DNase B*, anti-deoxyribonuclease B antibody; *anti-dsDNA*, anti–double-stranded DNA antibody; *anti-GBM*, glomerular basement membrane antibody; *ASO*, antistreptolysin O antibody; *C-ANCA*, cytoplasmic antineutrophil cytoplasmic antibody; *IgA*, immunoglobulin A; *IgG*, immunoglobin G; *P-ANCA*, perinuclear antineutrophil cytoplasmic antibody; *SLE*, systemic lupus erythematosus; *WHO*, World Health Organization.
From Ronco C et al: *Critical care nephrology*, ed 3, Philadelphia, 2019, Elsevier.

schistocytes on peripheral blood smear. These parameters may be normal in renal-limited thrombotic microangiopathy, which can only be diagnosed via biopsy.
• Blood cultures should be obtained from any febrile patient.

IMAGING STUDIES

• Chest radiograph: If opacities are present, consider diffuse alveolar hemorrhage as occurs with ANCA-associated vasculitis and anti-GBM disease (Goodpasture disease).
• Renal ultrasound to exclude structural causes of hematuria and proteinuria. A kidney size of <9 cm in sagittal length may indicate extensive scarring and a low likelihood of reversibility.
• Echocardiogram in patients with new cardiac murmurs or positive blood cultures to evaluate for endocarditis and pericardial effusion.
• Kidney biopsy with light, electron, and immunofluorescence microscopy.
• Biopsy of other affected organs if systemic vasculitis is suspected.

Rx TREATMENT

NONPHARMALOGIC THERAPY

• Low-sodium (i.e., 2 g sodium) diet if edema or hypertension is present
• Low-potassium diet if patient is hyperkalemic

ACUTE GENERAL Rx

• Acute management is specific to the type of GN and requires urgent nephrology consultation. The Kidney Disease Improving Global Outcome (KDIGO) guidelines for GN management provides evidence-based diagnostic and treatment strategies.
• Diuretics if edema and/or other antihypertensives if hypertension is present.

TABLE 2   Antigens Identified in Glomerulonephritis

Post-Streptococcal GN	Streptococcal Pyrogenic Exotoxin B, Plasmin Receptor
Anti-GBM disease	a3 type IV collagen (likely induced by molecular mimicry)
IgA nephropathy	Immune complex of anti-glycan antibodies and complement components
Membranous nephropathy	Phospholipase A_2 receptor (idiopathic), neutral endopeptidase in podocyte (congenital), thrombospondin type I domain-containing 7A (THSD7A),[12] exotosin 1 (EXT1) and exostosin 2 (EXT2), NELL1, Sema3B, PCDH7, and HBeAg (hepatitis associated). New antigens continue to be identified.
Staphylococcus aureus–associated GN	*Staphylococcus* superantigens induce polyclonal response; not necessarily antigen in glomeruli
Membranoproliferative GN	HCV and HBsAg in hepatitis-associated MPGN
ANCA-associated vasculitis	Proteinase 3 (C-ANCA) and myeloperoxidase (P-ANCA) in neutrophils; other "minor" antigens include lysosome-associated membrane protein 2 (LAMP2) on endothelial cells (likely induced by molecular mimicry to fimbriated bacterial antigens). Minor antigens are generally not associated with vasculitis.[13]

ANCA, Antineutrophil cytoplasmic antibody; *GBM*, glomerular basement membrane; *GN*, glomerulonephritis; *HBeAg*, hepatitis B virus early antigen; *HBsAg*, hepatitis B surface antigen; *HCV*, hepatitis C virus; *IgA*, immunoglobulin A; *MPGN*, membranoproliferative glomerulonephritis.
Adapted from Floege J et al: *Comprehensive clinical nephrology*, ed 4, Philadelphia, 2010; and Sethi S: New 'antigens' in membranous nephropathy, *J Am Soc Nephrol* 32:268-278, 2021.

• Correction of electrolyte abnormalities (hypocalcemia, hyperkalemia) and metabolic acidosis.
• Hemodialysis in patients with diuretic-resistant volume overload, refractory hyperkalemia, uremic symptoms, and severe metabolic acidosis. Plasma exchange therapy for antibody removal is indicated in select cases such as in patients with anti-GBM disease.
• Initial therapy for most patients with RPGN involves pulse methylprednisolone followed by daily oral prednisone, oral or intravenous immunosuppressant therapy such as cyclophosphamide or rituximab, and, in some settings, plasmapheresis.

CHRONIC Rx[14]

• Some types of GN have a relapsing and remitting course. Periodic monitoring of blood pressure, urinalysis, serum creatinine and blood urea nitrogen, serum albumin, and random urine protein-to-creatinine ratio are important to detect relapsing disease.
• ACE inhibitors or angiotensin II type 1 receptor blockers (ARBs) to reduce proteinuria. Mineralocorticoid receptor antagonists and SGLT2 inhibitors may also be considered for proteinuria reduction.
• Lipid management with lipid-lowering agents as indicated.
• Monitor for side effects related to immunosuppression such as infection, cytopenias,

TABLE 3 Pathologic Features of Immune Glomerular Diseases

Disease	Pathogenesis	LM	IF	EM
Membranous	In situ immune complex deposition (PLA$_2$R is antigen)	Capillary wall thickening	Capillary wall granular IgG and C3	Subepithelial deposits
IgA nephropathy	Abnormal IgA glycosylation	Mesangial hypercellularity	Mesangial dominant IgA (and some C3)	Mesangial deposits
Membranoproliferative glomerulonephritis (MPGN)	Immune complex deposition	Endocapillary hypercellularity, mesangial sclerosis, "double contouring"	Capillary wall IgG (less IgM) and C3	Subendothelial deposits
C3 glomerulonephritis (C3GN)	Dysregulation of alternative pathway of complement	Variable features, but often similar to MPGN	Capillary wall dominant C3 (less or no Igs)	Variable, but subendothelial deposits
Dense deposit disease (DDD)	Dysregulation of alternative pathway of complement	Variable, but often similar to MPGN or mesangial cell hypercellularity	Capillary wall dominant C3 (less or no Igs)	Dense deposits in GBM
Postinfectious glomerulonephritis	Immune complex deposition, planted or circulating antigen	Endocapillary hypercellularity	Capillary wall IgG and C3	Subepithelial "hump" deposits
Anti-GBM disease	Circulating anti-GBM antibodies (antigen is α3 chain of COL4)	Capillary wall necrosis and crescents	Capillary wall linear IgG and C3	No deposits, GBM ruptures
Pauci-immune glomerulonephritis	ANCAs (antineutrophil cytoplasmic antibodies)	Capillary wall necrosis and crescents	No or sparse Ig/C3 staining	No or sparse deposits
Lupus nephritis (Class I-VI)	Immune complex deposition	Variable, class-dependent	"Full-house" staining for all Igs, C3, and C1q	Numerous deposits typically (location is class-dependent)

COL4, Type IV collagen; *EM,* electron microscopy; *GBM,* glomerular basement membrane; *IF,* immunofluorescence; *Igs,* immunoglobulins; *LM,* light microscopy.
From McPherson RA, Pincus MR: *Henry's clinical diagnosis and management by laboratory methods,* ed 23, St Louis, 2017, Elsevier.

Diseases and Disorders

I

osteoporosis or osteopenia, GI ulcers, high blood pressure, and malignancy.
- Routine health maintenance with CDC recommended vaccinations for immunocompromised patients and/or patients with chronic kidney disease, and age-appropriate malignancy screening. Live vaccines are contraindicated in patients actively receiving immunosuppressant therapy.

DISPOSITION
- Prognosis is generally correlated to initial serum creatinine and degree of fibrosis on kidney biopsy.
- In general, prognosis is worse in patients with heavy albuminuria/proteinuria, low glomerular filtration rate at presentation, severe hypertension, and kidney biopsy-proven crescentic GN with high degree of crescents.

REFERRAL
Nephrology consultation for all patients with suspected GN. Urgent consultation is recommended if hyperkalemia, acidosis, or azotemia is present.

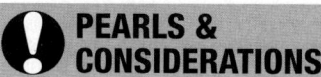

PEARLS & CONSIDERATIONS

COMMENTS
- Diagnosis of acute GN should be established by kidney biopsy if the biopsy results influence the treatment plan, especially with systemic illnesses, significant proteinuria (>500 mg/day), or increasing serum creatinine. Exploration for systemic illness, including infections, autoimmune disease, and malignancy is required along with careful history, physical examination, and serologic tests. Some patients with suspected GN may not require a kidney biopsy because of the success of supportive therapies (e.g., infection-related GN).
- Nephrology consultation should be obtained before initiating immunosuppressive therapy. ACE inhibitor or ARB therapy is essential for proteinuria reduction, unless contraindicated. SGLT2 inhibitors and mineralocorticoid receptor antagonists such as spironolactone have been added to ACE inhibitor treatment for greater proteinuria reduction.
- Regular monitoring for side effects of immunosuppressive drugs and complications of corticosteroids is necessary.
- Monitor lipids and treat persistent hyperlipidemia.

RELATED CONTENT
Glomerulonephritis (Patient Information)
Acute Kidney Injury (Related Key Topic)

REFERENCES
Available at eBooks.Health.Elsevier.com

AUTHORS: **NATHANIEL HOCKER, MD,** and **RUPALI AVASARE, MD**

BASIC INFORMATION

DEFINITION

Acute kidney injury (AKI) is defined as a rapid impairment in kidney function that results in oliguria and retention of nitrogenous products in the blood normally excreted by the kidneys, that is, azotemia. The decline in kidney function can result in volume overload and dysregulation of acid-base status and electrolytes. Current consensus criteria for diagnosis of AKI requires an increase in serum creatinine of 0.3 mg/dl within 48 h or 1.5 times baseline serum creatinine over 7 days, and/or a decline in urine in output to <0.5 ml/kg/h for 6 to 12 h. AKI is further graded by severity as described in Table 1.[1]

SYNONYMS

AKI
Acute renal failure (ARF)
Acute kidney failure

ICD–10 CM CODES	
N17.0	Acute kidney failure with tubular necrosis
N17.1	Acute kidney failure with acute cortical necrosis
N17.2	Acute kidney failure with medullary necrosis
N17.8	Other acute kidney failure
N17.9	Acute kidney failure, unspecified
N99.0	Postprocedural (acute) (chronic) kidney failure
O90.4	Postpartum acute kidney failure

EPIDEMIOLOGY & DEMOGRAPHICS[2]

- An estimated 20% of hospitalized patients and 60% of intensive care unit patients develop AKI.
- AKI occurs in 20% of patients with moderate sepsis and in >50% of patients with septic shock and positive blood cultures.
- More than 40% of hospital-associated AKI is iatrogenic.
- AKI in hospitalized patients is associated with increased hospital length-of-stay and cost.
- Most common cause of AKI in hospitalized patients is from intrinsic kidney failure due to acute tubular necrosis (ATN).
- Key risk factors for AKI include older age, preexisting chronic kidney disease, diabetes mellitus, and/or preexisting proteinuria.

PHYSICAL FINDINGS & CLINICAL PRESENTATION[3]

- The clinical presentation of AKI depends on the presence of any preexisting conditions, the underlying conditions, the precipitating event(s) that caused the AKI and the severity of AKI (Fig E1).
- Early or mild AKI is frequently asymptomatic.
- Frequent presenting symptoms include weakness, anorexia, generalized malaise, and nausea.
- Patients may develop oliguric or nonoliguric kidney injury.

TABLE 1 Consensus Acute Kidney Injury Definitions and Classification Systems

Serum Creatinine		Urine Output
RIFLE Criteria		
Risk	Increase in SCr to ≥1.5 times baseline *or* decrease in GFR by >25% within 7 days	<0.5 ml/kg/h for >6 h
Injury	Increase in SCr to >2 times baseline *or* decrease in GFR by >50% within 7 days	<0.5 ml/kg/h for >12 h
Failure	Increase in SCr to >3 times baseline *or* decrease in GFR by >75% within 7 days *or* increase in SCr to ≥4 mg/dl with an acute rise of 0.5 mg/dl	<0.3 ml/kg/h for >24 h *or* anuria for 12 h
Loss	Complete loss of kidney function requiring dialysis for >4 wk	
ESRD	Complete loss of kidney function requiring dialysis for >3 mo	
AKIN Criteria		
Stage 1	Increase in SCr by ≥0.3 mg/dl *or* increase in SCr to ≥1.5 times baseline within 48 h	<0.5 ml/kg/h for ≥6 h
Stage 2	Increase in SCr to >2 times baseline within 48 h	<0.5 ml/kg/h for ≥12 h
Stage 3	Increase in SCr to >3 times baseline within 48 h *or* increase in SCr to ≥4 mg/dl with a rise of 0.5 mg/dl within 24 h *or* initiation of dialysis	<0.3 ml/kg/h for ≥24 h *or* anuria for ≥12 h
KDIGO Criteria		
Stage 1	Increase in SCr by ≥0.3 mg/dl within 48 h *or* increase in SCr to ≥1.5 times baseline within 7 days	<0.5 ml/kg/h for ≥6 h
Stage 2	Increase in SCr to >2 times baseline within 7 days	<0.5 ml/kg/h for ≥12 h
Stage 3	Increase in SCr to >3 times baseline within 7 days *or* increase in SCr to ≥4 mg/dl *or* initiation of dialysis	<0.3 ml/kg/h for ≥24 h *or* anuria for ≥12 h

AKIN, Acute kidney injury network; *ESRD,* end-stage renal disease; *GFR,* glomerular filtration rate; *KDIGO,* kidney disease improving global outcomes; *RIFLE,* risk, injury, failure, loss, end-stage kidney disease; *SCr,* serum creatinine.
From Newman M et al: *Perioperative medicine,* ed 2, Philadelphia, 2022, Elsevier.

- Oliguria is defined as <400 to 500 ml of urine per 24 h. Anuria is frequently seen in ATN or bilateral obstructive uropathy.
- Physical examination should focus on evaluation of volume status, eliciting systemic signs of AKI, and findings supportive of kidney injury etiology.
- Clinical signs and symptoms are numerous; some key findings are highlighted:
  1. Peripheral edema from volume overload, heart failure, liver failure, or nephrotic syndrome
  2. Pulmonary edema
  3. Cardiac dysrhythmias
  4. Neurologic findings include altered mental status, delirium, lethargy, myoclonus, seizures, and asterixis
  5. Pruritus, uremic odor
  6. Flank pain
  7. Painless hematuria may be seen with glomerulonephritis (GN), whereas painful hematuria is more consistent with obstructive uropathy
  8. Pericardial effusion and/or pericardial rub
  9. Fever, skin rash, and arthralgia can be seen with systemic vasculitis
  10. Classic triad of fever, rash, and eosinophilia in the setting of AKI strongly implicates allergic interstitial nephritis (AIN). However, the simultaneous appearance of all three manifestations occurs in only 30% of cases. When AIN is considered

the cause of AKI, a careful review of medications is required

ETIOLOGY[3-6]

- **Prerenal:** Inadequate renal perfusion caused by hypovolemia, congestive heart failure (impaired cardiac output), cirrhosis (fluid third-spacing), sepsis (vasodilation), abdominal compartment syndrome, or other. Sixty percent of community-acquired cases of AKI are due to prerenal conditions.
- **Postrenal:** Bladder outlet obstruction (prostatic enlargement, urethral fibrosis), ureteral obstruction (stones, bladder masses, retroperitoneal fibrosis, ureteral fibrosis), or renal vein occlusion. With two functioning kidneys, bilateral obstruction is usually required to produce significant AKI. Postrenal causes of AKI account for 5% to 15% of community-acquired AKI.
- **Intrinsic renal:** ATN, AIN, and GN. Common causes of ATN include ischemia (e.g., hypotension or shock, postcardiac bypass, or aorta surgery), rhabdomyolysis, sepsis, drug toxicity (e.g., aminoglycosides, amphotericin, cisplatin), and iodinated radiocontrast-induced nephropathy. Contrast-induced nephropathy is the third most common cause of new-onset AKI in hospitalized patients. However, most of these cases have multiple confounding factors and are better characterized as contrast-associated nephropathy. AIN can develop after

exposure to medications, most commonly NSAIDs, antibiotics, and proton pump inhibitors. Microvascular diseases that cause AKI include thrombotic microangiopathies (e.g., thrombotic thrombocytopenic purpura, classic and atypical hemolytic-uremic syndrome, and preeclampsia) and cholesterol emboli.

- Causes of AKI are listed in Table 2.
- Nearly one third of AKI cases may be prevented or mitigated.

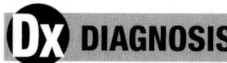 DIAGNOSIS

Table 3 summarizes useful clinical features, urinary findings, and confirmatory tests in the differential diagnosis of AKI.

DIFFERENTIAL DIAGNOSIS
Refer to "Etiology." Diagnostic tests to distinguish prerenal and renal AKI are described in Table 4. A diagnostic approach to patients with suspected AKI is shown in Fig. 2.

LABORATORY TESTS[1,3-5]
- Elevated serum creatinine.
- Standard estimating equations for glomerular filtration rate (GFR) require steady-state creatinine levels and are not recommended to estimate GFR during AKI.
- Elevated blood urea nitrogen (BUN): BUN-to-creatinine ratio is commonly >20:1 in prerenal azotemia, postrenal azotemia, and acute GN.
- BUN-to-creatinine ratio is <20:1 in acute interstitial nephritis and ATN.
- Hyperkalemia, hyperphosphatemia, and metabolic acidosis are common.
- Hypocalcemia with hyponatremia or hypernatremia may occur, depending on etiology.
- Urinalysis is the initial diagnostic evaluation. Prerenal and postrenal AKI are typically characterized by a normal urinalysis. Conversely, abnormal findings should prompt further workup for specific intrinsic causes of AKI that may require intervention. Hematuria and proteinuria imply GN; heavy (>3+) proteinuria is associated with leukocyturia and may signify AIN. Microscopic examination of urine sediment may facilitate diagnosis: Granular casts in ATN, dysmorphic red blood cells or red blood cell casts in acute GN, and white blood cell casts in AIN.
- In oliguric patients, obtain urine sodium and creatinine concentrations for determination of fractional excretion of sodium: $FE_{Na} = 100\% \times (U_{Na} \times P_{Cr})/(P_{Na} \times U_{Cr})$. $FE_{Na} <1\%$ occurs in prerenal AKI and >1% occurs in intrinsic AKI. FE_{Na} may be falsely elevated in patients taking diuretics or falsely low in several intrinsic renal conditions, including acute GN, contrast-induced nephropathy, and rhabdomyolysis. (U_{Na}, urinary sodium; U_{Cr}, urinary creatinine; P_{Cr}, plasma creatinine; P_{Na}, plasma sodium).
- Fractional excretion of urea (FE_{Urea}) can be used to assess renal dysfunction in AKI. FE_{Urea} is more useful than FE_{Na} during diuretic therapy. FE_{Urea} is calculated as follows: $FE_{Urea} = 100\% \times (U_{Urea} \times P_{Cr})/(P_{Urea} \times U_{Cr})$. If $FE_{Urea} <35\%$ prerenal AKI is likely, and if $FE_{Urea} >50\%$ intrinsic AKI is likely. (U_{Urea}, urinary urea; P_{Urea}, plasma urea).
- Urinary osmolality range of 250 mOsm/kg H_2O to 300 mOsm/kg H_2O in ATN (isosthenuria), <400 mOsm/kg H_2O in postrenal azotemia, and >500 mOsm/kg H_2O in prerenal azotemia and acute GN.
- In suspected GN (e.g., hematuria plus proteinuria), additional serologic testing may be warranted. Abnormal liver function tests and elevated inflammatory markers are nonspecific. Immune complex deposition disorders (e.g., infectious GN, lupus nephritis, cryoglobulinemic vasculitis) are characterized by

TABLE 2 Etiologies of Acute Kidney Injury

Prerenal Causes (Decreased Renal Blood Flow)	Intrinsic Renal Causes	Postrenal Causes
Hypovolemia	**Vascular: Large and Small Vessels**	**Ureteral Obstruction**
Renal losses (diuretics, osmotic agents, polyuria)	Renal vein obstruction (thrombosis, ventilation with high-level PEEP, abdominal compartment syndrome)	Tumor (intrinsic or extrinsic)
Gastrointestinal losses (vomiting, diarrhea)	Microangiopathy (thrombotic thrombocytopenic purpura, hemolytic-uremic syndrome, disseminated intravascular coagulation, preeclampsia)	Fibrosis
Cutaneous losses (burns, exfoliative syndromes)		Ligation during pelvic surgery
Hemorrhage	Malignant hypertension	**Bladder Neck Obstruction**
Pancreatitis	Scleroderma renal crisis	Benign prostatic hypertrophy
Decreased Cardiac Output	Transplant rejection	Prostate cancer
Congestive heart failure	Atheroembolic disease	Neurogenic bladder
Pulmonary embolism	**Glomerular**	Tricyclic antidepressants
Acute myocardial infarction	Antiglomerular basement membrane disease (Goodpasture syndrome)	Ganglionic blockers
Severe valvular heart disease	Antineutrophil cytoplasmic antibody-associated glomerulonephritis (Wegener granulomatosis)	Bladder tumor
Abdominal compartment syndrome	Immune complex glomerulonephritis, systemic lupus erythematosus, postinfectious cryoglobulinemia, primary membranoproliferative glomerulonephritis	Calculus
Renal artery obstruction (stenosis, embolism, thrombosis, dissection)	**Tubular**	Hemorrhage/clot
Systemic Vasodilation	Ischemic	**Urethral Obstruction**
Sepsis	Cytotoxic	Strictures
Anaphylaxis	Heme pigment (rhabdomyolysis, intravascular hemolysis)	Tumor
Anesthetics	Crystals (tumor lysis syndrome, seizures, ethylene glycol poisoning, vitamin C megadose, acyclovir, indinavir, methotrexate)	Phimosis
Drug overdose	Drugs (aminoglycosides, lithium, amphotericin B, pentamidine, cisplatin, ifosfamide, radiocontrast agents), synthetic cannabinoid use	Renal calcinosis
Afferent Arteriolar Vasoconstriction	**Interstitial**	Obstructed urinary catheter, ureteral stent, or ileal conduit
Hypercalcemia	Drugs (penicillins, cephalosporins, NSAIDs, proton pump inhibitors, allopurinol, rifampin, indinavir, mesalamine, sulfonamides, trimethoprim)	Pelvic trauma, retroperitoneal hematoma
Drugs (NSAIDs, amphotericin B, calcineurin inhibitors, orepinephrine, radiocontrast agents, aminoglycosides)	Infection (pyelonephritis, viral infection)	
Hepatorenal syndrome	**Systemic Disease**	
Efferent arteriolar vasodilation (angiotensin converting enzyme inhibitors, aldosterone receptor blockers)	Sjögren syndrome, sarcoidosis, systemic lupus erythematosus, lymphoma, leukemia, interstitial nephritis, uveitis	
Trauma	Calculus	

NSAIDs, Nonsteroidal antiinflammatory drugs; *PEEP,* positive end-expiratory pressure.
Modified from Cameron JL, Cameron AM: *Current surgical therapy,* ed 10, Philadelphia, 2011, Saunders.

TABLE 3 Useful Clinical Features, Urinary Findings, and Confirmatory Tests in the Differential Diagnosis of Acute Kidney Injury

Cause of Acute Kidney Injury	Some Suggestive Clinical Features	Typical Urinalysis Results	Some Confirmatory Tests
Prerenal azotemia	Evidence of true volume depletion (thirst, postural or absolute hypotension and tachycardia, low jugular venous pressure, dry mucous membranes and axillas, weight loss, fluid output greater than input) or decreased effective circulatory volume (e.g., heart failure, liver failure), treatment with NSAID, diuretic, or ACE inhibitor/ARB	Hyaline casts $FE_{Na} < 1\%$ $U_{Na} < 10$ mmol/L SG >1.018	Occasionally requires invasive hemodynamic monitoring; rapid resolution of AKI with restoration of renal perfusion
Diseases Involving Large Renal Vessels			
Renal artery thrombosis	History of atrial fibrillation or recent myocardial infarction, nausea, vomiting, flank or abdominal pain	Mild proteinuria Occasionally RBCs	Elevated LDH level with normal transaminase levels, renal arteriogram, MAG3 renal scan, MRA*
Atheroembolism	Usually age >50 yr, recent manipulation of aorta, retinal plaques, subcutaneous nodules, palpable purpura, livedo reticularis	Often normal Eosinophiluria Rarely casts	Eosinophilia, hypocomplementemia, skin biopsy, renal biopsy
Renal vein thrombosis	Evidence of nephrotic syndrome or pulmonary embolism, flank pain	Proteinuria, hematuria	Inferior venacavogram, Doppler flow studies, MRV*
Diseases of Small Renal Vessels and Glomeruli			
Glomerulonephritis or vasculitis	Compatible clinical history (e.g., recent infection), sinusitis, lung hemorrhage, rash or skin ulcers, arthralgias, hypertension, edema	RBC or granular casts, RBCs, white blood cells, proteinuria	Low complement levels; positive antineutrophil cytoplasmic antibodies, antiglomerular basement membrane antibodies, antistreptolysin O antibodies, anti-DNase, cryoglobulins; renal biopsy
HUS/TTP	Compatible clinical history (e.g., recent gastrointestinal infection, cyclosporine, anovulants), pallor, ecchymoses, neurologic findings	May be normal, RBCs, mild proteinuria, rarely RBC or granular casts	Anemia, thrombocytopenia, schistocytes on peripheral blood smear, low haptoglobin level, increased LDH, renal biopsy
Malignant hypertension	Severe hypertension with headaches, cardiac failure, retinopathy, neurologic dysfunction, papilledema	May be normal, RBCs, mild proteinuria, rarely RBC casts	LVH by echocardiography or ECG, resolution of AKI with BP control
Ischemic or Nephrotoxic Acute Tubular Necrosis			
Ischemia	Recent hemorrhage, hypotension, surgery often in combination with vasoactive medication (e.g., ACE inhibitor, NSAID)	Muddy-brown granular or tubular epithelial cell casts, $FE_{Na} > 1\%$, $U_{Na} > 20$ mmol/L SG 1.010	Clinical assessment and urinalysis usually inform diagnosis
Exogenous toxin	Recent contrast medium-enhanced procedure; nephrotoxic medications; certain chemotherapeutic agents often with coexistent volume depletion, sepsis, or chronic kidney disease	Muddy-brown granular or tubular epithelial cell casts $FE_{Na} > 1\%$, $U_{Na} > 20$ mmol/L SG 1.010	Clinical assessment and urinalysis usually inform diagnosis
Endogenous toxin	History suggestive of rhabdomyolysis (coma, seizures, drug abuse, trauma)	Urine supernatant tests positive for heme in absence of RBCs	Hyperkalemia, hyperphosphatemia, hypocalcemia, increased CK, myoglobin
	History suggestive of hemolysis (recent blood transfusion)	Urine supernatant pink and tests positive for heme in absence of RBCs	Hyperkalemia, hyperphosphatemia, hypocalcemia, hyperuricemia, and free circulating hemoglobin
	History suggestive of tumor lysis (recent chemotherapy), myeloma (bone pain), or ethylene glycol ingestion	Urate crystals, dipstick-negative proteinuria, oxalate crystals, respectively	Hyperuricemia, hyperkalemia, hyperphosphatemia (for tumor lysis); circulating or urinary monoclonal protein (for myeloma); toxicology screen, acidosis, osmolal gap (for ethylene glycol)
Diseases of the Tubulointerstitium			
Allergic interstitial nephritis	Recent ingestion of drug and fever, rash, loin pain, or arthralgias	White blood cell casts, white blood cells (frequently eosinophiluria), RBCs, rarely RBC casts, proteinuria (occasionally nephritic)	Systemic eosinophilia, renal biopsy
Acute bilateral pyelonephritis	Fever, flank pain and tenderness, toxic state	Leukocytes, occasionally white blood cell casts, RBCs, bacteria	Urine and blood cultures
Postrenal AKI	Abdominal and flank pain, palpable bladder	Frequently normal, hematuria if stones, prostatic hypertrophy	Plain abdominal radiography, renal ultrasonography, postvoid residual bladder volume, computed tomography, retrograde or antegrade pyelography

ACE, Angiotensin-converting enzyme; *AKI,* acute kidney injury; *ARB,* angiotensin receptor blocker; *BP,* blood pressure; *CK,* creatine kinase; *DNase,* deoxyribonuclease; *ECG,* electrocardiography; FE_{Na}, fractional excretion of sodium; *HUS,* hemolytic uremic syndrome; *LDH,* lactate dehydrogenase; *LVH,* left ventricular hypertrophy; *MAG3,* mercaptoacetyltriglycine; *MRA,* magnetic resonance angiography; *MRV,* magnetic resonance venography; *NSAID,* nonsteroidal antiinflammatory drug; *RBC,* red blood cell; *SG,* specific gravity; *TTP,* thrombotic thrombocytopenic purpura; U_{Na}, urinary sodium concentration.

*Contrast-enhanced MRA and MRV should be used with extreme caution in patients with AKI.

From Skorecki K et al: *Brenner & Rector's the kidney,* ed 10, Philadelphia, 2016, Elsevier.

TABLE 4 Diagnostic Tests to Distinguish Between Prerenal and Renal Acute Kidney Injury

Index	Prerenal Causes	Renal Causes
FE_{Na}	<1%	>2%
Urine sodium	<10 mmol/L	>40 mmol/L
Urine/plasma osmolality	>1.5	1-1.5
Renal failure index	<1	>2
BUN-to-serum creatinine ratio	>20	<10

BUN, Blood urea nitrogen; FE_{Na}, fractional excretion of sodium. Calculation of FE_{Na}: (Urine sodium × Plasma creatinine)/(Plasma sodium × Serum creatinine) ×100. Renal failure index: (Urine sodium × Urine creatinine)/Plasma creatinine.
From Cameron JL, Cameron AM: *Current surgical therapy*, ed 10, Philadelphia, 2011, Saunders.

decreased complement levels (C3, C4). Specific testing includes antinuclear antibodies (lupus), antineutrophil cytoplasmic antibodies (ANCA-associated vasculitis), antiglomerular basement membrane antibodies (Goodpasture disease), and cryoglobulins. Kidney biopsy is frequently required for diagnostic confirmation.

- Creatinine phosphokinase level is indicated if rhabdomyolysis is suspected; positive blood reaction on a urine dipstick with typically few or no red blood cells by microscopy may indicate myoglobinuria from rhabdomyolysis.
- Serum free light chain analysis, serum and urine protein electrophoresis, and serum and urine immunofixation electrophoresis for suspected multiple myeloma or other plasma cell dyscrasias. Myeloma can cause AKI via a variety of mechanisms, including tubular precipitation of filtered light chains (cast nephropathy), hypercalcemia, and amyloidosis, among others.
- Kidney biopsy may be indicated in patients with intrinsic kidney failure when considering specific therapy. The major indications for kidney biopsy include the following: Differential diagnosis of nephrotic syndrome, distinguishing lupus vasculitis from other vasculitides, distinguishing lupus membranous nephropathy from idiopathic membranous nephropathy, confirmation of hereditary nephropathies based on ultrastructure, diagnosis of rapidly progressive GN, distinguishing AIN from ATN, and separation of primary glomerulonephritides. In addition to establishing a diagnosis, biopsy may determine renal prognosis and guide direction of management. Severe interstitial fibrosis is associated with poor renal outcomes.
- Biomarkers of kidney injury have been explored for earlier diagnosis of AKI and to separate intrinsic from prerenal causes. Candidate markers include neutrophil gelatinase-associated lipocalin (NGAL), kidney-injury molecule 1 (KIM-1), and the product of tissue inhibitor of metalloprotein-ase-2 and insulin-like growth-factor binding protein-7 (TIMP2*IGFBP7).
- TIMP2*IGFBP7 is U.S. FDA approved for risk prediction of AKI. However, there remains little published experience with this test, and the clinical role remains undefined.

IMAGING STUDIES[1,5]

- ECG for arrhythmia detection, especially in hyperkalemia: Peaked T waves in precordial leads, widening QRS interval, and/or bradycardia with AV node blockade.
- Chest radiograph to detect signs of congestive heart failure and pulmonary renal syndromes that frequently present with alveolar hemorrhage (antiglomerular basement membrane or ANCA-associated vasculitis).
- Bladder scan to assess post-void residual urine when urinary obstruction is suspected.
- Kidney ultrasonography to determine kidney sizes (distinguishes acute from chronic kidney disease), presence of obstruction, and renal vascular status (Doppler study).

Rx TREATMENT

Management of AKI depends on the underlying etiology. Some conditions (e.g., GN) require specific therapy. The general focus of treatment for established AKI is supportive care and limiting additional injury. Fig. 3 illustrates an algorithm for management of AKI.

NONPHARMACOLOGIC THERAPY

- Withdraw nephrotoxic medications.
- Evaluate volume status and correct hypovolemia. Goal of therapy is to increase cardiac output and improve tissue perfusion.
- Avoid excessive fluid administration in patients who are nonvolume responsive.[1,5,6]
- Dietary modification: (1) Energy prescription (29 to 36 Kcal/kg/day), (2) potassium restriction (60 mmol/day), (3) sodium restriction (90 mmol/day), (4) phosphorus restriction (<800 mg/day), and (5) high biologic value protein (1.2 g/kg/day) depending on requirement for dialysis.[7]
- Daily weight to monitor for fluid retention, in addition to intake and output measurement.
- Modification of drug dosages or schedules of renally excreted medications. Dosing should consider the trajectory of renal function, during evolving and recovering AKI, and may require additional adjustments in patients who require dialysis.[8]

ACUTE GENERAL Rx

- Correct electrolyte abnormalities and metabolic acidosis.
- Administer loop diuretics for volume overload.
- Administer vasopressors for circulatory shock or vasodilators, when appropriate, to optimize cardiac output in congestive heart failure.

Specific treatment is variable and depends on cause of AKI.[8-12]

- Prerenal: Intravenous (IV) volume expansion with isotonic solutions in hypovolemic patients or those with shock. Balanced crystalloid solutions are preferable.
- Intrinsic kidney failure: Discontinue all potential nephrotoxins and treat condition(s) causing kidney failure. In severe AIN cases, consider a trial of corticosteroids. For acute noninfectious GN, high-dose pulse corticosteroids are first-line therapy, typically in conjunction with other immunomodulatory therapy and/or plasma exchange, depending on the clinical scenario.
- Postrenal: Eliminate cause of obstruction. Immediate bladder catheter insertion for suspected bladder outlet obstruction. This maneuver should precede the kidney ultrasonogram during the diagnostic workup. Percutaneous nephrostomy tubes or ureteral stents may be required for upper urinary tract obstruction.
- Hyperkalemia-related ECG changes: IV calcium if electrocardiographic changes are present; IV insulin and/or glucose to shift potassium into cells; and IV bicarbonate therapy when metabolic acidosis is present to shift potassium into cells. These three treatments are temporary, and definitive therapy requires potassium removal via the GI tract by cation exchangers or via the urinary tract by diuretics or dialytic therapy.

Dialysis in AKI:

- General indications for initiation of dialysis during AKI:
  1. Uremic symptoms (e.g., encephalopathy, pericarditis, seizures).
  2. Extracellular fluid volume overload refractory to medical management.
  3. Severe acid-base derangement(s) refractory to medical management.
  4. Significant electrolyte derangement(s) (e.g., hyperkalemia, hyponatremia) refractory to medical management.
- Among critically ill patients, kidney replacement therapy may be required despite an absence of other indications. Optimal timing of initiation of dialysis remains controversial and is not solely dependent on previous metabolic parameters. Multiple recent clinical trials have not shown that early dialysis in AKI is beneficial.
- Intermittent hemodialysis and continuous renal replacement therapy (CRRT) have similar outcomes for patients with AKI. However, CRRT is associated with greater hemodynamic stability and fluid removal compared to conventional intermittent hemodialysis. CRRT is employed in critically ill patients with hemodynamic instability.

ADJUNCTIVE Rx

- Monitoring of renal function parameters and electrolytes.
- Renally excreted drugs are adjusted according to creatinine clearance or GFR to prevent further kidney damage or other medication-related toxicities.
- Prevent further renal insult with appropriate volume expansion, particularly before contrast

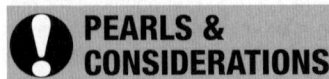

FIG. 2 Diagnostic approach to patients with suspected acute kidney injury (AKI). *AGN,* Acute glomerulonephritis; *AIN,* acute interstitial nephritis; *CT,* computed tomography; *Exog,* exogenous; *HUS/TTP,* hemolytic-uremic syndrome/thrombotic thrombocytopenic purpura. (From Floege J et al: *Comprehensive clinical nephrology,* ed 4, Philadelphia, 2010, Saunders.)

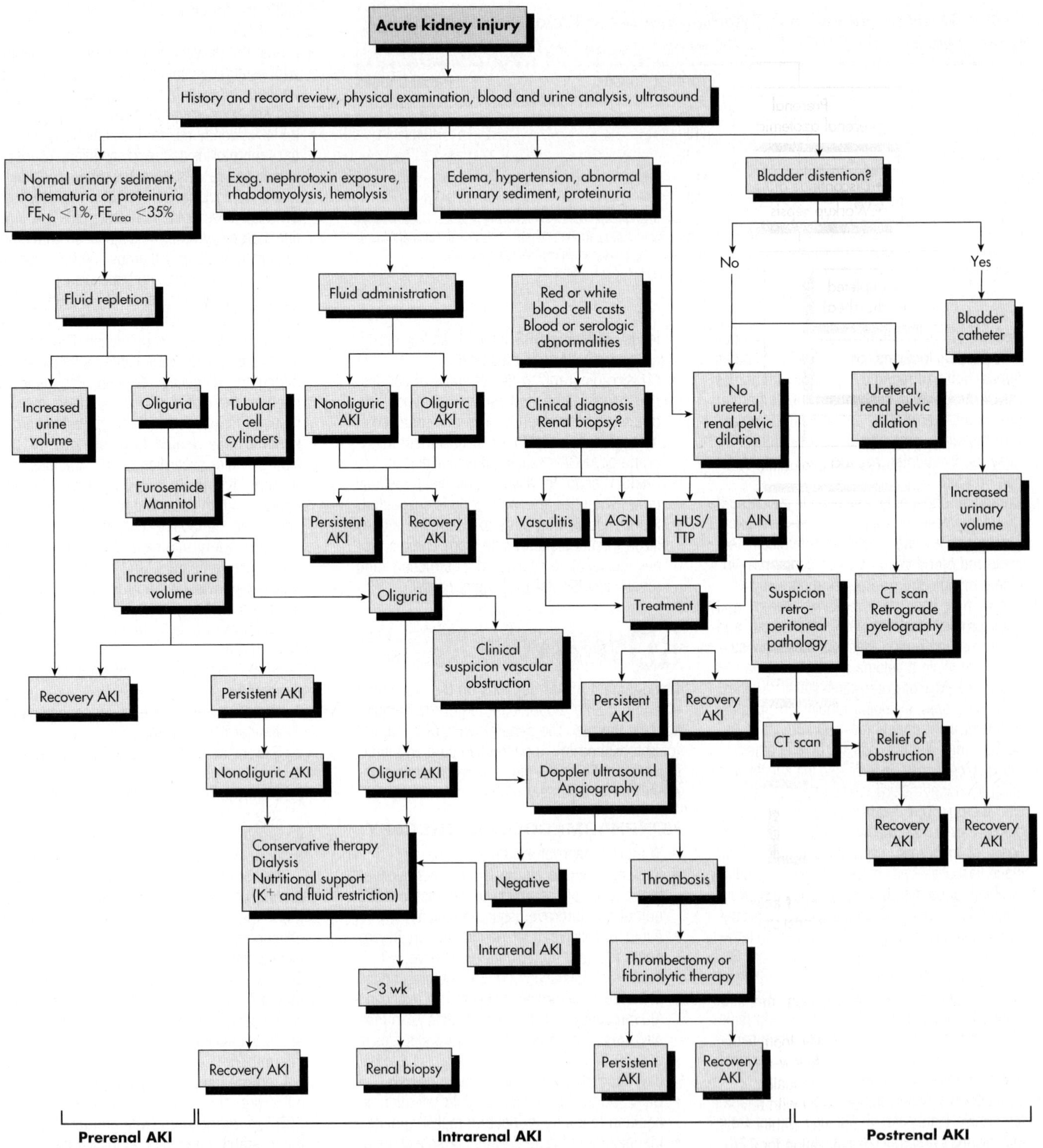

administration, and avoid nephrotoxic agents. Volume expansion with isotonic solutions is more effective than hydration with hypotonic solutions. Isotonic saline or bicarbonate-containing solutions are effective.

- Renal function recovery (ability to discontinue dialysis) varies from 50% to 75% in AKI survivors. Preexisting chronic kidney disease, longer duration of dialysis dependence, congestive heart failure, and older age are negative prognostic factors for renal function recovery.

- Overall mortality rate in AKI is nearly 25% and approaches 50% to 60% in patients who require acute dialysis.

- The combination of AKI and sepsis is associated with a mortality rate as high as 70%.

PEARLS & CONSIDERATIONS

- Patients with AKI are susceptible to infections and sepsis.

- In patients with community-acquired AKI, it is important to obtain a thorough medication

A

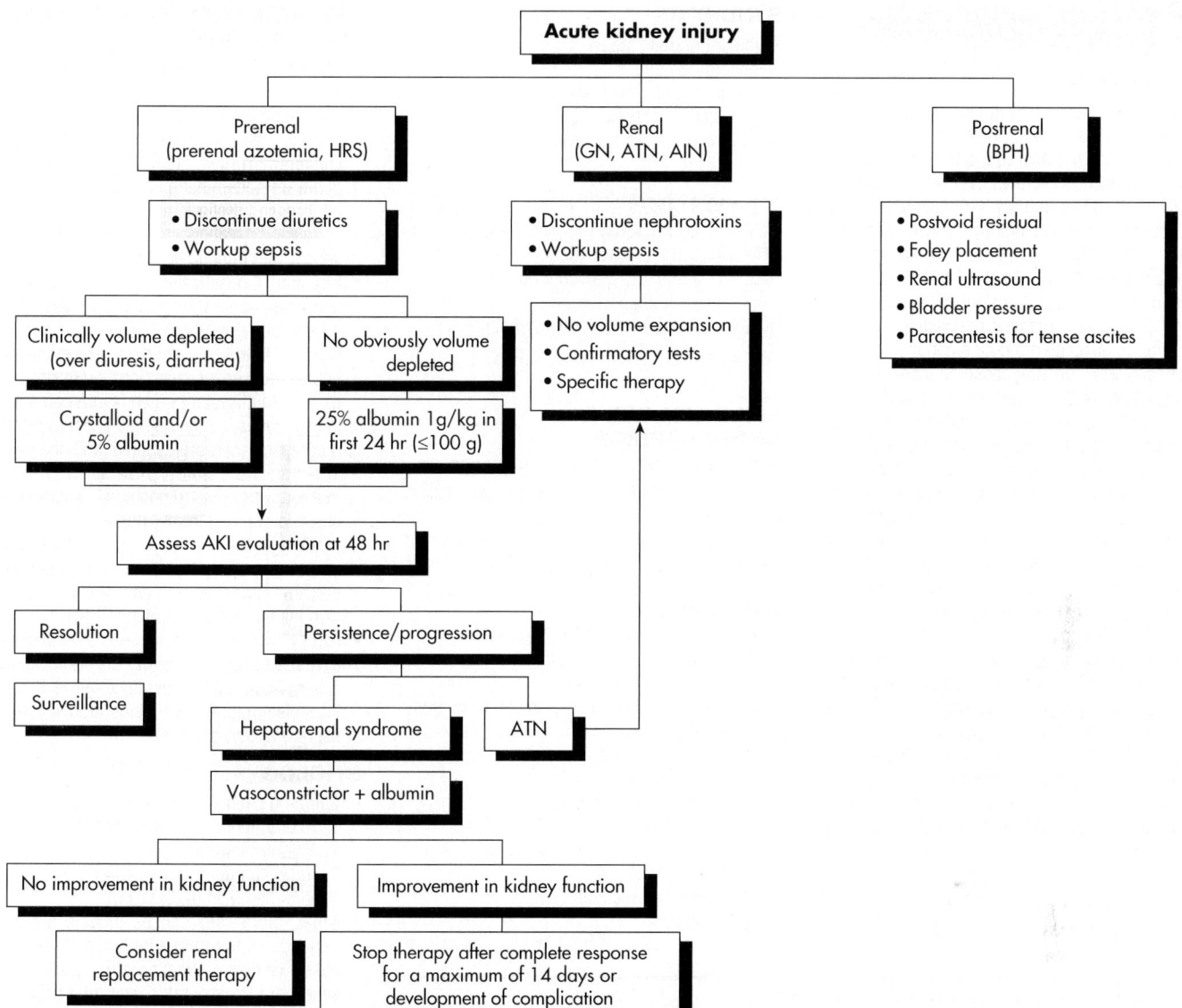

FIG. 3 Algorithm for management of acute kidney injury (AKI). *AIN,* Acute interstitial nephritis; *ATN,* acute tubular necrosis; *BPH,* benign prostatic hypertrophy; *GN,* glomerulonephritis; *HRS,* hepatorenal syndrome. (From Ronco C et al: *Critical care nephrology,* ed 3, Philadelphia, 2019, Elsevier.)

history, including nonprescription medications and supplements.
- AKI survivors are at risk for development of chronic kidney disease, and follow-up with monitoring of kidney function annually for at least 3 yr is recommended, even with apparent renal recovery. An initial visit within 3 mo after discharge from hospitalization for AKI is recommended.

However studies associating AKI with rapid subsequent loss of kidney function have been shown to have methodological limitations and after pre-AKI, eGFR, proteinuria, and other covariables are accounted for, the association between mild to moderate AKI and worsening subsequent loss of kidney function in patients with CKD has been found to be small.[13]

REFERENCES & SUGGESTED READINGS

Available at eBooks.Health.Elsevier.com.

RELATED CONTENT

Acute Renal Failure (Patient Information)
Chronic Kidney Disease (Related Key Topic)

AUTHOR: **JUNIOR UDUMAN, MD, MS**

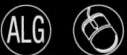
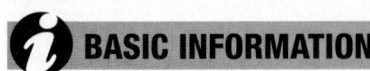 **BASIC INFORMATION**

DEFINITION

Acute liver failure (ALF) is defined as the rapid progression of liver dysfunction resulting in coagulopathy and altered mentation in patients without previously known liver disease. Practically, it is described as the constellation of acute severe hepatic injury (<26 wk); synthetic liver dysfunction, specifically coagulopathy (international normalized ratio [INR] >1.5); and any degree of mental alteration (encephalopathy) in a patient without preexisting cirrhosis and in the absence of acute alcoholic hepatitis. ALF can also be diagnosed in patients with preexisting liver disease, such as Wilson disease, vertically acquired hepatitis B, and autoimmune hepatitis (despite the possibility of cirrhosis in these patients), provided that diagnosis of these conditions was made within the preceding 26 wk.[1] Box 1 summarizes classifications of ALF. ALF must be distinguished from acute-on-chronic liver failure and acutely decompensated cirrhosis, two syndromes that pertain to acute deterioration in patients with preexisting chronic liver disease.[2] *Acutely decompensated cirrhosis* refers to the development of ascites, encephalopathy, gastrointestinal hemorrhage, or any combination of these disorders in patients with cirrhosis.[1] Acute-on-chronic liver failure is a syndrome where acute and severe hepatic derangements occur secondary to various insults in patients with chronic liver disease, including both cirrhotic and non-cirrhotic. It occurs in the context of intense systemic inflammation (e.g., infections or alcoholic hepatitis) and can be associated with single or multiorgan failure.[2,3]

SYNONYMS

Fulminant hepatic failure
Fulminant hepatitis
Fulminant hepatic necrosis
Acute hepatic necrosis
Acute and subacute necrosis of liver
ALF

ICD-10CM CODES
K72	Hepatic failure, not elsewhere classified
K72.0	Acute and subacute hepatic failure
K72.00	Acute and subacute hepatic failure without coma
K72.01	Acute and subacute hepatic failure with coma

EPIDEMIOLOGY & DEMOGRAPHICS

INCIDENCE: Affects approximately 2000 people/yr in U.S. and 1 to 8 people per million population in the U.K.[1]

PREDOMINANT SEX & AGE: Seen more often in women (90% of cases), often affects younger people

RISK FACTORS[1]:
- Intentional or inadvertent drug overdose
- Risk factors for viral hepatitis:
  1. Intravenous drug use
  2. Occupational exposure to blood or body fluids
  3. Blood transfusions
  4. Hemodialysis
  5. Intranasal cocaine use
  6. Imprisonment
  7. Travel to endemic hepatitis areas
- Previous alcohol use
- Hepatotoxic medications
- Critical illness

PHYSICAL FINDINGS & CLINICAL PRESENTATION[4]

- **Clinical Presentation** Initial symptoms of ALF are mostly nonspecific and depend on the etiology of liver injury. They include fatigue, lethargy, anorexia, and nausea/vomiting. Pruritus, jaundice, and right upper quadrant abdominal pain and distention may be present. Symptoms may also be more serious and consist of severe hypotension, sepsis, and hepatic encephalopathy.
- **Physical Examination** Findings include, by definition, abnormal neurologic findings of encephalopathy (Table 1). Other findings may include jaundice, asterixis, hepatomegaly, decreased hepatic mass on percussion, and ascites. Multisystem organ failure can ensue. In rare cases, as the hepatic encephalopathy progresses, cerebral edema and increased intracranial pressure can occur, with abnormal pupillary exam findings, hypertension, bradycardia, respiratory depression (Cushing triad), and loss of brain stem reflexes. Seizures secondary to increased intracranial pressure and hypoxia can occur. Vesicular skin lesions are suggestive of HSV.
- Family history of unexplained liver disease/cirrhosis should prompt slit lamp ocular examination for the identification of Kayser-Fleischer rings (copper rings around the iris seen in Wilson disease).

ETIOLOGY[4]

- Common causes in the Western world:
  1. Acetaminophen toxicity (46%)
  2. Indeterminate (14%)
  3. Idiosyncratic drug reaction (12%)
  4. Viral hepatitis (A, B) (10%)
- Other, more rare causes include alcoholic hepatitis, autoimmune hepatitis, Wilson disease, ischemic hepatopathy, Budd-Chiari syndrome, acute fatty liver of pregnancy, venoocclusive disease, toxin ingestion (e.g., mushroom poisoning [*Amanita phalloides*]), sepsis, infiltrative malignancy (breast cancer, lymphoma, myeloma, melanoma, small cell lung cancer), and other viruses (adenovirus, hepatitis E, herpes simplex virus [HSV]). Box 2 summarizes possible etiologies of liver failure.

LABORATORY FINDINGS[4]

- Coagulopathy is characteristic of patients with ALF, given decreased synthesis of clotting factors II, V, VII, IX, and X by the liver. Patients with ALF typically have a prolonged prothrombin time (INR >1.5), elevated transaminases, and elevated bilirubin, and may have a low platelet count (<150,000).
- Other possible laboratory findings can include an elevated blood urea nitrogen (BUN)/creatinine (studies show 30% to 50% also have acute kidney injury) and hypoglycemia (impairment of gluconeogenesis). Electrolyte disturbances, hyponatremia, hypophosphatemia, hypomagnesemia, hypokalemia, metabolic acidosis or respiratory alkalosis, elevated lactate dehydrogenase, and elevated ammonia.

BOX 1 Classifications of Acute Liver Failure

Trey and Davidson
Fulminant hepatic failure: Development of HE within 8 wk of onset of symptoms

British Classification
Acute liver failure (includes only patients with encephalopathy)

Subclassification Depending on the Interval between the Onset of Jaundice and HE
- Hyperacute liver failure: 0-7 days
- Acute liver failure: 8-28 days
- Subacute liver failure: 29-72 days
- Late-onset acute liver failure: 56-182 days

French Classification
- Acute hepatic failure: A rapidly developing impairment of liver function
- Severe acute hepatic failure: Prothrombin time or factor V concentration below 50% of normal with or without HE

Subclassification
- Fulminant hepatic failure: HE within 2 wk of onset of jaundice
- Subfulminant hepatic failure: HE between 3 and 12 wk of onset of jaundice

International Association for the Study of Acute Liver Failure
Acute liver failure (occurrence of HE within 4 wk after onset of symptoms)

Subclassification
- Acute liver failure—hyperacute: Within 10 days
- Acute liver failure—fulminant: 10-30 days
- Acute liver failure—not otherwise specified
- Subacute liver failure (development of ascites and/or HE from 5-24 wk after onset of symptoms)

HE, Hepatic encephalopathy.
From Vincent JL et al: *Textbook of critical care,* ed 7, Philadelphia, 2017, Elsevier.

TABLE 1 Features Distinguishing Acute Liver Failure from Chronic Hepatic Encephalopathy or Portal Systemic Encephalopathy

Feature	Acute Liver Failure	Portal Systemic Encephalopathy
History		
Onset	Usually acute	Varies; may be insidious or subacute
Mental state	Mania may evolve to deep coma	Blunted consciousness
Precipitating factor	Viral infection or hepatotoxin	Gastrointestinal hemorrhage, exogenous protein, drugs, uremia, infection
History of liver disease	No	Usually yes
Symptoms		
Nausea, vomiting	Common	Unusual
Abdominal pain	Common	Unusual
Signs		
Liver	Small, soft, tender	Usually large, firm, no pain
Nutritional state	Normal	Cachectic
Collateral circulation	Absent	May be present
Ascites	Absent	May be present
Laboratory Test		
Transaminases	Very high	Normal or slightly high
Coagulopathy	Present	Often present

From Jankovic J et al: *Bradley and Daroff's neurology in clinical practice,* ed 8, Philadelphia, 2022, Elsevier.

BOX 2 Etiologic Classification of Acute Liver Failure

Acetaminophen Toxicity
- Idiosyncratic drug injury

Infrequent Agents
- Isoniazid
- Valproate
- Halothane
- Phenytoin
- Sulfonamide
- Propylthiouracil
- Amiodarone
- Disulfiram
- Dapsone
- Bromfenac
- Troglitazone
- Zidovudine
- Lamivudine
- Lamotrigine
- Gatifloxacin
- Methotrexate

Miscellaneous Agents
- Ecstasy
- Cocaine
- Phencyclidine

Rare Agents
- Carbamazepine
- Ofloxacin
- Ketoconazole
- Lisinopril
- Nicotinic acid
- Labetalol
- Etoposide
- Imipramine
- Interferon alfa
- Flutamide
- Tolcapone
- Nefazodone
- Oral contraceptives

Combination Agents With Enhanced Hepatotoxicity
- Alcohol-acetaminophen
- Trimethoprim-sulfamethoxazole
- Rifampicin-isoniazid
- Amoxicillin-clavulanic acid

Viral Hepatitides
- Hepatitis A, B, C, D, E, G
- Human herpesvirus
- Cytomegalovirus
- Epstein-Barr virus
- Herpes simplex virus
- Varicella zoster virus
- Paramyxovirus
- Parvovirus B19
- Adenovirus
- Togavirus
- Parvovirus
- SEN virus
- TT virus
- Yellow fever virus

Toxins
- CCl_4
- *Amanita phalloides*
- Yellow phosphorus
- Herbal products

Vascular
- Ischemic
- Venoocclusive disease
- Budd-Chiari syndrome
- Malignant infiltration
- Non-Hodgkin lymphoma

Miscellaneous
- Wilson disease
- Autoimmune hepatitis
- Acute fatty liver of pregnancy
- Reye syndrome

From Vincent JL et al: *Textbook of critical care,* ed 7, Philadelphia, 2017, Elsevier.

DIAGNOSIS

DIFFERENTIAL DIAGNOSIS

- Severe acute hepatitis, also known as acute liver injury (including alcoholic hepatitis): Jaundice and coagulopathy without encephalopathy
- Acute-on-chronic liver failure (in patients with liver disease duration >26 wk)
- Cirrhosis (includes decompensated cirrhosis)
- Hepatocellular carcinoma
- Table 1 describes features distinguishing ALF from chronic hepatic encephalopathy or portal systemic encephalopathy

WORKUP (TABLE 2)[1,4-7]

- Fig. 1 describes an algorithm for evaluation of ALF.
- Clinical history is critical, but in the case of patients with severe encephalopathy, the history may be limited, and efforts should be made to obtain information from the patient's family. Important history components include medication use (6-mo history of prescriptions, over-the-counter medications, herbal supplements), alcohol use, recreational drug use, prior symptoms of jaundice, onset of symptoms, history of depression and prior suicide attempts, recent travel to endemic areas of viral hepatitis, sexual exposures, previous blood transfusions, family history of liver failure/disease, history of malignancy, or hypercoagulable state.
- Physical examination should include assessing for stigmata of chronic liver disease, as their presence has different diagnostic and management implications, and mental status. Grading of hepatic encephalopathy should be performed (Table 3). Perform an asterixis maneuver, consider psychometric tests (i.e., number connection test) to detect subtle degree of encephalopathy.
- Laboratory evaluation should be targeted to assess the severity of ALF, as well as its etiology. Early testing includes CBC, liver function tests (LFTs) including prothrombin time and INR, bilirubin, chemistry panel (sodium, potassium, chloride, bicarbonate, BUN, creatinine, glucose, magnesium, phosphate, calcium), arterial blood gas, arterial lactate, blood type and screen, acetaminophen level, ethanol level, toxicology screen, viral hepatitis serologies (hepatitis A immunoglobulin M [IgM], hepatitis B surface antigen, anti-hepatitis B core IgM, anti-hepatitis C antibody [IgM and IgG]), hepatitis C viral load (HCV RNA), anti-hepatitis E IgM and IgG, HSV-1 IgM and HSV polymerase chain reaction (PCR), Epstein-Barr virus DNA PCR, cytomegalovirus DNA PCR, anti-hepatitis D IgM and IgG, hepatitis D viral load (HDV RNA), ceruloplasmin level (as well as serum copper and 24-h urine copper if high suspicion), pregnancy test, arterial ammonia level, autoimmune markers (antinuclear antibody, anti-smooth muscle antibody, anti-liver kidney microsomal antibody type 1, total IgG levels), HIV-1, HIV-2, amylase, and lipase.

TABLE 2 Investigations in Acute Liver Failure

Investigation	Purpose	Suggested Frequency
Hematology		
Full blood examination	Anemia and thrombocytopenia for bleeding risk	Daily
Hemostatic parameters:		Daily
INR	Measure of hepatic insufficiency	Daily
Fibrinogen	Measure of hepatic insufficiency and bleeding risk	Daily
Blood film	Assess for hemolysis in Wilson disease and AIH	At presentation
Biochemistry		
Serum electrolytes	Management of Na$^+$, K$^+$	6-hourly
Liver function tests		Daily
AST, ALT	Assess hepatocyte injury and necrosis	Daily
Bilirubin, ALP, GGT	Assess hepatic insufficiency and cholestasis	Daily
Phosphate	Often low with liver failure, especially with CRRT	Daily
Creatinine	Measure of renal function	
Urea	Usually low in liver failure	Daily
Ammonia	Hyperammonemia associated with neurologic injury	Daily (at least)
Lactate	Measure of hepatic and circulatory failure	6-hourly
Blood glucose	Measure of hepatic insufficiency	6-hourly
Arterial blood gas analysis	Assess ventilation, oxygenation, and acid-base status	6-hourly
Acetaminophen concentration	Check for acetaminophen overdose in all ALF patients	At presentation
Copper studies	Ceruloplasmin low in Wilson disease	At presentation
β-hCG	Screen for pregnancy in female patients	At presentation
Lipase	Assess for pancreatitis	As indicated
Toxicologic screen	Assess for illicit drug use according to local practice	As indicated
Microbiology		
Serology		
Hepatotropic viruses	HAV, HBV, HDV, HEV as causes of ALF	At presentation
Nonhepatotropic viruses	EBV, CMV, HSV, VZV, parvovirus B19	At presentation
Microscopy and culture	Low threshold to assess for sepsis: blood, sputum, etc.	As indicated
Autoimmune markers		At presentation
ANA, ANCA, AMA, anti-LKM, anti-SM	Varying patterns in AIH	At presentation
Imaging		
Liver ultrasound with Doppler	Assess liver size, parenchyma, vascular integrity for Budd-Chiari	At presentation
Chest x-ray	Assess for pulmonary complications	Daily
CT brain	If evidence of trauma or focal neurologic deficits	As indicated
CT abdomen	Volumetric assessment of liver for prognosis	As indicated
Other		
ECG	Assess for toxidromes, arrhythmia, ischemia	Daily
EEG	Assess for possible seizure activity	As indicated
Liver biopsy	Assess for AIH or possible underlying cirrhosis	As indicated

ABG, Arterial blood gas; *ALP*, alkaline phosphatase; *ALT*, alanine transaminase; *ANA*, antinuclear antibody; *ANCA*, antineutrophil cytoplasmic antibody; *anti-LKM*, anti–liver kidney microsomal antibody; *anti-SM*, anti–Smith antibody; *APTT*, activated partial thromboplastin time; *ARDS*, acute respiratory distress syndrome; *AST*, aspartate transaminase; *b-hCG*, beta human chorionic gonadotrophin; *CMV*, cytomegalovirus; *EBV*, Epstein-Barr virus; *ECG*, electrocardiograph; *EEG*, electroencephalograph; *GGT*, gamma glutamyl transpeptidase; *HAV*, hepatitis A virus; *HBV*, hepatitis B virus; *HDV*, hepatitis D virus; *HEV*, hepatitis E virus; *HSV*, herpes simplex virus.
From Vincent JL et al: *Textbook of critical care*, ed 8, Philadelphia, 2024, Elsevier.

- Imaging studies include abdominal ultrasound with Doppler to evaluate for Budd-Chiari syndrome, portal hypertension, hepatic congestion, and hepatic steatosis. Cirrhosis cannot be diagnosed in the setting of ALF, as the liver may appear nodular in ALF due to massive necrosis. Consider cross-sectional imaging of the liver (triphasic CT, magnetic resonance cholangiopancreatography, or MRI with gadolinium), especially in patients with a history of malignancy, to rule out malignant infiltration. CT or MRI of the head should be considered to ensure no other causes for altered mental status.
- Prompt liver biopsy (via transjugular approach to decrease risk of bleeding) should be performed in cases in which:
  1. The etiology is unknown after the initial workup; *or*
  2. The etiology is thought to be secondary to autoimmune hepatitis, malignancy, or HSV.

COMPLICATIONS

Complications or progression of liver failure may result in cerebral edema due to increased intracranial pressure (in up to 40% of patients). Hypoglycemia and lactic acidosis are common complications of ALF, as well as acute kidney injury and pancreatitis (particularly in acetaminophen-induced ALF). Upper gastrointestinal hemorrhage is uncommon (in 1.5% of patients). Infections can occur due to impaired leukocyte function (in nearly 80% patients). High-output cardiac failure and acute respiratory distress syndrome can also occur. Hypotension occurs due to decreased oral intake as well as extravasation of fluid into extravascular space.

Ⓡˣ TREATMENT (BOXES 3 AND 4, TABLE 4)[1,4-6]

Broadly, the treatment of ALF should include:
- Identification of the etiology of liver injury, if possible, and specific treatment
- Symptomatic and supportive management and transfer to an intensive care unit (ICU) if necessary
- Early involvement of a liver specialist and transfer to a transplant center when required

NONPHARMACOLOGIC THERAPY[1,4-6]

- Initial treatment should focus on the patient's mental status and managing encephalopathy.
  1. Grade I encephalopathy may be managed on a medical ward (neuro vital signs q4h).
  2. Grade II, III, and IV encephalopathy should be managed in an ICU (with elevated head of the bed to 30 degrees). Grade III and IV encephalopathy require intubation and mechanical ventilation.
  3. Decreased stimulation is important (avoiding sedatives; dimly lit, quiet room; no audible monitor alarms).
- A liver specialist should be notified urgently, and arrangements should be made for imminent transfer to a transplant center. Early

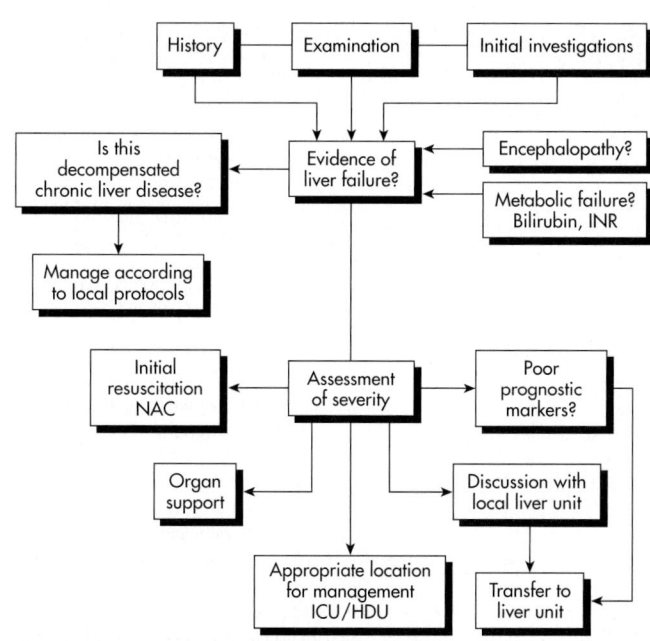

FIG. 1 Initial management of a patient presenting with liver failure. *HDU,* High-dependency unit; *ICU,* intensive care unit; *INR,* international normalized ratio; *NAC,* N-acetylcysteine. (From Parrillo JE, Dellinger RP: *Critical care medicine, principles of diagnosis and management in the adult,* ed 5, Philadelphia, 2019, Elsevier.)

TABLE 3 Grades of Encephalopathy

Grade	Description
I	Changes in behavior with minimal change in level of consciousness (mild confusion, slurred speech, disordered sleep)
II	Gross disorientation, drowsiness, possibly asterixis, inappropriate behavior
III	Marked confusion (stupor), incoherent speech, sleeping most of the time but rousable to vocal stimuli
IV	Comatose, unresponsiveness to pain, decorticate or decerebrate posturing

transport is important, as the patient transport risks increase or even preclude transfer in later stages of encephalopathy.
- Nutritional support should be initiated early. A daily intake goal of 60 g of protein (or amino acids 0.8 to 1.2 g/kg/day) is recommended to prevent catabolism of protein stores. Enteral feeding should be initiated in patients with grade III or IV encephalopathy.
- Fluid support should be initiated if patient is not tolerating oral intake, or signs of hypoperfusion are present. Crystalloid solutions (normal saline in hypotensive patients, normal saline + 75 mEq/L NaCO$_3$ in acidotic patients, normal saline + dextrose in hypoglycemic patients) can be used.

PHARMACOLOGIC TREATMENT[1,4-6]

- If encephalopathy progresses and cerebral edema develops leading to increased ICP, intravenous mannitol is recommended to reduce cerebral edema transiently. Prophylactic

BOX 3 Management of Fulminant Hepatic Failure

No sedation except for procedures
Minimal handling
Enteric precautions until infection ruled out
Monitor:
- Heart and respiratory rate
- Arterial BP, CVP
- Core/toe temperature
- Neurologic observations
- Gastric pH (>5.0)
- Blood glucose (>4 mmol/L)
- Acid-base
- Electrolytes
- PT, PTT
Fluid balance
- 75% maintenance
- Dextrose 10%-50% (provide 6-10 mg/kg/min)
- Sodium (0.5-1 mmol/L)
- Potassium (2-4 mmol/L)
Maintain circulating volume with colloid/FFP
Coagulation support only if required
Drugs:
- Vitamin K
- H$_2$ antagonist
- Antacids
- Lactulose
- N-acetylcysteine for acetaminophen toxicity
- Broad-spectrum antibiotics
- Antifungals
Nutrition
- Enteral feeding (1-2 g protein/kg/day)
- PN if ventilated

BP, Blood pressure; *CVP,* central venous pressure; *PT,* prothrombin time; *PTT,* partial thromboplastin time; *FFP,* fresh frozen plasma; *PN,* parenteral nutrition.
From Fuhrman BP, Zimmerman JJ: *Fuhrman and Zimmerman's pediatric critical care,* ed 4, Philadelphia, 2011, Mosby.

BOX 4 Hepatic Replacement Therapeutic Options Available to Patients With Fulminant Hepatic Failure

Liver Transplantation
- Cadaveric transplantation
- Whole liver
- Reduced-size liver
- Split liver
- Auxiliary partial liver
- Orthotopic position
- Heterotopic position
- Auxiliary whole liver
- Living-related transplantation
- Left lateral segment
- Left lobe
- Extended left lobe
- Right lobe

Artificial Liver Assist Devices
- Non–cell-based systems
- Charcoal hemoperfusion
- High-volume plasmapheresis
- Continuous high-frequency hemodiafiltration
- Molecular adsorbent recirculating system (MARS)
- Cell-based systems (bioartificial liver assist devices)
- Primary porcine hepatocytes
- Human hepatoblastoma cells
- Extracorporeal liver assist device (ELAD)

Hepatocyte Transplantation

From Vincent JL et al: *Textbook of critical care,* ed 7, Philadelphia, 2017, Elsevier.

hyperventilation is not recommended in patients with ALF. Serum sodium should be maintained between 140 to 150 mmol/L. In patients with the highest risk of cerebral edema, hypertonic saline is recommended.
- Phenytoin can be used to manage seizures. In patients not responding to phenytoin, short-acting benzodiazepines may be used.
- Sedative medications should be avoided, as they are not cleared well and may mask signs of worsening encephalopathy or cerebral edema.
- Lactulose and rifaximin are not routinely recommended for encephalopathy treatment; neomycin should be avoided due to concerns of nephrotoxicity.
- Broad-spectrum antibiotics should be started immediately if infection is suspected. Sources usually include respiratory, urinary, and blood; there is no evidence for empiric antibiotic treatment. Antifungals should be initiated if no initial improvement with antibiotics occurs.
- In the case of persistent hypotension, norepinephrine is the initial vasopressor of choice; vasopressin can be added as a second pressor to maintain mean arterial pressure (MAP) >75 mm Hg. Persistent hypotension despite fluid resuscitation and pressor support should prompt concern for adrenal insufficiency.
- If dialysis is required for renal support, continuous mode is recommended over intermittent hemodialysis.

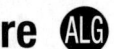
TABLE 4	General ICU Care of Acute Liver Failure Patients	
Intervention	**Suggested Target/Approach**	**Method/Examples**
Treatment for specific underlying etiology	Reversal of pathologic process and minimization of ongoing injury	• N-acetyl cysteine infusion for acetaminophen overdose • Withdrawal of hepatotoxic drugs • Nucleoside analogues for HBV • Penicillin or silibinin for *Amanita* mushroom poisoning • Urgent delivery of fetus for AFLP
Hemodynamic support	Hemodynamic parameters according to patient's clinical progress: • CVP 6-10 mm Hg • MAP 65-70 mm Hg • Even daily fluid balance	• Fluid administration • Vasoactive infusions (e.g., norepinephrine) • Low-dose corticosteroid administration if persisting shock
Sepsis care	• Low threshold for empiric broad-spectrum antibiotics if clinical suspicion of infection • Consider antifungal therapy if deterioration after several days of critical illness • Regular cultures of blood, urine, and sputum • Daily CXR	• Extended-spectrum β-lactams • Liposomal amphotericin or echinocandin antifungal therapy if deterioration after several days of critical illness
Respiratory support		• Intubate patients with high-grade encephalopathy • Avoid hypoventilation, especially during vulnerable periods such as during intubation, neuroimaging, and transfers
Renal support		• Ensure blood flow >200 ml/min • Use high exchange rates of lactate-free replacement fluid (40-50 ml/kg/h) • Turn off heater • Aim for blood ammonia within normal range • Monitor electrolytes (especially phosphate, potassium, magnesium) • Administer hypertonic saline by continuous infusion to avoid reduced serum osmolarity while on CRRT
Hematologic support	• Hb >7.0 g/dl • INR <6 • Platelet count >75 × 10^9/L • Fibrinogen >1.5 g/L	• Avoid treating isolated derangements in hemostatic parameters • Prophylactic FFP is not recommended before most procedures • Avoid extreme hypofibrinogenemia and thrombocytopenia • Administer vitamin K 10 mg IV daily • Use FFP, platelets, and cryoprecipitate if factor support is required
Metabolic/gastrointestinal/nutritional care	• Blood glucose 6-10 mmol/L • Stress ulcer prophylaxis • Enteral feeding	• Concentrated dextrose infusion via central line • H_2 blocker or PPI therapy • Enteral feeding via nasogastric tube

AFLP, Acute fatty liver of pregnancy; *CVP,* central venous pressure; *CXR,* chest x-ray; *FFP,* fresh frozen plasma; *Hb,* hemoglobin; *HBV,* hepatitis B virus; *INR,* international normalized ratio; *MAP,* mean arterial pressure; *PPI,* proton pump inhibitor.
From Vincent JL et al: *Textbook of critical care,* ed 8, Philadelphia, 2024, Elsevier.

• Patients should receive stress ulcer prophylaxis, given the risk of gastrointestinal bleeding.
• Routine correction of thrombocytopenia or INR correction are not recommended in the absence of bleeding. However, in the setting of clinical bleeding or the need for a procedure with a high bleeding risk, plasma or clotting factors are recommended. Vitamin K should be given routinely since in patients with ALF vitamin K deficiency is common.
• Part of the pharmacologic treatment will be specific to the suspected etiology of ALF.
• If acetaminophen is the known or suspected cause, an IV acetylcysteine protocol should be initiated. *N*-acetylcysteine is not harmful and dramatically alters the course in acetaminophen toxicity, so there should be a low threshold to start, particularly in young patients or those with no known cause of ALF.
• The most common regimens for NAC administration are the 21-h IV protocol and 72-h oral dosing protocol, though the 21-h IV protocol is preferred if there is established hepatic failure.[8]
• The 21-h IV protocol is:
  1. Loading dose: 150 mg/kg (maximum of 15 g in 200 ml D5W) over 60 min
  2. Second (maintenance) dose: 12.5 mg/kg/h over 4 h followed by
  3. Third dose: 6.25 mg/kg/h for 16 h
• A repeat acetaminophen level and alanine transaminase (ALT) should be checked at hour 18 of NAC treatment. If either the acetaminophen level or the ALT is elevated, the 16-h portion of treatment (6.25 mg/kg) should be extended and another ALT, INR, or acetaminophen level should be checked every 12 h. The acetylcysteine can be stopped once the acetaminophen level is undetectable, INR <2, or ALT is shown to be either normal or decreasing. Additional information on acetaminophen overdose is available in the topic "Acetaminophen Poisoning."

• *N*-acetylcysteine therapy outside of acetaminophen poisoning has been investigated, but evidence for the benefit is inconclusive. Studies have shown that using NAC in patients with non–acetaminophen-related acute liver failure significantly improved survival rate, posttransplant survival, and transplant-free survival.[9] However, routine use of NAC for acute liver failure is not currently recommended by practice guidelines and is center specific.[10]
• Liver support systems:
  1. Liver support systems have been trialed either to support the patient until the liver recovers or as a bridge to liver transplantation.
  2. High-volume plasma exchange can improve hepatic encephalopathy and transplant-free survival in a patient ineligible for liver transplantation, but no survival benefit has been shown for a patient undergoing liver transplantation with plasma

exchange compared with supportive therapy alone.[11]

3. The molecular absorbents recirculating system (MARS) is an artificial extracorporeal hepatic support system that allows albumin-bound toxins to be removed. MARS has been shown to improve hemodynamics and biochemical variables, and there is emerging evidence that MARS therapy is associated with higher transplant-free survival. However, the routine use of MARS is not currently recommended by practice guidelines.[12]

4. Bioartificial support systems in the form of hepatocytes (human or other mammalian origin) have also been used in cartridges as part of extracorporeal systems. These have not shown any benefit, with or without transplantation.

MONITORING[1,5]

- In patients with high-grade hepatic encephalopathy (HE) awaiting transplant, intracranial pressure (ICP) monitoring is recommended in centers with expertise in ICP monitoring.
- Measures used to monitor and control cerebral edema caused by acute liver failure are summarized in Box 5.
- Neurologic examination every 1 to 4 h is recommended in the absence of ICP monitoring.
- Patients with suspected acetaminophen toxicity should have LFTs monitored every 12 h. Otherwise, LFTs can be monitored daily.
- Chemistry panels and prothrombin time/INR should be monitored every 8 to 12 h. Correction of coagulopathy should be avoided because it can interfere with assessment of liver function. In the setting of life-threatening bleeding, fresh frozen plasma (FFP) and recombinant factor VIIa can be considered.

- Point-of-care glucose should be checked every 4 h initially to evaluate for hypoglycemia. If hypoglycemia is detected, dextrose should be added to crystalloid solution.
- Because of the increased risk of infection, daily urine, sputum, and blood cultures, as well as chest x-ray examinations, should be checked even in the absence of signs or symptoms of infection.

PROGNOSIS[1,4,5]

- Overall mortality from ALF is 30% to 40% and has improved significantly over the last 20 yr.
- Transplant-free survival in ALF in the setting of acetaminophen, hepatitis A, shock liver, and pregnancy-related disease is >50%; for all other causes of ALF, transplant-free survival is <25%.
- Higher-grade hepatic encephalopathy and renal dysfunction in non-acetaminophen ALF predict worse survival.
- Multiple models have been developed to predict spontaneous recovery in ALF patients (King's College criteria, Clichy criteria, MELD score, APACHE II score).
- The King's College criteria form the basis of the model most commonly used for prognostication (Table 5).
- Transplantation:
  1. Patients with ALF are given the highest priority for liver transplantation. ALF accounts for only 10% of the U.S. liver transplants.
  2. Contraindications to listing include medical history of irreversible brain injury, psychiatric illness severe enough to affect patients' survival or likelihood of compliance with medications, active sepsis, severe medical comorbidities including

malignancy, increasing dependence on ventilator/inotropic support, acute substance abuse, previous episodes of self-harm (>5 episodes), refractory mental illness, and inadequate family support.

3. For patients with alcoholic liver disease, many centers require a 6-mo abstinence period, but several transplant centers in North America and Europe have transplanted selected patients with alcoholic hepatitis who were unlikely to survive 6 mo.[13]

4. Mortality on the waiting list is 25%; 1-yr and 5-yr survival after transplantation are 73% and 67%, respectively.

5. Predictive criteria for death without emergency liver transplantation are summarized in Box 6.

❗ PEARLS & CONSIDERATIONS

- ALF is defined as severe hepatic injury (as evidenced by elevated liver enzymes) with INR >1.5 and hepatic encephalopathy occurring <26 wk before presentation in a patient with no prior history of liver disease.
- Close to half of ALF is caused by drug ingestion, usually acetaminophen.
- Given the potential rapidity of deterioration, referral must be made as soon as possible to a liver transplant center.
- There should be a low threshold to start N-acetylcysteine.
- Coagulopathy should not be corrected unless life-threatening bleeding occurs or it is recommended by the liver transplant hepatologist.

BOX 5   Measures Used to Monitor and Control Cerebral Edema Caused by Acute Liver Failure

1. Correction of metabolic abnormalities.
   - Electrolytes (Na, K, Cl, HCO3).
   - Acid-base (if patient is on mechanical ventilation, induce mild respiratory alkalosis).
   - Glucose (maintenance intravenous glucose infusion).
2. Avoid overtransfusion or overhydration.
   - Carefully match intake and output once patient is euvolemic.
   - Daily weight.
   - Avoid use of blood products unless indicated for ongoing bleeding and correction of coagulopathy or to maintain hemostasis when intracranial monitor has been placed. In the latter circumstance, the patient may require diuresis to avoid an excess in intravascular volume, especially from plasma.
3. Institute dialysis in patients in renal failure.
   - Continuous arteriovenous or venovenous hemodialysis is preferred over standard hemodialysis.
   - Avoid severe volume shifts, stabilize blood pressure, maintain euvolemia, correct electrolyte and acid-base abnormalities.
4. Mechanical ventilation (worsening encephalopathy, >grade II).
   - Main indication in liver failure is airway protection to prevent aspiration pneumonia.
   - Induce mild respiratory alkalosis (pH 7.45-7.50, pCO$_2$ 20-30 mm Hg).
   - Elevate head of bed 15-30 degrees.
   - Use sedation to avoid having the patient "fight the endotracheal (ET) tube."
5. Consider placement of intracranial pressure (ICP) monitor in the epidural space.
   - Should be considered when patients evolve from stage II (agitated confusion) to stage III (stuporous) encephalopathy.
   - Maintain adequate platelet count (>60,000) with platelet transfusions and INR <1.5 with fresh frozen plasma if necessary.
   - Mannitol is used to control ICP in patients with intact renal function or in those on dialysis. Mannitol is given in 0.5-1 g/kg doses. Serum electrolytes, glucose, and osmolarity should be checked every 4-6 h. If ICP is elevated, osmolarity <310, and Na <145, then give mannitol. Mannitol should be withheld if the patient has excessive serum osmolarity or significant hypernatremia.

From Vincent JL et al: *Textbook of critical care,* ed 8, Philadelphia, 2024, Elsevier.

TABLE 5 King's College Hospital Criteria for Liver Transplantation in Acute Liver Failure

Acetaminophen-Induced Acute Liver Failure	Non–Acetaminophen-Induced Acute Liver Failure
Arterial pH <7.3 (irrespective of grade of encephalopathy) *OR* Grade III or IV encephalopathy *and* Prothrombin time >100 sec *and* Serum creatinine >3.4 mg/dl	Prothrombin time >100 sec (irrespective of grade of encephalopathy) *OR* Any of three of the following variables (irrespective of grade of encephalopathy): • Age <10 yr or >40 yr • Etiology: Non-A hepatitis, non-B hepatitis, halothane hepatitis, idiosyncratic drug reactions • Duration of jaundice before onset of encephalopathy >7 days • Prothrombin time >50 sec • Serum bilirubin >18 mg/dl

Sec, Seconds.

BOX 6 Predictive Criteria for Death Without Emergency Liver Transplantation

King's college criteria[14]
Acetaminophen overdose
- Arterial pH <7.3 (irrespective of grade of encephalopathy) or
- PT >100 seconds (INR >6.5) and
- Serum creatinine >3.4 mg/dl (>300 µmol/L) and
- Patients with West Haven grade III and IV hepatic encephalopathy
Non–acetaminophen-induced liver injury
Acute form (delayed jaundice-encephalopathy <7 days):
- PT >100 seconds (INR >6.5) (irrespective of grade of encephalopathy) or any three of the following variables:
  - Aged <10 or >40 yr
  - Non-A, non-B hepatitis, halothane hepatitis, idiosyncratic drug reactions
  - Subacute form: delayed encephalopathy >7 days
  - Serum bilirubin 17.4 mg/dl (300 µmol/L)
  - PT >50 seconds
Clichy criteria[15]
- Grade III or IV encephalopathy and
- Factor V <20% in patients <30 yr or
- Factor V <30% in patients >30 yr
Liver biopsy[16]
- ≤60% necrosis on transjugular biopsy associated with ELT-free survival
Computed tomography[17]
- Liver volume <1000 cm³ predicts failure to achieve ELT-free survival for nonacetaminophen ALF

ELT, Emergency liver transplantation; *INR*, international normalized ratio; *PT*, prothrombin time.
From Vincent JL et al: *Textbook of critical care*, ed 8, Philadelphia, 2024, Elsevier.

RELATED CONTENT

Acetaminophen Poisoning (Related Key Topic)
Ascites (Related Key Topic)
Encephalopathy (Related Key Topic)

Hepatopulmonary Syndrome (Related Key Topic)
Hepatorenal Syndrome (Related Key Topic)

REFERENCES

Available at eBooks.Health.Elsevier.com

AUTHORS: **SIMRAN GUPTA, MD,** and **MAY MIN, MD**

Diseases
and Disorders

I

BASIC INFORMATION

DEFINITION

Acute respiratory distress syndrome (ARDS) is a form of noncardiogenic pulmonary edema that results from acute damage to the alveoli. It is characterized by diffuse infiltrative lung lesions with resulting interstitial and alveolar edema, severe hypoxemia, and respiratory failure.[1-3] The cardinal feature of ARDS, refractory hypoxemia, is caused by formation of protein-rich alveolar edema after damage to the integrity of the lung's alveolar-capillary barrier.

The initial definition of ARDS was based on the American–European Consensus Conference (AECC) from 1994 and included the following components:

- The syndrome must present acutely
- A ratio of Pao_2 to Fio_2 ≤200 regardless of the level of positive end-expiratory pressure (PEEP)
- The detection of bilateral pulmonary infiltrates on frontal chest x-ray examination.
- Absence of congestive heart failure (pulmonary artery wedge pressure [PAWP] ≤18 mm Hg or no clinical evidence of elevated left atrial pressure on the basis of chest x-ray examination or other clinical data).

The 2012 Berlin definition of ARDS (Table 1, Fig. 1) addresses some of the limitations of the AECC definition and establishes the criteria for ARDS:

- Timing: Within 1 week of a known clinical insult or new or worsening respiratory symptoms
- Chest imaging (chest x-ray examination or computed tomography [CT] scan): Bilateral opacities, not fully explained by effusions, lobar/lung collapse, or nodules
- Origin of edema: Respiratory failure not fully explained by cardiac failure or fluid overload. Need objective assessment (e.g., echocardiography) to exclude hydrostatic edema if no risk factors are present
- Oxygenation (if altitude is higher than 1000 m, the correction factor should be calculated as follows: [Pao_2/Fio_2 × {barometric pressure/760}]
- Mild: 200 mm Hg <Pao_2/Fio_2 ≤300 mm Hg with PEEP or continuous positive airway pressure (CPAP) ≥5 cm H_2O (this may be delivered noninvasively in the mild ARDS group)
- Moderate: 100 mm Hg <Pao_2/Fio_2 ≤200 mm Hg with PEEP or CPAP ≥5 cm H_2O
- Severe: Pao_2/Fio_2 ≤100 mm Hg with PEEP or CPAP ≥5 cm H_2O

SYNONYMS

ARDS
Adult respiratory distress syndrome
Acute lung injury

ICD-10CM CODE
J80   Acute respiratory distress syndrome

EPIDEMIOLOGY & DEMOGRAPHICS

- More than 150,000 ARDS cases per yr in the U.S.
- 7.1% of all patients admitted to an intensive care unit (ICU) and 16.1% of all patients on mechanical ventilation develop ARDS.
- An international study in 50 countries revealed that 10% of patients admitted to an ICU fulfilled criteria for ARDS, and 93% developed it within 48 h of admission. The study reinforced that ARDS is underrecognized.[4]
- Black, Hispanic, and other patients belonging to racial minority groups in the U.S. were observed to exhibit significantly higher in-hospital sepsis-related respiratory failure and associated mortality.[5]

PHYSICAL FINDINGS & CLINICAL PRESENTATION[6]

- Signs and symptoms:
  1. Dyspnea
  2. Chest discomfort
  3. Cough
  4. Anxiety
- Physical examination:
  1. Tachypnea
  2. Tachycardia
  3. Hypertension
  4. Paradoxic breathing and use of accessory muscles
  5. Coarse crepitations or crackles of both lungs
  6. Fever may be present if infection is the underlying etiology

ETIOLOGY (TABLES 2 AND 3)

- Sepsis (>40% of cases)
- Aspiration: Near-drowning, aspiration of gastric contents (>30% of cases)
- Trauma (>20% of cases)
- Pneumonia
- Multiple transfusions, blood products
- Drugs (e.g., overdose of morphine, methadone, heroin; reaction to nitrofurantoin)

TABLE 1   2012 Berlin Definition of Acute Respiratory Distress Syndrome (All Components Must Be Present)

Timing	Within 1 wk of a known clinical insult or new/worsening respiratory symptoms		
Chest imaging	Bilateral opacities: Not fully explained by effusions, lobar/lung collapse, or nodules		
Origin of edema	Respiratory failure not fully explained by cardiac failure or fluid overload; need objective assessment (e.g., echocardiography) to exclude hydrostatic edema if no risk factor for ARDS is present		
Oxygenation	*Mild ARDS*	*Moderate ARDS*	*Severe ARDS*
	200 < Pao_2/Fio_2 ≤300 with PEEP or CPAP ≥5 cm H_2O	100 < Pao_2/Fio_2 ≤200 PEEP ≥5 cm H_2O	Pao_2/Fio_2 ≤100 with PEEP ≥5 cm H_2O

ARDS, Acute respiratory distress syndrome; *CPAP,* continuous positive airway pressure; *PEEP,* positive end-expiratory pressure.
From Weinberger SE: *Principles of pulmonary medicine,* ed 7, Philadelphia, 2019, Elsevier.

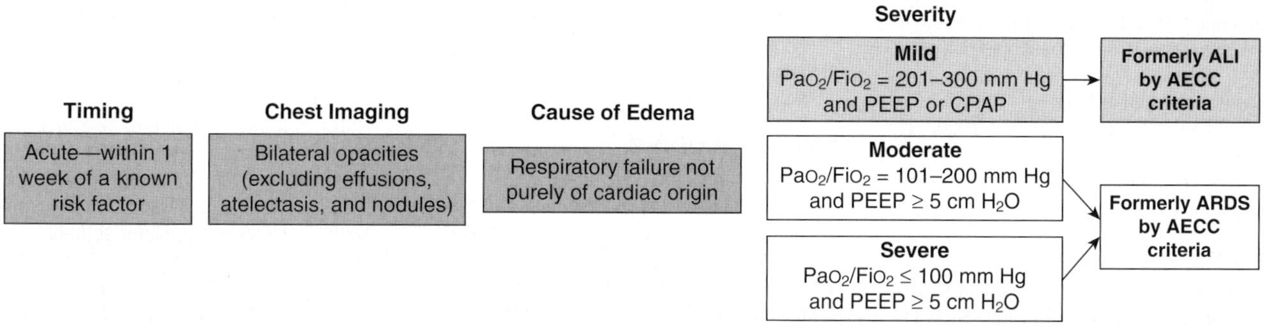

Severity

Timing	Chest Imaging	Cause of Edema	
Acute—within 1 week of a known risk factor	Bilateral opacities (excluding effusions, atelectasis, and nodules)	Respiratory failure not purely of cardiac origin	**Mild** Pao_2/Fio_2 = 201–300 mm Hg and PEEP or CPAP → Formerly ALI by AECC criteria
			Moderate Pao_2/Fio_2 = 101–200 mm Hg and PEEP ≥ 5 cm H_2O
			Severe Pao_2/Fio_2 ≤ 100 mm Hg and PEEP ≥ 5 cm H_2O → Formerly ARDS by AECC criteria

FIG. 1 The Berlin definition of ARDS. *AECC,* American–European Consensus Conference; *ALI,* acute lung injury; *ARDS,* acute respiratory distress syndrome; *CPAP,* continuous positive airway pressure; *FIO₂,* fraction of inspired oxygen; *PaO₂,* partial pressure of oxygen; *PEEP,* positive end-expiratory pressure. (From Vincent JL et al: *Textbook of critical care,* ed 8, Philadelphia, 2024, Elsevier.)

TABLE 2 Conditions Associated with Acute Respiratory Distress Syndrome by Possible Mechanisms of Injury

Direct Injury (Pulmonary)	Indirect Injury (Nonpulmonary)
Pneumonia (bacterial, viral [e.g., influenza, COVID-19])	Sepsis
	Major trauma
Aspiration	Multiple blood transfusions
Pulmonary contusion	Pancreatitis
Toxic inhalation	Cardiopulmonary bypass
Near-drowning	Drug overdose
Reperfusion injury (e.g., post–lung transplant)	Adverse effects of medication

COVID-19, Coronavirus disease 2019.
From Broaddus VC et al: *Murray & Nadel's textbook of respiratory medicine,* ed 7, Philadelphia, 2022, Elsevier.

TABLE 3 Risk Factors Associated with Development of Acute Lung Injury and Acute Respiratory Distress Syndrome

Direct Lung Injury	Indirect Lung Injury
Pneumonia	Sepsis
Aspiration of gastric contents	Multiple trauma
Pulmonary contusion	Cardiopulmonary bypass
Fat, amniotic fluid, or air emboli	Drug overdose
Near-drowning	Acute pancreatitis
Inhalational injury	Transfusion of blood products
Reperfusion pulmonary edema	

From Vincent JL et al: *Textbook of critical care,* ed 8, Philadelphia, 2024, Elsevier.

- Noxious inhalation (e.g., chlorine gas, high O_2 concentration)
- Postresuscitation
- Cardiopulmonary bypass
- Burns
- Pancreatitis
- Neuromuscular causes (Table 4)
- Alcohol abuse: History of chronic alcohol abuse significantly increases the risk of developing ARDS in critically ill patients

DIAGNOSIS

DIFFERENTIAL DIAGNOSIS (TABLE 5)
- Cardiogenic pulmonary edema
- Interstitial lung disease (acute interstitial pneumonia, nonspecific interstitial pneumonia, cryptogenic organizing pneumonia, acute eosinophilic pneumonia, hypersensitivity pneumonia, pulmonary alveolar proteinosis)
- Connective tissue diseases, such as polymyositis
- Diffuse alveolar hemorrhage
- Lymphangitic carcinomatosis from T-cell or B-cell lymphomas
- Drug-induced lung diseases (amiodarone, bleomycin)

WORKUP
The search for an underlying cause should focus on treatable causes (e.g., infections such as sepsis or pneumonia).
- Arterial blood gases (ABGs)
- Hemodynamic monitoring

- Bronchoalveolar lavage (selected patients)
- Transthoracic echocardiogram

LABORATORY TESTS
- ABGs:
  1. Initially: Varying degrees of hypoxemia, generally resistant to supplemental oxygen
  2. Respiratory alkalosis, decreased Pco_2
  3. Widened alveolar-arterial gradient
  4. Hypercapnia as the disease progresses
- Bronchoalveolar lavage:
  1. The most prominent finding is an increased number of polymorphonucleocytes.
  2. The presence of eosinophilia has therapeutic implications because these patients respond to corticosteroids.
- Blood and urine cultures
- Blood work:
  1. Increased or reduced white blood cell count with left shift if concomitant infectious process
  2. Normal or mildly elevated B-type natriuretic peptide level
  3. Increased lactate level if concomitant sepsis or septic shock

IMAGING STUDIES
Chest x-ray examination (Fig. 2).
- The initial chest x-ray examination might be normal in the initial hours after the precipitating event.
- Bilateral interstitial infiltrates are usually seen within 24 to 72 h; they often are more prominent in the bases and periphery.
- CT scan of chest: Bilateral diffuse, dense consolidations with air bronchograms.

- Chest ultrasound is emerging as a safe and inexpensive bedside tool for the evaluation of ARDS. Training in this modality, however, is needed prior to adoption as it carries a higher false-positive rate than conventional imaging formats.[7]

TREATMENT

NONPHARMACOLOGIC THERAPY
Treatment of ARDS is supportive. There is no specific pharmacotherapy for ARDS. Management principles are summarized in Table 6.
Hemodynamic monitoring:
- Can be used for the initial evaluation of ARDS (in ruling out cardiogenic pulmonary edema) and its subsequent management. However, a pulmonary catheter is not indicated in the routine management of ARDS. Trials have shown that clinical management involving the early use of pulmonary artery catheters in patients with ARDS did not significantly affect mortality and morbidity rates and may result in more complications as compared with a central venous catheter.
- Although no dynamic profile is diagnostic of ARDS, the presence of pulmonary edema, a high cardiac output, and a low pulmonary capillary wedge pressure (PCWP) is characteristic of ARDS.
- It is important to remember that partially treated intravascular volume overload and flash pulmonary edema can have the hemodynamic features of ARDS; filling pressures can also be elevated by increased intrathoracic pressures or with fluid administration; cardiac function can be depressed by acidosis, hypoxemia, or other factors associated with sepsis.
Ventilatory support:
- Noninvasive positive-pressure ventilation (NIPPV) (i.e., BiPAP) should only be used in selected cases in patients with hypoxic respiratory failure.
- A randomized multicenter, open-label trial showed that high-flow oxygen by nasal cannula increased ventilator-free days and reduced 90-day mortality compared with NIPPV in patients with hypoxemic respiratory failure without hypercapnia. Either modality should not delay intubation and mechanical ventilation initiation in patients with rapidly progressing clinical deterioration.
- Mechanical ventilation is generally necessary to maintain adequate gas exchange. Ventilatory strategy for patients with ARDS as proposed by the ARDS Network is summarized in Table 7. A low tidal volume and low plateau pressure ventilator strategy are recommended to avoid ventilator-induced injury. Assist-control is generally preferred initially with the following ventilator settings:
  1. Fio_2 1.0 (until a lower value can be used to achieve adequate oxygenation). When possible, minimize oxygen toxicity by maintaining Fio_2 at <60%.
  2. Tidal volume: Set initial tidal volume at 6 ml/kg of predicted body weight (PBW).

TABLE 4 Neuromuscular Causes of Acute Respiratory Failure

Location	Disorder	Associated Autonomic Dysfunction?
Spinal cord	Tetanus[4]	Frequent
Anterior horn cell	Amyotrophic lateral sclerosis	No
	Poliomyelitis	No
	Rabies	Frequent
	West Nile virus flaccid paralysis	No
Peripheral nerve	Guillain-Barré syndrome	Frequent
	Critical illness polyneuropathy	No
	Diphtheria	No, but cardiomyopathy and arrhythmias may occur
	Porphyria	Occasional
	Ciguatoxin (ciguatera poisoning)	Occasional
	Saxitoxin (paralytic shellfish poisoning)	No
	Tetrodotoxin (pufferfish poisoning)	No
	Thallium intoxication	No
	Arsenic intoxication	No
	Lead intoxication	No
	Buckthorn neuropathy	No
Neuromuscular junction	Myasthenia gravis	No
	Botulism[5]	Frequent
	Lambert-Eaton myasthenic syndrome	Yes, frequent dry mouth and postural hypotension
	Hypermagnesemia	No
	Organophosphate poisoning	No
	Tick paralysis	No
	Snake bite	No
Muscle	Polymyositis/dermatomyositis	No
	Acute quadriplegic myopathy	No
	Eosinophilia-myalgia syndrome	No
	Muscular dystrophies	No, but cardiac rhythm disturbances may occur
	Carnitine palmitoyl transferase deficiency	No
	Nemaline myopathy	No
	Acid maltase deficiency	No
	Mitochondrial myopathy	No
	Acute hypokalemic paralysis	No
	Stonefish myotoxin poisoning	No
	Rhabdomyolysis	No
	Hypophosphatemia	No

From Vincent JL et al: *Textbook of critical care,* ed 8, Philadelphia, 2024, Elsevier.

TABLE 5 Conditions That Mimic ARDS

	Findings on Chest Imaging	Potential Diagnostic Tests
Diffuse alveolar hemorrhage	Bilateral alveolar and ground-glass infiltrates	Bronchoscopy with bronchoalveolar lavage
Pulmonary alveolar proteinosis	Central and lower lung zone alveolar infiltrates, "bat wing" appearance, "crazy paving" on CT	High-resolution CT, bronchoscopy with bronchoalveolar lavage and PAS staining
Acute interstitial pneumonia	Bilateral alveolar and ground-glass infiltrates, septal thickening, traction bronchiectasis	No alternative cause of ARDS identified, open or thoracoscopic lung biopsy
Cryptogenic organizing pneumonia	Peripheral distribution of alveolar infiltrates, migratory infiltrates	Bronchoscopy with transbronchial lung biopsy
Acute exacerbation of idiopathic pulmonary fibrosis	Ground-glass opacities superimposed on peripheral, basilar fibrotic changes	CT demonstrating characteristic fibrotic changes

ARDS, Acute respiratory distress syndrome; *CT,* computed tomography; *PAS,* periodic acid–Schiff.
Adapted from Janz DR, Ware LB: Approach to the patient with the acute respiratory distress syndrome, *Clin Chest Med* 35(4): 685-696, 2014. From Vincent JL et al: *Textbook of critical care,* ed 8, Philadelphia, 2024, Elsevier.

Tidal volumes are reduced from 6 ml/kg of PBW to a minimum of 4 ml/kg if plateau airway pressures exceed 30 cm of water. The concept of using PBW is based on the fact that lung size depends most strongly on height and sex; PBW normalizes the tidal volume to lung size. Aim to maintain plateau pressure (P_{plat}) at <30 mm Hg PEEP 5 cm H_2O or greater (to increase lung volume and keep alveoli open).

3. PEEP should be increased in small increments of 3 to 5 cm H_2O to achieve acceptable arterial saturation (>0.9) with nontoxic Fio_2 values (<0.6) and acceptable airway plateau pressures (<30 to 35 cm H_2O). It is important to remember that an increase in PEEP may lower cardiac output and, despite improvement in Pao_2, may actually have a negative effect on tissue oxygenation (the major determinants of tissue oxygenation are hemoglobin, percent saturation, and cardiac output). The optimal level of PEEP remains unestablished.[8] Although higher levels of PEEP may help prevent life-threatening hypoxemia and be associated with lower hospital mortality in patients meeting criteria for ARDS, such benefit is unlikely in patients with less severe lung injury (Pao_2/Fio_2 >200) and a strategy of treating such patients with high PEEP levels may be harmful. A study published in 2017 demonstrated that the open lung approach increases mortality in patients with moderate to severe ARDS.[9]

4. Inspiratory flow: 60 L/min.

5. Ventilatory rate: High ventilatory rates of up to 35 breaths/min are often necessary in patients with ARDS to achieve the desired minute ventilation because of their increased physiologic dead space and smaller lung volumes. Patients must be monitored for excessive intrathoracic gas trapping (auto-PEEP or intrinsic PEEP) that can depress cardiac output.

- Permissive hypercapnia: To maintain a low plateau pressure, a low tidal volume is frequently required, leading to a reduced minute ventilation and hypoventilation with consequently a respiratory acidosis (elevated Pco_2 and reduced pH). Most patients (excluding patients with cerebral edema, acute coronary syndrome, seizures, cardiac arrhythmias, and so on) can tolerate a low pH without major consequences. Bicarbonate replacement is suggested when the pH falls to below 7.20.

- Sedation: Gamma-aminobutyric acid (GABA) receptor agonists (including propofol and benzodiazepines) have traditionally been the most commonly administered sedative drugs for ICU patients. Recent trials indicate that the alpha-2 agonist dexmedetomidine (Precedex) may have distinct advantages. At comparable sedation levels, dexmedetomidine-treated patients spent less time on ventilator, experienced less delirium, and developed less tachycardia and hypertension. The most notable adverse effect of dexmedetomidine was bradycardia.

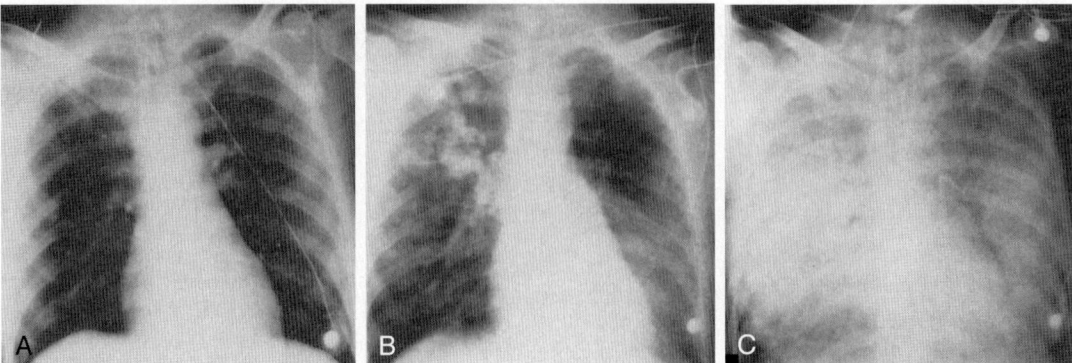

FIG. 2 Acute respiratory distress syndrome. X-ray of a young man who had sustained severe trauma and blood loss in a road traffic accident; the lungs cover a period of 5 days from a relatively normal x-ray **(A),** to bilateral infiltrates **(B),** to bilateral "whiteout" **(C),** accompanied by severe hypoxemia. A Swan-Ganz catheter for measurement of pulmonary artery "wedge" pressure (as a reflection of left atrial pressure) can be seen in situ on the x-ray film in **C.** The patient died shortly after the last film.

TABLE 6 ARDS Management Principles

Supportive Care

Supplemental oxygen to ensure adequate oxygenation

Lung-protective ventilation

- Volume and pressure limited
- Ensure ventilator synchrony
- Prone position if Pao_2/Fio_2 <150 despite protective ventilation

Reduce oxygen consumption if hypoxia is critical

Support adequate perfusion for other organs; focus on both cardiac output and blood pressure

Find and Treat Underlying Cause

Consider infections, mimics

Minimize Further Edema Accumulation

Seek lowest pulmonary microvascular pressure that maintains adequate perfusion

Diurese/reduce vascular volume while maintaining adequate perfusion

Avoid Harm

Volume- and pressure-limited ventilation strategy

Avoid both hypotension and volume overload

Goal-directed sedation with frequent reassessment

Avoid hyperoxia

Consider early physical rehabilitation

Seek and treat neuromuscular, cognitive, and psychological impairments during recovery

---

ARDS, Acute respiratory distress syndrome; *Fio₂,* fractional concentration of oxygen in inspired gas; *Pao₂,* partial pressure of arterial oxygen.
From Broaddus VC et al: *Murray & Nadel's textbook of respiratory medicine,* ed 7, Philadelphia, 2022, Elsevier.

- Neuromuscular blockade: The benefits of early continuous neuromuscular blockade in patients with ARDS who are receiving mechanical ventilation remains unclear. In a trial among patients with moderate-to-severe ARDS who were treated with a strategy involving a high PEEP, there was no significant difference in mortality at 90 days between patients who received an early and continuous infusion of the neuromuscular blocking agent cisatracurium and those who were treated with a usual-care approach with lighter sedation targets.[10,11]
- Discontinuing ventilation/extubation: Fig. 3 is an algorithm for assessing whether a patient is ready to be liberated from mechanical ventilation and extubated.

ACUTE GENERAL Rx

Identify and treat precipitating conditions:

- Blood and urine cultures and trial of antibiotics in presumed sepsis (routine administration of antibiotics in all cases of ARDS is not recommended).
- Prompt repair of bone fractures in patients with major trauma.
- Crystalloid resuscitation in pancreatitis.
- Fluid management: In most patients with ARDS, fluid restriction is associated with better outcomes than a liberal fluid policy. Optimal fluid and hemodynamic management of patients with ARDS should be patient specific; in general, administration of crystalloids is recommended if a downward trend in PCWP is associated with diminished cardiac index, resulting in pre-renal azotemia, oliguria, and relative tachycardia.[12]

- Positioning the patient: Changes in position can improve oxygenation by improving the distribution of perfusion to ventilated lung regions; repositioning (lateral decubitus positioning) should be attempted in patients with hypoxemia that is not responsive to other medical interventions. Placing patients with moderate and severe hypoxemia in a prone position may improve their oxygenation. A meta-analysis that included the recent trials by Guerin et al (see Suggested Readings) showed that in patients with severe ARDS, early application of prolonged (over 16 h/day) prone-positioning sessions significantly decreases 28-day and 90-day mortality.
- Corticosteroids: Routine use of corticosteroids in ARDS is not recommended; corticosteroids may be beneficial in patients with many eosinophils in the bronchoalveolar lavage fluid or in patients with severe pneumonia. Systemic infections should be ruled out or adequately treated before administration of corticosteroids. Use of methylprednisolone has not been shown to increase the rate of infectious complications but is associated with a higher rate of neuromuscular weakness. In addition, starting methylprednisolone therapy more than 2 wk after the onset of ARDS may increase the risk of death. Corticosteroids have been shown to beneficial in ARDS caused by SARS-Cov2 (COVID-19 virus).[7] This has renewed interest in the use of corticosteroids in other forms of ARDS.
- Nutritional support: Nutritional support, preferably administered by the enteral route, is necessary to maintain adequate colloid oncotic pressure and intravascular volume. The use of antioxidants and dietary oil supplements is still equivocal and cannot be recommended at this time.

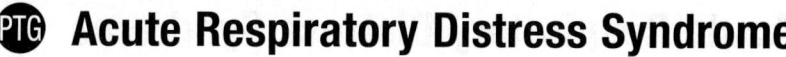
TABLE 7 Ventilator Management of Patients with ARDS

Calculate Predicted Body Weight (PBW)
- Males: PBW (kg) = 50 + 2.3 [(height in inches) − 60] or 50 + 0.91 [(height in cm) − 152.4]
- Females: PBW (kg) = 45.5 + 2.3 [(height in inches) − 60] or 45.5 + 0.91 [(height in cm) − 152.4]

Ventilator Mode
Volume assist/control until weaning

Tidal Volume (Vt)
- Initial Vt: 6 ml/kg predicted body weight
- Measure inspiratory plateau pressure (P_{plat}, 0.5 sec inspiratory pause) every 4 hours AND after each change in PEEP or Vt.
- If P_{plat} >30 cm H2O, decrease Vt to 5 or to 4 ml/kg.
- If P_{plat} <25 cm H2O and Vt <6 ml/kg PBW, increase Vt by 1 ml/kg PBW.

Respiratory Rate (RR)
- With initial change in Vt, adjust RR to maintain minute ventilation.
- Make subsequent adjustments to RR to maintain pH 7.30-7.45, but do not exceed RR = 35/min, and do not increase set rate if $PaCO_2$ <25 mm Hg.

I:E Ratio
- Acceptable range, 1:1-1:3 (no inverse ratio)

FiO$_2$, PEEP, and Arterial Oxygenation
Maintain PaO2 = 55-80 mm Hg or SpO2 = 88%-95% using the following PEEP/FiO2 combinations:

FiO$_2$	0.3-0.4	0.4	0.5	0.6	0.7	0.8	0.9	1
PEEP	5-8	8-14	8-16	10-20	10-20	14-22	16-22	18-25

Acidosis Management
- If pH <7.30, increase RR until pH ≥7.30 or RR = 35/min.
- If pH remains <7.30 with RR = 35, consider bicarbonate infusion.
- If pH <7.15, Vt may be increased (P_{plat} may exceed 30 cm H_2O).

Alkalosis Management
If pH >7.45 and patient is not triggering ventilator, decrease set RR but not below 6/min.

Fluid Management
- Once patients are out of shock, adopt a conservative fluid management strategy.
- Use diuretics or fluids to target a central venous pressure (CVP) of <4 mm Hg or a pulmonary artery occlusion pressure (PAOP) of <8 mm Hg.

Liberation From Mechanical Ventilation
- Daily interruption of sedation
- Daily screen for spontaneous breathing trial (SBT)
- SBT when all of the following criteria are present:
  (a) FiO$_2$ <0.40 and PEEP <8 cm H_2O
  (b) Not receiving neuromuscular blocking agents
  (c) Patient is awake and following commands
  (d) Systolic arterial pressure >90 mm Hg without vasopressor support
  (e) Tracheal secretions are minimal, and the patient has a good cough and gag reflex

Spontaneous Breathing Trial
- Place patient on 5 mm Hg pressure support with 5 mm Hg PEEP *or* T-piece.
- Monitor HR, RR, and oxygen saturation for 30-90 min.
- Extubate if there are no signs of distress (tachycardia, tachypnea, agitation, hypoxia, diaphoresis).

From Vincent JL et al: *Textbook of critical care*, ed 8, Philadelphia, 2024, Elsevier.

- Tracheostomy: Tracheostomy is warranted in patients requiring >2 wk of mechanical ventilation; discussion regarding tracheostomy should begin with patient (if alert and oriented) and/or family members/legal guardian after 5 to 7 days of ventilatory support. Early tracheostomy (within 4 days of admission to critical care) does not limit mortality and results in many unneeded procedures.[13]
- Some form of deep vein thrombosis prophylaxis is indicated in all patients with ARDS.
- Stress ulcer prophylaxis with sucralfate suspension (by nasogastric tube), or proton pump inhibitors (PO or intravenous [IV]) or histamine-2 blockers (PO or IV). Should be reserved for seriously ill patients who are at high risk for this complication.[14]

- The use of surfactant remains controversial. Patients who receive surfactant have a greater improvement in gas exchange in the initial 24-h period than patients who receive standard therapy alone; however, the use of exogenous surfactant does not improve survival.
- Table E8 summarizes rescue therapies, and Fig. 4 illustrates the management of acute respiratory failure from acute lung injury and ARDS.
- The SARS-CoV-2 virus first identified in 2019 can lead to severe ARDS. There was debate on whether ARDS caused by the virus merited special management. There is now consensus and sufficient evidence that it should not be treated differently than other ARDS resulting from other

etiologies. See the chapter on viral pneumonia.[15,16]

DISPOSITION
- Patients who survive ARDS are at risk of diminished functional capacity, mental illness, and decreased quality of life. Prognosis for ARDS varies with the underlying cause. Prognosis is worse in patients with chronic liver disease, nonpulmonary organ dysfunction, sepsis, and advanced age. ARDS survivors are at high risk for incident joblessness and substantial loss of wages, and 58% of those returning to work received disability.
- Elevated values of dead space fraction ([PaCO$_2$ >2 PeCO$_2$]/PaCO$_2$; normal is <0.3) is associated with an increased risk of death.

Approach to Discontinuing Ventilation/Extubation

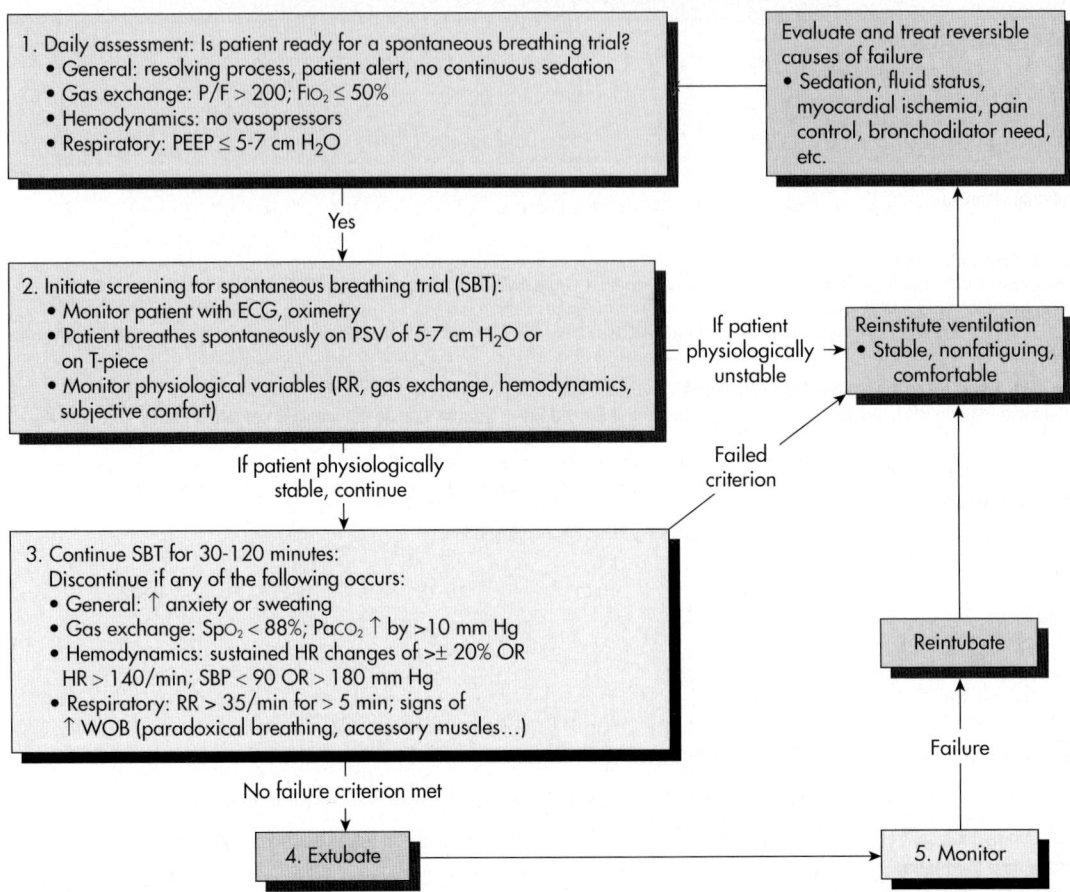

FIG. 3 Algorithm for assessing whether a patient is ready to be liberated from mechanical ventilation and extubated. *ECG,* Electrocardiogram; *HR,* heart rate; *Paco₂,* arterial partial pressure of carbon dioxide; *PEEP,* positive end-expiratory pressure; *P/F,* Pao₂/Fio₂; *PSV,* pressure support ventilation; *RR,* respiratory rate; *SBP,* systolic blood pressure; *Spo₂,* oxygen saturation based on pulse oximeter; *WOB,* work of breathing. (From Goldman L, Shafer AI: *Goldman-Cecil medicine,* ed 26, Philadelphia, 2020, Elsevier.)

- In ARDS, the percentage of potentially recruitable lung is variable and associated with the response to PEEP.
- Overall mortality rate varies between 32% and 45%. Most deaths are attributable to sepsis or multiorgan dysfunction rather than primary respiratory causes.
- Trials have shown that as compared with the current standard of care, a ventilator strategy using esophageal measures to estimate the transpulmonary pressure significantly improves oxygenation and compliance. Further trials will determine if this approach should be widely adopted.
- Other strategies for treatment of life-threatening refractory hypoxemia (inhaled nitric acid, extracorporeal membrane oxygenation [ECMO], high-frequency oscillatory ventilation, recruitment maneuvers) may improve oxygenation, but their impact on mortality remains unproven. Use of ECMO in combination with lung-protective ventilation was found to be

beneficial as a treatment strategy early in the course of ARDS related to H1N1 infection. Extracorporeal gas exchange may allow the use of low tidal volumes and lower levels of inspired oxygen and use of higher PEEP if desired. ECMO is costly and labor-intensive. The role and proper use of ECMO for patients with ARDS have not been clearly defined.[17,18]
- General indications for ECMO in severe cases of ARDS are:
  1. Severe hypoxemia (e.g., ratio of Pao₂ to Fio₂ <80 despite the application of high levels of PEEP [typically 15 to 20 cm H₂O]) for at least 6 h in patients with potentially reversible respiratory failure
  2. Uncompensated hypercapnia with acidemia (pH <7.15) despite the best accepted standard of care for management with a ventilator
  3. Excessively high-end inspiratory plateau pressure (>35 to 45 cm H₂O, according to the patient's body size) despite the best

accepted standard of care for management with a ventilator

REFERRAL

Surgical referral for tracheostomy (see "Acute General Rx").
Referral to ECMO team or center in severe cases when indicated.

RELATED CONTENT

Acute Respiratory Distress Syndrome (ARDS) (Patient Information)
Pneumonia, Viral (Related Key Topic)

REFERENCES

Available at eBooks.Health.Elsevier.com

AUTHOR: **JORGE MERCADO, MD**

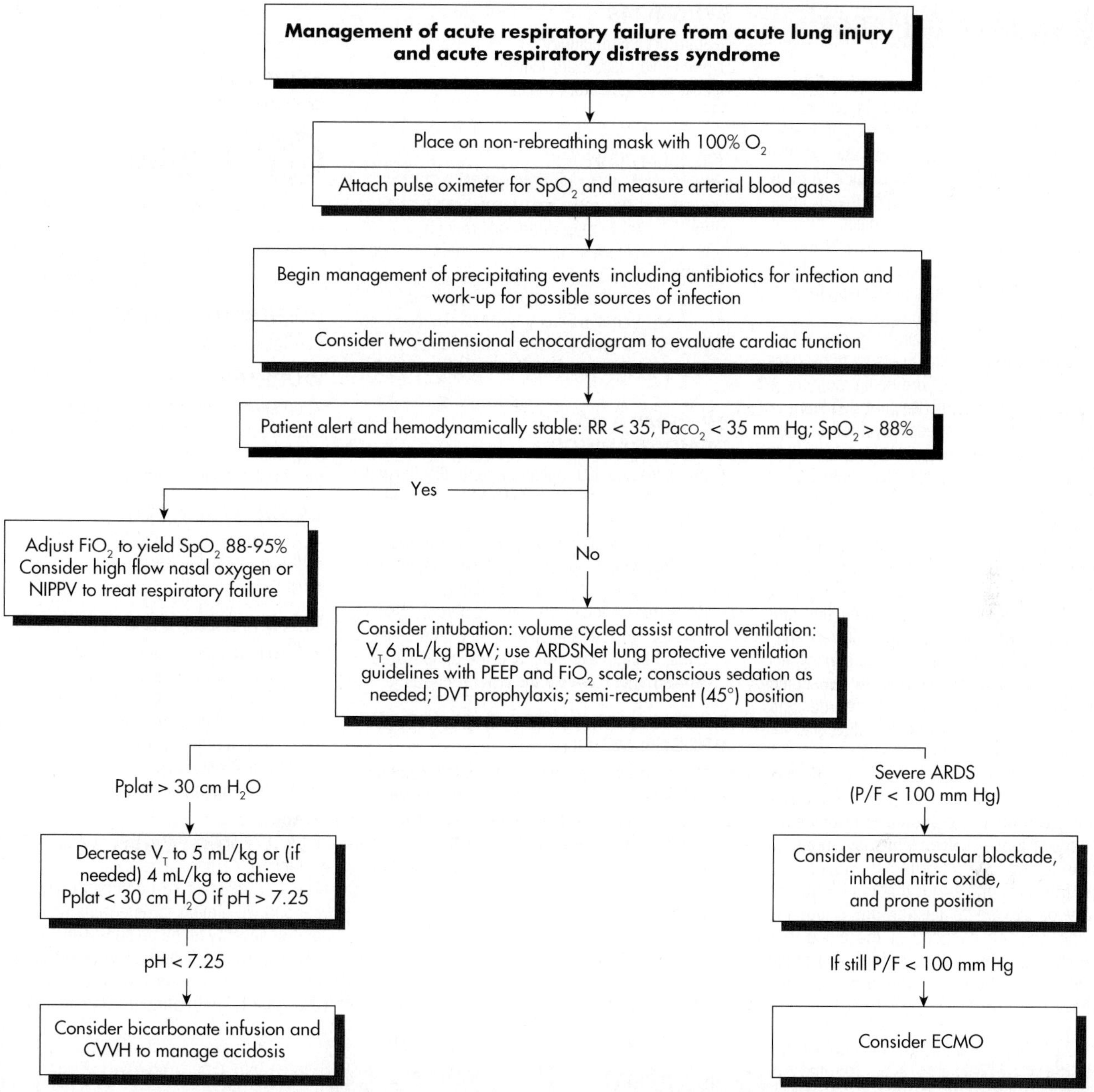

I

Management of acute respiratory failure from acute lung injury and acute respiratory distress syndrome

↓

Place on non-rebreathing mask with 100% O_2

Attach pulse oximeter for SpO_2 and measure arterial blood gases

↓

Begin management of precipitating events including antibiotics for infection and work-up for possible sources of infection

Consider two-dimensional echocardiogram to evaluate cardiac function

↓

Patient alert and hemodynamically stable: RR < 35, $Paco_2$ < 35 mm Hg; SpO_2 > 88%

— Yes —

Adjust FiO_2 to yield SpO_2 88-95%
Consider high flow nasal oxygen or NIPPV to treat respiratory failure

No

Consider intubation: volume cycled assist control ventilation: V_T 6 mL/kg PBW; use ARDSNet lung protective ventilation guidelines with PEEP and FiO_2 scale; conscious sedation as needed; DVT prophylaxis; semi-recumbent (45°) position

Pplat > 30 cm H_2O

Severe ARDS (P/F < 100 mm Hg)

Decrease V_T to 5 mL/kg or (if needed) 4 mL/kg to achieve Pplat < 30 cm H_2O if pH > 7.25

Consider neuromuscular blockade, inhaled nitric oxide, and prone position

pH < 7.25

If still P/F < 100 mm Hg

Consider bicarbonate infusion and CVVH to manage acidosis

Consider ECMO

FIG. 4 Management of acute respiratory failure from acute lung injury and acute respiratory distress syndrome. *CVVH,* Continuous venovenous hemofiltration; *DVT,* deep venous thrombosis; *ECMO,* extracorporeal membrane oxygenation; *NIPPV,* noninvasive positive pressure ventilation; *PBW,* predicted body weight; *PEEP,* positive end-expiration pressure; *P/F,* Pao_2/Fio_2; P_{plat}, plateau airway pressure; *RR,* respiratory rate; Spo_2, arterial oxygen saturation; *VT,* tidal volume. (From Goldman L, Shafer AI: *Goldman-Cecil medicine,* ed 26, Philadelphia, 2020, Elsevier.)

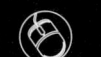
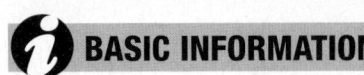 **BASIC INFORMATION**

DEFINITION

Respiratory failure is a condition in which the respiratory system fails in one or both of its gas exchanging functions (oxygenation and carbon dioxide elimination). There are two major types of acute respiratory failure (ARF): type I (hypoxemic) and type II (hypercapnic). In addition, type III (associated with atelectasis) and type IV (hypoperfusion of respiratory muscles in patients with shock) have also been described. Table 1 summarizes the classification of ARF.

Hypoxemic respiratory failure is characterized by a low arterial partial pressure of oxygen, usually <60 mm Hg while breathing room air. A major cause of hypoxemic respiratory failure is Acute Respiratory Distress Syndrome (see "ARDS" chapter), but other etiologies include heart failure and pneumonia. See Table E2 for list of potential etiologies for acute hypoxemic respiratory failure.

Hypercapnic respiratory failure is defined as an elevation in arterial partial pressure of carbon dioxide to >45 mm Hg. This is directly proportional to the rate of CO_2 production and inversely proportional to the rate of CO_2 elimination by the lungs. Both hypoxemia and hypercapnia can occur at the same time, depending on the location of the underlying disorder and mechanism. Table 3 summarizes etiologies for acute hypercapnic respiratory failure.

Respiratory failure can be acute or chronic. The acute presentation occurs within minutes to hours, whereas the chronic form develops over days or longer.[1] Hypoxemia is dangerous because it can lead to tissue hypoxia. Oxygen concentration is one factor that contributes to delivery of oxygen to tissues but is not the only one. Oxygen capacity of the blood, hemoglobin capacity, cardiac output, and blood flow also contribute to oxygenation of the tissues.

SYNONYMS

Respiratory insufficiency
Hypercarbic respiratory failure
Hypoxemic respiratory failure
ARF

ICD-10CM CODES
J96.00	Acute respiratory failure
J96.01	Acute respiratory failure with hypoxia
J96.02	Acute respiratory failure with hypercapnia
J96.90	Respiratory failure, unspecified
J96.91	Respiratory failure, unspecified with hypoxia
J96.92	Respiratory failure, unspecified with hypercapnia

EPIDEMIOLOGY & DEMOGRAPHICS

- An estimated 1.9 million patients discharged from acute care hospitals nationwide meet criteria for ARF.
- The peak incidence of ARF is in the winter months, when upper and lower respiratory tract infections are more prevalent.
- Comorbid conditions, including chronic disorders of the cardiac, pulmonary, neurologic, renal, hepatic systems, and the patient's advanced age, increase the risk of mortality.

PHYSICAL FINDINGS & CLINICAL PRESENTATION

- Hypoperfusion to brain occurs within seconds
- Decreased myocardial contractility, tachycardia early, bradycardia in late presentation
- Decreased diaphragmatic function
- Shift of the oxyhemoglobin dissociation curve to the right
- Physical symptoms:
  1. Dyspnea
  2. Somnolence
  3. Headaches
  4. Confusion
  5. Asterixis
  6. Coma

ETIOLOGY

See Tables E2 and 3.

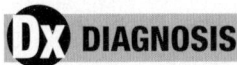 **DIAGNOSIS**

Diagnosis is made clinically according to physical examination findings and is confirmed by arterial blood gas. Table 4 summarizes common clues obtained from the history and physical examination.

DIFFERENTIAL DIAGNOSIS

See Tables E2 and 3.

WORKUP

After supportive therapy is initiated, a careful search for the underlying cause of the respiratory failure is critical, as this may have important implications on ultimate therapy.

LABORATORY TESTS

- Arterial blood gas (Fig. E1)
- Basal metabolic panel
- CBC

IMAGING STUDIES

- Chest imaging studies include:
  1. Chest x-ray examination
  2. Computed tomography scan of the chest (with angiography when suspecting pulmonary embolism)
  3. Chest ultrasound
  4. Ventilation perfusion scan

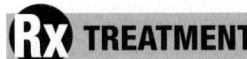 **TREATMENT**

The treatment of respiratory failure is initially supportive, aiming to determine first the acuity and/or severity of the presentation. Correction of the hypoxemia, hypercapnia, and management of the underlying etiology of the condition are essential to its treatment.[1] Potential indications

---

TABLE 1 Classification of Acute Respiratory Failure

	Type I	Type II	Type III	Type IV
Mechanism of Hypoxemia	Low FiO₂ ventilation/perfusion (V/Q) mismatch Shunting Reduced diffusing capacity	Hypoventilation	Shunting Hypoventilation V/Q mismatch	Hypoperfusion or inadequate oxygenation of peripheral tissues
Location of Pathologic Process	Inhaled air composition Alveolar-capillary unit Oxygen-carrying capacity of blood	Airway Central nervous system (CNS) Neuromuscular system Chest wall	Alveolar-capillary unit collapse with regional hypoventilation	Cardiovascular system Peripheral tissues
Clinical Syndromes	Cardiogenic pulmonary edema Acute respiratory distress syndrome Pneumonia Interstitial lung disease Pulmonary embolism Pulmonary hypertension Atelectasis Alveolar hemorrhage Carbon monoxide poisoning Anatomic shunts	Chronic obstructive pulmonary disease Asthma CNS depression (intoxication) CNS trauma or injury Neuromuscular disorders Skeletal disorders Obesity-hypoventilation syndrome	Thoracic or upper abdominal surgery or trauma Inadequate postoperative analgesia Pleural tumor or inflammation Trapped lung Subdiaphragmatic tumor or inflammation Obesity	Septic (distributive) shock Hypovolemic shock Cardiogenic shock Compromised cellular oxidation Hypermetabolic states

Fio₂, Fraction of inspired oxygen.
Modified from Jean-Louis V: *Intensive care medicine: annual update 2008,* Berlin Heidelberg, 2008, Springer-Verlag.

TABLE 3   Potential Causes of Acute Hypercapnic Respiratory Failure

Central Nervous System	Spinal Cord, Nerves, Muscle	Chest Wall, Thoracic Cage	Increased Dead Space
Medications (anesthetics and/or opioids)	Medications	Trauma	Obstructive airways disorders
Alveolar hypoventilation	Trauma	Kyphoscoliosis	Upper: Acute epiglottitis, foreign
Trauma	Myasthenia gravis	Flail chest	body aspiration, tracheal tumor
Meningoencephalitis	Guillain-Barré syndrome	Pleural disease	Lower: COPD, asthma, cystic
Localized tumors or vascular abnormalities of the medulla	Electrolyte abnormalities	Scleroderma	fibrosis
Strokes affecting medullary control centers		Morbid obesity	
Severe alkalosis		Ascites	
		Severe ileus	

COPD, Chronic obstructive pulmonary disease.

TABLE 4   Common Clues Obtained from the History, Symptoms, and Clinical Examination Findings That Can Help in the Initial Diagnostic Workup and Management of Acute Respiratory Failure

History and Symptoms	Signs on Physical Examination	Diagnosis
Cough, sputum, secretions	Rales or wheezing	Pneumonia, chronic obstructive pulmonary disease (COPD) exacerbation, bronchiectasis
Sudden onset of shortness of breath	Normal auscultation and percussion, possible signs of leg swelling to suggest deep vein thrombosis	Pulmonary embolism
History of heavy smoking	Wheezing, rhonchi	Emphysema, chronic bronchitis
Orthopnea, chest pain, paroxysmal nocturnal dyspnea	Arrhythmia, peripheral edema, jugular venous distention, peripheral hypoperfusion	Congestive heart failure or acute coronary syndrome
Trauma, aspiration, blood transfusions	Diffuse crackles	Acute respiratory distress syndrome
History of allergies, wheezing, or airway disease	Wheezing	Asthma, COPD
Exposure to heavy metals, handling of animals, dust or other significant environmental exposures	"Velcro" rales, clubbing	Chronic interstitial lung disease
Choking, aspiration, vomiting, dental procedures	Inspiratory stridor, poor air entry	Foreign body
Drug abuse	Constricted or dilated pupils, altered mental status, skin marks, perforated nasal septum, hypersalivation, decreased respiratory frequency	Central nervous system depression, intoxication
Exposure to a new drug/chemical or foods known to be allergenic	Swollen oral mucosa and tongue; stridor or wheezing	Angioedema, anaphylaxis
Progressive muscle weakness or immobility	Sensory abnormalities	Neuromuscular disorders
Trauma, procedures, inhalational injury	Absent breath sounds unilaterally, hypertympanic, tracheal deviation	Pneumothorax
Trauma, procedures	Absent breath sounds, dull on percussion, tracheal deviation	Hemothorax

From Vincent JL et al: *Textbook of critical care*, ed 8, Philadelphia, 2024, Elsevier.

for mechanical ventilation are summarized in Table 5.[2] The decision windows for noninvasive ventilation (NIV) or endotracheal intubation are illustrated in Fig. 2.

NONPHARMACOLOGIC THERAPY
- Hypoxemia may require treatment with supplemental oxygen, positive pressure support in the form of NIV, or mechanical ventilation.[3,4]
- Hypercapnia may require treatment with ventilatory support, NIV, or mechanical ventilation. The decision for either can be difficult and is primarily based on clinical presentation, severity of symptoms, comorbidities, and level of acid base derangement, as well as mental status.

- Contraindications to NIV include respiratory arrest, hemodynamic or cardiac instability, or inability to protect the airway.
- Monitoring carbon dioxide levels has not been standardized, but a change in symptoms and/or worsening in mental status can prompt a repeat in blood gas analysis.
- Worsening blood gas levels can be remediated with changes in the pressures on the noninvasive ventilator or by switching to a mechanical ventilator.

ACUTE GENERAL Rx
- Ventilatory support, either invasive (mechanical ventilation) or noninvasive, is often

required. Early clinical identification of failure is important to circumvent delayed intubation, and therefore careful monitoring is required.[5] Table 6 provides an overview of features of selected modes of mechanical ventilation. Potential advantages and disadvantages of each mode are summarized in Table 7.
- Compared with NIV, high-flow nasal oxygen (HFNO) as initial ARF management may improve several clinical outcomes. Compared with conventional oxygenation therapy, HFNO as postextubation management may reduce reintubation and improve patient comfort.[6,7]

TABLE 5 Potential Indications for Mechanical Ventilation

Physiologic Mechanism	Clinical Assessment	Normal Range	Value(s)/Finding(s) Supporting Need for Mechanical Ventilation
Hypoxemia	P(a-a)o$_2$ gradient (mm Hg)	25-65	>350
	Pao$_2$/Fio$_2$ ratio	425-475	<300
	Sao$_2$	98%	<90% despite supplemental oxygen
Hypercarbia/inadequate alveolar ventilation	Paco$_2$	35-45 mm Hg	Acute increase from patient's baseline pH <7.20 Mental status decline
Oxygen delivery/oxygen consumption imbalance	Elevated lactate	≤2.2 mg/dl	≥4 mg/dl despite adequate resuscitation
	Decreased mixed venous oxygen saturation	70%	<70% despite adequate acute resuscitation
Increased work of breathing	Minute ventilation	5-10 L/min	>15-20 L/min
	Dead space	0.15-0.30	≥0.5 (acute)
Inspiratory muscle weakness	NIP	80-100 cm H$_2$O	<20-30
	VC	60-75 ml/kg	<15-20
Acute decompensated heart failure	Jugular venous distention		Clinical judgment combined with the listed factors
	Pulmonary edema		
	Decreased EF		
Inadequate lung expansion	Vt (ml/kg)	5-8	<4-5
	VC (ml/kg)	60-75	<10-15
	Respiratory rate (breaths/min)	12-20	≥35

EF, Ejection fraction; *Fio$_2$,* fraction of inspired oxygen; *NIP,* negative inspiratory pressure; *P(a-a)o$_2$,* alveolar-arterial oxygen pressure difference; *Pao$_2$,* partial pressure of oxygen; *Paco$_2$,* partial pressure of carbon dioxide; *Sao$_2$,* arterial oxygen saturation; *VC,* vital capacity; *Vt,* tidal volume.
From Parrillo JE, Dellinger RP: *Critical care medicine: principles of diagnosis and management in the adult,* ed 5, Philadelphia, 2019, Elsevier.

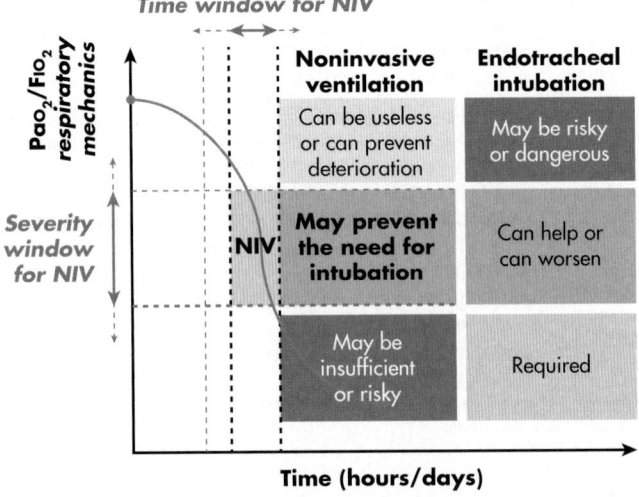

FIG. 2 The decision windows for noninvasive ventilation (NIV) or endotracheal intubation. There is an optimal window of time and severity of injury in which to consider NIV. As a patient worsens over time (see curve of patient course), one must consider whether the severity is appropriate for NIV or intubation and invasive mechanical ventilation. For the right level of severity, NIV can be valuable in offering needed support and perhaps preventing the need for intubation. If the severity worsens further, NIV may be insufficient or risky, and intubation may then be required. If the condition is mild, neither NIV nor invasive mechanical ventilation would be warranted. Unfortunately, there are no strictly objective criteria that delineate the windows of severity or of time for determining exactly when NIV should be used. *Fio$_2$,* Fraction of inspired oxygen; *Pao$_2$,* partial pressure of oxygen. (From Broaddus VC et al: *Murray & Nadel's textbook of respiratory medicine,* ed 7, Philadelphia 2022, Elsevier.)

TABLE 6 Overview of Features of Selected Modes of Mechanical Ventilation

Ventilator Mode	Trigger	Control	Cycling	Inspiratory Flow
Continuous mandatory ventilation	Time	Flow or pressure	Volume or time	Selected or decelerating
Volume control/assist control (VC/AC)	Patient or time	Flow	Volume	Square, decelerating, or sinusoidal
Pressure control/assist control (PC/AC)	Patient or time	Pressure	Time	Decelerating
Synchronized intermittent mandatory ventilation	Patient or time	Pressure for patient breaths Flow (VC) or pressure (PC) for ventilator breaths	Flow for spontaneous breaths Volume or time for ventilator breaths	Decelerating for spontaneous breath Square (VC), decelerating (VC or PC), sinusoidal for spontaneous breaths
Stand-alone pressure-support ventilation	Patient	None	Flow	Decelerating

From Parrillo JE, Dellinger RP: *Critical care medicine: principles of diagnosis and management in the adult,* ed 5, Philadelphia, 2019, Elsevier.

TABLE 7   Potential Advantages and Disadvantages of Selected Modes of Mechanical Ventilation

Mode	Advantage(s)	Disadvantage(s)
Controlled mechanical ventilation	Rests muscles of respiration	Requires use of heavy sedation/neuromuscular blockade
Assist volume control	Reduced work of breathing	Potential adverse hemodynamic effects
	Guarantees delivery of set tidal volume (unless peak pressure limit alarm is exceeded)	May lead to inappropriate hyperventilation and excessive inspiration pressures
Assist pressure control	Allows limitation of peak inspiratory pressures	Same as for assist volume control
		Potential hyperventilation or hypoventilation with lung resistance/compliance changes
Synchronized intermittent mandatory ventilation	Less interference with normal cardiovascular function	Increased work of breathing compared with assist control
		Patient may find it difficult to adjust to two different types of ventilator breaths
Stand-alone pressure-support ventilation	Patient comfort	Apnea alarm is only backup
	Improved patient-ventilator interaction	Variable patient tolerance
	Decreased work of breathing	

From Parrillo JE, Dellinger RP: *Critical care medicine: principles of diagnosis and management in the adult,* ed 5, Philadelphia, 2019, Elsevier.

- Certain diagnoses allow for management with noninvasive techniques. COPD exacerbation and cardiogenic pulmonary edema have been shown to respond favorably to noninvasive ventilation, such as CPAP, and prevent intubation.[8]

REFERRAL
Pulmonologist

RELATED CONTENT
Acute Respiratory Distress Syndrome (Related Key Topic)
Asthma (Related Key Topic)
Carbon Monoxide Poisoning (Related Key Topic)
Chronic Obstructive Pulmonary Disease (Related Key Topic)
Interstitial Lung Disease (Related Key Topic)
Pneumonia, Bacterial (Related Key Topic)
Pneumonia, Mycoplasma (Related Key Topic)
Pneumonia, *Pneumocystis jiroveci* (Related Key Topic)
Pneumonia, Viral (Related Key Topic)
Pulmonary Embolism (Related Key Topic)
Pulmonary Edema (Related Key Topic)

REFERENCES

Available at eBooks.Health.Elsevier.com.

AUTHOR: **JORGE MERCADO, MD**

BASIC INFORMATION

DEFINITION

An acute inability to urinate when the bladder is full. Acute urinary retention (AUR) is often, but not always, painful. The distended bladder may be palpable and percussible. AUR is distinct from chronic urinary retention, a condition in which patients can still void but chronically retain a significant volume of urine in the bladder after voiding.[1] Chronic urinary retention is generally not painful.

SYNONYMS

AUR
Urinary retention
Retaining urine

ICD-10CM CODES	
R33	Retention of urine
R33.8	Other retention of urine
R33.9	Retention of urine, unspecified

EPIDEMIOLOGY & DEMOGRAPHICS

INCIDENCE:

- One of the most common urologic emergencies.
- Typically occurs in aging men, especially those older than 60 yr. However, it may occur in any age group and in either sex.[1-3]
- Over a 5 yr period, AUR will occur in 10% of men older than 70 yr and in one third of men older than 80 yr. There is a near-linear increase in age-specific incidence for men ages 40 to 80 yr.[1,2]

PREVALENCE: Estimates are 40/100,000 men and 3/100,000 women. Prevalence increases as average lifespan increases.[1,2]

GENETICS: None known.

PHYSICAL FINDINGS & CLINICAL PRESENTATION

- Acute inability to pass urine or the tendency to pass only small amounts of urine.
- Pain and/or pressure in the lower abdomen and suprapubic region is typical. Low back pain may also occur. Pain may be absent, especially in older adults, patients with underlying neurologic disorders, and during chronic urinary retention.[1,2]
- Palpable and/or percussible bladder may be detected during abdominal examination in the suprapubic region.
- Suprapubic or bladder tenderness with deep palpation may be elicited.
- Increased urge to urinate with palpation of bladder (pressure applied to suprapubic region).
- Rarely, flank pain and costovertebral angle tenderness are present when high bladder pressures are transmitted to the ureters and kidney.
- Increased severity of lower urinary tract symptoms (LUTS), such as poor or intermittent urine stream, straining to pass urine, sudden urge to urinate, waking up many times at night to pass urine, increased frequency, and feeling of incomplete voiding, is

associated with increased AUR risk. Patients may complain of worsening LUTS prior to episode, including increased urinary urgency, incontinence, nocturia, stranguria, hesitancy, and intermittency. These symptoms usually develop between 1 day and a few weeks prior to AUR.[1]
- Patients with cognitive deficits or inability to communicate may present with restlessness, discomfort, confusion, and/or delirium.
- Acute kidney injury, electrolyte abnormalities, nausea, and lower extremity edema may be present with delayed presentation.[1,3-5]

ETIOLOGY

- Urinary retention generally results from one of three categories:
  1. Bladder outflow obstruction, as seen in benign prostatic hyperplasia (BPH), urethral stricture disease, malignancy, constipation, and gross hematuria where large clots can obstruct the urethra or bladder neck
  2. Disruption of detrusor muscle innervation in association with diabetic neuropathy, spinal cord injury, progressive neurologic pathologies, and bladder contractile dysfunction and decompensation secondary to prolonged outlet obstruction
  3. Bladder overdistension that leads to impaired contractility and may result from general anesthesia, epidural anesthesia, or anticholinergic use
- It is important to keep in mind that multiple processes may be at play leading to AUR, and there is usually a "triggering event" — the proverbial "last straw that broke the camel's back." For example, in an elderly patient with diabetes mellitus, diabetes-related neuropathy can lead to a weakened bladder contraction. With ongoing bladder outflow obstruction due to BPH, taking diphenhydramine (anticholinergic side effects) for a cold could "trigger" an AUR.[1,2]
- Triggering events could include anesthesia for surgical procedures (especially spinal, orthopedic, and urologic), trauma, medications (e.g., over-the-counter antihistamines and sympathomimetic agents commonly found in cough medications, anticholinergic drugs, and opioids), excessive fluid intake (e.g., alcohol), urinary tract infection, central nervous system insults (e.g., strokes, hemorrhage, spinal cord injuries), and severe constipation.
- In women, obstructive factors can include benign tumors (especially fibroid tumors); malignant tumors of pelvic, urethral, or vaginal origin; urethral strictures and urethral meatal stenosis; postpartum vulvar edema; and labial fusion. Pelvic organ prolapse, including cystocele, rectocele, and uterine prolapse, can also lead to urinary retention.[1,6]
- Infection including prostatitis, urethritis, cystitis, genital herpes, and herpes zoster may also contribute to AUR.
- AUR is common in the postoperative period when patients are less mobile, are constipated, or have received opioid medications.[1,2]

DX **DIAGNOSIS**

DIFFERENTIAL DIAGNOSIS

- AUR is typically self-evident to the cognitively intact patient and the treating physician.
- Chronic urinary retention.
- Pelvic masses, fluid collections, uterine fibroids, pregnancies, or ascites may be confused for a full bladder, particularly when using bedside ultrasonic bladder capacity-measuring instruments.

WORKUP

- History is focused on urologic symptoms: Dysuria, hematuria, baseline voiding symptoms (caliber and force of stream, nocturia, sensation of incomplete emptying, double-voiding, incontinence, hesitancy), past episodes of retention, surgical history (urologic and other surgical procedures, particularly recent ones), pelvic/perineal trauma, and urologic cancer.
- History should include a complete list of prescribed and over-the-counter medications and recent medication changes.
- Review of symptoms should include presence of fever, back pain, neurologic symptoms, and rash.
- Rectal examination for masses, fecal impaction, perineal and perianal sensation, prostate size, and sphincter tone.
- Genitourinary examination in men, with special attention for meatal stenosis and phimosis or paraphimosis.
- Pelvic examination in women to assess for evidence of pelvic organ prolapse(s).
- Neurologic examination, with particular evaluation for "saddle" anesthesia (i.e., cauda equina syndrome) and pelvic sensory or motor deficits to rule out an underlying neurologic cause.
- Gross hematuria should prompt consideration of genitourinary malignancy.

LABORATORY TESTS

- Electrolytes, blood urea nitrogen (BUN), and serum creatinine.
- Urinalysis and culture obtained via bladder or suprapubic catheterization.
- Prostate-specific antigen (PSA) testing is not helpful in AUR and may be falsely elevated after catheter placement. This test should not be routinely checked in the acute setting.[1]

IMAGING STUDIES

- Bladder ultrasound or a bedside post-void residual urine scan (bladder scan) can be diagnostic. Ascites, pelvic fluid collections, body habitus, and presence of surgical implants (e.g., reservoirs for inflatable penile prostheses or artificial urinary sphincters) may confound accurate volume measurement with these devices.[1,3]
- Renal ultrasound or abdominopelvic computed tomography (CT) may be obtained when there is kidney functional impairment and/or hydronephrosis is suspected.

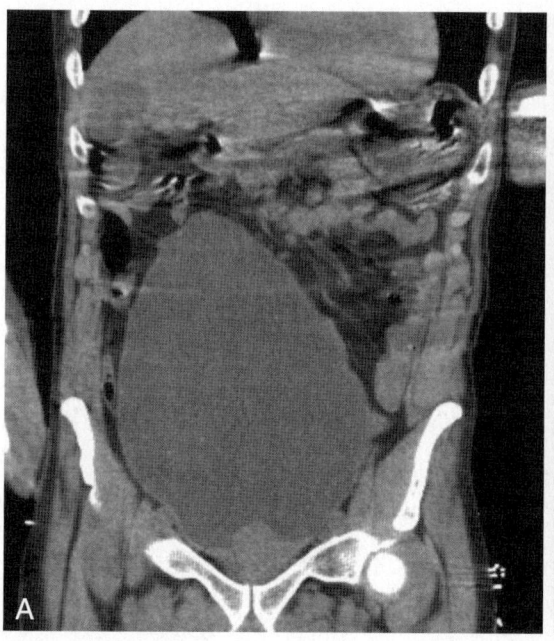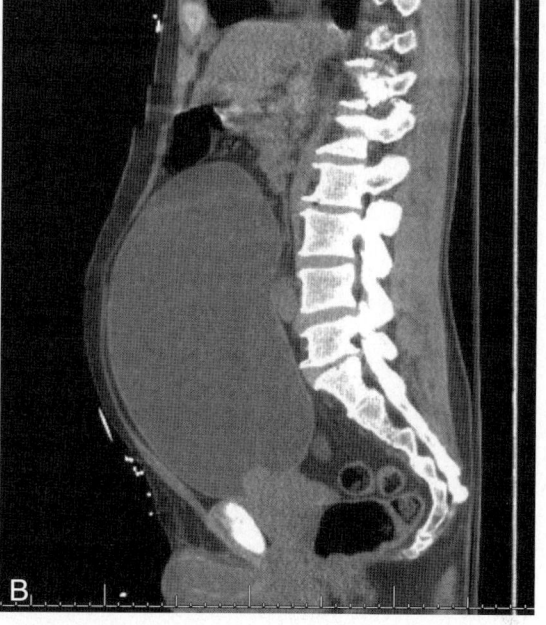

FIG. 1 Large-volume urinary retention. Computed tomography images of coronal view **(A)** and sagittal view **(B)** of greatly distended bladder. The bladder extends into the midabdomen and above the pubic symphysis. More than 2 L of urine were drained on bladder catheterization.

- Abdominal ultrasound or CT (Fig. 1) can be helpful when high volumes are measured by a bedside bladder scan but low volumes are returned upon bladder catheterization. This may also be helpful if there is suspicion of a pelvic mass.
- MRI may be obtained when a spinal cord problem is suspected.
- Evaluation of bladder function by urodynamic testing may be conducted after initial management, particularly in women with no evidence of anatomic obstruction or in patients with longstanding obstruction and/or other neurologic conditions that affect bladder contractility.
- X-rays are of limited utility in evaluating AUR, but may show underlying constipation.

Rx TREATMENT

ACUTE GENERAL Rx

- Bladder catheterization is both diagnostic and therapeutic, especially when the results of the bladder scan are unreliable due to a condition like ascites.
- Prompt bladder decompression and drainage is the initial management of AUR, generally by indwelling urethral catheterization. Coude-tip (angled-tip) catheters can facilitate catheter placement in men with large prostates.[1,3,4] Self-clean intermittent catheterization is an option for patients with sufficient dexterity, vision, and motivation.
- Urologic consultation is advised after recent genitourinary surgery or a history of urethral stricture disease or difficult urethral catheterizations.
- When urethral catheterization is not possible or is contraindicated, suprapubic catheter

placement or advanced endoscopic interventions may be required.[1,3,5]
- Postdecompression hematuria may develop shortly after bladder drainage from small vessel injury of the overstretched bladder wall. This complication is usually self-limiting.[1,4] It is important to observe the timing of post-decompression hematuria (shortly after catheterization) to differentiate it from initial hematuria.
- Monitor for postobstructive diuresis that results from a mixed osmotic and saline diuresis from salt and urea accumulation during the period of obstruction.[1,4]
- Avoid and/or discontinue medications that precipitate AUR (e.g., narcotics, anticholinergics, antihistamines).

CHRONIC Rx

- Alpha-blockers relax the muscle of the prostate and bladder neck, which allows urine to flow more easily. These drugs are effective for treatment of BPH symptoms in men. These agents also increase the success rate of early catheter removal and should be initiated, unless contraindicated. There is limited evidence to suggest benefit in women.[1]
- Tamsulosin (most commonly used alpha blocker for BPH) has a half-life of 15 h. It takes about 3 days to reach maximum concentration in the blood. As such, a voiding trial is reasonable 3 to 7 days after relief of obstruction in most patients.
- If feasible, discontinue medications that increase the risk of AUR.
- Correct constipation and increase patient mobility.
- Inability to void after 3 to 7 days of catheterization mandates urologic consultation with more intensive evaluation of AUR, including

possible cystoscopic evaluation and/or urodynamic studies.
- For patients who are unable to void after a voiding trial, either initiate clean intermittent catheterization, often two to three times a day, or have the urinary bladder catheter replaced.[1]

DISPOSITION

- Patients can be discharged home when close follow-up is feasible and progressive kidney injury and postobstructive diuresis are absent.[1,3-5]
- Hospital admission if patients have the following: sepsis; complicated urinary tract infection; acute kidney injury; severe postobstructive diuresis; hyperkalemia; acidemia or azotemia; or if AUR is from malignancy, hematuria, or spinal cord compression.[1,3-5]

REFERRAL

- Urologist, if initial bladder catheterization is unsuccessful, or in surgical scenarios of radical prostatectomy, transurethral resection of prostate, urethral stricture surgery, and other bladder/prostate surgeries
- Urologic referral for recurrent AUR in men
- Gynecologic referral is mandatory if a pelvic mass is identified as etiology of AUR in women
- Nephrology consultation if medical kidney disease is suspected

! PEARLS & CONSIDERATIONS

- AUR is often painful.
- Rapid bladder drainage is of paramount importance.
- Monitor for postobstructive diuresis and correct electrolyte abnormalities.
- Request urologic advice or referral for AUR after urologic surgery.

PREVENTION

- Avoid and/or treat constipation.
- Avoid and/or discontinue medications that precipitate AUR (e.g., narcotics, anticholinergics, antihistamines).
- Patients with BPH should be cautious regarding medications that may precipitate AUR, including antihistamines, sympathomimetics, sedatives, and anticholinergics. On a chronic basis, 5-α reductase inhibitors (e.g., finasteride, dutasteride) may reduce the risk of AUR in men with BPH and large prostates.

RELATED CONTENT

Benign Prostatic Hyperplasia (Related Key Topic)

REFERENCES

Available at eBooks.Health.Elsevier.com

AUTHORS: **SOHRAB ARORA, MD, MS, Mch** and **DAVID A. LEAVITT, MD**

BASIC INFORMATION

DEFINITION

Alcohol-associated hepatitis (ALD) is a severe, progressive, inflammatory, and cholestatic liver disease occurring in patients with long-term heavy alcohol use (60 to 80 g/day in men and 20 to 40 g/day in women). Main characteristics include rapid onset of jaundice, hepatomegaly, generalized malaise, and subtle systemic inflammatory response features. The clinical diagnosis of ALD and alcohol-associated hepatitis can be accurate; however, the diagnostic accuracy is increased by the use of liver biopsy. A consensus report from the National Institute on Alcoholism and Alcohol Abuse defined the clinical diagnosis of acute alcohol-associated hepatitis. This working definition of alcohol-associated hepatitis includes the onset of jaundice within 60 days of ongoing alcohol consumption of more than three drinks (~40g) per day for women and four drinks (~50 to 60g) per day for men for a minimum of 6 mo, a serum bilirubin level greater than 3 mg/dl, an elevated serum AST level (>50 IU/L), a serum AST:ALT ratio greater than 1.5, and no other obvious cause for hepatitis. This consensus statement proposed classifying patients with alcohol-associated hepatitis as definite when a liver biopsy was used to establish the diagnosis, probable when the clinical and laboratory features were present without potential confounding problems, and possible when confounding problems were present.[1]

SYNONYMS

ALD
Alcoholic Hepatitis
AH

ICD-10CM CODES
K70.10 Alcoholic hepatitis without ascites
K70.9 Alcoholic liver disease, unspecified

EPIDEMIOLOGY & DEMOGRAPHICS

- Approximately 2 million people in the U.S. (about 1% of the population) are affected by alcoholic liver disease.
- Alcohol-associated hepatitis accounts for 0.08% to 0.09% of admissions in the U.S. Almost 7% during their initial hospitalization and 40% of those with severe disease die within 6 mo of clinical presentation.[2]
- Typical presentation age: 40 to 50 yr. Majority occurs before age 60.
- Patients with alcoholic hepatitis typically drink more than 100 g of alcohol daily for two or more decades.
- Excessive alcohol intake is the third leading preventable cause of death in the U.S.

PREVALENCE: Various forms of ALD will develop in ~35% of patients with alcohol use disorder.[3]
PREDOMINANT SEX & AGE: The majority of patients are males. Males are two times as likely as women to abuse alcohol. However, women develop alcoholic hepatitis after a shorter time and smaller amount of alcoholic exposure than men.

RISK FACTORS: Drinking multiple alcohol types, drinking alcohol between meal times, poor nutrition, female gender, obesity, Hispanic ethnicity, long-term ingestion of >10 to 20 g/day of alcohol in women and >20 to 40 g/day in men
GENETICS: No genetic predilection for any one race. In the U.S., however, there is increased incidence in minority groups.

PHYSICAL FINDINGS & CLINICAL PRESENTATION

Common presenting symptoms include:
- Rapid onset of jaundice within 60 days of heavy alcohol consumption (>50 g/day) for at least 6 mo
- Jaundice with duration <3 mo
- Right upper quadrant abdominal/epigastric pain
- Nausea/vomiting
- Malaise
- Low-grade fever
- Anorexia
- Abdominal distention/pain (due to ascites)
- Weight loss or malnourishment
- Proximal muscle wasting and weakness
- Complications of liver impairment (GI bleed; confusion, lethargy, ascites)

Findings on physical examination include:
- Jaundice and ascites
- Hepatomegaly, with tender liver on palpation
- Fever (first exclude other causes of fever, such as spontaneous bacterial peritonitis, urinary tract infection [UTI], pneumonia)
- Asterixis (a flapping tremor)
- Splenomegaly
- Tachycardia/tachypnea
- Hypotension
- Peripheral edema
- Abdominal distention with shifting dullness (ascites)
- Hepatic bruit (may occur in >50% of patients)
- With coexistent cirrhosis, look for:
  1. Gynecomastia
  2. Proximal muscles wasting
  3. Spider angiomata
  4. Altered hair distribution

DIAGNOSIS

DIFFERENTIAL DIAGNOSIS
- Hepatitis B
- Hepatitis C
- Nonalcoholic steatohepatitis (NASH)
- Chronic pancreatitis
- Drug-induced liver injury
- Hemochromatosis
- Cholangitis

WORKUP
- Diagnosis of ALD is clinically supported by laboratory findings.
- The standard screening test for alcohol abuse is the Alcohol Use Disorders Identification Test (AUDIT).
- A thorough and detailed history is needed.
- Relevant questions may include:
  1. When patient started drinking
  2. Number of times patient drinks per day

  3. How many years of regular/daily drinking
  4. Types of alcohol
  5. Home or bar drinking
  6. Rehabilitation for drinking
  7. Social problems (e.g., arrest for public intoxication or driving under the influence, marital discord due to alcoholism)
  8. A typical patient may have a long history of excessive alcohol intake (>100 g of alcohol per day for at least 20 yr)
- Abdominal imaging with ultrasound (the imaging of choice) to rule out gallstones, biliary, and other liver diseases such as liver abscess or hepatocellular carcinoma.

LABORATORY TESTS

The best biomarkers of harmful ethanol use are γ-glutamyltransferase (GGT), aspartate aminotransferase (AST), ethyl glucuronide (ETG), and phosphatidyl ethanol.
- Only one third of hospitalized patients with fatty liver have laboratory abnormalities, which usually consist of mild increases in serum AST and ALT levels
- Elevated transaminase (aspartate aminotransferase [AST] >45 U/L but <500 U/L; however, some patients may not have elevations in ALT, AST in early phases)
- AST: Alanine aminotransferase [ALT] ratio ≥2:1
- S-bilirubin >5 mg/dl
- Increased prothrombin time [PT]/international normalized ratio [INR]
- Elevated GGT
- Carbohydrate-deficient transferrin (CDT) is a reliable marker for chronic alcoholism
- Elevated C-reactive protein [CRP is a good marker of alcoholic hepatitis]
- Electrolyte disorder (hypokalemia, hypomagnesemia, low zinc, hypophosphatemia)
- Hypoalbuminemia
- Hyperferritinemia
- CBC (may reveal leukocytosis with bandemia or anemia or thrombocytopenia); mean corpuscular volume (MCV) may be elevated
- Screening tests to rule out other conditions include checking:
  1. Hepatitis B surface antigen (HBsAg), hepatitis B core antibody (HB$_c$Ab) (IgM), hepatitis A antibody (IgM)
  2. Antihepatitis C antibody, hepatitis C ribonucleic acid (RNA)
  3. Ferritin-transferrin saturation
  4. Alpha-fetoprotein
  5. Alkaline phosphatase
- Laboratory criteria of severe alcoholic hepatitis are defined as:
  1. Maddrey Discriminant Function (MDF) score >32, which is calculated as follows: MDF = 4.6 × prothrombin time–control-prothrombin time + total bilirubin (mg/dl)
  OR
  2. Model for End-Stage Liver Disease (MELD) >21
  AND/OR
  3. Hepatic encephalopathy. There are other models for determining severity such as the Alcohol Hepatitis Histologic Score

(AHHS) or for prognostication such as the MELD + Lille combination models.

IMAGING STUDIES

Ultrasonography is the preferred imaging study. The earliest histologic change in alcohol-related liver disease is macrovesicular steatosis.

LIVER BIOPSY

- Liver biopsy is rarely needed
- Useful to:
  1. Confirm the diagnosis
  2. Evaluate the effect of coexisting disease
  3. Rule out cirrhosis
  4. Exclude other diagnoses (especially other causes of liver diseases, biliary obstruction, Budd-Chiari syndrome)
- Typical histologic findings include:
  1. Micro- or macrovesicular steatosis
  2. Hepatocyte injury (ballooning degeneration and focal hepatocyte necrosis)
  3. Mallory-Denk bodies (characteristic of alcoholic hepatitis)
  4. Perivenular fibrosis
  5. Portal and lobular inflammation with neutrophils or lymphocyte infiltration

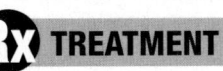

TREATMENT

Glucocorticoid therapy can result in dramatic improvement in survival in carefully selected patients with severe alcohol-associated hepatitis. Three factors limit its usefulness: (1) a number of patients are not candidates for therapy because of obvious contraindications; (2) a significant number of patients fail to respond; and (3) glucocorticoids have limited efficacy in patients with chronic kidney disease or acute kidney injury and do not appear to prevent the development of hepatorenal syndrome. Therefore, in patients who have contraindications to glucocorticoid therapy or any degree of renal disease, aggressive standard medical care with attention to factors such as nutrition, infection, and adequate perfusion should be pursued, and opportunities for clinical trials of LT should be considered. Table 1 lists the factors that should be taken into account in the approach to patients with suspected severe alcohol-associated hepatitis.[1] An algorithm for the management of patients with suspected alcohol-associated hepatitis is described in Fig. 1.

Treatment can be divided into three main components:
1. Determining the severity of the disease using Maddrey Discriminant Function (DF) and Model for End Stage Liver Disease (MELD)
2. Supportive care that includes lifestyle modifications and nutritional support
3. Pharmacologic therapy

LIFESTYLE MODIFICATIONS

- Abstinence, together with adequate nutritional support, is the cornerstone of management.
- Abstinence from alcohol (this improves both short- and long-term survival).
- Nonpharmacologic methods to promote abstinence include cognitive-behavioral therapy (CBT), Alcoholics Anonymous (AA) attendance, and motivational interviewing.

- Pharmacologic aids include using naltrexone, acamprosate, or baclofen.
- Monitor abstinence with breath test or urine drug screen (for use in past 3 days) or hair sample analysis for ethyl glucuronide (test alcohol intake within the last few months).
- Smoking cessation (to decrease oxidative stress).
- Treatment of substance abuse.

NUTRITIONAL SUPPORT

- Good nutrition is an essential part of treatment because many patients with ALD have severe protein-calorie malnutrition as well as deficiencies of trace minerals and several vitamins.
- Nutritional support includes:
  1. Liberal vitamin supplementation (especially thiamine, folic acid, vitamin K)
  2. Mineral supplementation **(but not iron)**
  3. Calorie counting is essential. A high calorie intake (1.2 to 1.4 times the normal resting intake) may be required
  4. Protein intake of 1.2 to 1.5 g/kg of ideal body weight per day will provide adequate support. **Exception: In patients with severe encephalopathy, protein restriction may be required**
  5. Fluid management

PHARMACOLOGIC THERAPY

Severe ALD may require treatment. Severity can be assessed by calculating the MELD score or MDF score or the Glasgow score.
- An MDF score ≥ 32 indicates significant or severe ALD (30-day mortality of 50%).

TABLE 1   Factors to Consider in the Approach to the Patient with Suspected Severe Alcohol-Associated Hepatitis

Initial Findings That Support a Diagnosis of Alcohol-Associated Hepatitis	
Clinical presentation	Prolonged heavy alcohol intake, recent-onset jaundice, malaise, ascites, edema, pruritus, fever, confusion/lethargy/agitation, asterixis, tender hepatomegaly, splenomegaly, pedal edema
Laboratory features	Abrupt rise in serum total bilirubin (>3 mg/dl), AST > ALT (usually > 2X ULN), GGTP > 100 U/ml, albumin < 3.0 g/L, INR > 1.5, leukocyte count > 12,000/mm³
Exclusion of Other Causes of Jaundice	
Autoimmune hepatitis	Exclude severe autoimmune hepatitis if first episode and/or clinical suspicion
DILI	Review detailed history of medication, supplements, pharmacy records Consult http://livertox.nih.gov
Ischemic hepatitis	Suspect if hypotension, septic shock, massive bleeding, or recent cocaine use
Mechanical obstruction	Rule out HCC, biliary obstruction, Budd-Chiari syndrome Perform Doppler abdominal US and, if indicated, MRI
Viral hepatitis	Rule out acute hepatitis A, B, C, or E, especially if first episode or high clinical suspicion
Treatment of Alcohol Abuse and Liver-related Complications	
Alcoholism	Consult addiction specialist Moderate withdrawal symptoms: baclofen Severe withdrawal symptoms: benzodiazepines, phenobarbital
Hepatic encephalopathy	Assess for precipitant: GI bleed, infection, medication nonadherence Treat underlying precipitant, add lactulose, rifaximin, zinc
Infection	Rule out pneumonia, cellulitis, SBP, urinary tract infection, meningitis Obtain chest film Broad-spectrum antibiotics, if indicated
Renal insufficiency	Early detection and close monitoring Volume expansion with albumin Consider IV albumin plus a vasoconstrictor if progressive hepatorenal syndrome

ULN, Upper limit of normal.
Feldman M et al: *Sleisenger and Fordtran's gastrointestinal and liver disease,* ed 11, Philadelphia, 2021, Elsevier.

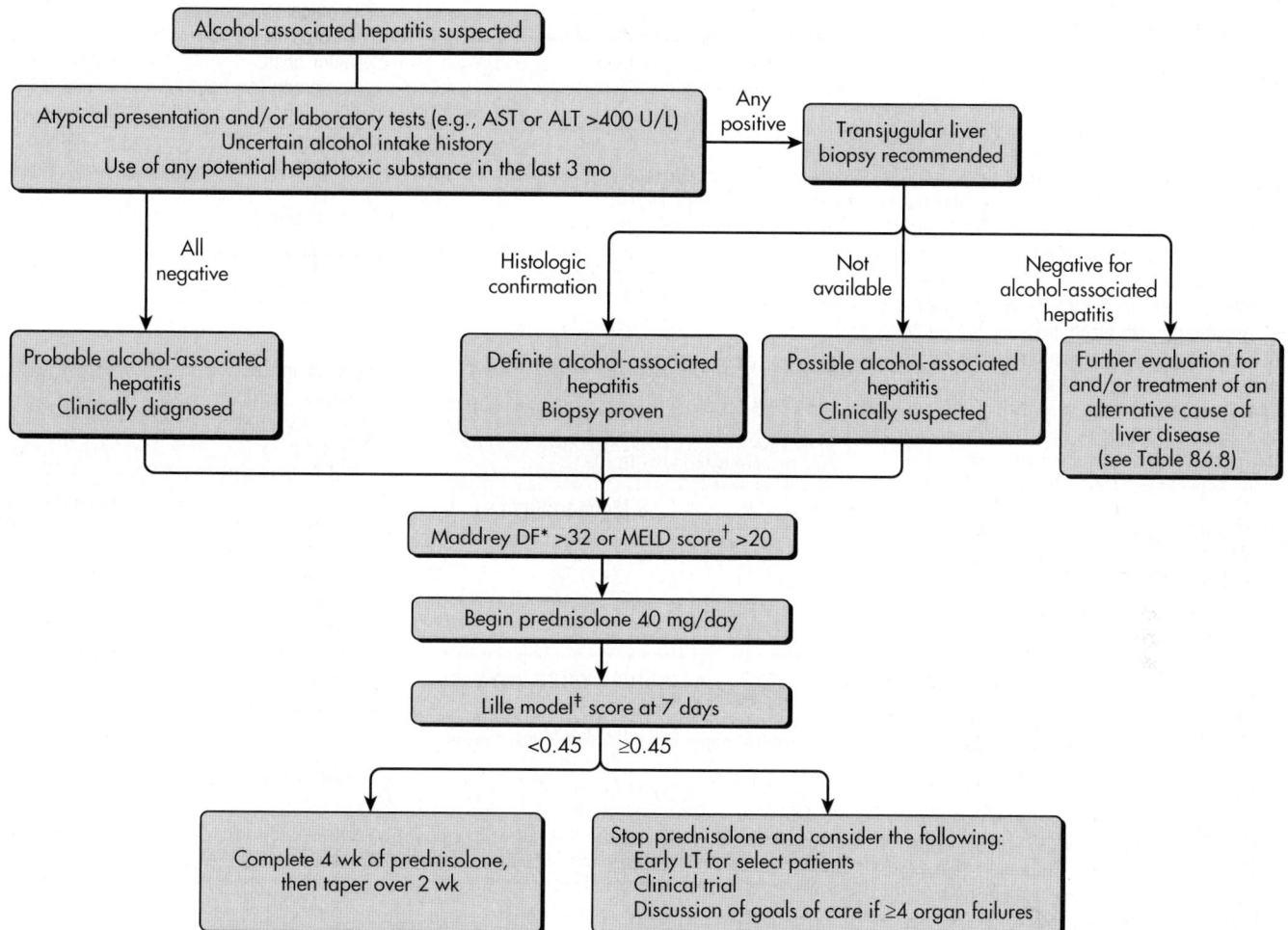

FIG. 1 Algorithm for the management of a patient with suspected alcohol-associated hepatitis. *The Maddrey discriminant function (DF) is calculated as follows: 4.6 (prothrombin time of patient − prothrombin time of control) + serum bilirubin level (in mg/dl). †The MELD score is based on the serum bilirubin level, international normalization ratio, and serum creatinine level. ‡The Lille model score is based on the patient's age, serum albumin, serum bilirubin, serum creatinine, and prothrombin time. Online calculators for these various models are available at http://www.lillemodel.com. (From Feldman M et al: *Sleisenger and Fordtran's gastrointestinal and liver disease*, ed 11, Philadelphia, 2021, Elsevier.)

- MELD score can easily be calculated (visit https://optn.transplant.hrsa.gov/resources/allocation-calculators/meld-calculator/). This score predicts short-term survival in patients with cirrhosis. A score >20 predicts increased short-term mortality.
- Glasgow score: Contains four variables (BUN, PT, WBC count, and bilirubin). A score ≥9 indicates increased mortality.

Indications for hospitalization include:
- MDF ≥32
- MELD >20
- Glasgow score >8
- Hepatic encephalopathy

Patients with severe ALD may be treated with glucocorticosteroids (prednisolone 40 mg/day for 28 days with a 2-wk taper). Glucocorticosteroids reduce hepatic injury, suppress inflammation, and promote liver regeneration. However, not all studies have demonstrated consistent therapeutic benefits for steroids, even in high-risk patients.[4] Prednisolone should be discontinued if bilirubin does not decrease by day 17. An alternative agent for patients with

contraindications to corticosteroids is pentoxifylline. Pentoxifylline is not effective in patients who do not respond to prednisone, and data supporting its use is weak.

LIVER TRANSPLANTATION
- Liver transplantation could be considered for patients with MELD >26 and unresponsive to steroids.
- Usually reserved for patients with end-stage liver disease. Patients whose hepatitis is not responding to medical therapy have a 6-mo survival rate of approximately 30%. Since most hepatitis deaths occur within 2 mo, early liver transplantation is attractive and associated with higher than 80% survival at 3 yr.
- Patients with ALD must be sober for at least 6 mo before they can be eligible for consideration for liver transplantation. However, transplantation candidates should not be based solely on 6 mo abstinence, and other factors, such as social support and need for rehabilitation, should be considered.

REFERRAL

Severe acute ALD may require intensive care unit (ICU) care and referral to different subspecialists:
- GI/hepatology (for patients with evidence of GI hemorrhage)
- Nutritional services
- Nephrology (for acute renal failure, hepatorenal syndrome)
- Neurology (for change in mental status, seizures)
- Infectious disease (for fever/leukocytosis)

PROGNOSIS
- Three prospective studies demonstrated that patients with mDF values of 32 or greater have a poor prognosis, with 1-mo mortality rates of 35% to 50% (Table 2). As a result, the MDF has been incorporated into the selection criteria for most therapeutic trials of patients with alcohol-associated hepatitis. The prognosis of patients with MDF values greater than or equal to 32 can be further stratified by the presence of encephalopathy and

development of acute kidney injury. Three other prognostic models, the MELD score, the Glasgow alcohol-associated hepatitis score, and the ABIC score, have been shown to predict survival in patients with severe alcohol-associated hepatitis (Tables 3-5). Although none is perfect, each of these models appears to be effective in selecting patients for medical therapy. The short-term survival of patients with MDF values less than 32 have ranged from 83% to 100% in various studies. To determine the prognosis of all patients with alcohol-associated hepatitis more accurately, a scoring system (ABIC) has been proposed that separates patients into three groups with predicted 3-mo survival rates of 25%, 70%, and 100% based on the patient's age, bilirubin, INR, and creatinine, respectively[1] (see Table 4).

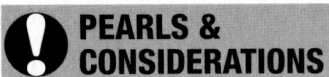

PEARLS & CONSIDERATIONS

COMMENTS

- Referral to substance abuse treatment programs may be helpful.
  1. Stress to patients that there are limited long-term drug treatments for ALD
  2. Maintaining good general nutrition is important.
  3. Advise patient about the risk of taking certain medications, especially acetaminophen.
- Periodic follow-up to monitor patient's response to check basic metabolic panel (BMP) and liver function tests (LFTs).
- Encourage alcohol abstinence. Abstinence improves long-term survival.
- If patient develops liver cirrhosis, check serum alpha-fetoprotein every 6 mo and liver ultrasound annually to rule out hepatocellular carcinoma.
- Vaccinate patient against hepatitis A and B viruses, pneumococci, influenza A virus, and routine adult vaccinations, if appropriate.

RELATED CONTENT

Alcoholic Hepatitis (Patient Information)

REFERENCES

Available at eBooks.Health.Elsevier.com.

AUTHOR: **FRED F. FERRI, MD**

TABLE 2 Correlation of the Maddrey Discriminant Function (DF)* with Prognosis in Alcohol-Associated Hepatitis

	Non-Severe Disease	Severe Disease
Score	<32	≥32
Short-term mortality rate (%)	10	30-60
Glucocorticoid therapy indicated	No	Yes

*DF = {4.6 × [prothrombin time (sec) − control prothrombin time (sec)]} + (serum bilirubin [mg/dl]).
From Feldman M et al: *Sleisenger and Fordtran's gastrointestinal and liver disease*, ed 11, Philadelphia, 2021, Elsevier.

TABLE 3 Correlation of the MELD Score* with 3-month Mortality Rate in Alcohol-Associated Hepatitis

Score	3-Mo Mortality (%)
22	10
29	30
33	50
38	80

*MELD = (0.957 × log [creatinine] + 0.378 × log[bilirubin] + 1.12 × log[INR] + 0.643) × 10.
From Feldman M et al: *Sleisenger and Fordtran's gastrointestinal and liver disease*, ed 11, Philadelphia, 2021, Elsevier.

TABLE 4 Correlation of the ABIC Score* and the 90-day Mortality Rate in Alcohol-Associated Hepatitis

Severity	90-Day Mortality (%)
Low (<6.71)	0
Intermediate (6.71-8.99)	30
High (≥9.0)	75

*ABIC score = (age × 0.1) + (serum bilirubin × 0.08) + (serum creatinine × 0.3) + (INR × 0.8).
From Feldman M et al: *Sleisenger and Fordtran's gastrointestinal and liver disease*, ed 11, Philadelphia, 2021, Elsevier.

TABLE 5 The Glasgow Alcohol-Associated Hepatitis Score

	POINTS		
Parameters	**1**	**2**	**3**
Age (yr)	<50	≥50	−
WBC count (10⁹/L)	<15	≥15	−
Blood urea nitrogen (mmol/L)	<5	≥5	−
Serum bilirubin level (μmol/L)	<125	125-250	>250
INR	<1.5	1.5-2.0	>2.0

The total score ranges from 5 to 12. A score ≥ 9 indicates a poor prognosis.

INR, International normalization ratio; *WBC*, white blood cell.
From Feldman M et al: *Sleisenger and Fordtran's gastrointestinal and liver disease*, ed 11, Philadelphia, 2021, Elsevier.

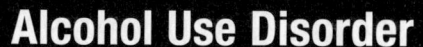

A

Diseases
and Disorders

 BASIC INFORMATION

DEFINITIONS

- "Standard drink": One standard drink is defined as 14 g of absolute ethanol that includes 12 oz of beer, 5 ounces of wine, or 1.5 oz of 80-proof spirits.[1]
- "Moderate drinking": Moderate drinking has been defined as two standard drinks per day for men and one drink per day for women and persons older than 65 yr.[2]
- "At-risk drinking": For men, *at-risk drinking* or *harmful alcohol use* is defined as more than 14 drinks/wk or more than four drinks/day. For women, at-risk drinking is defined as three or more drinks per day or seven or more drinks per wk.
- "Binge drinking": Binge drinking is defined as drinking enough within about 2 h to bring alcohol blood concentration up to 0.08 g/dl or higher. Typically, five or more standard drinks for men or four or more standard drinks for women.[2]
- "Alcohol use disorder (AUD)": Alcohol use disorder is a problematic pattern of alcohol use characterized by craving, use despite consequences, loss of control over intake, and physiologic dependence. It leads to clinically significant impairment or distress, and it is defined by the DSM-5-TR through specific diagnostic criteria and can be classified as mild, moderate, or severe.[3]
- "Alcohol withdrawal": The American Psychiatric Association[3] defines diagnostic criteria for *alcohol withdrawal* as follows:
  1. Cessation of (or reduction in) alcohol use that has been heavy and prolonged
  2. Two (or more) of the following, developing within several hours to a few days of cessation or reduction of alcohol use:
     a. Autonomic hyperactivity (e.g., sweating or pulse rate >100 beats/min)
     b. Increased hand tremor
     c. Insomnia
     d. Nausea and vomiting
     e. Transient visual, tactile, or auditory hallucinations or illusions
     f. Psychomotor agitation
     g. Anxiety
     h. Generalized tonic-clonic seizures
  3. The symptoms cause clinically significant distress or impairment in social, occupational, or other important areas of functioning
  4. The symptoms are not attributable to a general medical condition and are not better accounted for by another mental disorder.

SYNONYMS

Alcohol dependence
Alcohol abuse
Alcohol withdrawal syndrome
Alcoholism
AUD

ICD-10CM CODES
F10	Alcohol Related Disorders
F10.1	Alcohol abuse
F10.2	Alcohol dependence
F10.23	Alcohol dependence with withdrawal
F10.231	Alcohol dependence with withdrawal delirium
F10.25	Alcohol dependence with alcohol-induced psychotic disorder with delusions
F10.26	Alcohol dependence with alcohol-induced persisting amnestic disorder

EPIDEMIOLOGY & DEMOGRAPHICS

INCIDENCE (IN U.S.):
- Excessive alcohol use is responsible for 140,000 deaths annually.[4] A total of $249 billion in annual economic costs are attributed to the health effects of excessive alcohol use, which include injuries, violence, poisonings, unintended pregnancy and sexually transmitted illnesses (STIs), poor pregnancy outcomes, cancer, and cardiovascular and liver diseases.
- According to the National Survey on Drug Use and Health conducted in 2021, 133.1 million people aged 12 or older reported current alcohol use. Of those, 45.1% had binge drinking behavior over the past month. This was more prevalent in young adults aged 18 to 25.[5]
- Lifetime prevalence rates DSM-5-TR criteria for AUD among adults were estimated to be 29.1% overall with rates of mild, moderate, and severe symptoms being 8.6%, 6.6%, and 13.9%, respectively.[3]

PEAK INCIDENCE: Age at onset of AUD peaks in the late teens or early 20s, mean age of onset is estimated at 26.2 yr. Mean age of onset for mild AUD is 30.1 yr, for moderate is 25.9 yr, and for severe is 23.9 yr.[6]

PREVALENCE (IN U.S.):[3] 29.1% % of population ≥18 yr

PREDOMINANT SEX:[3]
- Lifetime risk for males 36.0%
- Lifetime risk for females 22.7%

RISK FACTORS:[3,8,9]
- Male sex
- Early life stress
- Permissive cultural attitudes toward drinking and intoxication
- Unemployment/low socioeconomic status
- Widowed/separated/divorced or never married
- Mood disorder (major depression, bipolar disorder)
- Addiction to another substance, including tobacco
- Limited support system

GENETICS: Family history and polygenic risk scores are independently associated with susceptibility for development of AUD.[7]

PHYSICAL FINDINGS & CLINICAL PRESENTATION

- Recurring minor trauma or falls
- GI bleeding from gastritis and/or varices
- Pancreatitis (acute and chronic)
- Liver disease
- Odor of alcohol on breath
- Signs of alcohol withdrawal
- Peripheral neuropathy
- Recent memory loss

ETIOLOGY

Social and genetic factors play key roles.

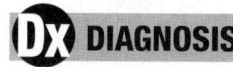 **DIAGNOSIS**

WORKUP

- The United States Preventive Services Task Force (USPSTF)[10] recommends that clinicians screen adults 18 yr and older for alcohol misuse and provide persons engaged in risky or hazardous drinking with brief behavioral counseling interventions to reduce alcohol misuse. Several screening tests (CAGE [Table 1], TWEAK, Single Alcohol Screening Question (SASQ), and Alcohol Use Disorders Identification Test-Concise [AUDIT-C; Table 2]) are available.
- The four-item CAGE (feeling need to **C**ut down, **A**nnoyed by criticism, **G**uilty about drinking, and need for an **E**ye-opener in the morning) is a popular screening test in primary care. A positive response should lead to further questioning. The sensitivity of the CAGE ranges from 43% to 94%, and its specificity ranges from 70% to 97% in the primary care setting.[11]
- The five-item TWEAK scale (**T**olerance, **W**orry, **E**ye-openers, **A**mnesia, [**K**] cut down) and the TACE questionnaire (**T**olerance, **A**nnoyance, **C**ut down, **E**ye-opener) are designed to screen pregnant women for alcohol misuse. They detect lower levels of alcohol consumption that may pose risks during pregnancy.
- A single-question screening about alcohol consumption in a day ("When was the last time you had more than X drinks in a day?"

TABLE 1 CAGE Questionnaire for Alcohol Problems Screening

C	Have you felt the need to Cut down on your drinking?
A	Have people Annoyed you by criticizing your drinking?
G	Have you ever felt bad or Guilty about your drinking?
E	Have you had a drink first thing in the morning to steady your nerves or to get rid of a hangover (i.e., an "Eye opener")?

From Stern TA et al: *Massachusetts General Hospital handbook of general hospital psychiatry*, ed 7, Philadelphia, 2018, Elsevier.

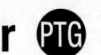
TABLE 2 AUDIT-C Questionnaire for Alcohol Problems Screening[a]

Question	Score
How often did you have a drink containing alcohol in the past year?	Never (0 points) Monthly or less (1 point) 2-4 times per month (2 points) 2-3 times per week (3 points) >4 times per week (4 points)
In the past year, how many drinks did you have on a typical day when you were drinking?	0-2 (0 points) 3-4 (1 point) 5-6 (2 points) 7-9 (3 points) 10 or more (4 points)
How often did you have six or more drinks on one occasion in the past year?	Never (0 points) Less than monthly (1 point) Monthly (2 points) Weekly (3 points) Daily or almost daily (4 points)

AUDIT-C, Alcohol Use Disorders Identification Test-Concise.
[a]AUDIT-C is scored 0-12, with score >4 (men) and >3 (women) considered positive for problematic drinking.

From Stern TA et al: *Massachusetts General Hospital handbook of general hospital psychiatry,* ed 7, Philadelphia, 2018, Elsevier.

[where X is five for men and four for women]) with the threshold set at "in the past 30 days" is 82% sensitive and 79% for unhealthy alcohol use, and 88% sensitive and 67% specific for detection of AUD.[12] This single question can also indicate frequency of binge drinking behavior, which would warrant further exploration.

- The three-question AUDIT-C is a shorter form of the 10-item AUDIT, and the questions center on the quantity and frequency of alcohol use. It asks how often someone has a drink containing alcohol, how many standard drinks containing alcohol one consumes on a typical day when one is drinking, and how often one has six or more drinks on one occasion. Scoring ranges from 0 to 4 on each question with a total score range of 0 to 12. A total score of 3 or higher for women and 4 or higher for men indicates harmful alcohol use and need for further assessment.
- AUD as defined by the DSM-5-TR[3] as a pattern of alcohol use causing significant impairment or distress as manifested by at least two of the following criteria within a 12-mo period: alcohol is often taken in larger amounts than intended; desire or unsuccessful efforts to cut down or control use; large amount of time spent in obtaining, using, or recovering from alcohol; cravings; alcohol use resulting in failure to fulfill major role obligations at work, school, or home; continued use despite persistent social or interpersonal problems caused by alcohol; important social, occupational, or recreational activities are given up or reduced because of use;

recurrent alcohol use in situations in which it is physically hazardous; continued use despite knowledge of physiologic or psychologic problem that is likely exacerbated by alcohol; tolerance (increased amounts of use to achieve intoxication or diminished effect with continued use of the same amount of alcohol) or alcohol withdrawal. The presence of two to three symptoms indicates mild AUD; four to five is moderate; and six or greater is severe. Severe or prolonged alcohol use can lead to neurologic sequelae (e.g., memory loss, peripheral neuropathy), liver manifestations (e.g., spider angiomata, palmar erythema, plethoric facies, hepatic and/or spleen enlargement, hypertension, jaundice, ascites, GI bleeding, or esophageal varices), or cardiologic sequelae (cardiomyopathy, atrial fibrillation).[13]

- Laboratory evaluation (see "Laboratory Tests").

LABORATORY TESTS

Laboratory tests alone do not diagnose alcohol use disorder, though may identify consequences of harmful alcohol use:

- Increased liver enzymes (aspartate aminotransferase [AST], alanine aminotransferase [ALT], γ-glutamyltransferase [GGT]; typically AST:ALT ratio of ≥2:1)
- Low albumin, hypophosphatemia, hypomagnesemia from malnutrition
- CBC may reveal low hemoglobin, anemia, pancytopenia, and/or elevated mean corpuscular volume from toxic effect of alcohol on erythrocyte development in nutritional deficiencies
- Stool for occult blood may be positive as a result of gastritis or variceal bleeding
- Low folate, vitamin B_{12}, vitamin B_6, vitamin B_1 levels

IMAGING STUDIES

Computed tomography (CT) or ultrasound of abdomen may reveal fatty liver disease or cirrhosis in advanced stages. Head imaging may be indicated if presentation involves trauma or neurologic signs.

Rx TREATMENT

NONPHARMACOLOGIC THERAPY

- Screening, Brief Interventions, and Referral for Treatment (SBIRT) should be implemented in primary care settings.[1,14] Screening scales are discussed above.
- Brief interventions such as 12-step facilitation, cognitive-behavioral therapy (CBT), and motivational interviewing can improve the chances of recovery in patients with alcohol use disorder and dependence.
- Acceptance and Commitment Therapy (ACT) is a third-wave CBT therapy that has shown some benefit in alcohol use disorder.[15]
- Referral to most intensive substance use care should be considered for individuals with severe alcohol use disorder.
- Depression, if present, should be treated at same time alcohol is withdrawn.

ACUTE GENERAL Rx

Alcohol withdrawal syndrome (AWS) occurs when a person stops ingesting alcohol after prolonged consumption. The severity of the syndrome depends on a patient's pattern and duration of alcohol use and the time from the patient's last alcohol ingestion. Blood ethanol level decreases by 20 mg/dl/h in a normal person. Alcohol withdrawal can range from minor discomfort requiring minimal medications to multisystem organ failure requiring intensive care treatment. There are four major withdrawal syndromes as discussed below. Table 3 summarizes medications for the treatment of alcohol use disorder. The cornerstone of treatment for alcohol withdrawal syndrome is the use of benzodiazepines, though barbiturates such as phenobarbital are sometimes used, as well as alpha-2 agonists such as clonidine in inpatient settings.

- **Mild/Early Withdrawal:**
  1. Time interval: Begin to see symptoms from 6 to12 h after the last drink.
  2. Manifestation: Tremors, mild agitation or anxiety, insomnia, headache, palpitations/tachycardia, diaphoresis, GI upset; symptoms are relieved by alcohol.
  3. Workup: CBC, electrolytes, glucose, blood urea nitrogen, creatinine, GGT, ALT, AST, serum vitamin B_{12} and folic acid.
  4. Treatment: minor withdrawal states can be self-limiting and resolve within 48 h if the patient does not have an excessive alcohol use history, clinical signs of excessive chronic alcohol use (as discussed in laboratory findings above), and does not have risk factors for development of more severe withdrawal states. Patients at risk for more severe withdrawal states should be admitted and managed in an inpatient setting.
  5. Candidates for outpatient detoxification should have a reasonable support system (e.g., reliable contact person) who can monitor progress and lack of any significant comorbid conditions (e.g., suicide risk, seizure disorder, coexisting benzodiazepine dependence, prior unsuccessful outpatient detoxification, pregnancy, cirrhosis) or risk factors for severe withdrawal (history of severe withdrawal symptoms, history of withdrawal seizures or delirium tremens, multiple previous detoxifications, concomitant psychiatric or medical illness, high levels of alcohol consumption [random blood alcohol level >200 mg/dl or history of >15 standard drinks per day], metabolic derangement, early withdrawal signs with elevated blood alcohol level, age >40).
  6. The Clinical Institute Withdrawal Assessment Scale for Alcohol, Revised (CIWA-Ar) scale can be used to measure the severity of alcohol withdrawal. It consists of 10 items: Nausea; tremor; autonomic hyperactivity; anxiety; agitation; tactile, visual, and auditory disturbances; headache; and disorientation. Each item is assigned a

TABLE 3   Medications for the Treatment of Alcohol Use Disorder

Medication	Dosage	Mechanism	Adverse Effects	Notes
Acamprosate[†]	666 mg 3 times daily	Glutamate-mediated neuronal hyperexcitability antagonist	Diarrhea, nausea/vomiting, myalgia, rash, dizziness, palpitations; rarely, renal impairment	Reduce dosage with renal insufficiency
Disulfiram[†]	250-500 mg daily	Inhibition of aldehyde dehydrogenase	Drowsiness, rash; rarely, hepatotoxicity, optic neuritis, peripheral neuropathy	Must be ≥12 h before last drink; avoid in patients with hepatic or cardiac impairment.
Naltrexone[†]	PO: 50-100 mg daily IM: 380 mg monthly	Opioid antagonist (reduce subjective reward)	Nausea, indigestion, headache, fatigue; rarely, hepatitis	Contraindicated if opioid use is present
Topiramate[*]	25-150 mg twice daily	Modulates GABA and antagonize glutamate receptors	Dizziness, drowsiness, fatigue, anorexia, cognitive dysfunction, anxiety, depression, paresthesia, nonanion gap metabolic acidosis, nephrolithiasis	Dose adjustment in kidney impairment; useful in concurrent migraine, seizures
Gabapentin[*]	600 mg 3 times daily	Modulates GABA activity	Dizziness, drowsiness, withdrawal if abruptly discontinued	Dose adjustment in kidney impairment; useful in concurrent anxiety, chronic pain, seizures

[†]Currently approved by FDA for the indication noted.
[*]Not FDA approved, off label use
IM, Intramuscular; *PO,* by mouth.

score from 0 to 7. For the category of "tremor," 0 indicates that tremor is not present and 7 that tremor is severe, even with arms not extended. The maximum total score is 67. Patients with mild AWS symptoms (CIWA-Ar score <8) can be monitored on an outpatient basis. Benzodiazepines are beneficial for most patients with a CIWA-AR score ≥8 and are strongly recommended in patients with substantial withdrawal symptoms (CIWA-Ar score >12). Patients with CIWA-Ar score of ≥15 should be admitted. Note that some patients will score highly on the CIWA due to subjective symptoms, even when not experiencing withdrawal. A modified CIWA using only objective findings (heart rate, systolic blood pressure, tremor, diaphoresis) is sometimes used instead.

7. Outpatient Treatment:
   a. The patient and support person(s) should be educated on withdrawal symptoms, time course, medication administration and side effects, and what to do if symptoms worsen. The patient should be assessed daily.
   b. Fixed dose regiment is preferred, small quantities are prescribed on each visit.
   c. Longer-acting benzodiazepines (e.g. chlordiazepoxide or diazepam) may be preferred due to decreased risk of rebound withdrawal in patients without liver disease (where the preferred agents would be lorazepam, oxazepam).
   d. Patients should also be prescribed thiamine and a multivitamin.
8. Inpatient treatment:
   a. In patients with mild to moderate withdrawal and without history of seizures, individualized benzodiazepine administration (rather than a fixed-dose regimen) results in lower benzodiazepine administration and avoids unnecessary sedation. CIWA-Ar monitoring every 4 h

with symptom-triggered lorazepam should be administered: for CIWA-Ar scores equal to or greater than 8, patient receives lorazepam 2 to 4 mg.
   b. Beta-adrenergic blockers: Beta-blockers are useful for controlling blood pressure and tachyarrhythmias. However, they do not prevent progression to more serious symptoms of withdrawal and, if used, should not be administered alone but in conjunction with benzodiazepines. Beta-blockers should be avoided in patients with contraindications to their use (e.g., bronchospasm, bradycardia, or severe congestive heart failure). Centrally acting alpha-adrenergic agonists such as clonidine ameliorate symptoms in patients with mild to moderate withdrawal but do not reduce delirium or seizures.
   c. Vitamin replacement: Thiamine 100 mg intravenous (IV) or intramuscular (IM) for at least 5 days plus oral multivitamins. The IV administration of glucose can precipitate Wernicke encephalopathy in patients with chronic alcohol use with thiamine deficiency; therefore thiamine administration should precede IV dextrose.
   d. Hydration PO or IV (high-caloric solution): If IV, glucose with Na^+, K^+, Mg^{2+}, and phosphate replacement prn.
   e. Social rehabilitation: Group therapy such as Alcoholics Anonymous; identification and treatment of social and family problems should be initiated during the patient's hospital stay.

• **Alcoholic Hallucinosis:**
1. Older term that has fallen out of favor due to overlapping usages and inconsistent definitions.
2. Time interval: 12 to 24 h after last drink.
3. Manifestations: Hallucinations usually are auditory, but hallucinations occasionally are visual, tactile, or olfactory; usually

there is no clouding of sensorium as in delirium.
4. Treatment: Most symptoms remit after 48 h, treatment should include treating alcohol withdrawal state.

• **Withdrawal Seizures:**
1. Time interval: Within 12 to 48 h after last drink, though have been described as early as 1 to 2 h
2. Risk factors: Preexisting seizure disorder, history of head trauma, history of previous alcohol withdrawal seizures
3. Manifestations: Tonic-clonic generalized convulsions with loss of consciousness; focal signs are usually absent
4. Workup: consider further investigation with CT scan of head and electroencephalography if indicated (e.g., presence of focal neurologic deficits, prolonged postictal confusion state). In addition, in a febrile patient who is having a seizure or altered mental state, a lumbar puncture is necessary
5. Treatment: Admission and benzodiazepines for seizure control
   a. Diazepam 2.5 mg/min IV or lorazepam 1 to 2 mg IV every 2 h until seizure is controlled (check for respiratory depression or hypotension) may be beneficial for prolonged seizure activity. Withdrawal seizures generally are self-limited. The use of other anticonvulsants for short-term treatment of alcohol withdrawal seizures is not recommended.
   b. Thiamine 100 mg IV, followed by IV dextrose, should also be administered.
   c. Electrolyte imbalances (increased Mg^{2+}, decreased K^+, increased or decreased Na^+, decreased PO_4^{3-}) that may exacerbate seizures should be corrected.

• **Delirium Tremens (DT):**
1. Time interval: Variable; usually 48 to 72 h after last drink, later onset has also been described

2. Risk Factors: History of alcohol withdrawal delirium, history of chronic daily alcohol use, age >40, concurrent medical/surgical illnesses, withdrawal symptoms in the context of elevated blood alcohol levels
3. Manifestations: Tachycardia, hypertension, hyperthermia, disorientation, visual hallucinations (other sensory hallucinations also occur), agitation, paranoid delusions; this is the most serious clinical presentation of alcohol withdrawal (mortality rate is approximately 15% in untreated patients).
4. Treatment:
   a. Admission
   b. Vital signs q30min (neurologic signs, if necessary)
   c. Use of lateral decubitus or prone position if restraints are necessary
   d. NPO: Nasogastric tube for abdominal distention may be necessary but should not be routinely used
   e. Laboratory studies: Same as for early alcohol withdrawal
   f. Vigorous hydration (4 to 6 L/day): IV with glucose (Na$^+$, K$^+$, PO$_4^{3-}$ and Mg^{2+} replacement [if patient has hypophosphatemia or hypomagnesemia])
   g. Vitamins: Thiamine 100 mg IV qd. The initial dose of thiamine should precede the administration of IV dextrose; multivitamins (may be added to the hydrating solution)
   h. Sedation: Control of agitation should be achieved with rapid-acting sedative-hypnotic agents in adequate doses to maintain light somnolence for the duration of delirium
      1) Initially: Lorazepam 2 to 5 mg IM/IV repeated prn
      2) Maintenance (individualized dosage): Chlordiazepoxide, 50 to 100 mg PO q4 to 6 h, lorazepam 2 mg PO q4h, or diazepam 5 to 10 mg PO tid; withhold doses or decrease subsequent doses if signs of oversedation are apparent
      3) Midazolam is also effective for managing DTs. Its rapid onset (sedation within 2 to 4 min of IV injection) and short duration of action (approximately 30 min) make it an ideal agent for titration in continuous infusion
   i. Treatment of seizures (as previously described)
   j. Diagnosis and treatment of concomitant medical, surgical, or psychiatric conditions

CHRONIC Rx

- See Table 3
- Pharmacotherapies for alcoholism include:
  1. Acamprosate is a synthetic compound with a chemical structure similar to the neurotransmitter γ-aminobutyric acid and the amino acid neuromodulator taurine. Its mechanism of action is not completely understood. It is indicated for the maintenance of abstinence from alcohol in patients with alcohol dependence who are abstinent at treatment initiation. It should be used only as part of a comprehensive psychosocial treatment program. It does not cause a disulfiram-like reaction as a result of ethanol ingestion. Dose is two 333-mg tablets tid. Treatment should be initiated as soon as possible after the period of alcohol withdrawal, when the patient has achieved abstinence, and should be maintained if the patient relapses. Avoid acamprosate if severe renal impairment is present.
  2. The long-acting opiate antagonist naltrexone inhibits the rewarding effects of alcohol. The starting dose is 25 mg/day, increased to 50 mg PO qd after 1 wk. An extended-release, once-monthly injection of naltrexone is also available and can be used along with psychosocial support to maintain alcohol abstinence. In patients with opioid dependence, naltrexone can precipitate acute withdrawal syndrome and should not be used at least 7 days from last opioid use. Avoid naltrexone if acute hepatitis, hepatic failure, or ongoing opioid use is present.
  3. Disulfiram (Antabuse): Dosage is 500 mg max qd for 1 to 2 wk, then 125 to 500 mg qd. It interferes with the metabolism of alcohol by inhibiting aldehyde dehydrogenase, causing an accumulation of acetaldehyde. It produces unpleasant symptoms (nausea, flushing, elevated blood pressure, headache, weakness) when alcohol is ingested. It is an older drug that is now rarely used.
  4. Topiramate, baclofen, or gabapentin can be offered as second line drugs; to patients with moderate to severe alcohol use disorder topiramate might be preferable.
  5. Avoid pharmacologic treatments in pregnant or breastfeeding women.

DISPOSITION

See "Referral."

REFERRAL

- To Alcoholics Anonymous or Adult Children of Alcoholics
- Family members to Al-Anon or Al-A-Teen
- Many cities have Salvation Army Adult Rehabilitation centers; all patients accepted, regardless of ability to pay

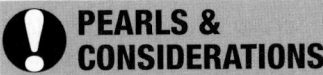

PEARLS & CONSIDERATIONS

COMMENTS

- Relative indications for inpatient alcohol detoxification are as follows: History of DT or withdrawal seizures, severe withdrawal symptoms, concomitant psychiatric or medical illness, pregnancy, multiple previous detoxifications, recent high levels of alcohol consumption, and lack of reliable support network.
- Detoxification is not a stand-alone treatment but should serve as a bridge to a formal treatment program for alcohol dependence.
- Acute management of alcohol withdrawal depends on the pattern of use and last drink.
- An effective strategy for the primary care physician is to screen patients for harmful alcohol use using scales and follow up the conversation with further exploration of stage of change in a nonjudgmental way.
- Alcohol-associated liver disease is among the most common liver diseases.

RELATED CONTENT

Alcohol Use Disorder (Patient Information)
Drug Use Disorder (Related Key Topic)
Alcoholic Hepatitis (Related Key Topic)
Substance Use Disorder (Related Key Topic)
Wernicke Syndrome (Related Key Topic)

AUTHORS: **FRANCISCO J. BARRERA, MD, SM** and **ASHIKA BAINS, MD, MS**

REFERENCES

Available at eBooks.Health.Elsevier.com

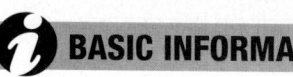
Diseases
and Disorders

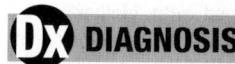 BASIC INFORMATION

DEFINITION

Dementia is a syndrome characterized by progressive loss of previously acquired cognitive skills, including memory, language, insight, and judgment. Alzheimer disease (AD) is thought to account for the majority of all cases of dementia.

ICD-10CM CODES
G30.0	Alzheimer disease with early onset
G30.1	Alzheimer disease with late onset
G30.8	Other Alzheimer disease
G30.9	Alzheimer disease, unspecified

EPIDEMIOLOGY & DEMOGRAPHICS

INCIDENCE: Risk doubles every 5 yr after the age of 65. The Chicago Health and Aging Population study found that the average annual incidence in people ages 65 and above was 2.3%, with Blacks having a significantly increased risk compared to Whites.[1]

PREVALENCE: Approximately 1/9 people (10.7%) ages ≥65 has Alzheimer dementia. Currently an estimated 6.5 million Americans have AD; 5% of the population between the ages of 65 and 74, 13.1% between 75 and 84, and 33.2% at ≥85 yr. Between 12% and 18% of Americans over age 60 are thought to have mild cognitive impairment (MCI).[2]

PREDOMINANT SEX: Females greater than males. In the U.S. 4 million women versus 2.5 million men are affected (12% of women, 9% of men ≥65).[2]

PHYSICAL FINDINGS & CLINICAL PRESENTATION
- Spouse or other family member, usually not the patient, notes insidious memory impairment.
- Patients have difficulties learning and retaining new information and handling complex tasks (e.g., balancing the checkbook) and have impairments in reasoning, judgment, spatial ability, and orientation (e.g., difficulty driving, getting lost away from home).
- Behavioral changes, such as mood changes and apathy, may accompany memory impairment. In later stages, patients may develop agitation and psychosis.
- Rare variants: Three rare variants are described and are discussed later:
  1. Posterior cortical atrophy
  2. Dysexecutive variant
  3. Logopenic progressive aphasia

(Dx) DIAGNOSIS

Diagnosis of AD has evolved with the development of biomarkers that indicate AD pathology in vivo such as brain amyloidosis and pathologic tau accumulation. The National Institute on Aging (NIA) and the Alzheimer Association (AA) recommended new diagnostic criteria and guidelines for AD in 2011, and these criteria were further revised in 2018 (Table 1). The NIA-AA criteria differed from prior DSM or NINDCS-ADRDA criteria in the following ways:

(1) They recommend AD be considered a disease well before the onset of symptoms by incorporating biomarkers in diagnosis, and (2) they define three distinct stages of AD: (1) *Preclinical* AD, in which there is measurable biologic evidence of AD pathology but no symptoms; (2) MCI due to AD, in which the patient experiences mild memory loss but experiences no functional impairment at home or work but demonstrates biomarker evidence of AD; and (3) *dementia* due to AD, in which the patient experiences cognitive decline causing functional impairment and demonstrates biomarker evidence of AD. The 2018 NIA-AA criteria define AD not as three clinical syndromes but as a biologic process defined by biomarkers indicating the presence of beta amyloid (A+), pathologic tau (T+), and neurodegeneration or neuronal injury (N+). Using the ATN system and clinical status together allows an entire study population to be characterized (Fig. 1).

Biomarkers have not been commonly used in the clinic but have invariably been used in AD clinical trials. However, with the advent of monoclonal antibodies targeting beta amyloid, biomarker-based diagnosis—especially in patients with early stage disease who may be eligible for new, disease modifying treatment—is becoming an important part of the diagnostic process. Biomarkers transform the diagnosis of AD into one that can be established definitively while the patient is still alive. In clinical practice, the diagnosis has been commonly made based on clinical history, a thorough physical and neurologic examination, and use of reliable and

TABLE 1 New Diagnostic Criteria

Criteria for Probable Alzheimer Disease	DSM-5 2013	NINCDS—ADRDA 2007	NIA-AA 2018
		RESEARCH CRITERIA	
Insidious onset	X	X	X
Onset over months to years		X	X
Progressive decline	X	X	X
Deficits are not explained by delirium or other medical or psychiatric conditions	X	X	X
Social/occupational impairment	X		X
Presence of episodic memory deficit	X	X	
Cognitive deficits in at least two domains	X		X
Neuropsychologic testing required for diagnosis?	Preferably	X	Only if routine history and mental status testing are inconclusive
Abnormal PET or MRI scan		Supportive feature*	Required if needed to show biomarker evidence of amyloidosis, tauopathy, neurodegeneration as part of the biomarker-based AT(N) diagnostic schema
Genetic markers?	X	Supportive feature*	For research purposes
	Required only if there is evidence of multiple causes and no clear evidence of progression and decline in memory and another cognitive domain		
Abnormal cerebrospinal fluid marker required?		Supportive feature*	Required if needed to show biomarker evidence of amyloidosis, tauopathy, neurodegeneration as part of the biomarker-based AT(N) diagnostic schema

DSM-5, Diagnostic and Statistical Manual of Mental Disorders, fifth edition; *MRI,* magnetic resonance imaging; *NIA-AA,* National Institute on Aging–Alzheimer's Association; *NINCDS-ADRDA,* National Institute of Neurological and Communicative Disorders and Stroke–Alzheimer's Disease and Related Disorders Association; *PET,* positron emission tomography.
*At least one supportive feature is required for diagnosis of probable AD.
Modified from Fillit HM: *Brocklehurst's textbook of geriatric medicine and gerontology,* ed 8, Philadelphia, 2017, Elsevier.

Biomarker Profile		Cognitive Stage		
		Cognitively Unimpaired	**Mild Cognitive Impairment**	**Dementia**
	A⁻ T⁻ (N)⁻	normal AD biomarkers, cognitively unimpaired	normal AD biomarkers with MCI	normal AD biomarkers with dementia
	A⁺ T⁻ (N)⁻	Preclinical Alzheimer pathologic change	Alzheimer pathologic change with MCI	Alzheimer pathologic change with dementia
	A⁺ T⁺ (N)⁻ / A⁺ T⁺ (N)⁺	Preclinical Alzheimer disease	Alzheimer disease with MCI (Prodromal AD)	Alzheimer disease with dementia
	A⁺ T⁻ (N)⁺	Alzheimer and concomitant suspected non-Alzheimer pathologic change, cognitively unimpaired	Alzheimer and concomitant suspected non-Alzheimer pathologic change with MCI	Alzheimer and concomitant suspected non-Alzheimer pathologic change with dementia
	A⁻ T⁺ (N)⁻ / A⁻ T⁻ (N)⁺ / A⁻ T⁺ (N)⁺	non-Alzheimer pathologic change, cognitively unimpaired	non-Alzheimer pathologic change with MCI	non-Alzheimer pathologic change with dementia

FIG. 1 Descriptive nomenclature: Syndromal cognitive staging combined with biomarkers. *AD,* Alzheimer disease; *MCI,* mild cognitive impairment. NOTE: Formatting denotes three general biomarker "categories" based on biomarker profiles: Those with normal AD biomarkers *(no color)*, those with non-AD pathologic change *(dark gray)*, and those who are in the Alzheimer continuum *(light gray)*. (From Clifford RJ Jr et al: NIA-AA research framework: toward a biological definition of Alzheimer's disease, *Alzheimer Dement* 14:535-562, 2018.)

BOX 1 Red Flags for an Alzheimer Disease Diagnosis

- Age <65yr
- Fluctuating level of consciousness (consider toxic-metabolic encephalopathy, dementia with Lewy bodies)
- Behavioral, emotional, or personality disturbances overshadowing cognitive impairment (consider frontotemporal dementia, HIV dementia)
- Rapidly (6-12 mo) progressive development (consider Creutzfeldt–Jakob disease, paraneoplastic limbic encephalitis, autoimmune encephalitis, HIV dementia, frontotemporal dementia)
- Presence of physical abnormalities:
  1. Gait impairment (consider vascular dementia, HIV dementia, NPH, chronic subdural hematomas, Parkinson disease and atypical Parkinsonian disorders)
  2. Lateralized signs, e.g., hemiparesis, spasticity, other corticospinal tract signs (consider vascular dementia)
  3. Movement disorders
  4. Myoclonus (consider Creutzfeldt–Jakob disease, paraneoplastic encephalitis)
  5. Rigidity, bradykinesia (parkinsonism) (consider dementia with Lewy bodies and Parkinson disease)

Modified from Kaufman DM et al: *Kaufman's clinical neurology for psychiatrists,* ed 9, Philadelphia 2023, Elsevier.

---

valid diagnostic criteria (i.e., DSM or NINDCS-ADRDA) such as the following:
- Loss of memory and one or more additional cognitive abilities (aphasia, apraxia, agnosia, or other disturbance in executive functioning)
- Impairment in social or occupational functioning that represents a decline from a previous level of functioning and results in significant disability
- Deficits that do not occur exclusively during the course of delirium
- Insidious onset and gradual progression of symptoms
- Cognitive loss documented by neuropsychologic tests
- No physical signs, neuroimaging, or laboratory evidence of other diseases that can cause dementia (i.e., metabolic abnormalities, medication or toxin effects, infection, stroke, Parkinson disease, subdural hematoma, or tumors)

Red flags for an AD diagnosis are summarized in Box 1.

DIFFERENTIAL DIAGNOSIS (TABLE 2)
- Other neurodegenerative dementia (Table 3):
  1. Primary age-related tauopathy
  2. Limbic predominant age-related TDP-43 encephalopathy (LATE)
  3. Argyrophilic grain disease
  4. Frontotemporal lobar degeneration
  5. Dementia with Lewy bodies
  6. Parkinson disease dementia
  7. Corticobasal syndrome
  8. Progressive supranuclear palsy
- Vascular cognitive impairment disorder (vascular dementia due to multiple strokes, severe small vessel changes, chronic vasculitis, or chronic subdural hematoma)
- Subjective memory loss
- Depression (pseudodementia) (Table 4)
- Neoplasm (benign or malignant brain tumor, leptomeningeal disease)
- Infection (HIV-associated dementia, neurosyphilis, progressive multifocal leukoencephalopathy [PML])
- Toxic/metabolic (EtOH, myxedema coma, subacute combined degeneration, pellagra, mercury exposure, drug effects)
- Organ failure (hepatic encephalopathy)

WORKUP
HISTORY & GENERAL PHYSICAL EXAMINATION:
- Medication lists should always be reviewed for drugs or home remedies that may cause mental status changes, especially anticholinergic medications, benzodiazepines, opiates, barbiturates, and neuroleptics.
- Patients should be screened for depression, because it can sometimes mimic dementia but often occurs as a coexisting condition and should be treated.
- On examination, look for signs of metabolic disturbance, presence of psychiatric features, or focal neurologic deficits.
- Symptoms and preserved abilities of Alzheimer dementia by disease stage are summarized in Table 5.

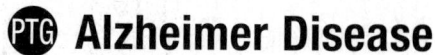
TABLE 2   Cognitive Disorders in Older Adults

Diagnosis (% of Dementias Attributable)	History	Physical Examination Findings	Imaging Findings	Comment
Normal aging changes (n/a)	Delayed retrieval (forgetting names, dates), slower processing (takes longer to learn new things). No functional limitations	None	Mild generalized cortical atrophy, mild ventricular enlargement. No focal findings	Patients may have white matter disease and/or prior lacunar infarcts related to HTN, DM, and cardiovascular disease, etc., but unrelated to memory complaints
Mild cognitive impairment (n/a)	Cognitive deficits beyond what is expected for age across one or more domains	None	Variable depending on etiology. Atrophy of medial temporal lobe and/or hippocampus (pre-Alzheimer disease)	Clinical course highly dependent on etiology. Amnestic MCI most likely to progress to dementia (50%) Neuropsychologic testing may help to clarify diagnosis
Alzheimer disease (67%)	Progressive memory loss and other cognitive deficits	Essentially normal in early stages Moderate: Patients may develop apraxia, aphasia	Medial temporal, parietal lobe, and/or hippocampal atrophy on MRI. Positivity on amyloid PET scan	Patients will occasionally present with unusual variants based on atypical neuroanatomic pathology; for example, fixed delusions or behavioral manifestations (dysexecutive variant) or prominent visual symptoms (posterior cortical atrophy)
Vascular dementia (20%, includes mixed dementia)	Prominent vascular risk factors, possible history of stroke/TIA, possible stepwise disease progression. Executive dysfunction may be prominent early symptom	Variable depending on distribution of disease	Cortical and subcortical infarcts and white matter disease	Commonly present in conjunction with Alzheimer disease— known as mixed dementia
Lewy body dementia and Parkinson dementia (15%)	Fluctuating cognition, well-formed visual hallucinations, REM sleep disorder, falls, sensitivity to neuroleptics	Orthostatic hypotension, postural instability, hyposmia, bradykinesia, resting tremor, rigidity	No specific findings on MRI. Positivity on dopamine transporter PET scan	Parkinson dementia occurs in patients with preexisting Parkinson disease of at least 1-yr duration, followed by onset of cognitive deficits
Frontotemporal dementia (<5%)	Two variants: Behavioral variant (50%) presents with progressive personality and behavioral changes Primary progressive aphasia presents with progressive language impairment	Frontal release signs	Frontal and temporal lobe atrophy	Executive function and episodic memory generally preserved in early stages of disease
Chronic traumatic encephalopathy (CTE, unknown)	History of multiple concussions and/or traumatic brain injury, most commonly in former athletes or military personnel. Concurrent behavioral changes and psychiatric disease common	None	Nonspecific white matter changes	Tauopathy in cortical and perivascular regions of the brain. CTE can only definitely be diagnosed by autopsy; there is currently no definitive clinical criteria for diagnosis
Rapidly progressive dementia (<1%)	Memory symptoms progressive over weeks to months	Variable depending on etiology Myoclonus/startle reflex suggestive of prion disease	Variable depending on etiology	Rapidly progressive dementias are rare and merit urgent referral to a neurologist Specialized testing should be based on patient-specific risk factors
Delirium (n/a)	Identifiable toxic, metabolic, or infectious etiology and/or precipitants (e.g., acute hospital admission). Rapid onset	Inattention, disorganized thinking, and/or altered level of consciousness. Fluctuating course	No specific findings	EEG will demonstrate acute slowing Generally reversible with correction of precipitant(s)

DM, Diabetes mellitus; *EEG,* electroencephalogram; *HTN,* hypertension; *MCI,* mild cognitive impairment; *MRI,* magnetic resonance imaging; *PET,* positron emission tomography; *REM,* rapid eye movement; *TIA,* transient ischemic attack.

From Warshaw G et al: *Ham's primary care geriatrics,* ed 7, Philadelphia, 2022, Elsevier.

TABLE 3 Features Distinguishing Alzheimer Disease and Frontotemporal Dementia

Feature	Alzheimer Disease	Frontotemporal Dementia
Age at onset (yr)	>65	53 (mean)
Memory impairments	Early, pronounced	Subtle, at least initially, with preserved visuospatial ability
Behavior abnormalities	None until middle or late stage	Early and prominent perseverative and compulsive behavior; hyperorality; impaired executive ability
Language impairment	Except for anomia, none until late stage	Paraphasias, anomia, decreased fluency
CT/MRI appearance	General atrophy, but especially parietal and temporal lobes	Frontal and temporal lobe atrophy
Histologic marker	Aβ accumulation	Tau accumulation

CT, Computed tomography; MRI, magnetic resonance imaging.
From Kaufman DM et al: Kaufman's clinical neurology for psychiatrists, ed 9, Philadelphia, 2023, Elsevier.

TABLE 4 Clinical Features of Delirium, Depression, and Alzheimer's Disease

	Delirium	Depression	Alzheimer's Disease
Onset of initial symptoms	Abrupt	Relatively discrete	Insidious
	Difficulty with attention and disturbed consciousness	Dysphoric mood or lack of pleasure	Memory deficits—verbal and/or spatial
Course	Fluctuating—over days to weeks	Persistent—usually lasting months if untreated	Gradually progressive, over years
Family history	Not contributory	May be positive for depression	May be positive for AD
Memory	Poor registration	Patchy/inconsistent	Recent > remote
Memory complaints	Absent	Present	Variable—usually absent
Language deficits	Dysgraphia	Increased speech latency	Confrontation naming difficulties
Affect	Labile	Depressed/irritable	Variable—may be neutral

From Stern TA: Massachusetts General Hospital handbook of general hospital psychiatry, ed 7, Philadelphia, 2018, Elsevier.

MENTAL STATUS TESTING: Brief mental status testing can be done easily and quickly in the office. Formal neuropsychologic testing offers more nuanced data about a patient's current cognitive and emotional function but is not required for straightforward cases. Formal neuropsychologic testing is indicated when patients present with atypical symptoms, have significant psychiatric comorbidities, and when patients' or families' report of cognitive dysfunction differs from findings on a bedside cognitive assessment. Also, neuropsychologic testing may be beneficial if there are concerns that in the future, the patient's testamentary capacity will be challenged.

Commonly used cognitive tests to detect dementia include the Folstein Mini-Mental State Examination (MMSE), the Mini-Cog test, and the Montreal Cognitive Assessment. A newer self-administered gerocognitive examination (SAGE) which patients complete by themselves, usually in 15 minutes is now available and consists of a validated 11-item instrument that compares favorably with MMSE and has the advantage of self-administration at home.[3] A meta-analysis examining the performance of commonly used screening tests for dementia identified 11 commonly used tests, with the MMSE having the most data. The combined sensitivity and specificity for detecting dementia were 0.81 and 0.89, respectively, for the MMSE and 0.91 and 0.86, respectively, for the Mini-Cog. Subgroup analysis revealed that only the Montreal Cognitive Assessment had comparable performance to the MMSE for detecting MCI with 0.89 sensitivity and 0.75 specificity.

The Mini-Cog (https://mini-cog.com/) is a 3-min instrument consisting of a 3-item recall test for memory and a simply scored clock drawing test. The Montreal Cognitive Assessment (MoCA, www.mocatest.org/) is a 30-point test that takes approximately 10 min to administer and includes tests of visuospatial function, attention, verbal recall, language, abstraction, and orientation. A score of 25 points or less (26 points if the patient has <12 yr of education) indicates cognitive impairment. The test is available in >35 languages, and multiple forms in English allow for repeated assessments over time. A summary of commonly used tests may be found in Table E6.

Mental status testing should include tests that assess the following cognitive functions:

- Orientation: Ask the patient to give the day, date, month, year, and place and to name the current president.
- Attention: Ask the patient to recite the months of the year forward and in reverse.
- Verbal recall: Ask the patient to remember three items; test for recall after a 1- and 5-min delay.
- Language: Ask the patient to write and then read a sentence; have the patient name both common and less common objects.
- Visuospatial: Ask the patient to draw a clock and to set the hands of the clock at 11:10.

Patients with AD typically have trouble with verbal recall in addition to experiencing visuospatial or language deficits. Attention is usually preserved until the later stages of AD, so consider alternative diagnoses in patients who perform poorly on tests of attention early in their disease. A summary of the pattern of cognitive deficits associated with different dementias and depression may be found in Table 7.

In addition to the common amnestic presentation, AD rarely presents as one of three rare nonamnestic syndromes that affect memory later in the course of the disease. These three rare presentations should also raise suspicion of another dementia type. A primary language variant presents as either logopenic expressive aphasia or progressive nonfluent aphasia and may be either a form of AD or of frontotemporal lobar degeneration. A primary visuospatial variant called posterior cortical atrophy presents with disturbances in complex visual processing and may be a form of either AD or dementia with Lewy bodies. An executive/behavioral variant presents with impaired executive function and/or behavior derangement and may represent either a frontal variant of AD or behavioral variant frontotemporal dementia.

LABORATORY TESTS (TABLE 8)
- CBC
- Serum electrolytes
- Glucose
- Blood urea nitrogen/creatinine
- Liver and thyroid function tests
- Serum vitamin B_{12}
- Syphilis serology (rapid plasma reagin [RPR]), if supported by clinical history
- HIV screening as appropriate
- Lumbar puncture if history or signs of cancer, infectious process, or unusual clinical presentation (e.g., rapid progression of symptoms)

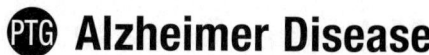
TABLE 5 Symptoms and Preserved Abilities of Alzheimer Dementia by Disease Stage Symptoms and Preserved Abilities by Cognitive Domain Across Various Stages of Alzheimer Dementia

	Mild	Moderate	Severe
Memory			
Symptoms	• Loss of short-term memory; may recall some aspects of important events • May lose enjoyment in reading because of difficulty following a story line	• Forgets entire events have occurred, some long-term memories remain • Repetitive questioning may become troublesome for caregivers	• Complete loss of short-term memory • May not recognize familiar individuals • Long-term memories fade
Preserved abilities	• May benefit from simple reminders, routines, and habits • May still derive enjoyment from reminiscing	• May still enjoy reminiscing with the assistance of visual or verbal stimulation	• Implicit memory may still be preserved • Familiar environments and persons may be comforting
Executive Function			
Symptoms	• Difficulty acting on desired goals, resulting in irritation • Judgment may be poor • Social graces may suffer • May demonstrate anhedonia or apathy	• Problem-solving ability very limited • Angry outbursts • Impulsive • Difficulty in new situations • Requires reminders or physical support to complete ADLs	• Requires assistance with all ADLs • Cannot independently set goals or act upon them • Gradual loss of motor abilities, including dysphagia
Preserved abilities	• Decision-making capacity is likely to be intact • Comprehension may increase if information presentation is adapted	• Capacity for simple, every-day decision making may be preserved, even if capacity for complex decision making is lost	
Language and Communication			
Symptoms	• Some word-finding difficulties	• More pronounced difficulty understanding written or spoken language • Difficulty making needs known	• Gradual loss of speech
Preserved abilities	• Can engage in conversations, but may require environmental supports, such as those recommended by speech and language pathologists		• Ability to communicate needs nonverbally through emotional expression or other cues (e.g., grimacing to indicate pain)
Sensory/Perceptual			
Symptoms	• Difficulty with interpreting complex visual figures or displays	• May develop hallucinations or delusions	• May react poorly to noxious stimulation from the environment
Preserved abilities	• Ability to follow and enjoy simplified visual displays		• May enjoy individually enhanced sensory environments • Tactile stimulation may be preferable to auditory or visual
	• May respond positively to interventions, such as personalized music		

ADLs, Activities of daily living.
From Warshaw G et al: *Ham's primary care geriatrics,* ed 7, Philadelphia, 2022, Elsevier.

• Electroencephalogram (EEG) if there is history of seizures, episodic confusion, rapid clinical decline, or suspicion of Creutzfeldt-Jakob disease
• Apolipoprotein E genotyping, measurement of CSF tau, and amyloid and functional imaging including positron emission tomography (PET [Fig E2]), single-photon emission computed tomography (SPECT), amyloid PET imaging, and tau PET imaging are not yet routinely used outside of clinical trials because insurers generally do not pay for these tests
• Brain biopsy is usually reserved for diagnoses such as prion disease and cerebral vasculitis. Generally performed postmortem

IMAGING STUDIES

• MRI (Fig. E3) to rule out hydrocephalus, cerebrovascular disease, and mass lesions, including subdural hematoma and to look for typical patterns of neurodegeneration (i.e., regional brain atrophy) such as hippocampal atrophy. CT can be used if MRI is contraindicated.

• Amyloid PET: The FDA has approved several agents for beta-amyloid PET imaging, including florbetapir, flutemetamol, and florbetaben. As with these other imaging agents, a positive amyloid scan does not establish a diagnosis of AD or any other cognitive disorder, but a negative scan indicating sparse to no amyloid plaques is inconsistent with a neuropathologic diagnosis of AD. A positive amyloid scan indicates the presence of moderate to frequent amyloid neuritic plaques; neuropathologic examination has shown this amount of amyloid plaque is present in AD patients but may also be present in individuals with other types of neurologic conditions as well as in cognitively normal older adults.
• Tau PET: The FDA has approved one agent for tau imaging: Flortaucipir. Flortaucipir is used to estimate the density and distribution of aggregated tau neurofibrillary tangles in adult patients with cognitive impairment under evaluation for AD. It is not indicated for use in patients undergoing evaluation for

chronic traumatic encephalopathy, which is also a tauopathy.

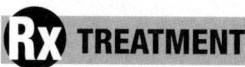 **TREATMENT**

NONPHARMACOLOGIC THERAPY

• Patient safety, including risks associated with impaired driving, wandering behavior, leaving stoves unattended, and accidents, must be addressed with the patient and family early and appropriate measures implemented.
• Wandering, hoarding, or hiding objects, repetitive questioning, withdrawal, and social inappropriateness often respond to behavioral therapies.
• Cognitive stimulation programs are beneficial for maintenance of cognitive function and improved self-reported quality of life in patients with mild to moderate AD.
• Person-centered care approach applied to care of people living with dementia is summarized in Table 9.

ACUTE GENERAL Rx

None

TABLE 7 Patterns of Cognitive Impairment by Domain and Dementia

	Episodic Memory	Attention	Language	Executive	Visuospatial		Behavioral Symptoms
Alzheimer disease	(I)		Simple (P) Divided (I)	Phonemic (P) Semantic (I) Naming (I)	(I)	Simple (P) Complex (I)	Early apathy, late psychotic symptoms
Mild cognitive impairment—amnestic	Immediate and Delayed recall (I) Recognition (I)		Simple (P) Divided (P)	(P)	(P)	(P)	(P)
Vascular dementia	Immediate and Delayed recall (V) Recognition (P)		Simple (P) Divided (I)	(I)	(I)	(P)	Depression
Behavioral variant FTLD	(V)		Simple (P) Divided (I)	(I)	(I)	(P)	Disinhibition, apathy, hyperorality, inappropriate social interaction
Semantic variant PPA	(P)		(P)	(I) Comprehension (I) Fluency	(P)	(P)(I) Visual agnosia	(P)
Nonfluent variant PPA	(P)		(P)	(I) Fluency (P) Comprehension, (I) Expressive speech	(P)	(P)	(P)
Parkinson disease dementia	(V) Immediate and Delayed recall (P) Recognition		(I)	(P)	(I)	(I)	Depression, possible hallucinations, psychomotor slowing
Dementia with Lewy bodies	(V) Immediate and Delayed recall (P) Recognition		(V)	(V)	(I)	(I)	Hallucinations, delusions
Depression	(V) Immediate and Delayed recall (P) Recognition		(V)	(V) Fluency (P) Naming	I/V	(P)	Psychomotor slowing, apathy

FTLD, Frontotemporal lobar degeneration; *I,* impaired; *P,* preserved; *PPA,* primary progressive aphasia; *V,* variable.
From Fillit HM: *Brocklehurst's textbook of geriatric medicine and gerontology,* ed 8, Philadelphia, 2017, Elsevier.

TABLE 8 Laboratory Evaluation of Patients with Dementia

Type of Study	Examples
Basic studies, excluding reversible with specific indication from history for causes of dementia or examination	• Complete blood count (CBC) • Chemistry or metabolic panel (SM-17) • Thyroid function tests (thyroid-stimulating hormone [TSH]) • Vitamin B_{12}, folate levels • Computed tomography (CT) or magnetic resonance imaging (MRI) • HIV testing • Sedimentation rate • Hemoglobin A1C (HbA1C) • Urinalysis • Chest x-ray • Urine or plasma for drugs or heavy metals
Adjuvant Studies to Aid Diagnosis	
Other tests as indicated by history or physical or neurologic examination	• Single-photon emission computed tomography (SPECT) • Positron emission tomography (PET) • Lumbar puncture with cerebrospinal fluid for β-amyloid

From Fillit HM: *Brocklehurst's textbook of geriatric medicine and gerontology,* ed 8, Philadelphia, 2017, Elsevier.

CHRONIC Rx

- Symptomatic treatment of memory disturbance (Table 10):
  1. Cholinesterase inhibitors (ChEIs [Table 11]): Donepezil (Aricept), galantamine (Razadyne), and rivastigmine (Exelon)
     a. FDA approved for the treatment of mild to moderate AD with the exception of donepezil, which is approved for mild, moderate, and severe dementia. Common side effects include vivid dreams, bradycardia, and GI side effects (nausea, diarrhea, and anorexia). GI side effects may be bothersome enough to require either a slower escalation of dosage or switching to another agent. The rivastigmine patch has lower rates of GI side effects than the oral agents. Table 12 summarizes some instruments used to monitor clinical response of AD to pharmacologic therapy.
  2. NMDA receptor antagonist: Memantine (Namenda)
     a. FDA approved for the treatment of moderate to severe AD. Common side effects include constipation, dizziness, or headache. Memantine is contraindicated in patients with renal insufficiency or history of seizures.
  3. Anti-amyloid monoclonal antibodies:
     a. Aducanumab (Aduhelm): Aducanumab was the first FDA-approved human immunoglobulin G1 (IgG1) monoclonal antibody targeting beta-amyloid. It targets aggravated forms of amyloid beta protein that accumulate in the brain of patients with AD. It is FDA-approved for MCI due to AD and mild dementia due to AD, and its approval was marked by controversy.
     b. Lecanemab is the second anti-amyloid monoclonal antibody approved by the FDA. It is a humanized IgG1 monoclonal antibody that binds to A β soluble protofibrils. It is also indicated for individuals with MCI due to AD and early dementia due to AD. Trials have shown that Lecanemab reduces markers of amyloid in early Alzheimer disease and results in moderately less decline on measures of cognition and function than placebo.[4]
     c. Anti-amyloid monoclonal antibodies can result in a potentially serious side effect called amyloid related imaging abnormalities (ARIA). ARIA can take two forms, ARIA-E (edema) and ARIA-H (hemosiderin deposition).
  4. ARIA-E is diagnosed when the MRI demonstrates focal cerebral vasogenic edema or sulcal effusions.
  5. ARIA-H is diagnosed with the development of microhemorrhage and/or superficial siderosis.

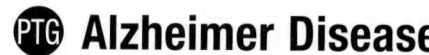
TABLE 9 Person-Centered Care Approach Applied to Care of People Living with Dementia

Key Component	Early Stage	Middle Stage	Late Stage
Develop a personalized, goal-oriented care plan, based on a thorough medical, functional, and social assessment	• Conduct a functional assessment, including sensory status, language abilities • Establish stage-appropriate, personally meaningful goals • Encourage advance care planning, including naming a surrogate decision maker • Discuss advantages and disadvantages of pharmacotherapy to help with cognitive or behavioral symptoms and monitor regularly for side effects		• Engage with family members and surrogate decision makers to interpret patient's nonverbal communication • If on ChE-I, consider discontinuation
Periodically review the person's goals and care plan to assess ongoing effectiveness and to address evolving goals	• Refer to community resources to promote the person's ongoing connection with and engagement in personally meaningful activities • Assess and address caregiver stress • Consider referral to senior centers or adult day programs to promote social engagement • In-home care services may be helpful		• Personalized music programs may be helpful • Hospice consultation may be indicated
Engage an interprofessional team that adapts its composition in response to the needs of the person living with dementia	• Care managers to refer to resources in community • SLP referral to teach caregivers supported communication approaches • PT/OT: In-home safety evaluation and customization of activities • Pharmacy to assist with deprescribing and simplification of medication regimen • Specialty referrals (psychiatry, dementia care clinics) for management of BPSD	• Care managers: Assist with symptom management, respite services • SLP consultation for assistance with supported communication approaches and feeding techniques • OT consultation to maximize functional independence	• Care managers: Assistance managing symptoms, referral for respite services • Palliative care or hospice consultation for symptom management and end-of-life care • OT sensory stimulation approaches to promote wellbeing
A specified team leader to facilitate information transfer, care coordination, and continuity	• Primary care provider or specialty-trained care manager, such as nurse specialist or social worker	• Primary care provider or specialty-trained care manager	• Primary care provider or hospice team

BPSD, Behavioral and psychologic symptoms of dementia; *CHe-I,* acetylcholinesterase inhibitors; *OT,* occupational therapy; *PT,* physical therapy; *SLP,* speech language pathology.
From Warshaw G et al: *Ham's primary care geriatrics,* ed 7, Philadelphia, 2022, Elsevier.

TABLE 10 Symptomatic Treatment of Memory Disturbance

	Initial Dose	Target Dose
Donepezil	5 mg qd for 4-6 wk	10 mg qd
Rivastigmine	1.5 mg bid with food, increase by 1.5 mg bid weekly	3-6 mg bid
Galantamine	4 mg bid with food, increase by 4 mg bid every 4 wk	8-12 mg bid
Memantine	5 mg qd, increase by 5 mg weekly	10 mg bid

bid, Twice daily; *qd,* once daily.

TABLE 11 Acetylcholinesterase Inhibitor Dosing

Drug	Initial Dose	Recommended Dose	Minimum Therapeutic Dose	Formulations
Donepezil	5 mg daily	10 mg daily	5 mg daily	5, 10, 23 mg
Galantamine IR	4 mg bid	12 mg bid	8 mg bid	4, 8, 12 mg
Galantamine ER	8 mg daily	24 mg daily	16 mg daily	8, 12, 24 mg
Rivastigmine	1.5 mg bid	6 mg bid	3 mg bid	1.5, 3, 4.5, 6 mg
Rivastigmine patch	4.6 mg daily	9.5 mg daily	9.5 mg daily	4.6, 9.5, 13.3 mg

bid, Twice daily.
Acetylcholinesterase inhibitor dosing and suggested titration intervals. From US Department of Veterans Affairs. *Pharmacy Benefits Management Services.* 2018 [cited October 15, 2019]. Available at: http://www.pbm.va.gov/. Note that medication doses can be increased every 4 wk as patient tolerates.
From Warshaw G et al: *Ham's primary care geriatrics,* ed 7, Philadelphia, 2022, Elsevier.

6. ARIA may be mild, moderate, or severe. Even severe ARIA may be asymptomatic.
7. Prescribing anti-amyloid monoclonal antibodies requires demonstrating the presence of amyloidosis using either CFS or amyloid PET. A baseline MRI is also required. ARIA usually occurs early in administration, and an MRI monitoring protocol must be used with this class of medication. Given the complexity of this medication and the restrictions surrounding Medicare reimbursement for these medications, patients should be referred to special centers with established protocols for the safe administration and monitoring of this medication.
• Symptomatic treatment of neuropsychiatric and behavioral disturbances (Table 13).
1. Depression, agitation, delusions, or hallucinations may respond to medications.

Brexpiprazole, a second generation antipsychotic drug was recently FDA approved for once daily treatment of agitation associated with dementia due to AD. It provides modest improvements in agitation symptoms but can cause serious adverse effects. It has not been compared with older second generation antipsychotic drugs that are available generically and have been used off label for many

Diseases and Disorders

I

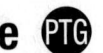

TABLE 12 Instruments Used to Monitor Clinical Response of Alzheimer Disease (AD) to Pharmacologic Therapy

Mini-Mental State Examination
- Global measure of cognition widely used by physicians and third-party caregivers
- Assesses orientation, registration, recall, language, and attention
- Uses a 30-point scale
- Requires ≈5-10 min to complete
- Sensitivity, 80%-90%; specificity, 80%
- Administered by psychometricians, nurses, and physicians
- AD typically advances by 3 points/yr

Clock Drawing
- Global measure of cognition widely used by physicians
- Multiple scoring systems with proven validity; sensitivity, 59%; specificity, 90%
- Assesses multiple cognitive domains in a single test
- 1-2 min to complete
- Minimal training to administer

Geriatric Depression Scale
- Evaluates depressive symptoms in patients
- Requires 5 min to complete
- Very useful in assessing depression in new patients and in follow-up
- Minimal training to administer
- Ease of administration has led to rapid spread in its use

From Fillit HM: *Brocklehurst's textbook of geriatric medicine and gerontology*, ed 8, Philadelphia, 2017, Elsevier.

TABLE 13 Treatment of Behavioral and Neuropsychiatric Symptoms

	Initial Dose	Maximum Dose
Atypical Antipsychotics		
Olanzapine	2.5 mg qd to bid, may increase by 2.5 mg as needed	7.5 mg bid
Quetiapine	25 mg bid, may increase by 25 mg every 2 days	250 mg tid
Antidepressants		
Sertraline	25-50 mg qd, may increase by 25 mg every wk	200 mg qd
Escitalopram	10 mg qd, may increase after 1 wk to 20 mg qd	10 mg qd

bid, Twice daily; *qd,* once a day.

years (Table 13). Nonpharmacologic treatments should always be tried first.
- A recent review and meta-analysis of cholinesterase inhibitors, memantine, and supplements determined that cholinesterase inhibitors and memantine slightly reduced short-term cognitive decline, and cholinesterase inhibitors slightly reduced reported functional decline, but differences versus placebo were of uncertain clinical importance. Evidence was mostly insufficient on drug treatment of behavioral and psychologic symptoms of dementia and on supplements for all outcomes.

DISPOSITION & REFERRAL
- Patients with complex or atypical presentations or challenging management issues should be referred to a neurologist, geriatric psychiatrist, or geriatrician with expertise in dementia.
- Patients early in the disease process who may be eligible for anti-amyloid monoclonal antibodies should be referred to a center with experience with these new drugs.
- Approximately one in eight hospitalized patients with AD who develop delirium will have at least one adverse outcome (e.g., institutionalization, cognitive decline, death) associated with delirium.

- Family education and support may help reduce need for skilled nursing facility and reduce caregiver stress, depression, and burnout.

PEARLS & CONSIDERATIONS

The physician should make a thorough search for the treatable causes of dementia. Current American Academy of Neurology practice parameters recommend:
- Treat cognitive symptoms of AD with ChEls.
- Treat depression.
- Treat agitation and psychosis using nonpharmacologic interventions first and use pharmacologic interventions at the lowest possible dose if other interventions have failed.
- Encourage caregivers to participate in educational programs and support groups.
In addition, refer patients with MCI or early AD to centers with experience with the new anti-amyloid monoclonal antibodies.

COMMENTS
- Ginkgo biloba is marketed widely as effective in delaying cognitive impairment; however, trials have shown that it is not effective in reducing the incidence of Alzheimer dementia or dementia overall.

- Higher midlife fitness levels seem to be associated with lower hazards of developing all-cause dementia later in life independent of cerebrovascular disease. Exercise also may slow the rate of functional deterioration in mild AD.
- Even moderate adherence to the MIND (the Mediterranean-DASH Intervention for Neurodegenerative Delay) diet, a hybrid of the Mediterranean and DASH diets specifically designed to optimize brain health, has been shown to reduce the incidence of AD.
- Strategies for prevention of dementia are summarized in Table 14.
- Antipsychotics should be used with extreme caution in treating dementia-related psychosis. All antipsychotics carry a warning from the FDA stating that the medication is not approved for dementia-related psychosis because elderly patients on either conventional or atypical antipsychotics experience an increased risk of death due to cardiovascular or infectious causes.
- Apolipoprotein E (APOE) is the main cholesterol-carrying molecule in the brain, and it exists in three allelic variants: E2, E3, and E4. The E3 allele is most common and has a neutral influence on developing AD, whereas the E2 allele, the rarest allele, may be protective against AD. The E4 allele increases the risk of developing AD and advances the age of first symptoms in those who experience the disease. However, neither E4 heterozygosity or homozygosity is required or sufficient to cause AD. Among Caucasians, E4 heterozygosity increases the risk of developing AD approximately threefold, whereas E4 homozygosity increases AD risk by approximately 15 times compared to the E3/E3 baseline. The APOE E4 allele is also associated with an earlier age of onset of AD. Because the benefits of genetic testing are often modest, and the tests themselves are often imprecise in identifying risk, the test is generally discouraged. Genes implicated in the development of AD are summarized in Table 15. Recent trials, however, reveal that the disclosure of APOE genotyping results to adult children of patients with AD did not result in significant short-term psychologic risks. Test-related distress was reduced among those who learned that they were *APOE4* negative. Persons with high levels of emotional distress before undergoing genetic testing are more likely to have emotional difficulties after disclosure.

For additional information for patients, families, and clinicians, contact the following organizations:
- Alzheimer's Association (http://www.alz.org/; 800-272-3900)
- Alzheimer's Disease Education and Referral Center (www.nia.nih.gov/Alzheimers; 800-438-4380)

REFERENCES
Available at eBooks.Health.Elsevier.com.

AUTHOR: **JOSEPH S. KASS, MD, JD, FAAN**

TABLE 14 Strategies for Prevention of Dementia

Recommendation	Quality of Evidence
Engage in physical activity	Moderate
In adults with **mild cognitive impairment,** engage in physical activity to slow cognitive decline	Low
Tobacco cessation	Low
Do not exceed maximum daily recommended amount of alcohol intake	Moderate[a]
Follow a healthy diet based on WHO recommendations[b]	Moderate[c]
Follow a Mediterranean diet	Moderate
Maintain a healthy weight	Low
Participate in cognitively stimulating activities or cognitive training	Low
Treatment of hypertension	High
Treatment of *diabetes mellitus*	Moderate
Treatment of dyslipidemia	Low

Strategies for Prevention of Dementia, as based on World Health Organization (WHO) 2019 Guidelines for Risk Reduction of Cognitive Impairment and Dementia.
[a]4 units of alcohol per wk for men, 7 units of alcohol per wk for women.
[b]Components include 5 daily servings of nonstarchy vegetables, <10% dietary intake of free sugars, <30% dietary intake of fats (preferentially unsaturated fats), <5 g daily of salt.
[c]Strength of evidence is variable based on individual dietary components.
From Warshaw G et al: *Ham's primary care geriatrics,* ed 7, Philadelphia, 2022, Elsevier.

TABLE 15 Genes Implicated in the Development of Alzheimer Disease

Gene	Comment
APP	>30 known mutations associated with EOAD; located on chromosome 21; associated with elevated risk of AD in Down syndrome
PSEN1	>150 known mutations associated with EOAD
PSEN2	<20 known mutations associated with EOAD
APOE	Three known alleles: • $\varepsilon 2$ – protective of LOAD • $\varepsilon 3$ – Neutral risk of LOAD • $\varepsilon 4$ – Increased risk of LOAD

AD, Alzheimer disease; *EOAD,* early-onset Alzheimer disease; *LOAD,* late-onset Alzheimer disease.
From Warshaw G et al: *Ham's primary care geriatrics,* ed 7, Philadelphia, 2022, Elsevier.

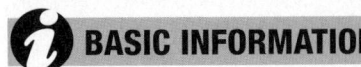 **BASIC INFORMATION**

DEFINITION

Amaurosis fugax is a temporary loss of monocular vision caused by transient retinal ischemia due to reversible occlusion within the ophthalmic artery or its branches. The ophthalmic artery is a branch of the internal carotid artery, and the central retinal artery is a branch of the ophthalmic artery.

ICD-10CM CODE	
G45.3	Amaurosis fugax

EPIDEMIOLOGY & DEMOGRAPHICS

INCIDENCE (IN U.S.): An uncommon but important presentation of carotid artery disease
PEAK INCIDENCE: Approximately 55 yr

PHYSICAL FINDINGS & CLINICAL PRESENTATION

- Onset is sudden, typically lasting seconds to minutes, and often accompanied by scotomas such as a shade or curtain being pulled over the front of the eye (usually downward).
- Vision loss can be complete, hemianopic, or quadratic.
- Acute stage: Cholesterol emboli may be seen in retinal artery (*Hollenhorst plaque*).

ETIOLOGY

- Usually embolic from either the internal carotid artery or the heart
- Cardiac embolus most commonly due to atrial fibrillation
- Internal carotid artery embolus will be apparent as carotid stenosis on carotid imaging such as computed tomography (CT) angiography, magnetic resonance (MR) angiography, or carotid ultrasound
- Giant cell arteritis (GCA) causing inflammation of retinal arteries
- Hyperviscosity syndromes, such as sickle cell disease, which causes ischemia in the vascular territory of the ophthalmic artery
- Hypercoagulable states
- Hypotension and resultant hypoperfusion due to cardiac failure, hypovolemia, reduced cardiac output from a dysrhythmia, or orthostatic hypotension
- Reversible cerebral vasoconstriction syndrome
- Idiopathic

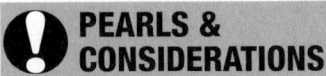 **DIAGNOSIS**

DIFFERENTIAL DIAGNOSIS

- Retinal migraine: In contrast to amaurosis, the onset of visual loss develops more slowly, usually over 15 to 20 min.
- Transient visual obscurations occur in the setting of papilledema due to elevated intracranial pressure; intermittent rises in intracranial pressure briefly compromise optic disc perfusion and cause transient visual loss lasting 1 to 2 sec. The episodes may be binocular. If the visual loss persists at the time of evaluation (i.e., vision has not yet recovered), then the differential diagnosis should be broadened to include:
  1. Anterior ischemic optic neuropathy: Arteritic (classically GCA) or nonarteritic
  2. Central retinal artery occlusion
  3. Branch retinal artery occlusion

WORKUP

- Workup should focus on embolic sources, but GCA should always be considered.
- Careful examination of retina; embolus may be visible and confirm the diagnosis (Fig. E1).
- Auscultation of arteries for carotid bruits.
- Examination of all pulses and for temporal artery tenderness.
- Inquire about symptoms of GCA (scalp tenderness, headache, fever, jaw claudication).
- Examine for signs of hemispheric stroke resulting from intracranial atherosclerosis (contralateral limb and facial weakness or sensory loss, aphasia, etc.).

LABORATORY TESTS

- CBC with erythrocyte sedimentation rate and C-reactive protein.
- Serum chemistries, including lipid profile and hemoglobin A1C.
- Cardiac enzymes and ECG.
- Hypercoagulable workup is discretionary based on younger age and history.

IMAGING STUDIES

- CT or MR angiography of head and neck preferred to examine carotid and intracranial vasculature. Carotid ultrasound if contraindication to MR or CT angiography.
- MRI of the brain with diffusion-weighted imaging to look for infarcts, especially those presenting with focal neurologic disturbances.
- Transthoracic echocardiography is indicated to screen for sources of emboli in patients with evidence of heart disease and in patients without an evident source for transient neurologic deficit. Transesophageal echocardiography is more sensitive for detecting cardiac sources of emboli (ventricular mural thrombus, atrial appendage, patent foramen ovale, aortic arch).
- Extended monitoring for atrial fibrillation if neither carotid stenosis nor GCA is found to be the etiology.

Rx **TREATMENT**

NONPHARMACOLOGIC THERAPY

- Diet (decrease saturated fatty acids and high-cholesterol foods)
- Exercise
- Cessation of tobacco use and illicit drug use

ACUTE GENERAL Rx

- Investigate as an emergency.
- Aspirin.
- If GCA is suspected, start prednisone and refer for temporal artery biopsy within 48 h (see "Giant Cell Arteritis" in Section I).

CHRONIC Rx

- Reduce risks by carotid endarterectomy if stenosis >50%. Carotid stenting may be performed in high-risk surgical candidates.
- Manage vascular risk factors such as hypertension, hyperlipidemia (statin therapy), diabetes, smoking cessation, etc.
- Antiplatelet therapy due to arterial atherosclerosis and postcarotid intervention; anticoagulation if etiology is atrial fibrillation.

DISPOSITION

Among patients with >50% carotid stenosis who do not undergo carotid endarterectomy, those who present with transient monocular blindness have an approximate 10% risk of stroke within 3 yr compared with an approximate 20% risk in patients who present with a hemispheric transient ischemic attack (TIA).

REFERRAL

- As with any TIA, emergent inpatient workup in a hospital that is a certified stroke center, if possible.
- If significant carotid stenosis, consider either carotid endarterectomy or carotid stenting for the following:
  1. Ipsilateral high-grade (≥70%) stenosis, but consider for ipsilateral stenosis of 50% to 69%
  2. Multiple TIAs despite medical therapy in the setting of high-grade or ulcerative disease

PEARLS & CONSIDERATIONS

- Cholesterol emboli in retinal arteries on fundoscopy confirm the diagnosis.
- Recognize that transient visual loss has multiple other causes.
- Refer to emergent evaluation like any other TIA.

RELATED CONTENT

Amaurosis Fugax (Patient Information)
Carotid Artery Stenosis (Related Key Topic)
Giant Cell Arteritis (Related Key Topic)
Transient Ischemic Attack (Related Key Topic)

AUTHORS: **NAOMI R. KASS, BA** and **JOSEPH S. KASS, MD, JD, FAAN**

BASIC INFORMATION

DEFINITION

Anaphylaxis is a severe allergic reaction that is rapid in onset and life-threatening. In anaphylaxis, immunoglobulin E (IgE)– and non–IgE-mediated systemic degranulation of mast cells causes respiratory, cardiovascular, GI, and/or mucocutaneous signs and symptoms.

SYNONYM

Anaphylactic reaction

ICD-10CM CODES

T78.2	Anaphylactic shock, unspecified, initial encounter
T78.00XA	Anaphylactic reaction due to unspecified food, initial encounter
T80.52XA	Anaphylactic reaction due to vaccination, initial encounter
T63.94XA	Toxic effect of contact with unspecified venomous animal, undetermined, initial encounter

EPIDEMIOLOGY & DEMOGRAPHICS

INCIDENCE: The incidence of anaphylaxis in the U.S. is 50 to 2000 episodes/100,000 persons with a lifetime prevalence of 1.6% to 5.1%. Incidence is on the rise with emergency department visits for anaphylaxis increasing by 101% between 2005 and 2014. Despite this increase, anaphylaxis-related fatalities remain stable at 0.7 per million adults/yr. Medications and insect stings are leading triggers in adults, whereas foods and insect stings are the leading triggers in children and adolescents.

Racial, economic (Box E1), and ethnic disparities exist in regard to anaphylaxis incidence and fatalities. In the United States, Black individuals have been found to have a higher risk of fatal food related anaphylaxis and worse outcomes when compared to White individuals.

RISK FACTORS: Atopy is a risk factor for anaphylaxis triggered by food, exercise, and latex. Risk factors for severe anaphylaxis include cardiovascular disease, asthma, older age, mast cell disorder, beta-blocker use, and ACE inhibitor use.

PHYSICAL FINDINGS & CLINICAL PRESENTATION (TABLE E1)

- Mucocutaneous: Urticaria, pruritus, skin flushing, angioedema (Table 2)
- Respiratory: Dyspnea, cough, wheezing, hypoxia, stridor, rhinitis
- Cardiovascular: Hypotension, tachycardia, weakness, dizziness, syncope, malaise, vascular collapse (Table 3)
- GI: Nausea, vomiting, diarrhea, dysphagia, abdominal pain

ETIOLOGY (BOX 2, TABLE E4)

Anaphylaxis results from a sudden systematic release of histamine and other inflammatory mediators from basophils and mast cells due to both IgE and non–IgE-mediated mechanisms. Virtually any substance may induce anaphylaxis.

In an acute setting, the cause of anaphylaxis is often unidentifiable (30% to 60% of cases):
- Foods and food additives: Peanuts, tree nuts, eggs, shellfish, fish, cow's milk, fruits, soy
  1. Alpha-1,3-galactose (alpha-gal): Lone star tick bite causes IgE sensitization to alpha-gal (carbohydrate moiety found in red meat) causing delayed anaphylaxis when consuming mammalian products
- Medications: Antibiotics (especially penicillins and sulfa-based agents), insulin, allergen extracts, opiates, vaccines, NSAIDs, contrast media, streptokinase, immunomodulators, intravenous (IV) iron
- Environmental exposures: Bee or wasp sting, snake venom, fire ant venom
- Blood products: Plasma, immunoglobulin, cryoprecipitate, whole blood
- Latex
- Exercise

Box 3 summarizes agents frequently associated with immune and nonimmune types of anaphylaxis.

DIAGNOSIS

DIFFERENTIAL DIAGNOSIS

- Allergic reaction
- Other causes of shock such as sepsis or pulmonary embolism
- Endocrine disorders (carcinoid, adrenal crisis, paradoxical pheochromocytoma)
- Systemic mastocytosis
- Serum sickness
- Severe asthma (the key clinical difference is the abrupt onset of symptoms in anaphylaxis vs. a history of progressive worsening of symptoms)
- Scombroid poisoning
- Localized angioedema
- Acute urticaria
- Presyncopal syndromes including vasovagal reactions
- Airway foreign body, vocal cord dysfunction
- Globus hystericus, anxiety disorder

WORKUP

Workup is aimed at ruling out other conditions that may mimic anaphylaxis. Given the potentially life-threatening nature of anaphylaxis, treatment should not be delayed. Clinical criteria for diagnosing anaphylaxis are summarized in Box 4.

LABORATORY TESTS

Laboratory evaluation is generally not helpful because anaphylaxis is a clinical diagnosis. Elevated serum and urine histamine levels and serum tryptase levels (measured 30 min to 2 h after symptom onset compared to baseline) can be useful for diagnosis of anaphylaxis, but the results of these tests are not usually available in the emergency setting and normal levels do not preclude the diagnosis.

IMAGING STUDIES

Are generally not helpful. Chest radiography for evaluation of foreign body aspiration or pulmonary pathology is indicated in patients with acute respiratory compromise. Consider ECG in all patients with sudden loss of consciousness or reports of chest pain or dyspnea and in any elderly patient. ECG in anaphylaxis usually reveals sinus tachycardia.

TREATMENT

NONPHARMACOLOGIC THERAPY

- Remove the trigger. Establish and protect airway. Provide supplemental O_2 if indicated.
- Rapidly establish IV access and administer IV fluids (i.e., normal saline).
- Cardiac monitoring is recommended.

ACUTE GENERAL Rx

- 0.3 to 0.5 mg intramuscular (IM) epinephrine (1:1000 concentration) should be rapidly administered for adults and children >30 kg in the anterolateral thigh. Any patient weighing over 50 kg should receive 0.5 mg IM. 0.01 mg/kg IM epinephrine (1:1000 concentration) should be administered for children <30 kg. IM administration is preferred because it provides more reliable and quicker rise to effective plasma levels. The dose may be repeated within minutes if symptoms do not improve.
- Adjunct therapies include histamine-1 H_1 and H_2 receptor antagonists such as diphenhydramine and famotidine. Although useful to improve cutaneous erythema and pruritus, H_1 antagonists are not effective in reversing upper airway obstruction, respiratory compromise, or hypotension and their onset of action is delayed 1 to 2 h.
- Corticosteroids are not useful in the acute episode because of their slow onset of action and have not been shown to decrease the risk of or prevent prolonged or biphasic anaphylaxis (recurrent anaphylaxis after complete improvement). Despite this they are commonly used in clinical practice and are considered secondary treatment.
- Vasopressor therapy with IV epinephrine (1:10,000 concentration) is indicated in patients with refractory hypotension/cardiovascular collapse despite crystalloid resuscitation and IM epinephrine. Small IV boluses of epinephrine can also be used in the periarrest state.
- Aerosolized β-agonists are useful to control bronchospasm.
- Patients taking β-blocking medications may be refractory to initial treatment; consider administration of IV glucagon.
- Treatment is the same in pregnant patients as specific recommendations in this population does not exist due to limited data. If hypotension is present, it is advised to lie the patient in the left lateral decubitus position to reduce compression on the vena cava.
- Table 5 summarizes drugs and other agents used in anaphylaxis therapy.
- Fig. E1 illustrates an algorithm for the management of a patient with severe anaphylaxis.

TABLE 2 Dynamics of Cardiovascular Abnormalities in Anaphylactic Shock

	At Onset of Reaction	Early Stage (Minutes) with No Treatment	Prolonged Shock
Blood pressure	↓	↓↓	↓↓↓
Pulse	↑	↑	↑↑
Cardiac output	↑	↓	↓↓
PVR	↓	→↓*	→↑↓*
Intravascular volume	→↓	↓	↓↓↓

Peripheral vascular resistance (PVR) can vary, likely depending on internal compensation response.
From LoVerde D et al: Anaphylaxis, *Chest* 153(2):528-543, 2018, https://doi.org/10.1016/j.chest.2017.07.033.

TABLE 3 Signs and Symptoms of Anaphylaxis: Frequency of Occurrence

Sign or Symptom	Percentage of Cases (%)
Cutaneous	>90
Urticaria and angioedema	85-90
Flush	45-55
Pruritus without rash	2-5
Respiratory	40-60
Dyspnea, wheeze	45-50
Upper airway angioedema	50-60
Rhinitis	15-20
Dizziness, syncope, hypotension	30-35
Abdominal	
Nausea, vomiting, diarrhea, cramping pain	25-30
Miscellaneous	
Headache	5-8
Substernal pain	4-6
Seizure	1-2

BOX 2 Causes of Anaphylaxis

IgE-dependent mechanisms
Drugs, Chemicals, and Biologic Agents
  Penicillins, cephalosporins, sulfonamides, muscle relaxants, vaccines, insulin, thiamine, protamine, gamma globulin, cis-carboplatin and doxorubicin, monoclonal antibodies cetuximab/rituximab, antivenoms, formaldehyde, ethylene oxide, chlorhexidine, semen

Foods
  Peanuts, tree nuts, shellfish, fin fish, milk, egg, fruits, vegetables, sesame, flour
  Hymenoptera sting venom, insect saliva, other venoms
  Bees, wasps, ants, hornets, ticks, triatoma "kissing bugs," snakes, scorpions, jellyfish

Natural Rubber Latex
Environmental
  Pollen, horse dander, hydatid cyst rupture

Non–IgE-Dependent Mechanisms
Physical factors
  Exercise, cold, heat, sunlight

Medications and Biologic Agents
  Opiates, aspirin and NSAIDs, ACE inhibitors, vancomycin, radiocontrast media, N-acetylcysteine, fluorescein

Food Additives
  Metabisulphite, tartrazine

Idiopathic
  Exclusion of all known causes including mastocytosis

Several mechanisms may coexist, such as exercise-induced following food.
Non–IgE-dependent mechanisms include complement activation, kinin production, or potentiation and direct mediator release.
ACE inhibitor use is an important cause of unexplained angioedema, occurring in up to 1:200 patients on these drugs; it may develop at any interval after starting (most commonly early on).
NOTE: Cross-reactivity is seen; both IgE-dependent and non–IgE-dependent reactions may occur with the same agent.
ACE, Angiotensin-converting enzyme inhibitors; *IgE,* immunoglobulin E; *NSAIDs,* nonsteroidal, antiinflammatory drugs.
From Cameron P et al: *Textbook of adult emergency medicine,* ed 5, Sydney, Australia, 2019, Elsevier.

DISPOSITION

- Patients with mild episodes should be observed for 1 h after resolution of symptoms. Patients with severe symptoms (cyanosis, pulse oxygen <92%, systolic blood pressure <90 mm Hg, confusion, loss of consciousness, incontinence), >1 dose of epinephrine, wide pulse pressure, unknown trigger, cutaneous signs or symptoms, and medication trigger in children should be observed for at least 6 h to monitor for biphasic anaphylaxis.

CHRONIC Rx

- Patients appropriate for discharge after remaining asymptomatic should have two epinephrine autoinjectors prescribed. Include instructions on when and how to use.

REFERRAL

- Referral to an allergist can be help determine a cause if unclear in the emergent setting.

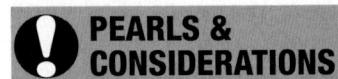

PEARLS & CONSIDERATIONS

COMMENTS

- Patient education regarding the nature of the illness and preventive measures is recommended. A documented history of previous anaphylactic episodes or known triggers is the most reliable method of identifying individuals at risk.
- Prescription for a prefilled epinephrine syringe (EpiPen or EpiPen Jr.) should be given, and the patient should be instructed on the use of this emergency kit, and to carry it with them at all times. School-aged children should keep an additional EpiPen at school with the appropriate staff.
- Patients should also be advised to carry or wear a MedicAlert ID describing substances that have caused anaphylaxis.
- Avoidance of radiologic contrast is also recommended in those who have had a prior reaction. However, pretreatment regimens with methylprednisolone or diphenhydramine, exist for those who have had contrast reactions in the past.
- Venom immunotherapy immediately after a sting is effective and recommended for up to 5 yr after the anaphylactic incident.

AUTHORS: **RORY MERRITT, MD, MEHP,** and **FAHAD ALI, MD**

BOX 3 Agents Frequently Associated with Immune and Nonimmune Types of Anaphylaxis

Immunologic Mechanisms
Immunoglobulin E (IgE)-mediated:
Food (nuts, shellfish, fruits, etc.)
Venoms (stinging insects)
Medications (β-lactam antibiotics, NSAIDs, neuromuscular blocking agents, etc.)
Natural rubber latex
Seminal fluid
Radiocontrast media (in some cases)

IgE-independent
Radiocontrast media (in most cases)
Dextrans
Monoclonal antibodies (rituximab)
Medications (β-lactam antibiotics, NSAIDs, etc.)
Natural rubber latex
Seminal fluid

Nonimmunologic Mechanisms
Medications (opioids, protamine, etc.)

IgE, Immunoglobulin E; *NSAIDs,* nonsteroidal antiinflammatory drugs.
From Parrillo JE, Dellinger RP: *Critical care medicine: principles of diagnosis and management in the adult,* ed 5, Philadelphia, 2019, Elsevier.

BOX 4 Clinical Criteria for Diagnosing Anaphylaxis

Anaphylaxis is highly likely when any one of the following three criteria is fulfilled:
1. Acute onset of an illness (minutes to several hours) with involvement of the skin, mucosal tissue, or both (e.g., generalized urticaria, itching or flushing, swollen lips/tongue/uvula) and at least one of the following:
   a. Respiratory compromise (e.g., dyspnea, wheeze/bronchospasm, stridor, reduced PEF, hypoxemia)
   b. Reduced blood pressure or associated symptoms of end-organ dysfunction (e.g., hypotonia collapse, syncope, incontinence)
OR
2. Two or more of the following that occur rapidly after exposure to a likely allergen for that patient (minutes to several hours):
   a. Involvement of the skin-mucosal tissue (e.g., generalized urticaria, itch/flush, swollen lips/tongue/uvula)
   b. Respiratory compromise (e.g., dyspnea, wheeze/bronchospasm, stridor, reduced PEF, hypoxemia)
   c. Reduced blood pressure or associated symptoms (e.g., hypotonia collapse, syncope, incontinence)
   d. Persistent gastrointestinal symptoms (e.g., crampy abdominal pain, vomiting)
OR
3. Reduced blood pressure after exposure to known allergen for that patient (minutes to several hours)
   a. Infants and children: Low systolic blood pressure (age-specific) or >30% decrease in systolic blood pressure
   b. Adults: Systolic blood pressure of <90 mm Hg or >30% decrease from that person's baseline

PEF, Peak expiratory flow.
From Sampson HA et al: Second symposium on the definition and management of anaphylaxis: summary report—Second National Institute of Allergy and Infectious Disease/Food Allergy and Anaphylaxis Network symposium, *J Allergy Clin Immunol* 117(2):391-397, 2006, https://doi.org/10.1016/j.jaci.2005.12.1303.

TABLE 5 Management of a Patient with Anaphylaxis

Treatment	Mechanism(s) of Effect	Dosage(s)	Comments; Adverse Reactions
Patient Emergency Management (Dependent on Severity of Symptoms)			
Epinephrine (adrenaline)	α_1-, β_1-, β_2-Adrenergic effects	0.01 mg/kg, up to 0.5 mg IM in lateral thigh Adrenaclick, Auvi-Q, EpiPen Jr./EpiPen: 0.15 mg IM for 8-25 kg 0.3 mg IM for 25 kg or more Epinephrine autoinjector: 0.1 mg for 7.5-15 kg 0.15 mg for 15-25 kg 0.3 mg for 25 kg or more	Tachycardia, hypertension, nervousness, headache, nausea, irritability, tremor
Cetirizine (liquid)	Antihistamine (competitive of H_1 receptor)	Cetirizine liquid: 5 mg/5 ml, 0.25 mg/kg, up to 10 mg PO	Hypotension, tachycardia, somnolence
Alternative: Diphenhydramine	Antihistamine (competitive of H_1 receptor)	1.25 mg/kg up to 50 mg PO or IM	Hypotension, tachycardia, somnolence, paradoxical excitement
Transport to an Emergency Facility			
Emergency Personnel Management (Dependent on Severity of Symptoms)			
Epinephrine (adrenaline)	α_1-, β_1-, β_2-Adrenergic effects	0.01 mg/kg, up to 0.5 mg IM in lateral thigh Epinephrine autoinjector: 0.1 mg for 7.5-15 kg 0.15 mg for 15-25 kg 0.3 mg for 25 kg or more 0.01 ml/kg/dose of 1:1,000 (vial) solution, up to 0.5 ml IM May repeat every 10-15 min For severe hypotension: 0.01 ml/kg/dose of 1:10,000 slow IV push	Tachycardia, hypertension, nervousness, headache, nausea, irritability, tremor
Supplemental Oxygen and Airway Management			
Volume Expanders			
Crystalloids (normal saline or Ringer lactate)		30 ml/kg in 1st h	Rate titrated against BP response If tolerated, place patient supine with legs raised
Colloids (hydroxyethyl starch)		10 ml/kg rapidly followed by slow infusion	Rate titrated against BP response If tolerated, place patient supine with legs raised
Antihistamines			
Cetirizine (liquid)	Antihistamine (competitive of H_1 receptor)	Cetirizine liquid: 5 mg/5 ml 0.25 mg/kg, up to 10 mg PO	Hypotension, tachycardia, somnolence
Alternative: Diphenhydramine	Antihistamine (competitive of H_1 receptor)	1.25 mg/kg, up to 50 mg PO, IM, or IV	Hypotension, tachycardia, somnolence, paradoxic excitement
Ranitidine	Antihistamine (competitive of H_2 receptor)	1 mg/kg, up to 50 mg IV Should be administered slowly	Headache, mental confusion
Alternative: Cimetidine	Antihistamine (competitive of H_2 receptor)	4 mg/kg, up to 200 mg IV Should be administered slowly	Headache, mental confusion
Corticosteroids			
Methylprednisolone	Antiinflammatory	Solu-Medrol (IV): 1-2 mg/kg, up to 125 mg IV Depo-Medrol (IM): 1 mg/kg, up to 80 mg IM	Hypertension, edema, nervousness, agitation
Prednisone	Antiinflammatory	1 mg/kg up, to 75 mg PO	Hypertension, edema, nervousness, agitation
Nebulized albuterol	β-Agonist	0.83 mg/ml (3 ml) via mask with O_2	Palpitations, nervousness, CNS stimulation, tachycardia; use to supplement epinephrine when bronchospasm appears unresponsive; may repeat
Postemergency Management			
Antihistamine		Cetirizine (5-10 mg qd) or loratadine (5-10 mg qd) for 3 days	
Corticosteroids		*Optional:* Oral prednisone (1 mg/kg up to 75 mg) daily for 3 days	

Preventive Treatment
Prescription for epinephrine autoinjector and antihistamine
Provide written plan outlining patient emergency management (may download form from http://www.aap.org or http://www.foodallergy.org)
Follow-up evaluation to determine/confirm etiology
Immunotherapy for insect sting allergy

Patient Education
Instruction on avoidance of causative agent
Information on recognizing early signs of anaphylaxis
Stress early treatment of allergic symptoms to avoid systemic anaphylaxis
Encourage wearing medical identification jewelry

BP, Blood pressure; *CNS,* central nervous system; *IM,* intramuscularly; *IV,* intravenously; *PO,* orally; *qd,* every day.
From Kliegman RM, Geme JS: *Nelson textbook of pediatrics,* Philadelphia, 2019, Elsevier.

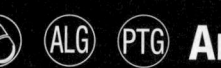
Diseases
and Disorders

I

BASIC INFORMATION

DEFINITION

Angina pectoris is a term used to describe a clinical syndrome, typically characterized by chest, jaw, shoulder, back, or arm discomfort that is caused by myocardial ischemia. This is most commonly related to atheromatous plaque in one or more than one large epicardial coronary artery; however, myocardial ischemia may occur in the absence of obstructive coronary artery disease (CAD), such as uncontrolled hypertension, microvascular disease, valvular heart disease, hypertrophic cardiomyopathy, coronary spasm, or endothelial dysfunction. Any situation that causes an imbalance in myocardial oxygen supply and demand can cause an angina syndrome. Angina can be classified as follows:

- Chronic stable angina, stable ischemic heart disease (SIHD), or chronic CAD:
  1. Predictable. Usually follows a precipitating event (e.g., climbing stairs, sexual intercourse, a heavy meal, emotional stress, cold weather)
  2. Generally, has the same severity as previous attacks; relieved by rest or by the customary dose of sublingual nitroglycerin.
  3. Caused by a fixed coronary artery obstruction secondary to atherosclerosis. The presence of one or more obstructions in major coronary arteries is likely; the severity of stenosis is usually >70%
- Unstable (rest, recent onset, crescendo angina; will be reviewed under "Acute Coronary Syndrome"):
  1. Rest angina: Angina occurring at rest and usually prolonged >20 min, occurring within 1 wk of presentation.
  2. Recent onset: Angina of at least CCS Class III severity occurring less than 2 mo after the onset of the symptoms.
  3. Crescendo angina: Previously diagnosed angina that is distinctly more frequent, longer in duration, or lower in threshold (i.e., increased by >1 CCS class within 2 mo of initial presentation to at least CCS Class III severity)
- Prinzmetal variant:
  1. Occurs at rest, common after cold exposure
  2. Cyclical in nature
  3. ECG finding of episodic ST-segment elevations
  4. Caused by coronary artery spasm with or without superimposed CAD
  5. Patients are more likely to develop ventricular arrhythmias
- Microvascular angina (syndrome X):
  1. Refers to patients with angina symptoms, positive exercise test, normal coronary angiograms, and no coronary spasm. Defective endothelium-dependent dilation in the coronary microcirculation contributes to the altered regulation of myocardial perfusion and the ischemic manifestations in these patients.
  2. Patients with chest pain and normal or nonobstructive coronary angiograms are

predominantly women, and many have a prognosis that is not as benign as commonly thought (2% risk of death or myocardial infarction [MI] at 30 days of follow-up).
- Refractory angina:
  1. Refers to patients who, despite optimal medical therapy with at least maximal doses, or as tolerated of two antianginal medications, in addition to aspirin, aggressive risk factor modification, such as smoking cessation, adequate control of hypertension, diabetes, and hyperlipidemia, still have both angina and objective evidence of ischemia
- Other:
  1. Angina due to aortic stenosis and idiopathic hypertrophic subaortic stenosis, cocaine-induced coronary vasoconstriction

FUNCTIONAL CLASSIFICATION

Stable angina should be classified using a grading system. The most commonly adopted is that of the Canadian Cardiovascular Society (CCS):
- Class I: Ordinary physical activity, such as walking or climbing stairs, does not cause angina. Angina occurs with strenuous, rapid, or prolonged exertion at work or recreation.
- Class II: Slight limitation of ordinary activity. Angina occurs on walking or climbing stairs rapidly; walking uphill; walking or stair climbing after meals, in cold, in wind, or under emotional stress; or only during the few hours after awakening. Angina occurs on walking more than two level blocks and climbing more than one flight of ordinary stairs at a normal pace and in normal conditions.
- Class III: Marked limitations of ordinary physical activity. Angina occurs on walking one to two level blocks and climbing one flight of stairs in normal conditions and at a normal pace.
- Class IV: Inability to carry on any physical activity without discomfort; anginal symptoms may be present at rest.

ICD-10CM CODES

I20.1	Angina pectoris with documented spasm
I20.8	Other forms of angina pectoris
I20.9	Angina pectoris, unspecified
I25.110	Atherosclerotic heart disease of native coronary artery with unstable angina pectoris
I25.111	Atherosclerotic heart disease of native coronary artery with angina pectoris with documented spasm
I25.118	Atherosclerotic heart disease of native coronary artery with other forms of angina pectoris
I25.119	Atherosclerotic heart disease of native coronary artery with unspecified angina pectoris
I25.700	Atherosclerosis of coronary artery bypass graft(s), unspecified, with unstable angina pectoris
I25.790	Atherosclerosis of other coronary artery bypass graft(s) with unstable angina pectoris
I25.791	Atherosclerosis of other coronary artery bypass graft(s) with angina pectoris with documented spasm
I25.798	Atherosclerosis of other coronary artery bypass graft(s) with other forms of angina pectoris
I25.799	Atherosclerosis of other coronary artery bypass graft(s) with unspecified angina pectoris

EPIDEMIOLOGY & DEMOGRAPHICS

- It is estimated that one in three adults in the U.S. (about 81 million) has some form of cardiovascular disease. Based on the NHANES survey 2007 to 2010, an estimated 15.4 million have coronary heart disease (CHD) of which 7.8 million have angina.[1]
- Angina is most common in middle-aged and elderly men. Among persons 60 to 79 yr of age, approximately 25% of men and 16% of women have CHD, and these figures rise to 37% and 23% among men and women >80 yr of age, respectively.
- The incidence of CHD and angina in women after menopause is similar to that of men.
- Although the survival rate has steadily improved over time, SIHD remains the number one cause of death in men and women (27% of deaths).
- The initial manifestation of ischemic heart disease is angina pectoris in 50%, and about 50% of patients presenting to the hospital with acute coronary syndrome have preceding angina.
- Two older population-based studies from Olmstead County, MN, and Framingham, MA, showed annual rate of MI in patients with symptomatic angina of 3% to 3.5%/yr.
- Within 12 mo of initial diagnosis, 10% to 20% of patients with diagnosis of stable angina progress to MI or unstable angina.

RISK FACTORS:
- Advanced age.
- Male sex.
- Genetic predisposition, family history of premature CAD in first-degree relatives (men <55 yr of age, and women <65 yr of age).
- Smoking (risk of first MI is increased by near threefold).
- Hypertension.
- Hyperlipidemia.
- Impaired glucose tolerance or diabetes mellitus.
- History of stroke or peripheral arterial disease.
- Chronic kidney disease (CKD).
- Metabolic syndrome.
- Physical inactivity.
- Obesity (body mass index [BMI] >30% over ideal). A higher BMI during childhood is also associated with an increased risk of CHD in adulthood.
- Entities that cause increased oxygen demand include hyperthermia (particularly if accompanied by volume contraction), hyperthyroidism, and cocaine or methamphetamine abuse.
- Cocaine is used by >5 million Americans regularly and is responsible for >64,000 emergency department (ED) evaluations

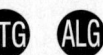
yearly to rule out myocardial ischemia. Cocaine causes sympathomimetic toxicity and not only increases myocardial oxygen demand but also induces coronary vasospasm and can cause infarction in young patients. Long-term cocaine use can cause premature development of SIHD.

- Severe uncontrolled hypertension causes increased myocardial oxygen demand and decreased subendocardial perfusion that increases left ventricular (LV) wall tension. Hypertrophic cardiomyopathy and aortic stenosis can induce even more severe LV hypertrophy and resultant wall tension.
- Other causes of increased myocardial oxygen demand are ventricular or supraventricular tachycardias. Ambulatory monitoring may be required to diagnose these.
- Entities that limit myocardial oxygen supply such as anemia may cause angina when the hemoglobin drops to <9 g/dl, and ST-T-wave changes (depression or inversion) can occur at levels <7 g/dl.
- Hypoxemia resulting from pulmonary disease (e.g., pneumonia, asthma, chronic obstructive pulmonary disease, pulmonary hypertension, interstitial fibrosis, or obstructive sleep apnea) can also precipitate angina.
- Polycythemia, leukemia, thrombocytosis, and hypergammaglobulinemia.
- Oral contraceptive and hormone replacement therapy use.
- Coronary artery calcium is associated with an increased risk of MI.
- Long-term use of NSAIDs.
- Exposure to air pollution from traffic (dilute diesel exhaust) promotes myocardial ischemia and is associated with adverse cardiovascular events.
- Low serum folate levels required for conversion of homocysteine to methionine are associated with an increased risk of fatal CHD. Hyperhomocysteinemia has a toxic effect on vascular endothelium and interferes with proliferation of arterial wall smooth muscle cells. Elevated plasma homocysteine level is a strong and independent risk factor for CHD events, especially in patients with type 2 diabetes mellitus.
- Elevated levels of highly sensitive C-reactive protein (hs-CRP, cardio CRP). Diseases associated with systemic inflammation can lead to accelerated atherosclerosis.
- Depression.
- Vasculitis.
- Elevated levels of lipoprotein-associated phospholipase A_2.
- Elevated fibrinogen levels.
- Low level of red blood cell glutathione peroxidase-1 activity.
- Radiation therapy.

PHYSICAL FINDINGS & CLINICAL PRESENTATION

- The assessment of chest pain should include quality, location, severity, and duration of pain; radiation; associated symptoms; provocative factors; and alleviating factors. Anginal pain can be described as "squeezing," "griplike,"

"suffocating," and "heavy," but it is rarely sharp or stabbing and typically does not vary with position or respiration. The classic Levine sign is placing a clenched fist over the precordium to describe the pain. Many patients do not, however, describe angina as frank pain but as tightness, pressure, or discomfort. Other patients, in particular women and older adults, can present with atypical symptoms such as nausea, vomiting, midepigastric discomfort, sharp (atypical) chest pain, dizziness, or syncope.

- Ischemic pain of more than 20 min duration should raise concern for possible acute coronary syndrome.
- Women are more likely than men to report atypical chest pain or discomfort (65% reported on Women's Ischemic Syndrome Evaluation [WISE] study).
- The elderly and diabetics may report symptoms other than chest pain, such as dyspnea, fatigue, or diaphoresis.

DIAGNOSIS

DIFFERENTIAL DIAGNOSIS

- Nonischemic cardiovascular: Aortic dissection, pericarditis
- Pulmonary: Pulmonary embolism, pneumothorax, pneumonia, pleuritis
- GI: Esophageal, esophagitis, spasm, reflux, biliary colic, cholecystitis, choledocholithiasis, cholangitis, peptic ulcer, pancreatitis
- Chest wall: Costochondritis, fibrositis, rib fracture, sternoclavicular arthritis, herpes zoster (before the rash)
- Psychiatric: Anxiety disorders, hyperventilation, panic disorder, primary anxiety, affective disorders (i.e., depression), somatoform disorders, thought disorders (i.e., fixed delusions)

WORKUP

- In patients with chest pain, the probability of CAD should be estimated on the basis of patient age, sex, cardiovascular risk factors, and pain characteristics.
- The most important diagnostic element is the history. Chest pain or left arm pain or discomfort occurring with exertion and relieved by rest in a patient with cardiovascular risk factors is consistent with a high likelihood of CAD.
- 2021 ACC/AHA/ASE chest pain guidelines recommending chest pain should be described clinically as cardiac chest pain, probable cardiac chest pain, and noncardiac chest pain.[1,2]
- Typical angina (definite) will have the following three features: (1) Substernal chest discomfort with a characteristic quality and duration, (2) provoked by exertion or emotional stress, and (3) relieved by rest and/or sublingual nitroglycerin.
- Noncardiac chest pain will have one or none of the previously listed features.
- Physical examination may be completely normal in many patients; however, certain findings may be helpful in the assessment of the

patient with suspected SIHD. Some findings may identify consequences of ischemia or possible causes of the anginal syndrome other than CAD. The presence of hypertension, arcus senilis, xanthelasma, carotid or peripheral bruits, and a prominent S4 are all physical signs that could raise concern for the presence of CAD. A murmur of mitral regurgitation may be a marker of an ischemic cardiomyopathy or transient ischemia. A murmur suggestive of hypertrophic cardiomyopathy or aortic stenosis may suggest a cause of angina other than CAD.

- The ultimate goal for an SIHD patient's evaluation is to identify high-risk CAD patients with minimal use of resources. In general, four common steps would help a clinician to assess high feature of SIHD. Those are (1) CAD risk assessment based on various classic risk factors, (2) functional capacity and stress test result, (3) LV and right ventricular (RV) function, and (4) coronary anatomy. Every patient does not need each of the modalities. HEART (history, ECG, age, risk factors, and troponin) score, ADAPT (Accelerated Diagnostic protocol to assess chest pain using troponins), and EDACS (emergency department ACS) score would be useful to risk-stratify patients prior to any ischemic testing. One should classify stable angina without history of CAD patients to low, intermediate, and high pretest probability or likelihood for CAD after assessment of comorbidities and atherosclerotic vascular disease risk factors. Consider functional capacity and stress test (ETT [exercise tolerance test], ETT-MIBI [ETT-myocardial perfusion imaging (multiplex ion beam imaging with dipyridamole/technetium sestamibi)] or stress echo) in intermediate pretest probability patients who are greater than 65 yr of age with suspecting obstructive CAD (>50% stenosis), and consider cardiac CT angiogram for less than 65 yr of age with suspecting nonobstructive CAD (<50% stenosis). Exercise testing (Fig. 1) is preferred to pharmacologic stress tests when possible. Functional capacity and stress test results categorize SIHD patients based on their risk of annual mortality. Patients with an estimated annual mortality of <1% classify as low risk, 1% to 3% are considered as intermediate risk, and >3% annual mortality belongs to high-risk patient population (please see "Coronary Artery Disease" chapter).[1,2]

LABORATORY TESTS

- Screen for hypertension, diabetes, and hyperlipidemia per routine guidelines.
- ECGs should be obtained during pain and when the patient is free of any discomfort. A normal resting ECG is not unusual in patients with SIHD; in patients who present with chest pain, 1% to 6% who have an acute MI will have a normal or nondiagnostic ECG.
- Chest x-ray examination PA and lateral if symptoms suggestive of heart failure, pericardial disease, aortic aneurysm/dissection.

- Cardio-CRP (hs-CRP): Its elevation is a relatively moderate predictor of CHD, and it adds prognostic information to that conveyed by the Framingham risk score.

EXERCISE TESTING AND IMAGING STUDIES (SEE "CORONARY ARTERY DISEASE" CHAPTER, FIG. 1)

- Exercise testing is used for diagnosis as well as prognosis of SIHD. If the patient is physically capable of performing at least moderate physical exercise, exercise stress testing (see Fig. 1) is useful because of the important

prognostic information obtained from exercise performance and the hemodynamic response. Risk stratification based on noninvasive testing is summarized in Table 1. Patients who have an intermediate likelihood of CAD, as patients in a low-risk or high-likelihood category are more likely to have a false-positive or false-negative result, respectively. Risk assessment is also indicated in patients with SIHD who are being considered for revascularization of known coronary stenosis of unclear physiologic significance. The exercise treadmill test is contraindicated in patients with presence of ST depression >0.5 mm or

Wolff-Parkinson-White syndrome, left bundle branch block, or pacemaker rhythm in baseline ECG.

- Stress echocardiography or stress testing with myocardial perfusion imaging may be employed when baseline electrocardiographic abnormalities are present that render the electrocardiographic response to exercise uninterpretable. Stress echocardiography has the advantage of higher specificity and a lower cost. Stress radionuclide perfusion imaging has a higher sensitivity, particularly for single-vessel coronary disease, and has a higher technical success rate. When

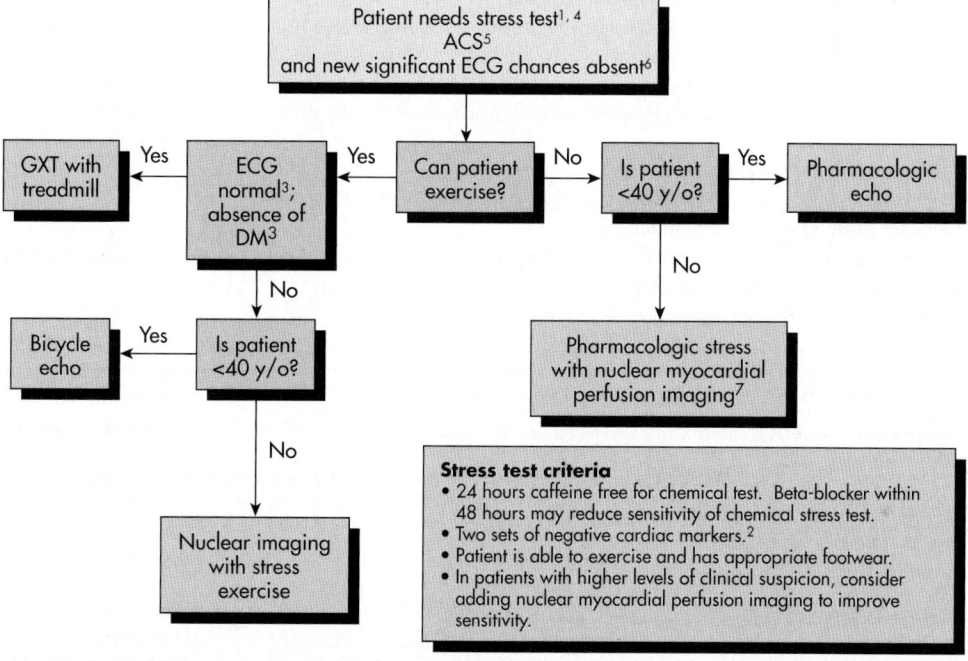

FIG. 1 Stress test algorithm. *ACS*, Acute coronary syndrome; *BBB*, bundle branch block; *DM*, diabetes mellitus; *ECG*, electrocardiogram; *echo*, echocardiography; *ED*, emergency department; *GTX*, graded exercise test; *LVH*, left ventricular hypertrophy; *NSTE*, non–ST-segment elevation; *NSTEMI*, NSTE myocardial infarction; *STE*, ST-segment elevation; *y/o*, years old. (From Adams JG et al: *Emergency medicine: clinical essentials*, ed 2, Philadelphia, 2013, Saunders.)

TABLE 1 Risk Stratification Based on Noninvasive Testing

High Risk (>3% Annual Risk for Death or Myocardial Infarction)
1. Severe resting left ventricular dysfunction (LVEF <35%) not readily explained by noncoronary causes
2. Resting perfusion abnormalities involving ≥10% of the myocardium without previous known MI
3. High-risk stress findings on the ECG, including:
   - ≥2-mm ST-segment depression at low workload or persisting into recovery
   - Exercise-induced ST-segment elevation
   - Exercise-induced VT/VF
4. Severe stress-induced LV dysfunction (peak exercise LVEF <45% or drop in LVEF with stress ≥10%)
5. Stress-induced perfusion abnormalities encumbering ≥10% of the myocardium or stress segmental scores indicating multiple vascular territories with abnormalities
6. Stress-induced LV dilation
7. Inducible wall motion abnormality (involving >2 segments or 2 coronary beds)
8. Wall motion abnormality developing at a low dose of dobutamine (≤10 mg/kg/min) or at a low heart rate (<120 beats/min)
9. Multivessel obstructive CAD (≥70% stenosis) or left main stenosis (≥50% stenosis) on CCTA

Intermediate Risk (1%-3% Annual Risk for Death or Myocardial Infarction)
1. Mild to moderate resting LV dysfunction (LVEF of 35%-49%) not readily explained by noncoronary causes
2. Resting perfusion abnormalities involving 5%-9.9% of the myocardium in patients without a history or previous evidence of MI
3. ≥1-mm ST-segment depression occurring with exertional symptoms
4. Stress-induced perfusion abnormalities encumbering 5%-9.9% of the myocardium or stress segmental scores indicating 1 vascular territory with abnormalities but without LV dilation
5. Small wall motion abnormality involving 1-2 segments and only 1 coronary bed
6. Single-vessel CAD with ≥70% stenosis or moderate CAD stenosis (50%-69% stenosis) in ≥2 arteries on CCTA

Low Risk (<1% Annual Risk for Death or Myocardial Infarction)
1. Low-risk treadmill score (score ≥5) or no new ST-segment changes or exercise-induced chest pain symptoms when achieving maximal levels of exercise
2. Normal or small myocardial perfusion defect at rest or with stress encumbering <5% of the myocardium*
3. Normal stress or no change in limited resting wall motion abnormalities during stress
4. No coronary stenosis >50% on CCTA

*Although the published data are limited, patients with these findings will probably not be at low risk in the presence of either a high-risk treadmill score or severe resting LV dysfunction (LVEF <35%).
CCTA, Cardiac computed tomography angiography; *LVEF,* left ventricular ejection fraction; *VF,* ventricular fibrillation; *VT,* ventricular tachycardia. Assessment of coronary artery calcium can also be used to contribute to risk assessment.
Modified from Fihn SD et al: ACCF/AHA/ACP/AATS/PCNA/SCAI/STS guideline for the diagnosis and management of patients with stable ischemic heart disease: a report of the American College of Cardiology Foundation/American Heart Association Task Force on Practice Guidelines, and the American College of Physicians, American Association for Thoracic Surgery, Preventive Cardiovascular Nurses Association, Society for Cardiovascular Angiography and Interventions, and Society of Thoracic Surgeons, *Circulation* 126:e354, 2012; In: Libby P et al: *Braunwald's heart disease, a textbook of cardiovascular medicine,* ed 12, Philadelphia, 2022, Elsevier.

the patient is unable to exercise adequately, pharmacologic stress testing (i.e., dobutamine, adenosine, regadenoson) may be used with these imaging modalities.

- A good predictor of risk for a patient with stable angina is the Duke treadmill score, which incorporates the patient's functional status (METS or time in minutes during the Bruce protocol), ST-segment depression in millimeters, and an angina index (yes or no). Patients with favorable Duke scores (>5) have a 5-yr survival rate of >97%; this is independent of other factors such as coronary anatomy and LV function.
- Echocardiography is indicated in patients with murmurs suggestive of aortic stenosis, hypertrophic cardiomyopathy, mitral regurgitation, mitral valve prolapse, previous MI, pathologic Q waves, complex ventricular arrhythmias, heart failure, hypertension, diabetes, and abnormal ECG.
- Cardiac computed tomography (CCTA; Fig. E2) is useful for the detection of subclinical CAD in asymptomatic patients with an intermediate Framingham 10-yr risk estimate of 10% to 20%. 2021 ACC/AHA/ASE chest pain guidelines recommend cardiac computed tomographic angiogram (cardiac CTA) as a front-line imaging modality in patients with

greater than 65 yr of age and stable angina. Trials comparing CCTA to invasive coronary angiography (ICA) in patients with stable angina have shown that an initial strategy of CCTA for anatomic imaging is associated with similar outcomes but fewer procedural complications and invasive angiograms.[3] CCTA detects and quantifies coronary calcium and evaluates the lumen and wall of the coronary artery. CCTA CT cost and radiation exposure are limiting factors to recommending widespread routine use of this marker. CCTA has an excellent negative predictive value to rule out severe CAD in the setting of active chest pain evaluation in the emergency room (ROMICAT-II trial). In 2018 the SCOT-HEART trial showed coronary CTA resulted in a lower risk of nonfatal MI than standard care alone (ETT) in stable angina patients. Myocardial perfusion imaging and noninvasive fractional flow ratio would be possible with cardiac CTA as well.

- Coronary artery calcium score is a strong predictor of incidence of CAD and provides predictive information in patients with low to intermediate pretest probability of CAD beyond that provided by standard risk factors. A score <100 indicates low risk and a score >400 high risk.

- Cardiac MRI, in addition to its use for diagnosis of arrhythmogenic right ventricular dysplasia, can also be used to assess myocardial perfusion and viability as well as function in patients unable to exercise. Additional studies are needed to determine the cost effectiveness of these studies in patients with ischemic cardiomyopathy.
- Invasive coronary angiography remains the gold standard for the identification of clinically significant CAD. Angiography is performed to define the location and extent of coronary disease; indicated in selected patients who are candidates for coronary revascularization (either coronary artery bypass graft [CABG] surgery or angioplasty).

🆁🆇 TREATMENT

Five fundamental overlapping strategies are recommended:
- Patient education: Support active participation of patients in the decision-making process of their treatment.
- Management of comorbid conditions that contribute to or worsen SIHD.
- Aggressive modification of preventable risk factors such as smoking cessation, weight

reduction in obese patients, regular aerobic exercise program (at least 30 to 60 min/day for 5 days per wk), correction of folate deficiency, reduced intake of saturated fats (to <7% of total calories) and trans-fatty acids (to <1% of total calories), low-sodium diet (<2 g/day), and teaching importance of medication adherence. Whole grains as the main form of carbohydrates, an abundance of fruits and vegetables, and adequate omega-3 fatty acids are optimal for prevention of SIHD.

- Evidence-based pharmacologic management to improve quality of life and survival.
- Use appropriate revascularization procedures to improve survival and long-term outcomes in selected patients.

PHARMACOLOGIC THERAPY (SEE "CORONARY ARTERY DISEASE")

Treatment can be classified based on medications that prevent MI and death.

- Aspirin reduces cardiovascular mortality and morbidity rates by 20% to 25% among patients with CAD. Appropriate dose is 75 to 162 mg/day in the absence of contraindications. It inhibits the enzyme cyclooxygenase and synthesis of thromboxane A2 and reduces the risk of adverse cardiovascular events by 33% in patients with unstable angina. Patients' intolerant to aspirin can be treated with clopidogrel or can undergo aspirin desensitization. Clopidogrel irreversibly blocks the P2Y12 adenosine diphosphate receptor on the platelet surface, thereby interrupting platelet activation and aggregation. Clopidogrel can be combined with ASA in high-risk patients with SIHD with low risk for bleeding complications or can be given alone in patients that are aspirin intolerant. Dose is 75 mg/day.
- Ticagrelor, in the PEGASUS-TIMI-54, reduced the risk of death, cardiovascular MI, or stroke in patients after 1 yr of MI. However, it is associated with an increased risk of bleeding when compared to placebo.
- Dipyridamole is not recommended as an antiplatelet therapy for the treatment of patients with SIHD.
- Beta-adrenergic blockers, which prevent MI and death, are first-line therapy in the management of angina pectoris. They achieve their major antianginal effect by decreasing myocardial oxygen demand in reducing heart rate and systolic blood pressure product, atrioventricular nodal conduction, and myocardial contractility, in this manner contributing to a reduction in angina onset, with improvement in the ischemic threshold during exercise and during the usual daily activities. Absent contraindications, they should be regarded as initial therapy for stable angina for all patients. Their dose should generally be adjusted to reduce the resting heart rate to 55 to 60 beats/min. Despite the difference among the available beta-blockers, they all seem to be equally efficacious in SIHD. Beta-blockers recommended for at least 2 to 3 yr after MI, and lifelong for patients with LV

ejection fraction of <40% with heart failure or prior MI.

- Nitrates cause venodilation and relaxation of vascular smooth muscle; the decreased venous return from venodilation decreases diastolic ventricular wall tension (preload) and thereby reduces mechanical activity (and myocardial oxygen consumption) during systole. Relaxation of vascular smooth muscle increases coronary blood flow and reduces systemic pressure. Dilation of the arterial wall will not be affected by plaque, but independent of an intact endothelium, leads to reduced resistance across the obstructed lumen. Nitroglycerin contributes to coronary blood flow redistribution by augmenting collateral flow and lowering ventricular diastolic pressure from areas of normal perfusion to ischemic zones. Nitroglycerin also has demonstrated antithrombotic and antiplatelet effects. Sublingual nitroglycerin or nitroglycerin spray should be prescribed to all patients with SIHD for immediate angina relief. Tolerance to nitrates can be minimized by avoiding sustained blood levels with a daily nitrate-free period (e.g., omission of bedtime dose of oral isosorbide dinitrate or 12 h on/ 12 h off transdermal nitroglycerin therapy). Nitrates are relatively contraindicated in patients with hypertrophic obstructive cardiomyopathy and should also be avoided in patients with severe aortic stenosis. Nitrates should not be used within 24 h of sildenafil (Viagra) or vardenafil (Levitra) or within 48 h of tadalafil (Cialis) because of the potential for hypotension.
- Calcium channel blockers are antiischemic medications that have no proven mortality benefit in SIHD. They improve myocardial oxygen supply by decreasing coronary vascular resistance and augmenting epicardial conduit vessel and systemic arterial blood flow. Myocardial demand is decreased by a reduction in myocardial contractility, systemic vascular resistance, and arterial pressure. They are first-line treatment when beta-blockers are contraindicated. They play a major role in preventing and terminating myocardial ischemia induced by coronary artery spasm. They are particularly effective in treating microvascular angina. All classes of calcium channel blockers reduce anginal episodes, increase exercise duration, and reduce use of sublingual nitroglycerin in patients with effort-induced angina. Short-acting calcium channel blockers should be avoided. Calcium channel blockers (particularly nondihydropyridine) should generally also be avoided in patients with CHF secondary to systolic dysfunction due to its negative inotropic effect.
- Ranolazine, which has been tested in four different studies with a total of 1737 patients (MARISA, CARISA, RAN080, and ERICA), inhibits the late inward sodium current, indirectly reducing the sodium-dependent calcium current during ischemic conditions and leading to improvement in ventricular diastolic tension and oxygen consumption. It

seems to increase the efficiency of energy production in the heart, maintaining cardiac function. Its antianginal and antiischemic effects do not depend on reductions in heart rate or blood pressure. It is indicated for treatment of chronic angina that is inadequately controlled with other antianginals. It represents a new class of drugs known as metabolic modulators and can be useful when prescribed as substitute for beta-blockers or in combination with them for relief of symptoms when initial treatment with beta-blockers is not successful or is contraindicated. Side effects include prolongation of QT interval. Low doses of diltiazem and verapamil should be used with ranolazine. The extended-release preparation reduces the frequency of angina, improves exercise performance, and delays the development of exercise-induced angina and ST-segment depression.

- ACE inhibition through changes in the physiologic balance between angiotensin II and bradykinin could contribute to the reductions in LV and vascular hypertrophy, atherosclerosis progression, plaque rupture, and thrombosis; the favorable changes in cardiac hemodynamics; and the improved myocardial oxygen supply/demand. It has been shown to be effective in reducing cardiovascular death, MI, and stroke in patients who are at risk for or who had vascular disease. They are indicated in patients with hypertension, diabetes, LVEF <40%, and CKD. Angiotensin receptor blockers (ARBs) can be given to patients with SIHD who are intolerant to ACE inhibitors and qualify for them.
- Use of high-intensity statin drugs is recommended in all patients with CAD. In late 2018 the American College of Cardiology (ACC) recommended an low density lipoprotein (LDL) goal of <70 mg/dl for secondary prevention of atherosclerotic cardiovascular disease. There is no LDL goal for primary prevention. The FDA approved PCSK9 (proprotein convertase subtilisin/kexin type 9) inhibitors (alirocumab and evolocumab) for heterozygous familial hypercholesterolemia in those who maximally tolerated statins. Newer 2018 lipid guidelines suggested starting PCSK9 inhibitor in very-high-risk atherosclerotic cardiovascular disease patients who did not meet the LDL goal on high-intensity statin and ezetimibe. One should always consider adding ezetimibe to high-intensity statin prior to initiation of PCSK9 inhibitor due to cost issues. Inclisiran, evinacumab, and bempedoic acid are reasonable nonstatin therapy alternatives in patients who are unable to tolerate statin and reach target LDL levels.
- Influenza vaccine is recommended for patients with SIHD on annual basis to prevent all-cause mortality, morbidity, and hospitalization caused by the exacerbation of underlying medical conditions produced by influenza.
- The EMPAREG OUTCOME, CANVAS, DECLARE-TIMI 58, and CREDENCE trial showed that SGLT2 inhibitors significantly reduce cardiovascular events in type 2 diabetic patients.

NEW MODALITIES FOR THE TREATMENT OF CHRONIC STABLE ANGINA PECTORIS

- Although a significant amount of progress has been made in the management of CAD with percutaneous coronary intervention (PCI) and CABG, many patients with the condition require additional therapeutic modalities for relief of symptoms and improvement in quality of life. This group of patients includes those with diffuse CAD who are not suitable for revascularization, patients with previous multiple PCIs or CABG limiting the chances for further revascularization, the lack of vascular conduits for CABG, severe LV systolic dysfunction in patients with previous CABG or PCI, and comorbidities that would render the patients at high risk for revascularization.
- The following pharmacologic agents have been used for the management of stable angina in combination with the standard protocol of nitrates, beta-blockers, calcium channel blockers, and ranolazine: High-dose statin therapy, trimetazidine, perhexiline, nicorandil, allopurinol, ivabradine, fasudil, and testosterone.
- Other, nonpharmacologic modalities that are highly experimental include stem cell therapy, therapeutic angiogenesis, and mechanical therapies such as external counter pulsation, spinal cord stimulation, transmyocardial laser revascularization, and coronary sinus reducing device.
- In TACT (Trial to Assess Chelation Therapy), ethylenediaminetetraacetic acid (EDTA) intravenous infusion resulted in significant decrease in total mortality, recurrent MI, stroke, coronary revascularization, or hospitalization for angina. Thus chelation therapy was upgraded from Class III (not recommended) to Class IIb in the 2014 SIHD guidelines. Allopurinol, a xanthine oxidase inhibitor, was shown to reduce myocardial oxygen demand per unit of cardiac output in patients with heart failure in a small crossover study of 65 patients given 600 mg of allopurinol daily for 6 wk. Allopurinol increased the median time to ST depression from 232 sec at baseline to 393 sec. Further and larger studies are necessary to recommend allopurinol as an adjunctive therapy for stable angina.
- Testosterone improves endothelial dysfunction and may be an effective antiangina agent. However, given the potential side effects, additional trials are necessary to recommend testosterone as an adjunctive drug for chronic angina.
- The value of enhanced external counter pulsation (EECP) was assessed with the MUST-EECP trial, which randomly assigned 139 outpatients with angina, documented CAD, and a positive stress test to 35 h of active EECP. The results indicated the following regarding EECP: (1) Was well tolerated; (2) exercise duration increased in both groups; (3) active EECP patients had a significant increase in time to 1-mm ST-segment depression, whereas there was no change in the inactive group; (4) more patients undergoing active EECP had a decrease in angina episodes, and fewer had

an increase in angina symptoms compared with the active group. These data corroborate similar data from multicenter registries. The American Heart Association, American College of Cardiology, Society for Cardiovascular Angiography and Interventions, American Thoracic Society, and Society of Thoracic Surgeons focused update states that EECP may be considered for relief of refractory angina.
- The following treatments have NOT been shown to be beneficial in reducing cardiovascular risk or improving clinical outcomes: Estrogen therapy, vitamin C, vitamin E, and beta-carotene supplementation; treatment of elevated homocysteine with folate or vitamins B_6 and B_{12}; chelation therapy; garlic; coenzyme Q10; selenium; and chromium.

REFERRAL

Revascularization:

- Revascularization methods should be formulated taking into consideration improved survival or improved symptoms. Revascularization includes either PCI (balloon angioplasty and stenting) or CABG. However, note that although the role of PCI is unquestionable in the presence of an acute MI, its role is not so clear in stable CAD. The utilization of PCI for stable CAD was reduced by 51.7% from 2007 to 2011, and hospitals with higher volumes of PCI had the largest reduction of these procedures.
- **To improve survival:**
  1. Perform CABG for patients with significant (>50% diameter stenosis) left main coronary artery stenosis, more than 70% diameter stenosis in proximal left anterior descending artery (LAD), or more than 70% diameter stenosis in three major epicardial vessels, >70% diameter stenosis in two major coronary arteries with severe or extensive myocardial ischemia, and in patients with mild to moderate LV systolic dysfunction (EF 35% to 50%) and significant multivessel CAD. Left internal mammary artery (LIMA) graft improves survival when used to bypass a proximal LAD artery stenosis. CABG is recommended in preference to PCI to improve survival in patients with multivessel CAD with Syntax score of >22 and multivessel CAD with diabetes, particularly if a LIMA graft to LAD is used.[2]
  2. PCI is reasonable as an alternative to CABG in selected stable patients (low or intermediate SYNTAX score and/or high STS score) with unprotected left main CAD, low risk of PCI procedural complications, and a high likelihood of good long-term outcome *and* clinical characteristics that predict a significantly increased risk of adverse surgical outcomes (e.g., STS-predicted risk of operative mortality >5).
- To improve symptoms:
  1. CABG or PCI to improve symptoms is beneficial in patients with one or more significant (>70% diameter) coronary artery stenosis amenable to revascularization and unacceptable angina despite

maximal medical treatment, or in whom increasing medical therapy cannot be implemented because of medication contraindications, adverse effects, or patient preferences. In 2017, ORBITA trial showed no significant improvement in angina score after PCI for optimally treated stable angina patients. However, 85% of study patients in placebo group underwent PCI within 6 wk after ORBITA trial completed. In 2020, the Ischemia trial showed no benefit with routine invasive therapy compared to conservative treatment in moderate to severe ischemia patients. However, this study excludes patients with ACS, severe and frequent symptoms, EF <35%, and left main stenosis. Hybrid coronary revascularization: LIMA-to-LAD artery grafting and of >1 non-LAD coronary artery can be used in patients who have an unfavorable aorta, have poor target vessels for CABG, have unsuitable graft conduits, or have unfavorable LAD for PCI.
- Compared with PCI, CABG is more effective in relieving angina and leads to fewer repeated revascularizations but has a higher risk for procedural stroke. Survival to 10 yr is similar for both procedures.
- Angioplasty and coronary stents (Fig. E3).
- PCI has an established place in treating angina but is not superior to intensive medical therapy to prevent MI and death in symptomatic or asymptomatic patients. Patients selected for PCI should also be candidates for CABG. Approximately 80% of patients show immediate benefit after PCI. The development of coronary stents has increased the number of patients who can be treated in the cardiac laboratory. Cardiac stents (Fig. E4) are currently used in nearly 95% of all patients with PCI lesions. The rate of restenosis is reduced by placing a stent electively in primary atheromatous lesions. The major limitations of stenting are subacute thrombosis, restenosis within the stent, bleeding complications when antiplatelets are used after stenting, and higher cost. The combination of aspirin and P2Y12 antagonists is effective in preventing coronary stent thrombosis and the duration of therapy depends on whether bare metal stents (BMS) or drug-eluting stents (DES) are used. Duration of dual antiplatelet therapy can be as short as 4 wk for BMS, but 6 to 12 mo of therapy is generally required for DES. This difference in duration is due to the lack of endothelium proliferation in DES initially. New drug-eluting stents with thin struts releasing limus-family analogs from durable polymers have lowered the risk of stent thrombosis compared with early-generation stents releasing sirolimus or paclitaxel. Current evidence supports the use of drug-eluting stents in most clinical settings without safety concerns (unless there are contraindications to use of dual antiplatelet therapy).[2]

PEARLS & CONSIDERATIONS

COMMENTS

- Although nitrate responsiveness is usually an integral part of a diagnostic strategy for SIHD, recent reports question its value and conclude that in a general population admitted for chest pain, relief of pain after nitroglycerin treatment does not predict active CAD and should not be used to guide diagnosis in the acute care setting.
- CABG is associated with higher long-term survival rates and lower rates of repeat revascularization than PCI and stenting; however, patients often prefer stenting because it is less invasive, involves a shorter hospital stay, and has a lower in-hospital mortality rate.

RELATED CONTENT

Angina (Patient Information)
Unstable Angina (Patient Information)

Acute Coronary Syndrome (Related Key Topic)
Coronary Artery Disease (Related Key Topic)
Myocardial Infarction (Related Key Topic)

AUTHOR: **MAHESWARA SATYA GANGADHARA RAO GOLLA, MD**

REFERENCES

Available at eBooks.Health.Elsevier.com.

BASIC INFORMATION

DEFINITION

- The mucocutaneous swelling caused by the release of vasoactive mediators is called urticaria and angioedema.[1]
- Urticaria causes edema of the superficial dermis.
- Angioedema is due to a transient increase in vascular permeability of the mucosal/submucosal or dermal/subcutaneous tissues resulting in tissue swelling.[2]

SYNONYMS

Angioneurotic edema
Hereditary angioedema (HAE)

ICD-10CM CODES

T78.3	Angioedema
D84.1	Angioedema, hereditary

EPIDEMIOLOGY & DEMOGRAPHICS

INCIDENCE: 100 to 3000/100,000 persons for urticaria and angioedema. Approximately 7.4% of the general population will experience angioedema alone.[3]

LIFETIME PREVALENCE: Approximately 25% of the population experiences urticaria and/or angioedema at some time during life. The prevalence of hereditary angioedema is one case/50,000 persons.[1,2,4,5]

DEMOGRAPHICS:

- Race: African Americans have higher rates of ACE inhibitor-induced angioedema.[6,7]
- Sex: hereditary angioedema (HAE) occurs more frequently in women than men.[6]
- Angioedema commonly occurs after adolescence in the third decade of life.[6]
- The mean age of onset of HAE is 8 to 12 yr and rarely occurs before 1 yr of age.[6]
- Angioedema can occur together with urticaria (40%) or alone (20%); the remaining 40% have urticaria alone.[6,8]

PHYSICAL FINDINGS & CLINICAL PRESENTATION

- Angioedema may be acute or chronic:
  1. Acute angioedema is defined as symptoms lasting ≤6 wk.
  2. Chronic angioedema is defined as symptoms lasting >6 wk.
- Angioedema is characterized by the following:
  1. Nonpruritic, nonpitting, burning, occasionally painful swelling of deep skin layers or submucosal membranes
  2. Poorly demarcated
  3. Commonly involve eyelids, lips (Fig. E1), tongue, and extremities
  4. Can involve the upper airway, causing respiratory distress
  5. Can involve the GI tract, leading to abdominal pain, nausea, vomiting, and diarrhea
  6. Resolves slowly within hours to a few days

ETIOLOGY

- Angioedema, with or without urticaria, is classified as histaminergic (mast cell mediated), bradykinin-mediated, or idiopathic nonhistaminergic.[8,9]
- Angioedema is primarily caused by immune activation with release of vasoactive mediators, resulting in postcapillary venule inflammation, vascular leakage, and edema in the deep layers of the dermis and subcutaneous tissue.
- Pathologically, angioedema has both immunologic- and nonimmunologic-mediated mechanisms (Fig. 2).
  1. Mast cell (histamine)-mediated angioedema has several pathogeneses. Immunoglobulin E–mediated angioedema results from antigen exposure (e.g., foods [milk, eggs, peanuts, shellfish] or drugs [beta-lactam antibiotics, quinolones, NSAIDs, phenytoin, recombinant tissue plasminogen activator]).[8-11] Opiates and muscle relaxers (succinylcholine) can directly activate mast cells. Complement-mediated angioedema involving immune complex mechanisms can also lead to mast cell activation that manifests as serum sickness.

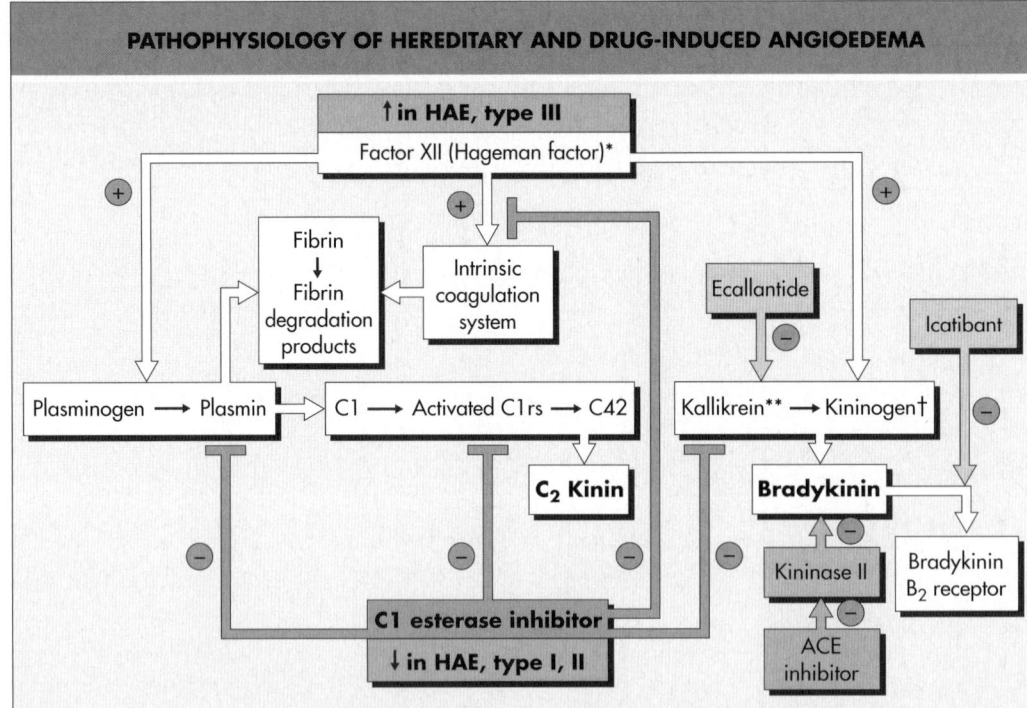

FIG. 2 Pathophysiology of hereditary and drug-induced angioedema. Angiotensin-converting enzyme *(ACE)* inhibitor-induced urticaria is believed to result from the inhibition of endogenous kininase and a subsequent increase in bradykinin. Icatibant and ecallantide have been approved for the emergency treatment of hereditary angioedema *(HAE)* as alternatives to C1 esterase inhibitor (C1-INH) concentrate (derived from human plasma) or recombinant C1-INH (derived from milk of transgenic rabbits). Icatibant, a decapeptide, is a specific bradykinin B2 receptor antagonist. Ecallantide, a 60-amino acid recombinant protein, selectively inhibits kallikrein. Off label, icatibant has been used to treat ACE inhibitor-induced angioedema. Two forms of C1-INH, one of which is administered intravenously and the other subcutaneously, are approved for prevention of attacks. Lanadelumab, a human monoclonal antibody that inhibits plasma kallikrein, received FDA approval for biweekly injections to prevent attacks. (From Bolognia J et al: *Dermatology,* ed 4, London, 2018, Elsevier Limited.)

*The active form of factor XII (Hageman factor) is XIIa.

**Kallikrein is formed from prekallikrein.

†High-molecular-weight.

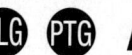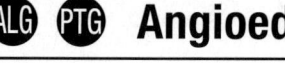

A

2. Hereditary angioedema is subdivided into three different groups: HAE with deficit C1-inhibitor (HAE-1), HAE with dysfunctional C1-inhibitor (HAE-2), and HAE with normal C1-inhibitor function (HAE nC1-INH). HAE-1 and HAE-2 result from autosomal dominant mutations in the *SERPING1* gene, which codes for C1 esterase inhibitor (C1-INH), a serine protease. C1-INH inhibits plasma kallikrein, a protease that cleaves kininogen and releases bradykinin. HAE nC1-INH encapsulates several different mutations that affect the contact activation system at different points, which are thought to potentiate bradykinin. Bradykinin increases capillary permeability and activates pain receptors.[2]

3. Acquired angioedema is usually associated with other diseases, most commonly B-cell lymphoproliferative disorders, but may also result from the formation of autoantibodies directed against C1-inhibitor protein.

4. ACE inhibitors increase kinin activity, which increases bradykinin and can lead to angioedema in select individuals.

5. Other causes of angioedema include infection (e.g., herpes simplex, hepatitis B, Coxsackie A and B, *Streptococcus, Candida, Ascaris,* and *Strongyloides*), insect bites and stings, stress, physical factors (e.g., cold, exercise, pressure, and vibration), connective tissue diseases (e.g., systemic lupus erythematosus, Henoch-Schönlein purpura), and idiopathic causes.[10,11]

Dx DIAGNOSIS

A detailed history and physical examination usually establish the diagnosis of angioedema. Extensive laboratory testing is of limited value.

DIFFERENTIAL DIAGNOSIS
- Anaphylaxis
- Contact dermatitis
- Cellulitis
- Lymphedema
- Arthropod bite
- Hypothyroidism

- Atopic dermatitis
- Mastocytosis
- Granulomatous cheilitis
- Bullous pemphigoid
- Urticaria pigmentosa
- Erythema multiforme
- Epiglottitis
- Peritonsillar abscess
- Parasite infection
- Superior vena cava syndrome
- Systemic capillary leak syndrome

WORKUP
- An extensive workup searching for the cause of angioedema is often unrevealing (40%).
- Workup, including diagnostic blood tests and allergy testing, is performed according to results of the history and physical examination. Fig. 3 illustrates an algorithm for the diagnosis of angioedema.

LABORATORY TESTS
- CBC, erythrocyte sedimentation rate, and urinalysis are sometimes helpful as part of the initial evaluation.

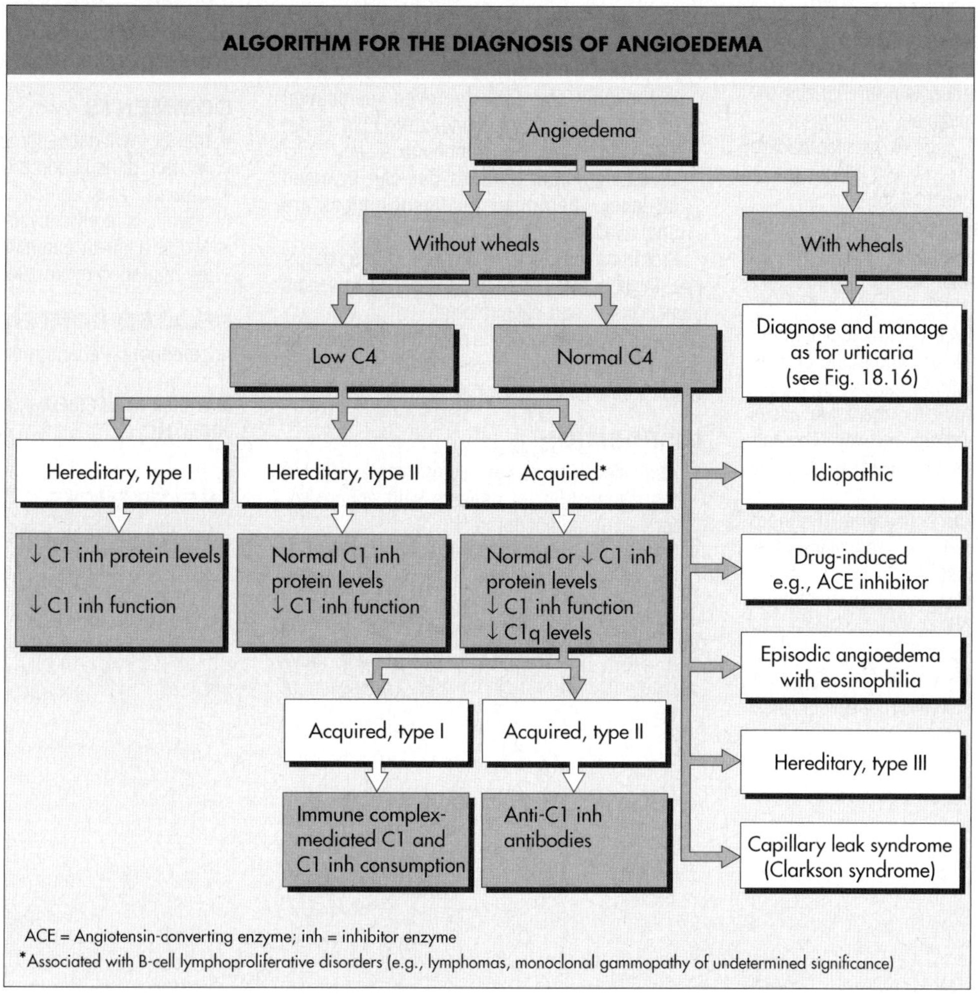

ALGORITHM FOR THE DIAGNOSIS OF ANGIOEDEMA

Angioedema
→ Without wheals / With wheals

Without wheals → Low C4 / Normal C4

With wheals → Diagnose and manage as for urticaria (see Fig. 18.16)

Low C4 → Hereditary, type I / Hereditary, type II / Acquired*

Hereditary, type I → ↓ C1 inh protein levels / ↓ C1 inh function

Hereditary, type II → Normal C1 inh protein levels / ↓ C1 inh function

Acquired* → Normal or ↓ C1 inh protein levels / ↓ C1 inh function / ↓ C1q levels

Acquired → Acquired, type I / Acquired, type II

Acquired, type I → Immune complex-mediated C1 and C1 inh consumption

Acquired, type II → Anti-C1 inh antibodies

Normal C4 → Idiopathic / Drug-induced e.g., ACE inhibitor / Episodic angioedema with eosinophilia / Hereditary, type III / Capillary leak syndrome (Clarkson syndrome)

ACE = Angiotensin-converting enzyme; inh = inhibitor enzyme
*Associated with B-cell lymphoproliferative disorders (e.g., lymphomas, monoclonal gammopathy of undetermined significance)

FIG. 3 Algorithm for the diagnosis of angioedema. Episodic angioedema with hypereosinophilia, along with weight gain and fever, is known as Gleich syndrome. *ACE,* Angiotensin-converting enzyme. (From Bolognia J et al: *Dermatology,* ed 4, London, 2018, Elsevier Limited.)

- Serum total tryptase is helpful in confirming mast cell–mediated anaphylaxis.
- C4 levels are usually reduced in acquired and hereditary angioedema (occurring without urticaria). If C4 levels are low, C1-INH levels and activity should then be obtained. There are isolated reports of hereditary angioedema with normal C4 levels but reduced C1-INH levels.
- Skin prick and in vitro sIgE (ImmunoCAP) testing may be done if food allergies are suspected.
- Skin biopsy can be considered in patients with chronic angioedema refractory to corticosteroid treatment.

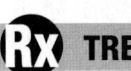 **TREATMENT**

NONPHARMACOLOGIC THERAPY

- Eliminate the offending agent
- Avoid triggering factors (e.g., cold, stress, certain medications, including ACE inhibitor)
- Cold compresses to affected areas

ACUTE GENERAL Rx

- Acute life-threatening angioedema involving the larynx is treated with the following. However, it should be noted that bradykinin-mediated angioedema will have minimal response to these medications.
  1. Epinephrine 0.3 mg in a solution of 1:1000 given subcutaneous
  2. Diphenhydramine 25 to 50 mg intravenous (IV) or intramuscular or cetirizine 10 mg IV (where available)
  3. Cimetidine 300 mg IV or famotidine 20 mg IV
  4. Methylprednisolone 125 mg IV
- Corticosteroids (prednisone 1 mg/kg/day for 5 days and then tapered over 7 days) may be used for symptomatic relief of refractory acute angioedema.
- Purified plasma-derived C1-INH replacement therapy is effective in treating acute attacks of hereditary angioedema caused by C1 inhibitor deficiency; however, there are cases of worsening angioedema as well. The following therapies are approved as abortive therapies for HAE.[2,8]
  1. Purified C1 inhibitor concentrate (Berinert)
  2. Icatibant (Firazyr), a bradykinin–B2-receptor antagonist
  3. Ecallantide (Kalbitor), a kallikrein inhibitor

CHRONIC Rx

- Maintenance therapy in mast cell–mediated, nonhereditary angioedema is H_1 antihistamines:
  1. Cetirizine 10 mg/day (may require up to 4× the FDA-approved dosing)
  2. Fexofenadine 180 mg/day (may require up to 4× the FDA-approved dosing)
  3. Levocetirizine 5 mg/day (may increase up to 10mg bid)
  4. Hydroxyzine 10 to 25 mg q6h
- H_2 antihistamines can be added to H_1 antihistamines:
  1. Cimetidine 400 mg bid
  2. Famotidine 20 mg bid
- Doxepin, a tricyclic antidepressant, can be added to H_1 and H_2 antihistamines.
- Omalizumab is an anti-IgE monoclonal antibody that has shown efficacy in cases refractory to antihistamines alone although is not FDA approved for isolated angioedema.
- Several classes of medication are FDA approved for long-term prophylaxis for HAE.[2,8] Androgens (danazol) are effective but are associated with many adverse effects. IV plasma-derived C1 inhibitors (Cinryze, Berinert) are safe and effective and may be used in patients who have frequent or severe attacks. Cost can be a limiting factor. A twice-weekly subcutaneous formulation (Haegarda/CSL830, CSL Behring) is approved by the FDA to treat HAE-1 and HAE-2 hereditary angioedema. Lanadelumab and berotralstat are kallikrein inhibitors that have recently received FDA approval for prophylaxis therapy of HAE.[8] Berotralstat is the only oral FDA-approved medication for HAE prophylaxis. Tranexamic acid is not FDA approved for prophylaxis and has several contraindications but can be used off-label when other treatment options are unavailable.[2,8]

Promising potential prophylactic therapies for HAE include two different prekallikrein inhibitors (donidalorsen and sebetralstat), which were effective in phase 2 trials, and a monoclonal antibody that inhibits activated factor XII (garadicamab), which was effective in a phase 3 trial.[8,12,13]

DISPOSITION

- Antihistamines achieve symptomatic relief in more than 85% of patients with nonhereditary acute angioedema.[14]
- For chronic nonhereditary angioedema, antihistamines remain the mainstay in therapy and systemic steroids should be reserved for severe or refractory cases.
- A small percentage of people will have recurrence of symptoms after completion of treatment.

- Chronic angioedema can last for months to years but possibly longer in the situation of HAE.

REFERRAL

Consultation with an allergist and/or dermatologist is recommended in patients with chronic angioedema, hereditary angioedema, and recurring angioedema.

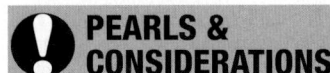 **PEARLS & CONSIDERATIONS**

ACE inhibitors can cause angioedema months or years after initiation.[15] Angiotensin receptor blockers (ARBs) can also cause angioedema, although the risk is substantially less than that of ACE inhibitors. Approximately 10% of patients with recurrent angioedema had ACE inhibitor exposure with median duration of 1 yr prior to symptom onset. Incidence rates per 1000 person-yr are 4.38 cases for ACE inhibitors, 1.66 cases for ARBs. The incidence rate is also very high for the direct renin inhibitor aliskiren (4.67). Starting the angiotensin receptor/neprilysin inhibitor sacubitril-valsartan (SV) was associated with a lower likelihood of angioedema compared to starting ACE inhibitors (hazard ratio 0.18; 95% confidence interval of 0.11 to 0.29).[7] There was no difference in angioedema risk between initiating SV vs. ARBs.

COMMENTS

- Identifying a cause for angioedema in patients is often difficult and met with frustration.
- Chronic angioedema, unlike acute angioedema, is rarely caused by an allergic reaction.
- HAE is a life-threatening condition and should be managed by an allergist.

RELATED CONTENT

Angioedema (Patient Information)

AUTHORS: **RYAN FRIEDMAN, MD**, and **SHYAM JOSHI, MD**

REFERENCES

Available at eBooks.Health.Elsevier.com.

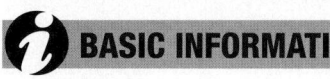
Diseases and Disorders

I

BASIC INFORMATION

DEFINITION

Aortic regurgitation (AR) is abnormal retrograde blood flow into the left ventricle from the aorta due to an inadequately closing aortic valve (AV). The inadequate closure of the valve can result from either disease of the ascending aorta (ex., dilation) and aortic root or disease of aortic valve leaflets. In addition, it can be acute or chronic in nature.

Stages of chronic aortic regurgitation:
- Stage A = at risk of aortic insufficiency (AI) without even trace AR (e.g., bicuspid AV, AV sclerosis, diseases of the ascending aorta, history of rheumatic heart disease, or infective endocarditis)
- Stage B = progressive AI with mild to moderate AR and preserved left ventricular ejection fraction (LVEF)
- Stage C = asymptomatic severe AR with preserved (stage C1) or reduced (stage C2) LVEF
- Stage D = symptomatic severe AR

SYNONYMS

Aortic insufficiency
AI
AR

ICD-10CM CODES
I35.1	Nonrheumatic aortic (valve) insufficiency
I35.2	Nonrheumatic aortic (valve) stenosis with insufficiency
I06.1	Rheumatic aortic insufficiency
I06.2	Rheumatic aortic stenosis with insufficiency
Q23.1	Congenital insufficiency of aortic valve

EPIDEMIOLOGY & DEMOGRAPHICS

Prevalence varies with severity of AR, age, and gender, as summarized in Table 1.
- Most common cause in the developing world is rheumatic heart disease.
- Most common causes in developed countries are aortic root dilation, congenital bicuspid aortic valve, and calcific valve disease.

TABLE 1 Prevalence of Aortic Regurgitation (AR)

Mild AR Prevalence	Males	Females
Age 50-59	3.7%	1.9%
Age 60-69	12.1%	6%
Age 70-83	12.2%	14.6%
Moderate-Severe AR Prevalence	**Males**	**Females**
Age 50-59	0.5%	0.2%
Age 60-69	0.6%	0.8%
Age 70-83	2.2%	2.3%

From Singh JP et al: Prevalence and clinical determinants of mitral, tricuspid, and aortic regurgitation (the Framingham Heart Study), *Am J Cardiol* 83:897, 1999.

- Infectious endocarditis (IE) is the most frequent cause of acute AR.

PHYSICAL FINDINGS & CLINICAL PRESENTATION

Clinical presentation varies depending on whether AR is acute or chronic. Chronic AR is well tolerated (except when secondary to IE), and patients remain asymptomatic for years. Common manifestations after significant deterioration of LVEF (Fig. 1) are dyspnea on exertion, syncope, chest pain, and congestive heart failure (CHF). The stages of chronic AR are summarized in Table 2. Acute severe AR manifests primarily with hypotension caused by a sudden fall in cardiac output and resultant cardiogenic shock. A rapid rise in left ventricular diastolic pressure results in a further decrease in coronary blood flow.

Physical findings in chronic AR:
- Widened pulse pressure (markedly increased systolic blood pressure with decreased diastolic blood pressure).
- Findings associated with widened pulse pressure:
  1. Bounding, "water hammer," or collapsing pulse (**Corrigan pulse**) can be palpated at the wrist or femoral artery and is caused by the rapid rise and sudden collapse of arterial pressure during late systole.
  2. Head "bobbing" with each heart beat (**de Musset sign**).
  3. "Pistol shot femorals" (**Traube sign**) describes a loud sound over the femoral artery with systole and diastole.
  4. Capillary pulsations (**Quincke sign**) may occur on the lips or at the base of the nail beds.
- A to-and-fro intermittent femoral murmur (**Duroziez sign**) may be heard with slight compression of the femoral arteries. Popliteal systolic pressure increased >20 mm Hg over the brachial systolic pressure (**Hill sign**); a 40 to 60 mm difference represents moderate AR and >60 mm difference, severe AR.
- Findings more of historical than practical interest, which are neither sensitive nor specific, include:
  1. **Mueller sign**—Systolic pulsations of the uvula
  2. **Becker sign**—Visible pulsations of the retinal arteries and pupils
  3. **Mayne sign**—More than a 15 mm Hg decrease in diastolic blood pressure with arm elevation from the value obtained with the arm in the standard position
  4. **Rosenbach sign**—Systolic pulsations of the liver
  5. **Gerhard sign**—Systolic pulsations of the spleen

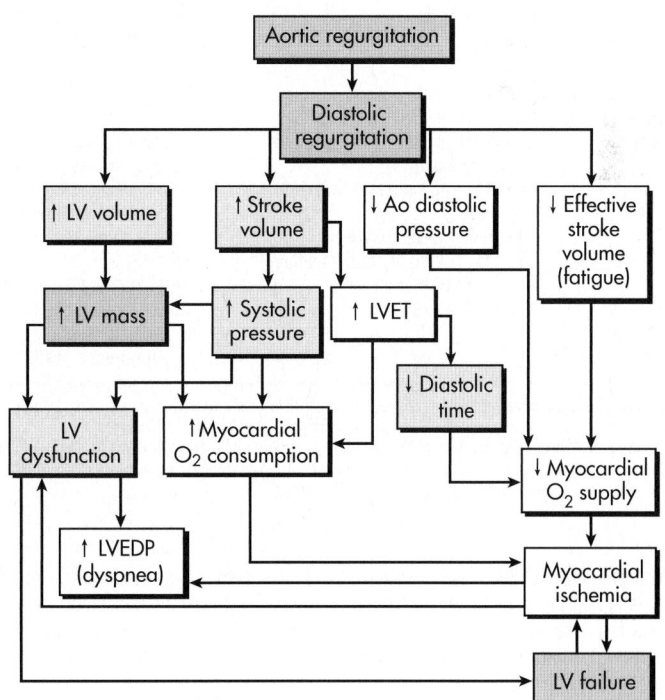

FIG. 1 Pathophysiology of aortic regurgitation. Regurgitation results in an increased left ventricular (*LV*) volume, increased stroke volume, increased aortic (*Ao*) systolic pressure, and decreased effective stroke volume. Increased LV volume results in an increased LV mass, which may lead to LV dysfunction and failure. Increased LV stroke volume increases systolic pressure and prolongation of LV ejection time (*LVET*). Increased LV systolic pressure results in a decrease in diastolic time. Decreased diastolic time (myocardial perfusion time), diastolic aortic pressure, and effective stroke volume lead to reduced myocardial O_2 supply. Increased myocardial O_2 consumption and decreased myocardial O_2 supply produce myocardial ischemia, which further impairs LV function. *LVEDP,* Left ventricular end-diastolic pressure. (From Boudoulas H, Gravanis MB: Valvular heart disease. In Gravanis MB [ed]: *Cardiovascular disorders: pathogenesis and pathophysiology,* St Louis, 1993, Mosby, p. 64.)

TABLE 2 Stages of Chronic Aortic Regurgitation

Stage	Definition	Valve Anatomy	Valve Hemodynamics	Hemodynamic Consequences	Symptoms
A	At risk of AR	Bicuspid aortic valve (or other congenital valve anomaly) Aortic valve sclerosis Diseases of the aortic sinuses or ascending aorta History of rheumatic fever or known rheumatic heart disease IE	AR severity none or trace	None	None
B	Progressive AR	Mild to moderate calcification of a trileaflet valve bicuspid aortic valve (or other congenital valve anomaly) Dilated aortic sinuses Rheumatic valve changes Previous IE	*Mild AR:* Jet width <25% of LVOT vena contracta <0.3 cm RVol <30 ml/beat RF <30% ERO <0.10 cm^2 Angiography grade 1+ *Moderate AR:* Jet width 25%-64% of LVOT Vena contracta 0.3-0.6 cm RVol 30-59 ml/beat RF 30%-49% ERO 0.10-0.29 cm^2 Angiography grade 2+	Normal LV systolic function Normal LV volume or mild LV dilation	None
C	Asymptomatic severe AR	Calcific aortic valve disease Bicuspid valve (or other congenital abnormality) Dilated aortic sinuses or ascending aorta Rheumatic valve changes IE with abnormal leaflet closure or perforation	*Severe AR:* Jet width ≥65% of LVOT Vena contracta >0.6 cm Holodiastolic flow reversal in the proximal abdominal aorta RVol ≥60 ml/beat RF ≥50% ERO ≥0.3 cm^2 Angiography grade 3+ to 4+ In addition, diagnosis of chronic severe AR requires evidence of LV dilation	*C1:* Normal LVEF (≥55%) and mild-to-moderate LV dilation (LVESD ≤50 mm) *C2:* Abnormal LV systolic function with depressed LVEF (<55%) or severe LV dilation (LVESD >50 mm or indexed LVESD >25 mm/m^2)	None; exercise testing is reasonable to confirm symptom status
D	Symptomatic severe AR	Calcific valve disease Bicuspid valve (or other congenital abnormality) Dilated aortic sinuses or ascending aorta Rheumatic valve changes Previous IE with abnormal leaflet closure or perforation	*Severe AR:* Doppler jet width ≥65% of LVOT Vena contracta >0.6 cm Holodiastolic flow reversal in the proximal abdominal aorta RVol ≥60 ml/beat RF ≥50% ERO ≥0.3 cm^2 Angiography grade 3+ to 4+ In addition, diagnosis of chronic severe AR requires evidence of LV dilation	Symptomatic severe AR may occur with normal systolic function (LVEF ≥55%), mild-to-moderate LV dysfunction (LVEF 40%-55%), or severe LV dysfunction (LVEF <40%). Moderate-to-severe LV dilation is present	Exertional dyspnea or angina, or more severe HF symptoms

AR, Aortic regurgitation; *ERO,* effective regurgitant orifice; *HF,* heart failure; *IE,* infective endocarditis; *LV,* left ventricle; *LVEF,* left ventricular ejection fraction; *LVESD,* left ventricular end-systolic dimension; *LVOT,* left ventricular outflow tract; *RF,* regurgitant fraction; *RVol,* regurgitant volume.
From Otto CM et al: 2020 ACC/AHA Guideline for the Management of Patients With Valvular Heart Disease: Executive Summary: a report of the American College of Cardiology/American Heart Association Joint Committee on Clinical Practice Guidelines [published correction appears in *Circulation* 143(5):e228, 2021] [published correction appears in *Circulation* 143(10):e784, 2021] *Circulation* 143(5):e35-e71, 2021, https://doi.org/10.1161/CIR.0000000000000932.

6. *Landolfi sign*—Pupil dilation and constriction with each heartbeat on the ocular exam
Cardiac auscultation reveals:
- Displacement of cardiac impulse downward and to the patient's left
- S$_3$ heard over the apex
- Decrescendo, blowing diastolic murmur heard along left sternal border (Fig. E2)
- Low-pitched apical diastolic rumble (*Austin Flint* murmur)—the precise etiology is uncertain, but it is generally believed to be related to increased velocity of mitral inflow consequent to the AR
- Early systolic ejection sound and systolic ejection murmur

In patients with acute aortic insufficiency, both the wide pulse pressure and the large stroke volume are absent. A short, blowing diastolic murmur may be the only finding on physical examination.

ETIOLOGY (BOX 1)
- Leaflet abnormalities:
  1. Infective endocarditis
  2. Rheumatic fibrosis (most common cause in developing countries)
  3. Trauma with valvular rupture
  4. Congenital heart disease (bicuspid aortic valve—most common cause in the U.S., sinus of Valsalva aneurysm)
  5. Myxomatous degeneration

  6. Calcific AV disease
  7. Drug-induced (fenfluramine, dexfenfluramine, pergolide, cabergoline)
  8. Systemic rheumatic disorders (ankylosing spondylitis, rheumatoid arthritis, systemic lupus erythematosus)
  9. Iatrogenic (e.g., Aortic balloon valvotomy)
- Aortic root or ascending aorta abnormalities:
  1. Annuloaortic ectasia
  2. Genetic syndromes (Ehlers-Danlos, Marfan)
  3. Trauma
  4. Ankylosing spondylitis
  5. Syphilitic aortitis
  6. Systemic hypertension
  7. Aortic dissection

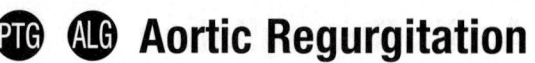

A

Diseases
and Disorders

I

Leaflet Abnormalities
Rheumatic disease
Aortic valve sclerosis and calcification
Congenital abnormalities (bicuspid, unicuspid, and quadricuspid valves; aortic regurgitation associated with discrete subaortic stenosis and ventricular septal defect)
Infective endocarditis
Myxomatous valve disease
Complicating balloon valvuloplasty and transcatheter aortic valve implantation
Rare causes (drugs, leaflet fenestration, irradiation, nonbacterial endocarditis, trauma)

Aortic Root Abnormalities
Chronic hypertension
Marfan syndrome
Annuloaortic ectasia
Aortic dissection
Ehlers-Danlos syndrome
Osteogenesis imperfecta
Atherosclerotic aneurysm
Syphilitic aortitis
Other systemic inflammatory disorders (giant cell aortitis, Takayasu disease, Reiter syndrome)

Combined Valve and Aortic Root Abnormalities
Bicuspid aortic valve
Ankylosing spondylitis

From Evangelista A et al: Aortic regurgitation: clinical presentation, disease stages, and management. In Otto CM, Bonow RO (eds.): *Valvular heart disease. A companion to Braunwald's heart disease,* ed 5, Philadelphia, 2021, Elsevier, pp. 179-196.

- Postprocedural AR, usually due to a paravalvular leak, occurs in 10% to 20% of patients undergoing transcatheter aortic valve replacement (TAVR). Patients with more than mild AR after TAVR have worse outcomes than those without AR.
- Moderate or severe AR is more common with the use of CoreValve TAVR device.
- Important predictors for developing post-TAVR aortic regurgitation include implantation depth, Agaston calcium score, and undersized valve.

Dx DIAGNOSIS

DIFFERENTIAL DIAGNOSIS
- Patent ductus arteriosus, pulmonary regurgitation, and other valvular abnormalities.
- The differential diagnosis of cardiac murmurs is described in Sections II and III.

WORKUP
- Echocardiogram, chest radiograph, ECG, cardiac magnetic resonance (CMR) imaging, and cardiac catheterization (selected patients)
- Medical history and physical examination focused on dyspnea on exertion, syncope, chest pain, and CHF

IMAGING STUDIES
- Chest radiography:
  1. Left ventricular hypertrophy (LVH) (chronic AR)
  2. Aortic dilation
  3. Normal cardiac silhouette with pulmonary edema: Possible in patients with acute AR
- ECG is not useful for diagnostic purposes but is commonly used in evaluation of patients with chronic AR to exclude associated arrhythmia. Typical findings on an ECG are LVH as a result of volume overload.
- Echocardiography (Fig. E3) is the main imaging modality to diagnose AR and assess left ventricular size and function. Quantification of the severity of regurgitation can be made either qualitatively by Doppler vena contracta width (severe if >0.6 cm) or quantitatively by effective regurgitant orifice area (severe if >0.30 cm^2), regurgitant volume (severe if >60 ml per/beat), and/or regurgitant fraction ≥50%.[1]
- Echocardiography can also be used for periodic monitoring of asymptomatic patients with normal LV systolic function and chronic AR.
- TTE (Class I) is indicated to assess severity and presence of AR in patients with bicuspid aortic valve or with known dilation of the aortic sinuses or ascending aorta.[1]
- TEE, CMR, or cardiac catheterization is indicated (class 1) in patients with moderate or severe AR and suboptimal echocardiographic images or discrepancy between TTE and clinical findings in order to assess AR severity, LV systolic function, and aortic size.[1,2]

Rx TREATMENT

NONPHARMACOLOGIC THERAPY
- Avoidance of competitive sports and heavy weight lifting if severe AR, patient is symptomatic, ejection fraction <50%, AR is associated with aortic root dilation
- Salt restriction
- Endocarditis prophylaxis is not recommended for chronic AR patients with native valves undergoing invasive procedures. However, antibiotic prophylaxis is recommended for patients with a prior history of infective endocarditis or a presence of prosthetic heart valve

ACUTE GENERAL Rx
- Emergent AV replacement (preferred) or repair for acute, severe AR[3]
- Intraaortic balloon pump is contraindicated
- Afterload reduction: ACE inhibitors and vasodilators (i.e., nitroprusside) in acute AR; diuretics for pulmonary edema
- Avoid beta-blockers that can prolong diastole
- Emergent surgical referral for cardiogenic shock

CHRONIC Rx
Management depends on whether patients are symptomatic and candidates for valve surgery. ACC/AHA guidelines for aortic valve replacement for chronic aortic regurgitation are summarized in Table 3 and Fig. 4.
- Symptomatic patients with severe AR who are candidates for valve surgery should proceed with valve replacement after medical optimization of heart failure.
- A trial comparing the outcomes of transcatheter aortic valve replacement (TAVR) with surgical aortic valve replacement (SAVR) in patients with pure aortic insufficiency (PAI) revealed no significant statistical difference in in-hospital mortality, fewer respiratory complications, acute kidney injuries, septic shock, and mechanical ventilation with TAVR but significantly more cardiopulmonary resuscitation and permanent pacemaker placements. TAVR could be considered for patients with PAI who are not candidates for surgery (Table 4).[4]
- Patients with severe AR who have LV systolic dysfunction and/or symptomatic but have a high and prohibitive surgical risk, guideline directed medical therapy is recommended including ACE inhibitors, ARBs, and sacubitril/valsartan.
- Other medical treatments for AR are based on limited studies. Beta-blocker use is controversial but has been associated with a higher survival rate in severe AR. Vasodilatory therapies (nifedipine and enalapril) have failed to show benefit in reducing the need for or delaying AV replacement in asymptomatic, severe AR with normal systolic function, but ACE/ARB therapy may indeed benefit moderate to severe AR.[5] Long-term vasodilator therapy with ACE inhibitors or nifedipine may be used in patients who have concomitant hypertension. There is no current definitive indication of medical therapy with afterload reduction for aortic regurgitation other than hypertension control specifically a systolic blood pressure >140 mm Hg.[1]
- Beta-blockers in combination with ACE inhibitors are reasonable in patients with symptomatic severe AR or LV dysfunction when surgery cannot be performed because of concomitant comorbidities. In a retrospective cohort study of 756 patients with chronic AR, beta-blocker therapy was associated with decreased mortality. Patients treated

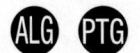
TABLE 3 American College of Cardiology/American Heart Association Guidelines for Aortic Valve Replacement (AVR) for Chronic Aortic Regurgitation (AR)

Class	Indication	LOE
I	AVR for symptomatic patients with severe AR regardless of LV systolic function (stage D).	B
	AVR for asymptomatic patients with chronic severe AR and LV systolic dysfunction (LVEF <55%) (stage C2).	B
	AVR for patients with severe AR (stage C or D) while undergoing cardiac surgery for other indications.	C
IIa	AVR is reasonable for asymptomatic patients with severe AR with normal LV systolic function (LVEF ≥55%), but severe LV dilation (stage C2, LVESD >50 mm).	B
	AVR is reasonable in patients with moderate AR (stage B) who are undergoing other cardiac surgery.	C
IIb	AVR may be considered for asymptomatic patients with severe AR and normal LV systolic function (stage C1, LVEF ≥55%) but severe LV dilation (LVEDD >65 mm) if surgical risk is low.*	C

*Particularly in the setting of progressive LV enlargement.
LOE, Level of evidence; *LV*, left ventricular; *LVEDD*, LV end-diastolic dimension; *LVEF*, LV ejection fraction; *LVESD*, LV end-systolic dimension.
From Zipes DP et al: *Braunwald's heart disease, a textbook of cardiovascular disease*, ed 11, Philadelphia, 2019, Elsevier.

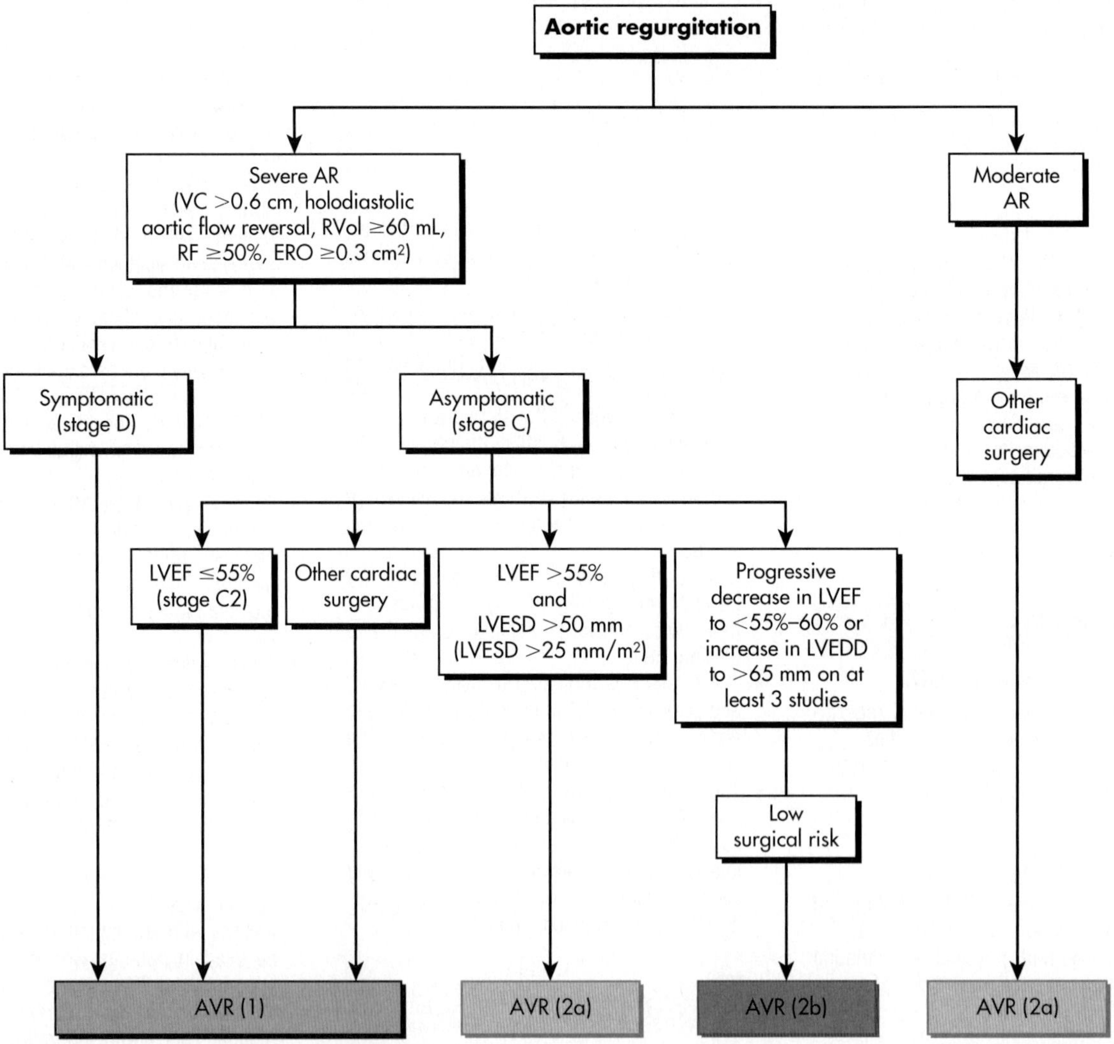

FIG. 4 Management of patients with chronic aortic regurgitation. *AR,* Aortic regurgitation; *AVR,* aortic valve replacement; *EDD,* end-diastolic dimension; *EF,* ejection fraction; *ERO,* effective regurgitant orifice; *ESD,* end-systolic dimension; *LV,* left ventricular; *RF,* regurgitant fraction; *RVol,* regurgitant volume; *VC,* vena contracta. (From Otto CM et al: 2020 AHA/ACC guideline for the management of patients with valvular heart disease: a report of the American College of Cardiology/American Heart Association Task Force on Practice Guidelines, *J Am Coll Cardiol,* 77:e25-e197, 2021.)

TABLE 4 Class 1 Recommendations for TAVR (ACC/AHA 2020 Guidelines)

COR	LOE	Recommendation
1	A	For symptomatic patients of any age with severe AS and a high or prohibitive surgical risk, TAVR is recommended if predicted post-TAVR survival is >12 mo with an acceptable quality of life
1	A	For symptomatic patients with severe AS who are >80 yr of age or for younger patients with a life expectancy <10 yr and no anatomic contraindication to transfemoral access, TAVR is recommended
1	A	For symptomatic patients with severe AS who are 65-80 yr of age and no anatomic contraindication to transfemoral access, after shared decision making, TAVR is an alternative to SAVR
1	B-NR	In asymptomatic patients with severe AS and an LVEF <50% who are ≤80 yr of age and no anatomic contraindication to transfemoral access, TAVR is an alternative to SAVR (preference according to age)

COR, Class of recommendation; *LOE,* level of evidence; *LVEF,* left ventricular ejection fraction; *NR,* nonrandomized.
From Otto CM et al: 2020 ACC/AHA guideline for the management of patients with valvular heart disease: a report of the American College of Cardiology/American Heart Association Joint Committee on Clinical Practice Guidelines, *J Am Coll Cardiol* 142(5):e72-e227, 2020.

with beta-blockers were more likely to be taking ACE inhibitors and dihydropyridine calcium channel blockers as well (53% vs. 40%). In the same study, patients treated with beta-blockers and undergoing AVR were also noted to have a mortality benefit.[6]
- Diuretics and sodium restriction for CHF.

REFERRAL

Surgical referral is reserved for the following patients:
- Patients with acute severe AR (i.e., infective endocarditis) and cardiogenic shock
- Symptomatic patients with severe AR regardless of LV systolic function (Class I)
- Patients with hemodynamically stable severe AR undergoing CABG or surgery on the aorta or other heart valves

- Evidence of systolic dysfunction with left ventricular ejection fraction of less than 55% and asymptomatic patients with chronic severe AR[7]
- Patients with moderate AR who are undergoing other forms of cardiac surgery
- Asymptomatic patients with severe AR and left ventricular ejection fraction >55% but with left ventricular dilation:
  1. Echocardiographic end-systolic dimension >50 mm (Class IIa level of evidence) *or;*
  2. Echocardiographic end-diastolic dimension >65 mm with low surgical risk (Class IIb)
- For patients with severe AR with increased surgical risk, off-label use of TAVR is also an option. Newer-generation TAVR valves such as JenaValve and J valve compared to early generation devices for native aortic

regurgitation had higher device success, less residual AI, and lower need for second valve implantation[8]

RELATED CONTENT

Aortic Insufficiency (Patient Information)
Transcatheter Aortic Valve Replacement (Related Key Topic)

REFERENCES

Available at eBooks.Health.Elsevier.com

AUTHOR: **SARTHAK KHARE, MD**

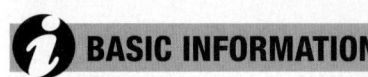

BASIC INFORMATION

DEFINITION

Aortic stenosis (AS) occurs with aortic valve thickening/calcification and is the most common adult valvular disease in developed nations. Symptoms typically appear when the valve orifice decreases to <1 cm² (normal orifice is 3 to 4 cm²). Criteria for severe AS include a valve area <1.0 cm², a mean gradient >40 mm Hg, or a peak velocity >4 m/sec (correlating with a peak gradient of 64 mm Hg). Doppler aortic jet velocities >5 m/sec is defined as very severe.[1]

SYNONYMS

Aortic valve stenosis
AS

ICD-10CM CODES	
I35.0	Nonrheumatic aortic (valve) stenosis
I35.2	Nonrheumatic aortic (valve) stenosis with insufficiency
Q23.0	Congenital stenosis of aortic valve

EPIDEMIOLOGY & DEMOGRAPHICS

- Aortic stenosis is the most common valve lesion in adults in North America and Europe.
- The prevalence demonstrates a strong relationship with age, affecting 0.2% between ages 50 and 59, 1.3% between 60 and 69, 3.9% between 70 and 79, and 9.8% between 80 and 89.

PHYSICAL FINDINGS & CLINICAL PRESENTATION

- Harsh mid-systolic, crescendo-decrescendo murmur (Fig. 1) best heard at base of heart and radiating into neck vessels; often associated with a thrill or ejection click; may also be heard well at the apex.
- Signs of severe AS include absent or diminished intensity of the second heart sound and/or slow-rising carotid upstroke with delayed amplitude (pulsus parvus et tardus), presence of S4, and a reverse splitting of the second heart sound.
- Early symptoms include decreased exercise tolerance, dyspnea on exertion, exertional dizziness or syncope, and exertional angina.
- Late symptoms include angina (secondary primarily to reduced coronary blood flow and increased total left ventricle [LV] oxygen demand), syncope, and heart failure.
- Table 1 summarizes the stages of valvular aortic stenosis.
- Pathophysiology: Antegrade velocities remain normal until the cross-sectional area of the left ventricular outflow tract (typically 3 to 4 cm²) is reduced by roughly half. At this point, secondary to the increased resistance, the left ventricle systolic pressure starts to increase, and the LV adapts with concentric hypertrophy. The hypertrophy allows for normalization of the wall stress and preservation of the ejection fraction, cardiac output, and

left ventricular end diastolic pressures despite the LV/peripheral arterial system pressure gradient.
- LV hypertrophy eventually leads to LV diastolic dysfunction, which may herald early symptoms. That said, symptoms generally do not begin until stenosis becomes severe (valve area <1.0 cm², a mean gradient >40 mm Hg, or a peak gradient >4 m/sec).
- For most patients, after becoming symptomatic, LV systolic function will begin to drop (decreased cardiac output and stroke volume) with development of signs and symptoms of overt heart failure. At this point, if a symptomatic severe AS patient does not undergo valve replacement, their mortality drastically increases.[1,2]
- Acquired von Willebrand disease is seen in approximately 20% of severe AS, which can lead to GI bleeding from angiodysplasia (Heyde syndrome) that resolves after aortic valve replacement.

ETIOLOGY

- Idiopathic calcification of the aortic valve (most common cause in North America and Europe, presents at ages 60 to 80)
- Rheumatic heart disease: Characterized by commissural fusion leaving a small central orifice (most common cause worldwide)
- Progressive stenosis of congenital unicuspid or bicuspid valve (found in 1% to 2% of the population, presents at ages <30 yr for unicuspid and at ages 40 to 60 for bicuspid valves)[3]
- Less common causes include rare metabolic disease (Fabry disease), systemic lupus erythematosus, radiation, end-stage

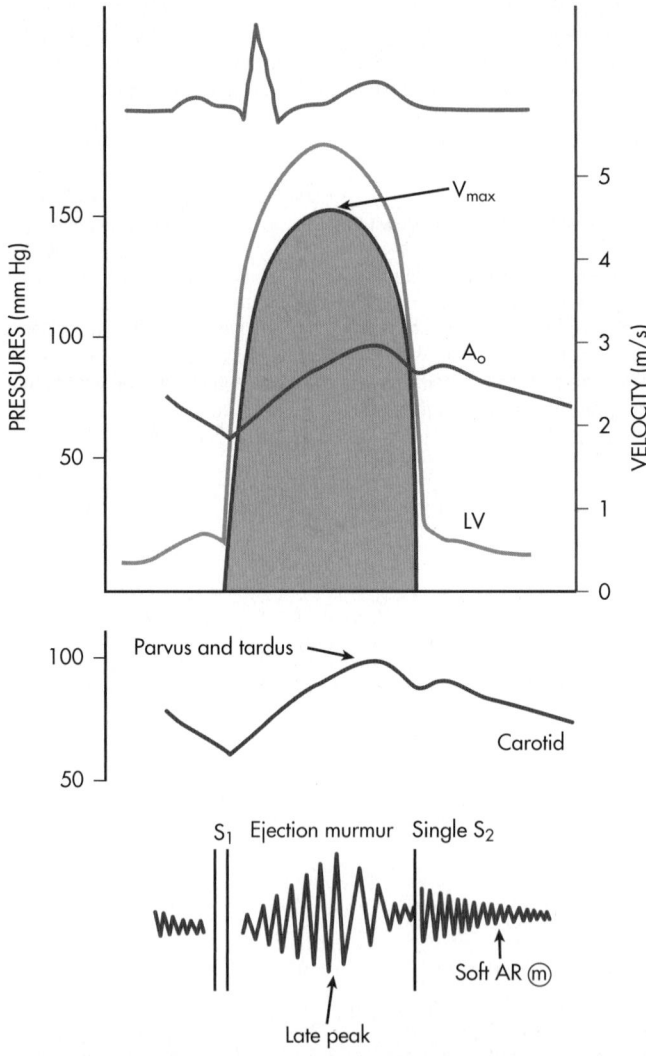

FIG. 1 Relationship between left ventricle *(LV)* and aortic *(Ao)* pressures and the Doppler aortic stenosis velocity curve *(in red)*. The pressure difference between the LV and aorta in systole is four times the velocity squared (the Bernoulli equation). Thus a maximum velocity *(V_{max})* of 4.3 m/sec corresponds to a maximum LV to Ao pressure difference of 74 mm Hg and a mean systolic gradient of 44 mm Hg. On physical examination, the slow rate of rise and delayed peak in the carotid pulse (or parvus and tardus) matches the contour of the aortic pressure waveform. The murmur corresponds to the Doppler velocity curve with a harsh crescendo-decrescendo late-peaking systolic murmur, best heard at the aortic region (upper right sternal border). Often, a soft, high-pitched diastolic decrescendo murmur of aortic regurgitation also is appreciated. *AR,* Aortic regurgitation. (From Libby P et al: *Braunwald's heart disease, a textbook of cardiovascular medicine,* ed 12, Philadelphia, 2022, Elsevier.)

TABLE 1 Stages of Valvular Aortic Stenosis

Stage	Definition	Valve Anatomy	Valve Hemodynamics	Hemodynamic Consequences	Symptoms
A	At risk of AS	Bicuspid aortic valve (or other congenital valve anomaly) Aortic valve sclerosis	Aortic V_{max} <2 m/sec	None	None
B	Progressive AS	Mild to moderate leaflet calcification of a bicuspid or trileaflet valve with some reduction in systolic motion or rheumatic valve changes with commissural fusion	*Mild AS:* Aortic V_{max} 2.0-2.9 m/sec or mean ΔP <20 mm Hg *Moderate AS:* Aortic V_{max} 3.0-3.9 m/sec or mean ΔP 20-39 mm Hg	Early LV diastolic dysfunction may be present Normal LVEF	None
C	Asymptomatic severe AS				
C1	Asymptomatic severe AS with preserved LVEF	Severe leaflet calcification or congenital stenosis with severely reduced leaflet opening	*Severe AS:* Aortic V_{max} ≥4 m/sec or mean ΔP ≥40 mm Hg AVA typically is ≤1 cm² (or AVAi ≤0.6 cm²/m²) Very severe AS is an aortic V_{max} ≥5 m/sec, or mean ΔP ≥60 mm Hg	LV diastolic dysfunction Mild LV hypertrophy Normal LVEF	None; exercise testing is reasonable to confirm symptom status
C2	Asymptomatic severe AS with LV dysfunction	Severe leaflet calcification or congenital stenosis with severely reduced leaflet opening	Aortic V_{max} ≥4 m/sec or mean ΔP ≥40 mm Hg AVA typically is ≤1 cm² (or AVAi ≤0.6 cm²/m²)	LVEF <50%	None
D	Symptomatic severe AS				
D1	Symptomatic severe high-gradient AS	Severe leaflet calcification or congenital stenosis with severely reduced leaflet opening	*Severe AS:* Aortic V_{max} ≥4 m/sec, or mean ΔP ≥40 mm Hg AVA typically is ≤1 cm² (or AVAi ≤0.6 cm²/m²), but may be larger with mixed AS/AR	LV diastolic dysfunction LV hypertrophy Pulmonary hypertension may be present	Exertional dyspnea or decreased exercise tolerance Exertional angina Exertional syncope or presyncope
D2	Symptomatic severe low-flow/low-gradient AS with reduced LVEF	Severe leaflet calcification with severely reduced leaflet motion	AVA ≤1 cm² with resting aortic V_{max} <4 m/sec, or mean ΔP <40 mm Hg Dobutamine stress echo shows AVA ≤1 cm² with V_{max} ≥4 m/sec at any flow rate	LV diastolic dysfunction LV hypertrophy LVEF <50%	HF, angina, syncope or presyncope
D3	Symptomatic severe low-gradient AS with normal LVEF or paradoxical low-flow severe AS	Severe leaflet calcification with severely reduced leaflet motion	AVA ≤1 cm² with aortic V_{max} <4 m/sec, or mean ΔP <40 mm Hg AVAi ≤0.6 cm²/m² Stroke volume index <35 ml/m² Measured when the patient is normotensive (systolic BP <140 mm Hg)	Increased LV relative wall thickness Small LV chamber with low-stroke volume. Restrictive diastolic filling LVEF ≥50%	HF, angina, syncope or presyncope

AR, Aortic regurgitation; *AS,* aortic stenosis; *AVA,* aortic valve area; *AVAi,* aortic valve area indexed to body surface area; *BP,* blood pressure; *HF,* heart failure; *LV,* left ventricle; *LVEF,* left ventricular ejection fraction; *ΔP,* pressure gradient; *V_{max},* maximum aortic velocity.
From Nishimura RA et al: 2014 AHA/ACCF guideline for the management of patients with valvular heart disease: a report of the American College of Cardiology Foundation/American Heart Association Task Force on Practice Guidelines. In Mann DL et al (eds.): *Braunwald's Heart Disease,* ed 10, Philadelphia, 2015, Elsevier.

renal disease, and obstructive vegetations/endocarditis may all cause early development of AS
- Genetic variation in the LPA locus, mediated by Lp(2) levels, is associated with aortic valve calcification across multiple ethnic groups and with incidental clinical aortic stenosis[4]

Dx DIAGNOSIS

DIFFERENTIAL DIAGNOSIS
- Hypertrophic cardiomyopathy
- Mitral regurgitation
- Ventricular septal defect
- Aortic sclerosis. Aortic stenosis is distinguished from aortic sclerosis by the degree of valve impairment. In aortic sclerosis, the valve leaflets are abnormally thickened but obstruction to outflow is absent or minimal

- Subvalvular membrane or supravalvular AS
- Stages of valvular AS
  1. Stage A = at risk of AS
  2. Stage B = progressive AS (formerly known as mild and moderate AS)
  3. Stage C = asymptomatic severe AS
  4. Stage D = symptomatic severe AS

WORKUP
- Echocardiography: The primary test for diagnosis (see "Imaging Studies")
- ECG: May demonstrate left ventricular hypertrophy and/or left atrial abnormality
- Chest radiograph: May demonstrate cardiomegaly. Poststenotic dilation of the ascending aorta may also be evident
- Cardiac catheterization in selected patients (see "Imaging Studies")
- Dobutamine challenge (for low-flow, low-gradient AS)[5]

IMAGING STUDIES
- Doppler echocardiography: Used to evaluate structure and anatomy of the valve. Hemodynamics can easily be assessed; allows calculation of both aortic valve area and estimation of pressure gradients to determine severity of AS (Fig. 2). Furthermore, allows evaluation of the LV size and function and pulmonary pressures.
- Chest x-ray examination:
  1. Poststenotic dilation of the ascending aorta
  2. Calcification of aortic cusps
  3. Rounding of left ventricle (LV) apex
- ECG:
  1. Left ventricular hypertrophy (found in 80% of patients)
  2. Left atrial enlargement
  3. Atrial fibrillation (in late disease)

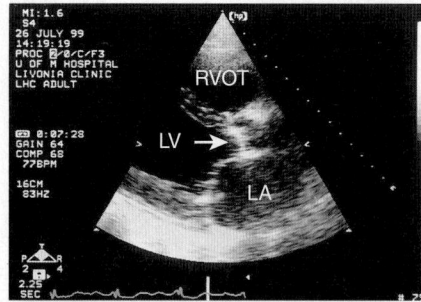

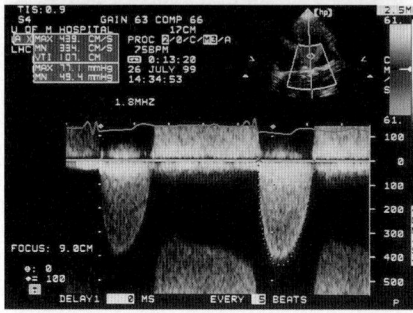

FIG. 2 Echocardiogram recorded in a patient with severe aortic stenosis. The *top panel* is a parasternal long-axis view recorded in systole. Left ventricular function is diminished. The aortic valve is markedly thickened and partially calcified. Its motion is markedly reduced, and in systole it appears that the valve occludes the orifice *(arrow)*. The *lower panel* is a continuous-wave Doppler recorded from the apex of the left ventricle along a line aimed through the stenotic aortic valve. Note the aortic stenosis signal below the zero crossing line. The peak velocity is 430 cm/sec, which corresponds to a maximum gradient of 77 mm Hg and a mean gradient of 49.4 mm Hg. *LA,* Left atrium; *LV,* left ventricle; *RVOT,* right ventricular outflow tract. (From Libby P et al: *Braunwald's heart disease, a textbook of cardiovascular medicine*, ed 12, Philadelphia, 2022, Elsevier.)

- Cardiac catheterization: Indicated in symptomatic patients awaiting aortic valve replacement (AVR) in order to detect coexisting coronary artery stenosis that may need treatment at the same time as aortic valve replacement. Cardiac catheterization can also be used to determine invasive aortic gradients (which may be underestimated on echocardiography).
- A computed tomography (CT) with contrast for imaging the aorta may be needed for annular sizing and aortic measurements, and if a transcatheter aortic valve replacement (TAVR) is planned, the CT scan is crucial to planning TAVR approach.[1]
- Exercise testing: Strongly encouraged for any patient with stage C "asymptomatic" severe AS to evaluate exercise tolerance and to look for a fall in systemic blood pressure while exercising. It should be performed under supervision and is contraindicated in symptomatic severe aortic stenosis.

Rx TREATMENT

GENERAL Rx
MEDICAL:
- Once symptomatic, the mainstay of treatment is replacement of the valve. AS is a surgical disease. Fig. 3 summarizes a treatment strategy for patients with severe AS.[1,6]
- Optimize loading conditions by keeping a normal volume status (gentle diuresis for volume overload as preload dependent) and controlling hypertension (HTN) but avoid vasodilators (nitrates); maintain sinus rhythm.
- In 2007, the AHA guidelines for prevention of infectious endocarditis were revised, and routine antibiotic prophylaxis to undergo dental or other invasive procedures is no longer recommended, unless the patient has prior endocarditis.[7]

INDICATIONS FOR AORTIC VALVE REPLACEMENT: Valve replacement is the treatment of choice in symptomatic patients because there is a 50% mortality rate at 2 yr with medical therapy alone. If a patient does not have a >1 yr life expectancy, then replacement should not be considered, but rather palliative therapies should be discussed. ACC/AHA guidelines for aortic valve replacement for aortic stenosis are summarized in Table 2.

Percutaneous balloon aortic valvuloplasty (BAV) serves best as palliative therapy in severely symptomatic patients who are not surgical candidates and as a bridge to therapy in patients not ready for TAVR/SAVR or a bridge to decision (for patients with unclear candidacy for TAVR/SAVR). Restenosis occurs in most adult patients within 6 mo, so BAV is not a long-term therapy. The 2020 updated ACC/AHA guidelines for choice of surgical vs. transcatheter treatment of aortic stenosis are summarized in Table 3.[1]

Valve replacement is a **Class I indication** for any patients with:
- Stage D1: Symptomatic severe AS
- Stage C2: Asymptomatic severe AS with LV ejection fraction (EF) <50%
- Stage C1 or C2: Asymptomatic severe AS undergoing CABG or surgery on the aorta or other heart valves

Valve replacement is a **Class IIa indication** for patients with:
- Stage D2: Low-flow/low gradient (with low ejection fraction <50%) with a positive low-dose dobutamine stress echo
- Stage D3: Symptomatic patients with low-flow/low gradient severe AS with a **normal LVEF** ≥50%, a valve area ≤1.0 cm², and a stroke volume index <35 ml/m²
- Stage C: Asymptomatic severe AS and abnormal blood pressure response (decrease in systolic blood pressure) or decreased exercise tolerance during exercise
- Stage C: Asymptomatic patients with critical AS (peak velocity >5 m/sec or mean pressure gradient >60 mm Hg) with low surgical risk

- Stage B: Patients with moderate AS who are undergoing cardiac surgery for other indications

Valve replacement is a **Class IIb indication** for patients with:
- Stage C: Asymptomatic severe AS in a low-risk patient showing rapid progression of disease (V_max >0.3m/sec/yr).
- When deciding replacement strategy, surgical aortic valve replacement (SAVR) vs. transcatheter aortic valve replacement (TAVR), in all cases a heart team approach is a Class I indication. TAVR is a catheter-based technology that allows for implantation of a prosthetic valve without open heart surgery, decreasing recovery time and hospital stay.
- Historically, the choice of SAVR vs. TAVR strategy had been driven by patient surgical risk. Primarily due to TAVR trial design, patients were classified by their STS-PROM score into four categories: Extreme surgical risk (absolute surgical contraindication), high surgical risk (STS-PROM score >8), intermediate surgical risk (STS-PROM score 4 to 8), and low surgical risk (STS-PROM score <4). As more data have been collected, the two approaches, SAVR vs. TAVR, appear to be more and more comparable with regard to valve durability. TAVR is associated with slightly lower mortality, shorter hospital length of stay, less bleeding, lower risk of transient or permanent atrial fibrillation, more rapid return to normal activities, and less pain postprocedure than SAVR.
- SAVR, on the other hand, has less need for permanent pacemaker placement, lower rate of valve reintervention, and is associated with a lower risk of paravalvular leak. As such, deciding between the two approaches now focuses on patient's age, anatomic contraindications for transfemoral TAVR, high risk or prohibitive surgical risk, the life expectancy of the patient, and the patient's values and preferences.

AVR criteria is listed in Table 2.
- For patients who are **>80 yr of age** or for younger patients with a life expectancy <10 yr and no anatomic contraindications to transfemoral TAVR, transfemoral TAVR is recommended in preference to SAVR.
- For patients who are **65 to 80 yr of age** and have no anatomic contraindications to transfemoral TAVR, either SAVR or transfemoral TAVR is recommended after shared decision making about the balance between expected patient longevity and valve durability.
- For patients who are **<65 yr of age** or have a life expectancy >20 yr, SAVR is recommended. For patients with a bicuspid valve, a heart team approach, as with all aortic valve replacements, is strongly advised.

DISPOSITION
- The presence of even mild symptoms is an indicator of poor survival for patients with AS. The average duration of symptoms before death is angina, 5 yr; syncope, 3 yr; CHF, 2 yr.

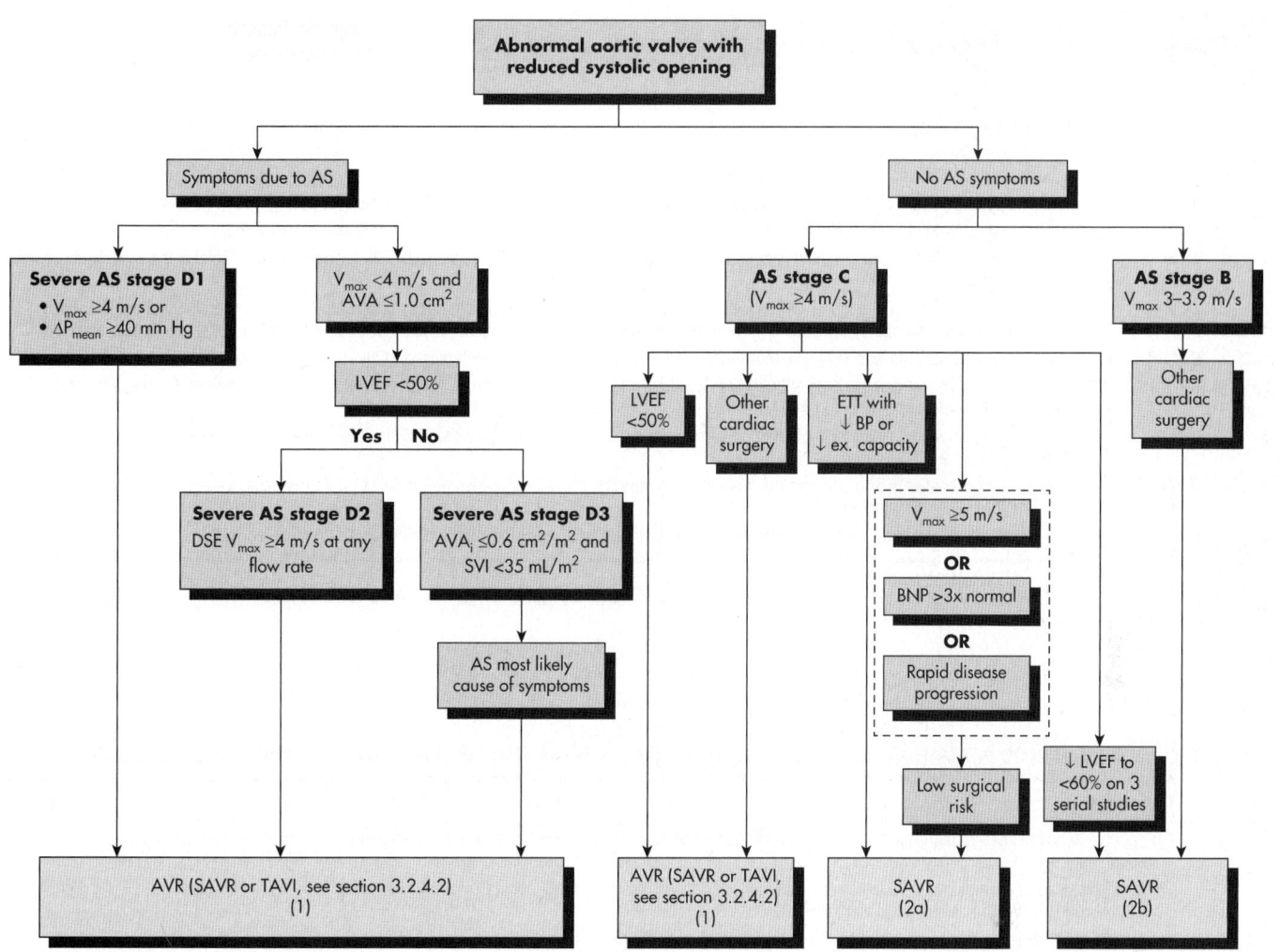

FIG. 3 Management strategy for patients with severe AS. Arrows show the decision pathways that result in a recommendation for AVR. Periodic monitoring is indicated for all patients in whom AVR is not yet indicated, including those with asymptomatic (Stage C) and symptomatic (Stage D) AS and those with low-gradient AS (Stage D2 or D3) who do not meet the criteria for intervention. *AS,* Aortic stenosis; *AVA,* aortic valve area; *AVAi,* aortic valve area index; *AVR,* aortic valve replacement; *BNP,* B-type natriuretic peptide; *BP,* blood pressure; *DPmean,* mean systolic pressure gradient between LV and aorta; *DSE,* dobutamine stress echocardiography; *ETT,* exercise treadmill test; *LVEF,* left ventricular ejection fraction; *SAVR,* surgical aortic valve replacement; *SVI,* stroke volume index; *TAVI,* transcatheter aortic valve implantation; *TAVR,* transcatheter aortic valve replacement; *V$_{max}$,* maximum velocity. (From Otto CM et al: 2020 AHA/ACC Guideline for the management of patients with valvular heart disease: a report of the American College of Cardiology/American Heart Association Task Force on Practice Guidelines, *JACC* 77(4):e25-197, 2021.)

- Approximately 75% of patients with symptomatic AS will die within 3 yr of symptom onset unless the aortic valve is replaced.

REFERRAL

- A heart team referral for valve replacement in all symptomatic AS patients (Class I indication). There are studies that are examining the presence of moderate or severe valvular calcification, together with a rapid increase in aortic jet velocity and elevated BNP, to identify patients with a very poor prognosis who should be considered for early valve replacement rather than delayed until symptoms develop. Additionally, patients with severe AS who are asymptomatic should be considered for exercise stress test to see if they are truly without symptoms (low exercise tolerance) or if the BP drops with exercise, both which would be indications for a heart team referral.

- In asymptomatic patients, Doppler echocardiography is recommended every 6 to 12 mo for severe aortic stenosis, every 1 to 2 yr for moderate disease, and every 2 to 3 yr for mild disease. Should have a low threshold to repeated echocardiogram for any change in symptoms or exam.
- Referral to cardiology should be considered in any patients with severe AS and in particular those with low-flow, low-gradient (low ejection fraction) symptomatic aortic stenosis for further workup (dobutamine stress echo).
- Balloon valvuloplasty is useful in infants and children or poor surgical candidates who do not have calcified valve apparatus; it can be done as an intermediate procedure to stabilize high-risk patients before surgery.
- Role of palliative care: If life expectancy with aortic valve replacement (SAVR or TAVR) is <1 yr **or** the patient's quality of life is

unlikely to improve after aortic valve replacement (due to coexisting significant comorbidities), palliative care consultation is extremely valuable as it focuses on shared decision making as well as improving quality of life without interruption of conservative medical therapy.[1]

RELATED CONTENT

Aortic Stenosis (Patient Information)
Transcatheter Aortic Valve Replacement (TAVR)
(Related Key topic)

AUTHORS: **AHMAD MUSTAFA, MD,** and **CRAIG L. BASMAN, MD, FACC, FSCAI**

REFERENCES

Available at eBooks.Health.Elsevier.com.

TABLE 2 Indications for Aortic Valve Replacement in Patients with Aortic Stenosis

COR	LOE	Recommendations
1	A	1. In adults with severe high-gradient AS (stage D1) and symptoms of exertional dyspnea, HF, angina, syncope, or presyncope by history or on exercise testing, AVR is indicated.
1	B-NR	2. In asymptomatic patients with severe AS and an LVEF <50% (stage C2). AVR is indicated.
1	B-NR	3. In asymptomatic patients with severe AS (stage C1) who are undergoing cardiac surgery for other indications, AVR is indicated.
1	B-NR	4. In symptomatic patients with low-flow, low-gradient severe AS with reduced LVEF (stage D2). AVR is recommended.
1	B-NR	5. In symptomatic patients with low-flow, low-gradient severe AS with normal LVEF (stage D3), AVR is recommended if AS is the most likely cause of symptoms.
2a	B-NR	6. In apparently asymptomatic patients with severe AS (stage C1) and low surgical risk, AVR is reasonable when an exercise test demonstrates decreased exercise tolerance (normalized for age and sex) or a fall in systolic blood pressure of ≥10 mm Hg from baseline to peak exercise.
2a	B-R	7. In asymptomatic patients with very severe AS (defined as an aortic velocity of ≥5 m/sec) and low surgical risk, AVR is reasonable.
2a	B-NR	8. In apparently asymptomatic patients with severe AS (stage C1) and low surgical risk, AVR is reasonable when the serum B-type natriuretic peptide (BNP) level is greater than three times normal.
2a	B-NR	9. In asymptomatic patients with high-gradient severe AS (stage C1) and low surgical risk. AVR is reasonable when serial testing shows an increase in aortic velocity ≥0.3 m/sec/yr.
2b	B-NR	10. In asymptomatic patients with severe high-gradient AS (stage C1) and a progressive decrease in LVEF on at least three serial imaging studies to <60%, AVR may be considered.
2b	C-EO	11. In patients with moderate AS (stage B) who are undergoing cardiac surgery for other indications. AVR may be considered.

AS, Aortic stenosis; *AVR,* aortic valve replacement; *HF,* heart failure; *LVEF,* left ventricular ejection fraction.
From Otto CM, et al. 2020 AHA/ACC guideline for the management of patients with valvular heart disease: a report of the American College of Cardiology/American Heart Association Task Force on Practice Guidelines, *J Am Coll Cardiol* 77:e25-e197, 2021.

TABLE 3 Updated 2020 ACC/AHA Guidelines for Choice of Surgical vs. Transcatheter Treatment of Aortic Stenosis (AS)

Class	Indication	LOE
I	For patients in whom TAVR or high-risk surgical AVR is being considered, members of a heart valve team should collaborate to provide optimal patient care.	A
	For symptomatic and asymptomatic patients with severe AS and any indication for AVR who are **<65 yr of age** or have a life expectancy >20 yr, SAVR is recommended. *(Modified 2020)*	A
	For symptomatic patients with severe AS who are **65 to 80 yr of age** and have no anatomic contraindication to transfemoral TAVI, either SAVR or transfemoral TAVI is recommended after shared decision making about the balance between expected patient longevity and valve durability. *(Modified 2020)*	A
	For symptomatic patients with severe AS who are **>80 yr of age** or for younger patients with a life expectancy <10 yr and no anatomic contraindication to transfemoral TAVI, transfemoral TAVI is recommended in preference to SAVR. *(Modified 2020)*	A
I	For patients with an indication for AVR for whom a bioprosthetic valve is preferred but valve or vascular anatomy or other factors are not suitable for transfemoral TAVI, SAVR is recommended. *(Modified 2020)*	A
I	For symptomatic patients of any age with severe AS and a high or prohibitive surgical risk, TAVI is recommended if predicted post-TAVI survival is >12 mo with an acceptable quality of life. *(Modified 2020)*	A
IIb	Percutaneous aortic balloon dilation may be considered as a bridge to surgical or transcatheter AVR in severely symptomatic/critically ill patients with severe AS.	C

ACC, American College of Cardiology; *AHA,* American Heart Association; *AVR,* aortic valve replacement; *LOE,* level of evidence; *TAVR,* transcatheter AVR.
From Otto CM et al: Guideline for the management of valvular heart disease, *JACC* 77(4):e25-197, 2021.

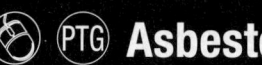

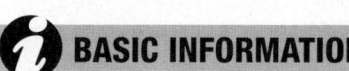 BASIC INFORMATION

DEFINITION

Asbestosis is a slow, progressive diffuse interstitial fibrosis as a consequence of dose-related inhalation exposure to fibers of asbestos in miners, millers, workers of asbestos textiles, and insulators. Clinically, the lung involvement is characterized by bilateral diffuse interstitial fibrosis, more pronounced in the lower lobes, and pleural thickening, leading to shortness of breath and dry cough.

Asbestos exposure can lead to the spectrum of pulmonary pathology, including pulmonary fibrosis; asbestos-related pleural plaque disease (ARPD), both focal and diffuse; and malignancies (lung cancer or mesothelioma).

ICD-10CM CODE
J61   Pneumoconiosis due to asbestos and other mineral fibers

EPIDEMIOLOGY & DEMOGRAPHICS

- 5 to 10 new cases per 100,000 persons per yr in the U.S.
- Prolonged interval (20 to 30 yr) between exposures to inhaled fibers and clinical manifestations of disease.
- Most common in workers over age 40 yr involved in the primary extraction of asbestos from rock deposits and in those involved in the fabrication and installation of products containing asbestos (e.g., naval shipyards in World War II; installation of floor tiles, ceiling tiles, acoustic ceiling coverings, wall insulation, and pipe coverings in public buildings).
- Smokers and heavy drinkers have the greatest risk of developing this disease.

PHYSICAL FINDINGS & CLINICAL PRESENTATION

- Insidious onset of shortness of breath and dry cough with exertion is usually the first sign of asbestosis.
- Dyspnea becomes more severe as the disease advances; with time, progressively less exertion is tolerated.
- Cough is frequent and usually paroxysmal, dry, and nonproductive. Hemoptysis is rare but reported. Scant mucoid sputum may accompany the cough in the later stages of the disease.
- Fine end-respiratory crackles (rales, crepitations) are heard more predominantly in the lung bases.
- Digital clubbing, edema, and jugular venous distention may be present.
- Advanced cases may have signs of right heart failure.

ETIOLOGY/PATHOGENESIS

Inhalation of asbestos fibers. The pathogenesis of pulmonary interstitial inflammation and fibrosis is related to immune mechanisms. Asbestosis is known to be associated with positive serum antinuclear antibody (ANA) and rheumatoid factor (RF). An important role of interleukin-1beta (IL-1beta) in the pathogenesis of asbestosis and its systemic autoimmune manifestations has been reported.

Asbestos-Related Pulmonary Manifestations[1]:
- *Pleural Plaques:* Pleural plaques are the most common manifestation of prior asbestos exposure. They are usually a radiographic finding, and they do not cause any pulmonary symptoms. Usual presentation 20 to 30 yr after exposure.
- *Diffuse Pleural Thickening (DPT):* It is usually due to involvement of the visceral pleura. Occurs few years after exposure. It is thought to be due to fibrosis from chronic pleural irritation from asbestos. It is a radiographic finding and usually does not cause symptoms.
- *Rounded Atelectasis:* Always adjacent to the pleura, and vessels and bronchi entering the area of collapse appear bent, forming a "comet tail," which is typical for rounded atelectasis. Usually is asymptomatic, but if presenting with pleural effusion should be investigated further to rule out malignancy or infection.
- *Benign Asbestos Pleural Effusion:* Usually unilateral, though Bilateral presentation can occur. These effusions often spontaneously resolve in a few months, but some may persist or recur for several years. Effusion usually exudative, with eosinophil predominance.
- *Asbestos-Related Interstitial Lung Disease:* Can be mild or can progress to diffuse pulmonary fibrosis. Needs to be differentiated from usual interstitial pneumonia (UIP) and other interstitial lung disease (ILD).
- *Asbestos-Associated Cancer:* Asbestos exposure is linked to increased risk of lung cancer and mesothelioma. Risk increases in smokers. Mesothelioma is associated with asbestos exposure, but the most common cancer associated with asbestos exposure is bronchogenic carcinoma.

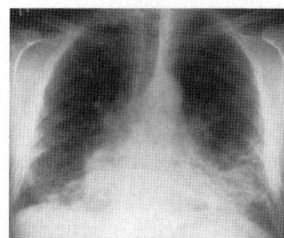 DIAGNOSIS

DIFFERENTIAL DIAGNOSIS
- Silicosis
- Siderosis, other pneumonoconioses
- Interstitial lung disease
- Lung cancer

WORKUP
- Documentation of exposure history
- Pulmonary function testing
- Diagnostic imaging studies

LABORATORY TESTS
- Generally not helpful
- Arterial blood gases: May show hypoxemia and/or hypercarbia in advanced stages

PULMONARY FUNCTION TESTING:
- Most often shows decreased vital capacity (VC), decreased total lung capacity (TLC), and decreased carbon monoxide gas transfer (DLco)
- FEV1 might be reduced in concomitant smokers

BRONCHOSCOPY WITH BRONCHOALVEOLAR LAVAGE:
- Clinical utility of bronchoscopy is limited. It can be helpful in ruling out infection, or hypersensitivity pneumonitis. Asbestos bodies are found in sputum and bronchoalveolar lavage (BAL) fluid of asbestos workers but utility in diagnosis of asbestos-related lung disease and progression is limited.

IMAGING STUDIES
- Chest x-ray (Fig. 1): Imaging findings associated with asbestos exposure may vary from benign pleural disease (including discrete plaques, pleural calcification, diffuse pleural thickening with blunting of costophrenic angles, and thickening of the interlobar fissure) to asbestosis (diffuse interstitial pulmonary fibrosis).
- CT scan of chest (Fig. 2): Typical findings of asbestosis on high-resolution CT of the chest include increased interstitial markings found mainly at the bases (Fig. 3). As the disease progresses, honeycombing is noted.

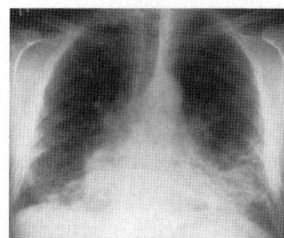

FIG. 1 Asbestosis. Posteroanterior radiograph shows coarse linear opacities at both lung bases obscuring the cardiac borders. (From McLoud TC: *Thoracic radiology: the requisites,* St Louis, 1998, Mosby.)

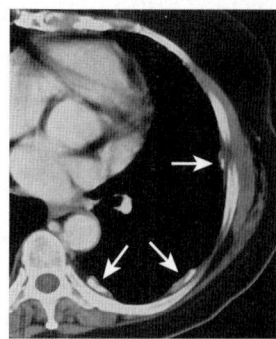

FIG. 2 Asbestos-related pleural plaques. Typical calcified pleural plaques *(arrows)* are visible. They are often internal to the ribs. (From Webb WR et al: *Fundamentals of body CT,* ed 4, Philadelphia, 2014, Saunders.)

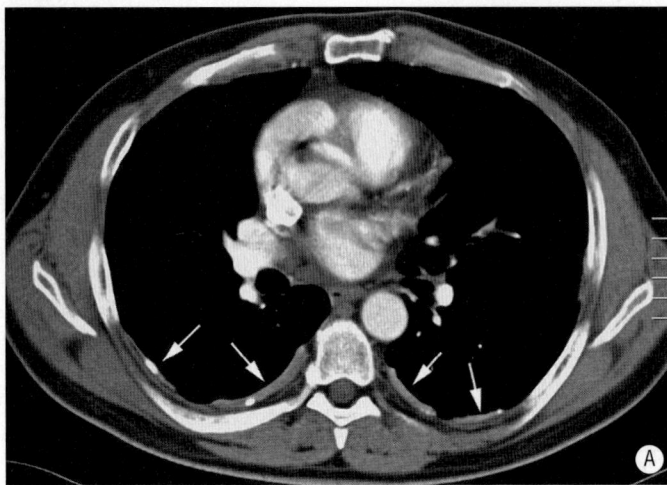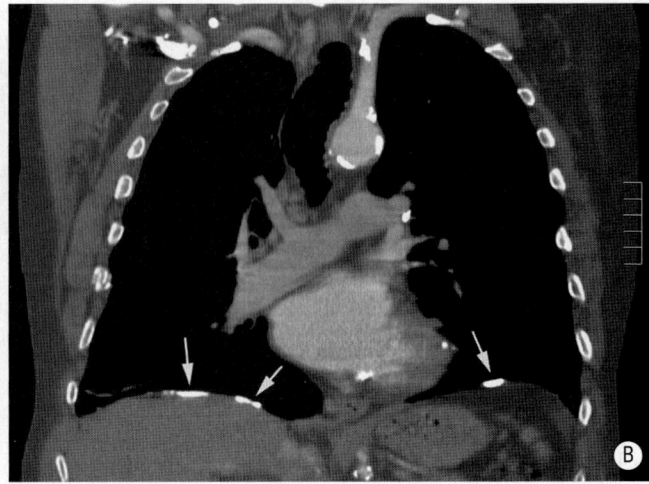

FIG. 3 Pleural plaques caused by asbestos exposure. (A) Axial and **(B)** coronal computed tomography. Pleural plaques are most commonly found along the lower thorax and on the diaphragmatic pleura *(arrows)*. They can partially or completely calcify or ossify. (From Adam A et al: *Grainger & Allison's diagnostic radiology,* ed 5, 2007, Churchill Livingstone: In Grant LA: *Grainger & Allison's diagnostic radiology essentials,* ed 2, London, 2019, Elsevier.)

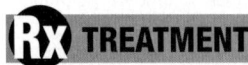 **TREATMENT**

NONPHARMACOLOGIC THERAPY

- Smoking cessation
- Exercise program to maximize available lung function. Pulmonary rehabilitation can be considered in advanced cases for improved cardiopulmonary capacity
- Supplemental oxygen on a PRN basis
- Removal of patient from further asbestos fiber exposure
- Prompt identification and treatment of respiratory infections
- Pneumococcal vaccination and annual influenza vaccination

PHARMACOLOGIC THERAPY

- There is no specific pharmacologic treatment for asbestosis.
- Some new data are coming out targeting IL-1beta therapy on the progression of lung fibrosis that suggest a new perspective for the treatment of systemic autoimmune features of asbestosis and, possibly, of lung involvement.[2]

DISPOSITION

- Death is usually from respiratory failure from cor pulmonale.
- Survival in patients after development of mesothelioma is 4 to 6 yr.
- Benign asbestos pleural effusions (BAPEs) are usually small and unilateral and occur years before the onset of interstitial disease.
- Diffuse pleural thickening and asbestosis are associated with increased risks of malignant peritoneal mesothelioma beyond the risk calculated to be associated with the degree of asbestos exposure.[3]
- None of the benign pleural diseases or ARPD was associated with an increased risk of malignant pleural mesothelioma.
- Asbestos increases the risk for development of lung cancer regardless of smoking status. The joint effect of asbestos and smoking is additive and depends in part on the presence of asbestosis. Patients with a history of tobacco smoking who have diffuse parenchymal disease secondary to asbestos, have a fortyfold increased risk of lung cancer compared to never-smokers. Asbestos workers who stop smoking experience a dramatic decline in lung cancer risk, which approaches that of nonsmokers after 30 yr.
- Low-dose chest CT scanning offers an excellent opportunity to detect early-stage lung cancers in asbestos-exposed workers.
- CT is more sensitive than radiography, CT without contrast generally suffices for evaluation, and PET scan (fluorodeoxyglucose-positron emission tomography) may have utility in patients with mesothelioma.

RELATED CONTENT

Asbestosis (Patient Information)

REFERENCES

Available at eBooks.Health.Elsevier.com.

AUTHOR: **IMRANA QAWI, MD**

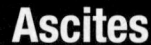

BASIC INFORMATION

DEFINITIONS

Ascites is a pathologic accumulation of fluid in the peritoneal cavity, most commonly due to portal hypertension caused by cirrhosis.

- **Diuretic-resistant ascites:** Ascites that cannot be mobilized or the early occurrence of ascites that cannot be prevented because of a lack of response to dietary sodium restriction and intensive diuretic treatment
- **Diuretic-intractable ascites:** Ascites that cannot be mobilized or the early recurrence of ascites that cannot be prevented because of the development of diuretic-induced complications that preclude the use of effective doses of diuretics
- Ascites may be graded according to the amount of fluid in the peritoneal cavity[1,2]:
  1. Grade 1 (mild ascites): Ascites only detectable by ultrasound
  2. Grade 2 (moderate ascites): Ascites with moderate symmetric abdominal distention
  3. Grade 3 (large ascites): Ascites with marked abdominal distention

SYNONYMS

Peritoneal cavity fluid
Hydroperitoneum
Hydroperitonia
Hydrops abdominis

ICD-10CM CODES

R18	Ascites
K70.11	Alcoholic hepatitis with ascites
K70.31	Alcoholic cirrhosis of liver with ascites
K71.51	Toxic liver disease with chronic active hepatitis with ascites
R18.8	Other ascites

EPIDEMIOLOGY & DEMOGRAPHICS

Ascites is the most common decompensation-defining complication of cirrhosis and is associated with worse prognosis. Ascites occurs at a rate of 7% to 10% annually in cirrhotic patients and occurs in ~60% of individuals with cirrhosis within 10 yr of diagnosis.[3] Cirrhosis is the cause of more than 80% of cases of ascites.[4]

PHYSICAL FINDINGS & CLINICAL PRESENTATION

- Important information to elicit within history:
  1. History of viral hepatitis
  2. Ongoing or previous heavy alcohol use
  3. Current or previous intravenous drug use and/or intranasal cocaine use
  4. Sexual history (e.g., unprotected sex with multiple partners, men who have sex with men)
  5. History of transfusions, tattoos, piercings, or incarceration
  6. Travel history and time spent in endemic regions for hepatitis
  7. Symptoms suggestive of peritoneal malignancy (e.g., weight loss, pain, palpable masses, rectal/vaginal bleeding)
  8. Other liver disease symptoms (e.g., increasing abdominal girth, jaundice, pruritus, confusion, pedal edema)
  9. Cardiac symptoms (e.g., pedal edema, shortness of breath, orthopnea, chest pain)
  10. Hypothyroid disease (fatigue, weight gain, constipation)
  11. History of ascites, prior treatment, large volume paracentesis (LVP) requirements and frequency
- Important physical exam findings:
  1. Protuberant abdomen (Fig. E1)
  2. Bulging flanks (can be present in obesity)
  3. Flank dullness to percussion (requires ~1500 ml of fluid)
  4. Fluid wave on abdominal exam
  5. Lower extremity edema
  6. Shifting dullness on abdominal exam
  7. Physical signs associated with liver cirrhosis: Spider angiomas, jaundice, loss of body hair, skeletal muscle wasting (sarcopenia), Dupuytren contracture, bruising, palmar erythema, gynecomastia, testicular atrophy, rectal varices, and caput medusa

ETIOLOGY

Pathophysiology of ascites (Fig. E2): Increased hepatic resistance to portal flow leads to portal hypertension. A portal pressure >12 mm Hg appears to be required for fluid retention.[5] The splanchnic vessels respond by increased secretion of nitric oxide, causing splanchnic artery vasodilation. Vasodilation appears also to be mediated by the translocation of enteric bacteria and bacterial products. Early in the disease, increased plasma volume and increased cardiac output compensate for this vasodilation. However, as the disease progresses, the effective arterial blood volume decreases, causing sodium and fluid retention through activation of the renin-angiotensin system. Over time, activation of the sympathetic system causes renal vascular perfusion to decrease and may lead to hepatorenal syndrome. The change in capillary pressure causes increased permeability and retention of fluid in the abdomen.[5] Principal causes of ascites formation categorized by underlying pathophysiology are summarized in Box E1.

Dx DIAGNOSIS

DIFFERENTIAL DIAGNOSIS

- Chronic parenchymal liver disease, leading to portal hypertension
- Acute liver failure
- Noncirrhotic portal hypertension (e.g., portal vein clot)
- Peritoneal carcinomatosis
- Cardiac disease (e.g., heart failure, constrictive pericarditis)
- Hepatic venous outflow obstruction (e.g., Budd-Chiari syndrome, IVC webs)
- Protein losing enteropathy
- Peritoneal tuberculosis
- Nephrotic syndrome
- Pancreatitis

WORKUP

Evaluation of patients with cirrhosis and a first episode of ascites is summarized in Box 2.

LABORATORY TESTS

- Initial evaluation should always include:
  1. Diagnostic paracentesis. Initial laboratory tests on ascitic fluid should include a cell count and differential, albumin, total protein, culture, and Gram stain. A serum-ascites albumin gradient (SAAG) should be calculated in all patients. The SAAG is measured by subtracting the level of albumin in the ascitic fluid from a concurrent serum albumin measurement: SAAG = serum albumin–ascites albumin.
     a. If the SAAG is greater than 1.1 g/dl, the cause of ascites can be attributed

---

BOX 2 Evaluation of Patients with Cirrhosis and a First Episode of Ascites

Evaluation of Liver Disease
- Standard blood tests: Liver function, coagulation parameters, CBC
- Abdominal US
- EGD
- Liver biopsy (selected cases)

Evaluation of Kidney Function
1. Serum creatinine level
2. Serum sodium and potassium levels
3. Urine sodium output (preferably 24-h urine collection)
4. Urine protein quantitation (preferably 24-h urine collection)

Ascitic Fluid Analysis
1. Polymorphonuclear leukocyte (neutrophil) count
2. Total protein and albumin concentrations
3. Bacterial culture (in blood culture bottles)
4. Other tests depending on clinical presentation: Glucose, LDH, amylase, triglycerides, cholesterol, cytologic examination, mycobacterial culture

From Feldman M et al: *Sleisenger and Fordtran's gastrointestinal and liver disease*, ed 11, Philadelphia, 2021, Elsevier.

to portal hypertension (e.g., cirrhosis, or post-sinusoidal elevated pressures as in Budd-Chiari syndrome or heart failure). A total ascitic protein level >2.5 g/dl may be indicative of cardiac ascites.[4]

  b. If SAAG is less than 1.1 g/dl, the cause of ascites is not portal hypertension (e.g., peritoneal carcinomatosis, tuberculous ascites, nephrotic syndrome). Optional tests on ascitic fluid that may aid in diagnosis include amylase, lactic dehydrogenase, acid-fast bacilli, and glucose levels.

  c. Cell count and differential: Ascitic fluid with greater than 250 neutrophils per cubic mm is diagnostic of spontaneous bacterial peritonitis (SBP).[4]

  d. Total ascitic fluid protein: Patients with protein concentration <1.5 g/dl have an increased risk of SBP.[1]

  e. Cytology: Obtain in patients with a high index of suspicion for associated malignancy.[2]

2. Aspartate aminotransferase, alanine transaminase, total and direct bilirubin, albumin, alkaline phosphatase, gamma-glutamyl transpeptidase.

3. CBC, coagulation studies (prothrombin time/INR).

4. Electrolytes, blood urea nitrogen (BUN), creatinine.

- Causes of ascites in the normal or diseased peritoneum by SAAG are summarized in Table 1.
- Fig. 3 illustrates an algorithm for the approach to the differential diagnosis of ascites.

IMAGING STUDIES

- Abdominal ultrasound (Fig. E4) is the most sensitive measure for detecting ascitic fluid; a computed tomography or MRI scan is a viable alternative. Doppler studies of portal and hepatic veins should be added to rule out vascular etiology of ascites.
- Endoscopy of the upper GI tract should be considered to evaluate for esophageal and gastric varices if ascites is secondary to portal hypertension.

(Rx) TREATMENT

NONPHARMACOLOGIC THERAPY

- Sodium-restricted diet (88 mmol/day or <2 g/day) is recommended for all patients with grade 2 ascites.
- Fluid restriction is only indicated in patients with hyponatremia (Na ≤125 mmol/L).
- All patients should be counseled on avoiding NSAIDs, ACE inhibitors, ARBs, alpha-adrenergic antagonists, and aminoglycoside antibiotics.

ACUTE GENERAL Rx

Patients with moderate-volume ascites causing only moderate discomfort may be treated on an outpatient basis with the following diuretic regimen:

- Spironolactone: Start at 50 to 100 mg/day and titrate up every 3 to 4 days to a maximum dose of 400 mg/day (monotherapy or combination therapy with furosemide).[2]
- Furosemide: Start at 40 mg/day and titrate up to 160 mg/day maximum (no role for monotherapy). A ratio of 40 mg/day of furosemide to 100 mg/day of spironolactone is an effective strategy in most patients but can be modified based on kidney function and electrolytes.[2]
- Monitor renal function and sodium levels carefully for signs of prerenal azotemia (in patients without edema, goal weight loss is 300 to 500 g/day; in patients with edema, goal weight loss is 800 to 1000 g/day). Furosemide alone is not recommended.[2]
- Measurement of the urinary sodium level can be helpful to identify noncompliance with dietary sodium restriction and diuretic therapy. Patients excreting more than 78 mmol of sodium/day (24-h urine) and not losing weight likely have nonadherence with low Na diet. Patients with low Na excretion, less than 78 mmol daily, require up titration of diuretics and evaluation of compliance.

Patients with large-volume ascites causing marked discomfort or impairment in activities of daily living may be treated in the outpatient setting with diuretic therapy alone or in combination with large-volume paracentesis.

- Large-volume paracentesis: Defined as >5L removed during a single paracentesis.
- Diuretic therapy until loss of fluid is noted (maximum spironolactone 400 mg daily and furosemide 160 mg daily).

  1. No difference in long-term mortality rate was found; however, paracentesis is faster, more effective, and associated with fewer adverse effects.[3]

  2. Patients receiving large-volume paracentesis (>5L) should receive albumin replacement therapy at the dose of 6 to 8 g/L of ascites removed to prevent

TABLE 1 Diagnosis of Ascites

CLASSIFICATION OF ASCITES BY SERUM ASCITES–ALBUMIN GRADIENT (SAAG)

SAAG High (≥1.1 g/dl)	SAAG Low (<1.1 g/dl)
Cirrhosis	Peritoneal carcinomatosis
Alcoholic hepatitis	Tuberculous peritonitis
Cardiac ascites	Pancreatic ascites
Massive liver metastases	Bile leak
Fulminant hepatic failure	Inflammation, e.g., systemic lupus erythematosus
Cirrhosis plus another cause	Nephrotic syndrome

CHARACTERISTICS OF PARACENTESIS FLUID

Etiology	Color	Saag (g/L)	RBCs	WBCs (Cells/Microl)	Cytology	Other
Cirrhosis	Straw	≥11	Few	<250		Protein <25 g/L
Infected ascites	Straw	≥11	Few	≥250 polymorphs or >500 cells		Positive culture
Neoplastic	Straw/hemorrhagic/mucinous	<11	Variable	Variable	Malignant cells	Protein >25 g/L
Tuberculosis	Clear/turbid/hemorrhagic	<11	High	>1000, 70% lymphocytes		Acid-fast bacilli + culture Protein >25 g/L
Cardiac failure	Straw	≥11	0	<250		Protein >25 g/L
Pancreatic	Turbid/hemorrhagic	<11	Variable	Variable		Amylase increased
Lymphatic obstruction or disruption	White	<11	0	0		Fat globules on staining

From Talley NJ et al: *Essentials of internal medicine*, ed 4, Chatswood NSW, 2021, Elsevier Australia.
RBC, Red blood cell; *WBC,* white blood cell.

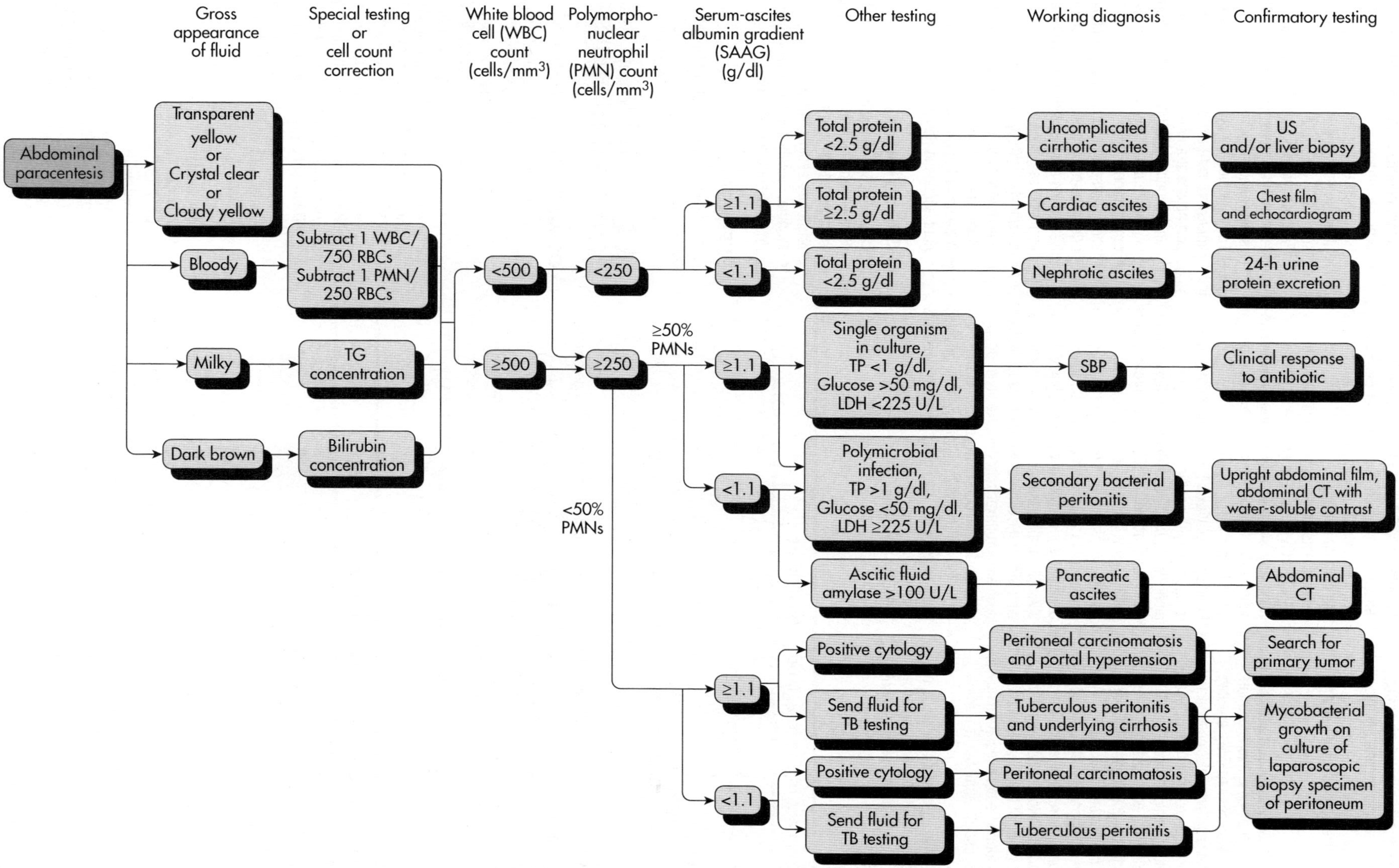

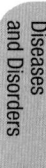

FIG. 3 Algorithm for the approach to the differential diagnosis of ascites. *LDH,* Lactic dehydrogenase; *PMN,* polymorphonuclear neutrophil; *RBC,* red blood cell; *TB,* tuberculosis; *TG,* triglyceride; *TP,* total protein; *U/L,* upper and lower; *US,* ultrasound. (From Feldman M et al: *Sleisenger and Fordtran's gastrointestinal and liver disease,* ed 10, Philadelphia, 2016, Elsevier.)

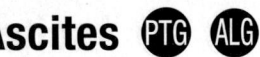
post-paracentesis circulatory dysfunction (PPCD).[2,6] Patients with renal dysfunction or hyponatremia should receive albumin for lower volumes as well.

Boxes 3 and 4 summarize ascites management.

CHRONIC Rx

- 5% to 10% of patients with large-volume ascites will be refractory to high-dose diuretic treatment.[1] Treatment strategies include repeated large-volume paracentesis with infusion of albumin every 2 to 4 wk or placement of a transjugular intrahepatic portosystemic shunt (TIPS).[3] TIPS evaluation should include echocardiogram, assessment for hepatic encephalopathy (HE), and characterization of liver impairment.
- Long-term albumin administration (40 g weekly) may improve mortality, reduce episodes of HE, and delay accumulation of ascites compared to standard medical therapy.[7] However, more research is needed before recommending the long-term use of albumin in routine management.[2]
- There are limited data on use of nonselective betablockers (NSBBs) in patients with diuretic-resistant ascites. Changes in mean arterial pressure (MAP) should be carefully monitored in patients on NSBBs, and these should be dose-reduced or stopped if substantial decrease in MAP is observed or systolic blood pressure is less than 90 mm Hg.[4]
- Patients known to have ascites should receive a diagnostic paracentesis if they develop any signs of SBP or upon any admission to the hospital even in the absence of these signs.
- Primary prophylaxis for SBP is recommended in patients with ascitic fluid protein <1.5 g/dl along with impaired renal function (creatinine ≥1.2 mg/dl or 106 micromol/L), BUN ≥25 mg/dl or 8.9 mmol/L or Na ≤130 mmol/L, or liver failure (Child-Pugh score ≥9 and bilirubin ≥3 mg/dl or 51 micromol/L).[2]
- Secondary prophylaxis for SBP should be instituted in all patients who were diagnosed with SBP in the form of a daily fluoroquinolone such as ciprofloxacin or norfloxacin, or double-strength trimethoprim-sulfamethoxazole.[2]
- Patients with known ascites who develop gastrointestinal bleeding should receive intravenous ceftriaxone for 7 days to prevent bacterial infections.

- Clinical use of vaptan agents is not currently recommended in cirrhotic patients.
- Oral midodrine 7.5 mg three times daily has been shown to increase urine volume, urine sodium, mean arterial pressure, and survival.[3]
- Peritoneovenous shunts or surgical portosystemic shunts have poor evidence and are not recommended.
- The Automated Low-Flow Ascites pump (not approved in North America) works by transporting small amounts of fluid from the peritoneal cavity to the bladder. Studies have shown improved symptoms and reduced LVP requirements.[3,8]
- Liver transplantation remains definitive management for cirrhosis with refractory ascites.[8] Referral to a transplant-capable center should be discussed.
- Diagnostic criteria of refractory ascites is outlined in Box 5. Its management is summarized in Table 2.
- A treatment approach to patients with malignant ascites is described in Fig. E5.

DISPOSITION

- Development of ascites signals a shift to decompensated cirrhosis and close follow-up is required. 2-yr mortality reaches 75% in refractory ascites cases.[3]
- Monitor closely for worsening liver function and development of SBP.

REFERRAL

Referral to hepatology at a transplant-capable center

PEARLS & CONSIDERATIONS

COMMENTS

- Prevalence of SBP in patients with ascites ranges between 10% and 30%.[6]
  1. Presence of at least 250 neutrophils per cubic millimeter of ascitic fluid is diagnostic; however, ascitic culture should be obtained for every diagnostic paracentesis where SBP is being considered.
  2. Gram-negative bacteria such as *E. coli* are the most common isolates.[6]
  3. Third-generation cephalosporins are the treatment of choice for most patients. There should be consideration of multidrug resistant organisms (MDRO) in patients with nosocomial infection, critical illness, or recent hospitalization. MDRO treatment may be tailored to local antimicrobiograms.
  4. Albumin improves survival in patients with SBP. Antibiotics should be administered with 1.5 g/kg albumin on treatment day 1 and 1.0 g/kg albumin on day 3 to prevent hepatorenal syndrome.[6]
  5. For patients diagnosed with SBP, a repeat diagnostic paracentesis may be obtained

---

BOX 3   Management of Grade 2 (Moderate) Ascites

Diet
- Low-sodium diet (80-120 mEq/day)

Diuretics
First episode of ascites:
Spironolactone, 100 mg/day; increase in a stepwise manner every 72 h according to treatment response to a maximum dose 400 mg/day
If no response or hyperkalemia develops, add furosemide, 40 mg/day, increasing in a stepwise manner to a maximum dose of 160 mg/day
Recurrent ascites:
Combination diuretic treatment with spironolactone and furosemide (same doses as above)

Monitoring
Daily body weight (recommended body weight loss is up to 0.5 kg/day in patients without edema and 0.5-1 kg/day in patients with ascites and edema)
Once ascites has been mobilized, continue a low-sodium diet and the minimum diuretic dose necessary to avoid reaccumulation of ascites

From Feldman M et al: *Sleisenger and Fordtran's gastrointestinal and liver disease*, ed 11, Philadelphia, 2021, Elsevier.

BOX 4   Management of Grade 3 (Tense) Ascites

Diet
- Low-sodium diet (80-120 mEq/day)

Large-Volume Paracentesis
- IV albumin should be administered (8 g per L of ascites removed)

Diuretics
The minimum diuretic dose necessary to avoid accumulation of ascites should be continued
If the patient has not received diuretic treatment previously, start with spironolactone, 100 mg/day, and furosemide, 40 mg/day
If the patient was receiving diuretic treatment, restart diuretics at a higher dose. If there is no response to treatment, assess the patient's sodium intake for adherence to a low-sodium diet, and increase the diuretic doses progressively to a maximum of spironolactone, 400 mg/day, and furosemide, 160 mg/day

From Feldman M et al: *Sleisenger and Fordtran's gastrointestinal and liver disease*, ed 11, Philadelphia, 2021, Elsevier.

BOX 5 Diagnostic Criteria of Refractory Ascites

Diuretic-Resistant Ascites
Ascites that cannot be mobilized or the early recurrence of which cannot be prevented because of a lack of response to sodium restriction and diuretic treatment

Diuretic-Intractable Ascites
- Ascites that cannot be mobilized or the early recurrence of which cannot be prevented because of the development of diuretic-induced complications that preclude the use of an effective diuretic dosage

Prior Treatment
- Patients must be on an intensive diuretic therapy (spironolactone 400 mg/day and furosemide 160 mg/day) for at least 1 wk and on a salt-restricted diet of <80 mEq/day

Other Definitions
Lack of response: Mean weight loss of <0.8 kg over 4 days and urinary sodium output less than sodium intake
Early ascites recurrence: Reappearance of grade 2 or 3 ascites within 4 wk of initial mobilization
Diuretic-induced hepatic encephalopathy: The development of encephalopathy in the absence of any other precipitating factor
Diuretic-induced renal impairment: An increase of the serum creatinine level by >100% to a value >2 mg/dl in a patient with ascites that is responding to treatment

From Feldman M et al: *Sleisenger and Fordtran's gastrointestinal and liver disease*, ed 11, Philadelphia, 2021, Elsevier.

TABLE 2 Management of Refractory Ascites

Definitions	Ascites That is not Eliminated Even With Maximum Diuretic Therapy
	Ascites that is not eliminated because maximum dosages of diuretics cannot be attained, given the development of diuretic-induced complications
Recommended therapy	Total paracentesis + IV albumin (7-9 g/L of ascites removed) if >5 L removed
	Continue with salt restriction and diuretic therapy as tolerated
Alternative therapy	TIPS for patients who require frequent paracenteses (every 1-2 wk) and whose CTP score is ≤11 or MELD <17
Peritoneovenous shunt for patients who are not candidates for TIPS or transplant	

Data from Garcia-Tsao G, Lim JK; Members of the Veterans Affairs Hepatitis C Resource Center Program: Management and treatment of patients with cirrhosis and portal hypertension: recommendations from the Department of Veterans Affairs Hepatitis C Resource Center Program and the National Hepatitis C Program, *Am J Gastroenterol* 104:1802-1829, 2009.
Data from European Association for the Study of the Liver. EASL Clinical Practice Guidelines for the management of patients with decompensated cirrhosis, *J Hepatol* 2018;69(2):406-460, 2018. Erratum in: *J Hepatol* 69(5):1207, 2018. In Vincent JL et al: *Textbook of critical care*, ed 8, Philadelphia, 2024, Elsevier.
CTP, Child-Turcotte-Pugh; *IV*, intravenous; *MELD*, model for end-stage liver disease; *TIPS*, transjugular intrahepatic portosystemic shunt.

at 48 h after initiation of antibiotics to assess for response. A decrease of total ascitic polymorphonuclear neutrophil (PMN) count by at least 25% from baseline PMN count is considered a response.[6]
6. By 1 yr post-SBP, 70% of patients have recurrence of SBP and should therefore receive ciprofloxacin 750 mg PO once/wk indefinitely for prophylaxis.[6]

PREVENTION
- Prevention of liver cirrhosis through avoidance of long-term use of alcohol, immunization against hepatitis A and B, and treatment of hepatitis C
- In cirrhotic patients, following a low-sodium diet (<2 g daily)

RELATED CONTENT
Ascites (Patient Information)
Cirrhosis (Related Key Topic)

REFERENCES
Available at eBooks.Health.Elsevier.com.

AUTHORS: **SIMRAN GUPTA, MD** and **MAY MIN, MD**

(i) BASIC INFORMATION

DEFINITION

Aspiration pneumonia refers to pulmonary infection of the lower airways and lung parenchyma resulting from entry of colonized oropharyngeal or upper gastrointestinal contents.[1] *Aspiration pneumonia* is considered part of the continuum that also includes community- and hospital-acquired pneumonias.[1] *Chemical pneumonitis* (or *aspiration pneumonitis*) refers to lung injury and inflammation resulting from entry of sterile substances toxic to the lower airways.

SYNONYMS

Pneumonia, aspiration
Aspiration pneumonitis

ICD-10CM CODE
J69.0   Pneumonitis due to inhalation of food and vomit

EPIDEMIOLOGY & DEMOGRAPHICS

INCIDENCE (IN U.S.):
- 7.1 cases per 10,000 people admitted to the hospital[2]
- 30.9 cases per 10,000 people admitted to the hospital >65 yr of age[2]

PREVALENCE (IN U.S.): Unknown (unreliable data)
PREDOMINANT SEX: Slight male predominance[2]
PREDOMINANT AGE: >65 yr
PEAK INCIDENCE: Elderly patients in hospitals or nursing homes[2,3]

PHYSICAL FINDINGS & CLINICAL PRESENTATION

- Symptoms develop within hours to a few days after aspiration event, though anaerobic infections can have a more subacute presentation.
- Clinical presentation ranges from minimal symptoms to fulminant respiratory failure.
- Symptoms can include dyspnea, diffuse wheeze, cough, hypoxia, tachypnea, tachycardia, sputum production, and fever.
- Lung exam may demonstrate wheezes, crackles, or rhonchi.

ETIOLOGY

Complex interaction of etiologies, ranging from chemical (often acid) pneumonitis after aspiration of sterile gastric contents (generally not requiring antibiotic treatment) to bacterial aspiration. Risk factors for aspiration pneumonia include vomiting, decreased consciousness, opiate abuse (Fig. 1), poor dentition, ineffective cough reflex or glottic closure, and gastroesophageal reflux disease.[4-11] Box 1 and Fig. E2 summarize risk factors for aspiration pneumonia.

COMMUNITY-ACQUIRED ASPIRATION PNEUMONIA:
- Most patients have a mixed infection with aerobic and anaerobic bacteria. The most common bacteria are Streptococcus pneumoniae, Staphylococcus aureus, Haemophilus influenzae, and Enterobacteriaceae.[12-14] Anaerobes (Peptostreptococcus, Fusobacterium nucleatum, Fusobacterium necrophorum, Prevotella, and Bacteroides species) are less frequently isolated.[15]
- High-risk groups: Age >65 yr; alcohol use; IV drug use; altered mental status; stroke victims; cardiac arrest; and patients with esophageal disorders, seizures, periodontal disease, or recent dental manipulations.[4-11]

HOSPITAL-ACQUIRED ASPIRATION PNEUMONIA:
- Causative organisms:
  1. Anaerobes listed above, although in many studies gram-negative aerobes (60%) and gram-positive aerobes (20%) predominate[13,16-18]
  2. *E. coli, P. aeruginosa, S. aureus* including MRSA, *Klebsiella, Enterobacter, Serratia,* *Proteus* spp., *H. influenzae, S. pneumoniae, Legionella,* and *Acinetobacter* spp. (sporadic pneumonias) in two thirds of cases
  3. Fungi, including *Candida albicans,* in <1%[19]
- High-risk groups: Seriously ill hospitalized patients (especially patients with coma, acidosis, alcohol use disorder, uremia, diabetes mellitus, nasogastric intubation, or recent antimicrobial therapy), who are frequently colonized with aerobic gram-negative rods; patients undergoing anesthesia; those with strokes, dementia, or swallowing disorders; patients >65 yr; and those receiving antacids or H$_2$ blockers, or proton pump inhibitors (but not sucralfate)

BOX 1   Risk Factors for Dysphagia and Aspiration Pneumonia

Cerebrovascular disease
Ischemic stroke
Hemorrhagic stroke
Subarachnoid hemorrhage
Degenerative neurologic disease
Alzheimer disease
Multiinfarct dementia
Parkinson disease
Amyotrophic lateral sclerosis (motor neuron disease)
Multiple sclerosis
Head and neck cancer
Oropharyngeal malignancy
Oral cavity malignancy
Esophageal malignancy
Other
Scleroderma
Diabetic gastroparesis
Reflux esophagitis
Presbyesophagus
Achalasia

From Vincent JL et al: *Textbook of critical care,* ed 8, Philadelphia, 2024, Elsevier.

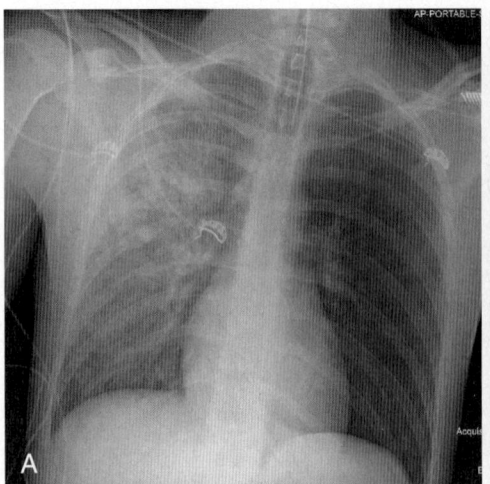
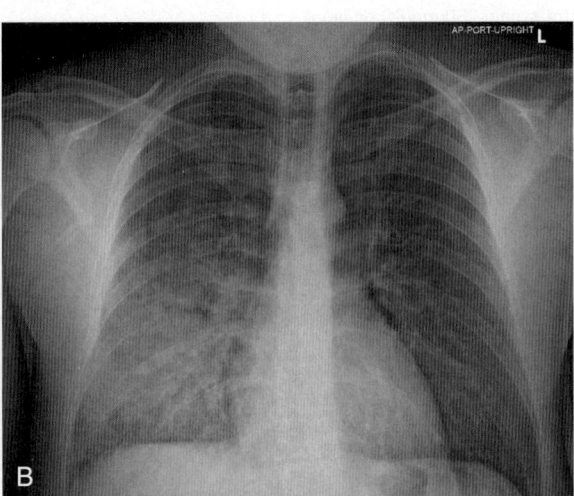

FIG. 1 Aspiration pneumonitis. A, Aspiration pneumonitis seen in a young male who presented after being found down with an opiate overdose. Note the asymmetric distribution of his infiltrates. **B,** Note the asymmetric distribution of the infiltrates, the presence of air bronchograms, and blurring of the hilar structures. (From Vincent JL et al: *Textbook of critical care,* ed 8, Philadelphia, 2024, Elsevier.)

- Hypoxic patients receiving concentrated O_2 have diminished ciliary activity, increasing risk for aspiration pneumonia

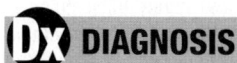 **DIAGNOSIS**

DIFFERENTIAL DIAGNOSIS
- Other necrotizing or cavitary pneumonias (especially tuberculosis, gram-negative pneumonias)
- See "Tuberculosis, Pulmonary"

WORKUP
- Chest x-ray
- Complete blood count (CBC), blood cultures
- Sputum Gram stain and culture
- Consideration of tracheal aspirate or bronchoscopy sample if intubated
- CT of chest if diagnosis is unclear or when suspecting complications

LABORATORY TESTS
- CBC: Leukocytosis often present
- Sputum Gram stain:
  1. Often useful when carefully prepared immediately after obtaining suctioned or expectorated specimen, examined by experienced observer.
  2. Only specimens with multiple white blood cells and rare or absent epithelial cells should be examined.
  3. Unlike other bacterial pneumonias (e.g., pneumococcal), multiple organisms may be present in aspiration pneumonia.
  4. Long, slender rods suggest anaerobes, though these organisms are difficult to isolate due to frequent contamination of sputum samples with oral flora.
  5. Sputum from pneumonia caused by acid aspiration may be devoid of organisms.
  6. Cultures should be interpreted in light of morphology of visualized organisms.

IMAGING STUDIES
- Chest x-ray may be negative early in the disease course.[20] It often reveals opacities in gravity-dependent lung regions. In an upright patient, opacities commonly affect the basal segments of the lower lobes. In a supine patient, opacities can involve the superior segment of the lower lobes, posterior right upper lobe, or the apicoposterior segment of the left upper lobe (Fig. E3). Chest x-ray can also demonstrate a pattern of diffuse lung involvement characteristic of acute respiratory distress syndrome. (See related content in "Acute Respiratory Distress Syndrome".)
- Aspiration pneumonia of several days' duration (or longer) may reveal necrosis (especially community-acquired anaerobic pneumonias) and even cavitation with air-fluid levels, indicating lung abscess.

Rx TREATMENT

NONPHARMACOLOGIC THERAPY
- Management to prevent repeated aspiration
- Ventilatory support if necessary
- Rehabilitative management: Physical, pulmonary, and dysphagia therapy combined with appropriate nutrition can reduce length of stay and mortality
- Fig. 4 illustrates a prevention and treatment algorithm for pulmonary aspiration

ACUTE GENERAL Rx
- **Chemical pneumonitis:** Acute aspiration of acidic gastric contents without bacteria may not require antibiotic therapy; initial treatment involves airway maintenance and management of bronchospasm and airway edema. Routine adjunctive treatment with glucocorticoids is not

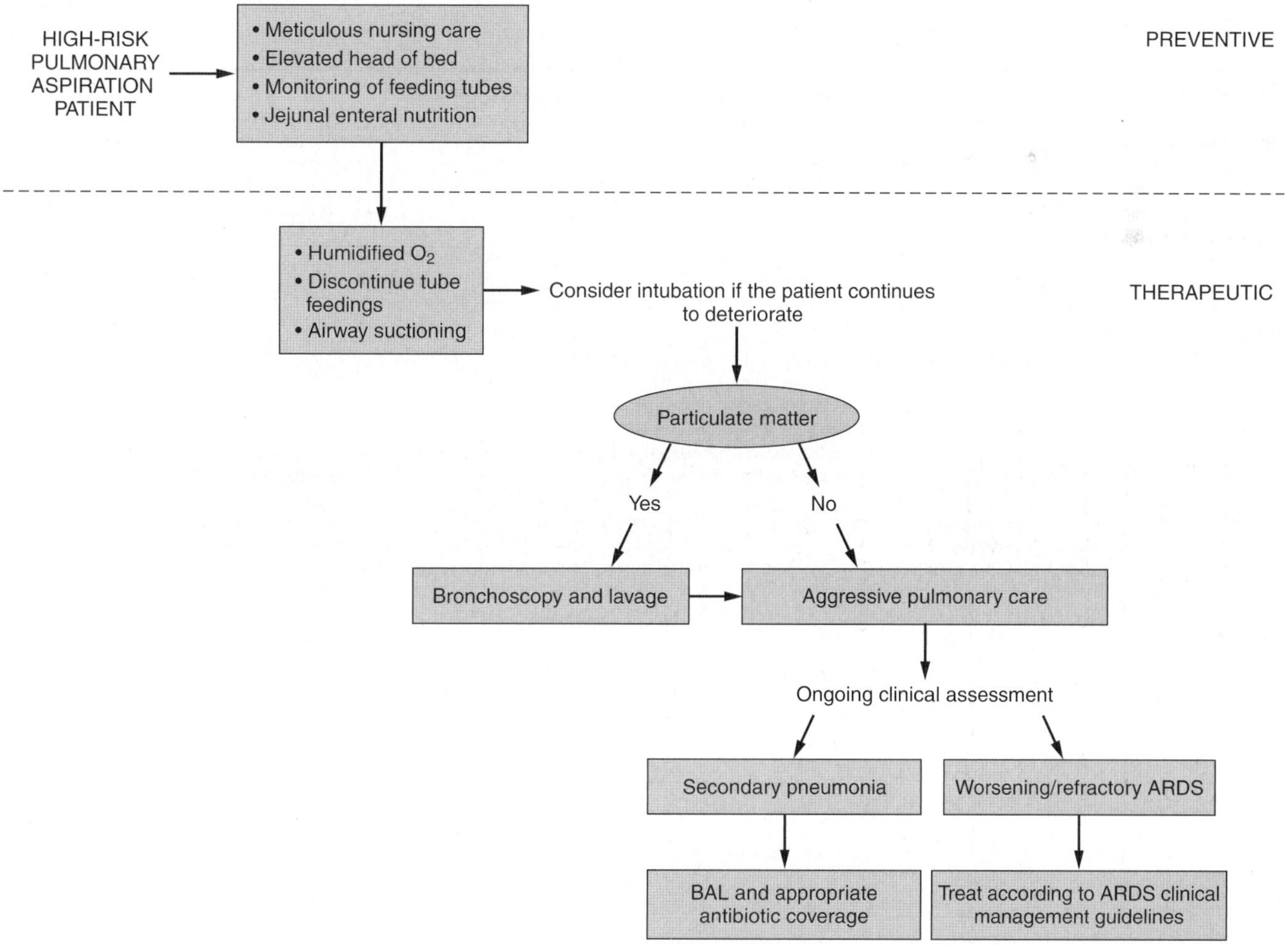

FIG. 4 Prevention and treatment algorithm for pulmonary aspiration. *ARDS,* Acute respiratory distress syndrome; *BAL,* bronchoalveolar lavage. (From Newman M et al: *Perioperative medicine,* ed 2, Philadelphia 2022, Elsevier.)

recommended. Empiric antibiotics may be considered in severe cases, but their ongoing use should be reassessed at 48 to 72 h.[1]

- **Aspiration pneumonia:** Antibiotic selection depends on the site of acquisition (long-term care facility, hospital, community), which modifies risk factors for infection with multidrug-resistant pathogens. Additionally, a history of treatment with broad-spectrum antibiotics in the past 90 days warrants empiric treatment for multidrug-resistant organisms.[21,22]

  1. Community-acquired aspiration pneumonia or hospital-acquired cases with low risk of multidrug-resistant pathogens: Ampicillin-sulbactam 1.5 to 3 g every 6 h IV, or amoxicillin-clavulanate PO 875 mg twice daily, or a fluoroquinolone (levofloxacin 750 mg IV or PO) is effective. Clindamycin (450 mg oral qid or 600 mg IV every 8 h) can be added to the other agent when the risk of predominantly anaerobic infection is high.

  2. Nursing home aspirations or hospital-acquired aspiration pneumonias with concerns for resistance: Broad-spectrum treatment with piperacillin-tazobactam 4.5 g q8h or 3.375 g q6h, cefepime 2 g q8h, levofloxacin 750 mg IV or PO once daily, imipenem 500 mg q6h or 1 g q8h, or meropenem 1 g q8h. The addition of vancomycin (15 mg/kg q12h IV) or linezolid (600 mg q12h PO or IV) is warranted if MRSA is suspected or known (e.g., documented nasal or respiratory colonization with MRSA).

     a. Knowledge of resident flora in the microenvironment of the aspiration within the hospital is crucial to intelligent antibiotic selection; consult infection control nurses or hospital epidemiologist.

     b. Confirmed *Pseudomonas* pneumonia in patients not in septic shock or at high risk of death can be treated with an antipseudomonal beta-lactam agent (piperacillin/tazobactam, cefepime, meropenem) or an antipseudomonal fluoroquinolone pending results of susceptibility testing. In severe cases, empiric two-drug combination therapy with an antipseudomonal beta-lactam agent and an antipseudomonal fluoroquinolone or an aminoglycoside is recommended. The choice of agents should be guided by the results of drug susceptibility testing when available.

DISPOSITION

Repeat chest x-ray in 6 to 8 wk in most patients.

PREVENTION

For patients with difficulty swallowing thin liquids, adding thickening agents to provide nectar-thick, pudding-thick, and honey-thick fluids is an option. Sitting patients upright when eating (and for some time afterward), chin tucking when swallowing, eating more slowly, and use of various swallowing maneuvers are additional techniques for prevention of aspiration in elderly and debilitated patients (Box 2).

REFERRAL

Consultation with infectious disease and/or pulmonary specialists recommended for patients with respiratory distress, hypoxia, ventilatory support, pneumonia in more than one lobe, necrosis or cavitation on chest x-ray, or for those not clinically responding to antibiotic therapy within 2 to 3 days.

RELATED CONTENT

Aspiration Pneumonia (Patient Information)

AUTHOR: **NARGES ALIPANAH-LECHNER, MD**

REFERENCES

Available at eBooks.Health.Elsevier.com.

BOX 2 Reducing Risk of Aspiration and Aspiration Pneumonia in Older Adults

Hand Feeding
- Provide a rest period (>30 min) before feeding time.
- Have the patient sit upright at 90 degrees or highest position allowed by medical condition.
- Avoid rushed or forced feeding; feeding by syringe is risky.
- Alternate liquids with solids.
- Recognize the high risks of sedatives, hypnotics, and other psychotropic medications, and try to wean or reduce dosages.
- Speech-language therapist referral: Evaluate patient for possible benefit of chin-down position when swallowing or of adjusting liquid viscosity; thickened liquids of varying types may improve swallowing in some patients (ice cream and Jell-O are considered thin liquids).

Tube Feeding
- *Note:* Both nasogastric and gastrostomy tube feeding may increase aspiration risks.
- Consider continuous feedings rather than intermittent (bolus) feedings.
- Keep backrest elevated at least 30 degrees during feedings, if possible.
- Consider pump-assisted feedings rather than gravity-controlled feedings.
- A gastric residual volume >200 ml during continuous feeding or before intermittent feedings may increase risk (but this remains controversial).[23]
- Prokinetic agents such as metoclopramide or erythromycin may improve feeding tolerance but are associated with their own serious potential side effects.
- Placing the feeding tube tip beyond the pylorus (jejunostomy, gastrojejunostomy) may reduce aspiration in some patients.
- Using colored dye in tube feeding is contraindicated (it was originally thought that adding coloring to liquid tube feeding formulas would help identify probable feeding aspiration if the dye was found after throat and pulmonary suctioning).

From Fillit HM: *Brocklehurst's textbook of geriatric medicine and gerontology*, ed 8, Philadelphia, 2017, Elsevier.

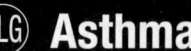
BASIC INFORMATION

DEFINITION

The National Asthma Education and Prevention Program (NAEPP) guidelines define asthma as "a chronic inflammatory disease of the airways in which many cells and cellular elements play a role: In particular mast cells, neutrophils, eosinophils, T lymphocytes, macrophages, and epithelial cells. In susceptible individuals, this inflammation causes recurrent episodes of coughing (particularly at night or early in the morning), wheezing, breathlessness, and chest tightness. The episodes are usually associated with widespread but variable airflow obstruction that is reversible either spontaneously or as a result of treatment." **Status asthmaticus,** or acute severe asthma, is a refractory state that does not respond to standard therapy such as inhaled beta-agonists or subcutaneous epinephrine. It may persist for several hours.

SYNONYMS

Bronchospasm
Reactive airway disease
Asthmatic bronchitis

ICD-10CM CODES

J45.20	Mild intermittent asthma, uncomplicated
J45.21	Mild intermittent asthma with (acute) exacerbation
J45.22	Mild intermittent asthma with status asthmaticus
J45.30	Mild persistent asthma, uncomplicated
J45.31	Mild persistent asthma with (acute) exacerbation
J45.32	Mild persistent asthma with status asthmaticus
J45.40	Moderate persistent asthma, uncomplicated
J45.41	Moderate persistent asthma with (acute) exacerbation
J45.42	Moderate persistent asthma with status asthmaticus
J45.50	Severe persistent asthma, uncomplicated
J45.51	Severe persistent asthma with (acute) exacerbation
J45.52	Severe persistent asthma with status asthmaticus
J45.901	Unspecified asthma with (acute) exacerbation
J45.902	Unspecified asthma with status asthmaticus
J45.909	Unspecified asthma, uncomplicated
J45.991	Cough variant asthma
J45.998	Other asthma

EPIDEMIOLOGY & DEMOGRAPHICS

- Asthma has been diagnosed in 7.7% of the population in the U.S. Its prevalence is steadily rising among patients older than 65 yr, African Americans, women, and persons living below the poverty level.
- It is estimated that 300 million people have asthma. An increase in prevalence to 400 million is anticipated by 2025.

- It accounts for around 440,000 hospitalizations and 1.8 million emergency department (ED) visits yearly in the U.S.
- It was previously more common in children, but given the increase of adult-onset asthma, it is now more common in adults (7.5% of children vs. 7.7% of adults).
- Overall, mortality secondary to asthma has declined in the U.S. to 10.5 per 1 million but has not changed for children ages 1 to 14 yr.
- 50% to 80% of children with asthma develop symptoms before 5 yr of age. Early childhood risk factors for asthma are described in Table 1. Box 1 summarizes risk factors for severe and fatal asthma in adults.

TABLE 1 Early Childhood Risk Factors for Persistent Asthma

Parental asthma
Allergy:
  Atopic dermatitis (eczema)
  Allergic rhinitis
  Food allergy
  Inhalant allergen sensitization
  Food allergen sensitization
Severe lower respiratory tract infection:
  Pneumonia
  Bronchiolitis requiring hospitalization
  Wheezing apart from colds
  Male sex
  Low birthweight
  Environmental tobacco smoke exposure
  Possible use of acetaminophen (paracetamol)
  Exposure to chlorinated swimming pools
  Reduced lung function at birth

From Kliegman RM et al: *Nelson textbook of pediatrics,* ed 19, Philadelphia, 2011, Saunders.

BOX 1 Risk Factors for Severe and Fatal Asthma in Adults

- History of prior nonfatal asthma attack
- Prior intubation
- Female sex
- Age >65 yr
- African American ethnicity
- Obesity
- Tobacco use
- Inhalational drug abuse
- Poorly controlled disease
- Poor recognition of dyspnea and other symptoms
- Steroid dependence
- H1N1 viral infection
- Misuse or lack of proper use of maintenance medications
- Psychiatric illness
- Lack of access to medical care
- Lack of ability to limit triggers (i.e., persistent exposure to pollutants, dust)
- Comorbid heart disease, obesity, and/or diabetes
- Bronchoalveolar lavage predominance of neutrophils, interleukin 8, and matrix metalloproteinase

From Parrillo JE, Dellinger RP: *Critical care medicine, principles of diagnosis and management in the adult,* ed 5, Philadelphia, 2019, Elsevier.

PHYSICAL FINDINGS & CLINICAL PRESENTATION

Physical examination findings vary with the stage and severity of asthma and may reveal a normal lung examination. Some degree of wheezing and prolonged expiratory phases of respiration are usually present with persistent or acute disease. Box 2 and Table 2 summarize signs and symptoms of severe asthma. Physical examination during status asthmaticus may reveal:

- Tachycardia and tachypnea
- Use of accessory respiratory muscles
- Pulsus paradoxus (inspiratory decline in systolic blood pressure >10 mm Hg)
- Absence of wheezing (silent chest) or decreased wheezing can indicate worsening obstruction
- Mental status changes: Generally secondary to hypoxia and hypercapnia and constitute an indication for urgent intubation
- Paradoxical abdominal and diaphragmatic movement on inspiration (detected by palpation over the upper part of the abdomen in a semirecumbent position) indicates diaphragmatic fatigue, another sign of impending respiratory crisis

ETIOLOGY

- The pathophysiology of asthma involves a complex interaction among various environmental and genetic factors (Figs. E1, E2, and E3). Genetic and phenotypic associations in asthma are described in Box 3.
- Allergic (atopic, extrinsic) asthma is triggered by various aeroallergens or nonallergic (nonatopic) nonspecific (e.g., dust, cigarette smoke, fumes, cold air, exercise) exposures in patients who are prone to develop immunoglobulin E (IgE) antibodies in response to various exposures.

BOX 2 Signs and Symptoms of Severe Asthma

- "Tripoding"—sitting upright and leaning forward
- Diaphoresis
- Use of accessory muscles
- Asynchronous accessory muscle use
- Air trapping and hyperinflation manifesting as decreased inspiratory stroke volume and pulsus paradoxus
- Peak flow <200 L/min and/or <30% predicted*
- FEV1 <1 L/min and/or <20% predicted*
- Evidence of barotrauma:
  1. Unilateral diminution in breath sounds
  2. Tracheal deviation
  3. Thoracic crepitus
  4. Signs of impending respiratory arrest:
  5. Altered mentation
  6. Cyanosis
  7. Hypoxia
  8. Hypercarbia
  9. Hemodynamic instability

*Silent chest.

From Parrillo JE, Dellinger RP: *Critical care medicine, principles of diagnosis and management in the adult,* ed 5, Philadelphia, 2019, Elsevier.

TABLE 2 Objective Findings in Asthma Assessment

Factor	Severe Asthma
Pulse rate (beats/min)	≥120
Respiratory rate (breaths/min)	≥30
Use of accessory muscles of respiration	If present, may indicate severe asthma; if absent, may have equally severe asthma in 50% of cases
ABG analysis (mm Hg)	$Pao_2 \leq 60$ or $Paco_2 \geq 42$ indicates severe asthma; all other values difficult to interpret unless PEF known
Pulmonary function studies	PEF measures the degree of airflow obstruction; most useful in assessing severity and guiding treatment decisions

ABG, Arterial blood gas; $Paco_2$, partial pressure of carbon dioxide in arterial blood; Pao_2, partial pressure of oxygen in arterial blood; PEF, peak expiratory flow rate.
From Walls RM et al: *Rosen's emergency medicine, concepts and clinical practice,* ed 10, Philadelphia, 2023, Elsevier.

TABLE 3 Factors That Contribute to Worsening Asthma Control and Coexisting Conditions

Contributing Factor	Proposed Intervention
Tobacco use	Encourage tobacco cessation and assist with both nonpharmacologic and pharmacologic methods to help patients quit smoking; discuss avoidance of secondhand smoke
GERD	Consider empiric therapy for symptomatic GERD Barium swallow or pH probe study to diagnose GERD Impedance study if nonacid reflux is suspected Referral to gastroenterology for evaluation and treatment Consider surgical management for refractory cases
Atopy and allergic rhinitis	Consider empiric therapy with nasal steroids, nasal and oral antihistamines, leukotriene antagonists Consider skin prick testing or specific IgE testing to guide allergen identification and avoidance Referral to allergist or otolaryngologist for evaluation Consider allergen immunotherapy
Nasal polyps and chronic sinusitis	Refer to otolaryngologist for evaluation and treatment Possible surgical intervention for refractory cases Consider aspirin desensitization for patients with nasal polyps and aspirin sensitivity
Vocal cord dysfunction*	Laryngoscopy to diagnose vocal cord dysfunction Referral to speech pathologist for evaluation and treatment
Obesity*	Encourage weight loss Consider bariatric surgery
Obstructive sleep apnea*	Referral for sleep study and initiate therapy for sleep apnea Referral to sleep specialist for complex cases
Psychologic factors*	Evaluate for anxiety and depression

*May coexist with asthma with overlapping symptoms.
GERD, Gastroesophageal reflux disease; Ig, immunoglobulin.
From Broaddus VC et al: *Murray & Nadel's textbook of respiratory medicine,* ed 7, Philadelphia, 2022, Elsevier.

- Factors that contribute to worsening asthma control and coexisting conditions are summarized in Table 3.
- A longitudinal epidemiologic cohort study of a prebirth cohort observed that maternal intake of foods commonly considered allergenic (peanut and milk) was associated with a decrease in allergy and asthma in the offspring. No dietary restrictions during pregnancy are therefore recommended for the prevention of allergies or asthma.
- Nonallergic (intrinsic) asthma commonly manifests as adult-onset asthma in response to respiratory tract infection or psychologic stress.
- Occupational exposure to certain organic or nonorganic agents can trigger asthma.
- Dampness and mold contribute to the risk of developing asthma; remediation of these in homes reduces asthma symptoms and medication use in adults.
- Exercise-induced asthma is seen most frequently in adolescents and manifests with bronchospasm after beginning of exercise and improves with discontinuation of exercise.
- Drug-induced asthma is associated with use of NSAIDs, β-blockers, sulfites, and certain foods and beverages.
- There is a strong association of the *ADAM 33* gene with asthma and bronchial hyperresponsiveness. Experimental, genetic, and clinical studies support an important role for type-2 inflammatory pathways in the pathogenesis of severe asthma. Atopic triggers

BOX 3 Genetic and Phenotypic Associations in Asthma

- ***ADAM33:*** Gene bronchoconstriction
- ***ORMDL3/GSDMB*** locus, chromosome 17q21: Childhood onset
- CpG portion of ***ACSL3:*** Associated with maternal exposure to automobile pollution
- ***IL33*** on chromosome 9
- ***IL2RB*** on chromosome 22

From Parrillo JE, Dellinger RP: *Critical care medicine, principles of diagnosis and management in the adult,* ed 5, Philadelphia, 2019, Elsevier.

stimulate Th2 cells to produce interleukin (IL)-5, IL-13, and IL-4, driving IgE synthesis, eosinophilia, and airway changes. IL-5 is felt to be the most specific cytokine in eosinophil regulatory pathways. Nonatopic triggers (e.g., smoke, viruses) also have a vital role in the type-2 inflammatory pathway. Type-2 innate lymphoid cells (ILC2) produce IL-5, IL-13 through release of damaged associated molecular patterns (DAMPs) from the respiratory epithelium.

- Damaged airway epithelium also releases innate immunity cytokines known as alarmins (TSLP, IL-25, IL-33). These airway epithelium cytokines initiate multiple type-2 inflammatory pathways in response to allergen and infection-driven inflammation. IL-33 and IL-25 are known to mainly activate ILC2s. Thymic stromal lipoproteins (TSLP), on the other hand, have been shown to promote antigen-presenting cells (APCs) that lead to the activation of T cells and B cells.

Ⓓ DIAGNOSIS

DIFFERENTIAL DIAGNOSIS (BOX 4)

- Postinfectious bronchitis
- Rhinitis with postnasal drip
- Paradoxical vocal fold motion (vocal cord dysfunction)
- Chronic obstructive pulmonary disease (COPD)
- Gastroesophageal reflux disease (GERD)
- Pneumonia and other respiratory tract infections
- Foreign body aspiration (most frequent in younger patients)
- Anxiety disorder
- Interstitial lung disease
- Hypersensitivity pneumonitis
- Heart failure
- Pulmonary embolism

WORKUP

- An algorithm for diagnosing asthma in adults is illustrated in Fig. 4. Diagnosis of asthma requires documentation of airway obstruction and some degree of reversibility.
- For symptomatic adults and children age >5 yr who can perform spirometry, pre- and postbronchodilator spirometry is the recommended test of choice.

BOX 4 The Differential Diagnosis of Asthma

Cardiac conditions
    Valvular heart disease
    Congestive heart failure
    COPD exacerbation
Pulmonary infection
    Pneumonia
    Allergic bronchopulmonary aspergillosis
    Löffler syndrome
    Chronic eosinophilic pneumonia
Upper airway obstruction
    Laryngeal edema
    Laryngeal neoplasm
    Foreign body
    Vocal cord dysfunction
Endobronchial disease
    Neoplasm
    Foreign body
    Bronchial stenosis
Pulmonary embolus
Cystic fibrosis
Carcinoid tumor
Allergic/anaphylactic reaction
Adverse drug reaction (ACE inhibitors)
Miscellaneous conditions
    Churg-Strauss syndrome
    GERD
    Hyperventilation with panic attack
    Noncardiogenic pulmonary edema
    Addison's disease
    Invasive worm infection

ACE, Angiotensin-converting enzyme; *COPD,* chronic obstructive pulmonary disease; *GERD,* gastroesophageal reflux disease.
From Walls RM et al: *Rosen's emergency medicine, concepts and clinical practice,* ed 10, Philadelphia, 2023, Elsevier.

- Airflow reversibility is defined as increase in forced expiratory volume in 1 sec (FEV_1 by at least 12% and 200 ml) after inhaling a short-acting bronchodilator.
- The degree of reversibility measured by spirometry correlates with airway inflammation, and patients with a high degree of reversibility have a greater risk of irreversible airflow obstruction in subsequent years.
- For children age <5 yr, spirometry is generally not feasible. Those with asthma symptoms should be treated as having suspected asthma after alternative diagnoses are ruled out.
- Negative spirometry results do not rule out asthma. Patients with high clinical suspicion should undergo bronchial challenge testing with methacholine or other specific agents.
- The clinician should evaluate for environmental causes (e.g., house dust mites, indoor pets) and exposure to other allergens or irritants (e.g., tobacco smoke.)
- In the absence of spirometry, variability of peak flow measurements can be used to diagnose asthma.

After diagnosis, the severity of asthma should be classified during the initial assessment before initiating therapy. Patients are divided into four groups based on the severity of their asthma symptoms and number of exacerbations. Initial severity assessment and therapy is summarized in Table 4.

- Once therapy is initiated, the emphasis for clinical management should be aimed at achievement of asthma control. The level of asthma control should be used to guide decisions either to maintain or adjust therapy.

- Schedule visits at 2- to 6-wk intervals for patients who are initiating therapy or who require a step up in therapy to achieve or regain asthma control. Schedule visits at 6- to 12-mo intervals after asthma control is achieved to monitor whether control is maintained. The interval will depend on factors such as the duration of asthma control or the level of treatment required, especially for patients who are on asthma biologic therapy. Consider scheduling visits at 3-mo intervals if step-down therapy is anticipated.

LABORATORY TESTS

- Arterial blood gases (ABGs) can be used during acute bronchospasm in staging the severity of an asthmatic attack:
  1. Mild: Decreased Pao_2 and $Paco_2$, increased pH
  2. Moderate: Decreased Pao_2, normal $Paco_2$, normal pH
  3. Severe: Marked decreased Pao_2, increased $Paco_2$, and decreased pH
- CBC: Leukocytosis with left shift may indicate the existence of bacterial infection. Elevated eosinophils point toward allergic component of asthma.
- Serum IgE and eosinophil levels help guide treatment for patients with severe persistent asthma and monitor response to treatment in this group.
- Spirometry is recommended at the initial assessment and at least every 1 to 2 yr after treatment is initiated and when the symptoms and peak expiratory flow have stabilized. Spirometry may be performed more

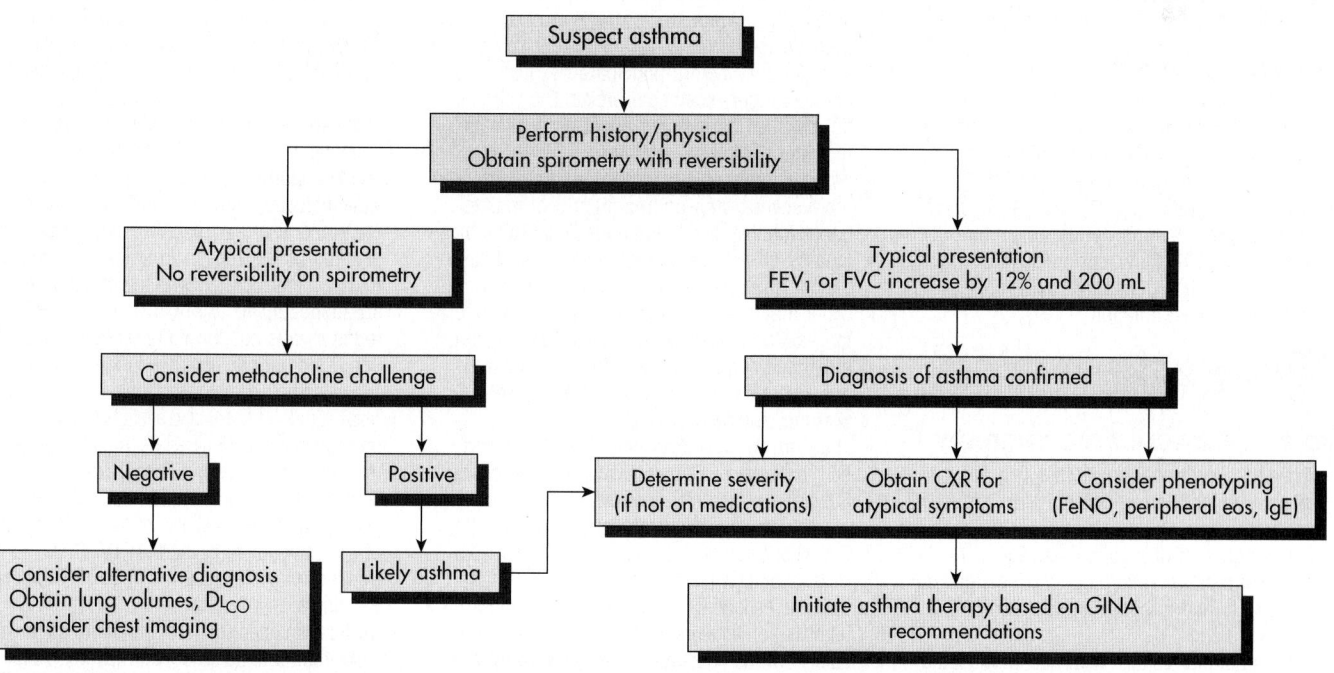

FIG. 4 Algorithm for diagnosing asthma in adults. The diagnosis of asthma is based on a careful personal history, physical examination, and lung function testing. Spirometry should be obtained in every patient in whom asthma is suspected. Other tests are useful when clinical features are atypical and to determine severity and asthma phenotype. *CXR,* Chest radiograph; *Dl_{CO},* diffusing capacity for carbon monoxide; *eos,* eosinophils; *FeNO,* fraction of exhaled nitric oxide; *FEV_1,* forced expiratory volume in 1 sec; *FVC,* forced vital capacity; *GINA,* Global Initiative for Asthma; *IgE,* immunoglobulin E. (From Broaddus VC et al: *Murray & Nadel's textbook of respiratory medicine,* ed 7, Philadelphia, 2022, Elsevier.)

TABLE 4 Initial Severity Assessments and Therapies in the Emergency Department

	Mild to Moderate	Severe
PEF (percentage predicted/personal best)	≥40%	Unable or <40%
Oxygen therapy	Maintain Sao$_2$ ≥90%	Maintain Sao$_2$ ≥90%
Nebulized Albuterol Solution		
Albuterol	2.5 mg every 20 min for up to three doses	5.0 mg every 20 min for three doses Continuous for 1 h if severe
Albuterol Metered-Dose Inhaler With Spacer		
Albuterol (90 μg/puff)	6-12 puffs every 20 min for up to three doses with supervision	Same for three doses (if able to do) with supervision
Ipratropium Therapy		
Nebulized solution	0.5 mg every 20 min for three doses (may mix with albuterol solution)	0.5 mg every 20 min for three doses (may mix with albuterol solution)
MDI (18 μg/puff) with spacer	8 puffs every 20 min for three doses	8 puffs every 20 min for three doses
Systemic Corticosteroids		
Oral (preferred)	40-50 mg of prednisone or prednisolone per day if no immediate response to albuterol	40-to 50 mg of prednisone or prednisolone per day
IV (unable to take orally or absorb)	125 mg of methylprednisolone per day	125 mg of methylprednisolone per day
IV magnesium sulfate	Not indicated	2 g over 20 min (or at rates of up to 1 g/min) if PEF ≤25% predicted

IV, Intravenous; *MDI,* metered-dose inhaler; *PEF,* peak expiratory flow rate; *Sao$_2$,* oxygen saturation in arterial blood.
From Broaddus VC et al: *Murray & Nadel's textbook of respiratory medicine,* ed 7, Philadelphia, 2022, Elsevier.

frequently, if indicated, based on severity of symptoms or lack of response to treatment.
- Peak expiratory flow rate (PEFR) can be used to assess severity of an acute exacerbation episode. Values should be compared with individual's personal best number (see "asthma action plan").
- Specific allergy testing may be helpful in a subgroup of patients.
- Fractional exhaled nitric oxide (FeNO) can be used to assess airway inflammation and to guide treatment and monitor response.

IMAGING STUDIES
- Chest x-ray examination: Usually normal, may show evidence of thoracic hyperinflation (e.g., flattening of the diaphragm, increased volume over the retrosternal air space).
- ECG: Tachycardia, nonspecific ST-T wave changes are common during an asthma attack; may also show cor pulmonale, right bundle branch block, right axial deviation, counterclockwise rotation.

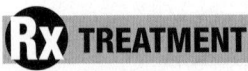 **TREATMENT**

NONPHARMACOLOGIC THERAPY
- Avoidance of triggering factors (e.g., salicylates, sulfites), environmental, or occupational triggers
- Encouragement of regular exercise
- Patient education regarding warning signs of an attack and proper use of medications (e.g., inhalers)
- Assess asthma control with use of validated questionnaires

GENERAL Rx
The 2007 NAEPP Guidelines for the Diagnosis and Management of Asthma and the 2020 Focused Updates to the Asthma Management Guidelines (see Tables 5 to 7) provide treatment algorithms by age groups with a step-up approach based on the severity of symptoms.

An approach to home management of acute asthma is described in Fig. E5. Selected inhaled medications used by patients with asthma are summarized in Table 8.
- Short-acting beta-selective adrenergic agonists (SABAs) administered by inhalation are the most effective therapy for quick relief of asthmatic symptoms. They are recommended for use only as needed for relief of symptoms or before anticipated exposure to known triggers such as exercise. They should not be used as a single agent except for intermittent asthma symptoms.
- When symptoms become more frequent or more severe, step-up treatment with maintenance inhalers is recommended (see Table 5).
- Inhaled corticosteroids (ICSs) are the mainstay of treatment for maintenance therapy.
- Other maintenance treatment options include long-acting beta-agonist (LABA), combination of inhaled corticosteroids and LABA, leukotriene receptor antagonist (LTRA), cromolyn, zileuton, and theophylline.
- There are several corticosteroid/LABA combination inhalers available (fluticasone/salmeterol [Advair], budesonide/formoterol [Symbicort], mometasone/formoterol [Dulera], and ICS/LABA fluticasone furoate 200 mcg and vilanterol 25 mcg inhalation powder [Breo Ellipta]). A large study investigating the safety of LABA and ICS combination inhalers confirmed their long-term safety and demonstrated a reduced risk of exacerbations and improved lung function, when compared with an equivalent dose of ICS alone. A trial[1] of albuterol–budesonide fixed–dose combination rescue inhaler for asthma revealed that the risk of severe asthma exacerbation was significantly lower with as-needed use of a fixed-dose combination of 180 mcg of albuterol and 160 mcg of budesonide than with as needed use of albuterol alone among patients with uncontrolled moderate-to-severe asthma who were receiving a wide range of inhaled glucocorticoid-containing maintenance therapies.
- Long-acting muscarinic antagonists (LAMAs): Studies have shown some degree of benefit when adding a LAMA to ICS + LABA in moderate to severe asthma. The LAMA tiotropium (Spiriva), which has been used for decades as a first-line treatment for COPD, is now approved for the treatment of asthma and is included in the most recent (2020) Global Initiative for Asthma (GINA) guidelines as a possible add-on at step 4. A systematic review including more than 7000 patients demonstrated the use of LAMA compared with placebo as an add-on to inhaled corticosteroids was associated with lower risk of exacerbation. Adding LAMA to a dual LABA-ICS regimen was not shown to reduce exacerbation rates but can improve lung function.
- Triple-therapy combination inhalers (corticosteroid/LABA/LAMA) are also available for the treatment of asthma (fluticasone furoate/vilanterol/umeclidinium [Trelegy Ellipta]). None of these combinations is approved or indicated for the initial treatment of asthma or for acute therapy of asthma symptoms by the FDA. There is no evidence that one product is more effective than the others.
- Oral corticosteroids are reserved as a last resort for maintenance therapy for recalcitrant cases.

IMMUNOLOGIC TARGETS
- Tezepelumab, a human monoclonal antibody to thymic stromal lymphopoietin (TSLP), is

TABLE 5 Stepwise Approach for Managing Asthma in Youths ≥12 Yr and Adults

Treatment	Intermittent Asthma Step 1	MANAGEMENT OF PERSISTENT ASTHMA IN INDIVIDUALS 12+ YR OF AGE				
		Step 2	Step 3	Step 4	Step 5	Step 6^
Preferred	PRN SABA	Daily low-dose ICS and PRN SABA or PRN concomitant ICS and SABA#	Daily and PRN combination low-dose ICS-formoterol#	Daily and PRN combination medium-dose ICS-formoterol#	Daily medium-dose ICS-LABA + LAMA and PRN SABA#	Daily high-dose ICS-LABA + oral systemic corticosteroid + PRN SABA
Alternative		Daily LTRA* and PRN SABA or cromolyn,* or nedocromil,* or zileuton,* or theophylline,* and PRN SABA	Daily medium-dose ICS and PRN SABA or Daily low-dose ICS-LABA, or daily low-dose ICS + LAMA,# or daily low-dose ICS + LTRA,* and PRN SABA or Daily low-dose ICS + theophylline* or zileuton,* and PRN SABA	Daily medium-dose ICS-LABA or daily medium-dose ICS + LAMA, and PRN SABA# or Daily medium-dose ICS + LTRA* or daily medium-dose ICS + theophylline,* or daily medium-dose ICS + zileuton,* and PRN SABA	Daily high-dose ICS + LTRA* or daily high-dose ICS + theophylline,* and PRN SABA	
		Steps 2-4: Conditionally recommend the use of subcutaneous immunotherapy as an adjunct treatment to standard pharmacotherapy in individuals >5 yr of age whose asthma is controlled at the initiation, build up, and maintenance phases of immunotherapy.#			Consider adding asthma biologics (e.g., anti-IgE, anti-IL-5, anti-IL-5R, anti-IL-4/IL-13)	

*Cromolyn, nedocromil, LTRAs (including zileuton and montelukast), and theophylline were not considered in the 2020 NAEPP update.
**The AHRQ systemic reviews that informed this report did not include studies that examined the role of asthma biologics. Thus this 2020 NAEPP update does not contain specific recommendations for the use of biologics in asthma in steps 5 and 6.
^Data on the use of LAMA therapy in individuals with severe persistent asthma (Step 6) were not included in the AHRQ systematic review, and thus no recommendation is made.
#Updated based on the 2020 guidelines. The stepwise approach is meant to assist, not replace, the clinical decision-making required to meet individual patient needs. If alternative treatment is used and response is inadequate, discontinue it and use the preferred treatment before stepping up. Zileuton is a less desirable alternative due to limited studies as adjunctive therapy and the need to monitor liver function. Theophylline requires monitoring of serum concentration levels. In step 6, before oral systemic corticosteroids are introduced, a trial of high-dose ICS + LABA + either LTRA, theophylline, or zileuton may be considered, although this approach has not been studied in clinical trials. Steps 1, 2, and 3 preferred therapies are based on Evidence A; step 3 alternative therapy is based on Evidence A for LTRA, Evidence B for theophylline, and Evidence D for zileuton. Step 5 preferred therapy is based on Evidence B. Step 6 preferred therapy is based on (EPR-2 1997) and Evidence B for omalizumab. Immunotherapy for steps 2-4 is based on Evidence B for house-dust mites, animal danders, and pollens; evidence is weak or lacking for molds and cockroaches. Evidence is strongest for immunotherapy with single allergens. The role of allergy in asthma is greater in children than in adults. Clinicians who administer immunotherapy or omalizumab should be prepared and equipped to identify and treat anaphylaxis that may occur. This information is directly abstracted from the 2007 NAEPP *Expert Panel Report 3: Guidelines for the diagnosis and management of asthma* and is not intended to promote or endorse any of the listed products. To access the complete 2007 *Expert Panel Report 3: Guidelines for the diagnosis and management of asthma*, go to https://www.nhlbi.nih.gov/sites/default/files/media/docs/asthsumm.pdf. The "2020 Focused Updates to the Asthma Management Guidelines: a report from the National Asthma Education and Prevention Program Coordinating Committee Expert Panel Working Group" can be found at https://www.nhlbi.nih.gov/sites/default/files/publications/AsthmaManagementGuidelinesReport-2-4-21.pdf.
EIB, Exercise-induced bronchospasm; *ICS*, inhaled corticosteroid; *LABA*, long-acting beta₂-agonist; *LTRA*, leukotriene receptor antagonist; *PRN*, as necessary; *SABA*, inhaled short-acting beta₂-agonist.
From 2020 Focused updates to the asthma management guidelines: a report from the National Asthma Education and Prevention Program Coordinating Committee Expert Panel Working Group. https://www.nhlbi.nih.gov/sites/default/files/publications/AsthmaManagementGuidelinesReport-2-4-21.pdf.

FDA approved as an add-on on therapy for adults and children aged 12 yr and older with severe asthma not controlled by their current asthma regimen.

- Dupilumab, a human monoclonal antibody to IL-4 and IL-13, is FDA approved for use in adult and pediatric patients >6 mo with moderate to severe asthma with an eosinophilic phenotype or with oral corticosteroid–dependent asthma.
- Mepolizumab (Nucala), a monoclonal antibody to IL-5, is approved by the FDA as an add-on for patients ≥12 yr with severe eosinophilic asthma that is uncontrolled.
- Reslizumab, another anti-IL-5 monoclonal antibody, has a similar indication for eosinophilic asthma and uses a higher eosinophil cutoff (≥400 µL) based on a greater predictive value for sputum eosinophilia.
- Benralizumab, a monoclonal anti-IL-5 receptor alpha antibody, is an additional FDA-approved add-on treatment to consider for patients >12 yr with persistent severe eosinophilic asthma.
- Omalizumab, an anti-IgE monoclonal antibody, is an FDA-approved add-on asthma treatment for moderate to severe persistent asthma in patients 6 yr of age and older with a positive skin test or in vitro reactivity to a perennial aeroallergen and symptoms that are inadequately controlled with inhaled corticosteroids.

BRONCHIAL THERMOPLASTY

Select patients with severe persistent asthma who have failed medical treatment may benefit from bronchial thermoplasty. This requires the insertion of a catheter via bronchoscopy and use of radiofrequency heat to reduce bronchial smooth muscle. Long-term follow-up data showed persistent reduction in asthma exacerbation and fewer ED visits over a period of 5 yr in carefully selected patients. FDA labeling is for "severe persistent asthma inadequately controlled on ICS + LABA."

OTHER MEDICATIONS

- Azithromycin: The AZISAST Trial randomized 109 patients on high-dose ICS/LABA (step 4 or 5 per GINA guidelines) to maintenance therapy with azithromycin or placebo. There was no benefit seen with azithromycin therapy regarding any of the primary outcomes, although a subgroup analysis showed that patients with noneosinophilic asthma had fewer exacerbations. This result suggests azithromycin may be an effective option for the neutrophilic/Th-1 phenotype, but more data are needed.
- Immunosuppressants such as methotrexate can decrease long-term steroid requirements; however, they have significant side effects, and there is no evidence of persistent therapeutic effect after discontinuation. Fig. 6 illustrates a process toward initiating biologic therapy.

SEVERE ASTHMA TREATMENT (ATS/ERS GUIDELINES)

- The American Thoracic Society (ATS) classification of "severe asthma" refers to patients who require high-dose inhaled or near-continuous oral glucocorticoid treatment to maintain asthma control.

Diseases and Disorders

I

TABLE 6 Stepwise Approach for Managing Asthma in Children 5 to 11 Yr

Treatment	Intermittent Asthma Step 1	MANAGEMENT OF PERSISTENT ASTHMA IN INDIVIDUALS 5-11 YR OF AGE				
		Step 2	Step 3	Step 4	Step 5	Step 6
Preferred	PRN SABA	Daily low-dose ICS and PRN SABA	Daily and PRN combination low-dose ICS-formoterol#	Daily and PRN combination medium-dose ICS-formoterol#	Daily high-dose ICS-LABA and PRN SABA	Daily high-dose ICS-LABA + oral systemic corticosteroid and PRN SABA
Alternative		Daily LTRA,* or cromolyn,* or nedocromil,* or theophylline,* and PRN SABA	Daily medium-dose ICS and PRN SABA or Daily low-dose ICS-LABA, or daily low-dose ICS + LTRA,* or daily low-dose ICS + theophylline,* and PRN SABA	Daily medium-dose ICS-LABA and PRN SABA or Daily medium-dose ICS + LTRA* or daily medium-dose ICS + theophylline,* and PRN SABA	Daily high-dose ICS + LTRA* or daily high-dose ICS + theophylline,* and PRN SABA	Daily high-dose ICS + LTRA* + oral systemic corticosteroid or daily high-dose ICS + theophylline* + oral systemic corticosteroid, and PRN SABA
		Steps 2-4: Conditionally recommend the use of subcutaneous immunotherapy as an adjunct treatment to standard pharmacotherapy in individuals >5 yr of age whose asthma is controlled at the initiation, build up, and maintenance phases of immunotherapy.			Consider omalizumab**,#	

*Cromolyn, nedocromil, LTRAs (including montelukast), and theophylline were not considered in the 2020 NAEPP update.

**Omalizumab was the only biologic mentioned in the NAEPP 2020 update.

#Updated based on the 2020 guidelines. The stepwise approach is meant to assist, not replace, the clinical decision-making required to meet individual patient needs. If alternative treatment is used and response is inadequate, discontinue it and use the preferred treatment before stepping up. Theophylline is a less desirable alternative due to the need to monitor serum concentration levels. Step 1 and step 2 medications are based on Evidence A. Step 3 ICS 1 adjunctive therapy and ICS are based on Evidence B for efficacy of each treatment and extrapolation from comparator trials in older children and adults—comparator trials are not available for this age group; steps 4-6 are based on expert opinion and extrapolation from studies in older children and adults. Immunotherapy for steps 2-4 is based on Evidence B for house-dust mites, animal danders, and pollens; evidence is weak or lacking for molds and cockroaches. Evidence is strongest for immunotherapy with single allergens. The role of allergy in asthma is greater in children than in adults. Clinicians who administer immunotherapy should be prepared and equipped to identify and treat anaphylaxis that may occur. This information is directly abstracted from the 2007 NAEPP *Expert Panel Report 3: Guidelines for the diagnosis and management of asthma* and is not intended to promote or endorse any of the listed products.

EIB, Exercise-induced bronchoconstriction; *ICS,* inhaled corticosteroid; *LABA,* long-acting beta₂-agonist; *LTRA,* leukotriene receptor antagonist; *prn,* as necessary; *SABA,* inhaled short-acting beta₂-agonist.

From 2020 Focused updates to the asthma management guidelines: a report from the National Asthma Education and Prevention Program Coordinating Committee Expert Panel Working Group. https://www.nhlbi.nih.gov/sites/default/files/publications/AsthmaManagementGuidelinesReport-2-4-21.pdf.

TABLE 7 Stepwise Approach for Managing Asthma in Children 0 to 4 Yr

Treatment	Intermittent Asthma Step 1	MANAGEMENT OF PERSISTENT ASTHMA IN INDIVIDUALS 0 TO 4 YR OF AGE				
		Step 2	Step 3	Step 4	Step 5	Step 6
Preferred	PRN SABA and At the start of RTI: Add short course daily ICS#	Daily low-dose ICS and PRN SABA	Daily medium-dose ICS and PRN SABA	Daily medium-dose ICS-LABA and PRN SABA	Daily high-dose ICS-LABA and PRN SABA	Daily high-dose ICS-LABA + oral systemic corticosteroid and PRN SABA
Alternative		Daily montelukast* or cromolyn,* and PRN SABA		Daily medium-dose ICS + montelukast* and PRN SABA	Daily high-dose ICS + montelukast* and PRN SABA	Daily high-dose ICS + montelukast* + oral systemic corticosteroid and PRN SABA
			For children age 4 yr only, see step 3 and step 4 on Management of Persistent Asthma in Individuals Ages 5-11 Yr diagram.			

*Cromolyn and montelukast were not considered for this updated and/or have limited availability for use in the United States. The FDA issued a Boxed Warning for montelukast in March 2020.

#Updated based on the 2020 guidelines. The stepwise approach is meant to assist, not replace, the clinical decision-making required to meet individual patient needs. If alternative treatment is used and response is inadequate, discontinue it and use the preferred treatment before stepping up. If clear benefit is not observed within 4-6 wk and patient/family medication technique and adherence are satisfactory, consider adjusting therapy or alternative diagnosis. Studies on children 0-4 yr are limited. Step 2 preferred therapy is based on Evidence A. All other recommendations are based on expert opinion and extrapolation from studies in other children. This information is directly abstracted from the 2007 NAEPP *Expert Panel Report 3: Guidelines for the diagnosis and management of asthma* and is not intended to promote or endorse any of the listed products.

ICS, Inhaled corticosteroid; *LABA,* long-acting beta₂-agonist; *LTRA,* leukotriene receptor antagonist; *PRN,* as needed; *RTI,* respiratory tract infection; *SABA,* inhaled short-acting beta₂-agonist;

From 2020 Focused updates to the asthma management guidelines: a report from the National Asthma Education and Prevention Program Coordinating Committee Expert Panel Working Group. https://www.nhlbi.nih.gov/sites/default/files/publications/AsthmaManagementGuidelinesReport-2-4-21.pdf.

TABLE 8 Selected Inhaled Medications Used by Patients with Asthma

Generic Name	Trade Name*	Dose/Puff	Dose as Puffs	Comments
Beta-Agonist Bronchodilators†				
Albuterol-MDI‡	AccuNeb, Proair HFA, Proventil HFA, Ventolin HFA, Airomir HFA, Salamol HFA	Varies from 90–200 μg	2 puffs as needed for asthma symptoms. Can be repeated every 4 h. 10–12 puffs in 24 h is the maximum dose. Use of more than 6 puffs/day should prompt medical consultation for asthma control.	All are metered-dose inhalers that deliver a fixed amount of medication per puff.
Albuterol-DPI	Ventolin, Asmasal, Salbulin	100 or 200 μg	1 puff as needed, otherwise same as albuterol MDI.	All are dry powder inhalers that deliver a fixed amount of medication per inhalation.
Albuterol solution	—	Varies from 0.63–5 mg/ml	Inhale while breathing till solution consumed. Need for more than 6 home treatments/day should prompt medical consultation.	This solution is for use with a liquid nebulizer driven by compressed gas. Mix the dose with a volume of sterile normal saline to achieve a nebulizer concentration of 0.63 mg/ml.
Levalbuterol-MDI	Xopenex HFA		Same as albuterol-MDI.	The isolated R-isomer of albuterol. Some studies show superiority to the racemic albuterol found in the MDIs listed above.
Levalbuterol-solution	Xopenex inhalation solution	0.63 mg/ml	Same as albuterol solution.	Nebulizer solution as noted for albuterol above.
Terbutaline-DPI	Bricanyl	250 or 500 μg	Same as albuterol-MDI.	Dry powder inhaler, uses patient generated effort to achieve airflow to disperse and deposit medication.
Terbutaline solution	Bricanyl inhalation solution	2.5 mg/ml	Same as albuterol.	The per dose amount is 2 ml with sterile saline added to achieve the requisite volume for the nebulizer used.
Long-Acting Anticholinergic Bronchodilator for Use in Severe Asthma				
Tiotropium bromide	Spiriva Respimat (MDI)	1.25 μg	2 puffs once/day.	For patients with asthma not controlled by β-agonist and inhaled glucocorticoid treatment.
Inhaled Glucocorticoids				
Beclomethasone	Beclovent, Clenil, Qvar, Asmabec	Comes in both MDI and DPI inhalers with amounts per puff varying from 50–400 μg	Adjust dose to achieve asthma control with a dose of 2 puffs twice/day. The maximum dose is 2 puffs twice daily of the highest strength.	Inhaled glucocorticoid with the longest use record. Although medication is generic, the inhaler type and propellant may be proprietary. Dose adjustments for patients in renal or hepatic failure are not needed.
Budesonide	Budelin, Pulmicort	Inhalers are all DPIs with amounts per dose 100–400 μg. Solution for nebulization is also available with amount of drug per treatment varies between 0.5–1.0 mg	Adjust dose to achieve asthma control with a dose of 2 puffs twice/day. The maximum dose is 2 puffs twice daily of the highest strength.	Dose adjustments for patients in renal or hepatic failure are not needed.
Fluticasone propionate	Flovent, Flixotide	MDIs with 50, 125, 250 μg dose strengths as well as packets for nebulization at 0.25 and 1.0 mg/ml	With MDI, start at low concentration and adjust dose to achieve asthma control with a dose of 2 puffs twice/day. The maximum dose is 2 puffs twice daily of the highest strength. With nebulizer, choose a concentration that gives asthma control when used twice daily.	Dose labels on U.S. marketed inhalers are 44, 110, and 220 μg/puff. The difference is the amount loaded in the metering chamber (outside of U.S.) vs the dose leaving the inhaler (U.S.). Dose adjustments for patients in renal failure not needed. In patients with hepatic failure, patients should be carefully monitored for steroid side effects and dose adjusted appropriately.
Ciclesonide	Alvesco	MDIs delivering 40, 80, or 160 μg	With MDI, start at low concentration and adjust dose to achieve asthma control with a dose of 2 puffs twice/day. The maximum dose is 2 puffs twice daily of the highest strength.	Dose adjustments for patients in renal or hepatic failure are not needed.
Flunisolide	Aerospan	80 μg	Start at 2 puffs twice/day and escalate as needed. 4 puffs twice/day is maximal dose.	Dose adjustments for patients in renal or hepatic failure are not needed.
Mometasone	Asmanex HFA	100 or 200 μg in HFA form; 110 or 220 μg in DPI form	Start with 200 (220) μg once/day (P.M. dosing suggested). Max dose is 800 (880) μg once daily. Titrate dose down as control is achieved.	Dose adjustments for patients in renal failure not needed. In patients with hepatic failure, patients should be carefully monitored for steroid side effects and dose adjusted appropriately.

Continued

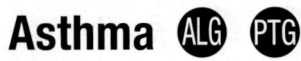
TABLE 8 Selected Inhaled Medications Used by Patients with Asthma—cont'd

Generic Name	Trade Name*	Dose/Puff	Dose as Puffs	Comments
Combination Inhalers Containing Both IGC and LABA§				
IGC = fluticasone propionate LABA = salmeterol	Advair, Seretide, AirFluSal, Sirdupla	Available as MDIs or DPIs. Each type contains a fixed dose of LABA with varying amounts of IGC. Exact amounts vary by inhaler type.	Start with 1 puff twice daily at the lowest dose of IGC that is effective for asthma control. Titrate up and down as symptom control requires. Max dose is 4 puffs of highest strength per day.	Dose adjustments for patients in renal failure not needed. In patients with hepatic failure, patients should be carefully monitored for steroid side effects and dose adjusted appropriately.
IGC = fluticasone propionate LABA = formoterol	Flutiform	Available only as MDIs. Each strength contains a fixed dose of LABA with varying amounts of IGC.	Start with 2 puffs twice daily at the lowest dose of IGC that is effective for asthma control. Titrate up and down as symptom control requires. Max dose is 4 puffs of highest strength per day.	Dose adjustments for patients in renal failure not needed. In patients with hepatic failure, patients should be carefully monitored for steroid side effects and dose adjusted appropriately. Not recommended for children under 12 yr.
IGC = budesonide 'LABA = formoterol	DuoResp, Symbicort, Bufoler	Available only as DPIs. Each strength contains a fixed dose of LABA with varying amounts of IGC. Exact amounts vary by inhaler type.	Start with 1 puff twice daily at the lowest dose of IGC that is effective for asthma control. Titrate up and down as symptom control requires. Max dose is 4 puffs of highest strength per day.	Dose adjustments for patients in renal or hepatic failure are not needed.
IGC = budesonide LABA = salmeterol	Busalair	Available only as DPIs. Each strength contains a fixed dose of LABA with varying amounts of IGC. Exact amounts vary by inhaler type.	Start with 1 puff twice daily at the lowest dose of IGC that is effective for asthma control. Titrate up and down as symptom control requires. Max dose is 4 puffs of highest strength per day.	Dose adjustments for patients in renal or hepatic failure are not needed.
IGC = mometasone LABA = formoterol	Dulera	Available only as MDIs. Each strength contains a 5-μg dose of formoterol with varying amounts of IGC. Exact amounts vary by inhaler type.	Start with 1 puff twice daily at the lowest dose of IGC that is effective for asthma control. Titrate up and down as symptom control requires. Max dose is 4 puffs of highest strength per day.	Dose adjustments for patients in renal or hepatic failure are not needed.
IGC = beclomethasone LABA = formoterol	Fostair MDI or DPI or Fostair Inhalation Solution	All contain 6 μg of formoterol with amounts of glucocorticoid varying from 100-200 μg.	Adjust IGC dose to achieve asthma control with a dose of 2 puffs twice/day.	Not available in the U.S.
IGC = fluticasone furoate LABA = vilanterol	Relvar Ellipta or Breo Ellipta	All forms contain 25 μg of vilanterol with amount of glucocorticoid varying from 92-184 μg.	Adjust IGC dose to achieve asthma control with a dose of 2 puffs once/day.	Bronchodilator effect of vilanterol onsets in about 15 min. Dose adjustments for patients in renal failure not needed. In patients with hepatic failure, patients should be carefully monitored for steroid side effects and dose adjusted appropriately.

*Not all products marketing each medication are listed.

†All are short acting with onset of effect 5-10 min and duration of effect 4-8 h. All patients with asthma should have a short-acting bronchodilator as a rescue inhaler to use for rescue from signs of airway obstruction.

‡The generic names albuterol and salbutamol are synonyms. Albuterol is used in the U.S. and salbutamol in many other countries.

§LABAs alone should not be used in patients with asthma.

DPI, Dry powder inhale; *HFA,* hydrofluoroalkane; *IGC,* inhaled glucocorticoid; *LABA,* long-acting β-agonist; *MDI,* metered-dose inhaler.

From Goldman L, Shafer AI: *Goldman-Cecil medicine,* ed 26, Philadelphia, 2020, Elsevier.

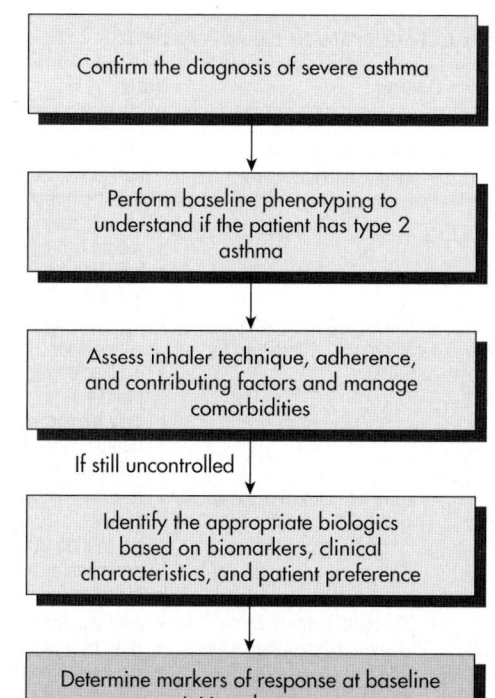

FIG. 6 **Recommended process toward initiating biologic therapy.** A diagnosis of severe asthma should be confirmed using objective measures of lung function, and evidence for type 2 asthma should be assessed. Before initiating biologic therapy, evaluate for comorbid conditions, alternative diagnoses, and poor inhaler technique or adherence. Measurement of type 2 biomarkers will help select initial therapy. Reassess for clinical response in 4 mo. (From Broaddus VC et al: *Murray & Nadel's textbook of respiratory medicine,* ed 7, Philadelphia, 2022, Elsevier.)

- In patients who do not achieve adequate control with the combination of a high-dose inhaled glucocorticoid and LABA, an additional controller medication such as an LTRA or LAMA is recommended.
- For patients with atopic severe asthma who have a serum IgE level of 30 to 700 IU/ml and documented sensitivity to a perennial allergen, adding omalizumab is recommended.
- For patients with severe asthma, frequent exacerbations, and an eosinophilic phenotype despite guideline-based therapy, consider add-on therapy with one of the anti-interleukin (IL)-5 antibodies, mepolizumab, reslizumab, benralizumab, or anti-IL-4α receptor antibody dupilumab. Table 9 summarizes FDA-approved biologics for treatment of moderate to severe asthma.
- A decision tree for selecting initial biologic therapy and assessment of response for severe asthma are illustrated in Figs. 7 and 8.
- Bronchial thermoplasty is approved for use in selected adults with severe asthma that is not well controlled with inhaled glucocorticoids and LABAs.
- Potential alternative and experimental therapies include immunomodulatory therapy and macrolide antibiotics.[a]

---

[a]Recent trials (AMAZES) in patients who have symptomatic asthma despite inhaled maintenance therapy have shown that azithromycin 500 mg 3 times/wk reduced exacerbations and improved quality of life.

- In the future, treatments tailored to asthma phenotypes may improve asthma outcomes.[a] Treatment of status asthmaticus is as follows:
1. Oxygen generally started at 2 to 4 L/min by nasal cannula or Venti-Mask at 40% Fio_2; further adjustments are made according to oxygen saturations.
2. Bronchodilators: Initiate treatment with albuterol nebulizer solution (0.63 mg/3 ml, 1.25 mg/3 ml, 2.5 mg/3 ml, or 5.0 mg/ml): 2.5 to 5 mg every 20 min over the first h, then 2.5 to 10 mg every 1 to 4 h as needed or 10 to 15 mg/h continuously. Other useful medications are levalbuterol nebulizer solution (0.31 mg/3 ml, 0.63 mg/3 ml, 1.25 mg/3 ml) and ipratropium nebulizer solution (0.25/ml [0.025%]).
3. Corticosteroids:
   a. Early administration is advised, particularly in patients using steroids at home.
   b. Patients may be started on systemic corticosteroids; methylprednisolone, prednisone, or prednisolone may be used. Dose range is from 40 to 80 mg/day in one or two divided doses, generally given until peak expiratory flow reaches 70% of predicted value.
   c. Generally for corticosteroid courses <1 wk; there is no need to taper the dose.
   d. IV hydration: Judicious use is necessary to avoid heart failure in elderly patients. Aggressive IV hydration is not recommended.

   e. IV antibiotics are indicated when there is suspicion of bacterial infection (e.g., infiltrate on chest radiograph, fever, or leukocytosis).
   f. Intubation and mechanical ventilation are indicated when previous measures fail to produce significant improvement. Table 10 summarizes treatment of life-threatening asthma. Recommendations for initial ventilator setting and subsequent ventilator adjustments based on Pplat (end-respiratory plateau pressure) and arterial pH in patients with severe asthma exacerbation are illustrated in Fig. 9.
   g. Discharge home from the ED is appropriate if the FEV_1 or PEF after treatment is 70% or greater of the personal best or predicted value and if there is sustained improvement in lung function and symptoms for at least 1 h.

Asthma in the workplace[2]:
- Work-related asthma (WRA) encompasses *Occupational Asthma* (OA) defined as asthma caused by a specific agent at the workplace (Tables 11 to 13) and *Work-Exacerbated Asthma* (WEA), which is asthma exacerbated by, but not caused by, nonspecific stimuli in the workplace (Fig. 10).
- OA should be suspected in every adult with new-onset asthma. Although the respiratory symptoms are similar to those encountered in *Non-Work-Related Asthma* (NWRA), in OA their appearance and severity are usually modulated by work exposure. Characteristics of WRA compared with NWRA and OA are summarized in Table 14.
- Advantages and limitations of diagnostic tests for occupational asthma are summarized in Table 15.

REFERRAL

Box 5 describes indications for referral to an asthma specialist.

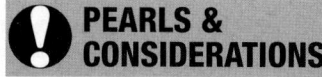

**PEARLS &
CONSIDERATIONS**

COMMENTS

- The differentiation of asthma from COPD can be challenging. A history of atopy and intermittent, reactive symptoms points toward a diagnosis of asthma, whereas smoking and advanced age are more indicative of COPD. Spirometry is useful in distinguishing asthma from COPD.
- In all asthma patients, it is important to treat or prevent comorbid conditions (e.g., rhinosinusitis, vocal cord dysfunction, gastroesophageal reflux disease). However, despite the presumed association between asthma and GERD, trials of PPIs in patients with poorly controlled asthma did not reveal any beneficial effects.
- According to the 2020 NAEPP guidelines, steps 3 and 4 had strong recommendations to use daily medium-dose ICS-formoterol not only as maintenance but also for as-needed therapy.
- Inhaled low-dose corticosteroids are the single most effective therapy for adult patients

TABLE 9 Summary of FDA-Approved Biologics for Treatment of Moderate to Severe Asthma

Biologic Agent	MOA	Patient Selection	Dosing	Notes
Omalizumab (Xolair) FDA approved in 2003	Humanized IgG1 antibody that binds to the Cε3 domain of free IgE and prevents it from binding to FcεR1	• Age ≥6 yr in the U.S. (≥12 yr in the U.K.) • IgE: 30-700 IU/ml • Allergic sensitization by skin prick or specific IgE testing	• 75-375 mg SC per IU every 2-4 wk based on age, weight, and IgE levels	• Highest efficacy in T2-high patients • Efficacy not based on IgE level or eosinophil count • Data from real-world studies demonstrate efficacy when dosed outside accepted weight and IgE levels • Indicated for *moderate to severe* allergic asthma
Mepolizumab (Nucala) FDA approved in 2015	Humanized IgG1 antibody that inhibits IL-5 from binding to the α-subunit of the IL-5 receptor complex on eosinophils	• ≥12 yr • Blood AEC of ≥150 cells/μL at the time of testing or ≥300 cells/μL in the previous yr • ≥300 cells/μL only in the U.K.	• 100 mg SC every 4 wk • 300 mg SC every 4 wk for EGPA	• Approved for home administration via the autoinjector • In clinic dosing using the lyophilized powder • Only biologic currently approved for EGPA • Demonstrated OCS-sparing effects • Indicated for severe eosinophilic asthma
Reslizumab (Cinqair) FDA approved in 2016	Humanized IgG4 antibody that inhibits IL-5 from binding to the α-subunit of the IL-5 receptor complex expressed on eosinophils	• Age ≥18 yr • Blood AEC ≥400 cells/μL in the previous yr	• 3 mg/kg IV infusion every 4 wk	• Response is better with higher eosinophil counts • No data on OCS-sparing effects; SC OCS dosing study was negative • Indicated for severe eosinophilic asthma
Benralizumab (Fasenra) FDA approved in 2017	Humanized recombinant IgG1 antibody that binds with high affinity to the α-subunit of the IL-5 receptor	• Age ≥12 yr • Blood AEC ≥300 cells/μL in the previous yr	• 30 mg SC every 4 wk for the first 3 doses then every 8 wk	• Available for prefilled autoinjector • Results in total depletion of eosinophils • Demonstrated OCS-sparing effects • Indicated for severe eosinophilic asthma
Dupilumab (Dupixent) FDA approved in 2018	Fully human monoclonal antibody to the α-unit of IL-4 receptor; blocks IL-4 and IL-13	• Age ≥12 yr • Moderate to severe asthma • Blood AEC ≥300 cells/μL in the previous yr • FeNO >25 ppb	• 200 mg or 300 mg SC every 2 wk after initial loading dose. No loading dose required for nasal polyps • 200 mg for moderate to severe persistent asthma, 300 mg for atopic dermatitis, nasal polyps and oral steroid-dependent asthma	• Home administration only • Antidrug antibody in 2%-5% patients • Indicated for nasal polyps, atopic dermatitis, and asthma (*moderate to severe* persistent eosinophilic asthma or oral steroid–dependent asthma regardless of T2 markers) • Demonstrated OCS-sparing effects • Exercise caution in patients with baseline eosinophils >1500 cells/μL due to transient elevation of eosinophils for 4 mo after initiation of therapy
Tezepelumab (Tezspire) FDA approved 2021	Human monoclonal antibody anti-TSLP that binds to TSLP	• Adults and children aged 12 yr and older • Severe asthma not controlled by their current asthma regimen	• Administer by subcutaneous injection • Recommended dosage is 210 mg administered once every 4 wk	• Is not available currently for home administration. • Most common adverse reactions (incidence ≥3%) are pharyngitis, arthralgia, and back pain.

AEC, Absolute eosinophil count; *EGPA,* eosinophilic granulomatosis with polyangiitis; *FDA,* Food and Drug Administration; *FeNO,* fraction of exhaled nitric oxide; *Ig,* immunoglobulin; *IL,* interleukin; *IU,* international units; *IV,* intravenous; *OCS,* oral corticosteroid; *SC,* subcutaneous.
From Broaddus VC et al: *Murray & Nadel's textbook of respiratory medicine,* ed 7, Philadelphia, 2022, Elsevier.

with asthma who require more than an occasional use of SABAs to control their asthma.
• Stepping down inhaled corticosteroids after asthma is well controlled has level A evidence.
• Leukotriene modifiers/receptor agonists represent a reasonable alternative in adults unable or unwilling to use corticosteroids; however, these agents are less effective than monotherapy with inhaled corticosteroids.
• Use of LABAs alone without use of a long-term asthma maintenance medication, such as an inhaled corticosteroid, is contraindicated. LABAs should also not be used in patients whose asthma is adequately controlled on low- or medium-dose inhaled corticosteroids. Continued use of LABAs may cause down-regulation of the beta-2 receptor with loss of the bronchoprotective effect from rescue therapy with a SABA.
• Patients who remain symptomatic despite inhaled corticosteroids benefit from the addition of LABAs. Trials in patients with poorly controlled asthma despite the use of inhaled glucocorticoids and LABAs have shown that the addition of tiotropium, a long-acting anticholinergic bronchodilator approved for treatment of COPD, increased the time to the first severe exacerbation and provided modest sustained bronchodilation.
• Therapy with systemic corticosteroids accelerates the resolution of acute asthma and reduces the risk of relapse. There is no evidence that doses >50 to 100 mg prednisone equivalent are beneficial.
• In patients with allergies and elevated serum immunoglobulin (Ig) E levels, use of anti-IgE therapy is beneficial.
• Bronchial thermoplasty may be considered in select patients with severe persistent asthma with recurrent exacerbations or ED visits.
• Biologic modifiers of the Th2 immune pathways (neutralizing monoclonal antibodies, receptor antagonists, soluble receptors) as well as epithelial-derived cytokines are potential options for the development of new treatments of severe asthma. Adjunct therapies for bronchospasm are summarized in Table 16.
• The response to treatment for asthma is characterized by wide individual variability. A functional glucocorticoid-induced transcript 1 gene *(GLCCI1)* variant is associated with substantial decrements in the response to inhaled glucocorticoids in patients with asthma. Another potential cause of the variability in response to treatment is heterogeneity in the role of IL-13 expression in the clinical asthma phenotype. Patients with asthma who have a certain biochemical signature are more likely to respond to an anti-IL-13 monoclonal antibody than those without such a signature. Identification of genetic variants can eventually lead to

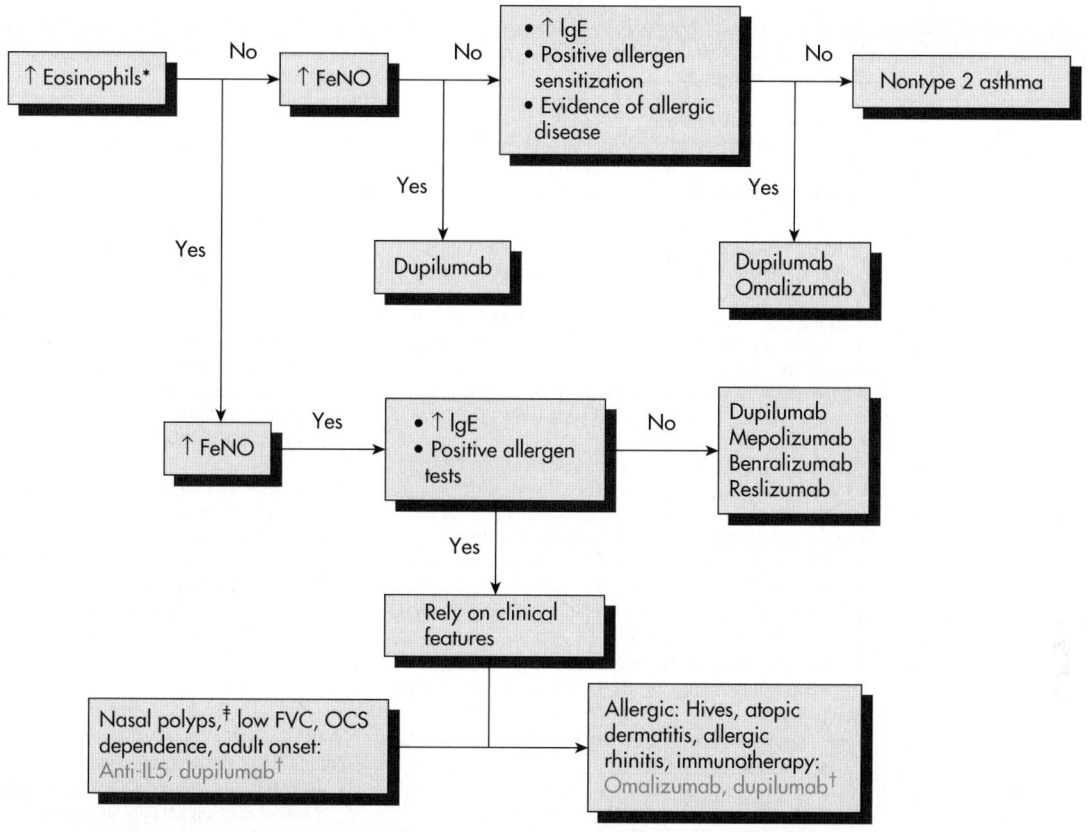

FIG. 7 Decision tree for selecting initial biologic therapy for severe asthma in patients with type 2 features. This algorithm is guided by high-quality evidence from clinical trials and supporting data. Medications are listed alphabetically, not in order of preference. Patients should have regular assessment of clinical benefit, and treatment should be adjusted until asthma control is achieved. *Increased eosinophils is defined by blood eosinophil counts >150-300/μL. Dupilumab should not be used for patients with >1500 eosinophils/μL. †At the time of publication, dupilumab is also FDA approved for use in nasal polyps and atopic dermatitis. Omalizumab is also FDA approved for use in chronic urticaria. ‡Nasal polyps predict an enhanced response to these T2 biologics when targeting asthma. The efficacy of each biologic for nasal polyps may differ. *FDA,* U.S. Food and Drug Administration; *FeNO,* fraction of exhaled nitric oxide; *FVC,* forced vital capacity; *IgE,* immunoglobulin E; *OCS,* oral corticosteroid. (From Broaddus VC et al: *Murray & Nadel's textbook of respiratory medicine,* ed 7, Philadelphia, 2022, Elsevier.)

Management based on response

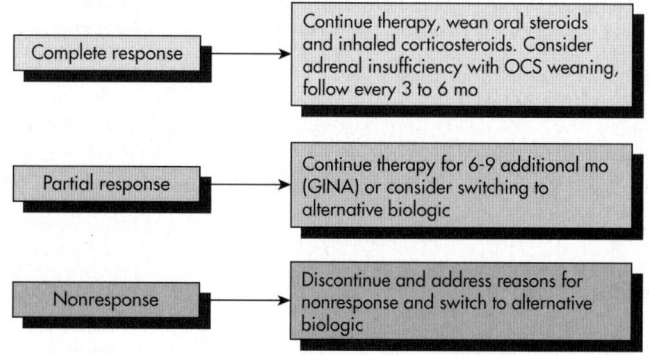

Consistently assess and document response markers: Asthma control, medication use, exacerbations, and biomarkers in all patients.

FIG. 8 Assessing response to biologic therapy. Before initiating biologic therapy, choose markers of response that will be monitored (e.g., exacerbations, oral corticosteroid use, asthma control, lung function, rescue bronchodilator use, patient comfort, and satisfaction). Most patients will experience at least a partial response to biologic therapy, 10%-15% will have no response, and a small proportion will have a complete response. Assess response continuously and adjust asthma medications and/or biologics based on response. *GINA,* Global Initiative for Asthma; *OCS,* oral corticosteroids. (From Broaddus VC et al: *Murray & Nadel's textbook of respiratory medicine,* ed 7, Philadelphia, 2022, Elsevier.)

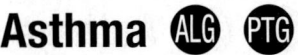

TABLE 10	Summary of Treatment for Life-Threatening Asthma	
Treatment	**Dose and Frequency**	**Comments**
Oxygen	1-3 L/min by nasal cannula Goal is to maintain oxygen saturation (Spo_2) >92% Use heated cascade humidifier to avoid dry air–induced bronchoconstriction	Transient drop in O_2 tension with beta-adrenergic therapy Avoid hyperoxia (may be associated with hypercarbia)
Bronchodilators		
Beta$_2$-selective agonists: Albuterol or salbutamol, levalbuterol	*Albuterol:* 2.5-5 mg (0.5-1 ml of 0.5% solution in 5 ml of normal* saline) by nebulizer every 20 min for 3 doses total (for optimal delivery, dilute aerosols to a minimum of 3 ml at gas flow of 6-8 L/min), followed by 2.5-10 mg q1-4h as needed, or 10-15 mg/h continuously; titration based on response and severity of symptoms *Albuterol MDI,* delivered with a spacer (each spacer dose takes 1-2 min; 90 μg/puff), 4-8 puffs every 20 min for 4 h, then q4h as needed *Albuterol:* 5-7.5 mg by jet nebulizer (each treatment takes 15-20 min) *Levalbuterol* (0.63 mg/3 ml and 1.25 mg/3 ml nebulizer): 1.25-2.5 mg every 20 min for 3 doses total, then 1.25-5 mg q1-4h as needed, or 5-7.5 mg/h continuous nebulization *Levalbuterol MDI* (45 μg/puff): 4-8 puffs every 20 min for 4 h, followed by q1-4h as needed	Beta$_2$-selective agonists are the cornerstone of therapy Continuous nebulization used for a majority of severely ill patients In study of continuous vs. intermittent therapy in severe exacerbations (excluding life-threatening asthma), no difference noted in pulmonary function improvement or need for hospitalization Lower frequency of side effects with continuous treatment Watch for hypokalemia, tremors, tachycardia, and lactic acidosis Oral or parenteral route: Loss of beta$_2$-selectivity MDI: 4 puffs of albuterol (0.36 mg) = 2.5 mg of albuterol nebulization Levalbuterol 0.63 mg = racemic albuterol 1.25 mg for efficacy and side effects *Intubated patients:* Nebulizers are less efficient in delivering doses to lower airways (6%-10%) than MDIs (11%)
Epinephrine	*Subcutaneous epinephrine* dose for adults: 0.3-0.5 ml of a 1:1000 dilution (1 mg/ml), depending on age and weight; repeat every 20 min for 3 doses total	
Terbutaline	*Subcutaneous terbutaline:* 0.25 mg; repeat every 20 min for 3 doses total	Terbutaline is the parenteral agent of choice in pregnancy For refractory life-threatening asthma: Intravenous epinephrine (high risk for cardiac events, infarction, and arrhythmias) or racemic epinephrine may be considered
Anticholinergics		
Ipratropium (for acute severe asthma warranting visit to emergency department)	*Ipratropium bromide:* 0.5 mg by nebulizer (0.25 mg/ml) every 20 min for 3 doses, then q2-4h as needed *Ipratropium MDI* (0.018 mg/puff): 4-8 puffs per treatment every 20 min for up to 3 h *Combinations:* Albuterol (2.5 mg/3 ml) + ipratropium (0.5 mg/3 ml): 3 ml every 20 min for 3 doses total, then as needed MDI delivering albuterol 90 μg + ipratropium 18 μg: 8 puffs every 20 min for up to 3 h	Ipratropium: Onset of action is slow (20 min), peak effectiveness at 60-90 min, no systemic side effects, improved lung function and reduced recovery time Use a handheld mouthpiece nebulizer (contamination of the ocular area with precipitation of narrow-angle glaucoma may occur if facemask is used for delivery of anticholinergic agent) Ipratropium may be combined with nebulized albuterol dose in the emergency room; no proven benefit shown in hospitalized patients
Corticosteroids: Prednisone, prednisolone, methylprednisolone	40-80 mg/day in 1 or 2 divided doses until peak expiratory flow reaches 70% of predicted or personal best FEV$_1$ or PEFR <50% Methylprednisolone 40 mg IV q6h or Hydrocortisone 200 mg IV	No advantage of higher doses No advantage of IV therapy over oral if absorption and gut transit are not impaired Total steroid course: 3-10 days, <1 wk; no need to taper steroids Inhaled steroids can be started at any time
Heliox	Helium-oxygen mixture (80-20 or 70-30) Routine use cannot be recommended at this time	Improves O_2 and aerosolized medication delivery to distal lung Decreases flow turbulence and resistance Lower gas density facilitates exhalation, reduces air trapping and intrinsic PEEP Improves pulmonary function in subgroup of patients with most severe airflow obstruction
Magnesium sulfate	2 g IV given over 20 min; may repeat Monitor magnesium levels Avoid in renal insufficiency	Bronchodilation from inhibition of the calcium channel and decreased acetylcholine release IV and inhaled or nebulized magnesium sulfate improves pulmonary function in acute severe asthma IV magnesium widely used as adjunct therapy

FEV$_1$, Forced expiratory flow in 1 second; *IV,* intravenous; *MDI,* metered-dose inhaler; *PEEP,* positive end-expiratory pressure; *PEFR,* peak expiratory flow rate.

From Parrillo JE, Dellinger RP: *Critical care medicine, principles of diagnosis and management in the adult,* ed 4, Philadelphia, 2014, Elsevier.

Diseases
and Disorders

I

INITIAL SETTINGS

Tidal volume (V_T)	7–8 mL/kg
Respiratory rate	12–14/min
Inspiratory flow rate	60 L/min
FiO_2	1.0
PEEP	0–5 cm H_2O

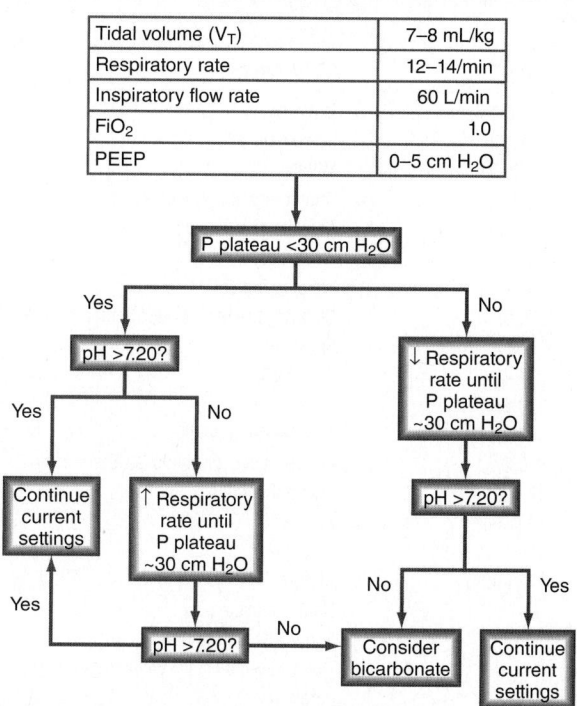

FIG. 9 Recommendations for initial ventilator settings and subsequent ventilator adjustments based on Pplat (end-inspiratory plateau pressure) and arterial pH in patients with severe asthma exacerbation. (From Vincent JL et al: *Textbook of critical care,* ed 8, Philadelphia, 2024, Elsevier.)

TABLE 11 Principal Agents Causing Occupational Asthma

Agent		Occupation or Industry
High-Molecular-Weight Agents		
Cereals, flour	Wheat, rye, barley, buckwheat	Flour mills, bakers, pastry makers
Latex	Proteins from the *Hevea* tree	Health care workers, laboratory technicians
Animals	Mice, rats, cows, seafood	Laboratory workers, farmers, seafood processing
Enzymes	α-Amylase, maxatase, alcalase, papain, bromelain, pancreatin	Baking product production, bakers, detergent production, pharmaceutical industry, food industry
Low-Molecular-Weight Agents		
Isocyanates	Toluene diisocyanate, methylene diphenyldiisocyanate, hexamethylene diisocyanate	Polyurethane production, plastic industry, insulation, molding, spray painting
Metals	Chromium, nickel, cobalt, platinum	Metal refinery, metal alloy production, electroplating, welding
Biocides	Formaldehyde, glutaraldehyde, quaternary ammonium compounds	Health care workers, cleaners
Persulfate salts	Hair bleach	Hairdressers
Acrylates	Cyanoacrylates, methacrylates, diacrylates, and triacrylates	Adhesives, dental and orthopedic materials, sculptured fingernails, printing inks, paints and coatings
Acid anhydrides	Phthalic, trimellitic, maleic, tetrachlorophthalic anhydrides	Epoxy resin workers
Reactive dyes	Reactive black 5, pyrazolone derivatives, vinyl sulfones, carmine	Textile workers, food industry workers
Woods	Red cedar, iroko, obeche, oak, and others	Sawmill workers, carpenters, cabinet and furniture makers

From Broaddus VC et al: *Murray & Nadel's textbook of respiratory medicine,* ed 7, Philadelphia, 2022, Elsevier.

TABLE 12 Frequency of Agents Causing Sensitizer-Induced Occupational Asthma According to a Large European Multicenter Study

HMW Agents	n (%)*	LMW Agents	n (%)*
Flour/grains	369 (31.3)	Isocyanates	206 (17.4)
Latex	36 (3.0)	Persulfate salts	78 (6.6)
Enzymes	26 (2.2)	Metals	42 (3.6)
Storage mites	12 (1.0)	Quaternary ammonium compounds	38 (3.2)
Rodents	11 (0.9)	Acrylate compounds	35 (3.0)
Cow dander	11 (0.9)	Wood dusts	35 (3.0)
Fish and seafood	8 (0.7)	Welding fumes	30 (2.5)
Insects and derived products	6 (0.5)	Cleaning products or disinfectants (NOS)	27 (2.3)
Ornamental plants	6 (0.5)	Epoxy resins	18 (1.5)
Molds	5 (0.4)	Aldehydes	17 (1.4)
Soybean flour	3 (0.2)	Drugs	16 (1.4)
Spices	3 (0.2)	Metalworking fluids	15 (1.3)
Vegetable gums	3 (0.2)	Resins, glues, or paints (NOS)	15 (1.3)
Various plant-derived products	26 (2.2)	Acid anhydrides	11 (0.9)
Various animals and derived products	18 (1.5)	Amines	10 (0.8)
		Colophony	4 (0.3)
Total:	543 (46.5)	Styrene	3 (0.2)
		Reactive dyes	2 (0.2)
		Triglycidyl isocyanurate	2 (0.2)
		Other low-molecular-weight agents (NOS)	21 (17.8)
		Total:	624 (52.9)

*Percentage of total identified agents ($n = 1167$); the causal agent was not precisely identified in 13 subjects.
HMW, High molecular weight; *LMW*, low molecular weight; *NOS*, not otherwise specified.
From Vandenplas O et al: Are high-and low-molecular-weight sensitizing agents associated with different clinical phenotypes of occupational asthma? *Allergy* 74:261-272, 2019.

TABLE 13 Potential Risk Factors for Occupational Asthma

Risk Factor	Evidence	Agents or Settings
Environmental Factors		
High level of exposure	Strong	HMW agents
	Moderate	LMW agents: Platinum salts, acid anhydrides, isocyanates
Cigarette smoking	Moderate	For IgE sensitization: Laboratory animals, snow crab, prawn, salmon, psyllium, green coffee, enzymes, acid anhydrides, platinum, reactive dyes
	Weak	For clinical OA: Laboratory animals, enzymes
Skin exposure	Weak	Isocyanates
Host-Related Factors		
Atopy	Strong	HMW agents
	Weak	LMW agents: Platinum, acid anhydrides
Genetic markers:		
HLA class II alleles	Moderate	LMW agents: Isocyanates, red cedar, acid anhydrides, platinum salts
		HMW agents: Laboratory animals, latex
Antioxidant enzymes*	Moderate	Isocyanates
SNPs of alpha-T catenin	Moderate	Isocyanates
TLR4 polymorphisms	Weak	Laboratory animals
IL-4 receptor alpha and IL-13 polymorphisms	Weak	Isocyanates
Preexisting nonspecific bronchial hyperresponsiveness	Moderate	HMW agents: Laboratory animals, flour, latex
Work-related rhinitis	Strong	Laboratory animals
Sex (female)	Weak	Snow crab processors

*Glutathione-*S*-transferase and *N*-acetyltransferase.
HLA, Human leukocyte antigen; *HMW*, high molecular weight; *IgE*, immunoglobulin E; *IL*, interleukin; *LMW*, low molecular weight; *OA*, occupational asthma; *SNPs*, single nucleotide polymorphisms, *TLR4*, Toll-like receptor-4.
From Broaddus VC et al: *Murray & Nadel's textbook of respiratory medicine*, ed 7, Philadelphia, 2022, Elsevier.

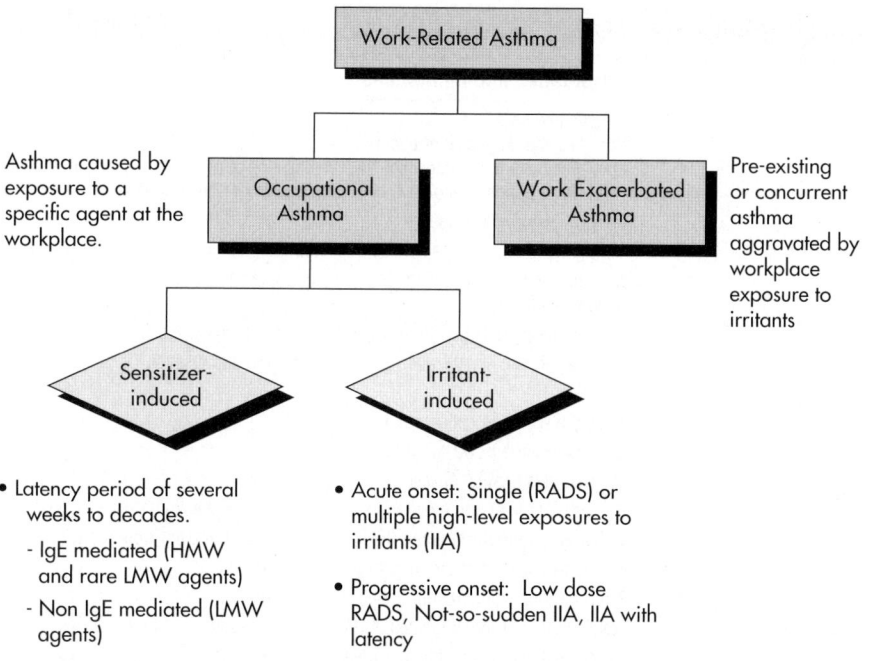

FIG. 10 Categorization of work-related asthma into subsets based on the cause and timing of the asthma. *HMW,* High molecular weight; *IgE,* immunoglobulin E; *IIA,* irritant-induced (occupational) asthma; *LMW,* low molecular weight; *RADS,* reactive airway dysfunction syndrome. (From Broaddus VC et al: *Murray & Nadel's textbook of respiratory medicine,* ed 7, Philadelphia, 2022, Elsevier.)

TABLE 14   Characteristics of Work-Exacerbated Asthma Compared with Non–Work-Related Asthma and Occupational Asthma

Characteristics	Compared with Adults with Non–Work-Related Asthma	Compared with Adults with Occupational Asthma
Sex	Similar,[3,4] or predominance of men in subjects with WEA[5]	Similar,[5] or greater number of women in subjects with WEA[8]
Age	Older[3,4]	Similar or younger[8]
Race	More nonwhite[3]	More nonwhite[8]
Education	Less[3]	N/A
Smoking habits	More likely to have smoked cigarettes[3]	More smokers[5]
Asthma severity	More asthma exacerbations requiring ED visits or hospitalizations in workers with WEA[5] More days with asthma symptoms, more severe asthma based on self-report[3]	Same number of asthma exacerbations requiring ED visits or hospitalizations[9] Greater need of ICS in subjects with WEA[9]
Functional characteristics	Similar FEV$_1$, PC$_{20}$[5]	Less PEF variability when at work in subjects with WEA compared with OA[10] PC$_{20}$ may be lower in subjects with WEA[11]
Airway inflammation	Neutrophilic inflammation inconsistently found depending on the study[6,7]	Less likely to have eosinophilic airway inflammation[7,9]

ED, Emergency department; *FEV$_1$,* forced expiratory volume in 1 second; *ICS,* inhaled glucocorticoids; *N/A,* not applicable; *OA,* occupational asthma; *PC$_{20}$,* provocative concentration of methacholine; *PEF,* peak expiratory flow; *WEA,* work-exacerbated asthma.
From Broaddus VC et al: *Murray & Nadel's textbook of respiratory medicine,* ed 7, Philadelphia, 2022, Elsevier.

TABLE 15 Advantages and Limitations of Diagnostic Tests for Occupational Asthma

Diagnostic Tests	Advantages and Limitations
Assessment of nonspecific bronchial hyperresponsiveness	Simple, low cost Confirms the diagnosis of asthma Low specificity for diagnosis of OA. The absence of airway hyperresponsiveness does not exclude the diagnosis of OA in patients who have been removed from the workplace
Immunologic tests	Easy to perform, low cost Commercial extracts are available (skin prick tests or specific IgE for HMW agents) Measurement of specific IgE available for some LMW agents (anhydrides, acids, isocyanates, aldehydes) but low sensitivity Lack of standardization for most occupational allergens except for latex Can identify the sensitization but not necessarily the disease
PEF monitoring	Low cost Requires workers' collaboration Low adherence ($<60\%$) Possible falsification of results Requires 2 wk at and away from work (not always possible) Impossible to perform when the worker has been removed from work No standardized method for interpreting the results Interpretation of the results requires experience
Specific inhalation challenges in the laboratory	Confirmation of the diagnosis of OA when test result is positive False-negative test results are possible Costly Available in only a few centers worldwide
Specific inhalation challenges at the workplace	Exclude diagnosis if negative when performed in the usual work conditions Require usual work conditions Costly
Noninvasive measures of airway inflammation	Sputum cell counts • Impossible to falsify • Bring additional evidence to the diagnosis of OA • Costly • Not widely available • Does not allow confirmation or exclusion of the diagnosis of OA by itself Exhaled NO • Easy to perform • Inconsistent results • Difficult to interpret • Affected by many different factors

HMW, High molecular weight; *IgE*, immunoglobulin E; *LMW*, low molecular weight; *NO*, nitric oxide; *OA*, occupational asthma; *PEF*, peak expiratory flow.
From Broaddus VC et al: *Murray & Nadel's textbook of respiratory medicine*, ed 7, Philadelphia, 2022, Elsevier.

BOX 5 Possible Indications for Referral to an Asthma Specialist

- Severe, acute asthma that has caused loss of consciousness, hypoxia, respiratory failure, convulsions, or near death
- Poorly controlled asthma as indicated by admission to a hospital, frequent need for emergency care, need for oral corticosteroids, absence from school or work, disruption of sleep, interference with quality of life
- Severe, persistent asthma requiring step 4 care (consider for patients who require step 3 care)
- Patient <3 yr who requires step 3 or 4 care (consider for patient <3 yr who requires step 2 care)
- Requirement for continuous oral corticosteroids or high-dose inhaled corticosteroids or more than two short courses of oral corticosteroids within 1 yr
- Need for additional diagnostic testing such as allergy skin testing, rhinoscopy, provocative challenge, complete pulmonary function testing, bronchoscopy
- Consideration for immunotherapy
- Need for additional education regarding asthma, complications of asthma and treatment of asthma, problems with adherence to management recommendations, or allergen avoidance
- Uncertainty of diagnosis
- Complications of asthma, including sinusitis, nasal polyposis, aspergillosis, severe rhinitis, vocal cord dysfunction, gastroesophageal reflux

Modified from National Asthma Education and Prevention Program, National Heart, Lung, and Blood Institute: *Expert panel report 2: guidelines for the diagnosis and management of asthma*, Bethesda, MD, 1997, National Institutes of Health, NIH publication No 97-4051.

A

TABLE 16 Adjunct Therapies for Bronchospasm

Nontraditional Therapy for Severe Bronchospasm	Comments
Intravenous beta₂-agonists	No data show any benefit in adding IV agent to nebulization Avoid IV isoproterenol owing to danger of myocardial toxicity
Oral or IV leukotriene receptor antagonists (LTRAs): Montelukast 10 mg oral daily, zafirlukast	Rapid bronchodilation in impending respiratory failure Improves pulmonary function within 10 min Oral LTRAs can be added as an adjunct in severe asthma
Noninvasive positive-pressure ventilation (NPPV)	NPPV reduces the need for endotracheal intubation in severe asthma exacerbation
Inhaled nitric oxide (NO) (adding 15 ppm to the inspiratory circuit)	Rapid improvement in ventilated patients with asthma refractory to medical treatment
Omalizumab (anti-IgE antibody)	Role in acute asthma is unstudied Improves asthma control in allergic asthmatics
General anesthetic agents: Isoflurane or halothane anesthesia IV thiopental, IV propofol, IV ketamine	Propofol relaxes the smooth muscles in arteries and veins and has bronchodilator effect
Plasma exchange (during pregnancy) Pumpless extracorporeal carbon dioxide removal Extracorporeal life support (ECLS)	Case reports of adjunct therapies; used as salvage therapy for life-threatening asthma
Glucagon	Rapid smooth muscle relaxant, short half-life; small study report
Nebulized DNase (dornase 2.5 mg via tracheal tube)	Case report of use in pregnant patient with rapid improvement
Bronchial lavage	Anecdotal reports: Exacerbates auto-PEEP, decreases oxygenation

IgE, Immunoglobulin E; *IV,* intravenous; *PEEP,* positive end-expiratory pressure.
From Parrillo JE, Dellinger RP: *Critical care medicine, principles of diagnosis and management in the adult,* ed 4, Philadelphia, 2014, Elsevier.

TABLE 17 Asthma Biomarkers and Associated Phenotypes as Predictors of Response to Specific Therapies

Biomarker	Asthma Phenotype	Predicts
Elevated exhaled nitric oxide (>50 ppb in adults, >35 ppb in children)	T2-high	Response to inhaled steroids
Sputum eosinophils >3%	T2-high	Response to inhaled steroids
Peripheral blood eosinophils (>0.3 × 10⁹/L or 300/µL)	T2-high	Response to anti-IL-5 therapy
Elevated total IgE >30 IU	Allergic/T2	Response to omalizumab
Allergy skin tests and elevated specific IgE	Allergic/T2	Response to immunotherapy, omalizumab
Lack of elevated peripheral and sputum eosinophils and low FeNO	T2-low	Response to tiotropium and macrolides (likely to be poor responders to steroids)

FeNO, Fraction of exhaled nitric oxide; *IgE,* immunoglobulin E; *T2,* type 2.
From Broaddus VC et al: *Murray & Nadel's textbook of respiratory medicine,* ed 7, Philadelphia 2022, Elsevier.

personalized asthma treatment. Asthma biomarkers and associated phenotypes as predictors of response to specific therapies are summarized in Table 17. Failure of pharmacologic treatment is often due to uncontrolled comorbid conditions (tobacco, allergic rhinitis, pollutants), poor inhaler technique, or lack of adherence to prescribed medication.

RELATED CONTENT

Asthma (Patient Information)
Asthma-COPD Overlap Syndrome (Related Key Topic)

AUTHORS: **LAREN TAN, MD, MBA,** and **DERRICK CLELAND, DO, MPH**

REFERENCES & SUGGESTED READINGS
Available at eBooks.Health.Elsevier.com.

BASIC INFORMATION

DEFINITION

Astrocytomas are neuroepithelial tumors arising from glial precursor cells called astrocytes. The distinction of different grades of astrocytoma provides important clinical prognostic information (Table 1). According to the World Health Organization (WHO) classification astrocytoma is classified as follows based on the histopathology:

- Grade I: Pilocytic astrocytoma
- Grade II: Diffuse astrocytoma
- Grade III: Anaplastic astrocytoma
- Grade IV: Glioblastoma
- Grades III and IV are considered high-grade astrocytomas or malignant

As per new WHO classification, glioblastoma (IDH wild type, CNS WHO grade 4) and astrocytoma (IDH mutant, CNS WHO grade 4) are considered two separate entities.

SYNONYM

Astroglial neoplasms

ICD-10CM CODE
C71.9 Malignant neoplasm of brain, unspecified

EPIDEMIOLOGY & DEMOGRAPHICS

- In 2022, there were an estimated 25,050 new cases and 18,280 deaths due to primary central nervous system (CNS) tumors in the U.S.,[1] of which astrocytomas constituted approximately 10% of cases according to the Central Brain Tumor Registry of the United States (CBTRUS).
- The incidence of primary CNS tumor is 6.4 cases per 100,000 persons per yr with age-adjusted death rate of 4.4 per 100,000 population, of which about 50% cases are that of glioblastoma.

PHYSICAL FINDINGS & CLINICAL PRESENTATION

- The presenting symptoms of astrocytoma partly depend on its location and rate of growth.
- Astrocytomas classically present with any one or more of the following features:
  1. Headache (not frequent) are associated with mass effect
  2. New-onset partial or generalized seizures (<50%)
  3. Nausea and vomiting, fatigue, weakness
  4. Focal neurologic deficit (cranial nerve palsy, hemiplegia, ataxia, visual loss, language alteration, etc.)
  5. Change in mood, memory, or mental status
  6. Papilledema (rare)

ETIOLOGY

- No agents have been definitively implicated in the causation of CNS tumors though risk factors can be identified in some patients. Farmers and petrochemical workers have a higher incidence of primary brain tumors, and CNS exposure to ionizing radiation is a known risk factor.
- Different hereditary syndromes are associated with increased risk and high frequency of astrocytoma.
  1. Neurofibromatosis type 1 is associated with increased frequency of astrocytoma.
  2. Inherited syndromes such as Lynch syndrome and Li-Fraumeni syndrome are associated with an increased frequency of malignant gliomas.

Gene and chromosomal alterations in astrocytoma:

- Alteration in p53, a tumor suppressor encoded by the *TP53* gene on chromosome 17p, plays a key role in the development of at least one third of all grades of astrocytoma. In high-grade astrocytomas, p53 function may be deregulated by alteration of other genes, including amplification of MDM2 or MDM4 and 9p deletions that result in loss of the p14 product of the *CDKN2A* gene.[2]
- Mutations of isocitrate dehydrogenase 1 gene *(IDH1)* occur in a large fraction of grade II and grade III astrocytomas as well as in other gliomas. IDH-mutated tumors have a *better* prognosis compared to IDH-wild type tumors.
- Gliomas can be defined into five molecular groups with the use of three alterations: Mutations in the *TERT* promoter, mutations in *IDH*, and codeletion of chromosome arms 1p and 19q (1p/19q codeletion).[3]

DIAGNOSIS

A provisional diagnosis of astrocytoma is made on clinical grounds and radiographic imaging studies. Tissue pathology is needed to establish the diagnosis and to grade the astrocytoma.

DIFFERENTIAL DIAGNOSIS

The differential diagnosis is vast and includes any cause of headache, seizures, change in mental status, and focal neurologic deficits.

WORKUP

- The imaging modality of choice is contrast-enhanced MRI, which can demonstrate anatomy and pathologic process in detail. Computed tomography (CT) scanning is reserved for patients who are unable or unwilling to get MRI. Biopsy with histologic confirmation is required to establish a diagnosis of astrocytoma.
- Stereotactic biopsy under CT or MRI guidance is reserved for tumors that are deeply seated, multicentric tumors, or diffuse nonfocal tumors where surgical resection is not practical. Major objectives of surgical resection are to maximally remove the tumor bulk, reduce tumor-associated mass effect and elevated intracranial pressure, and to provide tissue for pathologic analysis. Surgical resection is carried out in a manner that minimizes the risk to neurologic functioning. Surgery can also rapidly reduce the tumor bulk with potential benefits in terms of mass effect, edema, and hydrocephalus.

LABORATORY TESTS

- CBC
- Complete chemistry panel
- Coagulation testing (prothrombin time, partial thromboplastin time)

IMAGING STUDIES

MRI (Fig. 1) is the diagnostic imaging study of choice. MRI with contrast and magnetic resonance angiography are used to locate the margins of the tumor, distinguish vascular masses from tumors, and provide clear views of the posterior fossa. If MRI of the brain is contraindicated, head CT with contrast is the next best imaging, though low-grade astrocytoma may not be seen on CT scan.

TREATMENT

ACUTE GENERAL Rx

- Corticosteroids reduce cerebral edema and thus minimize secondary brain injury from cerebral retraction. Usually, dexamethasone

TABLE 1 Comparison of Astrocytoma Histopathology

	Pilocytic Astrocytoma	Diffuse Astrocytoma	Anaplastic Astrocytoma	Glioblastoma Multiforme
Malignant potential	Benign	Low grade	High grade	Very malignant
Age (approximate)	Children	Third or fourth decade	Fifth decade	Sixth decade
Location	Optic chiasm or hypothalamus > cerebellum > brainstem*	Hemispheres (cortex + white matter)	Hemispheres (cortex + white matter)	Hemispheres (cortex + white matter)
Enhancement	Mild	Mild	Moderate (ring)	Intense
Vasogenic edema	Minimal	Minimal	Moderate	Significant
Calcification	Common	Up to 20%	Occasional	Rare

*It is typically cystic with a mural nodule and located within the posterior fossa—it tends to be solid or lobulated when seen elsewhere.

From Grant LA et al: *Grainger & Allison's diagnostic radiology essentials*, ed 2, Philadelphia, 2019, Elsevier.

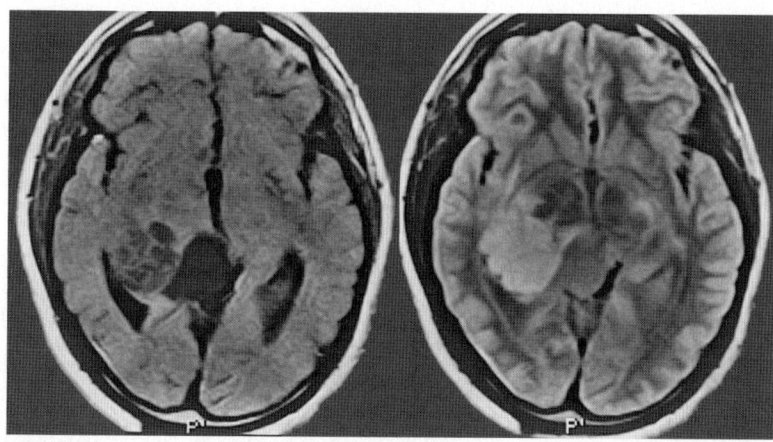

FIG. 1 Magnetic resonance image of a low-grade astrocytoma, demonstrating a hypointense right temporal lesion without contrast enhancement on T1 and hyperintense signal on T2. (From Goetz CG, Pappert EJ: *Textbook of clinical neurology*, Philadelphia, 1999, Saunders.)

is started immediately preoperatively in all primary CNS tumors (unless CNS lymphoma is suspected) and continued in the immediate postoperative period with tapering as quickly as possible.

- If there is increased intracranial pressure and impending herniation, patient should be started on intravenous (IV) mannitol, and mechanical ventilation with hyperventilation should be considered if there is depressed consciousness.
- The use of preoperative prophylactic anticonvulsants is less commonly indicated though the current practice patterns indicate widespread use of levetiracetam or phenytoin.

STAGE-SPECIFIC Rx

- Maximal surgical resection of the tumor, when feasible, is the mainstay of management of astrocytomas. Postoperative adjuvant radiotherapy and chemotherapy approaches are individualized based on pathologic and molecular characteristics of the tumor.
- Grade I astrocytomas are usually indolent, circumscribed tumors. Complete surgical resection is curative for these tumors. If complete surgical resection is not feasible due to tumor location (e.g., tumor in optic pathway, hypothalamus, and in deep midline structures), then asymptomatic patients can be observed in these cases until maximally safe resection is feasible upon progression. Unfortunately, despite aggressive near-total resection, delayed recurrence and eventual malignant transformation are common.
- In grade II astrocytoma, the extent of postoperative residual disease after maximal tumor resection is an important variable for time to first relapse. Postoperative chemotherapy (PCV regimen or temozolomide) concurrent with radiotherapy improves progression-free survival and overall survival. Watchful waiting is also an option. Newer IDH inhibitors (vorasidenib) are available for IDH mutant astrocytoma.[4]
- In grade III anaplastic astrocytoma, surgical resection followed by postoperative chemotherapy and radiotherapy is routinely used. Recent randomized clinical trials have

established a survival benefit with the use of concurrent chemotherapy (temozolomide or nitrosoureas).

- In grade IV glioblastoma, maximal surgical resection improves median survival. Concurrent temozolomide chemotherapy with radiotherapy followed temozolomide chemotherapy is recommended for patients whose tumors are MGMT-methylated and are less than 70 yr of age.[5] MGMT-unmethylated tumors have a worse prognosis and less benefit from temozolomide. For older individuals with poor performance status unable to tolerate combination therapy, short-course radiation or single-agent temozolomide is also an option.
- In the case of both recurrent and newly diagnosed glioblastoma, the use of tumor-treatment fields devices in conjunction with the use of temozolomide chemotherapy has demonstrated a survival benefit and is approved by the FDA.[6]

TREATMENT OF RECURRENT DISEASE

- For grade 1 astrocytoma, re-resection should be considered. For patients who have tumors that are not amenable to resection, chemotherapy or radiotherapy can improve recurrence-free survival, although the role of chemotherapy in adults remain controversial.
- For grade 2 astrocytoma, radiation therapy can be considered in the relapsed setting if not given in the adjuvant setting. Data on use of chemotherapy in low-grade gliomas in adults is sparse. Although the results are encouraging, the number of patients treated in these studies is small and there were many methodologic flaws in the studies. For recurrent grade III anaplastic astrocytoma treated with radiation therapy in the past, there is a role for chemotherapy. Nitrosoureas-based regimen and temozolomide have shown efficacy in this setting.
- The combination of irinotecan with bevacizumab or bevacizumab alone has been studied, and median survival is similar with either approach.

- Various targeted therapies are currently being studied in patients with recurrent glioblastoma. The combination of dabrafenib plus trametinib (BRAF and MEK inhibitors) has demonstrated clinical activity in patients with BRAF^{V600E}-mutation–positive recurrent or refractory high-grade glioma and low-grade glioma and was approved by the FDA in this setting.[7]
- Immune checkpoint inhibitors have been evaluated in the recurrent setting, and randomized studies have not shown any survival benefits compared to bevacizumab therapy. However, certain subsets of patients with recurrent glioblastoma multiforme (GBM) have demonstrated survival benefits when used in neoadjuvant approach or in hypermutated tumors.
- Autologous tumor lysate-loaded dendritic cell vaccine (DCVax-L) has been evaluated in addition to standard of care and resulted in statistically significant extension of survival for both newly diagnosed and recurrent GBM patients.[8] Chimeric antigen T-cells (CAR-T) directed against different antigens are being evaluated in patients with recurrent glioma.
- Low-intensity alternating electric fields are also being used for the treatment of recurrent glioblastoma.

PROGNOSIS

- Grade 1 astrocytoma has a good prognosis and is usually cured with surgical resection.
- Grade 2 astrocytoma has a median survival of about 7.5 yr with treatment.
- Grade 3 anaplastic astrocytoma has a median survival of approximately 5 yr. Patients with tumors that have IDH-mutation and 1p/19q co-deletion have superior survival compared with patients without deletion.
- Median survival of glioblastoma is approximately 14 mo. Primary glioblastomas are IDH-wild type and account for 90% of cases. Grade 4 astrocytomas, in contrast, are IDH-mutated, have typically evolved from low-grade gliomas, and have a much more protracted natural course than the primary cases.

REFERRAL

A multidisciplinary consultation with a neurosurgeon, radiation oncologist, and neurooncologist is required to assist in the diagnostic workup and to provide immediate and follow-up treatment.

RELATED CONTENT

Astrocytoma (Patient Information)
Brain Cancer (Patient Information)
Brain Neoplasm, Benign (Related Key Topic)
Brain Neoplasm, Glioblastoma (Related Key Topic)

REFERENCES
Available at eBooks.Health.Elsevier.com.

AUTHOR: **JOSEPH EDMUND, MD**

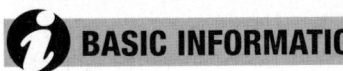

BASIC INFORMATION

DEFINITION

Atelectasis describes collapse of part or all of the lung with resultant volume loss. There are two major types of atelectasis.[1]

- Obstructive atelectasis: Most common and results from a blocked airway (e.g., mucous plug or tumor-obstructing airway) with resorption of the gas in the alveoli distal to the area of obstruction.
- Nonobstructive atelectasis: May result from several nonobstructive etiologies, including external compression from outside the lung (e.g., pleural effusion), abnormalities in surfactant leading to increased tendency for part of the lung to collapse, reduction in size of part of the lung due to scarring, and decreased ventilation of a portion of the lung.

ICD-10CM CODE
J98.11   Atelectasis

EPIDEMIOLOGY & DEMOGRAPHICS

- Postoperative patients and patients with lung or chest wall injury are at increased risk of atelectasis.
- Asbestos exposure increases risk for an entity called "rounded atelectasis."
- Occurs frequently in patients receiving mechanical ventilation.
- No known racial or sexual predilection for atelectasis.
- Dependent regions of the lung are more prone to atelectasis.

PHYSICAL FINDINGS & CLINICAL PRESENTATION

- Patient may be asymptomatic or may have cough, dyspnea, and decrease in oxygen saturations.
- Physical examination may disclose decreased or absent breath sounds over affected area, with dullness to percussion, decreased fremitus, and decreased vocal resonance.

ETIOLOGY

- Airway obstruction (e.g., endobronchial tumor, a lymph node, foreign bodies, mucous plug)
- Extrinsic bronchial compression (e.g., neoplasms, aneurysms of ascending aorta, enlarged left atrium)
- Pleural disease (e.g., pleural effusion, mesothelioma, rounded atelectasis, pneumothorax)
- Alveolar injury (e.g., toxic fumes, aspiration of gastric contents, infections, acute respiratory distress syndrome)
- Chest wall abnormalities (e.g., trauma, scoliosis, rib fracture, obesity)
- Impaired respiratory mechanics or decreased cough response (e.g., pain, postanesthetic effect, abdominal distention, neuromuscular disease)
- Trauma caused by shear force generated by repetitive expansion and collapse during positive-pressure ventilation (e.g., mechanical ventilation)

- Characteristic rounded atelectasis may be associated with prior asbestos exposure
- Table 1 summarizes anatomic causes of atelectasis

DIAGNOSIS

DIFFERENTIAL DIAGNOSIS

- Neoplasm
- Pneumonia
- Pleural effusion, pulmonary infarction
- Abnormalities of brachiocephalic vein and the left pulmonary ligament

WORKUP

- Chest x-ray (Fig. 1)
- Thoracic ultrasonography
- Chest computed tomography (CT) scan (prone positioning CT scan with improvement or reduction in atelectasis) may be used to differentiate from other etiology
- Bronchoscopy (in select patients) to assess for endobronchial obstruction

IMAGING STUDIES

- Chest x-ray often suggests the diagnosis.
- Ultrasonography helps differentiate atelectasis from effusion or consolidation.
- Chest CT scan is useful in patients with suspected endobronchial neoplasm or extrinsic bronchial compression. Prone images help differentiate true consolidation from dependent atelectasis.

TREATMENT

NONPHARMACOLOGIC THERAPY

- Deep breathing
- Mobilization of the patient: Encouraging out of bed in upright position, ambulation
- Incentive spirometry
- Tracheal suctioning in select patients (e.g., mechanical ventilation and tracheostomy)
- Mechanical airway clearance therapies for improving cough and clearance of secretions from airways:
  1. Positive expiratory pressure (PEP) devices (e.g., Acapella, Aerobika, TheraPEP)
  2. Cough assist devices

3. Chest physiotherapy with vest therapy, frequencer, or chest wall percussion
- Bronchoscopy might be helpful with mucous plug aspiration, removal of foreign body, or evaluation for endobronchial and peribronchial lesions

ACUTE GENERAL Rx

- Oxygen if indicated
- Positive-pressure breathing (continuous positive airway pressure by face mask, positive end-expiratory pressure for patients on mechanical ventilation)
- Use of mucolytic agents (e.g., acetylcysteine) or hypertonic saline if due to mucous plugging
- Bronchodilator therapy in selected patients
- Pain control in postoperative and trauma cases to facilitate deeper breathing
- Pleural drainage in cases of large effusions, hemothorax, or empyema

Prevention and treatment of postoperative atelectasis is illustrated in Fig. 2. Perioperative interventions including continuous positive end-expiratory pressure (PEEP) intraoperatively, noninvasive pressure support ventilation following extubation, and early implementation of physical therapy have been shown to reduce the incidence of postoperative atelectasis after thoracic surgery.[2]

CHRONIC Rx

- Guide therapy depending on the underlying etiology because some chronic atelectasis may not warrant treatment.
- Consider role of airway clearance therapies (e.g., flutter valve) and incentive spirometry.
- If significant endobronchial obstruction, may need to consider debulking of obstruction or possible placement of bronchial stent.
- If external compression (e.g., pleural effusion or mass) is leading to the atelectasis, then need to drain or remove the contributing source of the compression.

DISPOSITION

Prognosis varies with the underlying etiology.

REFERRAL

- If indicated, referral to pulmonary or interventional pulmonology (1) for bronchoscopy

TABLE 1   Anatomic Causes of Atelectasis

Cause	Clinical Examples
External compression on the pulmonary parenchyma	Pleural effusion, pneumothorax, intrathoracic tumors, diaphragmatic hernia
Endobronchial obstruction completely obstructing the ingress of air	Enlarged lymph node, tumor, cardiac enlargement, foreign body, mucoid plug, broncholithiasis
Intraluminal obstruction of a bronchus	Foreign body, asthma, granulomatous tissue, tumor, secretions including mucous plugs, bronchiectasis, pulmonary abscess, chronic bronchitis, acute laryngotracheobronchitis, plastic bronchitis
Intrabronchiolar obstruction	Bronchiolitis, interstitial pneumonitis, asthma
Respiratory compromise or paralysis	Neuromuscular abnormalities, osseous deformities, overly restrictive casts and surgical dressings, defective movement of the diaphragm, or restriction of respiratory effort

From Kliegman RM: *Nelson textbook of pediatrics,* ed 21, Philadelphia, 2020, Elsevier.

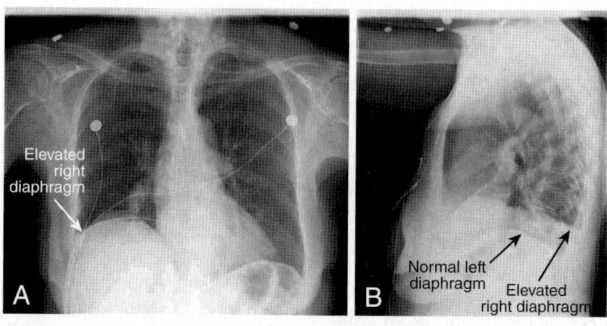

FIG. 1 Atelectasis with elevated diaphragm: An example of volume loss. The right hemidiaphragm in this patient appears elevated on both the posterior-anterior **(A)** and the lateral **(B)** views. Is this the correct interpretation of the x-ray, and if so, what is the cause? Consider the alternative interpretations. A subpulmonic pleural effusion would appear similar, as it would have the same density as liver, heart, and diaphragm and would layer over the diaphragm with the patient upright. This appears less likely in that a meniscus might be seen along the lateral chest wall with a pleural effusion but is not present here. In addition, a pleural effusion occupies space and might be expected to push the heart to the left, whereas in this case the heart may be slightly deviated to the right. Atelectasis of the lower right lung would result in volume loss, pulling the heart and hemidiaphragm into the space normally occupied by the lung. This is consistent with the observed features. An infiltrate in this location could explain the x-ray findings but appears less likely for similar reasons to those cited for effusion. Some simple maneuvers could narrow the differential diagnosis. Chest ultrasound, decubitus x-ray views, or CT could identify an effusion. (From Broder JS: *Diagnostic imaging for the emergency physician,* Philadelphia, 2011, Saunders.)

to evaluate for obstructing lesion as etiology for atelectasis, (2) for possible removal of foreign body, (3) to debulk or remove endobronchial tumor, or (4) to place endobronchial stent.

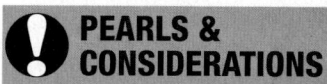 **PEARLS & CONSIDERATIONS**

COMMENTS

- Atelectasis after surgery and in most clinical presentations is most commonly benign. Patients should be educated that ambulation and frequent changes of position are helpful to reopen collapsed segments of lung. Sitting the patient upright in a chair is recommended to increase both volume and vital capacity relative to the supine position. Adequate pain control and early mobilization are paramount after surgical intervention or rib fractures.
- Additional diagnostic evaluation is indicated when clinical suspicion for bronchial obstruction or pleural disease.

RELATED CONTENT

Atelectasis (Patient Information)

REFERENCES

Available at eBooks.Health.Elsevier.com.

AUTHOR: **LORRIANA E. LEARD, MD**

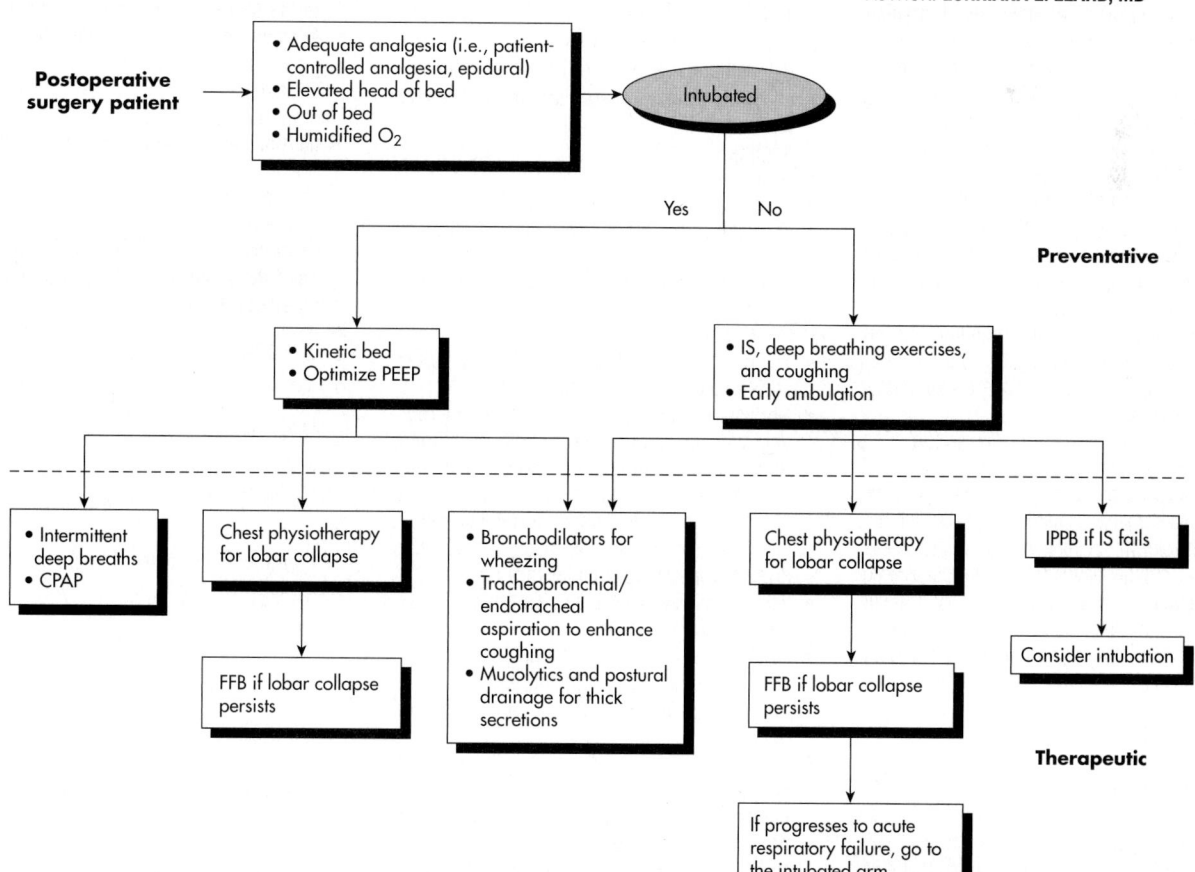

FIG. 2 Prevention and treatment algorithm for postoperative atelectasis. *CPAP,* Continuous positive airway pressure; *FFB,* flexible fiberoptic bronchoscopy; *IPPB,* intermittent positive-pressure breathing; *IS,* incentive spirometry; *PEEP,* positive end-expiratory pressure. (From Newman M et al: *Perioperative medicine,* ed 2, Philadelphia, 2022, Elsevier.)

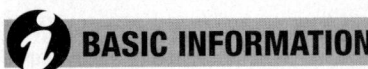 BASIC INFORMATION

DEFINITION

Atrial fibrillation (AF) is a supraventricular tachyarrhythmia characterized by disorganized and rapid atrial activation and uncoordinated atrial contraction. AF occurs when structural and/or electrophysiologic abnormalities alter atrial tissue to promote abnormal impulse formation and/or propagation. The ventricular rate is dependent on the conduction properties of the atrioventricular (AV) node, which can be influenced by vagal/sympathetic tone, medications, or disease of the AV node.

Multiple classification schemes have been used in the past to characterize AF. The current classification scheme (divided into three major types) used by the American College of Cardiology (ACC)/American Heart Association (AHA) guideline committee is as follows:

- Paroxysmal AF: More than one episode of AF that terminate spontaneously or with intervention within 7 days
- Persistent AF: Episodes of AF that last longer than 7 days
  1. Early-persistent AF: AF that has been continuous for longer than 7 days but fewer than 3 mo
  2. Long-standing persistent AF: AF that has persisted for longer than 1 yr, either because cardioversion has failed or because cardioversion has not been attempted
- Permanent AF: When patient and physician decide to stop pursuing restoring sinus rhythm
- In addition to the previous AF categories, which are mainly defined by episode timing and termination, the ACC/AHA/European Society of Cardiology (ESC) guidelines describe additional AF categories in terms of other characteristics of the patient:
  1. Lone atrial fibrillation (LAF): Generally refers to AF in younger patients without clinical or echocardiographic evidence of cardiopulmonary disease, diabetes, or hypertension
  2. Nonvalvular AF: Atrial fibrillation in the absence of moderate-to-severe mitral stenosis or in the presence of a mechanical heart valve
  3. Secondary AF: Occurs in the setting of a primary condition that may be the cause of the AF, such as acute myocardial infarction, cardiac surgery, pericarditis, myocarditis, hyperthyroidism, pulmonary embolism, pneumonia, or other acute disease. It is considered separately because AF is less likely to recur once the precipitating condition has resolved
  4. Silent AF: Asymptomatic AF diagnosed by an ECG or rhythm strip

SYNONYMS

AF
Paroxysmal atrial fibrillation (PAF)
AFib

ICD-10CM CODES
I48.0	Paroxysmal atrial fibrillation
I48.1	Persistent atrial fibrillation
I48.2	Chronic atrial fibrillation
I48.91	Unspecified atrial fibrillation

EPIDEMIOLOGY & DEMOGRAPHICS

- The prevalence of AF increases with age, from 2% in adults <65 to 9% of those >65 yr old.
- AF affects over 3 million people in the United States. AF is uncommon in infants and children and, when present, almost always occurs in association with structural heart disease.
- The incidence of AF is significantly higher in men than in women in all age groups (1.1% versus 0.8%). AF appears to be more common in whites than in blacks, who may have lower awareness of the disease.
- Stroke due to thromboembolism is the most common and dreaded complication of AF. The rate of ischemic stroke in patients with nonrheumatic AF averages 5% a yr, which is somewhere between 2 and 7× the rate of stroke in patients without AF. The risk of stroke is not due solely to AF; changes in the endothelium and elevated markers of inflammation that may contribute to thrombosis are found in patients with AF, regardless of their rhythm at the time. The attributable risk of stroke from AF is estimated to be 1.5% for those aged 50 to 59 yr, and it approaches 36% for those aged 80 to 89 yr.
- Table 1 summarizes the thromboembolic risk score.

PHYSICAL FINDINGS & CLINICAL PRESENTATION

Clinical presentation is variable:

- Palpitations, dizziness, or light-headedness
- Fatigue, weakness, or impaired exercise tolerance
- Angina
- Dyspnea
- Some patients are asymptomatic
- Cardiac auscultation revealing irregularly irregular rhythm
- Thromboembolic phenomenon such as stroke

ETIOLOGY

- The most frequent change in AF is the loss of atrial muscle mass and atrial fibrosis
- Fibrillation is presumed to be caused by multiple wandering wavelets, usually originating from the pulmonary veins. Both reentrant and focal mechanisms have been proposed. See Fig. 1 for mechanisms of atrial fibrillation. Fig. 2 illustrates an approach to selecting drug therapy for ventricular rate control
- Vascular causes: Hypertensive heart disease
- Valvular heart disease
- Pulmonary causes: Pulmonary embolism, chronic obstructive pulmonary disease, obstructive sleep apnea, carbon monoxide poisoning
- Structural cardiac disease: Hypertrophic cardiomyopathy, congestive heart failure, coronary artery disease, myocardial infarction, congenital heart disease (especially those that lead to atrial enlargement such as atrial septal defect)
- Pericarditis and myocarditis
- Arrhythmias: Atrial tachycardias and atrial flutters have been associated with atrial

fibrillation, as has Wolff-Parkinson-White syndrome
- Endocrine: Thyrotoxicosis, hyperthyroidism or subclinical hyperthyroidism, pheochromocytoma, obesity
- Surgery: Both cardiac and noncardiac
- Electrolytes: Hypokalemia, hypomagnesemia
- Systemic stress: Fever, anemia, hypoxia, sepsis, infections (e.g., pneumonia)
- Medications/toxins: Digitalis, adenosine, theophylline, amphetamines, cocaine, antihistamines, alcohol abuse and/or withdrawal, caffeine, steroidal antiinflammatory drugs (SAIDs), nonsteroidal antiinflammatory drugs (NSAIDs), Marine omega-3 fatty acids[1]
- Frequency of vigorous exercise is associated with an increased risk of developing AF in young men and joggers
- Porphyrias have been associated with autonomic dysfunction and increased risk of AF
- Patients with metabolic syndrome, excessive vitamin D intake, or excessive niacin intake have a higher risk of AF

Dx DIAGNOSIS

DIFFERENTIAL DIAGNOSIS

- Multifocal atrial tachycardia
- Atrial flutter
- Frequent atrial premature beats
- Atrial tachycardia
- AV nodal reentry tachycardia (AVNRT)
- Wolff-Parkinson-White syndrome

WORKUP

The evaluation of atrial fibrillation involves diagnosis, determination of the etiology, and

---

TABLE 1 CHA_2DS_2-VASc Score and Associated Increased Annual Risk for Stroke

C	Congestive heart failure	1
H	Hypertension	1
A	Age >75 yr	1
D	Diabetes	1
S	Stroke, TIA	2
V	Vascular disease	1
A	Age 65-74 yr	1
Sc	Sex (female)	1
Total score	Annual risk of stroke	
0	0.2%	
1	0.6%	
2	2.2%	
3	3.2%	
4	4.8%	
5	7.2%	
6	9.7%	
7	11.2%	
8	10.8%	
9	12.2%	

TIA, Transient ischemic attack.
From Warshaw G et al: *Ham's primary care geriatrics,* ed 7, Philadelphia, 2022, Elsevier.

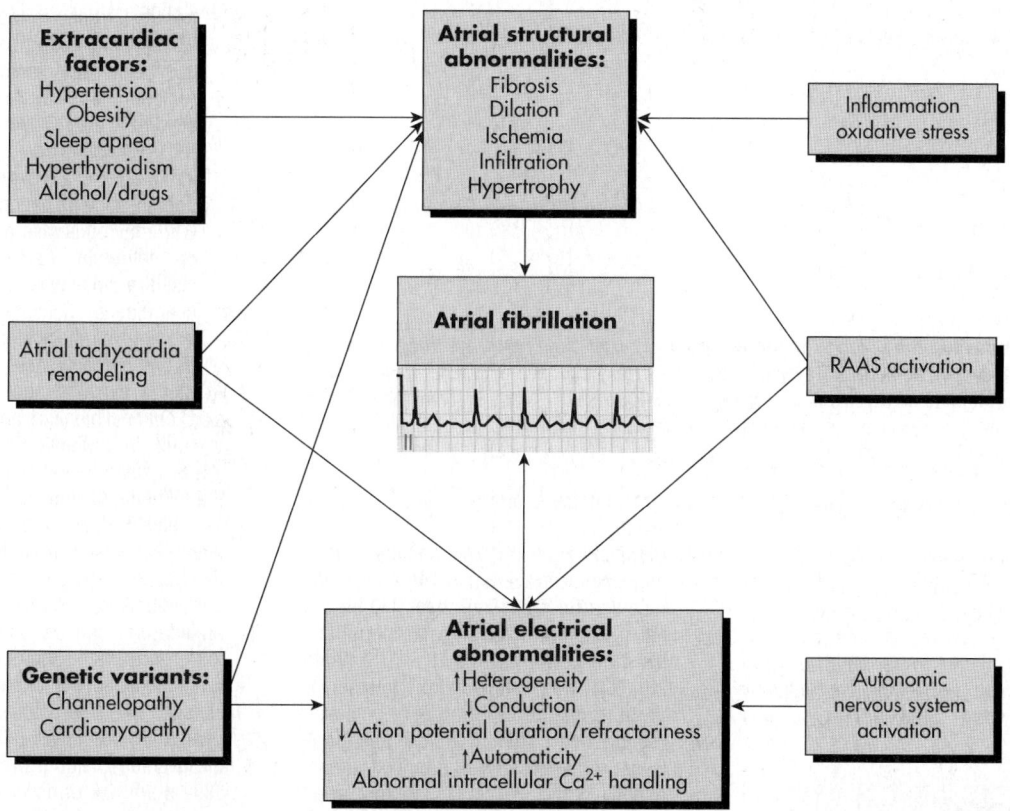

FIG. 1 Mechanisms of atrial fibrillation. Ca^{2+}, Ionized calcium; *RAAS*, renin-angiotensin-aldosterone system. (From Parrillo JE, Dellinger RP: *Critical care medicine, principles of diagnosis and management in the adult,* ed 5, Philadelphia, 2019, Elsevier.)

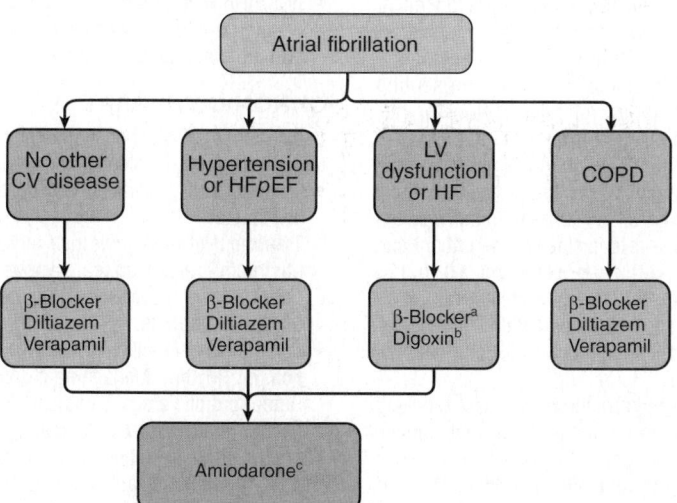

FIG. 2 Approach to selecting drug therapy for ventricular rate control. Drugs are listed alphabetically. **(A)** β-Blockers should be instituted after stabilization of patients with decompensated heart failure (HF). The choice of β-blocker (e.g., cardioselective) depends on the patient's clinical condition. **(B)** Digoxin is not usually first-line therapy. It may be combined with a β-blocker and/or a nondihydropyridine calcium channel blocker when ventricular rate control is insufficient and may be useful in patients with heart failure. **(C)** In part because of concern over its side effect profile, use of amiodarone for chronic control of ventricular rate should be reserved for patients who do not respond to or are intolerant of β-blockers or nondihydropyridine calcium antagonists. *COPD,* Chronic obstructive pulmonary disease; *CV,* cardiovascular; *HF,* heart failure; *HFpEF,* heart failure with preserved ejection fraction; *LV,* left ventricular. (From Parrillo JE, Dellinger RP: *Critical care medicine, principles of diagnosis and management in the adult,* ed 5, Philadelphia, 2019, Elsevier.)

classification of the arrhythmia. A minimal evaluation includes a history and physical examination, ECG, transthoracic echocardiogram, and case-specific laboratory work to rule out secondary AF.

LABORATORY TESTS
- Thyroid-stimulating hormone, free T_4
- Serum electrolytes
- Toxicity screen
- CBC count (looking for anemia, infection)
- Renal and hepatic function tests
- D-Dimer/CT scan of chest pulmonary embolism protocol (if the patient has risk factors to merit a pulmonary embolism workup)

IMAGING STUDIES
- ECG (Fig. E3)
- Absence of P waves
- Fibrillatory or F waves at the isoelectric baseline with varying amplitude, morphology, and intervals (Fig. 4)
- Irregular ventricular rate
- Echocardiography to rule out structural heart disease (evaluate ventricular size, thickness, and function, atrial size, pericardial disease, and valve function)
- Chest radiography (if pulmonary disease or congestive heart failure [CHF] is suspected)
- Transesophageal echocardiography (TEE): Helpful to evaluate for left atrial thrombus (particularly in the left atrium appendage) to guide cardioversion or ablation (if thrombus is seen, cardioversion should be delayed)
- CT and MRI: In patients with a positive D-dimer result, chest CT angiogram may be necessary to rule out pulmonary embolus. 3D imaging technologies (CT scan or MRI) are often helpful to evaluate atrial anatomy if AF ablation is planned
- 6-min walk test or exercise test: 6-min walk or exercise testing can help assess the adequacy of rate control. Exercise testing can also exclude ischemia prior to treatment of patients with class Ic antiarrhythmic drugs

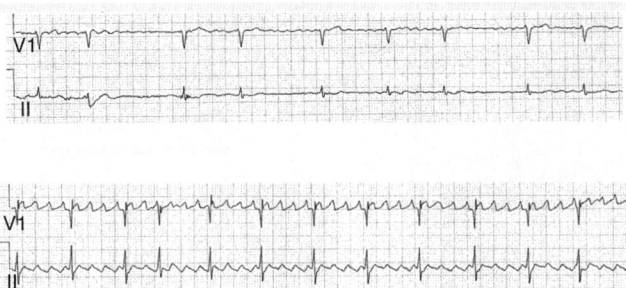

FIG. 4 Comparison between the F waves of atrial fibrillation *(top panel)* **and the flutter waves of atrial flutter** *(bottom panel)*. Note that F waves are variable in rate, shape, and amplitude, whereas flutter waves are constant in rate and all aspects of morphology. Shown are leads V1 and II. (From Libby P et al: *Braunwald's heart disease, a textbook of cardiovascular medicine*, ed 12, Philadelphia, 2022, Elsevier.)

and can be used to reproduce exercise-induced AF
- Sleep study (if sleep apnea is suspected)
- Holter monitor or event recorder if the diagnosis of AF is in question and to assess AF burden
- Electrophysiologic study: When initiation of AF is secondary to a supraventricular tachycardia, such as AVNRT or Wolff-Parkinson-White syndrome

Rx TREATMENT

ACUTE GENERAL Rx

New-onset AF:
- If the patient is hemodynamically unstable (hypotension, congestive heart failure, or angina), perform synchronized cardioversion after immediate conscious sedation with a rapid short-acting sedative (e.g., midazolam). The ACC/AHA recommendations for cardioversion of atrial fibrillation are summarized in Table 2. The likelihood of cardioversion-related clinical thromboembolism is low in patients with AF lasting <48 h. Patients with AF lasting >2 days have a 5% to 7% risk for clinical thromboembolism if cardioversion is not preceded by several weeks of anticoagulation therapy. However, if transesophageal echocardiography reveals no atrial thrombus, cardioversion may be performed safely after therapeutic anticoagulation has been achieved. Alternatively, patients can be safely anticoagulated for approximately 1 mo and then undergo cardioversion without transesophageal echocardiogram. Anticoagulant therapy should be continued for at least 1 mo after cardioversion to minimize the incidence of adverse thromboembolic events. It can be stopped after 1 mo as long as AF has not recurred if the patient is deemed low risk of stroke using the congestive heart failure, hypertension, age, diabetes, stroke/TIA, and vascular disease (CHA_2DS_2-VASc) scoring system (see Table 1).
- If the patient is hemodynamically stable, a rate-control strategy is typically pursued initially. ACC/AHA recommendations for pharmacologic rate control of atrial fibrillation are summarized in Table 3.

- Treatment options for rate control include the following:
1. Diltiazem 0.25 mg/kg (maximum of 25 mg) given intravenously (IV) over 2 min followed by a second dose of 0.35 mg/kg (maximum of 25 mg) 15 min later if the rate is not slowed to <100 beats/min. May then follow with IV infusion 10 mg/h (range, 5 to 15 mg/h) to achieve a resting heart rate of <100 beats/min. Onset of action after IV administration is usually within 3 min, with peak effect most often occurring within 10 min. After the ventricular rate is slowed, the patient can be changed to oral diltiazem 60 to 90 mg q4 to 6h. High doses of calcium channel blockers can exacerbate heart failure and thus should be used with caution in patients presenting with symptoms of heart failure or depressed ejection fraction.
2. Verapamil 2.5 to 5 mg IV initially, then 5 to 10 mg IV 10 min later if the rate is still not slowed to <100 beats/min. After the ventricular rate is slowed, the patient can be changed to oral verapamil 80 to 120 mg q6 to 8h. The main concern is hypotension and heart failure with this medication, and it should not be used in patients with CHF.
3. Esmolol and metoprolol are beta-blockers available in IV preparations that can be used. High doses of beta-blockers can have negative inotropic effects in heart failure and should be used with caution.
4. Digoxin is not a potent AV nodal blocking agent and has a potential for toxicity and therefore cannot be relied on for acute control of the ventricular response, but it may be used in conjunction with beta-blockers and calcium channel blockers. It may be a useful adjunct to a beta-blocker in the hypotensive or heart failure patient, which is not infrequent. When used, give 0.5 mg IV loading dose (slow) and then 0.25 mg IV 6 h later. A third dose may be needed after 6 to 8 h; the daily dose varies from 0.125 to 0.25 mg (decrease dosage in patients with renal insufficiency and elderly patients) depending on the heart rate and signs or symptoms of digoxin

toxicity. Toxicity is manifested by GI and visual complaints, atrial tachyarrhythmias, heart block, and ventricular tachycardia.
5. Amiodarone has a class IIa recommendation from the ACC/AHA/ESC for use as a rate-controlling agent for patients who are intolerant of or unresponsive to other agents, such as patients with heart failure who may otherwise not tolerate diltiazem or metoprolol. Caution should be exercised in those who are not receiving anticoagulation because amiodarone can promote cardioversion, thereby posing a thromboembolic risk.
- AV nodal blocking agents, particularly calcium channel blockers and digoxin, should be avoided in patients with Wolff-Parkinson-White syndrome and AF because, by blocking the AV node, AF impulses may be transmitted exclusively down the accessory pathway, which can result in ventricular fibrillation. If this happens, the patient will require immediate defibrillation. Procainamide, flecainide, or amiodarone can be used instead if Wolff-Parkinson-White syndrome is suspected.
- In the acute setting, pharmacologic cardioversion (e.g., ibutilide, dofetilide) is less commonly used than electrical cardioversion. A major disadvantage with pharmacologic cardioversion is the risk of development of ventricular tachycardia and other serious arrhythmias, especially due to acute prolongation of the QT interval.
- ACC/AHA recommendations for maintenance of sinus rhythm in patients with atrial fibrillation are summarized in Table 4.

CHRONIC THERAPY
- Avoidance of alcohol in patients with suspected excessive alcohol use.
- Treatment of underlying source or cause, if any found.
- Treatment of modifiable risk factors such as obstructive sleep apnea, hypertension, and obesity have been shown to decrease AF burden in patients.
- Per the Atrial Fibrillation Follow-up Investigation of Rhythm Management (AFFIRM) and Rate Control versus Electrical Cardioversion (RACE) trials, either rate control or rhythm control strategies show no difference in composite cardiovascular end points of death, CHF, bleeding, drug side effects, or thromboembolism. However, the more recent Early Treatment of Atrial Fibrillation for Stroke Prevention Trial (EAST-AFNET 4 trial) suggested that an initial rhythm control strategy may result in lower risk of the combined cardiovascular endpoint of death, stroke, or hospitalization. Both approaches require appropriate anticoagulation to reduce stroke risk.
- For patients without symptomatic AF, a rate-control strategy with calcium channel blockers, beta-blockers, or digoxin may be a reasonable option. The RACE 2 trial indicates that a lenient rate control strategy, with a target resting heart rate of <110 beats/min, is noninferior to a strict control strategy, with a target resting heart rate of

TABLE 2 ACC/AHA Recommendations for Cardioversion of Atrial Fibrillation

Class	Indication	Level of Evidence
Pharmacologic Cardioversion		
Class I (indicated)	Administration of flecainide, dofetilide, propafenone, or ibutilide is recommended for pharmacologic cardioversion of AF.	A
Class IIa (reasonable)	Administration of amiodarone is a reasonable option for pharmacologic cardioversion of AF.	A
	A single oral bolus dose of propafenone or flecainide ("pill-in-the-pocket") can be administered to terminate persistent AF outside the hospital once treatment has proved safe in the hospital for selected patients without sinus or AV node dysfunction, bundle branch block, QT interval prolongation, the Brugada syndrome, or structural heart disease. Before antiarrhythmic medication is initiated, a beta-blocker or nondihydropyridine calcium channel antagonist should be given to prevent rapid AV conduction in the event atrial flutter occurs.	C
	Administration of amiodarone can be beneficial on an outpatient basis in patients with paroxysmal or persistent AF when rapid restoration of sinus rhythm is not deemed necessary.	C
Class IIb (may be considered)	Administration of quinidine or procainamide might be considered for pharmacologic cardioversion of AF, but the usefulness of these agents is not well established.	C
Class III (not indicated)	Digoxin and sotalol may be harmful when used for pharmacologic cardioversion of AF and are not recommended.	A
	Quinidine, procainamide, disopyramide, and dofetilide should not be started out of the hospital for conversion of AF to sinus rhythm.	B
Direct-Current Cardioversion		
Class I (indicated)	When a rapid ventricular response does not respond promptly to pharmacologic measures for patients with AF with ongoing myocardial ischemia, symptomatic hypotension, angina, or heart failure, immediate R wave–synchronized direct-current cardioversion is recommended.	C
	Immediate direct-current cardioversion is recommended for patients with AF involving preexcitation when very rapid tachycardia or hemodynamic instability occurs.	B
	Cardioversion is recommended in patients without hemodynamic instability when symptoms of AF are unacceptable to the patient. In case of early relapse of AF after cardioversion, repeated direct-current cardioversion attempts may be made after administration of antiarrhythmic medication.	C
Class IIa (reasonable)	Direct-current cardioversion can be useful to restore sinus rhythm as part of a long-term management strategy for patients with AF.	B
	The patient's preference is a reasonable consideration in the selection of infrequently repeated cardioversions for the management of symptomatic or recurrent AF.	C
Class III (not indicated)	Frequent repetition of direct-current cardioversion is not recommended for patients who have relatively short periods of sinus rhythm between relapses of AF after multiple cardioversion procedures despite prophylactic antiarrhythmic drug therapy.	C
	Electrical cardioversion is contraindicated in patients with digitalis toxicity or hypokalemia.	C
Pharmacologic Enhancement of Direct-Current Cardioversion		
Class IIa (reasonable)	Pretreatment with amiodarone, flecainide, ibutilide, propafenone, or sotalol can be useful to enhance the success of direct-current cardioversion and to prevent recurrent AF.	B
	In patients who relapse to AF after successful cardioversion, it can be useful to repeat the procedure after prophylactic administration of antiarrhythmic medication.	C
Class IIb (may be considered)	For patients with persistent AF, administration of beta-blockers, disopyramide, diltiazem, dofetilide, procainamide, or verapamil may be considered, although the efficacy of these agents to enhance the success of direct-current cardioversion or to prevent early recurrence of AF is uncertain.	C
	Out-of-hospital initiation of antiarrhythmic medications may be considered in patients without heart disease to enhance the success of cardioversion of AF.	C
	Out-of-hospital administration of antiarrhythmic medications may be considered to enhance the success of cardioversion of AF in patients with certain forms of heart disease once the safety of the drug has been verified for the patient.	C
Prevention of Thromboembolism in Patients With Atrial Fibrillation Undergoing Cardioversion		
Class I (indicated)	For patients with AF of 48-h duration or longer, or when the duration of AF is unknown, anticoagulation (INR, 2.0-3.0) is recommended for at least 3 wk before and 4 wk after cardioversion, regardless of the method (electrical or pharmacologic) used to restore sinus rhythm.	B
	For patients with AF of more than 48-h duration requiring immediate cardioversion because of hemodynamic instability, heparin should be administered concurrently (unless contraindicated) by an initial intravenous bolus injection, followed by a continuous infusion in a dose adjusted to prolong the activated partial thromboplastin time to 1.5-2× the reference control value. Thereafter, oral anticoagulation (INR, 2.0-3.0) should be provided for at least 4 wk, as for patients undergoing elective cardioversion. Limited data support subcutaneous administration of low-molecular-weight heparin in this indication.	C
	For patients with AF of less than 48-h duration associated with hemodynamic instability (angina pectoris, myocardial infarction, shock, or pulmonary edema), cardioversion should be performed immediately, without delay, for prior initiation of anticoagulation.	C
Class IIa (reasonable)	During the 48 h after onset of AF, the need for anticoagulation before and after cardioversion may be based on the patient's risk of thromboembolism.	C
	As an alternative to anticoagulation before cardioversion of AF, it is reasonable to perform transesophageal echocardiography in search of thrombus in the left atrium or left atrial appendage.	B

Continued

TABLE 2 ACC/AHA Recommendations for Cardioversion of Atrial Fibrillation—cont'd

Class	Indication	Level of Evidence
	a. For patients with no identifiable thrombus, cardioversion is reasonable immediately after anticoagulation with unfractionated heparin (e.g., initiated by intravenous bolus injection and an infusion continued at a dose adjusted to prolong the activated partial thromboplastin time to 1.5-2× the control value until oral anticoagulation has been established with an oral vitamin K antagonist [e.g., warfarin] as evidenced by an INR ≥2.0).	B
	Thereafter, continuation of oral anticoagulation (INR, 2.0-3.0) is reasonable for a total anticoagulation period of at least 4 wk, as for patients undergoing elective cardioversion.	B
	Limited data are available to support the subcutaneous administration of a low-molecular-weight heparin in this indication.	C
	b. For patients in whom thrombus is identified by transesophageal echocardiography, oral anticoagulation (INR, 2.0-3.0) is reasonable for at least 3 wk before and 4 wk after restoration of sinus rhythm, and a longer period of anticoagulation may be appropriate even after apparently successful cardioversion because the risk of thromboembolism often remains elevated in such cases.	C
	For patients with atrial flutter undergoing cardioversion, anticoagulation can be beneficial according to the recommendations as for patients with AF.	C

ACC, American College of Cardiology; *AF,* atrial fibrillation; *AHA,* American Heart Association; *AV,* atrioventricular; *INR,* international normalized ratio.
From Libby P et al: *Braunwald's heart disease, a textbook of cardiovascular medicine,* ed 12, Philadelphia, 2022, Elsevier.

TABLE 3 ACC/AHA Recommendations for Pharmacologic Rate Control of Atrial Fibrillation

Class	Indication	Level of Evidence
Class I (indicated)	Measurement of the heart rate at rest and control of the rate with pharmacologic agents (either a beta-blocker or nondihydropyridine calcium channel antagonist, in most cases) are recommended for patients with persistent or permanent AF.	B
	In the absence of preexcitation, intravenous administration of beta-blockers (esmolol, metoprolol, or propranolol) or nondihydropyridine calcium channel antagonists (verapamil, diltiazem) is recommended to slow the ventricular response to AF in the acute setting, exercising caution in patients with hypotension or heart failure.	B
	Intravenous administration of digoxin or amiodarone is recommended to control heart rate in patients with AF and heart failure who do not have an accessory pathway.	B
	In patients who experience symptoms related to AF during activity, the adequacy of heart rate control should be assessed during exercise, adjusting pharmacologic treatment as necessary to keep the rate in the physiologic range.	C
	Digoxin is effective after oral administration to control the heart rate at rest in patients with AF and is indicated for patients with heart failure or left ventricular dysfunction and for sedentary individuals.	C
Class IIa (reasonable)	A combination of digoxin and either a beta-blocker or nondihydropyridine calcium channel antagonist is reasonable to control the heart rate both at rest and during exercise in patients with AF. The choice of medication should be individualized and the dose modulated to avoid bradycardia.	B
	It is reasonable to use ablation of the AV node or accessory pathway to control heart rate when pharmacologic therapy is insufficient or associated with side effects.	B
	Intravenous amiodarone can be useful to control heart rate in patients with AF when other measures are unsuccessful or contraindicated.	C
	When electrical cardioversion is not necessary in patients with AF and an accessory pathway, intravenous procainamide or ibutilide is a reasonable alternative.	C
Class IIb (may be considered)	When the ventricular rate cannot be adequately controlled both at rest and during exercise in patients with AF by a beta-blocker, nondihydropyridine calcium channel antagonist, or digoxin, alone or in combination, oral amiodarone may be administered to control the heart rate.	C
	Intravenous procainamide, disopyramide, ibutilide, or amiodarone may be considered for hemodynamically stable patients with AF involving conduction over an accessory pathway.	B
	When the rate cannot be controlled with pharmacologic agents or tachycardia-mediated cardiomyopathy is suspected, catheter-directed ablation of the AV node may be considered in patients with AF to control the heart rate.	C
Class III (not indicated)	Strict rate control (<80 beats/min at rest or <110 beats/min during 6-min walk) is not beneficial compared to a resting rate <110 beats/min in asymptomatic patients with persistent AF and an ejection fraction >40%, although uncontrolled tachycardia can lead to reversible left ventricular dysfunction over time.	B
	Digitalis should not be used as the sole agent to control the rate of ventricular response in patients with paroxysmal AF.	B
	Catheter ablation of the AV node should not be attempted without a prior trial of medication to control the ventricular rate in patients with AF.	C
	In patients with decompensated heart failure and AF, intravenous administration of a nondihydropyridine calcium channel antagonist may exacerbate hemodynamic compromise and is not recommended.	C
	Intravenous administration of digitalis glycosides or nondihydropyridine calcium channel antagonists to patients with AF and a preexcitation syndrome may paradoxically accelerate the ventricular response and is not recommended.	C

ACC, American College of Cardiology; *AF,* atrial fibrillation; *AHA,* American Heart Association; *AV,* atrioventricular.
From Libby P et al: *Braunwald's heart disease, a textbook of cardiovascular medicine,* ed 12, Philadelphia, 2022, Elsevier.

TABLE 4 ACC/AHA Recommendations for Maintenance of Sinus Rhythm in Patients with Atrial Fibrillation

Class	Indication	Level of Evidence
Class I (indicated)	Before initiation of antiarrhythmic drug therapy, treatment of precipitating or reversible causes of AF is recommended.	C
	Catheter ablation by an experienced operator is useful in selected patients with symptomatic paroxysmal AF who have failed treatment with an antiarrhythmic drug and have a normal or mildly dilated left atrium and normal or mildly reduced left ventricular function.	A
Class IIa (reasonable)	Pharmacologic therapy can be useful in patients with AF to maintain sinus rhythm and to prevent tachycardia-induced cardiomyopathy.	C
	Infrequent, well-tolerated recurrence of AF is reasonable as a successful outcome of antiarrhythmic drug therapy.	C
	Outpatient initiation of antiarrhythmic drug therapy is reasonable in patients with AF who have no associated heart disease when the agent is well tolerated.	C
	In patients with lone AF without structural heart disease, initiation of propafenone or flecainide can be beneficial on an outpatient basis in patients with paroxysmal AF who are in sinus rhythm at the time of drug initiation.	B
	Sotalol can be beneficial in outpatients in sinus rhythm with little or no heart disease, prone to paroxysmal AF, if the baseline uncorrected QT interval is shorter than 460 milliseconds, serum electrolyte values are normal, and risk factors associated with class III drug–related proarrhythmia are not present.	C
	Catheter ablation is a reasonable treatment of symptomatic persistent AF.	A
Class IIb (may be considered)	Catheter ablation may be reasonable for patients with symptomatic paroxysmal AF and significant left atrial dilation or significant left ventricular dysfunction.	A
Class III (not indicated)	Antiarrhythmic therapy with a particular drug is not recommended for maintenance of sinus rhythm in patients with AF who have well-defined risk factors for proarrhythmia with that agent.	A
	Pharmacologic therapy is not recommended for maintenance of sinus rhythm in patients with advanced sinus node disease or AV node dysfunction unless they have a functioning electronic cardiac pacemaker.	C

ACC, American College of Cardiology; *AF,* atrial fibrillation; *AHA,* American Heart Association.
From Libby P et al: *Braunwald's Heart Disease, a Textbook of Cardiovascular Medicine,* ed 12, Philadelphia, 2022, Elsevier.

<80 beats/min and an exercise heart rate of <110 beats/min. Most recent ACC/AHA guidelines, however, recommend targeting a heart rate <80 beats/min over a target of <110 beats/min.

- In patients with symptomatic AF, younger patients, or those with difficult to control heart rate, an attempt should be made to maintain sinus rhythm with antiarrhythmic agents. Options of antiarrhythmic agents include amiodarone, dronedarone (paroxysmal atrial fibrillation only without heart failure), dofetilide, flecainide, propafenone (contraindicated with structural heart disease), or sotalol. The decision of which strategy to follow should be best made in consultation with a cardiologist. Use of dronedarone should be avoided in patients with persistent or permanent atrial fibrillation because of worsened cardiovascular outcomes, especially in those with concomitant symptomatic heart failure (see Fig. 5 for a proposed algorithm to guide maintenance of sinus rhythm).

NONPHARMACOLOGIC THERAPY

- Catheter ablation of AF has become a common procedure for symptomatic drug-refractory or drug-intolerant patients. Sinus rhythm can be maintained long term in the majority of patients with paroxysmal atrial fibrillation (PAF) by circumferential pulmonary vein ablation performed in experienced centers. Established centers have reported success rates of 70% to 85% in patients with paroxysmal AF, but up to 50% of patients may require more than one ablation to achieve success. Complication rates are 4.5% in the largest international survey of hospitals performing this procedure. Success with persistent AF is much lower, with long-term success rates of 40% to 50% in many studies, and such patients often require more than one procedure. The most common techniques used to isolate the pulmonary veins are radiofrequency ablation and cryoballoon ablation, which have shown similar results for patients with PAF. Pulse field ablation is a newer technique currently in clinical trials.

- Pulmonary vein isolation is being increasingly used to treat AF in patients with heart failure. Trials have shown that pulmonary vein isolation is superior to AV node ablation with biventricular pacing in patients with heart failure who have drug-refractory AF. Pulsed field ablation which delivers mocrosecond high-voltage electrical fields may limit damage to tissues outside the myocardium. A recent trial among patients with paroxysmal AF receiving a catheter-based therapy found that pulsed field ablation was non-inferior to conventional thermal ablation with respect to freedom from a composite of initial procedure failure, documented atrial tachyarrhythmia after a 3-month blanking period, antiarrhythmic drug use, cardioversion, or repeat ablation and with respect to devise and serious adverse events at 1 year.[1b]

- AV nodal ablation with permanent pacemaker implantation may become necessary in some patients in whom rate and rhythm are difficult to control despite drugs and cardioversion, although it is generally used as a therapy of last resort.

- The Cox-Maze III surgical procedure, with its modifications creating electrical barriers to the macroreentrant circuits that are believed to underlie AF, is being performed with good results in some medical centers (preservation of sinus rhythm in 70% to 95% of patients without the use of long-term antiarrhythmic medication). Success rates are higher in paroxysmal than in persistent or permanent atrial fibrillation. Surgical ablation is often used for patients undergoing aortic or mitral valve surgery. As a stand-alone procedure, it is a Class IIb. Some centers perform surgical pulmonary vein isolation similar to this procedure using a mini-thoracotomy or video thoracoscopic "Mini-Maze" approach. Another surgical method is a pericardioscopic approach that allows extensive posterior wall ablation and, when combined with catheter ablation in a "hybrid" approach, has shown promising results for patients with persistent AF.

- It is important to understand that ablation therapy will not eliminate the need to take anticoagulant drugs. Even after ablation, patients with AF face increased risk of thromboembolic events and most electrophysiologists suggest lifelong anticoagulation for patients with elevated stroke risk score. Due to the increasing success rate of ablation, catheter-based therapy is considered the first-line treatment for paroxysmal AF patients intolerant or refractory to one medication or IIa for persistent patients.[2] It remains a IIb indication for patients in longstanding persistent atrial fibrillation.

STROKE PREVENTION (FIGS. E6 AND E7)

- The decision whether to pursue long-term anticoagulation must be made in light of the patient's risk for a cardioembolic event versus risk for a bleeding event. ACC/AHA recommendations for prevention of thromboembolism in atrial fibrillation are summarized in Table 5. In nonvalvular AF, CHA_2DS_2-VASc has superseded the $CHADS_2$ scoring system (C = congestive

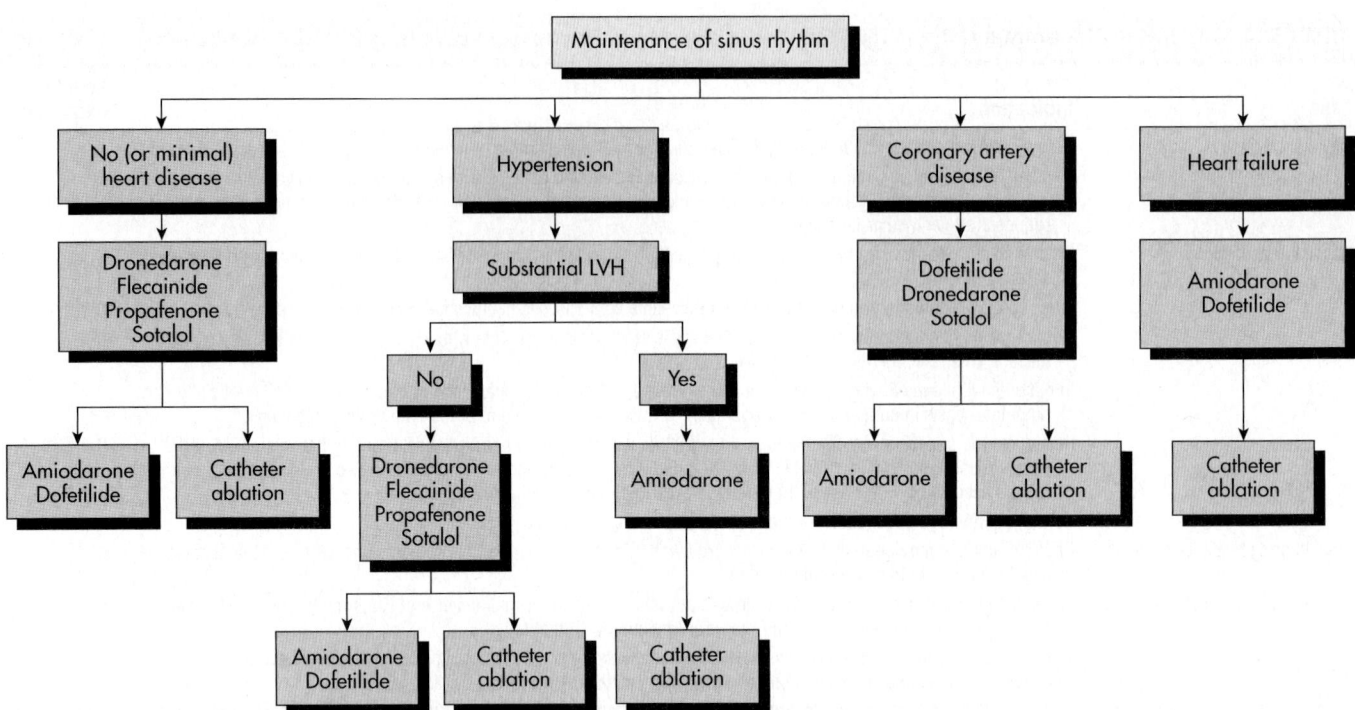

FIG. 5 Therapy to maintain sinus rhythm in patients with recurrent paroxysmal or persistent atrial fibrillation. Drugs are listed alphabetically and not in order of suggested use. The seriousness of heart disease progresses from left to right, and selection of therapy in patients with multiple conditions depends on the most serious condition present. *LVH*, Left ventricular hypertrophy. (From Wann LS et al: 2011 ACCF/AHA/HRS Focused update on the management of patients with atrial fibrillation [updating the 2006 guideline]: a report of the American College of Cardiology Foundation/American Heart Association Task Force on Practice Guidelines, *J Am Coll Cardiol* 57[2]:223-242, 2011.)

heart failure; H = hypertension; A = age [>75 yr is 2 points]; D = diabetes; S = stroke, transient ischemic attack, or thromboembolic disease [2 points]; V = vascular disease, A = age 65 to 74 yr; and Sc = sex category, with females getting 1 extra point). Patients with a CHA_2DS_2-VASc score of 0 are considered low risk, 1 to 2 are considered moderate risk, and >2 are considered high risk. Per guidelines, patients with a score of 0 do not merit anticoagulation. Patients with a score of 1 can be treated at the discretion of the physician with either aspirin or an oral anticoagulant (warfarin or a novel oral anticoagulant). Anticoagulation with either warfarin or a novel oral anticoagulant is recommended for all men with a $CHADS_2$-VASc score of 2 or above and women with a $CHADS_2$-VASc score of 3 or above. The available direct-acting oral anticoagulants (DOACs) are recommended over warfarin in DOAC-eligible patients with atrial fibrillation.[3]

- Increasing amounts of evidence now show that aspirin likely does not protect a person from stroke in AF and has recently been dropped from most of the ACC/AHA and European Atrial Fibrillation guidelines. Target INR for patients on warfarin with an indication for anticoagulation is 2 to 3 and should be diligently monitored to avoid risk of stroke versus bleeding. Patients with hypertrophic cardiomyopathy or thyrotoxicosis with AF also have a high risk of stroke and should be anticoagulated irrespective of their $CHADS_2$-VASc score.
- The DOACs include several factor Xa inhibitors (Table 6) and a direct thrombin inhibitor.
  1. Factor Xa inhibitors (apixaban, rivaroxaban, edoxaban) are also effective in reducing

stroke and systemic embolism in patients with atrial fibrillation. The Apixaban for Reduction in Stroke and Other Thromboembolic Events in Atrial Fibrillation (ARISTOTLE) trial in patients at high risk for stroke (mean $CHADS_2$ score 2.1) using apixaban, the Rivaroxaban Once Daily Oral Direct Factor Xa Inhibition Compared with Vitamin K Antagonism for Prevention of Stroke and Embolism Trial in Atrial Fibrillation (ROCKET AF) trial using rivaroxaban in patients with $CHADS_2$ score 3.5, and the Effective Anticoagulation with Factor Xa Next Generation in Atrial Fibrillation (ENGAGE-AF) trial using edoxaban in patients with a $CHADS_2$ score of at least 2, showed that these anticoagulants reduce the risk of stroke, systemic embolism, and serious bleeding compared with warfarin. Rivaroxaban showed noninferior efficacy to warfarin in prevention of thromboembolism. Apixaban showed superior stroke reduction, reduced bleeding events, and an overall mortality benefit when compared with warfarin. Edoxaban showed noninferiority to warfarin with respect to stroke and systemic embolism prevention, with lower rates of bleeding and death from cardiovascular causes, but benefit was limited to patients with moderately impaired renal function. Rivaroxaban and edoxaban are dosed once a day, and apixaban is dosed twice a day. A factor Xa reversal agent, andexanet alfa, has received FDA approval as a reversal for the anticoagulant effect of these agents.
  2. Dabigatran is a direct thrombin inhibitor indicated to reduce the risk of stroke and

systemic embolism in patients with non-valvular atrial fibrillation. In the RE-LY trial of 18,113 patients with mean $CHADS_2$ score of 2.1, dabigatran 110 mg bid was noninferior to warfarin, and 150 mg bid was superior to warfarin in prevention of thromboembolic events. Bleeding risk was similar to that of warfarin for both doses. Idarucizumab has been approved as a dabigatran reversal agent. Onset is immediate, and it provides full reversal for at least 24 h in most patients.
- The decision to anticoagulate should be made irrespective of whether the atrial fibrillation is paroxysmal, persistent, or permanent.
- For patients in whom anticoagulation with warfarin or other anticoagulants is contraindicated due to high bleeding risk (Table 7), left atrial appendage exclusion is an alternative. Several methods can be used, including the Lariat procedure and the AtriClip, but these are still considered unproven for stroke prevention in AF. The Watchman and Amulet devices are left atrial appendage occlusion devices approved by the FDA for stroke prevention specifically for patients with AF that require anticoagulation but have an appropriate reason to seek an alternative. Patients with surgical ligation of the left atrial appendage still have an indication for anticoagulation due to lack of clinical trials showing a stroke risk reduction and inconsistent techniques.
- Perioperative bridging anticoagulation in patients with AF: Current guidelines advise perioperative continuation of warfarin in low-risk patients ($CHADS_2$ score 0 to 2) and bridging anticoagulation only in those at

TABLE 5 ACC/AHA Recommendations for Prevention of Thromboembolism in Atrial Fibrillation

Class	Indication	Level of Evidence
Class I (indicated)	Antithrombotic therapy to prevent thromboembolism is recommended for all patients with AF, except those with lone AF or contraindications.	A
	The selection of the antithrombotic agent should be based on the absolute risks of stroke and bleeding and the relative risk and benefit for a given patient.	A
	For patients without mechanical heart valves at high risk of stroke, chronic oral anticoagulant therapy with a vitamin K antagonist is recommended in a dose adjusted to achieve the target intensity international normalized ratio (INR) of 2.0-3.0 unless contraindicated. Factors associated with highest risk for stroke in patients with AF are prior thromboembolism (stroke, transient ischemic attack, or systemic embolism) and rheumatic mitral stenosis.	A
	Anticoagulation with a vitamin K antagonist is recommended for patients with more than one moderate risk factor. Such factors include age ≥75 yr, hypertension, heart failure, impaired left ventricular systolic function (ejection fraction ≤35% or fractional shortening <25%), and diabetes mellitus.	A
	INR should be determined at least weekly during initiation of therapy and monthly when anticoagulation is stable.	A
	Dabigatran is a useful alternative to warfarin in patients with AF and risk factors for stroke who do not have a prosthetic heart valve or significant valve disease, a creatinine clearance <15 ml/min, or advanced liver disease.	B
	Aspirin, 81-325 mg daily, is recommended as an alternative to vitamin K antagonists in low-risk patients or in those with contraindications to oral anticoagulation.	A
	For patients with AF who have mechanical heart valves, the target intensity of anticoagulation should be based on the type of prosthesis, maintaining an INR of at least 2.5.	B
	Antithrombotic therapy is recommended for patients with atrial flutter as for those with AF.	C
Class IIa (reasonable)	For primary prevention of thromboembolism in patients with nonvalvular AF who have just one of the following validated risk factors, antithrombotic therapy with either aspirin or a vitamin K antagonist is reasonable, based on an assessment of the risk of bleeding complications, ability to safely sustain adjusted chronic anticoagulation, and the patient's preferences: Age ≥75 yr (especially in female patients), hypertension, heart failure, impaired left ventricular function, or diabetes mellitus.	A
	For patients with nonvalvular AF who have one or more of the following less well-validated risk factors, antithrombotic therapy with either aspirin or a vitamin K antagonist is reasonable for prevention of thromboembolism: Age 65-74 yr, female gender, or coronary artery disease. The choice of agent should be based on the risk of bleeding complications, ability to sustain adjusted chronic anticoagulation, and the patient's preferences.	B
	It is reasonable to select antithrombotic therapy by the same criteria irrespective of the pattern (i.e., paroxysmal, persistent, or permanent) of AF.	B
	In patients with AF who do not have mechanical prosthetic heart valves, it is reasonable to interrupt anticoagulation for up to 1 wk without substituting heparin for surgical or diagnostic procedures that carry a risk of bleeding.	C
	It is reasonable to reevaluate the need for anticoagulation at regular intervals.	C
Class IIb (may be considered)	In patients ≥75 yr at increased risk of bleeding but without frank contraindications to oral anticoagulant therapy, and in other patients with moderate risk factors for thromboembolism who are unable to safely tolerate anticoagulation at the standard intensity of INR 2.0-3.0, a lower INR target of 2.0 (range, 1.6-2.5) may be considered for prevention of ischemic stroke and systemic embolism.	C
	When surgical procedures require interruption of oral anticoagulant therapy for longer than 1 wk in high-risk patients, unfractionated heparin may be administered or low-molecular-weight heparin given by subcutaneous injection, although the efficacy of these alternatives in this situation is uncertain.	C
	After percutaneous coronary intervention or revascularization surgery in patients with AF, low-dose aspirin (<100 mg/day) and/or clopidogrel (75 mg/day) may be given concurrently with anticoagulation to prevent myocardial ischemic events, but these strategies have not been thoroughly evaluated and are associated with an increased risk of bleeding.	C
	In patients undergoing percutaneous coronary intervention, anticoagulation may be interrupted to prevent bleeding at the site of peripheral arterial puncture, but the vitamin K antagonist should be resumed as soon as possible after the procedure and the dose adjusted to achieve an INR in the therapeutic range. Aspirin may be given temporarily during the hiatus, but the maintenance regimen should then consist of the combination of clopidogrel, 75 mg daily, plus warfarin (INR, 2.0-3.0). Clopidogrel should be given for a minimum of 1 mo after implantation of a bare-metal stent, at least 3 mo for a sirolimus-eluting stent, at least 6 mo for a paclitaxel-eluting stent, and 12 mo or longer in selected patients, following which warfarin may be continued as monotherapy in the absence of a subsequent coronary event. When warfarin is given in combination with clopidogrel or low-dose aspirin, the dose intensity must be carefully regulated.	C
	In patients with AF younger than 60 yr without heart disease or risk factors for thromboembolism (lone AF), the risk of thromboembolism is low without treatment, and the effectiveness of aspirin for primary prevention of stroke relative to the risk of bleeding has not been established.	C
	In patients with AF who sustain ischemic stroke or systemic embolism during treatment with low-intensity anticoagulation (INR, 2.0-3.0), rather than add an antiplatelet agent, it may be reasonable to raise the intensity of the anticoagulation to a maximum target INR of 3.0-3.5.	C
	Clopidogrel plus aspirin may be considered in patients who cannot tolerate or who refuse an oral anticoagulant.	B
Class III (not indicated)	Long-term anticoagulation with a vitamin K antagonist is not recommended for primary prevention of stroke in patients younger than 60 yr without heart disease (lone AF) or any risk factors for thromboembolism.	C

ACC, American College of Cardiology; *AF,* atrial fibrillation; *AHA,* American Heart Association.
From Libby P et al: *Braunwald's heart disease, a textbook of cardiovascular medicine,* ed 12, Philadelphia, 2022, Elsevier.

Diseases and Disorders

I

TABLE 6 Characteristics of Non–Vitamin K Antagonists and Oral Anticoagulants

	Dabigatran	Apixaban	Edoxaban	Rivaroxaban
Mechanism	Oral direct thrombin inhibitor	Oral direct factor Xa inhibitor	Oral direct factor Xa inhibitor	Oral direct factor Xa inhibitor
Prodrug	Yes	No	No	No
Standard dose	150 mg twice daily	5 mg twice daily	60 mg once daily	20 mg once daily
Reduced dose	110 mg twice daily; 75 mg twice daily in U.S.	2.5 mg twice daily	30 mg once daily	15 mg once daily
Bioavailability	3%-7%	50%	62%	66% without food, 80%-100% with food
Renal clearance of absorbed dose	80%	27%	50%	35%
Plasma protein binding	35%	87%	55%	95%
Dialyzability	50%-60%	14%	Not available	Not available
Liver metabolism: CYP3A4 involved	No	Yes (25%)	Minimal (<4% of elimination)	Yes (18%)
Absorption with food	No effect	No effect	6%-22%	≥39%
Elimination half-life	12-17 h	12 h	10-14 h	5-9 h (young), 11-13 h (elderly)

From Hoffman R et al: *Hematology, basic principles and practice*, ed 8, Philadelphia, 2023, Elsevier.

TABLE 7 Risk Stratification for Bleeding: The HAS-BLED Score

Clinical Characteristic	Points
Hypertension	1
Abnormal renal/liver function	1 or 2
Stroke	1
Bleeding	1
Labile INRs	1
Elderly (age >65 yr)	1
Drugs or alcohol	1 or 2
Cumulative score	Range 0-9

Hypertension = systolic blood pressure >160 mm Hg; abnormal renal function = dialysis, transplant, creatinine >2.6 mg/dL or >200 μmol/L; abnormal liver function = cirrhosis or bilirubin >2× normal with AST/ALT/AP >3× normal; labile INR = unstable/high INRs, time in therapeutic range <60%; drugs = antiplatelet agents, nonsteroidal anti-inflammatory drugs; alcohol = eight or more drinks/wk.
ALT, Alanine aminotransferase; *AP*, alanine phosphatase; *AST*, aspartate aminotransferase; *INR*, international normalized ratio.
From Hoffman R et al: *Hematology, basic principles and practice*, ed 8, Philadelphia, 2023, Elsevier.

highest risk of thromboembolism (CHADS₂ score 5 to 6). The recent Bridging Anticoagulation in Patients who Require Temporary Interruption of Warfarin Therapy for an Elective Invasive Procedure or Surgery (BRIDGE) Study found that for patients who require procedure-related warfarin interruption, forgoing bridging anticoagulation was noninferior to perioperative bridging with low-molecular-weight heparin and decrease the risk of major bleeding. Based on this study, a no-bridging strategy is appropriate for lower-risk AF and minor procedures, but in high-risk patients having major surgery the answer remains debatable.

PROGNOSIS
- AF is associated with a 1.5- to 1.9-fold higher risk of death, which is in part due to the strong association between AF and thromboembolic events.

- AF is also independently associated with an increased risk of incident myocardial infarction, especially in women and blacks.
- Development of AF predicts heart failure and is associated with a worse New York Heart Association Heart Failure classification. AF may also worsen heart failure in individuals who are dependent on the atrial component of the cardiac output.
- AF in the setting of acute myocardial infarction was associated with a 40% increase in mortality compared to patients in sinus rhythm.
- ACC/AHA recommendations for special considerations in atrial fibrillation are summarized in Table 8.

DISPOSITION
Factors associated with maintenance of sinus rhythm after cardioversion include:
- Left atrium diameter <60 mm
- Absence of mitral valve disease
- Short duration of AF

REFERRAL
Refer to a cardiologist those patients in whom antiarrhythmic therapy or catheter-based/surgical intervention is being considered.

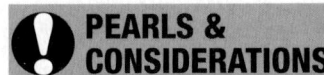 **PEARLS & CONSIDERATIONS**

COMMENTS
The number of patients anticoagulated in the United States is approximately half the number that should be anticoagulated for AF, resulting in a large burden of stroke. The exact burden of AF needed to trigger the need for anticoagulation is not known, though recent pacemaker trials have suggested that as little as 6 min confers significant stroke risk. Reversal agents for the new class of anticoagulation are now available: Idarucizumab for reversal of dabigatran; andexanet alfa for reversal of apixaban and rivaroxaban.
Perioperative management strategies: The risk of bleeding with surgical or invasive procedures in patients on oral anticoagulation are

summarized in Table 9. Perioperative management is outlined in Table 10.
The American Academy of Family Physicians and the American College of Physicians provide the following recommendations for the management of newly detected AF:
- Rate control with chronic anticoagulation is the recommended strategy for the majority of asymptomatic patients with chronic AF. Rhythm control has not been shown to be superior to rate control (with chronic anticoagulation) in reducing morbidity and mortality and may be inferior in some patient subgroups to rate control. Rhythm control is appropriate when based on other special considerations, such as patient symptoms, exercise tolerance, and patient preference.
- Patients with AF should receive chronic anticoagulation, unless they are at low risk for stroke as stated earlier or have specific contraindications.
- For patients with AF, the following drugs are recommended for their demonstrated efficacy in rate control during exercise and while at rest: Atenolol, metoprolol, diltiazem, and verapamil (drugs listed alphabetically by class). Digoxin is effective only for rate control at rest and therefore should be used only as a second-line agent for rate control in AF.
- For patients who elect to undergo acute cardioversion to achieve sinus rhythm in AF, both direct-current cardioversion and pharmacologic conversion are appropriate options in an otherwise healthy patient.
- Both transesophageal echocardiography with short-term prior anticoagulation followed by early acute cardioversion (in absence of intracardiac thrombus) with postcardioversion anticoagulation vs delayed cardioversion with preanticoagulation and postanticoagulation are appropriate management strategies for patients who elect to undergo cardioversion.
- Among patients with paroxysmal AF without previous antiarrhythmic drug treatment, ablation compared with antiarrhythmic drugs resulted in a lower rate of recurrent atrial tachyarrhythmias at 2 yr. However, recurrence was frequent in both groups.

TABLE 8 ACC/AHA Recommendations for Special Considerations in Atrial Fibrillation

Class	Indication	Level of Evidence
Postoperative Atrial Fibrillation		
Class I (indicated)	Unless contraindicated, treatment with an oral beta-blocker to prevent postoperative AF is recommended for patients undergoing cardiac surgery.	A
	Administration of AV nodal blocking agents is recommended to achieve rate control in patients who develop postoperative AF.	B
Class IIa (reasonable)	Preoperative administration of amiodarone reduces the incidence of AF in patients undergoing cardiac surgery and represents appropriate prophylactic therapy for patients at high risk for postoperative AF.	A
	It is reasonable to restore sinus rhythm by pharmacologic cardioversion with ibutilide or direct-current cardioversion in patients who develop postoperative AF, as advised for nonsurgical patients.	B
	It is reasonable to administer antiarrhythmic medications in an attempt to maintain sinus rhythm in patients with recurrent or refractory postoperative AF, as recommended for other patients who develop AF.	B
	It is reasonable to administer antithrombotic medication in patients who develop postoperative AF, as recommended for nonsurgical patients.	B
Class IIb (may be considered)	Prophylactic administration of sotalol may be considered for patients at risk for development of AF after cardiac surgery.	B
Acute Myocardial Infarction		
Class I (indicated)	Direct-current cardioversion is recommended for patients with severe hemodynamic compromise or intractable ischemia, or when adequate rate control cannot be achieved with pharmacologic agents in patients with acute myocardial infarction and AF.	C
	Intravenous administration of amiodarone is recommended to slow a rapid ventricular response to AF and to improve left ventricular function in patients with acute myocardial infarction.	C
	Intravenous beta-blockers and nondihydropyridine calcium antagonists are recommended to slow a rapid ventricular response to AF in patients with acute myocardial infarction who do not display clinical left ventricular dysfunction, bronchospasm, or AV block.	C
	For patients with AF and acute myocardial infarction, administration of unfractionated heparin by either continuous intravenous infusion or intermittent subcutaneous injection is recommended in a dose sufficient to prolong the activated partial thromboplastin time to 1.5-2× the control value, unless contraindications to anticoagulation exist.	C
Class IIa (reasonable)	Intravenous administration of digitalis is reasonable to slow a rapid ventricular response and to improve left ventricular function in patients with acute myocardial infarction and AF associated with severe left ventricular dysfunction and heart failure.	C
Class III (not indicated)	The administration of class IC antiarrhythmic drugs is not recommended in patients with AF in the setting of acute myocardial infarction.	C
Management of Atrial Fibrillation Associated with Wolff-Parkinson-White (WPW) Preexcitation Syndrome		
Class I (indicated)	Catheter ablation of the accessory pathway is recommended for symptomatic patients with AF who have WPW syndrome, particularly those with syncope due to rapid heart rate or those with a short bypass tract refractory period.	B
	Immediate direct-current cardioversion is recommended to prevent ventricular fibrillation in patients with a short anterograde bypass tract refractory period in whom AF occurs with a rapid ventricular response associated with hemodynamic instability.	B
	Intravenous procainamide or ibutilide is recommended to restore sinus rhythm in patients with WPW in whom AF occurs without hemodynamic instability in association with a wide QRS complex on the electrocardiogram (≥120-msec duration) or with a rapid preexcited ventricular response.	C
Class IIa (reasonable)	Intravenous flecainide or direct-current cardioversion is reasonable when very rapid ventricular rates occur in patients with AF involving conduction over an accessory pathway.	B
Class IIb (may be considered)	It may be reasonable to administer intravenous quinidine, procainamide, disopyramide, ibutilide, or amiodarone to hemodynamically stable patients with AF involving conduction over an accessory pathway.	B
Class III (not indicated)	Intravenous administration of digitalis glycosides or nondihydropyridine calcium channel antagonists is not recommended in patients with WPW syndrome who have preexcited ventricular activation during AF.	B
Hyperthyroidism		
Class I (indicated)	Administration of a beta-blocker is recommended to control the rate of ventricular response in patients with AF complicating thyrotoxicosis, unless contraindicated.	B
	In circumstances when a beta-blocker cannot be used, administration of a nondihydropyridine calcium channel antagonist (diltiazem or verapamil) is recommended to control the ventricular rate in patients with AF and thyrotoxicosis.	B
	In patients with AF associated with thyrotoxicosis, oral anticoagulation (INR, 2.0-3.0) is recommended to prevent thromboembolism, as recommended for AF patients with other risk factors for stroke.	C
	Once a euthyroid state is restored, recommendations for antithrombotic prophylaxis are the same as for patients without hyperthyroidism.	C
Management of Atrial Fibrillation During Pregnancy		
Class I (indicated)	Digoxin, a beta-blocker, or a nondihydropyridine calcium channel antagonist is recommended to control the rate of ventricular response in pregnant patients with AF.	C

Continued

TABLE 8 ACC/AHA Recommendations for Special Considerations in Atrial Fibrillation—cont'd

Class	Indication	Level of Evidence
	Direct-current cardioversion is recommended in pregnant patients who become hemodynamically unstable because of AF.	C
	Protection against thromboembolism is recommended throughout pregnancy for all patients with AF (except those with lone AF and/or low thromboembolic risk). Therapy (anticoagulant or aspirin) should be chosen according to the stage of pregnancy.	C
Class IIb (may be considered)	Administration of heparin may be considered during the first trimester and last month of pregnancy for patients with AF and risk factors for thromboembolism. Unfractionated heparin may be administered either by continuous intravenous infusion in a dose sufficient to prolong the activated partial thromboplastin time to 1.5-2× the control value or by intermittent subcutaneous injection in a dose of 10,000-20,000 units every 12 h, adjusted to prolong the midinterval (6 h after injection) activated partial thromboplastin time to 1.5× control.	B
	Despite the limited data available, subcutaneous administration of low-molecular-weight heparin may be considered during the first trimester and last month of pregnancy for patients with AF and risk factors for thromboembolism.	C
	Administration of an oral anticoagulant may be considered during the second trimester for pregnant patients with AF at high thromboembolic risk.	C
	Administration of quinidine or procainamide may be considered to achieve pharmacologic cardioversion in hemodynamically stable patients who develop AF during pregnancy.	C
Management of Atrial Fibrillation in Patients with Hypertrophic Cardiomyopathy (HCM)		
Class I (indicated)	Oral anticoagulation (INR, 2.0-3.0) is recommended in patients with HCM who develop AF, as for other patients at high risk of thromboembolism.	B
Class IIa (may be considered)	Antiarrhythmic medications can be useful to prevent recurrent AF in patients with HCM. Available data are insufficient to recommend one agent over another in this situation, but (a) disopyramide combined with a beta-blocker or nondihydropyridine calcium channel antagonist or (b) amiodarone alone is generally preferred.	C
Management of Atrial Fibrillation in Patients with Pulmonary Disease		
Class I (indicated)	Correction of hypoxemia and acidosis is the recommended primary therapeutic measure for patients who develop AF during an acute pulmonary illness or exacerbation of chronic pulmonary disease.	C
	A nondihydropyridine calcium channel antagonist (diltiazem or verapamil) is recommended to control the ventricular rate in patients with obstructive pulmonary disease who develop AF.	C
	Direct-current cardioversion should be attempted in patients with pulmonary disease who become hemodynamically unstable as a consequence of AF.	C
Class III (not indicated)	Theophylline and beta-adrenergic agonist agents are not recommended for patients with bronchospastic lung disease who develop AF.	C
	Beta-blockers, sotalol, propafenone, and adenosine are not recommended in patients with obstructive lung disease who develop AF.	C

ACC, American College of Cardiology; *AF,* atrial fibrillation; *AHA,* American Heart Association; *AV,* atrioventricular; *INR,* international normalized ratio.
From Libby P et al: *Braunwald's heart disease, a textbook of cardiovascular medicine,* ed 12, Philadelphia, 2022, Elsevier.

TABLE 9 Risk for Bleeding with Surgical or Invasive Procedures

Risk	Type of Procedure	Examples
Low	Nonvital organs involved, exposed surgical site, limited dissection, percutaneous access	Lymph node biopsy, dental extraction, cataract extraction, most cutaneous surgery, laparoscopic procedures, coronary angiography
Moderate	Vital organs involved, deep or extensive dissection	Laparotomy, thoracotomy, mastectomy, major orthopedic surgery, pacemaker insertion
High	Bleeding likely to compromise surgical result, bleeding complications frequent	Neurosurgery, ophthalmic surgery, cardiopulmonary bypass, prostatectomy or bladder surgery, major vascular surgery, renal biopsy, bowel polypectomy

TABLE 10 Perioperative Management Strategies for Patients on Chronic Oral Anticoagulant Therapy

Clinical Situation	Suggested Anticoagulation Management
Low bleeding-risk surgery (dental, cataract, skin)	• Consider reducing dose of warfarin to achieve an INR ≤2.0 • Consider holding dose of DOAC until after the procedure
Low thrombotic risk Aortic valve prosthesis without other thrombotic risk factors[a] *or* AF with low stroke risk *or* VTE >3 mo previously	• Stop warfarin 5 days prior to surgery, safe to operate when INR ≤1.5 • Hold DOACs for 5 half-lives—dabigatran for 2-3 days, rivaroxaban, apixaban, edoxaban for 2 days • Restart warfarin in evening of the day of surgery after hemostasis secured; restart DOACs on postoperative day 3 or 4 • Start prophylactic LMWH on the morning of the day after surgery and continue until INR >1.8 or full dose of DOACs resumed

Continued

TABLE 10 Perioperative Management Strategies for Patients on Chronic Oral Anticoagulant Therapy—cont'd

Clinical Situation	Suggested Anticoagulation Management
Moderate thrombotic risk Mitral or multiple valve prostheses *or* Aortic prosthesis with risk factors for thrombosis *or* AF at high stroke risk *or* VTE within past 3 mo	• Stop warfarin 5 days before surgery • Begin twice-daily LMWH in therapeutic doses starting 3 days before surgery with last dose at least 12 h prior to surgery • Hold DOACs for 5 half-lives—dabigatran for 3-4 days, rivaroxaban, apixaban, edoxaban for 2-3 days; no bridging • Restart warfarin in evening of the day of surgery after hemostasis secured; restart DOACs on postoperative day 3 or 4 • Start prophylactic LMWH on the morning of the day after surgery and continue until INR >1.8 or full dose of DOACs resumed

AF, Atrial fibrillation; *DOAC*, direct oral anticoagulant; *INR*, international normalized ratio; *LMWH*, low-molecular-weight heparin; *VTE*, venous thromboembolism.
[a]Risk factors include caged-ball or single tilting-disk valve, *AF*, history of stroke/transient ischemic attack or other embolic event, left ventricular failure, underlying hypercoagulable state including cancer.
From Hoffman R et al: *Hematology, basic principles and practice,* ed 8, Philadelphia, 2023, Elsevier.

Diseases and Disorders

I

• Among patients with atrial fibrillation who undergo packed cell volume, the risk of bleeding is lower among those who receive dual therapy with dabigatran and a $P2Y_{12}$ inhibitor (clopidogrel or ticagrelor) than among those who receive triple therapy with warfarin, a $P2Y_{12}$ inhibitor, and aspirin. Dual therapy has been shown to be noninferior to triple therapy with respect to the risk of thromboembolic events.[4]

• In patients with atrial fibrillation and stable coronary artery disease, rivaroxaban monotherapy is noninferior to combination therapy with rivaroxaban plus a single antiplatelet agent for efficacy and superior for safety.[5]

• In patients presenting to the ED with recent-onset, symptomatic atrial fibrillation, a wait-and-see approach is noninferior to early cardioversion in achieving a return to sinus rhythm at 4 wk.[6]

RELATED CONTENT

Atrial Fibrillation (Patient Information)

REFERENCES

Available at eBooks.Health.Elsevier.com

AUTHOR: **TANIA B. BABAR, MD**

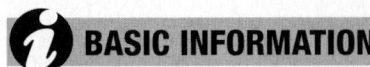
BASIC INFORMATION

DEFINITION

Typical atrial flutter is the term commonly applied to the atrial macroreentrant circuit that circulates around the tricuspid annulus in the right atrium. The critical isthmus of the circuit is the tissue between the inferior vena cava and the tricuspid annulus, and a more precise name for this arrhythmia is *cavotricuspid isthmus-dependent (CTI) atrial flutter,* or CTI flutter. Because of its anatomic and physiologic stability, the result is regular atrial depolarizations, typically at a rate of 250 to 350 beats/min. Regular, macroreentrant atrial arrhythmias at this rate that do not use the CTI are referred to as *atypical atrial flutter.* Because of the stability of atrial flutter, conduction through the atrioventricular node (AVN) is often predictable at a common mathematical denominator. For example, when the flutter rate is 300 beats/min, 2:1 conduction results in a ventricular rate of 150 beats/min. By extension, 3:1 conduction results in a ventricular rate of 100 beats/min, 4:1 in a rate of 75 beats/min, and 5:1 in a rate of 60 beats/min. If the regular atrial impulses conduct at a variable rate through the AVN, the result may be an irregular QRS pattern.

Table 1 summarizes the different types of atrial flutter and distinguishing features on scalar electrocardiography.

ICD-10CM CODES

I48.3	Typical atrial flutter
I48.4	Atypical atrial flutter
I48.92	Unspecified atrial flutter

EPIDEMIOLOGY & DEMOGRAPHICS

- Atrial flutter is the second most common sustained atrial tachyarrhythmia after atrial fibrillation, with an estimated 200,000 new cases annually in the U.S.
- Atrial flutter is common in patients with congestive heart failure, chronic obstructive pulmonary disease (COPD), pulmonary vascular disorders such as pulmonary embolism, or during the first wk after open heart surgery.
- Atrial flutter occurs more frequently with advancing age (5/100,000 age <50 vs 587/100,000 age >80 yr) and 2.5× more frequently in men than in women.
- Patients taking antiarrhythmics for chronic suppression of atrial fibrillation may present with atrial flutter.
- Atrial flutter is typically seen in patients with underlying structural heart disease and is uncommon in children or young adults without congenital heart disease.
- More than 50% of patients with atrial flutter will develop atrial fibrillation in 3 yr, and more than 80% will develop atrial fibrillation within 5 yr. This is important when considering treatment options for atrial flutter, especially anticoagulation.

CLASSIFICATION

Historically, the Wells classification designated atrial flutter as type I and type II. However, it is now recognized that tachycardias satisfying either of the definitions for type I or type II can be caused by reentrant circuits or by rapid focal atrial tachycardia, and this classification is infrequently used. Designating atrial flutter based on CTI dependence is more useful because of the management options (i.e., ablation). Type I CTI-dependent atrial flutter, also known as common atrial flutter or typical atrial flutter, has an atrial rate of 250 to 350 beats/min. The reentrant loop circles the tricuspid valve in the right atrium, passing through the CTI, a body of fibrous tissue in the lower atrium between the inferior vena cava and the tricuspid valve. CTI flutter can revolve around the tricuspid annulus in either direction (counterclockwise or clockwise) when viewing the tricuspid annulus en face.

- Counterclockwise atrial flutter is the more common type (~75%). The flutter waves are "sawtooth" and negative on the surface ECG leads II, III, and aVF; positive in V1; and negative in V6 (Fig. E1).
- Clockwise atrial flutter is less common (~25%): The reentry loop cycles in the opposite direction; thus the flutter waves are upright in leads II, III, and aVF; negative in V1; and positive in V6 (Fig. E2).
- Atypical atrial flutter is defined by absence of CTI dependence and may occur in patients with prior cardiac surgery, congenital heart disease, prior radiofrequency ablation (especially after left atrial ablation for atrial fibrillation) or may be idiopathic. One ECG feature is the lack of discordance of the flutter wave polarity between the inferior leads (leads II, III, and aVF) and V1. Flutter circuits in the left atrium (such as mitral annular flutter) often have upright flutter waves in all precordial leads.

PHYSICAL FINDINGS & CLINICAL PRESENTATION

- Palpitations
- Dizziness, light-headedness, syncope, or near syncope
- Angina
- Congestive heart failure
- Embolic phenomena from intracardiac thrombus

ETIOLOGY

- Age-related degenerative changes
- Rheumatic heart disease
- Congenital heart disease
- Left ventricular dysfunction or congestive heart failure
- Acute myocardial infarction (rarely)
- Thyrotoxicosis
- Pulmonary embolism

TABLE 1 Characteristics of Different Types of Atrial Flutter and Distinguishing Features on Scalar Electrocardiography

Type	Reentrant Circuit	ECG Pattern	Lead V1/V6
Typical counterclockwise	Tricuspid annulus dependent on the CTI	Sawtooth flutter wave; negative in II, III, and aVF	Positive V1, negative V6
Typical clockwise	Tricuspid annulus dependent on the CTI	"Inverse sawtooth"; positive and often notched in II, III, and aVF	Broad and negative in V1 (often notched) Positive in V6
Lower loop reentry	CTI	Usually similar to typical counterclockwise CTI flutter except subtle loss of terminal positive deflection in leads II, III, and aVF	Usually similar to typical counterclockwise
Upper loop reentry	Superior vena cava and upper crista terminalis	Similar to typical clockwise flutter	Similar to typical clockwise flutter
Right atrial free wall	Around areas of scar in lateral or posterior right atrium (caused by previous atrial surgery or spontaneously)	Variable	Typically negative or biphasic with terminal negative deflection in V1
Septal atrial flutter	Atrial septum, typically after previous surgery	Variable	Usually biphasic or isoelectric in V1
Mitral annular flutter	Around mitral annulus, often slow zone of block around PV interval; frequently occurs in setting of left atrial surgery or ablation	Variable; I, III, and aVF, often positive but low amplitude	Usually positive in V1 (or rarely isoelectric) and often broad
Postatrial fibrillation ablation/maze flutter	Variable; circuit involves previous ablations or scar in left atrium	Variable	Variable

aVF, Augmented vector foot; *CTI,* cavotricuspid isthmus; *PV,* pulmonary vein.
From Zipes DP: *Braunwald's heart disease, a textbook of cardiovascular medicine,* ed 11, Philadelphia, 2019, Elsevier.

- Mitral valve disease
- Cardiac surgery
- Chronic obstructive pulmonary disease
- Obesity
- Pericarditis
- Pulmonary hypertension
- Antiarrhythmic therapy use in patients with atrial fibrillation
- Other causes of right atrial enlargement
- Systemic infections (such as COVID-19)[1]

Dx DIAGNOSIS

DIFFERENTIAL DIAGNOSIS

- Atrial fibrillation
- Atrial tachycardia
- Supraventricular tachycardia:
  1. Atrioventricular node reentry
  2. Orthodromic reciprocating tachycardia (using a concealed bypass tract)
  3. Junctional ectopic tachycardia
  4. Wolff-Parkinson-White syndrome
- Sinus tachycardia

WORKUP

ECG (Fig. 3)
Laboratory evaluation
Assessment of CHA_2DS_2-VaSc score (Table 2)

LABORATORY TESTS

- Thyroid function studies
- Serum electrolytes, including renal and hepatic tests (anticipating antiarrhythmic therapy use)
- CBC and PT/INR values (anticipating anticoagulation therapy)

IMAGING STUDIES

- ECG:
  1. Absence of P waves.
  2. Typical CTI flutter has a regular, "sawtooth," or "F" (flutter) wave pattern without an isoelectric baseline in leads II, III, and aVF. There is discordance of the polarity of the flutter waves between the inferior leads and V1.
  3. There is rarely 1:1 atrioventricular (AV) conduction in atrial flutter (unless preexcitation is present, or patient is on an antiarrhythmic drug). Rather, AV conduction is usually in a 2:1 (see Fig. E1), 3:1, or 4:1 fashion, with corresponding usual ventricular rates of 150, 100, or 75 beats/min, respectively (assuming an atrial rate of 300 beats/min). With high vagal tone or AV block, ventricular rates may be slow in atrial flutter.

- Holter monitoring or event recorder to assess for presence of paroxysmal atrial flutter or to identify the arrhythmia if symptoms are nonspecific. These monitors can also identify triggering events, as well as rate control during tachycardia.
- Echocardiography (for new diagnoses) to evaluate for structural heart disease (atrial enlargement, left and right ventricular size, thickness, and function; atrial size, and valve function)
- Transesophageal echocardiography: Consider in the setting of cardioversion in the absence of an appropriate duration of anticoagulation to ascertain the absence of intracardiac (e.g., left atrial appendage) thrombi
- Electrophysiologic studies: Required for a precise diagnosis and for ablation
- Pulmonary vascular imaging (e.g., a CT scan with contrast) if a pulmonary embolism is suspected

Rx TREATMENT

ACUTE Rx OF UNSTABLE PATIENT

- Treatment choices are based on clinical circumstances. Fig. 4 describes an acute treatment of atrial flutter algorithm.[2] Table 3 summarizes atrial flutter therapy.
- In cases of electrocardiographic uncertainty, atrial flutter may be differentiated from SVT through vagal maneuvers that slow AV conduction (e.g., the Valsalva maneuver, carotid sinus massage) or the use of adenosine. These interventions may reveal flutter waves and help with a diagnosis, but they will not terminate atrial flutter.
- Direct current cardioversion is the treatment of choice for unstable patients. This may be successful with energies as low as 25 joules, but because 100 joules is virtually always successful, this may be a reasonable initial shock strength. If the electrical shock results in atrial fibrillation, a second shock at a higher energy level is used to restore normal sinus rhythm. Sedation of a conscious patient is highly recommended. After cardioversion, patients will need anticoagulation for at least 1 mo due to resultant atrial stunning from the presence of atrial flutter. Subsequent anticoagulation will depend on their stroke risk (CHA_2DS_2-VASc score; Table 2).
- Overdrive pacing in the atrium may also terminate atrial flutter. This method is especially useful in patients who have recently undergone cardiac surgery and still have temporary

atrial pacing wires and in patients who have an implanted pacemaker or defibrillator with an atrial lead.

ACUTE Rx OF STABLE PATIENT

- Proceed with either rate control or rhythm control strategy. Data are inconclusive on which strategy is more effective, but in general, atrial flutter is more difficult to rate-control than atrial fibrillation. Rhythm control is recommended in patients with debilitating symptoms or those who fail attempts at rate control. Atrial flutter may spontaneously convert to normal sinus rhythm with rate control strategy.
- For a rate control strategy: First-line agents are calcium channel blockers and beta-blockers. Digoxin and amiodarone may be used in those with borderline hypotension, decompensated congestive heart failure, and those unable to tolerate first-line agents.
- Avoid calcium channel blockers if known EF <40%.
- Digoxin has a narrow therapeutic window, and thus caution is recommended in patients with kidney impairment.
- Amiodarone use is typically a rhythm control agent but also has utility in rate control. It carries the risk of cardioverting a patient not on anticoagulation.
- A rhythm control strategy can be employed using either electrical or pharmacologic cardioversion.
- While electrical cardioversion is often successful, its effects are not durable. The rate of recurrence of atrial flutter with cardioversion alone is difficult to determine because most published data combine atrial flutter with atrial fibrillation. However, the recurrence rate is substantial, perhaps 50% at 1 yr.
- For pharmacologic cardioversion, intravenous ibutilide is a first-line medication in patients with normal systolic function and QT intervals. The success rate is approximately 60%, and it is more effective than procainamide, sotalol, or amiodarone. Oral flecainide (300 mg once) or oral propafenone (600 mg) may be used as well. Cardiac telemetry monitoring is required for 4 to 6 h after giving antiarrhythmic

TABLE 2 CHA_2DS_2-VASc Risk Score for Prediction of Stroke Risk in Atrial Fibrillation

Risk Factor	Points
CHF/LV dysfunction	1
Hypertension	1
Age ≥75 yr	2
Diabetes mellitus	1
Stroke/TIA/embolism	2
Vascular disease	1
Age 64-74 yr	1
Sex category (female)	1
Maximum score	9

CHF, Congestive heart failure; *LV*, left ventricular; *TIA*, transient ischemic attack.

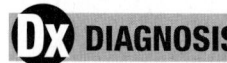

FIG. 3 Rhythm strip of atrial flutter. (From Cameron P: *Textbook of adult emergency medicine*, ed 5, Philadelphia, 2020, Elsevier.)

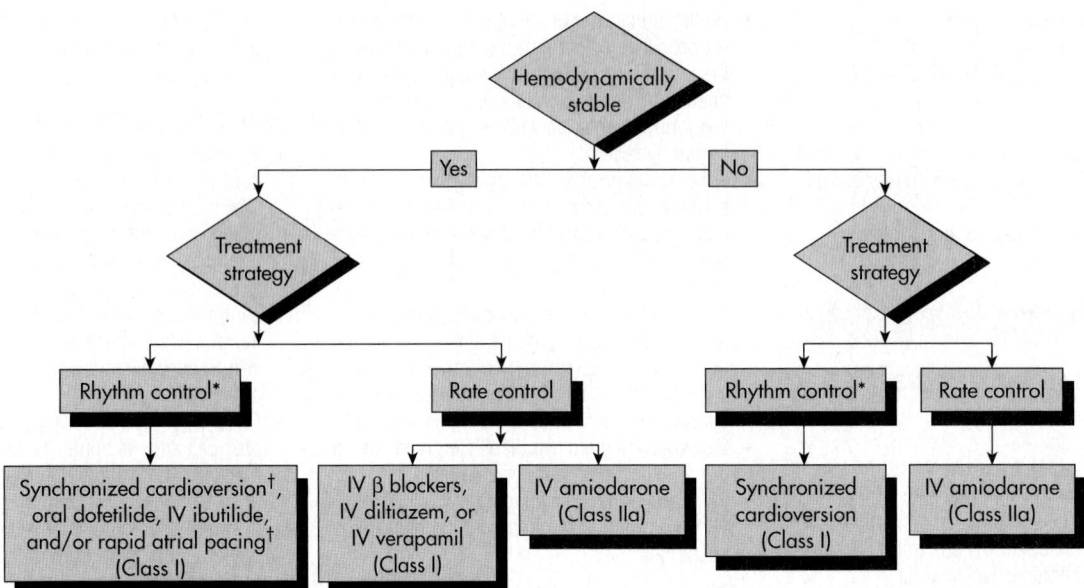

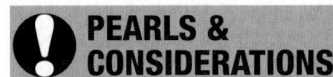

FIG. 4 Acute treatment of atrial flutter. *Anticoagulation as per guideline is mandatory. †For rhythms that break or recur spontaneously, synchronized cardioversion, or rapid atrial pacing is not appropriate. *IV*, Intravenous. (Reproduced with permission from Page RL et al: 2015 ACC/AHA/HRS guideline for the management of adult patients with supraventricular tachycardia, *JACC* 67[13]:e27-e115, 2016. In Olshansky B et al: *Arrhythmia essentials*, ed 2, Philadelphia, 2017, Elsevier.)

medications at these doses in patients receiving this therapy for the first time.

- Anticoagulation should be considered and initiated as discussed in the next section. Patients undergoing a rhythm control strategy may need prolonged anticoagulation or a TEE before cardioversion to rule out an intracardiac thrombus.

CHRONIC Rx

- Chronic treatment of atrial flutter is indicated to prevent symptoms and adverse remodeling of the heart (arrhythmia induced cardiomyopathy, AIC). This may either be in the form of a rate or rhythm control strategy although the latter is preferred because successful rhythm control can be achieved in >90% of cases through catheter ablation.
- Radiofrequency ablation is often offered as treatment for recurrent episodes of typical atrial flutter, but it is also highly effective for initial episodes. It has been shown to improve health-related quality of life.
- In those patients who fail, opt not to, or are not candidates for catheter ablation, electrical cardioversion followed by pharmacologic therapy to maintain sinus rhythm may be considered.
- Elective outpatient cardioversion or ablation can be performed either immediately preceded by transesophageal echocardiography (TEE) to evaluate the left atrium and the left atrial appendage for thrombus or after a period of at least 3 wk of documented therapeutic anticoagulation. At least 4 wk of anticoagulation should be administered after cardioversion or ablation, if not longer, depending on the overall thromboembolic risk of the patient as determined by the CHA_2DS_2-VASc score.
- Pharmacologic options to maintain sinus rhythm include dofetilide, amiodarone, flecainide, propafenone, or sotalol. The choice of antiarrhythmic therapy is dictated by the presence or

absence of underlying structural heart disease and other comorbidities (i.e., coronary artery disease, renal impairment, etc.). It is important to keep in mind that antiarrhythmic drugs carry the risk of toxicity and can also be proarrhythmic.

- In addition to rate or rhythm control of atrial flutter, stroke risk mitigation is also a vital part of atrial flutter management. Prophylactic anticoagulation should be addressed depending on stroke risk, guided by the CHA_2DS_2-VASc score. Antithrombotic therapy is recommended based on the same guidelines as in atrial fibrillation.[3] Anticoagulation should be considered for patients whose CHA_2DS_2-VASc score is ≥2 in men or ≥3 in women. Options for oral anticoagulants include warfarin (target INR 2-3) or direct oral anticoagulants (DOACs, e.g., dabigatran, rivaroxaban, apixaban, or edoxaban), although the latter is now recommended over the former (except for cases of moderate to severe mitral stenosis or mechanical heart valves). For patients with a CHA_2DS_2-VASc score of 1 (men) or 2 (women), prescribing an oral anticoagulant to reduce stroke risk may be considered (previous recommendation for aspirin was removed).[4] Left atrial appendage closure may also be an option in patients at high risk for bleeding with anticoagulation.
- Long-term anticoagulation after a successful flutter ablation should be a shared decision between patient and provider.

DISPOSITION

More than 85% of patients convert to regular sinus rhythm after cardioversion. Ablation success rates exceed 90%.

REFERRAL

Refer patients who are being considered for rhythm control of atrial flutter to a cardiac electrophysiologist, especially patients who are candidates for radiofrequency ablation.

❗ PEARLS & CONSIDERATIONS

COMMENTS

- The surface ECG is the best tool for recognizing atrial flutter and distinguishing atrial flutter from atrial fibrillation. The inferior leads (II, III, aVF) are the best for seeing the characteristic sawtooth pattern and V1 discordance can help identify typical atrial flutter.
- Ablation for typical atrial flutter is highly effective, straightforward, and relatively safe. It should be considered for patients with recurrent episodes and even for a first-ever episode.
- Patients with atrial flutter carry a significant risk for subsequent development of atrial fibrillation.
- Anticoagulation should be considered for all patients whose CHA_2DS_2-VASc score is ≥2 (men) or ≥3 (women). For patients with a CHA_2DS_2-VASc score of 1 (men) or 2 (women), risks and benefits should be considered on an individual basis. Long-term anticoagulation after successful flutter ablation should be a shared decision between patient and provider.
- Although anticoagulation recommendations for atrial flutter are identical to those for atrial fibrillation, studies suggest that the absolute risk of stroke is lower from atrial flutter than from fibrillation.

RELATED CONTENT

Atrial Flutter (Patient Information)
Atrial Fibrillation (Related Key Topic)

REFERENCES

Available at eBooks.Health.Elsevier.com.

AUTHORS: **EITAN S. FRANKEL, MD** and **DANIEL R. FRISCH, MD**

TABLE 3 Atrial Flutter Therapy	
Acute therapy for poorly tolerated AFL or continuous rapid ventricular rate	• If prolonged (i.e., >48-72 h), anticoagulation is required as cardioversion may be associated with thromboembolic risk. Anticoagulation guidelines for cardioversion are the same as for atrial fibrillation and may indicate need for a TEE for prolonged episodes. Adenosine and carotid massage can be used to help diagnose AFL masquerading as sinus rhythm. • First line: Electrical cardioversion under sedation with anticoagulation as necessary. Consider the length of the episode. • Second line: Ibutilide or procainamide may be attempted for conversion before electrical cardioversion attempts. Ibutilide may be 60%-70% effective if AFL has been present for <48 h. • Alternative: Rapid atrial pacing (esophageal, epicardial, or endocardial, depending on the situation). To pace terminate, pace for 10-15 sec at a rate of 10%-20% faster than rate of flutter. If ineffective, burst pace 10 beats/min faster at a time for 10-15 sec at a time until conversion to AF or sinus rhythm. When AF occurs, it is usually short lived and terminates spontaneously within 24 h. If persistent, electrical cardioversion can be attempted with or without antiarrhythmic drugs. Atrial fibrillation cannot be pace terminated. However, slower AFL (rate <350 bpm) of any flutter wave morphology can often be pace terminated. • Oral drug loading alone to terminate AFL is rarely useful. • If recurrent episodes, use class IC or III antiarrhythmic drugs until steady state is achieved, then attempt cardioversion. These drugs (particularly 1C drugs) may stabilize the flutter circuit. It may also create another form of AFL—"1C" AFL—from AF. Ablation remains first-line therapy, especially if AFL is isthmus dependent. • Consider ablation for cases of AFL. However, despite AFL ablation, AF may occur, especially in individuals with underlying structural heart disease. • AV nodal ablation, although not preferable, could be considered when ventricular rate control cannot be achieved and flutter cannot be ablated (e.g., in the presence of a left atrial appendage clot), or if symptomatic, refractory, and/or if associated with tachycardia-induced cardiomyopathy. This option may be considered in cases where individuals have multiple forms of nonablatable AFL or AF and especially for those who do have nonisthmus-dependent AFL.
Chronic prevention	• Consider radiofrequency catheter ablation early; it has become first-line therapy. • Drug therapy alone for pure AFL flutter is usually not effective. • If drug therapy is chosen, be guided by the presence/absence of structural heart disease. • If structural heart disease without CHF: Sotalol (often initiated in the hospital), dofetilide, amiodarone. • If structural heart disease with CHF: Amiodarone, dofetilide. • If no structural heart disease: Propafenone, flecainide, sotalol, dofetilide, or amiodarone, but propafenone or flecainide may need concomitant AV nodal blocking drugs to prevent 1:1 conduction. • If class I or III drugs are used, first control the ventricular response rate with an AV nodal blocking drug. Otherwise, the vagolytic effects of class IA drugs can enhance AV nodal conduction, and both 1A and 1C drugs can lead to AFL with 1:1 AV conduction.
Nonresponders with severe symptoms	• If typical AFL, radiofrequency ablation within the cavotricuspid isthmus is highly effective. • Atypical AFL is more difficult to ablate and depends on the location of reentrant circuit. Success rates are lower than that for typical AFL. It is more difficult when there is congenital heart disease, valve disease, or prior surgery in which significant areas of scar are present. • Ventricular rate control, antiarrhythmic drugs, or AV node ablation (less preferable) can be performed for atypical, nonablatable AFL. • If AV node ablation and pacing is performed and AFL is intermittent, mode-switching function should be programmed "ON."
MI	• If hemodynamic intolerance or ongoing refractory myocardial ischemia, emergent cardioversion. AFL may increase MVO2 due to rapid ventricular rate, causing further ischemia, diastolic dysfunction, and pulmonary congestion and edema. • If recurrent, IV amiodarone or procainamide. • Consider temporary antitachycardia pacing if recurrent and poorly tolerated.
Preoperative	• For cardiac surgery, convert AFL to NSR if adequate anticoagulation has been achieved, or ensure that ventricular response is well controlled. • If surgery is elective and AFL is chronic, antiarrhythmic drugs or catheter ablation may be considered. However, anticoagulation should be continued at least 4 wk after conversion of longer-term (>48 h) AFL prior to elective surgery. • For more urgent surgery in which anticoagulation cannot be used, consider rate control without cardioversion. • For short-duration (<48 h) AFL, DCC can be performed (may consider therapeutic anticoagulation before electrical cardioversion with surgical consultation as to risk).
Postoperative	• AFL occurs in 10%-20% of all patients after cardiac surgery; it typically occurs with AF. Incidence peaks at days 2-3. It is more common in older patients. It rarely occurs after other types of surgery. The AFL may resolve spontaneously; however, the rhythm can increase the length of hospital stay, exacerbate heart failure, slow the recovery process, and cause symptoms. • Control rate with β-adrenergic blocker if no CHF or bronchospastic disease and LVEF >40%. Diltiazem is often successful as a second-line drug, but use with caution in patients with a reduced LVEF. Digoxin for rate control is less effective but may be considered, particularly in patients with poor LV function. • IV amiodarone may be useful for persistent and poorly tolerated AFL; amiodarone or other antiarrhythmic drugs may be helpful for recurrent episodes. • Electrical cardioversion or atrial pace termination (if atrial pacing leads are present) is often successful, especially when employed early after the AFL onset. • Discontinue inotropic drugs, if possible.

AF, Atrial fibrillation; *AFL,* atrial flutter; *AV,* atrioventricular; *CHF,* congestive heart failure; *DCC,* direct current cardioversion; *IV,* intravenous; *LV,* left ventricle; *LVEF,* left ventricular ejection fraction; *MI,* myocardial infarction; *MVO₂,* myocardial oxygen consumption; *NSR,* normal sinus rhythm; *TEE,* transesophageal echocardiography.
From Olshansky B et al: *Arrhythmia essentials,* ed 2, Philadelphia, 2017, Elsevier.

BASIC INFORMATION

DEFINITION

Attention-deficit/hyperactivity disorder (ADHD) is a chronic disorder of two core symptoms: inattention and/or hyperactivity or impulsivity. Symptoms manifest in childhood, last at least 6 mo (persistent pattern), and cause functional impairment in multiple settings (e.g., school, home, with friends).[1,2] The diagnostic keys for ADHD are described in Table 1.

SYNONYMS

Hyperactivity
Attention deficit disorder (ADD)
Attention deficit disorder with hyperactivity
Attention deficit syndrome with hyperactivity
ADHD

ICD-10CM CODES
F90.0	Attention-deficit/hyperactivity disorder, predominantly inattentive type
F90.1	Attention-deficit/hyperactivity disorder, predominantly hyperactive/impulsive type
F90.2	Attention-deficit/hyperactivity disorder, combined type
F90.8	Attention-deficit/hyperactivity disorder, other type
F90.9	Attention-deficit/hyperactivity disorder, unspecified type

DSM-5-TR CODES
314.00	Predominantly inattentive presentation
314.01	Predominantly hyperactive-impulsive presentation

EPIDEMIOLOGY & DEMOGRAPHICS

PREVALENCE: 9% to 15% of school-age children (most prevalent neurodevelopmental disorder among children); up to 14% of adolescents and 3% to 5% of adults.[3,4] Children from families with low socioeconomic status and children with public insurance are diagnosed with ADHD at higher rates than their peers.

PREDOMINANT SEX: Among children, male predominance with ratio of 4:1 for the predominantly hyperactive type and 2:1 for the predominantly inattentive type.[5] Among adults, ratio is closer to 1:1 (sex difference may reflect referral bias).

PREDOMINANT AGE: Some symptoms must occur before age 12. Symptoms (especially hyperactivity symptoms) tend to diminish with age. Up to 80% continue to meet criteria in adolescence, and an estimated 35% to 65% have some symptoms in adulthood.[5]

PEAK INCIDENCE: Diagnosis is usually first made in school-age children (6 to 9 yr).

RISK FACTORS: Possible risk factors include in utero tobacco/alcohol/illicit substance exposure or hypoxia, low birth weight, prematurity, genetics, lead exposure (though most children with elevated lead levels do not develop ADHD), sleep deficiency, head trauma in young children, family dysfunction, low socioeconomic status.[6,7] Evidence supports possible association between dietary factors (e.g., refined sugar; food additives; food sensitivity; fatty acid, iron, and zinc deficiencies) and ADHD in a small percentage of patients. Two mechanisms have been described: Sensitivity to refined sugar and/or functional reactive hypoglycemia after sugar intake (release of stress hormones such as adrenaline).[8,9] A causal link between environmental toxins and ADHD has not been clearly established.

Up to 64% of children and adolescents with ADHD have comorbid neurodevelopmental and psychiatric disorders, such as autism-spectrum disorders (ASD), oppositional defiant disorder (ODD), depression, anxiety, and learning disabilities.[10]

GENETICS: Strong polygenetic component. First-degree relatives of patients with ADHD have 2 to 6× greater risk of ADHD relative to controls. Studies suggest potential involvement of several genes, including those associated with serotonin and glutamate transporters as well as dopamine metabolism, in addition to neuronal development. Genome-wide association studies suggest significant single nucleotide polymorphism (SNP) heritability in ADHD. SNPs can be used to create polygenic scores to predict risk of traits or identify symptoms, although currently this is only done in the research realm.[11,12]

NEUROANATOMY: Compared to non-ADHD children, those with ADHD have been found to have reductions in cerebral (smaller prefrontal cortex, reduced thickness of anterior cingulate cortex, bilateral corticofrontal thinning) and cerebellar volume, and increased gray matter in the posterior temporal and inferior parietal regions.[13,14] Functional brain imaging has evidenced those with ADHD have reduced global and local activation in the basal ganglia and anterior frontal lobe.[15] These deficits correlate with neuropsychiatric testing and suggest that patients with ADHD have impaired executive function and difficulties with response inhibition.[10]

PHYSICAL FINDINGS & CLINICAL PRESENTATION

- Three types:
  1. Predominantly inattentive: Difficulty organizing, planning, remembering, concentrating, starting/completing tasks; symptoms may not be present during preferred activities
  2. Predominantly hyperactive/impulsive: Restless, excessive fidgetiness, talkative, disruptive/intrusive, disinhibited, impatient
  3. Combined
- Usually diagnosed in elementary school when achievement is compromised, and behavioral problems are not tolerated. Children with academic underproductivity, problems with peer and family relations, or discipline issues are often referred for evaluation. Of the more than 6 million children in the U.S. who have ADHD, most have comorbid conditions (see the following) and nearly half use special education and mental health services.
- In adults, motoric hyperactivity is less common, but restlessness, edginess, and difficulty relaxing are often seen. Disorganization and difficulty completing tasks are other common complaints.
- Small differences in the structure and functioning of the brain are seen on neuroimaging, but these differences cannot be used to diagnose ADHD.

ETIOLOGY

Strongest evidence exists for genetic inheritance. Other theories include abnormal metabolism of brain catecholamines, delayed maturation of cerebral cortex, altered reward processing, and disrupted default mode network, as well as environmental factors (see earlier).[10] Catecholamine metabolism appears to play a role in ADHD pathogenesis, as noradrenergic pathways modulate higher cortical and executive functions, including attention, alertness, and vigilance.[10,16] Studies have also shown norepinephrine and dopamine systems in the prefrontal cortex contributing to the pathogenesis of ADHD.[10]

DX **DIAGNOSIS**

Diagnostic criteria for ADHD include symptoms of hyperactivity, impulsivity, and/or inattention that affect function and are present in more than one setting (e.g., academic, emotional, social). Diagnostic evaluation includes comprehensive medical, developmental, and psychosocial history.[1,2]

DIFFERENTIAL DIAGNOSIS

- Medical: Visual/hearing impairment, seizure disorder, head injury, sleep disorder, medication interactions, thyroid abnormalities, lead toxicity, movement disorders
- Psychiatric: Intellectual disability, specific learning disorder, autism spectrum disorder/development delay, major depressive disorder, bipolar disorder, disruptive mood dysregulation disorder, anxiety, obsessive-compulsive disorder, oppositional defiant disorder, intermittent explosive disorder, conduct disorder, posttraumatic stress disorder, reactive attachment disorder, and substance abuse disorder

---

TABLE 1 Diagnostic Keys for Attention-Deficit/Hyperactivity Disorder

1. Inattention
   a. Careless mistakes in schoolwork, work, or other activities
   b. Seems not to listen when spoken to directly
   c. Poor follow-through on schoolwork or chores
   d. Difficulty organizing
   e. Easily distracted by extraneous stimuli and is forgetful
2. Hyperactivity
   a. Trouble sitting still
   b. May act as if "driven by a motor"
   c. May talk excessively
3. Impulsivity
   a. Trouble holding back in class
   b. Trouble taking turns
   c. Interrupts

- Psychosocial: Mismatch of learning environment with ability, family dysfunction, abuse/neglect

WORKUP

- Clinical interview should include assessment of symptoms and have an impact on work/school and relationships; developmental history; personal and family psychiatric history, including substance abuse; social history, including family dysfunction; medical history, including personal or family history of cardiac conditions.
- Physical examination should be performed to investigate medical causes for symptoms, coexisting conditions, and contraindications to treatment. Special focus should be paid to evaluation of dysmorphic features, neurologic examination (including hearing and vision), and assessment for neurocutaneous findings.
- Information from collateral sources (parents, partners, teachers) is crucial to diagnosis. Many patients will not display symptoms during an office visit and may underreport or overreport symptoms.
- Self-rating scales and standardized symptom-specific questionnaires from collateral sources can help diagnose and assess response to treatment. The use of ADHD-specific rating scales over broader behavioral rating scales is associated with improved sensitivity and specificity.
- Laboratory or imaging studies should be undertaken only if indicated by history or physical examination.
- The FDA has approved a quantitative electroencephalogram test to aid in the diagnosis of ADHD in children, but sufficient evidence to support its routine use is lacking.
- Ancillary testing (e.g., neuropsychologic testing, including verbal and performance IQ/achievement testing and language evaluation, and mental health assessment) may be indicated based on clinical findings and may require referral.

Rx TREATMENT

NONPHARMACOLOGIC THERAPY

- The majority of studies comparing the efficacy of pharmacologic vs nonpharmacologic interventions demonstrate the superiority of pharmacologic treatments. Proposed interventions have included restrictive or elimination diets, artificial food color exclusions, free fatty acid supplementation, cognitive training, neurofeedback, and focused behavioral interventions, but these are not routinely recommended.[9,10]
- Studies on combined treatments have not shown significant improvements in core ADHD symptoms when behavioral treatments are added to stimulant medications. However, improvements in related areas such as parent-child relations, aggressiveness, teacher-rated social skills, and reaching achievement have been seen in combined treatment groups.[17]

- Prevailing opinion favors a multimodal approach in which nonpharmacologic behavioral therapies including parent-child behavioral therapy and social skills training can be used to target comorbid conditions or behaviors that have not responded to medication.
- Behavioral therapy/interventions alone are often considered when children are under 6 yr, symptoms and impairment are mild, if parents are opposed to or patients cannot tolerate medications, or if there is uncertainty or disagreement about the diagnosis (e.g., between parents and teachers).[17]
- Behavioral interventions (e.g., goal setting and rewards systems) show short-term efficacy and are endorsed by most national organizations. Time management and organizational skills appear useful. Social skills training may also be useful.
- Educational interventions are recommended. Children with ADHD are entitled to reasonable educational accommodations under a 504 Plan or the Individuals with Disabilities Education Act.
- Many support and advocacy groups provide education and other resources (e.g., Children and Adolescents with ADHD, National ADD Association, American Academy of Child and Adolescent Psychiatry).
- Psychotherapy such as cognitive therapy, play therapy, or insight-oriented therapy are unlikely to be useful in addressing the core symptoms of ADHD.[17]
- Digital therapeutics are emerging for the treatment of ADHD. One digital therapeutic, delivered through a video game format, has been approved by the FDA for treatment of ADHD.

ACUTE GENERAL Rx

- A 2021 meta-analysis of 29 studies evaluating the relative cost-effectiveness of pharmacologic and nonpharmacologic therapy in ADHD revealed strong cost-effectiveness for both interventions relative to placebo, with good evidence supporting a benefit for pharmacologic therapy in children and adolescents.[18]
- Most studies on treatment of ADHD are performed in children. Very few data exist that examine the effectiveness of pharmacologic vs nonpharmacologic therapies in adults throughout the life span.
- Mainstay of treatment is stimulant medication. Second-line therapies include antidepressants and alpha-agonists. Table 2 summarizes FDA-approved treatments for ADHD.[10]
- Stimulants:
  1. Release or block uptake of dopamine and norepinephrine.
  2. Include short- and long-acting methylphenidate, dextroamphetamine, and dextroamphetamine/amphetamine combinations (mixed amphetamine salts). A methylphenidate patch (Daytrana) is available, as is a pro-drug form of dextroamphetamine, lisdexamfetamine (Vyvanse), which is designed to limit the abuse potential. A long-acting oral suspension of methylphenidate (Quillivant XR), a long-acting chewable

tablet of methylphenidate (QuilliChew ER), a long-acting orally disintegrating tablet of mixed amphetamine preparation (Adzenys XR-ODT), and a long-acting liquid amphetamine preparation (Dyanavel XR) are also available. A fixed dose combination (Azstarys) of the stimulant dexmethylphenidate and the prodrug serdexmethylphenidate is a newer FDA approved once-daily treatment of ADHD in patients ≥6 yr.
  3. All stimulants are equally effective; however, not all patients improve with stimulants. Patients who do not respond well to one stimulant may respond to another.
  4. Do not cause euphoria or lead to addiction when taken as directed. However, selective norepinephrine reuptake inhibitors (atomoxetine, viloxazine; see below) should be considered as alternatives to stimulants in patients with a history of substance use disorders or those for whom a concern for diversion is warranted.
  5. Improve cognition, inattention, impulsiveness/hyperactivity, and driving skills. Limited impact on academic performance, learning, and emotional problems.
  6. Side effects are usually mild, reversible, and dose dependent, including anorexia, weight loss, sleep disturbances, increased heart rate and blood pressure, irritability, moodiness, headache, onset or worsening of motor tics, reduction of growth velocity (but not adult height). Do not worsen seizures in patients on adequate anticonvulsant therapy. Rebound of symptoms can occur with withdrawal of medication.
  7. Stimulants are associated with an increased risk of cardiovascular events and death. Patients should be carefully evaluated for cardiovascular disease before beginning therapy and be periodically monitored, including blood pressure checks, while they are treated. However, despite concerns regarding cardiovascular risk, these medications are generally safe. Recent studies have shown that among young and middle-aged adults, current or new use of ADHD medications, compared with nonuse or remote use, is not associated with an increased risk of serious cardiovascular events. Routine, pretreatment screening with ECGs is not currently recommended by the American Academy of Pediatrics or the American Academy of Child and Adolescent Psychiatry.
  8. There are reports of psychotic or manic symptoms (particularly hallucinations) associated with stimulant use in children and adolescents, emerging in <1% of treated children (1 in 400 to 1 in 600).
  9. Prenatal exposure to methylphenidate or amphetamines does not appear to be associated with overall increase in risk of major malformations. However, both have been associated with cardiac malformation with borderline statistically significant findings and low overall absolute risk.
- Atomoxetine (Strattera):
  1. Selective norepinephrine reuptake inhibitor.

TABLE 2	Select FDA-Approved Treatments for Attention-Deficit Hyperactivity Disorder			
Generic Name	**Brand Name**	**Formulations and Strengths**	**Duration of Behavioral Effect (h)**	**Comments**
Amphetamines				
D-amphetamine	Dexedrine	Tablets: 5, 10 mg	3-6	
	Dexedrine Spansule	Spansules: 5, 10, 15 mg		
	ProCentra	Oral solution: 5 mg/5 ml		
Mixed amphetamine/ dextroamphetamine	Adderall	Tablets: 5, 7.5, 10, 12.5, 15, 20, 30 mg	4-6	
	Adderall XR	Capsules: 5, 10, 15, 20, 25, 30 mg	8-10	Capsule with 1:1 ratio of IR to DR beads
	Evekeo	Tablets: 5, 10 mg	10	Racemic amphetamine sulfate, 1:1 D-amphetamine and L-amphetamine
	Dyanavel	Oral suspension: 2.5 mg/ml	8-13	Shake the bottle before administering the dose
Lisdexamfetamine dimesylate	Vyvanse	Capsules: 20, 30, 40, 50, 60, 70 mg	8-12	Inactive prodrug in which L-lysine is chemically bonded to D-amphetamine
Methylphenidates				
Methylphenidate	Ritalin	Tablets: 5, 10, 20 mg	3-4	
	Methylin	Tablets, chewable: 2.5, 5, 10 mg	3-4	
		Oral solution: 5 mg/5 ml, 10 mg/5 ml (500 ml)	3-4	
	Ritalin LA	Capsules: 10, 20, 30, 40 mg	8-9	Capsule with 1:1 ratio of IR beads to DR beads
	Metadate ER	Tablets: 10, 20 mg	5-8	
	Metadate CD	Capsules: 10, 20, 30 mg	8-9	Capsule with 3:7 ratio of IR beads to DR beads
	Concerta	Tablets: 18, 27, 36, 54 mg	8-12	Ascending profile, OROS technology
	Daytrana	Transdermal patch: 10, 15, 20, 30 mg/9 h	9	Delivery rate of 1.1, 1.6, 2.2, 3.3 mg/h for the patches, respectively, based on 9-h wear times in patients ages 6-12 yr
	Quillivant XR	Oral suspension: 25 mg/5 ml	8-12	Shake the bottle before administering the dose
	QuilliChew ER	Chewable tablets: 20, 30, 40 mg	8	
	Aptensio XR	Capsules: 10, 15, 20, 30, 40, 50, 60 mg	9-12	May be swallowed or opened and contents mixed into food
	Adhansia XR	Capsules: 25, 35, 45, 55, 70, 85 mg	IR portion: 1.5-2.5 DR portion: 8.5-16	IR layer with 20% of dose, controlled release layer with 80%
Dexmethylphenidate	Focalin	Tablets: 2.5, 5, 10 mg	IR: 0.5-4 XR: 6.5-12	d-Threo-enantiomer of methylphenidate, twice as potent as racemic methylphenidate; XR capsule contains IR component
	Focalin XR	Capsules: 5, 10, 20 mg		
Nonstimulant Medications				
Atomoxetine	Strattera	Capsules: 10, 18, 25, 40, 60, 80, 100 mg		Steady state requires 4-6 wk to see effect
Guanfacine	Intuniv	Tablets: 1, 2, 3, 4 mg	8	
Clonidine	Kapvay	Tablets: 0.1, 0.2 mg	12-24	
Digital Therapeutics				
Digital Attention Treatment	EndeavorRx			Video game platform, improves attention

DR, Delayed-release; *IR,* immediate-release; *OROS,* osmotic-controlled release oral delivery system.
Adapted from Stern TA et al: *Massachusetts General Hospital handbook of general hospital psychiatry,* ed 7, Philadelphia, 2018, Elsevier.

2. Generally felt to be less effective than stimulants, but a useful alternative in patients who have not tolerated or responded to stimulants or in the setting of patient or family substance abuse. A 2021 meta-analysis of the relative cost-effectiveness of different pharmacologic therapies found that all stimulant medications had a relative advantage as compared to placebo with the exception of atomoxetine, which did not have robust data supporting its relative cost-effectiveness, adding further support to this medication being used primarily as second-line therapy. Additionally, atomoxetine was found in a large network meta-analysis of 81 studies to be inferior to both methylphenidate and amphetamine salts in clinician-rated scales of ADHD in a population of more than 10,000 children.[17-19]

3. Efficacy and safety of use beyond 2 yr of treatment have not been studied. There have been reports of behavioral abnormalities and increased suicidality in children and adolescents.

4. Side effects: Gastrointestinal upset, sleep disturbance, decreased appetite, dizziness,

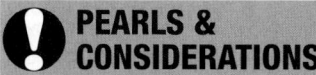

sexual side effects in men. Cardiovascular side effects have also been reported.

5. There have been rare reports of severe liver injury in adults and children.

- Antidepressants (bupropion, imipramine, desipramine, nortriptyline):
  1. May be useful in patients with coexisting psychiatric disorders
  2. Studies comparing efficacy versus stimulants are inconclusive
  3. Side effects: Arrhythmias, anticholinergic effects, lowering of seizure threshold, insomnia
- Alpha-2-adrenergic agonists (clonidine, guanfacine):
  1. Appear to be less effective than stimulants as a medication class, but may be used as an alternative therapy in cases of poor treatment response to stimulants or when side effects are intolerable (typically, sleep disturbances, irritability/aggression, overarousal).
  2. Extended-release formulations of guanfacine (Intuniv) and clonidine (Kapvay) have been approved by the FDA for treatment of ADHD in children ages 6 to 17 yr. A transdermal clonidine patch is also available.
  3. Potential side effects include sedation, fatigue, headache, bradycardia, hypotension, rebound hypertension, and depression.
- Use of medications, particularly stimulants (which are monitored under the Controlled Substance Act), requires frequent monitoring.
- Early initiation of pharmacologic therapy for ADHD has been shown to reduce the risk of comorbid psychiatric conditions in later life, with the strongest risk reduction in substance use disorders.[19]

- At this time, the FDA and the American Academy of Pediatrics recommend that direct-to-consumer pharmacogenetic tests should not be used to guide decision making regarding the safety, efficacy, or optimal dosing scheme of any medication for the treatment of ADHD.

DISPOSITION

- Although symptoms may change over time, for many patients ADHD represents a chronic condition that requires lifelong management. A 2021 meta-analysis of 12 high-quality studies revealed persistence of ADHD into adulthood in 43% of subjects.[19]
- A 2021 review of adult ADHD found that, for individuals for whom ADHD persisted from childhood to adulthood, 36% of subjects developed comorbid alcohol use disorder; 27% developed antisocial personality disorders; and 32% developed cannabis use disorder.[20]
- ADHD persisting into adulthood has been associated with an elevated relative risk of interaction with the criminal justice system, with a meta-analysis revealing 31% (CI 26% to 36%) of adult-persistent ADHD subjects experiencing conviction and/or jail time from criminal activity, largely attributable to comorbid substance use disorders.[19,20]
- Patients are at higher risk for academic underachievement, lower socioeconomic status, work and relationship difficulties, high-risk behavior, and psychiatric comorbidities.

REFERRAL

- Diagnosis complicated by difficult-to-treat comorbid neurodevelopmental and psychiatric disorders

- Lack of adequate response to stimulants/atomoxetine/alpha-adrenergic agents

⚠ PEARLS & CONSIDERATIONS

- The World Health Organization's Adult Self-Report Scale (ASRS) v1.1 has good sensitivity and adaptability to the primary care setting.
- ADHD has been associated with criminal behavior in some studies. Data analysis has shown that among patients with ADHD, rates of criminality are lower during periods when they receive ADHD medication.
- Recommendations for the diagnosis and management of ADHD have been published by the Centers for Disease Control and Prevention (http://www.cdc.gov/ncbddd/adhd/guidelines.html).

RELATED CONTENT

Attention Deficit Hyperactivity Disorder (ADHD) (Patient Information)

AUTHORS: **MARIA CAMILA VELEZ FLOREZ, MD** and **DANIEL CHAIT, MD, MEd**

REFERENCES

Available at eBooks.Health.Elsevier.com.

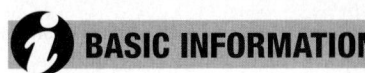

BASIC INFORMATION

DEFINITION

Autism spectrum disorder (ASD) is a neurodevelopmental syndrome that encompasses a continuum of developmental impairments in social communication and repetitive sensorimotor behaviors.

The diagnostic criteria for ASD can be found in the *Diagnostic and Statistical Manual of Mental Disorders,* Fifth Edition, Text Revision (DSM-5-TR) or the *International Classification of Diseases,* 11th Revision (ICD-11), both updated in 2022. Both frameworks include persistent impairment in several domains integral to social functioning, including language, nonverbal communication, social interactions, and repetitive and inflexible patterns of behavior, interests, or activities. Comorbid intellectual disability, neurologic and medical problems, and an increased risk of psychiatric disorders are frequently present; thus ASD diagnoses can be further characterized by the presence or absence of associated features, namely intellectual disability, language impairment, medical or genetic conditions, and catatonia.[1] Both core and associated features can vary dramatically among individuals, making ASD a highly heterogeneous syndrome.[2]

ASD has been strongly correlated with dozens of susceptibility genes, as well as both prenatal and perinatal risk factors. Despite advancements in our understanding of risk patterns, ongoing work is necessary to understand for whom, how, and when certain behavioral or pharmacologic treatments may be most efficacious. Overall, the prognosis of individuals with ASD has been improving as awareness, diagnostic accuracy, and treatments improve. Although most individuals with ASD will require additional supports and some may not be able to live independently, many are often able to integrate well into the community. Early intervention can be critical in ensuring that individuals with ASD can live without significant or debilitating symptoms in their lives.

SYNONYMS

ASD
Autism
Autistic disorder
Early infantile/child autism
Kanner autism
Asperger disorder
Pervasive developmental disorder (changed in ICD-11)

ICD-10CM CODE
F84.0   Autism spectrum disorder
DSM-5-TR CODE
299.00   Autism spectrum disorder

EPIDEMIOLOGY & DEMOGRAPHICS

INCIDENCE (IN U.S.): ASD afflicts an estimated 1% to 3% of children in the United States.

PREVALENCE (IN U.S.): Approximately 1 in 40 children.[3] Prevalence has risen over the past few decades; unclear if this trend is due to the inclusion of subthreshold cases, increased awareness of the disorder and diagnostic accuracy, or a true increase in the frequency of ASD.
PREDOMINANT SEX & AGE: Male:female ratio of ~3:1[4]
PEAK INCIDENCE: The majority of children with ASD are identified by age 4, generally for having failed to achieve developmental milestones for communication. However, gender as well as cognitive, linguistic, and adaptive functioning can affect ASD presentation and thus age of diagnosis.[3]
RISK FACTORS: Prenatal and perinatal risk factors for ASD include hypoxia-related obstetric complications, prenatal infections, maternal use of certain medications (e.g., valproic acid) during pregnancy, maternal health conditions (e.g., diabetes, hypertension, obesity, preeclampsia), advanced parental age, maternal multiparity, preterm birth, and congenital sensory deficits.[5,6] Other environmental factors include toxic exposures, such as significant exposure to air pollution (either during pregnancy or in the postnatal period) and heavy maternal smoking (≥20 cigarettes/day during pregnancy).[7]
GENETICS:
- ASD is highly heritable with an estimated heritability index of approximately 80%.[8]
- Concordance is estimated to be 13% for full siblings and dizygotic twins, and 59% for monozygotic twins.[8] Though the concordance rates for ASD vary widely across studies, they consistently increase with degree of relatedness.
- Polygenic and single nucleotide variants, copy number variants, tandem repeats, noncoding, and rare inherited variants have been identified.[9]
NEUROBIOLOGIC FACTORS: Neurobiologic studies (imaging, electrophysiology, autopsy) have demonstrated brain differences in ASD compared to non-ASD individuals. These include abnormal neural networks and different patterns of connectivity, cortical changes (e.g., enlargement of gray and white matter volumes), structural abnormalities (e.g., sulcal and gyral anatomy), and alternations in neurotransmitter systems such as serotonin and γ-aminobutyric-acid (GABA).[10,11]
ASSOCIATED CONDITIONS: Many neurodevelopmental conditions and genetic syndromes are comorbid with ASD. Approximately 20% to 50% of people with ASD have intellectual disability, 50% have attention-deficit/hyperactivity disorder (ADHD), 25% are associated with genetic syndromes, and 12% have epilepsy.[12] Table 1 includes many of the associated conditions and syndromes.[1-4,6,13]

PHYSICAL FINDINGS & CLINICAL PRESENTATION

- Common triad of marked impairment in social interactions (poor social-emotional reciprocity), impaired and atypical verbal and nonverbal communication, and repetitive and unusual behavior or play

- Marked impairment in the understanding and use of both verbal and nonverbal communication, including unchanging facial expression and lack of gestures during interactions
- Stereotypic behavior (e.g., hand flapping, body rocking) or language (e.g., echolalia)
- Perceptual hypersensitivity (i.e., auditory, tactile, olfactory, gustatory) and avoidance of novel stimuli; or perceptual hyposensitivity (e.g., abnormally high threshold for pain)
- Up to 20% of adolescents and adults with ASD display signs of catatonia

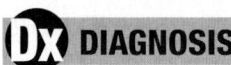 DIAGNOSIS

DIFFERENTIAL DIAGNOSIS

- Several psychiatric or neurodevelopmental disorders present with symptoms similar to those of ASD (e.g., ADHD, Tourette syndrome, selective mutism, catatonia, social phobia, obsessive/compulsive disorder, expressive language disorder, mixed receptive-expressive language disorder, stereotypic movement disorder, intellectual disability). Notable differences are present in age of onset and developmental trajectories.
- Social (pragmatic) communication disorder, introduced in DSM-5, is characterized by significant difficulties with verbal and nonverbal communication (but without restricted/repetitive interests and behaviors).
- Individuals with attachment disorders can present with language delays, cognitive delays, social difficulties, and stereotypies, often in the context of early childhood neglect.

WORKUP

- Gold standard includes assessments of detailed developmental history, family history, intellectual functioning, ASD symptomatology, and adaptive behaviors.
- The American Academy of Pediatrics (AAP) and the Centers for Disease Control and Prevention (CDC) recommend that all children be formally screened for ASD at 18 and 24 mo.

TABLE 1   Associated Conditions or Syndromes

Associated Conditions

Fragile X syndrome
Tuberous sclerosis
Angelman syndrome
Rett syndrome
Cohen syndrome
Cornelia de Lange syndrome
Neurofibromatosis type 1
Down syndrome
DiGeorge syndrome
Noonan syndrome
Klinefelter syndrome
Prader-Willi syndrome

- "Red flags" for critical delays in social communication development should be recognized and prompt evaluation for ASD (Table 2).
- Additional workup may include assessment of language functioning, neuropsychologic functioning, motor disorder evaluation, and psychiatric presentation.[14]
- Rule out underlying medical conditions, including genetic syndromes.

LABORATORY TESTS

- Phenylketonuria (PKU) screen (usually done at birth in the United States)
- Lead exposure screening
- School-based hearing screening may be sufficient in older children with ASDs and without significant language or learning deficits
- Karyotype, chromosome microarray analysis, and DNA testing
- Creatine kinase (CK) and thyroid-stimulating hormone (TSH) can be considered if there are motor concerns on physical examination

IMAGING STUDIES

- Electroencephalogram to diagnose coexisting seizure disorder if seizures are suspected or if language regression is present (e.g., Landau-Kleffner syndrome).
- Brain imaging is recommended if macrocephaly, microcephaly, or motor difficulties with increased tone are present on physical examination.[14]

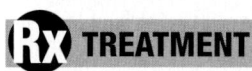 **TREATMENT**

NONPHARMACOLOGIC THERAPY

- Highly structured home and school environments
- Education for families and teachers. The Autism Speaks website may be helpful in this regard: https://www.autismspeaks.org

- Behavioral training program in both the home and school environments
- Special educational programs focused on language, communication, social, and life skills development (e.g., TEACCH)
- Applied behavioral analysis (ABA) (e.g., Discrete Trial Training)
- Applied Behavioral Analysis (ABA) procedures with social-emotional development (e.g., Pivotal Response Training, Floortime, Early Start Denver Model)
- Cognitive-behavioral therapy (CBT) has proven effective to ameliorate symptoms of anxiety in higher functioning individuals with ASD

ACUTE GENERAL Rx

- Only risperidone and aripiprazole are FDA-approved for the management of specific symptoms associated with ASD (i.e., irritability and aggression); many other medications are used off-label to target specific symptoms with varying degrees of evidence
- Obsessive or ritualistic behaviors: Selective serotonin reuptake inhibitors (SSRIs), atypical antipsychotics, valproic acid
- Aggression, irritability, self-injury: Atypical antipsychotics (e.g., risperidone, aripiprazole), alpha-2 agonists (e.g., clonidine), anticonvulsant mood stabilizers, opiate antagonist (self-injury only)
- Hyperactivity, impulsivity, inattention: Stimulants, alpha-2 agonists (e.g., clonidine), atypical antipsychotics
- Anxiety: SSRIs, buspirone, mirtazapine
- Mood lability: Valproic acid, carbamazepine, lithium, aripiprazole
- Depression: SSRIs, mirtazapine
- Catatonia: Use lorazepam and avoid antipsychotics, which can worsen catatonia; if unsuccessful, electroconvulsive therapy may be indicated

- Medications used to decrease specific symptoms associated with ASD are summarized in Table E3
- A placebo-controlled treatment of intranasal oxytocin therapy in children and adolescents with ASD showed no significant differences in measures of social or cognitive functioning over a period of 24 wk[15]

CHRONIC Rx

- Extended use of medications for acute management of comorbid psychiatric disorder
- Use of medications for comorbid medical conditions, including sleep problems and gastrointestinal (GI) problems
- Pharmacotherapy is palliative, not curative, for ASD

COMPLEMENTARY & ALTERNATIVE MEDICINE

- Preliminary evidence is available for effectiveness of melatonin in ameliorating sleep problems.[16]
- Very limited rigorous evidence is available on the effectiveness of complementary and alternative medicine, including nutritional interventions.[17]

DISPOSITION

- Most children will require some degree of assistance as adults.
- With early diagnosis and proper treatment/support, the prognosis for children without language and intellectual impairment is fair to very good despite lifelong symptoms.
- Best outcomes are associated with early identification and treatment, the development of oral communication skills, and the cognitive and behavioral capacity for inclusion in regular education settings with typically developing peers.
- Poorer outcomes include lack of joint attention by age 4, lack of functional speech by age 5, intellectual disability, seizures, comorbid medical or psychiatric syndromes, and pervasive lack of social relatedness.
- DSM-5-TR identifies qualifiers for three levels of severity to identify the magnitude of social and behavioral impairment and the support required to ensure the safety and well-being of the individual: Level 1 (requiring support), Level 2 (requiring substantial support), and Level 3 (requiring very substantial support).[2]

REFERRAL

Assistance may be needed in diagnosis (child psychiatrist, clinical psychologist, geneticist, pediatric neurologist, developmental pediatrician), symptom management (speech language pathologist, occupational therapist, behavioral therapist, clinical psychologist), parental teaching (clinical psychologist, psychiatric social worker), and intervention within the school system (educational advocate, attorney).

TABLE 2 Red Flags for Social Communication Development

Prompt evaluation should occur for any of the following:

No vocalizations by 6 mo: A parent should be able to have a reciprocal "conversation" by this age, consisting of at least several volleys back and forth.

No polysyllabic consonant babbling by 12 mo: At least some of these vocalizations should be directed at someone with communicative intent.

No gestures by 12 mo: The earliest gesture an infant learns is to raise his/her arms to request to be picked up, usually once sitting independently. Pointing should be with an isolated index finger, not the whole hand, and should be used "to request" or "to show," not just pointing at pictures in a book or pointing to have an adult label items. Any use of hand-over-hand by the child (e.g., putting a parent's hand on the cabinet door where the cookies are kept or using the parent's hand to point at pictures in a book) is a hallmark of ASD.

No spontaneous (not echoed) single words by 16 mo other than mama or dada: Spontaneous words must be beyond those used simply to label items and must be used by the child to communicate, to request, to show, or to share.

No spontaneous (not echoed) phrases by 24 mo or sentences by 36 mo: Spontaneous phrases and sentences must be used by the child to communicate, to request, to show, or to share.

Any loss of social communication abilities, including babbling, single words, phrases, response to name, social engagement, or gestures: If a parent reports their infant has decreased or stopped any social communication milestones, this is usually the hallmark of the onset of regression.

From Swaiman K et al: *Swaiman's pediatric neurology, principles and practice,* ed 6, Philadelphia, 2017, Elsevier.

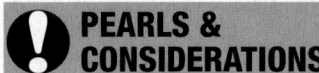

PEARLS & CONSIDERATIONS

- There is no scientific evidence of a relationship between childhood vaccination and the development of ASD.
- Evidence suggests that a disproportionate number of children with ASD suffer from a variety of medical problems, including sleep difficulties, GI problems, and oral health problems.
- Psychiatric comorbidities are very prominent across the life span, with estimated prevalence ranging from 40% to 70%.[13]

RELATED CONTENT

Autism (Patient Information)

AUTHORS: **ADRIANA CANTOS, MD** and **NICHOLAS OMID DANESHVARI, MD**

REFERENCES

Available at eBooks.Health.Elsevier.com

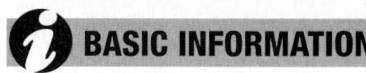
BASIC INFORMATION

DEFINITION

Autosomal dominant polycystic kidney disease (ADPKD) is the most common inherited form of kidney disease. ADPKD is a systemic, inherited disorder caused by sequence variations in the *PKD1* and *PKD2* genes in the majority of cases (approximately 93%). These sequence variations lead to fluid-filled cyst formation, proliferation, and growth in multiple organs, including the kidneys, liver, and pancreas. ADPKD is also associated with multiple gastrointestinal, connective tissue, and cardiovascular abnormalities.

SYNONYMS

Polycystic kidney disease
ADPKD
PKD
Hereditary polycystic kidney disease

ICD-10CM CODES	
Q61.3	Polycystic kidney, unspecified
Q61.2	Polycystic kidney, adult type
Q61.19	Other polycystic kidney, infantile type
Z82.71	Family history of polycystic kidney

EPIDEMIOLOGY & DEMOGRAPHICS

- Most common hereditary cause of chronic kidney disease (CKD) and end-stage renal disease (ESRD)
- Mendelian autosomal dominant disorder
- Each child of an affected parent has a 50% chance of inheriting a gene with sequence variations
- Affects all ethnic groups equally worldwide.
- ADPKD type 1: Approximately 78% of affected individuals with genetically resolved cases have a gene sequence variant located on chromosome 16 (*PKD1* gene).
- ADPKD type 2: Approximately 15% of affected individuals with genetically resolved cases have a gene sequence variant located on chromosome 4 (*PKD2* gene).
- ADPKD type 3: Increasing number of cases (nearly 7%) linked to gene sequence variations in the alpha glucosidase II gene *(GANAB)* located on chromosome 11q12.3.
- More recently, several additional gene variants have been identified that are associated with the ADPKD phenotype. These include *DNAJB11, ALG8, ALG9, ALG5,* and *IFT140.*
- Disease has 100% penetrance and does not skip generations.

INCIDENCE: ADPKD prevalence has been reported to be between 1 in 400 and 1 in 1000 live births, based on earlier studies from Denmark. The U.S. ADPKD prevalence has been reported in subsequent studies from Europe and Japan to be between 1 in 2525 and 1 in 4000. In a large diverse U.S. population, an estimated ADPKD prevalence of 42.6 per 100,000 persons was observed. Black and non-Hispanic White members had higher prevalence compared with Hispanic and Asian members. This cohort was established by an EHR-based approach.[1]

GENETICS: The majority of ADPKD cases stem from sequence variations in the *PKD1* gene, located on the short arm of chromosome 16. The gene encoding polycystin-1 protein (PC1) plays a vital role in cell-cell and cell-matrix interactions and primary ciliary function. Sequence variants of the *PKD1* gene lead to altered differentiation of epithelial cells and the abnormal phenotypic expression that characterizes ADPKD. ADPKD is less commonly (approximately 17%) caused by sequence variations in the *PKD2* gene, located on chromosome 4. The *PKD2* gene encodes the protein polycystin-2 (PC2) that is involved in intracellular calcium signaling. Patients with variants in *PKD2* typically have milder disease with later onset of hypertension, ESRD, and death. PC1 and PC2 form a single functional protein complex via interactions of their intracellular carboxy termini. Consequently, variants of either the *PKD1* or *PKD2* gene produce a similar phenotype that cannot be clinically distinguished.

8% of patients with ADPKD do not have either *PKD1* or *PKD2.* Other loci have been identified in patients with an ADPKD-like phenotype. Gene products of *GANAB, DNAJB11, AG5, AG8,* and *AG9* are involved in the glycosylation, folding, quality control, and trafficking of membrane and secreted proteins in the ER. Mutations in these genes result in defects in protein maturation and cell surface localization of PC1.

The *GANAB* gene is located on chromosome 11q12.3 and expressed in kidney and liver. The gene product plays an important role in PC1 maturation. Typically, ADPKD patients with *GANAB* gene variants have mild ADPKD and mild-to-severe polycystic liver disease.[2]

Sequence variations in *DNAJB11* have been identified in seven families. *DNAJB11* sequence variants result in impaired maturation of PC1. These patients develop renal insufficiency after the sixth decade of life. Phenotypic features differ from classic ADPKD caused by *PKD1* and *PKD2* variants. Multiple small cysts, normal size kidneys, and chronic interstitial fibrosis demonstrating features of autosomal dominant tubulointerstitial kidney diseases (ADTKD) are characteristic features of patients with *DNAJB11* variants.[3]

Pathogenic variants in *ALG5* have been identified in five families. All 23 affected members developed chronic kidney disease after the sixth decade of life, and eight members developed ESRD.[4]

Mutations in *ALG8* and *ALG9* are known to cause kidney and liver cysts. The kidney phenotype is considered to be mild.[5]

Monoallelic *IFT140* loss-of-function variants were found in 38 families.

IFT 40 encodes for the IFT 40 protein, which is a principal component of the IFT-A core complex. These core complex proteins belong to a group of proteins that are involved in intraflagellar transport within the cilia. IFT-A core complex proteins are involved in the retrograde trafficking of proteins within the cilium. Loss or disruption of ciliary function has been associated with a cystic phenotype.[6]

PHYSICAL FINDINGS & CLINICAL PRESENTATION

ADPKD is a systemic disorder, and symptoms relate primarily to kidney cyst burden or total kidney volume (TKV) and extrarenal involvement, including polycystic liver disease and vascular complications. TKV and kidney cyst volume increase exponentially with time and follow a patient-specific curvilinear increase.

RENAL MANIFESTATIONS

Most patients with ADPKD are relatively asymptomatic, particularly in the first three decades of life. A diagnosis of ADPKD is typically established by identification of an affected family member with asymptomatic screening (approximately 40% of cases) or renal imaging performed for clinical indications (pain, hematuria, infection, or stone). Patients may present with gross hematuria, flank mass/pain, polyuria/nocturia, fever due to a kidney or lower urinary tract infection, nephrolithiasis, or blood pressure elevation. Typically, more than half of patients will experience one of these complications by age 30. All of these complications represent manifestations of increased kidney cyst burden or TKV.

Acute flank pain can be caused by a kidney stone, kidney or liver cyst rupture, or hemorrhage. Chronic pain is typically due to enlarged kidneys. Gross hematuria occurs in 35% to 50% of patients by the age of 40 and associates with greater TKV. Gross hematuria may also result from spontaneous or traumatic cyst rupture into the collecting system. Less often, microscopic hematuria secondary to nephrolithiasis occurs. Nephrolithiasis occurs in approximately 27% of patients with ADPKD, due in part to low levels of urinary citrate, increased serum uric acid concentrations, and alterations in calcium oxalate and calcium phosphate supersaturation. Nephrolithiasis may present with acute flank pain with radiation to the groin, often with fever and hematuria, which is often microscopic.

Polyuria, nocturia, and increased thirst are manifestations of impaired urinary concentrating ability in ADPKD patients. Proteinuria is not a common feature (approximately 18% of adults and 27% of children) and is usually less than 1 g/day. However, detectable proteinuria and microalbuminuria correlate with increased TKV and more severe kidney disease.

Lower urinary tract infections are common in ADPKD and may not occur more frequently than in the general population. Renal cyst infections are specific to ADPKD, and patients typically present with localized flank pain, fever, and nausea and vomiting, similar to pyelonephritis.

CARDIAC MANIFESTATIONS

Hypertension occurs in 60% of patients with ADPKD before decline in kidney function, and it is diagnosed earlier in men than in women. Hypertension in ADPKD is due primarily to upregulation of the intrarenal renin-angiotensin-aldosterone system (RAAS). Hypertension strongly associates with increased cyst burden or TKV. Hypertension is a predictor of worse kidney outcomes and is associated with cardiovascular morbidity and mortality. Cardiac valvular abnormalities occur in

25% to 30% of ADPKD patients and include mitral valve prolapse and aortic regurgitation.

EXTRARENAL MANIFESTATIONS

- The prevalence of intracranial aneurysms (ICAs) in ADPKD is approximately 5% and increases to as high as 20% in patients who have a first-degree relative with a known intracranial aneurysm rupture.
- ICA rupture is a serious complication and may produce significant permanent morbidity or death. Routine ICA screening is recommended for patients with a family history of ICA or intracerebral bleed. Recently, smoking exposure and concurrent hypertension have been shown to associate with ICA in ADPKD. Screening is also recommended for ADPKD patients before major elective surgery, patients employed in high-risk occupations that would potentially place the lives of others at risk from a ruptured aneurysm (e.g., pilots, heavy machine operators), and patients with warning symptoms such as a sentinel headache.
- In addition to kidney cysts, cysts can develop in the liver, pancreas, and seminal vesicles. Hepatic cysts are the most common extrarenal manifestation and occur in nearly 85% of ADPKD patients by age 30. Liver cystic disease is typically asymptomatic and develops slightly later than kidney cysts in ADPKD. However, hepatic cysts can cause serious complications including pain, infection, bleeding, and biliary obstruction. Liver cysts continue to grow and expand even after ESRD occurs.
- Colonic diverticula and abdominal or inguinal hernias occur more frequently in ADPKD patients.
- Seminal vesical cysts have been reported to occur in up to 40% of men with ADPKD but are not associated with reduced fertility.
- Patients with ADPKD may be at an increased risk of developing liver, colon, and kidney cancer. However, there is sparse evidence on which to recommend any change in current cancer screening guidelines for ADPKD patients.

NATURAL HISTORY

- Patients with *PKD1* sequence variants typically have more severe disease progression than patients with *PKD2* sequence variants. The median age of onset of ESRD is 58 yr in patients with variation in the *PKD1* gene and 79 yr in patients with variation in *PKD2*.
- Patients with truncating *PKD1* gene alterations experience more severe disease progression than patients with nontruncating *PKD1* gene alterations. The median age of onset of ESRD is 55 yr in *PKD1* patients with truncating gene alterations and 67 yr with nontruncating gene alterations.[7]
- Other clinical risk factors associated with progressive kidney disease in ADPKD include male gender, onset of hypertension before 35 yr of age, gross hematuria before age 40 yr, proteinuria or microalbuminuria, increased urinary sodium excretion, and increased circulatory low-density lipoprotein cholesterol levels. However, all of these risk factors are mediated through cyst burden or TKV.

- Data from the Consortium of Radiologic Imaging Studies of Polycystic Kidney Disease (CRISP) indicate that a decline in renal blood flow and increases of TKV and cyst volume are strong predictors of future renal functional decline and progression to CKD stage 3.[8] A baseline height-adjusted TKV (htTKV) of 600 ml/min predicts the risk of developing CKD stage 3 within 8 yr.[9] Patients with ADPKD may be classified as 1A-1E based on the Mayo Clinic Imaging Classification of ADPKD that helps physicians identify patients with severe disease (www.mayo.edu/research/documents/pkd-center-adpkd-classification/doc-20094754 www.mayo.edu/research/documents/pkd-center-adpkd-classification/doc-20094754). This classification is based on annual growth rates estimated from age-based htTKV: <1.5% (1A); 1.5% to 3% (1B); 3% to 4.5% (1C); 4.5% to 6% (1D); and >6%/yr (1E).[10] This classification should only be applied in cases of ADPKD classified as typical ADPKD (i.e., large kidneys with extensive cysts scattered throughout both kidneys at ages 15 to 80 yr). Patients in class 1A are at a low risk for renal function decline. Patients in classes 1C-1E are at a high risk for progressive disease. For patients with the same gene type, GFR is predicted to decline faster by 0.89 ml/min/1.73 m² per yr for each step up in class from 1A to 1E. Patients in class 1E, on average, reach ESRD before age 50 yr.[11]
- A worldwide prospective observational study of patients with ADPKD demonstrated that a greater baseline htTKV is associated with low eGFR, greater likelihood of hypertension, kidney pain, hematuria, worse patient-reported health-related quality of life outcomes, decreased work productivity, and increased health care utilization.[12]
- Racial and ethnic disparities exist when it comes to outcomes in patients with ADPKD. Black and Hispanic individuals develop ESRD at a younger age. Mean age of onset of ESRD requiring renal replacement therapy was 57 yr, 55 yr, and 53 yr in White, Black, and Hispanic patients, respectively. Among Black and Hispanic patients predialysis care is much lower, they are less likely to choose home dialysis as the initial modality of choice, they have higher rates of central venous catheter use, they are less likely to receive preemptive transplant, and they have lower odds of transplant after dialysis initiation. Median time from being waitlisted to transplantation was longer, at 28 mo and 24 mo in Black and Hispanic patients as opposed to 15 mo among White patients.[13]

Dx DIAGNOSIS

- Ultrasound of the kidneys is the most commonly used imaging modality for screening and diagnosis. It is inexpensive, readily available, noninvasive, and free of radiation. Computed tomography (CT) and MRI are also used (Fig. E1), but typically in the setting of acute complications. CT scans (Fig. E2)

and MRI are more sensitive than ultrasound (Fig. E3), with cyst detection at <1 cm.
- The following diagnostic criteria are used for diagnosis of ADPKD in asymptomatic individuals at risk for development of disease (i.e., positive family history of ADPKD).[14]
- Individuals 15 to 39 yr of age: At least three unilateral or bilateral kidney cysts.
- Individuals 40 to 59 yr of age: At least two cysts in each kidney.
- Individuals older than 60 yr of age: At least four cysts in each kidney.
- For patients with no family history of ADPKD, there is no definitive number of cysts and/or cyst location that provides an unequivocal diagnosis. The diagnosis is strongly suspected when multiple and bilateral kidney cysts are present along with hepatic cysts. Currently, more than 20 bilaterally distributed cysts with a consistent phenotype is considered reliable for making a diagnosis.
- Genetic testing can be done to diagnose ADPKD when imaging results are equivocal and when a definitive diagnosis is required in a young, at-risk individual (e.g., potential living kidney donor or family planning).

DIFFERENTIAL DIAGNOSIS

- Multiple benign simple cysts
- Autosomal recessive polycystic kidney disease
- Familial juvenile nephronophthisis
- Medullary cystic or UMOD (uromodulin) disease
- Medullary sponge kidney
- Tuberous sclerosis
- von Hippel-Lindau syndrome
- Acquired cystic kidney disease
- Table 1 compares clinical features of cystic kidney diseases

LABORATORY TESTS

- Hemoglobin and hematocrit may be elevated because of increased erythropoietin production; however, these levels are usually similar to levels seen in other CKD patients.
- Urinalysis can show microscopic hematuria and proteinuria (rarely >1 g per day).
- With decreased kidney function, blood urea nitrogen and creatinine are elevated.
- Platelet counts can be mildly reduced in patients with extensive polycystic liver disease from splenic sequestration.
- Metabolic acidosis, hyperparathyroidism, and hyperphosphatemia are associated with CKD in ADPKD.

Rx TREATMENT

NONPHARMACOLOGIC THERAPY

Dietary intervention is prescribed to all ADPKD patients.

- Restriction of dietary salt (<2 g sodium per day) and calories is recommended. Post hoc analysis of the HALT-PKD trial in which all patients were instructed to follow a sodium-restricted diet (2.4 g per day) showed that greater urine sodium excretion was associated with kidney growth or increase in htTKV and more rapid renal function decline.[15]

TABLE 1 Comparison of Clinical Features of Cystic Kidney Diseases

Disease	Inheritance	Frequency	Gene Product	Age of Onset	Cyst Origin	Renomegaly	Cause of ESRD	Other Manifestations
ADPKD	AD	1:400-1000	Polycystin-1(PC1); Polycystin-2(PC2); Glucosidase II alpha subunit (GIIα); DnaJB11	20s and 30s	Anywhere (including Bowman capsule)	Yes	Yes (for PC1, PC2, or DnaJB11) No (for GIIα)	Liver cysts; Cerebral aneurysms; Hypertension; Mitral valve prolapse; Kidney stones; UTIs
ARPKD	AR	1:10,000-40,000	Fibrocystin/polyductin	First yr of life	Distal nephron, CD	Yes	Yes	Hepatic fibrosis; Pulmonary hypoplasia
ACKD	No	90% of ESRD patients at 8 yr	None*	Yr after onset of ESRD	Proximal and distal tubules	Rarely	No	None
Simple cysts	No	50% in those older than 40 yr	None**	Adulthood	Anywhere (usually cortical)	No	No	None
NPHP	AR	1:80,000	Nephrocystins (NPHP1–20)	Childhood or adolescence	Medullary DCT	No	Yes	Retinal degeneration; neurologic, skeletal, hepatic, cardiac malformations
ADTKD-UMOD	AD	Rare	Uromodulin	Adults	Cortico-medullary	No	Yes	Gout
ADTKD-MUC1	AD	Rare	Mucin-1	Adults	Cortico-medullary	No	Yes	None
ADTKD-REN	AD	Rare	Renin	Childhood	Cortico-medullary	No	Yes	Anemia, gout, hyperkalemia
ADTKD-HNF1B	AD; spontaneous	Rare	HNF1β	Childhood or adulthood	Cortico-medullary	Rarely	Variable	Early-onset diabetes, pancreatic hypoplasia, hypomagnesemia, hyperthyroidism, liver function abnormalities, gout, renal and urogenital anomalies, mental retardation, risk of renal cell carcinoma
MSK	No	1:5000-20,000	None*	30s	Medullary CD	No	No	Kidney stones
Tuberous sclerosis	AD	1:10,000	Hamartin (TSC1), tuberin (TSC2)	Childhood	Loop of Henle, DCT	Rarely	Rarely	Renal cell carcinoma, tubers, seizures, angiomyolipoma, hypertension
VHL syndrome	AD	1:40,000	VHL protein	20s	Cortical nephrons	Rarely	Rarely	Retinal angioma, CNS hemangioblastoma, renal cell carcinoma, pheochromocytoma
Oral-facial-digital syndrome-1	XD	1:250,000	OFD1 protein	Childhood or adulthood	Renal glomeruli	Rarely	Yes	Malformation of the face, oral cavity, and digits; liver cysts; mental retardation
HIPKD	AR	Rare	Phospho-mannomutase 2	Childhood	Renal glomeruli	Yes	Yes	Hypoglycemic seizures; occasional liver cysts
BBS	AR	1:65,000-160,000	BBS 1-18	Adulthood	Renal calyces	Rarely	Yes	Syndactyly and polydactyly, obesity, retinal dystrophy, male hypogenitalism, hypertension, mental retardation

ACKD, Acquired cystic kidney disease; *AD,* autosomal dominant; *ADPKD,* autosomal dominant polycystic kidney disease; *ADTKD,* autosomal dominant tubulointerstitial kidney disease; *AR,* autosomal recessive; *ARPKD,* autosomal recessive polycystic kidney disease; *BBS,* Bardet-Biedl syndrome; *CD,* collecting duct; *CNS,* central nervous system; *DCT,* distal convoluted tubule; *DnaJB11,* DnaJ homolog subfamily B member 11; *ESRD,* end-stage renal disease; *HIPKD,* PKD with hyperinsulinemic hypoglycemia; *HNF1β,* hepatocyte nuclear factor 1 β; *MSK,* medullary sponge kidney; *MUC1,* mucin-1; *NPHP,* nephronophthisis; *REN,* renin; *UMOD,* uromodulin; *UTI,* urinary tract infection; *VHL,* von Hippel-Lindau; *XD,* X-linked dominant.
*No known genetic susceptibility.
From Goldman L, Shafer AI: *Goldman-Cecil medicine,* ed 26, Philadelphia, 2020, Elsevier.

- Intracellular cyclic adenosine monophosphate (cAMP) contributes to cyst formation and growth in ADPKD. Circulating vasopressin stimulates renal cAMP production. Increasing water intake to greater than 3 L per day can suppress circulating vasopressin levels. Consequently, increasing water intake is recommended for all ADPKD patients with preserved kidney function. However, serum sodium should be monitored carefully in advanced CKD because patients are vulnerable to development of hyponatremia.

ACUTE GENERAL Rx

- The treatment of gross hematuria is typically supportive with bed rest (compress bleeding cyst), hydration, and analgesics without nonsteroidal antiinflammatory drugs. Antihypertensive medications should be stopped during this time.
- Extracorporeal shock wave lithotripsy (ESWL) has been used in patients with small obstructing kidney stones (<2 cm diameter) in the renal pelvis or calyces. There is some concern that residual stone fragments cause renal dysfunction. Percutaneous nephrolithotomy is a potentially safer option in certain cases.
- Infections are treated with antibiotics that penetrate cysts, including fluoroquinolones, trimethoprim/sulfamethoxazole, vancomycin, and rarely, chloramphenicol.
- New therapies affecting cyst growth.

CHRONIC GENERAL Rx

- In young individuals with preserved kidney function, the HALT-PKD trial showed that strict blood pressure control of <110/75 mm Hg was associated with a slower increase of TKV (15% slower over 5 yr), reduced urinary albumin excretion, and greater reduction of left ventricular mass index.[16]
- For ADPKD patients over the age of 35 yr or with renal dysfunction, the goal blood pressure is <130/80 mm Hg. For young, healthy patients with ADPKD and with intact kidney function, the goal blood pressure target can be <110/75 mm Hg.
- ACE inhibitors or angiotensin II type 1 receptor blockers are the drug of choice as first-line treatment for hypertension.
- Hyperlipidemia should be aggressively treated, and the low density lipoprotein (LDL) cholesterol target is <80 mg/dl.
- In a randomized, double-blind, placebo-controlled phase 2 trial involving 91 children and young adults with ADPKD, pravastatin was found to have a beneficial effect on htTKV, left ventricular mass index, and urinary albumin excretion. Over a 3-yr period, a 23% increase in htTKV was observed in the pravastatin group compared to 31% in the placebo group.[17]
- Statin therapy did not show any benefit in a post hoc analysis of the HALT-PKD trials. However, this study was not randomized, different statin drugs and doses were used, and only a small number of statin users were in this study.[18]
- Currently, statin use in the management of ADPKD is by physician choice. A larger, randomized controlled trial is required to study the effect of statins on cyst growth.
- Patients who progress to ESRD require renal replacement therapy. Both peritoneal dialysis and hemodialysis can be used as a bridge to kidney transplantation, but preemptive transplantation is preferred.

The complication rates after nephrectomy are higher with prekidney transplant nephrectomy compared with posttransplant nephrectomy. Blood transfusion during prekidney transplant nephrectomy may cause allosensitization and delay transplantation evaluation. Consequently, routine prekidney transplant nephrectomy is not recommended. Prekidney transplant unilateral or bilateral nephrectomy is recommended only in select patients with recurrent infections, recurrent or severe bleeding, renal cell carcinoma, and significant kidney enlargement causing limitation of daily activities and malnutrition.

TOLVAPTAN

- In a phase 3, double-blind, placebo-controlled, randomized trial (TEMPO 3:4 trial) involving 1450 patients with PKD and preserved kidney function, the vasopressin-receptor 2 antagonist tolvaptan significantly decreased kidney volume and slowed the decline in kidney function. The benefits of tolvaptan on TKV rate of increase and decline of kidney function are greater in patients with increased albuminuria. The benefits of tolvaptan on TKV were seen across CKD stages 1 to 3.[19]
- The effect of tolvaptan on delaying renal function decline was maintained for an additional 2 yr in the extension study, the TEMPO 4:4 trial, in which all participants were offered tolvaptan treatment for an additional 2 yr.[20]
- A second tolvaptan trial (REPRISE) examined the safety and efficacy of tolvaptan in more advanced ADPKD. This was a 12-mo, phase 3, randomized withdrawal, multicenter, placebo-controlled, and double-blind trial that included 1370 patients with estimated glomerular filtration rates (eGFR) between 25 and 65 ml/min/1.73 m^2. Tolvaptan-treated patients demonstrated a reduction in eGFR decline of 35% compared to placebo. Those receiving placebo lost 3.61 ml/min per 1.73 m^2 per yr. Tolvaptan-treated patients demonstrated an eGFR decline of 2.34 ml/min per 1.73 m^2 per yr, a statistically significant difference of 1.27 ml/min per 1.73 m^2 per yr. The beneficial effect of tolvaptan on renal function decline was established in all subgroups (<55 yr, men and women, and patients with CKD stages 3A, 3B, and 4). Beneficial effects were not present in subjects older than 55 yr. Firm conclusions cannot be made in this subgroup due to relatively smaller numbers.[21]
- Based on the above studies, on April 24, 2018, the FDA approved tolvaptan for treatment of ADPKD in adult patients at risk for rapidly progressing ADPKD.
- Patients at Mayo classes 1C-1E levels of cyst burden (faster rates of cyst growth) likely have rapidly progressive disease and should be considered for treatment with tolvaptan.

Treated individuals may experience polyuria, nocturia, abnormally frequent urination, and polydipsia. Post hoc analyses of the TEMPO 3:4 and TEMPO 4:4 trials suggest that drug effects are more pronounced early after drug initiation and in subjects with better kidney function. Appropriate hydration is essential to prevent thirst, dehydration, and hypernatremia.

- A minor eGFR reduction of 5% to 10% is anticipated after initiation of tolvaptan and eGFR reduction is reversible upon drug discontinuation. Tolvaptan dose reduction or withholding of the agent is recommended if a significant decline of eGFR of >20% is observed. Renal function testing should be carried out 2 and 4 wk after initiation of therapy, then monthly for the next 18 mo and every 3 mo afterward. To ensure that patients are maintaining hydration while on tolvaptan, plasma sodium concentration measurements must be obtained. Urinary osmolality can be used to assess treatment response and target drug dosing.
- Another important adverse event associated with tolvaptan is liver toxicity. Two patients in the TEMPO 3:4 trial (https://pubmed.ncbi.nlm.nih.gov/23121377/) and one patient in the TEMPO 4:4 trial (https://pubmed.ncbi.nlm.nih.gov/28379536/) developed serious drug-induced liver injury. In the REPRISE trial, liver adverse effects were greater in the tolvaptan group compared to placebo (5.6% vs. 1.2%). Because of the risks of serious liver injury, tolvaptan prescriptions are only available through a restricted distribution program called the Risk Evaluation and Mitigation Strategy (REMS). Under this program, liver function testing is done before initiation of treatment, at 2 wk and 4 wk after initiation, then monthly for the first 18 mo and every 3 mo afterward.

OTHER THERAPIES AFFECTING CYST GROWTH

- A small trial involving the somatostatin analogue octreotide long-acting repeatable depot showed that there was significantly less increase in TKV in the octreotide group than in the placebo group. Another randomized phase 3 trial involving 100 ADPKD patients with eGFRs between 15 and 40 ml/min per 1.73 m^2 demonstrated that a 3-yr treatment with octreotide long-acting release (octreotide LAR) significantly slowed kidney volume growth. Octreotide LAR did not affect GFR decline compared to placebo. However, fewer patients in the octreotide group than in the placebo group progressed to the combined endpoint of doubling of serum creatinine and ESRD (19% vs. 43%).[22] A 1-yr, randomized, placebo-controlled study of another somatostatin analogue, pasireotide long-acting release, demonstrated slow rates of increase of total liver and volumes.
- In a phase 2, randomized, double-blind, placebo-controlled study, the oral tyrosine kinase inhibitor bosutinib reduced kidney growth and preserved kidney function. However, medication-related adverse events (diarrhea, rash,

and pancreatitis) and acute declines in kidney function have limited the development of this therapy.[23] A phase 2 trial of another tyrosine kinase inhibitor, tesevatinib, is ongoing.

- Two randomized, double-blind trials investigating the mammalian target of rapamycin (mTOR) inhibitors, sirolimus and everolimus, did not show any effect on renal function in patients with ADPKD. The shorter duration of these trials and potentially inadequate dosing of the medications may have affected the outcome.[24,25]
- There is an increased accumulation of glycosphingolipids in patients who have ADPKD that is mediated via the mTOR pathway, which has been thought to worsen cystogenesis. A phase 2/3 study looking at the efficacy of the glycosphingolipid inhibitor venglustat was stopped after an interim analysis showed a lack of effect on kidney growth rate.
- Renal cyst formation and growth over time results in increased interstitial inflammation, oxidative stress, and fibrosis. Bardoxolone has antiinflammatory and antioxidant properties and is undergoing investigation in a phase 3 randomized trial as a possible treatment for ADPKD.
- Metformin, which has been widely used in the treatment of type 2 diabetes mellitus, has been shown to be effective in treating ADPKD in preclinical studies. Metformin activates adenosine monophosphate kinase (AMPK), which in turn leads to inhibition of mTORC1 and cystic fibrosis transmembrane regulator (CFTR), resulting in decreased cellular proliferation and fluid secretion. A recent phase 2 trial investigating the use of metformin in 97 patients with early-stage ADPKD (eGFR> 60 ml/min/1.73m^2) showed that this therapy is safe. However, only about one third of the patients tolerated the maximum dose of 2000 mg/day. Metformin did not show benefit in the exploratory secondary endpoints of

eGFR slope decline and annual percent change in htTKV. The short duration of the trial, inability to use the maximum dose in most patients due to gastrointestinal side effects, and inclusion of patients with mild disease (only 50% had Mayo Class 1C-1E) could have affected the outcomes.[26] A larger international phase 3 trial investigating the efficacy of metformin for ADPKD is being planned.

- Non-inactivated *PKD1* mRNA is inhibited by its 3'-UTR miR-17 motif, lowering the PC1 below a critical threshold. Medications targeting the miR-17 family rises PC1 levels by preventing inhibition of non-inactivated *PKD1* mRNA. Early stage clinical trials using therapeutics that inhibit the function of miR-17 are underway.[27]
- Growing evidence suggests that a metabolic defect exists in ADPKD that can contribute to cyst growth. Obesity and being overweight were strongly associated with the rate of progression in early stage PKD in the HALT-PKD cohort. In rodent models of ADPKD, caloric restriction, time-restricted feeding, and ketogenic diets have been shown to reduce cystic disease. Clinical trial data or human data are not available yet.
- A feasibility trial of a time-restricted feeding protocol that restricts eating to a feeding window of 8 h/day is being investigated in patients with ADPKD who are obese or overweight.
- In a retrospective uncontrolled observational study of ADPKD patients who self-initiated a ketogenic diet, 90% of patients reported significant weight loss; 64% reported lower blood pressure; 66% reported diet-related side effects, including fatigue, hunger, and keto flu; and 42% reported intermittent breaks in their dietary regimen every mo. 17% raised significant safety concerns largely to do with increased cardiovascular risk due to increases in total and low-density

lipoprotein cholesterol of 13 and 8.5 mg/dl, respectively.[28]

REFERRAL

- Patients with ADPKD should be referred at time of diagnosis to a nephrologist for ongoing care. Urology can also be consulted for patients with nephrolithiasis and recurrent episodes of gross hematuria or for consideration of nephrectomy before kidney transplantation.
- Genetic counseling should be offered if patients plan to start a family or are considering kidney screening examinations for children. Individuals at risk for ADPKD should undergo pretest and posttest counseling if ADPKD is discovered.

⚠ PEARLS & CONSIDERATIONS

- ADPKD is the most common, single, genetic cause of CKD.
- TKV increases exponentially over time, and the increase of TKV is a strong predictor of future kidney functional decline.
- Increasing water intake to >3 L per day is recommended for patients with ADPKD and preserved kidney function.
- Tolvaptan is recommended for patients with rapidly progressing ADPKD.
- Strict blood pressure control is recommended for all ADPKD patients.

RELATED CONTENT

Polycystic Kidney Disease (Patient Information)

REFERENCES

Available at eBooks.Health.Elsevier.com.

AUTHORS: **BHARATHI V. REDDY, MD** and **ARLENE CHAPMAN, MD**

A

Diseases and Disorders

I

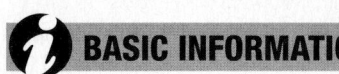
BASIC INFORMATION

DEFINITION
Babesiosis is a tick-transmitted protozoan disease of animals, caused by intraerythrocytic parasites of the genus *Babesia*. Humans are incidentally infected, resulting in a nonspecific febrile illness. The disease can be severe in immunocompromised hosts.

ICD-10CM CODE
B60.0   Babesiosis

EPIDEMIOLOGY & DEMOGRAPHICS
INCIDENCE (IN U.S.): From 2011 to 2015 the CDC was notified of 7612 cases of babesiosis. Cases were reported in 27 states, with 94.5% of cases occurring in seven states (Fig. E1). In 2017, there were 2350 reported cases in the U.S.
PREVALENCE (IN U.S.):
- In areas of high endemicity, seropositivity ranging from 9% (Rhode Island) to 21% (Connecticut)
- Highest number of reported cases in New York
PREDOMINANT SEX: Males (most likely through increased exposure to vectors during recreational or occupational activities)
PREDOMINANT AGE: Severity apparently increasing with age >50 yr or neonate
PEAK INCIDENCE: Spring and summer months, May through September
GENETICS: None known
CONGENITAL INFECTION: Definite evidence of vertical transmission
NEONATAL INFECTION: Many cases of perinatal transmission
BLOOD TRANSFUSION 7 ORGAN TRANSPLANT: Many instances. Blood donation screening for antibodies to and DNA from *B. microti* has been shown to significantly decrease the risk of transfusion-transmitted babesiosis.

PHYSICAL FINDINGS & CLINICAL PRESENTATION
- Incubation period is 1 to 4 wk; 6 to 9 wk, occasionally longer in transfusion-associated disease.
- Gradual onset of irregular fever, chills, diaphoresis, headache, myalgia, arthralgia, fatigue, and dark urine. Symptoms usually begin within 1 mo after tick bite and within 6 mo after transfusion of infected blood products. Fever is the most frequently reported clinical manifestation.
- On physical examination: Petechiae, frank or mild hepatosplenomegaly, and jaundice. Most patients have a normal physical examination.
- Infection with *B. divergens* (Europe) produces a more severe illness with a rapid onset of symptoms and increasing parasitemia progressing to massive intravascular hemolysis and renal failure.

ETIOLOGY
- Vector: Deer tick, *Ixodes scapularis* (Fig. E2) (also known as *I. dammini*).
  1. Feeds on rodents during the spring and summer while in its larval and nymphal stages and on deer as an adult.

2. Requires a blood meal to mature to each stage, hence human infection.
3. During the warmer months in endemic areas, humans are readily infected while engaging in outdoor activities.
4. Tick must attach for 36 to 72 h to transmit infection.
5. *Babesia* life cycle is illustrated in Fig. E3.
- *B. microti* and *B. divergens* account for most human infections. Table 1 compares causal agents and clinical manifestations of babesiosis.
- In the U.S., cases caused by *B. microti* are acquired on offshore islands of the northeastern coast, including Nantucket Island, Cape Cod, and Martha's Vineyard in Massachusetts; Block Island in Rhode Island; and Long Island, Fire Island, and Shelter Island in New York; as well as the nearby mainland, including Connecticut, Rhode Island, Massachusetts, New York, and New Jersey.
- Sporadic cases reported from California, Georgia, Maryland, Minnesota, Virginia, Wisconsin, and most recently the WA-1 strain from Washington state and the MO-1 strain from Missouri.
- *B. divergens* is implicated in human disease in Europe, where the disease remains rare and predominantly associated with asplenia.
- *B. venatorum* is emerging as an important pathogen in mainland China.
- Majority of cases of *B. microti* are asymptomatic.
- Is transmissible by transfusion of erythrocytes, or through red cell–contaminated platelets.
- Mixed infections (*B. microti* and *Borrelia burgdorferi*, the causative agent of Lyme disease) are estimated to occur in 50% (Rhode Island and Connecticut) to 60% (New York) of cases.

DIAGNOSIS

DIFFERENTIAL DIAGNOSIS
- Malaria
- Ehrlichiosis
- Leptospirosis
- Salmonellosis, including typhoid fever
- Acute viral hepatitis
- Hemorrhagic fevers
- Subacute bacterial endocarditis

WORKUP
Babesiosis should be suspected in any febrile patient living or traveling in an endemic area, irrespective of exposure history to ticks or tick bites, especially if asplenic. The hallmark of babesiosis is hemolysis with resulting anemia. Elevated liver enzymes, thrombocytopenia, and acute kidney injury may occur.

LABORATORY TESTS
- The preferred methods for diagnosing babesiosis are polymerase chain reaction (PCR) using whole blood specimens (babesia PCR) or blood parasite peripheral blood screen (BPARS).
- In experienced hands, sequential examination of Giemsa-stained thin smears is equally effective.

- Babesial DNA by PCR has comparable sensitivity and specificity to microscopic analysis of thin blood smears. PCR is more sensitive than smears at the onset of infection when parasite load may be minimal.
- Diagnosis is achieved serologically by indirect immunofluorescence assay (IFA) specific for *B. microti*.
  1. Assay is hampered by the inability to distinguish between exposed patients and those who are actively infected.
  2. Immunoglobulin G titer of ≥1:64 is indicative of seropositivity, whereas one ≥1:1024 is considered diagnostic of acute infection. Immunoglobulin M (IgM) titer of 1:64 is considered indicative of acute infection.
  3. IgM indirect immunofluorescent-antibody test may be highly sensitive and specific for diagnosis. IgM titer of ≥1:64 is considered indicative of acute infection.
- CBC may reveal mild to moderate thrombocytopenia and anemia, and/or reticulocytosis. The white blood cell (WBC) count may be normal, elevated, or low. Abnormally elevated serum chemistries, including creatinine, liver function profile, lactate dehydrogenase, and indirect and total bilirubin levels; haptoglobin is low.
- Urinalysis may reveal proteinuria and hemoglobinuria.
- Examination of Giemsa- or Wright-stained thin blood films for intraerythrocytic parasites (Fig. E4) (may need to examine 200 to 300 microscopic fields).
  1. In its classic, though infrequently seen, form a "tetrad" or "Maltese cross" composed of four daughter cells attached by cytoplasmic strands is observed.
  2. More commonly, smaller forms composed of a single chromatin dot are eccentrically located within bluish cytoplasm.
  3. Parasitized erythrocytes may be multiply infected but not enlarged.
  4. Extraerythrocytic forms may be seen.
  5. Gametocytes are *not* seen; this is a characteristic of malaria.

TREATMENT

NONPHARMACOLOGIC THERAPY
Supportive care with adequate hydration

ACUTE GENERAL Rx
- In patients with intact spleens: Predominantly asymptomatic or if symptomatic, generally self-limited.
- Therapy may be offered to any symptomatic patient. Table 2 summarizes treatment recommendations.
- Therapy is mandatory for the severely ill patient, especially if asplenic, elderly, or immunosuppressed. Combination of atovaquone 750 mg q12h and azithromycin 500 mg on day 1 and 250 mg/day thereafter for 7 to 10 days appears to be as effective as a regimen of clindamycin and quinine with fewer adverse reactions. This is the preferred regimen for mild disease.
- Combination of quinine sulfate 650 mg PO tid plus clindamycin 600 mg PO tid (600 mg

TABLE 1 Causal Agents and Clinical Manifestations of Babesiosis

Babesia Species	Geographic Distribution	Tick Vectors	Animal Reservoirs	Epidemiology	Clinical Manifestations
B. divergens	United Kingdom, Western Europe, Eastern Europe, Sweden, Russia; not reported in United States	*Ixodes ricinus*	Cattle, reindeer	Incubation, 1-4 wk. Occurs during summer months in cattle-raising regions Targets splenectomized or immunocompromised patients primarily	Fulminant course with high case-fatality rate Fever, rigors, headache, myalgia, jaundice, hemoglobinuria, hemolytic anemia, acute renal failure, multiorgan failure
B. microti	Parallels the U.S. Northeast endemic regions for *Borrelia burgdorferi*, especially the islands off New York, Massachusetts, Connecticut, and Rhode Island and focal areas in Connecticut, New Jersey, Wisconsin, and Minnesota	Deer ticks: *Ixodes dammini* and *Ixodes scapularis*	White-footed mouse (*Peromyscus leucopus*)	Incubation, 1-4 wk after tick bites or 4-9 wk after blood transfusions Transmission primarily by nymphal ticks Targets older, not necessarily immunocompromised patients, particularly severe in those immunocompromised by HIV infection, advanced age, coinfections with B. burgdorferi Seasonality parallels tick nymph activity; 80% of cases occur from May to August	Often asymptomatic in young, healthy patients Self-limited influenza-like febrile illness with onset of anorexia, malaise, and lethargy followed in 1 wk by high fever, diaphoresis, myalgias; mild splenomegaly and rarely hepatomegaly Later hemolysis, hemolytic anemia, thrombocytopenia, jaundice, acute renal failure, especially in the splenectomized, older adults, or the immunocompromised Complications include ARDS and DIC Case-fatality rate, 5%
MO-1 (a relative or subspecies of B. divergens)	Rural Missouri and Kentucky	*Ixodes dentatus* (rabbit tick)	Rabbits, birds	Incubation, 1-4 wk after tick bites Spring to autumn seasonality Targets the splenectomized, like B. divergens	Same as above—often asymptomatic, except in the splenectomized, who will develop high parasitemia and multiorgan failure
WA-1 (a relative or subspecies of B. gibsoni)	Rural Washington state	Ixodid ticks, including *Ixodes dentatus*	Unknown—wild canids and ungulates suspected	Incubation, 1-4 wk Targets the splenectomized, older adults, immunocompromised, premature infants May be transmitted by blood transfusion	Same as above—often asymptomatic, except in the splenectomized, who will develop high parasitemia and multiorgan failure
CA-1, CA-2, etc. subspecies (relatives or subspecies of mule deer and bighorn sheep *Babesia* species)	U.S. Pacific coast, primarily rural and semirural areas of California	Ixodid ticks	Unknown—mule deer and bighorn sheep suspected	Incubation, 1-4 wk Targets the splenectomized, elderly, immunocompromised, and premature infants	Same as above—often asymptomatic, except in the splenectomized, who will develop high parasitemia and multiorgan failure

ARDS, Acute respiratory distress syndrome; *DIC,* disseminated intravascular coagulation; *HIV,* human immunodeficiency virus.
From Bennett JE et al: *Mandell, Douglas, and Bennett's principles and practice of infectious diseases*, ed 9, Philadelphia, 2020, Elsevier.

parenterally qid) taken for 7 to 10 days. Severely ill patients are hospitalized and treated with clindamycin and quinine or azithromycin plus atovaquone.

- Exchange transfusions in addition to antimicrobial therapy: Successful treatment for severe infections in asplenic patients associated with high levels of *B. microti* or *B. divergens* parasitemia. Exchange transfusion is recommended for patients with >10% parasitemia but may be considered for any severely ill patient.
- Patients who experience relapse and patients who are immunocompromised may require a longer duration of therapy.
- Splenic rupture may occur in otherwise healthy young individuals; this manifests with severe abdominal pain and is diagnosed by CT scan.
- ARDS, CHF, DIC may complicate serious cases.

DISPOSITION

- Prognosis is usually good, and fatal outcomes are rare.
- Fatalities are 3% to 9% of hospitalized patients but 20% of transfusion associated or immunocompromised cases.

REFERRAL

- For prompt consultation with an infectious disease specialist if the diagnosis is acutely suspected, especially in the asplenic, elderly, or immunocompromised patient
- For hospitalization for the severely ill patient who may require exchange transfusions in addition to antibiotic therapy

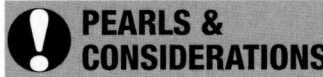 **PEARLS & CONSIDERATIONS**

COMMENTS

- Prevention of babesiosis in asplenic or immunocompromised hosts is best achieved by avoidance of areas where the vector is endemic, especially in May through September.
- *Babesia* may reactivate after splenectomy or immunosuppression in prior *Babesia* patients.
- If residence or travel in endemic areas is unavoidable, advise patients to perform daily cutaneous self-examination, wear light-colored clothing (to facilitate removal of ticks), tuck pants into socks, and apply tick repellent (diethyltoluamide and dimethyl phthalate) to skin or clothing.

- Advise a daily inspection for ticks in family pets (e.g., cats and dogs).
- Infection with *B. divergens,* especially in the asplenic patient, is often fatal.
- Concurrent cases of babesiosis and Lyme disease, *Anaplasma, Borrelia miyamotoi,* and Powassan virus have been documented—check for combined infection in severely ill patients.
- A combination of clindamycin and quinine has been successfully used to treat babesiosis during the third trimester of pregnancy without incurring apparent adverse effect on the fetus.
- In 2011 the CDC added babesiosis to the list of nationally notifiable diseases.
- Tick avoidance is paramount in prevention of babesiosis.

RELATED CONTENT

Babesiosis (Patient Information)

SUGGESTED READINGS

Available at eBooks.Health.Elsevier.com.

AUTHOR: **PATRICIA CRISTOFARO, MD**

TABLE 2 Treatment of Human Babesiosis

Species	Illness	Host[a]	First-Line Regimen[b]	Alternative Regimen[b]
Babesia microti	Mild		Atovaquone 750 mg q12h PO plus azithromycin 500 mg PO on day 1 and 250 mg/day PO from day 2 on; for 7-10 days[d]	
	Severe[c]	Immunocompetent	Atovaquone 750 mg q12h PO plus azithromycin 500 mg/day IV[e,f]; for 7-10 days[d]	Clindamycin 600 mg q6h IV plus quinine 650 mg q6-8h PO[f,g,h,i]; for same duration
		Immunocompromised and/or asplenic	Atovaquone 750 mg q12h PO plus azithromycin 500 mg/d IV[j]; for at least 6 consecutive wk, including 2 final wk during which parasites are no longer detected on blood smear[k,l]	Atovaquone 750 mg q12h PO plus clindamycin 600 mg q6h IV with or without azithromycin 500 mg/day IV[m,n]; for same duration
Babesia divergens	Mild	Immunocompetent	Clindamycin 600 mg q8h PO plus quinine 650 mg q6 to 8h PO; for 7-10 days[d,h]	Atovaquone 750 mg q12h PO plus azithromycin 500 mg PO on day 1 and 250 mg/day PO from day 2 on; for 7-10 days[d,n]
	Severe	Immunocompromised and/or asplenic	Immediate complete RBC exchange transfusion combined with clindamycin 600 mg q6h IV plus quinine 650 mg q6-8h PO; for 7-10 days[d,h]	

IV, Intravenously; PO, orally; RBC, red blood cell.

[a]Dosages are provided for treatment of adults. For pediatric cases, consider using atovaquone 20 mg/kg q12h PO (up to 750 mg/dose) plus azithromycin 5-10 mg/kg PO (up to 250-500 mg/dose), or clindamycin 7-10 mg/kg q6 to 8h IV or PO (up to 600 mg/dose) plus quinine 8 mg/kg q8h PO (up to 650 mg/dose).

[b]Atovaquone is available in a suspension form and should be taken with dietary fat to increase absorption.

[c]Consider partial or complete RBC exchange transfusion in cases of high-grade parasitemia (≥10%), severe anemia (hemoglobin <10 g/dL), or organ (pulmonary or renal) compromise.

[d]Duration may be extended if symptoms other than fatigue linger.

[e]Intravenous azithromycin may be replaced with oral azithromycin (250-500 mg/day) once the patient has improved.

[f]Recommended for the treatment of severe babesiosis in hospitalized patients.

[g]Intravenous clindamycin may be replaced with oral clindamycin (600 mg q8h) once the patient has improved.

[h]Because quinine carries a risk of QT segment prolongation and torsade de pointes, patients should be monitored by electrocardiography. In the setting of hepatic or renal disease, quinine serum levels should be monitored.

[i]If cardiac toxicity or untoward adverse effects occur, quinine can be replaced with oral atovaquone (750 mg q12h).

[j]Intravenous azithromycin can be replaced with oral azithromycin (500 mg/day) once the patient has improved. Higher doses of oral azithromycin (600-1000 mg/day) accelerate symptom resolution and parasite clearance.

[k]Blood smear is recommended to monitor resolution of infection in severely immunocompromised patients, but recent case reports support the use of a real-time polymerase chain reaction assay to ensure complete parasite clearance.

[l]Duration may vary. In a patient who had been treated with rituximab, parasite clearance was achieved after 27 mo of uninterrupted antimicrobial therapy. If asplenia is the only comorbidity, antimicrobial therapy may be shortened as long as clinical cure and parasite clearance are achieved in less than 4 wk.

[m]Prolonged administration of clindamycin places the patient at risk of Clostridioides difficile (formerly Clostridium difficile) infection.

[n]Atovaquone can be replaced with atovaquone-proguanil. Atovaquone-proguanil should be taken with dietary fat but should not be given to patients with severe renal impairment.

From Bennett JE et al: *Mandell, Douglas, and Bennett's principles and practice of infectious diseases,* ed 9, Philadelphia, 2020, Elsevier.

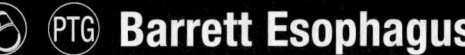
Diseases
and Disorders

I

BASIC INFORMATION

DEFINITION

Barrett esophagus occurs when the squamocolumnar junction is displaced ≥1 cm proximal to the gastroesophageal junction and the squamous lining of the lower esophagus is replaced by metaplastic columnar epithelium, which predisposes to the development of esophageal adenocarcinoma. Although cardia-type epithelium has been shown to predispose to esophageal cancer, the presence of intestinalized epithelium is still considered essential for the diagnosis. Recent data show that the absolute annual risk for esophageal carcinoma in Barrett esophagus is 0.12%, which is much lower than the assumed risk of 0.5% that is the basis for current surveillance guidelines.[1-3]

SYNONYMS

Esophagus, Barrett
Esophagus, columnar-lined
Ulcer, Barrett

ICD-10CM CODES
K22.70	Barrett esophagus without dysplasia
K22.710	Barrett esophagus with low-grade dysplasia
K22.711	Barrett esophagus with high-grade dysplasia
K22.719	Barrett esophagus with dysplasia, unspecified

EPIDEMIOLOGY & DEMOGRAPHICS

- Male:female ratio of 4:1.
- Mean age of onset is 40 yr, with a mean age range of diagnosis of 55 to 60 yr.
- Occurs more frequently in white and Hispanic individuals than in African American individuals, with a ratio of 10 to 20:1.
- Lower socioeconomic status (captured by household net worth) is associated with increased prevalence of Barrett esophagus.[4]
- Mean prevalence of 5% to 15% in patients undergoing endoscopy (esophagogastroduodenoscopy [EGD]) for symptoms of gastroesophageal reflux disease (GERD). It is estimated that 5.6% of adults in the U.S. have Barrett esophagus. The prevalence rate may be as low as ~1% in patients without risk factors and varies based on patient location (Western vs. non-Western countries) and number of risk factors.
- Independent risk factors include chronic reflux (>5 yr), hiatal hernia, age >50 yr, male sex, white ethnicity, smoking history, and intraabdominal obesity. A family history of at least one first-degree relative with Barrett esophagus or adenocarcinoma of the esophagus is associated with a threefold to fivefold increased risk of Barrett esophagus and esophageal adenocarcinoma.[5,6]

PHYSICAL FINDINGS & CLINICAL PRESENTATION

SYMPTOMS:
- Chronic heartburn
- Dysphagia with solid food
- Less frequent: Chest pain, hematemesis, melena
- Patients may be asymptomatic
- May be an incidental finding on EGD in patients without reflux symptoms

PHYSICAL FINDINGS:
- Nonspecific; can be completely normal
- Epigastric tenderness on palpation

ETIOLOGY:
- Metaplasia is thought to result from reepithelialization of esophageal tissue injured as a result of chronic GERD. Activation of proliferative and inflammatory pathways likely induces a molecular phenotypic reprogramming of progenitor cells to form intestinal epithelium (Figs. E1 and E2). Several candidate cells have been identified, including migrating gastric epithelial cells, residual embryonic cells, transitional columnar epithelium, or submucosal glands or ducts.[2,3,5,7]
- Patients with Barrett esophagus tend to have more severe esophageal motility disturbances (decreased lower esophageal sphincter pressure, ineffective peristalsis) and greater esophageal acid exposure on 24-h pH monitoring. Table 1 lists some physiologic abnormalities that have been reported in patients with Barrett and suggests how these abnormalities may contribute to GERD severity.
- Bile salts in the presence of acid may produce oxidative stress, induce reactive oxygen species, and alter transcriptional factor activity, all of which may induce the formation of Barrett epithelium, DNA damage, and dysplastic progression.
- Familial clustering of GERD and Barrett esophagus suggests a genetic predisposition. Early data suggest that patients who develop Barrett are genetically predisposed to a severe inflammatory response to GERD.
- One meta-analysis of genome-wide association studies identified eight risk loci associated with Barrett esophagus and esophageal adenocarcinoma. Candidate susceptibility loci include *CRTC1, BARX1,* and *FOXP1.*[8,9]
- Progression from metaplasia to dysplasia to carcinoma is associated with accumulating changes in gene structure and expression, including the caudal-related homeobox family of transcription factors *(CDX1* and *CDX2),* the embryonic transcription factor SOX2, and the tumor suppressors p16 *(CDKN2A)* and

TP53. Biomarkers and developing technology such as TissueCypher, an image analysis platform, may help better predict cancer progression compared to histology alone, though current studies show low sensitivity and specificity.
- Chromosomal deletions, duplications, and translocation are all potential early events in progression of Barrett esophagus to malignancy.[10] A recent study suggests c-MYC and HNF4A as transcriptional drivers of metaplasia.[11]
- A recent Australian study suggests the presence of four pathologic criteria (loss of surface maturation, mucin depletion, nuclear enlargement, and increase of mitosis), together, was associated with greater progression from low-grade dysplasia to high-grade dysplasia or adenocarcinoma.[12]
- Transcriptionally active high-risk human papillomavirus has been described in cohorts of patients with Barrett esophagus with dysplasia and esophageal adenocarcinoma.
- Patients with Barrett esophagus and esophageal adenocarcinoma may have a shift in the esophageal microbiome toward a gram-negative population, which may play a role in oncogenesis through the release of proinflammatory cytokines and activation of oncogenic transcriptional regulators such as nuclear factor-κB (NF-κB).[13,14]

DIAGOSIS

DIFFERENTIAL DIAGNOSIS
- GERD, uncomplicated
- Erosive esophagitis
- Gastritis
- Peptic ulcer disease
- Angina
- Malignancy
- Stricture or Schatzki ring

WORKUP
- The American Gastroenterological Association Medical Position Panel gave a weak recommendation for screening patients with multiple risk factors, including age over 50, male sex, white race, chronic GERD, hiatal hernia, elevated body mass index, and intraabdominal distribution of body fat.[15-17] An international consensus group suggested

TABLE 1 Proposed Physiologic Abnormalities Contributing to Gastroesophageal Reflux Disease in Patients With Barrett Esophagus

Abnormality	Potential Consequences
Extreme hypotension of the lower esophageal sphincter	Gastroesophageal reflux
Ineffective esophageal motility	Defective clearance of refluxed material
Gastric acid hypersecretion	Reflux of highly acidic gastric juice
Duodenogastric reflux	Esophageal injury caused by reflux of bile acids and pancreatic enzymes
Decreased salivary secretion of EGF	Delayed healing of reflux-damaged esophageal mucosa
Decreased esophageal pain sensitivity to refluxed caustic material	Failure to initiate therapy

EGF, Epidermal growth factor.

From Feldman M et al: *Sleisenger and Fordtran's gastrointestinal and liver disease,* ed 11, Philadelphia, 2021, Elsevier.

screening men over 60 with GERD symptoms for more than 10 yr. An American College of Gastroenterology (ACG) Clinical Guideline suggests that screening for Barrett esophagus may be considered in men with chronic (>5 yr) and/or frequent (weekly or more) symptoms of GERD and two or more risk factors for Barrett esophagus or esophageal adenocarcinoma. Risks factors include age >50 yr, white race, presence of central obesity, current or past history of smoking, and a confirmed family history of Barrett esophagus or a first-degree relative with esophageal adenocarcinoma.[2] An American Society for Gastrointestinal Endoscopy (ASGE) guideline stated that although there was insufficient evidence on the effectiveness of screening, if done, it should be performed for high-risk individuals, defined as patients with a family history of esophageal adenocarcinoma or Barrett esophagus or moderate-risk patients with GERD and one of the earlier-defined risk factors.[5,18] General population screening is not currently recommended as screening using current techniques may not improve mortality rates from adenocarcinoma.[15,16]

- EGD (Fig. E3, Fig. E4, Fig. E5) with biopsy is necessary for diagnosis. Ideally, this should be done by high-resolution white-light endoscopy using the Seattle protocol with biopsies of any lesions followed by four-quadrant biopsies for every 2-cm segment. If erosive esophagitis is present, patients should be treated to heal esophagitis with repeat endoscopy and biopsies 8 to 12 wk later to determine if underlying Barrett esophagus is present. ASGE and ACG recommend concurrent use of chromoendoscopy or virtual chromoendoscopy if available. Repeat endoscopy following initial normal screening endoscopy has low utility.
- Unsedated transnasal endoscopy and esophageal cytology devices (Cytosponge, EsophaCap, or Esocheck) may be acceptable alternatives to conventional endoscopy.[19] Wireless esophageal capsule endoscopy may detect Barrett esophagus but with too low a sensitivity and specificity to be recommended.[11] Imaging studies are not useful.
- Diagnosis requires the presence of metaplastic columnar epithelium at least 1 cm proximal to the gastroesophageal junction (Fig. E6). Longer-segment (≥3 cm) Barrett esophagus is more readily diagnosed (Fig. E7). Barrett esophagus may be described using the Prague criteria, documenting the circumferential and maximal length of involvement by a C and M score, though the Prague criteria are unreliable when Z line displacement is <1 cm.[20] Biopsy of a normal Z line or a Z line with <1 cm displacement is not recommended given the potential high false-positive rate of Barrett diagnosis, which can lead to unnecessary surveillance endoscopy.[21] The Paris classification may be used to report associated visible lesions.
- At least two expert GI pathologists should concur if any grade of dysplasia is diagnosed.[2,15] A recent meta-analysis demonstrated a change

in diagnosis in 55% of cases when reviewed by an expert pathologist, most commonly with indeterminate or low-grade dysplasia.[21]
- Intestinal metaplasia of the gastric cardia is not Barrett esophagus and does not have the same risk for malignancy.
- Biomarkers using tissue samples and, more recently, blood tests involving whole-genome sequencing and even breath tests for volatile organic compounds, and advanced imaging techniques, such as mutational load, fluorescence in situ hybridization, autofluorescence imaging, white light postprocessing algorithms, confocal laser endomicroscopy, and optical coherence tomography (recently incorporated into volumetric laser endomicroscopy), are being evaluated to assist with diagnosis and to better understand progression of disease, prediction of response to therapy, or prognosis.
- Recent advancements also have been made in artificial intelligence. One example from the United Kingdom involves 3D reconstruction of endoscopic images with which Prague criteria C and M scores have been determined with >97% accuracy.[22]
- Screening for *Helicobacter pylori* infection in patients with GERD and Barrett esophagus is not recommended.

Rx TREATMENT

The goal is to control GERD symptoms and maintain healed mucosa.

NONPHARMACOLOGIC THERAPY

Nonpharmacologic therapy includes lifestyle modifications; elevating head of bed; and avoiding chocolate, tobacco, caffeine, mints, and certain drugs (see "Gastroesophageal Reflux Disease").

ACUTE GENERAL Rx

- Proton pump inhibitors are the most effective treatment for GERD. Therapy should be titrated to control symptoms and/or to promote healing of endoscopic signs of disease.[23]
- If patient is asymptomatic and incidentally found to have Barrett esophagus, once-daily proton pump inhibitors should be prescribed, as they may reduce the risk of neoplastic progression. Increasing dosage to twice daily is only recommended if breakthrough symptoms arise.[15]

CHRONIC Rx

- Chronic acid suppression is recommended to control symptoms, maintain healing, and reduce neoplastic progression. For patients with Barrett esophagus, the benefits of the use of proton-pump inhibitors are thought to outweigh the potential risks.[15,22,24,25]
- Antireflux surgery may be considered for management of GERD and associated sequelae, but it has not been proven to be superior to medical therapy and has no clear role in the management of Barrett esophagus. Barrett patients continue to require endoscopic surveillance of their esophagus.

- When GERD is controlled by either medical or surgical therapy, ablation of metaplastic epithelium usually leads to replacement by normal squamous epithelium. Because only a minority of patients with Barrett esophagus progress to high-grade dysplasia or carcinoma, endoscopic eradication therapy (EET) is not recommended for the general population of patients with nondysplastic Barrett esophagus.[17,25,26]
- EET is becoming the treatment of choice for low-grade dysplasia and is the treatment of choice for high-grade dysplasia and intramucosal cancer.[2,12,26-28] Radiofrequency ablation or photodynamic therapy, combined with endoscopic mucosal resection (EMR) or endoscopic submucosal dissection (ESD) of visible mucosal irregularities, should be performed in conjunction with aggressive surveillance and eradication of all remaining Barrett epithelium. Endoscopic therapy is preferred over surgical treatment in properly staged individuals, given lower morbidity and mortality rates and similar long-term survival rates. These therapies may even be considered for patients with focal intramucosal carcinoma, if properly staged (T1 SM1 or lower). Radiofrequency ablation is currently first-line, and cryotherapy (carbon dioxide, liquid nitrogen, or nitric oxide) and argon plasma coagulation are being evaluated for the complete eradication of both dysplasia and intestinal metaplasia and reduced risk for disease progression. All these options run the risk for residual or buried metaplasia. Ultimate goals of therapy include both complete eradication of dysplasia (CE-D) and complete eradication of intestinal metaplasia (CE-IM). Even with CE-IM, recurrence has been documented in 5% to 39.5% of patients. Modalities for endoscopic treatment of Barrett esophagus are summarized in Table 2. Given the high rates of recurrence of Barrett esophagus, those who have undergone successful EET should then continue with endoscopic surveillance.[2]
- Surgical resection is definitive therapy and may be offered for multifocal high-grade dysplasia, carcinoma that has extended into the submucosa (T1 SM2 or 3), or patients with poorly differentiated carcinomas or with evidence of lymphovascular invasion. Surgery also may be considered in patients with resistant, progressive, or recurrent disease in the face of endoscopic therapy. Mortality appears to be lower with experienced surgeons operating in high-volume centers.
- Patients with cardiovascular risk factors may be considered for low-dose aspirin therapy for chemoprevention of esophageal adenocarcinoma. NSAIDs or NSAIDs combined with statins are potentially effective at reducing the risk of esophageal adenocarcinoma but are not currently recommended for use because of the risk of adverse effects.

DISPOSITION

- The relative risk of developing esophageal adenocarcinoma for a patient with Barrett

TABLE 2 Modalities for Endoscopic Treatment of Barrett Esophagus

OVERALL COMMENTS REGARDING ENDOSCOPIC ERADICATION THERAPY[34]

EET preferred to surveillance in LGD (conditional recommendation, low quality of evidence)

EET preferred to surveillance in HGD (strong recommendation, moderate quality of evidence)

EET preferred to surgery in HGD/IMC (strong recommendation, very low quality of evidence)

Endoscopic resection of visible lesions with ablation of residual segment preferred against endoscopic resection of entire BE segment (strong recommendation, low quality of evidence)

In patient with remission of IM after EET, surveillance is recommended against no surveillance (conditional recommendation, very low quality of evidence)

Intervention	Preparation	Training	Best practices	Quality indicators
Cap-assisted endoscopic mucosal resection	Healing of esophagitis preferred Ideal for nodules/visible lesions <1.0 cm in largest diameter	Moderate learning curve though techniques mirror that in large polypectomy and variceal banding[35]; studies indicate that competency varies widely but may be achieved after 25-75 procedures National/international gastrointestinal societies may provide educational/hands-on courses (highly recommended)	Accurate photo documentation and coding of procedure is important Preferred for resection of visible nodularity and lesions less than 1-1.5 cm in size	[a]Adequate sampling in adherence to the Seattle Protocol for any Barrett's segment not involved by nodules/visible lesions [a]Assessment/documentation of complications such as bleeding necessitating hospitalization or blood transfusion, perforation, or stricture formation
Endoscopic submucosal dissection	Healing of esophagitis preferred Ideal for nodules/visible lesions greater than 1.0-1.5 cm in largest diameter	Highest learning curve: Studies indicate that competency varies widely but may be achieved after 20-200 procedures[36] National/international gastrointestinal societies may provide educational/hands-on courses (highly recommended)	Accurate photo documentation and coding of procedure is important Preferred for resection of visible nodularity and lesions greater than 1-1.5 cm in size	[a]Adequate sampling in adherence to the Seattle Protocol for any Barrett's segment not involved by nodules/visible lesions [a]Assessment/documentation of complications such as bleeding necessitating hospitalization or blood transfusion, perforation, or stricture formation [*]Documentation and achievement of rates of en bloc and R0 resection
Radiofrequency ablation	Healing of esophagitis preferred	Mild-moderate learning curve; F[37]	Assessment of posttreatment damage is vital Multidisciplinary care for patient discomfort after procedures is recommended	[a]Adequate sampling in adherence to the Seattle Protocol for any Barrett's segment not involved by nodules/visible lesions [a]Assessment/documentation of complications such as bleeding necessitating hospitalization or blood transfusion, perforation, or stricture formation [a]Assessment of CRD/CRIM rates as well as recurrence rates
Cryotherapy	Healing of esophagitis preferred Spray cryotherapy requires venting tube to avoid gastric overdistension	No studies have specifically assessed learning curve outcomes	Important to assess posttreatment changes	[a]Adequate sampling in adherence to the Seattle Protocol for any Barrett's segment not involved by nodules/visible lesions [a]Assessment/documentation of complications such as bleeding necessitating hospitalization or blood transfusion, perforation, or stricture formation [a]Assessment of CRD/CRIM rates as well as recurrence rates
Hybrid APC	Healing of esophagitis is preferred Adequate washing of area to be treated is essential	No studies have specifically assessed learning curve outcomes	Important to assess post-treatment changes Alternative to RFA and cryoablation in those not responding to initial treatment	[a]Adequate sampling in adherence to the Seattle Protocol for any Barrett's segment not involved by nodules/visible lesions [a]Assessment/documentation of complications such as bleeding necessitating hospitalization or blood transfusion, perforation, or stricture formation [a]Assessment of CRD/CRIM rates as well as recurrence rates

[a]Overview of common interventions used in Barrett endoscopic eradication therapy.

From Vani JA et al: Quality in Barrett's esophagus: diagnosis and management, *Tech Innov Gastrointest Endosc* 24(4):364-380, 2022. https://doi.org/10.1016/j.tige.2022.01.009.

esophagus, as compared with the general population, is 11.3, a substantial drop from the relative risk of 30 or 40 estimated in earlier reports. The risk is greater in men and in patients with longer (≥3 cm) columnar-lined segments.

- The risk of progression to esophageal adenocarcinoma from untreated Barrett with low-grade dysplasia is ~0.5% per yr, and with high-grade dysplasia ranges from 6% to 19% per yr.
- In the United States and Europe, the Prague criteria are recommended as a means of risk

stratification and determination of the frequency surveillance endoscopy. However, adherence is extremely variable.[1,29,30]

- Prasad et al. developed a model to predict progression of Barrett esophagus to neoplasia ("Progression in Barrett's Oesophagus score") based on sex, smoking history, length of Barrett involvement, and histology.[31]

- Frequency of monitoring is controversial. No prospective studies have proved that endoscopic surveillance is cost effective or increases life expectancy. Similarly, there are no clear guidelines for when surveillance should be stopped, although the ACG suggests stopping with less than an expected 5-yr survival or when a patient is no longer fit enough to undergo endoscopy or EET.[2]

- Patients with Barrett esophagus currently undergo EGD and systematic four-quadrant biopsy ("Seattle protocol") using white light and chromoendoscopy at intervals determined by the presence and grade of dysplasia. Wide-area transepithelial sampling with computer-assisted 3D analysis (WATS-3D) may increase the detection of dysplasia. All visible mucosal abnormalities should undergo biopsy.[15,29]

  1. Patients without dysplasia should have follow-up every 3 to 5 yr ($\geq$3 cm or <3 cm Barrett involvement, respectively).[2]
  2. Patients indefinite for dysplasia require aggressive, intensified medical therapy and close follow-up and resampling within 6 mo.
  3. Patients with low-grade dysplasia should have aggressive antisecretory (proton pump inhibitor) therapy, repeat endoscopy within 2 to 6 mo, and either endoscopic ablation therapy or extensive mucosal sampling at 6 and then every 12 mo

thereafter. Patients with high-grade dysplasia should have expert confirmation and extensive mucosal sampling. Advanced imaging techniques should be used to localize all neoplastic lesions. This includes virtual chromoendoscopy, narrow-band imaging (NBI), blue laser imaging (BLI), and i-scan. A simple and inexpensive technique is the use of acetic acid spray, which turns Barrett epithelium white, before turning neoplastic lesions red after 30 to 40 sec. High-grade dysplasia with visible mucosal irregularities should be removed by EMR or ESD, followed by mucosal ablation. Consider intensive surveillance every 3 mo for at least 1 yr and then annually thereafter. Endoscopic treatment is preferred over intensive surveillance in patients with high-grade dysplasia.[32]

  4. The ACG recommends after complete eradication that surveillance endoscopy be performed at 1 yr and 2 yr for low-grade dysplasia, and 3, 6, 12 mo and annually for high-grade dysplasia.[2] This is less frequent than previously recommended.

- Patients should be treated aggressively for GERD before surveillance.

- A Nordic population-based cohort study demonstrated that a quarter of all esophageal carcinomas are detected within a year after a negative upper endoscopy in patients with newly diagnosed Barrett esophagus. The finding of high rates of post endoscopy esophageal adenocarcinoma (PEEC) and post endoscopy esophageal neoplasia (PEEN) would seem to undermine the goal of early cancer detection in Barrett esophagus. The reasons for this require further study.[33]

REFERRAL

- Consider EGD with biopsy in male or selected female patients with multiple risk factors who have not had previous EGD.
- Refer patients with GERD for evaluation if "red flag" symptoms are present (dysphagia, odynophagia, weight loss, vomiting, early satiety, GI bleeding, iron deficiency).
- Refer patients with biopsy-proved Barrett esophagus for surveillance.
- For those with low-grade or high-grade dysplasia, refer for ablative therapy with EMR or ESD if appropriate, followed by intensive surveillance. Esophageal resection may be considered.

RELATED CONTENT

Barrett Esophagus (Patient Information)
Esophageal Tumors (Related Key Topic)
Gastroesophageal Reflux Disease (Related Key Topic)

AUTHORS: **HARLAN G. RICH, MD, FACP, AGAF** and **NAVEENA SUNKARA, MD**

REFERENCES

Available at eBooks.Health.Elsevier.com.

Diseases and Disorders

I

BASIC INFORMATION

DEFINITION

Acute peripheral facial nerve (cranial nerve VII) palsy

SYNONYMS

Idiopathic facial paralysis
Facial nerve palsy

ICD-10CM CODE
G51.0   Bell palsy

EPIDEMIOLOGY & DEMOGRAPHICS

INCIDENCE: 13 to 34 cases per 100,000
PREDOMINANT SEX & AGE: Sexes are equally affected. The median age is 40.
PEAK INCIDENCE: Patients <70 yr and pregnant females, especially during the third trimester and first postpartum wk
RISK FACTORS: Diabetes and pregnancy

PHYSICAL FINDINGS & CLINICAL PRESENTATION

- Patients present with acute or subacute (hours to days) onset of unilateral facial paralysis with maximal weakness at 3 wk. Clinical findings are dependent on the location of facial nerve injury (Fig. 1) and involvement of associated branches. One third of patients demonstrate incomplete paralysis, and the remaining two thirds have complete paralysis. Recovery usually occurs within the first 6 mo.
- Patients may also present with variable involvement of taste over the anterior two thirds of the tongue and/or altered secretion of the lacrimal and salivary glands.
- Several systems of clinical measurement of facial nerve function have been devised. In the House-Brackmann system, grade I is normal function, grade VI is complete absence of facial motor function, and grades II to V are intermediate (Table 1). The major functional criteria of the House-Brackmann system—absolute movement, synkinesis, eye closure, asymmetry at rest, and absolute paralysis—can be utilized within the existing House-Brackmann framework to create unambiguous and nonoverlapping categories of progression of deficit correlated with each grade (Fig. 2).

ETIOLOGY

Most cases of Bell palsy are thought to be secondary to either a viral inflammatory or immune injury. Herpes simplex virus is thought to be the most common viral pathogen followed by herpes zoster. Other infectious causes include Epstein-Barr virus, cytomegalovirus, adenovirus, rubella, and mumps.

DIAGNOSIS

DIFFERENTIAL DIAGNOSIS

- Cortical stroke: Forehead and periorbital muscles are spared in stroke patients because of bilateral innervation of the upper face

- Brain stem stroke: Ipsilateral weakness in the upper and lower muscles of facial expression due to a stroke affecting the nucleus or fascicle of the seventh nerve
- Lyme disease: Facial nerve palsy is the most common cranial neuropathy associated with Lyme disease. In Lyme meningitis, facial nerve palsy may be unilateral or bilateral
- HIV
- Ramsay Hunt syndrome: Facial nerve paralysis associated with ipsilateral zoster oticus
- Parotid gland tumors
- Trauma/temporal bone fracture
- Meningeal processes:
  1. Infectious: Lyme disease, HIV, syphilis, leprosy, tuberculosis meningitis, fungal meningitis
  2. Inflammatory: Sarcoidosis, Sjögren syndrome, and Guillain-Barré syndrome and its variants
  3. Leptomeningeal carcinomatosis or lymphomatosis: Breast cancer, lung cancer, and lymphoma are most common
- Moebius syndrome
- Melkersson-Rosenthal syndrome

WORKUP

- Bell palsy is a clinical diagnosis.
- Additional workup may be necessary in patients with an uncertain diagnosis, complete seventh nerve injury, evidence of neurologic dysfunction in addition to seventh nerve injury, and lack of recovery.

LABORATORY TESTS

Laboratory tests are not typically recommended. However, if the diagnosis of Bell palsy is in question (e.g., bilateral facial nerve palsy, concern for a secondary etiology), then it is reasonable to pursue the following tests:

- Lyme antibody followed by Western blot for positive cases for confirmation. Consider lumbar puncture for CSF analysis for Lyme serologies. In areas with endemic Lyme disease routine testing for Lyme disease may be indicated in all patients with Bell palsy (16% prevalence of Lyme disease)[1]

- Glycosylated hemoglobin (HgA1C)
- HIV
- Rapid plasma reagin (RPR)

ELECTRODIAGNOSTIC TESTING

Electrodiagnostic testing may be performed 10 days to 2 wk after the onset of symptoms to assess the integrity of a motor unit and the degree of nerve damage. Facial motor response remains normal for the first 3 days following an injury and then rapidly decreases depending on the severity of the lesion. A facial motor study may be performed at 10 days and compared to the contralateral side. A motor response that is 10% the amplitude of the unaffected side on electrodiagnostic testing corresponds with 90% motor axon degeneration. One study found that patient recovery was poor when this critical value was reached.

IMAGING STUDIES

Imaging studies are not usually indicated.
- Brain MRI is indicated in certain cases, such as an upper motor neuron pattern (able to wrinkle forehead) where the temporalis branch of the facial nerve is spared to evaluate for stroke or other upper motor neuron (UMN) lesion.
- Brain MRI with gadolinium is indicated either when other cranial nerve palsies are present or when a meningeal process is suspected.
- Computed tomography (CT) scan of temporal bone is indicated in cases of either trauma or complete facial paralysis in which the surgeon is considering decompression.

TREATMENT (FIG. 3)

NONPHARMACOLOGIC THERAPY

- Reassurance that most patients will have a full recovery and that the patient did not sustain a stroke.
- Eye patch to prevent corneal drying/abrasion and subsequent ulceration. Patients may protect their eyes with Lacri-Lube at night and artificial tears during the day.

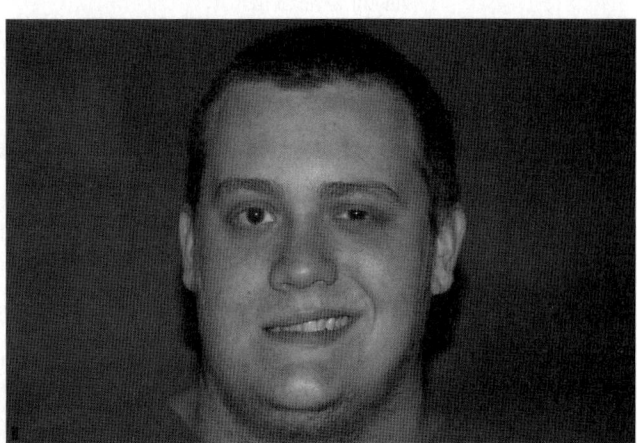

FIG. 1 Right facial palsy. On attempting to smile, there is little right facial action, the right palpebral fissure remains widened, and the right lower face fails to fully activate. (From Jankovic J et al: *Bradley and Daroff's neurology in clinical practice,* ed 8, Philadelphia, 2022, Elsevier.)

TABLE 1 House-Brackmann Facial Nerve Grading System

Grade	Description	Characteristics	At Rest	Forehead	Eye	Mouth
I	Normal	Normal facial function in all areas				
II	Mild dysfunction	Slight weakness noticeable on close inspection; may have very slight synkinesis	Normal symmetry and tone	Moderate to good function	Complete closure with minimum effort	Slight asymmetry
III	Moderate dysfunction	Obvious but not disfiguring difference between two sides; noticeable but not severe synkinesis, contracture, or hemifacial spasm	Normal symmetry and tone	Slight to moderate movement	Complete closure with effort	Slightly weak with maximum effort
IV	Moderately severe dysfunction	Obvious weakness and/or disfiguring asymmetry	Normal symmetry and tone	None	Incomplete closure	Asymmetric with maximum effort
V	Severe dysfunction	Barely perceptible motion only	Asymmetry	None	Incomplete closure	Slight movement
VI	Total paralysis	No movement				

From Flint PW et al: *Cummings otolaryngology, head and neck surgery,* ed 7, Philadelphia, 2021, Elsevier.

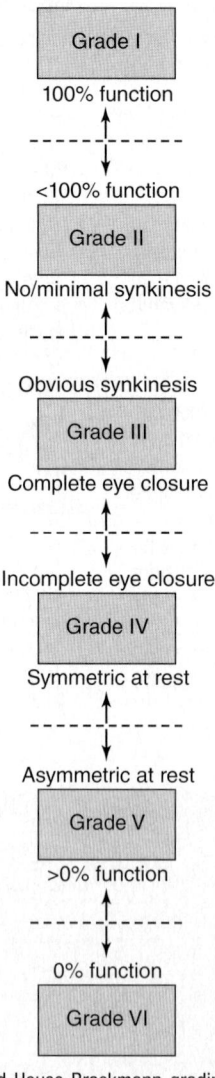

FIG. 2 Schematic diagram of a modified House-Brackmann grading scale—including the major functional criteria of absolute movement, synkinesis, eye closure, asymmetry at rest, and absolute paralysis—used in assigning unambiguous and nonoverlapping degrees of facial paralysis. (From Flint PW et al: *Cummings otolaryngology, head and neck surgery,* ed 7, Philadelphia, 2021, Elsevier.)

- Acupuncture with needle manipulation and strong stimulation has been shown to improve recovery after Bell palsy when compared to acupuncture without needle manipulation.[2]

ACUTE GENERAL Rx

- Corticosteroids started within 72 h will expedite speed and rate of recovery in most patients. Antiviral therapy alone has no benefit.
  1. Two high-quality randomized trials assessed efficacy of early (<72 h) treatment with glucocorticoids alone, antiviral therapy alone, and combination therapy in the treatment of Bell palsy. Glucocorticoids alone were effective, while antiviral therapy showed no benefit when given either alone or with concomitant glucocorticoid therapy.
  2. The largest study compared groups receiving the following treatments: (a) 60 mg prednisolone daily for 5 days, (b) 1000 mg valacyclovir three times daily for 1 wk, (c) combination therapy, and (d) placebo. All interventions were administered within 72 h of presentation.[1]
     a. Time to recovery, determined at a 1-yr follow-up appointment, was shortest in the group treated with prednisolone monotherapy.
     b. The efficacy of valacyclovir monotherapy did not differ from placebo, and no added benefit was seen with combination therapy.
- A 2016 Cochrane review found that high-quality evidence supported the use of corticosteroids with a number needed to treat of 10 to avoid one incomplete recovery.[2]
- A 2012 American Academy of Neurology evidence-based guideline update: Steroids and antivirals for Bell palsy concluded that Level A evidence supported offering patients with new-onset Bell palsy treatment with oral steroids to increase the probability of recovery of facial nerve function. Level C evidence supported offering these patients antivirals in addition to steroids, since the combination increases the

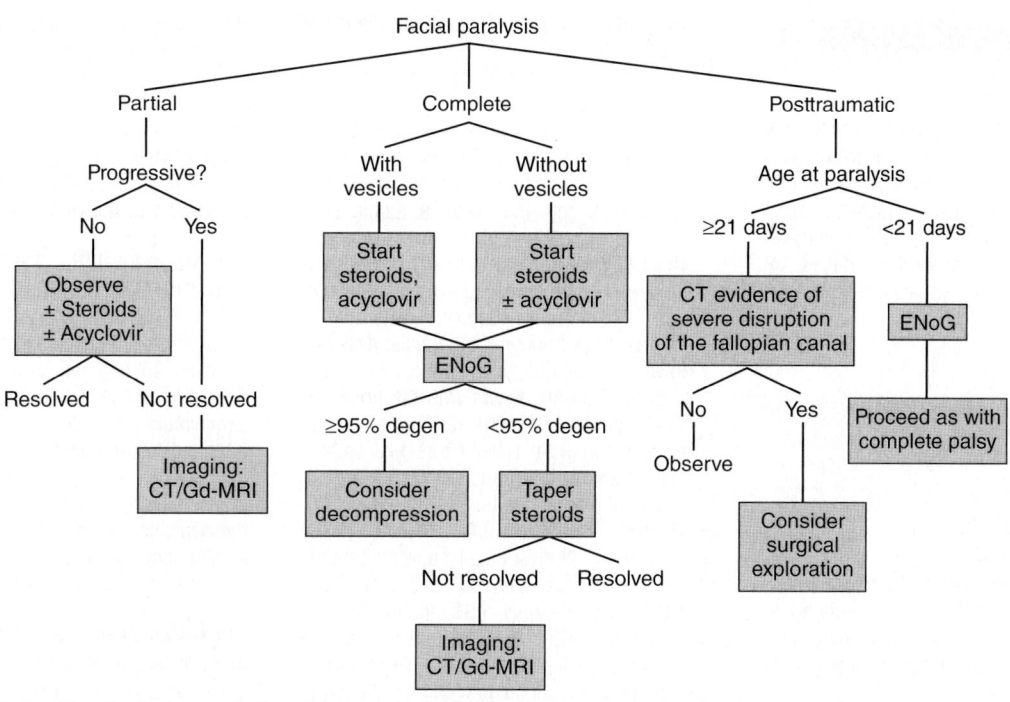

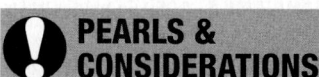

FIG. 3 Management algorithm for facial paralysis. *CT,* Computed tomography; *degen,* degeneration; *ENoG,* electroneuronography; *Gd,* gadolinium enhanced; *MRI,* magnetic resonance imaging. (From Flint PW et al: *Cummings otolaryngology, head and neck surgery,* ed 7, Philadelphia, 2021, Elsevier.)

probability of recovery of facial function. However, patients offered combination treatment should be counseled that antivirals have not been established as efficacious and any benefit is likely to be modest at best.[3]

Treatment regimens vary slightly but prednisone 60 mg/day for 5 days followed by a rapid taper over several days is one approach. Despite the lack of strong clinical evidence, some authors still recommend treatment with valacyclovir (1000 mg 3 times daily for 1 wk) in severe cases (i.e., level IV or greater on the House-Brackmann grading system). Eye care should include frequent lubrication of the affected eyelid and closure of the affected lid during sleep.

- Surgical decompression is not currently recommended.
  1. The 2001 American Academy of Neurology Practice Parameter concluded there was insufficient evidence to make any recommendation regarding surgical decompression for Bell palsy.
  2. This conclusion was further substantiated by a 2021 Cochrane systematic review, which looked at additional studies, again

citing insufficient evidence regarding surgical decompression for Bell palsy.[4]

CHRONIC Rx

Botulinum toxin may be used in cases of hemifacial spasm that may follow recovery from Bell palsy.

DISPOSITION

- Between 70% and 90% of patients with Bell palsy have a complete recovery within a few weeks.
- 85% show recovery after 3 wk. Prognosis is favorable if recovery is seen during this timeframe.
- 13% have slight sequelae, and 16% have residual weakness, synkinesis, or contracture.
- Recurrence rate is 7%, and the average time to recurrence is 10 yr.

REFERRAL

- Neurologist if clinical diagnosis is in question
- Ophthalmologist if concern for corneal abrasion or ulceration

⚠ **PEARLS & CONSIDERATIONS**

COMMENTS

- Assess wrinkling of forehead. If present on affected side, ensure that the facial weakness is not central.
- Assess for strength of eye closure. A patient with Bell palsy will have difficulty with ipsilateral eye closure, whereas a patient with a central lesion with have equal eye closure strength bilaterally.
- Assess for other cranial nerve deficits or long-tract signs because brain stem fascicular lesions of the seventh nerve can show peripheral facial pattern of weakness.

RELATED CONTENT

Bell Palsy (Facial Palsy) (Patient Information)

REFERENCES

Available at eBooks.Health.Elsevier.com.

AUTHOR: **JOSEPH S. KASS, MD, JD, FAAN**

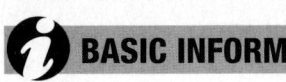 **BASIC INFORMATION**

DEFINITION

Benign paroxysmal positional vertigo (BPPV) is a labyrinthine disorder and is the most common cause of vertigo. It is characterized by paroxysms of brief spinning sensation accompanied by nystagmus that usually last less than a minute. These paroxysms are generally induced by changes in head position with respect to gravity.

SYNONYM

BPPV

ICD-10CM CODE
H81.1   Benign paroxysmal vertigo

EPIDEMIOLOGY & DEMOGRAPHICS

INCIDENCE: Incidence increases with advancing age. Unrecognized BPPV can be found in about 10% of certain geriatric populations, and there is a cumulative incidence of nearly 10% by age 80 yr.

PREVALENCE: Lifetime prevalence is 2.4%. Reported prevalence is 10.7% and 64 cases per 100,000 population. BPPV is by far the most common type of vertigo.

PREDOMINANT SEX & AGE: Female (2:1 to 3:1 ratio); peak onset: 50 to 60 yr

RISK FACTORS: Head trauma, inner ear surgery, viral labyrinthitis, Ménière disease, migraine. The majority are idiopathic.

GENETICS: Unknown

PHYSICAL FINDINGS & CLINICAL PRESENTATION

- Brief paroxysms of vertigo and nystagmus with certain head positions are seen in 70%.
- Episodes are typically triggered by head position changes such as getting in or out of bed, rolling over in bed, tilting the head forward, or bending forward.
- Episodes are brief, usually lasting 30 to 40 sec but can recur for several days or months.
- Usually no hearing abnormalities are present.
- Direction of nystagmus depends on the canal affected with reversal of direction being seen while sitting up, and fatigability with repeated testing.
- Rarely persistent vertigo and disequilibrium may be seen.
- The plane in which the eyes deviate as a result of vestibular stimulation depends on the combination of canals that are stimulated (Table 1). If only the posterior semicircular canal on one side is stimulated (as occurs with BPPV), a vertical-torsional deviation of the eyes can be observed, which is followed by a fast corrective response generated by the conscious brain in the opposite direction. However, if the horizontal canal is the source of stimulation (as occurs with the horizontal canal variant of BPPV [HC-BPPV]), a horizontal deviation with a slight torsional component (because this canal is slightly off the horizontal plane) results.

POSTERIOR SEMICIRCULAR CANAL (PSC): While posterior, horizontal, or superior semicircular canal can be affected as isolated or in different combinations, PSC involvement is most common (60% to 90%) and will be discussed in the following sections. Nystagmus is up-beating and torsional and can be elicited by the Dix-Hallpike maneuver.

DIX-HALLPIKE MANEUVER: With head turned to one side at an angle of 45 degrees, patient is moved rapidly from sitting to supine position with head hanging below the end of the table at an angle of 15 to 20 degrees. The posterior semicircular canal comes into the sagittal plane, and the free-floating otolith debris moves down and away from the ampulla. An up-beating and torsional nystagmus will be seen with the top poles of the eye beating toward the lower ear.

HORIZONTAL SEMICIRCULAR CANAL: Involvement may be underestimated as it may remit spontaneously. It produces either geotropic nystagmus beating toward the ground or apogeotropic nystagmus beating toward the ceiling when the head is turned to either side in the supine position. The nystagmus beats stronger toward the affected ear.

HEAD ROLL TEST FOR THE RIGHT HORIZONTAL SEMICIRCULAR CANAL (INDUCING GEOTROPIC NYSTAGMUS): Patient is moved from sitting to supine position, then head is rolled 90 degrees to the left. The otolithic debris moves away from the cupula of the horizontal semicircular canal, a left-beating geotropic nystagmus (toward the ground) is seen. Next the head is turned 90 degrees to the right—a right-beating stronger geotropic nystagmus is seen as otolithic debris moves toward the cupula of the right horizontal semicircular canal.

SUPINE HEAD ROLL TEST FOR THE RIGHT HORIZONTAL SEMICIRCULAR CANAL (INDUCING APOGEOTROPIC NYSTAGMUS): Patient is moved from sitting to supine position, then head is rolled 90 degrees to the left. This induces deflection of the cupula of the right horizontal semicircular canal due to otolithic debris near or attached to the cupula. A strong, right-beating apogeotropic nystagmus (toward the ceiling) is induced. Next, the head is turned 90 degrees in the opposite direction. Now the right horizontal semicircular canal cupula is deflected in the opposite direction and a weak, left-beating apogeotropic nystagmus results.

SUPERIOR SEMICIRCULAR CANAL: Involvement is rare as it is located uppermost in the labyrinth and so otolithic debris is unlikely to become trapped. A downbeat and torsional nystagmus where the top poles of the eye beat toward the lower ear is seen. Evaluating for central lesions is a must in these cases.

ETIOLOGY

The fundamental pathologic process is believed to be the movement of otolithic debris in the endolymph of the inner ear. The debris may be present in the cupula (cupulolithiasis) or free floating within the semicircular canal near the cupula (canalithiasis). Static head position changes with respect to gravity, causing the debris to move within the semicircular canal and creating a false sense of rotation.

DX DIAGNOSIS

Elicitation of a typical nystagmus with Dix-Hallpike is the standard for diagnosing posterior canal BPPV. However, 25% of symptomatic patients may not exhibit nystagmus. Appropriate referral to a neurologist or neuro-otologist should be considered in these cases.

TABLE 1 Physiologic Properties and Clinical Features of the Components of the Peripheral Vestibular System

Localization	Component(s)	Triggered Eye Movements	Common Clinical Conditions	Localizing Features
Semicircular Canals				
Posterior canal	PC	Vertical, torsional	BPPV-PC	Nystagmus
Anterior canal	AC	Vertical, torsional	BPPV-AC, SCD	Nystagmus, fistula test
Horizontal canal	HC	Horizontal ≥ torsional	BPPV-HC, fistula	Nystagmus
Vestibular Nerve				
Superior division	AC, HC, utricle	Horizontal > torsional	VN, ischemia	Nystagmus, head-thrust test
Inferior division	PC, saccule	Vertical, torsional	VN, ischemia	Nystagmus
Common trunk (cranial nerve 8)	AC, HC, PC, utricle, saccule	Horizontal > torsional	VN, VP, ischemia	Nystagmus, head-thrust test, auditory findings
Labyrinth	AC, HC, PC, utricle, saccule	Horizontal > torsional	EH, labyrinthitis	Nystagmus, auditory findings

AC, Anterior canal; *BPPV*, benign paroxysmal positional vertigo; *EH*, endolymphatic hydrops; *HC*, horizontal canal; *PC*, posterior canal; *SCD*, superior canal dehiscence; *VN*, vestibular neuritis; *VP*, vestibular paroxysmia.

From Jankovic J et al: *Bradley and Daroff's neurology in clinical practice*, ed 8, Philadelphia, 2022, Elsevier.

Fig. 1 shows a diagnostic algorithm for vertigo and dizziness.

DIFFERENTIAL DIAGNOSIS
- Vestibular neuritis
- Vestibular migraine
- Ménière disease
- Stroke
- Box 1 lists causes of vertigo with and without hearing loss
- Table 2 describes the differential diagnosis of true vertigo

WORKUP
- BPPV is a clinical diagnosis. Key elements in the initial dizziness history are summarized in Table E3.
- The Hallpike test, also known as the Dix-Hallpike test or the Nylen-Barany test, confirms the diagnosis of posterior canal BPPV, which is the most common variant. This test should be reserved for those patients suspected of triggered vertigo from head position change, and caution should be exercised in performing it in patients with acute vestibular syndrome (acute and constant dizziness, nausea or vomiting, unsteady gait, nystagmus, and intolerance to head motion lasting more than a day), whose main differential diagnosis includes vestibular neuritis and posterior circulation stroke. Thus if a patient is actively experiencing vertigo during history taking and there has been no immediate prior head movement, then the Hallpike test should not be performed because this history is inconsistent with BPPV, which requires head movement to elicit symptoms. The Hallpike test is performed with the patient sitting up. The examiner turns the patient's head 45 degrees to one side and then moves the patient from the upright seated position to a supine position with the head overhanging the edge of the gurney (Fig. 2). The patient is queried for the occurrence of vertigo, and the eyes are observed for nystagmus after a latency period of a few seconds. In a patient with classic posterior canal BPPV, the nystagmus usually lasts 5 to 30 sec and is combined with upbeating (the fast phase beats toward the forehead) and ipsilateral torsional (the top pole beating toward the downward ear) motion. The patient is then brought back up to the seated position, and the test is repeated with the head turned 45 degrees to the other side. Findings are summarized in Box 2.[1]

IMAGING STUDIES
To be obtained only when stroke remains high in the differential diagnosis

Rx TREATMENT
- BPPV usually resolves without treatment in 2 to 4 wk. Recurrences are common in the first yr, and long-term recurrence rates range from 30% to 50%.
- Nausea and vomiting may be treated symptomatically with medications.
- Canalith repositioning maneuvers (Epley and Semont maneuvers for the posterior canal) are effective. Fig. 3 shows a general management algorithm in approaching patients with dizziness and vertigo. The Epley maneuver is the main canalith-repositioning maneuver used to treat posterior semicircular canal BPPV.[1] These maneuvers are designed to "flush" otolithic debris out of the semicircular canals into the vestibule where they are resorbed. Epley maneuver for BPPV of the posterior canal is recommended as standard of care by the American Academy of Neurology and American Academy of Otolaryngology-Head and Neck Surgery. When patients do not respond, it may be related to the technique, or they may be refractory. There is no clear consensus on how many times the maneuver should be performed at a single visit. Many prefer to do it two or three times if nystagmus is still present with the second maneuver. Other maneuvers such as barbecue, Vannucchi-Asprella, and Gufoni are used to reposition debris in the horizontal semicircular canal and will not be discussed here.

EPLEY MANEUVER:
- Head is turned 90 degrees toward unaffected side. The head and trunk are then turned an additional 90 degrees in the same direction, so that the patient lies on the unaffected side with head pointing toward the floor. The otolithic debris moves in the same direction, producing a brief nystagmus. The patient is then moved to a sitting position, which allows the debris to fall out of the canal into the utricle through the common crus.
- Each position should be maintained for 30 sec or until the nystagmus or vertigo resolves. Sometimes nystagmus in the opposite direction is seen. It is prudent for patients to sit still in the upright position for about 15 min and then to walk cautiously.

NONPHARMACOLOGIC THERAPY
Transection of the ampullary nerve (singular nerve) and plugging of the involved canal are rarely performed for intractable and treatment-resistant cases.

ACUTE GENERAL Rx
- Canalith repositioning
- Vestibular suppressants such as antihistamines, benzodiazepines, and anticholinergics

---

BOX 1 Causes of Vertigo with and without Hearing Loss

Hearing Loss
Conductive
- Otitis media with effusion
- Chronic suppurative otitis media or cholesteatoma should be considered

Sensorineural
- Perilymphatic fistula
- Tumor
- Ménière disease
- Migraine headache
- Genetic syndromes
- Temporal bone fracture
- Vestibular concussion

No Hearing Loss
Acute Vertigo
- Perilymphatic fistula
- Benign positional vertigo
- Seizure
- Labyrinthitis

Recurrent or Chronic Vertigo
- Acoustic neuroma
- Multiple sclerosis

From Marx JA et al: *Rosen's emergency medicine: concepts and clinical practice*, ed 7, Philadelphia, 2010, Elsevier.

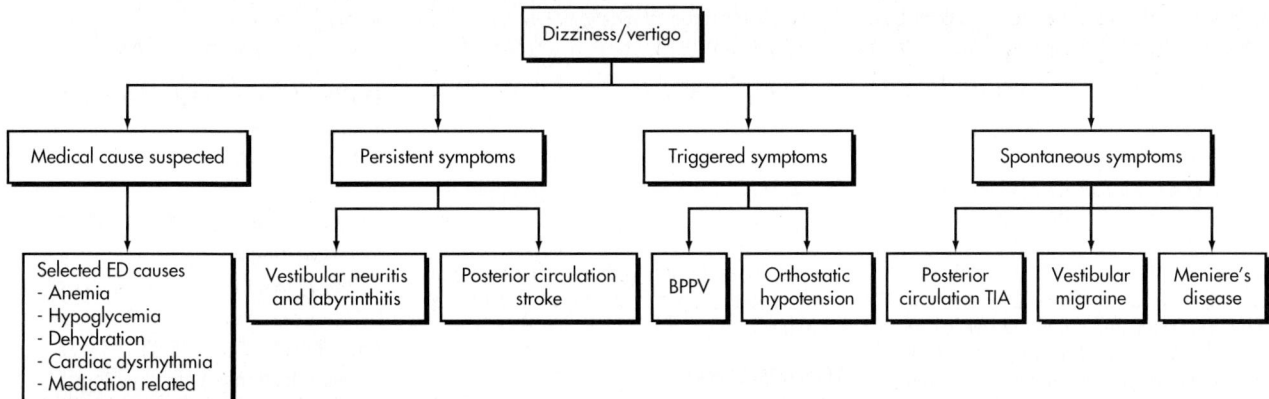

FIG. 1 Diagnostic algorithm for dizziness and vertigo. *BPPV,* Benign paroxysmal positional vertigo; *TIA,* transient ischemic attack. (From Walls RM et al: *Rosen's emergency medicine, concepts and clinical practice*, ed 10, Philadelphia, 2023, Elsevier.)

TABLE 2 Differentiating Benign Paroxysmal Positional Vertigo from Vestibular Neuritis/Labyrinthitis

	Benign Paroxysmal Positional Vertigo	Vestibular Neuritis/Labyrinthitis
Age	More common in older adults	More common in younger patients
Hearing loss	None	None in vestibular neuritis; hearing loss in labyrinthitis
Frequency of symptoms	Episodic (occurs with certain movements of the head)	Constant
Hallpike test	Positive usually on one side only with upbeat and torsional nystagmus and reproduction of vertigo symptoms	Symptoms may be worsened in head-hanging position (NOTE: It is advised not to administer Hallpike test in a patient with a clinical history consistent with vestibular neuritis or labyrinthitis.)
Head impulse test	Negative (NOTE: It is advised not to administer head impulse test in a patient with a clinical history consistent with BPPV.)	Positive (corrective saccade seen)
Epley maneuver	Highly effective	Ineffective
Recurrence	Frequent	Rare (2%-11%)

BPPV, Benign paroxysmal positional vertigo.
From Walls RM et al: *Rosen's emergency medicine, concepts and clinical practice,* ed 10, Philadelphia, 2023, Elsevier.

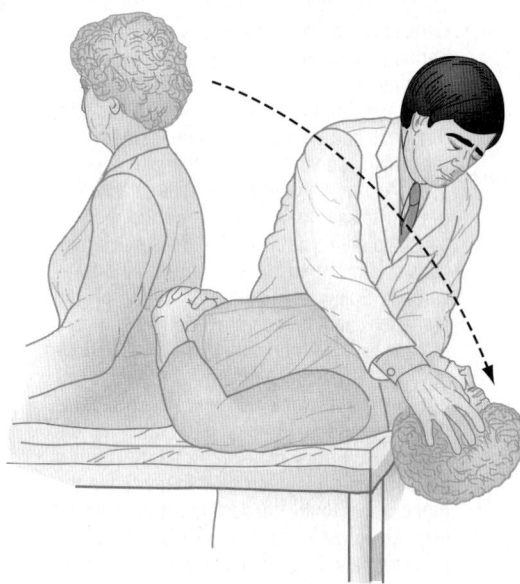

FIG. 2 Testing for positional vertigo and nystagmus. (From Walls RM et al: *Rosen's emergency medicine, concepts and clinical practice*, ed 10, Philadelphia, 2023, Elsevier.)

BOX 2 Classic Findings during Hallpike Test in Posterior Canal Benign Paroxysmal Positional Vertigo

Latency (delay in nystagmus and vertigo once in head-hanging position) of approximately 3-10 sec, although delay can take up to 30 sec on rare occasions
Reproduction of vertigo symptoms in head-hanging position
Upbeat (fast phase toward forehead) and torsional nystagmus (usually toward the downward ear)
Vertigo and nystagmus escalate in head-hanging position, then slowly resolve over 5-30 sec
Nystagmus and vertigo may reverse direction when patient returns to sitting position
Nystagmus and vertigo decrease with repeated testing (fatigability)

From Walls RM et al: *Rosen's emergency medicine, concepts and clinical practice,* ed 10, Philadelphia, 2023, Elsevier.

are commonly used to treat BPPV despite a lack of evidence for their effectiveness. Most vestibular suppressants are antiemetic medications (Table 4), which not only suppress nausea and vomiting but also decrease the sensation of vertigo. Meclizine (12.5 to 50 mg every 4 to 6 h) can exacerbate symptoms in patients with non-vertiginous types of dizziness. It should be reserved for patients with BPPV who have failed the Epley maneuver or for patients who have an alternative diagnosis of peripheral vertigo, such as vestibular neuritis. Transdermal scopolamine has shown disappointing results for treatment of peripheral vertigo but may be considered a third-line option.[1]

CHRONIC Rx

If multiple treatments are needed, patients should be instructed to perform the maneuvers at home.

REFERRAL

To a neuro-otologist, otolaryngologist, neurologist

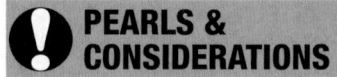

PEARLS & CONSIDERATIONS

- BPPV is a benign and self-limiting condition but can be disabling.
- Diagnosis is clinical, and canalith repositioning maneuvers are effective.

PATIENT & FAMILY EDUCATION

- Reassurance
- Fall precautions

REFERENCE & SUGGESTED READINGS

Available at eBooks.Health.Elsevier.com.

RELATED CONTENT

Ménière Disease (Related Key Topic)
Vestibular Neuronitis (Related Key Topic)

AUTHOR: **JOSEPH S. KASS, MD, JD, FAAN**

B

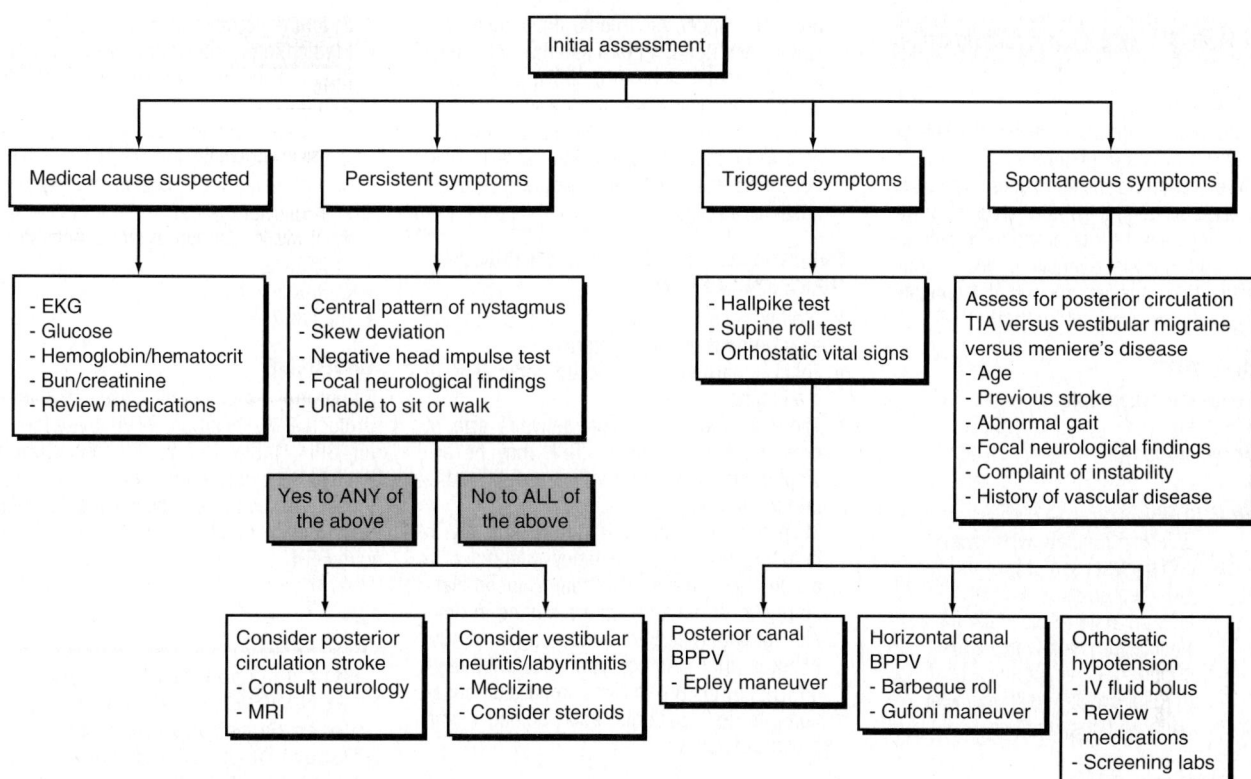

FIG. 3 **Management algorithm for dizziness and vertigo.** *BPPV,* Benign paroxysmal positional vertigo; *ECG,* electrocardiogram; *IV,* intravenous; *MRI,* magnetic resonance imaging; *TIA,* transient ischemic attack. (From Walls RM et al: *Rosen's emergency medicine, concepts and clinical practice,* ed 10, Philadelphia, 2023, Elsevier.)

Diseases and Disorders

I

TABLE 4	Medications for Acute Vertigo	
Drug	**Usual Starting Dosage**	**Antiemetic Action**
Promethazine (Phenergan)	12.5-25 mg IM, PO, PR (FDA boxed warning recommends IM over IV given risks of extravasation)	Moderate
Ondansetron (Zofran)	4 mg IV, SL/PO, IM	Prominent
Dimenhydrinate (Dramamine)	50-100 mg IM, IV, PO	Moderate
Prochlorperazine (Compazine)	5-10 mg IV, IM, PO, PR	Prominent
Droperidol (Inapsine)	0.625-2.5 mg IM	Prominent
Metoclopramide (Reglan)	5-10 mg IV, IM, PO	Prominent
Lorazepam (Ativan)	1-2 mg IV, IM, PO	Mild
Diazepam (Valium)	1 mg IV, IM, PO	Mild
Meclizine (Antivert)	12.5-50 mg PO	Mild
Scopolamine (Transderm-Scop)	0.2 mg transdermal patch	Moderate

IM, Intramuscular; *IV,* intravenous; *PO, per os* (by mouth); *PR,* per rectum; *SL,* sublingual.

From Walls RM et al: *Rosen's emergency medicine, concepts and clinical practice,* ed 10, Philadelphia, 2023, Elsevier.

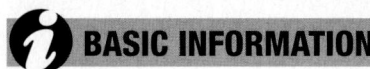

BASIC INFORMATION

DEFINITION

Benign prostatic hyperplasia (BPH) is the benign growth of the prostate, generally originating in the periureteral and transition zones, with subsequent obstructive and irritative voiding symptoms. Histologically, BPH refers to the proliferation of smooth muscle, epithelium, and stromal cells within the transition zone of the prostate that surrounds the proximal urethra.

SYNONYMS

Benign prostatic hypertrophy
BPH
Prostatic hypertrophy

ICD-10CM CODES

N40.1	Enlarged prostate with lower urinary tract symptoms
N40.0	Enlarged prostate without lower urinary tract symptoms
N40.3	Nodular prostate with lower urinary tract symptoms
N40.2	Nodular prostate without lower urinary tract symptoms

EPIDEMIOLOGY & DEMOGRAPHICS

- 80% of men have evidence of BPH by age 80 yr.
- Medical and surgical intervention for problems caused by BPH is required in <20% of males by age 75 yr.
- Transurethral resection of the prostate (TURP) is the tenth most common operative procedure (<400,000/yr in U.S.).
- 10% to 30% of men with BPH have occult prostate cancer. The incidence of metastatic

prostate cancer for middle-aged men was stable from 2004 to 2010 and then increased from 12 to 17 cases/100,000 from 2010 to 2018.[1] It is unclear if this increase was due to U.S. Preventive Services Task Force (USPSTF) recommendations against PSA screening in 2008 and 2012 or to more aggressive diagnostic strategies

PHYSICAL FINDINGS & CLINICAL PRESENTATION

- Digital rectal examination (DRE) reveals enlargement of the prostate.
- Focal enlargement may be indicative of malignancy.
- There is poor correlation between size of prostate, and symptoms (BPH may be asymptomatic if it does not encroach on the urethral lumen).
- Most patients with BPH report difficulty in initiating urination (hesitancy), decrease in caliber and force of stream, incomplete emptying of bladder often resulting in double voiding (need to urinate again a few minutes after voiding), postvoid "dribbling," and nocturia. Box 1 lists important questions to ask patients about bladder and prostate function.

ETIOLOGY

Multifactorial (Fig. E1); a functioning testicle is necessary for development of BPH (as evidenced by the absence in males who were castrated before puberty).

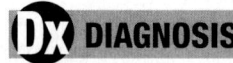 DIAGNOSIS

DIFFERENTIAL DIAGNOSIS

- Prostatitis
- Prostate cancer

- Strictures (urethral)
- Medications interfering with the muscle fibers in the prostate and also with bladder function:
  1. Opiates: Impaired autonomic function
  2. Decongestants: Increased sphincter tone
  3. Antihistamines: Decreased parasympathetic tone
  4. Tricyclic antidepressants: Anticholinergic effects
- Neurogenic bladder
- Bladder cancer

WORKUP

Symptom assessment (use of American Urological Association [AUA] Symptom Index for BPH [Table 1, Box 2]), laboratory tests. Postvoid residual measurement and uroflowmetry are optional assessment.[2] Fig. E2 describes a diagnostic approach to patients with BPH.

BOX 1 The IPSS Mnemonic "FUN WISE" Is a Reminder of the Seven Questions to Ask the Patient About Bladder and Prostate Function

F	Frequency
U	Urgency
N	Nocturia
W	Weak stream
I	Intermittency
S	Straining
E	Sensation of incomplete emptying

From Robertson RP et al: *DeGroot's endocrinology, basic science and clinical practice,* ed 8, Philadelphia, 2023, Elsevier.

TABLE 1 International Prostate Symptom Score (I-PSS)

Symptom	Not at All	Less Than 1 Time in 5	Less Than Half the Time	About Half the Time	More Than Half the Time	Almost Always	Total Score
Incomplete emptying: Over the past month, how often have you had a sensation of not emptying your bladder completely after you finished urinating?	0	1	2	3	4	5	
Frequency: Over the past month, how often have you had to urinate again <2 h after you finished urinating?	0	1	2	3	4	5	
Intermittency: Over the past month, how often have you found you stopped and started again several times when you urinated?	0	1	2	3	4	5	
Urgency: Over the past month, how often have you found it difficult to postpone urination?	0	1	2	3	4	5	
Weak stream: Over the past month, how often have you had a weak urinary stream?	0	1	2	3	4	5	
Straining: Over the past month, how often have you had to push or strain to begin urination?	0	1	2	3	4	5	
	None	1 Time	2 Times	3 Times	4 Times	5 or More times	
Nocturia: Over the past month, how many times did you most typically get up to urinate from the time you went to bed at night until the time you got up in the morning?	0	1	2	3	4	5	

Total I-PSS score =

BOX 2 IPSS (Out of 35)

Score	Correlation
0 to 7	Mildly symptomatic
8 to 19	Moderately symptomatic
20 to 35	Severely symptomatic

From Robertson RP et al: *DeGroot's endocrinology, basic science and clinical practice*, ed 8, Philadelphia, 2023, Elsevier.

LABORATORY TESTS

- Prostate-specific antigen (PSA): Protease secreted by epithelial cells of the prostate; elevated in 30% to 50% of patients with BPH. Testing for PSA increases detection rate for prostate cancer and tends to detect cancer at an earlier stage. However, the PSA test does not discriminate well between patients with symptomatic BPH and those with prostate cancer, particularly if the cancer is pathologically localized and curable. The test may also trigger additional evaluation, including ultrasound biopsy of the prostate. Asymptomatic men with PSA levels >2 ng/ml do not need annual testing. According to the AUA, PSA testing and DRE should be offered to any asymptomatic man >50 yr with a life expectancy of 10 yr. PSA testing can also be offered at an earlier age in men at higher risk of prostatic cancer (e.g., first-degree relatives with prostate cancer; African American race). The USPSTF currently recommends individualized screening decisions for men between ages 55 and 69 and advises against screening for older men.
- Measurement of "free" PSA is useful to assess the probability of prostate cancer in patients with normal DRE and total PSA between 4 and 10 ng/ml. In these patients the global risk of prostate cancer is 25%. However, if the free PSA is >25%, the risk of prostate cancer decreases to 8%, whereas if the free PSA is <10%, the risk of cancer increases to 56%. Free PSA is also useful to evaluate the aggressiveness of prostate cancer. A low free PSA percentage generally indicates a high-grade cancer, whereas a high free PSA percentage is generally associated with a slower-growing tumor.
- Elevated measurement of prostate cancer gene 3 *(PCA3)* in urine specimens collected after digital examination is helpful in deciding about prostate biopsy in men with elevated PSA (increased *PCA3* = increased likelihood of prostate cancer).
- Urinalysis, urine culture, and sensitivity to rule out infection (if suspected).
- Blood urea nitrogen and creatinine to rule out postrenal insufficiency.

IMAGING STUDIES

- In patients with elevated PSA levels, MRI of prostate is useful to guide decisions on whether to perform biopsies. MRI also facilitates biopsy of suspicious areas.[1]
- Transrectal ultrasound is inserted in patients with palpable nodules or significant elevation of PSA. It is also useful to estimate prostate size. BPH may also be evident in suprapubic ultrasound and MRI (Fig. E3).
- Uroflowmetry may be used to determine relative impact of obstruction on urine flow. Urethral pressure profile is useful to predict prostatic hypertrophy within the urethral lumen.
- Pressure flow studies, although invasive, are particularly helpful in patients whose history and/or examination suggest primary bladder dysfunction as a cause of symptoms of prostatism. They are also useful in patients for whom a distinction between prostatic obstruction and impaired detrusor contractility may affect the choice of therapy. However, pressure flow studies may not be useful in the workup of the usual patient with symptoms of prostatism.
- Postvoid residual urine measurement has not been proved useful in predicting the need for or response to treatment; it may be useful in monitoring the course of the disease in patients who elect nonsurgical treatment.
- Urethral cystoscopy is an option during later evaluation if invasive treatment is being planned.

Rx TREATMENT

NONPHARMACOLOGIC THERAPY
BEHAVIOR AND LIFESTYLE MODIFICATION:
- Avoidance of caffeine or any other foods that may exacerbate symptoms
- Avoidance of medications that may exacerbate symptoms (e.g., most cold and allergy remedies)

GENERAL Rx (BOX 3)
- Asymptomatic patients with prostate enlargement caused by BPH generally do not require treatment. Patients with mild to moderate symptoms are candidates for pharmacologic treatment (see the following). For patients who have specific complications from BPH, prostate surgery is usually the most appropriate form of treatment. However, surgery may result in significant complications (e.g., incontinence, infection).
- Alpha-blockers (e.g., tamsulosin, alfuzosin, doxazosin, prazosin, terazosin) relax smooth muscle of the bladder neck and prostate and can increase peak urinary flow rate. They have no effect on the size of the prostate. Alpha-1 blockers are useful in symptomatic patients to relieve symptoms of obstruction by causing relaxation of smooth muscle tone in the prostatic capsule, urethra, and bladder neck. Alpha blockers are associated with "inappropriate floppy iris syndrome," inquire above planned cataract surgery before prescribing.[1]
- Hormonal manipulation with finasteride, a 5-alpha-reductase inhibitor (ARI) that blocks conversion of testosterone to dihydrotestosterone, can be added to patients with prostate size estimated to be at least 30 cc to reduce the size of the prostate. Usual dose is 5 mg/day. Treatment requires ≥6 mo for maximal effect. ARI shrink the prostate by ~25%. Symptom improvement is slow typically requiring up to 6 mo for maximum effect.
- Dutasteride is also a 5-alpha-reductase inhibitor useful to decrease prostate size and improve urinary flow. In addition to inhibiting the isoform of 5-alpha-reductase located in the prostate, the medication inhibits a second isoform and reduces dihydrotestosterone formation in the skin and liver. Usual dose is 0.5 mg/day.
- Combination of an alpha-blocker and ARI is appropriate in patients responding poorly to one agent.
- Tadalafil 2.5 to 5 mg/day has been FDA-approved to treat patients with signs and symptoms of BPH and patients with both ED and signs and symptoms of BPH. Tadalafil can potentiate the hypotensive effect of alpha-blockers and should not be used in combination with alpha-blockers.
- The dietary supplement saw palmetto is commonly used for relief of symptoms of BPH. Recent trials using 160 mg of saw palmetto bid did not improve symptoms of BPH. This contrasts with the positive findings of many previous studies. Trials with higher dose-ranging protocols are currently in progress.
- A surgical referral is warranted if the BPH results in chronic kidney disease, refractory urinary retention, or recurrent urinary tract infection if there is concern for bladder or

---

BOX 3 Medical Management of BPH

5-Alpha-Reductase Inhibitors
Block conversion of testosterone to the more potent dihydrotestosterone (DHT)
Reduce prostate size, PSA level, and symptoms in 6 to 12 mo
Finasteride and dutasteride

Alpha-Adrenergic Receptor Antagonists
Relax prostate smooth muscle
Improve symptoms but do not reduce risk of urinary retention
Tamsulosin and silodosin—selective alpha1 blockers

Combination
5-alpha reductase inhibitor combined with an alpha blocker
Dutasteride/tamsulosin available as a single tablet

From Robertson RP et al: *DeGroot's endocrinology, basic science and clinical practice*, ed 8, Philadelphia, 2023, Elsevier.

---

prostate cancer, or if symptoms do not respond to medical therapy.[3]

- Some men with BPH also have "storage" symptoms such as frequency and urgency despite use of alpha blockers. Clinicians often adds antimuscarinic drugs (oxybutynin, tolterodine) to mitigate these symptoms. Trials have shown that addition of an antimuscarinic drug to a beta blocker will have minimal effects on urgency and frequency and will expose patients to significant side effects from the antimuscarinic agents. Complete bladder emptying should be confirmed by estimating post void residual before instituting antimuscarinic medications.[4]

- Prostatic urethral lift (PUL) is an outpatient treatment option for BPH.

- The prostatic urethral lift implant (UroLift) is an increasingly popular minimally invasive procedure for BPH. It is placed transurethrally at the site of obstruction to open the urethra by compressing the obstructing prostatic lobes and holding them permanently retracted with suture-based implants. Advantages are low risk for ejaculatory or erectile disfunction and use of local anesthesia or propofol sedation. Major disadvantage is 6% annual reintervention rate.

- TURP (Box 4) is the most commonly used surgical procedure for BPH. It is recommended for patients unresponsive to medical therapy who have renal insufficiency, recurrent UTIs, bladder stones, or gross hematuria. Transurethral incision of the prostate (TUIP), a procedure almost equivalent in efficacy, is limited to patients whose estimated resection tissue weight would be ≤30 g. TUIP can be performed in an ambulatory setting or during a 1-day hospitalization. Open prostatectomy is typically performed on patients with very large prostates.

- Laser therapy for BPH is a less invasive alternative to TURP; Yttrium Aluminum Garnett (YAG) laser enucleation has minimal effect on potency, libido, or patient satisfaction with his sex life and is associated with retrograde ejaculation. The main advantage over TURP is less risk of bleeding. However, recent studies indicate that at least in the initial 7 mo after surgery, TURP is moderately more effective than laser therapy in relieving symptoms of BPH.

- Transurethral needle ablation with radiofrequency to remove periurethral prostate tissue is being increasingly used in patients with prostate volume >60 ml and moderate symptoms. It has a low morbidity rate, but treatment failure is ~25% at 5 yr and <80% at 10 yr.

- Balloon dilation of the prostatic urethra is less effective than surgery for relieving symptoms but is associated with fewer complications. It is a reasonable treatment option for patients with smaller prostates and no middle lobe enlargement.

- Water vapor thermal therapy uses radiofrequency to create stored thermal energy in the form of steam. It should only be performed for patients with a prostate size between 30 and 80 cc. It can also be performed in-office under regional anesthesia. It has a high likelihood of presentation of sexual function.[3]

- Robotic waterjet treatment (aquablation) is performed using a high-velocity saline jet from a robotic handpiece placed transurethrally.

Can be used for those with small to medium prostate sizes from 30 to 80 cc. It has similar efficacy to TURP but confers less risk for ejaculatory dysfunction.[3]

- Surgery need not be the treatment of last resort for most patients; that is, patients need not undergo other treatments for BPH before they can have surgery. However, recommending surgery on the grounds that a patient's surgical risk will "only increase with age" is generally inappropriate.

DISPOSITION

With appropriate therapy, symptoms improve or stabilize in <70% of patients with BPH.

REFERRAL

Urology referral for patients with severe or intolerable symptoms and for any patient suspected of having prostate cancer (10% to 30% of men with BPH)

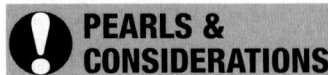

COMMENTS

- Emerging technologies for treating BPH, including prostatic artery embolization, transurethral holmium laser enucleation, transurethral electrovaporization, and transurethral microwave thermotherapy of the prostate, appear promising; however, long-term effectiveness has not yet been demonstrated.

- The increase in the use of pharmacologic management has resulted in <30% reduction in the total number of TURP procedures.

- Combined drug therapy for BPH with an alpha-blocker and a 5-alpha-reductase inhibitor is superior to monotherapy with either agent. After 1 yr of combination therapy, withdrawal of the alpha-blocker will usually not exacerbate symptoms.

- Treatment with 5-alpha-reductase inhibitors (finasteride, dutasteride) is associated with approximately 30% higher risk for developing type 2 diabetes.

RELATED CONTENT

Enlarged Prostate (Patient Information)

REFERENCES & SUGGESTED READINGS

Available at eBooks.Health.Elsevier.com.

AUTHOR: **FRED F. FERRI, MD**

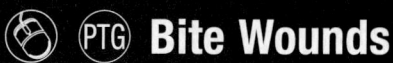
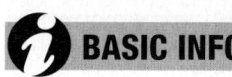 **BASIC INFORMATION**

DEFINITION

A bite wound can be animal or human, accidental, or intentional.

ICD-10CM CODES
S41.159A	Open bite of unspecified upper arm, initial encounter
T14.1	Open wound of unspecified body region
T01.9	Multiple open wounds, unspecified
S31.000A	Unspecified open wound of lower back and pelvis without penetration into retroperitoneum, initial encounter

EPIDEMIOLOGY & DEMOGRAPHICS

- Bite wounds account for 1% of emergency department visits, and about 2% of patients need hospitalization.
- More than 1 million bites occur in human beings annually in the U.S.
- Dog bites account for 85% to 90% of all bites and result in 10 to 20 fatalities yearly in the U.S.; most dog bite victims are children. Cat bites account for 10% to 20%. The animal typically is owned by the victim.
- Infection rates are highest for cat bites (30% to 50%), followed by human bites (15% to 30%) and dog bites (5%).
- The extremities are involved in 75% of bites.

PHYSICAL FINDINGS & CLINICAL PRESENTATION

- The appearance of the bite wound is variable (e.g., puncture wound, tear, avulsion).
- Cellulitis, lymphangitis, and focal adenopathy may be present in infected bite wounds.
- Patient may have fever and chills.

ETIOLOGY

- Increased risk of infection: Human and cat bites, closed-fist injuries, wounds involving joints, puncture wounds, face and lip bites, bites with skull penetration, bites in immunocompromised hosts.
- Mixed aerobes and anaerobes typically compose the bacteria in bite wounds. Most frequent infecting organisms:
  1. *Pasteurella* spp: Responsible for majority of infections within 24 h of dog *(P. canis)* and cat *(P. multocida, P. septica)* bites
  2. *Capnocytophaga canimorsus* (formerly DF-2 bacillus): A gram-negative organism responsible for late infection, usually after dog bites
  3. Gram-negative organisms *(Pseudomonas, Haemophilus):* Often found in human bites
  4. *Streptococcus* spp., *Staphylococcus aureus*
  5. *Eikenella corrodens* in human bites

Dx DIAGNOSIS

DIFFERENTIAL DIAGNOSIS

- Bite from a rabid animal (often the attack is unprovoked)
- Factitious injury

WORKUP

- Determination of the time elapsed since the patient was bitten, status of rabies immunization of the animal, and underlying medical conditions that might predispose the patient to infection (e.g., diabetes mellitus [DM], immunodeficiency).
- Documentation of bite site, notification of appropriate authorities (e.g., police department, animal officer).

- Table 1 summarizes management procedures for bite wounds.

LABORATORY TESTS

- Generally not necessary
- Hematocrit if there has been significant blood loss
- Wound cultures (aerobic and anaerobic) if there is evidence of sepsis or victim is immunocompromised; cultures should be obtained before irrigation of the wound but after superficial cleaning

IMAGING STUDIES

Radiographs are indicated when bony penetration is suspected or if there is suspicion of fracture or significant trauma; they are also useful for detecting foreign bodies (when suspected).

TABLE 1 Management of Bite Wounds

History

Animal Bite

Ascertain the type of animal, whether the bite was provoked or unprovoked, and the situation/environment in which the bite occurred. Follow rabies guidelines for details on management of bites that carry a risk of rabies.

Patient

Obtain information on antimicrobial allergies, current medications, splenectomy, liver disease, or other immunosuppressive conditions.

Physical Examination

Assess nerve and tendon function along with signs and symptoms of infection.

Culture

Obtain aerobic and anaerobic cultures from infected wounds.

Irrigation and Débridement

Irrigate with water and débride devitalized or necrotic tissue.

Radiographs

Plain radiographs should be obtained if bony penetration is highly possible; radiographs can also provide a baseline for future evaluation of osteomyelitis.

Wound Closure

Primary wound closure is usually not advocated unless wounds are extensive and closure is necessary for cosmetic or functional reasons, especially large facial or neck wounds or those overlying the joints. When possible, delayed primary closure or allowing the wound to close by secondary intention is recommended.

Antimicrobial Therapy

Early Presenting (Uninfected) Wounds

Provide antimicrobial therapy for (1) moderate-to-severe injuries, especially if preexisting edema or significant crush injury is present; (2) bone or joint space penetration; (3) deep hand wounds; (4) immunocompromised patients (including those with advanced liver disease, asplenia, or chronic steroid therapy); (5) wounds adjacent to a prosthetic joint; and (6) wounds in close proximity to the genital area. In most cases, coverage should include *Pasteurella* (*Eikenella* in human bites), *Staphylococcus, Streptococcus,* and anaerobes, including *Fusobacterium, Porphyromonas, Prevotella,* and *Bacteroides* species.

Infected Wounds

Cover *Pasteurella* (*Eikenella* in human bites), *Staphylococcus, Streptococcus,* and anaerobes, including *Fusobacterium, Porphyromonas, Prevotella,* and *Bacteroides* spp. The following oral antimicrobials can be considered in adults for most terrestrial animal and human bites:
- First choice: Amoxicillin-clavulanic acid 875/125 mg, 1 tablet by mouth twice daily
- Penicillin allergy:
  1. Metronidazole 500 mg, 1 tablet by mouth three times daily *plus* trimethoprim-sulfamethoxazole, 1 double-strength tablet by mouth twice daily
  2. Moxifloxacin 400 mg, 1 tablet by mouth daily
  3. Doxycycline 100 mg, 1 tablet by mouth twice daily
- In adults in whom intravenous antibiotics are deemed necessary, single antimicrobial choices can include ampicillin-sulbactam, cefoxitin, ertapenem, or moxifloxacin.
- Empirical regimens for marine- and freshwater-acquired infection should also cover *Vibrio* and *Aeromonas* species, respectively, with agents such as third-generation cephalosporins (e.g., cefotaxime) and fluoroquinolones.

Hospitalization

Indications can include signs and symptoms of systemic toxicity.

Continued

TABLE 1 Management of Bite Wounds—cont'd

Immunizations

Provide tetanus and rabies immunization, if indicated.

Elevation

Elevation may be required if preexisting edema is present.

Immobilization

For significant injures, consider immobilizing the extremity, especially the hands, with a splint.

Follow-Up

Patients should be reminded to follow up within 48 h or sooner for worsening or unresolved symptoms.

Reporting

Reporting the incident to a local health department may be required in selected cases.

From Bennett JE et al: *Mandell, Douglas, and Bennett's principles and practice of infectious diseases*, ed 9, Philadelphia, 2020, Elsevier.

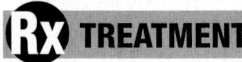

TREATMENT

NONPHARMACOLOGIC THERAPY

- Local care with débridement, vigorous cleansing, and saline irrigation of the wound; débridement of devitalized tissue
- High-pressure irrigation to clean bite wound and ensure removal of contaminants (e.g., use saline solution with a 30- to 35-ml syringe equipped with a 20-gauge needle or catheter with tip of syringe placed 2 to 3 cm above the wound)
- Avoid blunt probing of wounds (increased risk of infection)
- If the animal is suspected to be rabid: Infiltrate wound edges with 1% procaine hydrochloride, swab wound surface vigorously with cotton swabs and 1% benzalkonium solution or other soap, and rinse wound with normal saline

ACUTE GENERAL Rx

- Avoid suturing of hand wounds and any wounds that appear infected. Recommendations for bite wound closure and prophylactic antibiotics are noted in Table 2.
- Clenched fist injuries that develop after a punch to another's mouth usually require hospitalization, IV antibiotics, and evaluation by a hand specialist. Indications for admission after an animal bite are summarized in Box 1.
- Puncture wounds should be left open.
- Give antirabies therapy and tetanus immune globulin (250 to 500 units intramuscularly [IM] in limb contralateral to toxoid) and toxoid (adult or child older than 5 yr: 0.5 ml DT given IM, child <5 yr 0.5 ml DPT IM) as needed.
- Risk factors for bite wound infections are described in Table 3. Use empiric antibiotic therapy (Table 4) in high-risk wounds (e.g., cat bite, hand bites, face bites, genital area bites, bites with joint or bone penetration, human bites, immunocompromised host): Amoxicillin-clavulanate 875 to 1000 mg bid for 7 days or cefuroxime 500 mg bid for 7 days.
- In hospitalized patients, IV antibiotics of choice are cefoxitin 1 to 2 g q6h, ampicillin-sulbactam 1.5 to 3 g q6h, ticarcillin-clavulanate 3 g q6h, cefoxitin 2 g IV q8h, or ceftriaxone 1 to 2 g q24h.
- Penicillin allergy: Animal bite (doxycycline or moxifloxacin or trimethoprim-sulfamethoxazole with either clindamycin or metronidazole); human bite (moxifloxacin plus clindamycin, trimethoprim-sulfamethoxazole plus metronidazole).
- Prophylactic therapy for persons bitten by others with HIV and hepatitis B (see "Section V").

BOX 1 Indications for Admission after an Animal Bite

Structural
- Injury to deep structures (bones, joints, tendons, arteries, or nerves)
- Injuries requiring reconstructive surgery
- Injuries requiring general anesthesia for appropriate wound care

Infectious
- Rapidly spreading cellulitis
- Significant lymphangitis or lymphadenitis
- Evidence of sepsis
- Infection in patients at high risk for complications (see Table 3)
- Infections involving bones, joints, tendons
- Infection with failed outpatient therapy

From Walls RM et al: *Rosen's emergency medicine, concepts and clinical practice*, ed 10, Philadelphia, 2023, Elsevier.

- The comparative in vitro antimicrobial activity of selected oral antimicrobial agents against common bite wound pathogens is summarized in Table 5.

DISPOSITION

- Prognosis is favorable with proper treatment.
- Important prognostic factors are type and depth of wound, which compartments are entered, and pathogenicity of inoculated bacteria.
- Punctures that are difficult to irrigate adequately, carnivore bites over vital structures (arteries, nerves, joints), and tissue crushing that cannot be débrided have a worse prognosis.
- In general, human bites have a higher complication and infection rate than do animal bites.
- Nearly 50% of the anaerobic gram-negative bacilli isolated from human bite wounds may be penicillin resistant and beta-lactamase positive.

PREVENTION

Box 2 provides advice for avoiding the bites and attacks of common pets.

REFERRAL

- Hospitalization and IV antibiotic therapy for infected human bites; bites with injury to joints, nerves, or tendons; or any animal bites unresponsive to oral therapy.
- Human bites with tendon involvement should go to operating room for washout.
- In the outpatient setting, bite wounds should be reevaluated within 48 h to assess for signs of infection.

RELATED CONTENT

Animal and Human Bites (Patient Information)

AUTHOR: FRED F. FERRI, MD

TABLE 2 Recommendations for Bite Wound Closure and Prophylactic Antibiotics

Species	Suturing	Prophylactic Antibiotics
Dogs, coyotes, wolves	The majority except hands and feet	Hand and foot wounds High-risk wounds[a]
Cat	Face only	All wounds extending through the epidermis
Human	Face only (up to 24 h after the bite)	All wounds extending through the epidermis
Monkey	Face only (up to 24 h after the bite)	All wounds extending through the epidermis
Rodent	All (but rarely needed)	No
Ferret, pig, horse, camel, bear, big cats	Face only	All wounds extending through the epidermis

[a]High-risk wounds: Deep puncture wounds, crush injury or damage to deep structures, delayed presentation (>6 h), wounds closed primarily, and high-risk patients (see Table 3).
From Walls RM et al: *Rosen's emergency medicine, concepts and clinical practice*, ed 10, Philadelphia, 2023, Elsevier.

TABLE 3   Risk Factors for Bite Wound Infections

Factor	High Risk	Low Risk
Species	Cat (domestic and wild) Human Monkey Pig Camel Bear	Dog (excluding hands and feet) Rodent
Location of wound	Hand (especially clenched-fist injuries [CFIs]) Foot	Face Scalp
Wound type	Puncture Crush injury or damage to deep structures Presence of devitalized tissue Delayed presentation (more than 6 h) Closed primarily	Laceration Superficial
Patient characteristics	Age over 50 Diabetes Renal failure Liver disease Alcoholism Immune disorder Malnutrition Use of corticosteroids or other immunosuppressive medications Peripheral vascular disease Chronic edema of the bitten area	

From Walls RM et al: *Rosen's emergency medicine, concepts and clinical practice*, ed 10, Philadelphia, 2023, Elsevier.

TABLE 4   Suggested Antibiotic Regimens for Bite Wound Prophylaxis and Inpatient Treatment of Established Infections

Species	Prophylaxis	Inpatient Treatment of Established Infection
Dog and cat	Amoxicillin/clavulanate (Augmentin) 875/125 mg q12h for 5 days Ciprofloxacin, 500 mg BID for 7 to 14 days Moxifloxacin 400 mg po qd for 7 to 14 days Clindamycin 300 mg QID plus trimethoprim-sulfamethoxazole 160/800 mg BID for 7 to 14 days	Ampicillin/sulbactam (Unasyn) 1.5 g (1 g ampicillin plus 0.5 g sulbactam) to 3 g (2 g ampicillin plus 1 g sulbactam) q6h for 7-14 days Piperacillin/tazobactam (Zosyn) 3.375 g (3 g piperacillin and 0.375 g tazobactam) IV QID for 7-14 days Imipenem 500 mg IV q6h or 1 g IV q8h Meropenem 500 mg IV q8h Ertapenem 1 g/day IV/IM Ciprofloxacin or moxifloxacin plus metronidazole (Flagyl) 250-500 mg QID Ciprofloxacin 600 mg BID or 400 mg IV BID or moxifloxacin 400 mg PO/IV qd plus clindamycin 300 mg QID
Human and monkey	Amoxicillin-clavulanate 875/125 mg q12h Ciprofloxacin 500 mg twice per day or trimethoprim-sulfamethoxazole 160/800 mg BID plus clindamycin 300 mg QID	Ampicillin/sulbactam 1.5 g (1 g ampicillin plus 0.5 g sulbactam) to 3 g (2 g ampicillin plus 1 g sulbactam) q6h Imipenem 500 mg IV q6h or 1 g IV q8h Meropenem 500 mg IV q8h Ertapenem 1 g/day IV/IM Ceftriaxone 1 g IVPB BID plus metronidazole 250 to 500 mg TID Clindamycin 600 mg QID plus ciprofloxacin 500 mg BID or 400 mg IV BID
Rodent	Not recommended	
Ferret, pig, horse, bear, big cats, coyotes, wolves	Same as for cats and dogs	Same as for cats and dogs
Camel	Ciprofloxacin 500 mg q12h Ofloxacin 400 mg po q12h	Same as for cats and dogs

From Walls RM et al: *Rosen's emergency medicine, concepts and clinical practice*, ed 10, Philadelphia, 2023, Elsevier.

TABLE 5 Comparative In Vitro Antimicrobial Activity of Selected Oral Antimicrobial Agents against Common Bite Wound Pathogens

	Staphylococcus aureus[a]	Eikenella corrodens	Streptococcus	Haemophilus	Pasteurella	Anaerobes
Amoxicillin	−	+	v	v	v	v
Amoxicillin–clavulanic acid	v	+	+	+	+	+
Cephalexin	v	−	v	−	v	−
Cefaclor	v	−	v	v	v	−
Cefuroxime	v	v	v	v	v	−
Meropenem	v	+	+	+	+	+
Dicloxacillin	v	−	v	−	−	−
Erythromycin	v	−	v	−	v	−
Azithromycin	v	v	v	−	v	v
Clarithromycin	v	v	v	−	v	−
Trimethoprim-sulfamethoxazole	+	+	v	+	+	−
Moxifloxacin	+	+	+	+	+	+
Clindamycin	+	−	+	−	−	+

+, Active; −, poorly active or inactive; v, variable.
[a] Methicillin-resistant *S. aureus* can be a pathogen in bite wounds.
From Cherry JD et al: *Feigin and Cherry's textbook of pediatric infectious diseases,* ed 8, Philadelphia, 2019, Elsevier.

BOX 2 Advice for Avoiding the Bites and Attacks of Common Pets

Dogs
- Do not leave a young child alone with a dog.
- Never approach or try to pet an unfamiliar dog, especially if it is tied up or confined.
- Always ask the dog's owners if you can pet the dog.
- Do not lean over a dog or pet it directly on the head.
- Do not kiss a dog.
- Avoid quick or sudden movements that may startle a dog.
- Never pet or step over a sleeping dog.
- Never try to take a bone or toy away from a dog (other than your own dog).
- Know the appearance of an angry dog: Barking, growling, snarling with teeth showing, ears laid flat, legs stiff, tail up, and hair on the back standing up.
- Never step between two fighting dogs; if you need to separate them, use a bucket of water or a hose.
- Do not approach a female dog that is nursing her pups.
- Teach injury prevention advice to children from an early age.

Cats
- Be aware that some cats do not like prolonged petting.
- Know warning signs of an impending bite: Twitching of the tail, restlessness, and "intention" bites (i.e., the cat moves to bite but does not bite).

Ferrets
- Do not sell or adopt a ferret that is known to bite.
- Do not push your fingers through the wires of a ferret cage.
- Reach for a ferret from the side with the palm upward rather than from above.
- Do not handle food and then handle young ferrets without washing your hands first.
- Do not poke a ferret or pull on its tail or ears.
- Never leave a ferret alone with a child or infant.
- If a ferret bites and locks on very tightly, pour cold and fast-running water over its face.

From Auerbach P: *Wilderness medicine, expert consult,* premium edition—enhanced online features and print, Philadelphia, 2012, Elsevier.

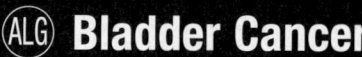
 BASIC INFORMATION

DEFINITION

Bladder cancer is a field change disease in which the entire urothelium from the renal pelvis to the urethra is susceptible to malignant transformation. The disease stages include non–muscle-invasive bladder cancer, muscle-invasive bladder cancer, and metastatic urothelial carcinoma.

ICD-10CM CODES

C67.9	Malignant neoplasm of bladder, unspecified
C79.11	Secondary malignant neoplasm of bladder
D09.0	Carcinoma in situ of bladder
D30.3	Benign neoplasm of bladder
D41.4	Neoplasm of uncertain behavior of bladder
D49.4	Neoplasm of unspecified behavior of bladder

EPIDEMIOLOGY & DEMOGRAPHICS

- In 2023, an estimated 82,290 new cases and 16,710 deaths occurred in the U.S.[1] It is the sixth most common malignancy in the U.S., with a median age of diagnosis of 69 yr in men and 71 yr in women.
- Globally, there were an estimated 573,200 new cases and 212,500 deaths in 2020.

PREDOMINANT SEX: It is three to four times more common in men than in women; lifetime risks are 1 in 26 for men and 1 in 88 for women.

PEAK INCIDENCE: Incidence increases with age: Higher after age 60 yr, uncommon in those younger than 40 yr.

RISK FACTORS:
Smoking:
- More than half of bladder cancers are related to smoking; there is a two- to threefold increase for subjects smoking >10 cigarettes per day.
- Smokers of higher tar and nicotine cigarettes as well as those who smoke unfiltered cigarettes have a higher risk.
- Pipe smokers have a lower risk of bladder cancer compared with cigarette smokers.
- Cigars, snuff, and chewing tobacco do not influence bladder cancer risk.

Diet:
- Diets rich in beef, pork, and animal fat increase risk of bladder cancer.
- Beer consumption has been linked to bladder cancer development as a result of the presence of nitrosamines in the beer.
- Medications: Long-term (>1 yr) use of pioglitazone and rosiglitazone.

GENETICS: Bladder cancer is multifactorial in etiology, involving both genetic and environmental interactions. Overall, approximately 20% to 25% of the male U.S. population with bladder cancer developed the disease due to occupational exposure.

DISTRIBUTION: The three types of bladder cancer are:
- Transitional cell carcinoma (93%),
- Squamous cell carcinoma (6%), and
- Adenocarcinoma (1%)

PATHOGENESIS: Two pathways exist for bladder cancer (TCC):
- Papillary superficial disease occasionally leading to invasive cancer (75% cases)
- Carcinoma in situ (CIS) and solid invasive cancer with high risk of disease progression (25% cases)

SUPERFICIAL CANCER:
- T_a: Papillary low-grade tumor with a high rate of recurrence; disease progression in 5%
- T_1: Higher-grade papillary tumor that infiltrates the lamina propria; often associated with flat CIS that may involve the urothelium diffusely; disease progression in 30% to 50%. This is subdivided into:
  1. T_{1a}: Penetration up to the muscularis mucosa; disease progression in 5%
  2. T_{1b}: Penetration through the muscularis mucosa; disease progression in 53%

FLAT CIS:
- Entirely separate pathway of cancer development manifested by dysplasia, which leads to the occurrence of poorly differentiated malignant cells that replace or undermine the normal urothelium and extend along the plane of the bladder wall. It penetrates the basement membrane and lamina propria in 20% to 30%

of cases and is associated with the development of solid tumor growth. A p53 defect occurs in 50% of these cases.

At presentation, 50% to 51% of cancers are in situ, 34% to 35% are localized to the bladder, 17% are regionally spread to the lymph nodes, and 4% to 5% present with distant metastases. Eighty percent of superficial TCC recur, with up to 30% progressing to a higher stage or grade. Younger patients most commonly develop low-grade papillary noninvasive TCC and are less likely to have recurrences when compared with older patients with similar lesions. Involvement of the upper tracts with tumor occurs in 25% to 50% of cases (see Table 1).

MOLECULAR EPIDEMIOLOGY: TCC is usually a field change disease with tumors arising at different times and sites in the urothelium, suggesting a polyclonal etiology. Non–muscle-invasive bladder cancer (NMIBC) and muscle-invasive bladder cancer (MIBC) are genetically different. NMIBC is characterized by a high frequency of FGFR oncogene mutations, leading to constitutive activation of the RAS/MAPK pathway. In MIBC, *TP53* gene mutations prevail. In general, mutations in *FGFR* and *TP53* are mutually exclusive, suggesting that NMIBC and MIBC develop along different oncogenic pathways. However, these mutations often occur simultaneously in stage pT_1 tumors that invade the connective tissue layer underlying the urothelium. Recently, somatic mutations in the *PIK3CA* oncogene, which encodes the catalytic

TABLE 1 2018 TNM Bladder Cancer Stage Classification

T stage	Description
T_X	Primary tumor cannot be assessed
T_0	No evidence of primary tumor
T_a	Noninvasive papillary carcinoma
T_{is}	Carcinoma in situ
T_1	Tumor invades lamina propria
T_2	Tumor invades muscularis propria
pT_{2a}	Tumor invades superficial muscularis propria (inner half)
pT_{2b}	Tumor invades deep muscularis propria (outer half)
T_3	Tumor invades perivesical tissue
pT_{3a}	Microscopic invasion
pT_{3b}	Macroscopic invasion (extravesical mass)
T_4	Tumor invades any of the following: Prostatic stroma, seminal vesicles, uterus, vagina, pelvic wall, abdominal wall
T_{4a}	Tumor invades prostatic stroma, uterus, vagina
T_{4b}	Tumor invades pelvic wall, abdominal wall
Regional lymph nodes (N)	
N_0	No lymph node metastasis
N_1	Single lymph node metastasis in true pelvis (perivesical, obturator, internal/external iliac, or sacral lymph node)
N_2	Multiple lymph node metastases in true pelvis (perivesical, obturator, internal/external iliac, or sacral lymph node metastasis)
N_3	Metastasis to the common iliac lymph nodes
Distant metastasis (M)	
M_0	No distant metastasis
M_1	Distant metastasis
M_{1a}	Distant metastasis limited to lymph nodes beyond the common iliacs
M_{1b}	Nonlymph-node distant metastases

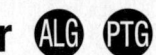

subunit p110α of class-IA PI3 kinase, were described in 13% to 27% of bladder tumors. Mutations in the *RAS* oncogenes (*HRAS*, *KRAS*, and *NRAS*) have also been found in 13% of bladder tumors and in all stages and grades; they are mutually exclusive with *FGFR3* mutations.

PHYSICAL FINDINGS & CLINICAL PRESENTATION

- Gross, painless hematuria
- Microhematuria
- Frequency, urgency, occasional dysuria
- With locally invasive to distant metastatic disease, the presentation can include:
  1. Abdominal pain
  2. Flank pain
  3. Lymphedema
  4. Renal failure
  5. Anorexia
  6. Bone pain

ETIOLOGY

Bladder cancer is a potentially preventable disease associated with specific etiologic factors:[2]

- Cigarette smoking is associated with 45% to 65% of cases. The risk of developing a TCC is two to four times higher in smokers, and that risk becomes equal to nonsmokers only after 12 to 15 yr of smoking abstinence. Smoking is associated with higher histologic grade and stage plus increase in the number and size of tumors
- Occupational exposures: Dye workers, textile workers, tire and rubber workers, petroleum workers
- Chemical exposure: O-toluidine, 2-naphthylamine, benzidine, 4-amino-biphenyl, and nitrosamines
- Exposure to herpes papilloma virus type 16

Squamous carcinomas are associated with:
- Schistosomiasis
- Urinary calculi
- Indwelling catheters
- Bladder diverticula

Miscellaneous causes:
- Phenacetin abuse
- Cyclophosphamide
- Pelvic irradiation
- Tuberculosis

Adenocarcinomas are associated with:
- Exstrophy
- Endometriosis
- Neurogenic bladder
- Urachal abnormalities
- As a secondary site for distant metastases from other organs (e.g., colon cancer)

Dx DIAGNOSIS

- History and physical examination
- Urinalysis
- Cystoscopy with bladder barbotage and biopsy. Fluorescence cystoscopy offers improvement in the detection of flat neoplastic lesions such as carcinoma in situ
- Transurethral resection of bladder tumor (TURBT)

- There is insufficient evidence to determine whether a decrease in mortality rate from bladder cancer occurs with hematuria testing, urinary cytology, or a variety of other tests on exfoliated urinary cells or other substances
- Urinary biomarkers: Six urinary biomarkers have been approved by the FDA for diagnosis on surveillance of bladder cancer[3]
  1. Quantitative nuclear matrix protein 22 (Alere NMP22)
  2. Qualitative NMP22 (BladderChek)
  3. Qualitative bladder tumor antigen (BTA stat)
  4. Quantitative BTA (BTA TRAK)
  5. Fluorescence in situ hybridization (FISH)
  6. Fluorescent immunohistochemistry (ImmunoCyt)

Generally, urinary biomarkers miss a substantial proportion of patients with bladder cancer and are subject to false-positive results in others. Accuracy is poor for low-stage and low-grade tumors.

DIFFERENTIAL DIAGNOSIS

- Urinary tract infection
- Frequency-urgency syndrome
- Interstitial cystitis
- Stone disease
- Endometriosis
- Neurogenic bladder

WORKUP

Fig. 1 illustrates a diagnostic and treatment algorithm for bladder cancer. Staging is summarized in Table 1.

LABORATORY TESTS

- Urine cytology.
- Urine telomerase: Telomerase activity in voided urine or bladder washings determined by the telomeric repeat amplification protocol (TRAP) assay. This test has been reported to accurately detect the presence of bladder tumors in men. It represents a potentially useful noninvasive diagnostic innovation for bladder cancer detection in high-risk groups such as habitual smokers or in symptomatic patients.

IMAGING STUDIES

- Renal ultrasound, retrograde pyelography, computed tomography (CT) scan, and MRI.
- One or a combination of studies can be used. In the absence of skeletal symptoms, bone scan is not recommended.

Rx TREATMENT

SURGICAL APPROACHES

- The goal of any resection should be the visual eradication of any tumor burden and the assurance of an adequate depth of resection.
- Initially, transurethral resection of bladder tumor (TURBT). Using cutting current, a loop electrode is used to resect the tumor inclusive of muscularis propria (Fig. E2). Histologically, bladder tumors frequently exhibit growth beyond the visible edge, and, as such, resection should include an approximate 2-cm margin of normal-appearing tissue.

Wide resection of tumors will ensure completeness, whether the tumor has a broad base or a tentacular growth pattern (Fig. E3).
- Loop biopsy of the prostatic urethra if high-grade TCC is suspected.
- If superficial disease, follow-up protocol with repeat TURBT and/or the use of intravesical agents is recommended.
- For advanced bladder cancer, radical cystectomy with urethrectomy (unless orthotopic diversion is planned), and either ileal loop conduit or orthotopic diversion.
- Results from a recent randomized trial demonstrated that patients who undergo robotic cystectomy have shorter hospital stays, fewer wound complications, fewer thromboembolic events, and overall improved short-term quality of life without any impact on overall survival.[4]

BLADDER PRESEVATION APPROACHES: After cystectomy for muscle-invasive disease, 50% or more of the patients will develop metastases. Most patients develop metastases at distant sites; a third of patients relapse locally. Bladder preservation is offered to individuals who refuse surgery or are not suitable radical cystectomy patients. Bladder-sparing protocols include extensive TURBT or partial cystectomy with external-beam or interstitial radiotherapy and systemic chemotherapy. Radiotherapy as a single treatment modality is not effective. The best predictor of successful bladder preservation is a complete response after the combination of initial TURBT and neoadjuvant chemotherapy with stages T_2 to T_{3a}.

INDICATIONS FOR PARTIAL CYSTECTOMY:

- Tumor within a bladder diverticulum
- Solitary, primary, and muscle-invasive or high-grade lesion of a region of the bladder that allows complete excision with adequate surgical margins
- Inability to adequately resect tumor by TURBT alone because of size or location
- Tumor overlying a ureteral orifice requiring ureteral reimplantation
- Biopsy of a radiation-induced ulceration
- Palliation of severe local symptoms
- Patient refusal of urinary diversion
- Poor-risk patient who is not a diversion candidate

CONTRAINDICATIONS:

- Multiple tumors
- CIS
- Cellular atypia on biopsy
- Prostatic invasion
- Invasion of the trigone
- Inability to achieve adequate surgical margins
- Prior radiotherapy
- Inability to maintain adequate bladder volume after resection
- Evidence of extravesical tumor extension
- Poor surgical risk

ACUTE GENERAL Rx

INDICATIONS FOR INTRAVESICAL CHEMOTHERAPY:

- High-grade tumor
- Tumor size <5 cm

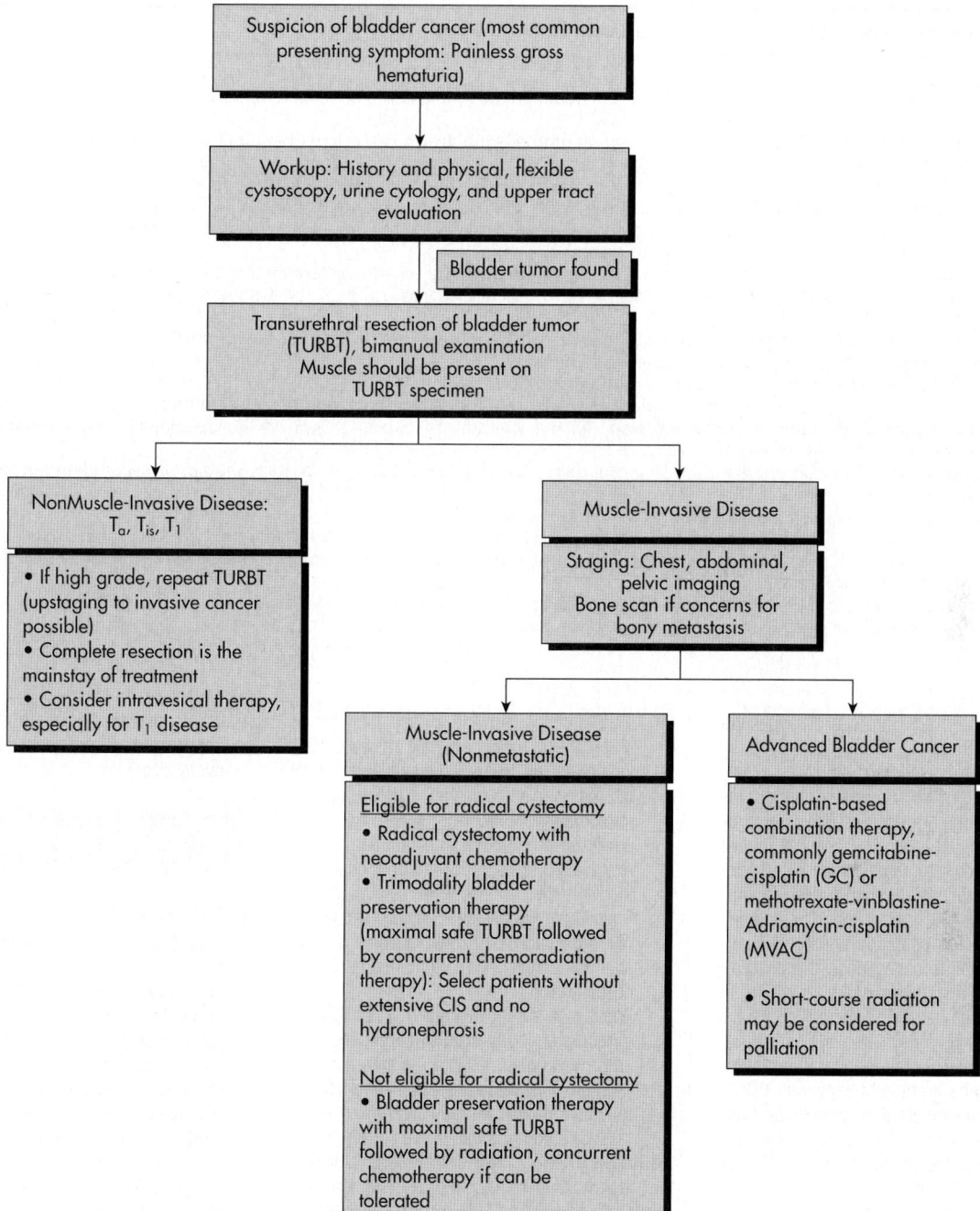

FIG. 1 Diagnostic and treatment algorithm for bladder cancer. *CIS,* Carcinoma in situ. (From Niederhuber JE: *Abeloff's clinical oncology,* ed 6, Philadelphia, 2020, Elsevier.)

- Multiple tumors
- Presence of CIS
- Positive urinary cytologic findings after a resection
- Incomplete tumor resection
Intravesical agents: Thiotepa, doxorubicin, mitomycin C, BCG, interferon, interleukin-2, keyhole-limpet hemocyanin, and gemcitabine. Photodynamic therapy with hematoporphyrin derivatives has also been used.

INDICATIONS FOR CYSTECTOMY:
- Large tumors not amenable to complete TURBT
- High-grade tumor
- Multiple tumors with frequent recurrences

- Diffuse CIS not responsive to intravesical chemotherapy
- Prostatic urethra involvement
- Irritative bladder symptoms with upper tract deterioration
- Muscle-invasive disease
- Disease outside the bladder

SYSTEMIC THERAPY:
- Nonmetastatic cancers:
  1. Cisplatin-based chemotherapy is used concurrently with radiotherapy in bladder preservation therapy approaches for resectable cases.
  2. Combination cisplatin-based chemotherapy regimens are used as perioperative

(neoadjuvant and adjuvant) therapy for locally advanced disease in conjunction with bladder resection.[5,6] Neoadjuvant chemotherapy, including dose-dense regimens, are associated with improved progression-free survival and higher rates of chemotherapy completion in comparison to the postoperative setting in this setting.
  3. Neoadjuvant immunotherapy has been associated with high rates of pathologic complete responses in early trials.
  4. In patients with high-risk muscle-invasive urothelial carcinoma who have undergone radical cystectomy, disease-free survival is

BOX 1 American Urological Association Guideline Recommendations

For all index patients:
- Standard: Physicians should discuss with the patient the treatment options and the benefits and harms, including side effects, of intravesical treatment.

For a patient who presents with an abnormal growth on the urothelium but who has not yet been diagnosed with bladder cancer:
- Standard: If the patient does not have an established histologic diagnosis, a biopsy should be obtained for pathologic analysis.
- Standard: Under most circumstances, complete eradication of all visible tumors should be performed.
- Standard: If bladder cancer is confirmed, periodic surveillance cystoscopy should be performed.
- Option: An initial single dose of intravesical chemotherapy may be administered immediately postoperatively.

For a patient with small volume, low-grade T_a bladder cancer:
- Recommendation: An initial single dose of intravesical chemotherapy may be administered immediately postoperatively.

For a patient with multifocal and/or large volume, histologically confirmed, low-grade T_a or a patient with recurrent low-grade T_a bladder cancer:
- Recommendation: An induction course of intravesical therapy with bacillus Calmette-Guérin or mitomycin C is recommended for the treatment of these patients with the goal of preventing or delaying recurrence.
- Option: Maintenance bacillus Calmette-Guérin or mitomycin C may be considered.

For a patient with initial histologically confirmed high-grade T_a, T_1, and/or carcinoma in situ bladder cancer:
- Standard: For patients with lamina propria invasion (T_1) but without muscularis propria in the specimen, repeat resection should be performed prior to additional intravesical therapy.
- Recommendation: An induction course of bacillus Calmette-Guérin followed by maintenance therapy is recommended for treatment of these patients.
- Option: Cystectomy should be considered for initial therapy in select patients.

For a patient with high-grade T_a, T_1, and/or carcinoma in situ bladder cancer that has recurred after prior intravesical therapy:
- Standard: For patients with lamina propria invasion (T_1) but without muscularis propria in the specimen, repeat resection should be performed prior to additional intravesical therapy.
- Recommendation: Cystectomy should be considered as a therapeutic alternative for these patients.
- Option: Further intravesical therapy may be considered for these patients.

improved with adjuvant use of nivolumab immunotherapy.[7]
- Metastatic or relapsed cancers:
  1. Combination cisplatin-based chemotherapy regimens are used as palliative therapy in fit patients. The most effective combination regimens include MVAC (cisplatin, methotrexate, vinblastine, doxorubicin) and GC (gemcitabine, cisplatin), which provide palliation and overall survival benefit. Recently, dose-dense MVAC chemotherapy given every 2 wk in fit patients has been demonstrated to have superior progression-free survival compared to the GC chemotherapy approach.
  2. Maintenance immunotherapy with PDL-1 inhibitor avelumab after completing first-line chemotherapy improves overall survival and is the standard of care for this group of patients.
  3. In patients who are ineligible to receive cisplatin-based chemotherapy regimens, the use of immune checkpoint inhibitors is the preferred first-line therapy option in patients with PD-L1–expressing tumors. Available agents include the PD-1 inhibitors (nivolumab, pembrolizumab) and PDL-1 inhibitors (atezolizumab, durvalumab, avelumab).
  4. Immunotherapy is used in patients who have failed at least one prior chemotherapy regimen and results in superior survival compared to conventional subsequent lines of chemotherapy.
  5. Alterations in the gene encoding fibroblast growth factor receptor (FGFR) are detected in 15% to 20% of cases of locally advanced or metastatic urothelial carcinoma.

Erdafitinib, a tyrosine kinase inhibitor of FGFR, has shown response rates of 40% in previously treated patients with FGFR alterations, and median survival of approximately 14 mo.[8]
  6. Enfortumab vedotin, an antibody drug conjugate consisting of a monoclonal antibody targeting nectin-4 conjugated to monomethyl auristatin E, has been approved for patients who do not respond to both chemotherapy and immune-checkpoint in-hibitors.[9]
  7. Sacituzumab govitecan is a TROP-2-directed antibody-drug conjugate that has improved outcomes in patients previously treated with platinum-based chemotherapy and immunotherapy and has received accelerated approval in this setting.[10]

RADIOTHERAPY: Conflicting reports suggest that superficial bladder cancer is more sensitive to radiotherapy. Only 20% to 30% of patients with invasive bladder cancer can be cured by external-beam radiation therapy alone. It is used in combination with surgery or with systemic agents to treat bladder cancer primarily in patients who are not surgical candidates or who refuse surgery. Combination chemotherapy (cisplatin) given concurrently with radiotherapy has shown significant improved locoregional control of bladder cancer in bladder-preservation strategies.

CHRONIC Rx

Follow-up Recommendations for Superficial Bladder Cancer:
- Cystoscopy, bladder barbotage, and bimanual examination every 3 mo for 2 yr, then every 6 mo for 2 yr, and annually thereafter.

- Upper tract studies are based on the risk of upper tract tumor development, generally every 2 to 5 yr.

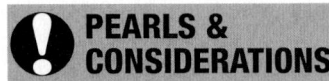

PEARLS & CONSIDERATIONS

COMMENTS

- Useful prognostic parameters for bladder tumor recurrence and subsequent progression are tumor grade, tumor depth, multifocal tumors, frequency of recurrence, tumor size, CIS, lymphatic invasion, papillary or solid tumor configuration.
- Currently, the incidence of occupational bladder cancer seems to be increasing faster in women than in men. Workers with aromatic amine exposure have the highest incidence, whereas those exposed to polycyclic aromatic hydrocarbons and heavy metals have the greatest mortality.
- The 5-yr survival for bladder cancer is 76%; it ranges from 96% for in situ, 70% for localized, 35% for regional, and 5% for distant cancers.
- Box 1 describes the American Urological Association Guideline Recommendations for bladder cancer.

RELATED CONTENT

Bladder Cancer (Patient Information)

REFERENCES

Available at eBooks.Health.Elsevier.com.

AUTHOR: **BHARTI RATHORE, MD**

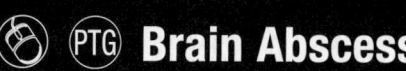
Disabilities
and Disorders

I

BASIC INFORMATION

DEFINITION

Brain abscesses are focal intracerebral infections that can arise as a result of trauma, neurosurgical procedures, local spread of infection (e.g., bacterial sinusitis, amoebic infection via the nasopharynx), or hematogenous spread of infection from extraneural sites (e.g., endocarditis).

ICD-10CM CODES
G06.0	Intracranial abscess and granuloma
B58.2	Toxoplasma meningoencephalitis
A18.89	Cerebral tuberculosis
A43.9	Nocardiosis

EPIDEMIOLOGY & DEMOGRAPHICS

INCIDENCE: Uncommon (reported incidence 0.4 to 0.9 cases/100,000 population; occurs ~2% as commonly as brain tumors).[1,2] More common in immunocompromised patients.
PREDOMINANT SEX: Men affected more than women (ratio 2:1 to 3:1)
PREDOMINANT AGE: Occurs at any age

PHYSICAL FINDINGS & CLINICAL PRESENTATION

- Classic triad: Fever, headache, and focal neurologic deficit (present in less than 20% of cases).[2,3]
- Clinical presentation is often due to the manifestations of the space-occupying lesion rather than to signs of systemic infection.
- Fever is present in only 24% to 58% of patients.[2-5]
- Headache is usually localized to the side of the abscess; onset can be gradual or severe; present in 55% to 75% of cases.[2,5]
- Focal neurologic findings (e.g., seizures, hemiparesis, aphasia, ataxia) depend on the location of the abscess and are seen in 23% to 48% of cases.[2,5]
- Presence of adjacent infections (dental abscess, otitis media, sinusitis, or postneurosurgical infection) may be a clue to the underlying source and potential pathogens involved.
- Table 1 describes common presenting findings of brain abscess.

ETIOLOGY

- The potential organisms involved in a brain abscess may be predicted based on the underlying source of infection (Table 2):
  1. Contiguous focus of infection (55% of all brain abscesses):
     a. Paranasal sinusitis: Occur in frontal lobe; streptococci (especially microaerophilic and anaerobic streptococci), *Bacteroides*, *Haemophilus*, and *Fusobacterium* spp.
     b. Otitis media/mastoiditis: Occur in temporal lobe and cerebellum; aerobic and anaerobic streptococci, *Enterobacteriaceae*, *Bacteroides*, and *Pseudomonas* spp.
     c. Dental infection: Occur in frontal lobe; mixed *Fusobacterium*, *Bacteroides*,

TABLE 1 Common Symptoms and Signs in Brain Abscess[a]

Symptom or Sign	Frequency (%)
Headache	49-97
Mental status changes	28-91
Focal neurologic deficits	20-66
Fever	32-79
Triad of headache, fever, and focal deficit	<50
Seizures	13-35
Nausea and vomiting	27-85
Nuchal rigidity	5-52
Papilledema	9-51

[a]The clinical presentation varies depending on size and location of the abscess.
Data from references 7-13.
From Bennett JE et al: *Mandell, Douglas, and Bennett's principles and practice of infectious diseases*, ed 9, Philadelphia, 2020, Elsevier.

Actinomyces, and *Streptococcus* spp. (especially *S. viridans*, *S. intermedius*, and anaerobic streptococci)
     d. Penetrating head injury: Site of abscess depends on site of wound; *Staphylococcus aureus*, aerobic streptococci, *Clostridium* spp., *Enterobacteriaceae*
     e. Postoperative infections after neurosurgery: *Staphylococcus epidermidis* and *S. aureus*, *Enterobacteriaceae*, and *Pseudomonas aeruginosa*
  2. Hematogenous spread from a distant site of infection (25% of all brain abscesses): Typically multiple abscesses present, often in middle cerebral artery distribution; infecting organism(s) depend on source
     a. Congenital heart disease: Streptococci, *Haemophilus* spp.
     b. Endocarditis: *S. aureus*, *Streptococcus viridans*

     c. Urinary tract: *Enterobacteriaceae*, *Pseudomonas*
     d. Intraabdominal: *Enterobacteriaceae*, *Bacteroides* spp, *Candida* spp.
     e. Lung: Streptococci, *Actinomyces* spp., *Fusobacterium* spp.
     f. Immunocompromised hosts: *Toxoplasma* spp., *Enterobacteriaceae*, *Nocardia* spp., *Listeria* spp., tuberculosis, fungi including *Aspergillus*, *Cryptococcus*, *Mucorales*
     g. Fungi are responsible for up to 90% of cerebral abscesses in solid organ transplant recipient
  3. Cryptogenic (unknown source): 20% of all brain abscesses

DIAGNOSIS

DIFFERENTIAL DIAGNOSIS (TABLE 3)

- Other parameningeal infections: Subdural empyema, epidural abscess, cavernous sinus thrombosis
- Embolic strokes in patients with bacterial endocarditis or valvular heart disease
- Mycotic aneurysm
- Acute hemorrhagic leukoencephalitis
- Parasitic infections: Toxoplasmosis, echinococcosis, cysticercosis
- Metastatic or primary brain tumors
- Cerebral infarction/stroke
- Central nervous system (CNS) vasculitis
- Chronic subdural hematoma
- Primary CNS lymphoma (HIV-infected patients) or posttransplant lymphoproliferative disorder (PTLD), transplant recipients

WORKUP

Physical examination, laboratory tests, imaging studies, cultures of blood and abscess contents

TABLE 2 Predisposing Conditions and Microbiology of Brain Abscess

Predisposing Condition	Usual Microbial Isolates
Otitis media or mastoiditis	Streptococci (anaerobic or aerobic), *Bacteroides* and *Prevotella* spp., *Enterobacteriaceae*
Sinusitis (frontoethmoid or sphenoid)	Streptococci, *Bacteroides* spp., *Enterobacteriaceae*, *Staphylococcus aureus*, *Haemophilus* spp.
Dental infection	Mixed *Fusobacterium*, *Prevotella*, *Actinomyces*, and *Bacteroides* spp., streptococci
Penetrating trauma or postneurosurgical	*S. aureus*, streptococci, *Enterobacteriaceae*, *Clostridiodes*
Lung abscess, empyema, bronchiectasis	*Fusobacterium*, *Actinomyces*, *Bacteroides*, and *Prevotella* spp., streptococci, *Nocardia* spp.
Bacterial endocarditis	*S. aureus*, streptococci
Congenital heart disease	Streptococci, *Haemophilus* spp.
Neutropenia	Aerobic gram-negative bacilli, *Aspergillus* spp., *Mucorales*, *Candida* spp., *Scedosporium* spp.
Transplantation	*Aspergillus* spp., *Candida* spp., *Mucorales*, *Scedosporium* spp., *Enterobacteriaceae*, *Listeria monocytogenes*, *Nocardia* spp., *Toxoplasma gondii*, *Mycobacterium tuberculosis*
HIV infection	*T. gondii*, *Nocardia* spp., *Mycobacterium* spp., *Listeria monocytogenes*, *Cryptococcus neoformans*

From Bennett JE et al: *Mandell, Douglas, and Bennett's principles and practice of infectious diseases*, ed 9, Philadelphia, 2020, Elsevier.

TABLE 3 Differential Diagnosis of CNS Infection and Tumor

	Brain Abscess	Bacterial Meningitis	Herpetic Encephalitis	Brain Tumor
History				
Headache	Severe, often focal	Severe, generalized	Mild to severe	Absent to severe
Focal defect	Often	Occasional	Occasional	Often
Progression	Days to weeks	Hours to days	Days	Days to months
Physical Examination				
Fever	Variable	>90%	>90%	Rare
Early focal signs	Often	Occasional	Occasional	Often
Pressure signs	Often	Rare	Occasional	Often
Extra-CNS infection	Often	Often	No	No
CT or MRI Scan				
Focal	Always[a]	No	Often	Always
Ring effect/onset	Often/late[b]	No	No	Often/early

[a]May be negative or nonspecific during first 48 h of illness.
[b]Development of abscess wall may be delayed by steroid therapy.
CNS, Central nervous system; *CT,* computed tomography; *MRI,* magnetic resonance imaging.
From Vincent JL et al: *Textbook of critical care,* ed 8, Philadelphia, 2024, Elsevier.

LABORATORY TESTS

- Computed tomography (CT) scans help localize lesions.
- White blood cell counts may be normal.
- Erythrocyte sedimentation rate may be normal.
- Lumbar puncture may be contraindicated based on location of the abscess(es) due to presence of increased intracranial pressure and the risk of herniation or intraventricular spread of infection. Lumbar puncture is helpful only in patients with suspicion of concurrent meningitis or abscess rupture into the ventricular system; the risk of herniation must be considered in all cases.
- The yield of Gram stain and culture of material aspirated at the time of surgical or stereotactic drainage is very high. Note that cultures may be negative if antibiotics are administered prior to the procedure; once a suspicion of brain abscess is raised, timely drainage and cultures should be a priority.
- Cultures of contiguous sites of infection should be considered (e.g., paranasal sinus, otitis, wounds from a neurosurgical procedure). These sites of infection may need surgical drainage to control the infection.[1,5,6]
- Blood cultures and cerebrospinal fluid cultures may identify the causative organism in up to 25% of patients.
- Abscess cultures and blood cultures in immunocompromised hosts should include staining and cultures for mycobacteria, fungi, and *Nocardia.*

IMAGING STUDIES

- CT scan with contrast enhancement (Fig. E1) or MRI with gadolinium can be used to detect brain abscess. MRI with gadolinium (Fig. E2) may provide more detailed images to differentiate between abscess and tumor or other mass. Diffusion-weighted imaging is helpful in differentiating brain abscess from cystic or necrotic brain tumors.[1]
- Serial CT scanning is recommended to follow the response to therapy.

Rx TREATMENT

ACUTE GENERAL Rx

- Effective treatment involves a combination of empiric antibiotic therapy and timely aspiration of the abscess for diagnosis and source control. If multiple abscesses are present, the largest of the abscesses (in noncritical sites) should be prioritized for aspiration and culture. If the patient is immunocompromised, cytology and mycobacterial and fungal cultures may be needed to make a definitive diagnosis. Common pathogens and empirical therapy for brain abscess are summarized in Table 4.
- If there is evidence of edema or mass effect on CT or MRI, treatment of elevated intracranial pressure is paramount.
  1. Hyperventilation of mechanically ventilated patients.
  2. Dexamethasone initially in a dosage of 10 mg intravenous (IV) followed by 4 mg IV q6h until symptoms of cerebral edema subside.[1] Steroids should be discontinued as soon as possible as they can delay effective immune response to infection and may interfere with antimicrobial delivery into abscess fluid.
  3. Mannitol 0.25 to 1 g/kg IV over 20 to 30 min q6 to 8h; maximum of 6 g/kg in 24 h.[1]
- Medical therapy is never a substitute for surgical intervention to relieve increased intracranial pressure. Neurologic deterioration usually mandates urgent surgical intervention.
- Steroids should be limited to patients with severe cerebral edema or midline shift.

MEDICAL Rx

If an abscess is <2.5 cm in diameter and the patient is neurologically stable, start empiric antibiotics and observe. Empiric antibiotic therapy should be guided by:[1,5]
- Suspicion of primary source
- Presence of single or multiple abscesses (suggesting hematogenous spread of underlying infection)

TABLE 4 Empiric Antimicrobial Therapy for Bacterial Brain Abscess

Predisposing Condition	Antimicrobial Regimen
Otitis media or mastoiditis	Metronidazole + third-generation cephalosporin[a]
Sinusitis (frontoethmoid or sphenoid)	Metronidazole + third-generation cephalosporin[a,b]
Dental infection	Metronidazole + third-generation cephalosporin[a]
Penetrating trauma or postneurosurgical	Vancomycin + third-generation or fourth-generation cephalosporin[a,c]
Lung abscess, empyema, bronchiectasis	Third-generation cephalosporin[a] + metronidazole + sulfonamide[d]
Bacterial endocarditis	Vancomycin[e]
Congenital heart disease	Third-generation cephalosporin[a]
Unknown	Vancomycin + metronidazole + third-generation or fourth-generation cephalosporin[a,c]

[a]Cefotaxime or ceftriaxone; the fourth-generation cephalosporin cefepime may also be used.
[b]Add vancomycin when infection caused by methicillin-resistant *Staphylococcus aureus* is suspected.
[c]Use ceftazidime or cefepime as the cephalosporin if *Pseudomonas aeruginosa* is suspected.
[d]Trimethoprim-sulfamethoxazole; include if *Nocardia* spp. is suspected.
[e]Additional agents should be added based on other likely microbiologic etiologies.
From Bennett JE et al: *Mandell, Douglas, and Bennett's principles and practice of infectious diseases,* ed 9, Philadelphia, 2020, Elsevier.

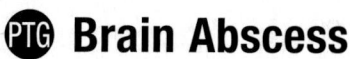

- Patient's underlying medical conditions (e.g., HIV infection, transplant recipient cyanotic, or valvular heart disease)
- Primary infection or contiguous source (Table 5):[1]
  1. Otitis media/mastoiditis, sinusitis: Third-generation cephalosporin (cefotaxime 2 g q4h IV or ceftriaxone 2 g q12h IV) plus metronidazole 15 mg/kg IV as a loading dose, then 7.5 mg/kg q8h IV, not to exceed 4 g/day
  2. Dental infection: Penicillin G (20 million to 24 million units per day IV in six divided doses) plus metronidazole (dose as above)
  3. Head trauma: Third- or fourth-generation cephalosporin (cefotaxime 2 g IV q4h or ceftriaxone 2 g IV q12h or cefepime 2 g IV q8h) plus vancomycin (30 mg/kg IV in two divided doses adjusted for renal function)
  4. Postoperative neurosurgery: Vancomycin (dose as above) plus ceftazidime (2 g IV q8h) or cefepime (2 g IV q8h), or meropenem (1 g IV q8h). Replace vancomycin with nafcillin (2g IV q4h) if susceptibility testing reveals methicillin-sensitive S. aureus

- Hematogenous spread (congenital heart disease, endocarditis, urinary tract, lung, or intraabdominal infection): Vancomycin (empiric therapy, dose as above) or nafcillin (if susceptibility testing reveals methicillin-sensitive S. aureus, dose as above) plus metronidazole plus third-generation cephalosporin (cefotaxime 2 g IV q4h or ceftriaxone 2 g IV q12h). Antibiotic therapy can be adjusted based on the etiology of the underlying infection, if known. Depending on the source, many experts advocate for anaerobic coverage, even with no documentation given suboptimal sensitivity of current culture techniques
- HIV-infected or immunocompromised patient[1]: Metronidazole plus a third-generation cephalosporin, antifungal, and/or antiparasitic agents
- Duration of antibiotic therapy is guided by the clinical course and serial CT scan findings; it is usually prolonged. Most experts recommend parenteral treatment for at least 4 to 8 wk, with serial neuroimaging to ensure adequate resolution. (Imaging weekly could be considered for first 2 wk of therapy, then every 2 wk until resolution.) Surgical therapy may be required for clinical failure (i.e., increasing size of abscess on imaging despite antibiotic therapy)[1]

Treatment of mycobacterial, fungal, Toxoplasma, and Nocardia infections may be for several months.

SURGICAL Rx

- Three indications for surgical intervention:
  1. Collect specimens for culture and sensitivity to guide antibiotic therapy
  2. Reduce mass effect
  3. Clinical failure with antibiotic therapy alone
- Stereotactic biopsy or aspirate of the abscess if surgically feasible
- Essential to selection of targeted antimicrobial coverage

TABLE 5 Antimicrobial Therapy for Brain Abscess[a]

Organism	Standard Therapy	Alternative Therapies
Bacteria		
Actinomyces spp.[b]	Penicillin G	Clindamycin
Bacteroides fragilis[b]	Metronidazole	Clindamycin
Enterobacteriaceae[b]	Third-generation cephalosporin[c]	Aztreonam, trimethoprim-sulfamethoxazole, fluoroquinolone, meropenem
Fusobacterium spp.[b]	Metronidazole	Clindamycin, meropenem
Haemophilus spp.[b]	Third-generation cephalosporin[c]	Aztreonam, trimethoprim-sulfamethoxazole
Listeria monocytogenes	Ampicillin or penicillin G[d]	Trimethoprim-sulfamethoxazole
Mycobacterium tuberculosis	Isoniazid + rifampin + pyrazinamide + ethambutol	
Nocardia spp.	Trimethoprim-sulfamethoxazole or sulfadiazine	Minocycline, imipenem, meropenem, third-generation cephalosporin,[c] amikacin, linezolid
Prevotella melaninogenica[b]	Metronidazole	Clindamycin, meropenem
Pseudomonas aeruginosa	Ceftazidime or cefepime	Aztreonam, fluoroquinolone, meropenem
Staphylococcus aureus		
Methicillin-sensitive	Nafcillin or oxacillin	Vancomycin
Methicillin-resistant	Vancomycin	Trimethoprim-sulfamethoxazole
Streptococcus anginosus (milleri) group, other streptococci[b]	Penicillin G	Third-generation cephalosporin,[c] vancomycin
Fungi		
Aspergillus spp.	Voriconazole	Liposomal amphotericin B, amphotericin B lipid complex, amphotericin B deoxycholate, itraconazole,[e] posaconazole[e]
Candida spp.	Liposomal amphotericin B,[f] amphotericin B lipid complex,[f] amphotericin B deoxycholate[f]	Fluconazole, voriconazole
Cryptococcus neoformans	Amphotericin B deoxycholate,[f] liposomal amphotericin B,[f] amphotericin B lipid complex[f]	Fluconazole
Mucorales	Liposomal amphotericin B, amphotericin B lipid complex, amphotericin B deoxycholate	Posaconazole,[e] isavuconazole[e]
Scedosporium apiospermum	Voriconazole	Itraconazole,[e] posaconazole[e]
Protozoa		
Toxoplasma gondii	Pyrimethamine + sulfadiazine	Pyrimethamine + clindamycin; trimethoprim-sulfamethoxazole; pyrimethamine + azithromycin, clarithromycin, atovaquone, or dapsone

[a]Choice of specific antimicrobial agents for standard therapy, or consideration of alternative therapies, should be based on in vitro susceptibility testing for pathogens for which testing can be performed.
[b]Depending on the pathogenesis of bacterial brain abscess (see text), these bacteria may be isolated as part of a mixed infection.
[c]Cefotaxime or ceftriaxone.
[d]Addition of an aminoglycoside should be considered.
[e]Consider for use in salvage therapy in nonresponding patients or in patients intolerant of amphotericin B–based therapies.
[f]Addition of flucytosine may be considered.
From Bennett JE et al: Mandell, Douglas, and Bennett's principles and practice of infectious diseases, ed 9, Philadelphia, 2020, Elsevier.

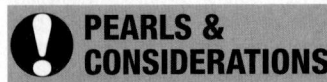
- Timing and choice of surgery depend on:
  1. Primary infection source
  2. Number and location of the abscesses
  3. Whether the procedure is diagnostic or therapeutic
  4. Neurologic status of the patient

DISPOSITION

- Prompt diagnostic consideration, early institution of appropriate antimicrobial therapy, and advanced neuroradiologic imaging have reduced the mortality rate from brain abscesses from 40% to 80% in the preantibiotic era to 10% to 20% at present.
- Morbidity is usually manifest as persistent neurologic sequelae (seizures, intellectual or behavioral impairment, motor deficits).

REFERRAL

Consultation with infectious disease and neurosurgery

PEARLS & CONSIDERATIONS

COMMENTS

- It is important to maintain a high index of suspicion because a brain abscess often presents with nonspecific symptoms.
- Rapid imaging and early institution of appropriate antimicrobial therapy improve patient morbidity and mortality.
- Neurosurgical consultation is mandatory.

PREVENTION

Because brain abscesses arise from either contiguous infections or hematogenously from a remote site, early and appropriate treatment of predisposing infections is paramount to prevent brain abscess.

RELATED CONTENT

Brain Abscess (Patient Information)

REFERENCES

Available at eBooks.Health.Elsevier.com.

AUTHOR: **STACI A. FISCHER, MD**

BASIC INFORMATION

DEFINITION

Brain neoplasms are a diverse group of primary (predominantly nonmetastatic) tumors arising from one of many different cell types within the central nervous system (CNS). Specific tumor subtypes and prognosis depend on the tumor cell of origin, certain genetic markers, and pattern of growth. The diffuse low-grade gliomas (LGGs) currently include World Health Organization (WHO) grade II astrocytomas and oligodendrogliomas. The histologic classification oligoastrocytoma is no longer appropriate in the era of molecular markers, though the diagnosis of *oligoastrocytoma, NOS* still exists when molecular data are not available.

SYNONYMS

Low-grade glioma (LGG)
Glioneuronal tumor
Meningioma
Primary brain tumor

ICD-10CM CODE	
D33.2	Benign neoplasm of brain, unspecified

EPIDEMIOLOGY & DEMOGRAPHICS

INCIDENCE: U.S. incidence rate of a new brain tumor is approximately 6.4/100,000 persons per year for all primary brain tumors (Table 1). One third of these are considered malignant and the remainder benign or borderline malignant. The incidence rate in children aged 0 to 19 yr is lower (5.6 per 100,000 children). Primary brain neoplasms account for ~2% of all cancers, with a disproportionate share of cancer morbidity and mortality. It is the most common cause of cancer death in children up to 15 yr.[1]

PREDOMINANT SEX & AGE: Slight male predominance of malignant brain tumors (8.0 vs. 5.5/100,000 person/yr). Men account for slightly less than half of cases of both benign and malignant brain tumors, as meningiomas have a higher incidence in women.

PEAK INCIDENCE: Depends on histology, though highest peak at ~age 50 yr.

RISK FACTORS: Exposure to ionizing radiation has been implicated in meningiomas, gliomas, and nerve sheath tumors. No convincing evidence has shown a link with trauma, occupation, cellular phone use, diet, or electromagnetic fields.

GENETICS: Molecular alterations in primary brain tumors are summarized in Table E2. Most primary CNS neoplasms are sporadic; 5% are associated with hereditary syndromes (Table 3) that predispose to neoplasia.[1] The most common of these include:

- Li-Fraumeni syndrome: *p53* mutation on chromosome 17q13, gliomas
- Von Hippel-Lindau: VHL, chromosome 3p25, hemangioblastoma
- Tuberous sclerosis: *TSC1/TSC2* (chromosome 9q34/16p13), subependymal giant cell astrocytoma
- Neurofibromatosis type 1: NF1, chromosome 17q11, neurofibroma, optic nerve glioma, low-grade glioma
- Neurofibromatosis type 2: NF2, chromosome 22q12, schwannoma, meningioma, ependymoma
- Retinoblastoma: pRB, chromosome 13q, retinoblastoma
- Gorlin syndrome: PTCH, chromosome 9q31, desmoplastic medulloblastoma
- Hereditary nonpolyposis colorectal cancer (HNPCC): Mismatch repair deficiency, high-grade gliomas

PHYSICAL FINDINGS & CLINICAL PRESENTATION

- In general, the location, size, and rate of growth will determine the symptoms and signs of a brain tumor.
- Headache is common and is the worst symptom in nearly half of all patients.[2] The headaches are usually a dull, constant pain that is often worse at night. Symptoms of increased intracranial pressure may also be present, including nausea and vomiting, and may worsen with changes in body position that increase thoracic pressure (coughing, sneezing, Valsalva maneuver). Papilledema is suggestive of obstructive hydrocephalus.
- Seizures occur in 33% of patients and are among the most common symptoms, particularly with brain metastases and low-grade gliomas.[2] The type of seizure and clinical presentation depend on the location of the brain tumor. Tumor-related seizures are typically repetitive and have similar presentation patterns (semiology). It is thought that patients with seizures typically have smaller tumors at the time of diagnosis compared with those with other symptoms, because the onset of seizures prompts an imaging study, leading to an earlier diagnosis.
- Focal neurologic signs and symptoms, including muscle weakness, sensory changes, or visual disturbances are also quite frequent. In addition, cognitive dysfunction, accompanied by changes in memory or personality, may be recounted, often in retrospect.

ETIOLOGY

Most cases are idiopathic, though specific chromosomal abnormalities have been implicated in some tumor types.

DIAGNOSIS

- Diagnosis is typically based on clinical presentation and imaging characteristics. Specifically, neuroimaging is critical for preoperative planning and tumor etiology.
- Tumors are best seen on brain MRI with and without contrast; calcifications are sometimes present. However, low-grade gliomas often do not enhance with contrast. Contrast enhancement is concerning for a higher-grade glioma.
- Benign and low-grade tumors, typically in the glioma family, are heterogeneous and are generally seen as an infiltrating hemispheric lesion.

DIFFERENTIAL DIAGNOSIS

- Stroke/cerebral hemorrhage
- Abscess/parasitic cyst
- Demyelinating disease: Multiple sclerosis, postinfectious encephalomyelitis
- Metastatic tumors
- Primary CNS lymphoma

WORKUP

Neuroimaging studies and pathologic sampling are the most important diagnostic modalities in evaluation of brain tumors and are critical for preoperative planning. Most recently updated in 2021, the fifth edition of the WHO Classifications of Tumors of the Central Nervous System highlighted the importance of integrated diagnosis

---

TABLE 1 Frequency of Primary Central Nervous System Tumors

CHILDREN (0-14 Yr)		ADULTS (≥15 Yr)	
Type	**Percentage**	**Type**	**Percentage**
Glioblastoma	20	Glioblastoma	50
Astrocytoma	21	Astrocytoma	10
Ependymoma	7	Ependymoma	2
Oligodendroglioma	1	Oligodendroglioma	3
Medulloblastoma	24	Medulloblastoma	2
Neuroblastoma	3	Neurilemmoma	2
Neurilemmoma	1	Pituitary adenoma	4
Craniopharyngioma	5	Craniopharyngioma	1
Meningioma	5	Meningioma	17
Teratoma	2	Pinealoma	1
Pinealoma	2	Hemangioma	2
Hemangioma	3	Sarcoma	1
Sarcoma	1	Others	5
Others	5	TOTAL	100
TOTAL	100		

From Goetz CG, Pappert EJ: *Textbook of clinical neurology*, Philadelphia, 1999, Saunders

TABLE 3 Hereditary Syndromes Associated with Brain Tumors

Syndrome	Associated CNS Tumors	Gene	Chromosomal Locus	Defective Protein and Normal Function
Neurofibromatosis type 1	Optic pathway gliomas, meningiomas, neuromas	NF1	17q11-12	Neurofibromin; GTPase-activating protein that negatively regulates Ras
Neurofibromatosis type 2	Bilateral acoustic neuromas, meningiomas, gliomas	NF2	22q12	Merlin; related to membrane cytoskeleton linker protein 4.1 superfamily
Tuberous sclerosis	Cerebral hamartomas	TSC1	9q34	Hamartin
	Subependymal giant cell astrocytoma (SEGA)	TSC2	16p13	Tuberin; associates with hamartin; both are involved in signaling downstream of Akt
von Hippel-Lindau syndrome	Hemangioblastomas	VHL	3p25-29	VHL protein; degrades HIF-1α
Li-Fraumeni syndrome	Malignant gliomas	TP53	17p13	p53; maintains genomic stability
Cowden syndrome	Meningiomas	PTEN	10q23	PTEN; lipid phosphatase, counters PI3 kinase activation
Gorlin syndrome (nevoid basal cell carcinoma syndrome)	Medulloblastomas	PTCH	9q22	Cell surface receptor; regulates normal brain development
Turcot syndrome	Medulloblastomas	APC	5q21	APC; part of Wnt/β-catenin signaling pathway
	Malignant gliomas	hMLH1	3p21	Involved in mismatch repair
	Malignant gliomas	PMS2	7p22	Involved in mismatch repair
Familial retinoblastoma	Pineoblastomas	RB	13q14	Rb protein; regulates entry into S phase
Ataxia-telangiectasia	CNS lymphoma	ATM	11q22-23	ATM protein; involved in DNA damage sensing
Multiple endocrine neoplasia syndrome 1	Pituitary adenomas	MEN1	11q13	Menin

APC, Adenomatous polyposis coli; *ATM*, ataxia-telangiectasia mutated; *CNS*, central nervous system; *GTPase*, guanosine triphosphatase.
From Niederhuber JE et al: *Abeloff's clinical oncology*, ed 6, Philadelphia, 2020, Elsevier.

using histology, immunohistochemistry, and molecular analysis for the diagnosis of tumors.[3]

LABORATORY TESTS

- Classically, histologic examination can provide the exact diagnosis. Additional features such as proliferative index, immunohistochemical stains, and electron microscopy can also be used to aid in diagnosis. However, the most recent diagnostic criteria now also demand molecular and genetic classifications (e.g., 1p19q codeletion for the diagnosis of oligodendrogliomas).
- The current classification schema for gliomas is based on molecular genetics and histologic criteria. Tumor histology/histologic diagnosis (World Health Organization [WHO] grading system) includes number of mitoses, capillary endothelial proliferation, and necrosis.
- Molecular genetic analysis of tumors is critical to classification of tumor type, stratification of treatments, and prognosis. Low-grade gliomas are divided into three categories based on molecular genetic findings based on the presence of an isocitrate dehydrogenase (IDH) mutation or 1p/19q codeletion.

The presence of both a 1p/19q codeletion and an IDH mutation indicates an oligodendroglioma. The presence of an IDH mutation (without a 1p/19q codeletion) with *TP53* and *ATRX* mutations indicates an astrocytoma. The other category of glioma lacks both an IDH mutation and a 1p/19q codeletion.

- A codeletion of 1p/19q bestows a favorable prognosis. Low-grade gliomas lacking an IDH mutation have a poorer prognosis, one comparable to glioblastoma.
- The presence of the following mutations can upgrade a histologically low-grade glioma to a high-grade glioma: *TERT* promoter mutation, *EGFR* mutation, gain of chromosome 7/loss of chromosome 10, CDKN2A/B homozygous loss.
- However, even tumors with benign histology can cause significant morbidity due to their location and effect on surrounding structures.

IMAGING STUDIES

- MRI with gadolinium enhancement is highly sensitive and permits visualization of the tumor with relation to the surrounding tissue. Specifically, enhancing tumor can be distinguished from surrounding edema. Low-grade tumors often present as an infiltrating lesion without mass effect. MRI is superior to computed tomography (CT) scanning for evaluating the meninges, subarachnoid space, and posterior fossa, and for defining relation to major intracranial vessels, although CT scanning is useful if calcification or hemorrhage is suspected. Fig. E1 shows the appearance of astrocytoma in imaging studies.
- Magnetic resonance spectroscopy can be used as a tool to help differentiate intracranial tumors from other intracranial processes using different chemical markers, usually in the setting of differentiating recurrence vs. radiation necrosis. For example, *N*-acetylaspartate is often decreased in brain tumors, whereas choline, a component of cell membranes, is often increased in brain tumors because of high cellular turnover.
- PET scan is helpful to distinguish neoplastic lesions (with high rate of metabolism) from other lesions such as demyelination or radiation necrosis (with a much lower metabolic rate). Such lesions take up greater amounts of glucose than surrounding tissues or tumors with slower metabolic rates. PET may be useful to help map functional areas of the brain before surgery or radiation.
- Functional MRI is now used as an adjunct in perioperative planning for patients whose lesion is in vital regions, such as those responsible for speech, language, and motor control.

Rx TREATMENT

NONPHARMACOLOGIC THERAPY

- Maximal surgical removal or debulking is the initial treatment of choice and provides tissue for diagnosis and molecular characterization. Maximal safe resection is often favored with a trend toward improved survival with this approach.[4]
- Biopsy alone is performed if the tumor is located in eloquent regions of brain or is inaccessible; this is essential for histopathologic diagnosis. Biopsy can be performed under CT or MRI guidance using stereotactic localization.
- If the tumor is benign (e.g., meningioma, acoustic neuroma), often no further therapy is required.

ACUTE GENERAL Rx (BOX 1)

Antiseizure medications have been used perioperatively and to control seizures resulting from focal lesions. Prophylactic use of anticonvulsants is not typically recommended without clear history of seizures.

CHRONIC Rx

- The decision to use chemotherapy and its timing (before, during, or after radiation therapy or surgery) is highly dependent on the age of the patient, grade of the tumor, and the amount of residual following surgery. In

BOX 1 Management of Supratentorial Astrocytomas

Grade I (pilocytic) astrocytomas: Surgery is curative. If residual tumor is seen on postoperative images, the patient should undergo a second craniotomy to resect the entire tumor. Radiation therapy and chemotherapy have limited usefulness for the treatment of these tumors. Radiation can be considered for recurrent or unresectable tumors.

Grade II (low-grade) astrocytoma: Surgery is the mainstay of therapy for tumors in noneloquent regions of brain. In patients younger than 40 yr who undergo gross total resection, no additional therapy is given. Incomplete resection is typically treated with radiation alone; however, increasing evidence suggests that chemotherapy improves survival.

Grade III astrocytoma (anaplastic astrocytoma) and grade IV gliomas (glioblastoma): Surgery is required to establish tissue diagnosis, preferably also with debulking. Chemotherapy is begun with temozolomide during radiation therapy and continued for six cycles after completion of the radiation regimen. The radiation dose generally is 60 Gy. Tumor tissue is sent for analysis of O^6-methylguanine DNA-methyltransferase (MGMT) promoter activity. Temozolomide is offered to all patients, however, regardless of promoter methylation status.

From Niederhuber JE et al: *Abeloff's clinical oncology,* ed 6, Philadelphia, 2020, Elsevier.

children, chemotherapy is often used to delay radiation therapy. In a recent trial in patients with grade II glioma who were younger than 40 yr of age and had undergone subtotal tumor resection or who were 40 yr of age or older, progression-free survival and overall survival were longer among those who received combination chemotherapy following radiation therapy than among those who received radiation therapy alone.[5]

- Radiation is useful for certain types of tumors and is often used if there is residual tumor after surgery; conventional radiation uses external beams over a period of weeks, whereas stereotactic radiosurgery delivers a single, high dose of radiation to a well-defined area (usually <1 cm). Long-term effects of radiation therapy include radiation necrosis (particularly of white matter), blood vessel hyalinization, secondary tumors (usually meningiomas, sarcomas, and malignant astrocytomas), and cognitive changes.[6]
- In patients with newly diagnosed grade III gliomas with IDH mutation but without 1p/19q codeletion, the use of radiation followed by adjuvant chemotherapy with temozolomide was associated with an overall survival benefit. This benefit was not seen when compared to concurrent use of temozolomide with radiation or with radiation therapy alone.[7]
- Recent trial results from the INDIGO trial suggest that utilization of an IDH inhibitor, vorasidenib, in patients with IDH-mutated low-grade glioma can improve progression-free survival, thus delaying further treatment.[8]
- Experimental therapies are continually in development and target molecular characteristics of tumors and signal transduction cascades involved in tumor growth. Some of these therapies involve antisense molecules, biologic agents, immunotherapies, or angiogenesis inhibitors. Intratumoral drug infusions and convection-enhanced delivery of novel agents are currently under study.

DISPOSITION

In general, younger age, high performance status, lower pathologic grade, the presence of an IDH mutation, and a 1p/19q codeletion have more favorable prognosis. For all histologic subtypes of brain tumors, pediatric and young adult patients have a better survival rate.

REFERRAL

- All cases warrant evaluation by a neuro-oncologist and neurosurgeon. Referral to a neurologist is indicated for management of seizures and headaches related to the tumor if there are no neuro-oncologists available.
- Patients should be evaluated for physical and occupational therapy.
- Children should undergo neuropsychologic evaluations and screening for learning disabilities.

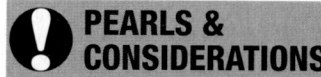
PEARLS & CONSIDERATIONS

COMMENTS

Molecular genetic characterization is important for diagnosis, therapeutic approach, and prognosis, for which mutations in IDH and the presence of a 1p/19q codeletion represented some of the critical genetic determinations. In general, younger age, high performance status, and lower pathologic grade have more favorable prognosis. For all histologic subtypes of brain tumors, pediatric and young adult patients have a better survival.

PATIENT & FAMILY EDUCATION

American Brain Tumor Association (www.abta.org)
National Brain Tumor Society (www.braintumor.org)
Pediatric Low-Grade Astrocytoma (PLGA) (https://akidsbraintumorcure.org)

RELATED CONTENT

Brain Cancer (Patient Information)
Astrocytoma (Related Key Topic)
Meningioma (Related Key Topic)

REFERENCES & SUGGESTED READINGS

Available at eBooks.Health.Elsevier.com.

AUTHOR: **LILY C. PHAM, MD**

BASIC INFORMATION

DEFINITION

- Glioblastoma (GBM) is the most aggressive primary brain tumor and is classified as WHO Grade IV in the World Health Organization's (WHO) classification system. GBM is diffusely infiltrative and has an astrocytic lineage. GBM is the most common brain and central nervous system (CNS) malignancy, accounting for 48.3% of malignant primary brain and CNS tumors, 54% of all gliomas, and 14.6% of all primary brain and CNS tumors.[1]
- GBM represents a molecularly heterogeneous disease with numerous subclassifications. GBMs comprise primary and secondary subtypes that evolve through different genetic pathways, affect patients at different ages, and have differences in outcomes. Primary *(de novo)* GBMs account for 80% of GBMs and occur in older patients (mean age 65 yr). Secondary GBMs develop from lower grade astrocytomas or oligodendrogliomas and occur in younger patients (mean age 45 yr).[2]
- With the recent changes to 2021 WHO Classification of Tumors of the Central Nervous System, diagnosis of a high-grade glioma or glioblastoma is dependent on both histology and molecular mutations. The term GBM is now outdated in favor of high-grade glioma, followed by specific mutations.[3]
- Overall prognosis for high-grade glioma is poor with median survival being 11 to 16 mo and 5-yr overall survival at 6.8%.[1]

ICD-10CM CODE
C71.9 Malignant neoplasm of brain, unspecified

EPIDEMIOLOGY & DEMOGRAPHICS

INCIDENCE: Based on the 2019 Central Brain Tumor Registry of the United States (CBTRUS) report, the average annual age-adjusted incidence rate (IR) of GBM is 3.22/100,000 population.[1]

PREDOMINANT SEX & AGE: GBM is primarily diagnosed at older ages, with the median age of diagnosis at 65 yr. It is uncommon in children, accounting for ~3% of all brain and CNS tumors reported among infants to 19-yr-olds. A higher incidence of GBM has been reported in men compared with women; the incidence rate is 1.58 times higher in males [3.97 vs. 2.53]. Caucasians have the highest incidence rates for GBM compared with any other race in the U.S.[1]

RISK FACTORS: Many genetic and environmental factors have been studied in GBM, but no risk factor that accounts for a large proportion of GBM has been identified. Like many cancers, the causes are sporadic. Factors associated with GBM risk are prior therapeutic radiation, decreased susceptibility to allergy, immune factors and immune genes, and some single nucleotide polymorphisms (SNPs) detected by genome-wide association studies (GWAS). There is no substantial evidence of GBM association with lifestyle characteristics such as cigarette smoking, alcohol consumption, drugs, or dietary exposure to N-nitroso compounds (cured or smoked meat or fish). Inconsistent and nondefinitive results have been published regarding the risk of glioma with use of mobile phones.[4]

PHYSICAL FINDINGS & CLINICAL PRESENTATION

Patients present with a variety of symptoms dependent of tumor location, including headache, seizures, symptoms of increased intracranial pressure, weakness, sensory deficits, and cognitive disturbances.

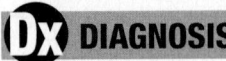 **DIAGNOSIS**

IMAGING STUDIES

Initial workup includes imaging studies. Brain MRI with and without contrast is the study of choice and demonstrates a contrast-enhancing tumor (Fig. 1). Functional MRI is now used as an adjunct modality in perioperative planning for patients whose lesion is in eloquent regions, such as those responsible for speech, language, and motor control.[5]

HISTOLOGY

- Pathologically, GBM is a high-grade astrocytoma characterized by hypercellularity, mitotic activity, nuclear atypia, pseudopalisading necrosis, and microvascular proliferation. Various molecular markers have been identified distinguishing GBM from other lower grade astrocytomas, as well as differentiating primary and secondary subtypes of GBM.[6]
- Recent C-IMPACT-NOW and 2021 WHO criteria also include various molecular markers for GBM that can predict a more GBM-like prognosis for lower grade gliomas, necessitating treatment similar to histologic GBMs. These markers include *TERT* promoter mutations, *EGFR* amplification, gain of chromosome 7/loss of chromosome 10, and *CDNK2A/B* homozygous loss.[3,7]

Rx TREATMENT

- GBM is an aggressive neoplasm with a median survival of 3 mo if untreated.
- Combined modality therapy with surgery, RT (Fig. 2), and chemotherapy has significantly improved survival of GBM patients. Treatment is complex and initially consists of maximal-safe

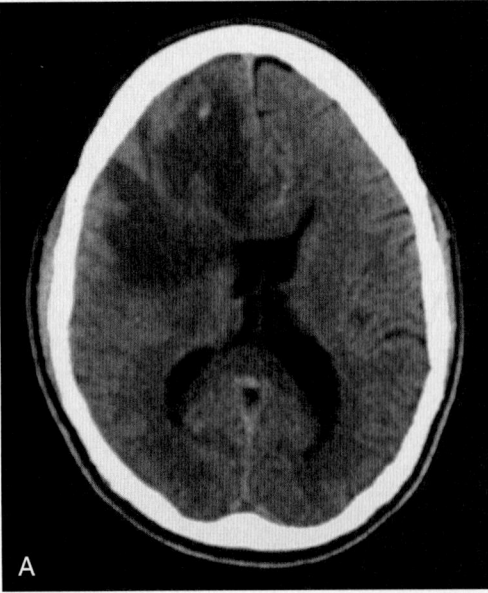
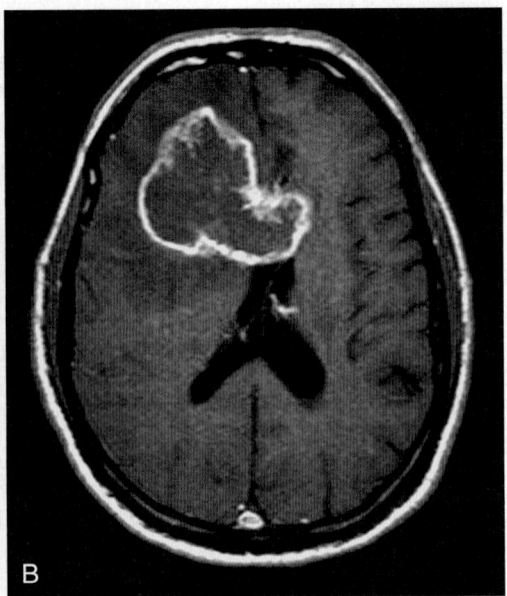

FIG. 1 Glioblastoma multiforme (astrocytoma World Health Organization grade IV/IV). A, On noncontrast computed tomography the mass cannot be clearly separated from the edema. **B,** A postgadolinium T1-weighted image shows an irregular rim of enhancement of this mass that crosses the midline via the corpus callosum. This 50-yr-old man presented with altered mental status. (From Soto JA, Lucey BC: *Emergency radiology: the requisites,* ed 2, Philadelphia, 2017, Elsevier.)

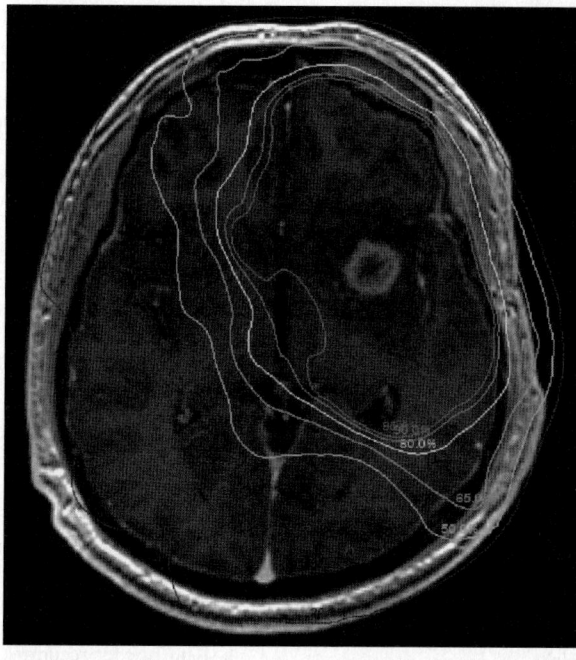

FIG. 2 Radiation planning magnetic resonance image in a patient with a left frontal glioblastoma. (From Jankovic J et al: *Bradley and Daroff's neurology in clinical practice*, ed 8, Philadelphia, 2022, Elsevier.)

surgical resection followed by RT with concurrent temozolomide (TMZ) chemotherapy, followed by 6 to 12 cycles of maintenance TMZ.[8]
- Surgical intervention has decompressive and cytoreductive effects, and there is increasing evidence of a significant survival advantage with complete resection.[9]
- Various emerging treatment modalities under investigation seem promising, including immunotherapy. Regression of glioblastoma after chimeric antigen receptor T-cell therapy has been reported. Intratumoral infusion of recombinant nonpathogenic polio-rhinovirus chimera (PVSRIPO) has improved survival rate in advanced stage glioblastoma.
- Symptomatic treatment includes corticosteroids to reduce cerebral edema, antiepileptic drugs for seizures, and analgesics for headache.

DISPOSITION

Survival: GBM has a poor prognosis with a low relative survival estimate; only a few patients reach long-term survival status of 2.5 yr, and 6.8% of patients survive 5 yr postdiagnosis. The relative survival for the first year after diagnosis is 35%, falls in the second year postdiagnosis to 13.7%, and continues to fall thereafter. Median survival of GBM postdiagnosis is 15 mo following standard therapy. Several variables affect the prognosis of GBM patients, including age, preoperative performance status, tumor location, preoperative imaging characteristics of the tumor, and the extent of resection.[1]

Prognostic molecular markers in GBM: All GBMs are WHO grade IV but exhibit significant genetic heterogeneity. Tumor subtypes, based on genetic alterations, exist within this larger homogeneous histologic category and carry prognostic significance. These markers include methylation status of the gene promoter for O^6-methylguanine-DNA methyltransferase (MGMT), isocitrate dehydrogenase enzyme 1/2 *(IDH1/2)* mutation, epidermal growth factor receptor (EGFR) overexpression and amplification, tumor protein *(TP53)* mutation, *ATRX* mutation and genetic losses of chromosomes.[10-12]
- Primary GBMs show EGFR amplification, phosphatase and tensin homolog gene *(PTEN)* mutations, and loss of heterozygosity (LOH) 10q, p16 deletions; less frequently shown are mouse double-minute 2 (MDM2) amplification, high frequency of telomerase reverse transcriptase (hTERT) promoter mutations, and absence of *IDH1* mutation.[11]
- The hallmark of secondary GBMs is *TP53*, alpha thalassemia/mental retardation syndrome X-linked *(ATRX)* and *IDH1* mutations, and LOH 10q.[10]
- The MGMT promoter is methylated in approximately 50% of newly diagnosed GBMs. MGMT methylation is more common in secondary than primary GBM (75% vs. 36%, respectively) and has prognostic and predictive significance of better overall survival in patients with GBM, irrespective of treatment choices.[12]
- *IDH1/2* mutations are far more common in grades II and III astrocytomas and oligodendrogliomas compared with GBMs, and more than 90% of the mutations involve *IDH1*. *IDH1/2* mutations are a selective molecular marker of secondary GBMs, help distinguish them from primary GBMs, and are a marker of more favorable prognosis in high-grade gliomas.[10-11]
- In GBMs, EGFR signaling promotes cell division, tumor invasiveness, and resistance to radiation therapy (RT) and chemotherapy. About 40% of all GBMs have EGFR amplification, and it is more common in primary as compared with secondary GBMs.[10-13]
- Mutation of the *TP53* gene has been found in 60% to 70% of secondary GBMs and 25% to 30% of primary GBMs, and it occurs more frequently in younger patients. Studies of *TP53* mutations as a prognostic marker have not been definitive.[13]
- *ATRX* is frequently mutated in grade II to III astrocytomas (71%), oligoastrocytomas (68%), and secondary GBMs (57%) but is infrequent in primary (4%) and pediatric GBMs (20%) as well as pure oligodendroglial tumors (14%). In a prospective cohort of patients with astrocytic tumors, those harboring *ATRX* loss had a significantly better prognosis than the ones that expressed *ATRX* and had IDH mutation.[10-13]
- *TERT* mutation is one of the most frequent genetic alterations in primary adult GBMs and is significantly higher in these tumors as compared with secondary adult or any pediatric GBMs. GBMs with *TERT* mutation have a shorter survival than those without *TERT* mutations. However, when adjusted for GBM subtype (primary and secondary), they do not have a significant impact on survival.[13]
- The presence of a *TERT* promoter mutation, *EGFR* amplification, and gain of entire chromosome 7 and loss of entire chromosome 10 in a histologically lower grade glioma is now classified as molecular grade IV high-grade glioma per the 2021 edition of the WHO Classification of Tumors of the Central Nervous System.[3]

REFERRAL

Treatment involves a multidisciplinary team approach including oncology, neurosurgery, neurology, and radiation oncology.

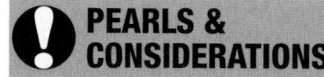

PEARLS & CONSIDERATIONS

COMMENTS
- Glioblastoma is an aggressive, infiltrative, primary brain cancer with a generally poor prognosis. The median survival is 15 mo with therapy.
- The mainstay of treatment for glioblastoma includes maximum surgical resection, radiation, and chemotherapy. Extent of resection is a prognostic factor in overall survival.
- To date, there are only two FDA-approved medications for the treatment of glioblastoma: Temozolomide and bevacizumab. Newer targeted therapies based on molecular mutations are under investigation in clinical trials.
- NCCN guidelines also offer tumor treatment field as a potential treatment option; however, this should be discussed with the patient's neuro-oncologist to properly evaluate the pros and cons.[14]

REFERENCES & SUGGESTED READING
Available at eBooks.Health.Elsevier.com.

AUTHOR: **LILY C. PHAM, MD**

BASIC INFORMATION

DEFINITION

A breast abscess is an acute inflammatory process resulting in the formation of a collection of purulent material (pus) in breast tissue. It is characterized by a painful, erythematous mass formation in the breast, occasionally draining through the overlying skin or through the nipple duct.

SYNONYMS

Subareolar abscess
Lactational or puerperal abscess

ICD-10CM CODES
091.111	Abscess of breast associated with pregnancy, first trimester
091.112	Abscess of breast associated with pregnancy, second trimester
091.113	Abscess of breast associated with pregnancy, third trimester
091.119	Abscess of breast associated with pregnancy, unspecified trimester
091.12	Abscess of breast associated with the puerperium
091.13	Abscess of breast associated with lactation

EPIDEMIOLOGY & DEMOGRAPHICS

INCIDENCE: Of all breast abscesses, 10% to 30% are lactational, developing as a complication of mastitis. Acute mastitis occurs in up to 10% of nursing mothers, with 1/15 of these women developing a breast abscess. Puerperal mastitis is more common in the initial breastfeeding months.

Non-lactational abscesses may develop as a complication of mastitis or cellulitis. Smoking, obesity, and diabetes are risk factors for non-lactational mastitis with a breast abscess. Other risk factors for non-lactational abscesses include rheumatoid arthritis, steroid treatment, and trauma. More recently, nipple piercing may also be associated with infection.

PHYSICAL FINDINGS & CLINICAL PRESENTATION

- Painful, erythematous induration involving breast and leading to fluctuant, possibly palpable abscess
- Systemic symptoms: Fever and malaise
- Note that mastitis and abscess can occur either sequentially or concurrently

ETIOLOGY

- Lactational abscess: Milk stasis (from blockage, fewer feedings, excess supply, weaning, etc.) and bacterial infection leading to mastitis and then to abscess, with *Staphylococcus aureus* (commonly methicillin-resistant *S. aureus* [MRSA]) the most common causative agent. Group A *Streptococcus*, group B *Streptococcus*,

and corynebacteriae are also commonly encountered.
- Subareolar abscess:
  1. Central ducts involved, with obstructive nipple duct changes leading to bacterial infection
  2. Cultured polymicrobial organisms, including anaerobes, staphylococci, streptococci, and others

DIAGNOSIS

DIFFERENTIAL DIAGNOSIS

- Galactocele
- Inflammatory breast cancer
- Advanced carcinoma with erythema, edema, and/or ulceration
- Tuberculous abscess (rare in the U.S.)
- Hidradenitis of breast skin
- Sebaceous cyst with infection
- Plugged milk duct

WORKUP

- Clinical examination
- Ultrasound to identify fluid collection, which can be used to guide treatment options such as facilitating aspiration
- If abscess suspected, referral to surgeon for incision, drainage, and biopsy

LABORATORY TESTS

- Perform culture and sensitivity test of abscess contents.
- For women who are lactating, culture of the breast milk may be used to guide selection of antibiotics if an aspirate is not obtained.
- If mammogram or ultrasound is required but prevented by discomfort, perform after treatment and subsequent resolution of abscess.
- Blood cultures are not typically necessary outside of the setting of severe infection (e.g., hemodynamic instability).

TREATMENT

NONPHARMACOLOGIC THERAPY

- Established abscesses may be treated with incision and drainage (I&D) or needle aspiration; the latter is usually with ultrasound guidance and typically requires multiple procedures for resolution
  1. High likelihood of patients treated with aspiration subsequently requiring I&D
- Biopsy of abscess cavity wall to exclude carcinoma

ACUTE GENERAL Rx

- Antibiotics: Generally targeting staphylococci (*S. aureus*) for lactational abscess. Recommended initial antibiotic therapy is nafcillin or oxacillin 2 g q4h IV or cefazolin 1 g q8h IV for 10 to 14 days. Alternative includes vancomycin 1 g IV q12h.
- Outpatient management with dicloxacillin 500 mg q6h PO or cephalexin 500 mg q6h

PO is reasonable for uncomplicated cases without suspicion for MRSA.
- If acute mastitis is identified and treated early without the development of an abscess, resolution without drainage is possible.
- Subareolar abscess: Broad-spectrum antibiotic treatment (e.g., cephalexin 500 mg PO QID or cefazolin 1 g q8h IV for 10 to 14 days for more severe infection) and drainage are needed to control acute phase. If an abscess is odoriferous, consider anaerobes as the most likely etiology and add metronidazole 500 mg PO/IV TID. Augmentin and clindamycin are reasonable alternatives in this situation.

CHRONIC Rx

Further surgical treatment for recurrences or fistula

DISPOSITION

- Lactational abscess: Possible to continue breastfeeding without risk of infection to the infant
- Subareolar abscess:
  1. High risk for recurrence or complication of fistula formation
  2. Incision and drainage often associated with poor cosmetic outcome
  3. Patient informed and referred to General Surgery for evaluation and treatment

REFERRAL

- If abscess drainage is required
- If subareolar abscess is involved, refer to surgery

PEARLS & CONSIDERATIONS

COMMENTS

Milk drainage (either by breastfeeding or pumping) is important for relief of discomfort in the setting of lactational infection and facilitates a reduction in the duration of symptoms and improved outcomes. It is appropriate to encourage women to continue breastfeeding following breast infection, even in the setting of incision and drainage.

It is important to rule out inflammatory breast cancer if a suspected breast infection does not respond to antibiotics, as infections of the breast can have similar clinical and mammographic appearance to inflammatory breast cancer.

RELATED CONTENT

Breast Abscess (Patient Information)
Breast Cancer (Related Key Topic)
Mastodynia (Related Key Topic)

SUGGESTED READINGS
Available at eBooks.Health.Elsevier.com.

AUTHORS: **AMANDA JONES, MD** and **ANTHONY SCISCIONE, DO**

BASIC INFORMATION

DEFINITION

Breast cancer is an epithelial carcinoma arising from the ducts (ductal) or the lobules (lobular) of the breast that is initially in situ and over time progresses to become invasive in nature.

CLASSIFICATION[1]

Carcinomas originate in the epithelium of the collecting ducts (ductal) or the terminal lobular ducts (lobular). Breast sarcomas are rare (<1% of primary cases) and arise from stromal or connective tissue. Tumor grade is based on tubule formation, nuclear pleomorphism, and mitotic counts using the Nottingham score to determine low, intermediate, or high grade.

Initially, breast carcinoma may be divided into in situ and invasive lesions (Table 1). Invasive ductal carcinoma (IDC) accounts for approximately 80% of invasive carcinomas while invasive lobular carcinoma (ILC) constitute 10% to 15% of cases. Other subtypes include mucinous, tubular, medullary, micropapillary, and papillary carcinomas. Both in situ and invasive carcinomas are often found in the same breast quadrant. Multifocal carcinomas are not uncommon, and bilateral breast carcinomas occur in 1% to 2% of new cases.

GENOMIC PROFILING[1]

Historically, the treatment of breast cancer was based on tumor histologic characteristics, axillary node status, tumor size, receptor patterns, and grade of differentiation. In addition to simplified histologic classification, a classification based on gene expression or profiling, including the presence of hormone receptors, has evolved. The genomic analysis of tumors has led to the molecular subtyping of breast cancers. Breast tumors are classified into five different molecular subtypes: Luminal-A and -B, basal, HER2, and normal.

TABLE 1 Simplified Classification of Breast Carcinoma Based on Histology

Type of Carcinoma	Percentage of All Cases Diagnosed
Ductal Carcinoma	
In situ	5
Infiltrating	70
Infiltrating with uniform histologic appearance	10
Medullary, Colloid, Comedo, Tubular, Papillary	
Lobular Carcinoma	
In situ	3
Infiltrating	9
Inflammatory carcinoma	2
Paget disease	1

From Gershenson DM et al: *Comprehensive gynecology,* ed 8, Philadelphia, 2022, Elsevier.

Basal-like tumors include triple-negative tumors, which are estrogen-, progesterone-, and HER2-negative by immunohistochemistry. A more aggressive subtype of triple-negative tumors, claudin-low tumors, has also been described. These divisions are detailed in Table 2.

ICD-10CM CODES
C50.911	Malignant neoplasm of unspecified site of right female breast
C50.912	Malignant neoplasm of unspecified site of left female breast
C50.919	Malignant neoplasm of unspecified site of unspecified female breast
C50.921	Malignant neoplasm of unspecified site of right male breast
C50.922	Malignant neoplasm of unspecified site of left male breast
C50.929	Malignant neoplasm of unspecified site of unspecified male breast

EPIDEMIOLOGY & DEMOGRAPHICS

- In 2023, there were an estimated 300,590 new patients and an estimated 43,700 deaths in the U.S.[2]
- Male breast cancers are rare (1% of all cases).
- Table 3 describes risk factors for breast cancer.
- Factors associated with a decreased risk for breast cancer are summarized in Table 4.
- Known genetic mutations in breast cancer are described in Table 5. Genetically defined group of women with *BRCA1* or *BRCA2* genes (Table 6) carry lifetime risk as high as 85%.

PHYSICAL FINDINGS & CLINICAL PRESENTATION

- Increasing number of small breast cancers are found by mammograms, in which case patients are usually asymptomatic or lack physical findings.
- Palpable lump or mass which can be self- or physician-detected.
- Skin and/or nipple retraction and skin edema, erythema, ulcer, satellite nodule.
- Nodal enlargement in axilla and supraclavicular areas.
- Nipple discharge may be serous or bloody.
- Generalized symptoms and signs, including fatigue, weight loss, jaundice, and anorexia, may be present in metastatic cases.

ETIOLOGY

- Endogenous and exogenous estrogen exposure is key to the development of receptor-positive breast cancer
- Molecular classification of breast cancer based on gene expression profiling has shown it to be of the following types:[3]
  1. Luminal A type: Endocrine responsive with favorable prognosis
  2. Luminal B type: Endocrine responsive with less favorable prognosis
  3. Normal type: Resemble normal epithelium and prognosis similar to luminal B type
  4. *HER2* amplified type: *HER2* gene amplification occurs in 15% to 20% of cases
  5. Basal type: hormone receptor and *HER2* negative cancers with poor prognosis
- Approximately 10% of all women with breast cancer have a germline mutation of *BRCA1, BRCA2, P53,* or other mutations
- Possibly interaction of ovarian estrogen, non-ovarian estrogen, estrogens of exogenous origin with breast tissue of varied carcinogenic susceptibility to develop cancer
- Other known or suspected variables: Childbearing, breastfeeding practice, diet, physical activity, body mass, alcohol intake

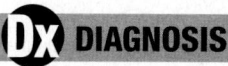 DIAGNOSIS

DIFFERENTIAL DIAGNOSIS

Benign disease is summarized in Table 7. Noninvasive neoplasms of the breast were previously broadly divided into two major types, LCIS and DCIS (Box 1). LCIS is no longer regarded as a neoplasm of the breast but is regarded as a risk factor for the development of breast cancer.

The following nonmalignant breast lesions can simulate breast cancer on both physical and mammogram examinations:
- Fibrocystic changes
- Fibroadenoma
- Hamartoma

WORKUP

- Initial workup:
  1. Mass and axillary nodal assessment by medical professional.
  2. Diagnostic mammogram followed by breast ultrasound for suspicious lesions.
  3. MRI (Fig. 1) detects suspicious lesions better than mammography in women with

TABLE 2 Classification of Breast Carcinoma Based on Gene Profiling and Hormone Receptor

Expression Type	Grade	Characteristic Behavior	Hormone Receptor Status*
Luminal A	Usually low grade	Good prognosis	E and P+
Luminal B	All grades	Mixed prognosis	E and P+, Her2 (Neu)+
Her2 (Neu)	Higher grades	Poor prognosis	E and P−, Her2 (Neu)+
Basal	Usually grade 3	Poor prognosis	Triple negative
Normal breast†	Usually low grade	Good prognosis	Triple negative

*E, Estrogen receptor; P, progesterone receptor.
†Normal breast does not express gene profiling of basal elements and myoepithelial gene expression.
From Gershenson DM et al: *Comprehensive gynecology,* ed 8, Philadelphia, 2022, Elsevier.

TABLE 3 Risk Factors for Breast Cancer

Risk Factor	Qualification	Relative Risk
Age	≤49 yr	2.0
	50-59 yr	2.3
	Age 60-69 yr	3.5
	≥70 yr	6.7
Geographic	Common in Western countries	
Age at menarche	>14 yr (low risk) vs. <12 yr	1.5
Age at first full-term pregnancy	<20 yr (low risk) vs. >30 yr	1.9-3.5
Late menopause	<45 yr (low risk) vs. >55 yr (high risk)	2.0
Hormone replacement therapy	No use vs. current	1.2
Contraceptive pill use	None vs. past or current use	1.07-1.2
Alcohol use	None vs. 2-5 drinks/day	1.4
Postmenopausal weight gain	Women with a higher body mass index (BMI)	1.1 per 5 BMI units
Bone density	Lowest vs. highest quartile	2.7-3.5
Nightshift work	Exposed to nightshift work	1.48
Smoking	History of smoking	1.10*
Benign breast disease	None vs. positive biopsy result	1.7
Breast density (as measured by mammography)	0% vs. ≥75%	1.8-6.0
Hyperplasia with atypia	None vs. positive biopsy result	3.7
Multiple relatives, not first degree, with breast cancer		
One first-degree relative with breast cancer (mother or sister)	None vs. yes	2.6
Two or more first-degree relatives	Increased risk if the cancers are premenopausal	
Deleterious *BRCA1/BRCA2* genes	Negative vs. positive	2.0-7.0
Mantle radiation for treatment of malignancy	Very high risk, which increases with age	

*Summary relative risk.
From Gershenson DM et al: *Comprehensive gynecology,* ed 8, Philadelphia, 2022, Elsevier.

TABLE 4 Factors Associated With a Decreased Risk for Breast Cancer

Demographic	Qualification	Relative Risk
Born and living outside Western countries		
Late menarche	After age 14	
Oophorectomy	Yes vs. no	0.3
Lactation	>16 mo vs. none	0.73
Parity	≥5 vs. 0	0.73
Postmenopausal body mass (kg/m²)	<22.9 vs. >30.7	0.63
Physical activity	Yes vs. no	0.70
Vitamin D	Low levels associated with risk	
Intake of vitamin D	Associated with decreased risk	
Olive oil and omega-3 fatty acids		
Low-fat diet	Results suggestive but not yet conclusive	
Aspirin	>1×/wk for ≥16 mo vs. no use	0.79

From Gershenson DM et al: *Comprehensive gynecology,* ed 8, Philadelphia, 2022, Elsevier.

dense breasts or inherited predisposition to breast cancer.[4] When MRI is used for screening, it should be used in addition to screening mammography. Although MRI is more sensitive than mammography, it may still miss some malignancies that a mammogram would detect. For routine MRI screening, the American Cancer Society has recommended a risk-adjusted model:
a. Annual screening beginning at age 30 yr for women at high lifetime risk for breast cancer development (approximately 20% to 25% or greater) (Box 2).
b. Discussion with physicians regarding the benefits and limitations of adding MRI screening for women at moderately increased lifetime risk (15% to 20%).
c. MRI is not recommended for women with a lifetime risk of developing breast cancer of less than 15%.
d. Table 8 summarizes guidelines for evaluation and treatment of nonpalpable ductal carcinoma in situ.

- Diagnosis:
  1. Positive aspiration cytology on a clinically and mammographically suspicious mass is highly accurate, but requires open biopsy confirmation.
  2. Stereotactic, ultrasound-guided core-needle biopsy procedures are accurate and have low complication rates. Indications for stereotactic core biopsy are summarized in Box 3. Box 4 describes contraindications to stereotactic core biopsy.
  3. Excisional surgical biopsy establishes diagnosis.

STAGING

Table 9 describes the pathologic staging of breast cancer.

IMAGING STUDIES

Mammograms (Fig. E2, Fig. E3): 30% to 50% of breast cancers are detected by screening mammograms as a spiculated mass, a mass with or without microcalcifications, or a cluster of microcalcifications. MRI is particularly useful in patients with breast implants and when there is a strong family history of breast cancer. MRI is better for assessing response to neoadjuvant chemotherapy and for identifying the primary tumor in patients presenting with axillary adenopathy.

- A trial comparing PET-CT to conventional staging (bone scan, CT of chest, abdomen and pelvis) in patients with clinical stage III or IIb ductal carcinoma who were being considered for curative-intent therapy revealed that patients were significantly more likely to be upstaged to stage IV (23% vs 11%) when using PET-CT, indicating that PET-CT is more likely to identify distant disease than conventional imaging.[1]

(Rx) TREATMENT

NONPHARMACOLOGIC THERAPY

- These approaches include various types of surgical resection and reconstruction (Box 5) as well as adjuvant radiotherapy.
- Early breast cancer: The primary therapy is usually surgical with a choice between modified radical mastectomy and breast-conserving treatments, and axillary staging with sentinel node biopsy or axillary dissection.
  1. Breast-conserving surgery removes the malignancy with a surrounding rim of grossly normal breast parenchyma. This procedure is depicted in Fig. E4, which shows the completed lumpectomy and skin incision for the axillary component of the procedure. The breast specimen that is removed is oriented and its edges are inked before sectioning. Specimen radiography should be performed for all nonpalpable lesions or if there are microcalcifications associated with the palpable tumor. If a margin appears to be close or is positive histologically on intraoperative assessment, re-excision to achieve a clear margin is required. Orientation of the surgical specimen

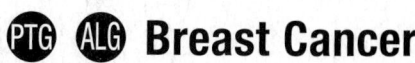

TABLE 5 Known Genetic Mutations in Breast Cancer and Their Management

Genetic Mutation	Breast Cancer Risk	Management
ATM	Increased by 15%-40%	Annual mammography starting at age 40 with consideration for breast tomosynthesis/magnetic resonance imaging (MRI)
BARD1	Limited evidence for increased risk but stronger for triple-negative breast cancer	Annual mammography starting at age 40 with consideration for breast tomosynthesis/MRI
BRCA1 BRCA2	Both carry increased absolute risk greater than 60%	Breast awareness starting at age 18 Clinical breast examination every 6-12 mo starting at age 25 yr Breast screening: Age 25-29 yr: Annual breast MRI screening with contrast or mammogram with consideration of tomosynthesis, only if MRI is unavailable or individualized based on family history if a breast cancer diagnosis before age 30 is present Age 30-75 yr: Annual mammogram with consideration of tomosynthesis and breast MRI screening with contrast Age >75 yr: Management should be individualized Consider risk-reducing mastectomy
BRIP1	Potential increase in risk	Management based on family history
CDH1	Increased absolute risk 41%-60%	Annual mammogram with consideration of tomosynthesis or breast MRI with contrast starting at age 30
CHECK2	Increased absolute risk 15%-40%	Annual mammography starting at age 40 with consideration for breast tomosynthesis/MRI
MSH2 MLH1 MSH6 PMS2 EPCAM	Limited evidence of increased risk, absolute risk is <15%	Management based on family history
NBN	Increased risk of breast cancer with variant 657del5	Management based on family history
NF1	Increased absolute risk 15%-40%	Annual mammography starting at age 30 with consideration for breast tomosynthesis/MRI
PALB2	Increased absolute risk 41%-60%	Annual mammography starting at age 30 with consideration for breast tomosynthesis/MRI Consider risk-reducing mastectomy
PTEN	Increased absolute risk 40%-60%	Breast awareness starting at age 18 Clinical breast examination every 6-12 mo starting at age 25 yr (or 5-10 yr before earliest known breast cancer in the family) Breast screening: Age 25-29 yr: Annual breast MRI screening with contrast or mammogram with consideration of tomosynthesis, only if MRI is unavailable or individualized based on family history if a breast cancer diagnosis before age 30 is present Age 30-75 yr: Annual mammogram with consideration of tomosynthesis and breast MRI screening with contrast Age >75 yr: Management should be individualized Consider risk-reducing mastectomy
RAD51C	Increased absolute risk 15%-40%	Management based on family history
RAD51D	Increased absolute risk 15%-40%	Management based on family history
STK11	Increased absolute risk 40%-60%	Annual mammography alternating with breast MRI every 6 mo starting at age 30 and clinical breast examination every 6 mo
TP53	Increased absolute risk >60%	Breast awareness starting at age 18 Clinical breast examination every 6-12 mo starting at age 20 yr Breast screening: Age 20-29 yr: Annual breast MRI screening with contrast or mammogram with consideration of tomosynthesis, only if MRI is unavailable or individualized based on family history if a breast cancer diagnosis before age 30 is present Age 30-75 yr: Annual mammogram with consideration of tomosynthesis and breast MRI screening with contrast Age >75 yr: Management should be individualized Consider risk-reducing mastectomy

From Gershenson DM et al: *Comprehensive gynecology*, ed 8, Philadelphia, 2022, Elsevier.

TABLE 6 Major Inherited Gene Mutation Syndromes Associated With Breast Cancer

Syndrome	Gene	Incidence	Lifetime Breast Cancer Risk	Associated Cancer Risks
BRCA1	BRCA1	1/500-1/1000	85%	Ovary and pancreas
BRCA2	BRCA2	Unclear	85%	Ovary and pancreas
Cowden	PTEN	1/100,000-1/200,000	50%	Thyroid and endometrium
Li-Fraumeni	TP53	1/20,000	90%	Sarcoma, brain, and leukemia

Other syndromes, including Peutz-Jeghers syndrome, ataxia telangiectasia, *CHEK2* gene mutation, and Fanconi syndrome, have much smaller lifetime risks with poorer penetrance.
From Gershenson DM et al: *Comprehensive gynecology*, ed 8, Philadelphia, 2022, Elsevier.

Diseases and Disorders

B

I

TABLE 7 American Board of Pathology Histologic Classification of Benign Disease

Histopathologic Findings	Approximate Relative Risk
Nonproliferative	No added risk
Cysts	
Duct ectasia	
Calcification	
Fibroadenoma	
Milk ductal epithelial hyperplasia	
Sclerosing adenosis	No added risk
Papillomatosis	Slight added risk
Radial scars	
Complex sclerosing lesions	?
Moderate florid hyperplasia	1.5:1-2:1
Atypical hyperplasia (ductal and lobular)	4:1
Extensive ductal involvement of atypical hyperplasia	7:1
Lobular carcinoma in situ	10:1
Ductal carcinoma in situ	10:1

From Niederhuber JE: *Abeloff's clinical oncology,* ed 6, Philadelphia, 2020, Elsevier.

BOX 1 Transverse Rectus Abdominis Muscle Flap Reconstruction

Indications
   Breasts of all sizes
   Breast ptosis
Relative contraindications
   Smoking
   Abdominal liposuction
   Previous abdominal surgery
   Pulmonary disease
   Obesity
Contraindications
   Previous abdominoplasty
   Patient unable to tolerate 4- to 6-wk recovery period
   Patient unable to tolerate longer procedure

From Townsend CM et al: *Sabiston textbook of surgery,* ed 21, St Louis, 2022, Elsevier.

allows focal re-excision of involved margins and improves the cosmetic result by reducing the amount of normal breast parenchyma that is excised.
2. Table 10 compares ductal versus lobular carcinoma in situ. Adjuvant treatment guidelines for patients with early-stage invasive breast cancer are described in Table 11.
3. Among patients with limited sentinel lymph nodes (SLN) who are treated with breast conservation and systemic therapy, survival with sentinel lymph node dissection (SLND) is not inferior to axillary lymph node dissection (ALND).[6]
4. DCIS: Local breast-conserving therapy (lumpectomy plus radiation therapy) or mastectomy followed by endocrine therapy in estrogen receptor-positive cases.

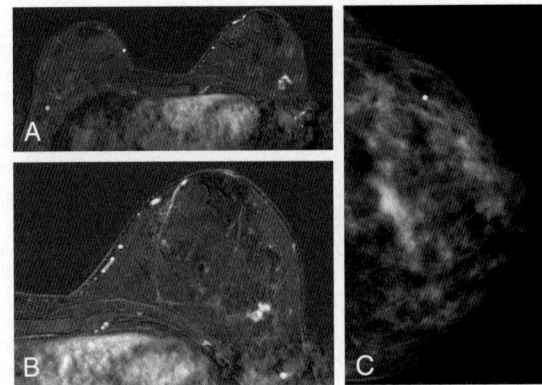

FIG. 1 A 42-yr-old woman with *BRCA2* mutation. Magnetic resonance imaging (MRI) screening showed a 1.2-cm invasive ductal cancer in the lower outer left breast seen only on MRI **(A and B)** and subsequently on second-look ultrasound. **C,** The mammogram showed only dense breast tissue. (From Cameron JL, Cameron AM: *Current surgical therapy,* ed 12, Philadelphia, 2017, Elsevier.)

BOX 2 American Cancer Society MRI Breast Cancer Screening Recommendations

Women at High Lifetime Risk (Risk Criteria for Breast Magnetic Resonance Imaging Screening. ≈20%-25% or Greater) of Breast Cancer
Known *BRCA1* or *BRCA2* gene mutation
First-degree relative with *BRCA1* or *BRCA2* gene mutation, but have not had genetic testing themselves
Lifetime risk of breast cancer of ≈20%-25% or greater
Radiation therapy to the chest between the ages of 10 and 30
Li-Fraumeni syndrome or Cowden syndrome or a first-degree relative with one of these syndromes
Women at Moderately Increased (15%-20%) Lifetime Risk
Lifetime risk of breast cancer of 15%-20% according to risk assessment tools based mainly on family history
Personal history of breast cancer, ductal carcinoma in situ, lobular carcinoma in situ, atypical ductal hyperplasia, or atypical lobular hyperplasia
Extremely dense breasts or unevenly dense breasts when viewed by mammograms

From Townsend CM et al: *Sabiston textbook of surgery,* ed 21, St Louis, 2022, Elsevier.

TABLE 8 Guidelines for Evaluation and Treatment of Nonpalpable Ductal Carcinoma In Situ

1. Careful multiview mammography with or without ultrasound and including magnification views
  • Document extent of disease
  • Identify other areas of microcalcification
2. Suspicious microcalcifications and densities cleared with needle localization biopsy
3. Specimen radiography with magnification techniques
4. Radiograph-directed histopathologic evaluation with orientation of specimen by surgeon using multicolored inked margins
5. Complete pathologic description to include:
  • Type of DCIS and size of tumor
  • Relation to microcalcifications
  • Distance of lesion from inked margins
  • Presence of multifocality
  • Presence or risk of microinvasion
6. Repeat mammography with magnification to confirm successful clearing of suspicious areas
7. Repeat breast excision if:
  • Residual microcalcifications are found
  • Margins are unacceptable

DCIS, Ductal carcinoma in situ.
From Niederhuber JE: *Abeloff's clinical oncology,* ed 6, Philadelphia, 2020, Elsevier.

• Invasive breast cancer: Mastectomy or lumpectomy, along with sentinel lymph node evaluation followed by radiation therapy for large tumors.
  1. Invasive breast cancer may require systemic therapy options including endocrine therapy and/or chemotherapy. Current guidelines use stage and biologic characteristics in the development of treatment recommendations to guide decisions regarding systemic therapy for breast cancer (Table 12). Endocrine therapy is

BOX 3   Indications for Stereotactic Core Biopsy

- Certain probably benign lesions, BI-RADS 3, depending on clinical suspicion, patient or physician preference, or when short-term follow-up is not practical
- Lesions suspicious, BI-RADS 4
- Lesions highly suspicious, BI-RADS 5
- New suspicious microcalcifications, developing asymmetries, or architectural distortions
- Nonpalpable asymmetry, focal asymmetry, or solid mass on mammogram not seen on ultrasound
- Mammographic lesions corresponding to suspicious areas of enhancement on MRI

BOX 4   Contraindications to Stereotactic Core Biopsy

- Patient unable to lie prone or cooperate
- Patient's weight
- Lesion location near nipple, too superficial to skin, or too posterior to chest wall
- Lesion mammographically occult
- Patient has severe kyphosis or movement disorders
- Lack of breast tissue thickness for adequate compression

recommended alone or after chemotherapy in patients with hormone-receptor positive tumors. Breast cancer intrinsic subtypes are summarized in Table 13. Treatment according to breast cancer subtypes is described in Table 14. Adjuvant hormone therapy with antiestrogen drugs reduces disease recurrence and mortality in women with breast cancer. Aromatase inhibitors (anastrozole, letrozole, exemestane, fulvestrant) decrease the agonist effect of estrogen by inhibiting estrogen synthesis and have become preferred first-line hormonal treatment agents over the selective estrogen receptor modulator tamoxifen.

2. The CDK inhibitor abemaciclib plus antiestrogen therapy is approved as adjuvant treatment for high-risk patients with hormone receptor–positive, HER2-negative, node-positive early breast cancer.[7]

3. The adjuvant use of the PARP inhibitor olaparib plus endocrine therapy improves disease-free survival in patients with germline *BRCA1/BRAC2* mutations.[8]

4. Standard *adjuvant chemotherapy* options used in the U.S. include AC (cyclophosphamide plus doxorubicin), AC-T (doxorubicin and cyclophosphamide followed by a taxane), and TC (docetaxel and cyclophosphamide) regimens. In patients with *HER2*-expressing cancers, standard adjuvant regimens also include the addition of trastuzumab and pertuzumab for 1-yr duration. Fig. E5 illustrates considerations for adjuvant chemotherapy in breast cancer.

5. *Neoadjuvant chemotherapy* (same regimens as used in the adjuvant setting) results in pathologic complete responses in significant number of cases, causes downstaging, provides an assessment of chemosensitivity, and provides no deleterious effect on survival.

- Early-stage triple-negative breast cancer: The PD-1 inhibitor pembrolizumab in combination with chemotherapy is used as neoadjuvant treatment and then continued as an adjuvant treatment after surgical resection.

1. The benefit of adjuvant chemotherapy or hormone therapy can be assessed by commercially available *multigene assays* (OncotypeDx, Mammaprint), which help in determining prognostic and predictive benefit associated with the use of both hormonal therapy and chemotherapy. The TAILORx trial supported the routine use of multigene assays to identify intermediate-risk score patients in which chemotherapy can be safely omitted.[9] Among premenopausal women with one to three positive lymph nodes and a recurrence score of 25 or lower based on the 21-gene breast cancer assay, those who received chemoendocrine therapy had longer invasive disease-free survival and distant relapse-free survival than those who received endocrine-only therapy, whereas postmenopausal women did not have any benefit from adjuvant chemotherapy.

2. *Metastatic breast cancer* is treated based on the extent of bone-only or visceral disease sites as well as the rate of symptomatic progression. All management of metastatic breast cancer is palliative. Table 15 summarizes median survival of patients with metastatic breast cancer by location of metastases.

3. Typically, bone-only metastatic disease is treated with upfront, sequential hormonal therapy with tamoxifen or aromatase inhibitors. The combination of CDK4/CDK6 inhibitors (palbociclib, ribociclib, abemaciclib) with aromatase inhibitors is typically used as up-front therapy and improves overall survival. Second-line therapy with aromatase inhibitor plus mTOR inhibitor everolimus is used.

4. In the case of *PIK3CA*-mutated, hormone-receptor-positive, *HER2*-negative advanced breast cancer who had received endocrine therapy previously, treatment with the combination of alpelisib plus fulvestrant prolonged progression-free survival, leading to the approval of this combination approach.[10] Commonly used cytotoxic chemotherapy and anti-*HER2* therapy drugs in metastatic breast cancer are summarized in Table 16.

5. Patients with progressive bone disease or those with visceral disease are treated with typically single-agent chemotherapy and occasionally with combination chemotherapy regimens. The chemotherapy agents are the same as those used in early stages of disease. Sequential chemotherapy with different classes of chemotherapy agents are usually used to provide palliation with improvement in survival and symptoms.

6. Patients whose tumors have germline *BRCA1/2* mutations can be treated with the PARP inhibitors olaparib or talazoparib.

7. Patients with triple-negative breast cancer whose tumors express the program death ligand-1 receptor derive a survival benefit with the use of the combination of immune checkpoint inhibitor pembrolizumab plus chemotherapy.[11]

8. Sacituzumab govitecan is an antibody–drug conjugate targeting the human trophoblast cell-surface antigen 2 (Trop-2), which is expressed in most breast cancers. Progression-free and overall survival were significantly longer with sacituzumab govitecan than with single-agent chemotherapy among relapsed triple-negative breast cancer patients.[12]

- *HER2*/neu-positive metastatic breast cancer:

1. The combination of monoclonal antibodies pertuzumab and trastuzumab plus taxane chemotherapy significantly improves the median overall survival to >5 yr.[13]

2. The antibody-drug conjugates TDM-1 and trastuzumab dexrutecan improve survival in this group of patients.[12]

3. For HER-2 low-expressing metastatic breast cancer, trastuzumab dexrutecan improves overall survival in comparison to chemotherapy.

4. The chimeric antibody margetuximab, which incorporates an engineered Fc region to increase immune activation, improves progression-free survival when used with chemotherapy in patients previously treated with two or more prior anti-*HER2*/neu therapies.

5. Oral *HER2*-directed inhibitors such as neratinib and tucatinib are active in previously treated patients with metastatic disease.

- The FDA has approved elacestrant, an oral estrogen receptor antagonist for treatment of *ER*-positive, *HER2*-negative, *ESR1*-mutated advanced or metastatic breast cancer in postmenopausal women or men who had disease progression following endocrine therapy.

TABLE 9 Pathologic Staging of Breast Cancer

T_X	**Primary Tumor Cannot Be Assessed**
T_0	No evidence of primary tumor
T_{is}	Carcinoma in situ
T_{is} (DCIS)	Ductal carcinoma in situ
T_{is} (LCIS)	Lobular carcinoma in situ
T_{is} (Paget)	Paget disease of the nipple NOT associated with invasive carcinoma and/or carcinoma in situ (DCIS and/or LCIS) in the underlying breast parenchyma. Carcinomas in the breast parenchyma associated with Paget disease are categorized based on the size and characteristics of the parenchymal disease, although the presence of Paget disease should still be noted
T_1	Tumor ≤20 mm in greatest dimension
T_{1mi}	Tumor ≤1 mm in greatest dimension
T_{1a}	Tumor >1 mm but ≤5 mm in greatest dimension
T_{1b}	Tumor >5 mm but ≤10 mm in greatest dimension
T_{1c}	Tumor >10 mm but ≤20 mm in greatest dimension
T_2	Tumor >20 mm but ≤50 mm in greatest dimension
T_3	Tumor >50 mm in greatest dimension
T_4	Tumor of any size with direct extension to the chest wall and/or to the skin (ulceration or skin nodules)
T_{4a}	Extension to chest wall, not including only pectoralis muscle adherence/invasion
T_{4b}	Ulceration and/or ipsilateral satellite nodules and/or edema (including peau d'orange) of the skin, which do not meet the criteria for inflammatory carcinoma
T_{4c}	Both T_{4a} and T_{4b}
T_{4d}	Inflammatory carcinoma
N_X	Regional lymph nodes cannot be assessed (e.g., previously removed)
N_0	No regional lymph node metastasis
N_1	Metastasis to movable ipsilateral level I, II axillary lymph node(s)
N_2	Metastases in ipsilateral level I, II axillary lymph nodes that are clinically fixed or matted or in clinically detected ipsilateral internal mammary nodes in the *absence* of clinically evident axillary lymph node metastasis
N_{2a}	Metastases in ipsilateral level I, II axillary lymph nodes fixed to one another (matted) or to other structures
N_{2b}	Metastases only in clinically detected ipsilateral internal mammary nodes and in the *absence* of clinically evident level I, II axillary lymph node metastases
N_3	Metastases in ipsilateral infraclavicular (level III axillary) lymph node(s), with or without level I, II axillary node involvement, or in clinically detected ipsilateral internal mammary lymph node(s) and in the *presence* of clinically evident level I, II axillary lymph node metastasis; or metastasis in ipsilateral supraclavicular lymph node(s), with or without axillary or internal mammary lymph node involvement
N_{3a}	Metastasis in ipsilateral infraclavicular lymph node(s)
N_{3b}	Metastasis in ipsilateral internal mammary lymph node(s) and axillary lymph node(s)
N_{3c}	Metastasis in ipsilateral supraclavicular lymph node(s)
M_0	No clinical or radiographic evidence of distant metastasis
$cM_{0(i+)}$	No clinical or radiographic evidence of distant metastases, but deposits of molecularly or microscopically detected tumor cells in circulating blood, bone marrow, or other nonregional nodal tissue that are no larger than 0.2 mm in a patient without symptoms or signs of metastases
M_1	Distant detectable metastases as determined by classic clinical and radiographic means and/or histologically proven >0.2 mm
G_X	Grade cannot be assessed
G_1	Low combined histologic grade (favorable)
G_2	Intermediate combined histologic grade (moderately favorable)
G_3	High combined histologic grade (unfavorable)

Stage Groupings in Breast Cancer

Stage	*T*	*N*	*M*
0	T_{is}	N_0	M_0
I_A	T_1	N_0	M_0
I_B	T_0-T_1	N_{1mi}	M_0
II_A	T_0-T_1	N_1	M_0
	T_2	N_0	M_0
II_B	T_2	N_1	M_0
	T_3	N_0	M_0
III_A	T_0-T_2	N_2	M_0
	T_3	N_1-N_2	M_0
III_B	T_4	N_0-N_2	M_0
III_C	Any T	N_3	M_0
IV	Any T	Any N	M_1

From Goldman L, Schafer AI: *Goldman's Cecil medicine,* ed 24, Philadelphia, 2012, Saunders; Amin MB, Edge SB, Greene FL, et al: *AJCC Cancer Staging Manual,* 8th ed. New York, 2018, Springer.

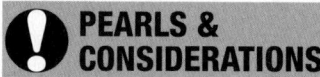

B

Diseases
and Disorders

I

BOX 5 Options for Breast Reconstruction

Autogenous
Abdominal-based flaps
Transverse rectus abdominis muscle (TRAM)
Single pedicle
Double pedicle
Free flap
Deep inferior epigastric perforator flap*

Latissimus dorsi musculocutaneous flap
Gluteal flap*
   Superiorly based
   Inferiorly based
Rubens flap*
Thoracoepigastric flap
Lateral thigh flap*
Breast-splitting procedure

Alloplastic
Silicone gel implant
Silicone implant with saline fill
Smooth wall
Textured wall
Round
Anatomic shaped

Combination procedures
Latissimus dorsi flap with implant
TRAM flap with implant

From Townsend CM et al: *Sabiston textbook of surgery,* ed 21, St Louis, 2022, Elsevier.

TABLE 10 Carcinoma In Situ: Lobular Versus Ductal

Feature	Lobular Carcinoma In Situ	Ductal Carcinoma In Situ
Age	Younger	Older
Palpable mass	No	Uncommon
Mammographic appearance	Not detected on mammography	Microcalcifications, mass
Immunophenotype	E-cadherin negative	E-cadherin positive
Usual manifestation	Incidental finding on breast biopsy	Microcalcifications on mammography or breast mass
Bilateral involvement	Common	Uncertain
Risk and site of subsequent breast cancer	25% risk for invasive breast cancer in either breast over remaining lifespan	At site of initial lesion; 0.5% risk/yr of invasive breast cancer in opposite breast
Prevention	Consider tamoxifen or raloxifene	Consider tamoxifen or raloxifene if estrogen-receptor positive
Treatment	Yearly mammography and breast examination	Lumpectomy ± radiation; mastectomy for large or multifocal lesions

From Goldman L, Schafer AI: *Goldman's Cecil medicine,* ed 24, Philadelphia, 2012, Saunders.

CHRONIC Rx

Follow-up after treatment of early breast cancer stages includes:

- Patient instruction in monthly breast self-examination.
- Regular clinical evaluations as delineated by medical oncologist or surgeon.
- Annual mammograms and breast MRI as indicated.
- Laboratory tests as indicated.
- Tumor markers and CT scans for surveillance are *not* recommended.
- Adjuvant therapy: In premenopausal women with hormone receptor–positive early breast cancer, use of aromatase inhibitor exemestane plus ovarian suppression, compared with tamoxifen plus ovarian suppression, significantly reduced recurrence. In postmenopausal women with hormone receptor–positive breast cancer, aromatase inhibitor therapy improves survival outcomes compared with tamoxifen. Women who take tamoxifen for 10 yr lower their recurrence risk by 25% and their dying of breast cancer risk by 27% compared with those who took it for just 5 yr. In postmenopausal women with hormone-receptor positive breast cancer, recent trial data showed that in women treated with 5 yr of adjuvant endocrine therapy, extending hormone therapy by 5 yr provided no benefit over a 2-yr extension but was associated with more bone fractures.
- Retrospective analyses suggest that occult lymph-node metastases are an important prognostic factor for disease recurrence or survival; however, recent data indicate that the magnitude of the difference in outcome at 5 yr is small (1.2 percentage points) and do not favor additional evaluation of initially negative sentinel nodes.
- Adding zoledronic acid to adjuvant endocrine therapy improves disease-free survival in premenopausal patients with estrogen-responsive early breast cancer.

REFERRAL

Referral to a multidisciplinary team consisting of a breast surgeon, reconstructive surgeon, medical oncologist, and radiation oncologist is necessary as soon as breast cancer is suspected.

⚠ PEARLS & CONSIDERATIONS

BREAST CANCER IN PREGNANCY AND LACTATION

- Frequency in women 40 yr or younger reported to be 15%
- May carry worse prognosis because disease discovery delayed by engorged and nodular breast changes and/or because disease progression more rapid in pregnancy
- Survival is similar to nonpregnant early-stage patients in same age group
- Expedient workup recommended, including mammography and sonography
- Choice of mastectomy or lumpectomy with axillary dissection for treatment
- Adjuvant chemotherapy and radiotherapy delayed until third trimester or after delivery
- Other contraindications to radiation are summarized in Box 6

DUCTAL CARCINOMA IN SITU (DCIS, INTRADUCTAL CARCINOMA) (SEE TABLE 10)

- Discovered by mammogram as cluster of microcalcifications and/or density
- Presents less often as a palpable mass or nipple discharge
- With widespread mammogram screening, DCIS accounts for 15% to 20% of all breast cancers
- Treated with lumpectomy with cure rates 98% to 99%
- Higher-risk cases require breast radiation and adjuvant hormone therapy
- Mastectomy is required with multifocal and/or high-grade DCIS

INFLAMMATORY CARCINOMA

- Rare, rapidly progressive, and often lethal form of breast cancer
- Presents as erythematous and edematous breast resembling mastitis
- Biopsy required, including that of the skin
- Treatment with upfront combination chemotherapy followed by surgery and radiotherapy

TABLE 11 Adjuvant Treatment Guidelines for Patients With Early-Stage Invasive Breast Cancer

Patient Group	Treatment
Hormone Receptor-Positive and HER2 Positive Breast Cancer	
<0.5 cm	Consider adjuvant endocrine therapy
0.6-1 cm	Adjuvant endocrine therapy
	Consider adjuvant chemotherapy and trastuzumab
>1 cm	Adjuvant endocrine therapy
	Adjuvant chemotherapy and trastuzumab
Node positive	Adjuvant endocrine therapy
	Adjuvant chemotherapy with pertuzumab and trastuzumab
Hormone Receptor-Positive and HER2 Negative Breast Cancer	
<0.5 cm	No adjuvant therapy
>0.5 cm	Adjuvant hormonal therapy
	Consider adjuvant chemotherapy based on 21-gene recurrence score
Node-positive	Adjuvant hormonal therapy + adjuvant chemotherapy
Hormone Receptor-Negative and HER2 Positive Breast Cancer	
<0.5 cm	Consider adjuvant chemotherapy and trastuzumab
0.6-1 cm	Consider adjuvant chemotherapy and trastuzumab
>1 cm	Adjuvant chemotherapy and trastuzumab
Node positive	Adjuvant endocrine therapy
	Adjuvant chemotherapy with pertuzumab and trastuzumab
Hormone Receptor-Negative and HER2 Negative Breast Cancer	
≤0.5 cm	No adjuvant therapy
0.6-1.0 cm	Consider adjuvant chemotherapy
>1 cm or node positive	Adjuvant chemotherapy

HER2, Human epidermal growth factor receptor 2.
Modified from National Comprehensive Cancer Network Guidelines. Available at www.nccn.org.

TABLE 12 Decision-Making for Systemic Therapy

Stage	Systemic Therapy	Comments
I (<1 cm)		
Hormone receptor–positive	Endocrine therapy ± chemotherapy	Consider genomic testing
Hormone receptor–negative	Consider chemotherapy	
HER-2–positive	Strongly consider trastuzumab and chemotherapy	
I (>1 cm)		
Hormone receptor–positive	Endocrine therapy ± chemotherapy	Consider genomic testing
Hormone receptor–negative	Chemotherapy	
HER-2–positive	Trastuzumab and chemotherapy	
II (Lymph Node–Negative)		
Hormone receptor–positive	Endocrine therapy ± chemotherapy	Consider genomic testing
Hormone receptor–negative	Chemotherapy	
HER-2–positive	Trastuzumab and chemotherapy	
II (Lymph Node–Positive), III		
Hormone receptor–positive	Chemotherapy + endocrine therapy	Endocrine therapy should be recommended for all patients
Hormone receptor–negative	Chemotherapy	Decision-making for chemotherapy may be influenced by results from ongoing clinical trials
HER-2–positive	Trastuzumab and chemotherapy	Consider neoadjuvant chemotherapy with dual HER-2–targeted therapy

HER-2, Human epidermal growth factor receptor 2.
From Townsend CM et al: *Sabiston textbook of surgery,* ed 21, St Louis, 2022, Elsevier.

- Prognosis is improved with 5-yr disease-free survival approaching 50% (Fig. E6)

COMMENTS

- The U.S. Preventive Services Task Force (USPSTF) now recommends against automatic "routine" screening of younger women (age range 40 to 49). The task force recommends biennial screening mammography for all middle-aged women (age range 50 to 74). It also states that current evidence is insufficient to assess the benefits and harms of screening mammography in older women (aged 75 and older). The task force also discourages women from performing breast self-examination. Several other U.S. organizations, such as the American Congress of Obstetricians and Gynecologists, however, still recommend annual screening beginning at age 40 yr. Breast cancer screening recommendations by organization are summarized in Table 17.
- The American Cancer Society screening guidelines are summarized in the following:[14]
  1. Women should continue screening mammography as long as their overall health is good and they have a life expectancy of 10 yr or longer. (Qualified recommendation)
  2. Women with an *average risk* of breast cancer should undergo regular screening mammography as below:
     a. Women should have the opportunity to begin annual screening between the ages of 40 and 44 yr. (Qualified recommendation)
     b. Women aged 45 to 54 yr should be screened annually. (Qualified recommendation)
     c. Women 55 yr and older should transition to biennial screening or continue screening annually (qualified recommendation).
- Women who are at *high risk* for breast cancer based on certain factors should get an MRI and a mammogram every year, typically starting at age 30 yr. This includes women who:
  1. Have a lifetime risk of breast cancer of about 20% to 25% or greater, according to risk assessment tools that are based mainly on family history.
  2. Have a known *BRCA1* or *BRCA2* gene mutation (based on genetic testing).
  3. Have a first-degree relative (parent, brother, sister, or child) with a *BRCA1* or *BRCA2* gene mutation and have not had genetic testing themselves.
  4. Had radiation therapy to the chest between the ages of 10 and 30 yr.
  5. Have Li-Fraumeni syndrome, Cowden syndrome, or Bannayan-Riley-Ruvalcaba syndrome, or have first-degree relatives with one of these syndromes.
- Physicians should be familiar with the risks and benefits of these various competing recommendations in order to better counsel patients.

TABLE 13 Breast Cancer Intrinsic Subtypes

Subtype	Characteristics	Markers
Luminal A	Low grade. High ER ~40% of all breast cancer Good prognosis	ER+, PR+, HER2–Low Ki-67 (<14%)
Luminal B	Higher grade. Lower ER ~20% of all breast cancer Poorer prognosis than luminal A	ER+, PR+/–, HER2+/–High Ki-67 (>14%)
HER2-enriched	High grade. Often node positive P53 mutations ~10%-15% of all breast cancer	ER–, PR–, HER2+
Basal-like	High proliferation. BRCA dysfunction ~15%-20% of all breast cancer Poor prognosis	ER–, PR–, HER2–CK5/6 Or EGFR+

CK, Cytokeratin; EGFR, epidermal growth factor receptor; ER, estrogen receptor; HER2, human epidermal growth factor receptor 2; PR, progesterone receptor.
From Cameron JL, Cameron AM: Current surgical therapy, ed 12, Philadelphia, 2017, Elsevier.

TABLE 14 Treatment According to Breast Cancer Subtype

Subtype	Treatment Response and Prognosis
Luminal A	Respond to endocrine therapy • Premenopausal: SERMs (tamoxifen) • Postmenopausal: AIs (exemestane, anastrozole, letrozole)
Luminal B	Response to endocrine therapy lower. Response to chemotherapy greater than luminal A
HER2-enriched	Respond to anti-HER2 agents (trastuzumab, pertuzumab, lapatinib)
Basal-like	No response to endocrine therapy or anti-HER2 agents. Chemotherapy only treatment outside of a clinical trial

AIs, Aromatase inhibitors; HER2, human epidermal growth factor receptor 2; SERMs, selective estrogen receptor modulators.
From Cameron JL, Cameron AM: Current surgical therapy, ed 12, Philadelphia, 2017, Elsevier.

TABLE 16 Commonly Used Cytotoxic Chemotherapy and Anti-HER2 Therapy Drugs in Metastatic Breast Cancer

Cytotoxic Chemotherapy

Albumin-bound paclitaxel
Capecitabine
Cisplatin
Carboplatin
Docetaxel
Doxorubicin
Epirubicin
Eribulin
Gemcitabine
Ixabepilone
Vinorelbine

Anti-HER2 Therapy

Ado-trastuzumab emtansine
Lapatinib
Pertuzumab
Trastuzumab

HER2, Human epidermal growth factor receptor 2.
From Niederhuber JE: Abeloff's clinical oncology, ed 6, Philadelphia, 2020, Elsevier.

TABLE 15 Median Survival in Months of Patients With Metastatic Breast Cancer by Location of Metastases

Location	Survival (Months)
Liver (>30% replacement)	3
Lung (lymphangitic)	3
Lung (nodular)	22
Skin	27
Bones	36+

From Townsend CM et al: Sabiston textbook of surgery, ed 21, St Louis, 2022, Elsevier.

BOX 6 Contraindications to Radiation

Absolute
Pregnancy

Relative
Systemic scleroderma
Active systemic lupus erythematosus
Prior radiation to breast or chest wall
Severe pulmonary disease
Severe cardiac disease (if tumor is left sided)
Inability to lie supine
Inability to abduct arm on affected side
p53 mutation

From Townsend CM et al: Sabiston textbook of surgery, ed 21, St Louis, 2022, Elsevier.

- Breast radiologic evaluation, evaluation of nipple discharge, and evaluation of palpable mass are described in Section III.
- Exposure of the heart to ionizing radiation during breast cancer radiotherapy increases risk of ischemic heart disease. The increased rate of ischemic heart disease begins within a few years of exposure and continues for at least 20 yr. The increase is proportional to the mean radiation dose to the heart.

RISK REDUCTION STRATEGIES
- Prophylactic bilateral mastectomy reduces the risk for invasive breast cancer by >90%.
- Counseling points for women with average risk interested in contralateral prophylactic mastectomy (CPM) are summarized in Box 7.
- Selective estrogen receptor modulators (SERM) reduce the incidence of hormone receptor-positive invasive breast cancer by 50%.
- Ovarian failure is a common toxic effect of chemotherapy. Administration of the gonadotropin-releasing hormone (GnRH) agonist goserelin appears to protect against ovarian failure, reducing the risk of early menopause and improving prospects for fertility.

REFERENCES
Available at eBooks.Health.Elsevier.com.

RELATED CONTENT
Breast Cancer (Patient Information)
Breast Cancer: For Men (Patient Information)
Breast Abscess (Related Key Topic)
Fibrocystic Breast Disease (Related Key Topic)

AUTHOR: **BHARTI RATHORE, MD**

B

Diseases and Disorders

I

TABLE 17 Breast Cancer Screening Recommendations by Organization

Organization	When to Initiate Screening	Frequency of Screening	When to Stop Screening
American Academy of Family Physicians (AAFP)	Follow U.S. Preventive Services Task Force (USPSTF) recommendations	Follow USPSTF recommendations	Follow USPSTF recommendations
American Cancer Society (ACS)	Opportunity to begin screening at ages 40-44 Regular screening starting at age 45	Annually from age 45-54 Biennially starting at age 55 with opportunity to continue annually	Continue screening mammography as long as overall health is good, and life expectancy is 10 yr or longer
American College of Obstetricians and Gynecologists (ACOG)	Annual screening starting at age 40	Annually	Not specified
American College of Physicians (ACP)	Individualized for women ages 40-49 Regular screening starting at age 50	Biennially	Age 75 yr or older Women of any age with life expectancy <10 yr
American College of Radiology (ACR)	Annual screening starting at age 40	Annually	Should be considered as long as the patient is in good health and is willing to undergo additional testing if an abnormality is detected
National Comprehensive Cancer Network (NCCN)	Annual screening starting at age 40	Annually	Upper age limit is not yet established Consider comorbid conditions limiting life expectancy (e.g., ≤10 yr) and whether therapeutic interventions are planned
U.S. Preventive Services Task Force (USPSTF)	Individualized for women ages 40-49 Regular screening beginning at age 50	Biennially	Insufficient evidence to recommend for or against screening at age 75 or older

From Niederhuber JE: *Abeloff's clinical oncology,* ed 6, Philadelphia, 2020, Elsevier.

BOX 7 Counseling Points for Women With Average Risk Interested in Contralateral Prophylactic Mastectomy (CPM)

- There is a low annual contralateral breast cancer risk in women with average risk factors.
- Risk of contralateral breast cancer is decreasing with use of adjuvant therapy.
- Removing the contralateral breast does not decrease the risk for developing distant metastases.
- Breast cancer does not commonly metastasize from one breast to the other.
- CPM does not improve breast cancer–specific survival.
- CPM does not decrease local recurrence.
- Contralateral breast cancers tend to be at a lower stage than the initial primary cancer.
- CPM increases the surgical complication risk.
- Choice of CPM may influence reconstruction options.
- There are alternatives to CPM, including chemoprevention and surveillance.

From Cameron JL, Cameron AM: *Current surgical therapy,* ed 12, Philadelphia, 2017, Elsevier.

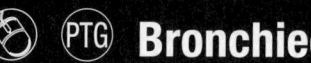
Diseases
and Disorders

I

BASIC INFORMATION

DEFINITION

Bronchiectasis is a chronic lung disease defined by permanent dilatation of bronchi and clinically marked by a syndrome of cough, sputum production, and recurrent exacerbations. Bronchiectasis disease is heterogenous in both etiology and natural history, but the common element is a vicious vortex that propagates disease due to inflammation, impaired mucociliary clearance, infection, and structural lung damage.[1] It can radiographically be divided into cylindric, varicose, and cystic subtypes, which often overlap and coexist, but may aid in diagnosis and overall prognosis.

ICD-10CM CODES
J47.0	Bronchiectasis with acute lower respiratory infection
J47.1	Bronchiectasis with (acute) exacerbation
J47.9	Bronchiectasis, uncomplicated
Q33.4	Congenital bronchiectasis

EPIDEMIOLOGY & DEMOGRAPHICS

- The incidence and prevalence of bronchiectasis are steadily rising globally.[2]
- In the U.S. and Europe, prevalence increases markedly with age, with peak incidence in those older than age 65, and is more common in women than in men.[3,4]
- The exact prevalence of bronchiectasis is unclear. In the U.S., the average annual prevalence was approximately 700 per 100,000 persons among Medicare beneficiaries between 2012 and 2014[5] and up to 566 per 100,000 persons in the United Kingdom around this time period.[6]
- There are multiple identified etiologies that can vary by geographic region, yet idiopathic continues to remain the most frequent diagnosis worldwide.[2]
- Table 1 summarizes conditions associated with the risk of bronchiectasis.

PHYSICAL FINDINGS & CLINICAL PRESENTATION

- Chronic cough, typically with expectoration of purulent sputum
- Frequent bronchitis or pneumonias requiring antibiotic treatment
- Generalized malaise and/or weight loss
- Fever and/or night sweats
- Hemoptysis
- Crackles, wheezing, or squeaks on lung exam
- Halitosis

ETIOLOGY

- Postinfectious (e.g., previous pneumonia, lung abscess, tuberculosis, nontuberculous mycobacterial infections, fungal infections, viral infections)
- Cystic fibrosis
- Ciliary dysfunction (primary ciliary dyskinesia, Kartagener syndrome)
- Chronic obstructive pulmonary diseases (e.g., chronic obstructive pulmonary disease [COPD], asthma)
- Impaired host defense (e.g., hypogammaglobulinemia, acquired immunodeficiency syndrome, chemotherapy)
- Localized airway obstruction (aspiration, congenital structural defects, foreign bodies, neoplasms)
- Inflammation (chronic gastroesophageal reflux disease [GERD], inflammatory pneumonitis, granulomatous lung disease, allergic aspergillosis)
- Congenital disorders such as tracheobronchomegaly (Mounier-Kuhn syndrome), cartilage deficiency (Williams-Campbell syndrome, Marfan syndrome), alpha-1 anti-trypsin deficiency
- Connective tissue and autoimmune diseases (Sjogren disease, ulcerative colitis, rheumatoid arthritis)
- Cellular pathophysiologic mechanism of bronchiectasis is illustrated in Fig. E1

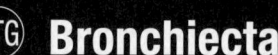 DIAGNOSIS

DIFFERENTIAL DIAGNOSIS

- Chronic bronchitis or chronic rhinosinusitis
- Chronic obstructive pulmonary disease

- Asthma
- Tuberculosis
- Interstitial fibrosis
- Chronic lung abscess
- Foreign body aspiration
- Cystic fibrosis
- Lung carcinoma
- Gastroesophageal reflux disease
- Diffuse panbronchiolitis
- Bronchiolitis obliterans

LABORATORY TESTS

- Pulmonary function tests with bronchodilators
- Sputum for Gram stain, culture and susceptibilities, and acid-fast bacteria
- Serum immunoglobulins (total immunoglobulin A [IgA], IgM, IgG and subclasses)
- Testing for allergic bronchopulmonary aspergillosis (serum IgE, precipitating IgG antibodies [precipitins] to *Aspergillus*, specific IgE antibodies to *Aspergillus*, *Aspergillus* skin test)
- CBC with differential (leukocytosis with left shift, anemia, eosinophilia)
- Alpha-1 antitrypsin level and phenotype
- Sweat test and/or CFTR genetic testing in patients with even low suspicion for cystic fibrosis
- Primary ciliary dyskinesia evaluation when suspected
- Antinuclear antibody (ANA), rheumatoid factor (RF) and anti–cytric citrullinated protein antibodies (CCP), anti–Sjogren syndrome antibodies (SSA/SSB) when driven by history or exam
- Serum anti-*Pseudomonas aeruginosa* (PA) IgG antibody testing is highly accurate to detect chronic PA colonization in bronchiectasis patients[7] and may be a marker of treatment response

IMAGING STUDIES

- Chest x-ray examination (Fig. 2 and Fig. E3) may be normal or have crowded lung markings, "tram-track" sign of dilated bronchi, or small cystic spaces at the base of the lungs.

TABLE 1 Conditions Associated with Bronchiectasis

Heritable Impaired Mucociliary Clearance	Inhalation	Postinfectious Conditions	Structural Abnormalities
Cystic fibrosis (classic or variant)	Aspiration	Childhood lower respiratory tract infections	Williams-Campbell syndrome
Primary ciliary dyskinesia	Gastroesophageal reflux	Protracted bacterial bronchitis	Mounier-Kuhn syndrome
Alpha1-antitrypsin deficiency	Toxic inhalation/thermal injury	Granulomatous infections	Marfan syndrome
		Necrotizing pneumonia	Sequestration
		Mycosis	Agenesis
			Hypoplasia

Idiopathic Inflammatory Disorders	Obstruction	Primary Immune Disorders	Miscellaneous
Sarcoidosis	Asthma	Humoral defects	Human immunodeficiency virus infection
Rheumatoid arthritis	Chronic obstructive pulmonary disease/emphysema	Cellular and/or mixed disorders	Yellow nail syndrome
Ankylosing spondylitis	Allergic bronchopulmonary aspergillosis	Neutrophil dysfunction	Radiation injury
Systemic lupus erythematosus	Foreign body	Other	
Sjogren syndrome	Tumor		
Inflammatory bowel disease	Extrinsic airway compression		
Relapsing polychondritis			

Adapted from Broaddus VC et al: *Murray & Nadel's textbook of respiratory medicine*, ed 7, Philadelphia, 2022, Elsevier.

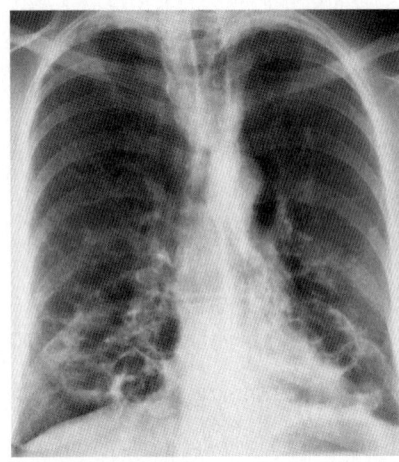

FIG. 2 Bronchiectasis. Multiple ring shadows, many containing air-fluid levels, are present throughout the lower zones of this patient with cystic bronchiectasis. (From Grant LA: *Grainger & Allison's diagnostic radiology essentials,* ed 2, Philadelphia, 2019, Elsevier.)

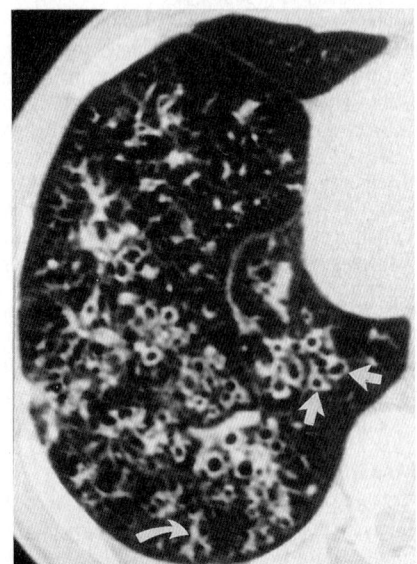

FIG. 4 Bronchiectasis. Computed tomography demonstrating dilated subsegmental bronchi. The bronchi are larger than the accompanying vessels with some demonstrating the "signet ring" sign *(arrows).* Plugging of peripheral bronchi is also evident *(curved arrow).* (From Grant LA: *Grainger & Allison's diagnostic radiology essentials,* ed 2, Philadelphia, 2019, Elsevier.)

- High-resolution computed tomography (CT) scan of the chest (Fig. 4 and Figs. E5 to E7) is the gold standard of diagnosis.
  1. The CT study should be noncontrast with the use of a 1- to 1.5-mm window every 1 cm with acquisition time of 1 sec.
  2. Findings include enlarged bronchoarterial ratio of >1.5 (normal 0.7), lack of tapering of an airway toward the periphery, ballooned cysts at the end of bronchi, and airway mucus impaction.
  3. Radiographic examples of different forms of bronchiectasis are illustrated in Fig. 8.

- Bronchoscopy may be helpful to evaluate hemoptysis, rule out obstructive lesions, removal of impacted mucus plugs, and obtain microbiologic data on respiratory pathogens when expectorated or induced sputum is not attainable.
- Table 2 summarizes diagnostic studies for the classification and management of patients with bronchiectasis.

BRONCHIECTASIS EXACERBATION

- Current international agreed definition[7] includes worsening in three or more of the following symptoms for at least 48 h in a patient with bronchiectasis:
  1. Cough
  2. Sputum volume and/or change in consistency; sputum purulence
  3. Breathlessness or exercise intolerance
  4. Fatigue and/or malaise
  5. Hemoptysis
- These should be assessed by a clinician to determine if treatment is required (see "Treatment")
- Consider sputum culture (with antibiotic susceptibility testing)
- Consider chest x-ray

Rx TREATMENT

NONPHARMACOLOGIC THERAPY

- Mucus clearance is essential and central to therapy: Low risk and shown to improve chronic symptoms of cough, breathlessness, and may reduce frequency of exacerbations. Techniques include active cycle breathing, positive expiratory pressure (e.g., Acapella, Aerobika), chest wall oscillation (i.e., vest therapy), oscillating and lung expansion therapy, trained autogenic drainage, and manual chest percussion (e.g., caregiver cupping hand with aggressive patting)
- Exercise, particularly aerobic and/or active breathing (e.g., yoga)
- Supplemental oxygen for hypoxemia
- Nocturnal positive pressure for hypercarbia in advanced disease

ACUTE GENERAL Rx

- At times of bronchiectasis exacerbation
  1. Increase airway clearance frequency, ensure adequate hydration, and use of bronchodilators when warranted.
  2. If changes in symptoms are more than 48 h, attempt to use antibiotic therapy based on the results of sputum Gram stain, culture, and susceptibility testing.
  3. If antibiotics are utilized, continue therapy for 14 days.
  4. In those with inadequate or inconclusive sputum test results, therapy can be based on knowledge of past culture growth, or empiric with doxycycline, trimethoprim-sulfamethoxazole, or amoxicillin/clavulanate if concerned for mixed etiologies.
- Admit to hospital for signs of respiratory distress, systemic symptoms, or inability to improve with oral outpatient therapy.

1. Initiate intravenous antibiotics.
2. Focus on mucus clearance, nutrition assessment, and physiotherapy.
3. Evaluate for hypoxemia and need for supplemental supplies prior to discharge.

COMPLEMENTARY & ALTERNATIVE MEDICINE

- Avoidance of tobacco
- Maintenance of proper nutrition and hydration
- Daily exercise
- Stress reduction
- Behavioral risk reduction of viral exposures
- Behavioral modifications to reduce gastroesophageal reflux

CHRONIC Rx

- Infections should be promptly identified and treated.
- Adults with bronchiectasis with a new isolation of *P. aeruginosa* should be offered eradication antibiotic treatment. This should not be offered to adults with bronchiectasis following new isolation of pathogens other than *P. aeruginosa.*[8]
  1. Measurement of serum anti-*Pseudomonas aeruginosa* (PA) IgG antibody may help predict success[9]
- Bronchodilators should be used before physiotherapy, including inhaled mucoactive drugs and inhaled antibiotics, in those with evidence of obstructive ventilatory defect or bronchospasm. This increases tolerability and optimizes delivery of medications in diseased areas of the lungs.
- Inhaled corticosteroids should not be offered to adults with isolated bronchiectasis or in those with concurrent COPD, as there is no proven benefit and a strong association of nontuberculous mycobacteria infection with their use. However, the diagnosis of bronchiectasis should not affect the use of inhaled corticosteroid in patients with comorbid asthma.
- Inhaled hyperosmolar agents (e.g., hypertonic saline) should be considered in conjunction with airway clearance in patients who have difficulty expectorating sputum.
- Inhaled mucolytics can be considered in those with difficulty expectorating sputum, poor quality of life, or where standard airway clearance has failed to control symptoms. However, rhDNase should not be offered to patients with bronchiectasis not related to cystic fibrosis as there is an associated decline in forced expiratory volume in the first second (FEV_1) and forced vital capacity in this population.[10]
- Macrolide thrice weekly should be offered for adults with bronchiectasis who have three or more exacerbations per year.[11]
- Immunoglobulin replacement should be considered in patients with selective immunoglobulin deficiency.

DISPOSITION

- Prognosis is variable with severity of the disease and underlying etiology of bronchiectasis. The bronchiectasis severity index,[12] and FACED

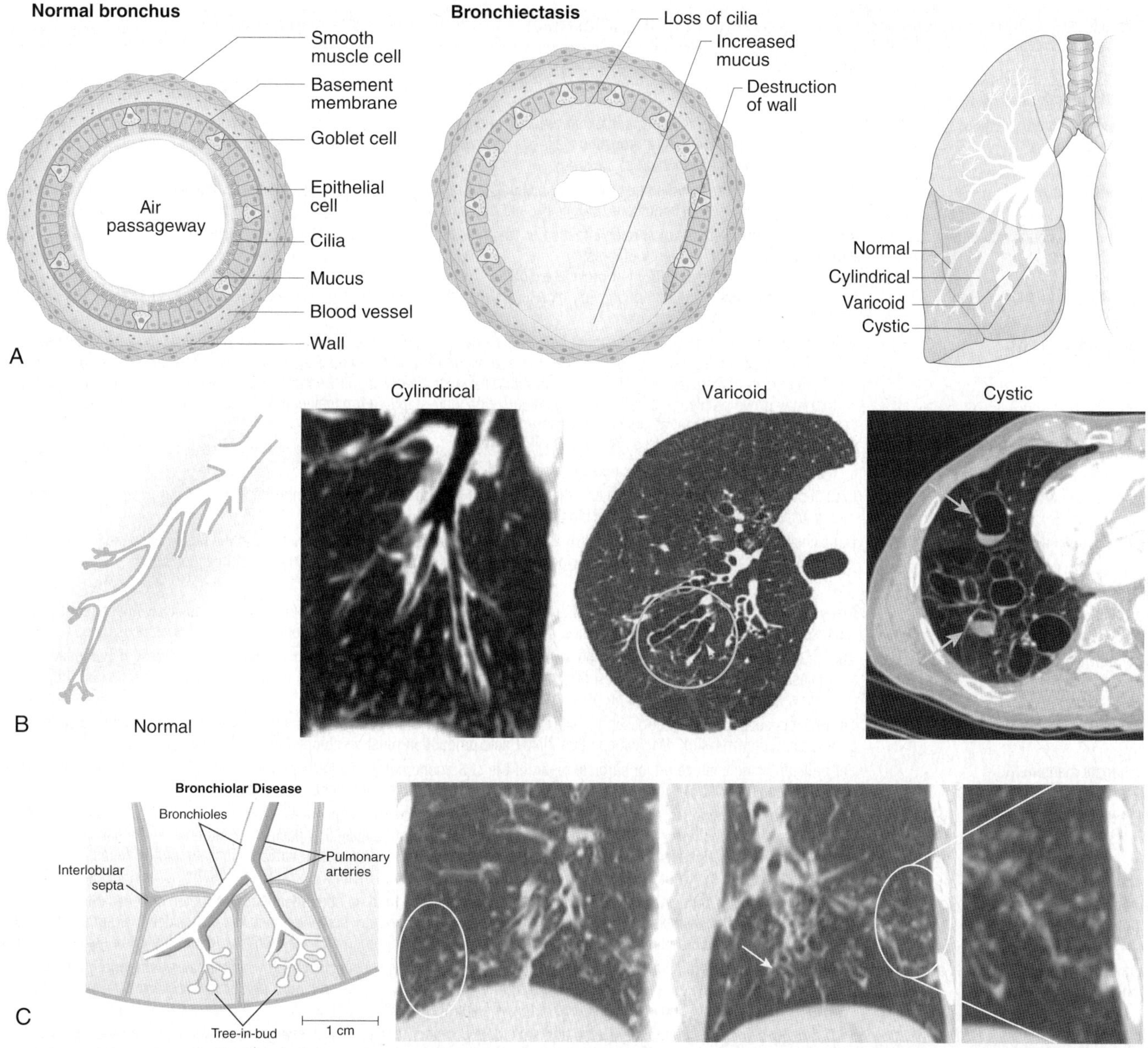

Normal bronchus

- Smooth muscle cell
- Basement membrane
- Goblet cell
- Epithelial cell
- Cilia
- Mucus
- Blood vessel
- Wall

Air passageway

A

Bronchiectasis

- Loss of cilia
- Increased mucus
- Destruction of wall

Normal
Cylindrical
Varicoid
Cystic

Cylindrical

Varicoid

Cystic

B

Normal

Bronchiolar Disease

- Bronchioles
- Pulmonary arteries
- Interlobular septa
- Tree-in-bud

1 cm

C

FIG. 8 Radiographic examples of different forms of bronchiectasis. A, The three top figures show a cross-section diagram of a normal airway, a bronchiectatic airway, and the three different forms of bronchiectasis on longitudinal view. **B,** The middle panel shows a diagram of a normal bronchial tree demonstrating usual tapering as the airway branches distally *(far left)* and axial computed tomography images showing cylindrical bronchiectasis *(middle left),* varicoid bronchiectasis *(middle right, yellow circle),* and cystic bronchiectasis *(arrows, far right).* **C,** The bottom panel shows a diagram of bronchiolitis *(left)* and a coronal computed tomography image *(right)* of inflammatory bronchiolitis manifested as tree-in-bud opacification *(white ovals)* (enlarged at far *right)* and bronchiectasis *(arrow)* in a patient with nontuberculous mycobacterial lung disease. (From Broaddus VC et al: *Murray & Nadel's textbook of respiratory medicine,* ed 7, Philadelphia, 2022, Elsevier.)

scores are helpful for the prediction of future hospitalization and mortality, respectively.[13]
- Pulmonary function declines at a faster rate in those with *Pseudomonas* colonization or frequent exacerbations.
- Concomitant rheumatoid arthritis or COPD is associated with worse prognosis.

REFERRAL

- Gastroenterology for evaluation of gastroesophageal reflux, esophageal motility disorders, and consideration of fundoplication when indicated to prevent progression of disease.
- Pulmonary rehabilitation may improve exercise capacity and should be considered when

there is significant breathlessness or new respiratory failure after exacerbation.[14]
- Embolization should be considered for recurrent hemoptysis.
- Surgical partial lung resection may be an option in patients with localized disease, severe disease unresponsive to medical therapy, or in patients with massive hemoptysis. Surgical resection of localized bronchiectasis is safe and improves quality of life.
- Referral for lung transplantation should be considered in the age-appropriate individual when FEV$_1$ is <30% predicted or there is a rapid decline, need for continuous supplemental oxygen, hypercarbia, recurrent hemoptysis not controlled

by embolization, increasing frequency or severity of exacerbations requiring intravenous antibiotics, or onset of pulmonary hypertension.

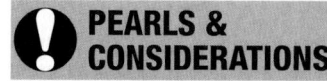

PEARLS & CONSIDERATIONS

COMMENTS

- Current clinical research is elucidating differential inflammatory endotypes, leading us closer to personalized targeted therapies.[15]
- The activity and quantity of neutrophil serine proteases are increased in the sputum of patients with bronchiectasis at baseline and

TABLE 2 Diagnostic Studies for the Classification and Management of Patients with Bronchiectasis

Test	Comments
Initial Diagnostic and Monitoring Studies	
Computed tomography lung scan (CTLS)	Definitive test for bronchiectasis, and aid in differentiation of pattern. Thin-section, high-resolution images may help detect subtle airway dilation before bronchial walls are grossly thickened. Contrast is generally not helpful and may, in fact, compromise the overall resolution of the study.
Pulmonary function tests (PFTs)	Comprehensive PFTs, including spirometry, bronchodilator responsiveness, lung volumes, and diffusion capacity aid in hints regarding predisposing conditions, prognosis, and management.
Complete blood count with differential	Anemia may reflect effects of chronic infection or blood loss (consider inflammatory bowel disorders). Leukocytosis may mark severity of infection. Eosinophilia may suggest ABPA/M or provide endotype.
ESR, C-reactive protein	Nonspecific markers of inflammation; very high levels may suggest underlying connective tissue disease or vasculitis. Can aid during treatment of exacerbations.
Routine sputum culture	Antibiotic therapy in bronchiectasis should generally be directed against specific pathogens and guided by in vitro susceptibility. Chronic infections with mucoid strains of *Pseudomonas aeruginosa* and *Staphylococcus aureus* may raise suspicions for CF and aid in management strategies. *Stenotrophomonas maltophilia* and *Burkholderia cepacia* are gram-negative bacilli that may prove problematic pathogens in patients with long-standing bronchiectasis. Of note, isolation of *B. cepacia* and *Helicobacter pylori* requires special laboratory techniques.
Mycobacterial sputum culture	Environmental mycobacteria such as *Mycobacterium avium* complex and *M. abscessus* are increasingly common. Presence can worsen symptoms and progress disease.
Fungal sputum culture	In patients with an asthmatic component, the presence of *Aspergillus* species (or other molds including *Pseudallescheria* or *Penicillium*) may be suggestive of etiology.
Immunoglobulin (Ig) levels	Deficiencies of IgG or IgA may promote bronchiectasis; IgG subclass deficiencies may also be a factor. Elevated levels of IgE may suggest ABPA or Job syndrome. Hyper-IgM may be associated, as well, with chronic infections.
Directed Diagnostic Studies	
CT scan of sinuses	Many patients with bronchiectasis also suffer chronic rhinosinusitis. The presence of extensive sinus involvement suggests possible CF, immunoglobulin deficiencies, or ciliary disorders. Optimal management entails aggressive sinus care.
Barium swallow (BaS)	The BaS may detect disturbed deglutition, esophageal diverticula, obstructing lesions (tumors or strictures), hypomotility, achalasia, hiatal hernias, or lower esophageal sphincter (LES) incompetence with reflux. The absence of reflux on a BaS, however, does not exclude this problem (see "pH probe").
pH probe	For patients suspected of gastroesophageal reflux, an 18- to 24-h study with a transnasal pH probe may identify, quantitate, and characterize reflux. Medications that inhibit acid production must be stopped before such tests.
Esophageal manometry	For patients being considered for surgical repair of the LES, manometry should be performed to determine that the esophagus generates sufficient pressure to propel food and liquids through the tightened sphincter.
Tailored hypopharyngography (TH)	TH is useful in detecting abnormalities of the initial phase of swallowing, deglutition. Persons particularly prone to problems include those with prior strokes, Parkinson disease, bulbar disorders including postpolio syndrome, and those with prior laryngeal or pharyngeal surgery. Note that some patients have gross aspiration without clinical manifestations (choking, coughing); this may occur in individuals with none of the above risk factors.
Sweat chloride, CF genotyping, and nasal potential differences	For bronchiectasis patients with bilateral disease, recurrent sinusitis, and no other identified risk factor, mild variants of CF appear should be considered. Sweat chloride is regarded as the primary screening test, but a considerable portion of adults with variants have borderline or normal results. Nasal potential difference may be useful for identifying CF in equivocal cases.
Alpha-1 antitrypsin (AAT) levels and phenotype	AAT anomalies appear to be a substantial risk factor for bronchiectasis, especially with white females. Abnormal proteinase inhibitor (Pi) phenotypes, even heterozygous patterns such as MS, appear to confer risk even with normal levels of AAT. Repletion of AAT may enhance resistance to lower respiratory tract infections.
Primary ciliary dyskinesia (PCD) evaluation	PCD is likely significantly underdiagnosed and should be considered with mid or lower lobe predominant disease, recurrent sinusitis, respiratory distress at birth, situs invertus, or no other identified risk factor of advanced disease. Although not universally available, consider nasal nitric oxide levels, nasal ciliated epithelium biopsy with transmission electron microscopy, and genetic evaluation with commercial sequencing.
Collagen vascular disease (CVD) serologies	Various CVDs may contribute to the risk for bronchiectasis, including RA, ankylosing spondylitis, and systemic lupus erythematosus. Thus, for patients with compatible histories or physical findings, assays for rheumatoid factor, aCCP, HLA-B27, ANA, SSA/Ro and/or SSB/La may provide insight into predisposing conditions.
Schirmer test	For patients with histories suggestive of "sicca syndrome" (dry eyes, dry mouth, oral ulcers), a positive Schirmer test may indicate the presence of either primary or secondary (associated with a CVD) Sjögren syndrome.

ABPA/M, Allergic bronchopulmonary aspergillosis/other mycoses; *ANA,* antinuclear antibody; *CF,* cystic fibrosis; *CT,* computed tomography; *ESR,* erythrocyte sedimentation rate; *HLA,* human leukocyte antigen; *NO,* nitric oxide; *PCD,* primary ciliary dyskinesia; *RA,* rheumatoid arthritis.

Adapted from Mason RJ: *Murray & Nadel's textbook of respiratory medicine,* ed 5, Philadelphia, 2010, Saunders.

increase further during exacerbations. A phase 2 trial revealed a reduction of neutrophil serine protease activity with brensocatib, an oral reversible inhibitor of dipeptidyl peptidase 1 (DPP-1), an enzyme responsible for the activation of neutrophil serine proteases.[16] There is an ongoing phase 3 trial of this agent, and prospective work on other immunomodulators.

- Patients with bronchiectasis are susceptible to nontuberculous mycobacterium pulmonary infection. Consider periodically screening using acid-fast bacillus sputum cultures and directly testing when there is a change in symptoms or clinical course.

PATIENT & FAMILY EDUCATION

Bronchiectasis and NTM 360 (COPD Foundation: www.bronchiectasisandntminitiative.org/)
Bronchiectasis Info and Research (https://bronchiectasisinfo.org/)

RELATED CONTENT

Bronchiectasis (Patient Information)

REFERENCES

Available at eBooks.Health.Elsevier.com.

AUTHOR: **B. SHOSHANA ZHA, MD, PhD**

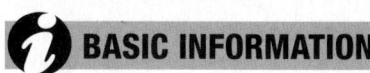
BASIC INFORMATION

DEFINITION

- Delayed conduction in the His-Purkinje system that meets criteria for right bundle branch block (RBBB), left bundle branch block (LBBB), or hemifascicular block. The latter can be either left anterior fascicular block (LAFB) or left posterior fascicular block (LPFB). Bifascicular block is a combination of RBBB and either LAFB or LPFB. All of these are categories of bundle branch block. Any delayed conduction that does not meet these criteria is not considered bundle branch block and instead categorized as intraventricular conduction delay (IVCD)[1,2] (see "Intraventricular Conduction Delay"). Repolarization abnormalities may be seen in multiple leads with LBBB and in leads V1 to V3 in RBBB. These include T wave inversion and ST segment depression in the opposite direction from the QRS complex. Fig. E1 illustrates a diagrammatic representation of fascicular blocks in the left ventricle. Table 1 and Table 2 summarize common diagnostic criteria for fascicular blocks and bundle branch blocks.
- The bundle branch block can be persistent or intermittent. Tachycardia-related aberrancy as well as bradycardia-related aberrancy has been described.

SYNONYMS

Fascicular block
Aberrancy
Conduction block
Conduction disturbance
Conduction delay
Conduction defect

ICD-10CM CODES
Bundle branch block (fascicular block):

I44.4	Anterior (left anterior fascicular block [LAFB])
I44.5	Posterior (left posterior fascicular block [LPFB])
I44.60	Hemiblock (hemifascicular block)
I44.7	Left (left bundle branch block [LBBB])
I45.10	Right (right bundle branch block [RBBB])
I45.2	Bilateral (bifascicular block)

EPIDEMIOLOGY & DEMOGRAPHICS

PREVALENCE: The estimated prevalence in the general population for any type of bundle branch block ranges between 0.2% and 3.4% and increases with age.
- Complete LBBB[3]: 0.4% in men age 50, increasing to 5.7% in men aged 80; 1.1% in women aged 50 to 80

- Complete RBBB[4,5]: 0.2% in men before age 30, 0.8% in men aged 50, 1.3% in men aged 80, 1.3% in women aged 50 to 80, and 2.3% in both men and women aged 60
- Incomplete RBBB[6,7]: 13.5% at age 20, decreasing to 3.4% at age 50

PREDOMINANT SEX & AGE: Bundle branch blocks are more common in men, and the incidence increases with age.

PEAK INCIDENCE: The cumulative incidence of any type of bundle branch block increases with age, being 1.5% at age 50 and reaching 18% at age 80.[4]

RISK FACTORS: Male gender, older age, structural heart disease, cardiomyopathy, and hypertension

GENETICS: Most cases of bundle branch block are not hereditary. The Brugada syndrome, an autosomal dominant genetic disorder, presents with pseudo-RBBB pattern but is not a true bundle branch block (see section on "Brugada Syndrome"). Hereditary bundle branch defect is an autosomal dominant genetic disease reported in Lebanon, mapped to the long arm of chromosome 19.

PHYSICAL FINDINGS & CLINICAL PRESENTATION

- RBBB may lead to a wide splitting of the second heart sound (S2). Either LBBB or RBBB can cause continuous splitting of S2 during respiration.
- Isolated bundle branch block is typically asymptomatic, but might reflect underlying heart disease, either in the conduction system or the surrounding cardiac tissues. Its existence can aggravate the clinical picture of the causal entity.
- In patients with heart failure, the presence of LBBB can cause ventricular dyssynchrony and worsen heart failure. LBBB or RBBB, when coexistent with coronary artery disease, diabetes, or heart failure, are markers for increased mortality.
- RBBB can be seen in pulmonary hypertension or acute pulmonary embolism; entities that increase the right ventricular afterload. The presence of bundle branch block can be associated with other conduction defects such as second or third degree atrioventricular (AV) block.
- Intermittent bundle branch block is predominantly rate-related, usually manifesting as RBBB during tachycardia or acute reduction of the R-R interval, which is common in atrial fibrillation.
- Bradycardia-dependent aberrancy, a phenomenon wherein bundle branch block appears or worsens at slower heart rates, has been described. For more, see later in the "Etiology" section.
- Alternating bundle branch block, wherein conduction delay alternates between RBBB and LBBB, is indicative of severe conduction system disease and often progresses to complete heart block.

ETIOLOGY

- Bundle branch block can arise from disease in the His-Purkinje conduction system or

---

TABLE 1 Common Diagnostic Criteria for Fascicular Blocks

Left Anterior Fascicular Block

Frontal plane mean QRS axis between −45 and −90 degrees
qR pattern in lead aVL, rS pattern in the inferior leads (II, III, aVF)
QRS duration <120 msec
Time to peak R wave in aVL ≥45 msec
Exclusion of other factors causing left axis deviation (e.g., left ventricular hypertrophy, inferior infarction)

Left Posterior Fascicular Block

Frontal plane mean QRS axis between +90 and +180 degrees
rS pattern in leads I and aVL with qR pattern in leads III and aVF
QRS duration <120 msec
Exclusion of other factors causing right axis deviation (e.g., right ventricular overload patterns, lateral infarction)

aVF, Augmented vector foot; *aVL*, augmented vector left.

Modified from Mann DL et al: *Braunwald's heart disease, a textbook of cardiovascular medicine*, ed 12, Philadelphia, 2022, Elsevier.

TABLE 2 Common Diagnostic Criteria for Bundle Branch Blocks

Complete Left Bundle Branch Block

QRS duration ≥130 msec
Broad, notched, or slurred R waves in leads I, aVL, V5, and V6
Small or absent initial R waves in right precordial leads (V1 and V2) followed by deep S waves
Negative T waves in leads with prominent S wave (usually V1-V3) may be seen but are not necessary for diagnosis
Absent septal Q waves in leads I, V5, and V6
Prolonged time to peak R wave (>60 msec) in leads V5 and V6

Complete Right Bundle Branch Block

QRS duration ≥120 msec
rsr′, rsR′, or rSR′ patterns in leads V1 and V2
The QRS complexes in leads V1-V3 may show secondary ST-T wave changes opposite in direction to the major QRS deflection
S waves in leads I and V6 ≥40 msec wide
Normal time to peak R wave in leads V5 and V6 but >50 msec in V1

aVF, Augmented vector foot; *aVL*, augmented vector left.

Modified from Mann DL et al: *Braunwald's heart disease, a textbook of cardiovascular medicine*, ed 12, Philadelphia, 2022, Elsevier.

from disease or fibrosis surrounding the conduction system (i.e., myocardial infarction). It can also be induced by antiarrhythmic drugs or by hyperkalemia. Selected causes of bundle branch block include: Intracardiac catheter manipulation, myocardial ischemia or infarction, myocarditis, cardiomyopathy, congenital heart disease, and Lenegre or Lev disease. RBBB in particular is associated with pulmonary hypertension and pulmonary embolism, whereas LBBB can be a consequence of an anterior myocardial infarction.

- Rate-related branch block in normal hearts is typically observed in tachycardia or in atrial fibrillation, particularly when a long R-R interval is followed by a shorter one. This is due to the Ashman phenomenon, wherein a long cycle length interval leads to a prolongation in the refractory period, resulting in a bundle branch block on the subsequent early beat. This is a common property of all cardiac tissues but more evident in the conduction system. Rate-related bundle branch block is usually seen as RBBB since the right bundle has a longer refractory period than the left bundle for the same heart rate.
- Bradycardia-dependent aberrancy is another observed phenomenon. This may occur due to the emergence of automaticity in a bundle branch block during diastole, leading to bundle branch block on a subsequent beat. Other possible explanations include inhibition by vagal tone or phase 4 block. In a phase 4 block, the cells have depleted their sodium reserves, leading to lower resting membrane potentials. This impedes cellular excitability, causing a conduction block.
- In patients with LBBB, detailed cardiac mapping has demonstrated that the site of block is in the proximal left conduction system in 64% of cases.[3]

Dx DIAGNOSIS

DIFFERENTIAL DIAGNOSIS
- Refer to Table 3.

- An accessory pathway can cause an appearance of RBBB or LBBB.
- If lead V1 is placed higher than the fourth intercostal space or more right than the parasternal area, the ECG can resemble incomplete RBBB.
- An inferior myocardial infarction can resemble left anterior fascicular block. In the inferior myocardial infarction, the inferior leads (II, III, aVF) will have qR or QS morphology, whereas in the left anterior fascicular block they will have rS morphology.
- Left posterior fascicular block can resemble lateral myocardial infarction, right ventricular hypertrophy, dextrocardia, or lateral accessory pathway.
- Accelerated idioventricular rhythm can resemble LBBB or RBBB, depending on the origin of the ectopic ventricular pacemaker.

WORKUP
- Carry out resting, ambulatory, and exercise electrocardiogram.
- Investigate potential coexisting comorbidities such as heart failure, myocardial infarction, and cardiomyopathies.
- Acute LBBB should prompt investigation for anterior myocardial infarction (Fig. 2), whereas acute RBBB warrants investigation for pulmonary hypertension, or pulmonary embolism (Fig. 3).
- Refer to Figs. 2 and 3 for illustrative examples of diagnostic evaluations for bundle branch block.

LABORATORY TESTS
- Standard laboratory testing appropriate for age, gender, and metabolic abnormalities.
- Electrolyte abnormalities and especially hyperkalemia should be excluded.
- If the cause of bundle branch block is suspected to be secondary to a pathologic entity, laboratory testing should be targeted accordingly. For example, cardiac biomarkers should be obtained if myocardial infarction is suspected; natriuretic peptides (BNP or NT-proBNP) can be used to assess for heart failure; or thyroid function tests can be used to investigate for hyperthyroidism and

hypothyroidism. If suspicions arise for an autoimmune or inflammatory cause such as rheumatic heart disease or myocarditis, tests for antinuclear antibody (ANA), anti–double-stranded DNA (anti-dsDNA), or rheumatoid factor might be relevant.

IMAGING STUDIES
Electrocardiogram (Figs. E4 and E5)

Rx TREATMENT

- Treatment should primarily focus on addressing the underlying cause (Tables 4 and 5). These may include management strategies for conditions like myocardial infarction, cardiomyopathies, hypertension, heart failure, and other pathologies that can lead to bundle branch block.
- Asymptomatic patients with an isolated bundle branch block usually do not require specific treatment.

NONPHARMACOLOGIC THERAPY
- In patients with bundle branch block and associated heart failure, particularly those with LBBB, New York Heart Association (NYHA) class II to IV symptoms, and a reduced ejection fraction (≤35%), options for cardiac resynchronization therapy (CRT) should be explored. In this setting, CRT with biventricular or His-bundle devices has been shown to improve symptoms and decrease mortality. Table 6 provides a summary guide to the recommended indications for CRT based on congestive heart failure (CHF) class, QRS duration, and presence or absence of an LBBB. The class of recommendation is based on the ACC/AHA recommendation system. This guide applies to patients with sinus rhythm and EF ≤35% despite optimal medical therapy.
- Patients with atrial fibrillation who otherwise meet the previous criteria have a Class IIA indication for CRT, provided that ventricular pacing is expected to be required a substantial proportion of the time.

TABLE 3 Differential Diagnosis of Bundle Branch Block

	RIGHT BUNDLE BRANCH BLOCK		LEFT BUNDLE BRANCH BLOCK		HEMIFASCICULAR BLOCK	
	Incomplete	Complete	Incomplete	Complete	Left Anterior Fascicular Block	Left Posterior Fascicular Block
QRS Axis	Normal	Normal	Normal or left	Normal or left	Left and >−45°	Right and >+90°
QRS Duration	<120 msec	>120 msec	<120 msec	>130 msec	<120 msec	<120 msec
I	qRs	Deep S	No q wave	Tall R wave, no q wave, no S wave	Positive QRS	rS
aVL	qRs	Deep S		Tall R wave, no q wave, no S wave	qR	rS
II, III, aVF					rS	qR
Precordial Leads	rSR′ in V1-V2, qRs in V5-V6	RsR′ in V1-V2, deep S in V5-V6	No q wave in V5-V6	QS or rS in V1-V2, tall R wave and no q wave or S wave in V5-V6	Poor R wave progression in V1-V3	
aVR	rsR′				Often tall R wave	

aVF, Augmented vector foot; *aVL,* augmented vector left; *aVR,* augmented vector right.

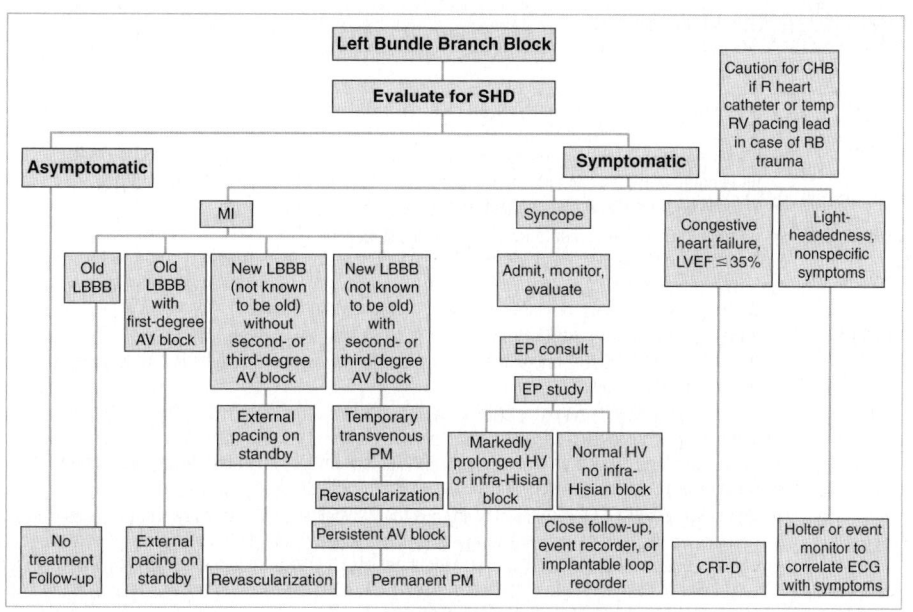

FIG. 2 Left bundle branch block. *AV,* Atrioventricular; *CHB,* complete heart block; *CRT-D,* cardiac resynchronization therapy combined with a defibrillator; *ECG,* electrocardiogram; *EP,* electrophysiology; *HV,* histoventricular; *LBBB,* left bundle branch block; *LVEF,* left ventricular ejection fraction; *MI,* myocardial infarction; *PM,* pacemaker; *RB,* right bundle; *RV,* right ventricular; *SHD,* structural heart disease (no overt evidence of myocardial, valvular, congenital, or coronary heart disease). (From Olshansky B et al: *Arrhythmia essentials,* ed 2, Philadelphia, 2017, Elsevier.)

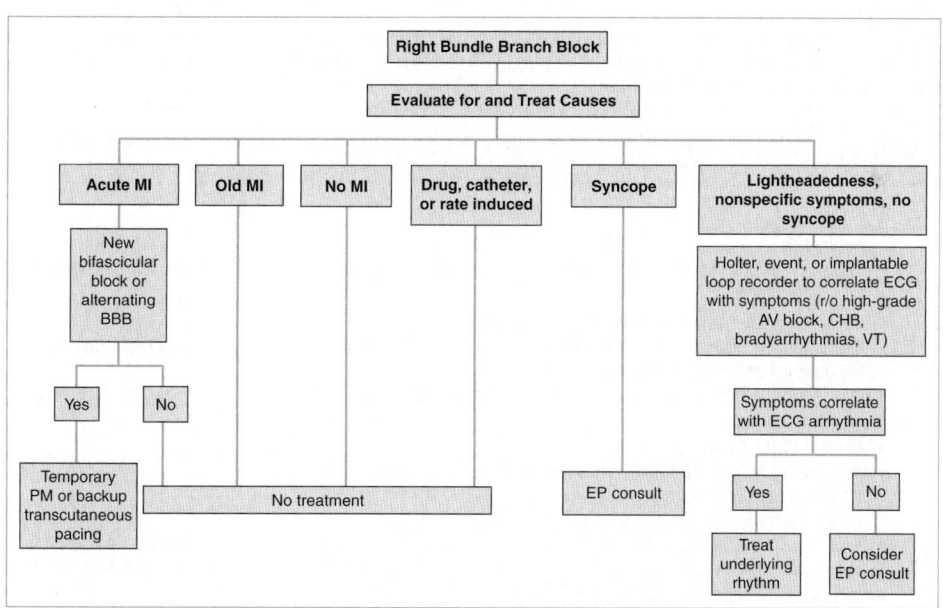

FIG. 3 Right bundle branch block. *AV,* Atrioventricular; *BBB,* bundle branch block; *CHB,* complete heart block; *ECG,* electrocardiogram; *EP,* electrophysiology; *MI,* myocardial infarction; *PM,* pacemaker; *VT,* ventricular tachycardia. (From Olshansky B et al: *Arrhythmia essentials,* ed 2, Philadelphia, 2017, Elsevier.)

- Permanent pacemaker is appropriate for patients with cardiac syncope or coexisting third degree, or Mobitz type II second degree AV block, when not due to a reversible cause.

ACUTE GENERAL Rx

In cases of acutely established bundle branch block, the underlying cause should be thoroughly investigated. For instance, in acute LBBB, anterior myocardial infarction should be investigated, whereas an acute RBBB typically calls for examination targeting pulmonary embolism.

CHRONIC Rx

Efforts should be made to optimize the management of any coexisting comorbidities such as coronary artery disease, heart failure, hyperkalemia, or diabetes.

DISPOSITION

There is no specific disposition plan for isolated bundle branch block. However, in the event of a new bundle branch block accompanied by associated symptoms, entities such as myocardial ischemia or infarction, myocarditis, and cardiomyopathy should be investigated prior to disposition. Pulmonary embolism should also be investigated in a new RBBB with suspecting symptoms.

REFERRAL

In selected patients at risk for sudden cardiac death such as Brugada syndrome, or in cases where a new bundle branch block is associated with acute symptoms, referral is indicated.

TABLE 4 Left Bundle Branch Block Management

Setting	Therapy
Asymptomatic normal LV function	• No therapy—rule out structural heart disease, ischemic heart disease. • Requires long-term follow-up. • If instrumentation of the right ventricle is planned, be ready to temporarily pace (preferably externally or via a temporary pacemaker wire) if transient traumatic RBBB with resultant complete AVB is induced. • Trauma to the right bundle can last from minutes to more than 24 h.
Symptomatic (syncope, lightheadedness)	• Admit, monitor, and evaluate for structural heart disease. • If syncope occurs, EP consultation and possible EP testing is indicated. • If HV interval is 100 msec or more or if infra-Hisian block is provoked with atrial pacing at rates of <160 bpm with or without procainamide challenge, implant a permanent pacemaker.
Symptomatic cardiomyopathy (CHF)	• If LVEF is 35% or less, NYHA class II, III, or IV heart failure symptoms are present with LBBB with QRS duration of more than 130 ms: CRT-D ICD implantation is indicated (may improve LV function, reduce heart failure symptoms, and reduce the risk of sudden death).
Myocardial infarction	• New (or not known to be old) LBBB: Revascularization with direct PTCA with or without stent. • Temporary pacemaker if second-degree or third-degree AVB is present. • New onset LBBB indicates extensive myocardial ischemia or infarction and is associated with worse prognosis. • Have external (transcutaneous) pacing on standby if no AVB is present.
Preoperative	• No therapy is required if the patient is asymptomatic, whether or not coronary artery disease or systolic dysfunction is present. • Cardiac workup (stress test, echocardiogram) to exclude structural heart disease if symptomatic. • LBBB is not per se an indication for treadmill testing. If stress testing is performed, imaging must accompany the test if the aim is to document the presence of obstructive coronary artery disease; imaging is not required if the aim of the stress test is the assessment of effort tolerance.
Postoperative	• No therapy if asymptomatic. • Common after aortic valve replacement (usually persistent) and after CABG (transient due to cardioplegia).
Alternating LBBB and RBBB	• Alternating BBB may be due to trifascicular disease. • Because of the high rate of progression to CHB, permanent pacemaker implantation is advised. • Alternating BBB may also be seen as a digitalis toxic rhythm, although in current practice this occurs only rarely.

AVB, Atrioventricular block; *BBB*, bundle branch block; *CABG*, coronary artery bypass graft; *CHB*, complete atrioventricular block; *CHF*, congestive heart failure; *CRT-D*, cardiac resynchronization and defibrillation therapy; *EP*, electrophysiology; *HV*, histoventricular; *ICD*, implantable cardioverter defibrillator; *LBBB*, left bundle branch block; *LV*, left ventricular; *LVEF*, left ventricular ejection fraction; *NYHA*, New York Heart Association; *PTCA*, percutaneous transluminal coronary angioplasty; *RBBB*, right bundle branch block.

From Olshansky B et al: *Arrhythmia essentials*, ed 2, Philadelphia, 2017, Elsevier.

TABLE 5 Right Bundle Branch Block Management

Setting	Therapy
Outpatient asymptomatic	• No therapy • May occur with instrumentation of the right ventricle (e.g., Swan-Ganz catheter) and trauma to the right bundle • Can last up to 24 h
Symptomatic (syncope)	• Admit the patient with RBBB who has syncope • If symptoms of syncope occur (may be related to AVB or VT), attempt to correlate symptoms with rhythm by Holter or event monitoring • Evaluate for underlying structural cardiac disease • Consider EP testing to assess AV conduction and the presence of inducible VT (present in up to 30% of symptomatic RBBB patients) if the patient is syncopal

MI	• Isolated RBBB: No therapy
	• RBBB with LAFB or LPFB (that is new or not known to be old) or alternating BBB:
	  • Temporary pacemaker
	  • Alternatively, placement of a transcutaneous pacing system
	• RBBB occurs in 3%-7% of MIs, often with LAFB, and usually because of anterior or anteroseptal infarction
	• The combination is less common in the current era of early revascularization via percutaneous techniques

Preoperative	• No therapy—temporary pacemaker not required • Perform cardiac evaluation to exclude other cardiovascular disease
Postoperative	• No treatment • Most common conduction disturbance in this setting
Alternating LBBB and RBBB	• Permanent pacemaker if not due to reversible cause

AV, Atrioventricular; *AVB*, atrioventricular block; *BBB*, bundle branch block; *EP*, electrophysiology; *LAFB*, left anterior fascicular block; *LBBB*, left bundle branch block; *LPFB*, left posterior fascicular block; *MI*, myocardial infarction; *RBBB*, right bundle branch block; *VT*, ventricular tachycardia.

From Olshansky B et al: *Arrhythmia essentials*, ed 2, Philadelphia, 2017, Elsevier.

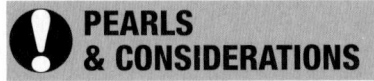

PEARLS & CONSIDERATIONS

COMMENTS

Bundle branch block can occur as a normal variant, particularly in younger individuals. A comprehensive history and physical exam are essential to identify associated cardiac abnormalities. An acute LBBB could be an indicator of anterior myocardial infarction, whereas acute RBBB might be due to pulmonary embolism. For patients suffering from heart failure with a depressed ejection fraction, cardiac resynchronization is beneficial in the presence of LBBB, but these benefits are not seen with RBBB. Finally, it is important to monitor patients with new bundle branch block for the potential development of higher degrees of heart block or other arrhythmias.

PREVENTION

Prevention primarily revolves around the management and modification of associated

TABLE 6 Recommended Indications for CRT Based on Congestive Heart Failure (CHF) Class, QRS Duration, and Presence or Absence of a Left Bundle Branch Block (LBBB)

| CHF Class | QRS 120-149 ms | | QRS >150 ms | |
	LBBB	Non-LBBB	LBBB	Non-LBBB
Class I	III	III	IIB (EF <30% in ischemic heart disease)	III
Class II	IIA	III	I	IIB
Class III	IIA	IIB	I	IIA
Class IVa	IIA	IIB	I	IIA

comorbidities such as optimization of heart failure, coronary artery disease, hypertension, and diabetes. Regular follow-up and adherence to prescribed medications, a heart-healthy diet, regular physical activity, and avoidance of tobacco and excessive alcohol can aid in preventing the development or progression of a bundle branch block.

PATIENT & FAMILY EDUCATION
Bundle branch block refers to a condition affecting the heart's electrical system. There are several types, but clinically the most important is the left bundle branch block in which one of the two main "wires" (called conduction pathways) in the heart is not functioning correctly. As a result, the heart's pumping chambers are squeezing out of sync. This can further impair the heart's ability to pump blood, particularly in individuals already dealing with heart failure. It is more common in older adults and individuals with serious heart disease.

RELATED CONTENT
Atrioventricular Dissociation (Related Key Topic)
Brugada Syndrome (Related Key Topic)
Heart Failure (Related Key Topic)
Intraventricular Conduction Delay (Related Key Topic)
Myocardial Infarction (Related Key Topic)
Pulmonary Embolism (Related Key Topic)

REFERENCES
Available at eBooks.Health.Elsevier.com.

AUTHORS: **IOANNIS KOULOURIDIS, MD, MSc** and **JOHN WYLIE, MD, FACC**

Diseases and Disorders

B

I

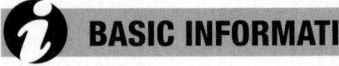

BASIC INFORMATION

DEFINITION

Calcium pyrophosphate dihydrate crystal deposition (CPPD) disease refers to the precipitation of calcium pyrophosphate dihydrate (CPP) in connective tissues that may be asymptomatic or may be associated with several clinical syndromes, including acute and chronic arthritis.[1] CPP was formerly abbreviated and commonly referred to as "CPPD," but the abbreviation is now reserved for "CPP deposition." Alternative names (Table 1) representing specific clinical or radiographic features of CPPD disease include pseudogout, chondrocalcinosis, and pyrophosphate arthropathy.[2]

Pseudogout/acute CPP crystal arthritis is used to describe acute attacks of CPP crystal-induced arthritis that clinically resembles the arthritis that is commonly encountered in gout.[3,4] The term *acute CPP crystal arthritis* is now preferred in place of *pseudogout*.

Chondrocalcinosis (CC) refers to radiographic calcification in hyaline cartilage and/or fibrocartilage and does not confirm the diagnosis of CPP-related arthritis as it can be present in other types of crystal deposition diseases or be asymptomatic.[2,5]

Pyrophosphate arthropathy is the term used for a chronic structural arthropathy related to CPP deposition.[2,5]

SYNONYMS

CPP crystal deposition disease
CPPD
Chondrocalcinosis (CC)
Pseudogout
Pyrophosphate arthropathy

ICD-10CM CODES
M11.2	Other chondrocalcinosis
M11.9	Crystal arthropathy, unspecified
M11.8	Other specified crystal arthropathies
M11.1	Familial chondrocalcinosis

EPIDEMIOLOGY & DEMOGRAPHICS

PREVALENCE:
- The epidemiology of CPPD crystal deposition is described in Table 2.[6]
- Most linked with advancing age (average age of 72).

RISK FACTORS:[7]
- Hyperparathyroidism
- Osteoarthritis
- Loop diuretic use

GENETICS: Familial forms

Associated with *ANKH* (ankylosis human) gene, which functions to transport inorganic pyrophosphate (PPi) out of cells, or the osteoprotegerin gene (TNFRSF11B)

Familial mutations can increase extracellular PPi levels and lead to onset of CPPD disease in the third or fourth decade of life

PHYSICAL FINDINGS & CLINICAL PRESENTATION

- *Acute CPP crystal arthritis/pseudogout:* Monoarticular attacks most commonly involve the knee and wrist but can be polyarticular (Fig. E1). Patients, especially the elderly, can have systemic manifestations such as fever and altered mental status and therefore diagnostic aspiration is essential to rule out septic arthritis. Situations that may trigger acute CPPD crystal arthritis are described in Box E1[6]
- Asymptomatic disease ("asymptomatic CPPD")
- Pseudogout (acute CPP crystal arthritis)
- Pseudo-RA (rheumatoid arthritis; chronic CPP crystal inflammatory arthritis): Symmetric polyarthritis
- Pseudo-OA (osteoarthritis), with or without superimposed acute attacks (OA with CPPD)
- Pseudo-neuropathic joint disease
- Spinal involvement causing spine stiffness associated with ankylosing spondylitis or diffuse idiopathic skeletal hyperostosis (DISH)
- Crowned-dens syndrome caused by crystal deposition in the ligamentum flavum of the cervical spine, either asymptomatic or spinal cord compression syndromes
- Pseudo-polymyalgia rheumatica (pseudo-PMR): Pain and stiffness in the neck and shoulder girdle mimicking PMR

ETIOLOGY

- Idiopathic
- Familial
- Trauma
- Metabolic and endocrine disorders (Table 3): Hyperparathyroidism, hypophosphatasia, hemochromatosis, hypomagnesemia, Gitelman syndrome, Bartter syndrome, gout, ochronosis, acromegaly, Wilson disease, familial hypocalciuric hypercalcemia, X-linked hypophosphatemic rickets[5,8]

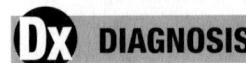 **DIAGNOSIS**

DIFFERENTIAL DIAGNOSIS

- Gouty arthritis (Table 4)
- Septic arthritis
- RA
- Osteoarthritis
- Spondyloarthritis (ReA, PsA)
- PMR

Table 5 describes metabolic diseases predisposing to CPPD disposition. Section II describes the differential diagnosis of acute monoarticular and oligoarticular arthritis and crystal-induced arthritides. An algorithm for evaluation and treatment of CPPD is shown in Fig. 2.[5]

LABORATORY TESTS

- Arthrocentesis will demonstrate the presence of weakly positive birefringent rhomboid-shaped crystals by compensated polarized light microscopy (Fig. E3).[5]
- Synovial fluid should always be analyzed for cell count with differential, crystals, Gram stain, and culture because acute CPP crystal arthritis/pseudogout and septic arthritis can coexist.

TABLE 1 Nomenclature of Calcium Pyrophosphate and Associated Syndromes

Definition	Old Terms	EULAR Recommendations	Preferred Term (Abbreviation)
Radiographic correlate of CPPD	Chondrocalcinosis, chondrocalcinosis articularis	Chondrocalcinosis	Chondrocalcinosis (CC)
Acute inflammatory arthritis caused by CPP crystals	Pseudogout	Acute CPP crystal arthritis	Acute CPP crystal arthritis
Calcium pyrophosphate dihydrate crystals	Calcium pyrophosphate dehydrate; calcium pyrophosphate dihydrate	Calcium pyrophosphate crystals	Calcium pyrophosphate crystals (CPP crystals)
All clinical syndromes associated with CPP crystals	Calcium pyrophosphate dihydrate deposition disease	None	Calcium pyrophosphate deposition disease (CPPD)
Chronic arthritis caused by CPP crystals ± inflammation	Calcium pyrophosphate dihydrate deposition disease: Pyrophosphate arthropathy; pseudorheumatoid arthritis; pseudoosteoarthritis	Chronic CPP crystal arthritis, OA with CPPD	Chronic CPP crystal arthritis, OA with CPPD
Deposition of calcium pyrophosphate crystals in joints or tissue with or without clinical symptoms	Calcium pyrophosphate dihydrate deposition	CPPD	Calcium pyrophosphate deposition (CPPD)

CPP, Calcium pyrophosphate; *CPPD,* calcium pyrophosphate dihydrate crystal deposition disease; *EULAR,* European League Against Rheumatism; *OA,* osteoarthritis.
From Hochberg MC et al: *Rheumatology,* ed 8, Philadelphia, 2023, Elsevier.

TABLE 2 Epidemiology of Calcium Pyrophosphate Dihydrate Crystal Deposition

Age Association	Rises With Age
Sex distribution	(F:M) 1:1
Chondrocalcinosis prevalence	8.1% (age range 63-93)
Pyrophosphate arthropathy prevalence	3.4% (age range 40-89)
Geography	Appears ubiquitous
Genetic associations	Mutations of *ANKH* gene on chromosome 5p (CCAL2) and unknown genes on chromosome 8q (CCAL1)

From Hochberg MC et al: *Rheumatology*, ed 5, St. Louis, 2011, Mosby.

TABLE 3 Diseases Associated With Calcium Pyrophosphate Dihydrate Crystal Deposition Disease

Disease	Strength of Evidence for a Link With CPPD	Recommended Testing
Hyperparathyroidism	Strong	Calcium, parathyroid hormone level
Hemochromatosis	Strong	Fe, TIBC, ferritin, C282Y
Hypophosphatasia	Strong	Alkaline phosphatase
Hypomagnesemia	Strong	Magnesium
Gout	Strong	Synovianalysis
Rheumatoid arthritis	Moderate	Clinical judgment
Osteoporosis	Moderate	Bone density if warranted

CPPD, Calcium pyrophosphate dihydrate crystal deposition disease; *TIBC*, total iron-binding capacity.
From Hochberg MC et al: *Rheumatology*, ed 5, St. Louis, 2011, Mosby.

TABLE 4 Differences Between Acute Gouty Arthritis and Acute Calcium Pyrophosphate Crystal Arthritis

Symptom or Sign	Acute Gout	Acute CPP Crystal Arthritis
Pattern of joint involvement	First MCP joint, other lower extremity joints	Knee, wrist, ankle, spine
Response to colchicine	Excellent in early attack	Variable
Blood in joint fluid	Unusual	Not unusual
Duration of attack	7-10 days	Days to weeks

CPP, Calcium pyrophosphate dihydrate; *MCP*, metacarpophalangeal.
From Hochberg MC et al: *Rheumatology*, ed 8, Philadelphia, 2023, Elsevier.

TABLE 5 Metabolic Diseases Predisposing to Calcium Pyrophosphate Dihydrate Crystal Deposition

	CC	Pseudogout	Chronic PA
Hemochromatosis	Yes	Yes	Yes
Hyperparathyroidism	Yes	Yes	No
Hypophosphatasia	Yes	Yes	No
Hypomagnesemia	Yes	Yes	No
Gout	Possibly	Possibly	No
Acromegaly	Possibly	No	No
Ochronosis	Yes	Yes	No
Familial hypocalciuric hypercalcemia	Possibly	No	No
X-linked hypophosphatemic rickets	Possibly	Possibly	Possibly

CC, Chondrocalcinosis; *PA*, pyrophosphate arthropathy.

- Evaluate for possible metabolic causes, especially in younger patients aged <55 yr or patients with florid polyarticular disease. Box 2 describes screening blood tests for metabolic diseases associated with CPPD crystal deposition.[6]

IMAGING STUDIES
- Radiographic clues to calcium pyrophosphate deposition disease are summarized in Box 3.
- Plain radiographs (Figs. E4, E5, and E6) often reveal CC located parallel to subchondral bone.[5]
  1. Classic locations for CC (see Fig. E1) include knee menisci (Fig. E7), wrist triangular fibrocartilage, symphysis pubis, and glenoid and acetabular labra.[5,9]
  2. Other locations can include MCP joints, wrist, patellofemoral joint, spine, and pelvis.

- Musculoskeletal ultrasound can detect deposition of CPP crystals within the hyaline cartilage and/or fibrocartilage. In contrast to urate crystal deposits in gout, CPP crystals often deposit within the substance of the hyaline cartilage and fibrocartilage, providing a means to distinguish CPP from urate deposition that occurs on the surface of the hyaline cartilage as seen in gout (Fig. E8).[9]
- Dual-energy CT (computed tomography) scan can differentiate mineral deposits through color-coded images and may aid in the diagnosis of CPPD from other crystal arthropathies.[9,10]

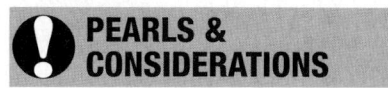

Rx TREATMENT

NONPHARMACOLOGIC THERAPY
General measures such as immobilization of inflamed joint

ACUTE GENERAL Rx[5]
- Monoarticular pseudogout:
  1. Aspiration followed by intraarticular corticosteroid injection (often superior to systemic treatment in the elderly)
- Polyarticular pseudogout:
  1. Oral corticosteroids, colchicine, or NSAIDs, if not contraindicated. A 2-day regimen comparing colchicine (1.5 mg on day 1 and 1 mg on day 2) versus prednisone (30 mg on days 1 and 2) showed similar short-term efficacy in a recent trial[5a]

CHRONIC GENERAL Rx[5]
Prophylaxis: Colchicine 0.6 mg twice daily or once daily as tolerated
- Pseudo-RA or refractory disease: Hydroxychloroquine or methotrexate
- Anakinra (Interleukin-1 receptor antagonist): Treatment and prophylaxis of polyarticular acute CPP crystal arthritis unresponsive to oral corticosteroids
- Treat underlying metabolic disease
- Management options for CPPD are summarized in Boxes E4 and E5

DISPOSITION
Structural joint damage may occasionally occur, requiring arthroplasty in rare cases.

REFERRAL
Rheumatology

! PEARLS & CONSIDERATIONS

COMMENTS
- Pseudogout is now referred to as acute CPP crystal arthritis.
- It primarily affects patients above 60 yr old and prevalence increases with age.
- CPPD has predilection for knees, wrists, hips, shoulders, and ankles.
- CPP crystals have rhomboid shape and positively birefringent.

C

Diseases and Disorders

I

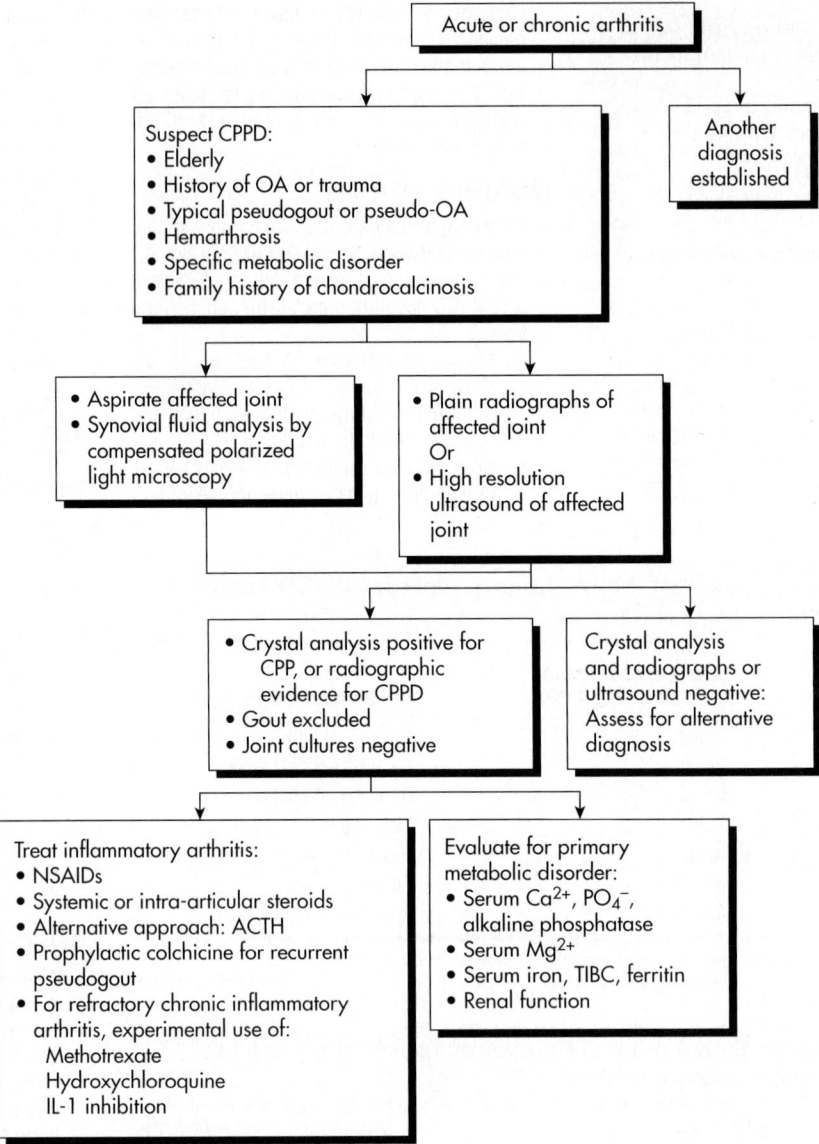

FIG. 2 Algorithm for evaluation and treatment of calcium pyrophosphate dihydrate disease. *ACTH,* Adrenocorticotropic hormone; *CPP,* calcium pyrophosphate dihydrate; *CPPD,* calcium pyrophosphate dihydrate crystal deposition; *IL,* interleukin; *NSAIDs,* nonsteroidal antiinflammatory drugs; *OA,* osteoarthritis; *TIBC,* total iron-binding capacity. (From Firestein GS et al: *Kelley and Firestein's textbook of rheumatology,* ed 10, Philadelphia, 2017, Elsevier.)

BOX 2 Screening Blood Tests for Metabolic Diseases Associated With Calcium Pyrophosphate Dihydrate Crystal Deposition

Calcium
Alkaline phosphatase
Magnesium
Ferritin, iron, transferrin
Liver function
Thyroid-stimulating hormone

From Hochberg MC et al: *Rheumatology,* ed 5, St Louis, 2011, Mosby.

BOX 3 Radiographic Clues to Calcium Pyrophosphate Deposition Disease

Chondrocalcinosis
Linear calcifications in tendons of knee, foot, plantar fascia
Large subchondral cysts
Severe joint destruction

From Hochberg MC et al: *Rheumatology,* ed 8, Philadelphia, 2023, Elsevier.

- Other medical conditions such as hyperparathyroidism, hemochromatosis, and hypomagnesemia can affect CPPD.
- Acute CPP crystal arthritis/pseudogout attacks have been reported to occur in the setting of surgical procedures, diuresis, bisphosphonate administration, and hyaluronate joint injections.
- Chronic CPPD can cause secondary osteoarthritis.

RELATED CONTENT

Pseudogout (Patient Information)
Gout (Related Key Topic)

REFERENCES

Available at eBooks.Health.Elsevier.com.

AUTHOR: **JINSEONG KIM, MD**

C

Diseases and Disorders

I

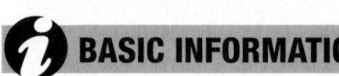 **BASIC INFORMATION**

DEFINITION

Severe and invasive diseases are caused by *Candida* infection. More than 15 different *Candida* spp. cause disease in humans, but at least 95% of invasive disease is caused by *C. albicans*, *C. glabrata*, *C. tropicalis*, *C. parapsilosis*, and *C. krusei*. These organisms cause serious disease referred to as invasive candidiasis. Invasive candidiasis embodies a variety of diseases caused by hematogenous spread of *Candida* to multiple viscera (e.g., kidney, brain, heart). These diseases include candidemia, disseminated candidiasis, meningitis, and endophthalmitis. Invasive candidiasis is a significant cause of morbidity and mortality for certain groups of patients. Further, invasive candidiasis is a very common fungus in patients with COVID-19. This coinfection can be associated with severe illness and death.

SYNONYM

Systemic candidiasis

ICD-10CM CODES	
B37.89	Other sites of candidiasis
B37.1	Pulmonary candidiasis
B37.2	Candidiasis of skin and nail
B37.5	Candidal meningitis
B37.6	Candidal endocarditis
B37.7	Candidal sepsis
B37.9	Candidiasis unspecified

EPIDEMIOLOGY & DEMOGRAPHICS

INCIDENCE:
- Invasive candidiasis is the most common fungal disease among hospitalized patients in the developed world. It is an important nosocomial infection. It affects over 250,000 people worldwide each year and causes more than 50,000 deaths.
- In the U.S., *Candida* spp. cause 8% to 10% of nosocomial bloodstream infections (fourth most common bloodstream infection). *C. albicans* is the most common cause of candidemia, but other non-*albicans* spp. have been implicated in recent years. These include *C. glabrata*, *C. parapsilosis*, *C. tropicalis*, and *C. krusei*. Incidence rates of candidemia are between 2 and 14 cases per 100,000 persons.
- *Candida auris* cases and transmission have seen a dramatic increase in the U.S. since it was first reported in 2016. The rise in echinocandin-resistant cases and evidence of transmission is significant because echinocandins are first-line therapy for invasive *Candida* infections, including *C. auris*.[1]

PREDOMINANT SEX & AGE: Equal between males and females; all ages are susceptible.

RISK FACTORS: Prolonged hospitalization and intensive care unit (ICU) stay, use of broad-spectrum antibiotics, prolonged indwelling of catheters (especially central venous catheters), acute and chronic renal failure, surgery requiring general anesthesia, cancer (e.g., solid neoplasms), transplantation (bone marrow or solid organ), recent chemotherapy/radiation therapy, use of immunosuppressive drugs, parenteral alimentation, use of internal prosthetic devices, organ transplant, hemodialysis, mechanical, surgical procedures

PHYSICAL FINDINGS & CLINICAL PRESENTATION

- History
  1. Fever unresponsive to broad-spectrum antibiotics
  2. History of prolonged indwelling intravenous (IV) catheter
  3. A personal history of any of the risk factors listed earlier
- Physical findings (general)
  1. Fever
  2. Hypotension
  3. Generalized malaise
  4. Tachycardia
  5. Change in mental status
  6. Signs of multiorgan system failure
- Specific diseases
  1. Candidemia
     a. A positive blood culture is the gold standard for the diagnosis of candidemia. Obtain blood cultures in patients suspected to have candidemia. *Candida* spp. must be isolated from at least one blood culture. A positive culture for *Candida* should be investigated thoroughly because of the increased risk of morbidity and mortality. Attributable mortality to candidemia in adults is 15% to 20%.
     b. Most common manifestation of invasive candidiasis.
     c. Physical examination may include fever, macronodular skin lesions, septic shock, *Candida* endophthalmitis.
  2. Disseminated candidiasis
     a. Seen in patients with neutropenia who have undergone cytotoxic chemotherapy for a hematologic malignancy
     b. Associated with multiple deep-organ infections or failure
     c. Blood culture positive
     d. Fever not responding to broad-spectrum antibiotics
     e. Physical examination: Discrete erythematous or palpable rash, sepsis/septic shock
  3. Endophthalmitis
     a. Iatrogenic/accidental or traumatic fungal infection of the eye (exogenous) or hematogenous seeding of the eye (endogenous); *C. albicans* accounts for about 90% of cases of endogenous endophthalmitis.
     b. Starts as choroidal lesion, progresses to vitreitis and endophthalmitis and eventually blindness.
     c. Physical examination shows fever. An early funduscopic examination by an ophthalmologist should be performed in all patients with candidemia. Funduscopic examination may show large and off-white cotton ball–like lesions with indistinct borders. Patients usually present with decreased visual acuity and occasional pain.

  4. *Candida* infection of the central nervous system
     a. Meningitis: *Candida* can spread hematogenously to the meninges during craniotomy or through ventriculoatrial/peritoneal shunts. Culture cerebrovascular fluid to establish diagnosis.
     b. Commonly found in long-term ICU patients.
     c. May manifest as meningitis, mycotic aneurysms, change in mental status.
     d. Physical examination reveals fever, neck rigidity, confusion, headache, and coma.
  5. Candidal musculoskeletal infections
     a. *Candida* infects the skeletal system, especially the joints as a result of trauma, joint injections, and other surgical interventions, such as IV drug use (hematogenous seeding).
     b. Previously uncommon; now relatively common probably because of increased frequency of candidemia and disseminated candidiasis.
     c. Knee and vertebral column (especially lumbosacral vertebral disks and vertebral bodies, which can lead to vertebral osteomyelitis, with or without diskitis) are involved.
     d. Physical examination is usually unremarkable but may show tenderness over involved area, fever, erythema, bone deformity, weight loss, and sometimes a draining fistulous tract.
  6. Candidal infections of the heart
     a. Usually found in patients with artificial heart valves, IV drug users, and patients with an indwelling central venous catheter
     b. May manifest as infective endocarditis, myocarditis, or pericarditis
     c. Physical examination reveals fever, hypotension, tachycardia, new or changing murmur, and signs and symptoms of heart failure
  7. Hepatosplenic candidiasis (chronic systemic candidiasis)
     a. Seen in patients with hematologic malignancy and neutropenia; usually develops during recovery from a neutropenic state (normally after undergoing myeloablative chemotherapy).
     b. On examination, patients have low-grade fever, right upper quadrant pain, palpable/tender liver, splenomegaly, and rarely jaundice.
     c. MRI/ultrasound (US)/computed tomography (CT) may reveal multiple focal abnormalities in the liver, spleen, and kidneys.
  8. *Candida* peritonitis
     a. Associated with GI surgery: Perforations, acute necrotizing pancreatitis, peritoneal dialysis. Pancreatic abscess, gangrenous cholecystitis, and common bile duct obstruction are other GI manifestations of *Candida* infection. *C. albicans* is the commonly isolated species in intraabdominal *Candida* infection.
     b. Clinical manifestations include fever, chills, abdominal pain; nausea, vomiting, constipation.

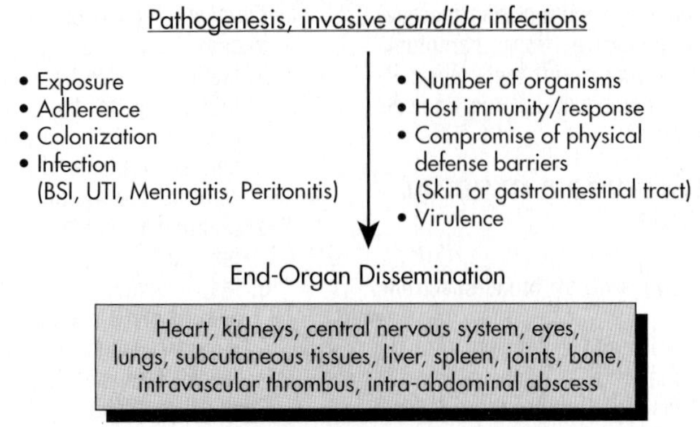

Pathogenesis, invasive *candida* infections

- Exposure
- Adherence
- Colonization
- Infection
  (BSI, UTI, Meningitis, Peritonitis)

- Number of organisms
- Host immunity/response
- Compromise of physical defense barriers (Skin or gastrointestinal tract)
- Virulence

↓

End-Organ Dissemination

Heart, kidneys, central nervous system, eyes, lungs, subcutaneous tissues, liver, spleen, joints, bone, intravascular thrombus, intra-abdominal abscess

FIG. 1 Pathogenesis of invasive candidiasis. *BSI*, Bloodstream infection; *UTI*, urinary tract infection. (From Cherry JD: *Feigin and Cherry's pediatric infectious diseases*, ed 8, Philadelphia, 2019, Elsevier.)

c. Physical examination reveals abdominal distention, abdominal pain, absent bowel sounds.
9. Other forms of invasive candidiasis
   a. *Candida* splenic abscess
   b. *Candida* cholecystitis
   c. Renal candidiasis
   d. Mediastinitis: Usually occurs after thoracic surgery. Clinical manifestations include chest wall erythema, sternal instability, and fever
   e. Empyema: Common in patients with malignancies
   f. Pneumonia (rare)
   g. Septic arthritis

ETIOLOGY

- Fig. 1 illustrates the pathogenesis of invasive candidiasis.
- Several species of *Candida* exist in nature.
- Medically significant include:
  1. *C. albicans:* Together with *C. glabrata,* they account for 70% to 80% of *Candida* in invasive candidiasis
  2. *C. glabrata:* Together with *C. albicans,* they account for 70% to 80% of *Candida* in invasive candidiasis
  3. *C. parapsilosis:* Associated with indwelling vascular catheters and prosthetic devices
  4. *C. tropicalis:* Especially in leukemic patients
  5. *C. krusei:* Resistant to fluconazole and ketoconazole

(Dx) DIAGNOSIS

DIFFERENTIAL DIAGNOSIS

- Sepsis (bacterial)
- Septic shock
- Cryptococcosis
- Aspergillosis

LABORATORY TESTS

- Laboratory studies are nonspecific. It is often necessary to perform several diagnostic tests to achieve maximum accuracy.
- High index of suspicion is needed.
- Candidemia/disseminated candidiasis: Candidemia represents the tip of the iceberg with respect to the more invasive forms of candidiasis. Central lines often contribute to the

propagation of candidemia. From the blood, infection can spread to almost any organ.
1. Blood culture is the gold standard of diagnosis. They are helpful but have low positive yield. Only 40% to 60% of patients with infection have positive culture. 95% of blood cultures that are positive for *Candida* spp. become positive within 96 h. *Candida* in a blood culture is *not* a contamination, and the source of the infection should be sought.
2. Diagnosis also can be made from normally sterile sites. Specific species identification is necessary because only 10% of known *Candida* spp. produce disease in humans.
3. The T2 magnetic resonance assay of whole blood can be performed on blood samples even after initiation of antifungal therapy.
4. Serum (1,3) beta-D-glucan detection assay: High specificity and high positive predictive value. It can also be used for diagnosing invasive candidiasis when blood cultures are negative.
5. New techniques allow for quick identification of *Candida* spp. in blood. These include:
   a. Peptide nucleic acid fluorescence in-situ hybridization (PAN-FISH).
   b. Matrix-assisted laser desorption ionization time-of-flight mass spectrometry (MALDI TOF MS).
- Hepatosplenic candidiasis (focal):
  1. Elevated serum alkaline phosphatase

IMAGING STUDIES

- Imaging studies are generally not required or useful.
- Ultrasound is useful for diagnosing hepatosplenic abscess. "Bull's eye or target lesions" are observed in the liver and spleen.
- CT scanning may be used to diagnose hepatosplenic candidiasis, as well as intraabdominal/renal abscesses.
- Transesophageal echocardiogram is useful to rule in or rule out *Candida* endocarditis.

(Rx) TREATMENT

- To successfully treat invasive *Candida* infection, it is important to start antifungal medication as early as possible. A small delay (~12 to 24 h) in

starting treatment may result in a significantly excessive mortality rate.
1. Do not dismiss *Candida* spp. as a contaminant when it is isolated in blood cultures or other sterile sites.
2. Before treatment, also consider removal of an intravenous catheter.
- Antifungals available include:
  1. Azoles (e.g., fluconazole, posaconazole, itraconazole, voriconazole). They inhibit the synthesis of ergosterol, a fungal cell component.
  2. Echinocandins (e.g., caspofungin, micafungin, anidulafungin). These are glucan synthesis inhibitors. Glucan is an important component of fungal cell walls. Most studies have provided reasonable support for echinocandins as treatment of choice for the majority of patients with invasive candidiasis.
  3. Polyenes (e.g., amphotericin B, lipid formulation of amphotericin, nystatin). Broad spectrum. Their mechanism of action is to increase cytoplasmic permeability.
  4. Antimetabolites (e.g., flucytosine). Flucytosine is deaminated to 5-fluorouracil in fungal cell. 5-Fluorouracil inhibits RNA and protein synthesis.
  5. Recently the FDA granted orphan drug designation approval of miltefosine for the treatment of invasive candidiasis.

TREATMENT PLANS (TABLES 1 AND 2)

CANDIDEMIA:

General principles:
- For documented candidemia, 2 wk of antifungal treatment after the first negative blood culture is recommended.
- In nonneutropenic patients, a dilated funduscopic examination in the first week of treatment is recommended.
- In neutropenic patients, delay above until neutrophil recovery because characteristic ocular findings may be delayed.
- Treatment depends on whether the patient is neutropenic or not.
  1. **Nonneutropenic adult patients:** The initial treatment is with an echinocandin (e.g., caspofungin 70 mg loading dose, then 50 mg/day IV *or* micafungin 100 mg/day IV). Alternatives include fluconazole 800 mg as loading dose, then 400 mg/day for at least 2 wk after clinical improvement or negative blood culture. Amphotericin B is equally efficacious.
  2. **Neutropenic adult patients:** An echinocandin is the drug of choice (e.g., caspofungin 70 mg IV loading dose, then 50 mg/day IV or micafungin 100 mg/day IV or anidulafungin 200 mg IV loading dose, then 100 mg IV all for at least 2 wk after clear blood culture and after clinical improvement. An alternative is fluconazole.
  3. **Preferred oral step-down therapy:** Neutropenic and nonneutropenic clinically stable patients can be transitioned to oral fluconazole (400 mg [6 mg/kg] daily) after about 5 to 7 days if they have:
     a. *Candida*-susceptible fluconazole *and*
     b. Negative blood cultures

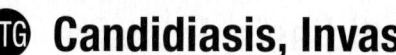

C

Diseases
and Disorders

I

TABLE 1 *Candida* Treatment Strategies

Indications	Primary Treatment	Alternative	Comments
Candidemia			
Nonneutropenic patients	An echinocandin[a]	Fluconazole: 800-mg (12-mg/kg) loading dose, then 400 mg (6 mg/kg) daily or LFAMB[b] or Voriconazole: 6 mg/kg twice daily for 2 doses, then 4 mg/kg twice daily	Fluconazole for patients who are clinically stable and have no prior azole exposure. Fluconazole can also be step-down therapy for patients who have susceptible isolates and blood cultures converted to negative.
Neutropenic patients	An echinocandin[a] or LFAMB[b]	Fluconazole: 800-mg (12-mg/kg) loading dose, then 400 (6 mg/kg) daily or Voriconazole: 6 mg/kg twice daily for 2 doses, then 4 mg/kg twice daily	An echinocandin is preferred. Fluconazole is step-down therapy for clinically stable patients with susceptible isolates and negative blood cultures. Voriconazole is used when additional coverage for mold is preferred.
Cardiovascular endocarditis	LFAMB[b] with or without 5-FC, 25 mg/kg qid or An echinocandin[c]	Step-down to fluconazole 400-800 mg (6-12 mg) daily for susceptible organism, patient clinically stable, negative blood cultures	Valve replacement is strongly recommended.
Central nervous system	LFAMB[b] with or without 5-FC, 25 mg/kg qid for several weeks	Fluconazole: 400-800 mg (6-12 mg) daily for susceptible organism after clinical improvement	Removal of prosthetic devices is strongly recommended.
Urinary tract			
Asymptomatic candiduria	Not indicated except in neonates and instrumentation of infected urinary tract		
Symptomatic cystitis	Fluconazole: 200 mg (3 mg/kg) daily for 2 wk	AMB-D: 0.3-0.6 mg/kg for 1-7 days or 5-FC: 25 mg/kg qid	Bladder irrigation with AMB-D, 50 mg/L, can be used for fluconazole-resistant species.
Renal parenchymal candidiasis	Fluconazole: 200-400 mg (3-6 mg/kg) daily for 2 wk or An echinocandin[a]	LFAMB[b] or AMB-D: 0.5-0.7 mg/kg daily with or without 5-FC 25 mg/kg qid[d] or 5-FC alone for 2 wk	
Ocular: chorioretinitis with or without vitritis	Fluconazole: 400-800 mg (6-12 mg/kg) daily or Voriconazole: 6 mg/kg IV q12h for 2 doses, then 4 mg/kg IV q12h	LFAMB: 3-5 mg/kg IV daily, with or without 5-FC, 25 mg/kg qid	Intravitreal AMB-D, 5-10 μg, or voriconazole, 100 μg. Often vitrectomy is used if 3-4+ vitritis or macular involvement is present.

AMB-D, Amphotericin B deoxycholate; *5-FC,* 5-fluorocytosine; *LFAMB,* lipid formulation of amphotericin B.
[a]Once-daily micafungin, 100 mg; caspofungin, 70-mg loading, then 50 mg; or anidulafungin, 200-mg loading, then 100 mg.
[b]Liposomal amphotericin B (AmBisome), 3-5 mg/kg daily, or amphotericin B lipid complex (Ablecet), 5 mg/kg daily.
[c]For initial therapy of *Candida* endocarditis, the 2016 guidelines recommend caspofungin, 150 mg; micafungin, 150 mg; or anidulafungin, 200 mg once daily.
[d]Strength of recommendations for 5-FC is weak.
From Bennett JE et al: *Mandell, Douglas, and Bennett's principles and practice of infectious diseases,* ed 9, Philadelphia, 2020, Elsevier.

DISSEMINATED CANDIDIASIS: Fluconazole is the drug of choice.

DISSEMINATED CANDIDIASIS WITH END-ORGAN INFECTION:
- Treatment is the same as for candidemia of nonneutropenic patients. In most cases, therapy is prolonged for at least 4 to 6 wk.
- The echinocandins are the first-line therapy.

OSTEOMYELITIS OR SEPTIC ARTHRITIS:
- Fluconazole 400 mg IV or PO *or*
- Caspofungin 50 mg/day IV *or*
- Micafungin 100 mg/day IV

ENDOCARDITIS:
- Caspofungin 50 to 150 mg/day *or*
- Micafungin 100 to 150 mg/day *or*
- Anidulafungin 100 to 200 mg/day

MYOCARDITIS:
- Lipid-based amphotericin B 3 to 5 mg/kg/day *or*
- Caspofungin 150 mg/day *or* micafungin 100 mg/day

ESOPHAGITIS:
- Caspofungin 50 mg/day IV
- Fluconazole 200 to 400 mg/day

PERICARDITIS: Lipid-based amphotericin B 3 to 5 mg/kg/day

SURGICAL CARE: Includes:
- Drainage
- Removal of any foreign bodies
- Surgical debridement
- Organ-specific care (e.g., valve replacement for endocarditis, splenectomy for splenic abscess, or vitrectomy for fungal endophthalmitis)

DISPOSITION
- Several factors affect prognosis: Infection site, degree of immune suppression, and how quickly diagnosis and therapy are initiated
- Overall mortality rate: 30% to 40%

REFERRAL
- Always involve an infectious disease specialist.
- Referral to specialist will depend on the organ involved. For example:
  1. Endocarditis will require a cardiothoracic surgeon.
  2. Endophthalmitis will require an ophthalmologist.

FOLLOW-UP CARE
- Prolonged periods, mainly in the hospital, of antifungal treatment may be necessary.

- Closely monitor patients on amphotericin B because of the high incidence of side effects. Check basic metabolic panel, magnesium, and CBC at least twice a week.

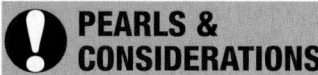 **PEARLS & CONSIDERATIONS**

PREVENTION
Basic preventive measures are similar to those used for nosocomial infections. This includes:
- Maximizing hand hygiene recommendations:
  1. Handwashing
  2. Using alcohol/chlorhexidine solution
- Adhering strictly to recommendations for placement and care of central lines and catheters
- Judicious use of antimicrobials
  1. Notes on *Candida auris*:
     a. The Centers for Disease Control and Prevention issued warnings in 2016 about the emergence of *C. auris,* a multidrug-resistant *Candida* sp. It is resistant to fluconazole and amphotericin B in 93% and 35% of patients, respectively.

TABLE 2 *Candida* Treatment: Other Indications

Indication	Primary Treatment	Alternative	Comment
Peritonitis	An echinocandin[a] or Fluconazole: 400-800 (6-12 mg/kg) daily or Voriconazole: 6 mg/kg q12h IV or PO, then 4 mg/kg q12h	LFAMB: 3-5 mg/kg daily	*Candida* recovered from an existing drain does not necessarily indicate peritonitis. Drains may become colonized. *Candida* from "freshly placed" drains usually requires treatment. Infected peritoneal dialysis catheters must be removed.
Chronic mucocutaneous candidiasis	Fluconazole or Itraconazole or Posaconazole	LFAMB: 3-5 mg/kg daily or An echinocandin (standard doses)	In severe cases, LFAMB may be necessary. After induction with a systemic antifungal for at least 4 wk, step-down suppressive therapy can be used with topical polyenes.
Oral thrush (mucocutaneous candidiasis)	Clotrimazole troches: 10 mg, dissolved slowly in mouth 5 times daily or Miconazole mucoadhesive buccal tablet: 50 mg placed on gum near canine tooth once daily for 7-14 days or Nystatin suspension: 100,000 U/ml, swish and swallow 4-6 ml 4 times daily; *or* 1-2 nystatin pastilles: 200,000 U each, dissolved slowly in mouth qid for 14 days or Fluconazole: 100-200 mg daily	Itraconazole solution: 200 mg daily or Posaconazole oral suspension: 100 mg bid on day 1, then 100 mg daily or Voriconazole: 200 mg bid or IV echinocandin[a] or AMB-D: 0.3 mg/kg daily	IV agents are reserved for refractory cases.
Candida esophagitis	Fluconazole: 200-400 mg IV or PO (3-6 mg/kg) daily for 14-21 days or An echinocandin[a] for 14-21 days	Itraconazole oral solution: 200 mg daily for 14-21 days or Posaconazole suspension: 400 mg bid for 14-21 days or Voriconazole: 200 mg bid or AMB-D: 0.3-0.7 mg/kg daily	IV agents are for refractory patients.
Candida vulvovaginitis	Multiple topical agents are available or Fluconazole: 150-mg single dose for mild disease; for severe acute vulvovaginitis, repeat 150 mg q72h for 2-3 doses	*Candida glabrata* unresponsive to azoles; boric acid gel capsule: 600 mg daily for 14 days	Fluconazole, 150-mg single dose weekly, has been used for recurrent disease.

AMB-D, Amphotericin B deoxycholate; *LFAMB,* lipid formulation of amphotericin B.
[a]Once-daily micafungin, 100 mg; caspofungin, 70-mg loading dose, then 50 mg; or anidulafungin, 200-mg loading dose, then 100 mg.
From Bennett JE et al: *Mandell, Douglas, and Bennett's principles and practice of infectious diseases,* ed 9, Philadelphia, 2020, Elsevier.

b. It has caused invasive health care-associated infections in many countries and has high mortality rates.
c. Initial treatment is with echinocandin. Patient should be closely followed with cultures.
d. Special infection control precautions should be followed for patients infected with or colonized by *C. auris.*

PROPHYLAXIS

Antifungal prophylaxis should be limited to patients in whom it has proved beneficial: Patients with GI anastomotic leakage, patients undergoing transplantation of the pancreas or small bowel, selected patients undergoing liver transplantation who are at high risk for candidiasis, and extremely low-birth-weight neonates in settings with a high incidence of neonatal candidiasis.

PATIENT & FAMILY EDUCATION

- Inform them about the risk factors for invasive candidiasis.
- Inform them of the seriousness of the disease and the associated high morbidity/mortality rates, thus requiring aggressive treatment.
- Side effects and toxicities associated with treatment.

RELATED CONTENT

Candidiasis (Patient Information)
Candidiasis, Cutaneous (Related Key Topic)

REFERENCE

Available at eBooks.Health.Elsevier.com.

AUTHOR: **FRED F. FERRI, MD**

BASIC INFORMATION

DEFINITION

Cannabinoid use disorder (CUD) refers to the inability to stop using cannabinoids despite causing harm or consequences, whether physiologic or psychologic.[1] CUD includes the use and abuse of natural cannabis as well as synthetic cannabinoids—more potent variations of natural cannabis that have increased in popularity in recent years.[2] First appearing in the 2000s, synthetic cannabinoids (often referred to as spice, K2, and kush) have since become the fastest-growing psychoactive drug with many new products being developed every year; over 177 new synthetic cannabinoids were developed in 2014.[3] These compounds act as full agonists at the CB1 receptor (the main cannabinoid receptor in the central nervous system), whereas THC found in natural cannabis acts as a partial agonist—synthetic cannabinoids thus produce similar but stronger effects as cannabis.[3]

CUD differs from other substance use disorders because of the widespread misbelief that cannabinoids are harmless and do not cause dependence or withdrawal.[1,4] As cannabis continues to be legalized for medical and recreational purposes, decreased stigma and increased access are possible contributors to increased prevalence of CUD.[4,5]

SYNONYMS

Cannabis use disorder
Cannabinoid dependence
Cannabis abuse
Marijuana abuse
CUD

ICD-10CM CODES	
F12.1	Mental and behavioral disorders due to use of cannabinoids: harmful use
F12.2	Mental and behavioral disorders due to use of cannabinoids: dependence syndrome
DSM-5-TR CODES	
305.20	Cannabis Use Disorder Moderate/Severe
304.30	Cannabis Use Disorder Mild

EPIDEMIOLOGY & DEMOGRAPHICS

As of 2016, of an estimated 192 million persons worldwide who had used cannabinoids in the previous year, 22.1 million people (11.5%) met criteria for CUD.[1] In the United States, an estimated 4.2 million people meet criteria for CUD in the past year as of 2015.[6]
INCIDENCE: Data on CUD incidence remains limited. One study by the National Survey on Drug Use and Health has illustrated an annual incidence of 2.7% in individuals >12 yr of age.[7]
PEAK INCIDENCE: Mean incidence of CUD is 21.7 yr.[4] When stratified by mild, moderate, and severe disease, mild CUD has a later mean incidence (23.1) than moderate (21.2) and severe (20.1) disease.[4]
PREVALENCE: Prevalence of 12-mo CUD was 2.5%.[4] Prevalence of lifetime CUD was 6.3%.[4]

Among regular cannabinoid users, lifetime prevalence of CUD is estimated at 9% to 30%,[8] with lifetime prevalence of moderate-severe CUD estimated at 8% to 12%.[6]
PREDOMINANT SEX & AGE: Odds of lifetime CUD were higher for men and young adults.[4] The mean age of onset of CUD was 21.7.[4]
GENETICS: Twin studies have found that genetic factors contribute to 59% in females and 51% in males to CUD.[1] Genes involved in CUD include *DRD2,* which is involved in dopamine regulation, and *CNR1,* which encodes cannabinoid receptors.[1] However, there have not been any reliable risk alleles detected.[1] Variations in the *CNR1* gene may predispose patients to cannabinoid-induced psychosis, though data remain limited.[3]
RISK FACTORS: Risk factors for progression to CUD include early onset of cannabinoid use; daily cannabinoid use; family history of use disorder; family members who use cannabis; lower socioeconomic status; poor academic performance; unstable or abusive family; co-use with tobacco; co-occurring mental health disorders including mood, anxiety, posttraumatic stress disorder (PTSD), and personality disorders; and other substance use disorder.[1,9] It is important to note that the majority of research has refuted the "gateway" hypothesis that cannabinoids work as a gateway to other illegal drugs.[10]

PHYSICAL FINDINGS & CLINICAL PRESENTATION

The high of ingestion can include euphoria, bonding with peers and pleasant perceptual disturbances with smoked effects beginning immediately.[9] Physical findings of recent cannabinoid use (within 2 h) include conjunctival injection, increased appetite, dry mouth, and tachycardia.[1] One physical finding that can indicate CUD is the presence of cannabinoid withdrawal, a common set of symptoms affecting up to half of regular users.[11] Cannabinoid withdrawal symptoms can occur 24 to 48 h after cessation and can include irritability, anxiety, changes in sleep patterns, depressed mood, and at least one physical symptom causing severe discomfort, such as headache, abdominal pain, or fever.[1] An additional finding that can indicate CUD is cannabinoid hyperemesis syndrome, in which patients present with cyclical vomiting and current or recent history of cannabinoid use.[1]

Cannabinoid use may also cause psychosis (referred to as cannabis-induced psychosis) and other negative psychiatric effects.[1,12] Synthetic cannabinoids in particular are more likely to cause harmful psychiatric symptoms (e.g., psychosis, anxiety, and panic attacks) than cannabis, and thus present a significant public health concern.[2] This is thought to occur because synthetic cannabinoids are more potent agonists of the cannabinoid receptors and lack cannabidiol (CBD), a non-intoxicating chemical found in natural cannabis that may act as a natural antipsychotic by blocking THC's binding to the CB1 receptor.[2]

ETIOLOGY

There are a variety of etiologies for beginning substance use that may lead to substance use disorder. Social influences, such as to conform to peers and for enjoyment or experimentation, are significant reasons for cannabinoid use in adolescents and young adults.[12] Others begin using cannabinoids for relaxation or for self-medication of mental illness, including depression, anxiety, and post-traumatic stress disorder (PTSD).[12] Additionally, psychosocial risk factors include lack of family/parental support in childhood, negative or traumatic life events, and poor social support increase risk of cannabinoid use.[1] Once a patient begins using cannabinoids, many genetic, psychosocial, and medical risk factors increase their risk of developing CUD, as stated earlier.

DIAGNOSIS

DIFFERENTIAL DIAGNOSIS

Differential diagnosis may include other substance use disorders; this can be differentiated through a thorough history and laboratory evaluation including toxicology screen and blood alcohol level.[12] Additionally, symptoms of CUD such as mood and thought disorder, anxiety, and psychosis may be similar to primary psychiatric disorders including depression, panic disorder, generalized anxiety disorder, or psychotic disorders such as schizophrenia.[1,12] Symptoms of these primary psychiatric disorders are present both before and after initial administration and cessation of cannabinoids, and time course can be obtained through thorough history, including collateral.[1,12]

WORKUP

The diagnosis of CUD is primarily a clinical one made through taking a history. CUD history is consistent with persistent cannabinoid use despite negative effects on social life, physical or mental health.[1] Cannabinoid-specific behavioral changes include impaired motor coordination and judgment, euphoria, anxiety, and social withdrawal.[1] Additionally, a thorough history can indicate the presence of amotivational syndrome, the presence of apathy and reduced self-efficacy in cannabinoid users.[13] Recent studies have found that cannabinoid use, but not alcohol or tobacco use, is a significant predictor of lower initiative and persistence.[13]

The screening question "In the past year, how often have you used cannabis or other cannabinoids?" may be beneficial for patients with higher baseline risk, including those with a history of incarceration or mental illness.[1] Diagnosis can be made if a patient meets 2 of 11 *The Diagnostic and Statistical Manual of Mental Disorders,* 5th Edition, Text Revision criteria with these symptoms causing impairment in functioning.[1] The number of these symptoms a patient meets can be used to measure the severity of CUD, with two or three symptoms classified as mild, four or five symptoms classified as moderate, and six or more classified as severe.[1]

Cannabinoid Use Disorder

LABORATORY TESTS

The diagnosis of CUD is made primarily by a thorough history. Although urine or blood testing for the THC metabolite delta-9-tetrahydrocannibinolic acid can indicate whether a patient is currently using cannabis, a positive result is not necessarily indicative of substance use disorder.[12] Because of increasing legality of cannabinoids, many commonly used urine toxicology screen no longer test for cannabis. Of note, many synthetic cannabinoids do not result on standard laboratory screens; mass spectroscopy has shown some promise in detecting synthetic cannabinoids but is expensive and may not detect newly developed compounds.[3] Laboratory tests to rule out other similarly appearing conditions, including heavy metals, electrolyte levels, and immunologic studies, may be warranted to rule out other causes.[12]

IMAGING STUDIES

Imaging is not necessary for diagnosis of CUD, though may be ordered to rule out other similarly appearing conditions.[12]

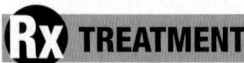 TREATMENT

NONPHARMACOLOGIC THERAPY

Effective nonpharmacologic therapies include cognitive-behavioral therapy (CBT) to teach coping and relapse-prevention skills, motivational-enhancement therapy (MET) to improve patients' motivation to decrease or stop cannabinoid use, and contingency management (CM) to offer incentives and reinforcement for decreasing or eliminating cannabinoid use.[8] For adolescent patients, family-based treatment options have the highest efficacy; however, CBT, MET, and brief interventions (such as motivational interviewing) also may be effective.[8] While private facilities exist to specifically treat cannabinoid use disorders, most public facilities, including most detoxification facilities, do not treat patients primarily using cannabinoids. Technology-driven interventions, involving these methods delivered via the internet or other technology medium, show similar efficacy for both adults and adolescents with both reduced cost and increased accessibility.[8]

ACUTE GENERAL Rx

Several widely used psychiatric medications may help with withdrawal symptom management in the acute setting, though many are not sufficient on their own for treatment of cannabinoid withdrawal and data on their effectiveness are not robust.[6] Symptoms of cannabinoid withdrawal tend to present within 1 wk of cessation of use[6] and can include irritability, anxiety, changes in sleep patterns, depressed mood, decreased appetite, and physical symptoms, including headache, abdominal pain, fever, chills, and tremors.[1,6] Mirtazapine may help with some withdrawal symptoms such as insomnia and decreased appetite but does not prevent relapse or improve mood.[6] Quetiapine has been found to help with sleep, improve appetite, and prevent weight loss, though it does not prevent relapse (similar to mirtazapine) and may paradoxically increase cravings.[6] Zolpidem may also assist with sleep difficulties during withdrawal, though the medication itself has some abuse and dependence potential.[6]

Administration of cannabinoid agonists represent an alternative approach to treating acute cannabis withdrawal, a paradigm similar to treatment of opioid and tobacco/nicotine use disorder.[11] The oral cannabinoid agonist dronabinol may help with global withdrawal symptoms, including craving, appetite and mood disturbances, and physical symptoms.[6,11] Nabilone, another synthetic cannabinoid with better bioavailability and efficacy, may reduce irritability and sleep disturbances during withdrawal,[6] though this evidence is mixed with other studies demonstrating no benefit.[11] Nabiximols, a cannabinoid agonist containing both THC and CBD administered via buccal spray, has beneficial effects on a variety of cannabinoid withdrawal symptoms including reducing cravings, irritability, and depression, with minor benefits in sleep and appetite disturbances, restlessness, and other physical symptoms.[6,11] In one study, nabiximols was shown to decrease the length of cannabis withdrawal in the inpatient setting by 2 days.[6] Pure CBD has also been shown to reduce withdrawal symptoms, particularly when administered at a higher dose of 800mg per day.[11]

CHRONIC Rx

Similarly to treatment for acute symptoms and withdrawal, there are currently no FDA-approved pharmacotherapies for CUD—much research is still in early stages and as such data are weak and occasionally contradictory.[6] Gabapentin has been shown to decrease both cravings and quantity of cannabinoid use in a small pilot study.[6] Topiramate also has been shown to decrease quantity of cannabinoid use in adolescents, though can be poorly tolerated and slower titration of the medication may be beneficial.[6] Quetiapine has been shown in one study to decrease the number days of cannabis use per week after 5 wk of treatment, with greater effect seen with longer treatment duration.[14]

Oral cannabinoid agonists represent another approach to chronic cannabis use disorder treatment. Although dronabinol may help with withdrawal symptoms as previously mentioned, it has not been shown to improve abstinence rates.[6,11] However, one study has shown a decrease in days of cannabis use per week after 3 wk of treatment with dronabinol (with greater effect seen with longer treatment duration), and this effect is also seen when combined with the alpha-2 agonist lofexidine.[14] Nabilone has shown weak and mixed results, with some studies illustrating a decrease cannabinoid use and relapse rates[6] while other studies have shown no effect on cannabis use.[11] In contrast, nabiximols has been shown to significantly reduce cannabis use, possibly due to the added effect of its non-intoxicating CBD component.[11] Long-term administration of naltrexone has been shown to decrease cannabis use and positive effects from cannabis, and N-acetylcysteine has shown encouraging data in decreasing cannabis use in adolescents and young adults.[6] CBD has also been shown to reduce cannabis use and improve abstinence.[11] As CBD is nonintoxicating, it may be safer than the above THC-containing products (especially for adolescents), offering lower potential for addiction and abuse and reduced risks of THC side effects such as cognitive impairment.[15] Administration of oxytocin has been shown to augment nonpharmacologic treatment approaches such as motivational enhancement therapy.[6]

COMPLEMENTARY & ALTERNATIVE MEDICINE

Of note, cannabinoids are often used as alternative medicine treatment for a variety of medical conditions. However, because cannabis is classified as a schedule I controlled substance by the FDA, research into the use of cannabis as alternative medicine is minimal and most research has been done with THC alone.[12] Medical cannabis as an industry is also significantly less evidence-based and highly regulated than traditional pharmaceuticals; dispensaries often make many decisions about strains used and dosing given based on opinion rather than rigorous clinical data.[12] Thus, providers prescribing medical cannabis should be aware that medical cannabis may not always be used as intended.[12]

DISPOSITION

The described treatments can be completed either on an outpatient or inpatient basis, depending on patient acuity.[6] Cannabinoid withdrawal does not pose a serious medical risk, and most people with CUD can be treated outpatient with supportive care.[1]

REFERRAL

Behavioral health referral for both medication and psychotherapeutic management is warranted for CUD treatment.[12] Because many individuals use cannabinoids as self-medication for pain, referral to neurology or pain management for an adequate and safer pain control regimen may also be warranted.[12] Additionally, referral to sleep medicine may be helpful for insomnia and other sleep disorders from chronic use or withdrawal.[12]

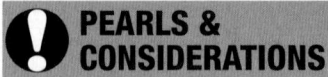 PEARLS & CONSIDERATIONS

COMMENTS

- CUD is much more prevalent than many might assume.
- CUD often co-occurs with other substance use disorders and mental health disorders, but the "gateway" hypothesis has largely been refuted.[10]

Although many treatments (pharmacologic and nonpharmacologic) show promise in helping with cannabinoid withdrawal and decreasing or stopping cannabinoid use, there are currently no FDA-approved therapies for CUD and treatment is largely up to provider discretion based on limited data from early-stage research.[6]

- Cannabinoid use is increasing, and the landscape of cannabinoid use and abuse is changing with its destigmatization and legalization.[16] New approaches to CUD prevention and treatment must be developed to adapt to this changing environment.

PREVENTION

With rates of adolescent cannabinoid use increasing (and now surpassing rates of tobacco use), effective prevention programs remain an important public health tool.[17] Many previous youth drug prevention campaigns using scare tactics and punishment have not been effective.[17] Instead, programs should provide scientifically accurate data about the risks and consequences of drug use (without overstating risks or equating all use with abuse), move beyond an abstinence-only framework, and contain strategies and information that adolescents find relatable.[17]

Recent cannabis legalization in many states provides a new landscape for CUD prevention.

Data on the effects of legalization are new and limited; however, increased legal cannabis availability (as measured by density of and proximity to legal cannabis dispensaries) has been linked to increased use.[16] This effect is especially pronounced among populations with lower pre-legalization use and access, such as women and young adults.[16] Increased availability may also be linked to increased negative cannabis-associated health outcomes including vomiting, psychosis, and cannabis-related pregnancy hospitalizations.[16] Thus, density limits for cannabis dispensaries and other availability restrictions may be a prudent policy measure in the wake of legalization.

PATIENT & FAMILY EDUCATION

With cannabinoid use increasing across many demographics and the widespread belief that cannabis is a harmless drug, patient education is an important tool for prevention of CUD. There is an inverse relationship between perception of risk and cannabis use; as such, psychoeducation is valuable for both prevention and treatment of CUD.[9] All patients should be educated about the risks of cannabinoid use, but especially those under the age of 21 who are especially susceptible to CUD and at higher risk of poor long-term outcomes thereof.[12] As with all other substances, pregnant patients should be educated about the harmful effects of cannabinoids on the fetus; this is especially important as cannabinoid use during pregnancy is increasing.[12]

RELATED CONTENT

Substance Use Disorder (Related Key Topic)
Synthetic Cannabinoids (Related Key Topic)
Medical Marijuana (Related Key Topic)

REFERENCES

Available at eBooks.Health.Elsevier.com.

AUTHORS: **SARANYA S. KHURANA, MD, MPH** and **DANIEL J. HARRIS, MD**

C

Diseases and Disorders

BASIC INFORMATION

DEFINITION

Dilated cardiomyopathy (DCM) is characterized by dilation and impaired contraction of one or both ventricles that is not wholly the result of hypertension, coronary atherosclerosis, valvular dysfunction, congenital, or other structural heart disease. As a result, the systolic function of the heart is impaired and may develop overt heart failure, atrial and/or ventricular arrhythmias, and sudden death. The disease is considered idiopathic if primary and secondary causes of heart disease are excluded.

SYNONYMS

Congestive cardiomyopathy
Idiopathic cardiomyopathy

ICD-10CM CODES	
B33.24	Viral cardiomyopathy
I11.0	Hypertensive heart disease with heart failure
I42.0	Dilated cardiomyopathy (includes congestive cardiomyopathy)
I42.9	Cardiomyopathy, unspecified (includes cardiomyopathy [primary] [secondary] NOS)
I43	Cardiomyopathy in diseases classified elsewhere
I50.20 to I50.9	(Unspecified, Acute, Chronic, or Acute on Chronic) + (systolic, diastolic, or combined) (congestive) heart failure
O90.3	Peripartum cardiomyopathy

EPIDEMIOLOGY & DEMOGRAPHICS

- The estimated age-adjusted prevalence of dilated cardiomyopathy in the United States general population is approximately 36 per 100,000 and a predilection for men with a male/female ratio of 3:1. The incidence is approximately 5 to 7 per 100,000 persons per year, although younger patients (<55 yr) were more frequently affected with an incidence up to 18/100,000.[1]
- African Americans have a threefold increased risk for developing DCM, irrespective of comorbidities or socioeconomic factors, compared with whites.
- DCM is the most common form of cardiomyopathy, comprising approximately 60% of all cardiomyopathies.
- Reports indicate that 30% to 40% of DCM cases are caused by pathogenic or likely pathogenic gene variants. More than 50 genes have been associated with DCM.[2]

PHYSICAL FINDINGS & CLINICAL PRESENTATION

Affected patients may present in a number of ways, and the etiology is most often elucidated with obtaining a focused history. The patient may display common symptoms of congestive heart failure, which may either be insidious or present suddenly. The patient also may be asymptomatic and the diagnosis made only by the incidental finding of cardiomegaly on a chest x-ray examination. Patients with DCM may also present with arrhythmias, thromboembolic disease secondary to left ventricular mural thrombus, and pregnancy-associated cardiomyopathy. Classic signs of heart failure include:

- Increased jugular venous pressure
- Narrow pulse pressure
- Pulmonary rales, hepatomegaly, peripheral edema
- S3, S4
- Mitral regurgitation, tricuspid regurgitation (less common)
- Pulsus alternans (sign of advanced ventricular dysfunction)

ETIOLOGY

DCM can be attributed to genetic and nongenetic causes, including hypertension, valve disease, inflammatory/infectious causes, and toxins.

- Idiopathic (often a viral infection that cannot be confirmed)
- Infections (viral [human herpesvirus 6, influenza, echovirus, cytomegalovirus, Coxsackie B, adenovirus, parvovirus, HIV], rickettsial, mycobacterial, toxoplasmosis, trichinosis, Chagas disease)
- Ischemic heart disease
- Alcoholism (15% to 40% of all cases in Western countries)
- Uncontrolled tachyarrhythmia ("tachycardia-mediated")
- Sleep apnea—obstructive or nonobstructive
- Cirrhotic (not necessarily alcohol-induced)
- End-stage renal disease–related
- Nutritional deficiencies (selenium, L-carnitine, thiamine)
- Peripartum—The diagnosis should be considered particularly in patients with symptoms of heart failure occurring from the last trimester of pregnancy to 6 mo postpartum particularly in patients above 35 yr of age, African American, preeclampsia, and multiple gestations
- Chemotherapeutic (anthracycline, doxorubicin, daunorubicin) or pharmacologic agents (antiretrovirals, phenothiazines) (see "Cardiomyopathy, Chemical-Induced")
- Substance abuse (cocaine, heroin, organic solvents "glue-sniffer's heart")
- Toxins (cobalt, lead, phosphorus, carbon monoxide, mercury), collagen-vascular disease (systemic lupus, rheumatoid arthritis, polyarteritis, dermatomyositis, sarcoidosis)
- Hereditary familial neuromuscular disorders (e.g., muscular dystrophy, myotonic dystrophy)
- Endocrine dysfunction (acromegaly, osteogenesis imperfecta, myxedema, thyrotoxicosis, diabetes)
- Hematologic (e.g., sickle cell anemia, hereditary sideroblastic anemias and thalassemias, hypereosinophilia, hereditary hemochromatosis)
- Stress-induced (i.e., takotsubo or broken heart syndrome)
- LV noncompaction
- Autoimmunity ("antiheart antibodies" [AHAs] [beta-1 adrenoceptor, alpha-myosin heavy chain, beta-myosin heavy chain, myosin light chain]) are hypothesized to cause DCM based on animal studies. Appears to be applicable to humans as AHAs can be detected in 38% of patients with an idiopathic DCM
- Over 60 genes have been associated with DCM in various studies. *TTN* truncating mutations (mutations in *TTN*, the gene encoding the sarcomere protein titin) are a common cause of dilated cardiomyopathy, occurring in approximately 25% of familial cases of idiopathic dilated cardiomyopathy and in 18% of sporadic cases. Pathogenic variants in the myosin heavy chain 7 (MYH7) have been described in 1% to 5.3% of DCM cases, making it one of the common genes in patients with DCM. Additional concerning genes include LMNA, and truncating FLNC variants[2-4]

DIAGNOSIS

Dilated cardiomyopathy is a diagnosis of exclusion, made after ruling out other potential causes of myocardial dysfunction.

DIFFERENTIAL DIAGNOSIS (TABLE 1)

- Coronary atherosclerosis, that is, left ventricular dysfunction secondary to ischemia and/or myocardial infarction
- Valvular dysfunction (especially aortic and mitral regurgitation)
- Other cardiomyopathies (restrictive, hypertrophic)
- Pulmonary disease (embolism, obstructive, restrictive)
- Pericardial abnormalities (constrictive pericarditis, tamponade)
- Hypothyroidism/myxedema
- Athlete's heart
- Chagas cardiomyopathy
- Familial dilated cardiomyopathy (inherited)

WORKUP

- Medical history: Emphasis on symptoms of dyspnea, orthopnea, paroxysmal nocturnal dyspnea, weight gain, palpitations, fatigue, or signs of systemic and pulmonary embolism, substance abuse history, and possible toxin exposures (especially occupational)
- Physical examination (see "Physical Findings & Clinical Presentation")
- Testing (see "Laboratory Tests" and "Imaging Studies" for more detail): Laboratory, chest x-ray, electrocardiogram (ECG), echocardiogram, cardiac catheterization; myocardial biopsy is not routinely recommended, unless acute myocarditis requiring immunosuppressive therapy is considered (e.g., giant cell myocarditis)

LABORATORY TESTS

- Chemistries/metabolites (deficiencies), renal function tests (renal dysfunction)
- Cardiac biomarkers (elevation of cardiac troponin or BNP): Persistently increased cardiac troponin T levels are a marker of poor outcome in cardiomyopathy patients

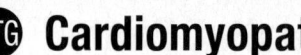

C

TABLE 1 Classification of Cardiomyopathies by Phenome and Genome

	PHENOME				GENOME	
Type	Morphology	Physiology	Pathology	Systemic Conditions, Clinical Features, Risk Factors	Nonsyndromic, Usually Single Gene	Syndromic
Dilated (DCM)	Dilation of LV or LV and RV with minimal or no wall thickening	Reduced contractility is the primary defect; variable degree of diastolic dysfunction	Myocyte hypertrophy; scattered fibrosis	Hypertension; alcohol; thyrotoxicosis, myxedema; persistent tachycardia; toxins (e.g., chemotherapy, especially anthracyclines); radiation	Diverse gene ontology with >30 genes implicated	Diverse array of associated conditions, especially muscular dystrophies: Emery-Dreifuss muscular dystrophy, limb-girdle muscular dystrophy, Duchenne/Becker muscular dystrophy; Laing distal myopathy; Barth syndrome; Kearns-Sayre syndrome; others[9-11]
Restrictive (RCM)	Usually normal chamber sizes; minimal to moderate wall thickening	Contractility normal or near-normal with a marked increase in end-diastolic filling pressure	Specific to type, diagnosis: amyloid, iron, glycogen storage disease, others	Endomyocardial fibrosis, amyloid, sarcoid, scleroderma, Churg-Strauss syndrome, cystinosis, lymphoma, pseudoxanthoma elasticum, hypereosinophilic syndrome, carcinoid	If not associated with systemic genetic disease, genetic cause usually from sarcomeric gene rare variants	Gaucher disease, hemochromatosis, Fabry disease, familial amyloidosis; mucopolysaccharidoses, Noonan syndrome
Hypertrophic (HCM)	Usually normal or reduced internal chamber dimension; wall thickening pronounced, especially septal hypertrophy	Systolic function increased or normal	Myocyte hypertrophy, classically with disarray	Severe hypertension can confound clinical, morphologic diagnosis	Rare variants of genes encoding sarcomeric proteins	Noonan syndrome, LEOPARD syndrome, Danon syndrome, Fabry disease, Wolff-Parkinson-White syndrome, Friedreich ataxia, MERRF, MELAS
Arrhythmogenic right ventricular cardiomyopathy (ARVC)	Scattered fibrofatty infiltration, classically of RV but also of LV; dilation of RV or LV, or both, is common but not universal	Ventricular arrhythmias (VT, VF) early or late, reduced contractility with progressive disease; can mimic DCM	Islands of fatty replacement; fibrosis	Palmoplantar keratoderma, wooly hair in Naxos syndrome	Rare variants of genes encoding proteins of desmosome	Naxos syndrome
Inflammatory	Normal or dilated without hypertrophy	Reduced systolic function	Inflammatory infiltrates	Hypereosinophilic syndrome, acute myocarditis		
Ischemic	Normal or dilated without hypertrophy	Reduced systolic function	Areas of infarcted myocardium	Hypercholesterolemia, hypertension, diabetes, cigarette smoking, family history	Familial hypercholesterolemia; other heritable lipid disorders	Familial hypercholesterolemia
Infectious	Normal or dilated without hypertrophy	Reduced systolic function	Specific to infection	Viral (especially acute myocarditis); protozoal (e.g., Chagas disease); bacterial, direct infection (e.g., Lyme disease) or from acute cellular toxicity as result of systemic toxins (e.g., *Streptococcus*, gram-negative, others)	Genetic predisposition to infection and/or variable response to infective agent	

LV, Left ventricle; *MELAS*, mitochondrial encephalopathy, lactic acidosis, and strokelike symptoms; *MERRF*, myoclonic epilepsy associated with ragged-red fibers; *RV*, right ventricle; *VF*, ventricular fibrillation; *VT*, ventricular tachycardia.
From Libby P et al: *Braunwald's heart disease, a textbook of cardiovascular medicine*, ed 12, Philadelphia, 2022, Elsevier.

- Endocrine (particularly thyroid)
- Iron studies (hemochromatosis, deficiency)
- Rheumatologic and inflammatory (ANA, ESR, CRP)
- Others as indicated (HIV, Lyme, neurohormonal)
- Anti–*T. cruzi* serology (Chagas)
- Genetic testing

IMAGING STUDIES
CHEST X-RAY:
- Cardiac silhouette enlargement (particularly left ventricle)
- Pulmonary vascular redistribution and congestion (Kerley B lines, cephalization of vasculature), pleural effusion (may appear as unilateral, most often on the right side)

ECG:
- ECG findings are typically nonspecific, and sinus tachycardia is usually a reflection of underlying heart failure. Large voltage in precordial leads and low voltage in limb leads may be seen in advanced disease
- Intraventricular conduction defects, left bundle branch block, or right bundle branch block

- Arrhythmias (atrial fibrillation, premature ventricular or atrial contractions, ventricular tachycardia)
- Echocardiogram (Fig. E1): Low ejection fraction with global hypokinesis
- Four-chamber enlargement (LV enlargement usually predominates)
- Mitral or tricuspid regurgitation ("secondary" regurgitation from tethering due to incomplete leaflet closure caused by ventricular dilation)

CARDIAC CATHETERIZATION:
- On initial presentation to exclude obstructive epicardial coronary artery disease

CARDIAC MAGNETIC RESONANCE IMAGING (CMRI):
- CMR with its tissue characterization properties aids in determining specific etiologies such as sarcoid and myocarditis, and directs further investigations and cause-specific treatment. Using a combination of T1 mapping, ECV fraction, and LGE helps in optimal risk stratification for patients with DCM.

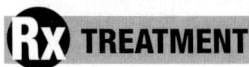 **TREATMENT**

NONPHARMACOLOGIC THERAPY
- Treatment of underlying disease (systemic lupus, alcoholism)
- Dietary sodium restriction (<2 g/day)
- Exercise training has been shown to be associated with reduced risk for hospitalization and death in patients with history of heart failure in limited trials; enrollment in a formal cardiac rehabilitation program may be beneficial in improving patient's functional status

ACUTE GENERAL Rx
- Identify and treat the etiology of the acute exacerbation, when able. A helpful mnemonic is FAILURE: Failure to take medications, Anemia/Arrhythmia, Ischemia/Infection/Infarction, Lifestyle (dietary indiscretion), Upregulation of cardiac output (hyperthyroidism or pregnancy), Renal failure, Embolus (pulmonary).
- Diuretics are indicated for all patients with current symptoms or history of heart failure and reduced left ventricular ejection fraction (LVEF) with evidence of volume overload (see "Physical Findings and Clinical Presentation") to improve symptoms. Although diuretics are the mainstay for treatment for heart failure exacerbations, it is important to note that diuretics have not been shown to improve mortality rates.
- Patients with associated coronary atherosclerosis (angina, ECG changes, reversible defects on myocardial perfusion imaging) may benefit from percutaneous or surgical revascularization.

CHRONIC Rx
- Diuretics as noted in "Acute General Rx."
- ACE inhibitors (and angiotensin receptor blockers) have been shown to have favorable effects on ventricular remodeling in patients with cardiomyopathy and a demonstrable mortality benefit in these patients. They also reduce afterload and improve cardiac output. Recommended in all patients with reduced LV systolic function (EF ≤40%), regardless of symptoms unless specific contraindications exist.
- Beta-blockers work by inhibiting the adverse effects of the sympathetic nervous system in patients with ventricular systolic dysfunction (EF ≤40%). *Only* carvedilol, long-acting metoprolol succinate, and bisoprolol have shown a mortality benefit in patients with LV systolic dysfunction. Unless specifically contraindicated, they should be started after the acute exacerbation has resolved and titrated to the maximum tolerated dose.
- Aldosterone antagonists (spironolactone and eplerenone) have shown mortality benefit along with a decreased rate of hospitalization for heart failure in patients with symptomatic heart failure and reduced LV systolic function (EF ≤35%). They should be used following label guidelines and with close monitoring of renal function and potassium.
- Hydralazine/nitrates improve both morbidity and mortality and should be considered in the following populations: African Americans with persistent NYHA class III or IV heart failure with an EF <40% on optimal medical therapy (beta-blocker and ACE or ARB) or for those unable to take ACE inhibitors or ARBs due to intolerance, hypotension, or renal insufficiency.
- Digoxin is used for its positive inotropic effects in heart failure due to systolic dysfunction. It has no mortality benefit but has been shown to improve patients' quality of life in appropriately selected patients.
- Angiotensin receptor–neprilysin inhibitor (ARNI), sacubitril-valsartan (LCZ696 or Entresto), approved in the U.S. in 2015, was developed to block harmful effects of renin-angiotensin-aldosterone system (RAAS) activation while raising levels of endogenous vasoactive peptides degraded by neprilysin, such as natriuretic peptides, bradykinin, and adrenomedullin. Used in place of an ACE inhibitor or angiotensin receptor blocker and on top of optimal medical therapy in patients with class II to IV heart failure and an EF of 40% or less was found to significantly reduce multiple heart failure end points, including death, hospitalizations, and CV death in comparison to enalapril.[4,5]
- SGLT2 inhibitors, dapagliflozin, and empagliflozin have been found to reduce the combined risk of cardiovascular death or hospitalization for heart failure in patients with reduced left ventricular ejection fraction <40% when added to GDMT in patients regardless of diabetes status. The FDA approved dapagliflozin in 2020 followed by approval of empagliflozin in 2021.[5-7]

Ivabradine was FDA approved in 2015 for patients with stable, symptomatic chronic heart failure with left ventricular ejection fraction ≤35% who are in sinus rhythm with resting heart rates ≥70 beats/min and either of the following: (1) are on maximally tolerated doses of beta-blockers or (2) have a contraindication to beta-blocker use. It acts by blocking the hyperpolarization-activated cyclic nucleotide-gated (HCN) channel responsible for the cardiac pacemaker I_f current, which regulates heart rate.[7,8]

DISPOSITION
- Annual mortality rate is 20% in patients with moderate heart failure, and it exceeds 50% in patients with severe heart failure. Once symptomatic, hospitalizations are frequent and readmission rates are high (>50% at 3 mo). A multispecialty treatment approach (e.g., primary care, cardiology, nutrition, and cardiac rehabilitation) is recommended.[8,9]
- Factors associated with an adverse outcome in dilated cardiomyopathy are described in Table 2.

REFERRAL
The current guidelines recommend ICD as a Class IIa indication for primary prevention in

TABLE 2 Factors Associated With an Adverse Outcome in Dilated Cardiomyopathy

Clinical	Noninvasive	Invasive
NYHA Class III/IV	Low LV ejection fraction	High LV filling pressures
Increasing age	Marked LV dilation	
Low exercise peak oxygen consumption	Low LV mass	
Marked intraventricular conduction delay	≥Moderate mitral regurgitation	
Complex ventricular arrhythmias	Abnormal diastolic function	
Abnormal signal-averaged ECG	Abnormal contractile reserve	
Evidence of excessive sympathetic stimulation	Right ventricular dilation or dysfunction	
Protodiastolic gallop (S₃)		
Elevated serum BNP		
Elevated uric acid		
Decreased serum sodium		

BNP, Brain natriuretic peptide; *ECG,* electrocardiogram; *LV,* left ventricular; *NYHA,* New York Heart Association.
From Hare JM: The dilated, restrictive, and infiltrative cardiomyopathies. In Bonow RO et al (eds): *Braunwald's heart disease—a textbook of cardiovascular medicine,* ed 9, St Louis, 2011, Saunders.

nonischemic DCM, symptomatic HF, and LVEF ≤35% after 3 mo of optimal medical therapy. Patients with LVEF <35%, left bundle branch block on ECG (QRS ≥0.13 sec), and persistent heart failure symptoms may benefit from cardiac resynchronization therapy via a biventricular device.

- Patients should be referred to genetic counseling concurrent with genetic testing.
- Consider heart transplantation for relatively young patients (there is no precise age threshold) free of other significant comorbid conditions who are unresponsive to medical therapy. Dilated cardiomyopathy is the reason for 45% of all heart transplantations in the U.S.

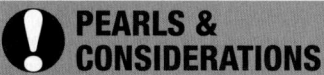

PEARLS & CONSIDERATIONS

COMMENTS

- Patients should be encouraged to restrict or eliminate alcohol and reduce sodium intake (<2 g daily).

- Patients may benefit from daily weight checks as a means of early detection of volume overload and decompensated heart failure.
- Vulnerability to cardiomyopathy among chronic alcohol abusers is partially genetic and related to the presence of the ACE DD genotype.
- Idiopathic dilated cardiomyopathy is often familial, and apparently healthy relatives may have latent, early, or undiagnosed disease. Echocardiographic evaluation of family members is recommended.
- Recent studies have shown Myocardial CD3+ T-lymphocyte count from EMB was an independent predictive biomarker for poor outcomes in DCM.[10]
- Genetic testing is recommended in all patients with familial DCM and should be considered in patients with sporadic DCM. Genetic testing is currently associated with the identification of a culprit variant of ~15% to 25% in patients with sporadic DCM and ~20% to 40% in patients with familial DCM.[3,4,11]

- Screening of asymptomatic first-degree family members of an individual with DCM can allow early detection of DCM, prompt initiation of treatment, and improvement in long-term outcome.
- Risk scores such as the Krakow DCM Risk Score and Madrid Genotype Score have been proposed to identify high-risk DCM patients and predict pathogenic genotypes in DCM patients respectively.[11,12]

RELATED CONTENT

Dilated Cardiomyopathy (Patient Information)
Cardiomyopathy, Chemical Induced (Related Key Topic)

AUTHORS: **SANA RIAZ, MBBS** and **JENNIFER BELL, MD**

REFERENCES

Available at eBooks.Health.Elsevier.com.

C

Diseases and Disorders

I

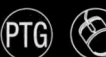

 BASIC INFORMATION

DEFINITION

Hypertrophic cardiomyopathy (HCM) is most commonly an autosomal dominant myocardial disorder characterized by myofibrillar disarray, fibrosis, and marked thickening (hypertrophy) of the left ventricular (LV) wall (≥15 mm), without dilation *not explained by another cardiac or systemic disorder*. The interventricular septum is the most common site of enlargement (Fig. E1), though hypertrophy may involve other focal regions or may be concentric. HCM may result in hemodynamically significant obstruction within the left ventricular outflow tract (LVOT) and/or impairment of the diastolic function of the left ventricle. However, about one-third of patients have no obstruction at rest or with provocation.

SYNONYMS

HCM
Hypertrophic cardiomyopathy
Idiopathic hypertrophic subaortic stenosis (IHSS)
Hypertrophic obstructive cardiomyopathy (HOCM)
Hypertrophic nonobstructive cardiomyopathy
Asymmetric septal hypertrophy (ASH)
Familial hypertrophic cardiomyopathy

ICD-10CM CODES
I42.1	Obstructive hypertrophic cardiomyopathy (includes hypertrophic subaortic stenosis)
I42.2	Other hypertrophic cardiomyopathy (includes nonobstructive hypertrophic cardiomyopathy)
I42.8	Other cardiomyopathies
I42.9	Cardiomyopathy, unspecified (includes cardiomyopathy [primary] [secondary] not otherwise specified)

EPIDEMIOLOGY & DEMOGRAPHICS

- Prevalence in the general population in the U.S., China, and Japan is estimated to be between 1/500 and 1/200 (the most common genetically transmitted cardiovascular disease).[1]
- HCM is the most common cause of sudden cardiac death in young athletes (more commonly among blacks).
- There is equal prevalence in men and women (probably underdiagnosed in women).
- Women with HCM have a worse prognosis.[2]
- It occurs across ethnicities (probably underdiagnosed in blacks).
- The mortality rate is ~1%/yr, as high as 2%/yr in children.[1]
- The most common form of the disease is familial (60% to 70% of cases), and it follows an autosomal dominant inheritance pattern with variable expression.
- Spontaneous mutations can also occur, accounting for ~20% of cases. It is otherwise indistinguishable from the familial form.
- A variant form seen in the elderly (5% to 10% of cases) has a better prognosis and is not typically associated with sudden cardiac death.

- The familial form is usually diagnosed in young patients. It is most often caused by a mutation in one of the contractile protein genes of the cardiac sarcomere. (See "Etiology" for more details.)
- Nonsarcomeric genetic mutations that cause storage disease (e.g., Fabry disease) have a similar clinical presentation.
- Apical HCM is a variant more common among Asians: As many as 41% of Chinese HCM and 15% of Japanese HCM patients. Clinically, there is no LVOT obstruction.

PHYSICAL FINDINGS & CLINICAL PRESENTATION

The clinical presentation of HCM varies widely. Patients may have subtle symptoms of progressive congestive heart failure (CHF). At the time of diagnosis, most patients are asymptomatic, referred, and diagnosed based on family history. HCM may be suspected based on abnormalities found on physical examination. Classic findings include:
- Harsh, systolic, crescendo–decrescendo murmur at the left sternal border or apex. The murmur increases with maneuvers that decrease venous return or LV size (Valsalva, standing) and decreases with those that increase venous return or afterload (squatting, hand grip, post-Valsalva release).
- Paradoxical splitting of S2 (if LV is present).
- S4 may be present.
- Double or triple LV apical impulse ("triple ripple"): Atrial contraction, early rapid ejection, and late slow ejection).
- Pulsus bisferiens (double pulsation on palpation of the carotid pulse).
Increased obstruction can occur with:
- Drugs: Digitalis, β-adrenergic stimulators (isoproterenol, dopamine, epinephrine), nitroglycerin, vasodilators, diuretics, alcohol, inhalation of amyl nitrate
- Hypovolemia
- Tachycardia
- Valsalva maneuver
- Standing position
Decreased obstruction is seen with:
- Drugs: β-adrenergic blockers, calcium channel blockers, disopyramide, α-adrenergic stimulators
- Volume expansion
- Bradycardia
- Hand-grip exercise
- Squatting position
- Release phase of the Valsalva maneuver
Clinical manifestations are as follows:
- Syncope or presyncope (usually seen with exercise)
- Angina
- Palpitations
- Sudden cardiac death
- Heart failure (typically with advanced stages): Dyspnea on exertion, orthopnea, edema, increased jugular venous pressure, paroxysmal nocturnal dyspnea

ETIOLOGY

- Genetic: Autosomal dominant trait with variable penetrance caused by mutations in multiple

genes encoding proteins of the cardiac sarcomere and calcium regulation. To date, >1400 mutations have been identified among at least 13 genes, with variable phenotypes, expressivity, and penetrance.[3] The most vigorous evidence indicates that eight genes are known to definitively cause HCM: Beta myosin heavy chain, myosin binding protein C, troponin T, troponin I, tropomyosin alpha-1 chain, actin, regulatory light chain, and essential light chain. HCM may be caused by a single mutation in one of two alleles; however, 5% of patients have at least two mutations. Sarcomeric protein gene mutations account for up to 60% of cases of HCM.[4]
- Metabolic: Most are autosomal recessive, but some are X-linked. Most commonly, they are due to Anderson-Fabry disease (a lysosomal storage disease). Other metabolic etiologies include the glycogen storage diseases Pompe and Danon, AMP-kinase (PRKAG2), and carnitine disorders.[5]
- Mitochondrial: These comprise autosomal dominant, autosomal recessive, X-linked, and maternally inherited traits. Most frequently, they are due to mutations in the respiratory chain protein complexes. The age of onset and severity of involvement are variable.
- Neuromuscular: These are most commonly associated with Friedreich ataxia but are also associated with *FHL1*.[5]
- Malformation syndromes: These etiologies include Noonan (formerly referred to as LEOPARD), Costello, and Cardiofaciocutaneous Syndrome.
- Amyloidosis includes familial ATTR, wild-type TTR (senile), and amyloid light-chain (AL) amyloidosis.
- Drug-induced: Tacrolimus, hydroxychloroquine, and steroids.
- Sporadic occurrence.

Dx **DIAGNOSIS**

DIFFERENTIAL DIAGNOSIS

- Hypertensive heart disease
- Valvular and subvalvular aortic stenosis
- Athlete's heart
- Infiltrative cardiomyopathy

WORKUP

- Medical history: Unexplained clinical manifestations and/or family history of sudden death.
- Physical examination: See "Physical Findings & Clinical Presentation."
- Genetic counseling with or without testing. All first-degree family members of HCM patients should undergo disease screening.
- ECG is abnormal in 75% to 95% of patients, although no pathognomonic findings exist. Typical findings include: LV hypertrophy (abnormally tall R waves in the precordial leads) in up to 80% of patients (Fig. E2).
- Echocardiography (Fig. 3) is usually diagnostic because the majority of patients have significant LV hypertrophy (see "Imaging Studies" for details) and should be repeated every 12 to 24 mo or as clinically indicated.

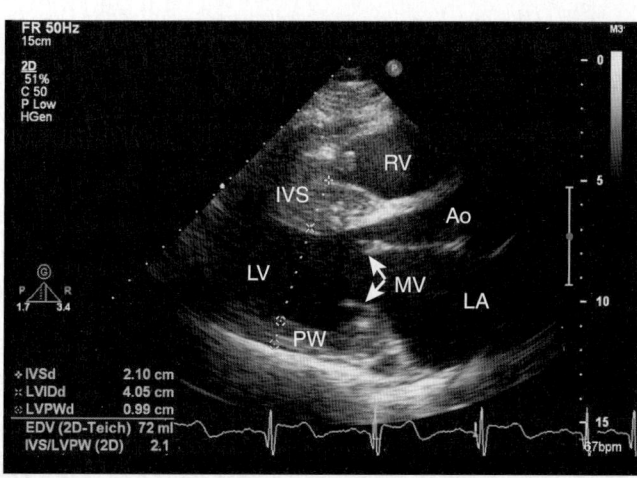

FIG. 3 Echocardiographic appearance of hypertrophic cardiomyopathy. Parasternal long-axis view from a patient with hypertrophic cardiomyopathy demonstrating asymmetric septal hypertrophy. The interventricular septum (marked by *arrow*) measures 2.1 cm; the posterior wall measures 0.99 cm. *Ao,* Aorta; *IVS,* interventricular septum; *LA,* left atrium; *LV,* left ventricle; *MV,* mitral valve; *PW,* posterior wall; *RV,* right ventricle. (From Issa Z et al: *Clinical arrhythmology and electrophysiology,* ed 2, Philadelphia, 2012, Saunders.)

- For patients suspected to have HCM and in whom echocardiography is inconclusive, cardiac magnetic resonance imaging (CMRI) can be performed for diagnosis clarification or risk stratification.[6]
- 24 to 48 h Holter monitoring to screen for potentially lethal ventricular arrhythmias (the principal cause of syncope or sudden death in obstructive cardiomyopathy) should be performed at the initial diagnosis and in patients who subsequently develop palpitations, lightheadedness, or syncope. The presence of these arrhythmias identifies patients who are candidates for implantable cardioverter-defibrillator (ICD) therapy.
- In the absence of significant LVOT obstruction, exercise testing is indicated at diagnosis and annually to evaluate for symptoms and response to exercise. A drop in systolic blood pressure by at least 20 mm Hg or failure to augment by at least 20 mm Hg with exercise are markers of poor prognosis. They are indicators for referral for myotomy/myomectomy. Cardiopulmonary exercise testing can provide objective evidence for worsening diseases but must be performed every 2 to 3 yr.
- Biomarkers of myocardial fibrosis in HCM include brain natriuretic peptide and high-sensitivity cardiac troponin T and I. Other laboratories include CBC, basic metabolic panel, liver function test, thyroid-stimulating hormone, serum protein electrophoresis, and urine protein electrophoresis free light chain ratio (kappa/lambda).
- Screening for sarcomere protein gene mutations in family members of patients with HCM can identify a broad subgroup with an increased propensity toward long-term impairment of LV function and adverse outcomes, irrespective of the myofilament (thick, intermediate, or thin) involvement.[5]
- Specific sarcomere mutation does not predict the prognosis or the risk of sudden death. In individuals with pathogenic mutations who

do not express the HCM phenotype, it is recommended to perform serial ECG, transthoracic echocardiogram (TTE), and clinical assessment at periodic intervals (12 to 24 mo in children and adolescents and 3 to 5 yr in adults), based on the patient's age and change in clinical status.
- Endomyocardial biopsy may be helpful to rule out diseases other than HCM if a diagnosis remains inconclusive after extensive testing.

IMAGING STUDIES
- Chest x-ray film may be normal or show cardiomegaly.
- Two-dimensional echocardiography is the hallmark of HCM diagnosis and assesses the severity of obstruction when present. LV wall thickness will usually be ≥15 mm (although some may be genetically positive, but phenotype negative), and most patients (up to 95%) will have asymmetric (ratio of septum thickness to LV wall thickness >1.3:1) LV wall hypertrophy. Symmetric LV hypertrophy is less common. The septum is most often affected, followed by the LV mid-cavity and apex. In apical HCM, the use of contrast to assess for apical aneurysms is suggested. In addition, 25% to 30% of patients will manifest systolic anterior motion (SAM) of the anterior leaflet of the mitral valve, causing obstruction of the LVOT and mitral regurgitation.[7] SAM produces a dynamic, eccentric, posteriorly directed jet of regurgitation. Transesophageal echocardiography should be considered if the underlying mechanism is unclear because intrinsic mitral pathology may alter the therapeutic approach. Two-dimensional strain imaging echocardiography is helpful for the differentiation of HCM and cardiac amyloidosis from other causes of ventricular wall thickening. Up to 80% of HCM patients also will have diastolic dysfunction as evidenced by pulsed mitral valve inflow pattern and tissue Doppler.

- CMRI or cardiac CT may be of diagnostic value when echocardiographic studies are technically inadequate. MRI is also useful in identifying unusual segmental hypertrophy undetectable by standard echocardiography and can detect myocardial replacement fibrosis (an independent predictor of adverse cardiac outcomes and ventricular arrhythmias) using late gadolinium enhancement. CMRI evaluation may be considered every 5 yr or every 2 to 3 yr in patients with progressive disease.[8]

Rx TREATMENT

NONPHARMACOLOGIC THERAPY
- Avoid volume depletion: An underfilled left ventricle causes a closer approximation of the hypertrophic interventricular septum and anterior mitral valve leaflet, worsening the outflow tract obstruction and mitral regurgitation, potentially leading to dizziness, hypotension, and/or syncope.
- Avoid medications that worsen dynamic LVOT obstruction.
- Exercise: The risk of sudden cardiac death is increased by exercise in certain high-risk athletes with HCM, and rapid heart rates may cause LV underfilling, as described earlier; therefore, participation in competitive sports and intense physical activity should be avoided. Low-to-moderate intensity recreational exercise is beneficial as part of a healthy lifestyle. For athletes with HCM, a comprehensive evaluation and shared discussion of potential risks of sports participation by an expert provider is recommended.
- Avoid alcohol: Alcohol use (even in small amounts) may increase LVOT obstruction. Other stimulants such as cocaine and other sympathomimetic recreational drugs should also be avoided.

ACUTE GENERAL Rx
- Therapy for HCM is directed at blocking the effect of catecholamines and generally avoiding vasodilator or diuretic agents that can exacerbate the dynamic LVOT obstruction.[3,7,9]
- Beta-blockers have beneficial effects on symptoms (principally dyspnea and chest pain) and exercise tolerance appear to be largely a result of a decrease in the heart rate with consequent prolongation of diastole and increased passive ventricular filling. By reducing the inotropic response, beta-blockers may also reduce myocardial oxygen demand and decrease the outflow gradient during exercise, when sympathetic tone is increased. Dose titration to a resting heart rate of less than 65 bpm is recommended.
- Nondihydropyridine calcium channel blockers (e.g., verapamil [preferred], or diltiazem) can also decrease LV outflow obstruction through a mechanism similar to beta-blockers. However, they are mainly second-line agents used in patients who cannot tolerate beta-blockers as they also theoretically have vasodilatory properties that may worsen severe outflow tract gradients.

- Disopyramide is an antiarrhythmic that is also a negative inotrope, resulting in further decrease in outflow gradient. It is sometimes used in combination with beta-blockers.
- Cardiac myosin inhibitors (mavacamten) in recent trials demonstrated efficacy in reduction of LVOT obstruction and improvement of symptoms in patients with obstructive HCM and was approved for use in 2022.[10,11]
- Prophylactic antibiotics before dental, GI, and genitourinary procedures are no longer recommended according to the American Heart Association (AHA) guidelines.
- Avoid use of digitalis, intravenous inotropes, dihydropyridine calcium channel blockers (e.g., nifedipine, amlodipine), nitrates, and vasodilators.
- Diuretics, ACE inhibitors, and angiotensin receptor blockers should be used with caution.
- Intravenous phenylephrine (or another pure vasoconstricting agent) is recommended for the treatment of acute hypotension in patients with obstructive HCM who do not respond to fluid administration.
- ICDs are a safe and effective therapy in HCM patients prone to ventricular arrhythmias. Patient selection for ICD placement is illustrated in Fig. 4. In their practice guidelines, the major cardiology societies (AHA/ACC/HRS) give a strong recommendation (Class I) for ICD implantation in all patients with HCM who have had an episode of sustained ventricular tachycardia or fibrillation. In addition, they endorse the prophylactic placement of an ICD (Class IIa recommendation) for patients with one or more of the major risk factors for sudden cardiac death (outlined in "Disposition"). In patients with reduced ejection fraction (EF) of ≤50%, an ICD placement may be beneficial (Class IIa).[8]
- Dual-chamber pacing may provide symptomatic relief of symptoms attributable to LVOT obstruction and refractory to medical therapy; however, the role is very limited (Class IIb indication per ACC/AHA/HRS guidelines).[8]
- Biventricular pacing for treatment of NYHA functional class II and III heart failure in HCM patients is generally reserved for patients with left bundle branch block, whose EF remained <50%, despite guideline-directed therapy.
- Systolic dysfunction in patients with HCM is defined as an EF of ≤50%, at which point medical therapy should follow guidelines for heart failure with reduced EF (ACE inhibitors, angiotensin II receptor blockers, beta-blockers, etc.).
- HCM patients are at an increased risk of atrial fibrillation (AF) as well as systemic thromboembolism. AF occurs in >20% of the HCM population. AF is an important source of symptoms, morbidity, and mortality and correlates to a worse prognosis. Anticoagulation for AF is indicated independent of CHA_2DS_2-VASc score and should aim for thromboembolic risk mitigation with direct-acting oral anticoagulants as a first-line option, a vitamin K antagonist as a second-line option, and symptom alleviation via rhythm (generally preferred due to poor tolerance of AF with HCM) or rate control.[8,12]
- Gene-silencing agents are under investigation as targeted treatment for HCM patients.[10,11]
- Fig. 5 illustrates management of symptoms in patients with hypertrophic cardiomyopathy.

DISPOSITION

HCM is not a static disease. Some adults may experience subtle regression in wall thickness, whereas others (~5% to 10%) paradoxically evolve into an end-stage cardiomyopathy resembling dilated cardiomyopathy, characterized by cavity enlargement, LV wall thinning, and systolic dysfunction. Patients with HCM are at increased risk for sudden death, especially if the onset of symptoms began during childhood. Severe LV outflow obstruction at rest is also a strong, independent predictor of severe symptoms of heart failure and death. ICD implantation for primary prevention should be considered if patients (particularly the young) have at least one of the following high-risk features:

- Personal history of sudden cardiac death or out of hospital cardiac arrest (major risk factor) (Class I)[8]
- Spontaneous sustained ventricular tachycardia or ventricular fibrillation (major risk factor) (Class I)[8]
- Family history of premature death in a first-degree relative possibly caused by HCM
- Unexplained syncope
- Nonsustained ventricular tachycardia during Holter monitoring
- Substantial septal hypertrophy (>30 mm)
- LV apical aneurysm
- Abnormal blood pressure response during exercise
- Increased delayed gadolinium enhancement on cardiac MRI

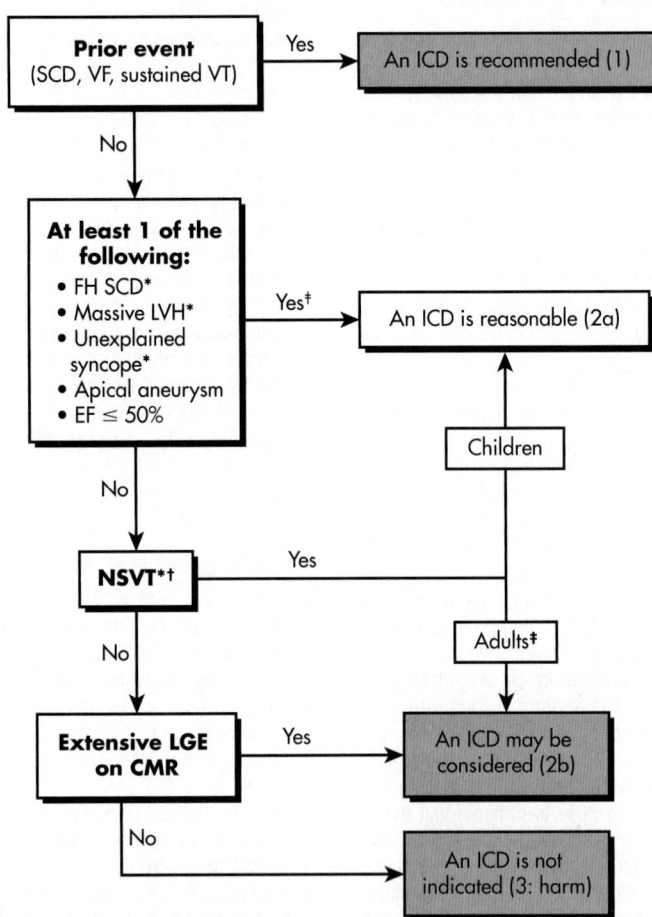

FIG. 4 Patient selection for ICD placement. *ICD decisions in pediatric patients with HCM are based on ≥1 of these major risk factors: family history of HCM SCD, NSVT on ambulatory monitor, massive LVH, and unexplained syncope. †It would seem most appropriate to place greater weight on frequent, longer, and faster runs of NSVT. ‡In patients >16 yr of age, 5-yr risk estimates can be considered to fully inform patients during shared decision-making discussions. *CMR*, Cardiovascular magnetic resonance; *EF*, ejection fraction; *FH*, family history; *HCM*, hypertrophic cardiomyopathy; *ICD*, implantable cardioverter-defibrillator; *LGE*, late gadolinium enhancement; *LVH*, left ventricular hypertrophy; *NSVT*, nonsustained ventricular tachycardia; *SCD*, sudden cardiac death; *VF*, ventricular fibrillation; *VT*, ventricular tachycardia. (Adapted from Ommen SR et al: AHA/ACC guideline for the diagnosis and treatment of patients with hypertrophic cardiomyopathy: a report of the American College of Cardiology/American Heart Association Joint Committee on Clinical Practice Guidelines, *J Am Coll Cardiol* 76[25]:e159-e240, 2020. In: Libby P et al: *Braunwald's heart disease, a textbook of cardiovascular medicine*, ed 12, Philadelphia, 2022, Elsevier.)

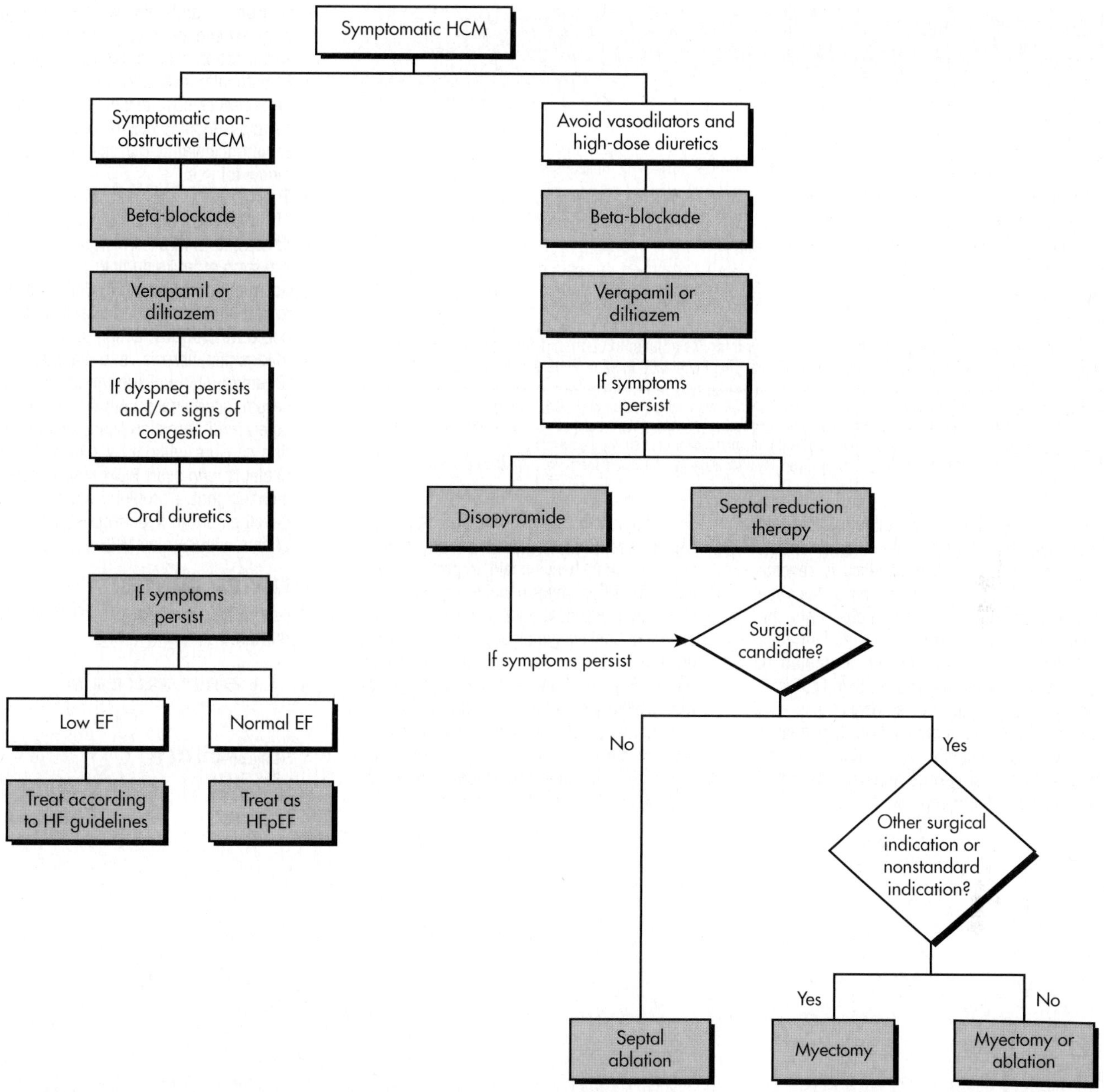

```
                    ┌──────────────────┐
                    │  Symptomatic HCM │
                    └──────────────────┘
```

FIG. 5 Management of symptoms in patients with hypertrophic cardiomyopathy. (From Libby P et al: *Braunwald's heart disease, a textbook of cardiovascular medicine,* ed 12, Philadelphia, 2022, Elsevier.)

REFERRAL

- Surgical treatment (septal myectomy involving resection of the basal septum) is now the gold standard for relieving outflow tract obstruction in patients with large outflow gradient (≥50 mm Hg) and moderate to severe symptoms unresponsive to medical therapy.[8,13] The risk for sudden death from arrhythmias is not altered by surgery. When this operation is performed by experienced surgeons in tertiary referral centers, the operative mortality rate is <1%, and many patients are able to achieve near-normal exercise capacity after surgery. Mitral valvuloplasty or plication in combination with myectomy may be necessary in <5% of patients. Risks of surgery include AV nodal block, ventricular septal defect, and aortic regurgitation (AR).

- Alcohol septal ablation is a nonsurgical alternative to reduce the size of the interventricular septum.[12] This can be done in patients with HCM refractory to pharmacologic treatment, particularly in those who are not candidates for myectomy due to high surgical risk or patient preference. This technique involves the injection of ethanol in a septal perforator branch of the left anterior descending coronary artery (Fig. E6), producing a controlled myocardial infarction of the interventricular septum, and thereby reducing septal mass and consequently the LVOT gradient. This method may lead to improvement in both subjective and objective measures of exercise capacity, but results are not as effective as surgery because they are associated with a high incidence of heart block, requiring

permanent pacing in ~25% of patients, and/or recurrence of obstruction and symptoms. This should be done only at centers with experienced operators.

- Refractory end-stage heart failure symptoms can be treated with an LV assist device, a biventricular assist device, or a heart transplant.

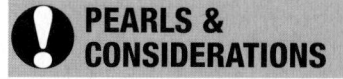

COMMENTS

- Clinical screening of first-degree relatives with two-dimensional echocardiography and ECG is indicated. Starting at the age of 12, periodic screening at 12- to 24-mo intervals is recommended for children of patients with

TABLE 1 Proposed Clinical Family Screening Strategies With Echocardiography or Cardiovascular Magnetic Resonance (and 12-Lead Electrocardiography) for Detection of HCM With Left Ventricular Hypertrophy*

Age <12 yr

Optional unless:

Malignant family history of premature death from HCM or other adverse complications

Competitive athlete in an intense training program

Onset of symptoms

Other clinical suspicion of early left ventricular hypertrophy

Age 12-21 yr†

Every 12-24 mo

Age >21 yr

Imaging at onset of symptoms, or possibly at 3- to 5-yr intervals at least through midlife; more frequent intervals for imaging are appropriate in families with malignant clinical course or history of late-onset HCM

*In family members who had not undergone genetic testing or in whom testing was unresolved or indeterminant.
†Age range takes into consideration individual variability in achieving physical maturity, and in some patients, screening may be justified at an earlier age; initial evaluation should be performed no later than early pubescence.
From Maron BJ et al: Genetics of hypertrophic cardiomyopathy after 20 years: clinical perspectives, *J Am Coll Cardiol* 60:705, 2012.

HCM and in competitive athletes. Periodic screening of first-degree adult family members not in competitive athletics is recommended at 3- to 5-yr intervals because hypertrophy may not be detected until the sixth decade of life. If the index patient does not have a definite pathogenic mutation, genetic testing of relatives is not indicated.

- Genetic counseling and screening (Fig. E7, Table 1) are recommended in first-degree relatives of patients with HCM. Genetic screening of first-degree relatives can refine or eliminate the need for periodic clinical screening. At least 13 genes are known to cause HCM: Cardiac myosin binding protein-C, beta-myosin heavy chain, troponin T, troponin I, alpha tropomyosin, actin regulatory light chain, and essential light chain. Clinical predictors of positive genotype, such as the presence of ventricular arrhythmias, age at diagnosis, degree of LV wall hypertrophy, and family history of HCM, may aid in patient selection for genetic testing and increase the yield of cardiac sarcomere gene screening. Currently, a mutation can be identified in 40% to 60% of all cases, sporadic or familial.[5,8,14]

- All HCM patients who wish to become pregnant should be given prenatal counseling about the risk of transmission (about 50%) to their offspring and followed at a tertiary care center specializing in high-risk pregnancies. Most patients with HCM tolerate pregnancy well due to the higher circulating blood volume.
- The mortality rate in HCM is approximately 1% to 2% per year.
- About one-third of HCM patients will not have a resting or labile outflow gradient (i.e., non-obstructive form of HCM). Still, it is important to note that lethal ventricular arrhythmias can occur without obstruction or symptoms.
- Myocardial fibrosis is a hallmark of HCM. (Biomarkers of collagen metabolism such as serum C-terminal propeptide of type I procollagen [PICP] are significantly higher in mutation carriers without LV hypertrophy and in subjects with overt HCM than in controls, indicating that a probiotic state precedes the development of hypertrophy of fibrosis identifiable with cardiac MRI).[15]

RELATED CONTENT

Hypertrophic Cardiomyopathy (Patient Information)

AUTHOR: **JEFFREY CHILCOTE II, MD**

REFERENCES

Available at eBooks.Health.Elsevier.com.

BASIC INFORMATION

DEFINITION

Restrictive cardiomyopathy is a rare form of cardiomyopathy that refers to either an idiopathic or a secondary myocardial disorder (in the absence of ischemic, hypertensive, valvular, or congenital heart disease) characterized by restrictive filling (Fig. E1). Other features include normal or reduced left ventricular (LV) and right ventricular (RV) volumes with diastolic dysfunction, and normal or near normal systolic LV and RV function.[1] Restrictive cardiomyopathy may result from inherited or acquired diseases, which are broadly classified into several groups such as infiltrative, storage disease, noninfiltrative, and endomyocardial. From a pathophysiologic perspective, the myocardium is abnormally stiff, resulting in decreased compliance, abnormal relaxation in diastole, and increased filling pressures.[2]

SYNONYMS

Idiopathic restrictive cardiomyopathy
Infiltrative cardiomyopathy

ICD-10CM CODES	
I43.1	Cardiomyopathy in metabolic diseases
D86.XX	Sarcoidosis-related codes
E83.11X	Hemochromatosis-related codes
E85.X	Amyloidosis-related codes
I42.5	Other restrictive cardiomyopathy
I42.8	Other cardiomyopathies
I42.9	Cardiomyopathy, unspecified

EPIDEMIOLOGY & DEMOGRAPHICS

- A relatively uncommon cardiomyopathy,[3] accounting for 5% of all primary myocardial diseases.
- Most frequently caused by amyloidosis, sarcoidosis, storage diseases or myocardial fibrosis (following open heart surgery, transplantation, or radiation).
- Patients classified as having "idiopathic" restrictive cardiomyopathy, in whom there is no clear underlying etiology, may have mutations in sarcomere components such as troponin T (TNNT2 gene), troponin I (TNNI3), alpha-actin (ACTC), and beta-myosin heavy chain (MYH7). Mostly inherited in an autosomal dominant pattern.
- Restrictive cardiomyopathy may represent an overlap with hypertrophic cardiomyopathy in many familial cases.

PHYSICAL FINDINGS & CLINICAL PRESENTATION

Restrictive cardiomyopathy presents with symptoms of progressive left-sided and right-sided heart failure:

- Fatigue, weakness (caused by low output as patients are unable to augment cardiac output by increasing heart rate [HR] without compromising ventricular filling).
- Progressively worsening exercise intolerance and dyspnea.

- Anginal chest pain can be seen (particularly in patients with amyloidosis) from myocardial compression of small coronaries and infiltrative deposition in intramural coronary arteries.
- Palpitations (atrial fibrillation is common), dizziness, or syncope (from orthostasis, heart block, or malignant arrhythmia).
- Edema, jugular venous distention.
- In later stages, there may be overt symptoms and signs of liver dysfunction (e.g., ascites, hepatomegaly).
- Kussmaul sign may be present (rise, or failure to fall, of the jugular veins on inspiration).
- On auscultation, murmurs of mitral or tricuspid regurgitation may be heard; an S3 may be present.
- Apical impulse may be palpable (can help distinguish it from constrictive pericarditis) and nondisplaced.
- There may be a prominent y-descent of the jugular venous pulse on jugular venous tracing caused by rapid ventricular filling in early diastole due to elevated atrial pressures.

ETIOLOGY

Disease may be classified according to pathophysiologic processes:

- Infiltrative:
  1. Amyloidosis (most common overall): The main types include AA, AL, and ATTR (transthyretin-mutated or wild type [commonly known as senile systemic]). AL amyloidosis (also called primary amyloidosis) is a rare plasma cell disorder with overproduction of monoclonal kappa or lambda light chain immunoglobulins that can misfold. AA amyloidosis (also called secondary amyloidosis) is a rare condition seen in the setting of chronic inflammatory states such as rheumatologic diseases, leading to excess production of amyloid fibrils. Wild-type TTR is produced primarily in the liver and is a protein tetramer that breaks into monomers and can deposit into tissues. Mutant TTR is due to a mutation in the TTR gene causing the tetramer protein to break down into monomers.
  2. Sarcoidosis (more commonly causing a dilated cardiomyopathy with regional wall motion abnormalities): A multisystem inflammatory disorder of unknown cause characterized by noncaseating granulomas. Sarcoidosis classically presents with bilateral hilar adenopathy, pulmonary infiltrates, and multiorgan involvement including cardiac, ocular/nervous system, renal, hepatic, and bone marrow. Nevertheless, asymptomatic cardiac involvement is fairly common, and cardiac involvement may precede other organ manifestation. Clinicians should consider the diagnosis of sarcoidosis in otherwise healthy young or middle-age patients who present with cardiac symptoms, conduction disorders, arrhythmias, or heart failure.
  3. Metabolic products such as cysteine (very rare).

- Noninfiltrative:
  1. Idiopathic (familial subtypes may have genetic overlap with hypertrophic cardiomyopathy[4])
  2. Scleroderma
  3. Diabetic cardiomyopathy
- Storage diseases:
  1. Hemochromatosis (more commonly associated with a dilated cardiomyopathy)
  2. Glycogen or other storage diseases (Gaucher, Hurler, Fabry—all rare)
- Endomyocardial:
  1. Endomyocardial fibrosis
  2. Hypereosinophilic syndrome (Loeffler syndrome)
- Iatrogenic:
  1. Drug related (anthracyclines, hydroxychloroquine, serotonin, ergotamine, busulfan, methysergide)
  2. Mediastinal radiation (for breast cancer, Hodgkin lymphoma, and other chest malignancies)
- Carcinoid heart disease
- Metastatic tumors

DIAGNOSIS

The diagnosis of idiopathic or primary restrictive cardiomyopathy is rare and is a diagnosis of exclusion. Diagnosis of restrictive cardiomyopathy relies on a constellation of clinical, laboratory, and imaging findings. The diagnosis of restrictive cardiomyopathy should be suspected in a patient with evidence of diastolic dysfunction with restrictive filling pattern on echocardiogram. Echocardiography-based 2-dimensional and Doppler are essential for determining diastolic dysfunction. Cardiac magnetic resonance (CMR) imaging can aid in the diagnostic process, but the use should be determined on an individual basis. Endomyocardial biopsy (EMB) may also be helpful for establishing a diagnosis.

DIFFERENTIAL DIAGNOSIS

- Constrictive pericarditis (see Table 1)
- Valvular dysfunction (especially aortic stenosis)
- Hypertrophic cardiomyopathy
- Hypertensive heart disease

WORKUP

- CBC with differential (to identify eosinophilia), electrolytes, iron studies, serum renal function studies, liver function tests, plasma brain natriuretic peptide (BNP), monoclonal protein studies, chest x-ray examination, electrocardiogram (ECG), echocardiogram
- Right and left heart catheterization, cardiac computed tomography (CT), and CMR imaging (in select cases)
- Nuclear imaging may be used to screen for ATTR amyloid deposition
- Aspiration biopsy of subcutaneous fat to detect amyloidosis[5]
- Endomyocardial biopsy if diagnostic confirmation needed
- BNP serum levels (>400 pg/ml): There are data suggesting that BNP levels are markedly elevated in restrictive cardiomyopathy but

TABLE 1 Differentiation Between Restrictive Cardiomyopathy and Constrictive Pericarditis

Type of Evaluation	Restrictive Cardiomyopathy	Constrictive Pericarditis
Physical examination	Kussmaul sign present Apical impulse may be prominent Regurgitant murmurs are common	Kussmaul sign may be present Apical impulse usually not palpable Pericardial knock may be present Pulsus paradoxus may be present
Electrocardiography	Low QRS voltage commonly seen in amyloidosis (but up to ¼ of amyloid patients may not have) Pseudoinfarction pattern Bundle branch blocks AV conduction disturbances Atrial fibrillation	Low QRS voltage Repolarization abnormalities
Chest radiography	Cardiomegaly may be present	Calcification of the pericardium may be present
Echocardiography	Marked enlargement of the atria Increased wall thickness (especially in amyloidosis) Valvular thickening (especially in hypereosinophilia)	Atria usually of normal size Normal wall thickness Pericardial thickening may be seen
Doppler echocardiography	Restrictive mitral inflow (dominant E wave with short deceleration time/interventricular relaxation time <70 ms, mitral inflow E/A ratio >2.5) No significant variation of transvalvular velocities with respiration Reversal of forward flow in hepatic veins during inspiration Low tissue Doppler velocities	Restrictive mitral inflow (dominant E wave with short deceleration time) Increased velocity of RV filling and decreased velocity of LV filling with inspiration; opposite with expiration; variation in velocity exceeds 25% Reversal of forward flow in hepatic veins during expiration Increased septal tissue Doppler velocities with below normal lateral velocities (annulus reversus)
Cardiac catheterization	Prominent atrial x and y descents (w sign) Dip-and-plateau appearance of ventricular diastolic pressure Diastolic pressures increased but not equalized (LV diastolic pressure higher than RV diastolic pressure) Ventricular concordance PA systolic pressure often >60 mm Hg	Prominent atrial x and y descents (w sign) Dip-and-plateau appearance of ventricular diastolic pressure Increase and equalization of diastolic pressures Discordance of RV and LV peak systolic pressures (with inspiration, RV systolic pressure increases and LV systolic pressure decreases) Ventricular discordance PA systolic pressure generally <50 mm Hg
Endomyocardial biopsy	May reveal specific cause of restrictive cardiomyopathy	No specific findings on endomyocardial biopsy Pericardial biopsy may reveal abnormality
Computed tomography, magnetic resonance imaging	Late gadolinium myocardial enhancement in certain conditions	Pericardial thickening >2 mm
Laboratory testing	BNP is elevated	BNP may be normal to slightly elevated

AV, Atrioventricular; *BNP*, brain natriuretic peptide; *LV*, left ventricular; *PA*, pulmonary artery; *RV*, right ventricular.
From Andreoli TE et al (eds): *Andreoli and Carpenter's Cecil essentials of medicine*, ed 8, Philadelphia, 2010, Saunders.

near normal in constrictive pericarditis, most likely resulting from the lack of myocardial stretching in constriction that is required for BNP release

- Genetic testing, including testing for transthyretin mutation in amyloidosis[6]

IMAGING STUDIES

- Chest x-ray examination:
  1. Ranges from normal cardiomediastinal silhouette to moderate cardiomegaly (primarily because of biatrial enlargement).
  2. Evidence of heart failure may be present.
  3. Presence of pericardial calcification favors alternative diagnosis of constrictive pericarditis.
- ECG:
  1. Nonspecific ST-T wave abnormalities are the most common finding. Voltage may be low in infiltrative etiologies such as amyloidosis.
  2. Frequent atrial and ventricular ectopy are often present. Atrial fibrillation may be present.
  3. High-degree atrioventricular block, intraventricular conduction delay may be seen in advanced cases.

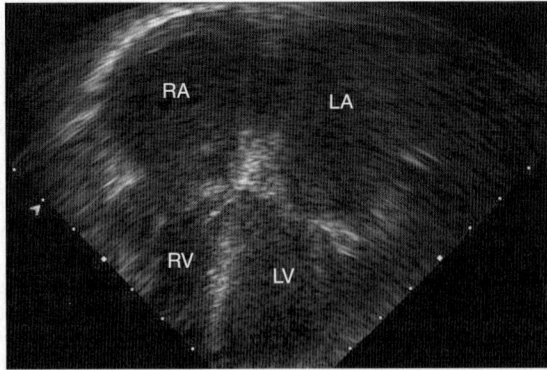

FIG. 2 Echocardiogram of a patient with restrictive cardiomyopathy. The optical four-chamber view shows the markedly enlarged right and left atria, compared to the normal-sized left and right ventricular chambers. *LA*, Left atrium; *LV*, left ventricle; *RA*, right atrium; *RV*, right ventricle. (From Kliegman RM: *Nelson textbook of pediatrics*, ed 21, Philadelphia, 2020, Elsevier.)

- Echocardiogram (Fig. 2):
  1. Biatrial enlargement almost always present.
  2. Wall thickness depends on etiology; often thickened in infiltrative disease.
  3. Myocardial appearance may be altered (speckled pattern with apical sparing suggestive of amyloidosis).[7]
  4. Ventricular chamber sizes and systolic function are often normal or reduced.
  5. Echo Doppler shows evidence of diastolic dysfunction (restrictive physiology). Tissue Doppler demonstrates low mitral annular velocities.
  6. Regional wall motion abnormalities seen in noncoronary artery distribution, aneurysms.

- Cardiac catheterization:
  1. Characteristic hemodynamic findings are a dip and plateau, or square-root sign, in the LV tracing in which a deep and rapid decline in ventricular pressure at the onset of diastole is immediately followed by rapid rise and plateau in early diastolic phase.
  2. To distinguish restrictive cardiomyopathy from constrictive processes (Fig. E3):
     a. Constrictive: Usually involves both ventricles and leads to equalization of diastolic pressures among all four cardiac chambers to within 5 mm Hg. There is discordance in RV and LV pressures generated during inspiration, which is due to increased ventricular interdependence and decreased left atrial filling (caused by a decreased gradient in inspiration between the pulmonary veins, which are outside the constrictive process and the left atrium).
     b. Restrictive cardiomyopathy: Impairs the left ventricle more than the right, often with left-sided end-diastolic pressures of 5 mm Hg greater than the right. The presence of increased pulmonary arterial systolic pressures is also suggestive of restrictive disease. Simultaneous RV and LV pressure tracings demonstrate concordant patterns during the respiratory cycle.
- Cardiac CT scan may be helpful to identify a thickened and calcified pericardium, consistent with constrictive pericarditis. However, ~80% of patients may not have thickened pericardium (so no thickening does not rule out the possibility of constrictive pericarditis).
- CMR imaging may also be useful to distinguish restrictive cardiomyopathy from constrictive pericarditis (thickness of the pericardium >4 mm in the latter).[8] CMR imaging is particularly helpful in the diagnosis of the amyloid or sarcoid variants and may have value in other variants as well. Late gadolinium enhancement can be seen with infiltrative diseases.
- Technetium pyrophosphate bone scintigraphy is useful in diagnosis of transthyretin cardiac amyloidosis and differentiates it from light chain amyloidosis.

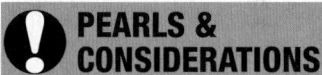

TREATMENT

NONPHARMACOLOGIC THERAPY
Congestive symptoms may respond to dietary sodium restriction (<2 g/day).

ACUTE GENERAL Rx
Treatment of volume overload and heart failure symptoms with diuretic therapy

CHRONIC Rx
- Treatment involves management of the underlying disease if it exists:
  1. Hemochromatosis may respond to repeated phlebotomy and iron chelators to decrease iron deposition in the heart.

  2. Sarcoidosis may respond to corticosteroid therapy.
  3. Primary amyloidosis may respond to chemotherapy (high-dose melphalan paired with dexamethasone, followed by autologous stem cell therapy or bortezomib-based regimens). ATTR may be treated with liver transplant or novel therapeutic agents that inhibit the rate-limiting step in the amyloidogenic process (i.e., tafamidis).
  4. Eosinophilic cardiomyopathy may respond to corticosteroid and cytotoxic drugs.
  5. There is no effective therapy for other causes of restrictive cardiomyopathy.
- Overall, the goal of treatment is to reduce symptoms by decreasing filling pressures while preserving cardiac output. Because there is currently no drug available to specifically act on myocardial relaxation, therapy centers on low-dose diuretics to lower the preload.
- Beta-blockers or calcium channel blockers have not been demonstrated to improve symptoms or alter the course of disease. Must be careful not to decrease HR too far, as this will affect cardiac output ($CO = HR \times$ stroke volume), and many patients are intolerant of their use for this reason. Beta-blockers should also be used with caution in patients without pacemakers with sarcoidosis who are at risk of AV block.
- ACE inhibitors (or angiotensin receptor blockers [ARBs]) and vasodilators should be avoided in patients with amyloidosis as they are poorly tolerated. Even small doses can trigger profound hypotension (probably due to associated autonomic neuropathy).
- Atrial fibrillation is common and patients with it or with a history of embolization should be anticoagulated. Tachycardia (of any cause) is poorly tolerated and a common cause of decompensation. Rate control is of paramount importance. Cardioversion in case of rapid atrial fibrillation should be considered. Of note, digoxin should be used with caution as it is potentially arrhythmogenic (particularly in patients with amyloidosis).
- Fibrosis of the cardiac conduction system may result in complete heart block presenting as dizziness or syncope (especially in amyloidosis) and pacemaker implantation may be required. The course of restrictive cardiomyopathy is variable and depends on the underlying etiology. Death usually results from heart failure or arrhythmias, and interventions aimed at addressing these are recommended.
  1. For the amyloid variant, an implantable cardiac defibrillator offers little prophylactic benefit beyond the ability to pace because the cause of sudden cardiac death is usually electromechanical disassociation.

COMPLEMENTARY & ALTERNATIVE MEDICINE
Patients will report taking various herbs and supplements, such as coenzyme Q, citing health benefit. However, none are evidence-based

therapies shown to improve symptoms or prognosis.

DISPOSITION
Prognosis varies with the etiology of the cardiomyopathy but is poor overall as disease is rarely detected before advanced stages. Most patients progress to end-stage heart failure.

REFERRAL
Cardiac transplantation and/or LV assist device (LVAD) implantation can be considered in patients with refractory heart failure symptoms unresponsive to medical management and idiopathic or familial restrictive cardiomyopathies. Transplantation is a final option for patients with treatment-refractory symptoms of heart failure and for whom long-term survival could be achieved.[9] Early workup and referral are paramount in these patients, as they have the highest waitlist mortality among transplant candidates with severe heart failure. After heart transplantation, there appears to be no significant difference in survival compared to other transplant subgroups.[10]

PEARLS & CONSIDERATIONS

COMMENTS
The prognosis for this condition remains poor despite advances in heart failure therapy. The majority of deaths among patients with idiopathic restrictive cardiomyopathy were cardiovascular in nature, attributable mainly to heart failure, sudden death, stroke, or malignant cardiac arrhythmia.

PREVENTION
Aside from managing diseases with known links to restrictive cardiomyopathy, the vast majority of cases cannot be prevented.

PATIENT & FAMILY EDUCATION
Patients and families should be counseled on the symptomatology, natural course, and prognosis of restrictive cardiomyopathy. As the disease progresses further, it is important to establish goals of care for palliation and to maximize quality of life.

RELATED CONTENT
Restrictive Cardiomyopathy (Patient Information)

AUTHOR: **XUAN YAO, MD**

REFERENCES
Available at eBooks.Health.Elsevier.com.

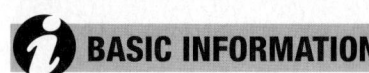

BASIC INFORMATION

DEFINITION

Carotid artery stenosis is narrowing of the carotid arterial lumen, typically as a result of atherosclerosis.

SYNONYM

Atherosclerotic disease of the carotid artery

ICD-10CM CODES	
I65.29	Occlusion and stenosis of unspecified carotid artery
I65.21	Occlusion and stenosis of right carotid artery
I65.22	Occlusion and stenosis of left carotid artery
I65.23	Occlusion and stenosis of bilateral carotid arteries

EPIDEMIOLOGY & DEMOGRAPHICS

INCIDENCE: 2.2 to 8/1000 persons/yr. The incidence of ischemic stroke has declined from about 2% to 1% annually,[1] presumably due to improved medical management over the past 20 yr.

PREVALENCE: 11 to 77/100,000 persons; it is estimated that 5/1000 persons aged 50 to 60 yr and 100/1000 persons >80 yr have carotid stenosis >50%. The incidence of carotid artery stenosis is unknown because screening is not routine. However, the incidence of transient ischemic attack (TIA), a common presenting symptom of carotid stenosis, is well known. Carotid artery stenosis may occur in the cervical portion of the common or internal carotid artery (extracranial carotid stenosis) or in the intracranial portion of the internal carotid artery. Intracranial internal carotid stenosis is a common cause of intracranial atherosclerotic disease (ICAD). Both extracranial and intracranial carotid stenosis is a common type of large vessel atherosclerotic disease. All forms of large vessel atherosclerotic disease, whether extracranial carotid or vertebral disease or ICAD, account for approximately 15% of all ischemic strokes, with carotid disease accounting for the majority of cases.[2]

PREDOMINANT SEX & AGE: Male:female ratio of 2:1.

PEAK INCIDENCE: Peak incidence is between 50 and 60 yr.

RISK FACTORS: Hypertension, dyslipidemia, diabetes mellitus, and smoking are the four major modifiable risk factors; age is the major nonmodifiable risk factor.

GENETICS: Multifactorial; twin studies (monozygotic vs. dizygotic) suggest a familial influence.

PHYSICAL FINDINGS & CLINICAL PRESENTATION

Patients with carotid artery stenosis are often asymptomatic, but many either have a carotid bruit or experience a TIA. Asymptomatic intracranial and extracranial carotid stenosis refer to the absence of ischemic events (TIA or ischemic stroke) within the territory of the stenosed artery or its branches.

- Carotid bruit: The presence of a carotid bruit is a better indicator of generalized atherosclerosis and is thus a better predictor of ischemic heart disease than future stroke.
- TIA: Carotid artery stenosis is classically heralded by ipsilateral transient monocular blindness (amaurosis fugax), contralateral numbness, or weakness or aphasia.

ETIOLOGY

- Atherosclerosis (most common)
- Aneurysm
- Arteritis
- Carotid dissection
- Fibromuscular dysplasia
- Postradiation necrosis
- Vasospasm

ANATOMIC ABNORMALITIES: Normally the right common carotid artery originates from the brachiocephalic artery, whereas the left common carotid artery originates at the arch of the aorta. The carotid arteries then rise through the neck and bifurcate at approximately C4 to form the external and internal carotid arteries. The extracranial segment of the internal carotid artery spans from the common carotid bifurcation up to the carotid canal, where it enters the skull base and then becomes the intracranial portion.

DIAGNOSIS

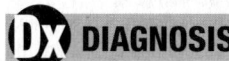

DIFFERENTIAL DIAGNOSIS

Aneurysm, arteritis, and carotid dissection

WORKUP

Systematic history, examination, and diagnostic studies to assess for carotid stenosis and other risk factors of TIA and stroke. Carotid artery stenosis is responsible for ~10% of all ischemic strokes.

LABORATORY TESTS

CBC, comprehensive metabolic panel, fasting lipid profile, prothrombin time/international normalized ratio, activated partial thromboplastin time, Hemoglobin A1C

IMAGING STUDIES

- Four imaging modalities are available for the evaluation of carotid artery stenosis (Table 1).
- Patients with TIA or stroke should be evaluated for carotid artery stenosis via carotid duplex (Fig. E1), magnetic resonance angiography (MRA), or computed tomography angiography (CTA). Diagnostic cerebral angiography may be obtained to confirm the degree of stenosis and plan for intervention (Fig. E2).
- CTA or MRA of the head and neck are the preferred noninvasive modalities for evaluation of intracranial circulation, with diagnostic cerebral angiography being the most accurate.
- The U.S. Preventive Services Task Force recommends against screening for asymptomatic carotid artery stenosis in the general adult population.
- Screening with carotid duplex may be considered in asymptomatic patients with carotid bruit, in those with multiple risk factors for atherosclerosis, or in those with known atherosclerotic disease at other sites such as coronary artery disease, peripheral arterial disease, or abdominal aortic aneurysms.
- Patients identified to have >50% stenosis on carotid duplex may be reimaged annually to assess progression and should have intensive medical management of vascular risk factors.
- Intracranial vs. extracranial carotid stenosis should be noted on imaging evaluation, as treatment options may differ.

TABLE 1 Imaging Modalities for Carotid Stenosis

Imaging Modality	Benefit	Drawback
Cerebral angiography	Gold standard Assesses plaque morphology Assesses presence of collaterals	Invasive High cost 4% incidence rate of complications 1% incidence rate of serious complications or death
Carotid duplex	Sensitive in detecting high-grade stenosis (>70%) Less invasive Lower cost	Can be limited by body habitus Technician dependent Overestimates degree of stenosis May not distinguish high-grade stenosis from complete occlusion
Magnetic resonance angiography (MRA)	Sensitive in detecting high-grade stenosis (>70%) Less operator dependent	Overestimates degree of stenosis Cannot be performed in patients who are critically ill, unable to tolerate supine positioning, have pacemaker or other ferromagnetic hardware, or are claustrophobic* Expensive Takes much longer to obtain compared with other modalities
Computed tomography angiography (CTA)	Sensitive for high-grade stenosis	Contraindicated in patients with serum creatinine concentration >1.5 mg/dl Uses ionizing radiation

*One study revealed that ~17% of patients are unable to tolerate MRA secondary to claustrophobia or are unable to lie still for procedure.

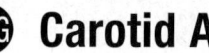

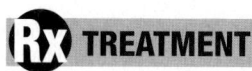 **TREATMENT**

ACUTE GENERAL Rx

- General medical therapy should be aimed at risk factor reduction (see "Stroke, Secondary Prevention"). Antiplatelet therapy plays an important role in the medical treatment. Three antiplatelet options are available for patients with carotid artery stenosis: ASA, ASA plus dipyridamole, or clopidogrel.
- Intracranial carotid stenosis treatment after a stroke or TIA was outlined in the SAMMPRIS (stenting and aggressive medical management for preventing recurrent stroke in intracranial stenosis) trial. SAMMPRIS recommendations included treatment with dual antiplatelet therapy (DAPT) using aspirin and clopidogrel for 90 days after an ischemic event, along with aggressive vascular risk factor modification (see "Stroke, Secondary Prevention") that included body mass index <25 kg/m² and moderate intensity exercise, followed by lifelong ASA monotherapy.
- Asymptomatic extracranial and intracranial carotid stenosis treatment is focused on lowering the risk of stroke. Treatment includes a statin, aspirin, and aggressive risk factor modification, and in selected cases surgical management.

NONPHARMACOLOGIC THERAPY

Carotid endarterectomy (CEA) and carotid angioplasty and stenting (CAS) (Fig. E3) are the two main revascularization options available in extracranial carotid artery stenosis. Recently a new modality of revascularization is also being explored, TCAR (transcarotid artery revascularization). TCAR refers to a combined surgical procedure consisting of open exposure of the vessel and an endovascular approach. The decision on which revascularization procedure to favor depends on whether the stenotic lesion is symptomatic as well as the degree of stenosis, medical comorbidities, operative risk of the patient, and experience and outcomes data of the proceduralist. Factors associated with increased risk from carotid artery surgery are summarized in Table 2.

In a trial involving asymptomatic patients with severe carotid stenosis who were not at high risk for surgical complications, stenting was noninferior to endarterectomy regarding the rate of the primary composite end point at 1 yr. In analyses that included up to 5 yr of follow-up, there were no significant differences between the study groups in the rates of non–procedure-related stroke, all stroke, and survival.

ASYMPTOMATIC EXTRACRANIAL AND INTRACRANIAL CAROTID STENOSIS: The benefit of surgical revascularization of the carotids (CEA or CAS) in asymptomatic patients is not well established. In the U.S., more than 90% of carotid artery interventions are performed in asymptomatic patients, although evidence suggests that up to 90% of these patients are undergoing an ultimately unnecessary and potentially harmful procedure. In contrast, the percentage of

TABLE 2 Factors Associated With Increased Risk From Carotid Artery Surgery

Anatomic Criteria
High cervical or intrathoracic lesion
Previous neck surgery or radiation therapy
Contralateral carotid artery occlusion
Previous ipsilateral carotid endarterectomy
Contralateral laryngeal nerve palsy
Tracheostomy

Medical Comorbidities
Age >80 yr*
Class III or IV congestive heart failure
Class III or IV angina pectoris
Left main coronary disease
Two- or three-vessel coronary artery disease
Need for open heart surgery
Ejection fraction ≤30%
Recent myocardial infarction
Severe chronic obstructive lung disease

*The risk for a cerebrovascular accident (stroke) with carotid artery stent placement is increased, and the risk for myocardial infarction with carotid endarterectomy is increased.

From Libby P et al: *Braunwald's heart disease, a textbook of cardiovascular medicine*, ed 12, Philadelphia, 2022, Elsevier.

interventions performed for asymptomatic stenosis is ~60% in Germany and Italy, 15% in Canada and Australia, and 0% in Denmark.

According to the most recent guidelines, revascularization procedures may be considered in asymptomatic patients with >70% stenosis if the anticipated perioperative risk is <3%, but surgery should be recommended only after considering medical comorbidities and life expectancy and after discussing the risks and benefits in detail with the patients. It is important to note that trials of CEA for asymptomatic carotid stenosis were performed before the era of aggressive medical management of vascular risk factors. Recently launched studies of asymptomatic carotid stenosis vs. aggressive contemporary medical management will answer lingering questions from older studies. In short, patients with asymptomatic stenosis of <50% should never undergo revascularization, but annual duplex surveillance may be undertaken, and aggressive vascular risk factor reduction must be implemented. Asymptomatic carotid stenosis of 50% to 69% warrants intensive vascular risk reduction only. Individuals with asymptomatic stenosis of 70% to 99% may undergo surgical evaluation, although the risk benefit ratio remains uncertain, but such individuals should be placed on maximal medical therapy. A chronically occluded carotid artery should not be revascularized, but intensive medical management of vascular risk factors is indicated.

SYMPTOMATIC EXTRACRANIAL CAROTID STENOSIS: In patients who have suffered a nondisabling ischemic stroke or TIA in the preceding 6 mo, surgical revascularization by CEA is recommended if the degree of carotid stenosis

is severe (70% to 99%) and if the anticipated rate of perioperative stroke or mortality is <6%. The number needed to treat to prevent one stroke in 2 yr is six.

In patients who have suffered a nondisabling ischemic stroke or TIA in the preceding 6 mo and who have moderate carotid stenosis (50% to 69%), CEA is recommended based on an assessment of the patient's age, sex, and comorbidities. To prevent one stroke in 5 yr, 15 patients with moderate carotid stenosis would have to undergo CEA. Factors to consider in recommending CEA for patients with moderate symptomatic carotid stenosis are age, sex, and comorbidities. The NASCET trial, which studied the efficacy of CEA vs. medical management for symptomatic carotid artery stenosis, suggested that women experience higher complication rates from CEA than men. However, the CREST trial, which compared CEA to carotid stenting, did not find a sex-related outcome difference between the two interventions in terms of primary outcome, which was the composite of stroke, myocardial infarction, or death during the periprocedural period or ipsilateral stroke within 4 yr. However, when periprocedural events are examined alone, CREST data suggest that the periprocedural risk of events seems to be higher in women who have CAS than those who undergo CEA, whereas men experience no significant difference in periprocedural risk. CREST also found that patients >70 yr did better with CEA than with carotid stenting. All patients undergoing CEA should be started on aspirin (ASA; 81 or 325 mg/day) and a high-dose statin before surgery. This therapy, along with blood pressure control and aggressive management of other vascular risk factors, should be continued indefinitely.

CAS can be an alternative to CEA in select patients considered to be at high surgical risk or with unfavorable neck anatomy for surgery.

CEA is preferred over CAS in older patients.

For patients undergoing CAS, dual antiplatelet therapy (DAPT) is recommended for a minimum of 30 days followed by single antiplatelet thereafter.

When feasible, early revascularization within 14 days after incident event should be undertaken unless there are definite contraindications. Data suggest that women with symptomatic lesions lose benefit of intervention if the intervention is delayed beyond 14 days after incident event, and the preferred intervention is CEA. For patients undergoing early intervention, CEA is associated with lower periprocedural complication rate than CAS.

Surgical revascularization is inappropriate for <50% stenosis, total carotid occlusion, or in patients with major disabling strokes.

DISPOSITION

Disposition and prognosis depend on several variables (Table 3): The degree of stenosis, the presence of symptoms, medication adherence, and the type of intervention, if any, performed.

ASYMPTOMATIC INTRACRANIAL CAROTID STENOSIS: Asymptomatic ICAD presents a low risk of stroke in its ipsilateral territory;

TABLE 3 Carotid Stenosis Management

Degree of Carotid Artery Stenosis	<50%	50%-69%	70%-99%
Asymptomatic	Medical management	Medical management	Medical management
		Inconclusive evidence base to favor surgical treatment. May be considered in select patients with >60% stenosis.*	CEA in highly selected patients*
Symptomatic	Medical management	CEA	CEA
		CAS can be an alternative	CAS can be an alternative

CAS, Carotid artery stenting; *CEA*, carotid endarterectomy.
*CEA can be considered in asymptomatic patients with >70% stenosis if the anticipated rate of perioperative complications (stroke, myocardial infarction, and death) is <3%, life expectancy is >5 yr, and the risks and benefits (including medical co-morbidities) have been discussed thoroughly with the patients and their families.

however, this risk is markedly increased in symptomatic patients (TIA, stroke). Therefore, the mainstay of treatment is aggressive risk factor modification.

SYMPTOMATIC INTRACRANIAL CAROTID STENOSIS: Symptomatic intracranial carotid stenosis is defined as the occurrence of an ischemic event in the stenotic vessel's territory. SAMMPRIS was not limited to carotid ICAD but extended to large vessel artery stenosis anywhere within the intracranial circulation. SAMMPRIS has established the treatment gold standard of DAPT for 90 days followed by aspirin monotherapy with concomitant aggressive risk factor modification. Currently, there is no role for oral anticoagulants in the treatment of ICAD associated stroke.

ICAD has proven to be a difficult entity to treat. If an ischemic event recurs in the same territory affected previously, the patient should be evaluated by an endovascular specialist, although interventions such as stenting of intracranial vessels remains controversial. Extracranial-intracranial bypass has largely been eliminated as a treatment option in ICAD.

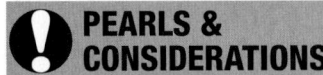

PEARLS & CONSIDERATIONS

The results of ongoing studies concerning the best treatment of patients with carotid artery stenosis may result in guideline changes.

SPECIAL CONSIDERATION

Some studies have shown that in patients with bilateral hemodynamically significant stenosis (>70%), blood pressure reduction resulted in worsened outcomes for stroke. These patients would likely be candidates for CEA.

Symptomatic women with severe carotid stenosis can be managed by CEA provided that the perioperative risk of the operators is low (4%). Although the periprocedural stroke risks may be increased in symptomatic women undergoing CAS, the choice of CAS or CEA should be tailored by subgroups. For example, women with restenosis or severe coronary disease may do best with CAS, whereas those >70 yr of age of having tortuous vessels are best off with CEA.

Both women and men with carotid stenosis should undergo aggressive medical management of cardiovascular risk factors in the periprocedural period and beyond for the rest of their lives regardless of whether they are undergoing revascularization.

Carotid artery occlusion (100% blockage), for which there is no routine treatment, was reexamined in the national Carotid Occlusion Surgery Study (COSS). Recently published results from the COSS trial demonstrate that superficial temporal artery to middle cerebral artery anastomosis does not provide an overall benefit for ipsilateral 2-yr stroke recurrence when compared to medical therapy alone.

PREVENTION

Prevention of carotid stenosis should include pursuit of a healthy lifestyle and management of risk factors for atherosclerosis.

SCREENING

The U.S. Preventive Services Task Force (USP-STF) recommends against screening for asymptomatic carotid stenosis in adults in the general population without a history of stroke or TIA.[3]

PATIENT & FAMILY EDUCATION

Patients should be counseled to pursue a healthy lifestyle including exercise and smoking cessation. In addition, patients should take an active role in controlling blood pressure and blood glucose.

RELATED CONTENT

Carotid Stenosis (Patient Information)
Transient Ischemic Attack (Related Key Topic)

REFERENCES AND SUGGESTED READINGS

Available at eBooks.Health.Elsevier.com.

AUTHORS: **NAOMI R. KASS, BA, CARLOS DE LA GARZA, MD,** and **SHAWN D. MOORE, MD**

BASIC INFORMATION

DEFINITION

Carpal tunnel syndrome (CTS) is a compression neuropathy of the median nerve as it passes under the transverse carpal ligament at the level of the wrist (Figs. E1 and E2). It is the most common compressive neuropathy.

SYNONYMS

CTS
Median nerve compression
Median neuropathy

ICD-10CM CODES

G56.0	Carpal tunnel syndrome, unspecified upper limb
G56.01	Carpal tunnel syndrome, right upper limb
G56.02	Carpal tunnel syndrome, left upper limb
G56.03	Carpal tunnel syndrome, bilateral upper limbs

EPIDEMIOLOGY & DEMOGRAPHICS

INCIDENCE: 3.8% of the general population (the most common entrapment neuropathy).
PREDOMINANT SEX: Females are affected two to five times as often as males.
PREDOMINANT AGE: 40 to 60 yr old

PHYSICAL FINDINGS & CLINICAL PRESENTATION

- Pain and paresthesias in the volar or palmar aspect of the thumb, index finger, middle finger, and radial half of the ring finger (Fig. E3), worse at night, with awakenings from sleep being common. Pain is related to nerve ischemia.
- *Tinel sign* at wrist: Tapping lightly over the median nerve on the volar surface of the wrist produces a tingling sensation radiating from the wrist to the hand.
- *Phalen sign* (Fig. E4): Reproduction of symptoms after 1 min of gentle, unforced wrist flexion.
- **Durkan test:** Direct continual pressure over the patient's carpal tunnel for 30 sec elicits symptoms.
- Thenar atrophy (Fig. E5) in long-standing cases with weakness of thumb abduction and opposition.
- Findings may be bilateral in up to 65% of patients.

ETIOLOGY

- Idiopathic in most cases—caused by increased pressure within the carpal tunnel leading to nerve ischemia.
- Commonly associated with diabetes, increased BMI, female gender, advancing age, pregnancy, hypothyroidism, rheumatologic disorders, amyloidosis, and autoimmune disorders.[1] Related orthopedic pathology includes trigger fingers.

- No objective relationship or causality between jobs with significant keyboard use and CTS, but specific occupations with repetitive impaction in the palm or use of vibratory tools may contribute to the development of CTS.[2,3]
- May also occur due to mass occupying lesions (tenosynovitis, gout, ganglion) or as a result of trauma (distal radius fractures, perilunate and lunate dislocations, etc.).
- Table E1 summarizes conditions associated with carpal tunnel syndrome.

DIAGNOSIS

DIFFERENTIAL DIAGNOSIS

- Cervical radiculopathy
- Cervical myelopathy
- Chronic tendinitis
- Pronator teres syndrome
- Anterior interosseous syndrome
- Complex regional pain syndrome
- Brachial plexopathy, thoracic outlet syndrome
- Polyneuropathy
- Other entrapment neuropathies
- Traumatic wrist injuries
- Vascular disorders (Raynaud syndrome)

IMAGING STUDIES

CTS is a clinical diagnosis, but imaging may assist workup in uncertain situations. Accumulating evidence suggests that diagnostic ultrasound may be almost as sensitive as nerve conduction velocity tests and may help identify the structural cause of nerve compression.[4] X-ray or MRI may be helpful in ruling out other conditions.

ELECTRODIAGNOSTIC STUDIES

Nerve conduction velocity tests (NCS) demonstrate impaired sensory conduction across the carpal tunnel and may help guide treatment based on the severity of median nerve compression. Electromyography may show active denervation muscle potentials. Specificity of NCS and electromyography for CTS is >95%, and sensitivity is >85%.[5]

TREATMENT

ACUTE GENERAL Rx

- Activity modification and ergonomic optimization (desk, keyboard)
- Nocturnal wrist splint has been shown to be effective by preventing prolonged wrist flexion or extension while sleeping
- No evidence for effectiveness of NSAIDs as a cure, but do provide short term pain relief
- Corticosteroid injection of carpal canal on ulnar side of palmaris longus tendon proximal to wrist crease (Figs. E6 and E7): Can be done with palpation or under ultrasound guidance
- Low-dose oral corticosteroids occasionally used but usually not effective

- Short-term benefit from ultrasound therapy (physical therapy modality)
- Carpal tunnel release may be indicated if inadequate response from nonoperative treatment; severe carpal tunnel syndrome diagnosed on EMG/NCS, or rapid progression of symptoms

DISPOSITION

Clinical course may have remissions and exacerbations. Some may progress from intermittent to persistent sensory complaints (numbness, tingling, paresthesia) and then to motor symptoms. In pregnancy, carpal tunnel symptoms may be secondary to fluid retention.[6] Symptoms can resolve spontaneously weeks after delivery.

REFERRAL

Surgical referral is needed if conservative treatment fails. Surgery (sectioning of transverse carpal ligament) is performed by open, endoscopic, or minimal incision techniques, with good long-term results. Carpal tunnel release is one of the most common surgeries performed, with approximately 400,000 conducted per yr with revision rates as low as 1.2% to 1.5%.[7]

PEARLS & CONSIDERATIONS

- The sensory changes of CTS spare the thenar eminence. This distinctive pattern occurs because the palmar cutaneous branch of the median nerve arises proximal to the wrist, passing superficial to the tunnel.
- Patients presenting with ring and small finger symptoms in addition to thumb, index, and middle finger symptoms may have underlying cervical spine pathology or concomitant median and ulnar nerve compression. An EMG/NCS can help better identify any sites of nerve compression.
- The role of repetitive hand or wrist use and workplace factors in the development of CTS remains controversial.
- Cross-sectional area of the median nerve may not have a prognostic role for patient's undergoing local steroid injection.[8]
- A recent study showed similar safety profile for open carpal tunnel releases performed in an office-based procedure room compared to an operating room.[9]

RELATED CONTENT

Carpal Tunnel Syndrome (Patient Information)

REFERENCES

Available at eBooks.Health.Elsevier.com.

AUTHORS: **MICHAEL M. SHIPP, MD, JONATHAN S. GE, ScB, LAUREN E. PIANA, MD,** and **MANUEL F. DASILVA, MD**

Celiac Disease

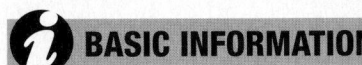

BASIC INFORMATION

DEFINITION

Celiac disease is a chronic autoimmune disease characterized by malabsorption and diarrhea precipitated by ingestion of food products containing gluten in genetically susceptible persons. Gluten is a protein complex found in wheat, rye, and barley.

SYNONYMS

Gluten-sensitive enteropathy
Celiac sprue
Nontropical sprue
CD

ICD-10CM CODE
K90.0   Celiac disease

EPIDEMIOLOGY & DEMOGRAPHICS

- The prevalence of celiac disease is 0.5% to 1% in the general population in North America and Western Europe and 5% in high-risk groups such as first-degree relatives of persons with the disease. The prevalence of celiac disease in the U.S. has increased fourfold over the past three decades, but the trend is flattening. The decline in undiagnosed celiac disease may reflect greater public and professional attention to gluten-related issues. Worldwide celiac disease affects 0.6% to 1% of the population. Celiac disease is significantly more common in persons with type 1 diabetes mellitus (DM) and is associated with greater risk of retinopathy and nephropathy in this population.
- Incidence is highest during infancy and the first 36 mo of life (after introduction of foods containing gluten), in the third decade (frequently associated with pregnancy and severe anemia during pregnancy), and in the seventh decade.
- There is a slight female predominance.
- The average age of diagnosis is in the fifth decade of life.
- The risk for celiac disease is 5% to 10% in newborn children of parents with the disease and nearly 20% in siblings.
- It is estimated that only 10% to 15% of persons with celiac disease in the U.S. have been diagnosed.

PHYSICAL FINDINGS & CLINICAL PRESENTATION

- Physical examination may be entirely within normal limits.
- Weight loss, dyspepsia, short stature, and failure to thrive may be noted in children and infants.
- Weight loss, fatigue, and diarrhea are common in adults.
- Abdominal pain, nausea, and vomiting are unusual.
- Pallor as a result of iron deficiency anemia is common.
- Atypical forms of the disease are being increasingly recognized and include osteoporosis, short stature, anemia, infertility, and

neurologic problems. Manifestations of calcium deficiency, such as tetany and seizures, are rare and can be exacerbated by coexistent magnesium deficiency.
- Angular cheilitis, aphthous ulcers, atopic dermatitis, and dermatitis herpetiformis are frequently associated with celiac disease.
- Table 1 summarizes the clinical spectrum of celiac disease.
- Table 2 summarizes extraintestinal manifestations of celiac disease.
- Disorders associated with celiac disease are summarized in Box 1.

ETIOLOGY

- Celiac sprue is considered an autoimmune-type disease, with tissue transglutaminase (tTG) suggested as a major autoantigen. It results from an inappropriate T-cell-mediated immune response against ingested gluten in genetically predisposed individuals who carry either HLA-DQ2 or HLA-DQ8 genes. There is sensitivity to gliadin, a protein fraction of gluten found in wheat, rye, and barley. In patients with celiac disease, immune responses to gliadin fractions promote an inflammatory reaction, mainly in the upper small intestine, manifested by infiltration of the lamina propria and the epithelium with chronic inflammatory cells and villous atrophy. The susceptibility to celiac disease may also be related to other environmental factors such as bacterial microbiome and reovirus infection. Table 3 summarizes biomarkers in the diagnosis of celiac disease and monitoring compliance to gluten-free diet.
- Seroconversion to celiac autoimmunity may occur at any time.
- Timing of introduction of gluten into the infant diet in children at risk remains inconclusive. Children initially exposed to gluten in the first 3 mo of life have a fivefold increased risk. Current recommendations are to delay introduction of gluten into the diet of a genetically susceptible infant until 4 to 6 mo of age while the mother continues to breastfeed.
- Trials involving randomized feeding intervention in infants at high risk for celiac disease have shown that as compared to placebo, the introduction of small quantities of gluten at 16 to 24 wk of age did not reduce the risk of celiac disease by 3 yr of age.

DIAGNOSIS

Diagnostic criteria for celiac disease require at least four out of five or three out of four if the HLA genotype is not performed:
1. Typical symptoms of celiac disease
2. Positivity of serum celiac disease immunoglobulin A (IgA) class autoantibodies at high titer
3. HLA-DQ2 or HLA-DQ8 genotypes
4. Celiac enteropathy at the small intestinal biopsy
5. Response to gluten-free diet

DIFFERENTIAL DIAGNOSIS

- Inflammatory bowel disease
- Laxative abuse

- Intestinal parasitic infestations
- Lactose intolerance
- Other: Irritable bowel syndrome, tropical sprue, chronic pancreatitis, Zollinger-Ellison syndrome, cystic fibrosis (children), lymphoma, eosinophilic gastroenteritis, short bowel syndrome, Whipple disease
- Intestinal lymphoma, tuberculosis, radiation enteritis, HIV enteropathy

LABORATORY TESTS

- IgA anti-tTG antibody by enzyme-linked immunosorbent assay (tissue transglutaminase [tTG] test) is the best screening serologic test for celiac disease. IgA antiendomysial antibodies (EMA) test is also a good screening test for celiac disease but is best used as a confirmatory test in cases of borderline positive results. In patients with IgA deficiency, the IgG deamidated gliadin peptide (DPG) test (deamidated gliadin peptides) can be used for diagnosis. Screening of close relatives is initially done with polymerase chain reaction (PCR) testing for HLA-DQ2 or HLA-DQ8. Those that are positive should then have serum tTG IgA screening. All diagnostic serologic testing for celiac disease should be performed before a gluten-free diet is initiated. Table 4 summarizes the sensitivity, specificity, and positive and negative predictive values of serologic tests for untreated celiac disease. High titers of tTG are an accurate marker for celiac disease and eliminate the need for biopsy.[1]
- Complete blood count, ferritin level: Iron deficiency anemia (microcytic anemia, low ferritin level) may be present.
- Celiac disease can lead to malabsorption: Screen for vitamin B_{12} level, folate level, vitamin D level, serum calcium, albumin, magnesium; vitamin B_{12} deficiency, vitamin D

TABLE 1   Clinical Spectrum of Celiac Disease

Symptomatic

Frank malabsorption symptoms: Chronic diarrhea, failure to thrive, weight loss

Extraintestinal manifestations: Anemia, fatigue, hypertransaminasemia, neurologic disorders, short stature, dental enamel defects, arthralgia, aphthous stomatitis

Silent

No apparent symptoms in spite of histologic evidence of villous atrophy

In most cases identified by serologic screening in at-risk groups (see "Laboratory Tests")

Latent

Subjects who have a normal histology, but at some other time, before or after, have shown a gluten-dependent enteropathy

Potential

Subjects with positive celiac disease serology but without evidence of altered jejunal histology

It might or might not be symptomatic

From Kliegman, RM: *Nelson textbook of pediatrics*, ed 21, Philadelphia, 2020, Elsevier.

TABLE 2 Extraintestinal Manifestations of Celiac Disease

Manifestation	Probable Cause(s)
Cutaneous	
Ecchymoses and petechiae	Vitamin K deficiency; rarely, thrombocytopenia
Edema	Hypoproteinemia
Dermatitis herpetiformis	Epidermal (type 3) tTG autoimmunity
Follicular hyperkeratosis and dermatitis	Vitamin A malabsorption, vitamin B complex malabsorption
Endocrinologic	
Short stature, delayed puberty	Malnutrition, hypothalamic-pituitary dysfunction
Amenorrhea, infertility, impotence	Malnutrition, hypothalamic-pituitary dysfunction, immune dysfunction
Secondary hyperparathyroidism	Calcium and/or vitamin D malabsorption with hypocalcemia
Hematologic	
Anemia	Iron, folate, or vitamin B_{12}, deficiency
Hemorrhage	Vitamin K deficiency; rarely, thrombocytopenia due to folate deficiency
Thrombocytosis, Howell-Jolly bodies	Hyposplenism
Hepatic	
Elevated liver biochemical test levels	
Autoimmune hepatitis	Lymphocytic hepatitis
Autoimmunity	
Muscular	
Atrophy	Malnutrition due to malabsorption
Weakness	Generalized muscle atrophy, hypokalemia
Neurologic	
Peripheral neuropathy	Deficiencies of vitamin B_{12} and thiamine; immune-based neurologic dysfunction
Ataxia	Cerebellar and posterior column damage
Demyelinating CNS lesions	Immune-based neurologic dysfunction
Seizures	Unknown
Skeletal	
Osteopenia, osteomalacia, and osteoporosis	Malabsorption of calcium and vitamin D, secondary hyperparathyroidism, chronic inflammation
Osteoarthropathy	Unknown
Pathologic fractures	Osteopenia and osteoporosis

tTG, Tissue transglutaminase.
From Feldman M et al: *Sleisenger and Fordtran's gastrointestinal and liver disease,* ed 11, Philadelphia, 2021, Elsevier.

BOX 1 Disorders Associated with Celiac Disease

Associated Conditions
Addison disease
Autoimmune hemolytic anemia
Autoimmune liver diseases
Bird-fancier's lung
Cavitary lung disease
Cystic fibrosis
Dermatitis herpetiformis
Diabetes mellitus type 1
Down syndrome
Epilepsy with cerebral calcification
Fibrosing alveolitis
Hypothyroidism or hyperthyroidism
Idiopathic pulmonary hemosiderosis
Immune thrombocytopenic purpura
Immunoglobulin (Ig)A deficiency
Iridocyclitis or choroiditis
Macroamylasemia
Microscopic colitis
Recurrent pericarditis
Sarcoidosis
Sjögren syndrome

Increased Morbidity After Celiac Disease Diagnosis
Cardiovascular: Ischemic heart disease, cerebrovascular disease, atrial fibrillation, dilated cardiomyopathy
Malignancy: Non-Hodgkin lymphoma, small intestinal adenocarcinoma
Respiratory: Chronic obstructive pulmonary disease, asthma, tuberculosis, influenza

Modified from Mulder CJ, Tytgat GN: Coeliac disease and related disorders, *Neth J Med* 31:286-299, 1987.

deficiency, hypomagnesemia, and hypocalcemia are not uncommon in celiac disease.

- Biopsy of the small bowel, considered the gold standard, has been questioned as a reliable and conclusive test in all cases. It may be reasonable in children with significant elevations of tTG levels (>100 U) to first try a gluten-free diet and consider biopsy in those who do not improve with diet. Repeat small-bowel biopsies are no longer required to show healing when there is a clear response to a gluten-free diet.
- The HLA-DQ2 allele is identified in >90% of patients with celiac disease, and HLA-DQ8 is identified in most of the remaining patients. These genes occur in only 30% to 40% of the general population. Their greatest diagnostic value is in their negative predictive value, making them useful when negative in ruling out the disease.

IMAGING STUDIES
- Consider bone density in newly diagnosed adult patients.

- Capsule endoscopy can be used to evaluate mucosa of the small intestine, especially if future innovations will allow mucosal biopsy.

Rx TREATMENT

NONPHARMACOLOGIC THERAPY
Patients should be instructed on a gluten-free diet (avoidance of wheat, rye, and barley). Safe grains (gluten-free) include rice, corn, oats, buckwheat, millet, amaranth, quinoa, sorghum, and teff (an Ethiopian cereal grain). The lowest amount of daily gluten that causes damage to the celiac intestinal mucosa is 10 to 15 mg/day. One slice of bread contains 1.6 g of gluten. Principles of initial dietary therapy for patients with celiac disease are summarized in Box 2.

GENERAL Rx
- Correct nutritional deficiencies with iron, folic acid, calcium, vitamin D, and vitamin B_{12} as needed.

- A diagnostic approach to patients with celiac disease who have persistent or recurrent symptoms is illustrated in Fig. 1.
- Prednisone 20 to 60 mg once a day gradually tapered is useful in refractory cases.
- Lifelong gluten-free diet is necessary. A referral to a nutritionist experienced in celiac disease and gluten-free diet is recommended at initial diagnosis.

DISPOSITION
- Prognosis is good with adherence to a gluten-free diet. Rapid improvement is usually seen within a few days of treatment. Healing of the intestinal damage typically occurs within 6 to 24 mo after initiation of the diet. Lack of response to gluten-free diet occurs in 5% of patients and is due to unintentional ingestion of gluten or presence of coexisting GI disorders such as inflammatory bowel disease (IBD), lactose or other carbohydrate intolerance, and pancreatic insufficiency.
- Serial antigliadin or antiendomysial antibody tests can be used to monitor the patient's adherence to a gluten-free diet.
- Repeat small-bowel biopsy after treatment generally reveals significant improvement. It is also useful to evaluate for increased risk of small-bowel T-cell lymphoma in these

TABLE 3 Biomarkers in the Diagnosis of Celiac Disease and Monitoring Compliance to Gluten-Free Diet

Biomarker	Method	Comments
Antireticulin antibodies—IgG/IgA	IFA (rat kidney)	Lack optimal sensitivity and specificity for routine diagnostic use
Total IgA	Quantitative nephelometry	Useful in ruling out IgA deficiency; specific IgG antibodies need to be tested in IgA-deficient individuals
Antigliadin antibodies—IgG/IgA	Quantitative EIA	Low sensitivity and specificity; useful in monitoring dietary compliance
Antideaminated gliadin antibodies—IgG/IgA	Quantitative EIA	Inferior performance relative to other diagnostic assays
Antiendomysial antibodies—IgG/IgA	IFA (rhesus monkey esophagus; human umbilical cord)	High sensitivity and specificity in CD; observer bias limits usefulness
Antitissue glutaminase—IgG/IgA	Quantitative EIA	Assays using purified human or recombinant human tTG are more sensitive than those using guinea pig tTG; useful in both diagnosis and monitoring dietary compliance
HLA-DQ2/HLA-DQ8	PCR-based assays	High negative predictive value; not affected by dietary gluten; found in ≈ 30% of general population

CD, Celiac disease; *EIA*, enzyme immunoassay; *IFA*, immunofluorescence; *IgA*, immunoglobulin A; *IgG*, immunoglobulin G; *PCR*, polymerase chain reaction; *tTG*, tissue transglutaminase.
From McPherson RA, Pincus MR: *Henry's clinical diagnosis and management by laboratory methods*, ed 23, Philadelphia, 2017, Elsevier.

TABLE 4 Sensitivity, Specificity, and Positive and Negative Predictive Values of Serologic Tests for Untreated Celiac Disease

Serologic Test	Sensitivity* (%)	Specificity* (%)	Positive Predictive Value (%)	Negative Predictive Value (%)
Immunoglobulin A Tissue Transglutaminase				
Endomysial antibody by indirect immunofluorescence assay	85-98	97-100	98-100	80-95
Guinea pig tTG ELISA	95-98	94-95	91-95	96-98
Human tTG ELISA	95-100	97-100	80-95	100
Antigliadin Antibodies (AGAs)				
IgA	75-90	82-95	28-100	65-100
IgG	69-85	73-90	20-95	41-88

AGA, Antigliadin antibodies; *ELISA*, enzyme-linked immunosorbent assay; *IgA*, immunoglobulin A; *IgG*, immunoglobulin G; *tTG*, tissue transglutaminase.
*Wide variations in test sensitivity and specificity rates are reported among different laboratories. (Stern M: Comparative evaluation of serologic tests for celiac disease: a European initiative toward standardization, *J Pediatr Gastroenterol Nutr* 31:513-519, 2000.)
From Feldman M et al: *Sleisenger and fortran's gastrointestinal and liver disease*, ed 10, Philadelphia, 2016, Elsevier.

patients, especially untreated patients. Some experts recommend a repeat biopsy only in selected patients who have an unsatisfactory response to a strict gluten-free diet; however, recent data (Lebwohl et al) show that the risk for lymphoproliferative malignancy (LPM) is affected by the results of follow-up intestinal biopsy performed to document mucosal healing. Increased risk for LPM in celiac disease is associated with the follow-up biopsy results, with a higher risk among patients with persistent villous atrophy. Follow-up biopsy may effectively stratify patients with celiac disease by risk for subsequent LPM.

ⓘ PEARLS & CONSIDERATIONS

COMMENTS
- The presence of dermatitis herpetiformis is pathognomonic for celiac disease.
- In close relatives, repeated serum tTG IgA testing may be useful in those with positive *HLA-DQ2* or *HLA-DQ8* tests because celiac disease may not manifest until later in life, and initial negative results do not preclude the possibility of future onset of celiac disease.
- Celiac disease should be considered in patients with unexplained metabolic bone disease, osteoporosis, transaminasemia, or hypocalcemia, because gastrointestinal symptoms are absent or mild. Clinicians should also consider testing children and young adults for celiac disease if unexplained weight loss, abdominal pain or distention, or chronic diarrhea is present.
- Screening for celiac disease is recommended in first-degree relatives. It should also be considered in patients with type 1 diabetes mellitus and in those with certain autoimmune disorders such as primary biliary cirrhosis, primary sclerosing cholangitis, autoimmune hepatitis, IBD, thyroid disease (hypothyroidism occurs in up to 15% of patients with celiac disease), systemic lupus erythematosus, rheumatoid arthritis, and Sjögren syndrome due to increased risk of celiac disease in these populations. Screening persons with Down syndrome or Turner syndrome has also been recommended.
- The prevalence of celiac disease in patients with dyspepsia is twice that of the general population. Screening for celiac disease should be considered in all patients with persistent dyspepsia.
- Patients with celiac disease have an overall risk of cancer that is almost twice that of the general population. The risk of adenocarcinoma of the small intestine is increased manifold compared with the risk in the general population. Celiac disease is also associated with an increased risk for non-Hodgkin lymphoma, especially of T-cell type and primarily localized in the gut. Lymphoma is 4 to 40 times more common, and death from lymphoma is 11 to 70 times more common in patients with celiac disease. Patients with refractory celiac disease are at greatest risk for T-cell lymphoma.

BOX 2 Principles of Initial Dietary Therapy for Patients with Celiac Disease

Avoid all foods containing wheat, rye, and barley gluten (pure oats usually safe).
Avoid malt unless clearly labeled as derived from corn.
Use only rice; corn; maize; buckwheat; millet; amaranth; quinoa; sorghum; potato or potato starch; soybean; tapioca; and teff, bean, and nut flours.
Wheat starch and products containing wheat starch should only be used if they contain less than 20 ppm gluten and are marked "gluten free."
Read all labels and study ingredients of processed foods.
Beware of gluten in medications, supplements, food additives, emulsifiers, or stabilizers.
Limit milk and milk products initially if there is evidence of lactose intolerance.
Avoid all beers, lagers, ales, and stouts (unless labeled gluten free).
Wine, most liqueurs, ciders, and spirits, including whiskey and brandy, are allowed.

Modified from Trier JS: Celiac sprue and refractory sprue. In Feldman M et al: *Sleisenger and Fortran's gastrointestinal and liver disease*, ed 10, Philadelphia, 2016, Elsevier.

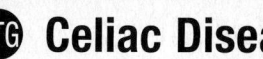

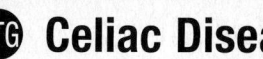

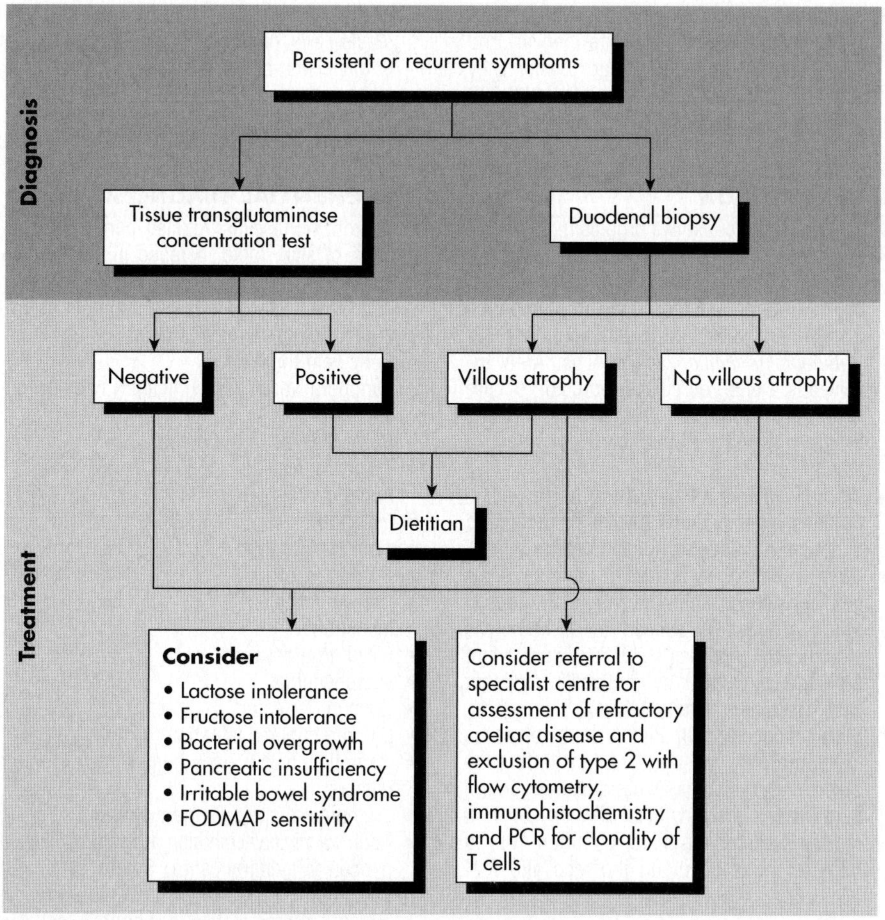

FIG. 1 Diagnostic approach to patients with celiac disease who have persistent or recurrent symptoms. Serologic and histologic assessment via tTG antibody measurement and duodenal biopsy, respectively, allow for identification of those patients for whom ongoing gluten exposure is likely; such patients would benefit from further follow-up with a dietitian. Among those with villus recovery and negative tTG testing, alternative causes for symptoms should be sought. Among patients with persistent villus atrophy and symptoms suggestive of malabsorption, refractory celiac disease should be considered and hematopathology for clonal T-cell rearrangement performed to identify those patients with refractory celiac disease type II. *tTG,* Tissue transglutaminase. (From Lebwohl B et al: Coeliac disease, *Lancet* 391[10115]: 70-81, 2018.)

- Patients with celiac disease who have followed a gluten-free diet for prolonged periods may not experience relapse of symptoms for several months after gluten is reintroduced.

RELATED CONTENT

Celiac Disease (Patient Information)
Dermatitis Herpetiformis (Related Key Topic)
Malabsorption (Related Key Topic)

SUGGESTED READING

Available at eBooks.Health.Elsevier.com

AUTHOR: **FRED F. FERRI, MD**

BASIC INFORMATION

DEFINITION

Cellulitis is an infection of the deep dermis and subcutaneous tissues characterized by erythema, warmth, and tenderness of the involved area. Diagnosis is made on the basis of history and physical examination.

SYNONYMS

Erysipelas (cellulitis generally caused by group A β-hemolytic streptococci [GABHS])
SSSIs (skin and skin structure infections)
ABSSSIs (acute bacterial skin and skin structure infections)

ICD-10CM CODES
H05.011	Cellulitis of right orbit
H05.012	Cellulitis of left orbit
H05.013	Cellulitis of bilateral orbits
H05.019	Cellulitis of unspecified orbit
H60.10	Cellulitis of external ear, unspecified ear
H60.11	Cellulitis of right external ear
H60.12	Cellulitis of left external ear
H60.13	Cellulitis of external ear, bilateral
K12.2	Cellulitis and abscess of mouth
L03.011	Cellulitis of right finger
L03.012	Cellulitis of left finger
L03.019	Cellulitis of unspecified finger
L03.031	Cellulitis of right toe
L03.032	Cellulitis of left toe
L03.039	Cellulitis of unspecified toe
L03.111	Cellulitis of right axilla
L03.112	Cellulitis of left axilla
L03.113	Cellulitis of right upper limb
L03.114	Cellulitis of left upper limb
L03.115	Cellulitis of right lower limb
L03.116	Cellulitis of left lower limb
L03.119	Cellulitis of unspecified part of limb
L03.211	Cellulitis of face
L03.221	Cellulitis of neck
L03.311	Cellulitis of abdominal wall
L03.312	Cellulitis of back [any part except buttock]
L03.313	Cellulitis of chest wall
L03.314	Cellulitis of groin
L03.315	Cellulitis of perineum
L03.316	Cellulitis of umbilicus
L03.317	Cellulitis of buttock
L03.319	Cellulitis of trunk, unspecified
L03.811	Cellulitis of head [any part, except face]
L03.818	Cellulitis of other sites
L03.90	Cellulitis, unspecified

EPIDEMIOLOGY & DEMOGRAPHICS

- Occurs most frequently in diabetics, immunocompromised hosts, and patients with venous and lymphatic compromise.
- Frequently found near skin breaks (trauma, surgical wounds [surgical site infections develop in 2% to 5% of all surgical procedures], ulcerations, tinea infections). Edema, animal or human bites, subadjacent osteomyelitis, and bacteremia are potential sources of cellulitis.
- Skin and soft-tissue infections account for >14 million outpatient visits per yr and $3.7 billion in ambulatory care costs. They also are responsible for more than 650,000 admissions in the U.S./yr.

PHYSICAL FINDINGS & CLINICAL PRESENTATION

Variable with the causative organism:
- Erysipelas (Fig. E1): Superficial-spreading, warm, erythematous lesion distinguished by indurated, elevated margin; lymphatic involvement, vesicle formation common.
- *Haemophilus influenzae* cellulitis: Area involved is a blue-red/purple-red color; occurs mainly in children; generally involves the face in children and the neck or upper chest in adults.
- *Vibrio vulnificus:* Larger hemorrhagic bullae, cellulitis, lymphadenitis, myositis; often found in critically ill patients in septic shock.
- Table 1 describes anatomic variants of or predispositions to cellulitis. Typically, nonpurulent cellulitis is caused by β-hemolytic streptococci, whereas cellulitis with purulent drainage is caused by methicillin-resistant *Staphylococcus aureus* (MRSA).
- Staphylococcal cellulitis: Area involved is erythematous, hot, and swollen; differentiated from erysipelas by nonelevated, poorly demarcated margin; local tenderness and regional adenopathy are common; up to 85% of cases occur on the legs and feet (Fig. E2).

ETIOLOGY

- Any disruption of the skin barrier provides a portal for pathogens to enter the skin and soft tissues
- Group A β-hemolytic streptococci (may follow a streptococcal infection of the upper respiratory tract). β-Hemolytic streptococci are implicated in most cases of nontraumatic cellulitis
- Staphylococcal cellulitis: Diabetics, athletes, men who have sex with men, people living in public housing, and incarcerated men are at greater risk for MRSA infection. A community-acquired MRSA strain, USA 300, is replacing nosocomial strains of MRSA in hospitals
- Intravenous (IV) drug use: MRSA, *Pseudomonas aeruginosa*
- *V. vulnificus:* Higher incidence in patients with liver disease (75%) and in immunocompromised hosts. *V. vulnificus* infection is the leading cause of death related to seafood consumption in the U.S.
- *Erysipelothrix rhusiopathiae:* Common in people handling poultry, fish, or meat
- *Aeromonas hydrophila:* Generally occurs in contaminated open wounds in fresh water
- Fungi *(Cryptococcus neoformans):* In immunocompromised granulopenic patients
- Gram-negative rods *(Serratia, Enterobacter, Proteus, Pseudomonas):* May be present in immunocompromised or granulopenic patients
- Hot tub exposure: *P. aeruginosa*; fish tank exposure: *Mycobacterium marinum*
- Bites: Human *(Eikenella corrodens),* dog *(Pasteurella multocida, C. canimorsus),* cat *(P. multocida),* rat *(Streptobacillus moniliformis)*

DIAGNOSIS

DIFFERENTIAL DIAGNOSIS

- Necrotizing fasciitis (reddish-purple discoloration of skin, rapid increase in size, woody induration and pale appearance rather than erythema, violaceous bullae, pain out of proportion to appearance, sepsis)
- Deep vein thrombosis
- Peripheral vascular insufficiency (venous stasis dermatitis)
- Paget disease of the breast
- Thrombophlebitis
- Acute gout
- Psoriasis
- *Candida* intertrigo
- Pseudogout
- Osteomyelitis
- Insect bite
- Fixed drug eruption
- Lymphedema
- Contact dermatitis
- Olecranon bursa infection
- Herpetic whitlow, early herpes zoster (before blisters)
- Erythema migrans (Lyme disease)
- Rare: *Vaccinia* vaccination, Kawasaki disease, pyoderma gangrenosum, Sweet syndrome, carcinoma erysipeloides, anaerobic myonecrosis, erythromelalgia, eosinophilic cellulitis (Well syndrome), familial Mediterranean fever

LABORATORY TESTS

- Laboratory testing is generally not required for the evaluation of cellulitis and uncomplicated soft tissue infections in the absence of comorbidities
- CBC with differential: Leukocytosis may be present but is a nonspecific finding
- Gram stain, culture (aerobic and anaerobic):
  1. Aspirated material from:
     a. Advancing edge of cellulitis
     b. Any vesicles
  2. Swab of any drainage material
  3. Punch biopsy (in selected patients)
- Blood cultures in hospitalized patients, patients with cellulitis superimposed on lymphedema, patients with buccal or periorbital cellulitis, and patients suspected of having a salt- or fresh-water source of infection. Bacteremia uncommon in cellulitis (positive blood cultures in 4% of patients)
- Antistreptolysin O (ASLO) titer (in suspected streptococcal disease)
- The cause of cellulitis remains unidentified in most patients. Patients with recurrent lower-extremity cellulitis (Fig. E2) should be inspected for tinea pedis. If found, it should be treated

IMAGING STUDIES

- Imaging is generally not necessary but may be helpful in suspected purulent soft tissue infections and osteomyelitis.

TABLE 1   Anatomic Variants of or Predispositions to Cellulitis

Anatomic Variant or Predisposition	Location	Likely Bacterial Cause
Periorbital cellulitis	Periorbital	*Staphylococcus aureus, Streptococcus pneumoniae,* group A streptococci
Buccal cellulitis	Cheek	*Haemophilus influenzae* type b
Cellulitis complicating body piercing	Ear, nose, umbilicus	*S. aureus,* group A streptococci
After mastectomy (with axillary node dissection)	Ipsilateral upper extremity	Nongroup A β-hemolytic streptococci
After lumpectomy (with limited axillary node dissection, breast irradiation)	Ipsilateral breast	Nongroup A β-hemolytic streptococci
After saphenous vein harvest for coronary artery bypass	Ipsilateral leg	Group A or nongroup A β-hemolytic streptococci
After radical pelvic surgery, radiation therapy	Vulva, inguinal areas, legs	Group B and group G streptococci
After liposuction	Thigh, abdominal wall	Group A streptococci, peptostreptococci
Postoperative (very early) wound infection	Abdomen, chest, hip	Group A streptococci
Injection drug use ("skin popping")	Extremities, neck	*S. aureus,* streptococci (groups A, C, F, G)*
Perianal cellulitis	Perineum	Group A streptococcus

*Other bacteria to consider based on isolation from skin or abscesses in this setting include *Enterococcus faecalis,* viridians group streptococci, coagulase-negative staphylococci, anaerobes (including *Bacteroides* and *Clostridium* spp.), and Enterobacteriaceae.
From Bennett JE et al: *Mandell, Douglas, and Bennett's principles and practice of infectious diseases,* ed 9, Philadelphia, 2020, Elsevier.

- Computed tomography or MRI in patients with suspected necrotizing fasciitis (deep-seated infection of the subcutaneous tissue that results in the progressive destruction of fascia and fat).

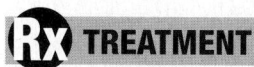 **TREATMENT**

NONPHARMACOLOGIC THERAPY

Immobilization and elevation of the involved limb. Cool sterile saline dressings to remove purulence from any open lesion. Support stockings in patients with peripheral edema.

ACUTE GENERAL Rx

Treatment should initially cover *Streptococcus* and methicillin-sensitive *S. aureus* and should be expanded for MRSA in patients with risk factors (e.g., IV drug users, residents of long-term care facilities, athletes, children, men who have sex with men, prisoners).

ERYSIPELAS:
- PO: Dicloxacillin 500 mg PO q6h or cephalexin 500 mg qid
- IV: Cefazolin 1 g q6 to 8h or nafcillin 1.0 or 1.5 g IV q4 to 6h

NOTE: Use vancomycin 1 g IV q12h in patients allergic to penicillin.

STAPHYLOCOCCAL CELLULITIS:
- PO: Dicloxacillin 250 to 500 mg qid.
- IV: Nafcillin 1 to 2 g q4 to 6h.
- Cephalosporins (cephalexin 500 mg qid) also provide adequate antistaphylococcal coverage, except for MRSA.
- Trimethoprim-sulfamethoxazole (160 mg/800 mg 1 PO bid) may be appropriate in outpatient mild MRSA infections. Use vancomycin 1.0 to 2.0 g IV qd or linezolid 0.6 g IV q12h in patients with moderate/severe

MRSA. Daptomycin (Cubicin), a cyclic lipopeptide, can be used as an alternative to vancomycin for complicated skin and skin structure infections. Usual dose is 4 mg/kg IV given over 30 min every 24 h. Telavancin is a new glycopeptide derivative of vancomycin effective for gram-positive skin and skin structure infections, including those caused by MRSA. Tedizolid is an oxazolidinone effective in ABSSSI as an alternative to linezolid. Ceftaroline fosamil (Teflaro) is a newer IV cephalosporin also effective against MRSA. Dalbavancin and tedizolid are two new drugs FDA-approved for skin and skin structure infections, including those caused by MRSA.
- Transition from IV to oral antibiotics for complicated staphylococcus infections is contingent on eradication of bacteremia and drainage of all purulent foci. Addressing substance use is imperative when injection drug use complicates the picture.[1]

H. INFLUENZAE CELLULITIS:
- PO: Cefixime or cefuroxime
- IV: Cefuroxime or ceftriaxone

VIBRIO VULNIFICUS:
- Doxycycline 100 mg IV bid + ceftazidime 2 g IV q8h or IV ciprofloxacin 400 mg bid. Mild cases treated with oral antibiotics (doxycycline 100 mg bid + ciprofloxacin 750 mg bid).
- IV support and admission into intensive care unit (mortality rate >50% in septic shock).

E. RHUSIOPATHIAE:
- Penicillin

A. HYDROPHILA:
- Aminoglycosides
- Chloramphenicol
- Complicated skin and skin structure infections in hospitalized patients can be treated with daptomycin (Cubicin) 4 mg/kg IV q24h

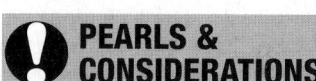 **PEARLS & CONSIDERATIONS**

- 16.6% of acute cellulitis cases are unresponsive to initial treatment mainly due to inappropriate antibiotic selection and dosing (weight-based dosing is preferred).
- Prophylactic antibiotics (e.g., dicloxacillin 500 mg bid or erythromycin 250 mg bid) are controversial but can be considered with patients with ≥4 episodes of cellulitis despite optimized control of risk factors. Recurrent cellulitis with no identifiable cause occurs in 22% of cases despite antibiotic prophylaxis.
- In patients with uncomplicated cellulitis in the outpatient setting, adding trimethoprim-sulfamethoxazole to cephalexin for MRSA coverage is unnecessary and does not increase the likelihood of clinical cure.
- In patients with chronic edema of the leg, daily use of compression garments on the leg can lower the incidence of recurrent cellulitis.

RELATED CONTENT

Cellulitis (Patient Information)
Erysipelas (Related Key Topic)
Necrotizing Fasciitis (Related Key Topic)

AUTHOR: **FRED F. FERRI, MD**

REFERENCE & SUGGESTED READINGS

Available at eBooks.Health.Elsevier.com.

BASIC INFORMATION

DEFINITION

Cervical cancer is the penetration of the basement membrane and infiltration of the stroma of the uterine cervix by malignant cells. The cancer arises from normal cervical epithelium through progressive development of low-grade and high-grade cervical intraepithelial lesions.[1]

ICD-10CM CODES
C53.8 Malignant neoplasm of overlapping sites of cervix uteri
C53.9 Malignant neoplasm of cervix uteri, unspecified
D06.7 Carcinoma in situ of other parts of cervix
D06.9 Carcinoma in situ of cervix, unspecified

EPIDEMIOLOGY & DEMOGRAPHICS

INCIDENCE: Per the World Health Organization, cervical cancer is the fourth most common malignancy in women. It is reported that nearly 9 out of 10 women who died of cervical cancer were in an underdeveloped region of the world.[2]
PREDOMINANCE: Higher incidence rates occur in developing countries. Among the U.S. population, Hispanics have a higher incidence than African Americans, who likewise have a higher incidence than Caucasians. Compared to Caucasian women, African American and Hispanic women have increased risk of late-stage diagnosis and worse disease progression.[3]
RISK FACTORS: The major risk factor is persistent infection with high-risk human papillomavirus (HPV; types 16 and 18 are the most oncogenic with 31, 33, 35, 45, 52, and 58 also considered high risk). Smoking, early age of coitarche, multiple sexual partners, immunocompromised state, nonbarrier methods of contraception, and multiparity are also risk factors.

PHYSICAL FINDINGS & CLINICAL PRESENTATION

In the early stages, cervical cancer associated with high-risk HPV may be asymptomatic. As the disease progresses, symptoms may include:
- Unusual vaginal bleeding, particularly postcoital (Fig. E1).
- Vaginal discharge and/or odor (watery, blood-tinged).
- Pelvic pain in early stage disease. In later stages, back pain or disrupted urination or defecation may occur.
- Advanced cases may present with lower-extremity edema or renal failure.
- In early stages, there may be little or no obvious cervical lesion; more advanced cases may have large, bulky, friable lesions (Fig. E2) encompassing majority of the vagina.[4]

ETIOLOGY

- Infection with high-risk HPV types is a necessary, although not sufficient, cause of almost all cases of cervical cancer. Persistent HPV infection leads to precancerous changes of the cervix known as cervical intraepithelial

neoplasia (CIN). CIN can progress to invasive cervical cancer.
- Both squamous cell and adenocarcinoma of cervix are associated with HPV infection (Table 1).
- More than 40 HPV types can infect the cervix. Most cases are believed to be linked to presence of HPV 16, 18, 31, 35, 39, 45, 51, 52, 56, 58, 59, and 68 by interaction of E6 and E7 oncoprotein on p53 gene product.[5]

DIAGNOSIS

DIFFERENTIAL DIAGNOSIS

- Cervical polyp or prolapsed uterine fibroid.
- Neoplasia metastatic from a separate primary neoplasia.
- Box 1 summarizes benign mimics of cervical adenocarcinoma.
- Box E2 summarizes the major categories of cervical carcinomas. Categories of squamous carcinoma are described in Box 3.
- Table 2 summarizes the differential diagnosis of squamous intraepithelial lesions.

WORKUP

- Thorough history and physical examination
- Pelvic examination with careful rectovaginal examination
- Table 3 summarizes the clinical evaluation of patients with newly diagnosed cervical cancer
- Cervical cancer screening includes options for either co-testing (PAP plus high risk HPV) or HPV primary testing. Compared with Pap testing, HPV testing has greater sensitivity for detection of CIN. Addition of HPV test for high-risk types to Pap test to screen women in mid-30s for cervical cancer reduces incidence of grade 2 or 3 CIN or cancer detected by subsequent screening examinations
- Colposcopy with directed biopsy and endocervical curettage
- International Federation of Gynecology and Obstetrics (FIGO) staging is described in Table 4

TABLE 1 Descriptive Categories of Low-Grade Squamous Intraepithelial Lesion and High-Grade Squamous Intraepithelial Lesion

	Descriptors	Human Papillomavirus	p16 Immunostaining
LSIL	CIN1, flat condyloma, mild dysplasia	HR (70%)	Usually diffuse
	Exophytic condyloma	LR	Negative or patchy
	Immature condyloma (papillary immature metaplasia)	LR	Negative or patchy
	Immature flat metaplastic LSIL	HR	Usually diffuse
HSIL	CIN2 or moderate dysplasia	HR (45% type 16)	Diffuse
	CIN3 or severe dysplasia/carcinoma in situ	HR (60% type 16)	Diffuse
	Keratinizing SIL	HR	Diffuse
	HSIL with immature metaplastic phenotype	HR	Diffuse
	Papillary carcinoma in situ	HR	Diffuse
	Adenosquamous carcinoma in situ	HR	Diffuse

CIN, Cervical intraepithelial lesion; *HR,* high risk; *HSIL,* high-grade squamous intraepithelial lesion; *LR,* low risk; *LSIL,* low-grade squamous intraepithelial lesion; *SIL,* squamous intraepithelial lesion.
From Crum CP et al: *Diagnostic gynecologic and obstetric pathology,* ed 3, Philadelphia, 2018, Elsevier.

BOX 1 Benign Mimics of Cervical Adenocarcinoma

Deep nabothian cysts, florid deep glands
Tunnel clusters
Endocervical gland hyperplasias
  Lobular hyperplasia
  Diffuse laminar hyperplasia
Adenomyoma of the endocervical type
Endocervicosis, florid cystic endosalpingiosis
Müllerian papilloma
Microglandular hyperplasia
Mesonephric hyperplasia
Ectopic prostate
Deep tubal metaplasia

From Crum CP et al: *Diagnostic gynecologic and obstetric pathology,* ed 3, Philadelphia, 2018, Elsevier.

BOX 3 Categories of Squamous Carcinoma

Squamous cell carcinoma
Large cell keratinizing (well-differentiated)
Large cell nonkeratinizing (moderately differentiated)
Small cell nonkeratinizing (poorly differentiated)
Lymphoepithelial-like carcinoma
Spindle cell (sarcomatoid) carcinoma
Verrucopapillary carcinomas
Papillary (squamotransitional) carcinoma
Verrucous carcinoma (rare)[a]
Condylomatous carcinoma[a]
Basaloid carcinomas[ab]

[a]In young women, an extensive (giant) condyloma must be excluded.
[b]May be associated with adenoid basal and adenoid cystic carcinomas, as well as carcinosarcomas.
From Crum CP et al: *Diagnostic gynecologic and obstetric pathology,* ed 3, Philadelphia, 2018, Elsevier.

LABORATORY TESTS
- CBC, chemistry profile
- Squamous cell carcinoma antigen in research setting
- Carcinoembryonic antigen

TABLE 2 Differential Diagnosis of Squamous Intraepithelial Lesions

Category	Mimic	Distinguishing Features
LSIL	Mucosal polyp (vaginal)	Minimal acanthosis, no koilocytosis
	Reactive epithelial changes	Mild superficial karyomegaly, occasional binucleated intermediate cells
	Postmenopausal changes	Superficial cell karyomegaly, cytoplasmic halos
HSIL	Immature reactive/repair	Basal hyperchromasia, uniform nuclear spacing and nuclear contour, nucleoli
	Immature metaplasia	Uniform maturation, minimal surface hyperchromasia
	Atrophy	No mitoses, uniform chromasia, nuclear density
	Atypical atrophy	Enlarged nuclei, uncommon
	Implantation site	Uniform and wide nuclear spacing, bizarre nuclei
	Endometrial histiocytes	Small, indented nuclei, granular cytoplasm, lack of polarity

HSIL, High-grade squamous intraepithelial lesion; *LSIL,* low-grade squamous intraepithelial lesion.
From Crum CP et al: *Diagnostic gynecologic and obstetric pathology,* ed 3, Philadelphia, 2018, Elsevier.

IMAGING STUDIES

- Chest x-ray examination
- Depending on stage, may need computed tomography (CT) scan, MRI (Fig. E3), PET/CT
- Table 3, intravenous pyelogram

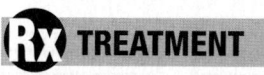 **TREATMENT**

NONPHARMACOLOGIC THERAPY

- FIGO stage I$_A$: Cone biopsy or simple hysterectomy
- FIGO stage I$_B$ or II$_A$: Type III radical hysterectomy and pelvic lymphadenectomy or pelvic radiation therapy. Minimally invasive radical hysterectomy is associated with shorter overall survival than open surgery among women with stage IA2 or IB2 cervical carcinoma[6,7]

TABLE 3 Clinical Evaluation of Patients with Newly Diagnosed Cervical Cancer

History	Review of Systems	General Physical Examination
Risk factors (STDs, smoking, OCPs, HIV), prior abnormal Pap tests, previous dysplasia, and treatment	Abnormal vaginal bleeding or discharge, pelvic pain, flank pain, sciatica, hematuria, rectal bleeding, anorexia, weight loss, bone pain	Peripheral lymphadenopathy
Evaluation	Common procedures (FIGO)	Alternative procedures
Invasive cancer	Cervical biopsy	Histologic diagnosis required
	Endocervical curettage	
	Cervical conization	
Tumor size; involvement of the vagina, bladder, rectum, and parametria	Pelvic examination under anesthesia	MRI of pelvis preferred over CT
Anemia	Complete blood count	—
Renal failure	Serum chemistries	—
Hematuria	Urinalysis	—
Bladder involvement	Cystoscopy with biopsy and urine cytology	CT, MRI pelvis
Rectal infiltration	Proctoscopy with biopsy	CT, MRI pelvis; barium enema
Hydronephrosis	IVP	Renal ultrasonography; CT abdomen
Pulmonary metastases	Chest radiography	CT chest; PET scan
Retroperitoneal lymphadenopathy	—	Lymphangiogram, CT, MRI, PET scan

CT, Computed tomography; *FIGO,* Federation of International Gynecologists and Obstetricians; *HIV,* human immunodeficiency virus; *IVP,* intravenous pyelography; *MRI,* magnetic resonance imaging; *OCP,* oral contraceptive pill; *PET,* positron emission tomography; *STD,* sexually transmitted disease.
From Disaia PJ et al: *Clinical gynecologic oncology,* ed 9, Philadelphia, 2017, Elsevier.

TABLE 4 Federation of International Obstetrics and Gynecology Staging of Cervical Cancer

Stage	Invasion	Prognosis 5-Yr Survival	Treatment
I$_{A1}$	Depth of invasion ≤3 mm and width ≤7 mm (includes early stromal invasion of up to 1 mm)	98%-99%	Local excision; if margins of a LLETZ/cone clear (i.e., no residual tumor or CIN) then conization is adequate, with no need for pelvic lymphadenectomy
I$_{A2}$	Depth of invasion 3.1-5 mm and width ≤7 mm	95%	Simple hysterectomy and pelvic lymphadenectomy. If fertility sparing required, large cone and lymphadenectomy
I$_{B1}$	Tumor confined to cervix and diameter <2 cm	90%-95%	Radical hysterectomy (and lymphadenectomy)
I$_{B2}$	Tumor confined to cervix and diameter ≥2 cm to <4 cm	80%	Chemo-radiotherapy
I$_{B3}$	Tumor confined to cervix and diameter ≥4 cm		Chemo-radiotherapy
II$_A$	Upper two thirds of vagina	70%-90%	Chemotherapy & radiotherapy
II$_B$	Upper two thirds of vagina plus parametrial disease but not up to pelvic wall	60%-70%	Chemo-radiotherapy
III$_A$	Lower third of vagina	30%-50%	Chemotherapy & radiotherapy
III$_B$	Pelvic sidewall and/or hydronephrosis		Chemo-radiotherapy
III$_C$	Involvement of pelvic and/or paraaortic lymph nodes		Chemo-radiotherapy
IV$_A$	Bladder, rectum	20%	Chemo-radiotherapy
IV$_B$	Beyond pelvis		

CIN, Cervical intraepithelial neoplasia; *LLETZ,* large loop excision of the transformation zone.
From Magowan BA: *Clinical obstetrics and gynecology,* ed 4, Philadelphia, 2019, Elsevier.

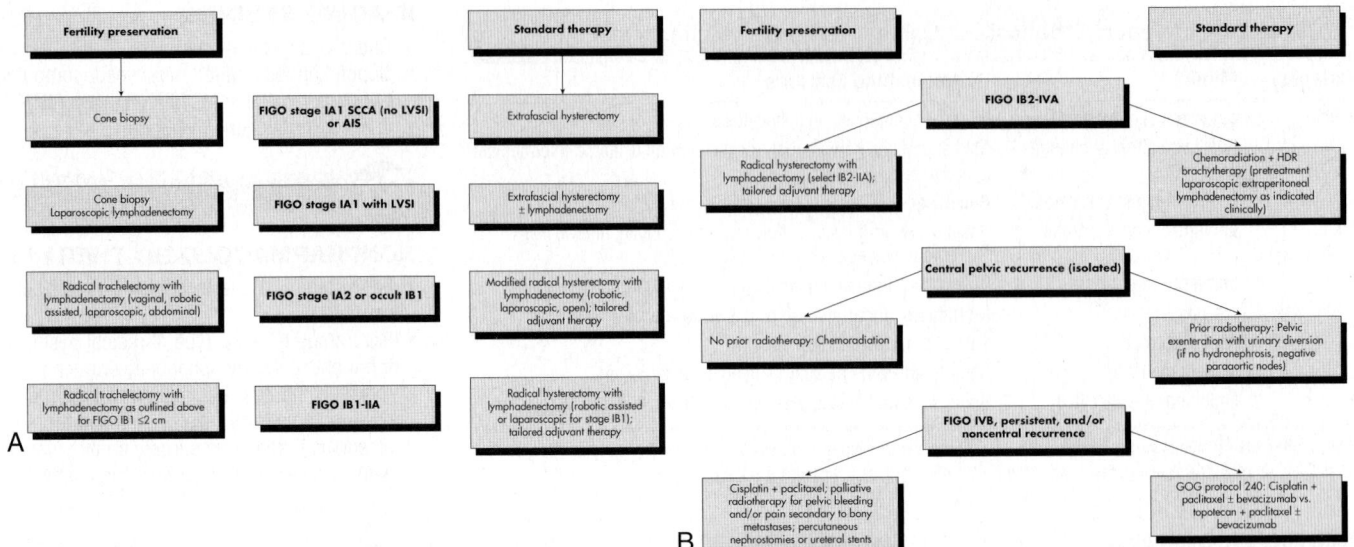

FIG. 4 A and **B,** Algorithm for therapy. *AIS,* Adenocarcinoma *in situ; FIGO,* Federation of International Gynecologists and Obstetricians; *GOG,* gynecologic oncology group; *HDR,* high-dose rate; *LVSI,* lymphovascular space invasion; *SCCA,* squamous cell carcinoma associated antigen. (From Disaia PJ et al: *Clinical gynecologic oncology,* ed 9, Philadelphia, 2017, Elsevier.)

- Advanced or bulky disease: Multimodality therapy (radiation, chemotherapy, and/or surgery); platinum use before radiation therapy[8]

ACUTE GENERAL Rx

- Table 4 summarizes treatment according to tumor stage. Fig. 4 describes a treatment algorithm for invasive cervical cancer.
- Chemotherapy is cisplatin-based. In advanced cases, cervical cancer may present with massive and acute vaginal bleeding requiring volume and blood replacement, vaginal packing or other hemostatic modalities, and/or high-dose local radiotherapy.
- A recent phase-3 trial[9] with cemiplimab, a fully human programmed cell death 1 (PD-1)-blocking antibody, showed significantly longer survival among patients with recurrent cervical cancer after first-line platinum-containing chemotherapy.

CHRONIC Rx

- Physical examination with Pap smear every 3 mo for 2 yr, every 6 mo for 3 to 5 yr, annually thereafter. Table 5 summarizes a proposed schedule for interval evaluation of cervical cancer after radiotherapy or surgery in asymptomatic patients
- Chest x-ray examination annually (optional)
- Other imaging done only as clinically indicated
- Localized pelvic recurrence may be treated and cured with pelvic exenteration[1]

DISPOSITION

Five-yr survival varies by stage:
- Stage I: 90% to 95%
- Stage II: 40% to 80%
- Stage III: <60%
- Stage IV: <15%

TABLE 5 Proposed Schedule for Interval Evaluation of Cervical Cancer after Radiotherapy or Surgery (Asymptomatic Patient*)

Year	Frequency	Examination
1	3 mo	Pelvic examination, Pap smear
	6 mo	Chest radiography, CBC, BUN, creatinine
	1 yr	IVP or CT scan with contrast
2	4 mo	Pelvic examination, Pap smear
	1 yr	Chest radiography, CBC, BUN, creatinine, IVP or CT scan with contrast
3-5	6 mo	Pelvic examination, Pap smear

*Symptomatic patients should have appropriate examination where indicated.
BUN, Blood urea nitrogen; *CBC,* complete blood count; *CT,* computed tomography; *IVP,* intravenous pyelogram; *Pap,* Papanicolaou. From Disaia PJ et al: *Clinical gynecologic oncology,* ed 9, Philadelphia, 2017, Elsevier.

Early detection by Pap smear is imperative for long-term improvements in survival. Cervical cancer screening guidelines are summarized in Table E6.

REFERRAL

Gynecologic oncologist for all invasive disease

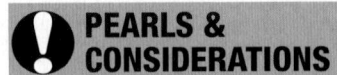

PEARLS & CONSIDERATIONS

- HPV vaccination is indicated in males and females age 9 to 26 yr for the prevention of cervical cancer caused by HPV types 6, 11, 16, and 18. HPV vaccination is over 90% effective in preventing infection and cervical cancer. There are now HPV vaccines that are effective against nine strains of high-risk HPV. Per the Centers for Disease Control and Prevention, those who are between the ages of 27 and 45 may now choose to be vaccinated, if they have not been already, depending on

their risk for new HPV infection. However, vaccination among this age range is less effective, as many have already been exposed to HPV.[10]
- Available evidence supports discontinuation of cervical cancer screening among women aged 65 yr or older who have had adequate screening and are not otherwise at high risk.
- Updated recommendations from the American College of Obstetricians and Gynecologists on screening for cervical cancer in average-risk women are in Table E7.

REFERENCES

Available at eBooks.Health.Elsevier.com.

RELATED CONTENT

Cervical Cancer (Patient Information)
Cervical Dysplasia (Related Key Topic)

AUTHORS: **LAUREN DAVIS RIVERA, MD, MSEd,** and **SUDESHNA CHATTERJEE-PAER, MD**

C

Diseases and Disorders

I

BASIC INFORMATION

DEFINITION

Cervical dysplasia refers to atypia of intraepithelial cells of the cervix that do not cross the basement membrane; it is a precursor to cervical cancer, though some atypia may spontaneously regress. It is most commonly caused by persistent infection with human papillomavirus (HPV), especially types 16, 18, 31, and 33, though other high-risk types exist. Characteristics of dysplasia include increased cellularity, nuclear abnormalities, and increased nuclear to cytoplasmic ratio. Fig. E1 is a diagram of cervical epithelium showing various terminologies used to characterize progressive degrees of cervical neoplasia. Fig. 2 provides a comparison of grading systems for cervical squamous dysplasia.

SYNONYMS

Atypical squamous cells of uncertain significance (ASCUS)

Low-grade squamous intraepithelial lesion (LSIL)

High-grade squamous intraepithelial lesion (HGSIL or HSIL)

Cervical atypia

Precancerous changes of the cervix

ICD-10CM CODES
N87.9	Dysplasia of cervix uteri, unspecified
R87.610	Atypical squamous cells of undetermined significance on cytologic smear of cervix (ASC-US)
R87.611	Atypical squamous cells cannot exclude high-grade squamous intraepithelial lesion on cytologic smear of cervix (ASC-H)
R87.612	Low-grade squamous intraepithelial lesion on cytologic smear of cervix (LGSIL)
R87.613	High-grade squamous intraepithelial lesion on cytologic smear of cervix (HGSIL)
R87.614	Cytologic evidence of malignancy on smear of cervix
R87.615	Unsatisfactory cytologic smear of cervix
R87.618	Other abnormal cytological findings on specimens from cervix uteri
R87.619	Unspecified abnormal cytological findings in specimens from cervix uteri
Z12.4	Encounter for screening for malignant neoplasm of cervix

EPIDEMIOLOGY & DEMOGRAPHICS

Dysplasia affects people in low-income countries at higher rates due to lower adoption of the HPV vaccine. Dysplasia occurs more frequently than cancer and is found in 2% to 5% of Pap smears.[1]

INCIDENCE:
- Incidence is changing over time since the introduction of the HPV vaccine and shifts in screening.
- Dysplasia and atypia: Age 25 to 35; cancer: Peak age 40 to 44 yr (8 cases/100,000 persons).[2]
- Abnormal Pap smear rate revealing dysplasia in approximately 1 in 20 Pap smears, though there is variation based on population risk factors. The false-negative rate approaches 40%.
- Age-adjusted incidence of severe dysplasia is 35 cases/100,000 persons.
- Approximately half of new cervical cancer cases had never been screened, and another 10% had not been screened in more than 5 yr.

RISK FACTORS:
- Persistent HPV infection, notably with high risk types: 16, 18, 31, 33

- Health care access: Lack of HPV vaccination, lack of access to screening, lack of prior Pap smear or HPV-based screening
- Sexual activity risks: Heterosexual coitus, coitus during puberty (transformation-zone metaplasia peak), multiple sexual partners, history of sexually transmitted disease (STD), "high-risk" male partner (HPV+)
- Medical comorbidity risks: HIV, other immunocompromising illnesses, other genital tract neoplasias, tuberculosis
- Exposure risks: Tobacco use, substance use, diethylstilbestrol (DES) exposure
- Low socioeconomic status
- Early first pregnancy

GENETICS:
- Germline mutations increasing the risk of cervical cancer have not been identified, though clusters of cases within families have been reported.[3]

PHYSICAL FINDINGS & CLINICAL PRESENTATION

- Dysplasia is most commonly diagnosed on routine screening, with HPV alone, cytology alone, or contesting.
- Signs and symptoms include abnormal vaginal bleeding, postcoital bleeding, abnormal discharge, vaginal irritation and itching, and pain with intercourse.
- Incidental findings of a mass in the cervix or lower uterine segment or pelvic lymphadenopathy can be found on exam or with imaging.
- Cervical lesions associated with dysplasia often are not visible to the naked eye; therefore, physical findings are best seen on colposcopy with 3% acetic acid-prepared or Lugol's solution.
- Colposcopic and exam findings: Leukoplakia (white lesions without dye), acetowhite epithelium, punctuation, mosaicism, abnormal vessels, abnormal transformation zone, and abnormal iodine uptake.

Histological features	Traditional system	WHO system	British Society for Cervical Cytology	Bethesda system
Atypical squamous cells not meeting the criteria for dysplasia	Mild atypia	Mild atypia	Borderline nuclear abnormality	Atypical squamous cells (ASC)
Koilocytes plus mild atypia	HPV infection	HPV infection	HPV plus borderline change	Low-grade squamous intraepithelial lesion (SIL)
Dysplasia limited to lower third of epithelium	Mild dysplasia	CIN 1	Mild dyskaryosis (low-grade dyskaryosis)	Low-grade SIL
Dysplasia limited to lower two-thirds of epithelium	Moderate dysplasia	CIN 2	Moderate dyskaryosis (high-grade dyskaryosis)	High-grade SIL
Dysplasia extending into upper third of epithelium	Severe dysplasia	CIN 3	Severe dyskaryosis (high-grade dyskaryosis)	High-grade SIL
Dysplasia of full thickness of epithelium	Carcinoma in situ	CIN 3	Severe dyskaryosis (high-grade dyskaryosis)	High-grade SIL

FIG. 2 Comparison of grading systems. *CIN,* Cervical intraepithelial neoplasia; *HPV,* human papillomavirus; *WHO,* World Health Organization. (From Young B et al: Female reproductive system. In *Wheater's basic pathology,* Philadelphia, 2011, Elsevier, pp. 216-315.)

- Histopathology findings: Increased cellularity, nuclear abnormalities, and increased nuclear-to-cytoplasmic ratio.
- Cervical intraepithelial neoplasia (CIN) develops in the "transformation zone" of the cervix. Cells shed from the surface may be sampled by a variety of devices, so that cells from both the endocervix and ectocervix can then be examined microscopically for cytologic abnormalities, termed dyskaryosis. Although dyskaryosis is a cytologic diagnosis (Fig. E3), the degree of dyskaryosis correlates, to some extent, with the degree of CIN, which is a histologic diagnosis (Fig. E4).

ETIOLOGY

- Strongly associated and initiated by oncogenic HPV infection (high-risk HPV types are 16, 18, 31, 33, 35, 45, 51, 52, 56, and 58; low-risk HPV types are 6, 11, 42, 43, and 44).
- Dysplasia associated with HPV infections, particularly high-risk HPV strains, is caused by alterations in gene expression by infected squamous cells. HPV-associated proteins E6 and E7 bind to and degrade and inactivate p53 and retinoblastoma protein, respectively, which alter DNA repair mechanisms.[3]
- Other causes include vaginal and cervical infections, recent intercourse, recent instrumentation of the cervix, postmenopausal changes, exogenous hormone use, radiation exposure, cervical polyps, cysts, and HPV infection. Most causes of atypia are not pathologic and will not lead to cervical cancer.

🅓🆇 DIAGNOSIS

DIFFERENTIAL DIAGNOSIS

- Metaplasia
- Hyperkeratosis
- Condyloma
- Nabothian cysts
- Microinvasive carcinoma
- Glandular epithelial abnormalities
- Vulvar intraepithelial neoplasm
- Vaginal intraepithelial neoplasm
- Metastatic tumor involvement of the cervix

WORKUP

- All patients with a cervix should be screened regularly for cervical cancer and dysplasia using either cytology alone, HPV testing alone, or a cotest depending on their risk. See screening guidelines in Table 1. Screening is more frequent in patients with a history of abnormal results or prior dysplasia.
- Patients without a cervix with a prior history of high-grade dysplasia (CIN II, III, or carcinoma in situ) require screening for 25 yr after treatment/excision or abnormality.
- Abnormal cytology and/or HPV positivity: Risk assessment using American Society for Colposcopy and Cervical Pathology (ASCCP) guidelines should be performed; colposcopy or immediate excisional treatment may be recommended; follow ASCCP treatment algorithm guidelines.
- Consider screening for sexually transmitted disease (gonorrhea, *Chlamydia,* herpes, HIV, HPV).
- Grossly evident or suspicious lesions should be referred for colposcopy and biopsy with endocervical curettage (ECC). Examination should include cervix, vagina, vulva, and anus; some patients qualify for immediate treatment; refer to ASCCP guidelines.
- For glandular cell abnormalities (AGCs): Refer for colposcopy and possible directed biopsy/ECC; strongly recommend endometrial sampling.
- In pregnancy: Abnormal cytology should be followed by colposcopy in the first trimester and at 28 to 32 wk; only high-grade lesions suspicious for carcinoma biopsied; ECC is contraindicated.

LABORATORY TESTS

- Primary HPV, primary cytology, or cotesting (cytology with HPV) depending on patient characteristics
- HPV DNA typing
- Colposcopy, directed cervical biopsy, and ECC (for indications see "Workup")
- As compared with Pap testing, HPV testing has greater sensitivity for the detection of intraepithelial neoplasia
- Gonorrhea and chlamydia screening should be offered at least annually, especially to high-risk groups and all patients <26 yr old
- HIV screening test if indicated (high-risk group or no HIV screen in past)
- Follow-up testing per ASCCP guidelines; see Table 1 for management

IMAGING STUDIES

- Not typically recommended for routine workup of cervical dysplasia. High-grade dysplasia with suspected invasive carcinoma can be evaluated clinically and with computed tomography (CT) C/A/P to evaluate for metastases.
- If advanced cancer is suspected, PET-CT scan can be considered.

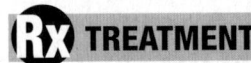 **TREATMENT**

UPDATED 2019 ASCCP RISK-BASED MANAGEMENT CONSENSUS GUIDELINES[1]

- Recommendations of colposcopy, treatment, or surveillance will be based on a patient's risk of CIN 3 or greater as determined by a combination of current results and past history.
- Repeat HPV testing or cotesting at 1 yr is recommended for patients with minor screening abnormalities indicating HPV infection with low

---

TABLE 1 Summary of Recommendations

Population	Recommended Screening Method	Management of Screen Results	Comments
<21 yr	No screening		
21-29 yr	Cytology alone every 3 yr; consider primary HPV testing in 25-29 yr with average risk	If normal results, routine screening. If cytology is abnormal, reflex HPV testing and typing should be performed on the same sample. Risk assessment of CIN3+ should be performed; if risk is 4% or greater, colposcopy or treatment are recommended. Refer to ASCCP.	Abnormal results require follow-up and more frequent surveillance.
30-65 yr	Any one of the following: Primary HPV testing every 5 yr Cotesting every 5 yr with HPV and cytology simultaneously performed Cytology alone every 3 yr (not preferred)	HPV-positive samples should be typed; cytology should be performed on the same sample for any high-risk HPV-positive specimen.	Abnormal results require follow-up and may require treatment.
>65 yr	No screening following adequate negative prior screening; requires ×3 consecutive negative cytology or ×2 consecutive negative contesting or high-risk HPV results within 10 yr before stopping screening	More older adults are finding new sexual partners, which may increase their risks of exposure.	Patients with a history of high-grade lesions or a more severe diagnosis should continue routine screening for at least 25 yr since last abnormal screen.
After TOTAL hysterectomy	No screening if no history of high-grade cervical precancerous lesions or cervical cancer	Not applicable.	Make sure all patients are up to date on cervical cancer screening before hysterectomy.

ACCP, American Society for Colposcopy and Cervical Pathology; *HPV,* human papillomavirus;
Modified from American College of Obstetricians and Gynecologists: Updated cervical cancer screening guidelines, ACOG Clinical. Available at https://www.acog.org/clinical/clinical-guidance/practice-advisory/articles/2021/04/updated-cervical-cancer-screening-guidelines.

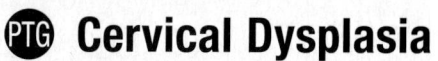
C

Diseases and Disorders

I

risk of underlying CIN 3+ (e.g., HPV-positive, low-grade cytologic abnormalities after a documented negative screening HPV test or cotest).

- Expedited treatment is recommended for patients with HSIL cytology.
  1. For nonpregnant patients 25 yr or older, expedited treatment, defined as treatment without preceding colposcopic biopsy demonstrating CIN 2+, is preferred when the immediate risk of CIN 3+ is ≥60% and is acceptable for those with risks between 25% and 60%.
  2. Expedited treatment is preferred for nonpregnant patients 25 yr or older with high-grade squamous intraepithelial lesion (HSIL) cytology and concurrent positive testing for HPV genotype 16 (i.e., HPV 16-positive HSIL cytology) and never or rarely screened patients with HPV-positive HSIL cytology regardless of HPV genotype.
  3. Shared decision-making should be used when considering expedited treatment, especially for patients with concerns about the potential impact of treatment on pregnancy outcomes.
- Excisional treatment is preferred to ablative treatment for histologic HSIL (CIN 2 or CIN 3) in the U.S. Excision is recommended for adenocarcinoma in situ (AIS).
- For CIN1, observation is preferred to treatment.
- Histopathology reports based on Lower Anogenital Squamous Terminology (LAST)/World Health Organization (WHO) recommendations for reporting histologic HSIL should include CIN 2 or CIN 3 qualifiers (i.e., HSIL [CIN 2] and HSIL [CIN 3]).
- All positive primary HPV screening tests, regardless of genotype, should have additional reflex triage testing performed from the same laboratory specimen (e.g., reflex cytology).
  1. Additional testing from the same laboratory specimen is recommended because the findings may inform colposcopy practice. For example, HPV 16-positive HSIL cytology qualifies for expedited treatment.
  2. HPV 16 or 18 infections have the highest risk for CIN 3 and occult cancer, so additional evaluation (e.g., colposcopy with biopsy) is necessary even when cytology results are negative.
  3. If HPV 16 or 18 testing is positive and additional laboratory testing of the same sample is not feasible, the patient should proceed directly to colposcopy.
- Continued surveillance with HPV testing or cotesting at 3-yr intervals for at least 25 yr is recommended after treatment and initial posttreatment management of histologic HSIL, CIN 2, CIN 3, or AIS.
- Continued surveillance at 3-yr intervals beyond 25 yr is acceptable for as long as the patient's life expectancy and ability to be screened are not significantly compromised by serious health issues.
  1. The 2012 guidelines recommended return to 5-yr screening intervals and did not specify when screening should cease. New evidence indicates that risk remains

elevated for at least 25 yr, with no evidence that treated patients ever return to risk levels compatible with 5-yr intervals.
- Surveillance with cytology alone is acceptable **only if** testing with HPV or cotesting is not feasible.
- Cytology alone is less sensitive than HPV testing for detection of precancer and therefore is recommended to be repeated more frequently. For surveillance of high-risk individuals as identified by abnormal screening results, cytology is recommended at 6-mo intervals; HPV testing or cotesting is recommended annually. Cytology is recommended annually when 3-yr intervals are recommended for HPV or cotesting.
- HPV assays that are FDA-approved for screening should be used for management according to their regulatory approval in the U.S. (NOTE: All HPV testing in this document refers to testing for high-risk HPV types only.)
  1. For all management indications, HPV mRNA and HPV DNA tests without FDA approval for primary screening alone should only be used as a cotest with cytology, unless sufficient, rigorous data are available to support use of these particular tests in management.

ACUTE GENERAL Rx
- If LSIL (formerly CIN 1), observation may be appropriate dependent on risk stratification
- If HSIL (formerly CIN 2 or CIN 3), excisional treatment

CHRONIC Rx
- Primary prevention: The HPV vaccination series should be offered to all patients beginning at age 9 through 26. Patients age 27 to 45 could benefit from vaccination, though vaccinating in this age group should be individualized.[4]
- Secondary prevention: Close monitoring of patients with a history of dysplasia or excisional treatment should be performed according to guidelines; smoking cessation should be encouraged.

DISPOSITION
- Because of the large number of women in high-risk groups, the prevalence of HPV, and the high false-negative Pap smear rate, routine screening should be strongly encouraged for all women, especially those with a history of cervical dysplasia.
- Success rates for treatment approach 80% to 90%.
- Detection of persistent dysplasia or recurrence requires careful follow-up.
- Cervical treatment can increase risk for poor obstetric outcomes (cervical incompetence with subsequent miscarriage or preterm birth), which requires careful consideration and discretion for use of loop electrosurgical excision procedure and cone biopsy in women desiring future childbearing.
- Appropriate counseling and informed consent are needed when considering any form of management of cervical dysplasia.

REFERRAL
- Patients with abnormal cytology or high-risk or untyped HPV positivity should be referred to a provider, preferably a trained obstetrician/gynecologist, who can appropriately treat the patient in an age-specific manner and also perform a colposcopy or excisional procedure if indicated as part of the new recommendations. Given the morbidity associated with both underevaluation and undertreatment, as well as reacting excessively to cytologic findings, a provider who is intimately familiar with ASCCP guidelines should be sought.
- An interactive application for phones and tablets made by ASCCP is available for a small fee to providers and can be helpful in determining follow-up and screening intervals.
- If treatment is required, patients should be referred to a gynecologist or gynecologic oncologist skilled in the diagnosis and treatment of preinvasive cervical disease.

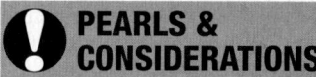 **PEARLS & CONSIDERATIONS**

COMMENTS
- Testing for human papillomavirus will identify 91% of the small proportion of women with posttreatment residual or recurrent disease, but a high proportion of all women who are tested will test positive and need colposcopy.
- HPV vaccination is recommended for males and females from ages 9 to 26. For individuals ages 27 through 45 yr who are not adequately vaccinated, HPV vaccination can be considered and administered with shared decision-making. Benefits of the vaccine in older age groups are lower due to decreased immunogenicity with age and preexposure and preexisting HPV infections.

PREVENTION
- Cervical cancer is an almost entirely preventable disease; all patients should be evaluated for eligibility for HPV vaccination; earlier vaccination in childhood is safe and associated with higher immunogenicity and efficacy. The vaccine is not recommended in pregnancy.
- Routine screening should be performed in all patients with a cervix; additional surveillance at more frequent intervals should be performed for patients with a history of cervical dysplasia.

RELATED CONTENT
Cervical Cancer (Related Key Topic)
Cervical Dysplasia (Patient Information)
Cervical Polyps (Related Key Topic)
Pap Smear Abnormalities (Patient Information)

AUTHORS: **ELLEN MYERS, MD** and **KELLY MCNAMARA, MD**

REFERENCES
Available at eBooks.Health.Elsevier.com.

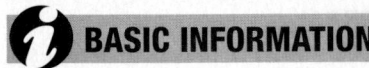 BASIC INFORMATION

DEFINITION

Genital infection with *Chlamydia trachomatis* (CT) is the most prevalent sexually transmitted disease in the U.S. In women, *Chlamydia* infection can result in cervicitis, acute urethral syndrome, endometritis, and pelvic inflammatory disease. These infections can, in turn, lead to ectopic pregnancy, infertility, and chronic pelvic pain (see "Pelvic Inflammatory Disease"). In men, CT infection may cause mucopurulent discharge, urethritis, epididymitis, and prostatitis. Both men and women can develop rectal CT infection, which is often asymptomatic but may manifest as proctitis. CT serovars L1-3 are associated a with a less common manifestation of CT, lymphogranuloma venerum (LGV). This is more commonly seen among men who have sex with men (MSM) and often manifests as proctocolitis with notable lymphadenopathy. Newborns born via an infected birth canal are at risk for conjunctivitis and pneumonia. A majority of individuals affected with CT are asymptomatic. Thus screening tests play an important role in detection of this infection to initiate treatment, impede disease sequelae, and prevent further transmission.[1-3]

ICD-10CM CODES

A56.2	Chlamydial infection of genitourinary tract, unspecified
A56	Other sexually transmitted chlamydial diseases
A56.0	Chlamydial infection of lower genitourinary tract
A56.00	Chlamydial infection of lower genitourinary tract, unspecified
A56.01	Chlamydial cystitis and urethritis
A56.02	Chlamydia vulvovaginitis
A56.09	Other chlamydial infection of lower genitourinary tract
A56.1	Chlamydial infection of pelviperitoneum and other genitourinary organs
A56.19	Other chlamydial genitourinary infection
A56.2	Chlamydial infection of genitourinary tract, unspecified
A56.3	Chlamydial infection of anus and rectum
A56.4	Chlamydial infection of pharynx
A56.8	Sexually transmitted chlamydial infection of other sites

EPIDEMIOLOGY & DEMOGRAPHICS

- *C. trachomatis* is the most commonly reported sexually transmitted disease in the U.S., with more than 1.6 million cases reported to the Centers for Disease Control and Prevention (CDC) in 2021. This represents a decreased in reported cases with 1.8 million cases reported in 2019. Rather than a decrease in disease, this is believed to represent lack of access to outpatient testing and treatment during the COVID-19 pandemic.[2]
- Regardless, many cases of CT infection are asymptomatic and likely remain undiagnosed. It is estimated that 10% of men and 5% to 30% of women have symptoms.[4]

- Age is a strong predictor for risk of CT infection. Individuals less than 25 yr old are the largest age group affected by *C. trachomatis*; 61% of reported *Chlamydia* infections were among individuals ages 15 to 24 yr.[2]
- *Chlamydia* conjunctivitis occurs in 18% to 44% of infants, and chlamydial pneumonia occurs in 3% to 16% of infants who are delivered by mothers with untreated CT infection at the time of delivery.[4]
- Pelvic inflammatory disease develops in 10% to 15% of women with untreated CT infections.[5]
- Untreated CT increases a person's risk of acquiring HIV.[4]
- In men, 15% to 55% of nongonococcal urethritis cases are caused by *C. trachomatis*.
- Anorectal *Chlamydia* infection can occur in partners who engage in anal sex and is more common among men who have sex with men. However, it can also occur in women with CT cervicitis and no history of anal sex.[4]
- Table 1 summarizes clinical characteristics of common *C. trachomatis* infections.

PHYSICAL FINDINGS & CLINICAL PRESENTATION

- Chlamydial infections are commonly asymptomatic. Clinical manifestations in symptomatic women affected with *C. trachomatis* may include vaginal discharge or irregular vaginal bleeding. Purulent discharge or cervicitis may be visualized on speculum examination. Easily induced endocervical bleeding can be noted on examination and is caused by inflammation of endocervical columnar epithelium. Untreated infection can ascend the reproductive tract, causing pelvic inflammatory disease. Clinical signs of pelvic inflammatory disease are cervical, uterine, or adnexal tenderness on examination. Complications of pelvic disease are ectopic pregnancy, infertility, and chronic pelvic pain.
- Symptoms in men may include dysuria or a mucopurulent penile discharge. A complication that can arise from CT infection in men is epididymitis, which manifests as unilateral testicular pain, hydrocele, or swelling of the epididymis. An untreated CT infection can also cause prostatitis in men. Prostatitis may present as urinary dysfunction, pain with ejaculation, and pelvic pain.
- Chlamydial conjunctivitis can be experienced by both men and women and is the result of conjunctiva exposed to infected genital secretions. CT infection can also cause proctitis or infection of the rectum in men and women. This usually presents with rectal pain, discharge, or bleeding. CT infection of the throat is usually asymptomatic in both men and women and not a usual cause of pharyngitis. Less frequent manifestations of CT infection may include perihepatitis (Fitz-Hugh–Curtis syndrome), reactive arthritis (Reiter syndrome), or LGV.
- Clinical manifestations and sequelae of *Chlamydia trachomitis* urogenital infections and patterns of transmission are illustrated in Fig. 1.

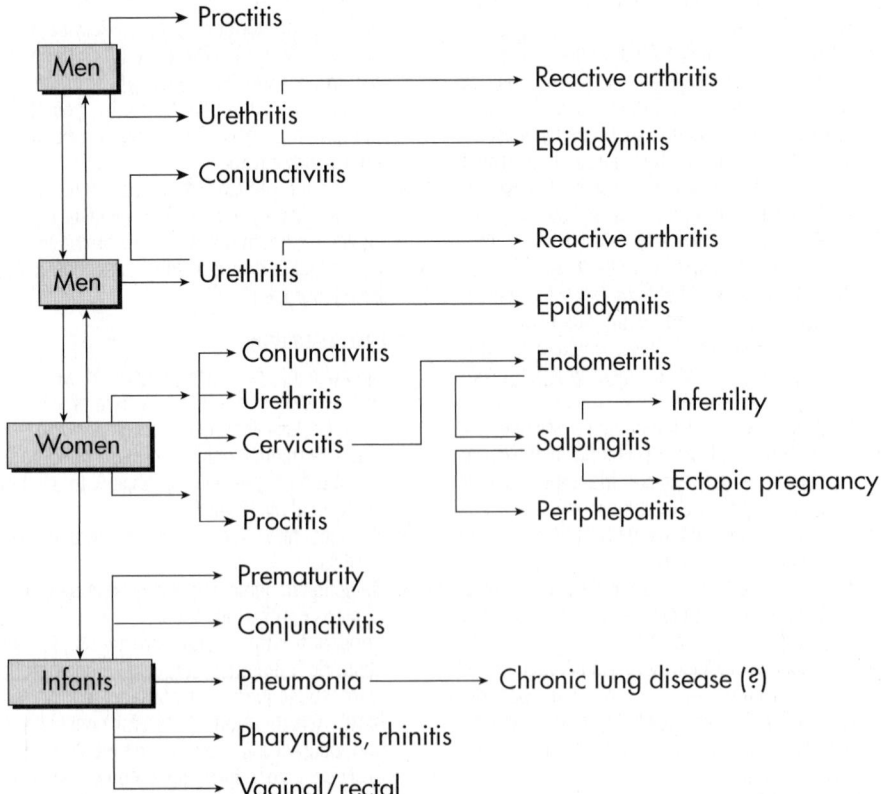

FIG. 1 Clinical manifestations and sequelae of *Chlamydia trachomatis* urogenital infections and patterns of transmission. (From Bennett JE et al: *Mandell, Douglas, and Bennett's principles and practice of infectious diseases*, ed 9, Philadelphia, 2020, Elsevier.)

TABLE 1   Clinical Characteristics of Common *Chlamydia trachomatis* Infections

	Infection	Symptoms and Signs	Presumptive Diagnosis	Definitive Diagnosis	Treatment
Men	Nongonococcal urethritis	Urethral discharge, dysuria	Urethral leukocytosis; no gonococci seen	Urine or urethral NAAT	Doxycycline, 100 mg PO bid, for 7 days
	Epididymitis	Unilateral epididymal tenderness, swelling; pain; fever, presence of NGU	Urine or urethral NAAT	Urethral leukocytosis; pyuria on urinalysis	STI likely: Ceftriaxone 500 mg (1 g for individuals weighing >150 kg) IM plus doxycycline, 100 mg PO bid, for 10 days
					If enteric organisms are suspected:
					Ceftriaxone, 500 mg (1 g for individuals weighing >150 kg) IM, plus levofloxacin, 500 mg bid for 10 days
	Proctitis (non-LGV)	Rectal pain, discharge and bleeding; history of receptive anal intercourse	≥1 PMN/OIF on rectal Gram stain; no gonococci seen	Urine or urethral NAAT; rectal culture or NAAT	Ceftriaxone, 500 mg (1 g for individuals weighing >150 kg) IM, plus doxycycline, 100 mg PO bid, for 7 days
	Lymphogranuloma venereum proctitis	Painful, tender inguinal lymphadenopathy, fever	"Groove sign"	Urine, urethral, lymph node, or rectal NAAT; rectal or lymph node culture; LGV-specific testing if available	Doxycycline, 100 mg PO bid, for 21 days
Women	Cervicitis	Mucopurulent cervical discharge; ectopy, easily induced bleeding	≥20 PMN/OIF on cervical Gram stain	Urine or cervical NAAT	Doxycycline, 100 mg PO bid, for 7 days
	Urethritis	Dysuria, frequency; no hematuria	Pyuria on UA; negative urine Gram stain and culture	Urine, cervical, or urethral NAAT	Doxycycline, 100 mg PO bid for 7 days
	Pelvic inflammatory disease	Lower abdominal pain, adnexal pain, cervical motion tenderness	Evidence of mucopurulent cervicitis	Urine or cervical NAAT	Outpatient: Ceftriaxone 500 mg IM as a single dose, plus doxycycline 100 mg PO bid for 14 days, with metronidazole, 500 mg PO bid for 14 days
Adults	Conjunctivitis	Ocular pain, redness, discharge; simultaneous genital infection	Gram stain of conjunctival swab negative for bacterial pathogens; PMNs on smear	DFA or NAAT on conjunctival swab	Doxycycline, 100 mg PO bid for 7 days
Newborns	Conjunctivitis	Ocular pain, redness, discharge; simultaneous genital infection	Gram stain of conjunctival swab negative for bacterial pathogens; PMNs on smear	DFA or NAAT on conjunctival swab; vagina, rectum, pharynx also often positive	Erythromycin base 50 mg/kg/day, PO divided into four doses daily for 14 days; evaluate and treat parents as well
	Pneumonia	Staccato cough, tachypnea, hyperinflation	Diffuse interstitial infiltrate, eosinophilia	Nasopharyngeal NAATs or culture; MIF serology (IgM)	Erythromycin base or ethylsuccinate 50 mg/kg/day, PO divided into four doses daily for 14 days; evaluate and treat parents as well

bid, Twice daily; *DFA,* direct fluorescent antibody; *IgM,* immunoglobulin M; *IM,* intramuscular; *LGV,* lymphogranuloma venereum; *MIF,* microimmunofluorescence; *MSM,* men who have sex with men; *NAAT,* nucleic acid amplification test; *NGU,* nongonococcal urethritis; *OIF,* oil immersion field; *PMN,* polymorphonuclear neutrophil; *PO,* by mouth; *STI,* sexually transmitted infection; *UA,* urinalysis.
From Bennett JE et al: Bennett JE et al: *Mandell, Douglas, and Bennett's principles and practice of infectious diseases,* ed 9, Philadelphia, 2020, Elsevier.

ETIOLOGY
- *C. trachomatis* consists of 15 serotypes
- Obligate, intracellular bacteria

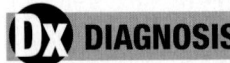 **DIAGNOSIS**

DIFFERENTIAL DIAGNOSIS

Differential diagnosis depends on presenting symptoms. Some of the common differentials are listed in the following:
- Candidiasis
- Conjunctivitis
- Ectopic pregnancy
- Endometriosis
- Gonorrhea
- Mycoplasma infection
- Pelvic inflammatory disease
- Trichomonas
- Urethritis
- Urinary tract infection

WORKUP

Individuals with signs and symptoms mentioned previously should be screened for CT infection. Because majority of CT infections are asymptomatic, routine screening should be offered to individuals at risk for CT infection. In women, screening reduces the rate of pelvic inflammatory disease. Annual screening is thus recommended for all sexually active women less than 25 yr of age and women at any age at risk for sexually transmitted infections. Risk factors include acquiring a new sexual partner, having more than one sexual partner or a nonmonogamous partner (includes individuals working in the sex industry), or having a history of sexually transmitted infection. Screening interval is determined by any new risk for exposure since the last negative screening. The CDC recommends CT screening for all pregnant women under the age of 25 and for any pregnant woman over the age of 25 who is at increased risk for acquiring CT at their initial prenatal care visit. These same pregnant women should be screened again during the third trimester. At a minimum, annual screening is also recommended for men who have sex with men and persons with HIV.[1,3]

LABORATORY TESTS
- Nucleic acid amplification tests (NAATs) are the gold standard for diagnosis because of their high sensitivity and specificity for the detection of CT infection. The FDA has approved these tests for male and female urine collection and for provider-collected endocervical, vaginal, and male urethral specimens.[1,3]
- Rectal and pharyngeal collection site specimens may be taken from individuals who engage in receptive anal and oral intercourse, but these collection sites are not FDA approved.
- Vaginal swabs are more sensitive than urine for the detection of CT and are often preferred. The sensitivity of vaginal swab vs. urine for CT has been estimated as 94.1% vs. 86.9%.[6]
- For best results, urine collection should be completed with a first-void urine sample.
- Self-collected vaginal swab samples for women have the same sensitivity and specificity as provider-collected samples.
- The same specimen can be used to test for *Chlamydia* and gonorrhea.
- Sexual partners of a person testing positive for CT infection should be treated if they had sexual contact with that individual within 60 days before onset of symptoms or CT diagnosis.
- Microscopy should not be used for *Chlamydia* diagnosis; however, >10 white blood cells per high-power field with a mucopurulent discharge can be a presumptive diagnosis.

TREATMENT

ACUTE GENERAL Rx

ADOLESCENTS & ADULTS: Nongonococcal urethritis, urethritis, cervicitis, conjunctivitis (except for lymphogranuloma venereum):
- Doxycycline 100 mg PO bid for 7 days

INFECTION IN PREGNANCY:
- Azithromycin 1 g PO single-dose therapy

ALTERNATIVE REGIMENS:
- Azithromycin 1 g PO × single-dose therapy *or*
- Levofloxacin 500 mg/day PO for 7 days
- Alternative regimen in pregnancy: Amoxicillin 500 mg PO tid for 7 days

NOTE: Azithromycin (Pregnancy Risk Category B) is generally considered safe and effective during pregnancy and with lactation. Doxycycline is contraindicated in pregnancy.

FOLLOW-UP:
- Observed single-dose therapy should be offered to individuals for whom compliance is a concern.

- To minimize disease transmission to partners, affected persons should be advised to refrain from sexual intercourse for 7 days after single-dose therapy, until completion of 7-day therapy, or until resolution of symptoms.
- To prevent reinfection, affected individuals should refrain from sexual intercourse until all of their partners have been treated.
- Re-collection by NAAT method in <4 wk from treatment can yield a false-positive result due to the sensitivity of this testing method.
- Both men and women treated for *Chlamydia* should be retested at approximately 3 mo after treatment to screen for reinfection. If patients do not return to clinical settings within 3 mo, rescreen the patient at the next presentation for clinical care.
- Pregnant women with *C. trachomatis* infection should have a test of cure 4 wk after treatment and should then be retested within 3 mo.

RECURRENT & PERSISTENT URETHRITIS: Retreat noncompliant patients with the above regimens. If patient was initially compliant, recommended regimens include metronidazole 2 g PO in single dose plus erythromycin base 500 mg PO qid for 7 days or erythromycin ethylsuccinate 800 mg PO qid for 7 days.

RECTAL *CHLAMYDIA*: A 7-day course of doxycycline (100 mg twice daily for 7 days) is superior to single-dose infection among men who have sex with men.[1]

REFERRAL

Refer to infectious disease specialist if persistent infection or gynecologist if salpingitis is suspected.

RELATED CONTENT

Cervicitis (Related Key Topic)
Urethritis, Gonococcal (Related Key Topic)
Gonorrhea (Related Key Topic)
Urethritis, Nongonococcal (Related Key Topic)
Pelvic Inflammatory Disease (Related Key Topic)

AUTHORS: **BETHANY K SEDERDAHL, MPH, MD** and **ANTHONY SCISCIONE, DO**

REFERENCES & SUGGESTED READINGS

Available at eBooks.Health.Elsevier.com.

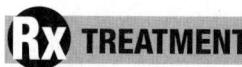

ℹ BASIC INFORMATION

DEFINITION

Cholecystitis is acute or chronic inflammation of the gallbladder generally caused by gallstones (>95% of cases).

SYNONYMS

Gallbladder attack
Biliary colic

ICD-10CM CODES
K81.9	Acute cholecystitis
K80.00	Calculus of gallbladder with acute cholecystitis without obstruction
K81.9	Cholecystitis, unspecified

EPIDEMIOLOGY & DEMOGRAPHICS

- Acute cholecystitis occurs most commonly in women during the fifth and sixth decades. Approximately 120,000 cholecystectomies are performed for acute cholecystitis annually in the U.S.
- The incidence of gallstones is 0.6% in the general population and much higher in certain ethnic groups (>75% of Native Americans by age 60 yr). Most patients with gallstones are asymptomatic. Of such patients, biliary colic develops in 1% to 4% annually.

PHYSICAL FINDINGS & CLINICAL PRESENTATION

- Pain and tenderness in the right hypochondrium or epigastrium; pain possibly radiating to the infrascapular region
- Palpation of the right upper quadrant eliciting marked tenderness and stoppage of inspired breath (Murphy sign)
- Guarding
- Fever (33%)
- Jaundice (25% to 50% of patients)
- Palpable gallbladder (20% of cases)
- Nausea and vomiting (>70% of patients)
- Fever and chills (>25% of patients)
- Medical history often revealing ingestion of large, fatty meals before onset of pain in the epigastrium and right upper quadrant

ETIOLOGY

- Gallstones (>95% of cases). Factors contributing to gallstone formation are illustrated in Fig. E1
- Ischemic damage to the gallbladder, critically ill patient (acalculous cholecystitis)
- Infectious agents, especially in patients with AIDS (cytomegalovirus, *Cryptosporidium*)
- Strictures of the bile duct
- Neoplasms, primary or metastatic
- Risk factors for cholelithiasis include age, obesity, female sex, rapid weight loss, ethnicity/race (Native American), use of contraceptives, pregnancy, diabetes mellitus, use of glucagon-like peptide-1 (GLP-1) receptor agonists,[1] hemolysis, total parenteral nutrition, biliary parasites

Dx DIAGNOSIS

DIFFERENTIAL DIAGNOSIS

- Hepatic: Hepatitis, abscess, hepatic congestion, neoplasm, trauma
- Biliary: Neoplasm, stricture, sphincter of Oddi dysfunction
- Gastric: Pelvic ulcer disease, neoplasm, alcoholic gastritis, hiatal hernia, nonulcer dyspepsia
- Pancreatic: Pancreatitis, neoplasm, stone in the pancreatic duct or ampulla
- Renal: Calculi, infection, inflammation, neoplasm, ruptured kidney
- Pulmonary: Pneumonia, pulmonary infarction, right-sided pleurisy
- Intestinal: Retrocecal appendicitis, intestinal obstruction, high fecal impaction, irritable bowel syndrome (IBS), inflammatory bowel disease (IBD)
- Cardiac: Myocardial ischemia (particularly involving the inferior wall), pericarditis
- Cutaneous: Herpes zoster
- Trauma
- Fitz-Hugh-Curtis syndrome (perihepatitis), ruptured ectopic pregnancy
- Subphrenic abscess
- Dissecting aneurysm
- Nerve root irritation caused by osteoarthritis of the spine

WORKUP

Workup consists of detailed history and physical examination coupled with laboratory evaluation and imaging studies. No single clinical finding or laboratory test is sufficient to establish or exclude cholecystitis without further testing. Acute acalculous cholecystitis is acute inflammation of the gallbladder in the absence of stones. The term acalculous cholecystitis has been questioned as incorrectly suggesting that the disease is simply cholecystitis without stones. Instead, the term necrotizing cholecystitis has been proposed to reflect the distinct etiology, pathology, and prognosis of the disease. The symptoms of acalculous biliary pain may be indistinguishable from those of cholelithiasis. For older adult patients at risk, a high index of suspicion for biliary tract sepsis is the best hope for early recognition and treatment. Table 1 delineates several diagnostic criteria for acute acalculous cholecystitis.

LABORATORY TESTS

- Leukocytosis (12,000 to 20,000) is present in >70% of patients.
- Elevated alkaline phosphatase, ALT, AST, bilirubin; bilirubin elevation >4 mg/dl is unusual and suggests presence of choledocholithiasis.
- Elevated amylase may be present (consider pancreatitis if serum amylase elevation exceeds 500 U).

IMAGING STUDIES

- Ultrasound of the gallbladder (Figs. 2 and E3) is the preferred initial test; it will demonstrate the presence of stones and also dilated gallbladder with thickened wall and surrounding edema in patients with acute cholecystitis.
- Nuclear imaging (HIDA scan) (Fig. E4) is useful for diagnosis of cholecystitis when sonogram is inconclusive: Sensitivity and specificity exceed 90% for acute cholecystitis. This test is only reliable when bilirubin is <5 mg/dl. A positive test result (absence of gallbladder filling within 60 min after the administration of tracer) will demonstrate obstruction of the cystic or common hepatic duct; the test will not demonstrate the presence of stones.
- Computed tomography (CT) scan of abdomen (Fig. E5) is useful in cases of suspected abscess, neoplasm, or pancreatitis.
- Plain radiograph of the abdomen generally is not useful because <25% of stones are radiopaque.

Rx TREATMENT

NONPHARMACOLOGIC THERAPY

Provide intravenous (IV) hydration; withhold oral feedings.

ACUTE GENERAL Rx

- Laparoscopic (percutaneous) cholecystectomy (PC) is considered the treatment of choice for most patients. The rate of conversion to open cholecystectomy is higher when laparoscopic cholecystectomy (CCY) is performed for acute cholecystitis rather than for uncomplicated cholelithiasis; conservative management with IV fluids and antibiotics (ampicillin-sulbactam 3 g IV q6h or piperacillin-tazobactam 4.5 g IV q8h) may be justified in some high-risk patients to convert an emergency procedure into an elective one with a lower mortality rate.
- Endoscopic retrograde cholangiopancreatography with sphincterotomy and stone extraction can be performed in conjunction with laparoscopic cholecystectomy for patients with choledochal lithiasis; approximately 7% to 15% of patients with cholelithiasis also have stones in the common bile duct.

DISPOSITION

- Prognosis is good; elective laparoscopic cholecystectomy can be performed as outpatient procedure.
- Hospital stay (when necessary) varies from overnight with laparoscopic cholecystectomy to 4 to 7 days with open cholecystectomy.
- Complication rate is approximately 1% (hemorrhage and bile leak) for laparoscopic cholecystectomy and <0.5% (infection) with open cholecystectomy.

REFERRAL

Surgical referral in all patients with acute cholecystitis

TABLE 1 Diagnostic Criteria for Acute Acalculous Cholecystitis

Technique	Findings
Clinical evaluation	Right upper quadrant tenderness, if present, supports the diagnosis but is lacking in 75% of cases
	Unexplained fever, hypotension, leukocytosis, or hyperamylasemia is frequently the only finding
US	Thickened gallbladder wall (>4 mm) in the absence of ascites and hypoalbuminemia (serum albumin <3.2 g/dl)
	Sonographic Murphy sign (maximum tenderness over the US-localized gallbladder)
	Pericholecystic fluid collection
	Bedside availability is a major advantage
CT	Thickened gallbladder wall (>4 mm) in the absence of ascites and hypoalbuminemia
	Pericholecystic fluid, subserosal edema (in the absence of ascites), intramural gas, or sloughed mucosa
	The best test for excluding other intra-abdominal diseases but requires moving the patient to a scanner
Hepatobiliary scintigraphy	Nonvisualization of the gallbladder with normal excretion of radionuclide into the bile duct and duodenum indicates a positive result for acute cholecystitis
	Results in critically ill, immobilized patients may be falsely positive because of viscous bile
	Better at excluding than confirming acute cholecystitis

CT, Computed tomography; *US,* ultrasound.
From Feldman M et al: *Sleisenger and Fordtran's gastrointestinal and liver disease,* ed 11, Philadelphia, 2021, Elsevier.

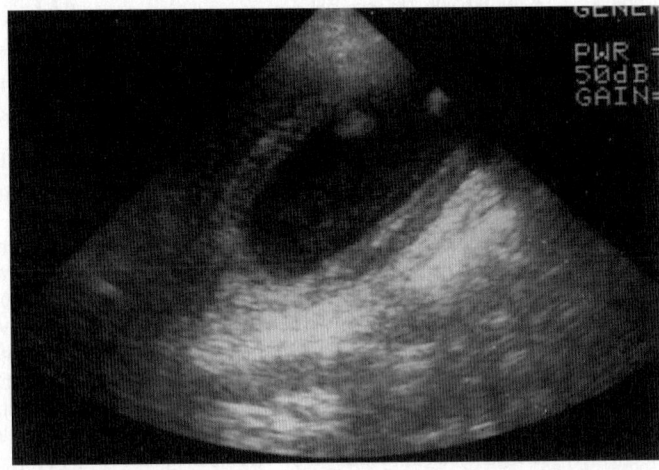

FIG. 2 Thickened gallbladder wall in acute cholecystitis. The gallbladder contains echogenic calculi. (From Grainger RG et al [eds]: *Grainger and Allison's diagnostic radiology,* ed 4, Philadelphia, 2001, Churchill Livingstone.)

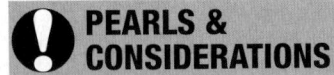

PEARLS & CONSIDERATIONS

COMMENTS

- Patients should be instructed that stones may recur in bile ducts.
- Gallbladder aspiration, in which all fluid visualized by ultrasound is aspirated, represents a nonsurgical treatment when patients who are at high operative risk develop acute cholecystitis. Salvage cholecystectomy is reserved for nonresponders.

REFERENCE & SUGGESTED READINGS

Available at eBooks.Health.Elsevier.com.

RELATED CONTENT

Gallbladder Attack (Cholecystitis) (Patient Information)
Cholangiocarcinoma (Related Key Topic)
Choledocholithiasis (Related Key Topic)
Cholelithiasis (Related Key Topic)
Cholangitis (Related Key Topic)
Functional Gallbladder Disorder (Related Key Topic)

AUTHOR: **FRED F. FERRI, MD**

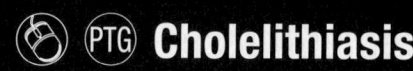

C

Diseases and Disorders

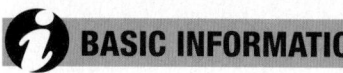 **BASIC INFORMATION**

DEFINITION

Cholelithiasis is the presence of stones in the gallbladder.

SYNONYM

Gallstones

ICD-10CM CODES	
K80.80	Other cholelithiasis without obstruction
K80.81	Other cholelithiasis with obstruction
K91.86	Retained cholelithiasis following cholecystectomy

EPIDEMIOLOGY & DEMOGRAPHICS

- Gallstone disease can be found in 12% of the U.S. population. Of these, 2% to 3% (500,000 to 600,000) are treated with cholecystectomies each year.
- Annual medical expenditures for gallbladder surgeries in the U.S. exceed $5 billion.
- Incidence of gallbladder disease increases with age. Highest incidence is in the fifth and sixth decades. Predisposing factors for gallstones are female sex, pregnancy, age >40 yr, family history of gallstones, obesity, ileal disease, oral contraceptives, diabetes mellitus, rapid weight loss, estrogen replacement therapy.
- Patients with gallstones have a 20% chance of developing biliary colic or its complications at the end of a 20-yr period. Significant predictors of gallstone-related events are large stone (>10 mm), presence of multiple stones, and female sex.

PHYSICAL FINDINGS & CLINICAL PRESENTATION (TABLE 1)

- Physical examination is entirely normal unless patient is having biliary colic; 80% of gallstones are asymptomatic.
- Typical symptoms of obstruction of the cystic duct include intermittent, severe, cramping pain affecting the right upper quadrant.
- Pain occurs mostly at night and may radiate to the back or right shoulder. It can last from a few minutes to several hours.

TABLE 1 Pathophysiology, Clinical Manifestations, Diagnosis, and Treatment of Gallstone Disease

	Biliary pain	Acute Cholecystitis	Choledocholithiasis	Cholangitis
Pathophysiology	Intermittent obstruction of the cystic duct No acute inflammation of the gallbladder	Impacted stone in the cystic duct Acute inflammation of the gallbladder Secondary bacterial infection in ≈50%	Stone passed from the gallbladder via the cystic duct or formed in the BD Intermitted obstruction of the BD	A stone in the BD causing bile stasis Bacterial superinfection of stagnant bile Early bacteremia
Symptoms	Severe, poorly localized, epigastric or right upper quadrant visceral pain growing in intensity over 15 min and remaining constant for 1-6 h, often with nausea Frequency of attacks varies from days to months Gas, bloating, flatulence, and dyspepsia are not related to stones	75% of cases are preceded by attacks of biliary pain Visceral epigastric pain gives way to moderately severe localized pain in the right upper quadrant, back, right shoulder, or, rarely, chest Nausea with some vomiting is frequent Pain lasting >6 h favors cholecystitis over biliary pain alone	Often asymptomatic Symptoms (when present) are indistinguishable from biliary pain Predisposes to cholangitis and acute pancreatitis	Charcot triad (pain, jaundice, and fever) is present in 70% of patients Pain may be mild and transient and is often accompanied by chills Mental confusion, lethargy, and delirium suggest sepsis
Physical findings	Mild-to-moderate epigastric/right upper quadrant tenderness during an attack, with mild residual tenderness lasting days Often, findings are normal	Fever, but usually to <102°F unless complicated by gangrene or perforation Right subcostal tenderness with inspiratory arrest (Murphy sign) Palpable gallbladder in 33% of patients, especially those having their first attack Mild jaundice in 20%; higher frequency in older adults	Often findings are completely normal if the obstruction is intermittent Jaundice with pain suggests stones; painless jaundice and a palpable gallbladder favor malignancy	Fever in 95%, right upper quadrant tenderness in 90% Jaundice in 80% Peritoneal signs in 15% Hypotension and mental confusion (forming Reynolds pentad in combination with Charcot triad) coexist in 15% and suggest gram-negative sepsis
Laboratory findings	Usually normal Elevated serum bilirubin, alkaline phosphatase, or amylase levels suggest coexisting BD stones	Leukocytosis with band forms is common Serum bilirubin level may be 2-4 mg/dl, and aminotransferase and alkaline phosphatase levels may be elevated even in the absence of a BD stone or hepatic infection Mild serum amylase and lipase elevations are seen even in the absence of pancreatitis If serum bilirubin is >4 mg/dl or amylase or lipase is markedly elevated, a BD stone should be suspected	Elevated serum bilirubin and alkaline phosphatase levels are seen with BD obstruction Serum bilirubin level >10 mg/dl suggests malignant obstruction or coexisting hemolysis A transient "spike" in serum aminotransferase and amylase (or lipase) levels suggests the passage of a stone	Leukocytosis in 80%, but the remainder may have a normal WBC count with or without band forms Serum bilirubin level is >2 mg/dl in 80% Serum alkaline phosphatase level is usually elevated Blood cultures are usually positive, especially during chills or a fever spike; 2 organisms are grown in cultures from half of patients
Diagnostic studies	US Oral cholecystography Meltzer-Lyon test	US Hepatobiliary scintigraphy Abdominal CT	ERCP EUS MRC Percutaneous THC	ERCP Percutaneous THC

Continued

TABLE 1 Pathophysiology, Clinical Manifestations, Diagnosis, and Treatment of Gallstone Disease—cont'd

	Biliary pain	Acute Cholecystitis	Choledocholithiasis	Cholangitis
Natural history	After the initial attack, 30% of patients have no further symptoms Symptoms develop in the remainder at a rate of 6% per year, and severe complications at a rate of 1%-2% per year	50% of cases resolve spontaneously in 7-10 days without surgery Left untreated, 10% of cases are complicated by a localized perforation and 1% by a free perforation and peritonitis	The natural history is not well defined, but complications are more common and more severe than for asymptomatic stones in the gallbladder	A high mortality rate if unrecognized, with death from septicemia Emergency decompression of the BD (usually by ERCP) improves survival dramatically
Treatment	Elective laparoscopic cholecystectomy, possibly with IOC ERCP for stone removal or BD exploration if IOC shows stones	Laparoscopic cholecystectomy, possibly with IOC if feasible; otherwise open cholecystectomy BD exploration or ERCP for stone removal if IOC shows stones	Stone removal at the time of ERCP, followed in most cases by early laparoscopic cholecystectomy	Emergency ERCP with stone removal or at least biliary decompression Antibiotics to cover gram-negative and possibly anaerobic organisms and *Enterococcus* spp. Subsequent cholecystectomy

BD, Bile duct; *CT*, computed tomography; *ERCP*, endoscopic retrograde cholangiopancreatography; *EUS*, endoscopic ultrasound; *IOC*, intraoperative cholangiography; *MRC*, magnetic resonance cholangiography; *THC*, transhepatic cholangiography; *US*, ultrasound; *WBC*, white blood cells.
From Feldman M et al: *Sleisenger and Fordtran's gastrointestinal and liver disease*, ed 11, Philadelphia, 2021, Elsevier.

- Symptoms of gallstone disease and its complications are described in Table 2 and Fig. E1.

ETIOLOGY

- 75% of gallstones contain cholesterol and are usually associated with obesity, female sex, and diabetes mellitus; mixed stones are most common (80%); pure cholesterol stones account for only 10% of stones and are the result of biliary supersaturation due to cholesterol secretion into the gallbladder and accelerated cholesterol nucleation and crystallization.
- 25% of gallstones are pigment stones (bilirubin, calcium, and variable organic material)

associated with hemolysis and cirrhosis. These tend to be black-pigmented stones that are refractory to medical therapy.
- 50% of mixed-type stones are radiopaque.

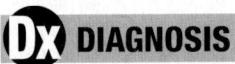 **DIAGNOSIS**

DIFFERENTIAL DIAGNOSIS

- Peptic ulcer disease
- Gastroesophageal reflux disease
- Irritable bowel disease
- Pancreatitis
- Neoplasms

- Nonnuclear dyspepsia
- Inferior wall myocardial infarction
- Hepatic abscess

LABORATORY TESTS

Generally normal unless patient has biliary obstruction (elevated alkaline phosphatase, bilirubin).

IMAGING STUDIES

- Ultrasound of the gallbladder (Figs. E2 and E3) will detect small stones and biliary sludge (sensitivity, 95%; specificity, 90%); the presence of dilated gallbladder with thickened wall is suggestive of acute cholecystitis.

TABLE 2 Symptoms of Gallstone Disease and Its Complications

Disease	Pathophysiology	Symptoms
Biliary colic	Transient gallstone impaction at the cystic duct or ampulla of Vater	Intermittent right upper quadrant pain associated with nausea or vomiting. Pain in the epigastrium or radiating to the right scapular tip. Episodes last 30 min to several hours with days or months between episodes.
Acute cholecystitis	Inflammation of the gallbladder caused by obstruction of the cystic duct. May occur in the presence or absence of bacterial superinfection	Patients appear ill and cannot take deep breaths. They have constant pain that lasts 30-60 min and worsens with movement. Persistent common bile duct impaction usually promotes vomiting. Physical examination demonstrates right upper quadrant tenderness with voluntary guarding and a positive Murphy sign (arrest of inspiration during deep palpation over the gallbladder).
Emphysematous cholecystitis	Infection with gas-producing bacteria such as *Escherichia coli*, *Clostridium perfringens*, and anaerobic streptococci	Symptoms are similar to those with acute cholecystitis. Gas may be seen on abdominal plain films or CT. Male diabetics are most commonly affected.
Chronic cholecystitis	Persistent inflammation and fibrosis of the gallbladder with poor motor and absorptive function	Patients are usually asymptomatic but may report multiple previous attacks of colic. Porcelain gallbladder develops from chronic inflammation and may progress to carcinoma.
Acalculous cholecystitis	Probably related to biliary stasis in the setting of critical illness and altered gastrointestinal motility	Seen in patients with traumatic injuries, burns, and critical illness, as well as in those receiving total parenteral nutrition. The mortality for this disorder is twice as high as that for acute calculous cholecystitis.
Gallbladder perforation	Stones erode through an inflamed and necrotic gallbladder wall. Stones may travel into the peritoneal cavity or cause adhesions between nearby structures. Bile peritonitis may develop	More than half of patients with gallbladder perforation have fever and a palpable right upper quadrant mass. Mortality in these patients is 30%.

CT, Computed tomography.
From Adams JG et al: *Emergency medicine, clinical essentials*, ed 2, Philadelphia, 2013, Elsevier.

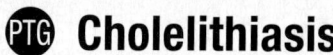

- Nuclear imaging (HIDA scan) can confirm acute cholecystitis (>90% accuracy) if gallbladder does not visualize within 4 h of injection and the radioisotope is excreted in the common bile duct.
- Common bile duct stones can be detected noninvasively by magnetic resonance cholangiopancreatography or invasively by endoscopic retrograde cholangiopancreatography (ERCP) and intraoperative cholangiography.

Rx TREATMENT

NONPHARMACOLOGIC THERAPY

Lifestyle changes (avoidance of diets high in polyunsaturated fats, weight loss in obese patients; however, avoid rapid weight loss)

ACUTE GENERAL Rx

- The management of gallstones is affected by the clinical presentation.
- Asymptomatic patients do not require therapeutic intervention. Proposed criteria for prophylactic cholecystectomy are described in Table E3.
- Surgical intervention is generally the ideal approach for symptomatic patients. Laparoscopic cholecystectomy is preferred over open cholecystectomy because of the shorter recovery period and lower mortality rate. Between 5% and 26% of patients undergoing elective laparoscopic cholecystectomy will require conversion to an open procedure. Most common reason is the inability to clearly identify the biliary anatomy.
- Laparoscopic cholecystectomy after endoscopic sphincterectomy is recommended for patients with common bile duct stones and residual gallbladder stones. Where possible, single-stage laparoscopic treatments with removal of duct stones and cholecystectomy during the same procedure are preferable. Percutaneous cholecystectomy is an alternative for patients who are critically ill with gallbladder empyema and sepsis.
- Patients who are not appropriate candidates for surgery because of coexisting illness or patients who refuse surgery can be treated with oral bile salts: Ursodiol or chenodiol. Candidates for oral bile salts are patients with cholesterol stones (radiolucent, noncalcified stones), with a diameter of ≤15 mm and having three or fewer stones. Candidates for medical therapy must have a functioning gallbladder and must have absence of calcifications on CT scans.
- Extracorporeal shock wave lithotripsy (ESWL) is another form of medical therapy. It can be used in patients with stone diameter of ≤3 cm and having three or fewer stones.

DISPOSITION

- Complicated gallstone events develop in 8% of patients with incidentally discovered gallstones after 17 yr.
- After ESWL, stones recur in approximately 20% of patients after 4 yr.
- Patients with at least one gallstone <5 mm in diameter have a greater than fourfold increased risk of presenting with acute biliary pancreatitis. A policy of watchful waiting in such cases is generally warranted.
- A potential serious complication of gallstones is acute cholangitis. ERCP and endoscopic sphincterectomy followed by interval laparoscopic cholecystectomy are effective in acute cholangitis.
- Uncommon complications of gallstone disease are summarized in Table 4.

RELATED CONTENT

Gallstones (Patient Information)
Cholecystitis (Related Key Topic)
Choledocholithiasis (Related Key Topic)

AUTHOR: **FRED F. FERRI, MD**

TABLE 4 Uncommon Complications of Gallstone Disease

Complication	Pathogenesis	Clinical Features	Diagnosis/Treatment
Emphysematous cholecystitis	Secondary infection of the gallbladder wall with gas-forming organisms (*Clostridium welchii, Escherichia coli,* and anaerobic streptococci) More common in older adult diabetic men; can occur without stones	Symptoms and signs similar to those of severe acute cholecystitis	Plain abdominal films may show gas in the gallbladder fossa US and CT are sensitive for confirming gas Treatment is with IV antibiotics, including anaerobic coverage, and early cholecystectomy High morbidity and mortality rates
Cholecystoenteric fistula	Erosion of a (usually large) stone through the gallbladder wall into the adjacent bowel, most often the duodenum, followed in frequency by the hepatic flexure, stomach, and jejunum	Symptoms and signs similar to those of acute cholecystitis, although sometimes a fistula may be clinically silent Stones >25 mm, especially in older adult women, may produce a bowel obstruction, or "gallstone ileus"; the terminal ileum is the most common site of obstruction Gastric outlet obstruction (Bouveret syndrome) may occur rarely	Plain abdominal films may show gas in the biliary tree and/or a small bowel obstruction in gallstone ileus, as well as a stone in the right lower quadrant if the stone is calcified Contrast upper GI series may demonstrate the fistula A fistula from a solitary stone that passes may close spontaneously Cholecystectomy and bowel closure are curative Gallstone ileus requires emergency laparotomy; the diagnosis is often delayed, with a resulting mortality rate of ≈20%
Mirizzi syndrome	An impacted stone in the gallbladder neck or cystic duct, with extrinsic compression of the common hepatic duct from accompanying inflammation or fistula	Jaundice and right upper quadrant pain	ERCP demonstrates dilated intrahepatic ducts and extrinsic compression of the common hepatic duct and possible fistula Preoperative diagnosis is important to guide surgery and minimize the risk of BD injury
Porcelain gallbladder	Intramural calcification of the gallbladder wall, usually in association with stones	No symptoms attributable to the calcified wall per se, but carcinoma of the gallbladder is a late complication in ≈20%	Plain abdominal films or CT show intramural calcification of the gallbladder wall Prophylactic cholecystectomy is indicated to prevent carcinoma

BD, Bile duct; *CT,* computed tomography; *ERCP,* endoscopic retrograde cholangiopancreatography; *GI,* gastrointestinal; *IV,* intravenous; *US,* ultrasound.
From Feldman M et al: *Sleisenger and Fordtran's gastrointestinal and liver disease,* ed 11, Philadelphia, 2021, Elsevier.

C

Diseases and Disorders

I

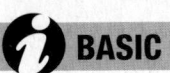

BASIC INFORMATION

DEFINITION

Chronic kidney disease (CKD) is diagnosed when there is evidence of kidney damage for more than 3 mo (urine albumin >30 mg/g creatinine, hematuria, or parenchymal abnormalities) and/or decreased kidney function (glomerular filtration rate [GFR] <60 ml/min per 1.73 m^2.[1] Advanced CKD, when GFR is <30 ml/min per 1.73 m^2, is characterized by accumulation of metabolic waste products in the blood, electrolyte abnormalities, mineral and bone disorders, and anemia. The pathophysiology of CKD and its manifestations are summarized in Table 1.

CLASSIFICATION

The 2012 Kidney Disease: International Global Outcomes classifies CKD with a C-G-A format: Cause (etiology), GFR (G1 to G5), and albuminuria (A1 to A3) by urine albumin-to-creatinine ratio. This format is recommended when documenting and discussing CKD. Fig. E1 depicts how CKD prognosis worsens with either increasing levels of albuminuria or declining GFR. Until now, most physicians used the 2009 CKD EPI (chronic kidney disease epidemiology collaboration) to calculate estimated glomerular filtration rate (eGFR), which took into account race. Recently in 2021, the joint NKF-ASN task force recommended the use of the new 2021 CKD EPI equation that excludes race from this calculation.

SYNONYMS

CKD
Chronic renal failure (CRF)
Chronic renal insufficiency (CRI)
Chronic renal disease (CRD)

ICD-10CM CODES
N18.1	Chronic kidney disease, stage G1
N18.2	Chronic kidney disease, stage G2
N18.30	Chronic kidney disease, stage G3 NOS
N18.31	Chronic kidney disease, stage G3a
N18.32	Chronic kidney disease, stage G3b
N18.4	Chronic kidney disease, stage G4
N18.5	Chronic kidney disease, stage G5
N18.6	End-stage renal disease
N18.9	Chronic kidney disease, unspecified

EPIDEMIOLOGY & DEMOGRAPHICS

- In the U.S., 37 million adults are estimated to have CKD, and approximately 90% do not know that they have diminished kidney function.[2] One in three U.S. adults is at risk for CKD.[2,3]
- Total Medicare spending on CKD and end-stage renal disease (ESRD) patients exceeds $120 billion USD. Accompanying chronic diseases such as diabetes and heart failure compound the cost of caring for these individuals, and CKD is considered a "cost multiplier," accounting for 25% of Medicare expenditures. Spending per patient-yr for

patients with all three chronic conditions of CKD, diabetes, and heart failure was more than twice as high ($40,516) as for patients with only CKD.[3]
- CKD will be the fifth highest cause of years of life lost world-wide by 2040.[4]
- Kidney transplantation represents the best option for kidney replacement therapy, offering greater longevity and quality of life while having the lowest overall cost. Mortality is significantly lower (48.9 per 1000) versus those on dialysis (160.8 per 1000).[2]

PHYSICAL FINDINGS & CLINICAL PRESENTATION

- Most patients with early CKD have no or few symptoms on physical exam
- Skin pallor, ecchymosis
- Sleep disorder
- Hypertension, edema, jugular venous distention
- Leg cramps, restless legs, peripheral neuropathy
- Emotional lability, depression, decreased cognitive function
- Uremic frost, odor, and fetor in severe cases
- Clinical presentation varies with the degree of kidney disease and its underlying etiology. Common symptoms are generalized fatigue, nausea, anorexia, pruritus, sleep disturbance, smell and taste disturbances, hiccoughs, and seizures

ETIOLOGY

- Diabetes mellitus
- Hypertension
- Glomerular disease
- Failed kidney transplant
- Interstitial nephritis (e.g., drug hypersensitivity, analgesic nephropathy)

TABLE 1 Pathophysiology of Chronic Kidney Disease

Manifestation	Mechanisms
Accumulation of nitrogenous waste products	Decrease in glomerular filtration rate
Acidosis	Decreased ammonia synthesis Impaired bicarbonate reabsorption Decreased net acid excretion
Sodium retention	Excessive renin production Oliguria
Sodium wasting	Solute diuresis Tubular damage
Urinary concentrating defect	Solute diuresis Tubular damage
Hyperkalemia	Decrease in glomerular filtration rate Metabolic acidosis Excessive potassium intake Hyporeninemic hypoaldosteronism
Renal osteodystrophy	Impaired renal production of 1,25-dihydroxycholecalciferol Hyperphosphatemia Hypocalcemia Secondary hyperparathyroidism
Growth retardation	Inadequate caloric intake Renal osteodystrophy Metabolic acidosis Anemia Growth hormone resistance
Anemia	Decreased erythropoietin production Iron deficiency Folate deficiency Vitamin B$_{12}$ deficiency Decreased erythrocyte survival
Bleeding tendency	Defective platelet function
Infection	Defective granulocyte function Impaired cellular immune functions Indwelling dialysis catheters
Neurologic symptoms (fatigue, poor concentration, headache, drowsiness, memory loss, seizures, peripheral neuropathy)	Uremic factor(s) Aluminum toxicity Hypertension
Gastrointestinal symptoms (feeding intolerance, abdominal pain)	Gastroesophageal reflux Decreased gastrointestinal motility
Hypertension	Volume overload Excessive renin production
Hyperlipidemia	Decreased plasma lipoprotein lipase activity
Pericarditis, cardiomyopathy	Uremic factor(s) Hypertension Fluid overload
Glucose intolerance	Tissue insulin resistance

From Kliegman RM: *Nelson textbook of pediatrics*, ed 21, Philadelphia, 2020, Elsevier.

- Obstructive nephropathies (e.g., nephrolithiasis, prostatic disease)
- Congenital disease (e.g., Alport syndrome, polycystic kidney disease)
- Vascular diseases (renal artery stenosis, hypertensive nephrosclerosis)
- Autoimmune disorders
- Acute kidney injury (AKI)

Dx DIAGNOSIS

GFR is considered the best overall index of kidney function, but it is not the only measure of kidney health. Although quantitation of albuminuria has been less widely adopted in clinical practice than assessment of eGFR, its evaluation is critical for determining a prognosis. When applying eGFR equations, one must appreciate that CKD is defined over a 3-mo interval (Table 2). Furthermore, changes in calculation of eGFR have been recommended by the NKF-ASN Task Force on Reassessing the Inclusion of Race in Diagnosing Kidney Diseases in April of 2021. This change involved excluding race when calculating eGFR in the CKD-EPI equation. Furthermore, the task force determined cystatin C should be combined with creatinine in the outpatient setting to determine a more complete evaluation of renal function.[5]

Therefore serum creatinine measurement, which all eGFR equations are based on, must be repeated and trended to establish a diagnosis of CKD. Furthermore, to properly trend the eGFR in a given individual, creatinine must be in a steady state of production. Albuminuria assesses kidney damage and complements the eGFR evaluation. Consequently, the National Kidney Foundation (NKF) and the American Society for Clinical Pathology (ASCP) advocate optimal screening for CKD in the primary care setting using the new "Kidney Profile" test. The Kidney Profile combines the following two measurements: eGFR with serum creatinine (CPT 82565) and urine albumin-to-creatinine ratio (ACR) (albumin, urine [e.g., microalbumin], quantitative: CPT 82043; and urine creatinine: CPT 82570). Patients with CKD have an elevated risk for cardiovascular disease, and results from combined eGFR and ACR testing can be a strong predictor of cardiovascular mortality and kidney failure risk.[3]

WORKUP

- Ultrasound: Evaluation for sagittal length, echogenicity, and anatomic abnormalities including causes of obstructive uropathy
- Kidney biopsy: Greatest diagnostic determination for AKI of unknown etiology and albuminuric disorders; generally, not performed when kidneys are small (<8.5 to 9.0 cm in length) or if CKD is advanced
- Table 3 provides evidence-based strategies to slow progression of CKD

LABORATORY TESTS

- Blood urea nitrogen (BUN) and serum creatinine: Serum creatinine is used to determine eGFR via multivariable (creatinine, age, sex) prediction equations normalized to a body surface area of $1.73 \ m^2$. eGFR calculators are available online (www.kidney.org/kls/professionals/gfr_calculator.cfm). The preferred eGFR equation is the new race-free eGFR 2021 Chronic Kidney Disease Epidemiology Collaboration (CKD–EPI).[5]
- Urinalysis: Biochemical identification of albumin and/or blood. Microscopy may demonstrate formed elements, including red blood cells, white blood cells, casts, and crystals. The five year risk for CKD is about 5% in people with persistent microscopic hematuria.[6]
- Serum chemistry: Sodium, potassium (elevated), chloride, and total carbon dioxide (primarily low bicarbonate), calcium (low), phosphorus (elevated), glucose (elevated), and uric acid (elevated). Parathyroid hormone (PTH) can be elevated in advanced CKD.
- Urinary protein excretion. A urine total protein-to-creatinine ratio $>1000 \ mg/g$ creatinine or albumin-to-creatinine ratio of $>500 \ mg/g$ creatinine generally indicates glomerular disease because tubular proteinuria is usually less than this threshold.[1]
- Special studies: Serum and urine immunoelectrophoresis (multiple myeloma), serum free light chains (monoclonal gammopathy of renal significance), antinuclear antibody (i.e., systemic lupus erythematosus), and other serologic tests for determination of etiology of glomerular disorders.[1]
- Cystatin C: A small protein biomarker used for determination of glomerular filtration. It is used to estimate GFR when a serum

creatinine-based eGFR determination is less accurate, i.e., HIV or malnutrition, or if a more precise eGFR is required.[5] The European Kidney Function Consortium (EKFC) EKFC eGFRcys equation, which has the same mathematical form as the EKFC eGFRcr equation but has a scaling factor for cystatin C that does not differ according to race or sex, has been reported to improve the accuracy of GFR assessment over that of commonly used equations.[7]

IMAGING STUDIES

- Ultrasound of kidneys and bladder for kidney length measurements (normal, 10 to 12 cm based on height) and to rule out cause of obstructive uropathy
- Plain radiographs of the aorta and extremities ordered for other reasons may reveal vascular and extraskeletal calcification

Rx TREATMENT

CKD typically progresses slowly. Therefore, even relatively small reductions of GFR loss can delay the onset of ESRD by years. For this reason, an aggressive, multiple risk factor intervention to slow GFR decline is warranted, except in patients with low ESRD risk. CKD treatment plan goals include reduction of albuminuria to the greatest extent possible and control of hypertension. Albuminuria reduction to less than 500 mg/day or more, often with inhibition of the renin-angiotensin-aldosterone system, and maintenance of blood pressure to $<130/<80$ mm Hg are the two most important aspects of treatment.[8]

NONPHARMACOLOGIC THERAPY

The Kidney Disease: Improving Global Outcomes organization recommends lowering protein intake in adults with CKD to 0.8 g/kg per day and eGFR below 30 ml/min per $1.73 \ m^2$, whereas high protein intake (>1.3 g/kg per day) should be avoided in adults with CKD at risk of progression. Table 4 describes nutritional recommendations for patients with CKD.[1]

- Referral to a dietitian for medical nutritional therapy for patients with eGFR <50 ml/min per $1.73 \ m^2$ is recommended and is a Medicare-covered service.
- Dietary restriction of sodium (~100 mmol/day), potassium (≤60 mmol/day), and phosphorus (<800 mg/day). Potassium restriction is recommended for those with or at risk for hyperkalemia only.
- Blood pressure: Current guidelines from the American College of Cardiology/American Heart Association and the National Kidney Foundation Kidney Disease Outcomes Quality Initiative recommend a goal blood pressure of $<130/<80$ mm Hg for diabetic and nondiabetic CKD.
- Contrast-enhanced magnetic resonance imaging (MRI): Gadolinium-based contrast media (GBCM) with group II agents should not be withheld regardless of renal function if MRI is deemed medically necessary.

TABLE 2 Criteria for Definition of Chronic Kidney Disease

Kidney Disease is defined as abnormalities of kidney structure or function, present for more than 3 mo, with implications for health. These may include the following:

Markers of kidney damage	Albuminuria (AER $\geq$30 mg/24 h; ACR $\geq$30 mg/g [$\geq$3 mg/mmol])
	Urine sediment abnormalities
	Electrolyte and other abnormalities caused by tubular disorders
	Abnormalities detected through histology
	Structural abnormalities detected through imaging
	History of kidney transplantation
Decreased GFR	GFR <60 ml/min per $1.73 \ m^2$

ACR, Urine albumin-to-creatinine ratio; *AER,* albumin excretion rate; *GFR,* glomerular filtration rate; *KD,* kidney disease.
From Kidney Disease Improving Global Outcomes (KDIGO) CKD Work Group: KDIGO 2012 clinical practice guideline for the evaluation and management of chronic kidney disease, *Kidney Int Suppl* 3:1-150, 2013. In Floege J et al: *Comprehensive clinical nephrology,* ed 7, Philadelphia, 2024, Elsevier.

TABLE 3 Evidence-Based Strategies to Slow the Progression of Kidney Disease

Risk Factor	Guideline-Concordant Treatment Goals and Recommended Agents	Certainty of Evidence	Strength of Recommendation
Overweight	Maintain a healthy weight (BMI 20-25 kg/m²)	D	1
Diet	Lower or maintain salt intake to <90 mmol/day (equivalent to <2 g sodium/day or <5 g sodium chloride/day)	C	1
	Low protein intake: 0.8 g/kg/day in adults with diabetes or without diabetes and CKD (G4-G5), with appropriate education	C (diabetes-related CKD); B (nondiabetic CKD)	2
Smoking	Smoking cessation	Not graded	1
Exercise	Encourage 30-60 min of aerobic exercise at least 5 times/wk	D	1
Proteinuria/albuminuria	Monitoring and follow up; treatment with ACE inhibitors/ARBs, with proteinuria >300 mg/24 h	B	1
Blood pressure	<130/80 mm Hg (diabetes or proteinuric CKD),[a] <140/80 mm Hg (nondiabetic or nonproteinuric CKD)	B	1
Diabetes	HbA$_{1c}$ <7% and use of newer agents (i.e., SGLT2 inhibitors may yield significant benefits for patients with CKD stages 1-4 with regard to CV and kidney outcomes)	A	1
Dyslipidemia	Use of lipid-lowering medications[b]	Not graded	
Metabolic acidosis	Bicarbonate supplementation with levels <20 mEq/L		
Other metabolic risk factors (elevated uric acid)	Insufficient evidence to support or refute the use of agents for hyperuricemia	Not graded	
Multifactorial risk modification/CV risk reduction	Multifactorial intervention strategy addressing BP control and CV risk (with secondary prevention measures, ASA, β-blockers, when appropriate); use of ACE inhibitors or ARBs, statins, and SGLT2 inhibitors where clinically indicated and appropriate	Not graded	

ACE, Angiotensin-converting enzyme; *ARB,* angiotensin-receptor blocker; *ASA,* acetylsalicylic acid; *BMI,* body mass index; *BP,* blood pressure; *CKD,* chronic kidney disease; *CV,* cardiovascular; *HbA$_{1c}$,* hemoglobin A$_{1c}$; *MI,* myocardial infarction; *SGLT2,* sodium-glucose cotransporter-2.
Strength of recommendation: 1, recommended for most patients; 2, suggested for the majority of people, but different choices will be appropriate for some patients; not graded: left to the discretion of care provider, guidance is based on common sense or the given topic does not allow adequate application of evidence.
Certainty of evidence: A, high; B, moderate; C, low; D, very low.
[a]Use of ACE inhibitors/ARBs recommended.
[b]"Fire-and-forget" strategy: a high-dose statin or moderate dose statin combined with ezetimibe recommended for all CKD patients aged >50 yr regardless of serum lipid levels. Patients aged 18-50 years should be treated if they have established CV disease, diabetes, or an estimated 10-yr risk of coronary death or nonfatal MI >10%.
From Floege J et al: *Comprehensive clinical nephrology,* ed 7, Philadelphia, 2024, Elsevier.

TABLE 4 Nutritional Recommendations in Chronic Kidney Disease

Recommendations are for typical patients but always should be individualized on the basis of clinical, biochemical, and anthropometric indices.

Daily Intake	Predialysis CKD	Hemodialysis	Peritoneal Dialysis
Protein (g/kg ideal BW) (see "KDOQI" for estimation of adjusted edema-free BW)	0.6-1.0 Level depends on the view of the nephrologist 1.0 for nephrotic syndrome	Min ≥1.1	Min 1.0-1.2
		Recommendations are in conjunction with an adequate energy intake. Requirements may be higher during illness because of multiple comorbidities or during acute periods of infection, including peritonitis.	
Energy (kcal/kg BW)	35 (younger than 60 yr) 30-35 (older than 60 yr)	35 (younger than 60 yr) 30-35 (older than 60 yr) 30-40 kcal/kg ideal BW	35 including dialysate calories (younger than 60 yr) 30-35 including dialysate calories (older than 60 yr)
Sodium (mmol)	<100 (more if salt-wasting)	<100	<100
Potassium	Reduce if hyperkalemic	Reduce if hyperkalemic	Reduce if hyperkalemic; potassium restriction is generally not required. May need to increase potassium intake if hypokalemic.
	If hyperkalemic, advice will take the form of decreasing certain foods (e.g., some fruits and vegetables) and giving information about cooking methods.		
Phosphorus	Reduce because of phosphate retention. Monitor levels. Advice will take the form of reducing certain foods (e.g., dairy, offal, some shellfish) and processed foods with high content of added phosphates and giving information about the timing of binders with high-phosphorus meals and snacks.		

Recommendations are for typical patients but always should be individualized based on clinical, biochemical, and anthropometric indices. *BW,* Body weight; *CKD,* chronic kidney disease; *KDOQI,* Kidney Disease Outcomes Quality Initiative.
From Floege J et al: *Comprehensive clinical nephrology,* ed 7, Philadelphia, 2024, Elsevier.

- Medications: Reviewed for potential toxicity and dosages adjusted based on eGFR.
- Resistance exercise training can preserve lean body mass and improve nutritional status and muscle function in patients with moderate CKD.

- Avoid iodinated radiocontrast media for eGFR <30 ml/min per 1.73 m². Prophylactic intravenous volume expansion with sodium chloride or sodium bicarbonate before dye exposure is equally effective and is usually recommended when eGFR <45 ml/min per 1.73 m².

- Smoking cessation.
- Nephrology referral: Late or delayed nephrology referral for patients with CKD is associated with greater burden and severity of comorbid disease and CKD complications, increased risk of hospitalization, reduced

BOX 1 Suggested Criteria for Referral of Patients With Chronic Kidney Disease to a Nephrologist

Referral Criteria

Grade of recommendation: 1, recommendation, evidence B

- Acute deterioration of kidney function
- GFR <30 ml/min/1.73 m^2
- Significant and sustained albuminuria (albumin:creatinine ratio ≥ 300 mg/g; equivalent to protein:creatinine ratio ≥500 mg/g or proteinuria ≥500 mg/24 h)
- CKD progression (sustained decrease in the GFR >5 ml/min/1.73 m^2 per yr or due to a change of category [from G1 to G2, from G2 to G3a, from G3a to G3b, from G3b to G4, or from G4 to G5] when the latter is accompanied by a GFR loss of ≥5 ml/min/1.73 m^2)[a]
- Microhematuria not explained by other causes, sediment with >20 RBCs/field, especially in the case of RBC casts
- Resistant high BP (not controlled with a combination of three antihypertensive drugs, including a diuretic)
- Persistent serum potassium abnormalities
- Recurrent nephrolithiasis
- Hereditary kidney disease

BP, Blood pressure; *CKD,* chronic kidney disease; *GFR,* glomerular filtration rate; *NSAIDs,* nonsteroidal antiinflammatory drugs; *RBCs,* red blood cells.

[a]Small fluctuations in GFR do not necessarily indicate progression. When the above progression criteria are detected, it is necessary to rule out potentially reversible exacerbation factors (progression vs. exacerbation) such as obstructive uropathy, volume depletion, situations of hemodynamic instability or use of NSAIDs, cyclooxygenase-2 inhibitors, nephrotoxic antibiotics, radiocontrast agents, or renin-angiotensin system blockers in certain hemodynamic conditions.

From KDIGO 2012 clinical practice guideline for the evaluation and management of chronic kidney disease. Kidney Int Suppl. 2013;3.

access to patient-centric home dialysis and kidney transplant, and reduced survival.[7] Criteria for referral are listed in Box 1.

- Referral for kidney transplantation evaluation should be considered for patients with eGFR <20 ml/min per 1.73 m^2, unless absolute contraindications are present (e.g., malignancy within the past year).
- Chronic kidney disease education to better inform the patient of various facets of the disease and modalities for dialysis is important.

ACUTE GENERAL Rx

- Angiotensin-converting enzyme inhibitors (ACEIs) and angiotensin II type 1 receptor blockers (ARBs) reduce cardiovascular risk and slow progression of CKD. Combining ACEI and ARB agents is not recommended because of increased risks of hyperkalemia and AKI. Elevation of serum creatinine 30% or more higher than baseline serum creatinine within 3 mo of initiating ACEI or ARB therapy is generally tolerated without complication(s) and does not indicate parenchymal injury or the need to dose adjust or discontinue drug therapy.
- The nonsteroidal mineralocorticoid-receptor antagonist finerenone is recommended in the revised 2022 KDIGO Guidelines for patients with type 2 DM and CKD (eGFR ≥25 mL/min) who have normal serum potassium levels and albuminuria despite a minimum tolerated dose of an ACE or ARB.[9]
- In 2019, the U.S. FDA approved canagliflozin, a sodium-glucose cotransporter (SGLT-2) inhibitor, the first novel treatment for type 2 diabetic kidney disease (DKD) in nearly 18 yr. Canagliflozin was effective in the CREDENCE clinical trial (Canagliflozin and Renal Events in Diabetes with Established Nephropathy Clinical Evaluation), which showed that canagliflozin

achieved its primary end point compared with placebo and reduced the renal-specific composite of progression to ESRD, doubling of serum creatinine, and renal or cardiovascular death. Canagliflozin had been previously shown to reduce the decline in eGFR and albuminuria in DKD. Another SGLT-2 inhibitor, dapagliflozin, substantially reduced the rate of progression of CKD and frequency of ESRD in patients with and without diabetes in the DAPA-CKD trial (Dapagliflozin and Prevention of Adverse Outcomes in Chronic Kidney Disease). Glucagon-like peptide 1 receptor agonists (GLP-1 RA) have shown similar improvements in cardiovascular and kidney outcomes in patients with type 2 diabetes; however, the renal end points were secondary outcomes. The SGLT-2 inhibitor class has been recommended especially for patients with CKD who also have heart failure, as salt and water loss occur from glucosuria. The SGLT-2 inhibitor empagliflozin is now FDA approved to reduce the risk of sustained eGFR decline, end-stage kidney disease, CV death, and hospitalization for heart failure in adults with CKD at risk of progression. GLP-1 RAs are especially recommended for atherosclerotic cardiovascular disease. The addition of chlorthalidone for CKD patients with difficult-to-treat hypertension may reduce blood pressure and proteinuria.[10,11]

- Erythropoiesis-stimulating agents (ESAs), such as epoetin alfa and beta and darbepoetin alfa, are administered to reduce the need for transfusions in CKD patients with anemia. A target hemoglobin of 9 to 11 g/dl is reasonable to avoid premature and excessive ESA use. Higher hemoglobin values have been associated with adverse cardiovascular events. Iron sufficiency should be present,

defined as transferrin saturation >20% and ferritin >100 ng/ml before ESA therapy is initiated.[1]

- Optimal diuretic therapy should be prescribed for edema or cardiopulmonary congestion, although it has not shown mortality benefit in CKD.
- ACEIs or ARBs retard progression of CKD and lower blood pressure but cause short-term reductions of GFR and increase serum potassium.
- Treat metabolic acidosis with oral sodium bicarbonate to attain a goal serum HCO$_3$ level of approximately 22 to 26 mmol/L.[1]
- Statin therapy, or a combination of statin and ezetimibe, is recommended in adults ≥50 yr with eGFRs <60 ml/min per 1.73 m^2. Lipid management focuses on absolute risk for coronary events, and there are no target cholesterol levels without any effect on GFR trajectory.
- Therapy of mineral and bone disease in patients with CKD targets normal serum calcium and phosphorus levels. Calcitriol and vitamin D analogs are for patients at CKD stages G4 to G5 and severe, progressive hyperparathyroidism.
- Hepatitis C: The 2022 updated 2022 KDIGO guidelines[12] recommended expanding treatment of hepatitis C with sofosbuvir-based regimens to patients with CKD glomerular filtration rate categories G4 and G5, including those receiving dialysis, expanding the donor pool for kidney transplant recipients by accepting HCV-positive kidneys regardless of the recipient's HCV status and initiating direct-acting antiviral treatment of HCV-infected patients with clinical evidence of glomerulonephritis without requiring kidney biopsy.
- Dietary phosphate restriction is recommended for nearly all CKD patients. For additional management of hyperphosphatemia, phosphate-binders are recommended. Calcium-based phosphate binders, although inexpensive, should be restricted if total serum calcium is >10.2 mg/dl or if serum phosphorus exceeds 6.0 mg/dl. Sevelamer carbonate and lanthanum carbonate are effective as phosphate binders but are more expensive. Two iron-based phosphate-binding agents, sucroferric oxyhydroxide and ferric citrate, are effective phosphate-binders.[13]
- Uremic pruritus: Difelikefalin, a selective agonist of kappa opioid receptors, reduces itch intensity in hemodialysis patients.[14]
- The U.S. Centers for Disease Control and Prevention's Advisory Committee on Immunization Practices recommends pneumococcal vaccination of individuals >19 yr at time of CKD diagnosis with 20-valent (PCV20) or both 15-valent strain (PCV15) and 23-valent strain (PPSV23) vaccines in sequence. An annual influenza vaccination for all persons aged ≥6 mo who do not have a contraindication is recommended. Individuals at high risk of progression of CKD with eGFRs <30 ml/min per 1.73 m^2 should be immunized against hepatitis B to ensure seroconversion.[15]

C

Diseases and Disorders

I

TABLE 5 Risk Factors Associated With the Initiation and Progression of Chronic Kidney Disease

Initiation Factors	Progression Factors
Systemic hypertension	Older age
Diabetes mellitus	Sex (male)
Cardiovascular disease	Race/ethnicity
Dyslipidemia	Genetic predisposition
Smoking	Poor BP control
Obesity/metabolic syndrome	Poor glycemic control
Hyperuricemia	Proteinuria
Low socioeconomic status	Cardiovascular disease
Nephrotoxin exposure: abuse of NSAIDs, analgesics, traditional herbal remedies; exposure to heavy metals, lead	Dyslipidemia
	Smoking
	Obesity/metabolic syndrome
	Hyperuricemia
	Low socioeconomic status
	Nephrotoxins (NSAIDs, contrast agents)
	Recurrent AKI events
	Metabolic acidosis

AKI, Acute kidney injury; *CKD,* chronic kidney disease; *NSAIDs,* nonsteroidal antiinflammatory drugs.
From Floege J et al: *Comprehensive clinical nephrology,* ed 7, Philadelphia, 2024, Elsevier.

- Initiation of dialysis: Early initiation of dialysis at eGFR 10 to 15 ml/min per 1.73 m² does not enhance survival compared with a symptom-driven strategy for initiation of dialysis at eGFR <8 to 10 ml/min per 1.73 m².
  1. Urgent indications: Uremic pericarditis, neuropathy, neuromuscular abnormalities, congestive heart failure, hyperkalemia, or seizure.
  2. Other indications: GFR 10 to 15 ml/min per 1.73 m² with progressive anorexia, weight loss, anuria, disordered sleep, pruritus, uncontrolled fluid gain with hypertension, and signs of heart failure.
  3. Nearly 4 million people worldwide currently rely on some form of dialysis for treatment of ESRD. Peritoneal dialysis accounts for approximately 11% of patients undergoing dialysis overall.

DISPOSITION

- Prognosis is influenced by CKD stage and burden of comorbid illness. Risk factors associated with the initiation and progression of chronic kidney disease are summarized in Table 5.
- Late nephrology referral or no referral to a nephrologist within 6 to 12 mo before a diagnosis of ESRD is established is associated with greater morbidity and mortality. Despite recommendations for early referral, nearly two thirds of CKD patients are referred late, and a majority of patients do not realize they live with CKD.
- *Choosing Wisely* is an American Board of Internal Medicine Foundation initiative (www.choosingwisely.org/societies/american-society-of-nephrology/) that promotes conversations between clinicians and patients by helping patients choose evidence-based care that avoids wasteful or unnecessary medical tests, treatments, and procedures.
- Genetic susceptibility for CKD is prominent in African Americans. Two high-risk alleles of apolipoprotein L1 predict more rapid CKD progression independent of diabetes, race, and lipid and nonlipid factors. Approximately 14% of African Americans have two risk alleles, and 38% have one risk allele.
- Kidney transplantation in selected patients improves survival. Whereas the 2-yr kidney graft survival rate for living-related donor transplantations is >80%, the 2-yr graft survival rate for cadaveric donor transplantation is approximately 70%.

REFERENCES

Available at eBooks.Health.Elsevier.com.

AUTHORS: **KLODIA M. HERMEZ, DO** and **SNIGDHA T. REDDY, MD**

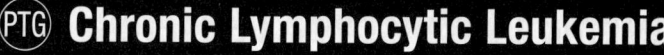
 BASIC INFORMATION

DEFINITION

Chronic lymphocytic leukemia (CLL) is a lymphoproliferative disorder characterized by proliferation and accumulation of mature-appearing neoplastic B cells.

SYNONYM

CLL

ICD-10CM CODES	
C91.10	Chronic lymphocytic leukemia of B-cell type not having achieved remission
C91.11	Chronic lymphocytic leukemia of B-cell type in remission
C91.12	Chronic lymphocytic leukemia of B-cell type in relapse

EPIDEMIOLOGY & DEMOGRAPHICS

- Most frequent form of leukemia in Western countries (20,160 new cases and 4410 deaths annually in the U.S.). Incidence rate is 4.7 per 100,000 person-yr, increasing to 17 cases per 100,000 at age 65. It is more common in patients with a family history of CLL or other lymphoid malignancy.
- Median age at diagnosis in the U.S. is 70 yr with male/female ratio of 2:1.
- CLL accounts for 1% of all cancers and 11% of all hematologic neoplasms. Because of its prolonged clinical course, over 200,000 individuals with CLL are estimated to live in the U.S.
- CLL may be preceded by monoclonal B-cell lymphocytosis—a premalignant, asymptomatic condition with less than 5000/mm^3 CLL-like cells circulating in the blood.
- CLL confined to the lymph nodes is less common and termed small lymphocytic lymphoma (SLL); SLL is biologically and therapeutically equivalent to CLL.

PHYSICAL FINDINGS & CLINICAL PRESENTATION

- At presentation most patients are asymptomatic. Many are diagnosed on the basis of incidentally discovered lymphocytosis.
- Symptoms include fatigue, recurrent infections (pneumonia, herpes zoster), enlarging lymph nodes.
- B symptoms (fever, weight loss, and drenching night sweats) occur in 10% of patients at presentation.
- Small diffuse lymphadenopathy and splenomegaly are typical findings on clinical examination, but they are absent in most patients at diagnosis.
- A minority of CLL patients (<10%) may develop autoimmune hemolytic anemia or immune thrombocytopenia at diagnosis or during the course of the disease.
- At a rate of 1% per yr, CLL may undergo a histologic transformation into an aggressive lymphoma (Richter transformation), characterized by a rapidly growing nodal mass, elevated LDH, and constitutional symptoms.

ETIOLOGY

Remains largely unknown. Accumulation of genetic defects causing resistance to apoptosis and chronic stimulation of the B-cell receptor by autoantigens or undefined microorganisms have been implicated.

Dx **DIAGNOSIS**

- The diagnosis of CLL requires presence of >5000/mm^3 clonal B cells, for >3 mo, with a characteristic immunophenotype on flow cytometry, which is essential for diagnosis.
- CLL cells are typically positive for CD5, CD19, CD23 and weakly positive for CD20, while they are negative for CD10, Cyclin D1, and CD103. In some cases, molecular studies for CLL-specific chromosomal alterations (deletion of chromosome 13q, 11q, 17p, or trisomy 12) may be helpful.
- Table 1 describes the evaluation of CLL patients at diagnosis.

DIFFERENTIAL DIAGNOSIS

- Few acute infections with lymphocytosis (mononucleosis, pertusis)
- Other lymphoproliferative disorders that involve blood (can be distinguished using flow cytometry): Follicular lymphoma, mantle cell lymphoma, splenic marginal zone lymphoma, prolymphocytic leukemia, adult T-cell lymphoma/leukemia, hairy cell leukemia (Table 2)
- Acute lymphocytic leukemia can be differentiated by presence of lymphoblasts rather than mature lymphocytes
- Persistent polyclonal B-cell lymphocytosis: A rare, benign condition affecting (predominantly female) middle-aged smokers

LABORATORY TESTS

- CBC demonstrates lymphocytosis with mature lymphocytes and characteristic "smudge cells" on the peripheral smear (Fig. E1); anemia and thrombocytopenia may be present in more advanced cases.
- Bone marrow examination is **not** indicated in most cases, except when differentiation between autoimmune cytopenias and marrow infiltration by CLL is difficult.
- Hypogammaglobulinemia and elevated lactate dehydrogenase may be present at the time of diagnosis.
- Cytogenetic evaluation (using fluorescent in situ hybridization, [FISH]), mutational status of the immunoglobulin heavy chain variable region (IGHV, unmutated gene with >98% homology indicates worse prognosis), and presence of TP53 mutations are essential for prognostic assessment and optimal treatment selection.
- Other prognostic markers include: High serum beta-2 microglobulin, presence of

---

TABLE 1 Evaluation of Chronic Lymphocytic Leukemia Patients at Diagnosis

History
- B symptom and fatigue assessment
- Infectious history assessment
- Occupational assessment for chemical exposure
- Familial history of CLL and lymphoproliferative disorders
- Preventive interventions for infections and secondary cancers

Physical Examination

Laboratory Assessment
- CBC with differential
- Morphology assessment of lymphocytes
- Chemistry, LFT enzymes, LDH
- Flow cytometry assessment to confirm immunophenotype of CLL
- Serum immunoglobulins
- Serum β$_2$M levels
- Interphase cytogenetics for del(17p13.1), del(11q22.3), del(13q14), del(6q21), and trisomy 12
- IGHV and TP53 mutational analysis
- Stimulated metaphase karyotype (if available)

Selected Tests under Certain Circumstances
- DAT, haptoglobin, reticulocyte count if anemia present
- CT scan if unexplained abdominal pain or enlargement present
- PET scan or biopsy (or both) if concern for a histologic transformation
- BM aspirate and biopsy if cytopenias unexplained by disease burden
- Familial counseling if first-degree relative with CLL

Teaching
- Varicella zoster identification instruction
- Skin cancer identification
- Disease education (Leukemia and Lymphoma Society)

B symptoms, Fever, night sweats, weight loss; *BM*, bone marrow; β$_2$M, beta-2 microglobulin; *CBC*, complete blood count; *CLL*, chronic lymphocytic leukemia; *CT*, computed tomography; *DAT*, direct antiglobulin test; *IGHV*, immunoglobulin heavy chain variable region; *LDH*, lactate dehydrogenase; *LFT*, liver function test; *PET*, positron emission tomography.
From Hoffman R et al: *Hematology, basic principles and practice*, ed 8, Philadelphia, 2023, Elsevier.

TABLE 2 Diseases That Can Mimic Chronic Lymphocytic Leukemia

- Follicular lymphoma
- Mantle cell lymphoma
- Marginal zone lymphoma (particularly splenic)
- Hairy cell leukemia (particularly variant)
- Acute lymphoblastic leukemia
- T-cell prolymphocytic leukemia
- Large granular natural killer or T-cell leukemia
- Persistent polyclonal B-cell lymphocytosis

From Hoffman R et al: *Hematology, basic principles and practice*, ed 8, Philadelphia, 2023, Elsevier.

CD38 or ZAP-70 (also associated with poor prognosis), complex karyotype, and additional somatic mutations associated with worse prognosis (*ATM, NOTCH1, SF3B1,* and *BIRC3* genes).

STAGING

Staging reflects the clinical burden of disease and aids assessment of prognosis and treatment decision making. The historical staging systems by Rai and Binet remain in clinical use. They use **only** physical examination and the CBC (i.e., no scans). The modified Rai system distinguishes three risk groups:

- Low risk (lymphocytosis alone, or stage 0)
- Intermediate risk (presence of lymphadenopathy, hepatomegaly, or splenomegaly, formerly stage I/II)
- High risk (presence of anemia with hemoglobin <11 g/dl, or thrombocytopenia with platelet count <100,000/mm³, formerly stage III/IV)

The Binet system divides CLL into three stages:

- Stage A: Involvement of <3 nodal areas (counting separately cervical, axillary, or inguinal lymph nodes, spleen, and liver)
- Stage B: Three or more areas involved
- Stage C: Presence of anemia (hemoglobin <10 g/dl) or thrombocytopenia (<100,000/mm³), independent of the areas involved

Prognosis in CLL can be determined using the CLL-International Prognostic Index (CLL-IPI), which includes five factors: 17p/*TP53* status, *IGVH* mutational status, serum beta-2-microglobulin, Rai/Binet stage (0/A vs. others), and age >65 yr. Overall 5-yr survival varies from 93% for the low-risk group to 23% for the very high-risk group (Table 3).

IMAGING STUDIES

Imaging studies (computed tomography [CT] or PET/CT scans) are not necessary for asymptomatic patients at diagnosis. They are obtained in case of clinical concerns for bulky internal adenopathy, Richter transformation, or prior to starting therapy.

℞ TREATMENT

- At present, there is no standard curative therapy for CLL, so treatment is only instituted for progressive or symptomatic disease (Table 4) with a goal of symptom relief and prolongation of life. However, novel therapies aim at achieving complete remissions with no detectable "minimal residual disease" (MRD, indicating less than 1:10,000 malignant B-cells in the marrow or blood).
- "Watchful waiting" (i.e., observation without therapy) is the optimal strategy for all early-stage, asymptomatic patients outside of clinical trials because early therapy provides no survival or quality-of-life benefit.[1]
- Chemotherapy is no longer routinely used in CLL because of inferior survival compared with novel targeted approaches.[2-4]
- Oral Bruton tyrosine kinase (BTK) inhibitors (ibrutinib, acalabrutinib, or zanubrutinib), or the BCL2 inhibitor venetoclax in combination with an anti-CD20 antibody obinutuzumab, are typically initiated for patients with symptoms related to disease, bulky adenopathy, rapidly increasing lymphocyte count, or progressive cytopenias.

ACUTE GENERAL Rx

- Although historically initial treatment was chosen depending on the patient's age, comorbidities, and CLL cytogenetics, BTK inhibitors or venetoclax/obinutuzumab are appropriate for most patients (Fig. 2).
- BTK inhibitors (ibrutinib, acalabrutinib, or zanubrutinib) are the most frequently used first-line therapy. Their downsides include lack of complete remissions and need for long-term daily drug therapy. The combination of venetoclax with obinutuzumab offers a time-limited alternative but is associated with a risk of tumor lysis syndrome. Three-drug combinations are currently studied as first-line therapy.
- BTK inhibitors are associated with diarrhea, arthralgias, and increased risk of infections; ibrutinib use can induce hypertension, atrial fibrillation, and occasional bleeding (particularly with concurrent anticoagulants).
- A recent phase 3 trial[5] in patient with released or refractory CLL comparing Zanubrutinib with Ibrutinib revealed longer profession-free survival and fewer cardiac events with Zanubrutinib.
- Recurrent CLL is often characterized by acquired deletion or mutation of the *TP53* gene and can be treated with a variety of salvage regimens:
  1. BTK inhibitors for patients who did not receive them as first line of treatment; third-generation noncovalent BTK inhibitors (pirtobrutinib) provide additional efficacy.
  2. Venetoclax alone or in combination with anti-CD20 antibody or a BTK inhibitor.
  3. Oral PI3K inhibitors (duvelisib, idelalisib).
  4. Anti-CD20 monoclonal antibodies: Obinutuzumab, rituximab, typically in combination with chemotherapy (bendamustine or fludarabine plus cyclophosphamide).
  5. Alemtuzumab (anti-CD52 monoclonal antibody).
  6. Palliative radiation therapy to bulky lymph nodes or spleen.
  7. Clinical trials of chimeric antigen receptor (CAR) T cells or bispecific antibodies.
- Allogeneic bone marrow transplantation is rarely offered to younger patients with recurrent, refractory disease.

CHRONIC Rx

Treatment of systemic complications:

- Tumor lysis syndrome may occur during initial or subsequent therapy (particularly venetoclax) but is extremely unlikely prior to treatment in CLL, even with high lymphocyte counts.

TABLE 3 Prognosis of Patients with CLL at the Time of Diagnosis, Stratified by the CLL-International Prognostic Index

Number of High Risk Factors	Risk Group	Percent of Patients	Median Time to First Chemotherapy	Overall Survival at 5 Yr
0-1	Low	38%	5-10 yr	93%
2-3	Intermediate	34%	4-5 yr	79%
4-6	High	23%	1-3 yr	63%
7-10	Very high	5%	<1 yr	23%

Risk factors include age >65 yr (1 point), stage Rai I-IV or Binet B-C (1 point), unmutated *IGVH* (2 points), beta-2-microglobulin >3.5 mg/L (2 points), or deletion 17p/*TP53* mutation (4 points). *CLL,* Chronic lymphocytic leukemia.

TABLE 4 Modified Indications for Treatment of Chronic Lymphocytic Leukemia

- Grade 2 or greater fatigue limiting life activities
- B symptoms persisting for ≥2 wk
- Lymph nodes >10 cm or progressively enlarging lymph nodes causing symptoms
- Spleen or liver with progressive enlargement or causing symptoms
- Anemia (hemoglobin <11 g/dl) referable to CLL
- Thrombocytopenia (platelets <100 × 10¹²/L) referable to CLL or ITP poorly responsive to traditional therapy
- Severe paraneoplastic process (e.g., autoimmune cytopenias, vasculitis, myositis) process related to CLL not responsive to traditional therapies

B symptoms, Fever, night sweats, weight loss; *AIHA,* Autoimmune hemolytic anemia; *CLL,* chronic lymphocytic leukemia; *ITP,* idiopathic thrombocytopenic purpura; *WBC,* white blood cell.
From Hoffman R et al: *Hematology, basic principles and practice*, ed 8, Philadelphia, 2023, Elsevier.

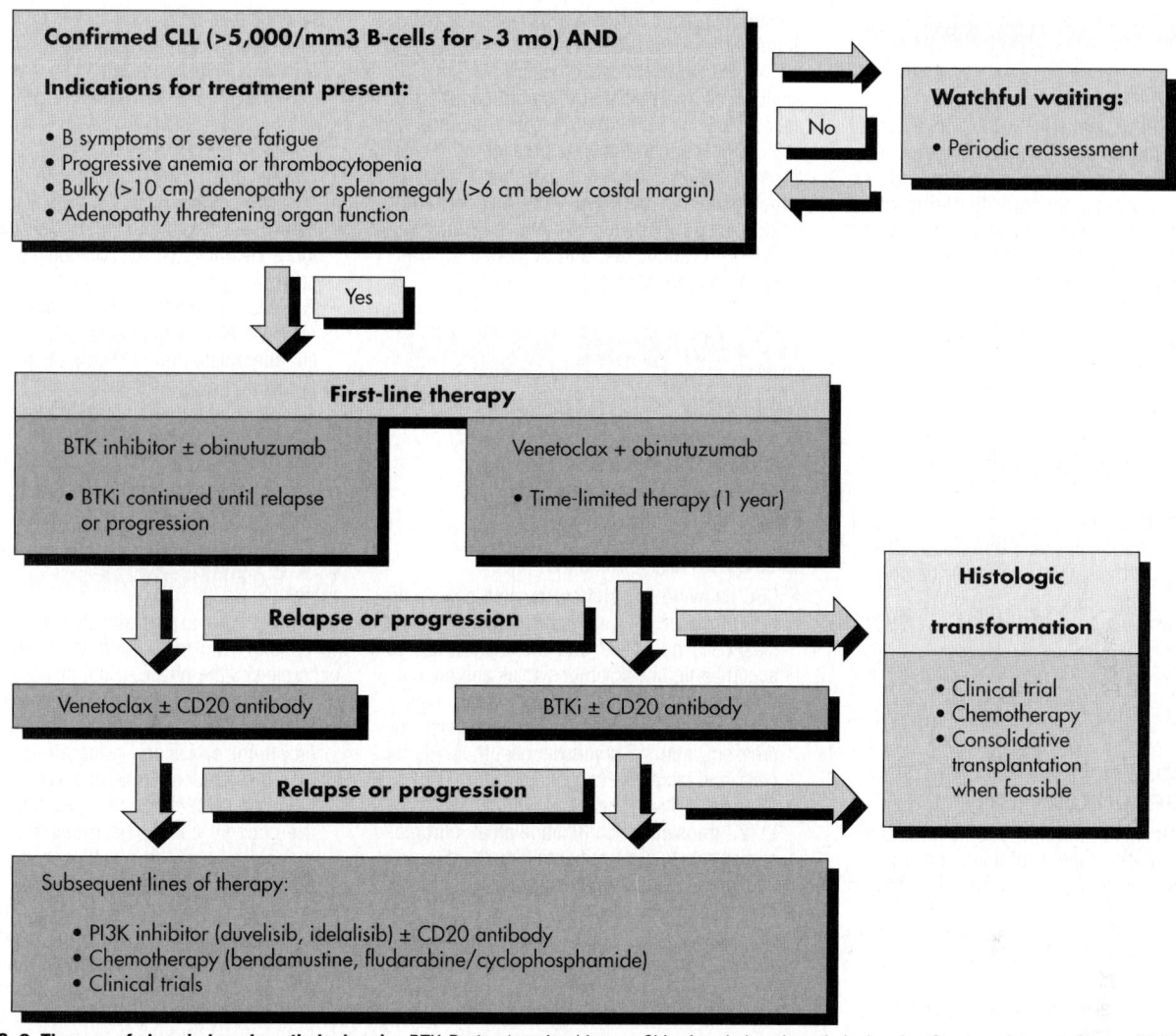

FIG. 2 Therapy of chronic lymphocytic leukemia. *BTK,* Bruton tyrosine kinase; *CLL,* chronic lymphocytic leukemia. (Courtesy Adam J. Olszewski, MD.)

Diseases and Disorders

I

- CLL patients are at increased risk of solid tumors and should adhere to age-appropriate screening modalities; skin cancers, including melanoma, are particularly common.
- Hypogammaglobulinemia is frequent in CLL and may cause recurrent infections, particularly pneumonias. Immunoglobulin supplementation (0.3 to 0.5 g/kg intravenous monthly or equivalent doses subcutaneous weekly) may prevent infections but has no effect on the course of CLL.
- Patients who had received chemoimmuno-therapy are at risk for opportunistic infections, including herpes zoster and *Pneumocystis jirovecii* pneumonia.
- Specific adverse effects of novel agents are commonly seen in clinical practice. Ibrutinib may cause hypertension, atrial fibrillation, chronic diarrhea, or hemorrhage, and must be held before surgical procedures. Venetoclax may cause tumor lysis syndrome and neutropenia.

- Autoimmune hemolytic anemia, thrombocyto-penia, and (rare) neutropenia may be treated with steroids, immunoglobulin, or immune suppression without CLL-directed therapy.
- CLL is a contraindication to administration of live vaccines (varicella zoster, mumps/measles/rubella, yellow fever, intranasal influenza). Patients should adhere to the recommended schedule of immunization against *Pneumococcus* and influenza.
- Patients with CLL are at increased risk of complications from COVID-19 and have lower probability of serologic response to COVID-19 vaccination.

DISPOSITION

Most patients have extended survival, though they may die from infectious complications of prior chemotherapy. Richter transformation is a residual source of mortality in the era of novel agents. Palliative treatment should be offered to patients who are no longer benefiting from aggressive therapy to avoid pervasive and futile treatment with distressing complications.
- Patients with CLL have poor outcomes after failure of covalent (BTK) inhibitor treatment. Pirtobrutinib, a highly selective, noncovalent (reversible) BTK inhibitor has shown efficacy in phase 1-2 trials in patients with heavily treated CLL who have received a covalent BTK inhibitor.[6]

REFERENCES
Available at eBooks.Health.Elsevier.com.

RELATED CONTENT
Chronic Lymphocytic Leukemia (Patient Information)

AUTHOR: **ADAM J. OLSZEWSKI, MD**

Chronic Myeloid Leukemia

BASIC INFORMATION

DEFINITION

Chronic myeloid leukemia (CML) is a clonal stem malignancy characterized by the presence of the Philadelphia chromosome, an acquired cytogenetic abnormality arising out of the reciprocal translocation of long arms of the *ABL* and *BCR* genes on chromosomes 9 and 22. The resultant *BCR:ABL* fusion oncogene is associated with the development of abnormal myeloid proliferation and accumulation of immature granulocytes.

SYNONYMS

Chronic granulocytic leukemia
Chronic myelogenous leukemia

ICD-10CM CODES
C92.10	Chronic myeloid leukemia, BCR/ABL-positive, not having achieved remission
C92.11	Chronic myeloid leukemia, BCR/ABL-positive, in remission
C92.12	Chronic myeloid leukemia, BCR/ABL-positive, in relapse

EPIDEMIOLOGY & DEMOGRAPHICS

- CML presents in the mid-50s range and accounts for 15% to 20% of adult leukemias.
- Incidence is 1 to 1.5 cases per 100,000 people annually.
- In 2023, an estimated 8930 new cases and 1310 deaths were estimated in the U.S.[1]

PHYSICAL FINDINGS & CLINICAL PRESENTATION

- Up to 50% patients are asymptomatic, with diagnosis based on abnormal blood counts.
- The initial chronic phase (CP-CML) has a myeloproliferative picture lasting months to years, which then evolves into an advanced phase (AP-CML) characterized by poor response to therapy and worsening cytopenias. Finally, it evolves into a terminal blast phase (BP-CML), resulting in acute leukemia (70% myeloid and approximately 30% lymphoid subtype). The criteria for accelerated and blast phases of CML are described in Table 1.
- Chronic phase symptomatic patients have fatigue, weight loss, early satiety, and left abdomen pain, and the examination can reveal splenomegaly. Occasionally, hyperleukocytosis and severe thrombocytosis can cause hyperviscosity-related symptoms.
- Accelerated phase patients usually have fevers, sweats, weight loss, abdomen pain, and progressive splenomegaly.
- Blast phase patients can additionally have bone pain; symptomatic anemia, infectious complications, and bleeding.

ETIOLOGY & PATHOLOGY

The etiology of CML is unclear, although radiation exposure has been linked in its development and an increased incidence has been noted in atomic bomb exposure survivors.

The Philadelphia chromosome results in most cases in a 210-kd translated oncoprotein called "p210 BCR-ABL1." This oncoprotein acts as a constitutively expressed defective tyrosine kinase. The downstream pathways affected include JAK/STAT, PI3K/AKT, and RAS/MEK; they involve cell growth, cell survival, inhibition of apoptosis, and activation of transcription factors.

DIAGNOSIS

DIFFERENTIAL DIAGNOSIS

- Splenic lymphoma
- Primary myelofibrosis
- Chronic neutrophilic leukemia
- Essential thrombocythemia

LABORATORY TESTS

- CBC showing left-shifted myeloid cells, with the presence of precursor polymorphonuclear cells, basophils, and eosinophils; can be accompanied by thrombocytosis and anemia.
- Bone marrow biopsy demonstrates hypercellularity with granulocytic hyperplasia, increased ratio of myeloid cells to erythroid cells, and increased megakaryocytes (Fig. E1).
- Bone marrow cytogenetics demonstrated the 9:22 translocation (Philadelphia chromosome) in >95% of patients (Fig. 2).
- Leukocyte alkaline phosphatase is markedly decreased (unlike other myeloproliferative disorders).
- *BCR-ABL* fusion transcripts can be measured using quantitative reverse transcription polymerase chain reaction (RT-PCR) technology using either peripheral blood or bone marrow; serial peripheral blood monitoring of transcript level is utilized at 3-mo intervals to determine molecular remission status.

RISK STRATIFICATION

- Chronic phase CML patients can be stratified into three categories: Low-, intermediate-, or high-risk, using the Sokal, Hasford (EURO), or more recently, the EUTOS long-term (ELTS) score.
- Patients developing secondary mutations have variable response to second- or third-line therapies; the *T315I* mutation is typically associated with resistance and is treated with allogeneic stem cell transplantation (SCT).

IMAGING STUDIES

Ultrasound or computed tomography scan of abdomen can be done.

TREATMENT

Treatment with a potential to either cure CML or prolong long-term survival should be used according to the phase of the disease.[2,3]

- Chronic phase: The therapeutic approach involves the use of either a first-generation (imatinib) or second-generation (dasatinib, nilotinib, or bosutinib) oral tyrosine kinase inhibitor (TKI). Imatinib mesylate binds to the canonic adenosine triphosphate (ATP)–binding site of the Abl kinase domain and blocks phosphorylation of tyrosine residues on substrate protein. Inhibiting phosphorylation prevents activation of signal transduction pathways that cause CML (Fig. E3). The decision to select a particular TKI is based on patient comorbidities, age, and

TABLE 1 Definitions of the Accelerated and Blastic Phases of Chronic Myeloid Leukemia

Criteria	MD Anderson Cancer Center[a]	International Bone Marrow Transplant Registry	World Health Organization
Accelerated Phase			
Percent blasts	15-29	10-29	10-19
Percent blasts + promyelocytes	≥30	≥20	NA
Percent basophils	≥20	≥20% (basophils + eosinophils)	≥20
Platelets (×10⁹/L)	<100	Unresponsive ↑, persistent ↓	<100 or >1000 unresponsive
Cytogenetics	CE	CE	CE not at diagnosis
WBCs	NA	Difficult to control, or doubling in <5 days	NA
Anemia	NA	Unresponsive	NA
Splenomegaly	NA	Increasing	NA
Other		Chloromas, myelofibrosis	Megakaryocyte proliferation, fibrosis

Blastic Phase

30% or more blasts; or extramedullary blastic disease, except for the World Health Organization classification, which requires 20% or more

CE, Clonal evolution; NA, not applicable; WBC, white blood cell.
[a]These criteria were also used in all the interferon-α and tyrosine kinase inhibitor studies.
From Niederhuber JE: *Abeloff's clinical oncology*, ed 6, Philadelphia, 2020, Elsevier.

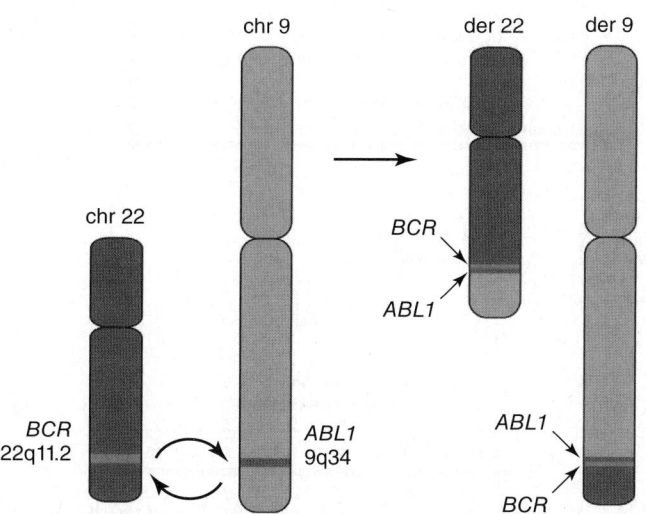

Philadelphia Chromosome
t(9;22)(q34;q11.2)

FIG. 2 The Philadelphia chromosome, der(22q), results from the reciprocal translocation of a portion of the *ABL1* gene on chromosome 9 at band q34 to the region of the *BCR* gene on chromosome 22 at band q11.2. In turn, a portion of *BCR* is translocated to chromosome 9 to the region of ABL1. In 5% to 10% of patients with chronic myeloid leukemia, cryptic or complex rearrangements result in a *BCR-ABL1* fusion gene, even though no Philadelphia chromosome is detected cytogenetically. (From Jaffe ES et al: *Hematopathology,* ed 2, Philadelphia, 2011, Saunders.)

TABLE 2 Approved Indications in Chronic Myeloid Leukemia

	Frontline	Salvage	Accelerated	Blastic
Imatinib	400 mg QD 340 mg/m² per day	400 mg QD (IFN failure)	600 mg QD (IFN failure)	600 mg QD (IFN failure)
Dasatinib	100 mg QD	100 mg QD A	140 mg QD A	140 mg QD A
Nilotinib	300 mg BID	400 mg BID A	400 mg BID A	—
Bosutinib	—	500 mg QD B	500 mg QD B	500 mg QD B
Ponatinib	—	45 mg QD B	45 mg QD B	45 mg QD B
Omacetaxine	—	1.25 mg/m² SC × 14 days every 28 days (induction), then × 7 days every 28 days C	1.25 mg/m² SC × 14 days every 28 days (induction), then × 7 days every 28 days C	—

A, Resistance or intolerance to prior therapies including imatinib; *B*, resistance or intolerance to prior tyrosine kinase inhibitors (TKIs); *BID*, twice daily; *C*, resistance or intolerance to two prior TKIs; *IFN*, interferon; *QD*, daily; *SC*, subcutaneously.
From Niederhuber JE: *Abeloff's clinical oncology,* ed 6, Philadelphia, 2020, Elsevier.

often formulary restrictions. Most patients obtain hematologic and cytogenetic remissions while major molecular remissions are observed in 25% to 60% cases.[4] Patients who lose their initial response, develop secondary mutations, or develop intolerance to therapy can be treated with newer third-generation TKIs (asciminib, ponatinib). Omacetaxine, a protein synthesis inhibitor, is also effective in patients who have previously received TKI therapy. The approved indications are summarized in Table 2. An

algorithm of the suggested treatment approach in CML is illustrated in Fig. 4.

- Second-generation TKIs (dasatinib, nilotinib, or bosutinib) are preferred for patients with an intermediate- or high-risk Sokal or Hasford score, especially for patients whose goal is to achieve a deep and rapid molecular response and eventual drug discontinuation for treatment-free remission (TFR).
- Some patients develop resistance to currently available TKI drugs. The ABL

myristoyl pocket (STAMP) inhibitor, asciminib, has demonstrated superiority over bosutinib in achieving molecular responses in patients previously treated with more than two other TKIs.[5]

- During therapy for chronic phase CML, treatment efficacy is monitored using serial RT-PCR to measure peripheral blood *BCR-ABL* transcripts every 3 to 6 mo.
- Accelerated phase: Patients are initially treated with second-generation TKIs but often require allogeneic SCT.
- Blast phase: Patients are initially treated with conventional induction chemotherapy as per the type of evolved acute leukemia and then subsequently undergo allogeneic SCT.
- Symptomatic hyperleukocytosis is treated with leukapheresis and hydroxyurea; allopurinol should be started to prevent urate nephropathy after the rapid tumor lysis.

DISPOSITION

- Response definition and monitoring are summarized in Table 3.
- Median survival for patients with chronic phase CML undergoing therapy with current TKIs is estimated to last 25+ yr.
- Median survivals for patients with accelerated and blast phase CML are 5 yr and 7 to 11 mo, respectively.
- Discontinuing oral TKI therapy can be attempted in chronic phase CML patients who have achieved deep, long-term molecular remissions can be considered in select cases; however, molecular relapses can occur in up to half the cases.[6] Criteria for TKI discontinuation include:
  1. Age >18 yr
  2. Chronic phase CML
  3. Prior TKI therapy for at least 3 yr
  4. Stable major molecular response >2 yr as documented on at least four occasions using quantitative RT-PCR assays performed more than 3 mo apart

Outcomes are better when treatment-free remission is attempted during first-line TKI therapy. Of patients who undergo treatment discontinuation, approximately half suffer molecular relapse and ultimately only 25% of all newly diagnosed patients attain long-term treatment-free remissions.

REFERRAL

To hematology physician

⚠ PEARLS & CONSIDERATIONS

- Chronic-phase CML patients should be risk-stratified at diagnosis to define prognosis upfront; patients achieving complete cytogenetic remission or major molecular remission by 12 mo have consistently superior long-term outcomes.
- Regular monitoring of molecular response using peripheral blood RT-PCR for *BCR:ABL* transcript levels is done every 3 to 6 mo for disease monitoring.

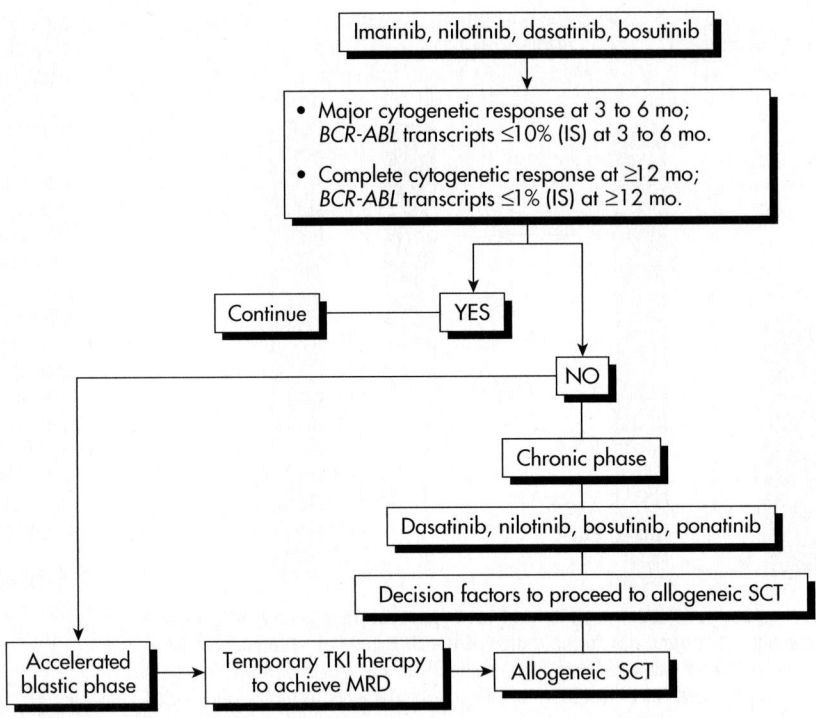

• Choice of salvage (TKI) depends on frontline TKI, and *BCR-ABL* mutation. If *T315I* mutation, only ponatinib is effective; if not available, use hydrea or chemotherapy, and proceed to allogeneic stem cell transplantation (SCT).

• In CML salvage the following are considered:

– If relapse in accelerated-blastic phase, use TKIs as temporary measure to achieve minimal residual disease (MRD) and proceed to allogeneic SCT.

– If relapse in chronic phase, choice of TKI based on mutations. Choice to continue on TKI indefinitely depends on presence of absence of clonal evolution, adverse mutations, and response to TKIs.

– Older patients (≥65 yr) and patients with poor matching donors may decide to continue TKIs in combination with hydroxyurea or other chemotherapy to gain several years of good quality of life, rather than opt for allogeneic SCT.

FIG. 4 Algorithm of the suggested treatment approach in chronic myeloid leukemia (CML). *TKI*, Tyrosine kinase inhibitor. (From Niederhuber JE: *Abeloff's clinical oncology*, ed 6, Philadelphia, 2020, Elsevier.)

TABLE 3 Response Definition and Monitoring		
Hematologic Response	**Cytogenetic Response**	**Molecular Response**
Complete: Platelet count <450 × 10⁹/L; WBC count <10 × 10⁹/L; differential without immature granulocytes and with less than 5% basophils; nonpalpable spleen	Complete: Ph⁺ 0 Major: Ph⁺ 1%-35% Minor: Ph⁺ 36%-65% Minimal: Ph⁺ 66%-95% None: Ph⁺ <95%	Complete: *BCR-ABL* transcripts nonquantifiable and nondetectable[a] Major: ≤0.10%

BCR-ABL to control gene ratio according to the proposed international scale for measuring molecular response, with a standardized "baseline," as established in the *IRIS* trial, taken to represent 100% on the international scale, and a 3-log reduction from the standardized baseline (major molecular response) fixed at 0.10%. *ABL*, Abelson leukemia virus; *BCR*, breakpoint cluster region; *Ph+*, Philadelphia chromosome positive; *WBC*, white blood cell.
[a]Qualified by the limit of sensitivity of the polymerase chain reaction assay employed.
From Hoffman R et al: *Hematology: basic principles and practice*, ed 7, Philadelphia, 2018, Elsevier.

• Allogeneic stem cell transplantation is a useful modality for blast-phase CML patients and chronic phase CML patients who develop resistance to multiple lines of standard TKI therapy.[7]

REFERENCES
Available at eBooks.Health.Elsevier.com.

AUTHOR: **RITESH RATHORE, MD**

Diseases
and Disorders

I

 BASIC INFORMATION

DEFINITION

- Chronic obstructive pulmonary disease (COPD) is a heterogenous lung condition characterized by persistent respiratory symptoms (cough, dyspnea, sputum production) and airflow obstruction that is persistent and often progressive. Although exposure to tobacco smoke is a key risk factor, nontobacco related risk factors account for up to 40% of the global burden of COPD. Exposure to biomass fuel and occupational exposure to industrial dust and chemicals play an important role in the developing and the developed world, respectively. Childhood and developmental factors may contribute to the pathophysiology of COPD, which is related to changes in the airways (bronchitis/bronchiolitis) and/or alveoli (emphysema).
- Acute exacerbations and comorbidities contribute to overall disease severity and prognosis.
- Traditionally, the spectrum of COPD has been described as encompassing *emphysema*, characterized by loss of lung elasticity and destruction of lung parenchyma with enlargement of air spaces, and *chronic bronchitis*, characterized by obstruction of small airways and productive cough >3 mo for more than 2 successive yr. Although emphysema and chronic bronchitis are commonly associated with COPD, neither make the diagnosis in isolation (without airflow obstruction) and may precede development of airflow obstruction. This group of patients with structural and physiologic abnormalities of COPD but without airflow obstruction are now called pre-COPD.
- COPD and asthma can coexist in an individual.[1] See Asthma and COPD Overlap.

SYNONYMS

COPD
Emphysema
Chronic bronchitis

ICD-10CM CODES

J44.9	Chronic obstructive pulmonary disease, unspecified COPD type
J42	Chronic bronchitis, unspecified chronic bronchitis type
J44.0	Chronic obstructive pulmonary disease with acute lower respiratory infection
J44.1	Chronic obstructive pulmonary disease with acute exacerbation
J43.0	Unilateral emphysema
J43.1	Panlobular emphysema
J43.2	Centrilobular emphysema
J43.8	Other emphysema
J43.9	Pulmonary emphysema, unspecified emphysema type

EPIDEMIOLOGY & DEMOGRAPHICS

- COPD affects about 14% of U.S. adults aged 40 to 79 yr. Global prevalence is estimated to be ~10% to 12%.
- COPD is equally common among males and females, but prevalence appears to be increasing among females. Females may have higher symptom burden, higher mortality, and lower lung function with similar smoking history and faster decline in lung function.[2]
- 10% to 20% of COPD in the U.S. is due to occupational or other exposure to particulate matter (air pollution), chemical vapors, irritants, and fumes; 80% to 90% is due to cigarette smoking.
- COPD is the third leading cause of death in the U.S. and worldwide.
- 16 million office visits, 500,000 hospitalizations, 126,000 deaths annually, and >$18 billion in direct health care costs annually can be attributed to COPD.
- People living in rural areas of the U.S. are at greater risk for COPD and COPD exacerbation-related mortality than those living in urban areas, independent of hospital rurality and volume.[3]

PHYSICAL FINDINGS & CLINICAL PRESENTATION

- The most common symptoms of COPD include chronic cough, sputum production, and dyspnea, which is typically exertional in the early stages. As these symptoms are nonspecific, misdiagnosis is not uncommon and both over and underdiagnosis has been reported. Objective confirmation of airflow obstruction using pulmonary function testing is required to establish a diagnosis of COPD.
- Dyspnea may be subtle in the early stages as some patients may not be aware of having readjusted their lifestyle to accommodate limitations from dyspnea early on, and clinicians may need to proactively elicit symptomatology.
- Cough may be present, initially in mornings ("smokers cough") before progressing to chronic cough and often productive of large amounts of sputum. Historically, patients with chronic bronchitis were classified as *"blue bloaters"*; the name is derived from the bluish tinge of the skin (as a result of chronic hypoxemia and hypercapnia) and from the frequent presence of peripheral edema (from cor pulmonale). In contrast, patients with emphysema who had a cachectic appearance, but pink skin color (adequate oxygen saturation) and dyspnea manifested by pursed-lip breathing and use of accessory muscles of respiration were classified as *"pink puffers."* These terms have fallen out of favor as they do not encompass the heterogeneity of COPD.
- As the disease progresses with increasing airflow obstruction, features of advanced COPD may become more evident with combinations of the following signs and symptoms:
  1. Cyanosis with chronic cough, tachypnea, tachycardia, and fatigue
  2. Dyspnea (persistent, progressive), pursed-lip breathing with use of accessory muscles for respiration, decreased breath sounds, wheezing
  3. Chronic sputum production

TABLE 1 Systemic Manifestations and Comorbidities of COPD

Cardiovascular	Infarction
	Arrhythmia
	Congestive heart failure
	Aortic aneurysm
Hypercoagulability	Stroke
	Pulmonary embolism
	Deep vein thrombosis
	Atrophy
Systemic	Weight loss
	Osteoporosis
	Skin wrinkling
	Anemia
	Fluid retention
Lung cancer	Depression

From Mason RJ: *Murray & Nadel's textbook of respiratory medicine*, ed 5, Philadelphia, 2010, Saunders.

  4. Chest wall abnormalities (hyperinflation, increased anteroposterior diameter of the chest, i.e., "barrel chest," protruding abdomen)
  5. Flattening of diaphragm
  6. Presence of clubbing should alert the clinician to look for other conditions such as lung cancer, interstitial lung disease (ILD), and bronchiectasis
  7. Cachexia
- Systemic manifestations and comorbidities of COPD are described in Table 1.
- Acute exacerbation of COPD is mainly a clinical diagnosis (in patients with established diagnosis of COPD) and generally manifests with worsening dyspnea, increase in sputum purulence, and increase in sputum volume. Exacerbations of other illnesses with similar presentations must be considered in the differential diagnosis (e.g., heart failure, ILD, bronchiectasis).
- Respiratory symptom status, however, is not a reliable indicator of the presence of airflow obstruction. Smokers with normal-range spirometry may report respiratory symptoms.[4] Computed tomography (CT) imaging of these symptomatic smokers may demonstrate similar abnormal findings as seen among those with COPD (pre-COPD).[5] In contrast, individuals with significant airflow obstruction may report minimal symptoms. Individuals with sedentary lifestyles may underestimate their symptoms, and careful history taking is important to elicit symptoms suggestive of COPD.

ETIOLOGY (FIG. 1)

- Tobacco exposure (Fig. E2)
- Occupational exposure to pulmonary toxins (e.g., dust, noxious gases, vapors, fumes, cadmium, coal, silica); the industries with the highest exposure risk are plastics, leather, rubber, and textiles
- Atmospheric pollution: Indoor (biomass fuel) and outdoor (air pollution)
- Alpha-1-antitrypsin deficiency (rare; <1% of COPD patients) (see Alpha-1-Antitrypsin Deficiency)
- Perinatal and childhood disadvantage factors affecting lung growth and development[6]

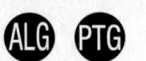

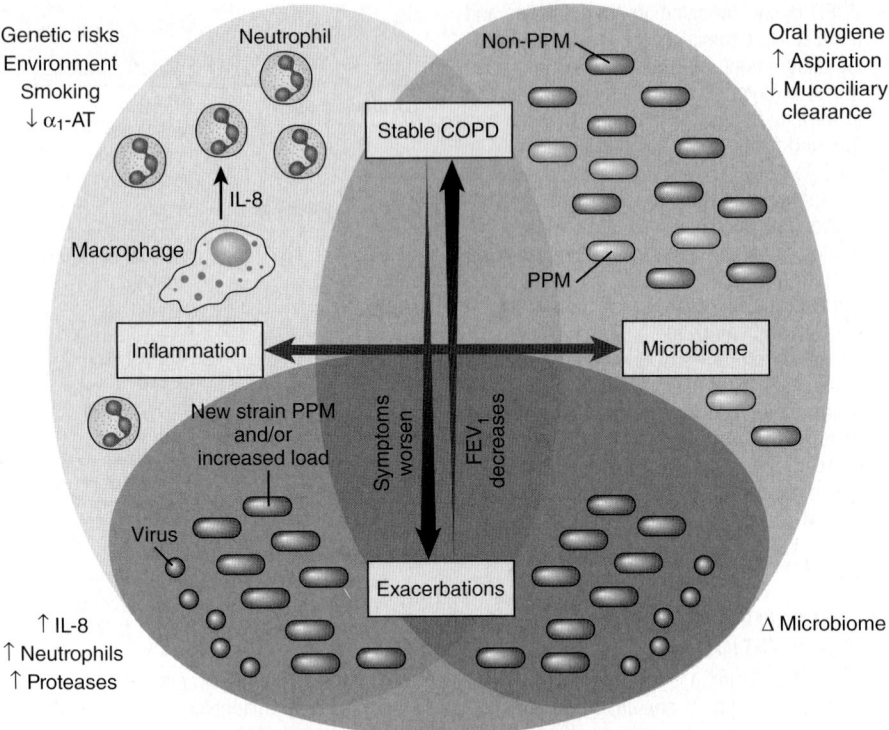

FIG. 1 Chronic obstructive pulmonary disease *(COPD)* pathophysiology. α_1-*AT*, α_1-Antitrypsin; *FEV$_1$*, forced expiratory volume in 1 sec; *IL-8*, interleukin-8; *PPM*, potentially pathogenic microorganism. (From Bennett JE et al: *Mandell, Douglas, and Bennett's principles and practice of infectious diseases*, ed 9, Philadelphia, 2020, Elsevier.)

Dx DIAGNOSIS

DIFFERENTIAL DIAGNOSIS

- Heart failure
- Asthma
- Tuberculosis, other respiratory infections
- Bronchiectasis
- Anemia
- Cystic fibrosis
- Neoplasm
- Pulmonary embolism
- Obliterative bronchiolitis
- Diffuse panbronchiolitis
- Sleep apnea, obstructive
- Hypothyroidism
- Neuromuscular disease

WORKUP

- Chest x-ray examination is seldom diagnostic but may demonstrate hyperinflation and may be useful to exclude an alternate diagnosis (e.g., congestive heart failure, tuberculosis).
- Pulmonary function testing (spirometry) (Fig. 3). Spirometry is the reference standard for diagnosing and assessing the severity of obstruction. Confirmation of airflow limitation measured by the ratio between forced expiratory volume in 1 sec (FEV$_1$) and forced vital capacity (FVC) is required to establish a diagnosis of COPD. A ratio <0.7 or lower than the lower limit of normal (LLN) in the presence of symptoms and risk factors establishes the diagnosis of COPD. GOLD guideline recommends repeat spirometry on a separate occasion when the ratio falls between 0.6 and 0.8.

- Oxygen saturation and arterial blood gases (useful in selected patients with FEV$_1$ <50% predicted, acute exacerbation, or hypoxia by pulse oximetry).
- Alpha-1-antitrypsin: All patients with COPD should be screened for alpha-1-antitrypsin deficiency.

LABORATORY TESTS

- CBC with differential: May reveal leukocytosis with left shift during acute exacerbation and secondary polycythemia in COPD with chronic hypoxia. Recent trials have shown that high blood eosinophils (including within the high-normal range) in COPD patients predicts response to corticosteroids. Prediction of treatment response remains imprecise, but inhaled corticosteroids (ICS) responsiveness begins to manifest at blood eosinophil counts >150 cells per cubic ml, with the best response seen at levels >300 cells per cubic ml.[7]
- Sputum may be purulent with bacterial respiratory tract infections. Sputum staining and cultures are usually reserved for cases refractory to antibiotic therapy. As the severity of disease progresses, some COPD patients' airways may become colonized by resistant microbes like *Pseudomonas* spp. And *Aspergillus* spp.
- Arterial blood gases: Normocapnia, mild to moderate hypoxemia may be present in mild to moderate COPD. Hypercapnia may develop as the disease becomes more severe. ABGs and pulse oximetry are usually used to determine if

a patient is a candidate for long-term oxygen therapy or if hypercapnia is present (ABGs).

- Pulmonary function testing (PFT) with measurement of forced vital capacity (FVC) and FEV$_1$: Spirometry should be obtained to diagnose airflow obstruction in clinically stable patients with respiratory symptoms. It should not be used to screen for airflow obstruction in individuals without respiratory symptoms. PFT results in COPD (Fig. 4) reveal abnormal diffusing capacity, increased total lung capacity and/or residual volume, and fixed reduction in FEV$_1$ in patients with emphysema; normal diffusing capacity and reduced FEV$_1$ are found in patients with chronic bronchitis. It is important to note that FEV$_1$ does not correlate well with individual patients' severity of dyspnea, exercise limitations, or health status. Evaluation of patients should also focus on symptom control and risk for adverse events in addition to FEV$_1$.
- Patients with COPD can generally be distinguished from asthmatics by presence of irreversible airflow obstruction measured by their incomplete response to a short-acting beta agonist and normal response to methacholine or other stimuli. However, many patients with COPD demonstrate significant response to bronchodilator (change in FEV$_1$ or FVC >10% relative to the predicted value, a recent change from previously defined criteria of >200 ml and 12%). Patients without a smoking history but with chronic asthmatic bronchitis may, over time, develop into COPD with airway obstruction that becomes irreversible.

ASSESSMENT

- After confirming obstruction by reduced FEV$_1$/ FVC ratio and grading the severity of obstruction using postbronchodilator FEV$_1$ (% reference) (Table 2), the Global Initiative for Chronic Obstructive Lung Disease (GOLD, Fig. 5, Table 3) assigns patients with COPD into three groups (A, B, and E) based on (1) a patient symptom score using one of two symptom questionnaires (CAT or mMRC), and (2) the number/severity of COPD exacerbations in 1 yr (see Table 3).
- In assessing the severity of COPD, the FEV$_1$ is limited by the fact that it does not take into account the systemic manifestations of COPD. Hence, it may predict survival at the population level but loses precision at an individual patient level. The BODE index (body mass index, degree of obstruction, dyspnea, and exercise capacity) has been proposed as a multidimensional scale to better assess morbidity and mortality associated with COPD at an individual level. It is better than the FEV$_1$ alone at predicting the risk of death from any cause and from respiratory causes among patients with COPD. In the BODE index, obstruction is measured by FEV$_1$ and dyspnea is measured by the modified Medical Research Council (MMRC) dyspnea questionnaire in a 6-min walk test. A score of 0 on the MMRC indicates that the individual is not troubled with breathlessness except with

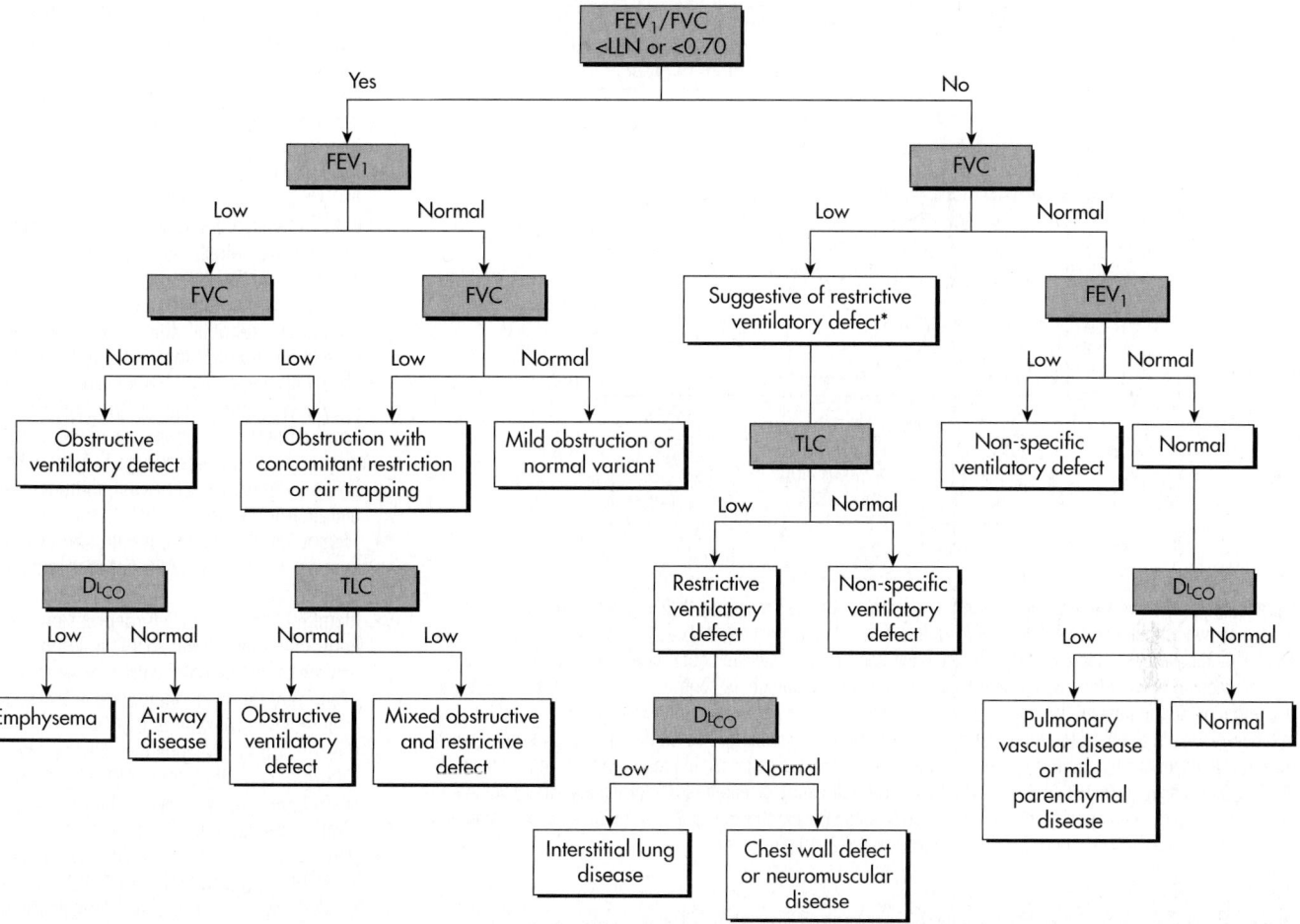

FIG. 3 Algorithm for interpretation of pulmonary function tests. The major pulmonary function tests include spirometry, lung volumes, and diffusing capacity. The figure provides a simplified schema for interpretation of common lung function patterns. Before interpreting lung function tests, evaluate the flow-volume and volume-time curves to ensure quality of the maneuver(s) and to identify patterns suggestive of obstructive ventilatory defect, restriction, or large airway obstruction. The first step in the interpretation is consideration of the forced expiratory volume in 1 sec *(FEV$_1$)* to the forced vital capacity *(FVC)* ratio. Low FEV$_1$ and low FVC will lead to a consideration of an obstructive ventilatory defect. Total lung capacity *(TLC)* is necessary for confirmation of a restrictive ventilatory defect. Diffusing capacity of carbon monoxide *(DL$_{CO}$)* helps assess presence of parenchymal disease in the setting of both obstructive and restrictive patterns; however, as noted in the text, the sensitivity and specificity of the DL$_{CO}$ for detection of emphysema, interstitial lung disease, or pulmonary vascular disease is not high near the lower limit of normal (LLN). Not infrequently, individuals have features of a mixed obstructive and restrictive pattern. A nonspecific pattern results when the FEV$_1$/FVC is normal and either the FEV$_1$ is low or the FVC is low and the TLC is normal. All patterns other than an obstructive ventilatory defect should be either confirmed or further evaluated with sequential testing as suggested in the schema. The schema gives a sequential approach that does not capture all combinations of test results. For combinations not represented (e.g., TLC < LLN and normal FVC, or DL$_{CO}$ and FEV$_1$ < LLN with normal FEV$_1$/FVC), the individual abnormalities may require further evaluation. *Low* indicates a value below the LLN; *normal* means at or above the LLN. *When FEV$_1$/FVC is above LLN and FVC is low but the FEV$_1$/FVC ratio is lower than expected—for example, considerably lower than the predicted value for the ratio—this can be interpreted as not clearly obstructive or restrictive. This pattern on spirometry alone should be investigated with further lung volume testing or imaging and followed closely. (From Broaddus VC et al: *Murray & Nadel's textbook of respiratory medicine*, ed 7, Philadelphia, 2022, Elsevier.)

strenuous exercise, 1 indicates shortness of breath when hurrying or walking up a slight hill, and 2 means the individual walks slower than people of the same age due to breathlessness or has to stop for breath when walking at own pace on level ground. A score of 3 means severe dyspnea because the person has to stop for breath after walking approximately 100 meters or after a few minutes on level ground, and a score of 4 indicates very severe dyspnea and is given when the individual is too breathless to leave the house or is breathless when dressing or undressing.

- A complete assessment of COPD entails recognition of comorbidities associated with the disease, especially those that present with similar symptoms leading to misdiagnosis of COPD, for example, congestive heart failure, cardiac arrhythmias, and ischemic heart disease or those that make symptom control difficult increasing the risk of exacerbation of COPD like anxiety/depression, gastroesophageal reflux disease (GERD), and obstructive sleep apnea. Skeletal muscle dysfunction and osteoporosis contribute to exercise intolerance in COPD patients. The number of comorbidities present in an individual incrementally increases mortality from COPD.[8]

IMAGING STUDIES

Chest x-ray examination:
- Hyperinflation with flattened diaphragm, tenting of the diaphragm at the rib, and increased retrosternal chest space (Fig. 6)

- Decreased vascular markings and bullae in patients with emphysema
- Thickened bronchial markings and enlarged right side of the heart in patients with chronic bronchitis

CT:
- CT scan is not routinely recommended in patients with COPD. It may be helpful in early detection of COPD. CT scan of the chest with volumetric assessment and dynamic functional mapping can detect early pathologic changes in the lung parenchyma (emphysema) and small airways (air trapping) in symptomatic smokers before the development of airflow obstruction.[4] CT scan is recommended for lung cancer screening and bronchial valve intervention for emphysema/

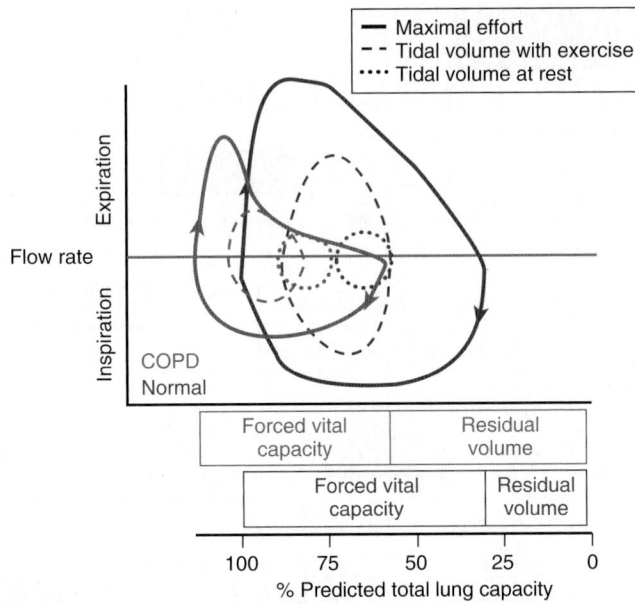

FIG. 4 Representative flow-volume loops in normal subjects *(red)* and COPD *(blue)*. Flow-volume tracings are shown at rest, with exercise *(dashed lines)*, and with maximal effort. The normal tracings demonstrate that the metabolic demands generated by exercise can be met with increased tidal volumes and frequency without reaching flow limitation, and that lung volumes do not change. In contrast, the patient with COPD has flow limitation during tidal breathing. Increasing tidal volumes and frequency limit expiratory time, and the flow limitation results in a failure to reach resting end-expiratory lung volume. The resulting increases in lung volumes, termed dynamic hyperinflation, are associated with an increased work of breathing and, hence, dyspnea. *CAT,* COPD Assessment Test; *COPD,* chronic obstructive pulmonary disease; *FEV1,* forced expiratory volume in 1 sec; *FVC,* forced vital capacity; *mMRC,* modified Medical Research Council Dyspnea Score. (From Goldman L, Shafer AI: *Goldman-Cecil medicine,* ed 26, Philadelphia, 2019, Elsevier.)

TABLE 2 Spirometric General Classification of Chronic Obstructive Pulmonary Disease (COPD)

Severity	FEV_1/FVC	FEV_1 % Predicted
GOLD 0: At risk	>0.7	≥80
Patients who:		
• Smoke or have exposure to pollutants		
• Have cough, sputum, or dyspnea		
• Have family history of respiratory disease		
GOLD 1: Mild COPD	≤0.7	≥80
GOLD 2: Moderate COPD	≤0.7	50-79
GOLD 3: Severe COPD	≤0.7	30-49
GOLD 4: Very severe COPD	≤0.7	<30

FEV_1, Forced expiratory volume in 1 sec; *FVC,* forced vital capacity; *GOLD,* Global Initiative for Chronic Obstructive Lung Disease criteria. From Bennett JE et al: *Mandell, Douglas, and Bennett's principles and practice of infectious diseases,* ed 9, Philadelphia, 2020, Elsevier.

air trapping. GOLD 2023 recommends a CT scan of the chest in patients with persistent exacerbations and in whom symptoms are out of proportion to airflow limitation severity.

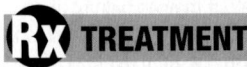 **TREATMENT**

Treatment of stable COPD is outlined in Fig. 7.

NONPHARMACOLOGIC THERAPY
- Smoking cessation and elimination of air pollutants.
- Vaccination: Pneumococcal, annual influenza, and SARS-CoV-2. Patients with COPD are at

increased risk of poor outcomes with COVID-19 infection, and COVID-19 vaccination per national guidelines is recommended.
- Supplemental oxygen, usually through a face mask/nasal cannula, to ensure oxygen saturation >90% as measured by pulse oximetry. Continuous oxygen therapy should be prescribed for patients with COPD who have resting arterial partial pressure of oxygen 55 mm Hg or less, or oxygen saturation 88% or less as measured by pulse oximetry. In patients with stable COPD and moderate resting desaturation (SpO_2 89% to 93%) or exercise-induced moderate desaturation (during the 6-min walk test, SpO_2 ≥80% for

≥5 min and <90% for ≥10 sec), long-term oxygen supplementation did not improve mortality or time to first hospitalization. Individual patient-related factors also should be considered while evaluating patients for oxygen supplementation.
- Pulmonary secretion clearance: Careful nasotracheal suction is indicated only in patients with excessive secretions and an inability to expectorate. Mechanical percussion of the chest as applied by a physical or respiratory therapist is ineffective in COPD.
- Pulmonary rehabilitation should be considered in all symptomatic COPD patients. Medicare will cover up to 36 sessions of pulmonary rehabilitation in COPD patients. Daily physical activity, at home or community settings, should be encouraged. Telerehabilitation may improve access to pulmonary rehabilitation in future.
- Weight loss in obese patients and nutritional support in underweight patients should be considered.
- Identification of anxiety/depression in patients diagnosed with COPD is important, as it may be associated with increased risk of exacerbations and decreased adherence to maintenance therapy of COPD.
- Use of continuous positive airway pressure (CPAP) in patients with COPD and obstructive sleep apnea, as it improves both survival and reduces hospital admissions.
- Home-based nocturnal noninvasive ventilation in select patients with severe COPD with hypercapnia may prevent recurrent hospitalizations.[9]

GENERAL Rx
- Pharmacologic treatment (Table 4) should be administered (Fig. 8) using the GOLD multimodal assessment tool. Current GOLD guidelines recommend treatment based on patient symptom burden and exacerbation risk (Table 5) irrespective of severity of obstruction by FEV_1.
- Pulmonary rehabilitation is recommended for patients in groups B and E.
- Patients in group A should receive a short-acting or long-acting anticholinergic or β_2-agonist for mild intermittent symptoms.
- Patients in group B should receive a combination long-acting anticholinergics and long-acting β_2-agonists.
- Patients in group E are at high risk of exacerbations and needs biomarker-based individualized treatment strategies. The initial choice is a combination of a long-acting anticholinergic and long-acting bronchodilator. If blood eosinophils are >300 cells/μl, a combination of a long-acting anticholinergic, long-acting bronchodilator and ICS should be considered. Adding ICS to inhaled regimens seems to have little or no effect when blood eosinophils are <100 cells/μl.
- Patients in group E who continue to have exacerbation despite above strategies should be considered for PDE4 inhibitor roflumilast (with chronic bronchitis) and/or chronic azithromycin (former smokers). Recently, dupilumab, a monoclonal antibody

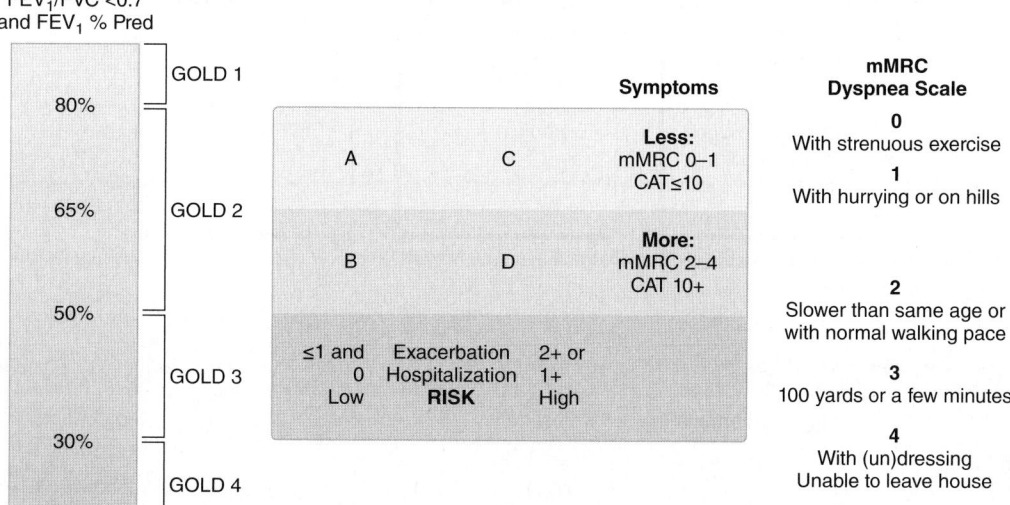

FIG. 5 GOLD Classification System for COPD. In addition to the severity of airflow obstruction (on the *left*), it incorporates symptoms and risk of exacerbation to create four groups: A, B, C, and D. Based on this new classification system, a COPD patient with FEV₁ 30% who had two exacerbations and has a CAT score of >10 will be categorized as GOLD Grade 3, Group D. Treatment is tailored according to the group, and GOLD grade is utilized to estimate prognosis. *CAT,* COPD Assessment Test; *COPD,* chronic obstructive pulmonary disease; *FEV1,* forced expiratory volume in 1 sec; *FVC,* forced vital capacity; *mMRC,* modified Medical Research Council Dyspnea Score; *Pred,* predicted. (Modified from https://goldcopd.org/wp-content/uploads/2023/03/GOLD-2023-ver-1.3-17Feb2023_WMV.pdf.)

TABLE 3   GOLD ABCD Assessment Tool

Moderate to severe exacerbation history	≥2 or ≥1 leading to hospital admission	C	D
	0 or 1 (not leading to hospital admission)	A	B
		Mild (mMRC or CAT)	Severe (mMRC or CAT)
		Symptoms burden	

The letter provides information about symptom burden and risk of exacerbation in addition to the airflow limitation severity classification that can be used to guide future therapy.
From Bennett JE et al: *Mandell, Douglas, and Bennett's principles and practice of infectious diseases,* ed 9, Philadelphia, 2020, Elsevier.

that blocks interleukin-13 (IL-13) and IL-4α subunit has been shown to be efficacious in this group.[10] It needs regulatory body approval before it can be available in the market. Another agent, Ensifentrine, a nebulized form of PDE3/PDE4 inhibitor, has shown promising results in two trials that awaits regulatory body approval.

- Bronchodilators are the mainstay of pharmacologic management of COPD. Bronchodilators improve symptoms, quality of life, and exercise tolerance and decrease incidence of exacerbations. Inhaled bronchodilators *should be offered* to all COPD patients with respiratory symptoms. Clinicians should base the choice of specific monotherapy on patient preference, cost, and adverse effect profile. Long-acting inhaled bronchodilators are superior to short-acting bronchodilators when taken as needed.

- Short-acting β₂-agonists (e.g., albuterol metered-dose inhaler 1 to 2 puffs q4 to 6h prn) or short-acting anticholinergic agents (e.g., ipratropium inhaler 2 puffs qid) are acceptable in patients with mild, variable symptoms. Anticholinergics (antimuscarinic agents) are also effective and are available in combination with albuterol (e.g., Combivent).

- Long-acting inhaled agents are preferred in patients with mild to moderate or continuous symptoms. Currently available inhaled long-acting antimuscarinic agents (LAMAs) are tiotropium (Spiriva), umeclidinium (Incruse), aclidinium (Tudorza), and glycopyrrolate (Seebri), revefenacin (Yupelri). Tiotropium is an excellent long-acting bronchodilator. It is very effective for long-term, once-a-day use. It has been shown to be superior to salmeterol, an inhaled long-acting β-agonist (LABA) in patients with moderate to severe COPD and may possibly slow the rate of decline in FEV₁. Although some trials have

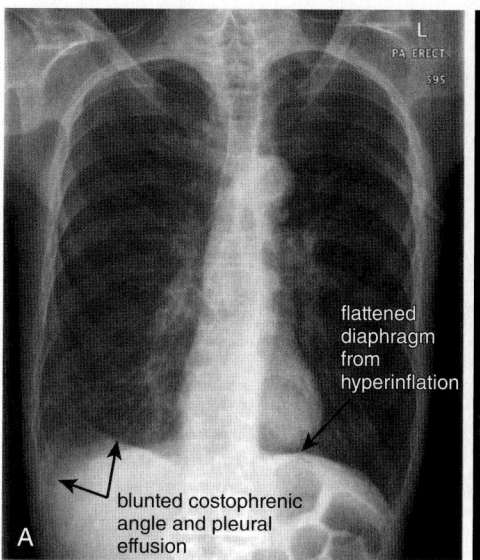

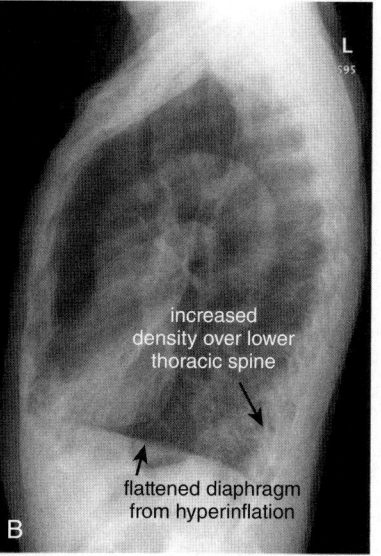

FIG. 6 Chronic obstructive pulmonary disease (COPD). A, Posterior-anterior (PA) upright chest x-ray. **B,** Lateral upright chest x-ray. This 63-yr-old man with a history of COPD presented with 2 wk of worsening cough with yellow sputum and dyspnea. His oxygen saturation was 87% in the emergency room. He has evidence of hyperinflation with flat diaphragm (particularly evident on the lateral x-ray) **(B).** The patient also has a blunted right costophrenic angle with an apparent effusion and increased densities in both the right and the left lung base **(A).** The lateral x-ray also shows increased density overlying the inferior thoracic spine, an abnormal spine sign. (From Broder JS: *Diagnostic imaging for the emergency physician,* Philadelphia, 2011, Saunders.)

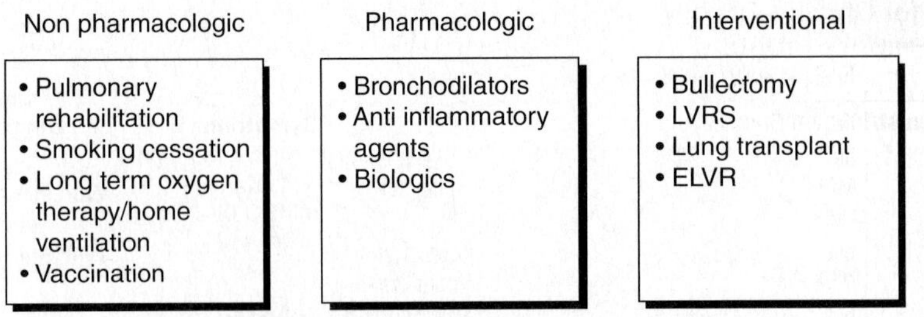

Chronic Obstructive Pulmonary Disease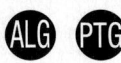

Non pharmacologic	Pharmacologic	Interventional
• Pulmonary rehabilitation • Smoking cessation • Long term oxygen therapy/home ventilation • Vaccination	• Bronchodilators • Anti inflammatory agents • Biologics	• Bullectomy • LVRS • Lung transplant • ELVR

FIG. 7 Treatment options for the management of stable chronic obstructive pulmonary disease. *ELVR*, Endoscopic lung volume reduction; *LVRS*, lung volume reduction surgery.

TABLE 4 Medications for Chronic Obstructive Pulmonary Disease

Drug(s)	Frequency/Formulation	Dosage	Side Effects
Long-Acting β-Agonists			
Salmeterol	qd DPI	50 μg	Palpitations, hypokalemia
Formoterol	bid Nebulizer	20 μg	
Indacaterol	qd DPI	75 μg	
Olodaterol	qd MDI	5 μg (2.5 μg/puff)	
Muscarinic Antagonists			
Aclidinium bromide	bid DPI	400 μg	Dry mouth Constipation
Tiotropium bromide	qd MDI DPI	5 μg (MDI) 18 μg (DPI)	Aggravation of narrow-angle glaucoma
Glycopyrronium	bid DPI	15.6 μg	
Umeclidinium	qd DPI	62.5 μg	
Ipratropium bromide	qd MDI	34 μg (17 μg/puff)	
Revefenacin	qd Nebulizer	175 μg	
Inhaled Corticosteroids			
Fluticasone	bid DPI	88-500 μg	Oropharyngeal candidiasis and hoarseness, and risk of pneumonia
Budesonide	bid DPI/nebulized	0.5-1 mg daily total 90-180 μg/actuation	
Beclomethasone	bid MDI	40-320 μg twice daily	
Mometasone	qd DPI	220-440 μg	
Flunisolide	bid MDI	220-440 μg twice daily	
Phosphodiesterase-4 inhibitors			
Roflumilast	Pill qd	250-500 μg	Diarrhea, nausea, and weight loss
Combination Inhalers			
Combination Long-Acting β-Agonist/Long-Acting Muscarinic Antagonist			
Formoterol/glycopyrrolate	bid MDI	9.6 μg formoterol/18 μg glycopyrrolate	Side effects of each constituent
Indacaterol/glycopyrrolate	bid DPI	27.5 μg indacaterol/15.6 μg glycopyrrola33t33e	
Olodaterol/tiotropium	qd MDI333	5 μg of each (2 puffs)	
Vilanterol/umeclidinium	qd DPI	25 μg vilanterol/62.5 μg umeclidinium	
Combination Short-Acting β-Agonist/Short-Acting Muscarinic Antagonist			
Albuterol/ipratropium	q4-6h	MDI Nebulizer	Side effects of each constituent

C

Diseases and Disorders

I

TABLE 4 Medications for Chronic Obstructive Pulmonary Disease—cont'd

Drug(s)	Frequency/Formulation	Dosage	Side Effects
Combination Long-Acting β-Agonist/Inhaled Corticosteroids			
Salmeterol/fluticasone	bid MDI DPI	14 μg salmeterol/55-232 μg fluticasone 50 μg/salmeterol/100-500 μg fluticasone	Side effects of each constituent
Formoterol/budesonide	bid MDI	9 μg formoterol/160-320 μg budesonide (two strengths available)	
Formoterol/mometasone	bid MDI	5 μg formoterol/100 or 200 μg mometasone; 2 inhalations per administration	
Vilanterol/fluticasone	qd DPI	25 μg vilanterol/100 μg fluticasone; one inhalation	
Combination Long-Acting β-Agonist/Long-Acting Muscarinic Antagonist/Inhaled Corticosteroids			
Vilanterol/umeclidinium/fluticasone	qd DPI	25 μg vilanterol/62.5 μg umeclidinium/100 μg fluticasone	Side effects of each constituent

bid, Twice daily; *DPI,* dry powder inhaler; *MDI,* metered-dose inhaler; *qd,* once daily.
From Goldman L, Shafer AI: *Goldman-Cecil medicine,* ed 26, Philadelphia, 2019, Elsevier.

shown higher hospitalization rates and mortality with tiotropium compared to LABAs, recent trials and meta-analyses have shown a reassuring safety profile of LAMAs in COPD.

- Salmeterol, formoterol, indacaterol, olodaterol, and vilanterol are available LABAs for long-term maintenance treatment of bronchospasm associated with COPD. Monotherapy with LABAs is not preferred. They are used in combination with LAMAs in COPD.
- LABAs and LAMAs in different combinations are now available on the market (umeclidinium/vilanterol [Anoro], tiotropium/olodaterol [Stiolto], indacaterol/glycopyrrolate [Utibron], glycopyrrolate/formoterol [Bevespi]). Although LAMAs and LABAs perform equally well for symptom control, LAMAs are generally preferred for symptom control and exacerbation reduction in COPD. Monotherapy with LABA is discouraged in COPD.
- Addition of inhaled steroids (fluticasone, budesonide, triamcinolone) is used to reduce exacerbations in patients with moderate to severe COPD. The role of ICS in COPD is evolving. Blood eosinophil count helps guide ICS therapy in COPD. Patients with blood eosinophil counts more than 300 cells per cubic milliliter and more than two exacerbations annually benefit the most from ICS therapy.[7] ICS therapy does not affect mortality among patients with COPD and is associated with a higher risk of pneumonia. ICS therapy is intended to be used as part of a combined regimen along with bronchodilators, and not as sole therapy (as can be used in asthma).
- Roflumilast: A selective oral PDE4 inhibitor useful to reduce the risk of COPD exacerbations in patients with severe COPD associated with chronic bronchitis and a history of exacerbations. It is not a bronchodilator and is not indicated for the relief of acute bronchospasm. It may be associated with adverse psychiatric reactions and should be avoided in patients with depression or hepatic impairment.
- Antibiotics (Fig. 9): For patients with frequent acute exacerbations of COPD despite optimal therapy with bronchodilators and ICS, long-term

use of the macrolide antibiotic azithromycin may be considered for its antiinflammatory properties. Prophylactic use of macrolide antibiotics (azithromycin 250 mg daily or thrice per week) has been shown to decrease the frequency of exacerbations and improve quality of life among selected patients with COPD; however, it may lead to hearing decrements in a small percentage of patients and increased prevalence of macrolide-resistant bacteria colonizing the airway. It should be avoided in patients with a long QT interval. Guidelines from the Global Initiative for Chronic Obstructive Lung Disease recommend 5 to 7 days of antibacterial therapy in patients with COPD exacerbation with increased dyspnea, increased sputum volume, and increased sputum purulence. Shorter antibiotic regimens (e.g., 2 days of levofloxacin) may be appropriate in COPD patients with mild-moderate exacerbations.[11]

- Systemic glucocorticoid therapy: Chronic systemic glucocorticoid therapy is generally not recommended even in severe COPD due to associated increase in mortality and morbidity.
- Triple therapy (LAMA plus LABA plus ICS [e.g., vilanterol/umeclidinium/fluticasone {Trelegy Ellipta}, budesonide/formoterol/glycopyrrolate {Breztri}]): Indicated in patients with COPD at high risk for exacerbations. Multiple recent clinical trials have demonstrated the efficacy of single inhaler triple therapy in patients with moderate to severe COPD in terms of reduction in exacerbation frequency and hospitalizations compared to dual agents like ICS/LABA and LAMA/LABA.[12] The greatest benefit occurs in patients with high eosinophil blood counts.
- During follow-up visits, symptom burden should be assessed by using objective questionnaires like COPD assessment tools (CATs). Medication side effects and inhaler compliance/technique should be assessed during each clinic visit.
- COPD patients with a cardiovascular indication for a beta-blocker should continue to receive the β-blocker therapy, including during an exacerbation. COPD patients should

not be started on a β-blocker therapy if there is no cardiovascular indication.

- Acute exacerbation of COPD (increase in sputum volume and purulence, worsening dyspnea) can be treated with:
1. Aerosolized β₂-agonists (e.g., metaproterenol nebulizer solution 5% 0.3 ml or albuterol nebulized 5% solution 2.5 to 5 mg).
2. Anticholinergic agents, which have equivalent efficacy to inhaled β-adrenergic agonists. Inhalant solution of ipratropium bromide 0.5 mg can be administered every 4 to 8 h.
3. Short courses of systemic corticosteroids have been shown to improve spirometric and clinical outcomes. Treatment failure occurs less often in patients who receive low-dose steroids than in those receiving high-dose parenteral steroids. Oral prednisone 40 mg/day for 5 days is generally effective. Longer courses confer no added benefit and increase the risk of pneumonia and mortality. Trials have shown that in patients with acute COPD exacerbations, systemic glucocorticoid treatment for 5 days is not inferior to treatment for 14 days.
4. Use of noninvasive positive pressure ventilation (NIPPV) decreases the risk of endotracheal intubation and decreases intensive care unit admission rates. Contraindications to its use are uncooperative patient, decreased level of consciousness, hemodynamic instability, inadequate mask fit, and severe respiratory acidosis. Increased airway pressure can be delivered by using inspiratory positive airway pressure, continuous positive airway pressure, or bilevel positive airway pressure, which combines the other modalities. When using NIPPV, the nasal mask is usually tolerated the best; however, patients must be instructed to keep their mouths closed while breathing with the nasal apparatus. Oxygen can be delivered at 10 to 15 L/min and started in spontaneous ventilation mode with an initial expiratory positive airway pressure setting

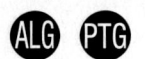

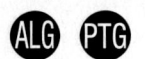

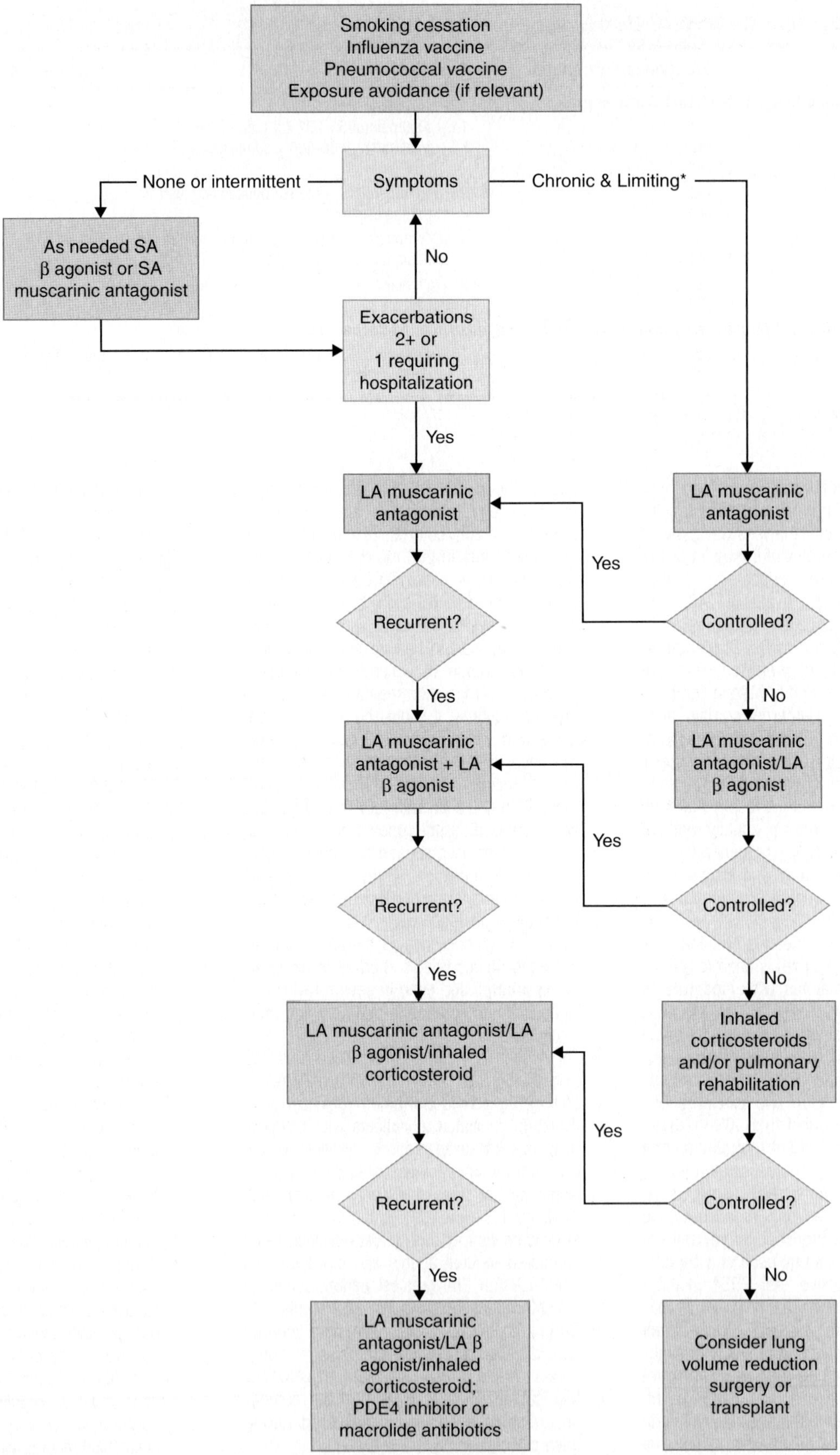

FIG. 8 Approach to the patient with chronic obstructive pulmonary disease. *Dyspnea causes the patient to walk slower than patients of the same age or to stop to catch their breath when walking at their own pace; patient stops for breath after walking 100 yards or less or after a few min; or patient is breathless when dressing or housebound due to dyspnea. *COPD,* Chronic obstructive pulmonary disease; *LA,* long acting; *PDE,* phosphodiesterase; *SA,* short acting. (From Goldman L, Shafer AI: *Goldman-Cecil medicine,* ed 26, Philadelphia, Elsevier, 2019.)

TABLE 5 Modified GOLD Treatment Recommendations According to Stable State Patient Group Category

Patient Group	First Choice	Second Choice	Alternative Choice
Pharmacologic Treatment Options			
A	SABA prn	LABA or LAMA	Theophylline
Symptoms low	or	or	
Exacerbation: 0 or 1 (not leading to hospital admission)	SAMA prn	SABA and SAMA	
B	LABA	LAMA and LABA	SABA and/or SAMA
Symptoms high	or		Theophylline
Exacerbation: 0 or 1 (not leading to hospital admission)	LAMA		
C	LAMA	LABA and ICS	PDE4 inhibitor
Symptoms low	or		SABA and/or SAMA
	LAMA and LABA		
Exacerbation: ≥2 or ≥1 leading to hospital admission			Theophylline
D	LAMA and LABA	ICS and LAMA	Carbocysteine
Symptoms high	or	or	Roflumilast
	LAMA and LABA and ICS	ICS and LABA and LAMA	
Exacerbation: ≥2 or ≥1 leading to hospital admission		or	Theophylline
		ICS and LABA and PDE-4 inhibitor	
		or	Azithromycin
		LAMA and LABA	
		or	
		LAMA and PDE-4 inhibitor	

Patient Group	Essential	Recommended	
Nonpharmacologic Treatment Options			
A	Smoking cessation	Physical activity	
		Influenza and pneumococcal vaccination; Tdap	
B-D	Smoking cessation	Physical activity	
	Pulmonary rehabilitation	Influenza and pneumococcal vaccination; Tdap	

Symptoms low = mMRC 0-1 or CAT <10. Symptoms high = mMRC ≥2 or CAT ≥10.
CAT, COPD Assessment Test; *GOLD,* Global Initiative for Chronic Obstructive Lung Disease criteria; *mMRC,* modified British Medical Research Council questionnaire; *ICS,* inhaled corticosteroid; *LABA,* long-acting β$_2$-adrenergic agonist; *LAMA,* long-acting muscarinic antagonist; *PDE-4,* phosphodiesterase type 4; *SABA,* short-acting β$_2$-adrenergic agonist; *SAMA,* short-acting muscarinic antagonist; *Tdap,* combined tetanus, diphtheria, and acellular pertussis vaccine.
Modified from Vogelmeier CD, Criner GJ, Martinez FJ, et al. Global strategy for the diagnosis, management, and prevention of chronic obstructive lung disease 2017 report: GOLD Executive Summary. *Eur Respir J.* 2017;49:1750214.

of 3 to 5 cm H_2O and an inspiratory positive airway pressure setting of up to 10 cm H_2O. Adjustments in these settings should be made in 2-cm H_2O increments. It is important to monitor patients with frequent vital sign measurements, arterial blood gases, or pulse oximetry. Intubation and mechanical ventilation may be necessary if previous measures fail to provide improvement.

5. Patients with severe exacerbations without prompt response to these therapies in the emergency room can be given a trial of a single dose of magnesium sulphate (2 g intravenous [IV] over 20 min). This has been shown to reduce hospitalization rates.[13]

6. IV aminophylline administration is controversial and not recommended.

7. Mucoactive agents (e.g., N-acetylcysteine) have not been consistently shown to be effective.

8. Guaifenesin may improve cough symptoms and mucus clearance; however, mucolytic medications are generally ineffective.

- ~50% of COPD exacerbations are caused by bacterial infection. Antibiotics are indicated in suspected bacterial respiratory infection (e.g., increased purulence and volume of phlegm).

1. *Haemophilus influenzae* and *Streptococcus pneumoniae* are frequent causes of acute bronchitis.

2. Oral antibiotics of choice are azithromycin, levofloxacin, amoxicillin-clavulanate, trimethoprim-sulfamethoxazole, doxycycline, and cefuroxime.

3. The two best predictors of potential benefit from antibiotics are purulent sputum and C-reactive protein (CRP) level >40 mg/L.

4. The role of procalcitonin-based protocols to guide antibiotics in COPD exacerbations is not clearly established.

- Fig. 10 illustrates the management of acute exacerbations of COPD. Guideline recommendations for hospital management of COPD exacerbations are described in Table 6. Indications for invasive mechanical ventilation are described in Box 1.

- Lung volume reduction surgery (LVRS) has been proposed as a treatment option for some patients with severe emphysema who have severe dyspnea despite optimal medical treatment. Overall it improves lung function, quality of life, and exercise capacity and reduces exacerbation rate with potential mortality benefit. LVRS is most beneficial in patients with both

predominantly upper-lobe emphysema and low baseline exercise capacity. Box 2 summarizes indications and contraindications for LVRS.

- Endoscopic lung volume reduction (ELVR) by endobronchial valve (EBV) placement via bronchoscopy to reduce lung volume with one-way valves that allow air to leave but not enter a lung segment has been FDA approved since June 2018.[14,15] It is most effective in patients who have evidence of severe air trapping and hyperinflation and lack collateral ventilation in the targeted lobe of the lung (Box 3).

- Lung transplant (see Box 2) should be considered in patients with advanced emphysema. Recommended referral criteria include[16]:

1. BODE score 5 to 6 with additional factor(s) present suggestive of increased risk of mortality:
   a. Frequent acute exacerbations
   b. Increase in BODE score >1 over past 24 mo
   c. Pulmonary artery to aorta diameter >1 on CT scan
   d. FEV_1 20% to 25% predicted

2. Clinical deterioration despite maximal treatment including medication, pulmonary

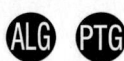
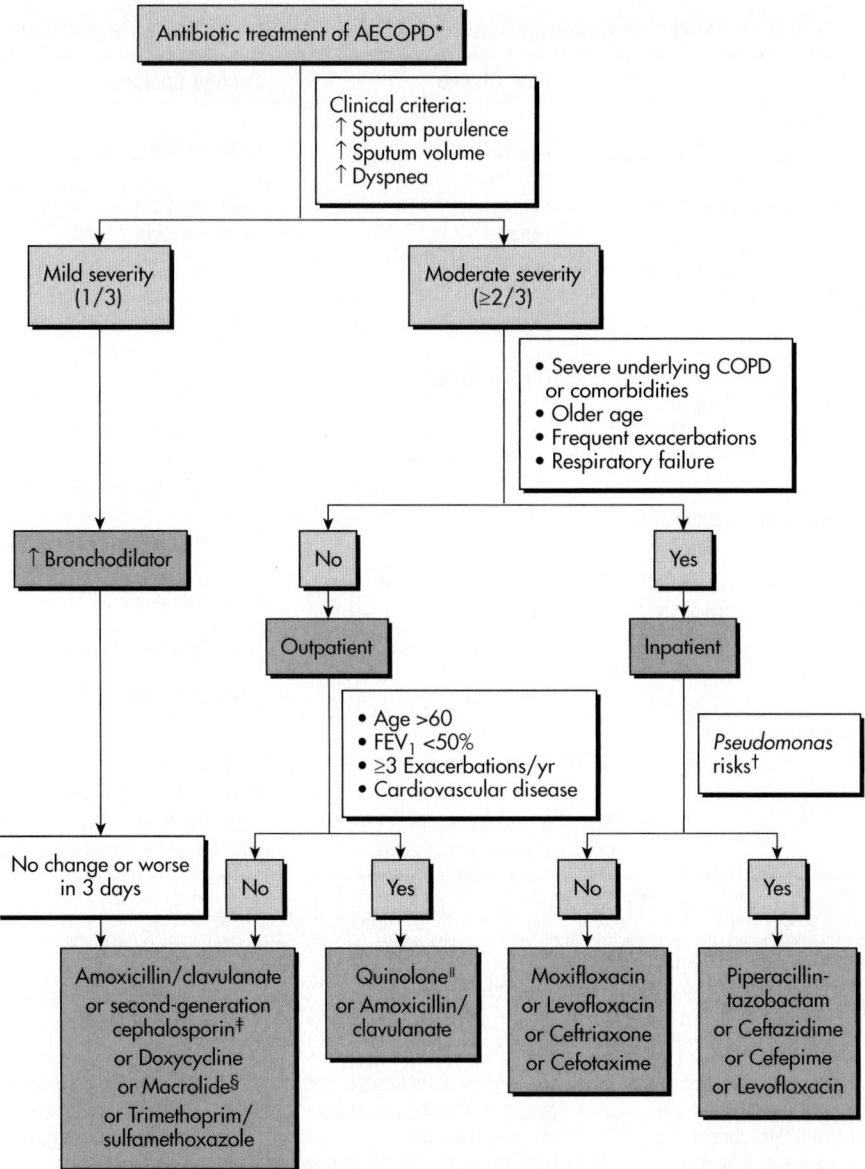

FIG. 9 Flowchart for antibiotic treatment decision in chronic obstructive pulmonary disease *(COPD)* **exacerbation.** *AECOPD*, Acute exacerbations of chronic obstructive pulmonary disease; *FEV₁*, forced expiratory volume in 1 sec. (From Bennett JE et al: *Mandell, Douglas, and Bennett's principles and practice of infectious diseases,* ed 9, Philadelphia, 2020, Elsevier.)

rehabilitation, oxygen therapy, and, as appropriate, nocturnal noninvasive positive pressure ventilation.

3. Poor quality of life unacceptable to the patient.

DISPOSITION

- After the initial episode of respiratory failure, 5-yr survival is ~25%.
- Development of cor pulmonale or hypercapnia and persistent tachycardia are poor prognostic indicators.

- Supplemental oxygen for patients with resting hypoxemia (defined as SpO_2 <89%) improves survival. The need for oxygen at rest may be the strongest predictor of mortality in chronic respiratory failure from COPD.
- Pulmonary rehabilitation, which includes strength and endurance training and education, nutritional, and psychosocial support, improves symptoms and exercise tolerance but is underutilized. Patients who initiate pulmonary rehabilitation within 90 days of discharge after hospitalization for COPD exacerbation are significantly less likely to be rehospitalized.[17]

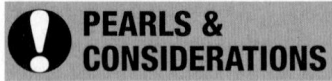

COMMENTS

- All patients with COPD should receive pneumococcal, annual influenza, and SARS-CoV-2 vaccines.
- Early antibiotic administration is associated with improved outcomes among patients hospitalized for acute exacerbations of COPD.
- Pulmonary artery enlargement as determined by a ratio of the diameter of the pulmonary

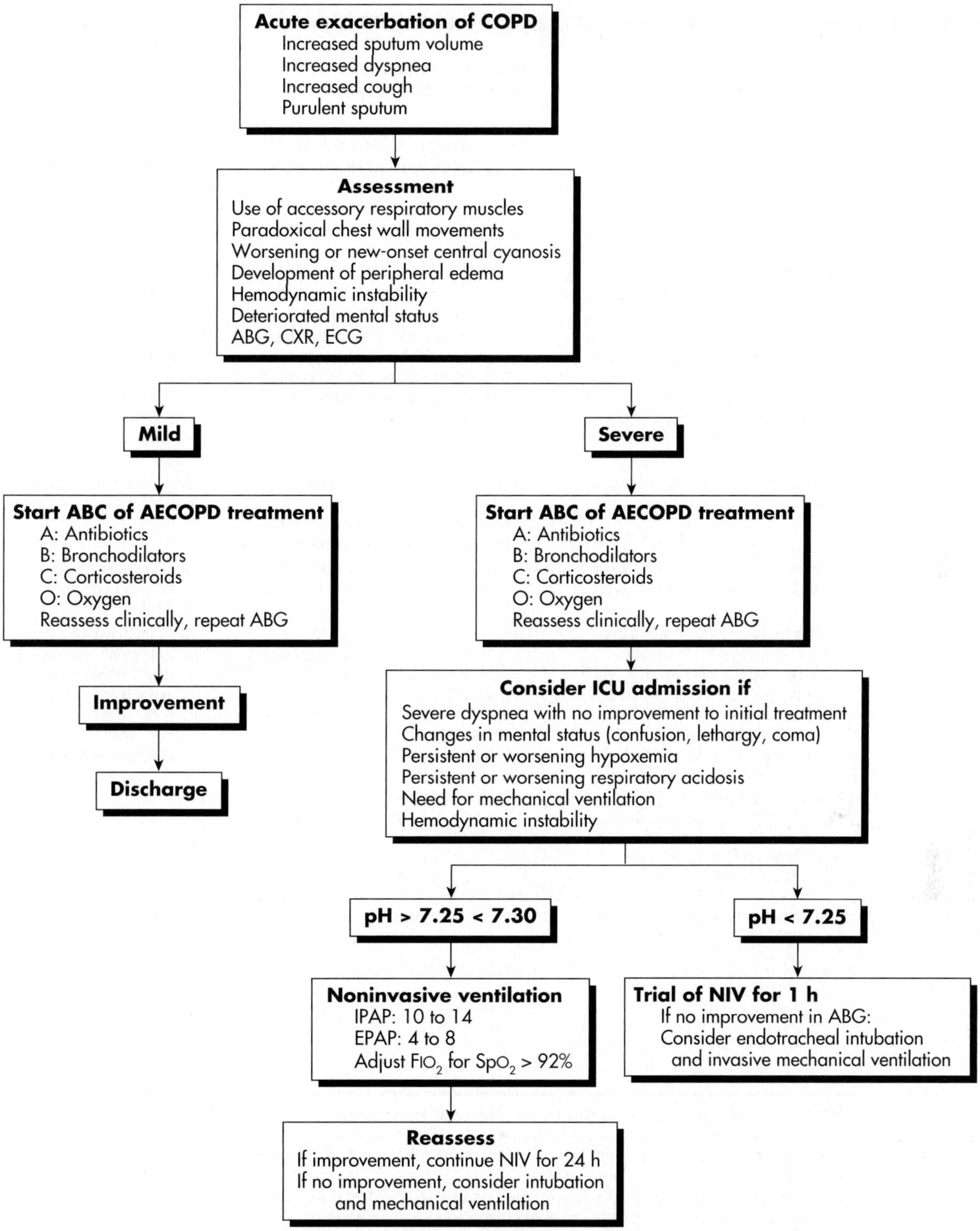

Acute exacerbation of COPD
Increased sputum volume
Increased dyspnea
Increased cough
Purulent sputum

Assessment
Use of accessory respiratory muscles
Paradoxical chest wall movements
Worsening or new-onset central cyanosis
Development of peripheral edema
Hemodynamic instability
Deteriorated mental status
ABG, CXR, ECG

Mild

Severe

Start ABC of AECOPD treatment
A: Antibiotics
B: Bronchodilators
C: Corticosteroids
O: Oxygen
Reassess clinically, repeat ABG

Start ABC of AECOPD treatment
A: Antibiotics
B: Bronchodilators
C: Corticosteroids
O: Oxygen
Reassess clinically, repeat ABG

Improvement

Discharge

Consider ICU admission if
Severe dyspnea with no improvement to initial treatment
Changes in mental status (confusion, lethargy, coma)
Persistent or worsening hypoxemia
Persistent or worsening respiratory acidosis
Need for mechanical ventilation
Hemodynamic instability

pH > 7.25 < 7.30

pH < 7.25

Noninvasive ventilation
IPAP: 10 to 14
EPAP: 4 to 8
Adjust FIO$_2$ for SpO$_2$ > 92%

Trial of NIV for 1 h
If no improvement in ABG:
Consider endotracheal intubation
and invasive mechanical ventilation

Reassess
If improvement, continue NIV for 24 h
If no improvement, consider intubation
and mechanical ventilation

FIG. 10 Management of acute exacerbations of chronic obstructive pulmonary disease. *ABG,* Arterial blood gas; *AECOPD,* acute exacerbations of chronic obstructive pulmonary disease; *COPD,* chronic obstructive pulmonary disease; *CXR,* chest x-ray; *ECG,* electrocardiogram; *EPAP,* expiratory positive airway pressure; *FIO$_2$,* fraction of inspired oxygen; *ICU,* intensive care unit; *IPAP,* inspiratory positive airway pressure; *NIV,* noninvasive ventilation; *SpO$_2$,* oxygen saturation measured by pulse oximetry. (From Parrillo JE, Dellinger RP: *Critical care medicine: principles of diagnosis and management in the adult,* ed 5, Philadelphia, 2019, Elsevier.)

C

Diseases
and Disorders

I

TABLE 6   Guideline Recommendations for Hospital Management of COPD Exacerbations

	Global Initiative for Chronic Obstructive Lung Disease[a]	American Thoracic Society/European Respiratory Society[b]	National Institute for Clinical Excellence[c]
Date of statement	2023	2017	2010
Diagnostic testing	Chest radiograph, oximetry, ABGs, ECG. Other testing as warranted by clinical indication.	Chest radiograph, oxygen saturation, ABGs, ECG, sputum Gram stain and culture.	Chest radiograph, ABG, ECG, complete blood count, sputum smear and culture, blood cultures if febrile.
Bronchodilator therapy	Inhaled short-acting β_2-agonist is recommended. Consider ipratropium if inadequate clinical response. Methylxanthines are not recommended due to increased side effect profiles.	Inhaled short-acting β_2-agonist and/or ipratropium with spacer or nebulizer, as needed.	Administer inhaled drugs by nebulizer or handheld inhaler. Specific agents and dosing regimens not specified. Consider theophylline if inadequate response to inhaled bronchodilators.
Antibiotics	Recommended if (1) increases in dyspnea, sputum volume, and sputum purulence all are present; (2) increase in sputum purulence along with increase in either dyspnea or sputum volume; or (3) need for assisted ventilation. See original document for complex treatment algorithm.	Base choice on local bacterial resistance patterns. Consider amoxicillin/clavulanate or respiratory fluoroquinolones. If *Pseudomonas* species and/or other *Enterobacteriaceae* are suspected, consider combination therapy.	Administer only if history of purulent sputum. Initiate with an aminopenicillin, a macrolide, or a tetracycline, taking into account local bacterial resistance patterns. Adjust therapy according to sputum and blood cultures.
Systemic corticosteroids	Daily prednisolone 30-40 mg (or its equivalent) orally for not more than 5-7 days.	Daily prednisone 30-40 mg orally for 10-14 days. Equivalent dose intravenously if unable to tolerate oral intake. Consider inhaled corticosteroids.	Daily prednisolone 30 mg (or its equivalent) orally for 7-14 days.
Supplemental oxygen	Maintain oxygen saturation >90%. Monitor ABGs for hypercapnia and acidosis.	Maintain oxygen saturation >90%. Monitor ABGs for hypercapnia and acidosis.	Maintain oxygen saturation within the individualized target range. Monitor ABGs.
Assisted ventilation	Indications for NPPV include severe dyspnea, acidosis (pH ≤7.35) and/or hypercapnia (PCO$_2$ >45 mm Hg), and respiratory rate >25 breaths/min. Contraindications to NPPV include respiratory arrest, hemodynamic instability, impaired mental status, copious bronchial secretions, and extreme obesity. Intubate if contraindication to NPPV or failure of NPPV (worsening ABGs or clinical status). Consider likelihood of recovery and patient's wishes and expectations before intubation.	Consider with pH <7.35 and PCO$_2$ >45-60 mm Hg and respiratory rate >24 breaths/min. Institute NPPV in a controlled environment, unless there are contraindications (e.g., respiratory arrest, hemodynamic instability, impaired mental status, copious bronchial secretions, and extreme obesity). Intubate If contraindication to NPPV or failure of NPPV (worsening ABGs or clinical status).	NPPV treatment of choice for persistent hypercapnic respiratory failure. Consider functional status, body mass index, home oxygen, comorbidities, prior ICU admissions, age, and FEV$_1$ when assessing suitability for intubation and ventilation.

ABGs, Arterial blood gases; *COPD,* chronic obstructive pulmonary disease; *ECG,* electrocardiogram; *FEV$_1$,* forced expiratory volume in 1 sec; *ICU,* intensive care unit; *PCO$_2$,* partial pressure of carbon dioxide; *NPPV,* noninvasive positive pressure ventilation.
[a]Data from https://www.goldcopd.org.
[b]Data from MacNee W: Standards for the diagnosis and treatment of patients with COPD: a summary of the ATS/ERS position paper, *Eur Respir J* 23:932-946, 2004.
[c]Data from https://www.nice.org.uk.

BOX 1   Indications for Invasive Mechanical Ventilation

Severe dyspnea, with use of accessory muscles and paradoxical abdominal motion
Respiratory frequency >35 breaths/min
Life-threatening hypoxemia (PaO$_2$ <40 mm Hg or PaO$_2$/FiO$_2$ <200 mm Hg)
Severe acidosis (pH <7.25) and hypercapnia (PaCO$_2$ >60 mm Hg)
Respiratory arrest
Somnolence, impaired mental status
Cardiovascular complications (hypotension, shock, heart failure)
Other complications: Metabolic abnormalities, sepsis, pneumonia, pulmonary embolism, barotrauma, massive pleural effusion
Noninvasive positive-pressure ventilation failure (or exclusion criteria)

FiO$_2$, Fraction of inspired oxygen; *PaCO$_2$,* partial pressure of carbon dioxide in arterial blood; *PaO$_2$,* partial pressure of oxygen in the arterial blood.
From Vincent JL et al: *Textbook of critical care,* ed 6, Philadelphia, 2011, Saunders.

BOX 2 Indications and Contraindications for Lung Volume Reduction Surgery and Lung Transplantation

Indications Common to Both Procedures
Emphysema with destruction and hyperinflation
Marked impairment (FEV$_1$ <35% predicted)
Marked restriction in activities of daily living
Failure of maximal medical treatment to correct symptoms

Contraindications to Both Procedures
Abnormal body weight (<70% or >130% of ideal)
Coexisting major medical problems increasing surgical risk
Inability or unwillingness to participate in pulmonary rehabilitation
Unwillingness to accept the risk of morbidity and mortality of surgery
Tobacco use within the past 6 mo
Recent or current diagnosis of malignant disease
Increasing age
Psychological instability, such as depression or anxiety disorder

Discriminating Conditions Favoring Lung Volume Reduction Surgery
Marked thoracic distention
Heterogeneous disease with obvious apical target areas
FEV$_1$ >20% predicted
Age between 60 and 70 yr

Discriminating Conditions Favoring Lung Transplantation
Diffuse disease without target areas
FEV$_1$ <20% predicted
Hypercapnia with PaCO$_2$ >55 mm Hg
Pulmonary hypertension
Age younger than 60 yr
α_1-Antitrypsin deficiency

FEV$_1$, Forced expiratory volume in 1 sec; *PaCO$_2$,* partial pressure of carbon dioxide in arterial blood.
From Sellke FW et al: *Sabiston & Spencer surgery of the chest,* ed 9, Philadelphia, 2016, Elsevier.

BOX 3 Selection Criteria for Endoscopic Lung Volume Reduction (ELVR) Procedure

Hetergenous or homogenous emphysema
FEV$_1$ 20%-50% predicted
Evidence of hyperinflation – TLC >100% and RV >175%
Little or absent collateral ventilation between the target and the ipsilateral lobes
Clinically stable but symptomatic despite maximal medical treatment
Adequate exercise capacity (6 min walk test >200 meters)
Absence of significant hypercapnia (>60 mm Hg) or hypoxia (<45 mm Hg on RA)
Absence of major cardiac comorbidities including pulmonary hypertension

FEV$_1$, Forced expiratory volume in 1 sec; *RA,* room air; *RV,* residual volume; *TLC,* total lung capacity.

artery to the diameter of the aorta [PA:A ratio] of >1 detected by CT is associated with severe exacerbations of COPD.
• The average person with COPD has one or two acute exacerbations each year.
• Eosinophilic airway inflammation may contribute to COPD exacerbations. Elevated blood eosinophil levels may be used to guide inhaled corticosteroid therapy in frequent exacerbators of COPD.
• Antieosinophilic targeted therapy with monoclonal antibody targeting IL-13 and IL-4 appears to be effective in a subgroup of COPD patients with high blood eosinophils.
• Current and former smokers (within 15 yr) with >30-pack-yr history of smoking should be assessed for lung cancer using annual low-dose CT.

RELATED CONTENT

Chronic Obstructive Pulmonary Disease (Patient Information)
Emphysema (Patient Information)
Alpha-1-Antitrypsin Deficiency (Related Key Topic)
Asthma-COPD Overlap (Related Key Topic)

REFERENCES

Available at eBooks.Health.Elsevier.com.

AUTHORS: **ANIL GHIMIRE, MD** and **VIPUL V. JAIN, MD, MS**

Diseases and Disorders

C

I

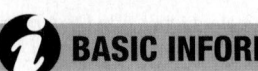 **BASIC INFORMATION**

DEFINITION

Chronic pancreatitis is a recurrent or persistent inflammatory process of the pancreas characterized by chronic pain and by pancreatic exocrine and/or endocrine insufficiency. It is classified anatomically as either large-duct disease or small-duct (minimal change) disease. Chronic pancreatitis can be classified as toxic-metabolic, idiopathic, genetic, autoimmune, related to recurrent and severe acute pancreatitis, and obstructive (Box 1).

ICD-10CM CODES
K86.1   Other chronic pancreatitis
K86.0   Alcohol-induced chronic pancreatitis

EPIDEMIOLOGY & DEMOGRAPHICS

- Chronic pancreatitis occurs in approximately 5 to 10 per 100,000 persons in industrialized countries and is usually associated with alcohol use, smoking, and certain gene mutations. It typically begins with recurrent painful bouts of pancreatitis followed by the insidious onset of chronic debilitating pain during the next 3 to 5 yr after an initial episode.[1]
- Average age at diagnosis is 35 to 55 yr; male:female ratio is 5:1.
- Annual incidence in the U.S. is 5 to 8 per 100,000 adults.
- Prevalence in the U.S. is 42 to 73 per 100,000 adults.[2]

PHYSICAL FINDINGS & CLINICAL PRESENTATION

- Persistent or recurrent epigastric and left upper quadrant pain (70% of patients) that may radiate to the back
- Tenderness over the pancreas, muscle guarding
- Significant weight loss
- Bulky, foul-smelling stools, greasy in appearance
- Epigastric mass (10% of patients)
- Jaundice (5% to 10% of patients)

ETIOLOGY

- Chronic alcoholism (most common cause)
- Obstruction (ampullary stenosis, tumor, trauma [with pancreatic duct stricture], pancreas divisum, annular pancreas)
- Tobacco
- Recurrent pancreatitis
- Vascular disease/ischemia
- Hypertriglyceridemia
- Chronic kidney disease
- Hereditary pancreatitis
- Severe malnutrition
- Idiopathic
- Untreated hyperparathyroidism (hypercalcemia)
- Mutations of the cystic fibrosis transmembrane conductance regulator (CFTR) gene and the TF genotype

---

BOX 1   Classification of Chronic Pancreatitis

Toxic-Metabolic
Alcohol
Tobacco
Hypercalcemia
Hypertriglyceridemia
Chronic renal failure

Idiopathic
Tropical calcific pancreatitis
    Fibrocalculous pancreatic diabetes
Early-onset idiopathic
Late-onset idiopathic

Genetic
Autosomal dominant
    Hereditary pancreatitis (PRSS1 mutations)
Autosomal recessive or modifier genes
    CFTR mutations
    SPINK1 mutations
    Chymotrypsin C mutations
    Claudin mutations
    Calcium sensing receptor gene
    Carboxy ethyl lipase
    Others

Autoimmune Pancreatitis
IgG4-related systemic disease, type 1
IgG4-related systemic disease, type 2

Recurrent and Severe Acute Pancreatitis
Postnecrotic (after severe necrotizing pancreatitis)
Vascular disease/ischemia

Obstructive
Benign pancreatic duct obstruction
    Traumatic stricture
    Stricture after severe acute pancreatitis
    Ampullary obstruction
    Sphincter of Oddi stenosis
    Celiac disease
    Crohn disease
    Duodenal wall cyst
    Pancreas divisum
Malignant pancreatic duct obstruction
    Ampullary carcinoma
    Duodenal carcinoma
    Pancreatic ductal adenocarcinoma
    Intraductal papillary mucinous neoplasm

Asymptomatic Pancreatic Fibrosis
Chronic alcohol use
Old age
Chronic kidney disease
Diabetes mellitus
Previous radiotherapy

Ig, Immunoglobulin G; *PRSS1,* protease serine 1 gene; *SPINK1,* serine protease inhibitor, Kazal Type 1 gene. From Feldman M et al: *Sleisenger and Fordtran's gastrointestinal and liver disease,* ed 11, Philadelphia, 2021, Elsevier.

- Other genetic mutations (cationic trypsinogen gene, chymotrypsinogen C gene, calcium-sensing receptor gene, claudin-2 gene, serine protease inhibitor, Kazal type 1 gene)
- ***Autoimmune pancreatitis (AIP)*** (Box 2)***:*** (5% of chronic pancreatitis cases): Presents clinically with jaundice (63% of patients) and abdominal pain (35%). Computed tomography (CT) may reveal diffusely enlarged pancreas, enhanced peripheral rim of hypoattenuation "halo," and low-attenuation mass in head of pancreas. Laboratory values reveal elevated serum immunoglobulin (Ig) G4, elevated serum Ig or gamma-globulin level, presence of antilactoferrin antibody (ALA), anticarbonic anhydrase (ACA) II level, antismooth-muscle antibody (ASMA), or antinuclear antibody (ANA)

- ***Sclerosing pancreatitis:*** A form of chronic pancreatitis characterized by infrequent attacks of abdominal pain, irregular narrowing of the pancreatic duct, and swelling of the pancreatic parenchyma; patients have high levels of serum immunoglobulins (IgG4); chronic sclerosing pancreatitis is also known as *autoimmune pancreatitis*

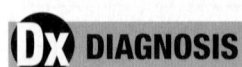 **DIAGNOSIS**

DIFFERENTIAL DIAGNOSIS

- Pancreatic cancer
- Peptic ulcer disease
- Cholelithiasis with biliary obstruction
- Malabsorption from other etiologies

BOX 2 Characteristics of Type 1 and Type 2 Autoimmune Pancreatitis

Feature	Type 1 AIP	Type 2 AIP
Histologic features	Lymphoplasmacytic infiltration Dense periductal infiltrate without damage to ductal epithelium Storiform fibrosis Obliterative phlebitis Abundant (>10 cells/HPF) IgG4-positive cells Fibroinflammatory process may extend to peripancreatic region	Lymphoplasmacytic and neutrophilic infiltration around ducts Destruction of duct epithelium by neutrophils (granulocytic epithelial lesion) Obliterative phlebitis rare No IgG4-positive cells
Average age at presentation	60-70 yr	40-50 yr, but may present in young adults and even children
Gender predominance	Male	Equal
Usual clinical presentations	Obstructive jaundice (75%) Acute pancreatitis (15%)	Obstructive jaundice (50%) Acute pancreatitis (33%)
Pancreatic imaging	Diffuse pancreatic enlargement (40%) Focal pancreatic enlargement (60%)	Diffuse pancreatic enlargement (15%) Focal pancreatic enlargement (85%)
IgG4	Elevated in serum (≈2/3 of patients) Positive in staining of involved tissues	Not associated
Other organ involvement	Biliary strictures Sialadenitis Retroperitoneal fibrosis Pseudotumors Kidney Lung Others	Not associated
Associated diseases		Inflammatory bowel disease
Long-term outcome	Frequent relapses	Rare or no relapse

From Feldman M et al: *Sleisenger and Fordtran's gastrointestinal and liver disease,* ed 11, Philadelphia, 2021, Elsevier.

TABLE 1 Available Diagnostic Tests for Chronic Pancreatitis

Tests of Pancreatic Structure	Tests of Pancreatic Function
EUS	Direct hormonal stimulation (with pancreatic stimulation by secretin or CCK or both): Using oroduodenal tube* Using endoscopy*
MRI with MRCP, with or without secretin stimulation	Fecal elastase
CT	Serum trypsinogen (trypsin)
ERCP	Fecal chymotrypsin
Abdominal US	Fecal fat
Plain abdominal film	Blood glucose level

Tests are listed in estimated order of decreasing sensitivity for each category.
CCK, Cholecystokinin; *CT,* computed tomography; *ERCP,* endoscopic retrograde cholangiopancreatography; *EUS,* endoscopic ultrasonography; *MRCP,* magnetic resonance cholangiopancreatography; *MRI,* magnetic resonance imaging.
*See text for explanations.
From Feldman M et al: *Sleisenger and Fordtran's gastrointestinal and liver disease,* ed 11, Philadelphia, 2021, Elsevier.

- Recurrent acute pancreatitis
- Renal insufficiency
- Intestinal ischemia or infarction
- Other: Crohn disease, gastroparesis, inflammatory bowel disease

WORKUP

Medical history with focus on alcohol use, laboratory tests, diagnostic imaging. Table 1 summarizes available diagnostic tests for chronic pancreatitis.

LABORATORY TESTS

- Serum amylase and lipase may be elevated (normal levels, however, do not exclude the diagnosis).
- Hyperglycemia, glycosuria, hyperbilirubinemia, and elevated serum alkaline phosphatase may also be present.

- Fecal elastase level: Simple, inexpensive and widely available. Levels below 50 mcg per gram of stool are indicative of steatorrhea. Levels between 51 and 200 mcg are below normal but can be due to several other disorders (IBD, renal failure, diabetes, watery diarrhea) and are not specific for steatorrhea.
- 72-h fecal fat determination over period of 48 or 72 h reveals excess fecal fat. This test is rarely performed and is generally available only in academic centers and major reference laboratories. It can be useful if the fecal elastase level and vitamin A or E levels are low but the patient does not exhibit the classic symptoms of steatorrhea.
- Secretin stimulation test is the best test for diagnosing pancreatic exocrine insufficiency. Pancreatic secretory function tests are summarized in Table 2.

- Lipid panel: Significantly elevated triglycerides can cause pancreatitis.
- Serum calcium: Hyperparathyroidism is a rare cause of chronic pancreatitis.
- Elevated levels of serum IgG4 are found in sclerosing pancreatitis and AIP.
- Elevated serum Ig or gamma-globulin level, presence of ALA, ACA II level, ASMA, or ANA in AIP.
- Decreased levels of serum fat-soluble vitamins (A and E) and other micronutrients (zinc, magnesium, and vitamin B_{12}).

IMAGING STUDIES

- Plain abdominal x-rays may reveal pancreatic calcifications (Fig. 1) in 25% of patients (95% specific for chronic pancreatitis).
- Ultrasound of abdomen may reveal duct dilation, pseudocyst, calcification, and presence of ascites.
- Contrast-enhanced CT scan of abdomen is the initial modality of choice. It is useful to detect calcifications (Fig. E2), evaluate for ductal dilation (Fig. E3), AIP, and rule out pancreatic cancer. CT in AIP reveals narrowed main pancreatic duct and a homogenous "sausage-shaped" pancreas.
- Magnetic resonance cholangiopancreatography (MRCP) and endoscopic ultrasonography (EUS) have similar specificity and sensitivity to CT.
- EUS (Fig. E4) has a sensitivity of 97% and a specificity of 60% for chronic pancreatitis and a very low complication rate; however, it is invasive and observer dependent. The diagnosis of chronic pancreatitis on EUS is summarized in Table E3. Fine-needle aspiration biopsy combined with EUS is also the

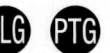
TABLE 2 Pancreatic Secretory Function Tests

Test	Description	Advantages	Disadvantages	Clinical Indications
Direct				
Secretin	Measurements of volume and HCO_3^- secretion into the duodenum after IV secretin	Provide the most sensitive and specific measurements of exocrine pancreatic function	Require duodenal intubation and IV administration of hormones; not widely available	Detection of mild, moderate, or severe exocrine pancreatic dysfunction
CCK	Measurements of duodenal outputs of amylase, trypsin, chymotrypsin, and/or lipase after IV CCK			
Secretin and CCK	Measurements of volume, HCO_3^-, and enzymes after IV secretin and CCK			
Indirect (Requiring Duodenal Intubation)				
Lundh test meal	Measurement of duodenal trypsin concentration after oral ingestion of a test meal	Does not require IV administration of hormones	Requires duodenal intubation, a test meal, and normal anatomy, including small intestinal mucosa; not widely available	Detection of moderate or severe exocrine pancreatic dysfunction when a direct test cannot be done (e.g., due to limited availability)
Indirect (Tubeless)				
Fecal fat	Measurement of fat in the stool after ingesting meals with a known amount of fat	Provides a quantitative measurement of steatorrhea	Requires sufficient dietary fat intake and collection of stool; only detects severe pancreatic dysfunction	Detection of severe exocrine pancreatic dysfunction and steatorrhea
Fecal chymotrypsin Fecal elastase 1	Measurement of chymotrypsin or elastase 1 in the stool	Do not require IVs, tubes, or administration of oral substrates	Insensitive for detecting mild or moderate dysfunction	Detection of severe exocrine pancreatic dysfunction
NBT-PABA Fluorescein dilaurate	Oral ingestion of NBT-PABA or fluorescein dilaurate with a meal, followed by measurements of PABA or fluorescein in serum or urine	Provide simple measurements for severe pancreatic dysfunction	Do not detect mild or moderate dysfunction; results may be abnormal in patients with small intestinal mucosal disease	Detection of severe exocrine pancreatic dysfunction

CCK, Cholecystokinin; *IV*, intravenous; *NBT-PABA*, N-benzoyl-ʟ-tyrosyl-*p*-aminobenzoic acid.
From Feldman M et al: *Sleisenger and Fordtran's gastrointestinal and liver disease*, ed 11, Philadelphia, 2021, Elsevier.

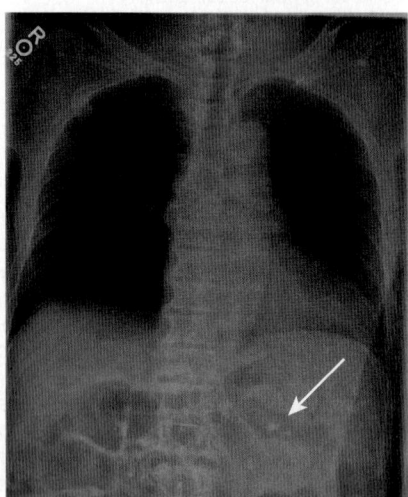

FIG. 1 A 51-yr-old man with chronic pancreatitis. A plain radiograph demonstrates multiple punctate foci of calcification overlying the expected location of the pancreas *(arrow)*, a finding consistent with chronic pancreatitis. (From Soto JA: *Emergency radiology, the requisites*, ed 2, 2017, Elsevier.)

preferred modality for evaluation of cystic or mass lesions to determine malignancy.
- MRCP is more expensive, takes longer, can miss calcification,[3] and is unsuitable for patients with claustrophobia.

- Endoscopic retrograde cholangiopancreatography (ERCP) (Fig. E5) had been traditionally used to evaluate for the presence of dilated ducts, strictures, pseudocysts, and intraductal stones; however, it is no longer recommended due to complications and availability of noninvasive imaging.

Rx TREATMENT

NONPHARMACOLOGIC THERAPY
- Avoidance of alcohol and tobacco
- Frequent, small-volume, low-fat meals

ACUTE GENERAL Rx
- Avoidance of narcotics if possible (simple analgesics or NSAIDs can be used). Fig. 6 describes an approach to the patient with painful chronic pancreatitis. Management of chronic pancreatitis focuses on treatment of symptoms.
- Treatment of steatorrhea with pancreatic supplements (e.g., Pancrease, Creon, pancrelipase titrated prn based on the amount of steatorrhea and patient's weight loss). Enzyme products for the treatment of chronic pancreatitis are summarized in Table 4. All non–enteric-coated enzymes should be used with acid-suppressing medications. Proton pump inhibitors and H_2 blockers reduce inactivation of the enzymes from gastric acid.

- Antioxidants (vitamin A, selenium, vitamin E) may be helpful for pain control in chronic pancreatitis.
- Percutaneous or via EUS celiac plexus blockade with corticosteroids or neurolysis with ethanol may provide temporary pain relief.
- Treatment of complications (e.g., type 1 diabetes mellitus).
- Autoimmune pancreatitis (AIP): Glucocorticoid therapy in patients with AIP and sclerosing pancreatitis can induce clinical remission and significantly decrease serum concentrations of IgG4, immune complexes, and the IgG4 subclass of immune complexes. Starting dose of oral prednisolone is 0.6 to 1.0 mg/kg/day tapered over 3 mo. Recurrent AIP is treated with glucocorticoids and immunomodulators (azathioprine, mycophenolate, mercaptopurine) or rituximab.

CHRONIC Rx
- Surgical intervention (e.g., distal pancreatectomy or pancreaticoduodenectomy) may be necessary in painful chronic pancreatitis to eliminate biliary tract disease and improve flow of bile into the duodenum by eliminating obstruction of pancreatic duct.[3]
- ERCP with endoscopic sphincterectomy and stone extraction and for treatment of pancreatic duct strictures is less invasive and more widely available than surgery and may be preferred as first-line treatment in painful chronic pancreatitis.

C

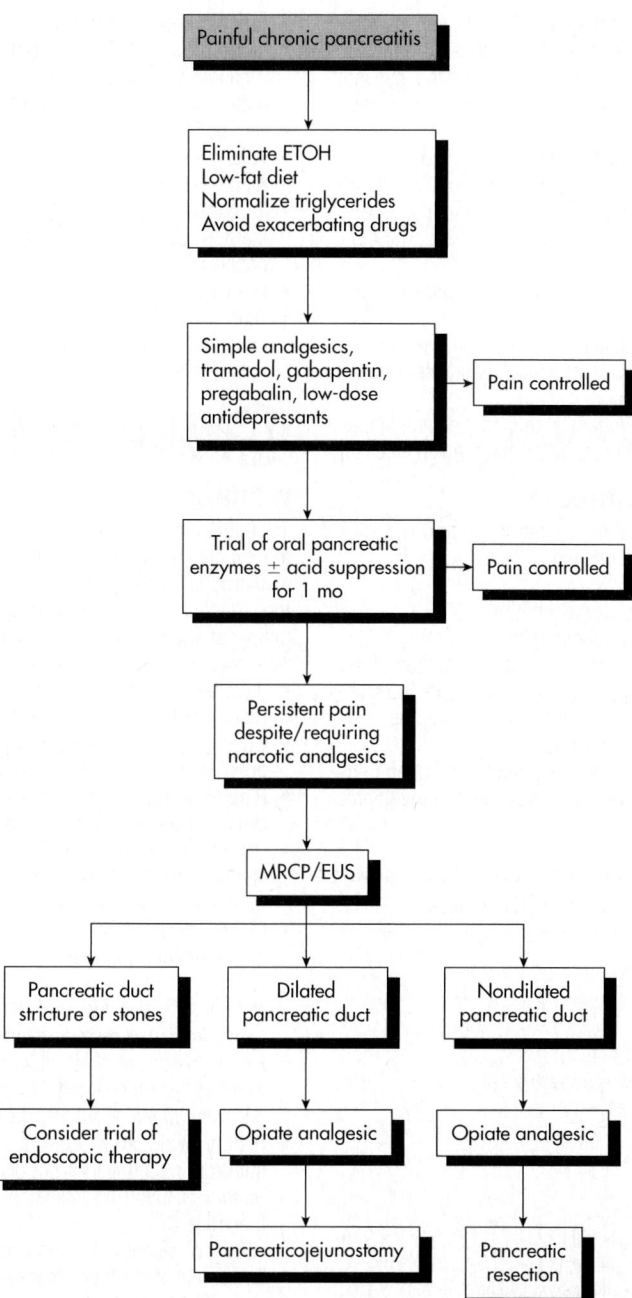

FIG. 6 Approach to the patient with painful chronic pancreatitis. *ETOH,* Alcohol; *EUS,* endoscopic ultrasound; *MRCP,* magnetic resonance cholangiopancreatography. (From Goldman L, Ausiello D [eds]: *Cecil textbook of medicine,* ed 24, Philadelphia, 2012, Saunders.)

- Percutaneous or EUS-guided celiac plexus blockade using glucocorticoids is effective in providing short-term pain relief in nearly half of patients.

DISPOSITION

- Long-term survival is poor (50% of patients die within 10 yr from chronic pancreatitis or malignancy).
- Prognosis is best in patients with recurrent acute pancreatitis resulting from cholelithiasis, hyperparathyroidism, or stenosis of the sphincter of Oddi.

REFERRAL

GI referral for ERCP, surgical referral in selected patients

RELATED CONTENT

Chronic Pancreatitis (Patient Information)
Malabsorption (Related Key Topic)
Pancreatitis, Acute (Related Key Topic)

REFERENCES & SUGGESTED READINGS

Available at eBooks.Health.Elsevier.com.

AUTHOR: **FRED F. FERRI, MD**

TABLE 4 Enzyme Products for the Treatment of Chronic Pancreatitis

Product	Formulation	Lipase Content per Pill or Capsule (USP units)
Creon	Enteric-coated capsule	3000; 6000; 12,000; 24,000; 36,000
Zenpep	Enteric-coated capsule	3000; 5000; 10,000; 15,000; 20,000; 25,000
Pancreaze	Enteric-coated capsule	4200; 10,500; 16,800; 21,000
Ultresa	Enteric-coated capsule	13,800; 20,700; 23,000
Pertzye	Enteric-coated with bicarbonate	8000; 16,000
Viokase	Non-enteric-coated tablet*	10,440; 20,880

The total dose of lipase per meal should be titrated based on response but usually requires at least 60,000 and usually 90,000 USP units (30,000 international units) of lipase per meal and one half that amount with snacks. The dose should be split equally during the meal and immediately after the meal.

*Non-enteric-coated agents require cotreatment with an histamine 2 receptor antagonist (H2RA) or proton pump inhibitor (PPI) to avoid denaturation of the enzymes by gastric acid.

From Feldman M et al: *Sleisenger and Fordtran's gastrointestinal and liver disease,* ed 11, Philadelphia, 2021, Elsevier.

Diseases and Disorders

I

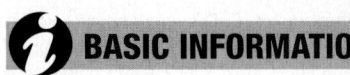

DEFINITION

Cirrhosis is defined histologically as the presence of irreversible fibrosis in the liver. It can be classified as micronodular, macronodular, or mixed; however, each form may be seen in the same patient at different stages of the disease, and this classification system has little utility in determining the underlying etiology of cirrhosis. Cirrhosis manifests clinically with portal hypertension, ascites and peripheral edema, hepatic encephalopathy, and variceal bleeding.

ICD-10CM CODES

K70.30	Alcoholic cirrhosis of liver without ascites
K70.31	Alcoholic cirrhosis of liver with ascites
K71.7	Toxic liver disease with fibrosis and cirrhosis of liver
K74.3	Primary biliary cirrhosis
K74.4	Secondary biliary cirrhosis
K74.5	Biliary cirrhosis, unspecified
K74.60	Unspecified cirrhosis of liver
K74.69	Other cirrhosis of liver
P78.81	Congenital cirrhosis (of liver)

EPIDEMIOLOGY & DEMOGRAPHICS

- Cirrhosis was the fourteenth-leading cause of death in the U.S. in 2015 and the thirteenth-leading cause of death globally. In the U.S., cirrhosis-related deaths increased 3.4% annually between 2009 and 2016.
- Alcohol abuse, hepatitis C, and nonalcoholic steatohepatitis are the major causes of cirrhosis in the U.S.
- Economic burden of cirrhosis in the U.S. exceeds $2 billion in direct costs and over $10 billion in indirect costs.

PHYSICAL FINDINGS & CLINICAL PRESENTATION

GENERAL: Fever (spontaneous bacterial peritonitis)
SKIN: Jaundice, palmar erythema, spider angiomata, ecchymosis (thrombocytopenia or coagulation factor deficiency), increased pigmentation (hemochromatosis), xanthomas (primary biliary cirrhosis), and diffuse pruritus. Cutaneous lesions often accompany cirrhosis and can be found in >40% of people with chronic alcoholism
EYES: Kayser-Fleischer rings (corneal copper deposition seen in Wilson disease; best diagnosed with slit lamp examination), scleral icterus
BREATH: Fetor hepaticus (breath has a sweet musty odor found in cirrhosis with hepatic failure)
CHEST: Possible gynecomastia in men
ABDOMEN: Tender or nontender hepatomegaly (congestive hepatomegaly), small, nodular liver (cirrhosis), palpable, nontender gallbladder (neoplastic extrahepatic biliary obstruction), palpable spleen (portal hypertension), dilated superficial periumbilical vein (caput medusae), venous hum auscultated over periumbilical veins (portal hypertension), ascites (portal hypertension, hypoalbuminemia), diffuse abdominal tenderness (spontaneous bacterial peritonitis)
RECTAL EXAMINATION: Hemorrhoids (portal hypertension), guaiac-positive stools (alcoholic gastritis, bleeding esophageal varices, peptic ulcer disease, bleeding hemorrhoids, portal gastropathy)
GENITALIA: Testicular atrophy in males (chronic liver disease, hemochromatosis)
EXTREMITIES: Pedal edema (hypoalbuminemia, anasarca), arthropathy (hemochromatosis), Dupuytren contractures
NEUROLOGIC: Asterixis (hepatic encephalopathy), choreoathetosis, dysarthria (Wilson disease)

ETIOLOGY (BOX 1)

- Chronic hepatitis B virus (HBV) and hepatitis C virus (HCV) infection
- Alcoholism
- Nonalcoholic steatohepatitis
- Primary biliary cholangitis
- Secondary biliary cirrhosis, obstruction of the common bile duct (stone, stricture, pancreatitis, neoplasm, sclerosing cholangitis)
- Autoimmune hepatitis
- Drugs with chronic hepatitis (e.g., acetaminophen, isoniazid, methotrexate, methyldopa)

BOX 1 Causes of Cirrhosis

Viral
- HBV
- HCV
- HDV

Autoimmune
- Autoimmune hepatitis
- PBC
- PSC

Toxic
- Alcohol
- Arsenic

Metabolic
- α_1 Antitrypsin deficiency
- Galactosemia
- Glycogen storage disease
- Hemochromatosis
- NAFLD and NASH
- Wilson disease

Biliary
- Atresia
- Stone
- Tumor

Vascular
- Budd-Chiari syndrome
- Cardiac fibrosis

Genetic
- CF
- Lysosomal acid lipase deficiency

Iatrogenic
- Biliary injury
- Drugs: High-dose vitamin A, methotrexate

From Feldman M et al: *Sleisenger and Fordtran's gastrointestinal and liver disease,* ed 11, Philadelphia, 2021, Elsevier.

- Chronic hepatic congestion (e.g., congestive heart failure [CHF], constrictive pericarditis, tricuspid insufficiency, thrombosis of the hepatic vein, obstruction of the vena cava)
- Hemochromatosis
- Wilson disease
- Alpha-1-antitrypsin deficiency
- Infiltrative diseases (amyloidosis, glycogen storage diseases, nonhepatocellular malignancies)
- Nutritional: Jejunoileal bypass
- Others: Parasitic infections (schistosomiasis), idiopathic portal hypertension, congenital hepatic fibrosis, systemic mastocytosis

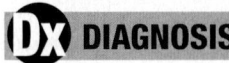

WORKUP

In addition to an assessment of liver function, the evaluation of patients with cirrhosis should also include an assessment of renal and circulatory function. Diagnostic workup is aimed primarily at identifying the most likely cause of cirrhosis. The history is extremely important:

- Alcohol abuse: Alcoholic liver disease
- History of hepatitis B or hepatitis C
- Obesity, type 2 diabetes mellitus, hyperlipidemia (nonalcoholic steatohepatitis)
- History of inflammatory bowel disease (IBD; primary sclerosing cholangitis)
- History of pruritus, hyperlipoproteinemia, and xanthomas in a middle-aged or elderly woman (primary biliary cholangitis)
- Erectile dysfunction, diabetes mellitus, hyperpigmentation, polyarthralgias (hemochromatosis)
- Neurologic disturbances (Wilson disease, hepatolenticular degeneration)
- Family history of "liver disease" (hemochromatosis [positive family history in 25% of patients], alpha-1-antitrypsin deficiency)
- History of recurrent episodes of right upper quadrant pain (biliary tract disease)
- History of blood transfusions, IV drug abuse (hepatitis C)
- History of repetitive hepatotoxic drug exposure
- Coexistence of other diseases with immune or autoimmune features (immune thrombocytopenic purpura, myasthenia gravis, thyroiditis, autoimmune hepatitis)
- Biopsy is the gold standard to diagnosis cirrhosis and is helpful when multiple etiologies are possible that might change management (autoimmune hepatitis, small duct primary sclerosing cholangitis, antimitochondrial antibody-negative primary biliary cholangitis, and infiltrative diseases such as lymphoma, amyloidosis, and granulomatous hepatitis). However, it is generally unnecessary if the clinical picture is highly suggestive of cirrhosis and management would not change. Biopsy can be useful in actively drinking patients with cirrhosis to distinguish between decompensated cirrhosis and cirrhosis with alcoholic hepatitis

LABORATORY TESTS

- Decreased hemoglobin and hematocrit, elevated mean corpuscular volume (Fig. E1).

Increased blood urea nitrogen (BUN) and creatinine (the BUN may also be "normal" or low if the patient has severely diminished liver function).

- Decreased sodium (dilutional hyponatremia), and decreased potassium (as a result of secondary aldosteronism or urinary losses). Evaluation of renal function should also include measurement of urinary sodium and urinary protein from 24-h urine collection. Acute kidney injury (AKI) occurs in up to 50% of hospitalized patients with cirrhosis and in 58% of such patients in the ICU[1] and may be due to renal hypoperfusion/hypovolemia, intrinisic kidney injury, or postrenal injury due to urinary obstruction.
- Decreased glucose in a patient with liver disease indicates severe liver damage.
- Other laboratory abnormalities:
  1. Alcohol-associated hepatitis and cirrhosis: Possible mild elevation of alanine aminotransferase (ALT) and aspartate aminotransferase (AST), usually <500 IU; AST> ALT (ratio >2:3).
  2. Extrahepatic obstruction: Possible moderate elevations of ALT and AST to levels <500 IU.
  3. Viral, toxic, or ischemic hepatitis: Extreme elevations (>500 IU) of ALT and AST.
  4. Transaminases may be normal despite significant liver disease in patients with jejunoileal bypass operations or hemochromatosis or after methotrexate administration.
  5. Alkaline phosphatase elevation can occur with extrahepatic obstruction, primary biliary cholangitis, and primary sclerosing cholangitis.
  6. Serum lactate dehydrogenase is significantly elevated in metastatic disease of the liver; lesser elevations are seen with hepatitis, cirrhosis, extrahepatic obstruction, and congestive hepatomegaly.
  7. Serum gamma-glutamyl transpeptidase is elevated in alcoholic liver disease and may also be elevated with cholestatic disease (primary biliary cholangitis, primary sclerosing cholangitis).
  8. Serum bilirubin may be elevated; urinary bilirubin can be present in hepatitis, hepatocellular jaundice, and biliary obstruction.
  9. Serum albumin: Significant liver disease results in hypoalbuminemia. Malnutrition

occurs in 20% to 60% of patients with cirrhosis.
- Prothrombin time/international normalized ratio (INR): Elevation in patients with liver disease indicates severe liver damage and poor prognosis. Table 1 summarizes hemostatic balance in liver disease.
  1. Presence of hepatitis B surface antigen implies acute or chronic hepatitis B.
  2. Presence of antimitochondrial antibody suggests primary biliary cholangitis, chronic hepatitis.
  3. Elevated serum copper, decreased serum ceruloplasmin, and elevated 24-h urine may be diagnostic of Wilson disease.
  4. Protein immunoelectrophoresis may reveal decreased α-1 globulins (alpha-1-antitrypsin deficiency), increased IgA (alcoholic cirrhosis), increased IgM (primary biliary cirrhosis), increased IgG (chronic hepatitis, cryptogenic cirrhosis).
  5. An elevated serum ferritin and increased iron saturation are suggestive of hemochromatosis.
  6. An elevated blood ammonia suggests hepatocellular dysfunction; serial values, however, are generally not useful in monitoring patients with hepatic encephalopathy because there is poor correlation between blood ammonia level and degree of hepatic encephalopathy.
  7. Serum cholesterol is elevated in cholestatic disorders.
  8. Antinuclear antibodies (ANA) may be found in autoimmune hepatitis.
  9. Alpha fetoprotein: Levels >1000 pg/ml are highly suggestive of hepatocellular carcinoma.
  10. Hepatitis C viral testing identifies patients with chronic hepatitis C infection.
  11. Elevated level of serum globulin (especially gamma-globulins) and positive ANA test may occur with autoimmune hepatitis.
  12. End-stage liver disease is characterized by decreased levels of most procoagulant factors with the notable exceptions of factor VIII and von Willebrand factor, which are elevated. Table 2 summarizes hemostatic indices in liver disease.

IMAGING STUDIES

- Ultrasonography is the initial procedure of choice. It can identify the size and shape of the liver (generally small and nodular in advanced cirrhosis) and can detect gallstones and dilation of bile ducts. The use of sonography on a periodic basis to screen for hepatocellular carcinoma in patients with cirrhosis should be considered.
- CT scan (Figs. 2 and 3) is useful for detecting mass lesions in liver and pancreas, assessing hepatic fat content, identifying idiopathic hemochromatosis, diagnosing Budd-Chiari syndrome early, assessing dilation of intrahepatic bile ducts, and detecting varices and splenomegaly. However, ultrasound is generally the preferred imaging modality of choice.
- MRI can be used to identify hemangiomas, hepatocellular carcinoma.
- Vibration-controlled transient elastography and magnetic resonance elastography are useful to assess advanced fibrosis. These noninvasive tests are less expensive and safer than biopsy and can be repeated over time to monitor disease progression.
- Technetium-99m sulfur colloid scanning is rarely used but can be useful for diagnosing cirrhosis (there is a shift of colloid uptake to the spleen and bone marrow), identifying hepatic adenomas (cold defect is noted), and diagnosing Budd-Chiari syndrome (there is increased uptake by the caudate lobe).
- Endoscopic retrograde cholangiopancreatography can be used for diagnosing periampullary carcinoma and common duct stones; it is also useful in diagnosing primary sclerosing cholangitis.
- Percutaneous transhepatic cholangiography is useful when evaluating patients with cholestatic jaundice and dilated intrahepatic ducts by ultrasonography; presence of intrahepatic strictures and focal dilation is suggestive of primary sclerosing cholangitis.

Rx TREATMENT

NONPHARMACOLOGIC THERAPY

- Avoid any hepatotoxins (e.g., ethanol, acetaminophen), improve nutritional status, vaccinate against hepatitis A and B if not already immune.
- Transjugular intrahepatic portosystemic shunt (TIPS, Fig. E4) in patients with recurrent variceal hemorrhage despite optimal medical therapy. Early use of TIPS is associated with significant reductions in treatment failure and in mortality in patients with cirrhosis who are hospitalized for acute variceal bleeding and are at high risk for treatment failure.
- Correction of malnutrition: Daily protein intake of 1.0 to 1.5 g per kg of body weight.

ACUTE GENERAL Rx

- Nonselective beta-blockers (nadolol, propranolol) in patients with cirrhosis and variceal hemorrhage, and some without hemorrhage but with high-risk bleeding features. Use with caution in patients with severe alcoholic

---

TABLE 1 Hemostatic Balance in Liver Disease

	Promotes Thrombosis	Promotes Bleeding
Primary hemostasis	• Increased vWF • Decreased ADAMTS13	• Thrombocytopenia • Platelet dysfunction
Secondary hemostasis	• Increased factor VIII • Decreased protein C, protein S, antithrombin	• Factor deficiencies: II, V, VII, IX, XI • Vitamin K deficiency • Hypofibrinogenemia • Dysfibrinogenemia
Fibrinolysis	• Reduced plasminogen • Increased PAI-1	• Reduced α2-antiplasmin, TAFI, factor XIII • Increased t-PA

ADAMST13, A disintegrin and metalloproteinase with thrombospondin; *PAI-1*, plasminogen activator inhibitor-1; *TAFI*, thrombin activatable fibrinolysis inhibitor; *t-PA*, tissue plasminogen activator; *vWF*, von Willebrand factor.
From Hoffman R et al: *Hematology, basic principles and practice*, ed 8, Philadelphia, 2023, Elsevier.

TABLE 2 Hemostatic Indices in Liver Disease

Laboratory Changes	PT	PTT	TCT	Fib	Clauss	Plt	Platelet Aggregation	FVII	DD	ELT
Thrombocytopenia	N	N	N	N	N	↓	N	N	N	N
Platelet dysfunction	N	N	N	N	N	N	Abnormal	N	N	N
Vitamin K deficiency[a]	↑	↑	N	N	N	N	N	↓	N	N
Factor deficiency	↑	↑	N	N	N	N	N	↓	N	N
Hypofibrinogenemia	N/↑	N/↑	↑	↓	↓	N	N	N	N	N
Dysfibrinogenemia	N/↑	N/↑	↑	N	↓	N	N	N	N	N
Hyperfibrinolysis	N/↑	N/↑	N/↑	N/↓	N/↓	N	N	↓	↑	↓
DIC	N/↑	N/↑	N/↑	↓	↓	↓	N	N/↓	↑	↓

Clauss, Clauss fibrinogen; *DD,* D-dimer; *DIC,* disseminated intravascular coagulation; *ELT,* euglobulin lysis time (measure of fibrinolysis); *Fib,* fibrinogen; *FVII,* factor VII functional assay; *N,* normal; *Plt,* platelet; *PT,* prothrombin time; *PTT,* partial thromboplastin time; *TCT,* thrombin clotting time.
[a]Differentiating between vitamin K deficiency and liver disease can be challenging with conventional laboratory tests. If available, performing a factor II assay with and without Echis venom (factor II biologic and factor II Echis) may be useful. Ecarin is derived from *Echis carinatus* snake venom and can activate prothrombin irrespective of γ-carboxylation. Factor II activity (biologic) is reduced in both vitamin K deficiency and liver disease. In contrast, the factor II Echis is reduced in liver disease but is normal in vitamin K deficiency.
From Hoffman R et al: *Hematology, basic principles and practice,* ed 8, Philadelphia, 2023, Elsevier.

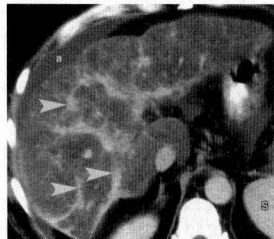

FIG. 2 Advanced cirrhosis with fatty infiltration. Delayed portal venous-phase computed tomography reveals that the liver is misshapen and nodular in contour. Parenchymal density that is significantly lower than that of the spleen *(S)* is indicative of fatty infiltration and continuing liver injury. Prominent scars and bands of fibrosis *(arrowheads)* are seen throughout the liver. Ascites *(a)* is present. (From Webb WR et al: *Fundamentals of body CT,* ed 4, Philadelphia, 2015, Saunders.)

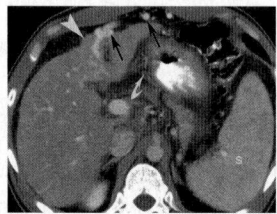

FIG. 3 Cirrhosis with portal hypertension. Postcontrast computed tomography reveals a liver that is nodular in contour *(arrowhead)* with patent enlarged paraumbilical veins *(black arrows)* and splenomegaly *(S),* findings indicative of portal hypertension. Mildly enlarged portosystemic collateral vessels *(curved arrow)* are also evident in the gastrohepatic ligament. (From Webb WR et al: *Fundamentals of body CT,* ed 4, Philadelphia, 2015, Saunders.)

hepatitis and decompensated cirrhosis with refractory ascites. Beta-blockers should be temporarily discontinued in patients with spontaneous bacterial peritonitis due to increased mortality and hepatorenal syndrome incidence.
- Pruritus due to liver disease may be treated with cholestyramine 4 g/day initially. Dose can be increased to 24 g/day as needed.
- Pain management: Avoid opiates (may precipitate or aggravate hepatic encephalopathy) and

NSAIDs (increased risk of gastrointestinal bleeding and renal failure). Low-dose tramadol and lidocaine patches are generally well tolerated.
- Sedatives: Benzodiazepines (lorazepam or oxazepam) may be used for alcohol withdrawal but should be avoided in patients with hepatic encephalopathy. Avoid benzodiazepines with liver metabolites (diazepam, chlordiazepoxide).
- Statins: Can be safely started and continued in patients with hyperlipidemia and/or nonalcoholic fatty liver disease.
- Proton pump inhibitors: Not routinely indicated; their use in patients with cirrhosis is associated with excess risk for spontaneous bacterial peritonitis and hepatic encephalopathy; avoid indiscriminate use of proton pump inhibitors (PPIs) in patients with cirrhosis.
- Antibiotics: Trimethoprim-sulfamethoxazole or ciprofloxacin/norfloxacin for spontaneous bacterial peritonitis prophylaxis in patients with a history of spontaneous bacterial peritonitis (SBP) an ascites protein concentration less than 1 g/dl, or history of variceal hemorrhage.
- Liver transplantation may be indicated in otherwise healthy patients (ages <65 yr) with severe cirrhosis and lack of contraindications. Contraindications to liver transplantation are AIDS, most metastatic malignancies, active substance abuse, uncontrolled sepsis, and uncontrolled cardiac or pulmonary disease.
- Causes of hepatic decompensation in cirrhosis are summarized in Box E2. Principal complications of cirrhosis are noted in Box 3 and Fig. 5.
- Treatment of complications of portal hypertension (ascites, esophagogastric varices, hepatic encephalopathy, spontaneous bacterial peritonitis, and hepatorenal syndrome; refer to these individual topics in Section I). The pathophysiology of ascites and renal dysfunction in patients with advanced cirrhosis is illustrated in Fig. 6.
- Fig. 7 summarizes the management of compensated and decompensated cirrhosis.
- Box 4 summarizes the management of coagulopathy in liver disease.

BOX 3 Principal Complications of Cirrhosis

Portal Hypertension
- Ascites
- Variceal bleeding

Malignancy
- Cholangiocarcinoma
- HCC

Bacterial Infections
- Bacteremia
- CDI
- Cellulitis
- Pneumonia
- SBP
- Urinary tract infection

Cardiopulmonary Disorders
- Cardiomyopathy
- Hepatic hydrothorax
- Hepatopulmonary syndrome
- Portopulmonary hypertension

GI Disorders
- GI bleeding
- Nonvariceal
- Variceal
- Protein-losing enteropathy
- Venous thrombosis

Renal Disorders
- Hepatorenal syndrome
- Other causes of acute kidney injury

Metabolic Disorders
- Adrenal insufficiency
- Hypogonadism
- Malnutrition
- Osteoporosis

Neuropsychiatric Disorders
- Depression
- Hepatic encephalopathy

Hematologic Disorders
- Anemia
- Hypercoagulability
- Hypersplenism
- Impaired coagulation

Unclear Etiology
- Erectile dysfunction
- Fatigue
- Muscle cramps

From Feldman M et al: *Sleisenger and Fordtran's gastrointestinal and liver disease,* ed 11, Philadelphia, 2021, Elsevier.

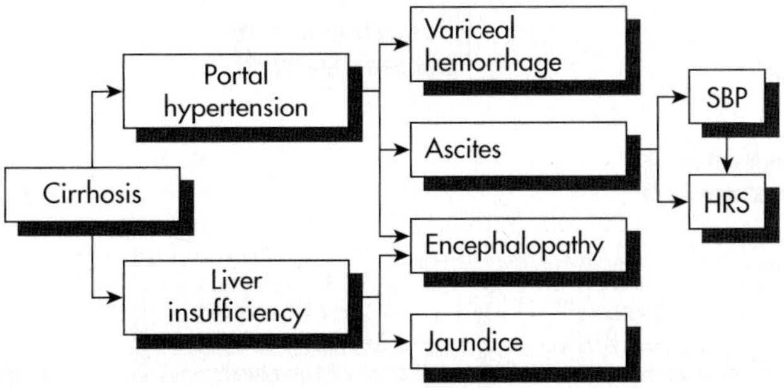

C

I

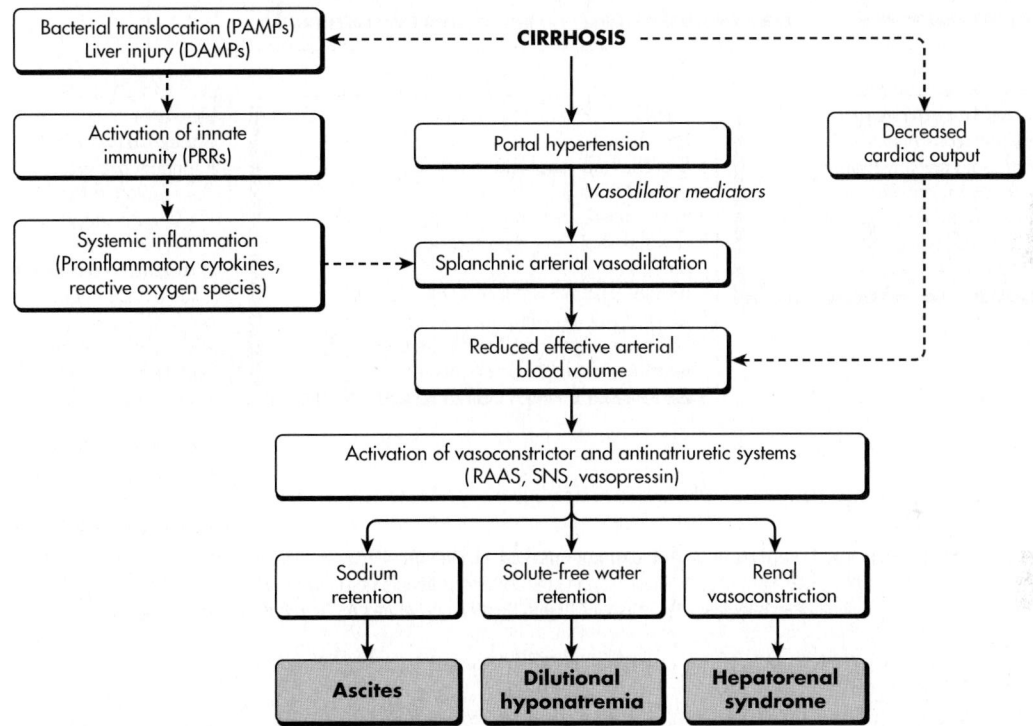

FIG. 5 Complications of cirrhosis result from portal hypertension or liver insufficiency. Varices and variceal hemorrhage are a direct consequence of portal hypertension. Ascites results from sinusoidal portal hypertension and can be complicated by infection (spontaneous bacterial peritonitis [SBP]) or renal dysfunction (hepatorenal syndrome *[HRS]*). Hepatic encephalopathy results from portosystemic shunting (i.e., portal hypertension) and liver insufficiency. Jaundice results solely from liver insufficiency. (From Goldman L, Schafer AI: *Goldman-Cecil medicine,* ed 26, Philadelphia, 2019, Elsevier.)

FIG 6 Pathophysiology of ascites and renal dysfunction in patients with advanced cirrhosis. Systemic circulatory dysfunction, characterized by splanchnic arterial vasodilatation, is the key mechanism leading to renal function abnormalities in cirrhosis. The development of effective arterial hypovolemia triggers activation of vasoconstrictor and antinatriuretic systems aimed at maintaining arterial pressure within normal limits. The activation of these systems has deleterious effects on the kidney and results in renal sodium retention, impairment of solute-free water excretion, and renal vasoconstriction that lead to the development of ascites, dilutional hyponatremia, and hepatorenal syndrome. At advanced stages of the disease (signified by the *dotted lines*), there is a decrease in cardiac output that also contributes to the decrease in effective blood volume. Finally, cirrhosis is associated with systemic inflammation triggered by pathogen-associated molecular patterns (PAMPs), derived from bacterial translocation, and damage-associated molecular patterns (DAMPs), from the injured liver, leading in turn to activation of innate immunity via pattern recognition receptors (PRRs). The release of inflammatory mediators contributes to further impairment of circulatory function. *RAAS,* Renin-angiotensin-aldosterone system; *SNS,* sympathetic nervous system. (From Feldman M et al: *Sleisenger and Fordtran's gastrointestinal and liver disease,* ed 11, Philadelphia, 2021, Elsevier.)

TREATMENT BASED ON SPECIFIC CAUSE OF CIRRHOSIS

- Remove excess body iron with phlebotomy and deferoxamine in patients with hemochromatosis.
- Remove copper deposits with D-penicillamine in patients with Wilson disease.
- Long-term ursodiol therapy will slow the progression of primary biliary cholangitis. It is, however, ineffective in primary sclerosing cholangitis.
- Glucocorticoids (prednisone 20 to 30 mg/day initially or combination therapy or prednisone and azathioprine) are useful in autoimmune hepatitis.
- Antivirals in chronic hepatitis C.

PROGNOSIS

- Prognosis varies with the etiology of the patient's cirrhosis and whether there is ongoing hepatic injury. Fig. 8 illustrates the natural history of cirrhosis. Patients with compensated cirrhosis (no associated complications or esophageal varices without bleeding) have a good prognosis with median survival over 12 yr.
- In patients with decompensated cirrhosis, the Model of End-stage Liver Disease with sodium (MELDNa) scoring (Table 3) is useful to predict 3-mo mortality and so is the main method of prioritizing patients awaiting liver

transplantation. It also has prognostic value following TIPS placement for patients with cirrhosis undergoing nontransplant surgeries. Mortality rate exceeds 80% in patients with hepatorenal syndrome.
- Regression of cirrhosis has been demonstrated after antiviral therapy in some patients with chronic hepatitis C. Regression is associated with decreased disease-related morbidity and improved survival.
- Cirrhosis is associated with an increased risk for hepatocellular carcinoma. However, the risk is low (1% 5-yr cumulative risk in alcoholic cirrhosis).

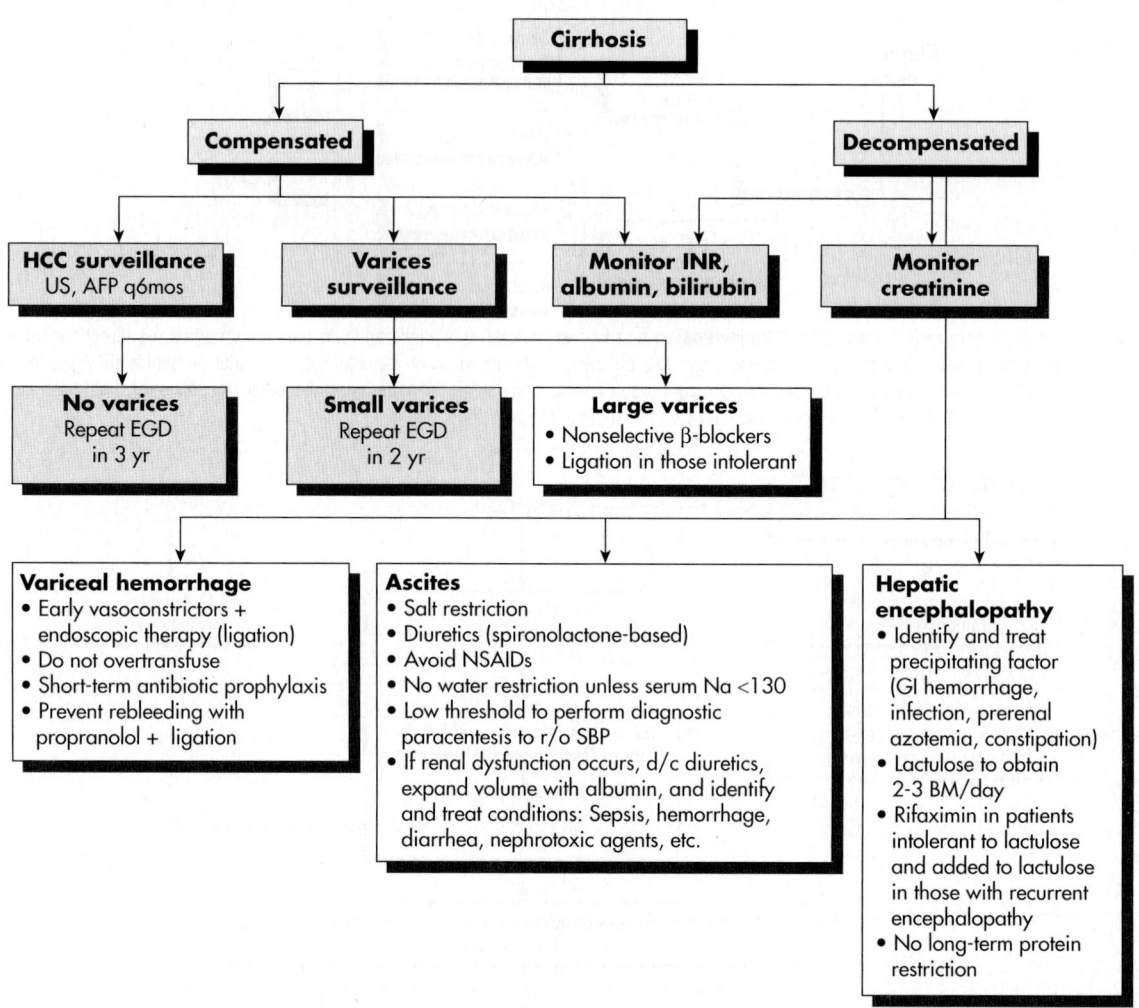

FIG. 7 Summary of the management of compensated and decompensated cirrhosis. *AFP,* α-Fetoprotein; *BM,* bowel movement; *d/c,* discontinue; *EGD,* esophagogastroduodenoscopy; *GI,* gastrointestinal; *HCC,* hepatocellular carcinoma; *INR,* international normalized ratio; *Na,* sodium; *NSAIDs,* nonsteroidal antiinflammatory drugs; *r/o,* rule out; *SBP,* spontaneous bacterial peritonitis; *US,* ultrasound. (From Goldman L, Schafer AI: *Goldman-Cecil medicine,* ed 26, Philadelphia, 2019, Elsevier.)

BOX 4   Management of Coagulopathy in Liver Disease

- Actively bleeding patients should be adequately resuscitated. Admission to the intensive care setting may be appropriate.
- Basic coagulation tests should be ordered to identify the cause of bleeding; these include CBC, PT (INR), PTT, thrombin clotting time, fibrinogen, D-dimer, FDP, and mixing studies. The need for more specialized tests will be dictated by the clinical situation and response to therapy.
- It is important to identify any localized source of bleeding (e.g., varices) amenable to procedural intervention to achieve hemostasis.
- A trial of 5-10 mg of vitamin K is reasonable in asymptomatic patients with prolonged PT and PTT but should be used with other therapies in actively bleeding patients.
- In patients with thrombocytopenia, platelet transfusions can be used, targeting platelet counts greater than 50 × 109 /L.
- In patients who can tolerate volume, FP 4-6 units (1000-1500 ml) given over 1-2 h can be used to replace coagulation factors. Coagulation parameters should be monitored to document effect and determine the timing and need for additional units.
- Dysfibrinogenemia or hypofibrinogenemia should be suspected if coagulation assays do not correct with FP or fibrinogen levels are low, respectively. Replacement can be attempted with 10-20 units of cryoprecipitate while following laboratory results.
- Patients who are intravascularly overloaded or who do not respond to FP should be considered for rFVIIa. Low doses of rFVIIa (25-50 μg/kg) are generally used, and repeated doses may be required because of the short rFVIIa half-life of 2-3 h. rFVIIa may be most suitable as a temporizing measure to enable invasive procedures or hemostasis to be achieved by other means. Avoid use in the setting of DIC.

From Hoffman R et al: *Hematology: basic principles and practice,* ed 7, Philadelphia, 2018, Elsevier.

C

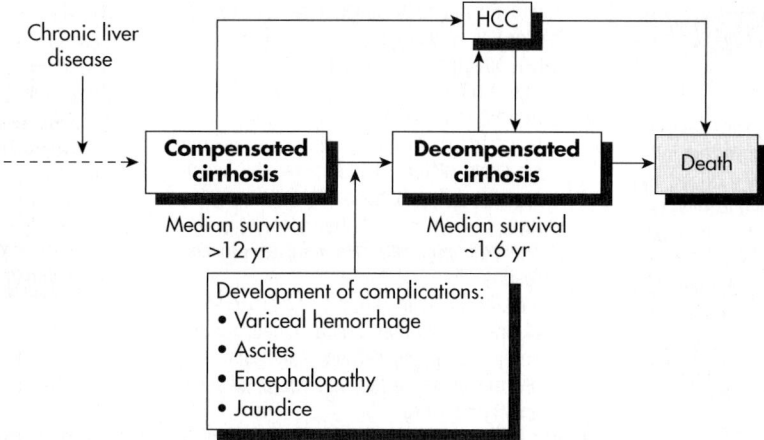

FIG. 8 Natural history of cirrhosis. Any chronic liver disease will lead to cirrhosis. Initially, cirrhosis will be compensated (median survival, >12 yr), but once complications (ascites, variceal hemorrhage, encephalopathy, jaundice) develop, it becomes decompensated (median survival, 1.6 yr). Hepatocellular carcinoma (HCC) can develop at any stage and precipitate decompensation and death. (From Goldman L, Schafer AI: *Goldman-Cecil medicine,* ed 26, Philadelphia, 2019, Elsevier.)

TABLE 3 The Two Most Commonly Used Scoring Systems in Cirrhosis

1. CHILD-TURCOTTE-PUGH (CTP) SCORE (RANGE, 5-15)

	Points Ascribed		
Parameters	**1**	**2**	**3**
Ascites	None	Grade 1-2 (or easy to treat)	Grade 3-4 (or refractory)
Hepatic encephalopathy	None	Grade 1-2 (or induced by a precipitant)	Grade 3-4 (or spontaneous)
Bilirubin (mg/dl)	<2	2-3	>3
Albumin (g/dl)	>3.5	2.8-3.5	<2.8
Prothrombin time (seconds > control) or INR	<4	4-6	>6
	<1.7	1.7-2.3	>2.3

CTP classification: Child A: Score of 5-6; Child B: Score of 7-9; Child C: Score of 10-15

2. MODEL OF END-STAGE LIVER DISEASE (MELD) SCORE (RANGE, 6-40)

$[0.957 \times LN \text{ (creatinine in mg/dl)} + 0.378 \times LN \text{ (bilirubin in mg/dl)} + 1.12 \times LN \text{ (INR)} + 0.643] \times 10$

MELD-Na is calculated first by determining the traditional MELD $(MELD_{(0)})$; if the initial $MELD_{(i)}$ score is 12 or greater, the score is adjusted by incorporating the serum sodium value $[MELD_{(0)} + 1.32 \times (137 - Na) - [0.033 \times MELD(i) \times (137 - Na)]]$

INR, International normalized ratio; *LN,* natural logarithm.
From Goldman L, Schafer AI: *Goldman-Cecil medicine,* ed 26, Philadelphia, 2019, Elsevier.

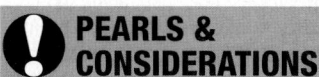 **PEARLS & CONSIDERATIONS**

COMMENTS

- Thrombocytopenia and advanced Child-Pugh classes (see Table 3) are associated with the presence of varices. These factors are useful to identify cirrhotic patients who benefit most from referral for endoscopic screening for varices.
- A combination of endoscopic and drug therapy reduces overall and variceal rebleeding in cirrhosis more than either therapy alone.

- PPI use, but not H_2RA use, is associated with risk for serious infections in patients with decompensated cirrhosis.
- In patients with compensated cirrhosis and clinically significant hypertension beta-blockers reduced a composite of decompensation or death.
- Patients with cirrhosis require pneumococcal vaccination, influenza, herpes zoster, tDAP, MMR, varicella, and hepatitis A and B vaccination.[2]

RELATED CONTENT

Cirrhosis (Patient Information)
Ascites (Related Key Topic)

Esophageal Varices (Related Key Topic)
Hepatic Encephalopathy (Related Key Topic)
Hepatopulmonary Syndrome (Related Key Topic)
Hepatorenal Syndrome (Related Key Topic)
Spontaneous Bacterial Peritonitis (Related Key Topic)
Primary Biliary Cholangitis (Related Key Topic)

REFERENCES & SUGGESTED READINGS

Available at eBooks.Health.Elsevier.com.

AUTHOR: **DAVID J. LUCIER JR., MD, MBA, MPH**

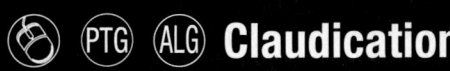
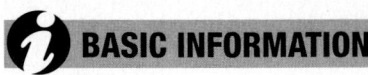

DEFINITION

Claudication can be defined as pain, fatigue, discomfort, or cramping due to vascular origin in a muscle group that is consistently induced by activity and is relieved with rest. Claudication results from inadequate blood flow to the target muscle group, which is not able to meet increased metabolic demand, resulting in a supply-and-demand mismatch because of peripheral arterial disease (PAD). Intermittent vascular claudication is more common in the lower extremities but can also affect the upper extremities.[1-3]

SYNONYM

Intermittent claudication

ICD-10CM CODES

I70.211	Atherosclerosis of native arteries of extremities with intermittent claudication, right leg
I70.212	Atherosclerosis of native arteries of extremities with intermittent claudication, left leg
I70.213	Atherosclerosis of native arteries of extremities with intermittent claudication, bilateral legs
I70.219	Atherosclerosis of native arteries of extremities with intermittent claudication, unspecified extremity
I70.311	Atherosclerosis of unspecified type of bypass graft(s) of the extremities with intermittent claudication, right leg
I70.312	Atherosclerosis of unspecified type of bypass graft(s) of the extremities with intermittent claudication, left leg
I70.313	Atherosclerosis of unspecified type of bypass graft(s) of the extremities with intermittent claudication, bilateral legs
I70.319	Atherosclerosis of unspecified type of bypass graft(s) of the extremities with intermittent claudication, unspecified extremity
I70.719	Atherosclerosis of other type of bypass graft(s) of the extremities with intermittent claudication, unspecified extremity

EPIDEMIOLOGY & DEMOGRAPHICS

- Symptomatic claudication in Western countries affects 5% to 6% of patients between the ages of 55 and 74.[1-3] A higher percentage of patients qualify for PAD by ankle-brachial index testing but remain asymptomatic.[4]
- PAD, which includes both symptomatic claudication and asymptomatic disease, is estimated to affect more than 230 million people around the world.[4]
- The prevalence of PAD is higher in women than men. The mechanism underlying this is not fully understood, but conventional risk factors do not fully account for the excess risk for PAD in women.[1]
- At-risk patients for PAD include:[2]
  1. Age ≥65 yr
  2. Age 50 to 64 yr with risk factors for atherosclerosis, including diabetes mellitus, smoking history, hyperlipidemia, hypertension, or family history of PAD
  3. Age <50 yr, with diabetes mellitus and one additional risk factor for atherosclerosis
  4. Individuals with known atherosclerotic disease in another vascular bed, for example, coronary, carotid, subclavian, renal, mesenteric artery, or abdominal aortic aneurysm (AAA)
- Risk factors associated with development of PAD are similar to coronary atherosclerosis (CAD) (odds ratio 2.6) and include increasing age, cigarette smoking (odds ratio 2.7), hypertension (odds ratio 1.6), diabetes mellitus (odds ratio 1.9), and hypercholesterolemia (odds ratio 1.2). In addition, patients with chronic kidney disease, metabolic syndrome, and elevated levels of C-reactive protein, lipoprotein(a), and homocysteine are at increased risk. Nontraditional risk factors include race/ethnicity, with African American patients being at higher risk. Hispanics also have similar to slightly higher rates of PAD compared to non-Hispanic whites.[4,5]
- There is a strong correlation among PAD, CAD, carotid artery stenosis, and generalized cerebrovascular disease. Individuals with known atherosclerotic disease in one vascular bed are likely to have disease in another.[2,4,5]
- The American College of Cardiology/American Heart Association (ACC/AHA) guidelines suggested the following distribution of clinical presentation of PAD in patients ≥50 yr of age[4]:
  1. Asymptomatic: 20% to 50%
  2. Atypical leg pain: 40% to 50%
  3. Classic intermittent claudication: 10% to 35%
  4. Critical limb ischemia with threatened limb: 1% to 2%

PHYSICAL FINDINGS & CLINICAL PRESENTATION

- The ACC/AHA and the European Society of Cardiology (ESC) described in detail the various physical and clinical findings to diagnose and manage appropriately.[2] The severity of symptoms varies with degree of PAD, collateral blood supply, and exertional demands.
- Classic symptoms include exertional calf pain, which limits the patient's activity and resolves within a few minutes of resting. Claudication can also typically present in the buttock and hip, thigh, calf, or foot, with one or more of the following signs or symptoms, depending on the level and degree of peripheral stenosis:[2,4,6]
  1. Diminished or absent pedal pulses
  2. Bruit over the distal aorta, iliac, or femoral arteries
  3. Pallor of the distal extremities and cool to the touch upon elevation
  4. Rubor with prolonged capillary refill upon dependent positioning
  5. Trophic changes, including hair/nail loss and muscle atrophy
  6. Nonhealing ulcers, necrotic tissue, and gangrene
  7. Weakness, numbness, or heaviness in the lower extremities
- True vascular claudication must be distinguished from "pseudoclaudication," which can be caused by severe venous obstruction or insufficiency, chronic compartment syndrome, spinal stenosis, osteoarthritis, and inflammatory muscle diseases. The characteristic features of pseudoclaudication that distinguish it from claudication are summarized in Table 1. Table 2 illustrates the differential diagnosis of intermittent claudication.[6]
- Location of pain usually corresponds to analogous anatomy:[6]
  1. Buttock and hip: Aortic or iliac disease
  2. Thigh: Aorta, iliac, or common femoral artery
  3. Upper two thirds of calf: Superficial femoral artery
  4. Lower one third of calf: Popliteal artery
  5. Foot: Tibial or peroneal artery
- Asymptomatic PAD is typically diagnosed by screening studies (exercise ankle brachial index, lower-extremity ultrasound) or incidentally on physical examination. Patients who are at significant risk for PAD often have multiple comorbidities that can alter their presentation. In the PARTNERS program report, 47% of those with a new diagnosis of PAD had no history of leg symptoms, 47%

TABLE 1 Distinguishing Characteristics Between Pseudoclaudication and Claudication

	Claudication	Pseudoclaudication
Characteristics	Limb cramping, tightness, fatigue	Similar to claudication with numbness
Location of discomfort	Lower extremity involving buttock, hip, thigh, calf, foot	Similar to claudication
Induced by exercise	Yes	Variable
Reproducible with distance walked	Consistent	Variable
Occurs with standing	No	Yes
Actions which provide relief	Stand	Sit
Time to relief	<5 min	≥30 min

C

TABLE 2 Differential Diagnosis of Intermittent Claudication

	Intermittent Claudication	Venous Claudication	Neurogenic Claudication
Quality of pain	Cramping	Aching, heaviness, tightness	"Pins and needles" sensation going down the leg, weakness
Onset	Gradual, consistent	Gradual; can, however, be immediate	Can be immediate
Relieved by	Stopping walking	Activity, elevation of leg	Sitting down, stooping, flexion at the waist
Location	Muscle groups (e.g., buttocks, thigh, calf)	Entire leg, worse in calf	Poorly localized, but can affect whole leg
Legs affected	Usually one	Usually one	Often both

From Swartz MH: *Textbook of physical diagnosis,* ed 7, Philadelphia, 2014, Saunders.

Diseases and Disorders

I

had atypical symptoms, and only 6% had classic symptoms.[7]

- Symptoms of intermittent claudication classically start distally within a muscle group (below the stenosis) and then ascend with continued activity.[6]
- Rest pain that occurs with leg elevation and is paradoxically relieved by walking may suggest severe PAD.[6]
- Critical limb ischemia may present as tissue ulceration and gangrene, which require prompt intervention.[4,6]

ETIOLOGY

The primary cause of claudication is peripheral atherosclerosis, resulting in a stenosis that impedes blood flow beyond the level necessary to meet the metabolic demand of limb muscles first with activity and then ultimately at rest. Other etiologies include neuropathy, musculoskeletal or degenerative disease, compartment or entrapment syndrome, vasculitis, and embolic events.[4]

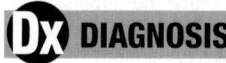 **DIAGNOSIS**

DIFFERENTIAL DIAGNOSIS[4]

- Spinal stenosis (neurogenic or pseudoclaudication)
- Musculoskeletal disorders: Arthritis or myositis
- Degenerative osteoarthritic joint disease, predominantly of the lumbar spine and hips
- Chronic compartment or popliteal artery entrapment syndrome
- Peripheral neuropathy
- Sciatica
- Atheromatous embolization and deep venous thrombosis, superficial thrombophlebitis
- Vasculitis: Thromboangiitis obliterans, Takayasu, or giant cell arteritis
- Symptomatic Baker cyst
- Venous claudication
- Raynaud phenomenon

WORKUP

History and physical findings suggest the diagnosis of claudication and noninvasive studies help confirm the diagnosis.
- Careful physical examinations include:[4,6]
  1. Measurement of blood pressure in both arms and notation of asymmetry
  2. Palpation and recording of carotid pulses, upstroke, amplitude, and presence of bruits
  3. Auscultation and palpation of abdomen for bruits, aortic pulsation, and diameter

4. Palpation of brachial, radial, ulnar, femoral, popliteal, dorsalis pedis, and posterior tibial pulses. Pulse intensity should be recorded as follows: 0, absent; 1+, diminished; 2+, normal; 3+, bounding
5. Auscultation of femoral arteries for the presence of bruits
6. Extremities should be inspected for color, temperature, integrity of the skin, hair loss, and hypertrophic nails

- Measurement of resting ankle-brachial index (ABI) should be considered first-line test in patients at risk for PAD.[2-4]
- An ABI is the ratio of higher ankle systolic pressure (between the dorsalis pedis and posterior tibial arteries) of each leg to the higher systolic pressure of either arm (brachial artery).[1,2]
- When measuring ABI, brachial pressures in both arms should be taken to avoid underestimating pressure due to subclavian artery stenosis.[2]
- The severity of PAD is based on the resting ABI[3,4]:
  1. Severe PAD: <0.4
  2. Moderate PAD: 0.4 to 0.69
  3. Mild PAD: 0.70 to 0.90
  4. Borderline: 0.91 to 0.99
  5. Normal: 1.00 to 1.40
  6. Noncompressible: >1.40
- ABI ≤0.90 has 75% sensitivity and 86% specificity in the detection of PAD.[3]
- A low ABI has been shown to be an independent predictor of mortality.[2,4]
- A high ABI (>1.4) may represent significant PAD caused by arterial wall stiffening. In such cases, measuring a toe-brachial index (TBI) can increase the sensitivity of testing, as highly calcified arteries are incompressible and may have an elevated ABI. A toe-brachial index <0.7 is considered abnormal and diagnostic of PAD.[7]
- Borderline resting ABI (>0.90 and ≤1.40) in patients with exertional leg symptoms should undergo exercise treadmill ABI testing to evaluate for PAD. This can help differentiate claudication from pseudoclaudication. If post treadmill ABI is normal, alternative causes of leg pain should be considered.[4]
- Progression of PAD is considered to have occurred if a decrease in ABI of 0.15 occurs while the patient is on treatment.[4,8]
- If a patient has a history concerning for PAD but a normal ABI, and if the clinician is concerned about a potential false-negative finding, performing an exercise stress ABI

can potentially demonstrate lower-extremity PAD.[2,4]
- If after exercise, ABI reading decreases by more than 20% or an ankle pressure decreases by 30 mm Hg, the patient should be considered to have significant PAD.[4]
- Segmental systolic pressures are measured at the level of the thigh, calf, ankle, metatarsal, and toes. Normally, successive segments have <20 mm Hg difference in pressures. If the gradient is >20 mm Hg, a significant stenosis is suspected in the interval vascular segment.[6]

IMAGING STUDIES

- Duplex ultrasound can be used to assess occlusion location, length, and patency of the distal arterial system or prior grafts; it is a good choice for initial imaging and surveillance monitoring after revascularization.[4]
- In patients with prior infrainguinal venous bypass grafts, the long-term patency should be evaluated at regular intervals using a duplex ultrasound approximately 4 to 6 wk postprocedure, 6 and 12 mo after graft placement, and then yearly.[4]
- Magnetic resonance angiography (MRA) and computed tomography angiography (CTA) are effective for imaging of the aorta and peripheral lower-extremity arteries above the knee. MRA has almost replaced catheter-based angiography, with 90% sensitivity and 97% specificity in identification of hemodynamically significant stenosis in the lower extremities.[4]
- MRA and CTA are useful to define the anatomy and assist in planning percutaneous and surgical revascularization; however, the utility of each is decreased by necessity of gadolinium contrast and noniodinated contrast agents, respectively.
- Angiography (Fig. 1) remains the gold standard for diagnosing PAD, particularly below the knee.

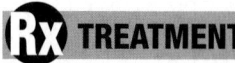 **TREATMENT**

Treatment of PAD includes two aspects. The first aspect is to address symptoms of a specific lesion, and the second is to manage the patient's increased cardiovascular risk to optimize outcomes.

NONPHARMACOLOGIC THERAPY

- Smoking cessation is of paramount importance. Smokers and former smokers should

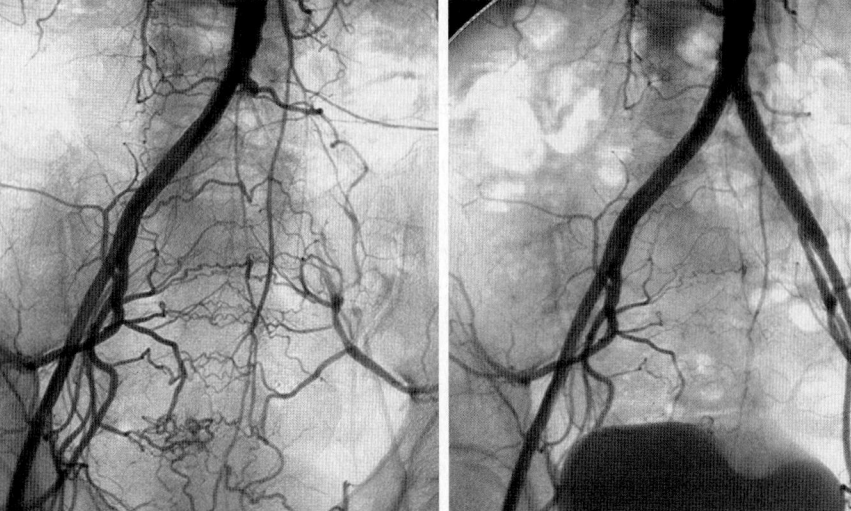

FIG. 1 Angiogram of the distal abdominal aorta and iliac arteries demonstrates an occluded left common iliac artery with extensive collateral circulation from contralateral internal iliac artery *(left panel),* **which resolved after successful stent implantation** *(right panel).* (Images courtesy Bart Domatch, MD, Radiology Department, University of Texas, Southwestern Medical Center, Dallas, Texas. From Andreoli TE et al: *Andreoli and Carpenter's Cecil essentials of medicine,* ed 8, Philadelphia, 2010, Saunders.)

be asked about tobacco use status at every visit and offered pharmacotherapy, counseling, and/or referred to smoking cessation programs (Class I, A).[4]

- Aggressive risk factor modification for hypertension, dyslipidemia, and diabetes mellitus, including diet, weight loss, and lifestyle counseling, is recommended (Fig. 2).
- Supervised exercise training should be performed as a first-line therapy for a minimum of 30 to 45 min, in sessions performed at least 3 times per wk, for a minimum of 12 wk.[4,9-11]
- Supervised exercise training programs under direct supervision in a hospital or outpatient facility and structured exercise are recommended for all patients with PAD. This has been shown to increase maximal walking distance, pain-free walking distance, and the 6-min walking distance. It typically requires 4 to 6 wk for patients to notice improvement.[4,9]
- Structured or home-based walking exercise program may be considered as an alternative treatment modality, but it has not been shown to be as efficacious. It can be combined with group-mediated cognitive behavioral intervention that can significantly improve endurance and physical activity for patients unable or unwilling to participate in supervised exercise training.[9,11]
- Lifestyle therapy in conjunction with exercise can be as, or more, effective than pharmacologic therapy and in some cases more effective than stent revascularization.[4,10]
- Intermittent mechanical compression appears to be an effective noninvasive treatment alternative for patients with intermittent claudication.[2,4]

ACUTE GENERAL Rx

Revascularization by an endovascular or surgical approach is usually reserved for patients with symptoms refractory to medical therapy or those with impending critical limb ischemia.[4]

CHRONIC Rx

- One antiplatelet agent, either aspirin 81 mg daily or clopidogrel 75 mg daily, should be initiated for symptomatic patients and those undergoing endovascular or surgical revascularization (Class I, A).[4]
- Dual antiplatelet therapy is recommended after infrainguinal stenting and carotid artery stenting for at least 1 mo (Class IIa, C) and single agent afterward.[4]
- Asymptomatic patients with PAD (ABI ≤0.90) without claudication symptoms may benefit from the addition of an antiplatelet agent (Class IIa, C), either aspirin or clopidogrel, as there is an increased cardiovascular risk in this subgroup.[4]
- Statin medications are indicated for all patients with PAD (Class I, A).[2,4]
  1. Low-density lipoprotein (LDL) cholesterol level of less than 100 mg/dl is recommended.
  2. A goal LDL cholesterol level of less than 70 mg/dl is recommended for patients with PAD and high risk for coronary atherosclerotic disease.
  3. Although new lipid guidelines have been published, the guidelines did not specifically address patients with PAD; therefore numerical targets can be considered. In those unable to reach the targets, a reduction in LDL >50% should be approached at a minimum.
- Antihypertensive therapy with beta-adrenergic blocking drugs and/or ACE inhibitors should be administered to all hypertensive patients with PAD to reduce the risk of myocardial infarction (MI), stroke, congestive heart failure, and cardiovascular death.[2,4]

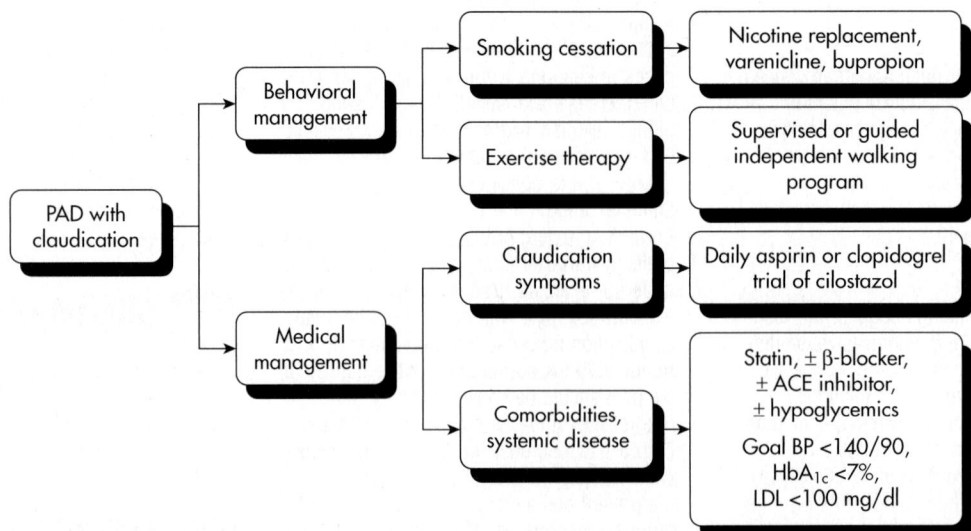

FIG. 2 Algorithm for revascularization in the management of claudication. *ACE,* Angiotensin-converting enzyme; *BP,* blood pressure; *HbA$_{1c}$,* hemoglobin A$_{1c}$; *LDL,* low-density lipoprotein; *PAD,* peripheral arterial disease. (From Cameron JL, Cameron AM: *Current surgical therapy,* ed 12, Philadelphia, 2017, Elsevier.)

- Cilostazol 100 mg bid may be used in conjunction with aspirin or clopidogrel. It has been shown to increase walking distance by 50% to 67% in symptomatic patients (Class I, A).[2,4] Cilostazol increases cyclic adenosine monophosphate (cAMP) levels, upregulates nitrous oxide (NO), and upregulates growth factors and chemokines that stimulate angiogenesis. Of note, cilostazol is contraindicated in patients with heart failure.[1]
- Anticoagulation with vitamin K antagonists is generally not recommended to reduce the risk of cardiovascular ischemic events in patients with PAD as there is increased morbidity with no mortality benefit. Its use to improve patency after bypass is uncertain (Class III, A).[2,4]
- Newer anticoagulants such as factor Xa inhibitors with improved safety profiles such as rivaroxaban have been shown to significantly reduce acute limb ischemia and improve mortality in patients with symptomatic PAD. Rivaroxaban may be considered alone or with aspirin 81 mg daily in patients under the age of 75 who are not at high risk of bleeding (data from the VOYAGER PAD and COMPASS trial).[12]
- Among patients with intermittent claudication, a single randomized controlled trial has shown a 24-wk treatment with ramipril resulted in significant increases in pain-free and maximum treadmill walking times compared with placebo.[13]
- Pentoxifylline is not effective for treatment of claudication. In a review of 24 studies with over 3000 participants, results remained unclear, and a randomized control trial showed no difference between pentoxifylline and placebo; thus this is not recommended as a treatment for claudication.[14]
- In patients with type 2 diabetes, a secondary analysis of the BARI 2D trial showed that an insulin-sensitizing approach (metformin, thiazolidinediones) reduces the risk of developing PAD when compared to insulin-providing therapy (glipizide, insulin). These patients also have lower rates of revascularization and amputation.[15]
- Patients who are tobacco smokers should be strongly advised to quit smoking at every visit and offered either varenicline or bupropion along with nicotine replacement therapy in the absence of any contraindications. Patients with PAD should avoid tobacco smoke exposure at work, at home, and in public places.[16]
- Novel agents, such as protease-activated receptor-1 (e.g., vorapaxar), added to existing antiplatelet therapy may have some benefit in decreasing acute limb-related ischemic events; however, its association with a risk of moderate to severe bleeding makes its benefits uncertain at this time.[2]
- Fig. 3 summarizes the nonoperative management of claudication.
- Revascularization through either a percutaneous or surgical approach is indicated in patients with lifestyle-limiting claudication and inadequate response to goal-directed medical therapy. It is also indicated in those with nonhealing ulcers or gangrene and in select patients with functional disability. Before such revascularization, each patient should have[4]:
1. Participated in a supervised exercise training program and been given goal-directed medical therapy.
2. Received comprehensive risk factor modification, including smoking cessation and optimal management of comorbidities.
3. Significant disability with either the inability to perform normal work or a serious impairment of other activities important to the patient.
4. Lower-extremity PAD lesion anatomy amenable to revascularization defined as low risk with high probability of initial and long-term success.

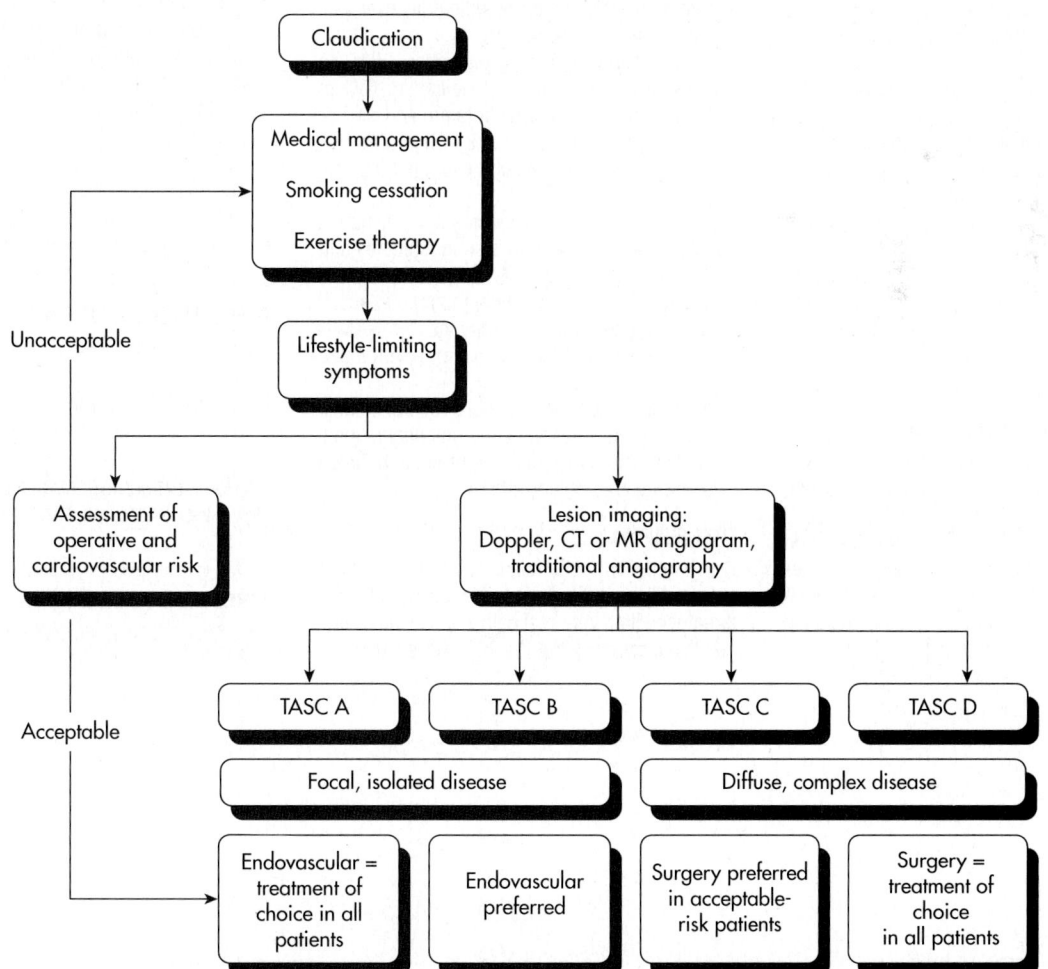

FIG. 3 Nonoperative management of claudication. *CT,* Computed tomography; *MR,* magnetic resonance; *TASC,* TransAtlantic Inter-Society Consensus class. (From Cameron JL, Cameron AM: *Current surgical therapy,* ed 12, Philadelphia, 2017, Elsevier.)

- Common procedures include:[2,4]
  1. Percutaneous balloon angioplasty can be used for long lesions or diffuse disease and has initial success rate of 90% but >60% restenosis rate over 12 mo. Balloon angioplasty combined with stenting is primarily used on discrete stenotic lesions in the iliac or femoropopliteal arteries.
  2. Aortoiliofemoral reconstruction or bypass or infrainguinal bypass (e.g., femoropopliteal, femorotibial).
  3. Endovascular intervention is recommended as the preferred revascularization technique for iliac and femoropopliteal arterial lesions. In the LEVANT II trial, endovascular stenting had greater primary patency rate than balloon angioplasty in patients with claudication at 12 mo.
  4. Stenting is an effective primary therapy for common and external iliac artery stenosis and occlusions. However, it is not recommended in the femoral, popliteal, or tibial arteries due to a low success rate except to salvage suboptimal balloon dilation.
  5. Percutaneous femoropopliteal bypass is FDA approved for patients with symptomatic femoropopliteal lesions 20 cm to 45 cm in length with chronic total occlusions or diffuse stenosis >70% who may be suboptimal candidates for surgical or endovascular treatment options based on DETOUR trial.[17]
  6. In severe, nonreversible cases with gangrene, amputation may be required.
- Endovascular procedures should not be performed in patients with PAD solely to prevent progression to critical limb ischemia, as reported rates of amputation or progression to critical limb ischemia are <10% to 15% over 5 yr or more, and increased mortality rate associated with claudication is usually the result of cardiovascular events rather than limb-related events.[4]

COMPLEMENTARY & ALTERNATIVE MEDICINE

- A meta-analysis found that over 12 to 24 wk, ginkgo biloba increased pain-free walking distance by 34 m compared with placebo,[18] although the benefit is not well established according to ACC/AHA guidelines. A subsequent prospective trial over 4 mo showed modest but insignificant increase in maximal treadmill walking time over placebo.[19]
- Naftidrofuryl, a serotonin receptor inhibitor, available in Europe and other parts of the world, had shown some efficacy in improving claudication symptoms in small trials.[20]
- B-complex vitamin supplementation to lower homocysteine levels for prevention of cardiovascular events in patients with PAD is not recommended (HOPE-2 trial).[21]
- Hormone replacement therapy has been shown to decrease the incidence of peripheral artery disease as measured by ankle-arm index after 1 yr of treatment in postmenopausal women (Rotterdam trial),[22] although it may be associated with increased risk of thrombotic complications when initiating therapy. Available data are conflicting.[23]
- Prior studies have shown that propionyl-L-carnitine, L-arginine, oral vasodilators, prostaglandins, and chelation therapy are ineffective in the treatment of intermittent claudication.[24-28]
- Acupuncture has shown some improvement in symptom relief and functional capacity in small studies but mainly in neurogenic claudication or mild peripheral arterial disease.[29]

PROGNOSIS

- It is unusual for intermittent claudication to progress to ischemic leg or limb loss, especially with aggressive use of conservative treatments, risk factor modification, exercise, and smoking cessation.[30]
- Among patients with claudication, 70% to 80% remain with stable claudication, 10% to 20% with worsening symptoms, and critical limb ischemia in 1% to 2% in 5 yr. The risk for nonfatal cardiovascular event is 20% and death is 15% to 30%.[30]
- The 5-yr risk for development of ischemic ulceration in patients treated for diabetes and with ABI <0.5 was 30% compared with only 5% in patients without either characteristic.[30]
- A screening duplex ultrasound for AAA is recommended for patients with symptomatic PAD.[31]
- All patients with PAD should receive annual influenza vaccination based on observational studies that have demonstrated a reduced cardiovascular event rate.[2,4]

REFERRAL

Consultation with physicians specializing in vascular medicine is recommended for patients with threatened limb loss, rest pain, nonhealing ulcers, functional disability from pain, and gangrene.

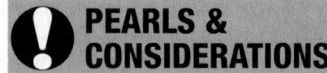

PEARLS & CONSIDERATIONS

- Approximately 70% of patients with peripheral vascular disease will have concomitant coronary artery disease.
- β-Blockers may worsen claudication symptoms in some patients, although their underuse is associated with excess cardiovascular death. Reviews of available data suggest that β-blockers are likely safe to use in patients with coronary artery disease and intermittent claudication. Patients with intermittent claudication are less likely to receive beta-blocker therapy after a myocardial infarction. Those who do not receive post-MI beta-blockers have at least a threefold higher mortality.[32,33]
- Patients with peripheral vascular disease may benefit from secondary cardiovascular prevention with clopidogrel versus aspirin more so than other high-risk patients.[2]
- PAD can be asymptomatic or with atypical symptoms, and a thorough history, physical exam, and clinical suspicion based on medical comorbidities may help guide therapy before lifestyle-limiting claudication or limb ischemia develops.[2-6]

COMMENTS

- Claudication is a marker for generalized atherosclerosis, and patients have a higher risk of death from cardiovascular events than from limb loss. Patients with PAD experience diminished overall quality of life similar to patients diagnosed with coronary artery or cerebrovascular disease.
- The ABI is more closely associated with exercise tolerance and severity of disease in persons with PAD rather than intermittent claudication or other leg symptoms.

RELATED CONTENT

Poor Circulation (Claudication) (Patient Information)
Peripheral Artery Disease (Related Key Topic)

AUTHORS: **EMIN ZARGARIAN, MD** and **PRANAV M. PATEL, MD, FACC, FAHA, FSCAI**

REFERENCES

Available at eBooks.Health.Elsevier.com.

C

Diseases
and Disorders

I

BASIC INFORMATION

DEFINITION

C. difficile infection (CDI) is the occurrence of diarrhea and bowel inflammation associated with antibiotic use caused by *Clostridioides difficile,* an anaerobic gram-positive, spore-forming, toxin-producing bacillus transmitted through the fecal-oral route. CDI can manifest clinically in several forms ranging from fulminant diarrhea and leukocytosis associated with pseudomembranous colitis, mild to severe acute diarrhea, short-term colonization seen typically in health care facilities, and recurrent CDI within 60 days after initial treatment occurring in 20% to 30% of cases.

SYNONYMS

Antibiotic-induced colitis
Pseudomembranous colitis
CDI

ICD-10CM CODE
A04.7 Enterocolitis due to *Clostridium difficile*

EPIDEMIOLOGY & DEMOGRAPHICS

- Cephalosporins are the most frequent offending agent in CDI because of their high rates of use.
- The antibiotic with the highest incidence is clindamycin (10% incidence of CDI with its use).
- Since 1996, the incidence of CDI has more than doubled. Severity of CDI has also increased due to the emergence of an epidemic virulent strain (NAP1/BI/027). CDI is the most common infectious cause of health care-associated diarrhea in adults. In the U.S. *C. difficile* is responsible for nearly half a million infections per yr and is associated with approximately 29,000 deaths/yr.
- Nosocomial CDI quadruples the cost of hospitalizations and increases annual expenditures by $4 and $6 billion in the U.S.
- Asymptomatic carriage of *C. difficile* is identified in more than 20% of patients hospitalized without diarrhea.

PHYSICAL FINDINGS & CLINICAL PRESENTATION

- Abdominal tenderness (generalized or lower abdominal)
- Fever
- In patients with prolonged diarrhea, poor skin turgor, dry mucous membranes, and other signs of dehydration may be present

ETIOLOGY

C. difficile colonizes the large intestines and releases two protein exotoxins (TcdA and TcdB) that cause colitis. The histopathology of pseudomembranous colitis consists of a significant polymorphonuclear infiltrate, a fibrinous exudate, and epithelial damage (Fig. E1). Infection is transmitted by spores that are resistant to antibiotics, heat, and acid. The NAP1 strain is predominant

TABLE 1   Risks for Development of *Clostridioides difficile* Infection

- Any antibiotic versus no antibiotic:
  1. Number of antibiotics (risk increases with number)
  2. Days of antibiotics (increased risk with increased days)
- Type of antibiotic:
  1. *Highest risk:* Clindamycin, fluoroquinolones, cephalosporins of second generation and higher
  2. *Moderate risk:* Penicillins, macrolides, penicillin β-lactamase inhibitors, carbapenems, vancomycin, metronidazole
  3. *Lower risk:* Aminoglycosides, tetracyclines, trimethoprim, sulfonamides, rifampin
- Proton pump inhibitors and histamine type 2 blockers
- Patient age (increased risk with increased age of the patient)
- Prior hospitalization
- Severity of underlying illness
- Abdominal surgery
- Nasogastric tube
- Duration of hospitalization
- Long-term care residency

From Bennett JE et al: *Mandell, Douglas, and Bennett's principles and practice of infectious diseases,* ed 9, Philadelphia, 2020, Elsevier.

among patients with *C. difficile* infection, whereas asymptomatic patients are more likely to be colonized with other strains. Risk factors (Table 1) for *C. difficile*:

- Administration of antibiotics: Can occur with any antibiotic, but occurs most frequently with clindamycin, cephalosporins, ampicillin, and fluoroquinolone
- Prolonged hospitalization
- Advanced age
- Abdominal surgery
- Underlying disease (malignancy, renal failure, debilitated status)
- Hospitalized, tube-fed patients are at risk for *C. difficile*-associated diarrhea. Clinicians should consider testing for *C. difficile* in tube-fed patients with diarrhea unrelated to the feeding solution
- Proton pump inhibitor (PPI) and H_2 blocker therapy increases risk of CDI and recurrent CDI. Risk is 1.7-fold higher with PPIs

DIAGNOSIS

The clinical signs of CDI generally include diarrhea, fever, and abdominal cramps after use of antibiotics. Although a history of recent antibiotic use is common, it is not a requirement for diagnosis.

CLASSIFICATION

The American College of Gastroenterology (ACG), the Infectious Diseases Society of America (IDSA), and the European Congress of Clinical Microbiology and Infectious Diseases (ECCMID) classify CDI as:
- Mild/moderate
  1. Diarrhea but no signs or symptoms of severe or fulminant CDI (ACG)

  2. White blood cell (WBC) $<15 \times 10^9$/L, serum creatinine <1.5 mg/dl (IDSA)
  3. Stool frequency <4 times daily, no signs of severe colitis (ECCMID)
- Severe
  1. Serum albumin <3 g/dl and WBC $>1.5 \times 10^9$/dl or abdominal tenderness (ACG)
  2. WBC $\geq15 \times 10^9$/L, serum creatinine >1.5 mg/dl (IDSA)
  3. Fever $>38.5°$ C, rigors, hemodynamic instability (ECCMID)
- Fulminant
  1. Hypotension or fever ≥38.5, or ileus, mental status change, and organ failure WBC $\geq35 \times 10^9$/L, hypotension, intensive care unit admission (ACG)
  2. Hypotension or shock, ileus, megacolon (IDSA)
  3. Peritoneal signs, ileus WBC $>16 \times 10^9$/L, elevated serum lactate increase in serum creatinine ($\geq1.5 \times$ baseline) (ECCMID)

DIFFERENTIAL DIAGNOSIS

- Gastrointestinal bacterial infections (e.g., *Salmonella, Shigella, Campylobacter, Yersinia*)
- Enteric parasites (e.g., *Cryptosporidium, Entamoeba histolytica*)
- Inflammatory bowel disease
- Celiac sprue
- Irritable bowel syndrome
- Ischemic colitis
- Antibiotic intolerance

WORKUP

- All patients with diarrhea accompanied by current or recent antibiotic use should be tested for *C. difficile*. *C. difficile* stool tests are positive in 3% of outpatients and up to 29% of inpatients without signs of infection. Testing and treatment for CDI is not recommended in asymptomatic individuals.
- Sigmoidoscopy (without cleansing enema) may be necessary when the clinical and laboratory diagnosis is inconclusive, and the diarrhea persists.
- In antibiotic-induced pseudomembranous colitis, the sigmoidoscopy often reveals raised white-yellow exudative plaques adherent to the colonic mucosa pseudomembranes (Fig. E2). These are seen more commonly in severe CDI.

LABORATORY TESTS (TABLE 2)

- Stool test for *C. difficile* toxin: Enzyme-linked immunosorbent assay for *C. difficile* toxins A and B. The latter is used most widely in the clinical setting. It has a sensitivity of 85% and a specificity of 100%.
- *C. difficile* toxin can be detected by cytotoxin tissue culture assay (cytotoxin assay, gold standard for identifying *C. difficile* toxin in stool specimen). This test is difficult to perform, and results are not available for 24 to 48 h.
- Fecal leukocytes (assessed by microscopy or lactoferrin assay) are generally present in stool samples.
- Complete blood count usually reveals leukocytosis. A sudden increase in white blood

TABLE 2 Endoscopic and Stool Diagnostic Tests for *Clostridioides difficile* and Its Toxins

Test	Sensitivity (%)	Specificity (%)	Comment
Colon endoscopy	~50	100	Sensitivity and specificity are for detection of PMC
Cell cytotoxicity	77-86	97-99	The less sensitive of two gold standards compared with toxigenic culture
EIA for toxin A	67-92	93-99	Versus cell cytotoxicity
EIA for toxin B	60-89	93-99	Versus toxigenic culture
EIA for GDH	71-100	67-99	Compared with stool culture for *C. difficile*
Toxigenic culture for *C. difficile*	95-100	96-100	The more sensitive of two gold standards compared with cell cytotoxicity
Nucleic acid amplification test (PCR and LAMP)	88-100	88-97	Versus toxigenic culture
			Most sensitive rapid single test available but also expensive
Two-step GDH testing[a]	56-90	81-97	Discrepancy between GDH and toxin test is 13%-19%
Three-step GDH testing[b]	83-100	93-100	

EIA, Enzyme immunoassay; *GDH,* glutamate dehydrogenase; *LAMP,* loop-mediated isothermal amplification; *NAAT,* nucleic acid amplification test; *PCR,* polymerase chain reaction; *PMC,* pseudomembranous colitis.

[a]Two-step GDH testing: EIA for GDH and EIA for toxins A and B.
[b]Three-step GDH testing: EIA for GDH and EIA for toxins A and B, arbitrated by NAAT for discrepancies.
From Bennett JE et al: *Mandell, Douglas, and Bennett's principles and practice of infectious diseases,* ed 9, Philadelphia, 2020, Elsevier.

cells to >30,000/mm^3 may be indicative of fulminant colitis.

- Laboratory indicators of **severe CDI** are leukocyte count >15,000/mm^3, serum creatinine ≥1.5 times baseline level, serum albumin <2.5 g/dl.

IMAGING STUDIES
- Abdominal film (flat plate and upright) is useful in patients with abdominal pain or evidence of obstruction on physical examination.
- Computed tomography can demonstrate typical findings of colonic wall thickening, dilatation,

and the so-called *accordion sign* (thickened haustral folds and trapped contrast material, ascites, or pericolonic stranding [Fig. E3]).

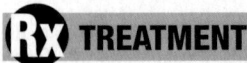 **TREATMENT**

NONPHARMACOLOGIC THERAPY
- Discontinue offending antibiotic.
- Fluid hydration and correction of electrolyte abnormalities.
- Probiotics to restore natural defense mechanisms may be useful as adjuvant therapy; however, evidence is limited. Probiotic trials have failed to show benefit in preventing *C. difficile*-associated diarrhea.
- Fecal microbiota transplantation (FMT) is an excellent treatment modality for recurrent CDI. It replaces the altered gut flora to allow colonization resistance. Trials have shown that it is more effective than vancomycin and may become standard treatment for recurrent CDI. Recent trials have shown that donor stool administered via colonoscopy are safe and more efficacious than autologous FMT in preventing further CDI episodes.

ACUTE GENERAL Rx (TABLE 3)
- Vancomycin 125 mg PO qid for 10 days can be used as initial treatment in patients with non-severe or severe CDI. Patients with fulminant CDI will require 500 mg qid for 10 days.

TABLE 3 Current Therapy for *Clostridioides difficile* Infection Based on Severity and Recurrence

CDI Type	Antibiotic	Dose[a]	Alternatives
C. difficile (nonsevere)	Vancomycin, or	125 mg PO qid × 10 days	If vancomycin or fidaxomicin is not available or contraindicated, metronidazole 500 mg PO tid × 10 days
	Fidaxomicin	200 mg PO bid × 10 days	
C. difficile (severe[b])	Vancomycin, or	125 mg PO qid × 10 days	None
	Fidaxomicin	200 mg PO bid × 10 days	
C. difficile (severe complicated or fulminant)	Vancomycin +	500 mg PO qid × 10-14 days	Tigecycline, 50 mg IV bid × 10-21 days in place of metronidazole
	Metronidazole	500 mg IV q8h × 10-14 days	Additional vancomycin via rectal retention enema, 500 mg in 100 ml normal saline q6h if complete ileus present
			Surgical colectomy or ileostomy
C. difficile (first recurrence)	Vancomycin, or	125 mg PO qid × 10 days if metronidazole was used for the initial episode	None
	Vancomycin taper and pulse, or	125 mg PO qid × 10 days, bid for 1 wk, qd for 1 wk, and then every 2 or 3 days for 2-8 wk if standard vancomycin was used for the initial episode	
	Fidaxomicin	200 mg PO bid × 10 days if vancomycin was used for the initial episode	
C. difficile (>1 recurrence)	Vancomycin taper and pulse, or	125 mg PO qid × 10 days, bid for 1 wk, qd for 1 wk, and then every 2 or 3 days for 2-8 wk	None
	Vancomycin/rifaximin, *or*	Vancomycin 125 mg PO qid × 10 days followed by rifaximin 400 mg PO tid × 20 days	
	Fidaxomicin, *or*	200 mg PO bid × 10 days	
	Fecal microbiota transplantation[c]		

[a]All randomized trials have compared 10-day treatment courses, but some patients (particularly those treated with metronidazole) may have delayed response to treatment and clinicians should consider extending treatment duration to 14 days in those circumstances.
[b]The criteria proposed for defining severe or fulminant CDI are based on expert opinion. These may need to be reviewed in the future upon publication of prospectively validated severity scores for patients with CDI.
[c]The opinion of the panel is that appropriate antibiotic treatments for at least two recurrences (i.e., three CDI episodes) should be tried prior to offering fecal microbiota transplantation.
Adapted from Bennett JE et al: *Mandell, Douglas, and Bennett's principles and practice of infectious diseases,* ed 9, Philadelphia, 2020, Elsevier.

- Fidaxomicin 200 mg bid for 10 days has shown noninferiority to vancomycin and a lower rate of CDI recurrence (25% with vancomycin vs. 15% with fidaxomicin); however, its higher cost is a limiting factor. Fidaxomicin can be used for initial treatment of nonsevere or severe CDI or for recurrence of CDI if vancomycin was used for initial treatment.
- Metronidazole 500 mg PO qid for 10 days can be used in low risk patients with mild disease if oral vancomycin or fidaxomicin are not available or contraindicated. A significant rise in clinical failure has been seen with metronidazole over the past decade, especially in patients with the BI/NAP/027 strain.
- Fulminant CDI treatment consists of high-dose vancomycin with or without IV metronidazole. In patients with ileus the addition of rectal vancomycin should be considered.
- Treatment of first recurrence should include a different regimen from initial treatment. Options include standard dose fidaxomicin, pulsed and extended fidaxomicin (200 mg PO bid × 5 days, then 200 mg once every other day for 20 days), if vancomycin was used for initial treatment. If fidaxomicin was used initially, standard oral vancomycin and pulsed and tapered oral vancomycin (125 mg PO qid × 10 to 14 days, then tapered) is appropriate.
- FMT: When standard treatment has failed, intestinal microbiota transplantation (IMT) is an effective alternative therapy (eradication rate is 94%). It involves infusing intestinal microorganisms (in a suspension of healthy donor stool) into the intestine of a sick patient via enema, oral capsule, gastroscope/colonoscope, or nasojejunal tube to restore the microbiota. In patients with recurrent *C. difficile* infection, FMT by oral capsule has been shown to be noninferior to transplantation by colonoscopy for recurrence at 12 wk. Trials comparing fresh vs. frozen fecal microbiota transplantation have shown equal efficacy.
- The human monoclonal antibody bezlotoxumab has been FDA-approved for use with antibacterial drug treatment to reduce recurrence of CDI. Cost is a limiting factor.

SURGICAL MANAGEMENT

- Indications: CDI unresponsive to medical therapy, fulminant colitis
- Clinical features: Colonic distention, severe abdominal pain/tenderness, systemic inflammatory response syndrome. Diarrhea may be absent because of ileus
- Surgical approaches:
  1. Traditional (subtotal or total colectomy), high mortality (50%)
  2. Colon-sparing (loop ileostomy with intraoperative colonic lavage using warmed polyethylene glycol solution via the ileostomy and instillations of postoperative vancomycin flushes via the ileostomy); lower mortality compared to traditional approach

CHRONIC Rx

- Judicious future use of antibiotics to prevent recurrences (e.g., avoid prolonged antibiotic therapy).
- Probiotics have been shown mildly effective in reducing the risk for CDI among patients prescribed antibiotics. They should not be used in immunocompromised or severely debilitated patients.
- Alcohol-based hand gels are inadequate for eradication of spores. They are inferior to soap and water for eradication of spores.
- Gastric acid suppression with PPIs increases risk of CDI. Preferential use of H_2RA should be considered in these patients.

DISPOSITION

- CDI recurrence after an initial episode is 20% to 25% regardless of initial treatment with metronidazole or vancomycin. Risk factors for development of recurrent CDI are summarized in Table 4. Each recurrence increases risk of repeat episodes (65% chance of recurrence after three CDI episodes). Recurrent CDI usually represents relapse rather than reinfection, no matter how long between episodes (Fig. E4). Recurrent episodes are best treated with a prolonged course of oral vancomycin followed by rifaximin (400 mg PO tid × 20 days) and fecal microbiota transplantation.

TABLE 4   Risk Factors for Development of Recurrent *Clostridioides difficile* Infection

Any prior episodes of *C. difficile* infection, particularly severe infection
Antibiotic use (concomitant or post-*C. difficile* infection treatment, or both)
Age ≥65 yr
Prolonged or recent stay in health care facility
High severity of Horn index for underlying illness
Immunosuppression
Proton pump inhibitor use
Infection with NAP1/BI/027 strain
Absence of an antitoxin A antibody response

From Bennett JE et al: *Mandell, Douglas, and Bennett's principles and practice of infectious diseases*, ed 9, Philadelphia, 2020, Elsevier.

- Fecal microbiota therapy (FMT) after CDI treatment is now FDA approved for patients with multiple episodes. Beginning 2 to 4 d after completion of CDI treatment, dosing consists of four capsules (Vowst™) administered orally, once daily for 3 d, prior to the first meal of the day. Magnesium citrate (or polyethylene glycol electrolyte solution if renal dysfunction is present) is administered the day before the first dose.[1] A rectally administered FMT (REBYOTA®) is also FDA approved for prevention of additional recurrances of CDI. Cost and formulary are major barriers to use of FMT.
- Hospital-acquired CDI is independently associated with an increased risk of in-hospital death. All hospitalized patients with CDI should be placed in contact isolation at least until resolution of diarrhea.

RELATED CONTENT

Clostridium difficile Infection (Patient Information)

AUTHOR: **FRED F. FERRI, MD**

REFERENCE & SUGGESTED READINGS

Available at eBooks.Health.Elsevier.com.

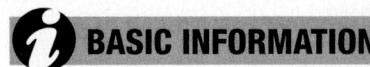 **BASIC INFORMATION**

DEFINITION

The term *cluster headache* refers to attacks of severe, unilateral pain associated with ipsilateral cranial autonomic symptoms and/or restlessness. An attack typically manifests as a sharp/stabbing orbital, supraorbital, and/or temporal pain lasting 15 to 180 min, occurring up to eight times a day over a span of weeks to months. Attacks associated with one or more ipsilateral cranial autonomic symptoms, including forehead and facial sweating, miosis, ptosis, eyelid edema, conjunctival injection, lacrimation (Fig. 1), nasal congestion, or rhinorrhea. Most patients are restless and/or agitated during an attack.

SYNONYMS

Ciliary neuralgia
Erythromelalgia of the head
Erythroprosopalgia of Bing
Headache, cluster
Histaminic cephalalgia
Horton headache
Petrosal neuralgia
Sluder neuralgia
Sluder syndrome

ICD-10-CM CODES
G44.001	Cluster headache syndrome, unspecified, intractable
G44.009	Cluster headache syndrome, unspecified, not intractable
G44.011	Episodic cluster headache, intractable
G44.019	Episodic cluster headache, not intractable
G44.021	Chronic cluster headache, intractable
G44.029	Chronic cluster headache, not intractable

EPIDEMIOLOGY & DEMOGRAPHICS

INCIDENCE: Estimated to occur in <1% of the population
PREDOMINANT SEX: Occurs three to four times more commonly in males than in females

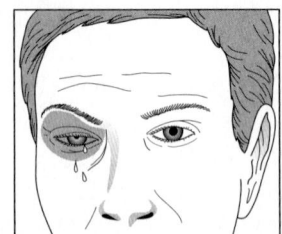

FIG. 1 This 43-yr-old man with cluster headaches suffers from nightly right-sided unrelenting, severe, stabbing unilateral periorbital pain for 45 min to 3 h accompanied by ipsilateral tearing and nasal discharge, along with ptosis and miosis (a partial Horner syndrome). Note that the ptosis prompts compensatory elevation of the eyebrow. (From Kaufman DM et al: *Kaufman's clinical neurology for psychiatrists*, ed 9, Philadelphia 2023, Elsevier.)

PREDOMINANT AGE: Peak age of onset is between 20 and 40 yr
GENETICS: May be inherited in up to 20% of cases, although uncertainty exists over the mode or modes of inheritance

PHYSICAL FINDINGS & CLINICAL PRESENTATION

- In most patients, attacks are nocturnal and provoked by alcohol ingestion.
- Attacks have an abrupt onset with pain escalating to maximal intensity over 5 to 15 min and a similarly abrupt cessation.
- Most attacks last 45 to 90 min.
- Attacks may occur in clusters separated by pain-free remission periods (episodic cluster headache) or occur without a remission period (chronic cluster headache).
- Pain is accompanied by ipsilateral forehead and facial sweating, miosis, ptosis, eyelid edema, conjunctival injection, lacrimation, nasal congestion, or rhinorrhea.
- Symptoms remain ipsilateral during the attack but may switch sides during subsequent attacks.
- Patients are agitated and active during an attack in contrast to migraine sufferers.
- Permanent partial Horner syndrome in 5% of patients, otherwise examination is normal.

ETIOLOGY

The exact pathophysiology remains unknown; however, activation of the posterior hypothalamic gray matter and the trigeminal-autonomic reflex via hypothalamic-trigeminal nucleus connection is the most widely accepted theory.

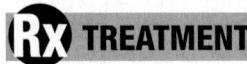 **DIAGNOSIS**

Per the *International Classification of Headache Disorders,* 3rd edition, the diagnosis of cluster headache requires all of the following:
- At least five attacks of severe or very severe unilateral orbital, supraorbital, and/or temporal pain lasting 15 to 180 min
- Frequency of attacks between one every other day to eight per day
- Presence of a sense of restlessness or agitation and/or ≥1 of the following (ipsilateral):
  1. Conjunctival injection and/or lacrimation
  2. Nasal congestion and/or rhinorrhea
  3. Eyelid edema
  4. Forehead and facial sweating
  5. Miosis and/or ptosis
- Episodic cluster headache: attacks fulfilling criteria for cluster headache occurring in bouts (cluster periods) lasting from 1 wk to 1 yr that are separated by attack-free intervals lasting ≥3 mo
- Chronic cluster headache: attacks fulfilling criteria for cluster headache occurring for ≥1 yr without an attack-free interval of ≥3 mo

DIFFERENTIAL DIAGNOSIS

- Primary headaches
  1. Migraine
  2. Other trigeminal autonomic cephalalgias
  3. Primary stabbing headache

- Secondary headaches
  1. Trigeminal neuralgia
  2. Temporal arteritis
  3. Acute-angle glaucoma
- Postherpetic neuralgia
- Venous sinus thrombosis
- Carotid-cavernous fistula or other cavernous sinus lesions
- Section II describes the differential diagnosis of headaches

WORKUP

Diagnosis is made clinically. Box 1 summarizes useful questions to ask patients with headaches.

IMAGING STUDIES

- None, unless history or examination suggests focal neurologic deficit or headaches change in character or are of new onset.
- MRI of the brain and/or vascular imaging may be necessary to exclude structural lesions, secondary headaches, and/or alternative diagnoses in patients with refractory symptoms.

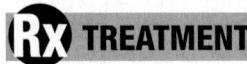 **TREATMENT**

NONPHARMACOLOGIC THERAPY

- Avoidance of triggers (e.g., alcohol, histamine, nitroglycerin, and tobacco) during clusters

ABORTIVE Rx (TABLE 1)

- Inhalation of 100% oxygen by face mask at a flow rate ≥12 L/min for 15 min aborts the attack in 60% to 80% of patients.
- Subcutaneous or nasal triptans (e.g., sumatriptan, zolmitriptan) will alleviate pain within 20 min in approximately 75% of patients. Only injectable and nasal formulations achieve a response that is rapid enough to be efficacious.
- Galcanezumab-gnlm is the first FDA-approved medication for episodic cluster headache in adults. First approved for migraine, this injectable medication is a humanized monoclonal antibody that blocks the binding of calcitonin gene-related peptide (CGRP) to the CGRP receptor. It reduces the average number of cluster headaches per week from baseline compared to placebo.
- Non-invasive vagus nerve stimulator, approved by the FDA for acute prevention of episodic cluster headache, may be particularly useful in patients with multiple daily attacks.
- Cafergot, octreotide, intranasal lidocaine, or intravenous (IV) dihydroergotamine may abort an attack or prevent one if given just before a predictable episode.
- NSAIDs such as indomethacin may be effective in prolonged attacks, although attacks typically resolve before oral analgesics can take effect.

PROPHYLACTIC Rx

- Patients with chronic cluster headache should start prophylactic treatment at increasing doses until good control is achieved then continue

---

BOX 1   Useful Questions to Ask the Patient With Headache

- How many types of headache do you have?
- When and how did each type begin?
- If the headaches are episodic, what is the frequency and duration?
- How long does it take for your headaches to reach maximal intensity?
- How long do your headaches last?
- When do the headaches tend to occur, and what factors trigger your headaches?
- Where does your pain start, and how does it evolve?
- What is the quality of your pain?
- How severe is your pain?
- Is the pain steady or pulsating (throbbing), or both?
- Are there symptoms that herald the onset of your headache?
- What are they, when do they begin, and how long do they last?
- Are there symptoms that accompany your headaches?
- Do you get nauseated with your headaches?
- Does light and/or noise bother you a lot more when you have a headache than when you do not?
- Do your headaches limit your ability to work, study, or participate in other activities?
- Does anything aggravate your pain (e.g., exertion)?
- Are your headaches getting better or worse or are they about the same?
- What treatments have been used to treat the headaches, both acutely and preventively?
- What helps your pain?
- Is there a family history of headaches?
- What previous testing have you had?
- Do you have other medical or neurologic problems?
- What do you think might be causing your headaches?
- How disabling are your headaches?
- Why are you seeking help now?

From Jankovic J et al: *Bradley and Daroff's neurology in clinical practice,* ed 8, Philadelphia, 2022, Elsevier.

TABLE 1   Treatment of Cluster Headaches

Medication	Dosage and Route Administered	Comments
Acute Treatment		
First-Line		
Sumatriptan	6 mg SQ	
Oxygen	At least 6-12 L/ min	
Second-Line		
Octreotide	100 micrograms SQ	GI symptoms
Metoclopramide	10 mg IV	Dystonic reaction
Discharge Treatment		
Dexamethasone	10 mg IM or IV	Most efficacious dose unknown
Verapamil	240-480 mg/day PO in 2-4 divided doses	May cause constipation, use cautiously if BP or HR are low
Melatonin	10 mg qHS	Well tolerated

From Walls RM et al: *Rosen's emergency medicine, concepts and clinical practice,* ed 10, Philadelphia, 2023, Elsevier.

treatment indefinitely, whereas those with episodic cluster headache may only require prophylaxis for the duration of the cluster period.
- Preventive therapy should begin with verapamil. Alternative treatment options are also listed below.
- Verapamil: Starting daily dose is 240 mg in three divided doses (more effective than extended release), but may be increased up to 960 mg/day. First-degree atrioventricular (AV) block may develop with escalating doses, so ECG should be checked.

- Topiramate: Up to 50 mg bid; can be used as add-on to verapamil.
- Lithium: Start with 300 mg once daily, going up to maintenance dose of 900 to 1200 mg/day, with frequent monitoring and adjustment to maintain therapeutic serum level of 0.4 to 1 mEq/L. Equally effective as verapamil, but with more side effects.
- Galcanezumab: 300 mg monthly during the cluster period.
- Melatonin: 10 mg per night. Evidence is weak and comes from scattered case reports.

- Prednisone: 60 mg/day orally for 1 wk followed by taper; headaches can return during taper.
- Ergotamine tartrate: 3 to 4 mg/day during clusters.
- Greater and lesser occipital nerve blocks (with lidocaine or bupivacaine) and steroid injections (Depo-Medrol, dexamethasone, or triamcinolone) may shorten the cluster period in patients with refractory symptoms. Consensus guidelines from the American Headache Society have been published recently.
- There is emerging evidence for benefit of a sphenopalatine ganglion block that may be available at some centers for both treatment and prophylaxis of cluster attacks.
- Neuromodulation may be considered in patients with persistent symptoms (daily or almost daily attacks for ≥2 yr) despite extensive medication trials. Per the current American Headache Society guidelines, options include sphenopalatine ganglion stimulation (level B evidence: Probably effective), occipital nerve stimulation (insufficient date but probably effective), and hypothalamic deep brain stimulation (level B evidence: Probably ineffective). Patient selection is key.

DISPOSITION
Headache-free periods tend to increase with increasing age.

REFERRAL
Refractory cluster headaches may require referral to a headache specialist.

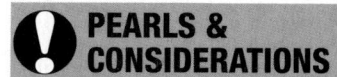

PEARLS & CONSIDERATIONS

COMMENTS
- Cluster headache may be episodic (attacks occurring in bouts lasting up to 1 yr that are separated by symptom-free intervals) and chronic (attacks occurring for ≥1 yr without remission).
- Episodic cluster headache is six times more common than the chronic form.
- Home oxygen therapy is reasonable for cluster headache sufferers.

SUGGESTED READINGS
Available at eBooks.Health.Elsevier.com.

RELATED CONTENT
Cluster Headaches (Patient Information)

AUTHORS: **OMAIR SHAKIL, MD, MPH** and **JOSEPH S. KASS, MD, JD, FAAN**

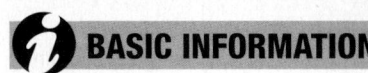 **BASIC INFORMATION**

DEFINITION

Colon cancer (CC) is a malignant neoplasm arising from the luminal surface of the large bowel with locations including the cecum and ascending colon (25% to 30%), transverse colon (10% to 13%), as well as descending and rectosigmoid colon (40% to 42%).

ICD-10CM CODES
C18	Malignant neoplasm of colon
C18.2	Malignant neoplasm of colon, ascending colon
C18.4	Malignant neoplasm of colon, transverse colon
C18.6	Malignant neoplasm of colon, descending colon
C18.7	Malignant neoplasm of colon, sigmoid colon
C19	Malignant neoplasm of rectosigmoid junction

EPIDEMIOLOGY & DEMOGRAPHICS

- Colorectal cancer (CRC) is the fourth most common cancer and the second leading cause of cancer deaths in the U.S. (estimated 153,020 new cases and 52,550 deaths in 2023).[1] Of these, two-thirds of new cases will be colon cancers, accounting for an estimated 106,970 new cases in 2023.
- Distant metastatic disease is present in 18% to 22% of patients at time of diagnosis.
- Worldwide, CRC is the third most common cancer and accounted for an estimated 1.9 million new cases and approximately 900,000 deaths in 2020. The highest incidence is in North America, Australasia, Europe, and South Korea.
- The peak incidence is in the seventh decade of life. The lifetime risk for development is 1 in 17, with 90% of cases occurring after age 50 yr.
- An alarming increase in cases of early onset CRC, defined as diagnosis in patients younger than 50 yr of age, has occurred in the U.S. and other high income countries over the past few decades.[2]

RISK FACTORS (TABLE 1):
- Hereditary polyposis syndromes
- Familial polyposis (high risk)
- Gardner syndrome (high risk)
- Turcot syndrome (high risk)
- Peutz-Jeghers syndrome (low to moderate risk)
- Inflammatory bowel disease (IBD), both ulcerative colitis and Crohn disease
- Family history of "cancer family syndrome"
- Heredofamilial breast cancer and colon carcinoma
- Pelvic irradiation history
- First-degree relatives with colorectal carcinoma
- Age >45 yr

- Dietary factors (diet high in fat or red meat, alcohol use, low vegetable intake)
- Hereditary nonpolyposis colon cancer (HNPCC): Autosomal dominant disorder characterized by early age of onset (mean age 44 yr) and right-sided or proximal CC, synchronous and metachronous CC, mucinous and poorly differentiated CC; accounts for 1% to 5% of all cases; Criteria for diagnosis of HNPCC are summarized in Table 2
- Previous endometrial or ovarian cancer, particularly when diagnosed at an early age

PHYSICAL FINDINGS & CLINICAL PRESENTATION

- Physical examination may be completely unremarkable.
- Palpable abdominal masses may indicate metastasis or complications of cancer (abscess, intussusception, volvulus).
- Abdominal distention and tenderness may be suggestive of colonic obstruction.
- Hepatomegaly may be indicative of hepatic metastasis.

ETIOLOGY

Colon cancer can arise through either of two mutational pathways: Microsatellite instability or chromosomal instability. Germline genetic mutations are the basis of inherited CC syndromes; an accumulation of somatic mutations in a cell is the basis of sporadic CC. Figs. 1 and E2 illustrates the molecular carcinogenesis of CC. Approximately 10% to 15% of CRC lack one or more mismatch repair enzymes (mismatch repair deficient [dMMR]-CRC).

Dx **DIAGNOSIS**

DIFFERENTIAL DIAGNOSIS
- Diverticular disease
- Strictures or adhesions
- IBD
- Infectious or inflammatory lesions
- Arteriovenous malformations
- Metastatic carcinoma
- Extrinsic masses (cysts, abscesses)

WORKUP

The clinical presentation of CC may consist of nonspecific symptoms (weight loss, anorexia, malaise) or of specific symptoms related to mass effect or bleeding. It is useful to divide colon cancer symptoms into those usually associated with the right- or left-sided cancers because the clinical presentation can vary with the location.

- Right side of colon:
  1. Anemia (from chronic blood loss).
  2. Abdominal pain may be present, or the patient may be completely asymptomatic.
  3. Bleeding is often missed because blood is mixed with feces.
  4. Obstruction and constipation are unusual because of the large right-sided lumen and more liquid stools.
- Left side of colon:
  1. Change in bowel habits (constipation, diarrhea, tenesmus, pencil-thin stools).
  2. Bleeding may be detected due to bright red blood coating the surface of the stool.
  3. Intestinal obstruction is frequent because of the small left-sided lumen.

CLASSIFICATION & STAGING (TABLE 3)

The American Joint Committee on Cancer 8th edition classification is below:
1. Confined to the mucosa-submucosa (stage I)
2. Invasion of muscularis propria (stage II)
3. Local node involvement (stage III)
4. Distant metastasis (stage IV)

TNM Classification:

Stage	TNM Classification
I	T_{1-2}, N_0, M_0
II$_A$	T_3, N_0, M_0
II$_B$	T_{4a}, N_0, M_0
II$_C$	T_{4b}, N_0, M_0
III$_A$	$T_{1-2}, N_1, M_0; T_1, N_{2a}, M_0$
III$_B$	$T_{3-4a}, N_1, M_0; T_{2-3}, N_{2a}, M_0; T_{1-2}, N_{2b}, M_0$
III$_C$	$T_{4a}, N_{2a}, M_0; T_{3-4a}, N_{2b}, M_0; T_{4b}, N_{1-2}, M_0$
IV$_A$	T(any), N(any), M_{1a}
IV$_B$	T(any), N(any), M_{1b}
IV$_C$	T(any), N(any), M_{1c}

TABLE 1 Recognized Risk Factors for Colorectal Cancer

Family History
- Colorectal cancer (CRC)
- Inherited syndromes (e.g., familial adenomatous polyposis [FAP])
- Racial and ethnic background (e.g., African American, Ashkenazi Jews)

Personal History
- Age
- Male sex
- Previous colonic polyps or CRC
- History of inflammatory bowel disease
- Diabetes mellitus

Lifestyle
- Obesity
- High consumption of alcohol
- Diet high in red meat and fat, low in fiber

From Niederhuber JE: *Abeloff's clinical oncology*, ed 6, Philadelphia, 2020, Elsevier.

TABLE 2 Criteria for Diagnosis of Hereditary Nonpolyposis Colon Cancer (HNPCC)

Amsterdam Criteria[a]
- At least three relatives have colorectal cancer, and all of the following are present:
  1. One is a first-degree relative (parent, sibling, or child) of the other two
  2. At least two successive generations are involved
  3. At least one relative had colorectal cancer when he or she was younger than 50
  4. Familial adenomatous polyposis has been excluded

Revised Bethesda Guidelines[b]

(Indicates tumors to select for microsatellite instability testing)

- Colorectal cancer in a patient younger than 50 yr
- A second synchronous or metachronous colorectal cancer or cancer associated with HNPCC
- Presence of high-level microsatellite instability histologically in a patient younger than 60 yr
- One or more first-degree relatives with either colorectal cancer or HNPCC-associated tumor diagnosed at younger than 50 yr
- Colorectal cancer in two or more first- or second-degree relatives with HNPCC-related tumors at any age

Either all of the Amsterdam criteria or one of the Bethesda criteria is used to identify an individual at risk of HNPCC

- HNPCC-associated tumors include endometrial, gastric, ovarian, pancreatic, ureter, renal pelvis, biliary tract, small bowel, and brain

[a]Vasen HF et al: New clinical criteria for hereditary nonpolyposis colorectal cancer (HNPCC, Lynch syndrome) proposed by the International Collaborative group on HNPCC, *Gastroenterology* 116:1453-1456, 1999.
[b]Umar A et al: Revised Bethesda Guidelines for hereditary nonpolyposis colorectal cancer (Lynch syndrome) and microsatellite instability, *J Natl Cancer Inst* 96:261-268, 2004.
From Niederhuber JE: *Abeloff's clinical oncology,* ed 6, Philadelphia, 2020, Elsevier.

LABORATORY TESTS

- Positive fecal occult blood test (FOBT): Many primary care physicians use single digital FOBT as their primary screening test. Single FOBT has low specificity for detecting human hemoglobin, is a poor screening method (sensitivity, 4.9%), and is inappropriate by itself since negative results do not decrease the odds of advanced neoplasia. The American College of Gastroenterology recommends the fecal immunochemical test (FIT), which measures intact human globin protein (as opposed to heme) in the stool and detects more advanced adenomas than FOBT.
- Fecal DNA testing is a screening method that detects colonic cells shed into the fecal stream that possess specific genetic or epigenetic changes. The technique has a reported sensitivity of 97% and a specificity of 90% for CRC stages I to III. In trials involving asymptomatic persons at average risk, multitarget stool DNA testing detects significantly more cancers than FIT but has more false-positive results. High cost and rate of false positives are the main obstacles inhibiting broader adoption of fecal DNA testing.

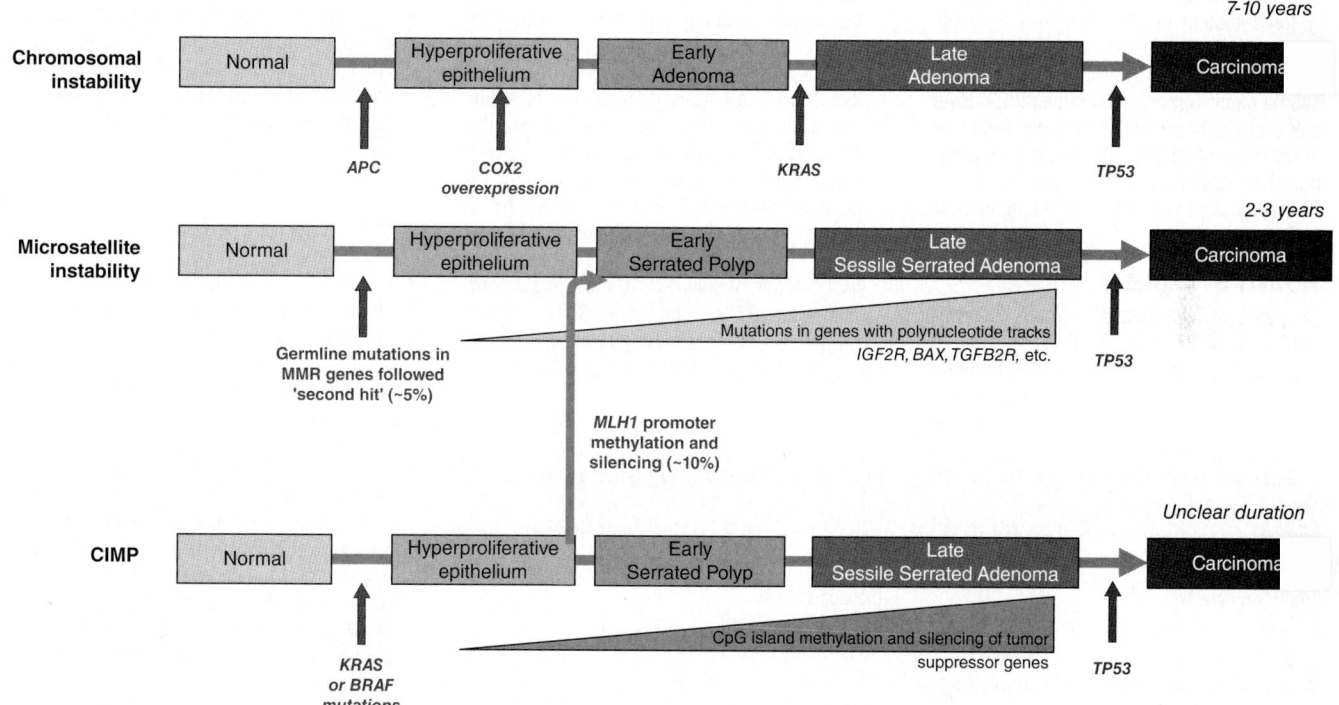

FIG. 1 Multistep models of colorectal cancer based on underlying genetic instability. As shown on the left, there are three major pathways: chromosomal instability *(top pathway)*, microsatellite instability *(middle pathway)*, and the CpG island methylation, or *CIMP (lower pathway)*. The progression from normal colonic epithelium to carcinoma is associated with the acquisition of several genetic and epigenetic alterations. In the chromosomal instability pathway *(top pathway)*, these alterations include the early loss of *APC*, followed by activation of oncogenes (e.g., *KRAS*) through a point mutation and inactivation of tumor suppressor genes (e.g., *APC*, *TP53*) through a point mutation or deletion. An increasing aggregate number of mutations can be correlated with progression from early benign adenoma to cancer, as reflected by analysis of polyps by size. In the microsatellite instability model *(middle pathway)*, mutations in DNA mismatch repair *(MMR)* genes create a mutator phenotype in which mutations accumulate in specific target genes. Tumors develop much more rapidly through this pathway than through the chromosomal instability pathway (2-3 yr compared to 7-10 yr). Germline mutations in *MMR* genes account for 5% of all colorectal tumors. In the *CIMP* pathway *(lower pathway)*, the initiating event is hypothesized to be a *BRAF* or *KRAS* activating mutation that somehow triggers extensive CpG island methylation, particularly of gene promoters, resulting in gene silencing. Among the potential gene targets is *MLH1*, a component of the MMR pathway, and when silenced as part of the *CIMP* pathway, the tumor evolves along a similar molecular as microsatellite unstable cancers (MSI-H). Sporadic *MLH1* methylation and silencing accounts for nearly 10% of sporadic colorectal cancers. Alternatively, serrated adenomas arising in the *CIMP* pathway can undergo a pathway similar to that of chromosomal instability to become microsatellite stable tumors. (From Feldman M et al: *Sleisenger and Fordtran's gastrointestinal and liver disease,* ed 11, Philadelphia, 2021, Elsevier.)

TABLE 3 World Health Organization Classification of Colorectal Carcinoma

- Adenocarcinoma
- Cribriform comedo-type adenocarcinoma
- Medullary carcinoma
- Micropapillary carcinoma
- Mucinous adenocarcinoma
- Serrated adenocarcinoma
- Signet ring cell carcinoma
- Adenosquamous carcinoma
- Spindle cell carcinoma
- Squamous cell carcinoma
- Undifferentiated carcinoma
- Neuroendocrine carcinoma (NEC):
  1. Large NEC
  2. Small NEC
- Mixed adenoneuroendocrine carcinoma

From Niederhuber JE: *Abeloff's clinical oncology*, ed 6, Philadelphia, 2020, Elsevier.

- Molecular markers (Table 4) including abnormal DNA from cancerous cells can be detected in stool. FIT combined with stool DNA test (FIT-DNA) has been approved by the FDA for colorectal screening. One study showed that one-time FIT-DNA had a higher sensitivity for detection of CRC than one-time FIT alone (92.3% vs. 73.8%), but specificity was lower (86.6% vs. 94.9%).[3]
- Plasma carcinoembryonic antigen (CEA) level is not useful for screening because it can be increased in nonmalignant conditions (smoking, IBD, alcoholic liver disease). A normal CEA result does not exclude the diagnosis of CRC.

IMAGING STUDIES

- Colonoscopy with biopsy (primary assessment tool): The 2023 American College of Physicians (ACP) guidelines recommend screening colonoscopy beginning at age 50, to be repeated every 10 yr in average-risk patients. Screening is recommended in African Americans beginning at age 45 yr. Persons with only one first-degree relative with CRC or advanced adenomas diagnosed at 60 yr or older may be screened as at average risk. The ACP recommends that clinicians stop screening in adults over age 75 yr or in adults with a life expectancy of <10 yr. The 2021 U.S. Preventive Services Task Force (USPSTF) guidelines expanded routine colonoscopy screening to between ages 45 and 75 yr while not routinely recommending it in persons older than 75 yr, and not recommending at all in persons older than 85 yr. If persons between the ages of 75 and 85 yr have never undergone screening, the decision about screening should be individualized according to health status.[4] In addition, the American College of Gastroenterology (ACG) and the American Cancer Society (ACS) both recommend expanded screening eligibility starting at age 45 in routine-risk patients.[5] Table 5 describes CRC screening and surveillance recommendations.
- Computed tomography colonoscopy (CTC) and virtual colonoscopy (VC) use helical (spiral) CT scanning to generate a 2D or 3D virtual colorectal image (Fig. E3). CTC does not require sedation, but, like optical colonoscopy, it requires some bowel preparation (either bowel cathartics or ingestion of iodinated contrast medium with meals during the 48 h before CT) and air insufflation. It also involves substantial exposure to radiation. In addition, patients with lesions detected by VC will require traditional colonoscopy. Compared with colonoscopy, CTC sensitivity for detection of polyps >10 mm ranges from 70% to 96%, and specificity ranges from 72% to 96%. CTC has replaced double-contrast barium enema as the radiographic screening alternative when patients decline colonoscopy.
- Capsule endoscopy allows visualization of the colonic mucosa but is not recommended as a screening procedure because its sensitivity for detecting colonic lesions is low compared with colonoscopy.
- CT scanning of the abdomen (Fig. E4), pelvis, and chest assists in preoperative staging.
- PET scanning (Fig. E5) can display functional information and is accurate in the detection of primary cancer and distant metastases. Colonography composed of a combined modality of PET and CT is a newer diagnostic modality that can provide whole-body tumor staging in a single session.

Rx TREATMENT

GENERAL Rx

- Surgical resection is the definitive and curative upfront treatment for stages I to III CC. Selected patients (high-risk stage II, all stage III) are recommended to receive adjuvant chemotherapy. Microsatellite instability can be used alongside clinicopathologic factors in stage II and III CC to guide adjuvant therapy (Fig. 6).
- The standard chemotherapy regimen for adjuvant therapy of resected CC is the combination of oxaliplatin with 5-fluorouracil (FOLFOX) or capecitabine (CAPOX) for a period of 3 to 6 mo. Older patients (>75 yr) and patients with significant comorbidities have more toxicity with combination chemotherapy; treatment with single-agent fluoropyrimidine therapy is a reasonable option in these patients.
- In stage II CC, adjuvant chemotherapy provides a modest improvement in overall survival by 3% to 4%, with current 5-yr survival rates in the 80% range. As such, current guidelines recommend consideration of adjuvant chemotherapy only in high-risk stage II patients.
- In stage III CC, the magnitude of survival benefit is significantly higher with adjuvant combination chemotherapy with 5-yr overall survival rates in the 70% range with wide variation in the subgroups. More recent data have revealed that low-risk stage III CC patients may have equivalent survival with adjuvant multiagent chemotherapy of only 3 mo in duration.
- Recently, preoperative combination chemotherapy for operable stage III CC has demonstrated marked histopathologic down-staging, fewer incomplete resections, and better 2-yr disease control in a randomized controlled setting. Also, histologic regression after chemotherapy strongly predicts a lower postoperative recurrence risk and can guide postoperative therapy.[6,7]
- Circulating tumor DNA levels have been utilized to make informed treatment decisions in patients with stage II CC. A ctDNA-positive result after surgery prompted chemotherapy use while patients who were ctDNA-negative

TABLE 4 Molecular Biomarkers Used in Clinical Standard-of-Care Decision Making in Colorectal Cancer

Biomarker	Purpose
APC mutation detection	Diagnosis of FAP
MMR protein expression *(MSH2, MLH1, MSH6, PMS2)*	Diagnosis of HNPCC
MSI analysis	
MMR mutation detection *(MSH2, MLH1, MSH6, PMS2)*	
BRAF mutation detection	
MYH mutation detection	Diagnosis of MYH-associated polyposis
LKB1, SMAD4, BMPR1A, PTEN mutation detection	Diagnosis of hamartomatous polyp syndromes
KRAS mutation analysis	Molecular stratification for treatment with EGFR inhibitors
BRAF mutation analysis	
Thymidylate synthase protein expression	Identification of response to 5-FU
MSI	Identification of response to 5-FU
Gene expression signature	Prognostication
PD-1	Stratification for response to PD-L1 blockade

EGFR, Epidermal growth factor receptor; *FAP*, familial adenomatous polyposis; *5-FU*, 5-fluorouracil; *HNPCC*, hereditary nonpolyposis colorectal cancer; *MMR*, mismatch repair; *MSI*, microsatellite instability.
From Niederhuber JE: *Abeloff's clinical oncology*, ed 6, Philadelphia, 2020, Elsevier.

TABLE 5 Colorectal Cancer (CRC) Screening and Surveillance Recommendations*

Indication	Recommendations
Average risk	ACP guidelines: Beginning at age 50 yr**: Colonoscopy every 10 yr; computed tomographic colonography every 5 yr; flexible sigmoidoscopy every 5 yr; double-contrast barium enema every 5 yr; stool blood testing annually or stool; DNA testing acceptable but not preferred USPSTF, ACS, and ACG guidelines: Starting above recommendations for testing beginning at age 45 yr
One or two first-degree relatives with CRC at any age or adenoma at age <60 yr	Colonoscopy every 5 yr beginning at age 40 yr, or 10 yr younger than earliest diagnosis, whichever comes first
Hereditary nonpolyposis CRC	Genetic counseling and screening.[†] Colonoscopy every 1-2 yr beginning at age 25 yr and then yearly after age 40 yr[‡]
Familial adenomatous polyposis and variants	Genetic counseling and testing.[†] Flexible sigmoidoscopy yearly beginning at puberty[‡]
Personal history of CRC	Colonoscopy within 1 yr of curative resection; repeat at 3 yr and then every 5 yr if normal
Personal history of colorectal adenoma	Colonoscopy every 3-5 yr after removal of all index polyps
Inflammatory bowel disease	Colonoscopy every 1-2 yr beginning after 8 yr of pancolitis or after 15 yr if only left-sided disease

ACG, American College of Gastroenterology; *ACP,* American College of Physicians; *ACS,* American Cancer Society; *DNA,* deoxyribonucleic acid; *USPSTF,* U.S. Preventative Services Task Force.
*Recommendations proposed by the American Cancer Society and U.S. Multi-Society Task Force on Colorectal Cancer; recommendations for average-risk patients also endorsed by the American College of Radiology.
**Screening colonoscopy at age 45 recommended by USPSTF.
[†]Whenever possible, affected relatives should be tested first because of potential false-negative results.
[‡]Screening recommendation for individuals with positive or indeterminate tests as well as for those who refuse genetic testing.

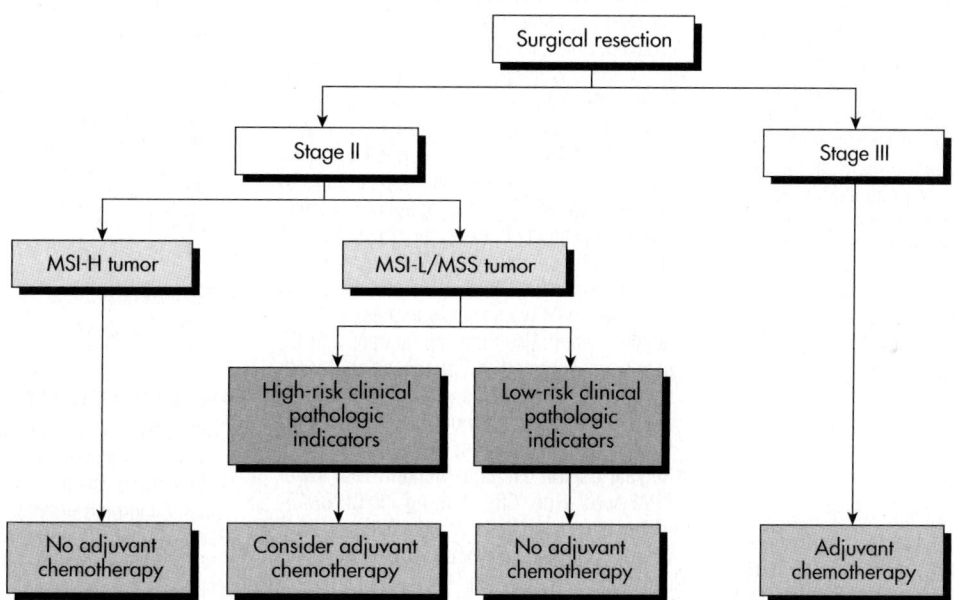

FIG. 6 Proposed algorithm for using microsatellite instability *(MSI)* **alongside clinicopathologic factors in stages II and III colorectal cancer.** ASCO guidelines: Inadequate samples nodes, T4 lesions, perforation, poorly differentiated histology. *MSI-H,* High-level microsatellite instability; *MSI-L/MSS,* low-level microsatellite instability/microsatellite stability. (From Niederhuber JE: *Abeloff's clinical oncology,* ed 6, Philadelphia, 2020, Elsevier.)

were not treated. The results showed that a ctDNA-guided approach reduced adjuvant chemotherapy use without compromising recurrence-free survival.[8]

- The outlook for patients with metastatic and relapsed CC has improved dramatically in the past few years. Median overall survival in patients with unresectable metastatic CC now is in the 30- to 36-mo range with modern chemotherapeutic regimens. In patients with limited, resectable metastases in sites such as the liver, the 5-yr median overall survival is in the 50% range.

- Chemotherapy agents used in the metastatic setting include 5-fluorouracil (5-FU), capecitabine,

irinotecan, oxaliplatin, and mitomycin. Chemotherapy regimens using a combination of antimetabolite (5-FU or capecitabine) in combination with either oxaliplatin or irinotecan form the backbone of systemic chemotherapy.

- Molecularly targeted therapy against the epidermal growth factor receptor (EGFR) and the angiogenesis pathway are used in combination with the chemotherapy backbone in metastatic CC. Antiangiogenic agents (bevacizumab, aflibercept, and ramucirumab) and the EGFR receptor blockers (cetuximab and panitumumab) are utilized in combination with standard chemotherapy regimens in metastatic CC patients.

- Among patients with refractory metastatic colorectal cancer, phase 3 trials have shown that treatment with trifluridine-tripiracil (FTD-TPI) plus bevacizumab resulted in longer survival than FTD-TPI alone.[9]

- The oral multitargeted kinase inhibitor regorafenib and the oral antimetabolite drug TAS-102 provide modest survival benefit in patients who have failed standard chemotherapy.

- Patients with tumors harboring BRAF mutations can now have improved survival with the use of combination molecularly targeted therapy consisting of encorafenib, binimetinib, and cetuximab.[10]

- The liver is generally the initial and most common site of CC metastases. Resection of liver-limited metastases followed by systemic combination chemotherapy is curative in more than 30% of selected patients. Metastasectomy of limited pulmonary metastases can also be considered in selected cases.
- Unresectable multiple liver metastases are often approached by locoregional therapeutic approaches such as transarterial chemoembolization, selective internal radiation therapy using yttrium-90 brachytherapy, or hepatic arterial infusional chemotherapy.
- In patients with pathologically confirmed microsatellite instability in their cancers (see Fig. 6), the checkpoint inhibitors (pembrolizumab, nivolumab) are effective options after failure of standard therapies and have been recently approved in this setting. Recent data have shown that upfront treatment with pembrolizumab is superior to conventional chemotherapy and results in doubling of progression-free survival in newly diagnosed patients with microsatellite instability-driven cancers.[11] Smaller studies have shown benefit with dual immunotherapy combination of nivolumab and ipilimumab. A phase 3 trial combining the KRAS G12C inhibitor sotorasib with panitumumab, an epidermal growth factor receptor (EGFR) inhibitor in patients with chemorefractory metastatic colorectal cancer resulted in longer progression-free survival than standard treatment.[12]
- Reviews of randomized systemic therapy trials in metastatic CC have demonstrated that right-sided cancers are associated with shorter overall survival when compared with left-sided cancers.

CHRONIC Rx

Follow-up is indicated with:
- Physician visits with a focus on clinical and disease-related history, directed physical examination, coordination of follow-up, and counseling every 3 to 4 mo for the first 3 yr and then every 6 mo for 2 yr.
- Colonoscopy at end of first yr, then after 3 yr, and subsequently every 5 yr.
- Malignant potential and surveillance of colonic polyps is summarized in Table E6.

- Baseline CEA level, if elevated, can be used after surgery as a measure of completeness of tumor resection. It is used to monitor tumor recurrence and is obtained every 3 to 6 mo for up to 5 yr.

DISPOSITION

The 5-yr survival rate varies with the stage of the carcinoma:

TNM Stage	5-yr Survival Rate (%)
I	>90
II$_{A-C}$	60-85
III$_{A-C}$	25-65
IV	5-10

- Overall, the 5-yr disease-free survival rate for resected CC has increased from 50% to 63% during the past two decades.
- Pathologic, molecular, and clinical features that may affect prognosis in patients with colon cancer are summarized in Table 7.
- High-frequency microsatellite instability (MSI-H) in CC is independently predictive of a relatively favorable outcome and reduces the likelihood of metastases.
- In patients with high-risk stage II and with stage III CC, there is improved 5-yr survival among patients treated with adjuvant chemotherapy.
- Expression patterns of microRNA are systemically altered in colon adenocarcinomas. High miR-21 expression is associated with poor survival and poor therapeutic outcome.
- The optimal timing from surgery to initiation of adjuvant chemotherapy is 4 to 8 wk. A longer time to initiation of adjuvant chemotherapy is associated with worse survival rates.
- Regular aspirin use after the diagnosis of CC has been reported to be associated with lower risk for CRC-specific and overall mortality, especially among individuals with tumors that overexpress cyclooxygenase-2. Regular aspirin use is associated with lower BRAF-wild type CRC but not with BRAF-mutated cancer risk. All aspirin doses starting with 75 mg daily had similar effects on CRC incidence and mortality.[13]

REFERRAL

Multidisciplinary referral to colorectal surgery or surgical oncology, medical oncology, radiation oncology

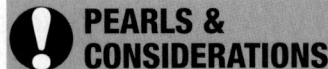

PEARLS & CONSIDERATIONS

COMMENTS

- Metastases of tumor cells to regional lymph nodes is the single most important prognostic factor in patients with colon cancer.
- Decreased fat intake to 30% of total energy intake, increased fiber through fruit and vegetable consumption may reduce CRC risk.
- Chemoprophylaxis with aspirin (81 mg/day) reduces the incidence of colorectal adenomas in persons at risk.[11]
- The National Cancer Institute has published consensus guidelines for universal screening for HNPCC in patients with newly diagnosed CRC. Tumors in mutation carriers of HNPCC typically exhibit microsatellite instability, a characteristic phenotype caused by expansion or contraction of short nucleotide repeat sequences. These guidelines (Bethesda Guidelines) are useful for selective patients for microsatellite instability testing. Screening patients with newly diagnosed CRC for HNPCC is cost effective, especially if the benefits to their immediate relatives are considered.
- The use of either annual or biennial FOBT significantly reduces the incidence of CRC.
- The detection of mutations in the *APC* gene from stool samples is a promising new modality for early detection of colorectal neoplasms.

REFERENCES

Available at eBooks.Health.Elsevir.com.

RELATED CONTENT

Colon Cancer (Patient Information)
Familial Adenomatous Polyposis and Gardner Syndrome (Related Key Topic)
Lynch Syndrome (Related Key Topic)
Peutz-Jeghers Syndrome and Other Polyposis Syndromes (Related Key Topic)

AUTHOR: **RITESH RATHORE, MD**

TABLE 7 Pathologic, Molecular, and Clinical Features that May Affect Prognosis in Patients with Colorectal Cancer

Feature or Marker	Effect on Prognosis
Pathologic	
Surgical-Pathologic Stage	
Depth of colon wall penetration	Increased penetration diminishes prognosis
Number of regional nodes involved by tumor	Greater number of involved nodes diminishes prognosis
Positive circumferential resection margin	Diminishes prognosis
Residual tumor after resection	Diminishes prognosis
Isolated microscopic tumor cells in regional lymph nodes	May diminish prognosis
Tumor Morphology and Histology	
Degree of differentiation	Well-differentiated tumors have a better prognosis than poorly differentiated lesions
Mucinous (colloid) or signet-ring cell histology	Diminishes prognosis
Scirrhous histology	Diminishes prognosis
Invasion	
Venous	Diminishes prognosis
Lymphatic	Diminishes prognosis
Perineural	Diminishes prognosis
Other Features	
Local inflammation and immunologic reaction	Improves prognosis
Tumor morphology	Polypoid or exophytic tumors have a better prognosis than ulcerating or infiltrating lesions
Tumor DNA content	Increased DNA content (aneuploidy) diminishes prognosis
Tumor size	No effect in most studies
Molecular	
Loss of heterozygosity at chromosome 18q (DCC, DPC4)	Diminishes prognosis
Loss of heterozygosity at chromosome 17p (TP53)	Diminishes prognosis
Loss of heterozygosity at chromosome 8p	Diminishes prognosis
Increased labeling index for p21WAF/CIP1 protein	Improves prognosis
Microsatellite instability	Improves prognosis
Mutation in BAX gene	Diminishes prognosis
Mutation in K-ras codon 12 or 13 or NRAS	Lack of response to anti-EGFR therapy
Mutation in BRAF (BRAF V600E)	Diminishes prognosis
Mutation in PI3K (PIK3CA)	Improved response to aspirin chemoprevention
Clinical	
Diagnosis in asymptomatic patients	May improve prognosis
Duration of symptoms	No demonstrated effect
Rectal bleeding as a presenting symptom	Improves prognosis
Colon obstruction	Diminishes prognosis
Colon perforation	Diminishes prognosis
Tumor location	Prognosis may be better for colonic than for rectal tumors Prognosis may be better for left colonic than right colonic tumors
Age <30 yr	Diminishes prognosis
High preoperative CEA level	Diminishes prognosis
Distant metastases	Markedly diminishes prognosis
Tumor regression grade	Complete eradication of tumor after preoperative therapy may improve prognosis

EGFR, EGF receptor.
From Feldman M et al: *Sleisenger and Fordtran's gastrointestinal and liver disease,* ed 11, Philadelphia, 2021, Elsevier.

BASIC INFORMATION

DEFINITION

Concussion is a mild traumatic brain injury (TBI) manifesting with self-limited symptoms at the less severe end of the brain injury spectrum.

The Fifth International Conference on Concussion in Sport (2016) defines sports-related concussion as *a traumatic brain injury induced by biomechanical forces* caused by a direct blow to the head, face, neck, or elsewhere on the body with an impulsive force transmitted to the head. (However, this definition is also applicable to concussion in general.) This injury results in the rapid onset of short-lived, spontaneously resolving neurologic impairment. In some cases, signs and symptoms evolve over several minutes to hours. Although neuropathologic changes may result, the acute clinical signs and symptoms largely reflect a functional disturbance rather than brain structural injury, and therefore no abnormality is seen on standard structural neuroimaging studies. A range of clinical signs and symptoms may develop that may or may not involve loss of consciousness. Resolution of the clinical and cognitive features typically follows a sequential course, but in some cases symptoms may be prolonged. The clinical signs and symptoms cannot be explained by drug, alcohol, or medication use, other injuries (such as cervical injuries, peripheral vestibular dysfunction, etc.), or other comorbidities (e.g., psychological factors or coexisting medical conditions).

SYNONYM

Mild traumatic brain injury (mTBI)

ICD-10CM CODES
S06.0	Concussion
S06.0X0A	Concussion without loss of consciousness, initial encounter
S06.0X0D	Concussion without loss of consciousness, subsequent encounter
S06.0X0S	Concussion without loss of consciousness, sequela
S06.0X1A	Concussion with loss of consciousness of 30 min or less, initial encounter
S06.0X9A	Concussion with loss of consciousness of unspecified duration, initial encounter

EPIDEMIOLOGY & DEMOGRAPHICS

INCIDENCE: 3.8 million sports- and recreation-related concussions occur each year in the U.S. It is estimated that as many as 50% of concussions go unreported.

PREVALENCE: Each year, U.S. emergency departments treat an estimated 135,000 sports- and recreation-related TBIs, including concussions, among children ages 5 to 18.

PREDOMINANT SEX & AGE:
- Children and teens are more likely to get a concussion and take longer to recover than adults.

- Limited studies have shown that in sports that are played by both men and women, women are at more risk of sustaining a concussion. In males the incidence is highest in football, followed by hockey, and in females, soccer. Player contact is the most common cause.

RISK FACTORS:
- Participating in high-impact sports and recreational activities
- Previous history of concussion
- Athletes with a body mass index (BMI) >27 kg/m² and those who train <3 h/wk
- Individuals who sustain a sports-related concussion and continue playing immediately after the injury require nearly twice as much time to recover as those who are removed immediately
- Military personnel

PHYSICAL FINDINGS & CLINICAL PRESENTATION

Common neurologic examination findings include nystagmus, changes in gait, balance abnormalities, truncal ataxia, gait ataxia, increased posture sway, saccadic eye movements with smooth pursuit, memory deficits, amnesia, disorientation, and emotional lability (Table 1).

ETIOLOGY

- Occurs when rotational or angular acceleration forces are applied to the brain, resulting in shear strain of the underlying neural elements, including altered autonomic function and impaired control of cerebral blood flow
- May be associated with a blow to the skull; however, direct impact to the head is not required

Dx DIAGNOSIS

DIFFERENTIAL DIAGNOSIS

- Migraine
- Cervical strain
- Posttraumatic vestibular injury

WORKUP

- There is no definitive diagnostic test for concussion. A standardized protocol (Table 2) can help first responders identify more subtle mental status changes. Physical exam should

TABLE 1 Common Symptoms of Sports-Related Concussion

Somatic	Cognitive	Neurobehavioral
Headache	Disorientation/confusion,	Lethargy/fatigue
Dizziness	Feeling "in a fog" or "hazy"	Drowsiness
Photophobia	Lack of attention/focus	Hypersomnia/insomnia
Phonophobia	Distractibility	Sadness/depression
Blurred vision/diplopia	Memory deficits	Anger
Nausea		Nervousness/irritability
		"Not feeling right"

Physical	Cognitive	Neurobehavioral
Loss of consciousness	Disorientation/confusion	Personality changes
Loss of awareness	Memory impairment	Irritability/violent outburst
Blank stare/dazed look	Slowed reaction time or processing speed	Depression
Seizure	Attention deficit	Emotional lability
Vomiting	Impaired comprehension	
Dysarthria/slurred speech	Problems with concentration	
Ataxia/discoordination		

From Jankovic J et al: *Bradley and Daroff's neurology in clinical practice,* ed 8, Philadelphia, 2022, Elsevier.

TABLE 2 Standardized Assessment of Concussion

Task	Possible Score
Orientation	
Month, date, day of week, year, time (1 point for each correct answer)	0-5
Immediate Memory	
Patient repeats a 5-word list spoken by examiner; 3 trials (1 point for each word correctly remembered)	0-15
Concentration	
Digits backward; 3-, 4-, 5-, and 6-digit strings (1 point for each digit string correctly repeated backward)	0-4
Months of the year in reverse order (1 point for repeating backward in correct sequence)	0-1
Delayed Memory Recall	
Patient repeats the 5 words from Immediate Memory test (1 point for each word correctly recalled)	0-5
TOTAL SCORE	0-30

From Goldman L, Shafer AI: *Goldman-Cecil medicine,* ed 26, Philadelphia, 2020, Elsevier.

TABLE 3 Grading of Concussion

Grade	Cantu System	American Academy of Neurology System
1 (Mild)	A. PTA <30 min B. No LOC	A. Transient confusion B. No LOC C. Symptoms resolved in <15 min
2 (Moderate)	A. LOC <5 min, or B. PTA >30 min	As above, but symptoms last >15 min (still *no* LOC) (PTA is common)
3 (Severe)	A. LOC ≥5 min, or B. PTA ≥24 h	*Any* LOC, whether brief (seconds) or prolonged

LOC, Loss of consciousness; *PTA,* posttraumatic amnesia.
From Jankovic J et al: *Bradley and Daroff's neurology in clinical practice,* ed 8, Philadelphia, 2022, Elsevier.

include smooth pursuits (examiner moves finger horizontally across field of vision), saccades, gaze instability, near point of convergence, accommodation, and balance. Patients with loss of consciousness or post-traumatic convulsive seizures should be transported to the emergency department. Concussions are graded according to the severity of symptoms: Presence or absence of loss of consciousness and time (more or less than 15 min) for resolution of symptoms (Table 3).

- Sideline assessment:
  1. No athlete with a suspected concussion should return to play that day.
  2. Neurologic assessment using a standardized tool, such as SCAT-3 (Sports Concussion Assessment Tool), which includes the BESS (Balance Error Scoring System), Maddocks Questions, and SAC (Standardized Assessment of Concussion).
  3. Monitor for deterioration; no athlete should be left alone.
- Office assessment:
  1. History focused on current symptoms. Consider using Postconcussion Symptom Checklist. According to the Consensus Statement on Concussion in Sport issued by the Fifth International Conference on Concussion in Sport, the following domains should be investigated when considering a diagnosis of sports-related concussion. A problem in one domain in the proper historical context should raise concern for sports-related concussion.
     a. Symptoms: Somatic (e.g., headache), cognitive (e.g., feeling like in a fog), and/or emotional symptoms (e.g., lability)
     b. Physical signs (e.g., loss of consciousness, amnesia, neurologic deficit)
     c. Balance impairment (e.g., gait unsteadiness)
     d. Behavioral changes (e.g., irritability)
     e. Cognitive impairment (e.g., slowed reaction times)
     f. Sleep/wake disturbance (e.g., somnolence, drowsiness)
  2. Neurologic exam
     a. Gait/balance testing. Consider the Balance Error Scoring System (BESS)
     b. Cerebellar coordination: Finger-to-nose testing (tested on SCAT-3 card)
     c. Convergence of Accommodative Sufficiency

- Neurocognitive testing:
  1. Computer-based programs, such as ImPACT, ANAM, CogSport
  2. Neuropsychiatric testing administered by a neuropsychologist
- When used in combination, symptom assessment, balance assessment, and neurocognitive testing provide a sensitivity of >90% for the identification of concussion.
- Consider the Buffalo Concussion Treadmill Test, which identifies physiologic dysfunction in concussion, rules out other diagnoses, and can quantify a safe level of activity in concussion recovery.

IMAGING STUDIES

- Computed tomography (CT) imaging is not universally indicated and should be considered on an individual basis. It is indicated in any athlete with a rapidly changing or focal neurologic exam or with a suspected intracranial bleed.
- Consider following PECARN guidelines.

Rx TREATMENT

ACUTE GENERAL Rx

- Removal from game
- Physical rest
  1. No return to play until asymptomatic for at least 24 h.
  2. Follow the return-to-play guidelines (Table 4).
  3. There is no evidence to support prolonged rest in concussed athletes longer than several weeks (see "Postconcussive Syndrome"). Prolonged inactivity after concussion has been linked to negative health effect. Light aerobic activity that avoids risk for reinjury decreases concussion symptoms, suggesting that low-level physical activity postconcussion might be beneficial.
- Cognitive rest to limit symptoms
  1. Limit screen time to less than 2 h/day.
  2. Academic accommodations at school. Consider return to school for half-days when tolerating 2 h of work at home.
  3. Encourage good sleep hygiene.

CHRONIC Rx

See "Postconcussive Syndrome."

DISPOSITION

- Physiologic recovery is slower than symptomatic recovery. Protocols involving a symptom-free waiting period before return to play are warranted. Table 4 summarizes recommendations on returning to play after a concussion. CDC protocols for managing return to activities after concussion are described in Table 5. Physical and cognitive rest are the cornerstones of initial concussion management, with

TABLE 4 Guidelines for the Management of Sport-Related Concussion*

Symptoms	First Concussion	Second Concussion
Grade 1: No loss of consciousness, transient confusion, resolution of symptoms and mental abnormalities in <15 min[†]	Remove from play Examine at 5-min intervals May return to play if symptoms disappear and results of mental function examination return to normal within 15 min	Allow return to play after 1 wk if there are no symptoms at rest or with exertion
Grade 2: As above but with mental symptoms for ≥15 min	Remove from play and disallow play for rest of day Examine for signs of intracranial lesion at sidelines and obtain further examination by a trained person on same day Allow return to play after 1 wk if neurologic examination is nonconcerning	Allow return to play after 2-wk period of no symptoms at rest or with exertion Remove from play for season if imaging shows abnormality
Grade 3: Any loss of consciousness	Perform thorough neurologic examination in hospital and obtain imaging studies when indicated Assess neurologic status daily until postconcussive symptoms resolve or stabilize Remove from play for 1 wk if loss of consciousness lasts seconds or for 2 wk if it lasts minutes; must be asymptomatic at rest and with exertion to return to play	Withhold from play until symptoms have been absent for at least 1 mo

*These guidelines reflect consensus opinion, are not evidence-based, and are under revision. Adapted from the American Academy of Neurology guidelines.
[†]Testing includes orientation, repetition of digit strings, recall of word list at 0 and 5 min, recall of recent game events, recall of current events, pupillary symmetry, finger-to-nose and tandem-gait tests, Romberg test, and provocative testing for symptoms with a 4-yd (3.5-m) sprint, five push-ups, and five knee bends.
From Jankovic J et al: *Bradley and Daroff's neurology in clinical practice,* ed 8, Philadelphia, 2022, Elsevier.

TABLE 5 Protocol for Return to Sport after Concussion

Return-to-play protocol follows a stepwise progress with each step taking ≥24 h. The athlete should continue to the next level if asymptomatic at the current level.
1. Back to regular activities such as school.
2. Light aerobic exercise such as walking or stationary cycling; no weight lifting.
3. Moderate activity such as jogging, brief running, moderate-intensity stationary biking, moderate-intensity weightlifting (less than their prior weightlifting routine).
4. Heavy, noncontact physical activity such as sprinting/running, regular weightlifting routine, noncontact sport specific drills.
5. Practice and full contact.
6. Competition.

From Centers for Disease Control and Prevention: Managing return to activities, 2018. Available at https://www.cdc.gov/headsup/providers/return_to_activities.html.

subsequent gradual return to school and physical activities. Repeated concussions, especially within days or weeks, carry a significant risk of permanent brain injury (second impact syndrome).

- If concussion symptoms occur with activity at one level, the athlete should stop the activity, rest until symptoms resolve, and then restart his or her progression at the level that did not elicit symptoms.
- There are no evidence-based guidelines for disqualifying or retiring an athlete from sport after a concussion. Each case should be individually considered.

REFERRAL

Referral to sports-medicine physician, neuropsychology, or concussion center is indicated if there is concern about the timing of return to contact or collision sport. Referral is also indicated in patients with preexisting neurologic disorders such as migraines, depression, or anxiety and in those who have had multiple concussions.

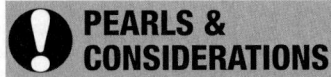

PEARLS & CONSIDERATIONS

PREVENTION
- Preparticipation evaluations for all athletes.
- Preparticipation neurocognitive and balance testing to establish a baseline.
- There is currently no evidence to support the use of concussion prevention headbands or mouth guards.
- Spontaneous recovery from acute concussion ranges from 1 to 2 wk in adults and up to 4 wk in adolescents.

PATIENT & FAMILY EDUCATION
Centers for Disease Control and Prevention: https://www.cdc.gov/TraumaticBrainInjury/get_the_facts.html.

RELATED CONTENT
Concussion (Patient Information)
Postconcussion Syndrome (Related Key Topic)
Traumatic Brain Injury (Related Key Topic)

SUGGESTED READINGS
Available at eBooks.Health.Elsevier.com.

AUTHOR: **JOSEPH S. KASS, MD, JD, FAAN**

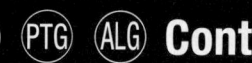

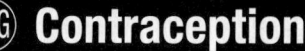

C

Diseases and Disorders

I

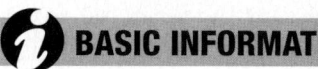

DEFINITION

Contraception refers to the various modalities that a sexually active person uses to prevent pregnancy. These options can be either medical or nonmedical and used by all genders. There are numerous options, and this chapter should not be considered to be fully comprehensive of every option. The options are as follows:
- No contraception (unprotected intercourse); failure rate 85% both typical use and perfect use
- Abstinence: Failure rate 0%
- Withdrawal: Failure rate with perfect use, 4%; with typical use, 19%
- Rhythm method (natural family planning)
  1. Failure rate with perfect use, 1% to 9%; with typical use, 20%
  2. Lactation amenorrhea method (LAM): 0.5% to 2.0% failure rate in the first 6 mo after delivery when exclusively breastfeeding and amenorrheic
- Barriers
  1. Male condom: Failure rate with perfect use, 3%; with typical use, 12%
  2. Female condom: Failure rate with perfect use, 5.1%; with typical use, 12.4%; FDA labeling states 25% failure rate
  3. Diaphragm and cervical cap: Failure rate 5% to 9% in nulliparous women, 20% in multiparous women
  4. Spermicides (aerosols, foam, jellies, creams, tabs): Failure rate with perfect use, 3%; with typical use, 21%
  5. New contraceptive gel (Phexxi): Failure rate with perfect use 7%, 14% with typical use
- Combined hormonal contraceptives
  1. Oral pill (various estrogen/progestin combinations): Failure rate with perfect use, <1%; with typical use, 3%
  2. Vaginal ring (NuvaRing): Failure rate Pearl index, 0.77
  3. Contraceptive patch: Failure rate, 0.4% to 0.7%
- Progesterone only pill ("Mini pill")
  1. Norethindrone: Failure rate with typical use, 1.1% to 13.2%. Requires precise timing of daily use for effectiveness
  2. New option drospirenone (Slynd): Failure rate of 4% based on one study
- Hormonal implants and injectables
  1. Nexplanon (etonogestrel) single rod subdermal implant: Failure rate of 0.05%
  2. Depo-Provera (medroxyprogesterone acetate): Failure rate, 0.3% in first year of use
- Emergency contraception (EC)
  1. Combined estrogen-progesterone regimen: Decreases pregnancy rate by 74% or more with women treated within 72 h of coitus
  2. Progestin-only method "Plan B": 2.2% pregnancy rate
  3. Selective progesterone receptor modulator (ulipristal acetate): 1.4% pregnancy rate
  4. Copper IUD: 0.1% pregnancy rate, most effective option

- Intrauterine device (IUD) or intrauterine system (IUS)
  1. Copper T (380-A): Hormone Free. Failure rate with perfect use, 0.6%; with typical use, 0.8%
  2. Levonorgestrel (LNG) IUD
  3. 52 mg LNG IUD (Mirena and Liletta): 1-yr failure rate, 0.1% to 0.2%, 5-yr cumulative failure rate 0.5% to 1.1%
  4. 19.5 LNG IUD (Kyleena): 5-yr cumulative failure rate, 0.6% to 1.6%
  5. 13.5 LNG IUD (Skyla): First year Pearl index, 0.48
- Female sterilization (tubal ligation): Failure rate with perfect use, 0.2%; with typical use, 3%
- Male sterilization (vasectomy): Failure rate of 0.1% in first year

SYNONYMS

Birth control
Family planning

ICD-10CM CODES	
Z30	Encounter for contraceptive management
Z30.0	Encounter for general counseling and advice on contraception
Z30.011	Encounter for initial prescription of contraceptive pills
Z30.012	Encounter for prescription of emergency contraception
Z30.013	Encounter for initial prescription of injectable contraceptive
Z30.014	Encounter for initial prescription of intrauterine contraceptive device
Z30.015	Encounter for initial prescription of vaginal ring hormonal contraceptive
Z30.016	Encounter for initial prescription of transdermal patch hormonal contraceptive device
Z30.017	Encounter for initial prescription of implantable subdermal contraceptive
Z30.018	Encounter for initial prescription of other contraceptives
Z30.09	Encounter for other general counseling and advice on contraception
Z30.2	Encounter for sterilization
Z30.4	Encounter for surveillance of contraceptives
Z30.430	Encounter for insertion of intrauterine contraceptive device

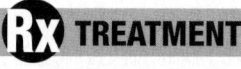

WORKUP

- To help facilitate method selection for the patient, we recommend obtaining the below information and consulting with Centers for Disease Control and Prevention Medical Eligibility Criteria.
  1. Thorough medical and surgical history
  2. Obstetric history (was fertility desired with conception?)

  3. Gynecologic history, including:
     a. History of previous sexually transmitted diseases
     b. Previous difficulties with contraception
     c. Frequency of intercourse
  4. Family history
- Table E1 summarizes when to start using contraceptive methods.
- Examinations and tests needed before initiation of contraceptive methods described in Table 2.
- Recommendations for routine follow-up after contraceptive initiation summarized in Table E3.

LABORATORY TESTS

- Pap smear should be done as routine and is not required before initiation of contraception
- Chlamydia and gonorrhea screening when appropriate
- Pregnancy test if suspected pregnancy

Rx TREATMENT

NONPHARMACOLOGIC THERAPY

- Male condoms
  1. 95% latex (rubber), 5% polyurethane, or natural membrane (lamb's intestine does not block transmission of sexually transmitted infections).
  2. Proper use: Place on an erect penis and leave ½-inch empty space at the tip of the condom; use with nonoil-based lubricants.
  3. Effectiveness is increased when used with spermicides.
  4. Main advantage: Condoms are the only method shown to reduce HIV transmission.
- Female condoms
  1. Composed of polyurethane, with one end open and one end closed
  2. Proper use: Place closed end over cervix, open end hanging out of vagina to cover penis and scrotum
  3. Highly effective against HIV
- Spermicides
  1. Types: Nonoxynol, octoxynol
  2. Forms: Jellies, creams, foams, suppositories, tablets, soluble films
  3. Proper use: Put in immediately before intercourse; may be used with other barrier methods
- New contraceptive gel
  1. Phexxi: Nonhormonal and works by lowering pH of vagina
  2. Proper use: Place in vagina up to 1 h before intercourse; may be used with other barrier methods
- Diaphragm and cervical cap
  1. Must be fitted by practitioner, used with contraceptive gels, and refitted with weight gain or loss of 4.5 kg. Must also be refitted after pregnancy.
  2. Diaphragm sizes: 50 to 105 mm; cervical cap sizes 26, 28, and 30 mm.
  3. The correct fit allows the woman to remain ambulatory without feeling the device.
  4. Proper use of diaphragm: Put in immediately before intercourse and keep in for

TABLE 2 Examinations and Tests Needed Before Initiation of Contraceptive Methods

Examination or Test	Cu-IUD and LNG-IUD	Implant	Injectable	CHC	POP	Condom	Diaphragm or Cervical Cap	Spermicide
Examination								
Blood pressure	C	C	C	A[a]	C	C	C	C
Weight (BMI) (weight [kg]/height [m]²)	—[b]	—[b]	—[b]	—[b]	—[b]	C	C	C
Clinical breast examination	C	C	C	C	C	C	C	C
Bimanual examination and cervical inspection	A	C	C	C	C	C	A[c]	C
Laboratory Test								
Glucose	C	C	C	C	C	C	C	C
Lipids	C	C	C	C	C	C	C	C
Liver enzymes	C	C	C	C	C	C	C	C
Hemoglobin	C	C	C	C	C	C	C	C
Thrombogenic mutations	C	C	C	C	C	C	C	C
Cervical cytology (Papanicolaou test)	C	C	C	C	C	C	C	C
STD screening with laboratory tests	—[d]	C	C	C	C	C	C	C
HIV screening with laboratory tests	C	C	C	C	C	C	C	C

BMI, Body mass index; *CDC*, Centers for Disease Control and Prevention; *CHC*, combined hormonal contraceptive; *Cu-IUD*, copper-containing intrauterine device; *HIV*, human immunodeficiency virus; *LNG-IUD*, levonorgestrel-releasing intrauterine device; *POP*, progestin-only pill; *STD*, sexually transmitted disease; *U.S. MEC*, U.S. Medical Eligibility Criteria for Contraceptive Use.

[a]In instances in which blood pressure cannot be measured by a provider, blood pressure measured in other settings can be reported by the woman to her provider.

[b]Weight (BMI) measurement is not needed to determine medical eligibility for any methods of contraception because all methods can be used (U.S. MEC 1) or generally can be used (U.S. MEC 2) among obese women. However, measuring weight and calculating BMI at baseline might be helpful for monitoring any changes and counseling women who might be concerned about weight change perceived to be associated with their contraceptive method.

[c]A bimanual examination (not cervical inspection) is needed for diaphragm fitting.

[d]Most women do not require additional STD screening at the time of IUD insertion. If a woman with risk factors for STDs has not been screened for gonorrhea and chlamydia according to CDC's *STD Treatment Guidelines* (https://www.cdc.gov/std/treatment), screening can be performed at the time of IUD insertion, and insertion should not be delayed. Women with current purulent cervicitis or chlamydial infection or gonococcal infection should not undergo IUD insertion (U.S. MEC 4).

From Curtis KM et al: U.S. selected practice recommendations for contraceptive use, 2016, *MMWR Recomm Rep* 65(4):1-66, 2016.

6 h after intercourse; must not remain in the vagina for longer than 24 h.
5. Proper use of cervical cap: Fit over the cervix exactly; must not remain in place for longer than 48 h.
- Lactation amenorrhea method (LAM)
  1. Three criteria must be met for this method to be effective: Exclusive breastfeeding (~ every 3 h), amenorrhea, and must be within 6 mo postpartum.
  2. If patient begins supplementing with formula, pumping and feeding by bottle, has any vaginal bleeding, or once infant is 6 mo old, recommend alternative contraception.
  3. Not a common practice in the U.S. but may be used with another method, such as the progesterone-only pill.
- Withdrawal
  1. Withdrawal of the penis from the vagina before ejaculation
  2. Depends on self-control, but there is a high typical use failure rate
- Rhythm method
  1. Symptothermal type: Mucus method and ovulation pain combined with basal body temperature
  2. Ovulation (Billings method): Takes into account mucus quality
  3. Basal body temperature method: Uses biphasic temperature chart
  4. Depends on awareness of physiology of male and female reproductive tracts
     a. Sperm viable in vagina for 2 to 7 days
     b. Ovum lifespan 24 h

- Sterilization
  1. Male
     a. Vasectomy to interrupt vas deferens and block passage of sperm to seminal ejaculate
     b. Scalpel and nonscalpel techniques available
     c. More easily performed procedure than female sterilization and does not require general anesthesia
  2. Female
     a. Leading method of birth control in U.S. in women older than 30 yr
     b. Interrupts fallopian tubes, blocking passage of ovum proximally and sperm distally through tube
     c. Methods: Bilateral salpingectomy, tubal ligation via removal of segment of fallopian tube, fulguration, application of clips (Filshie, Hulka) or band (Falope Ring)
     d. Essure: Tubal occlusion through hysteroscopic placement of microinserts into the fallopian tubes. Has been removed from the market

ACUTE GENERAL Rx

- Combination oral contraceptives
  1. Standard administration: Taken daily for 21 to 24 days, placebo or pill-free interval of 4 to 7 days
  2. Alternative regimen: Extended or continuous administration of active pills
  3. Less than 50 mcg ethinyl estradiol in most common combination oral contraceptives; progestins most commonly used in combination pills are norethindrone, levonorgestrel, norgestrel, norethindrone acetate, ethynodiol diacetate, norgestimate, or desogestrel
  4. Triphasic combination oral contraceptives (give varying doses of progestin and estrogens throughout cycle), monophasic oral contraceptives (offer same dose of progestin and estrogen throughout cycle), estrophasic pill (constant progesterone with variation of estrogen throughout the cycle)
  5. If pill taken with antibiotics, efficacy is affected by inadequate GI absorption in most cases; only rifampin truly reduces pill's effectiveness
  6. Increased body weight decreases effectiveness
     a. Table E4 describes oral contraceptive formulations available in the U.S. Guidelines for use of combination estrogen-progestin contraceptives in women 35 yr of age and older are described in Table E5.
     b. Fig. E1 describes recommended actions after late or missed combined oral contraceptives.
     c. Recommended actions after vomiting or diarrhea while using combined oral contraceptives are described in Fig. E2.
     d. Medical disorders with contraindicated contraceptive options are described in Table E6.
     e. Table E7 summarizes absolute and relative contraindications to combined hormonal contraceptives.

- Mini pill
  1. Progestin only; no placebo pills or pill-free intervals.
  2. May cause irregular bleeding because of the lack of estrogen effect on the lining of the uterus
  3. Table E8 provides a summary and recommendations for progestin-only oral contraceptive use
- Hormonal implants and injectables
  1. Nexplanon
     a. Single etonogestrel-secreting device that is inserted underneath the skin
     b. The most effective contraceptive available
     c. Approved by FDA in 2006 and effective over 3-yr period
  2. Depo-Provera
     a. Medroxyprogesterone acetate given every 3 mo in IM injection form
     b. Major side effect: Irregular bleeding; can also affect bone density
     c. Fertility return possibly delayed up to 1 yr or longer after last injection
     d. Table E9 provides a summary and recommendations for depot medroxyprogesterone acetate (DMPA) use
- Emergency contraception (EC)
  1. Done on emergency basis, if no contraceptive method used or failure of birth control (e.g., condom breakage or missed doses)
  2. Methods:
     a. Hormonal methods:
        (1) Levonorgestrel is available either as two 0.75-mg tablets taken 12 h apart (next choice) or as a 1.5-mg tablet taken once (Plan B, one step). It is indicated for emergency contraception to be used within 72 h after unexpected intercourse. It can be obtained OTC by women >15 yr of age and by prescription by younger patients. May be less effective in overweight and obese women.
        (2) Ulipristal (Ella) is a progesterone-receptor agonist/antagonist available by prescription only. It is a 30-mg, single-dose tablet and can be taken up to 5 days after unexpected intercourse. More effective than Plan B. Requires a prescription.
        (3) Combined estrogen-progesterone pills (Yuzpe regimen): In general, involves a first dose of 4 to 6 tablets (to achieve a dose of 100 to 120 mcg of ethinyl estradiol and 0.5 to 0.6 mg of levonorgestrel), followed by a second dose of 4 to 6 tablets 12 h later. Less effective option.
     b. Nonhormonal method: Copper IUD inserted within 5 days of coitus. Requires an office visit and insertion by trained provider.
- IUD
  1. Device inserted into uterus to prevent sperm and ovum from uniting in fallopian tube, thickens cervical mucous

  2. Types available in the U.S.:
     a. ParaGard (Copper T/380-A): A polyethylene T wrapped with a fine copper wire effective for 10 yr
     b. Mirena LNG IUD: A T-shaped system with a chamber that contains levonorgestrel. Releases 20 mcg/day. Recently approved for 8 yr
     c. Liletta LNG IUD: Lower cost. Releases 18.6 mcg/day. Recently approved for 6 yr
     d. Kyleena LNG IUD: Releases 9.8 mcg/day. Approved for 5 yr
     e. Skyla LNG IUD: Slightly smaller device and lowest dose of levonorgestrel (may cause more irregular bleeding). Releases 8 mcg/day. Approved for 3 yr
- Vaginal ring
  1. Types available in the U.S.:
     a. NuvaRing
        (1) Provides daily dose of 120 mcg of etonogestrel and 15 mcg ethinyl estradiol
        (2) Stays in vagina 3 wk and is removed the fourth for a contraceptive-free interval analogous to the placebo pills in combined oral contraceptive pills
        (3) 1 ring used per menstrual cycle
        (4) Increased body weight decreases effectiveness/combination oral contraceptive, but may have higher risk of DVT
  2. Recommended actions after delayed insertion or reinsertion with combined vaginal ring are described in Fig. E3
     a. Annovera
        (1) Provides daily dose of 150 mcg segesterone acetate and 13 mcg ethinyl estradiol
        (2) Stays in vagina 3 wk (21 days) and is removed the fourth for a contraceptive-free interval analogous to the placebo pills in combined oral contraceptive pills
        (3) 1 ring used for 13 menstrual cycles; on average, 1 yr per user
     b. Increased body weight decreases effectiveness/combination oral contraceptive, but may have higher risk of DVT
- Contraceptive patch
  1. Each patch contains 6 mg norelgestromin and delivers an estimated continuous systemic dose of 150 mcg norelgestromin and 15 mcg of ethinyl estradiol daily
  2. Worn 3 out of 4 wk
  3. Increased body weight decreases effectiveness
  4. Concern for increased risk of thromboembolic events
  5. Ortho Evra brand discontinued; Xulane (generic) available in the U.S.
  6. Recommended actions after delayed application or detachment with combined hormonal patch are described in Fig. E4

CHRONIC Rx

- With all the previously mentioned types of birth control, annual follow up visits are recommended, or as necessary, if problems arise.

- Pap smear should be completed per ASCCP guidelines.
- Sexually transmitted infection cultures should be performed as indicated.
- Patients with medical problems are followed up approximately every 6 mo when taking hormonal therapy.

DISPOSITION

- Follow up yearly or more frequently according to patient's side effects.
- Tailor birth control to patient according to different needs or side effects present at different times in life, notably bleeding profile, weight changes, and mood fluctuations. Effective counseling also requires an understanding of a woman's preference and medical risks, benefits, side effects, and contraindications of each contraceptive method.

REFERRAL

- If patient is medically complex, refer to a gynecologist for guidance on safe options.

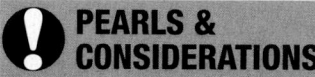

PEARLS & CONSIDERATIONS

- The most effective option is the one the person chooses to use, as they are more likely to use their chosen method correctly and consistently.
- Educate all patients at risk for pregnancy about the option for emergency contraception if needed.

COMMENTS

- With hormonal contraception, if neurologic or cardiac symptoms arise, stop method immediately, evaluate, and refer to internist when appropriate.
- The effectiveness of long-acting reversible contraception (IUDs and implants) is superior to that of contraceptive pills, patch, or ring and is not altered in adolescents and young women.
- Management of women with bleeding irregularities while using contraception is described in Fig. E5.
- The FDA has approved Opill, a progestin-only oral contraceptive that contains norgestrel for sale over-the-counter without a prescription. Dosage is one 0.075 mg tablet taken at the same time each day. It is intended to provide an accessible option for prevention of pregnancy.

SUGGESTED READINGS
Available at eBooks.Health.Elsevier.com

RELATED CONTENT
Contraception (Patient Information)
Emergency Contraception (Related Key Topic)

AUTHORS: **SIRI M. HOLTON, MD** and **SNEHA PARANANDI, MD**

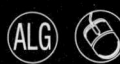
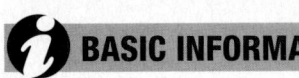 **BASIC INFORMATION**

DEFINITION

Coronary artery disease (CAD) is a clinical syndrome caused by plaque buildup (atherosclerosis) in the wall of the arteries that supply blood to the heart. Atherosclerosis can be defined as the narrowing of the artery as a result of plaque formation in the setting of lipid accumulation inside the arterial walls. CAD is silent in early stages and can progress to angina pectoris or acute coronary syndrome.

This topic addresses only stable CAD. Acute coronary syndromes (ACSs) and myocardial infarction (MI) are addressed as separate topics elsewhere.

SYNONYMS

Atherosclerotic heart disease
CAD
Chronic stable angina
Stable ischemic heart disease
Coronary arteriosclerosis

ICD-10CM CODES	
I25.0	Atherosclerotic cardiovascular disease
I25.1	Atherosclerotic heart disease
I25.10	Atherosclerotic heart disease of native coronary artery without angina pectoris
I25.110	Atherosclerotic heart disease of native coronary artery with unstable angina pectoris
I25.111	Atherosclerotic heart disease of native coronary artery with angina pectoris with documented spasm
I25.118	Atherosclerotic heart disease of native coronary artery with other forms of angina pectoris
I25.119	Atherosclerotic heart disease of native coronary artery with unspecified angina pectoris

EPIDEMIOLOGY & DEMOGRAPHICS

INCIDENCE:

- For persons who are 40 yr old, the lifetime risk of developing CAD is 49% in men and 32% in women. The risk increases with age in both men and women; however, the incidence in women lags behind that seen in men by approximately 10 yr.
- The incidence in premenopausal women is relatively low, whereas the incidence increases significantly in postmenopausal women.
- The initial presentation in men is more likely to be that of an MI, whereas women often present initially with angina.

PREVALENCE: It is estimated that 16.5 million Americans ≥20 yr of age have CAD. There is a slight male predominance at 55%, with incidence increasing with age. CAD prevalence is 7.9% for men and 5.1% for women.[1]

RISK FACTORS: The most prevalent risk factors include tobacco use, diabetes mellitus, hypertension, hyperlipidemia, obesity, family history, age, male sex, and peripheral vascular disease. Coronary plaque, especially noncalcified plaque, is more prevalent and extensive in HIV-infected men, independent of CAD risk factors.[2,3]

PHYSICAL FINDINGS & CLINICAL PRESENTATION

- Left anterior chest discomfort is often described as squeezing, heavy pressure, and burning. Associated symptoms include fatigue, dyspnea, weakness, lightheadedness, nausea, diaphoresis, altered mental status, and syncope.
- Discomfort that radiates to the neck, jaw, shoulder, and arm (left more than right) is common.
- Typical angina is exertional, resolves with rest after 3 to 5 min, and rarely lasts more than 30 min.
- Women and diabetes may not present with classic symptoms but may manifest more frequently with dyspnea or GI complaints.
- Discomfort is elicited by physical exertion, emotional stress, cold exposure, consumption of a large meal, and smoking.
- Early coronary disease is asymptomatic.
- Stigmata of atherosclerosis may include xanthelasma, tendon xanthomata, and evidence of peripheral vascular disease such as claudication and diminished peripheral pulses.

ETIOLOGY

The process of atherosclerosis begins when the endothelium is damaged or dysfunctional by a variety of different pathways/disease states: Hypertension, hyperlipidemia, trauma, toxins from drugs or tobacco use, or endothelial dysfunction sometime thought to be related to genetics. When the endothelium is dysfunctional, low-density lipoprotein (LDL) cholesterol circulating in the blood begins to accumulate within the intima. As the cholesterol accumulates within this plaque precursor, it begins to oxidize over time, which subsequently signals monocytes to migrate into the intima and convert to macrophages—this accumulation is known as a fatty streak. The macrophage cells enlarge and engulf cholesterol but can become overwhelmed and subsequently undergo apoptosis, leaving behind foam cells (the remnants of cholesterol-filled macrophages), as well as releasing inflammatory cytokines. Atherogenesis is further propagated by this resultant cellular necrosis within the forming plaque, promoting inflammatory mediator expression, intimal thickening, and migration of more macrophage cells.

Initially atheromatous plaques develop in an outward direction (otherwise known as positive remodeling), with enlargement of the external radius of the artery, thereby maintaining the inner luminal diameter and thus blood flow. Luminal obstruction and vascular calcification are both later stages of atherogenesis. As the process

continues, a well-defined core of extracellular lipids form—the collection is, at this stage, called an atheroma or fibrous plaque. Signals from the apoptotic macrophages prompt smooth muscle cell migration from the media, accelerating plaque formation by multiple actions, including secretion of collagen and elastin forming a protein fibrous cap, deposition of calcium, and releasing signals for neovascularization. By this time in the formation of the atheroma, the internal elastin membrane has become dysfunctional, allowing the passage of smooth muscle cells and perforations of neovascularization. Due to the previously mentioned changes and thickening of the intimal layer, there can be luminal narrowing, which reduces flow and ultimately can lead to symptoms of ischemia. This process of atherosclerosis occurs over many years.[4]

DX DIAGNOSIS

DIFFERENTIAL DIAGNOSIS OF ACUTE CHEST PAIN

- Cardiovascular causes
  1. Acute coronary syndrome
  2. Aortic dissection
  3. Pericarditis
  4. Coronary arterial vasospasm
- Pulmonary causes
  1. Pulmonary embolism
  2. Pneumonia
  3. Pleuritis
  4. Pneumothorax
- Gastrointestinal causes
  1. Esophageal spasm
  2. Esophagitis
  3. GERD
- Chest wall causes
  1. Rib fracture
  2. Sternoclavicular arthritis
  3. Herpes zoster
  4. Costochondritis
- Psychiatric causes
  1. Anxiety disorders

WORKUP

See Fig. E1. ACC/HFA guidelines for stress testing and advanced imaging are summarized in Tables 1 to 3.

LABORATORY TESTS

- Focused metabolic studies to rule out noncardiac causes (basic metabolic panel, liver function tests).
- CBC count can help rule out anemia-related chest discomfort.
- Fasting cholesterol panel is important in assessment of lipid-related risk factors.
- Hemoglobin A1c is important to follow glycemic control.
- High-sensitivity C-reactive protein.

IMAGING STUDIES

- When choosing the appropriate imaging study, one must keep in mind the patient's

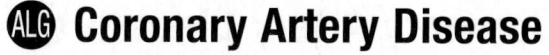

TABLE 1 ACC/AHA Guidelines for Stress Testing and Advanced Imaging for Initial Diagnosis in Patients With Suspected Stable Ischemic Heart Disease Who Require Noninvasive Testing

Test	EXERCISE STATUS		ECG INTERPRETABLE		PRETEST PROBABILITY OF ISCHEMIC HEART DISEASE			Recommendation	Level of Evidence
	Able	Unable	Yes	No	Low	Intermediate	High		
Patients Able to Exercise									
Exercise ECG	X		X			X		I	A
Exercise ECG with MPI or echo	X			X		X	X	I	B
Exercise ECG	X		X		X			IIa	C
Exercise ECG with MPI or echo	X		X			X	X	IIa	B
Pharmacologic stress CMR	X			X		X	X	IIa	B
CCTA	X		Either			X		IIb	B
Exercise echo	X		X			X		IIb	C
Pharmacologic stress with nuclear MPI, echo, or CMR	X		X			Any		III	C
Exercise stress with MPI	X		X		X			III	C
Patients Unable to Exercise									
Pharmacologic stress with nuclear MPI or echo		X	Either			X	X	I	B
Pharmacologic stress echo		X	Either		X			IIa	C
CCTA		X	Either		X	X		IIa	B
Pharmacologic stress CMR		X	Either			X	X	IIa	B
Exercise ECG		X		X		Any		III	C
Other Reasons for Cardiac Computed Tomography Angiography									
Continued symptoms after normal test results Inconclusive stress test results Unable to undergo stress test	Either		Either			X		IIa	C
CAC	Either		Either		X			IIb	C

ACC/AHA, American College of Cardiology/American Heart Association; CAC, coronary artery calcium (imaging); CCTA, coronary computed tomography angiography; CMR, cardiac magnetic resonance; ECG, electrocardiography; echo, echocardiography; MPI, myocardial perfusion imaging.
From Zipes DP: *Braunwald's heart disease: a textbook of cardiovascular medicine*, ed 11, Philadelphia, 2019, Elsevier.

TABLE 2 ACC/AHA Guidelines for Stress Testing and Advanced Imaging for Patients With Known Stable Ischemic Heart Disease Who Require Noninvasive Testing for Risk Assessment

Test	EXERCISE STATUS		ECG INTERPRETABLE		Additional Considerations	Recommendation	Level of Evidence
	Able	Unable	Yes	No			
Patients Able to Exercise							
Exercise ECG	X		X			I	B
Exercise ECG with MPI or echo	X			X	Abnormalities other than LBBB or ventricular pacing	I	B
Exercise ECG with MPI or echo	X		X			IIa	B
Pharmacologic stress CMR	X			X		IIa	B
CCTA	X			X		IIb	B
Pharmacologic stress imaging or CCTA	X		X			III	C
Patients Unable to Exercise							
Pharmacologic stress with nuclear MPI or echo		X	Either			I	B
Pharmacologic stress CMR		X	Either			IIa	B
CCTA		X	Either		Without previous stress test	IIa	C
Regardless of Ability to Exercise							
Pharmacologic stress with nuclear MPI or echo	Either			X	LBBB present	I	B
Exercise or pharmacologic stress with nuclear MPI, echo, or CMR	Either		Either		Known coronary stenosis being considered for revascularization	I	B
CCTA	Either		Either		Indeterminate result of functional testing	IIa	C
	Either		Either		Unable to undergo stress imaging	IIb	C
	Either		Either		Alternative to invasive coronary angiography when functional testing indicates moderate to high risk	IIb	C
Multiple stress tests or cardiac imaging at the same time	Either		Either			III	

ACC/AHA, American College of Cardiology/American Heart Association; CCTA, coronary computed tomography angiography; CMR, cardiac magnetic resonance; ECG, electrocardiography; echo, echocardiography; LBBB, left bundle branch block; MPI, myocardial perfusion imaging.
From Zipes DP: *Braunwald's heart disease: a textbook of cardiovascular medicine*, ed 11, Philadelphia, 2019, Elsevier.

TABLE 3 ACC/AHA Guidelines for Coronary Angiography to Assess Risk in Patients With Known or Suspected Stable Ischemic Heart Disease

Class	Indication	Level of Evidence
I (indicated)	Patients with SIHD who have survived sudden cardiac death or potentially life-threatening ventricular arrhythmia should undergo coronary angiography to assess cardiac risk.	B
	Patients with SIHD in whom symptoms and signs of heart failure develop should be evaluated to determine whether coronary angiography should be performed for risk assessment.	B
	Coronary arteriography is recommended for patients with SIHD whose clinical characteristics and results of noninvasive testing indicate a high likelihood of severe IHD and when the benefits are deemed to exceed risk.	C
IIa (good supportive evidence)	Coronary angiography is reasonable to further assess risk in patients with SIHD who have depressed LV function (EF <50%) and moderate-risk criteria on noninvasive testing with demonstrable ischemia.	C
	Coronary angiography is reasonable to further assess risk in patients with SIHD and inconclusive prognostic information after noninvasive testing or in patients for whom noninvasive testing is contraindicated or inadequate.	C
	Coronary angiography for risk assessment is reasonable for patients with SIHD who have unsatisfactory quality of life because of angina, have preserved LV function (EF >50%), and have intermediate-risk criteria on noninvasive testing.	C
III (no benefit)	Coronary angiography for risk assessment is not recommended in patients with SIHD who elect not to undergo revascularization or who are not candidates for revascularization because of comorbid conditions or individual preferences.	B
	Coronary angiography is not recommended to further assess risk in patients with SIHD who have preserved LV function (EF >50%) and low-risk criteria on noninvasive testing.	B
	Coronary angiography is not recommended to assess risk in patients who are at low risk according to clinical criteria and who have not undergone noninvasive risk testing.	C
	Coronary angiography is not recommended to assess risk in asymptomatic patients with no evidence of ischemia on noninvasive testing.	C

ACC/AHA, American College of Cardiology/American Heart Association; *EF,* ejection fraction; *IHD,* ischemic heart disease; *LV,* left ventricle; *SIHD,* stable ischemic heart disease.
From Zipes DP: *Braunwald's heart disease: a textbook of cardiovascular medicine,* ed 11, Philadelphia, 2019, Elsevier.

baseline activity levels and baseline electrocardiography (ECG) findings. In general, an exercise-based stress test yields a better idea of the patient's ischemic burden. Furthermore, each imaging modality focuses on a different element within the ischemia cascade. The ischemia cascade suggests that, with coronary artery luminal narrowing, there is a progression of findings as the demand for oxygen-carrying hemoglobin overwhelms the delivered blood supply. The ischemia cascade: Perfusion defect > diastolic dysfunction > systolic dysfunction > ECG changes and finally chest pain. See Tables 1 and 2 for further guidance on appropriate stress testing.

- ECG is important for assessing ischemia or prior infarct.
- Echocardiogram to assess left ventricular ejection fraction (LVEF) and the presence of wall motion abnormalities.
- Exercise treadmill test (ETT) is the gold standard to assess physiologic cardiac stress response in a patient with low or intermediate risk if the patient is able to exercise and has an "interpretable" baseline ECG (normal, right bundle branch block [RBBB], left ventricular hypertrophy [LVH] without repolarization abnormalities, <1 mm ST depression at rest). ETT provides high sensitivity but poor specificity. Therefore, if ETT is positive, further imaging studies may be obtained.

- Stress tests combined with imaging (exercise stress echo [Fig. E2] or exercise myocardial perfusion study) are the next best options if ETT cannot be performed because of physical limitation, if baseline ECG is uninterpretable or if ETT is positive.
- Although not used for angina or in an acute setting, a coronary artery calcium score can be used to improve CVD risk classification (Table 4). The coronary artery calcium (CAC) is estimated from a noncontrast computed tomography (CT; Fig. E3) scan. Normal coronary arteries do not have plaques or calcium, and the normal score is 0. A CAC score of 300 or higher, or 75th percentile or higher for age, sex, and ethnicity is considered a high

TABLE 4 Potential Uses of Coronary Artery Calcium Testing

Population	Purpose	Clinical Indications/Details
Asymptomatic persons without established ASCVD	Screening among *select* low- and borderline-risk patients	- CAC testing may be useful for risk assessment, particularly if this will impact the use of preventive therapies - Individuals who may benefit from such testing include those with strong family history of premature CAD or systemic inflammatory disease
	Shared decision making among *selected* borderline- and intermediate-risk adults in whom the decision regarding statin use is uncertain	- In intermediate-risk or selected borderline-risk adults (i.e., 10-yr ASCVD risk of 5%-20%), if the decision about statin use remains uncertain, it is reasonable to use a CAC score in the decision to withhold, postpone, or initiate statin therapy (see Fig. E4)
	Shared decision making among *select* high-risk adults who are unable to tolerate statin therapy	- In select high-risk adults who do not have known ASCVD and are unable to tolerate statin therapy, CAC testing may be reasonable for further risk stratification if this could impact the use of additional therapies (e.g., PCSK9 inhibitors)
Symptomatic persons with no known CAD	Low-risk patients with suspected CAD	- CAC testing may be useful to identify low-risk patients who have a low likelihood of obstructive CAD versus those with CAC >0 who may benefit from additional testing
Symptomatic persons with no known CAD	As add-on to other functional testing techniques	- Among individuals who do not have known CAD, who are referred for an ischemic evaluation, add-on CAC testing may be useful to determine the presence and severity of coronary plaque

From Libby P et al: *Braunwald's heart disease: a textbook of cardiovascular medicine,* ed 12, Philadelphia, 2022, Elsevier.

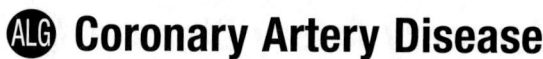

risk. According to the recent ACC/AHA guidelines, CAC is most appropriate among adults with an estimated 10-yr ASCVD risk <7.5% in whom questions remain about whether statin therapy is indicated. (Figs. E4 and E5) A CAC score >75th percentile for age, sex, and ethnicity is considered high risk and would justify revising a patient's risk upward.[5]

- Cardiac computed tomography angiography (CCTA, Fig. E6) can be considered as an alternative to stress testing. CCTA has excellent negative predictive value for obstructive CAD. CCTA may also identify plaque, which may change management (i.e., addition of a statin).
- Those with high-risk features (Box 1) should undergo invasive coronary angiography to assess coronary anatomy for revascularization.
- Coronary angiography is useful for both diagnostic and therapeutic interventions if there is evidence of significant ischemia by noninvasive assessment or progressive symptoms despite optimal medical therapy (as in the following).[6,7]

Rx TREATMENT

- See Fig. E7. Table 5 summarizes ACC/AHA guidelines for risk factor modification. Risk factors, clinical influences, and treatment considerations in older patients with CAD are illustrated in Figs. E8, E9, and Tables 6 and 7).
- Successful treatment of CAD entails minimizing the likelihood of major adverse cardiac events, which include death, MI, need for emergent coronary artery bypass grafting, or target lesion revascularization, while maximizing health and function.

NONPHARMACOLOGIC THERAPY
LIFESTYLE MODIFICATION:
- ≥150 min/wk of moderate-intensity activity or ≥75 min/wk of vigorous-intensity activity or a combination thereof (for adults) as one of the seven components of ideal cardiovascular health.
- A Mediterranean diet with a focus on vegetables, fruit, fish, whole grains, and olive oil has proven to reduce cardiovascular events to a degree greater than low-fat diets and equal to or greater than the benefit observed in statin trials.[8]
- Smoking cessation.
- Weight reduction can reduce various risk factors with improved lipid, blood pressure, and glycemic control.

THERAPEUTIC INTERVENTIONS: Coronary angiography with percutaneous coronary intervention (PCI) or coronary artery bypass graft (CABG) for patients on optimal medical therapy with persistent symptoms.

ACUTE GENERAL Rx
- Rest
- Sublingual nitroglycerin if rest does not provide adequate relief

CHRONIC Rx
- Antianginal therapy:
  1. Nitrates (isosorbide mononitrate and isosorbide dinitrate). These medications treat ischemia by venodilation to decrease preload, dilate epicardial coronary arteries, and recruit coronary collaterals. Furthermore, they attenuate platelet aggregation. Although they do not influence survival or decrease cardiovascular death in patients with chronic CAD, they do lower the rate of angina frequency and increase time

to ischemic ECG findings on treadmill testing.
  2. Beta-adrenergic antagonists (metoprolol, atenolol, carvedilol, or any other beta-blockers with the exception of those with intrinsic sympathomimetic activity). These medications work to relieve angina by decreasing myocardial oxygen demand by reducing heart rate, blood pressure, and contractility.
  3. Calcium channel blockers (CCBs; amlodipine or verapamil). The antianginal efficacy of CCBs is comparable to beta-blockers.
  4. Ranolazine. This is a selective inhibitor of late sodium influx into myocytes, which leads to decreased myocardial contractility. It can be used in combination with beta-blockers and significantly reduces frequency of angina and increases exercise duration and time to onset of angina. Although it rarely may cause QT prolongation, it has not been linked to any clinically important arrhythmias.[9]
  5. May benefit from combination therapy of the above.
- Antiplatelet therapy:
  1. Aspirin therapy (81 mg/day).[10] In regard to primary prevention the 2021 U.S. Preventive Services Task Force (USPSTF) recommendation statement on the use of low-dose aspirin for middle-age people (ages 40 to 59) with a 10-yr cardiovascular risk ≥10% states that the decision should be an individual one and respect professional judgment and patient preference. For age ≥60 the USPSTF recommends against low-dose aspirin for primary prevention.[11]
  2. Clopidogrel for those intolerant to aspirin therapy.
  3. Combination of aspirin and clopidogrel does not reduce cardiovascular events in stable CAD.[12]
  4. Antiplatelet drugs such as prasugrel and ticagrelor are used for ACS and do not have a recommended role in patients with stable CAD.
- Statins:
  1. HMG-CoA reductase inhibitors (statins) with high-intensity therapy for a target LDL reduction of >50% if safely achieved in high-risk patients; if not a candidate for high-intensity therapy, patient should receive at least moderate-intensity statin therapy that lowers LDL by 30% to 50%.
- PCSK9 inhibitors:
  1. This is a novel class of monoclonal antibodies that inhibit proprotein convertase subtilisin/kexin type 9. They cause dramatic reductions in LDL cholesterol and have been shown to reduce cardiovascular events. They are generally reserved for patients with familial hypercholesterolemia and patients with established vascular disease with LDL above goal despite maximal tolerated dose of statin.[13]
- Colchicine: In a randomized trial involving patients with chronic coronary disease, the risk of cardiovascular events was 31% lower

---

BOX 1   Noninvasive Risk Stratification

High Risk (>3% Annual Mortality Rate)
1. Severe resting left ventricular dysfunction (LVEF <35%)
2. High-risk treadmill score (≤−11)
3. Severe exercise left ventricular dysfunction (exercise LVEF <35%)
4. Stress-induced large perfusion defect (particularly if anterior)
5. Stress-induced multiple perfusion defects of moderate size
6. Large, fixed perfusion defect with LV dilation or increased lung uptake (thallium-201)
   a. Stress-induced moderate perfusion defect with LV dilation or increased lung uptake (thallium-201)
   b. Echocardiographic wall motion abnormality (involving >2 segments) developing at low dose of dobutamine (≤10 mg/kg/min) or at a low heart rate (<120 beats/min)
   c. Stress echocardiographic evidence of extensive ischemia

Intermediate Risk (1%-3% Annual Mortality Rate)
1. Mild/moderate resting left ventricular dysfunction (LVEF 35%-49%)
2. Intermediate-risk treadmill score (score between −11 and <5)
3. Stress-induced moderate perfusion defect without LV dilation or increased lung intake (thallium-201)
4. Limited stress echocardiographic ischemia with a wall motion abnormality only at doses of dobutamine involving ≤2 segments

Low Risk (<1% Annual Mortality Rate)
1. Low-risk treadmill score (≥5)
2. Normal or small myocardial perfusion defect at rest or with stress
3. Normal stress echocardiographic wall motion or no change of limited resting wall motion abnormalities during stress

TABLE 5 ACCF/AHA Guidelines for Risk Factor Modification

Class	Indication	Level of Evidence
Lipid Management		
I (indicated)	1. Lifestyle modifications, including daily physical activity and weight management, are strongly recommended for all patients with SIHD.	B
	2. Dietary therapy for all patients should include reduced intake of saturated fats (to <7% of total calories), trans fatty acids (to <1% of total calories), and cholesterol (to <200 mg/day).	B
	3. In addition to therapeutic lifestyle changes, a moderate or high dose of a statin should be prescribed in the absence of contraindications or documented adverse effects.	A
IIa (good supportive evidence)	4. For patients who do not tolerate statins, LDL cholesterol–lowering therapy with bile acid sequestrants, niacin, or both is reasonable.	B
Blood Pressure Management		
I (indicated)	1. All patients should be counseled about the need for lifestyle modification: Weight control; increased physical activity; alcohol moderation; sodium reduction; and emphasis on increased consumption of fresh fruits, vegetables, and low-fat dairy products.	B
	2. In patients with SIHD and a BP of 140/90 mm Hg or higher, antihypertensive drug therapy should be instituted in addition to or after a trial of lifestyle modifications.	A
	3. The specific medications used for the treatment of high BP should be based on specific patient characteristics and may include ACE inhibitors and/or beta-blocking agents, as well as the addition of other drugs such as thiazide diuretics or calcium channel blocking agents if needed to achieve a goal BP of less than 140/90 mm Hg.	B
Diabetes Management		
IIa (good supportive evidence)	1. For selected individual patients, such as those with a short duration of diabetes mellitus and a long life expectancy, a goal hemoglobin A1c (HbA1c) of 7% or less is reasonable.	B
	2. A goal HbA1c between 7% and 9% is reasonable for certain patients according to age, history of hypoglycemia, presence of microvascular or macrovascular complications, or presence of coexisting medical conditions.	C
IIb (weak supportive evidence)	3. Initiation of pharmacotherapy interventions to achieve a target HbA1c might be reasonable.	A
III (not indicated)	4. Therapy with rosiglitazone should not be initiated in patients with SIHD.	C
Physical Activity		
I (indicated)	1. For all patients, clinicians should encourage 30-60 min of moderate-intensity aerobic activity at least 5 days and preferably 7 days/wk, supplemented by an increase in daily lifestyle activities (e.g., walking breaks at work, gardening, household work) to improve cardiorespiratory fitness and move patients out of the least-fit, least-active, high-risk cohort (bottom 20%).	B
	2. For all patients, risk assessment with a physical activity history and/or an exercise test is recommended to guide prognosis and prescription.	B
	3. Medically supervised programs (cardiac rehabilitation) and physician-directed, home-based programs are recommended for at-risk patients at first diagnosis.	A
IIa (good supportive evidence)	4. It is reasonable for clinicians to recommend complementary resistance training at least 2 days/wk.	C
Weight Management		
I (indicated)	1. BMI and/or waist circumference should be assessed at every visit, and clinicians should consistently encourage weight maintenance or reduction through an appropriate balance of lifestyle physical activity, structured exercise, caloric intake, and formal behavioral programs when indicated to maintain or achieve a BMI of between 18.5 and 24.9 kg/m² and a waist circumference of less than 102 cm (40 in) in men and less than 88 cm (35 in) in women (less for certain racial groups).	B
	2. The initial goal of weight loss therapy should be to reduce body weight by approximately 5%-10% from baseline. With success, further weight loss can be attempted if indicated.	C
Smoking Cessation		
I (indicated)	1. Smoking cessation and avoidance of exposure to environmental tobacco smoke at work and home should be encouraged for all patients with SIHD. Follow-up, referral to special programs, and pharmacotherapy are recommended, as is a stepwise strategy for smoking cessation (Ask, Advise, Assess, Assist, Arrange, Avoid).	B
Management of Psychologic Factors		
IIa (good supportive evidence)	1. It is reasonable to consider screening patients with SIHD for depression and to refer or treat when indicated.	B
IIb (weak supportive evidence)	2. Treatment of depression has not been shown to improve cardiovascular disease outcomes but might be reasonable for its other clinical benefits.	C
Alcohol Consumption		
IIb (weak supportive evidence)	1. In patients with SIHD who drink alcohol, it might be reasonable for nonpregnant women to have 1 drink (4 oz of wine, 12 oz of beer, or 1 oz of spirits) a day and for men to have 1 or 2 drinks a day unless alcohol is contraindicated (such as in patients with a history of alcohol abuse or dependence or those with liver disease).	C
Exposure to Air Pollution		
IIa (good supportive evidence)	1. It is reasonable for patients with SIHD to avoid exposure to increased air pollution to reduce their risk for cardiovascular events.	C

ACE, Angiotensin-converting enzyme; *ACC/AHA,* American College of Cardiology/American Heart Association; *BMI,* body mass index; *BP,* blood pressure; *LDL,* low-density lipoprotein; *SIHD,* stable ischemic heart disease.
From Zipes DP: *Braunwald's heart disease: a textbook of cardiovascular medicine,* ed 11, Philadelphia, 2019, Elsevier.

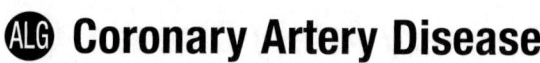
TABLE 6 ACC/AHA Atherosclerotic Cardiovascular Disease Risk Enhancers Used in the ACC/AHA Guidelines

Family history of premature ASCVD (men <55 yr, women <65 yr)

Primary hypercholesterolemia (LDL-C ≥160 mg/dl [4.1 mmol/L]; non-HDL-C ≥190 mg/dl [4.9 mmol/L])

Chronic kidney disease (eGFR 15-59 ml/min/1.73 m², not on dialysis or kidney transplant)

Metabolic syndrome

Conditions specific to women (e.g., preeclampsia, premature menopause)

Chronic inflammatory conditions (especially rheumatoid arthritis, lupus, psoriasis, HIV)

High-risk race/ethnicity (e.g., South Asian ancestry)

Lipids/Biomarkers

Persistently elevated triglycerides (≥175 mg/dl [2 mmol/L], fasting or nonfasting)

In selected individuals if measured:

hsCRP ≥2 mg/L

Lipoprotein(a) ≥50 mg/dl or ≥125 nmol/L

Apolipoprotein B ≥130 mg/dl

Ankle-brachial index <0.9

ACC, American College of Cardiology; *AHA,* American Heart Association; *ASCVD ,* atherosclerotic cardiovascular disease.
From Libby P et al: *Braunwald's heart disease: a textbook of cardiovascular medicine,* ed 12, Philadelphia, 2022, Elsevier.

among those who received 0.5 mg of colchicine once daily than among those who received placebo.[14,15]

- Glucagon-like peptide 1 receptor agonists (GLP-1RAs) and sodium-glucose co-transporter-2 (SGLT2) inhibitors reduce cardiovascular mortality. GLP-1RAs reduce stroke, and SGLT2 inhibitors reduce heart failure hospitalization and are preferred agents in patients with diabetes who also have, or are at high risk for, CV disease.[16,17]

CORONARY ARTERY REVASCULARIZATION

- Patients with symptoms refractory to optimal medical therapy as above or those with high clinical stress testing or an angiographic risk profile and suitable coronary anatomy may benefit from revascularization with either PCI or CABG surgery.[18] ACC/AHA guidelines for revascularization are summarized in Tables E8 and 9.

TABLE 7 Summary of the European Dyslipidemia Guidelines

CVD Risk Estimation

- Risk estimation (e.g., SCORE) is recommended for asymptomatic adults aged >40 yr without evidence of CVD, DM, CKD, FH, or LDL-C >4.9 mmol/L (>190 mg/dl). IC
- High- and very high-risk individuals (CVD, DM, moderate-to-severe renal disease, very high-risk factors, FH, or a high SCORE risk) are a priority for advice and management of all risk factors. IC

Lipid Analyses for CVD Risk Estimation

- **Total cholesterol** for estimation of total risk of CVD. IC
- **HDL-C** for further refining risk estimation. IC
- **LDL-C** is the primary lipid analysis method for screening, diagnosis, and management. IC
- **TGs** are recommended in routine lipid analysis. IC
- **Non-HDL-C** is recommended for risk assessment, particularly if high TGs, DM, obesity, or very low LDL-C.IC
- **Apolipoprotein B** is recommended for risk assessment, particularly in people with high TGs, DM, obesity, MetS, or very low LDL-C. Can be used as an alternative to LDL-C, if available, as the primary measurement for screening, diagnosis, and management, and may be preferred over non-HDL-C in people with high TGs, DM, obesity, or very low LDL-C. IC

Treatment Goals for LDL-C in Primary Prevention

- In individuals at very high risk, LDL-C reduction ≥50% and an LDL-C goal of <1.4 mmol/L (<55 mg/dl). IC
- In individuals at high risk, LDL-C reduction ≥50% and LDL-C goal of <1.8 mmol/L (<70 mg/dl). IA

CKD, Chronic kidney disease; *CVD,* cardiovascular disease; *FH,* familial hypercholesterolemia; *SCORE,* Systematic Coronary Risk Evaluation, predicting fatal cardiovascular events.
From Libby P et al: *Braunwald's heart disease: a textbook of cardiovascular medicine,* ed 12, Philadelphia, 2022, Elsevier.

TABLE 9 ACC/AHA Guidelines for Revascularization to Improve Symptoms in Patients with Significant Anatomic (>50% Left Main or >70% Nonleft Main Coronary Artery Disease) or Physiologic (Fractional Flow Reserve <0.80) Coronary Artery Stenoses

Clinical Setting	Recommendation		Level of Evidence
≥1 significant stenosis amenable to revascularization and unacceptable angina despite GDMT	I	CABG or PCI	A
≥1 significant stenoses and unacceptable angina in whom GDMT cannot be implemented because of medication contraindications, adverse effects, or patient preferences	IIa	CABG or PCI	C
Previous CABG with ≥1 significant stenosis associated with ischemia and unacceptable angina despite GDMT	IIa	PCI	C
	IIb	CABG	C
Complex 3-vessel CAD (e.g., SYNTAX score ≥22) with or without involvement of the proximal LAD artery and a good candidate for CABG	IIa	CABG preferred over PCI	B
Viable ischemic myocardium that is perfused by coronary arteries that are not amenable to grafting	IIb	TMR as an adjunct to CABG	B
No anatomic or physiologic criteria for revascularization	III	CABG or PCI	C

ACC/AHA, American College of Cardiology/American Heart Association; *CABG,* coronary artery bypass graft; *GDMT,* guideline-directed medical therapy; *LAD,* left anterior descending; *PCI,* percutaneous coronary intervention; *SYNTAX,* synergy between PCI with taxus and cardiac surgery; *TMR,* transmyocardial revascularization.
From Zipes DP: *Braunwald's heart disease: a textbook of cardiovascular medicine,* ed 11, Philadelphia, 2019, Elsevier.

- ACC/AHA class I indications for bypass surgery in chronic CAD patients include the following:
  1. High-grade (>50%) left main CAD
  2. Left main CAD-equivalent anatomy including >70% luminal stenosis in the left anterior descending artery and left circumflex arteries. CABG is also recommended over PCI when high complexity CAD is present. PCI is reasonable in selected patients if equivalent revascularization is possible
  3. Three-vessel disease with LVEF <50%
  4. Single- or two-vessel CAD with a large area of viable myocardium at risk
  5. Severe angina despite medical therapy if CABG can be performed with acceptable risk
- PCI has not been shown to reduce long-term rates of MI and death in patients with stable chronic CAD and therefore has no class I indications in this group. PCI is suitable in patients with suitable anatomy with refractory or lifestyle-limiting angina who have failed optimal medical therapy. Trials such as COURAGE, ORBITA, and ISCHEMIA have demonstrated no significant difference between optimal medical therapy and PCI in overall survival, MI, and ACS in patients with stable CAD. However, there is ~30% crossover to PCI in patients who are managed with optimal medical therapy alone.[7,19]
- The SYNTAX trial compared PCI to CABG in patients with stable angina. The trial used a numerical score based on qualitative plaque features on angiography with a primary composite endpoint of stroke, mortality, and MI (MACCE). In patients with low burden of CAD (SYNTAX <22) there was no difference between PCI and CABG up to 5 yr. In patients with intermediate burden (SYNTAX 23-32) there was no difference in MACCE at 5 yr (but a decrease in MI and/or revascularization). In patients with high burden of CAD (SYNTAX >33) it showed that surgical revascularization was associated with a lesser risk MACCE.[20]
- Patients with diabetes and multivessel CAD involving the left anterior descending artery should undergo CABG instead of PCI.[21]
- Trials continue to support CABG as superior to PCI in diabetic patients (BARI 2D, FREEDOM) with multivessel CAD and should remain the revascularization strategy of choice in this patient population.

DISPOSITION

- Risk estimators for cardiovascular events in patients without known CAD are summarized in Table 10.
- CAD is a common chronic condition with which many patients can live for years with good symptom control on optimal medical therapy.

REFERRAL

To a cardiovascular disease specialist

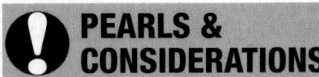

COMMENTS

- The transition from stable CAD to unstable angina must be carefully monitored. Symptoms of concern include more frequent episodes of chest pain, exertional dyspnea, chest pain that is less responsive to nitroglycerin, or first episode of chest pain. Regarding unstable angina, please refer to section on ACSs.
- ACC/AHA guidelines for follow-up noninvasive testing are summarized in Tables 11 and 12.

REFERENCES

Available at eBooks.Health.Elsevier.com.

RELATED CONTENT

Coronary Artery Disease (Patient Information)
Acute Coronary Syndrome (Related Key Topic)
Angina Pectoris (Related Key Topic)
Hypercholesterolemia (Related Key Topic)
Hyperlipoproteinemia, Primary (Related Key Topic)
Myocardial Infarction (Related Key Topic)

AUTHORS: **AHMAD MUSTAFA, MD** and
CRAIG L. BASMAN, MD, FACC, FSCAI

TABLE 10 Risk Estimators for Cardiovascular Events in Patients Without Known Coronary Artery Disease

Clinical Risk Estimator	Purpose of Risk Estimator	Limitations	Web or Mobile App Available
ASCVD Risk Estimator	10-yr risk of ASCVD event (CV death, MI, stroke)	Not validated for patients ≥80 yr old, excludes family history	Yes
Framingham Risk Score	Estimates risk for CV death, MI, stable and unstable angina	Excludes family history	Yes
MESA Risk Score	10-yr risk for CV death, MI, cardiac arrest, coronary revascularization	Excludes family history	Yes
Reynolds CVD Risk Score	Estimate risk for CV death, MI, stroke, revascularization	Does not account for treatment of hypertension	Yes
Adult Treatment Panel (ATP) III	Estimate risk for death or MI	Excludes DM or family history	Yes

ASCVD, Atherosclerotic cardiovascular disease; *CV,* cardiovascular; *DM,* diabetes mellitus; *MESA,* Multi-Ethnic Study of Atherosclerosis; *MI,* myocardial infarction.
From Warshaw G et al: *Ham's primary care geriatrics,* ed 7, Philadelphia, 2022, Elsevier.

TABLE 11 ACC/AHA Guidelines for Follow-Up Noninvasive Testing in Patients With Known Stable Ischemic Heart Disease: New, Recurrent, or Worsening Symptoms (Not Consistent With Unstable Angina)

Test	EXERCISE STATUS		ECG INTERPRETABLE		Additional Considerations	Recommendation	Level of Evidence
	Able	Unable	Yes	No			
Patients Able to Exercise							
Exercise ECG	X		X			I	B
Exercise ECG with MPI or echo	X			X		I	B
Exercise ECG with MPI or echo	X		Either		Previous requirement for imaging or known to be at high risk for multivessel CAD	IIa	B

Continued

TABLE 11 ACC/AHA Guidelines for Follow-Up Noninvasive Testing in Patients With Known Stable Ischemic Heart Disease: New, Recurrent, or Worsening Symptoms (Not Consistent With Unstable Angina)—cont'd

Test	EXERCISE STATUS		ECG INTERPRETABLE		Additional Considerations	Recommendation	Level of Evidence
	Able	Unable	Yes	No			
Pharmacologic stress MPI, echo, or CMR	X		X			III	C
Patients Unable to Exercise							
Pharmacologic stress with nuclear MPI or echo		X	Either			I	B
Pharmacologic stress CMR		X	Either			IIa	B
Exercise ECG		X		X		III	C
Regardless of Ability to Exercise							
CCTA	Either		Either		To assess patency of coronary stent or bypass graft ≥3 mm in diameter	IIb	C
	Either		Either		In absence of known moderate or severe calcification and to assess coronary stent <3 mm in diameter	IIb	C
	Either		Either		Known moderate or severe calcification or assessment of stent <3 mm in diameter	III	C

ACC/AHA, American College of Cardiology/American Heart Association; *CAD,* coronary artery disease; *CCTA,* cardiac computed tomography angiography; *CMR,* cardiac magnetic resonance; *ECG,* electrocardiography; *echo,* echocardiography; *MPI,* myocardial perfusion imaging.
From Zipes DP: *Braunwald's heart disease, a textbook of cardiovascular medicine,* ed 11, Philadelphia, 2019, Elsevier.

TABLE 12 ACC/AHA Guidelines for Follow-Up Noninvasive Testing in Patients With Known Stable Ischemic Heart Disease: Asymptomatic or Stable Symptoms

Test	EXERCISE STATUS		ECG INTERPRETABLE		Pretest Probability of Ischemia	Additional Considerations	Recommendation	Level of Evidence
	Able	Unable	Yes	No				
Exercise or pharmacologic stress with MPI, echo, or CMR at ≥2-yr intervals		X		X	Previous evidence of silent ischemia or at high risk for recurrent event	Unable to exercise, uninterpretable ECG, or incomplete revascularization	IIa	C
Exercise ECG at ≥1-yr intervals	X		X		Previous silent ischemia or at high risk for recurrent event		IIb	C
Exercise ECG	X		X		No previous silent ischemia and not at high risk for recurrent events		IIb	C
Exercise or pharmacologic stress imaging or CCTA	Either	Either				<5-yr intervals after CABG or <2 yr intervals after PCI	III	C

From Zipes DP: *Braunwald's heart disease: a textbook of cardiovascular medicine,* ed 11, Philadelphia, 2019, Elsevier.

ACC/AHA, American College of Cardiology/American Heart Association; *CABG,* coronary artery bypass graft; *CCTA,* cardiac computed tomography angiography; *CMR,* cardiac magnetic resonance; *ECG,* electrocardiography; *echo,* echocardiography; *MPI,* myocardial perfusion imaging; *PCI,* percutaneous coronary intervention.

(i) BASIC INFORMATION

DEFINITION
Crohn disease (CD) is an inflammatory disease of the bowel of unknown etiology, most commonly involving the terminal ileum and manifesting primarily with diarrhea, abdominal pain, fatigue, and weight loss.

SYNONYMS
CD
Regional enteritis
Inflammatory bowel disease (IBD)

ICD-10CM CODES
K50.00	Crohn disease of small intestine without complications
K50.011	Crohn disease of small intestine with rectal bleeding
K50.012	Crohn disease of small intestine with intestinal obstruction
K50.013	Crohn disease of small intestine with fistula
K50.014	Crohn disease of small intestine with abscess
K50.018	Crohn disease of small intestine with other complication
K50.019	Crohn disease of small intestine with unspecified complications
K50.10	Crohn disease of large intestine without complications
K50.111	Crohn disease of large intestine with rectal bleeding
K50.112	Crohn disease of large intestine with intestinal obstruction
K50.113	Crohn disease of large intestine with fistula
K50.114	Crohn disease of large intestine with abscess
K50.118	Crohn disease of large intestine with other complication
K50.119	Crohn disease of large intestine with unspecified complications
K50.80	Crohn disease of both small and large intestine without complications
K50.811	Crohn disease of both small and large intestine with rectal bleeding
K50.812	Crohn disease of both small and large intestine with intestinal obstruction
K50.813	Crohn disease of both small and large intestine with fistula
K50.814	Crohn disease of both small and large intestine with abscess
K50.818	Crohn disease of both small and large intestine with other complication
K50.819	Crohn disease of both small and large intestine with unspecified complications
K50.90	Crohn disease, unspecified, without complications
K50.911	Crohn disease, unspecified, with rectal bleeding
K50.912	Crohn disease, unspecified, with intestinal obstruction
K50.913	Crohn disease, unspecified, with fistula
K50.914	Crohn disease, unspecified, with abscess
K50.918	Crohn disease, unspecified, with other complication
K50.919	Crohn disease, unspecified, with unspecified complications

EPIDEMIOLOGY & DEMOGRAPHICS
PREVALENCE:
- Annual incidence ranges from 3 to 20 cases per 100,000.
- Median age of onset is 30 yr.
- Crohn disease has two peaks, the first between age 20 and 30 yr and the second a smaller peak around 50 yr.

PHYSICAL FINDINGS & CLINICAL PRESENTATION
- Physical exam findings vary depending on disease location and severity
- Abdominal tenderness, mass, or distention
- Chronic or nocturnal diarrhea
- Weight loss, fever, night sweats
- Hyperactive bowel sounds in patients with partial obstruction, bloody diarrhea
- Delayed growth and failure of normal development in children
- Perianal and rectal abscesses, perianal fistulas (Fig. E1), anal tags (Fig. E2), multiple sinuses and scarring (Fig. E3), mouth ulcers, cobblestone appearance of oral mucosa (Fig. E4), and atrophic glossitis
- Extraintestinal manifestations (Table 1): Joint swelling and tenderness, hepatosplenomegaly, erythema nodosum (Fig. E5), pyoderma gangrenosum (Fig. E6), clubbing, tenderness to palpation of the sacroiliac joints
- Symptoms may be intermittent, with varying periods of remission
- Overall, 45% to 50% of patients have ileocolonic inflammation, 30% have isolated small bowel disease, 20% have isolated colonic disease, and 5% have isolated upper GI or perianal manifestations

ETIOLOGY
Unknown. Pathophysiologically, Crohn disease involves an immune system dysfunction.

(Dx) DIAGNOSIS

DIFFERENTIAL DIAGNOSIS
- Ulcerative colitis (Table 2)
- Infectious diseases (tuberculosis, *Yersinia, Salmonella, Shigella, Campylobacter*)
- Parasitic infections (amebic infection)
- Pseudomembranous colitis
- Ischemic colitis in elderly patients
- Lymphoma
- Colon carcinoma
- Diverticulitis
- Radiation enteritis
- Collagenous colitis
- Fungal infections (*Histoplasma, Actinomyces*)
- Anorectal and colon diseases, formerly referred to as gay bowel syndrome
- Carcinoid tumors
- Celiac sprue
- Mesenteric adenitis

LABORATORY TESTS
- Decreased hemoglobin and hematocrit from chronic blood loss, effect of inflammation on bone marrow, and malabsorption of vitamin B_{12}
- Hypokalemia, hypomagnesemia, hypocalcemia, and low albumin in patients with chronic diarrhea
- Vitamin B_{12} and folate deficiency
- Elevated erythrocyte sedimentation rate and CRP
- Positive anti-*Saccharomyces cerevisiae* antibodies
- Elevated INR (due to vitamin K malabsorption)
- Fecal calprotectin has been reported as useful in screening of patients with suspected IBD. Based on a pretest probability of 32% in adults, an abnormal calprotectin test result increases the posttest probability to 91%, and a normal result reduces the probability of IBD to 3%. False elevations may occur with other gastrointestinal diseases such as bacterial, viral, and protozoal causes of infective diarrhea

ENDOSCOPIC EVALUATION
Endoscopic features of Crohn disease include asymmetric and discontinued disease, deep longitudinal fissures, cobblestone appearance, and presence of strictures (Fig. E7). Crypt distortion and inflammation are also present. Granulomas may be present.

IMAGING STUDIES
- CT of abdomen (Fig. E8) may show thickening of the terminal ileum and is helpful in identifying abscesses, fistulas (Fig. E9), and other complications.
- Magnetic resonance enterography (MRe) is superior to other imaging modalities in its ability to distinguish active from chronic fibrotic disease. It is, however, more expensive.
- In 10% to 15% of patients with IBD, a clear distinction between ulcerative colitis (UC) and Crohn disease cannot be made. In general, Crohn disease can be distinguished from ulcerative colitis by the presence of transmural involvement and the frequent presence of noncaseating granulomas and lymphoid aggregates on biopsy.

(Rx) TREATMENT

- The medical management of Crohn disease is based on disease activity. Medical therapy used in Crohn disease is summarized in Table 3.
- According to Hanauer and Sanborn, disease activity can be defined as follows:
  1. Mild to moderate disease: The patient is ambulatory and able to take oral alimentation. There is no dehydration, high fever, abdominal tenderness, painful mass, obstruction, or weight loss of >10%.
  2. Moderate to severe disease: Either the patient has not responded to treatment for mild to moderate disease or has more pronounced symptoms, including fever,

TABLE 1 Extraintestinal Manifestations of Disease in Patients with Inflammatory Bowel Disease[1-4]

Manifestation	Description	Epidemiology	Correlation With Active Bowel Disease	Treatment
Erythema nodosum	Painful, tender, raised, red nodules, often found on the anterior lower legs	1%-9% UC 6%-15% CD 5:1 female-male	90% associated with active bowel disease	Resolves with treatment of active bowel disease
Pyoderma gangrenosum	Ulcers on lower limbs, trunk, and adjacent to surgical stomas	0.5%-2% IBD	Not associated with active bowel disease[5]	Immunosuppressive therapy; occasionally shows spontaneous resolution
Aphthous ulcers	Oral ulcerations in buccal mucosa	20%-30% CD 20% UC	Associated with active bowel disease Associated with ocular and articular symptoms	Resolves with treatment of active bowel disease
Uveitis	Eye pain, redness, loss of visual acuity, floaters	3:1 female-male	Anterior uveitis: 30% associated with erythema nodosum Posterior uveitis: 90% associated with arthritis, particularly ankylosing spondylitis	Topical corticosteroids; systemic immune suppressants for severe cases
Episcleritis	Eye redness, irritation, and watering	5%-8% IBD 3:1 female-male	Associated with active bowel disease	Resolves with treatment of active bowel disease or topical corticosteroid therapy
Primary sclerosing cholangitis	Recurrent biliary sepsis, abdominal pain, pruritus, complications of portal hypertension and end-stage liver disease	3%-5% UC[6] Male preponderance	Not associated with active bowel symptoms; associated with colorectal cancer	Supportive therapy, management of complications of disease

CD, Crohn's disease; *IBD,* inflammatory bowel disease; *UC,* ulcerative colitis.
From Hochberg MC et al: *Rheumatology,* ed 8, Philadelphia, 2023, Elsevier.

TABLE 2 Crohn's Disease and Ulcerative Colitis

	Symptoms/Characteristics	Gastrointestinal Involvement	Endoscopic Findings	Pathologic Features
Crohn's disease	Abdominal pain, nonbloody diarrhea, perianal and internal fistulas More common in active smokers	Can involve intestine from mouth to anus	Skip lesions, serpiginous or deep ulcerations, strictures, fistulas, small bowel involvement	Transmural inflammation, noncaseating granulomas, skip lesions
Ulcerative colitis	Bloody diarrhea, tenesmus More common in nonsmokers and former smokers	Involves colon only	Superficial erosions or smaller ulcerations, continuous involvement from rectum to proximal colon	Continuous histologic inflammation from rectum to proximal colon

From Hochberg MC et al: *Rheumatology,* ed 8, Philadelphia, 2023, Elsevier.

significant weight loss, abdominal pain or tenderness, intermittent nausea and vomiting, or significant anemia.

3. Severe fulminant disease: Either the patient has persistent symptoms despite outpatient steroid therapy or has high fever, persistent vomiting, evidence of intestinal obstruction, rebound tenderness, cachexia, or evidence of an abscess.

4. Remission: The patient is asymptomatic or without inflammatory sequelae, including patients responding to acute medical intervention.

NONPHARMACOLOGIC THERAPY

- Nutritional supplementation is needed in patients with advanced disease. Total parenteral nutrition may be necessary in selected patients.
- Low-residue diet is necessary when obstructive symptoms are present.
- If diarrhea is prominent, increased dietary fiber and decreased fat in the diet are sometimes helpful.

- Psychotherapy is useful for situational adjustment crises. A trusting and mutually understanding relationship and referral to self-help groups are very important because of the chronicity of the disease and the relatively young age of the patients.
- Avoid oral feedings during acute exacerbation to decrease colonic activity: A low-roughage diet may be helpful in early relapse.

ACUTE GENERAL Rx

- Glucocorticoids play a central yet vexing role in the treatment of CD. Although their efficacy and rapid induction of clinical improvement are well established, repeated use or prolonged exposure leads to significant side effects. They have been the mainstay for treating moderate to severe active Crohn disease (Fig. 10). Corticosteroids are usually tapered over approximately 2 to 3 mo. Some patients require a low dose for a prolonged period of maintenance. Patients responding to glucocorticoids are transitioned to immunomodulators as their glucocorticoid is tapered.

- Steroid analogues are locally active corticosteroids that target specific areas of inflammation in the gastrointestinal tract. Budesonide is available as a controlled-release formulation and is approved for mild to moderate active Crohn disease involving the ileum and/or ascending colon. The adult dose is 9 mg qd for a maximum of 8 wk.
- Immunosuppressants such as azathioprine or mercaptopurine are used for maintenance of remission. Methotrexate is an alternative agent.
- Metronidazole 500 mg qid may be useful for colonic fistulas and treatment of mild to moderate active Crohn disease. Ciprofloxacin 1 g qd has also been found to be effective in decreasing disease activity.
- TNF inhibitors are agents useful to induce remission and maintain remission in patients with moderate to severe Crohn disease. Infliximab, a chimeric monoclonal antibody targeting tumor necrosis factor-α, is effective in the treatment of enterocutaneous fistulas and was the first biologic response modifier shown to be effective in CD. This medication

TABLE 3 Medical Therapy Used in Crohn Disease (CD)

Drug	Release Site	Treatment of CD	Side Effects
Oral 5-Aminosalicylates			
Sulfasalazine	Colon	Oral mesalamine for the treatment of mild CD but is at best minimally effective compared with placebo, and less effective than budesonide or corticosteroids	Rash, nausea, vomiting, headache, alopecia, and hypersensitivity reaction resulting in worsening diarrhea can occur
Mesalamine (mesalazine)	Distal ileum, colon		
Mesalamine (mesalazine) (controlled-release)	Duodenum, jejunum, ileum, colon		Severe adverse events such as interstitial nephritis, pancreatitis and pneumonitis can rarely occur
Olsalazine	Colon	Sulfasalazine is not useful because colonic bacteria need to cleave the drug, so it is of no benefit for small intestinal disease	
Balsalazide	Colon		
Topical 5-Aminosalicylates			
Mesalamine (mesalazine) enema	Rectum, sigmoid	Topical mesalamine should only be used for distal colonic CD as adjunctive therapy to systemic therapy	
Mesalamine (mesalazine) suppository	Rectum		
Antibiotics			
Ciprofloxacin	Systemic	Antibiotics are not used for the treatment of CD except for perianal CD	Ciprofloxacin: Tendonitis and rupture
Metronidazole			Metronidazole: Neuropathy
Amoxicillin/clavulanic acid			Amoxicillin/clavulanic acid: Hepatitis
Rifaximin			
Corticosteroids			
Budesonide (Entocort)	Small intestine, right colon	Induction of remission in mild-to-moderate CD involving the distal ileum and/or right colon. Not used for maintenance	High first-pass metabolism. More favorable side-effect profile than prednisone
Prednisone	Systemic	Induction of remission in mild-to-moderate CD. Not effective for maintenance of remission	Infection, diabetes mellitus, osteoporosis, osteonecrosis, cataracts, glaucoma, and myopathy. Increased risk of mortality, mood and sleep disturbance
Methylprednisolone	Systemic	Induction of remission in severe CD. Not used for maintenance	As for prednisone
Immunomodulators			
6-Mercaptopurine	Systemic	Effective for maintaining a steroid-induced remission of CD. Not used for induction	Allergic reactions, pancreatitis, myelosuppression, nausea, infections, hepatotoxicity, and malignancy, in particular lymphoma
Azathioprine	Systemic		
Methotrexate	Systemic	Effective at maintaining steroid-induced remission in moderate-to-severe CD. Not used for induction	Rash, nausea, diarrhea, myelosuppression, hepatic fibrosis, and rarely hypersensitivity pneumonitis
Biologics			
Anti-TNF:			
Infliximab	Systemic	Have been approved for the induction and maintenance of moderate-to-severe CD	Infections (tuberculosis, fungal infections), autoantibody formation, psoriasis, drug-induced lupus
Adalimumab	Systemic	Also used for fistulizing and perianal disease	Infusion reactions (infliximab), injection-site reaction (adalimumab and certolizumab), delayed hypersensitivity reaction (infliximab)
Certolizumab pegol	Systemic (second-line, less effective)	Combination therapy with immunomodulators is superior to monotherapy	Lymphoma (higher in combination therapy with immunomodulator)
Antiinterleukin therapy:			
Ustekinumab	Systemic anti-IL12/23	Second line	Nasopharyngitis (10%)
Risankizumab	Systemic IL 23 antagonist	Induction and maintenance	Upper respiratory infections, headache, arthralgias
Antiintegrin therapy:			
Natalizumab	Systemic	Effective in the induction and maintenance of remission in moderate-to-severe CD. Second-line to other biologics due to possibly causing progressive multifocal leukoencephalopathy (PML)	Infusion reaction, hepatotoxicity, infections, and autoantibody formation
Vedolizumab	Systemic	Effective in the induction and maintenance of remission in moderate-to-severe CD	Headache, infections, abdominal pain, infusion reactions

Modified from Talley NJ et al: *Essentials of internal medicine*, ed 4, Chatswood, NSW, 2021, Elsevier Australia.

can induce clinical improvement in 80% of patients with Crohn disease refractory to other agents. It can be used in combination with other medications such as azathioprine in patients with severe Crohn disease. A PPD test should be done before using this medication. Adalimumab and certolizumab are other TNF inhibitors also effective in inducing remissions and may be useful in adult patients with Crohn disease who cannot tolerate infliximab or have symptoms despite receiving infliximab therapy. Efficacy is better when an anti-TNF is used together with an immunomodulator.

- Natalizumab, a selective adhesion-molecule inhibitor, has been reported to be effective in increasing the rate of remission and response in patients with active Crohn disease. It is effective for patients in whom anti-TNF therapy has been unsuccessful. Prior to using natalizumab, serologic testing

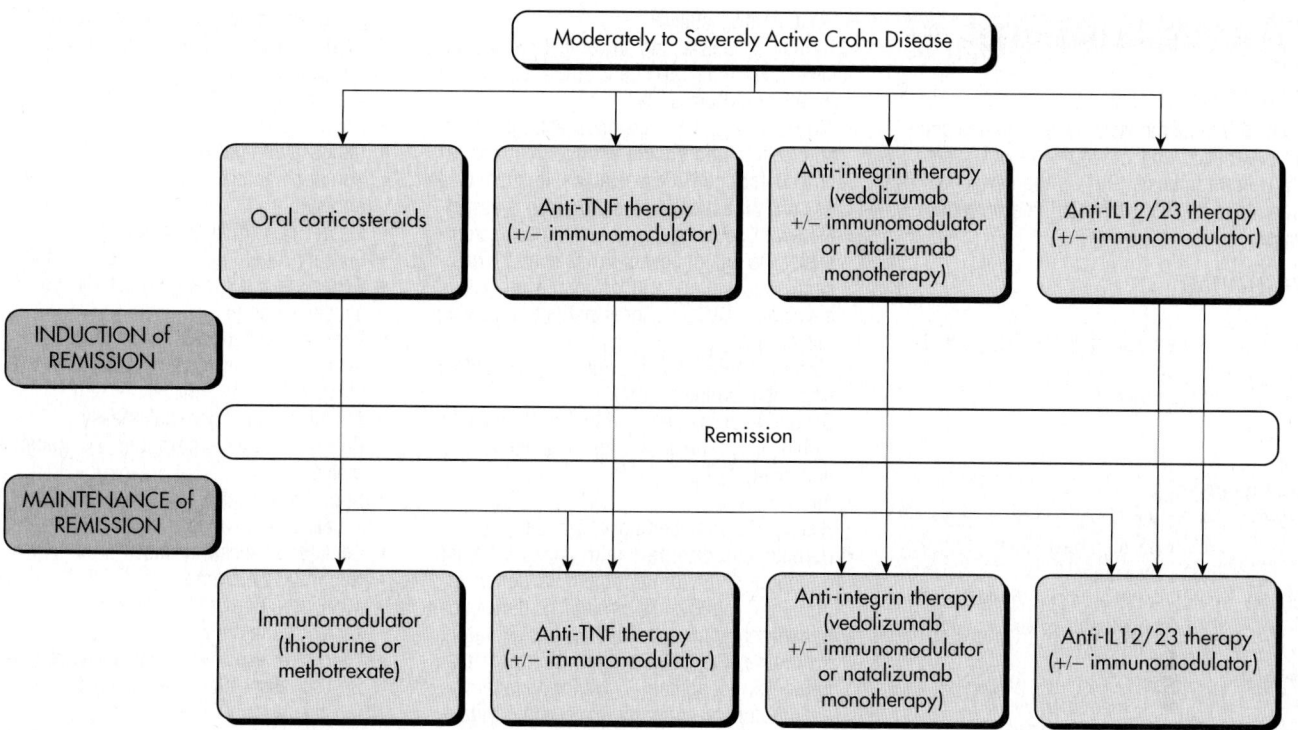

FIG. 10 Algorithm for management of moderately to severely active Crohn disease. (From Feldman M et al: *Sleisenger and Fordtran's gastrointestinal and liver disease,* ed 11, Philadelphia, 2021, Elsevier.)

should be done for JC virus, which causes multifocal leukoencephalopathy (PML), and if the patient is seronegative, the risk of PML from natalizumab is low. Vedolizumab is another IV integrin receptor antagonist recently FDA approved for moderate to severe Crohn disease patients who have not responded to or cannot tolerate standard treatment. Vedolizumab use is not associated with high risk of PML. Ustekinumab, a monoclonal antibody to the P_4O subunit of interleukin-12 and interleukin-23, has shown efficacy for induction and maintenance therapy for Crohn disease. It has been FDA-approved for moderate to severely active Crohn disease unresponsive to immunomodulators or corticosteroids or a tumor necrosis factor inhibitor.

- Hydrocortisone enema bid or tid is useful for proctitis.

- Most patients who have anemia associated with Crohn disease respond to iron supplementation. Erythropoietin is useful in patients with anemia refractory to treatment with iron and vitamins.

CHRONIC Rx

- Monitor disease activity with symptom review and laboratory evaluation (complete blood count and sedimentation rate).
- Liver tests and vitamin B_{12} levels monitored on a yearly basis.

DISPOSITION

There is no cure for CD, and most patients require at least one surgical resection. One tenth of patients have prolonged remission, three quarters have a chronic intermittent disease course, and one eighth have an unremitting course. Patients with IBD are at increased risk of colon cancer.

REFERRAL

Surgical referral is needed for complications such as abscess formation, obstruction, fistulas, toxic megacolon, refractory disease, or severe hemorrhage. Approximately 40% to 50% of patients will require some type of bowel surgery within the first 5 yr of Crohn disease. A conservative surgical approach is necessary because surgery is not curative. Multiple surgeries may also result in short bowel syndrome.

REFERENCES & SUGGESTED READINGS

Available at eBooks.Health.Elsevier.com.

RELATED CONTENT

Crohn Disease (Patient Information)

AUTHOR: **FRED F. FERRI, MD**

Deep Vein Thrombosis

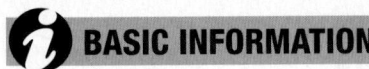

BASIC INFORMATION

DEFINITION

Venous thromboembolism is any thromboembolic event occurring within the venous system. Deep vein thrombosis (DVT) is the development of thrombi in the deep veins of the extremities or pelvis.

SYNONYMS

DVT
Venous thromboembolism (VTE) (VTE includes DVT and pulmonary embolism [PE])
Deep venous thrombosis
VTE

ICD-10CM CODES

I82.401	Acute embolism and thrombosis of unspecified deep veins of right lower extremity
I82.402	Acute embolism and thrombosis of unspecified deep veins of left lower extremity
I82.403	Acute embolism and thrombosis of unspecified deep veins of lower extremity, bilateral
I82.621	Acute embolism and thrombosis of deep veins of right upper extremity
I82.622	Acute embolism and thrombosis of deep veins of left upper extremity
I82.623	Acute embolism and thrombosis of deep veins of upper extremity, bilateral

EPIDEMIOLOGY & DEMOGRAPHICS

- Annual incidence of VTE is 0.1% to 0.27%, affecting up to 5% of the population during their lifetimes.
- The risk of recurrent thromboembolism is higher among men than women.
- In the U.S., there are approximately 900,000 DVT events annually. About 5% to 15% of persons with untreated DVT die from pulmonary embolism.
- Venous thromboembolism occurs in nearly 2 cases per 1000 pregnancies and is a leading cause of maternal mortality and morbidity.

PHYSICAL FINDINGS & CLINICAL PRESENTATION

- Pain and swelling of the affected extremity
- In lower extremity DVT: Leg pain on dorsiflexion of the foot *(Homan sign)*
- Physical examination may be unremarkable in early DVT

ETIOLOGY

The etiology is often multifactorial (prolonged stasis, coagulation abnormalities, vessel wall trauma [Fig. 1]).
The following are risk factors for DVT (Table 1):
- Prolonged immobilization (>3 days)

- Postoperative state
- Trauma to pelvis and lower extremities for lower extremity DVT; central line placement for upper extremity DVT
- Birth control pills, high-dose estrogen therapy; conjugated equine estrogen but not esterified estrogen is associated with increased risk of DVT; estrogen plus progestin is associated with doubling the risk of venous thrombosis. The use of bevacizumab is also significantly associated with an increased risk of developing DVT in cancer patients receiving this drug
- Visceral cancer (lung, pancreas, alimentary tract, genitourinary tract)
- Occult cancer is detected in 1 in 20 patients within a yr of receiving a diagnosis of unprovoked VTE
- Age >60 yr
- History of thromboembolic disease
- Hematologic disorders (e.g., factor V Leiden mutation [FVL], antithrombin III deficiency, protein C deficiency, protein S deficiency, heparin cofactor II deficiency, sticky platelet syndrome, G20210A prothrombin mutation, lupus anticoagulant, dysfibrinogenemias, anticardiolipin antibody, hyperhomocysteinemia, concurrent homocystinuria, high levels of factors VIII, XI, and single nucleotide polymorphisms [SNPs] such as CYP4V2). A classification of hypercoagulable states is described in Table 2
- Pregnancy and early puerperium
- Obesity (BMI >30)
- Congestive heart failure
- Surgery, fracture, or injury involving lower leg or pelvis
- Plaster cast immobilization
- Surgery requiring >30 min of anesthesia
- Gynecologic surgery (particularly gynecologic cancer surgery)
- Recent travel (within 2 wk, lasting ≥2 h). Every 2 h spent traveling increases VTE risk by 18%
- Smoking and abdominal obesity
- Central venous catheter or pacemaker insertion
- Superficial vein thrombosis (10% risk of DVT within 3 mo), varicose veins
- Collagen vascular disease
- Nephrotic syndrome
- Myeloproliferative disorders
- Testosterone therapy
- Long-term exposure to particulate air pollution is also associated with altered coagulation function and DVT risk
- Varicose veins
- NSAIDs and hormonal contraceptives[1]

TABLE 1 Increased Predisposition to Venous Thrombosis With Coexisting Risk Factors

Thrombotic Factor	Relative Risk (%)
OCP use	2-4
Hyperhomocysteinemia	2.5
FVL heterozygous	3-10
FVL heterozygous + HRT	15
FVL heterozygous + OCP use	30-40
FVL heterozygous + pregnancy	35
FVL homozygous	79
FVL homozygous + OCP use	100
Prothrombin gene mutation	1-5
Prothrombin gene mutation + FVL	6-10
Prothrombin gene mutation + OCP use	16
Protein C, S, ATIII deficiencies + OCP use	10

ATIII, Antithrombin III; *FVL*, factor V Leiden; *HRT*, hormone replacement therapy; *OCP*, oral contraceptive pill.
From Talley NJ et al: *Essentials of internal medicine*, ed 4, Chatswood, NSW, 2021, Elsevier Australia.

TABLE 2 Classification of Hypercoagulable States

Hereditary	Mixed	Acquired
Loss of Function		
Antithrombin deficiency	Hyperhomocysteinemia	Advanced age
Protein C deficiency		Previous venous thromboembolism
Protein S deficiency		Surgery
Gain of function		Immobilization
Factor V Leiden		Obesity
Prothrombin gene mutation		Cancer
Elevated factor VIII, IX, or XI levels		Pregnancy, puerperium
		Drug-induced: L-asparaginase, hormonal therapy

From Libby P et al: *Braunwald's heart disease, a textbook of cardiovascular medicine*, ed 12, Philadelphia, 2022, Elsevier.

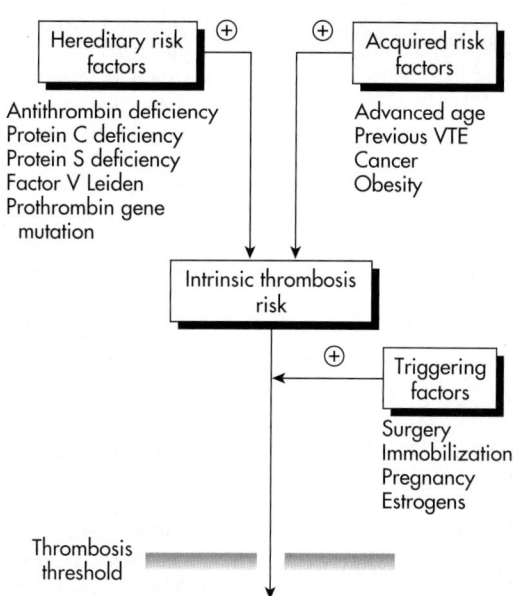

FIG. 1 Thrombosis threshold. Hereditary and acquired risk factors combine to create an intrinsic risk for thrombosis in each individual. This risk is increased by extrinsic triggering factors. If the intrinsic and extrinsic forces exceed a critical threshold at which thrombin generation overwhelms protective mechanisms, thrombosis occurs. *VTE,* Venous thromboembolism. (From Libby P et al: *Braunwald's heart disease, a textbook of cardiovascular medicine,* ed 12, Philadelphia, 2022, Elsevier.)

LABORATORY TESTS

- Laboratory tests are not specific for DVT.
- Baseline prothrombin time (INR), partial thromboplastin time, and platelet count should be obtained on all patients.
- D-dimer testing is sensitive but not specific for DVT. A negative result (D-dimer <0.5 mcg/ml) can exclude the diagnosis in a patient with low probability of DVT, but a positive result (≥0.5 mcg/ml) mandates additional testing with venous ultrasonography.
- Laboratory evaluation of young patients with DVT, patients with recurrent thrombosis without obvious causes, and those with a family history of thrombosis should include protein S (both total and free PS), protein C, fibrinogen, antithrombin III level, lupus anticoagulant, anticardiolipin antibodies, anti-b2 glycoprotein1, factor V Leiden, factor VIII, factor IX, and fasting plasma homocysteine levels. It is important to remember that the lupus anticoagulant assay and antithrombin, protein C, protein S, and dysfibrinogenemia testing cannot be properly interpreted if a patient is already on warfarin, whereas anticardiolipin antibody test, prothrombin G20210A, factor VII:C, factor V Leiden, and PT polymorphism can be performed when a patient is on warfarin.

Dx DIAGNOSIS

DIFFERENTIAL DIAGNOSIS

- Postphlebitic syndrome
- Superficial thrombophlebitis
- Ruptured Baker cyst
- Cellulitis, lymphangitis, Achilles tendinitis
- Hematoma
- Muscle or soft tissue injury, stress fracture
- Varicose veins, lymphedema
- Arterial insufficiency
- Abscess
- Claudication
- Venous stasis

WORKUP

- The clinical diagnosis of DVT is inaccurate. Pain, tenderness, swelling, or color changes are not specific for DVT.
- Clinical prediction rules can be used to establish pretest probability of DVT (Fig. 2). The Wells prediction rules for DVT and for pulmonary embolism are described in Table 3. These rules perform better in younger patients without a history of DVT and in those without comorbidities. In younger patients without associated comorbidities and a low pretest probability using Wells criteria and a negative high-sensitivity D-dimer test, the diagnosis of DVT can be reasonably excluded.
- Compression ultrasonography (CUS; Fig. E3) is preferred as the initial study to diagnose DVT in patients with intermediate to high pretest probability. An initial negative test limited to the proximal leg should be repeated after 5 days (if the clinical suspicion of DVT persists) to exclude DVT that is propagating proximally from the calf. Comprehensive

ultrasonography (whole-leg CUS) is a more extensive test that examines the deep veins from the inguinal ligament to the level of the malleolus. Literature reports indicate that it may be safe to withhold anticoagulation after negative results on comprehensive duplex ultrasonography in nonpregnant patients with a suspected first episode of symptomatic DVT of the leg.

IMAGING STUDIES

- Compression ultrasonography (CUS) is generally preferred as the initial study because it is noninvasive and can be repeated serially (useful to monitor suspected acute DVT); it offers good sensitivity for detecting proximal vein thrombosis (in the popliteal or femoral vein). Its disadvantages are poor visualization of deep iliac and pelvic veins and poor sensitivity in

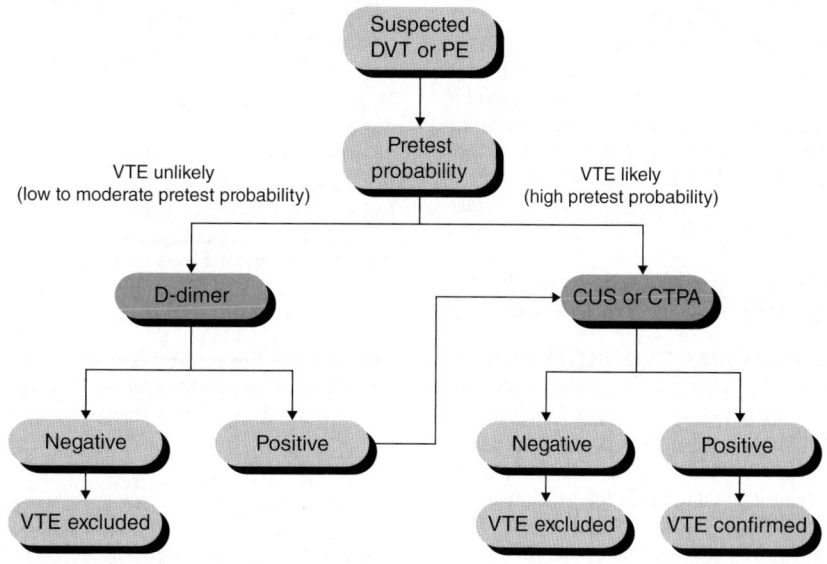

FIG. 2 Diagnostic approach in patients with suspected deep vein thrombosis *(DVT)* or pulmonary embolism *(PE).* The first step is an assessment of the pretest probability using a validated DVT or PE clinical prediction model. Patients categorized as venous thromboembolism *(VTE)* unlikely (low or moderate pretest probability) should undergo D-dimer testing. A negative D-dimer excludes the diagnosis, whereas those with a positive D-dimer test result or those categorized as VTE likely (high pretest probability) should undergo diagnostic imaging with compression ultrasound *(CUS)* or computed tomography pulmonary angiography *(CTPA)* to rule out or confirm DVT and PE, respectively. (From Hoffman R et al: *Hematology, basic principles and practice,* ed 8, Philadelphia, 2023, Elsevier.)

TABLE 3 Wells Scoring Scheme for Pre-Test Probability of Deep Vein Thrombosis*

Clinical Feature	Points
Risk Factors	
Active cancer	1
Paralysis, paresis, or recent plaster immobilization of the lower extremities	1
Recently bedridden >3 days or major surgery, within 4 wk	1
Signs	
Localized tenderness along the distribution of the deep venous system	1
Entire leg swollen	1
Asymmetric calf swelling (>3 cm difference, 10 cm below tibial tuberosity)	1
Asymmetric pitting edema	1
Collateral superficial veins (nonvaricose)	1
Alternative Diagnosis	
Alternative diagnosis as likely or more likely than deep venous thrombosis	−2

*Interpretation of score: High probability if 3 points or more, moderate probability if 1 or 2 points, and low probability if 0 points or less.
From Wells PS et al: Value of assessment of pretest probability of deep-vein thrombosis in clinical management, *Lancet* 350:1795-1798, 1997. In McGee S: *Evidence-based physical diagnosis,* ed 4, Philadelphia, 2018, Elsevier.

isolated or nonocclusive calf vein thrombi. Whole-leg compression ultrasound can generally exclude proximal and distal DVT in a single evaluation. Withholding anticoagulation following a single negative whole-leg CUS is associated with a relatively low risk of venous thromboembolism (3.5% of inpatients will develop DVT) during a 3-mo follow-up.

- Contrast venography (Fig. E4) is the gold standard for evaluation of DVT of the lower extremity. It is, however, invasive and painful and rarely used in clinical practice. Additional disadvantages are the increased risk of phlebitis, new thrombosis, renal failure, and hypersensitivity reaction to contrast media; it also gives poor visualization of the deep femoral vein in the thigh and the internal iliac vein and its tributaries.
- Magnetic resonance direct thrombus imaging (MRDTI) is an accurate noninvasive test for diagnosis of DVT. It is particularly useful in suspected DVT patients with leg casts, which prevent CUS, and in pregnant patients with positive D-dimer and negative CUS. Current limitations are its cost and lack of widespread availability.

℞ TREATMENT

NONPHARMACOLOGIC THERAPY

- Gradual resumption of normal activity. Immobility promotes stasis and propagation of DVT. Patients should get up and walk as tolerated. The theoretic risk that ambulation may dislodge thrombi in the legs, precipitating PE, is unfounded.
- Patient education on anticoagulant therapy and associated risks.

ACUTE GENERAL Rx

- Direct oral anticoagulants (DOACs) apixaban or rivaroxaban are preferred as monotherapy for initial treatment of DVT. These newer anticoagulants (Table 4) are noninferior to warfarin, do not require periodic lab monitoring,

and have a relatively low bleeding risk. They are preferred agents for extended treatment of venous thromboembolism if cost is not a significant issue. Among direct acting anticoagulants, rivaroxaban is associated with greater risk of gastrointestinal bleeding.[2]

- When apixaban or rivaroxaban are not available or contraindicated, initial treatment of DVT requires therapeutic doses of heparin (low-molecular-weight heparin [LMWH] or unfractionated). LMWH is preferred due to ease of administration, less hemorrhage, and significantly fewer deaths. Unfractionated heparin is preferred in patients with renal insufficiency because LMWH is predominantly excreted in the urine.
- LMWH is generally administered for 5 to 7 days. Recommended dose of enoxaparin is 1 mg/kg q12h SC. Once-daily fondaparinux, a synthetic analogue of heparin, is also as effective and safe as twice-daily enoxaparin in the initial treatment of patients with symptomatic DVT. Once systemic anticoagulation is initiated, vitamin K antagonist warfarin is initiated. Warfarin is titrated to maintain an INR between 2 and 3. After ≥5 days, heparin is stopped and warfarin is continued as monotherapy. Warfarin is also recommended for patients with antiphospholipid syndrome since these patients have increased risk of thrombosis and stroke when treated with rivaroxaban or apixaban.[3]
- Outpatient treatment of DVT is appropriate for patients without thrombophilic conditions or substantial comorbidity. Exclusions from outpatient treatment of DVT (Box 1) include patients with potential high complication risk (e.g., active or high risk of bleeding, hemoglobin <7, platelet count <50,000, guaiac-positive stool, recent cerebrovascular accident or noncutaneous surgery, noncompliance).
- Compression stockings are effective in reducing the incidence of postthrombotic syndrome and should be used starting within 1 mo of proximal DVT and continued for at least 1 yr after diagnosis.
- Insertion of an inferior vena cava filter to prevent pulmonary embolism is recommended in patients with contraindications to anticoagulation (e.g., hemorrhagic stroke, active internal bleeding, pregnancy), HIT in a

TABLE 4 Comparison of Dabigatran, Rivaroxaban, Apixaban, and Edoxaban

	Dabigatran	Rivaroxaban	Apixaban	Edoxaban
Target	Thrombin (IIa)	Factor Xa	Factor Xa	Factor Xa
Active drug	No	Yes	Yes	Yes
Onset time (h)	0.5-2	2-4	3-4	1-3
Half-life (h)	12-17	5-13	~12	10-14
Renal excretion (%)	80	33	27	50

Modified from Hoffman R et al: *Hematology, basic principles and practice,* ed 8, Philadelphia, 2023, Elsevier.

BOX 1 Contraindications to Outpatient Treatment of Venous Thromboembolism[a]

- Active or high risk of bleeding
- Recent surgery (within 7 days)
- Cardiopulmonary instability
- Severe symptomatic venous obstruction
- High risk of pulmonary embolism
- Thrombocytopenia (platelets <50,000/μL)
- Other medical or surgical condition requiring inpatient management
- Medical noncompliance
- Geographic or telephone inaccessibility
- Poor hepatic function (international normalized ratio ≥1.5)
- Unstable renal function (e.g., rising serum creatinine)
- Poor home health care support environment

[a]Not an at-inclusive list.
From Niederhuber JE: *Abeloff's clinical oncology,* ed 6, Philadelphia, 2020, Elsevier.

D

I

patient with an active VTE/PE, recurrent PE despite adequate anticoagulant therapy, emergent surgery in patient with DVT, presence of free-floating iliofemoral thrombus, lower IVC thrombosis (incipient embolization), and chronic pulmonary (thromboembolic) hypertension with limited pulmonary reserve. Table 5 summarizes indications for IVC filter placement.

- Potential harms associated with IVC filters include migration, vessel penetration, excess DVT risk, fracture.
- Thrombolytic therapy (streptokinase) can be used in rare cases (unless contraindicated) in patients with extensive iliofemoral venous thrombosis and a low risk of bleeding. There are concerns about hemorrhagic complications related to the large doses of thrombolytics required in systemic thrombolysis for DVT (2% to 10% risk of major hemorrhagic complications).
- Other treatment modalities for DVT include surgical thrombectomy and catheter-directed thrombolysis (CDT). Thromboreduction by surgical thrombectomy is effective but invasive and expensive. CDT is also invasive, carries a bleeding risk, and will generally require ICU admission.

CHRONIC Rx

- The optimal duration of anticoagulant therapy varies with the cause of DVT and the patient's risk factors. The risk of recurrence is low if VTE is provoked by surgery, intermediate if provoked by a nonsurgical risk factor, and high if unprovoked. These risks should determine whether patients with VTE should undergo short-term vs. indefinite treatment.
- Therapy for 3 mo is generally satisfactory in patients with reversible risk factors (low-risk group). A high D-dimer level measured after 3 mo of anticoagulation in patients with

unprovoked DVT should favor a longer duration of therapy. The American College of Chest Physicians Guidelines suggests that patients with first unprovoked VTE receive indefinite anticoagulation unless their bleeding risk is high.

- The risk of recurrence in patients with a first unprovoked VTE who have negative D-dimer results is not low enough to justify stopping anticoagulant therapy in men but may be low enough in some cases to justify stopping therapy in women who were taking estrogen at the time of initial VTE.
- Anticoagulation for 6 mo is recommended for patients with idiopathic venous thrombosis or medical risk factors for DVT (intermediate-risk group). About 20% of patients with unprovoked venous thromboembolism have a recurrence within 2 yr after the withdrawal of oral anticoagulant therapy. Use of daily low-dose aspirin after discontinuation of anticoagulant treatment may provide a modest reduction in DVT risk.
- Indefinite anticoagulation is necessary in patients with DVT associated with active cancer; long-term anticoagulation is also indicated in patients with inherited thrombophilia (e.g., deficiency of antithrombin III, protein C or S antibody), high factor VIII levels, antiphospholipid antibody, and those with recurrent episodes of idiopathic DVT (high-risk group). Long-term anticoagulation should also be considered in the presence of comorbidities such as paroxysmal nocturnal hemoglobinuria (PNH), SLE (especially with nephrotic syndrome), some myeloproliferative disorders, IBD, and Cushing syndrome.
- Measurement of D-dimer after withdrawal of oral anticoagulation may be useful to estimate the risk of recurrence in selected patients. In patients with a first unprovoked DVT, positive D-dimer test results after cessation

of anticoagulation predict recurrence, regardless of test timing or patient's age. Patients with a first spontaneous DVT and a D-dimer level <250 mg/ml after withdrawal of oral anticoagulation have a low risk of DVT recurrence. Risk is lower in women than in men. In patients who have completed at least 3 mo of anticoagulation for a first episode of unprovoked DVT and after approximately 2 yr of follow-up, a negative D-dimer result is associated with a 3.5% annual risk of recurrent disease, whereas a positive D-dimer result is associated with an 8.9% annual risk for recurrence. Hence, elevated D-dimer levels would be an indication for prolonged therapy (for 1 or 2 more yr at a minimum).

- The presence of residual thrombosis on ultrasonography when anticoagulant therapy is discontinued is also associated with an increased risk for subsequent recurrent DVT; tailoring the duration of anticoagulation on the basis of the persistence of residual thrombi on ultrasonography may reduce the rate of recurrent DVT. Additional trials are needed before this approach can be adapted for all patients.
- Patients with DVT and pulmonary embolism are at high risk of recurrence whenever anticoagulation is discontinued; therefore, many experts recommend prolonged anticoagulation in this population group, especially if other risk factors for recurrence are present.

! PEARLS & CONSIDERATIONS

COMMENTS

- The prevalence of occult cancer is low among patients with a first unprovoked venous embolism. Routine screening with computed tomography (CT) of the abdomen and pelvis does not provide a clinically significant benefit.
- When using heparin, there is a risk of heparin-induced thrombocytopenia (HIT) (with unfractionated more so than with LMWH). Platelet count should be obtained initially and repeated every 3 days while on heparin.
- Therapeutic options for cancer-associated venous thromboembolism are summarized in Box 2. DOACs are more effective and more cost-effective than LMWH for treating cancer-associated thrombosis (CAT).[4]
- Isolated Deep Vein Thrombosis of the Calf: The American College of Chest Physicians Guidelines suggest (1) anticoagulation in patients with severe symptoms or risk factors for proximal extension, and (2) repeat sonogram in 2 wk in lower risk patients and anticoagulation only in those patients whose DVTs extend proximally. However, a recent trial[5] comparing anticoagulation and serial ultrasound management in calf thrombosis suggests benefits of anticoagulation over ultrasound surveillance along for DVT of the distal lower extremity.
- In-hospital risk factors for venous thromboembolism and bleeding: The Padua Prediction

---

TABLE 5 Indications for Inferior Vena Cava Filter Placement

	Indications for IVC Filter Placement	Examples
1.	DVT and contraindication to anticoagulation (A)	Hemorrhage while on anticoagulation
2.	DVT and failure of anticoagulation (A)	Recurrent DVT or PE despite anticoagulation, inability to achieve or maintain adequate anticoagulation
3.	DVT and low cardiopulmonary reserve or high mortality risk from possible PE (R)	Severe pulmonary hypertension, right heart failure, known large right-to-left shunt
4.	Populations with very high risk for PE (R)	Some postbariatric, orthopedic, or neurosurgical patients or multitrauma patients. Patients with expected prolonged immobilization
5.	High risk for life-threatening PE (R)	Large, unstable (free-floating) IVC clot
6.	DVT and high fall risk (R)	
7.	Prophylaxis during catheter-directed thrombolysis of DVT (R)	

There are two absolute indications for IVC filter placement: First, if the patient is at risk for PE (i.e., DVT) but for whatever reason he/she is not a candidate for systemic anticoagulation (i.e., hemorrhage); and second, if the patient developed a PE, new DVT, or an extension of DVT while on proper anticoagulation. There are a number of relative indications for filter placement. They are presented in rows 3 through 7. In every case the decision to place a filter compels careful consideration of the risks and benefits and may require multidisciplinary input. *(A),* Absolute; *DVT,* deep vein thrombosis; *IVC,* inferior vena cava; *PE,* pulmonary embolism; *(R),* relative.

From Cameron JL, Cameron AM: *Current surgical therapy,* ed 12, Philadelphia, 2017, Elsevier.

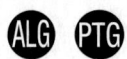

BOX 2   Therapeutic Options for Cancer-Associated Venous Thromboembolism (VTE)

Acute VTE Treatment Options
- Unfractionated heparin: 80 units/kg intravenous bolus followed by 18 units/kg/h infusion adjusted to aPTT ratio
- Dalteparin, 200 units/kg subcutaneously every 24 h
- Enoxaparin, 1 mg/kg subcutaneously every 12 h
- Tinzaparin, 175 units/kg subcutaneously every 24 h
- Fondaparinux, 5-10 mg subcutaneously every 24 h (5 mg for weight <50 kg, 7.5 mg for weight 50-100 kg, and 10 mg for weight >100 kg)
- Initial rivaroxaban dose 15 mg twice daily; switch to 20 mg once daily after 3 wk
- Dabigatran 150 mg bid after 5 days of parenteral agent
- Apixaban 10 mg bid × 7 days followed by 5 mg bid
- Edoxaban 60 mg once daily after 5 days of parenteral agent
- Vena caval filter

Chronic VTE Treatment Options
- Dalteparin, 200 units/kg subcutaneously every 24 h for 1 mo then 150 units/kg subcutaneously every 24 h
- Enoxaparin, 1 mg/kg every 12 h or 1.5 mg/kg subcutaneously every 24 h
- Tinzaparin, 175 units/kg subcutaneously every 24 h
- Vitamin K antagonists (e.g., warfarin) adjusted for an INR of 2-3
- Rivaroxaban 20 mg once daily; consider 10 mg once daily if appropriate
- Dabigatran 150 bid after 5 days of parenteral agent
- Apixaban 10 mg bid initial × 7 days followed by 5 mg bid
- Edoxaban 60 mg once daily after 5 days of parenteral agent
- Vena cava filter

From Niederhuber JE: *Abeloff's clinical oncology,* ed 6, Philadelphia, 2020, Elsevier.

Score is the most widely used risk assessment tool to aid clinicians in deciding whether to administer VTE prophylaxis to hospitalized medical patients. It has a point scoring system based on 11 variables (Table 6). A score of 4 or more points denotes a high risk for developing VTE. A simpler validated risk assessment model, developed at Intermountain Medical Center in Utah, predicts high risk if a patient has at least one of the following four risk factors: (1) previous VTE, (2) a medical indication for bed rest, (3) a peripherally inserted central venous catheter, or (4) cancer. Pharmacologic thromboprophylaxis is generally withheld if the bleeding risk is excessively high due to threatened, active, or recent major bleeding or thrombocytopenia.[6]

- Prophylaxis of DVT: Recommended in all patients at risk (e.g., low-molecular-weight heparin [enoxaparin 30 mg SC bid or fondaparinux 2.5 mg SC daily] after major trauma, postsurgery of hip and knee; enoxaparin 40 mg SC qd post-abdominal surgery in patients with moderate to high DVT risk; gradient elastic stockings alone or in combination with intermittent pneumatic compression [IPC] boots following neurosurgery). Graduated compression stockings (GCSs) are effective for preventing air-travel-related DVT and in reducing the risk of DVT in patients hospitalized for conditions other than stroke. The type of GCSs is also important because proximal DVT occurs more often in patients with stroke who wear below-knee stockings than in those who wear high-length stockings. The new oral anticoagulants (rivaroxaban, apixaban, etc.) are effective for thromboprophylaxis after THR and TKR. However, their clinical benefits over LMWH are marginal. Betrixaban is the first FDA-approved once-daily oral direct factor Xa inhibitor for prophylaxis of VTE in adults hospitalized for an acute medical illness with risk factors for VTE and moderately or severely restricted mobility. Apixaban appears to be as effective as LMWH for thromboprophylaxis in cancer patients but poses similar risk of bleeding and should be used with caution in patients with GI malignancies, thrombocytopenia, or renal impairment. Common regimens for venous thromboembolism prevention are summarized in Table 7. In patients with extremity fractures that have been treated operatively or with any pelvic or acetabular fracture, thromboprophylaxis with aspirin is noninferior to LMWH in preventing death and is associated with incidence of DVT, pulmonary embolism, and low mortality.[7] Box 3 describes traditional absolute and relative contraindications to pharmacologic

TABLE 6   Padua Prediction Score for Identification of Hospitalized Patients at Risk for Venous Thromboembolism

Risk Factor	Scoring
Cancer	3
Previous VTE	3
Immobility	3
Thrombophilia	3
Trauma/surgery	2
Age ≥70 yr	1
Heart/respiratory failure	1
Acute MI or stroke	1
Infection/rheumatologic disorder	1
Obesity	1
Hormonal treatment	1

High risk for developing pulmonary embolism is defined as 4 score points or greater.
VTE, Venous thromboembolic.
From Libby P et al: *Braunwald's heart disease, a textbook of cardiovascular medicine,* ed 12, Philadelphia, 2022, Elsevier.

TABLE 7   Common Regimens for Venous Thromboembolism Prevention

Condition	Prophylaxis
Hospitalization with medical illness	Unfractionated heparin 5000 units SC bid or tid or
	Enoxaparin 40 mg SC qd or
	Dalteparin 2500 units or 5000 units SC qd or
	Fondaparinux 2.5 mg SC qd with normal renal function (in patients with a heparin allergy such as heparin-induced thrombocytopenia) or
	Rivaroxaban 10 mg qd started at hospital discharge and continued for 5 wk
General surgery	Unfractionated heparin 5000 units SC bid or tid or
	Enoxaparin 40 mg SC qd or
	Dalteparin 2500 or 5000 units SC qd
Major orthopedic surgery	Warfarin (target INR 2.5) or
	Enoxaparin 30 mg SC bid or
	Enoxaparin 40 mg SC qd or
	Dalteparin 2500 or 5000 units SC qd or
	Fondaparinux 2.5 mg SC qd or
	Rivaroxaban 10 mg qd or
	Aspirin 81 mg BID or
	Rivaroxaban 10 mg qd for 5 days and then aspirin 81 mg daily thereafter
	Dabigatran 220 mg qd or
	Apixaban 2.5 mg twice daily

bid, Twice daily; *INR,* international normalized ratio; *qd,* every day; *SC,* subcutaneous; *tid,* three times a day.
From Libby P et al: *Braunwald's heart disease, a textbook of cardiovascular medicine,* ed 12, Philadelphia, 2022, Elsevier.

BOX 3 Traditional Absolute and Relative Contraindications to Pharmacologic and Mechanical Venous Thromboembolism Prophylaxis[a]

Contraindications to Pharmacologic Prophylaxis
- Active, recent, or high risk of clinically significant bleeding
- Thrombocytopenia (platelet count <50,000/μL)
- Systemic coagulopathy (e.g., disseminated intravascular coagulation, international normalized ratio >1.4, or activated partial thromboplastin time ratio >1.2, excluding lupus inhibitors)
- Known congenital bleeding disorders (e.g., hemophilia A or B and von Willebrand disease)
- Known functional acquired or congenital platelet disorder (e.g., Bernard-Soulier syndrome and uremic platelet dysfunction)
- Heparin-induced thrombocytopenia (for unfractionated or low-molecular-weight heparin)

Contraindications to Mechanical Prophylaxis
- Acute or recent deep venous thrombosis (within 3 mo)
- Arterial insufficiency in target limb
- Open lower extremity wound

[a]List not inclusive.
From Niederhuber JE: *Abeloff's clinical oncology,* ed 6, Philadelphia, 2020, Elsevier.

and mechanical venous thromboembolism prophylaxis.
- Recurrent Thromboembolism: The risk of recurrent venous thromboembolism in heterozygous carriers of factor V Leiden and a first spontaneous venous thromboembolism is similar to that of noncarriers of factor V Leiden; therefore, heterozygous patients should receive secondary thromboprophylaxis for a similar length of time as patients without factor V Leiden. Prediction of VTE recurrence in patients with prior unprovoked VTE is summarized in Table E8. Management of recurrent venous thromboembolism in patients with cancer is summarized in Table 9.
- Postthrombotic Syndrome: Approximately 20% to 50% of patients with DVT develop postthrombotic syndrome characterized by leg edema, pain, venous ectasia, skin induration, and ulceration. Patients with extensive DVT and those with more severe postthrombotic manifestations 1 mo after DVT have poorer long-term outcomes. Recent trials have shown that compression stockings after DVT do not prevent postthrombotic syndrome.
- Exercise following DVT is reasonable because it improves flexibility of the affected leg and does not increase symptoms in patients with postthrombotic syndrome.
- Upper Extremity DVT: It is less common than lower extremity DVT and is seen more frequently in patients requiring central venous catheters or wires. It confers risk for mortality, recurrent thromboembolic events, and postthrombotic syndrome similar to that of lower extremity DVT. It is classified as primary upper extremity DVT (Paget-Schroetter syndrome), defined as a thrombus in the axillary and subclavian veins in absence of identifiable thrombosis risk factors. It accounts for 20% of upper extremity DVT cases and may be due to an underlying anatomic abnormality at the thoracic outlet in combination with local hypercoagulability due to venous stretching or perivascular fibrosis from recurrent venous compression. Secondary upper extremity DVT is defined as any DVT related to a predisposing factor (e.g., insertion of central venous catheter, wires, or other devices; malignancy). In patients with secondary upper extremity DVT, removal of the catheter is not routinely recommended but is warranted if there is a catheter malfunction or infection, if anticoagulation therapy is contraindicated or has failed, or if the catheter is no longer needed. Anticoagulation therapy in upper extremity DVT consists of use of vitamin K antagonists, except in patients with cancer, for whom LMWH is preferred. Optimal duration of anticoagulation treatment in upper extremity DVT is 3 to 6 mo (including in those in whom a central catheter has been removed).
- DVT Therapy in Pregnancy: Vitamin K antagonists such as warfarin are contraindicated in pregnancy. Low-molecular-weight heparins are safe and effective. Typical agents used in pregnancy include dalteparin (200 IU per kg of body weight daily or 100 IU per kg twice daily) or enoxaparin (1.5 mg per kg daily or 1 mg per kg twice daily).
- Management of bleeding in patients taking anticoagulants is illustrated in Fig. 5.
- Reversal of Anticoagulation: Vitamin K (1 mg PO or 2 mg IV) can be used to reverse elevated INR (3 to 6) from warfarin when elective or urgent procedures are needed. The administration of vitamin K can take more than 24 h to fully restore vitamin K-dependent coagulation factors II, VII, IX, and X. The American College of Chest Physicians recommends the following guidelines for managing elevated INRs or bleeding in patients receiving vitamin A antagonist therapy:
  1. INR between 4.5 and 10 and no significant bleeding: Omit dose and monitor the next day, routine use of vitamin K is not recommended.
  2. INR >10 and no significant bleeding: Hold vitamin K antagonist, give 5 to 10 mg orally of vitamin K. Monitor the next day and use additional vitamin K if necessary. Resume therapy at lower dose when INR becomes therapeutic.
  3. Serious bleeding at any elevation of INR: Hold vitamin K antagonist and supplement with prothrombin complex concentrates (PCC). Give vitamin K (10 mg by slow intravenous [IV] infusion over 30 min to reduce the risk of anaphylaxis. Vitamin K1 can be repeated every 12 h. PCC composition in the U.S. (3-factor PCC) includes clotting factors II, IX, and X but minimal amounts of factor VII (unlike PCC products available outside of the U.S. [4-factor PCC], which have a significant amount of factor VII). In order to replace the low

TABLE 9 Management of Recurrent Venous Thromboembolism in Patients With Cancer

Causes	Management
Extrinsic vascular compression (causes sluggish flow)	Relieve vascular compression due to tumor, nodal masses, or anatomic abnormalities (i.e., May-Thurner syndrome/iliac vein compression, thoracic outlet syndrome) with surgical decompression, vascular stents, or other
Intrinsic vascular obstruction	Remove central venous catheter or devices responsible for sluggish flow
Trousseau syndrome	Switch to LMWH
Heparin-induced thrombocytopenia	Discontinue unfractionated or LMWH and start a direct thrombin inhibitor (preferred) or fondaparinux
Therapeutic resistance	If the patient is taking warfarin, switch to LMWH
	If the patient is taking LMWH, check to ensure the correct full weight-based dose is being used, switch to twice-daily dosing (if administration is once daily), consider checking LMWH (anti-Xa) level, initiate an empiric 25% dose increase, or switch to fondaparinux

LMWH, Low-molecular-weight heparin.
From Niederhuber JE: *Abeloff's clinical oncology,* ed 6, Philadelphia, 2020, Elsevier.

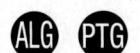

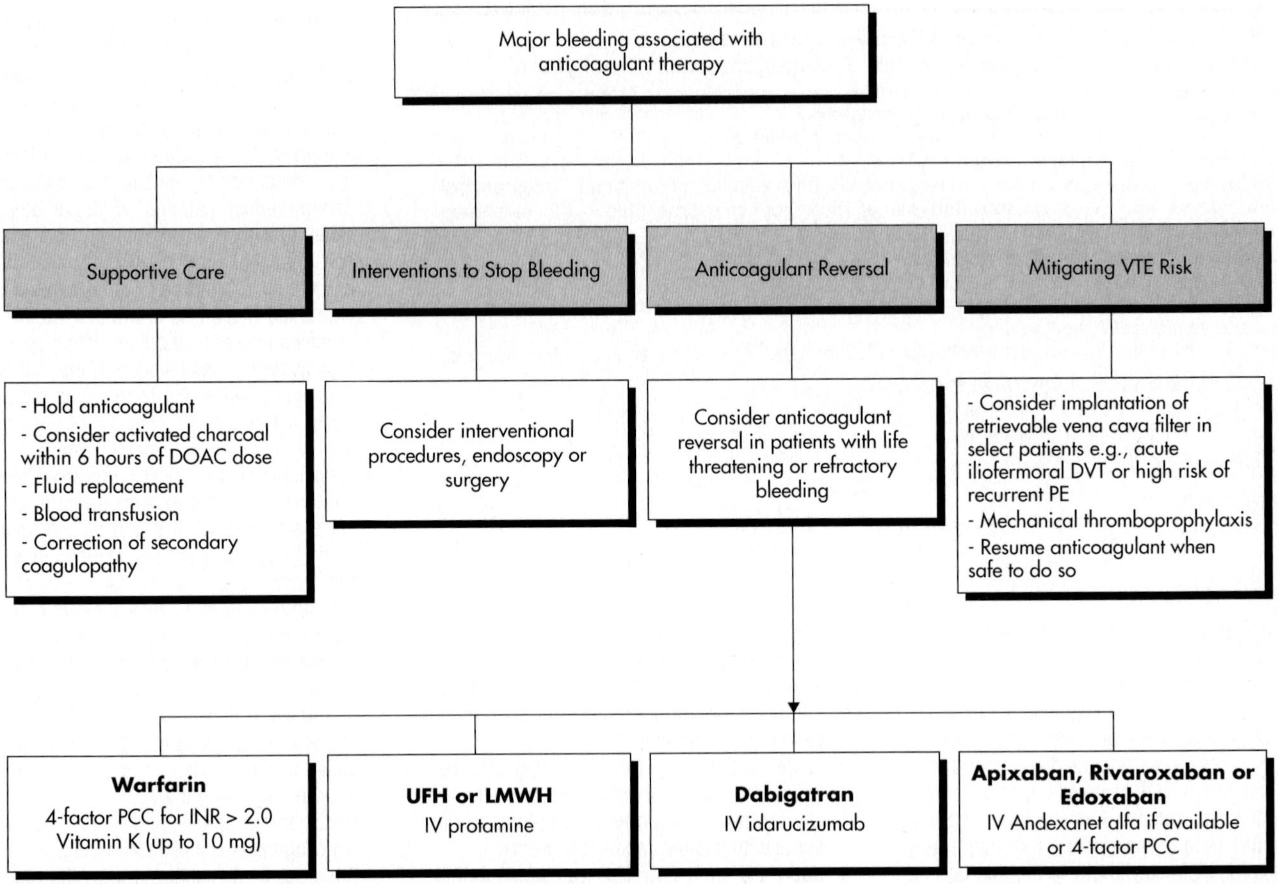

Major bleeding associated with anticoagulant therapy

Supportive Care	Interventions to Stop Bleeding	Anticoagulant Reversal	Mitigating VTE Risk
- Hold anticoagulant - Consider activated charcoal within 6 hours of DOAC dose - Fluid replacement - Blood transfusion - Correction of secondary coagulopathy	Consider interventional procedures, endoscopy or surgery	Consider anticoagulant reversal in patients with life threatening or refractory bleeding	- Consider implantation of retrievable vena cava filter in select patients e.g., acute iliofermoral DVT or high risk of recurrent PE - Mechanical thromboprophylaxis - Resume anticoagulant when safe to do so

Warfarin 4-factor PCC for INR > 2.0 Vitamin K (up to 10 mg)	**UFH or LMWH** IV protamine	**Dabigatran** IV idarucizumab	**Apixaban, Rivaroxaban or Edoxaban** IV Andexanet alfa if available or 4-factor PCC

FIG. 5 Management of bleeding in patients taking anticoagulants. *DOAC,* Direct oral anticoagulant; *FEIBA,* factor eight inhibitor bypass agent; *LMWH,* low-molecular-weight heparin; *PCC,* prothrombin concentrate complex; *UFH,* unfractionated heparin. (From Hoffman R et al: *Hematology, basic principles and practice,* ed 8, Philadelphia, 2023, Elsevier.)

factor VII, some clinicians in the U.S. will also give fresh frozen plasma (FFP) in addition to vitamin K and PCC in patients with life-threatening warfarin-related bleeding.
- Specific Reversal Agents for Nonvitamin K Antagonist Anticoagulants (Table 10):
    1. Idarucizumab, an antibody fragment given at a dose of 5 g IV, has been shown to completely reverse the anticoagulant effect of dabigatran within minutes.
    2. The anticoagulant activity of factor Xa inhibitors apixaban, rivaroxaban, and edoxaban can be rapidly reversed with IV administration of andexanet alfa.
    3. These reversal agents are very expensive (over $20,000 for each use).

REFERENCES & SUGGESTED READINGS
Available at eBooks.Health.Elsevier.com.

RELATED CONTENT
Deep Vein Thrombosis (DVT) (Patient Information)
Antiphospholipid Antibody Syndrome (Related Key Topic)
Hypercoagulable State (Related Key Topic)
Postthrombotic Syndrome (Related Key Topic)
Pulmonary Embolism (Related Key Topic)
Upper Extremity Deep Vein Thrombosis (Related Key Topic)

AUTHOR: **FRED F. FERRI, MD**

TABLE 10 Reversal Agents for Direct Oral Anticoagulants

Feature	Idarucizumab	Andexanet Alfa	Ciraparantag
Structure	Humanized antibody fragment	Recombinant human factor Xa variant	Synthetic, small cationic molecule
Mass (Da)	47,776	39,000	573
Mechanism of action	Binds dabigatran with high affinity	Competes with factors Xa (and IIa) for binding	Binds via hydrogen bonding
Target	Dabigatran	Rivaroxaban, apixaban, edoxaban, and heparins	Dabigatran, rivaroxaban, apixaban, edoxaban, and heparins
Administration	Intravenous bolus	Intravenous bolus followed by a 2-h infusion	Intravenous bolus
Measurement of reversal	Activated partial thromboplastin time, diluted thrombin time, or ecarin clotting time or chromogenic assay	Calibrated antifactor Xa assays	Whole-blood clotting time
Elimination	Renal (catabolism)	Not reported	Not reported
Cost	$3500 per dose in the U.S.	Unknown; likely to be at least as much as idarucizumab	Likely to be low

From Libby P et al: *Braunwald's heart disease, a textbook of cardiovascular medicine,* ed 12, Philadelphia, 2022, Elsevier.

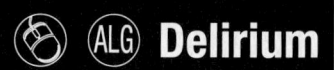

D

I

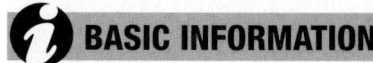 **BASIC INFORMATION**

DEFINITION

The American Psychiatric Association's *Diagnostic and Statistical Manual,* 5th edition (DSM-5), defines delirium as:
- Disturbance of consciousness with reduced ability to focus, sustain, or shift attention.
- The disturbance develops over a short period of time (usually hours to days) and tends to fluctuate during the course of a day.
- An additional disturbance in cognition (e.g., memory deficit, disorganization, language, visuospatial ability, or perception).
- A change in cognition or development of a perceptual disturbance that is not better accounted for by a preexisting, established, or evolving dementia.
- There is evidence from history, physical exam, or lab findings that the disturbance is caused by medical condition, substance intoxication or withdrawal (i.e., due to a drug of abuse or to a medication), or exposure to a toxin, or is due to multiple etiologies.

SYNONYMS

Acute confusional state
Toxic or metabolic encephalopathy

THEORIES REGARDING PATHOPHYSIOLOGY

- Neuroinflammation, with increased permeability of the blood-brain barrier
- Acetylcholine deficiency
- Other neurotransmitter imbalances, including excesses of norepinephrine, serotonin, and, most important, dopamine

CLASSIFICATION

Hyperactive, hypoactive, and mixed subtype

ICD-10CM CODES	
F05	Delirium, not induced by alcohol and other psychoactive substances
F05.9	Delirium, unspecified
F06.0	Organic hallucinosis
F05.8	Other delirium
F05.0	Delirium not superimposed on dementia
F05.1	Delirium superimposed on dementia

EPIDEMIOLOGY & DEMOGRAPHICS

Nearly 30% of older patients experience delirium at some time during the hospital course. In older surgical patients, the risk varies from 10% to 50%. Hypoactive is more common. Predisposing factors for delirium among older adults hospitalized for a medical or surgical illness are summarized in Table 1. Delirium is the most common mental disorder in patients with medical illness. Any age, race, or gender can be affected. Predisposing factors for the development of delirium during hospitalization are summarized in Table 2. Pediatric delirium is often missed but remains important because delirium is associated with longer hospital stays, decreased cognitive performance, and increased mortality. Risk factors include extremes of age, severe pain, illicit substance use, surgery, dementia, and kidney or liver failure (Table 3).

PHYSICAL FINDINGS & CLINICAL PRESENTATION

- One of the earliest symptoms is change in level of awareness and ability to focus, sustain, or shift attention. Symptoms may differ both among patients and within one patient. Family members or caregivers report that the patient "isn't acting quite right." Symptoms may include poor attention, sleepiness, agitation, or psychosis.
- Acuteness of presentation helps in differentiating delirium with dementia. Change in

---

TABLE 1 Predisposing Factors for Delirium Among Older Adults Hospitalized for a Medical or a Surgical Illness

Risk Factor	Odds Ratio (OR) Range[a]	The Delirium Vulnerability Scale
Cognitive impairment:	3.5-5	Choose one score only
• Chart diagnosis of dementia	2-4	3 points
• MMSE <24	4	2 points
• Prior history of delirium		1 point
Current history of depression	2-4	1 point
Current history of alcohol abuse	3-6.5	2 points
Current and untreated hearing loss	2	1 point
Current and untreated vision loss	2-3.5	1 point
Need assistance in two basic activities of daily living	2.5	1 point
Current use of anticholinergic	1.5-2.7	2 points
Dehydration defined by BUN/creatinine >21:1	1.8-2	1 point
Sodium abnormality (Na <130 or Na >150)	2-4	1 point
Vascular risk factors: history of:	2.3	Choose a score of 1 point if at least one risk factor was present (maximum score is also 1 point)
• Hypertension	1.3-2.9	
• Congestive heart failure	1.3	
• Diabetes mellitus	2.2	
• Cerebrovascular accident	1.4	
• Atrial fibrillation		
Admitted for		
• Urgent surgical repair of hip fracture	3	2 points
• Elective aortic aneurysm repair	6	3 points
Total Points		_____ (range 0-17)
Interpretation:	Risk category	Probability of developing delirium[b]
• 0-1 point	Low	<5%
• 2-3 points	Mild	5%-20%
• 4-7 points	Moderate	21%-40%
• >7 points	Severe	>40%

BUN, Blood urea nitrogen; *MMSE,* Mini-Mental State Examination.
[a]OR estimates were based on review of the literature.
[b]Delirium probability estimates for each risk category were based on a literature review and the authors' clinical and research experiences. The delirium vulnerability scale has not been validated in a prospective cohort study.
From Warshaw G et al: *Ham's primary care geriatrics,* ed 7, Philadelphia, 2022, Elsevier.

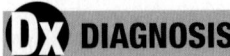

TABLE 2 Precipitating Factors for the Development of Delirium During Hospitalization for Medical or Surgical Illness

Precipitating Factor	Odds Ratio (OR)
Use of physical restraints	4.4
Malnutrition	4
Using more than three new medications during hospitalization	2.9
Use of bladder catheterization	2.4
Exposed to any iatrogenic event	1.9
Intraoperative hypotension (at least 31% drop in mean perioperative BP or a SBP ≤80 mm Hg)	1.4
Postoperative Hct <30%	1.7
Untreated postoperative pain	5.4-9
Use of anticholinergic drug	1.5-2.7

BP, Blood pressure; *Hct*, hematocrit; *SBP*, systolic blood pressure.
From Warshaw G et al: *Ham's primary care geriatrics*, ed 7, Philadelphia, 2022, Elsevier.

TABLE 3 Mnemonic for Risk Factors for Delirium and Agitation

I Watch Death	Delirium
Infection	**D**rugs
Withdrawal	**E**lectrolyte and physiologic abnormalities
Acute metabolic	**L**ack of drugs (withdrawal)
Trauma/pain	**I**nfection
Central nervous system pathology	**R**educed sensory input (blindness, deafness)
Hypoxia	**I**ntracranial problems (CVA, meningitis, seizure)
Deficiencies (vitamin B_{12}, thiamine)	**U**rinary retention and fecal impaction
Endocrinopathies (thyroid, adrenal)	**M**yocardial problems (MI, arrhythmia, CHF)
Acute vascular (hypertension, shock)	
Toxins/drugs	
Heavy metals	

CHF, Congestive heart failure; *CVA*, cerebrovascular accident; *MI*, myocardial infarction.
From Vincent JL et al: *Textbook of critical care*, ed 6, Philadelphia, 2011, Saunders.

cognition, perceptual problems (such as visual, auditory, or somatosensory hallucination usually with lack of insight), memory loss, disorientation, difficulty with speech and language. It is important to ascertain from family member or caregivers the patient's level of functioning before onset of delirium.
- Elderly patients with delirium often do not look sick, but patients with delirium are sick by definition.
- Hyperactive delirium represents only 25% of cases, with the others having hypoactive (quiet) delirium.
- There is often a prodrome phase that later blends into hypoactive delirium or erupts into an agitated confusional state.
- Physical examination should be performed, focusing on signs of infection, dehydration, or chronic disease that may be exacerbated. Vital signs are key. Consider using the Mini-Mental Status Exam or the Montreal Cognitive Assessment.
- Fig. 1 describes an algorithm for evaluation of mental status changes in an older patient.
- Table 4 summarizes delirium assessment tools.

ETIOLOGY

Can be multifactorial; often falls into one of the following categories (Table 5):
- Drugs: Benzodiazepines are the worst offenders, but other drugs such as narcotics, anticholinergics, beta-blockers, steroids, nonsteroidal antiinflammatory drugs, digoxin, cimetidine can cause delirium; also, withdrawal states such as alcohol withdrawal or benzodiazepine withdrawal can cause delirium
- Infection or inflammation
- Metabolic: Kidney or liver failure, thyroid, adrenal, or glucose dysregulation, anemia, vitamin deficiency such as Wernicke encephalopathy or vitamin B_{12} deficiency, inborn metabolic errors such as porphyrias or Wilson disease
- Stress: Surgery, sleep problems, pain, fever, hypoxia, anesthesia, environmental changes, fecal or urinary retention, burns
- Fluids, electrolytes, nutrition (FEN): Dysregulation of calcium, magnesium, potassium, or sodium; dehydration; volume overload; altered pH
- Brain disorder: Central nervous system (CNS) infection, head injury, hypertensive encephalopathy

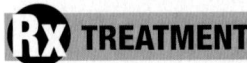 DIAGNOSIS

DIFFERENTIAL DIAGNOSIS
- Primary psychiatric illness
- Focal syndromes
- Dementia
- Sundowning
- Nonconvulsive status epilepticus

Remember, delirium may coexist with any of the listed conditions. Table 6 summarizes the differential diagnosis of delirium. Tables 7 and 8 describe clinical factors that help differentiate delirium and dementia from psychiatric disease. Potentially life-threatening causes of delirium are described in Table 9.

LABORATORY TESTS
- Complete blood count, electrolytes, liver function tests, ammonia, drug levels (digoxin, lithium)
- Toxicology screen, urinalysis, urine culture
- Thyroid function tests, vitamin B_{12}, and folate levels
- Rapid plasma reagin for syphilis, blood, urine, and spinal fluid culture
- Arterial blood gas
- Lumbar puncture is mandatory when cause of delirium is not obvious

IMAGING STUDIES
- Consider head CT (to look for bleed, trauma, tumor, atrophy, dementia, stroke)
- Chest radiograph (to look for tumor, infection)

ELECTROENCEPHALOGRAM
To exclude seizure, confirm diagnosis of metabolic encephalopathy

TREATMENT

NONPHARMACOLOGIC THERAPY
- The most important consideration is to keep the patient safe by using a variety of methods, including frequent reorientation.
- A quiet, restful, simplified environment with cues to time and location such as clock or calendar is helpful, as well as consistent staff providing both personal and medical care. If possible, encourage familiar family members and friends to keep the patient company.
- Early mobilization and minimized use of physical restraints (use of physical restraints if necessary to ensure safety).
- Visual and hearing aids for patients with these impairments.

ACUTE GENERAL Rx
- Reverse any treatable cause, such as volume repletion for patients with dehydration, antibiotics for urinary tract infection.
- Antipsychotic agents should not be used routinely for preventing or treating delirium. Pharmacologic treatment with antipsychotic agents should be initiated only when symptoms are severe, dangerous, or cause significant distress to the patient. In general these agents are similarly effective and the choice

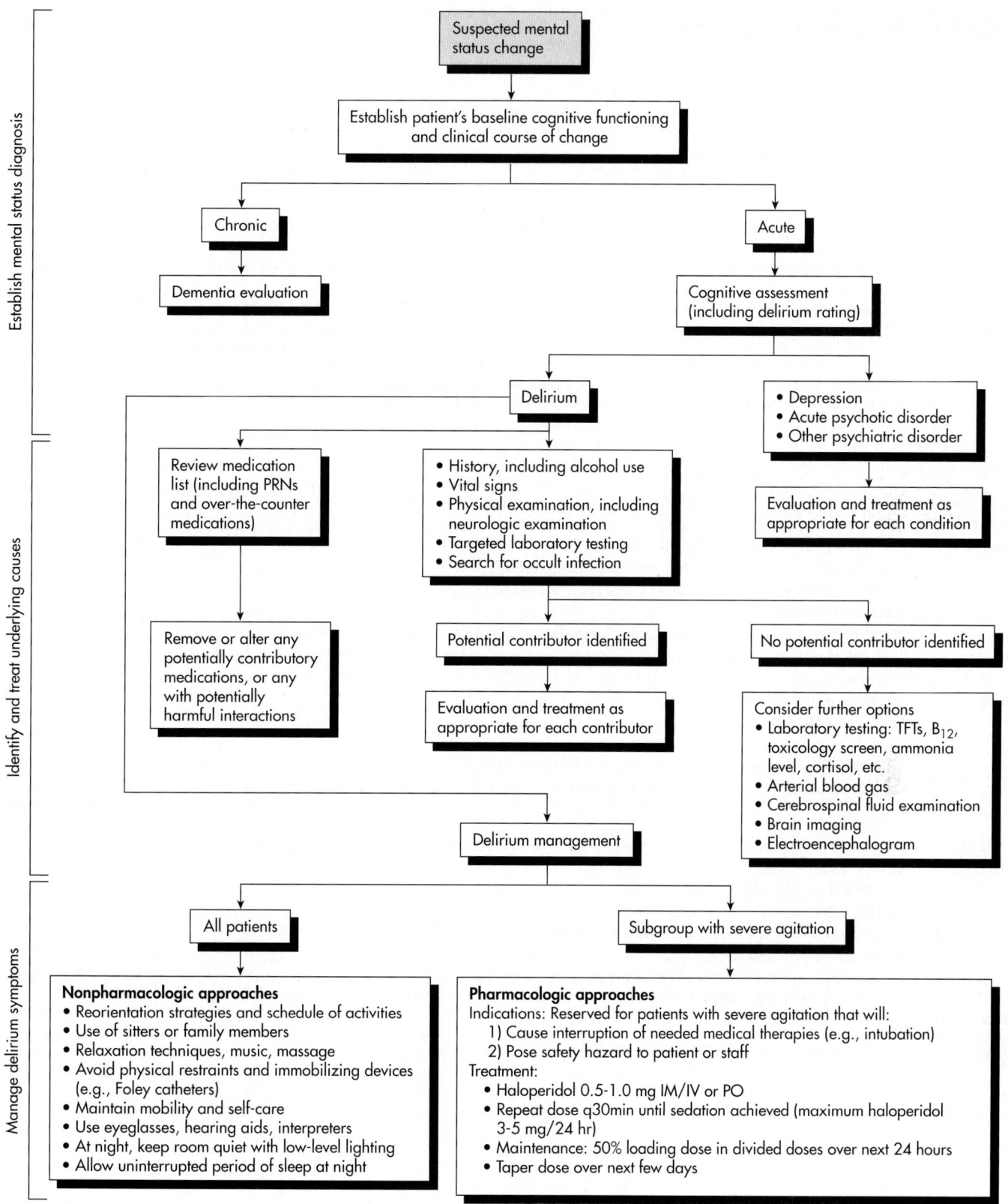

FIG. 1 Algorithm for evaluation of suspected mental status change in an older patient. *IM,* Intramuscular; *IV,* intravenous; *NG,* nasogastric; *PO,* by mouth; *PRN,* as needed; *TFTs,* thyroid function tests. (Modified from Goldman L, Ausiello D [eds]: *Cecil textbook of medicine,* ed 24, Philadelphia, 2012, Saunders.)

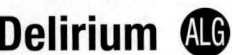

TABLE 4 Delirium Assessment Tools

Tool	Structure	Notes
Confusion Assessment Method (CAM)	Full scale of 11 items Abbreviated algorithm targeting four cardinal symptoms	Intended for use by nonpsychiatric clinicians
Confusion Assessment Method for the Intensive Care Unit (CAM-ICU)	Algorithm targeting four cardinal symptoms	Designed for use by nursing staff in the ICU
Intensive Care Delirium Screening Checklist (ICDSC)	8-item screening checklist	Bedside screening tool for use by nonpsychiatric physicians or nurses in the ICU
Delirium Rating Scale (DRS)	Full scale of 10 items Abbreviated 7- or 8-item subscales for repeated administration	Provides data for confirmation of diagnosis and measurement of severity
Delirium Rating Scale—Revised–98 (DRS-R-98)	16-item scale that can be divided into a 3-item diagnostic subscale and a 13-item severity subscale	Revision of DRS is better suited to repeat administration
Memorial Delirium Assessment Scale (MDAS)	10-item severity rating scale	Grades severity of delirium once diagnosis has been made
Neecham Confusion Scale	10-item rating scale	Designed for use by nursing staff and primarily validated for use in elderly populations in acute medical or nursing home setting

From Stern TA et al: *Massachusetts General Hospital handbook of general hospital psychiatry,* ed 7, Philadelphia, 2017, Elsevier.

TABLE 5 Major Causes of Delirium

Metabolic	Electrolytes: Hypo/hypernatremia, hypo/hypercalcemia, hypo/hypermagnesemia, hypo/hyperphosphatemia
	Endocrine: Hypo/hyperthyroidism, hypo/hypercortisolism, hypo/hyperglycemia
	Cardiac encephalopathy, hepatic encephalopathy, uremic encephalopathy
	Hypoxia and hypercarbia
	Vitamin deficiencies: Vitamin B_{12}, nicotinic acid, folic acid. Most notably Wernicke encephalopathy from thiamine deficiency
	Toxic and industrial exposures: Carbon monoxide, organic solvent, lead, manganese, mercury, carbon disulfide, heavy metals
	Porphyria
Toxic	Intoxication and overdose
	Serotonin syndrome
	Malignant neuroleptic syndrome
	Withdrawal: Alcohol, benzodiazepines, barbiturates, amphetamines, cocaine, coffee, phencyclidine, hallucinogens, inhalants, meperidine, and other narcotics
	Drugs: Anticholinergic, benzodiazepines, opiates, antihistamines, antiepileptics, muscle relaxants, dopamine agonists, monoamine oxidase inhibitors, levodopa, corticosteroids, fluoroquinolone and cephalosporin antibiotics, beta-blockers, digitalis, lithium, clozapine, tricyclic antidepressants, calcineurin inhibitors
Infectious	Urinary tract infection, pneumonia, sepsis, meningitis, encephalitis, Creutzfeldt-Jakob and other prion diseases
Neurologic	Vascular: Ischemic stroke, intracerebral or subarachnoid hemorrhage, vasculitis
	Autoimmune and paraneoplastic encephalitldes
	Neoplastic: Brain tumors, carcinomatous meningitis
	Seizure related: Postictal state, nonconvulsive status epilepticus
	Trauma: Concussion, subdural hematoma
Perioperative	Surgery: Thoracic (cardiac and noncardiac), vascular, and hip replacement, anesthetic and drug effects, hypoxia and anemia, hyperventilation, fluid and electrolyte disturbances, hypotension, embolism, infection or sepsis, untreated pain, fragmented sleep, sensory deprivation or overload
Miscellaneous	Hyperviscosity syndromes

From Jankovic J et al: *Bradley and Daroff's neurology in clinical practice,* ed 8, Philadelphia, 2022, Elsevier.

TABLE 6 Differential Diagnosis of Delirium

General Cause	Specific Cause
Vascular	Hypertensive encephalopathy Cerebral arteriosclerosis Intracranial hemorrhage or thrombosis Emboli from atrial fibrillation, patent foramen ovale, or endocarditic valve Circulatory collapse (shock) Systemic lupus erythematosus Polyarteritis nodosa Thrombotic thrombocytopenic purpura Hyperviscosity syndrome Sarcoid Posterior reversible encephalopathy syndrome (PRES) Cerebral aneurysm
Infectious	Encephalitis Bacterial or viral meningitis, fungal meningitis (cryptococcal, coccidioidal, *Histoplasma*) Sepsis General paresis Brain, epidural, or subdural abscess Malaria Human immunodeficiency virus Lyme disease Typhoid fever Parasitic (*Toxoplasma,* trichinosis, cysticercosis, echinococcosis) Behçet syndrome Mumps
Neoplastic	Space-occupying lesions, such as gliomas, meningiomas, abscesses Paraneoplastic syndromes Carcinomatous meningitis
Degenerative	Dementias Huntington disease Creutzfeldt-Jakob disease Wilson disease
Intoxication	Chronic intoxication or withdrawal effect of drugs, including sedative-hypnotics, opiates, tranquilizers, anticholinergics, dissociative anesthetics, anticonvulsants
Neurophysiologic	Epilepsy Postictal states Complex partial status epilepticus
Traumatic	Intracranial bleeds Postoperative trauma Heat stroke Fat emboli syndrome
Intraventricular	Normal-pressure hydrocephalus
Vitamin Deficiency	Thiamine (Wernicke-Korsakoff syndrome) Niacin (pellagra) B_{12} (pernicious anemia)
Endocrine/Metabolic	Diabetic coma and shock Uremia Myxedema Hyperthyroidism Parathyroid dysfunction Hypoglycemia Hepatic or renal failure Porphyria Severe electrolyte or acid/base disturbances Cushing or Addison syndrome Sleep apnea Carcinoid Whipple disease
Autoimmune	Autoimmune encephalitides Steroid-responsive encephalopathy associated with thyroiditis (SREAT)/Hashimoto encephalopathy Systemic lupus erythematosus Multiple sclerosis
Poisoning	Heavy metals (lead, manganese, mercury) Carbon monoxide Anticholinergics Other toxins
Anoxia	Hypoxia and anoxia secondary to pulmonary or cardiac failure, anesthesia, anemia
Psychiatric	Depressive pseudodementia, catatonia, Bell mania

From Stern TA et al: *Massachusetts General Hospital handbook of general hospital psychiatry,* ed 7, Philadelphia, 2017, Elsevier.

TABLE 7 Clinical Factors That Help Differentiate Delirium and Dementia From Psychiatric Disease

Characteristic	Delirium	Dementia	Psychiatric Illness
Symptoms			
Age at onset	<12 or >40 yr	Usually elderly, >50 yr	13-40 yr
Onset	Acute	Gradual or insidious	Gradual
Symptom course	Rapid, fluctuating	Stable and progressive	Stable
Duration	Days to weeks	Months to years	Months to years
Reversibility	Usually	Rarely	Rarely
History			
Past medical history	Substance abuse, medical illness	Comorbid conditions of aging	Previous psychiatric history
Family history	Unusual	History of dementia	History of psychiatric illness
Physical Examination			
Vital signs	Usually abnormal	Usually normal	Usually normal
Involuntary activity	May have tremors, asterixis, etc.	None unless coexistent disease	None
Mental Status			
Affect	Emotional lability	Flat affect with advanced disease	Flat affect
Orientation	Usually impaired	Impaired with advanced disease	Rarely impaired
Attention	Impaired	Slow to focus	Disorganized
Hallucinations	Primarily visual	Rare	Primarily auditory
Speech	Slow, incoherent, dysarthric	Usually coherent	Usually coherent
Consciousness	Decreased to impaired	Normal (clear)	Alert
Intellectual function	Usually impaired	Impaired	Intact

From Adams JG et al: *Emergency medicine, clinical essentials,* ed 2, Philadelphia, 2013, Elsevier.

TABLE 8 Special Problems in the Differential Diagnosis of Delirium[a]

Clinical Feature	Delirium	Dementias	Stroke With Wernicke Aphasia	Schizophrenia	Depression
Course	Acute onset; hours, days, or more	Insidious onset[b]; months or years; progressive	Sudden onset; chronic, stable deficit	Insidious onset, 6 mo or more; acute psychotic phases	Insidious onset, at least 2 wk, often months
Attention	Markedly impaired attention and arousal	Normal early; impairment later	Normal	Normal to mild impairment	Mild impairment
Fluctuation	Prominent in attention arousal; disturbed day/night cycle	Prominent fluctuations absent; lesser disturbances in day/night cycle	Absent	Absent	Absent
Perception	Misperceptions; illusions and pareidolias; hallucinations, usually visual, fleeting; paramnesia	Perceptual abnormalities much less prominent[c]; paramnesia	Normal	Hallucinations, auditory with personal reference	May have mood-congruent hallucinations
Speech and language	Abnormal clarity, speed, and coherence; disjointed and dysarthric; misnaming; characteristic dysgraphia	Early anomia; empty speech; abnormal comprehension	Prominent paraphasias and neologisms; empty speech; abnormal comprehension	Disorganized, with a bizarre theme	Decreased amount of speech
Other cognition	Disorientation to time, place; recent memory and visuospatial abnormalities	Disorientation to time, place; multiple other higher cognitive deficits	No other necessary deficits	Disorientation to person; concrete interpretations	Mental slowing; indecisiveness; memory retrieval difficulty
Behavior	Lethargy or delirium; non-systematized delusions; emotional lability	Disinterested; disengaged; disinhibited; delusions and other psychiatric symptoms	Paranoia possibly ensuing	Systematized delusions; paranoia; bizarre behavior	Depressed mood; anhedonia; lack of energy; sleep and appetite disturbances
Electroencephalogram	Diffuse slowing; low-voltage fast activity; specific patterns	Normal early; mild slowing later	Normal	Normal	Normal

[a]The characteristics listed are the usual ones and are not exclusive.
[b]Patients with vascular dementia may have an abrupt decline in cognition.
[c]Patients with dementia with diffuse cortical Lewy bodies often have a fluctuating mental status and hallucinations.
From Jankovic J et al: *Bradley and Daroff's neurology in clinical practice,* ed 8, Philadelphia, 2022, Elsevier.

TABLE 9 Potentially Life-Threatening Causes of Delirium

Condition	Diagnostics	Treatment
Wernicke's encephalopathy	Clinical triad: Change in mental status, gait instability, ophthalmoplegia	Thiamine 500 mg IM (may see improvement over the course of hours)
Hypoxia	Oxygen saturation/ABGs	Treat etiology, give oxygen
Hypoglycemia	Blood glucose	PO/IV administration of glucose, dextrose, sucrose, or fructose
Hypertensive encephalopathy	Blood pressure	Antihypertensive medication
Hyperthermia/hypothermia	Temperature	Cooling or warming interventions
Infectious process (e.g., sepsis, bacteremia, subacute bacterial endocarditis)	Infectious disease work-up	Treat infectious agent or site
Intracerebral hemorrhage	MRI/CT	Per hemorrhage type or location
Meningitis/encephalitis	LP, MRI	Antibiotic medication, immunotherapy
Metabolic (e.g., chemical derangements, renal failure, hepatic failure, thyroid dysfunction)	Laboratory investigations	Per derangement
Poisoning/toxic reaction (e.g., environmental exposures, medications, alcohol, illicit substances)	Toxicology panel	Per toxin
Status epilepticus	EEG	Anticonvulsants and/or IV benzodiazepines

ABGs, Arterial blood gases; *CT,* computed tomography; *EEG,* electroencephalogram; *IM,* intramuscular; *IV,* intravenous; *LP,* lumbar puncture; *MRI,* magnetic resonance imaging; *PO,* oral (per os).
From Stern TA: *Massachusetts General Hospital handbook of general hospital psychiatry,* ed 7, Philadelphia, 2018, Elsevier.

among them is usually made on the basis of side effects. Haloperidol is the least sedating but has a high risk of extrapyramidal side effects; quetiapine has the fewest side effects but is highly sedating.

- Haloperidol can be used with caution to control agitation, with doses ranging from 0.25 to 2 mg intramuscularly/intravenously (IM/IV) twice daily, repeating the dose every 20 to 30 min until patient has calmed and using lower doses for the elderly. An IV haloperidol protocol used at Massachusetts General Hospital in agitated delirious patients is described in Table E10.
- Most antipsychotics can prolong the QT interval and increase the risk of torsades de pointes. The effect is greatest with IV haloperidol and least with aripiprazole. Aripiprazole is available in tablets, solution, and injection. Starting dose is 1 mg twice a day.
- Risperidone 0.5 mg twice daily (off-label use, non-FDA approved) can also be used with caution with a slow increase to desired dose, not to exceed 1.0 to 2.0 mg.
- Avoid benzodiazepines and meperidine. Drug toxicity accounts for approximately 30% cases of delirium.

CHRONIC Rx

Delirium is not a chronic condition; if assessing a more long-term mental status change, consider other diagnoses.

DISPOSITION

Requires frequent monitoring often necessitating hospital level of care to ensure safety and assess cause.

REFERRAL

Consider neurologic or psychiatric consultation if not improved in several days or in complicated cases.

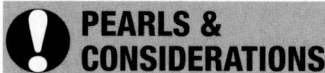 **PEARLS & CONSIDERATIONS**

COMMENTS

- Although benzodiazepines are frequently used in hospitalized patients for sedation and are the mainstay of therapy for alcohol withdrawal, they must be used with caution in the elderly because they can have a paradoxical effect on agitation.
- The use of atypical antipsychotics in managing patients with postoperative delirium has increased over the past decade due to the perception that they are less harmful than haloperidol; however, a recent study[1] in older patients did not show any major difference in in-hospital adverse events between atypical antipsychotics and haloperidol.

PREVENTION (TABLE 11)

- Avoid polypharmacy as much as possible.
- Optimize chronic medical conditions.
- Provide frequent reorientation and a soothing environment for high-risk patients (e.g., lights on during the day, off at night; open curtains during the day so patient can see the weather).
- In patients over 70 without dementia, regular exercise has been associated with lower risk for developing delirium, and early return to physical activity can improve outcomes in ill patients.

PATIENT & FAMILY EDUCATION

Inform about the above preventive techniques, especially polypharmacy risks.

REFERENCE & SUGGESTED READINGS

Available at eBooks.Health.Elsevier.com.

RELATED CONTENT

Delirium Tremens (Related Key Topic)

AUTHOR: **FRED F. FERRI, MD**

TABLE 11 Priorities (Consensus, Evidence-Based, and Speculative) for the Prevention, Management, and Advancement of the Treatment of Delirium

Community-Based Prevention	Hospital-Based Prevention	Hospital-Based Management	Postdischarge Management	Clinical Research Opportunities
Hospital avoidance strategies	Implementation of basic standards (e.g., screening for delirium) Minimization of iatrogenesis[a]	Implementation of basic standards (e.g., review of medications)[a]	Responsive, proportionate, and holistic follow-up[a]	Pragmatic research into optimizing care delivery
Identification and management of frailty	Multicomponent interventions to address frailty[b] Reorientation[b] Nutrition[b] Multidisciplinary care[a] Physiologic correction[b] Sensory optimization[b] Minimization of ward transfers[a] Avoidance of polypharmacy[b]	Multicomponent interventions to address frailty[a] Reorientation[a] Nutrition[a] Multidisciplinary care[a] Physiologic correction[a] Sensory optimization[a] Minimization of ward transfers[a] Reduction of drug burden[a]	Identification and management of frailty Reduction and cessation of antipsychotics	The interaction between frailty, interventions to ameliorate frailty, and delirium Transference from basic science models to trials of newer therapies Validation of delirium models using advanced imaging
Pleiotropic interventions (e.g., exercise/nutrition)	Monitor and promote early mobilization[b]	Monitor and promote early mobilization[a]	Review of the primary triggers for delirium and other state variables (e.g., mobility)	Delirium, mobility, and response to physical therapy
Early diagnosis and management of dementia	Screening for dementia[a]	Screening for delirium resolution and residual cognitive impairment	Screening for subsyndromal delirium or dementia[a]	The interaction between dementia, including non-Alzheimer dementia, and delirium
Education of nursing home facilities and staff	Education of nursing and medical staff[a]	Education of medical and nursing staff[a]	Caregiver support and education	The role of education of nonmedical staff, families,[c] and general public using multimedia solutions
Integrated geriatric care for planned major surgery	Targeted drug treatments (e.g., melatonin for sleep disturbance)[a] Family-based screening/ reorientation[b]	Delirium units Supported early discharge Family-based screening/ reorientation[a] Management in the nursing home with CGA capability	Adaptive and versatile methods of follow-up such as telemedicine	The role of novel and targeted interventions and models of care supported by assistive technologies
Public health awareness	Audit of care and cycle of care improvement[a]	Audit of care and cycle of care improvement[a]	Public health awareness/NGO engagement	Development of key indicators in the management of delirium

CGA, Comprehensive geriatric assessment; *NGO,* nongovernmental organization.
[a]Consensus role.
[b]Evidence-based role.
[c]Speculative role.
From Fillit HM: *Brocklehurst's textbook of geriatric medicine and gerontology,* ed 8, Philadelphia, 2017, Elsevier.

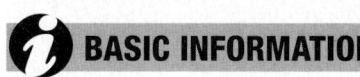

BASIC INFORMATION

DEFINITION

Dementia with Lewy bodies (DLB) is a neurodegenerative dementia occurring concurrently with or within 1 yr (either before or after) of the onset of parkinsonism. DLB also has other core features, including fluctuations in attention and alertness and recurrent vivid visual hallucinations. Diagnostic criteria for dementia syndrome associated with Lewy body pathology are described in Table 1. Patients generally respond to cholinesterase inhibitors, are very sensitive to the adverse effects of neuroleptics, and are less responsive to levodopa compared with Parkinson disease (PD) patients.

SYNONYMS

DLB
Lewy body dementia
Diffuse Lewy body disease
Lewy body type senile dementia
Cortical Lewy body disease

ICD-10CM CODE
G31.83   Dementia with Lewy bodies

EPIDEMIOLOGY & DEMOGRAPHICS

INCIDENCE: Accounts for 10% to 15% of all dementias. DLB is the second most common neurodegenerative cause of dementia after Alzheimer disease (AD) and is the third most common cause of dementia when vascular dementia is included in the tally.

PREVALENCE: Estimated 0.7% of individuals >65 yr.

PREDOMINANT SEX & AGE:
- Sex: Male predominance
- Mean age of onset: 75 yr. On average, 10 yr greater for dementia with Lewy bodies (DLB) than PD

PEAK INCIDENCE: Affects individuals in their sixth decade or older.

RISK FACTORS:
- Male sex
- Advanced age

GENETICS:
- Most cases are sporadic with a discordance among monozygotic twins, suggesting that either environmental or other epigenetic factors may play a major role in the incidence of DLB.
- Copy number variation of the alpha-synuclein gene *(SNCA)* has been reported in families with DLB. Rare autosomal dominant variants in *LRRK2* have also been reported. These genes are associated with PD and PD dementia in addition to DLB, suggesting a common molecular etiology with a spectrum of clinical phenotypes.
- The *APOE* ε4 allele has a higher prevalence in DLB than in control individuals, suggesting heightened disease risk conferred by the allele. Conversely, the *APOE* ε2 allele is enriched in control individuals, suggesting a neuroprotective role, or at least the lack of a deleterious effect, for the allele.
- Other factors include glucocerebrosidase genetic mutations, high prevalence of Lewy bodies with presenilin-1 mutations, and polymorphisms of the coding region for the synuclein genes.

PHYSICAL FINDINGS & CLINICAL PRESENTATION

- Importance of recognizing DLB relates to its pharmacologic management, including responsiveness to cholinesterase inhibitors, sensitivity to the adverse effects of neuroleptics, and relative unresponsiveness to levodopa.
- The diagnostic criteria for DLB have been revised several times. The latest revision, the Fourth Consensus Report of the DLB Consortium, was published in 2017 and is the basis for the diagnostic information outlined later. [1]
- The presence of dementia is absolute requirement for the diagnosis. The dementia is insidious in onset with a neuropsychologic profile of early impairments in visuoperceptual, attentional, and executive functions, with relative sparing early on of episodic memory (in contradistinction to ADs, in which impairment in episodic memory is a hallmark early finding). Memory impairment typically ensues as the disease progresses.

TABLE 1   Revised Criteria for the Clinical Diagnosis of Probable and Possible Dementia with Lewy Bodies (DLB)

Essential for a diagnosis of DLB is dementia, defined as a progressive cognitive decline of sufficient magnitude to interfere with normal social or occupational functions, or with usual daily activities. Prominent or persistent memory impairment may not necessarily occur in the early stages but is usually evident with progression. Deficits on tests of attention, executive function, and visuoperceptual ability may be especially prominent and occur early.

Core Clinical Features (The First Three Typically Occur Early and May Persist Throughout the Course.)
- Fluctuating cognition with pronounced variations in attention and alertness.
- Recurrent visual hallucinations that are typically well formed and detailed.
- REM sleep behavior disorder, which may precede cognitive decline.
- One or more spontaneous cardinal features of parkinsonism: bradykinesia (defined as slowness of movement and decrement in amplitude or speed), rest tremor, or rigidity.

Supportive Clinical Features
- Severe sensitivity to antipsychotic agents; postural instability, repeated falls, syncope or other transient episodes of unresponsiveness; severe autonomic dysfunction, such as constipation, orthostatic hypotension, urinary incontinence; hypersomnia; hyposmia; hallucinations in other modalities; systematized delusions; apathy, anxiety, and depression.

Indicative Biomarkers
- Relative preservation of medial temporal lobe structures on CT/MRI scan.
- Generalized low uptake on SPECT/PET perfusion/metabolism scan with reduced occipital activity ± the cingulate island sign on FDG-PET imaging.
- Prominent posterior slow-wave activity on EEG with periodic fluctuations in the pre-alpha/theta range.

Probable DLB Can be Diagnosed if:
1. Two or more core clinical features of DLB are present, with or without the presence of indicative biomarkers, or
2. Only one core clinical feature is present but with one or more indicative biomarkers.

Probable DLB Should Not Be Diagnosed on the Basis of Biomarkers Alone.
Probable DLB Can be Diagnosed if:
1. Only one core clinical feature of DLB is present, with no indicative biomarkers evidence, or
2. One or more indicative biomarkers is present but there are no clinical features.

DLB is Less Likely:
1. In the presence of any other physical illness or brain disorder, including cerebrovascular disease, sufficient to account in part or in total for the clinical picture, although these do not exclude a DLB diagnosis and may serve to indicate mixed or multiple pathologies contributing to the clinical presentation, or
2. If parkinsonian features are the only core clinical feature and appear for the first time at a state of severe dementia.

DLB should be diagnosed when dementia occurs before or concurrently with parkinsonism. The term Parkinson disease dementia (PDD) should be used to describe dementia that occurs in the context of well-established Parkinson disease. In a practice setting, the term that is most appropriate to the clinical situation should be used, and generic terms such as Lewy body disease are often helpful. In research studies in which distinction needs to be made between DLB and PDD, the existing 1-yr rule between the onset of dementia and parkinsonism continues to be recommended.

CT, Computed tomography; *EEG,* electroencephalogram; *FDG-PET,* fluorodeoxyglucose-positron emission tomography; *MRI,* magnetic resonance imaging; *PET,* positron emission tomography; *REM,* rapid eye movements; *SPECT,* single-photon emission computerized tomography.
From McKeith IG et al: Diagnosis and management of dementia with Lewy bodies: fourth consensus report of the DLB Consortium, *Neurology* 89(1):88-100, 2017.

- In addition to dementia, DLB has four core clinical features. For the diagnosis of probable DLB, the patient should have dementia plus either two core clinical features or one core clinical feature and one indicative biomarker. Possible DLB can be diagnosed in a patient with dementia who manifests only one core clinical feature or has no core clinical features but has one or more indicative biomarkers of the disease.
- Core clinical features:
  1. Fluctuations in cognition with marked variations in attention and alertness level
  2. Recurrent well formed, vivid visual hallucinations
  3. Rapid eye movement (REM) sleep behavior disorder (RBD), which may precede the cognitive decline by several years
  4. Parkinsonian motor features, which include at least one of the following: bradykinesia, rest tremor, or rigidity
     a. NB: The dementia either precedes the onset of parkinsonism or begins at the same time. For research purposes, 1 yr is used as the time in which dementia and parkinsonism should be appear. Because the first three core features often precede the onset of parkinsonism, at the time of diagnosis, parkinsonian may not have yet manifested.
- Supportive clinical features:
  1. Severe neuroleptic sensitivity
  2. Repeated falls
  3. Unexplained syncope or other episodes of nonresponsiveness
  4. Severe autonomic dysfunction
  5. Hyposmia
  6. Hallucinations other than visual
  7. Systematized delusions
  8. Apathy, anxiety, and depression
- Biomarkers:
  1. Indicative biomarkers
     a. Reduced dopamine transporter uptake in the basal ganglia demonstrated by single-photon emission computerized tomography (SPECT) or PET.
     b. Low uptake on 123iodine-MIBG myocardial scintigraphy
     c. Polysomnographic confirmation of REM sleep without atonia
  2. Suggestive biomarkers
     a. Relative preservation of medial temporal lobe structures on computed tomography/MRI scan.
     b. Generalized low uptake on SPECT/PET perfusion/metabolism scan with reduced occipital activity ± the cingulate island sign on fluorodeoxyglucose (FDG)-PET imaging.
     c. Prominent posterior slow-wave activity on electroencephalogram (EEG) with periodic fluctuations in the pre-alpha/theta range.

ETIOLOGY

- *SNCA* encodes for a protein normally found at the synapse with a role in vesicle production. In its insoluble form, *SNCA* aggregates into Lewy bodies found at the cortical and subcortical levels.

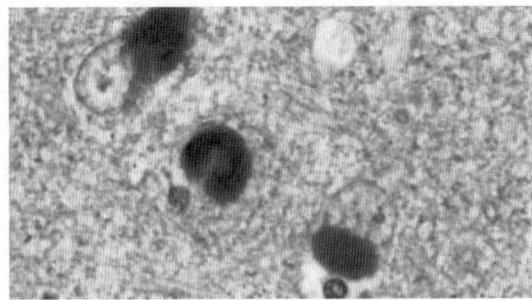

FIG. 1 Cortical Lewy bodies present in cerebral cortex, as opposed to Parkinson disease without dementia, in which Lewy bodies are found in the substantia nigra. Immunostain for alpha synuclein is characteristic for Lewy body immunohistologic profile. (From MacDonald AB: Spirochetal cyst forms in neurodegenerative disorders, hiding in plain sight, *Med Hypotheses* 67[4]:819-832, 2006.)

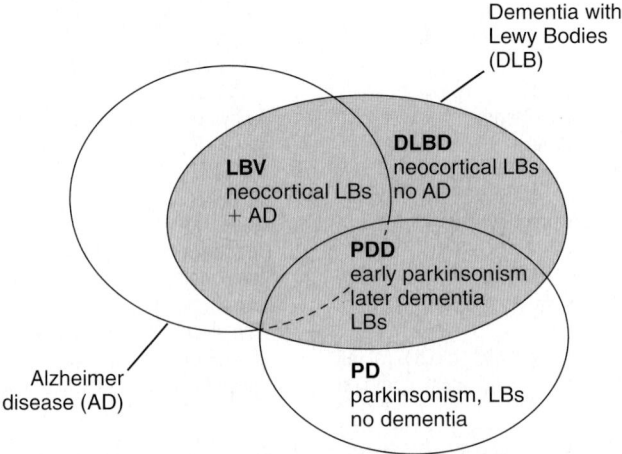

FIG. 2 Relationships among Alzheimer disease (AD), the three subtypes of dementia with Lewy bodies (DLB), and Parkinson disease (PD). Parkinsonism refers to the clinical symptoms of PD (hypokinesia, tremor, and muscular rigidity). *DLBD,* Diffuse Lewy body disease; *LBs,* Lewy bodies; *LBV,* Lewy body variant of Alzheimer disease; *PD,* Parkinson disease; *PDD,* Parkinson disease dementia. (From Lewis KA et al: Abnormal neurites containing C-terminally truncated α-synuclein are present in Alzheimer's disease without conventional Lewy body pathology, *Am J Pathol* 177[6]:3037-3050, 2010.)

- Lewy bodies (Fig. 1) are round, eosinophilic, intracytoplasmic inclusions in the nuclei of neurons.
- Cortical Lewy bodies are found in deep cortical layers of the anterior frontal and temporal lobes, the cingulate gyrus, and insula.
- As in PD, Lewy bodies aggregate in the following structures: Substantia nigra, locus coeruleus, raphe nuclei, nucleus basalis of Meynert, and brain stem nuclei.
- Fig. 2 shows the relationships among the subtypes of dementia.
- Many patients with DLB also have evidence of amyloidosis typical of AD. These patients often have a worse cognitive profile than pure DLB, with a cognitive phenotype typical of both AD (episodic memory loss) and DLB (inattention, executive dysfunction, and visuospatial dysfunction).

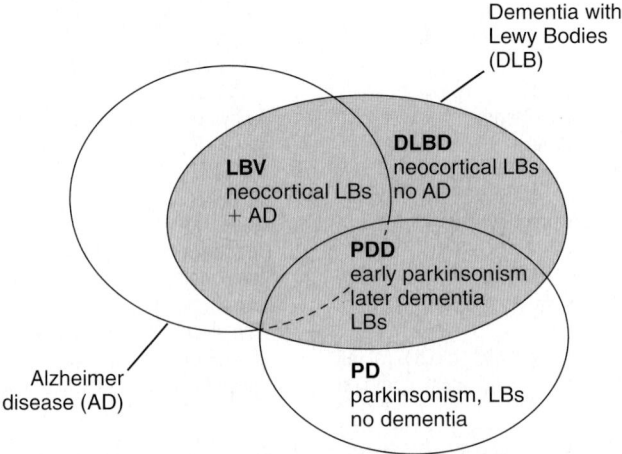 DIAGNOSIS

DIFFERENTIAL DIAGNOSIS

- Diagnosis of DLB when dementia occurs before or concurrently with extrapyramidal features—arbitrarily set as the "1-yr rule" vs.

PD with dementia, which occurs in the setting of well-established PD.
- Dementia: AD, vascular dementia, frontotemporal dementia. However, some patients have pathologic overlap of AD and DLB or DLB and vascular dementia.
- Parkinsonian features: Parkinson disease dementia, progressive supranuclear palsy (PSP), corticobasal syndrome (CBS), and multisystem atrophy (MSA).
- Rapidly progressive form: Creutzfeldt-Jakob disease (CJD). Lack of cerebellar signs and lack of typical CJD MRI may help distinguish DLB from classic CJD (but not variant form of CJD).
- Psychiatric features: Late-onset psychosis or depression with psychotic features.
- Hallucinations with fluctuations in consciousness: Temporal lobe epilepsy (TLE) or delirium due to toxic/metabolic or autoimmune derangement.

WORKUP

- MRI of the brain to evaluate for structural causes of dementia and exclude MRI features of vascular dementia or CJD.
- Lumbar puncture to rule out underlying chronic infections, only if there are atypical features.

- EEG if there is concern about TLE. However, both DLB and TLE may show nonspecific slowing or periodic complexes (see supportive biomarkers above).
- DaTScan [Ioflupane (123I)] imaging is a SPECT scan preceded by injection of a radiopharmaceutical that detects the loss of functional dopaminergic neuron terminals in the striatum, reflecting underlying PD or DLB.

LABORATORY TESTS

Rule out other potential reversible causes for dementia, including CBC, complete metabolic panel, thyroid-stimulating hormone, and B_{12}. Consider rapid plasma reagin and HIV testing as well.

IMAGING STUDIES

- MRI typically shows a relative preservation of the hippocampi and medial temporal lobe volumes (in contrast to AD), but generalized atrophy and white matter changes may be present.
- Generalized low uptake on SPECT/PET perfusion/metabolism scan with reduced occipital activity ± the cingulate island sign on FDG-PET imaging.

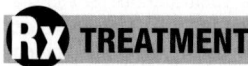

TREATMENT

Patient and caregiver education about benefits, side effects, and limitations of treatment is very important. Caregivers may be encouraged to avoid neuroleptics unless the psychotic features either trouble or endanger the patient. If neuroleptics must be used, typical neuroleptics must be avoided.

NONPHARMACOLOGIC THERAPY

- Social interaction and environmental novelty may improve cognitive dysfunction and psychiatric features often exacerbated by low levels of arousal and attention
- Behavioral methods, such as avoiding previously exposed environmental triggers known to cause anxiety, agitation, or aggression
- Physical therapy, mobility aids, and daily exercise

ACUTE GENERAL Rx

Atypical neuroleptic for disabling, persistent, bothersome (to the patient) psychotic features despite initiation of a cholinesterase inhibitor. A very low dose of an atypical antipsychotic (quetiapine 12.5 mg/day) may be started after patient/caregiver education regarding the sensitivity to neuroleptics. However, all neuroleptics do carry a boxed warning from the FDA about the increased mortality risk associated with neuroleptic use in patients with dementia. Patients and/or caregivers should be informed of this risk and allowed to balance the risk against the perceived benefit.

CHRONIC Rx

- Cholinesterase inhibitors for cognitive and behavioral symptoms. Rivastigmine (6 to 12 mg/day PO or 9.5 mg/day by transdermal patch) has shown in a randomized controlled trial (RCT) to significantly reduce anxiety, delusions, and hallucinations, as well as significantly improved performance on neuropsychologic testing.
- PD medications for disabling parkinsonian features. Carbidopa/levodopa is reported to be more effective with fewer side effects than dopamine agonists, which have higher rates of psychotic symptoms. Begin at a low dose—25/100 mg three times a day—and slowly titrate over several weeks as tolerated and according to response.
- Selective serotonin reuptake inhibitors are commonly used for depression.
- If REM sleep disorder remains disabling (or patient has not responded to an atypical antipsychotic initiated for psychosis), a trial of low-dose clonazepam (0.25 to 0.5 mg) or melatonin (3 mg) at bedtime remains an option.
- Orthostatic hypotension may be aided by nonpharmacologic therapy such as supportive stockings or pharmacologically by midodrine, fludrocortisone, or droxidopa.
- Memantine demonstrated an improvement in clinical global measure and remains well tolerated but may worsen hallucinations or delusions.
- Avoid anticholinergics (including tricyclic antidepressants), benzodiazepines, and typical neuroleptics, as they can trigger delirium and worsen symptoms.

DISPOSITION

- Survival resembles the progression of AD, but a minority of cases may have a rapid disease course.
- Progression in cognitive decline, similar to AD, by approximately 10%/yr on cognitive testing.

REFERRAL

DLB requires a multidisciplinary approach including the general practitioner, neurologist, neuropsychologist, and/or neuropsychiatrist.

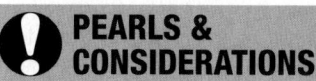

PEARLS & CONSIDERATIONS

COMMENTS

- Clinical presentation helps differentiate DLB from AD. AD presents with early signs of anterograde episodic memory loss without the benefit of cues on neuropsychologic testing because of cortical atrophy at the medial temporal lobe region.
- Vascular dementia may also present with evidence of frontal-subcortical features but typically without the core features listed in the criteria above.
- Bed partners may report that individuals with DLB "act out their dreams," sometimes violently, leading to sleeping in separate beds. This history may indicate REM sleep behavior disorder. A history of REM sleep behavior may precede the diagnosis by many years. However, REM sleep behavior does not necessarily lead to DLB, but can be premonitory of any alpha synucleinopathy, including PD and multiple system atrophy.

PATIENT & FAMILY EDUCATION

- Visual hallucinations (VHs) typically consist of innocuous, well-formed, detailed images of animate figures. These are classically labeled Lilliputian because the hallucinatory images are often relatively small. Unless VH lead to a potential threat to self or others, avoid antipsychotics due to the sensitivity of neuroleptics. Family/friends are often more alarmed by the VH than the patient with DLB.
- Apathy is a common clinical feature of DLB and mimics changes in mood, including depression or excessive daytime somnolence. These features are often noticed by family/friends.

REFERENCE

Available at eBooks.Health.Elsevier.com.

AUTHOR: **JOSEPH S. KASS, MD, JD, FAAN**

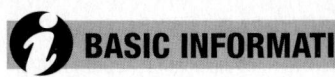

DEFINITION

Major depressive disorder (MDD) is an episodic, frequently recurring syndrome. The diagnosis requires that five of nine criteria be present for 2 wk. One of these nine criteria must be either a persistent depressed mood or pervasive anhedonia (loss of interest or pleasure in all, or almost all, usual interests or activities). Other symptoms include sleep disturbance (insomnia, hypersomnia, or interrupted sleep), appetite loss/gain or weight loss/gain, fatigue, psychomotor retardation or agitation, difficulty concentrating or indecisiveness, feelings of guilt or worthlessness, and recurrent thoughts of death or suicidal ideation.

SYNONYMS

MDD
Unipolar affective disorder
Clinical depression
Melancholia
Manic-depressive illness, depressed type
Depressive episode

Codes depend on whether the episode is single or recurrent, and also on clinical severity.

ICD-10CM CODES

F32.9	Depressive episode, unspecified
F33.0	Recurrent depressive episode, current episode mild
F33.1	Recurrent depressive disorder, current episode moderate
F33.2	Recurrent depressive disorder, current episode severe without psychotic symptoms
F33.3	Recurrent depressive disorder, current episode severe with psychotic symptoms
F33.4	Recurrent depressive disorder, currently in remission
F33.9	Recurrent depressive disorder, unspecified

DSM-5-TR CODES

296.21	Single episode
296.22	Single episode, moderate
296.23	Single episode, severe
296.24	Single episode, with psychotic features
296.31	Recurrent, mild
296.32	Recurrent, moderate
296.33	Recurrent severe
296.34	Recurrent, with psychotic features

EPIDEMIOLOGY & DEMOGRAPHICS

PREVALENCE (IN U.S.): Point prevalence of MDD in a community sample is 3% of men, 4.5% to 9.3% of women, and 3.2% of children.[1] 12-mo prevalence is 7.2% in men, 13.4% in women.[2] Patients with chronic medical illness have two- to threefold higher rates of MDD than age- and gender-matched patients.[3] The lifelong prevalence of a major depressive disorder among 13- to 18-yr-olds is 11% in the U.S. with a 12-mo prevalence of 7.5%.[2]

PREDOMINANT SEX: Lifetime risk female:male ratio 1.7:1.[2] Adolescent girls have both higher rates and more severe episodes of depression than their male counterparts.[1]

PREDOMINANT AGE: Mean age of onset of first episode is 26 to 29, though prevalent in all ages.[4]

PEAK INCIDENCE: 25 to 40 yr; 13% of postpartum women.[5]

LIFETIME RISK (IN U.S.): 15% of men, 26% of women.

GENETICS:

- Clear evidence of familial predominance.
- Prevalence is two to three times greater among first-degree relatives.
- Concordance among monozygotic twins 46%.[6]
- Several studies have documented associations between various genes and increased risk for MDD, but there remains no established pattern of inheritance.

PHYSICAL FINDINGS & CLINICAL PRESENTATION

- Clinical evaluation facilitated by organizing the major symptoms into four hallmarks: (1) Depressed mood, (2) anhedonia, (3) physical symptoms (sleep disturbance, appetite problem, fatigue, psychomotor changes), and (4) psychologic symptoms (difficulty concentrating or indecisiveness, guilt or worthlessness, and suicidal ideation).
- A stressful life event, typically a serious loss, may trigger a depressive episode. *The Diagnostic and Statistical Manual of Mental Disorders, 5th edition, Text Revision,* recommends that clinical judgment be used to determine if depression in the context of a loss should be diagnosed as a major depressive episode, normal grief, prolonged grief disorder, demoralization, or adjustment disorder.
- Somatic complaints such as pain, fatigue, insomnia, dizziness, headache, or GI problems occur in more than two-thirds of patients presenting to primary care with underlying MDD.
- Comorbid psychiatric disorders are often present. Anxiety disorders are the most common comorbid conditions.
- An episode of MDD can include psychotic features, which may be associated with mood-congruent delusional thinking (paranoid, nihilistic, and melancholic themes).
- May be associated with active suicidal ideation, including intent or plan, or a passive wish for death.
- May be underdiagnosed in elderly patients, with signs and symptoms attributed to normal aging or cognitive impairment.
- May be underdiagnosed in medically ill patients, with signs and symptoms attributed to medical illness or considered appropriate reaction to medical condition.

ETIOLOGY

- Genetic and environmental experiences, and their interaction, each contribute.
- Significant psychosocial stressors, including losses, trauma, and ramifications of adverse childhood events, often trigger MDD, particularly for index episodes.

- Numerous biologic correlates have been identified, though none is considered causative or diagnostic. Genes that influence the production and reuptake of serotonin, norepinephrine, dopamine, and glutamate, as well as nerve cell growth in brain regions underlying memory and emotional processing, are of greatest interest[7]. Abnormalities in brain regions underlying executive functioning, emotion regulation, and reward processing, as well as irregularities in functional connectivity have been identified.
- Cognitive risk factors include a pessimistic style of explaining negative events, a tendency to ruminate, and biases in processing emotional information and events.

DIAGNOSIS

DIFFERENTIAL DIAGNOSIS

- Time-course and symptomatology can distinguish MDD from persistent depressive disorder (formerly known as "dysthymia"), premenstrual dysphoric disorder, and substance-induced mood disorder.
- Anxiety disorders, posttraumatic stress disorder (PTSD), obsessive compulsive disorder (OCD), substance use disorders, and personality disorders often present with depressive symptoms or coexist with major depressive disorder.
- Important to determine if a depressive episode is part of major depression or part of bipolar disorder, which entails carefully screening for a history of manic symptoms.
- Important to distinguish from adjustment disorder. Depression in the context of a stressful life event is diagnosed as major depressive disorder if the symptom criteria are met and adjustment disorder if the symptom criteria are not met. Psychotherapy, rather than medication, is the treatment mainstay for adjustment disorder.
- Demoralization can overlap significantly with MDD, including prominent neurovegetative symptoms. Demoralization frequently lacks anhedonia and is directly related to an ongoing stressor (like a medical illness) from which escape is not seen as likely.
- Grief and bereavement, including prolonged grief disorder, can overlap with MDD. If symptoms meet criteria for MDD, MDD should still be diagnosed even in the setting of recent loss.
- Approximately 10% to 15% of depressive episodes are caused by general medical illnesses, such as Alzheimer disease, Parkinson disease, stroke, end-stage renal failure, cardiac disease, HIV infection, and cancer.[3]
- Some medical conditions can present with depressive symptoms (e.g., hypothyroidism, hyperthyroidism, pancreatic cancer, and neurosyphilis).
- Depression can coexist with dementia, though depression-related cognitive dysfunction (formerly known as "pseudodementia") must also be considered in such populations.

D

I

WORKUP

- Careful medical history is required to rule out nonpsychiatric etiology. Tables 1, 2, and 3 summarize common psychologic/cognitive, behavioral, physical, and somatic symptoms encountered in unipolar depressive disorders.

TABLE 1 Unipolar Depressive Disorders: Common Psychological and Cognitive Symptoms

Depressed mood
Lack of interest or motivation
Inability to enjoy things
Lack of pleasure (anhedonia)
Apathy
Irritability
Anxiety or nervousness
Excessive worrying
Reduced concentration or attention
Memory difficulties
Indecisiveness
Reduced libido
Hypersensitivity to rejection or criticism
Reward dependency
Perfectionism
Obsessiveness
Ruminations
Excessive guilt
Pessimism
Hopelessness
Feelings of helplessness
Cognitive distortions (e.g., "I am unlovable")
Preoccupation with oneself
Hypochondriacal concerns
Low or reduced self-esteem
Feelings of worthlessness
Thoughts of death or suicide
Thoughts of hurting other people

From Stern: *Massachusetts General Hospital handbook of general hospital psychiatry*, ed 7, Philadelphia, 2018, Elsevier.

TABLE 2 Unipolar Depressive Disorders: Common Behavioral Symptoms

Crying spells
Interpersonal friction or confrontation
Anger attacks or outbursts
Avoidance of anxiety-provoking situations
Social withdrawal
Avoidance of emotional and sexual intimacy
Reduced leisure-time activities
Development of rituals or compulsions
Compulsive eating
Compulsive use of the internet or video games
Workaholic behaviors
Substance use or abuse
Intensification of personality traits or pathologic behaviors
Excessive reliance or dependence on others
Excessive self-sacrifice or victimization
Reduced productivity
Self-cutting or mutilation
Suicide attempts or gestures
Violent or assaultive behaviors

From Stern: *Massachusetts General Hospital handbook of general hospital psychiatry*, ed 7, Philadelphia, 2018, Elsevier.

TABLE 3 Unipolar Depressive Disorders: Common Physical and Somatic Symptoms

Fatigue
Leaden feelings in arms or legs
Difficulty falling asleep (early insomnia)
Difficulty staying asleep (middle insomnia)
Waking up early in the morning (late insomnia)
Sleeping too much (hypersomnia)
Frequent naps
Decreased appetite
Weight loss
Increased appetite
Weight gain
Sexual arousal difficulties
Erectile dysfunction
Delayed orgasm or inability to achieve orgasm
Pains and aches
Back pain
Musculoskeletal complaints
Chest pain
Headaches
Muscle tension
Gastrointestinal upset
Heart palpitations
Burning or tingling sensations
Paresthesias

From Stern: *Massachusetts General Hospital handbook of general hospital psychiatry*, ed 7, Philadelphia, 2018, Elsevier.

- Physical examination reveals no specific diagnostic signs of depression, though psychomotor changes can be observed.
- Mental status examination.
- Self-report scales can assist in screening.
- Commonly used validated screening tools include the 15-item Geriatric Depression Scale in the elderly and the Patient Health Questionnaire (PHQ)-2 and PHQ-9. The PHQ-2 has a 97% sensitivity and 67% specificity in adults. If it is positive for depression, the PHQ-9 should be administered. The PHQ-9 has a 78% sensitivity and 87% specificity for depression in adults.[8]

LABORATORY TESTS

- Research is under way to identify biomarkers that may be useful in diagnosis; no laboratory studies are diagnostic at present.
- The following can assist in ruling out other confounding issues:
  1. Routine blood chemistry evaluation
  2. CBC with differential
  3. Thyroid function studies
  4. Vitamin D and B_{12} levels

IMAGING STUDIES

With unusual presentations (e.g., associated with new-onset severe headache, focal neurologic signs, a cognitive or sensory disturbance), the following may be performed:

- Electroencephalogram (EEG) (diffuse slowing indicates metabolic encephalopathy)
- Anatomic brain imaging (computed tomography scan or MRI)

Rx TREATMENT

NONPHARMACOLOGIC THERAPY

- Good evidence exists that cognitive-behavioral therapy (CBT) is as effective as antidepressant medication in achieving significant reduction or remission. Meta-analysis indicates that combining psychotherapy with medication is modestly more effective than either modality alone.[9]
- Various third-wave forms of CBT (e.g., acceptance and commitment, mindfulness-based [MBCT], and dialectical behavioral [DBT]), as well as traditional CBT, have demonstrated efficacy in numerous studies.
- Problem-solving and interpersonal psychotherapies are comparably efficacious.
- Growing evidence indicates that internet-based CBT and brief therapy interventions integrated into primary care to expand access to therapy are efficacious, with some studies finding comparable efficacy to standard length interventions.
- By 12 wk or earlier, psychotherapy and medication approaches are equally effective.
- Augmentation of standard depression treatment with CBT to address insomnia was found to significantly improve response rates.
- Official treatment guidelines recommend that medication be used as the first-line treatment for patients with severe depression, although some studies have found equal efficacy of medication and psychotherapy in the treatment of severe depression.
- Factors, including history of adverse childhood events, presence of precipitant stressful life events, family psychiatric history, the presence of anhedonia, and depression severity, may affect treatment response and risk of recurrence. Numerous genetic and neurobiologic variables that predict treatment response have been identified, particularly in combination with one another or with clinical characteristics. However, at present, there are no universally accepted markers that can aid clinicians in matching individuals to specific medications or interventions.

ACUTE GENERAL Rx

- Concurrent medical or psychiatric illnesses, history of prior response, cost, patient preference, and side effects should be considered when selecting initial treatment.
- Antidepressants are helpful in approximately 60% to 70% of cases, though sustained remission rates are lower.[5]
- Selective serotonin reuptake inhibitors (SSRIs) are generally first-line. According to the Sequenced Treatment Alternatives to Relieve Depression (STAR-D) trial, approximately 30% achieve remission with the first prescribed medication after 3 mo of treatment.[6] Another 25% to 30% respond to treatment but do not achieve remission. Treatment-refractory patients may be switched to another SSRI or another class of medication may be more helpful, offered adjunctive medication such as bupropion, or referred for evidence-based

counseling. Approximately 25% more patients will achieve remission with this secondary intervention.

- According to a network meta-analysis of 21 antidepressants, escitalopram, mirtazapine, paroxetine, and sertraline had higher response and lower dropout rates than other antidepressants, and all antidepressants were more effective than placebo.[10]
- Response to antidepressants for many patients is seen as early as 2 wk, and among patients showing little to no response, the odds of later response decrease the longer patients remain unimproved, particularly with antidepressant monotherapy.[11] Conversely, rapid response to treatment predicted improved outcomes in multiple studies.
- Antidepressants may transiently increase suicidality and aggression in patients under 25, an important side effect to discuss prior to treatment initiation. Other side effects include GI distress, sexual dysfunction, sleep disturbance, and weight gain. Characteristics of commonly used antidepressant drugs are summarized in Table E4.
- To date, there are no data to support combining antidepressants as first-line treatment. There is also no clear advantage to switching medications within vs. across different classes, or to switching vs. augmentation.
- Treatment should be continued for 4 to 9 mo after the full remission of depressive symptoms.[12]
- Electroconvulsive therapy (ECT) is the most effective means available for the treatment of severe, refractory depression. Transcranial magnetic stimulation (TMS) has also shown evidence of efficacy, though the magnitude of effects is more variable and overall smaller than ECT. Research is under way to investigate mechanisms to increase the efficacy of TMS.[13]
- Antipsychotic medication should be added for psychotic depression. Antipsychotic medication has also been shown to be helpful in augmenting antidepressants for nonpsychotic depression, and it may be beneficial for individuals with mixed manic-depressive features, although more research is needed.
- The Veterans Affairs (VA) Augmentation and Switching Treatments for Improving Depression Outcomes (VAST-D) trial found that switching to the antipsychotic aripiprazole resulted in statistically significant, though modest, improvement in remission rates compared with switching or augmenting with an antidepressant, although greater side effects resulted.[12]
- In older adults with treatment-resistant depression, augmentation of existing antidepressants with aripiprazole improves well-being

significantly more over 10 wk than a switch to bupropion and is associated with a numerically higher incidence of remission.[14]
- Intravenous ketamine has been found to be rapidly effective in treatment-resistant and suicidal depression.[15] Intranasal esketamine (Spravato) is approved for use in treatment-resistant depression. A recent trial comparing ketamine versus ECT for nonpsychotic treatment-resistant major depression revealed that ketamine is noninferior to ECT as therapy for treatment-resistant major depression without psychosis.[16] Further research is needed to determine whether positive effects are maintained, as effectiveness appears to fade without repeated use.
- Early data from open-label trials of psilocybin for treatment-resistant depression suggest sustained improvement of depressive symptoms at 3 and 6 mo, though the first randomized trial directly comparing psilocybin vs. conventional pharmacologic treatment for depression did not show a significant difference.[17]

CHRONIC Rx

Long-term treatment, in some cases lifelong, is recommended for multiple depressive episodes, an episode duration longer than 2 yr, a severe episode or significant suicidality, or a strong family history of severe depression or bipolar disorder.

COMPLEMENTARY & ALTERNATIVE MEDICINE

St. John's wort *(Hypericum perforatum)* is sold as a dietary supplement in the United States and is used for depression in the community. It is not consistently effective and should not be used in combination with antidepressants given the possibility of severe serotonin-related side effects, as well as effects on the metabolism of other drugs.

DISPOSITION

- Major depressive disorder is often a relapsing and remitting illness.
- Additional episodes are experienced by >50% of patients after one episode, with each additional episode linked to increased risk for subsequent episodes.[6]
- Without treatment, episodes last an average of 6 to 12 mo; risk of recurrence higher without treatment.[6]
- For many depressed individuals, subthreshold residual symptoms are present between episodes and define the majority of an individual's course of depression. Such symptoms may lead to impairment and warrant prolonged treatment.

REFERRAL

- If treatment-refractory
- If patient is suicidal or psychotic
- For suspected bipolar depression

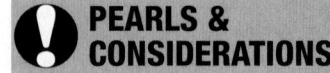

COMMENTS

- All threats of suicide should be taken very seriously. Clinicians can use the mnemonic SAL: Is the method **s**pecific? Is it **a**vailable? Is it **l**ethal?
- Rule out bipolar affective disorder before initiating antidepressant medication. Screening scales for bipolar disorder can be helpful in primary care settings to identify patients at increased risk for bipolar disorder. Antidepressants can induce mania in susceptible patients.
- Comorbid or diagnostically related entities such as OCD, generalized anxiety, and PTSD, while sometimes difficult to differentiate from MDD, share similar pharmacologic and therapy-based treatment principles.
- Various rating scales (e.g., Montgomery-Asberg Depression Rating Scale [MADRS], Hamilton Rating Scale for Depression [HAM-D], Beck Depression Inventory [BDI]) are available for diagnostic screening and to measure improvement over time.
- A two-question screener (PHQ2) is as effective as longer instruments. A positive answer to either question warrants a full assessment:
  1. Over the past 2 wk, have you ever felt down, depressed, or hopeless?
  2. Over the past 2 wk, have you felt little interest or pleasure in doing things?
- Depression screening programs without treatment programs are unlikely to improve depression outcomes.
- Strict monitoring of patients who initiate antidepressant therapy is necessary both for safety and to ensure optimal treatment. Use of self-report scales to measure symptom severity is helpful in monitoring outcomes and may result in improved outcomes.

REFERENCES
Available at eBooks.Health.Elsevier.com.

RELATED CONTENT
Depression (Patient Information)
Bipolar Disorder (Related Key Topic)

AUTHOR: **RACHEL L. MACLEAN, MD**

BASIC INFORMATION

DEFINITION

- Diabetes mellitus (DM) refers to a syndrome of hyperglycemia resulting from many different causes (see "Etiology"). It is broadly classified into type 1 (T1DM) and type 2 DM (T2DM). The terms *insulin-dependent* and *non–insulin-dependent* diabetes are obsolete because when a person with type 2 diabetes needs insulin, he or she remains labeled as type 2 and is not reclassified as type 1. Immune-mediated type 1 DM (type 1A) represents 5% to 10% of newly diagnosed diabetics. Tables 1 and 2 provide a general comparison of the two types of DM. One difference is that type 1 has usually complete or near-total knockout of insulin reserves mediated solely by immunogenic responses from carriers of certain genotypes, whereas type 2 is of polygenetic origin and may have patients who may start with hyperinsulinemia but have insulin resistance and through environmental factors such as diet and sedentary lifestyle leads to an imbalance between glucagon and insulin levels, resulting in combination of causes toward hyperglycemia. (Fig. 1)
- Some type 1 diabetics also may exhibit high levels of glucagon, and not all type 1 diabetics have complete islet cell destruction.
- The classification of diabetes also includes:
  1. **LADA**: Latent autoimmune diabetes of adult onset (sometimes called type 1.5 DM). These individuals are typically not insulin dependent initially and are often misclassified as having type 2 DM.
  2. **MODY**: Maturity onset diabetes of youth. These have various genetic expressions and can be classified into various subtypes:
     a. MODY 1, 2, 3, 4, and 5 (with 3 being most prevalent: 70% incidence with HNF-1-alpha [12q24] genetic expression).
     b. MODY 7 and 8 (rare).
  3. Ketosis-prone diabetes: Relapsing/remitting beta cell function with slow deterioration over time. It presents with ketoacidosis requiring insulin, then regains beta cell function, and patient is able to discontinue insulin. This for is most common under age 40, in those of African or Afro-Caribbean origin, and in obese or overweight patients.
  4. Secondary diabetes:
     a. Pancreatic disease or resection (e.g., cystic fibrosis)
     b. Chronic excessive corticosteroid exposure or Cushing syndrome
     c. Glucagonoma
     d. Acromegaly
     e. Other rare genetic disorders (e.g., mitochondrial diabetes MELAS syndrome).
  5. Rare autoimmune (e.g., type A and B insulin resistance syndrome).
  6. A classification of diabetes mellitus is shown in Box 1.
- Diabetes mellitus can be diagnosed by the following tests:
  1. A hemoglobin A_{1C} (HbA$_{1C}$) value $\geq$6.5% is considered diagnostic for diabetes. This test is preferred because of ease of administration and reliability.
  2. A fasting plasma glucose (FPG) $\geq$126 mg/dl, which should be confirmed with repeat testing on a different day. Fasting is defined as no caloric intake for at least 8 h.
  3. An oral glucose tolerance test (OGTT) with a plasma glucose $\geq$200 mg/dl 2 h after a 75 g (100 g for pregnant women) glucose load.
  4. Symptoms of hyperglycemia and a casual (random) plasma glucose $\geq$200 mg/dl are also indicative of DM. Classic symptoms of hyperglycemia include polyuria, polydipsia, and unexplained weight loss. At the time of diagnosis as a diabetic, B-cell function is at 25% to 30%.
- Individuals with glucose levels higher than normal but not high enough to meet the criteria for diagnosis of DM are considered to have "prediabetes," the diagnosis of which is made as follows:
  1. A fasting plasma glucose 100 to 125 mg/dl; this is referred to as *impaired fasting glucose.*
  2. After OGTT, a 2-h plasma glucose of 140 to 199; this is referred to as *impaired glucose tolerance.* Patients with impaired glucose tolerance or prediabetes have B-cell function at 50% of normal.
  3. A hemoglobin A_{1C} value of 5.7% to 6.4%.
- Table 3 describes diagnostic categories for DM and at-risk states.

SYNONYMS

IDDM (insulin-dependent diabetes mellitus)
NIDDM (non–insulin-dependent diabetes mellitus)
Type 1 diabetes mellitus (insulin-dependent diabetes mellitus)
Type 2 diabetes mellitus (non–insulin-dependent diabetes mellitus)
LADA (latent autoimmune diabetes of adult)
MODY (mature onset diabetes of youth)

TABLE 1 Characteristic Comparison of Type 1 Versus Type 2 Diabetes Mellitus

Characteristic	Type 1	Type 2
Nature Very different	Autoimmune disorder marked by destruction of insulin-producing beta cells and loss of insulin production	A disorder of insulin deficiency involving an interplay between both pancreatic and extrapancreatic contributions to disease
Symptoms Partial overlap	Rapid onset; very high to extremely high blood glucose levels; polyphagia; polydipsia, polyuria; ketoacidosis	Mild to moderate onset; modest to high elevations in blood glucose; mild polydipsia/polyuria; fatigue; visual changes/headache
Onset Very different	Sudden (symptoms for days to weeks)	Slower onset (symptoms for months to years)
Risk factors Typically different but overlap	Family history of autoimmune disease but particularly type 1 diabetes mellitus (tenfold increased risk vs. general population)	Overweight/obese; poor diet; sedentary lifestyle; ethnicity (higher in African Americans, Hispanics); family history of type 2 diabetes mellitus; history of gestational diabetes
Onset age Typically different but overlap	Typically early life through adolescence but can occur at any age	Typically adults but trending toward earlier age of onset
Treatment strategy Typically different	Absolute requirement for insulin (multiple daily injections or insulin pump); self-management lifestyle modification (monitor food types, exercise, etc.)	Dietary modifications and exercise alongside oral agents (for most); increasingly greater percentage of patients require insulin over time
Can it be prevented? Very different	Not at present (subject of major research efforts); future cases can be predicted by autoantibodies and genetics	Yes, for more than half of potential cases, with dietary modifications and exercise
Can it be reversed? Very different	Not at present (subject of major research efforts)	No, but for a limited few; patients can see disease managed and risk for complications reduced through diet modifications, exercise; growing evidence for disease improvements through combination therapies
Complications Mostly similar, but some variation	Acute emergencies of hypoglycemia and ketoacidosis leading to hypoglycemic unawareness; chronic effects of hyperglycemia can lead to retinopathy, nephropathy, neuropathy, cardiovascular disease, etc.	Acute emergencies of hypoglycemia and ketoacidosis leading to hypoglycemic unawareness; chronic effects of hyperglycemia can lead to retinopathy, nephropathy, neuropathy, cardiovascular disease, etc.

From Melmed S et al: *Williams textbook of endocrinology,* ed 14, Philadelphia, 2020, Elsevier.

Diseases and Disorders

TABLE 2   Characteristics of Type 1 and Type 2 Diabetes Mellitus

	Type 1 Diabetes	Type 2 Diabetes
Frequency	5%-10%	90%-95%
Age of onset	Any, but most common in children and young adults	More common with advancing age, but can occur in children and adolescents
Risk factors	Genetic, autoimmune, environmental	Genetic, obesity, sedentary lifestyle, race/ethnicity, hypertension, dyslipidemia, polycystic ovarian syndrome
Pathogenesis	Destruction of pancreatic beta cells, usually autoimmune	No autoimmunity Insulin resistance and progressive insulin deficiency
C-peptide levels	Very low or undetectable	Detectable
Prediabetes	Autoantibodies (GAD65, IA-2, IAA, ZnT8) may be present	Autoantibodies absent
Medication therapy	Insulin absolutely necessary; multiple daily injections or insulin pump	Oral agents and/or noninsulin injectable hypoglycemic drugs Insulin commonly needed
Therapy to prevent or delay onset of diabetes	Teplizumab	Lifestyle (weight loss and increased physical activity) Oral medications (metformin, acarbose) may be helpful

Modified from McPherson RA, Pincus MR: *Henry's clinical diagnosis and management by laboratory method*, ed 23, St Louis, 2017, Elsevier.

EPIDEMIOLOGY & DEMOGRAPHICS

- DM affects 9% to 10% of the U.S. population. Prevalence rates vary considerably by race/ethnicity. T1DM accounts for approximately 5% of diagnosed diabetes cases and is defined by the presence of one or more autoimmune markers.
- In the U.S., the overall pediatric incidence of T1DM is approximately 25 per 100,000 per yr. Incidence a varies according to age (peaking in the pubertal years, ages 10 to 14), season (winter more than summer), geographic location (Finland and other Nordic countries more than equatorial regions), and race and ethnic group (U.S. non-Hispanic White persons more than Native Americans).[1]

- Risk factors for type 1 DM are summarized in Table 4.
- There are three stages of type 1 DM. Patients in stage 1 have two or more diabetes-related autoantibodies, and those in stage 2 have developed asymptomatic dysglycemia but have normal other metabolic indices and do not require insulin treatment. Stage 3 is symptomatic clinical disease. Teplizumab is an anti-CD3 monoclonal antibody recently FDA approved to delay the onset of stage 3 type 1 DM in patients ≥8 yr old who have stage 2 type 1 DM.[2]
- While incidence of diabetes in adolescents is mostly type 1, the rate of type 2 being diagnosed in adolescents has increased by 1.5 times in certain given areas. This seems to correlate with the epidemic of pediatric obesity.
- Table 5 summarizes epidemiologic determinants of and risk factors for type 2 DM. Interacting genetic, biologic, behavioral, and environmental factors involved in the pathogenesis of type 2 SM are illustrated in Figs. E2 and E3.
- Incidence rate increases with age, varying from 2% in persons age 20 to 44 yr to 18% in persons 65 to 74 yr. T2DM can have a long presymptomatic phase, leading to a 4- to 7-yr delay in diagnosis. In the U.S. 1.2 million

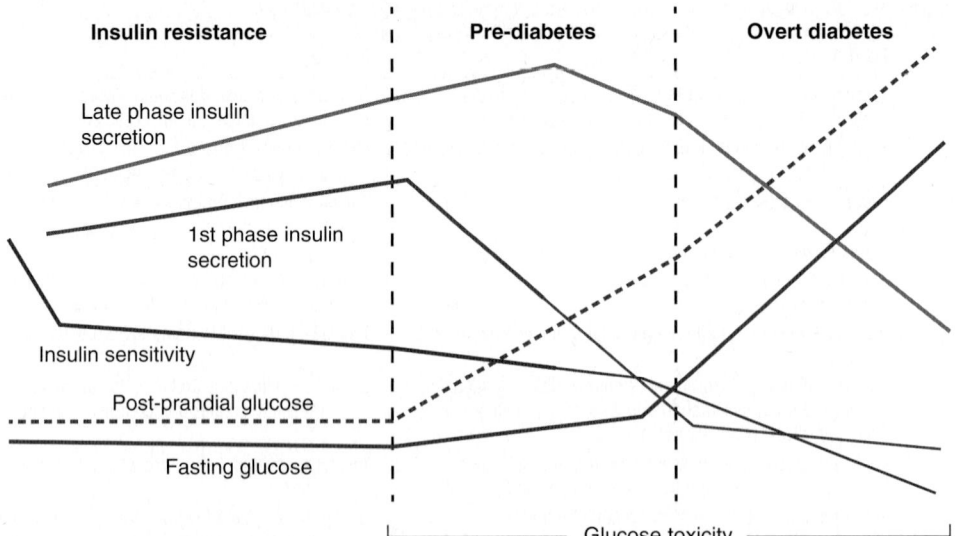

FIG. 1 The metabolic evolution of type 2 diabetes (T2D). The development of T2D begins with the insulin resistance phase, where increased first- and second-phase insulin secretion compensates for a decrease in insulin sensitivity in muscle and liver, sufficient to maintain normoglycemia. In the prediabetes phase, insulin secretion becomes inadequate to maintain normoglycemia. First-phase insulin secretion is abrogated, with a rise in postprandial glucose followed by a decline in second-phase insulin secretion and the appearance of impaired fasting glucose. The diabetes phase features overt hyperglycemia accompanied by progressive β cell exhaustion. In both the prediabetes and diabetes phases, glucose toxicity at the level of the pancreatic β cell contributes to reductions in glucose-induced insulin secretion. (From Robertson RP et al: *DeGroot's endocrinology, basic science and clinical practice*, ed 8, Philadelphia, 2023, Elsevier.)

BOX 1 Classification of Diabetes Mellitus

- Type 1 diabetes (beta cell destruction, usually leading to absolute insulin deficiency)
  1. Immune mediated
  2. Idiopathic
- Type 2 diabetes (may range from predominantly insulin resistance with relative insulin deficiency to a predominantly secretory defect with insulin resistance)
- Other specific types
  a. Genetic defects of beta cell function
     (1) Chromosome 12, HNF-1α (MODY3)
     (2) Chromosome 7, glucokinase (MODY2)
     (3) Chromosome 20, HNF-4α (MODY1)
     (4) Chromosome 13, insulin promoter factor-1 (IPF-1; MODY4)
     (5) Chromosome 17, HNF-1β (MODY5)
     (6) Chromosome 2, NeuroD1 (MODY6)
     (7) Mitochondrial DNA
     (8) Others
  b. Genetic defects in insulin action
     (1) Type A insulin resistance
     (2) Leprechaunism
     (3) Rabson-Mendenhall syndrome
     (4) Lipoatrophic diabetes
     (5) Others
  c. Diseases of the exocrine pancreas
     (1) Pancreatitis
     (2) Trauma/pancreatectomy
     (3) Neoplasia
     (4) Cystic fibrosis
     (5) Hemochromatosis
     (6) Fibrocalculous pancreatopathy
     (7) Others
  d. Endocrinopathies
     (1) Acromegaly
     (2) Cushing syndrome
     (3) Glucagonoma
     (4) Pheochromocytoma
     (5) Hyperthyroidism
     (6) Somatostatinoma
     (7) Aldosteronoma
     (8) Others
  e. Drug or chemical induced
     (1) Vacor
     (2) Pentamidine
     (3) Nicotinic acid
     (4) Glucocorticoids
     (5) Thyroid hormone
     (6) Diazoxide
     (7) β-Adrenergic agonists
     (8) Thiazides
     (9) Dilantin
     (10) γ-Interferon
     (11) Others
  f. Infections
     (1) Congenital rubella
     (2) Cytomegalovirus
     (3) Others
  g. Uncommon forms of immune-mediated diabetes
     (1) "Stiff-man" syndrome
     (2) Antiinsulin receptor antibodies
     (3) Others
  h. Other genetic syndromes sometimes associated with diabetes
     (1) Down syndrome
     (2) Klinefelter syndrome
     (3) Turner syndrome
     (4) Wolfram syndrome
     (5) Friedreich ataxia
     (6) Huntington chorea
     (7) Laurence-Moon-Biedl syndrome
     (8) Myotonic dystrophy
     (9) Porphyria
     (10) Prader-Willi syndrome
     (11) Others
- Gestational diabetes mellitus

From McPherson RA, Pincus MR: *Henry's clinical diagnosis and management by laboratory method*, ed 23, St Louis, 2017, Elsevier.

TABLE 3 Diagnostic Categories*: Diabetes Mellitus and At-Risk States

Fasting Plasma Glucose Level	2-H (75-G) OGTT RESULT		
	<140 mg/dl	140-199 mg/dl	≥200 mg/dl
<100 mg/dl	Normal	IGT[†]	DM
100-125 mg/dl	IFG[†]	IGT[†] *and* IFG[†]	DM
≥126 mg/dl	DM	DM	DM
HbA$_{1C}$ Level	<5.7%	5.7-6.4%	≥6.5%
	Normal	High-risk[†]	DM

DM, Diabetes mellitus; *HbA$_{1C}$*, glycosylated hemoglobin; *IFG*, impaired fasting glucose; *IGT*, impaired glucose tolerance; *OGTT*, oral glucose tolerance test.

*These diagnostic categories are based on the combined fasting plasma glucose level and a 2-h, 75-g oral glucose tolerance test (OGTT) result. Note that a confirmed random plasma glucose level of 200 mg/dl or higher in the appropriate clinical setting is diagnostic of diabetes and precludes the need for further testing.

[†]May be referred to as prediabetes.

From Goldman L, Schafer AI: *Goldman's Cecil medicine*, ed 24, Philadelphia, 2012, Saunders.

new cases of diabetes are diagnosed each yr, and 86 million have prediabetes. Currently, 30 million Americans have diabetes; with this current trend, it is predicted that by 2050, 1 out of 3 Americans will be diabetic.
- Diabetes accounts for 8% of all legal blindness in the U.S. and is the leading cause of end-stage renal disease (ESRD). Approximately 40% of patients in a given dialysis center are diabetic.
- Patients with diabetes are two to four times more likely than nondiabetic patients to experience development of cardiovascular disease (CVD).

PHYSICAL FINDINGS & CLINICAL PRESENTATION

- Physical examination varies with the presence of complications and may be normal in early stages.
- Diabetic retinopathy:
  1. Nonproliferative (background diabetic retinopathy):
     a. Initially: Microaneurysms, capillary dilation, waxy or hard exudates, dot and flame hemorrhages, arteriovenous shunts
     b. Advanced stage: Microinfarcts with cotton wool exudates, macular edema
  2. Proliferative retinopathy: Characterized by formation of new vessels, vitreous hemorrhages, fibrous scarring, and retinal detachment
- Cataracts and glaucoma occur with increased frequency in patients with diabetes.
- Diabetic macular edema: Swelling of the macula leading to loss of sharp vision in this part of the eye. People with this disorder usually already have retinopathy but may present separately as well.
- Diabetic neuropathy:
  1. Distal sensorimotor polyneuropathy:
     a. Symptoms include paresthesia, hyperesthesia, or burning pain involving bilateral distal extremities in a "stocking glove" distribution. This can progress to motor weakness and ataxia
     b. Physical examination may reveal decreased pinprick sensation, decreased sensation to light touch, decreased vibration sense, and loss of proprioception. Motor disturbances such as decreased deep tendon reflexes and atrophy of interosseous muscles can also be seen
  2. Autonomic neuropathy:
     a. GI disturbances: Esophageal motility abnormalities, gastroparesis, diarrhea (usually nocturnal):
        (1) Increased gastric emptying seen in type 2
        (2) Decreased gastric emptying seen in type 1
     b. Genitourinary (GU) disturbances: Neurogenic bladder (hesitancy, weak stream, and dribbling), impotence
     c. Cardiovascular (CV) disturbances: Orthostatic hypotension, tachycardia, decreased heart rate variability (HRV). Decreased HRV is associated with increased cardiac mortality, independent of ejection fraction
  3. Polyradiculopathy: Painful weakness and atrophy in the distribution of ≥1 contiguous nerve root
  4. Mononeuropathy involving cranial nerves III, IV, or VI or peripheral nerves can also occur
- Diabetic nephropathy: Pedal edema, pallor, weakness, uremic appearance
- Nephrotic syndrome: Proteinuria, hypertriglyceridemia, edema
- Nephritis: Progressive degeneration of nephrons focal glomerulosclerosis

TABLE 4 Risk of Type 1 Diabetes Mellitus

Group	Childhood Annual Incidence
U.S. general population	0.3% (15-25/100,000)
Offspring	1%
Sibling	3.2% (through adolescence); 6% lifetime
Dizygotic twin	6%
Mother	2%
Father	4.6%
Both parents	~10%
Monozygotic twin	50%, but incidence varies with age of index twin

From Melmed S et al: *Williams textbook of endocrinology*, ed 14, Philadelphia, 2020, Elsevier.

TABLE 5 Epidemiologic Determinants of and Risk Factors for Type 2 Diabetes Mellitus

Genetic Factors
Genetic markers
Family history

Demographic Characteristics
Age
Ethnicity

Behavioral and Lifestyle-Related Risk Factors
Obesity (including distribution of obesity and duration)
Physical inactivity
Diet
Stress
Westernization, urbanization, modernization
Medications
Shift work

Metabolic Determinants and Intermediate-Risk Categories of Type 2 Diabetes
Impaired glucose tolerance
Insulin resistance
Gestational diabetes
Offspring of women with diabetes during pregnancy
Intrauterine malnutrition or overnutrition
Microbiome composition

From Melmed S et al: *Williams textbook of endocrinology*, ed 14, Philadelphia, 2020, Elsevier.

Type IV renal tubular acidosis, hyperkalemic nephropathy, interstitial nephritis, causing hyporeninemic hypoaldosteronism. It is important to keep in mind that NSAIDs, ACE inhibitors, trimethoprim, and heparin can all reduce aldosterone and can cause or exacerbate the condition. 50% of patients on dialysis have diabetes as primary diagnosis; whereas glycemia is important to prevent nephropathy, the most significant contributing factor is hypertension.

- Foot ulcers: Occur in 15% of individuals with diabetes (annual incidence rate 2%) and are the leading causes of hospitalization; they are usually secondary to a combination of factors, including peripheral vascular insufficiency, repeated trauma (unrecognized because of sensory loss), and superimposed infection.
  1. Patient symptoms are usually less than would be expected from clinical findings, due to loss of sensation related to peripheral neuropathy.
  2. Comprehensive foot exams include visual inspection, assessment of pedal pulses, and assessment of protective sensation using a 10-g monofilament to test sensation.
  3. Prevention of foot ulcers in an individual with diabetes includes strict glucose control, patient education, prescription footwear, intensive podiatric care, and evaluation for surgical interventions.
  4. Foot examination should be done annually on all diabetics.
- Neuropathic arthropathy (Charcot joints): Bone or joint deformities from repeated trauma (secondary to peripheral neuropathy; Fig. E4).
- Necrobiosis lipoidica diabeticorum: Plaque-like reddened areas with a central area that fades to white-yellow, found on the anterior surfaces of the legs (Fig. E5); in these areas, the skin becomes very thin and can ulcerate easily.
- Other diabetic skin manifestations with diabetes include:
  1. Scleroderma diabeticorum: Thickening of skin and epidermis giving skin a "leather-like texture"; typically affects type 2, mainly on upper back and neck.

2. Dermatitis herpetiformis: Diffuse petechial rash associated with gluten insensitivity.
3. Vitiligo: Associated with type 1 and type 2 and affects skin coloration due to autoimmune reaction to pigmentation (at times may be associated with adrenal insufficiency, especially in type 1 patients). Patients should use SPF 30 sunscreen to prevent sunburn.
4. Acanthosis nigricans: Darkening of skin folds in neck and axilla, at times raised and velvety, thought to be associated with insulin resistance; other conditions such as Cushing and acromegaly can have this as well.
5. Diabetic dermopathy: Appears as shiny round or oval lesions on thin skin of the lower extremity, also known as "shin spots"; these are usually not painful and do not require treatment.
6. Eruptive xanthomatosis: Associated with uncontrolled blood sugars and extremely high triglycerides. There is a high risk for pancreatitis in patients with this finding; treatment is aimed at lowering blood sugars with insulin and fibrates.
7. Digital sclerosis: Skin on toes fingers and hands become waxy, thick, and tight, with joint stiffness; treatment is aimed at lowering blood sugars and encouraging use of lotions and moisturizers.
8. Bullosis diabeticorum: Rare disorder manifesting with blisters on hands, forearms, toes, and feet, usually painless. Lesions generally heal on their own.
- Box 2 summarizes cutaneous associations with diabetes mellitus.

ETIOLOGY

IDIOPATHIC DIABETES:

Type 1 DM: Results from autoimmune β-cell destruction, usually leading to absolute insulin deficiency (Fig. 6).
- Hereditary factors:
  1. Islet cell antibodies (found in 90% of patients within the first yr of diagnosis)
  2. Higher incidence of human leukocyte antigen (HLA) types DR3, DR4
  3. 50% concordance rate in identical twins
- Environmental factors: Viral infection (possibly coxsackievirus, mumps virus)

Type 2 DM: Results from insulin resistance and a progressive defect in insulin secretion (Fig. E7).
- Hereditary factors: 90% concordance rate in identical twins
- Environmental factors: Obesity, sedentary lifestyle, high carbohydrate content in food

DIABETES SECONDARY TO OTHER FACTORS:
- Hormonal excess: Cushing syndrome, acromegaly, glucagonoma, pheochromocytoma
- Drugs: Glucocorticoids, diuretics, oral contraceptives
- Insulin receptor unavailability (with or without circulating antibodies)
- Pancreatic disease: Pancreatitis, pancreatectomy, hemochromatosis, cystic fibrosis
- Genetic syndromes: Maturity onset diabetes of the young (MODY, monogenetic diabetes accounting for 2% to 5% of diabetes), familial

BOX 2 Some Cutaneous Associations with Diabetes Mellitus

Established or Probable Association
Necrobiosis lipoidica (NL) diabeticorum
Diabetic dermopathy
Diabetic bullae
Acanthosis nigricans
Acrochordons (skin tags)
Scleroderma diabeticorum
Limited joint mobility and waxy skin syndrome
Partial lipodystrophy
Malignant otitis externa
Neuropathic leg ulcers
Perforating disorders
Eruptive xanthomas
Hemochromatosis
Carotenemia
Pruritus
Xerosis and anhidrosis
Yellow nails, koilonychia
Increased susceptibility to infections:
Candida albicans
Staphylococcus aureus
Group A β-hemolytic streptococcus
Pseudomonas aeruginosa
Dermatophytes (tinea pedis, onychomycosis)
Corynebacterium minutissimum (erythrasma)

Possible Association
Disseminated granuloma annulare
Vitiligo

hyperlipidemias, myotonic dystrophy, lipoatrophy
- Gestational diabetes (GDM): Diabetes diagnosed during pregnancy that is due to pregnancy-related insulin resistance

Dx DIAGNOSIS

DIFFERENTIAL DIAGNOSIS
- Diabetes insipidus
- Stress hyperglycemia
- Diabetes secondary to hormonal excess, drugs, pancreatic disease

LABORATORY TESTS
- Diagnosis of DM is made on the basis of the following tests:
  1. Fasting glucose ≥126 mg/dl on two occasions
  2. Non-FPG ≥200 mg/dl and symptoms of DM
  3. OGTT (75 g glucose load for nonpregnant individuals) with 2-h value >200 mg/dl
  4. Glycosylated hemoglobin (HbA$_{1c}$) ≥6.5%. HbA$_{1c}$ level reflects average glycemia over previous 3 mo or longer. In known diabetics, this test should be performed at least twice yearly in stable patients and more frequently when therapy changes or patients are not meeting glycemic goals. HbA$_{1c}$ alone does not provide a measure of glycemic variability or hypoglycemia and is affected by the presence of hemoglobin variants, hemolysis, or blood loss
- Measurement of autoantibodies glutamic acid decarboxylase (GAD65) and tyrosine

phosphatase IA-2 are useful in suspected immune mediated type 1 DM (strong association).
- Screening for prediabetes and diabetes in asymptomatic patients (see Table 6):
  1. Should be considered in adults of any age who are overweight (body mass index [BMI] >25 kg/m²) or obese (BMI >30) and who have one or more additional risk factors for diabetes.
  2. In those who are without these risk factors, testing should begin at age 45 yr.
  3. If screen is normal, repeat testing should be carried out at least at 3-yr intervals.
  4. ADA recommends screening all Asian Americans with BMI 23 or higher every 2 yr.
- Detection and diagnosis of gestational diabetes mellitus (GDM):
  1. Screen for GDM using risk factor analysis and use of an OGTT. Pregnant women who are not known to have diabetes should be screened for gestational diabetes at 24 to 28 wk gestation with a "1-step" strategy with 75 g oral glucose tolerance test or a "2-step" approach with a 50-g (nonfasting) screen followed by a 100-g oral glucose tolerance test for those who screen positive. A diagnosis of GDM is made if any of the following levels of plasma glucose are exceeded: ≥92 mg/dl (5.1 mmol/L) when fasting, ≥80 mg/dl (10 mmol/L) at 1 h, or ≥153 mg/dl (8.5 mmol/L) at 2 h.
  2. Women with GDM should be screened for diabetes 6 to 12 wk postpartum and should be followed with subsequent

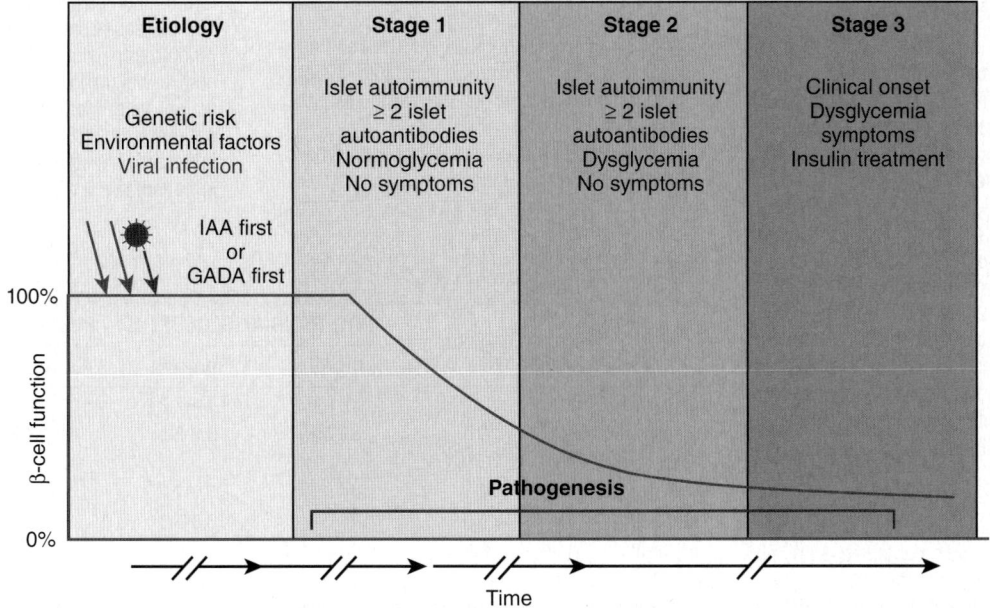

FIG. 6 Etiology and pathogenesis of autoimmune type 1 diabetes (T1D). The etiology is genetic and environmental, in yet unknown combinations. Biomarkers of two different endotypes are autoantibodies appearing either against insulin autoantibody *(IAA)* or glutamic acid decarboxylase autoantibody *(GADA)* first. The pathogenesis is initiated by islet autoimmunity to two or more autoantibodies (IAA, GADA, or autoantibodies against islet antigen-2 or Zn transporter 8) but normoglycemia and no symptoms (stage 1). Two or more autoantibodies remain, but dysglycemia develops (stage 2). The clinical onset is defined by dysglycemia (hyperglycemia), diabetes symptoms, and insulin requirement (stage 3). The loss of functional β cell mass is illustrated as a continuous variable, but the rate of loss varies between individuals dependent on the age at the first appearing islet autoantibody in combination with genetic and environmental (e.g., additional viral infections) factors. Dependent on the endotype of first-appearing autoantibody, time represents months to years. (From Robertson RP et al: *DeGroot's endocrinology, basic science and clinical practice*, ed 8, Philadelphia, 2023, Elsevier.)

TABLE 6 Criteria for Diabetes Screening in Asymptomatic Individuals

- Testing should be considered in all adults who are overweight (BMI >25 kg/m²*) and have additional risk factors:
  1. Physical inactivity
  2. A first-degree relative with diabetes
  3. High-risk ethnic population (e.g., African American, Hispanic American, Native American, Asian American, Pacific Islander)
  4. Delivered a baby weighing more than 9 lb or diagnosed with gestational diabetes mellitus
  5. Systemic hypertension (blood pressure >140/90 mm Hg or on antihypertensive therapy)
  6. High-density lipoprotein cholesterol level <35 mg/dl or triglyceride level >250 mg/dl
  7. Polycystic ovary syndrome
  8. Hemoglobin A_{1C} ≥5.7%, impaired glucose tolerance or impaired fasting glucose on prior testing
  9. Other clinical conditions associated with insulin resistance (e.g., severe obesity, acanthosis nigricans)
  10. History of cardiovascular disease
- If none of the above criteria are present, screening for diabetes should begin at age 45 yr
- If the results are normal, screening should be repeated at least every 3 yr. Depending on initial results and risk status, more frequent testing may need to be considered

*In some ethnic groups, such as Asians, at-risk body mass index (BMI) may be lower.
Modified from American Diabetes Association: Diagnosis and classification of diabetes mellitus, *Diabetes Care* 33(Suppl 1):S14, 2010; and from Goldman L, Schafer AI: *Goldman's Cecil medicine*, ed 24, Philadelphia, 2012, Saunders.

screening for the development of diabetes or prediabetes at least every 3 yr. A woman who had GDM during pregnancy has 50% risk of developing diabetes later in life; this is dependent on ethnicity (e.g., Pima Indians, Hispanic, African American).

- Screening for diabetic nephropathy:
  1. Screening should be done at diagnosis and then yearly for type 2 diabetes and 5 yr after diagnosis, then yearly in type 1 diabetes. 18% of type 1 DM may have early kidney changes, and future guidelines may change screening to 1 yr after diagnosis if poorly controlled, then annually for both type 1 and type 2.
  2. Screening can be performed using an albumin:creatinine ratio (microalbumin) in a random spot urine collection or by measurement of a 24-h urine collection for albumin and creatinine clearance. The urine albumin to creatinine ratio (ACR) is independently associated with mortality at all levels of estimated glomerular filtration rate (eGFR) in older adults with diabetes.
  3. The diagnosis of microalbuminuria (ACR 30 to 299 mg/24 h) should be based on 2 to 3 elevated levels within a 3- to 6-mo period because there is a marked variability in day-to-day albumin excretion. Patients with overt macroalbuminuria (>300 mg albumin/24 h or albumin: creatinine ratio >300) should be followed by urine protein:creatinine ratio.
- A fasting serum lipid panel, serum creatinine, and electrolytes should be obtained yearly on all adult patients with diabetes.
- Self-monitoring of blood glucose (SMBG) is crucial for assessing the effectiveness of the management plan. The frequency and timing of SMBG varies with the needs and goals of each patient. In most patients with type 1 DM and pregnant women taking insulin, SMBG is recommended at least 3 times/day. In patients with type 2 DM not on insulin, recommendations are unclear for SMBG, but testing once or twice/day is acceptable in most patients. Glycemic control is best evaluated when SMBG is combined with HbA_{1C} testing.

- Continuous glucose monitoring (CGM; Fig. E8) is now starting to play a more prominent role in reducing the number of fingersticks. Dexcom CGM has been approved by FDA for use by patients to adjust insulin based on CGM readings. Randomized trials in persons with type 1 DM and high glycated hemoglobin levels have shown that the use of intermittently scanned CGMs with optional alarms for high and low blood glucose levels results in significantly lower glycated hemoglobin levels than levels monitored by fingerstick testing.[3]
- The use of insulin pump and CGM readings and computer software can adjust insulin automatically (known as the "artificial pancreas").
- CGM can also be used in patients with type 2 on multiple daily injections.

- Limitations of CGM are that it cannot predict accuracy of blood glucose when <70 mg/dl.
- Screening for thyroid dysfunction (TSH level), vitamin B_{12} deficiency, and celiac disease should be considered in type 1 diabetes due to the increased frequency of other autoimmune diseases in these individuals.
- Consider screening for autoimmune polyendocrine syndromes (APS-2):
  1. APS-2: Most commonly known as Schmidt syndrome, heterogeneous not linked to one gene (HDLA-DQ2, HDLA-DQ8, AND HLA-DR4). Patients can have IDDM, hyperthyroidism, other autoimmune conditions, B_{12} deficiency, and myasthenia.

(Rx) TREATMENT

- Glycemic goals in adult diabetics are summarized in Table 7.
- Type 1 diabetes requires immediate initiation of insulin therapy. Newer biochemically modified insulins have duration of action ranging from 24 h of basal insulin level to ultrarapid duration for glycemic control at meal or snack times.[1]
- In type 1 diabetes, intensive glycemic control (HbA_{1C} <7) has been shown in randomized controlled trials (RCT) to reduce the risk of microvascular (neuropathy, retinopathy, nephropathy) and macrovascular (cardiovascular events) complications.
- Type 2 DM: Glucose-lowering medications are summarized in Table 8. The ADA and European Association for the Study of Diabetes recommend lifestyle intervention (diet and exercise) and metformin initiation. Metformin decreases hepatic glucose production and increases secretion of GLP-1. Metformin monotherapy does not cause hypoglycemia and is weight neutral or can cause modest weight loss. Metformin is contraindicated in patients with eGFR <30 ml/min/1.73 m², and initiation of metformin is not recommended in patients with eGFR 30-45 ml/min/1.73 m².

TABLE 7 Glycemic Goals in Adults*

	Hemoglobin A_{1C} (%)	PREPRANDIAL GLUCOSE		POSTPRANDIAL GLUCOSE**	
		mg/dl	mmol/L	mg/dl	mmol/L
ADA[†]: Adults	<7.0[‡]	80-130	4.4-7.2	<180	<10.0
Pregnant adults	<6.0	60-99	3.3-5.5	100-129	5.6-7.2
Older Adults:					
Healthy	<7.5	90-130	5.0-7.2	90-150	5.0-8.3
Intermediate	<8.0	90-150	5.0-8.3	100-180	5.6-10.0
Poor health	<8.5	100-180	5.6-10.0	110-200	6.1-11.1
AACE[§,¶]	≤6.5	≤110	≤6.1	≤140	<7.8

*Youth <18 yr of age: Goal hemoglobin A_{1C} <7.5%.
**1 to 2 h after beginning a meal for adults, except bedtime for older adults.
[†]ADA, American Diabetes Association (2015); Chiang et al (2014).
[‡]Lower goals may be appropriate for selected individuals if this can be accomplished safely (without significant hypoglycemia). Higher goals may be appropriate in some individuals (e.g., with a history of severe hypoglycemia, limited life expectancy, advanced complications, extensive comorbid conditions, or long-standing diabetes in whom the goal is difficult to achieve with appropriate education, monitoring, and therapies, including insulin).
[§]AACE, American Association of Clinical Endocrinologists, 2015.
[¶]For patients without concurrent serious illness and at low hypoglycemia risk.
From McPherson RA, Pincus MR: *Henry's clinical diagnosis and management by laboratory method*, ed 23, St Louis, 2017, Elsevier.

TABLE 8 Glucose-Lowering Medications

Class	HbA1c Reduction	Effect on Weight	Primary Side Effects	Contraindications
Metformin	1%-2%	Neutral	Gastrointestinal	eGFR <30 ml/min/1.73 m²
Sulfonylurea	1%-2%	1- to 3-kg gain	Hypoglycemia	Type 1 diabetes
Thiazolidinedione	0.5%-1%	2- to 4-kg gain	Fluid retention, bone fracture	Heart failure
Glucagonlike peptide 1 receptor agonist	0.5%-1.5%	Weight loss variable—up to 7 kg (semaglutide)	Gastrointestinal in nature	Gastroparesis; some still concerned about pancreatitis
Sodium glucose cotransporter 2 inhibitor	0.5%-0.7%	2- to 4-kg loss	Genital mycotic infection, urinary tract infection	Type 1 diabetes
Dipeptidyl peptidase 4 inhibitors	0.5%-0.8%	Neutral	Nothing consistent	Heart failure with saxagliptin

eGFR, Estimated glomerular filtration rate.
From Robertson RP et al: *DeGroot's endocrinology, basic science and clinical practice*, ed 8, Philadelphia, 2023, Elsevier.

Therapy can be augmented with additional agents (including early initiation of insulin therapy) to achieve adequate glycemic control. The choice of a second antihyperglycemic agent should be based on the presence of comorbid disorders such as heart failure, atherosclerotic cardiovascular disease, chronic kidney disease, and obesity. A proposed approach for earlier initiation of insulin therapy for patients with type 2 DM is illustrated in Fig. 9.

- Table 9 summarizes American College of Cardiology/American Heart Association (ACC/AHA) recommendations for primary prevention of CVD in patients with diabetes. Recommendations for secondary prevention of CVD are described in Table 10.
- It is important to remember that tight glycemic control may burden patients with complex treatment programs, hypoglycemia, weight gain, and costs. Clinicians should individualize HbA1c targets so that they are reasonable and reflect patients' personal and clinical contexts and their informed values and preferences. A target HbA1c <7 is reasonable for motivated new diabetic patients with long life expectancies, whereas less stringent controls (HbA1c 7.5 or higher) may be reasonable in elderly patients with limited life expectancy and elevated risk of hypoglycemia. The American Geriatrics Society recommends a general goal for glycated hemoglobin in older adults of 7.5% to 8.0%. Higher HbA1c targets (8% to 9%) are appropriate for older adults with multiple comorbidities, poor health, and limited life expectancy.[4]
- In type 2 diabetes, intensive glycemic control (HbA1c <7) has been shown in RCT to reduce the risk of microvascular complications. While intensive glucose control reduced the risk of some CVD outcomes (such as nonfatal MI), it did not reduce the risk of cardiovascular death or all-cause mortality and increased the risk of severe hypoglycemia.

NONPHARMACOLOGIC THERAPY

- Diet: The ADA does not recommend a special diet. However, newly diagnosed diabetics who are overweight or obese should be counseled to lose at least 5% of their body

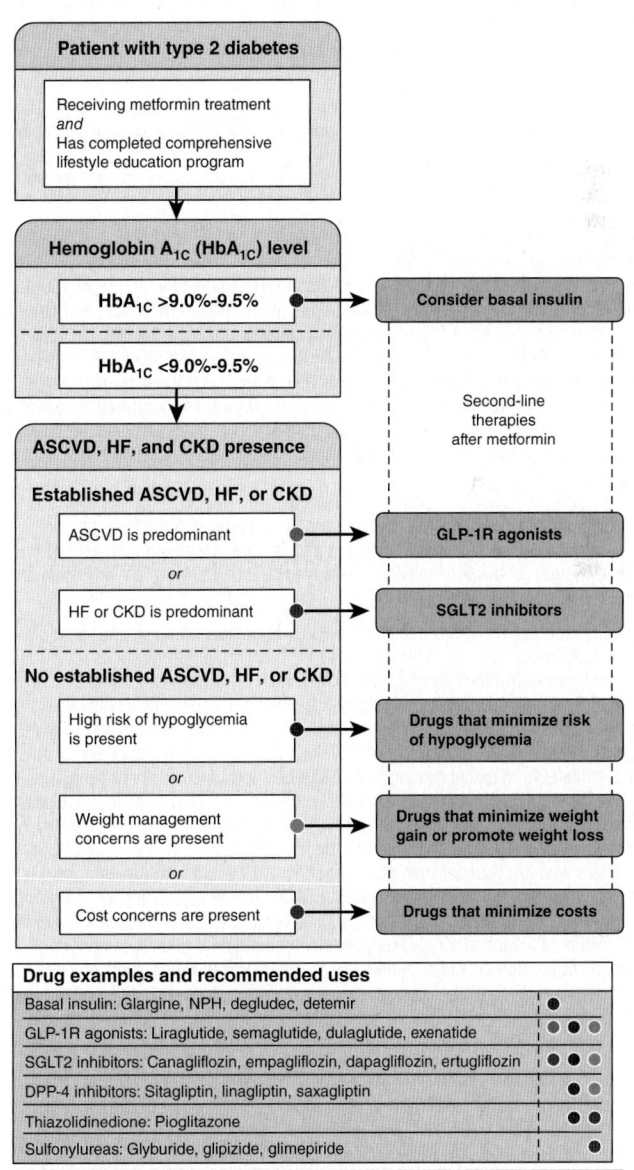

ASCVD indicates atherosclerotic cardiovascular disease; CKD, chronic kidney disease; DPP-4, dipeptidyl peptidase 4; GLP-1R, glucagon-like peptide 1 receptor; HF, heart failure; NPH, neutral protamine Hagedorn; SGLT2, sodium glucose cotransporter 2.

FIG. 9 Proposed approach for earlier initiation of insulin therapy for patients with type 2 diabetes. (From Robertson RP et al: *DeGroot's endocrinology, basic science and clinical practice*, ed 8, Philadelphia, 2023, Elsevier.)

TABLE 9 American College of Cardiology Foundation/American Heart Association Recommendations for Primary Prevention of Cardiovascular Disease in People with Diabetes

Lifestyle Management

Weight

Structured programs that emphasize lifestyle changes such as reduced fat (<30%-35% of daily energy) and total energy intake and increased regular physical activity, along with regular participant contact, can produce long-term weight loss on the order of 5%-7% of starting weight, with improvement in BP.

For persons with elevated plasma triglycerides and reduced HDL-C, improved glycemic control, moderate weight loss (5%-7% of starting weight), dietary saturated fat restriction, increased physical activity, and modest replacement of dietary carbohydrate (5%-7%) by either monounsaturated or polyunsaturated fats may be beneficial.

Medical Nutrition Therapy

To achieve reductions in LDL-C:
- Saturated fats should be less than 7% of energy intake.
- Dietary cholesterol intake should be less than 200 mg/day. Intake of *trans* unsaturated fatty acids should be less than 1% of energy intake.
- Total energy intake should be adjusted to achieve body weight goals.

Total dietary fat intake should be moderated (<30%-35% of total calories) and should consist mainly of monounsaturated or polyunsaturated fat.

Ample intake of dietary fiber (≥14 g/1000 calories consumed) may be of benefit.

If individuals choose to drink alcohol, daily intake should be limited to one drink for adult women and two drinks for adult men. One drink is defined as 12 ounces (oz) of beer, 4 oz of wine, or 1.5 oz of distilled spirits. Alcohol ingestion increases caloric intake and should be minimized when weight loss is the goal.

Individuals with elevated plasma triglyceride levels should limit intake of alcohol because it may exacerbate hypertriglyceridemia.

In both normotensive and hypertensive persons, a reduction in sodium intake may lower BP. The goal should be to reduce sodium intake to 1200-2300 mg/day (50-100 mmol/day), equivalent to 3000-6000 mg/day sodium chloride.

Physical Activity

To improve glycemic control, assist with weight loss or maintenance, and reduce risk for CVD, at least 150 min of moderate-intensity aerobic physical activity or at least 90 min of vigorous aerobic exercise per wk is recommended. The physical activity should be distributed over at least 3 days per wk, with no more than 2 consecutive days without physical activity.

For long-term maintenance of major weight loss, a larger amount of exercise (7 h of moderate or vigorous aerobic physical activity per wk) may be helpful.

Blood Pressure

BP should be measured at every routine diabetes visit. Patients found to have SBP ≥130 mm Hg or DBP ≥80 mm Hg should have BP confirmed on a separate day.

Patients with diabetes should be treated to achieve SBP at least <140 mm Hg and DBP <90 mm Hg, and for patients who can tolerate without adverse symptoms, targets can be as low as SBP <130 mm Hg and DBP <80-85 mm Hg. Patients with SBP of 130-139 mm Hg or DBP of 80-89 mm Hg should initiate lifestyle modification alone (weight control, increased physical activity, alcohol moderation, sodium reduction, and emphasis on increased consumption of fresh fruits, vegetables, and low-fat dairy products) for a maximum of 3 mo. If, after these efforts, targets are not achieved, treatment with pharmacologic agents should be initiated.

Patients with hypertension (SBP ≥140 mm Hg or DBP ≥90 mm Hg) should receive drug therapy in addition to lifestyle and behavioral therapy.

All patients with diabetes and hypertension should be treated with a regimen that includes either an ACE inhibitor, or if intolerant to an ACE inhibitor, an ARB. If one class is not tolerated, the other should be substituted. Other drug classes demonstrated to reduce CVD events in patients with diabetes—dihydropyridine calcium channel blockers, thiazide diuretics (chlorthalidone and indapamide), and β-blockers—should be added, in listed order of preference, as needed to achieve BP targets.

If ACE inhibitors, ARBs, or diuretics are used, kidney function and serum potassium levels should be monitored within the first 3 mo. If BP is stable, follow-up could occur every 6 mo thereafter.

Multidrug therapy generally is required to achieve BP targets.

In elderly hypertensive patients, BP should be lowered gradually to avoid complications.

Orthostatic measurement of BP should be performed in people with diabetes and hypertension when clinically indicated.

Patients not achieving target BP despite multidrug therapy should be referred to a physician specializing in the care of patients with hypertension.

Lipids

In adult patients with diabetes, lipid levels should be measured at least annually and more often if needed to achieve goals. In adults with diabetes who are younger than 40 with low-risk lipid values (LDL-C <100 mg/dl, HDL-C >50 mg/dl, triglycerides <150 mg/dl), lipid assessments may be repeated every 2 yr.

Lifestyle modification deserves primary emphasis in all individuals with diabetes. Patients should focus on the reduction of saturated fat and cholesterol intake, weight loss (if indicated), and increases in dietary fiber and physical activity. These lifestyle changes have been shown to improve the lipid profile in patients with diabetes. In persons with diabetes who are older than 40 yr, without overt CVD, statin therapy should be considered for primary prevention with recommendation to use at least moderate-dose and ideally intense-dose statins, independent of baseline LDL-C levels. On maximally tolerated statin, the goal is an LDL-C level <100 mg/dl (2.6 mmol/L), and ideally <70 mg/dl (1.8 mmol/L) for those at highest CVD risk. If LDL-lowering drugs are used, a reduction of at least 50% in LDL-C levels should be obtained.

If baseline LDL-C is <100 mg/dl, statin therapy should be initiated based on risk factor assessment and clinical judgment. Major risk factors in this category include age, sex, race/ethnicity, cigarette smoking, hypertension (BP >140/90 mm Hg or use of antihypertensive medication), high total cholesterol and low HDL-C (<40 mg/dl), and family history of premature CHD (CHD in male first-degree relatives ≤55 yr of age; CHD in female first-degree relatives ≤65 yr of age).

In people with diabetes who are younger than 40, without overt CVD, but who are estimated to be at increased risk for CVD either by clinical judgment or by risk calculator, at least moderate-intensity statin therapy is recommended, with an LDL-C goal of <100 mg/dl.

Combination therapy with LDL-lowering drugs (e.g., statins, ezetimibe, PCSK9 inhibitors) and fibrates or niacin may be necessary to achieve lipid targets, but to date, only the addition of ezetimibe to statin therapy has proven incremental CV outcomes benefit.

Beyond the consensus of therapeutic lifestyle intervention, the ADA and AHA guidelines have evolved significantly over recent years, no longer recommending pharmacologic treatment of low HDL-C or high triglyceride levels, except for those with extremely high fasting triglyceride levels, to consider fish oil or a fibrate to mitigate pancreatitis risk.

Tobacco

All patients with diabetes should be asked about tobacco use status at every visit.

Every tobacco user should be advised to quit.

The tobacco user's willingness to quit should be assessed.

The patient can be assisted by counseling and by developing a plan to quit.

Follow-up, referral to special programs, or pharmacotherapy (including nicotine replacement and bupropion) should be incorporated as needed.

Antiplatelet Agents

The ADA and AHA recommend aspirin therapy (75-162 mg/day) for primary prevention in patients with diabetes at increased CV risk (e.g., estimated 10-yr risk >10%), including most age ≥50 yr who have additional risk factors (e.g., family history of CVD, hypertension, smoking, dyslipidemia, albuminuria). In contrast, the ESC/EASD guidelines discourage aspirin for primary prevention in patients with diabetes, except for those estimated to be at the very highest CV risk, in whom such use may be considered.

People with aspirin allergy, bleeding tendency, existing anticoagulant therapy, recent gastrointestinal bleeding, and clinically active hepatic disease are poor candidates for aspirin, especially for primary prevention. Other antiplatelet agents may be a reasonable alternative for patients with high risk.

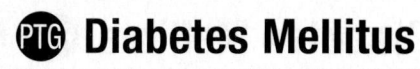

TABLE 9 American College of Cardiology Foundation/American Heart Association Recommendations for Primary Prevention of Cardiovascular Disease in People with Diabetes—cont'd

Glycemic Control

The HbA_{1C} goal for most patients with diabetes in general is less than 7% in the absence of CVD, with higher targets such as 8% (or higher) endorsed for patients with moderate to severe CVD or other serious comorbidities.

Type 1 Diabetes Mellitus

At present, all of the recommendations listed above for patients with type 2 DM appear to be appropriate for those with type 1 DM as well.

ACE, Angiotensin-converting enzyme; *ADA,* American Diabetes Association; *AHA,* American Heart Association; *ARB,* angiotensin receptor blocker; *BP,* blood pressure; *CHD,* coronary heart disease; *CV,* cardiovascular; *CVD,* cardiovascular disease; *DBP,* diastolic blood pressure; *DM,* diabetes mellitus; *EASD,* European Association for the Study of Diabetes; *ESC,* European Society of Cardiology; *HbA_{1C},* glycosylated hemoglobin; *HDL-C,* high-density lipoprotein cholesterol; *LDL-C,* low-density lipoprotein cholesterol; *SBP,* systolic blood pressure.

Data are from Fox CS et al: Update on prevention of cardiovascular disease in adults with type 2 diabetes mellitus in light of recent evidence: a scientific statement from the American Heart Association and the American Diabetes Association, *Circulation* 132:691-718, 2015; Ryden L et al: ESC guidelines on diabetes, pre-diabetes, and cardiovascular diseases developed in collaboration with the EASD. The Task Force on Diabetes, Pre-diabetes, and Cardiovascular Diseases of the European Society of Cardiology (ESC) and developed in collaboration with the European Association for the Study of Diabetes (EASD), *Eur Heart J* 34:3035-3087, 2013; ADA Standards of Medical Care in Diabetes—2016: abridged for primary care providers, *Diabetes Care* 34:3-21, 2016; Inzucchi SE et al: Management of hyperglycemia in type 2 diabetes, 2015: a patient-centered approach—update to a position statement of the American Diabetes Association and the European Association for the Study of Diabetes, *Diabetes Care* 38:140-149, 2013; and Stone NJ et al: 2013 ACC/AHA guideline on the treatment of blood cholesterol to reduce atherosclerotic cardiovascular risk in adults: a report of the American College of Cardiology/American Heart Association Task Force on Practice Guidelines, *Circulation* 129(Suppl 2):S1-S45, 2014; In Libby P et al: *Braunwald's heart disease, a textbook of cardiovascular medicine,* ed 12, Philadelphia, 2022, Elsevier.

TABLE 10 American College of Cardiology Foundation/American Heart Association Recommendations for Secondary Prevention of Cardiovascular Disease Specific to Patients with Diabetes

Class	Indication	Level of Evidence
I	Care for diabetes should be coordinated with the patient's primary care physician and/or endocrinologist.	C
	Lifestyle modifications including daily physical activity, weight management, blood pressure control, and LDL cholesterol management are recommended for all patients with diabetes.	B
	ACE inhibitors (or ARBs for those with ACE inhibitor intolerance) should be started and continued indefinitely in patients with diabetes, unless contraindicated.	A
	Use of aldosterone blockade in post-MI patients without significant kidney dysfunction or hyperkalemia is recommended in patients who are already receiving therapeutic doses of an ACE inhibitor and β-blocker, who have a left ventricular ejection fraction ≤40% and diabetes.	A
IIa	Metformin is an effective first-line pharmacotherapy and can be useful if not contraindicated.	A
	Individualizing the intensity of blood glucose–lowering interventions based on the individual patient's risk for hypoglycemia during treatment is reasonable.	C
IIb	Initiation of pharmacotherapy interventions to achieve target HbA_{1C} may be reasonable.	A
	A target HbA_{1C} of ≤7% may be considered, whereas the ADA/EASD endorse a target ≥8% for those with moderate to severe CVD.	C
	Less stringent HbA_{1C} goals may be considered for other patients with a history of severe hypoglycemia, limited life expectancy, advanced microvascular complications, or extensive comorbidity, or those in whom the goal is difficult to attain despite intensive therapeutic interventions.	C

ACE, Angiotensin-converting enzyme; *ADA,* American Diabetes Association; *ARB,* angiotensin receptor blocker; *CVD,* cardiovascular disease; *EASD,* European Association for the Study of Diabetes; *HbA_{1C},* glycosylated hemoglobin; *LDL,* low-density lipoprotein; *MI,* myocardial infarction.

Data are from Fox CS et al: Update on prevention of cardiovascular disease in adults with type 2 diabetes mellitus in light of recent evidence: a scientific statement from the American Heart Association and the American Diabetes Association, *Circulation* 132:691-718, 2015; Ryden L et al: ESC guidelines on diabetes, pre-diabetes, and cardiovascular diseases developed in collaboration with the EASD. The Task Force on Diabetes, Pre-diabetes, and Cardiovascular Diseases of the European Society of Cardiology (ESC) and developed in collaboration with the European Association for the Study of Diabetes (EASD), *Eur Heart J* 34:3035-3087, 2013; ADA Standards of Medical Care in Diabetes—2016: abridged for primary care providers, *Diabetes Care* 34:3-21, 2016; Inzucchi SE et al: Management of hyperglycemia in type 2 diabetes, 2015: a patient-centered approach—update to a position statement of the American Diabetes Association and the European Association for the Study of Diabetes, *Diabetes Care* 38:140-149, 2015; and Stone NJ et al: 2013 ACC/AHA guideline on the treatment of blood cholesterol to reduce atherosclerotic cardiovascular risk in adults: a report of the American College of Cardiology/American Heart Association Task Force on Practice Guidelines, *Circulation* 129(Suppl 2):S1-S45, 2014; In Libby P et al: *Braunwald's heart disease, a textbook of cardiovascular medicine,* ed 12, Philadelphia, 2022, Elsevier.

weight. Consultation with a registered dietitian is recommended.

1. Calories:
   a. The patient with diabetes can be started on 15 calories/lb of ideal body weight; this number can be increased to 20 calories/lb for an active person and 25 calories/lb if the patient does heavy physical labor.
   b. The calories should be distributed as 45% to 65% carbohydrates, <30% fat, with saturated fat limited to <7% of total calories, and 10% to 30% protein (protein intake of 0.8 g protein/kg body weight/day for patients not treated with dialysis). Daily cholesterol intake should not exceed 300 mg.
   c. The emphasis should be on complex carbohydrates rather than simple and refined starches, and on polyunsaturated instead of saturated fats in a ratio of 2:1.
   d. The glycemic index compares the increase in blood sugar after the ingestion of simple sugars and complex carbohydrates with the increase that occurs after the absorption of glucose; equal amounts of starches do not give the same increase in plasma glucose (pasta equal in calories to a baked potato causes less of an increase than the potato); thus it is helpful to know the glycemic index of a particular food product.

2. Fiber: Insoluble fiber (bran, celery) and soluble globular fiber (pectin in fruit) delay glucose absorption and attenuate the postprandial serum glucose peak.
   a. They also appear to reduce the increased triglyceride level often present in patients with uncontrolled diabetes. A diet high in fiber should be emphasized

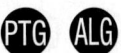

(20 to 35 g/day of soluble and insoluble fiber).

b. Diet programs: In 2015, a meta-analysis review of all research revealed that weight loss was equal no matter which diet program patients were involved in.

c. However, the only data to show evidence-based prevention of diabetes in prediabetics was the "Mediterranean diet."

d. The Mediterranean diet also showed a significant decrease in the percentage of established diabetics from needing insulin in the future and significant benefit in reducing cardiovascular events.

3. Other principles:

a. Modest sodium restriction to less than 2000 mg/day. If hypertension is present, restrict to <2400 mg/day; if nephropathy and hypertension are present, restrict to <2000 mg/day.

b. Moderation of alcohol intake recommended (≤2 drinks/day in men, ≤1 drink/day in women).

c. Nonnutritive artificial sweeteners are acceptable in moderate amounts.

d. However, it has been shown that artificial sweeteners may actually increase insulin resistance by affecting the action of insulin at receptor level.

- Exercise: Increases the cellular glucose uptake by increasing the number of insulin receptors. The following points must be considered:

1. Exercise program must be individualized and built up slowly. Consider beginning with 15 min of low-impact aerobic exercise three times per wk and increasing the frequency and duration to 30 to 45 min of moderate aerobic activity (50% to 70% of maximum age predicted heart rate) to 3 to 5 days/wk.

a. In the absence of contraindications, resistance training three times per wk should be encouraged.

2. Insulin is more rapidly absorbed when injected into a limb that is then exercised, and this can result in hypoglycemia.

3. Physical activity can result in hypoglycemia if medication dose or carbohydrate consumption is not modified. Ingestion of additional carbohydrates is recommended if preexercise glucose levels are <100 mg/dl.

4. Diabetes prevention program: Low-fat diet with exercise reduced diabetes by 58%. This encompassed diet of 1200 to 1800 kcal/day <30% from fat, exercise unsupervised and supervised, akin to brisk walking >150 min/wk of moderately intensity physical activity.

- Weight loss: To ideal body weight if the patient is overweight. Recent trials have shown that although weight loss has many positive health benefits for people with type 2 DM, such as slower decline in mobility, it does not reduce the number of cardiovascular events.

- Screening for nephropathy, neuropathy, and retinopathy: Annual serum creatinine and urine albumin excretion; initial comprehensive eye examination and at least annually thereafter.

- Diabetes self-management education: Could also address psychosocial issues.

- Self-monitoring of blood glucose should occur three to four times per day for patients using multiple insulin injections or on insulin pump therapy.

- Perform HbA$_{1C}$ at least two times a year in patients who are meeting treatment goals and who have stable glycemic control.

1. HbA$_{1C}$ quarterly in patients whose therapy has changed or who are not meeting glycemic goals.

2. The HbA$_{1C}$ goal for nonpregnant adults in general is <7%.

3. In the elderly, those with comorbidities, or those at risk for complications from hypoglycemia, a more moderate glycemic target (HbA$_{1C}$ 7 to 8) may be appropriate.

4. In elderly patients (>80 yr of age) with average life expectancy of 5 yr, a target HbA$_{1C}$ <8.0 is reasonable. In patients >80 yr with comorbidities and life expectancy of 3 yr, a target HbA$_{1C}$ of <9.0 may be appropriate.

GENERAL Rx

- Type 1 DM: Lifelong insulin therapy is required for persons with type 1 DM. It should consist of basal coverage, prandial coverage, and supplemental insulin for correction of hyperglycemia. Initial total insulin dosing ranges from 0.4 to 1.0 U/kg/day, 50% of which is basal insulin and 50% prandial insulin. Examples of insulin regimens used in type 1 DM are described in Table 11.

- Type 2 DM: When the previous measures fail to normalize the serum glucose, oral hypoglycemic agents should be added to the regimen in T2DM. Treatment options in patients with type 2 diabetes should be tailored to try to target core diabetic defects and apply therapies that lower HbA$_{1C}$ in a weight-neutral or weight-lowering fashion if possible; of course, cost of therapies needs to be considered as well. Contemporary guidelines stress the importance of a multifactorial approach that targets not only dysglycemia but also hypertension, dyslipidemia, and hypercoagulability.[5] Clinical features of commonly used oral antihyperglycemic agents are summarized in Table 12. Commonly used injectable agents other than insulin are described in Table 13.

- **Metformin:** The primary mechanism of metformin is to decrease hepatic glucose production and improve insulin sensitivity. Because metformin does not produce hypoglycemia when used as a monotherapy, it is preferred initially for most patients. Metformin can reduce A$_{1C}$ by 1.0% to 1.5%. It is contraindicated in patients with severe renal insufficiency with an estimated glomerular filtrate rate <30 ml/min. Starting metformin in patients with GFR between 30 and 45 ml/min is also not recommended. The excess risk for lactic acidosis is however negligible in patients with mild to moderate reductions in kidney function.[5,6]

- When metformin alone does not achieve the desired A$_{1C}$ goal, the choice of a second drug is dictated by the comorbidities.

1. For example, an SLGT2 inhibitor is preferred in patients with heart failure (HF) or chronic kidney disease (CKD). In patients with cardiovascular disease (CVD) or at high risk for CVD, a preferred drug would be a glucagon-like peptide-1 (GLP-1) receptor agonist or a sodium-glucose cotransporter 2 (SGLT2) inhibitor; in obese patients, tirzepatide or an GLP-1 agent would be preferred. Whereas in most patients without HF, CVD, CKD, or obesity, lowering the HbA$_{1C}$ while minimizing hypoglycemia is the main goal of therapy and can be achieved with dipeptidylpeptidase-4 (DPP-4) inhibitors, GLP-1 agonists, SGLT-2 inhibitors.

- **GLP-1 agonists:** Dulaglutide (Trulicity), semaglutide (Ozempic, Rybelsus), liraglutide (Victoza), exenatide (Byetta, Bydureon), and

---

TABLE 11 Examples of Insulin Regimens Used in Type 1 Diabetes

Intensive Insulin Regimens

Multiple Daily Injections

- Long-acting insulin given once daily, and rapid-acting insulin given at meals, snacks, and periodically to correct high blood sugars

Continuous Subcutaneous Insulin Infusion via Insulin Pump

- Rapid-acting insulin given at basal rate (rate can vary throughout the day) and as a bolus at meals, snacks, and as needed to correct high blood sugars
- Rapid-acting insulin given via pump according to automated insulin delivery algorithm and based on continuous glucose monitoring

Simplified Insulin Regimens

Multiple Daily Injections

- Long-acting insulin given once daily, NPH given at breakfast, and rapid-acting insulin given at breakfast and dinner (may be used when lunchtime insulin dosing is logistically difficult; lunch carbohydrate intake must be consistent)
- NPH given twice daily (breakfast and bedtime), and rapid-acting insulin given at meals
- NPH and rapid- or short-acting insulin given twice daily (breakfast and dinner)
- Premixed insulin (70/30, 75/25, 50/50) given twice daily (breakfast and dinner)

From Melmed S et al: *Williams textbook of endocrinology*, ed 14, Philadelphia, 2020, Elsevier.

TABLE 12 Clinical Features of Commonly Used Oral Antihyperglycemic Agents

Classes and Specific Agents (Commercial Names)	Commonly Used Dosages	Contraindications	Side Effects	%HbA$_{1c}$ Reduction as First or Second Therapy
Biguanide				
Metformin (Glucophage)	500-1000 mg bid	T1D, DKA eGFR <30	Nausea, diarrhea, abdominal pain	1-2
Metformin-ER	500-1000 mg bid	Severe cardiac, hepatic disease	Vitamin B$_{12}$ deficiency	
Secretagogue				
Glipizide (Glucotrol)	5-20 mg bid	T1D, DKA	Hypoglycemia	1-2
Glipizide-ER	2.5-10 mg daily		Weight gain	
Gliclazide (Diamicron)	80-160 bid			
Gliclazide-MR	30-120 daily			
Glimepiride (Amaryl)	0.5-4 mg daily			
Glyburide (Micronase et al)	2.5-10 mg bid			
Repaglinide (Prandin)	0.5-2 mg tid			
Nateglinide (Starlix)	60-120 mg tid			
Thiazolidinedione				
Pioglitazone (Actos)	15-30 mg daily	T1D, DKA	Weight gain	0.75-1.5
Rosiglitazone (Avandia)	4-8 mg daily	Symptomatic heart failure	Edema	
			Fractures	
DPP4 inhibitor[a]				
Sitagliptin (Januvia)	25-100 mg daily	T1D, DKA	Hypersensitivity	0.5-1
Vildagliptin (Galvus)	50 mg daily or bid			
Saxagliptin (Onglyza)	2.5-5 mg daily			
Linagliptin (Tradjenta)	5 mg daily			
Alogliptin (Nesina)	6.25-25 mg daily			
α-Glucosidase inhibitor[b]				
Acarbose (Precose)	25-50 mg tid	T1D, DKA	Flatulence, diarrhea, abdominal discomfort	0.5-1
Miglitol (Glyset)	25-50 mg tid			
SGLT inhibitor				
Canagliflozin (Invokana)	100-300 mg daily	T1D, DKA eGFR <30	Urinary frequency	0.5-1
Dapagliflozin (Farxiga)	5-10 mg daily		Urogenital infections	
Empagliflozin (Jardiance)	10-25 mg daily		Nausea, diarrhea	
Ertugliflozin (Steglatro)	5-15 mg daily		Hypotension	
Bile-acid sequestrant				
Colesevelam (Welchol)	Six 625-mg tabs daily	T1D, DKA	Constipation	0.5-1
		Pancreatitis, intestinal disease, hypertriglyceridemia		
Dopamine agonist				
Bromocriptine (Cycloset)	1.6-4.8 mg daily	T1D, DKA	Somnolence, dizziness, hypotension	0.5-1

bid, Twice daily; *DKA*, diabetic ketoacidosis; *eGFR*, estimated glomerular filtration rate; *ER*, extended release; *HbA$_{1c}$*, glycosylated hemoglobin; *MR*, modified release; *tid*, three times daily.
[a]The DPP4 inhibitors listed here are approved in the U.S. and/or the European Union. Other DPP4 inhibitors are available in certain countries, including anagliptin (Suiny), evogliptin (Suganon), gemigliptin (Zemiglo), gosogliptin (SatRx), omarigliptin (Marizev), teneligliptin (Tenelia), trelagliptin (Zafatek), and vildagliptin (Galvus).
[b]Acarbose and miglitol are available in the United States and the European Union. Voglibose (Basen et al) is available in other countries.
From Melmed S et al: *Williams textbook of endocrinology*, ed 14, Philadelphia, 2020, Elsevier.

lixisenatide (Adlyxin). These injectable agents are incretin mimetics that stimulate release of insulin from pancreatic beta cells and can be used as adjunctive therapy for patients with T2DM. GLP-1 agonists are not indicated in T1DM and are contraindicated in patients with severe renal impairment. Average A$_{1c}$ reduction is 1.0% to 2.0%. Advantages are weight loss, no hypoglycemia when used as monotherapy and reduced incidence of cardiovascular events and nephropathy. Side effects include injection site reactions, GI side effects (nausea, diarrhea, vomiting), increased risk of pancreatitis and thyroid C-cell carcinoma. Cost is a barrier to their use.
- **Dual GIP/GLP-1 agonists:** Tirzepatide (Mounjaro) is a novel, once weekly, injectable peptide with agonist activity at both the GIP and GLP-1 receptors. It increases insulin

secretion, decreases glucagon secretion, increases insulin sensitivity, delays gastric emptying, and reduces food intake. In randomized trials in patients with type 2 diabetes, tirzepatide reduced A$_{1c}$ and body weight more than semaglutide, insulin degludec (Tresiba), or insulin glargine (Lantus).[7] Average weight loss is 7 to 13 Kg. The most common side effects included GI adverse events (nausea, vomiting, diarrhea, abdominal pain). A$_{1c}$ reduction is 2.0% to 2.5%.
- **Sodium-glucose cotransporter 2 (SGLT$_2$) inhibitors:** Canagliflozin (Invokana), dapagliflozin (Farxiga), empagliflozin (Jardiance), and sotagliflozin (Zynquista). These medications decrease glucose reabsorption, increase urinary glucose excretion, and lower HbA$_{1c}$ 0.5% to 1.0%). Empagliflozin has been shown to slow progression of renal disease in type 2

diabetics with CVD. SGLT$_2$ inhibitors reduce the risk of hospitalization for heart failure or death from cardiovascular disease among patients with stable heart failure. Sotagliflozin therapy initiated before or shortly after discharge in patients with diabetes and recent worsening heart failure resulted in a significantly lower total number of deaths from cardiovascular causes and hospitalizations and urgent visits for heart failure vs. placebo in a recent trial.[8] Potential advantages include weight loss (up to 3.5% of BMI) and mild lowering of blood pressure (2 to 4 mm Hg). Side effects include increased risk of genital mycotic infections, urinary tract infections, and volume depletion. Renal function should be evaluated before starting SGLT$_2$ inhibitors and periodically thereafter. Temporary discontinuation of these meds is recommended in

TABLE 13 Clinical Features of Commonly Used Injectable Agents Other than Insulin

Types and Generic Names (Commercial Names)	Administration	Main Effects	Contraindications	Side Effects
Short-acting GLP1 agonist				
Exenatide (Byetta)	5-10 μg bid before breakfast and dinner	Postprandial glucose control and weight loss	T1D DKA	Nausea, diarrhea, abdominal pain
Lixisenatide (Adlyxin)	10-20 μg daily before breakfast		Pancreatitis History medullary carcinoma	Pancreatitis?
Long-acting GLP1 agonist				
Liraglutide (Victoza)	0.6-1.8 mg daily	Basal glucose control and weight loss	T1D	Nausea, diarrhea, abdominal pain
Dulaglutide (Trulicity)	0.75 or 1.5 mg weekly		DKA	
Extended-release exenatide (Bydureon)	2 mg weekly		Pancreatitis	Pancreatitis?
Semaglutide (Ozempic)	0.5 or 1 mg weekly		History medullary carcinoma	
Fixed-dose GLP1/insulin combination				
Liraglutide/degludec (Xultophy)	Daily, titrated	Glucose and weight control	T1D	Hypoglycemia
Lixisenatide/glargine (Soliqua)	Daily before breakfast, titrated		DKA Pancreatitis	Nausea, diarrhea, abdominal pain
			History medullary carcinoma	Pancreatitis?
Amylin agonist				
Pramlintide (Symlin)	tid before meals in T1D or T2D requiring prandial insulin	Postprandial glucose control and weight loss	Confirmed gastroparesis	Nausea Abdominal pain Hypoglycemia

DKA, Diabetic ketoacidosis.

From Melmed S et al: *Williams textbook of endocrinology,* ed 14, Philadelphia, 2020, Elsevier.

cases of reduced oral intake or fluid loss. Higher cost and limited drug formulary availability are limiting factors.

- **DPP-4 inhibitors:** Sitagliptin (Januvia), linagliptin (Tradjenta), saxagliptin (Onglyza), vildagliptin (Galvus and others), and alogliptin (Nesina, Vipidia). These medications raise blood incretin levels, thereby inhibiting glucagon release and lowering blood glucose levels. When used alone or with metformin, they do not cause hypoglycemia. They have modest efficacy (hemoglobin A_{1C} reductions of 0.5% to 1%, neutral effect on weight). Linagliptin does not require a dosage adjustment in renal insufficiency. Sitagliptin can be used in any degree of kidney disease but needs to be dosed based on GFR and creatinine levels.

- **Thiazolidinediones (pioglitazone and rosiglitazone)** increase insulin sensitivity and have been used in the therapy of type 2 diabetes. A_{1C} reduction is 1.0% to 1.5%. Serum transaminase levels should be obtained before starting therapy and monitored periodically. Thiazolidinediones, in general, result in moderate weight gain and increase the risk for heart failure and osteoporosis/fractures. Rosiglitazone has an FDA black box warning for heart failure exacerbations and myocardial ischemia. Pioglitazone and rosiglitazone cause increased incidence of bladder cancer. Use thiazolidinediones with caution with calcium channel blockers, especially amlodipine (can cause fluid retention and edema).

- **Acarbose and miglitol:** These agonists inhibit pancreatic amylase and small intestinal glucosidases, thereby delaying carbohydrate absorption in the gut and reducing associated postprandial hyperglycemia. The major side effects are flatulence, diarrhea, and abdominal cramps.

- **The meglitinides nateglinide and repaglinide and the bile acid sequestrant colesevelam** can also be used to lower glucose levels but are expensive and generally poorly tolerated.

- **Pramlintide** is a synthetic analog of human amylin, which is synthesized by pancreatic beta cells and cosecreted with insulin in response to food intake. It suppresses glucagon secretion and slows stomach emptying and can be used as an adjunctive treatment for patients with T1DM or T2DM who inject insulin at mealtime. Nausea is its major side effect. This therapy has been largely replaced with use of GLP-1 analogs.

- **Sulfonylureas:** Sulfonylureas interact with ATP-sensitive potassium channels in the beta-cell membrane to increase insulin secretion and work best when given before meals. They reduce A_{1C} by 1.0% to 1.5%. All sulfonylureas are contraindicated in patients who are allergic to sulfa. Use of sulfonylureas confers a greater risk of hypoglycemia than the other agents. Preferred agents in this class are glimepiride and glipizide. Sulfonylureas are now being considered for use as last or later resort or when cost is of major concern for the patient and when other therapies cannot be incorporated or are contraindicated.

- Combination therapy of various hypoglycemic agents is commonly used when dual therapy results in inadequate glycemic control.

1. **Insulin** is indicated for the treatment of all T1DM and for T2DM patients whose condition cannot be adequately controlled with diet and oral agents. The American College of Endocrinology and the American Association of Clinical Endocrinologists recommend initiation of insulin therapy in patients with type 2 diabetes and an initial HbA_{1C} level >9%, or if the diabetes is uncontrolled despite optimal oral glycemic therapy. Insulin therapy may be initiated as augmentation, starting at 0.1 to 0.2 unit/kg of body weight, or as replacement, starting at 0.6 to 1.0 unit/kg. Tables 14 and 15 summarize onset, peak, and duration of action of currently available insulin preparations. The risks of insulin therapy include weight gain, hypoglycemia, and in rare cases, allergic or cutaneous reactions.

2. Replacement insulin therapy should mimic normal release patterns.
   a. Approximately 50% to 60% of daily insulin can be given as a long-acting insulin (NPH, Ultralente, glargine, detemir) injected once or twice daily.
   b. The remaining 40% to 50% can be short-acting (regular) or rapid-acting (lispro, aspart, glulisine) to cover mealtime carbohydrates and correct increased current glucose levels.
   c. NPH and older basal insulins can be mixed with rapid-acting insulins like Humalog and regular; all newer basal insulins cannot be mixed in one syringe.
   d. Basal-bolus regimens are now preferred on injection of long-acting basal at bedtime or in AM to target fasting glycemia between 80 and 130, and rapid-acting mealtime insulins to target lower postprandial blood glucose <140 mg/dl.
   e. New combinations of basal insulins with GLP-1 analogs are now available:
      (1) Soliqua: Combines glargine insulin and lixisenatide in one pen. Patients

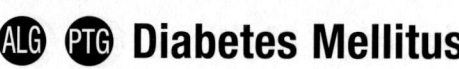

TABLE 14 Insulin Types and Action Profiles

Product	Onset of Action	Peak Action	Duration	
Rapid acting	Aspart (*Novolog* [Novo Nordisk, Princeton, NJ]) Lispro (*Humalog U-100* [Eli Lilly, Indianapolis, IN], *Humalog U-200* [Eli Lilly, Indianapolis, IN], *Admelog* [Sanofi, Bridgewater, NJ]) Glulisine (*Apidra* [Sanofi, Bridgewater, NJ])	10-30 min	30-180 min	3-5 h
	Aspart (*Fiasp* [Novo Nordisk, Princeton, NJ])	2.5 min	40-50 min	
	Insulin human (*Afrezza* [MannKind, Westlake Village, CA]) inhalation powder	12 min	35-45 min	1.5-3 h
Short acting	Regular U-100 (*Humulin R U-100* [Eli Lilly, Indianapolis, IN]) Regular U-100 (*Novolin R* [Novo Nordisk, Princeton, NJ]) Regular U-500 (*Humulin U-500*)	30-60 min	2-4 h	U-100: Up to 10 h U-500: Up to 24 h
Intermediate acting	NPH (*Humulin N*) NPH (*Novolin N*)	2-4 h	4-8 h	12-18 h
Long acting	Detemir (*Levemir* [Novo Nordisk, Princeton, NJ]) Glargine (*Lantus* [Sanofi, Bridgewater, NJ], *Basaglar* [Eli Lilly, Indianapolis, IN], Toujeo U-300 [Sanofi, Bridgewater, NJ]) Degludec (*Tresiba U-100* [Novo Nordisk, Princeton, NJ], *Tresiba U-200*)	2-4 h	Minimal	Detemir: 12-24 h Glargine: Up to 24 h Degludec: Up to 48 h
Premixed	70/30 (NPH/Aspart) (*Novolog 70/30*) 70/30 NPH/Regular (*Humulin 70/30*) 75/25 (NPH/Lispro) (*Humalog 75/25*) 50/50 (NPH/Lispro) (*Humalog 50/50*) [Other combinations may be available in Europe.]	5-60 min	Dual	12-18 h

---

TABLE 15 Clinical Features of Commonly Used Insulins

Types and Generic Names (Commercial Names)	Onset of Action (min)	Time to Peak (h)	Duration (h)	Administration
Rapid Acting				
Aspart (Fiasp)	<5	0.5-1.5	3-5	Just before or just after meals
Aspart (Novolog)	10-20	0.5-1.5	3-5	0-15 min before or just after meals
Lispro (Humalog)	10-20	0.5-1.5	3-5	
Glulisine (Apidra)	10-20	0.5-1.5	3-5	
Short Acting				
Regular human (Humulin R, Novolin R)	30-45	2-4	4-8	15-30 min before meals
Intermediate Acting				
NPH (Humulin N, Novolin N)	60-120	4-8	12-20	Once or twice daily
Long Acting				
Detemir (Levemir)	60-120	6-10	16-24	Usually once daily
Glargine (Lantus, Basaglar)	60-120	No pronounced peak	~24	
Degludec (Tresiba)	60-120	No pronounced peak	Up to 72	
Premixed				
70/30 NPH/R (Humulin 70/30, Novolin 70/30)	30-40	4-8	12-20	Usually twice daily, 0-30 min before meals
75/25 Protamine-lispro/lispro (Humalog Mix 70/30)	10-20	4-8	12-20	
70/30 Protamine-aspart/aspart (Novolog Mix 70/30)	10-20	4-8	12-20	
50/50 Protamine-lispro/lispro (Humalog Mix 50/50)	10-20	4-8	12-20	
50/50 Protamine-aspart/aspart (Novolog Mix 50/50)	15-60	4-8	12-20	
Concentrated				
U-500 Human regular (Humulin U-500)	30-45	6-12	12-24	Twice daily
U-200 Degludec (Tresiba U-200)	60-120	No pronounced peak	>24	Once daily
U-300 Glargine (Toujeo 300 U/ml)	60-120	No pronounced peak	Up to 72	Once daily

From Melmed S et al: *Williams textbook of endocrinology*, ed 14, Philadelphia, 2020, Elsevier.

---

taking <30 units start at 15 units and patient taking >30 units start at 30 units and are titrated every 3 to 4 days until fasting blood glucose levels are between 80 and 130 mg/dl. One should not exceed 60 units of glargine insulin.

(2) Xultophy 100/3.6 is degludec insulin and liraglutide combination in one pen. Dosing is based on Tresiba dose. Patients start at 16 units and increase by 2 units every 5 to 7 days to target fasting glycemia between 80 and 130 mg/dl, and dose cannot exceed 50 units. The use of this combination may eliminate or reduce prandial insulin needs and limits weight gain caused by insulin.

- Continuous subcutaneous insulin infusion (CSII, or insulin pump [see Fig. E8]) provides

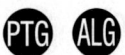
comparable or slightly better control than multiple daily injections. It should be considered for diabetes presenting in childhood or adolescence and during pregnancy. The guidelines for insulin pump therapy from the American Association of Diabetes Educators include "frequent and unpredictable fluctuations in blood glucose" and "patient perceptions that diabetes management impedes the pursuit of personal or professional goals." Use of insulin pumps are today coupled with CGM monitoring and with software in which the computer is making the automatic adjustments to glucose levels, constituting what is referred to as an "artificial pancreas." This allows for fewer fluctuations of glycemia. Newer hybrid closed-loop systems combine an insulin pump, a continuous glucose monitoring device, and control algorithms that automate insulin delivery to maintain glucose levels within predetermined ranges and avoid hypoglycemia or hyperglycemia.[1]

- Antiplatelet therapy: Low-dose aspirin (ASA; 81 mg/day) has been proven to lower the risk of subsequent myocardial infarction, stroke, or vascular death in secondary prevention studies. The ADA recommends low-dose aspirin for primary prevention in diabetic patients with one additional cardiovascular risk factor, including age older than 50 yr, cigarette smoking, hypertension, obesity, albuminuria, hyperlipidemia, and family history of coronary artery disease. Clopidogrel can be used in patients with atherosclerotic cardiovascular disease (ASCVD) and a documented aspirin allergy. The ADA does not recommend aspirin therapy in diabetics younger than 50 yr of age at low risk for coronary artery disease.
- Lipid management: Measure fasting lipid profile at least annually in adults.
  1. All patients with diabetes with one or more additional risk factors for CVD should be on statin therapy together with lifestyle modification regardless of baseline lipid levels.
  2. Diabetic patients aged 40 to 75 with LDL cholesterol of 70 to 189 mg/dl and without clinical ASCVD should receive at least moderate-intensity statin therapy and consider high-intensity statin therapy if 10-yr ASCVD risk is ≥7.5%.
  3. Ezetimibe can be added to moderate-intensity statin therapy in those who cannot tolerate high-intensity statin therapy.
  4. Combination therapy with statin and fenofibrate is not recommended but may be considered in those with triglyceride levels equal or greater than 204 mg/dl. If triglycerides are not at goal with combination of statin and fibrate, then prescription fish oil is advised if triglyceride levels still exceed 300 mg/dl.
  5. PCK-9 inhibitors may be considered in diabetics with CAD risk when statins are insufficient and in those who cannot tolerate statins, have had cardiovascular events, and cannot achieve A_{1c} to target goal.
- Hypertension: Antihypertensive therapy is recommended to keep systolic blood pressure

(BP) <140 and diastolic BP <90 mm Hg. Use of ACE inhibitors or angiotensin receptor blockers (ARBs) to decrease albuminuria and for prevention of progression of kidney disease should be considered regardless of presence of hypertension. Combination therapy with an ACE inhibitor and an ARB should be avoided due to increased risk of adverse effects among patients with diabetic nephropathy. In older adults a treatment goal of <130/70 mm Hg is not recommended due to higher mortality and morbidity.

- Bariatric surgery should be considered in adults with BMI >35 kg/m² and type 2 diabetes, especially if the diabetes is difficult to control with lifestyle and pharmacologic therapy. Five-yr outcome data showed that, among patients with type 2 DM and a BMR of 27 to 43, bariatric surgery plus intensive medical therapy was more effective than intensive medical therapy alone in decreasing, or in some cases resolving, hyperglycemia.[9]
- Hypoglycemia—a plasma glucose concentration low enough to cause symptoms or signs—is a rare occurrence in individuals without diabetes but is common in sulfonylurea-, glinide-, or insulin-treated diabetes.
- The plasma glucose concentration is normally maintained in a relatively narrow range, 72 to 144 mg/dl (4.0 to 8.0 mmol/L), owing to a fine balance between glucose influx (exogenous glucose delivery and endogenous glucose production) and glucose efflux (glucose utilization by insulin-sensitive tissues, such as the skeletal muscle, and insulin-insensitive tissues, particularly the brain).
- A classification of hypoglycemia in diabetics is shown in Table 16. Hypoglycemia results from an imbalance between glucose influx and glucose efflux due to either excessive glucose removal from the circulation, deficient glucose delivery into the circulation, or both.
- Hypoglycemia in diabetes is typically the result of the interplay of therapeutic hyperinsulinemia and compromised defenses against falling

glucose levels resulting in hypoglycemia-associated autonomic failure (HAAF), including defective glucose counterregulation and impaired awareness of hypoglycemia (Fig. E10).

- An attenuated sympathoadrenal response to falling glucose levels, the key feature of HAAF, is induced by recent antecedent hypoglycemia, sleep, or prior exercise, and is reversible by short-term scrupulous avoidance of hypoglycemia.
- Iatrogenic hypoglycemia is associated with both morbidity and fatality in type 1 and type 2 diabetes mellitus. Risk factors for hypoglycemia are summarized in Table 17. Treat hypoglycemia in a conscious person with glucose tab or gel 15 to 20 g and intramuscular injection of glucagon if unconscious. Patient and family members should be instructed on the administration of glucagon for individuals at significant risk for severe hypoglycemia. A sick day management protocol for diabetic patients is described in Box 3.

DISPOSITION

- Diabetic retinopathy occurs in nearly 15% of patients with diabetes after 15 yr of diagnosis and increases 1%/yr after diagnosis. Glycemic, lipid, and blood pressure controls are essential to reduce the risk and progression of diabetic retinopathy. An annual comprehensive eye exam by an ophthalmologist or optometrist should begin at the time of diagnosis for those with T2DM and after 5 yr in those with T1DM. Retinal laser photocoagulation and vitrectomy are effective treatment modalities. Prevention is best accomplished by strict glucose and BP control. Early blockade of the renin-angiotensin system has been shown to slow progression of retinopathy in patients with type 1 diabetes.
- The frequency of neuropathy in patients with type 2 diabetes approaches 70% to 80%. It can be subdivided into sensorimotor neuropathy and autonomic neuropathy. Duloxetine, a selective serotonin and norepinephrine reuptake inhibitor, is effective and FDA approved

TABLE 16 Classification of Hypoglycemia in Diabetes

Clinical Classification	Definition
Severe hypoglycemia	An event requiring the assistance of another person to actively administer carbohydrate, glucagon, or other resuscitative actions. Plasma glucose measurements may not be available during such an event, but neurologic recovery attributable to the restoration of plasma glucose to a normal level is considered sufficient evidence that the event was induced by a low plasma glucose concentration.
Documented symptomatic hypoglycemia	An event during which typical symptoms of hypoglycemia are accompanied by a measured plasma glucose concentration of ≤70 mg/dl (3.9 mmol/L).
Asymptomatic hypoglycemia	An event not accompanied by typical symptoms of hypoglycemia but with a measured plasma glucose concentration of ≤70 mg/dl (3.9 mmol/L).
Probable symptomatic hypoglycemia	An event during which symptoms typical of hypoglycemia are not accompanied by a plasma glucose determination but were presumably caused by a plasma glucose concentration of ≤70 mg/dl (3.9 mmol/L).
Pseudohypoglycemia	An event during which the person with diabetes reports any of the typical symptoms of hypoglycemia and interprets those as indicative of hypoglycemia, with a measured plasma glucose concentration that is >70 mg/dl (3.9 mmol/L) but is approaching that level.

From Melmed S et al: *Williams textbook of endocrinology*, ed 14, Philadelphia, 2020, Elsevier.

TABLE 17 Risk Factors for Hypoglycemia in Diabetes

Conventional Risk Factors: Absolute or Relative Insulin Excess

Insulin or insulin secretagogue doses are excessive, ill timed, or of the wrong type.
Exogenous glucose delivery is decreased (e.g., after missed meals, during the overnight fast).
Glucose utilization is increased (e.g., during exercise).
Endogenous glucose production is decreased (e.g., after alcohol ingestion).
Sensitivity to insulin is increased (e.g., after weight loss, with improved fitness or improved glycemic control, in the middle of the night).
Insulin clearance is decreased (e.g., with renal failure).

Risk Factors for Hypoglycemia-Associated Autonomic Failure

Absolute endogenous insulin deficiency.
A history of severe hypoglycemia, impaired awareness of hypoglycemia, or both, and recent antecedent hypoglycemia, prior exercise, or sleep.
Aggressive glycemic therapy per se (lower HbA$_{1C}$ levels, lower glycemic goals, or both).

HbA$_{1C}$, Glycosylated hemoglobin.
From Melmed S et al: *Williams textbook of endocrinology,* ed 14, Philadelphia, 2020, Elsevier.

BOX 3 Sick Day Management Protocol for Diabetic Patients

Examples of "Sick Day" Scenarios
- Feeling sick or presence of fever for 2 days or longer without getting better
- Vomiting or diarrhea for more than 6 h

Management
General Measures
- Check blood sugar levels at least every 4 h, but when values are changing quickly, check more often.
- Check urine or blood ketones.
- Modify usual insulin regimen according to a plan developed by the diabetes physician or team.
- Maintain adequate food and fluid intake. If your appetite is poor, aim for consumption of 50 g of carbohydrate every 3-4 h. If you are nauseous, high-carbohydrate liquids, such as regular (not diet) soft drinks or juice, or frozen juice bars, sherbet, pudding, creamed soups, or fruit-flavored yogurt usually are tolerated. Broth also is a good alternative.

Taking Medications When You Are Sick
- If you are eating: Continue taking your pills for diabetes or your insulin. Your blood sugar may continue to rise because of your illness.
- If you are nauseous or vomiting or otherwise cannot take your medicines:
  1. Continue to take your long-acting insulin (Lantus, Levemir, NPH).
  2. Call your doctor and discuss whether you need to adjust your short- or rapid-acting insulin dose (regular, lispro [Humalog], aspart [Novolog], glulisine [Apidra]) or your other diabetes medicines.

Examples of When to Call Physician or Diabetes Team
- If glucose levels are higher than 240 mg/dl despite taking extra insulin according to a sick day plan
- If you take diabetes pills and blood sugar is still above 240 mg/dl before meals and remains there for more than 24 h
- If symptoms/signs develop that might signal diabetic ketoacidosis or dehydration, such as dizziness, trouble breathing, fruity breath, or dry and cracked lips or tongue

From Parrillo JE, Dellinger RP: *Critical care medicine: principles of diagnosis and management in the adult,* ed 5, Philadelphia, 2019, Elsevier.

for relief of diabetic peripheral neuropathy. Pregabalin and gabapentin (900 to 3600 mg/day) are also effective for the symptomatic treatment of peripheral neuropathic pain. Topical capsaicin, 5% lidocaine transdermal patches, amitriptyline, and carbamazepine are also modestly effective. Use of high-dose vitamin combination of B$_{12}$, B$_6$ with alpha lipoic acid may help with nerve preservation and worsening of neuropathy, but will have no immediate effect on pain.
- Diabetic gastroparesis is most often seen in patients who have had diabetes for at least 10 yr and typically have retinopathy, neurop-

athy, and nephropathy. Major manifestations are postprandial fullness, nausea, vomiting, and bloating. Pharmacologic therapy involves prokinetic agents (metoclopramide). Endoscopic injection of botulinum toxin into the pylorus and gastric electrical stimulation (using electrodes placed laparoscopically in the muscle wall of the stomach antrum and connected to a neurostimulator) represent newer approaches to nonpharmacologic therapy.
- Nephropathy: The first sign of renal involvement in patients with DM is most often microalbuminuria, which is classified as incipient nephropathy. Before the current period of

intensive glycemic control and blood pressure with ACE inhibitors and angiotensin receptor blockade, it was suggested that 25% to 45% of diabetic patients would develop clinically evident renal disease (proteinuria) and 4% to 17% would progress to end-stage renal disease. In the current era of intensive glycemic and blood pressure control and ACE/ARB use, clinically evident diabetic nephropathy has declined to 9% and end-stage renal disease 2% to 7%. Use of ACE inhibitor or ARB is not recommended in diabetics with normal blood pressure, no microalbuminuria (urine albumin to creatinine ratio less than 30 mg/g creatinine) and normal renal function (eGFR >60 ml/min/1.73 m^2).
- Infections are generally more common in patients with diabetes because of multiple factors, such as impaired leukocyte function, decreased tissue perfusion secondary to vascular disease, repeated trauma because of loss of sensation, and urinary retention secondary to neuropathy.
- Prevention/delay of type 2 diabetes: Fewer than 10% of older adults with prediabetes progress to diabetes in 6.5 yr.[10] Patients with prediabetes should achieve weight loss of 5% to 10% of body weight and increase physical activity to at least 150 min/wk of moderate activity such as walking. Metformin therapy may be considered in those at high risk, especially if they have hyperglycemia (HbA$_{1C}$ ≥6) despite lifestyle interventions.
- The Mediterranean diet has been shown to prevent type 2 diabetes in patients with prediabetes and can delay the need of insulin use in type 2 diabetes in up to 50% of patients.
- Use of metformin in prediabetics can prevent onset of diabetes in up to 30% of patients, independent of diet.

REFERRAL
- Patients with diabetes should be advised to have annual ophthalmologic examinations. In T1DM, ophthalmologic visits should usually begin 5 yr after diagnosis, whereas T2DM patients should be seen from disease onset. Fig. 11 illustrates a flow chart useful in determining the timing of initial ophthalmic examination after a diagnosis of diabetes mellitus.
- Podiatric care can significantly reduce the rate of foot infections and amputations in patients with DM. Noninfected neuropathic foot ulcers require debridement and reduction of pressure.
- Nephrology consultation in all cases of proteinuria, hyperkalemia, uncontrolled BP, and when GFR has decreased to <30 ml/min/1.73 m^2.

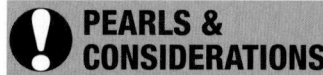 **PEARLS & CONSIDERATIONS**

COMMENTS
- Because normalization of serum glucose level is the ultimate goal, every patient with diabetes should measure his or her blood glucose with commercially available glucometers unless contraindicated by senility or blindness.

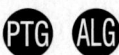

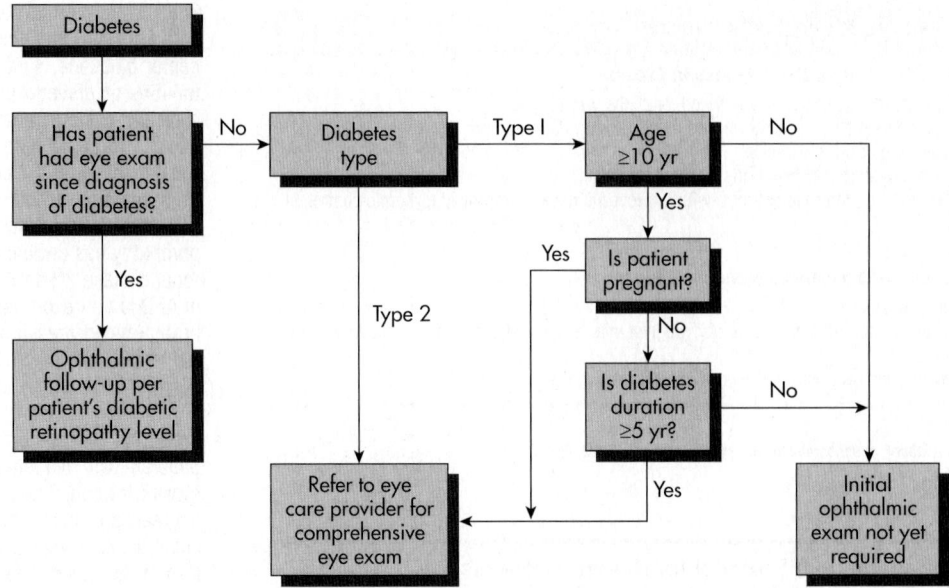

FIG. 11 Schematic flow chart of major principles involved in determining the timing of initial ophthalmic examination after a diagnosis of diabetes mellitus. These are minimal recommended times. Ocular symptoms, complaints, or other associated medical issues can necessitate earlier evaluation. Guidelines are regularly reevaluated based on new study results. (From Melmed S et al: *Williams textbook of endocrinology*, ed 14, Philadelphia, 2020, Elsevier.)

- Continuous glucose monitoring is now commercially available for all types of diabetics on multiple daily injections of insulin. The advantage of CGM is that it not only gives a patient a value, but it shows a rate of change at that moment and predicts impending hyperglycemia or hypoglycemia, allowing a patient to react appropriately. Among patients with poorly controlled type 2 DM treated with basal insulin without prandial insulin, CGM, as compared with blood glucose meter monitoring results in significantly lower HbA$_{1c}$ levels.[10]
- Underinsured children and those with psychiatric illness are at greater risk for acute complications in T1DM and require frequent monitoring and aggressive risk management with diet, exercise, and periodic laboratory evaluation.
- Significant sustained weight loss using bariatric surgery has been reported as effective in achieving remission of type 2 diabetes in morbidly obese patients. Bariatric surgery may be considered for adults with BMI >35 kg/m^2 and T2DM, especially if diabetes or associated comorbidities are difficult to control with lifestyle and pharmacologic therapy.
- Cigarette smoking predicts incident type 2 diabetes. For a smoker at risk for diabetes, smoking cessation should be coupled with strategies for diabetes prevention and early detection.
- Glycemic control in hospitalized patients: The American College of Physicians (ACP) recommends against using intensive insulin therapy to strictly control blood glucose in nonsurgical intensive care unit (SICU)/medical intensive care unit (MICU) in patients with or without DM. The ACP recommends a target blood glucose level of 130 to 180 mg/dl if insulin therapy is used.
- Studies have shown that tight glycemic control in SICU patients can reduce infection rates and ICU stay. This was not seen in MICU patients. However, there is evidence showing that patients using continuous intravenous insulin infusions to keep tight glycemic control after open heart surgery reduces sternal wound infection rates.
- Having diabetes for longer than 10 yr is associated with doubled risk for dementia at age 70.[10]

REFERENCES

Available at eBooks.Health.Elsevier.com.

RELATED CONTENT

Diabetes Mellitus Type 1 (Patient Information)
Diabetes Mellitus Type 2 (Patient Information)
Diabetic Foot (Related Key Topic)
Diabetic Gastroparesis (Related Key Topic)
Diabetic Ketoacidosis (Related Key Topic)
Diabetic Polyneuropathy (Related Key Topic)
Diabetic Retinopathy (Related Key Topic)
Gestational Diabetes Mellitus (Related Key Topic)
Hyperglycemic Hyperosmolar Syndrome (Related Key Topic)

AUTHORS: **FRANK B. D'ALESSANDRO, MD** and **FRED F. FERRI, MD**

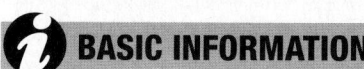
Diseases
and Disorders

I

BASIC INFORMATION

DEFINITION

Diabetic foot infections (DFIs) are a common and potentially serious problem in persons with diabetes. They usually arise from either a skin ulceration that occurs secondarily to peripheral neuropathy or in a wound caused by some form of trauma. The infection usually involves one or more bacteria and can spread to contiguous tissues including bone, causing an osteomyelitis.

SYNONYMS

Diabetic foot ulcer
Diabetic foot infection
DFI

ICD-10CM CODES
E11.621	Type 2 diabetes mellitus with foot ulcer
E10.5	Diabetes mellitus with peripheral circulatory complications
E10.6D	Diabetes mellitus with other specific complications

EPIDEMIOLOGY & DEMOGRAPHICS

INCIDENCE: DFIs are the most common cause of hospitalizations for diabetic patients. They account for 20% of all hospital admissions. Nearly one in six patients will die within 1 yr of their infection.

PREVALENCE: The lifetime risk of developing a foot ulcer in patients with diabetes is 34%,[1] and more than 50% of wounds become infected.[7] In fact, the most common diabetes-related complication leading to hospitalization and lower limb amputation is diabetic foot infection.[2-4] Indeed, seconds count, as every 1.2 sec someone develops a diabetic foot ulcer (DFU), every 7 sec around the world someone dies from diabetes, and every 20 sec an amputation is performed.[5]

PREDOMINANT SEX & AGE: Females greater than males.

PEAK INCIDENCE: More common in Hispanics, African Americans, and Native Americans due to increased rates of diabetes in those populations.

RISK FACTORS:
- Diabetes greater than 10 yr
- Poor glucose control
- Peripheral neuropathy: Altered protective sensation and altered pain response
- Diabetic angiopathy: Atherosclerotic obstruction of larger vessels leading to peripheral vascular disease
- Evidence of increased local pressure: Callus or erythema

PHYSICAL FINDINGS & CLINICAL PRESENTATION

- Based on guidelines by Infectious Diseases Society of America, infection is present if obvious purulent drainage and/or the presence of two or more signs of inflammation:
  1. Erythema
  2. Pain
  3. Tenderness
  4. Warmth
  5. Induration
- Systemic signs of infection include:
  1. Anorexia, nausea/vomiting
  2. Fever, chills, night sweats
  3. Change in mental status and recent worsening of glycemic control
- An earlier and commonly used classification system was originally proposed by Wagner (Table 1).
- An update to the Wagner system was introduced at the University of Texas (UT), San Antonio (Table 2), U.S. While similar to Wagner in its first three categories, this later system eliminated grades 4 and 5 and added stages A-D for each of the grades. The UT system was the first diabetic foot ulcer classification to be validated. UT system grades:
- Grade 0: Pre- or postulcerative (Stages A to D)
- Grade 1: Full-thickness ulcer not involving tendon, capsule, or bone (Stages A to D)
- Grade 2: Tendon or capsular involvement without bone palpable (Stages A to D)
- Grade 3: Probes to bone (Stages A to D)
- Stage:
  1. A: Noninfected
  2. B: Infected
  3. C: Ischemic
  4. D: Infected and ischemic

ETIOLOGY

- Neuropathy plays an important role in the development of bone and joint abnormalities in patients with diabetes. These deformities lead to biomechanical changes and the formation of high-pressure areas, which increases the risk of ulceration (Fig. 1). Furthermore, changes in foot biomechanics, combined with limited joint mobility, may result in structural deformities, including hallux abducto valgus, claw- and hammertoes, and abnormalities of the metatarsophalangeal joints. Patients with hammertoes are vulnerable to even minor shoe trauma, and contracted toes cause increased retrograde pressure along the plantar metatarsals. In addition, irregular osseous changes and midfoot collapse owing to Charcot neuroarthropathy, as well as severe flatfoot, equinus, and other knee or back problems, may contribute to increased biomechanical stress encountered by the foot, worsen the degree of ulceration, and/or inhibit proper healing.[6,7]
- Most diabetic foot infections are polymicrobial (can involve five to seven different bacteria) and depend on the extent of involvement.
- Superficial infections are likely due to gram-positive skin bacteria:
  1. *Staphylococcus aureus,* includes methicillin-resistant *S. aureus* (MRSA)
  2. *Streptococcus agalactiae* (group B streptococcus) and *Streptococcus pyogenes* (group A streptococcus)
  3. Coagulase-negative *Staphylococcus*
- Infections that are deep, chronically infected, or previously treated are likely to be polymicrobial:
  1. Include above bacteria plus enterococci, gram-negative rods including *Pseudomonas aeruginosa* and anaerobes
  2. With gangrene, can expect more anaerobic bacteria such as *Clostridia* and *Bacteroides* species
  3. Patients with multiple admissions can have more resistant bacteria such as extended-spectrum beta-lactamase (ESBL)-type

TABLE 1 Wagner Diabetic Foot Ulcer Classification System

Grade	Description
0	No ulcer, but high-risk foot (e.g., deformity, callus, insensitivity)
1	Superficial full-thickness ulcer
2	Deeper ulcer, penetrating tendons, no bone involvement
3	Deeper ulcer with bone involvement, osteitis
4	Partial gangrene (e.g., toes, forefoot)
5	Gangrene of whole foot

Modified from Oyibo S et al: A comparison of two diabetic foot ulcer classification systems: the Wagner and the University of Texas wound classification systems, *Diabetes Care* 24:84-88, 2001. In Melmed S et al: *Williams textbook of endocrinology,* ed 14, Philadelphia, 2020, Elsevier.

TABLE 2 University of Texas Wound Classification System

Stage	Grade 0	Grade 1	Grade 2	Grade 3
A	Preulcer or postulcer lesion; no skin break	Superficial ulcer	Deep ulcer to tendon or capsule	Wound penetrating bone or joint
B	+ Infection	+ Infection	+ Infection	+ Infection
C	+ Ischemia	+ Ischemia	+ Ischemia	+ Ischemia
D	+ Infection and ischemia	+ Infection and ischemia	+ Infection and ischemia	+ Infection and ischemia

Modified from Armstrong DG et al: Validation of a diabetic wound classification system. The contribution of depth, infection, and ischemia to risk of amputation, *Diabetes Care* 12:855-859, 1998. In Melmed S et al: *Williams textbook of endocrinology,* ed 14, Philadelphia, 2020, Elsevier.

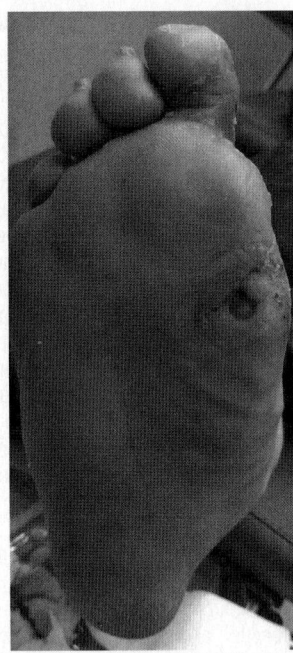

FIG. 1 Bone and joint abnormalities in the diabetic foot can result in the formation of high-pressure areas, increasing the risk of ulceration. (From Robertson RP et al: *DeGroot's endocrinology, basic science and clinical practice*, ed 8, Philadelphia, 2023, Elsevier.)

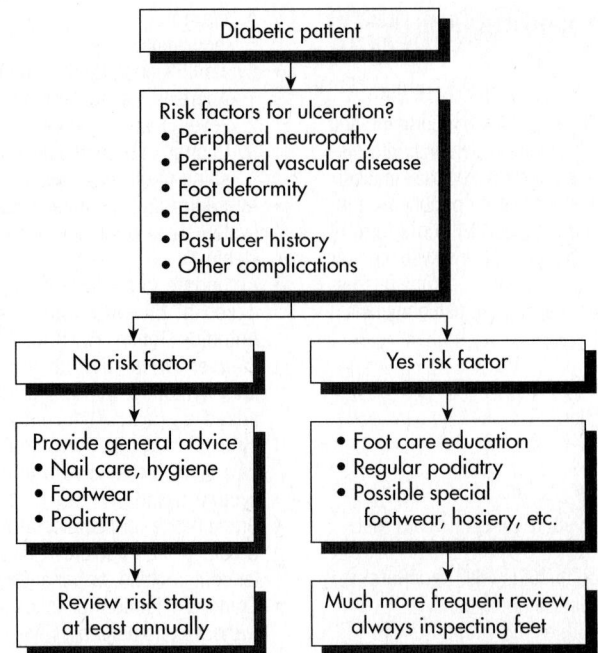

FIG. 2 Simple algorithm for risk screening in the diabetic foot. (From Melmed S et al: *Williams textbook of endocrinology*, ed 14, Philadelphia, 2020, Elsevier.)

resistant gram-negative rod bacteria, MRSA, and *Acinetobacter*

Dx DIAGNOSIS

DIFFERENTIAL DIAGNOSIS

Other inflammatory conditions that can mimic diabetic foot infections include:
- Crystal-associated arthritis such as gout
- Trauma
- Acute Charcot arthropathy from long-standing diabetes
- Venous stasis ulcers
- Deep vein thrombosis

WORKUP

Evaluation of a patient with a DFI involves determining the extent and severity of the infection, identifying the underlying factors that predispose to the infection, and determining the microbiologic etiology. An algorithm for risk screening in the diabetic foot is illustrated in Fig. 2.

PHYSICAL EXAMINATION

- Vital signs: Fever, chills, hypotension, tachycardia can be present.
- Detailed wound description: Length, width, and depth of wound, consistency of drainage, character of wound base: Granular fibrous necrotic.
- Determination of osteomyelitis: Highly likely if bone visible. A positive probe test to bone has a sensitivity of 66% and specificity of 85% in diagnosing bone infection.
- Necrotizing infections may present with cutaneous bullae, soft tissue gas, foul odor, and skin discoloration (Fig. E3).

- Severe infections may present with gangrene (Fig. E4), tissue necrosis, and evidence of tissue ischemia (Fig. E5), all of which may be limb threatening.

LABORATORY TESTS

Important to obtain at baseline and to assess response to therapy:
- Fewer than 50% of patients have an elevated white blood count.
- Determine blood urea nitrogen/creatinine (BUN/Cr), acidosis, hemoglobin A_{1c}, and blood sugar.
- Acute phase reactants: Sed rate and C-reactive protein (CRP) are markers for inflammation.
- Sed rate >70 increases probability of bone infection.
- Serum prealbumin and albumin are markers for nutritional status and ability to heal.
- An ulcer size larger than 2 cm^2 is indicative of osteomyelitis.
- Gram stains and cultures: Superficial cultures should not be obtained as they may contain colonizing bacteria; instead deep tissue cultures (aerobic and anaerobic) should be obtained.

IMAGING STUDIES

- Plain film x-ray evaluates bones and soft tissues and can detect presence of tissue gas, which would represent an emergent situation (Fig. 6).
- Osteomyelitis appears as radiolucencies, periosteal reaction, and destructive changes. Plain films are 67% specific and 60% sensitive for osteomyelitis.
- Bone scan: Indium-111 or technetium-99 can distinguish acute and chronic infections.
- Computed tomography and MRI: MRI is the most sensitive and specific test to detect osteomyelitis and abscess formation.

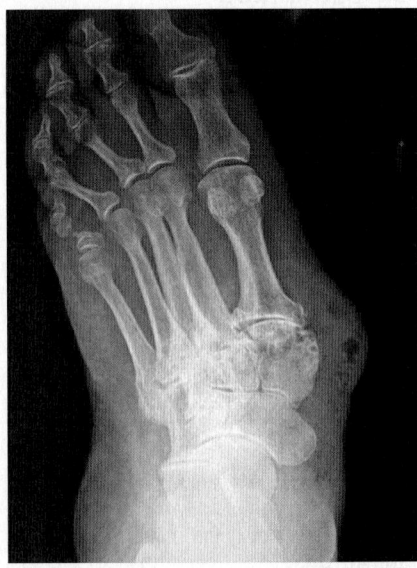

FIG. 6 X-ray. Significant soft tissue swelling in midfoot with numerous gas bubbles seen in the soft tissues.

OTHER DIAGNOSTIC TESTS

- Annual noninvasive vascular studies: Ankle brachial index (ABI): <0.90 or >1.30 indicates peripheral arterial disease
- Transcutaneous oxygen (TcPO2) tension measurements: Predictive of wound healing failure at levels below 25 mm Hg

Rx TREATMENT

Empiric antibiotic regimen should be started based on likely pathogens suspected and severity of disease. Wound management and debridement including surgical consultation are important as well.

NONPHARMACOLOGIC THERAPY

- Good nutrition will promote wound healing.
- Glycemic control will promote healing.
- Fluid and electrolyte balance will improve healing.

ACUTE GENERAL TREATMENT

WOUND MANAGEMENT:

- Debridement of callus and necrotic tissues by wound care specialist or surgeon and at times may require multiple debridements.
- Wound dressing: To absorb exudates and promote healing. Many products are available, but none has been proven superior and include:
  1. Enzymes
  2. Gels
  3. Hydrocolloids
  4. Antiseptics containing iodine or silver salts
  5. Honey
- Relieve pressure on the foot: Casts or special shoes.
- Amputation or revascularization procedures such as angioplasty or bypass grafting may be necessary.

ANTIBIOTIC MANAGEMENT:

- Prior to receiving culture results an empiric antibiotic regimen should be started as soon as possible to cover skin bacteria, gram-negative rods, and anaerobes. Options for intravenous (IV) therapy include:
  1. Piperacillin-tazobactam: 3.375 g IV q6h with normal kidney function. Will cover gram-negative rods including *Pseudomonas aeruginosa,* streptococci, anaerobes, and *Staphylococcus aureus.* Adjust dose based on CrCl.
  2. Meropenem: 1 g IV q8h with normal kidney function has comparable coverage as piperacillin-tazobactam. Similar agents include imipenem and doripenem.
  3. Third-generation cephalosporin such as cefepime, 2 g IV q8h, or ceftriaxone, 2 g IV qd, have excellent gram-negative coverage, and for anaerobic coverage add metronidazole, 500 mg IV q8h, or clindamycin 900 mg IV q8h. Cefepime will cover *Pseudomonas aeruginosa,* but ceftriaxone will not.
  4. For penicillin-allergic patients a combination of ciprofloxacin, 400 mg IV q12h, plus metronidazole or clindamycin is an option.

Aztreonam is another option for gram-negative rod coverage, 2 g IV q8h.

  5. If MRSA is suspected, need to add IV vancomycin, 15 to 20 mg/kg IV q8 to 12h, depending on age and CrCl and follow through levels to keep above 15. Other options include daptomycin, 4 mg/kg IV qd, which does not have to be adjusted for CrCl, or linezolid, 400 to 600 mg IV q12h.
  6. If VRE is suspected, options include tigecycline, 100-mg IV load dose, then 50-mg IV q12h, which also covers MRSA and gram-negative rods but not *Pseudomonas aeruginosa* or can use daptomycin or linezolid.
  7. If ESBL gram-negative bacteria are suspected, then options include meropenem or ertapenem, 1 g IV qd.
  8. Once culture results are known, can tailor antibiotics to more specific agent.
- Oral antibiotics used for milder infections include amoxicillin-clavulanate, 875 mg PO q12h, which will cover gram-negative rods, streptococci, and anaerobes, or ciprofloxacin plus metronidazole or clindamycin. Bactrim will cover MRSA and methicillin-susceptible *Staphylococcus aureus* and some gram-negative rods.

The expert panel on diabetic foot infection (DFI) of the International Working Group on the Diabetic Foot conducted a systematic review. Results of comparisons of different antibiotic regimens generally demonstrated that newly introduced antibiotic regimens appeared to be as effective as conventional therapy.

CHRONIC TREATMENT

- Length of therapy: Highly variable depending on the severity of the infection. In general, 2 to 4 wk of antibiotics is sufficient. If bone infection suspected or documented, may need 4 to 8 wk of antibiotics, preferably IV via a peripherally inserted central line (PICC line).
- Surgical debridement may also be necessary for several weeks.

COMPLEMENTARY MEDICINE

- Hyperbaric oxygen (HBO): Used as an adjunct to antibiotics, debridement, and revascularization in the therapy of chronic, nonhealing wounds associated with diabetes. Evidence of effectiveness is conflicting. HBO acts by:
  1. Inducing vasoconstriction and reducing vasogenic edema
  2. Facilitating fibroblast activity, angiogenesis, and wound healing

  3. Killing anaerobic bacteria and augmenting neutrophil bactericidal activity
- Negative pressure wound therapy (wound vac): Controlled, subatmospheric pressure applied to an open wound can accelerate healing and closure.
  1. An open cell foam insert is cut to fit the open wound and then secured under a clear, vapor-permeable, plastic dressing.
  2. Tubing extends from the sponge to a disposable collection canister.
  3. A portable pump applies 125 mm Hg of controlled suction to the system. The subatmospheric pressure (suction) is equally distributed across the open wound and evacuates stagnant fluid from the wound.

DISPOSITION

- Following up on sed rates, CRP, BUN/CR, and levels of vancomycin if that antibiotic used.
- Surgical or wound center care follow-up.
- HBO usually involves multiple sessions over several weeks.
- Wound vac is applied for weeks and requires periodic nursing follow-up.
- The risk of death at 5 yr for a patient with a diabetic foot ulcer is two to five times as high as the risk for a patient with diabetes without a foot ulcer.

REFERRAL

- Infectious disease consultant for antibiotic management
- Surgeon or wound care center for surgical treatments
- Endocrinologist for good diabetes care
- Vascular surgeon for angioplasty or bypass procedures

PEARLS & CONSIDERATIONS

- In a meta-analysis of randomized controlled trials on the outcome of DFIs, there was a 22.7% treatment failure rate.
- Patients should be advised to seek prompt medical attention as these infections can progress rapidly to gangrene.

REFERENCES & SUGGESTED READINGS

Available at eBooks.Health.Elsevier.com.

AUTHOR: **GLENN G. FORT, MD, MPH**

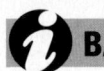 **BASIC INFORMATION**

DEFINITION

Gastroparesis is a syndrome characterized by objectively delayed gastric emptying in the absence of a mechanical obstruction of the stomach. It is associated with the cardinal symptoms of nausea, vomiting, early satiety, belching, bloating, and/or upper abdominal pain. It is commonly associated with longstanding, poorly controlled diabetes.

SYNONYMS

Gastroparesis diabeticorum
Gastrointestinal autonomic neuropathy
Delayed gastric emptying

ICD-10CM CODE
K31.84   Diabetic gastroparesis

EPIDEMIOLOGY & DEMOGRAPHICS

- Age-adjusted incidence of gastroparesis is 2.4 per 100,000 person-year for men and 9.8 per 100,000 person-year for women. The age-adjusted prevalence of definite gastroparesis is 9.6 per 100,000 persons for men and 38 per 100,000 persons for women.
- Gastroparesis is seen more commonly in women, and there is no known genetic predisposition to the disease.
- There are certain risk factors for development of gastroparesis, and diabetes is the most frequently recognized systemic disease. However, the most common form is idiopathic, where no detectable primary underlying abnormality is found. The idiopathic form accounts for approximately 50% of the patients with delayed gastric emptying.
- Other risk factors include:
  1. Postviral, especially rotavirus and Norwalk virus
  2. Medications including narcotics, calcium channel blockers, and tricyclic antidepressants
  3. Postsurgical
  4. Neurologic illnesses, such as multiple sclerosis, brain stem stroke, or tumor, etc.
  5. Autoimmune GI dysmotility
  6. Others such as mesenteric ischemia, scleroderma

PHYSICAL FINDINGS & CLINICAL PRESENTATION

- Patients with gastroparesis present with nausea, vomiting (vomitus may contain food ingested a few hours earlier), abdominal pain, early satiety, postprandial fullness, bloating, and in severe cases, weight loss. Although abdominal pain is a frequent symptom in patients with gastroparesis, it is rarely the predominant symptom.
- Interestingly, in patients with diabetes as the cause for gastroparesis, severe retching and vomiting are more commonly reported.
- Symptoms of gastroparesis are more pronounced in patients with type 1 diabetes, as compared with patients with type 2 diabetes.

- Physical examination findings may include epigastric distention or tenderness, but not guarding or rigidity. A succussion splash may be heard on auscultation by gently rocking the patient.

ETIOLOGY

- Diabetic gastroparesis is thought to result from impairment of neural control of gastric function. Various mechanisms of nerve injury include inflammatory changes to the autonomic ganglia or dropout of myelinated fibers involving the vagus nerve.
- Acute hyperglycemia has been found to have effects on the gastric sensory and motor functions by causing altered gastric electrical activity. It can also result in relaxation of the proximal stomach and decreased pressure in the antrum and pylorus. All of these processes can contribute to the retardation of gastric emptying.
- Achieving euglycemia can correct the gastric emptying delay.
- The effect of chronic hyperglycemia on the stomach is less clear, but there is some evidence that gastric emptying of meals is slower in patients with high glycated hemoglobin levels.

Dx **DIAGNOSIS**

DIFFERENTIAL DIAGNOSIS

- Functional dyspepsia[1]
- Gastric outlet obstruction
- Cyclic vomiting syndrome
- Chronic use of cannabinoids
- Irritable bowel syndrome
- Rumination syndrome
- Eating disorders such as anorexia nervosa and bulimia

WORKUP

- Thorough history and physical examination.
  1. An associated history of poorly controlled blood sugars may be present.
  2. A history of retinopathy, nephropathy, and neuropathy may be present in association with diabetes.
- All medications that can delay gastric emptying should be stopped before formal workup.

LABORATORY TESTS

No specific labs are needed to confirm the diagnosis, but the following can help to arrive at diagnosis:
- Hemoglobin A_{1c} (HbA_{1c})
- Thyroid-stimulating hormone (TSH)
- Total protein/albumin
- Hemoglobin
- Vitamin B_{12}
- Antinuclear antibody titers

IMAGING STUDIES

- Initial imaging should be done to rule out a mass causing mechanical obstruction.
  1. Upper GI endoscopy is first line.
  2. Computed tomography (CT) enterography vs. magnetic resonance (MR) enterography

may also be done to rule out mechanical obstruction from a small-bowel mass.
  3. Barium follow-through if CT or MR enterography unavailable.
- Food retained after overnight fasting may be suggestive of gastroparesis.
- After a mechanical obstruction has been ruled out, scintigraphic gastric emptying should be done as a confirmatory test.
  1. It is the simplest and most cost-effective test.
  2. Documenting the presence of delayed gastric emptying and assessing its severity is best done by measuring the delay in gastric emptying of solids.
  3. Patient is asked to ingest a standard, low-fat meal.
  4. Abnormal gastric emptying is defined as >10% gastric retention of solid food at 4 h and/or >60% at 2 h.
- ^{13}C breath test can also be used to measure gastric emptying.
  1. Not as sensitive as the scintigraphy method
- An alternative testing modality, called the *wireless motility capsule,* is as sensitive and specific as scintigraphy, but it is rather expensive and has not been shown to offer any added clinical information that scintigraphy has already provided.
  1. It is an ingestible, wireless capsule that measures pH, pressure, and temperature as it traverses the GI tract. Gastric emptying of the capsule occurs with phase III of the migrating motor complex, signifying completion of the postprandial phase.

Rx **TREATMENT**

- Diabetic gastroparesis is not progressive, and treatment is mainly directed toward alleviating patient symptoms. Exacerbating factors must be corrected as well.
- Patients can have a calorie-deficient diet, along with deficiencies in minerals and vitamins.

NONPHARMACOLOGIC THERAPY

- Nonpharmacologic therapy is considered the initial management for gastroparesis. This includes provision of nutritional support along with dietary modifications.
  1. Oral nutrition is preferred in mild disease. Diet should include small meals that are low in fiber (low-residue) and fat.
  2. In patients who cannot tolerate solids, meals can be homogenized and liquid meals supplemented with vitamins.
  3. Avoidance of carbonated beverages is recommended because these can lead to symptoms of bloating.
  4. Alcohol and tobacco smoking should also be stopped because these also delay gastric emptying.
  5. For patients with severe disease, a feeding jejunostomy tube may be considered. A successful trial of a nasojejunal feeding tube should precede placement.
  6. Optimize glucose and electrolyte levels.

ACUTE GENERAL Rx

- Prokinetic agents can be used to improve gastric motility. Ideally, these should be administered 10 to 15 min before meals.
  1. Metoclopramide and erythromycin are both available in intravenous and liquid form, which makes medication administration, tolerance, and efficacy more acceptable if patient symptoms are severe. Metoclopramide should generally not be used for over 12 wk because of the risk of tardive dyskinesia.
  2. The FDA has approved a nasal spray formulation of metoclopramide called Gimoti for diabetic gastroparesis in adults. Cost is a limiting factor.
  3. Domperidone is only available in the U.S. through investigational drug application due to increased risk of QT interval prolongation and arrhythmias.
- Antiemetic agents may also be needed for symptom relief in the acute setting.
  1. Phenothiazines, such as promethazine.
  2. 5-HT3 antagonists, such as ondansetron.
  3. Neurokinin receptor antagonist, such as aprepitant.
  4. Scopolamine patch.
- Intravenous fluid resuscitation may be required if signs or symptoms of dehydration are present due to persistent nausea and vomiting.
- Correct hyperglycemia even in the acute setting because delayed gastric emptying can be quickly corrected in the immediate setting.
- Discontinue medications that may delay gastric emptying.
  1. Pain medications.
     a. Avoid opioids.
     b. Tramadol may be used; however, one study showed that although gastric emptying was improved, colonic transit time was delayed.
  2. Incretin-based therapies and glucagon-like peptide 1 (GLP-1) analogues have been shown to retard gastric emptying.

CHRONIC Rx

- Metoclopramide should not be used for more than 12 wk unless the benefits outweigh the risks. Side effects include restlessness, anxiety, QT prolongation, and extrapyramidal effects such as dystonia and tardive dyskinesia.
- Erythromycin use is limited to 4 wk because longer use leads to tachyphylaxis. Similar effect is seen with the higher dose (250 mg) vs. a lower dose (40 mg).
- Pain management may need to be addressed for patients receiving chronic opioids.
  1. Low-dose tricyclic antidepressants, selective serotonin reuptake inhibitors, and pregabalin can be used as alternatives for long-term pain control.
- Endoscopic intrapyloric injection of botulinum toxin may be considered.
  1. Not shown to improve symptoms associated with diabetic gastroparesis but does have a modest effect on improving gastric emptying.
  2. Not approved as a mainstay treatment modality.
- Gastric electrical stimulation via a gastric electrical neurostimulator can be offered to patients with diabetic gastroparesis.
  1. Shown to improve symptom severity and gastric emptying.
  2. Approved as a humanitarian exemption device for patients with refractory symptoms.
- Surgical intervention.
  1. Venting gastrostomy, gastrojejunostomy, pyloroplasty, and gastrectomy are available.
  2. Rarely employed and is reserved for patients with severe, debilitating disease.

COMPLEMENTARY & ALTERNATIVE MEDICINE

- Dietary modifications as described earlier
- Acupuncture
- Autonomic retraining

PEARLS & CONSIDERATIONS

COMMENTS

- Diabetic gastroparesis does not change over time, and it occurs with both liquids and digestible solids as well as with indigestible food residues. However, impaired gastric emptying of indigestible solids may be an earlier abnormality.[2]
- Gastroparesis can be one of the consequences of chronic, poorly controlled diabetes.
- Symptoms of nausea, vomiting, bloating, early satiety, and abdominal pain in a patient with chronic, poorly controlled diabetes should prompt the possibility of gastroparesis.
- The diagnostic study of choice is gastric scintigraphy, performed by the nuclear medicine department.
- Discontinue all medications that can slow gastric emptying, especially opioids.
- Improve blood sugar control and avoid hyperglycemia.
- Antiemetics with prokinetic properties, such as metoclopramide, are most helpful in relieving nausea and vomiting, in both the acute and chronic presentations.
- Refer to gastroenterology for consideration of botulinum toxin injection or gastric neurostimulator placement if patients have poorly controlled and refractory disease.

PREVENTION

Focus on improved glycemic control in the long term.

PATIENT & FAMILY EDUCATION

- Gastroparesis Patient Association for Cures and Treatments (G-PACT)
- Association of Gastrointestinal Motility Disorders, Inc. (AGMD)

REFERENCES

Available at eBooks.Health.Elsevier.com.

RELATED CONTENT

Diabetes Mellitus (Key Related Topic)
Diabetic Polyneuropathy (Key Related Topic)

AUTHOR: **HUSSAIN R. KHAWAJA, MD, FACP**

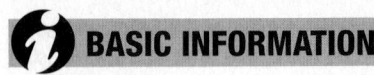

BASIC INFORMATION

DEFINITION

Diabetic ketoacidosis (DKA) is a life-threatening complication of diabetes mellitus. It results from an absolute or relative insulin deficiency that results in insulin resistance when paired with counterregulatory hormone and free fatty acid excess. DKA is characterized by the presence of an anion gap metabolic acidosis, ketonemia, and usually hyperglycemia.

SYNONYM

DKA

ICD-10CM CODES

E13.10	Diabetic ketoacidosis
E10.10	Type 2 diabetes mellitus with other specified complication
E10.11	Diabetic ketoacidosis with coma associated with type 1 diabetes mellitus
E08.10	Diabetes mellitus due to underlying condition with ketoacidosis without coma
E08.11	Diabetes mellitus due to underlying condition with ketoacidosis with coma
E13.11	Diabetic ketoacidosis with coma

EPIDEMIOLOGY & DEMOGRAPHICS

DKA is the most common hyperglycemic emergency among patients with type 1 (T1D) and type 2 diabetes (T2D), and may be the initial presentation in about 25% to 40% of those with T1D. In the past decade, the frequency of DKA has increased in the U.S., with more than 160,000 hospital admissions in 2017.[1] Social and racial-ethnic disparities are remarkable, with Black race/ethnicity and lower income individuals at heightened risk of DKA.[2] DKA most commonly occurs in individuals with T1D, with about one third of cases occurring in those with T2D. Those with ketosis-prone T2D are especially vulnerable. Overall, prevalence of DKA has increased, yet mortality has decreased to <5%, which is significantly lower than mortality from hyperglycemic hyperosmolar syndrome. Mortality from DKA in children and adolescents is most commonly due to cerebral edema, whereas in adults it is usually related to the precipitating illness (e.g., sepsis, cardiac or central nervous system ischemia, pneumonia). Older adult patients may present with multiple comorbidities that can complicate DKA even further.[3] The most common precipitating factor for DKA in older adults is related to insulin therapy nonadherence and underlying comorbidities. These patients often present with sepsis and, frequently, with atrial fibrillation. The combination of diabetes and atrial fibrillation increases morbidity and mortality associated with atrial fibrillation. In addition, older adult patients may be prescribed antipsychotic medications for underlying dementia, and this combination has been associated with a higher incidence of DKA admissions.

PHYSICAL FINDINGS & CLINICAL PRESENTATION

- Polyuria, polydipsia, polyphagia, weight loss, weakness
- Signs of dehydration (tachycardia, hypotension, dry mucous membranes, sunken eyes, poor skin turgor)
- Nausea, vomiting, abdominal tenderness, ileus
- Mental obtundation (can range from full alertness to coma)
- Tachypnea with air hunger (Kussmaul respirations)
- Fruity breath (caused by acetone)
- Evidence of precipitating factors (e.g., ischemia or infection)

ETIOLOGY

Hyperglycemia occurs from relative insulinopenia for the degree of transient insulin resistance plus an increase in counterregulatory hormones, which leads to increased hepatic gluconeogenesis and glycogenolysis. The resulting lipolysis and fatty acid oxidation produce ketonemia and metabolic acidosis. Both hyperglycemia and ketonemia result in an osmotic diuresis, which can lead to hypovolemia and subsequent decline in renal function. The pathophysiology of diabetic ketoacidosis is illustrated in Fig. 1.

DKA can be precipitated by various conditions:

- Infection (commonly of the respiratory tract, such as COVID-19, or the urinary tract or skin)
- Insulin deficiency (undiagnosed diabetes, medication nonadherence/inadequacy, insulin pump malfunction/disconnect, diabulimia)
- Inflammatory conditions (e.g., acute pancreatitis)
- Ischemia/infarction (e.g., myocardial infarction, stroke, bowel ischemia)
- Severe extracellular fluid volume depletion
- Drugs (e.g., steroids; thiazides; atypical antipsychotics; SGLT2 inhibitors; alcohol; sympathomimetics, including cocaine; and cancer treatment involving immune checkpoint inhibitors)

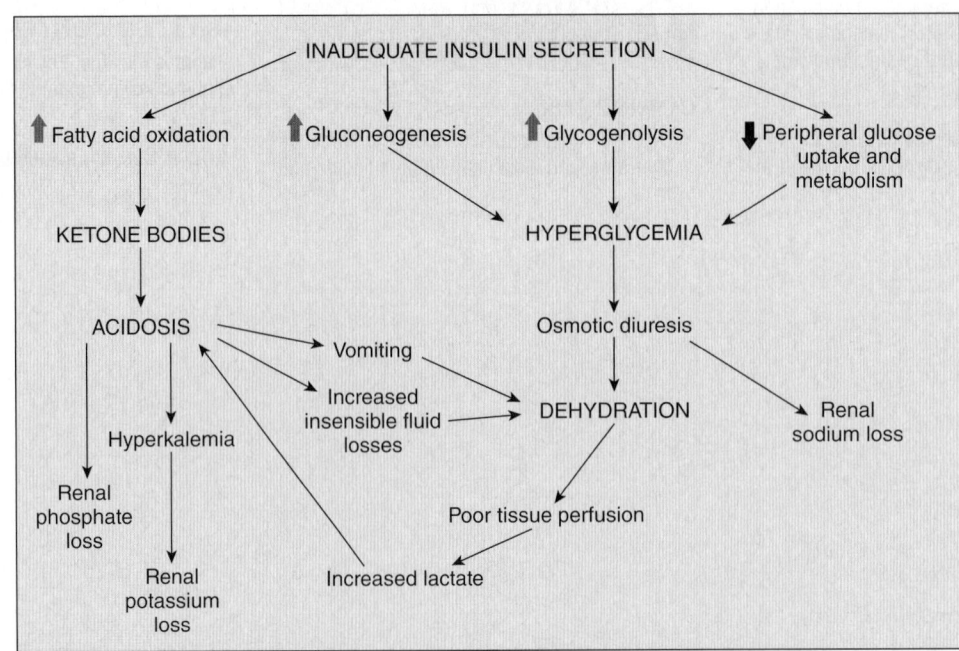

FIG. 1 Pathophysiology of diabetic ketoacidosis. (From Marcdante KJ et al: *Nelson essentials of pediatrics,* ed 9, Philadelphia, 2023, Elsevier.)

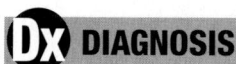 **DIAGNOSIS**

DIFFERENTIAL DIAGNOSIS[4]

- Hyperosmolar nonketotic state
- Alcoholic/starvation ketoacidosis
- Lactic acidosis
- Acute kidney injury/chronic kidney disease
- Metabolic acidosis caused by exogenous poisons (e.g., methanol, ethylene glycol, paraldehyde)
- Salicylate poisoning
- Hypovolemic or septic shock

WORKUP

After initial history is obtained, perform physical examination, including evaluation of airway, breathing, circulation, mental status, volume status, and signs suggestive of precipitating event(s). Diagnostic criteria for DKA are summarized in Table 1.

LABORATORY TESTS

- Serum glucose level: Generally >250 mg/dl. However, "euglycemic DKA" (EDKA) presenting with glucose <200 to 250 can occur in 10% of patients with DKA (e.g., exogenous insulin injection en route to hospital, food restriction, administration of an SGLT inhibitor [SGLTi],[5] pregnancy—a ketosis-prone state, prolonged fasting, h/o bariatric surgery, gastroparesis, insulin pump failure, cocaine intoxication, chronic liver disease, and glycogen storage disease).
- Arterial blood gas (demonstrating metabolic acidosis): Arterial pH <7.30 (<7.00 in severe cases).
- Serum beta hydroxybutyrate and urine ketones: Positive (beta hydroxybutyrate >3 mmol/L; ≥2+ urine ketones).
- Serum electrolytes:
  1. Serum bicarbonate concentration: <15 mmol/L (mild DKA may reduce levels to <18 mmol/L).
  2. Serum potassium concentration: Levels may initially measure as normal or high from extracellular shift with insulin deficiency and hyperosmolality. However, overall total body potassium depletion occurs from urinary losses and vomiting.
  3. Serum sodium concentration: May be low, normal, or high. Hyperglycemia increases plasma osmolality, which attracts intracellular water to the extracellular compartment and decreases the serum sodium level.[6] Correct the serum sodium concentration (Table 2): Add 1.6 mmol/L to the measured serum sodium level for every 100 mg/dl increase of serum glucose >100 mg/dl and <400 mg/dl, and then increase the sodium level by 4 mmol/L for each glucose increment of 100 mg/dl above 400 mg/dl.
  4. Serum calcium, magnesium, and phosphorus: May be significantly low and may decrease further with DKA treatment.
  5. Anion gap (see Table 2): Na − (Cl + HCO₃). Anion gap is increased (>10 mmol/L) from elevated ketones.
  6. Blood urea nitrogen (BUN) and creatinine: Generally, reveals acute kidney injury.
- Hemoglobin A1c if not performed within the preceding 3 mo.
- CBC with differential: May indicate underlying infection (leukocytosis >25,000/mm³),[4] inflammatory condition, or hemoconcentration. A leukocytosis of 10,000 to 15,000/mm³ is expected from the stress of illness alone.[7]
- Urinalysis, urine/blood cultures: As indicated based on exam findings.
- Pregnancy test: Perform in all female patients of reproductive age. DKA in pregnancy bodes significant fetal morbidity and mortality.[8]
- Lipase/liver enzymes: Obtain if abdominal pain is present. Elevated lipase can occur without underlying pancreatitis.

IMAGING STUDIES

ECG, chest x-ray examination, and other imaging studies as indicated to evaluate the precipitating cause(s).

Rx TREATMENT

NONPHARMACOLOGIC THERAPY

- Monitor mental status, vital signs, and urine output hourly until improved.
- Monitor serum glucose hourly and serum electrolytes, BUN, and creatinine every 2 to 4 h until DKA resolves.

ACUTE GENERAL Rx (FIG. 2)[4]

FLUID REPLACEMENT: Fluid therapy is initiated to expand volume and restore renal perfusion. On average, patients with DKA may have a typical total body water deficit of 100 ml/kg (up to 8 to 10 L).[9] In the absence of cardiac compromise or severe kidney impairment, infuse 0.9% normal saline (NS) at an initial rate of 1 to 1.5 L/h (alternatively, use 15 to 20 ml/kg per hour) for the first 1 to 2 h. The subsequent fluid choice depends on patient hemodynamics, electrolytes, and urinary output. If corrected serum sodium is normal or high, infuse 0.45% NS at 250 to 500 ml/h. If corrected serum sodium is low, continue 0.9% NS at a similar rate. Once serum glucose decreases to 200 mg/dl, add 5% dextrose to the intravenous (IV) fluid. The recommended sodium decline is 0.5 mmol/L per hour and should not surpass 10 to 12 mmol/L per day. Hyperglycemia (>250 mg/dl) resolves sooner than ketoacidosis (6 vs. 12 h, respectively).

A meta-analysis of three randomized trials[10] comparing normal saline to balanced electrolyte solutions (e.g., lactated Ringer's solution) in adults hospitalized with DKA showed that patients who received balanced solutions had shorter time to DKA resolution by 3 h. Additional trials with larger

---

TABLE 1 Diagnostic Criteria for Diabetic Ketoacidosis and Hyperglycemic Hyperosmolar State

DIAGNOSTIC CRITERIA AND CLASSIFICATION

	Diabetic Ketoacidosis			Hyperglycemic Hyperosmolar State
	Mild	*Moderate*	*Severe*	
Plasma glucose (mg/dL)	>250	>250	>250	>600
Arterial pH	7.25-7.30	7.00-≤7.24	<7.00	>7.30
Serum bicarbonate (mEq/L)	15-18	10-≤15	<10	>15
Urine ketone	Positive	Positive	Positive	Small
Serum ketone	Positive	Positive	Positive	Small
Effective serum osmolality	Variable	Variable	Variable	>320 mOsm/kg
Anion gap	>10	>12	>12	<12
Alteration in sensorium or mental obtundation	Alert	Alert/drowsy	Stupor/coma	Stupor/coma

From Robertson RP et al: *DeGroot's endocrinology, basic science and clinical practice*, ed 8, Philadelphia, 2023, Elsevier.

TABLE 2 Useful Formulas for the Evaluation of Diabetic Ketoacidosis and Hyperglycemic Hyperosmolar State

1. Calculation of anion gap (AG): $AG = [Na^+] - [Cl^- + HCO_3^-]$

2. Total and effective serum osmolality: $Total = 2[Na^+] + \dfrac{glucose\ (mg/dL)}{18} + \dfrac{BUN\ (mg/dL)}{2.8}$

3. $Effective = 2[Na^+] + \dfrac{glucose\ (mg/dL)}{18}$

4. Corrected serum sodium: $Corrected\ [Na^+] = \dfrac{1.6 \times (mg/dL) - 100}{100} + [measured\ Na^+]$

   Total body water (TBW) deficit: $TBW\ deficit = [weight\ (kg) \times 0.6] - \dfrac{corrected\ Na^+ - 1}{140}$

BUN, Blood urea nitrogen.
From Robertson RP et al: *DeGroot's endocrinology, basic science and clinical practice*, ed 8, Philadelphia, 2023, Elsevier.

D

Diseases and Disorders

I

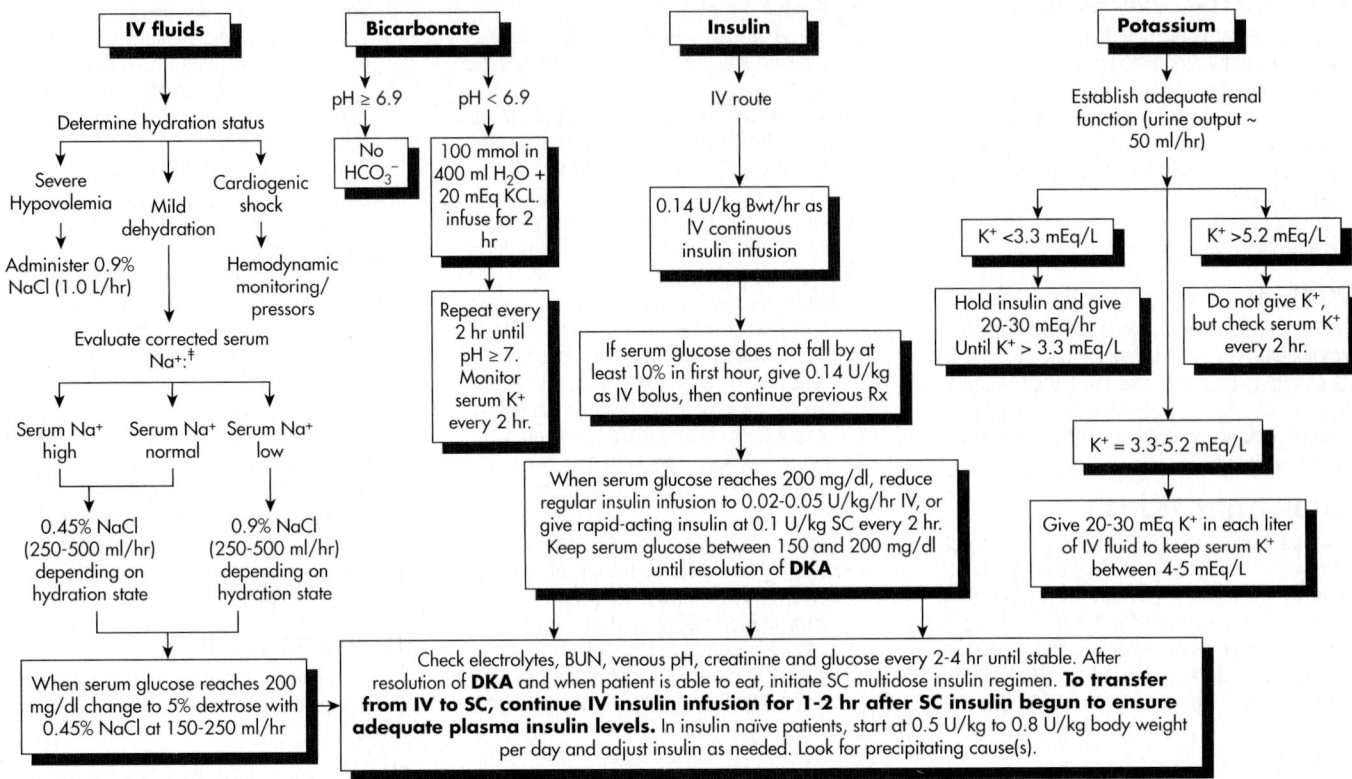

FIG. 2 **Management of diabetic ketoacidosis.** *BUN*, Blood urea nitrogen; *DKA*, diabetic ketoacidosis; *ECG*, electrocardiogram; *IV*, intravenous; *Rx*, prescription; *SC*, subcutaneous. (From Nyenwe EA et al: The evolution of diabetic ketoacidosis: an update of its etiology, pathogenesis, and management, *Metabolism* 65[4]:507-521, 2016.)

patient base should help determine if current guidelines for fluid resuscitation in DKA should include balanced crystalloid solutions.

INSULIN ADMINISTRATION: Insulin should not be started until after initiation of IV fluid resuscitation and correction of hypokalemia. Once these are addressed, administer initial bolus of IV regular insulin 0.1 units/kg followed by 0.1 units/kg per hour infusion or a continuous infusion of 0.14 units/kg per hour without initial bolus. If the serum glucose declines by less than 50 to 75 mg/dl in the first hour, increase insulin infusion rate hourly until a steady glucose decline is seen. After the serum glucose reaches 200 mg/dl and until DKA resolves, maintain the serum glucose concentration between 150 and 200 mg/dl by decreasing the insulin infusion to 0.02 to 0.05 units/kg per hour, or deliver subcutaneous rapid-acting insulin at 0.1 units/kg every 2 h. An alternative to IV insulin includes use of subcutaneous rapid-acting insulin for those presenting with mild-to-moderate DKA. Potential candidates for subcutaneous insulin include those patients who are alert, do not require admission to a critical care area, have a pH >7.0, are able to tolerate oral intake, and have a bicarbonate level of at least 10 mEq/L. Subcutaneous rapid-acting insulin can be given as an

initial bolus of 0.3 units/kg, followed by maintenance doses of 0.2 units/kg every 2 h. Once blood glucose is <250 mg/dl, administer 0.05 to 0.1 units/kg every 2 h until DKA resolves. If anion gap is not closed within 12 h, the patient should be switched to an IV insulin infusion.

POTASSIUM REPLACEMENT: Insulin therapy shifts potassium intracellularly, frequently causing hypokalemia. If the serum potassium concentration at presentation is between 3.3 and 5.2 mmol/L, infuse 20 to 30 mmol of potassium chloride (KCl) with each liter of IV fluid to maintain serum potassium at 4 to 5 mmol/L. If serum potassium is <3.3 mmol/L, withhold insulin until the serum potassium level is >3.3 mmol/L, and replace potassium by administering KCl infusion at 20 to 30 mmol/h. If the serum potassium level at presentation is >5.2 mmol/L, monitor the level every 2 h without replacement.

BICARBONATE REPLACEMENT: The administration of bicarbonate in DKA is generally not recommended. Bicarbonate does not improve time to resolution of acidosis or discharge, although adverse effects are associated with severe metabolic acidosis (decreased cardiac contractility, cerebral vasodilation). In adult patients with pH <6.9, administer 100 mmol (2 ampules) of sodium bicarbonate in 800 ml of

sterile water (isotonic solution) with 20 mmol KCl at 200 ml/h for 2 h until venous pH is >7.0. If pH is still <7 after infusion, repeat infusion every 2 h until pH is >7.

PHOSPHATE REPLACEMENT: Phosphate replacement is not routinely recommended, although phosphorus concentrations decrease with insulin administration. In patients with cardiac dysfunction, respiratory depression, or anemia and serum phosphorus <1 mg/dl, add 20 to 30 mmol/L of potassium phosphate to IV fluids to prevent diaphragmatic muscle weakness.

TRANSITION TO SUBCUTANEOUS INSULIN: Resolution of DKA occurs when blood glucose is <200 mg/dl and two of the following occur: Venous pH >7.3, serum bicarbonate >15 mmol/L, and anion gap ≤12 mmol/L. At this point, patients can transition to subcutaneous insulin but may remain on IV insulin if they have had nothing by mouth. Subcutaneous intermediate- or long-acting insulin should be overlapped with IV insulin by 2 to 4 h to maintain adequate insulin levels and prevent rebound hyperglycemia. When this transition occurs before a meal, the patient may receive a dose of prandial insulin with short- or rapid-acting analogues together with the basal insulin, and the IV insulin may be discontinued in an hour. In patients with a known history of controlled diabetes, their home insulin regimens may be resumed. In patients with known poorly controlled diabetes, the subcutaneous insulin dose can be determined based on stable insulin drip requirements. Insulin-naïve patients may be started on basal-bolus insulin therapy by calculation of total daily dose of 0.5 to 0.8 units/kg (split as half-basal and half-bolus; administer one third of total bolus for each meal) or by stable insulin drip requirements. Further subcutaneous insulin dose titration is based on blood glucose results. Resolution of glucotoxicity and the inciting condition(s) will decrease insulin requirements

DISPOSITION

In general, patients with DKA should be admitted to an intensive care unit with an insulin infusion. Those with mild DKA may be treated with rapid-acting insulin analogues under observation and then discharged. Timely follow-up with primary care or endocrinology is important, preferably with an appointment made before discharge, as over 40% of patients may be readmitted within 2 wk of hospital discharge.

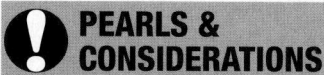

PEARLS & CONSIDERATIONS

COMMENTS

- DKA is the initial presentation of diabetes in 15% to 20% of adults and 30% to 40% of children. This underscores the importance of educating patients, families, and school administrators regarding early symptoms of diabetes with the aim of early diagnosis.
- Ketosis-prone diabetes, also referred to as Flatbush diabetes, is found more often in certain ethnic populations, including African American and Asian patients, among others.[4,5] Initial therapy with insulin is required

for acute management; however, diet alone or oral hypoglycemic agents can be used to achieve glycemic control without the need of insulin.

- The development of EDKA is characterized by normal or modestly elevated blood sugars with anion gap metabolic acidosis, ketonemia, and ketonuria.[11] Management is similar to DKA management. Mainstays of treatment involve correction of electrolytes and dehydration with IV fluids. However, higher percentages of dextrose (10% or 20%) are used to allow for concomitant high-dose insulin required to correct the acidosis.[5] If the patient is taking an SGLTi, stop immediately. Patients may resume SGLTi therapy only after DKA has resolved and if the patient is feeling well and discusses their condition with their primary outpatient managing physician.
- DKA in patients with end-stage renal disease (ESRD) is relatively uncommon secondary to decreased insulin clearance. In fact, low glomerular filtration rate increases the risk for hypoglycemia. However, when patients with ESRD develop DKA, special management considerations are needed.[7,12] These patients are usually anuric and do not produce an osmotic diuresis, negating the need for aggressive volume repletion. Vigorous volume resuscitation in this case may lead to volume overload, pulmonary edema, and respiratory distress. Anuric patients with ESRD do not have urinary potassium loss, thus making potassium replacement unnecessary. Similarly, phosphorus supplementation is not required. In fact, in severe acidosis, transcellular potassium shifts for hydrogen may produce hyperkalemia, prompting some providers to request immediate dialysis. Insulin therapy alone for hyperglycemia may also correct hyperkalemia without the need for dialysis. During DKA in patients with ESRD, dialysis is generally only recommended if there are hyperkalemia-induced electrocardiographic manifestations. A precipitous drop in serum glucose from an insulin infusion and hemodialysis may result in rapid tonicity shifts, predisposing to cerebral edema. Thus hemodialysis is typically delayed until the serum glucose is corrected. Due to increased risk for hypoglycemia, patients with ESRD require careful and preemptive insulin reduction from the hospital DKA protocol.
- Address affordability of insulin before discharge. Consider use of neutral protamine Hagedorn (NPH) insulin and regular or aspart insulin for as little as $25 per vial/pen (ReliOn™)
- Proper instructions for hypoglycemia prevention and management, insulin storage, dosing, meal timing, preparation before injection (e.g., resuspension of NPH), and use of delivery system (syringe/vial, pen, insulin pump) are essential.

PREVENTION

Many cases of DKA can be prevented by effective patient education and communication. Education of patients regarding sick day management includes early communication with the health care provider, continuing insulin during illness, checking ketones, and continuing an easily digestible liquid diet that contains carbohydrates.

REFERENCES

Available at eBooks.Health.Elsevier.com.

RELATED CONTENT

Diabetes Mellitus (Related Key Topic)
Hyperglycemic Hyperosmolar Syndrome (Related Key Topic)

AUTHOR: **JESSICA E. SHILL, MD**

D

I

BASIC INFORMATION

DEFINITION

Diabetic nephropathy (DN) is a chronic kidney disease defined by structural and functional changes that develop as a result of microvascular complications associated with long-standing or poorly controlled diabetes. The clinical presentation includes albuminuria, hypertension (HTN), and progressive reduction in renal function. This is demonstrated histologically as glomerular basement membrane thickening, mesangial matrix expansion, foot process effacement, arteriolar hyalinosis, microaneurysms, nodular glomerulosclerosis (Kimmelstiel-Wilson lesion), and tubulointerstitial fibrosis.[1]

SYNONYMS

Diabetic kidney disease
DN

ICD-10CM CODES

E10.21	Type 1 diabetes mellitus with diabetic nephropathy
E11.21	Type 2 diabetes mellitus with diabetic nephropathy

EPIDEMIOLOGY & DEMOGRAPHICS

INCIDENCE: Diabetes is present in 10% of the U.S. population. DN occurs in approximately 40% of patients who have diabetes for more than 10 yr.[2]

PREVALENCE: DN develops in approximately 30% of patients with type 1 diabetes (T1D) and 40% of patients with type 2 diabetes (T2D). DN is the leading cause of chronic kidney disease (CKD) and end-stage renal disease (ESRD) worldwide. Among incident ESRD patients in the U.S., diabetes is present in about 60.6%.[2,3]

PREDOMINANT SEX & AGE: Male patients and older age.

RISK FACTORS:[2]
- Male
- Older age
- Race: People of African descent, American Indian, Hispanic, Asian/Pacific Islander
- Family history of DN
- Hyperglycemia
- Hypertension
- Obesity
- Diabetic retinopathy
- Smoking
- Hyperlipidemia
- Early-onset T2D
- Low socioeconomic status

GENETICS: Polygenetic. Patients with a first-degree relative with DN are at increased risk.

PHYSICAL FINDINGS & CLINICAL PRESENTATION

- Peripheral edema
- Foamy urine
- Weight gain or weight loss
- Hypertension
- Diabetic retinopathy
- Microalbuminuria/proteinuria

- Decline in estimated glomerular filtration rate (eGFR)

ETIOLOGY

- DN develops as a result of microvascular complications associated with long-standing diabetes. (Box 1)
- DN is characterized by histologic changes (Fig. E1), including glomerular basement membrane thickening, mesangial matrix expansion, foot process effacement, arteriolar hyalinosis, microaneurysms, nodular glomerulosclerosis (Kimmelstiel-Wilson nodules), and tubulointerstitial fibrosis. These changes lead to urine albumin/protein excretion and decreased eGFR.[1,2]
- The pathophysiology leading to DN (Fig. 2) includes the generation of advance glycation end products, elaboration of growth factors, hemodynamic changes, and hormonal changes resulting in the release of reactive oxygen species and inflammatory mediators such as tumor necrosis factor-A (TNF-A), interleukin-1 (IL-1), and IL-6. These changes lead to glomerular hyperfiltration, glomerular hypertension, renal hypertrophy, and altered glomerular composition, which manifest as albuminuria, hypertension, and progressive decline in renal function.[1,4]

DIAGNOSIS

DIFFERENTIAL DIAGNOSIS[5]

- Hypertensive nephrosclerosis
- Focal segmental glomerulosclerosis
- Amyloidosis and light chain deposition disease
- Immunoglobulin A nephropathy
- Membranous nephropathy

WORKUP

- Workup should include thorough history and physical examination with focus on duration of diabetes, degree of hyperglycemia, presence of complications (including retinopathy), and appropriate laboratory testing (Fig. E3, Box 2). Stages of DN are illustrated in Fig. 4.

LABORATORY TESTS

CKD is defined as abnormality of kidney structure or function, present for >3 mo. CKD is

---

BOX 1   Natural History of Diabetic Kidney Disease

- Estimated glomerular filtration rate (eGFR) decline is faster in association with albuminuria, especially macroalbuminuria, but may also occur in nonalbuminuric patients.
- The natural history of diabetic kidney disease (DKD) appears to be similar in both types of diabetes.
- Patients with DKD are more likely to have anemia compared with patients with nondiabetic chronic kidney disease at comparably reduced levels of eGFR.
- Insulin resistance in patients with diabetes contributes to lower parathyroid hormone levels with an increased predisposition to adynamic bone disease.

From Robertson RP et al: *DeGroot's endocrinology, basic science and clinical practice*, ed 8, Philadelphia, 2023, Elsevier.

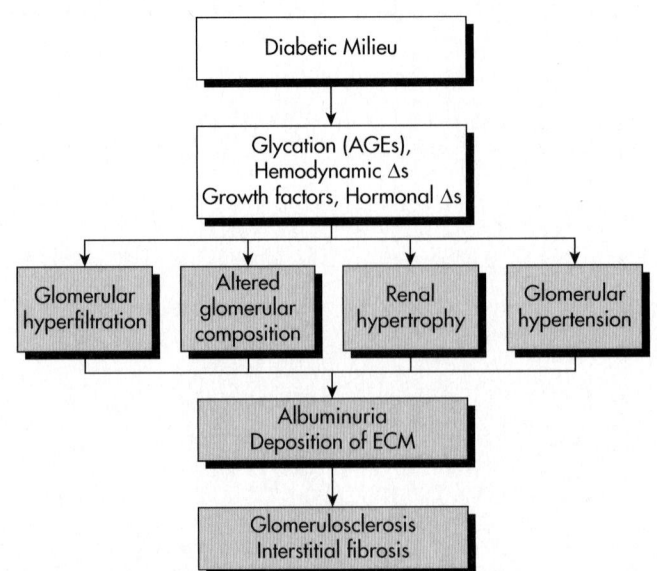

FIG. 2 Pathophysiology. *AGEs,* Advanced glycation end products; *ECM,* extracellular matrix. (From Umanath K et al: Update on diabetic nephropathy, *Am J Kidney Dis* 71:884, 2018.)

BOX 2 Diagnosis of Diabetic Kidney Disease

- Diabetic kidney disease (DKD) is diagnosed by microalbuminuria (urine albumin-to-creatinine ratio [UACR] 30-300 mg/g), macroalbuminuria (UACR >300 mg/g), estimated glomerular filtration rate (eGFR) <60 mL/min/1.73 m^2, or a combination of high albuminuria and low eGFR that persists for at least 3 mo in a person with diabetes.
- Annual screening for DKD is recommended within 5 yr of a diagnosis of type 1 diabetes mellitus and beginning at the time of diagnosis of type 2 diabetes mellitus.
- If there is a change in clinical status (progression to a more advanced chronic kidney disease category) or medications that can impact UACR and/or eGFR (renin angiotensin system inhibitor or sodium-glucose cotransporter 2 inhibitor), then UACR and eGFR should be measured more frequently (every 3-6 mo).
- Referral to a nephrologist is recommended if there is need for further diagnostic evaluation or management guidance, or if the eGFR is <30 mL/min/1.73 m^2.

From Robertson RP et al: *DeGroot's Endocrinology, Basic Science and Clinical Practice*, ed 8, Philadelphia, 2023, Elsevier.

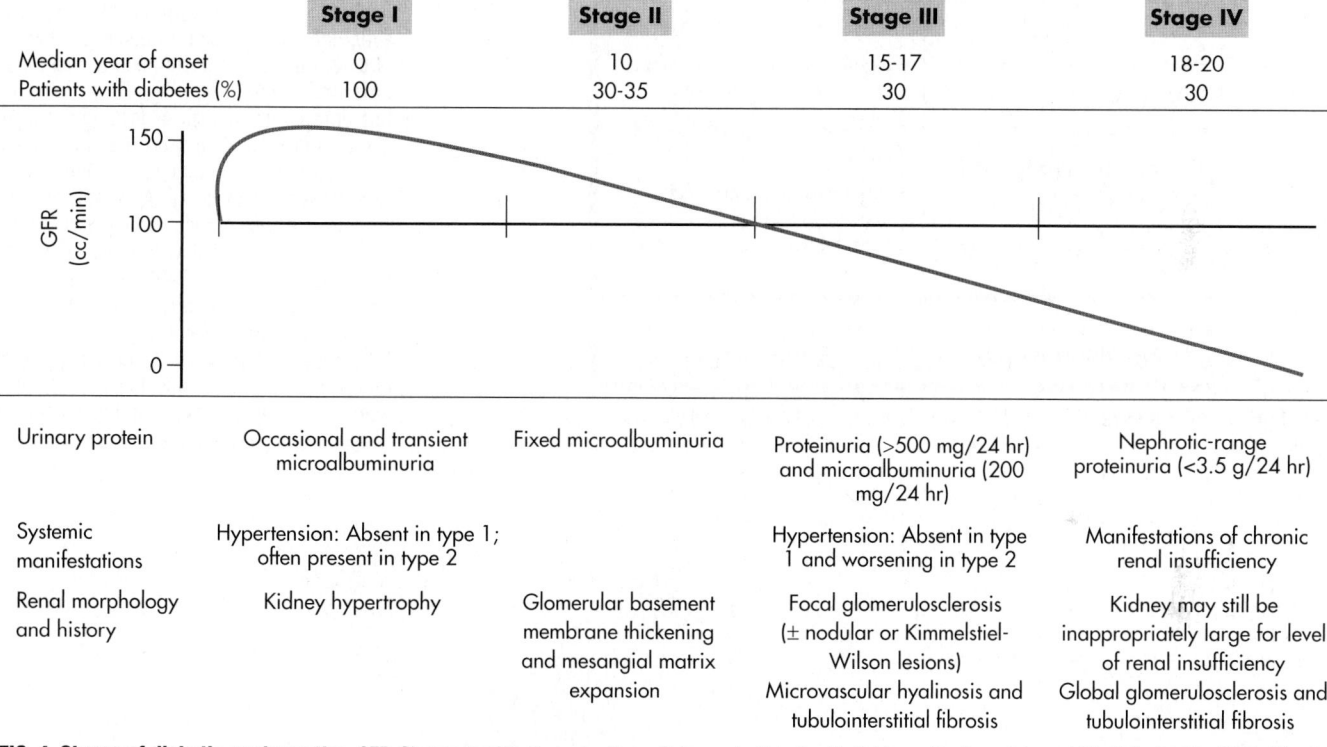

FIG. 4 Stages of diabetic nephropathy. *GFR,* Glomerular filtration rate. (From Goldman L, Schafer AI: *Goldman-Cecil medicine,* ed 26, Philadelphia, 2020, Elsevier.)

classified based on eGFR and albuminuria. Risk of CKD progression, cardiovascular events, and mortality increases with increasing albuminuria or decreasing eGFR. The KDIGO Heat Map guide frequency of laboratory monitoring, treatment, and referral to nephrology is shown in Fig. E5.

- Urine albumin-to-creatinine ratio (ACR)
  1. Microalbuminuria (moderately increased albuminuria) is defined as 30 to 299 mg/g and macroalbuminuria (severely increased albuminuria) is defined as >300 mg/g.
  2. Screening should be performed annually in patients with T1D with >5-yr duration and annually for patients with T2D from its onset.[2]
  3. Confirm microalbuminuria with 2 to 3 elevated levels within a 3- to 6-mo period.
  4. Early morning urine sample is recommended to identify albuminuria. Prolonged standing, heavy exercise, urinary

tract infection, uncontrolled hyperglycemia, and acute illness can cause transient albuminuria.
  5. In T1D, microalbuminuria occurs 5 to 10 yr from onset.
  6. In T2D, up to 25% of patients with DN may have little or no proteinuria.
- eGFR <60 ml/min/1.73 m^2
- Other tests
  1. Electrolytes
  2. Lipid profile

IMAGING STUDIES

- Renal ultrasound may help identify disease because kidney volume increases by an average of 15% with the onset of diabetes.
- Renal biopsy is confirmatory but is reserved only for patients with atypical features. Atypical features include rapid decline in eGFR (>5 ml/min/1.73 m^2 per yr), overt proteinuria without prior microalbuminuria, active

urine sediment, or features to suggest other systemic disease.[5] Microscopic hematuria with isomorphic erythrocyturia may be seen with DN. In T2D, DN can be present from the onset, whereas in T1D it typically develops after 5 yr. In general, diabetic patients with albuminuria, retinopathy, and progressive decline of kidney function do not require kidney biopsy (Fig. 6).

Rx TREATMENT

See Fig. 7[6] and Table 1 for comprehensive management of DN.

NONPHARMACOLOGIC THERAPY

- Smoking cessation
- Weight loss
- Regular exercise, moderate-intensity physical activity for cumulative duration of at least

150 min per week or to level compatible with cardiovascular and physical tolerance.

- Dietary modification, including a low-carbohydrate, low-fat diet while maintaining a protein intake of 0.8 g protein/kg/day in CKD and 1.0 to 1.2 g protein/kg/day in patients treated by dialysis.

ACUTE GENERAL Rx

- Early identification and an aggressive multipronged approach of treatment of DN is key to slowing progressive disease (Table E2). Fig. 8 illustrates the management of DN before the onset of renal failure.

- Glycemic control with a goal A_{1c} ranging from <6.5% to <8% is recommended by the Kidney Disease: Improving Global Outcomes (KDIGO) Diabetes Work Group 2020. The A_{1c} goal should be individualized, with a lower A_{1c} goal in patients with shorter duration of diabetes, younger age, early-stage CKD, absence of complications, presence of hypoglycemic awareness, and a longer life expectancy. Glycemic control delays microvascular complications and progression of DN.[7]

- First-line treatment for glycemic management in DN should include metformin and sodium-glucose cotransporter-2 inhibitor (SGLT2i). SGLT2i is recommended for T2D, CKD with eGFR >20 ml/min/1.73m². Once initiated it can be continued until dialysis or transplant. Risk of hypoglycemia with SGLT2i monotherapy remains low.[8]

- Glucagon-like peptide-1 receptor agonists (GLP1 RA) should be considered in patients who have not reached glycemic goals despite use of metformin and SGLT2i or are intolerant to those medications. GLP1RA is preferentially used in patients with obesity, T2D, and CKD as they promote weight reduction. GLP1RA should not be used in combination with dipeptidyl peptidase-4(DPP-4) inhibitors.[7]

- The ideal blood pressure goal is debatable. The current KDOQI guideline recommends a goal blood pressure <130/80 mm Hg; however, the Eighth Joint National Committee (JNC 8) guidelines recommend a goal blood pressure <140/90 mm Hg.

- Use of renin-angiotensin-aldosterone system (RAAS) blockers should be the cornerstone of hypertension management. Angiotensin type 1 receptor blockers (ARB) and ACE inhibitors (ACE-I) reduce proteinuria, lower blood pressure, and slow progression of DN. Combination therapy of ARB and ACE-I is not recommended due to greater risk of hyperkalemia and acute kidney injury.

- Dihydropyridine calcium channel blocker or diuretics can also be considered as first-line agents for hypertension management in absence of significant albuminuria.

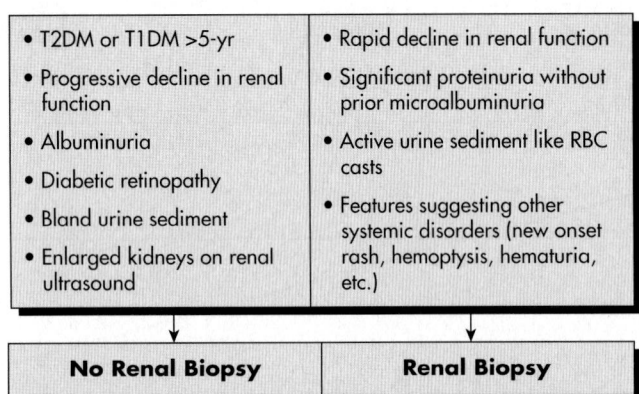

- T2DM or T1DM >5-yr
- Progressive decline in renal function
- Albuminuria
- Diabetic retinopathy
- Bland urine sediment
- Enlarged kidneys on renal ultrasound

- Rapid decline in renal function
- Significant proteinuria without prior microalbuminuria
- Active urine sediment like RBC casts
- Features suggesting other systemic disorders (new onset rash, hemoptysis, hematuria, etc.)

No Renal Biopsy | **Renal Biopsy**

FIG. 6 Role of renal biopsy. *RBC*, Red blood cell; *T1DM*, type 1 diabetes mellitus; *T2DM*, type 2 diabetes mellitus.

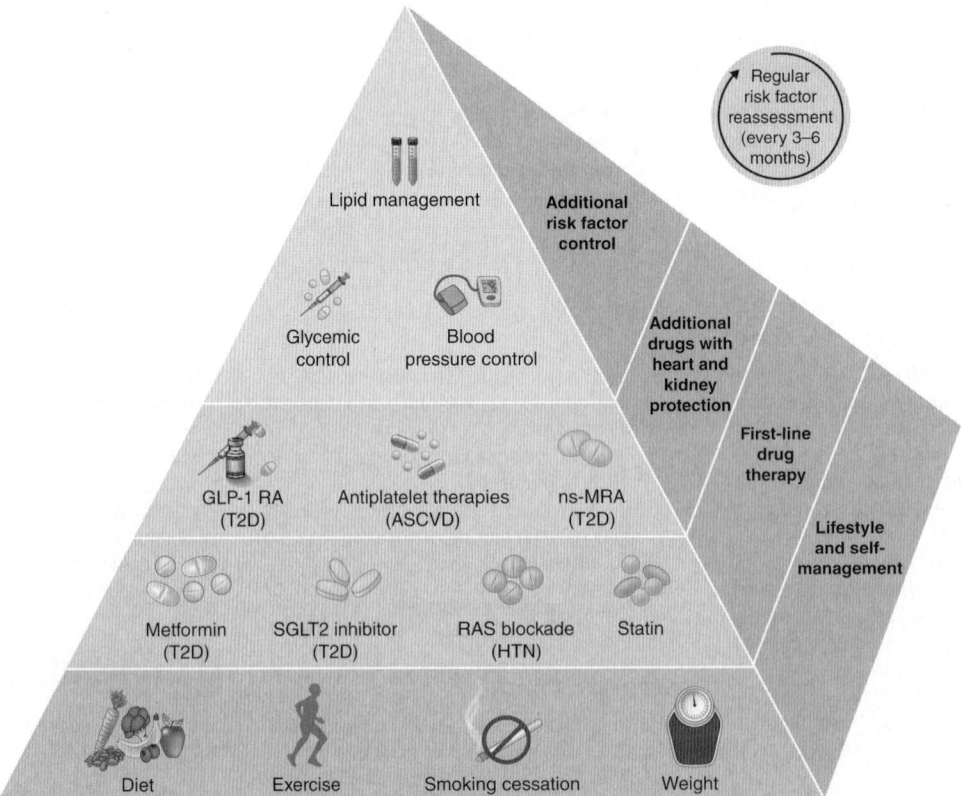

Regular risk factor reassessment (every 3–6 months)

Additional risk factor control

Lipid management

Glycemic control Blood pressure control

Additional drugs with heart and kidney protection

GLP-1 RA (T2D) Antiplatelet therapies (ASCVD) ns-MRA (T2D)

First-line drug therapy

Metformin (T2D) SGLT2 inhibitor (T2D) RAS blockade (HTN) Statin

Lifestyle and self-management

Diet Exercise Smoking cessation Weight

Diabetes with CKD

FIG.7 Kidney heart risk factor management in diabetes with chronic kidney disease *(CKD).* (From Kidney Disease: Improving Global Outcomes (KDIGO) Diabetes Work Group: KDIGO 2022 clinical practice guideline for diabetes management in chronic kidney disease, *Kidney Int* 102(5S):S1-S127, 2022. https://doi.10.1016/j.kint.2022.06.008.)

- Nonsteroidal mineralocorticoid receptor antagonists (MRAs) such as finerenone have shown cardiovascular and kidney benefits, and are recommended for patients with T2D, CKD with eGFR >25 ml/min/1.73m², residual albuminuria >30 mg/g despite RAAS blockers, and normal serum potassium. Serum potassium should be measured at 1 mo and every 4 mo while on therapy.[9]
- Cardiovascular events, including death, occur more frequently than ESRD; therefore statin is recommended in all patients with T1D or T2D and CKD, with moderate intensity for primary prevention and high intensity for patients with known atherosclerotic cardiovascular disease.[8]

CHRONIC Rx

- Identify anemia in CKD. Patients with DN are twice as likely to develop anemia compared to patients with nondiabetic CKD and may need treatment with erythropoiesis-stimulating agents.[2]

- Identify CKD bone and mineral disorder, especially adynamic bone disease, which develops more often with DN.[2]
- Fig. 9 illustrates the management of DN after the onset of renal failure.
- Patients with DN should have timely referral for kidney transplantation and vascular access evaluation as eGFR declines to 20 ml/min/1.73 m².
- Type IV renal tubular acidosis from hyporeninemic hypoaldosteronism and hyperkalemia is common in DN, especially with RAAS blockade and MRAs. Treatment with low-potassium diet, diuretics, sodium bicarbonate, and/or GI cation exchangers may be required.
- Fig. 10 illustrates the management of DN after the onset of clinical proteinuria.
- Treatment options for ESRD in patients with diabetes are summarized in Table 3.

DISPOSITION

- DN should ideally be monitored every 3 to 6 mo with assessment of blood pressure, eGFR, potassium, and ACR.
- Patients with DN with severe albuminuria and decreased eGFR have poor prognosis and are at higher risk of cardiovascular events and death.
- The 5-yr survival rate of patients with diabetes and ESRD is ~30%.

TABLE 1 Treatment of Diabetic Nephropathy

Stage I	Tight glucose control BP control—consider use of ACE-I or ARB
Stage II	Tight glucose control ACE-I or ARB
	BP control
	Smoking cessation
	Weight reduction
	Exercise
	Annual eye examination
Stage III	ACE-I or ARB BP control
	Restriction of dietary protein (to 0.8 g/kg/day of ideal body weight)
	Antihyperlipidemic medications
Stage IV	Treat manifestations of nephrotic syndrome and chronic renal insufficiency. Prepare for renal replacement therapy, including prevention of abnormalities in calcium and phosphorus metabolism and prevention of anemia by early use of erythropoietin

ACEI, Angiotensin-converting enzyme inhibitor; *ARB,* angiotensin-receptor blocker; *BP,* blood pressure.
From Goldman L, Schafer AI: *Goldman-Cecil medicine,* ed 26, Philadelphia, 2020, Elsevier.

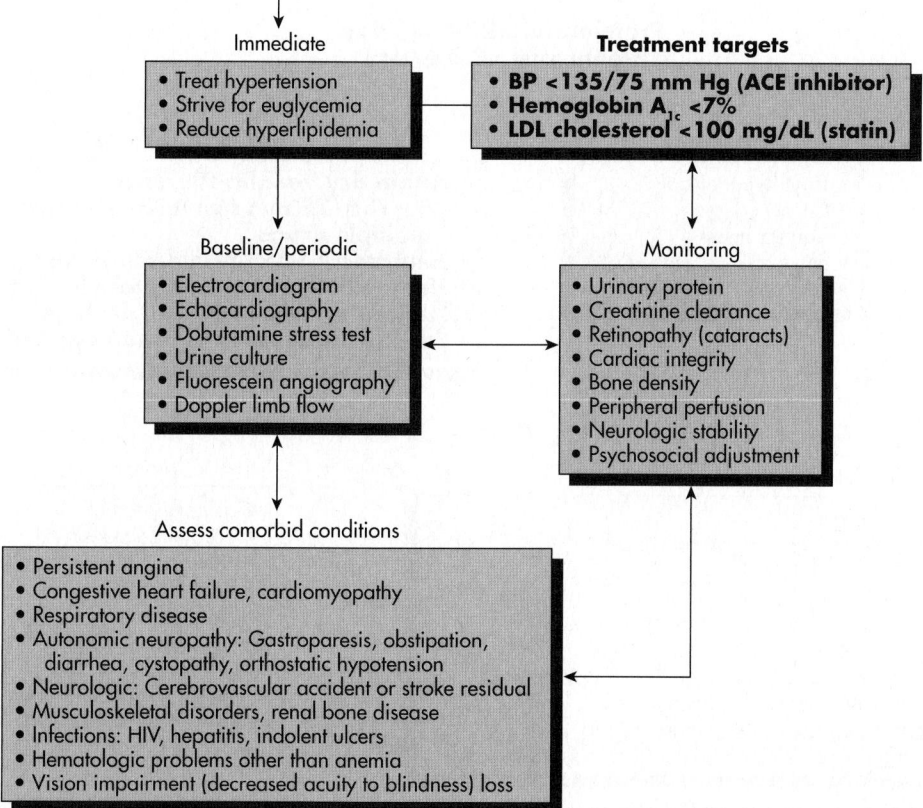

Microalbuminuria: 31–299 mg/day

Immediate
- Treat hypertension
- Strive for euglycemia
- Reduce hyperlipidemia

Treatment targets
- **BP <135/75 mm Hg (ACE inhibitor)**
- **Hemoglobin A$_{1c}$ <7%**
- **LDL cholesterol <100 mg/dL (statin)**

Baseline/periodic
- Electrocardiogram
- Echocardiography
- Dobutamine stress test
- Urine culture
- Fluorescein angiography
- Doppler limb flow

Monitoring
- Urinary protein
- Creatinine clearance
- Retinopathy (cataracts)
- Cardiac integrity
- Bone density
- Peripheral perfusion
- Neurologic stability
- Psychosocial adjustment

Assess comorbid conditions
- Persistent angina
- Congestive heart failure, cardiomyopathy
- Respiratory disease
- Autonomic neuropathy: Gastroparesis, obstipation, diarrhea, cystopathy, orthostatic hypotension
- Neurologic: Cerebrovascular accident or stroke residual
- Musculoskeletal disorders, renal bone disease
- Infections: HIV, hepatitis, indolent ulcers
- Hematologic problems other than anemia
- Vision impairment (decreased acuity to blindness) loss

FIG. 8 Flow chart illustrating the management of diabetic nephropathy before the onset of renal failure. *ACE,* Angiotensin-converting enzyme; *BP,* blood pressure; *HIV,* human immunodeficiency virus; *LDL,* low-density lipoprotein. (From Melmed S et al: *Williams textbook of endocrinology,* ed 14, Philadelphia, 2020, Elsevier.)

Diseases and Disorders

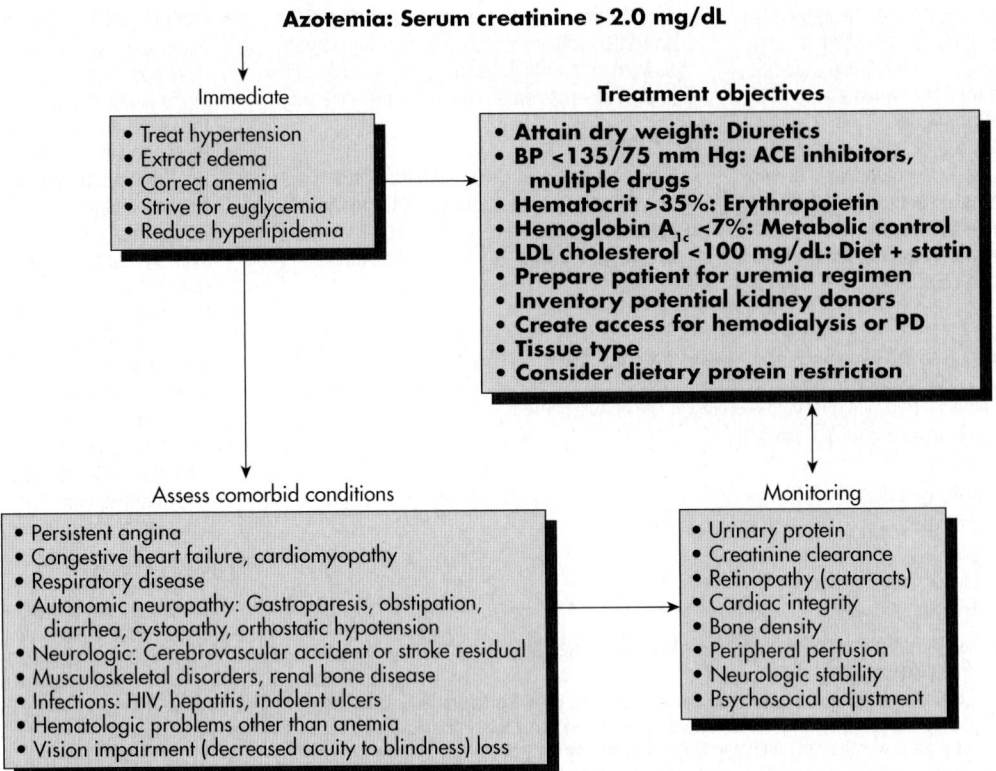

FIG. 9 Flow chart illustrating the management of diabetic nephropathy after onset of renal failure. *ACE,* Angiotensin-converting enzyme; *BP,* blood pressure; *HIV,* human immunodeficiency virus; *LDL,* low-density lipoprotein; *PD,* peritoneal dialysis. (From Melmed S et al: *Williams textbook of endocrinology,* ed 14, Philadelphia, 2020, Elsevier.)

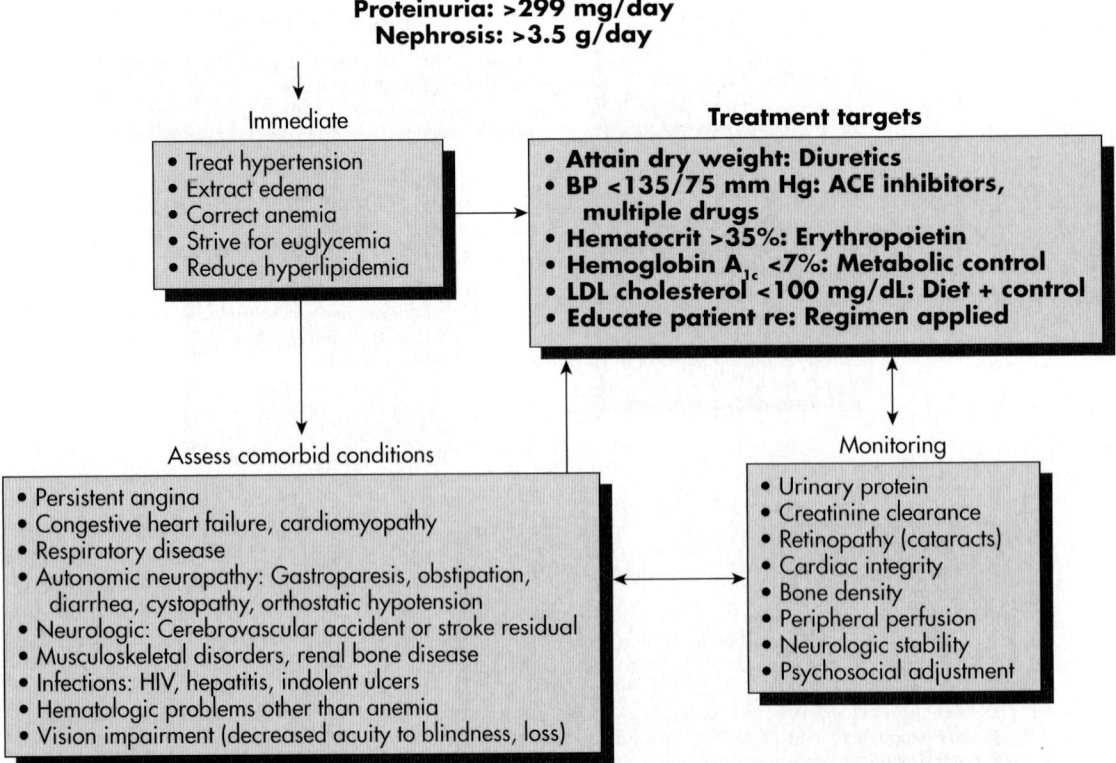

FIG. 10 Flow chart illustrating the management of diabetic nephropathy after the onset of clinical proteinuria. *ACE,* Angiotensin-converting enzyme; *BP,* blood pressure; *HIV,* human immunodeficiency virus; *LDL,* low-density lipoprotein. (From Melmed S et al: *Williams textbook of endocrinology,* ed 14, Philadelphia, 2020, Elsevier.)

TABLE 3 Options in Therapy for End-Stage Renal Disease in Patients with Diabetes

Variable	Peritoneal Dialysis	Hemodialysis	Kidney Transplantation
Extensive extrarenal disease	No limitation	No limitation except for hypotension	Excluded in cardiovascular insufficiency
Geriatric patients	Limited by frailty, cognitive dysfunction; patient treatment satisfaction greater with assisted peritoneal dialysis	No limitation	Arbitrary exclusion as determined by program
Complete rehabilitation	Rare, if ever	Very few patients	Common as long as graft functions
Death rate	Much higher than for nondiabetic patients	Much higher than for nondiabetic patients	About the same as for nondiabetic patients
First-year survival rate	~75%	~75%	>90%
First-year morbidity rate	~15 days in hospital	~12 days in hospital	Weeks to months hospitalized
Survival to second decade	Almost never	<5%	~1 in 5
Progression of complications	Usual and unremitting; hyperglycemia and hyperlipidemia	Usual and unremitting; might benefit from metabolic control	Interdicted by functioning pancreas plus kidney; partially ameliorated by correction of azotemia
Special advantage	Can be self-performed; avoids swings in solute and level of intravascular volume	Can be self-performed; efficient extraction of solute and water in hours	Cures uremia; freedom to travel
Disadvantages	Peritonitis; hyperinsulinemia; hyperglycemia, hyperlipidemia; long hours of treatment; more days hospitalized than with either hemodialysis or transplantation	Blood access a hazard for clotting, hemorrhage, and infection; cyclic hypotension, weakness, aluminum toxicity, amyloidosis	Cosmetic disfigurement, hypertension, personal expense for cytotoxic drugs; induced malignancy; HIV (human immunodeficiency virus) transmission
Patient acceptance	Variable, usual compliance with passive tolerance for regimen	Variable; often noncompliant with dietary, metabolic, or antihypertensive components of regimen	Enthusiastic during periods of good renal allograft function; exalted when pancreas proffers euglycemia
Relative cost	Most expensive over long run	Less expensive than kidney transplantation in the first year; subsequent years more expensive	Pancreas plus kidney engraftment most expensive uremia therapy for diabetics; after first year, kidney transplantation alone is lowest cost option

From Melmed S et al: *Williams textbook of endocrinology*, ed 14, Philadelphia, 2020, Elsevier.

REFERRAL

- Nephrology for CKD management
- Endocrinology for glycemic control
- Podiatry for foot care in the setting of neuropathy/peripheral vascular disease
- Ophthalmology for retinopathy management
- Dietitian for specific dietary counseling

❗ PEARLS & CONSIDERATIONS

- DN is the leading cause of CKD and ESRD worldwide. Early identification and an aggressive multipronged approach toward treatment of DN are key to slow its progression. Timely referral for renal transplant and vascular access evaluation as they progress to ESRD are essential.
- DN is characterized by specific histologic findings; however, the diagnosis usually is made without renal biopsy with the presence of clinical indicators, including long duration of disease (usually >5 yr) and presence of other complications of the disease (albuminuria, retinopathy).
- RAAS blockage is a vital component of DN treatment. After initiation of RAAS blockage, chemistry panel should be monitored in 2 to 4 wk to identify hyperkalemia or acute kidney injury. DN should ideally be monitored every 3 to 6 mo with assessment of blood pressure, eGFR, potassium, and ACR. Contraception should be advised in women at child-bearing age who are receiving ACE-I or ARB therapy and discontinued when pregnant.
- Accuracy of HbA1C as measure of glycemic control declines in advanced CKD (G4-G5) and dialysis. Continuous glucose monitoring or self-monitoring of blood glucose can improve glycemic control in these patients.[6]
- Insulin and many oral diabetes medications are metabolized and cleared by kidneys and need dose adjustment with decline in renal function. Metformin is contraindicated with eGFR <30 ml/min/1.73 m^2 and should be limited to <1000 mg/day in patients with eGFR <45 ml/min/1.73 m^2 because of its association with lactic acidosis. Monitor for vitamin B12 deficiency when on metformin for more than 4 yr. [8]
- SGLT2i and GLP-1 RA have been shown in recent trials to reduce all-cause mortality, cardiovascular mortality, nonfatal myocardial infarction, and kidney failure. SGLT2i can extend benefits in CKD patients even without T2DM. They are preferred as first-line agents along with metformin for glycemic management of diabetic kidney disease.[6,7,10]
- SGLT2i carry a risk of genital mycotic infections and diabetic ketoacidosis. These medications should be withheld during times of prolonged fasting, surgery, and critical illness.
- Transient reduction in eGFR up to 30% with introduction of RASi, SGLT2i, and MRAs should not lead to discontinuations of these medications.
- Diuretic dose reduction should be considered in patients at risk of hypovolemia before SGLT2i initiation.
- Patients with DN are at risk for acute kidney injury and should be counseled to avoid nephrotoxins such as NSAIDs and contrast studies.

PREVENTION

Treatment of risk factors, including blood pressure, blood sugar, and obesity.

PATIENT & FAMILY EDUCATION

Diabetes and Chronic Kidney disease by National Kidney Foundation (http://www.kidney.org/sites/default/files/docs/diabckd_stg5.pdf)

RELATED CONTENT

Diabetes Mellitus (Related Key Topic)

REFERENCES

Available at eBooks.Health.Elsevier.com.

AUTHOR: **YUVRAJ SHARMA, MD**

BASIC INFORMATION

DEFINITION

Diabetic polyneuropathy is a distal symmetric polyneuropathy (DSPN) characterized by numbness, tingling, pain, or weakness that affects the nerves in a stocking-and-glove pattern, beginning in the distal extremities. DSPN leads to substantial pain, morbidity, and impaired quality of life. A number of different classification schemes exist for diabetic neuropathy (Table 1, Box 1)

SYNONYMS

DSPN
Distal symmetric polyneuropathy
Diabetic peripheral neuropathy

ICD-10CM CODES

E11.40	Type 2 diabetes mellitus with diabetic neuropathy, unspecified
E11.41	Type 2 diabetes mellitus with diabetic mononeuropathy
E11.42	Type 2 diabetes mellitus with diabetic polyneuropathy
E11.43	Type 2 diabetes mellitus with diabetic autonomic (poly)neuropathy
E11.44	Type 2 diabetes mellitus with diabetic amyotrophy
E11.49	Type 2 diabetes mellitus with other diabetic neurologic complication

EPIDEMIOLOGY & DEMOGRAPHICS

PREVALENCE: The prevalence of diabetic polyneuropathy varies from approximately 5% to 100% in patients with diabetes mellitus in population-based studies. It is the most common form of peripheral neuropathy in the Western world.[1]
RISK FACTORS: Patients with poor glycemic control; other features of metabolic syndrome, such as hypertension, hypertriglyceridemia, and obesity; diabetic nephropathy; or retinopathy are at increased risk.[1]

PHYSICAL FINDINGS & CLINICAL PRESENTATION

- Patients most commonly experience numbness and tingling, but they may also experience either feelings of tightness or a sensation of heat or cold.[2]
- Pain is common, is often worst at night, and can be burning, aching, shooting, or lancinating in nature.[2]
- Sensory symptoms begin in the feet and may slowly ascend over months to years. Symptoms in the hands do not generally occur until symptoms in the lower extremities have reached the level of the knees. In more severe cases, the symptoms can spread to the trunk and head.[2]
- Neurologic examination reveals early loss of small-fiber modalities resulting in decreased pinprick and temperature sensation and later involvement of large-fiber modalities leading to a reduction in vibratory and proprioceptive sensation. Ankle reflexes are usually reduced or absent, and more proximal reflexes may also become involved as the neuropathy progresses. Strength is usually normal, but there can be some motor involvement leading to mild weakness and atrophy, which is usually limited to intrinsic foot muscles and ankle dorsiflexors.

ETIOLOGY

The precise etiology is unknown but most likely involves a complex interaction of metabolic derangements and microvascular insults occurring in the setting of diabetes.

DIAGNOSIS

DIFFERENTIAL DIAGNOSIS

Although diabetes is the leading cause of peripheral neuropathy in developed countries, there are numerous other causes requiring further investigation(s).

WORKUP

- A thorough history and neurologic examination are essential to confirm features consistent with a diabetic polyneuropathy and exclude other features suggesting alternative diagnoses.
- For some patients, neuropathy may be the presenting feature of previously undiagnosed diabetes.
- Electrodiagnostic evaluation to include nerve conduction studies and electromyography can be helpful in confirming the presence, extent, and severity of a neuropathy.
- Patients with DSPN typically have a reduction of amplitudes and slowing of conduction velocities involving sensory and possibly motor nerves in a length-dependent and symmetric fashion.
- Electromyographic examination of distal muscles may reveal fibrillation potentials, positive sharp waves, and large motor unit action potentials, all suggestive of denervation and reinnervation.
- Electrodiagnostic testing may be negative if the neuropathy is limited to small fiber involvement.
- Neither skin biopsy nor nerve biopsy is necessary in the vast majority of cases.
- Fig. 1 describes a diagnosis and treatment algorithm of diabetic autonomic neuropathy.

LABORATORY TESTS

- Fasting blood sugar, hemoglobin A1c, and 2-h oral glucose tolerance tests should all be considered in patients with peripheral neuropathy without a known history of diabetes.
- A focused laboratory evaluation for other common or potentially treatable causes of neuropathy is also indicated: CBC, comprehensive metabolic panel to include electrolytes and liver function tests, vitamin B_{12} and folate levels, thyroid function tests, serum protein electrophoresis with immunofixation.
- Additional laboratory tests can be considered, based on either history or exam findings suggesting other underlying diagnoses, such as antinuclear antibodies, extractable nuclear antigens, antineutrophil cytoplasmic antibodies, rheumatoid factor, HIV, hepatitis B and C, and cryoglobulins.

IMAGING STUDIES

Imaging is not necessary unless there is concern for an alternative or coexisting process based on the history and examination.

TABLE 1 Clinical Symptoms and Signs of DSPN

	Large Myelinated Nerve Fibers	Small Nerve Fibers
Function	Pressure, balance	Nociception; protective sensation
Symptoms	Numbness Tingling Poor balance	Pain: Burning Electric shocks Stabbing pain
Examination (clinically diagnostic)	Ankle reflexes Reduced Abolished Vibration perception* Reduced Absent 10-g monofilament* Reduced Absent Proprioception impaired	Thermal (cold/hot) discrimination* Reduced Absent Pinprick sensation* Reduced Absent

*Documented impairment/loss of symmetry, as well as a distal to proximal pattern.
From Robertson RP et al: *DeGroot's endocrinology, basic science and clinical practice,* ed 8, Philadelphia, 2023, Elsevier.

BOX 1 Clinical Classification of Diabetic Neuropathies

Symmetric
- Diabetic polyneuropathy
- Diabetic autonomic neuropathy
- Painful diabetic neuropathy

Asymmetric
- Diabetic radiculoplexopathy
- Diabetic thoracic radiculoneuropathy
- Mononeuropathies
- Carpal tunnel syndrome
- Ulnar neuropathy at the elbow
- Peroneal neuropathy at fibular head
- Cranial neuropathies

From Fillit HM: *Brocklehurst's textbook of geriatric medicine and gerontology,* ed 8, Philadelphia, 2017, Elsevier.

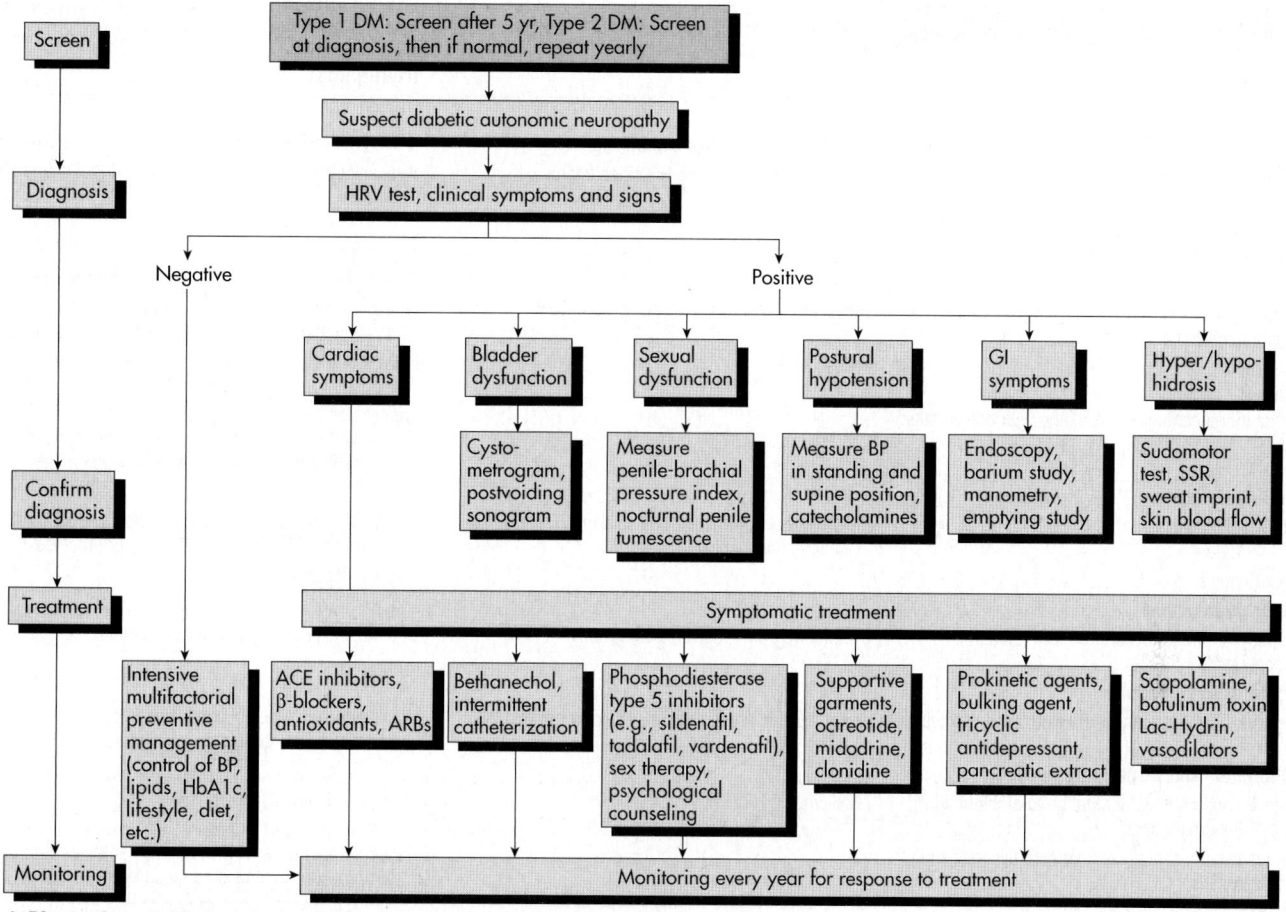

FIG. 1 Diagnosis and treatment algorithm of diabetic autonomic neuropathy. *ACE,* Angiotensin-converting enzyme; *ARBs,* angiotensin receptor blockers; *BP,* blood pressure; *DM,* diabetes mellitus; *GI,* gastrointestinal; *HbA1c,* glycohemoglobin; *HRV,* heart rate variability; *SSR,* sympathetic skin response. (Modified from Larsen PR et al [eds]: *Williams textbook of endocrinology,* ed 11, Philadelphia, 2008, Saunders.)

Rx TREATMENT

CHRONIC Rx

- Table 2 summarizes clinical features, diagnosis, and treatment of diabetic autonomic neuropathy.
- Glycemic control: The primary treatment for diabetic polyneuropathy is effective glycemic control, as this may either improve or at least slow progression of the neuropathy.
- Symptomatic management: Another aspect of treatment is the symptomatic management of pain and paresthesias. The American Academy of Neurology, the American Association of Neuromuscular and Electrodiagnostic Medicine, and the American Academy of Physical Medicine and Rehabilitation have together developed an evidence-based guideline for the treatment of painful diabetic neuropathy. Pregabalin, an anticonvulsant, is the only agent in the guideline that has been established as effective for painful diabetic neuropathy.[3] Other probably effective agents are listed in the following:
  1. Topical agents: Lidocaine 5% patch can be applied to painful areas for 12 h a day, capsaicin 0.075% applied qid
  2. Anticonvulsants: Gabapentin (100 to 1200 mg tid), pregabalin (50 to 100 mg tid), carbamazepine (100 mg bid)
  3. Antidepressants: Amitriptyline (10 to 100 mg qhs), nortriptyline (25 to 150 mg qhs), duloxetine (60 to 120 mg/day)
  4. Tramadol (50 mg qid as needed) can be a useful adjunctive analgesic
- Fig. 2 describes a treatment algorithm for neuropathic pain after exclusion of nondiabetic etiologies and stabilization of glycemic control.

DISPOSITION

The distal sensory loss of diabetic polyneuropathy places patients at increased risk of trauma to the extremities, with the potential for ulceration and infection that could ultimately require amputation if not attended to in a timely fashion.

REFERRAL

- A neurologist can assist in the diagnosis and management of diabetic polyneuropathy.
- Patients with diabetic polyneuropathy should also be evaluated at least annually by a podiatrist and ophthalmologist.
- Progression of diabetic polyneuropathy can be minimized by paying close attention to strict glycemic control as well as other risk factors such as hypertension and obesity.

! PEARLS & CONSIDERATIONS

COMMENTS

- For many patients, either DSPN or another form of diabetic neuropathy may be the initial presentation of previously undiagnosed diabetes.
- In addition to regular visits with podiatry, patients with diabetic polyneuropathy should be educated on aggressive foot hygiene and the importance of examining their own feet.
- Cannabidiol (CBD) use for reduction of chronic pain has markedly increased over the past decade, but overall quality of evidence in patients with painful neuropathy remains low.[4]

PATIENT & FAMILY EDUCATION

The following website is recommended: https://www.mayoclinic.com/health/diabetic-neuropathy/DS01045

REFERENCES

Available at eBooks.Health.Elsevier.com.

AUTHOR: **LYDIA SHARP, MD**

TABLE 2 Clinical Features, Diagnosis, and Treatment of Diabetic Autonomic Neuropathy

Symptoms	Tests	Treatments
Cardiac		
Resting tachycardia, exercise intolerance	HRV, MUGA thallium scan, MIBG scan	Graded supervised exercise, ACE inhibitors, β-blockers
Postural hypotension, dizziness, weakness, fatigue, syncope	HRV, supine and standing BP, catecholamines	Mechanical measures, clonidine, midodrine, octreotide, erythropoietin
Gastrointestinal		
Gastroparesis, erratic glucose control	Gastric emptying study, barium study	Frequent small meals, prokinetic agents (metoclopramide, domperidone, erythromycin)
Abdominal pain, early satiety, nausea, vomiting, bloating, belching	Endoscopy, manometry, electrogastrogram	Antibiotics, antiemetics, bulking agents, tricyclic antidepressants, pyloric botulinum toxin, gastric pacing
Constipation	Endoscopy	High-fiber diet, bulking agents, osmotic laxatives, lubricating agents
Diarrhea (often nocturnal alternating with constipation)		Soluble fiber, gluten and lactose restriction, anticholinergic agents, cholestyramine, antibiotics, somatostatin, pancreatic enzyme supplements
Sexual Dysfunction		
Erectile dysfunction	H&P, HRV, penile-brachial pressure index, nocturnal penile tumescence	Sex therapy, psychological counseling, phosphodiesterase inhibitors, PGE_1 injections, devices or prostheses
Vaginal dryness		Vaginal lubricants
Bladder Dysfunction		
Frequency, urgency, nocturia, urinary retention, incontinence	Cystometrogram, postvoid sonography	Bethanechol, intermittent catheterization
Sudomotor Dysfunction		
Anhidrosis, heat intolerance, dry skin, hyperhidrosis	Quantitative sudomotor axon reflex, sweat test, skin blood flow	Emollients and skin lubricants, scopolamine, glycopyrrolate, botulinum toxin, vasodilators
Pupillomotor and Visceral Dysfunction		
Blurred vision, impaired adaptation to ambient light, Argyll-Robertson pupil	Pupillometry, HRV	Care with driving at night
Impaired visceral sensation: Silent MI, hypoglycemia unawareness		Recognition of unusual presentation of MI, control of risk factors, control of plasma glucose levels

ACE, Acetylcholinesterase; *BP,* blood pressure; *H&P,* history and physical examination; *HRV,* heart rate variability; *MI,* myocardial infarction; *MIBG,* metaiodobenzylguanidine; *MUGA,* multigated angiography; *PGE*1, prostaglandin E_1.
From Melmed S et al: *Williams textbook of endocrinology,* ed 12, Philadelphia, 2011, Saunders.

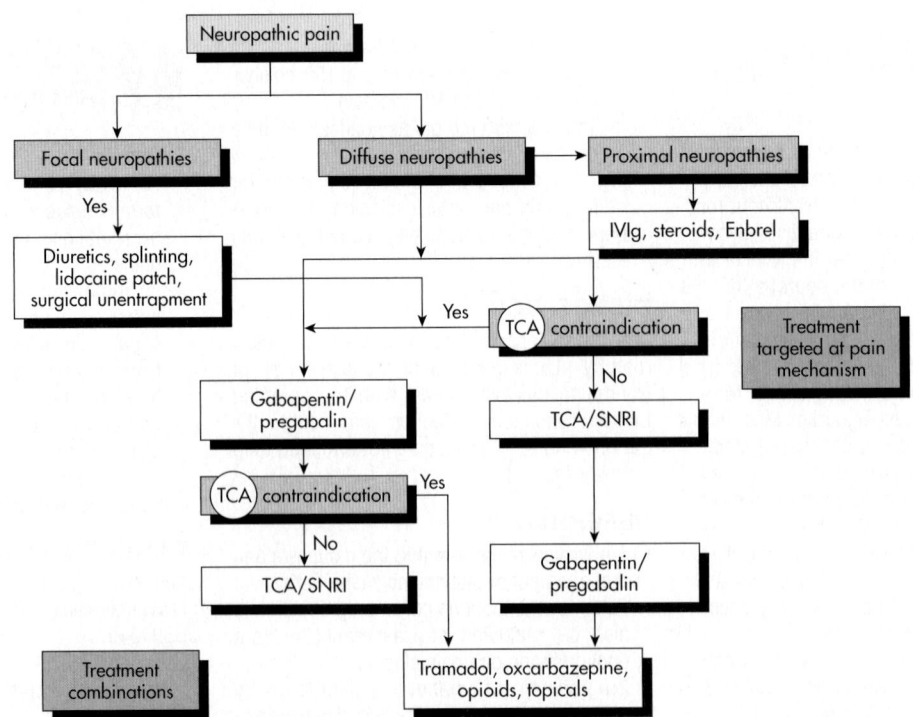

FIG. 2 Treatment algorithm for neuropathic pain after exclusion of nondiabetic etiologies and stabilization of glycemic control. *IVIg,* Intravenous immune globulin; *SNRI,* serotonin-norepinephrine reuptake inhibitors; *TCA,* tricyclic antidepressants. (From Melmed S et al: *Williams textbook of endocrinology,* ed 12, Philadelphia, 2011, Saunders.)

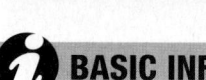 **BASIC INFORMATION**

DEFINITION

Diabetic retinopathy (Fig. 1) is a microvascular abnormality of the retina resulting in microaneurysms (Fig. E2), retinal hemorrhages, lipid exudates (Fig. E3), macular edema, and neovascular vessel growth (Fig. E4) and can ultimately end in blindness. Diabetic retinopathy can be classified into two stages: Nonproliferative (mild, moderate, and severe) and proliferative. A glossary and abbreviations pertinent to diabetic eye disease are described in Table E1.

SYNONYMS

Nonproliferative diabetic retinopathy (NPDR)
Proliferative diabetic retinopathy (PDR)
Diabetic macular edema (DME)

ICD-10CM CODES

E08.311	Diabetes mellitus due to underlying condition with unspecified diabetic retinopathy with macular edema
E08.319	Diabetes mellitus due to underlying condition with unspecified diabetic retinopathy without macular edema
E08.321	Diabetes mellitus due to underlying condition with mild nonproliferative diabetic retinopathy with macular edema
E08.329	Diabetes mellitus due to underlying condition with mild nonproliferative diabetic retinopathy without macular edema
E08.331	Diabetes mellitus due to underlying condition with moderate nonproliferative diabetic retinopathy with macular edema
E08.339	Diabetes mellitus due to underlying condition with moderate nonproliferative diabetic retinopathy without macular edema
E08.341	Diabetes mellitus due to underlying condition with severe nonproliferative diabetic retinopathy with macular edema
E08.349	Diabetes mellitus due to underlying condition with severe nonproliferative diabetic retinopathy without macular edema
E08.351	Diabetes mellitus due to underlying condition with proliferative diabetic retinopathy with macular edema
E08.359	Diabetes mellitus due to underlying condition with proliferative diabetic retinopathy without macular edema

EPIDEMIOLOGY & DEMOGRAPHICS

INCIDENCE (IN U.S.):
- After 20 yr of diabetes mellitus, nearly 99% of patients with type 1 and 60% with type 2 disease demonstrate some degree of diabetic retinopathy.
- A leading preventable cause of blindness in the U.S. between the ages of 20 and 74 yr.
- There are approximately 8000 new cases of diabetic retinopathy–induced blindness each year in the U.S.

PREVALENCE (IN U.S.):
- Prevalence of retinopathy increases with duration of diabetes. Found in 18% of people diagnosed with diabetes for 3- to 4-yr duration and in up to 80% of diabetics with a diagnosis of ≥15 yr.
- In the U.S., the prevalence of diabetic macular edema (the most common cause of vision impairment) is 4%, or approximately 750,000 people.
- Prevalence of diabetic retinopathy in patients 40 and older is 28.5%, or approximately 4.4 million people.
- The number of Americans with diabetic retinopathy is expected to nearly double, from 7.7 million to over 13 million between 2010 and 2050. Expected to triple in the Hispanic population.
- A significant proportion of people live with undiagnosed diabetes.

PREDOMINANT SEX: Males and females affected equally.
PREDOMINANT AGE: ≥30 yr.
GENETICS:
- The development of diabetes involves the interaction of genetic and nongenetic factors.
- Type 1 has an autoimmune basis, resulting in destruction of beta islet cells and has strong human leukocyte antigen associations.

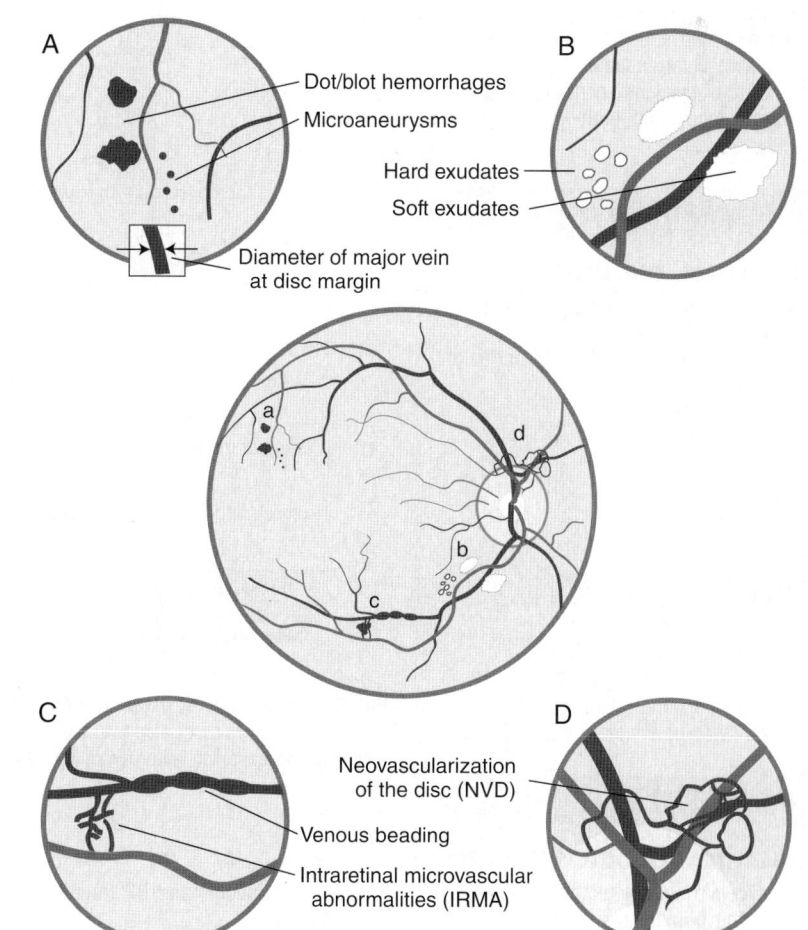

FIG. 1 Types of diabetic retinopathy. The center figure depicting the fundus of a patient with diabetic retinopathy is surrounded by four enlarged views, each labeled with a letter *(a to d)* corresponding to specific locations on the center figure. **A,** Microaneurysms and dot and blot hemorrhages. The diameter of microaneurysms is less than the width of a major vein at the disc margin (reproduced in *square inset*). **B,** Hard and soft exudates. **C,** Venous beading and intraretinal microvascular abnormalities *(IRMA)*. **D,** Neovascularization, which may be located within one disc diameter of the optic disc *(NVD)* or elsewhere (NVE). Although both IRMA and neovascularization represent the formation of new blood vessels, IRMA are confined to the layers of the retina, whereas neovascularization is on the inner surface of the retina or vitreous. (From McGee S: *Evidence-based physical diagnosis*, ed 4, Philadelphia, 2018, Elsevier.)

- Type 2 has genetic predisposition, but the specific genes are not yet well characterized.

PHYSICAL FINDINGS & CLINICAL PRESENTATION

- Microaneurysms
- Hemorrhages
- Cotton-wool spots
- Lipid exudates
- Macular edema
- Neovascularization
- Retinal detachment (in advanced cases)
- Vitreous hemorrhage
- In early cases, patient may not report a visual disturbance

ETIOLOGY

Prolonged hyperglycemia results in basement membrane thickening in retinal capillaries with subsequent loss of pericytes and endothelial decompensation resulting in breakdown of the blood–retina barrier and capillary occlusion, ischemia, and serum leakage (Fig. 5). This leads to the clinical findings of dot hemorrhages, microaneurysms, lipid exudate, and edema. Upregulation of vascular endothelial growth factor (VEGF) and other cytokines contributes to vascular incompetence and promotes growth of neovascular tissue.

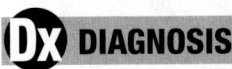 **DIAGNOSIS**

DIFFERENTIAL DIAGNOSIS

- Branch or central retinal vein occlusion
- Hypertensive retinopathy
- Ocular ischemic syndrome (carotid occlusion)
- Radiation retinopathy
- Retinal macroaneurysm
- Sickle cell retinopathy
- Valsalva retinopathy
- Lupus
- Retinal vasculitis
- Terson syndrome

WORKUP

- Fundus photography
- Optical coherence tomography
- Optical coherence angiography
- Fluorescein angiogram (Fig. E6)
- Laboratory workup if indicated based on DDx

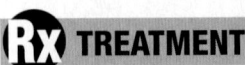 **TREATMENT**

NONPHARMACOLOGIC THERAPY

- Tight glycemic control remains the cornerstone in the primary prevention of diabetic retinopathy, particularly in type 1 as seen in the Diabetes Control and Complications Trial (DCCT) and less so in type 2 as seen in the United Kingdom Prospective Diabetes Study (UKPDS) and more recently in the Action to Control Cardiovascular Risk in Diabetes Trial (ACCORD). ADA guidelines recommend A1c <7.0.
- Intensive lowering of blood pressure was shown in UKPDS but not ACCORD to reduce progression of diabetic retinopathy. ADA guidelines recommend BP target of <140/90 mm Hg.
- Lipid lowering results in reduction of retinopathy progression (ACCORD Trial).
- Laser treatment (photocoagulation) for proliferative disease or noncenter involving macular edema. The International Classification of Diabetic Macular Edema (DME) is described in Table E2.
- Table 3 summarizes classification and management of diabetic retinopathy. A diabetic retinopathy and macular edema examination and treatment flow chart for nonpregnant patients is illustrated in Fig. E7 and Fig. E8 for pregnant patients.

ACUTE GENERAL Rx

- Intravitreal pharmacotherapy with anti-VEGF agents (e.g., bevacizumab, ranibizumab, aflibercept, brolucizumab, and faricimab) and/or corticosteroids is the standard of care for patients with center-involved diabetic macular edema.
- Bevacizumab is not FDA-approved for diabetic retinopathy but is the least costly and most commonly used initial treatment. In a

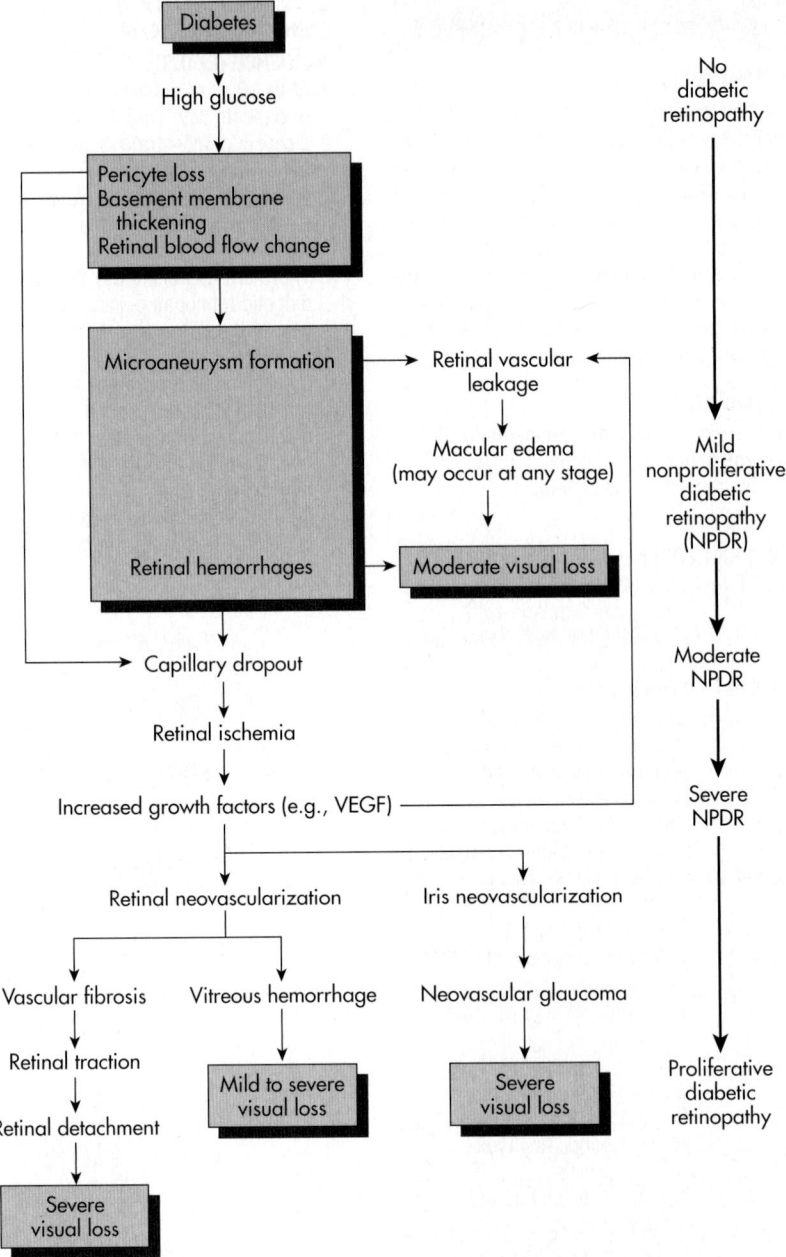

FIG. 5 Pathogenesis of diabetic retinopathy. This schematic flow chart represents the major preclinical and clinical findings associated with the full spectrum of diabetic retinopathy and macular edema. *VEGF,* Vascular endothelial growth factor. (From Melmed S et al: *Williams textbook of endocrinology,* ed 14, Philadelphia, 2020, Elsevier.)

TABLE 3 Abbreviated Early Treatment Diabetic Retinopathy Study (ETDRS) Classification of Diabetic Retinopathy

Category/Description	Management
Nonproliferative diabetic retinopathy (NPDR)	
No DR	Review in 12 mo
Very mild NPDR	Review most patients in 12 mo
Microaneurysms only	
Mild NPDR	
Any or all of: Microaneurysms, retinal hemorrhages, exudates, cotton wool spots, up to the level of moderate NPDR. No intraretinal microvascular anomalies (IRMA) or significant beading	Review range 6-12 mo, depending on severity of signs, stability, systemic factors, and patient's personal circumstances
Moderate NPDR	
• Severe retinal hemorrhages (more than ETDRS standard photograph 2A: About 20 medium to large per quadrant) in 1-3 quadrants or mild IRMA	Review in approximately 6 mo
• Significant venous beading can be present in no more than 1 quadrant	Proliferative diabetic retinopathy (PDR) in up to 26%, high-risk PDR in up to 8% within a year
• Cotton wool spots commonly present	
Severe NPDR	
The 4–2–1 rule; one or more of:	Review in 4 mo
• Severe hemorrhages in all 4 quadrants	PDR in up to 50%, high-risk PDR in up to 15% within a year
• Significant venous beading in 2 or more quadrants	Consider panretinal photocoagulation
• Moderate IRMA in 1 or more quadrants	
Very severe NPDR	
Two or more of the criteria for severe NPDR	Review in 2-3 mo
	High-risk PDR in up to 45% within a year
Proliferative diabetic retinopathy (PDR)	
Mild–moderate PDR	
New vessels on the disc (NVD) or new vessels elsewhere (NVE), but extent insufficient to meet the high-risk criteria	Treatment considered according to severity of signs, stability, systemic factors, and patient's personal circumstances such as reliability of attendance for review. If not treated, review in up to 2 mo
High-risk PDR	
• New vessels on the disc (NVD) greater than ETDRS standard photograph 10A (about 1/3 disc area)	Treatment advised (see text)
• Any NVD with vitreous hemorrhage	Should be performed immediately when possible, and certainly same day if symptomatic presentation with good retinal view
• NVE greater than 1/2 disc area with vitreous hemorrhage	

DR, Diabetic retinopathy.
From Bowling B: *Kanski's clinical ophthalmology, a systematic approach,* ed 8, Philadelphia, 2016, Elsevier.

trial of treatment of moderate vision loss due to diabetic macular edema involving the center of the macula, there was no significant difference in visual outcomes over a 2-yr period between aflibercept monotherapy and treatment with bevacizumab first with a switch to aflibercept in case of a suboptimal response.[1]
• Corticosteroid is generally reserved for anti-VEGF-resistant macular edema.
• Laser therapy: Panretinal laser photocoagulation (Fig. E9) reduces the risk of severe visual loss in patients with proliferative retinopathy.
• Focal laser reduces risk of moderate visual loss by 50% in patients with clinically significant macular edema.
• Vitrectomy for traction retinal detachment or vitreous hemorrhage.

CHRONIC Rx
• Monthly anti-VEGF injections until macular edema has resolved followed by extension of interval and close monitoring with optical coherence tomography
• Both ranibizumab (Lucentis) and aflibercept (Eylea) have been FDA-approved for treatment of diabetic retinopathy in patients with macular edema

• Repeated laser treatments may be necessary
• Diet and exercise; good medical control of disease, blood pressure, and cholesterol

DISPOSITION
• Retinal examination should be performed on all routine medical visits. Referral if abnormality seen.
• Routine annual eye examination in all patients with diabetes.

• Prognosis is improved with early diagnosis and treatment.
• Recommendations for primary care providers regarding eye care for diabetic patients are summarized in Table 4.

REFERRAL
Refer to ophthalmologist immediately on finding retinal abnormality to institute early treatment.

TABLE 4 Recommendations for Eye Care for Diabetic Patients

Primary care physician informs the patient at the time of diagnosis of diabetes that:
• Ocular complications are associated with diabetes and may threaten sight
• Timely detection and treatment may reduce the risk for decreased vision
Referral to an eye doctor competent in diabetes eye care:
• All patients 10-30 yr of age who have had diabetes for 5 or more years
• In patients in whom diabetes was diagnosed when older than 30 yr of age, examination at the time of diagnosis or shortly thereafter
Referral to an ophthalmologist:
• All women with insulin-dependent diabetes mellitus planning pregnancy within 12 mo, in the first trimester, and thereafter at the discretion of the ophthalmologist
• Patients found to have reduced corrected visual acuity, elevated intraocular pressure, and any other vision-threatening ocular abnormalities

From Robertson RP et al: *DeGroot's endocrinology, basic science and clinical practice,* ed 8, Philadelphia, 2023, Elsevier.

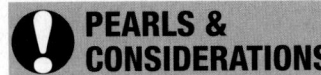

! PEARLS & CONSIDERATIONS

COMMENTS

- Early treatment of severe nonproliferative and proliferative retinopathy may minimize complications and visual loss.
- Tight blood sugar control in type 1 patients significantly reduces the probability of developing new-onset retinopathy as well as progression of existing retinopathy.
- Retinopathy is an independent risk marker for cardiovascular disease in patients with type 2 DM.
- Presence and severity of diabetic retinopathy correlates with diabetic nephropathy. Proliferative diabetic retinopathy in particular is a significant independent marker of incident nephropathy.

REFERENCE & SUGGESTED READINGS

Available at eBooks.Health.Elsevier.com.

RELATED CONTENT

Diabetic Retinopathy (Patient Information)
Diabetes Mellitus (Related Key Topic)

AUTHOR: **ROBERT H. JANIGIAN JR., MD**

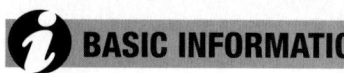

BASIC INFORMATION

DEFINITION

Disseminated intravascular coagulation (DIC) is an acquired thromboembolic disorder characterized by generalized activation of the clotting pathways, which results in the intravascular formation of fibrin and, ultimately, thrombotic occlusion of small and midsize vessels, resulting in end-organ damage.

SYNONYMS

Consumptive coagulopathy
DIC
Defibrination syndrome

ICD-10CM CODE
D65   Disseminated intravascular coagulation [defibrination syndrome]

EPIDEMIOLOGY & DEMOGRAPHICS

About 1% of hospitalized patients may have evidence of DIC. There is no predilection for age or gender. More than 50% of cases are associated with gram-negative sepsis or other septicemic infections, and up to 35% of patients with severe sepsis have DIC.

PHYSICAL FINDINGS & CLINICAL PRESENTATION

DIC occurs in acute and chronic forms and can present with bleeding, thrombosis, or laboratory evidence of clotting cascade activation and fibrinolysis without evident clinical sequelae. Acute DIC is more common and predominantly manifests as bleeding complications. The risk of bleeding increases with worsening thrombocytopenia and is fivefold higher when the platelet count is below $<50 \times 10^9$/liter. Sudden procoagulant exposure can prompt coagulation cascade activation and platelet consumption, resulting in thrombosis. In contrast, chronic DIC more frequently causes thrombotic complications. The diagnosis of chronic DIC can be challenging, as the PT and PTT are often normal. Multiple pathways are involved in DIC pathophysiology, ultimately leading to consumptive coagulopathy and thrombosis. These include (1) thrombin generation due to the release of tissue factor or other procoagulants, (2) suppression of physiologic anticoagulant (e.g., protein C/S or antithrombin insufficiency), (3) impaired fibrinolysis characterized by an increased level of plasminogen activator inhibitor type 1 (PAI-1) and fibrin degradation products, and (4) activation of inflammatory pathways.

Multiple organs may be involved with DIC, and clinical presentations may vary. They can include:
- Central nervous system: Altered mental status, transient neurologic deficits
- Cardiovascular: Hypotension, tachycardia
- Respiratory: Hypoxia, dyspnea, localized rales, and acute respiratory distress syndrome
- GI: Intestinal bleeding, bowel infarction
- Genitourinary: Oliguria, anuria, uremia, acidosis, metrorrhagia
- Skin: Wound site bleeding, epistaxis, gingival bleeding, hemorrhagic bullae, petechiae, ecchymosis, purpura, skin necrosis

ETIOLOGY

DIC results from the aberrant and generalized activation of the clotting system, resulting in simultaneous formulation of coagulation and fibrinolysis. As a result of increased thrombus generation in the small and medium vessels, clotting factors and platelets are consumed more rapidly than the synthetic function of the liver and bone marrow, respectively. Diseases associated with DIC are summarized in Box E1. Severe infection is the most common inciting etiology; an extensive list of other triggers is known, including:
- Infections (e.g., gram-negative sepsis, Rocky Mountain spotted fever, COVID-19, malaria, viral or fungal infection)
- Obstetric complications (e.g., fetal demise, amniotic fluid embolism, toxemia, abruptio placentae, septic abortion, preeclampsia/eclampsia, placenta previa, uterine atony)
- Tissue trauma (e.g., polytrauma, burns, hypothermia rewarming)
- Malignancy (e.g., adenocarcinomas [GI, prostate, lung, breast], especially mucin-producing cancers, lymphoproliferative/myeloproliferative; DIC is a hallmark of acute promyelocytic leukemia and a leading cause of mortality)
- Quinine, cocaine-induced rhabdomyolysis
- Liver failure
- Acute pancreatitis
- Transfusion reactions
- Respiratory distress syndrome
- Toxins (snake bites, amphetamine overdose)
- Other: Systemic lupus erythematosus (SLE), vasculitis, aneurysms, polyarteritis, hemangiomas with thrombocytopenia, and consumptive coagulopathy (Kasabach-Merritt syndrome)

DIAGNOSIS

DIFFERENTIAL DIAGNOSIS

- Hepatic necrosis: Normal or elevated factor VIII concentrations
- Vitamin K deficiency: Normal platelet count
- Hemolytic uremic syndrome: Coagulation assays are usually normal
- Thrombotic thrombocytopenic purpura: Low ADAMTS13 activity
- Renal failure, SLE, sickle cell crisis, dysfibrinogenemia
- HELLP syndrome (**h**emolysis, **e**levated **l**iver function tests, and **l**ow **p**latelets)
- COVID-19 related coagulopathy: Elevated fibrinogen, SARS-CoV-2 PCR positive

WORKUP

The diagnostic workup includes laboratory testing to characterize the coagulopathy and its severity and exclude conditions noted in the differential diagnosis (Table 1, Box 2). Additional workup is guided by the clinical scenario and may include distinguishing DIC progression (acute vs. chronic), chief manifestations (thrombotic or hemorrhagic), and extent (localized or systemic).

LABORATORY TESTS

- Peripheral blood smear generally shows red blood cell fragments (schistocytes) and low platelet counts.
- Coagulation testing: Diagnostic characteristics of DIC are decreased fibrinogen level, thrombocytopenia; and increased prothrombin time (PT), partial thromboplastin time (PTT), thrombin time (TT), fibrin split products, and D-dimer.
- Coagulopathy secondary to DIC must be differentiated from other coagulopathies that result from the underproduction of clotting factors, including liver disease or vitamin K deficiency.
  1. Vitamin K deficiency manifests with prolonged PT but normal PTT, TT, platelet, and

TABLE 1   Differential Diagnosis of Prolonged aPTT and PT in Suspected Disseminated Intravascular Coagulation

Test Result	Cause
PT prolonged, aPTT normal	Factor VII deficiency Mild vitamin K deficiency Mild liver insufficiency Low doses of vitamin K antagonists
PT normal, aPTT prolonged	Factor VIII, IX, or XI deficiency Unfractionated heparin Inhibitory antibody and/or antiphospholipid antibody Factor XII or prekallikrein deficiency
Both PT and aPTT prolonged	Factor X, V, II, or fibrinogen deficiency Severe vitamin K deficiency Vitamin K antagonists Global clotting factor deficiency Decreased synthesis: Liver failure Increased loss: Massive bleeding, DIC

aPTT, Activated partial thromboplastin time; *DIC,* disseminated intravascular coagulation; *PT,* prothrombin time.
From Hoffman R et al: *Hematology: basic principles and practice,* ed 8, Philadelphia, 2023, Elsevier.

fibrinogen levels; PTT may be elevated in severe cases.
2. Patients with liver disease have abnormal PT and PTT; TT and fibrinogen are usually normal unless severe disease is present; platelets are typically normal unless splenomegaly is present.
3. Factor VIII is not synthesized exclusively by the liver. It can differentiate between DIC, where it is low, and coagulopathy of liver disease, where it is normal or elevated.

IMAGING STUDIES

Imaging studies are generally not helpful. Imaging may help identify sequelae of DIC, including chest radiographs to exclude infectious processes in patients with pulmonary symptoms such as dyspnea, cough, or hemoptysis.

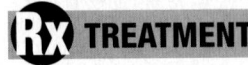 **TREATMENT**

ACUTE GENERAL Rx

- Correcting and eliminating the underlying cause is often sufficient to halt DIC (e.g., antimicrobial therapy for infection, removal of necrotic bowel, evacuation of uterus in obstetric emergencies).
- Patients with bleeding should be given replacement therapy with fresh frozen plasma (FFP) and platelets:
   1. FFP 10 to 15 ml/kg can normalize the international normalized ratio.
   2. Platelet transfusions are given when the platelet count is <10,000 (or higher if significant bleeding is present).
   3. Cryoprecipitate 1 U/5 kg is given for low fibrinogen. It can also be provided for preventing bleeding in patients with fibrinogen levels <100 mg/dl.
- Patients with extensive thrombosis (e.g., in acute promyelocytic leukemia, purpura fulminans, acral ischemia) require anticoagulation despite thrombocytopenia and abnormal coagulation parameters. Heparin therapy using unfractionated heparin with a lower PTT goal than is used in venous thrombosis may be helpful to increase the neutralization of thrombin. Low-molecular-weight heparin also may be used in this scenario.

- The mainstays of supportive treatment of DIC are summarized in Box E3.

DISPOSITION

The mortality rate in severe DIC exceeds 75%. The high mortality rate is often due to the severity of the underlying trigger and complications, including acute renal failure, intracerebral bleeding, shock, or cardiac tamponade.

REFERRAL

Hematology consultation is recommended in all cases of severe DIC and DIC with hemorrhagic or thrombotic complications.

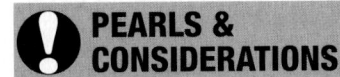 **PEARLS & CONSIDERATIONS**

COMMENTS

The treatment of chronic DIC is controversial. Low-dose subcutaneous heparin and/or combination antiplatelet agents such as aspirin and dipyridamole may be helpful.

RELATED CONTENT

Disseminated Intravascular Coagulation (Patient Information)

AUTHORS: **SOHAIP KABASHNEH, MD** and **PATAN GULTAWATVICHAI, MD**

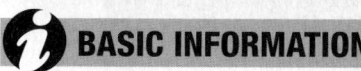
BASIC INFORMATION

DEFINITION

- Colonic diverticula are herniations of mucosa and submucosa[1] through the muscularis (Fig. E1). They are generally found along the colon's mesenteric border at the site where the vasa recta penetrates the muscle wall (anatomic weak point).
- *Diverticulosis* is the asymptomatic presence of multiple colonic diverticula (Fig. E2).
- *Diverticulitis* is an inflammatory process or localized perforation of diverticulum.

SYNONYMS

Diverticulosis
Diverticulitis
Diverticular hemorrhage

ICD-10CM CODES
K57.30   Diverticulosis of large intestine without perforation or abscess without bleeding
K57.32   Diverticulitis of large intestine without perforation or abscess without bleeding
K57.31   Diverticulosis of large intestine without perforation or abscess with bleeding

EPIDEMIOLOGY & DEMOGRAPHICS

- Incidence of diverticulosis in the general population is 35% to 50%. Prevalence of diverticulosis increases with ages (<10% under age 40 to over 50% in those >85).
- Diverticulosis is more common in Western countries, affecting >30% of people >40 yr and >50% of people >70 yr.
- Approximately 20% of patients with diverticula have an episode of diverticulitis.

PHYSICAL FINDINGS & CLINICAL PRESENTATION

- Physical examination in patients with diverticulosis is generally normal.
- Painful diverticular disease can present with left lower quadrant (LLQ) pain, often relieved by defecation; location of pain may be anywhere in the lower abdomen because of the redundancy of the sigmoid colon.
- An estimated 10% to 16% of patients with acute diverticulitis present with complicated disease (i.e., abscess or fistula formulation, perforation, or hemorrhage).
- Diverticulitis can cause muscle spasm, guarding, and rebound tenderness predominantly affecting the LLQ. Factors associated with diverticulitis are pain localized to left lower quadrant and exacerbated by movement, left-lower-quadrant tenderness on examination, fever 38.5° C (101.3° F) or higher, absence of vomiting, age >50 yr, and history of one or more episodes of diverticulitis.

ETIOLOGY

- Diverticular disease is believed to be secondary to low intake of dietary fiber.

- There are reports of a pathogenetic role for inflammation in diverticulitis that may be similar to that of irritable bowel syndrome (IBS), inflammatory bowel disease (IBD), or both, based on common histologic findings such as granulomas, infiltrating lymphocytes, tumor necrosis factor (TNF), histamine, and matrix metalloproteinases.

DIAGNOSIS

DIFFERENTIAL DIAGNOSIS

- IBS
- IBD
- Colorectal cancer
- Endometriosis
- Ischemic colitis
- Bowel obstruction/volvulus
- Urinary tract disorders (urolithiasis, hydronephrosis)
- Infections (pseudomembranous colitis, appendicitis, pyelonephritis, pelvic inflammatory disease [PID])
- Lactose intolerance
- Celiac disease
- Epiploic appendagitis
- Gynecologic disorders (ectopic pregnancy, menstrual irregularities, dyspareunia, endometriosis)
- Cholecystitis, biliary disease

LABORATORY TESTS

- White blood cell (WBC) count in diverticulitis reveals leukocytosis with left shift.
- Microcytic anemia can be present in patients with chronic bleeding from diverticular disease. Mean corpuscular volume (MCV) may be elevated in acute bleeding secondary to reticulocytosis.
- Urinalysis is useful to exclude urinary causes of pain.
- Pregnancy test is indicated in women of child-bearing age.
- Electrolytes and liver enzymes are useful in ruling out biliary causes of pain.
- C reactive protein (CRP) levels of 50 mg/L or greater is common in acute diverticulitis.

PROCEDURES: Colonoscopy should be avoided during acute diverticulitis due to the risk of perforation. It can generally be performed after 6 wk to rule out the presence of cancer and IBD. The American College of Physicians (ACP) does not recommend colonoscopy for those with uncomplicated diverticulitis, whereas the American College of Gastroenterology (AGA) recommends colonoscopy after a first episode of uncomplicated diverticulitis.

IMAGING STUDIES

- If clinical features are highly suggestive of diverticulitis, imaging studies are generally not necessary. It is reasonable to forgo a CT scan in patients in whom there is less diagnostic uncertainty, including previous episodes of diverticulitis, and are reliable and have a close follow up arranged.[2] Computed tomography (CT) is recommended by the ACP

when there is diagnostic uncertainty.[1] Unlike the ACP, the AGA recommends CT scanning routinely for patients who have never had an imaging-confirmed diagnosis of acute diverticulitis.

- A CT scan of the abdomen and pelvis (Fig. E3 and E4) with intravenous (IV) and luminal contrast is the preferred radiologic examination to diagnose acute diverticulitis. It can also diagnose diverticulosis and alternative diagnoses are identified in about half of the cases.[3] CT has a sensitivity of 93% to 97% and a specificity approaching 100% for diverticulitis. Typical findings are thickening of the bowel wall, fistulas, or abscess formation. CT may also reveal other disease processes (e.g., perforated diverticulitis [Fig. 5], appendicitis, tubo-ovarian abscess, Crohn disease) accounting for lower abdominal pain. In the Hinchey classification scheme based on CT results (Box 1), stage Ia indicates uncomplicated diverticulitis, whereas stages Ib (pericolic or mesenteric abscess in proximity to the primary inflammatory process), II (intraabdominal abscess distant from primary inflammatory process or pelvic/retroperitoneal abscess), III (generalized purulent peritonitis), and IV (generalized fecal peritonitis) indicate complicated diverticulitis. Ultrasonography and MRI can also be used. Abdominal ultrasonography has a 90% sensitivity and specificity for acute diverticulitis. MRI is also highly sensitive and specific for acute diverticulitis.
- Evaluation of suspected diverticular bleeding (Fig. 6):
  1. Arteriography if the bleeding is faster than 1 ml/min (advantage: The possible infusion of vasopressin directly into the arteries supplying the bleeding, as well as selective arterial embolization; disadvantages: Its cost and invasive nature)
  2. Technetium-99m sulfa colloid
  3. Technetium-99m labeled red blood cell (can detect bleeding rates as low as 0.12 to 5 ml/min)

TREATMENT

NONPHARMACOLOGIC THERAPY

- Increase in dietary fiber intake and regular exercise to improve bowel function. However, recent studies have challenged the common view that fiber intake protects against diverticulosis.
- Oral diet of clear liquids is recommended until pain resolves in cases of mild uncomplicated diverticulitis.
- Nothing by mouth (NPO) and IV hydration in severe diverticulitis; nasogastric (NG) suction if ileus or small bowel obstruction is present.
- Emergent surgery is required for perforation, peritonitis, or uncontrolled sepsis.

ACUTE GENERAL Rx
TREATMENT OF DIVERTICULITIS:
- Mild uncomplicated diverticulitis (75% of cases of diverticulitis): Antibiotics should be

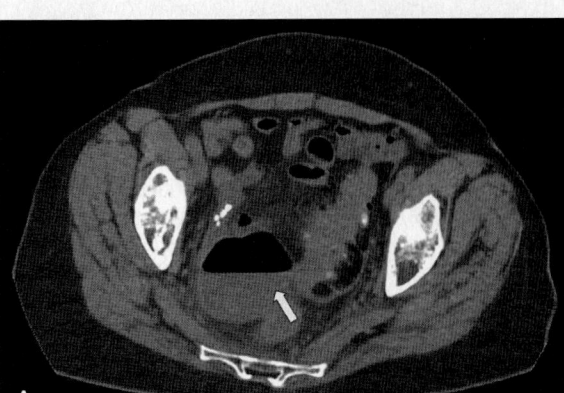 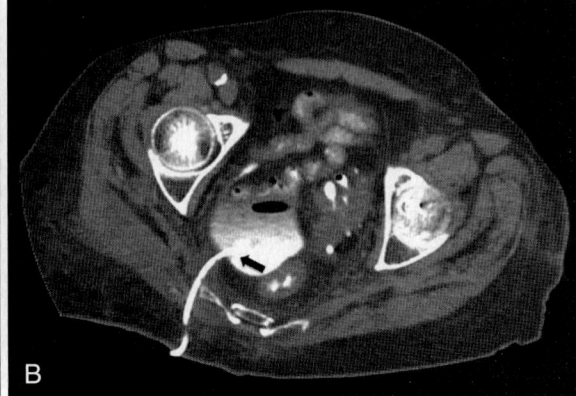

FIG. 5 Computed tomographic scans of abdomen-pelvis. A, Perforated diverticulitis: pelvic collection with an air-fluid level *(white arrow).* **B,** Same patient after interventional percutaneous drain placement of the diverticular abscess *(black arrow).* (From Bennett JE et al: *Mandell, Douglas, and Bennett's principles and practice of infectious diseases,* ed 9, Philadelphia, 2020, Elsevier.)

BOX 1   Hinchey Classification of Diverticulitis

1a. Pericolonic phlegmon and inflammation without fluid collection
1b. Pericolonic abscess <4 cm
2. Pelvic abscess or abscess >4 cm
3. Purulent peritonitis
4. Feculent peritonitis

From Walls RM et al: *Rosen's emergency medicine, concepts and clinical practice,* ed 10, Philadelphia, 2023, Elsevier.

---

used selectively rather than routinely.[4] Indications for antibiotic use in uncomplicated diverticulitis include WBC count over 15,000/mm,[4] C-reactive protein over 140 mg/L. Presence of fluid collection or lung segment of inflammation on CT scan, immunosuppression, or presence of comorbidities.[1] When indicated, broad-spectrum PO antibiotics (Box 2) (e.g., amoxicillin-clavulanate 875 mg/125 mg PO bid, or combinations of ciprofloxacin 500 mg PO bid and metronidazole 500 mg q6h).[4] Liquid diet for 7 to 10 days is also commonly prescribed. Trials have shown no benefit of IV vs. oral antibiotics and similar outcomes when using a 4-day course instead of a 7-day course of antibiotics. Other randomized trials and cohort studies have shown that antibiotics are not as beneficial or necessary as previously thought in cases of mild diverticulitis.[3] Other modalities such as 5-aminosalicylate products and probiotics remain controversial and of unclear benefit.

- Mild to moderate complicated diverticulitis, in-patient treatment: Single-agent therapy with ertapenem 1 mg IV every 24 h, ticarcillin-clavulanic acid 200 to 300 mg/kg per day divided doses every 6 h, or moxifloxacin 400 mg IV every 24 h for 4 to 7 days. Combination therapy of cefazolin (1 to 2 mg every 8 h) or levofloxacin (750 mg every 24 h) plus metronidazole (500 mg every 8 h) is also effective.
- Severe complicated diverticulitis: NPO and aggressive IV antibiotic therapy (Box 3)

1. Imipenem-cilastatin 500 mg IV q6h *or*
2. Piperacillin-tazobactam 4.5 g IV q8h *or*
3. Meropenem 1 g IV q8h *or*
4. Doripenem 500 mg IV q8h
5. Cefepime 2 g IV q8h or ciprofloxacin 400 mg IV q12h each in combination with metronidazole 500 mg IV q8h

- Surgical treatment (laparoscopic preferred over open colectomy) consisting of resection of involved areas and reanastomosis (if feasible); otherwise, a diverting colostomy with reanastomosis is performed when infection has been controlled. The need for surgery as well as its optimal timing is unclear, and surgery is no longer considered necessary after a couple of episodes of diverticulitis. Surgery may be considered in patients with:

1. Repeated episodes of diverticulitis (≥3 episodes within 2 yr), or those with persistent "smoldering" episodes (i.e., lasting >3 mo). However clinicians should not recommend segmental colectomy based solely on the number of diverticulitis episodes, and decisions regarding partial colectomy should reflect the patient's disease severity, operative risk, and patient's preference[2]
2. Poor response to appropriate medical therapy (failure of conservative management)
3. Abscess or fistula formation
4. Obstruction
5. Peritonitis: Colonic resection with a Hartmann pouch is the procedure of choice in critically ill patients with generalized peritonitis
6. Immunocompromised patients, first episode in young patient (<40 yr old)
7. Inability to exclude carcinoma (10% to 20% of patients diagnosed with diverticulosis on clinical grounds are subsequently found to have carcinoma of the colon)

DIVERTICULAR HEMORRHAGE:
- Bleeding is painless and stops spontaneously in the majority of patients (60%); it is usually caused by erosion of a blood vessel by a fecalith present within the diverticular sac.
- Medical therapy consists of blood replacement and correction of volume and any clotting abnormalities.

- Colonoscopic treatment with epinephrine injections, bipolar coagulation, or both may prevent recurrent bleeding and decrease the need for surgery. Endoclips (Fig. E7) can also be used to stop the bleeding.
- Surgical resection is necessary if bleeding does not stop spontaneously after administration of 4 to 5 U of packed red blood cells (PRBCs) or recurs with severity within a few days; if attempts at localization are unsuccessful, total abdominal colectomy with ileoproctostomy may be indicated (high incidence of rebleeding if segmental resection is performed without adequate localization).

DISPOSITION
- The risk of recurrence among patients with uncomplicated diverticulitis is 32% to 36%. Most patients with diverticulitis respond well to antibiotic management and bowel rest. Up to 30% of patients with diverticulitis will eventually require surgical management.
- Diverticular bleeding can recur in 15% to 20% of patients within 5 yr.

REFERRAL
- Colonoscopy is recommended in patients with clinical diagnosis of complicated left-sided diverticulitis who have not had recent colonoscopy. The procedure should be done a minimum of 6 to 8 wk after symptoms resolve.[5]
- Clinicians should discuss elective surgery to prevent recurrent diverticulitis after initial treatment in patients who have had uncomplicated diverticulitis that is persistent or recurs frequently or complicated diverticulitis.[5]

REFERENCES & SUGGESTED READINGS

Available at eBooks.Health.Elsevier.com.

RELATED CONTENT

Diverticular Disease (Patient Information)
Diverticulitis (Patient Information)
Diverticulosis (Patient Information)

AUTHOR: **FRED F. FERRI, MD**

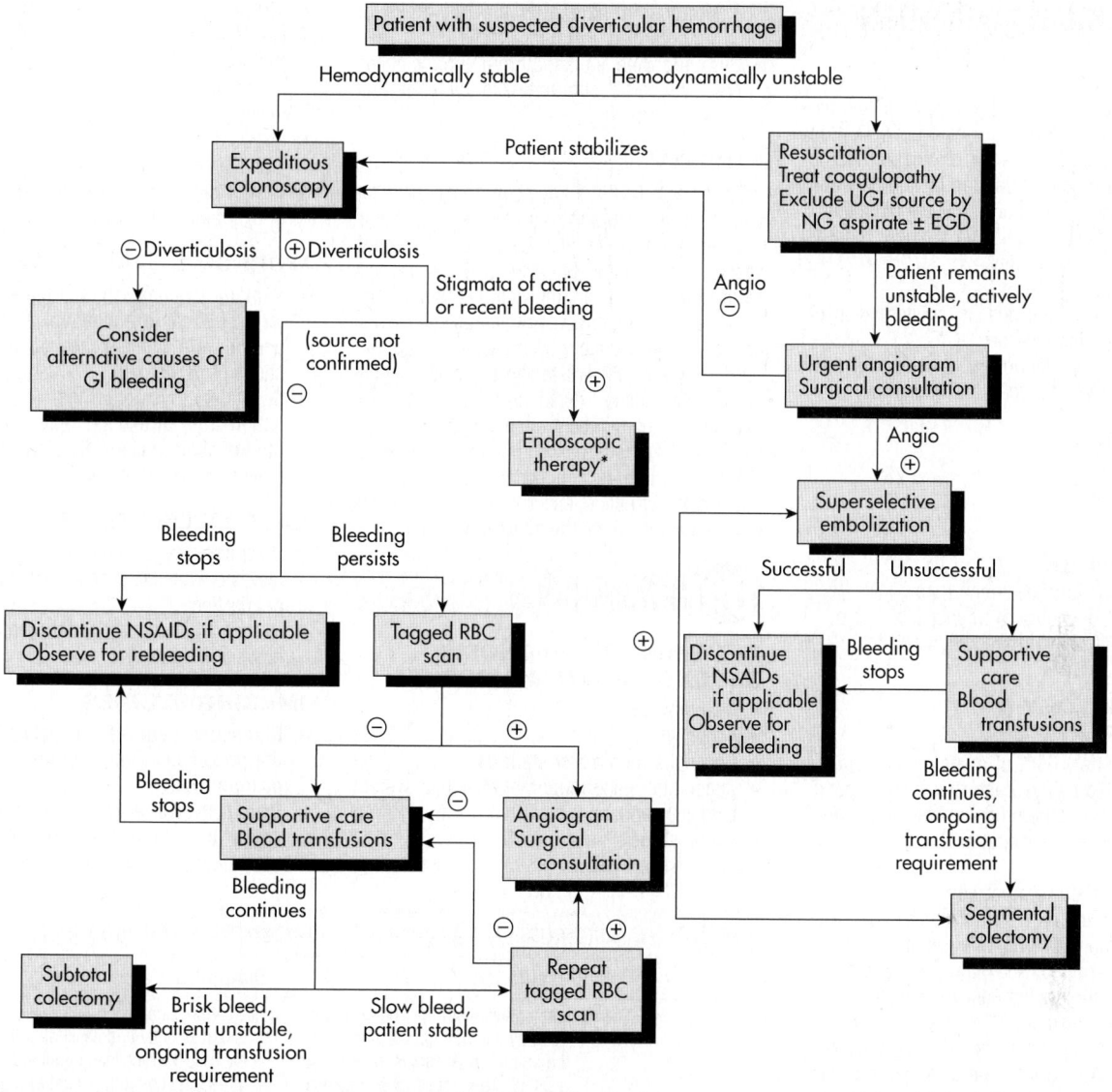

FIG. 6 Algorithm for the management of patients with suspected diverticular hemorrhage. *Angio*, Angiogram; *EGD*, esophagogastroduodenoscopy; *GI*, gastrointestinal; *NG*, nasogastric; *NSAID*, nonsteroidal antiinflammatory drug; *RBC*, red blood cell; *UGI*, upper GI. *Endoscopic therapy may consist of epinephrine injection alone or in combination with other therapies, such as heater probe coagulation, bipolar coagulation, endoclips, fibrin sealant, and band ligation. (From Feldman M et al: *Sleisenger and Fordtran's gastrointestinal and liver disease*, ed 11, Philadelphia, 2021, Elsevier.)

BOX 2 Oral Therapy for Uncomplicated Diverticulitis

Ciprofloxacin, 500 mg PO bid *and* metronidazole, 500 mg PO q8h
or
Amoxicillin-clavulanate, 875 mg-125 mg PO bid

bid, Twice a day; *PO*, by mouth (per os); *q*, every. From Walls RM et al: *Rosen's emergency medicine, concepts and clinical practice*, ed 10, Philadelphia, 2023, Elsevier.

BOX 3 Intravenous Antibiotic Coverage for Bowel Flora

Mild to Moderate Infection
- Pediatric:
  1. Metronidazole 7.5 mg/kg IV q6h AND ceftriaxone 50 mg/kg IV once daily OR
  2. Gentamicin 2.5 mg/kg IV q8h AND metronidazole 7.5 mg/kg IV q6h
- Adult:
  1. Metronidazole 500 mg IV q8h *plus*
  2. Ceftriaxone 1 g IV q24h *or*
  3. Ciprofloxacin, 400 mg IV q12h *or*
  4. Levofloxacin 750 mg IV q24h *or*
  5. Ampicillin-sulbactam, 3g IV q6h

Severe/Complicated Infection
Piperacillin/tazobactam 3.375 g IV q6h or 4.5 g (100 mg/kg) IV q8h OR
Metronidazole 500 mg IV q8h (7.5 mg/kg IV q6h) PLUS Cefepime 2 g (50 mg/kg) IV q12h OR
Ertapenem, 1g IV q24h (weight-based dose in pediatrics: 15 mg/kg/dose IV bid) *or* imipenem/cilastatin, 500 mg IV q6h (weight-based dose in pediatrics: 60 to 100 mg/kg/day divided q6h) *or* meropenem, 1 g IV q8h (weight-based dose in pediatrics: 20 mg/kg/dose IV q8h)

bid, Twice a day; *IV*, intravenous; *q*, every.
From Walls RM et al: *Rosen's emergency medicine, concepts and clinical practice*, ed 10, Philadelphia, 2023, Elsevier.

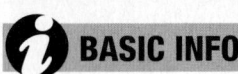 **BASIC INFORMATION**

DEFINITION

Dysmenorrhea is painful cramps of uterine origin that occur during a menstrual period, in absence of other pathology originating in the pelvis. Prevalence is estimated to vary between 45% and 95%. Dysmenorrhea is the most common gynecologic condition in women, regardless of age and nationality.

Types of dysmenorrhea:
- Primary dysmenorrhea is menstrual pain without organic disease.
- Secondary dysmenorrhea is menstrual pain associated with an identifiable disease.

SYNONYMS

Menstrual cramps
Painful periods

ICD-10CM CODES
N94.3	Primary dysmenorrhea
N94.5	Secondary dysmenorrhea
N94.6	Dysmenorrhea, unspecified

EPIDEMIOLOGY & DEMOGRAPHICS

- Approximately 50% of menstruating women are affected by dysmenorrhea, with approximately 10% of them having severe dysmenorrhea with incapacitation for 1 to 3 days per mo.
- Dysmenorrhea is most common in the age group 20 to 24 yr, with prevalence rates approaching 90% for this group.[1]
- Primary dysmenorrhea may appear 6 to 12 mo after ovulatory menstrual cycles begin.
- Secondary dysmenorrhea may occur at any time after menarche, but it may arise in a woman's 30s to 40s due to a causative underlying condition. The woman may also complain of dyspareunia, menorrhagia, intermenstrual bleeding, or postcoital bleeding.

PHYSICAL FINDINGS & CLINICAL PRESENTATION

- Sharp, crampy, midline, lower abdominal pain without a lower quadrant or adnexal component but possible radiation to the lower back and upper thighs
- Unremarkable pelvic examination in nonmenstruating patient
- Accompanying symptoms: Nausea, vomiting, headaches, anxiety, fatigue, diarrhea, fainting, and abdominal bloating
- Cramps usually lasting <24 h and seldom lasting >2 to 3 days
- Secondary dysmenorrhea
  1. Dyspareunia is a common complaint.
  2. Adolescents may report abnormal uterine bleeding, midcycle or acyclic pain, renal anomaly, lack of response to empiric medical treatment, dyspareunia, severe or worsening dysmenorrhea since menarche.[1]
  3. Bimanual pelvic-abdominal examination may demonstrate uterine or adnexal tenderness, fixed uterine retroflexion,

uterosacral nodularity, a pelvic mass, or an enlarged, irregular uterus.
- Dysmenorrhea is distinct from chronic pelvic pain, which is characterized by pain that lasts >6 mo[1]

ETIOLOGY

Prostaglandin $F_{2\alpha}$ is a key agent responsible for dysmenorrhea. It stimulates uterine contractions and cervical stenosis (narrowing) and increases vasopressin release. Behavior and psychologic factors have also been implicated in the etiology of primary dysmenorrhea. Primary dysmenorrhea only occurs in ovulatory cycles and is thought to be due to elevated prostaglandins and leukotrienes.[1] Secondary dysmenorrhea is usually caused by endometriosis, adenomyosis, leiomyomas (Fig. E1), and, less commonly, intrauterine device (IUD) use, or congenital or acquired outflow tract obstruction, including cervical stenosis or tissue band across the internal os (Fig. E2).

DIAGNOSIS

DIFFERENTIAL DIAGNOSIS: SECONDARY DYSMENORRHEA

- Adenomyosis
- Adhesions
- Cervical structures or stenosis
- Congenital malformation of Müllerian system
- Ectopic pregnancy
- Endometriosis
- Imperforate hymen
- IUD use
- Leiomyomas
- Ovarian cysts
- Pelvic congestion syndrome
- Pelvic inflammatory disease
- Polyps
- Transverse vaginal septum
- Table 1 summarizes the differential diagnosis of dysmenorrhea in adolescents

WORKUP & EVALUATION

- Primary dysmenorrhea: Characteristic history, physical examination, and ultrasound normal with the absence of an identifiable cause of pelvic pain
- Secondary dysmenorrhea: Physical examination and ultrasound may reveal vaginal/uterine abnormalities, fibroids, adenomyosis, polyps, endometriomas

LABORATORY TESTS

- No specific tests diagnostic for dysmenorrhea
- Elevated white blood cell count in the presence of infection
- Human chorionic gonadotropin to rule out ectopic pregnancy

IMAGING STUDIES

- Ultrasound scan of the pelvis to evaluate the presence of leiomyomas, adenomyosis, ovarian cysts
- Saline ultrasonography to assess the uterine cavity to rule out endometrial polyps or submucosal or intraluminal leiomyomas

TABLE 1 Differential Diagnosis of Dysmenorrhea in Adolescents

	Presentation	Diagnosis
Primary	Crampy pelvic pain may be accompanied by aching/heaviness in lower back and upper thighs, nausea, emesis, diarrhea, headache, mastalgia, fatigue, and dizziness; symptoms begin at or shortly before onset of menstrual flow and last 1-3 days.	Normal physical exam; internal exam only for sexually active adolescents. Ultrasound can be reserved for those patients with atypical presentations (e.g., onset at menarche) or those whose pain does not respond to NSAIDs and hormonal therapy.
Endometriosis and adenomyosis[a]	**Increasingly severe dysmenorrhea despite adequate therapy;** pain exacerbated during menses can occur acyclically as well.	Increased risk in patients with obstructive anomalies and possibly bleeding disorders; however, most teenagers with endometriosis have normal anatomy and bleeding indices; diagnosis is made visually during surgery. *Found in up to 69% of adolescents who underwent laparoscopy for persistent pelvic pain.*
Müllerian anomalies with partial outflow obstruction	**Pain begins at or shortly after menarche** and occurs with bleeding; presence of **known renal tract anomaly** (often coexists with Müllerian anomaly).	Pelvic ultrasound will demonstrate uterine anomalies (e.g., rudimentary uterine horn); MRI may be required to identify some lesions (e.g., obstructed hemivagina). *Found in 8% of adolescents who underwent laparoscopy for persistent pelvic pain.*
Pelvic inflammatory disease	Abrupt onset of dysmenorrhea more severe than baseline in a sexually active adolescent; presentation can range from mild discomfort to acute abdomen.	Clinical diagnosis made by findings of uterine or adnexal tenderness on bimanual pelvic examination; supporting features include dysuria, dyspareunia, **vaginal discharge,** fever, and increased white blood cell count.
Pregnancy complication	Coincident pain and bleeding may be misdiagnosed as dysmenorrhea.	Urine test positive for human chorionic gonadotropin.

MRI, Magnetic resonance imaging; *NSAID,* nonsteroidal antiinflammatory drug.
[a]Adenomyosis is the presence of endometrial tissue within the uterine myometrium.
Bold entries indicate "red flags" for diagnosis.
From Kliegman RM: *Nelson textbook of pediatrics,* ed 21, Philadelphia, 2020, Elsevier.

D

I

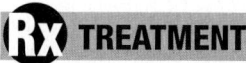 **TREATMENT**

NONPHARMACOLOGIC THERAPY

- Applying heat to the lower abdomen with hot compresses, heating pads, or hot water bottles seems to offer some relief.
- Offer reassurance that this is a treatable condition.

ACUTE GENERAL Rx

- Treatment of dysmenorrhea is summarized in Table 2
- NSAIDs such as ibuprofen 400 to 600 mg q4 to 6h or naproxen sodium 500 mg q12h
  1. Beginning 1 to 2 days before menstruation until cycle day 2 or 3[1]
- Oral contraceptives cyclically or continuously (taking only active pills), primarily in women with primary dysmenorrhea
- The levonorgestrel-containing IUD is increasingly being used to ameliorate symptoms of dysmenorrhea. Pain improvement has been shown in many cases to be even better than oral contraceptive pills
- Vitamin D supplements (research ongoing)[1]
- Magnesium supplements (research ongoing)
- Thiamine supplements (research ongoing)
- Fish oil supplements (research ongoing)
- Secondary dysmenorrhea: Treatment directed to the specific underlying condition

CHRONIC Rx

Acupuncture and transcutaneous electrical nerve stimulation may be tried. Nontraditional approaches such as acupuncture have been tried, with relief in some patients. However, there is not enough evidence to support the use of yoga, acupuncture, or massage. In cases in which medical therapy has not worked, laparoscopy or other surgical treatments should be considered depending on the secondary cause of the dysmenorrhea. However, if primary dysmenorrhea is suspected, surgical management is not preferred.[1] The levonorgestrel IUD has been shown to effectively reduce pain in women with primary dysmenorrhea.

DISPOSITION

The majority of patients are satisfactorily treated with good outcomes. If improvement from therapies is not achieved in 3 to 6 mo, providers may consider secondary causes of dysmenorrhea or patient compliance. Possible chronic complications with primary dysmenorrhea that has not been adequately treated can lead to anxiety and depression. With certain causes of secondary dysmenorrhea, infertility can become a problem.

REFERRAL

If a secondary cause of dysmenorrhea is revealed, refer to the appropriate specialist for further medical or surgical treatment (e.g., gynecologist, urogynecologist, reproductive endocrinologist, pain management center).

REFERENCE
Available at eBooks.Health.Elsevier.com.

RELATED CONTENT

Dysmenorrhea (Patient Information)
Dyspareunia (Related Key Topic)
Endometriosis (Related Key Topic)
Premenstrual Dysphoric Disorder (Related Key Topic)
Premenstrual Syndrome (Related Key Topic)

AUTHOR: **LAUREN C. ROBY, MD**

TABLE 2 Treatment for Dysmenorrhea

	Medication	Regimen	Comments
NSAIDs for up to 5 days	Ibuprofen, 200 mg	2 tablets PO q4-6h	Over-the-counter.
	Naproxen sodium, 275 mg	550 mg loading dose, then 275 mg PO q6h	Patients may prefer the equivalent 550 mg PO q12h dosing regimen.
	Celecoxib (cyclooxygenase [COX]-2 inhibitor)[a]	400 mg, then 200 mg PO q12h prn pain	Can be used for patients with von Willebrand disease.
Hormonal contraception	Combined oral contraceptive pills or vaginal ring	Continuous hormone regimens (vs. standard 21 hormone days followed by 7 placebo days) may offer better relief but may increase the risk of unexpected intermenstrual bleeding	The data favoring rings and pills over the combined hormone patch for this indication are sparse; treatment can be based on patient preference.
	Progestin-only methods	DMPA 150 mg IM or 104 mg SC q3 mo; levonorgestrel intrauterine device for up to 5 yr; etonogestrel implant for up to 3 yr	DMPA has potential side effects of weight gain and interference with expected bone density increase during adolescence, as well as a higher discontinuation rate than LARC methods.
Gonadotropin-releasing hormone agonist	Depot leuprolide	11.25 mg IM q3 mo	Consider for patients with presumed endometriosis not responsive to hormonal methods; add-back hormones are recommended to prevent bone loss.

DMPA, Depot medroxyprogesterone acetate; *IM,* intramuscular; *LARC,* long-acting reversible contraceptive; *NSAIDs,* nonsteroidal antiinflammatory drugs; *PO,* by mouth; *prn,* as needed; *SC,* subcutaneous.
[a]This medication may cause serious cardiovascular and GI events. Use with caution in patients with impaired renal or liver function, heart failure, or a history of GI bleeding or ulcer. Full prescribing information can be found at http://www.accessdata.fda.gov/drugsatfda_docs/label/2011/020998s033,021156s003lbl.pdf.
From Kliegman RM: *Nelson textbook of pediatrics,* ed 21, Philadelphia, 2020, Elsevier.

BASIC INFORMATION

DEFINITION

Early pregnancy loss is an intrauterine pregnancy that is determined to be nonviable via an empty gestational sac or a sac containing an embryo or fetus without fetal heart activity before 13 wk 0 days of pregnancy.

SYNONYMS

Spontaneous abortion
Miscarriage

ICD-10CM CODE

O03.9   Complete or unspecified spontaneous abortion without complication

EPIDEMIOLOGY & DEMOGRAPHICS

INCIDENCE:
- ~15% to 25% of all pregnancies
- ~80% of pregnancy losses overall are early and occur in the first trimester
- The incidence of clinically known early pregnancy loss increases with age:
  1. 9% to 17% between ages 20 to 30
  2. 20% at age 35
  3. 40% at age 40
  4. 80% at age 45

PREDOMINANT SEX & AGE: Affects females postmenarche and premenopause

RISK FACTORS:
- Advanced maternal age (with a positive correlation between age and risk)
- Prior early pregnancy loss

GENETICS: Over two thirds of early pregnancy losses before 12 wk estimated gestational age are associated with chromosomal abnormalities. The most frequent are autosomal trisomies. Thrombophilias associated with pregnancy loss are summarized in Box 1.

PHYSICAL FINDINGS & CLINICAL PRESENTATION

- Vaginal bleeding
- Uterine cramping

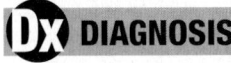 DIAGNOSIS

DIFFERENTIAL DIAGNOSIS

- Viable intrauterine pregnancy
- Pregnancy of unknown location
- Ectopic pregnancy
- Molar pregnancy
- Vaginal trauma

WORKUP

Thorough history and physical examination
- Timing, quantity, and quality of symptoms
- Abdominal and pelvic examination
- Studies
- Diagnosis through combination of laboratory studies and imaging: Serum β-hCG, ultrasonography

LABORATORY TESTS

- Serial serum β-hCG measurements in addition to serial ultrasound can be helpful in

differentiating possible ectopic, molar, resolution of spontaneous abortion, or viable intrauterine gestation.
- Depending on the specific clinical circumstances and how much diagnostic certainty the patient desires, a single serum β-hCG test or ultrasound examination likely insufficient to confirm diagnosis of early pregnancy loss.

IMAGING STUDIES

- Ultrasonography is the preferred modality to verify the presence of a viable intrauterine gestation, with specific guidelines for diagnosis of the status of the pregnancy (Table 1).
- A fetal heart rate <100 bpm at 5 to 7 wk gestation, in addition to subchorionic hemorrhage is suggestive of EPL.
- Further evaluation in 7 to 10 days is indicated.
- Box 2 summarizes the Society of Radiologists in Ultrasound Guidelines for Transvaginal Ultrasonographic Diagnosis of Early Pregnancy Loss.

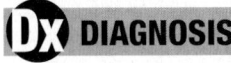 TREATMENT

NONPHARMACOLOGIC THERAPY

- Expectant management with adequate follow-up
- Surgical evacuation with adequate follow-up

PHARMACOLOGIC THERAPY

- Oral mifepristone and vaginal or buccal misoprostol
- Decreases time to expulsion, increases rate of complete expulsion without need for surgical intervention

- Consider only in women without infection, hemorrhage, severe anemia, or a history of bleeding disorders
- Follow up with ultrasound in 7 to 14 days to confirm complete passage of tissue or with serial serum β-hCG measurements

ACUTE GENERAL Rx

- Women who are Rh(D) negative should receive Rhogam
- 200 mg oral mifepristone, followed by 800 μg of misoprostol (vaginally, within 0 to 72 h or buccally, 24 to 48 h later) is considered to be the most effective regimen
- May repeat misoprostol dose as needed within 7 days if there is no response to the first dose
- If mifepristone not available, may administer 800 μg vaginal misoprostol alone with repeat dose as clinically indicated

DISPOSITION

- Complete passage of tissue may be noted via follow-up ultrasound in 7 to 14 days.
  - Absence of gestational sac and endometrial thickness <30 mm are often used as clinical criteria.
- Thickened endometrial stripe not an indication for surgical management in asymptomatic women.
- If fetal tissue is not visible on ultrasonography or ultrasonography is unavailable, serial serum β-hCG measurements may be used instead.
- May additionally consider standardized follow-up phone calls and urine pregnancy tests if ultrasonography is unavailable; however, no standardized protocol to guide use of these methods.

BOX 1   Thrombophilias Associated with Pregnancy Loss

Antiphospholipid antibodies—anticardiolipin, lupus anticoagulant, and anti-β2 glycoprotein
Antithrombin III deficiency
Elevated factor VIII levels
Factor V Leiden mutation
MTHFR mutations[a]
Plasminogen activator inhibitor-1 deficiency
Protein C deficiency
Protein S deficiency
Prothrombin G2021OA mutation
Thrombocytosis (thrombocythemia—platelet counts >750,000)

[a]Methylenetetrahydrofolate reductase mutations. (Mild hyperhomocysteinemia is technically not a thrombophilia, though it may be associated with thrombosis. Many laboratories include testing for the mutations in thrombophilia panels.)
From Gershenson DM et al: *Comprehensive gynecology,* ed 8, Philadelphia, 2022, Elsevier.

TABLE 1   Ultrasound Findings in Early Pregnancy

Ultrasound Findings	Gestational Age from LMP (days)	Approximate hCG (IU)	Approximate Risk of Pregnancy Loss[a]
Gestational sac	23-29	1500	<12%
Yolk sac	32-45	5000	<9%[b]
Embryonic disc	35-45		<8%
Fetal cardiac activity	>42 with CRL × 5 mm	13,000-15,000	<8%
Embryo 2 cm with heart rate	56		<2%

CRL, Crown-rump length; *hCG,* human chorionic gonadotropin; *LMP,* last menstrual period.
[a]If no vaginal bleeding.
[b]If the gestational sac is 10 mm.
From Gershenson DM et al: *Comprehensive gynecology,* ed 8, Philadelphia, 2022, Elsevier.

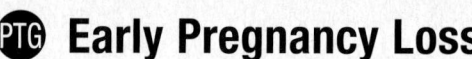

BOX 2 Society of Radiologists in Ultrasound Guidelines for Transvaginal Ultrasonographic Diagnosis of Early Pregnancy Loss[a]

Findings Diagnostic of Early Pregnancy loss[b]
Crown-rump length of ≥7 mm and no heartbeat
Mean sac diameter of ≥25 mm and no embryo
Absence of embryo with heartbeat 2 wk or more after a scan that showed a gestational sac without a yolk sac
Absence of embryo with heartbeat ≥11 days after a scan that showed a gestational sac with a yolk sac

Findings suggestive, but not diagnostic, of early pregnancy loss[c]
Crown-rump length of <7 mm and no heartbeat
Mean sac diameter of 16 to 24 mm and no embryo
Absence of embryo with heartbeat 7 to 13 days after an ultrasound scan that showed a gestational sac without a yolk sac
Absence of embryo for ≥6 wk after last menstrual period
Empty amnion (amnion seen adjacent to yolk sac, with no visible embryo)
Enlarged yolk sac (>7 mm)
Small gestational sac in relation to the size of the embryo (<5 mm difference between mean sac diameter and crown-rump length)

[a]Criteria are from the Society of Radiologists in Ultrasound Multispecialty Consensus Conference on early first trimester diagnosis of miscarriage and exclusion of a viable intrauterine pregnancy, October 2012.
[b]These are the radiologic criteria only and do not replace clinical judgment.
[c]When there are findings suspicious for early pregnancy loss, follow-up ultrasonography at 7 to 10 days to assess the pregnancy for viability is generally appropriate.
Data from American College of Obstetricians and Gynecologists et al: Practice bulletin no. 150: early pregnancy loss, *Obstet Gynecol* 125(5):1258-1267, 2015.

COMPLEMENTARY & ALTERNATIVE MEDICINE
No evidence-based recommendations

REFERRAL
No further workup generally is recommended until after the second consecutive clinical early pregnancy loss; however, patients should follow up with their routine OB/GYN.

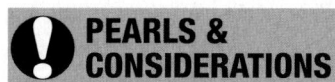 **PEARLS & CONSIDERATIONS**

COMMENTS
It is imperative to differentiate early pregnancy loss from other etiologies before initiating treatment at the risk of disruption of a normal viable intrauterine pregnancy, pregnancy complications, or birth defects.

PREVENTION
No evidence-based interventions have been proven to prevent early pregnancy loss. Women who have experienced at least three prior pregnancy losses, however, may benefit from progesterone therapy in the first trimester.

PATIENT & FAMILY EDUCATION
Patient education material can be obtained from local women's health clinics and also from the American College of Obstetricians and Gynecologists. Patients should follow up with their primary OB/GYN after pregnancy loss.

RELATED CONTENT
Miscarriage (Patient Information)
Ectopic Pregnancy (Key Related Topic)
Molar Pregnancy (Key Related Topic)
Vaginal Bleeding During Pregnancy (Key Related Topic)

AUTHORS: **SIRI M. HOLTON, MD** and **SNEHA PARANANDI, MD**

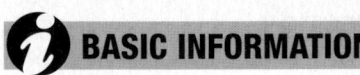 **BASIC INFORMATION**

DEFINITION

Eclampsia is the occurrence of new-onset tonic-clonic, focal, or multifocal seizures in the absence of other causative conditions in pregnant or postpartum women. It is often, but not always, associated with other signs and symptoms of preeclampsia. Atypical eclampsia occurs at <20 wk of gestation or as much as 23 days postpartum.

SYNONYM

Seizures of pregnancy

ICD-10CM CODES
015.00	Eclampsia in pregnancy, unspecified trimester
015.02	Eclampsia in pregnancy, second trimester
015.03	Eclampsia in pregnancy, third trimester
015.1	Eclampsia in labor
015.2	Eclampsia in the puerperium
015.9	Eclampsia, unspecified as to time period

EPIDEMIOLOGY & DEMOGRAPHICS

INCIDENCE: Based on a World Health Organization multicountry survey, the global prevalence of eclampsia is reported to be 0.3%. Although preeclampsia is a known risk factor for eclampsia, studies have shown that only 1.9% and 3.2% of patients with preeclampsia and severe preeclampsia, respectively, went on to develop eclampsia.
RISK FACTORS: Risk factors for eclampsia include multifetal gestation (3.6% in twin gestation), molar pregnancy, nonimmune hydrops fetalis, uncontrolled hypertension, preexisting hypertension, renal disease, systemic lupus, and preexisting heart disease.
GENETICS: Increased incidence with a first-degree relative (sister or mother) having had eclampsia.

PHYSICAL FINDINGS & CLINICAL PRESENTATION

- Eclampsia, or a seizure associated with pregnancy or postpartum, commonly begins as facial twitching that then spreads into a generalized tonic-clonic state lasting 60 to 90 sec, with cessation of respiration followed by a post-ictal period of amnesia, agitation, and confusion.
- The most common symptoms preceding eclampsia are persistent occipital or frontal headaches (80%), visual disturbance such as blurred vision or photophobia (45%), epigastric pain (20%), and altered mental status.
- 40% have severe hypertension, 40% have mild to moderate hypertension, and 20% are normotensive.
- Generalized edema with rapid weight gain (>2 lb/wk) may precede eclampsia.
- >17% are completely asymptomatic before seizure with no prior documentation of elevated blood pressure or proteinuria.

ETIOLOGY

The proposed common pathway relates to initial abnormal placentation leading to arterial resistance, vasoconstriction, and ischemia, which causes release of mediators of oxidative stress such as free radicals and cytokines. Endothelial damage to the cerebral vasculature ensues and an imbalance of angiogenic factors leads to abnormalities in the autoregulation of cerebral blood flow. This may involve transient vasospasm, ischemia, cerebral hemorrhage, and edema occurring by a mechanism involving hypertensive encephalopathy, decreased colloid osmotic pressure, and prostaglandin imbalance.

Dx DIAGNOSIS

DIFFERENTIAL DIAGNOSIS

- Preexisting seizure disorder
- Metabolic abnormalities (hypoglycemia, hyponatremia, hypocalcemia)
- Substance abuse
- Head trauma
- Cerebral infection (meningitis, encephalitis)
- Intracranial hemorrhage thrombosis, ischemia, or infarction
- Amniotic fluid embolism
- Space-occupying brain lesions or neoplasms
- Pseudoseizure
- Postdural puncture syndrome
- Hypertensive encephalopathy
- Posterior reversible encephalopathy syndrome (often seen in eclampsia)
- Vasculitis, angiopathy
- Thrombotic thrombocytopenic purpura

Atypical presentations such as prolonged post-ictal state; status epilepticus; gestational age <20 wk or >48 h postpartum; or signs of meningitis, substance abuse, severe uncontrolled hypertension, or seizures despite therapeutic levels of magnesium sulfate therapy should prompt a search for other seizure etiologies, including but not limited to those listed earlier.

WORKUP

- Laboratory tests and common findings
  1. Proteinuria: Severe (49%), mild to moderate (29%), absent (22%)
  2. Hematocrit: Elevated as a result of hemoconcentration
  3. Platelet count: Decreased in HELLP syndrome (hemolysis, elevated liver enzymes, and low platelet count)
  4. Liver function tests elevated in HELLP syndrome
  5. Blood urea nitrogen and creatinine: Elevated with renal involvement
- Rule out other causes of seizures during pregnancy:
  1. Serum electrolytes, glucose, calcium
  2. Toxicology profile
  3. Arterial blood gas: Maternal acidemia and hypoxia
  4. Imaging studies: Computed tomography (CT) scan or MRI indicated in atypical presentation (suspected intracerebral bleeding or focal neurologic deficit)

5. >90% of patients will have findings consistent with posterior reversible encephalopathy syndrome on MRI
6. Abnormal findings, including cerebral edema, hemorrhage, and infarction, are apparent in 50% of patients

Rx TREATMENT

ACUTE GENERAL Rx

- Elevate bed side rails, place patient in the lateral decubitus position (physical restraints may be necessary).
- Suction oropharyngeal secretions and vomitus and maintain airway to prevent aspiration.
- Administer adequate oxygenation.
- Obtain intravenous (IV) access.
- Initiate or continue continuous fetal heart monitoring.
- Magnesium sulfate should be administered. Give magnesium sulfate 6 g IV load over 20 min, then 2 g/h maintenance, for treatment and recurrent seizure prophylaxis. Adjust maintenance dose for renal insufficiency. If there is no IV access, give 10 g intramuscularly (IM) (5 g to each buttock). Phenytoin has been used as an alternative in patients in whom magnesium sulfate is contraindicated (e.g., heart block, myasthenia gravis).
- If repeated convulsions, give an additional 2 g IV over 3 to 5 min, as ~10% to 15% of patients will have a second seizure after initial loading dose.
- Monitoring parameters required on magnesium include creatinine function, urine output, and deep tendon reflexes. Clinical signs of progressive Mg^{2+} toxicity, such as loss of reflexes, should also be followed. If magnesium toxicity is suspected, check magnesium level (therapeutic range 4 to 7 mEq/L). If serum level >9.6 mg/dl, stop infusion. Respiratory and cardiac arrest occur at extremely high magnesium levels. Antidote for toxicity is IV calcium gluconate 10 ml of 10% solution over 3 min with IV furosemide to expedite excretion.
- If persistent seizures despite magnesium treatment, give sodium amobarbital 250 mg IV over 3 min, thiopental, or phenytoin 1250 mg IV over 25 min.
- Treat blood pressure (BP) >160 mm Hg systolic or BP >110 mm Hg diastolic with one of the following: Hydralazine 5 to 10 mg IV, and if persistent at 20 min, an additional 10 mg; labetalol hydrochloride 20, 40, 80 mg IV every 10 min if persistent, until a total maximum total dose of 300 mg; or immediate release nifedipine 10 to 20 mg orally every 20 min, if no IV access, to a total dose of 180 mg/day. If maximum dose of one medication is reached, add another medication to reach goal of BP >160 mm Hg systolic or BP >110 mm Hg diastolic.
- Evaluate patient for delivery; if signs of maternal or fetal deterioration are present, urgent or emergent delivery is indicated immediately following maternal stabilization, typically with cesarean delivery (C-section).

E

CHRONIC Rx

- After immediate stabilization of the mother is achieved, the next priority becomes optimization of adequate oxygenation, hemodynamics, and laboratory abnormalities, such as associated coagulopathies.
- Consider delivery timing; although eclampsia alone is not an indication for delivery, it is important to consider include gestational age, labor course, obstetric history, and fetal presentation in determining mode and urgency of delivery. If greater than 34 wk gestation, timely delivery is warranted once maternal stabilization is achieved. Give antenatal corticosteroids if 24 to 34 wk, and if 34 to 36-6/7 wk or 23-0/7 to 24 wk consider steroids. If unfavorable cervix and <30 wk of gestation, consider cesarean delivery; otherwise, consider induction.
- Controlled epidural is the anesthesia of choice for labor or cesarean delivery.
- Avoid general anesthesia in uncontrolled hypertension to minimize risk of catastrophic cerebral events.
- Continue magnesium sulfate through delivery process and for 24 h postpartum or for at least 24 h after the last convulsion.

DISPOSITION

- The maternal mortality rate for eclampsia averages 5% to 6%. Morbidity rate is 25%, including placental abruption (10%), disseminated intravascular coagulation, maternal apnea with fetal asphyxia, aspiration pneumonia, pulmonary edema (4%), renal failure, cardiopulmonary arrest, and coma.
- There is an increased risk of fetal death, neonatal death, preterm birth, and small-for-gestational-age birth.
- In patients with eclampsia, the risk of recurrence of eclampsia in a subsequent pregnancy is about 2% and the risk of preeclampsia is ~25%. The use of daily low-dose aspirin initiated at 12 to 16 wk and continuing until delivery may decrease that risk.

REFERRAL

Because of the potential for serious permanent maternal and fetal sequelae, all cases should be managed by a team approach of obstetrician, maternal and fetal medicine, neonatologist, and intensivist.

SUGGESTED READINGS
Available at eBooks.Health.Elsevier.com.

RELATED CONTENT
Eclampsia (Patient Information)
HELLP Syndrome (Related Key Topic)
Preeclampsia (Related Key Topic)

AUTHOR: **COURTNEY PFEUTI, MD**

Diseases
and Disorders

I

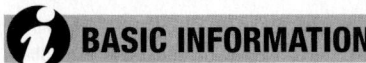

DEFINITION

An ectopic pregnancy (EP) occurs when a fertilized ovum implants outside the endometrial cavity.[1]

SYNONYMS

Tubal pregnancy (95%)
Interstitial (cornual) pregnancy (2%)[2]
Ovarian pregnancy (1% to 3%)
Abdominal pregnancy (0.03% to 1%)
Cervical pregnancy (0.5%)
Cesarean scar pregnancy (1% to 3%, 6% of all EP in women with prior cesarean)
Heterotopic pregnancy (1/4000 to 1/30,000, but 1/100 after in vitro fertilization)[1]

ICD-10CM CODES	
O00.9	Ectopic pregnancy, unspecified
O00.0	Abdominal pregnancy
O00.1	Tubal ectopic pregnancy
O00.2	Ovarian ectopic pregnancy
O00.8	Other ectopic pregnancy

EPIDEMIOLOGY & DEMOGRAPHICS

- 1% to 2% of pregnancies; represents 3% of pregnancy-related deaths.[3]
- Ectopic pregnancy causes 80% of first trimester deaths.[4]
- African American patients have a 1.5-fold higher risk.

PREVALENCE (IN U.S.): Accounts for up to 18% of women presenting to the emergency room with vaginal bleeding or abdominal pain.[1] Currently over 100,000 reported cases/yr.

RISK FACTORS: Prior ectopic, altered tubal anatomy, prior pelvic infection (pelvic inflammatory disease, tuboovarian abscess, salpingitis), prior tubal surgery, prior cesarean delivery, current intrauterine device use, assisted reproductive techniques, infertility, cigarette use, age >35, multiple lifetime sexual partners, diethylstilbestrol (DES) exposure in utero. Half of patients with EP have no risk factors.[1]

PHYSICAL FINDINGS & CLINICAL PRESENTATION

- The classic presentation of EP includes the triad of abnormal vaginal bleeding, pelvic pain, and an adnexal mass
- Abdominal tenderness: 95%
- Adnexal tenderness: 87% to 99%
- Amenorrhea or abnormal vaginal bleeding: 75%
- Peritoneal signs: 71% to 76%
- Adnexal mass: 33% to 53%
- Enlarged uterus: 6% to 30%
- Shoulder pain: 10%
- Tissue passage: 6% to 7%
- Shock: 2% to 17%

ETIOLOGY

- Anatomic obstruction to zygote passage
- Abnormalities in tubal motility
- Transperitoneal migration of the zygote

DIAGNOSIS

DIFFERENTIAL DIAGNOSIS

- Corpus luteum cyst
- Rupture or torsion of ovarian cyst, especially hemorrhagic
- Threatened or incomplete abortion
- Pelvic inflammatory disease/tuboovarian abscess
- Appendicitis
- Degenerating uterine fibroids
- Endometrioma or dermoid cyst
- Hydrosalpinx
- Gestational trophoblastic disease
- Heterophile antibodies[1]

WORKUP

- Consider in all patients with a positive pregnancy test and abdominopelvic pain
  1. Fig. 1 describes a diagnostic approach to suspected EP.
- Transvaginal ultrasound (Fig. E2 [*bottom*]).
  1. Intrauterine gestational sac with a yolk sac should be visible between 5 and 6 wk of gestation regardless of whether there are one or multiple gestations. If uncertain dating, use quantitative human chorionic gonadotropin (qhCG) levels to guide expected findings.
- ~70% EP are tubal. Fig. E2 *(top)* describes potential sites of ectopic implantations.
- Obtain qhCG level. Consider progesterone level if ultrasound inconclusive. Type and screen if presents with vaginal bleeding. Give Rhogam if Rh-negative status on initial presentation of vaginal bleeding with positive pregnancy test even if diagnosis inconclusive.
- Laparoscopy (Fig. E3) in equivocal situations and possibly for treatment.
- If pregnancy is not desired or determined to be nonviable, uterine aspiration can identify intrauterine location of chorionic villi.

LABORATORY TESTS

- Quantitative human chorionic gonadotropin (qhCG): Check on initial presentation to enable interpretation of initial ultrasound. If qhCG >6000 mIU/ml, should see intrauterine pregnancy (IUP) on abdominal scan; qhCG >3500 mIU/ml for transvaginal ultrasound. Inability to see IUP at or above these levels raises concern for ectopic. Multiple gestation may take longer to visualize, however, due to increased qhCG levels.[1]
- 25% to 50% of EP presents as a pregnancy of unknown location (PUL), in which initial ultrasound does not show a pregnancy in the uterus or the fallopian tube. Serial measurement of qhCG, obtained every 48 h, can help distinguish between an IUP, resolving miscarriage, or EP. The expected rate of qhCG rise varies by the initial starting qhCG. For an initial qhCG level <1500 mIU/ml, the expected rate of increase is 49%, compared to 40% for an initial qhCG level between 1500 and 3000 mIU/ml, and a 33% increase for an initial qhCG >3000 mIU/ml. However, some EPs will have a normal appearing

qhCG rise, and some will still rupture despite decreasing qhCG.[1]
- A single progesterone level <5 ng/ml has 99% specificity to predict nonviable pregnancy with inconclusive sonographic findings, but this cannot distinguish EP from failed IUP.
- Dropping hemoglobin/hematocrit may be associated with tubal rupture with internal hemorrhage or possible miscarriage.

IMAGING STUDIES

- Ultrasound: Presence of an intrauterine yolk sac makes EP extremely unlikely. However, if the patient used assisted reproductive technologies, a heterotopic pregnancy (EP with concurrent IUP) is possible. Repeat ultrasound within 10 to 14 days after presentation may identify the location of a pregnancy that was not identified initially.
- Findings on ultrasound in EP include:
  1. Empty uterus (i.e., no yolk sac or fetal pole; a pseudosac in uterus may appear similar to a gestational sac). May have trilaminar endometrium pattern[2]
  2. Adnexal mass ("ring of fire" appearance, can typically distinguish EP appearance from corpus luteum by tubal vs ovarian location)
  3. Enlarged hysterotomy scar with thin anterior uterine wall, may bulge beyond uterine contour or have negative sliding sign
  4. Free fluid in cul-de-sac or Morison's pouch
  5. Yolk sac and/or fetal pole in tube or extrauterine cardiac activity in adnexa

TREATMENT

NONPHARMACOLOGIC THERAPY

Surgery performed via laparoscopy is preferred; however, laparotomy is appropriate if patient is very unstable or if poor visualization during laparoscopy. Ruptured EP is managed surgically, as life-threatening intraabdominal hemorrhage may ensue. Transfuse blood as indicated.

- Salpingostomy, removing EP with tubal conservation, has benefit if patient only has one remaining tube preoperatively and desires future fertility, but will require postoperative serial monitoring of qhCG. Otherwise, randomized controlled trials and Cochrane Review suggest there is no difference in fecundity rate between salpingostomy and salpingectomy, and future fertility is not significantly different for surgical vs. medical therapy.[2,4]
- Salpingectomy, removal of affected fallopian tube, is the standard surgical procedure and preferred in the following circumstances:
  1. Ruptured tube
  2. Recurrent EP in the same tube
  3. Uncontrolled hemorrhage
  4. Future fertility not desired
- Direct injection of chemotherapy into a nontubal EP by laparoscopy, ultrasound guidance, or hysteroscopy. Direct injection of methotrexate (MTX), and possibly potassium chloride (KCl) if cardiac activity, may be performed

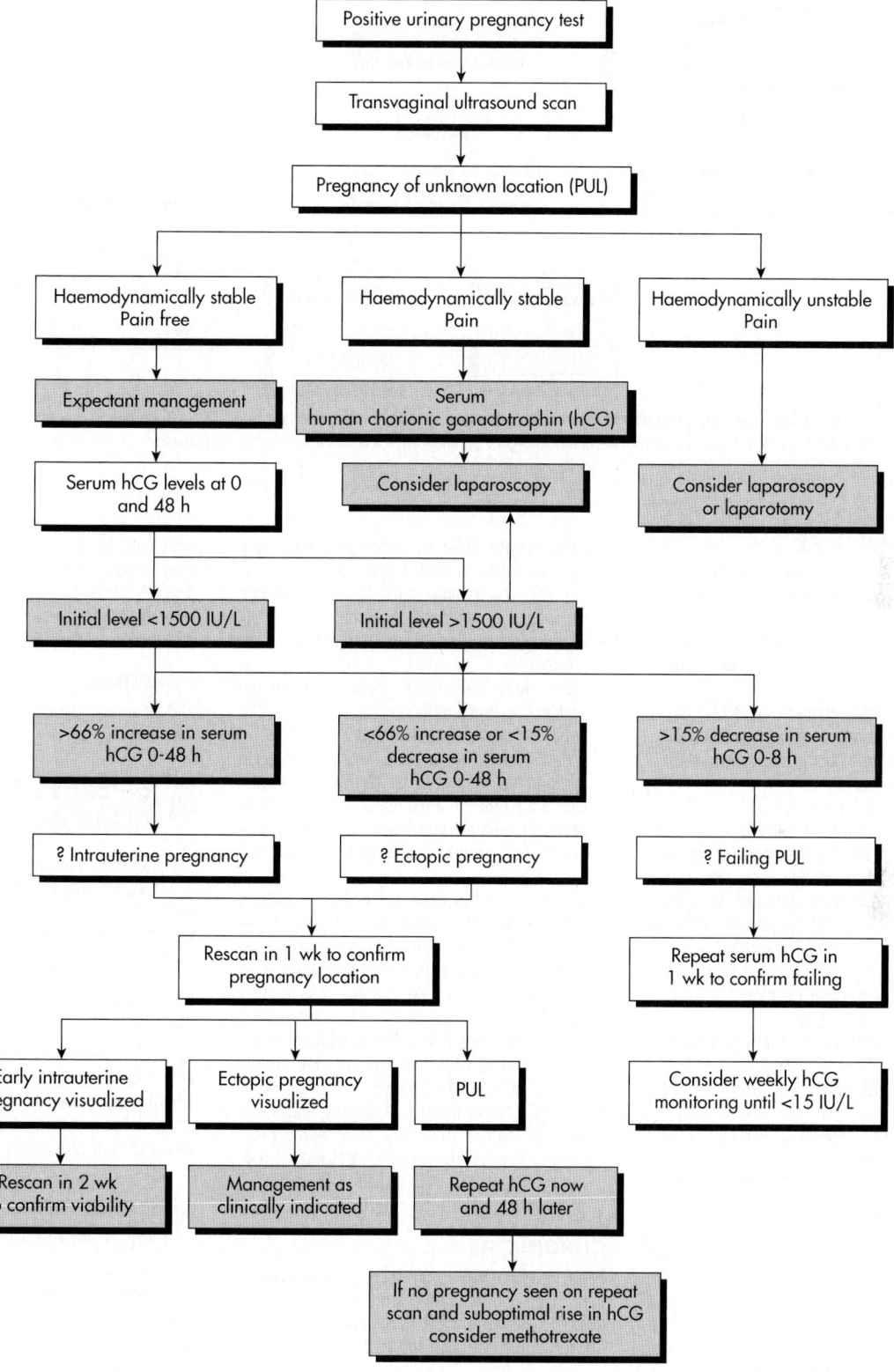

FIG. 1 Algorithm for managing suspected ectopic pregnancy. (From Magowan BA: *Clinical obstetrics & gynecology*, ed 4, Philadelphia, 2019, Elsevier.)

when the pregnancy is in a high-morbidity location, such as the cervix, cesarean delivery scar, or cornua.[3,5] A possible algorithm for use of MTX vs. surgery for ectopic pregnancy is illustrated in Fig. 4.

- Cervical and cesarean scar pregnancies may be managed with a combination of MTX

administration, laparoscopic and/or hysteroscopic techniques, ultrasound-guided suction curettage, uterine artery embolization (UAE), laparotomy, and possible hysterectomy. Vasopressin and UAE reduce bleeding. Systemic MTX as monotherapy is not recommended for cesarean scar EP.[5]

- Ovarian EP is managed surgically. Interstitial EP is also more safely managed surgically due to proximity to uterine vessels with 2.5% mortality in case of rupture.[3,2]
- Expectant management is only appropriate in asymptomatic cases with significant spontaneous qhGC decrease from an initial low level.

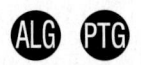
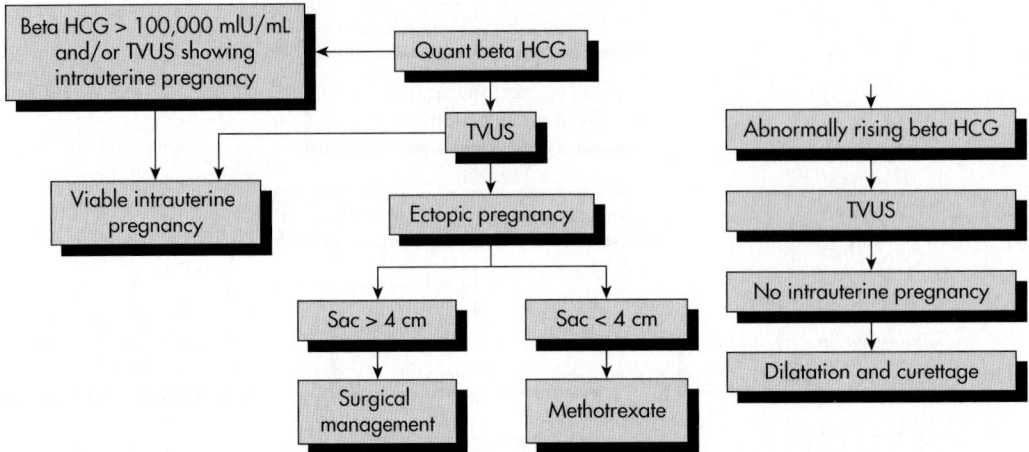

FIG. 4 Possible algorithm for use of methotrexate vs. surgery for ectopic pregnancy. *HCG,* Human chorionic gonadotropin; *Quant,* quantitative; *TVUS,* transvaginal ultrasound. (From Gershenson DM et al: *Comprehensive gynecology,* ed 8, Philadelphia, 2022, Elsevier.)

ACUTE GENERAL Rx

- Medical management with intramuscular (IM) MTX, a folic acid antagonist, is a safe option for tubal EP if the patient is stable. Check labs prior to administration (CBC, comprehensive metabolic panel). Future fertility is not affected.
- Absolute contraindications:
  1. Hemodynamically unstable; ruptured EP
  2. Patient unable to comply with follow-up
  3. Immunodeficiency
  4. Intrauterine pregnancy
  5. Medical contraindication to MTX includes clinically relevant hepatic or renal disease, as well as preexisting blood dyscrasias (thrombocytopenia, leukopenia, or significant anemia), as MTX is directly toxic to hepatocytes and renally excreted
  6. Breastfeeding, active pulmonary disease, or active peptic ulcer disease
- Relative contraindications:
  1. EP >4 cm mass as imaged by transvaginal ultrasound
  2. qhCG >5000 mIU/ml (up to 14% failure rate)
  3. Presence of embryonic cardiac activity (high failure rate)
  4. Refusal to accept blood products in case of failure and subsequent hemorrhage from rupture
- Most common regimen is single-dose IM MTX at a dose of 50 mg/m^2 per body surface area and is administered on day 1. May require second dose or surgical intervention if qhCG increases or plateaus (<15% drop) when comparing values from day 4 and 7. If qhCG does not decrease after two doses, consider surgical management.
- Success rate of single-dose protocol approximately 88% vs. multidose protocol, which is 92%. Single dose is associated with less adverse effects. Initial serum qhCG level is the best prognostic indicator of treatment success of single-dose protocol.
- Rupture during MTX treatment ranges from 7% to 14%.
- Other MTX regimens include multidose protocol ± leucovorin rescue.
- Avoid intercourse and heavy exercise to avoid trigger of rupture, alcohol due to symptom masking, and folic acid (prenatal vitamins) due to decreased MTX effectiveness, as well as sun exposure and NSAIDs due to increased toxicity until MTX treatment is complete.[3]
- Methotrexate adverse effects (AE) include nausea, vomiting, stomatitis, diarrhea, elevated LFTs, abdominal pain, and nephrotoxicity. Rare adverse effects of pneumonitis or alopecia can occur. AE resolve 3 to 4 days after MTX discontinued.[2]
- Ultrasound surveillance of resolution is not indicated because findings do not predict rupture or time to resolution.[1]
- The FDA recommends avoiding pregnancy until at least 1 ovulatory cycle after MTX.[1] Some experts recommend delaying pregnancy for at least 3 mo after MTX due to prolonged persistence in human tissue.[1]

CHRONIC Rx

Persistent EP results from residual trophoblastic tissue or secondary implantation after salpingostomy. There is a 5% incidence of persistent EP with conservative treatment.

DISPOSITION

If diagnosed and treated early (before rupture), prognosis is excellent for good recovery. Monitor qhCG weekly and use reliable contraception until qhCG is negative. With subsequent pregnancies, perform early ultrasound to confirm IUP and follow qhCG as indicated. There is a 10% recurrence rate for EP; however, this rate increases to 25% after two prior EPs.[1]

REFERRAL

Should obtain gynecologic consultation if EP is suspected.

ⓘ PEARLS & CONSIDERATIONS

Any patient who presents with vaginal bleeding, abdominal pain, or both with a positive pregnancy test and no prior documented IUP needs to be assessed for ectopic pregnancy. Do not assume that contraceptive use means pregnancy test will be negative.

PREVENTION

Absolute risk of EP is reduced by use of contraception, so although likelihood of EP is increased with IUD failure, the risk of EP is still lower overall due to contraceptive effectiveness.[3] Use of condoms reduces tubal exposure to infection, which also lowers future risk.

REFERENCES

Available at eBooks.Health.Elsevier.com.

RELATED CONTENT

Ectopic Pregnancy (Patient Information)
Spontaneous Abortion (Related Key Topic)
Vaginal Bleeding During Pregnancy (Related Key Topic)

AUTHORS: **LISA BIRD, MD** and **NIMA R. PATEL, MD, MS**

BASIC INFORMATION

DEFINITION

Human monocytic ehrlichiosis (HME) and human granulocytic anaplasmosis (HGA) are tick-borne rickettsial diseases. Ehrlichiosis is the generic name for infections caused by both *Ehrlichia* and *Anaplasma* genera. Table 1 describes the agent, vector, and geographic prevalence of these diseases. In addition to the U.S., some cases have occurred in Europe.

SYNONYMS

Human granulocytic ehrlichiosis (HGE)
Ehrlichiosis
Human monocytic ehrlichiosis (HME)
Human monocytotropic ehrlichiosis
Human granulocytic anaplasmosis (HGA)
Human granulocytotropic ehrlichiosis
Anaplasmosis
Human granulocytropic anaplasmosis

ICD-10CM CODES

A77.40	Ehrlichiosis, unspecified
A77.41	*Ehrlichiosis chaffeensis* [*E. chaffeensis*]
A77.49	Other ehrlichiosis

EPIDEMIOLOGY & DEMOGRAPHICS

INCIDENCE (IN U.S.): Highest overall incidence in Rhode Island (36.5/1 million), New York, New Jersey, Connecticut, Wisconsin, Minnesota, and northern California; >3000 cases identified in the United States since 2006. Greater than 5700 cases of HGA in 2017 alone. Prevalence of HME can approach 660/100,000 persons in an epidemic event.
PREDOMINANT SEX: Males:females 2:1.
PREDOMINANT AGE: Most severe disease 50 to 70 yr.
PEAK INCIDENCE: Occurs throughout the year, with peak incidence between May and July and again in September.

PHYSICAL FINDINGS & CLINICAL PRESENTATION

- Symptoms of ehrlichiosis typically appear after a median of 9 days (range 5 to 14 days) after a tick bite
- Most common initial symptoms
  1. Fever (96%)
  2. Chills, rigor
  3. Headache (72%)
  4. Myalgia
- Subsequent symptoms
  1. Anorexia, nausea
  2. Arthralgia
  3. Cough
  4. Confusion (meningoencephalitis in 20% of patients with HME)
  5. Abdominal pain
  6. Rash (erythematous to pustular) <30% in HME, uncommon in HGA
- Complications
  1. Hepatitis
  2. Interstitial pneumonitis; acute respiratory distress syndrome
  3. Neurologic complications in HME—seizures, coma, meningoencephalitis
  4. Renal and respiratory failure
  5. Heart failure and pericardial effusions, including tamponade
  6. Demyelinating polyneuropathy
  7. Toxic shock–like syndrome
  8. Life-threatening opportunistic infections, usually HGA-herpes simplex virus, aspergillus, candida
  9. Hemophagocytic lymphohistiocytosis (HLH)
- Clinical and laboratory abnormalities in HME and HGA are summarized in Table 2.

ETIOLOGY

- The causative agents are *Ehrlichia chaffeensis* for HME, *Anaplasma phagocytophilum* for HGA, and *Ehrlichia ewingii* for HGE.
- Vector:
  1. Almost certainly tick-borne, recently confirmed to be rarely transmitted by infected blood (including nosocomial infection). Perinatal and transplant transmission have been documented.
  2. HGA transmitted by *Ixodes scapularis* ticks in the northeastern states and HME by *Amblyomma americanum* (Lone Star tick) ticks in the south central, southeastern, and mid-Atlantic states. Fig. E1 illustrates the life cycles of HME (with *Ehrlichia chaffeensis*) and human granulocytic ehrlichiosis (anaplasmosis).
  3. Tick exposure reported in >90% of patients, with ~60% reporting tick bite.
  4. May also be transmitted by blood transfusion or solid organ transplant.
- Mammalian host: Deer, horses, dogs, white-footed mice, cattle, sheep, goats, bison.
- Host inflammatory and immune responses define final spectrum of disease beyond granulocytes, including hepatitis, interstitial pneumonitis, and nephritis with mild azotemia.
- Between 6% and 21% of patients with HGA also have serologic evidence of other *Ixodes* spp. tick-borne diseases: Lyme disease or babesiosis.
- Recovery is usual outcome; fatality rate of HGE is about 2% to 3%.
- HGA fatality <1%.
- Intensive care unit care required: 7%.

DIAGNOSIS

DIFFERENTIAL DIAGNOSIS

- Rocky Mountain spotted fever
- Colorado tick fever
- Q fever
- Relapsing fever
- Babesiosis
- Leptospirosis
- Lyme disease
- Tularemia
- Typhoid fever, paratyphoid fever
- Brucellosis
- Viral hepatitis
- Meningococcemia
- Infectious mononucleosis
- COVID-19
- Hematologic malignancy
- Thrombotic thrombocytopenic purpura (TTP)
- Table 3 describes clinical clues suggesting a diagnosis of a tick-borne illness manifesting as a nonspecific febrile illness

WORKUP

- Acute blood samples for Giemsa-stained smears; buffy coat if possible
- CBC (leukopenia, thrombocytopenia), liver function (elevated), blood urea nitrogen/creatinine
- Acute serum samples for serology: Antibodies are seldom detected at time of acute infection (they usually appear 2 to 4 wk following clinical illness)
- Chest x-ray examination (selected cases with respiratory symptoms)
- Bone marrow rarely needed

LABORATORY TESTS

- Polymerase chain reaction (PCR) to facilitate early diagnosis: Detection of *Ehrlichia/Anaplasma* DNA in blood or cerebrospinal fluid by PCR (Table E4)
- Giemsa-stained smear demonstrating morulae of the organism within granulocytes or monocytes (Figs. E2 and E3)
- Sensitivity of smear ~80% for HGA but ≤20% for HME
- CBC: Progressive leukopenia and thrombocytopenia with nadir near day 7
- C-reactive protein concentration is generally elevated
- Liver function tests: Increase in hepatic transaminases, lactate dehydrogenase, and alkaline phosphatase
- Elevated plasma creatinine concentration may be seen
- Serologic titer (IFA) >80 or fourfold increase in titer to antigen

IMAGING STUDIES

- Chest x-ray examination may show interstitial pneumonitis (unusual)
- MRI of the brain in cases of encephalitis

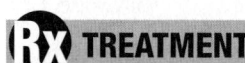 TREATMENT

ACUTE GENERAL Rx

- Immediate therapy in order to limit extent of acute illness and complication
- Doxycycline: 100 mg twice a day for 7 to 14 days is therapy of choice for adults and children >8 yr (4 mg/kg/day in two divided doses)
- Doxycycline is now recommended as well for children aged <8 yr
- Rifampin: 300 mg twice a day for 7 to 10 days; can be used in pregnancy and for children <8 yr at 10 mg/kg twice per day
- Most patients defervesce within 24 to 48 h given appropriate treatment

PROGNOSIS

Poor prognostic indicators include:
- Advanced age or immunosuppression
- Concomitant chronic illness (such as diabetes mellitus, collagen-vascular disease)
- Diagnostic delay

TABLE 1 Human Ehrlichioses and Anaplasmosis

	Human Monocytotropic Ehrlichiosis	Human Granulocytotropic Ehrlichiosis	Human Granulocytotropic Anaplasmosis
Former disease nomenclature	Human monocytic ehrlichiosis	Human granulocytic ehrlichiosis	Human granulocytic ehrlichiosis
Causative agent(s)	*Ehrlichia chaffeensis*	*Ehrlichia ewingii, Ehrlichia cani*—one asymptomatic human case reported in Venezuela	*Anaplasma phagocytophilum*
Leukocyte targets	Monocytic cell phagosomes	Neutrophil phagosomes	Granulocyte-neutrophil phagosomes
Tick vectors	*Amblyomma americanum* (lone star ticks)	*Amblyomma americanum* (lone star ticks), *Dermacentor variabilis* (American dog ticks)	*Ixodes persulcatus* complex (American deer ticks)—*I. scapularis, I. ricinus, I. pacificus*
Animal reservoirs	White-tailed deer, coyotes, dogs	White-tailed deer, dogs	Rodents, deer, ruminants, horses
U.S. regional distribution	Southeastern and south central United States	South central United States	Northeastern United States, upper Midwest, northern California
U.S. regional prevalence	2-5 cases/100,000	≤10% of presumed HME cases have *E. ewingii* infections in south central United States	50-60 cases/100,000; high seroprevalence rates in children (>20%) who have had subclinical infections
Seasonal occurrences	April-September, peaking in July	Spring-fall	May-July
Incubation periods (wk)	1-4	1-4	1-4
Modes of transmission	Tick bite, blood product transfusion	Tick bite, blood product transfusion	Tick bite, blood product transfusion, nosocomial
Frequently presenting clinical manifestations	Fever, malaise, headache, myalgias, rash in <40%	Same initial manifestations, but much milder, except in immuno-compromised individuals	Fever, malaise, headache, myalgias; rarely rash
Laboratory abnormalities	Leukopenia, thrombocytopenia, transaminitis	Leukopenia, thrombocytopenia, transaminitis	More pronounced and prolonged leukopenia, thrombocytopenia, transaminitis
Potential complications, especially in immunocom-promised individuals	Meningoencephalitis, acute renal and respiratory failure, hepatitis, myocarditis	Milder and less likely, except in patients immunocompromised by HIV/AIDS, organ transplantation, prolonged corticosteroid therapy	May be significant in immunocompromised patients with high fevers, seizures, confusion, hemorrhagic diathesis, rhabdomyolysis, shock, acute tubular necrosis, adult respiratory distress syndrome; some specific CNS compli-cations may include eighth nerve palsy, brachial plexopathy, demyelinating polyneuropathy
Case-fatality rate (CFR)	3%, higher in immunocompromised individuals	No deaths reported	0.5%, higher CFR in immunocompromised individuals
Recommended confirmatory diagnostic tests	Wright-stained peripheral blood smears with characteristic intracytoplasmic morulae in monocytes, DNA detection by PCR assay, culture	Wright-stained peripheral blood smears with characteristic intra-cytoplasmic morulae in neutro-phils, DNA detection by PCR	Wright-stained peripheral blood smears with characteristic intracytoplasmic aggregates in neutrophils, DNA detection by PCR assay, increased immunofluorescent antibodies in initial and paired serum samples
Current antibiotic resistance	Fluoroquinolones	Fluoroquinolones	Fluoroquinolones
Currently recommended antibiotic therapy, adults	Doxycycline, 100 mg PO bid, or tetracy-cline, 250-500 mg PO qid, for minimum of 3 days after defervescence to maximum of 14-21 days	Doxycycline, 100 mg PO bid, or tetra-cycline, 250-500 mg PO qid, for minimum of 3 days after deferves-cence to maximum of 14-21 days	Doxycycline, 100 mg PO bid, or tetracycline, 250-500 mg PO qid for minimum of 3 days after defervescence to maximum of 14-21 days
Currently recommended antibiotic therapy, children	Doxycycline, 4.4 mg/kg PO bid, or tetracycline, 25-50 mg/kg PO qid, for minimum of 3 days after defervescence to maximum of 14-21 days	Doxycycline, 4.4 mg/kg PO bid, or tet-racycline, 25-50 mg/kg PO qid, for minimum of 3 days after deferves-cence to maximum of 14-21 days	Doxycycline, 4.4 mg/kg PO bid, or tetracycline, 25-50 mg/kg PO qid, for minimum of 3 days after defervescence to maximum of 14-21 days

bid, Twice daily; *CNS,* central nervous system; *DNA,* deoxyribonucleic acid; *HME,* human monocytotropic ehrlichiosis; *HIV/AIDS,* human immunodeficiency virus infection/acquired immunodeficiency syndrome; *PCR,* polymerase chain reaction; *PO,* by mouth; *qid,* four times a day.

From Bennett JE et al: *Mandell, Douglas, and Bennett's principles and practice of infectious diseases,* ed 9, Philadelphia, 2020, Elsevier.

- Delayed onset of specific antibiotic therapy
- Concomitant HIV or organ transplant status

DISPOSITION
Repeat CBC every 2 to 4 wk until normal.

REFERRAL
For consultation with infectious diseases specialist in suspected cases

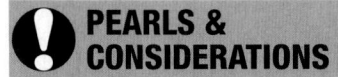 **PEARLS & CONSIDERATIONS**

- A new pathogenic *Ehrlichia* species, closely related to *E. muris,* has been identified in

Minnesota and Wisconsin. Organism-specific PCR and serologic testing can be used for identification.
- Duration of time tick must be attached to produce illness as few as 4 h.
- Delay in antibiotic treatment results in poorer outcome. Antibiotic treatment should be initi-ated as soon as infection is suspected.
- PCR is advised on newborn if mother was infected during pregnancy.

REFERENCES & SUGGESTED READINGS
Available at eBooks.Health.Elsevier.com.

RELATED CONTENT
Anaplasmosis (Patient Information)

AUTHOR: **PATRICIA CRISTOFARO, MD**

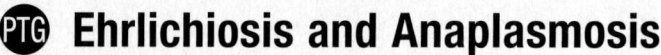

TABLE 2 Clinical and Laboratory Abnormalities in Human Monocytotropic Ehrlichiosis (HME) and Human Granulocytotropic Anaplasmosis (HGA)

SIGN, SYMPTOM, OR LABORATORY FINDING	HME MEDIAN % WITH ABNORMAL FINDING (IQR)[a]	HGA MEDIAN % WITH ABNORMAL FINDING (IQR)[b]
Fever	96 (95-99)	100 (94-100)
Headache	72 (69-72)	82 (60-96)
Myalgia	73 (63-75)	73 (61-82)
Malaise	77 (73-80)	97 (92-99)
Nausea	57 (56-59)	40 (35-52)
Vomiting	47 (37-56)	22 (17-35)
Diarrhea	25 (20-31)	20 (13-25)
Rash	26 (21-34)	5 (3-10)
Cough	28 (26-31)	27 (21-33)
Confusion/mental status changes	20 (19-22)	17 (17-18)
Leukopenia	60 (60-71)	63 (53-76)
Thrombocytopenia	79 (68-88)	80 (61-90)
Anemia	50 (38-54)	40 (14-48)
Elevated AST/ALT	88 (86-91)	80 (69-98)
Elevated creatinine	29	49 (25-71)
Elevated C-reactive protein	data not available	96 (83-100)

ALT, Alanine aminotransferase; *AST,* aspartate aminotransferase; *IQR,* interquartile range.
[a]HME meta-analysis data from references 1-8.
[b]HGA meta-analysis data from references 9-32.
From Bennett JE et al: *Mandell, Douglas, and Bennett's principles and practice of infectious diseases,* ed 9, Philadelphia, 2020, Elsevier.

TABLE 3 Clinical Clues (History, Physical Examination, or Laboratory) Suggesting the Diagnosis of a Tick-Borne Illness Manifesting as a Nonspecific Febrile Illness[a]

Disease	Clues
Anaplasmosis	Faint rash possible Low white blood cell or platelet count Elevated hepatic transaminases
Babesiosis	Findings of hemolysis History of splenectomy Presence of faint rash, hepatomegaly, or splenomegaly
Lyme disease	Careful skin examination for any rash consistent with erythema migrans Bradycardia from heart block Associated seventh nerve palsy or lymphocytic meningitis
Colorado tick fever	Saddle-back fever curve
Rocky Mountain spotted fever	Maculopapular or petechial rash Normal white blood cell count or low platelet count Hyponatremia Peripheral edema
Relapsing fever	Recurring episodes of fever with afebrile intervals
Tularemia	Acrally located ulcer Regional lymphadenopathy Possible associated pneumonia

[a]Apart from an epidemiologic context suggesting a tick-borne disease.

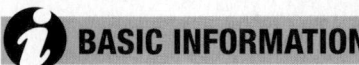
🛈 BASIC INFORMATION

DEFINITION
Infection of the pleural space, identified by aspiration of frank pus, positive Gram stain, and/or positive pleural fluid cultures.

SYNONYMS
Infected pleural effusion
Purulent pleural effusion
Pleural sepsis

ICD-10CM CODES
J90	Pleural effusion
A16.5	Empyema due to tuberculosis
J86	Pyothorax

EPIDEMIOLOGY & DEMOGRAPHICS
- The incidence and mortality rates of pleural infections have increased globally over the past decades.[1,2]
- Pleural infections occur in a bimodal distribution. Historically the most affected groups have been children and adults aged 65 to 74 yr. Males are affected twice as often as women, and risk factors include diabetes, substance use disorders, rheumatologic disease, poor dentition and aspiration.[1]
- Empyema is usually a complication of community-acquired pneumonia due to gram-positive aerobic organisms such as Streptococcus spp. or Staphylococcus spp. However, an empyema can develop from hematogenous spread of infection, iatrogenic inoculation from thoracic procedures, chest tubes, or trauma.[3]
- Pneumonias also can have associated pleural effusions that are either simple or complex and can be distinguished by loculations on imaging or through biochemical analysis of pleural fluid (low pH or glucose).
- Long-term sequelae from infected pleural effusions stem from the formation of a pleural rind and nonexpandable lung, which may require surgery.

PHYSICAL FINDINGS & CLINICAL PRESENTATION
- The clinical presentation of pleural infection may be indistinguishable from pneumonia with fevers, cough, dyspnea, malaise, and pleuritic chest pain. Elderly patients may not present with classic symptoms, but rather anemia, fatigue, and failure to thrive.
- There should be an increased suspicion for empyema if clinical signs of sepsis persist despite initiation of appropriate antibiotics.
- Rarely, empyema can manifest as slowly enlarging chest wall masses or form a fistula (e.g., empyema necessitans).
- Physical findings of empyema are those of pleural effusion: Decreased breath sounds and dullness to percussion over the involved part of the thorax. Systemic signs include fever, tachycardia, leukocytosis, and warmth and erythema over the involved area.

ETIOLOGY
Pleural bacteriology differs based on setting.
Community acquired:
- Streptococcus spp. (e.g., S. milleri, S. pneumoniae)
- Staphylococcus aureus
- Haemophilus influenzae
- Oral anaerobic bacteria (e.g., Bacteroides fragilis, Prevotella spp., Fusobacterium nucleatum, and Peptostreptococcus)
- Legionella spp.
- Mycobacterium tuberculosis
- Actinomyces spp.
Hospital acquired:
- Methicillin-resistant Staphylococcus aureus (MRSA)
- Methicillin-susceptible Staphylococcus aureus (MSSA)
- Gram-negative anaerobes

🄓🅧 DIAGNOSIS

- The initial diagnosis of a pleural infection includes clinical signs and symptoms of a respiratory infection and chest imaging suggestive of a pleural effusion.
- Ultrasonography provides additional information regarding the size and complexity of the effusion, which aids in guiding the safety and appropriateness of further fluid sampling.
- In the case of empyema, pleural fluid analysis may also guide the need for additional nonpharmacologic treatment, such as chest tube placement or intraleural fibrinolytic therapy.
- Clinical risk scores may also be used to prognosticate patients with infected pleural effusions.[4]

DIFFERENTIAL DIAGNOSIS
- See Pleural Effusion
- Uninfected parapneumonic effusion
- Lung abscess (Fig. 1)
- Heart failure
- Malignancy
- Tuberculous pleurisy
- Collagen vascular disease (particularly rheumatoid lung and systemic lupus erythematosus)

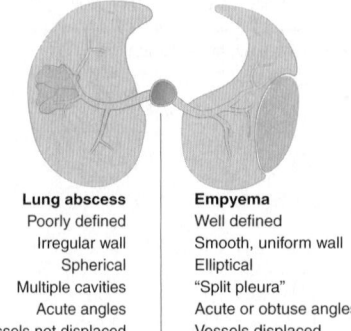

Lung abscess	Empyema
Poorly defined	Well defined
Irregular wall	Smooth, uniform wall
Spherical	Elliptical
Multiple cavities	"Split pleura"
Acute angles	Acute or obtuse angles
Vessels not displaced	Vessels displaced

FIG. 1 Empyema versus lung abscess. (From Webb WR et al: *Fundamentals of body CT*, ed 4, Philadelphia, 2015, Saunders.)

LABORATORY TESTS
- Pleural fluid: Cell count and differential, LDH, glucose, pH, protein
- Serum: LDH, protein, CBC with differential, C-reactive protein (CRP)
- Blood and pleural fluid cultures: Pleural fluid cultures identify pathogens in only 60% of cases; yield increases when pleural fluid is collected in culture bottles containing growth medium
- Pleural fluid analysis in the acute phase of empyema is a neutrophilic-predominant exudate: Pleural to serum protein ratio >0.5, pleural to serum LDH >0.6, pleural fluid LDH >2/3 the upper limit of normal serum LDH
- Blood urea nitrogen (BUN) and albumin: 3-mo survival prognostic calculators incorporating BUN, age, purulence, infection source, serum albumin have been developed (RAPID score)[4]
- When tuberculous pleurisy is suspected, adenosine deaminase ADA is highly sensitive study that can aid in the diagnosis[5]

IMAGING STUDIES
- Chest x-ray (Fig. 2, A)
- Lateral decubitus view to establish the presence of free fluid in the pleural space
- Computed tomography (CT) (Fig. 2, B) to establish the presence of fluid loculation, underlying mass lesions, and other intrathoracic pathology
- Ultrasound to evaluate effusion complexity, procedure planning, and effusion surveillance (Fig. 3)

🅡🅧 TREATMENT

NONPHARMACOLOGIC THERAPY
- Chest tube placement is indicated if any of the following are present: Aspiration of frank pus, pleural glucose <50 mg/dl, pleural pH <7.2.
- Chest tube placement is recommended in the setting of persistent clinical signs of sepsis despite initiation of appropriate antibiotics.
- Early instillation of thrombolytic agents (tPA and DNAse) has been shown to reduce treatment failure and need for surgical intervention;[6,7] however, it may be associated with higher adverse events.
- Open decortication, video-assisted thoracoscopic surgery (VATS), or pleuroscopy may be required in cases where the lung remains unexpandable, or source control is not obtained through conservative measures.
- Empyema tube.

ACUTE GENERAL Rx
- Maintenance of drainage (Fig. E4) until source control is achieved.
- Antibiotics directed at suspected or proven bacterial or fungal pathogens. Initial regimens include cefotaxime or ceftriaxone for suspected S. pneumoniae or group A Streptococcus, nafcillin or oxacillin for suspected methicillin-sensitive S. aureus, vancomycin or linezolid for suspected MRSA, ceftriaxone for suspected H. influenzae,

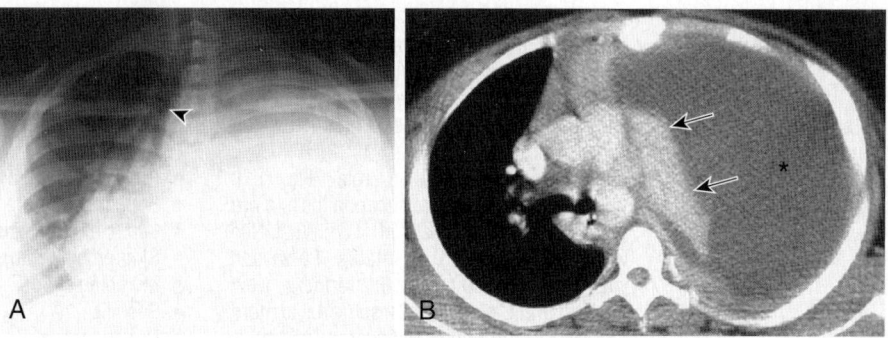

FIG. 2 Empyema and pneumonia in a teenager. A, Chest radiograph shows opacification of the left thorax. Note shift of mediastinum and trachea *(arrowhead)* to right. **B,** Thoracic computed tomography scan shows massive left pleural effusion *(asterisk).* Note the compression and atelectasis of the left lung *(arrows)* and shift of the mediastinum to the right. (From Kliegman RM et al: *Nelson textbook of pediatrics,* ed 19, Philadelphia, 2011, Saunders.)

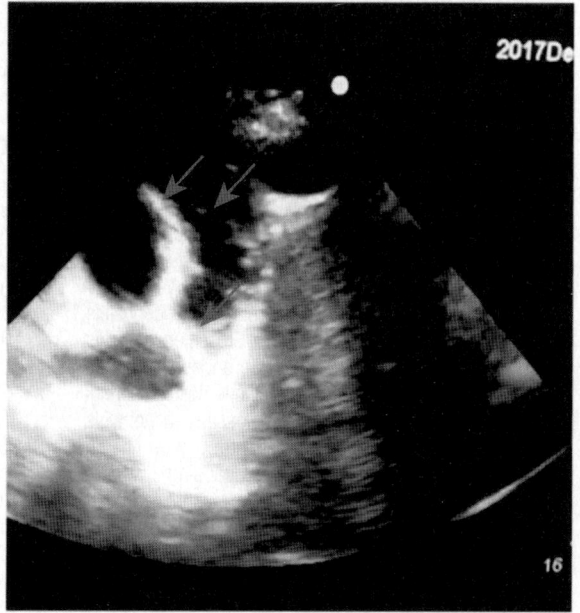

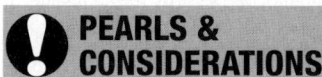

FIG. 3 An ultrasound image of a loculated parapneumonic effusion. The *arrows* show fibrinous septations. (From Gardecki J et al: Scan the lung: point-of-care ultrasound of a pulmonary consolidation with loculated pleural effusion, *Am J Emerg Med* 37[2]:377, 2019.)

and piperacillin-tazobactam when suspecting anaerobes. Other agents with excellent anaerobic coverage include clindamycin, carbapenem antibiotics such as meropenem and ertapenem, and ampicillin-sulbactam. These agents also have excellent gram-negative coverage.

CHRONIC Rx

- Pleural decortication may be indicated if sufficient pleural drainage cannot be accomplished using nonsurgical methods

or if lung reexpansion is limited due to a pleural rind.[8]
- Lung function should be monitored following completion of therapy.

DISPOSITION

Hospitalization with supplemental oxygen or ventilatory support if clinically indicated.

REFERRAL

Consultation by infectious diseases, pulmonary, or thoracic surgery specialists as needed.

! PEARLS & CONSIDERATIONS

Chest tube sizes (large vs. small bore) are of equal efficacy for empyema drainage.

REFERENCES

Available at eBooks.Health.Elsevier.com.

AUTHORS: **ADALI MARTINEZ, MD, MPH** and **YARON B. GESTHALTER, MD**

 **BASIC INFORMATION**

DEFINITION

Acute viral encephalitis is an acute febrile syndrome with evidence of meningeal involvement and of derangement of the function of the cerebrum, cerebellum, or brain stem.

SYNONYMS

Arboviral encephalitis
Brain stem encephalitis
Acute necrotizing encephalitis
Rasmussen encephalitis
Encephalitis lethargica

ICD-10CM CODES

A86	Unspecified viral encephalitis
A83.0	Japanese encephalitis
A83.1	Western equine encephalitis
A83.2	Eastern equine encephalitis
A83.3	St Louis encephalitis
A83.4	Australian encephalitis
A83.5	California encephalitis
A83.8	Other mosquito-borne viral encephalitis
A83.9	Mosquito-borne viral encephalitis, unspecified
A84.8	Other tick-borne viral encephalitis
A84.9	Tick-borne viral encephalitis, unspecified
A85.0	Enteroviral encephalitis
A85.1	Adenoviral encephalitis
A85.2	Arthropod-borne viral encephalitis, unspecified
A85.8	Other specified viral encephalitis
A92.31	West Nile virus infection with encephalitis
B00.4	Herpesviral encephalitis
B01.11	Varicella encephalitis and encephalomyelitis
B02.0	Zoster encephalitis
B05.0	Measles complicated by encephalitis
B06.01	Rubella encephalitis
B10.01	Human herpesvirus 6 encephalitis
B10.09	Other human herpesvirus encephalitis
B26.2	Mumps encephalitis
B94.1	Sequelae of viral encephalitis
G04.00	Acute disseminated encephalitis and encephalomyelitis, unspecified
G04.81	Other encephalitis and encephalomyelitis
G04.90	Encephalitis and encephalomyelitis, unspecified
G05.3	Encephalitis and encephalomyelitis in diseases classified elsewhere

EPIDEMIOLOGY & DEMOGRAPHICS

INCIDENCE (IN U.S.): About 20,000 cases/yr are reported to the CDC. West Nile infection is the most common arbovirus encephalitis in the U.S. being reported in 49/50 states in 2021 with 2445 cases and 165 deaths (6.8%). Each year in the U.S. approximately seven patients are hospitalized for encephalitis per 100,000 population.

PREVALENCE (IN U.S.):
- Arbovirus infections are transmitted by mosquitoes and thus cause infection when mosquitoes are active, especially summer and fall. Herpes simplex infections can occur at any time.
- Geography also plays a role (Fig. E1): Whereas Eastern equine encephalitis is more likely on the East Coast of U.S., West Nile virus has spread to 48 states. Powassan virus is more common in northern New England and Canada. La Crosse virus is more common in the upper Midwestern and mid-Atlantic and southeastern states.

PREDOMINANT SEX: Male = female
PREDOMINANT AGE: Any age
PEAK INCIDENCE: Any age, but children and older adults are more likely to have significant morbidity
GENETICS: No specific genetic or congenital predisposition

ETIOLOGY

- Can be caused by a host of viruses (Table E1), with herpes simplex the most common virus identified
- Arboviruses transmitted by mosquitoes include Eastern equine encephalitis, Western equine encephalitis, St Louis encephalitis, Venezuelan equine encephalitis, California virus encephalitis, Japanese B encephalitis, La Crosse encephalitis, Murray Valley and West Nile encephalitis. Tick-borne diseases (Table 2) include Russian spring-summer encephalitis, Powassan encephalitis, and other lesser known agents
- Also implicated: Rabies-causing agents, cytomegalovirus, Epstein-Barr, varicella-zoster, echo virus, mumps, adenovirus, coxsackie, rubeola, and herpes viruses
- Meningoencephalitis: Acute retroviral infection from HIV
- In the U.S., the most commonly identified etiologies are herpes simplex virus, West Nile virus, and the enteroviruses

PHYSICAL FINDINGS & CLINICAL PRESENTATION

- Initially, fever and evidence of meningeal irritation
- Headache and stiff neck
- Later, development of signs of cortical dysfunction: Lethargy, coma, stupor, weakness, seizures, facial weakness, as well as brainstem findings
- Cerebellar findings: Ataxia, nystagmus, hypotonia, myoclonus, cranial nerve palsies, and abnormal tendon reflexes
- Patients with rabies: Hydrophobia, anxiety, facial numbness, psychosis, coma, or dysarthria
- Rarely, movement disorders, such as chorea, hemiballismus, or dystonia
- Recall of a prodromal viral-like illness (this finding is not at all uniform)
- Skin/mucous membrane findings suggesting specific viral central nervous system diseases are described in Table 3
- Table 4 summarizes other specific findings associated with viruses causing central nervous system disease

Dx **DIAGNOSIS**

DIFFERENTIAL DIAGNOSIS

- Bacterial infections: Brain abscess, toxic encephalopathies, tuberculosis
- Protozoal infections
- Behçet syndrome
- Lupus encephalitis
- Sjögren syndrome
- Multiple sclerosis
- Syphilis
- Cryptococcus
- Toxoplasmosis
- Brucellosis
- Leukemic or lymphomatous meningitis
- Other metastatic tumors
- Lyme disease
- Cat-scratch disease
- Vogt-Koyanagi-Harada syndrome
- Mollaret meningitis
- Autoimmune encephalitis (Table 5)

WORKUP (BOX 1)

- Lumbar puncture to reveal pleocytosis, usually lymphocytic, although neutrophils may be seen early on
- Usually, elevated cerebrospinal fluid (CSF) protein
- Normal or low CSF glucose
- In herpes simplex encephalitis: Red blood cells and xanthochromia
- Selected tests on CSF fluid in viral encephalitis are described in Table 6
- Electroencephalogram changes showing periodic high-voltage sharp waves in the temporal regions and slow wave complexes suggestive of herpes encephalitis (Fig. E2)
- Computed tomography (CT) scan and MRI (Fig. 3) to reveal edema and hemorrhage in the frontal and temporal lobes
- Temporal lobe involvement suggests herpes simplex encephalitis (Fig. E4)
- Basal ganglia and thalami are areas involved as generally seen in Eastern equine encephalitis
- With West Nile infection, MRI changes have shown changes in basal ganglia, thalami, mesial temporal structures, brain stem, and cerebellum
- Arboviral infections suspected during outbreaks in specific areas
- Rising titers of neutralizing antibodies from the acute to the convalescent stage demonstrated but often not helpful in the acutely ill patient
- Polymerase chain reaction (PCR) that amplifies DNA from the CSF for herpes simplex encephalitis
- Rarely, brain biopsy to assist in the diagnosis; viral culture of cerebral tissue obtained if biopsy done
- Classic herpetic skin lesions suggestive of herpes encephalitis
- In diagnosing arboviral encephalitis:
  1. Presence of antiviral immunoglobulin M within the first few days of symptomatic disease; detected and quantified by enzyme-linked immunoassay

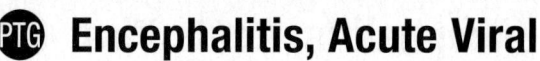
E

Diseases and Disorders

I

TABLE 2 Representative Tick-Borne Encephalitis Viruses

Virus Name	Family Taxonomy	Geographic Distribution	Tick Vectors	Wild Animal Reservoirs
Central European tick-borne encephalitis virus (TBEV-Eu)	Flaviviridae	Europe, except Iberian Peninsula	Ixodid ticks, especially *Dermacentor marginatus, Ixodes persulcatus,* and *Ixodes ricinus*	Mammals: especially rodents, including hedgehogs, wood mice, and voles; also deer and other ungulates, birds, and domestic livestock, especially goats
Deer tick virus	Flaviviridae	U.S. New England states (Connecticut, Massachusetts, New York)	*Ixodes scapularis*	Deer
Far Eastern TBEV (TBEV-FE)	Flaviviridae	Eastern Russia, China to far eastern Japan	*I. persulcatus*	Mammals: rodents, including hedgehogs, wood mice, voles; also birds, deer, other ungulates, and domestic livestock, especially goats
Langat virus	Flaviviridae	Malaysia	Ixodid ticks	Mammals: monkeys, rodents
Louping ill virus	Flaviviridae	U.S., Scotland	Ixodid ticks	Sheep
Powassan encephalitis virus	Flaviviridae	Canada, U.S. Northeast, far eastern Russia	*Ixodes* spp., particularly *I. scapularis, I. cookei; Dermacentor andersoni*	Mammals: rodents, skunks, and other medium-sized mammals, especially woodchucks
Siberian (Russian) spring-summer TBEV (TBEV-Sib)	Flaviviridae	Russia	*Ixodes* spp., particularly *I. persulcatus, I. ricinus*	Mammals: rodents, including hedgehogs, wood mice, voles; also birds, deer, other ungulates, and domestic livestock, especially goats
Turkish sheep encephalitis virus	Flaviviridae	Turkey	Ixodid ticks	Sheep
Bhanja virus	Bunyaviridae	Eastern Europe, Russia, central and West Africa	*Dermacentor* spp.; *Haemaphysalis intermedia*	Cattle, sheep, goats, hedgehogs
Crimean-Congo hemorrhagic fever virus	Bunyaviridae	Asia, Eastern Europe, Africa, Middle East	*Hyalomma marginatum, Hyalomma anatolicum*	Mammals: many domestic animals (buffalo, camels, cattle, goats, sheep), rabbits, rodents (hedgehogs), birds

From Bennett JE et al: *Mandell, Douglas, and Bennett's principles and practice of infectious diseases,* ed 9, Philadelphia, 2020, Elsevier.

TABLE 3 Skin/Mucous Membrane Findings Suggesting Specific Viral Central Nervous System Diseases

Exanthem or Mucous Membrane Change	Viral Agent	Specific Changes
Vesicular eruption	Enterovirus (A71)	"Hand, foot, and mouth disease": Macules/papules/vesicles on palms, soles, buttocks
	Herpes simplex	Grouped small (3 mm) vesicles on an erythematous base
	Varicella-zoster virus	Zoster: Vesicles in dermatomal distribution Primary VZV: Multiple vesicles, papules, pustules in various stages of eruption
Maculopapular eruption	Epstein-Barr virus	Diffuse maculopapular eruption following ampicillin treatment
	Measles	Diffuse maculopapular erythematous eruption beginning on face/chest and extending downward
	HHV-6	Roseola: Diffuse maculopapular eruption following 4 days of high fever
	Colorado tick fever	Maculopapular rash in 50%
	LCMV	Occasionally occurs with lymphadenopathy
	WNV, ZIKV	Diffuse erythematous maculopapular rash on chest and arms
Erythema multiforme	*(Mycoplasma)*	Many types of rash
Confluent macular rash	Parvovirus	Confluent erythema over cheeks ("slapped cheeks") followed by lacy reticular rash over extremities (late)
Purpura	Parvovirus	Rare "stocking glove" syndrome: Purpuric lesions on distal extremities
Pharyngitis	Enterovirus	Herpangina: Vesicles on soft palate
	Adenovirus	Pharyngitis, conjunctivitis
Conjunctivitis	St Louis encephalitis	Conjunctivitis
	ZIKV	Conjunctivitis
	Adenovirus	Conjunctivitis with pharyngitis (see above)

HHV-6, Human herpesvirus type 6; *LCMV,* lymphocytic choriomeningitis virus; *VZV,* varicella-zoster virus; *WNV,* West Nile virus; *ZIKV,* Zika virus.
From Jankovic J et al: *Bradley and Daroff's neurology in clinical practice,* ed 8, Philadelphia, 2022, Elsevier.

TABLE 4 Other Specific Findings Associated With Viruses Causing Central Nervous System Disease

Finding	Viruses
Alopecia	LCMV
Arthritis	LCMV, parvovirus, chikungunya
Biphasic illness	LCMV, Colorado tick fever
Lymphadenopathy	LCMV, mumps, HIV
Mastitis	Mumps
Mononucleosis	HCMV, EBV, CMV
Myelitis	WNV, St Louis encephalitis virus, VZV, EBV, HSV-1, CMV, herpes B virus, LCMV, EV-D68, EV-A71
Myocarditis/pericarditis	Enterovirus, (mumps, LCMV)
Orchitis/oophoritis	Mumps (LCMV, EBV)
Paresthesias	Colorado tick fever, LCMV, rabies
Parotitis	Mumps (LCMV)
Pneumonia	Influenza, parainfluenza, SARS-CoV2
Retinitis	HCMV, WNV, ZIKV (congenital)
Tremors, myoclonus	Arbovirus (e.g., WNV), EV-A71
Urinary retention	St Louis encephalitis virus, VZV, HCMV, HSV, herpes B virus, LCMV (see myelitis causing viruses)

EBV, Epstein-Barr virus; *EV*, enterovirus; *HCMV*, human cytomegalovirus; *HSV*, herpes simplex virus type; *LCMV*, lymphocytic choriomeningitis virus; *VZV*, varicella-zoster virus; *WNV*, West Nile virus; *ZIKV*, Zika virus.
From Jankovic J et al: *Bradley and Daroff's neurology in clinical practice*, ed 8, Philadelphia, 2022, Elsevier.

TABLE 5 Clues to an Autoimmune Versus Infectious Etiology for Encephalitis

Clues to an Autoimmune Etiology	Clues to an Infectious Etiology
Symptoms: Predominantly psychiatric (especially early and at an unusual age for initial presentation)	**Symptoms:** Broader, including fever,[a] headache, obtundation, meningismus
Onset: Subacute (days to weeks)	**Onset:** Often precipitous[a] (hours to days)
Medical history: Personal or family history of organ- or non–organ-specific autoimmune disorder	**Medical history:** Immunocompromised state
Serum: Systemic markers of autoimmunity (e.g., elevated ANA or TPO antibodies) and/or identification of a neural autoantibody	**Serum:** Markedly elevated[a] ESR and/or CRP, tests (cultures, ELISAs, PCR, western blots, antibodies, blood smears) identifying specific microbes
Cancer status: History of or concurrent malignancy	**Cancer status:** Generally N/A, unless immunocompromised (e.g., from chemotherapy)
CSF studies: Elevated WBC (usually <100 cells/μL), protein (usually <100 mg/dl), IgG index, oligoclonal bands, synthesis rate, and/or identification of a neural autoantibody	**CSF studies:** Elevated WBC (usually >100 cells/μL[a]), protein (usually >100 mg/dl), elevated RBC and/or xanthochromia possible, decreased glucose, tests (cultures, ELISAs, PCR, western blots, antibodies, smears) identifying specific microbes
EEG: Focal abnormalities	**EEG:** No particular pattern; could have triphasics
MRI brain: T2/FLAIR hyperintensities, rarely enhancement	**MRI brain:** T2/FLAIR hyperintensities (may be symmetric), more often has enhancement, may have leptomeningeal or spinal cord involvement, may have mass effect, may have blood
PET brain: Areas of hyper/hypometabolism	**PET brain:** Not typically done
Therapy: Response to immunosuppression	**Therapy:** Response to antimicrobials

ANA, Antinuclear antibody; *CRP*, C-reactive protein; *CSF*, cerebrospinal fluid; *EEG*, electroencephalography; *ELISA*, enzyme-linked immunosorbent assay; *ESR*, erythrocyte sedimentation rate; *FLAIR*, fluid attenuation inversion recovery; *IgG*, immunoglobulin G; *MRI*, magnetic resonance imaging; *N/A*, not applicable; *PCR*, polymerase chain reaction; *PET*, positron emission tomography; *RBC*, red blood cell count; *TPO*, anti-thyroperoxidase antibody; *WBC*, white blood cell count.
[a]May not apply to immunocompromised patients.
From Stern TA: *Massachusetts General Hospital handbook of general hospital psychiatry*, ed 7, 2018, Philadelphia, Elsevier.

2. Unusual to recover an arbovirus from the blood or CSF

LABORATORY TESTS

- Aside from the lumbar puncture, most other laboratory studies are nonspecific.
- Skin lesions and urine may be cultured for herpes simplex and CMV.

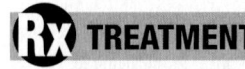 **TREATMENT**

ACUTE GENERAL Rx

- Supportive care, frequent evaluation, and neurologic examination
- Ventilatory assistance for patients who are moribund or at risk for aspiration
- Avoidance of infusion of hypotonic fluids to minimize the risk of hyponatremia
- For patients who develop seizures: Anticonvulsant therapy and follow-up in a critical care setting
- For comatose patients:
  1. Aggressive care to avoid decubitus ulcers, contractures, and deep vein thrombosis
  2. Close attention to weights, input/output, and serum electrolytes
- Acyclovir 30 mg/kg/day intravenous total dose divided in q8h intervals for 14 days for herpes simplex encephalitis
- Short courses of corticosteroids to control brain edema and prevent herniation
- In patients with suspected rabies:
  1. Human rabies immune globulin (HRIG) should be given at a dose of 20 U/kg.
  2. Active immunization may be stimulated by rabies vaccine, which is grown on a human diploid cell line (HDCV) and has reduced the number of doses needed to five.
  3. If suspect animal is a dog or cat and can be found, observe closely for 10 days to detect rabid behavior; any significant illness in the animal should promptly initiate humane sacrifice of the animal with the brain submitted to local or state health departments for pathology and immunologic testing for rabies. Any wild animal suspected of rabies should be humanely sacrificed, if possible, and submitted for rabies testing immediately.
  4. If signs are seen, animal should be euthanized and its brain examined for signs of rabies.
- No specific pharmacologic therapy for most other viral pathogens

CHRONIC Rx

Some patients may develop permanent neurologic sequelae; these patients will benefit from intensive rehabilitation programs, including physical, occupational, and speech therapy.

DISPOSITION

- Patients with suspected encephalitis of any cause should generally be admitted for initial

BOX 1   Diagnostic Algorithm

All Cases

CSF
- WBC count with differential, RBC count, protein, glucose
- Gram stain and bacterial culture
- Herpes simplex virus: 1/2 PCR (if test available, consider HSV CSF IgG and IgM in addition)
- VZV PCR (sensitivity may be low; if test available, consider VZV CSF IgG and IgM in addition)
- Enterovirus PCR

Blood/Serum
- Routine blood culture
- Epstein-Barr virus (EBV) antibodies (if positive for acute infection, check CSF EBV PCR)
- Hold acute serum and collect convalescent serum 10-14 days later for paired antibody testing

Respiratory, Stool
- Enterovirus PCR (respiratory, stool)
- Enterovirus (stool)

Conditional

Host Factors
- Neonate: Herpes simplex virus-2 PCR (CSF), swabs of skin vesicles, mouth, nasopharynx, conjunctivae, and rectum (viral culture)
- ≤3 yr: Parechovirus PCR (CSF and respiratory)
- Immunocompromised: Cytomegalovirus, human herpesvirus-6/7, JC virus, human immunodeficiency virus PCR (CSF)

Season and Exposure
- Summer/fall: West Nile virus (WNV) IgM (CSF, serum), WNV IgG (paired serum), and other appropriate arboviruses as geographically relevant
- Cat (particularly if with seizures and paucicellular CSF): *Bartonella* antibody (serum)

- Animal bite exposure: Rabies test[a]
- Rodent exposure: LCM antibody (serum)
- Tick and/or camping exposure: *Rickettsia* spp., antibody (serum), *Anaplasma phagocytophila* antibody (serum)
- Swimming or diving in brackish water: *Naegleria fowleri* (wet mount)[a]
- If history of sexual activity: Herpes simplex virus-2 (CSF PCR)

Signs and Symptoms
- Psychotic component or movement disorder: Anti-NMDAR antibody (CSF and serum), and abdominal ultrasound evaluation for teratoma
- Vesicular rash: Varicella zoster virus PCR (CSF)
- Rapid decompensation (especially with bite history or foreign travel): Rabies test[a]
- Respiratory (during influenza season): Influenza PCR (respiratory)
- Diarrhea and seizure (especially young child): Rotavirus (check stool for antigen), if positive then rotavirus PCR (CSF)

Laboratory Features
- CSF protein >100 mg/dl or CSF glucose less than two-thirds peripheral glucose and/or lymphocytic pleocytosis:
  1. Mycobacterial tuberculosis: Culture (CSF, respiratory), place PPD, and check IGRA, chest radiograph, fungal culture (CSF)
  2. Fungal (specific types depend on geographic residence and/or travel to endemic areas): Culture CSF *and* check antibody and antigen
  3. *Balamuthia mandrillaris*: Contact health department/CDC for assistance with testing
- CSF eosinophilia: *Baylisascaris procyonis* antibody

Travel
- Consider consultation with public health department concerning specific diseases such as arboviruses, rabies, and other diseases

[a]Contact health department for assistance with testing.
From Cherry JD et al: *Feigin and Cherry's pediatric infectious diseases,* ed 8, Philadelphia, 2019, Elsevier.

TABLE 6   Selected Tests for Viral Encephalitis

Organism/Syndrome	Test	Comment
West Nile Virus		
West Nile encephalitis	IgM in CSF	Diagnostic of CNS invasive disease or acute flaccid paralysis
Herpes Simplex Virus Type 1		
Herpes simplex encephalitis	PCR in CSF	Sensitive and specific in the acute phase
	CSF–serum antibody ratio	Useful 2 wk to 3 mo after onset
Herpes Simplex Virus Type 2		
Neonatal encephalitis	PCR in CSF	Confirmatory, high sensitivity
Relapsing meningitis	PCR in CSF	Sensitive and specific in first 3 days of illness
Varicella-Zoster Virus		
Meningoencephalitis	PCR in CSF	Confirmatory when used with clinical and spinal fluid findings; sensitivity unclear
Epstein-Barr Virus		
EBV encephalitis	PCR in CSF	Suggests CNS invasion by virus
JC Virus		
Progressive multifocal leukoencephalopathy	PCR in CSF	Diagnostic but incompletely (70%) sensitive
Cytomegalovirus		
CMV ventriculitis	PCR in CSF	Sensitive and specific

CMV, Cytomegalovirus; *CNS,* central nervous system; *CSF,* cerebrospinal fluid; *EBV,* Epstein-Barr virus; *IgM,* immunoglobulin M; *PCR,* polymerase chain reaction.
From Goldman L, Schafer AI: *Goldman's Cecil medicine,* ed 24, Philadelphia, 2011, Saunders.

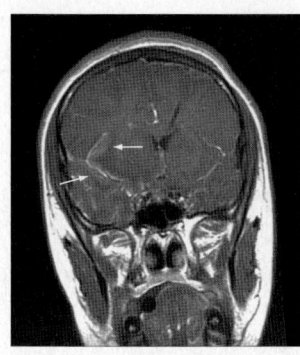

FIG. 3 Gadolinium-enhanced, T1-weighted brain MRI in a teenager with herpes simplex virus encephalitis. The scan shows gadolinium enhancement in the right insular cortex *(arrows)*. (From Swaiman KF et al: *Swaiman's pediatric neurology: principles and practice,* ed 6, Philadelphia, 2017, Elsevier.)

diagnostic workup and specific treatment (if available).
• Long-term management of patients with significant neurologic sequelae from encephalitis (e.g., memory defects, depression, difficulty with organization of thoughts, movement disorders) may benefit from rehabilitation services, home care, or nursing home placement.

REFERRAL
• To a neurologist for initial workup and management
• To an infectious disease specialist for diagnostic and therapeutic plan
• To a rehabilitation service for long-term evaluation and convalescent services

! PEARLS & CONSIDERATIONS

• West Nile virus encephalitis occurs primarily in elderly patients >65 yr of age.
• Rabies may occur months after contact with the rabid animal, and the exposure (especially bat rabies) may have been seemingly insignificant and even inapparent.
• Experimental therapies are worthy of consideration for some forms of viral encephalitis (e.g., immune plasma, ribavirin, interferons), and expert consultation should be obtained early on for possible treatment interventions with promising experimental therapies.
• A rare form of autoimmune encephalitis related to NMDA receptor antibody after infection by herpes simplex can be treated with steroids.[1]

REFERENCE & SUGGESTED READINGS
Available at eBooks.Health.Elsevier.com.

RELATED CONTENT
Herpes Encephalitis (Patient Information)
Rabies (Related Key Topic)
West Nile Virus Infection (Related Key Topic)

AUTHOR: **GLENN G. FORT, MD, MPH**

Diseases and Disorders

I

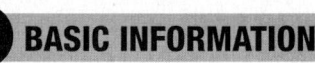 **BASIC INFORMATION**

DEFINITION

Encephalopathy is a clinical syndrome of global cognitive impairment characterized by impaired arousal, inattention, and disorientation.

SYNONYMS

Acute confusional state
Altered mental status

ICD-10CM CODES

E51.2	Wernicke encephalopathy
G04.30	Acute necrotizing hemorrhagic encephalopathy, unspecified
G04.31	Postinfectious acute necrotizing hemorrhagic encephalopathy
G04.32	Postimmunization acute necrotizing hemorrhagic encephalopathy
G04.39	Other acute necrotizing hemorrhagic encephalopathy
G92	Toxic encephalopathy
G93.40	Encephalopathy, unspecified
G93.41	Metabolic encephalopathy
G93.49	Other encephalopathy
I67.4	Hypertensive encephalopathy
I67.83	Posterior reversible encephalopathy syndrome
J10.81	Influenza due to other identified influenza virus with encephalopathy
J11.81	Influenza due to unidentified influenza virus with encephalopathy
P91.60	Hypoxic ischemic encephalopathy (HIE), unspecified
P91.61	Mild hypoxic ischemic encephalopathy (HIE)
P91.62	Moderate hypoxic ischemic encephalopathy (HIE)
P91.63	Severe hypoxic ischemic encephalopathy (HIE)

EPIDEMIOLOGY & DEMOGRAPHICS

PREVALENCE: 1.1% of adults in the general population >55 yr, 10% to 40% of hospitalized elderly, and 60% of nursing home patients >75 yr; 100,000 to 200,000 cases annually with anoxic encephalopathy

RISK FACTORS: Advanced age; cancer; AIDS; terminal illness; bone marrow transplant; postoperative state; poor nutritional status; acute or chronic cardiac, pulmonary, renal, or hepatic dysfunction; history of previous insult to the brain; epilepsy; drug abuse; alcoholism; overtreatment and undertreatment of pain; use of anticholinergics, benzodiazepines, opioids, barbiturates, and neuroleptics

PHYSICAL FINDINGS & CLINICAL PRESENTATION

- Common to all encephalopathies is a fluctuating level of arousal, poor attention, and dysfunction of other cognitive domains. Table 1 summarizes stages of encephalopathy in chronic liver disease.
- Some patients may appear agitated and others lethargic.

- Delusions (fixed false beliefs) and hallucinations are common.
- Asterixis (negative myoclonus) is common.
- Other physical findings, such as fever, ascites, jaundice, or tachycardia, may vary depending on the underlying cause of encephalopathy.
- Because toxins and metabolic disturbances are common causes of encephalopathy, the history should focus on exposure to toxins, especially medications with anticholinergic effects, and symptoms suggesting a concurrent illness such as a urinary tract infection, pneumonia, sepsis, meningitis, or encephalitis. Clinical events precipitating hepatic encephalopathy in patients with cirrhosis are summarized in Box 1.

ETIOLOGY

The final common pathway of all causes of encephalopathy is widespread neuronal dysfunction from either a structural or functional cause. Many conditions are reversible and carry a good prognosis if treated in a timely manner.

- Organ failure: Hepatic encephalopathy (Fig. 1), uremia, hypoxia, hypercapnia
- Infection: Systemic (e.g., urinary tract, pneumonia, sepsis) or involving the central nervous system (CNS) (e.g., meningitis, encephalitis)
- Toxin ingestion or withdrawal: Special consideration should be paid to alcohol, cannabis and other recreational drugs, benzodiazepines, anticholinergics, neuroleptics, and antibiotics (e.g., fluoroquinolones, cefepime, metronidazole, ertapenem)
- Electrolyte disturbances: Hypernatremia, hyponatremia, hypercalcemia

- Metabolic disorders: Acidosis, alkalosis, inborn errors of metabolism
- Endocrinopathy: Diabetic ketoacidosis, hyperglycemic hyperosmolar state, hypoglycemia, thyroid storm, myxedema, adrenal insufficiency, hyperadrenalism
- Neoplasm: Tumors of the CNS, primary or metastatic; paraneoplastic limbic encephalitis
- Nutritional deficiency, mostly in alcoholics and chronically ill patients, such as vitamin B_1 deficiency (Wernicke encephalopathy)
- Seizures: Postictal state, nonconvulsive status epilepticus, complex partial seizures, absence seizures
- Trauma: Concussion, contusion, subdural hematoma, epidural hematoma, diffuse axonal injury
- Vascular: Ischemic and hemorrhagic strokes, aneurysmal subarachnoid hemorrhage, cerebral vasculitis, cerebral venous sinus thrombosis
- Anoxic brain injury
- Psychiatric disease: Acute psychosis, mania, catatonia
- Acute demyelinating disease: Acute disseminated encephalomyelitis, tumefactive multiple sclerosis
- Other autoimmune diseases: Autoimmune encephalitis (e.g., anti-NMDA receptor encephalitis), lupus cerebritis, cerebral vasculitis (primary angiitis of the CNS or a secondary cerebral vasculitis)
- Other: Posterior reversible encephalopathy syndrome (PRES), hypertensive encephalopathy, postoperative status, sleep deprivation

---

TABLE 1 Stages of Encephalopathy in Chronic Liver Disease (West Haven Criteria)

Stage	Clinical Signs
Stage I	Mental slowness, euphoria or anxiety, shortened attention span, impaired calculating ability
Stage II	Lethargy or apathy, inappropriate behavior, personality change, more obvious problems with calculations
Stage III	Lethargic, somnolent, marked confusion and disorientation, but responds to verbal stimuli
Stage IV	Coma, patient may or may not respond to noxious stimuli

Patients with chronic liver disease rarely, if ever, demonstrate cerebral edema, regardless of the stage of encephalopathy.
From Vincent JL et al: *Textbook of critical care,* ed 8, Philadelphia, 2024, Elsevier.

BOX 1 Clinical Events Precipitating Hepatic Encephalopathy in Patients With Cirrhosis

Gastrointestinal hemorrhage
Infection (including spontaneous bacterial peritonitis)
Sepsis
Dehydration
Imbalance of electrolytes or acid-base
Renal failure
Drugs, toxins, medications (especially sedative-hypnotics or opioids)
Illicit substances
Alcohol
Dietary indiscretion (excessive protein intake)

From Vincent JL et al: *Textbook of critical care,* ed 8, Philadelphia, 2024, Elsevier.

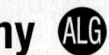

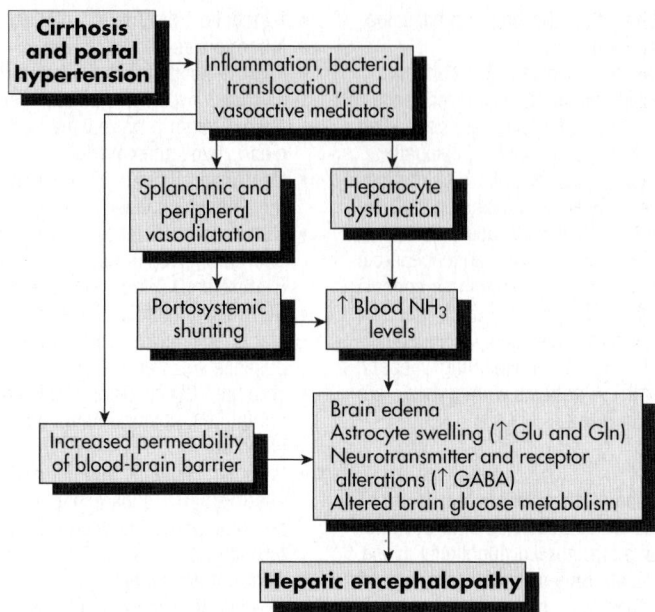

FIG. 1 Proposed pathophysiology of hepatic encephalopathy. *GABA,* Gamma-aminobutyric acid; *Gln,* glutamine; *Glu,* glutamate; *NH₃,* ammonia. (From Feldman M et al: *Sleisenger and Fordtran's gastrointestinal and liver disease,* ed 11, Philadelphia, 2021, Elsevier.)

IMAGING STUDIES

The following imaging and diagnostic studies may be indicated depending on history and physical examination:
- Chest radiograph to rule out pneumonia
- Head computed tomography (CT) to rule out intracranial hemorrhage, hydrocephalus, tumors
- Brain MRI with and without contrast and with diffusion-weighted images for suspected encephalitis, tumors, acute strokes, or acute autoimmune processes
- Magnetic resonance angiography/venography for strokes, arterial dissection, cerebral venous sinus thrombosis
- Conventional angiography for CNS vasculitis and aneurysms
- Electroencephalogram (EEG): Evaluate for sub-clinical status epilepticus

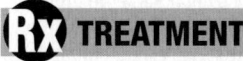 **TREATMENT**

The encephalopathy itself is a symptom of these underlying problems. In general, it is best to avoid treating the symptom of encephalopathy with antipsychotics or sedatives. The best approach is to treat the underlying toxic or metabolic disturbance.
- Thiamine supplementation.
- Glucose for hypoglycemia.
- Antibiotics in cases of infections (choose an agent with good CNS penetration in cases of primary CNS infections; to prevent exacerbation of underlying problem, ensure also that the agent is not associated with causing encephalopathy, if possible).
- Insulin in hyperglycemic conditions (e.g., diabetic ketoacidosis, hyperosmolar nonketosis, and sepsis).
- Correct electrolyte disturbances properly.
- Treat organ failure and its sequelae; for example, implement appropriate therapy for hyperammonemia and uremia.
- Ensure hemodynamic stability (blood pressure and heart rate).
- Eliminate medications that can cause or exacerbate encephalopathy: Anticholinergic drugs, benzodiazepines and other sedative-hypnotics, neuroleptics, and opioids.
- Consider acute intoxication with, or withdrawal from, drugs or alcohol and treat withdrawal appropriately.
- Consider serotonin syndrome and neuroleptic malignant syndrome in the appropriate clinical setting.

RELATED CONTENT

Delirium (Related Key Topic)
Encephalitis, Acute Viral (Related Key Topic)
Hepatic Encephalopathy (Related Key Topic)

AUTHOR: **JOSEPH S. KASS, MD, JD, FAAN**

DIAGNOSIS

DIFFERENTIAL DIAGNOSIS

Differential diagnosis for encephalopathy is broad. It is typically helpful to distinguish toxic/metabolic causes from primary neurologic causes.
- Dementia: Distinguished from encephalopathy by a history of slowly progressive cognitive decline over time (fluctuating cognitive function is rare except in dementia with Lewy bodies)
- Hypersomnia
- Aphasia: Distinguished from encephalopathy by the fact that aphasia is a specific disorder of language rather than a global disturbance of cognitive function
- Depression
- Psychosis: Some overlap with encephalopathy because delusions and hallucinations may be common to both. Patients with a primary thought disorder such as schizophrenia will have altered reality testing but should maintain orientation
- Mania
- Unaware wakefulness (vegetative state) or minimally conscious state: Patients appear awake (eyes are open) but exhibit either no evidence of consciousness or minimal or fluctuating evidence of consciousness
- Akinetic mutism: These patients do not talk and do not move; there is little fluctuation in their state, and there is no asterixis or other focal deficit
- Locked-in syndrome: May be distinguished from encephalopathy by the presence of fixed neurologic deficits (e.g., paralysis of all four limbs); however, the patient is aware of his or her environment

WORKUP

The best tool in the evaluation of encephalopathy is a good history and physical examination, including a neurologic examination, which will help tailor the remainder of the diagnostic workup. Interview family members and other providers to identify preceding events, medication changes, and medical history. Evaluate for focal neurologic deficits.

LABORATORY TESTS

- Comprehensive metabolic panel, amylase, lipase, ammonia, thyroid-stimulating hormone, B₁₂
- CBC with differential
- Drug screen and alcohol level (must order ethylene glycol separately if suspected)
- Lumbar puncture if meningitis, encephalitis, autoimmune process, or subarachnoid hemorrhage with negative imaging is suspected
- HIV, rapid plasma reagin (RPR)
- Urinalysis and microscopy, urine culture, blood cultures
- Arterial blood gases

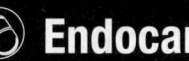
Diseases
and Disorders

I

 BASIC INFORMATION

DEFINITION

Infective endocarditis (IE) is an infection of the endocardial surface of the heart or mural endocardium. Box 1 describes the modified Duke criteria for the diagnosis of infective endocarditis.

ACUTE ENDOCARDITIS: Usually caused by *Staphylococcus aureus, Streptococcus pyogenes, Streptococcus pneumoniae,* and *Neisseria* organisms; classic clinical presentation of high fever, positive blood cultures, vascular and immunologic phenomenon

SUBACUTE ENDOCARDITIS: Usually caused by viridans streptococci in the presence of valvular pathology; less toxic, often indolent presentation with lower fevers, night sweats, fatigue

ENDOCARDITIS IN INJECTION DRUG USERS: Often involving *S. aureus* or *Pseudomonas aeruginosa* with variation that may be geographically influenced; tricuspid or multiple valvular involvement; high mortality rate of 50% to 60%

PROSTHETIC VALVE ENDOCARDITIS (EARLY): Usually caused by *S. aureus* (leading cause of prosthetic valve endocarditis [PVE]) within 2 mo of valve replacement; other organisms include *S. epidermidis,* gram-negative bacilli, diphtheroids, *Candida* organisms

PROSTHETIC VALVE ENDOCARDITIS (LATE): Typically develops >60 days after valvular replacement; involved organisms similar to early prosthetic valve endocarditis, including viridans streptococci, enterococci, and group D streptococci

NOSOCOMIAL ENDOCARDITIS:

- Secondary to intravenous catheters, total parenteral nutrition lines, pacemakers; coagulase-negative staphylococci, *S. aureus,* and streptococci most common.
- Non-HACEK (*Haemophilus* spp., *Aggregatibacter* spp., *Cardiobacterium hominis, Eikenella corrodens,* and *Kingella* spp.) gram-negative bacillus endocarditis is not primarily a disease of injection drug users. More than half of all cases are associated with health care contact.

SYNONYMS

IE
Bacterial endocarditis
Subacute bacterial endocarditis (SBE)
Endocarditis
Infective endocarditis

ICD-10CM CODES
I33.0 Acute and subacute infective endocarditis
I33.9 Acute endocarditis, unspecified

EPIDEMIOLOGY & DEMOGRAPHICS

INCIDENCE (IN U.S.): Yearly incidence is 15 cases/100,000 persons and is increasing as a result of medical interventions in the elderly and an increase in implanted cardiac devices

NOSOCOMIAL ENDOCARDITIS: 14% to 28% of cases

PREVALENCE (IN U.S.): 0.3 to 3 cases/1000 hospital admissions. 40,000 to 50,000 new cases per yr in the U.S.

BOX 1 Modified Duke Criteria for the Diagnosis of Infective Endocarditis[a]

Major Criteria
- Positive blood cultures for infective endocarditis
- Typical microorganism for infective endocarditis from two separate blood cultures in the absence of a primary focus: *Streptococcus viridans, Streptococcus bovis*
- HACEK group: *Haemophilus* spp, *Actinobacillus actinomycetemcomitans, Cardiobacterium hominis, Eikenella corrodens,* and *Kingella kingae*
- Community-acquired *Staphylococcus aureus* or enterococci
- Persistently positive blood cultures, defined as recovery of a microorganism consistent with infective endocarditis from blood cultures drawn more than 12 h apart or all of three or the majority of four or more separate blood cultures, with first and last drawn at least 1 h apart
- Single positive blood culture for *Coxiella burnetii* or antiphase IgG antibody titer >1:800

Evidence for Endocardial Involvement
- TTE (TEE in prosthetic valve) showing oscillating intracardiac mass on a valve or supporting structures, in the path of regurgitant jet or on implanted material, in the absence of an alternative anatomic explanation, *or*
- Abscess, *or*
- New partial dehiscence of prosthetic valve

Minor Criteria
- Predisposition (e.g., prosthetic valve, intravenous drug use)
- Fever: 38° C (100.4° F)
- Vascular phenomena
- Immunologic phenomena
- Microbiologic evidence: Positive blood culture but not meeting major criteria

[a]Adapted from Li JS et al: Proposed modifications to the Duke criteria for the diagnosis of infective endocarditis, *Clin Infect Dis* 30:633-638, 2000.
From Ballinger A: *Kumar & Clark's essentials of clinical medicine,* ed 6, Edinburgh, 2012, Saunders.

PREDOMINANT SEX: Male > female
PREDOMINANT AGE: 45 to 65 yr
PEAK INCIDENCE: Females: Often <35 yr old; males: 45 to 65 yr old
ENDOCARDITIS TRENDS: From 1998 through 2013 the population of patients with prosthetic valve endocarditis increased from 2% to 13.8%, as did cardiac device-related endocarditis, from 1.3% to 4.1%, whereas native valve endocarditis decreased from 74.5% to 68.4%.

PHYSICAL FINDINGS & CLINICAL PRESENTATION

- Clinical manifestations of infective endocarditis are described in Table 1 and Table 2.
- Fever may be variable in presentation; may be high, hectic, or absent.
- Fever, chills, fatigue, and rigors occur in 25% to 80% of patients.
- Heart murmur may be absent in right-sided endocarditis.
- Embolic phenomenon with peripheral manifestations is found in 50% of patients.
- Skin manifestations include petechiae, Osler nodes (Fig. E1), splinter hemorrhages, Janeway lesions (Fig. E2).
- Splenomegaly is more common with subacute course.

ETIOLOGY

Staphylococcal infection is now the leading cause of native or prosthetic valve infection. Variation in incidence may occur that is influenced by the patient's risk for developing infection. Table E3 summarizes the microbiology of infective endocarditis. Risk factors include hemodialysis (8%), intravenous (IV) drug use (10%), mitral regurgitation (43%), aortic regurgitation (26%), and rheumatic heart disease (3.3%).

TABLE 1 Symptoms in Infective Endocarditis

Symptom	Patients Affected (%)
Fever	80-95
Chills	40-70
Weakness	40-50
Malaise	20-40
Sweats	20-40
Anorexia	20-40
Headache	20-40
Dyspnea	20-40
Cough	20-30
Weight loss	20-30
Myalgia/arthralgia	10-30
Stroke	10-20
Confusion/delirium	10-20
Nausea/vomiting	10-20
Edema	5-15
Chest pain	5-15
Abdominal pain	5-15
Hemoptysis	5-10
Back pain	5-10

From Libby P et al: *Braunwald's heart disease: a textbook of cardiovascular medicine,* ed 12, Philadelphia, 2022, Elsevier.

The risk for IE varies for invasive dental procedures and by antibiotic prophylaxis (AP). A recent cohort study[1] revealed that AP was given in only 33% of procedures that fit American Heart Association guidelines for AP and in 3% of those that did not. High-risk patients given AP were 8 to 11 times less likely to develop IE after invasive dental procedures.

TABLE 2 Physical Findings in Infective Endocarditis

Finding	Patients Affected (%)
Fever	80-90
Heart murmur	75-85
New murmur	10-50
Changing murmur	5-20
Central neurologic abnormality	20-40
Splenomegaly	10-40
Petechiae/conjunctival hemorrhage	10-40
Splinter hemorrhages	5-15
Janeway lesions	5-10
Osler nodes	3-10
Retinal lesion or Roth spot	2-10

From Libby P et al: *Braunwald's heart disease: a textbook of cardiovascular medicine,* ed 12, Philadelphia, 2022, Elsevier.

ACUTE ENDOCARDITIS:
- *S. aureus* (MSSA and MRSA)
- *Staphylococcus lugdunensis*
- *Streptococcus pneumoniae*
- Streptococcal spp and groups A through G
- *Haemophilus influenzae*

SUBACUTE ENDOCARDITIS:
- Viridans streptococci (alpha-hemolytic) including nutritionally variant species:
   1. *Abiotrophia* spp and Granulicatella spp
- *Streptococcus bovis* (now called *S. gallolyticus*)
- Enterococci
- *S. aureus*

ENDOCARDITIS IN INJECTION DRUG USERS:
- *S. aureus*
- *P. aeruginosa*
- *Candida* spp
- Enterococci

PROSTHETIC VALVE ENDOCARDITIS (EARLY):
- *Staphylococcus epidermidis*
- *S. aureus*
- Gram-negative bacilli
- Group D streptococci

PROSTHETIC VALVE ENDOCARDITIS (LATE):
- *S. epidermidis*
- Viridans streptococci
- *S. aureus*
- Enterococci and group D streptococci

NOSOCOMIAL ENDOCARDITIS:
- Coagulase-negative staphylococci
- *S. aureus*
- Streptococci: Viridans, group B, enterococcus

HACEK ORGANISMS:
- Fastidious gram-negative bacilli
- *Haemophilus parainfluenzae*
- *Haemophilus aphrophilus*
- *Aggregatibacter actinomycetemcomitans*
- *Cardiobacterium hominis*
- *Eikenella corrodens*
- *Kingella kingae*

OTHER UNUSUAL PATHOGENS:
- Q fever: *Coxiella burnetii*
- *Bartonella henselae* (etiologic agent of cat scratch disease)
- *Tropheryma whipplei* (Whipple disease)

RISK FACTORS:
- Poor dental hygiene
- Long-term hemodialysis
- Diabetes mellitus
- HIV infection
- Mitral valve prolapse

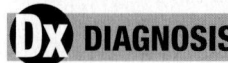 **DIAGNOSIS**

DIFFERENTIAL DIAGNOSIS
- Brain abscess
- Fever of unknown origin
- Pericarditis
- Meningitis
- Rheumatic fever
- Osteomyelitis
- Salmonella
- Tuberculosis
- Bacteremia
- Pericarditis
- Glomerulonephritis

WORKUP

Physical examination to evaluate for the previous physical findings followed by laboratory testing (see "Laboratory Tests"). Fig. 3 describes a diagnostic evaluation of suspected endocarditis. The modified Duke criteria for diagnosis of endocarditis defines "major criteria" as persistently positive blood cultures of organisms typical of endocarditis or endocardial involvement (new valvular regurgitation or positive echocardiogram). "Minor criteria" are defined as presence of predisposing condition or injection drug use, fever, embolic vascular pneumonia (e.g., glomerulonephritis, rheumatoid factor), or positive blood cultures not meeting major criteria. Definite endocarditis is two major criteria or one major criterion and three minor criteria or five minor criteria or presence of organisms by culture or histologic examination of a vegetation.

LABORATORY TESTS
- Blood cultures: Three sets in first 24 h (Table 4 describes causes of culture-negative endocarditis)
- More culturing if patient has received prior antibiotic
- CBC (anemia possibly present, subacute)
- White blood cell (leukocytosis is higher in acute endocarditis)
- Erythrocyte sedimentation rate and C-reactive protein (elevated)
- Positive rheumatoid factor (subacute endocarditis)
- Proteinuria, hematuria, red blood cell casts
- Serologies or polymerase chain reaction (PCR) for more unusual pathogens (*B. henselae, C. burnetii,* etc.)

IMAGING STUDIES
- Echocardiogram: Two-dimensional. Transthoracic echocardiography (TTE; Fig. E4) is noninvasive and more easily available but has less-than-optimal sensitivity (50% to 80%) for endocarditis.
- Transesophageal echocardiography (TEE): More sensitive in detecting vegetations and

preferred diagnostic modality. It is especially helpful with prosthetic valves or in detecting perivalvular disease (Fig. E5). Echocardiographic features that suggest potential need for surgical intervention are summarized in Table 5.
- Electrocardiogram: Look for cardiac conduction abnormalities, injury pattern, or evidence of pericarditis—any such new findings are suggestive of myocardial abscess.

TREATMENT

Initial intravenous (IV) antibiotic therapy (before culture results) is aimed at the most likely organism. The American Heart Association has developed guidelines based on the most frequently encountered bacteria. Tables 6 through 10 summarize treatment recommendations.
- **Native valve endocarditis** caused by penicillin-susceptible *S. viridans, S. gallolyticus* (previously called *S. bovis*), and other streptococci (minimum inhibitory concentrate [MIC] of penicillin ≤0.12 mcg/ml): Pen G 12 to 18 million U IV q24h continuous or divided q4h for 4 wk **or** ceftriaxone 2 g IV or intramuscular (IM) q day for 4 wk for penicillin-allergic patients. Vancomycin at 30 mg/kg per 24 h in two equally divided doses assuming normal kidney function, for 4 wk.
- **Native valve endocarditis** caused by strains of viridians streptococci and *S. gallolyticus (S. bovis)* relatively resistant to penicillin (MIC >0.12 mcg/ml): Pen G: 24 million units/24 h IV either continuously or in four or six equally divided doses for 4 wk **or** ceftriaxone 2 g/24 h IV or IM for 4 wk **plus** gentamicin 3 mg/kg/24 h IV or IM in one dose or in two or three equally divided doses for 2 wk **or** monotherapy with vancomycin 30 mg/kg/24 h IV in two equally divided doses for 4 wk not to exceed 2 g/24 h unless concentrations in serum too low.
- Native valve endocarditis due to *Staphylococcus:*
   1. **MSSA:** Nafcillin (or oxacillin) 12 g/24 h IV in four or six equally divided doses for 6 wk **plus** optional addition of gentamicin 3 mg/kg/24 h IV or IM in two or three equally divided doses for 3 to 5 days **or** cefazolin 6 g/24 h IV in three equally divided doses for 6 wk, **plus** optional addition of gentamicin 3 mg/kg/24 h IV or IM in two or three equally divided doses for 3 to 5 days. A newer antibiotic daptomycin has an indication for right-sided endocarditis with MSSA at 6 mg/kg IV q24h.
   2. **MRSA:** Vancomycin 30 mg/kg/24 h in 2 equally divided doses for 6 wk; not to exceed 2 g/24 h unless concentrations in serum are low.
- For culture-negative native valve endocarditis one of the following regimens is suggested: Ampicillin-sulbactam: 12 g/24 h IV in four equally divided doses for 4 to 6 wk **plus** gentamicin 3 mg/kg/24 h IV or IM in three equally divided doses for 4 to 6 wk **or** vancomycin

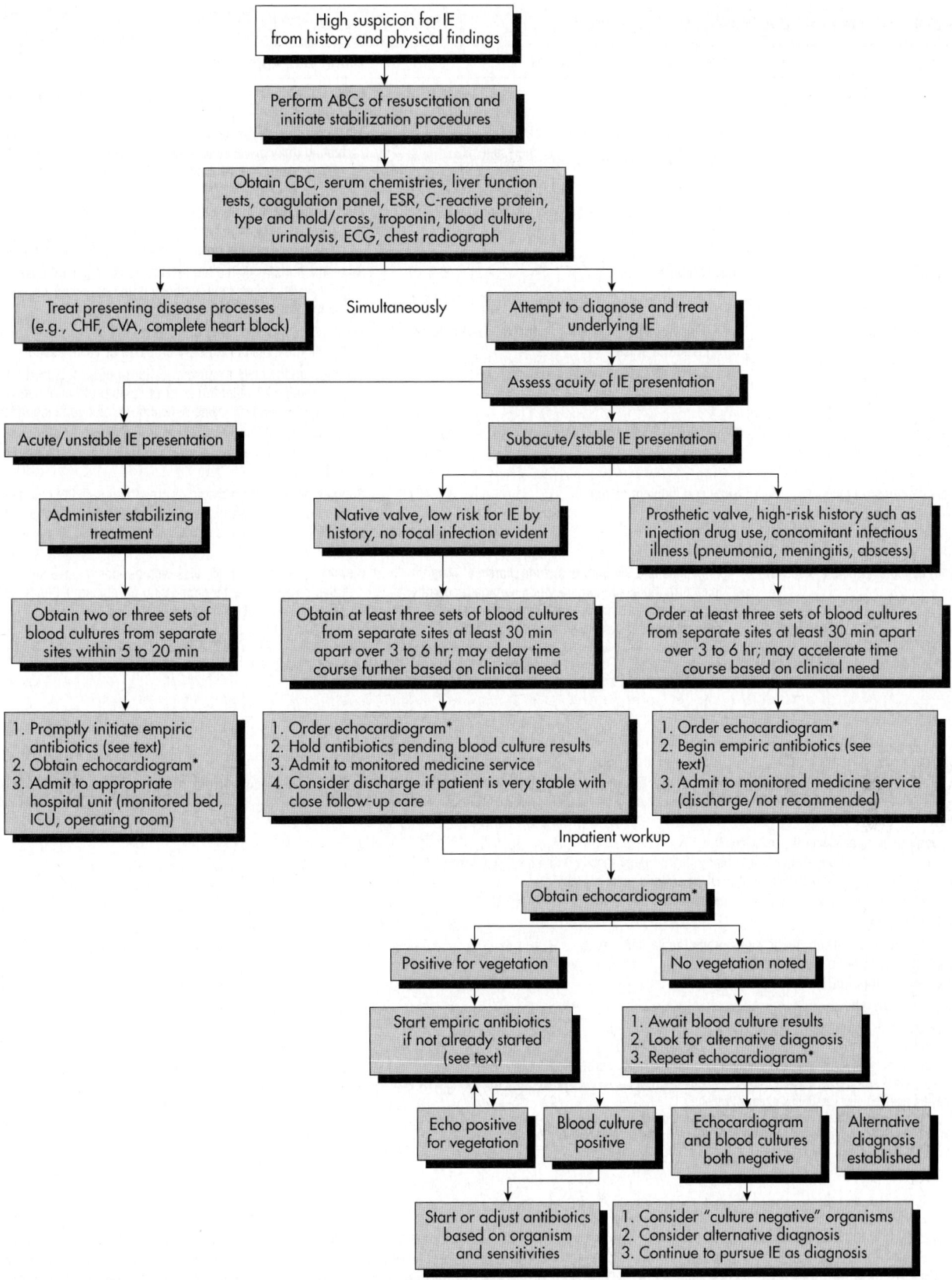

FIG. 3 Diagnostic algorithm for the emergency department management of patients in whom infective endocarditis *(IE)* is suspected. Echocardiography can be performed via either the transthoracic *(TTE)* or transesophageal *(TEE)* technique. TEE is more invasive but is more sensitive for detecting vegetations and complications of IE, such as perivalvular abscesses; it is recommended for prosthetic valves; for situations in which optimal visualization by TTE will be difficult, such as emphysema and morbid obesity; for high suspicion of IE but normal TTE findings; and for high suspicion of a complication of IE, such as perivalvular abscess. Normal findings with either technique do not exclude IE if clinical suspicion is high. Echocardiograms can be repeated in an attempt to identify problems such as vegetations and abscesses that may not be noted initially. *ABCs,* Airway, breathing, and circulation; *CBC,* complete blood count; *CHF,* congestive heart failure; *CVA,* cerebrovascular accident; *ECG,* electrocardiogram; *ESR,* erythrocyte sedimentation rate; *ICU,* intensive care unit. (From Adams JG et al: *Emergency medicine: clinical essentials,* ed 2, Philadelphia, 2013, Elsevier.)

TABLE 4 Causes of Culture-Negative Endocarditis

Organism	Epidemiology and Exposures	Diagnostic Approaches
Aspergillus and other noncandidal fungi	Prosthetic valve	Lysis-centrifugation technique; also culture and histopathologic examination of any emboli
Bartonella spp	*B. henselae:* Exposure to cats or cat fleas *B. quintana:* Louse infestation; homelessness, alcohol abuse	Most common cause of culture-negative IE in U.S.; serologic testing (may cross-react with *Chlamydia* spp.); PCR assay of valve or emboli is best test; lysis-centrifugation technique may be useful
Brucella spp	Ingestion of unpasteurized milk or dairy products; livestock contact	Blood cultures ultimately become positive in 80% of cases with extended incubation time of 4-6 wk; lysis-centrifugation technique may expedite growth; serologic tests are available
Chlamydia psittaci	Bird exposure	Serologic tests available but exhibit cross-reactivity with *Bartonella;* monoclonal antibody direct stains on tissue may be useful; PCR assay now available
Coxiella burnetii (Q fever)	Global distribution; exposure to unpasteurized milk or agricultural areas	Serologic tests (high titers of antibody to both phase 1 and phase 2 antigens); also PCR assay on blood or valve tissue
HACEK spp	Periodontal disease or preceding dental work	Although traditionally a cause of culture-negative IE, HACEK spp are now routinely isolated from most liquid broth continuous monitoring blood culture systems without prolonged incubation times
Legionella spp	Contaminated water distribution systems; prosthetic valves	Serology available; periodic subcultures onto buffered charcoal yeast extract medium; lysis-centrifugation technique; PCR assay available
Nutritionally variant streptococci	Slow and indolent course	Supplemented culture media or growth as satellite colonies around *Staphylococcus aureus* streak; antimicrobial susceptibility testing often requires processing specialized microbiology laboratory
Tropheryma whipplei (Whipple disease)	Typical signs and symptoms include diarrhea, weight loss, arthralgias, abdominal pain, lymphadenopathy, central nervous system involvement; IE may be present without systemic symptoms	Histologic examination of valve with periodic acid-Schiff stain; valve cultures may be done using fibroblast cell lines; PCR assay on vegetation material

HACEK, *Haemophilus* spp, *Aggregatibacter* spp, *Cardiobacterium hominis, Eikenella corrodens,* and *Kingella* spp; IE, infective endocarditis; PCR, polymerase chain reaction.
From Bennett JE et al: *Mandell, Douglas, and Bennett's principles and practice of infectious diseases,* ed 9, Philadelphia, 2020, Elsevier.

TABLE 5 Echocardiographic Features That Suggest Potential Need for Surgical Intervention

Vegetation

Persistent vegetation after systemic embolization
Anterior mitral valve leaflet vegetation, particularly if it is highly mobile with size >10 mm[a]
One or more embolic events during the first 2 wk of antimicrobial therapy[a]
Increase in vegetation size despite appropriate antimicrobial therapy[a,b]

Valvular Dysfunction

Acute aortic or mitral insufficiency with signs of ventricular failure[b]
Heart failure unresponsive to medical therapy[b]
Valve perforation or rupture[b]

Perivalvular Extension

Valvular dehiscence, rupture, or fistula[b]
New heart block[b,c]
Large abscess or extension of abscess despite appropriate antimicrobial therapy[b]

[a]Surgery may be required because of risk of embolization.
[b]Surgery may be required because of heart failure or failure of medical therapy.
[c]Echocardiography should not be the primary modality used to detect or monitor heart block.
From Libby P et al: *Braunwald's heart disease: a textbook of cardiovascular medicine,* ed 12, Philadelphia, 2022, Elsevier.

30 mg/kg/24 h IV in two equally divided doses for 4 to 6 wk; not to exceed 2 g/24 h unless concentrations in serum low **plus** gentamicin 3 mg/kg/24 h IV or IM in three equally divided doses for 4 to 6 wk **plus** ciprofloxacin 1000 mg/24 h PO or 800 mg/24 h IV in two equally divided doses for 4 to 6 wk.

- For treatment of native valve endocarditis due to HACEK organisms: Ceftriaxone 2 g/24 h IV or IM in one dose for 4 wk **or** ampicillin-sulbactam 12 g/24 h IV in four equally divided doses for 4 wk **or** ciprofloxacin 1000 mg/24 h PO or 800 mg/24 h IV in two equally divided doses for 4 wk.

- **Patients with prosthetic valves** endocarditis:
  1. Methicillin-susceptible strains: Nafcillin or oxacillin 12 g/24 h IV in six equally divided doses for at least 6 wk **plus** rifampin 900 mg/24 h IV or PO in three equally divided doses for at least 6 wk **plus** gentamicin 3 mg/kg IV or IM in two or three equally divided doses for 2 wk.
  2. Methicillin-resistant strains: Vancomycin 30 mg/kg/24 h in two equally divided doses for at least 6 wk **plus** rifampin 900 mg per 24 h IV or PO in three equally divided doses for at least 6 wk **plus** gentamicin 3 mg/kg/24 h IV or IM in two or three equally divided doses for 2 wk.

TABLE 6 Therapy of Native Valve Endocarditis Caused by Highly Penicillin-Susceptible Viridans Group Streptococci and *Streptococcus gallolyticus*

Regimen	Dosage[a] and Route	Duration (wk)	Class	LOE	Comments
Aqueous crystalline penicillin G sodium	12-18 million U/24 h IV either continuously or in four or six equally divided doses	4	IIa	B	Preferred in most patients >65 yr of age or patients with impairment of 8th cranial nerve function or renal function
Or					
Ceftriaxone sodium	2 g/24 h IV/IM in one dose	4	IIa	B	
Aqueous crystalline penicillin G sodium	12-18 million U/24 h IV either continuously or in six equally divided doses	2	IIa	B	2-wk regimen not intended for patients with known cardiac or extracardiac abscess or for those with creatinine clearance of <20 ml/min, impaired 8th cranial nerve function, or *Abiotrophia, Granulicatella* or *Gemella* spp infection; gentamicin dosage should be adjusted to achieve peak serum concentration of 3-4 μg/ml and trough serum concentration of <1 μg/ml when three divided doses are used; there are no optimal drug concentrations for single daily dosing[c]
Or					
Ceftriaxone sodium	2 g/24 h IV/IM in one dose	2	IIa	B	
Plus					
Gentamicin sulfate[b]	3 mg/kg/24 h IV/IM in one dose	2			
Vancomycin hydrochloride[d]	30 mg/kg/24 h IV in two equally divided doses, not to exceed 2 g/24 h unless concentrations in serum are inappropriately low	4	IIa	B	Vancomycin recommended only for patients unable to tolerate penicillin or ceftriaxone; vancomycin dosage should be adjusted to a trough concentration range of 10-15 μg/ml

Minimum inhibitory concentration (MIC) ≤0.12 μg/ml.
IM, Intramuscular; *IV,* intravenous; *LOE,* level of evidence; *MIC,* minimum inhibitory concentration.
[a]Dosages recommended are for patients with normal renal function.
[b]Other potentially nephrotoxic drugs (e.g., nonsteroidal antiinflammatory drugs) should be used with caution in patients receiving gentamicin therapy.
[c]Data for once-daily dosing of aminoglycosides for children exist, but no data for treatment of infective endocarditis (IE) are available.
[d]Vancomycin dosages should be infused over at least 1 h to reduce the risk of histamine-release "red man" syndrome.

TABLE 7 Therapy of Native Valve Endocarditis Caused by Strains of Viridans Group Streptococci and *Streptococcus gallolyticus* Relatively Resistant to Penicillin

Regimen	Dosage[a] and Route	Duration (WK)	Class	LOE	Comments
Aqueous crystalline penicillin G sodium	24 million U/24 h IV either continuously or in four to six equally divided doses	4	IIa	B	Patients with endocarditis caused by penicillin-resistant (MIC ≥0.5 μg/ml) strains should be treated with regimen recommended for enterococcal
Or					
Ceftriaxone sodium	2 g/24 h IV/IM in one dose	4	IIa	B	
Plus					
Gentamicin sulfate[b]	3 mg/kg/24 h IV/IM in one dose	2			
Vancomycin hydrochloride	30 mg/kg/24 h IV in two equally divided doses, not to exceed 2 g/24 h, unless serum concentrations are inappropriately low	4	IIb	C	Vancomycin[c] therapy recommended only for patients unable to tolerate penicillin or ceftriaxone therapy

Minimum inhibitory concentration (MIC) >0.12 μg/ml to <0.5 μg/ml.
IM, Intramuscular; *IV,* intravenous; *LOE,* level of evidence.
[a]Dosages recommended are for patients with normal renal function.
[b]See Table 6 for appropriate dosage of gentamicin.
[c]See Table 6 for appropriate dosage of vancomycin.
From Libby P et al: *Braunwald's heart disease: a textbook of cardiovascular medicine,* ed 12, Philadelphia, 2022, Elsevier.

Antibiotic therapy after identification of the organism should be guided by susceptibility testing, preferably by formal testing by MIC.

DISPOSITION

- The patient may need outpatient IV antibiotic therapy, and arrangements need to be made to ensure safe vascular access and continuity of care with outpatient IV therapy team.
- Long-term follow-up is essential after therapy has ended; relapse of endocarditis may occur.
- Prophylaxis with antibiotics will be needed before dental procedures as a previous episode of endocarditis increases the risk of recurrent

endocarditis associated with transient bacteremia from dental procedures.

REFERRAL

- To an infectious disease specialist
- To a cardiologist or a cardiac surgeon if evidence of heart failure, refractory infection, myocardial abscess, valve disruption, or major embolic events occur
- The timing and indications for surgical intervention to prevent systemic embolism in infective endocarditis remain controversial. Trials have shown that early surgery in patients with infective endocarditis and large vegetations

significantly reduced death and embolic events by decreasing the risk of systemic embolism

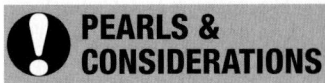

PEARLS & CONSIDERATIONS

- Serologies and/or PCR exist for more unusual zoonotic causes of endocarditis such as *B. henselae* (cat exposure), *C. burnetii* (farm animals), *Brucella* spp (unpasteurized milk or cheese), and *T. whipplei* (soil and farm animals).
- 1-yr mortality has not improved and remains at 30%.

Diseases and Disorders

I

TABLE 8 Therapy for Endocarditis of Prosthetic Valves or Other Prosthetic Material Caused by Viridans Group Streptococci and *Streptococcus gallolyticus*

Regimen	Dosage[a] and Route	Duration (wk)	Class	LOE	Comments
Penicillin-Susceptible Strain (MIC ≤0.12 μg/ml)					
Aqueous crystalline penicillin G sodium	24 million U/24 h IV either continuously or in four to six equally divided doses	6	IIa	B	Penicillin or ceftriaxone together with gentamicin has not demonstrated cure rates superior to those for monotherapy with penicillin or ceftriaxone for patients with highly susceptible strain; gentamicin should not be administered to patients with creatinine clearance of <30 ml/min.
Or					
Ceftriaxone	2 g/24 h IV/IM in one dose	6	IIa	B	
With or without					
Gentamicin sulfate[b]	3 mg/kg/24 h IV/IM in one dose	2			
Vancomycin hydrochloride[c]	30 mg/kg per 24 h IV in two equally divided doses	6	IIa	B	Vancomycin therapy recommended only for patients unable to tolerate penicillin or ceftriaxone.
Penicillin—Relatively or Fully Resistant Strain (MIC >0.12 μg/ml)					
Aqueous crystalline penicillin sodium	24 million U/24 h IV either continuously or in four to six equally divided doses	6	IIa	B	
Or					
Ceftriaxone	2 g/24 h IV/IM in one dose	6	IIa	B	
Plus					
Gentamicin sulfate	3 mg/kg/24 h IV/IM in one dose	6			
Vancomycin hydrochloride	30 mg/kg/24 h IV in two equally divided doses	6	IIb	C	Vancomycin therapy is recommended only for patients unable to tolerate penicillin or ceftriaxone.

IM, Intramuscular; *IV*, intravenous; *LOE*, level of evidence; *MIC*, minimum inhibitory concentration.
[a]Dosages recommended are for patients with normal renal function.
[b]See Table 6 for appropriate dosage of gentamicin.
[c]See text and Table 6 for appropriate dosage of vancomycin.
Reprinted with permission *Circulation*. 132:1435-1486, 2015. ©2015 American Heart Association, Inc.

TABLE 9 Therapy for Endocarditis Caused by Staphylococci in the Absence of Prosthetic Materials

Regimen	Dosage[a] and Route	Duration (wk)	Class	LOE	Comments
Oxacillin-Susceptible Strains					
Nafcillin or oxacillin[b]	12 g/24 h IV in four to six equally divided doses	6	IIa	B	For complicated right-sided IE and for left-sided IE; for uncomplicated right-sided IE, 2 wk (see text)
For penicillin-allergic (nonanaphylactoid type) patients:					Consider skin testing for oxacillin-susceptible staphylococci and questionable history of immediate-type hypersensitivity to penicillin
Cefazolin	6 g/24 h IV in three equally divided doses	6	IIa	B	Cephalosporins should be avoided in patients with anaphylactoid-type hypersensitivity to β-lactams; vancomycin should be used in these cases[c]
Oxacillin-Resistant Strains					
Vancomycin[b]	30 mg/kg/24 h IV in two equally divided doses	6	IIa	B	Adjust vancomycin dosage to a trough serum concentration of 10-15 μg/ml (see text for vancomycin alternatives)

IE, Infective endocarditis; *IV*, intravenous; *LOE*, Level of evidence.
[a]Dosages recommended are for patients with normal renal function.
[b]Penicillin G 24 million U/24 h IV in four to six equally divided doses may be used in place of nafcillin or oxacillin if strain is penicillin-susceptible (minimum inhibitory concentration. ≤0.1 μg/ml) and does not produce beta-lactamase.
[c]For specific dosing adjustment and issues concerning vancomycin, see Table 6 footnotes.
Reprinted with permission *Circulation*. 132:1435-1486, 2015. ©2015 American Heart Association, Inc.

COMMENTS
- For endocarditis prophylaxis refer to Section V.
- In regard to antibiotic prophylaxis before dental procedures in patients with orthopedic implants, the 2013 guidelines from the American Academy of Orthopedic Surgeons (AAOS) and the American Dental Association (ADA) advises clinicians to consider discontinuing the practice of routinely prescribing prophylactic antibiotics for patients with hip and knee prosthetic joint implants undergoing dental procedures.

- Viridans streptococcus are a large group of commensal bacteria that are either alpha-hemolytic on blood agar plates or nonhemolytic. Common members of this family include *S. mutans, S. anginosus, S. mitis, S. sanguis, S. oralis,* and *S. salivarius.* These tend to be oral/dental flora and most highly penicillin susceptible.
- Trials have shown that in patients with endocarditis in the left side of the heart who were in stable condition, changing to oral antibiotic treatment was noninferior to continued intravenous antibiotic treatment. Additional trials will be necessary before changing current parenteral antibiotic guidelines to include oral antibiotic regimens.

REFERENCE & SUGGESTED READINGS
Available at eBooks.Health.Elsevier.com.

RELATED CONTENT
Endocarditis (Patient Information)

AUTHOR: **GLENN G. FORT, MD, MPH**

TABLE 10 Therapy for Endocarditis of Prosthetic Valves or Other Prosthetic Material Caused by Staphylococci

Regimen	Dosage[a] and Route	Duration (wk)	Class	LOE	Comments
Oxacillin-Susceptible Strains					
Nafcillin or oxacillin	12 g/24 h IV in six equally divided doses	≥6	IIa	B	Penicillin G 24 million U/24 h IV in four to six equally divided doses may be used in place of nafcillin or oxacillin if strain is penicillin susceptible (MIC ≤0.1 µg/ml) and does not produce beta-lactamase; vancomycin should be used in patients with immediate-type hypersensitivity reactions to beta-lactam antibiotics (see Table 6 for dosing guidelines); cefazolin may be substituted for nafcillin or oxacillin in patients with nonimmediate hypersensitivity reactions to penicillins
Plus					
Rifampin	900 mg/24 h IV/PO in 3 equally divided doses	≥6			
Plus					
Gentamicin[b]	3 mg/kg/24 h IV/IM in two or three equally divided doses	2			
Oxacillin-Resistant Strains					
Vancomycin	30 mg/kg/24 h in two equally divided doses	≥6	IIa	B	Adjust vancomycin to achieve a trough serum concentration of 10-15 µg/ml (see text for gentamicin alternatives)
Plus					
Rifampin	900 mg/24 h IV/PO in three equally divided doses	≥6			
Plus					
Gentamicin	3 mg/kg/24 h IV/IM in two or three equally divided doses	2			

IM, Intramuscular; *IV,* intravenous; *LOE,* level of evidence; *MIC,* minimum inhibitory concentration; *PO,* oral.
[a]Dosages recommended are for patients with normal renal function.
[b]Gentamicin should be administered in close proximity to vancomycin, nafcillin, or oxacillin dosing.
Reprinted with permission *Circulation.* 132:1435-1486, 2015. ©2015 American Heart Association, Inc.

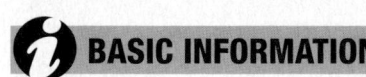

BASIC INFORMATION

DEFINITION

Endometrial cancer, also called endometrial carcinoma (EC), is cancer of the endometrium, which is the lining of the uterus. Traditionally, EC was divided into two types: Type 1, which is estrogen-driven, and type 2, which is not estrogen driven. However, EC is now more commonly subdivided into different types based on histology—how the cells appear under the microscope (Box 1).

Most endometrial cancers, >87%, are adenocarcinomas with endometrioid cancer being the most common type of adenocarcinoma (Table 1).

Histologic types include:
- Endometroid Carcinoma: Adenocarcinoma and adenocarcinoma variants
- Mucinous adenocarcinoma
- Serous adenocarcinoma
- Clear cell adenocarcinoma
- Undifferentiated carcinoma
- Neuroendocrine tumors
- Mixed carcinoma

SYNONYMS

Uterine cancer (some forms)
Carcinoma of the endometrium
EC

ICD-10CM CODES
C54.1	Malignant neoplasm of endometrium
C54.9	Malignant neoplasm of corpus uteri, unspecified
C55	Malignant neoplasm of uterus, part unspecified

EPIDEMIOLOGY & DEMOGRAPHICS

INCIDENCE:
- In 2021, 66,570 new cases of uterinc cancer are predicted in the U.S. The rate of new cases of EC was 28.1 per 100,000 based on 2014 to 2018 cases. Incidence was greater among white and black women compared with American Indian/Alaska Native, Hispanic, and Asian Pacific Islander women. It is the most common gynecologic malignancy in the U.S. and the most common type of cancer that affects the female reproductive organs.

BOX 1   Endometrial Primary Adenocarcinomas

Typical endometrioid adenocarcinomas
Adenocarcinoma with squamous elements
Clear cell carcinoma
Serous carcinoma
Secretory carcinoma
Mucinous carcinoma
Squamous carcinoma

From Gershenson DM et al: *Comprehensive gynecology,* ed 8, Philadelphia, 2022, Elsevier.

- Unlike most cancers in the U.S., endometrial cancer is rising in both incidence and associated mortality.

PREDOMINANT SEX & AGE:
- Median age at diagnosis: 63 yr
- Median age of death from EC: 70 yr

RISK FACTORS:
- Age: Most cases are diagnosed in postmenopausal women, with a median age of 63 yr.
- Estrogen exposure/hormone imbalance: Whether from early menarche, late menopause, diabetes, nulliparity, tamoxifen use, polycystic ovary syndrome, or unopposed estrogen therapy, the more exposure the endometrium has to estrogen, the more a woman's risk of developing EC increases.
- Obesity: Body mass index of 25 or greater is a major risk factor for EC.
- Genetics: Lynch syndrome increases the risk of EC (and ovarian, colon, and other types of cancers). Cowden syndrome: Relative risks can be found in Table 2.

PHYSICAL FINDINGS & CLINICAL PRESENTATION
- Abnormal uterine bleeding or postmenopausal bleeding in 90%
- Pyometra or hematometra
- Abnormal Pap smear: Endometrial cells, atypical glandular cells, or adenocarcinoma
- Incidental finding at hysterectomy

ETIOLOGY

Endogenous or exogenous chronic unopposed estrogen stimulation of the endometrium

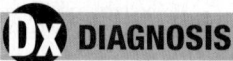 **DIAGNOSIS**

DIFFERENTIAL DIAGNOSIS
- Endometrial atypical hyperplasia
- Other genital tract malignancy
- Uterine polyps
- Atrophic vaginitis
- Granulosa cell tumor
- Fibroid uterus
- Adenomyosis

TABLE 1   Pathogenetic Subsets of Endometrial Carcinoma

Parameter	Type I	Type II
Age	50s-60s	60s-70s
Obesity	Common	Uncommon
Estrogenic stimuli	Common	Uncommon
Endometrium	Anovulatory	Atrophic
Precursor	Endometrial intraepithelial neoplasia	Presumed EmGD
Transition	Slow	Unknown
Type	Endometrioid	Papillary serous or mixed
Molecular genetics	MSI, *PTEN* mutation; loss of PAX2	p53 mutation, 1p deletions; loss of PAX2
Familial	Hereditary nonpolyposis colonic cancer syndrome	
Spread	Lymph nodes	Peritoneum
Concurrent ovarian	Common	Uncommon
Prognosis	Good	Poor

EmGD, Endometrial glandular dysplasia; *MSI,* microsatellite instability.
From Crum CP et al: *Diagnostic gynecologic and obstetric pathology,* ed 3, Philadelphia, 2018, Elsevier.

TABLE 2   Risk Factors for Endometrial Cancer

Factor	Relative Risk
Overweight (lbs):	
• 20-50	3.0
• 50+	10.0
Nulliparous:	
• vs. one child	2.0
• vs. five children	5.0
Late menopause (>52 vs. 49 yr)	2.4
Diabetes mellitus	2.7
Unopposed estrogen therapy	6.0
Tamoxifen therapy	2.0
Sequential oral contraceptives	7.0
Combination oral contraceptives	0.5
Cowden syndrome (*PTEN* mutation)	Three- to fivefold increased risk
Hereditary nonpolyposis colonic cancer syndrome	40%-60% lifetime risk
Family member with endometrial cancer	3.4

From Crum CP et al: *Diagnostic gynecologic and obstetric pathology,* ed 3, Philadelphia, 2018, Elsevier.

E

WORKUP

- Complete history and physical examination
- Endometrial biopsy or dilation and curettage (Table 3)
- Assessment of operative risk
- Staging (Tables 4 and 5)
- Fig. 1 is a diagnostic algorithm for diagnosing endometrial carcinoma for women with abnormal uterine bleeding

LABORATORY TESTS

- Complete blood count
- Prothrombin time and partial thromboplastin time if bleeding is heavy
- Chemistry profile including liver function tests
- Consider CA-125 level

IMAGING STUDIES

- Chest x-ray
- Computed tomography (CT) scan if concern for metastatic disease, and/or pelvic ultrasound (Fig. E2)
- Transvaginal ultrasound (Fig. E3) in postmenopausal women with vaginal bleeding

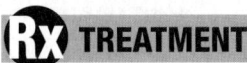 TREATMENT

NONPHARMACOLOGIC THERAPY

- Surgery is the mainstay of treatment, with or without adjuvant radiation and/or chemotherapy, depending on tumor histology, stage, and grade. Laparoscopic surgery for early-stage EC is as safe and effective as laparotomy. Robotic laparoscopy procedures have increased significantly in recent years for this indication.
- Surgery generally consists of pelvic washings, total hysterectomy and bilateral salpingo-oophorectomy, selective pelvic and periaortic lymphadenectomy, and omental biopsy depending on stage, grade, and histology.
- Brachytherapy and/or teletherapy are added in an advanced stage.

- Chemotherapy (carboplatin, paclitaxel) may be used for patients with high-risk endometrial cancer. Hormonal therapy (progestins alone or in combination with tamoxifen, selective estrogen-receptor modulators, aromatase inhibitors, synthetic steroid derivatives, and gonadotropin-releasing hormone analogues) may also be considered in cases where palliation, rather than cure, is the main intent of treatment, or in patients with multiple coexisting medical conditions who may not be surgical candidates.
- Hormonal therapy, commonly a levonorgestrel intrauterine device, is an option for some young women with early-stage, low-grade EC who wish to preserve fertility. This choice should be discussed with a gynecologic oncologist.

ACUTE GENERAL Rx

- A thorough workup should be completed before any therapy for EC.
- Surgery hysterectomy with bilateral salpingo-oophorectomy is the treatment of choice.

CHRONIC Rx

- Physical and pelvic examination every 3 mo for 2 yr, then every 6 mo for 2 yr, and annually thereafter with imaging as clinically indicated

---

TABLE 3 Differential Diagnosis of Endometrial Carcinoma (Curettings)

Parameter	Mimicking	Differential Diagnosis
Gland architecture	Cancer	Telescoping artifact; stromal collapse breakdown; sectioning artifacts
	Benign	Microglandular mucinous carcinoma; surface endometrioid carcinoma
Nuclear atypia	Cancer	Surface or glandular repair; Arias-Stella changes (hormonal therapy); radiation effect
Papillary changes	Cancer	Exfoliation artifact; stromal breakdown with papillary changes; papillary syncytial changes
	Benign	Papillary mucinous carcinoma

From Crum CP et al: *Diagnostic gynecologic and obstetric pathology,* ed 3, Philadelphia, 2018, Elsevier.

TABLE 4 National Comprehensive Cancer Network Treatment Guidelines for Endometrial Carcinoma After Comprehensive Surgical Staging

Stage I_A

Grade 1 without ARF	Observe
Grade 1 with ARF	Observe or VBT
Grade 2 or 3 without ARF	Observe or VBT
Grade 2 or 3 with ARF	Observe or VBT and/or pelvic RT

Stage I_B

Grade 1 without ARF	Observe
Grade 1 with ARF	Observe or VBT
Grade 2 without ARF	Observe or VBT
Grade 2 with ARF	Observe or VBT and/or pelvic RT
Grade 3 without ARF	Observe or VBT and/or pelvic RT
Grade 3 with ARF	Observe or VBT and/or pelvic RT ± chemotherapy

Stage II

Grade 1	VBT and/or pelvic RT
Grade 2	Pelvic RT and VBT
Grade 3	Pelvic RT and VBT ± chemotherapy

Stage III_A — Chemotherapy ± pelvic RT or tumor-directed RT ± chemotherapy or pelvic RT ± VBT

Stage III_B-III_C — Chemotherapy and/or tumor-directed RT

Stage IV_A-IV_B — Chemotherapy ± RT

ARF, Adverse risk factors (age, positive lymphovascular space invasion, tumor size, lower uterine or cervical involvement); *RT,* radiation therapy; *VBT,* vaginal brachytherapy.
From Niederhuber JE: *Abeloff's clinical oncology,* ed 6, Philadelphia, 2020, Elsevier.

TABLE 5 Revised FIGO Staging for Endometrial Cancer (adopted 2009)

Stages*	Characteristic
I	Tumor confined to the corpus uteri
I_A	No or less than half myometrial invasion
I_B	Invasion equal to or more than half of the myometrium
II	Tumor invades cervical stroma but does not extend beyond the uterus[†]
III	Local or regional spread of the tumor
III_A	Tumor invades serosa of the corpus uteri or the adnexa[‡]
III_B	Vaginal or parametrial involvement[‡]
III_C	Metastases to pelvic or paraaortic lymph nodes[‡]
III_C1	Positive pelvic nodes
III_C2	Positive paraaortic lymph nodes with or without positive pelvic lymph nodes
IV	Tumor invades bladder or bowel mucosa, or distant metastasis
IV_A*	Tumor invasion of bladder or bowel mucosa
IV_B	Distant metastases, including intraabdominal or inguinal lymph nodes

FIGO, Fédération Internationale de Gynécologie et d'Obstétrique (International Federation of Gynecology and Obstetrics).
* G1, G2, or G3.
[†]Endocervical glandular involvement should be considered only as stage I and no longer as stage II.
[‡]Positive cytology has to be reported separately without changing the stage.
From Lobo RA et al: *Comprehensive gynecology,* ed 7, Philadelphia, 2017, Elsevier.

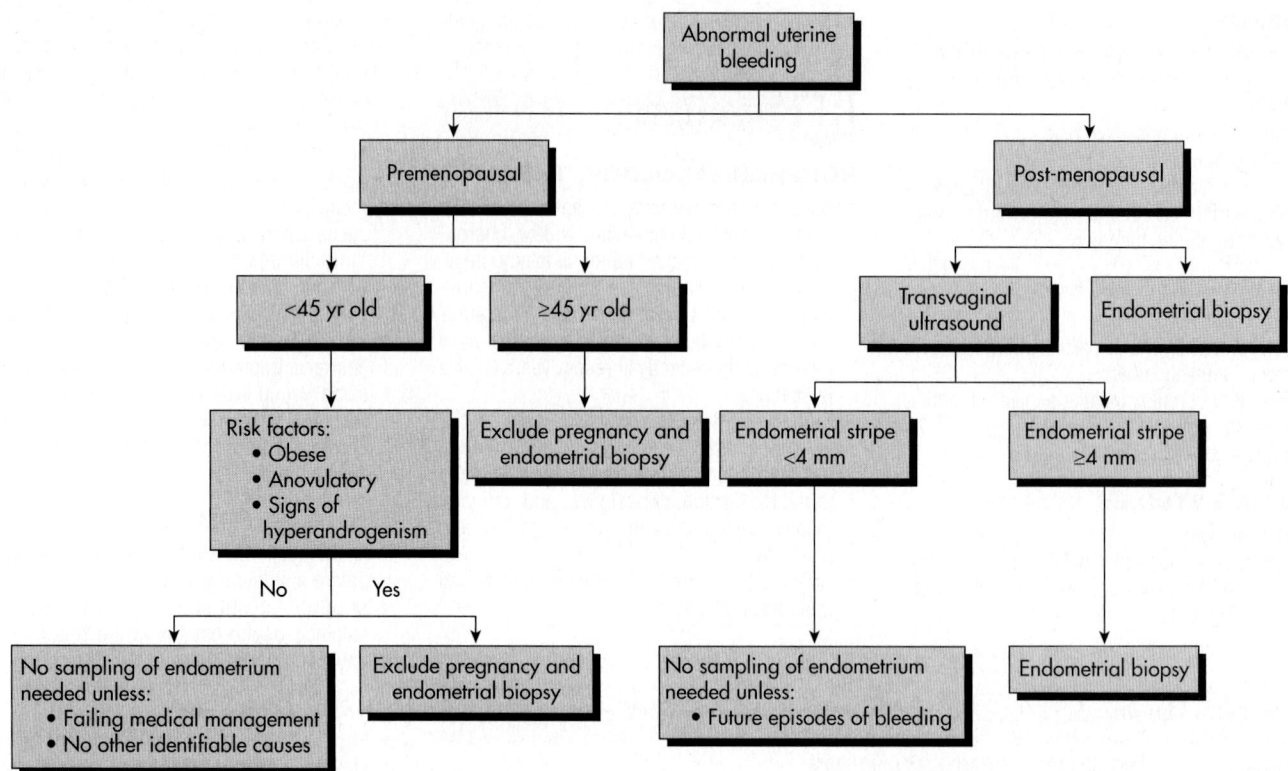

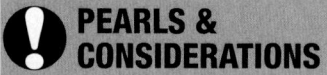

FIG. 1 Diagnostic algorithm to diagnose endometrial carcinoma for women with abnormal uterine bleeding. (From Niederhuber JE: *Abeloff's clinical oncology,* ed 6, Philadelphia, 2020, Elsevier.)

- Hormone replacement (combination) a consideration in low-risk patients (stage I or early stage II)

DISPOSITION

- Survival is generally defined by the stage of the disease and histology.
- The majority of cases present early, and the 5-yr survival is generally good (Fig. E4).
- Some histologic types (clear cell, papillary serous) have worse survival rates, as they tend to be more aggressive with higher rates of metastatic disease at the time of diagnosis.

PEARLS & CONSIDERATIONS

Any woman with postmenopausal bleeding or abnormal uterine bleeding with risk factors for endometrial cancer needs evaluation by a gynecologist and either endometrial biopsy and/or pelvic ultrasound. When endometrial cancer is diagnosed, the patient should be cared for by a gynecologic oncologist and undergo surgical staging in a minimally invasive procedure when possible.

RELATED CONTENT

Endometrial Cancer (Patient Information)
Abnormal Uterine Bleeding (Related Key Topic)
Uterine Malignancy (Related Key Topic)

AUTHORS: **EMILY SAUCK, DO, MBA** and **ANTHONY SCISCIONE, DO**

BASIC INFORMATION

DEFINITION

Endometriosis is defined as the presence of functioning endometrial glands and stroma-like tissue outside the uterine cavity (Fig. E1). It is an estrogen-dependent condition that causes dysmenorrhea and pelvic pain. It causes a chronic inflammatory reaction, often causing formation of adhesions in the abdomen and pelvis.

ICD-10CM CODES
N80.9	Endometriosis, unspecified
N80.0	Endometriosis of uterus
N80.1	Endometriosis of ovary
N80.2	Endometriosis of fallopian tube
N80.3	Endometriosis of pelvic peritoneum
N80.4	Endometriosis of rectovaginal septum and vagina
N80.5	Endometriosis of intestine
N80.6	Endometriosis in cutaneous scar
N80.8	Other endometriosis

EPIDEMIOLOGY & DEMOGRAPHICS

PREVALENCE:
- Reproductive-age women: 10%
- Women with dysmenorrhea: 40% to 60%
- Subfertile women: 25% to 50%
- 30% to 50% of women with endometriosis are infertile[1]
- In symptomatic adolescents undergoing laparoscopy, 64% were found to have endometriosis[2]
- Incidence peaks between ages 25 and 45 yr

MOST COMMON AGE AT DIAGNOSIS: 25 to 29 yr

GENETICS:
- Familial association: If first-degree relative is affected, the patient has a seven- to tenfold increased risk of having the disease.
- Polygenic-multifactorial inheritance pattern.

PHYSICAL FINDINGS & CLINICAL PRESENTATION

- Classic triad is dysmenorrhea, dyspareunia, and infertility.
- Presence of pelvic pain does not correlate with the total area of endometriosis (stage of disease), type of lesion, or volume of disease, but is correlated with the depth of infiltration.
- Other symptoms include abnormal bleeding (premenstrual spotting, menorrhagia), cyclic abdominal pain, irritable bowel syndrome, dyschezia, dysuria, hematuria, and urinary frequency.
- Rare manifestations: Catamenial hemothorax, bloody pleural effusion, massive ascites occurring during menses, kidney and brain lesions.
- Most severe discomfort is associated with lesions >1 cm in depth.
- Bimanual examination may reveal tender uterosacral ligaments, cul-de-sac nodularity, induration of the rectovaginal septum, fixed retroversion of the uterus, adnexal mass, and generalized or localized tenderness.

ETIOLOGY[3]
- Retrograde menstruation theory: Retrograde flow of sloughed endometrial cells through fallopian tubes to surrounding pelvic structures (Sampson theory)
- Coelomic metaplasia theory: Transformation of multipotential cells of the coelomic epithelium into endometrium-like cells
- Vascular dissemination theory: Transport of endometrial cells to distant sites by the uterine vascular and lymphatic systems
- Autoimmune disease theory: Disorder of immune surveillance allows growth of endometrial implants
- Molecular mechanisms in endometriosis are illustrated in Fig. E2
- Genes and gene products aberrantly expressed in endometrium from women with endometriosis are summarized in Table 1

DIAGNOSIS

DIFFERENTIAL DIAGNOSIS
- Ectopic pregnancy
- Acute appendicitis
- Chronic appendicitis
- Pelvic inflammatory disease (PID)
- Pelvic adhesions
- Ruptured hemorrhagic cyst
- Hernia
- Irritable bowel syndrome
- Uterine leiomyomata
- Adenomyosis
- Nerve entrapment syndrome
- Interstitial cystitis
- Musculoskeletal disorders

WORKUP
- Thorough history and physical examination, including pelvic ultrasound.
- Definitive diagnosis of endometriosis can be made only by histologic confirmation during surgery (gold standard).
- Fig. 3 illustrates a diagnostic and management algorithm for endometriosis.

SURGICAL STAGING
- American Society for Reproductive Medicine classification system for endometriosis (ASRM revised 1996) is the most widely accepted staging system
- Value: Uniform recording of operative findings
- Limitations
  1. Does not correlate well with the symptoms of pain, dyspareunia, or infertility
  2. Not a good predictor of successful pregnancy after treatment

Stage I	Minimal
Stage II	Mild
Stage III	Moderate
Stage IV	Severe

LABORATORY TESTS
Cancer antigen 125 (CA125): Limited overall value in the diagnosis of endometriosis
- Also elevated in ovarian epithelial neoplasm, myomas, adenomyosis, acute PID, ovarian cysts, pancreatitis, chronic liver disease, menstruation, and pregnancy

TABLE 1 Anatomic Distribution of Endometriosis

Common Sites	Rare Sites
Ovaries	Umbilicus
Pelvic peritoneum	Episiotomy scar
Ligaments of the uterus	Bladder
Sigmoid colon	Kidney
Appendix	Lungs
Pelvic lymph nodes	Arms
Cervix	Legs
Vagina	Nasal mucosa
Fallopian tubes	Spinal column

From Gershenson DM et al: *Comprehensive gynecology*, ed 8, Philadelphia, 2022, Elsevier.

- CA125 value >35 U/ml: Positive predictive value of 0.58 and a negative predictive value of 0.96 for the presence of endometriosis

IMAGING STUDIES
- Pelvic ultrasound
  1. Ultrasound characteristics may suggest endometriomas versus other benign or malignant ovarian conditions.
  2. Persistent solid or cystic-solid ovarian masses require definitive tissue diagnosis with laparoscopy.
- MRI
  1. Highly accurate in detecting endometriomas
  2. Limited sensitivity in detecting diffuse pelvic endometriosis, especially if sessile lesions
- CT scan may show adnexal masses of varying density (Fig. 4)

TREATMENT (TABLE 2)

NONPHARMACOLOGIC THERAPY
Expectant management (observation for 6 to 12 mo) for stage I or stage II endometriosis-associated infertility. Evaluation should take place if the patient meets the diagnostic criteria for infertility.

ACUTE GENERAL Rx
NSAIDs for symptomatic relief of dysmenorrhea.

CHRONIC Rx[4]
PHARMACOLOGIC MANAGEMENT: Estrogen-progesterone:
- Mechanism of action is decidualization and atrophy of endometrial tissue
- Continuous use of combination oral contraceptives for minimum of 6 mo and continuing indefinitely

Progestins:
- Mechanism of action is decidualization and atrophy of endometrial tissue
- Medroxyprogesterone acetate 10 to 30 mg orally daily
- Norethindrone acetate 5 mg orally daily or twice daily
- Levonorgestrel orally or levonorgestrel-releasing intrauterine system
- Comparison with danazol: Progestins cost less, have a more tolerable side-effect profile, and have comparable efficacy with

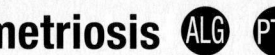
Diagnostic laparoscopy (describe using standard proforma, take photos)

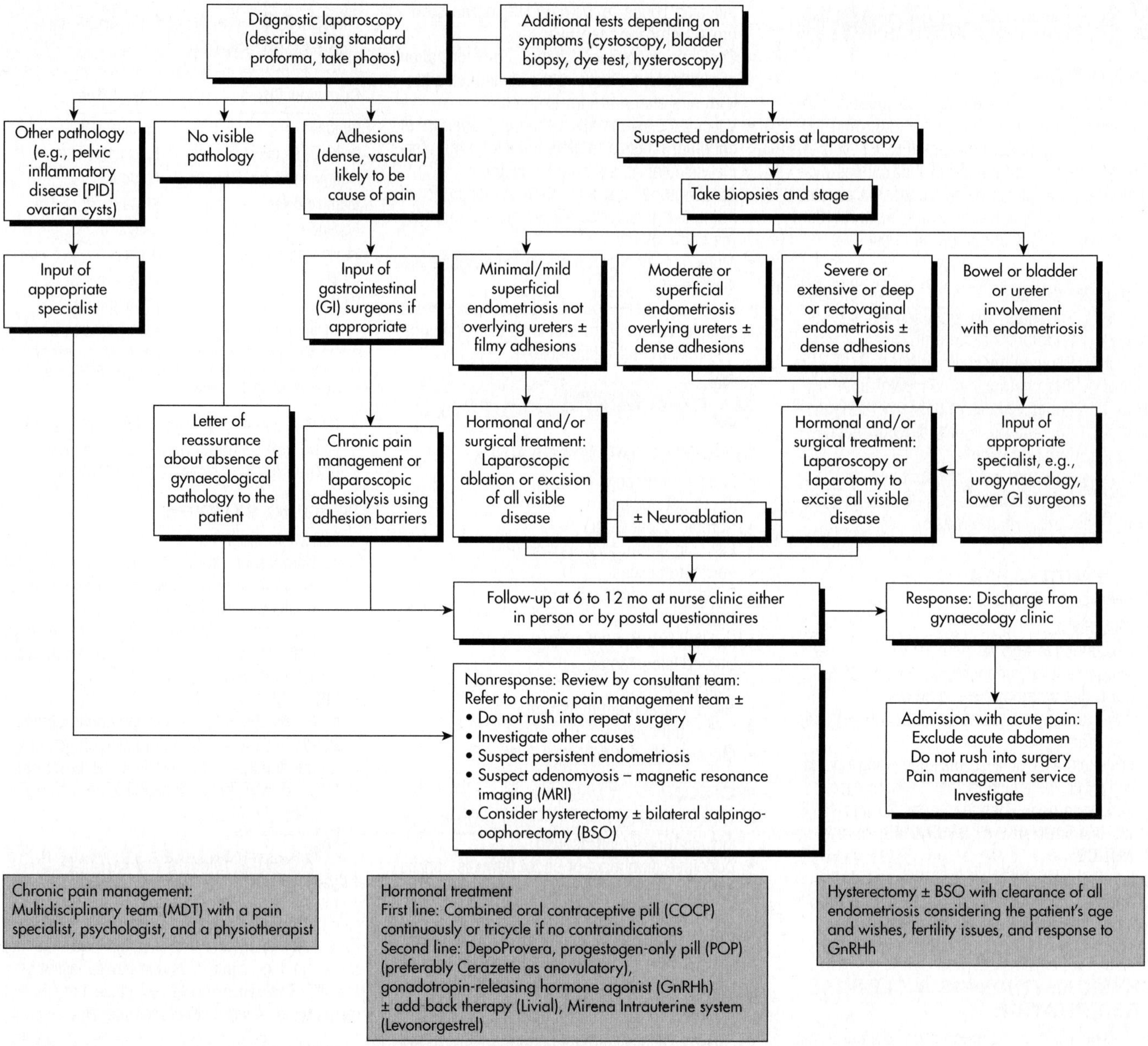

Additional tests depending on symptoms (cystoscopy, bladder biopsy, dye test, hysteroscopy)

Other pathology (e.g., pelvic inflammatory disease [PID] ovarian cysts)

No visible pathology

Adhesions (dense, vascular) likely to be cause of pain

Suspected endometriosis at laparoscopy

Take biopsies and stage

Input of appropriate specialist

Input of gastrointestinal (GI) surgeons if appropriate

Minimal/mild superficial endometriosis not overlying ureters ± filmy adhesions

Moderate or superficial endometriosis overlying ureters ± dense adhesions

Severe or extensive or deep or rectovaginal endometriosis ± dense adhesions

Bowel or bladder or ureter involvement with endometriosis

Letter of reassurance about absence of gynaecological pathology to the patient

Chronic pain management or laparoscopic adhesiolysis using adhesion barriers

Hormonal and/or surgical treatment: Laparoscopic ablation or excision of all visible disease

± Neuroablation

Hormonal and/or surgical treatment: Laparoscopy or laparotomy to excise all visible disease

Input of appropriate specialist, e.g., urogynaecology, lower GI surgeons

Follow-up at 6 to 12 mo at nurse clinic either in person or by postal questionnaires

Response: Discharge from gynaecology clinic

Nonresponse: Review by consultant team: Refer to chronic pain management team ±
• Do not rush into repeat surgery
• Investigate other causes
• Suspect persistent endometriosis
• Suspect adenomyosis – magnetic resonance imaging (MRI)
• Consider hysterectomy ± bilateral salpingo-oophorectomy (BSO)

Admission with acute pain: Exclude acute abdomen Do not rush into surgery Pain management service Investigate

Chronic pain management: Multidisciplinary team (MDT) with a pain specialist, psychologist, and a physiotherapist

Hormonal treatment
First line: Combined oral contraceptive pill (COCP) continuously or tricycle if no contraindications
Second line: DepoProvera, progestogen-only pill (POP) (preferably Cerazette as anovulatory), gonadotropin-releasing hormone agonist (GnRHh) ± add back therapy (Livial), Mirena Intrauterine system (Levonorgestrel)

Hysterectomy ± BSO with clearance of all endometriosis considering the patient's age and wishes, fertility issues, and response to GnRHh

FIG. 3 An example of a management pathway for patients with endometriosis after laparoscopy. (From Magowan BA: *Clinical obstetrics and gynecology*, ed 4, Philadelphia, 2019, Elsevier.)

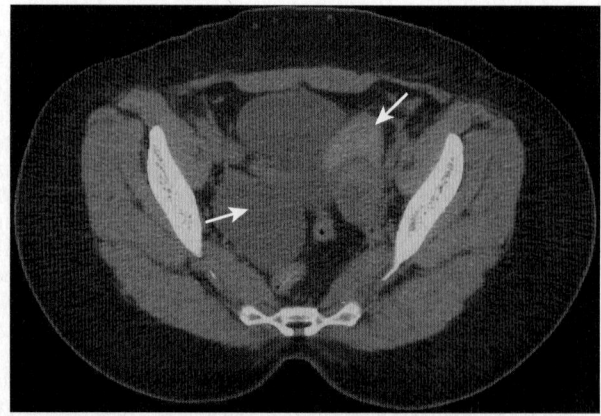

FIG. 4 Computed tomography scan demonstrates adnexal masses of varying density, subsequently proven to be endometriomas. (From Fielding JR et al: *Gynecologic imaging*, Philadelphia, 2011, Saunders.)

| TABLE 2 | Therapies for Endometriosis |

Medical

Hormonal

Oral contraceptives (cycling, noncycling)

Long-acting progestins (levonorgestrel intrauterine system, Depo-Provera, other)

Danazol

GnRH agonists (nafarelin, leuprolide acetate)

GnRH antagonists (elagolix)

Selective progesterone receptor modulators

Other

Nonsteroidal antiinflammatory drugs

Immunotherapy

Surgical

Conservative Therapy:

Laparoscopic ablation

Laparoscopic excision

Abdominal presacral neurectomy

Laparoscopic presacral neurectomy

Definitive Therapy

Hysterectomy/bilateral salpingo-oophorectomy

GnRH, Gonadotropin-releasing hormone.
From Robertson RP et al: *DeGroot's endocrinology: basic science and clinical practice,* ed 8, Philadelphia, 2023, Elsevier.

regard to pain relief and so are often the first-line drug. Very little justification for the use of danazol

Gonadotropin-releasing hormone (GnRH) agonists:
- Induce medical menopause by downregulating HPO axis, which results in hypoestrogenism
- Use usually limited to 6 to 12 mo due to hypoestrogenic effects such as osteopenia or osteoporosis but can be given longer in certain circumstances, particularly when paired with estrogen add-back therapy. Referral to specialist strongly advised
- Leuprolide acetate depot 3.75 mg intramuscularly (IM) monthly or 11.25 mg IM q3mo or nafarelin 400 mcg nasal puffs bid or goserelin 3.6 mg subcutaneously (SC) monthly
- Add-back therapy for protection against vasomotor symptoms and bone loss: Norethindrone acetate 5 mg PO daily alone or in combination with conjugated estrogen 0.625 mg orally daily
- Add-back therapy allows GnRH agonist use to be extended to 1 yr based on limited studies available
- Elagolix is an oral GnRH antagonist that provides partial to nearly complete estrogen suppression. Dosage is 150 mg once daily or 200 mg twice daily. It is effective in improving dysmenorrhea and nonmenstrual pain but is associated with hypoestrogenic side effects (hot flashes, hyperlipidemia, decreased bone density)[5]

Alternative therapies for inhibition of estrogen action currently under investigation are:
- Aromatase inhibitors: Anastrozole, letrozole
- SERM: Raloxifene
- Agents enhancing cell-mediated immunity are cytokines (interleukin-12 and interferon-α2b)
- Immunomodulators (loxoribine, levamisole)
- Antiinflammatory: Pentoxifylline

SURGICAL MANAGEMENT: Conservative:
- Laparoscopic removal of endometriotic implants by excision, electrocautery, or laser

- Directed at treating pain unresponsive to first-line medical treatment and/or enhancing fertility.
- Cystectomy for endometrioma (Fig. E5); must remove cyst wall to be effective long-term.
- Laparoscopic uterosacral nerve ablation (LUNA) for midline pain such as dysmenorrhea or dyspareunia (evidence does not support its use).
- Unless pregnancy is desired, patient is started on GnRH agonist therapy or continuous OCP immediately after surgery.

Definitive:
- Total abdominal hysterectomy with bilateral salpingo-oophorectomy and complete excision or ablation of endometriosis.
- Thorough abdominal exploration to ensure removal of all disease.
- Must be prepared to manage possible gastrointestinal and urinary tract endometriosis.
- 90% effective in pain relief; patient must be counseled that pain relief is not guaranteed.
- Estrogen replacement therapy (ERT) to be considered in all women undergoing definitive surgical management; after ERT, recurrence rate is 0% to 5% in women with endometriosis confined to the pelvis, but 18% in women with bowel involvement.
- Concern for malignant degeneration exists in implants if unopposed estrogen is used after definitive surgical therapy.

MANAGEMENT OF ENDOMETRIOSIS-ASSOCIATED INFERTILITY: Conservative surgery:
- Yields significantly higher pregnancy rate than does expectant management, in part due to correction of mechanical factors such as adhesions

Assisted reproductive technologies:
- Can be used to circumvent unknown mechanism of endometriosis-associated infertility.
- Superovulation with ovulation induction agents or gonadotropins results in threefold pregnancy rate over expectant management.

- Further improvement with intrauterine insemination combined with superovulation.
- In vitro fertilization (IVF) offers highest success rate compared with other treatments. If fallopian tubes are obstructed or severely damaged due to endometriosis, or if there is stage III or IV endometriosis, recommendation is to proceed directly to IVF.

DISPOSITION

Tends to recur unless definitive surgery is performed and should be considered a chronic condition. If conservative, fertility-sparing surgery is performed, then medical suppression is necessary after laparoscopy to prevent recurrence.

REFERRAL

To a reproductive endocrinologist for advanced surgical management or infertility management

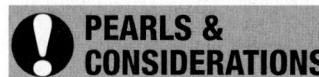 **PEARLS & CONSIDERATIONS**

COMMENTS

Patient information can be obtained through the following organizations: Endometriosis Association, https://endometriosisassn.org/, 8585 North 76th Place, Milwaukee, WI 53223, 414-355-2200 or 800-992-ENDO; American Society for Reproductive Medicine Patient Resources, https://www.asrm.org/resources/patient-resources/

REFERENCES

Available at eBooks.Health.Elsevier.com.

RELATED CONTENT

Endometriosis (Patient Information)
Dysmenorrhea (Related Key Topic)
Dyspareunia (Related Key Topic)

AUTHOR: **EMELIA ARGYROPOULOS BACHMAN, MD, FACOG**

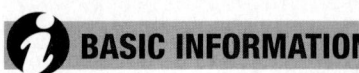 **BASIC INFORMATION**

DEFINITION

Per the Centers for Medicare and Medicaid Services, end-stage kidney disease (ESKD) is a medical condition in which a person's kidneys cease functioning on a permanent basis leading to the need for long-term dialysis or kidney transplantation to maintain life. Increasingly, the term ESKD is used instead of end-stage renal disease (ESRD) because the word "kidney" is more recognizable than "renal" to the lay public.

SYNONYMS

ESKD
Dialysis dependency
Renal replacement therapy
Chronic irreversible renal failure

ICD-10CM CODES
N18.6 End-stage renal disease
Z99.2 Dependence on renal dialysis
Z94.0 Kidney transplant status

EPIDEMIOLOGY & DEMOGRAPHICS

INCIDENCE: According to the U.S. Renal Data System (USRDS), there were ~130,522 incident cases of ESKD in the U.S. in 2020.[1]
- 84% of incident individuals began renal replacement therapy (RRT) with hemodialysis (HD).[1]
- 13% of incident individuals began RRT peritoneal dialysis (PD).[1]
- 3% of incident individuals began RRT with a preemptive kidney transplant.[1]
- Since 2010, there has been a steady increase in incident PD cases.[1]
- There is a significant cost difference among modalities, with average inflation-adjusted Medicare spending for HD at $95,932/person per yr (PPPY) versus PD at $81,525 PPPY.[1]

The incidence of ESKD differs among countries; the highest frequencies are in Taiwan, U.S., Singapore, Republic of Korea, Thailand, Japan, and the Phillipines.[1]
PREVALENCE: Per USRDS, there were 557,838 prevalent maintenance dialysis patients in 2020. The number of prevalent cases has increased by ~20,000 annually until 2019, when the COVID pandemic resulted in increased mortality and growth half the historical norm, leading to a decrease in prevalence in 2020.[1]
- 88% of all prevalent maintenance dialysis in the U.S. were treated by HD (97.5% at an in-center facility and 2.5% at home).[1]
- 12% of all prevalent maintenance dialysis patients were treated by PD.[1]

ESKD prevalence varies greatly by country, with Hong Kong, El Salvador, and Colombia having the highest PD utilization at 64%, 44%, and 22% respectively. Only in Denmark, Canada, Finland, Hong Kong, and England/Wales/Northern Ireland is home HD use >2%.[1]
PREDOMINANT SEX & AGE: The incidence and prevalence of ESKD increases with age, but individuals can experience ESKD at any age. Older patients are more likely to receive dialysis

with HD than PD. Men had a 64.6% higher adjusted ESKD incidence than women in 2020.[1]
RISK FACTORS: Risk factors for the development of ESKD include proteinuria, higher body mass index, diabetes mellitus, high blood pressure, higher serum creatinine, male sex, lower educational status, and African American descent.[2]
GENETICS: Genome-wide association studies have shown several genes that are associated with the development of chronic kidney disease (CKD) and progression to ESKD. The *APOL1* gene is most strongly implicated. Single-nucleotide variants of the following genes are associated with greater risk for the development of ESKD: *UMOD, PRKAG2, ANXA9, DAB2,* and *SHROOM3*.[3]

PHYSICAL FINDINGS & CLINICAL PRESENTATION

Most patients with CKD are asymptomatic at time of diagnosis. However, some patients may present with symptoms such as gross hematuria, "foamy urine," nocturia, flank pain, or decreased urine output.[4] Patients with advanced CKD may present with signs and symptoms of uremia, which may include hypertension, edema, uremic frost, asterixis, ankle clonus, altered mentation, pallor, peripheral neuropathy, coma, and pericardial friction rub. Classic uremic symptoms include anorexia, dysgeusia, aversion to meat, nausea or vomiting, hiccups, pruritus, weight loss, reversal of sleep cycles, restless legs, and loss of energy.[5]

ETIOLOGY

The most common causes of ESKD in the U.S. are, in order of frequency, diabetes, hypertension, glomerulonephritis, and cystic diseases.[1]

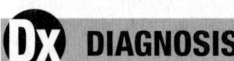 **DIAGNOSIS**

WORKUP

The diagnosis of ESKD is made within the setting of CKD manifesting as an elevated serum creatinine concentration and decreased glomerular filtration rate, typically <15 ml/min/1.73 m[2].[6] RRT is initiated when uremia, volume overload refractory to diuretic therapy, or electrolyte abnormalities refractory to medical therapy is present. The workup of CKD is discussed elsewhere (see "Chronic Kidney Disease"). The ongoing workup to assess the consequences of ESKD include measures of anemia, iron metabolism, metabolic acidosis, and mineral and bone disease.[7]

LABORATORY TESTS

Laboratory tests that warrant monitoring in ESKD include electrolytes, blood urea nitrogen, creatinine, glucose, calcium, phosphorus, intact parathyroid hormone (PTH), 25-hydroxyvitamin D, lipid panel, CBC with reticulocyte count, serum iron, transferrin saturation, and ferritin.[6]

Rx **TREATMENT**

- A kidney transplant is often the treatment of choice for ESKD, compared with a lifetime on dialysis. Patients should be assessed for kidney transplant eligibility and referred for kidney transplant evaluation when possible.
- A patient who requires HD will require vascular access for dialysis that is typically an arteriovenous fistula, graft or HD catheter (Table 1).
  1. An arteriovenous fistula or graft is the preferred access and should be monitored regularly to ensure its patency. If vascular access clotting is identified, prompt vascular access intervention is recommended.[8]
  2. The most common arteriovenous fistulas are radiocephalic, brachiocephalic, and brachiobasilic. Patients with CKD and ESKD are encouraged to preserve veins in their nondominant upper extremities by avoiding unnecessary venipunctures and intravenous lines, including central venous catheters and peripherally inserted central catheters.[8]
  3. A subcutaneously tunneled HD catheter is placed in a major vein.[8]
- Patients who require dialysis have two primary options for RRT: HD and PD (Table 2).
  1. In HD, the bloodstream is cannulated and diverted through a hemodialyzer that filters the plasma. A countercurrent flow of dialysate enriched in bicarbonate and other minerals and glucose removes uremic toxins (Table 3).[5]
     a. Dialysis is effective only for the clearance of non–protein-bound molecules.[5]
     b. Blood flow rate varies from 300 to 500 ml/min. Dialysate flow rate ranges from 500 to 800 ml/min.[5]
     c. Small solutes such as potassium will equilibrate quickly, whereas larger solutes such as beta 2-microglobulin equilibrate more slowly.[5]

TABLE 1 Hemodialysis Vascular Access

Vascular Access	Description	Benefits	Drawbacks
Tunneled catheter	Subcutaneously tunneled under skin to reduce contamination by skin flora	Immediate use	High infection risk High thrombosis risk
Arteriovenous graft	Synthetic tube connecting artery to vein	Ready to use when swelling resolves (~2 wk) Able to use in most patients	High stenosis/thrombosis rate Moderate infectious risk
Arteriovenous fistula	Vein cross-cut attached end-to-side to artery High-pressure flow dilates and thickens vein	Lowest infectious risk Longest lasting with lowest thrombosis risk	Maturation time Primary patency

TABLE 2 Advantages, Disadvantages, and Dialysis Prescription for End-Stage Renal Disease

	Peritoneal Dialysis	Hemodialysis
Access	Abdominal wall insertion of plastic catheter into the peritoneum Limitations: Swimming and bathing can be contraindicated. Previous abdominal surgery can be a contraindication; rarely, a patent pleuro-peritoneal canal exists	Arteriovenous fistula, usually in the forearm
Timing	Daily exchanges, either every 6 h (CAPD), or attached to an overnight (continuous) cycling machine (8 h) (CCPD); no nondialysis days	5-7 h every second or third day; in some circumstances, daily or overnight hemodialysis can be offered (e.g., pregnancy); some nondialysis days
Complications	Peritonitis (usually staphylococcal) Poorer exchange rates over time Peritoneal sclerosis in the long term	Bleeding from insertion sites Fistula aneurysm formation Recirculation or "steal" phenomenon Poor flow rates and technical difficulties Fistula thrombosis or infection Progressive neurologic disease
Compelling indications		Pregnancy Congestive cardiac failure Unstable coronary artery disease
Other considerations	Bulky home stores	Adequate space for machines at home Adequate plumbing, good-quality water supply
2-yr Patient survival	77%	60%-80%
2-yr Technique survival	64%	60%-80%

CAPD, Continuous ambulatory peritoneal dialysis; *CCPD*, continuous cycling peritoneal dialysis.
From Talley NJ et al: *Essentials of internal medicine,* ed 4, Chatswood, NSW, 2021, Elsevier Australia.

TABLE 3 Composition of Typical Hemodialysis and Peritoneal Dialysis Solutions

Component	Concentration in Hemodialysis Solutions	Concentration in Peritoneal Dialysis Solutions
Sodium	135-145 mEq/L	132 mEq/L
Potassium	1-3 mEq/L	0 mEq/L
Calcium	2.5-3.5 mEq/L	2.5-3.5 mEq/L
Chloride	95-110 mEq/L	95-105 mEq/L
Magnesium	0.5-1 mEq/L	0.5 mEq/L
Bicarbonate	32-40 mEq/L	
Lactate		35-40 mEq/L
Acetate	2.5-5 mEq/L	
Glucose	200 mg/dl	1500-4250 mg/dl

d. The volume of ultrafiltrate (plasma without protein) that is removed is determined clinically.[5]

2. In PD, the blood flow originates from the vascular parietal and visceral peritoneum, with the peritoneal membrane representing the "dialysis" membrane. Peritoneal dialysate is dextrose-based and hypertonic. The hypertonicity produces ultrafiltration. The concentration of dextrose is varied to increase or decrease ultrafiltration per clinical requirements.[9] Icodextrin is a polydispersed glucose polymer with an average molecular weight of 16,800 Da.

In contrast to glucose, it does not diffuse across the peritoneal membrane. Icodextrin facilitates a sustained colloid osmotic gradient (unlike crystalloid osmosis seen with glucose-based solutions) across the peritoneal membrane. This solution is suited for use during the longest exchange in PD and achieves a greater net ultrafiltration (UF) during the long dwell compared with conventional dextrose-based PD solutions.[9]

a. A tunneled catheter is placed through the abdominal wall. Peritoneal dialysate is infused into the peritoneum and

left to dwell as solute transfer occurs via convection or diffusion across concentration gradients.[9]

b. PD can be performed manually throughout the day or overnight via an automated cycler device.[9,10]

• In patients who require RRT, withholding treatment has substantial risk.
1. Patients with late-stage CKD are hypertensive in 60% to 90% of cases. If hypertension is untreated, the risks for accelerated heart disease and/or stroke increase.[5]
2. Hyperkalemic patients have increased risk of sudden cardiac death. Metabolic acidosis may increase risk for cardiovascular failure and bone demineralization.[6]
3. Patients with untreated uremia may manifest neuromuscular irritability, including seizures or confusion, altered mentation, and coma.[5]
4. Uremia may cause platelet dysfunction and increased risk for bleeding.[5]

• In addition to RRT, management of patients with ESKD involves treatment of anemia in CKD, disorders of bone and mineral metabolism, and cardiovascular disease. Targets in management of the dialysis patient are summarized in Table 4.
1. Patients receiving dialysis experience anemia for several reasons, including erythropoietin deficiency, GI bleeding, functional and absolute iron deficiency, increased red blood cell fragility, and blood loss from HD.[11]
   a. Management of anemia in CKD depends on the primary causative factor.
   b. Iron utilization is estimated by ferritin ($>$100 ng/ml) and transferrin saturation ($>$20%). Patients who do not meet both of these criteria are first treated with intravenous iron or a trial of oral iron. Intravenous iron may be administered without a trial of oral iron. In patients who are iron replete, erythropoiesis-stimulating agents are used to increase hemoglobin.[12] Randomized controlled trials demonstrate an association between increased cancer death and stroke with attainment of hemoglobin levels $>$11 g/dl. The target hemoglobin range for a dialysis patient is 9.0 to 11.0 g/dl, and these are not absolute criteria.[11]

• Patients with ESKD are at risk for several different metabolic bone disorders.
1. Secondary hyperparathyroidism of renal origin occurs in the majority of individuals who require RRT. This disorder is aggravated by concurrent metabolic acidosis. The intact PTH level is characteristically elevated in these individuals.[13]
2. The gold standard diagnosis for establishing a histologic diagnosis of bone disease is bone biopsy. Bone lesion parameters are characterized as turnover, mineralization, and volume.[14]
3. ESKD in patients who do not undergo bone biopsy is managed by measuring serologic markers, calcium, phosphate, and intact PTH.[14]

TABLE 4 Targets in Management of the Dialysis Patient

Management of:	Targets
Anemia	Hemoglobin 110-120 g/L In the setting of adequate iron stores; uremia leads to poor iron absorption, so parenteral iron is often required
Hyperphosphatemia	Phosphate <1.6 mmol/L
Calcium and PTH	Calcium: High normal range PTH: 15-30 pmol/L
Cholesterol, LDL, and triglycerides	Total cholesterol: <4.5 mmol/L LDL: <2.5 mmol/L Triglycerides: <2.0 mmol/L
Blood pressure	<140/90 mm Hg
Access	Good-quality access with aseptic approach to use
Dialysis adequacy	Reasonable urea concentrations in between dialysis, controlled potassium concentration, no episodes of fluid overload and, ultimately, control of symptoms

LDL, Low-density lipoprotein; *PTH,* parathyroid hormone.
From Talley NJ et al: *Essentials of internal medicine,* ed 4, Chatswood, NSW, 2021, Elsevier Australia.

4. Adynamic bone disease occurs more frequently in ESKD patients with diabetes. Typically, the intact PTH level is low (<150 pg/ml). PD confers a greater risk for adynamic bone disease. Patients undergoing HD are at greatest risk for osteitis fibrosis cystica and mixed lesions.[13]
5. Osteopenia.
- ESKD is considered a coronary heart disease equivalent with enhanced risk of mortality from cardiovascular causes. However, data are lacking regarding the efficacy of cardiovascular risk modification.
  1. Studies of statin therapy in patients with ESKD have not shown a reduction in cardiovascular mortality. Initiation of statin therapy after beginning RRT is not recommended.[7]
  2. Levels of cardiac biomarkers such as troponin-I and N-terminal pro–B-type natriuretic peptide (NT-proBNP) are frequently and chronically elevated in ESKD. Interpretation of these biomarkers must be considered within the context of clinical findings.[7]
- Because multiple medications are renally excreted or nephrotoxic, careful attention must be paid to choice and dosing of medications. Commonly used medications that should be used with caution in ESKD include low-molecular-weight heparin, morphine, oxycodone, gabapentin, pregabalin, digoxin, bisphosphonates, sodium glucose cotransport inhibitors, metformin, and electrolyte-containing solutions, including milk of magnesium, magnesium citrate, aluminum hydroxide, and magnesium hydroxide.[7]
- Management of ESKD in the intensive care unit is summarized in Table E5.

DISPOSITION

Morbidity and mortality remain exceptionally high for patients who require RRT.

Dialysis patients in 2020 had a mortality rate of 186 deaths/1000 person-yr.[1] Until 2020, this rate has been improving, with net reductions in all-cause mortality from 186.4/1000 person-yr in 2010 to 162.7 in 2019 for HD patients and from 152.3 to 129.8/1000 person-yr in the same time period for PD patients.[1] However, in 2020 there was a relative increase in mortality for both HD and PD patients (to 190.1/1000 person-yr and 155.8/1000 person-yr, respectively), in large part due to the COVID-19 pandemic, which was the third-leading cause of death among patients treated with in-center HD in 2020.[1]

- HD patients have greater earlier mortality, and PD patients have greater delayed mortality.[1]
- 5-yr survival probability rates for incident ESKD patients with disease onset in 2015 are 41.7% for HD patients and 46.5% for PD patients. The difference in survival rates is likely related to patient-selection factors rather than differences between modalities.[1]

REFERENCES

Available at eBooks.Health.Elsevier.com.

RELATED CONTENT

Chronic Kidney Disease (Related Key Topic)

AUTHORS: **BLAIRE BYG, MA** and **ANKUR SHAH, MD**

BASIC INFORMATION

DEFINITION

Eosinophilic esophagitis (EoE) is a chronic antigen- and immune-mediated disease of the esophagus, characterized by three criteria:

- Inflammation secondary to eosinophilic infiltration within the esophagus (confirmed with at least 15 eosinophils per high power field [HPF] detected on biopsy of mucosa taken at proximal and distal esophagus)
- Symptoms related to esophageal dysfunction are present
- Other etiologies of esophageal eosinophilia or dysphagia are ruled out

Remission of EoE is defined as repeat endoscopy with <15 eosinophils per HPF and does not always correlate with symptom resolution.

SYNONYMS

Esophageal eosinophilia
EoE
EE

ICD-10CM CODE
K20.0   Eosinophilic esophagitis

EPIDEMIOLOGY & DEMOGRAPHICS[1,2]

INCIDENCE (IN U.S.): 1 to 20 new cases/100,000 inhabitants/yr
PREVALENCE: Between 13 and 49 cases/100,000 inhabitants
PREDOMINANT SEX: Male predominance (ratio ~3:1)
PREDOMINANT AGE: Peak of disease activity at age 35 to 39
PEAK INCIDENCE: Older children; in adults, ages 30 to 50
RISK FACTORS: Genetic, host immune, and environmental (see "Genetics"). Allergy-mediated reactions play a significant role in the pathophysiology of EoE via food antigen–driven T helper 2 cells.
GENETICS:

- Association between thymic stromal lymphopoietin *(TSL)* gene mutation and risk for EoE
- Higher risk in those with homozygous pattern for the mutation
- *TSL* gene found on Yp11.3 chromosome
- Association with polymorphism on eotaxin-3 (CCL-26)

PHYSICAL FINDINGS & CLINICAL PRESENTATION

- Adults: Dysphagia to solid foods, food impaction, heartburn, noncardiac chest pain, increased time to consume meals, concurrent atopic diseases (asthma, eczema, rhinitis, atopic dermatitis, seasonal/food allergies)
- Children: Vomiting, regurgitation, nausea, epigastric/abdominal pain, chest pain, water brash, globus, decreased appetite, gagging, choking, refusal of food, possible atopy, failure to thrive
- Often associated with asthma, rhinitis, dermatitis, and other atopic conditions

ETIOLOGY

The immunopathogenesis of the disease is characterized by type 2 helper T (Th2)-cell inflammation involving T cells; eosinophils; mast cells; and the cytokines interleukin-4, interleukin-5, interleukin-13, and thymic stromal lymphopoigen.[3]

DIAGNOSIS

DIFFERENTIAL DIAGNOSIS

- Gastroesophageal reflux disease
- Eosinophilic gastritis, gastroenteritis, or colitis with esophageal involvement
- Celiac disease
- Achalasia and other motility disorders
- Schatzki ring or esophageal webs
- Crohn disease
- Pill esophagitis
- Drug hypersensitivity reactions
- Hypereosinophilic syndrome
- Infectious (fungal/viral)
- Graft-versus-host disease
- Vasculitis/pemphigus/connective tissue diseases

WORKUP

- Esophagogastroduodenoscopy (EGD) with at least two to four biopsy samples from distal and mid/proximal esophagus after a proton pump inhibitor (PPI) trial.
- Confirmation: Persistence of symptoms *and* ≥15 eosinophils/HPF on pathology (Fig. E1) although esophagus is normal in ~5% to 10% of patients.
- Other histologic findings can include basal zone hyperplasia, dilated intracellular spaces, and subepithelial fibrosis.
- Endoscopic findings can include white mucosal papules, which represent eosinophilic microabscesses, linear furrows, esophageal narrowing with stricture, mucosal tearing, firm resistance during esophageal biopsy, esophageal trachealization (Fig. E2), esophageal rings, or felinization of esophagus. Felinization of the esophagus is a radiologic term used to describe 1- to 2-mm transverse folds found circumferentially along the entire lumen of the esophagus that appear transiently on EGD and barium studies, possibly attributed to thickened and contracted muscularis mucosae.

LABORATORY TESTS

- 40% to 50% have elevated peripheral eosinophilia.
- 50% to 60% have elevated serum immunoglobulin E (IgE) levels.

IMAGING STUDIES

Esophagram can reveal rings and strictures. In one study 26% of esophageal strictures <15 mm in diameter were detected on esophagram but missed on endoscopy.[4] Despite this finding, esophagram is not routinely used in evaluation of EoE.

TREATMENT

NONPHARMACOLOGIC THERAPY

Three strategies of dietary therapy:

- Empiric six-food elimination diet (eliminates milk, soy, egg, wheat, nuts, and seafood), for patients with response, foods can be reintroduced one at a time for 6 wk
- Total elimination of all food allergens with elemental or amino acid–based formula
- Targeted elimination diet guided by allergy testing, typically skin prick testing or patch testing
- Elimination of food antigens with an elemental diet leads to resolution of esophageal eosinophilia in about 68% of patients[5]

Dysphagia due to a stricture associated with EoE should prompt consideration for endoscopic dilation. Multiple dilations may be required to achieve optimal outcome.

ACUTE GENERAL Rx[6,7]

Two strategies for medical therapy:

- An 8-wk trial of high-dose PPI therapy can be considered as a primary therapy in order to rule out esophageal eosinophilia due to gastroesophageal reflux disease (GERD).
  1. Repeat EGD can be considered after 8 wk to evaluate for histologic response.
  2. Most recent estimates indicate about two thirds of patients fail to respond.[5]
- Recommended pharmacologic treatment for EoE includes a trial of topical glucocorticoids via metered-dose inhaler or oral viscous budesonide, which have been shown to be equally effective.[8]
  1. Swallowed fluticasone 220 mcg/day in a divided dose 4× a day (adult dosing)
     a. Delivered by metered-dose inhaler without a spacer.
     b. Medication is sprayed into the patient's mouth and then swallowed.
     c. Patient should *not* inhale when the medication is being delivered.
     d. Patient should not eat or drink for 30 to 60 min after administration.
  2. Swallowed budesonide 2 mg/day, typically in divided doses
     a. Administered as viscous slurry: Mixing 1 mg/2 ml nebulizer ampules with sucralose (five 1-g packets per 1 mg of budesonide).
     b. Patient should not eat or drink for 30 to 60 min after taking the budesonide suspension.
     c. Can also be administered using a nebulizer: Patient then instructed to swallow accumulated liquid.
     d. Budesonide orodispersible formulation uses saliva for drug delivery increasing exposure to the esophageal surface of the drug.
        (1) Most recent estimates indicate about one third of patients fail to respond.[5]
        (2) Although rare, patients should be monitored for local viral/fungal infections and adrenal suppression.

(3) Currently systemic steroids are not recommended for the treatment of EoE.

3. Dupilumab (300 mg every 1 to 2 wk) is an effective FDA approved treatment for patients refractory to PPEs, swallowed steroids, and elimination diets. Histologic remission is acheived in 60% of patients after 24 wk of treatment with dupilumab.[9]

CHRONIC Rx

- In general, patients should be maintained on whichever therapy worked to decrease incidence of complications from inflammation such as esophageal strictures. However, there is a paucity of data examining the efficacy of maintenance use of PPI and dietary elimination.[5]
  1. If patient is responsive to PPI therapy, patient can be continued on PPI therapy.
  2. If patient responsive to dietary elimination, patient should be continued with slow addition of different food types as tolerated.
  3. If patient is responsive to topical steroids, continue steroids at lowest possible dose. A recent trial revealed that in EoE budesonide orodispersible tablets maintained remission at 48 wk.[1]

- If lack of response to initial therapy:
  1. Assess compliance.
  2. Restrict diet further.
  3. Increase steroid dose or consider alternative steroid.
     a. Switch from dietary modification to steroid therapy and vice versa.
     b. Reevaluate diagnosis and secondary causes of esophageal eosinophilia (see "Differential Diagnosis" earlier).
     c. Weekly subcutaneous injections of dupilumab (IL-4 alpha antagonist) improve histology and dysphagia symptoms in patients nonresponsive to PPI treatment.[10]
- Chronic histologic and symptomatic surveillance is recommended, although no optimal time interval has been proposed.

DISPOSITION

Follow-up by gastroenterologist is important to gauge progression or regression of disease.

REFERRAL

Referrals to gastroenterologists, allergists, and dieticians allow for a multidisciplinary approach to diagnosis and management of EoE.

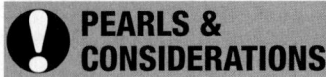

PEARLS & CONSIDERATIONS

COMMENTS

- Topical steroids and/or elimination diet are mainstay treatments for EoE.
- PPI-responsive esophageal eosinophilia (PPI-REE), which requires a PPI trial to be ruled out, is no longer in the algorithm for diagnosing EoE[10]; a PPI trial for treatment of GERD presenting with eosinophilia should be considered.
- Endoscopic surveillance of disease with or without symptoms is important to prevent further disease.
- Esophageal dilation is indicated in patients with dysphagia due to EoE-mediated strictures.

REFERENCES

Available at eBooks.Health.Elsevier.com.

RELATED CONTENT

Gastroesophageal Reflux Disease (Related Key Topic)

AUTHORS: **AZFAR K. NIAZI, MD** and **ZILLA HUSSAIN, MD**

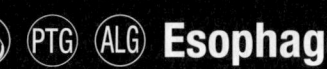
Diseases and Disorders

I

BASIC INFORMATION

DEFINITION

Esophageal tumors include benign and malignant neoplasms of the esophageal mucosa and wall. Carcinomas of the esophageal epithelium, both squamous cell carcinoma and adenocarcinoma (including adenoacanthoma, mucoepidermoid, and adenoid cystic), are the most common tumors of the esophagus. Rare esophageal tumors include both malignant (spindle cell, small cell, sarcoma, lymphoma, melanoma, and choriocarcinoma) and benign neoplasms (leiomyoma, papilloma, and fibrovascular polyps). One can also develop metastatic disease from a cancer that originated in another organ, but this is very rare. Breast cancer, lung cancer, and melanoma would be the most likely culprits. Other cancers can directly extend to the esophagus from the larynx, pharynx, lung, thyroid, or stomach. Approximately 15% of esophageal tumors arise in the proximal esophagus, 50% in the middle third of the esophagus, and 35% in the lower third. Tumors involving the esophageal-gastric junction are usually staged and treated as esophageal cancers if the tumor epicenter is no more than 2 cm into the proximal stomach. Tumors in the upper two thirds are usually squamous cell cancers, and tumors in the lower third are usually adenocarcinomas. The incidence of superficial esophageal cancers is increasing. These invade no deeper than the submucosa.

ICD-10CM CODES
C15.X	Malignant neoplasm of the esophagus (X defines location)
C15.3	Malignant neoplasm of upper third of esophagus
C15.4	Malignant neoplasm of middle third of esophagus
C15.5	Malignant neoplasm of lower third of esophagus
D00.2	Carcinoma of esophagus, in situ

EPIDEMIOLOGY & DEMOGRAPHICS

INCIDENCE: It is the eighth most common cancer worldwide and the seventh leading cause of cancer deaths. Rates are increasing every decade and are highest in the Asian esophageal cancer belt, extending from the Caspian Sea to northern China, with certain high-incidence pockets in Finland, Ireland, southeast Africa, and northwest France. Incidence has increased sixfold since 1975. Foods including cured meats and spicy regional fare likely play a role in certain areas. Increasing substance abuse with tobacco and alcohol also coincides with a rise in esophageal cancers. Rates of squamous cell carcinoma are decreasing while those of adenocarcinomas are dramatically increasing. The direct causes of squamous cell carcinoma most commonly include tobacco and alcohol abuse. Epithelial dysplasia usually occurs, which progresses to carcinoma in situ. Adenocarcinomas

are usually the result of gastroesophageal reflux disease (GERD) and obesity. The mucosa of the esophagus undergoes intestinal metaplasia. Genetic alterations occur and perpetuate during proliferation.

PREVALENCE: In the U.S., there were an estimated 21,560 new cases in 2022 and 16,120 deaths making it the eighth leading cause of death by cancer. The disease is much more common in men (79%) than women (21%) and carries a 75% mortality rate. The majority of cases are diagnosed at an advanced stage (unresectable or metastatic disease), which makes curing more difficult.

PREDOMINANT RACE, SEX, & AGE: In the U.S., squamous cell esophageal cancer is more common among African Americans compared to whites, whereas adenocarcinoma more common in whites. The highest male:female ratio is in the Hispanic population. Usually develops in fifth to seventh decades of life and is associated with a lower socioeconomic status.

GENETICS: Increasing evidence shows that genetics may play a role by increasing susceptibility to esophageal cancer. One well-identified disease associated with esophageal cancer is tylosis (focal nonepidermolytic palmoplantar keratoderma), linked to loss of heterozygosity on chromosome 17q. Familiar clustering of Barrett esophagus and the recent identification of germline mutations in affected sibling pairs support a genetic link to esophageal adenocarcinoma. Also, up to 25% of esophageal adenocarcinomas can have overexpression of *HER2*, which can lead to the use of targeted therapy (trastuzumab and pertuzumab) in the treatment plan.

PHYSICAL FINDINGS & CLINICAL PRESENTATION

Symptoms and signs:
- Dysphagia (74%): Initially with solid foods, gradually progresses to semisolids and liquids
- Chest pain
- Unintentional weight loss of short duration.
- Hoarseness: Suggests recurrent laryngeal nerve involvement
- Odynophagia
- Cervical adenopathy: Usually involving supraclavicular lymph nodes
- Dry cough: Suggests tracheal involvement
- Aspiration pneumonia: Caused by fistula between the esophagus and trachea
- Iron deficiency anemia: Related to chronic GI blood loss
- Massive hemoptysis or hematemesis from the invasion of vascular structures
- Advanced disease spreads to lymph nodes, liver, lungs, peritoneum, and pleura
- Hypercalcemia: Associated with squamous cell carcinoma from secretion of a parathyroid-like tumor peptide

ETIOLOGY

The pathogenesis of esophageal cancers is attributable to chronic recurrent oxidative damage from any of the following etiologic agents, which cause inflammation, and esophagitis, increased cell turnover, and, ultimately, initiation of the carcinogenic process.

ETIOLOGIC AGENTS:
Squamous cell carcinoma
- Excess alcohol consumption is strongly associated with squamous cell esophageal cancer in the U.S.; hard liquor is associated with a higher incidence than wine or beer
- Tobacco and alcohol synergistically increase risk for squamous cell cancer
- Other ingested carcinogens:
  1. Nitrates (converted to nitrites): South Asia, China
  2. Smoked opiates: Northern Iran
  3. Fungal toxins in pickled vegetables
  4. Betel nut chewing
- Mucosal damage
  1. Long-term exposure to extremely hot tea (>70° C [158° F])
  2. Ingestion of lye or extremely acidic solutions, including reflux of stomach acid
- Radiation-induced strictures
- Achalasia: Incidence of esophageal cancer is seven times greater in this population
- Host susceptibility as a result of precancerous lesions:
  1. Plummer-Vinson syndrome (Paterson-Kelly): Glossitis with iron deficiency
  2. Congenital hyperkeratosis and pitting of palms and soles (tylosis)
- Human papillomavirus infection (types 16 and 18) has been detected in squamous cell carcinoma of the esophagus, sometimes associated with p53 tumor suppressor gene mutations
- Possible relationship with prolonged bisphosphonates (≥10 prescriptions, or >3 yr use)
- Possible association with celiac sprue or dietary deficiencies molybdenum, selenium, zinc, vitamin A

ADENOCARCINOMA:
- The incidence of adenocarcinoma is continually rising.
- Smoking increases risk of adenocarcinoma, particularly in patients with Barrett.
- Obesity, hiatal hernia, and diets lacking in fresh fruit and vegetables and high in fat (particularly from red meat and processed foods) increase risk.
- Chronic GERD leading to Barrett metaplasia and adenocarcinoma via immune cell infiltration and production of inflammatory mediators and reactive oxygen species. The annual rate of transformation from Barrett to adenocarcinoma is <0.5%.
- *Helicobacter pylori* infection may reduce risk of adenocarcinoma but can increase risk of lymphoma.

DIAGNOSIS

DIFFERENTIAL DIAGNOSIS
- Achalasia
- Scleroderma of the esophagus
- Diffuse esophageal spasm
- Esophageal rings and webs

LABORATORY TESTS

CBC, blood chemistry, and liver enzymes should be obtained at diagnosis. No biomarkers are

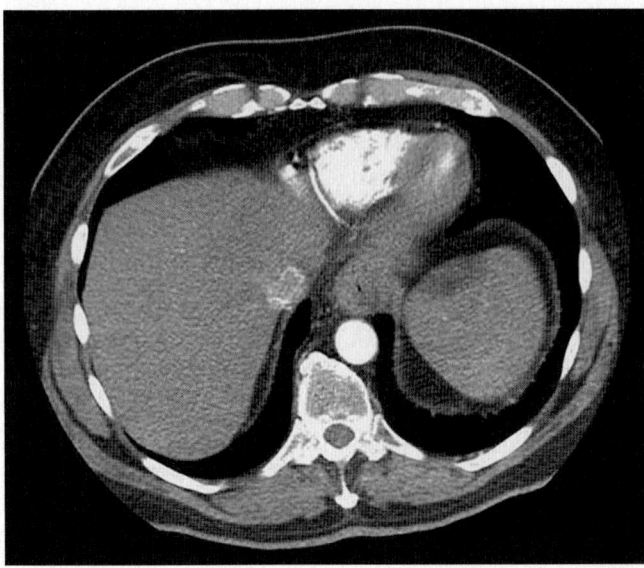

FIG. 2 Computed tomography of the chest showing abnormal thickening of the esophagus suggestive of malignancy. (From Cameron JL, Cameron AM: *Current surgical therapy,* ed 12, Philadelphia, 2017, Elsevier.)

currently recommended to diagnose, monitor, or predict outcomes. While both the carcinoembryonic antigen (CEA) and cancer antigen (CA)-19-9 can be elevated in patients with esophageal cancer (up to 70%), the sensitivity is low (18% to 35%) and there is no proven predictive value.

IMAGING STUDIES

Imaging studies are important not only for diagnosis but for accurate staging:

- Esophagogastroduodenoscopy (EGD) (Fig. E1) should be performed initially to visualize all tumors and allow histopathologic confirmation.
- Endoscopic inspection of the larynx, trachea, and bronchi may identify concomitant cancers of head, neck, and lung ("triple endoscopy").
- Endoscopic ultrasound (EUS) (see Fig. E1) appears to be the most accurate method for locoregional staging: To determine the depth of tumor invasion and to assess for and possibly obtain fine needle aspiration biopsies of suspicious lymph nodes. EUS is superior to computed tomography (CT) (Fig. 2) or PET for assessment of both T and N status. It is highly accurate for celiac nodal status, though slightly lower for other regional lymph nodes due to difficulty accessing the node without traversing the tumor. Obstructing lesions may preclude EUS assessment.
- PET CT has become the standard of care along with EUS, for the most accurate staging. These modalities can determine tumor spread for preoperative staging. Obtaining the PET/CT scan before EUS has several advantages. The PET/CT scan may demonstrate distant metastatic disease, eliminating the need for the patient to undergo EUS. The PET/CT scan may also identify a suspicious lymph node that can be specifically examined and sampled during the EUS procedure (Fig. E3).
- Bronchoscopy should be considered for proximal and middle third esophageal tumors to assess for direct tracheal invasion.

- CT scans of the chest and abdomen are useful for restaging patients after initial therapy.

STAGING

Table 1 describes the TNM staging system for cancer of the esophagus from the American Joint Committee on Cancer Criteria. The depth of invasion of the tumor defines the T status (Fig. E4). High-grade dysplasia includes malignant cells confined to the epithelium by the basement membrane and is by definition noninvasive (Tis). T1a tumors invade the lamina propria or muscularis mucosa, whereas T1b tumors invade into the submucosa. T2 tumors invade the muscularis propria, and T3 tumors invade the adventitia but not surrounding structures. T4a tumors invade adjacent structures that are usually resectable (diaphragm, pleura, and pericardium). T4b tumors invade adjacent structures that are typically unresectable (trachea and aorta). Fig. 5 illustrates an algorithm for staging thoracic esophageal cancer.

(Rx) TREATMENT

ALL STAGES OF ESOPHAGEAL CANCER

Although the histology of esophageal cancer can differ, most studies have combined tissue types in exploring treatment options. The histology develops secondary to differing pathogenesis and causative agents with tumor biology likely playing a role through varying mutations. The likelihood of response and prognosis can differ as well. However, as there is a lack of data on how histology should dictate the treatment approach, we generally attack this cancer in a uniform manner as most studies have suggested the optimum benefit be obtained through a neoadjuvant chemoradiation approach followed by surgery when applicable in up to stage III disease.

TABLE 1 TNM Staging System for Cancer of the Esophagus (American Joint Committee on Cancer Criteria)

Primary Tumor (T)*

T_X	Primary tumor cannot be assessed
T_0	No evidence of primary tumor
T_{is}	High-grade dysplasia[†]
T_1	Tumor invades lamina propria, muscularis mucosae, or submucosa
T_{1a}	Tumor invades lamina propria or muscularis mucosae
T_{1b}	Tumor invades submucosa
T_2	Tumor invades muscularis propria
T_3	Tumor invades adventitia
T_4	Tumor invades adjacent structures
T_{4a}	Resectable tumor invading pleura, pericardium, or diaphragm
T_{4b}	Unresectable tumor invading other adjacent structures, such as aorta, vertebral body, trachea, etc.

Lymph Node (N)‡

N_X	Regional lymph nodes cannot be assessed
N_0	No regional lymph node metastasis
N_1	Metastasis in 1-2 regional lymph nodes
N_2	Metastasis in 3-6 regional lymph nodes
N_3	Metastasis in 7 or more regional lymph nodes

Distant Metastasis (M)

M_X	Metastasis cannot be assessed
M_0	No distant metastasis
M_1	Distant metastasis

TNM, Tumor, node, metastases.
*(1) At least maximal dimension of the tumor must be recorded and (2) multiple tumors require the T(m) suffix.
[†]High-grade dysplasia includes all noninvasive neoplastic epithelia that was formerly called carcinoma in situ.
[‡]Number must be recorded for total number of regional nodes sampled and total number of reported nodes with metastasis.
From Edge S et al (eds): *AJCC cancer staging manual,* ed 7, New York, 2010, Springer.

COMBINATION THERAPY: CHEMORADIOTHERAPY FOLLOWED BY SURGICAL RESECTION: Induction chemotherapy, given before chemoradiation for patients with locally advanced but still possibly resectable disease, has been administered with good results. However, no studies have shown this approach superior to chemoradiation alone. Standard fractionation 3D-RT is utilized in chemoradiotherapy.

- Chemotherapy is most often given with concurrent radiotherapy. Chemotherapy acts as a radiosensitizer and makes tumor cells more vulnerable to the effects of ionizing radiation, thus improving tumoricidal effects on cancer. Neoadjuvant chemoradiotherapy followed by surgery is the most common approach for patients with resectable disease but is employed primarily for patients with stage IIA or higher disease. Five-yr survival is improved with a neoadjuvant approach (39%) versus surgery alone (16%). Several trials have now shown that preoperative therapy improves

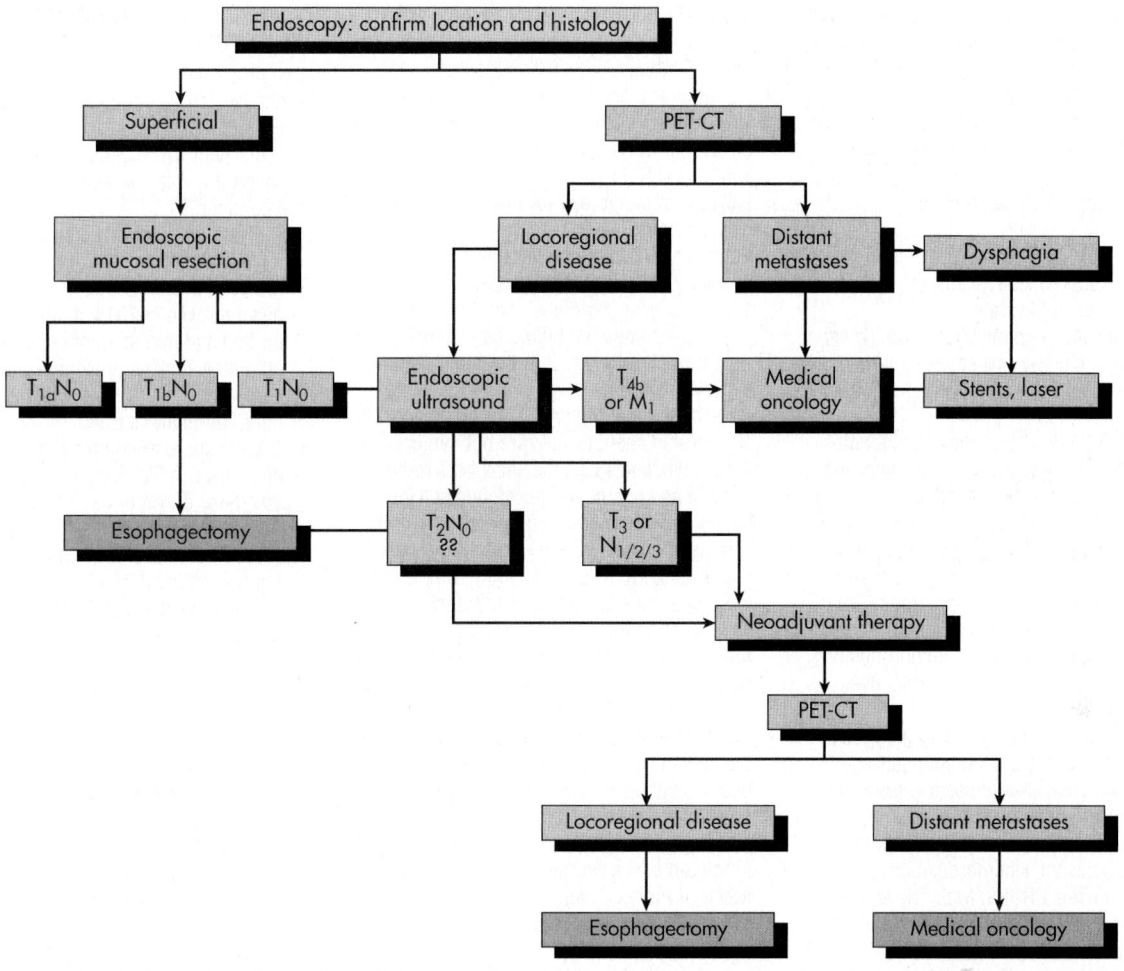

FIG. 5 An algorithm for staging a thoracic esophageal cancer patient. Metastatic disease must always be confirmed by pathologic evaluation of the tissue in question. *PET-CT,* Positron emission tomography–computed tomography. (From Sellke FW et al: *Sabiston & Spencer surgery of the chest,* ed 9, Philadelphia, 2016, Elsevier.)

survival among patients with potentially curable esophageal or esophagogastric junction cancer. Neoadjuvant chemotherapy alone is another option for locally advanced disease, but results are not as good as with neoadjuvant chemoradiotherapy.

- Chemoradiotherapy followed by surgery should be offered to late stage I ($T_{1b}N_0$ or higher), stage II, and stage III esophageal cancer patients as the current standard of care. In several studies, this approach significantly improved local control, reduced recurrence, and reduced mortality compared with surgery alone in patients with resectable esophageal cancer. This also increases the chance of an R0 resection. Trimodality therapy is the preferred treatment for most esophageal cancers.
- Chemoradiotherapy alone may be offered as definitive treatment for patients who are not surgical candidates, and some of these patients may be cured.
- Combination chemotherapy using a platinum doublet (platinum agent plus second agent) can achieve significant tumor reduction in 30% to 60% of patients. Cisplatin, oxaliplatin, or carboplatin is usually given with 5-FU (5-fluorouracil) or paclitaxel to obtain the

desired tumoricidal effects. Other chemotherapeutic agents with activity in esophageal cancer include docetaxel and irinotecan.
- Capecitabine in combination with either cisplatin or oxaliplatin is as effective as 5-FU in the neoadjuvant or definitive treatment setting and can be substituted.
- Neoadjuvant chemoradiotherapy can result in a 50% pCR for patients with squamous pathology and 25% PCR for those with adenocarcinoma. Consequently, the need for resection in these patients is unclear. To establish a CR short of resection, the patient would need EGD with EU and biopsies. In patients whom surgery is a high risk secondary to comorbidities, those with squamous pathology may opt to defer on surgery if all biopsies are negative.
- Complications of chemoradiotherapy primarily include mucositis, nausea, vomiting, diarrhea, myelosuppression, nephrotoxicity, ototoxicity, neurotoxicity with peripheral neuropathy, esophageal stricture, esophageal rupture, trachea-esophageal fistula (6%), and radiation pneumonitis. These can occur to varying degrees and are certainly more significant in the elderly and those with significant comorbidities.

- Postoperative adjuvant chemoradiotherapy should be offered to node-positive patients who underwent surgical resection without neoadjuvant chemoradiotherapy.

SURGICAL RESECTION:
- Surgical resection of both squamous cell and adenocarcinoma of the middle esophagus and lower third of the esophagus is an acceptable initial modality for local and resectable disease (early stage I and stage II) in the absence of widespread metastases detected by CT-PET and transesophageal ultrasound (T_1 and T_2 tumors). Gastric pull-through or colonic interposition typically is used to provide luminal continuity.
- The optimal timing of surgery following neoadjuvant chemoradiotherapy is approximately 5 to 7 wk, though some patients may require more time to improve nutrition.
- Endoscopic mucosal resection may replace radical surgical resection in patients with dysplasia and some small early tumors with no lymph node involvement (T_{is} or T_{1a}), but a recent Cochrane review found no studies comparing endoscopic resection vs. surgery. Endoscopic mucosal resection may be beneficial for patients who are poor surgical candidates. It may be performed in conjunction

with ablative therapies, including radiofrequency ablation, thermal ablation techniques, laser ablation, argon plasma coagulation, or photodynamic therapy. Electrocoagulation (electrofulguration) is also being used and may aid in the relief of esophageal blockage.

- Complications of surgery, including endoscopic resection and local therapy:
  1. Esophageal rupture.
  2. Anatomic fistula (usually with colon interposition, subphrenic abscesses).
  3. Respiratory complications.
  4. Cardiovascular complications are most common, including myocardial infarction, cerebrovascular accident, and pulmonary embolism.
  5. Mortality is lower and clinical outcomes are better at high-volume hospitals and with minimally invasive surgery.
  6. Hybrid minimally invasive esophagectomy has been reported to have a lower incidence of intraoperative and postoperative major complications, specifically pulmonary complications, than open esophagectomy, without compromising overall and disease-free survival over a 3-yr period.[1]

Despite adequate preoperative staging, 25% of patients initially treated with surgical resection will have microscopically positive resection margins and are upstaged at the time of surgery. This has led to the majority of patients receiving neoadjuvant chemoradiotherapy as demonstrated in the CROSS Trial. The median disease-free survival for this group of patients was significantly prolonged as compared with the surgery-alone group. Death from recurrent cancer was decreased by 9% in the neoadjuvant group as well. The benefit of neoadjuvant therapy resulted in a 13% survival advantage at 10-yr follow-up, consistent regardless of histologic subtype.

For patients who receive no neoadjuvant therapy and undergo resection and are found to have positive margins or node-positive disease, adjuvant therapy is strongly recommended in an attempt to prevent progression. There is likely a benefit for chemoradiotherapy with positive margins, but the role of chemotherapy alone vs. chemoradiotherapy in node-positive patients is unclear. If combination therapy is likely to be tolerated, it should be considered.

PRETREATMENT PATIENT PREPARATION: The patient needs to stop smoking and drinking alcohol if at all possible. Before neoadjuvant or definitive chemoradiotherapy, the patient should have placement of an intravenous access device and a feeding tube (J-tube is preferable before surgical resection). Poor nutrition and weight loss will continue during neoadjuvant therapy and needs to be minimized.

RADIATION THERAPY:

- Squamous cell carcinoma is more radiosensitive than adenocarcinoma. Radiotherapy achieves good local control but is generally only used as monotherapy in a palliative mode for obstructive symptoms in patients with unresectable or advanced cancer or those with multiple comorbidities that limit

treatment. It is best used for cervical esophageal tumors, but response rates are best when combined with chemotherapy.

- Radiotherapy in the preoperative/neoadjuvant setting is taken to a total dose of 40 to 50 Gy. For definitive therapy, the dose range is 60 to 66.6 Gy.
- Palliative radiotherapy for bone metastasis is also effective.
- Complications of radiotherapy: Can best be avoided by 3D conformal therapy.
  1. Esophageal stricture, fistula formation, radiation-induced pulmonary fibrosis, and transverse myelitis are the most common adverse events.
  2. Radiotherapy-induced cardiomyopathy and skin changes are rare but can occur. It is difficult to shield the heart from radiation as these organs are positioned so close.
- Intensity modulated radiation therapy (IMRT) can also be used for the treatment of esophageal cancers. It is associated with a more favorable toxicity profile. Very few studies have been completed to date using chemotherapy with IMRT and is therefore not considered a standard approach at this time for neoadjuvant therapy.
- Brachytherapy: This is also an option for patients in a palliative mode. It provides high-dose radiation to a localized area and may prevent the need for a stent in patients with dysphagia. Its use is very limited in prior irradiated tissue for fear of fistula and perforation of the esophagus.
- Laser therapy and stents can also be considered for palliative care.

TREATMENT OF UNRESECTABLE, LOCALLY ADVANCED, OR METASTATIC DISEASE

- Combination chemotherapy regimens as a rule have a higher response rate than single-agent therapy. Response rates can be as high as 50% but that does not always translate into prolonged survival.
- Neoadjuvant chemotherapy regimens can also be utilized in locally advanced or metastatic settings. Oxaliplatin is now preferred over cisplatin for a more favorable toxicity profile with similar efficacy. This combined with 5-FU can yield response rates shown in several studies of up to 50%. The most widely used regimen in metastatic disease, both squamous cell and adenocarcinoma, is FOLFOX. Immunotherapy with either nivolumab or pembrolizumab is now also usually added to a metastatic regimen. Patients with MSI-H/dMMR tumors (independent of PD-L1 status) should be treated with immunotherapy and can receive this alone as first line treatment in the metastatic setting. Capecitabine can be substituted for 5-FU in these regimens. Other acceptable doublet regimens include carbo/taxol and cisplatin/docetaxel.
- Another useful regimen in second-line treatment would include Ramucirumab and paclitaxel for EGJ adenocarcinoma.

TARGETED MOLECULAR THERAPY

Two drugs have been approved for adenocarcinoma of the esophagus. Ramucirumab is a VEGF inhibitor, and trastuzumab is effective in cancers with overexpression of *HER2*. There is no apparent role for either drug in squamous cell carcinoma.

- Ramucirumab is a recombinant monoclonal IgG1 antibody that is a vascular endothelial growth factor receptor 2 (VEGFR-2) antagonist approved in 2014. It inhibits ligand proliferation and migration of endothelial cells and ultimately inhibits angiogenesis. Indicated for second-line therapy in with paclitaxel or as third line monotherapy.
- Trastuzumab, in combination with oxaliplatin and 5-FU (FOLFOX), is considered the standard of care as first-line therapy for metastatic esophageal cancer in patients with HER2 overexpressing adenocarcinoma. Approximately 22% of adenocarcinomas will overexpress the type II epidermal growth factor receptor HER2. The overall response rate is 47%.
- Fam-trastuzumab deruxtecan-nxki (Enhertu) was approved in 2021 for the treatment of metastatic gastric and gastroesophageal adenocarcinoma as monotherapy for patients who have received a prior trastuzumab-based regimen. This is an HER2-directed antibody and topoisomerase inhibitor conjugate drug that demonstrated statistically significant ORR and OS in patients who progressed on at least two prior chemo regimens, including trastuzumab, 5-FU, and a platinum-containing regimen.
- Entrectinib and larotrectinib are also approved for neurotrophic-tropomyosin receptor kinase (NTRK) gene fusion–positive tumors. These are selective tyrosine kinase inhibitors. The NTRK gene fusion and amplification is much more common in adenocarcinoma, but in both types of histology, less than 1% of tumors have this molecular marker.

IMMUNOTHERAPY IN ESOPHAGEAL CANCER

- Drugs constitute a class that act as an immune checkpoint inhibitor that targets programmed death ligand 1 (PD-1).
- Patients at high risk of recurrent disease following neoadjuvant chemoradiation and surgery who undergo an R0 resection have been found to benefit from 1 yr of adjuvant immunotherapy with nivolumab, regardless of PD-L1 status.
- Nivolumab and pembrolizumab have shown varying response rates of 10% to 25% in patients who have progressive/metastatic disease and failed traditional therapy with at least one prior chemotherapy regimen. Both pembrolizumab and nivolumab are now approved in the U.S. for treatment of esophageal cancer. These appear to be most effective in patients with squamous cell histology, but adenocarcinomas also respond regardless of PD-L1 status. A recent open-label phase 3 trial of adults with previously

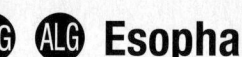

untreated, unresectable, recurrent, or metastatic esophageal squamous cell carcinoma revealed that both first-line treatment with nivolumab plus chemotherapy and first-line treatment with nivolumab plus ipilimumab resulted in significantly longer overall survival than chemotherapy alone in patients with advanced esophageal squamous-cell carcinoma with no new safety signals identified.[2]

- Patients with MSI-H– and dMMR-positive tumors are more likely to respond to immunotherapy.

FOLLOW-UP CARE

The majority of recurrences develop within 12 mo of diagnosis. Clinical monitoring, lab tests, imaging, and endoscopic evaluations where appropriate (especially in Barrett esophagus), are performed for postoperative surveillance, without clear benefit of earlier detection or decreased mortality. For patients who have undergone definitive therapy, endoscopic surveillance should be performed every 3 mo for the first yr, and then at least annually. Palliative procedures such as endoscopic dilation, endoscopic ablation, endoscopic mucosal resection, photodynamic therapy, brachytherapy, feeding tube insertion, or placement of expandable metal stents or polyvinyl prostheses to bypass tumors have all been used for unresectable patients. The morbidity and mortality associated with resection in patients with advanced disease and/or for palliation argues against offering surgery to most of these patients.

SURVIVORSHIP

- Overall 5-yr survival for all stages at presentation is 20% (39% for localized disease, 21% for regional disease, and 4% for distant disease).

- Endoscopic therapy for highly selected stage 0 or stage I patients with disease limited to the submucosa may have 5-yr survival rates of 70% to 90%.
- Surgical resection without neoadjuvant treatment: 5-yr survival rate is 5% to 30%, with higher survival (45% to 50%) in early-stage cancers.
- Radiation therapy without chemotherapy or surgery: 5-yr survival rate of 6% to 20%.
- Chemoradiotherapy without surgery: 5-yr survival up to 30%.
- Combined trimodality treatment: 45% to 50% 5-yr survival rates (all stages of disease).
- Patients with metastatic disease have median survivals of less than 1 yr with palliative chemotherapy.

REFERRAL

- To gastroenterologist for endoscopy for patients with dysphagia, odynophagia, unexplained weight loss, or for palliative care
- To medical oncologist for evaluation of preoperative chemotherapy and care of the metastatic patient
- To radiation oncologist for palliative therapy if tumor is actively bleeding, unresectable, or if obstruction is present
- To hospice if appropriate

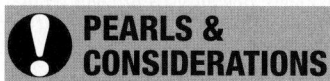

COMMENTS

More than 50% of patients with esophageal cancer are diagnosed when the disease is metastatic or unresectable.

PREVENTION

- A diet high in fruits, vegetables, and antioxidants may be associated with lower risk of esophageal cancer.
- Avoid tobacco and excessive alcohol use.
- Avoid ingested toxins known to cause esophageal cancers.
- Aspirin may have a chemopreventive role in Barrett esophagus but is only currently recommended for patients with other (e.g., cardiac) indications.
- No evidence that vitamins, Chinese herbs, or green tea prevents esophageal cancer.
- Screening the general population is not recommended. If Barrett esophagus is detected, regularly scheduled surveillance endoscopies are necessary, with consideration for radiofrequency or other ablation therapy if dysplasia is detected.

PATIENT & FAMILY EDUCATION

Provide education and support about the likely prognosis because most esophageal cancers are diagnosed at an advanced stage.

REFERENCES

Available at eBooks.Health.Elsevier.com.

RELATED CONTENT

Esophageal Cancer (Patient Information)
Barrett Esophagus (Related Key Topic)

AUTHOR: **ANTHONY G. THOMAS, DO, FACP**

E

Diseases
and Disorders

I

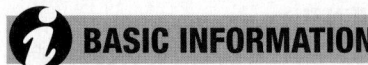

BASIC INFORMATION

DEFINITION

Esophageal varices are dilated submucosal veins that occur in patients with underlying portal hypertension, function as a shunt between the portal venous and systemic venous circulation, and can result in severe upper GI hemorrhage.

ICD-10CM CODES
I85.00 Esophageal varices without bleeding
I85.01 Esophageal varices with bleeding

EPIDEMIOLOGY & DEMOGRAPHICS

INCIDENCE:
- Esophageal varices: 5% to 15% per yr in patients with cirrhosis
- Hemorrhage:
  1. One third of all patients with varices will develop hemorrhage.
  2. Variceal hemorrhage occurs in 25% to 40% of patients with cirrhosis.
  3. The risk of bleeding from varices is approximately 15% at 1 yr.
  4. Survivors of an episode of active bleeding have a 70% risk of recurrent hemorrhage within 1 yr.

PREVALENCE: Approximately 50% of patients with cirrhosis have varices at the time of diagnosis.

RISK FACTORS: Cirrhosis, low platelet count, and advanced Child-Pugh class, hepatitis C with advanced fibrosis

PHYSICAL FINDINGS & CLINICAL PRESENTATION

- Often asymptomatic until acute upper GI hemorrhage: Hematemesis, hypovolemia
- No physical findings specific for esophageal varices
- Stigmata of cirrhosis and portal hypertension may be evident: Palmar erythema, telangiectasias, gynecomastia, testicular atrophy, jaundice, caput medusae, lower extremity edema, ascites, splenomegaly, hemorrhoids, asterixis

ETIOLOGY

- Portal hypertension results from obstruction to portal venous outflow, and varices subsequently develop in order to decompress the hypertensive portal vein and return blood to the systemic circulation.
- Varices may appear when portal vein pressures rise above 10 to 12 mm Hg.
- Cirrhosis is the most common cause of portal hypertension.

DIAGNOSIS

DIFFERENTIAL DIAGNOSIS

- Budd-Chiari syndrome, cirrhosis, portal vein thrombosis, schistosomiasis, Wilson disease
- Other causes of upper GI bleeding: Duodenal or gastric ulcers, gastric cancer, Mallory-Weiss tear

WORKUP

Upper endoscopy (Fig. E1), laboratory tests, and imaging

LABORATORY TESTS

- CBC:
  1. Anemia (blood loss, nutritional deficiencies, alcohol myelosuppression)
  2. Thrombocytopenia (hypersplenism, alcohol myelosuppression)
- Renal function panel:
  1. Blood urea nitrogen: Often increased in setting of upper GI bleeding
  2. Creatinine: Often elevated by hypovolemia, monitor for hepatorenal syndrome
  3. Sodium: Dilutional hyponatremia
- Heme-positive stools
- Type and crossmatch: In preparation for blood transfusion
- International normalized ratio/prothrombin time (INR/PT) and partial thromboplastin time (PTT): Coagulation factors produced in liver and may be prolonged in liver disease or impairment
- Liver function tests: Alanine transaminase (ALT)/aspartate aminotransferase (AST) may be normal in cirrhotic patients due to long-standing fibrosis; elevated alkaline phosphatase and a direct hyperbilirubinemia may be present if cholestatic liver disease is present
- Serum albumin: Severe liver disease results in hypoalbuminemia

IMAGING STUDIES

Invasive:
- Esophagogastroduodenoscopy (EGD) (upper endoscopy):
  1. In all patients with cirrhosis, screen for the presence or absence of varices and determine subsequent risk for variceal hemorrhage.
  2. In patients with small varices (<5 mm) repeat EGD in 2 yr (unless decompensation occurs).
  3. In patients with compensated cirrhosis who do not have varices, screening is repeated every 2 to 3 yr.
  4. In patients with decompensated cirrhosis (ascites, hepatic encephalopathy, variceal hemorrhage, or jaundice), it is repeated every year or at the time of first decompensation.
  5. Emergently performed if there is evidence of acute upper GI bleeding to diagnose and treat variceal hemorrhage.

Noninvasive:
- Esophagography with barium can diagnose esophageal varices (Fig. E2).
- Capsule endoscopy can also diagnose esophageal varices, although sensitivity is not yet established.
- Computed tomography (CT) scan (Fig. E3).

TREATMENT

NONPHARMACOLOGIC THERAPY

- Endoscopic variceal ligation (Fig. E4) is an alternative to nonselective β-blockers for primary prophylaxis against variceal hemorrhage.

It is also used in patients unable to tolerate β-blockers
1. Typically for patients with medium or large varices at highest risk for hemorrhage (Child-Pugh B/C or red wale markings viewed on endoscopy)
2. Usually two to four sessions
3. May not be a permanent solution because varices can recur after initial eradication
4. Associated with significant complications, including hemorrhage from banding-induced ulcerations
   a. Therefore should be performed by endoscopists with expertise in prophylactic banding
   b. First surveillance endoscopy 1 to 3 mo after obliteration, then every 6 to 12 mo indefinitely

ACUTE GENERAL Rx

- Variceal hemorrhage: Acute hemodynamic resuscitation with packed red blood cell transfusion, correct coagulopathy and thrombocytopenia, airway protection and intubation as necessary, antibiotics (ceftriaxone or norfloxacin) for SBP prophylaxis, octreotide maintained for 2 to 5 days in conjunction with endoscopic therapy. The use of balloon tamponade in the control of active variceal bleeding should be a last resort when other forms of therapy are not available or fail to achieve hemostasis. Balloon tamponade (Fig. E5) should be used only as a temporary means of stabilization and a bridge to a more definitive form of therapy.
- EGD to treat bleeding esophageal varices by esophageal band ligation or sclerotherapy (Fig. 6).

CHRONIC Rx

Primary prophylaxis (Fig. 7):
- Nonselective β-blockers such as propranolol (20 mg twice daily), nadolol (40 mg once daily), or carvedilol (6.25 mg twice daily)
  1. Increase as tolerated for goal heart rate of approximately 55 beats/min
  2. Blocks the adrenergic dilatory tone in mesenteric arterioles, resulting in unopposed alpha-adrenergic mediated vasoconstriction and therefore a decrease in portal inflow

Secondary prophylaxis (Fig. E8):
- All patients with compensated cirrhosis who have bled from esophageal varices should receive esophageal band ligation and β-blockers, unless β-blockers are contraindicated.
  1. Transjugular intrahepatic portosystemic shunt or surgical shunt may be performed if bleeding from esophageal varices continues or recurs despite this dual therapy.
- For patients with decompensated cirrhosis there is evidence, although limited, against the use of prophylactic β-blockers due to the risk for increased mortality.

REFERRAL

Consultation with a gastroenterologist is recommended in all patients with cirrhosis or portal hypertension in order to screen for esophageal varices.

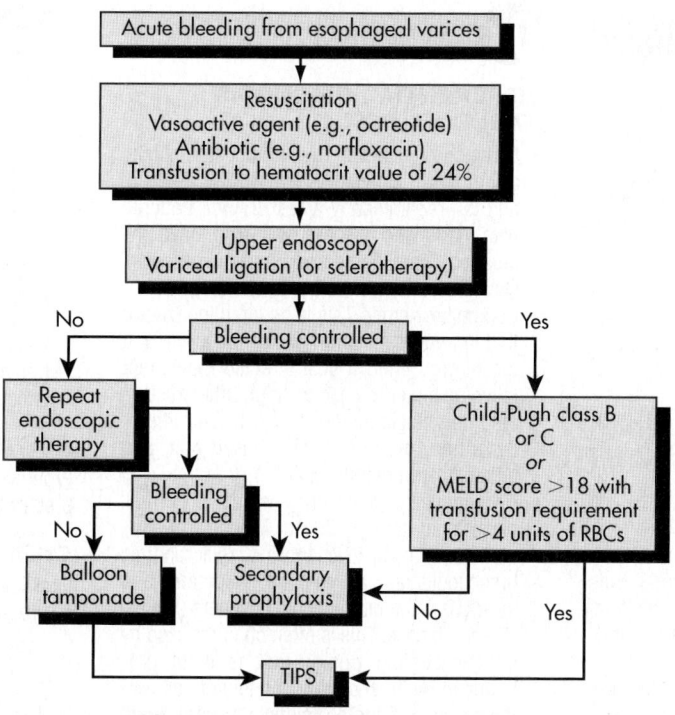

FIG. 6 Algorithm for the management of bleeding esophageal varices. *MELD,* Model end state liver disease; *RBC,* red blood cell; *TIPS,* transjugular intrahepatic portosystemic shunt. (From Feldman M et al: *Sleisenger and Fordtran's gastrointestinal and liver disease,* ed 11, Philadelphia, 2021, Elsevier.)

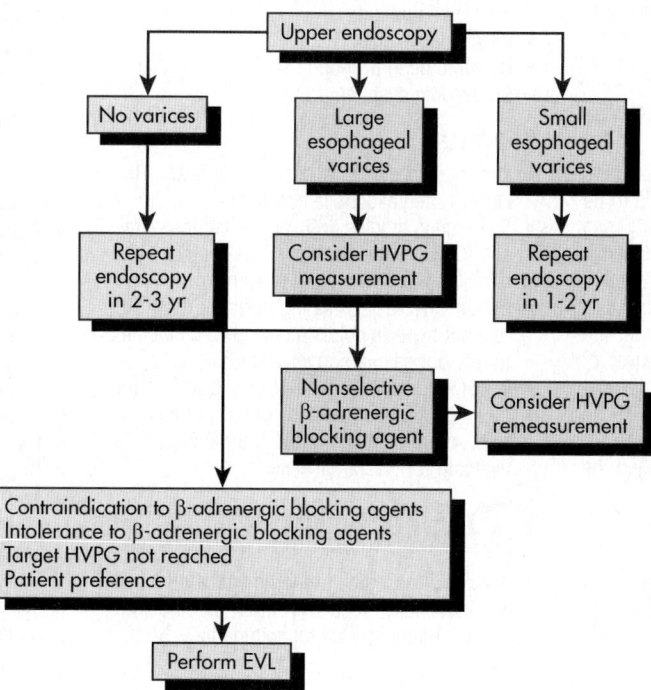

FIG. 7 Algorithm for the primary prophylaxis of esophageal variceal bleeding in patients with cirrhosis. The hepatic vein pressure gradient *(HVPG)* may be measured in patients with large varices before a nonselective β-adrenergic blocking agent is started and remeasured 1 mo after the maximum tolerated dose of the β-blocker is reached. The goal of treatment is to reduce the HVPG to <12 mm Hg or by ≥20%. *EVL,* Endoscopic variceal ligation. (From Feldman M et al: *Sleisenger and Fordtran's gastrointestinal and liver disease,* ed 10, Philadelphia, 2016, Elsevier.)

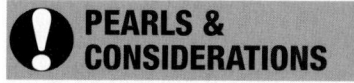

PEARLS & CONSIDERATIONS

Besides variceal size, risk factors for variceal hemorrhage include Child-Pugh class B/C or variceal red wale markings on endoscopy.

RELATED CONTENT

Cirrhosis (Related Key Topic)
Portal Hypertension (Related Key Topic)

AUTHOR: **FRED F. FERRI, MD**

Essential Tremor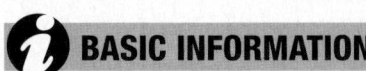

BASIC INFORMATION

DEFINITION

An isolated tremor syndrome of bilateral upper limb action tremor that occurs with at least 3 yr duration, with or without tremor in other locations and the absence of other neurologic signs such as dystonia, ataxia, or parkinsonism.[1]

SYNONYMS

Benign essential tremor
Familial tremor

ICD-10CM CODE
G25.0   Essential tremor

EPIDEMIOLOGY & DEMOGRAPHICS

- Prevalence of essential tremor (ET) was 0.32% in the general population. The total number of people suffering from ET worldwide was 24.91 million in 2020.[2]
- More common in males than in females across the whole life span.
PREDOMINANT AGE: Bimodal age at onset with peaks occurring in the 20s and 60s.[3]
GENETICS: 30% to 70% of patients have a positive family history of this disorder, and first-degree of relatives of patient with ET are ~4.7 times more likely to have ET than controls.[4]

PHYSICAL FINDINGS & CLINICAL PRESENTATION

- Essential tremor is characterized by a bilateral action tremor of 6 to 12 Hz that tends to be more prominent on one side of the body than the other. In approximately 50% of patients, the tremor also worsens with intention (Fig. E1), specifically at the termination of a goal-directed movement. This can be seen at the very end of the finger-to-nose maneuver or while drinking from a glass. The tremor can be found in the upper extremities (90% to 95%), head (30%), legs (10% to 15%), or voice (20%), and is usually absent when the affected body part is at rest.
- In addition to the kinetic tremor, a postural tremor may be seen when the patient holds the body part against gravity. The postural tremor is usually most noticeable at the wrist and is usually of lower amplitude than the kinetic tremor.
- Patients with essential tremor may also have gait ataxia on tandem walk and may report a history of increased falls or near falls.
- No other neurologic abnormalities are found on examination.
- Symptoms worsen over time and with emotional distress, fatigue, or the use of caffeine or other stimulants and improve with intake of small amounts of alcohol.[5]

ETIOLOGY

Often an inherited disease in an autosomal dominant pattern. Sporadic cases without a family history can occur.

DIAGNOSIS

DIFFERENTIAL DIAGNOSIS (TABLE 1 & BOX 1)

- Parkinson disease: The tremor is usually asymmetric, especially early in the disease, and is predominantly a rest tremor. Patients with Parkinson disease will also have increased tone, decreased facial expression, slowness of movement, and shuffling gait.
- Cerebellar tremor: This is an intention tremor that increases steadily right before arriving at the target during a goal-directed movement (such as finger to nose testing). Other associated neurologic abnormalities include ataxia, dysarthria, dysmetria, wide-based gait, and difficulty with tandem gait.
- Drug-induced: Many drugs enhance normal, physiologic tremor. These include caffeine, nicotine, lithium, levothyroxine, β-adrenergic bronchodilators, amiodarone, valproate, and selective serotonin reuptake inhibitors (SSRIs).
- Wilson disease: This is often characterized by a wing-beating tremor that is most pronounced with shoulders abducted, elbows flexed, and fingers pointing toward each other. Usually there are other neurologic abnormalities including dysarthria, dystonia, and Kayser-Fleischer rings on ophthalmologic examination.
- Physiologic tremor.
- Dystonic head tremor.
- Spasmodic dysphonia.

WORKUP

- Essential tremor is a clinical diagnosis. Review of medications is essential.
- All imaging studies (MRI, computed tomography [CT]) are unnecessary unless other neurologic abnormalities are present.
- Obtain thyroid-stimulating hormone (TSH) to rule out hyperthyroidism and ionized calcium to rule out calcium abnormalities.
- In patients younger than 40 yr old with other neurologic abnormalities, order ceruloplasmin, serum copper, and 24-h urine copper to evaluate for Wilson disease.

TREATMENT

Treatment of essential tremor is indicated when it is functionally impairing. First-line medications can reduce tremor magnitude by ~50%.[6]

NONPHARMACOLOGIC THERAPY

- Stress management.
- Minimization of caffeine use if consumption is correlated with worsened symptoms.
- Wrist weights and use of weighted utensils may be helpful in reducing tremor amplitude during feeding.
- Consumption of small quantities of alcohol at social functions, although the symptom relief may be short in duration and may be followed by tremor rebound.
- A recent trial using MRI-guided focus ultrasound thalamotomy found it effective in reducing hand tremor in patients with essential tremor. Side effects included sensory and gait disturbances.

ACUTE GENERAL Rx

Propranolol (20 to 40 mg) may be used in preparation for specific event.

CHRONIC Rx

First-line therapy:
- Propranolol:
  1. Dose: Typical starting dose is 60 or 80 mg/day. The usual therapeutic dose is 160 mg/day.
  2. Side effects: Relative contraindications in asthma, heart block, unstable heart failure, bradycardia, hypotension, and type 1 diabetes.
- Primidone:
  1. Dose: 12.5 to 25 mg every night at bedtime (qhs). Increase by 12.5 to 25 mg/day every wk. Usual therapeutic dose is between 62.5 and 750 mg/day (assuming side effects are tolerated).
  2. Side effects: Sedation and nausea are common at treatment initiation.
- Topiramate:
  1. Dose: 25 mg qhs, may titrate up to by 25 mg per wk in twice a day (bid) dosing to maximum of 400 mg (200 mg bid)
  2. Side effects: Paresthesia, reduced appetite, weight loss, somnolence, concentration/attention difficulty, and memory difficulty
Second-line therapy:
- Propranolol + Primidone
- Gabapentin:
  1. Dose: 300 mg tid. Usual therapeutic dose is 1200 to 3600 mg/day in three divided doses
- Benzodiazepines (i.e., alprazolam)
  1. Alprazolam dose: 0.125 to 1.5 mg/day in divided dose

TABLE 1	Overlapping Features of Various Types of Tremor		
Feature	**Parkinson Syndrome**	**Cerebellar Tremor**	**Essential Tremor**
Present at rest	Yes	No	No
Increased tone	Yes	No	No
Decreased tone	No	Yes	No
Postural abnormality	Yes	Yes	No
Head involvement	Yes	Yes	Yes
Intentional component	No	Yes	Yes
Incoordination	No	Yes	No

From Remmel KS et al: *Handbook of symptom-oriented neurology*, ed 3, St Louis, 2002, Mosby.

BOX 1 Classification and Differential Diagnosis of Tremor

Resting Tremors
PD
Other parkinsonian syndromes (less common)
Midbrain (rubral) tremor (Holmes tremor): Rest < postural < intention
WD (also acquired hepatocerebral degeneration)
Essential tremor

Postural Tremors
Physiologic tremor
Exaggerated physiologic tremor; these factors can also aggravate other forms of tremor:
Stress, fatigue, anxiety, emotion
Endocrine: Hypoglycemia, thyrotoxicosis, pheochromocytoma
Drugs and toxins: Adrenocorticosteroids, β-agonists, dopamine agonists, amphetamines, lithium, tricyclic antidepressants, neuroleptics, theophylline, caffeine, valproic acid, alcohol withdrawal, mercury ("hatter's shakes"), lead, arsenic, others
Essential tremor (familial or sporadic)
Primary writing tremor and other task-specific tremors
Orthostatic tremor
With other CNS disorders:
PD (postural tremor, reemergent tremor, associated essential tremor)
Other akinetic-rigid syndromes
Idiopathic dystonia, including focal dystonias
With peripheral neuropathy:
Charcot-Marie-Tooth disease (called the *Roussy-Lévy syndrome*)
Other peripheral neuropathies
Cerebellar tremor

Intention Tremors
Diseases of cerebellar outflow (dentate nuclei, interpositus nuclei, or both, and superior cerebellar peduncle):
MS, trauma, tumor, vascular disease, WD, acquired hepatocerebral degeneration, drugs, toxins (e.g., mercury), others

Miscellaneous Rhythmic Movement Disorders
Functional/psychogenic tremor
Rhythmic movements in dystonia (dystonic tremor, myorhythmia)
Rhythmic myoclonus (segmental myoclonus, e.g., palatal or branchial myoclonus, spinal myoclonus), myorhythmia
Oscillatory myoclonus
Asterixis
Clonus
Epilepsia partialis continua
Hereditary chin quivering
Spasmus nutans
Head bobbing with third ventricular cysts
Nystagmus

CNS, Central nervous system; *MS,* multiple sclerosis; *PD,* Parkinson disease; *WD,* Wilson disease.
From Jankovic J et al: *Bradley and Daroff's neurology in clinical practice,* ed 8, Philadelphia, 2022, Elsevier.

- Focal botulinum toxin injections[7]
  1. Effective for essential head tremor
  2. Side effect: Transient weakness rarely disabling

SURGICAL Rx

Thalamic deep brain stimulation (or possibly thalamotomy) contralateral to side of tremor is reserved for resistant tremor or for patients who do not tolerate drug therapy. Surgical ablation of the ventral intermediate nucleus of the thalamus with use of magnetic resonance-guided focused ultrasound is also an available option for severe refractory ET.[8]

DISPOSITION

Patients should be reassured that the condition is not associated with other neurologic disabilities; however, it can become functionally disabling over time.

REFERRAL

This is a condition that can be treated initially by the primary care physician; however, if patient fails first-line therapies, the patient should be referred to a neurologist for other drug trials and discussion of possible surgical options.

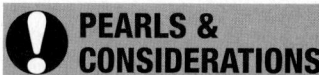

PEARLS & CONSIDERATIONS

- Essential tremor is the most common of all movement disorders. It is characterized by an action tremor that increases at the end of goal-directed movement.
- In addition to motor dysfunction, essential tremor can cause significant psychologic impact on patients in social situations.

REFERENCES

Available at eBooks.Health.Elsevier.com.

AUTHORS: **NAOMI R. KASS, BA, IBRAHIM Z. D. NOORBHAI, MD,** and **FARIHA JAMAL, MD**

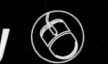
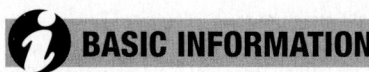 **BASIC INFORMATION**

DEFINITION

Exocrine pancreatic insufficiency (EPI) is a condition characterized by a deficiency in pancreatic digestive enzymes resulting in inadequate digestion of fats, carbohydrates, and proteins. The most common cause of EPI is chronic pancreatitis (CP) in adults and cystic fibrosis (CF) in children. Clinically, EPI commonly results in fat malabsorption and is characterized by steatorrhea, weight loss, and maldigestion. In mild cases, it may be asymptomatic or result in mild abdominal discomfort with normal appearing bowel movements.[1]

SYNONYMS

Pancreatic insufficiency
EPI
Fat malabsorption

ICD-10CM CODE
K86.81   Exocrine pancreatic insufficiency

EPIDEMIOLOGY & DEMOGRAPHICS

PREVALENCE: EPI occurs in 20% to 30% of patients after acute pancreatitis and 60% to 90% of patients within 10 to 12 yr of chronic pancreatitis diagnosis. It is present in 90% of patients with CF. For chronic pancreatitis, which has an estimated prevalence 50 per 100,000 persons, this equates to ~164,000 cases in the U.S. alone.[1] EPI occurs commonly in patients with diabetes mellitus (DM) with prevalence as high as 50% with estimates of severe EPI occurring in 5% to 30% of patients with type I DM and 5% to 15% of patients with type 2 DM.[1,2]

PREDOMINANT SEX & AGE: Demographic data strictly for EPI are lacking; however, chronic pancreatitis is the most common cause of EPI and has a slight male predominance (55%) with a mean age of diagnosis of 45 yr. Given the natural history of EPI as noted above, this would equate to a typical age of onset of approximately 55 to 57 yr old.[1]

RISK FACTORS:
- Pancreatitis (chronic and acute)
- Cystic fibrosis (CF)
- Surgery (i.e., pancreaticoduodenectomy, gastrectomy, esophagectomy)
- Toxin exposure (tobacco, alcohol, antiretroviral medication)
- Pancreatic adenocarcinoma
- Neuroendocrine neoplasm (with or without treatment with somatostatin analogs)
- Ductal obstruction (congenital or acquired)
- Genetic predisposition (including CF and Shwachman-Diamond syndrome)
- History of autoimmune disorders (type 1 diabetes mellitus, inflammatory bowel disease, Sjögren syndrome)
- Type 2 DM
- Celiac disease

PHYSICAL FINDINGS & CLINICAL PRESENTATION

Many patients may be asymptomatic or only present with mild symptoms. Clinically significant EPI may not appear until 90% of pancreatic enzyme production has been lost. Symptoms may include bloating, belching, and steatorrhea (stools often described as loose, greasy, foul-smelling, floating or sticking to the toilet bowl, and pale or clay-colored). The clinical features may mimic and coexist with common gastrointestinal conditions (e.g., irritable bowel syndrome [IBS], small-intestinal bacterial overgrowth [SIBO], celiac disease), which may delay diagnosis. Patients often limit dietary fat intake to avoid or reduce steatorrhea. Severity depends on the degree of pancreatic loss and can be categorized into mild or moderate-to-severe disease as follows:
- Mild disease
  1. Asymptomatic
  2. Normal bowel movements
  3. Mild abdominal discomfort
  4. Bloating
- Moderate-to-severe disease
  1. Chronic diarrhea
  2. Excessive weight loss
  3. Excessive flatulence
  4. Abdominal pain/bloating
  5. Voluminous and foul-smelling stools
  6. Fatty food intolerance
  7. Failure to thrive in children
  8. Steatorrhea (stool fat >6 g/day)
  9. Edema (as a result of protein malnutrition and hypoalbuminemia)
  10. Fat-soluble vitamin deficiencies (rare):
      a. Vitamin A (impaired night vision)
      b. Vitamin D (osteoporosis, metabolic bone disease, hyperparathyroidism, hypocalcemia)
      c. Vitamin E (neuropathy, anemia)
      d. Vitamin K (ecchymosis)

ETIOLOGY

EPI usually results from CP in adults or CF in children leading to fibrosis, necrosis, or lack of function of pancreatic acinar cells. It is also a common, self-limited occurrence in patients recovering from severe acute pancreatitis, with the severity of symptoms correlating with the degree of pancreatic necrosis. Causative factors can generally be classified into pancreatic and extrapancreatic conditions (Table 1).[1]

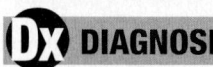 **DIAGNOSIS**

EPI is a clinical diagnosis for those with a history of pancreatic disease. For those without a history of pancreatic disease, but symptoms consistent with EPI, workup can include both indirect and direct measures of pancreatic function. Indirect measures include measurement of pancreatic enzymes in the stool or serum. Direct measures include endoscopic evaluation and collection of pancreatic fluids after administration of secretagogues. Although testing can be helpful in clarifying a diagnosis, there is no consensus on a diagnostic algorithm.[1,3]

DIFFERENTIAL DIAGNOSIS

The following conditions may present in a manner similar to EPI:
- Celiac disease
- Irritable bowel syndrome (IBS)
- Inflammatory bowel disease (IBD)
- SIBO
- Short bowel syndrome
- Infectious diarrhea, i.e., giardiasis
- Vasoactive intestinal peptide tumors

WORKUP

- A complete history, physical examination, and laboratory evaluation are essential to making the diagnosis and excluding other common causes of diarrhea and weight loss.
- Complete electrolyte panel to detect hypokalemia, hypocalcemia (in setting of vitamin D deficiency), hypomagnesemia, and metabolic acidosis from malabsorption and gastrointestinal losses.
- Genetic testing for cystic fibrosis transmembrane conductance regulator (CFTR) mutations should be carried out in the pediatric population.
- CBC may reveal anemia from iron, vitamin B_{12}, or folate deficiencies.
- Prolonged prothrombin times may be elevated because of vitamin K malabsorption.
- Alternative causes of maldigestion should be investigated, such as infection with *Giardia lamblia,* celiac serology, liver disease, and SIBO tests.

TABLE 1 Etiologies of Exocrine Pancreatic Insufficiencies

Pancreatic	Extrapancreatic
Acute/chronic pancreatitis (alcohol abuse, trauma, hereditary, idiopathic)	Celiac disease
Pancreatic cancer	Inflammatory bowel disease
Pancreatic, ampullary, and duct obstruction	Autoimmune pancreatitis
Cystic fibrosis	Zollinger-Ellison syndrome
Diabetes mellitus type 1 or 2	Gastrointestinal surgeries (gastrectomy, gastric bypass, extensive small-bowel surgery)
Shwachman-Diamond syndrome (EPI with anemia, neutropenia, and bony abnormalities)	
Hemochromatosis	
Sjögren's syndrome	

EPI, Exocrine pancreatic insufficiency.

LABORATORY TESTS

Direct and indirect pancreatic function tests are available to diagnose EPI.[1,3]

- **Indirect:** Measures the level of pancreatic enzymes or the consequences of exocrine insufficiency.
  1. **Fecal elastase-1 (FE-1):** The most sensitive and specific test of pancreatic function in both adults and children. This enzyme is minimally degraded during intestinal transit, so it is a good marker of pancreatic function. The FE-1 test measures enzymatic production of FE-1 and can be used to screen for moderate-to-severe EPI with high sensitivity. FE-1 levels >200 μg/g are normal, levels of 100 to 200 μg/g are considered mild, and levels <100 μg/g are severe for EPI. Patients with borderline levels should undergo repeat testing if necessary.[4] Liquid stool can lead to falsely low levels due to dilution.
  2. **Fecal chymotrypsin:** Sensitive and specific test of pancreatic function. Variably degraded during transit in the intestinal lumen.
  3. **Serum trypsinogen:** Reflects pancreatic acinar cell mass. Highly sensitive for severe EPI when levels <20 ng/ml. This test is not commonly employed in clinical practice.
  4. **^{13}C-Triglyceride breath test:** Monitors the digestion of isotope-labeled fat meal to reflect absorption and metabolization of product.
- **Direct:** The most sensitive and specific diagnostic tests for the diagnosis of EPI are invasive. Tests use hormonal secretagogues (CCK, secretin, or CCK-secretin) to stimulate the pancreas and then collect duodenal fluid to measure secretory content.
  1. **Double-lumen gastroduodenal (Dreiling) collection tube:** Placement of an orogastroduodenal tube with one lumen collecting pancreatic juices and the other suctioning from the stomach to prevent acid contamination. Placement is cumbersome and time consuming and requires fluoroscopy to confirm the proper locations. Serial measurements of bicarbonate are obtained over 1 h. Severe EPI is reflected by a peak bicarbonate concentration of <50 mEq/L.
  2. **Endoscopic pancreatic function test:** Endoscopic procedure performed under sedation for the collection of duodenal fluid. Generally, it is better tolerated by patients than Dreiling collection. A peak bicarbonate concentration <80 mEq/L is considered abnormal for 1-h testing.

IMAGING STUDIES

- Computed tomography (CT): First-line imaging study of choice. Permits visualization of the pancreas for evaluation of calcifications, cysts, deformation/obstruction of bile ducts, pancreatic/peripancreatic tumors, fibrosis, and parenchyma loss.
- Magnetic resonance cholangiopancreatography (MRCP): Provides 3D imaging of the pancreatic-biliary ductal system.[1]
- Endoscopic ultrasound has not been shown to be diagnostic for EPI, although it can better assess the morphology of the pancreas in those with suspected chronic pancreatitis.[3]

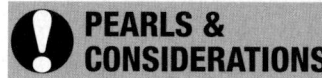 **TREATMENT**

The management of EPI includes dietary and lifestyle modifications, as well as pancreatic enzyme replacement therapy (PERT) and vitamin supplementation, to relieve maldigestion-related symptoms and restore normal nutritional health. Unfortunately, the disease is often underdiagnosed and subsequently undertreated, despite data showing that in certain circumstances, such as pancreatic malignancy, PERT can improve quality of life and lead to a longer life expectancy. Underlying diseases leading to EPI should also be treated.[1]

NONPHARMACOLOGIC THERAPY

Nutritional therapy aims to relieve maldigestion-related symptoms and ensure normal nutritional status. Patients should be encouraged to consume small and frequent meals. In addition, patients should abstain from consuming alcohol and smoking. Limiting dietary fat has not been shown to improve outcomes.[5]

PHARMACOLOGIC THERAPY

Oral administration of pancreatic enzyme replacements (Table 2) is the method of choice for treatment of EPI. The aim of PERT is to compensate for the deficiencies of normal pancreatic enzyme secretion and increase fat absorption. Doses are individually tailored and depend upon residual pancreatic function and fat content of the meal, but usually start at 25,000 to 40,000 IU of lipase in the form of enteric-coated mini-microspheres per main meal. PERT improves malabsorption of fat and protein and helps to relieve symptoms of abdominal pain, steatorrhea, and flatulence with studies reporting over 80% response to treatment.[6] Inadequate responses can be managed by either dose escalation or the addition of proton pump inhibitors or H_2 antagonists to prevent acid inactivation of lipase.[7]

Pediatric patients with EPI due to CF have shown improvement in pancreatic function with treatment of CFTR modulator, such as ivacaftor.[5]

DISPOSITION

- Consider further evaluation in patients with persistent weight loss and steatorrhea despite pancreatic enzyme replacement therapy.
- Patients diagnosed with EPI should also get a DEXA scan to evaluate for osteoporosis or osteopenia.

REFERRAL

- Consultation with a gastroenterologist can help expedite diagnosis and rule out alternate diagnoses.
- Referral to a nutritionist can aid the patient with malnutrition and alleviate symptoms.

PEARLS & CONSIDERATIONS

- The pancreas has an important role in the digestion of all nutrients, in particular, fats.
- EPI is a condition related to decreased pancreatic enzyme release resulting from loss of pancreatic parenchyma, inadequate pancreatic stimulation, pancreatic duct obstruction, or pancreatic enzyme inactivation.
- Common symptoms of EPI include weight loss, steatorrhea, and abdominal bloating.
- Timely diagnosis and adequate treatment with PERT therapy by the clinician is crucial because delay may impair growth in children, lead to adverse outcomes of malnutrition, and can increase morbidity and mortality in patients of all ages.
- Individualized dietary advice together with the appropriate PERT are the cornerstones of EPI therapy.

TABLE 2 Enzyme Products for the Treatment of Chronic Pancreatitis

Product	Formulation	Lipase Content per Pill or Capsule (USP Units)
Creon	Enteric-coated capsule	3000; 6000; 12,000; 24,000; 36,000
Zenpep	Enteric-coated capsule	3000; 5000; 10,000; 15,000; 20,000; 25,000
Pancreaze	Enteric-coated capsule	4200; 10,500; 16,800; 21,000
Ultresa	Enteric-coated capsule	13,800; 20,700; 23,000
Pertzye	Enteric-coated with bicarbonate	8000; 16,000
Viokase	Nonenteric-coated tablet*	10,440; 20,880

USP, United States Pharmacopeia.

The total dose of lipase per meal should be titrated based on response but usually requires at least 60,000 and usually 90,000 USP units (30,000 IU) of lipase per meal and half that amount with snacks. The dose should be split equally during the meal and immediately after the meal.

*Nonenteric-coated agents require cotreatment with an H_2 receptor antagonist or proton pump inhibitor to avoid denaturation of the enzymes by gastric acid.

REFERENCES AND SUGGESTED READINGS

Available at eBooks.Health.Elsevier.com.

RELATED TOPICS

AUTHORS: **SARAH ZAINELABDIN, MD** and **ROSS W. HILLIARD, MD, FACP**

Diseases and Disorders

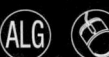
BASIC INFORMATION

DEFINITION

Febrile seizures are seizures that occur in febrile children (fever of at least 38° C [100.4° F]) between the ages of 6 mo and 5 yr in the absence of infection of the central nervous system (CNS), metabolic disturbance, or history of neonatal seizures or a previous unprovoked seizure. Febrile seizures are subdivided into two categories: Simple and complex. Simple febrile seizures last <15 min, are generalized (without a focal component), and occur once in a 24-h period, whereas complex febrile seizures are prolonged (>15 min), show focal neurologic signs, or occur more than once in 24 h.

SYNONYMS

Febrile convulsions
Seizures, febrile

ICD 10-CM CODE
R56.0   Febrile convulsions

EPIDEMIOLOGY & DEMOGRAPHICS

INCIDENCE: Febrile seizures are the most common seizures of childhood. 2% to 5% of children will have a febrile seizure by age 5 yr. Simple febrile seizures represent 65% to 90% of febrile seizures.
PREVALENCE: Represents up to 18% of all pediatric epilepsy syndromes.
PREDOMINANT SEX & AGE: Slightly more common in boys than in girls.
PEAK INCIDENCE: 6 mo to 5 yr.
RISK FACTORS: Family history and viral infections.
GENETICS: Febrile seizures tend to occur in families. Although clear evidence exists for a genetic basis of febrile seizures, the mode of inheritance is unknown.

PHYSICAL FINDINGS & CLINICAL PRESENTATION

Children with febrile seizures have normal physical and neurologic examinations.

ETIOLOGY

Viral infections are a common cause of a fever that triggers febrile seizures. Febrile seizures are likely multifactorial, with genetic and environmental factors.

DIAGNOSIS

DIFFERENTIAL DIAGNOSIS
- CNS infection (i.e., meningitis)
- Epilepsy

WORKUP
- It is important to first investigate whether an underlying infection exists. Fig. 1 describes guidelines for febrile seizure evaluation.
- In patients with simple self-limited febrile seizures with rapid return to consciousness and a normal neurologic examination, further workup is not routinely recommended.
- In patients with complex febrile seizures, laboratory workup and brain imaging are recommended.
- Electroencephalogram (EEG) is not routinely recommended in the evaluation of a neurologically healthy child with simple febrile seizures.

LABORATORY TESTS
- Routine blood workup (CBC with differential, complete metabolic panel [CMP], electrolytes) and blood and urine cultures are often performed, but there is no evidence that these tests are necessary for identifying the cause of a simple febrile seizure.
- Lumbar puncture should be performed in children with febrile seizures and signs and symptoms of meningitis (e.g., neck stiffness, Kernig sign, Brudzinski sign) or if the patient history or examination suggests the presence of meningitis or other intracranial infection.
- In infants 6 to 12 mo of age with febrile seizures, lumbar puncture is an option if they have not received the recommended *Haemophilus influenzae* type b (Hib) or pneumococcal vaccinations or if their immunization status is unknown.
- Lumbar puncture is also considered an option in children with febrile seizures pretreated with antibiotics.

IMAGING STUDIES
- MRI of the brain is not required in the routine evaluation of patients with simple febrile seizures.
- Imaging of the brain should be considered in children with complex febrile seizures and in children with focal neurologic deficits.
- Computed tomography (CT) scans of the head should be avoided in children, if possible, due to exposure to radiation and the relative low yield of the test compared with MRI. CT scans of the head are reserved for neurologic emergencies and are dose-adjusted for weight in children.

TREATMENT

NONPHARMACOLOGIC THERAPY
Not applicable

ACUTE GENERAL Rx
Febrile seizures do not usually require antiepileptic drug treatment.

CHRONIC Rx
No chronic treatment for febrile seizures is recommended.

DISPOSITION
- Treatment is not recommended.
- Febrile seizures should stop by age 5.
- Risk of recurrence in the first 2 yr after an initial febrile seizure is 15% to 70%.

COMPLEMENTARY & ALTERNATIVE MEDICINE
Not applicable

REFERRAL
Patients with recurrent febrile seizures need to be referred for a consultation by a pediatric neurologist.

PEARLS & CONSIDERATIONS

COMMENTS
- It is crucial to find out the etiology of the fever and to treat it appropriately.
- Patients with seizures and fever after age 5 are not classified as febrile seizures.

PREVENTION
Antipyretics do not reduce the recurrence risk of febrile seizures. However, fever should be treated and worked up independently of the diagnosis of febrile seizures.

PATIENT & FAMILY EDUCATION
- Children with febrile seizures do not need antiepileptic drug treatment.
- Patient education and information can be obtained at the Epilepsy Foundation: www.epilepsyfoundation.org/. Parents should be reassured that children without underlying developmental problems will usually not have lasting neurologic effects from febrile seizures.

AUTHOR: **PATRICIO SEBASTIAN ESPINOSA, MD, MPH, FAAN**

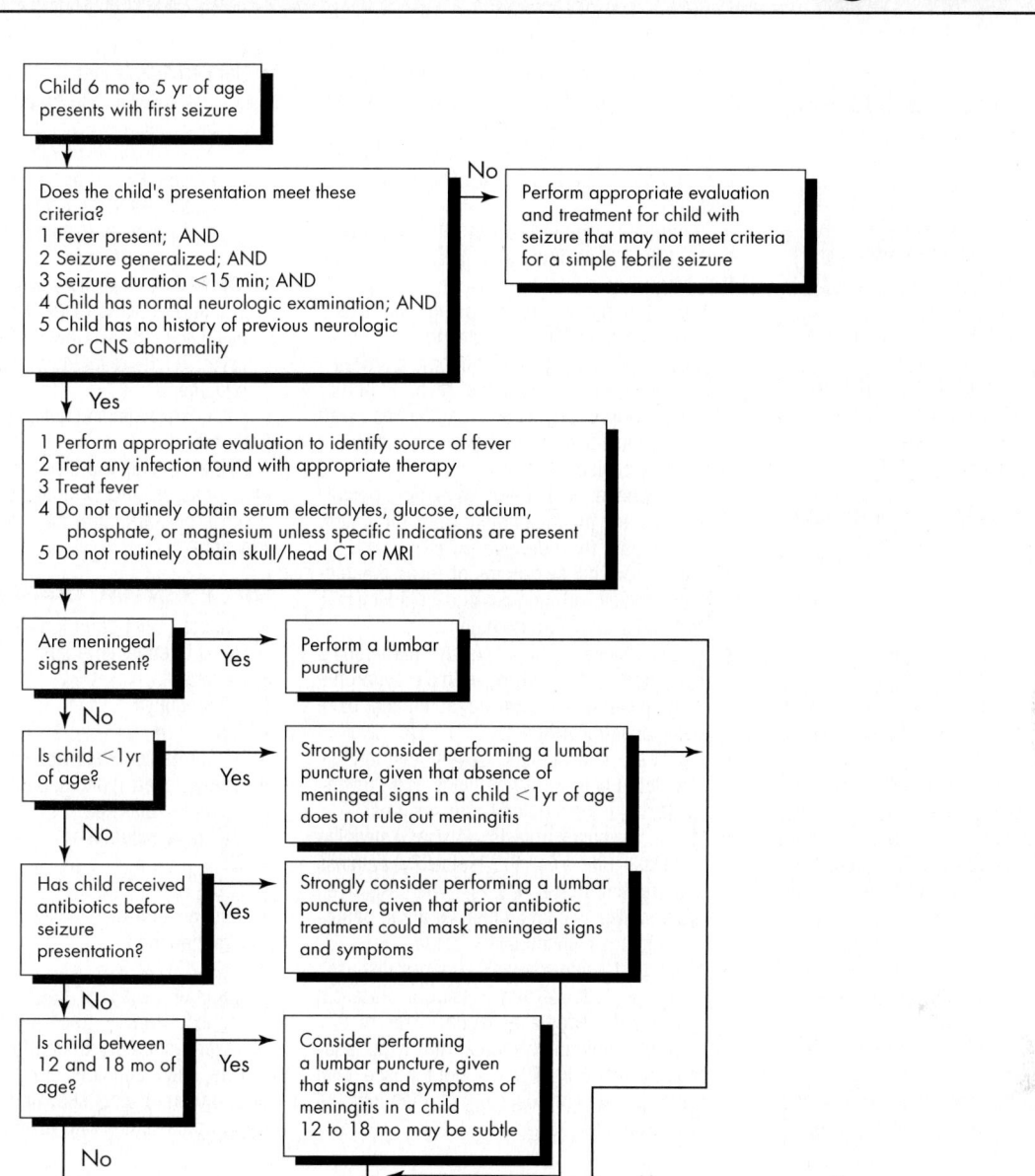

FIG. 1 Guidelines for febrile seizure evaluation. *CNS,* Central nervous system; *CT,* computed tomography; *EEG,* electroencephalogram; *MRI,* magnetic resonance imaging. (From Custer JW, Rau RE: *The Harriet Lane handbook,* ed 18, St Louis, 2009, Mosby.)

DEFINITION

A traveler who returns from a foreign country with a fever or develops a fever within 1 mo of returning.[1]

EPIDEMIOLOGY & DEMOGRAPHICS

Around 3% and up to 11% of patients returning from short periods of travel abroad report a febrile illness. Studies from the United States and Europe reveal that approximately 43% to 79% of travelers fall ill during or after traveling to a developing or newly industrialized country. In certain travel clinics, fever was the chief complaint in 28% of ill travelers who presented upon return home. Mortality is between 0.2% and 0.5%. The specific cause of fever may not be diagnosed in up to 25% of patients. [1,2]

Incidence is dependent on location and timing of travel. Risk factors include extremes of age and those who are immunocompromised.

PHYSICAL FINDINGS & CLINICAL PRESENTATION[1,3]

A detailed history of the travel must be obtained, including areas of travel, activities, sleeping arrangements, pre-travel immunizations, comorbidities, and use of malaria prophylaxis. Incubation period and time to symptom onset can assist with differential (Table 1). Additionally, skin findings may be particularly useful for diagnosis (Table 2).

Common causes of fever in returning travelers and their associated symptoms include the following:[1,3]

- Malaria: Abrupt rigors, relapsing high fevers, diaphoresis, malaise, headaches, myalgias, abdominal pain, nausea, vomiting, diarrhea
- Dengue fever ("breakbone fever"): Abrupt fever, severe myalgias, headaches with retro-orbital pain, maculopapular blanching rash, petechiae
- Chikungunya: High fever, myalgias, polyarthralgia, and maculopapular rash. Difficult to differentiate from dengue fever
- Zika: Prodromal symptoms of fever, maculopapular rash, arthralgias, and conjunctivitis. Up to 80% are asymptomatic
- Enteric fevers (typhoid fever, paratyphoid fever, travelers' diarrhea): Clinical syndrome of sustained fever, anorexia, abdominal pain, malaise, and diarrhea
- Japanese encephalitis: Asian distribution, associated with rural rice fields. High fevers, headache, nuchal rigidity, and seizures
- African trypanosomiasis (African sleeping sickness): Bite from the tsetse fly, painless chancre that grows for 2 to 3 wk. Associated with malaise, wasting, behavioral and neurologic changes, encephalitis, coma
- American trypanosomiasis (Chagas disease): Spread by reduviid bug (kissing or assassin bug). Painful edema at wound near mouth, unilateral periorbital edema, and lymphadenopathy for 2 to 4 wk. Latent phase with nerve destruction causing cardiac and GI manifestations

- Hemorrhagic fevers:
  1. Yellow fever: Classic presentation of jaundice, black emesis, albuminuria. May also have conjunctival injection, facial flushing, and relative bradycardia
  2. Ebola: Fever, myalgia, and abdominal pain that progress to hemorrhage, shock, and end-organ failure
- Middle East respiratory syndrome (MERS-CoV) and severe acute respiratory syndrome coronaviruses (SARS-CoV-1 and SARS-CoV-2): Fever, acute respiratory distress syndrome, pneumonia

Table 3 groups infections by common clinical findings.

Table 4 summarizes the constellations of exposures and clinical presentations suggestive of particular diagnoses in returning travelers.

DIFFERENTIAL DIAGNOSIS[1,3]

- Malaria (most common cause of fever after travel to endemic areas)
- Dengue
- Chikungunya
- Zika
- Hemorrhagic fevers: Yellow fever, Ebola
- Enteric fever: Typhoid, paratyphoid
- Travelers' diarrhea
- Meningococcemia
- TB
- Acute HIV
- Trypanosomiasis
- Viral hepatitis
- SARS-CoV-2
- Common causes of fever that are not travel-related: Urinary tract infection, upper and lower respiratory tract infections

One must consider travel location, activities, endemic diseases, and local outbreaks. Geographic region will assist with differential

---

TABLE 1 Incubation Periods of Common Travel-Related Infections*

Short Incubation (<10 days)	Medium Incubation (10-21 days)	Long Incubation (>21 days)
Malaria	Malaria	Malaria
Arboviruses including dengue, yellow fever, Japanese encephalitis	Flaviviruses: Tick-borne encephalitis and Japanese encephalitis	Schistosomiasis
		Tuberculosis
Hemorrhagic fevers: Lassa, Ebola, South American arenaviruses	Hemorrhagic fevers: Lassa, Ebola, Crimean-Congo	Acute HIV infection
	Acute HIV infection	Viral hepatitis
Respiratory viruses including severe acute respiratory syndrome	Typhoid and paratyphoid	Filariasis
	Giardia	*Rickettsia:* Q fever
Typhoid and paratyphoid	*Rickettsia:* Flea-borne, louse-borne, and scrub typhus, Q fever, spotted fevers (rare)	Secondary syphilis
Bacterial enteritis		Epstein-Barr virus including mononucleosis
Rickettsia: Spotted fever group—Rocky Mountain spotted fever, African tick typhus, Mediterranean spotted fever, scrub typhus, Q fever	Cytomegalovirus	Amebic liver disease
	Toxoplasma	Leishmaniasis
	Amebic dysentery	*Brucella*
Bacterial pneumonia including *Legionella*	Histoplasmosis	Bartonellosis (chronic)
Relapsing fever	*Brucella*	Babesiosis
Amebic dysentery	Leptospirosis	Rabies
Meningococcemia	Babesiosis	West African trypanosomiasis (chronic)
Brucella (rarely)	Rabies	Cytomegalovirus
Leptospirosis	East African trypanosomiasis (acute)	
Fascioliasis	Hepatitis A (rarely)	
Rabies (rarely)	Measles	
African trypanosomiasis (acute), East African (rarely)		

HIV, Human immunodeficiency virus.

* Diseases that commonly have variable incubation periods are shown more than once. However, most diseases may rarely have an atypical incubation period, and this is not shown here.

From Bennet et al: *Mandell, Douglas, and Bennet's principles and practice of infectious diseases,* ed 8, Philadelphia, 2015, Elsevier.

TABLE 2   Skin Lesions in Returned Travelers

Linear	Cutaneous Larva Migrans (*Ancylostoma* spp.)	Pruritic Serpiginous Lesions That Advance Slowly
	Larva currens	Urticarial linear lesions moving faster due to cutaneous migration of *Strongyloides stercoralis* filariform larvae
	Phytophotodermatitis	Noninfectious lesion due to interaction of natural psoralens (in lime juice spilled on skin) that interacts with UV radiation
Macular	Generalized	Consider drug reactions
	Localized	Consider tinea corporis or tinea versicolor
	Leprosy	Hypopigmented macular lesions with hypoesthesia or peripheral nerve enlargement
Maculopapular	With fever	Arbovirus: Dengue, chikungunya, measles, rubella, parvovirus, EBV, CMV, HIV, syphilis
		VHF
		Rickettsial infection
Nodular	Bacterial skin infection (staphylococcal/streptococcal)	May follow bug bites; pyoderma, impetigo, abscess formation, erysipelas, cellulitis, lymphangitis, or ulceration
	Gnathostomiasis	Migratory panniculitis common in Southeast Asia, less in Africa and Latin America
	Myiasis	Painful "boil"-like lesions in Africa (*Cordylobia anthropophaga*); or Latin America (*Dermatobia hominis*)
	Tungiasis (*Tunga penetrans*)	Nodular pale subcutaneous lesion with central dark spot
Papular	Insect bites most common	Grouped papules due to bed bug and flea bites
	Endemic mycoses	Histoplasmosis, penicilliosis
	Onchocerciasis (sub-Saharan Africa)	Generalized pruritic papular dermatitis
	Scabies	Regional or generalized pruritic papular rash
Ulcerative	Anthrax	Necrotic ulcer surrounded by edema
	Buruli ulcer (*Mycobacterium ulcerans*)	Destructive ulcer with undermining edges
	Chancre	*Trypanosoma brucei rhodesiense*: Occurs 48 h after tsetse fly bite; itchy, painful red/purple nodule, 2-5 cm diameter which ulcerates, with surrounding edema and associated lymphadenopathy
	Cutaneous leishmaniasis	Chronic, usually painless ulcer unless superinfected, with heaped-up margins on exposed skin surfaces, in travelers from high-risk areas, including Latin America, Mediterranean, Middle East, Asia, and parts of Africa
	Rickettsial infection such as African tick-bite fever or scrub typhus	Eschar: Dark, scabbed lesion at site of insect bite
	Ulceroglandular tularemia	Papule develops at site of inoculation with fever onset; becomes vesicular and pustular, then ulcerates. Tender, associated with painful lymphadenitis

CMV, Cytomegalovirus; *EBV,* Epstein-Barr virus; *HIV,* human immunodeficiency virus; *UV,* ultraviolet; *VHF,* viral hemorrhagic fever.
From Spec A et al: *Comprehensive review of infectious diseases,* Philadelphia, 2019, Elsevier.

TABLE 3   CDC: Clinical Findings and Select Associated Infectious Diseases

Common Clinical Findings	Infections to Consider After Tropical Travel
Fever and rash	Dengue, chikungunya, Zika, spotted fever or typhus group rickettsioses, typhoid fever (skin lesions may be sparse or absent), acute HIV infection, measles, varicella, mononucleosis, parvovirus B19, meningococcemia (lesions usually sparse)
Fever and abdominal pain	Typhoid fever, hepatitis, other viral syndrome, traveler's diarrhea, amebic liver abscess
Undifferentiated fever and normal or low white blood cell count	Dengue, rickettsial infections (scrub typhus, spotted fevers without rash), typhoid fever, chikungunya, Zika, acute HIV infection, early-stage viral hemorrhagic fevers, other viral infections
Fever and hemorrhage	Viral hemorrhagic fevers (e.g., dengue, yellow, Ebola, Lassa fever), meningococcemia, leptospirosis, spotted fever group (rickettsial infections)
Fever and arthralgia or myalgia (sometimes persistent)	Chikungunya, dengue, Zika, Ross River virus, muscular sarcocystosis, trichinellosis
Fever and eosinophilia	Acute schistosomiasis, drug hypersensitivity reaction, fascioliasis, sarcocystosis, trichinellosis, angiostrongyliasis, and other parasitic infections
Fever and respiratory symptoms/ pulmonary infiltrates	Influenza and other common bacterial and viral pathogens, legionellosis, tuberculosis, acute schistosomiasis, Q fever, leptospirosis, Middle East respiratory syndrome, acute histoplasmosis, or coccidioidomycosis, psittacosis, melioidosis, pneumonic plague
Fever and altered mental status/CNS involvement	Cerebral malaria, arboviral encephalitides (Jap. encephalitis, West Nile virus), meningococcal meningitis, eosinophilic meningitis (angiostrongyliasis), rabies, East African trypanosomiasis, scrub typhus, tickborne encephalitis, rabies
Fever and jaundice	Acute viral hepatitis (A, B, C, E), yellow fever and other viral hemorrhagic fevers, severe malaria, leptospirosis
Mononucleosis syndrome	EBV, CMV, toxoplasmosis, acute HIV
Fever persisting >2 wk	Malaria, typhoid fever, EBV, CMV, toxoplasmosis, acute HIV, acute schistosomiasis, brucellosis, tuberculosis, Q fever, visceral leishmaniasis (rare)
Fever with onset >6 wk after travel	Plasmodium vivax or ovale malaria, acute hepatitis (B, C, E), tuberculosis, amebic liver abscess, melioidosis, African trypanosomiasis, visceral leishmaniasis

CMV, Cytomegalovirus; *CNS,* central nervous system; *EBV,* Epstein-Barr virus; *HIV,* human immunodeficiency virus; *WBC,* white blood cells.
From Centers for Disease Control and Prevention: Travelers' health. Available at www.cdc.gov/travel/.

TABLE 4 Constellations of Exposures and Clinical Presentations Suggestive of Particular Diagnoses in Returned Travelers*

Exposure Scenario	Distinctive Findings	Diagnosis
Any exposure in any area with documented malaria transmission	Fever with or without any other finding	Malaria
Most tropical countries	Fever and altered mental status	Malaria, meningococcal meningitis, rabies, West Nile virus
Budget travel to India, Nepal, Pakistan, or Bangladesh	Insidious onset, high unremitting fever, toxic patient, paucity of physical findings	Enteric fever due to *Salmonella typhi* or *Salmonella paratyphi*
Freshwater recreational exposure in Africa	Fever, eosinophilia, hepatomegaly, negative malaria smear	Acute schistosomiasis (Katayama fever)
Bitten by *Aedes aegypti* in Central America, Southeast Asia, or the South Pacific	Fever, headache, myalgia, diffuse macular rash, mild to moderate thrombocytopenia	Dengue
Bitten by *A. aegypti* or *Aedes albopictus* in India, Malaysia, Singapore, the Caribbean, or an island in the Indian Ocean	Fever, headache, myalgia, diffuse macular rash, arthralgia, tenosynovitis often followed by chronic polyarthritis after the fever resolves	Chikungunya fever
Hunting or visiting game reserves in southern Africa	Fever, eschar, diffuse petechial rash	African tick typhus due to *Rickettsia africae*
Travel to Southeast Asia	Fever, eschar, diffuse petechial rash	Scrub typhus due to *Orientia tsutsugamushi*
Hiking, biking, swimming, rafting with exposure to fresh surface water	Fever, myalgia, conjunctival suffusion, mild to severe jaundice, variable rash	Leptospirosis
Cruise, elderly traveler	Influenza-like illness	Influenza A or B
Outdoor exposure anywhere in the Americas	Large, single furuncular lesion anywhere on body, with sense of movement inside	Myiasis due to *Dermatobia hominis* (botfly)
Clothing washed or dried out of doors in Africa	Multiple furuncular lesions around clothing contact points with skin	Myiasis due to *Cordylobia anthropophaga* (tumbu fly)
New sexual partner during travel	Fever, rash, mononucleosis-like illness	Acute human immunodeficiency virus infection
Travel to any developing country or to Western Europe	Coryza, conjunctivitis, Koplik spots, rash	Measles
Longer visit to humid areas of Africa, the Americas, or Southeast Asia	Asymptomatic eosinophilia or with periodic cough or wheezing	Strongyloidiasis
Sand fly bite in tropical areas	Painless skin ulcer with clean, moist base in exposed area	Cutaneous leishmaniasis
Resort hotel in southern Europe, ± exposure to whirlpool spas	Pneumonia	Legionnaires' disease
Explored a cave in the Americas	Fever, cough, retrosternal chest pain, hilar adenopathy	Histoplasmosis
Ingestion of unpasteurized goat cheese	Chronic fever, fatigue	*Brucella melitensis*
Long trip to West/Central Africa	Afebrile, intensely pruritic, evanescent truncal maculopapular rash	Onchocerciasis
Long trip to West/Central Africa	Migratory localized angioedema or swellings over large joints, eosinophilia	Loiasis
Safari to game parks of East Africa	Fever, nongenital chancre, fine macular rash	East African trypanosomiasis
Travel to Australia	Fever, fatigue, polyarthritis	Ross River virus
Farming areas of India and Southeast Asia	Fever, altered mental status, paralysis	Japanese encephalitis
Forested areas of central and eastern Europe and across Russia	Fever, altered mental status, paralysis	Tick-borne encephalitis
Rodent exposure in West Africa	Fever, sore throat, jaundice, hemorrhagic manifestations	Lassa fever
Ingestion of sushi, ceviche, or raw freshwater fish	Migratory nodules in truncal areas with overlying erythema or mild hemorrhage	Gnathostomiasis
Returning Hajj pilgrim or family contact	Fever, meningitis	Meningococcal meningitis
Ingestion of snails, fish, or shellfish in Asia or Australia	Eosinophilic meningitis	Angiostrongyliasis, gnathostomiasis
Diabetic or compromised host with exposure to moist terrain in Asia or Australia	Fever, sepsis, pneumonia or multifocal abscesses	Melioidosis
Summertime exposure to rodent droppings in Scandinavia	Fever with decreased renal function	Puumala virus
Ingestion of undercooked meat of any animal in any country	Fever, facial edema, myositis, increased creatine phosphokinase, massive eosinophilia, normal erythrocyte sedimentation rate	Trichinosis
Unvaccinated, returning from sub-Saharan Africa or forested areas of Amazonia	Fever, jaundice, proteinuria, hemorrhage	Yellow fever
Exposure to farm animals	Pneumonia, mild hepatitis	Q fever
Possible tick exposure almost anywhere	Fever, headache, rash, conjunctival injection, hepatosplenomegaly	Tick-borne relapsing fever
Poor hygienic conditions with possible body louse exposure in Ethiopia or Sudan	Fever, headache, rash, conjunctival injection, hepatosplenomegaly	Louse-borne relapsing fever

*The table includes illnesses of travelers (listed first) as well as less common diseases with presentations that should suggest the possibility of the appropriate diagnosis. Many diseases have a spectrum of presentation, and the table describes the most common presentations of these diseases. Many diseases have a spectrum of geographic origins, and the table describes the most common exposures seen in daily practice.

From Bennet et al: *Mandell, Douglas, and Bennet's principles and practice of infectious diseases*, ed 8, Philadelphia, 2015, Elsevier.

diagnosis. Table E5 pairs regions with common tropical diseases.

LABORATORY TESTS[3]

Consider:
- CBC
- Comprehensive metabolic panel
- Prothrombin time/international normalized ratio, partial thromboplastin time
- Urinalysis
- Blood, urine stool cultures
- Cerebrospinal fluid analysis, Gram stain, culture
- Rapid HIV screen
- Serial blood smears q8 to 12h over 2 days
- Specific serology for suspected infections
- SARS-CoV-2 Test

IMAGING STUDIES

Not usually required, but consider as clinically indicated:
- Chest x-ray
- Upright abdominal x-ray
- Computed tomography (CT): Head
- CT: Abdomen and pelvis

Rx TREATMENT

Pretravel prevention should focus on proper vaccinations and prophylactic medications. Post-travel treatment is dependent on the specific disease. Treatment ranges from supportive care to intravenous antibiotics. Treatment for the more common causes of fever in travelers is listed below, with an emphasis on malaria, given its prevalence:[2]

- Malaria, uncomplicated *Plasmodium falciparum* or species not identified:
  1. Artemether-lumefantrine (Coartem) 1 tab is 20 mg artemether/120 mg lumefantrine 3-day treatment schedule, 6 doses total
     a. Day 1: 1 dose PO followed by a second dose 8 h later
     b. Days 2 and 3: 1 dose PO bid
     c. 5 to <15 kg: 1 tab per dose
     d. 15 to <25 kg: 2 tabs per dose
     e. 25 to <35 kg: 3 tabs per dose
     f. 35 kg and up: 4 tabs per dose
  2. Malarone (atovaquone/proguanil): 250 mg atovaquone/100 mg proguanil
  3. Malarone 4 tabs PO daily for 3 days
  4. Quinine sulfate: 542 mg base (650 mg salt) PO q8h for 3 to 7 days *plus*
     a. Doxycycline 100 mg PO q12h for 7 days *or*
     b. Tetracycline: 250 mg PO qid for 7 days *or*
     c. Clindamycin: 20 mg base/kg/day PO divided tid for 7 days

  5. Mefloquine (not suggested as first-line treatment due to high incidence of neuropsychiatric side effects; high resistance in Southeast Asia): 684 mg base (750 mg salt) PO initial dose, 456 mg base (500 mg salt) PO 6 to 12 h after the first dose; total dose: 1250 mg salt
  6. For pediatric dosing, refer to CDC treatment table

- Severe malaria:
  1. Artesunate: 2.4 mg/kg per dose IV; administer 1 dose at 0, 12, 24, and 48 h for a total of 4 doses
  2. Followed by one of the following:
     a. Coartem: Treatment as above
     b. Doxycycline (clindamycin in pregnant patients): Treatment as above if patient can tolerate PO, otherwise administer 100 mg IV q12h and switch to oral doxycycline as soon as patient can take oral medication; for IV use, avoid rapid administration. Treatment course is 7 days
     c. Clindamycin: Treatment as above unless patient cannot tolerate PO, then 10 mg base/kg IV loading dose followed by 5 mg base/kg IV q8h; switch to PO clindamycin as soon as possible; treatment course is 7 days
     d. Mefloquine, if there is no other option

- Dengue: Supportive care, fever and pain control, prevent dehydration
  1. NSAIDs and aspirin contraindicated due to increased bleeding risk
  2. Acetaminophen or paracetamol q6h
  3. Cool compresses or ice compresses, bath if necessary

- Chikungunya: Supportive care, acetaminophen is the preferred first-line treatment in patients traveling to dengue endemic areas until dengue can be ruled out thus similar to dengue. After dengue is ruled out, NSAIDs, corticosteroids, and physical therapy might help lessen symptoms in those with persistent joint pain.

- Typhoid fever: Fluoroquinolone (ciprofloxacin), third-generation cephalosporins (cefixime or ceftriaxone), azithromycin. Duration varies based on severity

- Travelers' diarrhea: Ciprofloxacin, azithromycin

- Hemorrhagic viruses: Supportive care, typically

DISPOSITION

Disposition depends on the specific disease, severity of disease, and possibility of transmission, and can range from outpatient treatment to ICU level of care

REFERRALS

- Infectious disease consultation
- Contact CDC or local health department for recommendations pertaining to endemic diseases and treatment
- Some medical treatments and diagnostic testing must be sent to and from the CDC
- Mandatory reporting of some diseases to the CDC

! PEARLS & CONSIDERATIONS

- Differential depends on the geography and the patient's individual risk factors (e.g., pre-travel immunizations, comorbidities, activities).
- Until demonstrated otherwise, some travel medicine experts recommend assuming that all febrile travelers coming from malaria-endemic regions have malaria until proven otherwise.
- Keep a broad differential of other common sources of fever (e.g., urinary tract infections, respiratory tract infections) until a specific diagnosis is made.

PREVENTION

Check the CDC website and the Yellow Book for pretravel vaccinations.[2,4]

PATIENT & FAMILY EDUCATION

Visit Travelers' Health at https://wwwnc.cdc.gov/travel/ for further information.[4]

REFERENCES

Available at eBooks.Health.Elsevier.com.

RELATED CONTENT

Brucellosis (Related Key Topic)
Dengue Fever (Related Key Topic)
Histoplasmosis (Related Key Topic)
Human Immunodeficiency Virus (Related Key Topic)
Leishmaniasis (Related Key Topic)
Malaria (Related Key Topic)
Measles (Rubeola) (Related Key Topic)
Q Fever (Related Key Topic)
Rabies (Related Key Topic)
Salmonellosis (Related Key Topic)
Trichinellosis (Related Key Topic)
West Nile Virus Infection (Related Key Topic)
Yellow Fever (Related Key Topic)
Zika Virus (Related Key Topic)

AUTHORS: **JAMES ELLIOTT COOPER, MD** and **ABIGAIL COSGROVE, MD**

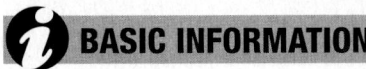

DEFINITION

Fibromyalgia (FM) is a syndrome characterized by chronic, widespread musculoskeletal pain without evidence of soft tissue inflammation. Key features include chronic fatigue, sleep disruption, cognitive disturbance, and psychiatric and somatic symptoms. FM can be considered a centralized pain state, with research suggesting that it is a disorder of pain regulation.

SYNONYMS

The term "fibrositis" is no longer used because there is no evidence of connective tissue inflammation in FM.

ICD-10CM CODE	
M79.7	Fibromyalgia

EPIDEMIOLOGY & DEMOGRAPHICS

Worldwide, the prevalence of FM is estimated to be between 2% and 8%, increasing with age. FM is most commonly diagnosed in women between ages 40 and 60 yr but can affect all ages and populations.[1]

PHYSICAL FINDINGS & CLINICAL PRESENTATION

Patients with FM often report the following symptoms:

- Chronic (>3 mo) widespread (affecting both sides of the body, above and below the waist, and involving the axial spine) musculoskeletal pain with tenderness to palpation of at least 11 of the 18 specific tender points associated with FM[2]
- Cognitive disturbances
- Fatigue and sleep disturbances
- Psychiatric symptoms (e.g., anxiety, depression)
- Headache (present in more than half of patients with FM; includes migraine and tension-type headaches)
- Paresthesias
- Associated disorders: Irritable bowel syndrome, interstitial cystitis/painful bladder syndrome

On physical examination, patients with FM can have tenderness, in particular soft tissue locations called tender points. Examination of tender points requires that the examiner be familiar with the areas to palpate and that they apply enough pressure (4 kg/cm^2 or enough to whiten the nail bed of the examiner's fingertips).

ETIOLOGY

Although the exact cause of FM is unknown, its etiology is thought to be multifactorial:

- Genetic and environmental factors may play a role. Evidence suggests that ascending and descending pain pathways operate abnormally, resulting in central amplification of pain signals.[3] Familial associations of FM provide the strongest evidence that reflects both these factors.

- In those predisposed, FM may be precipitated by physical or psychologic stress such as abuse, injury from accidents, illnesses (including autoimmune disorders), infections, and surgical procedures.
- Psychosocial, neuroendocrine, hormonal, and sociocultural factors also influence symptom expression.[4]

PATHOGENESIS

Much remains to be discovered about the pathogenesis of FM, although significant advances have been made over the past few decades. Researchers have shown that biochemical, metabolic, and immunoregulatory abnormalities exist in patients with FM. Hence, this condition is now believed to be neurosensory in nature.

- Augmented pain and sensory processing are hallmarks, resulting in diffuse pain, allodynia (pain brought on by nonpainful stimuli), and hyperalgesia (more intense and prolonged pain perception).[5]
- Brain imaging studies have demonstrated evidence of increased activation in pain processing networks, suggesting abnormal hyperactivity of pain detection and processing pathways.
- Afflicted persons show altered physiologic responses to painful stimulation at spinal and supraspinal levels.
- Brain neuroimaging studies have identified differences in brain structure, neurochemical concentrations, and functional brain networks in FM compared with control subjects. PET scans have revealed widespread activation of glial cells in the cortex, particularly in the frontal and parietal lobes.[6]
- Pain augmentation may also result from a loss of tonic inhibition by descending inhibitory pathways from the brain to the spinal cord.[7]

DIAGNOSIS

DIFFERENTIAL DIAGNOSIS

The presence of any of the disorders below does not necessarily exclude a diagnosis of FM because it can coexist with many conditions:

- Other functional somatic or "central sensitivity" syndromes: Myofascial pain, chronic fatigue syndrome, irritable bowel syndrome, headache/migraines, chronic pelvic and bladder pain disorders, and temporomandibular disorder
- Disorders that can mimic FM and must be ruled out include metabolic (e.g., hypothyroidism), infectious, and neurologic disorders
- Arthritis and rheumatic diseases (e.g., rheumatoid arthritis, systemic lupus erythematosus, osteoarthritis, Sjögren syndrome)
- Myalgias and other muscle disease (e.g., inflammatory and metabolic myopathies)
- Mood and anxiety disorders
- Sleep disorders (e.g., sleep apnea, restless leg syndrome)
- Neurologic disorders
- Medications: Statin-induced muscle pain, opioid-induced hyperalgesia[8]

WORKUP

A thorough history, physical examination, and appropriately selected laboratory or imaging studies can usually differentiate FM from connective tissue or other systemic diseases.

- Chronic (>3 mo) widespread pain is the hallmark symptom of FM, but fatigue, tenderness, depression/anxiety, nonrestorative sleep, cognitive difficulties ("fibrofog"), and functional impairment are other key symptoms.
- The 1990 ACR FM Classification Criteria used for clinical studies:
  1. Chronic, widespread pain in all four quadrants of the body and the axial skeleton
  2. Pain on digital palpation of at least 11 of 18 tender points
- The 2010 ACR diagnostic criteria for FM do not require a tender point examination; other disorders that would otherwise explain musculoskeletal pain must be excluded (Table 1).
- A diagnostic screening tool (Fibromyalgia Diagnostic Screen) developed by Arnold et al[9] was found to accurately screen for FM. This tool includes a patient self-reported questionnaire and an abbreviated physical examination with targeted lab tests.
- The most recent FM diagnostic criteria are by ACTION-APS Pain Taxonomy (AAPT), an international working group.[10] To fulfill AAPT criteria for FM, a patient is required to have a history of at least 3 mo of widespread pain in at least six of nine possible pain sites, and moderate to severe sleep disturbance or fatigue.

LABORATORY TESTS

- Selective use of ancillary tests complements the history and physical examination in diagnosis of FM. Testing should be highly focused on the exclusion of FM mimickers or suspected concurrent diseases.
- Complete blood cell count, routine chemistries, thyroid-stimulating hormone (TSH), 25-hydroxy vitamin D level (low levels can cause muscle pain), vitamin B$_{12}$ level (low levels can cause fatigue and pain), iron studies (low levels can cause fatigue and depressive symptoms), and magnesium levels (low levels can cause muscle spasms).
- Erythrocyte sedimentation rate (ESR) and C-reactive protein (CRP) are generally normal.
- Routine testing for antinuclear antibody (ANA) and/or rheumatoid factor should be avoided unless history and physical examination suggest an autoimmune disease.

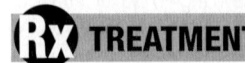 TREATMENT

GENERAL Rx

The goal in treating patients with fibromyalgia is to reduce the main symptoms of the syndrome (musculoskeletal pain, fatigue, depression, anxiety, poor sleep). The revised Fibromyalgia Impact Questionnaire (FIQR) (Fig. E1) is useful to assess functional status as well as overall impact and fibromyalgia symptoms.

- Challenging to treat; best approach may be combination of drug and nondrug therapies.

F

I

TABLE 1 2010 Fibromyalgia Diagnostic Criteria

Criteria

A patient satisfies diagnostic criteria for fibromyalgia if the following three conditions are met:
1. Widespread pain index (WPI) 7 and symptom severity (SS) scale score of 5 or WPI 3-6 and SS scale score of 9.
2. Symptoms have been present at a similar level for at least 3 mo.
3. The patient does not have a disorder that would otherwise explain the pain.

Ascertainment

1. WPI: Note the number of areas in which the patient has had pain over the past week. In how many areas has the patient had pain?

Score will be between 0 and 19.

Shoulder girdle, left	Hip (buttock, trochanter), left	Jaw, left	Upper back
Shoulder girdle, right	Hip (buttock, trochanter), right	Jaw, right	Lower back
Upper arm, left	Upper leg, left	Chest	Neck
Upper arm, right	Upper leg, right	Abdomen	
Lower arm, left	Lower leg, left		
Lower arm, right	Lower leg, right		

2. SS scale score:

Fatigue

Waking unrefreshed

Cognitive symptoms

For each of the three symptoms above, indicate the level of severity over the past week using the following scale:

0, No problem

1, Slight or mild problems, generally mild or intermittent

2, Moderate, considerable problems, often present at a moderate level

3, Severe: Pervasive, continuous, life-disturbing problems

Considering somatic symptoms in general, indicate whether the patient has:*

0, No symptoms

1, Few symptoms

2, A moderate number of symptoms

3, A great deal of symptoms

The SS scale score is the sum of the severity of the three symptoms (fatigue, waking unrefreshed, cognitive symptoms) plus the extent (severity) of somatic symptoms in general. The final score is between 0 and 12.

*Somatic symptoms that might be considered include muscle pain, irritable bowel syndrome, fatigue or tiredness, thinking or memory problems, muscle weakness, headache, pain or cramps in the abdomen, numbness or tingling, dizziness, insomnia, depression, constipation, pain in the upper abdomen, nausea, nervousness, chest pain, blurred vision, fever, diarrhea, dry mouth, itching, wheezing, Raynaud phenomenon, hives or welts, ringing in ears, vomiting, heartburn, oral ulcers, loss of or change in taste, seizures, dry eyes, shortness of breath, loss of appetite, rash, sun sensitivity, hearing difficulties, easy bruising, hair loss, frequent urination, painful urination, and bladder spasms.

Adapted from Wolfe F et al: The American College of Rheumatology preliminary diagnostic criteria for fibromyalgia and measurement of symptom severity, *Arthritis Care Res* 62:600-610, 2010.

- Nonpharmacologic (Table E2): There is evidence to support exercise (aerobic, strengthening, and stretching exercises), cognitive behavioral therapy, physical therapy, and patient education (e.g., regarding the disease, importance of good sleep and hygiene). However there is little high-quality, adequately powered evidence to support the various therapy classes.[11]
- FM can be due to abnormalities in many different neurotransmitter systems; thus, approaches and treatment responses may vary.
- Pharmacologic therapies for fibromyalgia are summarized in Table 3.

- Best evidence for tricyclics (low-dose amitriptyline, cyclobenzaprine), serotonin-norepinephrine reuptake inhibitors (milnacipran, duloxetine), gabapentinoids (gabapentin, pregabalin).
- Second-tier drug classes include selective serotonin reuptake inhibitors (SSRIs).
- "Start low, go slow" approach is best to avoid side effects, which are common.
- Medication adherence is generally poor.
- A metanalysis of commonly used medications revealed that amitriptyline had the greatest improvement in insomnia and overall quality of life, duloxetine (120 mg/day) provided the greatest reduction in pain and depression and treatment was modestly effective for fatigue and pain.[12]
- There is no evidence that acetaminophen, NSAIDs, or corticosteroids are effective in FM.
- The only analgesic that has demonstrated some efficacy in FM has been tramadol; can consider for treatment-resistant cases.
- Avoid narcotic use. Opioid use and abuse may aggravate chronic widespread pain.
- The pain and symptoms of FM can wax and wane, vary in physical location and in intensity day-to-day; many patients continue to have chronic pain and fatigue regardless of therapy.
- Disability rates vary from 10% to 30%.

REFERRAL

Referral to rheumatology, neurology, mental health professionals, physical medicine and rehabilitation, including physical therapy (PT). Multidisciplinary team approach is generally most helpful.

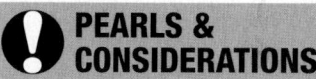 **PEARLS & CONSIDERATIONS**

- Fibromyalgia is a neurosensory disorder whereby affected individuals have abnormal central nociceptive processing.
- Diagnosis is based on the presence of chronic musculoskeletal pain in the absence of physical or laboratory evidence of inflammation and any other condition that would explain the symptoms.
- Treatment options are varied, but a combination of drug and nondrug options is likely to provide optimal results.
- Myofascial pain syndrome may represent a localized form of FM. It is associated with trigger points (rather than tender points as seen in FM). Some patients with myofascial pain syndrome may progress to FM.

COMMENTS

FM occurs frequently in patients with some rheumatic diseases, such as rheumatoid arthritis, ankylosing spondylitis, and systemic lupus erythematosus, in which prevalence of FM may reach 20%.[13]

REFERENCES

Available at eBooks.Health.Elsevier.com.

RELATED CONTENT

Fibromyalgia (Patient Information)

AUTHOR: **LUCA KATZ, BA**

TABLE 3 Pharmacologic Therapies for Fibromyalgia

Treatment	Cost	Specifics	Evidence level	Side Effects	Suggestions
Pharmacologic therapies		Pharmacologic therapy is best chosen based on the predominant symptoms and initiated in low dose with slow dose escalation.	5, Consensus		• Some practitioners find that getting patients on a drug regimen that helps improve symptoms before initiating nonpharmacologic therapies can help improve compliance.
Tricyclic compounds		• Amitriptyline 10-70 mg qhs • Cyclobenzaprine 5-20 mg qhs	1, A	Dry mouth, weight gain, constipation, "groggy" or drugged feeling	• When effective, can improve a wide range of symptoms, including pain, sleep, bowel, and bladder symptoms. • Taking these drugs several hours before bedtime improves side effect profile.
Serotonin norepinephrine reuptake inhibitors	Duloxetine is generic, milnacipran not	• Duloxetine, 30-120 mg/day • Milnacipran, 100-200 mg/day	1, A	Nausea, palpitations, headache, fatigue, tachycardia, hypertension	• Warning patients about transient nausea, taking with food, and slowly increasing dose can increase tolerability. • Milnacipran might be slightly more noradrenergic than duloxetine and thus potentially more helpful for fatigue and memory problems, but it is also more likely to cause HTN.
Gabapentinoids	Gabapentin is generic, pregabalin not	Gabapentin 800-2400 mg/day in divided doses Pregabalin up to 600 mg/day in divided doses	1, A	Sedation, weight gain, dizziness	Giving most or all of the dose at bedtime can increase tolerability.
γ-Hydroxybutyrate	Available for treating narcolepsy, cataplexy	GHB 4.5-6.0 g per night in divided doses	1, A	Sedation, respiratory depression, and death	Shown to be efficacious but not approved by U.S. FDA because of safety concerns.
Low-dose naltrexone	Low	4.5 mg/day	Two small single center RCTs		
Cannabinoids	NA	Nabilone 0.5 mg PO qhs-1.0 mg bid	1, A	Sedation, dizziness, dry mouth	No synthetic cannabinoid is approved in the U.S. for treatment of pain.
Selective serotonin reuptake inhibitors (SSRIs)	SSRIs that should be used in FM (see Suggestions) are all generic	Fluoxetine, sertraline, paroxetine	1, A	Nausea, sexual dysfunction, weight gain, sleep disturbance	Older, less selective SSRIs may have some efficacy in improving pain, especially at higher doses that have more prominent noradrenergic effects. Newer SSRIs (citalopram, escitalopram, desvenlafaxine) are less effective or ineffective as analgesics.
NSAIDs		No evidence of efficacy Can be helpful to treat comorbid "peripheral pain generators"	5, D	GI, renal, and cardiac side effects	Use the lowest dose for the shortest period of time to reduce side effects.
Opioids		Tramadol with or without acetaminophen, 50-100 mg every 6 h No evidence of efficacy for stronger opioids	5, D	Sedation, addiction, tolerance, opioid-induced hyperalgesia	There is increasing evidence that opioids are less effective for treating chronic pain than previously thought, and their risk-benefit profile is worse than other classes of analgesics.

bid, Twice a day; *FDA*, U.S. Food and Drug Administration; *FM*, fibromyalgia; *GHB*, gammahydroxybutyrate; *GI*, gastrointestinal; *HTN*, hypertension; *NSAIDs*, nonsteroidal antiinflammatory drugs; *PO*, oral; *qhs*, at bedtime; *RCT*, randomized controlled trial.
From Hochberg MC et al: *Rheumatology*, ed 7, Philadelphia, 2019, Elsevier.

F

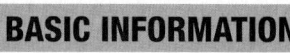 **BASIC INFORMATION**

DEFINITION

In 2017, the International League Against Epilepsy (ILAE) revised its classification of seizures. This article uses this updated nomenclature for focal seizures. Focal seizures (previously known as partial seizures) are caused by electrical discharges that originate in one hemisphere of the brain and cause symptoms based on the neuronal area they affect. There are two subtypes of focal seizure, categorized based on whether the seizures affect consciousness.

- Focal aware seizure (previously simple partial seizure): Does not impair awareness. Patients will be able to accurately state who they are and what is going on in their surroundings during a seizure but may not be aware they are having a seizure.
- Focal impaired awareness seizure (previously complex partial seizure): A seizure that impairs a patient's awareness for any part of the seizure.

These two subtypes of focal seizure can be further classified by whether they initially cause motor or nonmotor symptoms, as well as if they evolve into bilateral tonic-clonic seizures (previously known as secondary generalized tonic-clonic seizures).

SYNONYMS

Simple partial seizures
Seizures, partial
Partial seizures

ICD-10CM CODES
G40.0 Localization-related (focal) (partial) idiopathic epilepsy and epileptic syndromes with seizures of localized onset
G40.109 Localization-related (focal) (partial) symptomatic epilepsy and epileptic syndromes with simple partial seizures, not intractable, without status epilepticus

EPIDEMIOLOGY & DEMOGRAPHICS

INCIDENCE: 30 to 50 cases per 100,000 persons per year
PREVALENCE: Five to eight cases per 1000 persons
PREDOMINANT SEX & AGE: No gender preference

PHYSICAL FINDINGS & CLINICAL PRESENTATION

- Patients with focal seizures usually have normal physical and neurologic examinations when in a nonseizure state; however, if their seizures are secondary to a structural abnormality, such as a stroke or brain tumor, they will have a neurologic exam consistent with the area of central nervous system (CNS) structural damage.
- During focal aware seizures, patients are conscious. They will be able to correctly state their name and accurately describe their surroundings. Patients with focal impaired

awareness seizures will not be able to correctly state this information.
- Both focal seizure types can be further classified by their initial presenting symptoms.
  1. Focal seizures with initial motor symptoms include clonic (regularly spaced, rhythmic jerking), myoclonic (irregular jerking), hyperkinetic (thrashing or pedaling), tonic (increased tone), and atonic (loss of tone) seizures, as well as automatisms (lip smacking, fumbling of fingers). To avoid confusion, automatisms also can be seen in absence seizures, a type of nonmotor generalized seizure that will not be discussed here.
  2. Focal seizures with initial nonmotor symptoms include autonomic (e.g., changes in heart rate, blood pressure, sweating), sensory (e.g., changes in taste, smell, hearing, tactile sensation), emotional (sudden onset of emotions such as fear, anxiety, pleasure, etc.), or cognitive (e.g., change in language ability, thinking, feelings of déjà vu) changes and behavioral arrest (cessation of movement or talking) seizures.
- All focal seizures have the possibility of evolving into bilateral tonic-clonic seizures. These are distinct from generalized seizures, which are not discussed in this article, but which do not have a focal point of origin.
- Patients with focal seizures can experience postictal weakness/paralysis that usually resolves within 24 h (Todd paralysis). However, persistent focal neurologic deficits may also be indicative of a new structural brain lesion.

ETIOLOGY
- The etiology of focal seizures can be either genetic or due to an acquired neurologic injury.
- Frequent causes of focal seizures are tumors, stroke, CNS infections (neurocysticercosis among others), arteriovenous malformations (AVMs), cavernous malformations, traumatic brain injury, cortical dysplasia, and structural abnormalities.

Dx DIAGNOSIS

DIFFERENTIAL DIAGNOSIS
- Transient ischemic attack
- Movement disorders
- Psychogenic nonepileptic spells
- Migraines
- The differential diagnosis of nonepileptic events is summarized in Table 1. Table E2 summarizes clinical characteristics that help distinguish epileptic from nonepileptic events

WORKUP
Electroencephalogram (EEG). Ambulatory EEG and/or video EEG recommended for patients with diagnostic uncertainty

LABORATORY TESTS
Routine blood workup (comprehensive metabolic panel [CMP], CBC, glucose, electrolytes, thyroid-stimulating hormone) and urine toxicology may be considered in appropriate clinical situations.

IMAGING STUDIES
- In the absence of contraindications, MRI with contrast using a defined epilepsy protocol is preferred over computed tomography (CT) due to its increased sensitivity to both acute and remote causes of seizure.
- However, in the setting of acute trauma, acute focal deficit, or if there is concern for a space-occupying lesion, a noncontrast CT may be obtained first, followed later by an MRI.

Rx TREATMENT

- Almost all antiepileptic drugs are approved for focal seizures, either as monotherapy or as adjunct therapy. Carbamazepine traditionally has been the standard initial drug treatment for focal seizures. However, newer antiepileptic drugs have better side effect profiles.

TABLE 1 Differential Diagnosis of Nonepileptic Events

General Medical Conditions
- Transient ischemic attack (TIA)
- Complicated migraine
- Syncope
- Hypoglycemia
- Parasomnia (e.g., rapid eye movement [REM], behavior disorder, or night terrors)
- Narcolepsy
- Myoclonus (from metabolic disturbance)

Psychiatric Causes
- Conversion disorder
- Somatic symptom disorder
- Dissociative disorder
- Panic disorder (simulating focal seizures)

Volitional Deception
- Factitious disorder (goal is to maintain the sick role)
- Malingering (goal is to obtain secondary gain, e.g., disability income)

From Stern TA et al: *Massachusetts General Hospital handbook of general hospital psychiatry*, ed 7, Philadelphia, 2018, Elsevier.

- Lamotrigine, levetiracetam, and oxcarbazepine are effective and well-tolerated antiepileptic drugs for treating focal seizures.
- Eslicarbazepine is indicated for the treatment of focal-onset seizures as either monotherapy or adjunctive therapy. The recommended initial dose of eslicarbazepine is 400 mg once daily. Increase the dose in weekly increments of 200 mg, based on clinical response and tolerability, to a recommended maintenance dose of 800 to 1600 mg once daily.
- Lacosamide is indicated as either monotherapy or adjunctive therapy in patients with focal-onset seizures. The initial recommended dose is 50 mg twice daily; increase at weekly intervals by 50 mg twice daily, up to a recommended maintenance dose of 150 to 200 mg twice daily.
- Patients who continue to have seizures despite a trial of two antiepileptic drugs at adequate doses should be referred for evaluation for epilepsy surgery. Surgical treatments (e.g., temporal lobectomy in mesial temporal sclerosis) may be indicated in refractory cases of focal seizures.

GENERAL Rx

- Several factors should be considered when deciding to initiate antiseizure drug therapy after a first-time unprovoked seizure. An unprovoked seizure is one that was not caused by a toxic or metabolic disturbance, acute head trauma, or an acute stroke.
- According to evidence-based guidelines and several randomized trials, the greatest risk for seizure recurrence is in the first 2 yr after the first unprovoked seizure. Clinical factors increasing seizure recurrence include epileptiform discharges on EEG, a history of brain injury, a significant abnormality found on brain imaging (e.g., tumor, scarring, old stroke), and an initial nocturnal seizure.
- Immediate Initiation of antiseizure medications after a first-time unprovoked seizure reduces the 2-yr risk of seizure recurrence by approximately 35%. However, it does not significantly impact long-term outcomes, as patients who were started on antiepileptic medication after their first seizure and those started after their second seizure had similar rates of long-term seizure remission.
- A patient with a first unprovoked seizure with risk factors for seizure recurrence may be started on an antiseizure medication.

- In a patient with a first unprovoked seizure with a normal neurologic exam who does not have risk factors for seizure recurrence, drug therapy may be deferred until after a second unprovoked seizure.
- Recurrent seizures and seizures with abnormal studies may require treatment in the form of other medications, consideration of surgery, or with approved medical devices.

DISPOSITION

- Response to treatment often depends on the etiology of the focal seizures.
- 47% of patients become seizure free with monotherapy and 67% with polytherapy.
- Patients who do not respond to two drugs should be referred to an epilepsy center for consideration of surgical treatment.
- Patients should not drive until seizure free in accordance with local laws and regulations.
- Patients should avoid situations that may cause injuries or accidents in the event of a seizure, such as climbing ladders, swimming unsupervised, or taking baths (rather than showers).
- Many antiepileptic drugs also affect vitamin D absorption or metabolism, prompting attention to patients' bone health.
- All patients with epilepsy are at higher risk for depression and should be screened.
- Women of childbearing potential should be counseled about contraception and the importance of planning for pregnancy to optimize both obstetric and fetal outcomes.

REFERRAL

Patients with epilepsy and seizures should be referred for a consultation by a neurologist, preferably one with a special interest in epilepsy.

PEARLS & CONSIDERATIONS

- Focal seizures can be divided into those that impair awareness and those that do not. In both categories, seizures will initially have either motor or nonmotor symptoms. Sometimes, focal seizures can evolve into bilateral tonic-clonic seizures.
- Initial workup should include EEG, MRI with and without contrast (if possible), CMP, and CBC. Other lab tests may be ordered based on clinical suspicion to rule out systemic or provoked causes of seizures.

- Drug therapy after a patient's first unprovoked seizure is recommended for those who have EEG or MRI abnormalities, or a history of brain trauma or surgery.
- Carbamazepine has traditionally been the initial drug treatment for focal seizures. However, lamotrigine, levetiracetam, oxcarbazepine, and many other antiepileptic medications are equally useful for treatment and have fewer side effects. The patient's comorbidities and childbearing potential should be considered when prescribing antiseizure medication.
- Women of childbearing potential should be advised about the potential teratogenicity of antiseizure medications and should be encouraged to use effective birth control. Some antiseizure medications such as carbamazepine reduce the efficacy of oral contraceptive pills, whereas estrogen-containing compounds can reduce the efficacy of lamotrigine. Folic acid supplementation is also reasonable in the event of an unplanned pregnancy and in women planning pregnancy.
- All patients with seizures should be counseled about driving laws in their state of residence.

PREVENTION

- Sleep deprivation and alcohol consumption should be avoided.
- Medication adherence is compulsory to prevent seizure recurrence.

PATIENT & FAMILY EDUCATION

- Patient education and information can be obtained at the Epilepsy Foundation: http://www.epilepsyfoundation.org/.
- Patients should be counseled on general seizure precautions such as driving, swimming, bathing, and heights.
- Women of childbearing potential should be counseled about the importance of effective birth control and the need to plan pregnancies in order to optimize both fetal and maternal health.

RELATED CONTENT

Focal Motor Seizures (Patient Information)

AUTHOR: **JOSEPH S. KASS, MD, JD, FAAN**

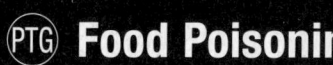

F

Diseases and Disorders

I

 BASIC INFORMATION

DEFINITION

Food poisoning is an illness caused by ingestion of food contaminated by bacteria and/or bacterial toxins. A foodborne disease outbreak is defined as two or more cases of a similar illness resulting from ingestion of a common food.

SYNONYMS

Enterotoxin-poisoning
Epidemic vomiting disease

ICD-10CM CODE
A05.9   Bacterial foodborne intoxication, unspecified

EPIDEMIOLOGY & DEMOGRAPHICS

INCIDENCE (IN U.S.):

- The Centers for Disease Control and Prevention estimates that each year one in six Americans will experience a foodborne illness.
- Approximately 800 foodborne disease outbreaks are reported in the U.S. each year, accounting for approximately 15,000 illnesses, 800 hospitalizations, and 20 deaths. Outbreak-associated foodborne illnesses are only a small subset of the estimated 9.4 million foodborne illnesses that occur annually in the U.S.
- Majority of identifiable causes are bacterial, although more than 250 known diseases can be transmitted through food.

PREDOMINANT AGE: Varies with specific agent.
PEAK INCIDENCE: Varies with specific organism
- Summer: *Staphylococcus aureus, Salmonella, Shigella* spp.
- Summer and fall: *Clostridium botulinum, Vibrio parahaemolyticus.*
- Spring and fall: *Campylobacter jejuni.*
- Winter: *Clostridium perfringens, Yersinia enterocolitica.*

NEONATAL INFECTION: Rare but severe with *Shigella* and *Salmonella* spp.

PHYSICAL FINDINGS & CLINICAL PRESENTATION

- Any combination of GI symptoms and fever. Orthostatic pulse and blood pressure changes should be noted
- Specific organisms suspected on the basis of the incubation period and predominant symptoms (Table 1), although a great deal of overlap exists
  1. Short incubation period (1 to 6 h): Involve the ingestion of preformed toxin; noninvasive.
     a. *S. aureus:* Nausea, profuse vomiting, and abdominal cramps common; diarrhea possible, but fever uncommon; usually resolves within 24 h; foods implicated in outbreaks include meats, mayonnaise, and cream pastries.
     b. *B. cereus:* Two forms, a short incubation (emetic) form (characterized by vomiting and abdominal cramps in virtually all patients, diarrhea in one third of patients, fever uncommon) and a

long incubation (diarrheal) form; illness usually mild, resolves within 12 h; unrefrigerated rice most often implicated as vehicle. Other sources include gravy, meats, stews, vanilla, and sauces.
  2. Moderate incubation period (8 to 16 h): Involves the in vivo production of toxin; noninvasive.
     a. *C. perfringens:* Severe crampy abdominal pain and watery diarrhea common; fever and vomiting unlikely; symptoms usually resolving within 24 h; outbreaks invariably related to cooked meat or poultry that is allowed to cool without refrigeration; most cases in the fall and winter months. *C. perfringens* is the third most common cause of foodborne illness in the United States.
     b. *B. cereus:* Diarrheal (or long incubation) form most commonly beginning with diarrhea, abdominal cramps, and occasionally vomiting; fever uncommon; usually resolves within 24 h; the responsible food is usually fried rice.
  3. Long incubation period (>16 h): Some toxin-mediated, some invasive.
- Toxin-producing organisms include
  1. *C. botulinum:* Should be considered when a diarrheal illness coincides with or precedes paralysis; severity of illness related to the quantity of toxin ingested; characteristic cranial nerve palsies progressing to a descending paralysis; fever usually absent; usually associated with home-canned foods.
  2. Enterotoxigenic *E. coli* (ETEC): Most common cause of travelers' diarrhea; after 1- to 2-day incubation period, abdominal cramps and copious diarrhea occur; vomiting and fever uncommon; usually resolves after 3 to 4 days; vehicle usually unbottled water or contaminated salad or ice
  3. Enterohemorrhagic *E. coli* (EHEC): Can cause severe abdominal cramps and watery diarrhea, which may eventually become bloody; bacteria (strain O157:H7) are noninvasive; no fever; illness may be complicated by hemolytic-uremic syndrome; associated with contaminated beef (especially hamburger), unpasteurized milk or juice. Table 2 summarizes the various strains of diarrheagenic *E. coli*
  4. *V. cholerae:* Varies from a mild, self-limited illness to life-threatening cholera; diarrhea, nausea and vomiting, abdominal cramps, and muscle cramps; no fever; severe cases may progress to shock and death within hours of onset; survivors usually have resolution of symptoms in 1 wk; U.S. cases are either imported or result from ingestion of imported food
- Invasive organisms include
  1. *Salmonella:* Associated most often with nontyphoidal strains; incubation period generally 12 to 48 h; nausea, vomiting, diarrhea, and abdominal cramps typical; fever possible; outbreaks of gastroenteritis related to contaminated poultry, meat, and dairy products

  2. *Shigella:* Asymptomatic infection possible, but some with fever and watery diarrhea that may progress to bloody diarrhea and dysentery; with mild illness, usually self-limited, resolves in a few days; with severe illness, may develop complications; transmission usually from person to person but can occur via contaminated food or water
  3. *C. jejuni:* The most common foodborne bacterial pathogen; incubation period is about 1 day, then a prodrome of fever, headache, and myalgias; intestinal phase marked by diarrhea associated with fever, malaise, and abdominal pain; diarrhea mild to profuse and bloody; usually resolves in about 7 days, but relapse is possible; associated with undercooked meats and poultry, unpasteurized dairy products, and drinking from freshwater streams
  4. *Y. enterocolitica* and *Y. pseudotuberculosis:* Infrequent causes of enteritis in the United States; children affected more often than adults; fever, diarrhea, and abdominal pain lasting 1 to 3 wk; some with mesenteric adenitis that mimics acute appendicitis; contaminated food or water is usually responsible
  5. *V. parahaemolyticus:* In the United States, most outbreaks in coastal states or on cruise ships during the summer months; incubation period usually >1 day, followed by explosive watery diarrhea in the majority of cases; nausea, vomiting, abdominal cramps, and headache also common; fever less common; usually resolves by 1 wk; related to ingestion of seafood
  6. Enteroinvasive *E. coli* (EIEC): A rare cause of disease in the United States; high incidence of fever and bloody diarrhea; may resemble bacillary dysentery
  7. *V. vulnificus:* May cause serious, often fatal illness in persons with chronic liver disease; GI symptoms usually absent, but fever, chills, hypotension, and hemorrhagic skin lesions possible; patients with liver disease or at increased risk of developing liver disease should avoid eating raw oysters

ETIOLOGY

- Table 3 describes pathogenic mechanisms in bacterial foodborne disease.
- Classically categorized as either inflammatory (invasive) or noninflammatory.
  1. Noninflammatory: *B. cereus, S. aureus, C. botulinum, C. perfringens, V. cholerae,* enterotoxigenic *E. coli* (ETEC), and enterohemorrhagic *E. coli* (EHEC); toxin-producing organisms that are noninvasive; fecal leukocytes are not seen
  2. Inflammatory: *Campylobacter,* enteroinvasive *E. coli* (EIEC), *Salmonella, Shigella, V. parahaemolyticus,* and *Yersinia;* cause disease by invasion of intestinal tissue; fecal leukocytes are seen

TABLE 1 Foodborne Disease Agents and Clinical Presentation

Usual Incubation Periods	Causative Agent	CLINICAL ILLNESS			Epidemiologic and Laboratory Diagnosis
		Fever	Diarrhea	Vomiting	
5 min-6 h (usually <3 h)	Chemical or toxin	Rare	Occasional	Common	Demonstration of toxin or chemical from food or epidemiologic incrimination of food
1-6 h (usually <1 h)	*Staphylococcus aureus* enterotoxin	Rare	Occasional	Profuse	Isolation of organisms in food (>10⁵/g)/vomitus/stool; detection of entero-toxin in food
	Bacillus cereus emetic toxin	Rare	Occasional	Profuse	Isolation of organisms in food (>10⁵/g)/vomitus/stool
6-24 h	*Clostridium perfringens* enterotoxin	Rare	Typical	Occasional	Isolation of organisms or toxin from food (10⁵/g) or stools of ill persons, epidemiologic incrimination of food; detection of enterotoxin in food
	B. cereus enterotoxin	Rare	Typical	Occasional	
12-72 h	*Clostridium botulinum*	Clinical syndrome compatible with botulism	Constipation more common		Isolation of organism or toxin from food (10⁵/g) or stools; demonstration of toxin in serum or food
16-96 h	*Shigella*	Common	Typical, often bloody	Occasional	Isolation of organism from clinical specimens from two or more ill persons; isolation of organism from epidemiologically implicated food
	Nontyphoidal *Salmonella*	Common	Typical	Occasional	
	Enteroinvasive *E. coli* (EIEC)	Common	Typical, may be bloody	Occasional	
	Enteropathogenic *E. coli* (EPEC)	Occasional	Typical	Occasional	
	Enterotoxigenic *E. coli* (ETEC)	Rare	Typical	Rare	
	Vibrio parahaemolyticus; V. cholerae enterotoxin	Occasional	Typical	Occasional	
1-3 days	Caliciviruses (noroviruses) Rotavirus	Occasional	Typical	Common	Antigen detection (enzyme immunoassay) in stool; immune electron microscopy of stool; detection of viral RNA in stool or vomitus by PCR
1-10 days	*Yersinia*	Uncommon	Typical, severe abdominal pain	Uncommon	Isolation of organisms from food or clinical specimens of ill persons
2-10 days	*Campylobacter jejuni*	Common	Typical, often bloody	Uncommon	Isolation of organisms from food or clinical specimens of ill persons
1-11 days	*Cryptosporidium*	Occasional	Common	Occasional	Demonstration of oocysts in stool or in small bowel biopsy of ill persons; demonstration of organism in epidemiologically implicated food
	Cyclospora	Occasional	Common	Occasional	Demonstration of parasite in stool or in small bowel biopsy of ill persons; demonstration of organism in epidemiologically implicated food
	Giardia intestinalis	Occasional	Common	Occasional	Demonstration of parasite in stool or in small bowel biopsy of ill persons; demonstration of organism in epidemiologically implicated food
2 days-weeks	*Bacillus anthracis*	Common	Typical	Frequent	Isolation of organism from blood or contaminated meat
1-7 days	*E. coli* O157:H7 and other Shiga toxin–producing *E. coli*	Uncommon	Typical	Frequent	Isolation of organism from food or stool or identification of toxin in stools of ill persons
3-60 days, usually 7-14	*Salmonella typhi*	Common	Diarrhea or constipation	Uncommon	Isolation of organisms from food or clinical specimens of ill persons
7-21 days	*Brucella* spp.	Common	Common	Rare	Isolation of organisms from blood or bone marrow culture of ill persons; fourfold increase in standard agglutination titer overall several weeks or single titer 1:160 in person with compatible clinical syndrome
1-4 wk	*Giardia lamblia*	Rare	Common	Rare	Stool for ova and parasite examination enzyme immunoassay
2 days-8 wk	*Trichinella spiralis*	Common	Common	Common	Serology, muscle biopsy

PCR, Polymerase chain reaction; *RNA,* ribonucleic acid.
From Cherry JD et al: *Feigin and Cherry's pediatric infectious diseases,* ed 8, Philadelphia, 2019, Elsevier.

TABLE 2 Diarrheagenic *Escherichia coli*

Strains	Pathogenic Mechanisms	Persons Affected	Clinical Features
DAEC	Diffuse adherence to Hep-2 cells	Children in developing countries	Watery diarrhea (acute) and persistent diarrhea
EAEC	Aggregative adherence to Hep-2 cells	Children in developing countries	Watery diarrhea (acute) and persistent diarrhea
STEC O157:H7 Non-O157:H7 O104:H4*	Shiga toxins 1 and 2	Children and adults Persons who ingest contaminated food, especially hamburger (outbreaks)	Watery diarrhea Bloody diarrhea (classic)
EIEC	Epithelial cell invasion	Children and adults	Watery diarrhea Dysentery
EPEC Typical Atypical	Attaching and effacing Bundle-forming pilus, attachment and effacement lesions or atypical adherence pattern	Children	Watery diarrhea (acute) Persistent diarrhea
ETEC	Heat-labile and/or heat-stable toxin Adherence	Children in developing countries; travelers	Watery diarrhea

DAEC, Diffusely adhering *Escherichia coli*; *EAEC*, enteroaggregative *E. coli*; *EIEC*, enteroinvasive *E. coli*; *EPEC*, enteropathogenic *E. coli*; *ETEC*, enterotoxigenic *E. coli*; *STEC*, Shiga toxin–producing *E. coli*.
From Feldman M et al: *Sleisenger and Fordtran's gastrointestinal and liver disease*, ed 11, Philadelphia, 2021, Elsevier.

TABLE 3 Pathogenic Mechanisms in Bacterial Foodborne Disease

Preformed Toxin	Toxin Production in Vivo	Tissue Invasion	Toxin Production and/or Tissue Invasion
Staphylococcus aureus *Bacillus cereus* (short incubation) *Clostridium botulinum*	*Clostridium perfringens* *B. cereus* (long incubation) *C. botulinum* (infant botulism) Enterotoxigenic *Escherichia coli* *Vibrio cholerae* O1 or O139 *V. cholerae* non-O1 Shiga toxin–producing *E. coli*	*Campylobacter jejuni* *Salmonella* *Shigella* Invasive *E. coli*	*Vibrio parahaemolyticus* *Yersinia enterocolitica*

From Mandell GL et al: *Principles and practice of infectious diseases*, ed 6, Philadelphia, 2005, Churchill Livingstone.

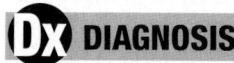 **DIAGNOSIS**

DIFFERENTIAL DIAGNOSIS

Gastroenteritis caused by viruses (Norwalk, Noro, or rotavirus), parasites *(Amoeba histolytica, Giardia lamblia),* or toxins (ciguatoxins, mushrooms, heavy metals)

LABORATORY TESTS

- Watchful waiting is often the most appropriate option, and ancillary testing is usually not necessary.
- In severe or persistent cases, stool test for fecal leukocytes may help narrow the differential diagnosis.
  1. Send stool for culture and for ova and parasites.
  2. Send stool for *C. difficile* toxin in patients with current or recent antibiotic use.
  3. Note: Some pathogens are not identified on routine stool culture; laboratory should be advised if *Yersinia, C. botulinum, Vibrio,* or enterohemorrhagic *E. coli* (O157:H7) are suspected.
  4. Finding *B. cereus, C. perfringens,* or *E. coli* in stool is of little value, because these may be part of the normal bowel flora.
  5. Stool cultures are positive in less than 40% of cases.
  6. Newer techniques such as polymerase chain reaction (PCR) testing provide a more rapid and reliable determination of specific pathogens.

- If botulism suspected, send food, serum, and stool for toxin assay.
- Blood cultures should be considered for all febrile patients.
- Consider toxic megacolon (identified on plain abdominal sonography).
- Consider sigmoidoscopy to obtain tissue and histology in hospitalized patients with bloody diarrhea.
- Consider lactoferrin measurement if an inflammatory etiology is suspected.

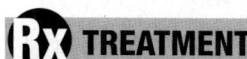 **TREATMENT**

NONPHARMACOLOGIC THERAPY

Adequate rehydration is the mainstay of therapy.

ACUTE GENERAL Rx

- Most cases of acute infectious diarrhea are viral, and antibiotics are not indicated.
- Gastroenteritis caused by the following bacterial organisms requires no antimicrobial treatment: *B. cereus, S. aureus, C. perfringens, V. parahaemolyticus, Yersinia,* and enterohemorrhagic and enteroinvasive *E. coli.*
- The usual cause of travelers' diarrhea is enterotoxigenic *E. coli.* Although usually a self-limited illness, antibiotics can shorten the course in patients with fever or dysentery.
  1. Azithromycin 1000 mg in a single oral dose or
  2. SMX/TMP one DS tab bid for 3 days or
  3. Ciprofloxacin 500 mg PO bid for 3 days

- The mainstay of therapy for cholera is fluid replacement. Antibiotics should be given to decrease shedding and duration of illness.
  1. Doxycycline 300 mg in a single dose or 100 mg PO bid for 3 days
  2. SMX/TMP 1 DS tab bid for 3 days
- Treatment is not indicated for *Salmonella* gastroenteritis. Patients who are at high risk of developing bacteremia may be treated for 48 to 72 h (see "Salmonellosis").
- Although shigellosis tends to be a self-limited illness, antibiotics shorten the course of illness and may limit transmission of the illness (see "Shigellosis").
- Those with moderate or severe *Campylobacter* diarrhea may benefit from treatment.
  1. Azithromycin 500 mg qd for 3 days or
  2. Erythromycin 500 mg PO qid for 5 days or
  3. Ciprofloxacin 500 mg PO bid for 5 days
- *V. vulnificus* sepsis should be treated with
  1. Doxycycline 100 mg intravenous (IV) bid for 2 wk
  2. Ceftazidime 2 g IV q8h for 2 wk
- For suspected botulism, antitoxin should be administered early (see "Botulism").
- Table 4 summarizes antibiotic therapy for nonsevere infections with common bacterial enteropathogens in immunocompetent adults.

CHRONIC Rx

Patients with *Salmonella* infections may become carriers and may require treatment (see "Salmonellosis").

TABLE 4 Antibiotic Therapy for Nonsevere Infections with Common Bacterial Enteropathogens in Immunocompetent Adults

Organism	Recommended Antibiotic(s)	Alternative Antibiotic(s)
Shigella Species		
Shigella infection (non-dysenteriae; for Shigella dysenteriae type 1, see text)	Ciprofloxacin 500 mg twice daily (or levofloxacin 500 mg daily) × 3 days	Azithromycin 500 mg-1 g daily 3-5 days TMP/SMX 160 mg/800 mg twice daily, if sensitive, × 3 days
Salmonella Species		
Enterocolitis, uncomplicated	Not usually recommended (see text)	Can consider in areas of high fluoroquinolone quinolone resistance; azithromycin 1 g daily × 5 days
Typhoid and enteric fevers*	Ciprofloxacin 500 mg twice daily (or ofloxacin 400 mg twice daily) × 7-14 days Ceftriaxone 2-3 g IV daily × 7-14 days	
Campylobacter Species		
Campylobacter jejuni	Not usually required Ciprofloxacin 500 mg twice daily × 3 days	Azithromycin 500 mg-1 g × 3-5 days
Yersinia enterocolitica		
Enterocolitis, uncomplicated	Not usually required	An aminoglycoside (parenteral) tetracycline 500 mg 4 times daily × 5 days TMP/SMX 160 mg/800 mg twice daily × 5 days Ciprofloxacin 500 mg twice daily × 5 days Doxycycline 100 mg twice daily × 5 days
Escherichia coli†		
Enterotoxigenic	Endemic disease; usually self-limited, supportive care (see text). Travelers' diarrhea: Ciprofloxacin 500 mg twice daily × 3 days Rifaximin 200 mg 3 times daily × 3 days	Azithromycin 500 mg-1 g daily × 3-5 days TMP/SMX 160 mg/800 mg twice daily, if sensitive, × 3 days
Shiga toxin–producing	Unclear if antibiotics are effective; may be harmful	
Vibrio Species		
Vibrio cholerae	Doxycycline 300 mg × 1 dose	Ciprofloxacin 1 g × 1 dose Azithromycin 1 g × 1 dose Tetracycline 500 mg every 6 h × 3 days
Vibrio parahaemolyticus	Usually not required; no controlled trials	As for V. cholerae

IV, Intravenous; *TMP/SMX,* trimethoprim/sulfamethoxazole.

Note: All antibiotics are administered orally unless otherwise indicated. Recommendations are given for treatment of mild/moderate infections only. Treatments for complicated infections or severely ill, bacteremic, or immunocompromised patients are not listed above and may differ from treatments for mild disease.

*For severe typhoid fever, consider the addition of glucocorticoids (dexamethasone 3 mg/kg × 1, then 1 mg/kg every 6 h × 48 h) to parenteral antimicrobial therapy. Antimicrobial sensitivity testing is required. Fluoroquinolones (e.g., ciprofloxacin) should not be used as empiric therapy in Asia or other areas with high fluoroquinolone resistance.

†Enteropathogenic, enteroaggregative, and diffusely enteroadherent *E. coli* are omitted from this table because these types are defined in research laboratories and are not diagnosed in routine clinical practice. Enteroinvasive *E. coli* presenting as inflammatory diarrhea should be treated empirically as for *Shigella* spp.

From Feldman M et al: *Sleisenger and Fordtran's gastrointestinal and liver disease,* ed 11, Philadelphia, 2021, Elsevier.

DISPOSITION
- Most infections are self-limited and do not require therapy.
- In immunocompromised host or patient with underlying disease, serious complications are possible.
- Postinfectious syndromes are important with some infections.
  1. Reiter syndrome: *Salmonella, Shigella, Campylobacter, Yersinia* spp.; more common in genetically susceptible host (HLA-B27+)
  2. Guillain-Barré syndrome: *Campylobacter* spp.

REFERRAL
If more than a mild illness

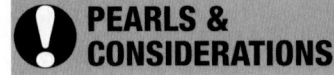 **PEARLS & CONSIDERATIONS**

COMMENTS
- Grossly underreported and undiagnosed
- All cases to be reported to the local health department
- Table E5 summarizes control and prevention measures of foodborne diseases

RELATED CONTENT
Bacterial Food Poisoning (Patient Information)
Salmonellosis (Related Key Topic)
Botulism (Related Key Topic)
Shigellosis (Related Key Topic)

AUTHOR: **GLENN G. FORT, MD, MPH**

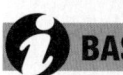
BASIC INFORMATION

DEFINITION

Frontotemporal dementia (FTD), also known as Frontotemporal Lobar Degeneration (FTLD), is an umbrella term that encompasses three distinct syndromes: Behavioral variant FTD (bvFTD), semantic dementia (SD), and progressive non-fluent aphasia (PNFA). All three syndromes are marked by frontal and/or temporal lobe atrophy; however, they manifest with different clinical presentations. The most common subtype is bvFTD, which is marked by changes in behavior and personality with disinhibition, lack of empathy, and the breaking of social norms. SD is characterized by a loss of word comprehension and meaning, and PNFA presents with agrammatic, nonfluent speech.

SYNONYMS

FTD
FTLD
Frontotemporal lobar degeneration (FTLD) is the term used for the neuropathologic findings seen in the different FTD syndromes.
Pick disease: This term was historically used to refer to FTD. However, it is now strictly a neuropathologic diagnosis for patients found to have Pick bodies at autopsy, as very few diagnoses of FTD are associated with these neuropathologic findings.

ICD-10CM CODES
G31.0	Frontotemporal dementia
G31.01	Pick disease
G31.09	Other frontotemporal dementia

EPIDEMIOLOGY & DEMOGRAPHICS

The current data on epidemiology of FTD are variable due to misdiagnosis and underreporting.

The following data are estimations obtained through systematic reviews.
INCIDENCE: The estimated annual incidence is 2.7 to 4.1 per 100,000 persons.
PREVALENCE: The estimated point prevalence is 15 to 22 per 100,000 persons.
PREDOMINANT SEX & AGE: There is a nearly equal distribution by sex, and the average age of presentation is 58 yr.
GENETICS: Approximately 40% of FTD cases have a positive family history, and several genes (Table 1) have been associated with the development of familial FTD. The most common are mutations in *C9ORF72, MAPT,* and *GRN* (Table 2).

PHYSICAL FINDINGS & CLINICAL PRESENTATION

- The early stage of bvFTD is characterized by changes in behavior and personality. Patients display a lack of insight into these changes, and family members may initially think they are either suffering a midlife crisis or experiencing a new-onset psychiatric disorder. Therefore, careful history-taking is required.
- Behavioral changes include disinhibition, impulsivity, distractibility, violation of social norms (such as offensive, insensitive, or inappropriate sexual remarks; inappropriate behaviors; inappropriately explicit or personal conversations; or encroachment on the personal space of others), as well as increased irritability and impulsive criminal behavior (such as shoplifting or violating traffic laws).
- Patients also display decreased ability to empathize with others, insensitivity to the needs and emotions of their loved ones, and detachment in their personal relationships.
- Apathy and inertia are also common symptoms, with possible development of immobility as the disorder progresses.
- Other associated symptoms that may develop are changes in language and speech (verbal aspontaneity, stereotyped phrases,

mutism in late stages), repetitive motor movements, or hyperphagia, especially for sweet foods.
- Physical exam findings for bv FTD can include abnormal cognition (e.g., clock drawing test [Fig. 1]), upper and/or lower motor neuron signs, dysarthria, dysphagia, and pseudobulbar affect. Some patients meet criteria for both FTD and amyotrophic lateral sclerosis. This overlap is typically related to a C9ORF72 mutation.
- Although behavioral changes can also occur in the other FTD syndromes of SD and PNFA, these two primarily have language deficits that precede the behavioral changes.
  1. SD is characterized by a gradual loss of the knowledge of words, objects, and concepts, with preservation of speech fluency and syntax.
  2. PNFA is characterized by effortful, nonfluent speech, word-finding difficulties, and agrammatism, with preservation of single-word comprehension.

Dx DIAGNOSIS

Diagnosis of bvFTD is primarily clinical, with neuroimaging, genetics, and pathology required for further confirmation. In 2011, the International Behavioral Variant FTD Consortium (FTDC) developed revised criteria for the diagnosis of bvFTD (Table 3).
- In summary, six core symptoms of bvFTD were identified. The presence of any three is sufficient to diagnose *possible* bvFTD.
- Diagnosis of *probable* bvFTD requires meeting the following three conditions: The patient (1) meets diagnostic criteria for possible bvFTD, (2) experiences a significant functional decline, and (3) has imaging showing frontal and/or anterior temporal atrophy or hypoperfusion.
- Diagnosis of *definitive* bvFTD can be made only in a patient with possible or probable

TABLE 1 Clinical, Genetic, and Pathologic Correlations in Frontotemporal Lobar Degeneration

Clinical Presentation	% of FTLD	Associated Genes	COMORBIDITIES					NEUROPATHOLOGIC SUBTYPES				
			Parkinsonism	MND	IBM PDB		FTLD-tau	FTLD-TDP	FTLD-FUS	FTLD-UPS	FTLD-ni
bvFTD	57%		+	+	+/−		++	++	+	+/−	+/−
		C9orf72	+ +	+	+ +			Type B > A		+/−	
		GRN	+	+				Type A			
		MAPT	+	+			+				
		VCP	+/−		+/−	+		Type D			
		CHMP2B	+/−	+/−	+/−					+	
nfvPPA	24%		+		+/−		++	+			
		C9orf72	+								
		GRN	++	+				Type A			
		MAPT	+	+			+				
svPPA	19%		+/−		+/−		+/−	++ (Type C)			
		Rarely genetic									

Number of plus signs (+) signifies relative frequency of the observation; +/− indicates rare observation. *bv,* Behavioral variant; *FTD,* frontotemporal dementia; *FTLD,* frontotemporal lobar degeneration; *FUS,* fused in sarcoma; *IBM,* inclusion body myopathy; *MND,* motor neuron disease; *nfv,* agrammatic or nonfluent variant; *ni,* no inclusions; *PDB,* Paget disease of the bone; *PPA,* primary progressive aphasia; *sv,* semantic variant; *TDP,* TAR DNA-binding protein; *UPS,* ubiquitin-proteasome system.
From Fillit HM: *Brocklehurst's textbook of geriatric medicine and gerontology,* ed 8, Philadelphia, 2017, Elsevier.

TABLE 2 Gene Mutations Associated with Frontotemporal Dementia

Gene	Chromosome	Protein	Protein Function	Mode of Inheritance	Mutation Frequency in Familial FTD	Mutation Frequency in Sporadic FTD	Age of Onset (Mean, Range)
C9ORF72	9p21.2	Unknown	Unknown	AD	21%	6%	50s (mid 20-80s)
MAPT	17q21.31	Microtubule-associated tau protein	Microtubule stabilization and assembly	AD	6.3%	1.5%	Mid-50s (20-80s)
GRN	17q21.31	Progranulin	Activates signaling cascades for development, inflammation, and wound repair	AD	5%-15%	5%	60s (mid 30-80s)

AD, Autosomal dominant; *FTD,* frontotemporal dementia.
From Deleon J, Miller BL: Frontotemporal dementia. In Daniel CK et al (eds): *Handbook of clinical neurology,* ed 148, Philadelphia, 2018, Elsevier, pp. 409-430.

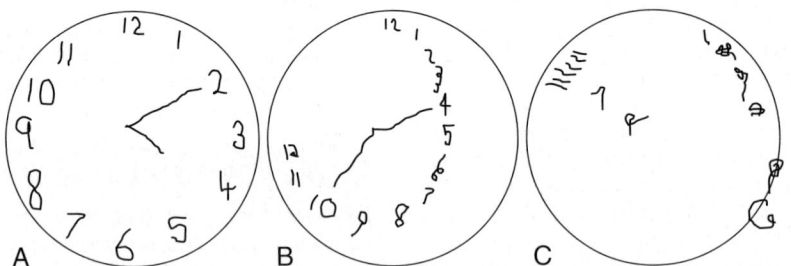

FIG. 1 The clock drawing test. The patient is provided with a circular outline and asked to draw the numbers as they appear on the face of a clock. Once the numbering is complete, the patient is asked to set the hands to a particular time (often "ten past" the hour to test if the patient can suppress the impulse to include the number *10*). **A,** This drawing demonstrates good planning and use of space. **B,** This drawing features some impulsiveness because the numbers are drawn out without regard for actual location, and the time "ten past four" is represented by hands pointing to the digits *10* and *4*. Note the perseveration indicated by the extra loops on the digits *3* and *6*. Impulsiveness and perseveration indicate frontal lobe dysfunction. **C,** This drawing demonstrates gross disorganization, although the patient took several minutes to draw the clock and believed it to be a good representation. (From Stern TA: *Massachusetts General Hospital handbook of general hospital psychiatry,* ed 7, 2018, Philadelphia, Elsevier.)

bvFTD, plus either (1) pathologic evidence of FTLD on biopsy or postmortem exam or (2) presence of a known causal genetic mutation.

DIFFERENTIAL DIAGNOSIS

- Other neurodegenerative disorders, including Alzheimer disease (AD), Parkinson disease, dementia with Lewy bodies, corticobasal syndrome, progressive supranuclear palsy, and chronic traumatic encephalopathy
- Psychiatric disorders (bipolar disorder, schizophrenia, obsessive-compulsive disorder, depression, personality disorders)
- Spontaneous low intracranial pressure with sagging of the front lobes
- Chronic subdural hematomas, especially frontal
- Central nervous system (CNS) tumors in the prefrontal cortex or compressing the prefrontal cortex
- Metabolic disturbances or nutritional deficiencies (thyroid disease, B₁₂ deficiency)
- Substance abuse/toxicities (ethanol, drugs of abuse, heavy metal poisoning)
- Infections (chronic meningitis, HIV-associated dementia, neurosyphilis)
- Cerebrovascular disease (stroke, vascular dementia, lacunar infarctions)
- Autoimmune encephalitis, sarcoidosis

WORKUP

- Careful history-taking with specific attention paid to initial symptoms, time course, progression of symptoms, family history, psychiatric history, and other medical history
- Comprehensive neurologic physical exam to help rule out other CNS etiologies
- Use of the International Behavioral Variant FTD Criteria for diagnosis (Table 3)
- Genetic testing for causal mutations of FTD *(C9ORF72, MAPT,* and *GRN)*
- Medication review (especially drugs that may alter mental status, such as anticholinergics, opiates, benzodiazepines, barbiturates, and neuroleptics)
- Neuropsychologic tests of executive function, memory, and social cognition to evaluate for other neurodegenerative disorders
- Psychiatric evaluation to rule out psychiatric disorders

LABORATORY TESTS

- CBC, serum electrolytes, glucose, blood urea nitrogen (BUN)/creatinine, liver function tests
- Cerebrospinal fluid (CSF) analysis for infection and measurement of CSF tau and amyloid

(which can help differentiate between FTD and AD—not typically measured in clinical practice)
- Vitamin B₁₂, thyroid function tests, HIV, and syphilis screening
- Urine toxicity screen
- In vivo histopathology:
  1. Almost all cases of FTLD have one of the following protein inclusions found on pathologic examination: TAR DNA-binding protein with molecular weight 43 kDa (TDP-43), microtubule-associated protein tau (MAPT), or fused-in-sarcoma protein (FUS).

IMAGING STUDIES

- In general, structural MRI and computed tomography (CT) will show gray matter atrophy in the frontal and/or temporal lobes, anterior cingulate cortex, and insula with variation in distribution between the different FTD subtypes.
  1. Patients with bvFTD specifically will usually show right greater than left-sided atrophy in the orbitofrontal, anterior cingulate, anterior insular, and anterior temporal cortices.
  2. SD is associated with atrophy in the temporal poles (left greater than right), and PNFA with atrophy in the left perisylvian region.
- A normal MRI scan does not exclude FTD, because changes may not be seen in early stages of the disorder. In these cases, SPECT or FDG-PET can be used to visualize areas of hypoperfusion/hypometabolism.

℞ TREATMENT

- No disease-modifying drugs currently exist for the treatment of FTD. With advances in the understanding of FTD pathophysiology and genetics, however, new therapies such as antisense oligonucleotides and tau-specific antibodies are being investigated for their efficacy in treating or altering the progression of the syndrome and may see eventual clinical application.
- Current management of FTD is aimed at management of behavioral symptoms through both pharmacologic and nonpharmacologic means.

TABLE 3   International Consensus Criteria for Behavioral Variant FTD

Must be present for any FTD clinical syndrome:
- Shows progressive deterioration of behavior and/or cognition by observation or history

Possible bvFTD
- Three of the features (A-F) must be present; symptoms should occur repeatedly, not just as a single instance:
  A. Early (3 yr) behavioral disinhibition
  B. Early (3 yr) apathy or inertia
  C. Early (3 yr) loss of sympathy or empathy
  D. Early (3 yr) perseverative, stereotyped, or compulsive/ritualistic behavior
  E. Hyperorality and dietary changes
  F. Neuropsychologic profile: Executive function deficits with relative sparing of memory and visuospatial functions

Probable bvFTD
- All the following criteria must be present to meet diagnosis:
  A. Meets criteria for possible bvFTD
  B. Significant functional decline
  C. Imaging results consistent with bvFTD (frontal and/or anterior temporal atrophy on CT or MRI or frontal hypoperfusion or hypometabolism on SPECT or PET)

Definite bvFTD
- Criteria A and either B or C must be present to meet diagnosis:
  A. Meets criteria for possible or probable bvFTD
  B. Histopathologic evidence of FTLD on biopsy at post mortem
  C. Presence of a known pathogenic mutation

Exclusion criteria for bvFTD
- Criteria A and B must both be answered negatively; criterion C can be positive for possible bvFTD but must be negative for probable bvFTD:
  A. Pattern of deficits is better accounted for by other nondegenerative nervous system or medical disorders
  B. Behavioral disturbance is better accounted for by a psychiatric diagnosis
  C. Biomarkers strongly indicative of Alzheimer disease or other neurodegenerative process

Additional features
- Presence of motor neuron findings suggestive of motor neuron disease
- Motor symptoms and signs similar to corticobasal degeneration and progressive supranuclear palsy
- Impaired word and object knowledge
- Motor speech deficits
- Substantial grammatical deficits

bvFTD, Behavioral variant frontotemporal dementia; *CT,* computed tomography; *FTD,* frontotemporal dementia; *FTLD,* frontotemporal lobar degeneration; *MRI,* magnetic resonance imaging; *PET,* positron emission tomography; *SPECT,* single-photon emission computed tomography.
From Rascovsky K et al: Sensitivity of revised diagnostic criteria for the behavioural variant of frontotemporal dementia TT, *Brain* 134:1-22, 2011.

NONPHARMACOLOGIC THERAPY

- Due to the impulsivity and the risk for injury seen in bvFTD, discussions with family members about driving, the patient's access to finances, and safety of the physical environment should be conducted early in management.
- For patients with motor symptoms, regular exercise and physical therapy are helpful.
- Speech therapy is helpful for patients with language deficits.
- Diet counseling can aid in prevention of weight gain in patients with hyperphagia.

ACUTE GENERAL Rx

None

CHRONIC Rx

- There are conflicting reports of the efficacy of several medications in the symptomatic treatment of FTD. These include selective serotonin reuptake inhibitors (SSRIs), serotonin and norepinephrine reuptake inhibitors, and antipsychotics.
- SSRIs have the most consensus for their benefit in the management of FTD. They have been shown to help decrease the severity of disinhibition, impulsivity, eating disorders, and repetitive behaviors.
- The use of antipsychotics is controversial, but they are sometimes given to control symptoms of aggression, agitation, and psychosis. However, patients with FTD are also at an increased risk for extrapyramidal side effects due to poorly functioning dopaminergic pathways and thus are usually used only when SSRIs are not successful.

DISPOSITION

- Patients with FTD benefit from having the social support and specialized care offered in dementia-focused care homes and skilled nursing facilities.
- The range and severity of behaviors seen in FTD can put a great burden on family and friends. Education, counseling, and connection with social support or referral to a dementia-focused care home can help reduce caregiver stress.

REFERRAL

Patients who have severe or complex presentations should be referred to a neurologist with expertise in dementia or neurodegenerative disorders.

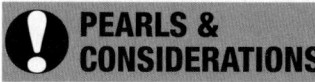

PEARLS & CONSIDERATIONS

FTD is a complex neurologic disorder with a wide variety of presenting symptoms. The most common syndrome seen is bvFTD; therefore patients with gradual-onset changes in personality, disinhibition, and increased impulsivity should be investigated for FTD. Therapy is aimed at management of the behavioral symptoms, most commonly through the use of SSRIs. Social support and dementia-specific care facilities are helpful for both patients and family members.

PATIENT & FAMILY EDUCATION

The Association for Frontotemporal Degeneration (https://www.theaftd.org; 866-507-7222)

SUGGESTED READINGS
Available at eBooks.Health.Elsevier.com.

RELATED CONTENT

Alzheimer Disease (Related Key Topic)
Parkinson Disease (Related Key Topic)
Dementia with Lewy Bodies (Related Key Topic)

AUTHOR: **JOSEPH S. KASS, MD, JD, FAAN**

BASIC INFORMATION

DEFINITION

Gastric cancer is an adenocarcinoma arising from the stomach and is histologically subdivided into intestinal and diffuse types; the diffuse type is more common in women and young patients, whereas the intestinal type is predominantly related to environmental factors (smoking; diet high in smoked, salted, and pickled food; nitrates and nitrites) and ethnicity (Asian and Pacific descent).

The classification of gastric adenocarcinoma by depth of invasion is illustrated in Fig. 1.

SYNONYMS

Gastric adenocarcinoma
Stomach cancer
Linitis plastica

ICD-10CM CODES

C16	Malignant neoplasm of stomach
C16.0	Malignant neoplasm of cardia of stomach
C16.1	Malignant neoplasm of stomach
C16.2	Malignant neoplasm of body of stomach
C16.3	Malignant neoplasm of pyloric antrum
C16.5	Malignant neoplasm of lesser curvature of stomach, unspecified
C16.6	Malignant neoplasm of greater curvature of stomach, unspecified
C16.8	Malignant neoplasm of overlapping sites of stomach

EPIDEMIOLOGY & DEMOGRAPHICS

- Gastric cancer is the sixth most common cancer worldwide, with an estimated 1,089,103 new cases in 2020, mostly (70%) occurring in developing countries, especially in Asia. It is the second-leading cause of cancer-related deaths worldwide, with an estimated 768,793 deaths in 2020.
- In the U.S., an estimated 26,500 new cases and 11,130 deaths were predicted in 2023.[1]
- The incidence and mortality rate of gastric cancer is 6.7 and 3.4, respectively, per 100,000 persons in the U.S. The incidence of distal stomach tumors has greatly declined, while that of proximal tumors of the cardia and fundus continues increasing.
- Gastric cancer is more common in male patients >65 yr.
- The male:female ratio is 3:2.
- Hereditary diffuse gastric cancer (HDGC) is autosomal-dominant, develops in the young (average age 37 yr), and germline truncating mutations in the tumor-suppressor E-cadherin gene *(CDH1)* are found in up to 50% cases. *CDH1* mutation carriers have an 80% lifetime risk of developing gastric cancer.[2]
- Increased gastric cancer risk is seen with Lynch syndrome, familial adenomatous polyposis (FAP), Peutz-Jeghers, juvenile polyposis syndrome, and hyperplastic gastric polyps.

PHYSICAL FINDINGS & CLINICAL PRESENTATION

- History may reveal postprandial fullness, significant weight loss (70% to 80%), nausea/vomiting (20% to 40%), dysphagia (20%), and dyspepsia unrelieved by antacids; epigastric discomfort, usually lessened by fasting and exacerbated by food intake, is also common.
- Epigastric or abdominal mass (30% to 50%), epigastric pain.
- Iron deficiency anemia and hemoccult-positive stools due to tumor bleeding.
- Hard, nodular liver may indicate metastatic disease to the liver.
- Ascites, lymphadenopathy, or pleural effusions may indicate metastases.

ETIOLOGY

- Chronic *Helicobacter pylori* gastritis. Gastric cancer develops in persons infected with *H. pylori* but not in uninfected persons. Persons with gastric ulcers, nonulcer-related dyspepsia, and gastric hyperplastic polyps are at risk, whereas those with *H. pylori* infection and duodenal ulcer are not at risk. Eradication of *H. pylori* reduces gastric cancer risk.[2]
- Germline pathogenic variants in nine genes *(APC, ATM, BREA1, BRCA2, CDH1, MLH1, MSH2, MSH6,* and *PALB2)* are associated with risk of gastric cancer. Persons with *H. Pylori* infection and a pathogenic variant have a higher cumulative risk of gastric cancer than noncarriers infected with *H. pylori.*[3]
- Patients with severe gastric atrophy, corpus-predominant gastritis, intestinal metaplasia, and pernicious anemia are at increased risk.
- Tobacco abuse, heavy alcohol consumption.
- Food additives (nitrosamines), smoked foods, occupational exposure to heavy metals, rubber, asbestos.
- Box 1 summarizes risk factors for gastric adenocarcinoma.

Dx DIAGNOSIS

DIFFERENTIAL DIAGNOSIS

- Gastric lymphoma (5% of gastric malignancies)
- Hypertrophic gastritis
- Peptic ulcer
- Reflux esophagitis

WORKUP

Upper endoscopy (Fig. E2) with biopsy will confirm diagnosis. Endoscopic ultrasonography in combination with PET/computed tomography (CT) scanning and operative lymph node dissection can be used in accurate tumor staging and aids in treatment planning. A general staging and treatment strategy for gastric adenocarcinoma is illustrated in Fig. 3. Table 1 and Fig. 1 describe staging systems for gastric carcinoma.

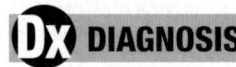

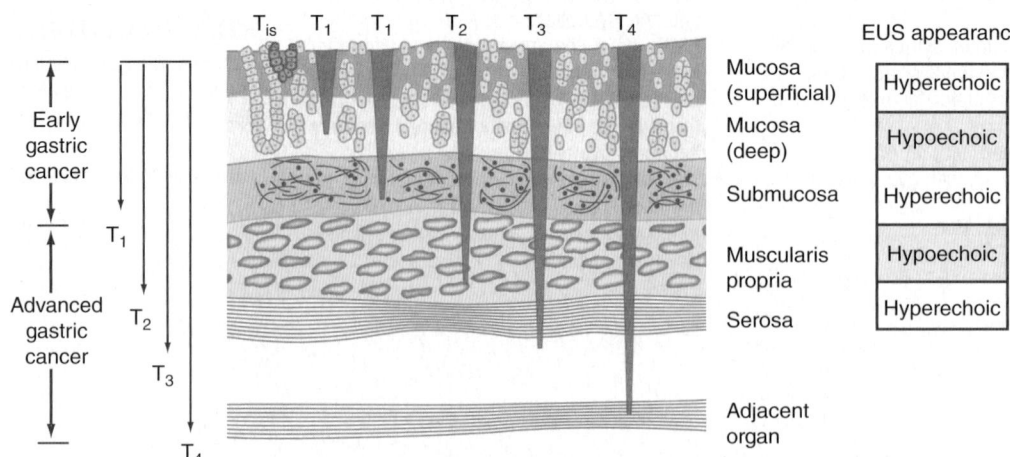

FIG. 1 Classification of gastric adenocarcinoma by depth of invasion (T classification). In the TNM classification, T denotes depth of invasion: T_{is} designates carcinoma in situ; T_1 tumors are confined to the mucosa (T_{1a}) and submucosa (T_{1b}); T_2 tumors invade the muscularis propria but not the serosa; T_3 tumors penetrate the subserosal connective tissue without involving the visceral peritoneum or contiguous structures; and T_4 tumors invade the serosa (visceral peritoneum) and may involve adjacent organs and tissues. In early gastric cancer, the disease is confined to the mucosa and submucosa (T_1), regardless of nodal involvement. (From Feldman M et al: *Sleisenger and Fordtran's gastrointestinal and liver disease,* ed 11, Philadelphia, 2021, Elsevier.)

BOX 1 Risk Factors for Gastric Adenocarcinoma

Definite
Adenomatous gastric polyps*
Chronic atrophic gastritis
Cigarette smoking
Dysplasia*
EBV
History of gastric surgery (esp. Billroth II)*
Hp infection
Intestinal metaplasia
Genetic factors
    Family history of gastric cancer (first-degree relative)*
    Familial adenomatous polyposis (with fundic gland polyps)*
    Hereditary nonpolyposis colorectal cancer*
    Juvenile polyposis*
Peutz-Jeghers syndrome*

Probable
High salt intake
History of gastric ulcer
Obesity (adenocarcinoma of the cardia only)
Pernicious anemia*
Regular aspirin or other NSAID use (protective)
Snuff tobacco use

Possible
Diet high in nitrates
Heavy alcohol use
High ascorbate intake (protective)
High intake of fresh fruits and vegetables (protective)
Low socioeconomic status
Ménétrier disease
Statin use (protective)

Questionable
High green tea consumption (protective)
Hyperplastic and fundic gland polyps

*Surveillance for cancer is recommended in patients with this risk factor.
EBV, Epstein-Barr virus; Hp, Helicobacter pylori; NSAID, nonsteroidal antiinflammatory drug.
From Feldman M et al: Sleisenger and Fordtran's gastrointestinal and liver disease, ed 11, Philadelphia, 2021, Elsevier.

TABLE 1 TNM Staging Criteria and Stages for Gastric Carcinoma Based on AJCC Eighth Edition

T Category	T Criteria
$T_X T_0 T_{is} T_1 T_{1a} T_{1b} T_2 T_3 T_4 T_{4a}$	Primary tumor cannot be assessed
	No evidence of primary tumor
	Carcinoma in situ: Intraepithelial tumor without invasion of the lamina propria, high-grade dysplasia
	Tumor invades the lamina propria, muscularis mucosae, or submucosa
	Tumor invades the lamina propria or muscularis mucosae
	Tumor invades the submucosa
	Tumor invades the muscularis propria
	Tumor penetrates the subserosal connective tissue without invasion of the visceral peritoneum or adjacent structures
	Tumor invades the serosa (visceral peritoneum) or adjacent structures
	Tumor invades the serosa (visceral peritoneum)

N Category	N Criteria
$N_X N_0 N_1 N_2 N_3 N_{3a}$	Regional lymph node(s) cannot be assessed
	No regional lymph node metastasis
	Metastasis in one or two regional lymph nodes
	Metastasis in three to six regional lymph nodes
	Metastasis in seven or more regional lymph nodes
	Metastasis in 7-15 regional lymph nodes

M Category	M Criteria
$M_0 M_1$	No distant metastasis
	Distant metastasis

Stage	pT	pN	M
Stage 0	T_{is}	N_0	M_0
Stage IA	T_1	N_0	M_0
Stage IB	$T_1 T_2$	$N_1 N_0$	$M_0 M_0$
Stage IIA	$T_1 T_2 T_3$	$N_2 N_1 N_0$	$M_0 M_0 M_0$
Stage IIB	$T_1 T_2 T_3 T_{4a}$	$N_{3a} N_2 N_1 N_0$	$M_0 M_0 M_0 M_0$
Stage IIIA	$T_2 T_3 T_{4a} T_{4b}$	$N_{3a} N_2 N_1$ or $N_2 N_0$	$M_0 M_0 M_0 M_0$
Stage IIIB	$T_1 T_2 T_3 T_{4a} T_{4b}$	$N_{3b} N_{3b} N_{3a} N_{3a} N_1$ or N_2	$M_0 M_0 M_0 M_0 M_0 M_0$
Stage IIIC	$T_3 T_{4a} T_{4b}$	$N_{3b} N_{3b} N_{3a}$ or N_{3b}	$M_0 M_0 M_0$
Stage IV	Any T	Any N	M_1

AJCC, American Joint Committee on Cancer; TNM, tumor, node, metastasis.

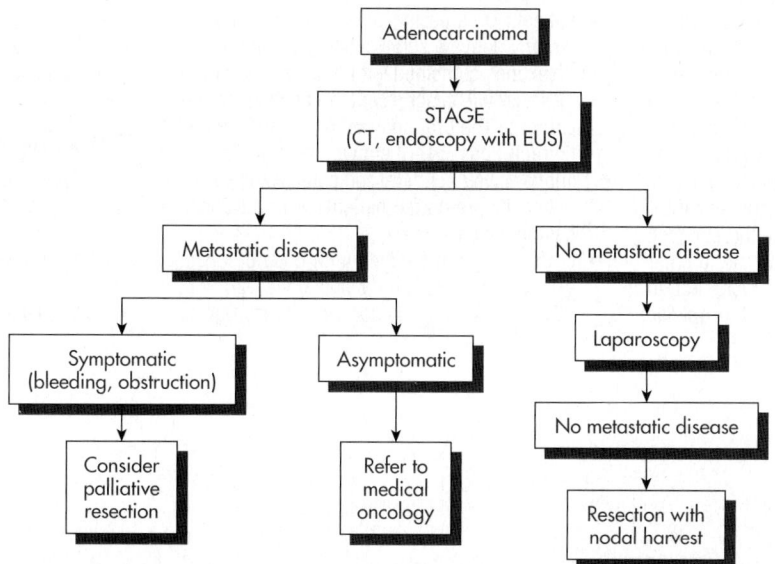

FIG. 3 General staging and treatment strategy for gastric adenocarcinoma. CT, Computed tomography; EUS, endoscopic ultrasound. (From Townsend CM et al: Sabiston textbook of surgery, ed 21, St Louis, 2022, Elsevier.)

LABORATORY TESTS

- CBC reveals microcytic anemia.
- Hemoccult-positive stools are detected.
- Chemistry panel can reveal hypoalbuminemia or abnormal liver enzymes in patients with metastasis to the liver.
- Up to 25% of gastric cancers overexpress the HER2/neu receptor, which can be detected by immunohistochemistry as a standard practice.
- Mutation-specific predictive genetic testing by polymerase chain reaction for truncating mutations in *CDH1* is recommended in families of patients with familial diffuse cancer because gastric cancer develops in three of every four carriers of a mutant *CDH1* gene. Genetic abnormalities in gastric adenocarcinoma are summarized in Table E2.

IMAGING STUDIES

- Chest and abdomen PET/CT scan to evaluate for metastases.
- Endoscopic ultrasound (EUS) is recommended as part of the staging workup for gastric cancer if there is no evidence of metastatic disease. It provides the most accurate evaluation of the depth of tumor invasion and assessment of perigastric lymph node involvement.

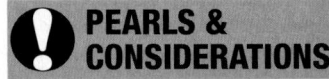

TREATMENT

The overall treatment strategy is dependent on tumor stage (early vs. locally advanced vs. metastatic) with surgery being the mainstay of therapy for nonmetastatic cases.

ACUTE GENERAL Rx

- Gastrectomy: Most curable tumors can be removed with adequate margins by subtotal gastrectomy; total gastrectomy is required in proximal cancers or large disease extent. The preferred treatment for lesions arising in the body or antrum of the stomach is a radical distal subtotal resection (Fig. E4), which removes approximately 80% of the stomach, along with the first portion of the duodenum, the gastrohepatic and gastrocolic omenta, and the nodal tissue adjacent to the celiac axis. Extensive or proximal cancers require a total gastrectomy to achieve an adequate proximal gastric margin (Fig. E5). If total gastrectomy is necessary, a splenectomy is sometimes performed, particularly in gastric cancers of the proximal third of the stomach and tumors of the body near the greater curvature. These cancers are more apt to metastasize to lymph nodes in the splenic

hilum that cannot be completely excised without a splenectomy. Routine splenectomy is no longer practiced due to increased complications.
- Laparoscopic distal gastrectomy with extended D2 lymphadenectomy is comparable to open surgery in terms of relapse-free survival for patients with locally advanced gastric cancer and is a potential standard treatment option for locally advanced gastric cancer.[4]
- Palliative gastrectomy (in cases of major bleeding or obstruction) can be performed in selected advanced cases. Gastric outlet obstruction can be addressed by either gastrojejunostomy or endoscopic stenting.
- Perioperative chemotherapy: In patients with operable, locally advanced, gastric cancer, perioperative chemotherapy decreases tumor size and tumor stage while improving progression-free and overall survival. Currently, the FLOT regimen (5-fluorouracil [5-FU], leucovorin, oxaliplatin, docetaxel) is used with four cycles administered prior to and after resection.[5]
- Similarly, perioperative chemotherapy with oxaliplatin plus S-1 chemotherapy was demonstrated to have better survival than adjuvant CAPOX (capecitabine, oxaliplatin) chemotherapy in a randomized study underscoring the value of perioperative, multimodal approach in these patients.[6]
- Postoperative chemotherapy: Combination chemotherapy with FOLFOX (5-FU, leucovorin, oxaliplatin) or CAPOX regimens is utilized; radiotherapy is reserved for high-risk patients (positive margins, extracapsular spread) only.
- Recurrent/metastatic cancer: The use of combination chemotherapy in combination with immune checkpoint inhibitor therapy results in improved overall survival. The use of platinum plus fluoropyrimidine chemotherapy in combination with either pembrolizumab or nivolumab has shown to improve overall survival in randomized trials.[7]
- Patients progressing after first-line chemotherapy derive a survival benefit with the use of taxanes combined with antivascular endothelial growth factor receptor-2 antibody ramucirumab. The oral antimetabolite, trifluridine/tipiracil, has been shown to significantly improve overall survival compared with placebo in heavily pretreated patients with advanced gastric cancer.
- In the subset of patients with gastric cancer expressing *HER2-2/neu* oncogene (20% to 25% cases), the addition of trastuzumab to

systemic chemotherapy prolongs overall survival. Improved overall survival rates are seen in patients when treated with trastuzumab deruxtecan (an antibody drug conjugate [ADC]) when compared to conventional salvage chemotherapy approaches.[8]
- CLDN18.2 is a tight junction protein exclusively expressed in normal gastric mucosa cells and demonstrated in up to 38% of gastric and gastroesophageal adenocarcinomas. Zolbetuximab, a monoclonal antibody targeting CLDN18.2, was evaluated in combination with capecitabine and oxaliplatin (CAPOX) or 5-FU and oxaliplatin (FOLFOX) as first-line treatment for CLDN18.2-positive, locally advanced unresectable or metastatic cases and demonstrated improved both progression free- and overall survival.[9] FDA approval is awaited.
- Immunotherapy with program death receptor-1 antibodies (nivolumab, pembrolizumab) has been shown to improve survival in previously treated patients with high-MSI tumors.
- Treatment algorithms for newly diagnosed gastric or gastroesophageal junction cancer are illustrated in Figs. E6 and E7.

DISPOSITION

- Median survival rate of metastatic or recurrent gastric carcinoma is 12 to 15 mo overall.
- The 5-yr survival rate for early gastric cancers is >35%.

PEARLS & CONSIDERATIONS

COMMENTS

- Gastrectomy patients will need vitamin B_{12} replacement. They are also at risk for dumping syndrome and should be advised to ingest frequent, small meals.
- Prophylactic gastrectomy should be considered in young, asymptomatic carriers of germline truncating *CDH1* mutations who belong to families with highly penetrant heredity diffuse gastric cancer.
- Gastric cancer screening for average-risk patients is not recommended in the U.S.

REFERENCES
Available at eBooks.Health.Elsevier.com.

RELATED CONTENT
Stomach Cancer (Patient Information)

AUTHOR: **RITESH RATHORE, MD**

BASIC INFORMATION

DEFINITION

Gastric outlet obstruction (GOO) is a mechanical obstruction involving the distal stomach or proximal duodenum resulting in delayed gastric emptying. It is not a single entity but rather can be the result of a variety of causes.

SYNONYMS

Pyloric obstruction
Stenosis of the pylorus
GOO

ICD-10CM CODE
K31.5   Obstruction of the duodenum

EPIDEMIOLOGY & DEMOGRAPHICS

INCIDENCE: Accurate statistics on incidence are not available. It is postulated that GOO has decreased over the past several decades due to improved treatment options for peptic ulcer disease, which is historically the leading cause for GOO. More recent data suggest that up to 50% to 80% of new cases are cancer related.[1,2]

RISK FACTORS:
- History of pancreatic or gastric malignancy
- Untreated peptic ulcer disease
- Chronic NSAID use
- *Helicobacter pylori* infection

PHYSICAL FINDINGS & CLINICAL PRESENTATION
- Signs of dehydration (tachycardia, hypotension, dry mucous membranes) are often present.
- Malnutrition may be evident depending on the chronicity of the obstruction.
- Epigastric tenderness may be present.
- Abdominal distention/tympanic mass in epigastric area or left upper quadrant (LUQ).
- Succession splash may be heard with a stethoscope placed on the abdomen while the patient rocks side to side. It has a low sensitivity and is positive if present 3 h after a meal, which suggests retained gastric contents.
- Sister Mary Joseph nodule (a periumbilical node) or Virchow's node (a left supraclavicular node) may be palpated in the setting of metastatic gastric cancer.

Patients with GOO often present with postprandial nonbilious vomiting, epigastric pain, nausea, easy satiety, and weight loss, though the presentation may differ depending on the cause of the obstruction. Patients with malignancy as the underlying cause often present with a more acute onset of symptoms, whereas those with peptic ulcer disease have more chronic symptoms. Physical examination findings most commonly include signs of dehydration and malnutrition, as well as abdominal tympanic distention and epigastric tenderness.

ETIOLOGY
- Historically, the most common cause of GOO was peptic ulcer disease; however, with the availability of proton pump inhibitors and treatment to eradicate *H. pylori* infection, this has been drastically reduced. Malignancy now accounts for the majority of cases, most frequently pancreatic adenocarcinoma with spread to the duodenum or stomach, or gastric cancer. Other rarer malignant causes include advanced gallbladder carcinoma or cholangiocarcinoma, gastric lymphoma, malignancy of the duodenum, ampullary cancer, and gastric carcinoid.
- Benign causes include peptic ulcer disease, caustic ingestion, stricture and scarring from NSAIDs or postsurgery, acute or chronic pancreatitis, and pancreatic pseudocysts. Rare causes include gastric obstructing polyps, bezoars, or volvulus, Bouveret syndrome (gallstone in the proximal duodenum), congenital annular pancreas, or infiltrative disease from Crohn, amyloid, or tuberculosis (Table 1).

DIAGNOSIS

Diagnosis is based on clinical presentation, imaging, and often endoscopy with biopsy.

DIFFERENTIAL DIAGNOSIS

It is important to exclude motility causes such as gastroparesis from diabetes, medications, or viral infections. The primary differential diagnosis to be considered in GOO is in determining the causes of the obstruction. See Table 1.

WORKUP

During the initial workup of GOO, it is important assess hydration and nutrition status and to determine the underlying cause. Consider the following:
- CBC, electrolytes, abdominal computed tomography (CT) scan, and upper endoscopy

LABORATORY TESTS

Laboratory tests are not diagnostic but should include a CBC and electrolytes.
- Electrolytes may reveal evidence of contraction alkalosis and hypokalemia, especially in the setting of repeated vomiting.
- The CBC may show evidence of anemia in a patient with underlying malignancy that may become more apparent after fluid replacement.

IMAGING STUDIES
- Abdominal x-rays are often not diagnostic but may reveal a significant gastric bubble.
- CT scan of abdomen (Fig. 1) may reveal gastric distention, mass, and evidence of malignant spread. This should be ordered without oral contrast if upper endoscopy is anticipated.
- Upper endoscopy is usually needed for both diagnostic and therapeutic purposes. This should occur after nasogastric tube placement and suction to remove gastric contents to reduce the chance of aspiration during the procedure. Endoscopy can determine the location and extension of the obstruction and may offer a diagnosis through biopsy.

TREATMENT

The general management of GOO consists of hydration, correcting metabolic abnormalities, pain management, and alleviating the obstruction.

NONPHARMACOLOGIC THERAPY
- Nothing by mouth (NPO) and nasogastric tube for gastric decompression
- Intravenous fluids using isotonic saline with potassium replacement
- Nutritional support

BENIGN CAUSES:
- Management of the obstruction depends on the underlying cause. The following recommendations are for GOO from peptic ulcer disease, the most common benign cause of GOO. Patients with rarer, benign causes of GOO may benefit from some of the following interventions as well, but treatment will be more specifically tailored to the underlying cause and decided with consultations from gastroenterology and surgery.
- GOO can be initially managed with 48 to 72 h of gastric decompression, fluid replacement, correction of metabolic abnormalities, and acid suppression. *H. pylori* infection should

---

TABLE 1   Causes of Gastric Outlet Obstruction

Benign	Malignant
Peptic ulcer disease	Pancreatic cancer
Gastric polyps	Gastric cancer
Caustic ingestion	Gallbladder carcinoma
Stricture/scarring from NSAIDs, radiation, postsurgical	Cholangiocarcinoma
	Gastric lymphoma
Acute or chronic pancreatitis	Ampullary cancer
Pancreatic pseudocyst	Duodenum cancer
Bouveret syndrome (gallstone in the proximal duodenum)	Gastric carcinoid
Congenital annular pancreas	
Infiltrative disease (Crohn, amyloid, tuberculosis)	
Bezoars	

NSAIDs, Nonsteroidal antiinflammatory drugs.

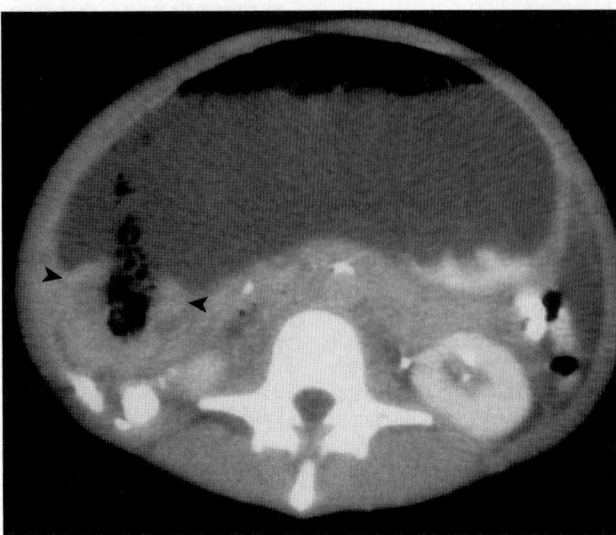

FIG. 1 Gastric outlet obstruction: Cancer of the antrum. A markedly distended stomach with an air-fluid level is seen on computed tomography. In this case, a mass in the distal end of the antrum is apparent *(arrowheads)*. (From Grainger RG et al [eds]: *Grainger & Allison's diagnostic radiology: a textbook of medical imaging*, ed 4, St Louis, 2001, Churchill Livingstone.)

be treated if appropriate. If this approach is unsuccessful, endoscopic dilation or surgery should be considered.

ENDOSCOPIC BALLOON DILATION: Endoscopic balloon dilation (EBD) is most commonly indicated in patients with GOO from peptic ulcer disease. It results in a lasting response in 70% to 80% of patients; however, narrow strictures often need gradual dilations performed in a stepwise fashion over several sessions. Recurrent stenosis requiring two or more dilations is an indication for surgery.

SURGICAL INTERVENTIONS:
- The goals of surgery include alleviating the obstruction and suppressing acid secretion.
- Surgical inventions such as laparoscopic antrectomy or distal gastrectomy with vagotomy, vagotomy with drainage via pyloroplasty, and laparoscopic gastrojejunostomy are potential options.

ENDOSCOPIC ULTRASOUND-GUIDED GASTRO-ENTEROSTOMY: Endoscopic ultrasound-guided gastroenterostomy (EUS-GE) is emerging as a

potential treatment option for benign (and malignant) GOO and might be associated with fewer adverse effects, fewer recurring symptoms, and decreased need for subsequent interventions compared with other techniques. However, further research is necessary to determine optimal technique and to directly compare the efficacy of EUS-GE with other endoscopic procedures and surgical options.[3,4]

MALIGNANT CAUSES: Management of malignant GOO depends on the type and extent of the underlying malignancy. General therapeutic options include endoscopic stenting, surgical resection or bypass, gastrostomy with possible feeding tube placement, and EUS-GE. Surgery is the treatment of choice when resection can be potentially curative. A laparoscopic approach is recommended based on current guidelines from the American Gastroenterological Association as this results in less blood loss and fewer days of hospitalization.[5] Consultation with gastroenterology, surgery, oncology, and palliative care can guide treatment decisions.

ACUTE GENERAL Rx
- Proton pump inhibitors to decrease gastric secretions
- Antiemetics to treat nausea
- Pain management
- Eradication of *H. pylori* infection, if applicable

CHRONIC Rx
- Avoidance of nonsteroidal antiinflammatory medications
- Proton pump inhibitors

DISPOSITION
Prognosis depends on the underlying cause of the GOO.

REFERRAL
Gastroenterology should be consulted for initial diagnostic and therapeutic options with consultations from surgery, oncology, and palliative care as needed.

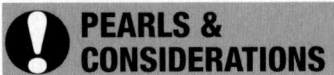

PEARLS & CONSIDERATIONS

COMMENTS
- Malignancy should be considered as the primary cause until proven otherwise.
- All patients, regardless of cause, benefit from a proton pump inhibitor.

REFERENCES
Available at eBooks.Health.Elsevier.com.

RELATED CONTENT
Pancreatic Cancer (Related Key Topic)
Gastric Cancer (Related Key Topic)
Peptic Ulcer Disease (Related Key Topic)
Gallbladder Cancer (Related Key Topic)

AUTHOR: **FRED F. FERRI, MD**

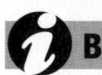
BASIC INFORMATION

DEFINITION

Gastroesophageal reflux disease (GERD) is a motility disorder characterized primarily by heartburn and caused by the reflux of gastric contents into the esophagus. A current definition is a condition that develops when the reflux of stomach contents causes at least two heartburn episodes per week and/or complications. Table 1 describes a classification system for esophagitis.

SYNONYMS

Peptic esophagitis
Reflux esophagitis
GERD

ICD-10CM CODES
K21.9	Gastroesophageal reflux disease without esophagitis
R12	Heartburn

EPIDEMIOLOGY & DEMOGRAPHICS

- GERD is one of the most prevalent GI disorders. It is the most common GI diagnosis recorded during visits to outpatient clinics. From 18% to 28% of adults are affected.
- The estimated prevalence of GERD is 13.3% of the population worldwide and 15.4% in North America. Costs related to GERD in the U.S. are estimated at $10 billion annually.[1]
- Nearly 7% of persons in the United States have heartburn daily, 20% have it monthly, and 60% have it intermittently. Incidence in pregnant women exceeds 80%.
- Nearly 20% of adults use antacids or over-the-counter H_2 blockers at least once a week for relief of heartburn.
- The phenotypic presentations of GERD include nonerosive reflux disease (in 60% to 70% of patients), erosive esophagitis (in 30%), and Barrett esophagus (in 5% to 12%).[1]

PHYSICAL FINDINGS & CLINICAL PRESENTATION

- Physical examination: Generally unremarkable
- Clinical signs and symptoms: Heartburn, dysphagia, sour taste, regurgitation of gastric contents into the mouth

TABLE 1 Los Angeles Endoscopic Classification System for Esophagitis

Grade A	One or more mucosal breaks confined to folds, ≤5 mm
Grade B	One or more mucosal breaks >5 mm confined to folds but not continuous between the tops of mucosal folds
Grade C	Mucosal breaks continuous between tops of ≥2 mucosal folds but not circumferential
Grade D	Circumferential mucosal break

From Feldman M et al: *Sleisenger and Fordtran's gastrointestinal and liver disease,* ed 11, Philadelphia, 2021, Elsevier.

- Chronic cough and bronchospasm
- Chest pain, laryngitis, early satiety, abdominal fullness, and bloating with belching
- Dental erosions in children

ETIOLOGY

- Incompetent lower esophageal sphincter (LES) (Fig. E1)
- Medications that lower LES pressure (calcium channel blockers, alpha-adrenergic antagonists, nitrates, theophylline, anticholinergics, sedatives, prostaglandins)
- Foods that lower LES pressure (chocolate, yellow onions, peppermint). Table 2 summarizes modulators of lower esophageal sphincter (LES) pressure
- Tobacco abuse, alcohol, coffee
- Pregnancy
- Gastric acid hypersecretion
- Hiatal hernia (controversial) present in >70% of patients with GERD; however, most patients with hiatal hernia are asymptomatic
- Obesity is associated with a statistically significant increase in the risk for GERD symptoms, erosive esophagitis, and esophageal carcinoma

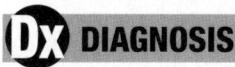 DIAGNOSIS

DIFFERENTIAL DIAGNOSIS

- Peptic ulcer disease
- Unstable angina
- Esophagitis (from infections such as herpes, *Candida*), medication induced (doxycycline, potassium chloride), eosinophilic esophagitis
- Esophageal spasm (nutcracker esophagus)
- Cancer of esophagus

WORKUP

- Aimed at eliminating the conditions noted in the differential diagnosis and documenting

the type and extent of tissue damage (Fig. E2). Generally, when symptoms of GERD are typical and the patient responds to therapy, there is no need for further diagnostic tests to verify the diagnosis.

- Upper GI endoscopy (Fig. E3) is useful to document the type and extent of tissue damage in persistent GERD and to exclude eosinophilic esophagitis and potentially malignant conditions such as Barrett esophagus. The American College of Physicians recommends endoscopy in the setting of GERD in people with heartburn and alarm symptoms (dysphagia, bleeding, anemia, weight loss, and recurrent vomiting). It is also indicated in people with GERD symptoms that persist despite a therapeutic trial of 4 to 8 wk of bid proton pump inhibitor (PPI) therapy in patients with severe erosive esophagus after a 2-mo course of PPI therapy to assess healing and rule out Barrett esophagus.

LABORATORY TESTS

- 24-h esophageal pH monitoring with transnasal catheter or a 48-h wireless capsule are sensitive diagnostic tests to assess the degree of acid exposure in the esophagus in patients not responding to acid-reducing therapy; however, they are not practical and generally not done. They are useful in patients with atypical manifestations of GERD, such as chest pain or chronic cough.
- High-resolution esophageal manometry is indicated in patients with refractory reflux in whom surgical therapy is planned.
- *Helicobacter pylori* testing is not indicated in GERD.

An upper GI series is useful in patients unwilling to have endoscopy or with medical contraindications to the procedure. It can identify

TABLE 2 Modulators of Lower Esophageal Sphincter (LES) Pressure

	Increase LES Pressure	Decrease LES Pressure
Hormones/peptides	Gastrin	CCK
	Motilin	Secretin
	Substance P	Somatostatin
		Vasoactive intestinal peptide
Neural agents	α-Adrenergic agonists	α-Adrenergic antagonists
	β-Adrenergic antagonists	β-Adrenergic agonists
	Cholinergic agonists	Cholinergic antagonists
Foods and nutrients	Protein	Chocolate
		Fat
		Peppermint
Other factors	Antacids	Barbiturates
	Baclofen	Calcium channel blockers
	Cisapride	Diazepam
	Domperidone	Dopamine
	Histamine	Meperidine
	Metoclopramide	Morphine
	Prostaglandin $F_{2\alpha}$	Prostaglandins E_2 and I_2
		Serotonin
		Theophylline

CCK, Cholecystokinin.
From Feldman M et al: *Sleisenger and Fordtran's gastrointestinal and liver disease,* ed 11, Philadelphia, 2021, Elsevier.

ulcerations and strictures; however, it may miss mucosal abnormalities. Only one third of patients with GERD have radiographic signs of esophagitis on an upper GI series.

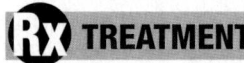 **TREATMENT**

NONPHARMACOLOGIC THERAPY

- Lifestyle modifications with avoidance of foods (e.g., citrus- and tomato-based products, onions, spicy foods, carbonated beverages, mint, chocolate, fried foods) and drugs that exacerbate reflux (e.g., caffeine, β-blockers, calcium channel blockers, α-adrenergic agonists, theophylline)
- Avoidance of tobacco and alcohol use
- Elevation of head of bed (4 to 8 in) with blocks
- Avoidance of lying down for at least 2 h after eating or drinking, especially after late or large evening meals
- Weight reduction to BMI <25, decreased fat intake
- Avoidance of clothing that is tight around the waist
- A trial in women revealed that adherence to diet and lifestyle changes reduced the risk of GERD to half compared with women who adhered to none[2]

GENERAL Rx

- An empiric 8-wk trial of a PPI given once/day is recommended for patients with classic heartburn and regurgitation but no alarm symptoms. PPIs should be taken 30 to 60 min before a meal because they bind to protein pumps that have been stimulated by meals.[3]
- PPIs (esomeprazole 40 mg qd, omeprazole 20 mg qd, lansoprazole 30 mg qd, rabeprazole 20 mg qd, pantoprazole 40 mg qd, or dexlansoprazole 30 mg) are generally safe, tolerated, and highly effective in most patients (Table E3). Omeprazole and esomeprazole are inhibitors of CYP2C19 and can increase serum concentrations of phenytoin and diazepam. Concomitant use of clopidogrel should also be avoided with omeprazole and esomeprazole. Increased risk of pneumonia has been documented in hospitalized patients. Long-term use of PPIs has been associated with increased risk of osteoporosis, and patients should be warned about an increased risk of fractures with long-term use. Use of PPIs in patients with cirrhosis increases risk of spontaneous bacterial peritonitis and hepatic encephalopathy. Rare side effects of PPIs include acute interstitial nephritis, hypomagnesemia, and QT prolongation.
- H₂ blocker (famotidine 40 mg qhs) can be used but is generally much less effective than PPIs.

- Antacids may be useful for relief of mild symptoms; however, they are generally ineffective in severe cases of reflux.
- Prokinetic agents (metoclopramide) are indicated only when PPIs are not fully effective. They can be used in combination therapy; however, side effects limit their use.
- Combination of PPE with an agent that reduces esophageal sphincter relaxation (baclofen) plus a neuromodulator (desipramine) may be tried in patients with refractory heartburn before considering surgery.
- For refractory cases: Think first, cut last. Some patients will respond to twice-daily PPIs or as-needed addition of a H₂ receptor blocker at bedtime. However, clinicians should be vigilant for alternative conditions that may be mistaken for GERD (e.g., achalasia).[3] Surgery with Nissen fundoplication (Fig. E4). Potential surgical candidates should have reflux esophagitis documented by esophagogastroduodenoscopy and normal esophageal motility as evaluated by manometry. Surgery generally consists of reduction of hiatal hernia when present and placement of a gastric wrap around the gastroesophageal (GE) junction (fundoplication). Although laparoscopic fundoplication is now widely used, long-term medical therapy is a better choice for most patients who are willing to remain on daily acid-reduction medication. In patients preferring surgical intervention, surgery should not be advised with the expectation that patients with GERD will no longer need to take antisecretory medications or that the procedure will prevent esophageal cancer among those with GERD and Barrett esophagus. Approximately 17.7% of patients who undergo primary laparoscopic antireflux surgery will experience recurrent gastroesophageal reflux requiring long-term medication use or secondary antireflux surgery. Risk factors for recurrence are older age, female sex, and comorbidity.
- Endoscopic radiofrequency heating of the GE junction (Stretta procedure) is a treatment modality for GERD patients unresponsive to traditional therapy. Its mechanism of action remains unclear. Endoscopic gastroplasty (EndoCinch procedure) is also aimed at treating GERD. Initial results appear encouraging; however, long-term studies are needed before recommending these procedures.
- Lifestyle modification must be followed for life because GERD is generally an irreversible condition in most patients.

DISPOSITION

- Recurrence of reflux is common if treatment is discontinued. Preliminary trials have shown that in patients with severe reflux esophagitis successfully treated with PPI therapy, stopping PPI medication was associated with T lymphocyte–predominant esophageal inflammation and

basal cell and papillary hyperplasia without loss of surface cells.
- The majority of patients respond well to therapy. In patients with chronic GERD, long-term outcomes are similar between medical therapy with PPIs and antireflux surgery. Prolonged use of PPIs is associated with increased risk of fractures of hip, wrist, and spine; increased risk of diarrhea from *Clostridioides difficile;* pneumonia; and possible iron deficiency from impaired iron absorption. PPIs also block the effects of clopidogrel by inhibiting cytochrome P450 2C19 isozyme. Therefore all PPIs (other than pantoprazole) should be avoided in patients using clopidogrel. H₂ blockers can be used for patients with GERD taking clopidogrel.
- Postsurgical complications occur in nearly 20% of patients (dysphagia, gas, bloating, diarrhea, nausea). Long-term follow-up studies also reveal that within 3 to 5 yr, 52% of patients who had undergone antireflux surgery are taking antireflux medications again.

REFERRAL

- There is a strong and probably causal relation between symptomatic prolonged and untreated GERD, Barrett esophagus, and esophageal adenocarcinoma. GI referral for upper endoscopy is needed when there are concerns about associated peptic ulcer disease, Barrett esophagus, or esophageal cancer. Patients with GERD and normal mucosa on initial endoscopy are diagnosed with "nonerosive GERD." Unlike erosive esophagitis and esophageal metaplasia (Barrett Esophagus), nonerosive GERD is not associated with increased risk of gastric cancer.[4]
- Patients with Barrett esophagus should undergo surveillance endoscopy with mucosal biopsy every 2 yr or less because the risk of developing adenocarcinoma of esophagus is at least 30 times greater than that of the general population.
- Testing and treating for *Helicobacter pylori* in patients with GERD has not been shown to improve symptoms.
- All children with dental erosions should be evaluated for GERD.

REFERENCES & SUGGESTED READINGS

Available at eBooks.Health.Elsevier.com.

RELATED CONTENT

Gastroesophageal Reflux Disease (GERD) (Patient Information)
Achalasia (Related Key Topic)
Barrett Esophagus (Related Key Topic)
Dysphagia (Related Key Topic)

AUTHOR: **FRED F. FERRI, MD**

BASIC INFORMATION

DEFINITION

Gestational diabetes mellitus (GDM) is hyperglycemia occurring during the second or third trimester in absence of a prepregnancy diagnosis of type 1 or type 2 diabetes. GDM has been defined as carbohydrate intolerance that is first discovered during pregnancy. However, it is now recognized that it is a heterogeneous disorder: Some women diagnosed with GDM have preexisting unrecognized glucose intolerance, and many have subtle metabolic disturbances.[1]

Screening for gestational diabetes mellitus in pregnant women without additional diabetic risk factors after 24 wk gestation is a grade B recommendation by the U.S. Preventive Services Task Force (USPSTF). In the U.S., a two-step approach to screening is commonly used between 24 and 28 wk gestation and is currently endorsed by the American College of Obstetricians and Gynecologists (ACOG) and the National Institutes of Health (NIH). The International Association of Diabetes in Pregnancy Study Group has recommended a simplified, one-step approach for screening and diagnosing GDM, which has been endorsed by the American Diabetes Association since 2011, with the acknowledgment that the one-step approach increases the prevalence of GDM without clear evidence of benefit. Pregnant women with diabetes mellitus (DM) (gestational or preexisting) are classified according to White classification (Table 1).

SYNONYMS

Gestational diabetes
Diet-controlled gestational diabetes (A1)
Medication-treated gestational diabetes (A2)

ICD-10CM CODES
O24.410	Gestational diabetes mellitus in pregnancy, diet controlled
O24.414	Gestational diabetes mellitus in pregnancy, insulin controlled
O24.419	Gestational diabetes mellitus in pregnancy, unspecified control
O99.810	Abnormal glucose complicating pregnancy

EPIDEMIOLOGY & DEMOGRAPHICS

INCIDENCE: Approximately 9% of pregnant women in the U.S. will be diagnosed with GDM using the two-step approach and 17% using the one-step approach.

PREDOMINANT SEX & AGE: Women of childbearing age; increased risk is observed in women >35 yr.

RISK FACTORS (BOX 1):
- Overweight or obesity (defined as body mass index greater than 25 or greater than 23 in Asian Americans)
- Family history of GDM or type 2 diabetes, particularly in first-degree relatives
- Polycystic ovarian syndrome
- Multiple gestation

TABLE 1 White Classification for Pregnant Women with Diabetes (Gestational or Preexisting)

Class	Description
A1	DM diagnosed during pregnancy and controlled by diet
A2	DM diagnosed during pregnancy and requiring medication
B	Insulin-requiring DM diagnosed before pregnancy, age >20 yr, lasting <10 yr
C	Insulin-requiring DM, onset at age 10-19 yr, with a duration 10-19 yr
D	Onset >10 yr or duration >20 yr, or associated with hypertension or background retinopathy
F	DM with renal disease
H	DM with coronary artery disease
R	DM with proliferative retinopathy
T	DM with renal transplant

DM, Diabetes mellitus.

- Hypertensive disorder of pregnancy or chronic hypertension
- Chronic systemic steroid use
- History of macrosomia in prior pregnancy
- Personal history of abnormal glucose tolerance or GDM in previous pregnancy
- Hispanic, Native American, African American, Asian, or Pacific Islander ethnicity
- Advanced maternal age (over age 35)
- Unexplained perinatal loss or malformation in previous or current pregnancy may be suggestive of preexisting diabetes

GENETICS: Higher rate in women with a family history of GDM or type 2 diabetes in a first-degree relative; specific human leukocyte antigen (HLA) alleles (DR3 or DR4) predispose to the development of DM after pregnancy.

PHYSICAL FINDINGS & CLINICAL PRESENTATION

Suspect GDM if:
- Fetal size greater than dates on Leopold or increased fundal height measurement
- Ultrasound findings of fetal macrosomia (especially enlarged abdominal circumference) or polyhydramnios

- Marked maternal obesity or weight gain above expected range
- Acanthosis nigricans (as underlying insulin resistance increases risk)
- Symptoms of diabetes
- Glucosuria
- Hemoglobin A1c ≥5.7 in the first trimester

ETIOLOGY

Pregnancy is associated with a small decrease in insulin sensitivity up to wk 7, then an increase in insulin sensitivity up to wk 18, and then a twofold to threefold increase in insulin resistance up to term. Diabetes in pregnancy, also known as hyperglycemia in pregnancy (HIP), is generally divided into diabetes that predated the pregnancy (type 1 diabetes mellitus [T1DM], type 2 diabetes mellitus [T2DM], secondary forms of diabetes, and monogenic diabetes) and hyperglycemia that is first detected in pregnancy (Fig. E1). Hyperglycemia that is first detected in pregnancy includes those with likely preexisting diabetes that was undiagnosed. Hence, hyperglycemia that is first detected in pregnancy is classified into "overt diabetes in pregnancy" (ODIP) and "gestational diabetes mellitus" (GDM). In this classification, ODIP refers to women who had an oral glucose tolerance test (OGTT) result meeting the nonpregnant criteria for diabetes, and GDM refers to the milder form of HIP.[3] This classification assumes that women with ODIP are at higher risk of adverse pregnancy outcomes and are more likely to have diabetes postpartum, but this is not always the case. In reality, it is increasingly recognized that diabetes in pregnancy represents a spectrum, from preexisting T1DM and T2DM to GDM, which classically was thought to develop toward the end of the second trimester.[1]

During normal pregnancy, several mechanisms contribute to increased insulin resistance. Placental secretion of human placental lactogen (hPL) decreases maternal insulin sensitivity, decreases maternal glucose utilization, and increases lipolysis, all to ensure adequate glucose availability to the growing fetus. Maternal pancreatic beta cells are increased in order to secrete additional insulin to compensate for the increased circulating blood glucose. Insulin resistance is also exacerbated by an increase in

BOX 1 Risk Factors for Gestational Diabetes

Women at greatest risk of gestational diabetes mellitus include those:
- Over 40 yr of age
- With a family history of type 2 diabetes mellitus (first-degree relative with diabetes or a sister with gestational diabetes mellitus)
- Who are overweight (defined as pre-pregnancy body mass index of >35 kg/m² (moderate risk factor if body mass index 25-35 kg/m²)
- Of racial background including Asian, Middle Eastern, Polynesian, Melanesian or Māori, African American, Indian subcontinent, and Indigenous Australian
- With a previous history of gestational diabetes (moderate risk factor)
- With a previous adverse obstetric outcome such as macrosomia (birth weight more than 4500 g or >90th percentile), shoulder dystocia, or polyhydramnios
- With previously elevated blood glucose level
- With polycystic ovarian syndrome
- On certain medications (e.g., corticosteroids)

From Talley NJ et al: *Essentials of internal medicine,* ed 4, Chatswood, NSW, 2021, Elsevier Australia.

Diseases and Disorders

I

maternal adipose deposition, decreased exercise, and increased caloric intake. GDM occurs when maternal insulin secretion cannot meet the increased glucose burden, resulting in carbohydrate intolerance and hyperglycemia.

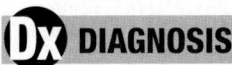 **DIAGNOSIS**

DIFFERENTIAL DIAGNOSIS

Preexisting type 1 or 2 DM not previously diagnosed

WORKUP

- History with focus on personal medical history, prior pregnancy history, and family history
- Routine prenatal examination
- Laboratory evaluation (see "Laboratory Tests")

LABORATORY TESTS

- Exclude preexisting diabetes.
- For women with risk factors for preexisting diabetes but without an existing diagnosis (see "Diagnosis"), consider early pregnancy screening for undiagnosed type 2 diabetes at the first prenatal visit. This early screen can be performed using the same two-step screening process as is used for gestational diabetes, though alternative testing strategies such as a 2-h glucose tolerance test with a 75-g glucose load or a hemoglobin A1c measurement are also reasonable. If initial screen in these patients is normal, repeat screen should be performed at 24 to 28 wk. If initial screen in these patients is abnormal, it would be suggestive of preexisting type 2 diabetes or underlying insulin resistance.
- A diagnosis of diabetes is made if a woman meets any of the following criteria: Fasting plasma glucose >126 mg/dl, A1c >6.5%, random plasma glucose >200 mg/dl. The authors consider a first-trimester A1c of ≥5.7 suggestive of preexisting insulin resistance and would be inclined to monitor closely for hyperglycemia.
- Two-step approach:
  1. For screening without risk factors, a 1-h, nonfasting 50-g oral glucose tolerance test (OGTT) is appropriate. If the result is abnormal (≥130 mg/dl, as defined by Carpenter and Coustan), a 3-h, 100-g oral glucose tolerance test is performed. The diagnosis of GDM is made if two or more of the following glucose values are met or exceeded:
     a. Fasting: 95 mg/dl
     b. 1-h plasma glucose: 180 mg/dl
     c. 2-h plasma glucose: 155 mg/dl
     d. 3-h plasma glucose: 140 mg/dl
  2. If one of four values on 3-h glucose tolerance test is abnormal, consider repeat testing in 1 mo, recommend a low-carbohydrate diet immediately and consider consultation with a nutritionist. At least one study has demonstrated increased perinatal risk in women with only one of four abnormal values on 3-h OGTT.
- One-step approach:
  1. Like the two-step, a one-step screening is performed at 24 to 28 wk on all pregnant

patients who have not been previously diagnosed with diabetes. This is a 2-h, 75-g oral glucose tolerance test performed after an overnight, 8-h fast. A diagnosis of GDM is made if one or more of the following values are met or exceeded:
  a. Fasting: ≥92 mg/dl
  b. 1-h plasma glucose ≥180 mg/dl
  c. 2-h plasma glucose ≥153 mg/dl
- After pregnancy, women with GDM have an increased risk of developing diabetes during their lifetime. Women with GDM should be screened at or after 6 wk postpartum with a 75-g, 2-h GTT to diagnose type 2 diabetes using the same criteria as nonpregnant patients. Alternatively, an HgbA1c can be performed at or after 12 wk postpartum.

IMAGING STUDIES

For women with gestational diabetes diagnosed at 24 to 28 wk gestation, the authors perform ultrasounds for growth every 3 wk from the time of diagnosis to monitor fetal size. We also initiate antenatal fetal surveillance by 32 wk gestation due to the risk of stillbirth associated with gestational diabetes (see "Imaging Studies"). Clinicians should consider local standards of care.

Rx **TREATMENT**

NONPHARMACOLOGIC THERAPY

- Glucose monitoring:
  1. Four times daily: Fasting and 2-h postprandial (defined as 2 h after the start of each meal)
  2. Goals: Fasting <95 mg/dl; 2-h postprandial <120 mg/dl
  3. Can also use 1-h postprandial goal of <140 mg/dl
- Dietary modifications for glycemic control:
  1. Follow a low-carbohydrate diet; avoid sugar and concentrated sweets; and eat small, frequent meals (three meals with two snacks is often recommended).
  2. Complex carbohydrates should be consumed over simple carbohydrates to prevent glucose fluctuations.
  3. Diet should adequately meet the needs of pregnancy (following sublist) while restricting carbohydrates to 33% to 40% of daily calories. Caloric needs in pregnancy:
     a. BMI <30: 30 kcal/kg/day
     b. BMI >30: 25 kcal/kg/day
     c. BMI >40: 12 to 14 kcal/kg/day
  4. Regular moderate exercise, defined as 30 min five times per wk.
  5. Ongoing nutrition counseling throughout pregnancy.

PHARMACOLOGIC Rx

Initiate if >20% of glucose values are elevated after trial of diet control:
- Insulin: Considered the gold standard in GDM management
  1. There are no randomized controlled trials on insulin regimens, and therapy is largely guided by expert opinion.

2. Insulin is the only FDA-approved medication for GDM (Pregnancy Class B) and does not cross the placenta.
3. Insulin may be started first line or added when oral medications have failed to achieve glycemic control. The authors consider factors such as the degree of hyperglycemia, obstacles to medication adherence, and gestational age at time of diagnosis (with early-onset diagnosis more likely to progress and require insulin) when initiating therapy. The ADA recommends insulin as first-line pharmacotherapy for GDM, and ACOG (2017) mirrors this recommendation (Level A).
4. Regardless of insulin regimen initiated, blood glucose values should be reviewed frequently, and the regimen adjusted and customized to optimize each woman's blood glucose levels, using a single agent or combination of long, intermediate, and/or short-acting insulins.
5. One commonly used regimen:
   a. Insulin 0.7 to 1.0 U/kg/day subcutaneous (based on current pregnant weight), with two thirds of the total daily dose given in the morning and one third of the total daily dose given in the evening.
   b. One third of each dose is given as short-acting insulin and the remaining two thirds as long-acting insulin.
- Oral hypoglycemics:
  1. Oral antidiabetic agents continue to be used in the management of GDM, despite a lack of FDA approval for this indication.
  2. Several recent studies have examined the potential benefits and harms of metformin and glyburide, comparing them with the gold-standard insulin and with each other. Metformin (compared with insulin) has been demonstrated to decrease maternal glucose levels, maternal weight gain, and the risk of gestational hypertension. Evidence grows that it may decrease the risk of preeclampsia as well. Although known to cross the placenta, concerns about the long-term risk in exposed offspring have been mitigated by at least one recent study showing no neurodevelopmental differences with intrauterine exposure to metformin vs. insulin. Meanwhile, recent meta-analyses have demonstrated worse neonatal outcomes with the use of glyburide compared with insulin. With both metformin and glyburide, many women go on to require insulin therapy.
  3. As of 2017, ACOG states that "in women who decline insulin therapy or for those women whom the obstetrician or obstetric care provider believes the patient will be unable to safely administer insulin, metformin is a reasonable second-line choice" (Level B);[3,4] ACOG also suggests that glyburide should not be recommended as a first-line agent due to a failure to achieve equivalent outcomes to insulin in most studies (also Level B).
  4. Metformin: Begin at 500 mg PO nightly or bid, and titrate up to a maximum of 2500 mg daily in divided doses.

5. Glyburide: Begin at 2.5 mg qd, and titrate up to a maximum of 20 mg qd (10 mg bid). Increase dose as needed by 2.5 to 5 mg/wk.

ANTENATAL TESTING

Antepartum testing is recommended for women with pregestational diabetes and gestational diabetes. There is no consensus regarding initiation, frequency, or modality of antepartum testing in gestational diabetes, and this should be guided by local standards.

For patients with GDMA2, the authors typically begin weekly nonstress test/amniotic fluid level beginning at 32 wk or when medications are initiated. We occasionally will progress to twice-weekly surveillance for patients with poor glucose control.

For patients with GDMA1, less frequent testing or delayed initiation of testing may be considered, as increased rates of stillbirth have not been observed in these women before 40 wk of gestation. However, clinicians should consider local standards of care.

For patients with preexisting or poorly controlled diabetes, vascular complications, or concomitant hypertension, the authors perform twice-weekly NST/AFI beginning at 28 wk. We will consider hospital admission to obtain glycemic control in patients with signs of poor glucose control.

TIMING & ROUTE OF DELIVERY

- Women with preexisting diabetes should be induced at 39 wk.
- Women with GDMA2 may also be induced at 39 wk unless otherwise indicated, with decisions regarding induction guided by local standards of care.
- In women with GDMA1, ACOG supports expectant management of up to 40 and 6/7 wk with appropriate antepartum testing.
- Counsel regarding elective cesarean delivery at or after 39 wk if estimated fetal weight is over 4500 g.
- Consider delivery earlier than 39 wk if poor glycemic control or other medical indications such as growth restriction or preeclampsia.

INTRAPARTUM MANAGEMENT

- Goal is normoglycemia (80 to 120 mg/dl) using insulin and D5 lactated Ringer intravenous (IV) fluid if needed.
- Monitor glucose every 1 to 2 h in active labor.
- Preparation for shoulder dystocia.
- If on glyburide, discontinue in labor or 12 h before a scheduled induction.
- If on insulin, consider decreased long-acting insulin by one third to one half before scheduled induction. Most experts recommend holding insulin entirely the morning of a scheduled cesarean delivery.

POSTPARTUM MANAGEMENT

- Class A2: Check fasting blood glucose level before discharge; if abnormal, continue checking at home and schedule early follow-up with primary care physician to confirm diagnosis of DM.
- 6-wk postpartum visit: Screen for impaired glucose tolerance and diabetes with a 75-g, 2-h glucose tolerance test. Alternatively, an HgbA1c or 3 fasting blood glucose levels may be performed at or after 12 wk postpartum. Unfortunately, screening for overt DM within 12 wk postpartum occurs in only one third of women with GD.[5]
- If no evidence of DM, screen annually for DM and counsel on risk factor modification.

REFERRAL

- Nutritionist
- Maternal-fetal medicine
- Diabetes educator
- Nurse care manager, when available

COMPLICATIONS

- Maternal: Preeclampsia, future type 2 DM or GDM, operative delivery
- Fetal: Polyhydramnios, macrosomia, congenital malformations, shoulder dystocia, birth trauma, intrauterine fetal demise
- Neonatal: Hypoglycemia, hypocalcemia, hyperbilirubinemia, polycythemia, perinatal death, respiratory distress, future obesity, and DM

⊘ PEARLS & CONSIDERATIONS

- **One-step vs two-step test for diagnosing GDM:** Despite more diagnosis of gestational diabetes with the one-step approach, trials have demonstrated no significance between group differences in the risks of the primary outcomes relating to perinatal and maternal complications. Using the one-step approach results in additional fetal testing (including fetal nonstress testing) and additional treatment (including initiation of insulin) with no significant improvement in pregnancy outcomes for the newborn or mother.
- A recent trial comparing lower vs. higher glycemic criteria for diagnosis of gestational diabetes revealed that using the lower glycemic criterion (FBS of at least 92 mg per deciliter [≥5.1 mmol per L], a 1 h level of at least 180 mg per deciliter [≥10.0 mmol per L], or a 2 h level of at least 153 mg per deciliter [≥8.5 mmol per L]) did not result in a lower risk or a large-for-gestational-age infant than use of the higher standard glycemic criteria.[2]
- Trials have shown that although treatment of mild gestational DM did not significantly reduce the frequency of a composite outcome that included stillbirth or perinatal death and several neonatal complications, it did reduce the risks of fetal overgrowth, shoulder dystocia, cesarean delivery, and hypertensive disorders.
- Lactation improves maternal glucose metabolism and may prevent or delay the development of type 2 DM following GDM. Higher lactation intensity and longer duration are independently associated with lower 2-yr incidences of DM after a GDM-affected pregnancy.

PREVENTION

Regular exercise, maintenance of ideal body weight, and high-fiber low-glycemic diet

REFERENCES & SUGGESTED READINGS

Available at eBooks.Health.Elsevier.com.

RELATED CONTENT

Gestational Diabetes (Patient Information)
Diabetes Mellitus (Related Key Topic)

AUTHORS: **TERESA C. LOGUE, MD, MPH** and **ANTHONY SCISCIONE, DO**

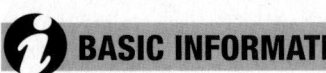 **BASIC INFORMATION**

DEFINITION

Gonorrhea is a sexually transmitted bacterial infection with a predilection for columnar and transitional epithelial cells. It commonly manifests as urethritis, cervicitis, or salpingitis. Infection may be asymptomatic. It differs between males and females in course, severity, and ease of recognition.

SYNONYMS

Gonococcal urethritis
Gonococcal vulvovaginitis
Gonococcal cervicitis
Gonococcal bartholinitis
GC

ICD-10CM CODES
A54.9	Gonococcal infection, unspecified
O98.211	Gonorrhea complicating pregnancy, first trimester
O98.212	Gonorrhea complicating pregnancy, second trimester
O98.213	Gonorrhea complicating pregnancy, third trimester
O98.219	Gonorrhea complicating pregnancy, unspecified trimester
O98.22	Gonorrhea complicating childbirth
O98.23	Gonorrhea complicating the puerperium
A54.03	Gonococcal cervicitis, unspecified
A54.00	Gonococcal infection of lower genitourinary tract, unspecified

EPIDEMIOLOGY & DEMOGRAPHICS

- The disease is common worldwide, affects both sexes and all ages, especially younger adults; highest incidence is in inner-city areas. Per Centers for Disease Control and Prevention (CDC) reports, approximately 1.6 million new cases were found in the U.S. in 2018, with more than half found in young people ages 15 to 24 yr. Gonorrhea is the second most-commonly reported communicable disease.
- Asymptomatic anterior urethral carriage may occur in 12% to 50% of cases in men.
- Asymptomatic in 50% to 80% of cases in women. Most common dissemination is by mucosal passage to fallopian tubes, resulting in pelvic inflammatory disease (PID) in 10% to 15% of infected women. Hematogenous spread may result in septic arthritis and skin lesions. Conjunctivitis rarely occurs but may result in blindness if not rapidly treated. Infection can occur in both men and women in oropharynx and anorectally.
- The World Health Organization (WHO) reported 78 million new cases of gonorrhea worldwide among adults in 2012.

PHYSICAL FINDINGS & CLINICAL PRESENTATION

- Males: Purulent discharge from anterior urethra (Fig. E1), with dysuria appearing 2 to 7 days after infecting exposure. May have rectal infection causing pruritus, tenesmus, and discharge, or may be asymptomatic.
- Females: Initial urethritis or cervicitis may occur a few days after exposure, frequently mild. Infections may be asymptomatic or may not produce recognizable symptoms until complications have occurred. In approximately 20% of cases, uterine invasion occurs after menstrual period with signs and symptoms of endometritis, salpingitis, or pelvic peritonitis. The patient may have purulent discharge or inflamed Skene or Bartholin glands.
- Classic presentation of acute gonococcal PID is fever, abdominal and adnexal tenderness, and, often, absence of purulent discharge. Physical examination may be normal if asymptomatic. Disseminated gonococcal infection (DGI) may manifest with petechial or pustular acral skin lesions (Fig. E2), asymmetric polyarthralgia, tenosynovitis, or oligoarticular septic arthritis. The infection is occasionally complicated by perihepatitis and, rarely, endocarditis or meningitis.

ETIOLOGY

- *Neisseria gonorrhoeae* is also known as gonococcus. Plasmids coding for β-lactamase render some strains resistant to penicillin or tetracycline. There is an increasing frequency of chromosomally mediated resistance to penicillin, tetracycline, fluoroquinolones, and cefoxitin. In the Far East, high-level resistance to spectinomycin is endemic.
- There are a rising number of cases of quinolone-resistant *N. gonorrhoeae* worldwide, with the expected number to rise in the U.S. from importation.
- Men who have sex with men are vulnerable to the emerging threat of antimicrobial-resistant *N. gonorrhoeae.*

DIAGNOSIS

DIFFERENTIAL DIAGNOSIS

- Nongonococcal urethritis (NGU)
- Nongonococcal mucopurulent cervicitis
- *Chlamydia trachomatis*
- *Trichomonas vaginalis*

WORKUP

Diagnosis depends on bacteriologic investigation. Culture and nucleic acid amplification tests (NAAT) are available for the detection of genitourinary infection with *N. gonorrhoeae.*

- NAATs are preferred testing modalities for the detection of genitourinary infection with *N. gonorrhoeae.* The performance of NAATs with respect to overall sensitivity, specificity, and ease of specimen transport is better than that of any other tests available for the diagnosis of gonococcal infections. NAATs should be used to detect gonorrhea except in cases of child sexual assault involving boys and rectal and oropharyngeal infections in prepubescent girls. When evaluating a potential gonorrhea treatment failure, case culture and susceptibility testing might be required. NAATs allow testing of the widest variety of specimen types, including endocervical swabs, vaginal swabs, urethral swabs (men), and urine (from both men and women).
- Culture: Gonorrhea culture on Thayer-Martin medium (organism is fastidious; requires aerobic conditions with increased carbon dioxide atmosphere; incubate ASAP). Culture has a sensitivity of 95% or more for urethral specimens from men with symptomatic urethritis and 80% to 90% for endocervical infection in women. Gram-negative intracellular diplococci are diagnostic in male urethral smears (Fig. E3). There is a false-negative rate of 60% to 70% in female cervical or urethral smears.
  1. Concomitant serologic testing for syphilis for all patients
  2. Concomitant *Chlamydia* testing for all patients
  3. Offer of HIV testing and counseling to all patients

LABORATORY TESTS

- First-catch urine (or genital swab) sample NAAT is the preferred screening and diagnostic test for gonorrhea. These tests have largely replaced collecting culture in many settings where persons are screened for asymptomatic genital infection. These tests are not more sensitive than culture for detecting *N. gonorrhoeae* in cervical or urethral specimen; however, they have specificities >99% and retain sensitivity when used to test voided urine or self-collected vaginal swabs.
- Gonorrhea culture on Thayer-Martin medium (organism is fastidious; requires aerobic conditions with increased carbon dioxide atmosphere; incubate ASAP). Culture has a sensitivity of 95% or more for urethral specimens from men with symptomatic urethritis and 80% to 90% for endocervical infection in women.
- Nonamplified DNA probe tests are less sensitive than culture or NAATs and are not useful in the diagnosis of rectal or pharyngeal infection or for testing urine; however, they are inexpensive, readily available, and offered in many laboratories in combination assays for *C. trachomatis.*
- Concomitant serologic testing for syphilis on all patients.
- Concomitant *Chlamydia* testing on all patients.
- Offer of HIV testing and counseling to all patients.

TREATMENT (TABLE 1)

ACUTE GENERAL Rx

For treatment of uncomplicated urogenital, rectal, or pharyngeal gonorrhea, the CDC recommends a single 500-mg intramuscular (IM) dose of ceftriaxone. For persons weighing ≥150 kg (300 lbs), a single 1-g IM dose of ceftriaxone should be administered. If chlamydial infection has not been excluded, doxycycline 100 mg orally twice a day for 7 days is recommended.

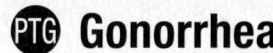

TABLE 1 Options for the Treatment of Gonorrhea[a]

Uncomplicated Infection of the Cervix, Urethra, and Rectum
- Ceftriaxone, 250 mg IM single dose *and*
- Azithromycin, 1 g PO single dose

Infection of the Pharynx
- Ceftriaxone, 250 mg IM single dose *and*
- Azithromycin, 1 g PO single dose

Conjunctivitis (Not Ophthalmia Neonatorum)

Ceftriaxone, 1 g IM single dose

Disseminated Gonococcal Infection

Ceftriaxone, 1 g IM or IV every 24 h for 24-48 h[b] after improvement, with switch to oral therapy for completion of 1 wk total antibiotic therapy, including cefixime, 400 mg PO twice daily

Meningitis and Endocarditis

Ceftriaxone, 1-2 g IV every 12 h for 10-14 days (meningitis) or ≥4 wk (endocarditis)

Ophthalmia Neonatorum

Ceftriaxone, 25-50 mg/kg IV or IM in a single dose, not to exceed 125 mg[c]

IM, intramuscular; *IV,* intravenous.

[a]Patients should abstain from sex for 1 wk after single-dose treatment. Test of cure for pharyngeal infection is recommended at 14 days if the ceftriaxone regimen is not used.

[b]Ceftriaxone administered IM may be reconstituted in 1% lidocaine solution to minimize injection pain. Alternative parenteral regimens include cefotaxime, ceftizoxime, and spectinomycin. See www.cdc.gov/std/treatment for specific regimens.

[c]Topical antibiotic therapy alone is inadequate for treatment of ophthalmia neonatorum.

Modified from Centers for Disease Control and Prevention: Sexually transmitted diseases treatment guidelines, 2015, *MMWR Morb Mortal Wkly Rep* 64:60-68, 2015; and Centers for Disease Control and Prevention: Sexually transmitted diseases (STDs): treatment and screening. Available at www.cdc.gov/std/treatment.

When ceftriaxone cannot be used for treating urogenital or rectal gonorrhea because of cephalosporin allergy, a single 240-mg IM dose of gentamicin, plus a single 2-g oral dose of azithromycin is an option. GI symptoms, primarily vomiting within 1 h of dosing, have been reported among 3% to 4% of treated persons. If administration of IM ceftriaxone is not available, a single 800-mg oral dose of cefixime is an alternative regimen. However, cefixime does not provide as high or sustained bactericidal blood levels as does ceftriaxone, and demonstrates limited treatment efficacy for pharyngeal gonorrhea.

When gonococcal expedited partner therapy (provision of prescriptions or medications for the patient to give to a sex partner without the health care provider first examining the partner) is permissible by state law and the partner is unable or unlikely to seek timely treatment, the partner may be treated with a single 800-mg oral dose of cefixime, provided that concurrent chlamydial infection in the patient has been excluded. Otherwise, the partner may be treated with a single 800-mg oral dose of cefixime plus oral doxycycline 100 mg twice daily for 7 days.

In cases of suspected cephalosporin treatment failure, clinicians should obtain relevant clinical specimens for culture and antimicrobial susceptibility testing, consult an infectious disease specialist or STD clinical expert (https://www.stdccn.org/external) for guidance in clinical management, and report the case to the CDC through state and local public health authorities within 24 h. Health departments should prioritize notification and culture evaluation for the patient's sex partner(s) from the preceding 60 days for those with suspected cephalosporin treatment failure or persons whose gonococcal isolates demonstrate reduced susceptibility to cephalosporins.

A test-of-cure is unnecessary for persons with uncomplicated urogenital or rectal gonorrhea who are treated with any of the recommended or alternative regimens. However, for persons with pharyngeal gonorrhea, a test-of-cure is recommended, using culture or nucleic acid amplification tests 7 to 14 days after initial treatment, regardless of the treatment regimen. Because reinfection within 12 mo ranges from 7% to 12% among persons previously treated for gonorrhea, those who have been treated should be retested 3 mo after treatment, regardless of whether they believe their sex partners were treated. If retesting at 3 mo is not possible, clinicians should retest within 12 mo after initial treatment.

Treatment of arthritis and arthritis-dermatitis syndrome:
- Recommended regimen: Ceftriaxone 1 g IM or intravenous (IV) every 24 h plus azithromycin 1 g orally as a single dose
- Alternative regimens: Cefotaxime 1 g IV every 8 h or ceftizoxime 1 g IV every 8 h *plus* azithromycin 1 g orally in a single dose

PREGNANCY: Pregnant women infected with *N. gonorrhoeae* in whom *Chlamydia* has been excluded should be treated with ceftriaxone 500 mg IM as a single dose for persons weighing <150 kg (300 lbs) or 1 g of IM ceftriaxone for persons weighing ≥150 kg (300 lbs). If *Chlamydia* has not been excluded, these patients should also receive azithromycin 1 g PO as a single dose. When cephalosporin allergy or other considerations preclude treatment and spectinomycin is not available, consultation with an ID specialist is recommended.

DISPOSITION
- All sexual partners should be identified, examined, tested, and receive presumptive treatment.
- Patients should be counseled to avoid unprotected intercourse with partners for 1 wk after all partners have completed treatment.
- Men or women who have been treated for gonorrhea should be retested in 3 mo because of risk of reinfection. If they are unable to be retested in 3 mo, then they should be retested when they next present to care within 12 mo of their care.

REFERRAL

PID requiring hospitalization, disseminated gonococcal infection

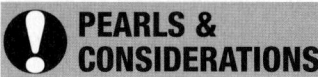

PEARLS & CONSIDERATIONS

COMMENTS
- This is a reportable disease.
- The proportion of gonorrhea cases in heterosexual men who are fluoroquinolone resistant (QRNG) has reached 6.7%, an elevenfold increase from 0.6% in 2001. Fluoroquinolone antibiotics are no longer recommended to treat gonorrhea in the U.S.
- The use of azithromycin as the second antimicrobial is preferred over doxycycline in areas of high prevalence of tetracycline resistance.
- The U.S. Preventive Services Task Force (USPSTF) recommends screening for gonorrhea in sexually active females younger than 25 yr and in women 25 and over who are at increased risk for infection (multiple partners, new partner, partner who has concurrent partners). The USPSTF also concludes that the current evidence is insufficient to assess the balance of benefits and harms of screening for gonorrhea in men.
- High-intensity counseling on sexual risk reduction has been shown to reduce sexually transmitted infections (STIs) in primary care and related settings.

SUGGESTED READINGS
Available at eBooks.Health.Elsevier.com.

RELATED CONTENT
Gonorrhea (Patient Information)
Cervicitis (Related Key Topic)
Chlamydia Genital Infections (Related Key Topic)
Pelvic Inflammatory Disease (Related Key Topic)
Urethritis, Gonococcal (Related Key Topic)

AUTHORS: **ANTHONY SCISCIONE, DO** and **ELLA STERN, MD**

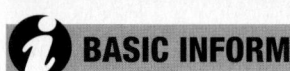 **BASIC INFORMATION**

Gout refers to a group of disease states caused by deposition of monosodium urate (MSU) in tissue, resulting from prolonged hyperuricemia. Clinical manifestations of gout include acute and chronic arthritis, soft tissue inflammation, tophus formation, gouty nephropathy, and nephrolithiasis. Untreated hyperuricemia in patients with gout may lead to chronic destructive deforming arthritis.

ICD-10CM CODES
M10	Gout
M10.0	Idiopathic gout
M10.1	Lead-induced gout
M10.2	Drug-induced gout
M10.3	Gout due to impairment of renal function
M10.4	Other secondary gout
M10.9	Gout, unspecified

EPIDEMIOLOGY & DEMOGRAPHICS

PREVALENCE: Self-reported prevalence in the U.S. is estimated at 3.9% of adults.[1] In the U.S., gout has been diagnosed in more than 10 million adults.[2]

PREDOMINANT SEX: Male:female ratio ~4:1. However, the prevalence of gout among women has increased in past decade. Compared with men, gout in women is more likely to be associated with diabetes, coronary heart disease, and chronic kidney disease.[3]

PREDOMINANT AGE: 30 to 50 yr in men; >60 yr in women

ETIOLOGY

- Gout is caused by inflammation resulting from MSU crystal deposition. The primary risk factors for MSU deposition are hyperuricemia, although local factors such as temperature, pH, and mechanical stress may play a role. Figs. E1, E2, and E3 illustrate the pathophysiology of gout.
- Hyperuricemia and gout develop from excessive uric acid production, a decrease in the renal excretion of uric acid, or both.
- Primary hyperuricemia results from an inborn error of metabolism and may be attributed to several biochemical defects.
- Secondary hyperuricemia may develop as a complication of acquired disorders (e.g., leukemia) or as a result of the use of certain drugs (e.g., diuretics). Consumption of alcohol, especially beer, increases the risk of gout, and fructose-rich beverage intake is associated with hyperuricemia. Gout promoters and inhibitors are summarized in Table 1.

PHYSICAL FINDINGS & CLINICAL PRESENTATION

ACUTE GOUT:
- Rapid onset of pain and swelling and erythema of a distal joint and/or periarticular soft tissue. Box 1 summarizes clinical pearls in acute gout attacks.

- May present as monoarthritis of any joint. Acute gout of the first metatarsophalangeal (MTP) joint is known as *podagra*.
- 10% to 15% of attacks are polyarticular.
- Spontaneous resolution occurs over days to weeks.

CHRONIC TOPHACEOUS GOUT (FIG. E4):
- Insidious onset of painless arthritis and soft tissue swelling
- Distal small joints characteristic
- May be confused with nodal osteoarthritis
- Box 2 summarizes clinical pearls in chronic gout

Dx DIAGNOSIS

DIFFERENTIAL DIAGNOSIS OF ACUTE GOUT
- Septic arthritis, cellulitis
- Pseudogout, calcium pyrophosphate crystal deposition disease
- Trauma

DIFFERENTIAL DIAGNOSIS OF CHRONIC GOUT
- Osteoarthritis (OA; especially nodal OA in women)
- Rheumatoid arthritis
- Psoriatic arthritis

Section II describes the differential diagnosis of acute monoarticular and oligoarticular arthritis.

WORKUP
Arthrocentesis and examination of synovial fluid

LABORATORY TESTS
- Uric acid: All patients with gout are hyperuricemic at some time, but during an acute attack the serum uric acid may be normal or low.
- Synovial aspirate: Usually cloudy and markedly inflammatory in nature (elevated white blood cells). Urate crystals in fluid are needle shaped and strongly negatively birefringent under polarized microscopy[4] (Fig. E5).
- CBC: Neutrophilic leukocytosis often present.
- Inflammatory markers: Erythrocyte sedimentation rate and C-reactive protein often elevated.

IMAGING STUDIES
- Plain radiography for diagnosis and evaluation. No typical findings in early gouty arthritis, but late disease is associated with characteristic punched-out marginal erosions (Fig. E6) and overhanging edges.
- Musculoskeletal ultrasound has been shown to be an effective means of detecting monosodium urate crystal deposition. Ultrasound can differentiate urate crystals that are found on the surface of articular cartilage from calcium pyrophosphate deposition disease (CPPD) crystals that are seen within the substance of the cartilage (Fig. E7). Double contour sign can be seen.[5]
- Dual-energy computed tomography (DECT) allows for color-coded images and detection of gout deposits and may be beneficial if there is difficulty in establishing the diagnosis.

TABLE 1	Gout Promoters and Inhibitors*	
Crystal formation	Seed nucleus (particulate)
	Immunoglobulin
	Phagocytes
	Low temperature
	Low pH
	Cation concentration
	Intraarticular dehydration
	Other (unknown) macromolecules
Triggering the acute flare (local factors)	Rapid change in urate level
	Microcrystal release
	IgG coat (apolipoproteins B, E inhibitory)
	Complement activation (classical, alternate, MAC)
	Inflammasome activation
	Cytokine and chemokine release
	Endothelial activation (e-selectin, ICAM-1, VCAM-1)
	Local trauma
Presence of susceptible phagocytes, mast cells (systemic events)	Surgery, trauma
	Infections, other intercurrent systemic illness
	Alcohol, dietary intake
	Drugs that raise or lower circulating urate level

ICAM-1, Intercellular adhesion molecule 1; *Ig*, immunoglobulin; *MAC*, membrane attack complex; *VCAM-1*, vascular cell adhesion molecule 1.

*A diverse array of proteins and other mediators have been identified on the surfaces of urate crystals. In addition to their proinflammatory effect through opsonizing existing crystals, immunoglobulin M (IgM) and immunoglobulin G (IgG) antibodies may promote crystal formation by providing a stable molecular platform for crystal nucleation and growth. Apolipoproteins are antiinflammatory molecules that coat crystals. The characteristics of the phagocytes encountering the crystals may be crucial; macrophages that are more differentiated are less likely to elicit proinflammatory cytokines.

From Hochberg MC et al: *Rheumatology*, ed 8, Philadelphia, 2023, Elsevier.

BOX 1   Acute Gout: *Clinical Pearls*

- Abrupt and rapid onset
- Maximal symptom intensity at 8-12 h
- Attacks often come on at night or early morning
- Most commonly monoarticular in men during first attack
- Metatarsophalangeal joint is first affected in 50% of cases; other commonly affected joints: Ankle, heel, knee, wrists, and hands
- Joints are red, hot, swollen, and exquisitely tender
- Attacks resolve within days to weeks without treatment

From Hochberg MC et al: *Rheumatology,* ed 8, Philadelphia, 2023, Elsevier.

BOX 2   Chronic Gout: *Clinical Pearls*

- Pattern of symptom changes: Time between attacks shortens; more joints may be involved
- Tophaceous disease may result in a destructive arthropathy
- Tophaceous deposits may be bothersome and cause marked reduction in quality of life
- Increased risk for nephrolithiasis
- Associated with comorbidities such as metabolic syndrome, diabetes mellitus, chronic kidney disease, cardiovascular disease, hyperlipidemia, and obesity

From Hochberg MC et al: *Rheumatology,* ed 8, Philadelphia, 2023, Elsevier.

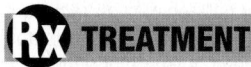 **TREATMENT**

TREATMENT OPTIONS FOR ACUTE GOUT (TABLE E2 & TABLE 3)

- Nonsteroidal antiinflammatory medication.
  1. Indomethacin 75 mg bid
  2. Ibuprofen 800 mg tid
  3. Naproxen 500 mg bid
  4. Celecoxib 200 mg bid
- Low-dose colchicine (less toxic, as effective as traditional high-dose colchicine): 1.2 mg PO, followed by 0.6 mg PO 1 h later, then 0.6 mg/day or bid. Dose for renal function.[6]
- Intraarticular corticosteroid injection (treatment of choice for monoarticular large joint attack): Triamcinolone acetonide 40 mg or equivalent for knee.

- Systemic corticosteroid therapy: Prednisone 40 mg PO for 3 days, then taper over 10 days (limited evidence currently, but studies have shown efficacy).[7]

TREATMENT OF HYPERURICEMIA IN PATIENTS WITH GOUT

The American College of Rheumatology, as well as most international rheumatology guidelines, recommend that every patient with gout who has tophi, more than two attacks of gout per year, chronic kidney disease, or nephrolithiasis be treated with pharmacologic urate-lowering therapy. Serum uric acid should be monitored on a regular basis and urate-lowering therapy intensified until a target of less than 6 mg/dl is reached. In most cases, urate-lowering therapy should be continued for life. Fig. E8 summarizes pharmacologic serum urate–lowering treatment.[1]

The American College of Physicians Guidelines recommends a more conservative approach based on recurrence of symptoms. These guidelines have been criticized for ignoring the progressive nature of gout and perpetuating the well-documented underuse and under-dosing of urate-lowering therapy.

NONPHARMACOLOGIC THERAPY

Lifestyle and dietary modification should always be a component of therapy for patients with gout, but this is rarely effective without concomitant pharmacologic urate-lowering therapy, as dietary modification can lower uric acid only about 1 mg/dl. Recommendations include reducing ingestion of red meat, kidney, liver, yeast extract, shellfish, and overall protein along with restricting alcohol intake. Discontinuation of diuretic therapy may help lower serum uric acid. Women with normal weight and best adherence to dietary approaches to stop hypertension (DASH) diet have a 68% lower risk for gout than women who are overweight or obese and are least adherent to the DASH diet.[3]

PHARMACOLOGIC TREATMENT OF SYMPTOMATIC HYPERURICEMIA

ALLOPURINOL: Allopurinol is very effective and safe when used properly. Correct dosing and patient compliance are essential elements in the prevention of erosive and tophaceous gout. Patients with renal insufficiency are at increased risk for allopurinol hypersensitivity, which manifests as fever, rash, and hepatitis occurring most commonly in the first 3 mo of therapy. The rash may progress to life-threatening toxic epidermal necrolysis if not recognized early.

Traditionally, therapy with allopurinol is initiated several weeks after the acute attack has resolved. However, initiation of allopurinol at presentation may improve long-term compliance without reducing the efficacy of acute treatment. The initial dose should be low (≤100 mg/day depending on creatinine clearance) in

TABLE 3   Treatment of Gout

Acute Gout	Interval Gout	Treatment of Hyperuricemia
NSAIDs (preferred): Indomethacin 50 mg qid or ibuprofen 800 mg tid (or other NSAID in full doses). Contraindicated in patients with renal insufficiency and gastrointestinal disorders *Or* **Colchicine, oral:** 1.2 mg followed by a second dose of 0.6 mg 1 h later Contraindicated in patients with renal insufficiency and gastrointestinal disorders *Or* **Intraarticular steroids** (Treatment of choice for large joint monoarthritis): Triamcinolone 40 mg or equivalent for knee *Or* **Systemic steroid therapy** (for patients in whom NSAIDs and colchicine are contraindicated) Prednisone 30-50 mg/day PO or in divided doses. May use lower dose in diabetic or postsurgical patients	**Colchicine, oral:** 0.6-1.2 mg/day as prophylaxis against recurrent attacks **NSAIDs may also be used for prophylaxis** **Hypouricemic agent:** Indicated for patients with recurrent attacks despite prophylaxis, severe hyperuricemia, presence of tophi, urolithiasis, or gouty arthritis **Other:** Weight loss, reduce alcohol (especially beer), diet low in seafood, red meat, organ meat, and fructose	**Colchicine, oral:** 0.6-1.2 mg/day for 4-6 wk before initiating hypouricemic therapy and for several months afterward to prevent recurrent attacks during initiation of hypouricemic therapy *And* **Allopurinol:** Initial dose 100 mg/day in patients with renal insufficiency or very high uric acid levels. Increase dose as needed to attain uric acid less than 6 mg/dl *Or* **Uricosuric agent** (Use only in patients with good renal function and <600 mg uric acid in a 24-h collection): Probenecid, 0.5-1 g bid, or sulfinpyrazone 100 mg tid or qid **Other:** Consider febuxostat for patients allergic to allopurinol and the addition of lesinurad in patients resistant to xanthine oxidase inhibitors. Pegloticase may be useful for selected patients with severe tophaceous gout

bid, Twice a day; *NSAID,* nonsteroidal antiinflammatory drug; *PO,* by mouth; *qid,* four times a day; *tid,* three times a day.

patients with renal insufficiency and those with very high uric acid levels.[8] High initial doses are associated with increased incidence of allopurinol hypersensitivity. The serum uric acid should be reevaluated after 4 to 6 wk of therapy, and the allopurinol dose adjusted to reduce the serum uric acid to <6 mg/dl. The most common therapeutic dosage of allopurinol is 300 mg/day, but the dose may be increased by 50 to 100 mg every 2 to 3 wk until the target serum uric acid level is achieved. There is evidence that increasing allopurinol doses in patients with renal insufficiency does not result in significant toxicity, but concurrent use with statins and colchicine is associated with a higher incidence of adverse effects. Some authors have reported using doses as high as 800 mg/day without excess toxicity. It is recommended that patients of Han Chinese, Thai, and Korean ancestry be tested for HLA-B*5801 before initiating allopurinol as these individuals are at high risk of allopurinol hypersensitivity if this allele is present.[1]

FEBUXOSTAT: Febuxostat is a xanthine oxidase inhibitor that has been shown to be more potent than allopurinol 300 mg/day for reducing serum uric acid. The chemical structure of febuxostat is different from allopurinol, making cross-reactive allergy unlikely. The metabolism of febuxostat is primarily hepatic, which obviates the need for dose adjustments because of renal insufficiency. Some cases of hepatic toxicity have been reported, and it is recommended that liver function tests be monitored. Febuxostat may help preserve renal function in patients with chronic kidney disease (CKD) but has not been tested in patients with severe renal failure.[1]

The primary indication for febuxostat is demonstrated allergy to allopurinol. The cost of febuxostat may be as much as 40 times that of allopurinol, and there is some evidence suggesting that febuxostat may be associated with higher cardiovascular and all-cause mortality than allopurinol in patients with cardiovascular risk factors. In 2019 the FDA added a boxed warning for increased risk of death with febuxostat.[9]

PROBENECID: Uricosuric agents may be used in patients with good renal function and urinary uric acid <600 mg in a 24-h collection. Probenecid can be used in patients with intolerance to xanthene-oxidase inhibitors. Compliance is poor due to the necessity of taking the drug more often than once daily.[1]

LESINURAD: Lesinurad is a URAT1 and OAT4 inhibitor approved by the FDA in 2015 for gout-associated hyperuricemia unresponsive to xanthine oxidase inhibitor monotherapy, to be taken in combination with a xanthine oxidase inhibitor.[10] This drug was withdrawn in 2019 because of business-related reasons without safety concerns noted.

PEGLOTICASE: Intravenous PEGylated uricase is FDA approved for treatment of severe refractory tophaceous gout. It is a PEGylated recombinant mammalian uricase that rapidly degrades urate when given intravenously. Use is limited by very high cost and potential toxicities, including frequent gout flares and anaphylaxis. Rasburicase is a nonpegylated uricase used in tumor lysis syndrome and is not indicated for gout treatment.[11]

REFERRAL

- Rheumatologist if diagnosis is not clear or therapy is complicated
- Podiatrist for management of pedal complications

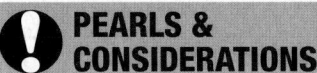

! PEARLS & CONSIDERATIONS

- Adherence to a healthful dietary pattern reduces risk of gout. A recent study revealed that women with normal weight and best adherence to the DASH diet (dietary approaches to stop hypertension) had 68% lower risk for gout than did women who were overweight and were nonadherent to the DASH diet.[12]

- Sodium-glucose cotransporter-2 (SGLT2) inhibitors currently FDA approved for type 2 diabetes and heart failure have been shown to reduce gout-related outcomes. This drug action may be related to antiinflammatory offsets through elevated circulating levels of ketone bodies and interleukin-2 beta secretion.[13]
- The interleukin-1 receptor antagonist anakinra (Kineret) is an effective off-label agent for treatment of gout in complex patients with contraindications to standard therapies. One study found 75% of patients using the biologic saw a partial or complete abatement of symptoms within 4 days.[14]
- Do not stop allopurinol during hospitalizations, surgery, or acute attacks unless there is evidence of drug allergy. The dosage of allopurinol should be adjusted in patients with acute kidney injury.

PATIENT & FAMILY EDUCATION

It is essential that patients, families, physicians, and other members of the health care team appreciate the importance of compliance with a daily allopurinol regimen if recurrent flares and progression to chronic arthritis and tophi are to be avoided. Allopurinol should be discontinued only for symptoms suggesting hypersensitivity; otherwise, it should be continued during flares, medical illnesses, and surgical procedures.[15]

REFERENCES

Available at eBooks.Health.Elsevier.com.

RELATED CONTENT

Gout (Patient Information)
Hyperuricemia (Related Key Topic)

AUTHORS: **JOSE P. GARCIA, MD** and **ANTHONY M. REGINATO, MD, PhD**

ℹ BASIC INFORMATION

DEFINITION

Graves disease is a hypermetabolic state caused by circulating immunoglobulin G (IgG) antibodies that bind to and activate the G-protein–coupled thyrotropin receptor. This activation stimulates follicular hypertrophy and hyperplasia, causing thyroid enlargement as well as increases in thyroid hormone production. It affects the thyroid, ocular muscles, and shin. It is characterized by thyrotoxicosis, diffuse goiter, and infiltrative ophthalmopathy (edema and inflammation of the extraocular muscles and an increase in orbital connective tissue and fat); infiltrative dermopathy characterized by lymphocytic infiltration of the dermis; accumulation of glycosaminoglycans; and occasionally edema.

SYNONYM

Thyrotoxicosis

ICD-10CM CODES
E05.00	Thyrotoxicosis with diffuse goiter without thyrotoxic crisis or storm
E05.01	Thyrotoxicosis with diffuse goiter with thyrotoxic crisis or storm

EPIDEMIOLOGY & DEMOGRAPHICS

INCIDENCE & PREVALENCE: Graves disease is the most common cause of hyperthyroidism. It affects 3% of women and 0.5% of men during their lifetime. There is a slight increased incidence among young African Americans. The annual incidence of Graves disease–associated ophthalmopathy is 16 cases/100,000 women and 3 cases/100,000 men. It is more common in Whites than Asians. Cigarette smoking is a risk factor.

PREDOMINANT AGE: Peak incidence is between 30 and 60 yr.

GENETICS: Patients often report a family history of Hashimoto thyroiditis, Graves disease, or other autoimmune conditions. Increased prevalence of *HLA-B8* and *HLA-DR3* in Whites with Graves disease. Concordance rate is 20% among monozygotic twins.

PHYSICAL FINDINGS & CLINICAL PRESENTATION (TABLES 1 & 2)

- Diffusely enlarged thyroid. Thyroid bruit may be present. Cervical lymphadenopathy also may be present.
- Elevated systolic blood pressure with a widened pulse pressure.
- Tachycardia, palpitations, tremor, hyperreflexia.
- Exophthalmos (50% of patients) (Figs. E1 and E2), lid retraction (lid lag), in which contraction of the levator palpebrae muscles of the eyelids show immobility of the upper eyelid with downward rotation of the eye.
- Nervousness, weight loss (weight gain in 10% of patients), heat intolerance, pruritus, muscle weakness, atrial fibrillation.
- Increased sweating, brittle nails, clubbing of fingers.
- Localized infiltrative dermopathy (1% to 2% of patients) is most frequent over the anterolateral aspects of the legs, commonly over the pretibial area (pretibial myxedema) but can be found at other sites (especially after trauma). It is nonpitting and indurated. It is typically patchy with a peau d'orange appearance to the skin.
- Men may have gynecomastia, reduced libido, and erectile dysfunction. Women often have irregular menses.

ETIOLOGY

Autoimmune etiology: Thyrotropin receptor antibodies (TRAb) mediated activation of thyroid-stimulating hormone receptor (TSHR). The activity of the thyroid gland is stimulated by the action of T cells, which induce specific B cells to synthesize antibodies against TSHRs in the follicular cell membrane. An overview of the pathogenesis of Graves orbitopathy is illustrated in Fig. E3.

ⓓ DIAGNOSIS

DIFFERENTIAL DIAGNOSIS

- Anxiety disorder
- Premenopausal state
- Thyroiditis
- Other causes of hyperthyroidism (e.g., toxic multinodular goiter, toxic adenoma)
- Other: Metastatic neoplasm, diabetes mellitus, pheochromocytoma

WORKUP

- The diagnosis is made clinically in most instances. The clinical assessment of the patient with Graves orbitopathy is summarized in Tables 3 and 4.

TABLE 1	Clinical Features of Graves Orbitopathy
Clinical Features	**Pathophysiology and Clinical Significance**
Gritty or foreign body sensation, light sensitivity (photophobia), excess tearing	Ocular surface irritation resulting from increased evaporative loss and/or impaired tear film formation because of proptosis or eyelid abnormalities
	May mimic other common ocular conditions, e.g., allergic conjunctivitis, dry eye disease
Eyelid swelling and redness Conjunctival swelling (chemosis) and redness Caruncle or plica swelling Gaze-evoked pain or spontaneous retrobulbar pain Elevated intraocular pressure	Reflect orbital inflammation and congestion
Upper eyelid retraction	Sympathetic activation of Muller's muscle Synkinetic activity of levator palpebrae superioris with superior rectus that tries to overcome the tight inferior rectus Inflammation, degeneration, and scarring of eyelid structures
Lower eyelid retraction/displacement	Correlates with the degree of proptosis Lower lid retractors apparently unaffected in Graves orbitopathy
Lid lag	Defined as a static phenomenon in which the upper eyelid assumes and maintains a higher position (relative to its position in primary gaze) with the eye in downgaze
Von Graefe's sign	Defined as a dynamic phenomenon in which the upper eyelid fails to descend smoothly and lags behind the eyeball during the course of downgaze
Lagophthalmos	Incomplete eyelid closure because of eyelid abnormalities and significant proptosis Predisposes to exposure keratopathy, especially when Bell's phenomenon is defective owing to tight inferior rectus
Diplopia and squint	The proliferation of orbital fibroblasts (de novo adipogenesis, secretion and accumulation of hydrophilic glycosaminoglycans) and inflammatory infiltration lead to enlargement of extraocular muscles, resulting in restrictive (instead of paralytic) strabismus
Proptosis	Expanded volume of retrobulbar structures pushes the eyeball forward Globe subluxation may occur in extreme proptosis
Visual loss	Watch out for sight-threatening Graves orbitopathy

From Robertson RP et al: *DeGroot's endocrinology: basic science and clinical practice*, ed 8, Philadelphia, 2023, Elsevier.

TABLE 2 Signs and Symptoms of Graves Hyperthyroidism

Symptoms
- Hyperactivity, irritability
- Heat intolerance and sweating
- Palpitations
- Dysphoria
- Fatigue and weakness
- Weight loss with increased appetite
- Diarrhea
- Polyuria
- Oligomenorrhea, loss of libido

Signs
- Tachycardia
- Atrial fibrillation in the elderly
- Tremor
- Goiter
- Warm, moist skin
- Muscle weakness, proximal myopathy
- Lid retraction or lag
- Exophthalmos
- Gynecomastia

From Robertson RP et al: *DeGroot's endocrinology: basic science and clinical practice,* ed 8, Philadelphia, 2023, Elsevier.

- The diagnostic workup includes a detailed medical history followed by laboratory and imaging studies and ECG. Patients often present with anxiety, heat intolerance, menstrual dysfunction, increased appetite, and weight loss. Elderly patients can have an atypical presentation (apathetic hyperparathyroidism). For additional information, refer to the topic "Hyperthyroidism."

LABORATORY TESTS
- Increased free thyroxine (T_4) and free triiodothyronine (T_3)
- Decreased thyroid-stimulating hormone
- Measurement of thyroid-stimulating antibodies (TSI) and TRAb
- Table E5 summarizes assays of TSHR antibody nomenclature and indications

IMAGING STUDIES
- 24-h radioactive iodine uptake (RAIU): Increased homogeneous uptake.
- Computed tomography (CT; Fig. E4 and Fig. E5) or MRI of the orbits is useful if there is uncertainty about the cause of ophthalmopathy.

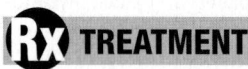

Rx TREATMENT

NONPHARMACOLOGIC THERAPY
- Patient education and discussion of therapeutic options.
- Smoking cessation: Smoking is associated with an increased risk of progression of Graves ophthalmopathy.

ACUTE GENERAL Rx
- Advantages and disadvantages of treatment options for Graves hyperthyroidism are summarized in Table E6. Intravenous glucocorticoids have been the most commonly used immunosuppressants in the treatment of active moderate-to-severe Graves orbitopathy (Table 7).
- Antithyroid drugs (thionamides, ATDs) to inhibit thyroid hormone synthesis or peripheral conversion of T_4 to T_3:
  1. Methimazole or propylthiouracil (PTU) are available. Methimazole is generally preferred because it has a longer half-life, allowing for once-daily dosing. PTU is preferred during pregnancy.
  2. Side effects: Skin rash (3% to 5%), arthralgias, myalgias, granulocytopenia (0.5%); rare side effects: Aplastic anemia, hepatic necrosis (PTU), cholestatic jaundice.
  3. Thionamide antithyroid drug therapy results in a remission in 40% to 50% of patients treated for 12 to 18 mo.
- Radioactive iodine (RAI):
  1. Treatment of choice for patients >21 yr and younger patients who have not achieved remission after 1 yr of ATD therapy.
  2. Contraindicated during pregnancy and lactation.

TABLE 3 Clinical Assessment of Patient with Graves Orbitopathy

SEVERITY MEASURES (USING THE MNEMONIC NO SPECS)

NO SPECS Class	Item	Method
0. No signs or symptoms		
1. Only signs, no symptoms	Lid aperture	With ruler in midline in mm
2. Soft tissue involvement	Eyelid and conjunctiva swelling and redness	Inspection, color pictures[a]
3. Proptosis	Exophthalmos	Hertel in mm
4. Extraocular muscle involvement	Eye muscle motility	Impaired elevation, abduction
	Diplopia	Subjective grading[b]
5. Corneal involvement	Keratitis, ulcer	Fluoresceine
6. Sight loss caused by optic nerve involvement	Dysthyroid optic neuropathy (DON)	Visual acuity, color vision, visual fields, optic disc

ACTIVITY MEASURES (USING THE CLINICAL ACTIVITY SCORE [CAS])

Inflammatory Sign	Item	Score
Pain	Spontaneous retrobulbar pain	1
	Pain on up gaze, side gaze, or down gaze	1
Redness	Redness of the eyelids	1
	Redness of the conjunctiva	1
Swelling	Swelling of the eyelids	1
	Swelling of the caruncle and/or plica	1
	Chemosis	1
Maximum CAS Score (assessed momently)		*7*
Impaired function	Increase in proptosis ≥2 mm in 1-3 mo	1
	Decrease of ≥8 degrees in eye muscle motility in any direction in 1-3 mo	1
	Decrease in visual acuity of more than one line on the Snellen chart (using pinhole) in 1-3 mo	1
Maximum CAS Score (assessed over time)		*10*

CAS, Clinical activity score.
[a]Color atlas in Dickinson AJ, Perros P: Controversies in the clinical evaluation of active thyroid-associated orbitopathy: use of a detailed protocol with comparative photographs for objective assessment, *Clin Endocrinol (Oxf)* 55:283-303, 2001.
[b]Intermittent diplopia = at awakening or when tired; inconstant diplopia = at extremes of gaze; constant diplopia = in primary or reading position.
From Melmed S et al: *Williams textbook of endocrinology,* ed 14, Philadelphia, 2020, Elsevier.

TABLE 4 Diagnosis of Dysthyroid Optic Neuropathy

Clinical Features	Examples of Diagnostic Test	Frequency in Dysthyroid Optic Neuropathy	Remarks
Reduced BCVA	Snellen chart	82%	• No single BCVA threshold can exclude DON, and 20% of cases have BCVA >0.67
Reduced color vision	Ishihara test	83%	• One of the most specific features • Can be present even if BCVA appears normal
RAPD	Swinging flashlight test	44%	• Possible only in unilateral DON or bilateral DON with significant asymmetry
Papilloedema	Fundoscopy	40%	• One of the most specific features • Optic disc pallor (present only in ~4%) may be observed in long-standing severe optic nerve dysfunction
Visual field defect	Automated perimetry	64%	• Most common patterns include central scotoma, an arcuate or altitudinal defect
Abnormal electrophysiology	Visual-evoked potentials	73% (↑ latency) 53% (↓ amplitude)	• Helpful to exclude DON if unequivocally normal • Interference by thyroid dysfunction and lack of reference range in elderly may make interpretation difficult • Time-consuming and not widely available
Apical crowding on imaging	CT or MRI orbits	95%	• Apical crowding is quantified by assessing the degree of perineural fat effacement on coronal images at the orbital apex • Less commonly imaging shows no apical crowding but reveals optic nerve stretching ± tenting at posterior eyeball because of severe proptosis

• Expert opinion suggests that DON can be diagnosed if papilloedema (after excluding alternative causes) is present or if two of the following features are present: impaired visual acuity or color vision, RAPD, and visual field defect.
• A U.S. group developed a mathematical formula, the Columbia thyroid eye disease-compressive optic neuropathy diagnostic formula (CTD formula), which helps guide clinicians in accurately diagnosing DON. The parameters include visual acuity, color vision, RAPD, visual field defect, ocular dysmotility, and proptosis. However, this has not been prospectively validated.

BCVA, Best corrected visual acuity; *CT,* computed tomography; *DON,* dysthyroid optic neuropathy; *MRI,* magnetic resonance imaging; *RAPD,* relative afferent pupillary defect.
From Robertson RP et al: *DeGroot's endocrinology: basic science and clinical practice,* ed 8, Philadelphia, 2023, Elsevier.

3. After radioactive therapy there may be an acute elevation of thyroid antibody titers and exacerbation of ocular symptoms in 15% to 20% of patients.
4. Post–radioactive iodine therapy glucocorticoid prophylaxis is summarized in Table 8.
• Surgery: Near-total thyroidectomy. Indications: Obstructing goiters despite RAI and ATD therapy, patients who refuse RAI and cannot be adequately managed with ATDs, and pregnant women inadequately managed with ATDs. Complications of surgery include hypoparathyroidism (4%) and vocal cord paralysis (1%).
• Adjunctive therapy: Beta-adrenergic receptor blockers (e.g., atenolol 50 to 100 mg/day) to alleviate the beta-adrenergic symptoms of hyperthyroidism (tachycardia, tremor); contraindicated in patients with bronchospasm.
• Graves ophthalmopathy: Methylcellulose eye drops to protect against excessive dryness, sunglasses to decrease photophobia, intraocular and systemic high-dose corticosteroids for severe exophthalmos. Worsening of ophthalmopathy after RAI therapy is often transient and can be prevented by the administration of prednisone. Other treatment options include antiinflammatory and immunosuppressive agents, radiation, and corrective surgical procedures. The administration of the antioxidant selenium (100 μg PO bid) has been recently reported as effective in improving quality of life, reducing ocular involvement, and slowing progression of the disease in patients with mild Graves orbitopathy. Its mechanism of action is believed to be an effect on the oxygen free radicals and cytokines that play a pathogenic role in Graves orbitopathy. Inhibition of the insulin-like growth factor I receptor (IGF-IR) is a new therapeutic strategy to combat the underlying autoimmune etiology of ophthalmopathy. Trials with teprotumumab, a human monoclonal antibody inhibitor of IGF-IR, in patients with active, moderate-to-severe ophthalmopathy have shown effectiveness in reducing proptosis.[1]
• Dermopathy and acropachy: Topical corticosteroids are often used but are generally ineffective. Trials using rituximab infusion for dermopathy have shown striking improvement.

CHRONIC Rx

Patients undergoing treatment with ATDs should be seen every 1 to 3 mo until euthyroidism is achieved and every 3 to 4 mo while they are receiving ATDs.

DISPOSITION

• ATDs induce sustained remission in <60% of cases.
• The incidence of hypothyroidism after RAI is >50% within the first year and 2% per year thereafter.

• Complications of surgery include hypothyroidism (28% to 43% after 10 yr), hypoparathyroidism (4%), and vocal cord paralysis (1%).
• Successful treatment of hyperthyroidism requires lifelong monitoring for the onset of hypothyroidism or the recurrence of thyrotoxicosis.
• RAI therapy is followed by the appearance or worsening of ophthalmopathy more often than is therapy with methimazole, particularly in patients who are cigarette smokers. It can be prevented with the administration of prednisone 0.5 mg/kg body weight per day starting 2 to 3 days after RAI, continued for 1 mo, then tapered off over 2 mo.
• Mild to moderate ophthalmopathy often improves spontaneously. Severe cases can be treated with high-dose glucocorticoids, orbital irradiation, or both. Orbital decompression may be used in patients with optic neuropathy and exophthalmos (see "Hyperthyroidism").

REFERENCES

Available at eBooks.Health.Elsevier.com.

RELATED CONTENT

Graves Disease (Patient Information)
Hyperthyroidism (Related Key Topic)

AUTHOR: **FRED F. FERRI, MD**

TABLE 7 Intravenous Glucocorticoid Use in Graves Orbitopathy—Regimen, Monitoring, and Absolute Contraindications

Regimen according to Graves orbitopathy (GO) status	• Active moderate-to-severe GO 1. Intravenous methylprednisolone 500 mg weekly for six doses, then 250 mg weekly for six doses 2. Cumulative dose 4.5 g, 12-wk course • Active moderate-to-severe GO with diplopia or severe proptosis 1. Intravenous methylprednisolone 750 mg weekly for six doses, then 500 mg weekly for six doses 2. Cumulative dose 7.5 g, 12-wk course • Dysthyroid optic neuropathy ("hit hard and short") 1. Intravenous methylprednisolone 750 mg alternate day for seven doses (2 wk) (if dysthyroid optic neuropathy resolves), then 500 mg weekly for five doses 2. Cumulative dose 7.75 g, 7-wk course
Monitoring and precautions	• Before treatment: 1. Check fasting blood glucose, liver function test, and markers for viral hepatitis 2. Ensure stable control of hypertension and diabetes mellitus if any • During treatment: 1. Monitor fasting blood glucose, liver function test, and blood pressure at least every other week 2. Observe for mood changes or mental disturbance • Adjunctive treatments: 1. Proton pump inhibitors (to prevent peptic ulcer) if needed
Absolute contraindications	• Recent viral hepatitis or significant hepatic dysfunction • Severe cardiovascular disease(s) • Uncontrolled severe hypertension or unstable diabetes mellitus • Active psychiatric disorders

From Robertson RP et al: *DeGroot's endocrinology: basic science and clinical practice,* ed 8, Philadelphia, 2023, Elsevier.

TABLE 8 Post–Radioactive Iodine Therapy Glucocorticoid Prophylaxis for Patients with Graves Hyperthyroidism

INDICATIONS ACCORDING TO DIFFERENT SCENARIOS

Graves Orbitopathy (GO) Status	Other Risk Factors[a] Present?	Radioactive Iodine Therapy (RAI) as One of the Possible Treatment Options?	GLUCOCORTICOID PROPHYLAXIS INDICATED?	
			ATA 2016[b]	ETA 2018[c]
No preexisting GO	No	Yes	No	No
No preexisting GO	Yes	Yes	Insufficient data for recommendation	Yes
Inactive mild-to-severe GO	No	Yes	No	No
Inactive mild-to-severe GO	Yes	Yes	No	Yes
Active mild GO	No	Yes	Yes, consider risk-benefit ratio	Yes
Active mild GO	Yes	Yes	Yes	Yes
Active moderate-to-severe GO or sight-threatening GO		No, RAI should be avoided		

REGIMENS OF GLUCOCORTICOID PROPHYLAXIS

Regimen	Dosing	When to Start?	Remarks
Standard-dose oral prednisone	0.4-0.5 mg/kg body weight daily for 4 wk, then taper over 8 wk	1-3 days after RAI	• Most well-validated regimen
Low-dose oral prednisone	0.2-0.3 mg/kg body weight daily, reduce by 2.5-5 mg every 7-14 wk, total 6 wk	1 day after RAI	• Not consistently effective • Better reserved for low-risk patients (e.g., mild or absent GO)
Intravenous methylprednisolone	500 mg weekly for 2 wk, then 250 mg weekly for 2 wk	2 days after RAI	• Equally effective but associated with less insomnia and gastric symptoms when compared with standard-dose oral prednisone

[a]High serum thyroid-stimulating hormone receptor antibody titer (>5-fold cutoff), acute or severe hyperthyroidism (high serum free T_3 >3- to 5-fold), active smoking, recent-onset hyperthyroidism (duration <5 yr), or delayed correction of post-RAI hypothyroidism.
[b]2016 American Thyroid Association Guidelines for Diagnosis and Management of Hyperthyroidism and Other Causes of Thyrotoxicosis[2]
[c]2018 European Thyroid Association Guideline for the Management of Graves' Hyperthyroidism[3]
From Robertson RP et al: *DeGroot's Endocrinology, basic science and clinical practice,* ed 8, Philadelphia, 2023, Elsevier.

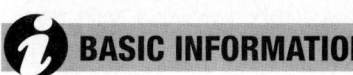
BASIC INFORMATION

DEFINITION

Head and neck squamous cell carcinoma is a malignant disease entity that arises from the epithelium of the mucosal surfaces of the upper aerodigestive tract and accounts for nearly 90% of head and neck cancers. This disease results from exposure to carcinogens and from the accumulation of genetic alterations. The workup and management of these patients depends on the specific subsite of the aerodigestive tract in the head and neck from which the primary tumor arises. These subsites are the oral cavity, oropharynx, nasopharynx, hypopharynx, and larynx. Cutaneous malignancies, thyroid neoplasms, and salivary gland neoplasms also occur in the head and neck but are beyond the scope of this chapter.

SYNONYMS

HNC
Head and neck cancer
HNSCC

ICD-10CM CODES	
C00-C14	Malignant neoplasms of lip, oral cavity, and pharynx
C30	Malignant neoplasm of nasal cavities, middle ear, and accessory sinuses
C32	Malignant neoplasm of larynx
C77.0	Secondary and unspecified malignant neoplasm of lymph nodes of head, face, and neck

EPIDEMIOLOGY & DEMOGRAPHICS

INCIDENCE:
- U.S. annual incidence of head and neck cancer (90% of which is squamous cell carcinoma) is ~62,000 persons/yr.
- Annual mortality is ~13,000 persons/yr.
- Accounts for ~3% of all cancers in the U.S. and >1.5% of all cancer deaths.
- Head and neck cancer was the seventh most common cancer worldwide in 2018.
- Human papillomavirus (HPV)-associated squamous cell carcinoma of the head and neck accounts for 5% to 20% of all HNSCCs, and 40% to 90% of those that arise in oropharynx.
- Incidence of all forms of HNSCC is on the decline, except oropharyngeal squamous cell carcinoma, which is increasing in incidence, likely related to the rise in human papilloma virus (HPV) associated HNSCC.

PREDOMINANT SEX & AGE: Male:female ratio is approximately 3:1. Risk increases significantly over the age of 40.

PEAK INCIDENCE: Sixth decade of life.

RISK FACTORS: The two most strongly implicated risk factors associated with HNSCC are tobacco and alcohol use. These carcinogens place the entire epithelium of the upper respiratory tract at risk for multiple primary tumors via a process known as field cancerization. More

recently, a new subset of HNSCC caused by the HPV has been increasing in prevalence. HPV 16 is the most common genotype detected. Patients are more likely to be white middle-aged men, nonsmokers, with minimal alcohol use and higher socioeconomic status.

GENETICS: Research is ongoing in genetic factors that lead to the development and progression of HNSCC. Tumor-suppressor genes, including *p53*, *NOTCH1*, and *CDKN2A*, among others, have been shown to harbor mutations in patients with HNSCC.

PHYSICAL FINDINGS & CLINICAL PRESENTATION

- Presenting signs and symptoms are related to local effects of the primary tumor, regional spread, metastatic disease, or paraneoplastic phenomena:
  1. Oral cavity, oropharynx, hypopharynx: Painful mass or ulceration (Fig. E1), dysphagia, odynophagia, weight loss
  2. Larynx: Hoarseness, voice change, shortness of breath, stridor
  3. Nasal cavity, paranasal sinus, nasopharynx: Referred otalgia, conductive hearing loss from middle ear effusion, epistaxis, cranial nerve palsies
  4. All sites: Cranial nerve palsies, painless neck mass from regional metastases to cervical lymph nodes. Most common site of distant metastases is the lung, with bone and liver being much less common
- Physical examination: A thorough examination of the head and neck, including cranial nerve examination, otoscopy, inspection and palpation of oral cavity, oropharynx, and neck, and general physical examination:
  1. Concerning examination findings: Unilateral middle ear effusion, ulcerated mass of the oral cavity (Fig. E2) or oropharynx, trismus, painless neck mass

ETIOLOGY

Exposure to carcinogens, including tobacco and alcohol, causes genetic alterations in the epithelium of mucosal surfaces lining the upper aerodigestive tract, leading to malignant transformation of epithelial cells. HPV-associated HNSCC is a direct result of the carcinogenic effects of the virus and is not related to alcohol and tobacco use. Primary nasopharyngeal carcinoma has a weak association with tobacco and alcohol and is endemic to southern China, Southeast Asia, and northern Africa. There is a strong association between Epstein-Barr virus infection and primary nasopharyngeal carcinoma.

Dx DIAGNOSIS

DIFFERENTIAL DIAGNOSIS

Lymphoma, primary salivary gland malignancy, thyroid malignancy, benign tumors of the upper aerodigestive tract, metastases

WORKUP

Initial workup includes a full physical examination, indirect and/or direct laryngoscopy, imaging

studies of the head and neck as well as the chest and/or body to assess for metastases, laboratory tests as indicated, and referral to a head and neck cancer specialist.

Additional workup by head and neck cancer specialist:
- Flexible fiberoptic laryngoscopy or mirror laryngoscopy
- Biopsy of the tumor in office or under anesthesia
- Fine-needle aspiration (FNA) and biopsy for patient who presents with a suspicious neck mass
- Panendoscopy with biopsy under anesthesia, which may include direct laryngoscopy, esophagoscopy, and/or bronchoscopy

LABORATORY TESTS

CBC, coagulation studies, electrolytes, ECG, liver function tests (albumin, transaminases, alkaline phosphatase), thyroid-stimulating hormone (TSH)

IMAGING STUDIES

- Computed tomography (CT) scan of the neck with contrast: Necessary to evaluate extent of primary tumor and nodal metastases in neck (Fig. E3)
- MRI of head and neck (optional): Useful for nasopharyngeal, infratemporal fossa, temporal bone, parotid, parapharyngeal, skull base, or intracranial involvement
- Chest x-ray examination or CT chest with contrast: To evaluate for lung metastases
- PET/CT (Fig. E4): Highlights areas in the body with increased metabolic uptake. Useful initially to assess extent of primary tumor, location of unknown primary tumor, cervical metastases, distant metastases, and second primary tumors. Can be used to monitor for recurrence in the posttreatment setting

STAGING

Staging is based on the tumor, node, metastasis (TNM) staging system provided by the AJCC (Table 1). Staging varies depending on the head and neck subsite that is involved. Any nodal metastasis in the neck automatically classifies as advanced disease (stage III or IV). Distant metastases place patients at stage IVC. The exception to this is HPV-positive cancer of the oropharynx, in which the most recent staging system allows for a patient to be classified as low as stage II even with cervical nodal metastases given the excellent response to treatment and prognosis for these tumors.

Rx TREATMENT

- Treatment consists of surgery, radiation, chemotherapy, or a combination of any or all of the three modalities. The goal is to use as few modalities as possible to minimize side effects of treatment without compromising oncologic success.
  1. Surgery (Fig. E5): Complete surgical resection of the primary tumor along with unilateral or bilateral neck dissections to remove involved or potentially involved lymph nodes as clinically indicated.

TABLE 1 TNM Staging System for Cutaneous Squamous Cell Carcinoma of the Head and Neck

T: Primary Tumor

T_X	Primary tumor cannot be assessed
T_{is}	Carcinoma in situ
T_1	Tumor <2 cm in greatest dimension
T_2	Tumor ≥2 cm, but <4 cm in greatest dimension
T_3	Tumor ≥4 cm in maximum dimension or minor bone erosion or perineural invasion[a]
T_4	Tumor with gross cortical bone/marrow, skull base invasion and/or skull base foramen invasion
T_{4a}	Tumor with gross cortical bone/marrow invasion
T_{4b}	Tumor with skull base invasion and/or skull base foramen involvement

N: Regional Lymph Nodes

Clinical N (cN)

N_X	Regional lymph nodes cannot be assessed
N_0	No regional lymph node metastasis
N_1	Metastasis in single ipsilateral lymph node, ≤3 cm in greatest dimension and ENE(−)
N_2	Metastasis in single ipsilateral lymph node, >3 cm but not >6 cm in greatest dimension and ENE(−); or in multiple ipsilateral lymph nodes, none >6 cm in greatest dimension; or in bilateral or contralateral lymph nodes and ENE(−), none >6 cm in greatest dimension and ENE(−)
N_{2a}	Metastasis in single ipsilateral lymph node, >3 cm but no >6 cm in greatest dimension and ENE(−)
N_{2b}	Metastasis in multiple ipsilateral lymph nodes, none >6 cm in greatest dimension and ENE(−)
N_{2c}	Metastasis in bilateral or contralateral lymph nodes, none >6 cm in greatest dimension and ENE(−)
N_3	Metastasis in lymph node, >6 cm in greatest dimension and ENE(−); or metastasis in any node(s) and clinically overt ENE [ENE(+)]
N_{3a}	Metastasis in a lymph node >6 cm in greatest dimension and ENE(−)
N_{3b}	Metastasis in any node(s) and ENE(+)

Pathologic N (pN)

N_X	Regional lymph nodes cannot be assessed
N_0	No regional lymph node metastasis
N_1	Metastasis in single ipsilateral lymph node, ≤3 cm in greatest dimension and ENE(−)
N_2	Metastasis in single ipsilateral lymph node, ≤3 cm in greatest dimension and ENE(+), or >3 cm but not >6 cm in greatest dimension and ENE(−); or metastases in multiple ipsilateral lymph nodes, none >6 cm in greatest dimension and ENE(−); or in bilateral or contralateral lymph nodes, none >6 cm in greatest dimension and ENE(−)
N_{2a}	Metastasis in single ipsilateral lymph node, ≤3 cm in greatest dimension and ENE(+), or a single ipsilateral node >3 cm but not >6 cm in greatest dimension and ENE(−)
N_{2b}	Metastasis in multiple ipsilateral lymph nodes, none >6 cm in greatest dimension and ENE(−)
N_{2c}	Metastasis in bilateral or contralateral lymph nodes, none >6 cm in greatest dimension and ENE(−)
N_3	Metastasis in lymph node, >6 cm in greatest dimension and ENE(−); or in a single ipsilateral node >3 cm in greatest dimension and ENE(+), or multiple ipsilateral, contralateral, or bilateral nodes, any with ENE(+)
N_{3a}	Metastasis in a lymph node >6 cm in greatest dimension and ENE(−)
N_{3b}	Metastasis in a single ipsilateral node >3 cm in greatest dimension and ENE(+), or multiple ipsilateral, contralateral, or bilateral nodes, any with ENE(+)

Note: A designation of *U* or *L* may be used for any N category to indicate metastasis above the lower border of the cricoid *(U)* or below the lower border of the cricoid *(L)*. Similarly, clinical and pathologic ENE should be recorded as ENE(−) or ENE(+).

M: Metastasis

M_0	No distant metastasis
M_1	Present distant metastasis

Staging for Cutaneous Squamous Cell Carcinoma

Stage 0	T_{is}	N_0	M_0
Stage I	T_1	N_0	M_0
Stage II	T_2	N_0	M_0
Stage III	T_3	N_0	M_0
Stage III	T_1	N_1	M_0
Stage III	T_2	N_1	M_0
Stage III	T_3	N_1	M_0
Stage IV	T_1	N_2	M_0
Stage IV	T_2	N_2	M_0
Stage IV	T_3	N_2	M_0
Stage IV	Any T	N_3	M_0
Stage IV	T_4	Any N	M_0
Stage IV	Any T	Any N	M1

ENE, Extranodal extension; *TNM,* tumor, node, metastasis.

[a]Deep invasion is defined as invasion beyond the subcutaneous fat or >6 mm (as measured from the granular layer of adjacent normal epidermis to the base of the tumor); perineural invasion for T_3 classification is defined as tumor cells within the nerve sheath of a nerve lying deeper than the dermis or measuring ≥0.1 mm in caliper or manifesting with clinical or radiographic involvement of named nerves without skull base invasion or transgression.

From Amin MB et al: *American Joint Committee on Cancer staging manual,* ed 8, Chicago, 2017, Springer.

2. Radiation: Allows for easier access to poorly exposed tumors such as those of the larynx, oropharynx, nasopharynx, or hypopharynx. Disadvantages include lengthy, time-intensive treatment course, xerostomia, pain, and higher surgical morbidity if salvage surgery is needed.

3. Chemotherapy: Useful only as an adjuvant to radiation therapy or for palliation. Single-agent cisplatin therapy is widely accepted in the U.S. as a standard for chemoradiation regimens for head and neck cancers of any site. Major toxicities include nausea, vomiting, renal toxicity, ototoxicity, and myelosuppression.

4. Reconstruction: Performed with the goal of optimizing functional and cosmetic outcomes. Options include primary closure, local flaps, regional flaps, skin grafts, and microvascular free flaps from other parts of the body (e.g., radial forearm, fibula, anterolateral thigh, latissimus, etc.).

ACUTE GENERAL Rx

- Early-stage disease (stage I or II):
  1. Single-modality treatment with surgery or radiation alone may be appropriate for early-stage head and neck cancer. The choice between one or the other depends on the specific subsite of the head and neck that is involved and the side effects profile for each modality.
  2. Treatment of the potentially involved lymph nodes in the neck with either neck dissection or radiation is controversial and depends on the clinical scenario and the judgment of the treatment team.

- Locoregionally advanced disease (stage III or IV):
  1. In general, these patients have large tumors >4 cm and/or cervical nodal metastases. Treatment typically involves multimodality therapy with either surgery followed by radiation therapy or upfront chemoradiation alone. Depending on the presence of certain adverse pathologic features of the surgical specimen, adjuvant chemoradiation may be necessary. If chemoradiation is the initial treatment modality, surgery may be needed in the adjuvant setting for residual or recurrent disease.
  2. Laryngeal cancers are the exception where select advanced disease with T_3 or N_1 tumors can be managed with single-modality therapy with surgery or radiation alone.
  3. Nasopharyngeal cancer is also an exception. This is not a surgical disease. Managed primarily by radiation to primary site and neck for early-stage disease. Chemoradiation is primary treatment for advanced disease. Surgery is reserved for recurrent or residual disease of primary site or neck following radiation therapy.
- Metastatic disease (stage IVC):
  1. Palliation of symptoms is the primary goal of treatment.
- All patients should be counseled on smoking cessation and avoidance of alcohol.

DISPOSITION

- Prognosis depends on the specific subsite of the head and neck that is involved. Overall 5-yr survival rate for head and neck squamous cell carcinoma is about 55%. This varies with 5-yr survival rates for carcinoma of the lip as high as 89.7% and carcinomas of the hypopharynx as low as ~30%.
- Patients are followed on a regular basis multiple times a year by a head and neck cancer specialist. After a 5-yr disease-free survival, patients are followed on a yearly basis.

REFERRAL

Referral should be made to an otolaryngologist or oral surgeon who specializes in head and neck cancer.

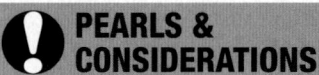 **PEARLS & CONSIDERATIONS**

PREVENTION

- Encourage all patients to cease using tobacco and to limit alcohol consumption.
- Examine the oral cavity and palpate the neck during the annual physical examination. Workup any suspicious masses or lesions.

PATIENT & FAMILY EDUCATION

- ENT Health: https://www.entnet.org/content/head-and-neck-cancer
- National Cancer Institute: https://www.cancer.gov/types/head-and-neck

RELATED CONTENT

Laryngeal Carcinoma (Related Key Topic)
Oral Cancer (Related Key Topic)

SUGGESTED READINGS
Available at eBooks.Health.Elsevier.com.

AUTHOR: **LOUIS F. INSALACO, MD**

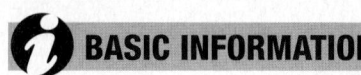
BASIC INFORMATION

DEFINITION

Complete heart block (CHB) is the absence of electrical impulse transmission from the atria to the ventricles when atrioventricular (AV) junction is not physiologically refractory, because of a functional or anatomic impairment of the conduction system, resulting in a bradycardia characterized by AV dissociation. It may be acquired or congenital. CHB can be permanent or reversible. Degenerative changes are the most common cause of CHB.[1]

SYNONYMS

Third-degree AV block
CHB
Complete AV block

ICD-10CM CODE
I44.2	Atrioventricular block, complete

EPIDEMIOLOGY & DEMOGRAPHICS

- The prevalence of CHB is 0.04%.
- The prevalence of CHB increases with age.

PHYSICAL FINDINGS & CLINICAL PRESENTATION

Physical examination may be normal. Cannon A waves may appear in the jugular vein periodically due to the right atrium contracting (against closed tricuspid valve) during ventricular systole. Patients may present with the following clinical manifestations:

- Dizziness, palpitations
- Syncope or presyncope (due to reduced cardiac output)
- Fatigue, shortness of breath, and impaired exercise tolerance
- Mental status changes
- Congestive heart failure
- Angina pectoris
- Some patients may be asymptomatic (e.g., congenital CHB, fast junctional escape rhythm)
- Sudden cardiac arrest

ETIOLOGY

- Fibrosis or sclerosis of the conduction system, Lenègre and Lev diseases[2]
- Acute myocardial infarction (MI)—inferior (14%) or anterior (2%) wall of patients, usually within 24 h
- Drug effect (digitalis, calcium channel blockers, beta-blockers, amiodarone, adenosine)
- Cardiomyopathy and myocarditis (rheumatic fever, diphtheria, viruses, toxoplasmosis, syphilis, COVID-19)
- Bacterial endocarditis with paravalvular abscess formation (e.g., AV endocarditis)
- Infiltrative processes of the myocardium (amyloidosis, sarcoidosis, scleroderma, tumor)[3]
- Metabolic abnormalities (hyperkalemia, hypoxia, hypothyroidism)
- Lyme carditis, rheumatoid nodules, polymyositis, Chagas disease
- Neuromuscular disorders (Becker muscular dystrophy, myotonic muscular dystrophy)
- Congenital (birth from mothers with systemic lupus, large atrial septal defect, and AV canal defects)
- Familial: SCN5 sodium channel mutations have been associated with CHB
- Iatrogenic (cardiac surgery, catheter ablation of arrhythmias, percutaneous coronary intervention). Transcatheter aortic valve implantation (TAVI) is frequently associated with new conduction abnormalities (2% to 8%); patients with preexisting right bundle branch block are at increased risk of CHB (resolves over time in most patients)
- Paroxysmal due to phase 4 block of the His-Purkinje system

DIAGNOSIS

DIFFERENTIAL DIAGNOSIS

- The differential diagnosis includes lesser degree of AV block, automatic accelerated junctional rhythms, and nonconducted premature atrial contractions.
- The atrial rate must be faster than the ventricular rate (more As than Vs), and the junctional or ventricular rate is regular. Episodes of AV dissociation with an accelerated ventricular or junctional pacemaker overtaking the sinus node can often mimic heart block on a single ECG.

WORKUP

- Workup such as routine laboratory tests, cardiac biomarkers, and cardiac imaging should be dictated by the clinical circumstances.
- ECG: Diagnostic of the disease (Figs. 1 and 2):
  1. P waves are present with a regular atrial rate that is faster than the ventricular rate.
  2. P waves are not related to the QRS complexes. The PR intervals are variable.
  3. RR intervals are regular.
  4. QRS complexes may be narrow with a rate of 40 to 60 beats/min (block proximal to His bundle) or wide with a rate of <40 beats/min (block distal to His bundle), depending on the location of the block in the conduction system.
  5. Complete AV block can result from block at the level of AV node, within the His bundle, or distal to it, in the Purkinje system.

TREATMENT

ACUTE GENERAL Rx

- Initial treatment should focus on the hemodynamic stability and symptoms of the patient.
- Fig. 3 illustrates the evaluation and management of third-degree AV block.
- Consider temporary pacemaker insertion if ventricular escape rate is slow (<40 beats/min) and associated with symptoms or hemodynamic compromise as well as wide QRS escape rhythms, which can be unstable, and

QT prolongation above 500 ms, increasing the risk of torsades de pointes ventricular tachycardias.

- CHB as a complication of inferior MI usually only requires temporary pacing; however, CHB because of anterior MI often requires permanent pacing due to direct injury to the conduction system (Table 1).
- Acquired CHB usually requires pacing, but patients with congenital CHB often have sufficiently rapid escape rhythm to prevent symptoms and avoid permanent pacemaker implantation.
- Withdraw AV-nodal blocking agents if any.
- Short-term therapy (until adequate pacing therapy is established):
  1. Vagolytic agents such as atropine may be used to increase the rate of the escape rhythm (for AV nodal level blocks).
  2. Catecholamines such as isoproterenol transiently used for a CHB at any site (use with extreme caution or not at all in patients with coronary artery disease or in patients with digitalis toxicity).
  3. Percutaneous external cardiac pacing (use only in emergent, unstable situation as it is uncomfortable for patients and may not always reliably capture the ventricle).
- Drugs cannot be relied on to increase heart rate (HR) for more than several hours or days without side effects; therefore, temporary or permanent pacemaker insertion is indicated.
- Symptomatic CHB in the absence of a condition that is likely to resolve is an American College of Cardiology (ACC)/American Heart Association (AHA)/Heart Rhythm Society (HRS) Class I indication for permanent pacemaker (PPM) placement.
- Class I indications for PPM placement in asymptomatic patients according to the ACC/AHA guidelines include:[1]
  1. Patients in sinus rhythm, with asystolic pauses greater than or equal to 3.0 sec or an escape rate <40 beats/min, or with an escape rhythm that is below the AV node
  2. Patients with atrial fibrillation and bradycardia with one or more pauses of at least 5 sec or longer
  3. After catheter ablation of the AV junction
  4. If cardiomegaly or left ventricular dysfunction is present with ventricular rates of 40 beats/min or faster
  5. Postoperative CHB that is not expected to resolve
  6. Symptomatic AV block because of guideline-directed medical therapy for which there is no alternative treatment with strong evidence of therapy benefit (beta-blockers in coronary artery disease [CAD] or heart failure with reduced ejection fraction [HFrEF])
  7. When it is associated with neuromuscular diseases, such as Erb dystrophy (limb-girdle muscular dystrophy), Kearns-Sayre syndrome, myotonic muscular dystrophy, and peroneal muscular atrophy
  8. CHB present during exercise in the absence of myocardial ischemia

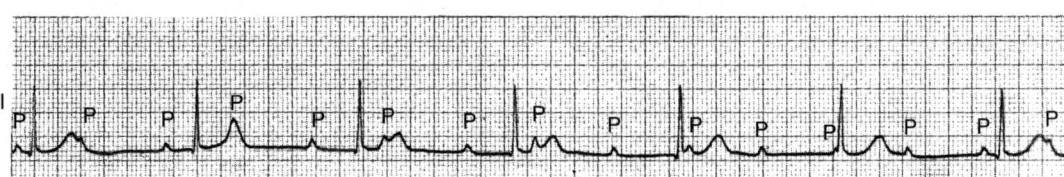

FIG. 1 Third-degree (complete) atrioventricular heart block is characterized by independent atrial *(P)* and ventricular (QRS) activity. The atrial rate is always faster than the ventricular rate. The PR intervals are completely variable. Some P waves fall on the T wave, distorting its shape. Others may fall in the QRS complex and be "lost." Notice that the QRS complexes are of normal width, indicating that the ventricles are being paced from the atrioventricular junction.

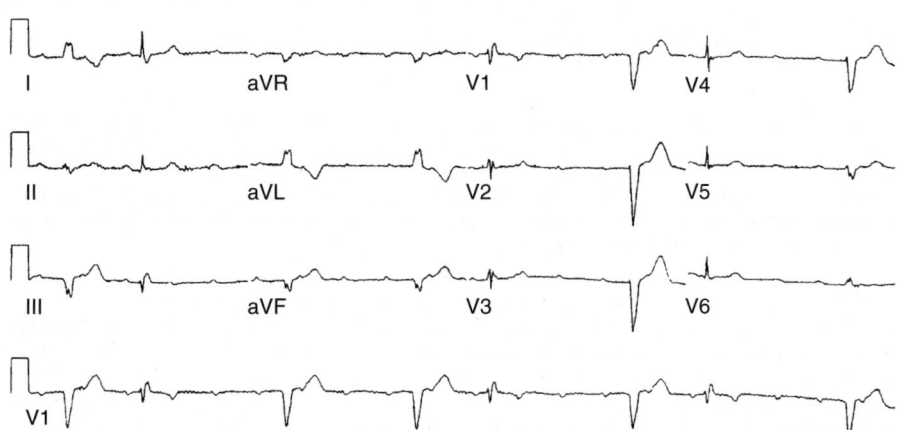

FIG. 2 High-grade atrioventricular block. Note that only three P waves conducted to the ventricle in the whole tracing. Conducted P waves were associated with normal PR intervals and right bundle branch block, a finding suggesting infranodal block. All other P waves were blocked, and ventricular escape rhythm with a left bundle branch block pattern is observed. Note that the block is not caused by retrograde concealment in the atrioventricular node or His-Purkinje system from the ventricular escape complexes because the conducted P waves occurred at a short cycle following the escape complexes. *aVF,* Augmented vector foot; *aVL,* augmented vector left; *aVR,* augmented vector right. (From Issa Z et al: *Clinical arrhythmology and electrophysiology,* ed 2, Philadelphia, 2012, Saunders.)

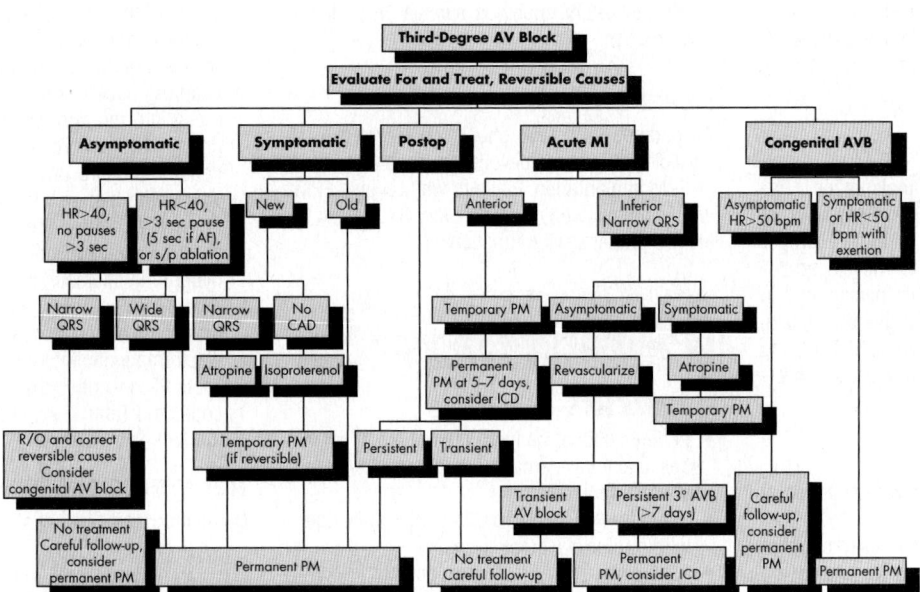

FIG. 3 Evaluation and management of third-degree atrioventricular *(AV)* block. *AF,* Atrial flutter; *AVB,* atrioventricular block; *bpm,* beats per minute; *CAD,* coronary artery disease; *HR,* heart rate; *ICD,* implantable cardioverter defibrillator; *MI,* myocardial infarction; *PM,* pacemaker; *R/O,* rule out; *s/p,* after. (From Olshansky B et al: *Arrhythmia essentials,* ed 2, Philadelphia, 2017, Elsevier.)

TABLE 1	Indications for Pacing in AV Block

Class I

1. Third-degree or advanced second-degree AV block at any anatomic level associated with any one of the following conditions:
   a. Symptoms (including heart failure) or ventricular arrhythmias attributable to AV block *(Level of Evidence: C)*
   b. Arrhythmias and other medical conditions that require drugs that result in symptomatic bradycardia *(Level of Evidence: C)*
   c. Documented periods of asystole >3.0 sec, any escape rate <40 beats/min, or any escape rhythm below the AV junction (e.g., a wide QRS morphology) in awake, asymptomatic patients in sinus rhythm *(Level of Evidence: C)*
   d. A documented period of asystole >5 sec in awake, asymptomatic patients in atrial fibrillation *(Level of Evidence: C)*
   e. After catheter ablation of the AV junction *(Level of Evidence: C)*
   f. Postoperative AV block that is not expected to resolve after cardiac surgery *(Level of Evidence: C)*
   g. Neuromuscular diseases, such as myotonic muscular dystrophy, Kearns–Sayre syndrome, Erb (limb-girdle) dystrophy, and peroneal muscular atrophy, with or without symptoms of bradycardia *(Level of Evidence: B)*
2. Asymptomatic third-degree AV block at any anatomic site with an average awake ventricular rate >40 beats/min in patients with cardiomegaly or left ventricular dysfunction or if the site of block is below the AV node *(Level of Evidence: B)*
3. Second-degree or third-degree AV block during exercise in the absence of myocardial ischemia *(Level of Evidence: C)*
4. Symptomatic second-degree AV block regardless of type or site of block *(Level of Evidence: B)*

Class IIa

1. Persistent third-degree AV block at any anatomic site with an average ventricular rate >40 beats/min in asymptomatic adult patients in the absence of cardiomegaly *(Level of Evidence: C)*
2. Asymptomatic second-degree AV block at intra- or infra-His levels found at electrophysiologic study *(Level of Evidence: B)*
3. First-degree or second-degree AV block with symptoms similar to those of pacemaker syndrome or hemodynamic compromise *(Level of Evidence: B)*
4. Asymptomatic type II second-degree AV block with a narrow QRS. When type II second-degree AV block occurs with a wide QRS, including isolated right bundle branch block, pacing becomes a Class I recommendation *(Level of Evidence: B)*

Class IIb

1. AV block due to drug use or toxicity when the block is expected to recur even after withdrawal of the drug *(Level of Evidence: B)*
2. Neuromuscular diseases, such as myotonic muscular dystrophy, Kearns–Sayre syndrome, Erb (limb-girdle) dystrophy, and peroneal muscular atrophy with any degree of AV block (including first-degree AV block), with or without symptoms of bradycardia *(Level of Evidence: B)*

Class III

1. Asymptomatic first-degree AV block *(Level of Evidence: B)*
2. Asymptomatic type I second-degree AV block at supra-His (i.e., the AV node) level or another site or not known to be intra- or infra-Hisian by electrophysiologic study *(Level of Evidence: C)*
3. AV block expected to resolve and unlikely to recur (e.g., drug toxicity, Lyme disease, or transient increases in vagal tone or during hypoxia in sleep apnea in the absence of symptoms) *(Level of Evidence: B)*

AV, Atrioventricular.
From Bonow RO et al: *Braunwald's heart disease: a textbook of cardiovascular medicine,* ed 11, Philadelphia, 2019, Saunders.

- Therapy is directed toward the underlying etiology if there is a reversible source (i.e., intravenous [IV] antibiotics for Lyme disease).
- Table 2 summarizes the management of CHB.

CHRONIC Rx

Dual-chamber pacemaker implantation. Patients with a pacemaker need regular follow-up and pacemaker monitoring to ensure proper device functioning. Interest has developed recently in placing the ventricular pacing lead in the His bundle region or left bundle region, which can result in a narrow-paced QRS and may prevent ventricular dyssynchrony associated with traditional RV pacing.[4]

DISPOSITION

- Mortality is highest in the neonatal period in congenital CHB.
- Prognosis is favorable after insertion of a pacemaker and is related to the underlying etiology of complete AV block (e.g., myocardial infarction, cardiomyopathy).

- Nonrandomized studies have shown that PPM insertion improves survival in patients with CHB.

REFERRAL

All patients with CHB should be referred to a cardiologist for consideration of temporary and/or PPM implantation. Patients who receive PPM should be followed routinely every 6 to 12 mo to ensure proper device functioning.

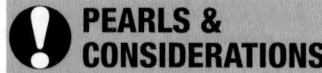
PEARLS & CONSIDERATIONS

COMMENTS

- Patients should be instructed to avoid activities that may damage the pacemaker (e.g., contact sports).
- Patients should be followed by cardiologist with routine pacemaker check.
- Pacemaker manufacturers do not recommend any special restrictions regarding proximity to typical household items.

- All pacemaker manufacturers offer pacemakers that are MRI compatible. Older pacemaker models and leads may have a strong relative contraindication for MRI.
- Leadless pacemakers that are implanted directly into the right ventricle using a special delivery system are available for special indications and are primarily used for patients who are at high risk for traditional pacemakers and do not require dual-chamber pacing.
- Some medical procedures, such as lithotripsy, hyperbaric chamber, and electrocautery used during surgery, may require pacemaker programming and testing perioperatively to avoid electromagnetic interference.
- Table E3 describes the five-letter pacemaker code, and Table 4 summarizes common permanent pacemakers.

RELATED CONTENT

Complete Heart Block (Patient Information)

REFERENCES

Available at eBooks.Health.Elsevier.com.

AUTHOR: **MOHAMMAD TARAWNEH, MD**

TABLE 2 Complete Heart Block Management

Setting	Therapy
Asymptomatic–Acquired	<ul><li>Rule out reversible causes, including: 1. Hyperkalemia. 2. Acute inferior MI. 3. Digoxin toxicity. 4. Excess calcium channel blocker therapy. 5. Lyme disease.</li><li>If HR <40 beats/min, first-line therapy is a permanent DDD pacemaker.</li><li>Temporary pacing is indicated if heart rate <40 beats/min.</li><li>The patient has impaired hemodynamics, and if permanent, pacing cannot be accomplished expeditiously.</li><li>The CHB has an identifiable and reversible cause, while awaiting recovery.</li><li>Temporary transvenous pacing must be used with caution in patients with any escape rhythm, particularly if wide QRS complex and slow.</li><li>Overdrive suppression can occur rapidly.</li><li>If the rate of escape rhythm >40 beats/min, permanent pacemaker insertion is controversial.</li><li>Temporary pacing is to be avoided in asymptomatic patients whose ventricular rates are >40 beats/min, especially if the QRS complex is narrow.</li><li>CHB due to radio frequency ablation of the AV junction to control ventricular response rate in atrial fibrillation requires permanent pacing.</li><li>May occur even if the patient is asymptomatic from a slow ventricular rate (40 beats/min) that may be quite stable over time.</li><li>Acquired CHB is associated with a poor short-term prognosis (>50% mortality in the first 6-12 mo after diagnosis).</li><li>If irreversible, pacing is indicated.</li></ul>
Symptomatic	<ul><li>A permanent pacemaker is indicated.</li><li>Temporary pacing is indicated if permanent pacing cannot be done expeditiously or if CHB has an identifiable and reversible cause (e.g., drug overdose).</li></ul>
Congenital	<ul><li>Usually associated with a narrow QRS complex with an escape rhythm arising in the AVN.</li><li>Patients are usually asymptomatic.</li><li>In patients who are asymptomatic, the indications for a pacemaker are controversial.</li><li>Patients will need close follow-up, at least annually, for evaluation of symptoms suggesting chronotropic incompetence.</li><li>If symptomatic bradycardia, a permanent pacemaker is indicated.</li><li>If rate is consistently <50 beats/min and does not increase with exercise (chronotropic incompetence), a permanent pacemaker is indicated.</li><li>Myocardial infarction If symptomatic bradycardia, a temporary pacemaker is indicated.</li><li>If CHB block occurs in the setting of an anterior infarction, permanent pacing is indicated if AVB persists.</li><li>CHB in inferior MI is generally in the AVN.</li><li>There is usually no need for a permanent pacemaker, as it usually resolves.</li><li>If it does not resolve, a permanent pacemaker may be indicated in some cases.</li></ul>
Preoperative	<ul><li>Permanent pacemaker first, unless the surgery is emergent.</li><li>If surgery is emergent, insert a temporary pacemaker preoperative with the plan for a permanent pacemaker after surgery.</li></ul>
Postoperative	<ul><li>Transcutaneous or temporary transvenous pacing.</li><li>A permanent pacemaker is indicated if there is permanent damage to the AV conduction system (e.g., after aortic valve surgery or VSD repair).</li></ul>

AV, Atrioventricular; *AVB,* atrioventricular block; *AVN,* atrioventricular node; *CHB,* complete atrioventricular block; *DDD,* dual chamber; *HR,* heart rate; *MI,* myocardial infarction; *VSD,* ventricular septal defect.

From Olshansky B et al: *Arrhythmia essentials,* ed 2, Philadelphia, 2017, Elsevier.

TABLE 4 Common Permanent Pacemakers

Code	Indication	Advantages	Disadvantages
VVI	Intermittent backup pacing; inactive patient	Simplicity; low cost	Fixed rate; risk of pacemaker syndrome
VVIR	Atrial fibrillation	Rate responsive	Requires advanced programming
DDD	Complete heart block	Atrial tracking restores normal physiology	No rate responsiveness; requires two leads and advanced programming
DDDR	Sinus node dysfunction; for rate responsiveness atrioventricular block and need	Universal pacer; all options available by programming	Complexity, cost, programming, and follow-up evaluation

From Marx JA et al: *Rosen's emergency medicine: concepts and clinical practice,* ed 8, Philadelphia, 2014, Saunders.

BASIC INFORMATION

DEFINITION

Second-degree heart block or second-degree atrioventricular (AV) heart block is characterized by a failure of one or more, but not all, atrial impulses to conduct to the ventricles. The block may be at any level of the AV conduction system. In both types of second-degree heart block, the sinus rate will continue at regular intervals, resulting in a constant sinus rate. When more than one atrial impulse is present for each ventricular complex, the rhythm may be described as a ratio of the number of atrial impulses to the number of ventricular complexes. Electrocardiographically there are three types of second-degree block:

- Mobitz I (Wenckebach):
  1. Characterized by a progressive prolongation of the PR interval prior to a blocked nonconducted beat and a shorter PR interval after that blocked beat; the conducted impulse will generally be narrow. The cycle may repeat periodically, leading to "grouped beating."
  2. Site of block is usually AV node (proximal to the His bundle).
- Mobitz type II:
  1. Characterized by fixed PR intervals before and after blocked beats and may be associated with a wide QRS morphology (right bundle branch block [RBBB] or left bundle branch block [LBBB] patterns).
  2. Site of block is usually infranodal, especially when QRS is wide.
  3. It has a greater propensity for progressing to third-degree AV block.
- Pure 2:1 conduction patterns cannot be reliably classified as Mobitz type I or type II because there are not enough P waves to characterize prolongation of the PR interval.
- Intrahisian block can also occur in the setting a short PR interval and a narrow QRS.

SYNONYMS

Wenckebach block (Mobitz type I block)
Mobitz type II block
AV block

EPIDEMIOLOGY & DEMOGRAPHICS

Mobitz type I block is more common and may occur in individuals with heightened vagal tone

or as a side effect of medications, such as β-blockers or calcium channel blockers.

PHYSICAL FINDINGS & CLINICAL PRESENTATION

- Patients with Mobitz type I are usually asymptomatic. Patients with either type may feel palpitations or the feeling of "missing a beat." Sudden loss of consciousness without warning (Adams-Stokes attack) can occur in patients with Mobitz type II; however, it is much more common in patients with complete heart block.
- Type I block: There is gradual decrease in the intensity of the first heart sound with widening of the a-c interval in the central venous waveform, ending in a pause, and an a wave not followed by a v wave in the neck along with an irregular pulse.
- Type II block: The first heart sound retains a constant intensity, with intermittent ventricular pauses and a wave not followed by v waves in the neck. There is an irregular pulse for most times with intermittent pauses.

ETIOLOGY

- High vagal tone (young patients, athletes at rest)
- Degenerative changes in the AV conduction system
- Ischemia at the AV nodes (type I with inferior wall myocardial infarction [MI] and type II with anterior wall MI)
- Drugs (digitalis, quinidine, procainamide, adenosine, calcium channel blockers [nondihydropyridines], β-blockers)
- Cardiomyopathies, collagen vascular diseases, infiltrative diseases (amyloidosis, sarcoidosis, hematochromatosis)
- Myocarditis/endocarditis (infectious, e.g., Lyme disease, Chagas disease; and noninfectious, e.g., systemic lupus erythematosus)
- Hyperkalemia, hypermagnesemia
- Hypothyroidism
- Prior cardiac valve surgery
- Catheter trauma, catheter ablation for arrhythmias

DIAGNOSIS

DIFFERENTIAL DIAGNOSIS

The ECG easily and reliably distinguishes Mobitz type I from Mobitz type II block and from other conduction abnormalities. It should be distinguished from the less common phenomenon of second-degree sinoatrial node exit block.

Mobitz type I block with a normal QRS complex tends to be benign and usually does not progress to more advanced forms of AV conduction within a short period of time because the disease is mostly confined to within the AV node. Mobitz type II block often precedes the development of Adams-Stokes syncope, symptoms are frequent, prognosis is compromised, and progression to third-degree AV block is common and sudden. Thus, type II second-degree AV block with a wide QRS typically indicates diffuse conduction system disease involving even the infranodal His-Purkinje system.[1,2]

WORKUP

ECG, ambulatory monitoring (Holter or external loop recorders) in selected patients

- Mobitz type I (Fig. 1) ECG shows:
  1. Sequential and gradual prolongation of PR interval leading to a nonconducted P wave
  2. Shortened PR interval following the pause as compared with the pre-pause PR interval
  3. Progressive shortening of the R-R interval prior to nonconducted atrial impulse
  4. Usually see "grouped beating" pattern
- Mobitz type II ECG shows (Fig. 2):
  1. Fixed duration of PR interval with constant P-P and R-R intervals
  2. Sudden nonconducted P wave
  3. Abnormal QRS duration or fascicular blocks are common
- In 2:1 AV block (Fig. 3), it cannot be determined based on the 12-lead ECG whether there is Mobitz type I or type II AV block, although a wide QRS complex is suggestive of Mobitz type II:
  1. Administering atropine can improve AV conduction if the AV block is type I or within the AV node; however, if it is infranodal (i.e., type II), the increased sinus rate caused by atropine may worsen the ratio of AV conduction, resulting in worsening bradycardia.
  2. Exercise stress testing may function in the same way as atropine above. If the disease is confined to the AV node, it may improve with exercise, but in cases of Mobitz type II AV block, the degree of AV block will worsen.
  3. Carotid sinus stimulation and other vagal maneuvers may worsen the AV block if it is at the level of the AV node (i.e., Mobitz type I) but will paradoxically improve the ratio of AV conduction by slowing down the sinus rate if it is a Mobitz type II or infranodal AV block.
  4. An algorithm for evaluation of patients with 2:1 AV block is illustrated in Fig. 4.

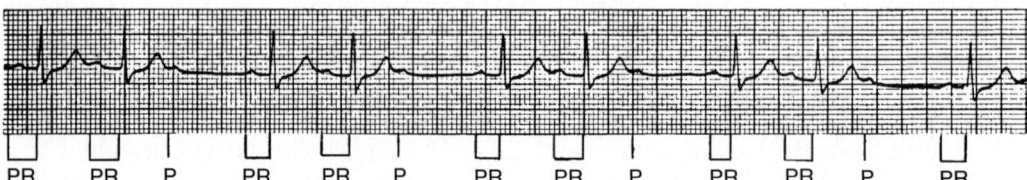

FIG. 1 Wenckebach (Mobitz type I) second-degree atrioventricular block. Notice the progressive increase in PR intervals, with the third P wave in each sequence not followed by a QRS. Wenckebach block produces a characteristically syncopated rhythm with grouping of the QRS complexes (group beating).

Rx TREATMENT

NONPHARMACOLOGIC THERAPY

Elimination of drugs that may induce AV block such as digoxin, β-blockers, and calcium channel blockers

ACUTE GENERAL Rx

- Treatment is usually not necessary unless the resting heart rate is <40 beats per min (bpm) while awake.
- If symptomatic (e.g., dizziness), atropine 1 mg (may repeat once after 5 min) may be tried to increase AV conduction; if no response, trial of dobutamine or isoproterenol may be helpful prior to insertion of a pacemaker.
- Atropine:[1]
  1. Reduces heart block due to hypervagotonia but not due to AV node ischemia
  2. Does not increase infranodal conduction (third-degree and second-degree AV block that is below the AV node)
  3. Should be used with caution in Mobitz type II AV block due to possible paradoxical decrease in heart rate (as atrial rate increases, AV conduction decreases)
  4. Is ineffective in heart transplantation patients
- If associated with anterior wall MI and wide QRS complex, consider insertion of a temporary pacemaker.
- Indications for permanent pacemaker (PPM) implantation by American College of Cardiology (ACC)/American Heart Association (AHA)/Heart Rhythm Society (HRS) 2019 guidelines:[3]
  1. Second-degree AV block with associated symptomatic bradycardia regardless of the type or site of the block (class I; level of evidence: B)
  2. Second-degree AV block provoked by exercise in the absence of myocardial ischemia (class I; level of evidence: C)
  3. Asymptomatic second-degree AV block at intra- or infra-His levels found at electrophysiologic study (class IIa; level of evidence: B)
  4. First- or second-degree AV block with symptoms similar to those of pacemaker syndrome or hemodynamic compromise (class IIa; level of evidence: B)
  5. Asymptomatic type II second-degree AV block with a wide QRS, including isolated right bundle branch block (class I; level of evidence: B)
  6. PPM is not indicated for asymptomatic type I second-degree AV block at supra-His

Lead V1

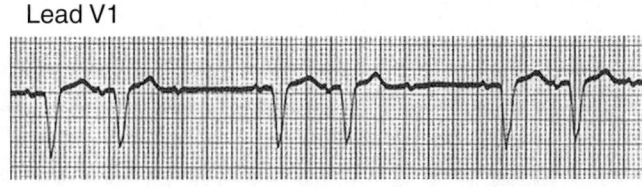

2nd degree AV block (type II) with LBBB

FIG. 2 Mobitz type II atrioventricular *(AV)* block with left bundle branch block *(LBBB).* Note the fixed P-P intervals with no change in PR intervals followed by a sudden nonconducted P wave. The LBBB indicates infranodal disease in the His-Purkinje system that is suggestive of Mobitz type II block.

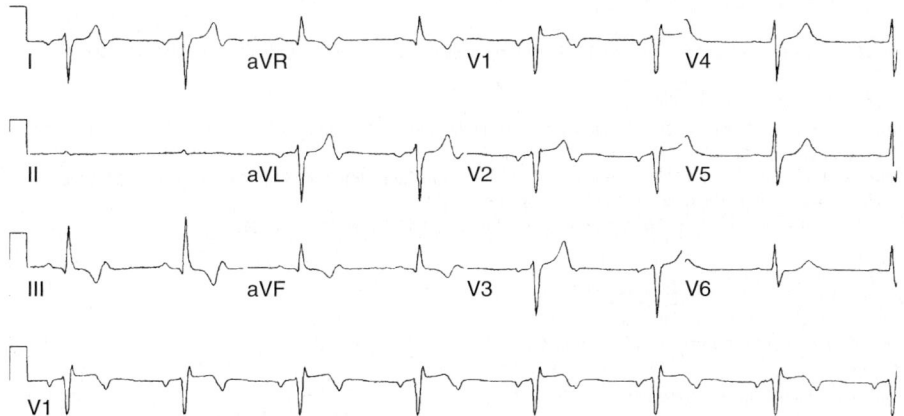

FIG. 3 Second-degree 2:1 atrioventricular block. Notice the short PR interval during conducted complexes and the wide QRS complexes, suggesting block in the His-Purkinje system. (From Issa Z et al: *Clinical arrhythmology and electrophysiology,* ed 2, Philadelphia, 2012, Saunders.)

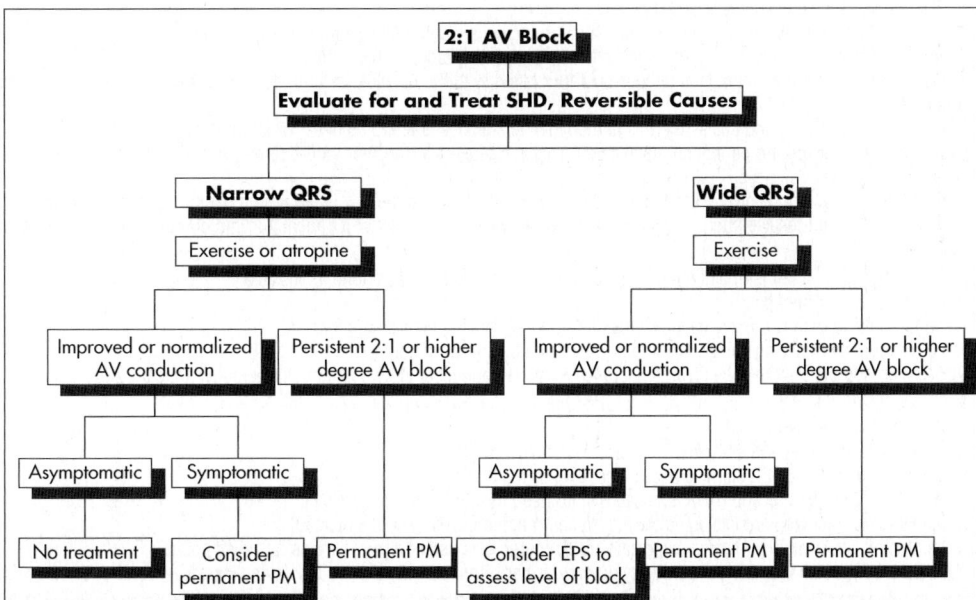

FIG. 4 Evaluation and management of 2:1 AV block. *AV,* Atrioventricular; *EPS,* electrophysiology study; *PM,* pacemaker; *SHD,* structural heart disease (no overt evidence of myocardial, valvular, congenital, or coronary heart disease). (From Olshansky B et al: *Arrhythmia essentials,* ed 2, Philadelphia, 2017, Elsevier.)

(AV node) level or that which is not known to be intra- or infra-Hisian (class III; level of evidence: C)

7. In patients with AV block who have indication for permanent pacing with left ventricular ejection fraction (LVEF) between 36% to 50% and are expected to require ventricular pacing more than 40% of the time, it is reasonable to choose pacing methods that maintain physiologic ventricular activation (e.g., CRT or His bundle pacing) over right ventricular pacing

- Table 1 summarizes the management of Mobitz type I second-degree AV block.
- Table 2 summarizes the management of Mobitz type II second-degree AV block.

DISPOSITION

Prognosis is good with insertion of a pacemaker.

REFERRAL

Referral for pacemaker insertion (see "Acute General Rx")

TABLE 1 Mobitz Type I Second-Degree Atrioventricular Block Management

Setting	Therapy
Outpatient— Asymptomatic	• Treadmill testing will help assess chronotropic competence (if this rhythm is not related to myocardial ischemia), as well as enhance AVN conduction, thereby reducing the degree of Wenckebach block (e.g., from 5:4 to 8:7 or producing first-degree AVB only). • Holter monitoring can assess the degree and level of AVB and the persistence of the problem during activities of daily living and any diurnal variation. • If the QRS duration is wide and Holter monitoring or stress testing suggests infranodal block, an electrophysiology study may help to confirm the level of AVB. • If block is demonstrated to be intra- or infra-Hisian, permanent pacemaker implantation is reasonable, even in an asymptomatic patient. • On occasion, intra-Hisian block can be demonstrated in a patient with a narrow, normal-appearing QRS complex by the production of higher degrees of AV block during treadmill testing with the increase in sinus rate. • No therapy. • If not due to reversible cause (e.g., drugs or transient damage to the AV node from Lyme disease) and the QRS duration is normal, as more advanced or complete heart block rarely develops. • There may be increased risk of syncope and symptoms in the future.
Outpatient— Symptomatic	• Some AV nodal blocking drugs (digoxin, β-adrenergic blockers, calcium blockers) may be the cause and should be reduced or stopped, if possible, and then only if severe symptomatic bradycardia occurs. • If older or at high risk for structural heart disease, consider an echocardiogram to assess LV function (even if no physical findings are present). • If due to a correctable cause such as AV nodal blocking drugs, stop the drug, if possible. • If there is a wide QRS or bundle branch block, it is possible that Wenckebach can be due to a block below the AV node (in the His-Purkinje system). • In this case, permanent pacemaker implantation is indicated. • Acutely, intravenous atropine or oral theophylline usually increases conduction through the AV node. • These may paradoxically decrease ventricular rate and increase the degree of block if the block is below the bundle of His. • Permanent pacemaker implantation is indicated if symptomatic second-degree AVB is not otherwise correctable.

Myocardial infarction	• Is often reversed during thrombolysis or angioplasty
	• May also appear for the first time concomitantly with these procedures
	• Transient in nature
	• Temporary DDD pacing for the following:
	  1. Persistent low heart rate (<40 bpm)
	  2. Low cardiac output
	  3. Ischemia
	  4. Refractory hypotension
	  5. Symptoms of light headedness and dizziness
	• Atropine or theophylline may reverse the block but can cause unwanted tachycardia during drug administration.
	• These drugs are only rarely indicated except at the time of presentation of the patient.
	• Atypical AV block is more common in inferior-posterior MIs due to the Bezold-Jarisch reflex and the effect of increased vagal tone on the AV node.
	• This is usually transient, and unless there is hemodynamic collapse, there is no need for a temporary pacemaker.
	• Rarely is there a need for a permanent pacemaker. This is true even if transient third-degree (complete) AV block occurs, as high degrees of block tend to resolve over 5-7 days.
	• If the AV block does not resolve but the ventricular rate is >40 bpm, no therapy is required if patient is asymptomatic.
	• If the block does not resolve after 7 days and/or the ventricular rate is <40 or if patient is symptomatic, a permanent pacemaker is indicated.

Preoperative	• Assess drugs given and their need; stop offending drugs that enhance vagal tone, if possible. • If no symptoms, no therapy. • If symptomatic and no reversible causes, provide temporary pacing before surgery. • Need for permanent pacing can be accomplished in the postoperative setting. • Atropine or isoproterenol may be given to increase AV node conduction if symptomatic or hemodynamically significant.
Postoperative	• Rare after CABG but, if it occurs, consider an offending drug or transient ischemia to the AV node. • No therapy is generally needed. • If associated with wide QRS complex, consider block below the His. • If it persists, consider an EP study to assess the level of the block. • If patient is asymptomatic and block is above His, no need for permanent pacemaker. • If patient is symptomatic or block is below the His, permanent pacemaker is indicated. • If the block is associated with valve (especially aortic) surgery, consider direct damage to the AV node. • If persistent, a pacemaker is indicated for symptoms or persistent slow rate (<40 bpm or no increase in rate with exercise).

AV, Atrioventricular; *AVB,* atrioventricular block; *AVN,* atrioventricular node; *bpm,* beats per minute; *CABG,* coronary artery bypass graft; *DDD,* dual-chamber; *EP,* electrophysiology; *LV,* left ventricular; *MI,* myocardial infarction.

From Olshansky B et al: *Arrhythmia essentials,* ed 2, Philadelphia, 2017, Elsevier.

TABLE 2	Mobitz Type II Second-Degree Atrioventricular Block Management
Setting	**Therapy**
Outpatient— Asymptomatic	• Risk for complete heart block and death is significant (approximately 50%). • A dual-chamber permanent pacemaker is recommended as the pacing system of choice. Consider conduction system pacing if high burden of pacing and depressed EF. • Admit the patient for a permanent pacemaker and place on a cardiac monitor. • In the absence of symptoms or progressive (higher-degree AVB), there is no need for a temporary pacemaker before permanent pacemaker implantation. • Avoid atropine. • Evaluate for the presence of underlying cardiac disease, such as infiltrative processes (e.g., amyloid) or MI.
Outpatient— Symptomatic	• Dual-chamber permanent pacemaker implantation is indicated. • Admit the patient and place on a cardiac monitor. • If symptomatic or hemodynamically detrimental ventricular bradycardia is present, a temporary pacemaker is indicated if a permanent system cannot be placed expeditiously. • Do not give atropine because this may worsen the AVB and produce a slower ventricular rate. • Exercise, sinus tachycardia, and catecholamines also can worsen the degree of block by enhancing AV nodal conduction and impinging on the refractory period of the His-Purkinje system.
Myocardial infarction	• Place temporary pacemaker. • Mobitz type II second-degree AVB is associated with a high rate of heart failure in this setting. • A permanent pacemaker is indicated if the AVB is persistent because the risk of complete heart block is >50%. • Long-term prognosis may not be improved. • Avoid the use of antiarrhythmic drugs (including lidocaine) in the absence of a pacemaker, unless there is sustained ventricular tachyarrhythmia, as these drugs may worsen the degree of AVB. • Do not give atropine. • Mobitz type II second-degree AVB has a lower (albeit not known with certainty) incidence in the current early revascularization era, but if present or of new onset may improve with time, in rare cases, when persistent, a pacemaker will likely be needed.
Preoperative	• Place permanent pacemaker. • If urgent or emergent surgery, place a temporary pacemaker with the plan for a permanent pacemaker after surgery. • If CABG, epicardial atrial and ventricular wires can be placed, with temporary pacing as standby, until a permanent transvenous pacemaker can be placed. • It is best to place the permanent pacemaker after CABG or other cardiac surgery as leads otherwise tend to dislodge. • If endocarditis, temporary pacemaker until infection resolves and after cardiac surgery. • Avoid antiarrhythmic drugs and atropine.
Postoperative	• If bradycardia, temporary pacing (via epicardial wires, if present, after cardiac surgery). • Temporary Mobitz type II AV block may resolve after cardiac surgery. • It may be due to trauma near the His-Purkinje system (e.g., with aortic valve surgery, where left bundle branch block is a not-infrequent accompaniment). • Persistent (e.g., more than 3-5 days) Mobitz type II block will require permanent pacing. • No antiarrhythmic drugs should be given unless an adequate backup ventricular pacing is available. • Endocarditis with abscess near the septum can destroy the His-Purkinje system. • Despite surgical repair, permanent pacing will likely be required. • For patients having tricuspid valve replacement, an endocardial lead can occasionally be placed across a porcine bioprosthesis without producing tricuspid regurgitation but should be avoided if there is a mechanical valve. • Tricuspid valve repair (e.g., annuloplasty) should not pose a problem in positioning a right ventricular lead.

AV, Atrioventricular; AVB, atrioventricular block; CABG, coronary artery bypass graft; MI, myocardial infarction.
From Olshansky B et al: *Arrhythmia essentials*, ed 2, Philadelphia, 2017, Elsevier.

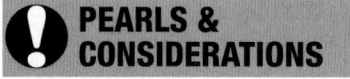

PEARLS & CONSIDERATIONS

COMMENTS
Patients with symptomatic Mobitz type II should be referred for a pacemaker. Asymptomatic patients should be referred if the AV block worsens with exercise and should be followed up routinely for potential development of high-grade AV block.[3]

REFERENCES
Available at eBooks.Health.Elsevier.com.

RELATED CONTENT
Second-Degree Heart Block (Patient Information)

AUTHOR: **ALEEM I. MUGHAL, MD, FHRS**

BASIC INFORMATION

DEFINITION

Heart failure (HF) is a complex clinical syndrome that can result from any structural or functional cardiac disorder that impairs the ability of the ventricle to fill with or eject blood. The cardinal manifestations of HF are dyspnea, fatigue, and fluid retention. The pathophysiology of HF (Fig. 1) is related to progressive activation of the neuroendocrine system to compensate for decreased effective circulating volume (Table 1), leading to total body volume overload and circulatory insufficiency.[1] These events culminate in the development of pulmonary congestion as well as peripheral edema. Specifically, the renin-angiotensin-aldosterone system (RAAS) is implicated; once activated, it can lead to volume expansion (sodium retention) and cardiac fibrosis (mediated through angiotensin II). Another recognized mechanism is disordered adrenergic stimulation as a key component of progression of disease. The term *congestive heart failure* (CHF) usually denotes a volume-overloaded status as a result of HF. Given that not all patients have volume overload at the time of the evaluation, *congestive heart failure* should be distinguished from the broader term *heart failure*.[1]

CLASSIFICATION: The American College of Cardiology/American Heart Association (ACC/AHA) describes the following four stages of HF.[2] This staging model was designed to emphasize the evolution and progression of HF over a continuum and the preventability of HF in at-risk patients.

- Stage A: Patients at high risk (e.g., with hypertension, atherosclerotic disease, diabetes mellitus, metabolic syndrome, cytotoxin, family history) for HF but without structural heart disease or symptoms of HF
- Stage B: Patients with structural heart disease (e.g., left ventricular [LV] dysfunction) but without symptoms of HF
- Stage C: Patients with structural heart disease with prior or current symptoms of HF
- Stage D: Patients with refractory HF requiring specialized interventions

In addition to the ACC/AHA stages described above, the New York Heart Association (NYHA) defines four functional classes of HF designed to describe the symptoms of stage C and D HF.[3] The functional classes are intended to assess the symptoms of HF and may fluctuate with therapy. It should be noted that current guidelines employ the functional classes to aid in determination of appropriate treatment.

- Asymptomatic or symptomatic only at activity levels that would limit normal individuals
- Symptomatic with ordinary exertion (e.g., 2 city blocks or 1 flight of stairs in a faster than usual pace)
- Symptomatic with less than ordinary exertion (e.g., less than 2 city blocks or 1 flight of stairs)
- Symptomatic at rest

Table 2 compares the ACC/AHA and the NYHA classification. Table 3 describes a simplified classification and common clinical characteristics of patients with acute HF.

TERMINOLOGY:

- Although HF has traditionally been classified as systolic vs. diastolic, this was dependent on the imaging modality used. With noted variation in the observed systolic function between studies, the ejection fraction serves as a better marker. HF is now categorized into *HF with reduced ejection fraction* (HFrEF) and *HF with preserved ejection fraction* (HFpEF). Other common classifications include right-sided vs. left-sided and high-output vs. low-output.[1] Systolic HF or HFrEF is defined by the presence of impaired contractility of the LV, as measured by ejection fraction (EF) ≤40% with clinical signs or symptoms of HF. In contrast, HFpEF has been described as evidence (clinical) of HF with an EF ≥50% with or without evidence of diastolic dysfunction. HF with mid-range ejection fraction (HFmrEF) is a newer concept, in which LVEF is between 41% and 49%. The term HFpEF improved is also sometimes used, used to describe patients who previously had HFrEF with an improvement in their EF.[4]
- Right-sided HF denotes peripheral signs and symptoms of HF without evidence of pulmonary congestion, as opposed to left-sided HF, which typically manifests with pulmonary congestion and subsequent signs and symptoms of right-sided HF.[1] The most common cause of right-sided HF is left-sided HF. High-output HF involves signs and symptoms of HF but features an elevated cardiac output unable to meet the abnormally high metabolic demands of peripheral tissues and is the result of myriad systemic disorders (e.g., systemic arteriovenous fistulas, hyperthyroidism, anemia). The term *acute decompensated HF* (ADHF) refers to worsening of signs or symptoms of HF due to a wide range of causes. Of note, HF is not equivalent to cardiomyopathy or LV dysfunction. These latter terms describe the possible structural or functional reasons for the development of HF, whereas HF is a clinical syndrome characterized by specific symptoms and signs.

SYNONYMS

HF
Congestive heart failure
CHF
Cardiac failure
Cardiogenic shock
Cardiogenic pulmonary edema

ICD-10CM CODES	
I50.9	Heart failure, unspecified
I50.20	Unspecified systolic (congestive) heart failure
I50.21	Acute systolic (congestive) heart failure
I50.22	Chronic systolic (congestive) heart failure
I50.23	Acute on chronic systolic (congestive) heart failure
I50.30	Unspecified diastolic (congestive) heart failure
I50.31	Acute diastolic (congestive) heart failure
I50.32	Chronic diastolic (congestive) heart failure
I50.33	Acute on chronic diastolic (congestive) heart failure
I50.40	Unspecified combined systolic (congestive) and diastolic (congestive) heart failure
I50.41	Acute combined systolic (congestive) and diastolic (congestive) heart failure
I50.42	Chronic combined systolic (congestive) and diastolic (congestive) heart failure
I50.43	Acute on chronic combined systolic (congestive) and diastolic (congestive) heart failure

EPIDEMIOLOGY & DEMOGRAPHICS

- There is variability in the reported demographics of HF due to heterogeneous definitions and classifications of HF. Incidence rate is lowest among White women and highest among Black men. African Americans have the highest risk for HF of the demographic groups with Blacks having a higher 5-yr mortality rate than Whites.[1]
- The lifetime risk of developing HF is 20% for Americans ≥40 yr of age.
  1. In the U.S., HF incidence has largely remained stable over the past several decades, with >650,000 new HF cases diagnosed annually.[2]
  2. Based on NHANES data, from 2013 to 2016, an estimated 6.2 million Americans ≥20 yr of age had HF. This represents an increase from an estimated 5.7 million U.S. adults with HF from 2009 to 2012.[5]
  3. Projections show that the prevalence of HF will increase 46% from 2012 to 2030, resulting in >8 million people ≥18 yr of age with HF.[6]
  4. There has been an increase in the prevalence of HF in the population over time. This is primarily due to improved treatment of hypertension and valvular and coronary disease, allowing patients to survive an early death only to later develop HF.[6]
- HF is primarily a condition of the elderly. Approximately 80% of patients hospitalized with HF are older than 65 yr. HF is the most common inpatient diagnosis in the U.S. for patients aged >65 yr.[6]
- HF incidence increases with age, rising from approximately 20 per 1000 individuals 65 to 69 yr to >80 per 1000 individuals among those >85 yr. Before age 75, the incidence of HF is higher in males, but both sexes are equally affected after this age cutoff.[5]
- In the U.S., 809,000 hospital discharges and 2.3 million emergency department visits/physician visits were associated with HF in 2016, which is a decline compared with 1.02 million hospital discharges in 2006.[5,6]
- Prevalence: 6.2 million persons in the U.S. and an estimated 26 million persons worldwide. The prevalence of HF is rising, especially in the elderly, particularly due to aging

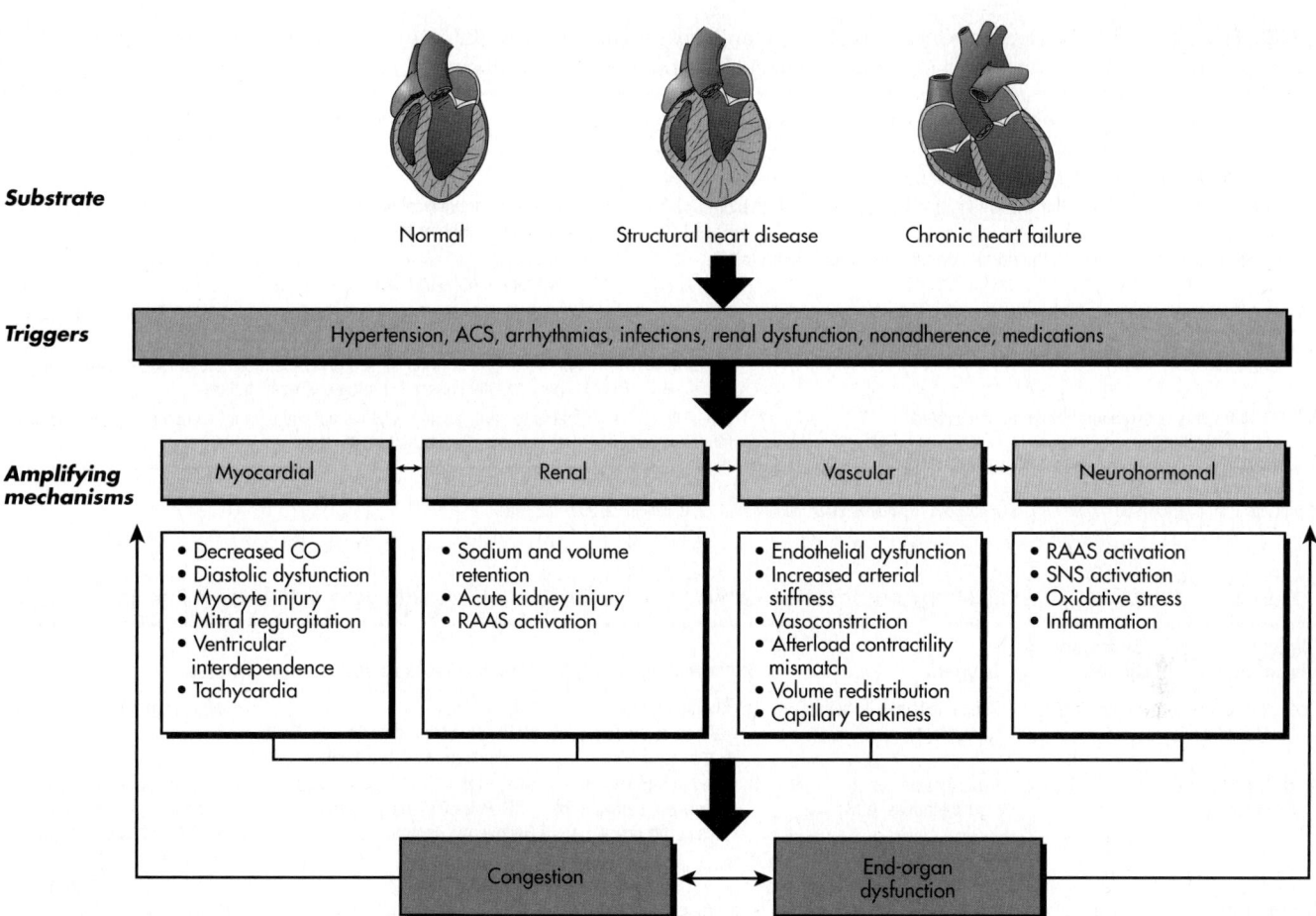

FIG. 1 Schematic of the pathophysiology of acute heart failure. *ACS,* Acute coronary syndrome; *CO,* cardiac output; *RAAS,* renin-angiotensin-aldosterone; *SNS,* sympathetic nervous system. (From Libby P et al: *Braunwald's heart disease: a textbook of cardiovascular medicine,* ed 12, Philadelphia, 2022, Elsevier.)

TABLE 1 Compensatory Mechanisms in Heart Failure

Compensatory Response	Stimuli	Beneficial Effects	Adverse Effects	Potential Pharmacologic Interventions
Renin-angiotensin system activation	↓CO/BP ↓Renal blood flow ↑β-Adrenergic activity	Maintain vital organ perfusion through vasoconstriction and sodium retention	↑Afterload → worsened LV function Adverse LV remodeling (apoptosis, myocyte hypertrophy)	ACE inhibitors ARBs
Adrenergic activation	↓CO/BP	↑CO through ↑ in heart rate and contractility ↑BP	↑Ischemia ↑Afterload → worsened LV function ↑LVEDP → pulmonary congestion Adverse LV remodeling (apoptosis, myocyte hypertrophy)	β-Adrenergic blocking agents
Renal salt and water retention	↑Antidiuretic hormone ↑Norepinephrine ↑Angiotensin II ↑Aldosterone ↓Renal blood flow	↑Preload → ↑Stroke volume and CO	Pulmonary and systemic congestion Adverse LV remodeling	Diuretics Aldosterone inhibitors ACE inhibitors, ARBs β-Adrenergic blocking agents
↑Natriuretic peptide secretion	Volume expansion (atrial stretch)	Diuresis Natriuresis Partial inhibition of renin-angiotensin system and norepinephrine	None known	Natriuretic peptides

ACE, Angiotensin-converting enzyme; *ARB,* angiotensin receptor blocker; *BP,* blood pressure; *CO,* cardiac output; *LV,* left ventricular; *LVEDP,* left ventricular end-diastolic pressure.
From Sellke FW et al: *Sabiston & Spencer surgery of the chest,* ed 9, Philadelphia, 2016, Elsevier.

of the population and improved survival from other conditions.[5]

- The estimated (direct and indirect) cost of HF in the U.S. was >$40 billion in 2012, with over half of these costs spent on hospitalizations. The mean cost of HF-related hospitalizations is

$23,077 per patient and is higher when HF was a secondary rather than the primary diagnosis.[5]

- HFrEF and HFpEF each make up about half of the overall HF burden of hospitalized HF events, half are in patients with HFrEF and the other half in patients with HFpEF.[7]

- The presence of ADHF services as an important juncture in the progression of HF, indicative of a worsening clinical course with increased risk of mortality and rehospitalization. An average hospitalization length for HF in the United States ranges around 4 to 5 days

TABLE 2 American College of Cardiology/American Heart Association (ACC/AHA) Stages of Heart Failure (HF) Compared to the New York Heart Association (NYHA) Functional Classification

ACC/AHA Stages of Heart Failure		NYHA Functional Classification	
A	At high risk for HF but without structural heart disease or symptoms of heart failure.	None	
B	Structural heart disease but without signs or symptoms of heart failure.	I	No limitation of physical activity. Ordinary physical activity does not cause symptoms of heart failure.
C	Structural heart disease with prior or current symptoms of heart failure.	I	No limitation of physical activity. Ordinary physical activity does not cause symptoms of heart failure.
		II	Slight limitation of physical activity. Comfortable at rest, but ordinary physical activity results in symptoms of heart failure.
		III	Marked limitation of physical activity. Comfortable at rest, but less than ordinary activity causes symptoms of heart failure.
D	Refractory heart failure requiring specialized interventions.	IV	Unable to carry on any physical activity without symptoms of heart failure, or symptoms of heart failure at rest.

HF, Heart failure.
From Libby P et al: *Braunwald's heart disease: a textbook of cardiovascular medicine,* ed 12, Philadelphia, 2022, Elsevier.

TABLE 3 Simplified Classification and Common Clinical Characteristics of Patients with Acute Heart Failure

Clinical Classification	Symptom Onset	Triggers	Signs and Symptoms	Clinical Assessment	Course
Decompensated heart failure	Usually gradual	Noncompliance, ischemia, infections	Peripheral edema, orthopnea, dyspnea on exertion	SBP: Variable CXR: Often clear despite elevated filling pressures	Variable, high rehospitalization rate
Acute hypertensive heart failure	Usually sudden	Hypertension, atrial arrhythmias, ACS	Dyspnea (often severe), tachypnea, tachycardia, rales common	SBP: High (>180/100 mm Hg) CXR with pulmonary edema Hypoxemia common	High acuity, but patient often responds quickly to therapy with vasodilators, noninvasive ventilation Postdischarge mortality is low
Cardiogenic shock	Variable	Progression of advanced HF or major myocardial insult (e.g., large AMI, acute myocarditis)	End-organ hypoperfusion; oliguria, confusion, cool extremities	SBP: Low or low normal LV function usually severely depressed RV dysfunction common Laboratory evidence of end-organ dysfunction (renal, hepatic)	High inpatient mortality Poor prognosis unless readily reversible cause or mechanical support, transplantation

ACS, Acute coronary syndrome; *AMI,* acute myocardial infarction; *CXR,* chest x-ray film; *LV,* left ventricular; *RV,* right ventricular; *SBP,* systolic blood pressure.
From Zipes DP: *Braunwald's heart disease: a textbook of cardiovascular medicine,* ed 11, Philadelphia, 2019, Elsevier.

but carries a 1-yr mortality rate of ~30%, over threefold of an increase from chronic, stable HF that does not require hospitalization.[8,9]

RISK FACTORS: Several conditions are associated with an increased risk of developing HF. If these are identified and treated appropriately, it may be possible to delay, if not prevent, the onset of HF and also reduce rates of decompensations.[4]

- Hypertension: The incidence of HF is higher in patients with higher blood pressures, older age of the hypertensive patient, and in patients who have been hypertensive for longer.
- Diabetes mellitus: The incidence of HF is increased in patients with diabetes mellitus, independent of the presence of structural heart disease.
- Metabolic syndrome: Appropriately treating hypertension, diabetes mellitus, and dyslipidemia can decrease the incidence of HF.
- Atherosclerotic disease: Patients with atherosclerotic disease are likely to develop HF.

PHYSICAL FINDINGS & CLINICAL PRESENTATION

The clinical and physical examination findings should be given the highest priority when determining the diagnosis of HF (Fig. 2). These signs and symptoms are dependent on the severity of disease, precipitant factors, comorbid conditions, and whether the HF symptoms are predominantly right-sided or left-sided. Clues in the patient's history when evaluating HF are summarized in Table 4.

- Common clinical manifestations are:[2]
  1. Dyspnea on exertion, that can progress to dyspnea at rest, caused by increasing pulmonary vascular congestion
  2. Orthopnea, caused by increased venous return in the recumbent position and further elevated pulmonary venous pressure
  3. Paroxysmal nocturnal dyspnea (PND) resulting from multiple factors including increased venous return in the recumbent position, decreased Pao$_2$, and decreased adrenergic stimulation of myocardial function during sleep
  4. Nocturnal angina resulting from increased myocardial oxygen demand (secondary to increased venous return in the recumbent position causing increased preload) in patients with concomitant coronary artery disease (CAD)

  5. *Cheyne-Stokes respiration* (alternating phases of apnea and hyperventilation) caused by prolonged circulation time from lungs to brain as a result of impaired cardiac output
  6. Fatigue, lethargy, and decreased functional capacity resulting from low cardiac output and hypoperfusion of peripheral tissues
  7. Lack of appetite and nausea, early satiety or a poor appetite
  8. Table 5 summarizes common presenting symptoms and signs of decompensated HF
- Physical examination (Table 6):[2]
  1. Fine pulmonary crackles, wheezes, tachypnea, hypoxia (due to elevated pulmonary pressures). Crackles may be absent in chronic and long-standing high pulmonary venous pressure because it allows for lymphatic drainage in the lungs to increase.
  2. Tachycardia and narrowed pulse pressure (due to increased sympathetic tone)
  3. S$_3$ gallop, paradoxic splitting of S$_2$, jugular venous distention, peripheral edema in

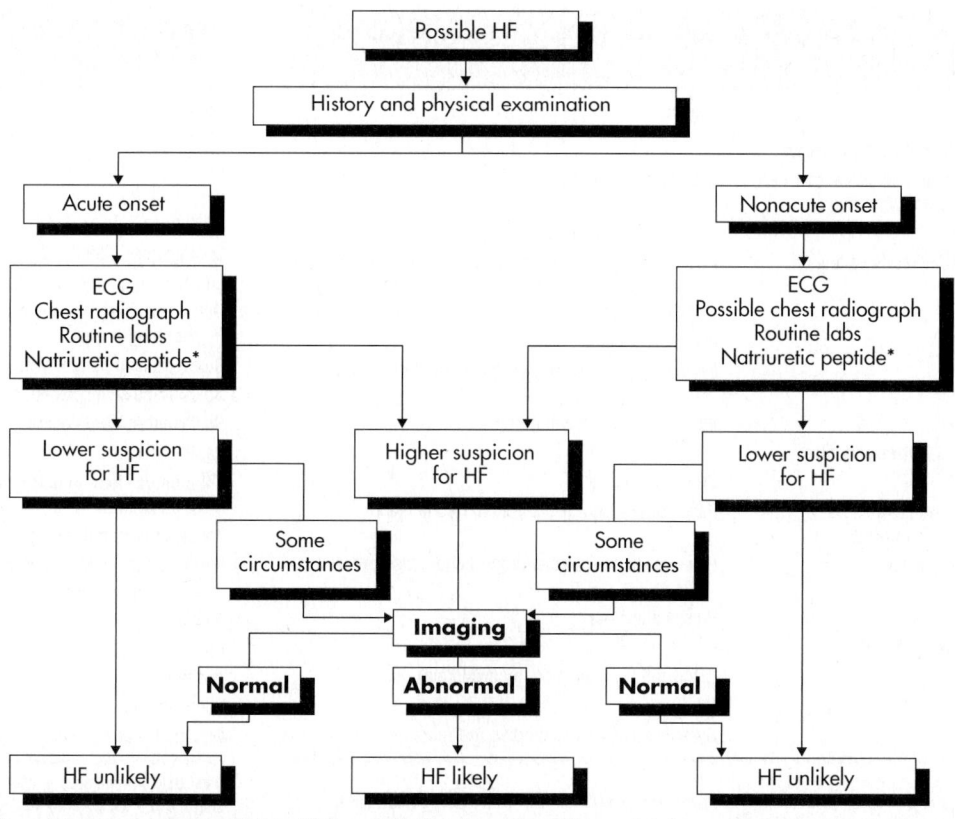

FIG. 2 Flow chart for the evaluation of patients with heart failure (HF). The diagnosis of HF is made using a combination of clinical judgment and initial and subsequent testing. Following thorough history and physical examination together with initial diagnostic testing, imaging (such as with echocardiography *[ECG]*) may still be necessary in ambiguous cases to definitively identify or exclude the diagnosis. (From Libby P et al: *Braunwald's heart disease, a textbook of cardiovascular medicine,* ed 12, Philadelphia, 2022, Elsevier.)

TABLE 4	Using the Medical History to Assess the Heart Failure Patient

Symptoms Associated With Heart Failure Include:

1. Fatigue
2. Shortness of breath at rest or during exercise
3. Dyspnea
4. Tachypnea
5. Cough
6. Diminished exercise capacity
7. Orthopnea
8. Paroxysmal nocturnal dyspnea
9. Nocturia
10. Weight gain/Weight loss
11. Edema (of the extremities, scrotum, or elsewhere)
12. Increasing abdominal girth or bloating
13. Abdominal pain (particularly if confined to the right upper quadrant)
14. Loss of appetite or early satiety
15. Cheyne-Stokes respirations (often reported by the family rather than the patient)
16. Somnolence or diminished mental acuity

Historical Information That Is Helpful in Determining if Symptoms Are Due to Heart Failure Include:

1. A past history of heart failure
2. Cardiac disease (e.g., coronary artery, valvular or congenital disease, previous myocardial infarction)
3. Risk factors for heart failure (e.g., diabetes, hypertension, obesity)
4. Systemic illnesses that can involve the heart (e.g., amyloidosis, sarcoidosis, inherited neuromuscular diseases)
5. Recent viral illness or history of HIV or Chagas disease
6. Family history of heart failure or sudden cardiac death
7. Environmental and/or medical exposure to cardiotoxic substances
8. Substance abuse
9. Noncardiac illnesses that could affect the heart indirectly (including high output states such as anemia, hyperthyroidism, arteriovenous fistulae)

From Libby P et al: *Braunwald's heart disease: a textbook of cardiovascular medicine,* ed 12, Philadelphia, 2022, Elsevier.

dependent tissues, congestive hepatomegaly, ascites, and hepatojugular reflux (due to volume overload)
4. Perioral and peripheral cyanosis, decreased capillary refill, pulsus alternans, and cool extremities (due to decreased cardiac output)
- Six common clinical presentations identified by European Society of Cardiology of Acute Heart Failure Syndromes:[10]
  1. ADHF presenting with hypertension (SBP >160): The hypertension leads to increased afterload causing pulmonary vascular congestion
  2. Worsening or decompensation of chronic HF
  3. Flash pulmonary edema
  4. Cardiogenic shock
  5. Acute coronary syndrome (ACS) and ADHF
  6. Isolated RV failure
- Each of these scenarios may require different therapies to effectively stabilize and treat the patient

Acute precipitants of HF decompensation include nonadherence with salt restriction or medications (most common cause), any acute systemic illness, infection, arrhythmias (e.g., atrial fibrillation), ischemia or infarction, uncontrolled hypertension, new medications (e.g., negative inotropic agents such as calcium channel blockers/antiarrhythmic agents),

TABLE 5 Common Presenting Symptoms and Signs of Decompensated Heart Failure

Symptoms	Signs
Predominantly Related to Volume Overload	
Dyspnea (exertional, paroxysmal nocturnal dyspnea, orthopnea, or at rest); cough; wheezing	Rales, pleural effusion
Foot and leg discomfort	Peripheral edema (legs, sacral)
Abdominal discomfort/bloating; early satiety or anorexia	Ascites/increased abdominal girth; right upper quadrant pain or discomfort; hepatomegaly/splenomegaly; scleral icterus
	Increased weight
	Elevated jugular venous pressure, abdominojugular reflux
	Increasing S3, accentuated P2
Predominantly Related to Hypoperfusion	
Fatigue	Cool extremities
Altered mental status, daytime drowsiness, confusion, or difficulty concentrating	Pallor, dusky skin discoloration, Hypotension
Dizziness, pre-syncope, or syncope	Pulse pressure (narrow)/proportional pulse pressure (low)
	Pulsus alternans
Other Signs and Symptoms of AHF	
Depression	Orthostatic hypotension (hypovolemia)
Sleep disturbances	S4
Palpitations	Systolic and diastolic cardiac murmurs

AHF, Acute heart failure.
From Libby P et al: *Braunwald's heart disease: a textbook of cardiovascular medicine,* ed 12, Philadelphia, 2022, Elsevier.

TABLE 6 Physical Findings of Heart Failure

Tachycardia
Extra beats or irregular rhythm
Narrow pulse pressure or thready pulse[a]
Pulses alternans[a]
Tachypnea
Cool and/or mottled extremities[a]
Elevated jugular venous pressure
Dullness and diminished breath sounds at one or both lung bases
Rales, rhonchi, and/or wheezes
Apical impulse displaced leftward and/or inferiorly
Sustained apical impulse
Parasternal lift
Third and/or fourth heart sound (either palpable and/or audible)
Tricuspid or mitral regurgitant murmur
Hepatomegaly (often accompanied by right upper quadrant discomfort)
Ascites
Presacral edema
Anasarca[a]
Pedal edema
Chronic venous stasis changes

[a]Indicative of more severe disease.
From Libby P et al: *Braunwald's heart disease; a textbook of cardiovascular medicine,* ed 12, Philadelphia, 2022, Elsevier.

NSAIDs, renal dysfunction, toxins (e.g., ethanol and anthracyclines), surgery, or valvular catastrophe.[10]

ETIOLOGY

LEFT VENTRICULAR FAILURE: The dichotomy of whether HF occurs in the setting of preserved or reduced LV systolic function plays an important role in treatment strategies. Patients with HFpEF may have significant abnormalities in active relaxation and passive stiffness of the LV as well as valvular disease. HfrEF denotes poor pump function.[10]

- Abnormal LV systolic function:
  1. CAD (acute or chronic ischemia, myocardial infarction [MI], LV aneurysm), the most common cause of cardiomyopathy in the U.S., comprising 50% to 75% of HF patients
  2. Increased afterload or pressure overload (severe hypertension, aortic stenosis)
  3. Increased preload or volume overload (mitral regurgitation, aortic regurgitation)
  4. Cardiomyopathy: Idiopathic, infiltrative (nonischemic)
  5. Infectious (Chagas, myocarditis)
  6. Infiltrative (amyloidosis, sarcoidosis, hemochromatosis)
  7. Toxins (ethanol, cocaine, anthracyclines)
  8. Tachycardia induced (e.g., with atrial fibrillation)
- Preserved LV systolic function (Table 7):[11]
  1. Impaired relaxation (myocardial ischemia, diabetes mellitus, metabolic syndrome)
  2. Tachyarrhythmia (featuring reduced diastolic filling time)

  3. Restrictive cardiomyopathy (myocardial stiffness, such as hypereosinophilic syndrome, amyloidosis, hemochromatosis)
  4. High cardiac output (thiamine deficiency, anemia, thyrotoxicosis, arteriovenous malformations)
  5. Increased afterload (uncontrolled hypertension, aortic stenosis, hypertrophic obstructive cardiomyopathy)
  6. Hypervolemia (oliguric renal failure, iatrogenic)

RIGHT VENTRICULAR FAILURE:
- Left-sided HF
- Chronic hypoxemic pulmonary disease
- Valvular heart disease (mitral stenosis or regurgitation)
- Pulmonary embolism
- Primary pulmonary hypertension
- Right-to-left shunts that cause systemic hypoxemia (e.g., large patent foramen ovale and tetralogy of Fallot)
- Left-to-right shunts that cause volume overload (e.g., atrial and ventricular septal defects)
- Bacterial endocarditis (right-sided)
- Right ventricular infarction

ⒹⓍ DIAGNOSIS

DIFFERENTIAL DIAGNOSIS
- Chronic obstructive pulmonary disease, asthma
- Cirrhosis
- Nephrotic syndrome
- Venous insufficiency
- Pulmonary embolism

- Acute respiratory distress syndrome
- Pneumonia, flu, and COVID-19
- Heroin overdose

WORKUP
- ACC/AHAA guidelines for initial and serial evaluation of HF are summarized in Table E8.
- Blood work (to diagnose potentially reversible causes, identify comorbidities, and assess disease severity):[2]
  1. CBC (to evaluate for anemia, infections), urinalysis, blood urea nitrogen, creatinine, electrolytes (worsening hyponatremia is a marker of disease severity and is associated with higher mortality rates), liver enzymes (hepatic congestion), thyroid function (especially in the elderly or patients with comorbid atrial fibrillation or known thyroid disease).
  2. Fig. E3 illustrates the use of biomarkers in HF. B-type natriuretic peptide (BNP) is a cardiac neurohormone secreted from the ventricles in response to elevated LV end-diastolic pressure. While the sensitivity is low in asymptomatic patients, low BNP level has a negative predictive value up to 90% in symptomatic patients. An elevated BNP correlates with severity of disease and parallels closely morbidity and mortality outcome measures. N-terminal-pro-BNP (NT-pro-BNP) is the cleavage remnant of BNP. It has a longer half-life and is renally cleared, making it susceptible to alterations in renal function. A level of <300 pg/ml has an age-independent 98% negative predictive

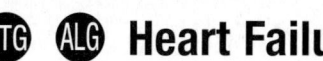

TABLE 7 Mechanisms/Factors Contributing to the Pathophysiology of Heart Failure with Preserved Ejection Fraction

Cardiovascular

LV Structure

Concentric remodeling, LV hypertrophy

LV Function

Diastolic dysfunction: Abnormal relaxation, decreased recoil, abnormal filling, decreased distensibility, increased diastolic pressure

Systolic dysfunction: Abnormal midwall and long-axis shortening, decreased twist

Hemodynamic load

Increased afterload and filling load

Heterogeneity

Dyssynergy, dyssynchrony

Left atrial structure and function

Increased LA volume and stiffness, decreased LA reservoir function, passive conduit function and active booster pump function

Ischemia

Subendocardial and microvascular disease, impaired coronary, pulmonary, and peripheral flow reserve

Rate and rhythm abnormalities

Chronotropic incompetence, atrial fibrillation, supraventricular tachycardia

Vascular dysfunction

Arterial stiffening, endothelial dysfunction

Cardiomyocyte

Abnormal calcium homeostasis ($\uparrow$ diastolic calcium or $\downarrow$ rate of calcium reuptake $\rightarrow$ incomplete or impaired relaxation)

Sarcolemmal calcium channels (Na^+/Ca^{2+} exchanger and calcium pump)

Sarcoplasmic reticulum Ca^{2+}ATPase (SERCA) abundance and function

Proteins modifying SERCA activity: Phospholamban, calmodulin, calsequestrin abundance, and phosphorylation state

Sarcoplasmic reticulum calcium release channels

Energetics ($\downarrow$ ATP or $\uparrow$ ADP slows actin-myosin cross-bridge release) ADP/ATP ratio, ADP and P_i concentration, phosphocreatine shuttle function

Proteins regulating cross-bridge formation and calcium sensitivity

Troponin C: Calcium binding

Troponin I: Phosphorylation state

Cytoskeletal proteins

Microtubules (increased density) $\rightarrow$ $\uparrow$ diastolic stiffness

Titin isoforms ($\uparrow$ noncompliant isoform and phosphorylation state) $\rightarrow$ $\uparrow$ diastolic stiffness

Extracellular Matrix

Collagen structure, geometry, content, collagen I/III ratio

Collagen homeostasis, synthesis, postsynthetic processing, posttranslational crosslinking, degradation

Basement membrane proteins

Bioactive proteins and peptides: MMP/TIMP, SPARC, TGF-β

Fibroblast structure, function, phenotype

Myofibroblast transdifferentiation

Extracardiac

Extrinsic forces (RV-LV interaction and pericardial constraint)

Peripheral muscle and ergoreflex dysfunction

Pulmonary hypertension (secondary to chronic pulmonary venous hypertension)

Neurohormonal activation

Comorbid conditions (renal dysfunction, anemia, chronic lung disease)

ADP, Adenosine diphosphate; ATP, adenosine triphosphate; LA, left atrium; LV, left ventricle; RV, right ventricle; SPARC, secreted protein, acidic and rich in cysteine [osteonectin]; TGF, transforming growth vector.
From Mann DL et al: *Braunwald's heart disease,* ed 10, Philadelphia, 2015, Elsevier.

---

value. There are new data to suggest that BNP screening and early intervention with risk factor modification in patients at risk of developing HF may prevent development of left ventricular dysfunction (class IIa recommendation). Natriuretic peptide biomarkers are also useful (class IA recommendation) both for diagnosis in patients presenting with dyspnea and for prognosis in patients with acute decompensated HF and chronic HF. Measurement of baseline levels of natriuretic peptide biomarkers on admission to the hospital is useful to establish a prognosis

in acutely decompensated HF, and pre-discharge natriuretic peptide level can be useful to establish a postdischarge prognosis. There are insufficient data to recommend natriuretic peptide biomarker–guided therapy or serial measurements for the purpose of reducing hospitalization or deaths. ACC/AHA/HFSA guidelines for the use of biomarkers in HF are summarized in Table 9.

3. Cardiac biomarkers may be elevated if ischemia is the precipitant factor. However, slight elevations are very common and may not always be due to obstructive

coronary artery disease. These elevations could be due to subendocardial ischemia (due to increased end-diastolic pressure resulting in decreased perfusion leading to oxygen supply-demand mismatch) and necrosis, or cardiomyocyte damage from the inflammatory cytokines or oxidative stress. Impaired renal function is very common, and decreased clearance of the biomarkers can contribute to their elevation. Therefore these elevations should be interpreted in the context of the clinical setting. Despite that, in patients with ADHF, a positive cardiac troponin test (from whatever mechanism) is associated with worse prognosis.

4. Screening for dyslipidemia and glucose intolerance, which are risk factors for CAD.

5. If hemochromatosis is suspected (specifically in Northern European patients), consider checking a transferrin saturation and ferritin level.

6. Consider HIV testing in high-risk patients and COVID-19 testing in all patients.

- ECG:[2]
  1. Look for signs of prior MI, chamber enlargement, hypertrophy, heart block, arrhythmia, and evidence of pericardial effusion.
  2. More than 25% of patients with HF have some form of intraventricular conduction abnormality that manifests as an increased QRS duration. The most common pattern seen is left bundle-branch block.
- Chest x-ray examination (Fig. 4):[2]
  1. Evaluate for pulmonary venous congestion, pulmonary edema, pleural effusion, cardiomegaly, chamber dilation, and Kerley B lines.
- Echocardiography:[2]
  1. Plays a critical diagnostic role in patients with HF and is useful in assessment of systolic, diastolic function in addition to assessment of valvular structure and function.
- Exercise stress testing:[2]
  1. May be useful in evaluating concomitant ischemic etiologies and assessment of degree of disability in stable compensated patients.
- Cardiac catheterization:[2]
  1. Left heart catheterization can help to identify coronary artery disease as a cause of HF. Right heart catheterization can help to evaluate intracardiac filling pressures, estimates of valvular areas, presence of intracardiac shunts, and calculation of hemodynamic properties such as cardiac output, systemic vascular resistance, and pulmonary artery wedge pressure to further guide management.
- Cardiac MRI:[2]
  1. Useful modality in accurately estimating EF (with less interstudy variability than conventional 2D echocardiography). MRI is also useful in excluding pericardial disease, identifying infiltrative disease, and assessing viability in cases of HF caused by underlying ischemic heart disease.

TABLE 9 ACC/AHA/HFSA Guidelines for Use of Biomarkers in Heart Failure

Class		Level of Evidence
Biomarkers for Prevention of HF		
IIa	For patients at risk of developing HF, natriuretic peptide biomarker–based screening can be useful to prevent the development of left ventricular dysfunction (systolic or diastolic) or new-onset HF.	B-R
Biomarkers for Diagnosis		
I	In patients presenting with dyspnea (acute or chronic), measurement of natriuretic peptide biomarkers is useful to support a diagnosis or exclusion of HF.	A
Biomarkers for Prognosis or Added Risk Stratification		
I	Measurement of BNP or NT-proBNP is useful for establishing prognosis or disease severity in chronic HF.	A
I	Measurement of baseline levels of natriuretic peptide biomarkers and/or cardiac troponin on admission to the hospital is useful to establish a prognosis in acutely decompensated HF.	A
IIa	During an HF hospitalization, a predischarge natriuretic peptide level can be useful to establish a postdischarge prognosis.	B-NR
IIb	In patients with chronic HF, measurement of other clinically available tests, such as biomarkers of myocardial injury or fibrosis, may be considered for additive risk stratification.	B-NR

ACC, American College of Cardiology; *AHA,* American Heart Association; *BNP,* B-type natriuretic peptide; *HF,* heart failure; *HFSA,* Heart Failure Society of America; *NT-proBNP,* N-terminal pro-B-type natriuretic peptide.
From Zipes DP: *Braunwald's heart disease: a textbook of cardiovascular medicine,* ed 11, Philadelphia, 2019, Elsevier.

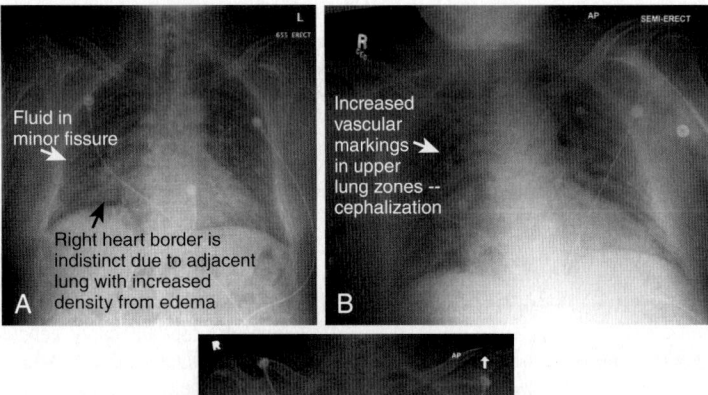
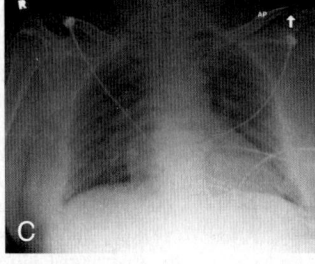

FIG. 4 Congestive heart failure. Mild left ventricular hypertrophy with restricted filling, ejection fraction >55%, and no pericardial effusion. This 63-yr-old man with coronary artery disease, chronic renal insufficiency, and diastolic heart failure (ejection fraction >55%) presented multiple times for dyspnea (**A, B,** and **C,** first through third clinical presentations). Each of these three radiographs shows signs of moderate pulmonary edema. The diaphragms and costophrenic angles are clear, suggesting no pleural effusion. The right heart border in all three images is indistinct because of interstitial edema in these locations. Portions of the left heart border are also indistinct. The upper lung fields have a hazy appearance indicating mild edema. Fluid is visible in the minor fissure on all three images. Does the similarity of these radiographs mean that edema is not the cause of the patient's dyspnea? No, he simply presented with pulmonary edema on all three occasions. (From Broder JS: *Diagnostic imaging for the emergency physician,* Philadelphia, 2011, Saunders.)

Ⓡ TREATMENT (FIG. 5)

NONPHARMACOLOGIC GENERAL MEASURES

- Assess the etiology and severity of disease. Educate the patient and family about the nature of the disorder. Assess the home setting and if patient has social support to ensure compliance, especially for patients with dementia.

- Identify and correct precipitating factors (e.g., increased sodium load, medication noncompliance, ischemia, infections, anemia, thyrotoxicosis) and address lifestyle modification (e.g., smoking and alcohol cessation, weight reduction, avoiding use of NSAIDs). Anemia is common in patients with HF. In patients with NYHA class II and III symptoms and iron deficiency, intravenous (IV) iron replacement may be reasonable to improve functional status and quality of life (class IIb recommendation).[12,13] Treatments with erythropoiesis-stimulating agents (ESAs) have not shown improved clinical outcomes in patients with systolic HF and mild-to-moderate anemia and are thus not recommended.[14] Table E10 describes ACC/AHA guidelines for treating patients at high risk for development of HF.

- Review list of medications and discontinue the ones that can contribute to HF (e.g., NSAIDs, antiarrhythmic drugs, calcium channel blockers, thiazolidinediones).[2]

- Dietary sodium restriction of <2 g/day is commonly recommended to patients with HF and is endorsed by many guidelines.[2]

- Restrict fluid intake to <2 L/day in patients with hyponatremia.[2]

- Caloric supplementation should be provided to patients with advanced HF with weight loss and muscle wasting due to cardiac cachexia. Weight loss may reflect cachexia caused by the higher total energy expenditure associated with HF compared with that of healthy sedentary subjects. The diagnosis of cardiac cachexia independently predicts a worse prognosis.[10]

- For patients with coexisting obstructive sleep apnea, continuous positive airway pressure (CPAP) may be reasonable after polysomnography (class IIb recommendation).[2]

- Exercise training (or regular physical activity) is recommended as safe and effective for patients with class I to III HF who are able to participate to improve functional status (class I recommendation). Cardiac rehabilitation is unfortunately an underused preventive measure, although it has been shown to reduce morbidity and mortality. Intensive cardiac rehabilitation can be useful in clinically stable patients with HF to improve functional capacity, exercise duration, health-related quality of life, and mortality (class IIa recommendation). Home-based cardiac rehabilitation is also an equally effective alternative if patients cannot participate in regular cardiac rehabilitation.[2]

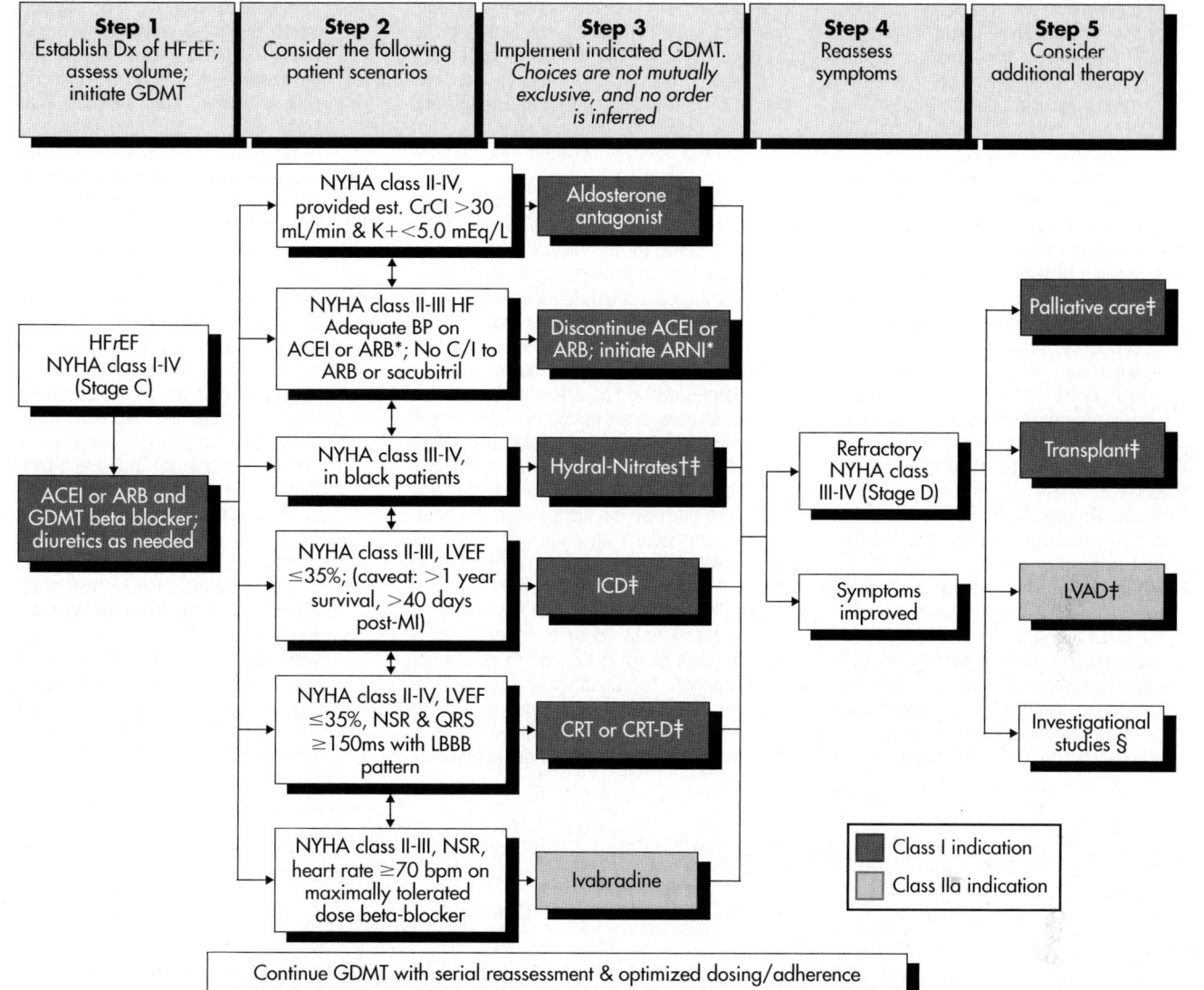

| Step 1
Establish Dx of HFrEF;
assess volume;
initiate GDMT | Step 2
Consider the following
patient scenarios | Step 3
Implement indicated GDMT.
*Choices are not mutually
exclusive, and no order
is inferred* | Step 4
Reassess
symptoms | Step 5
Consider
additional therapy |

FIG. 5 Treatment algorithm Stage C and D heart failure with a reduced ejection fraction. For all medical therapies, dosing should be optimized and serial assessment exercised. (Key: *See text for important treatment directions. †Hydral-Nitrates *green box:* The combination of ISDN/HYD with ARNI has not been robustly tested. BP response should be carefully monitored. ‡See 2013 ACC/AH heart failure guidelines. §Participation in investigational studies is also appropriate for stage C, NYHA class II and III HF. *ACEI,* Angiotensin-converting enzyme inhibitor; *ARB,* angiotensin receptor blocker; *ARNI,* angiotensin receptor neprilysin inhibitor; *BP,* blood pressure; *bpm,* beats per minute; *C/I,* contraindication; *CrCl,* creatinine clearance; *CRT-D,* cardiac resynchronization therapy–device; *Dx,* diagnosis; *GDMT,* guideline-directed management and therapy; *HF,* heart failure; *HFrEF,* heart failure with reduced ejection fraction; *ICD,* implantable cardioverter-defibrillator; *ISDN/HYD,* isosorbide dinitrate hydral-nitrates; *K+,* potassium; *LBBB,* left bundle branch block; *LVAD,* left ventricular assist device; *LVEF,* left ventricular ejection fraction; *MI,* myocardial infarction; *NSR,* normal sinus rhythm; *NYHA,* New York Heart Association. (From Yancy CW et al: 2017 ACC/AHA/HFSA focused update of the 2013 ACCF/AHA guideline for the management of heart failure: a report of the American College of Cardiology/American Heart Association Task Force on Clinical Practice Guidelines and the Heart Failure Society of America, *J Am Coll Cardiol* 2017;70[6]:776.)

- Pneumococcal vaccination, annual influenza vaccination.[2]
- ACC/AHA guidelines for treatment of asymptomatic left ventricular systolic dysfunction are summarized in Table E11.

TREATMENT OF ADHF

- Four phases in treatment of ADHF:
  1. 1st phase: Initial stabilization and management (Table E12)
  2. 2nd phase: Inpatient hospital care (Table E13)
  3. 3rd phase: Early discharge planning and care
  4. 4th phase: Early postdischarge care

- 1st phase: Initial stabilization and management
  1. Short-term goals: Hemodynamic stabilization, stabilization of respiratory status, symptom relief, optimization of tissue perfusion, and recognition of more immediately life-threatening conditions (e.g., arrhythmias, valvular catastrophe, MI, cardiac tamponade). Initial therapy of ADHF is contingent on appropriate determination of clinical scenario.[1]
  2. Management as per clinical scenario
     a. ADHF-associated hypertension: Goal is afterload reduction and decrease of systemic hypervolemia. Mode of treatment: Diuresis (IV loop diuretics) and vasodilators

(acutely nitrates and morphine followed by treatment with ACE inhibitors or angiotensin receptor blockers [ARBs]).
     b. Worsening or decompensation of chronic HF (HFrEF or HFpEF): Goal is control of volume status. Treatment is accomplished with vasodilators and diuretics.[10]
     c. Flash pulmonary edema: Goal is afterload reduction (vasodilators such as nitrates acutely), respiratory status stabilization, and diuresis (IV loop diuretics). Rate control can be initiated in patients with atrial fibrillation or tachyarrhythmias as it may improve cardiac filling and function.[10]

d. Cardiogenic shock: Goal is hemodynamic stabilization. Treatment consists of inotropes + vasopressors ± mechanical circulatory support ± emergent revascularization if indicated.[10]

e. ACS and ADHF: Goal is hemodynamic stabilization + emergent restoration of coronary perfusion. See "Acute Coronary Syndrome."

f. Isolated RV failure: Goals are identification of etiology: (1) Valvular, (2) pulmonary hypertension, and (3) primary RV failure secondary to ischemia. Treatment: Depends on etiology, either corrective surgery vs. treatment of pulmonary hypertension (endothelin antagonists, calcium channel blockers, phosphodiesterase inhibitors) vs. coronary reperfusion therapies.[10]

ACUTE PHARMACOLOGIC TREATMENTS:

- Vasodilators (Table 14) are appropriate in most patients with ADHF (contraindicated in cardiogenic shock and severe aortic stenosis or right-sided HF).
  1. Nitroglycerin (0.4 to 0.8 mg sublingually every 3 to 5 min, or by IV infusion starting at 0.2 to 0.4 mcg/kg/min with subsequent up titration) may be administered in the emergency setting until relative hypotension ensues. Nitrates are contraindicated after use of phosphodiesterase inhibitors such as sildenafil due to risk of hypotension.[10]
  2. Sodium nitroprusside (0.1 to 0.2 mcg/kg/min as an IV infusion) is a potent vasodilator with balanced venous and arteriolar effects that usually requires hemodynamic monitoring with an arterial line and may precipitate coronary steal and thiocyanate toxicity (elevated risk in renal failure).[10]
  3. When given intravenously, loop diuretics (Table 15) have an immediate vasodilator effect that provides clinical relief of symptoms before diuresis begins. Due to gut edema and unpredictable patterns of absorption, oral formulations may become less effective. Therefore, IV formulation should be used in the acute setting.[10] Studies showed no difference in outcome when using bolus dosing vs. continuous IV infusion.[15] Administration of smaller doses of short-acting loop diuretics multiple times daily is preferable to a single large dose because the kidneys can avidly reabsorb sodium after the initial diuresis. However, if a certain dose is not adequate to force diuresis, the dose, rather than the frequency, should be increased until a single effective dose is reached; more frequent doses can be added as needed. Therefore, monitoring of urine output, renal function, and electrolytes is key. The addition of a distal tubule inhibitor such as metolazone or chlorothiazide 30 min prior to loop diuretic dosing has a synergistic effect and often enhances diuresis because it inhibits sodium reabsorption in the distal segment in the face of increased sodium delivery from the loop. There is some evidence that also suggests that using 3 days of acetazolamide in patients who are known to be on diuretics at home can decrease time of hospitalization and time to decongestion and euvolemia. Diuretics should be used with caution in patients with aortic stenosis.

- Inotropic agents are used for temporary hemodynamic support in cardiogenic shock, but they have not been shown to improve survival. Many of these agents have serious associated adverse events including myocardial necrosis and malignant arrhythmias.[16]
  1. Dobutamine (starting at 2.5 to 5 mcg/kg/min) can be used for inotropic support but is associated with increased myocardial oxygen demand and cardiac arrhythmias and may result in hypotension from decreased systemic vascular resistance.
  2. Milrinone (37.5 to 75 mcg/kg loading dose, followed by 0.375 to 0.75 mcg/kg/min) can be used as a vasodilator and inotropic agent, but is associated with increased oxygen demand and cardiac arrhythmias, and may result in hypotension from decreased systemic vascular resistance.

TABLE 14 Intravenous Vasoactive Agents for the Treatment of Acute Heart Failure

Intravenous Medication	Initial Dose	Effective Dose Range[a]	Comments
Vasodilators			
Nitroglycerin; glyceryl trinitrate	20 μg/min	40-400 μg/min	Hypotension, headache; Tolerance with continuous use after 24 h
Isosorbide dinitrate	1 mg/h	2-10 mg/h	Hypotension, headache; Tolerance with continuous use within 24 h
Nitroprusside	0.3 μg/kg/min	0.3-5 μg/kg/min (usually <4 μg/kg/min)	Caution in patients with active myocardial ischemia; Hypotension; cyanide side effects (nausea, dysphoria); thiocyanate toxicity; light sensitive
Nesiritide[b]	2 μg/kg bolus with 0.010-0.030 μg/kg/min infusion[c]	0.010-0.030 μg/kg/min	Up-titration: 1 μg/kg bolus, then increase infusion rate by 0.005 μg/kg/min no more frequently than every 3 h, up to a maximum of 0.03 μg/kg/min) Hypotension, headache (less than with organic nitrates)
Inotropes			
Dobutamine	1-2 μg/kg/min	2-20 μg/kg/min	For inotropy and vasodilation; Hypotension, tachycardia, arrhythmias; ? mortality
Dopamine	1-2 μg/kg/min	2-4 μg/kg/min	For inotropy and vasodilation; Hypotension, tachycardia, arrhythmias; ? mortality
	4-5 μg/kg/min	5-20 μg/kg/min	For inotropy and vasoconstriction; Tachycardia, arrhythmias; ?mortality
Milrinone	25-75 μg/kg bolus over 10-0 min[c] followed by infusion	0.10-0.75 μg/kg/min	For vasodilation and inotropy; Hypotension, tachycardia, arrhythmias; Renal excretion; ?mortality
Enoximone[b]	0.25-0.75 mg/kg	1.25-7.5 μg/kg/min	For vasodilation and inotropy; Hypotension, tachycardia, arrhythmias; ? mortality
Levosimendan[b]	12-24 μg/kg bolus over 10 min[a] followed by infusion	0.5-2.0 μg/kg/min	For vasodilation and inotropy; active metabolite present for approximately 84 h; Hypotension, tachycardia, arrhythmias; ?mortality
Epinephrine		0.05-0.5 μg/kg/min	For vasoconstriction and inotropy; Tachycardia, arrhythmias, end-organ hypoperfusion; ?mortality
Norepinephrine		0.2-1.0 μg/kg/min	For vasoconstriction and inotropy; Tachycardia, arrhythmias, end-organ hypoperfusion; ?mortality

Use higher dose range for chronic diuretic use, renal insufficiency, and severe volume overload. Diuretic naïve patients should receive lower doses, initially.
[a]In general, titration of medication is accomplished by doubling of dose with careful monitoring for adverse effects.
[b]Not approved for use in all countries.
[c]Some clinicians do not administer a bolus dose, so as to decrease the risk of hypotension. Bolus not recommended in patients with hypotension.
From Libby P et al: *Braunwald's heart disease, a textbook of cardiovascular medicine*, ed 12, Philadelphia, 2022, Elsevier.

TABLE 15 Diuretics for Treating Fluid Retention in Chronic Heart Failure

Drug	Initial Daily Dose(S)	Maximum Total Daily Dose	Duration of Action
Loop Diuretics[a]			
Bumetanide	0.5-1.0 mg once or twice	10 mg	4-6 h
Furosemide	20-40 mg once or twice	600 mg	6-8 h
Torsemide	10-20 mg once	200 mg	12-16 h
Ethacrynic acid	25-50 mg once or twice	200 mg	6 h
Thiazide Diuretics[b]			
Chlorothiazide	250-500 mg once or twice	1000 mg	6-12 h
Chlorthalidone	25 mg once	100 mg	24-72 h
Hydrochlorothiazide	25 mg once or twice	200 mg	6-12 h
Indapamide	2.5 mg once	5 mg	36 h
Metolazone	2.5-5.0 mg once	5 mg	12-24 h
Potassium-Sparing Diuretics			
Amiloride	5.0 mg once	20 mg	24 h
Triamterene	50-100 mg twice	300 mg	7-9 h
AVP Antagonists			
Satavaptan	25 mg once	50 mg once	NS
Tolvaptan	15 mg once	60 mg once	NS
Lixivaptan	25 mg once	250 mg twice	NS
Conivaptan (IV)	20 mg IV loading dose followed by	100 mg once	7-9 h
	20 mg continuous IV infusion/day	40 mg IV	
Sequential Nephron Blockade			
Metolazone	2.5-10 mg once plus loop diuretic		
Hydrochlorothiazide	25-100 mg once or twice plus loop diuretic		
Chlorothiazide (IV)	500-1000 mg once plus loop diuretic		

Unless indicated, all doses are for oral diuretics.
IV, Intravenous; *mg,* milligrams; *NS,* not specified.
[a]Equivalent doses: 40 mg furosemide = 1 mg bumetanide = 20 mg torsemide = 50 mg of ethacrynic acid.
[b]Do not use if estimated glomerular filtration is less than 30 ml/min or with cytochrome 3A4 inhibitors.
Modified from Hunt SA, et al. ACC/AHA 2005 guideline update for the diagnosis and management of chronic heart failure in the adult: a report of the American College of Cardiology/American Heart Association Task Force on Practice Guidelines, *J Am Coll Cardiol* 46:e1-e82, 2005. In Libby P et al: *Braunwald's heart disease: a textbook of cardiovascular medicine,* ed 12, Philadelphia, 2022, Elsevier.

- Renal replacement therapy or ultrafiltration (can be used as an alternative to pharmacologic diuresis in ADHF when renal function is significantly compromised).[2]
- ACE inhibitors or ARBs, if part of a patient's chronic medication regimen, should be continued in the absence of hypotension, acute renal failure, or hyperkalemia.[10]
- β-blockers, if part of a patient's chronic medication regimen, may be continued or reduced in dosage in mild exacerbations of HF but should be discontinued in patients with hypotension or those requiring inotropic support. β-blockers should not be initiated in patients who are not on chronic β-blocker therapy until euvolemia is achieved unless used for rate control.[10]
- Morphine sulfate can cause venodilation and thus reduce cardiac preload. It may be used to reduce patient work of breathing and anxiety, but recent retrospective studies have suggested increased incidence of mechanical ventilation and in-hospital mortality in patients who received morphine.[10]
- If ADHF with preserved EF is suspected, therapy is usually aimed at relief of symptoms and correction of any potential precipitating etiologies (e.g., tachycardia, hypertension, ischemia). Treatment generally involves diuretics to reduce pulmonary congestion with caution to not overdiurese given the need for elevated filling pressures in these patients to ensure adequate stroke volume and cardiac output. Nitrates may be useful in providing symptomatic relief but may precipitate hypotension. Ventricular rate should be controlled in the presence of atrial fibrillation, which, at rapid rates, is poorly tolerated in patients with impaired diastolic filling. Negative inotropic agents such as β-blockers and calcium channel blockers can be used with caution.[2] ACC/AHA/HSFA guidelines for treatment of patients with stage C HF and preserved left ventricular ejection fraction are summarized in Table E16.
- Nesiritide (recombinant brain natriuretic protein) does not reduce morbidity or mortality (ASCEND-HF trial).[17]
- 2nd phase of ADHF treatment: Inpatient hospital care.
  1. This phase of treatment includes further diuresis and stabilization of volume status (Table 17). The patient should be carefully brought to euvolemia with daily volume status and electrolyte monitoring. The patient should also be transitioned to oral diuretics when stabilized. While inpatient, the patient should have his/her medical and device management optimized with the therapies discussed later.
- 3rd phase: Early discharge planning and care.
  1. The patient should be transitioned to oral diuretics and be placed on optimum outpatient maintenance therapy. If the patient was on IV inotropic therapy, oral regimens should be adjusted while these infusions are tapered off. Prolonged physiologic effects of these IV inotropic agents after their discontinuation before discharge may mask the inadequate diuretic regimen and intolerance to the vasodilator doses. This can result in readmission, especially with milrinone due to its long half-life that can be further prolonged by the common coexisting impaired renal function. Therefore it may be recommended that patients who received inotropic infusions remain hospitalized for at least 48 h after inotropic agents are discontinued and optimize the oral regimen.
- 4th phase: Early postdischarge care.
  1. The patient will require reevaluation and constant monitoring in order to avoid another episode of ADHF. Emphasis should be placed on importance of compliance with instructions regarding dietary restrictions

TABLE 17 Therapeutic Approaches for Volume Management in Acute Heart Failure (AHF)

Severity of Volume Overload	Diuretic	Dose (mg)	Comments
Moderate	Furosemide, or	20-40, or up to 2.5 times oral dose	IV administration preferable in symptomatic patients
	Bumetanide, or	0.5-1.0	Titrate dose according to clinical response.
	Torsemide	10-20	Monitor Na$^+$, K$^+$, creatinine, BP
Severe	Furosemide, or	40-160, or 2.5 times oral dose 5-40 mg/h infusion	Intravenously
	Bumetanide, or	1-4/0.5-2 mg/h infusion (max, 2-4 mg/h, limit 2-4 h)	Bumetanide and torsemide have higher oral bioavailability than furosemide, but IV administration preferable in AHF.
	Torsemide	20-100/5-20 mg/h	
	Ultrafiltration	200-500 ml/h	Adjust ultrafiltration rate to clinical response; monitor for hypotension; consider hematocrit sensor.
Refractory to loop diuretics	Add HCTZ, or	25-50 twice daily	Combination with loop diuretic may be better than very high dose of loop diuretics alone.
	Metolazone, or	2.5-10 once daily	Metolazone more potent if creatinine clearance <30 ml/min
	Chlorothiazide, or	250-500 mg IV 500-1000 mg PO	
	Spironolactone	25-50 once daily	Spironolactone best choice if patient not in renal failure and normal or low serum K$^+$, although may not be very potent
In case of alkalosis	Acetazolamide	0.5	Intravenously
Refractory to loop diuretics and thiazides	Add dopamine (renal vasodilation), or dobutamine or milrinone (inotropic agent) Ultrafiltration, or hemodialysis if coexisting renal failure		

BP, Blood pressure; *IV,* intravenous; *HCTZ,* hydrochlorothiazide; *PO,* by mouth.
From Libby P et al: *Braunwald's heart disease: a textbook of cardiovascular medicine,* ed 12, Philadelphia, 2022, Elsevier.

and daily body weight monitoring. Early follow-up should be scheduled as well as outpatient electrolyte monitoring if required after medication adjustments.

CHRONIC TREATMENT OF HFREF
The goals of HF therapy are clinical improvement followed by stabilizing, slowing, or even reversing deterioration in myocardial function, and ultimately a reduction in risk of morbidity (including hospitalization rates) and mortality.[2]
- ACE inhibitors:[18]
  1. Reduce morbidity and mortality.
  2. Produce both venous and arterial vasodilation acutely, thereby reducing both preload and afterload.
  3. Potential mechanism of long-term benefit is attenuation of RAAS activation and decreased myocardial remodeling and fibrosis.
  4. Used as first-line therapy for asymptomatic LV dysfunction (LVEF <40%) and symptomatic systolic HF (ACC/AHA grades A to D).
  5. Therapy should be initiated at low doses to prevent hypotension and rapidly titrated to higher doses as tolerated.
  6. Contraindications to the use of ACE inhibitors are renal insufficiency (creatinine clearance <30 ml/min), bilateral renal artery stenosis, hyperkalemia, hypotension, or adverse reactions (e.g., angioedema).
- ARBs:[19]
  1. Receptor antagonists to the angiotensin II receptor.

  2. Clinical trials have not shown any superiority compared to ACE inhibitors in patients with systolic HF (LVEF <40%).
  3. Reserved for patients who are ACE inhibitor intolerant.
  4. Combination therapy with ARBs and ACE inhibitors is generally not recommended.
  5. Have a similar contraindication profile to ACE inhibitors. Routine combined use of an ACE inhibitor, ARB, and aldosterone antagonist is potentially harmful for patients with HFrEF.
- Angiotensin receptor–neprilysin inhibitor (ARNI) (valsartan/sacubitril):[20,21]
  1. First-line therapy if affordable and side effects are tolerable.
  2. Neprilysin is an enzyme that degrades natriuretic peptides, bradykinin, adrenomedullin, and other vasoactive peptides.
  3. In a randomized controlled trial (PARADIGM-HF)[20] that compared valsartan/sacubitril with enalapril in symptomatic patients with HFrEF tolerating an adequate dose of either ACE inhibitor or ARB, the ARNI reduced the composite end point of cardiovascular death or HF hospitalization significantly, by 20%. Additionally, in another randomized controlled trial (PIONEER—HF),[21] in HFrEF patients hospitalized with decompensated HF, initiation of valsartan/sacubitril caused a greater reduction in NT-proBNP concentration than enalapril. Rates of adverse

effects did not significantly differ between the two groups.
  4. In patients with chronic symptomatic HFrEF NYHA class II or III who tolerate an ACE inhibitor or ARB, replacement by an ARNI is recommended to further reduce morbidity and mortality (class I).
  5. ARNI should not be administered concomitantly with ACE inhibitors or within 36 h of the last dose of an ACE inhibitor (class III: Harm).
  6. ARNI should not be administered to patients with a history of angioedema (class III: Harm).
  7. ARNI has not shown additional benefit over ARB in patients with preserved ejection fraction and is not indicated in this group of patients.
- β-Adrenergic blockers (β-blockers):[22-24]
  1. Reduce morbidity and mortality. Such benefits observed with bisoprolol (CIBIS II trial),[22] metoprolol succinate (MERIT-HF trial),[23] and carvedilol (COPERNICUS trial).[24]
  2. Benefit is believed to be conferred by blockade of sympathetic effects of neurohormonal stimulation due to HF.
  3. Are considered first-line therapy for symptomatic patients with systolic HF (NYHA class ≥II and LVEF <35%).
  4. Only carvedilol, bisoprolol, and metoprolol succinate (long acting) have been approved for the medical treatment of chronic HF; these agents are generally started in patients judged to be euvolemic

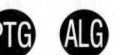 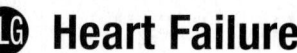

and dosage is to be slowly up titrated as tolerated.

5. Adverse effects include worsening HF (due to negative inotropic effects), fatigue, dizziness, bradycardia, hypotension, and bronchospasm.

- Aldosterone receptor antagonists:[25-27]
  1. Reduce morbidity and mortality.
  2. Indicated in patients with NYHA class II-IV HF, with LVEF ≤35%, already treated with ACE inhibitors and β-blockers without significant renal insufficiency or hyperkalemia. Patients with NYHA class II should have a history of prior cardiovascular hospitalization or elevated plasma natriuretic peptide levels to be considered for aldosterone receptor antagonists. Creatinine should be ≤2.5 mg/dl in men or ≤2.0 mg/dl in women (or estimated glomerular filtration rate >30 ml/min/1.73 m²), and potassium should be <5.0 mEq/L. They are also indicated for post-MI patients with EF ≤40% who have either symptomatic HF or diabetes mellitus.
  3. Spironolactone may cause gynecomastia, galactorrhea, and hyperkalemia (especially in patients with baseline renal insufficiency or type 4 renal tubular acidosis). It has been best studied in chronic HF with NYHA class III to IV symptoms (RALES study).[25]
  4. Eplerenone is associated with fewer endocrine side effects and has especially been studied in post myocardial infarction left ventricular dysfunction (EPHESUS trial)[26] and in chronic systolic HF with only class II symptoms (EMPHASIS-HF trial).[27]
  5. Inappropriate use of aldosterone receptor antagonists is potentially harmful because of life-threatening hyperkalemia or renal insufficiency when serum creatinine is >2.5 mg/dl in men or >2.0 mg/dl in women (or estimated glomerular filtration rate <30 ml/min/1.73 m²), and/or potassium >5.0 mEq/L.
- Sodium-Glucose Cotransporter 2 (SGLT2) Inhibitor:[28-32]
  1. SGLT2 inhibitors are known to lower blood sugar in patients with type 2 diabetes mellitus. However, they also possess properties associated with natriuresis, decreased fluid retention and edema, decreased RAAS activation, decreased sympathetic nervous system, reduced inflammation, and reduced oxidative stress. Thus, they are associated with improved cardiac structure and function (decreased preload, reduced remodeling/fibrosis, improved systolic function). They are also associated with improved endothelial function and overall improved vascular function.
  2. Currently used SGLT2 inhibitors include empagliflozin, canagliflozin, dapagliflozin, and ertugliflozin.
  3. Dapagliflozin has been shown to reduce cardiovascular deaths and hospitalizations in patients with NYHA class II, III, or IV HF

(LVEF ≤40%) regardless of the presence or absence of diabetes (DAPA-HF).[29]

  4. Empagliflozin has been shown to reduce HF hospitalizations and cardiovascular deaths in patients with HF with both reduced ejection fraction (EMPEROR-Reduced)[30] and preserved ejection fraction (EMPEROR-Preserved).[31]
  5. According to the new HF guidelines, in patients with symptomatic chronic HFrEF (EF≤40%), SGLT2i are now recommended to reduce hospitalization for HF and cardiovascular mortality, irrespective of the presence of type 2 diabetes (class I recommendation).[2] In patients with HFrEF, the new guidelines support the combination use of ARNI, β-blocker, MRA, and SGLT2 inhibitor as a new therapeutic standard.
- Diuretics:[33]
  1. They are used to maintain euvolemia and to improve symptoms as discussed previously.
  2. Although data on diuretic efficacy are limited, a meta-analysis of a few small trials found that they were associated with reduction in mortality as well as reduced hospitalization for HF.
  3. Of note, loop diuretics with better bioavailability, such as torsemide and bumetanide, may be used in diuretic-resistant patients but are generally more expensive.
  4. The ADVOR trial[34] revealed that the addition of acetazolamide, a carbonic anhydrase inhibitor that reduces proximal tubular sodium, to loop diuretics can improve the efficiency of loop diuretics and lead to faster decongestion in patients with acute decompensated HF with volume overload.
- Combination of isosorbide dinitrate and hydralazine:[35]
  1. Cause venous (nitrates) and arteriolar (hydralazine) vasodilation resulting in decreased preload and afterload.
  2. The combination of hydralazine and isosorbide dinitrate is recommended to reduce morbidity and mortality for patients self-described as African Americans with NYHA class III to IV HFrEF receiving optimal therapy with ACE inhibitors and β-blockers, unless contraindicated.
  3. A combination of hydralazine and isosorbide dinitrate can be useful to reduce morbidity or mortality in patients with current or prior symptomatic HFrEF who cannot be given an ACE inhibitor or ARB because of drug intolerance, hypotension, or renal insufficiency, unless contraindicated.
  4. Adverse effects of nitrates include hypotension, headaches, and tolerance as well as reflex tachycardia and lupus-like syndrome with hydralazine.
- Digoxin:[36]
  1. Positive inotropic and negative chronotropic drug that works by inhibition of the sodium-potassium transmembrane exchange pump and through its vagomimetic action.

  2. Commonly used in patients with concomitant atrial fibrillation.
  3. Has been shown to reduce HF-related hospitalizations but does not confer any mortality benefit (DIG trial).[36] However, there is evidence suggesting that digoxin may actually have an effect on survival that varies with the serum digoxin level; survival was improved when the level was between 0.5 and 0.8 ng/ml (most often in men) and significantly worsened when it was ≥1.2 ng/ml and >0.9 mg/ml in women.
  4. Caution must be used in patients with abnormal renal function to avoid digoxin toxicity and life-threatening arrhythmia. Avoid hypokalemia because potassium competes with digoxin on the same site of the Na⁺-K⁺-ATPase pump.
- I$_f$ channel inhibitor (ivabradine):[37]
  1. Ivabradine is a new therapeutic agent that selectively inhibits the I$_f$ current in the sinoatrial node, providing heart rate reduction.
  2. Ivabradine can be beneficial to reduce HF hospitalization for patients with symptomatic (NYHA class II-III) stable chronic HFrEF (LVEF ≤35%) who are receiving guideline-directed therapy, including a β-blocker at maximum tolerated dose, and who are in sinus rhythm with a heart rate of 70 bpm or greater at rest (class IIa).
- Cardiac resynchronization therapy (CRT):[38]
  1. Improves morbidity and mortality rates in selected patients.
  2. The presence of a bundle-branch block or other intraventricular conduction delay (IVCD) can cause ventricular dyssynchrony, which induces regional loading disparities and reduces the efficiency of ventricular contraction, thereby further impairing the systolic function of a failing ventricle.
  3. CRT is indicated for patients who have LVEF ≤35%, sinus rhythm, left bundle-branch block with a QRS duration of 150 ms or greater, and NYHA class II, III, or ambulatory IV symptoms on guideline-directed medical therapy. CRT is NOT indicated in patients whose functional status and life expectancy are limited predominantly by chronic noncardiac conditions. Life expectancy should be >1 yr.
  4. In the appropriate subset of patients, CRT in addition to optimal medical therapy has been shown in numerous clinical trials to improve symptoms by at least one NYHA class, improve 6-min walk distance and quality of life, reduce rate of HF-related hospitalization, and reduce rate of all-cause and cardiovascular mortality.
  5. ACC/AHA guidelines for cardiac resynchronization therapy are summarized in Table E18.
- Implantable cardioverter-defibrillators (ICDs):[2,39]
  1. Sudden cardiac death (SCD) is a common cause of death in patients with HF in both ischemic and nonischemic cardiomyopathies. Ventricular tachycardia (VT)

degenerating into ventricular fibrillation (VF) is the culprit in the majority of patients with SCD, although bradyarrhythmias do also occur with less frequency.

2. ICD therapy is recommended for primary prevention of SCD to reduce total mortality in selected patients with nonischemic dilated cardiomyopathy or ischemic heart disease at least 40 days post-MI with LVEF ≤35% and NYHA class II or III symptoms on chronic guideline-directed medical therapy, who have reasonable expectation of meaningful survival for >1 yr.

3. Patients with HF who survive an episode of sudden cardiac arrest or experience sustained VT in the presence of LVEF <35% are at high risk for future arrhythmic events and SCD and obtain a mortality benefit from ICD placement for secondary prevention, with or without adjunctive therapies such as antiarrhythmic drugs, radiofrequency ablation, surgery, or transplant.

4. ACC/AHA guidelines for indications for implantable cardioverter-defibrillators are summarized in Table E19.

- In the absence of an indication (e.g., atrial fibrillation), routine use of anticoagulation is currently not recommended in patients with HF. Even with the increased risk for LV thrombus formation in dilated cardiomyopathy and subsequent thromboembolization, data are conflicting about benefits of antithrombotic (antiplatelet or anticoagulant) therapy for primary prevention to reduce thromboembolic events or mortality in patients with systolic HF who are in sinus rhythm (SOLVD, V-HeFT, SAVE, HELAS, and WASH trials). It may be reasonable to consider anticoagulation for secondary prevention in patients with HF who had a prior thromboembolic event; however, risks and benefits should be carefully assessed.
- Antiplatelet agents are recommended for patients with concomitant CAD.
- Statins are not beneficial as adjunctive therapy when prescribed solely for the diagnosis of HF in the absence of other indications for their use.
- Calcium channel blocking drugs are not recommended as routine treatment for patients with HFrEF.
- Omega-3 polyunsaturated fatty acid supplementation is reasonable to use as adjunctive therapy in patients with NYHA class II to IV symptoms and HFrEF or HFpEF, unless contraindicated, to reduce mortality and cardiovascular hospitalizations.
- Percutaneous coronary intervention (PCI) or surgical revascularization should be considered in patients with HF and significant CAD who are revascularization candidates.
- In general, quadruple therapy, if tolerated, is recommended as foundational therapy. If all four therapies (ARNI, β-blocker, MRA, SGLT2 inhibitor) are initiated simultaneously at low doses, all pathways are blocked to some degree, and this results in rapid improvement of mortality and health status as well as rapid reduction of HF hospitalizations. Some

therapies offer further incremental benefit with increased doses (particularly ARNI and β-blocker), so if a patient tolerates quadruple therapy, doses can be increased to maximally tolerated doses.

- The following drugs can be added in selected patients in the absence of contraindications:
  1. Aldosterone antagonists improve survival in NYHA class II with LVEF <30% or NYHA class III-IV with EF <35%. Kidney function should be stable with eGFR ≥30 ml/min and potassium <5 mEq/L.
  2. Combination of hydralazine with a nitrate in patients (particularly African Americans) with a reduced EF.
  3. Digoxin reduces hospitalizations for HF and controls HR in atrial fibrillation. It can also help control symptoms.

CHRONIC TREATMENT OF HFpEF

- To date, there is a relative dearth of clinical trials examining effective chronic treatment strategies in this subset of patients with HFpEF. Current therapies are mainly for symptomatic relief. ACC/AHA guidelines for treatment of patients with end-stage JF are summarized in Table E20.
- Therapy mainly centers on relief of volume overload with judicious diuretic use (Table 17), treatment of ischemia via coronary revascularization (Table E21), management of atrial fibrillation, controlling heart rate and blood pressure to prevent acute decompensation, and restriction of sodium and fluid to prevent volume overload.
- Recently, SGLT2 inhibitor has shown to reduce the combined risk of worsening HF or cardiovascular death among patients with HF and a mildly reduced or preserved ejection fraction.[40]
- Diuretics should be used for relief of symptoms due to volume overload in patients with HFpEF.
- The use of β-blocking agents, ACE inhibitors, and ARBs in patients with hypertension is reasonable to control blood pressure in patients with HFpEF.
- The use of ARBs might be considered to decrease hospitalizations for patients with HFpEF.
- Aldosterone antagonists may be used in appropriate patients with HFpEF (EF >45%, elevated BNP or HF admission in the past year, potassium <5.0 mEq/L, estimated glomerular filtration rate >30 and creatinine <2.5 mg/dl) to decrease hospitalizations (class IIb recommendation).
- Routine use of nitrates or phosphodiesterase-5 inhibitors to increase activity or quality of life in patients with HFpEF is not recommended as there is no benefit.
- There is no evidence to support routine use of nutritional supplements, and they are not recommended for patients with HFpEF.
- Surgical options (Table E22) for contributing critical aortic stenosis, constrictive pericarditis, and hypertrophic cardiomyopathy (HCM) should be entertained in appropriate patients.

- In patients with comorbidities including anemia, hypertension, and sleep apnea, the following recommendations are made:
  1. IV iron replacement in patients with NYHA class II and III HF and iron deficiency (ferritin <100 ng/ml or 100 to 300 ng/ml with transferrin saturation <20%) to improve functional status and quality of life (class IIb recommendation).
  2. Titration of medical therapy to attain systolic blood pressure <130 mm Hg is recommended in patients with HFrEF and hypertension, as well as in patients with HFpEF and persistent hypertension after treatment of volume overload (class I recommendation).
  3. A formal sleep assessment should be obtained in patients with NYHA class II to IV HF with suspicion of sleep-disordered breathing. Continuous positive airway pressure should be used in patients with HF and obstructive sleep apnea to improve sleep quality and daytime sleepiness (class IIb recommendation).

DISPOSITION

- Coordination of care is essential in patients with chronic HF.
- Annual mortality of systolic HF ranges from 10% in stable patients with mild symptoms to 50% in patients with NYHA class IV disease (a mortality rate rivaling some malignancies). The Seattle Heart Failure Model provides an accurate estimate of 1-, 2-, and 3-yr survival before and after different therapies. This model can be useful to assess the need for LV assist device implantation or urgent transplantation. The calculator is available online at http://depts.washington.edu/shfm/.
- Cardiac transplantation has a 5-yr survival rate of ~70% and represents a viable option in selected patients. Fig. E6 describes an algorithm for evaluation of potential heart transplant recipient.[41]
- The use of an LV assist device (LVAD) in patients with advanced HF can result in a clinically meaningful survival benefit and improve quality of life in patients who are not candidates for cardiac transplantation.[41,42] There are two approved uses of LVADs specifically as a bridge to transplant and as destination therapy. There are two major categories of LVAD pulsatile flow devices vs. continuous flow devices. Continuous flow devices are associated with increased survival as destination therapy as compared to medically managed controls (REMATCH trial).[40]

REFERENCES & SUGGESTED READING
Available at eBooks.Health.Elsevier.com.

RELATED CONTENT
Heart Failure (Patient Information)

AUTHORS: **HUSAM ABU-NEJIM, MD, VISHNU KADIYALA, MD,** and **ARAVIND RAO KOKKIRALA, MD, FACC**

BASIC INFORMATION

DEFINITION

Heat exhaustion and heat stroke are part of a continuum of heat-related illness, and unless factors leading to heat exhaustion are corrected swiftly, affected patients can progress to heat stroke.

- **Heat exhaustion:** An illness resulting from prolonged, heavy activity in a hot environment with subsequent dehydration, electrolyte depletion, and rectal temperature >37.8° C (100° F) but ≤40° C (104° F).
- **Heat stroke:** A life-threatening heat illness characterized by extreme hyperthermia (core temperature >40° C [104.0° F]), dehydration, multiorgan failure, and neurologic manifestations. Heat stroke can be further subdivided into "exertional heat stroke" occurring in generally healthy individuals undergoing strenuous physical activity in warm conditions and "nonexertional heat stroke" often seen in elderly and/or debilitated patients with impaired thermal regulations due to illness or medications (see "Etiology").

SYNONYMS

Heat illness
Hyperthermia

ICD-10CM CODES
T67.5	Heat exhaustion, unspecified
T67.0	Heatstroke and sunstroke
T67.1	Heat syncope
T67.2	Heat cramp
T67.3	Heat exhaustion, anhydrotic
T67.6	Heat fatigue, transient

EPIDEMIOLOGY & DEMOGRAPHICS

INCIDENCE (IN U.S.): Incidence of heat stroke is approximately 20 cases/100,000 population.
PREDOMINANT AGE: Heat exhaustion and stroke occur more frequently in elderly patients, especially those taking diuretics or medications that impair heat dissipation (e.g., phenothiazines, anticholinergics, antihistamines, β-blockers). Table 1 describes factors predisposing to serious heat illness.

PHYSICAL FINDINGS & CLINICAL PRESENTATION

HEAT EXHAUSTION:
- Generalized malaise, weakness, headache, muscle and abdominal cramps, nausea, vomiting, hypotension, tachycardia.
- Rectal temperature is usually normal.
- Sweating is usually present.

HEAT STROKE:
- Neurologic manifestations (seizures, tremor, hemiplegia, coma, psychosis, other bizarre behavior).
- Evidence of dehydration (poor skin turgor, sunken eyeballs).
- Tachycardia, hyperventilation.
- Skin is hot, red, and flushed.
- Sweating is often (not always) absent, particularly in elderly patients.

- Classic heat stroke generally develops slowly over days and occurs predominantly in older persons and in those with chronic illness. Clinically heat stroke can be divided into three phases: A hyperthermic neurologic acute phase, a hematologic-enzymatic phase (peaking 24 to 48 h after the event), and a late renal-hepatic phase (if clinical symptoms are sustained for 96 h or longer).[1] Exertional heat stroke is more common in young, healthy persons; has a more rapid onset; and is associated with higher core temperatures. Table 2 compares classic and exertional heat stroke. Box 1 summarizes organ dysfunction seen in patients with heat stroke

ETIOLOGY

- Exogenous heat gain (increased ambient temperature)
- Increased heat production (exercise, infection, hyperthyroidism, drugs)

TABLE 1 Factors Predisposing to Serious Heat Illness

Individual Factors
Lack of acclimatization
Low physical fitness
Excessive body weight
Dehydration
Advanced age
Young age

Health Conditions
Inflammation and fever
Viral infection
Cardiovascular disease
Diabetes mellitus
Gastroenteritis
Rash, sunburn, and previous burns to large areas of skin
Seizures
Thyroid storm
Neuroleptic malignant syndrome
Malignant hyperthermia
Sickle cell trait
Cystic fibrosis
Spinal cord injury

Drugs
Anticholinergic properties (atropine)
Antiepileptic (topiramate)
Antihistamines
Glutethimide (Doriden)
Phenothiazines
Tricyclic antidepressants
Amphetamines, cocaine, "ecstasy"
Ergogenic stimulants (e.g., ephedrine, ephedra)
Lithium
Diuretics
β-Blockers
Ethanol

Environmental Factors
High temperature
High humidity
Little air motion
Lack of shade
Heat wave
Physical exercise
Heavy clothing
Air pollution (nitrogen dioxide)

From Goldman L, Schafer AI: *Goldman's Cecil medicine,* ed 24, Philadelphia, 2012, Saunders.

TABLE 2 Characteristics of Classic versus Exertional Heatstroke

Exertional	Classic
Healthy	Predisposing factors or medications
Younger	Older
Exercise	Sedentary
Sporadic	Heat wave occurrence
Diaphoresis	Anhidrosis
Hypoglycemia	Normoglycemia
DIC	Mild coagulopathy
Rhabdomyolysis	Mild CK level elevation
Acute renal failure	Oliguria
Marked lactic acidosis	Mild acidosis
Hypocalcemia	Normocalcemia

CK, Creatine kinase; *DIC,* disseminated intravascular coagulation.

From Walls RM et al: *Rosen's emergency medicine, concepts and clinical practice,* ed 10, Philadelphia, 2023, Elsevier.

BOX 1 Organ Dysfunction Seen in Patients with Heat Stroke

Encephalopathy
Rhabdomyolysis
Acute renal failure
Acute respiratory distress syndrome
Myocardial injury
Hepatocellular injury
Intestinal ischemia and infarction
Pancreatic injury
Hemorrhagic complication (e.g., disseminated intravascular coagulation)

From Adams JG et al: *Emergency medicine, clinical essentials,* ed 2, Philadelphia, 2013, Elsevier.

- Impaired heat dissipation (high humidity, heavy clothing, neonatal or elderly patients, drugs [phenothiazines, anticholinergics, antihistamines, butyrophenones, amphetamines, cocaine, alcohol, β-blockers])
- Diuretics, laxatives
- In infants a major risk factor is confinement in a closed car
- Fig. E1 describes the pathophysiology of heat stroke

DIAGNOSIS

DIFFERENTIAL DIAGNOSIS (BOX 2)
- Infections (meningitis, encephalitis, sepsis)
- Head trauma
- Epilepsy
- Thyroid storm
- Acute cocaine intoxication
- Malignant hyperthermia
- Heat exhaustion can be differentiated from heat stroke by the following:
  1. Essentially intact mental function and lack of significant fever in heat exhaustion
  2. Mild or absent increases in creatine phosphokinase (CPK), aspartate aminotransferase (AST), lactate dehydrogenase

BOX 2 Differential Diagnoses of Heatstroke

- Central nervous system hemorrhage
- Toxins, drugs
- Seizures
- Malignant hyperthermia
- Exercise-induced hyponatremia
- Neuroleptic malignant syndrome
- Serotonin syndrome
- Thyroid storm
- High fever, sepsis
- Encephalitis, meningitis

From Walls RM et al: *Rosen's emergency medicine, concepts and clinical practice,* ed 10, Philadelphia, 2023, Elsevier.

TABLE 3 Medications Associated with Heat Stroke

Drug Class	Examples
Anticholinergics	Atropine
	Benztropine
	Oxybutynin
	Scopolamine
Antidepressants	Tricyclics
Antiemetics	Metoclopramide
	Prochlorperazine
	Promethazine
Antiepileptics	Topiramate
	Zonisamide
Antihistamines	All
Antihypertensives	β-blockers
	Calcium channel blockers
Antipsychotics	All
Diuretics	Hydrochlorothiazide
	Furosemide
	Spironolactone
Ergogenic aids	Anabolic steroids
	Creatine
	Ephedra
Sympathomimetics	Amphetamines
	Cocaine
	Methylphenidate

From Walls RM et al: *Rosen's emergency medicine, concepts and clinical practice,* ed 10, Philadelphia, 2023, Elsevier.

(LDH), and alanine aminotransferase (ALT) in heat exhaustion

WORKUP

- Heat stroke: Comprehensive history with focus on medications associated with heat stroke (Table 3), physical examination, and laboratory evaluation (Box 3, see Table 2).
- Heat exhaustion: Clinical diagnosis (Box 4). In most cases, laboratory tests not necessary for diagnosis.

LABORATORY TESTS

Laboratory abnormalities may include the following:
- Elevated blood urea nitrogen (BUN), creatinine, hematocrit
- Hyponatremia or hypernatremia, hyperkalemia or hypokalemia

BOX 3 Heatstroke: Diagnosis

- Exposure to heat stress, endogenous or exogenous
- Signs of severe central nervous system dysfunction (coma, seizures, delirium)
- Core temperature usually >40.5° C (105° F), but may be lower
- Hot skin common, and sweating may persist
- Marked elevation of hepatic transaminase levels

From Walls RM et al: *Rosen's emergency medicine, concepts and clinical practice,* ed 10, Philadelphia, 2023, Elsevier.

BOX 4 Heat Exhaustion: Diagnosis

- Vague malaise, fatigue, headache
- Core temperature often normal; if elevated, <40° C (104° F)
- Mental function essentially intact; no coma or seizures
- Tachycardia, orthostatic hypotension, clinical dehydration (may occur)
- Other major illness ruled out
- If in doubt, treat as heatstroke

From Walls RM et al: *Rosen's emergency medicine, concepts and clinical practice,* ed 10, Philadelphia, 2023, Elsevier.

- Elevated LDH, AST, ALT, CPK, bilirubin
- Lactic acidosis, respiratory alkalosis (from hyperventilation)
- Myoglobinuria, hypofibrinogenemia, fibrinolysis, hypocalcemia

℞ TREATMENT (TABLE E4)

- Treatment of heat exhaustion consists primarily of placing the patient in a cool, shaded area and providing rapid hydration and salt replacement (Box 5).
  1. Fluid intake should be at least 2 L q4h in patients without history of congestive heart failure.
  2. Salt replacement can be accomplished by using one-quarter teaspoon of salt or two 10-grain salt tablets dissolved in 1 L of water.
  3. If intravenous (IV) fluid replacement is necessary, young athletes can be given normal saline IV (3 to 4 L over 6 to 8 h); in elderly patients, consider using 5% dextrose in ½ normal saline IV with the rate titrated to cardiovascular status.
- Patients with heat stroke should undergo rapid cooling (Box 6).
  1. Remove the patient's clothes and place the patient in a cool and well-ventilated room.
  2. If patient is unconscious, position on his or her side and clear the airway. Protect airway and augment oxygenation (e.g., nasal O₂ at 4 L/min to keep oxygen saturation >90%).

BOX 5 Heat Exhaustion: Management

- Rest
- Cool environment
- Assessment of volume status—orthostatic changes, blood urea nitrogen level, hematocrit, serum sodium concentration
- Fluid replacement—normal saline to replete volume if the patient is orthostatic; replace free water deficits slowly to avoid cerebral edema
- Healthy young patients are usually treated as outpatients; consider admission if the patient is older, has significant electrolyte abnormalities, or would be at risk for recurrence if discharged

From Walls RM et al: *Rosen's emergency medicine, concepts and clinical practice,* ed 10, Philadelphia, 2023, Elsevier.

BOX 6 Cooling Modalities to Lower Body Temperature in Heatstroke

Preferred
- Evaporative cooling with large circulating fans and skin wetting
- Ice water immersion

Adjuncts
- Ice packs to axillae and groin
- Cooling blanket
- Peritoneal lavage (unproven efficacy in humans)
- Rectal lavage
- Gastric lavage
- Cardiopulmonary bypass

From Walls RM et al: *Rosen's emergency medicine, concepts and clinical practice,* ed 10, Philadelphia, 2023, Elsevier.

3. Monitor body temperature every 5 min. Measurement of the patient's core temperature with a rectal probe is recommended. The goal is to reduce the body temperature to 39° C (102.2° F) in 30 to 60 min. Advantages, disadvantages, and efficacy of various cooling methods are described in Table 5.
4. Spray the patient with a cool mist and use fans to enhance airflow over the body (rapid evaporation method).
5. Immersion of the patient in ice water, stomach lavage with iced saline solution, IV administration of cooled fluids, and inhalation of cold air are advisable only when the means for rapid evaporation are not available. Immersion in tepid water (15° C [59° F]) is preferred over ice water immersion to minimize risk of shivering.
6. Use of ice packs on axillae, neck, and groin is controversial because they increase peripheral vasoconstriction and may induce shivering.

TABLE 5 Advantages, Disadvantages, and Efficacy of Various Cooling Methods

Cooling Method	Advantages	Disadvantages	Effectiveness
Antipyretics		Can worsen liver or renal injury	Not effective (the temperature set-point is not elevated in hyperthermia) Not effective in controlling pathologic inflammation
Evaporative cooling	Noninvasive, easy to monitor, readily available	Labor-intensive—requires constant moistening of skin	Comparison studies show the cooling rate on average to be slower than immersion Published rate range: 0.05-0.31° C/min (32.09-32.56° F/min)
Immersion	Noninvasive, rapid	Cumbersome, poorly tolerated, safety questionable if comorbid conditions present, monitoring difficult, shivering and vasoconstriction	Comparison studies show the cooling rate on average to be faster than evaporation Published rate range: 0.04-0.35° C/min (32.07-32.63° F/min)
Immersion of the hands and forearms	Noninvasive, easy to perform in the field	Shivering and vasoconstriction	Slower cooling but appropriate for mildly ill patients, such as those with heat exhaustion
Ice packing	Noninvasive, readily available	Shivering and vasoconstriction, poorly tolerated	Less effective than immersion or evaporation Some authorities recommend using both evaporation and ice
Cold gastric or peritoneal lavage	Very rapid	Invasive, cumbersome (cold sterile saline needed for peritoneal lavage)	In canine studies, questionably faster than evaporation or immersion
Dantrolene	In theory, decreases heat production by inhibiting muscle contraction		No clear efficacy; it may be more effective for exertional than for classic heat stroke
Benzodiazepines	Treatment of shivering to decrease heat production and heat-induced seizures	Sedation	Whether treatment increases cooling is unknown but may make cooling treatments tolerable Also effective for heat-related seizures

From Adams JG et al: *Emergency medicine: clinical essentials*, ed 2, Philadelphia, 2013, Elsevier.

7. Antipyretics are ineffective because the hypothalamic set point during heat stroke is normal despite the increased body temperature.
8. Intubate a comatose patient, insert a Foley catheter, and start nasal O_2. Continuous ECG monitoring is recommended.
9. Insert at least two large-bore IV lines and begin IV hydration with normal saline or Ringer lactate.
10. Draw initial laboratory studies: Electrolytes, CBC, blood urea nitrogen, creatinine, AST, ALT, CPK, LDH, glucose, prothrombin time (international normalized ratio), partial thromboplastin time, platelet count, Ca^{2+}, lactic acid, and arterial blood gases.
11. Treat complications as follows:
    a. Hypotension: Vigorous hydration with normal saline or Ringer lactate
    b. Convulsions: Diazepam 5 to 10 mg IV (slowly)
    c. Shivering: Chlorpromazine 10 to 50 mg IV
    d. Acidosis: Use bicarbonate judiciously (only in severe acidosis)
- Observe for evidence of rhabdomyolysis and hepatic, renal, or cardiac failure and treat accordingly.

DISPOSITION
Most patients recover completely within 48 h. Central nervous system injury is permanent in 20% of cases. Mortality rate can exceed 30% in patients with prolonged and severe hyperthermia. Delayed access to cooling is the leading cause of morbidity and mortality in persons with heat stroke.

REFERENCE
Available at eBooks.Health.Elsevier.com.

RELATED CONTENT
Heat Exhaustion and Heat Stroke (Patient Information)
Acute Kidney Injury (Related Key Topic)
Rhabdomyolysis (Related Key Topic)

AUTHOR: **FRED F. FERRI, MD**

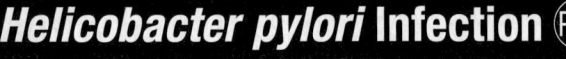
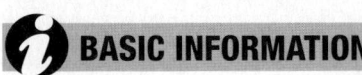 **BASIC INFORMATION**

DEFINITION

Infection of the human gastric mucosa with the organism *Helicobacter pylori,* a spiral-shaped gram-negative organism with unique features that allow it to survive in the hostile gastric environment.

SYNONYMS

H. pylori infection

ICD-10CM CODE

B96.81 *Helicobacter pylori* [*H. pylori*] as the cause of diseases classified elsewhere

EPIDEMIOLOGY & DEMOGRAPHICS

H. pylori is the most common chronic bacterial infection in human beings, probably affecting 50% of the Earth's population in all age groups, as well as 30% to 40% of the U.S. population. In developing nations, infection is acquired at an earlier age and occurs more frequently (70% prevalence in Africa).

PHYSICAL FINDINGS & CLINICAL PRESENTATION

- *H. pylori* causes histologic gastritis in all affected individuals. The majority of cases are asymptomatic and unlikely to proceed to serious consequences.
- *H. pylori* is a causative agent in peptic ulcer disease (PUD), gastric adenocarcinoma, and gastric mucosa–associated lymphoid tissue lymphoma, as well as a risk factor for iron deficiency anemia and likely chronic idiopathic thrombocytopenic purpura. It may manifest with the signs and symptoms of these disorders, including abdominal pain, bloating, anorexia, and early satiety. Table 1 and Fig. 1 describe association of *H. pylori* infection and disease states.
- "Alarm symptoms" that should prompt more immediate and aggressive workup include weight loss, dysphagia, protracted nausea or vomiting, anemia, melena, and palpable abdominal mass, particularly in older individuals.

ETIOLOGY

- Route of acquisition is unknown but is presumed to be person to person by fecal-oral or possibly oral-oral transmission.
- The majority of cases are acquired in childhood. Socioeconomic status and living conditions in childhood affect risk of acquisition of infection. These factors include housing density, number of siblings, overcrowding, sharing a bed, and lack of running water.
- Iatrogenic transmission has been documented.
- *H. pylori* does not invade gastroduodenal tissue but disrupts the mucous layer, causing

the underlying mucosa to be more vulnerable to acid peptic damage.
- It is unclear what differentiates the subset of patients with *H. pylori* who go on to develop ulcers or cancer.

TABLE 1 Association of *Helicobacter pylori* with Common Pathologic Lesions of the Upper Gastrointestinal Tract and with Nongastrointestinal Diseases

Lesion	Association with *H. pylori*
Chronic diffuse superficial gastritis	Nearly always associated[1,2]
Type A (pernicious anemia) gastritis	Negative association[3,4]
NSAID gastropathy	Negative or no association[5]
Acute erosive gastritis (e.g., alcohol, aspirin)	No association[1]
Gastric ulceration	Commonly observed in patients who are not ingesting NSAIDs or aspirin[3,6-8]
Duodenal ulceration	Usually associated with idiopathic lesions (non–drug induced, non–Zollinger-Ellison syndrome)[6,8-10]
Gastric adenocarcinoma	Positively associated with (noncardia) cancers of the gastric body and antrum[11-16]
Gastric lymphoma	Strongly associated with MALT-type B-cell lymphomas[17,18]
Idiopathic thrombocytopenic purpura	Often associated[19-21]
Nonulcer dyspepsia	Little or no association[22-26]
Gastroesophageal reflux disease	Presence of *cag*+ strains has protective association[27,28]
Barrett's esophagus	May colonize distalmost gastric epithelium in patients with gastric colonization[1]; presence of *cag*+ strains has protective association[27]
Adenocarcinoma of the esophagus	Presence of *cag*+ strains has protective association[15,29,30]
Childhood asthma and related allergic disorders (allergic rhinitis, eczema, and skin sensitization)	Presence of *cag*+ strains has protective association[31-34]

MALT, Mucosa-associated lymphoid tumor; *NSAID,* nonsteroidal antiinflammatory drug.
From Bennett JE et al: *Mandell, Douglas, and Bennett's principles and practice of infectious diseases,* ed 9, Philadelphia, 2020, Elsevier.

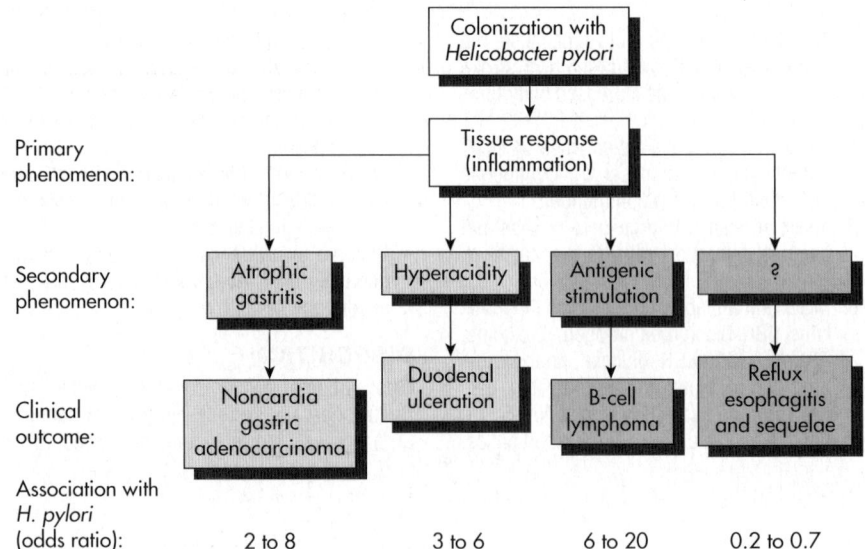

FIG. 1 Association of *Helicobacter pylori* colonization and disease states. After *H. pylori* acquisition, virtually all persons develop persistent colonization that lasts for life. Colonization induces tissue responses termed *chronic gastritis.* This process affects gastric physiology, including glandular structure, acid secretion, and antigen processing, which in turn affect disease risk. Colonization with *H. pylori* increases the risk for certain diseases (duodenal ulcer, gastric ulcer, noncardiac gastric adenocarcinoma, and B-cell lymphomas) but appears to decrease the risk for gastroesophageal reflux disease and its complications, including Barrett esophagus, and adenocarcinoma of the esophagus or gastric cardia. (From Bennett JE et al: *Mandell, Douglas, and Bennett's principles and practice of infectious diseases,* ed 9, Philadelphia, 2020, Elsevier.)

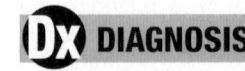 **DIAGNOSIS**

DIFERENTIAL DIAGNOSIS

- Infection with *H. pylori* should be considered in the face of PUD, gastric cancer, gastritis, and gastric mucosa–associated lymphoid tissue (MALT) lymphoma.

- *H. pylori* should be considered in the differential diagnosis of upper GI tract disease, along with nonulcer dyspepsia, reflux esophagitis, biliary tract disease, gastroparesis, pancreatitis, ischemic bowel, and unexplained iron deficiency anemia.

WORKUP

- Workup is indicated in patients with active PUD, a history of documented peptic ulcer, or gastric MALT lymphoma, as well as those with immune thrombocytopenic purpura (ITP), and otherwise unexplained iron deficiency. The role of routine screening in high-risk populations is not clear. However, numerous studies suggest that *H. pylori* eradication is protective against progression of premalignant gastric lesions. Consider testing those starting long-term NSAID, low-dose aspirin, or proton pump inhibitor (PPI) therapy. Routine identification and treatment of *H. pylori* in cases of nonulcer dyspepsia, gastroesophageal reflux disease (GERD), and in asymptomatic individuals in populations at high risk for gastric cancer is considered controversial. There is insufficient evidence to advocate screening in asymptomatic first-degree relatives of gastric cancer patients. A test-and-treat strategy may be used in patients younger than 55 with uncomplicated dyspepsia who have no alarm symptoms.
- Results of testing must be interpreted in relation to the individual patient's likelihood of *H. pylori* infection based on demographic risk factors. In the U.S. population, increased probability of infection exists in African Americans, Hispanics/Latinos, immigrants from developing nations, patients with poor socioeconomic status, Native Americans from Alaska, and persons >50 yr.
- Routine screening for *H. pylori* is not indicated in asymptomatic patients who are at low risk of infection.

- Infected patients with functional dyspepsia often benefit from treatment and should be evaluated for *H. pylori*.

LABORATORY TESTS (TABLE 2)

- Testing may be invasive or noninvasive depending on the need for endoscopy for other indications. There is no indication for endoscopy solely to diagnose *H. pylori*.
- Tests for *H. pylori* are differentiated as active or passive. Active tests provide direct evidence that *H. pylori* infection is currently present and include urea breath testing and stool antigen testing. Passive testing, which includes all serologic testing for *H. pylori*, detects the presence of antibodies to the organism. It is limited by its inability to distinguish between active current infection and prior infection that has resolved.
- Tests that use urease as a marker (urea breath and stool antigen tests and biopsy for urease activity) may result in false-negative results in patients taking antibiotics, bismuth, or antisecretory therapy, as well as those with active ulcer bleeding. Patients should be off antibiotics for 4 wk and off protein pump inhibitors for 2 wk before urea breath or stool antigen testing.
- When diagnostic endoscopy is indicated (for suspicion or follow-up of PUD or gastric MALT), antral biopsy should be tested for urease activity. If urease testing is likely to show a false-negative result because of recent PPI, bismuth, or antibiotic use, or active ulcer bleeding, the sample should undergo histologic examination.
- In cases in which biopsy is not indicated, urea breath testing or stool antigen testing is indicated to evaluate for active infection. Urea breath testing is slightly more expensive than stool antigen testing, but both costs are in the modest range. Choice can be made based on patient preference and availability. The sensitivities and specificities of these two tests are similar (>90%), but sensitivity

may be reduced in the face of active upper GI bleed or recent PPI use.

- Serologic testing should be avoided, although it may be useful in low-risk patients in areas with low prevalence to confirm lack of infection. In this situation, positive results should be confirmed with an active testing method.

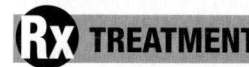 **TREATMENT**

ACUTE GENERAL Rx

- Test only patients whom you intend to treat if positive (see "Workup"). At this time, the value of eradicating *H. pylori* infection has been clearly demonstrated in patients with PUD or gastric MALT lymphoma.
- The optimal antibiotic regimen remains undefined. In addition to efficacy, side effects, cost, and ease of administration must be considered.
- Due to increasing resistance to clarithromycin, decisions regarding appropriate regimens should take into account local rates of clarithromycin resistance, as well as any prior macrolide exposure for the patient. Clarithromycin resistance can be assumed to be >15% in the U.S. unless local resistance information is available.
- The following regimens may be considered for first-line therapy:
  1. Quadruple therapy: PPI (esomeprazole 20 mg, lansoprazole 30 mg, pantoprazole 40 mg, omeprazole 40 mg, or rabeprazole 20 mg, all given bid), with twice-daily clarithromycin (500 mg), amoxicillin (1 g bid), and metronidazole 500 mg bid for 10 to 14 days.
  2. Bismuth quadruple therapy: PPI twice daily (see earlier) combined with bismuth subsalicylate (Pepto-Bismol and others) 262 or 525 mg four times daily, as well as tetracycline (500 mg qid) and metronidazole (250 mg qid or 500 mg tid-qid) for

---

TABLE 2   Modalities for *Helicobacter pylori* Diagnosis

Modality	Advantages	Disadvantages
Endoscopy with biopsy	Permits inspection of pathology; allows detection of ulcers, neoplasms	Invasive, expensive, time consuming
Culture	Permits determination of antimicrobial susceptibilities and pathogenic features of isolates	Not optimally sensitive in most laboratories. Requires several days for results
Histology	Generally more sensitive than culture. Allows direct visualization of organism and extent and nature of tissue involvement.	Gastritis may be patchy, and biopsy may be performed on wrong area. Insensitivity to detect small numbers of organisms. Requires several days for results
Urease detection	Rapid; most positive results seen within 2 h	Increased sensitivity requires longer incubation. May have false-positive results with bacterial overgrowth
Serology	Noninvasive, rapid, quantitative, inexpensive	No determination of lesions or pathology, no antimicrobial susceptibility. Not rapidly responsive to therapy
Urea breath tests	Relatively noninvasive, relatively rapid, quantitative, rapidly responsive to therapy. Most valuable for assessing response to eradication therapy after 4-8 wk	Involves expensive instrumentation or administration of radioisotopes. More invasive and less convenient than serology. No determination of lesions or pathology, no antimicrobial susceptibility
Stool antigen tests	Relatively noninvasive, relatively rapid, rapidly responsive to therapy. Most valuable for assessing response to eradication therapy after 6-8 wk	Not quantitative. Requires stool specimen, relatively expensive for developing countries. No determination of lesions or pathology, no antimicrobial susceptibility

From Bennett JE et al: *Mandell, Douglas, and Bennett's principles and practice of infectious diseases*, ed 9, Philadelphia, 2020, Elsevier.

10 to 14 days. This is now recommended as first-line therapy in areas of high clarithromycin resistance and in patients with penicillin allergy.

- Fixed-dose combinations of omeprazole, amoxicillin, rifabutin (Talicia), and others are now available for treatment of *H. pylori* infection in adults. They may improve compliance, but cost and formulary are significant limiting factors.
- Rifabutin triple therapy (rifabutin, amoxicillin, and PPI) is also available as an alternative option for first-line empiric treatment.
- Vonoprazan (a potassium-competitive acid blocker) has been FAD approved for *H. pylori* treatment in combination with amoxicillin (Voquezna Dual Pak) and with amoxicillin and clarithromycin (Voquezna Triple Pak).
- Current guidelines recommend extended treatment of 10 to 14 days.
- Recent guidelines suggest multiple other regimens that can be considered based on local resistance patterns and patient's allergy profile.
- Prior exposure to a macrolide or metronidazole, for any reason, is associated with increased resistance. A preferable regimen would include medications to which the patient has not been previously exposed.
- Diarrhea and abdominal cramping are commonly observed with many of the regimens. (Probiotics may diminish this effect.) Other side effects may include a metallic taste with metronidazole or clarithromycin, neuropathy, seizures, and disulfiram-like reaction with metronidazole, diarrhea with amoxicillin, photosensitivity with tetracycline, and *Clostridium difficile* infection with any antibiotic exposure. Bismuth may cause black stool

and constipation. Tetracycline is contraindicated in pregnant patients.
- 20% of patients may not respond to initial therapy. It is important to reinforce compliance. Second-line therapy should avoid antibiotics used in initial treatment and should include either bismuth-containing quadruple therapy or levofloxacin-containing triple therapy (regardless of local clarithromycin resistance patterns). When possible, management of those who do not respond to two courses of therapy should be guided by antimicrobial sensitivity testing (endoscopy with biopsy for cultures and sensitivity).

CHRONIC Rx

- It is essential to document clearance of infection after the completion of treatment. Repeat testing is generally performed 1 mo after completion of antibiotics and at least 2 wk after cessation of PPI therapy.
- Active tests such as urea breath test and stool antigen testing should be used. They are equally accurate in confirming eradication, and either may be used depending on availability and patient preference.
- Serology does not reliably revert to undetectable levels after treatment and should not be used to determine eradication.

DISPOSITION

Consider further evaluation in patients with recurrent symptoms after appropriate treatment.

REFERRAL

- Patients with gastric MALT lymphoma should be followed by a gastroenterologist and oncologist with expertise in the care of lymphoid neoplasms.

- Patients with dyspepsia who have tested positive for *H. pylori* and failed two courses of treatment should be referred for endoscopy and biopsy for culture and sensitivity.

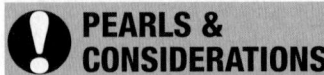

PEARLS & CONSIDERATIONS

- It remains unclear whether *H. pylori* eradication reduces the risk of progression to gastric cancer.
- Outcomes in PUD and gastric MALT lymphoma are improved with treatment of associated *H. pylori* infection.
- Tests that provide direct evidence of active *H. pylori* infection (urea breath and stool antigen testing) are preferred. These may result in false-negative results in patients taking antibiotics, bismuth, or antisecretory agents, which should be stopped at an appropriate time interval before testing.
- Be aware of high-risk populations in low-prevalence settings, including immigrants from Mexico, South America, Southeast Asia, and Eastern Europe.

REFERENCES & SUGGESTED READINGS

Available at eBooks.Health.Elsevier.com.

RELATED CONTENT

Helicobacter pylori Infection (Patient Information)
Gastritis (Related Key Topic)
Peptic Ulcer Disease (Related Key Topic)

AUTHOR: **FRED F. FERRI, MD**

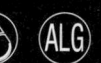 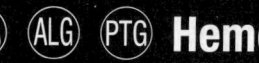
BASIC INFORMATION

DEFINITION

Hemochromatosis is an autosomal recessive disorder that disrupts the body's regulation of iron and is characterized by increased accumulation of iron in various organs (adrenals, liver, pancreas, heart, testes, kidneys, pituitary) and eventual dysfunction of these organs if not treated appropriately.

SYNONYMS

Bronze diabetes
Hereditary hemochromatosis (HH)

ICD-10CM CODES
E83.110	Hereditary hemochromatosis
E83.111	Hemochromatosis due to repeated red blood cell transfusions
E83.118	Other hemochromatosis
E83.119	Hemochromatosis, unspecified

EPIDEMIOLOGY & DEMOGRAPHICS

INCIDENCE: In whites, approximately 1/385 persons.
PREDOMINANT SEX & AGE: Generally diagnosed in men in their fifth decade. Diagnosis in females is generally not made until 10 to 20 yr after menopause.
GENETICS: Most common genetic disorder in North European ancestry. It affects 1 in every 150 to 220 persons of Northern European descent. Homozygosity for the *C282Y* mutation is now found in approximately 5/1000 persons of European descent.

PHYSICAL FINDINGS & CLINICAL PRESENTATION

- In earlier stages, patients completely asymptomatic and diagnosed due to abnormal laboratory tests
- Hepatic dysfunction leading to hepatomegaly, fibrosis, and eventually cirrhosis
- Noninflammatory arthropathy (Fig. E1)
- Gonadal insufficiency leading to loss of libido and testicular atrophy
- Diabetes mellitus: Risk greater in patients with family history
- Iron-induced cardiac disease resulting in cardiomyopathy, heart failure, and arrhythmias
- Skin pigmentation
- Clinical complications of iron overload are illustrated in Fig. E2

ETIOLOGY

- Hemochromatosis results from a failure in the regulation of the key liver-derived iron regulatory hormone hepcidin to respond to increasing iron stores. Hemochromatosis is caused by several genetic disorders, the majority of which result in loss-of-function mutations in regulatory components of hepcidin synthesis.[1] The majority of the patients diagnosed with hemochromatosis have mutation in the *HFE* gene and are either homozygous

for the *C282Y* mutation (*C282Y/C282Y*) or compound heterozygote for the *C282Y* mutation and either the mutation *H63D* (*C282Y/H63D*) or less commonly the *S65C* (*C282Y/S65C*).
- The remainder of the patients are classified as non–*HFE*-associated hemochromatosis.

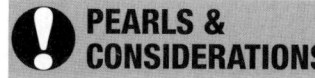 DIAGNOSIS

DIFFERENTIAL DIAGNOSIS

- Hereditary anemias with defect of erythropoiesis
- Cirrhosis, chronic liver disease, porphyria cutanea tarda
- Repeated blood transfusions
- Table 1 summarizes hereditary causes of iron overload

WORKUP

Medical history, physical examination, and laboratory evaluation should be focused on affected organ systems (see "Physical Findings & Clinical Presentation"). Fig. 3 outlines evaluation for possible hereditary hemochromatosis in an individual with negative family history. Liver biopsy is the gold standard for diagnosis; it reveals iron deposition in hepatocytes, bile ducts, and supporting tissues.

LABORATORY TESTS

Hemochromatosis may be characterized by elevations in serum transferrin saturation, ferritin levels, or hematologic measures. Since iron-related laboratory measurements vary, a sustained elevation must be documented on multiple occasions.[1]

- Transferrin saturation is the best screening test. Values >45% have a sensitivity of 94% in men and 73% in women for detection of *C282Y* homozygosity and are an indication for further testing.
- Elevated serum ferritin (about 300 mcg/L in men and above 200 mcg/L in women) has a sensitivity of 88% in men and 57% in women[1] and is good evidence of iron overload, but other causes like chronic inflammatory conditions, malignancy, and so forth need to be ruled out as ferritin is also an acute phase reactant.
- Genotypical screening for *C282Y* and *H63D* mutation in *HFE* gene should be done in patients with high transferrin saturation, elevated ferritin, or both.
- Liver biopsy (Fig. E4) is the gold standard but is not needed in somebody who has a persistently elevated transferrin saturation, elevated ferritin, or both.
- Hepatic iron index can help differentiate between various causes of iron overload.
- Elevated aspartate aminotransferase, alanine aminotransferase, and alkaline phosphatase are seen.
- Hyperglycemia is common in advanced stages.
- Endocrine abnormalities (decreased testosterone, luteinizing hormone, follicle-stimulating hormone) are noted.
- Table 2 describes laboratory findings in patients with hereditary hemochromatosis.

IMAGING STUDIES

Routine radiologic imaging is not needed. MRI (Fig. E5) may show low signal intensity in the liver and can be used to estimate hepatic iron concentration. Liver elastography is useful to estimate the degree of fibrosis.

TREATMENT

The goal of therapy is the removal of excess iron and maintaining it at a normal or near-normal level. Phlebotomy is first-line treatment. The goal is to reduce serum ferritin to 50 to 100 mg/ml. Box 1 summarizes the treatment of *HFE*-related hereditary hemochromatosis.

NONPHARMACOLOGIC THERAPY

Phlebotomy is the treatment of choice.

ACUTE GENERAL Rx

- The timing and frequency of phlebotomy needs to be individualized for each patient.
- For patients with heavy iron overload, twice-weekly phlebotomies should be started. In most patients, weekly phlebotomy is adequate.
- The effectiveness of treatment is monitored by periodic ferritin measurement. The goal is to bring ferritin level below 50 ng/ml.
- Patients with iron overload due to transfusion-dependent anemias may not tolerate phlebotomy. For these patients, iron chelation may be needed.
- The chelating agent deferoxamine has to be given daily as a 9- to 12-h IV or subcutaneous infusion, and compliance is difficult.
- The oral chelating agent deferasirox (Exjade) is effective but should not be used in patients with high-risk myelodysplastic syndrome because it can cause renal impairment, hepatic impairment, or GI hemorrhage, which can be fatal.

CHRONIC Rx

After the ferritin has been brought to <50 ng/ml, phlebotomy is needed on an as-needed basis to keep the ferritin at that level.

DISPOSITION

- Serum ferritin measurement is the most useful prognostic indicator of disease severity.
- Prognosis is good if phlebotomy is started early (before onset of cirrhosis or diabetes mellitus); women can have the full phenotypic expression of the disease, including cirrhosis, and also should be aggressively treated.

REFERRAL

For liver biopsy if diagnosis is uncertain

PEARLS & CONSIDERATIONS

COMMENTS

- Persons who are homozygous for the *HFE* gene mutation *C282Y* comprise 85% to 90% of phenotypically affected individuals. Patients

TABLE 1 Hereditary Iron Overload Disorders

Disorder	Gene, Chromosome Location	Inheritance	Plasma Transferrin Saturation	Plasma Ferritin	Iron Deposition Sites	Clinical Manifestations
Hereditary hemochromatosis, *HFE*-associated (type 1; OMIM235200)	*HFE*, 6p21	Autosomal recessive	Early increase; >45%	Later increase after third decade of life	Parenchymal iron overload affecting hepatocytes, heart, pancreas, other organs	Liver and heart disease, diabetes, gonadal failure, arthritis, skin pigmentation
Hereditary hemochromatosis, *TFR2*-associated (type 3; OMIM604250)	*TFR2*, 7q22	Autosomal recessive	Early increase; >45%	Later increase after third decade of life	Parenchymal iron overload affecting hepatocytes, heart, pancreas, other organs	Liver and heart disease, diabetes, gonadal failure, arthritis, skin pigmentation
Juvenile hemochromatosis, hemojuvelin-associated (type 2A; OMIM 602390)	*HJV*, 1q21	Autosomal recessive	Early increase; >45%	Increased by second decade of life	Parenchymal iron overload affecting hepatocytes, heart, pancreas, other organs	As for hereditary hemochromatosis, but liver involvement less prominent
Juvenile hemochromatosis, hepcidin-associated (type 2B; OMIM613313)	*HAMP*, 19q13	Autosomal recessive	Early increase; >45%	Increased by second decade of life	Parenchymal iron overload affecting hepatocytes, heart, pancreas, other organs	As for hereditary hemochromatosis, but liver involvement less prominent
Hemochromatosis, *DMT1*-associated (OMIM 206100)	*SCL11A2*, 12q13	Autosomal recessive	Early increase; >45%	Normal to moderately elevated	Hepatic iron overload, predominantly in hepatocytes	Severe microcytic anemia, liver dysfunction
Atransferrinemia (OMIM 209300)	*TF*, 3q22	Autosomal recessive	No plasma transferrin	Increased	Parenchymal iron overload affecting hepatocytes, heart, pancreas; no iron stores in bone marrow or spleen	Transfusion-dependent iron-deficiency anemia, growth retardation, poor survival
Aceruloplasminemia (OMIM 604290)	*CP*, 3q24-q25	Autosomal recessive	Decreased	Increased	Marked iron accumulation in basal ganglia, liver, pancreas	Diabetes, progressive neurologic disease, retinal degeneration
Hemochromatosis, ferroportin-associated, with impaired iron export (type 4A; OMIM606069)	*SLC40A1*, 2q32	Autosomal dominant	Remains normal or low	Early increase	Predominantly macrophage iron deposition	None
Hemochromatosis, ferroportin-associated, with hepcidin resistance (type 4B; OMIM606069)	*SLC40A1*, 2q32	Autosomal dominant	Early increase; >45%	Early increase	Parenchymal iron overload affecting hepatocytes, heart, pancreas, other organs	Similar to *HFE*-associated hemochromatosis

From Hoffman R et al: *Hematology, basic principles and practice*, ed 7, Philadelphia, 2018, Elsevier.

who are heterozygous for both *C282Y* and *H63D* generally do not have clinically evident disease unless coexisting factors (e.g., excessive alcohol intake) are present.

- Patients with hemochromatosis and serum ferritin levels <1000 ng/ml are unlikely to have cirrhosis. Liver biopsy to screen for cirrhosis may be unnecessary in such patients.
- Cirrhotic patients must be periodically monitored (ultrasound or computed tomography scan) because of their increased risk of hepatocellular carcinoma.
- *HFE* gene testing for *C282Y* mutation is a cost-effective method of screening relatives

of patients with hereditary hemochromatosis. The American College of Gastroenterology recommends genotyping persons who have abnormal iron screening tests and first-degree relatives of those identified with *C282Y* homozygosity.

- Established cirrhosis, hypogonadism, destructive arthritis, and insulin-dependent diabetes mellitus secondary to hemochromatosis cannot be reversed with repeated phlebotomy, but their progress can be slowed.
- In patients who are heterozygous for *C282Y* or *H63D* mutation, clinically meaningful iron overload does not develop.

- Screening for hepatocellular carcinoma is reserved for those with hereditary hemochromatosis and cirrhosis.

REFERENCE

Available at eBooks.Health.Elsevier.com.

RELATED CONTENT

Hemochromatosis (Patient Information)

AUTHOR: **FRED F. FERRI, MD**

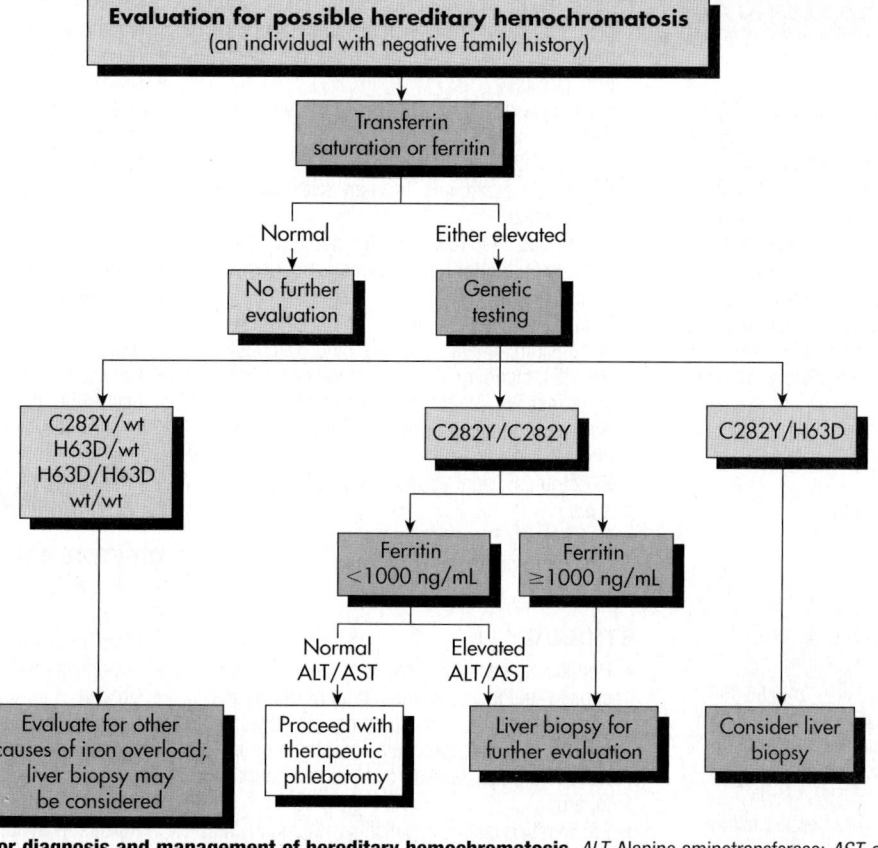

FIG. 3 Proposed algorithm for diagnosis and management of hereditary hemochromatosis. *ALT,* Alanine aminotransferase; *AST,* aspartate aminotransferase; *wt,* wild-type (normal). (From Goldman L, Schafer AI: *Goldman-Cecil medicine,* ed 27, Philadelphia, 2024, Elsevier.)

TABLE 2 Laboratory Findings in Patients with Hereditary Hemochromatosis

Measurements	Normal Subjects	PATIENTS WITH HEREDITARY HEMOCHROMATOSIS	
		Asymptomatic	Symptomatic
Blood (Fasting)			
Serum iron level (μg/dl)	60-180	150-280	180-300
Serum transferrin level (mg/dl)	220-410	200-280	200-300
Transferrin saturation (%)	20-45	45-100	80-100
Serum Ferritin Level (ng/ml)			
Men	20-200	150-1000	500-6000
Women	15-150	120-1000	500-6000
Genetic (*HFE* Mutation Analysis)			
C282Y/C282Y	wt/wt‡	C282Y/C282Y	C282Y/C282Y
C282Y/H63D*	wt/wt	C282Y/H63D	C282Y/H63D
Liver			
Hepatic Iron Concentration			
μg/g dry weight	300-1500	2000-10,000	8000-30,000
μmol/g dry weight	5-27	36-179	140-550
Hepatic iron index†	<1	1 to >1.9	>1.9
Liver Histology			
Perls Prussian blue stain	0, 1+	2+ to 4+	3+, 4+

*Compound heterozygote.
†Calculated by dividing the hepatic iron concentration (in μmol/g dry weight) by the age of the patient (in yr). With the increased use of genetic testing in patients with iron overload, the specificity of the hepatic iron index has diminished.
‡wt/wt: Wild type (normal).
From Goldman L, Schafer AI: *Goldman-Cecil medicine,* ed 24, Philadelphia, 2012, Elsevier

BOX 1 Treatment of *HFE*-Related Hereditary Hemochromatosis

Perform phlebotomy of 500 ml (1 unit) of whole blood weekly unless the hematocrit value drops below 37%.
Check the transferrin saturation and ferritin levels at 2- to 3-mo intervals to monitor response (optional).
When the iron stores are depleted (ferritin 50 to 100 ng/ml and transferrin saturation <50%), proceed to maintenance phlebotomy of 1 unit of whole blood every 2-3 mo. Aim to keep the transferrin saturation <50%; if successful, the ferritin level should remain between 50 and 100 ng/ml.

From Feldman M et al: *Sleisenger and Fordtran's gastrointestinal and liver disease,* ed 11, Philadelphia, 2021, Elsevier.

BASIC INFORMATION

DEFINITION

Hepatic encephalopathy is a neuropsychiatric syndrome occurring in patients with severe impairment of liver function and consequent accumulation of toxic products not metabolized by the liver. It is characterized by gradual impairment of the ability to perform mental tasks and to react to external stimuli. Fig. 1 illustrates the hepatic encephalopathy grades in acute liver failure. **Minimal hepatic encephalopathy** refers to patients with hepatic cirrhosis and mild cognitive impairment, but no history of overt encephalopathy.

SYNONYMS

Hepatic coma
Portal systemic encephalopathy
HE

ICD-10CM CODES

G92	Toxic encephalopathy
G93.40	Encephalopathy, unspecified
G93.41	Metabolic encephalopathy
K70.40	Alcoholic hepatic failure without coma
K70.41	Alcoholic hepatic failure with coma
K72.0	Acute and subacute hepatic failure
K72.00	Acute and subacute hepatic failure without coma
K72.01	Acute and subacute hepatic failure with coma
K72.1	Chronic hepatic failure
K72.10	Chronic hepatic failure without coma
K72.11	Chronic hepatic failure with coma
K72.9	Hepatic failure, unspecified
K72.90	Hepatic failure, unspecified without coma
K72.91	Hepatic failure, unspecified with coma
K91.82	Postprocedural hepatic failure

EPIDEMIOLOGY & DEMOGRAPHICS

INCIDENCE & PREVALENCE: Hepatic encephalopathy occurs in >40% of all cases of cirrhosis.

PHYSICAL FINDINGS & CLINICAL PRESENTATION

Hepatic encephalopathy can be classified by clinical stages described in Table 1. Other widely used scales are the four score criteria and the West Haven criteria. The West Haven criteria for grading hepatic encephalopathy is as follows:

- Grade (0): No abnormalities noted
- Grade (1): Unawareness (mild), euphoria or anxiety, shortened attention span, impairment of calculation ability, lethargy, or apathy
- Grade (2): Disorientation to time, obvious personality change, inappropriate behavior
- Grade (3): Somnolence to stupor, responsiveness to stimuli, gross disorientation, bizarre behavior
- Grade (4): Coma

The physical examination in hepatic encephalopathy varies with the stage and may reveal the following abnormalities:

- Skin: Jaundice, palmar erythema, spider angiomata, ecchymosis, dilated superficial periumbilical veins (caput medusae) in patients with cirrhosis
- Eyes: Scleral icterus, Kayser-Fleischer rings (Wilson disease)
- Breath: Fetor hepaticus
- Chest: Gynecomastia in men with chronic liver disease
- Abdomen: Ascites, small nodular liver (cirrhosis), tender hepatomegaly (congestive hepatomegaly)
- Rectal examination: Hemorrhoids (portal hypertension), guaiac-positive stool (alcoholic gastritis, bleeding esophageal varices, peptic ulcer disease, bleeding hemorrhoids)
- Genitalia: Testicular atrophy in males with chronic liver disease
- Extremities: Pedal edema from hypoalbuminemia
- Neurologic: Flapping tremor (asterixis), obtundation, coma with or without decerebrate posturing

ETIOLOGY

- Hepatic encephalopathy is thought to be caused mainly by accumulation of unmetabolized ammonia. The shunting of ammonia into the systemic circulation results in neuronal dysfunction leading to hepatic encephalopathy
- Precipitating factors in patients with underlying cirrhosis (upper gastrointestinal bleeding, hypokalemia, hypomagnesemia, analgesic and sedative drugs, sepsis, alkalosis, increased dietary protein)
- Acute fulminant viral hepatitis
- Drugs and toxins (e.g., isoniazid, acetaminophen, diclofenac and other NSAIDs, statins, methyldopa, loratadine, propylthiouracil, lisinopril, labetalol, halothane, carbon tetrachloride, erythromycin, nitrofurantoin, troglitazone, herbal products, flavocoxid)
- Reye syndrome
- Shock and/or sepsis
- Fatty liver of pregnancy
- Metastatic carcinoma, hepatocellular carcinoma
- Other: Autoimmune hepatitis, ischemic veno-occlusive disease, sclerosing cholangitis, heat stroke, amebic abscesses

DIAGNOSIS

DIFFERENTIAL DIAGNOSIS

- Delirium caused by medications or illicit drugs
- Cerebrovascular accident, subdural hematoma
- Meningitis, encephalitis
- Hypoglycemia
- Uremia
- Cerebral anoxia
- Hypercalcemia
- Metastatic neoplasm to brain
- Alcohol withdrawal syndrome/Wernicke-Korsakoff syndrome
- Hyponatremia
- Postictal state

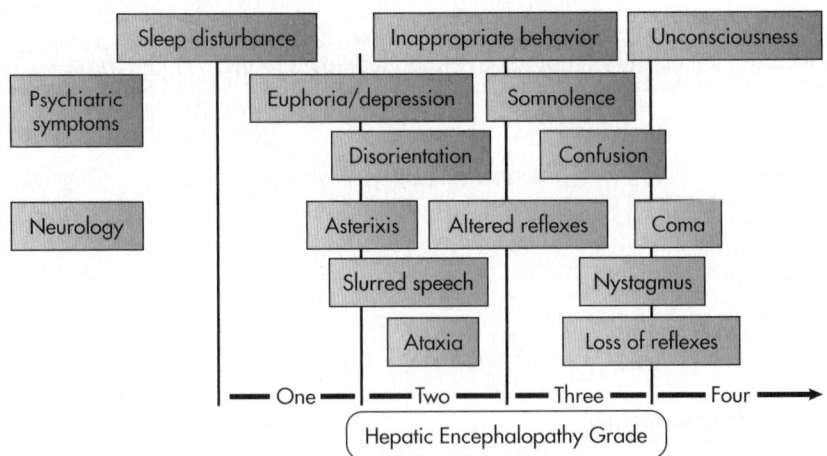

FIG. 1 Hepatic encephalopathy grade in acute liver failure. (From Parrillo JE, Dellinger RP: *Critical care medicine: principles of diagnosis and management in the adult,* ed 4, Philadelphia, 2014, Elsevier.)

TABLE 1 Stages of Encephalopathy in Chronic Liver Disease (West Haven Criteria)

Stage	Clinical Signs
Stage I	Mental slowness, euphoria or anxiety, shortened attention span, impaired calculating ability
Stage II	Lethargy or apathy, inappropriate behavior, personality change, more obvious problems with calculations
Stage III	Lethargic, somnolent, marked confusion and disorientation but responds to verbal stimuli
Stage IV	Coma, patient may or may not respond to noxious stimuli

Patients with chronic liver disease rarely, if ever, demonstrate cerebral edema, regardless of the stage of encephalopathy.
From Vincent JL et al: *Textbook of critical care,* ed 8, Philadelphia, 2024, Elsevier.

H

Diseases
and Disorders

I

WORKUP

Hepatic encephalopathy should be considered in any patient with cirrhosis who presents with neuropsychiatric manifestations. Exclude other etiologies with comprehensive history (obtained from patient, relatives, and others), physical examination, and laboratory and imaging studies. A pertinent history should include exposure to hepatitis, ethanol intake, drug history, exposure to toxins, intravenous (IV) drug abuse, measles or influenza with aspirin use (Reye syndrome), and history of carcinoma (primary or metastatic). Minimal hepatic encephalopathy may not be obvious on clinical examination but can be detected with neurophysiologic and neuropsychiatric testing (Table 2).

LABORATORY TESTS

- Alanine aminotransferase, aspartate aminotransferase, bilirubin, alkaline phosphatase, glucose, calcium, electrolytes, blood urea nitrogen, creatinine, albumin
- Complete blood count, platelet count, prothrombin time, partial thromboplastin time
- Serum and urine toxicology screen in suspected medication or illegal drug use
- Blood and urine cultures, urinalysis
- Venous ammonia level. Measurement of serum ammonia level is useful in the evaluation of acute liver failure because levels correlate with the severity of encephalopathy and elevated levels are predictive of severe encephalopathy and cerebral edema. It is not useful for the evaluation or screening of hepatic encephalopathy in patients with chronic liver disease because it can neither rule in nor rule out hepatic encephalopathy, and levels do not correlate with the degree of encephalopathy
- Arterial blood gases

IMAGING STUDIES

CT scan or MRI of the brain may be useful in selected patients to exclude other etiologies when diagnosis is unclear.

Rx TREATMENT

NONPHARMACOLOGIC THERAPY

- Identification and treatment of precipitating factors (Box 1).
- Restriction of protein intake is ill-advised and not necessary since normal protein intake does not appear to exacerbate hepatic encephalopathy.

ACUTE GENERAL Rx

The approach to patients with high grade hepatic encephalopathy is shown in Fig. 2. Table 3 summarizes the management of fulminant hepatic failure.

Reduction of colonic ammonia production:

- Lactulose 25 ml twice daily initially; dose is subsequently adjusted depending on clinical response to achieve production of three bowel movements daily. IV ornithine aspartate should be considered for those not responding to lactulose.
- The oral antibiotic rifaximin (550 mg PO bid) is effective in reducing the risk of recurrent hepatic encephalopathy in patients with

---

BOX 1 Clinical Events Precipitating Hepatic Encephalopathy in Patients with Cirrhosis

Gastrointestinal hemorrhage
Infection (including spontaneous bacterial peritonitis)
Sepsis
Dehydration
Imbalance of electrolytes or acid-base
Renal failure
Drugs, toxins, medications (especially sedative-hypnotics or narcotics)
Illicit substances
Alcohol
Dietary indiscretion (excessive protein intake)

From Vincent JL et al: *Textbook of critical care*, ed 8, Philadelphia, 2024, Elsevier.

---

cirrhosis and preventing post TIPS hepatic encephalopathy. It can be taken with lactulose, and the combination of lactulose and rifaximin is superior to lactulose alone in reversing hepatic encephalopathy. Rifaximin has also been shown to be effective in improving psychometric performance and health-related quality of life in patients with minimal hepatic encephalopathy. It is well tolerated but expensive.[1]
- Probiotics (e.g., one capsule containing 112.5 billion viable lyophilized bacteria tid) might also be beneficial in altering gut flora to reduce ammonia production.

Treatment of cerebral edema:
- Cerebral edema is often present in patients with acute liver failure, and it accounts for nearly 50% of deaths. Monitoring intracranial pressure by epidural, intraparenchymal, or subdural transducers and treatment of cerebral edema with mannitol (100 to 200 ml of 20% solution [0.3 to 0.4 g/kg of body weight]) given by rapid IV infusion are helpful in selected patients (e.g., potential transplantation patients).
- Fig. 3 illustrates the management of a sustained rise in intracranial pressure in liver failure.
- Dexamethasone and hyperventilation (useful in head injury) are of little value in treating cerebral edema from liver failure.

CHRONIC Rx

- Avoidance of any precipitating factors (e.g., high-protein diet, medications).
- Consideration of liver transplantation in selected patients with progressive or recurrent encephalopathy (Box 2). Liver transplantation remains the only curative therapeutic option.

DISPOSITION

Prognosis varies with the underlying etiology of the liver failure and the grade of encephalopathy (generally good for grades 1 or 2; poor for grades 3 or 4). Without proper therapy, the survival rate at 1 yr is 42% and decreases to 23% at 3 yr.

REFERRAL

The early stages of hepatic encephalopathy can be managed in the outpatient setting, whereas stages III or IV require hospital admission.

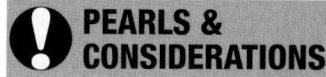 **PEARLS & CONSIDERATIONS**

COMMENTS

- Trials have shown that adding IV albumin to lactulose may improve outcomes in severe hepatic encephalopathy by reducing oxidative stress through reduction of levels of circulating cytokines and endotoxins.
- Long-acting benzodiazepines should not be used to treat anxiety and sleep disorders in patients with cirrhosis, as they may precipitate encephalopathy.
- Patients not responding to supportive therapy should be evaluated for liver transplantation.

TABLE 2 Neuropsychiatric Tests Used to Evaluate Hepatic Encephalopathy

Cerebral Function	Test
Learning and delayed recall	Story Memory Test
	Figure Memory Test
Concentration	Digit Vigilance Test
Fine motor coordination	Grooved Pegboard
Sequential procedures	Trail Making Test
Problem solving	Wisconsin Card Sorting Test
Attention	WAIS-R* Digit Symbol Subtest
Vocabulary	WAIS-R Vocabulary Subtest
Verbal fluency skills	Controlled Oral Word Association
	Animal Naming
Auditory comprehension	Complex Material
Visual-spatial analysis	WAIS-R Block Design Subtest
Psychological function	MMPI-2†

* WAIS-R, Wechsler Adult Intelligence Scale–Revised.
† MMPI-2, Minnesota Multiphasic Personality Inventory.
From Vincent JL et al: *Textbook of critical care*, ed 8, Philadelphia, 2024, Elsevier.

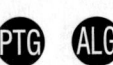

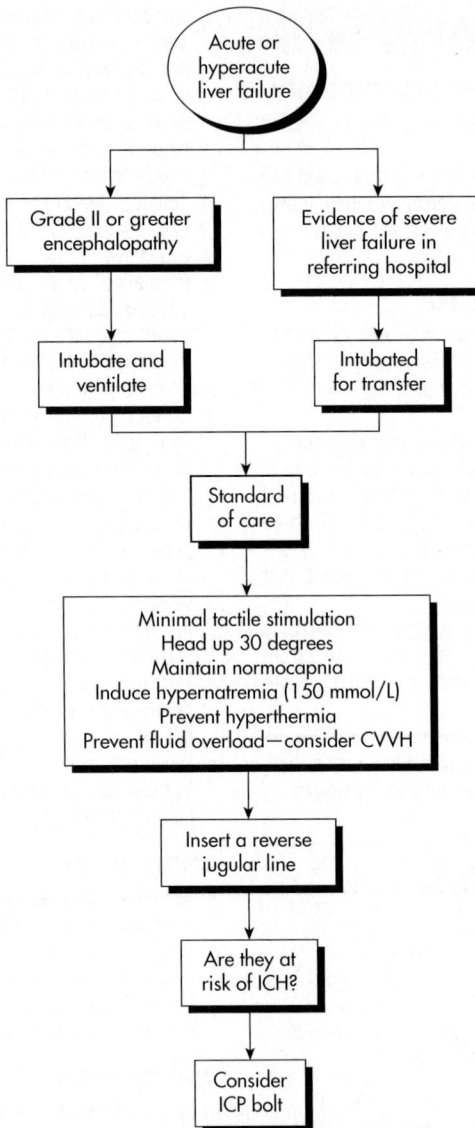

FIG. 2 Initial management of patient with high-grade encephalopathy. *CVVH,* Continuous venovenous hemofiltration; *ICH,* intracranial hypertension; *ICP,* intracranial pressure. (From Parrillo JE, Dellinger RP: *Critical care medicine: principles of diagnosis and management in the adult,* ed 5, Philadelphia, 2019, Elsevier.)

TABLE 3 Management of Fulminant Hepatic Failure

No sedation except for procedures
Minimal handling
Enteric precautions until infection ruled out
Monitor:
1. Heart and respiratory rate
2. Arterial BP, CVP
3. Core/toe temperature
4. Neurologic observations
5. Gastric pH (>5.0)
6. Blood glucose (>4 mmol/L)
7. Acid-base
8. Electrolytes
9. PT, PTT
Fluid balance:
1. 75% maintenance
2. Dextrose 10%-50% (provide 6-10 mg/kg/min)
3. Sodium (0.5-1 mmol/L)
4. Potassium (2-4 mmol/L)
Maintain circulating volume with colloid/FFP coagulation support only if required
Drugs:
1. Vitamin K
2. H_2 antagonist
3. Antacids
4. Lactulose
5. N-acetylcysteine for acetaminophen toxicity
6. Broad-spectrum antibiotics
7. Antifungals
Nutrition:
1. Enteral feeding (1-2 g protein/kg/day)
2. PN if ventilated

BP, Blood pressure; *CVP,* central venous pressure; *FFP,* fresh frozen plasma; *PN,* parenteral nutrition; *PT,* prothrombin time; *PTT,* partial thromboplastin time.
From Fuhrman BP et al: *Pediatric critical care,* ed 4, Philadelphia, 2011, Saunders.

- Not all patients with cirrhosis develop hepatic encephalopathy. It has been shown that 40% of persons with cirrhosis and minimal hepatic encephalopathy do not develop overt hepatic encephalopathy in long-term follow-up. There are genetic factors associated with development of hepatic encephalopathy in patients with cirrhosis. Genetic analyses have shown that glutaminase TACC and CACC haplotypes are linked to the risk for overt hepatic encephalopathy.

REFERENCE & SUGGESTED READINGS
Available at eBooks.Health.Elsevier.com.

RELATED CONTENT

Encephalopathy (Patient Information)
Cirrhosis (Related Key Topic)
Hepatic Encephalopathy (Related Key Topic)

AUTHOR: **FRED F. FERRI, MD**

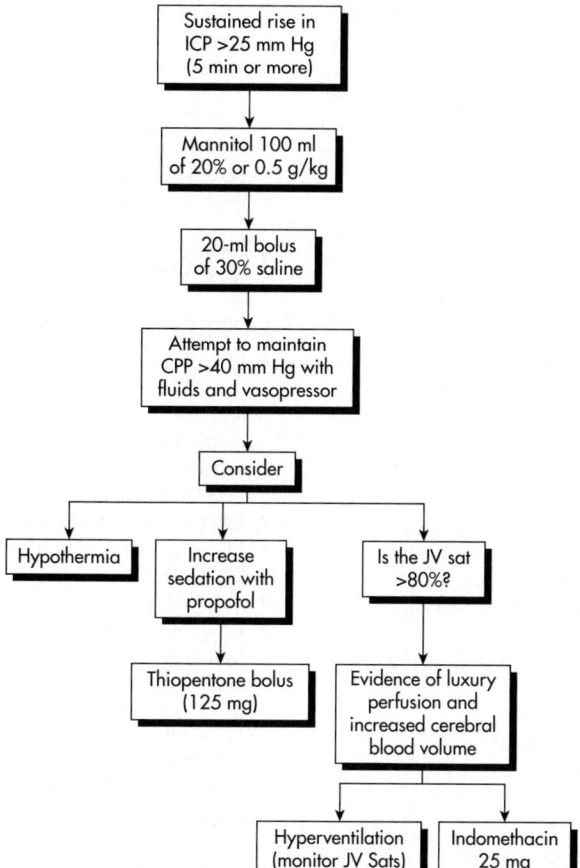

FIG. 3 Management of a sustained rise in intracranial pressure. *CPP,* Cerebral perfusion pressure; *ICP,* intracranial pressure; *JV,* jugular venous; *Sats,* saturation. (From Parrillo JE, Dellinger RP: *Critical care medicine: principles of diagnosis and management in the adult,* ed 5, Philadelphia, 2019, Elsevier.)

BOX 2 Various Prognostic Criteria Used for Liver Transplantation in Patients with Fulminant Hepatic Failure

King's College Criteria

Acetaminophen overdose:
- Arterial pH <7.3 (irrespective of grade of encephalopathy) or
- PT >100 sec (INR >6.5)
- Serum creatinine >3.4 mg/dl (>300 μmol/L)
- Patients with grade III and IV hepatic encephalopathy

Nonacetaminophen liver injury:
- PT >100 sec (INR >6.5) (irrespective of grade of encephalopathy) or any three of the following variables:
  1. Age <10 or >40 yr
  2. Non-A, non-B hepatitis, halothane hepatitis, idiosyncratic drug reactions
  3. Jaundice >7 days before onset of encephalopathy
  4. Serum bilirubin 17.4 mg/dl (300 μmol/L)
  5. PT >50 sec

Cliché Criteria

Factor V <20% in persons <30 yr or both of the following:
- Factor V <30% in patients >30 yr
- Grade III or IV encephalopathy

Serum Gc Globulin Levels
Decreasing Gc levels due to dying hepatocytes

Serum α-Fetoprotein Level
Serial increase from day 1 to day 3 has shown correlation with survival

Liver Biopsy
70% necrosis is discriminant of 90% mortality

From Vincent JL et al: *Textbook of critical care,* ed 6, Philadelphia, 2011, Saunders.

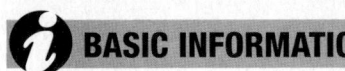

BASIC INFORMATION

DEFINITION
Hepatitis A is generally an acute self-limiting infection of the liver by an enterically transmitted picornavirus, hepatitis A virus (HAV). Infection may range from asymptomatic to fulminant hepatitis.

SYNONYMS
Infectious hepatitis
Short incubation hepatitis
Type A hepatitis
HAV (hepatitis A virus)

ICD-10CM CODES
B15.0   Hepatitis A with hepatic coma
B15.9   Hepatitis A without hepatic coma

EPIDEMIOLOGY & DEMOGRAPHICS
INCIDENCE:
- Hepatitis A occurs worldwide, affecting 1.4 million people annually and accounting for 20% to 40% of cases of viral hepatitis in the U.S. It is the most common cause of viral hepatitis worldwide.
- The seroprevalence increases with age, ranging from 10% in individuals aged <5 yr to 74% in those aged >50 yr.
- In the U.S., average disease rate was ~15 cases/100,000 persons/yr before routine vaccination of all children in certain states. The incidence after 2005 is about 1 case/100,000. There were 18,846 reported cases in the U.S. in 2019.
- The incidence is relatively higher in some regions in the U.S., including Arizona, Alaska, California, Idaho, Nevada, New Mexico, Oklahoma, Oregon, South Dakota, and Washington.
- At-risk groups include:
  1. Residents and staff of group homes
  2. Children and employees of day care centers
  3. People who engage in oral-anal contact, regardless of sexual orientation
  4. Intravenous (IV) drug abusers
  5. Travel to endemic areas
  6. Areas of overcrowding, poor sanitation, inadequate sewage treatment

PREVALENCE:
- Approximately three fourths of the U.S. population has serologic evidence of prior infection.
- Anti-HAV prevalence has an inverse relation to income and household size.

PREDOMINANT SEX: None, except higher infection rates seen in men who have sex with men who engage in oral–anal contact.

PREDOMINANT AGE & PEAK INCIDENCE:
- In areas of high rates of hepatitis A, virtually all children are infected while younger than 10 yr, but disease is rare.
- In areas of moderate rates of hepatitis A, disease occurs in late childhood and young adults.
- In areas of low rates of hepatitis A, most cases occur in young adults.

INCUBATION PERIOD: Averages 30 days (15 to 50)

PHYSICAL FINDINGS & CLINICAL PRESENTATION
- Infection with HAV may have acute or subacute presentation, icteric or anicteric. Severity of illness seems to increase with age (90% of infection in children aged <5 yr may be subclinical).
- The incubation period of HAV is 2 to 6 wk.
- A preicteric, prodromal phase of approximately 1 to 14 days; 15% no apparent prodrome. Symptoms are usually abrupt in onset and may include anorexia, fatigue, malaise, nausea, vomiting, fever, headache, and mild abdominal pain.
- Less common symptoms are chills, myalgias, arthralgias, upper respiratory symptoms, constipation, diarrhea, pruritus, urticaria.
- Jaundice occurs in >70% of patients. Patients older than 30 yr are more likely than younger individuals to have jaundice.
- The icteric phase is preceded by dark urine.
- Bilirubinuria is typically followed a few days later by clay-colored stools and icterus.

PHYSICAL EXAMINATION:
- Jaundice: Peaks in severity 2 wk after onset
- Hepatomegaly
- Splenomegaly
- Cervical lymphadenopathy
- Evanescent rash
- Petechiae
- Cardiac arrhythmias

COMPLICATIONS:
- Cholestasis
- Fulminant hepatitis
- Arthritis
- Myocarditis
- Optic neuritis
- Transverse myelitis
- Thrombocytopenic purpura
- Aplastic anemia
- Red cell aplasia
- Henoch-Schönlein purpura
- Immunoglobulin A (IgA) dominant glomerulonephritis

ETIOLOGY
- Caused by HAV, a 27-nm, nonenveloped, icosahedral, positive-stranded ribonucleic acid (RNA) virus.
- Transmission is fecal-oral route, from person to person. Transmission occurs with close contact or with food- or water-borne outbreaks with inadequately purified water or cooked foods. Recent outbreaks have involved green onions and tomatoes.
- Parenteral transmission is considered rare.
- Vertical transmission has also been reported.

DIAGNOSIS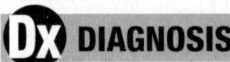

DIFFERENTIAL DIAGNOSIS
- Other hepatitis virus (B, C, D, E): Characteristics of the main hepatitis viruses are described in Table 1. Serology and polymerase chain reaction (PCR) test results are summarized in Table 2
- Infectious mononucleosis
- Cytomegalovirus infection
- Herpes simplex virus infection
- Leptospirosis
- Brucellosis
- Drug-induced liver disease
- Ischemic hepatitis
- Autoimmune hepatitis

WORKUP
- IgM antibody specific for HAV
- Liver function tests; ALT and AST elevations are sensitive for liver damage but not specific for HAV
- Elevated erythrocyte sedimentation rate (ESR)
- CBC; may find mild lymphocytosis

LABORATORY TESTS
- Diagnosis confirmed by IgM anti-HAV; it is detectable in almost all infected patients at presentation and remains positive for 3 to 6 mo
- A fourfold rise in titer of total antibody (IgM and IgG) to HAV confirms acute infection
- HAV detection in stool and body fluids by electron microscopy
- HAV RNA detection in stool, body fluids, serum, and liver tissue
- ALT and AST usually more than 8 times normal in acute infection
- Bilirubin usually 5 to 15 times normal

TABLE 1   Characteristics of the Main Hepatitis Viruses

	HAV	HBV	HCV	HDV	HEV
Family	Picornavirus	Hepadnavirus	Flavivirus	Incomplete	Calicivirus
Nucleic acid	RNA	DNA	RNA	RNA	RNA
Diameter (nm)	27	42	32	36	34
Incubation period (wk)	2-6	6-24	2-26	6-9	2-10
Spread					
Feces	Yes	No	No	No	Yes
Blood	Uncommon	Yes	Yes	Yes	No
Sexual	Uncommon	Yes	Uncommon	Yes	?
Vertical	No	Yes	Uncommon	Yes	No
Chronic infection	No	Yes	Yes	Yes	No
Vaccine	Available	Available	Nil	Nil	Nil

HAV, Hepatitis A virus; *HBV,* hepatitis B virus; *HCV,* hepatitis C virus; *HDV,* hepatitis D virus; *HEV,* hepatitis E virus.
From Cameron P et al: *Textbook of adult emergency medicine,* ed 5, 2019, Australia, Elsevier.

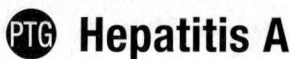

TABLE 2 Diagnostic Blood Tests: Serology and Viral Polymerase Chain Reaction

HAV	HBV	HCV	HDV	HEV
Acute/Active Infection				
Anti-HAV IgM (+)	Anti-HBc IgM (+)	Anti-HCV (+)	Anti-HDV IgM (+)	Anti-HEV IgM (+)
Blood PCR positive*	HBsAg (+)	HCV RNA (+) (PCR)	Blood PCR positive	Blood PCR positive*
	Anti-HBs (−)		HBsAg (+)	
	HBV DNA (+) (PCR)		Anti-HBs (−)	
Past Infection (Recovered)				
Anti-HAV IgG (+)	Anti-HBs (+)	Anti-HCV (+)	Anti-HDV IgG (+)	Anti-HEV IgG (+)
	Anti-HBc IgG (+)†	Blood PCR (−)	Blood PCR (−)	Blood PCR (−)
Chronic Infection				
N/A	Anti-HBc IgG (+)	Anti-HCV (+)	Anti-HDV IgG (+)	N/A
	HBsAg (+)	Blood PCR (+)	Blood PCR (−)	
	Anti-HBs (−)		HBsAg (+)	
	PCR (+) or (−)		Anti-HBs (−)	
Vaccine Response				
Anti-HAV IgG (+)	Anti-HBs (+)	N/A	N/A	N/A
	Anti-HBc (−)			

HAV, Hepatitis A virus; *HBc*, hepatitis B core; *HBs*, hepatitis B surface; *HBsAg*, hepatitis B surface antigen; *HBV*, hepatitis B virus; *HCV*, hepatitis C virus; *HDV*, hepatitis D virus; *HEV*, hepatitis E virus; *Ig*, immunoglobulin; *N/A*, not applicable; *PCR*, polymerase chain reaction.
* Research tool.
† Still poses a risk for reactivation.
From Kliegman RM: *Nelson textbook of pediatrics*, ed 21, Philadelphia, 2020, Elsevier.

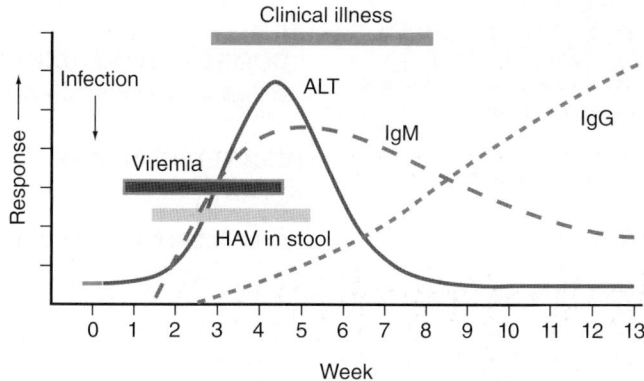

FIG. 1 Immunologic, virologic, and biochemical events during the course of a typical hepatitis A virus *(HAV)* infection. *ALT,* Alanine transaminase; *IgG,* immunoglobulin G; *IgM,* immunoglobulin M. (From Cherry JD et al: *Feigin and Cherry's pediatric infectious diseases,* ed 8, Philadelphia, 2019, Elsevier.)

- Alkaline phosphatase minimally elevated, but higher level in cholestasis
- Albumin and prothrombin time are generally normal; if elevated, they may herald hepatic necrosis
- Fig. 1 illustrates the typical course of hepatitis A

IMAGING STUDIES
- Rarely useful
- Sonogram (fulminant hepatitis)

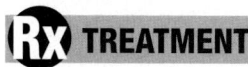 TREATMENT
- Usually self-limited
- Supportive care
- Those with fulminant hepatitis may require hospitalization and treatment of associated complications
- Activity as tolerated
- Advise to avoid alcohol and hepatotoxic drugs

- Patients with fulminant hepatitis should be assessed for liver transplantation

CHRONIC Rx
No chronic HAV and no chronic carrier state. The majority of patients have resolution of symptoms and liver abnormalities within 3 mo.

DISPOSITION
- Follow-up as outpatient.
- Most patients recover within 3 mo of infection, although 5% to 10% of patients will experience a relapse in the first 6 mo.
- HAV is a self-limited infection and does not cause chronic hepatitis.

REFERRAL
- To a hepatologist if severe, fulminant hepatitis develops

- To a transplant surgeon if liver transplant becomes a consideration for fulminant hepatitis and liver failure

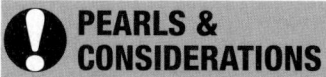 PEARLS & CONSIDERATIONS

- All cases of hepatitis A should be reported to the public health authorities because food-borne or water-borne outbreaks may occur, and public health efforts (mass vaccination or immunoglobulin therapy) may prevent secondary cases.
- Hepatitis A is a common illness in internationally traveled and developing countries. Pretravel vaccination is strongly recommended for travelers who are HAV susceptible. Table 3 summarizes recommendations for preexposure use of hepatitis A virus vaccine. Updated dosage recommendations are described in Table 4.
- Handwashing is important because the hepatitis A virus may survive for up to 4 h on the fingertips.
- There have been significant recent outbreaks of hepatitis A in the U.S. In 2016 to 2019 there was an increase of cases by 294% vs. cases in 2013 to 2015. This was mostly among the homeless, IV drug abusers, men having sex with men, and individuals who consumed certain imported food items. In 2023 there were six cases in Washington State associated with frozen strawberries.

PREVENTION
- Improvement in hygiene and sanitation
- Heating food
- Avoidance of water and foods from endemic area

PASSIVE IMMUNIZATION
- Immunoglobulin provides protection against HAV through passive transfer of antibody.
- Preexposure prophylaxis indicated for people traveling to endemic areas with immune globulin (Ig 0.02 or 0.06 ml/kg given intramuscularly [IM]) who have not received or cannot receive the hepatitis A vaccine before departure. The lower dose is effective for up to 3 mo, and the higher dose is effective for up to 5 mo.
- Postexposure prophylaxis (PEP): For individuals with a recent exposure to hepatitis A who have not received the vaccine, postexposure prophylaxis is warranted with either immunoglobulin (Ig 0.02 ml/kg given IM) or a single dose of the hepatitis A vaccine within 2 wk of the exposure. For healthy persons ages 12 mo to 40 yr of age, a single dose of the hepatitis A vaccine should be given. Children <12 mo, adults >40 yr of age, and persons who have chronic liver disease and who are immunocompromised should receive immunoglobulin.

ACTIVE IMMUNIZATION
- There are several inactivated and attenuated hepatitis vaccines; only the inactivated

TABLE 3 Recommendations for Routine Preexposure Use of Hepatitis A Virus Vaccine

Group	Comments
Children	Vaccine should be given to all children at age 1 yr (12-23 mo).* Vaccination of children 2-18 yr may also be warranted.[†]
International travelers[‡]	IG may be given in addition to or instead of vaccine; children <12 mo should receive IG.
Close contacts of newly arriving international adoptees	All persons who anticipate close personal contact (e.g., household contact or regular babysitter) during the first 60 days after arrival
Men who have sex with men	Includes adolescents
Illicit drug users	Includes adolescents
Persons with chronic liver disease, such as those with hepatitis B or C	Increased risk of fulminant hepatitis A with HAV infection
Persons receiving clotting factor concentrates	
Persons who work with HAV in research laboratory settings	

HAV, Hepatitis A virus; *IG,* immunoglobulin.
*Hepatitis A vaccine is not licensed for children <12 mo.
[†] States and communities with existing vaccination programs for children aged 2 to 18 yr are encouraged to maintain these programs. Catch-up vaccination for this age group may be warranted elsewhere in the context of ongoing outbreaks among children.
[‡] Persons traveling to Canada, Western Europe, Japan, Australia, or New Zealand are at no greater risk than in the U.S.
From Bennett JE et al: *Mandell, Douglas, and Bennett's principles and practice of infectious diseases,* ed 8, Philadelphia, 2015, Saunders.

TABLE 4 Indications and Updated Dosage Recommendations for GamaSTAN S/D Human Immune Globulin for Preexposure and Postexposure Prophylaxis Against Hepatitis A Infection

Indication	Updated Dosage Recommendation
Preexposure prophylaxis	
Up to 1 mo of travel	0.1 ml/kg
Up to 2 mo of travel	0.2 ml/kg
2 mo of travel or longer	0.2 ml/kg (repeat every 2 mo)
Postexposure prophylaxis	0.1 ml/kg

From Kliegman RM et al: *Nelson textbook of pediatrics,* ed 21, Philadelphia, 2020, Elsevier.

vaccines are currently available for use, and they have been found to be safe and highly immunogenic: HAVRIX or VAQTA. These can be used in adults and children older than 12 mo. They are given as a two-dose regimen 6 mo to 1 yr apart. A combined hepatitis A and hepatitis B vaccine called TWINRX is also available.

- Protective antibody levels were reached in 94% to 100% of adults 1 mo after the first dose; similar results have been found for children and adolescents.
- Theoretic analyses of antibody levels estimate duration of immunity to be 10 to 20 yr.
- Vaccine should be considered for persons who are at risk. Those traveling to or working in endemic areas, men who have sex with men, illegal drug users, persons with chronic liver disease, and children in areas with high rates of hepatitis A infection.
- The Advisory Committee on Immunization Practices recommends routine hepatitis A vaccination for all children beginning at 12 to 23 mo of age. Simultaneous administration of MMR and HCPA vaccines is recommended for infants aged 6 to 11 mo traveling internationally. The travel-related dose for infants aged 6 to 11 mo should not be counted toward the routine two-dose series.

SUGGESTED READINGS
Available at eBooks.Health.Elsevier.com.

RELATED CONTENT
Hepatitis A (Patient Information)

AUTHOR: **GLENN G. FORT, MD, MPH**

ℹ️ BASIC INFORMATION

DEFINITION

Hepatitis B is an infection of the liver parenchymal cells caused by the hepatitis B virus (HBV).

SYNONYMS

Serum hepatitis
Long incubation (30 to 180 days) hepatitis HBV
HBV

ICD-10CM CODES

B16	Acute hepatitis B
B16.0	Acute hepatitis B with delta-agent with hepatic coma
B16.1	Acute hepatitis B with delta-agent without hepatic coma
B16.2	Acute hepatitis B without delta-agent with hepatic coma
B16.9	Acute hepatitis B without delta agent and without hepatic coma
B18.0	Chronic viral hepatitis B with delta-agent
B18.1	Chronic viral hepatitis B without delta-agent
B19.1	Unspecified viral hepatitis B
B19.10	Unspecified viral hepatitis B without hepatic coma
B19.11	Unspecified viral hepatitis B with hepatic coma

EPIDEMIOLOGY & DEMOGRAPHICS

INCIDENCE:

- In U.S. overall incidence is ~1.1 cases/100,000.
- Much higher incidence in Europe (~1 million new cases annually) and in areas of high endemicity.
- In the U.S., transmission is mainly horizontal (percutaneous and mucous membrane exposure to infectious blood and other body fluids [e.g., sexual transmission, either homosexual or heterosexual]); also from needle sharing among drug abusers; occupational exposure to contaminated blood and blood products; persons receiving transfusions of blood and blood products; and hemodialysis patients.

NOTE: Improved screening of blood and blood products has greatly reduced, although not eliminated, the risk of posttransfusion HBV infection.

- In areas of high endemicity, transmission is largely vertical (perinatal): HBV exists in the blood and body fluids. Perinatal transmission from HBsAg-positive mothers is as high as 90% unless immunoprophylaxis is given.

PREVALENCE:

- An estimated 296 million people have chronic hepatitis B, of whom 221 million live in low- and middle-income countries.[1] North America, Western Europe, and Australia are areas of low prevalence, <2%. In the U.S. an estimated 800,000 to 2.2 million people have chronic HBV infection. About two thirds of them are unaware that they are infected.
- Africa, Asia, and the Western Pacific region are areas of high prevalence, ≥8%.

- Southern and Eastern Europe have intermediate rates, 2% to 7%.
- Chronically infected persons, those with positive HBsAg for >6 mo, represent the major source of infection.
- As many as 95% of infants and children aged <5, who typically have subclinical acute infection, will become chronic HBV carriers.
- Adults are more likely to have clinically evident acute infection, but only 1% to 5% will develop chronic infection.
- ~0.1% of patients with acute infection will develop fulminant acute hepatitis resulting in death.

PREDOMINANT SEX:

- Predominant in males because of increased intravenous (IV) drug abuse, homosexuality.
- Females more commonly terminate in chronic carrier state.

PREDOMINANT AGE: 20 to 45 yr

PEAK INCIDENCE: 30 to 45 yr of age, at rates of 5% to 20%

GENETICS: Neonatal infection:
- Rare in the U.S.
- High (up to 90%) in areas of high endemicity (only 5% to 10% of perinatal infections occur in utero).

PHYSICAL FINDINGS & CLINICAL PRESENTATION

- The incubation period of HBV infection is 4 to 24 wk. HBV infection presents as acute hepatitis in a minority of patients
- Patients often present with nonspecific symptoms
- Profound malaise (Fig. E1)
- Many asymptomatic cases
- Prodrome:
  1. 15% to 20% serum sickness (urticaria, rash, arthralgia) during early HBsAg
  2. HBsAg-Ab complex disease (polyarteritis nodosa–arthritis, arteritis, glomerulonephritis)
- Hepatomegaly (87%) with right upper quadrant tenderness:
  1. Hepatic punch tenderness
  2. Splenomegaly: Rare (10% to 15%)
- Jaundice (30% of patients), dark urine, with occasional pruritus
- Variable fever (when present, generally precedes jaundice and rapidly declines following onset of icteric phase)
- Spider angiomata: Rare; resolves during recovery
- Rare polyarteritis nodosa, cryoglobulinemia

ETIOLOGY

- Caused by HBV (42-nm hepadnavirus with an outer surface coat [HBsAg], inner nucleocapsid core [HBcAg; HBeAg]; DNA polymerase; and partially double-stranded DNA genome). There are eight genotypes (A to H) based on nucleotide sequence. The prevalence of each genotype varies widely.
- Transmission by parenteral route (needle use, tattooing, ear piercing, acupuncture, transfusion of blood and blood products, hemodialysis, sexual contact), perinatal transmission.

- Infection may result from contact of infectious material with mucous membranes and open skin breaks (e.g., HBV is stable and can be transmitted from toothbrushes, utensils, razors, baby toys, assorted medical equipment [respirators, endoscopes]).
- Oral intake of infectious material may result in infection through breaks in the oral mucosa.
- Food or water are virtually never found to be sources of HBV infection.
- Infection occurs primarily in liver, where necrosis probably results from cytotoxic T-cell response, direct cytopathic effect of HBcAg (core antigen), high-level HBsAg (surface antigen) expression, or coinfection with delta (D) hepatitis virus (RNA delta core within HBsAg envelope).
- Recovery (>90%):
  1. Fulminant hepatitis occurring in <1% (especially if coinfected with hepatitis D); 80% fatal
  2. Unusual (5%) prolonged acute disease for 4 to 12 mo, with recovery
  3. Overall fatality increases with age and viral inoculation (e.g., transfusions)
- Chronic hepatitis B (CHB) infection (1% to 2%), four phases:
  1. Immune-tolerant phase: A highly replicative/low-inflammatory phase in which HBV DNA levels are high (typically >1 million IU/ml), alanine aminotransferase (ALT) levels are normal, and biopsy samples have minimal signs of significant inflammation or fibrosis.
     a. This phase can persist for years, especially in those infected prenatally. More than 90% of perennial infection develop into chronic infection.
     b. With age there is a likely transformation to an HBeAg-positive immune-active phase.
  3. HBeAg-positive immune-active phase: Elevated ALT and HBV DNA levels in conjunction with liver injury (≥20,000 IU/ml). Median age of onset is 30 yr in those infected at a young age. Biopsy will show moderate to severe inflammation or fibrosis.
  4. Inactive CHB phase: HBV DNA levels are low or undetectable (<2000 IU/ml), ALT levels are normal, and anti-HBe is present. Biopsy shows minimal necroinflammation but variable fibrosis.
  4. HBeAg-negative immune reactivation phase: Elevated ALT and elevated HBV DNA (≥2000 IU/ml). Biopsy will show moderate to severe necroinflammation and fibrosis.
- Table 1 summarizes causes of hepatitis flares in patients with CHB.
- The most feared complications of CHB are cirrhosis and hepatocellular carcinoma (HCC), which kill more than 300,000 people/yr globally. One quarter to one third of patients will go on to develop these complications. The risk of developing HCC appears to be greatest among individuals with the highest serum levels of HBV DNA.

TABLE 1 Causes of Hepatitis Flares in Patients with Chronic Hepatitis B

Cause of Flare	Comment
Spontaneous	Factors that precipitate viral replication are unclear
Immunosuppressive therapy	Flares are often observed during withdrawal of the agent; preemptive antiviral therapy is required
Antiviral therapy for HBV	
Interferon	Flares are often observed during the second to third mo of therapy in 30% of patients; may herald virologic response
Nucleoside analog	
During treatment	Flares are no more common than with placebo
Drug-resistant HBV	Severe consequences can occur in patients with advanced liver disease
On withdrawal	Flares are caused by the rapid reemergence of wild-type HBV; severe consequences can occur in patients with advanced liver disease
HIV treatment	Flares can occur as a result of the direct toxicity of HAART or with immune reconstitution; HBV increases the risk of antiretroviral drug hepatotoxicity
Genotypic variation	
Precore and core promoter mutants	Fluctuations in serum ALT levels are common with precore mutants
Superinfection with other hepatitis viruses	May be associated with suppression of HBV replication

ALT, Alanine aminotransferase; *HAART,* highly active antiretroviral therapy; *HBV,* hepatitis B virus; *HIV,* human immunodeficiency virus.
From Feldman M et al: *Sleisenger and Fordtran's gastrointestinal and liver disease,* ed 11, Philadelphia, 2021, Elsevier.

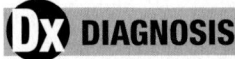 **DIAGNOSIS**

DIFFERENTIAL DIAGNOSIS

- Acute disease confused with other viral hepatitis infections (A, C, D, E)
- Any viral illness producing systemic disease and hepatitis (e.g., yellow fever, Epstein-Barr virus (EBV), cytomegalovirus (CMV), HIV, rubella, rubeola, coxsackie B, adenovirus, herpes simplex or zoster)
- Nonviral causes of hepatitis (e.g., leptospirosis, toxoplasmosis, alcoholic hepatitis, drug-induced [e.g., acetaminophen, INH], toxic hepatitis [carbon tetrachloride, benzene])

WORKUP

- Acute serum specimen for hepatitis B serology (HBsAg, HBsAb, HBcAb, HBeAg, HBeAb), HBDNA by polymerase chain reaction (PCR)
- Life function tests (LFTs)
- CBC
- Liver biopsy: Rarely indicated for diagnosis of fulminant viral hepatitis, chronic hepatitis, cirrhosis, carcinoma

LABORATORY TESTS

- Diagnosis of acute HBV infection is best confirmed by immunoglobulin M (IgM) HBcAb in acute or early convalescent serum or by HBDNA by PCR.
  1. Generally, IgM present during onset of jaundice
  2. Coexisting HBsAg
- HBsAg and IgG-HBcAb during acute jaundice are strongly suggestive of remote HBV infection and another cause for current illness (Fig. 2).
- HBsAb alone is suggestive of immunization response.
- With recovery, HBeAg is rapidly replaced by HBeAb in 2 to 3 mo, and HBsAg is replaced by HBsAb in 5 to 6 mo.
- In chronic HBV hepatitis, HBsAg and HBeAg are persistent without corresponding Ab.

- In chronic carrier state, HBsAg is persistent, but HBeAg is replaced by HBeAb.
- HBcAb develops in all outcomes.
- HBeAg correlation with highest infectivity; appearance of HBeAb heralds recovery.
- LFTs:
  1. ALT and AST: Usually more than eight times normal (often 1000 U/L) at onset of jaundice (minimal acute ALT/aspartate aminotransferase [AST] rises often followed by chronic hepatitis or hepatocellular carcinoma)
  2. Bilirubin: Variably elevated in icteric viral hepatitis
  3. Alkaline phosphatase: Minimally elevated (one to three times normal) acutely.
- Albumin and prothrombin time:
  1. Generally normal
  2. If abnormal, possible harbinger of impending hepatic necrosis (fulminant hepatitis)
- White blood cell (WBC) and erythrocyte sedimentation rate (ESR): Generally normal.

IMAGING STUDIES

- Sonogram to document rapid reduction in liver size during fulminant hepatitis or mass in hepatocellular carcinoma
- FibroScan (transient elastography): A noninvasive specialized ultrasound test to quantify liver fibrosis without liver biopsy

℞ **TREATMENT**

NONPHARMACOLOGIC THERAPY

- Symptomatic treatment as necessary
- Activity as tolerated
- High-calorie diet preferred; often best tolerated in morning

ACUTE GENERAL Rx

- In most cases of acute HBV infection, no treatment is necessary; >90% of adults will spontaneously clear infection.
- Hospitalization advisable for any patient in danger from dehydration caused by poor

oral intake, whose prothrombin time (PT) is prolonged, who has rising bilirubin level >15 to 20 μg/dl, or who has any clinical evidence of hepatic failure. Table 2 summarizes indications for prompt or urgent treatment of hepatitis B.
- IV therapy needed (rarely) for hydration during severe vomiting.
- Avoid hepatically metabolized drugs.
- No therapeutic measures are beneficial.
- Steroids not shown helpful.

CHRONIC Rx

- Selection of patients for treatment of chronic hepatitis B is summarized in Table 3. Treatment of chronic HBV infection is dependent on which phase the patient is found to be in:
  1. Therapy is warranted for patients in immune-active CHB stage (HBeAg negative or HbeAg positive) to decrease the risk of liver-related complications. Treatment options include:
  2. Nucleoside analogues:
     a. Entecavir: A nucleotide analogue. Dose 0.5 to 1 mg/day, suppresses HBV DNA replication and improves liver inflammation and fibrosis.
     b. Tenofovir disoproxil: 300 mg/day, is another nucleotide analogue. A newer formulation, tenofovir alafenamide (Vemlidy) 25 mg/day, has less renal and bone toxicity in long-term use.
     c. Other nucleotide agents: Lamivudine, telbivudine, and adefovir are less frequently used due to issues of resistance.
     d. Cure rates with nucleotide agents are between 1% and 12%, and thus most patients will require treatment indefinitely but are considered first line of therapy.
  3. Pegylated interferon alfa:
     a. Pegylated interferon 2a: 180 μg subcutaneously weekly for 48 wk. This will lead to seroconversion rates of 20% to 30% (HBeAg to anti-HBe), and 65% of

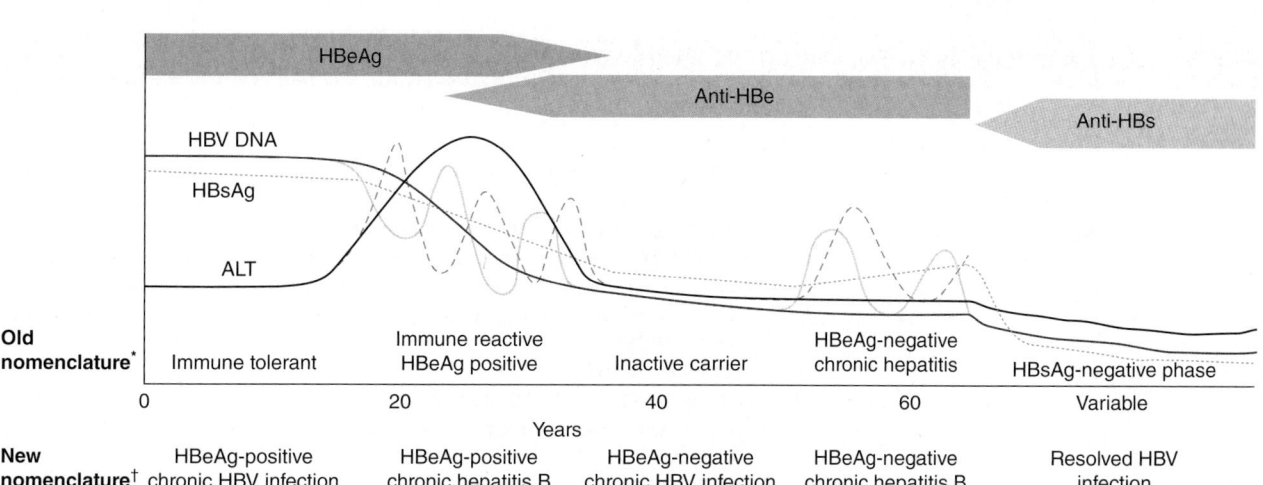

A

	HBeAg-positive		HBeAg-negative		HBsAg-negative
	Chronic HBV infection	**Chronic hepatitis B**	**Chronic HBV infection**	**Chronic hepatitis B**	**Resolved HBV infection**
HBsAg	High	High/ intermediate	Low	Intermediate	Negative
HBV DNA	≥10^7 IU/mL	10^4-10^7 IU/mL	<2000 IU/mL[‡]	≥2000 IU/mL	Undetectable
ALT	Normal	Elevated	Normal	Elevated[§]	Normal
Liver disease	None/minimal	Moderate/severe	None	Moderate/severe	None
Old terminology	Immune tolerant	Immune reactive HBeAg positive	Inactive carrier	HBeAg-negative chronic hepatitis	HBsAg-negative phase

B

FIG. 2 Natural history of and new nomenclature for patients with chronic HBV infection. The course is shown graphically in *A*, and the criteria for each phase are shown in *B*. Particularly in patients who are infected early in life, the first phase is *HBeAg-positive chronic HBV infection* (previously known as the immune tolerant phase). After decades of normal serum ALT and high HBV DNA levels, this phase evolves to *HBeAg-positive chronic hepatitis B* (previously known as the immune reactive phase) of variable duration. In this phase, there is active viral replication (high serum HBVDNA levels) and inflammation (high serum ALT levels) and an indication for antiviral therapy. Ultimately, patients enter a spontaneous or therapeutically induced phase of *HBeAg-negative chronic HBV infection* (previously known as the inactive carrier state), with minimal disease activity, which can last indefinitely. At the time of HBeAg seroconversion, however, immunologic pressure may select for a viral mutant (precore, core promoter, or both), which is incapable of producing HBeAg antigen. Viral and serum ALT levels typically fluctuate during this phase of *HBeAg-negative chronic hepatitis B*, and antiviral treatment is usually indicated. The last phase, which is the *HBsAg-negative phase* (previously known as the occult HBV infection phase) is characterized by negative HBsAg in serum and the presence of antibodies to HBcAg (anti-HBc), with or without detectable antibodies to HBsAg (anti-HBs). This phase is considered functional cure of HBV infection. If the patient has not entered this phase and is not treated, late disease complications often occur. The relative time dimensions of each phase are shown; note that there may be significant overlap of features among the various phases. *Anti-HBe,* antibody to HBeAg; *HBeAg,* hepatitis B e antigen; *HBsAg,* hepatitis B surface antigen. [†]European Association for the Study of the Liver. Electronic address: easloffice@easloffice.eu. EASL 2017 Clinical Practice Guidelines on the management of hepatitis B virus infection, *J Hepatol* 67:370-98, 2017. [‡]HBV DNA levels can be between 2000 and 20,000 IU/ml in some patients without signs of chronic hepatitis. [§]Persistently or intermittently, based on the traditional upper limit of normal (~40 IU/L). (Data from Lok AS et al: Hepatitis B cure: from discovery to regulatory approval, *J Hepatol* 67:847-61, 2017.)

TABLE 2 Indications for Prompt or Urgent Treatment of Hepatitis B

	Indications	**Preferred Agent**	**Principal Supportive Data**
Cirrhosis*			
Decompensated	Clinical stabilization; minimizing risk for recurrence after transplant	Entecavir (0.5 mg) or tenofovir (300 mg)[†]	Open label; multiple large case series
Borderline compensated	Forestalling disease progression; avoidance of transplantation	As above	Undefined
Well compensated	As above	As above	Randomized controlled trials
Acute Liver Failure			
HBV reactivation	Minimizing further liver injury; reducing risk of recurrence after liver transplantation, if needed	Entecavir (0.5 mg) or tenofovir (300 mg)[†]	Open label with comparison with historical controls
Severe acute hepatitis	Minimizing further liver injury and enhancing full recovery	Consider lamivudine or telbivudine[‡]	Small case series

HBV, Hepatitis B virus.
*It has been the author's (RP) practice to use maintenance antiviral therapy for all hepatitis B surface antigen (HBsAg)-positive patients with cirrhosis to prevent reactivation of hepatitis B.
[†]Daily dose should be adjusted according to the patient's renal function, as indicated in the manufacturer's recommendations.
[‡]Either agent can be used if the anticipated duration of therapy is ≤6 mo.
From Feldman M et al: *Sleisenger and Fordtran's gastrointestinal and liver disease,* ed 10, Philadelphia, 2016, Elsevier.

TABLE 3 Selection of Patients for Treatment in Chronic Hepatitis B

HBeAg	HBV DNA[a]	ALT[b]	Treatment Strategy
+	>20,000 IU/ml	<2 × ULN	Observe patient
			Consider liver biopsy or noninvasive measurement of liver disease if age > 40, ALT > 1 but <2 × ULN, family history HCC, HIV positive; treat if moderate-to-severe inflammation or fibrosis
+	>20,000 IU/ml	>2 × ULN	Observe 3-6 mo for spontaneous HBeAg seroconversion before treatment
			Treatment with PEG IFN-α (48 wk) or NUC (indefinite in most; minimum 6-12 mo after HBeAg seroconversion)
−	>20,000 IU/ml	>2 × ULN	Treatment with NUC (end point not defined; likely indefinite) PEG IFN-α (48 wk) second line
−	>2000 IU/ml	1 to <2 × ULN	Consider liver biopsy or noninvasive measurement of liver disease and treatment if moderate-to-severe inflammation or fibrosis
−	>2000 IU/ml	<ULN	Observe; treat if HBV DNA or ALT increase
±	+	Cirrhosis	Compensated: treat with NUC if HBV DNA detectable
			Decompensated: NUC; consider liver transplantation
±	−	Cirrhosis	Compensated: observe
			Decompensated: consider liver transplantation

ALT, Alanine aminotransferase; anti-HBe, antibody to hepatitis e antigen; DNA, deoxyribonucleic acid; HBeAg, hepatitis B e antigen; HBV, hepatitis B virus; HCC, hepatocellular carcinoma; HIV, human immunodeficiency virus; NUC, nucleoside or nucleotide; PEG IFN-α, pegylated interferon-α; ULN, upper limit of normal.
[a]Conversion factor to copies/ml = 5.6 (20,000 IU/ml is approximately 10^5 copies/ml).
[b]Also use moderate-to-severe necroinflammation on liver biopsy as guide.
Modified from Terrault N et al: AASLD Guidelines for the treatment of chronic hepatitis B, *Hepatology* 63:261-283, 2016.

patients will have HBV DNA <2000 IU/ml off therapy, but cure rates remain low at 3% to 7% and has significant side effects: Bone marrow suppression and exacerbation of existing neuropsychiatric symptoms, including depression. Candidates for interferon therapy should not have significant psychiatric disease, cardiac disease, cytopenia, seizure disorder, autoimmune disease, or pregnancy.

4. Therapy is not warranted in adults with immune-tolerant CHB. LFTs should be checked every 6 mo to look for conversion to immune-active or inactive status.

   a. Therapy may be warranted for select adults >40 with normal ALT and elevated HBV DNA (≥1 million IU/ml) with liver biopsy showing significant necroinflammation or fibrosis.

5. HBeAg-positive adults without cirrhosis who seroconvert to anti-HBe on therapy with entecavir or tenofovir disoproxil can discontinue treatment after a period of treatment consolidation.

6. It is recommended that patients receive indefinite therapy with entecavir or tenofovir disoproxil if HBeAg-negative immune-active CHB is present, unless there is a competing rationale for treatment discontinuation.

7. Adults with compensated cirrhosis and low levels of viremia (<2000 IU/ml) should be treated with entecavir or tenofovir disoproxil to reduce the risk of decompensation, regardless of ALT level.

DISPOSITION

- Follow-up as outpatient
- Acute disease: Infection will resolve (defined as clearance of hepatitis B surface antigen within 6 mo) in 90% of adult patients
- Rare fatalities (fulminant hepatitis)

- Possible chronic carrier state, cirrhosis, hepatocellular carcinoma
- Cure of HBV is an unrealistic goal for most patients with chronic infection because only a few patients will become HBsAb with current treatment modalities
- Without intervention, deaths from chronic hepatitis B are expected to peak at 1.14 million by 2035[1]

REFERRAL

To infectious disease specialist and gastroenterologist for consultation regarding fulminant hepatitis or prolonged cholestasis, for cases of uncertain etiology, or for treatment of CAH

⚠ PEARLS & CONSIDERATIONS

- The American Association for the Study of Liver Diseases (AASLD) recommends that in men infected with hepatitis B, liver cancer screening begin at age 40 and in women infected with hepatitis B, liver cancer screening begin at age 50.
- Other high-risk groups for the development of liver cancer include persons born of Asian/Pacific Islander descent, persons born in Africa, persons coinfected with hepatitis C, hepatitis D, or HIV, and persons with a family history of liver cancer and individuals with cirrhosis.

COMMENTS

- Virus and HBsAg in high titers in blood for 1 to 7 wk before jaundice and for a variable time thereafter.
- Screening (HBV surface antigen [HBsAg], HBV core antigen antibody, antibody to HBsAg) should be offered to high-risk groups.
- Transmission is possible during entire period of HBsAg (and especially during HBeAg) in serum.

- Universal precautions should be followed for all contacts with blood or secretions/excretions contaminated with blood.
- Antiviral therapy is recommended in pregnancy to reduce perinatal transmission if HBsAg positive and HBV DNA >200,000 IU/ml. Can use tenofovir disoproxil, lamivudine, or telbivudine. Tenofovir may be preferred because it has a better resistance profile, and there are more safety data in pregnant women with hepatitis B. Fig. 3 describes an algorithm for the treatment of hepatitis B surface antigen (HBsAg)-positive mothers during pregnancy.
- Preventing before exposure:
  1. Lifestyle changes.
  2. Meticulous testing of blood supply (although some chronically infected, infectious donors are HBsAg negative).
  3. Sterilization via steam or hypochlorite.
  4. Hepatitis B vaccine for high-risk groups given intramuscularly (IM) in deltoid to induce HBsAb (response should be confirmed) is protective (>90% effective). Yeast-derived HBsAg vaccines include: Recombivax HB (10 mcg HBsAg/ml) and Engerix-B (20 μg HBsAg/ml), each as a three-dose series over 6 mo. An alternative vaccine is the two-dose hepatitis B virus vaccine (HEPLISAV-B) that uses a novel immunostimulatory adjuvant for use in adults ≥18 yr old, administered at 0 and 1 mo. Table E4 summarizes doses and schedules of licensed Hepatitis B vaccines.
  5. Recommendation for universal childhood immunization with doses at birth, 1 mo, and 6 mo.
  6. The U.S. Advisory Committee on Immunization Practices has recommended universal hepatitis B vaccination for adults between the ages of 19 and 59 yr and has liberalized the recommendation for vaccination of adults who are 60 yr

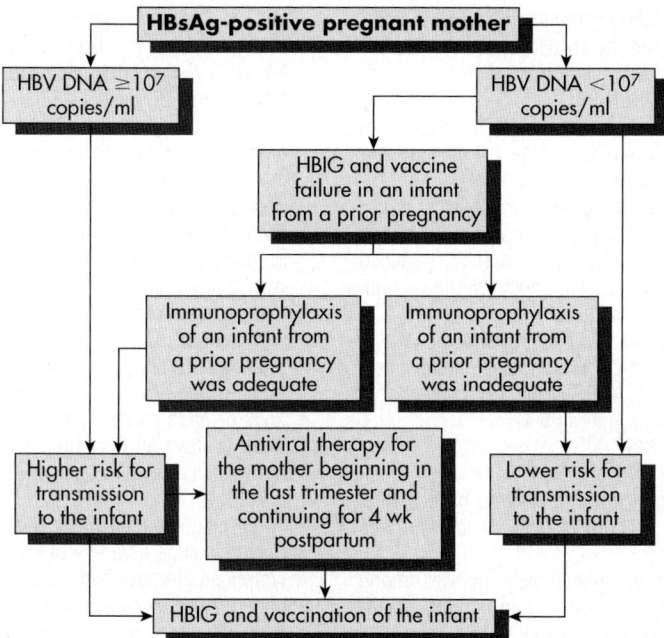

FIG. 3 Algorithm for the treatment of hepatitis B surface antigen (HBsAg)-positive mothers during pregnancy. The goal of treatment in highly viremic mothers is to lower the serum HBV DNA level by several $\log_{10}$ IU/ml by the time of delivery to minimize the chance of newborn infection. The choice of antiviral agent is less important if treatment of the mother is not needed long term. In the event that the treatment needs to be continued after delivery, the patient should be started on a high-genetic-barrier drug initially or switched to one immediately after delivery. See text for further details about drug selection. *DNA,* Deoxyribonucleic acid; *HBIG,* hepatitis B immune globulin; *HBV,* hepatitis B virus. (From Feldman M et al: *Sleisenger and Fordtran's gastrointestinal and liver disease,* ed 11, Philadelphia, 2021, Elsevier.)

or older with risk factors for hepatitis B. The committee has also proposed universal one-time hepatitis B screening for all adults (>18 yr).[1]

- Prevention after exposure:
  1. HBV hyperimmune globulin (HBIG) (0.06 ml/kg IM) given immediately after needle-stick, within 14 days of sexual exposure, or at birth, followed by HBV vaccination. A second dose of HBIG is given in 28 days for those refusing vaccine or vaccine nonresponders.
  2. Standard immune globulin: Nearly as effective as HBIG.
- Preventive therapy with entecavir or tenofovir disoproxil for patients who test positive for HBsAg and are undergoing chemotherapy may reduce the risk for HBV reactivation and HBV-associated morbidity and mortality.
- Hepatitis B prophylaxis is described in Section V.
- Table 5 summarizes interpretation of serologic markers and serum DNA in hepatitis B.
- The U.S. Preventive Services Task Force (USPSTF) recommends screening for hepatitis B infection in adolescents and adults of high risk. Patients at high risk include the following:
  1. People born in countries or area with HBV prevalence ≥2%
  2. People who were not vaccinated at birth and were both in the U.S. to parents who were born in countries or areas with prevalence >8%
  3. HIV-positive people
  4. Intravenous drug users
  5. Men who have sex with men
  6. People who live in households with, or have sex with, HBV-positive people

REFERENCE & SUGGESTED READINGS
Available at eBooks.Health.Elsevier.com.

RELATED CONTENT
Hepatitis B (Patient Information)

AUTHOR: **GLENN G. FORT, MD, MPH**

TABLE 5 Interpretation of Serologic Tests in Hepatitis B

Test	Acute Hepatitis B	Immunity Through Infection[a]	Immunity Through Vaccination	Chronic Hepatitis B
HBsAg	+	−	−	+
Anti-HBs	−	+	+	−
HBeAg	+	−	−	±[b]
Anti-HBe	−	±	−	±
Anti-HBc	+	+	−	+
IgM anti-HBc	+	−	−	−
HBV DNA	+	−	−	+
ALT	Elevated	Normal	Normal	Normal or elevated

ALT, Alanine aminotransferase; *anti-HBc,* antibody to hepatitis B core antigen; *anti-HBe,* antibody to hepatitis B e antigen; *anti-HBs,* antibody to hepatitis B surface antigen; *DNA,* deoxyribonucleic acid; *HBeAg,* hepatitis B e antigen; *HBsAg,* hepatitis B surface antigen; *HBV,* hepatitis B virus; *IgM,* immunoglobulin M.
[a]On occasion, individuals with past infection have isolated anti-HBc only. The presence of an isolated immunoglobulin G anti-HBc may indicate a window period during acute infection or remote prior infection with loss of HBsAg or anti-HBs. In such cases an HBV DNA test may prove useful.
[b]Chronic hepatitis B with a precore mutant is HBeAg− and anti-HBe+.
From Bennett JE et al: *Mandell, Douglas, and Bennett's principles and practice of infectious diseases,* ed 9, Philadelphia, 2020, Elsevier.

BASIC INFORMATION

DEFINITION

Hepatitis C is a liver parenchymal infection caused by hepatitis C virus (HCV).

SYNONYM

Transfusion-related non-A, non-B hepatitis

ICD-10CM CODES
B17.1	Acute hepatitis C
B17.10	Acute hepatitis C without hepatic coma
B17.11	Acute hepatitis C with hepatic coma
B18.2	Chronic viral hepatitis C
B19.20	Unspecified viral hepatitis C without hepatic coma
B19.21	Unspecified viral hepatitis C with hepatic coma

EPIDEMIOLOGY & DEMOGRAPHICS

Hepatitis C infection is the most common chronic blood-borne infection in the U.S. About 3% of baby boomers test positive for the virus. The Centers for Disease Control and Prevention (CDC) now in 2022 recommends:

- One-time, routine, opt out HCV testing for all individuals aged 18 or older (I,B).
- One-time HCV testing should be performed for all persons <18 yr with activities, exposures, or conditions or circumstances associated with an increased risk of HCV infection (I,B).
- Prenatal HCV testing as part of routine prenatal care is recommended with each pregnancy (I,B).
- Periodic repeat HCV testing should be offered to all persons with activities, exposures, or conditions or circumstances associated with an increased risk of HCV exposure (IIa,C).
- Annual HCV testing is recommended for all persons who inject drugs, for HIV infected men who have unprotected sex with men, and all men who have sex with men taking preexposure prophylaxis (PrEP) (IIa,C).
- Regardless of age or setting prevalence, all persons with risk factors should be tested for hepatitis C with periodic testing while risk factors persist.
- Any person who requests hepatitis C testing should receive it, regardless of disclosure risk, because many persons might be reluctant to disclose stigmatizing risk.
  The U.S. Preventive Services Task Force (USPSTF) recommends screening of all adults 18 to 79 yr for hepatitis C infection.

INCIDENCE: HCV infects more than 185 million individuals worldwide. Approximately 20% of patients chronically infected with HCV progress to cirrhosis.

- 150,000 new cases/yr (37,500 symptomatic; 93,000 later chronic liver disease; 30,700 cirrhosis). The incidence of acute HCV has declined substantially over the past 30 yr (from 7.4/100,000 to 0.7/100,000).
- ~9000 of these ultimately die of HCV infection; most common (40%) cause of nonalcoholic liver disease in the U.S.

PREVALENCE (IN U.S.):
- Overall prevalence of anti-HCV antibody is 1% to 1.2% (an estimated 2.7 million persons nationwide).
- Highest prevalence in hemophiliacs transfused before 1987 and users of injection drugs, 72% to 90%. Over past 30 yr, blood transfusion as a risk factor declined from 15% of cases to 1.9%.
- Among low-risk groups, prevalence 0.6%.

PREDOMINANT SEX: Slight male predominance.
PREDOMINANT AGE: Highest prevalence in 30- to 49-yr age group (65%).
PEAK INCIDENCE:
- 20 to 39 yr of age.
- African Americans and Whites have similar incidence of acute disease; Hispanics have higher rates.
- Prevalence is substantially higher among non-Hispanic Blacks than among non-Hispanic Whites.

GENETICS: Neonatal infection is rare; increased risk with maternal HIV-1 coinfection.

PHYSICAL FINDINGS & CLINICAL PRESENTATION

- Symptoms usually develop 7 to 8 wk after infection (range of 2 to 26 wk), but 70% to 80% of cases are subclinical.
- 10% to 20% report acute illness with jaundice and nonspecific symptoms (abdominal pain, anorexia, malaise).
- Fulminant hepatitis may rarely occur during this period.
- After acute infection, 15% to 25% have complete resolution (absence of HCV RNA in serum, normal alanine aminotransferase [ALT]).
- Progression to chronic infection is common, 50% to 84%. 74% to 86% have persistent viremia; spontaneous clearance of viremia in chronic infection is rare. 60% to 70% of patients will have persistent or fluctuating ALT levels; 30% to 40% with chronic infection have normal ALT levels.
- 15% to 20% of those with chronic HCV will develop cirrhosis over a period of 20 to 30 yr; in most others, chronic infection leads to hepatitis and varying degrees of fibrosis. Table 1 summarizes factors associated with progression of hepatic fibrosis in patients with chronic HCV infection. Table 2 describes factors associated with cirrhosis in persons with hepatitis C infection.
- 0.4% to 2.5% of patients with chronic infection develop hepatocellular carcinoma (HCC).
- 25% of patients with chronic infection continue to have an asymptomatic course with normal liver function tests (LFTs) and benign histology.
- In chronic HCV infection, extrahepatic sequelae include a variety of immunologic and lymphoproliferative disorders (e.g., cryoglobulinemia, membranoproliferative glomerulonephritis, and possibly Sjögren syndrome, autoimmune thyroiditis, polyarteritis nodosa, aplastic anemia, lichen planus, porphyria cutanea tarda, B-cell lymphoma, others).
- Direct antiviral treatment should be initiated without delay in patients with clinically significant extrahepatic manifestations of chronic HCV infection. Studies have shown a close link between treatment-induced, sustained viral clearance and a low risk of extrahepatic manifestations of HCV infection.[1]
- Fig. 1 illustrates the natural history of HCV infection.

ETIOLOGY

- Caused by HCV (single-stranded RNA flavivirus). HCV genotype 1 accounts for about 75% of HCV in the U.S. Genotypes 2 and 3 account for about 20% to 25% of infections, genotype 4 for 6%, and genotypes 5 and 6 for about 1%.

TABLE 1 Factors Associated with Progression of Hepatic Fibrosis in Patients with Chronic Hepatitis C Virus Infection

Established	Possible	Not Associated
Age >40 yr	Increased hepatic iron concentration	Viral genotype
Alcohol consumption	Male gender	Viral load
Hepatitis B virus coinfection	Serum ALT level	
HIV coinfection		
Immunosuppressed state		
Insulin resistance		
Marijuana use		
Obesity		
Schistosomiasis		
Severe hepatic necroinflammation		
Smoking		
White race		

ALT, Alanine aminotransferase; *HIV,* human immunodeficiency virus.
From Feldman M et al: *Sleisenger and Fordtran's gastrointestinal and liver disease,* ed 11, Philadelphia, 2021, Elsevier.

TABLE 2 Factors Associated with Cirrhosis in Persons with Hepatitis C Infection

Factor	Impact	Comment
Environmental		
Alcohol use	+4	The importance of minimal alcohol ingestion (<20 g/day) has not been established
Host		
HIV infection	+4	Increasingly important as HIV-related survival improves; may be masked by competing mortality
HBV infection	+3	Strong effect when HBsAg positive; relatively uncommon
Age	+4	Strong effect; increases as low as 40 yr. Hard to distinguish from infection duration
Body mass index	+2	Associated with metabolic syndrome
Duration of HCV infection	+3	Cirrhosis is rare before 10 yr
HLA type	+1?	HLA B54 is correlated with increased risk of cirrhosis; DRB1*0301 with lack of cirrhosis
Viral		
Quasi-species complexity	+1	Cross-sectional studies cannot assess causality, and complexity may be confounded by duration of infection
HCV genotype 1	+1?	Genotype 1b in some, but not other studies, could be confounded by longer duration of 1b infections
Quantitative measures of viremia (serum or plasma HCV RNA level)	+2	Not always detected or lost in multivariate analysis of age or HIV

HCV, Hepatitis C virus; *HIV,* human immunodeficiency virus; *HLA,* human leukocyte antigen; *RNA,* ribonucleic acid.
From Bennett JE et al: *Mandell, Douglas, and Bennett's principles and practice of infectious diseases,* ed 9, Philadelphia, 2020, Elsevier.

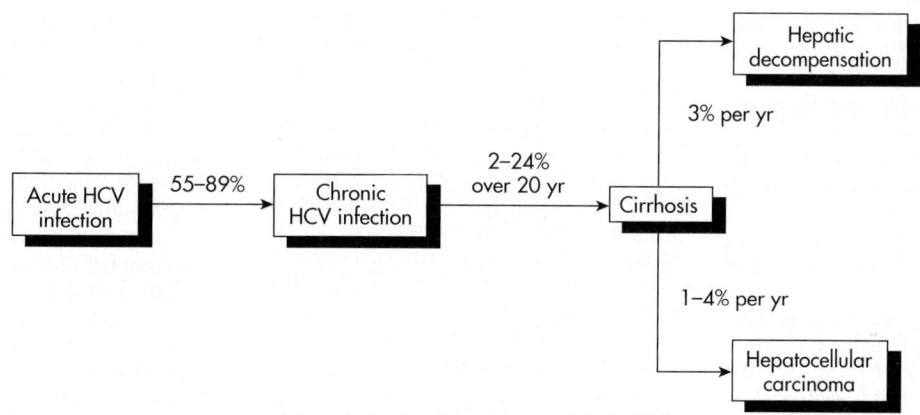

FIG. 1 Natural history of HCV infection. Hepatic decompensation includes ascites, hepatic encephalopathy, variceal hemorrhage, hepatorenal syndrome, or hepatic synthetic dysfunction. *HCV,* Hepatitis C virus. (From Feldman M et al: *Sleisenger and Fordtran's gastrointestinal and liver disease,* ed 11, Philadelphia, 2021, Elsevier.)

- Most HCV transmission is parenteral.
- In the U.S., advances in screening of blood and blood products have made transfusion-related HCV infection rare (the risk is estimated to be 0.001% per unit transfused).
- Injecting-drug use accounts for most HCV transmission in the U.S. (60% of newly acquired cases, 20% to 50% of chronically infected persons).
- Occupational needlestick exposure from an HCV-positive source has a seroconversion rate of 1.8% (range 0% to 7%).
- Nosocomial transmission rates (from surgery and procedures such as colonoscopy and hemodialysis) are extremely low.
- Sexual transmission and maternal-fetal transmission are infrequent (estimated at 5%).
- No identifiable risk in 40% to 50% of community-acquired hepatitis C, but snorting of cocaine by shared use of straw or rolled-up paper has been identified as a risk factor because it causes microscopic bleeding of nasal mucosa.

- HCV infection may stimulate production of cytotoxic T lymphocytes and cytokines (INF-γ), which probably mediate hepatic necrosis.

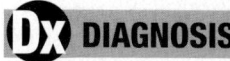 **DIAGNOSIS**

DIFFERENTIAL DIAGNOSIS
- Other hepatitis viruses (A, B, D, E).
- Other viral illnesses producing systemic disease (e.g., yellow fever, Epstein-Barr virus, cytomegalovirus, HIV, rubella, rubeola, coxsackie B, adenovirus, herpes simplex virus, herpes zoster virus).
- Nonviral hepatitis (e.g., leptospirosis, toxoplasmosis, alcoholic hepatitis, drug-induced hepatitis [acetaminophen, isoniazid], toxic hepatitis).

WORKUP
- Acute hepatitis C antibody, viral genotyping, viral titers.
- LFTs, CBC.

NOTE: ALT is an easy and inexpensive test to monitor infection and efficacy of therapy. However, ALT levels may fluctuate or even be normal in active or chronic infection and even with cirrhosis, and ALT may remain elevated even after clearance of viremia.

- Liver biopsy with histologic staging had been the gold standard for assessing the degree of disease activity and the likelihood of disease progression and also to help rule out other causes of liver disease but is less used with advent of newer technologies.
- Transient elastography (FibroScan) is a noninvasive specialized ultrasound assessment that quantifies liver fibrosis and corresponds it to the equivalent in the METAVIR scoring system traditionally used in liver biopsies. It is being increasingly used in place of liver biopsy in most institutions.

LABORATORY TESTS
- Diagnosis of acute hepatitis C is often by exclusion, because it takes 6 wk to 12 mo to

develop anti-HCV antibody (70% positive by 6 wk, 90% positive by 6 mo).

- Diagnostic tests include serologic assays for antibodies and molecular tests for viral particles.
  1. Enzyme immunoassay is the test for anti-HCV antibody:
     a. The current version can detect antibody within 4 to 10 wk after infection.
     b. False-negative rate in low-risk populations is 0.5% to 1%.
     c. False negatives also occur in immune-compromised persons, HIV-1, renal failure, HCV-associated essential mixed cryoglobulinemia.
     d. False positives in autoimmune hepatitis, paraproteinemia, and persons with no risk factors.
- The recombinant immunoblot assay that was previously recommended as a follow-up to positive antibody test is no longer available. The CDC now recommends that anyone who tests positive for HCV antibodies receive a follow-up HCV RNA test.
- Qualitative and quantitative HCV RNA tests using polymerase chain reaction (PCR): Lower limit of detection is <43 IU/ml.
- Used to confirm viremia and to assess response to treatment.
- Qualitative PCR useful in patients with negative enzyme immunoassay in whom infection is suspected.
- Quantitative tests use either branched-chain DNA or reverse transcription PCR; the latter is more sensitive.
- Viral genotyping can distinguish among genotypes 1, 2, 3, 4, 5, and 6, which is helpful in choosing therapy; most of these tests use PCR. Genotypes 1, 2, 3, and 4 predominate in the U.S. and Europe (genotype 1 is especially common in North America [60% to 75% of hepatitis C infections in the U.S.]).
- FibroSure score uses a combination of six serum markers of liver function plus age and sex in a patented algorithm to generate a measure of fibrosis and necroinflammatory activity in the liver as a quantitative surrogate marker for the corresponding METAVIR scoring system.
- LFTs: ALT and AST may be elevated to more than eight times normal in acute infection; in chronic infection ALT may be normal or fluctuate.
- Bilirubin may be 5 to 10 times normal.
- Albumin and prothrombin time generally normal; if abnormal, may be harbinger of impending hepatic necrosis.
- WBC and erythrocyte sedimentation rate (ESR) are generally normal.
- HIV testing. Infection with HCV is seen in 15% to 30% of individuals with HIV infection due to shared risk factors.
- All patients infected with HCV should be tested for hepatitis B. HBV vaccination is recommended for susceptible individuals, because HBV reactivation may occur during treatment of HCV with direct-acting antiviral therapy.

IMAGING STUDIES

- Transient elastography (FibroScan) to quantify liver fibrosis as an absolute score. Some insurance companies use this score as a basis to determine eligibility for treatment.
- Sonogram: Rapid liver size reduction during fulminant hepatitis or mass in HCC.

Rx TREATMENT

NONPHARMACOLOGIC THERAPY

Activity and diet as tolerated; avoid saw palmetto and green tea leaf herbs.

ACUTE GENERAL Rx

- Supportive care
- Avoid hepatically metabolized drugs

CHRONIC Rx

Response to therapy is influenced by HCV genotype. Recommendations for the treatment of hepatitis C in adults are changing constantly as new therapies come to the market. The advent of direct-acting antiviral agents (DAAs) has drastically changed treatment options and improved cure rates to >95%. The most up-to-date guidance is available at the website www.hcvguidelines.org. The following is a brief summary of the guidelines based on genotype. Newer agents containing fixed-dose combinations of DAA drugs have been approved for HCV infections caused by any of the six major HCV genotypes in patients without cirrhosis or with compensated cirrhosis. These agents are Mavyret (combination of glecaprevir, an HCV NS3/4A protease inhibitor; and pibrentasvir, an NS5A inhibitor) and Vosevi (combination of the NS5B nucleotide polymerase inhibitor sofosbuvir, the NS5A inhibitor velpatasvir, and the NS3/4A protease inhibitor voxilaprevir). Both agents are approved for use in treatment-experienced patients, and Mavyret is also approved for treatment-naïve patients. Currently, these treatment regimens are expensive and are covered by most insurance plans.

Genotype 1a: Options for treatment-naïve patients without cirrhosis, listed by level of evidence:
- Daily fixed-dose combination of glecaprevir (300 mg)/pibrentasvir (120 mg) (Mavyret) for 8 wk. Rating: Class I, Level A
- Daily fixed-dose combination of ledipasvir (90 mg)/sofosbuvir (400 mg) (Harvoni) for 12 wk. Rating: Class I, Level A. (Can also use this regimen for only 8 wk for patients who are non-Black, HIV-uninfected, and whose HCV RNA level is <6 million IU/ml. Rating: Class I, Level B.)
- Daily fixed-dose combination of sofosbuvir (400 mg)/velpatasvir (100 mg) (Epclusa) for 12 wk. Rating: Class I, Level A
- Alternative regimen: Daily fixed-dose combination of elbasvir (50 mg)/grazoprevir (100 mg) (Zepatier) for 12 wk and in those who do not have baseline NS5A RAVs (amino acid substitutions at 28, 30, 31, or 93 that confer resistance to elbasvir). Rating: Class I, Level A

Genotype 1a: Options for treatment-naïve patients with compensated cirrhosis:
- Daily fixed-dose combination of glecaprevir (300 mg)/pibrentasvir (120 mg) [Mavyret] for 8 wk. Rating: Class I, Level B. Use 12 wk if HIV-hepatitis C coinfected

- Daily fixed-dose combination of ledipasvir (90 mg)/sofosbuvir (400 mg) [Harvoni] for 12 wk. Rating: Class I, Level A
- Daily fixed-dose combination of sofosbuvir (400 mg)/velpatasvir (100 mg) [Epclusa] for 12 wk. Rating: Class I, Level A
- Alternative: Daily fixed-dose combination of elbasvir (50 mg)/grazoprevir (100 mg) [Zepatier] and in those in whom no baseline NS5A RAVs for elbasvir are detected for 12 wk. Rating: Class I, Level A

Genotype 1b: Treatment-naïve patients without cirrhosis:
- Daily fixed-dose combination of elbasvir (50 mg)/grazoprevir (100 mg) [Zepatier] for 12 wk. Rating: Class I, Level A
- Daily fixed-dose combination of glecaprevir (300 mg)/pibrentasvir (120 mg) [Mayvret] for 8 wk. Rating: Class I, A. Use 12 wk if HIV-hepatitis C coinfected
- Daily fixed-dose combination of ledipasvir (90 mg)/sofosbuvir (400 mg) [Harvoni] for 12 wk. Rating: Class I, Level A. (Can treat for 8 wk in patients who are non-Black, HIV-uninfected, and whose HCV RNA level is <6 million IU/ml. Class I, Level B.)
- Daily fixed-dose combination of sofosbuvir (400 mg)/velpatasvir (100 mg) [Epclusa] for 12 wk. Rating: Class I, Level A

Genotype 1b: Treatment-naïve patients with compensated cirrhosis:
- Daily fixed-dose combination of elbasvir (50 mg)/grazoprevir (100 mg) [Zepatier] for 12 wk. Rating: Class I, Level A
- Daily fixed-dose combination of glecaprevir (300 mg)/pibrentasvir (120 mg) [Mavyret] for 8 wk. Rating: Class I, Level B. Use 12 wk if HIV-hepatitis C coinfected
- Daily fixed-dose combination of ledipasvir (90 mg)/sofosbuvir [Harvoni] for 12 wk. Rating: Class I, Level A
- Daily fixed-dose combination of sofosbuvir (400 mg)/velpatasvir (100 mg) [Epclusa] for 12 wk. Rating: Class I, Level A

Genotype 2: Treatment-naïve regimens without cirrhosis:
- Daily fixed-dose combination of glecaprevir (300 mg)/pibrentasvir (120 mg) [Mavyret] for 8 wk. Rating: Class I, Level A
- Daily fixed-dose combination of sofosbuvir (400 mg)/velpatasvir (100 mg) [Epclusa] for 12 wk. Rating: Class I, Level A

Genotype 2: Treatment-naïve patients with compensated cirrhosis:
- Daily fixed-dose combination of sofosbuvir (400 mg)/velpatasvir (100 mg) [Epclusa] for 12 wk. Rating: Class I, Level A
- Daily fixed-dose combination of glecaprevir (300 mg)/pibrentasvir (120 mg) for 8 wk. Rating: Class I, Level B. Use 12 wk if HIV-hepatitis C coinfected

Genotype 3: Treatment-naïve patients without cirrhosis:
- Daily fixed-dose of glecaprevir (300 mg)/pibrentasvir (120 mg) for 8 wk. Rating: Class I, Level A
- Daily fixed-dose combination of sofosbuvir (400 mg)/velpatasvir (100 mg) [Epclusa] for 12 wk. Rating: Class I, Level A

Genotype 3: Treatment-naïve patients with compensated cirrhosis:
- Daily fixed-dose combination of glecaprevir (300 mg)/pibrentasvir (120 mg) [Mavyret] for 8 wk. Rating: Class I, Level B
- Daily fixed-dose combination of sofosbuvir (400 mg)/velpatasvir (100 mg) [Epclusa] for patients without baseline NS5A RAS Y93H for velpatasvir for 12 wk. Rating: Class I, Level A
- Alternative regimens:
  1. Daily fixed-dose combination of sofosbuvir (400 mg)/velpatasvir (100 mg) with weight-based ribavirin for patients with baseline NS5A RAS Y93H for velpatasvir for 12 wk. Rating: IIa, Level A
  2. Daily fixed-dose combination of sofosbuvir (400 mg)/velpatasvir (100 mg) [Epclusa]/voxilaprevir (100 mg) for patients with baseline NS5A RAS Y93H for velpatasvir for 12 wk. Rating: Class IIa, Level B

Genotype 4: Treatment-naïve patients without cirrhosis:
- Daily fixed-dose combination of glecaprevir (300 mg)/pibrentasvir (120 mg) [Mavyret] for 8 wk. Rating: Class I Level A
- Daily fixed-dose combination of sofosbuvir (400 mg)/velpatasvir (100 mg) [Epclusa] for 12 wk. Rating: Class I, Level A
- Daily fixed-dose combination of elbasvir (50 mg)/grazoprevir (100 mg) [Zepatier] for 12 wk. Rating: Class I, Level A
- Daily fixed-dose combination of ledipasvir (90 mg)/sofosbuvir (400 mg) [Harvoni] for 12 wk. Rating: Class I, Level A

Genotype 4: Treatment-naïve patients with compensated cirrhosis:
- Daily fixed-dose combination of sofosbuvir (400 mg)/velpatasvir (100 mg) [Epclusa] for 12 wk. Rating: Class I, Level A
- Daily fixed-dose combination of glecaprevir (300 mg)/pibrentasvir (120 mg) [Mavyret] for 8. Rating: Class I, Level B. Use 12 wk if HIV-hepatitis C coinfected
- Daily fixed-dose combination of elbasvir (50 mg)/grazoprevir (100 mg) [Zepatier] for 12 wk. Rating: Class IIa, Level B
- Daily fixed-dose combination of ledipasvir (90 mg)/sofosbuvir (400 mg) [Harvoni] for 12 wk. Rating: Class IIa, Level B

Genotypes 5 and 6: Treatment-naïve patients with and without compensated cirrhosis:
- Daily fixed-dose combination of glecaprevir (300 mg)/pibrentasvir (120 mg) [Mavyret] for 8 wk Rating: Class I, Level A. Use 12 wk if HIV-hepatitis C coinfected
- Daily fixed-dose combination of sofosbuvir (400 mg)/velpatasvir (100 mg) [Epclusa] for 12 wk. Rating: Class I, Level B
- Daily fixed-dose combination of ledipasvir (90 mg)/sofosbuvir (400 mg) [Harvoni] for 12 wk. Rating: Class IIa, Level B

Drug interactions can be significant with these regimens. With DAA regimens, viral loads are measured at 4 wk into the therapy to monitor success and at the end of therapy. A final viral load is measured 12 wk after completing the treatment, and, if undetectable, the patient is considered to have a sustained virologic response (SVR), which equates to a cure.

For *patients with decompensated cirrhosis,* there are also guidelines per genotype as well. (Treatment is based on genotype and whether the patient is able to use ribavirin or is ribavirin ineligible.) A regimen exists for patients with decompensated cirrhosis and genotype 1 to 6 in whom prior sofosbuvir or NS5A inhibitor-based treatment failed: Ledipasvir (90 mg)/sofosbuvir (400 mg) [Harvoni] with low initial dose of ribavirin (600 mg; increase as tolerated) for 24 wk (IIc) or sofosbuvir (400 mg)/velpatasvir (100 mg) [Epclusa] with weight-based ribavirin for 24 wk (IIc).

Determination of cirrhosis: Liver biopsy is not required. A patient is presumed to have cirrhosis if they have a FIB-4 Score >3.25 or any of the following findings from a previously performed test:
- Transient elastography indicating cirrhosis (e.g., FibroScan stiffness >12.5 kPA)
- FibroSure score >0.58 warrants treatment by most insurers. A score of 0.72 to 0.74 equals to a stage 3 METAVIR and >0.74 stage 4 cirrhosis
- Clinical evidence of cirrhosis (liver nodularity and/or splenomegaly on imaging, platelet <150,000/mm^3
- Prior liver biopsy showing cirrhosis

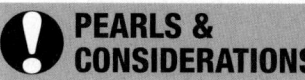

$$\text{FIB-4 Score} = \frac{\text{Age (Years)} \times \text{AST Level (U/L)}}{\text{Platelet count } (10^9/L) \times \sqrt{\text{ALT}\left(\frac{U}{L}\right)}}$$

Fibrosis-4 (FIB-4) Calculator

In 2017, a new salvage regimen was approved: Once-daily Vosevi (fixed-dose combination of 100-mg voxilaprevir [HCV NS3/4A protease inhibitor] plus 400-mg sofosbuvir and 100-mg velpatasvir. Eligible patients include:
- Genotypes 1, 2, 3, 4, 5, or 6 in patients previously treated with a regimen containing an NS5A inhibitor for 12 wk. (NOTE: In clinical trials, prior experience with NS5A inhibitors included daclatasvir, elbasvir, ledipasvir, ombitasvir, or velpatasvir.)
- Genotype 1a or 3 in patients previously treated with sofosbuvir without an NS5A inhibitor for 12 wk. (NOTE: In clinical trials, prior treatment experience included sofosbuvir with or without any of the following: Peginterferon alfa/ribavirin, ribavirin, HCV NS3/4A protease inhibitors: Boceprevir, simeprevir, or telaprevir.)
- Liver transplantation:
  1. Hepatitis C is the main indication for liver transplantation in the U.S.
  2. It is the only option for patients with deteriorating HCV-related cirrhosis and for some patients with HCC.
  3. Recurrent infection occurs in almost all patients with progressive fibrosis and cirrhosis; as many as 20% progress to cirrhosis within 5 yr posttransplant.
  4. There are regimens to treat HCV infection in post-liver transplant patients and will depend on whether patient is treatment naïve or experienced, genotype, and whether patient has compensated or decompensated cirrhosis.

DISPOSITION
- The absence of HCV RNA in blood 12 wk after completion of treatment is considered a cure. There is no need to check HCV antibodies because they will remain positive indefinitely.
- SVR after treatment among HCV-infected persons at any stage of fibrosis is associated with reduced HCC.
- Periodic abdominal ultrasonography for HCC screening (with or without alpha-fetoprotein testing) every 6 mo is recommended in patients with cirrhosis even after obtaining virologic cure.

REFERRAL
- To a hepatologist or infectious disease specialist for treatment for hepatitis C in patients who have been previously treated or for treatment failures with DAA agents.
- To a transplant surgeon for consideration of liver transplant if indicated.

! PEARLS & CONSIDERATIONS
- The American Association for the Study of Liver Diseases (AASLD) and Infectious Diseases Society of America (IDSA) recommend HCU screening for all adults (age ≥18 y) and all pregnant people during each pregnancy.[2]
- More rapid progression of disease in persons who drink alcohol regularly, persons of advanced age at time of infection, and those coinfected with other viruses (HIV, hepatitis B). All persons with identified HCV infection should receive a brief alcohol screening and intervention as clinically indicated.
- Regression of cirrhosis has been demonstrated after antiviral therapy in some patients with chronic hepatitis C. Regression is associated with decreased disease-related morbidity and improved survival.
- The presence of interleukin (IL)-28B and human leukocyte antigen (HLA) class II is independently associated with spontaneous resolution of HCV infection, and single nucleotide polymorphism IL-28B and DQB1*03:01 may explain ~15% of spontaneous resolution of HCV infection.
- In 2021 the FDA-approved Epclusa (sofosbuvir and velpatasvir) to treat hepatitis C in children 6 yr and older or weighing at least 37 lb (17 kg) with any of the six genotypes without cirrhosis or with mild cirrhosis. Epclusa with ribavirin was approved in the same population for severe cirrhosis.

REFERENCES & SUGGESTED READINGS
Available at eBooks.Health.Elsevier.com.

RELATED CONTENT
Hepatitis C (Patient Information)

AUTHOR: **GLENN G. FORT, MD, MPH**

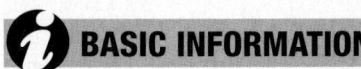 **BASIC INFORMATION**

DEFINITION

Hepatocellular carcinoma (HCC) is a malignant neoplasm of hepatocytes, and 85% of cases occur in patients who have been diagnosed with cirrhosis.

SYNONYMS

Hepatoma
HCC

ICD-10CM CODES
C22.0   Malignant neoplasm of liver and intrahepatic bile ducts

EPIDEMIOLOGY & DEMOGRAPHICS

HCC is the seventh most common cancer worldwide (~905,000 new cases/yr) and the second most common cause of cancer deaths (~830,000 deaths/yr). Incidence varies worldwide:

INCIDENCE:
- Peaks in fifth and sixth decades in Western countries, earlier in areas with perinatal hepatitis B transmission.
- Incidence has grown in the U.S. due to chronic hepatitis C, nonalcoholic fatty liver disease (NAFLD), metabolic syndrome, obesity, and diabetes mellitus.
  1. During the past two decades, the incidence in the U.S. doubled, and HCC is the fastest rising cause of cancer-related deaths in the U.S.
  2. In 2023, an estimated 41,210 new cases and 29,380 deaths occurred in the U.S.[1] The incidence in the U.S. is expected to increase to 56,000 cases by 2030.
  3. The greatest proportional increase has been among Hispanics and whites between 45 and 60 yr of age.
  4. The mean age of diagnosis is approximately 65 yr.

PREVALENCE: Areas with high rates of hepatitis B and C (East Asia, sub-Saharan Africa) have highest incidence.

PREDOMINANT SEX: Male:female ratios are between 2:1 and 4:1.

RISK FACTORS:
- Chronic hepatitis B infection accounts for 50% of all cases and most childhood cases
- Chronic hepatitis C infection markers are found in 80% to 90% of patients with HCC in Japan and 30% to 50% in the U.S.
- Cirrhosis from other causes: Alcoholic liver disease, nonalcoholic steatohepatitis, primary biliary cirrhosis, hemochromatosis, α1-antitrypsin deficiency, and autoimmune hepatitis
- Hepatotoxins: Aflatoxin B1
- Systemic diseases affecting the liver: Tyrosinemia
- Obesity and diabetes mellitus

PHYSICAL FINDINGS & CLINICAL PRESENTATION

- One third of patients are asymptomatic.
- Abdominal pain may be the initial presentation.
- Signs of underlying cirrhosis and portal hypertension are often present.

- Previously compensated cirrhosis with new ascites, encephalopathy, jaundice, or bleeding.
- Paraneoplastic syndromes (hypoglycemia, erythrocytosis, hypercalcemia, severe diarrhea, dermatomyositis) may be present. Box 1 summarizes paraneoplastic syndromes associated with hepatocellular carcinoma.
- Table 1 summarizes symptoms and signs of hepatocellular carcinoma.

Dx **DIAGNOSIS**

DIFFERENTIAL DIAGNOSIS

- Metastatic cancers to liver
- Intrahepatic cholangiocarcinoma
- Benign liver neoplasms (adenomas, focal nodular hyperplasia, and hemangiomas)
- Focal fatty infiltration

WORKUP

- History regarding risk factors
- Physical examination with attention to signs of chronic liver disease
- Laboratory evaluation and imaging studies
- Imaging studies: Ultrasound for initial testing; 3-phase computed tomography (CT) scan or dynamic contrast-enhanced MRI

LABORATORY TESTS

- Liver function tests.
- α-Fetoprotein (AFP) levels can be elevated in 70% of patients. An AFP level >400 ng/ml is highly suggestive of HCC; however, elevations may not be seen in up to 40% of patients with small lesions (1 to 2 cm).
- Paraneoplastic syndromes may cause hypercalcemia, hypoglycemia, and polycythemia.
- Elevated serum HBV DNA level (≥10,000 copies/ml) is a strong independent predictor of HCC development.

IMAGING STUDIES

Ultrasound (US), CT scan (Fig. E1), or MRI. US is most commonly used as a screening test for HCC in high-risk patients every 6 mo. Fig. E2

BOX 1   Paraneoplastic Syndromes Associated with Hepatocellular Carcinoma

Carcinoid syndrome
Hypercalcemia
Hypertension
Hypertrophic osteoarthropathy
Hypoglycemia
Neuropathy
Osteoporosis
Polycythemia (erythrocytosis)
Polymyositis
Porphyria
Sexual changes—isosexual precocity, gynecomastia, feminization
Thyrotoxicosis
Thrombophlebitis migrans
Watery diarrhea syndrome

From Feldman M et al: *Sleisenger and Fordtran's gastrointestinal and liver disease,* ed 10, Philadelphia, 2016, Elsevier.

---

shows a laparoscopic view of a cirrhotic liver with a nodular hepatoma.

The following imaging modalities are recommended based on US findings:
- Hepatic lesion <1 cm needs to be followed with a repeat US every 3 mo to ensure the lesion does not change in size. If stable for 24 mo, the interval for US can be increased to every 6 mo.
- Hepatic lesion >1 cm needs further confirmatory imaging with either a CT scan or an MRI scan. If the chosen imaging modality shows characteristics typical of HCC (hypervascular in the arterial phase with washout in the portal venous or delayed phase) the diagnosis of HCC is confirmed with no need for additional diagnostic testing or biopsy. If the imaging modality is inconclusive or atypical for HCC, then the alternate imaging test must be performed. If the second imaging modality is also inconclusive, an image-guided biopsy is recommended.

BIOPSY: Percutaneous biopsy under ultrasound or CT scan is obtained in the event that imaging studies are nondiagnostic or atypical for HCC, or if no cirrhosis is present. Negative biopsy results should be followed and the hepatic nodule reassessed every 3 to 6 mo until it is no longer seen, enlarges, or shows diagnostic characteristics.

SCREENING: Screening high-risk patients with US every 6 mo is currently recommended to identify early-stage HCC.[2] The added use of AFP increases detection rate but also increases false-positive results. The use of AFP alone has limited sensitivity and specificity. Patients on transplant waiting lists should be regularly screened for HCC because in the U.S. the development of HCC gives increased priority for liver transplantation. Screening for HCC is recommended in the following groups:
- Hepatitis B carriers (HBsAg positive): Asian males >40 yr, Asian females >50 yr, all cirrhotic hepatitis B carriers, family history of

---

TABLE 1   Symptoms and Signs of Hepatocellular Carcinoma

Symptom	Frequency (%)
Abdominal pain	59-95
Weight loss	34-71
Weakness	22-53
Abdominal swelling	28-43
Nonspecific GI symptoms	25-28
Jaundice	5-26
Sign	
Hepatomegaly	54-98
Ascites	35-61
Fever	11-54
Splenomegaly	27-42
Wasting	25-41
Jaundice	4-35
Hepatic bruit	6-25

GI, Gastrointestinal.

From Feldman M et al: *Sleisenger and Fordtran's gastrointestinal and liver disease,* ed 10, Philadelphia, 2016, Elsevier.

HCC, and North American blacks/Africans older than age 20 yr
- Cirrhosis (nonhepatitis B): Hepatitis C, alcoholic cirrhosis, hemochromatosis, primary biliary cirrhosis, and possibly α1-antitrypsin deficiency, autoimmune hepatitis, and non-alcoholic steatohepatitis

STAGING: The commonly used Barcelona Clinic Liver Cancer (BCLC) staging system includes patient performance status, cancer symptoms, number and size of nodules, and liver function.[3,4] The TNM staging classification is described in Table 2.

Treatment is determined according to stage (Fig. 3):
- Early stage (A): Asymptomatic single tumor 5 cm or 3 nodules, each ≤3 cm
- Intermediate stage (B): Patients with tumors that exceed early criteria but do not yet show cancer-related symptoms, vascular invasion, or metastases
- Advanced stage (C): Patients with mild cancer-related symptoms and/or vascular invasion or extrahepatic spread
- End-stage (D): Patients with advanced, symptomatic disease

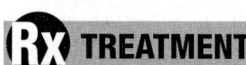 **TREATMENT**

- Treatment options for hepatocellular carcinoma are summarized in Table 3. Fig. 4 describes a treatment algorithm for HCC.

- Early stage: Curative treatment (surgical resection or liver transplantation).
- Patients who have a single lesion can be offered surgical resection if they are noncirrhotic or have cirrhosis with well-preserved liver function, normal bilirubin, and no significant portal hypertension.
- In surgically resected HCC patients with microvascular invasion, the use of adjuvant FOLFOX chemotherapy via hepatic arterial infusion chemotherapy (HAIC) results in improved disease-free survival.[5]
- Liver transplantation is an effective option for patients with HCC corresponding to the Milan criteria (Table 4). Living donor transplantation can be offered for HCC if the waiting time is expected to be long. Local ablation is safe and effective therapy for patients who cannot undergo resection or as a bridge to transplantation. With these options, survival at 5 yr ranges from 50% to 70%.
- Radiofrequency ablation (RFA) is used in patients with early HCC who are not surgical candidates, and very high local control rates at 2 yr are obtained (>90%), but eventual recurrence rates can approach 70% at 5 yr.
- Intermediate stage:
  1. Transarterial chemoembolization (TACE) is recommended as first-line, noncurative therapy for nonsurgical patients with large/multifocal HCC who do not have vascular invasion or extrahepatic spread.
  2. Transarterial use of selective internal radiation therapy (SIRT) with yttrium-90 radiolabeled glass microspheres is an alternative to traditional TACE approaches in this setting. Median survivals exceed 2 yr.
- Advanced stage: Multiple options for advanced HCC have been approved recently including targeted therapy, antiangiogenic therapy, and immunotherapy.[3,4]
- First-line therapy:
  1. In treatment-naïve patients with advanced HCC or recurrent HCC, the use of TACE followed by the oral multikinase inhibitor lenvatinib confers a survival benefit compared to TACE alone.[6]
  2. Sorafenib and lenvatinib are oral multikinase inhibitors, which are both approved as standard first-line therapy options based on overall survival improvement.
  3. In untreated patients, the immune checkpoint inhibitor atezolizumab combined with the antiangiogenic antibody bevacizumab improves overall survival compared to sorafenib and is a standard of care.[7]
  4. Dual immunotherapy with the combination of tremelimumab and durvalumab improves survival in untreated patients with unresectable HCC.[8]
- Second-line therapy:
  1. In previously treated patients, the oral multikinase inhibitors regorafenib and cabozantinib improve overall survival.
  2. Immune checkpoint inhibitors nivolumab and pembrolizumab improve overall survival. Dual immunotherapy with ipilimumab and nivolumab improves overall survival in patients previously treated with sorafenib and up to 29% survival is reported at 5 yrs.
  3. The antiangiogenic antibody ramucirumab improved survival in patients previously treated with sorafenib.

DISPOSITION

- For resectable HCC, the 5-yr survival after liver transplantation is 50% to 70% and 30% to 50% with surgical resection. For unresectable HCC, the overall prognosis is poor.
- Tumor size is an independent prognostic factor for resected small HCC (≤50 mm in diameter). Patients with tumors of 0 to 35 mm diameter have a better 60-mo HCC specific survival rate than do those with larger tumors (36 to 50 mm).

REFERRAL

Multidisciplinary gastrointestinal cancer team comprised of gastroenterology, transplant surgery, surgical oncology, interventional radiology, medical oncology, and radiation oncology

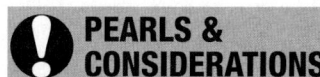 **PEARLS & CONSIDERATIONS**

- Universal hepatitis B vaccination in children in endemic areas has been shown to decrease the incidence of HCC.

TABLE 2 Hepatocellular Carcinoma TNM Staging Classification and Milan Criteria for Liver Transplantation

T Stage	
T_x	The primary tumor is not assessable
T_0	No tumor is present
T_1	A single tumor (of any size) without blood vessel invasion
	T_{1a}: Solitary tumor <2 cm (greatest dimension) without vascular invasion
	T_{1b}: Solitary tumor >2 cm (greatest dimension) without vascular invasion
T_2	A single tumor >2 cm *with* vascular invasion or multiple tumors (none >5 cm)
T_3	Multiple tumors, any more >5 cm
T_4	Tumor(s) invading a major branch of the portal or hepatic vein with direct invasion of adjacent organs including the diaphragm (other than gallbladder) or with perforation of the visceral liver peritoneum

N Stage

N_x	The lymph nodes are not assessable
N_0	There is no regional nodal involvement
N_1	There is regional nodal involvement

M Stage

M_0	There is no distant tumor spread
M_1	There is distant tumor spread

Milan Criteria for Liver Transplantation

1 tumor ≤5 cm in diameter, or

Up to 3 tumors ≤3 cm in diameter

+ No vascular invasion

+ No extrahepatic disease

Note

The tumor/node/metastasis (TNM) staging classification does not consider the background liver function, which is often impaired in cirrhosis and will affect treatment options and prognosis. Other staging systems consider both disease extent and liver function, but have not been compared accurately against one another:
- Barcelona Clinic Liver Cancer (BCLC) system
- Cancer of the Liver Italian Program (CLIP) system
- Okuda system

From Grant LA: *Grainger & Allison's diagnostic radiology essentials*, ed 2, Philadelphia, 2019, Elsevier.

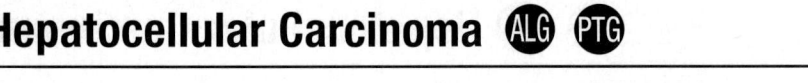

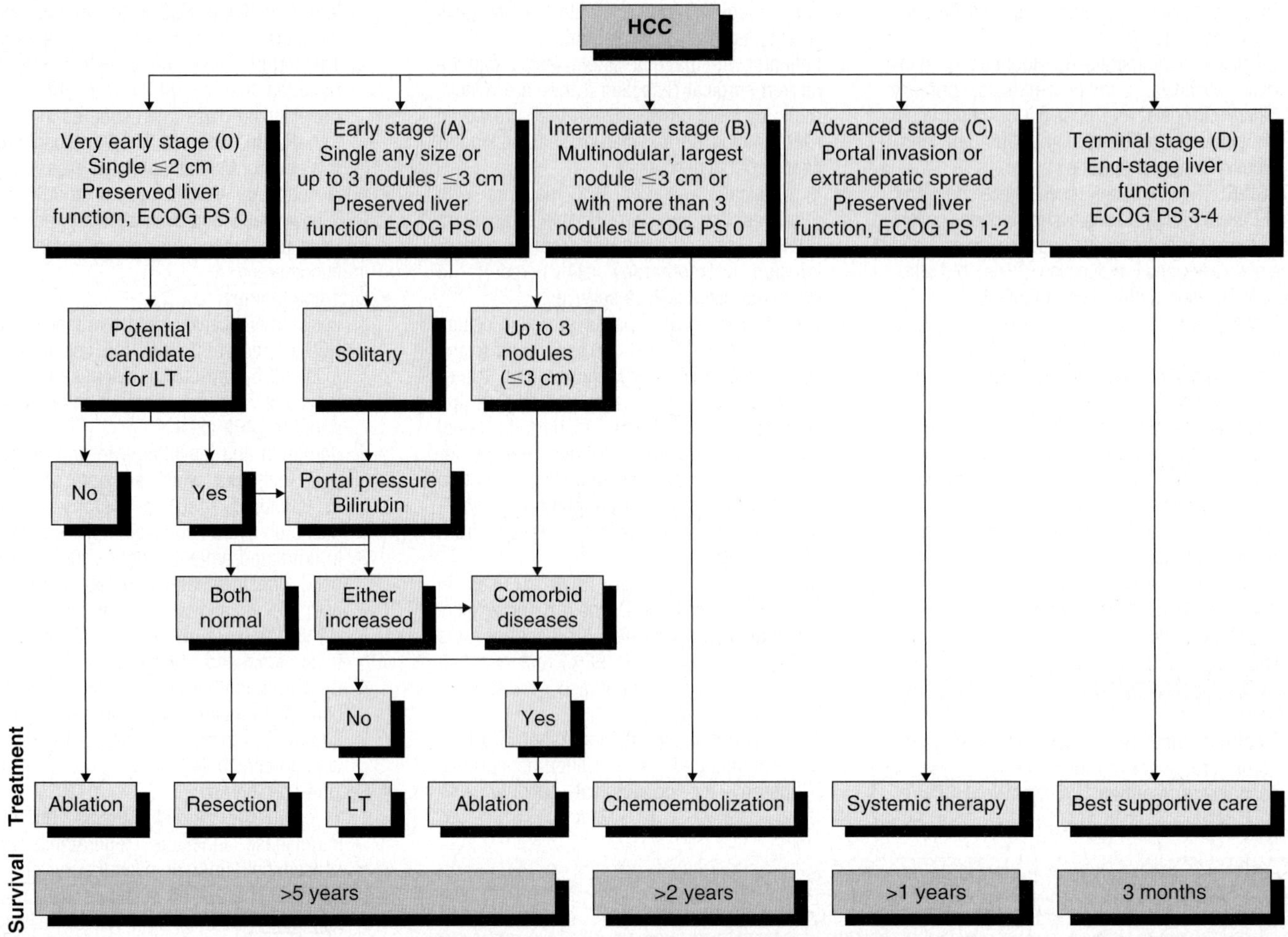

HCC

| Very early stage (0) Single ≤2 cm Preserved liver function, ECOG PS 0 | Early stage (A) Single any size or up to 3 nodules ≤3 cm Preserved liver function ECOG PS 0 | Intermediate stage (B) Multinodular, largest nodule ≤3 cm or with more than 3 nodules ECOG PS 0 | Advanced stage (C) Portal invasion or extrahepatic spread Preserved liver function, ECOG PS 1-2 | Terminal stage (D) End-stage liver function ECOG PS 3-4 |

Potential candidate for LT

Solitary

Up to 3 nodules (≤3 cm)

No Yes

Portal pressure Bilirubin

Both normal Either increased Comorbid diseases

No Yes

Treatment

| Ablation | Resection | LT | Ablation | Chemoembolization | Systemic therapy | Best supportive care |

Survival

| >5 years | >2 years | >1 years | 3 months |

FIG. 3 Barcelona Clinic Liver Cancer (BCLC) staging classification and treatment schedule with associated expected survival. Staging is based on tumor size and spread, the patient's Eastern Cooperative Oncology Group (ECOG) performance status (PS) on a scale of 0 (good) to greater than 2 (poor), and liver function as assessed by the Child-Pugh class. Patients with very early (*stage 0*) HCC are optimal candidates for surgical resection. Patients with early (*stage A*) HCC are candidates for radical therapy (resection, deceased-donor LT, or live-donor LT, or local ablation via percutaneous ethanol injection or radiofrequency ablation). Patients with intermediate (*stage B*) HCC benefit from transarterial chemoembolization. Patients with advanced HCC, defined as the presence of macroscopic vascular invasion, extrahepatic spread, or cancer-related symptoms (PS 1 or 2) (*stage C*), benefit from sorafenib or lenvatinib as first-line and regorafenib or nivolumab as second-line therapy. Patients with end-stage disease (*stage D*) should receive symptomatic treatment. The treatment strategy will transition from one stage to another when treatment fails or is contraindicated. (Adapted from Forner A et al: Hepatocellular carcinoma, *Lancet* 391:1301-1314, 2018.)

TABLE 3   Treatment Options for HCC

Modality	Comments
Surgical resection	Curative but limited to noncirrhotic patients and cirrhotic patients without portal hypertension May be technically difficult High recurrence rate
LT	Successful in selected patients (Milan criteria) Requires lifelong immunosuppression Expensive and not available worldwide
Radiofrequency ablation or ethanol injection	Potentially curative for small tumors, including multiple tumors High recurrence rate
Transarterial chemoembolization	Prolongs survival in unresectable tumors if hepatic function is preserved; not curative
Chemotherapy	No clear benefit; palliative only Drug toxicity is common
Targeted molecular therapies	Sorafenib is the first such agent shown to improve patient survival Improvement in patient survival with lenvatinib is similar to that with sorafenib Regorafenib, cabozantinib, and ramucirumab (if AFP >400 ng/ml) improve survival after sorafenib failure
Immune checkpoint inhibitors	Nivolumab and pembrolizumab are associated with improved survival after failure of or intolerance to sorafenib

From Feldman M et al: *Sleisenger and Fordtran's gastrointestinal and liver disease,* ed 11, Philadelphia, 2021, Elsevier.

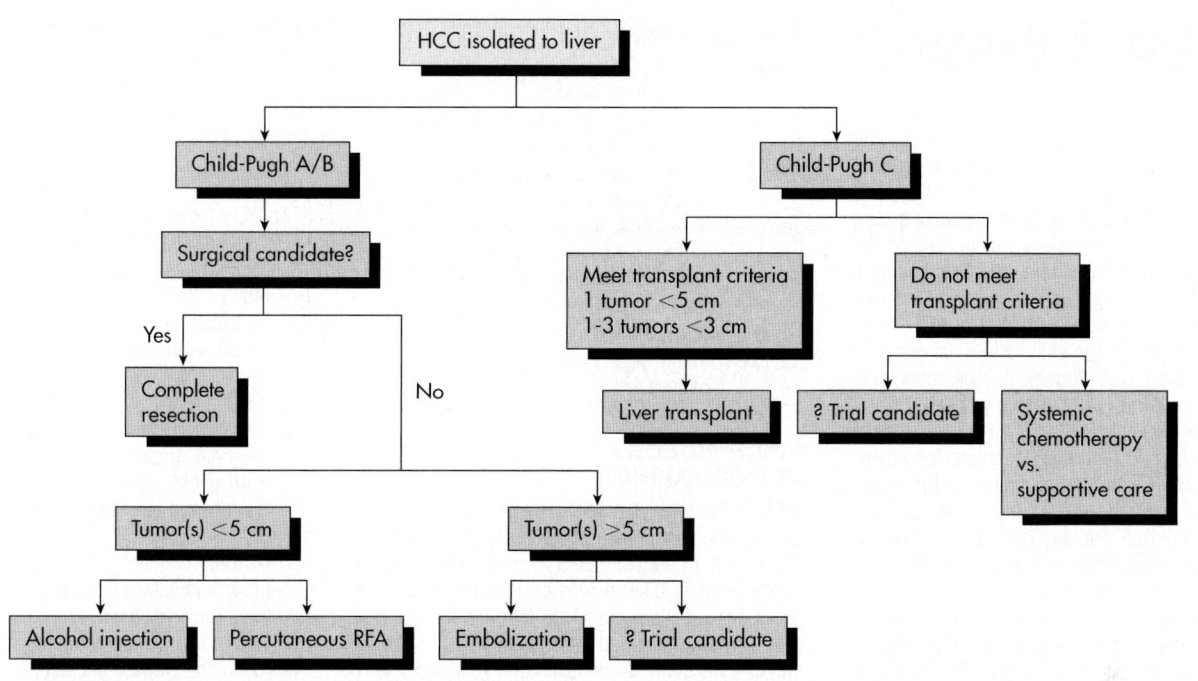

FIG. 4 Treatment algorithm for hepatocellular carcinoma (HCC). *RFA,* Radiofrequency ablation. (From Bruix J, Sherman M: AASLD: management of hepatocellular carcinoma: an update, *Hepatology* 53[3]:1020-1022, 2011.)

TABLE 4 Milan Criteria of Eligibility for Liver Transplantation

Presence of a tumor ≤5 cm in diameter in patients with single hepatocellular carcinomas
Or
≤3 Tumor nodules, each 3 cm or less in diameter, in patients with multiple tumors

From Cameron JL, Cameron AM: *Current surgical therapy,* ed 10, Philadelphia, 2011, Saunders.

- Treatment of patients with chronic hepatitis B–associated cirrhosis with lamivudine reduces the incidence of HCC. Treatment with entecavir in chronic hepatitis B-HCC can improve hepatic function and MELD score.

- HCC screening is recommended in high-risk patients because curative therapies are available only for small and early HCC.
- Patients diagnosed with HCC with an AFP >1000 are at increased risk for recurrence after transplantation regardless of tumor size.

- Low-dose daily aspirin use has been associated with less progression of liver disease in patients with chronic hepatitis B or C and lower HCC risk in those patients.

REFERENCES

Available at eBooks.Health.Elsevier.com.

RELATED CONTENT

Liver Cancer (Patient Information)

AUTHOR: **BHARTI RATHORE, MD**

BASIC INFORMATION

DEFINITION

Hereditary breast and ovarian cancer syndrome (HBOC) patients carry a significant cancer-associated alteration in the *BRCA1* and/or *BRCA2* gene. These genetic mutations can confer a heightened risk of malignancy in the breast, ovary, fallopian tube, and peritoneum in women and an elevated risk of prostate and breast cancer in men. Additionally, the risk of pancreatic cancer and skin cancer are elevated for both men and women. Another condition, Lynch syndrome or hereditary nonpolyposis colorectal cancer (HNPCC), is associated with an increased risk of endometrial cancer and ovarian cancer in women and cancer of the colon, stomach, pancreas, and small bowel in both women and men. Patients with Lynch syndrome carry significant pathogenic alterations in one of five genes, as noted below.

The cancer risk to those who test positive for these genetic mutations is significantly greater than the cancer risk associated with those who test negative—both in the general population and in those patients with a personal and/or family cancer history. Frequently, a cancer that is associated with a heritable genetic mutation presents at a younger age than that seen in the general population can be a relatively rarer type of cancer and/or affect multiple same-side family members. Identifying carriers can significantly reduce the morbidity and mortality of the patient and close family members.

SYNONYMS

HBOC
Hereditary breast and ovarian cancer syndrome
Lynch syndrome/hereditary nonpolyposis colorectal cancer (HNPCC)
Hereditary cancer syndrome

ICD-10CM CODES

Z15.01 Genetic susceptibility to malignant neoplasm of breast
Z15.02 Genetic susceptibility to malignant neoplasm of ovary
Z80.3   Family history of malignant neoplasm of breast
Z80.41 Family history of malignant neoplasm of ovary
Z80.49 Family history of malignant neoplasm of other genital organs (uterus, vagina, for example)
Z84.81 Family history of carrier of genetic disease

EPIDEMIOLOGY & DEMOGRAPHICS

INCIDENCE: Overall, an estimated 6% to 10% of gynecologic cancers are heritable. Approximately 7% to 10% of the estimated 276,480 (American Cancer Society 2020 estimate) new breast cancer cases annually are likely to be associated with heredity. Inherited pathogenic *BRCA 1, 2* mutations account for an estimated 11% to 15% of the estimated 21,750 (American Cancer Society 2020 estimate) annual new ovarian cancer cases. Less than 1% of the general population has a pathogenic mutation in the *BRCA 1* or *2* gene. As noted above, Lynch syndrome–associated mutations increase ovarian and uterine cancer as well as colorectal (up to 5% of colorectal cancers are considered heritable), pancreatic, and gastric cancers. This article will, however, focus on gynecologic disease. Tables 1 and 2 summarize genes associated with hereditary breast and ovarian cancer predisposition.

PREDOMINANT SEX & AGE: Although females are predominantly affected, males who carry deleterious mutations in *BRCA 1, 2* are at a significantly higher risk for cancer. Both sexes can transmit the altered gene to their offspring.

RISK FACTORS: *BRCA1* and *BRCA2* mutations can generate a greater risk of breast cancer than other well-established factors such as increased breast density, history of atypical ductal or lobular hyperplasia, nulliparity, obesity, and family history.

Up to 37% of breast cancer patients and 100% of ovarian/tubal/peritoneal cancer patients are at risk for hereditary breast and ovarian cancer syndrome.

Hereditary breast and ovarian cancer syndrome (HBOC):
- Individuals with *BRCA1, BRCA2* mutations (Fig. 1)
- Red flags (not an exhaustive list) for possible HBOC include personal or family history of:
  1. Personal breast cancer diagnosed at ≤45 yr old
  2. Triple-negative breast cancer (ER-, PR-, Her2-)
  3. Ovarian cancer: Very important factor (mostly papillary serous)
  4. Male breast cancer
  5. Two primary breast cancers
  6. Ashkenazi Jewish ancestry
  7. Breast cancer with ≥2 relatives with an HBOC-associated cancer (breast, ovary, prostate, pancreatic cancers)
  8. A previously identified HBOC mutation
  9. Two or more close relatives with breast cancer, one of whom was diagnosed at age 50 or younger
  10. Three or more HBOC-associated cancers at any age

GENETICS: The transmission pattern is autosomal dominant. A child whose father or mother has a *BRCA* mutation has a 50% chance of inheriting that genetic mutation.

NOTE: One half of *BRCA* carriers inherit the mutation from their father.
- Early onset of cancer may be a more important red flag than the number of affected

---

TABLE 1 Genes Associated with Hereditary Breast Cancer Predisposition

Gene	Syndrome	Relative Risk of BC	BC Risk by Age 80 Yr	Associated Cancers
High Penetrance				
BRCA1	HBOC	~15-30	70%	Ovarian, other
BRCA2	HBOC	~10-20	70%	Ovarian, pancreatic, prostate, other
p53	Li-Fraumeni syndrome	100	50% by 60 yr	Soft tissue sarcoma, osteosarcoma, brain tumors, adrenocortical carcinoma, leukemia, other
PTEN	Cowden syndrome	No reliable estimate	70%-80%	Thyroid (follicular and rarely papillary) endometrial, genitourinary, other
	Bannayan-Riley-Ruvalcaba syndrome			
	Proteus			
	Proteus-like syndrome			
STK11	Peutz-Jeghers syndrome	No reliable estimate	30% by age 60	Small intestine, colorectal, uterine, testicular and ovarian sex chord tumors, other
CDH1	Hereditary diffuse gastric carcinoma	~3.25	39%	Lobular breast, diffuse gastric, other
Lower or Moderate Penetrance				
ATM (heterozygote)	Ataxia-telangiectasia in homozygotes	~3	30	Undefined in heterozygotes
CHK2 (CHEK2)	Li-Fraumeni variant	1.5-3	20%-30%	Undefined
PALB2	None known	5	~40	Undefined in heterozygotes

BC, Breast cancer; *HBOC,* hereditary breast and ovarian cancer syndrome.
From Niederhuber JE: *Abeloff's clinical oncology,* ed 6, Philadelphia, 2020, Elsevier.

TABLE 2 Genes Associated with Hereditary Ovarian Cancer Predisposition

Gene	Syndrome	Relative Risk of OC	OC Risk by Age 80 Yr	Associated Cancers
High Penetrance				
BRCA1	Hereditary breast ovarian cancer syndrome	~50	~40%	Breast, other
BRCA2	Hereditary breast ovarian cancer syndrome	~8	11%-26%	Breast, pancreas, prostate, other
MLH1 MSH2 MSH6 PMS2 EPCAM	Lynch syndrome	~4	~20%	Colon Uterine Stomach Small intestine Urinary tract Pancreatic Possible other sites
Lower or Moderate Penetrance				
RAD51C	None	~5	~6%	Undefined Autosomal recessive Fanconi anemia
RAD51D	None	~12	~14%	Undefined Autosomal recessive Fanconi anemia

OC, Ovarian cancer.
From Niederhuber JE: *Abeloff's clinical oncology*, ed 6, Philadelphia, 2020, Elsevier.

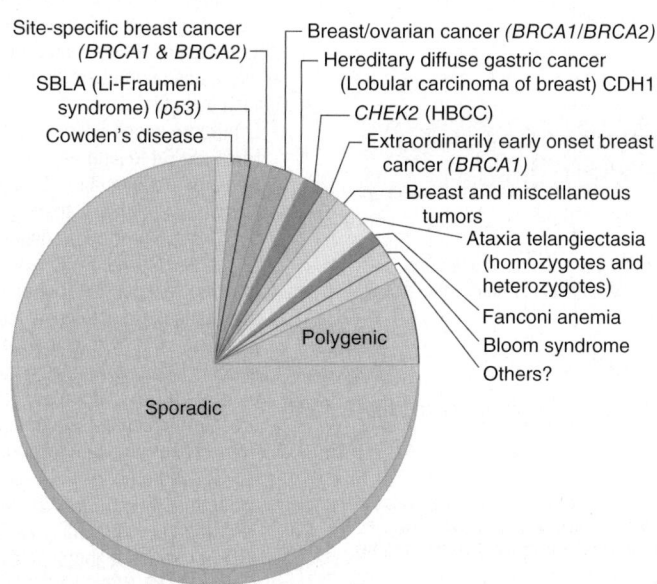

FIG. 1 Schematic depicting heterogeneity in breast cancer. *HBCC,* Hereditary breast and colorectal cancer; *SBLA,* sarcoma, breast and brain tumors, leukemia, laryngeal and lung cancer, and adrenal cortical carcinoma. (From Goldman L, Schafer AI: *Goldman's Cecil medicine,* ed 24, Philadelphia, 2012, Saunders.)

family members, especially if the number of family members is small to begin with.
- Testing criteria (Tables 3 and 4), as per National Comprehensive Cancer Network (NCCN) guidelines, may differ from the red flags noted previously.
- Family history extends to first-, second-, and third-degree relatives.
- Consider Lynch syndrome–associated cancers (e.g., colorectal, gastric, brain, pancreas, small bowel, skin, ureter, renal pelvis, GI polyps), as Lynch syndrome is also associated with ovarian and uterine (endometrial) cancer.
- BRCA stands for BReast CAncer.
  1. The majority (84%) of the approximately 7% of breast cancers and 14% of ovarian cancers that result from a heritable mutation are due to a BRCA1 (52%) and BRCA2 (32%) gene mutation.
  2. By age 70, in comparison to the 7.3% risk of breast cancer in the general population, or approximately double that risk if one has an affected first-degree relative, BRCA1 and BRCA2 mutation carriers have up to an 87% reported risk of developing breast cancer. As opposed to a general-population risk of 2% for developing a second breast primary within 5 yr of the initial diagnosis, women with HBOC mutations have a 12% to 27% risk. This risk climbs to a reported 50% *(BRCA2)* and up to 64% *(BRCA1)* by age 70.
  3. By age 70, in contrast to the 0.7% risk of ovarian cancer in the general population, there is a reported risk of up to 27% to 63% for *BRCA2* and *BRCA1* mutation carriers, respectively. The risk for ovarian cancer within 10 yr of a breast cancer diagnosis is 6.8% *(BRCA2)* to 12.7% *(BRCA1)* as opposed to a general-population risk of less than 1.0%.
  4. Men with HBOC have an up to tenfold increased risk for breast cancer and a more than twofold increase in prostate cancer in comparison to the general-population risk. In men, the *BRCA2* mutation increases this cancer risk more than the *BRCA1* mutation. In fact, the breast cancer risk for a male with a *BRCA2* mutation is up to 80 times the risk seen in the general population.
  5. Both men and women have an elevated risk (up to sevenfold) for pancreatic cancer (*BRCA2* >1) and for melanoma (2.5-fold increase with *BRCA2* + *status*).
  6. Ashkenazi Jewish ancestry is associated with founder mutations 187delAG *(BRCA1)*, 5382insC *(BRCA1)*, and 6174delT *(BRCA2)*, which confer a significantly elevated risk for breast and ovarian cancer. As opposed to the 1 in 400 risk in the general population, 1 in 40 individuals of Ashkenazi Jewish descent have a *BRCA 1* or *2* mutation.

Lynch syndrome (hereditary nonpolyposis colorectal cancer [HNPCC]):
- Individuals with MLH1, MSH2, MSH6, PMS2, EPCAM mutations.
- By age 70, Lynch syndrome carriers have—in addition to an increased risk for colorectal, gastric, hepatobiliary, urinary tract, small bowel, brain, skin, and pancreatic cancers—up to an approximately twentyfold increase in ovarian cancer (4% to 12% risk vs. the general-population risk of 0.7%) and up to an approximately fortyfold increase in uterine cancer (25% to 60+% risk vs. the general-population risk of 1.6%).
- The previously listed genes and others (e.g., PTEN, TP53, CDH1, STK11) that are found less frequently are considered high-penetrance genes, as they can increase the relative risk of their respective syndromes by greater than four- to fivefold.
- Other, more moderate-penetrant genes (e.g., CHEK2, ATM, PALB2, BRIP1, RAD51C, RAD51D), that is, those that are associated with a two- to fourfold increase in the relative risk of cancer, should be considered when assessing risk and ordering genetic tests.
- More than 12 known gene mutations are associated with an elevated risk for breast cancer, and a similar number are associated with an elevated risk for ovarian cancer. As such, screening for BRCA1, BRCA2 alone will miss these mutations.
- In addition to established deleterious mismatch repair gene mutations, gene alterations that are categorized in the literature as emerging risk mutations are also associated with hereditary gynecologic and other cancers.

TABLE 3   Testing Criteria for Breast and Ovarian Cancer Syndrome*

Individual from a family with a known deleterious *BRCA1* or *BRCA2* gene mutation
Personal history of breast cancer plus one or more of the following:
- Diagnosed at ≤45 yr of age
- Diagnosed at ≤50 yr of age with
  - An additional breast cancer primary
  - At least one close blood relative with breast cancer at any age
  - At least one close relative with pancreatic cancer
  - At least one close relative with prostate cancer
  - An unknown or limited family history
- Diagnosed at age 60 with
  - Triple-negative breast cancer
- Diagnosed at any age with
  - At least one close blood relative with breast cancer before 50 yr of age
  - At least two close blood relatives with breast cancer at any age
  - At least one close relative with pancreatic cancer
  - At least two close blood relatives with prostate cancer
  - A close female blood relative with ovarian cancer
  - An individual of ethnicity associated with a higher mutation frequency
- Personal history of ovarian cancer
- Personal history of male breast cancer
- Personal history of prostate cancer at any age with a close relative with breast, ovarian, or pancreatic cancer at any age
- Personal history of pancreatic cancer and Ashkenazi Jewish ancestry
- Family history meeting any of the above criteria
See NCCN guidelines for the most up-to-date and detailed description for counseling and testing.

*For more detailed information, see the National Comprehensive Cancer Network (NCCN) guidelines.
From Disaia PJ et al: *Clinical gynecologic oncology,* ed 9, Philadelphia, 2017, Elsevier.

TABLE 4   National Comprehensive Cancer Network (NCCN) Guidelines for Recommending Genetic Testing for *BRCA1* or *BRCA2* Mutations*

Personal history of breast cancer and one or more of the following:
- Diagnosed at age ≤45 yr
- Diagnosed with at least two breast cancer primaries (bilateral, separate ipsilateral), the first at age 50 yr
- Diagnosed at age ≤50 yr with one or more close relatives[†] with breast cancer (prostate or pancreatic) at any age
- Diagnosed with triple-negative breast cancer at age ≤60 yr
- Diagnosed at any age with one or more close relatives with breast cancer at age ≤50 yr
- Diagnosed at any age with two or more close relatives at any age
- Diagnosed at any age with one or more close relatives with invasive ovarian cancer (including fallopian tube and primary peritoneal) at any age
- Diagnosed at any age with two or more close relatives with pancreatic and/or prostate cancer
- Having a close male relative with breast cancer at any age

*Individuals with a limited or unknown family history may have an underestimated probability of a familial gene mutation detection.
[†]Close relative pertains to first-, second-, or third-degree blood relatives on the same side (either maternal or paternal) of the family.
From Disaia PJ et al: *Clinical gynecologic oncology,* ed 9, Philadelphia, 2017, Elsevier.

PHYSICAL FINDINGS & CLINICAL PRESENTATION

- Present at a younger age
- Bilaterality more likely
- Multiple primaries in one individual

ETIOLOGY

Hereditary cancers are typically due to a tumor suppression gene mutation that interferes with DNA repair thus allowing an otherwise potentially avoidable cancer to develop. This is distinct from familial cancers in which there is no isolated gene mutation. Such cancers appear in the family more frequently than that which would be statistically seen in the general population. Non-genetic factors such as lifestyle habits and environmental influences contribute to cancer risk as well.

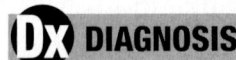 **DIAGNOSIS**

DIFFERENTIAL DIAGNOSIS

- General (sporadic) population or familial basis for the cancer in question—when the genetic testing is negative.
- Hereditary cancer is more likely to present at a younger age, to span a number of generations, to affect more family members than would be expected (if a large enough family), be associated with a suspicious familial pattern, and to include some rarer (ovary, male breast cancer, pancreatic cancer, for example) presentations.
  In addition to the more common syndromes listed previously, consider Cowden *(PTEN),* Peutz-Jeghers *(STK11),* Li-Fraumeni *(TP53),* and others (Table 5).

WORKUP

Family history questionnaire (revisited during subsequent visits), patient and family interviews, genetic counseling/risk assessment (including tools such as Tyrer-Cuzick/Gail/Claus models), and tailored cancer screening and genetic testing. Tablet-based intake questionnaires and computer algorithms are increasingly being used to identify at-risk patients.

LABORATORY TESTS

- A simple blood or saliva sample drawn in the office or a lab, after informed consent, is needed. This specimen should be sent to a reliable laboratory recognized nationally for its genetic cancer testing accuracy (technologic and interpretative), reporting format, and the support staff ability and availability for consultation, office counseling, and testing integration. Look for a laboratory that has published peer-reviewed data and has an accurate classification methodology that relies on an extensive database. Realize that these labs are not FDA approved and that CLIA certification, while needed, relies on just in-house data. Remember also that most patients get tested only once in their lifetime, and so accuracy is imperative. Update testing should be offered as appropriate and available.
- Options include:
  1. Syndrome specific (limited): For example, HBOC-*BRCA* testing (including large rearrangement detection); Lynch syndrome; founder mutation testing (187delAG, 5382insC, 6174delT)—Ashkenazi Jewish population (occasionally recommended as the first test for this population); single-site testing (if a previously identified gene mutation is known in the family); cancer specific, for example, breast cancer panel—*BRCA 1, 2* with/without reflex to broader panel (i.e., sequential testing).
  2. Comprehensive panel testing: Can include HBOC syndrome *(BRCA1, BRCA2),* Lynch syndrome *(MLH1, MSH2, MSH6, PMS2, EPCAM),* Li-Fraumeni *(TP53),* Cowden *(PTEN),* Peutz-Jeghers *(STK11), PALB2, CHEK2, ATM, BRIP1, RAD51C,* and others (30+ genes).
- Choice of the test is generally based on personal/family history, although thoroughness of the risk assessment may be limited by attempting to choose a gene test based on history/phenotype alone.
- Comprehensive panel testing has been shown to increase mutation detection. It can aid in test selection when patients qualify for more than one syndrome/cancer-specific test, and it can be used to capture a potentially broader view of risk. There may be a concern, however, for detecting and managing discovered mutations that are not clinically actionable at that time.
- Categories of results include (1) positive or negative (or more nuanced categories) for a deleterious mutation or (2) a genetic variant of uncertain significance, in which a cancer risk is not yet established or ruled out. Genetic testing companies will notify the ordering provider as

TABLE 5 Summary of Syndromes with Malignant Manifestations Associated with Breast and Ovarian Cancer

Syndrome	Breast Cancer	Ovarian Cancer	Endometrial Cancer	Colon Cancer	Other Types of Cancer
Hereditary breast and ovarian cancer	X	X			Pancreatic, prostate, and melanoma
Lynch		X	X	X	Gastric, ureteral, biliary, pancreatic, glioblastoma, renal pelvis
Li-Fraumeni	X			X	Sarcomas, brain, adrenocortical
Cowden	X		X	X	Benign mucocutaneous lesions, thyroid, gastrointestinal hamartomas
Peutz-Jeghers	X	X		X	Cervical adenoma malignum, gastrointestinal hamartomas, pancreatic, gastric, small bowel
Hereditary diffuse gastric cancer	X				Gastric, colorectal

Data from National Comprehensive Cancer Network. Breast Cancer: NCCN Evidence Blocks. Version 2.2019. NCCN Clinical Practice Guidelines in Oncology [after login]. Fort Washington, PA: NCCN; 2019 and Hampel H et al: A practice guideline from the American College of Medical Genetics and Genomics and the National Society of Genetic Counselors: referral indications for cancer predisposition assessment. Guideline Development Group, American College of Medical Genetics and Genomics Professional Practice and Guidelines Committee, and National Society of Genetic Counselors Practice Guidelines Committee, *Getet Med* 17:70-87, 2015. In American College of Obstetricians and Gynecologists, Committee Opinion, Number 793, December 2019.

to an update in category, as new data becomes available. It is critical that the classification of these variants is accurate.

IMAGING STUDIES

Screening transvaginal pelvic ultrasonography, annual mammography, annual MRI (when breast cancer risk is 20% or more based on Tyrer-Cuzick or other breast cancer risk screening models)

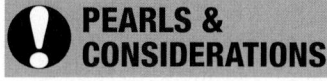

TREATMENT & RISK REDUCTION

- Heightened surveillance, judicious chemoprevention, and prophylactic surgery have been associated with improved outcomes.
- Surveillance includes patient breast awareness, clinician and self-breast exam, mammography, MRI, transvaginal ultrasonography, and CA-125 blood testing, for example.
- Chemopreventive approaches have been shown to reduce the risk of ovarian cancer by up to 60% (with an oral contraceptive) and risk of contralateral breast cancer by as much as 53% (with tamoxifen).
- In HBOC patients, prophylactic total mastectomy can reduce the risk of breast cancer by 90%, and a bilateral salpingo-oophorectomy, after childbearing or by age 40, can reduce the risk of ovarian cancer by up to 96% and the risk of breast cancer by up to 68%.
- Consider preimplantation genetic diagnosis in conjunction with in vitro fertilization.

REFERRAL

If services are needed beyond one's practice or comfort level, consider consulting with knowledgeable genetic counselors, gynecologists, gynecologic oncologists, breast surgeons, and gastroenterology specialists, among others.

PEARLS & CONSIDERATIONS

- Be vigilant. Be motivated by the risks: Women with these mutations are approximately 10 times more likely to develop breast cancer and 20 to 30 times more likely to develop ovarian cancer. **Look for red flags during every encounter**, regardless of the patient's chief complaint or scheduled visit type and inquire and regularly update information about the patient's personal and family history of cancer. Consider that approximately 10% of general practice patients have a significant family history. Supply a printed family history questionnaire. Always consider your patient's cancer risk, especially when charting a new treatment course or planning a surgical procedure. Oftentimes, a more comprehensive approach should be taken if a patient proves to be a mutation carrier.
- Adjust the age at which screening/treatment is initiated and the frequency of the visits depending on the age of the youngest affected family member, the at-risk cancer site, and the carrier status of the patient.
- Encourage input from the patient during the screening, workup, follow-up, and treatment.
- Recommend that the patient verify any questionable family history, collect appropriate family documentation/testing, and involve her family in the process. This involvement can include advising, counseling, and testing for close relatives.
- Focus counseling and testing (if appropriate) those family member(s) who, if tested, would render genetic testing of progeny/other family members less necessary. Testing an affected family member is oftentimes the most appropriate, efficient, cost-effective, and informative approach.
- Genetic testing can more accurately predict risk and enable a more tailored management approach than relying on one's family history alone. Be mindful that there may be other, although as yet unidentified, mutations at the root of one's patient's personal or family cancer history. Thus periodic update testing, as appropriate, is paramount.
- Refer to your professional societies and the NCCN for screening and surveillance/imaging/treatment guidelines. Don't hesitate to engage the assistance of a genetic counselor, gynecologist, oncologist, breast surgeon, and/or a gastroenterologist during this initial phase and, subsequently, as needed.
- Involve other appropriate specialists in the patient's short- and long-term care depending on the at-risk anatomic systems.
- Remember that *BRCA1*- and *BRCA2*-positive men are at a significantly higher risk for breast and prostate cancer, as well as skin and pancreatic cancer.
- Consider prophylactic bilateral (nerve- and nipple-sparing, if appropriate) mastectomy and bilateral salpingo-oophorectomy in high-risk patients.
- Encourage high-risk patients to complete childbearing at a younger age and consider, as appropriate, subsequent prophylactic bilateral salpingo-oophorectomy and menopause hormone therapy options.
- Recommend prophylactic bilateral salpingectomy for at-risk premenopausal patients during any other surgical procedure—once childbearing is complete. Consider assistive reproductive options, as appropriate.
- Genetic information cannot be used as the basis for a "preexisting condition" with regard to health insurance or employment, according to federal and state laws. However, it may play a role with respect to life insurance, disability insurance, and long-term care insurance.
- While insurance coverage generally is available, panel testing reimbursement may occasionally be challenged. Vocalize and document your support of the appropriate testing and management, with both your patient and her or his insurance company. Enlist the assistance of your local professional society, as needed.
- There may be a medical-legal risk if a failure to identify and/or genetically counsel or test a high-risk patient and/or her family results in a delay in the diagnosis or worsened prognosis of breast or ovarian cancer. The provider, laboratory, and the insurance company/employer may have legal exposure for failing

to order testing, for providing inaccurate results, or for denial of coverage, respectively.

- Being aware of a patient's cancer risk facilitates initiation of those preventive screenings and management strategies that have been shown to reduce the likelihood of cancer and improve early cancer detection rates. This can be of tremendous benefit both for the patient and family.

PREVENTION

Consider appropriate screening and surveillance (awareness/physical exam by patient and health care provider, imaging studies, diagnostic procedures/lab studies, counseling, and genetic testing) as well as prophylactic surgery and chemopreventive measures. Reassess at each subsequent office visit.

A new blood test (Galleri) designed to detect and locate up to 50 different cancers in asymptomatic patients using DNA sequencing to uncover abnormal cell-free DNA methylation patterns has been recently introduced on the market. This may serve to identify those larger groups of nongenetic cancers allowing earlier evaluation and treatment and ideally a better prognosis.

PATIENT & FAMILY EDUCATION

Always encourage patients to revisit their personal and family history and to update this information with all of their health care providers and their family members. Recommend that patients initiate discussions with their family members and other health care providers in an ongoing effort to reduce their and their loved ones' risk of heritable cancer.

Refer to NCCN guidelines (www.nccn.org) and national specialty society recommendations.

RELATED CONTENT

Breast Cancer (Related Key Topic)
Lynch Syndrome (Related Key Topic)
Ovarian Cancer (Related Key Topic)

AUTHOR: **DAVID I. KURSS, MD, FACOG, NCMP**

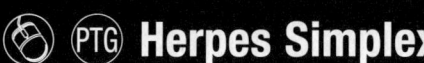

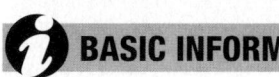 BASIC INFORMATION

DEFINITION

Herpes simplex is a viral infection caused by the herpes simplex virus (HSV). HSV-1 is associated primarily with oral infections, and HSV-2 causes mainly genital infections. However, either type can infect any site. After the primary infection, the virus enters the nerve endings in the skin directly below the lesions and ascends to the dorsal root ganglia, where it remains in a latent stage until it is reactivated.

SYNONYMS

Genital herpes
Herpes labialis
Herpes gladiatorum
Herpes digitalis
Oral herpes

ICD-10CM CODES

A60	Anogenital herpesviral (herpes simplex) infections
A60.04	Herpesviral vulvovaginitis
B00	Herpesviral (herpes simplex) infections
B00.1	Herpesviral vesicular dermatitis
B00.82	Herpes simplex myelitis
B00.9	Herpesviral infection, unspecified
P35.2	Congenital herpesviral (herpes simplex) infection

EPIDEMIOLOGY & DEMOGRAPHICS

- More than 85% of adults have serologic evidence of HSV-1 infection. The seroprevalence of adults with HSV-2 in the U.S. is 25%; however, only approximately 20% of these persons recall having symptoms of HSV infection.
- Most cases of eye or digital herpetic infections are caused by HSV-1.
- Worldwide, more than 400 million persons have genital herpes caused by HSV-2. In the U.S., 1 in 5 adults is infected with HSV-2, and 1 million new infections occur yearly.
- Frequency of recurrence of HSV-2 genital herpes is higher than HSV-1 oral labial infection.
- The frequency of recurrence is lowest for oral labial HSV-2 infections.
- The incidence of complications from herpes simplex (e.g., herpes encephalitis) is highest in immunocompromised hosts.
- Male circumcision significantly reduces the incidence of HSV-2.

PHYSICAL FINDINGS & CLINICAL PRESENTATION

PRIMARY INFECTION:

- Symptoms occur from 3 to 7 days after contact (respiratory droplets, direct contact).
- Constitutional symptoms include low-grade fever, headache and myalgias, regional lymphadenopathy, and localized pain.
- Pain, burning, itching, and tingling last several hours.
- Grouped vesicles, usually with surrounding erythema, appear and generally ulcerate or crust within 48 h (Fig. E1).

- The vesicles are uniform in size (differentiating it from herpes zoster vesicles, which vary in size). Scattered erosions covered with exudate may be noted on genitals (Fig. E2).
- During the acute eruption the patient is uncomfortable; involvement of lips and inside of mouth (Fig. E3) may make it unpleasant for the patient to eat; urinary retention may complicate involvement of the genital area.
- Lesions generally last from 2 to 6 wk and heal without scarring.

RECURRENT INFECTION:

- Generally caused by alteration in the immune system; fatigue, stress, menses, local skin trauma, and exposure to sunlight are contributing factors.
- The prodromal symptoms (fatigue, burning and tingling of the affected area) last 12 to 24 h.
- A cluster of lesions generally evolves within 24 h from a macule to a papule and then vesicles surrounded by erythema; the vesicles coalesce and subsequently rupture within 4 days, revealing erosions covered by crusts.
- The crusts are generally shed within 7 to 10 days, revealing a pink surface.
- The most frequent location of the lesions is on the vermilion border of the lips (HSV-1), the penile shaft or glans penis and the labia (HSV-2), buttocks (seen more frequently in women), fingertips (herpetic whitlow), and trunk (may be confused with herpes zoster).
- Rapid onset of diffuse cutaneous herpes simplex (eczema herpeticum) may occur in certain atopic infants and adults. It is a medical emergency, especially in young infants, and should be promptly treated with acyclovir.
- Herpes encephalitis, meningitis, and ocular herpes can occur in patients with immunocompromised status and occasionally in normal hosts.

ETIOLOGY

HSV-1 and HSV-2 are both DNA viruses.

DX DIAGNOSIS

DIFFERENTIAL DIAGNOSIS

- Impetigo
- Behçet syndrome
- Coxsackie virus infection
- Syphilis, chancroid, granuloma inguinale (Table 1)
- Stevens-Johnson syndrome
- Herpangina
- Aphthous stomatitis
- Varicella
- Herpes zoster

WORKUP

Diagnosis is based on clinical presentation. Laboratory evaluation confirms diagnosis.

LABORATORY TESTS

- Direct immunofluorescent antibody slide tests provide a rapid diagnosis.
- Viral culture is the most definitive method for diagnosis; results are generally available in 1 or 2 days. The lesions should be sampled

during the vesicular or early ulcerative stage; cervical samples should be taken from the endocervix with a swab.
- Pap smear will detect HSV-infected cells in cervical tissue from women without symptoms.
- Serologic tests for HSV: Immunoglobulin (Ig) G and IgM serum antibodies. Antibodies to HSV occur in 50% to 90% of adults. The presence of IgM or a fourfold or greater rise in IgG titers indicates a recent infection (convalescent sample should be drawn 2 to 3 wk after the acute specimen is drawn).
- Tzanck smear is a readily available test that will demonstrate multinucleated giant cells. However, it is not a highly sensitive test.

RX TREATMENT

- Herpes genitalis: Because no cure exists for herpes genitalis, treatment is focused on reducing the number of recurrences through suppressive therapy and on promoting rapid healing when a recurrence is present. In addition, treatment aims to reduce infectivity by reducing viral shedding and to reduce complications, such as urinary retention and aseptic meningitis. Tables 2 and 3 summarize antiviral chemotherapy for HSV infection.
- Herpes labialis: Antiviral therapy shortens the duration of discomfort/pain, hastens healing, and reduces viral shedding, thereby reducing dissemination of HSV. Treatment should be initiated ideally in the prodromal stage and no later than 48 h from the onset of lesions to obtain maximal clinical effect. Oral antiviral agents for herpes labialis include docosanol, famciclovir, and valaciclovir, and they are superior to topical antiviral agents. Topical acyclovir, penciclovir, and docosanol are optional treatments for recurrent herpes labialis, but they are less effective than oral treatments.

DISPOSITION

Most patients recover from the initial episode or recurrences without complications; immunocompromised hosts are at risk for complications (e.g., disseminated herpes simplex infection, herpes encephalitis).

REFERRAL

- Hospital admission in patients with herpes encephalitis or herpes meningitis and in immunocompromised hosts with diffuse herpes simplex infection
- Ophthalmology referral in patients with suspected ocular herpes

! PEARLS & CONSIDERATIONS

COMMENTS

- Provide patient education regarding transmission of HSV.
- Condom use offers significant protection against HSV-1 infection in susceptible women.
- Patients should be instructed on the use of condoms for sexual intercourse and on

TABLE 1 Features of Sexually Transmitted Infections Characterized by Genital Ulcers

	Syphilis	Genital Herpes	Chancroid	Granuloma Inguinale (Donovanosis)
Agent	*Treponema pallidum*	HSV-1, HSV-2	*Haemophilus ducreyi*	*Klebsiella granulomatis*
Incubation	10-90 days	2-14 days	1-10 days	8-80 days
Systemic findings	Primary syphilis: Uncommon Secondary syphilis: Fever, rash, malaise, anorexia, arthralgia, lymphadenopathy	Headache, fever, malaise, myalgia (40%-70%)	None	Local spread only
Inguinal lymphadenopathy	Late, bilateral, nontender, no suppuration	Early, bilateral, tender, no suppuration	Early, rapid, tender, and unilateral; suppuration likely (bubo)	Lymphatic obstruction
Primary lesion	Papule	Vesicle	Papule to pustule	Subcutaneous nodule
Ulcer Characteristics				
Number	Usually 1	Multiple	<3	>1, may coalesce
Edges	Distinct	Reddened, ragged	Sharply demarcated, serpiginous borders	Rolled, distinct
Depth	Shallow	Shallow	Shallow	Raised
Base	Red, smooth	Red, smooth	Necrotic	Beefy red, clean
Secretion	Serous	Serous	Purulent	None
Induration	Firm	None	None	Firm
Pain	None	Usual	Often	None
Diagnosis				
Serology	MHA-TP or FTA-ABS; VDRL or RPR	Seroconversion (primary infection only)	None	None
Isolation	No in vitro test; rabbit testes inoculation	Culture	Swab of ulcer on selective medium, node aspirates usually sterile	None
Microscopic	Dark-field examination	PCR or fluorescent antibody staining	Gram-negative coccobacilli	Staining of ulcer biopsy material for Donovan bodies
Treatment	*Early (primary, secondary and early latent)*: Benzathine penicillin G (2.4 million U IM) once *Late latent (>1 yr duration)*: Benzathine penicillin G (2.4 million U IM) weekly × 3 doses	Acyclovir *or* famciclovir *or* valacyclovir	Aspirate or excise fluctuant nodes Incision and drainage of buboes >5 cm Azithromycin *or* ceftriaxone *or* ciprofloxacin *or* erythromycin	Doxycycline *or* azithromycin

FTA-ABS, Fluorescent treponemal antibody–absorption; *HSV*, herpes simplex virus; *IM*, intramuscular; *MHA-TP*, microhemagglutination assay-*Treponema pallidum*; *PCR*, polymerase chain reaction; *RPR*, rapid plasma reagin; *VDRL*, Venereal Disease Research Laboratory.
From Marcdante KJ et al: *Nelson essentials of pediatrics*, ed 9, Philadelphia 2023, Elsevier.

avoiding kissing or sexual intercourse until lesions are crusted. Pericoital application of tenofovir gel, an antiretroviral vaginal gel, has also been shown to reduce the risk of HSV-2 in women. This may be useful in regions of the world where use of condoms is shunned.

- Patients should also avoid contact with immunocompromised hosts or neonates while lesions are present.
- Proper handwashing techniques should be explained.
- Patients with herpes gladiatorum (cutaneous herpes in athletes involved in contact sports) should be excluded from participation in active sports until lesions have resolved.
- Many new HSV-2 infections are asymptomatic. Since HSV-2 antibody tests have become commercially available, an increasing number of persons have learned that they have genital herpes through serologic testing. Persons with asymptomatic HSV-2 infection shed virus in the genital tract less frequently than persons with symptomatic infection, but much of the difference is attributable to less frequent genital lesions because genital lesions are accompanied by frequent viral shedding. The U.S. Preventive Services Task Force (USPSTF) recommends against routine serologic screening for genital HSV infection in asymptomatic adolescents and adults, including those that are pregnant.
- Suppressive treatment of HSV-2 infection lowers the incidence of genital lesions by 70% to 80% but cuts the rate of HSV-2 transmission to uninfected partners by only 50%.
- Pregnancy: Antiviral prophylaxis with acyclovir is recommended from 36 wk of gestation until delivery in women with a history of genital herpes. Elective cesarean delivery should be performed in laboring patients with active lesions to decrease the risk of neonatal herpes.
- Trials involving investigational herpes simplex vaccine have found it to be effective in preventing HSV-1 genital disease and infection, but not in preventing HSV-2 disease or infection.

RELATED CONTENT

Genital Herpes (Patient Information)
Oral Herpes (Patient Information)
Herpes Simplex Keratitis (Related Key Topic)

AUTHOR: **FRED F. FERRI, MD**

TABLE 2 Topical and Oral Antiviral Medications Used for Herpes Simplex Virus Infections*

Drug	Formulation	Regimen	Indication/Comment
Topical			
Acyclovir	5% cream (2 g, 5 g)	Apply 5 times/day	Recurrent HL; A: ≥12 yr; 4 days; Rx
	5% ointment (15 g, 30 g)	Apply 6 times/day	Initial GH, localized HSV; A: Adults; 7 days; Rx
Penciclovir	1% cream (1.5 g, 5 g)	Apply q2h (awake)	Recurrent HL; A: ≥12 yr; 4 days; Rx
Docosanol	10% cream (2 g)	Apply 5 times/day	HL; A: ≥12 yr; treat until healed; OTC
Oral (all Rx)			
Acyclovir	200-mg capsule		A: ≥2 yr
	400-mg, 800-mg tablet		
	200-mg/5-ml susp		
		200 mg 5 times/day	Initial GH; 10 days
		200 mg 5 times/day	Recurrent GH; 5 days
		400 mg 2 times/day	Suppression, recurrent GH; up to 12 mo, then reevaluate
Famciclovir	125-, 250-, 500-mg tablet		A: ≥18 yr
		1500-mg single dose	Recurrent HL
		1000 mg 2 times/day	Recurrent GH; 1 day
		250 mg 2 times/day	Suppression, recurrent GH; up to 12 mo
Valacyclovir	500-mg, 1-g caplet		A: Adults and ≥12 yr for HL
		1 g 2 times/day	Initial GH; 10 days
		500 mg 2 times/day	Recurrent GH; 3 days
		500 mg-1 g once daily	Suppressive GH
		2 g 2 times/day	HL; 1 day; both adults and children ≥12 yr

A, Approved; *GH,* genital herpes; *HL,* herpes labialis; *HSV,* herpes simplex virus; *OTC,* over-the-counter; *Rx,* by prescription.
*Approved indications and regimens listed; often used off-label.
From Paller AS, Mancini AJ: *Hurwitz clinical pediatric dermatology: a textbook of skin disorders of childhood and adolescence,* ed 5, Philadelphia, 2016, Elsevier.

TABLE 3 Antiviral Treatment for Herpes Simplex Virus in the Nonpregnant Patient

| Indication | ANTIVIRAL AGENT | | |
	Valacyclovir	Acyclovir	Famciclovir
First clinical episode	1000 mg bid, 7-10 days	400 mg tid; or 200 mg five times/day, 7-10 days	250 mg tid, 7-10 days
Recurrent episodes	1000 mg daily, 5 days; or 500 mg bid, 3 days	800 mg bid, 5 days; or 800 mg tid, 2 days	125 mg bid, 5 days 500 mg once then 250 mg bid, 2 days; 1000 mg bid, 1 day
Daily suppressive	1000 mg daily (≥10 recurrences/yr) or 500 mg daily (≤9 recurrences/yr)	400 mg bid	250 mg bid

bid, Twice per day; *tid,* three times per day.
Data from Workowski KA, Bolan GA: Centers for Disease Control and Prevention: sexually transmitted diseases treatment guidelines, 2015, *MMWR Recomm Rep* 64(RR-03):1-137, 2015; Gershenson DM et al: *Comprehensive gynecology,* ed 8, Philadelphia, 2022, Elsevier.

BASIC INFORMATION

DEFINITION

Herpes zoster is a disease caused by reactivation of the varicella-zoster virus, with spread of the virus alone from the sensory nerve to the dermatome. After the primary infection (chickenpox), the virus becomes latent in the dorsal root ganglia and reemerges when there is a weakening of the immune system (as a result of disease or advanced age). Over 90% of the adult U.S. population is latently infected with varicella zoster virus. Reactivation of latent varicella zoster virus (VZV) produces the clinical syndrome herpes zoster (shingles), which manifests as a unilateral eruption along a single dermatome and is usually preceded by prodromal pain and paresthesia. The eruption lasts around 7 to 10 days and progresses from erythematous macules and papules to vesicles, then pustules, and finally crusts over.

SYNONYMS

Shingles
HZ

ICD-10CM CODES

B02g	Herpes zoster
B02.0	Zoster encephalitis
B02.1	Zoster meningitis
B02.30	Zoster ocular disease, unspecified
B02.31	Zoster conjunctivitis
B02.32	Zoster iridocyclitis
B02.33	Zoster keratitis
B02.34	Zoster scleritis
B02.39	Other herpes zoster eye disease
B02.7	Disseminated zoster
B02.8	Zoster with other complications
B02.9	Zoster without complications

EPIDEMIOLOGY & DEMOGRAPHICS

- Herpes zoster occurs during the lifetime of 10% to 20% of the population. There are approximately 1 million cases annually in the U.S. The incidence of herpes zoster has increased fourfold over the past six decades.
- There is an increased incidence in immunocompromised patients (chemotherapy, radiotherapy, immunosuppression due to corticosteroids, AIDS, DM, malignancy), the elderly (most common after age 60) (Fig. 1), and children who acquired chickenpox when younger than 2 mo.

PHYSICAL FINDINGS & CLINICAL PRESENTATION

- Pain generally precedes skin manifestation by 3 to 5 days and is generally localized to the dermatome that will be affected by the skin lesions.
- Constitutional symptoms are often present (malaise, fever, headache).
- The initial rash consists of erythematous maculopapules generally affecting one dermatome (thoracic region in majority of

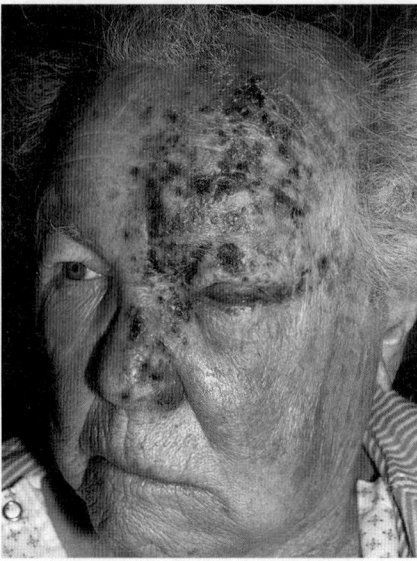

FIG. 1 Herpes zoster, involvement of the V1 dermatome. (From James WD et al: *Andrews' diseases of the skin: clinical dermatology,* ed 12, Philadelphia, 2016, Elsevier.)

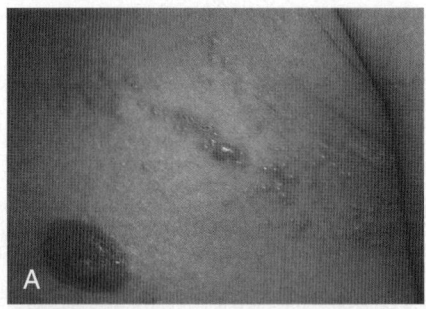

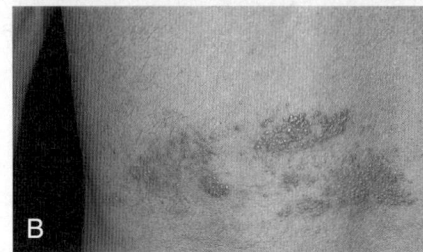

FIG. 2 A and **B,** Herpes zoster lesions in T3 distribution. (From Swartz MH: *Textbook of physical diagnosis,* ed 7, Philadelphia, 2014, Saunders.)

cases [Fig. 2]). Typically, the rash does not cross the midline. Some patients (<30%) may have scattered vesicles outside the affected dermatome. In rare cases the rash can be generalized (Fig. E3).
- The initial maculopapules evolve into vesicles and pustules by the third or the fourth day.
- The vesicles have an erythematous base (Fig. E4), are cloudy, of various sizes (a distinguishing characteristic from herpes simplex, in which the vesicles are of uniform size), and may have a classic appearance of grouped vesicles (Fig. 5).
- The vesicles subsequently become umbilicated and then form crusts that generally fall off within 3 wk; scarring may occur.

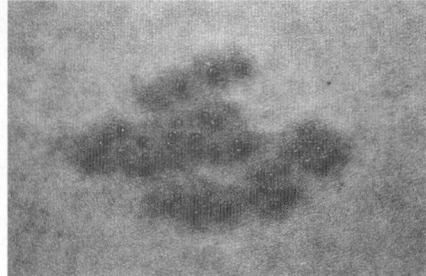

FIG. 5 Herpes zoster. Classic appearance of grouped vesicles. (From White GM, Cox NH [eds]: *Diseases of the skin: a color atlas and text,* ed 2, St Louis, 2006, Mosby.)

- Pain during and after the rash is generally significant. Postherpetic neuralgia occurs after herpes zoster in approximately one third of patients aged 60 yr and older and can persist for months or years.
- Secondary bacterial infection with *Staphylococcus aureus* or *Streptococcus pyogenes* may occur.
- Regional lymphadenopathy may occur.
- Herpes zoster may involve the trigeminal nerve (most frequent cranial nerve involved); involvement of the first division of the trigeminal nerve is known as "herpes zoster ophthalmicus" and can result in blindness. The appearance of blisters on the tip of the nose (Hutchinson sign) is a common manifestation of herpes zoster ophthalmicus. Involvement of the geniculate ganglion can cause facial palsy and a painful ear, with the presence of vesicles on the pinna and external auditory canal (Ramsay Hunt syndrome).
- Pain typical of herpes zoster in the absence of cutaneous lesions, known as "Zoster sine herpete," is rare.

ETIOLOGY

Reactivation of varicella virus (human herpes virus III)

DIAGNOSIS

DIFFERENTIAL DIAGNOSIS

- Rash: Herpes simplex and other viral infections, contact dermatitis
- Pain from herpes zoster: May be confused with acute myocardial infarction, pulmonary embolism, pleuritis, pericarditis, renal colic

WORKUP

The diagnosis of herpes zoster is usually made by the characteristic dermatomal presentation.

LABORATORY TESTS

Laboratory tests are generally not necessary. In cases where the clinical diagnosis is not obvious, PCR testing for varicella zoster virus has high sensitivity and specificity. It is readily available and results can usually be obtained in less than 24 h. Other laboratory studies for diagnosis of herpes zoster include viral culture, direct fluorescent antibody (DFA), and serologic testing.

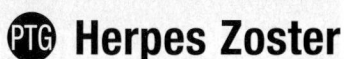

H

I

Rx TREATMENT

NONPHARMACOLOGIC THERAPY

- Wet compresses (using Burow solution or cool tap water) applied for 15 to 30 min 5 to 10 times a day may be useful to break vesicles and remove serum and crust. Then carefully pat dry.
- Care must be taken to prevent any secondary bacterial infection by keeping cutaneous lesions clean and dry.

ACUTE GENERAL Rx[1]

- Acyclovir, valacyclovir, and famciclovir are guanosine analogs that are phosphorylated by thymidine kinase to a triphosphate form that inhibits viral deoxyribonucleic acid (DNA) polymerase. The oral bioavailability of the antivirals determines the number of daily administrations. Patient compliance tends to decrease as the number of daily administrations increases. Oral antiviral agents can shorten the disease course and help prevent postherpetic neuralgia. They can decrease acute pain, inflammation, and vesicle formation when treatment is begun within 72 h of onset of rash. Treatment options are:
  1. Valacyclovir 1000 mg tid for 7 days
  2. Famciclovir 500 mg tid for 7 days
  3. Acyclovir 800 mg 5 times daily for 7 to 10 days

Acyclovir-resistant VZV infections have been reported in immunocompromised patients (i.e., acquired immune deficiency syndrome [AIDS], transplant patients). In these cases, foscarnet (given intravenously 40 mg/kg three times daily) can be used as an alternative.

- The role of corticosteroids in herpes zoster is controversial. Many physicians prescribe them to improve rash healing and reduce pain severity; however, a Cochrane review failed to show sufficient evidence to support the use of corticosteroids for the prevention of postherpetic neuralgia. Corticosteroids can be considered in older patients within 72 h of clinical presentation or if new lesions are still appearing if there are no contraindications to their use. Initial dose is prednisone 60 mg/day decreased by 5 mg/day until finished.
- Immunocompromised patients and patients with herpes zoster complicated by CNS involvement should be treated with intravenous (IV) acyclovir 10 to 15 mg/kg q8h in 1-h infusions for 7 days, with close monitoring of renal function and adequate hydration; vidarabine (continuous 12-h infusion of 10 mg/kg/day for 7 days) is also effective for treatment of disseminated herpes zoster in immunocompromised hosts.
- Patients with AIDS and transplant recipients may develop acyclovir-resistant varicella-zoster; these patients can be treated with foscarnet (40 mg/kg IV q8h) continued for at least 10 days or until lesions are completely healed.
- **Postherpetic neuralgia (PHN):** Pain management is especially difficult with conventional analgesics in zoster patients who develop PHN. Calcium channel $\alpha2$-δ ligands (gabapentin and pregabalin), tricyclic antidepressants, opioids, topical lidocaine, selective serotonin and norepinephrine reuptake inhibitors (duloxetine and venlafaxine), and topical capsaicin have been shown to reduce the pain associated with PHN. Of these medications, only gabapentin, pregabalin, 5% lidocaine patch, and 8% capsaicin patch have been approved by the Food and Drug Administration (FDA) specifically for the treatment of PHN. Adding gabapentin to an antiviral in patients with acute herpes zoster appears to significantly reduce the incidence of PHN. Gralise, a once-daily medication for the treatment of postherpetic neuralgia, is an extended-release form of gabapentin that not only has been shown to significantly decrease PHN pain scores but may also be associated with fewer side effects than its immediate-release counterpart. FDA has also approved Horizant, gabapentin enacarbil, for the once-daily therapy of PHN.

DISPOSITION

- The incidence of postherpetic neuralgia (defined as pain that persists more than 90 days after onset of rash) increases with age (<30% by age 40 yr, >70% by age 70 yr); antivirals reduce the risk of postherpetic neuralgia.
- Incidence of disseminated herpes zoster is increased in immunocompromised hosts (e.g., 15% to 50% of patients with active Hodgkin disease).
- Immunocompromised hosts are also more prone to neurologic complications (encephalitis, myelitis, cranial and peripheral nerve palsies, acute retinal necrosis). The mortality rate is 10% to 20% in immunocompromised hosts with disseminated zoster.
- Motor neuropathies occur in 5% of all cases of zoster; complete recovery occurs in >70% of patients.
- Rates of HZ recurrence are more frequent than previously reported and are comparable to rates of first HZ occurrence in immunocompetent individuals.

REFERRAL

- Hospitalization for IV acyclovir in patients with disseminated herpes zoster.
- Patients with herpes zoster ophthalmicus should be referred to an ophthalmologist.
- Consultation with an otolaryngologist is advisable in patients with Ramsey Hunt syndrome.
- Vaccination: In the absence of the herpes zoster vaccine, persons who live to 85 yr of age have a 50% risk of herpes zoster. Immunocompetent adults ≥50 yr (including those who have already received Zostavax) are appropriate candidates for recombinant varicella zoster virus vaccine (Shingrix). It consists of two doses 2 to 6 mo apart and is preferred over Zostavax for herpes zoster prevention. Adults who are VZV seronegative (never had varicella) should be immunized against varicella with two doses of varicella vaccine (Varivax). Despite its efficacy and safety, use of this vaccine remains low (<8% of potential recipients).

PEARLS & CONSIDERATIONS
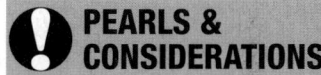

REFERENCE & SUGGESTED READING

Available at eBooks.Health.Elsevier.com.

RELATED CONTENT

Shingles (Patient Information)
Postherpetic Neuralgia (Related Key Topic)
Ramsey Hunt Syndrome (Related Key Topic)

AUTHOR: **FRED F. FERRI, MD**

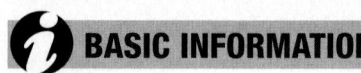 **BASIC INFORMATION**

DEFINITION

Hodgkin lymphoma is a malignant disorder arising from germinal center B cells and characterized histologically by the presence of multinucleated giant cells (Reed-Sternberg cells) in a mixed inflammatory background.

ICD-10CM CODES

C81.90	Hodgkin lymphoma, unspecified, unspecified site
C81.00	Nodular lymphocyte predominant Hodgkin lymphoma, unspecified site
C81.10	Nodular sclerosis classical Hodgkin lymphoma, unspecified site
C81.20	Mixed cellularity classical Hodgkin lymphoma, unspecified site
C81.30	Lymphocyte depleted classical Hodgkin lymphoma, unspecified site
C81.79	Other classical Hodgkin lymphoma, extranodal and solid organ sites
C81.90	Hodgkin lymphoma, unspecified, unspecified site
C81.91	Hodgkin lymphoma, unspecified, lymph nodes of head, face, and neck
C81.92	Hodgkin lymphoma, unspecified, intrathoracic lymph nodes
C81.93	Hodgkin lymphoma, unspecified, intra-abdominal lymph nodes
C81.94	Hodgkin lymphoma, unspecified, lymph nodes of axilla and upper limb
C81.95	Hodgkin lymphoma, unspecified, lymph nodes of inguinal region and lower limb
C81.96	Hodgkin lymphoma, unspecified, intrapelvic lymph nodes
C81.97	Hodgkin lymphoma, unspecified, spleen
C81.98	Hodgkin lymphoma, unspecified, lymph nodes of multiple sites
C81.99	Hodgkin lymphoma, unspecified, extranodal and solid organ sites

EPIDEMIOLOGY & DEMOGRAPHICS

- There is a bimodal age distribution (15 to 34 yr and >50 yr).
- Incidence is 2.5 in 100,000 cases; >8800 new cases of Hodgkin lymphoma diagnosed annually in the U.S.
- Concordance for Hodgkin lymphoma in identical twins suggests that a genetic susceptibility underlies Hodgkin lymphoma in young adulthood.
- There is association between certain human leukocyte antigen (HLA) haplotypes, especially HLA-A1.
- There is an increased risk in smokers and HIV-infected individuals.

PHYSICAL FINDINGS & CLINICAL PRESENTATION

- Painless palpable lymphadenopathy is the most common presenting symptom.
- The most common site of involvement is the neck region.

- Fever and night sweats: Fever in a cyclical pattern (days or weeks of fever alternating with afebrile periods) is known as Pel-Ebstein fever.
- Unexplained weight loss, generalized malaise.
- Persistent, nonproductive cough.
- Lymph node pain associated with alcohol ingestion often because of heavy eosinophil infiltration of the tumor sites is relatively uncommon.
- Generalized pruritus.
- Hepatosplenomegaly.
- Other: Superior vena cava syndrome, spinal cord compression (rare), erythema nodosum (very rare), ichthyosis (very rare).

ETIOLOGY

- Evidence implicating Epstein-Barr virus remains controversial.
- Cigarette smoking has also been implicated.
- Many recent studies reveal that the malignant Hodgkin/Reed-Sternberg cells are pre-apoptotic germinal center B cells that acquire genomic perturbations that prevent their effective elimination and create the microenvironment of ineffective immune reaction that sustains their survival.

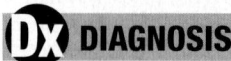 **DIAGNOSIS**

DIFFERENTIAL DIAGNOSIS

- Non-Hodgkin lymphoma
- Sarcoidosis and other rare nonmalignant lymphadenopathies (e.g., Kikuchi-Fujimoto disease, Castleman disease)
- Infections (e.g., cytomegalovirus, Epstein-Barr virus, toxoplasmosis, HIV, tuberculosis)
- Drug reaction

WORKUP

Diagnosis is confirmed by lymph node biopsy. The World Health Organization classifies Hodgkin lymphoma into two groups: Classic Hodgkin lymphoma (CHL; 95%) and nodular lymphocyte-predominant Hodgkin lymphoma (NLPHL; 5%). Classic Hodgkin lymphoma has four main histologic subtypes based on the type of immune infiltrate surrounding the Hodgkin/Reed-Sternberg cells, but they do not have major clinical or prognostic relevance: Nodular sclerosis (Fig. E1), mixed cellularity (Fig. E2), lymphocyte rich, and lymphocyte depleted. NLPHL is a separate disease with differing histopathologic and clinical characteristics, and specific therapy more resembling that for non-Hodgkin lymphomas.

Nodular sclerosis occurs mainly in young adulthood, whereas the mixed cellularity type is more prevalent after age 50 yr. Table 1 summarizes key features of Hodgkin lymphomas.

Staging: Table 2 describes the Ann Arbor/Cotswold staging classification.

Proper staging requires the following:
- Detailed history (with documentation of "B symptoms") and physical examination
- Excisional biopsy with histologic, immunophenotypic, and immunohistochemical analysis
- Laboratory evaluation (CBC, erythrocyte sedimentation rate [ESR], blood urea nitrogen,

creatinine, liver function tests, albumin, lactate dehydrogenase, HIV test), immunophenotypic markers
- PET/CT scan of the chest, abdomen, and pelvis (Fig. 3)
- Unilateral bone marrow biopsy in selected patients (rarely indicated)

Box 1 summarizes recommended staging procedures for Hodgkin lymphoma.

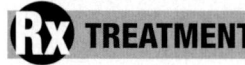 **TREATMENT**

ACUTE GENERAL Rx

The main therapeutic modality includes chemotherapy with treatment selection and duration depending on stage and other risk factors (Table 3). Patients are generally assigned to one of the three risk groups: Early favorable (stage 1 or 2 without risk factors), early unfavorable (stage 1 or 2 with risk factors), or advanced (stage 3 or 4). In the U.S., chemotherapy is the standard treatment for early favorable or unfavorable Hodgkin lymphoma, with the infrequent addition of involved site radiotherapy. Chemotherapy (Table 4) is used for advanced-stage disease with radiotherapy in selected patients, mainly in those with bulky disease.

Many oncologists use the combination of doxorubicin, bleomycin, vinblastine, and dacarbazine (ABVD). ABVD does not cause infertility or stem cell damage and can be used in patients with HIV infection. The four drugs comprising ABVD are administered intravenously, on day 1 and 15 of 28-day cycles, which are typically not delayed for asymptomatic cytopenias. Modifications to this treatment paradigm include the substitution of bleomycin with alternative agents, because bleomycin is associated with pulmonary toxicity, or intensification with the addition of other chemotherapies.

Patients with early favorable CHL (i.e., stage 1 or 2 with fewer than three nodal sites of involvement, no B symptoms, bulky or extranodal disease, and baseline ESR <50) can be treated with either four cycles of ABVD alone or two cycles followed by 20 Gy of involved-field radiation therapy.

Patients with early unfavorable Hodgkin lymphoma (stage 1 or 2 with the aforementioned risk factors) typically receive four cycles of ABVD plus involved-site radiotherapy to 30 Gy. Extended chemotherapy alone, in the absence of bulky disease, is an alternative approach, especially in younger women who may have increased risk of breast cancer after radiation therapy. The risk of disease recurrence is higher in patients who receive chemotherapy alone, but there may be no difference in overall survival.

Advanced-stage CHL is typically treated with one of the three regimens: ABVD, dose-escalated bleomycin, etoposide, doxorubicin hydrochloride (Adriamycin), cyclophosphamide, vincristine (Oncovin), procarbazine, and prednisone (BEACOPP), or BV-AVD. ABVD is typically given as six monthly cycles, though patients who achieve a complete metabolic response on a restaging PET-CT performed after two cycles may omit further bleomycin,

TABLE 1 Key Features of Histologic Subtypes of Hodgkin Lymphoma

Lymphoma (% of Cases)	Demographics, Clinical Presentation	Morphology	Cell Surface Markers
Nodular sclerosis (70%)	M = F, <30 yr with mediastinal mass, occasional spleen or lung involvement; 40% have B symptoms; most patients present with stage II disease	Broad bands of collagen, nodules of lymphoid tissue with aggregates of HRS cells and lacunar cells, multinucleated variants	CD15, CD30, CD45-EBV in 1%-40%
Mixed cellularity (20%)	M > F; median age, 38 yr; peripheral lymphadenopathy common, spleen, BM; B symptoms common; patients often stage III or IV	Classic HRS cells in mixture of lymphocytes, plasma cells, eosinophils, histiocytes	CD15, CD30, CD45-EBV in 75%
Lymphocyte-rich (~5%)	M > F, older age; peripheral lymphadenopathy; B symptoms rare; most patients with stage I or II disease	Scattered classic HRS cells among numerous small lymphocytes; nodular growth pattern	CD15, CD30; Oct2 and BOB.1 vary; J-chain absent; EBV in 40%-75%
Lymphocyte depleted (<1%)	M > F; median age, 30-37 yr; B symptoms, advanced stage common; associated with HIV; poor prognosis	Classic HRS cells common with paucity of background lymphocytes; pleomorphic HRS cells mimic sarcoma	CD15, CD30, CD45-EBV positive in HIV-affected patients
Nodular, lymphocyte predominant (NLPHL, 5%)	M > F, 30-50 yr, with peripheral lymphadenopathy	Mononuclear cells with convoluted nuclei (popcorn or L&H cells) loosely aggregated in nodules of small B cells	CD45, CD20, bcl-6, J-chain, Oct-2, BOB.1, EBV absent in LP cells

BM, Bone marrow; *CHL,* classical Hodgkin lymphoma; *EBV,* Epstein-Barr virus; *F,* female; *HIV,* human immunodeficiency virus; *HRS,* Hodgkin Reed-Sternberg; *L&H,* lymphocytic and histiocytic; *LP,* lymphoplasmacytic; *M,* male.
From McPherson RA, Pincus MR: *Henry's clinical diagnosis and management by laboratory methods,* ed 23, St Louis, 2017, Elsevier.

TABLE 2 Cotswold-Modified Ann Arbor Staging System for Hodgkin Lymphoma

Stage	Criteria
I	Disease affecting a single lymph node region or lymphoid structure (e.g., spleen, thymus, Waldeyer ring)
II	Disease affecting two or more discrete lymph node regions confined to the same side of the diaphragm
III	Disease affecting two or more discrete lymph node regions or lymphoid structures on both sides of the diaphragm
IV	Disease that has spread to one or more extranodal sites (that do not meet the criteria for E) or extralymphatic structure including involvement of the bone marrow, liver, or lungs
Designation	**Criteria**
A	Absence of B symptoms[a]
B	Presence of B symptoms[a]
S	Involvement of the spleen
E	Single extranodal site or involvement of an extranodal site that is contiguous to an involved nodal region
X	Bulky disease as defined as >1/3 mediastinum at its widest part or a nodal mass >10 cm at its greatest diameter

[a]B symptoms: Constitutional symptoms including night sweats, fevers, or weight loss (>10% over 6 mo).
From Hoffman R et al: *Hematology: basic principles and practice,* ed 8, Philadelphia, 2023, Elsevier.

continuing with four cycles of AVD. BEACOPP is an intensified regimen. It results in better initial tumor control, but the long-term survival may not significantly differ from that with ABVD, and the rate of complications is higher (including 3% rate of treatment-related death, secondary leukemias, and universal infertility).

BV-AVD is a combination of brentuximab vedotin (a CD30-targeting antibody-drug conjugate) and doxorubicin, vinblastine, and dacarbazine. In patients with previously untreated stage III or IV classic Hodgkin lymphoma,[1] this regimen provides a small but statistically significant benefit in overall survival compared with ABVD, although with higher rates of neutropenia and neuropathy.

Nivolumab-AVD is a combination of an immune checkpoint inhibitor (via PD-1 blockade), and doxorubicin, vinblastine, and dacarbazine. In patients with previously untreated stage III or IV classic Hodgkin lymphoma, this regimen provides improved progression-free survival compared to BV-AVD. Initial reports show lower rates of immune toxicity with this regimen compared to prior therapies containing nivolumab for other malignancies. These data remain immature, but Nivo-AVD may ultimately replace BV-AVD and ABVD as the first-line standard of care.

- Recommendations for the primary treatment of Hodgkin lymphoma outside of clinical trials are described in Table 5.
- Patients who experience recurrent or refractory disease typically receive second-line (salvage) chemotherapy followed by consolidative autologous stem cell transplantation, although in some cases radiation therapy can be used.
- Patients who experience recurrent Hodgkin lymphoma after second-line treatment can receive further effective treatment using targeted immunotherapy.
- Brentuximab vedotin is an anti-CD30 antibody drug conjugate associated with an overall response rate of 75% in relapsed/refractory Hodgkin lymphoma. It also can be used as a maintenance therapy for high-risk patients undergoing autologous stem cell transplantation.
- Checkpoint inhibitors are monoclonal antibodies targeting the programmed death 1 (PD-1) molecule (present on T cells) or its ligands (present on Hodgkin/Reed-Sternberg cells). This group includes agents such as nivolumab and pembrolizumab, which are both approved for treatment of relapsed/refractory Hodgkin lymphoma. The overall response rate to nivolumab among patients with Hodgkin lymphoma who relapsed after autologous stem cell transplant and posttransplant brentuximab vedotin was 65%. The overall response rate to pembrolizumab among patients with Hodgkin lymphoma relapsing after ≥3 lines of therapy was 69%.

DISPOSITION
- Classic Hodgkin lymphoma is cured in >95% of patients with early favorable disease, about 85% of those with early unfavorable

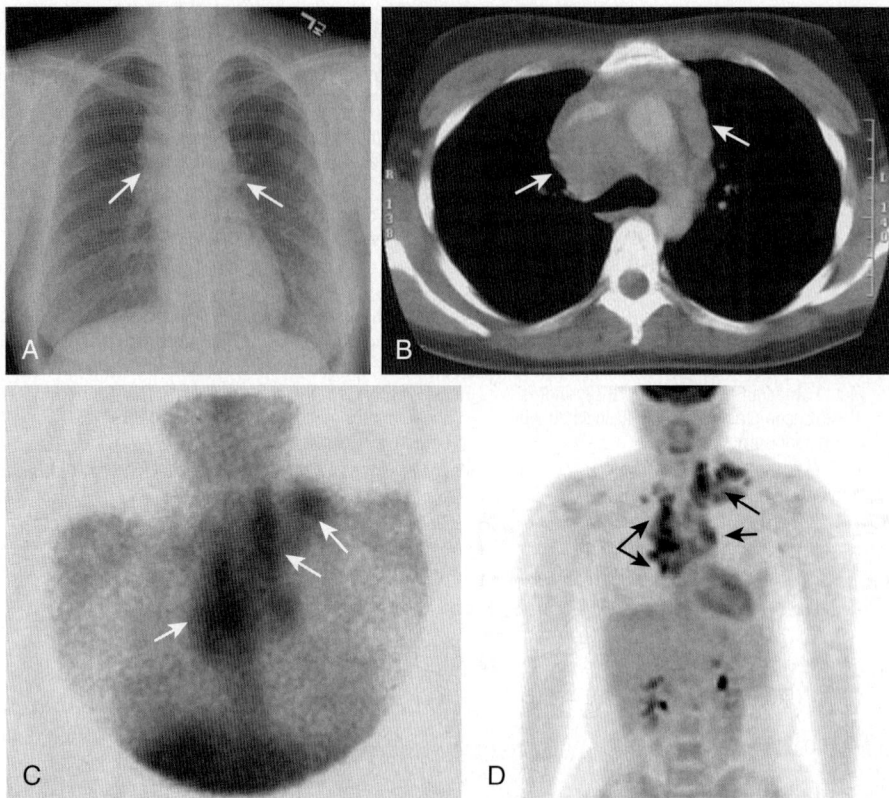

FIG. 3 Imaging of Hodgkin lymphoma. Bulky Hodgkin disease as seen on chest radiograph **(A)**, CT of the chest **(B)**, gallium scan **(C)**, and PET **(D)**. The *arrows* indicate sites of disease. Note that the PET and CT scans provide more detailed information than the chest radiograph and gallium scan. (From Goldman L, Schafer AI: *Goldman's Cecil medicine,* ed 24, Philadelphia, 2012, Saunders.)

BOX 1 Recommended Staging Procedures for Hodgkin Lymphoma

The following staging procedures are recommended for the initial workup of Hodgkin lymphoma:
1. Adequate surgical biopsy reviewed by an experienced hematopathologist
2. Cytologic examination of any effusion in selected cases
3. Detailed history, with attention to the presence or absence of systemic symptoms, and a careful physical examination, emphasizing node chains, size of the liver and spleen, and inspection of Waldeyer ring
4. Routine laboratory tests: Complete blood cell count, erythrocyte sedimentation rate, liver and kidney function tests, and HIV serology
5. Neck, chest, and abdominal CT imaging fused with 18-fluorodeoxyglucose (FDG) PET scan (Fig. 3)

From Goldman L, Schafer AI: *Goldman's Cecil medicine,* ed 24, Philadelphia, 2012, Saunders.

TABLE 3 Standard Treatment Approach According to Prognostic Group

Early-favorable HL	Combined modality therapy • 2-4 cycles of chemotherapy followed by involved-field radiotherapy
Early-unfavorable HL (intermediate-stage)	Combined modality therapy • 4-6 cycles of chemotherapy followed by involved-field radiotherapy
Advanced HL	Extensive chemotherapy • 6 cycles of chemotherapy ± consolidation with localized radiotherapy

HL, Hodgkin lymphoma.
From Hoffman R et al: *Hematology: basic principles and practice,* ed 8, Philadelphia, 2023, Elsevier.

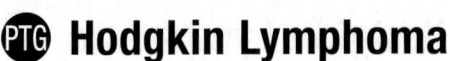

TABLE 4 Standard Chemotherapy Regimens for the Treatment of Advanced Hodgkin Lymphoma

Regimen	Drugs	Route	Schedule
ABVD	Adriamycin 25 mg/m^2	IV	Day 1 and 15
	Bleomycin 10 mg/m^2	IV	Day 1 and 15
	Vinblastine 6 mg/m^2	IV	Day 1 and 15
	Dacarbazine 375 mg/m^2	IV	Day 1 and 15
			Every 28 days
BEACOPP (escalated)	Bleomycin 10 mg/m^2	IV	Day 8
	Etoposide 200 mg/m^2	IV	Day 1-3
	Adriamycin 35 mg/m^2	IV	Day 1
	Cyclophosphamide 1250 mg/m^2	IV	Day 1
	Vincristine 1.4 mg/m^2	IV	Day 8
	Procarbazine 100 mg/m^2	PO	Days 1-7
	Prednisolone 40 mg/m^2	PO	Days 1-14
	G-CSF	SC	From day 8
			Every 21 days
A2VD (AVD with Brentuximab vedotin)	Adriamycin 25 mg/m^2	IV	Day 1 and 15
	Brentuximab vedotin 1.2 mg/kg	IV	Day 1 and 15
	Vinblastine 6 mg/m^2	IV	Day 1 and 15
	Dacarbazine 375 mg/m^2	IV	Day 1 and 15
	G-CSF	SC	
			Every 28 days

G-CSF, Granulocyte colony-stimulating factor.
From Hoffman R et al: *Hematology: basic principles and practice,* ed 8, Philadelphia, 2023, Elsevier.

disease, and 75% to 80% of those with advanced-stage disease.
- Stage is the principal prognostic factor, although in advanced-stage disease, the International Prognostic Score can further stratify prognosis (Table 6).
- Unlike escalated BEACOPP, ABVD is not associated with a risk of leukemia.
- Mediastinal irradiation increases the risk of subsequent cardiac disease, including valvular and pericardial disease, accelerated coronary artery disease, and conduction abnormalities.
- Radiation therapy increases the risk of developing secondary solid tumors, especially breast cancer in women younger than age 30 yr.
- Table 7 describes potential late complications of Hodgkin lymphoma treatment and appropriate clinical responses and preventive strategies during survivorship phase.
- Late effects associated with conventional therapy for Hodgkin lymphoma are summarized in Table 8.

REFERRAL
- To surgery for lymph node biopsy
- Fertility clinic for sperm banking
- Hematology/oncology
- Radiation oncology, in selected cases

TABLE 5 Recommendations for the Primary Treatment of Hodgkin Lymphoma Outside of Clinical Trials

Group	Stage	Recommendation
Early favorable	CS I-II A, no RFs	2 cycles ABVD + ISRT (20 Gy) (or 3-4 cycles or ABVD alone)
Early unfavorable	CS I-II A/B + RFs	4-6 cycles ABVD ±30 Gy for nonbulky disease 4-6 cycles ABVD + 30 Gy for bulky disease
Advanced stages	CS IIB + RFs, CS III A/B, CS IV A/B	6 cycles ABVD (deescalated to AVD among patients with negative PET after 2 cycles); 6 cycles BV-AVD BEACOPP-escalated *or* BEACOPP-14 ± RT, 20-30 Gy for residual tumor (PET positive) and/or bulky disease

ABVD regimen, doxorubicin, vinblastine, bleomycin, and dacarbazine; *BEACOPP-baseline* regimen, bleomycin, etoposide, doxorubicin, cyclophosphamide, vincristine, procarbazine, and prednisone; *BEACOPP-escalated* regimen, bleomycin, etoposide, doxorubicin, cyclophosphamide, vincristine, procarbazine, prednisone, and G-CSF; *BEACOPP-14* regimen, bleomycin, etoposide, doxorubicin, cyclophosphamide, vincristine, procarbazine, prednisone, and G-CSF; *BV-AVD,* brentuximab, vedotin, doxorubicin, vinblastine, and dacarbazine; *CS,* clinical stage; *IF,* involved field; *ISRT,* involved-site radiation therapy; *MOPP* regimen, mechlorethamine, Oncovin (vincristine), procarbazine, and prednisone; *PET,* positron emission tomography; *RF,* risk factors; *RT,* radiation therapy; *Stanford V* regimen, nitrogen mustard, doxorubicin, vinblastine, bleomycin, vincristine, etoposide, and prednisone.

TABLE 6 International Prognostic Score (IPS) for Advanced Hodgkin Lymphoma

No. of Prognostic Factors	% of Patients	5-yr FFP (%)	5-yr OS (%)
0-1 (low-risk)	29	79	90
2-3 (intermediate-risk)	52	64	80
4-7 (high-risk)	19	47	59

FFP, Freedom from progression; *OS,* overall survival.
From Hoffman R et al: *Hematology: basic principles and practice,* ed 8, Philadelphia, 2023, Elsevier.

TABLE 7 Potential Late Complications of Hodgkin Lymphoma Treatment and Appropriate Clinical Responses and Preventive Strategies

Risk/Problem	Incidence/Response
Dental caries	Neck or oropharyngeal irradiation can cause decreased salivation. Patients should have careful dental care follow-up and should make their dentist aware of the previous irradiation.
Hypothyroidism	Thyroid irradiation during curative therapy for Hodgkin lymphoma leads to hypothyroidism in >50% of patients. All patients whose TSH level becomes elevated should be treated with lifelong thyroxine replacement in doses sufficient to suppress TSH levels to low normal. This is also necessary to ensure that the radiation-damaged thyroid is not subjected to long-term stimulation by thyroid-stimulating hormone, which can increase the risk of thyroid neoplasm.
Infertility	ABVD is not known to cause permanent gonadal toxicity, although oligospermia for 1-2 yr after treatment is common. Direct or scatter radiation to gonadal tissue can cause infertility, amenorrhea, or premature menopause, but this seldom occurs with the current fields used for the treatment of Hodgkin lymphoma. Thus with the current chemotherapy regimens and radiation fields used, most patients will not develop these problems. In general, after treatment, women who continue menstruating are fertile, but men require semen analysis to provide a specific answer. High-dose chemoradiotherapy and hematopoietic stem cell transplantation almost always cause permanent infertility in both genders, although some young women occasionally recover fertility.
Impaired immunity to infections	Hodgkin lymphoma and its treatment can lead to lifelong impairment of full immunity to infection. All patients should be given annual influenza immunization and pneumococcal immunization every 5 yr. Patients whose spleen has been irradiated or removed should also be immunized against meningococcal types A and C and *Haemophilus influenzae* type B. As for all adults, diphtheria, tetanus, and COVID-19 immunizations should be kept up-to-date.
Secondary neoplasms	Although uncommon, certain secondary neoplasms occur with increased frequency in patients who have been treated for Hodgkin lymphoma. These include acute myelogenous leukemia, thyroid, breast, lung, and upper GI carcinoma and melanoma, and cervical carcinoma in situ. It is appropriate to screen for these neoplasms for the rest of the patient's life because they might have lengthy induction periods. Women who undergo breast irradiation before age 30 benefit from intensified breast cancer screening using MRI.

ABVD, Adriamycin, bleomycin, vinblastine, dacarbazine; *GI,* gastrointestinal; *MRI,* magnetic resonance imaging; *TSH,* thyroid-stimulating hormone.
From Abeloff MD: *Clinical oncology,* ed 3, Philadelphia, 2004, Saunders.

TABLE 8 Late Effects Associated With Conventional Therapy for Hodgkin Lymphoma

Common Therapeutic Exposures	Potential Late Effects
Anthracyclines	Cardiomyopathy, arrhythmias, subclinical left ventricular dysfunction, secondary AML or MDS
Corticosteroids	Cataracts, osteopenia, osteoporosis, avascular necrosis
Bleomycin	Pulmonary dysfunction
Vincristine, vinblastine	Peripheral neuropathy, Raynaud phenomenon
Procarbazine, mechlorethamine, dacarbazine	Hypogonadism, infertility, secondary AML or MDS
Cyclophosphamide	Hypogonadism, infertility, hemorrhagic cystitis, dysfunctional voiding, bladder malignancy, secondary AML or MDS
Mantle irradiation	Hypothyroidism, premature cardiovascular disease, cardiac valvular disease, cardiomyopathy, arrhythmias, carotid artery disease, scoliosis or kyphosis, second malignant neoplasm in radiation field (e.g., thyroid, breast), pulmonary dysfunction
Inverted Y irradiation	Hypogonadism, infertility, adverse pregnancy outcome, second malignant neoplasm in radiation field (e.g., GI)
Splenectomy	Acute life-threatening infections
Blood products	Chronic viral hepatitis, HIV

AML, Acute myeloid leukemia; *HIV,* human immunodeficiency virus; *MDS,* myelodysplastic syndrome.
From Hoffman R et al: *Hematology: basic principles and practice,* ed 8, Philadelphia, 2023, Elsevier.

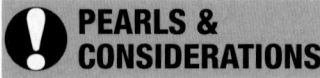

PEARLS & CONSIDERATIONS

COMMENTS
- Young male patients should consider sperm banking before the initiation of therapy even though the risk of infertility with ABVD is low. Symptomatic males, particularly with advanced-stage Hodgkin lymphoma, may have disease-related oligospermia at diagnosis.

- Chemotherapy with or without involved-field radiotherapy should be the standard treatment for Hodgkin lymphoma with early-stage disease. Chemotherapy is the standard of care for advanced stage.
- After failure of ABVD therapy, >60% of patients who have had a relapse and ~30% of patients with initially refractory lymphoma can be cured with subsequent therapy.
- Classic Hodgkin lymphoma has the highest rate of response to immunotherapy with checkpoint inhibitors among all human cancers. These treatments are actively investigated for first-line therapy.

REFERENCE & SUGGESTED READINGS
Available at eBooks.Health.Elsevier.com.

RELATED CONTENT
Hodgkin Lymphoma (Patient Information)

AUTHOR: **ARI PELCOVITS, MD**

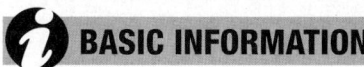

BASIC INFORMATION

DEFINITION

The human immunodeficiency virus (HIV) is a retrovirus that is responsible for causing acquired immunodeficiency syndrome (AIDS). HIV infection does not necessarily mean a person has AIDS. Table 1 summarizes surveillance case definition for HIV.

SYNONYMS

HIV

AIDS: The result of progressive HIV infection in which a person has a weakened immune system and meets specific diagnostic criteria (See "Acquired Immunodeficiency Syndrome" in Section I and Table 2.)

ICD-10CM CODE

B20   Human immunodeficiency virus (HIV) disease

EPIDEMIOLOGY & DEMOGRAPHICS (IN U.S.)

- An estimated 1.2 million people in the U.S. are infected with HIV, and approximately 14% of them do not know they are infected.[1]
- Worldwide each year, an estimated 1.3 million persons living with HIV become pregnant. The vast majority of pregnant persons living with HIV reside in low- and middle-income countries with limited access to antiviral therapy (ART) and in the absence of ART, 15% to 30% of infants born to persons with HIV acquire HIV antenatally or perinatally, with additional transmission during breast feeding.[2]
- There are ~38,000 new HIV diagnoses each year, according to the Centers for Disease Control and Prevention (CDC).[1]
- Incidence is highest among gay, bisexual, and other men who have sex with men (MSM) and African American/Black and Hispanic/Latino populations.

PREDOMINANT RISK GROUPS:

- Gay, bisexual, and other MSM is the group most affected by HIV.
- MSM account for approximately two thirds of all new diagnoses each year, according to the CDC.[1]
- HIV disproportionately affects MSM of younger age and African American/Black and Hispanic/Latino background.
- Heterosexual transmission accounts for ~25% of new HIV diagnosis. Injection drug use accounts for ~6% to 7%.
- Table 3 summarizes risk factors associated with sexual transmission of HIV.

RACIAL DATA:

- African American/Black individuals account for >40% of all new HIV diagnoses despite being 12% of the U.S. population.[1]
- Hispanics/Latinos account for >25% of all new HIV diagnoses despite being 18% of the U.S. population.

GENETICS:

FAMILIAL DISPOSITION

Individuals with deletions in the CCR5 gene are immune from infection with macrophage tropic virus (the predominant virus in sexual transmission).[3] Other genetic variants may contribute to rapid progression or long-term control of the virus once infected. One in 300 individuals infected with HIV is an "elite controller," which means they are able to maintain a normal CD4 count and undetectable viral load through immune control.[4]

CONGENITAL INFECTION

- Fewer than 100 children a year <13 yr receive a diagnosis of perinatally acquired HIV, according to the CDC.[5]
- No specific congenital abnormalities are associated with HIV infection, although there is a higher risk of spontaneous abortion and low birth weight.

NEONATAL INFECTION

- May occur during delivery or via breastfeeding
- Typically asymptomatic
- All pregnant women should be tested for HIV and, if positive, take anteretrovirals (ARVs)[6]

PHYSICAL FINDINGS & CLINICAL PRESENTATION

- Signs and symptoms are variable with stage of disease (Fig. 1).
- Acute HIV infection (0 to 3 mo, usually within several weeks)[7]:
  1. Causes a self-limited mononucleosis-like illness in 50% to 80% of individuals, characterized by fever, sore throat, lymphadenopathy, headache, and a rash resembling roseola. Individuals may also be asymptomatic.

TABLE 2 Surveillance Definitions of AIDS-Defining Conditions

Opportunistic Infections:
- *Pneumocystis jiroveci (carinii)*
- *Mycobacterium avium* complex
- *Mycobacterium tuberculosis*
- Toxoplasmosis
- Candidiasis: Esophageal and systemic
- Histoplasmosis
- Cryptococcosis
- Cryptosporidiosis and isosporiasis
- Leishmaniasis
- Cytomegalovirus disease
- Recurrent bacterial infections (≥2 episodes/yr)

Lymphomas

Kaposi Sarcoma

Cervical Cancer

AIDS Dementia Syndrome

Wasting Syndrome

AIDS, Acquired immunodeficiency syndrome.
From Hoffman R et al: *Hematology: basic principles and practice,* ed 7, Philadelphia, 2018, Elsevier.

TABLE 3 Risk Factors Associated with Sexual Transmission of HIV

Sexually transmitted infections
1. Ulcerative or nonulcerative diseases
- Genital tract inflammation
- HIV disease
  1. Higher viral loads
  2. Lower CD4+ levels
  3. Acute HIV infection
  4. Lack of effective antiretroviral therapy
  5. Lack of heterozygosity or homozygosity for the inactivating 32-base pair deletion in the chemokine receptor gene (CCR5)
- Anatomic factors
  1. Lack of circumcision
  2. Cervical ectopy
  3. Leukocytospermia
  4. Hormonal contraception
- Sexual practices
  1. Receptive anal intercourse
  2. Sexual activity during menses
  3. Bleeding during intercourse (disruption of vaginal mucosa through trauma)
  4. Lack of barrier protection
- HIV viral features
  1. Syncytium formation
  2. Certain viral clades

From Bennett JE et al: *Mandell, Douglas, and Bennett's principles and practice of infectious diseases,* ed 9, Philadelphia, 2020, Saunders.

TABLE 1 Surveillance Case Definition for HIV Infection in Adults and Adolescents (Age >13 yr)

Stage	Laboratory Evidence	Clinical Evidence
Stage 1	Laboratory confirmation of HIV infection and CD4+ T-lymphocyte count of ≥500 cells/μl or CD4+ T-lymphocyte percentage of ≥29%[a]	No AIDS-defining condition (see Table 2)
Stage 2	Laboratory confirmation of HIV infection and CD4+ T-lymphocyte count of 200-499 cells/μl or CD4+ T-lymphocyte percentage of 14%-28%[a]	No AIDS-defining condition (see Table 2)
Stage 3	Laboratory confirmation of HIV infection and CD4+ T-lymphocyte count of <200 cells/μl or CD4+ T-lymphocyte percentage of <14%[a]	Documentation of an AIDS-defining condition with laboratory confirmation of HIV infection (see Table 2)
Stage unknown	Laboratory confirmation of HIV infection and no information on CD4+ T-lymphocyte count or percentage	No information on presence of an AIDS-defining condition

AIDS, Acquired immunodeficiency syndrome.
[a]The CD4+ T-lymphocyte percentage is a percentage of the total lymphocyte count.
From Hoffman R et al: *Hematology, basic principles and practice,* ed 7, Philadelphia, 2018, Elsevier.

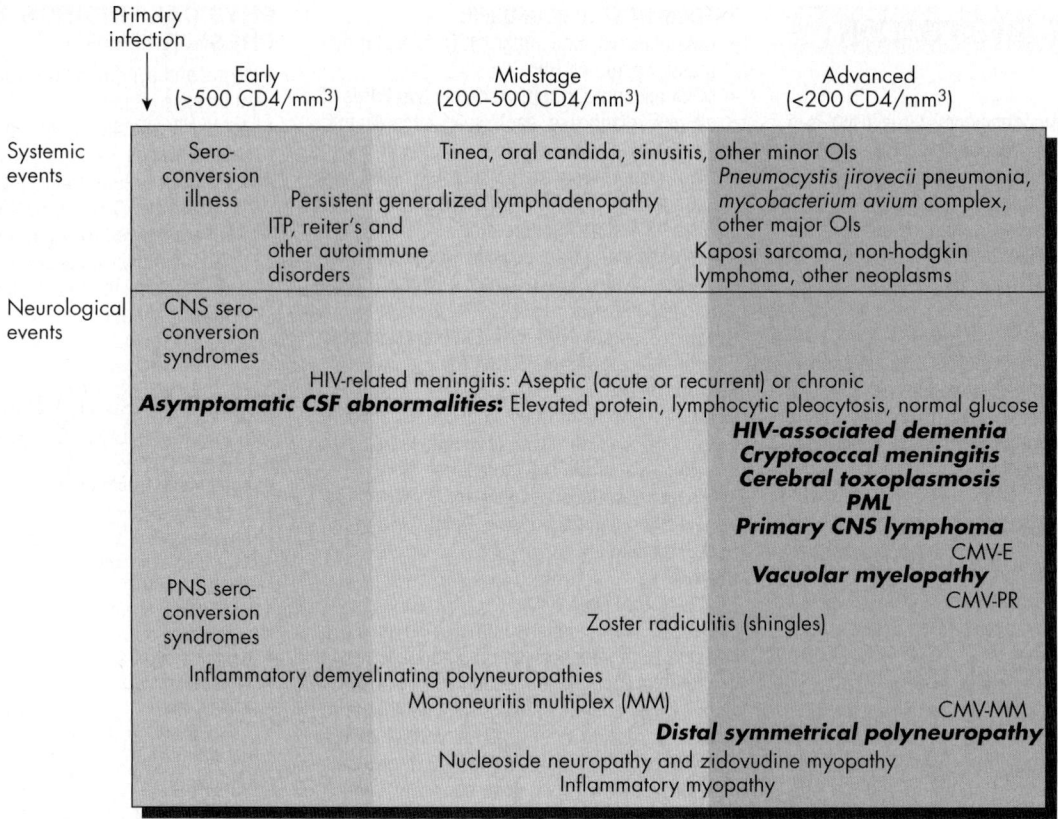

FIG. 1 Systemic and neurologic events in human immunodeficiency virus (HIV) infection. Temporal sequence is approximate and indicates the increasing risk of systemic and neurologic complications as HIV infection advances. *CMV-E*, Cytomegalovirus encephalitis; *CMV-PR*, CMV polyradiculitis; *CNS*, central nervous system; *CSF*, cerebrospinal fluid; *ITP*, idiopathic thrombocytopenic purpura; *OIs*, opportunistic infections; *PML*, progressive multifocal leukoencephalopathy; *PNS*, peripheral nervous system. (From Jankovic J et al: *Bradley and Daroff's neurology in clinical practice*, ed 8, Philadelphia, 2022, Elsevier.)

2. In a minority of acute cases, aseptic meningitis, Bell palsy, or peripheral neuropathy may occur.
3. Opportunistic infections such as thrush or *Pneumocystis jiroveci* pneumonia (PJP) may occur.

- Chronic HIV infection is usually characterized by a prolonged asymptomatic "latent" phase without symptoms followed by nonspecific symptoms of lymphadenopathy, fatigue, weight loss, diarrhea, and skin changes, including seborrheic dermatitis, localized herpes zoster, and/or fungal infection.
- Advanced disease is characterized by AIDS-associated diseases, including infections and malignancies (see specific disorders). Anemia may be multifactorial (Table 4).
- HIV infection in women may be associated with lower levels of viral load at comparable degrees of immunosuppression when compared with men. Furthermore, women may, on average, have higher CD4 counts at the time of HIV diagnosis.
- Another special consideration in women infected with HIV is the high incidence of human papillomavirus (HPV) coinfection and risk for cervical cancer. HIV-positive women should be screened for cervical cancer at time of initial HIV diagnosis and annually thereafter if Pap testing is normal.[8] If the results of three

consecutive Pap tests are normal, then follow-up testing can occur every 3 yr. HPV vaccination is also recommended in men and women 9 to 26 yr who are HIV positive (three doses at 0, 1 to 2, and 6 mo). For adults aged 27 to 45 yr, clinicians should discuss and may consider HPV vaccination in persons who are most likely to benefit.

- Coinfection with HIV and hepatitis C virus (HCV) is common because of similar transmission risk. Hepatitis C is most commonly transmitted by contaminated needles or blood exposure. HCV can be transmitted sexually, but the risk is low. Patients with HIV and HCV progress faster to cirrhosis. Patients may already have signs of advanced liver disease at the time of diagnosis.

ETIOLOGY

- HIV is a single-stranded ribonucleic acid (RNA) retrovirus (Fig. E2) that is categorized as type 1 or 2.
- HIV-1 was derived from transmission of a simian immunodeficiency virus (SIV) from chimpanzees in Central Africa; HIV-2 was derived from an SIV found in sooty mangabey monkeys from West Africa.[9]
- HIV-1 is the predominant pathogenic retrovirus in human populations; HIV-2 has limited distribution (primarily West Africa) and tends

to progress less rapidly than HIV-1. HIV-2 should be considered in individuals from West Africa or whose sexual partners are from West Africa.

- HIV is transmitted by sexual contact, shared needles, blood transfusion, or from mother to child during pregnancy, delivery, or breastfeeding.
- Primary target of infection: CD4 lymphocytes.

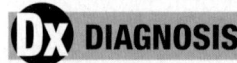 **DIAGNOSIS**

DIFFERENTIAL DIAGNOSIS

- Acute HIV infection: Often diagnosed or confused with mononucleosis or other respiratory viral infections
- Late symptoms: Similar to those produced by other wasting/chronic illnesses such as neoplasms, tuberculosis (TB), disseminated fungal infection (such as *Candida*), malabsorption, or depression
- HIV-related encephalopathy: Confused with Alzheimer disease or other causes of chronic dementia (cognitive impairment in HIV infection is described in another chapter in Section I); myelopathy and neuropathy possibly resembling other demyelinating diseases such as multiple sclerosis
- Direct central nervous system (CNS) involvement: Manifests as encephalopathy,

---

TABLE 4 Etiology of Anemia in Human Immunodeficiency Virus

HIV Related

HIV Infection

- Anemia of chronic disease
- Blunted production/response to erythropoietin
- Suppression of CFU-GEMM (HIV/inflammatory cytokines)

Neoplasms Infiltrating BM

Non-Hodgkin lymphoma, KS, Hodgkin lymphoma

Infections of the BM

- Parvovirus B19
- Atypical mycobacteria (MAI/MAC)
- *Mycobacterium tuberculosis*
- *Histoplasma*
- CMV

Medications Causing Decreased Production	Medications Causing Hemolysis
- RT inhibitors	- Indinavir
- Ganciclovir	- Bactrim and dapsone in G6PD deficiency
- Bactrim	
- Amphotericin B	

HIV Unrelated

- B$_{12}$ and/or folic acid deficiencies
- Iron deficiency caused by chronic blood loss

BM, Bone marrow; *CFU-GEMM,* colony-forming unit–granulocyte, erythrocyte, macrophage, megakaryocyte; *CMV,* cytomegalovirus; *G6PD,* glucose-6-phosphate dehydrogenase; *KS,* Kaposi sarcoma; *MAC,* Mycobacterium avium complex; *MAI,* Mycobacterium avium-intracellulare; *RT,* reverse transcriptase.
From Hoffman R et al: *Hematology, basic principles and practice,* ed 7, Philadelphia, 2018, Elsevier.

myelopathy, or neuropathy in advanced cases. Table 5 summarizes neuromuscular syndromes in HIV infection

- Renal failure, rheumatologic disorders (Table 6), thrombocytopenia, or cardiac abnormalities (Table E7) may be seen in association with HIV-1

WORKUP

Diagnosis is established by testing for HIV-1 or HIV-2 antibodies in the blood. The CDC recommends routine testing for patients in all health care settings unless the patient declines (opt-out screening). This includes routine testing of pregnant women. It is also recommended that separate written consent should no longer be required, although by law this is being addressed on a state-by-state basis. Generally, all persons aged 13 to 64 yr should undergo HIV testing at least once and more frequently (at least once a year) if risk factors.[10] For individuals who may be at higher risk (e.g., men who are having sex with multiple other men), 3 to 6 mo is recommended.

An FDA-approved at-home rapid HIV screening test is available. It uses swabs of oral fluids from upper and lower gums. A positive test requires confirmatory testing. Clinicians should be aware of the "window period" (i.e., an antibody test may take up to 3 mo to become "reactive" in a person with newly acquired HIV infection).

LABORATORY TESTS

HIV antibodies are detected by a two-step technique:

- An initial screening test (i.e., either an antibody/antigen test or an antibody test).
- Confirmation of an initial positive screening test with more specific assays. The classic confirmatory test is the Western blot, but other modalities may be used. Fig. E3 illustrates the laboratory diagnosis of HIV infection.
- Screening antibody tests generally measure HIV-1 and HIV-2 antibodies. Confirmatory tests will generally differentiate between HIV-1 and HIV-2 as well. However, commercial viral load assays (HIV RNA polymerase chain reaction [PCR]) are specific only for HIV-1 in the United States.
- Fourth-generation antibody/antigen tests can detect the "p24" antigen, which is present early in HIV infection and can be used to diagnose HIV earlier than previous generations. An HIV RNA PCR still should be sent if acute HIV infection is suspected.
- Baseline viral resistance testing (e.g., genotype) is recommended for all newly diagnosed patients with HIV to guide choice of ART.
- The CD4 count and HIV viral load (e.g., HIV RNA PCR) should be measured in all patients.
- The CD4 count is a marker of current immune status. Table E8 describes the World Health Organization (WHO) immunologic classification for established HIV infection.
- The HIV RNA PCR (viral load) is predictive of disease progression.

TABLE 5 Neuromuscular Syndromes in Human Immunodeficiency Virus Type 1 Infection

Diagnosis	Disease Stage	Clinical Features	Diagnostic Studies	Treatment
AIDP	Early > late	Weakness more than sensory loss	CSF: ↑ WBCs	Early: IVIG, steroids, plasmapheresis
CIDP			↑↑ Protein	Late: Consider ganciclovir/foscarnet
			NCS: Demyelination	
MM	Early or late	Multiple painful mononeuropathies	NCS: Multifocal axonal neuropathy	Early: None
			Biopsy: Inflammation/vasculitis	Late: Steroids/cyclophosphamide
			CMV	Ganciclovir/foscarnet
Nucleoside Neuropathy	Any stage	Distal sensory loss Neuropathic pain	NCS: Distal axonopathy Increased serum lactate	Nucleoside withdrawal
DSPN	Late	Distal sensory loss Neuropathic pain	NCS: Distal axonopathy	NSAIDs, capsaicin AED, tricyclics
PP	Late	Progressive flaccid paraparesis, urinary dysfunction, LS pain	CSF: Increased WBCs (PMNs), CMV PCR+	Ganciclovir/foscarnet Cidofovir
DILS	Late	Sjögren syndrome, distal motor and sensory loss, pain	NCS: Axonal neuropathy Biopsy: CD8+ T cells, HIV-1	Zidovudine/ART Steroids
Zidovudine Myopathy	Any stage	Proximal weakness Myalgias	EMG: ± irritative Biopsy: Ragged red fibers	Zidovudine withdrawal
Polymyositis	Any stage	Proximal weakness Myalgias	EMG: ± irritative Biopsy: Inflammatory infiltrates	Steroids, IVIG Immunosuppressants
ALS-like	Late	Weakness, dysphagia	EMG: Neurogenic	ART

AED, Antiepileptic drug; *AIDP,* acute inflammatory demyelinating polyneuropathy; *ALS,* amyotrophic lateral sclerosis; *ART,* antiretroviral therapy; *CIDP,* chronic inflammatory demyelinating polyneuropathy; *CMV,* cytomegalovirus; *CSF,* cerebrospinal fluid; *DILS,* diffuse infiltrative lymphocytosis syndrome; *DSPN,* distal sensory polyneuropathy; *EMG,* electromyography; *IVIG,* intravenous immunoglobulin; *LS,* lumbosacral; *MM,* mononeuritis multiplex; *NCS,* nerve conduction studies; *NSAID,* nonsteroidal antiinflammatory drug; *PCR,* polymerase chain reaction; *PMNs,* polymorphonuclear leukocytes; *PP,* progressive polyradiculopathy; *WBCs,* white blood cells.
From Bennett JE et al: *Mandell, Douglas, and Bennett's principles and practice of infectious diseases,* ed 8, Philadelphia, 2015, Saunders.

TABLE 6 Rheumatic Diseases Associated with or Occurring in Patients with HIV Infection

Unique to HIV Infection
- Diffuse infiltrative lymphocytosis syndrome
- HIV-associated arthritis
- Zidovudine-associated myopathy
- Painful articular syndrome

Encountered in HIV-Infected Patients
- HIV-associated reactive arthritis
- Polymyositis
- Psoriatic arthritis
- Polyarteritis nodosa
- Giant cell arteritis
- Hypersensitivity angiitis
- Granulomatosis with polyangiitis
- Henoch-Schönlein purpura
- Behçet's disease
- Infectious arthritis (bacterial, fungal)

Ameliorated by HIV Infection but Worsening or Reappearing with IRIS
- Rheumatoid arthritis
- Systemic lupus erythematosus
- Sarcoidosis

IRIS, Immune reconstitution inflammatory syndrome.
From Firestein GS et al: *Firestein & Kelley's textbook of rheumatology*, ed 11, Philadelphia, 2021, Elsevier.

- Rapid serologic tests have been increasingly used and are useful in specific settings: Occupational exposures, pregnant women in labor without previous testing, and patients in high seroprevalence areas (for immediate results). Specimens are either blood or saliva, and results are given within 1 to 20 min. Although sensitivity is high (99%), false-positive tests are more common in low seroprevalence populations. Thus all positive results must be confirmed with standard serology.
- Early during infection (i.e., acute HIV infection), standard antibody tests may be negative ("window period"). The fourth-generation antibody/antigen test reduces this window period. The standard for diagnosing HIV during acute infection is by testing for HIV RNA (viral load).
- Table E9 compares the WHO and CDC staging systems.

Rx TREATMENT

NONPHARMACOLOGIC THERAPY
Maintenance of adequate nutrition

ACUTE GENERAL Rx
Acute management of opportunistic infections and malignancies (see "AIDS-associated disorders," "Pneumonia, *Pneumocystis jiroveci (carinii);*" "Cryptococcosis;" "Tuberculosis, Pulmonary;" "*Cryptosporidium* Infection;" "Toxoplasmosis;" etc., elsewhere in this text)

CHRONIC Rx
All HIV-infected patients should be considered for ART regardless of CD4 cell count. The benefit of ART is well established in preventing progression to AIDS and associated opportunistic infections. Furthermore, individuals who are on ART and undetectable are highly unlikely to transmit HIV to others (i.e., "Treatment as Prevention"). Identifying individuals with HIV as soon as possible and prescribing ART is the basis of effective public health approaches to addressing HIV. Updated guidelines are available for further recommendations.[11]

- Therapy is strongly recommended for all patients with established HIV infection regardless of the CD4 count. Most people with chronic HIV infection are asymptomatic. ART is recommended regardless of CD4 cell counts. The recommendations are due to the safety and benefit of newer antivirals in preventing AIDS and decreasing both morbidity and mortality. Earlier treatment may also help reduce transmission of the virus to others due to reductions in viral loads.
- ART generally consists of using a three-drug regimen to treat HIV infection. Classes of antiretrovirals include:[12]
  1. Nucleoside/nucleotide reverse transcriptase inhibitor (NRTI): Zidovudine (AZT), lamivudine (3TC), emtricitabine (FTC), tenofovir disoproxil fumarate (TDF), tenofovir alafenamide (TAF), and abacavir (ABC)
  2. Protease inhibitors (PI): Lopinavir/ritonavir, atazanavir, fosamprenavir, darunavir, saquinavir, and tipranavir. These PIs may be "boosted" by ritonavir or cobicistat to increase levels
  3. Nonnucleoside reverse transcriptase inhibitors (NNRTI): Nevirapine, efavirenz, etravirine, doravirine, or rilpivirine
  4. Integrase inhibitors (II): Raltegravir, elvitegravir, bictegravir, dolutegravir, and cabotegravir
  5. Fusion inhibitors: Enfuvirtide (T-20). This drug is administered through subcutaneous injections and is only used as part of a salvage regimen for individuals who have failed multiple other regimens
  6. CCR5 inhibitors: Maraviroc. Before using this drug, a viral trophism assay should be checked to determine if the virus uses the CCR5 coreceptor to infect cells. If the virus uses the CXCR4 coreceptor, this drug will not be effective
  7. Postattachment inhibitors: Ibalizumab. Blocks CD4 receptors that HIV needs to enter cells with
  8. Attachment inhibitors: Fostemsavir. Binds to the gp120 protein on the outer surface of HIV, preventing HIV from entering CD4 cells
- Adding a fourth drug to the three-drug regimen does not improve viral suppression or outcomes and is not recommended. Treatment interruptions based upon CD4 responses appear harmful in recent comparative studies versus standard continuous treatment protocols and should be avoided. Antiretroviral regimens for initial therapy are summarized in Table 10.
- Typical dosing regimen consists of two NRTIs and either an NNRTI, PI, or II. IIs are now the preferred third drug because of tolerability. Data support inclusion of lamivudine or emtricitabine as one of the two NRTIs.
- Two-drug regimens with specific antiretroviral medications may be an option in certain situations. Dolutegravir/lamivudine is the preferred option in appropriate clinical situations in which it is preferable to avoid other NRTIs such as abacavir and tenofovir-based regimens. Dolutegravir/lamivudine is not recommended for individuals with a higher viral load (>500,000 copies/ml), hepatitis B virus (HBV) and HIV coinfection, or when results of genotypic resistance testing are unavailable.
- Individuals with drug-resistant HIV may be on more complex and atypical regimens. Consultation with an HIV specialist is recommended.
Standard NRTIs include:
- Tenofovir disoproxil fumarate/emtricitabine 1 tablet once daily. Individuals with underlying renal dysfunction or requiring other nephrotoxic agents may be at increased risk of renal toxicity while taking tenofovir. TDF may also be associated with reductions in bone mineral density.
- Tenofovir alafenamide/emtricitabine 1 tablet once daily. TAF is a newer formulation of TDF with less nephrotoxicity and bone mineral density effects but may lead to increased weight gain. Both TDF/FTC and TAF/FTC are recommended components of the initial regimen (with a "backbone" medication). TDF should be avoided in patients with a creatinine clearance (CrCl) <60 ml/min. TAF should be avoided in patients with a CrCl <30 ml/min.
- Abacavir/lamivudine 1 tablet once daily. Abacavir may be associated with increased risk of myocardial infarction. Before using this drug, individuals should be checked for human leukocyte antigen (HLA)-B*5701. Individuals with this allele are at higher risk of serious hypersensitivity reactions, and this drug should be avoided.
- Zidovudine/lamivudine 1 tablet twice daily. Once widely prescribed; now rarely used due to lower efficacy compared with tenofovir-emtricitabine; zidovudine is associated with lipoatrophy and anemia, as well as GI and CNS side effects.
Standard backbone regimens include:
- Integrase inhibitors: (these are now considered first line):
  1. Bictegravir (50 mg once daily): Fixed-dose combination of bictegravir with the NRTIs TAF and FTC
  2. Dolutegravir (50 mg once daily): Fixed-dose combination of dolutegravir and the NRTIs abacavir and lamivudine for once-daily treatment of HIV-1 infection. HLA-B*5701 should be checked first
  3. Elvitegravir: Given with cobicistat (booster) and tenofovir/emtricitabine in a fixed-dose combination
  4. Raltegravir (400 mg twice a day). Has a lower barrier to resistance, and other IIs should be considered first

TABLE 10 Which Antiretroviral Regimen to Choose for Initial Therapy

Preferred Regimens	Comments
Integrase inhibitor-based regimen Bictegravir/TAF/FTC	Use abacavir only in individuals who are HLA-B*5701 negative. Dolutegravir/3TC should not be used in individuals with HIV RNA >500,000 copies/ml, HBV coinfection, or in whom ART is to be started before the results of HIV genotypic resistance testing for reverse transcriptase or HBV testing are available.
Dolutegravir + TDF/FTC or TAF/FTC Dolutegravir/ABC/3TCDolutegravir/3TC PI-based regimen Darunavir/r or Darunavir/c (once daily) + TDF/FTC or TAF/FTC	Use if there is a concern for drug resistance.
Preferred regimen for pregnant women ABC/3TC or TDF/FTC plus raltegravir or darunavir/r or atazanavir/r	TDF should be avoided in renal impairment.

Alternative Regimens	Comments
INSTI-based regimens Raltegravir + TDF/FTC or TAF/FTC Elvitegravir/cobicistat/TDF/FTC Elvitegravir/cobicistat/TAF/FTC RAL + ABC/3TC	
NNRTI-based regimens (in alphabetical order) DOR/TDF/3TC or DOR + TAF/FTC EFV/TDF/FTC or EFV + TAF/FTC RPV/TDF/FTC or RPV/TAF/FTC	EFV should not be used with caution in the first trimester of pregnancy or in women trying to conceive. NVP should not be used in patients with moderate to severe hepatic impairment (Child-Pugh B or C). Should not be used in women with pretreatment CD4 >250 cells/mm^3 or men with CD4 >400 cells/mm^3. ABC should not be used in patients who test positive for HLA-B*5701.
PI-based regimens (in alphabetical order) ATV/r or ATV/c + TDF/FTC or TAF/FTC DRV/c or DRV/r + ABC/3TC	Use with caution in patients with high risk of cardiovascular disease or with pretreatment HIV. RNA >100,000 copies/ml. Once-daily LPV/r is not recommended in pregnant women.

3TC, Lamivudine; *ABC*, abacavir; *ART*, antiretroviral therapy; *ATV*, atazanavir; *DOR*, doravirine; *DRV*, darunavir; *EFV*, efavirenz; *FPV*, fosamprenavir; *FTC*, emtricitabine; *HLA*, human leukocyte antigen; *INSTI*, integrase strand transfer inhibitor; *LPV*, lopinavir; *MRV*, maraviroc; *NNRTI*, nonnucleoside reverse transcriptase inhibitor; *NVP*, nevirapine; *PI*, protease inhibitor; *r*, low dose ritonavir; *RAL*, raltegravir; *RNA*, ribonucleic acid; *RVP*, rilpivirine; *TAF*, tenofovir alafenamide; *TDF*, tenofovir disoproxil fumarate. The following combinations in the recommended list are available as fixed-dose combination formulations: ABC/3TC, EFV/TDF/FTC, LPV/r, TDF/FTC, RPV/TDF/FTC, and ZDV/3TC.
Modified from DHHS Panel on Antiretroviral Guidelines for Adults and Adolescents: *Guidelines for the use of antiretroviral agents in adults and adolescents with HIV,* Washington, DC, Department of Health and Human Services.

- NNRTIs:
  1. Efavirenz 600 mg daily: Should be used in caution in women in the first trimester or those who are contemplating pregnancy.
  2. Rilpivirine: Given with tenofovir and emtricitabine as part of a fixed-dose combination.
  3. Nevirapine 200 mg two times a day: Avoid with CD4 count >250 in men and >350 cells/mm^3 in women because of the risk of hepatitis. Rarely used.
  4. Etravirine 200 mg two times a day: This drug is generally used in patients for whom other regimens have failed. Etravirine retains activity in many patients who have developed resistance against efavirenz and nevirapine.
- PIs (ritonavir boosted):
  1. Darunavir and ritonavir (800 mg and 100/day): This is considered a preferred PI regimen within the U.S. Department of Health and Human Services (DHHS) guidelines with either tenofovir disoproxil fumarate or TAF and emtricitabine.
  2. Atazanavir and ritonavir (300 mg and 100 mg) 2 tablets a day: Lower pill burden but use with caution in combination with acid-reducing agents (can alter absorption).
  3. Lopinavir and ritonavir (200 mg/50 mg) 2 tablets twice a day (or 4 tablets once a day): Most likely to cause diarrhea and has the greatest negative effect on triglyceride levels; less commonly used.
  4. Fosamprenavir and ritonavir (700 mg and 100 mg) 2 tablets twice a day (or 4 tablets once a day): Cannot take fosamprenavir with sulfa allergy; less commonly used.

  5. Saquinavir and ritonavir: Saquinavir is no longer recommended for initial treatment of any patient and should be prescribed only in consultation with a specialist.
- All these drugs have their own unique, as well as class-specific, side effects and require careful follow-up to achieve optimal antiviral effects. Compliance with the drug regimen and tolerance of common side effects are critically important to maintain drug efficacy. Antiviral response should be monitored by baseline HIV viral load and CD4 count and repeat measurement at 2 and 4 wk into treatment and then periodically (every 3 to 6 mo) to ensure viral suppression.
- All patients should have genotypic resistance testing upon entry into medical care and before initiation of ART.
- In experienced patients, an antiretroviral regimen should be constructed based on past antiretroviral use and the results of genotypic or phenotypic testing.
- Patients with a CD4 count <200/mm^3 should be given preventive therapy for PJP (Table 11).
- Evaluation of chronic diarrhea in patients with HIV is described in the "Acquired Immunodeficiency Syndrome" topic in Section I.
- Criteria for discontinuing and restarting opportunistic infection prophylaxis for adults and adolescents with HIV infection is described in Table 12.
- HIV infection in a pregnant woman poses special challenges and considerations. Appropriate and timely ART given to mother and newborn has been shown to dramatically reduce the risk of perinatal transmission of HIV.

The goal of therapy is to achieve an undetectable viral load. For HIV-infected pregnant women who are already receiving ART: (1) Continue therapy if suppressing viral replication, but avoid use of efavirenz in the first trimester (substitution is recommended in the first trimester); (2) if viremia on therapy, genotypic testing is recommended. For HIV-infected pregnant women who have never received ART: (1) All women should start on ART as soon as possible. Most antiretrovirals are safe in pregnancy; however, efavirenz should be avoided because of possible teratogenicity (Class D), DDI and D4T should be avoided (potential of lactic acidosis), and some protease inhibitors may be dose-altered in pregnancy. Nevirapine should not be initiated in an antiretroviral-naive pregnant patient with CD4 counts >250 cells/mm^3 because of the risk of hepatotoxicity. (2) Women who do not need ART for their own health should also initiate three-drug therapy but may do so at the end of the first trimester.
- Preferred ART medications during pregnancy include:
  1. NRTIs: TDF/FTC, TDF/3TC, or ABC/3TC
  2. INSTI: Raltegravir; dolutegravir can be used after the first trimester; limited data with bictegravir. Elvitegravir should not be used in pregnancy because of inadequate drug concentrations
  3. PIs: ATV/r or DRV/r
- ART should continue through the baby's birth. Zidovudine should also be given intravenously to the woman at the time of labor if the woman has an HIV RNA >1000 copies/ml or

TABLE 11 Criteria for Discontinuing and Restarting Opportunistic Infection Prophylaxis for Adults and Adolescents with Human Immunodeficiency Virus Infection

Opportunistic Infection	Criteria for Discontinuing Primary Prophylaxis	Criteria for Restarting Primary Prophylaxis	Criteria for Discontinuing Secondary Prophylaxis/Chronic Maintenance Therapy	Criteria for Restarting Secondary Prophylaxis/Chronic Maintenance Therapy
Pneumocystis pneumonia (PJP)	CD4+ count >200 cells/mm³ for >3 mo in response to ART	CD4+ count <200 cells/mm³	CD4+ count increased from <200 cells/mm³ to >200 cells/mm³ for ≥3 mo in response to ART If PJP is diagnosed when CD4+ count >200 cells/mm³, prophylaxis should probably be continued for life regardless of CD4+ count rise in response to ART	CD4+ count <200 cells/mm³, or if PCP recurred at a CD4+ count >200 cells/mm³
Toxoplasma gondii encephalitis (TE)	CD4+ count >200 cells/mm³ for >3 mo in response to ART	CD4+ count <100-200 cells/mm³	Successfully completed initial therapy, remain asymptomatic of signs and symptoms of TE, and CD4+ count >200 cells/mm³ for >6 mo in response to ART	CD4+ count <100 cells/mm³
Microsporidiosis	Not applicable	Not applicable	No signs and symptoms of nonocular microsporidiosis and CD4+ count >200 cells/mm³ for >6 mo in response to ART Patients with ocular microsporidiosis should be on therapy indefinitely regardless of CD4+ count	No recommendation
Disseminated *Mycobacterium avium* complex (MAC) disease	CD4+ count >100 cells/mm³ for ≥3 mo in response to ART	CD4+ count <50 cells/mm³	If fulfill the following criteria: Completed ≥12 mo therapy, and no signs and symptoms of MAC, and have sustained (≥6 mo) CD4+ count >100 cells/mm³ in response to ART	CD4+ count <50 cells/mm³
Bartonellosis	Not applicable	Not applicable	If fulfill the following criteria: Received 3-4 mo of treatment CD4+ count >200 cells/mm³ for ≥6 mo Certain specialists would discontinue therapy only if *Bartonella* titers have also decreased by fourfold	No recommendation
Mucosal candidiasis	Not applicable	Not applicable	If used, reasonable to discontinue when CD4+ count >200 cells/mm³	No recommendation
Cryptococcal meningitis	Not applicable	Not applicable	If fulfill the following criteria: Completed course of initial therapy Remain asymptomatic of cryptococcosis CD4+ count ≥200 cells/mm³ for >6 mo in response to ART Certain specialists would perform a lumbar puncture to determine if cerebrospinal fluid is culture and antigen negative before stopping therapy	CD4+ count <100 cells/mm³
Histoplasma capsulatum infection	If used, CD4+ count >150 cells/mm³ for 6 mo on ART	For patients at high risk for acquiring histoplasmosis, restart at CD4+ count ≤150 cells/mm³	If fulfill the following criteria: Received itraconazole for ≥1 yr. Negative blood cultures CD4+ count >150 cells/mm³ for ≥6 mo in response to ART Serum *Histoplasma* antigen <2 units	CD4+ count ≤150 cells/mm³
Coccidioidomycosis	If used, CD4+ count ≥250 cells/mm³ for ≥6 mo	If used, restart at CD4+ count <250 cells/mm³	**Only for patients with focal coccidioidal pneumonia:** Clinically responded to ≥12 mo of antifungal therapy CD4+ count >250 cells/mm³ Receiving ART Suppressive therapy should be continued indefinitely, even with increase in CD4+ count on ART for patients with diffuse pulmonary, disseminated, or meningeal diseases	No recommendation

H

TABLE 11 Criteria for Discontinuing and Restarting Opportunistic Infection Prophylaxis for Adults and Adolescents with Human Immunodeficiency Virus Infection—cont'd

Opportunistic Infection	Criteria for Discontinuing Primary Prophylaxis	Criteria for Restarting Primary Prophylaxis	Criteria for Discontinuing Secondary Prophylaxis/Chronic Maintenance Therapy	Criteria for Restarting Secondary Prophylaxis/Chronic Maintenance Therapy
Cytomegalovirus retinitis	Not applicable	Not applicable	CD4+ count >100 cells/mm³ for >3-6 mo in response to ART. Therapy should be discontinued only after consultation with an ophthalmologist, taking into account magnitude and duration of CD4+ count increase, anatomic location of the lesions, vision in the contralateral eye, and the feasibility of regular ophthalmologic monitoring. Routine (every 3 mo) ophthalmologic follow-up is recommended for early detection of relapse or immune restoration uveitis	No recommendation
Isospora belli infection	Not applicable	Not applicable	Sustained increase in CD4+ count to >200 cells/mm³ for >6 mo in response to ART and without evidence of *I. belli* infection	No recommendation

ART, Antiretroviral therapy.

Modified from Centers for Disease Control and Prevention: Guidelines for prevention and treatment of opportunistic infections in HIV-infected adults and adolescents. Recommendations from CDC, the National Institutes of Health, and the HIV Medicine Association of the Infectious Diseases Society of America, *MMWR* 58(RR-4):1-CE4, 2009.

TABLE 12 Prophylaxis to Prevent First Episode of HIV-Related Opportunistic Disease

Pathogen	Indication	First Choice	Alternative
Pneumocystis jiroveci pneumonia (PJP, previously referred to as *Pneumocystis carinii*, PCP)	CD4+ count <200 cells/mm³ or oropharyngeal candidiasis CD4+ <14% or history of AIDS-defining illness CD4+ count >200 but <250 cells/mm³ if monitoring CD4+ count every 1-3 mo is not possible	Trimethoprim-sulfamethoxazole (TMP-SMX) double-strength PO daily; *or* single-strength daily	TMP-SMX 1 double-strength PO 3 times weekly; *or* dapsone 100 mg PO daily or 50 mg PO bid; *or* aerosolized pentamidine 300 mg via Respirgard II nebulizer every month; *or* atovaquone 1500 mg PO daily
Toxoplasma gondii encephalitis	*Toxoplasma* IgG–positive patients with CD4+ count <100 cells/mm³ Seronegative patients receiving PCP prophylaxis not active against toxoplasmosis should have *Toxoplasma* serology retested if CD4+ count declines to <100 cells/mm³ Prophylaxis should be initiated if seroconversion occurred	TMP-SMX, 1 double-strength PO daily	TMP-SMX 1 double-strength PO 3 times weekly; *or* TMP-SMX 1 single-strength PO daily; *or* dapsone 50 mg PO daily + pyrimethamine 50 mg PO weekly + leucovorin 25 mg PO weekly; *or* dapsone 200 mg PO weekly + pyrimethamine 75 mg PO weekly + leucovorin 25 mg PO weekly
Mycobacterium tuberculosis infection (TB) (treatment of latent TB infection or LTBI)	(1) Diagnostic test for LTBI, no evidence of active TB, and no prior history of treatment for active or latent TB (2) Diagnostic test for LTBI, but close contact with a person with infectious pulmonary TB and no evidence of active TB (3) A history of untreated or inadequately treated healed TB (i.e., old fibrotic lesions) regardless of diagnostic tests for LTBI and no evidence of active TB	Isoniazid (INH) 300 mg PO daily or 900 mg PO twice weekly for 9 mo—both plus pyridoxine 25 mg PO daily; *or* for persons exposed to drug-resistant TB, selection of drugs after consultation with public health authorities	Rifampin (RIF) 600 mg PO daily × 4 mo; *or* rifabutin (dosage depends on ART regimen). Be careful of drug interactions with these medications (PIs and NNRTIs) Isoniazid (15 mg/kg rounded up to the nearest 50 or 100 mg; 900 mg maximum) and rifapentine (10-14.0 kg 300 mg; 14.1-25.0 kg 450 mg; 25.1-32.0 kg 600 mg; 32.1-49.9 kg 750 mg; ≥50.00 kg 900 mg maximum) once weekly for a total of 3 mo
Disseminated *Mycobacterium avium* complex (MAC) disease	CD4+ count <50 cells/mm³—after ruling out active MAC infection	Azithromycin 1200 mg PO once weekly; *or* clarithromycin 500 mg PO bid; *or* azithromycin 600 mg PO twice weekly	RFB 300 mg PO daily (dosage adjustment based on drug-drug interactions with antiretroviral therapy); rule out active TB before starting RFB

Continued

TABLE 12 Prophylaxis to Prevent First Episode of HIV-Related Opportunistic Disease—cont'd

Pathogen	Indication	First Choice	Alternative
Streptococcus pneumoniae infection	CD4+ count >200 cells/mm³ and no receipt of pneumococcal vaccine in the past 5 yr. CD4+ count <200 cells/mm³—vaccination can be offered In patients who received polysaccharide pneumococcal vaccination (PPV) when CD4+ count <200 cells/mm³ but has increased to >200 cells/mm³ in response to antiretroviral therapy	A single dose of PCV13 followed by a single dose of PPSV23 at least 8 wk later. A second dose of PPSV23 should be given 5 yr after the initial PPSV23 dose	
Influenza A and B virus infection	All HIV-infected patients	Inactivated influenza vaccine 0.5 ml IM annually	
Histoplasma capsulatum infection	CD4+ count ≤150 cells/mm³ and at high risk because of occupational exposure or live in a community with a hyperendemic rate of histoplasmosis (>10 cases/100 patient-yr)	Itraconazole 200 mg PO daily	
Coccidioidomycosis	Positive IgM or IgG serologic test result in a patient from a disease-endemic area; and CD4+ count <250 cells/mm³	Fluconazole 400 mg PO daily itraconazole 200 mg PO bid	
Varicella-zoster virus (VZV) infection	*Preexposure prevention:* Patients with CD4+ count ≥200 cells/mm³ who have not been vaccinated, have no history of varicella or herpes zoster, or who are seronegative for VZV NOTE: Routine VZV serologic testing in HIV-infected adults is not recommended *Postexposure—close contact with a person who has active varicella or herpes zoster* For susceptible patients (those who have no history of vaccination or of either condition, or are known to be VZV seronegative)	*Preexposure prevention:* Primary varicella vaccination (Varivax), 2 doses (0.5 ml SC) administered 3 mo apart. If vaccination results in disease because of vaccine virus, treatment with acyclovir is recommended *Postexposure therapy:* Varicella-zoster immune globulin (VariZIG) 125 IU per 10 kg (maximum of 625 IU) IM, administered within 96 h after exposure to a person with active varicella or herpes zoster NOTE: As of June 2007, VariZIG can be obtained only under a treatment IND (1-800-843-7477, FFF Enterprises)	VZV-susceptible household contacts of susceptible HIV-infected persons should be vaccinated to prevent potential transmission of VZV to their HIV-infected contacts Alternative postexposure therapy: Postexposure varicella vaccine (Varivax) 0.5 ml SC × 2 doses, 3 mo apart if CD4+ count >200 cells/mm³; *or* preemptive acyclovir 800 mg PO 3×/day for 5 days These two alternatives have not been studied in the HIV population
Human papillomavirus (HPV) infection	Women aged 11-26 yr. Men aged 11-26 yr	HPV quadrivalent vaccine 0.5 ml IM mo 0, 2, and 6	
Hepatitis A virus (HAV) infection	HAV-susceptible patients with chronic liver disease or who are injection-drug users, or men who have sex with men. Certain specialists might delay vaccination until CD4+ count >200 cells/mm³	Hepatitis A vaccine 1 ml IM ×2 doses—at 0 and 6-12 mo IgG antibody response should be assessed 1 mo after vaccination; nonresponders should be revaccinated	
Hepatitis B virus (HBV) infection	All HIV patients without evidence of prior exposure to HBV should be vaccinated with HBV vaccine, including patients with CD4+ count <200 cells/mm³ *Patients with isolated anti-HBc:* Consider screening for HBV DNA before vaccination to rule out occult chronic HBV infection	Hepatitis B vaccine IM (Engerix-B 20 μg/ml or Recombivax HB 10 μg/ml) at 0, 1, and 6 mo anti-HBs should be obtained 1 mo after completion of the vaccine series	Some experts recommend vaccinating with 40-μg doses of either vaccine
	Vaccine nonresponders: Defined as anti-HBs <10 IU/ml 1 mo after a vaccination series For patients with low CD4+ count at the time of first vaccination series, certain specialists might delay revaccination until after a sustained increase in CD4+ count with antiretroviral therapy	Revaccinate with a second vaccine series	Some experts recommend revaccinating with 40-μg doses of either vaccine

AIDS, Acquired immunodeficiency syndrome; *ART,* antiretroviral therapy; *HB,* hepatitis B; *Ig,* immunoglobulin; *IM,* intramuscular; *IND,* investigational new drug; *NNRTI,* nonnucleoside analog reverse transcriptase inhibitor; *PI,* protease inhibitors; *PO,* by mouth; *RFB,* rifabutin.
Modified from Centers for Disease Control and Prevention: Guidelines for prevention and treatment of opportunistic infections in HIV-infected adults and adolescents: recommendations from CDC, the National Institutes of Health, and the HIV Medicine Association of the Infectious Diseases Society of America, *MMWR* 58(RR-4):1-CE4, 2009.

there is a concern for poor adherence, regardless of whether it is an existing component of her three-drug regimen. In women with viral loads persistently >1000 copies/ml despite appropriate ART, cesarean section may further lower risk of transmission. For women with HIV RNA <1000 copies/ml zidovudine (AZT) should also be given to the newborn for the first 6 wk of life. If HIV RNA levels are >1000 copies/ml, infants should receive combination ART, which may include zidovudine, lamivudine, and nevirapine for 6 wk. Mothers should completely avoid nursing.

DISPOSITION

- Ongoing care consisting of frequent medical evaluations and monitoring of CD4 counts and HIV viral loads
- Long-term care focused on providing up-to-date ART and prophylaxis of PJP and other opportunistic infections, as well as early detection of complications
- Ongoing assessment for cardiovascular risk and other primary prevention interventions
- Screening for hepatitis A, B, and C. Treatment when indicated. Drugs such as TDF and lamivudine have activity against both HIV and hepatitis B and may be used in patients with coinfection
- Vaccinations including hepatitis A and B (when susceptible), pneumococcus (PCV13 and PPSV23), tetanus/diphtheria/pertussis, meningococcal, and influenza. COVID-19 vaccination is also safe to administer at all CD4 cell counts. Box 1 summarizes vaccinations in HIV-positive adults
- Yearly screening for other sexually transmitted infections (chlamydia, gonorrhea, and syphilis). This includes trichomonas in women and extragenital testing for chlamydia and gonorrhea (i.e., pharyngeal and rectal) in MSM
- Consideration of AIDS (lymphomas, HPV) and non-AIDS related (screening for general population, age-specific cancers)

REFERRAL

To a physician knowledgeable and experienced in the management of HIV infection and its complications. According to 2018 CDC surveillance data, only 78% of patients are linked to care within 30 days after diagnosis, and a

---

BOX 1 Vaccination in HIV-Positive Adults

Generally Avoid
- Bacille Calmette-Guérin (BCG)
- Oral polio
- Oral typhoid

Avoid if CD4+ Cells <200
- Yellow fever
- Measles
- Varicella-zoster virus (VZV)

Give Routinely
- Tetanus/diphtheria (or Tdap)
- Hepatitis A/B
- *Streptococcus pneumoniae*
- *Haemophilus influenzae* type B (Hib)
- Meningococcal
- Influenza, yearly

Give if Indicated for Travel
- Typhoid Vi
- Meningococcal
- Polio, inactivated polio vaccine (IPV)
- Rabies
- Japanese encephalitis
- Tick-borne encephalitis

From Auerbach P: *Wilderness medicine, expert consult, premium edition—enhanced online features and print*, Philadelphia, 2012, Saunders.

sustained viral suppression is achieved in only 55% to 60% of persons (and a smaller percentage of infected adolescents and young adults) with diagnosed HIV.[13]

PREVENTION

- TDF/FTC or TAF/FTC may be used as preexposure prophylaxis (PrEP). Individuals who are HIV negative may take TDF/FTC or TAF/FTC once a day to prevent HIV infection. TDF/FTC as PrEP has been demonstrated to be effective in MSM, heterosexuals, and injection drug users. Importantly, TAF/FTC as PrEP has been shown to be effective in MSM and transwomen but not for cisgender women. Individuals on PrEP should be monitored every 3 mo for renal dysfunction, HIV status, other STIs, and adherence. The FDA has approved Apretude, an intramuscular extended-release (ER) formulation of the integrase strand transfer inhibitor (INSTI) cabotegravir (CAB-LA) for use every 2 mo to prevent

---

sexually acquired HIV-1 infection in at-risk adolescents and adults. Recent trials have shown that CAB-LA is superior to daily oral TDF-FTC in preventing HIV infection among MSM and transgender women.
- Postexposure prophylaxis (PEP) is an effective prevention intervention for individuals exposed to HIV infection, either occupationally or through a sexual exposure. PEP should be taken within 72 h of an exposure and continued for 28 days. Baseline HIV status, renal function, hepatitis B/C, and liver function should be assessed. The recommended first-line regimen is TDF/FTC or TAF/FTC once daily plus raltegravir 400 mg PO twice daily or dolutegravir 50 mg once daily. The FDA has approved Cabenuva, an extended-release formulation of cabotegravir copackaged with an extended-release formulation of rilpivirine. As a once-monthly IM regimen for adults with HIV-1 infection who are virologically suppressed (HIV-1 RNA <50 copies/ml) on a stable antiretroviral regimen without history of treatment failure and without resistance to either drug.

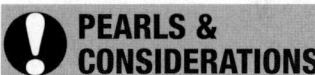

PEARLS & CONSIDERATIONS

COMMENTS

- ART should be initiated in all HIV-infected individuals regardless of CD4 cell counts.
- ART in combination with avoidance of breastfeeding and elective cesarean section in women with viremia reduces risk for mother-to-child transmission.

REFERENCES & SUGGESTED READINGS

Available at eBooks.Health.Elsevier.com.

RELATED CONTENT

Human Immunodeficiency Virus (HIV) Infection (Patient Information)
Acquired Immunodeficiency Syndrome (Related Key Topic)

AUTHOR: **PHILIP A. CHAN, MD, MS**

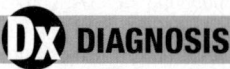 BASIC INFORMATION

DEFINITION

Hydronephrosis, Greek for "water inside the kidney," is an anatomic dilation of the collecting system of the kidneys (renal pelvis and/or calyces). When combined with ureteric dilation, the term hydroureteronephrosis is used. *Hydronephrosis is a structural finding, not a specific diagnosis, and is not synonymous with obstruction.*[1,2] Etiologically, hydronephrosis can result from obstruction to antegrade urine flow (kidney>ureter/s>bladder>urethra), retrograde reflux of urine across the ureterovesical junction (vesicoureteral reflux, VUR), or simply too much urine for the ureters to handle (as in pathologic diuresis states).

SYNONYMS

Pelviectasis
Caliectasis
Pelvocaliectasis
Pyelocaliectasis

ICD-10CM CODES

N13.1	Hydronephrosis with ureteral stricture, not elsewhere classified
N13.2	Hydronephrosis with renal and ureteral calculous obstruction
N13.30	Unspecified hydronephrosis
N13.39	Other hydronephrosis
Q62.0	Congenital hydronephrosis
Q62.11	Hydronephrosis with ureteropelvic junction obstruction

EPIDEMIOLOGY & DEMOGRAPHICS

Prevalence derived from multiple autopsy series ranges from 2% to 4%,[3] with subjects ranging from neonates to geriatric patients. Antenatal hydronephrosis is one of the most common findings in prenatal ultrasound scans, affecting up to 5% of pregnancies, with 30% to 40% persisting postnatally.[4] Of these, 40% will resolve spontaneously. Hydronephrosis in children is often caused by congenital and structural abnormalities of the kidneys and ureters, such as ureteropelvic junction obstruction or vesicoureteral reflux. Hydronephrosis in adults is often a result of obstruction of one or both kidneys, usually caused by stones, tumors, infections, and trauma. Stones are the most common cause of upper urinary tract obstruction.[2,3] In adults 20 to 60 yr old, hydronephrosis is more common in women, secondary to pregnancy/gynecologic causes. During pregnancy, physiologic hydronephrosis (more commonly on the right) occurs in up to 90% of cases, is often asymptomatic, and typically resolves postpartum. In older patients (age >60 yr), obstruction from prostate enlargement and obstruction from malignancy are the most common causes.[1,2]

PHYSICAL FINDINGS & CLINICAL PRESENTATION

Hydronephrosis may present as an asymptomatic, incidental finding during imaging performed for another purpose. Symptoms often indicate an element of obstruction. Presentation depends on etiology (obstruction, reflux), degree of obstruction (complete or partial), duration (acute or chronic), anatomic factors (unilateral or bilateral; intrinsic or extrinsic to the ureter), underlying comorbidities (diabetes mellitus, immunocompromised, postoperative states, etc.), and the presence of superimposed urinary tract infection.

HISTORY:
- Pain is usually present along the flank, with radiation toward the ipsilateral groin or lower abdominal quadrant. If onset is sudden and severe, consider a ureteral stone. Ureteral stone also should be a differential for males presenting with penile/ipsilateral testicular pain and benign genital examination/scrotal ultrasound. If pain is induced by diuresis (e.g., following consumption of alcohol or caffeine), consider ureteropelvic junction obstruction (Dietl crisis). When obstruction is subacute to chronic, symptoms may be vague, less intense, or absent, and may wax and wane in severity (renal colic). Extrinsic compression (e.g., malignancy-associated compression of ureters or retroperitoneal fibrosis) usually has a more insidious onset compared with intrinsic obstruction (e.g., ureteral stone or blood clot).
- Nausea and vomiting are typically associated with acute obstruction, usually from an intrinsic process.
- Oliguria/anuria may occur with complete, bilateral obstruction, or with an obstructed solitary kidney.
- Urinary symptoms are often absent unless there is an associated condition, including urinary tract infection, distal ureteral stone, or urinary retention. These voiding symptoms include dysuria, urinary urgency, and, frequency, hematuria, pelvic pressure, and discomfort.
- Hematuria may indicate a stone, urinary tract infection, or malignancy.
- The site of obstruction can relate to the presentation, with upper tract obstruction frequently presenting with flank pain, whereas lower tract obstruction is often associated with obstructive voiding symptoms, such as straining, frequency, sensation of incomplete emptying, dribbling, and/or slow urinary stream.

PHYSICAL EXAMINATION: A complete physical examination is warranted but may not be helpful in the assessment of hydronephrosis. Special attention should be paid to the following:
- Blood pressure.
- Palpable abdominal mass: Rare, except in children or thin patients with massive hydronephrosis. Costovertebral angle tenderness is typically not a reliably present (or absent) finding. An enlarged, often palpable and percussible bladder is the most common lower abdominal "mass."
- Complete genitourinary and pelvic examination:
  1. Pelvic examination will assess for pelvic masses or pelvic organ prolapse, which is rarely associated with ureteral obstruction.
  2. Digital rectal examination will assess for prostatic abnormality or rectal mass.
  3. Genital examination (bedside or via cystoscopy) may show meatal stenosis/urethral stricture disease.
  4. Residual urine volume may demonstrate incomplete emptying of the bladder. Residual urine volume can be evaluated indirectly by bedside ultrasonography or directly by bladder catheterization.

ETIOLOGY

Hydronephrosis can be caused by extrinsic or intrinsic factors relative to the urinary tract (Table 1). Causes may be grouped as congenital or acquired.

DX DIAGNOSIS

DIFFERENTIAL DIAGNOSIS

Diagnostic workup depends on age, acuity of presentation, associated symptoms, and if hydronephrosis was diagnosed incidentally.

LABORATORY TESTS[1]

- Evaluation of kidney function: Blood urea nitrogen and creatinine. If azotemia is present, bilateral obstruction or unilateral obstruction of a solitary kidney is present.
- Electrolyte abnormalities: Hyponatremia or hypernatremia, hyperkalemia, and low bicarbonate concentration. Calculation of fractional excretion of sodium (FeNa) or fractional excretion of urea (FEUrea) can help provide clues to etiology of acute kidney injury.[1]
- Urinalysis and sediment examination: White blood cells, red blood cells, or bacteria in the appropriate setting (e.g., infection, stones). Urine microscopy facilitates crystal identification, which may suggest urinary stone disease. The sediment may be normal in obstructive renal disease.
- Urine culture: Urinalysis or presentation suggests urinary tract infection.

IMAGING STUDIES[2]

- Ultrasound is an excellent initial screening test, especially for children and pregnant women, with evaluation of the kidneys, portions of the ureters, bladder wall, bladder volume, and contour of the collecting system and ureters. Point-of-care ultrasound provides early, rapid imaging and aids patient triage and justification for additional imaging.[5] Ultrasound is >90% sensitive and specific for hydronephrosis. Although not definitive, the absence of ureteral jets on ultrasound may be an indirect sign of upstream obstruction (Fig. E1).
- Abdominal plain film or KUB (kidney, ureter, and bladder) x-rays have limited diagnostic value unless conducted with ultrasound and may demonstrate radiopaque kidney or ureteral stones.
- Abdominal computed tomography (CT) scan without intravenous contrast medium localizes sites of obstruction (Figs. E2 and E3), especially if an ureteral calculus is the cause

TABLE 1 Hydronephrosis: Differential Diagnoses

Obstructive

Intrinsic to the urinary tract	*Ureter:* Ureteropelvic junction obstruction, ureterovesical junction obstruction, stricture, tumor, ureterocele, stone, blood clot, sloughed papilla, infection, hyperplastic polyp
	Bladder: Malignancy, stone, bladder neck obstruction, urine retention, neurogenic lower urinary tract dysfunction
	Prostate: Benign prostatic enlargement, prostatitis, abscess, prostate malignancy
	Urethra: Stricture, stone, diverticulum, malignancy, posterior urethral valves, phimosis
Extrinsic to the urinary tract	**Reproductive system:**
	Uterus: Pregnancy, prolapse, fibroids, malignancy
	Ovary: Malignancy, cyst, abscess
	Vascular system:
	Aneurysm: Abdominal aorta, iliac vessel
	Aberrant vessels: Ureteropelvic junction
	Venous: Retrocaval ureter, ovarian vein syndrome
	Gastrointestinal system:
	Inflammatory bowel disease, GI malignancy, abscesses, cysts
	Diseases of the retroperitoneum:
	Retroperitoneal fibrosis
	Retroperitoneal malignancy (primary or metastatic deposits)
	Hematoma
	Lymphocele
	Iatrogenic injury

Nonobstructive

	Vesicoureteral reflux
	Extrarenal pelvis
	Pyelonephritis
	Pathologic diuresis (diabetes insipidus, postobstructive diuresis)

GI, Gastrointestinal.

of obstruction. A normal ureteral width by unenhanced CT is 2 to 3 mm wide in adults. If kidney function is normal, CT urography (without and then with contrast, and with delayed images of the ureters) provides anatomic information and is the modality of choice for assessment of upper tract tumors or incidental hydronephrosis.

- Magnetic resonance urogram (MRU) is an alternative to contrast-enhanced CT that provides detail, but MRI cannot directly detect a stone. Severely impaired renal function may preclude gadolinium administration. MRI may be used when other tests are inconclusive or contraindicated (e.g., pregnancy, chronic kidney disease, radiocontrast media allergy).
- Antegrade or retrograde ureterogram/pyelogram is an invasive procedure used when CT or MRI scans with radiocontrast media are contraindicated (e.g., contrast allergy, renal impairment).
- Voiding cystourethrography (VCUG) evaluates for possible vesicoureteral reflux and/or bladder neck or urethral obstruction.
- Radioisotope renography (diuretic renography, Tc-99m MAG3 renogram) is a functional procedure that provides differential renal function and determines presence of clinically significant obstruction.[1]

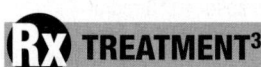 **TREATMENT**[3]

ACUTE GENERAL Rx

- Analgesics (NSAIDs vs. opioid analgesics, based on clinical situation), antiemetics, and fluids for treatment of pain, nausea, and vomiting
- Antibiotics for urinary tract infection/pyelonephritis

Specific management:

- Management depends on presence of obstruction, etiology, and location of hydronephrosis. Prompt treatment of infection and relief of obstruction prevent long-term loss of kidney function. Chronic renal obstruction from any cause may produce permanent functional deterioration. Renal recovery depends on duration and severity of obstruction.
- General principles include the following:
  1. Routine outpatient evaluation for hydronephrosis is appropriate in asymptomatic or minimally symptomatic patients with no infection, electrolyte derangements, or acute kidney injury.
  2. Surgical treatment is aimed at relieving obstruction when hydronephrosis is associated with urinary tract infection, acute kidney injury, uncontrollable pain, or nausea and vomiting. Surgical treatment is also indicated with complete urinary

obstruction from a bilateral obstructing process or unilateral obstruction in a solitary kidney.
  3. Urethral catheter or suprapubic catheter placement is indicated for bladder outlet obstruction. Monitor patients for postobstructive diuresis after relief of obstruction.
  4. Ureteral stenting is carried out for decompression of one or both kidneys. Percutaneous nephrostomy tubes are an alternative to ureteral stenting and may be required in the setting of extrinsic ureteral compression or when ureteral stenting is not possible or fails.

REFERRAL

Prompt referral is paramount in the setting of severe symptoms, infection, or impaired renal function.

- Urology for diagnostic and/or therapeutic procedures (pediatric urologist for antenatal or postnatal hydronephrosis)
- Oncology for diagnosed neoplasm
- Gynecology for pregnancy or if female pelvic anatomy is involved
- Nephrology for electrolyte/acid-base disturbances

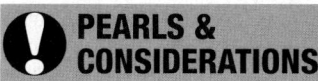 **PEARLS & CONSIDERATIONS**

COMMENTS

- Hydronephrosis is not a primary disorder, and an underlying etiology must be sought.
- Children often have congenital causes; adults generally have acquired intrinsic or extrinsic causes.
- There are obstructive and nonobstructive causes of hydronephrosis. Further evaluation can be performed without specialty consultation with a CT urogram, magnetic resonance urogram, or diuretic renogram.
- Prompt renal decompression is critical when hydronephrosis is associated with infection, severe kidney injury, and/or electrolyte abnormalities.

PREVENTION

Timely and appropriate management of acute kidney obstruction prevents long-term kidney damage. Hydronephrosis may persist after relief of the obstructing cause.

REFERENCES

Available at eBooks.Health.Elsevier.com.

AUTHORS: **EMILY CHAN BRODOWSKY, MD** and **DAVID A. LEAVITT, MD**

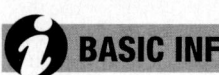 **BASIC INFORMATION**

DEFINITION
Hypercholesterolemia refers to a blood cholesterol measurement ≥200 mg/dl.

SYNONYMS
Hyperlipidemia
Hypercholesteremia
Dyslipidemia
Type II familial hyperlipoproteinemia

ICD-10CM CODE
E78.0   Pure hypercholesterolemia

EPIDEMIOLOGY & DEMOGRAPHICS
- More than 105 million (37% of) adults in the U.S. have total blood cholesterol levels higher than 200 mg/dl. Of this group, more than 36 million adults have extremely high-risk cholesterol levels over 240 mg/dl (13%).
- For men over the age of 20, approximately 48% of White men, 45% of Black men, and 50% of Hispanic men have high blood cholesterol.
- For women over the age of 20, approximately 50% of White women, 42% of Black women, and 50% of Hispanic women have hypercholesterolemia.
- Prevalence of hypercholesterolemia increases with age.
- According to National Health and Nutrition Examination Survey (NHANES) data approximately 47% of adults had at least one of three risk factors for cardiovascular disease—uncontrolled high blood pressure, uncontrolled high levels of low-density lipoproteins (LDL) cholesterol, or current smoking.

PHYSICAL FINDINGS & CLINICAL PRESENTATION
- A detailed medication history should be performed because some medications may affect lipid levels (e.g., thiazides, corticosteroids, β-blockers, and estrogens).
- The physical examination should include measurements of body mass index and blood pressure (BP), thyroid and liver assessments, and examining peripheral pulses including carotids for bruits.
- Physical findings, particularly in the familial forms may include:
  1. Tendon xanthomas
  2. Xanthelasma
  3. Arcus corneae
  4. Arterial bruits (young adulthood)

ETIOLOGY
PRIMARY:
- Genetics
- Obesity
- Dietary intake
SECONDARY:
- Hypothyroidism
- Diabetes mellitus (DM)
- Nephrotic syndrome
- Obstructive liver disease: Hepatoma, extrahepatic biliary obstruction, primary biliary cirrhosis

- Alcohol or tobacco use
- Dysgammaglobulinemia (multiple myeloma, systemic lupus erythematosus)
- Drugs: Oral contraceptives, progesterone, corticosteroids, thiazide diuretics, β-blockers, androgenic steroids, retinoic acid derivatives, protease inhibitors

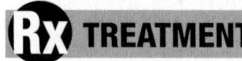 **DIAGNOSIS**

DIFFERENTIAL DIAGNOSIS
- Always consider underlying secondary causes for the elevated cholesterol.
- Patients with very high LDL cholesterol usually have genetic forms of hypercholesterolemia (see "Hyperlipoproteinemia, Primary"). Early detection of these cases and family testing to identify similarly affected relatives is important.
- Metabolic syndrome:
  1. A constellation of lipid and nonlipid risk factors of a metabolic origin
  2. Diagnosed when three or more of the following are present: Abdominal obesity (waist circumference >40 in for men and >35 in for women); fasting triglycerides >150 mg/dl; HDL <40 mg/dl in males and <50 mg/dl in females; systolic BP >130 mm Hg and diastolic BP >85 mm Hg; fasting glucose >110 mg/dl

WHO SHOULD BE SCREENED:
- The American Association of Clinical Endocrinologists (AACE) recommends screening of patients >20 yr of age for elevated cholesterol every 5 yr, males >45 yr and females >55 yr of age every 1 to 2 yr, and >65 yr of age every yr up to 75 yr of age regardless of coronary artery disease (CAD) risk status. Patients above 75 yr of age with multiple CAD risk factors should continue to get screened annually.
- The United States Preventive Services Task Force (USPSTF) supports routine screening for men aged >35 yr and women aged >45 yr by measurement of nonfasting total and HDL cholesterol alone. The USPSTF finds insufficient evidence to recommend for or against general lipid screening in children and adolescents.[1] This conclusion runs counter to the recommendation from the American Academy of Pediatrics (AAP), American College of Cardiology (ACC), and the American Heart Association (AHA) all of whom endorse screening children at ages 9 to 11 and adolescents at ages 17 to 21 y.
- In 2010 the USPSTF recommended routine screening for overweight and obese persons aged <20 yr.
- In 2011, American College of Cardiology (ACC)/American Heart Association (AHA) recommended screening for hypertriglyceridemia by a nonfasting measurement. A nonfasting level of <200 mg/dl is commensurate with an optimal level of <100 mg/dl, and no further testing is required. However, a nonfasting level of >200 mg/dl warrants further testing with a fasting lipid profile.

LABORATORY TESTS
- Obtain a lipid profile. A fasting lipid panel has been traditionally preferred over a nonfasting

lipid profile; however, this recommendation has come into question, and expert consensus statements from Canada and Europe recommend nonfasting lipid testing as the new standard for lipid measurement. In nonfasting patients, triglyceride levels ≥175 mg/dl should be considered elevated as compared with <150 mg/dl for fasting panels. Fasting lipid panels are preferred for patients with triglycerides over 400 mg/dl.
- Lipoprotein(a) [Lp(a)]: Current U.S. guidelines suggest that Lp(a) may be used as a "risk-enhancing factor" to support statin prescription, in concert with other factors and shared decision-making, among primary prevention patients aged 40 to 75 yr with an estimated 10-yr risk for atherosclerotic cardiovascular disease (ASCVD) of 5.0% to 19.9%.[2]
- Perform a workup for secondary causes if clinically indicated, such as thyroid-stimulating hormone, metabolic profile, liver function tests (LFTs), and fasting glucose.

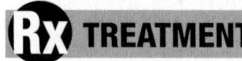 **TREATMENT**

NONPHARMACOLOGIC THERAPY
- First-line treatment: Dietary therapy can result in 5% to 15% reduction in LDL cholesterol level
- Composition of the **TLC diet:**
  1. Total fat 25% to 30% of total calories
  2. Polyunsaturated fat up to 10% of total calories
  3. Monounsaturated fat up to 20% of total calories
  4. Saturated fats <7% of total calories
  5. Carbohydrate 50% to 60% of total calories
  6. Protein 15% of total calories
  7. No more than 200 mg/day of cholesterol
  8. Fiber 20 to 30 g/day
- Increased physical activity: Encourage 30 min of moderately intense physical activity, four to six times a wk (e.g., brisk walking, riding stationary bike, water aerobics)
- Maintenance of a healthy weight
- Avoidance of tobacco products
- Counseling on CAD risk factors (Table 1)
- Plant-based diets (including stanol-containing margarines, oat bran, and nuts) have shown effectiveness in controlling lipids

ACUTE GENERAL Rx
No acute treatment needed

TABLE 1   Risk Factors for Heart Disease

1. Cigarette smoking
2. Hypertension (BP ≥140/90 mm Hg or on medications)
3. Low HDL cholesterol (<40 mg/dl)*
4. Family history of premature CHD (<55 yr in first-degree male relative or <65 yr in first-degree female relative)
5. Age (men ≥45 yr, women ≥55 yr)

BP, Blood pressure; *CHD*, congenital heart disease; *HDL*, high-density lipoprotein cholesterol.
*HDL cholesterol >60 mg/dl counts as a negative risk factor; its presence removes one risk factor from the total count.

BOX 1 2013 ACC/AHA Summary of Key Recommendations for the Treatment of Blood Cholesterol to Reduce ASCVD Risk in Adults

- Heart-healthy lifestyle habits should be encouraged for all individuals
- The appropriate intensity of statin therapy should be initiated or continued
  1. Clinical ASCVD*
     a. Age 75 yr or less and no safety concerns: High-intensity statin (class I, level A)
     b. Age 75 yr or safety concerns: Moderate-intensity statin (class I, level A)*
  2. Primary prevention: Primary LDL-C 190 mg/dl or greater
     a. Rule out secondary causes of hyperlipidemia (class I, level B)
     b. Age 21 yr or older: High-intensity statin (class I, level B)
     c. Achieve at least a 50% reduction in LDL-C (class IIa, level B)
     d. LDL-C lowering nonstatin therapy may be considered to further reduce LDL-C (class IIb, level C)
  3. Primary prevention: Diabetes, 40 to 75 yr of age, and LDL-C 70 to 189 mg/dl
     a. Moderate-intensity statin (class I, level A)
     b. Consider high-intensity statin when 7.5% or greater 10-yr ASCVD risk using the Pooled Cohort Equations (class IIa, level B)‡
  4. Primary prevention: No diabetes, 40 to 75 yr of age, and LDL-C 70 to 189 mg/dl
     a. Estimate 10-yr ASCVD risk using the Risk Calculator based on the Pooled Cohort Equations in those *not* receiving a statin; estimate risk every 4 to 6 yr (class I, level B)
     b. To determine whether to initiate a statin, engage in a clinician-patient discussion of the potential for ASCVD risk reduction, adverse effects, drug-drug interactions, and patient preferences
     c. Reemphasize heart-healthy lifestyle habits and address other risk factors (class IIa, level C)
        (1) 7.5% or greater 10-yr ASCVD risk: Moderate- or high-intensity statin (class I, level A)
        (2) 5% to 7.5% 10-yr ASCVD risk: Consider moderate-intensity statin (class IIa, level B)
        (3) Other factors may be considered: LDL-C 160 mg/dl or greater, family history of premature ASCVD, hs-CRP 2.0 mg/L or greater, CAC score 300 Agatston units or greater, ABI less than 0.9, or lifetime ASCVD risk (class IIb, level C)
  5. Primary prevention when LDL-C is less than 190 mg/dl and age is less than 40 or more than 75 yr, or less than 5% 10-yr ASCVD risk
     a. Statin therapy may be considered in selected individuals (class IIb, level C)
  6. Statin therapy is not routinely recommended for individuals with NYHA class II-IV heart failure or who are receiving maintenance hemodialysis
- Regularly monitor adherence to lifestyle and drug therapy with lipid and safety assessments
  1. Assess adherence, response to therapy, and adverse effects within 4 to 12 wk following statin initiation or change in therapy (class I, level A)
     a. Measure a fasting lipid panel (class I, level A)
     b. Do not routinely monitor ALT or CK unless symptomatic (class IIa, level C)
     c. Screen and treat type 2 diabetes according to current practice guidelines. Heart-healthy lifestyle habits should be encouraged to prevent progression to diabetes (class I, level B)
     d. Anticipated therapeutic response: Approximately 50% or greater reduction in LDL-C from baseline for high-intensity statin and 30% to 50% for moderate-intensity statin (class IIa, level B)
        (1) Insufficient evidence for LDL-C or non–HDL-C treatment targets from RCTs
        (2) For those with unknown baseline LDL-C, an LDL-C less than 100 mg/dl was observed in RCTs of high-intensity statin therapy
     e. Less than anticipated therapeutic response:
        (1) Reinforce improved adherence to lifestyle and drug therapy (class I, level A)
        (2) Evaluate for secondary causes of hyperlipidemia if indicated (class I, level A)
        (3) Increase statin intensity, or if on maximally tolerated statin intensity, consider addition of nonstatin therapy in selected high-risk individuals (class IIb, level C)§
  2. Regularly monitor adherence to lifestyle and drug therapy every 3 to 12 mo once adherence has been established. continue assessment of adherence for optimal ASCVD risk reduction and safety (class I, level A)
- In individuals intolerant of the recommended intensity of statin therapy, use the maximally tolerated intensity of statin (class I, level B). If there are muscle or other symptoms, establish that they are related to the statin (class IIa, level B)

ABI, Ankle brachial index; *ACC*, American College of Cardiology; *AHA*, American Heart Association; *ALT*, alanine transaminase; *ASCVD*, atherosclerotic cardiovascular disease; *CAC*, coronary artery calcium; *CK*, creatine kinase; *hs-CRP*, high sensitivity C-reactive protein; *LDL-C*, low-density lipoprotein cholesterol; *MI*, myocardial infarction; *NYHA*, New York Heart Association; *RCTs*, randomized clinical trials; *TIA*, transient ischemic attack.
*Clinical ASCVD includes acute coronary syndromes, history of MI, stable or unstable angina, coronary or other arterial revascularization, stroke, TIA, or peripheral arterial disease presumed to be of atherosclerotic origin.
‡These factors may include primary LDL-C of 160 mg/dl or greater or other evidence of genetic hyperlipidemias; family history of premature ASCVD with onset at less than 55 yr of age in a first-degree male relative or at less than 65 yr of age in a first-degree female relative; hs-CRP 2 mg/L or greater; CAC score 300 Agatston units or greater or 75th percentile or greater for age, sex, and ethnicity; ABI less than 0.9; or lifetime risk of ASCVD. Additional factors that might aid in individual risk assessment could be identified in the future.
§High-risk individuals include those with clinical ASCVD, an untreated LDL-C 190 mg/dl or greater, suggesting genetic hypercholesterolemia, or individuals with diabetes 40 to 75 yr of age and LDL-C 70 to 189 mg/dl.
From 2013 ACC/AHA guideline on the treatment of blood cholesterol to reduce atherosclerotic cardiovascular risk in adults: a report of the American College of Cardiology/American Heart Association Task Force on Practice Guidelines, *J Am Coll Cardiol* 63(25 Pt B):2889-2934, 2014.

TABLE 2 Atherosclerotic Cardiovascular Disease

1. Coronary heart disease: Acute coronary syndromes, history of myocardial infarction, stable or unstable angina, coronary or other arterial revascularization
2. Stroke or transient ischemic attack
3. Peripheral arterial disease

CHRONIC Rx

- Box 1 summarizes the key recommendations for the treatment of blood cholesterol to reduce ASCVD risk in adults.
- The guidelines identify four high-risk groups that benefit from statin therapy:
  1. Patients with clinical ASCVD (Table 2, Fig. 1)
  2. LDL ≥190 mg/dl
  3. DM aged 40 to 75 yr and LDL 70 to 189 mg/dl

  4. 10-yr risk for ASCVD ≥7.5% and LDL 70 to 189 mg/dl
- The 10-yr risk of ASCVD is calculated with the risk calculator available at http://my.americanheart.org/cvriskcalculator.
- ASCVD events are reduced by using the maximum tolerated statin intensity in the aforementioned groups shown to benefit the most (Tables 3 and 4).

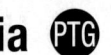

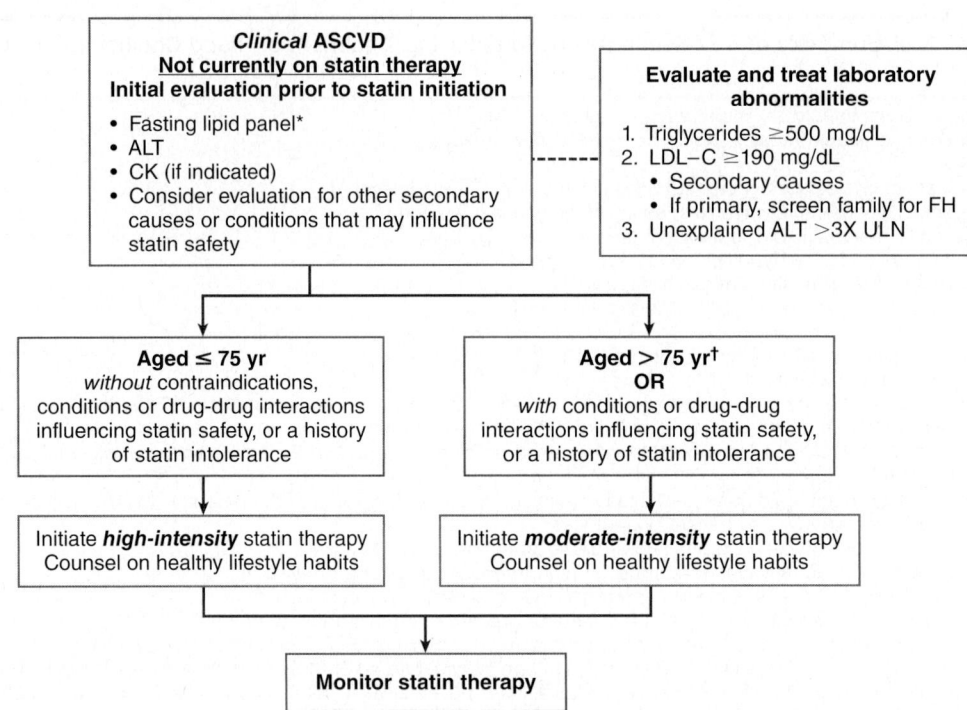

FIG. 1 Initiating statin therapy in individuals with clinical ASCVD. *Fasting lipid panel is preferred. In a nonfasting individual, a nonfasting non–HDL-C >220 mg/dl may indicate genetic hypercholesterolemia that requires further evaluation or a secondary etiology. If nonfasting triglycerides are >500 mg/dl, a fasting lipid panel is required. †It is reasonable to evaluate the potential for ASCVD benefits and for adverse effects and to consider patient preferences in initiating or continuing a moderate- or high-intensity statin in individuals with ASCVD >75 yr of age. *ALT,* Alanine transaminase; *ASCVD,* atherosclerotic cardiovascular disease; *CK,* creatine kinase; *FH,* familial hypercholesterolemia; *HDL-C,* high-density lipoprotein cholesterol; *LDL-C,* low-density lipoprotein cholesterol; *ULN,* upper limit of normal. (Modified from Stone NJ et al: 2013 ACC/AHA guideline on the treatment of blood cholesterol to reduce atherosclerotic cardiovascular risk in adults: a report of the American College of Cardiology/American Heart Association Task Force on Practice Guidelines, *J Am Coll Cardiol,* 2013. In Libby P et al: *Braunwald's heart disease, a textbook of cardiovascular medicine,* ed 10, Philadelphia, 2015, Elsevier.)

TABLE 3 Statin Benefit Groups and Recommended Therapy

Statin Benefit Group	High Intensity	Moderate Intensity	Additional Testing
Clinical ASCVD	Yes	Consider[†]	None
Primary LDL-C >190 mg/dl	Yes	Consider[†]	None
Diabetes without ASCVD and 10-yr risk ≥7.5%*	Yes	Consider[†]	None
Diabetes without ASCVD and 10-yr risk <7.5%*	Consider[‡]	Yes	Case by case
Primary prevention and 10-yr risk ≥7.5%*	Consider[‡]	Yes	Case by case
Primary prevention and 10-yr risk <7.5%*	Consider[‡]	Consider[‡]	Case by case

ASCVD, Atherosclerotic cardiovascular disease; *LDL-C,* low-density lipoprotein cholesterol.
*Based on Pooled Cohort Risk Equations.
[†]If age >75 yr or not candidate for high intensity.
[‡]If abnormal high-sensitivity C-reactive protein, coronary artery calcium, ankle-brachial index, lifetime risk.
From Boyden TF et al: Implementing new guidelines in the management of blood cholesterol, *Am J Med* 127:705, 2014.

- Additional factors such as C-reactive protein >2 mg/L, primary LDL >160, genetic hyperlipidemias, family history of premature coronary heart disease (CHD), ankle-brachial index <0.9, and coronary artery calcium score (CAD) assessed with computed tomography may be used in patients who are not in one of four statin benefit groups and for whom a decision to initiate statin therapy is otherwise unclear. Statins are generally beneficial in patients at intermediate risk and selected patients with borderline risk who have a calcium score that is 100 or higher or who are in the 75th percentile or higher for their age, sex, and race. Statins should also

be considered in persons with scores of 1 to 99, particularly if they are age 55 yr or older.
- Percent reduction in LDL cholesterol is used as a guide to compliance and adherence to therapy in the 2018 AHA/ACC Revised Clinical Practice Guidelines (Fig. E2). Studies have shown that compared with less intensive LDL-C lowering, more intensive lowering reduces all-cause mortality and cardiovascular mortality; patients with higher baseline LDL-C have greater benefit.
- Moderate-intensity statin therapy should be continued for individuals >75 yr of age for secondary prevention. However, factors such as comorbidities, safety, and priorities of care

should be considered before initiating statins for primary prevention of ASCVD.
- Adherence to lifestyle and to statin therapy should be reiterated with patients before the addition of a nonstatin drug.
- High-risk patients with a suboptimal response to statins who are unable to tolerate a recommended intensity or who are completely statin intolerant may benefit from the addition of a nonstatin cholesterol-lowering agent such as ezetimibe and/or Protein Convertase Subtilisin/Kexin 9 (PCSKS 9) inhibitor to reduce risk for major cardiovascular events.[3] Combination therapies for LDL are summarized in Table 5.

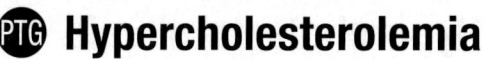

TABLE 4 High-, Moderate-, and Low-Intensity Statin Therapy*

	Daily Dose		
Statin Therapy	High Intensity† ↓LDL-C ≥50%	Moderate Intensity‡ ↓LDL-C 30<50%	Low Intensity§ ↓LDL-C <30%
Atorvastatin	**(40ǁ)-80 mg**	**10** *(20)* **mg**	
Rosuvastatin	**20** *(40)* **mg**	*(5)* **10 mg**	
Simvastatin		**20-40 mg¶**	*10 mg*
Pravastatin		**40** *(80)* **mg**	**10-20 mg**
Lovastatin		**40 mg**	**20 mg**
Fluvastatin		*80 mg (Fluvastatin XL)*	**20-40 mg**
Fluvastatin		**40 mg****	
Pitavastatin		**2-4 mg**	*1 mg*

FDA, U.S. Food and Drug Administration; *LDL-C*, low-density lipoprotein cholesterol; *XL*, extended-release.

*Individual responses to statin therapy varied in randomized, controlled trials and vary in clinical practice. A less-than-average response may have a biologic basis. Statins and dosages in bold were reduced in major cardiovascular events in randomized, controlled trials. Statins and doses in italics were approved by the FDA but were not tested in randomized, controlled trials.

†Daily dose decreases LDL-C levels by an average of ≥50%.

‡Daily dose decreases LDL-C levels by an average of 30 to <50%.

§Daily dose decreases LDL-C levels by an average of <30%.

ǁEvidence from 1 randomized, controlled trial only; down-titration if patient is unable to tolerate atorvastatin, 80 mg.

¶Although simvastatin, 80 mg, was evaluated in randomized, controlled trials, the FDA recommends against initiation of or titration to 80 mg of simvastatin because of increased risk for myopathy and rhabdomyolysis.

**Twice daily.

Reprinted with permission of the authors: Stone NJ et al: 2013 ACC/AHA guideline on the treatment of blood cholesterol to reduce atherosclerotic cardiovascular risk in adults: a report of the American College of Cardiology/American Heart Association Task Force on Practice Guidelines, *J Am Coll Cardiol* 63(25, Part B):2889-2934, 2014.

- Ezetimibe inhibits cholesterol absorption in the intestine, whereas statins inhibit cholesterol production primarily in the liver. Ezetimibe is not as effective as most statins, but will reduce LDL by 15% to 22%. It can reduce the risk of heart attacks and strokes when taken alongside a statin, but there is little evidence it can do this if used on its own.
- PCSK9 binds to LDL receptors on hepatocytes, promotes receptor degradation, and prevents LDL-C clearance from the circulation thereby increasing serum concentrations of LDL-C. PCSK9 monoclonal antibody inhibitors alirocumab (Praluent), evolocumab (Repatha), and inclisiran (Leqvio), a PCSK9-directed small interfering RNA, are currently indicated as adjunct to diet and maximally tolerated statin therapy for the treatment of adults with heterozygous familial hypercholesterolemia or clinical atherosclerotic cardiovascular disease, who require additional lowering of LDL cholesterol. PCSK9 inhibitors lower risk for ischemic cardiovascular events in persons with stable CAD and elevated atherogenic lipoproteins despite statin therapy. These medications are administered by subcutaneous injection and are expensive.
- The management of metabolic syndrome includes weight reduction, increased physical activity, and treatment of hypertension, elevated triglycerides, and low HDL cholesterol.
- According to recent studies, each 40 mg/dl reduction in LDL cholesterol by statin therapy confers a 20% reduction in ASCVD. In other words, a relative risk reduction of 30% in ASCVD by moderate-intensity therapy and 45% by high-intensity therapy has been approximated.
- Recent trials have shown that bempedoic acid, an inhibitor of ATP citrate lyase, reduces LDL cholesterol. The addition of bempedoic acid to maximally tolerated statin therapy did not lead to a higher incidence of overall adverse events than placebo and led to significant lowering of LDL cholesterol.
- Recent trials have shown that bempedoic acid, an inhibitor of ATP citrate lyase, reduces LDL cholesterol. The use of bempedoic acid in statin intolerant patients or the addition of bempedoic acid to maximally tolerated statin therapy did not lead to a higher incidence of overall adverse events than placebo and led to significant lowering of LDL cholesterol. However recent clinical trials[4] have shown that bempedoic acid when used alone does not reduce the risk of cardiovascular death or death from any cause.
- Table 6 summarizes oral drugs affecting lipoprotein metabolism.

DISPOSITION & FOLLOW-UP

- Baseline LFT testing should be done before initiation of statin therapy and as clinically indicated thereafter.
- Creatine kinase level monitoring is not recommended unless a patient reports muscle weakness or myalgias.
- Statin therapy should be monitored by repeating a lipid profile within 4 to 12 wk after initiation of therapy.
- Counseling about behavioral lifestyle changes and risk factors for CHD should be provided at every follow-up visit.
- Adverse effects of statin-associated diabetes vary by statin intensity: One excess case of diabetes per 1000 treated individuals with moderate-intensity statin and three excess cases of diabetes per 1000 treated individuals with high-intensity statin per year has been reported. Myopathy and hemorrhagic stroke incidence is around one excess case per 10,000 treated individuals.

- Per new guidelines, those who develop diabetes during statin therapy should be advised to continue moderate to high intensity statins to reduce their risk of ASCVD events and should adhere to a heart-healthy diet, engage in physical activity, cease tobacco use, and maintain a healthy body weight (Table 6).
- Regarding choice of statin, Atorvastatin and Rosuvastatin are preferred in most patients with moderate to high; hypercholesterolemia for patients on simvastatin with moderate to high. Maintain patients on 80 mg daily of simvastatin only if they have been taking this dose for 12 or more mo without evidence of muscle toxicity. Do not start new patients on simvastatin 80 mg. Place patients who do not meet their LDL goal on simvastatin 40 mg on alternative LDL-C-lowering treatment(s) to reach goal.

REFERRAL

Patients with rare lipid disorders, hyperlipoproteinemias, patients resistant to treatment, on complex regimens, and with evidence of disease progression despite treatment should be referred to a lipid specialist.

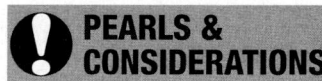 **PEARLS & CONSIDERATIONS**

COMMENTS

- New features in the 2018 clinical practice guidelines compared to the 2013 guidelines support the addition of nonstatin medications (ezetimibe or PCSK9 inhibitors) to statin therapy for secondary prevention in patients at very high risk. In primary prevention, a clinical patient risk discussion is strongly recommended before a decision is made about statin treatment. Among intermediate-risk patients, identification of risk-enhancing factors and coronary calcium testing is recommended when considering the use of a statin.
- Familial hypercholesterolemia (FH) is characterized by elevated cholesterol concentrations early in life. Untreated FH is associated with premature cardiovascular disease in adulthood. Screening can detect FH in children, and lipid-lowering treatment in childhood can reduce lipid concentrations in the short term, with little evidence of harm. A 20-yr follow-up study of statin therapy has shown that initiation of statin therapy during childhood in patients with FH slows the progression of carotid intima media thickness and reduces the risk of cardiovascular disease in adulthood.
- The American Academy of Pediatrics (AAP) guideline recommends consideration toward pharmacologic treatment for children with LDL >190 mg/dl or >160 mg/dl if other risk factors are present.
- *HDL cholesterol efflux capacity* refers to the ability of HDL to accept cholesterol from macrophages, which is a key step in reverse cholesterol transport. It is inversely associated with the incidence of cardiovascular events and may be a useful biomarker when added to traditional risk factors.

TABLE 5 Combination Therapies for LDL

Statin plus ezetimibe	Ezetimibe added to a statin may further reduce LDL by 20% or more and reduce triglycerides by 7%-13%. The combination provides equivalent LDL reduction to a fourfold increase in statin dose. Daily ezetimibe added to a low-dose statin given 2-3 times/wk can improve tolerance. Combination pills containing statin and ezetimibe are available. Most common side effects reflect those of the individual drugs. Combination ezetimibe and simvastatin has been shown to decrease cardiovascular events in patients with renal disease and acute coronary syndrome.
Statin and PCSK9 inhibitors	This combination is the most effective known treatment for hypercholesterolemia. There are no known negative interactions between these two therapies. This combination reduces CHD events more than statin alone.
Statin plus bile acid sequestrants	Bile acid sequestrants in combination with statins further decrease LDL from 24% to 60%. Cholestyramine and colestipol can interfere with the absorption of statins. Colesevelam does not affect statin absorption. The statin-colesevelam combination is not ideal for patients with high triglycerides but may be useful in those with type 2 diabetes mellitus because colesevelam reduces glycemia.
Statin plus niacin	Adding niacin to a statin can lower LDL by 10% to 20%, in addition to beneficial effects on triglycerides. When used in combination with a statin, the maximum dose of niacin should be 2000 mg/day. This combination in subjects with already low LDL levels did not reduce CHD events.
Bile acid sequestrants plus niacin	Before the availability of statins, bile acid sequestrants plus niacin were used to lower LDL in high-risk patients. The availability of colesevelam and extended-release niacin has made this combination tolerable for many patients who are unable to use statins.
Ezetimibe plus bile acid sequestrants	Ezetimibe inhibits cholesterol absorption, and sequestrants enhance cholesterol excretion through conversion to bile acids. The combination can have additive effects. This combination is useful for patients who cannot take statins.

CHD, Coronary heart disease; *LDL,* low-density lipoprotein; *PCSK9,* proprotein convertase subtilisin/kexin type 9.
From Melmed S et al: *Williams textbook of endocrinology,* ed 14, St Louis, 2019, Elsevier.

TABLE 6 Drugs Affecting Lipoprotein Metabolism

Drug Class	Agents and Daily Doses	Lipid/Lipoprotein Effects	Side Effects	Contraindications
HMG-CoA reductase inhibitors (statins)	Lovastatin (10-40 mg) Pravastatin (10-80 mg) Simvastatin[†] (5-80 mg) Fluvastatin (20-40 mg) Atorvastatin (10-80 mg) Rosuvastatin (5-40 mg) Pitavastatin (2-4 mg)	LDL↓ 20%-60% HDL↑ 5%-15% TG↓ 7%-30%	Myalgias, myositis Increased liver enzymes New-onset diabetes (with intensive therapy) Unproven concerns about memory loss	Active or chronic liver disease Pregnancy Concomitant use of certain drugs*
Bile acid sequestrants	Colestipol (5-20 g) Colesevelam[‡] (2.6-3.8 g) Cholestyramine (4-16 g)	LDL↓ 15%-30% HDL↑ 3%-5% TG No change or increase	Gastrointestinal distress, constipation, drug interaction, hypertriglyceridemia Decreased absorption of fat-soluble vitamins	TG >300 mg/dl GI motility disorder
Omega-3 fatty acids	Fish oils (4-6 g)	TG↓ 45% HDL↑ 13%	Increased bleeding time Nausea	Caution with anticoagulant therapy
Nicotinic acid	Immediate release (niacin) (1.5-3 g) Extended release (Niaspan) (1-2 g)	LDL↓ 5%-25% HDL↑ 15%-35% TG↓ 20%-50%	Flushing Hyperglycemia Hyperuricemia (or gout) Upper GI distress Hepatotoxicity	Chronic liver disease Severe gout Diabetes Peptic ulcer disease Pregnancy/lactation
Fibric acids	Gemfibrozil (600 mg bid) Fenofibrate (45-145 mg)	LDL↓ 5%-20% HDL↑ 10%-20% TG↓ 20%-50%	Dyspepsia Gallstones Myopathy (especially with concomitant use of gemfibrozil and statins)	Severe renal disease (dose adjustment for fenofibrate) Severe hepatic disease Caution with statins Can worsen LDL cholesterol
Ezetimibe (cholesterol absorption inhibitor)	Ezetimibe (10 mg)	LDL↓ 18% HDL↑ 1% TG↓ 8%	Abdominal pain; myalgias	Liver disease Avoid with resins and fibrates

GI, Gastrointestinal; *HDL,* high-density lipoprotein; *HMG-CoA,* 3-hydroxy-3-methylglutaryl coenzyme A; *LDL,* low-density lipoprotein; *TG,* triglyceride.
*Cyclosporine, macrolide antibiotics, various antifungal agents, and cytochrome P-450 inhibitors (fibrates and niacin should be used with appropriate caution).
†Dosages of simvastatin 80 mg are no longer recommended. Potential interactions with amlodipine and ranolazine warrant doses ≤2 mg daily.
‡Colesevelam reduces glucose and A1c ;0.5% and has been approved for treatment of diabetes with dyslipidemia.
Modified from The National Cholesterol Education Program, *JAMA* 285:2486, 2001. In Boyden TF et al: Implementing new guidelines in the management of blood cholesterol, *Am J Med* 127:705, 2014.

- There are currently no pharmacologic therapies approved to reduce Lp(a) and ASCVD risk. Although PCSK9 monoclonal antibodies reduce Lp(a), they are not approved for use among individuals who meet LDL cholesterol targets. Niacin modestly reduces Lp(a) but may not further reduce ASCVD risk in addition to statins.[5,6]

REFERENCES & SUGGESTED READINGS

Available at eBooks.Health.Elsevier.com.

RELATED CONTENT

High Cholesterol (Patient Information)

Coronary Artery Disease (Related Key Topic)
Hyperlipoproteinemia, Primary (Related Key Topic)
Statin-Induced Muscle Syndrome (Related Key Topic)

AUTHOR: **FRED F. FERRI, MD**

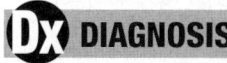

H

I

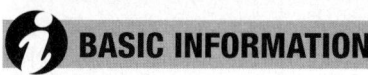 **BASIC INFORMATION**

DEFINITION

Hypercoagulable state is an inherited or acquired condition associated with an increased risk of thrombosis. A classification of hypercoagulable states is described in Table 1.

SYNONYM

Thrombophilia

ICD-10CM CODES
D68.5	Primary thrombophilia
D68.6	Other thrombophilia
D68.8	Other specified coagulation defects
D68.9	Coagulation defect, unspecified

EPIDEMIOLOGY & DEMOGRAPHICS

INCIDENCE, PREVALENCE, & PREDOMINANT SEX & AGE: See Table 2. Significant variations in the prevalence rates and thrombotic risks for hypercoagulable states are reported. This may reflect geographic variation in the prevalence of genetic defects, different populations, or the presence of other unidentified thrombophilic risk factors. When thrombosis occurs, it is often associated with an acquired risk factor (e.g., surgery, pregnancy, oral contraceptive [OCP] use).

RISK FACTORS: Family history of thrombosis, increasing age, tobacco use, immobility, surgery, prior history of deep vein thrombosis (DVT), pregnancy, hormone replacement therapy, trauma, connective tissue disease, underlying malignancy, medications (megestrol acetate, tamoxifen, oral contraceptives). Potential prothrombotic states are summarized in Table 3.

PHYSICAL FINDINGS & CLINICAL PRESENTATION

- Inherited thrombophilia is usually associated with venous thromboembolism (VTE), most commonly DVT[1]
- Some acquired thrombophilias are associated with arterial thrombosis[1]
- Pregnancy complications[1]
- Medical conditions associated with increased risk of thrombosis

ETIOLOGY

- Thrombosis is often a multifactorial process with genetic, environmental, and acquired factors. Table E4, Table E5, Table E6, and Table E7 describe causes of acquired and inherited deficiencies in antithrombin, protein C, and protein S.
- All thrombotic factors ultimately lead to blood flow stasis, endothelial damage, or change in blood constituents to cause thrombosis. These three components of thrombosis are known as the Virchow triad.

- Thrombotic risk increases with use of OCPs or hormone replacement therapy (HRT) and during the pregnancy/postpartum period.[1]
- Adverse pregnancy outcomes may be caused by thrombosis of the uteroplacental circulation.

DIAGNOSIS

DIFFERENTIAL DIAGNOSIS

INHERITED: Factor V Leiden (FVL) mutation:[2-4]
- Autosomal-dominant mutation with incomplete penetrance
- Causes activated protein C resistance (APCR); 90% of APCR is caused by FVL mutation
- Most common inherited thrombophilia; accounts for 40% to 50% of cases

TABLE 3 Potential Prothrombotic States

Congenital

Deficiency of anticoagulants
AT-III, protein C or protein S, plasminogen
Resistance to cofactor proteolysis
Factor V Leiden
High levels of procoagulants
Prothrombin 20210 mutation
Damage to endothelium

Acquired

Obstruction to flow indwelling lines
Pregnancy
Polycythemia/dehydration
Immobilization
Injury
Trauma, surgery, exercise
Inflammation
IBD, vasculitis, infection, Behçet syndrome
Hypercoagulability
Malignancy
Antiphospholipid syndrome
Nephrotic syndrome
Oral contraceptives
L-Asparaginase

Rare Other Entities

Congenital dysfibrinogenemia
Acquired
Paroxysmal nocturnal hemoglobinuria
Thrombocythemia
Vascular grafts

AT-III, Antithrombin III; *IBD,* inflammatory bowel disease.
From Kliegman, RM: *Nelson textbook of pediatrics,* ed 19, Philadelphia, 2011, Saunders.

TABLE 1 Classification of Hypercoagulable States

Hereditary	Mixed	Acquired
Loss of Function		
Antithrombin deficiency	Hyperhomocysteinemia	Previous venous thromboembolism
Protein C deficiency	Obesity	Pregnancy, puerperium
Protein S deficiency	Cancer	Drug-induced:
		Heparin-induced thrombocytopenia
		Prothrombin complex concentrates
		L-Asparaginase
		Hormonal therapy
Gain of Function		
Factor V Leiden	Postoperative	
Prothrombin FII G20210A	Myeloproliferative disorders	
Elevated factor VIII, IX, or XI		

From Hoffman R et al: *Hematology, basic principles and practice,* ed 8, Philadelphia, 2023, Elsevier.

TABLE 2 Hypercoagulable Conditions

	Prevalence in General Population (%)	Prevalence in Population with Thrombosis (%)	A/V Events	Relative Risk of Thrombosis
FVL mutation	5% of Whites; rare in non-Whites	12%-40%	V	Heterozygous: 3-7; homozygous: 80
Prothrombin G20210A mutation	3% of Whites; rare in non-Whites	6%-18%	V	3
AT deficiency	0.02%	1%-3%	V	20-50
PC deficiency	0.2%-0.4%	3%-5%	V	7-15
PS deficiency	0.03%-0.1%	1%-5%	V	5-11
Antiphospholipid antibody syndrome	1%-2%	5%-21%	V + A	2-11

A, Arterial; *AT,* antithrombin; *FVL,* factor V Leiden; *PC,* protein C; *PS,* protein S; *V,* venous.

- Risk of VTE is sevenfold greater in heterozygous carriers compared with noncarriers; however, the risk increases to 30-fold in heterozygous carriers who use OCP compared with noncarriers who do not use OCP
- Risk of VTE is increased 100-fold in homozygous women who use OCP
- May be associated with cardiovascular disease in select high-risk subgroups

Prothrombin G20210A mutation:[5-8]
- Autosomal-dominant mutation with incomplete penetrance
- OC use in heterozygous carriers is associated with a sixfold increased risk of VTE compared with noncarriers not using OCPs
- May be associated with cardiovascular disease in select high-risk subgroups and young patients with ischemic stroke
- Causes increased mRNA accumulation and protein synthesis, leading to elevated prothrombin plasma concentrations

Protein C, protein S, antithrombin (AT) deficiency:[5,9]
- Autosomal-dominant inheritance; many mutations identified for each of these conditions
- Decreased level (type I deficiency) or abnormal function (type II deficiency)
- First episode of thrombosis is usually in young adults

Protein C and protein S[9,10] deficiency:
- Homozygous condition is very rare; usually associated with lethal thrombosis in infancy
- Associated with warfarin-induced skin necrosis, which occurs secondary to depletion of vitamin K–dependent anticoagulant factors sooner than procoagulant factors in the first few days of therapy

AT deficiency:[10]
- Most thrombogenic of the inherited thrombophilias; 50% lifetime risk of thrombosis.
- Homozygous condition is very rare, probably not compatible with normal fetal development.
- Arterial thrombosis can occur rarely.
- Can cause heparin resistance.

Other possible causes: Non-O blood group, dysfibrinogenemia, elevated thrombin-activatable fibrinolysis inhibitor, elevated factor IX and factor XI levels

ACQUIRED: Antiphospholipid antibody syndrome (APS):[10]
- Most common cause of acquired thrombophilia
- Can present as arterial or venous thrombosis, recurrent pregnancy loss, and adverse pregnancy outcomes
- Thromboembolic events occur in up to 30% of population; high risk of recurrent thrombosis (up to 70% reported)
- See "Antiphospholipid Antibody Syndrome" for more information

Conditions associated with increased risk of thrombosis:
- Prior thrombosis
- Trauma
- Medical illness: Heart failure, respiratory failure, infection, diabetes mellitus, obesity, nephrotic syndrome, inflammatory bowel disease
- Chronic hemolysis–paroxysmal nocturnal hemoglobinuria, atypical hemolytic uremic syndrome, sickle cell anemia

- Pregnancy (sixfold increased risk of VTE), postpartum, OCP use (fourfold increased risk, higher risk with third-generation OCPs), transdermal contraceptive patch, HRT (twofold increased risk), tamoxifen, raloxifene
- Immobilization, travel
- Surgery (especially orthopedic), central venous catheters
- Hyperviscosity syndromes
- Myeloproliferative neoplasms
- Malignancy: Disease or treatment related
- Heparin-induced thrombocytopenia and thrombosis
- Smoking

WORKUP

- History (presence of conditions or use of medications predisposing to thrombosis, family history of thrombosis), physical examination, laboratory tests, imaging studies. Routine investigations to evaluate a patient with thrombosis are summarized in Box 1.
- Age-appropriate cancer screening.
- No consensus exists regarding screening for thrombophilia; few cost-effectiveness or outcomes data are available. Thrombophilia screening is probably overused, as results usually do not change management.[1]
- Thrombophilia screening is not recommended for primary prevention of VTE; some advocate testing prior to OCP use or pregnancy in women with a strong family history of thrombosis or thrombophilia.[1,11,12] Box 2 summarizes recommendations regarding when to perform a thrombophilia screen. Essential tests for thrombophilia screening are described in Box 3.
- Screening not recommended if VTE was associated with an identified risk factor. A possible exception is thrombosis associated with pregnancy, the postpartum period, or with OCP use.[1,11,12]
- Reasonable to pursue workup for VTE with weak triggers, a strong family history, and

female family members of childbearing age; consider testing for FVL, prothrombin G20210A mutation, protein C, protein S, and AT deficiency. Consider testing for APS if extensive DVT or pulmonary embolism (PE).[1,11,12]
- Unprovoked VTE:
  1. Screen individuals for APCR, prothrombin G20210A mutation, protein C, protein S, AT deficiency, and APS if any of the following are present: <50 yr of age at first episode of thrombosis + strong family history of thrombosis or female family member of childbearing age, thrombosis in unusual anatomic location (cerebral veins or splanchnic veins; if splanchnic veins, consider testing as well for myeloproliferative neoplasms [MPN] and paroxysmal nocturnal hemoglobinuria [PNH]).[1]
  2. Screen all others for APS.[1]
- Arterial thrombosis: Screen for APS.[1]

NOTE: Routine screening for factor VIII level or hyperhomocysteinemia is not recommended.[10]

TIMING OF WORKUP: Ideally >2 wk after discontinuation of vitamin K antagonists (VKA) and >2 days after discontinuation of direct oral anticoagulant (DOAC) (except for APS, which requires prolonged anticoagulation).[1]

NOTE: Acute thrombosis, anticoagulation, pregnancy, and many medical conditions can affect the results and must be considered in the timing and interpretation of the workup.[1,12]

LABORATORY TESTS

- Initial workup: CBC with peripheral smear, electrolytes, calcium, creatinine, blood urea nitrogen (BUN), liver function tests, prothrombin time/partial thromboplastin time, prostate-specific antigen (in men aged >50 yr), urinalysis.[10]
- NOTE: Genetic counseling and written informed consent should be obtained before genetic testing. Abnormal nongenetic tests should be repeated after 6 wk to decrease false-positive results.[13]

BOX 1 Routine Investigations to Evaluate a Patient with Thrombosis

Test	Abnormality	Diagnostic Information
Complete blood count	Elevated hematocrit Increased white count Increased platelet count Leukopenia Thrombocytopenia	Myeloproliferative disorder (e.g., essential thrombocythemia, polycythemia vera); may be found in paroxysmal nocturnal hemoglobinuria; if associated with heparin administration, consider heparin-induced thrombocytopenia
Blood film	Leukoerythroblastic changes	Underlying neoplasm invading bone marrow
Liver function tests	Abnormal tests	May point to malignancy
Renal function	Impaired renal function	Assess prior to anticoagulation with heparin, low-molecular-weight heparin or new oral anticoagulants
Urinalysis	Proteinuria	Nephrotic syndrome; may be associated with venous thromboembolism or renal vein thrombosis
PT and aPTT	Prolonged PT and aPTT	To enable safe anticoagulation to proceed if required Need to exclude lupus anticoagulant

aPTT, Activated partial thromboplastin time; *PT,* prothrombin time.
From Hoffman R et al: *Hematology, basic principles and practice,* ed 8, Philadelphia, 2023, Elsevier.

BOX 2 When to Perform a Thrombophilia Screen

Clinical Scenario
- First episode of unprovoked venous thromboembolism in individuals younger than 40 yr of age
- Thrombosis in an unusual site (e.g., cerebral or mesenteric thrombosis)
- Two or more first-degree relatives with unprovoked thrombosis
- Three or more early pregnancy losses, or one or more fetal deaths after 10 wk gestation

From Hoffman R et al: *Hematology, basic principles and practice*, ed 8, Philadelphia, 2023, Elsevier.

BOX 3 Essential Tests for Thrombophilia Screening

- Basic coagulation screen
  1. International normalized ratio (INR): To exclude warfarin effect—warfarin will lower protein C and S levels
  2. Activated partial thromboplastin time (aPTT): To exclude heparin effect—heparin will lower antithrombin levels
- Functional assay for antithrombin (with heparin to detect type II defects)
- Functional assay for protein C
- Functional assay for protein S (immune assays for total and free protein S)
- APC resistance assay: With genetic test for factor V Leiden for confirmation of abnormal results
- Genetic test for *FIIG 20210A* gene mutation
- Anticardiolipin and β_2-glycoprotein-1 antibodies (IgG and IgM) and lupus anticoagulant assay

From Hoffman R et al: *Hematology: basic principles and practice*, ed 8, Philadelphia, 2023, Elsevier.

- APC-resistance assay tests for factor V Leiden mutation. Presence of lupus anticoagulant causes false positives. Follow-up positive result with a confirmatory genetic test.[10]
- Prothrombin G20210A mutation testing.[10]
- AT, protein C, and protein S deficiency: Functional assays are initial tests, then follow up positive result with antigenic assay to determine the type of deficiency. Note that antigenic assays for protein S should measure free and total levels. The functional assays for protein C and S deficiency testing may be falsely low in the presence of APCR or elevated factor VIII level and falsely high if lupus anticoagulant is present.[10]
- APS: Any one of the following found elevated on two occasions at least 12 wk apart: Lupus anticoagulant, anticardiolipin antibodies (IgG/IgM isotype), or anti–β_2-glycoprotein-I antibodies (IgG/IgM isotype).[10]

IMAGING STUDIES

Chest radiograph and other tests as appropriate to diagnose thrombosis and rule out associated conditions.

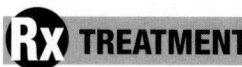 **TREATMENT**

NONPHARMACOLOGIC THERAPY

OC/HRT use and smoking should be avoided.[1]
PROPHYLAXIS:
- Prophylactic anticoagulation in high-risk situations.[1]
- Patients with AT deficiency may benefit from antithrombin concentrates in high-risk situations.[14]
- Pregnancy prophylaxis: Timing and intensity of therapy are based on the patient's risk

(genetic or acquired defect and clinical history). Women with thrombophilia and recurrent adverse pregnancy outcomes may benefit from prophylaxis with heparin (low-molecular-weight heparin most commonly used) and low-dose aspirin.[11]

ACUTE GENERAL Rx

Initial therapy is the same as for individuals with and without thrombophilia, with exceptions for protein C, AT deficiency, and APS as detailed in the following:
Venous thrombosis:
- DOACs such as Xa inhibitors (rivaroxaban and apixaban) have been FDA-approved for treatment in acute DVT and are currently recommended as first-line therapy. They have been found to be noninferior to warfarin, appear easier to use with fewer drug interactions, and have a trend toward less major bleeding.[15]
- In patients unable to take DOACs, begin low-molecular-weight heparin (LMWH) and warfarin simultaneously. Continue heparin for at least 5 days and until international normalized ratio (INR) is therapeutic for 2 consecutive days; continue warfarin for at least 3 mo. Aim for INR of 2 to 3. Unfractionated heparin (UH) or fondaparinux (factor Xa inhibitor) may be used as alternatives to LMWH. LMWH is preferred over UH (except in patients with massive pulmonary embolism, increased risk of bleeding, or renal failure) because of equivalent or superior effectiveness and a better safety profile.
- Thrombophilia is not associated with a higher risk of recurrent VTE during warfarin therapy, with the exception of cancer patients in whom LMWH for 3 to 6 mo is associated with

lower rates of recurrence than warfarin therapy.[15]
- In pregnancy, anticoagulate with heparin throughout pregnancy and for at least 6 wk postpartum. Minimum duration of anticoagulation should be 6 mo. LMWH is preferred over UH. Warfarin may be used postpartum.[9]
- Consider thrombolysis or thrombectomy in patients with massive pulmonary embolism or large proximal lower extremity DVT.[15]
Protein C deficiency:
- Warfarin-induced skin necrosis: Discontinue warfarin, give vitamin K, and start heparin anticoagulation. Consider protein C replacement with protein C concentrate or fresh frozen plasma. Warfarin may be restarted at a low dose (2 mg daily for 3 days and increase by 2 to 3 mg daily until target INR is reached). Continue heparin for at least 5 days and until warfarin-induced anticoagulation is achieved.
AT deficiency:
- AT concentrates may be used if difficulty achieving anticoagulation (heparin resistance), severe thrombosis, or recurrent thrombosis despite adequate anticoagulation.[9]
APS:
- Warfarin is superior to rivaroxaban in patients with APS. The RAPS trial randomized patients with triple positive APS to receive either rivaroxaban or warfarin and found significantly higher rates of thrombosis in the rivaroxaban group. A subsequent trial noted increased endogenous thrombin potential (a marker of less effective anticoagulation) in APS patients switched to rivaroxaban following initial VKA therapy compared to those continued on warfarin. This study was not powered to assess clinical efficacy. If a patient with triple positive APS is on DOAC, it is recommended to transition them to VKA therapy.[15]
Arterial thrombosis:
- Anticoagulation and evaluation for thrombolysis or surgery.

CHRONIC Rx

- Optimal duration of anticoagulation remains unknown. Length of therapy may be individualized by assessing the risk of recurrence. Residual thrombosis (on ultrasonography) or elevated d-dimer levels after completion of anticoagulation are associated with an increased risk of recurrence. With these findings, consider prolonging anticoagulation.
- Must consider risk and benefit; risk of major bleeding 2% to 3% annually in general population on anticoagulation but higher in the elderly (7% to 9% per yr). Long-term anticoagulation is usually not indicated given the low risk of recurrent thrombosis for most conditions and the bleeding risk associated with anticoagulation.
- Indefinite anticoagulation considered if any of the following:
  1. Life-threatening thrombosis or thrombosis at an unusual site
  2. More than a single genetic defect
  3. Presence of AT deficiency or APS
  4. Unprovoked DVT or PE with low bleeding risk

TABLE 8 Management of Women with a History of Venous Thrombosis During Pregnancy and the Puerperium

Clinical History	Thrombophilia	Antepartum	Postpartum[a]
Prior VTE due to a transient risk factor	No	Surveillance	Yes
Prior VTE due to pregnancy or estrogens	Yes or no	Prophylactic LMWH	Yes
Prior idiopathic VTE	Yes or no	Prophylactic LMWH	Yes
Recurrent VTE	Yes or no	Treatment dose LMWH	Resume long-term anticoagulation
No prior VTE Positive family history	Antithrombin deficiency; homozygous FII G20210A; or Factor V Leiden; or dual heterozygosity for both mutations	Prophylactic or intermediate dose LMWH	Yes

LMWH, Low-molecular-weight heparin; *VTE,* venous thromboembolism.
[a]Postpartum prophylaxis involves a 6-wk course of prophylactic doses of LMWH or dose-adjusted warfarin (target INR: 2.0-3.0).
From Hoffman R et al: *Hematology, basic principles and practice,* ed 8, Philadelphia, 2023, Elsevier.

5. >1 Provoked DVT or PE with low bleeding risk
- Patients with active cancer may benefit from indefinite anticoagulation.

DISPOSITION
Depends on underlying condition

REFERRAL
Hematology, maternal-fetal medicine, obstetric medicine

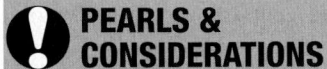

PEARLS & CONSIDERATIONS

COMMENTS
- Women with thrombophilic defects but no prior history of venous thromboembolism, or family history of the same, likely do not require antepartum prophylaxis or postpartum treatment, but definitive data are lacking. A summary of these recommendations is provided in Table 8.
- DOACs and warfarin therapy effectively reduce the risk of recurrent VTE; when therapy is discontinued VTE risk increases.
- Warfarin is preferred over DOAC for triple positive APS patients based on the data showing rivaroxaban to be inferior to warfarin in this population.[15]
- Previous episode of VTE is a major risk factor for recurrence regardless of the presence of thrombophilia. Risk is greatest in the first 2 yr after thrombosis. 40% of all patients with

unprovoked VTE have recurrence within 5 yr.[1]
- Genetic risk factors for thrombosis in non-white patients remain largely unknown.
- Interpreting workup: Many medical conditions cause acquired abnormalities.
  1. Acute thrombosis may be associated with lupus anticoagulant, increased anticardiolipin antibodies, and elevated factor VIII levels.[10]
     a. Heparin therapy: Antithrombin levels decrease by up to 30%; can affect lupus anticoagulant testing depending on available assay[10]
     b. Warfarin therapy: Cannot measure protein C and protein S (levels and function decrease); antithrombin levels may increase; can affect lupus anticoagulant testing
     c. Acute thrombosis: Antithrombin level, protein C, and protein S levels may be falsely lowered[10]
  2. Protein C, protein S, and antithrombin levels decrease with surgery, liver disease, disseminated intravascular coagulation, and chemotherapy. Protein C level also decreases with severe infection but levels increase with age and hyperlipidemia. Protein S and antithrombin levels also decrease with nephrotic syndrome, pregnancy, and estrogen therapy (HRT, OCs).[10]
  3. APCR is increased with pregnancy, estrogen therapy (HRT, OCs), and certain cancers; elevated factor VIII level and antiphospholipid antibodies can cause APCR.[10]

PREVENTION
Evidence is equivocal in regard to the effectiveness of compression stockings in preventing postthrombotic syndrome.

PATIENT & FAMILY EDUCATION
National Blood Clot Alliance
120 White Plains Road, Suite 100
Tarrytown, NY 10591
https://www.stoptheclot.org/contact.htm
National Collaborative Outreach Project of the Blood Clot Outreach Program at the Hemophilia and Thrombosis Center University of North Carolina at Chapel Hill
https://www.clotconnect.org/about-clot-connect/about
Factor V Leiden Resources
https://www.fvleiden.org/resources/index.html
APS Foundation of America, Inc.
P.O. Box 801
LaCrosse, WI 54602-0801
https://www.apsfa.org/

REFERENCES
Available at eBooks.Health.Elsevier.com.

RELATED CONTENT
Thrombophilia (Patient Information)
Antiphospholipid Antibody Syndrome (Related Key Topic)
Deep Vein Thrombosis (Related Key Topic)
Pulmonary Embolism (Related Key Topic)

AUTHORS: **SOVIJJA POU, MD** and **JOHN L. REAGAN, MD**

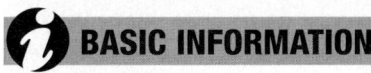
BASIC INFORMATION

DEFINITION

Hyperemesis gravidarum refers to a severe and persistent form of nausea and vomiting in pregnancy. While no precise criteria exist to define hyperemesis, it may be characterized by at least a 5% weight loss from prepregnancy weight, dehydration, ketonuria, and electrolyte imbalance. Typical onset occurs at wk 4 to 8 of pregnancy, continuing through wk 14 to 16 of pregnancy.

ICD-10CM CODES
O21.0 Mild hyperemesis gravidarum
O21.1 Hyperemesis gravidarum with metabolic disturbance

EPIDEMIOLOGY & DEMOGRAPHICS

INCIDENCE: 0.3% to 3% of pregnancies
RISK FACTORS: Women with increased placental mass, including molar pregnancy or multiple gestation, family history or personal history of hyperemesis gravidarum, prior miscarriage, nulliparity, young age, hyperthyroidism, gastrointestinal disorders, vestibular disease, motion sickness, long interpregnancy interval, and supertaster status. Alcohol use, smoking, and anosmia may be protective. A female fetus increases the risk by 1.27-fold.
GENETICS: A genetic predisposition may exist; hyperemesis gravidarum is more common among first-degree relatives of those diagnosed with the condition, and certain placental protein gene variants associated with hyperemesis have been identified.

PHYSICAL FINDINGS & CLINICAL PRESENTATION

- Weight loss of more than 5% from pregravid weight
- Symptoms: Nausea, vomiting, spitting, enhanced olfactory senses, food and/or fluid intolerance, lethargy
- Signs: Poor skin turgor, dry mucous membranes, hypotension, tachycardia
- Complications include inadequate caloric and nutritional intake, dehydration, and electrolyte abnormalities, including hyponatremia, hypocalcemia, hypokalemia, and, in severe cases, hypochloremic metabolic acidosis or Wernicke encephalopathy from thiamine deficiency. Severe hyperemesis gravidarum also has been shown to correlate with higher rates of anxiety and depression

ETIOLOGY

Unknown, but likely multifactorial. Theories include interactions between hCG and the thyroid, gestational hyperestrogenemia, and gastric dysrhythmias.

DIAGNOSIS

DIFFERENTIAL DIAGNOSIS

- Gastrointestinal conditions: Gastroenteritis, gastroparesis, biliary tract disease, hepatitis, intestinal obstruction, peptic ulcer disease, appendicitis, inflammatory bowel disease
- Genitourinary tract conditions: Pyelonephritis, nephrolithiasis
- Metabolic disease: Hyperthyroidism, hyperparathyroidism, diabetic ketoacidosis, cannabinoid hyperemesis syndrome, porphyria, adrenal insufficiency
- Neurologic conditions: Pseudotumor cerebri, vestibular lesions, migraines, tumors of the central nervous system, cyclic vomiting syndrome
- Miscellaneous: Drug toxicity or intolerance, psychogenic
- Pregnancy-related conditions: Acute fatty liver of pregnancy, preeclampsia

WORKUP

Diagnosis is one of exclusion. History and physical examination along with laboratory tests to rule out other causes of vomiting should be performed.

LABORATORY TESTS

- Basic metabolic panel (BMP) may reveal hyponatremia, hypokalemia, low serum urea.
- Urinalysis may show elevated specific gravity, ketonuria, or proteinuria.
- Liver enzymes (alanine transaminase [ALT] typically more elevated than aspartate aminotransferase [AST], both usually reaching only two to three times the upper limit of normal).
- Serum bilirubin (<4 mg/dl).
- Serum amylase or lipase (up to 5× greater than normal).
- CBC may show an increase in hematocrit from volume depletion.
- Magnesium and calcium may be low.
- Thyroid-stimulating hormone and free T_4 (transient hyperthyroidism occurs in two thirds of women with hyperemesis gravidarum; this is biochemical hyperthyroidism that usually resolves by 18 wk of gestation; testing and treatment should not be undertaken without additional clinical evidence of intrinsic thyroid disease).

IMAGING STUDIES

- Ultrasound to evaluate for multiple gestation or molar pregnancy
- If the patient is having associated pain, a right upper quadrant ultrasound may be indicated to evaluate biliary tract disease

TREATMENT

NONPHARMACOLOGIC THERAPY

- Prevention with prenatal vitamins before conception
- Avoidance of foods and smells that trigger nausea
- Ginger (200 to 500 mg q8h)
- Protein-heavy meals
- Frequent small meals, every 1 to 2 h
- Reassurance and support, in some cases intensive cognitive-behavioral therapy

ACUTE GENERAL Rx

- Pyridoxine (vitamin B₆) 10 to 25 mg PO q8h
- Doxylamine 12.5 to 25 mg qhs
- Pyridoxine (10 mg)/doxylamine (10 mg) combination, starting with two tablets qhs and adding an additional one tablet every A.M. and one tablet every P.M. if needed
- Antiemetics including promethazine, prochlorperazine, metoclopramide, and ondansetron have been shown to be generally safe and effective in improving pregnancy outcome
- Corticosteroids (methylprednisolone, prednisone) may be considered after 10 wk of gestation
- Intravenous (IV) fluid and electrolyte administration if evidence of deficiency is found
- Thiamine prior to dextrose administration to avoid Wernicke encephalopathy
- Restart oral intake gradually no less than 48 h after vomiting has stopped

CHRONIC Rx

- If unable to tolerate oral intake, consider replacing with enteral or parenteral feeding
- Repeated IV fluid and electrolyte replacement can be conducted through outpatient visits

COMPLEMENTARY & ALTERNATIVE MEDICINE

- Supportive psychotherapy
- Acupuncture
- Acupressure with use of a wrist band

DISPOSITION

- Infants born from pregnancies complicated by hyperemesis may have a higher risk of being small for gestational age or low birth weight than those not; however, this may be limited to infants of women who have experienced significant weight loss in the setting of hyperemesis.
- Women with hyperemesis gravidarum should be counseled that they have a higher risk than other women of developing similar symptoms in future pregnancies.

PEARLS & CONSIDERATIONS

COMMENTS

Nausea and vomiting in early pregnancy are associated with psychosocial morbidity.

RELATED CONTENT

Hyperemesis Gravidarum (Patient Information)

AUTHORS: **T. CAROLINE BANK, MD** and **MARWAN MA'AYEH, MD**

BASIC INFORMATION

DEFINITION

Hyperglycemic hyperosmolar syndrome (HHS) is a life-threatening complication of diabetes mellitus characterized by marked hyperglycemia, dehydration, electrolyte derangements, and hyperosmolality with or without mental obtundation, all in the absence of significant ketoacidosis. The main drivers of HHS are extreme hyperglycemia and resultant osmotic diuresis.[1]

SYNONYMS

HHS
Hyperosmolar hyperglycemic syndrome
Diabetic hyperosmolar syndrome
Hyperglycemic hyperosmolar nonketotic syndrome
Hyperglycemic hyperosmolar nonketotic coma
Hyperosmolar hyperglycemic state
Nonketotic hyperosmolar syndrome

ICD-10CM CODES
E08.00	Diabetes mellitus due to underlying condition with hyperosmolarity without nonketotic hyperglycemic-hyperosmolar coma (NKHHC)
E08.01	Diabetes mellitus due to underlying condition with hyperosmolarity with coma
E09.00	Drug or chemical induced diabetes mellitus with hyperosmolarity without nonketotic hyperglycemic-hyperosmolar coma (NKHHC)
E09.01	Drug or chemical induced diabetes mellitus with hyperosmolarity with coma
E11.00	Type 2 diabetes mellitus with hyperosmolarity without nonketotic hyperglycemic-hyperosmolar coma (NKHHC)
E11.01	Type 2 diabetes mellitus with hyperosmolarity with coma
E13.00	Other specified diabetes mellitus with hyperosmolarity without nonketotic hyperglycemic-hyperosmolar coma (NKHHC)
E13.01	Other specified diabetes mellitus with hyperosmolarity with coma

EPIDEMIOLOGY & DEMOGRAPHICS[1-4]

HHS is a rare condition that most commonly affects patients with type 2 diabetes mellitus, and it may be the first presentation of diabetes. Approximately 20% of patients have no history of diabetes. Onset of HHS is slower than that of diabetic ketoacidosis (DKA). Older adults with new-onset diabetes or those who have poorly controlled type 2 diabetes and are predisposed to extracellular fluid volume depletion (dehydration) are at increased risk for HHS. Mortality from HHS is estimated at 5% to 20%, a greater mortality rate than for diabetic ketoacidosis. Prognosis is determined by several factors, including age, degree of dehydration, and presence of other comorbidities. While mild ketosis and acidosis may present in HHS, progression to DKA is uncommon, yet reasons why remain unclear. Mixed DKA-HHS can occur (DKA criteria with elevated osmolality) and bodes a greater mortality than for either DKA or HHS alone. Social and racial-ethnic disparities are noted with Black race/ethnicity and lower-income individuals at heightened risk of HHS.

PHYSICAL FINDINGS & CLINICAL PRESENTATION[2]

- Polyuria, polydipsia, weight loss, weakness
- Mental status changes that can range from full alertness to coma
- Focal neurologic signs (e.g., hemiplegia, hemianopsia) or seizures (focal or generalized), aphasia, visual hallucinations
- Symptoms of coexisting illnesses or comorbidities that may have precipitated the event
- Signs of extracellular fluid volume depletion, including dry mucous membranes, poor skin turgor, sunken eyes, hypotension, and tachycardia
- Normothermia or hypothermia despite the presence of infection, due to peripheral vasodilation

ETIOLOGY

HHS can be precipitated by various conditions.[2]
- Infection is the most common precipitant (especially pneumonia, urinary tract infections, and COVID-19)
- Insulin deficiency (undiagnosed diabetes, inadequate insulin, or medication nonadherence)
- Inflammatory conditions (e.g., acute pancreatitis, acute cholecystitis)
- Ischemia/infarction (e.g., myocardial infarction, stroke, bowel ischemia)
- Kidney failure
- Severe dehydration (e.g., burns, heat stroke)
- Drugs (e.g., steroids, thiazides, beta blockers, atypical/conventional antipsychotics, sympathomimetics including cocaine, alcohol, and pentamidine)

A relative insulin deficiency provides enough insulin to inhibit significant ketogenesis but is insufficient to inhibit hepatic gluconeogenesis and glycogenolysis or to promote peripheral glucose uptake, resulting in consequent hyperglycemia. With underlying illness, counterregulatory hormone excess leads to further blood glucose elevation. The resultant extreme hyperglycemia leads to osmotic diuresis.[5,6] If adequate hydration is not maintained, dehydration and worsening renal function ensue. In patients with inadequate fluid intake due to altered thirst mechanisms or the inability to access fluids, as may be seen in older adults, the risk of severe dehydration further increases. Diminished renal filtration further impairs glucose excretion, thus exacerbating the hyperglycemia, dehydration, and hyperosmolality and increasing the risk for cardiovascular collapse.

DIAGNOSIS

DIFFERENTIAL DIAGNOSIS
- Diabetic ketoacidosis
- Stroke (especially in older adults with neurologic abnormalities)
- Hypovolemic or septic shock
- Encephalopathy

WORKUP

After an initial history is obtained, perform a physical examination that includes immediate evaluation of airway, breathing, circulation, mental status, volume status, and signs suggestive of a precipitating event, including infection, myocardial infarction, or stroke.

LABORATORY TESTS
- Hyperglycemia: Blood glucose >600 mg/dl (Box 1)[7]
- Serum osmolality: Usually >320 mOsm/kg (a useful indicator of severity[1])
- Complete metabolic panel: Serum creatinine, blood urea nitrogen (BUN), electrolytes, glucose
- Serum sodium: May be low, normal, or high. Hyperglycemia increases plasma osmolality that translocates intracellular water to the extracellular compartment, decreasing serum sodium. Serum sodium can be corrected by adding 1.6 mmol/L to the measured serum sodium level for every 100 mg/dl increase in serum glucose >100 mg/dl and <400 mg/dl, and then increase the sodium level by 4 mmol/L for each glucose increment of 100 mg/dl above 400 mg/dl.[8] Marked osmotic diuresis induced by hyperglycemia may cause the serum sodium level to be normal or high
- Serum potassium and phosphate: Total body potassium and phosphate deficits typically occur due to urinary losses from osmotic diuresis. However, these levels may be acutely normal or high due to extracellular shift secondary to insulin deficiency and hyperosmolality
- Anion gap and serum lactate: Anion gap may be normal or elevated in the setting of lactic acidosis
- Arterial blood gas: pH >7.30
- Serum and urine ketones: Negative or small
- Serum bicarbonate: >15 mmol/L

BOX 1 Diagnostic Testing Criteria for Patients with Hyperglycemic Hyperosmolar State[7]

Glucose higher than 600 mg/dl
Normal pH (classically, however, patients are often mildly acidotic)
No significant ketosis*
Serum osmolarity
- >320 mOsm/L with any mental status changes, *or*
- >350 mOsm/L

From Adams JG et al (eds): *Emergency medicine: clinical essentials*, ed 2, Philadelphia, 2013, Saunders.

- Hemoglobin A1c (if not performed in past 3 mo)
- Complete blood count with differential. May indicate presence of underlying infection (leukocytosis >25,000/mm^3), inflammatory condition, hemoconcentration. A leukocytosis of 10,000 to 15,000/mm^3 is expected from the stress of illness alone[2]
- Urinalysis, urine/sputum/blood cultures as indicated based on physical exam findings to evaluate the precipitating illness and other comorbidities

IMAGING STUDIES

Electrocardiogram (ECG), chest radiograph, and other imaging studies as indicated to evaluate the precipitating causes

℞ TREATMENT
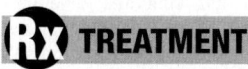

ACUTE GENERAL Rx (FIG. E1)[2,5,6]

Aggressive fluid resuscitation, intravenous insulin, and electrolyte correction are the mainstays of treatment. The initial goal of HHS treatment includes restoring the water deficit with intravenous fluids. This will help to normalize the plasma hyperosmolality, improve renal perfusion and insulin resistance, reduce the counterregulatory hormone release, and eventually correct hyperglycemia. Selecting the appropriate type of fluid is important to prevent complications related to dysnatremia. Improper management of plasma sodium concentration and plasma osmolality during treatment of HHS has been associated with the life-threatening complication of cerebral edema.

AGGRESSIVE INTRAVENOUS FLUID REPLACEMENT: Due to trivial ketonemia and the insulin sensitivity of most HHS patients, initial treatment is intravenous fluid alone without insulin. Insulin used prior to intravenous hydration or early in resuscitation risks a precipitous drop in serum osmolality. In the absence of cardiac compromise or end-stage renal disease, infuse 0.9% normal saline (NS) at an initial rate of 1 L/h for the first h. This is then followed by adjustments in the rate of infusion based on electrolyte values and hemodynamics. A lower rate of 250 to 500 ml/h may be adequate in the absence of severe dehydration. If the corrected serum sodium is elevated, 0.45% NS may be infused instead. Reassess corrected sodium needs by frequent checks and calculation. Recommended sodium decline is 0.5 mmol/L/h and should not surpass 10 to 12 mmol/L per day. Use measured or calculated osmolality to guide the rate of fluid resuscitation for gradual normalization of osmolality. Recommended serum osmolality decline is 3 mOsm/kg per h. Once serum glucose decreases to 300 mg/dl,

change the intravenous fluid to 5% dextrose with 0.45% NS at 150 to 250 ml/h.

INSULIN: Once glucose is no longer significantly improving with fluids alone, reassess patient's fluid status and initiate intravenous insulin. Administer initial bolus of intravenous regular insulin 0.1 units/kg followed by 0.1 units/kg per h infusion or a continuous infusion of 0.14 units/kg per h without initial bolus. If serum glucose declines by less than 50 to 75 mg/dl in the first hour, increase the insulin infusion rate every hour until a decline is noted. Once the serum glucose reaches 300 mg/dl, decrease the insulin infusion rate to 0.02 to 0.05 units/kg per h to maintain serum glucose between 200 and 300 mg/dl until resolution of HHS.

POTASSIUM REPLACEMENT: Insulin therapy shifts potassium intracellularly, frequently causing hypokalemia. If serum potassium at presentation is between 3.3 and 5.2 mmol/L, infuse 20 to 30 mmol of potassium chloride (KCl) with each liter of intravenous fluid to maintain serum potassium between 4 and 5 mmol/L. If the serum potassium concentration at presentation is <3.3 mmol/L, replace potassium by administering KCl infusion at 20 to 30 mmol/h, and withhold insulin until the serum potassium concentration is >3.3 mmol/L. If the serum potassium at presentation is >5.2 mmol/L, monitor serum potassium level every 2 h without intravenous potassium supplementation.

PHOSPHORUS & MAGNESIUM REPLACEMENT:

- Phosphorus and magnesium replacement are not routinely recommended. There are no studies of the utility of phosphate administration during treatment of HHS. Very low phosphorus levels may limit adenosine triphosphate (ATP) generation, thus limiting adequate diaphragm function. In patients with cardiac dysfunction, respiratory depression, or anemia and serum phosphate <1 mg/dl, add 20 to 30 mmol/L potassium phosphate to intravenous fluids.
- Monitor serum glucose hourly and serum electrolytes, BUN, and creatinine every 2 to 4 h until resolution of HHS.

TRANSITION TO SUBCUTANEOUS INSULIN: Normalization of serum osmolality and mental status indicates resolution of HHS. At this point, a transition to subcutaneous insulin should be performed. Overlap the initiation of subcutaneous intermediate- or long-acting insulin and discontinuation of intravenous insulin by 2 to 4 h to ensure adequate insulin levels and prevent rebound hyperglycemia. In patients with a known history of diabetes, their home insulin regimen may be initiated if adequate prior to presentation. In patients with poorly controlled diabetes, the subcutaneous insulin dose can be determined based on their stable insulin drip

requirement. Insulin-naive patients may be started on basal-bolus insulin therapy either by calculation of total daily dose of 0.5 to 0.8 units/kg (split as half-basal and half-bolus; administer one-third total bolus for each meal) or by their individual stable insulin drip requirements. Further subcutaneous insulin dose titration is based on subsequent blood glucoses. Resolution of glucotoxicity and inciting condition(s) will decrease insulin requirements. The underlying infection/inflammatory condition or precipitating event must be adequately treated.

CHRONIC Rx

Most patients will need insulin at discharge, at least short term. Patients whose diabetes was previously well controlled on oral agents may resume oral therapy after blood glucose stabilization by insulin.

DISPOSITION

Most patients require treatment in an emergency care setting, such as the intensive care unit or in a step-up facility.

ⓘ PEARLS & CONSIDERATIONS
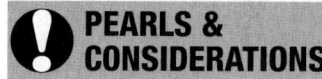

COMMENTS

- When patients with end-stage renal disease experience development of HHS, special management considerations are needed.[9] Aggressive fluid resuscitation is unnecessary in anuric end-stage renal disease patients, because most patients cannot produce the osmotic diuresis associated with normal kidney function. Note that urinary potassium and phosphorus losses will not occur, thereby limiting the need for supplementation. Lower continuous insulin infusion rates are required in patients with end-stage renal disease because of decreased insulin clearance. Hemodialysis is typically delayed until serum glucoses are corrected. Precipitous decreases in serum glucose from insulin administration and hemodialysis may result in rapid shifts in tonicity, predisposing cerebral edema.
- Education of the patient, family, and caregivers at long-term care facilities regarding optimal glycemic control, limiting modifiable risk factors for HHS, and prevention of dehydration is paramount.

REFERENCES

Available at eBooks.Health.Elsevier.com.

AUTHOR: **JESSICA E. SHILL, MD**

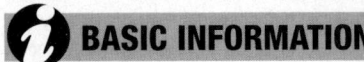

BASIC INFORMATION

DEFINITION

Abnormal elevation of serum potassium (K^+) concentration. It is associated with either normal or altered total body stores of potassium. Normal serum K^+ is 3.5 to 5.0 milliequivalents per liter (mEq/L). Hyperkalemia is defined as being mild (5.1 to 6.0 mEq/L), moderate (6.0 to 7.0 mEq/L), and severe (>7.0 mEq/L). Serum K^+ >7 mEq/L can lead to significant hemodynamic and neurologic consequences. Levels of K^+ >8.5 mEq/L can cause respiratory paralysis or cardiac arrest and can be rapidly fatal if untreated.

SYNONYM

Hyperpotassemia

ICD-10CM CODE
E87.5   Hyperpotassemia

EPIDEMIOLOGY & DEMOGRAPHICS

INCIDENCE & PREVALENCE:[1,2]

- Overall incidence and prevalence of hyperkalemia in the general population is unknown.
- Rarely detected in the general population, hyperkalemia is encountered in 2.6% of emergency department visits and 3.5% of hospital admissions.
- Patients with chronic kidney disease (CKD) have the highest prevalence of hyperkalemia, at approximately 10%. Increased risk depends on underlying conditions, including end-stage kidney disease (ESKD), acute kidney injury (AKI), cardiovascular disease (CVD), diabetes mellitus (DM), metabolic acidosis (especially nonanion gap acidosis), and medications such as renin-angiotensin-aldosterone system inhibitors (RAASi), mineralocorticoid receptor antagonists (MRA), and other potassium-sparing diuretics.
- The prevalence of an ICD-10 diagnosis for hyperkalemia was 14.6%.

PREDOMINANT SEX & AGE:[1]

- More common with increasing age due to increased prevalence of etiologic factors such as CKD, DM, CVD, and concomitant use of medications that predispose to hyperkalemia.
- Lower socioeconomic groups also have an increased prevalence, where monitoring of drug therapy and control of DM and hypertension may be inadequate.

RISK FACTORS:[3] Usually multifactorial, associated with various combinations of kidney failure (often oliguric), potassium supplementation, drugs that impair kidney potassium excretion, and movement of potassium out of cells due to hyperglycemia or inorganic metabolic acidosis.

Primary risk factor is CKD, especially if glomerular filtration rate (GFR) is <15 to 20 ml/min/1.73 m^2, more commonly associated with diabetes mellitus types 1 and 2 or urinary tract obstruction with nephropathy (especially if there is interstitial nephritis).

Medications associated with hyperkalemia:

- Potassium-sparing diuretics (e.g., spironolactone, triamterene, amiloride, eplerenone, finerenone)
- NSAIDs
- ACE inhibitors (ACEIs)
- Angiotensin II type 1 receptor blockers (ARBs)
- Angiotensin receptor Neprilysin inhibitor (ARNI)
- Direct renin inhibitors
- Calcineurin inhibitors (cyclosporine, tacrolimus, and voclosporin)
- Pentamidine
- Digoxin toxicity, particularly in CKD patients
- Trimethoprim-containing medications
- Heparin
- Ketoconazole
- Metyrapone
- β-blockers
- Succinylcholine
- Penicillin
- Herbs
- Dietary salt substitutes

Additional risk factors:

- Male sex
- Not Black
- DM
- CVD
- Congestive heart failure (CHF)
- AKI
- CKD
- Metabolic acidosis (hyperchloremic, non-anion gap)
- Urinary obstruction
- Total parenteral nutrition

GENETICS: Syndromes associated with hyperkalemia include:

- Pseudohypoaldosteronism type 1 (autosomal recessive)
- Pseudohypoaldosteronism type 2 (autosomal dominant; familial hyperkalemic hypertension, i.e., Gordon syndrome):
  1. Rare inherited form of hyperkalemia characterized by hypertension, hyperchloremic metabolic acidosis, and hyperkalemia with normal GFR
  2. Sequence variants of several genes that are involved in renal tubular sodium, potassium, or chloride transport
  3. All forms respond to treatment with thiazide-like diuretics
- Hyperkalemic periodic paralysis (autosomal dominant)
  1. Genetic sequence variant resulting in flaccid, generalized weakness and hyperkalemia
- Glomerulopathy with fibronectin deposits (autosomal dominant)
  1. Unknown genetic variant that produces proteinuria, hypertension, and type 4 renal tubular acidosis (RTA)
- Disorders of steroid metabolism and mineralocorticoid receptors:
  1. 21-hydroxylase deficiency with low aldosterone level
  2. Aldosterone synthase deficiency with low aldosterone level
  3. Congenital mineralocorticoid (aldosterone) receptor defect (exceedingly rare)
- Congenital hypoaldosteronism (autosomal recessive):
  1. Genetic variant associated with low aldosterone and salt wasting

2. Increased serum ratio of 18-hydroxycorticosterone to aldosterone
- Nephronophthisis:
  1. Manifestations include bilaterally enlarged kidneys, inflammatory portal fibrosis, and development of ESKD
- Disorders of chloride homeostasis (autosomal recessive):
  1. Genetic variant causing isolated hyperchlorihidrosis with excessive salt-wasting in sweat resulting in severe hyponatremic dehydration and hyperkalemia

PHYSICAL FINDINGS & CLINICAL PRESENTATION[4]

Most patients presenting with hyperkalemia are asymptomatic, with the abnormal laboratory parameter discovered inadvertently. Symptoms, when present, are nonspecific and primarily related to neuromuscular or cardiac dysfunction.

- Muscle paralysis
- Dyspnea
- Palpitations
- Chest pain
- Nausea or vomiting
- Paresthesias

Aside from bradycardia, the physical exam usually does not alert the examiner to a diagnosis of hyperkalemia. Flaccid paralysis and/or depressed or absent deep tendon reflexes may be detected.

ETIOLOGY (TABLE 1, BOX 1)

- Total body potassium content is approximately 3200 mEq and is primarily an intracellular ion (predominantly in muscle cells) with only 2% (70 mEq) residing in the extracellular space.
- Potassium is maintained in a narrow range of normal (3.8 to 5.0 mEq/L) by redundant and highly efficient homeostatic mechanisms that simultaneously control internal potassium ion redistribution while regulating net potassium excretion. When a defect occurs in one or both of these two processes, a net rise in extracellular potassium occurs, resulting in hyperkalemia.
- The kidney is responsible for regulation of potassium reabsorption and excretion (95%). Kidney failure or failure of tubular potassium secretion are the typical reasons for hyperkalemia.
- CKD is the most important predisposing condition for hyperkalemia due to a reduction of glomerular filtration. Patients with progressive CKD should consume a potassium-restricted diet. Low-sodium intake may be compensated by an increase in salt-substitute (containing potassium chloride) intake that may inadvertently increase potassium intake. AKI is commonly accompanied by hyperkalemia. Hyperkalemia in AKI may originate from or be exacerbated by a potassium load from increased tissue breakdown that may occur with rhabdomyolysis, GI bleeding, or blood transfusions with outdated blood. These processes can often result in the development of severe and life-threatening hyperkalemia.

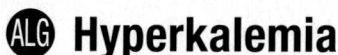

H

I

TABLE 1 Causes of Hyperkalemia

High Intake of K⁺ Ions
- Only if there is also a disorder leading to a low rate of excretion of K⁺ ions

Shift of K⁺ Ions Out of Cells
- Tissue breakdown (e.g., crush trauma, rhabdomyolysis, tumor lysis), exhausting exercise, after seizures, status epilepticus
- Na/K-ATPase problem
  1. Tissue hypoxia
  2. Lack of a stimulus (e.g., lack of insulin [e.g., patients with DKA], inhibition of insulin release by α-adrenergic surge, use of nonselective β-blockers)
  3. Inhibition of Na/K-ATPase (e.g., by drugs, e.g., digoxin)
- α-Adrenergic surge (causing inhibition of the release of insulin or a direct effect to cause a shift of K⁺ ions out of cells)
- Hyperosmolality (e.g., administration of mannitol)
- Metabolic acidosis due to acids that cannot be transported on the monocarboxylic acid cotransporter (e.g., HCl, citric acid)
- Increase K⁺ efflux from cells (administration of succinylcholine, fluoride intoxication)
- Hereditary causes (e.g., hyperkalemic periodic paralysis)

Diminished K⁺ Ion Loss in the Urine
- Advanced chronic renal insufficiency
- Drugs that interfere with renal K⁺ ion excretion
  1. Drugs that cause acute renal failure or acute interstitial nephritis
  2. Drugs that interfere with the renin–angiotensin-aldosterone axis (e.g., nonsteroidal anti-inflammatory drugs, direct renin blockers, ACE inhibitors, angiotensin receptor blockers)
  3. Drugs that inhibit aldosterone synthesis (e.g., heparin, ketoconazole)
  4. Aldosterone receptor blockers (e.g., spironolactone, eplerenone)
  5. Drugs that block ENaC in the CDN (e.g., amiloride, trimethoprim)
  6. Drugs the interfere with activation of ENaC via proteolytic cleavage (e.g., nafamostat mesylate)
- Diminished electrogenic reabsorption of Na⁺ ions in the CDN
  1. Very low delivery of Na⁺ ions to the CDN
  2. Some patients with hyporeninemic hypoaldosteronism
  3. Low levels of aldosterone (e.g., Addison's disease)
  4. Genetic disorders involving the aldosterone receptor or ENaC (type I pseudohypoaldosteronism)
- Increased electroneutral reabsorption of Na⁺ ions in DCT or CDN
  1. Increased reabsorption of Na⁺ and Cl⁻ ions in the DCT (e.g., familial hypertension with hyperkalemia [WNK 4 or WNK1 mutations]), drugs (e.g., calcineurin inhibitors), and some patients with diabetic nephropathy and hyporeninemic hypoaldosteronism
  2. Increased electroneutral reabsorption of Na⁺ and Cl⁻ ions in the CDN due to increased parallel activity of pendrin and NDCBE (e.g., some patients with hyporeninemic hypoaldosteronism)

ACE, Angiotensin-converting enzyme; *Cl*, chloride; *CDN*, cortical distal nephron; *DCT*, distal convoluted tubule; *DKA*, diabetic ketoacidosis; *ENaC*, epithelial sodium channels; *K*, potassium; *Na*, sodium; *NDCBE*, sodium-driven chloride/bicarbonate exchanger.
From Kamel SK, Halpertin ML: *Fluid, electrolyte, and acid-base physiology*, ed 5, Philadelphia, 2017, Elsevier.

BOX 1 Five Most Common Causes of Hyperkalemia

- Spurious elevation: Hemolysis due to drawing or storing of the laboratory sample or post-blood sampling leak from markedly elevated white blood cells, red blood cells, or platelets
- Renal failure: Acute or chronic
- Acidosis: Diabetic ketoacidosis (DKA), Addison disease, adrenal insufficiency, type 4 renal tubular acidosis
- Cell death: Rhabdomyolysis, tumor lysis syndrome, massive hemolysis or transfusion, crush injury, burn
- Drugs: Acute digitalis overdose, succinylcholine, angiotensin-converting enzyme inhibitors, angiotensin receptor blockers, nonsteroidal antiinflammatory drugs (NSAIDs), spironolactone, amiloride, potassium supplementation

From Walls RM et al: *Rosen's emergency medicine, concepts and clinical practice*, ed 10, Philadelphia, 2023, Elsevier.

- DM with insulin deficiency and/or hypertonicity with hyperglycemia.
- CVD, especially myocardial infarctions, left ventricular hypertrophy, and CHF, are often associated with various pharmacologic interventions that may induce or worsen hyperkalemia. CVD in association with CKD contributes to the development of hyperkalemia.
- Renin-angiotensin-aldosterone system inhibitors (RAASi), potassium-sparing diuretic administration, or digoxin in association with CKD may produce hyperkalemia in up to 10% of treated individuals vs. 2% of non-CKD patients. In patients at risk for hyperkalemia, dual RAASi therapy should not be used.

- β_2-receptor blockers, digoxin, heparin: The potassium elevation is generally small with mild increase, from 0.2-0.5 mEq/L.
- CHF. Risk for hyperkalemia is strongly associated with stage of CKD and use of spironolactone, especially in addition to a RAASi medication.

Dx DIAGNOSIS

DIFFERENTIAL DIAGNOSIS

Hyperkalemia develops through three mechanisms: Impaired cellular potassium redistribution, decreased renal potassium secretion, and increased potassium intake. In the presence of normal renal and adrenal function, it is difficult to ingest sufficient potassium to become hyperkalemic. Consequently, hyperkalemia is rarely seen in people without advanced CKD, unless supervening factors are present. The differential diagnosis is listed in Table 2.

WORKUP

Fig. 1 illustrates a clinical approach to hyperkalemia. The following steps should be followed in the workup of hyperkalemia:

- Rule out pseudohyperkalemia: An in vitro phenomenon caused by mechanical release of potassium from cells during phlebotomy or specimen processing. This may be encountered with severe leukocytosis (>70,000/cm³), thrombocytosis (platelet count >500,000 cm³), prolonged fist-clenching during phlebotomy, and use of a small-bore needle. The diagnosis is made when serum K⁺ exceeds the plasma K⁺ by >0.5 mEq/L (>0.5 mmol/L). Contamination with potassium-EDTA in some specimen tubes can spuriously increase plasma potassium, and the diagnostic clue is a low plasma calcium concentration.
- If there is no predisposition for hyperkalemia, repeat laboratory testing before treatment is undertaken.
- ECG for electrocardiographic signs of hyperkalemia. ECG changes may not follow a classical progression pattern, described below:
  1. Early ECG changes are seen with serum K⁺ of 5.5 to 6.5 mEq/L: Peaked T waves (Fig. 2), especially in precordial leads; shortened QT interval; and variable ST segment depression
  2. Serum K⁺ >6.5 mEq/L: Widening QRS complex with intraventricular conduction delay (QRS >120 milliseconds that does not meet the criteria for right or left bundle branch block)
  3. Serum K⁺ >7 mEq/L: Decreased P wave amplitude with increased PR interval and development of bradycardia (atrioventricular node block)
  4. Serum K⁺ >8.0 mEq/L: Absence of P waves and progressive widening of QRS that merges with T wave (sine wave), followed by ventricular fibrillation or asystole

In patients on chronic maintenance hemodialysis with hyperkalemia, T wave tenting was nonpredictive of serum potassium, especially in older adults and in patients with DM. There have

TABLE 2 Differential Diagnosis of Hyperkalemia

- Pseudohyperkalemia
- Cellular redistribution from intra- to extracellular space
  1. Mineral acid acidosis (not endogenous organic acidosis)
     a. Hyperkalemia inhibits ammoniagenesis, reducing net acid secretion and compounding metabolic acidosis
  2. Hypertonicity (hyperglycemia, sucrose, mannitol)
  3. DM: Insulin deficiency
  4. Hyperkalemic periodic paralysis
  5. Beta$_2$-adrenergic antagonists
  6. Alpha-adrenergic agonists
  7. Drugs
     a. Glucagon
     b. Digoxin overdose
     c. Aminocaproic acid-A
     d. Tetrodotoxin
     e. Succinylcholine
  8. Rebound after labile
  9. Extreme exercise
  10. Crush and tissue injury
      a. Rhabdomyolysis
      b. Hemolysis
      c. Tumor lysis syndrome
- Decreased renal excretion
  1. CKD
     a. Use of nonsteroidal antiinflammatory drugs (NSAIDs)
  2. ESKD
  3. Type 4 renal tubular acidosis
     a. Diabetes mellitus
     b. Obstructive nephropathy
     c. Amiloride
     d. Trimethoprim
     e. Pentamidine
     f. Succinylcholine (muscle depolarizing anesthetic)
     g. Volume depletion
     h. HIV infections
- Excess intake (rare except in advanced CKD or ESKD)
  1. Salt substitute (typically, KCl)
  2. Potassium-enriched foods (melons, citrus juice, raw coconut juice [44.3 mmol/L], Noni juice [56 mmol/L])
  3. Riverbed clay (red clay) very enriched, with 100 mEq K/100 g clay
- Mineralocorticoid deficiency (Addison disease)
  1. Hypoaldosteronism: Primary or secondary
  2. HIV infection
- Defect of tubular function or voltage defect resulting in hyperkalemia and hypertension:
  1. Genetic
     a. Pseudohyperaldosteronism type 2
- Also known as familial hyperkalemic hypertension or Gordon syndrome
  1. Acquired
     a. Calcineurin inhibitors (tacrolimus and cyclosporine)

CKD, Chronic kidney disease; *DM*, diabetes mellitus; *ESKD*, end-stage kidney disease; *KCl*, potassium chloride.

even been case reports of severe hyperkalemia with no ECG changes.

- Examine for the symptoms or physical findings of hyperkalemia and order basic studies:
  1. ECG
  2. CBC and platelet count
  3. Basic metabolic profile with a calculated estimated GFR (eGFR) (CKD alone should not develop hyperkalemia until eGFR is <20 to 25 ml/min per 1.73 m^2)
  4. Urine potassium and sodium concentrations
  5. Depending on history and results of initial laboratory testing, the following treatments may be indicated:
     a. Serum glucose concentration to rule out hypertonicity
     b. Digoxin level, as applicable **ALG**
     c. Arterial or venous blood gas, if acidosis is suspected
     d. Urinalysis with microscopy
     e. Serum cortisol and aldosterone levels after other common causes are ruled out
     f. Serum uric acid and phosphorus concentration to rule out tumor lysis syndrome
     g. Serum creatinine phosphokinase (CPK), calcium, and phosphorus measurements for rhabdomyolysis
- Accurate assessment of kidney function by eGFR or calculated GFR to define AKI or CKD stage and risk of hyperkalemia and acid-base status, especially if a hyperchlore-mic, nonanion gap metabolic acidosis is present.
- Hyperchloremic, nonanion gap metabolic acidosis associated with hyperkalemia is usually a type 4 RTA, with hyporeninemic hypoaldosteronism, which is common with urinary tract outlet obstruction, diabetic kidney disease, and acute or chronic kidney disorders involving the tubules.
- Determine presence of a renal origin for hyperkalemia using the urine potassium concentration as renal or endogenous vs. exogenous, with nephrology consultation as required.

LABORATORY TESTS

- Serum electrolytes, blood urea nitrogen, and creatinine
- Urinalysis and urine protein-creatinine ratio
- Serum and plasma potassium levels
- Serum and urine creatinine levels
- Cortisol level
- Aldosterone level
- 18-Hydroxycorticosterone level

IMAGING STUDIES

- Ultrasound of the kidneys and bladder
- Computed tomography scan of the kidneys, ureters, and bladder

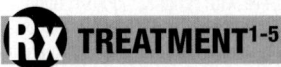 **TREATMENT**[1-5]

- The treatment of severe hyperkalemia requires three tasks carried out in close succession:
  1. Reverse any electrocardiographic changes caused by the hyperkalemia to prevent a fatal arrhythmia (calcium)
  2. Redistribute potassium into cells (insulin, albuterol, and sodium bicarbonate when there is metabolic acidosis)
  3. Removal of the potassium from the body (sodium polystyrene sulfonate, zirconium cyclosilicate, patiromer, or dialysis)
- Supportive measurements such as pacing, and pressors do not work in the setting of severe hyperkalemia. In acute, severe, life-threatening hyperkalemia, the approach is divided into two components. First, stabilize the myocardium to prevent a fatal arrhythmia. Giving intravenous (IV) calcium is cardioprotective in the setting of hyperkalemia, commonly reversing all hyperkalemic ECG changes within seconds of administration. However, it does not decrease the potassium levels; therefore other therapies are needed to reduce the potassium level.
- Before giving calcium, make sure digoxin toxicity is not present, as calcium administration can be fatal in the face of digoxin-induced hyperkalemia.
- Treatment intensity is directly related to the rapidity with which hyperkalemia developed, absolute potassium level, and evidence for toxicity by symptoms, neuromuscular examination, and ECG changes. The more rapid the rise in potassium, the higher the level; the more severe the cardiotoxicity depicted by the ECG changes, the more aggressive the therapy should be.

NONPHARMACOLOGIC THERAPY

- The mainstay of therapy should be educating the patient and the family regarding a low-potassium diet (<3 g/day), as well as providing a list of high-potassium foods to avoid.
- Maintaining adequate extracellular fluid volume and prevention of volume depletion,

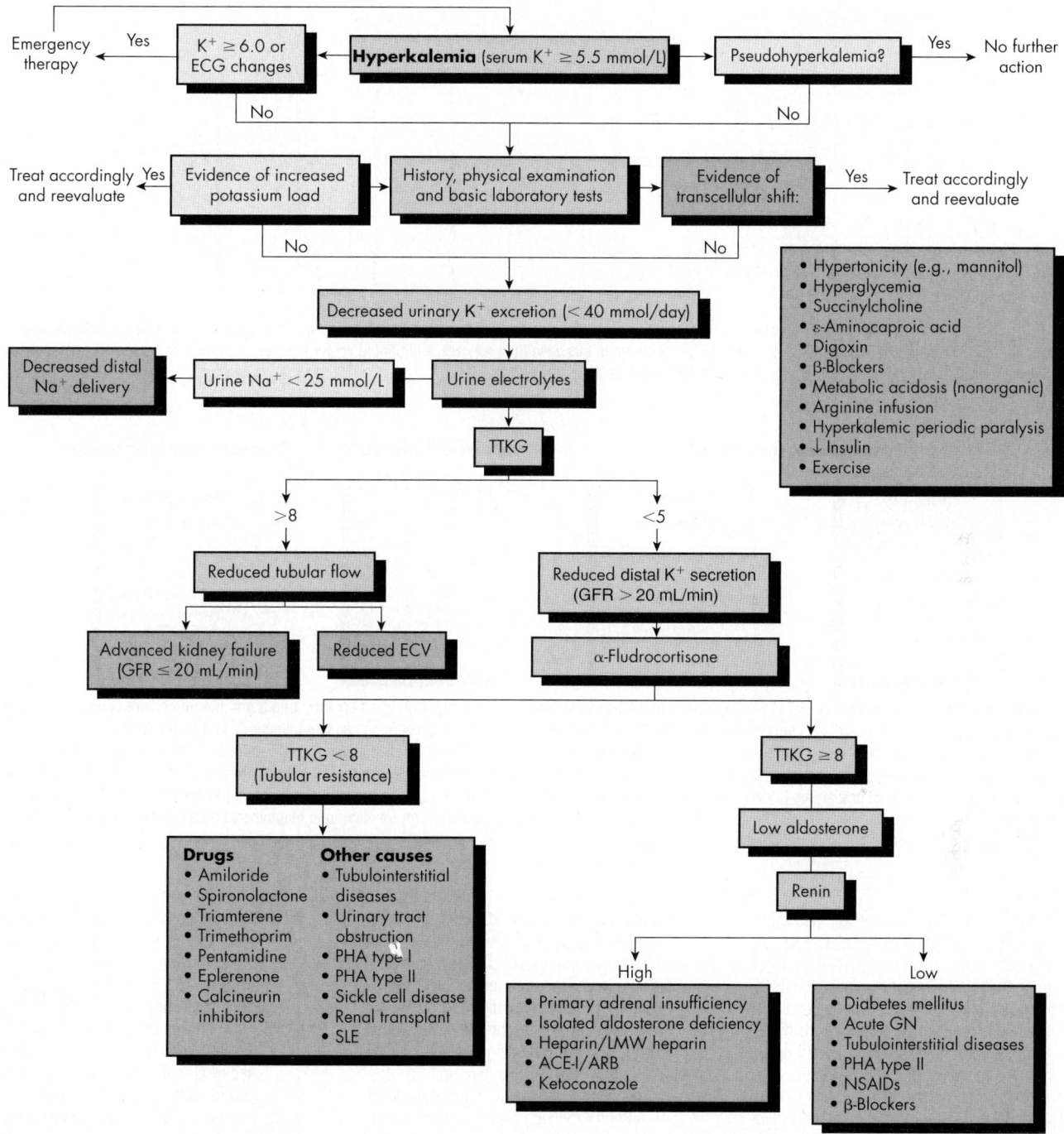

FIG. 1 Clinical approach to hyperkalemia. *ACE-I,* Angiotensin-converting enzyme inhibitor; *ARB,* angiotensin II type 1 receptor blocker; *CCD,* cortical collecting duct; *ECG,* electrocardiogram; *ECV,* effective circulatory volume; *GFR,* glomerular filtration rate; *GN,* glomerulonephritis; *HIV,* human immunodeficiency virus; *K,* potassium; *LMW heparin,* low-molecular-weight heparin; *Na,* sodium; *NSAID,* nonsteroidal antiinflammatory drug; *PHA,* pseudohypoaldosteronism; *SLE,* systemic lupus erythematosus; *TTKG,* transtubular potassium gradient. (From Skorecki K et al: *Brenner & Rector's the kidney,* ed 10, Philadelphia, 2016, Elsevier.)

which limits potassium excretion by the kidney.
- Increasing patient awareness of hyperkalemia including use of educational tools facilitating communication about hyperkalemia (e.g., https://www.kidney.org/atoz/content/what-hyperkalemia).

ACUTE GENERAL Rx

In patients with severe hyperkalemia, treatment (Fig. 3) is as follows:[6,7]

- IV calcium (Fig. 4) to ameliorate cardiac toxicity (if not digoxin toxic).
  1. 10% calcium gluconate or calcium chloride (gluconate preferred).
  2. 10 ml of 10% solution IV over 10 min (repeat in 5 min if not effective or arrhythmia recurs).
- Identify and remove sources of potassium intake.
- IV glucose and insulin infusion to enhance cellular uptake of potassium.

1. Make sure to closely monitor glucose every hour for several hours for hypoglycemia, especially in patients with advanced CKD.
- Correct severe acidosis with IV sodium bicarbonate.
- Consider beta-adrenergic agonist therapy (e.g., nebulized albuterol, 10 mg via Venturi mask). Preferred over alkali therapy in patients with CKD.
- Increase potassium excretion with administration of loop diuretic IV or cation-exchange medications mentioned previously.

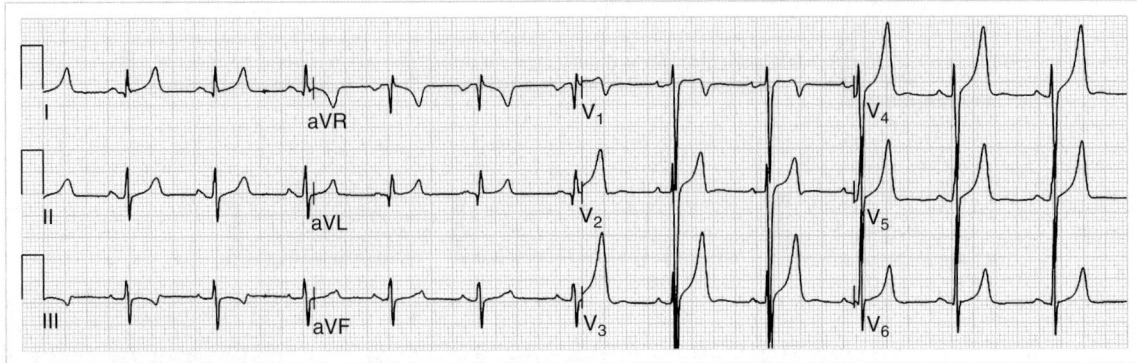

FIG. 2 Tall peaked T waves with hyperkalemia. This 12-lead electrocardiogram shows the tented T waves that are commonly seen in mild to moderate degrees of hyperkalemia. Tented T waves of hyperkalemia need not be tall, although in this case they are. *aVF,* Augmented vector foot; *aVL,* augmented vector left; *aVR,* augmented vector right. (From Olshansky B et al: *Arrhythmia essentials,* ed 2, Philadelphia, 2017, Elsevier.)

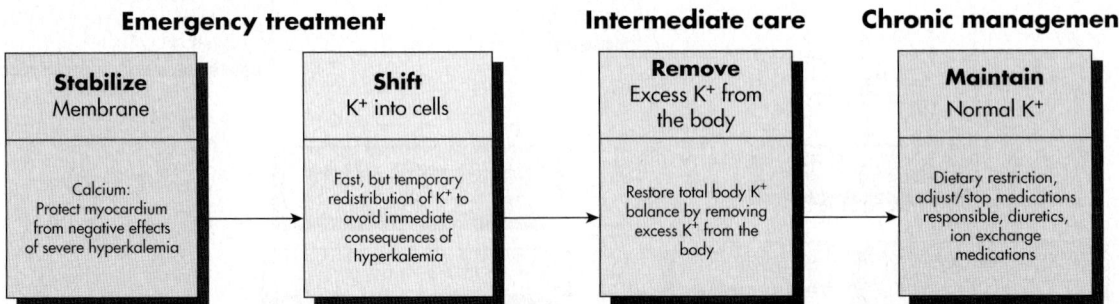

FIG. 3 Management of hyperkalemia. Here is the approach to managing severe hyperkalemia. During emergency treatment, the immediate concern is to stabilize the membranes to protect the myocardium from the negative effects of severe hyperkalemia by administering calcium gluconate. In the next few minutes, the priority is to shift potassium *(K⁺)* into the cells with a fast but temporary redistribution of K⁺ to avoid immediate consequences of hyperkalemia. This is accomplished with insulin and β₂-adrenergic receptor agonists. In the following hours to days, intermediate care is focused on removing the K⁺ from the body and restoring total K⁺ balance with potassium binders, loop diuretics, or dialysis. Sodium bicarbonate may be used to shift K⁺ into cells when metabolic acidosis is the cause of hyperkalemia. Once total body K⁺ balance is achieved, attempts to identify the underlying cause follow and developing long-term management plans including a low-potassium diet, discontinuation, or modification of RAAS inhibitors, and the use of the newer potassium binders.

1. Medications that increase potassium excretion in addition to IV saline and loop diuretics, such as an aldosterone analogue (e.g., 9-alpha fludrocortisone acetate [Florinef]) in patients with hyporeninemia or hypoaldosteronism or patients with hyperkalemia who have solid organ transplant and are on calcineurin inhibitor (CNI).
- Emergency dialysis for refractory hyperkalemia, defined as ongoing hyperkalemia unresponsive to conservative measures.
- After correction of hyperkalemia, long-term management should be initiated to maintain normal potassium. Measures include dietary potassium restriction, adjusting/stopping medications associated with hyperkalemia, and/or administration of newer ion exchange resins such as sodium zirconium cyclosilicate and patiromer. The use of sodium polystyrene sulfate has greatly decreased due to lack of data demonstrating consistent efficacy and because newer agents are available (i.e., patiromer and zirconium cyclosilicate).

CHRONIC Rx

In the presence of a moderate elevation of potassium and no ECG abnormalities:

- Correct origin of increased potassium (e.g., inhibited excretion or increased intake)
- Increase potassium excretion with a diuretic or potassium ion exchange medication (Table 3).
  1. Sodium polystyrene sulfonate (SPS) is a polymeric cation-exchange resin (dose: 15 to 30 g up to four times daily).
     a. Sodium ion exchanger and is nonselective for potassium, also having affinity for calcium and magnesium ions.
     b. Lacking long-term use studies, with only one small 7-day randomized clinical study performed.
     c. Short-term efficacy is inconsistent with variable onset of action (hours to days).
     d. Reported adverse events include intestinal ischemia and colonic necrosis (rare, 16 or 23 events per 1000 person-yr). FDA added warning label to SPS regarding concomitant use of sorbitol (historically used to prevent constipation) and the risk of colonic necrosis and other serious GI adverse events. Concomitant use of sorbitol with SPS is currently not recommended.
     e. Long-term use can result in hypocalcemia and hypomagnesemia, and levels should be monitored intermittently.

f. Medications can potentially bind other medications, so should not be taken for 3 h before or after dosing.
2. Patiromer is a nonreabsorbed oral calcium-containing potassium-binding polymer suspension (dose: 8.4 to 25.2 g daily).
   a. Shown to lower serum potassium in hyperkalemia associated with diabetic nephropathy and CHF on RAASi.
   b. Calcium is the ion exchanger (not sodium), and it can form calcium carbonate in the colon and affect absorption of some medications, especially ciprofloxacin, levothyroxine, and metformin. Administer at least 3 h before or after all oral medications.
   c. Can bind magnesium and may be associated with hypomagnesemia. Magnesium monitoring is recommended with long-term use.
3. Sodium zirconium cyclosilicate is a nonabsorbed inorganic polymer that selectively exchanges potassium for sodium and hydrogen ions (Initial dose: 10 g, three times daily for up to 48 h. Subsequent dose: 5 g every other day to 15 g daily for long-term use).
   a. Sodium is the exchanged ion and may be associated with sodium overload

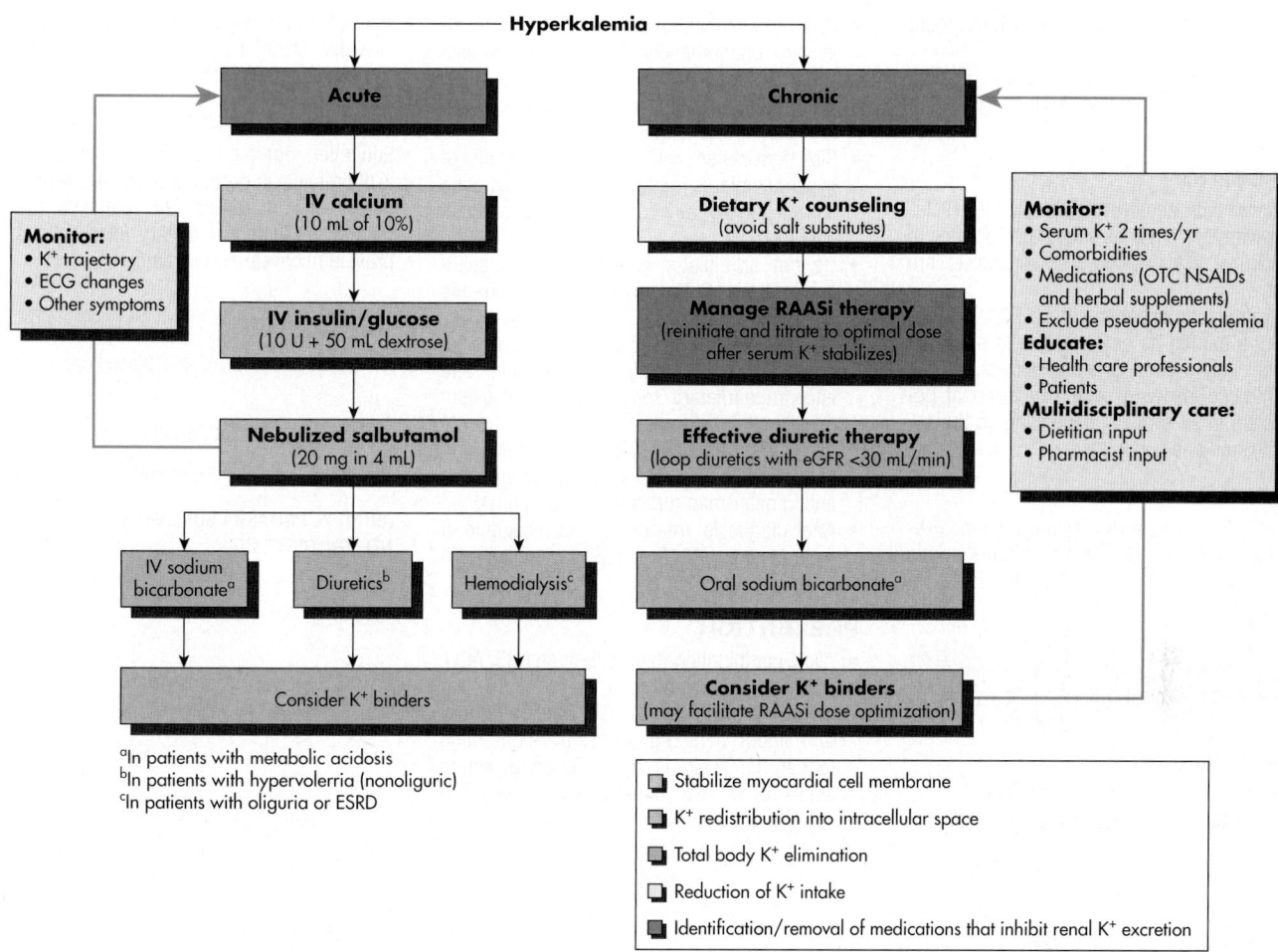

FIG. 4 Algorithm for treatment of hyperkalemia. Treatment options for the management of acute and chronic hyperkalemia. In patients with acute hyperkalemia, intravenous *(IV)* calcium reduces membrane excitation in cardiac tissue within 1 to 3 min, while insulin and b-agonists redistribute potassium *(K⁺)* to the intracellular space (30 to 60 min) but do not reduce total body K⁺. b-Agonists have a short duration of effect (2 to 4 h), and glucose must be administered with insulin to prevent hypoglycemia. Sodium bicarbonate use, which promotes K⁺ elimination through increased urinary K⁺ excretion, is limited to patients with metabolic acidosis, and effective diuretic therapy depends on residual kidney function. Hemodialysis increases total K⁺ elimination and may be used for resistant acute hyperkalemia. *ECG,* Electrocardiography; *eGFR,* estimated glomerular filtration rate; *ESRD,* end-stage renal disease; *NSAIDs,* nonsteroidal antiinflammatory drugs; *OTC,* over-the-counter; *RAASi,* renin-angiotensin-aldosterone system inhibition. (From Palmer BF et al: Clinical management of hyperkalemia, *Mayo Clin Proc* 96(3):749, 2021.)

TABLE 3 Available Potassium Ion Exchange Resins

	Sodium Polystyrene Sulfonate	Patiromer	Sodium Zirconium Cyclosilicate
Dosage	15-30 g One to four times daily	8.4 g, 16.8 g, or 25.2 g Once daily	10 g, 3 times daily for up to 48 h; then 5 g every other day to 15 g daily
Counterion	Sodium	Calcium	Sodium
Average daily sodium load	1500-12,000 mg	0 mg	400-2400 mg
Concomitant dose separation with other oral medications	3-h separation	3-h separation	2-h separation

if large doses are used for a prolonged time.

b. Agent is taken at least 2 h before or after all oral medications.

Patiromer and sodium zirconium cyclosilicate are much more palatable and predictable, and efficacy has been demonstrated in clinical trials compared to SPS. The use of the newer potassium binders is often limited by the formularies available to some patients depending

on their insurance, often leaving SPS as the only viable choice.

Management of nonurgent hyperkalemia:
- Discontinue or reduce medications that interfere with potassium excretion.
  1. Stop RAASi (special care if in combination)
  2. Stop spironolactone, eplerenone, amiloride, and triamterene
  3. Stop all NSAIDs and COX-2 inhibitors
  4. Herbal medicine: Stop Chan su and Noni juice, if applicable

5. Modify CNI therapy, if feasible
- Prescribe a low-potassium diet (70 mEq/day).
- Administer a loop diuretic or thiazide (CNI-induced hyperkalemia).
- If serum bicarbonate is <22 mmol/L, administer sodium bicarbonate tablets (650 mg tablet [7.8 mmol per tablet]) or Shohl solution (sodium citrate [1 mmol per ml] 3 to 60 ml twice per day).
- Patiromer or sodium zirconium cyclosilicate avoids use of SPS for chronic hyperkalemia.

1. Neither agent is used for severe/urgent hyperkalemia.

- Continuation of a RAASi may be possible when using patiromer or sodium zirconium cyclosilicate.

DISPOSITION

- Patients with acute symptomatic hyperkalemia with ECG changes should be admitted to a hospital in a monitored bed/intensive care unit.
- Asymptomatic patients with no ECG changes can be treated as outpatients and educated extensively regarding a low-potassium diet, with close follow-up including a repeat potassium in 24 to 48 h, depending on the severity, and one week later.

REFERRAL

Patients with associated hypertension, proteinuria, CKD, or persistent hyperkalemia should be referred to a nephrologist for evaluation.

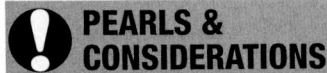

COMMENTS

- Rule out hemolysis of blood samples.
- If a spurious result is suspected, repeat the test.

- Rule out pseudohyperkalemia, defined as an in vitro phenomenon in which the ex vivo serum potassium level in the specimen tube is elevated, but the in vivo plasma potassium is in the normal range.
- Risk associated with comparable levels of hyperkalemia is higher in individuals with normal kidney function compared to those with CKD.
- Do not administer IV calcium or insulin/dextrose if no ECG changes for hyperkalemia are seen.
- Provide education regarding avoidance of rich potassium-containing foodstuffs and encourage dietary restriction of potassium (avoid salt substitutes).
- Evaluate for urinary obstruction, especially in patients with diabetes (neurogenic bladder) and in older men (prostatic hypertrophy).
- After diagnosis, treatment, and resolution of hyperkalemia, RAASi should be reinitiated if medically indicated prior.

PREVENTION

- Avoid combination therapies of an ARB, ACEI, or direct renin inhibitor.
- In patients with type 4 RTA, provide education about avoiding potassium-containing foodstuffs, avoiding travel to areas where such foods are common, and avoiding volume depletion.

- In CKD patients or patients with type 4 RTA, avoid using salt substitutes that contain potassium chloride.

PATIENT & FAMILY EDUCATION

Education regarding potassium content of foods is of practical importance. A certified renal nutritionist should review the patient's medical records for potential dietary interventions and provide necessary education.

REFERENCES

Available at eBooks.Health.Elsevier.com.

RELATED CONTENT

Chronic Kidney Disease (Related Key Topic)

AUTHORS: **PRIYASHA SURI, MD** and **NELSON KOPYT, DO**

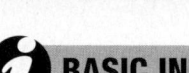

BASIC INFORMATION

DEFINITION

- Primary hyperlipoproteinemia is a group of genetic disorders of the lipid transport proteins in the blood that manifests as abnormally elevated levels of cholesterol, triglycerides, or both in the serum of affected patients.
- Usually defined as total cholesterol, low-density lipoprotein (LDL), triglycerides, or lipoprotein A levels above 90th percentile or high-density lipoprotein (HDL) or apo A-1 levels below the 10th percentile for the general population. Fig. E1 illustrates the structure of lipoproteins. Plasma lipoprotein composition is described in Table 1.

SYNONYM

Hyperlipidemia

ICD-10CM CODES
E78.0	Pure hypercholesterolemia
E78.2	Mixed hyperlipidemia
E78.1	Pure hyperglyceridemia
E78.4	Other hyperlipidemia
E78.3	Hyperchylomicronemia

EPIDEMIOLOGY & DEMOGRAPHICS

INCIDENCE: The most common types are lipoprotein A excess, hypertriglyceridemia, and combined hyperlipidemia.

- Incidence of heterozygous familial hypercholesterolemia: 1:500
- Incidence of homozygous familial hypercholesterolemia: 1:1 million
- Familial hypercholesterolemia: Autosomal dominant disorder
- Familial combined hyperlipidemia: Possibly an autosomal dominant disorder
- Multifactorial predilection: Apparent in majority of affected individuals

GENETICS:

- Familial lipoprotein lipase deficiency: Autosomal recessive, resulting in an elevation in the plasma chylomicrons and triglycerides
- Familial apoprotein CII deficiency: Autosomal recessive, resulting in increased serum chylomicrons, very low-density lipoprotein (VLDL), and hypertriglyceridemia
- Familial type 3 hyperlipoproteinemia: Single-gene defect requiring contributory factors to manifest
- Familial hypercholesterolemia: Autosomal dominant defect of the LDL receptor, resulting in an elevated serum cholesterol level and normal triglycerides. HoFH is the most severe form of the disease. LDL levels can reach over 500 mg/dl and can cause death in childhood
- Familial hypertriglyceridemia: Common, autosomal dominant defect resulting in elevated VLDL and triglycerides
- Multiple lipoprotein–type hyperlipidemia: Autosomal dominant, manifesting as isolated hypercholesterolemia, isolated hypertriglyceridemia, or hyperlipidemia
- Polygenic hypercholesterolemia: Multifactorial

- Polygenic hyperalphalipoproteinemia: Autosomal dominant or polygenic, causing an elevated HDL
- A classification of lipoprotein disorders and their clinical findings and management are summarized in Table 2

PHYSICAL FINDINGS & CLINICAL PRESENTATION

- Familial lipoprotein lipase deficiency: Recurrent bouts of abdominal pain in infancy, eruptive xanthomas, hepatomegaly, splenomegaly, lipemia retinalis
- Familial apoprotein CII deficiency: Occasional eruptive xanthomas
- Familial type 3 hyperlipoproteinemia: Xanthoma striata palmaris or tuberoeruptive xanthomas, xanthelasmas, arterial bruits at a young age, gangrene of the lower extremities at a young age
- Familial hypercholesterolemia: Tendon xanthomas, arcus corneae, xanthelasma
- Familial hypertriglyceridemia: Associated obesity; eruptive xanthomas (Fig. E2) can develop with exacerbations

ETIOLOGY

- Genetic defects causing lipid abnormalities
- Environmental influences, including diet, drugs, and alcohol intake

DIAGNOSIS

DIFFERENTIAL DIAGNOSIS

Secondary causes of hyperlipoproteinemias:

- Hypothyroidism
- Diabetes mellitus
- Pancreatitis
- Autoimmune hyperlipoproteinemia
- Nephrotic syndrome
- Biliary obstruction; Table E3 describes the differential diagnosis of hyperlipidemia and dyslipidemia

WORKUP

- Family history for premature cardiac disease
- Personal history of recurrent pancreatitis
- Detailed physical examination

LABORATORY TESTS

- Standard lipid profile; Table 4 summarizes laboratory findings in lipid disorders
- If normal, further testing with measurement of lipoprotein A, apo B, and apo A-1
- Lipoprotein electrophoresis and ultracentrifugation (for phenotypic classification). Clinically relevant apolipoproteins are summarized in Table E5.
- Workup for secondary causes: Thyroid-stimulating hormone, fasting glucose, liver function, renal function, urinary protein

TREATMENT

NONPHARMACOLOGIC THERAPY

- Cornerstone of treatment: Dietary therapy
  1. TLC diet (therapeutic lifestyle changes): See "Hypercholesterolemia" topic

- Risk factor reduction includes smoking cessation, treatment of hypertension, exercise
- Familial lipoprotein lipase deficiency and familial apoprotein CII deficiency: Fat-free diet
- Remainder of cases, except those with polygenic hyperalphalipoproteinemia: Fat- and cholesterol-restricted diets
- Nonpharmacologic interventions can include LDL apheresis and liver transplantation

ACUTE GENERAL Rx

No acute treatment is needed.

CHRONIC Rx

- Medications commonly used to treat hyperlipidemias are summarized in Table 6. Table 7 differentiates statins based on potency.
- Familial lipoprotein lipase deficiency, polygenic hyperalphalipoproteinemia, or familial apoprotein CII deficiency: No chronic drug therapy.
- Familial type 3 hyperlipoproteinemia: Usually responds well to secondary causes being treated and diet therapy; if not, fibric acids may be tried.
- Familial hypercholesterolemia: Statins, bile acid sequestrants, or niacin. Ezetimibe and proprotein convertase subtilisin/Kexin type 9 (PCSK9 inhibitors) can be added to statins to achieve LDL goals.[1] PCSK9 binds to LDL receptors on hepatocytes, promote receptor degradation, and prevent LDL-C clearance from the circulation thereby increasing serum concentrations of LDL-C. PCSK9 monoclonal antibody inhibitors alirocumab (Praluent), evolocumab (Repatha), and inclisiran (Leqvio), a PCSK9-directed small interfering RNA, are currently indicated as adjunct to diet and maximally tolerated statin therapy for the treatment of adults with heterozygous familial hypercholesterolemia or clinical atherosclerotic cardiovascular disease, who require additional lowering of LDL cholesterol. PCSK9 inhibitors lower risk for ischemic cardiovascular events in persons with stable CAD and elevated atherogenic lipoproteins despite statin therapy. These medications are administered by subcutaneous injection and are expensive.
- Familial hypertriglyceridemia: Fibric acids (fenofibrate), niacin, omega-3 PUFA-containing fish oil capsules. Icosapent ethyl, a highly purified eicosapentaenoic acid ester, has been shown to lower triglyceride levels and cardiovascular risk in patients with hypertriglyceridemia. Icosapent ethyl (Vascepa) is indicated as an adjunct to diet to relieve triglyceride levels in adult patients with severe ($\geq$500 mg/dl) hypertriglyceridemia. It is also indicated as an adjunct to maximally tolerated statin therapy to reduce the risk of myocardial infarction, stroke, coronary revascularization, and unstable angina requiring hospitalization in adult patients with elevated triglyceride levels ($\geq$150 mg/dl) and established cardiovascular disease or diabetes mellitus and two or more additional risk factors for cardiovascular disease.

TABLE 1 Plasma Lipoprotein Composition and Apolipoproteins

	Origin	Density (g/ml)	Size (nm)	% Protein	[Cholesterol] in Plasma mg/dl (mmol/L)*	[Triglyceride] in Fasting Plasma (mmol/L)†	Major Apo	Other Apo
Chylomicrons‡	Intestine	<0.95	100-1000	1-2	0.0	0	B48	A-I, Cs
Chylomicron remnants‡	Chylomicron metabolism	0.95-1.006	30-80	3-5	0.0	0.0	B48, E	A-I, A-IV, Cs
VLDL	Liver	<1.006	40-50	10	4-15 mg% (0.1-0.4)	15-100 mg% (0.2-1.2)	B100	A-I, Cs
IDL	VLDL	1.006-1.019	25-30	18	4-12 mg% 0.1-0.3	10-25 mg% (0.1-0.3)	B100, E	
LDL	IDL	1.019-1.063	20-25	25	50-130 mg% (1.5-3.5)	15-35 mg% (0.2-0.4)	B100	
HDL	Liver, intestine	1.063-1.210	6-10	40-55	35-62 mg% (0.9-1.6)	10-15 mg% (0.1-0.2)	A-I, A-II	A-IV
Lp(a)	Liver	1.051-1.082	25	30-50			B100, (a)	

Apo, Apolipoprotein; *HDL*, high-density lipoprotein; *IDL*, intermediate-density lipoprotein; *LDL*, Low-density lipoprotein; *Lp(a)*, lipoprotein(a); *VLDL*, very-low-density lipoprotein.
*In mmol/L; for mg/dl, multiply by 38.67.
†In mmol/L; for mg/dl, multiply by 88.5.
‡In the fasted state, serum (or plasma) should not contain chylomicrons or their remnants.
From Libby P et al: *Braunwald's heart disease, a textbook of cardiovascular medicine*, ed 12, Philadelphia, 2022, Elsevier.

TABLE 2 Disorders of Lipids: Clinical Findings and Management

Disorder	Xanthomas	Cardiovascular	Gastrointestinal	Neurologic	Ophthalmologic	Other Findings	Management
Type I	Eruptive, tendinous, xanthelasmas	None	Acute abdomen, hepatosplenomegaly, pancreatitis	None	Lipemia retinalis, retinal vein occlusion	Diabetes, lipemic plasma	Diet, plasmapheresis
Type II	Planar, especially intertriginous, tendinous, tuberous	Generalized atherosclerosis	None	None	Arcus cornea	None	Type IIa: Bile acid sequestrants, statins, niacin, fish oil / Type IIb: Statins, niacin, fibrate
Type III	Planar, especially palmar, tuberous	Atherosclerosis	None	None	None	Abnormal glucose tolerance, hyperuricemia	Statins, fibrate
Type IV	Eruptive, tuberous	Atherosclerosis	Acute abdomen, hepatosplenomegaly, pancreatitis	None	Lipemia retinalis	Obesity	Statins, fibrate, niacin
Type V	Eruptive, tuberous	Atherosclerosis	Acute abdomen, hepatosplenomegaly, pancreatitis	None	Lipemia retinalis	Obesity, hyperinsulinemia	Niacin, fibrate
Tangier	Macular rash, foam cells in biopsies	Atherosclerosis	Acute abdomen, hepatosplenomegaly	Peripheral neuropathy	Corneal infiltration	Enlarged orange tonsils, lymphadenopathy	
Apolipoprotein A-I and C-III deficiency	Planar and tendon xanthomas, foam cells in biopsies	Atherosclerosis	Normal	Normal	Corneal clouding	None	
HDL deficiency with planar xanthomas	Planar xanthomas, foam cells in biopsies	Atherosclerosis	Hepatomegaly	Normal	Corneal opacity	None	

HDL, High-density lipoprotein.
From Paller AS, Mancini AJ: *Hurwitz clinical pediatric dermatology: a textbook of skin disorders of childhood and adolescence*, ed 5, St. Louis, 2016, Elsevier.

- Multiple lipoprotein–type hyperlipidemia: Drug therapy aimed at the predominant lipid abnormality noted.
- Recent data suggest in patients with lipoprotein abnormalities that treatment goals should be based on non-HDL cholesterol rather than LDL cholesterol.
- The FDA has approved mipomersen and lomitapide in patients with homozygous familial hypercholesterolemia already taking maximum doses of other lipid-lowering drugs. Both medicines are hepatotoxic and very expensive.
- Trials with bempedoic acid, an inhibitor of adenosine triphosphate citrate lyase that lowers LDL cholesterol, have shown to significantly lower LDL when bempedoic acid was added to maximally tolerated statin therapy. Bempedoic acid is approved for use alone (Nexletol) and in a fixed-dose combination with ezetimibe (Nexlizet) as an adjunct to diet and maximally tolerated statin therapy in adults with heterozygous familial hypercholesterolemia or established ASCVD who require additional LDL-C lowering.

DISPOSITION

- Those with polygenic hyperalphalipoproteinemia: Excellent prognosis for longevity
- Those with familial hypercholesterolemia, familial type 3 hypercholesterolemia, or multiple lipoprotein–type hyperlipidemia: Even with

TABLE 4 Laboratory Findings in Lipid Disorders

Disorder	Inheritance	OMIM No.	Prevalence	Cholesterol	Triglycerides	VLDL	Chylomicrons	LDL	HDL	Serum	Cause
Type I	AR		1/million	↑	↑↑↑	↑	↑	↓	↓↓↓	Creamy top	
a: Familial hyperchylomicronemia		239600, 246650, 615947									a. Deficiency from mutations in lipoprotein lipase; *LMF1; GPIHBP1*
b: Familial apoprotein C2 or A-V deficiency		207750, 133650									b. Deficient ApoC-2 or ApoA-5 (see Type V)
c: —		118830									c. LP lipase inhibitor in blood
Type II			1 in 500 for heterozygotes	↑	NI or ↑	↑	NI	↓	↓	Clear	
a: Familial hypercholesterolemia	AD	143890, 144010, 603776									LDL receptor defect in 60%-80%; *APOB, PCSK9,* each <5%
	AR	603813									*LDLRAP1*
b: Familial combined hyperlipidemia	AD, AR	144250	1 in 100							Clear	Polygenic Decreased LDL receptor and ApoB-100 dysfunction
Type III Familial dysbetalipoproteinemia	AR	107741	1 in 10,000	↑	↑	↑	↑	↓	NI	Turbid	ApoE-2 synthesis
Type IV Familial hypertriglyceridemia	AD	144600	1 in 100	↑	NI↑	↑	NI	↓	↓↓	Turbid	Renal disease, diabetes
Type V	AR	144650	Very rare	↑	↑↑↑	↑	↑	↓	↓↓↓	Creamy top, turbid bottom	Apo A-V (ApoA-5) deficiency

AD, Autosomal dominant; *Apo,* apolipoprotein; *AR,* autosomal recessive; *HDL,* high-density lipoprotein; *LDL,* low-density lipoprotein; *LP,* lipoprotein; *NI,* normal; *OMIM,* Online Mendelian Inheritance in Man; *VLDL,* very low-density lipoprotein; ↑, increased; ↓, decreased.

From Paller AS, Mancini AJ: *Hurwitz clinical pediatric dermatology: a textbook of skin disorders of childhood and adolescence,* ed 5, St. Louis, 2016, Elsevier.

aggressive treatment, at high risk for accelerated atherosclerosis and coronary artery disease

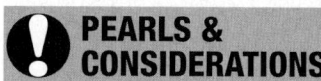 **PEARLS & CONSIDERATIONS**

COMMENTS

- Patient information is available through the American Heart Association.

- Lipid-lowering drug therapy is recommended for children ≥10 yr whose LDL-C levels remain extremely elevated after 6 mo to 1 yr of dietary modification. Drug therapy also can be considered for children with LDL-C levels of ≥190 mg/dl.
- Most dyslipidemia interventions require lifelong treatment and at least 6-12 mo to significantly reduce the risk of cardiovascular events.

REFERENCE & SUGGESTED READINGS

Available at eBooks.Health.Elsevier.com.

RELATED CONTENT

Hypercholesterolemia (Related Key Topic)

AUTHOR: **FRED F. FERRI, MD**

TABLE 6 Current Lipid-Lowering Medications

Generic Name	Trade Name	Recommended Dose Range
Statins		
Atorvastatin	Lipitor	10-80 mg
Fluvastatin	Lescol	20-80 mg
Lovastatin	Mevacor	20-80 mg
Pitavastatin	Livalo	2-4 mg
Pravastatin	Pravachol	10-40 mg
Rosuvastatin	Crestor	10-40 mg
Simvastatin	Zocor	10-80 mg
ATP-Citrate Lyase Inhibitor		
Bempedoic acid	Nexletol	180 mg
PCSK9 Inhibitors		
Evolocumab	Repatha	140 mg every 2 wk or 420 mg once monthly
Alirocumab	Praluent	75 mg every 2 wk or 300 mg once monthly
Inclisiran	Leqvio	300 mg twice yearly
Cholesterol Absorption Inhibitor		
Ezetimibe	Zetia (Ezetrol)	10 mg
Bile Acid Absorption Inhibitors		
Cholestyramine	Cholestyramine	Cholestyramine
Colestipol	Colestipol	Colestipol
Colesevelam	Colesevelam	Colesevelam
Fibrates		
Bezafibrate	Bezalip	400 mg
Fenofibrate	Tricor, Trilipix Lipidil (Micro, EZ)	40-200 mg
Gemfibrozil	Lopid	600-1200 mg
Niacin	Niacin	1-3 g
Nicotinic acid	Niaspan	1-2 g

From Libby P et al: *Braunwald's heart disease, a textbook of cardiovascular medicine*, ed 12, Philadelphia, 2022, Elsevier.

TABLE 7 Expected Decrease in Low-Density Lipoprotein Cholesterol in Response to Statins

Drug	MEAN REDUCTION BY DOSE: % CHANGE FROM BASELINE				
	5 mg	10 mg	20 mg	40 mg	80 mg
Rosuvastatin	−40%	−46%	−52%	−55%	—
Atorvastatin	—	−37%	−43%	−48%	−51%
Simvastatin	−26%	−30%	−38%	−41%	−47%
Lovastatin	—	−21%	−27%	−31%	−40%
Pravastatin	—	−20%	−24%	−30%	−36%
Fluvastatin	—	—	−22%	−25%	−35%
Ezetimibe alone		−20%			
Bile acid sequestrants (Cholestyramine, Colestipol, Colesevelam): add a mean 15% decrease					

Adapted from Grundy SM et al: 2018 AHA/ACC/AACVPR/AAPA/ABC/ACPM/ADA/AGS/APhA/ASPC/NLA/PCNA guideline on the management of blood cholesterol: a report of the American College of Cardiology/American Heart Association Task Force on Clinical Practice Guidelines, *J Am Coll Cardiol* 73(24):e285-e350, 2019; and Mach F et al: Adverse effects of statin therapy: perception vs. the evidence—focus on glucose homeostasis, cognitive, renal and hepatic function, haemorrhagic stroke and cataract, *Eur Heart J* 39(27):2526-2539, 2019. In: Libby P et al: *Braunwald's heart disease, a textbook of cardiovascular medicine*, ed 12, Philadelphia, 2022, Elsevier.

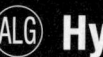
Diseases
and Disorders

I

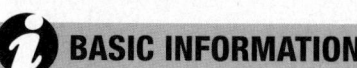 **BASIC INFORMATION**

DEFINITION

Hypernatremia is a clinical disorder that results from net water deficit (i.e., dehydration). It is identified when the serum sodium concentration (S_{Na}) exceeds the upper limit of the normal range (145 mEq/L). Hypernatremia does not reflect the net total body sodium content or extracellular fluid volume status. Consequently, patients with hypernatremia may be hypovolemic, hypervolemic, or normovolemic.

SYNONYMS

Hyperosmolality
Hypertonicity
High serum sodium concentration
Dehydration hyponatremia

ICD-10CM CODES
E87.0 Hyperosmolality and/or hypernatremia
E86.0 Dehydration/volume depletion

EPIDEMIOLOGY & DEMOGRAPHICS

The prevalence of hypernatremia varies based on the defined population and clinical setting. In the outpatient setting, hypernatremia occurs at the extremes of age. The prevalence among adults is 0.7% while prevalence among elderly is 2.6%.[1] Almost 60% of cases develop in hospitalized patients, and approximately 80% of these cases occur in intensive care units.[2]

Among noncritical hospitalized patients, the prevalence of hypernatremia is 0.2% to 2.5%.[2,3] The incidence is greater in critically ill and older adult patients, and the prevalence ranges from 10% to 26% in the hospitalized population.[2,3] The severity of hypernatremia correlates with mortality.[2] In patients with COVID-19, hypernatremia is noted in as high as 10%, and these patients have a twofold increased risk of death.[2,4]

RISK FACTORS:

- Age >60 yr
- Sex
- Acute kidney injury on admission
- Altered mental status
- Mechanical ventilation
- Enteral tube feeding
- Negative fluid balance
- Hyperglycemia
- Hypertonic solution administration (e.g., bicarbonate or mannitol)
- Hypokalemia
- Hypercalcemia
- Underlying polyuric disorders

PHYSICAL FINDINGS & CLINICAL PRESENTATION

- Symptoms generally correlate with severity of hypernatremia, how rapidly hypernatremia developed (Figs. 1 and 2), and the underlying cause.

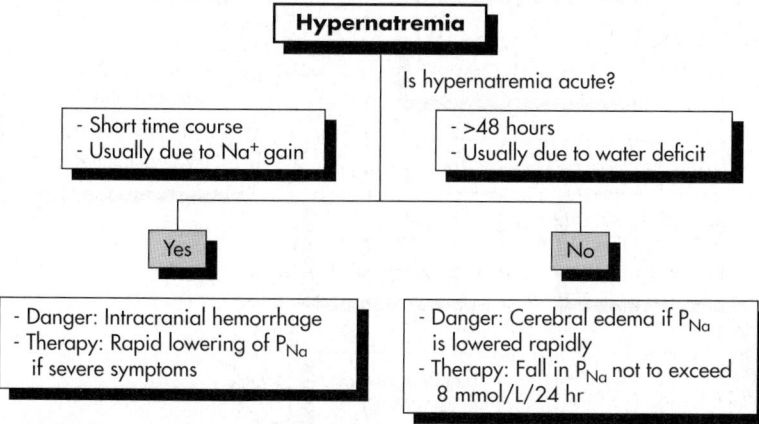

FIG. 1 Emergencies associated with hypernatremia. The emergencies in patients with acute hypernatremia are caused by brain cell shrinkage and resultant rupture of blood vessels, leading to focal intracerebral and subarachnoid hemorrhages. The danger in the patient with chronic hypernatremia is a rapid and large fall in the PNa, which results in brain cell swelling and possibly brain herniation. (From Kamel SK, Halpertin ML: *Fluid, electrolyte, and acid-base physiology*, ed 5, Philadelphia 2017, Elsevier.)

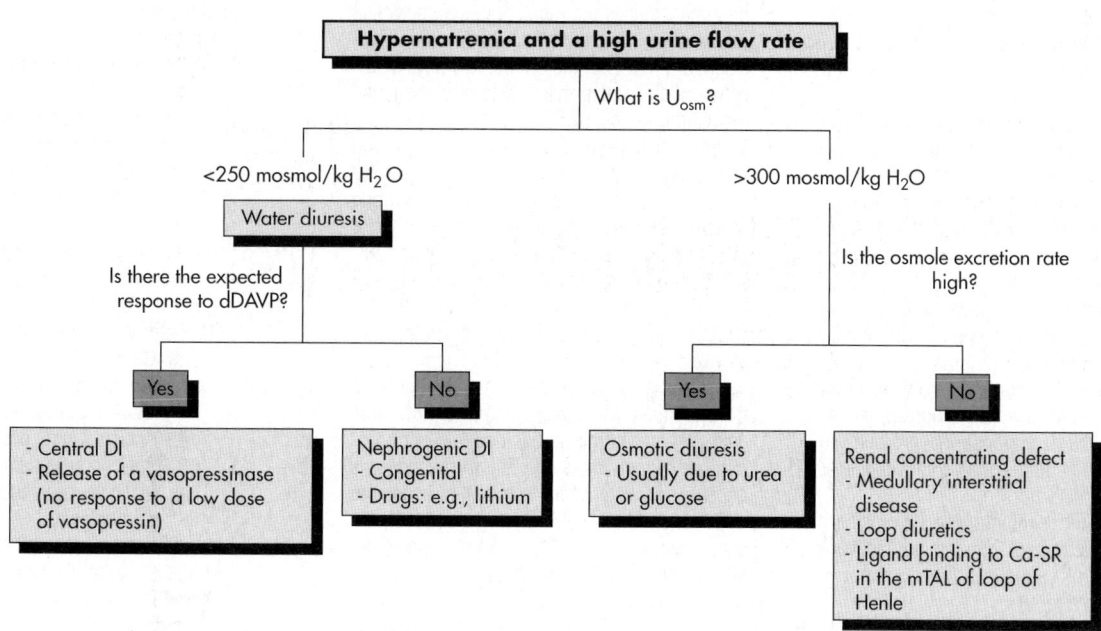

FIG. 2 Hypernatremia with a high urine flow rate. The first step is to determine whether the water loss is caused by a water diuresis or an osmotic diuresis, or whether there is a renal concentrating defect. The principal tools are assessment of the U_{osm} (urine osmolality) and calculation of the osmole excretion rate. In a patient with central diabetes insipidus *(DI)* or a water diuresis caused by the release of a vasopressinase, U_{osm} should rise to a value that is higher than the P_{osm} (plasma osmolality) in response to the administration of deamino-D-arginine vasopressin *(dDAVP)*. If not, nephrogenic DI is the basis of the water diuresis. A value of the U_{osm} that is higher than 300 mosmol/kg H_2O suggests that the basis of hypernatremia is an osmotic diuresis if the osmole excretion rate is appreciably higher than 1000 mosmol/day or a renal concentrating defect if the osmole excretion rate is not high. Examples of ligand binding to the calcium sensing receptor *(Ca-SR)* in the medullary thick ascending limb *(mTAL)* of the loop of Henle include calcium ions in a patient with hypercalcemia, cationic drugs (e.g., gentamicin, cisplatin). (From Kamel SK, Halpertin ML: *Fluid, electrolyte, and acid-base physiology*, ed 5, Philadelphia 2017, Elsevier.)

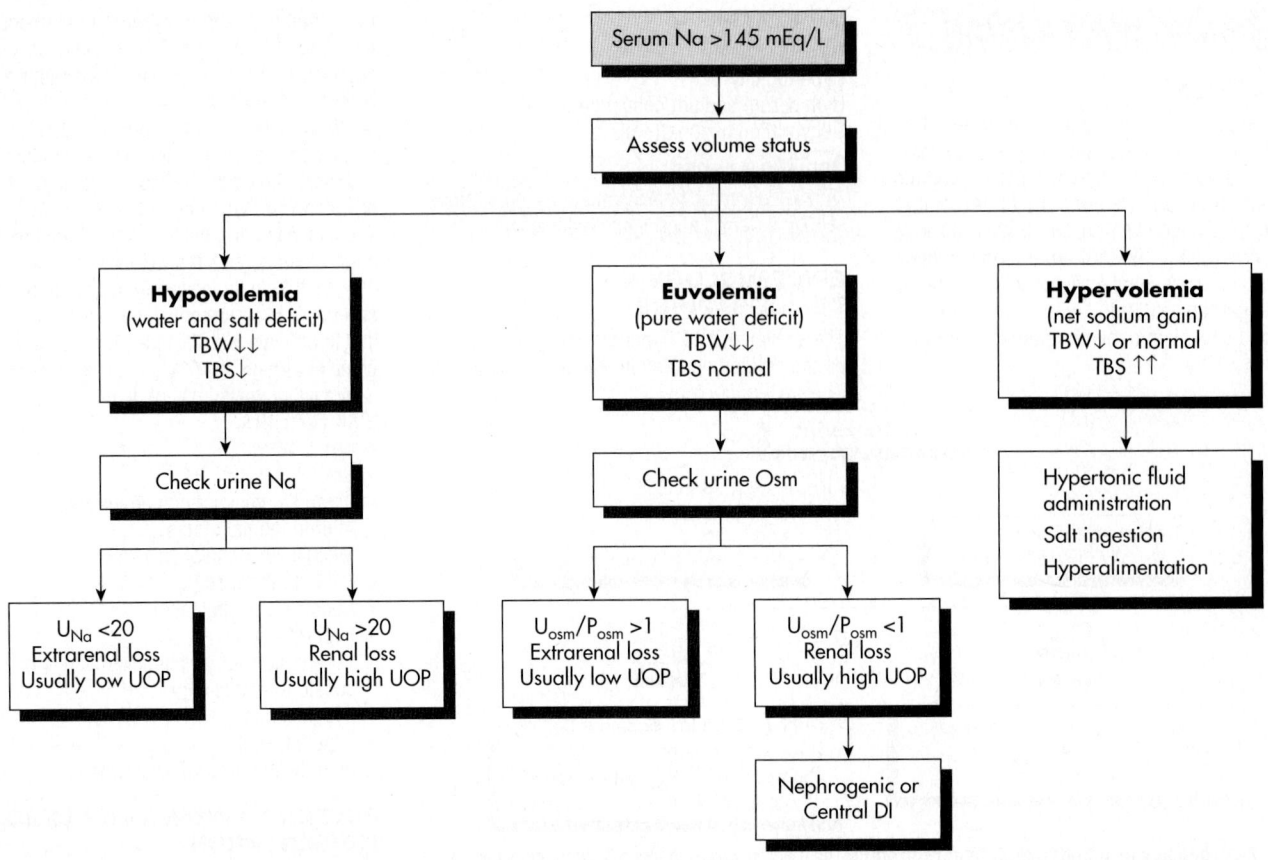

FIG. 3 Diagnostic approach to hypernatremia. *DI,* Diabetes insipidus; *Na,* sodium; *Osm,* osmolality; *TBS,* total body salt; *TBW,* total body water; *UOP,* urine output; U$_{osm}$, urine osmolality; P$_{osm}$, plasma osmolality. (Adapted from Gilbert SJ, Weiner DE: *National Kidney Foundation primer on kidney disease,* ed 6, Philadelphia, 2017, Saunders.)

- In mild hypernatremia, symptoms can include generalized muscle weakness, fatigue, restlessness, anorexia, nausea, and vomiting.[5]
- With severe hypernatremia, symptoms can begin with lethargy and irritability and progress to confusion, seizures, and rarely, coma.[5]
- In extreme scenarios, particularly in infants, hypernatremia-induced brain cell shrinkage can lead to intracranial bleeding from vascular stretching.[6,7]
- Polydipsia and polyuria may be present in certain types of hypernatremia, such as with diabetes insipidus (DI).[6]
- Key elements of the history should focus on water intake, fluid loss, urine output, insensible losses, thirst response, accessibility to water, and medications that could cause or be associated with thirst.[6]
- Clinicians should evaluate the extracellular fluid volume status of patients to facilitate determination of cause and management of hypernatremia (Fig. 3).

ETIOLOGY

- The etiology of hypernatremia is understood through the Edelman equation (refer to "Hyponatremia"). S$_{Na}$ closely approximates the ratio of total exchangeable body (TB) cations (sodium and potassium, TB$_{Na}$ + TB$_{K}$) to total body water (TBW).[8]
- Serum [Na] = S$_{Na}$ = (TB$_{Na}$ + TB$_{K}$)/TBW.[8]

- Hypernatremia is the result of net water deficit or excessive sodium intake.[8] Renal water regulation and thirst stimuli are the key physiologic components that prevent hypernatremia and maintain homeostasis.[8]
- To prevent hypernatremia, water is retained and urine is concentrated by the kidneys under the influence of antidiuretic hormone or arginine vasopressin (AVP). Impairment of AVP secretion, reduction of the corticomedullary concentration gradient, or inability of AVP to stimulate water reabsorption leads to excessive renal water loss and hypernatremia.[8]
- Elevated plasma osmolality from hypernatremia triggers the hypothalamic thirst response.[8] If water intake exceeds water loss or net solute gain, hypernatremia is avoided.[8] Hypernatremia develops when the thirst response is impaired or when there is a lack of access to water, a common circumstance for mechanically ventilated patients, infants, and older adults who may have cognitive impairment(s) and physical limitation(s).[7,8]

Hypernatremia can be classified in the following manner:

- Excessive water loss[1]
  1. GI losses
     a. Vomiting or nasogastric losses
     b. Ileostomy
     c. Pancreaticobiliary fistula
     d. Diarrhea
     e. Laxatives

  2. Renal losses[1]
     a. Osmotic diuresis
        (1) Osmotic diuretics (mannitol, sorbitol, glycine)
        (2) Glucosuria (hyperglycemia, SGLT2 inhibitor administration)
        (3) Urea diuresis (e.g., steroid use, high-protein diet, hypercatabolic state)
        (4) Postobstructive and post–acute tubular necrosis (post-ATN) diuresis
     b. Water diuresis[1,9]
        (1) Central diabetes insipidus (CDI)
           (a) Genetic
              i. Autosomal dominant
              ii. Autosomal recessive
           (b) Acquired (e.g., posttrauma, iatrogenic, craniopharyngioma, metastatic cancers, encephalitis)
           (c) Sarcoidosis
           (d) Langerhans cell histiocytosis
           (e) Eosinophilic granulomatosis
        (2) Nephrogenic diabetes insipidus (NDI)[10]
           (a) Genetic
              i. Arginine vasopressin receptor 2 *(AVPR2)* or aquaporin 2 *(AQP2)* gene sequence variants
              ii. Autosomal dominant polycystic kidney disease
              iii. Familial hypocalciuric hypercalcemia from renal

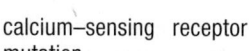

calcium–sensing receptor mutation
  (b) Acquired
    i. Chronic kidney disease
    ii. Post-ATN diuresis
    iii. Hypokalemia
    iv. Hypercalcemia (diverse causes)
    v. Drugs (e.g., lithium, amphotericin, ifosfamide, demeclocycline)
    vi. Gestation (increased placental vasopressinase)
- Impaired water intake[6]
  1. Adipsia or hypodipsia
    a. Septo-optic dysplasia
    b. Craniopharyngioma
  2. Impaired access to water
    a. Mechanical ventilation
    b. Dementia
    c. Cognitive impairment
- Excessive sodium intake[6]
  1. Hypertonic saline or sodium bicarbonate administration
  2. Salt tablet excess ingestion
  3. Saltwater drowning

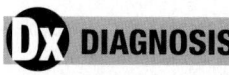 DIAGNOSIS

DIFFERENTIAL DIAGNOSIS

Hypernatremia is a clinical result of net water deficit as a result of dehydration.[11] Conversely, volume depletion occurs as a result of net loss of total body sodium and water that reduces the extracellular fluid and intravascular volumes.[11,12] The combination of dehydration and volume depletion has management implications. For example, normovolemic hypernatremia is caused by pure water loss, and the appropriate volume of water replacement is adequate treatment.[12,13] This strategy is not appropriate in hypovolemic hypernatremia because volume electrolytes (sodium and potassium) and water losses also require replacement.[12,13]

WORKUP

- Workup: Detailed history and physical examination. Historical features that reveal volume depletion and/or dehydration are critical and include a family history of DI and medication or drug use that enhances renal water excretion.[13]
- Hospitalized patients: Frequent monitoring of cumulative fluid intake and fluid losses is mandatory. The most common cause is replacement of total net fluid loss with 0.9% saline.[6,12]
- Hypernatremia in adults: Usually develops from net water loss and inability to access water (e.g., altered mentation, mechanical ventilation).[6] If access to water is not restricted, etiologies that impair thirst center function should be considered.
- In the presence of polyuria, the underlying etiology should be sought.

LABORATORY TESTS[8]

- Serum chemistry: Serial S_{Na} measurements based on clinical scenario (e.g., 2 to 12 h). Frequent monitoring maintains the correction rate of S_{Na} at recommended levels. Derangements of other electrolyte and renal parameters frequently accompany hypernatremia.
- Urine osmolality (U_{osm}): With a normal hypothalamic-pituitary-kidney axis, a plasma osmolality (P_{osm}) elevation of $\geq 1\%$ induces AVP secretion and increases urine concentration (U_{osm} exceeds P_{osm}, typically >600 to 700 mOsm/kg). Accordingly, U_{osm} distinguishes central or nephrogenic DI from the presence of extrarenal water loss.
  1. Low U_{osm} (<300 mOsm/kg) suggests hypernatremia from CDI or NDI. After an initial diagnostic workup is conducted, differentiation between CDI and NDI is required (see "Diabetes Insipidus" chapter).

2. High U_{osm} typically occurs from extrarenal water losses.
- Urine sodium (U_{Na}) and urine potassium (U_K): U_{Na} assists in the determination of intravascular volume (see Fig. 3). The sum of U_{Na} and U_K quantify urine electrolyte-free water clearance to guide therapy, as explained later. Electrolyte-free water has no effective osmolality (tonicity) at equilibrium and is water composed of no electrolytes with or without urea. Urinary parameters should be monitored every 12 to 24 h until S_{Na} is adequately corrected.

℞ TREATMENT

- Treatment of hypernatremia requires replacement of the existing water deficit and of ongoing daily electrolyte-free water losses.
- Volume replacement generally precedes replacement of water deficit.
- A stepwise approach to the therapy of hypernatremia is depicted in Fig. 4.
  1. Step 1: Determine rate of S_{Na} correction.[5,13]
    a. Although the exact risk is unknown, overcorrection of chronic hyponatremia (>48 h) may induce serious neurologic consequences, namely cerebral edema.
    b. Based on clinical data from infants and critically ill adults, chronic hypernatremia should not be corrected faster than 10 to 12 mEq/L/day, or an average of 0.5 mEq/L/h. This rate would apply to most nonhospitalized older adult patients because hypernatremia develops over several days.
    c. In rare individuals with acute hypernatremia (e.g., intentional or accidental massive sodium ingestions), the S_{Na} may be rapidly corrected (within 24 h) to normal S_{Na} levels. The rate of correction should be no less than 0.25 mmol/h, as prolonged hypernatremia is associated with mortality risk.

- Step 1: Identify rate of correction.
- Step 2: Calculate free water deficit.

$$\text{Water deficit} = \text{TBW} \left[\frac{\text{Current } S_{Na} - \text{Desired } S_{Na}}{\text{Desired } S_{Na}} \right]$$

- Step 3: Choose fluid replacement regimen.

$$\text{Change in } S_{Na} = \frac{\text{Infusate Na} - \text{Current } S_{Na}}{\text{TBW} + 1}$$

- Step 4: Assess ongoing water losses.
  - Urinary water losses estimated by free water clearance

$$C_{\text{electrolyte-free}} = V \left[1 - \frac{U_{Na} + U_K}{S_{Na}} \right]$$

  - Insensible water losses approximately 15-20 mL/kg/day
- Step 5: Determine underlying cause.

FIG. 4 Approach to treatment of hypernatremia. $C_{electrolyte-free}$, Electrolyte-free water clearance; *Na,* sodium; S_{Na}, serum sodium; *TBW,* total body water; U_K, urine potassium; U_{Na}, urine sodium; *V,* urine volume. (Adapted from Gilbert SJ, Weiner DE: *National Kidney Foundation primer on kidney disease,* ed 6, Philadelphia, 2017, Saunders.)

2. Step 2: Calculate free water deficit[6,8]
   a. Free water deficit is the volume of free water required to correct the current S_{Na} to the target S_{Na}. This is estimated by the Adrogué-Madias formula:
      (1) Water deficit = TBW × [(Current S_{Na}/Target S_{Na}) − 1].
   b. For the preceding formula, TBW is the estimated TBW. TBW estimates are 50% to 60% of lean body weight in men and women. Target S_{Na} is the S_{Na} that should be achieved in a 24-h period as determined in Step 1.
3. Step 3: Choose fluid replacement regimen[6,8]
   a. With a pure water deficit, the water deficit of Step 2 should be replaced by enteral water or intravenous D_5W.
   b. When possible, the enteral route should be used during hydration therapy to avoid rapid glucose water infusions that may induce hyperglycemia and produce an osmotic diuresis. This pathophysiologic sequence may occur, as D_5W infusion rates are increased to greater than 300 ml/h.
   c. The rate of water replacement (ml/h) is obtained by dividing the calculated water deficit volume by 24 h. It is essential that the ongoing rate of water loss (e.g., urine losses, stool losses) be addressed simultaneously.
   d. Because hypovolemia is present in more than 50% of cases of hypernatremia, concurrent volume replacement with isotonic fluid should be administered (0.9% sodium chloride or lactated Ringer's solution, as required). An alternative strategy is to use a single infusion of 0.45% saline solution that replaces salt and water along with potassium deficits. For example, 1 L of 0.45% NaCl adds 500 ml of water and 500 ml of 0.9% NaCl to the TBW.
   e. The change in S_{Na} with 1 L of a particular replacement fluid can be predicted by the Adrogué-Madias formula:
      (1) Change in S_{Na} = ($Na_{infusate}$ − current S_{Na}) / (TBW + 1).
   f. This formula applies to the one-time administration of a 1-L infusate with a sodium concentration ($Na_{infusate}$). $Na_{infusate}$ concentrations for 0.45% saline, 0.9% saline, and 3% saline are 77, 154, and 513 mEq/L, respectively.
4. Step 4: Assess ongoing water losses[6,8]
   a. Ongoing daily water losses (skin, stool, and respiratory tract) must be calculated and treated simultaneously. Failure to account for these losses leads to an undercorrection of hypernatremia.
   b. Urinary losses are estimated by the electrolyte-free water clearance equation shown in Fig. 4.
   c. Insensible water losses can be estimated as 15 to 20 ml/kg/day.

Evaluate for any underlying cause of hypernatremia and treat accordingly. If hypernatremia occurs with hypervolemia, use loop diuretics to remove excess sodium.[8] However, diuretic therapy will also increase water losses that must be accounted for.

Repeat Steps 1 to 4 until S_{Na} is reduced to approximately 140 to 145 mEq/L.

The preceding method represents guidance based on classical estimating equations and periodic monitoring of clinical parameters and is key to achievement of the target S_{Na}.

DISPOSITION

Management of hypernatremia generally warrants inpatient admission because patients have underlying conditions that impair the thirst response.

REFERRAL

Nephrology consultation for management of hypernatremia and evaluation of underlying causes is appropriate. Endocrinology consultation may be warranted if DI is suspected.

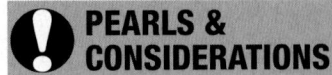

❗ PEARLS & CONSIDERATIONS

COMMENTS

- Hypernatremia is a water-deficit problem associated with impaired thirst and/or inability to obtain water.
- Hypernatremia has morbid consequences, including mortality.
- Hypernatremia may present with hypovolemia, and the latter is usually treated first.
- The S_{Na} correction rate includes determination of the water deficit plus ongoing water losses.

REFERENCES

Available at eBooks.Health.Elsevier.com.

AUTHOR: **LALATHAKSHA KUMBAR, MD**

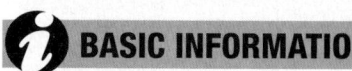
BASIC INFORMATION

DEFINITION

Normal blood pressure (BP) in adults can be defined as systolic BP <120 mm Hg and diastolic BP <80 mm Hg. Elevated BP is defined as systolic BP between 120 and 129 mm Hg or diastolic BP <80 mm Hg. Hypertension (HTN) can be divided into (1) stage 1: Systolic BP from 130 to 139 mm Hg or diastolic BP from 80 to 89 mm Hg and (2) stage 2: Systolic BP ≥140 mm Hg or diastolic BP ≥90 mm Hg. This definition is based on accurate measurements and average of ≥2 readings on ≥2 occasions.

SYNONYMS

HTN
Essential hypertension
Idiopathic hypertension
High BP

ICD-10CM CODES

I10	Essential (primary) hypertension
I15.0	Renovascular hypertension
I15.1	Hypertension secondary to other renal disorders
I15.2	Hypertension secondary to endocrine disorders
I15.8	Other secondary hypertension
I15.9	Secondary hypertension, unspecified
O10.919	Unspecified pre-existing hypertension complicating pregnancy, unspecified trimester
I67.4	Hypertensive encephalopathy

EPIDEMIOLOGY & DEMOGRAPHICS

- In the U.S., 50% of people aged 60 to 69 yr and ~75% of people >70 yr of age are affected by HTN. Worldwide, it is estimated that 41% of people ages 35 to 70 yr have HTN, and only 46.5% of them are aware of it.
- Peak prevalence increases with age and is highest among non-Hispanic Black adults in the U.S.
- HTN is linked with a higher risk of heart attack, stroke, heart failure, and kidney disease.

PHYSICAL FINDINGS & CLINICAL PRESENTATION

Physical examination may be entirely within normal limits, except for the presence of elevated BP. A proper initial physical examination on a hypertensive patient should include the following:
- The BP should be measured with an appropriately sized cuff (bladder of the cuff should cover at least two thirds of the circumference of the arm) and taken in both arms (the higher of the readings being used). Table 1 describes BP cuff size and error in measurement.
- The BP should be measured twice on each visit and separated by at least 1 to 2 min to allow the return of trapped blood.

- The patient should be seated in a calm environment for at least 5 min with the arm in which BP is measured rested on support level with the heart.
- Postural BP change should always be recorded in the elderly to diagnose postural hypotension. This is assessed by taking BP in supine (after 5-min rest) and standing (after 2 min) positions. A drop of ≥20 mm Hg in systolic, a drop of ≥10 mm Hg diastolic BP, or symptoms of cerebral hypoperfusion is suggestive of postural (orthostatic) hypotension.
- A diagnosis of HTN may be established if the BP is markedly elevated (>180/110 mm Hg) or has evidence of end organ damage; otherwise such a diagnosis should wait until BP is found elevated on more than two readings on more than two different occasions.
- Nonoffice (home, workplace, 24-h ambulatory) BP determination to establish the pattern of HTN (sustained, "white coat," or "masked" HTN) in selected patients.
- Measure heart rate, height, weight, body mass index, and waist circumference.
- Some general clinical clues for when to screen for secondary HTN include:
  1. Severe or resistant HTN
  2. An acute rise in BP developing in a patient with previous stable BP
  3. Age less than 30 yr, nonobese, non-Black with no family history of HTN
  4. Sudden onset or accelerated HTN
  5. Age of onset before puberty. If above is suspected, additional tests for secondary HTN should be done, including renin, aldosterone, cortisol levels, 24-h urine metanephrines, and serum catecholamines
- Physical examination should include searching for secondary causes, and sequelae of HTN.
- Examine skin for the presence of café-au-lait spots (neurofibromatosis), uremic appearance (renal failure), and violaceous striae (Cushing syndrome).
- Perform careful funduscopic examination; check for papilledema, retinal exudates, hemorrhages, arterial narrowing, arteriovenous compression.
- Examine neck for carotid bruits, distended neck veins, and enlarged thyroid gland.

- Perform extensive cardiopulmonary examination: Check for a laterally displaced point of maximal intensity, an S3 or S4, and valvular murmurs.
- Palpate abdomen for renal masses (pheochromocytoma, polycystic kidneys), and auscultate for bruit over the aorta and renal arteries.
- Examine arterial pulses (dilated or absent femoral pulses and BP greater in upper extremities than lower extremities suggest aortic coarctation).
- Look for truncal obesity (Cushing syndrome) and pedal edema (congestive heart failure [CHF]).
- Table 2 provides a guide to evaluation of identifiable causes of HTN.
- Table 3 summarizes clinical clues to guide the investigation in young patients with hypertension that has a potentially hereditary cause.

ETIOLOGY

- Essential (primary) HTN (85%)
- Drug induced or drug related (5%)
  1. NSAIDs
  2. Oral contraceptives
  3. Corticosteroids
- Renal HTN (5%)
  1. Renal parenchymal disease (3%)
  2. Renovascular HTN (RVH) (<2%)
- Endocrine (<2%) (Table 4)
  1. Primary aldosteronism (at least 5%)
  2. Pheochromocytoma (0.2%)
  3. Cushing syndrome and long-term steroid therapy (0.2%)
  4. Hyperparathyroidism or thyroid disease (0.2%)
- Coarctation of the aorta (0.2%)
- Causes of secondary hypertension are summarized in Box 1

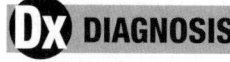 **DIAGNOSIS**

WORKUP

- The objective for the initial evaluation of HTN is to establish the diagnosis and stage of HTN. Table 5 summarizes initial laboratory evaluation of the hypertensive patient

TABLE 1 Blood Pressure Cuff Size and Error in Measurement*

	ARM CIRCUMFERENCE		
Cuff Bladder Size	28 cm or less	29-42 cm	43 cm or more
Regular (12 × 23 cm)	Accurate	Overestimates SBP by 4-8 mm Hg DBP by 3-6 mm Hg	Overestimates SBP by 16-17 mm Hg DBP by 10-11 mm Hg
Large (15 × 33 cm)	Underestimates SBP by 2-3 mm Hg DBP by 1-2 mm Hg	Accurate	Overestimates SBP by 5-7 mm Hg DBP by 2-4 mm Hg
Thigh (18 × 36 cm)	Underestimates SBP by 5-7 mm Hg DBP by 1-3 mm Hg	Underestimates SBP by 5-7 mm Hg DBP by 2-4 mm Hg	Accurate

DBP, Diastolic blood pressure reading; *SBP*, systolic blood pressure reading.
Overestimation means that hypertension may be diagnosed in someone with normal blood pressure; *underestimation* means that the blood pressure reading may be normal in someone who actually has high blood pressure. See text for further discussion.
From McGee S et al: *Evidence-based physical diagnosis*, ed 4, Philadelphia, 2018, Elsevier.

TABLE 2 Guide to Evaluation of Identifiable Causes of Hypertension

Suspected Diagnosis	Clinical Clues	Diagnostic Testing
Chronic kidney disease	Estimated GFR <60 ml/min/1.73 m² Urine albumin-to-creatinine ratio ≥30 mg/g	Renal sonography
Renovascular disease	New elevation in serum creatinine, marked elevation in serum creatinine with ACEI or ARB, drug-resistant hypertension, flash pulmonary edema, abdominal, or flank bruit	Renal sonography (atrophic kidney), CT or MR angiography, invasive angiography
Coarctation of the aorta	Arm pulses > leg pulses, arm BP > leg BP, chest bruits, rib notching on chest radiography	MR angiography, TEE, invasive angiography
Primary aldosteronism	Hypokalemia, drug-resistant hypertension	Plasma renin and aldosterone, 24-h urine aldosterone and potassium after oral salt loading, adrenal vein sampling
Cushing syndrome	Truncal obesity, wide and blanching purple striae, muscle weakness	1 mg dexamethasone-suppression test, urinary cortisol after dexamethasone, adrenal CT
Pheochromocytoma	Paroxysms of hypertension, palpitations, perspiration, and pallor; diabetes	Plasma metanephrines, 24-h urinary metanephrines and catecholamines, abdominal CT or MR imaging
Obstructive sleep apnea	Loud snoring, large neck, obesity, somnolence	Polysomnography

ACEI, Angiotensin-converting enzyme inhibitor; *ARB,* angiotensin receptor blocker; *BP,* blood pressure; *CT,* computed tomography; *GFR,* glomerular filtration rate; *MR,* magnetic resonance; *TEE,* transesophageal echocardiography.
From Goldman L, Schafer AI: *Goldman's Cecil medicine,* ed 24, Philadelphia, 2012, Saunders.

- Gather office and nonoffice BP readings, assess presence of target organ damage (TOD), assess the level of global cardiovascular disease risk, and produce a plan for individualized monitoring and therapy
- Patient counseling and education should be prominent features of the initial evaluation
- Pertinent history:
  1. Age of onset of HTN, previous antihypertensive therapy
  2. Family history of HTN, stroke, cardiovascular disease
- Diet, salt intake, caffeine, alcohol, drugs (e.g., oral contraceptives, NSAIDs, decongestants, steroids)
- Occupation, lifestyle, pain, socioeconomic status, psychologic factors
- Other cardiovascular risk factors: Hyperlipidemia, obesity, diabetes mellitus
- Symptoms of secondary HTN:
  1. Headache, palpitations, excessive perspiration (possible pheochromocytoma)
  2. Weakness, polyuria (consider hyperaldosteronism)
  3. Claudication of lower extremities (seen with coarctation of aorta)
  4. Loud snoring, daytime somnolence, morning confusion (may warrant evaluation for sleep apnea)

LABORATORY TESTS
- Routine laboratory tests recommended before initiating therapy include:
  1. Urinalysis with microscopic evaluation; for signs of glomerulopathy
  2. Basic metabolic panel and calcium; for signs of kidney damage, hypokalemia (primary aldosteronism and Cushing syndrome), hypercalcemia (hyperparathyroid)
  3. CBC
  4. Screening for coexisting diseases that may adversely affect prognosis; hemoglobin

A_{1c} or fasting glucose level, serum lipid panel
  5. Optional tests include measurement of urinary albumin or albumin/creatinine ratio

IMAGING STUDIES
- Electrocardiogram (ECG): Check for presence of left ventricular hypertrophy (LVH) with strain pattern.
- Renal duplex ultrasonography, computed tomography (CT) angiography, or magnetic resonance angiography of the renal arteries in suspected renovascular hypertension (renal artery stenosis) may be considered.

🆁🆇 TREATMENT

NONPHARMACOLOGIC THERAPY
Lifestyle modifications (the initial treatment of hypertension should focus on lifestyle modifications [Table 6]):
- Weight loss if overweight (target body mass index [BMI] <25).
- Limit alcohol intake to 1 oz of ethanol per day (<2 drinks/day) in men or 0.5 oz (<1 drink/day) in women.
- Regular aerobic exercise (at least 30 min/day on most days).
- Reduce sodium intake to <100 mmol/day (<1.5 g of sodium/day).
- Maintain adequate dietary potassium (>3500 mg/day) intake in patients with normal kidney function.
- Smoking cessation.
- The BP reduction seen ranges from 2 to 20 mm Hg, most significant with substantial weight loss and the implementation of the Dietary Approaches to Stop Hypertension (DASH) eating plan, which relies on a diet high in fruits and vegetables, moderate in low-fat dairy products, and low in animal protein but with

substantial amount of plant protein from legumes and nuts.

ACUTE GENERAL Rx
- Multiple recent consensus documents regarding BP goals and when to initiate treatment have been published. Antihypertensive medications are summarized in Table 7. Antihypertensive choices in the setting of cardiovascular comorbidity are described in Table 8.
  1. For low-risk adults (no atherosclerotic cardiovascular disease [ASCVD] or 10-yr cardiovascular disease [CVD] risk <10%) with stage 1 hypertension, management should start with nonpharmacologic therapy. If BP remains uncontrolled after 3 to 6 mo, then consider starting pharmacologic therapy.[1]
  2. For adults with confirmed hypertension and known CVD or 10-yr ASCVD event risk of 10% or higher, a BP target of less than 130/80 mm Hg is recommended.[2]
  3. For adults with confirmed hypertension without additional markers of increased CVD risk, a BP target of less than 130/80 mm Hg may be reasonable.
- In addition, initiation of therapy recommendations is as follows:
  1. Use of BP-lowering medication is recommended for primary prevention of CVD in adults with no history of CVD and with an estimated 10-yr ASCVD risk, <10% and stage 2 HTN.
  2. Use of BP-lowering medications is recommended for secondary prevention of recurrent CVD events in patients with clinical CVD and for primary prevention in adults with an estimated 10-yr ASCVD risk of 10% or higher and stage 1 HTN.
  3. Initiate antihypertensive drug therapy with two first-line agents of different classes for adults with stage 2 HTN and BP more than 20/10 mm Hg higher than their target.

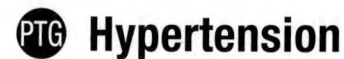
Diseases and Disorders

I

TABLE 3 Clinical Clues to Guide the Investigation in Young Patients with Hypertension That Has a Potentially Hereditary Cause

Specific Conditions	Possible Causes of Familial Hypertension	Clinical Clues
Catecholamine-Producing Tumors		
Pheochromocytoma/paraganglioma	Familial cases are responsible for <30% of cases, including MEN2A and MEN2B, von Hippel-Lindau disease, neurofibromatosis, and familial paraganglioma syndromes (SDH complex mutations)	Paroxysmal palpitations, headaches, diaphoresis, pale flushing; syndromic features of any of the associated disorders
Neuroblastomas (adrenal) Aortic or renovascular lesions	1%-2% of neuroblastomas are familial	
Coarctation of the aorta	Overrepresented in families but no familial distribution	Asymmetry between upper- and lower-extremity BP, radial-formal pulse delay; associated with Turner syndrome, Williams syndrome, and bicuspid aortic valve
Renal artery stenosis caused by fibromuscular dysplasia or inherited arterial wall lesions	<10% familial with AD pattern	Abnormal renal vascular imaging results; vascular disease in the carotid territory at an early age; common in neurofibromatosis and Williams syndrome; also present in tuberous sclerosis, Ehlers-Danlos syndrome, and Marfan syndrome
Parenchymal kidney disease GN	Alport disease (X-linked, AR, or AD), familial IgA nephropathy (AD with incomplete penetrance)	Proteinuria, hematuria, low eGFR
PKD	ADPKD type 1 or 2, ARPKD	Multiple renal cysts (as few as three in patients under 30 yr)
Adrenocortical disease Glucocorticoid-remediable aldosteronism (familial hyperaldosteronism type I)	AD chimeric fusion of the 11β-hydroxylase and aldosterone synthase genes	Cerebral hemorrhages at young age, cerebral aneurysms; mild hypokalemia; high plasma aldosterone, low renin
Familial hyperaldosteronism	AD; unknown defect	Severe type 2 hypertension in early adulthood; high plasma aldosterone, low renin; no response to glucocorticoid treatment
Familial hyperaldosteronism type III	AD; unknown defect	Severe hypertension in childhood with extensive target-organ damage; high plasma aldosterone, low renin; marked bilateral adrenal enlargement
Congenital adrenal hyperplasia	AR mutations in 11β-hydroxylase or 21-hydroxylase	Hirsutism, virilization; hypokalemia and metabolic alkalosis; low plasma aldosterone and renin
Monogenic Primary Renal Tubular Defects		
Gordon syndrome	AD mutations of *KLHL3, CUL3, WNK1*, and *WNK4*; AR mutations of *KLHL3*	Hyperkalemia and metabolic acidosis with normal renal function
Liddle syndrome	AD mutations of the epithelial sodium channel	Hypokalemia and metabolic alkalosis; low plasma aldosterone and renin
Apparent mineralocorticoid excess	AD mutation in 11β-hydroxysteroid dehydrogenase type 2	Hypokalemia and metabolic alkalosis; low plasma aldosterone and renin
Geller syndrome Hypertension-brachydactyly syndrome	AD mutation in the mineralocorticoid receptor AD mutations in the phosphodiesterase E3A enzyme	Hypokalemia and metabolic alkalosis; low plasma aldosterone and renin; increased BP during pregnancy or exposure to spironolactone
Unknown Mechanisms		
Hypertension-brachydactyly syndrome	AD	Short fingers (small phalanges) and short stature; brain stem compression from vascular tortuosity in the posterior fossa
Essential Hypertension		
	Polygenic	When obesity or metabolic syndrome is present, the likelihood of essential hypertension is higher

AD, Autosomal dominant; *ADPKD,* autosomal dominant polycystic kidney disease; *AR,* autosomal recessive; *ARPKD,* autosomal recessive polycystic kidney disease; *BP,* blood pressure; *eGFR,* estimated glomerular filtration rate; *GN,* glomerulonephritis; *IgA,* immunoglobulin A; *MEN,* multiple endocrine neoplasia; *PKD,* polycystic kidney disease; *SDH,* succinate dehydrogenase.
From Skorecki K et al: *Brenner and Rector's the kidney,* ed 10, Philadelphia, 2016, Elsevier.

4. Patients with diabetes mellitus and chronic kidney disease are considered high risk.
5. In the general non-Black population, preferred initial agents are thiazide-type diuretics, ACE inhibitors (ACEI), calcium channel blockers (CCBs), or angiotensin receptor blockers (ARBs). ACEI or ARBs are preferred initial agents in diabetics and those with chronic kidney disease (CKD) in this population.[3]
6. Preferred initial agents in the Black population (including diabetics) are thiazide-type diuretics or CCBs.

7. When selecting drugs, try to give once per day dosages to improve compliance. Also consider the cost of the medication, metabolic and subjective side effects, and drug-drug interactions.
- The major advantages and limitations of each class of drugs are described as follows:
  1. Thiazide diuretics:
     a. Advantages: Inexpensive, once-daily dosing. Useful in edematous states, CHF, chronic renal disease, elderly patients (decreased incidence of hip fractures in elderly patients)

b. Disadvantages: Significant adverse metabolic effects (hypokalemia), increased risk of cardiac arrhythmias, sexual dysfunction, gout flares, possible adverse effects on lipids and glucose levels
  2. β-Blockers:
     a. Advantages: Ideal in hypertensive patients with ischemic heart disease or status post myocardial infarction (MI); favored in hyperkinetic, young patients (resting tachycardia, wide pulse pressure, hyperdynamic heart) and stable CHF patients

TABLE 4 Adrenocortical Causes of Hypertension

Low Renin and High Aldosterone

Primary Aldosteronism
- Aldosterone-producing adenoma (APA)—30% of cases
- Bilateral idiopathic hyperplasia (IHA)—60% of cases
- Primary (unilateral) adrenal hyperplasia—2% of cases
- Aldosterone-producing adrenocortical carcinoma—<1% of cases
- Familial hyperaldosteronism (FH)
  1. FH type I (*CYP11B1/CYP11B2* germline chimeric gene)—<1% of cases
  2. FH type II (APA or IHA; germline *CLCN2* mutations)—<6% of cases
  3. FH type III (germline *KCNJ5* mutations)—<1% of cases
  4. FH type IV (germline *CACNA1H* mutations)—<0.1% of cases
- Ectopic aldosterone-producing adenoma or carcinoma—<0.1% of cases

Low Renin and Low Aldosterone
- Congenital adrenal hyperplasia
  1. 11β-Hydroxylase deficiency
  2. 17α-Hydroxylase deficiency
- Deoxycorticosterone-producing tumor
- Primary cortisol resistance
- Apparent mineralocorticoid excess (AME)/11β-HSD 2 deficiency
  1. Genetic
  2. Type 1 AME
  3. Type 2 AME
- Acquired
  1. Licorice or carbenoxolone ingestion (type 1 AME)
  2. Cushing syndrome (type 2 AME)

Cushing Syndrome
- Exogenous glucocorticoid administration—most common cause
- Endogenous
  1. ACTH-dependent—85% of cases
     a. Pituitary
     b. Ectopic
  2. ACTH-independent—15% of cases
     a. Unilateral adrenal disease (adenoma or carcinoma)
  1. Bilateral adrenal disease
     a. Bilateral adenoma
     b. Macronodular hyperplasia
     c. Primary pigmented nodular adrenal disease (rare)

ACTH, Corticotropin; HSD, hydroxysteroid dehydrogenase.
From Melmed S et al: *Williams textbook of endocrinology*, ed 14, 2019, Elsevier.

b. Disadvantages: Adverse effect on quality of life (increased incidence of fatigue, depression, impotence), bronchospasm, hypoglycemia, peripheral vascular disease, adverse effects on lipids, masking of signs and symptoms of hypoglycemia in diabetics
3. Calcium antagonists:
   a. Advantages: Helpful in hypertensive patients with ischemic heart disease. Generally favorable effect on quality of life; can be used in patients with bronchospastic disorders, renal disease, peripheral vascular disease, metabolic disorders, and salt sensitivity. CCBs'

BOX 1 Causes of Secondary Hypertension

Endocrine Causes
Epinephrine excess
Aldosterone excess
Thyroid disease
Pregnancy

Vascular Causes
Coarctation of the aorta
Renal artery stenosis
Atherosclerosis (smokers, diabetes mellitus, advancing age)

Renal Disease
Inherited
Inflammation—glomerulonephritis
Diabetes mellitus
Drug reactions
Renal tumors (renal cell carcinoma, reninoma)

Medication-Induced
NSAIDs
Corticosteroids
Analgesics
Ethanol
Cyclosporine (ciclosporin)
SSRIs
Oral contraceptives

Malignancy-Related
Skin lesions such as endothelinomas
PTH- and PTHRP-producing cancers
Anti–VEGF-related cancer treatment
Adrenal tumors
Multiple endocrine neoplasia

NSAIDs, Nonsteroidal antiinflammatory drugs; *PTH,* parathyroid hormone; *PTHRP,* parathyroid hormone-related peptide; *SSRIs,* selective serotonin reuptake inhibitors; *VEGF,* vascular endothelial growth factor.
From Talley NJ et al: *Essentials of internal medicine*, ed 4, Chatswood, NSW, 2021, Elsevier Australia.

BP-lowering effect is independent of Na+ intake.
   b. Disadvantages: Diltiazem and verapamil should be avoided in patients with CHF caused by systolic dysfunction because of their negative inotropic effects; pedal edema may occur with nifedipine and amlodipine; constipation can be severe in elderly patients receiving verapamil. CCB-related edema is positional in nature and improves with lying position; additional strategies include switching CCB classes, reducing dosage, giving the medication later in the day, and adding a venodilator (nitrates, an ACE, or an ARB); diuretics may improve edema, but at the expense of a reduction in plasma volume.
4. ACE inhibitors:
   a. Advantages: First-line therapy for patients with left ventricular dysfunction, helpful in prevention of diabetic renal disease; effective in decreasing LVH, and remodeling.
   b. Disadvantages: Dry cough is a frequent side effect (5% to 20% of patients); hyperkalemia may occur in patients with diabetes or severe renal insufficiency; hypotension may occur in volume-depleted patients; increased

risk of renal failure in patients with renal artery stenosis; contraindicated in pregnancy.
5. ARBs:
   a. Advantages: Well tolerated, favorable impact on quality of life; useful in patients unable to tolerate ACE inhibitors because of persistent cough and in CHF and diabetic patients; single daily dose. An episode of renal insufficiency with ACE inhibitors does not rule out future therapy with an ARB unless high-grade bilateral renal artery stenosis exists.
   b. Disadvantages: Hypotension may occur in volume-depleted patients; hyperkalemia; risk of renal failure in renal artery stenosis; contraindicated in pregnancy.
6. Alpha-adrenergic blockers:
   a. Advantages: No adverse effect on blood lipids or insulin sensitivity; helpful in benign prostatic hypertrophy.
   b. Disadvantages: Postural hypotension, sedation; syncope can be avoided by giving an initial low dose at bedtime. Generally considered third- or fourth-line agent.
7. Central alpha-antagonists:
   a. Oral clonidine mainstay of therapy for hypertensive urgencies because of the ease of administration and relative safety.
   b. Transdermal clonidine; useful in management of labile HTN, the hospitalized patient who cannot take medications by mouth, and patients subject to early-morning BP surges. At equivalent doses, transdermal clonidine is more apt to precipitate salt and water retention than is the case with oral clonidine.
   c. Dose beyond 0.4 mg causes fatigue, sedation, dry mouth, salt and water retention, and rebound HTN upon abrupt termination of the medication.
8. Combined α- and β-adrenergic receptor blockers:
   a. Labetalol, nebivolol, and carvedilol: Use is reserved to treat complicated hypertensive patient when an antihypertensive effect beyond β-blockade is sought. Intravenous (IV) labetalol is used for hypertensive emergencies. Carvedilol is shown to have less adverse effect on glycemic control than metoprolol and to reduce urinary protein excretion in hypertensive diabetic patients.
9. Direct-acting smooth muscle relaxant: Hydralazine
   a. Advantages: Beneficial in Black patients when used with isosorbide dinitrate.
   b. Disadvantages: May lead to reflex tachycardia, worsening ischemia (best used with nitrates), at higher doses or with renal failure can lead to a reversible drug-induced lupus.

TABLE 5 Initial Laboratory Evaluation of the Hypertensive Patient to Investigate the Presence of Comorbid Conditions, Secondary Causes, or Established Target-Organ Damage

Test	Clinical Usefulness
Serum creatinine (and estimated glomerular filtration rate)	Assessment of renal function. Identifies parenchymal kidney disease as a possible secondary cause as well as established TOD.
Serum potassium	Low potassium (of renal origin) suggests mineralocorticoid excess (primary or secondary), glucocorticoid excess, Liddle syndrome. High potassium with normal renal function suggests Gordon syndrome. Low levels raise caution about the use of thiazides and loop diuretics. High levels preclude the use of ACEIs, ARBs, renin inhibitors, and potassium-sparing diuretics.
Serum sodium	If high, suggests primary aldosteronism. If low, alerts to the need to avoid thiazide diuretics.
Serum bicarbonate	If high, suggests aldosterone excess (primary or secondary). If low with normal renal function, suggests Gordon syndrome (with high potassium) or primary hyperparathyroidism (with high calcium).
Serum calcium	If high, suggests primary hyperparathyroidism.
Serum glucose	Identifies prediabetes or diabetes. In the appropriate setting, suggests glucocorticoid excess, pheochromocytoma, or acromegaly.
Lipid profile	Identifies hyperlipidemia.
Hemoglobin/hematocrit	If high, in the absence of other hematologic abnormalities or underlying lung disease, suggests sleep apnea.
Urinalysis*	Proteinuria and hematuria identify a possible secondary cause (glomerulonephritis). Proteinuria can also be a marker of TOD.
Electrocardiogram	Identifies left ventricular hypertrophy, old myocardial infarction, or other ischemic changes. Identifies conduction abnormalities that may preclude the use of β-blockers or nondihydropyridine CCBs.

ACEI, Angiotensin-converting enzyme inhibitor; *ARB,* angiotensin receptor blocker; *CCB,* calcium channel blocker; *TOD,* target-organ damage.
The most recent guidelines do not recommend blood urea nitrogen (BUN) measurement alone.
* Some organizations recommend screening microalbuminuria as a more sensitive tool to identify early renal injury.
From Skorecki K et al: *Brenner and Rector's the kidney,* ed 10, Philadelphia, 2016, Elsevier.

TABLE 6 Effects of Lifestyle Modifications on Blood Pressure

Lifestyle Modification	Specifics	Level of Evidence	Approximate Reduction in Systolic Blood Pressure
Weight loss	Maintain BMI <25 kg/m^2	A	5-20 mm Hg per 10 kg weight loss
Physical activity	At least 30 min per day	A	~5 mm Hg
Reduce salt intake	Limit sodium to 2.4 g per day	A	~5 mm Hg
Heart-healthy diet, such as DASH	Low-fat diet with fruits and vegetables	A	~11 mm Hg
Potassium supplementation	Preferably as part of dietary modification	A	~4 mm Hg
Stop smoking		A	1-6 mm Hg
Moderation of alcohol consumption	Limit alcohol to ≤2 drinks/day for men and ≤1 drink/day for women	A	~4 mm Hg

A, Supported by one or more high quality randomized trials; *BMI,* body mass index, *DASH,* Dietary Approaches to Stop Hypertension.
Modified from Whelton PK et al: 2017 ACC/AHA/AAPA/ABC/ACPM/AGS/APhA/ASH/ASPC/NMA/PCNA guideline for the prevention, detection, evaluation, and management of high blood pressure in adults: a report of the American College of Cardiology/American Heart Association Task Force on Clinical Practice Guidelines, *J Am Coll Cardiol* 71:e127-e248, 2018. In Warshaw G et al: *Ham's primary care geriatrics,* ed 7, Philadelphia, 2022, Elsevier.

10. Renin inhibitors: Newest class of antihypertensives (Aliskiren)
    a. Advantages: Generally well tolerated; once-daily dosing; can be used alone or in combination with other antihypertensive agents (avoid combining with ACE inhibitors or ARBs given increase of hyperkalemia).
    b. Disadvantages: Contraindicated in pregnancy; should not be used in patients with impaired renal function; excessive cost; paucity of cardiovascular outcomes data showing benefit.

TREATMENT OF RENOVASCULAR HYPERTENSION: The therapeutic approach varies with the cause of the renovascular hypertension (RVH) (refer to "Renal Artery Stenosis" for additional information).
- Young patients with fibromuscular dysplasia refractory to medical therapy can be treated with percutaneous transluminal renal angioplasty (PTRA).
- Medical therapy is advisable in elderly patients with atheromatous RVH; useful agents are:
  1. β-Blockers: Highly effective in patients with elevated plasma renin
  2. ACE inhibitors: Highly effective; however, should be avoided in patients with bilateral renal artery stenosis or with a solitary kidney and renal artery stenosis
  3. Diuretics: Often used in combination with ACE inhibitors
- Surgical revascularization: A recent trial revealed that renal-artery stenting does not confer a significant benefit with respect to the prevention of clinical events when added to comprehensive, multifactorial medical therapy in people with atherosclerotic renal-artery stenosis and hypertension or CKD.

HTN DURING PREGNANCY:
- HTN complicates 5% to 12% of all pregnancies.
- The American Obstetrical Committee defines BP of 130/80 mm Hg as the upper limit of normal at any time during pregnancy.
- A rise of 30 mm Hg systolic or 15 mm Hg diastolic is also considered abnormal regardless of the absolute values obtained.
- Hypertension during pregnancy can be from chronic HTN, gestational HTN, preeclampsia or preeclampsia superimposed on chronic HTN. It is important to distinguish the etiology because the risk to mother and fetus is much greater in preeclampsia.

  In pregnant women with mild chronic hypertension, a strategy of targeting a blood pressure of less than 140/90 mm Hg is associated with better pregnancy outcomes than a strategy of reserving treatment only for severe hypertension, with no increase in the risk of small-for-gestational-age birth weight.[4]
- Treatment of chronic HTN during pregnancy is as follows:
  1. Initial treatment with conservative measures (proper nutrition, limited physical activity).
  2. When drug therapy is necessary, initiation of methyldopa, hydralazine, labetalol, or nifedipine is preferred. Table 9 summarizes drugs used to treat hypertension in pregnancy.
  3. ACE inhibitors can cause fetal and neonatal complications; their use should be avoided in pregnancy.
  4. The safety of CCBs remains unclear.
  5. Diuretics should be used only if there is a specific reason for initiating and maintaining their use (e.g., HTN associated with severe fluid overload or left ventricular dysfunction).

MALIGNANT HTN, HYPERTENSIVE EMERGENCIES, AND HYPERTENSIVE URGENCIES: Definitions:
- Malignant HTN occurs with HTN when there are grades III and IV retinopathy (exudates, hemorrhages, and papilledema).
  1. The rate of BP rise is a critical factor in the development of malignant HTN.

TABLE 7 Antihypertensive Drugs

Drug Class	Mechanism of Action	Possible Adverse Effects
Thiazide-like diuretics Chlorthalidone Hydrochlorothiazide Indapamide Potassium-sparing diuretics Triamterene Spironolactone	Inhibit sodium and chloride reabsorption in the kidney, reducing intravascular volume and peripheral vascular resistance	Volume depletion hypotension, hyponatremia, hypokalemia, hypomagnesemia, hyperuricemia (gout), hyperglycemia, renal impairment
Angiotensin-converting enzyme inhibitors (ACE inhibitors) Benazepril Captopril Fosinopril Lisinopril Ramipril	Inhibits ACE, interfering with conversion of angiotensin I to angiotensin II, reducing vasoconstriction	Hyperkalemia (with impaired renal function), cough, angioedema, rash, renal impairment, altered taste
Angiotensin II receptor blockers (ARB) Candesartan Irbesartan Losartan Valsartan	Antagonizes angiotensin II AT1 receptors, reducing vasoconstriction	Hyperkalemia, renal impairment Do not use an ACE inhibitor and an ARB simultaneously
Beta-Blockers		Sinus bradycardia, heart block, fatigue, bronchospasm, hyperglycemia, confusion. Not recommended as first-line agents unless the patient has ischemic heart disease or heart failure
Beta₁ Selective Metoprolol	Selectively antagonizes β-1 adrenergic receptors	
Dual acting Carvedilol Labetalol	Antagonizes α-1, β-1, and β-2 adrenergic receptors	
Calcium channel blockers—Nondihydropyridines Diltiazem Verapamil	Prolong AV node refractory period and have negative inotropic effect; less effective as vasodilators	Sinus bradycardia, heart block, heart failure, rash, GERD, constipation, gingival hyperplasia
Calcium channel blockers—Dihydropyridines Amlodipine Felodipine Nicardipine Nifedipine	Inhibit calcium influx, relaxing vascular smooth muscle and decreasing peripheral resistance causing vasodilation with little or no negative effect upon cardiac contractility or AV nodal conduction	Peripheral edema
Alpha-adrenergic agonists, centrally acting Methyldopa Clonidine	Stimulates α-2 adrenergic receptors centrally	Sedation, dry mouth, constipation. Avoid in older adults because of central nervous system adverse effects
Alpha₁ selective adrenergic antagonists, peripherally acting Doxazosin Prazosin Terazosin	Antagonizes peripheral α-1 adrenergic receptors	Orthostatic hypotension. Consider in patients with benign prostatic hypertrophy

GERD, Gastroesophageal reflux disease.
From Warshaw G et al: *Ham's primary care geriatrics,* ed 7, Philadelphia, 2022, Elsevier.

TABLE 8 Antihypertensive Choice in the Setting of Cardiovascular Comorbidity

Compelling Indication	Diuretic	BB	ACEI	ATRA	CCB	ALDO ant
Heart failure	✓	✓	✓	✓		✓
Post-myocardial infarction		✓	✓			✓
High risk of coronary artery disease	✓	✓	✓		✓	
Diabetes	✓	✓	✓	✓	✓	
Chronic kidney disease			✓		✓	
Recurrent stroke prevention	✓		✓			

ACEI, Angiotensin-converting enzyme inhibitor; *ALDO ant,* aldosterone antagonist; *ATRA,* angiotensin II receptor antagonist; *BB,* beta-adrenoceptor antagonist; *CCB,* calcium-channel blocker.
From Talley NJ et al: *Essentials of internal medicine,* ed 4, Chatswood, NSW, 2021, Elsevier Australia.

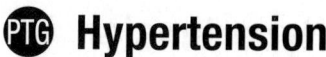

TABLE 9 Drugs Used to Treat Hypertension in Pregnancy

Drug	Starting Dose	Maximum Dose	Comments
Acute Treatment of Severe Hypertension			
Hydralazine	5-10 mg IV every 20 min	20 mg*	Avoid in cases of tachycardia and persistent headaches
Labetalol	20-40 mg IV every 10-15 min	220 mg*	Avoid in women with asthma or congestive heart failure
Nifedipine	10-20 mg PO every 30 min	50 mg*	Avoid in case of tachycardia and palpitations
Long-Term Treatment of Hypertension			
Methyldopa	250 mg bid	4 g/day	
Labetalol	100 mg bid	2400 mg/day	
Nifedipine	10 mg bid	120 mg/day	
Thiazide diuretic	12.5 mg bid	50 mg/day	

bid, Twice daily; *IV*, intravenous.
*If desired blood pressure levels are not achieved, switch to another drug.
From Gabbe SG: *Obstetrics,* ed 6, Philadelphia, 2012, Saunders.

2. Complications and mortality rates are much higher in malignant HTN compared with essential HTN.
3. Requires immediate BP reduction (not necessarily into normal ranges) to prevent or limit target organ disease.

- Hypertensive emergencies occur when the BP elevation is >180 mm Hg systolic and/or >120 mm Hg diastolic without evidence of new or progressive organ dysfunction. It requires rapid lowering of BP to prevent end-organ damage.
- Hypertensive urgencies are BP elevations >180 mm Hg systolic and/or >120 mm Hg diastolic with end-organ damage that should be corrected within 24 h of presentation.
  1. Most clinicians suggest lowering the BP to <160 mm Hg/<100 mm Hg or to a level no more than 30% lower than the patient's baseline BP.

Therapy: The choice of therapeutic agents varies with the cause. IV medications are preferred in hypertensive emergencies.

- Nitroprusside is the drug of choice in hypertensive encephalopathy, HTN and intracranial bleeding, malignant HTN, HTN and heart failure, dissecting aortic aneurysm (used in combination with propranolol); its onset of action is immediate. Because it is metabolized to cyanide, patients should be carefully monitored for toxicity (mental status changes, acidemia).
- Fenoldopam is a vasodilator agent useful for the short-term (up to 48 h) management of severe HTN when rapid but quickly reversible reduction of BP is required. It should be avoided in patients with glaucoma.
- Other commonly used agents are the IV CCBs nicardipine and clevidipine (useful for urgent treatment of HTN in the ICU or operating room), the β-blocker esmolol (useful in aortic dissection or postoperative HTN), labetalol (combined β-adrenergic and α-blocker useful in patients with coronary disease), phentolamine (useful for catecholamine-related emergencies), IV nitroglycerin (used in patients with cardiac ischemia and hypertensive

crisis), and hydralazine (used for hypertensive emergencies in pregnancy).
- Table 10 summarizes IV medications useful in hypertensive crisis.
  The following are important points to remember when treating hypertensive emergencies:
- Introduce a plan for long-term therapy at the time of the initial emergency treatment.
- Agents that reduce arterial pressure can cause the kidney to retain sodium and water; therefore, the judicious administration of diuretics should accompany their use.
- The initial goal of antihypertensive therapy is not to achieve a normal BP, but rather to gradually reduce the BP; cerebral hypoperfusion may occur if the mean BP is HTN in patients with CKD.

HTN MANAGEMENT IN THE NEUROLOGIC-NEUROSURGICAL ICU: Guidelines for BP management in the most common conditions treated in the neurologic-neurosurgical intensive care unit are summarized in Table 11.

![icon] **PEARLS & CONSIDERATIONS**

COMMENTS

- "Masked hypertension" refers to the detection of HTN with home or ambulatory monitoring. Up to 40% of patients with BP less than 140/90 mm Hg in the office may have masked hypertension. Automated BP monitors are useful to screen for masked HTN.
- "White coat hypertension" is defined as an elevated BP during medical office examination, whereas BP is in the normal range while at home. Its prevalence is as high as 30% among patients with an elevated BP in the office. These patients are at increased risk for overt HTN.
- For patients with HTN, every 20/10 mm Hg increase in BP doubles the risk of cardiovascular events.
- Most patients will require at least two medications for BP control.

- If BP is greater than 20/10 mm Hg above goal, therapy should be initiated with two drugs.
- Resistant HTN: HTN is considered resistant if the BP cannot be reduced below target levels in patients who are compliant with an optimal triple-drug regimen that includes a diuretic. Terms *refractory* and *resistant* are used interchangeably. Causes include pseudohypertension, measurement artifact, medication nonadherence, volume overload, and secondary HTN.
  1. Pseudohypertension in elderly: Hardened and sclerotic artery is not compressible; hence, falsely elevates BP measurement artifact
  2. Measurement artifact: BP taken incorrectly (small cuff, improper support)
- Renal sympathetic denervation: A blinded trial did not show a significant reduction of systolic BP in patients with resistant hypertension 6 mo after renal artery denervation as compared with a sham control.[5]
- Barriers to BP control: System issues, provider issues, patient issues, and behavior issues. The rate at which physicians adopt recommended changes based on evidence-based findings can be quite slow and has been properly described as "clinical inertia."
- Indications for specialist referral for patients with HTN are described in Table 12.
- U.S. guidelines for the treatment of HTN recommend the following:[2]
  1. Use of BP-lowering medication for secondary prevention in patients with cardiovascular disease and average SBP ≥130 mm Hg or DBP ≥80 mm Hg, and for primary prevention in adults with an estimated 10-yr ASCVD risk of >10% and an average SBP ≥130 mm Hg or DBP ≥80 mm Hg.
  2. In patients with no history of cardiovascular disease and an estimated 10-yr ASCVD risk <10%, BP-lowering medication is recommended for those with an average SBP ≥140 mm Hg or an average DBP ≥90 mm Hg.

REFERENCES

Available at eBooks.Health.Elsevier.com.

RELATED CONTENT

High Blood Pressure (Patient Information)
High Blood Pressure—Child (Patient Information)
Eclampsia (Related Key Topic)
Pheochromocytoma (Related Key Topic)
Preeclampsia (Related Key Topic)
Renal Artery Stenosis (Related Key Topic)

AUTHOR: **TANIA B. BABAR, MD**

H

Diseases and Disorders

I

TABLE 10 Treatment of Hypertensive Crisis: Intravenous Medications

Drug Name and Mechanism of Action	Indications/Advantages/Dose	Disadvantages/Adverse Effects/Metabolism Cautions
Sodium Nitroprusside Nitric oxide compound; vasodilation of arteriolar and venous smooth muscle Increases cardiac output by decreasing afterload	Useful in most hypertensive emergencies Onset of action immediate, duration of action 1-2 min Dose: 0.25 µg/kg/min Maximum dose: 8-10 µg/kg/min	Contraindicated in high-output cardiac failure, congenital optic atrophy. Anemia and liver disease at risk of cyanide toxicity: Acidosis, tachycardia, change in mental status, almond smell on breath. Risk of thiocyanate toxicity with renal disease: Psychosis, hyperreflexia, seizure, tinnitus. Cautious use with increased intracranial pressure. Do not use maximum dose for >10 min. Crosses the placenta.
Nitroglycerin Directly interacts with nitrate receptors on vascular smooth muscle Primarily dilates venous bed Decreases preload	Use with symptoms of cardiac ischemia, perioperative hypertension in cardiac surgery Initial dose: 5 µg/min Maximum dose: 100 µg/min	Contraindicated in angle-closure glaucoma, increased intracranial pressure. Blood pressure decreased secondary to decreased preload, cardiac output—avoid when cerebral or renal perfusion compromised. Caution with right ventricular infarct.
Labetalol β- and α-Adrenergic blockade α:β-Blocking ratio is 1:7	Onset of action 2-5 min, duration 3-6 h Bolus 20 mg, then 20-80 mg every 10 min for maximum dose 300 mg Infuse at 0.5-2 mg/min	Avoid in bronchospasm, bradycardia, congestive heart failure, greater than first-degree heart block, second/third trimester pregnancy. Use caution with hepatic dysfunction, inhalational anesthetics (myocardial depression). Enters breast milk.
Esmolol Cardioselective β1-adrenergic blocking agent	Use with aortic dissection Use during intubation, intraoperative, and postoperative hypertension Onset of action 60 sec, duration 10-20 min, 200-500 µg/kg/min for 4 min, then infuse 50-300 µg/kg/min	See labetalol. Not dependent on renal or hepatic function for metabolism (metabolized by hydrolysis in red blood cells).
Fenoldopam Postsynaptic dopamine-1 agonist; decreases peripheral vascular resistance; 10 times more potent than dopamine as vasodilator	May be advantageous in kidney disease, increases renal blood flow, increases sodium excretion, no toxic metabolites Initial dose: 0.1 µg/kg/min, with titration every 15 min No bolus	Contraindicated in glaucoma (may increase intraocular pressure) or allergy to sulfites; hypotension, especially with concurrent β-blocker. Check serum potassium every 6 h. Concurrent acetaminophen may significantly increase blood levels. Dose-related tachycardia.
Hydralazine Primarily dilates arteriolar vasculature	Primarily used in pregnancy/eclampsia Dose: 10 mg every 20-130 min; maximum dose 20 mg Decreases blood pressure in 10-20 min Duration of action 2-4 h	Reflex tachycardia; give β-blocker concurrently. May exacerbate angina. Half-life 3 h, affects blood pressure for 100 h. Depends on hepatic acetylation for inactivation.
Phentolamine α-Adrenergic blockade	Used primarily to treat hypertension from excessive catecholamine excess (e.g., pheochromocytoma) Dose: 5-15 mg Onset of action 1-2 min, duration 3-10 min	β-Blockade is generally added to control tachycardia or arrhythmias. As in all catecholamine excess states, β-blockers should never be given first, as the loss of β-adrenergically mediated vasodilation will leave α-adrenergically mediated vasoconstriction unopposed and result in increased pressure.
Nicardipine Dihydropyridine calcium channel blocker; inhibits transmembrane influx of calcium ions into cardiac and smooth muscle	Onset of action 10-20 min, duration 1-4 h Initial dose: 5 mg/h to maximum of 15 mg/h	Avoid with congestive heart failure, cardiac ischemia. Adverse effects include tachycardia, flushing, headache.
Clevidipine Short-acting dihydropyridine calcium channel antagonist	Initial dose: 1 mg/h; can be increased to 21 mg/h	Reduces blood pressure without affecting cardiac filling pressures or causing reflex tachycardia.
Enalaprilat Angiotensin-converting enzyme inhibitor	Onset of action 15-20 min, duration 12-24 h Dose: 1.25-5 mg every 6 h	Response not predictable, with high renin states may see acute hypotension. Hyperkalemia in setting of reduced glomerular filtration rate. Avoid in pregnancy.
Trimethaphan Nondepolarizing ganglionic blocking agent; competes with acetylcholine for postsynaptic receptors	Used in aortic dissection Dose: 0.5-5 mg/min	Does not increase cardiac output. No inotropic cardiac effect. Disadvantages include parasympathetic blockade, resulting in paralytic ileus and bladder atony and development of tachyphylaxis after 24-96 h of use.

From Vincent JL et al: *Textbook of critical care*, ed 7, Philadelphia, 2017, Elsevier.

TABLE 11 Guidelines for Blood Pressure Management in the Most Common Conditions Treated in the Neurologic-Neurosurgical Intensive Care Unit

Diagnosis	Recommendation
Acute ischemic stroke	Establish and maintain BP <185/110 mm Hg before receiving intravenous thrombolysis
	Keep <180/105 mm Hg if thrombolysis
	Treat only BP >220/120 mm Hg if no thrombolysis
	Keep <180/105 mm Hg following endovascular clot retrieval
Intracerebral hemorrhage	Keep SBP <180 and MAP <130 mm Hg
	(ideal SBP <160 mm Hg)
Subarachnoid hemorrhage	Keep SBP <160 mm Hg before aneurysm treated
	Do not lower BP after aneurysm treated
Traumatic brain injury	Keep adequate MAP to maintain CPP 60-70 mm Hg
	Suggested SBP goals: >100 mm Hg (ages 50-69 yr) or >110 mm Hg (ages 15-49 yr)

BP, Blood pressure; *CPP,* cerebral perfusion pressure; *MAP,* mean arterial pressure; *SBP,* systolic blood pressure.
From Jankovic J et al: *Bradley and Daroff's neurology in clinical practice,* ed 8, Philadelphia, 2022, Elsevier.

TABLE 12 Indications for Specialist Referral for Patients with Hypertension

Urgent Treatment Needed

Accelerated hypertension (severe hypertension with grade III-IV retinopathy)

Particularly severe hypertension (>220/120 mm Hg)

Impending complications (e.g., transient ischemic attack, left ventricular failure)

Possible Underlying Cause

Any clue in history or examination of a secondary cause (e.g., hypokalemia with increased or high-normal plasma sodium)

Elevated serum creatinine

Proteinuria or hematuria

Sudden onset or worsening of hypertension

Young age (any hypertension <20 yr; needing treatment <30 yr)

Therapeutic Problems

Multiple drug intolerances

Multiple drug contraindications

Persistent nonadherence or nonconcordance

Special Situations

Unusual blood pressure variability

Possible white coat hypertension

Hypertension in pregnancy

From Floege J et al: *Comprehensive clinical nephrology,* ed 4, Philadelphia, 2010, Saunders.

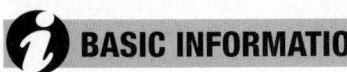

BASIC INFORMATION

DEFINITION

Hyperthyroidism is a hypermetabolic state resulting from excess thyroid hormone. Thyrotoxicosis is a general term for excess circulating and tissue hormone levels.

SYNONYM

Thyrotoxicosis

ICD-10CM CODES

E05.00	Thyrotoxicosis with diffuse goiter without thyrotoxic crisis or storm
E05.01	Thyrotoxicosis with diffuse goiter with thyrotoxic crisis or storm
E05.10	Thyrotoxicosis with toxic single thyroid nodule without thyrotoxic crisis or storm
E05.11	Thyrotoxicosis with toxic single thyroid nodule with thyrotoxic crisis or storm
E05.20	Thyrotoxicosis with toxic multinodular goiter without thyrotoxic crisis or storm
E05.21	Thyrotoxicosis with toxic multinodular goiter with thyrotoxic crisis or storm
E05.30	Thyrotoxicosis from ectopic thyroid tissue without thyrotoxic crisis or storm
E05.31	Thyrotoxicosis from ectopic thyroid tissue with thyrotoxic crisis or storm
E05.40	Thyrotoxicosis factitia without thyrotoxic crisis or storm
E05.41	Thyrotoxicosis factitia with thyrotoxic crisis or storm
E05.80	Other thyrotoxicosis without thyrotoxic crisis or storm
E05.81	Other thyrotoxicosis with thyrotoxic crisis or storm
E05.90	Thyrotoxicosis, unspecified without thyrotoxic crisis or storm
E05.91	Thyrotoxicosis, unspecified with thyrotoxic crisis or storm
E06.2	Chronic thyroiditis with transient thyrotoxicosis

EPIDEMIOLOGY & DEMOGRAPHICS

INCIDENCE & PREVLANCE:

- Hyperthyroidism affects 2% of women and 0.2% of men in their lifetimes.
- Toxic multinodular goiter usually occurs in women >55 yr and is more common than Graves disease in the elderly.

PHYSICAL FINDINGS & CLINICAL PRESENTATION

- Patients with hyperthyroidism generally present with tachycardia, tremor, hyperreflexia, anxiety, irritability, emotional lability, panic attacks, heat intolerance, sweating, increased appetite, diarrhea, weight loss, menstrual dysfunction (oligomenorrhea, amenorrhea). Presentation may be different in elderly patients (see the following).
- Patients with Graves disease may present with exophthalmos, lid retraction, and lid lag (Graves ophthalmopathy). The following signs and symptoms of ophthalmopathy may be present: Blurring of vision, photophobia, increased lacrimation, double vision, and deep orbital pressure. Clubbing of fingers associated with periosteal new bone formation in other skeletal areas (Graves acropachy) and pretibial myxedema may also be noted.
- Clinical signs of hyperthyroidism in the elderly may be masked by manifestations of coexisting disease (e.g., new-onset atrial fibrillation, exacerbation of congestive heart failure).

ETIOLOGY (TABLE 1)

- Graves disease (diffuse toxic goiter): 80% to 90% of all cases of hyperthyroidism; Graves disease results from the action of thyroid-stimulating antibodies (TSAbs) that bind to and activate the thyroid-stimulating hormone (TSH)-Receptors
- Toxic multinodular goiter (Plummer disease)
- Toxic adenoma
- Iatrogenic and factitious
- Transient hyperthyroidism (subacute thyroiditis, Hashimoto thyroiditis)
- Rare causes: Hypersecretion of TSH (e.g., pituitary neoplasms), struma ovarii, ingestion of large amount of iodine in a patient with preexisting thyroid hyperplasia or adenoma

TABLE 1 Causes of Hyperthyroidism

I. Excessive TSH-Receptor Stimulation

Graves disease (TRAb)
Pregnancy-associated transient hyperthyroidism (hCG)
Trophoblastic disease (hCG)
Familial gestational hyperthyroidism (mutant TSH receptor)
TSH-producing pituitary adenoma

II. Autonomous Thyroid Hormone Secretion

Multinodular toxic goiter (somatic mutations)
Solitary toxic thyroid adenoma (somatic mutation)
Congenital activating TSH-receptor mutation (genomic mutation)

III. Destruction of Follicles with Release of Hormone

Subacute de Quervain thyroiditis (virus infection)
Painless thyroiditis/postpartum thyroiditis (hashitoxicosis—autoimmune)
Acute thyroiditis (bacterial infection)
Drug-induced thyroiditis (amiodarone, interferon-γ)

IV. Extrathyroidal Sources of Thyroid Hormone

Iatrogenic overreplacement with thyroid hormone
Excessive self-administered thyroid medication
Food and supplements containing excessive thyroid hormone
Functional thyroid cancer metastases
Struma ovarii

hCG, Human chorionic gonadotropin; *TRAb,* thyrotropin-receptor antibodies; *TSH,* thyroid-stimulating hormone (thyrotropin).
From Melmed S et al: *Williams textbook of endocrinology,* ed 14, St Louis, 2019, Elsevier.

(Jod-Basedow phenomenon), hydatidiform mole, carcinoma of thyroid, amiodarone therapy

DIAGNOSIS

DIFFERENTIAL DIAGNOSIS

- Anxiety disorder
- Pheochromocytoma
- Metastatic neoplasm
- Diabetes mellitus
- Premenopausal state

WORKUP

Suspected hyperthyroidism requires laboratory confirmation and identification of its etiology because treatment varies with cause. A detailed medical history will often provide clues to the diagnosis and etiology of the hyperthyroidism. Fig. 1 describes a diagnostic approach to suspected hyperthyroidism.

LABORATORY TESTS

- Elevated free thyroxine (T_4)
- Elevated free triiodothyronine (T_3): Generally not necessary for diagnosis
- Low TSH (unless hyperthyroidism is a result of the rare hypersecretion of TSH from a pituitary adenoma). Serum TSH is the best test for diagnosis of thyrotoxicosis
- Thyroid autoantibodies: Thyroglobulin and thyroid peroxidase antibodies occur in up to 80% of patients with Graves disease. They are useful in selected cases to differentiate Graves disease from toxic multinodular goiter (absent thyroid antibodies)

IMAGING STUDIES

- 24-h radioactive iodine uptake (RAIU) is useful to distinguish hyperthyroidism from iatrogenic thyroid hormone synthesis (thyrotoxicosis factitia) and from thyroiditis (Box 1).
- An overactive thyroid shows increased uptake, whereas a normal underactive thyroid (iatrogenic thyroid ingestion, painless or subacute thyroiditis) shows normal or decreased uptake.
- The RAIU results also vary with the etiology of the hyperthyroidism:
  1. Graves disease: Increased homogeneous uptake
  2. Multinodular goiter: Increased heterogeneous uptake
  3. Hot nodule: Single focus of increased uptake
- RAIU is also generally performed before the therapeutic administration of radioactive iodine to determine the appropriate dose.

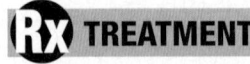 TREATMENT

NONPHARMACOLOGIC THERAPY

Patient education regarding thyroid disease and discussion of the therapeutic options. Avoidance of strenuous physical exercise, caffeine, and tobacco in patients with uncontrolled thyrotoxicosis. Patients should be informed that radioiodine, antithyroid drugs, and surgery are all reasonable

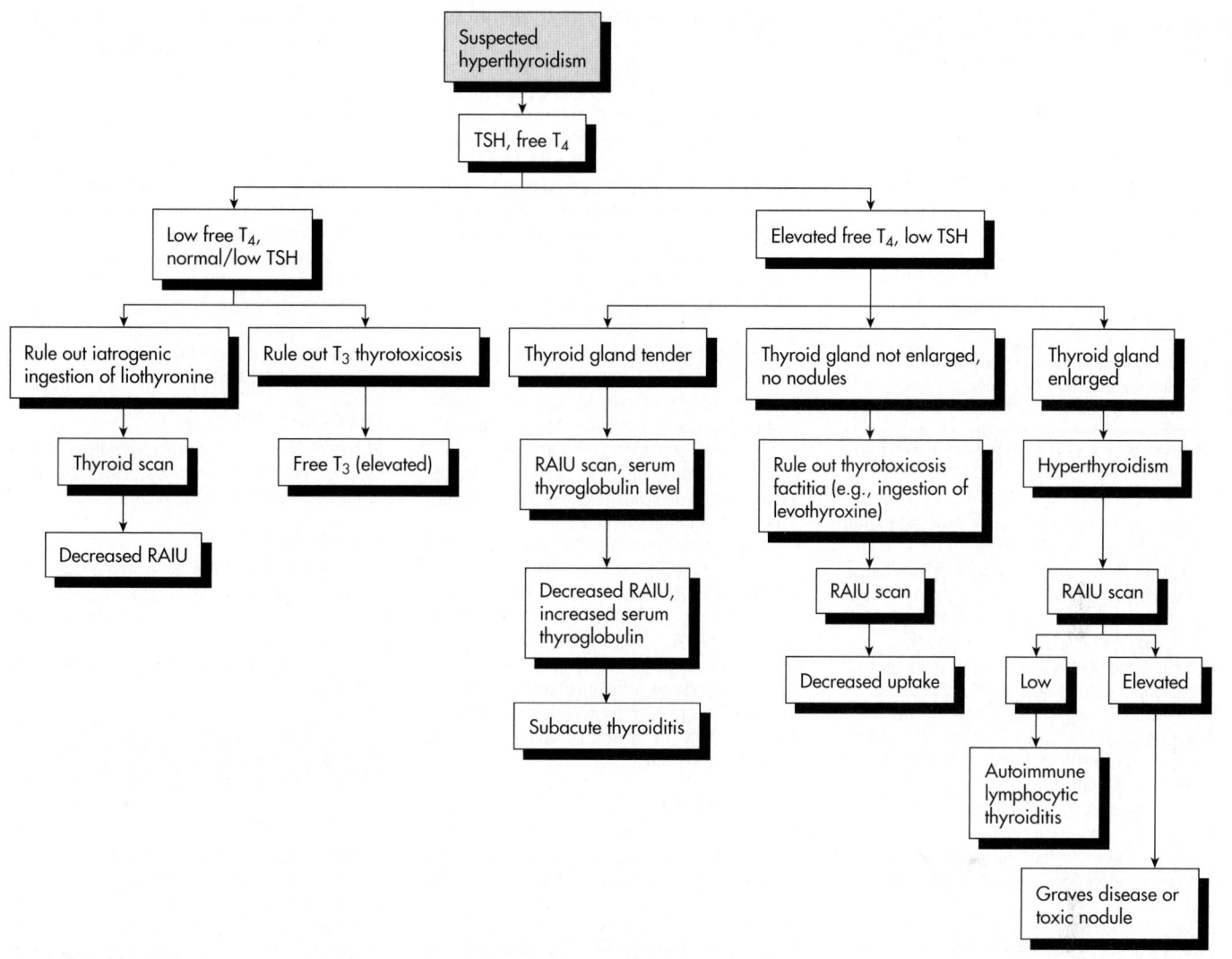

FIG. 1 Hyperthyroidism. *RAIU*, Radioactive iodine uptake; *TSH*, thyroid-stimulating hormone.

BOX 1   Differentiation of Causes of Hyperthyroidism According to Pattern of Radionucleotide Uptake

Reduced Uptake	Generalized Increased Uptake	Focal Increased Uptake
• Thyroiditis	• Graves disease	• Toxic multinodular goiter
• Exogenous thyroxine	• Excess thyroid-stimulating hormone stimulation	• Hyperfunctioning adenoma
• Iodine loading		
• Ectopic thyroid hormone secretion (struma ovarii)		

From Talley NJ et al: *Essentials of internal medicine,* ed 4, Chatswood, NSW, 2021, Elsevier Australia.

---

treatment options for hyperthyroidism. It is crucial for the physician to have a detailed discussion with the patient about the benefits and risks relative to lifestyle, patients' values, and coexisting conditions.

ACUTE GENERAL Rx

ANTITHYROID DRUGS (THIONAMIDES) (TABLES 2 AND 3): Propylthiouracil (PTU) and methimazole inhibit thyroid hormone synthesis by blocking production of thyroid peroxidase (PTU and methimazole) or inhibit peripheral conversion of T_4 to T_3 (PTU). Methimazole is favored by most endocrinologists because of the potential for hepatic failure with PTU. PTU is preferred in pregnant women during the first trimester because methimazole has been associated with aplasia cutis and with choanal and esophageal atresia. CBC and differential should be obtained before their use.
- Dosage: Methimazole 15 to 30 mg/day given as a single dose; PTU 50 to 100 mg PO q8h.
- Antithyroid drugs can be used as the primary form of treatment or as adjunctive therapy before radioactive therapy or surgery or afterward if the hyperthyroidism recurs.

- Side effects (Table 4): Skin rash (3% to 5% of patients), arthralgias, myalgias, granulocytopenia (0.5%). Rare side effects are aplastic anemia, hepatic necrosis from PTU, cholestatic jaundice from methimazole.
- When antithyroid drugs are used as primary therapy, they are usually given for 6 to 18 mo; prolonged therapy may cause hypothyroidism. Monitor thyroid function every 2 mo for 6 mo, then less frequently.
- The use of antithyroid drugs before radioiodine therapy is best reserved for patients in whom exacerbation of hyperthyroidism after radioactive iodine therapy is hazardous (e.g., elderly patients with coronary artery disease or significant coexisting morbidity). In these patients the antithyroid drug can be stopped 2 days before radioactive iodine therapy, resumed 2 days later, and continued for 4 to 6 wk.

RADIOIODINE THERAPY (RADIOACTIVE IODINE [RAI]):[131]
- RAI is the treatment of choice for patients age >21 yr and younger patients who have not achieved remission after 1 yr of antithyroid drug therapy. RAI is also used in

TABLE 2 Mechanism of Action of Thionamide Antithyroid Drugs

- Intrathyroidal inhibition of:
  1. Iodine oxidation/organification
  2. Iodotyrosine coupling
  3. Thyroglobulin biosynthesis
  4. Follicular cell growth
- Extrathyroidal inhibition of T_4/T_3 conversion (propylthiouracil)
- Immunologic effects:
  1. Direct effects on both intrathyroidal T cells and human leukocyte antigen class II expression by thyrocytes
  2. Increase numbers of suppressor T cells and decrease intrathyroidal activated T cells
  3. Inhibit proinflammatory mediator release, including oxygen radicals, by thyroid cells

From Robertson RP et al: *DeGroot's endocrinology, basic science and clinical practice*, ed 8, Philadelphia, 2023, Elsevier.

hyperthyroidism caused by toxic adenoma or toxic multinodular goiter.

- Contraindicated during pregnancy (can cause fetal hypothyroidism) and lactation. Pregnancy should be excluded in women of child-bearing age before RAI is administered.
- A single dose of RAI is effective in inducing a euthyroid state in nearly 80% of patients.
- There is a high incidence of post-RAI hypothyroidism (>50% within first yr and 2%/yr thereafter); these patients should be frequently evaluated for the onset of hypothyroidism. There is a modest but significant excess risk for thyroid cancer and excess mortality risk for breast cancer and other solid cancer with RAI treatment.[1]

SURGICAL THERAPY (SUBTOTAL THYROIDECTOMY):

- Indicated in obstructing goiters, in any patient who refuses RAI and cannot be adequately managed with antithyroid medications (e.g., patients with toxic adenoma or toxic multinodular goiter), and in pregnant patients who cannot be adequately managed with antithyroid medication or develop side effects to them. Thyroidectomy can also be considered as primary therapy in refractory cases of amiodarone-induced hyperthyroidism. Thyroidectomy is not indicated for low RAIU hyperthyroidism.
- Patients should be rendered euthyroid with antithyroid drugs before surgery.
- Complications of surgery include hypothyroidism (28% to 43% after 10 yr), hypoparathyroidism, and vocal cord paralysis (1%).
- Most patients should be started on replacement doses of levothyroxine (1.7 mcg/kg/day) before discharge from hospital.
- Hyperthyroidism recurs after surgery in 10% to 15% of patients.

ADJUNCTIVE THERAPY: Propranolol alleviates the beta-adrenergic symptoms of hyperthyroidism; initial dose is 20 to 40 mg PO q6h; dosage is gradually increased until symptoms are controlled. Major contraindications to propranolol are congestive heart failure and bronchospasm. Diagnosis and treatment of thyrotoxic storm are also discussed in Section I.

CHRONIC Rx

- Patients undergoing treatment with antithyroid drugs should be seen every 1 to 3 mo until euthyroidism is achieved and every 3 to 4 mo while they remain on antithyroid therapy. After treatment is stopped, periodic monitoring of thyroid function tests with TSH is recommended every 3 mo for 1 yr, then every 6 mo for 1 yr, then annually.
- Orbital decompression surgery can be used to correct Graves orbitopathy. The administration of the antioxidant selenium (100 mcg PO bid) has been recently reported as effective in improving quality of life, reducing ocular involvement, and slowing progression of the disease in patients with mild Graves orbitopathy. Its mechanism of action is believed to be an effect on the oxygen free radicals and cytokines that play a pathogenic role in Graves orbitopathy.

DISPOSITION

Successful treatment of hyperthyroidism requires lifelong monitoring for the onset of hypothyroidism or the recurrence of thyrotoxicosis.

REFERRAL

- Endocrinology referral is recommended at the time of initial diagnosis and during treatment.
- Surgical referral in selected patients (see "Surgical Therapy").
- Hospitalization of all patients with thyrotoxic storm.

❗ PEARLS & CONSIDERATIONS

COMMENTS

- Elderly hyperthyroid patients may have only subtle signs (weight loss, tachycardia, fine skin, brittle nails). This form is known as ***apathetic hyperthyroidism*** and manifests with lethargy rather than hyperkinetic activity. An enlarged thyroid gland may be absent. Coexisting medical disorders (most commonly cardiac disease) may also mask the symptoms. These patients often have unexplained

TABLE 3 Pharmacology and Pharmacokinetics of Thionamide Antithyroid Drugs

	Methimazole	Propylthiouracil
Absorption	Rapid	Rapid
Bioavailability	~100%	~100%
Peak serum level	60-120 min	60 min
Serum half-life	6-8 h	90 min
Thyroidal concentration	5×10^{-5} mol/L	Unknown
Thyroidal turnover	Slow	Moderate
Duration of action	>24 h	8-12 h
Serum protein binding	Nil	>75%
Crosses placenta	++	+
Levels in breast milk	++	+
Volume of distribution	40 L	20 L
Excretion	Renal	Renal
Metabolism during illness		
• Renal	Nil	Nil
• Liver	Prolonged	Nil
Potency	10-50	1
Normalization T_3/T_4	6 wk	12 wk
Adverse events (AE, %)	15	20
Agranulocytosis (%)	0.6	1.8
Cross-reaction of AE (%)	13.8	15.2
Compliance	High	Fair
Costs	Low	Moderate

From Robertson RP et al: *DeGroot's endocrinology, basic science and clinical practice*, ed 8, Philadelphia, 2023, Elsevier.

TABLE 4 Adverse Events of Thionamide Antithyroid Drugs

Common (1%-5%)
- Skin rash
- Urticaria
- Arthralgia
- Fever
- Transient mild leukopenia

Rare (0.2%-0.5%)
- Gastrointestinal
- Abnormalities of taste and smell
- Agranulocytosis (within the first 90 d)

Very Rare
- Hepatitis (propylthiouracil, PTU)—avoid in children!
- Vasculitis, lupus-like (PTU)
- Aplastic anemia (PTU)
- Thrombocytopenia (PTU)
- Hypoglycemia (antiinsulin antibody) (PTU)
- Cholestatic jaundice (methimazole)
- Pancreatitis (?)

From Robertson RP et al: *DeGroot's endocrinology, basic science and clinical practice*, ed 8, Philadelphia, 2023, Elsevier.

congestive heart failure, worsening of angina, or new-onset atrial fibrillation resistant to treatment. See the topic "Graves Disease" for additional information on diagnosis and treatment.

- **Subclinical hyperthyroidism** is defined as a normal serum-free thyroxine and free triiodothyronine levels with a TSH level suppressed below the normal range and usually undetectable. Prevalence in the general population is 1% to 2%. These patients usually do not present with signs or symptoms of overt hyperthyroidism. Subclinical hyperthyroidism is associated with an increased risk of atrial fibrillation and heart failure in older adults. Treatment options include observation or a therapeutic trial of low-dose antithyroid agents for 6 mo to attempt to induce remission. The American Thyroid Association and the American Association of Clinical Endocrinologists recommend treatment of patients with TSH levels <0.1 mIU if they are older than 65 or have associated comorbidities (osteoporosis, heart failure).

- *Thyrotoxic periodic paralysis (TPP)* is a hyperthyroidism-related hypokalemia and muscle-weakening condition resulting from a sudden shift of potassium into cells. Many patients do not have other symptoms of hyperthyroidism. Typical presentation involves an Asian adult male with acute fatigue and muscle weakness initially presenting in the lower extremities. Physical examination reveals decreased deep tendon reflexes, hypertension, and tachycardia. ECG often reveals U waves, high QRS voltage, and first-degree atrioventricular block. Additional laboratory testing reveals normal acid-base state, hypokalemia with low urinary potassium excretion (spot urinary potassium concentration <20 mEq/L from potassium shift into cells), hypophosphatemia, hypophosphaturia, and hypercalciuria. Electromyography during attacks shows low-amplitude compound muscle action potential of the tested muscle. Therapy consists of cautious potassium supplementation (increased risk of rebound hyperkalemia). Use of nonselective β-blockers (e.g., propranolol) to counteract hyperadrenergic activity, which may be causing TPP, may also be useful.

HYPERTHYROIDISM IN PREGNANCY

In otherwise healthy women, a biochemical diagnosis of overt hyperthyroidism can be made in 0.7% to 0.9%, and another 1.0% to 2.1% of women can be diagnosed with subclinical hyperthyroidism. However, from a clinical perspective, two major subtypes of overt hyperthyroidism should be distinguished. First, the majority of women with gestational hyperthyroidism will present with a physiologic form of transient biochemical hyperthyroidism (also referred to as gestational transient thyrotoxicosis). This is caused by high hCG concentrations, which typically peak between 8 and 12 wk of pregnancy and are higher in IVF and twin pregnancies. Most of these women have no or mild (transient) thyrotoxic symptoms and rarely require symptomatic treatment (i.e., propranolol). Trophoblastic diseases, partial and complete hydatidiform moles, and choriocarcinoma are other rare causes of hCG-mediated (but pathologic) hyperthyroidism in pregnancy. Non–hCG-mediated hyperthyroidism, the second major type of overt hyperthyroidism in pregnancy, is caused by Graves disease or, less commonly, autonomous thyroid hormone production (toxic adenoma or multinodular toxic goiter). Non–hCG-mediated hyperthyroidism during pregnancy is rare and can be further categorized as preexisting Graves disease (estimated prevalence 0.5%), new-onset Graves disease (0.05%), and autonomous thyroid hormone production (0.1%).

When untreated, the vast majority of women with Graves disease will present with overt biochemical abnormalities and thyrotoxic symptoms. Overt hyperthyroidism from Graves disease is associated with a high risk of adverse outcomes such as preeclampsia, preterm birth, low birth weight, and maternal heart failure. The clinical presentation of women with hyperthyroidism because of a toxic nodule or toxic multinodular goiter is more heterogeneous. In some cases, the additional hCG stimulation of pregnancy causes only transient hyperthyroidism, while preconception hyperthyroidism because of nodular disease may be more severe and in some cases necessitate treatment with antithyroid drugs, surgery, or radioablation therapy.

Although some clinical clues, including the personal and family past medical history, preconception onset of symptoms, goiter, or ophthalmopathy, can raise suspicion for Graves hyperthyroidism, biochemical evaluation is the key to diagnosis (Fig. E2). Typically, Graves hyperthyroidism in pregnancy presents with an FT_4 concentration greater than 1.5 times the upper limit of normal and relatively high T_3 concentrations but, most important, markers of autoimmunity in the form of positive serum thyroid-stimulating immunoglobulin or TSH receptor antibody (TRAb). Because new-onset Graves disease during pregnancy is very rare, some physicians prefer to perform a targeted approach to TRAb testing, whereas others prefer a universal testing approach in women with hyperthyroidism during pregnancy. In rare cases of a suspected nonpalpable toxic (T_3-producing) adenoma, thyroid ultrasound may be useful, although there is a high baseline risk of thyroid incidentaloma of up to 33%. Thyroid ultrasound cannot be used to distinguish physiologic, hCG-mediated hyperthyroidism from Graves hyperthyroidism.[2]

REFERENCES
Available at eBooks.Health.Elsevier.com.

RELATED CONTENT
Hyperthyroidism (Patient Information)
Graves Disease (Related Key Topic)
Thyrotoxic Storm (Related Key Topic)

AUTHOR: **FRED F. FERRI, MD**

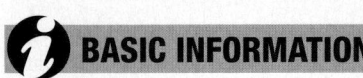

BASIC INFORMATION

DEFINITION

Hypoglycemia refers to abnormally low blood glucose levels in circulating plasma. It is defined as a glucose value <70 mg/dl (3.9 mmol/L). "Serious hypoglycemia" refers to values <54 mg/dl (3.0 mmol/L). "Severe hypoglycemia" is any glucose value necessitating external assistance to correct it. "Reactive hypoglycemia" refers to symptoms of hypoglycemia with plasma glucose value >70 mg/dl. A multitude of scenarios can lead to this potentially fatal condition.[1]

SYNONYMS

Glycopenia
Low blood glucose
Low blood sugar
HG

ICD-10CM CODES

E10.641	Type 1 diabetes mellitus with hypoglycemia with coma
E10.649	Type 1 diabetes mellitus with hypoglycemia without coma
E11.641	Type 2 diabetes mellitus with hypoglycemia with coma
E11.649	Type 2 diabetes mellitus with hypoglycemia without coma
E13.641	Other specified diabetes mellitus with hypoglycemia with coma
E13.649	Other specified diabetes mellitus with hypoglycemia without coma
E16.1	Other hypoglycemia
E16.2	Hypoglycemia, unspecified

EPIDEMIOLOGY & DEMOGRAPHICS

- Most commonly seen in patients with diabetes mellitus (DM).[1,2]
- More common in type 1 DM. Estimated that glucose levels may be as low as 50 to 60 mg/dl ~10% of the time in type 1 DM.[1,3]
- Although less prevalent than type 1, absolute cases of hypoglycemia are more prevalent in patients with type 2 DM secondary to the significantly larger population of people with type 2 DM. Rates of severe hypoglycemic episodes in type 1 DM range from 115 to 320 episodes/100 patient yr. Rates for type 2 DM range from 35 to 70 episodes/100 patient yr.[2,3]
- Elderly adults with DM are at higher risk of hypoglycemia due to alterations in adaptive physiologic responses to low glucose levels. In addition, this patient population has comorbidities, including cognitive and functional decline, that interfere with rapid identification and response to hypoglycemic episodes. Elderly patients are more likely to be hospitalized for insulin-related hypoglycemia than younger cohorts.[2]

PHYSICAL FINDINGS & CLINICAL PRESENTATION[1]

- Symptoms are often nonspecific.
- Early symptoms include sweating, pallor, anxiety, palpitations, hunger, and tremor.
- Late symptoms with lower plasma glucose levels include seizures, altered mental status, and coma.
- Profound or prolonged hypoglycemic episodes can cause irreversible brain injury, cardiopulmonary arrest, and death.
- Older adults may present with atypical symptoms: Nausea, unsteadiness, falls, or transient ischemia that can delay diagnosis.[2]

ETIOLOGY (BOX 1)

- Systemic glucose balance and effects of circulating hormones on endogenous production and use of glucose are described in Table 1. Physiologic responses to decreasing plasma glucose concentrations are summarized in Table 2
- Medications (Table 3) are the most common cause of hypoglycemia.[1,2] Common examples include beta-blockers, indomethacin, sulfonylureas, levofloxacin, and trimethoprim
- Most common causes include hyperinsulinemia due to therapeutic treatment with exogenous insulin and/or insulin secretagogues (sulfonylureas [SU] and meglitinides [MG]). Medication taken without appropriate exogenous glucose intake, and the increased insulin sensitivity that occurs with weight loss, may also result in hypoglycemic episodes[2]
- Alcohol use leading to lack of endogenous glucose production[1,2]
- Critical illness
  1. Organ failure (hepatic, cardiac, or renal)
  2. Sepsis (urinary tract infection and pneumonia are common precipitators in the elderly population)
- Hormone deficiency (cortisol, glucagon, and epinephrine)
- Endogenous hyperinsulinism (insulinoma, functional β-cell disorders, insulin autoimmune hypoglycemia)
- Rare fatal episodes thought to be secondary to ventricular arrhythmias

DIAGNOSIS[1]

Characterized by Whipple triad:
- Symptoms potentially explained by hypoglycemia
- Low blood glucose levels during the symptoms
- Relief of symptoms with administration of glucose or glucagon

DIFFERENTIAL DIAGNOSIS

Hypoglycemic symptoms in the presence of normal plasma glucose levels (>70 mg/dl) point to other etiologies: Postprandial syndrome, stroke, sepsis, seizure/post-ictal state, cardiac disease, psychiatric disease, metabolic disorders (hyperthyroidism, pheochromocytoma), **and** drug intoxication.[1]

WORKUP

- If Whipple triad is positive, the next step is consideration of the patient's medical status.[1]
- Iatrogenic factors are the most common causes of hypoglycemia in hospitalized patients (NPO status, feeding times, glucose-lowering medications, and interactions between medications).[1]
- Detailed history, including past medical history, a thorough medication history, and timing of hypoglycemia (in regard to meals and medications).

BOX 1 Causes of Hypoglycemia

Postprandial Hypoglycemia (Reactive)
- Postoperative rapid gastric emptying (alimentary hyperinsulinism)
- Fructose intolerance
- Galactosemia
- Leucine intolerance
- Idiopathic

Fasting Hypoglycemia
- Overuse of glucose
- Elevated insulin levels
- Exogenous insulin (therapeutic, factitious)
- Oral hypoglycemic (therapeutic, factitious)
- Islet cell disorders (adenoma, nesidioblastosis, cancer)
- Excessive islet cell function (prediabetes, obesity)
- Antibodies to endogenous insulin
- Normal to low insulin levels
- Ketotic hypoglycemia
- Hypermetabolic state (sepsis)
- Rare extrapancreatic tumors
- Carnitine deficiency

Underproduction of Glucose
- Hormone deficiencies (growth hormone, glucagon, hypoadrenalism)
- Enzyme disorders
- Glycogen metabolism (glycogen phosphorylase, glycogen synthetase)
- Hexose metabolism (glucose-6-phosphatase, fructose-1,6-biphosphatase)
- Glycolysis, Krebs cycle (phosphoenolpyruvate carboxykinase, pyruvate carboxylase, malate dehydrogenase)
- Alcohol and probably other drugs
- Liver disease (cirrhosis, fulminant hepatic failure)
- Severe malnutrition

From Jankovic J et al: *Bradley and Daroff's neurology in clinical practice,* ed 8, Philadelphia, 2022, Elsevier.

TABLE 1 Systemic Glucose Balance[a] and Effects of Circulating Hormones on Endogenous Production and Use of Glucose

Source of Glucose Influx or Efflux	HORMONAL EFFECTS		
	Insulin	Glucagon	Epinephrine
Glucose Influx into the Circulation			
Exogenous glucose delivery			
Endogenous glucose delivery			
In liver: Glycogenolysis and gluconeogenesis	↓	↑	↑
In kidneys: Gluconeogenesis	↓		↑
Glucose Efflux Out of the Circulation			
Ongoing brain glucose utilization			
Variable glucose utilization by other tissues (e.g., muscle fat, liver, kidneys)	↑		↓

[a]Total glucose influx = total glucose efflux.
From Melmed S et al: *Williams textbook of endocrinology,* ed 14, Philadelphia, 2019, Elsevier.

TABLE 2 Physiologic Responses to Decreasing Plasma Glucose Concentrations

Response	Glycemic Threshold[a] (mmol/L [mg/dl])	Physiologic Effects	Role in Prevention or Correction of Hypoglycemia (Glucose Counterregulation)
↓ Insulin	4.4-4.7 (80-85)	↓ R_a (↑ R_d)	Primary glucose regulatory factor, first defense against hypoglycemia
↑ Glucagon	3.6-3.9 (65-70)	↑ R_a	Primary glucose counterregulatory factor, second defense against hypoglycemia
↑ Epinephrine	3.6-3.9 (65-70)	↓ R_a, ↑ R_c	Involved, critical when glucagon is deficient, third defense against hypoglycemia
↓ Cortisol and growth hormone	3.6-3.9 (65-70)	↓ R_a, ↓ R_c	Involved, not critical
Symptoms	2.8-3.1 (50-55)	↑ Exogenous glucose	Prompt behavioral defense (food ingestion)
↓ Cognition	<2.8 (50)	—	(Compromises behavioral defense)
↓ Brain glucose metabolism	<2.8 (50)	—	—

R_a, Rate of glucose appearance, glucose production by the liver and kidneys; R_c, rate of glucose clearance by insulin-sensitive tissues; R_d, rate of glucose disappearance, glucose utilization by insulin-sensitive tissues such as skeletal muscle (no direct effect on central nervous system glucose utilization).
[a]Arterialized venous, not venous, plasma glucose concentrations.
From Melmed S et al: *Williams textbook of endocrinology,* ed 14, Philadelphia, 2019, Elsevier.

TABLE 3 Diagnostic Approach to an Adult with Documented Fasting Hypoglycemia

1. Consider the most likely disorders (drugs, critical illness, endocrine deficiency, non–β cell tumor, and insulinoma) while supporting the plasma glucose concentration if necessary.
2. Examine the history, physical examination, and available laboratory data for clinical clues to include or exclude the above categories.

Cause	Response
Insulin- or sulfonylurea-treated diabetes	Adjust the therapeutic regimen
Use of other drugs known or suspected to cause hypoglycemia	Discontinue use of the drug
Hepatic, renal, or cardiac failure; sepsis; or inanition	Treat the underlying disorder
Anorexia, weight loss, change in skin pigmentation, known pituitary or adrenocortical disease, hypotension, hyponatremia, hyperkalemia	Evaluate for adrenocortical/pituitary insufficiency
Known non–β cell tumor, mass on examination or imaging studies	Check for high IGF-2 or IGF-2:IGF-1 ratio

3. In the absence of clinical clues, consider medication error, endogenous hyperinsulinism, and surreptitious or malicious insulin secretagogue or insulin administration.

IGF, Insulin-like growth factor.
From Robertson RP et al: *DeGroot's endocrinology, basic science and clinical practice,* ed 8, Philadelphia, 2023, Elsevier.

• Special attention should be given to chronic diseases that can precipitate hypoglycemia such as severe hepatitis or cirrhosis, recurrent infections (diabetic foot ulcers, urinary tract infection, pneumonia), advanced heart disease, and chronic renal disease with a glomerular filtration rate <60.[2]

LABORATORY TESTS

• An algorithm for recognition and evaluation of hypoglycemia is described in Fig. E1. Table 4 describes a diagnostic approach to an adult with documented fasting hypoglycemia.
• If the etiology is not apparent after a thorough history, the following testing is appropriate:

FASTING SAMPLES: If symptoms witnessed when fasting, with verified low blood glucose levels, consider the following laboratory tests: Plasma glucose, β-hydroxybutyrate (BHOB), insulin, C-peptide, proinsulin, screen for SU and MG metabolites.[1]

POSTPRANDIAL SAMPLES:
• Plasma glucose, insulin, C-peptide, and proinsulin before ingestion of the meal and every 30 min thereafter for 5 h.[1]
• Only evaluate the samples drawn when glucose levels are <60 mg/dl.
• If a patient has a presentation consistent with Whipple triad, then measure SU, MG, and antibodies to insulin.[1]

72-H FAST: (Tables 5, 6)[1]
• Collect blood specimens for measurement of plasma glucose, insulin, C-peptide, proinsulin, and BHOB every 6 h until the glucose concentration is <60 mg/dl.
• Increase frequency of sampling to every 1 to 2 h.
• Insulin, C-peptide, and proinsulin are only relevant in specimens in which plasma glucose concentration is <60 mg/dl.
• The fast should be ended when any of the following occurs:
  1. The plasma glucose concentration is <45 mg/dl.
  2. The patient has symptoms or signs of hypoglycemia.
  3. 72 h has elapsed.
  4. The plasma glucose concentration is <55, and Whipple triad has been documented on a prior occasion.
• Insulin antibodies are also measured, but are unneeded during the hypoglycemic state.

IMAGING STUDIES[1]

If hypoglycemia is suspected secondary to an insulinoma or malignancy, transabdominal ultrasound (US), computed tomography scan, or endoscopic US can be used to aid in the diagnosis and for staging purposes.

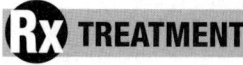 TREATMENT

NONPHARMACOLOGIC THERAPY[1]

• Recognition of signs and symptoms and self-monitoring of blood glucose are especially important in insulin-deficient patients.
• Avoiding drugs that can exacerbate hypoglycemia (e.g., alcohol) if episodes occur repeatedly.

TABLE 4 Drug-Induced Hypoglycemia

Drugs Capable of Causing Hypoglycemia by Themselves
- Antidiabetic drugs
- Insulin
- Sulfonylureas
- Benzoic acid derivatives (meglitinide)

Other
- Alcohol
- Salicylates
- Propranolol
- Pentamidine
- Sulfonamides
- Vacor rodenticide
- Quinine/quinidine
- Propoxyphene
- Para-aminobenzoic acid
- Perhexiline

Drugs That Probably Cause Hypoglycemia Only in Combination with Insulin/Sulfonylurea/Benzoic Acid Derivatives or Under Special Circumstances (e.g., malnutrition, infection, renal insufficiency)
- Biguanides
- Angiotensin-converting enzyme
- Phenylbutazone
- Lidocaine
- Warfarin (Coumadin)
- Ranitidine, cimetidine
- Doxepin
- Danazol
- Azopropazone
- Oxytetracycline
- Clofibrate, benzofibrate
- Colchicine
- Ketoconazole
- Chloramphenicol
- Haloperidol
- Monoamine oxidase inhibitors
- Thalidomide
- Orphenadrine
- Selegiline
- Abenzolene
- Flecainide
- Fluoxetine
- Clomipramine
- Indomethacin
- Chloroquine

From Robertson RP et al: *DeGroot's endocrinology, basic science and clinical practice*, ed 8, Philadelphia, 2023, Elsevier.

TABLE 5 Sample Protocol for a 72-H Fast

Admit before the evening meal. Discontinue all nonessential medications. Insert an intravenous line for blood sampling.

Begin blood sampling (plasma glucose, insulin, C-peptide) just before the meal and continue every 30 min for 6 h and thereafter every 2 to 3 h.

Sampling should also include sulfonylureas/meglitinides. Additional studies could include morning cortisol, insulin antibodies, and/or IGF-2 based on clinical suspicion and do not necessarily require hypoglycemia.

Patient may consume calorie- and caffeine-lacking liquids and should ambulate.

The fast is ended at 72 h or earlier if the patient has a plasma glucose level <45 mg/dl (2.5 mmol/L) with symptoms or <55 mg/dl (3.1 mmol/L) with prior Whipple's triad or if 72 h have elapsed.

At the end of the fast, draw samples for all the above measurements and inject 1 mg of glucagon intravenously and measure plasma glucose at 10, 20, and 30 min.

IGF-1, Insulin-like growth factor-1.
From Robertson RP et al: *DeGroot's endocrinology, basic science and clinical practice*, ed 8, Philadelphia, 2023, Elsevier.

- Bedtime snacks if hypoglycemia occurs at night.
- In situations caused by tumor etiologies (e.g., islet cell, insulinoma, and nonislet cell), definitive treatment may require surgical removal.

PHARMACOLOGIC THERAPY[1,4]

- Treating the underlying etiology that exacerbates hypoglycemia (e.g., infection, proper diabetic regimen, proper diabetic diet)
- Fast-acting carbohydrates (e.g., glucose tablets, hard candy, intravenous [IV] dextrose infusion)
- Pure glucose (dextrose) if caused by insulin secretagogue in addition with α-glucosidase inhibitor
- In severe hypoglycemia with seizure activity, 25 g of 50% dextrose IV or 0.5 to 1.0 mg intramuscular/subcutaneous glucagon
- In persistent hypoglycemia after IV dextrose therapy, consider sulfonylurea overdose or insulin pump malfunction. If an insulin pump is present, remove it. If sulfonylurea overdose is suspected, treat with IV dextrose infusion and octreotide 50 to 100 μg every 6 to 12 h for adults, followed by 1 to 2 μg/kg every 6 to 12 h[4]
- Fig. 2 describes a management algorithm for hypoglycemia

REFERRAL

- Most **episodes** of hypoglycemia can be managed by primary care physicians by adjusting medications.
- If the cause is not clear, then endocrinology referral is recommended.
- Severe symptomatic hypoglycemia **requires** emergent treatment.

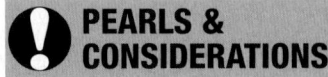 **PEARLS & CONSIDERATIONS**

- Hypoglycemia causes severe **morbidity and mortality** if not dealt with promptly and effectively.
- Hypoglycemia is very common in patients with DM, especially type 1 DM, and most commonly it is a side effect of medication(s).
- Elderly patients with DM are at higher risk for serious hypoglycemic episodes and can initially present with atypical symptoms.
- In patients who are hospitalized, the etiology is often multifactorial.
- Clinically important hypoglycemia is uncommon in nondiabetic patients, and evaluation for a hypoglycemic disorder in these patients should only occur if the Whipple triad is met.
- Pediatric hypoglycemia: A classification of hypoglycemia in infants and children is summarized in Table E7.

REFERENCES & SUGGESTED READINGS

Available at eBooks.Health.Elsevier.com.

RELATED CONTENT

Diabetes Mellitus (Related Key Topic)
Insulinoma (Related Key Topic)

AUTHORS: **BENJAMIN E. HOOK, MD** and **TRACY LEIGH LEGROS, MD, PhD**

TABLE 6 Interpretation of a 72-H Fast

Diagnosis	Symptoms or Signs	Plasma Glucose (mg/dL)	Plasma Insulin (μU/mL)	Plasma C-Peptide (nmol/L)	β-Hydroxybutyrate	Autoimmune Antibodies	IGF-mediated	Oral Agent Screen
Normal	No	<55	<3	<0.2	>2.7	−	N	−
Endogenous hyperinsulinism	Yes	<55	>3	>0.2	<2.7	−	N	−
Factitious insulin	Yes	<55	>3	<0.2	<2.7	−	N	−
Factitious oral agent	Yes	<55	>3	>0.2	<2.7	−	N	+
Non–islet cell tumor	Yes	<55	<3	<0.2	<2.7	−	↑	−
Autoimmune disorder	Yes	<55	>>3	>>0.2	<2.7	+	N	−

IGF, Insulin-like growth factor; *N*, normal.
From Robertson RP et al: *DeGroot's endocrinology, basic science and clinical practice,* ed 8, Philadelphia, 2023, Elsevier.

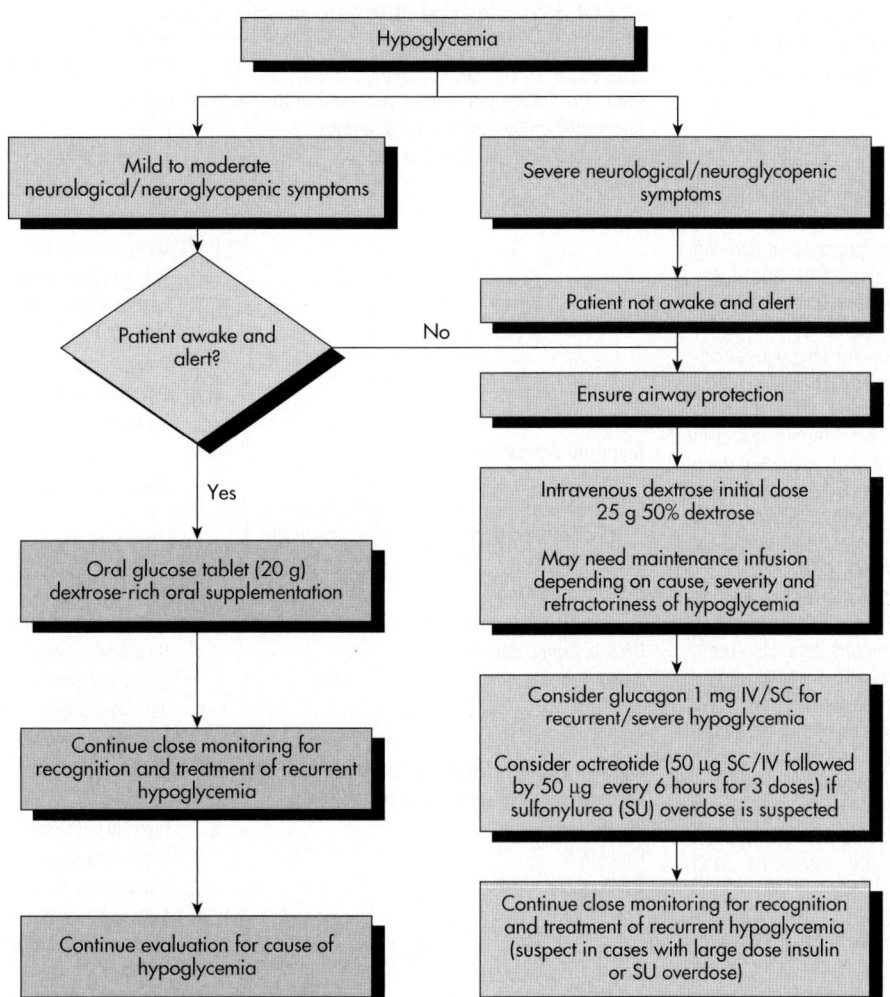

FIG. 2 Management of hypoglycemia. *IV*, Intravenous; *SC*, subcutaneous. (From Vincent JL et al: *Textbook of critical care,* ed 7, Philadelphia, 2017, Elsevier.)

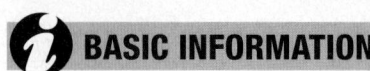
BASIC INFORMATION

DEFINITION

Male hypogonadism is a clinical syndrome involving subnormal testosterone levels and/or impaired sperm production due to dysfunction at one or both levels of the hypothalamic-pituitary-testicular axis.

SYNONYM

Testicular dysfunction

ICD-10CM CODES

E23.0	Hypopituitarism
E23.1	Drug-induced hypopituitarism
E29	Testicular dysfunction
E29.1	Testicular hypofunction
E29.8	Other testicular dysfunction
E29.9	Testicular dysfunction, unspecified
E89.3	Postprocedural hypopituitarism

EPIDEMIOLOGY & DEMOGRAPHICS

INCIDENCE: Hypogonadism is the most common clinical disorder of the testis. Incidence is unclear due to the many possible underlying factors, nonspecificity of symptoms, and questions relating to the adequacy of a diagnostic serum total testosterone threshold.

PREVALENCE: Prevalence of hypogonadism increases with aging, obesity, diabetes mellitus, and other comorbidities. The average decrease in serum total testosterone levels in aging men is 1% to 2% per yr. Prevalence rises to 23% among men in their 70s. However, in population-based surveys of community-dwelling middle-aged and older males, prevalence of hypogonadism is approximately 6%.

RISK FACTORS: These are many and include genetic abnormalities; the aging process; pituitary and testicular lesions and disorders; medications; drug abuse; HIV disease; acute illnesses; chronic cardiac, hepatic, renal, and pulmonary diseases; cancer; ionizing radiation; chemotherapy; obesity; and malnutrition.

GENETICS: Genetic abnormalities underlie a number of hypogonadal disorders including Klinefelter syndrome, Noonan syndrome, hemochromatosis, Kallmann syndrome, and Prader-Willi syndrome.

PHYSICAL FINDINGS & CLINICAL PRESENTATION

Sexual (Specific):
- Decrease in frequency of erections
- Erectile dysfunction
- Decrease in libido
- Decreased fertility
- Small or shrinking testes
- Gynecomastia
- Diminished sexual hair
- Hot flushes and sweats

Neuropsychologic (Less Specific):
- Depression
- Inability to concentrate
- Diminished motivation and vitality
- Decrease in self-confidence

- Diminished energy and stamina
- Sleep disturbances

Physical Features and Findings:
- Diminished capacity for physical activity
- Decrease in physical endurance and performance
- Diminished muscle mass and strength
- Increase in body fat
- Decrease or loss of axillary and pubic hair and decrease in shaving frequency
- Fine wrinkling over the lateral aspects of the face
- Breast enlargement with or without tenderness
- Change in consistency and decrease in size of testes

- Fragility fractures
- Anemia

ETIOLOGY

- The importance of a careful history and examination cannot be overstated to determine the etiology of possible hypogonadism. Primary hypogonadism is a result of a decrease in testicular testosterone secretion and/or a decrease in spermatogenesis with an associated increase in gonadotropin levels as in Klinefelter syndrome, cryptorchidism, and following orchitis, testicular trauma, chemotherapy, and irradiation. The causes of primary hypogonadism are summarized in Table 1.

TABLE 1 Causes of Primary Hypogonadism

Common Causes	Uncommon Causes
Androgen Deficiency and Impairment of Sperm Production	
Congenital or Developmental Disorders	
Klinefelter syndrome (XXY) and variants	Myotonic dystrophy
	Uncorrected cryptorchidism
	Noonan syndrome
	Bilateral congenital anorchia
	Polyglandular autoimmune syndrome
	Testosterone biosynthetic enzyme defects
	CAH (TART)
	Complex genetic syndromes
	Down syndrome
	LH receptor mutation
Acquired Disorders	
Bilateral surgical castration or trauma	Orchitis
Drugs (spironolactone, ketoconazole, abiraterone, enzalutamide, alcohol, chemotherapy agents)[a]	
Ionizing radiation	
Systemic Disorders	
Chronic liver disease (hepatic cirrhosis)[a,b]	Malignancy (lymphoma, testicular cancer)
Chronic kidney disease[a,b]	Sickle cell disease[b]
Aging[b]	Spinal cord injury
	Vasculitis (polyarteritis)
	Infiltrative disease (amyloidosis, leukemia)
Isolated Impairment of Sperm Production or Function	
Congenital or Developmental Disorders	
Cryptorchidism	Myotonic dystrophy
Varicocele	Sertoli cell–only syndrome
Y chromosome microdeletions	Primary ciliary dyskinesia
	Down syndrome
	FSH receptor mutation
Acquired Disorders	
Orchitis	Environmental toxins
Ionizing radiation	
Chemotherapy agents	
Thermal trauma	
Systemic Disorders	
Acute febrile illness	Spinal cord injury
Malignancy (testicular cancer, Hodgkin disease)[b]	
Idiopathic azoospermia or oligozoospermia	

CAH, Congenital adrenal hyperplasia; *FSH,* follicle-stimulating hormone; *LH,* luteinizing hormone; *TART,* testicular adrenal rest tumor.
[a]Functional causes that are potentially reversible with discontinuation of offending medication, or with liver or renal transplantation.
[b]Combined primary and secondary hypogonadism.
From Melmed S et al: *Williams textbook of endocrinology,* ed 14, Philadelphia, 2019, Elsevier.

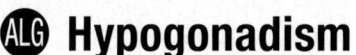

- Secondary hypogonadism is due to hypothalamic-pituitary dysfunction, which results in a decrease in testosterone levels and/or spermatogenesis with gonadotropin levels that are subnormal or inappropriately within the normal range. Table 2 summarizes causes of secondary hypogonadism.

- Combined primary and secondary hypogonadism is a result of deficits at both the level of the hypothalamic-pituitary axis and testes with variable gonadotropin levels depending upon the predominance of the level of the defect.

TABLE 2 Causes of Secondary Hypogonadism

Common Causes	Uncommon Causes
Androgen Deficiency and Impairment of Sperm Production	
Congenital or Developmental Disorders	
Constitutional delayed puberty	CHH due to genetic mutations
Hemochromatosis	CHH, idiopathic (IHH)
	Kallmann syndrome
	Congenital adrenal hypoplasia
	Isolated LH deficiency, LHβ mutations
	Complex genetic syndromes
Acquired Disorders	
Hyperprolactinemia[a]	Hypopituitarism
Opioids[a]	
Androgenic anabolic steroids, progestins, estrogen excess[a]	
GnRH agonist or antagonist[a]	
	Pituitary or hypothalamic tumor
	Surgical hypophysectomy, pituitary or cranial irradiation
	Vascular compromise, traumatic brain injury
	Granulomatous or infiltrative disease
	Infection
	Pituitary stalk disease
	Lymphocytic or autoimmune hypophysitis
	Acquired IHH
Systemic Disorders	
Glucocorticoid excess (Cushing syndrome)[a,b]	Chronic systemic illness[a,b]
Chronic organ failure[a,b]	Spinal cord injury
Chronic liver disease (hepatic cirrhosis), chronic kidney disease, chronic lung disease, chronic heart failure[a]	Transfusion-related iron overload (β-thalassemia)[a]
Chronic systemic illness[a,b]	
Type 2 diabetes mellitus[a]	Sickle cell disease
Malignancy[a]	Cystic fibrosis
Rheumatic disease (rheumatoid arthritis)[a]	
HIV disease[a]	
Starvation,[b] malnutrition,[b] eating disorders, endurance exercise[a]	
Morbid obesity, obstructive sleep apnea[a]	
Acute and critical illness[a]	
Aging (comorbid illnesses associated with aging)[a,b]	
Isolated Impairment of Sperm Production or Function	
Congenital or Developmental Disorders	
	Congenital adrenal hyperplasia (21-hydroxylase deficiency, 11β-hydroxylase deficiency)
	Isolated FSH deficiency, FSHβ mutations
Acquired Disorders	
Testosterone, androgenic anabolic steroids	Androgen- or hCG-secreting tumors
Malignancy (Hodgkin disease, testicular cancer)[b]	Hyperprolactinemia

CHH, Congenital hypogonadotropic hypogonadism; *FSH,* follicle-stimulating hormone; *GnRH,* gonadotropin-releasing hormone; *hCG,* human chorionic gonadotropin; *HIV,* human immunodeficiency virus; *IHH,* idiopathic hypogonadotropic hypogonadism; *LH,* luteinizing hormone.
[a]Functional causes that are potentially reversible or treatable with discontinuation of offending medication, treatment of underlying cause of gonadotropin suppression or organ transplantation.
[b]Combined primary and secondary hypogonadism.
From Melmed S et al: *Williams textbook of endocrinology,* ed 14, Philadelphia, 2019, Elsevier.

Dx DIAGNOSIS (FIG. 1)

DIFFERENTIAL DIAGNOSIS

Hypogonadotropic or Secondary Hypogonadism:
- Pituitary dysfunction: Hypopituitarism, functioning or nonfunctioning pituitary tumor, lymphocytic hypophysitis, infiltrative disease as with sarcoidosis, hemochromatosis, and histiocytosis X
- Hyperprolactinemia: Prolactinoma, medication-related, chronic kidney disease
- Genetic: Kallmann syndrome with anosmia, Prader-Willi syndrome with morbid obesity
- Acute and chronic illnesses; malnutrition; emotional disorders; HIV; sleep apnea; aging; malignancies; obesity; and renal, hepatic, pulmonary, and cardiac diseases
- Opioids, central nervous system (CNS): Active medications, glucocorticoid excess, and GnRH analogues (androgen deprivation therapy)

Hypergonadotropic or Primary Hypogonadism:
- Genetic: Klinefelter syndrome, Noonan syndrome, myotonic dystrophy
- Gonadal damage due to drugs, alcohol, radiation, chemotherapy, trauma
- Congenital anorchia (vanishing testis syndrome)
- Cryptorchidism
- Mumps orchitis, HIV orchitis
- Diabetes mellitus
- Hodgkin disease
- Aging

Combined Primary and Secondary Hypogonadism:
- Hemochromatosis, sickle cell disease, thalassemia
- Alcoholism, glucocorticoid therapy, aging
- Chronic cardiac, hepatic, renal, pulmonary diseases, and HIV disease

WORKUP

- Determine the presence or absence of male hypogonadism on the basis of history, clinical manifestations and findings, and documentation of consistently low serum total testosterone levels and/or abnormal seminal fluid analysis.
- Morning serum total testosterone levels should be measured on at least two or three occasions for confirmation of diagnosis and when necessary followed by measurement of serum free or bioavailable testosterone.
- Serum follicle-stimulating hormone (FSH) and luteinizing hormone (LH) levels are measured to determine whether hypogonadism is primary, secondary, or a result of combined defects of the hypothalamic-pituitary axis and testis. The cause of testosterone deficiency should be definitively determined before initiation of testosterone replacement therapy.
- Hormonal assessment of gonadal status should not be done during an acute or subacute illness.

LABORATORY TESTS

- Serum total testosterone is tightly bound to sex hormone binding globulin (SHBG) and weakly bound to circulating albumin. 0.5% to 3% of serum total testosterone is unbound or free.

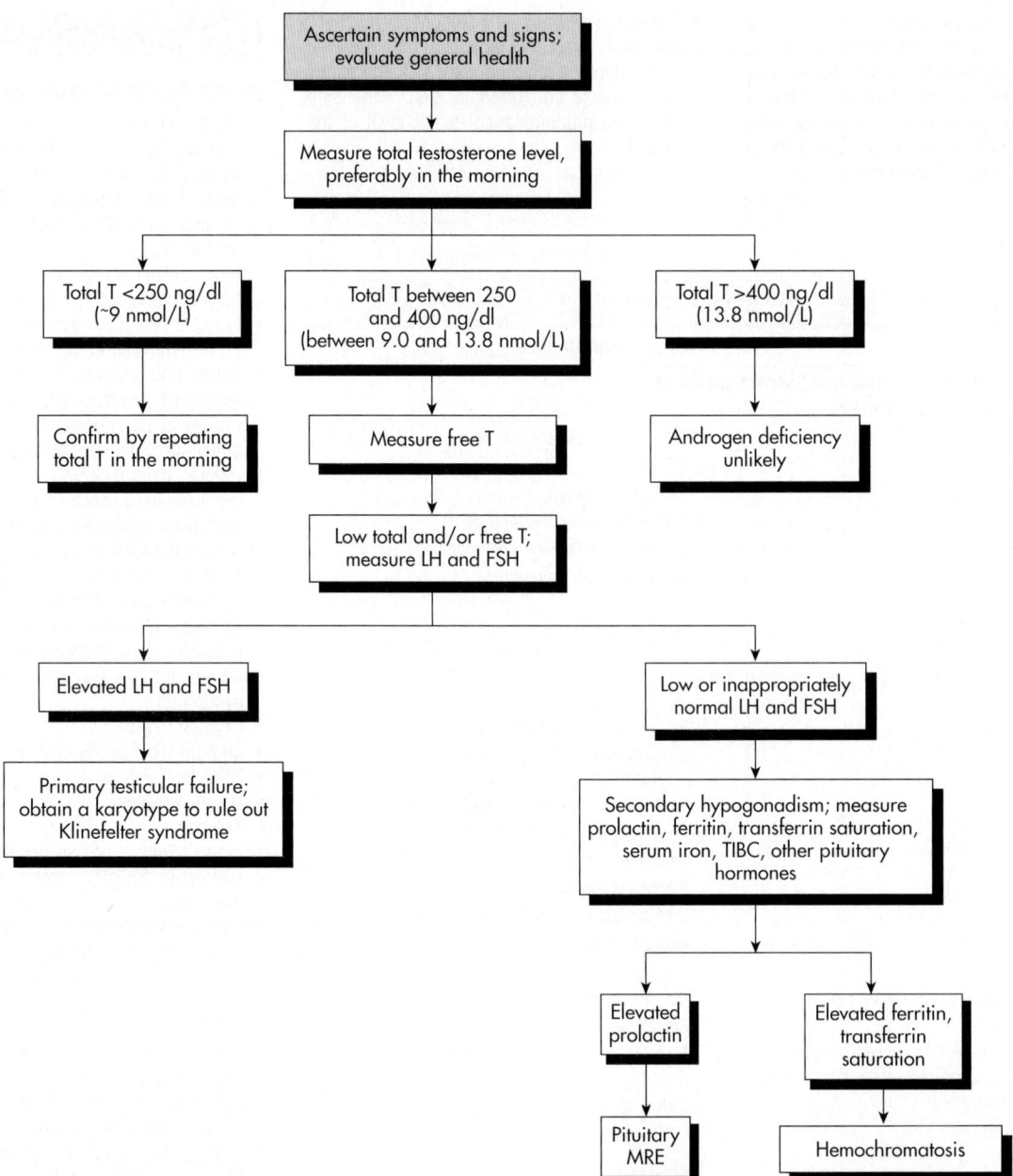

FIG. 1 Algorithm showing an approach for the diagnostic evaluation of adult men suspected of having androgen deficiency. *FSH,* Follicle-stimulating hormone; *LH,* luteinizing hormone; *MRE,* magnetic resonance elastography; *T,* testosterone; *TIBC,* total iron-binding capacity. (From Shalender B, Shehzad B: Diagnosis and treatment of hypogonadism in men, *Best Pract Res Clin Endocrin* 25:251-270, 2011.)

- Liquid chromatography tandem mass spectrometry assays for total serum testosterone are more accurate than immunoassays.
- Bioavailable testosterone refers to unbound testosterone plus the testosterone that is loosely bound to albumin.
- Free testosterone, if necessary, is best measured by equilibrium dialysis or centrifugal ultrafiltration.
- An SHBG measurement is helpful in determining the adequacy or normality of a serum total testosterone measurement. Conditions that lower SHBG include obesity, protein-losing states, androgens, hypothyroidism, and familial SHBG deficiency. Increases in SHBG occur in those with hyperthyroidism,

hepatitis, cirrhosis, and HIV disease, aging, and by estrogens.
- The lower limit of normal for serum total testosterone in a healthy young male is approximately 240 to 950 ng/dl and a low-normal serum free testosterone in a young normal male is 5 to 20 ng/dl. Serum total testosterone in a healthy young male ranges from 300 to 1000 ng/dl and normal free testosterone ranges from 5 to 20 ng/dl.
- Serum total testosterone levels can vary from day to day, and there is a diurnal rhythm in young normal males with morning levels that are higher by approximately 20% to 25% as compared with levels in the afternoon.

- In elderly males, the diurnal rhythm is diminished with levels approximately 10% lower in the afternoon as compared with morning levels.
- Serum FSH and LH measurements are important in delineating primary, secondary, and combined hypogonadism.
- Hypogonadal symptoms are more likely to be seen in those with total serum testosterone levels of less than 230 ng/dl for young normal males. Serum total testosterone levels of <150 ng/dl are unequivocally low.
- Transient suppression of total serum testosterone may occur during acute illness, in males that are being treated with glucocorticoid, in those taking opiates or CNS-active medications, in those with malnutrition or

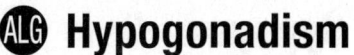
poor eating habits, and during excessive physical exercise.

- Quantity and quality of sperm counts and activity can vary in a significant way for a variety of reasons. Therefore, in assessing fertility, seminal fluid analysis should be done on two or more occasions, each separated by 2 or more wk, and on semen collected within an hour of ejaculation after more than 2 days of abstinence.
- Depending on the clinical picture and examination, other studies may be necessary, including a karyotype analysis, for example, for Klinefelter syndrome, or serum prolactin measurement for patients with possible hyperprolactinemia, which may be drug-induced, related to a prolactinoma, or to chronic renal disease.

IMAGING STUDIES

In males with severe androgen deficiency with low serum gonadotropin levels, increased serum prolactin levels, hypopituitarism, severe headaches, and visual defects, an MRI of the pituitary would be appropriate. In males with hypogonadism and a history of fractures, dual energy x-ray absorptiometry measurements of spine and hip should be obtained to further delineate the status of the skeletal system.

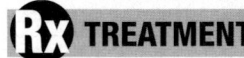 **TREATMENT**

Testosterone replacement therapy is indicated when patients have symptoms and signs of hypogonadism and serum testosterone levels that are consistently subnormal with levels of <250 ng/dl. The goal of replacement therapy is to restore serum testosterone levels to within the normal range of values and to have a positive effect on the constellation of hypogonadal symptoms and signs. Subnormal spermatogenesis, if present in such patients, is not affected by testosterone therapy. In patients with hypogonadotropic or secondary hypogonadism, chorionic gonadotropin and/or GnRH therapy can optimize spermatogenesis, whereas, generally in patients with primary hypogonadism, subnormal spermatogenesis and infertility are irreversible.

NONPHARMACOLOGIC THERAPY

- Weight reduction, especially when it appears to be a major factor underlying male hypogonadism

- Discontinuation of anabolic steroids, CNS-active medications, and narcotic abuse
- Surgery or radiation therapy for patients with a pituitary functioning or nonfunctioning tumor with visual field abnormality and headaches who are not candidates for further medical therapy or have been unsuccessfully treated with medication
- Surgery indicated for chronic gynecomastia and, occasionally, in cases with recent-onset gynecomastia that has not responded to testosterone replacement therapy

CHRONIC Rx

Testosterone formulations (Table 3):

- Parenteral testosterone preparations: Testosterone enanthate (generic) and testosterone cypionate (Depo-Testosterone and generic) 150 to 200 mg are injected intramuscularly every 2 wk. Following injections, there are appreciable fluctuations in serum testosterone, with levels rising within the first several days and a subsequent decrease to normal and in some cases to below normal at the end of the 2 wk. As a result of the varying levels of testosterone, patients may have related

TABLE 3	Overview of Available Testosterone Preparations			
Route of Administration	Formulation	Starting Dose/Interval	Advantages	Disadvantages
Intramuscular injections	Testosterone enanthate	250 mg Every 2-3 wk	Relatively inexpensive Flexibility of dosing	Requires IM injections Excursions in T concentrations may be associated with fluctuating symptoms
	Testosterone cypionate	250 mg Every 2-3 wk	Relatively inexpensive Flexibility of dosing	Requires IM injections Excursions in T concentrations may be associated with fluctuating symptoms
	Testosterone propionate (not available in U.S.)	50-100 mg Every 3-5 days		Frequent IM injections, not suited for chronic treatment T concentrations fluctuate
	Mix of testosterone esters (Sustanon)	One vial 250 mg Every 2-3 wk	Relatively inexpensive Flexibility of dosing	Regular IM injections Excursions in T concentrations may be associated with fluctuating symptoms
	Testosterone undecanoate	1000 mg at wk 0 and 6, and then every 12 wk United States: 750 mg at wk 0 and 4, and then every 10 wk	Infrequent administration	Local discomfort after IM injection of large volume (3 or 4 ml) Coughing/dyspnea within 15-30 min of injection in small number of patients (15-19/1000 injections)
Subcutaneous implants	Implantable pellets (only available in U.S. and Australia)	150-450 mg every 3 mo or 600-1200 mg every 6 mo	Infrequent administration Relatively stable T concentrations	Requires minor surgical insertion Pellets may extrude Local hematoma or infection rarely
Subcutaneous injections	Testosterone enanthate	75 mg Once weekly	Ease of application	Increased blood pressure, injection site reactions, headache
Transdermal	T patch (only available in some countries)	2 or 4 mg per patch 4 mg every 24 h	Ease of application	Skin irritation
	T gel	Available as 1%, 1.62%, 2% gel in unit-dose packets or via a metered-dose pump system Dose dependent on the formulation: 50 mg for 1% T gel; 81 mg for T 1.62%; 60 mg for 2% T gel Once daily	Ease of application Flexibility of dosing	Risk of transfer to female partner or child Variable T concentrations from day to day
	T solution (Axiron)	60 mg 1-2 times/day in the axillae		Risk of transfer to female partner or child Variable T concentrations from day to day

Continued

TABLE 3 Overview of Available Testosterone Preparations—cont'd

Route of Administration	Formulation	Starting Dose/Interval	Advantages	Disadvantages
Oral	Testosterone undecanoate capsules (not available in U.S.)	40-80 mg/capsule 2-3 times/day	Convenient administration Avoids first-pass metabolism	Short half-life, requires multiple daily dosing Ingestion with fatty meal Fluctuating T levels due to variable absorption
	Modified testosterone undecanoate	237 mg/capsule 2 times/day	Ingestion with regular meal Avoids first-pass metabolism	Twice-daily administration
	Testosterone buccal bioadhesive tablet	30 mg/tablet 2 times/day	Avoids first-pass metabolism	Local gum irritation Alteration of taste No dose titration
Intranasal	Nasal gel	One pump of 5.5 mg per nostril 3 times/day	Rapid absorption Avoids first-pass metabolism	Local nasal side effects Multiple applications per day

From Robertson RP et al: *DeGroot's endocrinology, basic science and clinical practice*, ed 8, Philadelphia, 2023, Elsevier.

symptoms. Adjustments in dose and dosing interval may help to alleviate the serum fluctuations and clinical symptoms. Testosterone undecanoate (AUEFD-ENDO) is an injectable depot formulation FDA-approved for male hypogonadism. The recommended dosage is 750 mg injected intramuscularly at 0 and 4 wk, and then every 10 wk thereafter.

- Topical testosterone preparations:
  1. Testosterone adhesive patch (Androderm) delivers 2.5 or 5 mg of testosterone when applied nightly to the back, abdomen, upper arms, or thighs. Serum testosterone levels rise to within normal range in a few hours after application and, thereafter, are relatively stable. Daily doses of up to 10 mg may be necessary.
  2. Testosterone 1% gels (AndroGel and Testim). AndroGel is available in 2.5 g and 5 g gel units that deliver 2.5 mg and 5 mg of testosterone, respectively. The gel is applied daily in the morning by hand over the shoulder, upper arms, or abdomen. Adjustments in dose to 7.5 g or 10 g of gel may be necessary to optimize serum testosterone levels. AndroGel (1.62%) pump is also available for daily application. Testim is available in 5-g and 10-g tubes and with morning applications over the shoulders or arms delivers 5 mg and 10 mg of testosterone, respectively. Both AndroGel and Testim provide relatively stable serum testosterone levels. Two new transdermal formulations, Fortesta and Axiron, are now available and are applied daily by metered dose pumps. With these preparations, care is necessary to avoid skin-to-skin contact exposure with others.
- Testosterone pellets: Three to six pellets of testosterone each containing 75 mg of testosterone are surgically inserted subcutaneously every 3 to 6 mo and provide relatively stable serum testosterone levels.
- Testosterone undecanoate (Jatenzo) is an oral testosterone formulation approved for patients with hypogonadism associated with structural or genetic etiologies, and it is not indicated in men with age-related hypogonadism.

BOX 1 Contraindications for Testosterone Replacement Therapy

- Desire for fertility in the near future
- Untreated and treated breast cancer
- Untreated, locally advanced or metastatic prostate cancer
- Unevaluated palpable prostate nodule
- Unevaluated PSA >4 ng/ml (>3 ng/ml in men with high risk for prostate cancer, e.g., Black Americans or men with affected first-degree relatives)
- Severe lower urinary tract symptoms (IPSS >19)
- Hematocrit >48%-50%
- Thrombophilia
- Severe congestive heart failure
- Recent myocardial infarction or stroke
- Untreated sleep apnea

IPSS, International Prostate Symptom Score.
From Robertson RP et al: *DeGroot's endocrinology, basic science and clinical practice,* ed 8, Philadelphia, 2023, Elsevier.

RISKS & ADVERSE EFFECTS

- Contraindications to testosterone therapy (Box 1) include prostate cancer, breast cancer, chronic obstructive pulmonary disease, untreated obstructive sleep apnea, congestive heart failure, and polycythemia. Relative contraindications include severe benign prostatic hyperplasia, hematocrit ≥50% at baseline, sleep apnea, and severe congestive heart failure.
- Patients on chronic testosterone therapy need to be followed carefully with prostate and prostate-specific antigen assessments and hematocrit measurements for possible excessive induction of erythrocytosis, initially at 3 to 6 mo and at regular intervals thereafter. Table 4 summarizes monitoring during testosterone treatment.
- Current testosterone use for 6 mo or shorter is associated with 63% higher risk for venous thromboembolism (VTE). VTE risk peaks during the first 6 mo and declines to 25% thereafter.
- A clinical trial involving over 5,000 men (age range 45 to 80, mean age 63) receiving testosterone replacement found no significant differences between testosterone replacement and placebo in regards to cardiovascular events.[1]

- A randomized trial[2] evaluating testosterone treatment and fractures in men with hypogonadism revealed that testosterone is associated with a modest increase in fractures.

REFERRAL

Endocrinology for full endocrine and metabolic assessment and therapy. Urology for further assessment and follow-up of the prostate and for evaluation and therapy of erectile dysfunction. Neurosurgery for evaluation and possible surgery for a pituitary lesion. Plastic surgery for chronic gynecomastia. Reproductive endocrinology for those with an infertility problem.

❗ PEARLS & CONSIDERATIONS

COMMENTS

- Do not screen men "routinely" for hypogonadism. Screening men with nonspecific symptoms of hypogonadism (e.g., decreased energy) is also not recommended. Screening should be limited to men with specific signs and symptoms of hypogonadism.
- Male hypogonadism is an important and frequently encountered problem that requires a complete medical history, examination, and

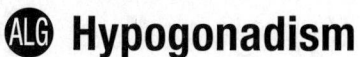

TABLE 4 Monitoring During Testosterone Treatment

Parameter	Timing	Further Management
Measures of Efficacy		
Symptoms and signs of androgen deficiency	At baseline, after 3-12 mo, and then yearly	Continue testosterone treatment in men with clinical improvement and no adverse effects. Consider discontinuing testosterone treatment in men if no clinical improvement.
BMD	For men at high risk for fracture, BMD before treatment; for men with osteoporosis or minimal-trauma fracture, BMD after 1-2 yr	Institute appropriate treatment for men with osteoporosis, including calcium and vitamin D.
Serum testosterone	*Testosterone ester injection:* After 3-6 mo, measured midway between injections or at end of dosing interval (if androgen deficiency symptoms are present at that time) *Testosterone patch:* After 3-4 wk, at 8-10 h after application *Testosterone gel:* After 2 wk, at any time after application *Buccal testosterone:* After 4-6 wk, at any time after application (preferably in the morning) *Testosterone pellets:* At end of dosing interval *Oral testosterone undecanoate:* After 1 wk, at 3-5 h after oral dose *Testosterone undecanoate injection:* At end of dosing interval	Adjust dose or dosing interval to achieve serum testosterone concentrations in the mid-normal range.
Adverse Effects		
Hematocrit	At baseline, after 3-6 mo, and then yearly	If hematocrit is >54%, stop or reduce dosage of testosterone until hematocrit declines to normal and reinitiate testosterone at a lower dosage. Investigate for a hypoxic condition such as obstructive sleep apnea or chronic lung disease.
PSA level, with or without DRE (using shared decision making, i.e., if a patient desires prostate cancer screening after discussion of risks and benefits of PSA screening and monitoring), in men >50 yr (>40 if risk factors for prostate cancer)	At baseline, after 3-6 mo, and then according to accepted guidelines	Urologic evaluation with any of the following: • Confirmed PSA >4 ng/ml any time during testosterone treatment • PSA increase >1.4 ng/ml within 12 mo of testosterone treatment • Palpable abnormality (nodule or induration) on DRE • Worsening of lower urinary tract symptoms (e.g., IPSS score >19)
Obstructive sleep apnea (snoring, witnessed apnea, daytime somnolence, unexplained erythrocytosis, worsening hypertension or edema)	At baseline, after 3-12 mo, and then yearly	Evaluate for obstructive sleep apnea or adjustment of CPAP settings. Evaluate for other causes of hypoxia.
Formulation-specific adverse effects	At baseline, after 3-6 mo, and then yearly	Discontinue and switch to another formulation.
Testosterone ester injections	Discomfort, bleeding, or hematoma with IM injections Fluctuations in energy, mood, libido Allergy to oil vehicle (rare)	Reinstruct on the self-injection site technique. Consider shortening the injection interval if the nadir testosterone level is low.
Testosterone patch	Skin irritation Adhesion to skin	Coadministration of corticosteroid cream may reduce skin irritation.
Testosterone gel	Contact transfer to others Skin dryness at site of application	Reinstruct on washing hands and covering application area after gel dries or showering 4-6 h after application, avoiding prolonged skin-to-skin contact of application site with women and children.
Buccal testosterone tablets	Gum irritation or inflammation Poor adhesion to gums Altered or bitter taste	Reinstruct on proper application and reassure to complete an adequate trial with the correct technique.
SC testosterone pellets	Pellet extrusion Implantation-site infection, bleeding, fibrosis	Reimplant pellets. Treat infection with appropriate drainage and antibiotics.

BMD, Bone mineral density; *CPAP,* continuous positive airway pressure; *DRE,* digital rectal examination; *IM,* intramuscular; *IPSS,* International Prostate Symptom Score; *PSA,* prostate-specific antigen; *SC,* subcutaneous.
From Melmed S et al: *Williams textbook of endocrinology,* ed 14, Philadelphia, 2019, Elsevier.

H

Diseases
and Disorders

I

hormonal assessment to determine whether a patient has hypogonadism and requires testosterone replacement therapy. Treated patients need to be seen on a regular basis to avoid possible testosterone adverse effects. Patients requiring testosterone replacement should have testosterone, prostate specific antigen, and hematocrit levels monitored.

- Trials to evaluate the effects of testosterone treatment in older men revealed that in symptomatic men 65 yr of age or older, raising testosterone concentrations for 1 yr from moderately low to the mid-normal range had a moderate benefit with respect to sexual function and some benefit with respect to mood and depressive symptoms but no benefit with respect to vitality or walking distance.
- Controversy exists regarding the safety of testosterone replacement therapy following reports of increased risk of cardiovascular events. However, a recent trial among men with androgen deficiency dispensed testosterone prescriptions revealed lower risk of cardiovascular outcomes over a median follow-up of 3.4 yr.
- Clinical trials have also demonstrated that testosterone replacement in men with low testosterone increases volumetric bone mineral density and estimated bone strength more in trabecular than peripheral bone and more in the spine than the hip.

REFERENCES & SUGGESTED READINGS

Available at eBooks.Health.Elsevier.com.

AUTHOR: **FRED F. FERRI, MD**

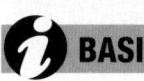
BASIC INFORMATION

DEFINITION[1]

Hypokalemia is defined as serum potassium less than 3.5 mEq/L. Severe and life-threatening hypokalemia is defined when potassium levels are <2.5 mEq/L. In outpatient populations undergoing laboratory testing, mild hypokalemia can be found in almost 14%. It can be caused by multiple factors, including medications, medical conditions, fluid loss, and/or low dietary potassium intake. Normal daily potassium intake is 40 to 120 mEq per day, about 80% of which is then excreted in the urine. The kidney can lower potassium excretion to a minimum of 5 to 25 mEq per day in the presence of potassium depletion.[2] Thus, decreased intake alone rarely causes significant hypokalemia. This was demonstrated in a study of normal individuals in whom lowering potassium intake to 20 mEq per day was associated with a reduction in serum potassium from 4.1 mEq/L at baseline to 3.5 mEq/L.[3] Distal potassium secretion is regulated by the amount of sodium in the lumina of the distal and collecting tubules, flow of urine in these segments of the nephron, and the aldosterone activity. Serum potassium in and of itself is an important factor in the regulation of aldosterone activity. The kidneys are the major regulator of external potassium homeostasis (or balance); therefore, excessive loss through the kidneys or retention because of loss of excretory function of the kidneys eventually leads to hypokalemia or hyperkalemia.

However, a low potassium intake can add to the severity of potassium depletion when another cause of hypokalemia is superimposed.[4]

SYNONYMS

Low potassium
Renal potassium wasting

ICD 10-CM CODE
E87.6   Hypokalemia

EPIDEMIOLOGY & DEMOGRAPHICS[1,5,6]

INCIDENCE: Depends on patient population; patients with normal kidney function who are not receiving medications have <1% incidence of hypokalemia.

PREVALENCE: In the outpatient population undergoing laboratory testing, mild hypokalemia can be found in almost 14%. Furthermore, as many as 20% of hospitalized patients are found to have hypokalemia, but this is clinically significant in only 4% to 5%. Severe hypokalemia is relatively uncommon. Approximately 80% of patients who are receiving diuretics become hypokalemic, while many patients with hypokalemia can also have an associated systemic disease.[7-9] The prevalence of unprovoked hypokalemia was reported to be 2.2% for African Americans and 0.3% for European Americans.[10] In a cohort study of acutely admitted medical patients, hypokalemia was present in 16.8% of patients, with plasma [K+] levels <2.9 mmol/L occurring in 3.3% of patients.[11]

PREDOMINANT SEX & AGE: There are no significant differences in prevalence between males and females.[7] Hypokalemia is seen more in older (age >65) hypertensive females being treated with potassium-losing diuretics. Prevalence of unprovoked hypokalemia for African Americans in the Atherosclerosis Risk in Communities (ARIC) cohort was more than five times that for European Americans.[10]

RISK FACTORS: Chronic kidney disease, heart failure, certain gastrointestinal disorders, and diuretic use

GENETICS: Hypokalemia caused by genetic disorders is rare. Some genetic causes of hypokalemia include congenital adrenal hyperplasia (11-beta hydroxylase or 17-alpha hydroxylase), Barter syndrome, Gitelman syndrome, and Liddle syndrome.

PHYSICAL FINDINGS & CLINICAL PRESENTATION[1]

Potassium is an essential electrolyte that maintains resting membrane potential affecting fluid balance, nerve function, and muscle function.

Hypokalemia can cause muscle weakness, muscle cramps, fatigue, lethargy, cardiac arrhythmias, hypertension, constipation, numbness, paresthesias, insulin resistance, and hypertension. Severe hypokalemia can lead to rhabdomyolysis, myoglobinuria, and respiratory muscle weakness. Hypokalemia can lead to a variety of cardiac arrhythmias and electrocardiogram (ECG) abnormalities such as premature atrial complex, premature ventricular beats, sinus bradycardia, paroxysmal atrial or junctional tachycardia, atrioventricular block, and ventricular tachycardia or fibrillation.

The severity of these symptoms can vary based on the degree of hypokalemia and the cause of hypokalemia. ECG changes may include depression of the ST segment, decrease in the amplitude of the T wave, and increase in the amplitude of U waves that occur at the end of the T interval, and prolongation of the QT interval. Fig. 1 demonstrates U waves seen on ECG in hypokalemia.

ETIOLOGY[1,4,8,12-17]

There are many causes of hypokalemia; they have been categorized into the following groups:

• *Decreased Intake of Potassium:* The average dietary intake of potassium ranges from 70 to 140 mmol in the U.S. Hypokalemia due to poor intake of potassium is seen in individuals with poor nutrition or on restrictive diets. Some examples of potassium-rich foods include bananas, potatoes, avocados, tomatoes, spinach, mushrooms, fish, and yogurt.

• *Increased Urinary Losses:* In a balanced state of body potassium, 80% of potassium intake is excreted by the kidneys. Urinary potassium is for the most part secretory potassium. Distal potassium secretion is regulated by the amount of sodium in the lumen of the distal and collecting tubules, flow of urine in these segments of the nephron, and the aldosterone activity. Serum potassium in and of itself is an important factor in the regulation of aldosterone activity.[4] This excretion of potassium can be enhanced through diuretics, loss of gastric secretions, hypomagnesemia,

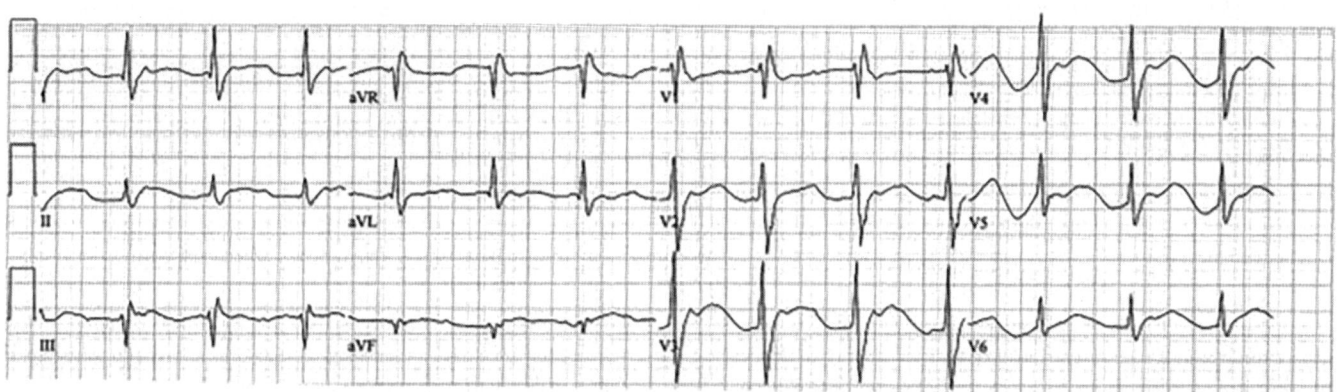

FIG. 1 ECG manifestations of hypokalemia. 12-lead ECG in a patient with severe hypokalemia with so-called "giant" U waves, particularly in V3-V5 where the U wave masks the preceding T wave and after P wave. (From Diercks DB et al: Electrocardiographic manifestations: electrolyte abnormalities, *J Emerg Med* 27(2):153-160, 2004. https://doi.org/10.1016/j.jemermed.2004.04.006.)

nonreabsorbale anions, kidney disorders (RTA type 1 or 2), salt-wasting nephropathies, or increased urinary output.

- *Transcellular Shifts:* Potassium is naturally stored inside cells. Movement of potassium from inside the cell into the extracellular space is dependent on the sodium-potassium-ATPase channel. This Na-K-ATPase exchanges three potassium ions for two sodium ions to move sodium outside the cell and potassium inside the cell. This generates an electrical gradient allowing for a passive efflux of potassium when channels are open. Specifically, insulin, epinephrine, glucocorticoids, aldosterone, and/or alkalosis will shift potassium into a cell, which can cause hypokalemia.
- *Gastrointestinal Losses:* In a balanced state of body potassium, 15% of potassium intake is excreted by the gastrointestinal tract.[4] Loss of potassium through the gastrointestinal tract can be seen in vomiting and diarrhea. The use of laxatives can also lead to further potassium loss as well as medications that bind potassium in the gastrointestinal tract.
- *Magnesium Deficiency:* Deficiency in magnesium can lead to potassium wasting through inhibition of ROMK channels in the thick ascending limb in the loop of Henle. It has been estimated that 50% of clinically significant hypokalemia is associated with hypomagnesemia.
- *Endocrine Disorders:*
  1. Primary hyperaldosteronism can be seen in aldosterone-secreting adenomas, adrenal carcinomas, hyperplasia of the zona glomerulosa, and exogenous aldosterone secretion. Aldosterone will lead to sodium retention and potassium excretion by the principal cells in the collecting duct. Hyperaldosteronism is also comminate with hypertension.
  2. Cushing syndrome can be iatrogenic or from a pituitary adenoma. The excess cortisol production in Cushing syndrome will bind to mineralocorticoid receptors and act like aldosterone, which will lead to hypokalemia.
  3. Insulinoma can cause hypokalemia through intracellular shift of potassium.
- *Renal Dysfunction:* The kidney plays a major role in potassium homeostasis.
  1. Type 1 distal renal tubular acidosis (RTA)—there is a defect in the hydrogen/potassium ATPase pump, leading to excretion of potassium.
  2. Type 2 RTA—there is a defect in the sodium/hydrogen antiporter and the sodium bicarbonate cotransporter leading to excess bicarbonate loss in the urine. This will result in osmotic diuresis leading to potassium excretion.
  3. Hypokalemia can also be seen in chronic kidney disease due to medication side effects (discussed later).
- *Genetic Conditions:*
  1. Liddle syndrome has a defect in the epithelial sodium channel (ENaC) in the collecting duct causing inappropriate

sodium resorption. This facilitates potassium and hydrogen loss in the urine leading to hypokalemia and metabolic alkalosis.
  2. Bartter syndrome has a defect in the sodium/chloride transport in the thick ascending loop of Henle. This leads to loss of sodium and chloride in the urine. A compensatory mechanism leads to aldosterone release, which will resorb sodium in exchange for potassium secretion in the distal tube.
  3. Gittleman syndrome has a genetic mutation in the *SLC12A3* gene, which encodes for a thiazide-sensitive sodium-chloride cotransporter in the distal convoluted tubule. This defect leads to hypokalemic hyperchloremic metabolic alkalosis with hypercalciuria and hypomagnesemia.
  4. Familial periodic paralysis is a subtype of a group of rare muscle weakness disorders. Mutations occur in genes associated with the dihydropyridine-sensitive calcium channel, which is responsible for sodium and calcium transport in the muscles. This leads to abnormal uptake of potassium in the muscle cells leading to hypokalemia.
  5. Congenital adrenal hyperplasia (11-beta hydroxylase or 17-alpha hydroxylase) can cause mineralocorticoid excess. This will lead to sodium retention and potassium excretion by the principal cells in the collecting duct. Hyperaldosteronism is also comminate with hypertension.
- *Medications:*
  1. Antimicrobials—nafcillin, ampicillin, penicillin, aminoglycosides, amphotericin B, and foscarnet
  2. Diuretics—acetazolamide, bumetanide, chlorthalidone, ethacrynic acid, furosemide, indapamide, metolazone, thiazides, and torsemide
  3. Bicarbonate
  4. Laxatives
  5. Insulin
  6. Mineralocorticoids
  7. Beta-2 receptor agonists—albuterol, ephedrine, epinephrine, formoterol, isoproterenol, pseudoephedrine, terbutaline, and salmeterol
  8. Xanthine
  9. Cisplatin
  10. Toluene
- *Other:*
  1. Chronic licorice and gan cao ingestion can lead to hypokalemia through inhibition of 11B-hydroxysteroid dehydrogenase, which will lead to overproduction of cortisol.
  2. Potassium can also be excreted through other bodily fluids such as sweat. Excessive sweating can also lead to hypokalemia.
- Pseudohypokalemia is most commonly caused by acute leukemia. The large number of leukocytes will uptake potassium into the cells when blood is stored in a collection vial. This can be identified by checking the

potassium (which will be normal) in samples stored at 4° C (39° F).

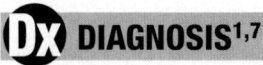

DIAGNOSIS[1,7]

DIFFERENTIAL DIAGNOSIS

Malnutrition, laxative abuse/use, primary hyperaldosteronism, hyperthyroidism/thyrotoxicosis, hypocalcemia, metabolic alkalosis, chronic alcohol abuse, insulinoma, beta-blocker toxicity, magnesium deficiency, and Cushing syndrome

WORKUP[1,7,18]

Obtain serum potassium, most often through a metabolic profile. The evaluation of hypokalemia is summarized in Fig. 2. Pseudohypokalemia and hypomagnesemia should be excluded prior to ordering additional tests.

An electrocardiogram (ECG) can be ordered to assess for cardiac arrhythmias and potential digoxin toxicity. ECG findings consistent with hypokalemia include flattening of the T waves, U waves, ventricular arrhythmias, and prolonged QT interval. U waves can be seen in Fig. 1.[19]

LABORATORY TESTS

- Arterial blood gas or venous blood gas to evaluate for alkalosis, which will be seen in hyperaldosteronism, Cushing syndrome, and Liddle syndrome
- Urine drug screen to screen for diuretics and/or stimulants
- Serum renin, aldosterone, and cortisol. Primary hyperaldosteronism will have an elevated morning aldosterone to renin ration >20 to 1
- Serum insulin and C peptide levels
- Pituitary imaging to evaluate for Cushing syndrome
- Urine sodium, chloride, potassium, and osmols to evaluate for laxative use
- Complete blood count (CBC) with differential to assess leukocyte count to rule out pseudo-hypokalemia
- Genetic tests for the congenital disorders: 17-beta hydroxylase enzyme assay

IMAGING STUDIES

When indicated, can consider
- Adrenal CT to rule out adrenal adenoma
- Brain MRI to rule out pituitary adenoma

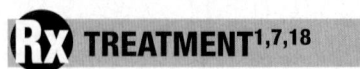

TREATMENT[1,7,18]

NONPHARMACOLOGIC THERAPY

- Increase potassium in diet. Some examples of potassium-rich foods include bananas, potatoes, avocados, tomatoes, spinach, mushrooms, fish, and yogurt.
- Discontinue medications or behaviors causing potassium loss.
- Surgical intervention may be needed in the setting of adrenal adenoma or intestinal obstruction causing emesis.

ACUTE GENERAL Rx (FIG. 3)[20]

- It is important to identify the underlying cause of hypokalemia.

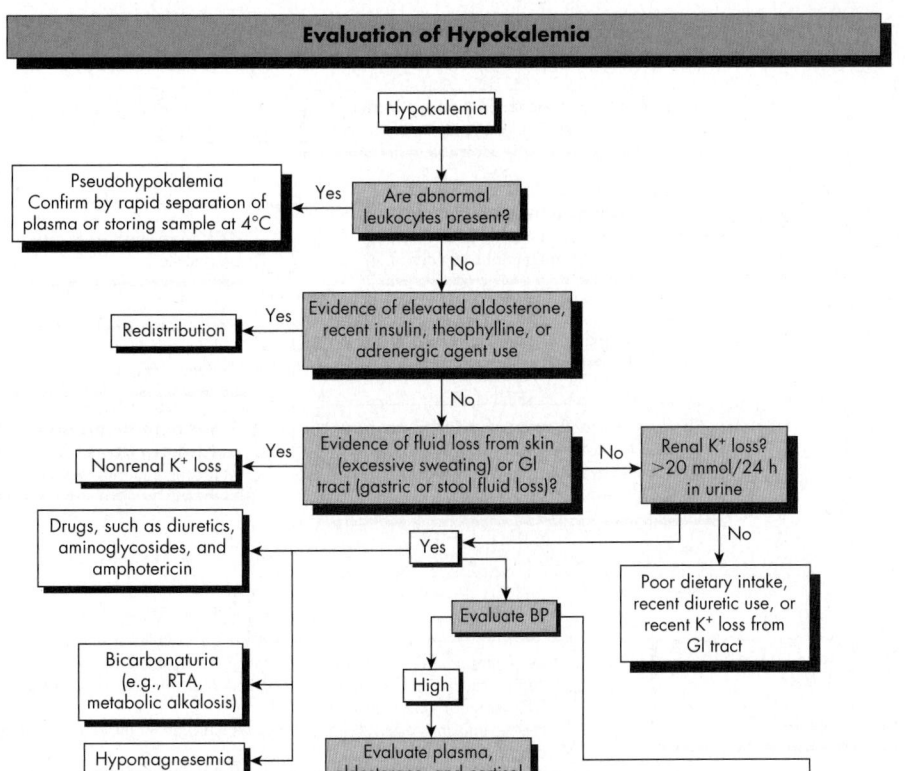

FIG. 2 Diagnostic evaluation of hypokalemia. *BP*, Blood pressure; *GI*, gastrointestinal; *GRA*, glucocorticoid-remediable aldosteronism; *RTA*, renal tubular acidosis. (From Johnson RJ et al: *Comprehensive clinical nephrology*, Philadelphia, 2023, Elsevier Health Sciences.)

- Correct hypomagnesemia.
- Replace potassium with potassium chloride or potassium bicarbonate, for a goal serum potassium around 4.0 mEq/L.
  1. If potassium is less than 2.5 mEq/L or if the patient is unable to tolerate oral intake, then initiate potassium replacement with intravenous (IV) potassium.
- Beta blockers such as propranolol have been used in select cases, when increased sympathetic tone is thought to be the predominant cause of hypokalemia (as in hypokalemic thyrotoxic periodic paralysis).
- When hypokalemia occurs in the setting of uncontrolled diabetes or in diabetic ketoacidosis or a hyperosmolar hyperglycemic state, it is important to correct potassium prior to initiating insulin therapy.
- It is important to monitor serum potassium during replacement, especially when hypokalemia is severe or associated with ECG changes. Watch for rebound hyperkalemia when hypokalemia is caused by transcellular shifts.

CHRONIC Rx

Oral potassium replacement, potassium-sparing diuretics, and ACEIs/ARBs can be used to maintain potassium levels.

COMPLEMENTARY & ALTERNATIVE MEDICINE

Increase oral intake of magnesium if hypomagnesemia is the cause of hypokalemia.

DISPOSITION

Several studies have shown that even mild hypokalemia is associated with increased long-term mortality.

REFERRAL

- Refer to nephrology if renal tubular potassium wasting is suspected.
- Refer to endocrinology if Cushing syndrome, hyperaldosteronism, or congenital adrenal hyperplasia is suspected.
- Refer to surgery if insulinoma, obstructive GI mass, adrenal adenoma, or renal artery stenosis is diagnosed.

- Refer to psychiatry if laxative abuse, alcohol abuse, or an eating disorder is suspected.
- Refer to nutrition for counseling on dietary potassium and magnesium intake.

❗ PEARLS & CONSIDERATIONS

COMMENTS

- Potassium chloride is a large pill and often difficult for patients to swallow. Consider powdered form or liquid form for patients with difficulty swallowing pills.
- IV potassium chloride is a vesicant and may need a central line for higher infusion rates.

PREVENTION

Ensure proper potassium supplementation when prescribing diuretics.

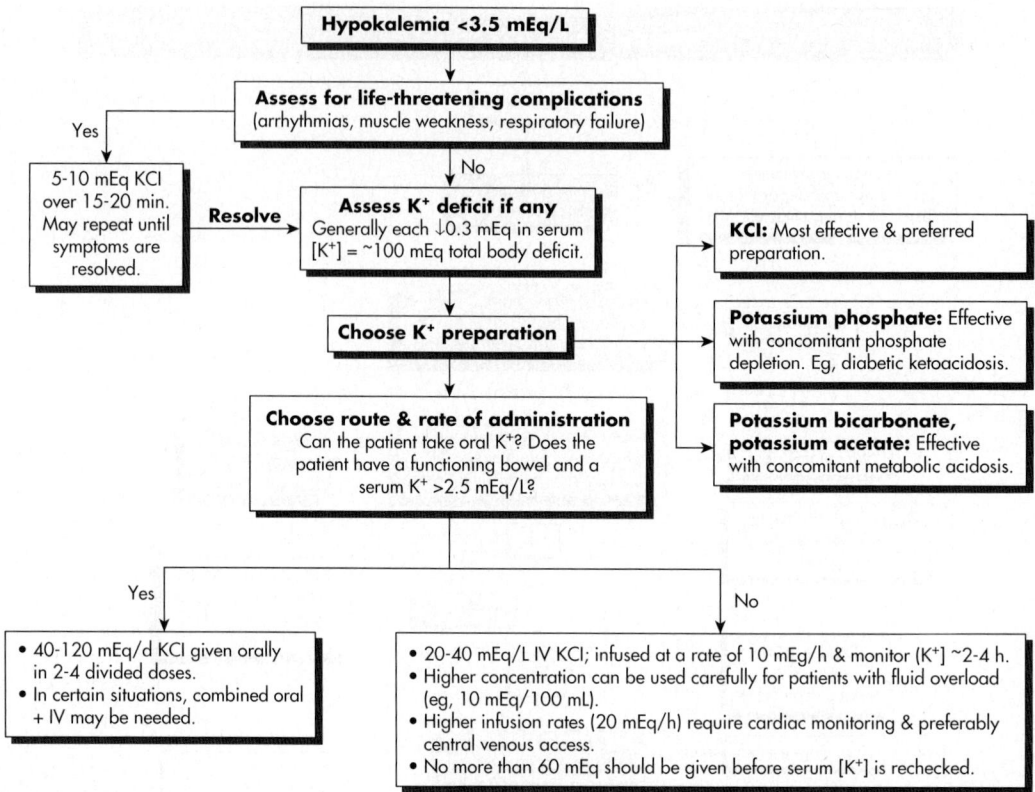

FIG. 3 General principles of hypokalemia management. These steps should be helpful in most cases of hypokalemia; however, clinical judgment should be exercised when applying it to individual patients. Serum potassium (K⁺) concentration generally should not be checked until 1 h after an intravenous *(IV)* dose is given (2 h after an oral dose). Parenteral potassium should be avoided except in the urgent conditions listed and transitioned to oral preparations as soon as possible. Serum potassium levels should be monitored carefully, especially in patients with kidney or cardiac disease. *KCl,* Potassium chloride.

REFERENCES

Available at eBooks.Health.Elsevier.com.

AUTHORS: **STEFANI THOMPSON, MD** and
SANDEEP SOMAN, MD, FNKF, FAMIA

BASIC INFORMATION

DEFINITION

An osmole is a solute that attracts water across a semipermeable membrane. Tonicity or effective osmolality refers to the direction of water flux with plasma water as the referent solution. Net water flow into the central nervous system (CNS) from plasma is a hypotonic state and from the CNS to plasma is a hypertonic state. Solutes that rapidly equilibrate between intracellular fluid (ICF) and extracellular fluid (ECF) compartments are ineffective osmoles because no net water movement between compartments occurs.

Hyponatremia is defined as a measured plasma or serum sodium concentration (S_{Na}) less than the lower limit of normal (<130 to 135 mmol/L). Since clinical manifestations of hyponatremia are due to hypotonicity, appropriate clinical management depends on distinguishing the majority of patients with hypotonic hyponatremia from those who are hypertonic or isotonic. Isotonic hyponatremia, also known as pseudohyponatremia, is due solely to a laboratory artifact (vide infra). The reader should be aware that some textbooks still incorrectly use the term "pseudohyponatremia" to refer to hypertonic hyponatremia. Hyponatremia is used synonymously with hypotonic hyponatremia in this chapter. References to pseudohyponatremia and hypertonic hyponatremia are specifically identified by these terms.

If the hyponatremia has developed over a period of less than 48 h, it is called acute hyponatremia. If it is known that hyponatremia has been present for 48 h or more, or if the duration is unclear, it is referred to as chronic hyponatremia. This is especially important when determining therapeutic approach.

SYNONYMS

Low serum sodium concentration
Hypo-osmolality

ICD-10CM CODE
E87.1 Hypo-osmolality and hyponatremia

EPIDEMIOLOGY & DEMOGRAPHICS

PREVALENCE: The prevalence of hyponatremia varies widely according to setting and population age. In the general U.S. population dataset of the National Health and Nutrition Examination Survey (NHANES), the overall prevalence was 1.72%.[1] One study of emergency department patients reported a prevalence of 2.3% in patients 16 to 21 yr old and 16.9% in patients >80 yr. Following surgery for traumatic hip fracture, the incidence of moderate (<135 mmol/L) and severe (<130 mmol/L) postoperative hyponatremia was 27% (95% confidence interval [CI], 21.7% to 32.5%) and 9% (95% CI, 5.7% to 12.8%), respectively. The prevalence was reported at approximately 8% in stable, older outpatients and 18% to 20% in sick or frail populations. The overall incidence at or during hospital admission is comparable. Higher rates are noted in patients admitted for congestive heart failure (CHF) or cirrhosis and in older adult patients admitted for fragility fractures.

PREDOMINANT SEX & AGE: Prevalence of hyponatremia was significantly higher in women in the NHANES dataset (2.09%; $P = 0.004$) and increased with age.[1]

RISK FACTORS: In NHANES, hyponatremia was more common in participants with hypertension, diabetes, coronary artery disease, stroke, chronic obstructive pulmonary disease, cancer, and psychiatric disorders, and less common in participants with no comorbidities (1.04%; $P < 0.001$).[1] A significant risk of death was associated with hyponatremia in unadjusted (hazard ratio [HR], 3.61; $P < 0.001$) and adjusted Cox models (HR 2.43; $P < 0.001$). The incidence in outpatients who were using thiazide diuretics was 15.1%, with a HR of 4.95 (95% CI, 4.12 to 5.96). Reported frequencies of hyponatremia in outpatients taking selective serotonin reuptake inhibitors or selective norepinephrine reuptake inhibitors varied widely, between 0.5% and 32%.

GENETICS: The hyponatremic disorder referred to as nephrogenic syndrome of inappropriate antidiuresis (SIAD), is caused by rare familial gain-of-function sequence variants of the V2 vasopressin receptor (V2R) gene. Activation of variant receptors located in the renal collecting duct produces overt hyponatremia in infancy.[2]

PHYSICAL FINDINGS & CLINICAL PRESENTATION

- Critical history includes detailed assessment of dietary fluid, protein, and electrolyte consumption; GI and insensible losses of fluid and electrolytes; urine output; and changes in weight, medication use, and behavior or cognition. Recent medical procedures involving irrigation of tissue beds (e.g., transurethral prostatectomy or hysteroscopy with endometrial resection), participation in marathons or other strenuous endurance exercise, or attendance at "rave" parties where illicit use of 3,4-methylenedioxy-methamphetamine (MDMA, or ecstasy) is common should be noted.[3] Comorbid conditions that increase the risk of hyponatremia include malignancy, CNS or pulmonary disease, adrenal insufficiency, CHF, liver disease, and nephrotic syndrome.
- The etiology of hyponatremia may affect the clinical presentation directly and/or by its effect on the extracellular fluid volume (ECFV) and exchangeable Na (TB_{Na}). Hypovolemia and hypervolemia (respectively, decreased or increased total ECFV and TB_{Na}) are identified by conventional clinical criteria (including clinical exam demonstrating edema, ascites, and pulmonary congestion and hemodynamic variables) but specifically does not refer to intravascular volume. If available, vector bioimpedance analysis has been shown to further increase accuracy.[4] Specific manifestations of the precipitating cause or underlying diseases may be evident (e.g., fever and delirium following the use of MDMA, stigmata of alcoholism or malnutrition, fever and/or localizing symptoms related to pneumonia or other pulmonary disease, or headaches and visual field defects from an intracranial mass).
- Neurologic symptoms predominate as the direct clinical manifestations of acute and/or severe hyponatremia, mainly due to astrocyte swelling. Compensatory processes that reduce cerebral edema by extrusion of electrolytes, amino acids, and carbohydrates from brain cells take 24 h to become fully active and up to 7 days to reach completion. Therefore patients who develop hyponatremia over less than 24 to 48 h have the highest degree of brain swelling, the most severe neurologic symptoms, and greatest risk of permanent or fatal brain injury. Postpubertal, premenopausal women appear to undergo cerebral compensation more slowly, placing them at greater risk from acute hyponatremia.[5]
- Acute hyponatremia may result in nausea and malaise as S_{Na} approaches 130 mmol/L or less. Headache, lethargy, obtundation, neurogenic pulmonary edema, and/or seizures may occur when S_{Na} is <120 mmol/L. In the most severe cases, death from brain stem herniation can occur.[6]
- Chronic hyponatremia rarely presents with life-threatening clinical manifestations. However, subtler neurologic disturbances such as ataxia, short-term memory deficits, fatigue, lethargy, and nausea have been commonly reported. Muscular weakness and elevated creatine kinase and even rhabdomyolysis may occur. Chronic hyponatremia has also been associated with increased risk of falls, fractures, and osteoporosis in older patients. In addition, hyponatremia has been associated with increased risk of cardiovascular complications and mortality in a diverse group, including older outpatients, general hospital-admitted patients, and patients admitted for stroke, subarachnoid hemorrhage, CHF, cirrhosis, pneumonia, hip fracture, and liver transplantation.[7-9]

ETIOLOGY

- Hypotonic hyponatremia: The S_{Na} after correction for hyperglycemia (or the effects of exogenous effective osmoles such as mannitol or sorbitol) closely approximates the ratio of exchangeable total body cations (sodium and potassium, $TB_{Na} + TB_K$) to total body water (TBW).[10]
  1. Serum [Na] = S_{Na} = ($TB_{Nae} + TB_{Ke}$)/ TBW
  2. The term *exchangeable* means that sodium or potassium ions can easily enter or exit from their compartment(s), respectively, which are the ECF and ICF spaces. TB_{Na} is the main determinant of ECF volume, and TB_K is the principal determinant of ICF volume.
  3. Hypotonic hyponatremia results from a decrease of the numerator, increase of the denominator.
- ECFV depletion (disproportionately greater decrease of TB_{Na} and/or TB_K than TBW)
  1. GI losses with intake of hypotonic fluids

2. Renal losses (diuresis, tubulopathies) with intake of hypotonic fluid
3. Cerebral/renal salt wasting
- Normovolemic hyponatremia (normal ECFV and TB_{Na})[3]
  1. SIAD (see "Syndrome of Inappropriate Antidiuresis")
  2. Medications (thiazide diuretics, selective and nonselective serotonin reuptake inhibitors, narcotics, MDMA/ecstasy, carbamazepine, cyclophosphamide, nicotine, desmopressin, phenothiazines, terlipressin)
  3. Pain, nausea, stress
  4. Marathon running or other endurance exercise[11]
  5. Primary polydipsia
  6. Solute-limited water excretion (tea-and-toast diet, beer potomania)
  7. Adrenal insufficiency
  8. Reset osmostat
  9. Severe potassium deficiency with normal total body sodium
- Hypervolemic hyponatremia (disproportionately greater increase in TBW than increased TB_{Na}) is associated with decreased effective arterial blood volume.
  1. Nephrotic syndrome
  2. Cirrhosis
  3. Congestive heart failure

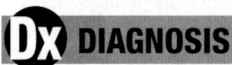 **DIAGNOSIS**

DIFFERENTIAL DIAGNOSIS

- **Pseudohyponatremia:** This is a laboratory artifact of decreasing prevalence and magnitude, rarely lowering falsely the S_{Na} by more than 5 mEq/L. Since it is an in vitro, not an in vivo phenomenon, no net water movement into the CNS occurs.[12] Serum osmolality is normal in pseudohyponatremia *only* if the other determinants of calculated serum osmolality are normal (i.e., serum concentrations of glucose and blood urea nitrogen [BUN]). Many clinicians misunderstand this and incorrectly diagnose pseudohyponatremia whenever they encounter low S_{Na} with "normal" serum osmolality (275 to 295 mOsm/L) as measured by freezing point depression with a low S_{Na}. By far, the most common cause for this situation is the combination of hypotonic hyponatremia with an elevated serum glucose or BUN. The more reliable method for diagnosing pseudohyponatremia is to calculate the serum osmolal gap, normally less than 10 mOsm/kg H_2O.
  1. Serum osmolal gap (mOsm/kg H2O) = Lab-measured S_{Osm} − Calculated-S_{Osm}
  2. Calculated-S_{Osm} = [2 × S_{Na} (mmol/L) + BUN (mg/dl)/2.8 + Glucose (mg/dl)/18 + Ethanol (mg/dl)/4.6]
  3. This calculated difference increases to abnormal values when the serum sodium used to compute calculated osmolality is artifactually low.
  4. Note that BUN and ethanol are ineffective osmoles that do not alter S_{Na}, while glucose is an effective osmole that shifts

water from ICF to ECF and lowers S_{Na} by approximately 1.6 mEq/L for each increase of 100 mg/dl upto a concentration of 400 mg/dl. Above blood glucose concentration of 400 mg/dl, an average correction factor for S_{Na} of 2.4 mmol/L for each increase of 100 mg/dl was more accurate.[13]
  5. Normally, the plasma solid (protein and lipid) phase occupies approximately 7% of plasma volume. S_{Na} is reported as milliequivalents (mEq) of sodium per liter of plasma. Certain pathologic conditions (elevated serum total protein/paraproteinemia most commonly, and severe hypercholesterolemia especially when associated with lipoprotein-X) increase the ratio of the solid phase to the aqueous phase. These conditions may artifactually reduce the S_{Na} measurement because the volume of water, and therefore the number of sodium ions per volume of plasma, is reduced, despite a normal concentration of sodium in plasma water. When pseudohyponatremia is suspected, measurement of S_{Na} by direct ion-selective electrode potentiometry of undiluted plasma (e.g., by blood gas analyzer) is recommended.[12]
- **Hypertonic hyponatremia:** Small solutes such as glucose (in absence of insulin), mannitol, and sorbitol accumulate to higher concentrations in the ECF than in the ICF and shift water from the ICF to the ECF compartment. Since the ICF has a very low sodium concentration (10 to 15 mmol/L), S_{Na} is diluted and hyponatremia occurs. With hyperglycemia, a decrease in S_{Na} of 1.6 mmol/L occurs for each increment of serum glucose of 100 mg/dl.[14]

WORKUP

- Fig. E1 illustrates the initial steps in the clinical approach to the patient with hyponatremia.
- A diagnostic approach to the patient with chronic hyponatremia is described in Fig. E2.
- A comprehensive history should include details of medication use, drug abuse, psychiatric disorders, exercise habits, prior S_{Na} measurements, diet, external fluid losses, volume and composition of oral and intravenous (IV) fluid intake, and any suggestion of disorders associated with hyponatremia (e.g., disorders of the lungs, CNS, heart, kidney, liver, or adrenal gland; malignancies; diabetes mellitus; nausea; vomiting; pain; or stress).
- Comprehensive physical examination including careful review of vital signs, weight, intake and outputs; evidence of increased ECFV (e.g., edema, ascites, pulmonary congestion, or pleural effusions), volume contraction, and evidence of comorbid diseases listed previously (e.g., abnormal pulmonary, neurologic or cardiovascular exam, or hepatomegaly).

LABORATORY TESTS

- Serum glucose to diagnose and adjust for hyperosmolar hypernatremia and osmolar-induced shifts of water from ICF to ECF.

- Serum potassium: Potassium is the principal intracellular cation. Because S_{Na} = (TB_{Na} + TB_K)/TBW, decreases in TB_K lower S_K and S_{Na}.[10]
- Random urine osmolality and 24-h urine volume: U_{osm} <100 mOsm/kg H_2O usually indicates appropriate suppression of antidiuretic hormone (ADH), suggesting diagnoses of solute-limited water excretion, primary polydipsia, or a reset osmostat (if S_{Na} is below the patient's altered setpoint). U_{osm} ≥100 mOsm/kg H_2O generally indicates that ADH is present. However, U_{osm} approximately 300 mOsm/kg is frequently encountered in patients using loop diuretics regardless of ADH level, and even higher osmolality can be seen during osmotic diuresis. The latter is characterized by total urine osmolar excretion >900 mOsm/day. However, in both cases urinary ([Na] + [K]) equals approximately 60 to 90 mmol/L, resulting in significant electrolyte-free water (EFW) loss.
- Random urine sodium (U_{Na}), and urine potassium (U_K): U_{Na} <20 mmol/L indicates stimulation of the renin angiotensin aldosterone system due to decreased ECFV or decreased effective arterial blood volume. Urine potassium losses should be calculated and replaced during therapy.
- Specific testing for comorbid diseases listed previously as clinically indicated (e.g., fasting morning cosyntropin-stimulated serum cortisol level and brain natriuretic peptide).

IMAGING STUDIES

Not routinely required. Computed tomography or MRI may be indicated in the presence of specific symptoms, a diagnosis of an associated etiology, or an evaluation of an associated delirium coincident with acute hyponatremia.

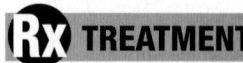 **TREATMENT**

NONPHARMACOLOGIC THERAPY

Hyponatremic patients excrete less EFW than they ingest or receive. Moderate fluid restriction (10 to 15 ml/kg) is indicated while patients are hyponatremic, especially if EFW excretion remains impaired. Diets high in protein, sodium, and potassium increase urine osmolar load and increase free water excretion.

ACUTE GENERAL Rx

- Acute (hypotonic) hyponatremia is defined as developing in less than 48 h. Changes in brain cell volume in patients with hyponatremia are illustrated in Fig. E3. Acute hyponatremia results in larger increases in brain water content than equivalent chronic changes in S_{Na} due to lack of brain cell adaptation to hypotonicity. Consequently, correction of acute hyponatremia is a medical emergency and mandates an increase in S_{Na} of 4 to 6 mmol/L within the initial 1 to 3 h of therapy, depending on severity of symptoms and acuity of S_{Na} elevation.[7-9] Iatrogenic cases, classically in children or premenopausal women receiving perioperative hypotonic fluids, are fortunately rare now. These circumstances can present with headache or nausea prior to the onset of severe symptoms and require emergent correction (Fig. 4). Acute hyponatremia is rare in patients with high ECFV.

- Controlled increases of S_{Na} at a rapid rate nearly always require hypertonic saline: Recommended rate of correction in severe acute hyponatremia is an increase in S_{Na} of 3 to 6 mmol/L in the first hour. Consultation with a nephrologist or other expert clinician in the management of severe acute hyponatremia should be undertaken. In normovolemic patients, furosemide 20 to 40 mg IV may be used concurrently with hypertonic saline to prevent complications of acute ECFV expansion, although the additional loss of EFW may result in more rapid increases in S_{Na}.

- Regardless of type of treatment, acute, severe hyponatremia requires monitoring in an intensive care setting with frequent measurements of S_{Na}, urine volume, and U_{osm} until patients are neurologically stable and S_{Na} approaches the lower normal range.

CHRONIC Rx

- Chronic hyponatremia develops over 48 h or more: The risk of cerebral edema is minimized via adaptive loss of intracellular electrolytes and organic osmolytes (i.e., beta taurine, myoinositol, and others). In contrast, the risk of osmotic demyelination syndrome caused by overly rapid correction of the S_{Na} increases.[15] A recommended target for correction of hyponatremia in this setting is 6 to 8 mmol/L per day.[7-9]

- Hypovolemia with chronic hyponatremia: Usual clinical practice is administration of

0.9% saline to restore ECFV. The direct effect of isotonic solutions on S_{Na} is negligible. However, eventual reestablishment of euvolemia can be expected to suppress ADH that may trigger rapid increases in S_{Na} resulting from high urinary EFW loss. Administration of desmopressin (DDAVP) may prevent or arrest overly rapid correction of chronic hyponatremia.[16,17] Regardless of volume status, administration of DDAVP with quantitatively determined volumes of D_5W to lower S_{Na} back to safe concentrations following overly rapid correction has been shown to prevent or reverse osmotic demyelination syndrome.[18]

- Overcorrection of S_{Na}: The risk of overly rapid correction is greatest for hyponatremic patients with low solute intake (tea-and-toast diets or beer potomania). These patients typically have $U_{osm} < 100$ mOsm/kg H_2O with

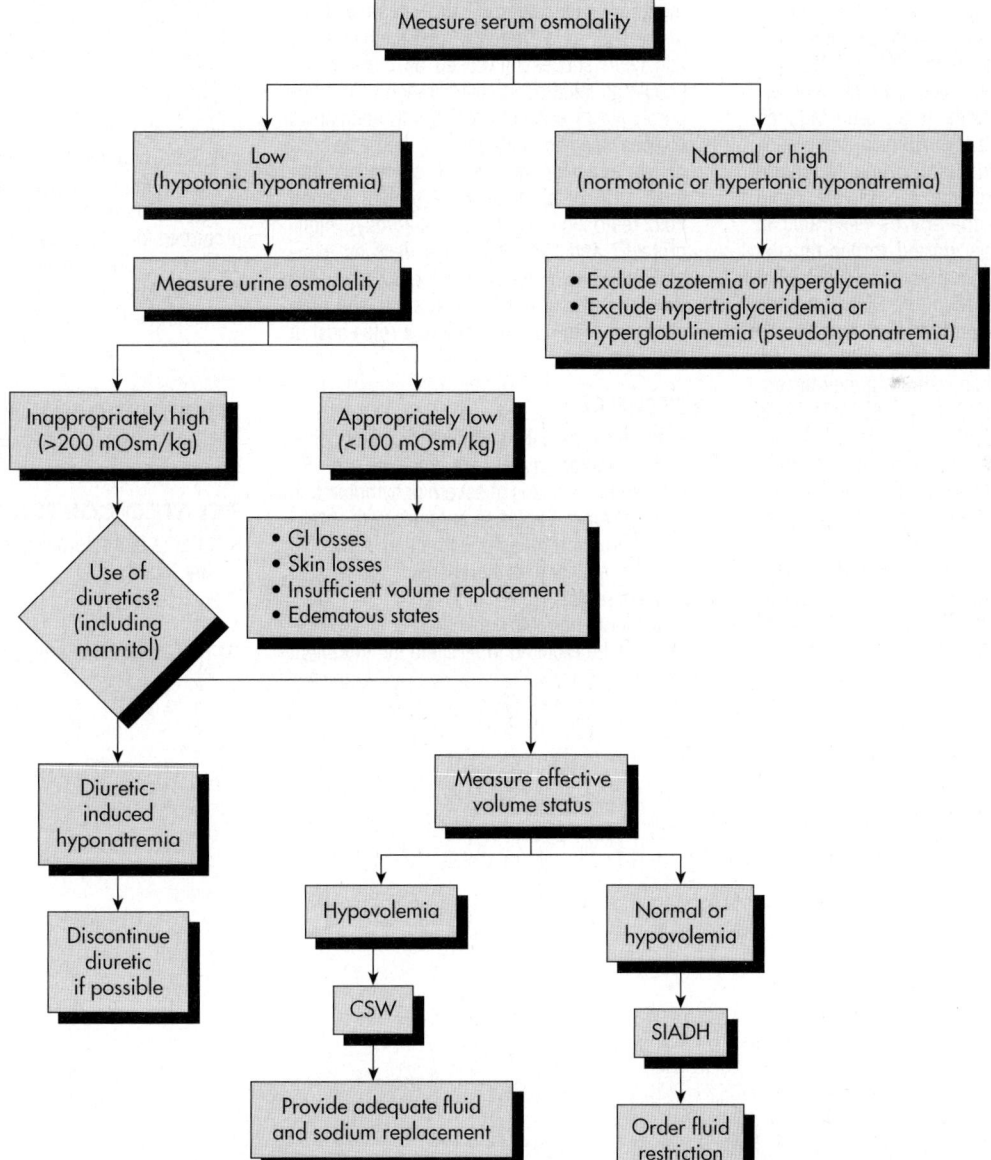

FIG. 4 Algorithm for the diagnosis and management of hyponatremia in critically ill neurologic patients. *CSW,* Cerebral salt-wasting; *GI,* gastrointestinal; *SIADH,* syndrome of inappropriate secretion of antidiuretic hormone. (From Jankovic J et al: *Bradley and Daroff's neurology in clinical practice,* ed 8, Philadelphia, 2022, Elsevier.)

ADH suppression. Reflex administration of IV saline is contraindicated: 1 L of IV 0.9% saline (308 mOsm/L) supplies an osmolar load sufficient for excretion in up to 3 to 6 L of hypotonic urine in the absence of ADH. The preferred treatment of this situation is fluid restriction and dietary supplementation to supply appropriate quantities of protein and electrolytes. If needed, small quantities of 0.9% saline can be given quantitatively to augment oral intake. If rapid urinary water loss occurs during treatment of hyponatremia (i.e., >200 ml/h for 2 or more h), there is a concern for overcorrection of S_{Na}. In this situation, free water equivalent (as 5% dextrose IVPB) can be provided and/or electrolyte free water excretion in the urine may be therapeutically blunted by DDAVP to prevent and/or ameliorate overcorrection of S_{Na}.

- The treatment of normovolemic patients is covered in detail in the "Syndrome of Inappropriate Antidiuresis" chapter and is only briefly reviewed here.[2] The goal of therapy in these patients is to reduce TBW in a controlled fashion maintaining TB_{Na} and TB_K. Some patients with chronic normovolemic hyponatremia (e.g., drug-induced etiologies or primary polydipsia) have self-limited abnormalities and primarily require monitoring to prevent excessively rapid correction. Active therapy as described in the chapter can be started to shorten the hospital stay or if the offending drug cannot be discontinued. If required, DDAVP can be administered intermittently to temporarily block further losses of free water to slow the overall rate of correction. If overcorrection occurs, oral and/or IV hypotonic fluids may be quantitatively administered to actively lower the serum sodium.[15-17] Other disorders may only slowly resolve the condition and require more active therapy as delineated in "Syndrome of Inappropriate Antidiuresis," consisting of either a direct V2 receptor antagonist or a loop diuretic combined with replacement of electrolytes lost during diuresis.

DISPOSITION

- Patients with symptomatic or severe hyponatremia require monitoring in an intensive care unit setting until the S_{Na} is stabilized at a safe level. Periodic monitoring of serum sodium, urine volume, and urine osmolality and electrolytes is required, with adjustments in therapy as outlined previously as needed.
- Potential contributing causes should be evaluated and treated appropriately.
- Risk of recurrence depends primarily on the nature of the underlying disorders present. Hypovolemic hyponatremia (e.g., diarrhea- or diuretic-induced electrolyte and water losses) or drug-induced SIAD generally do not recur if the offending medication is discontinued or if GI losses are not chronic. Older patients or patients with alcohol-use disorders with solute-limited diuresis due to low electrolyte and protein intake may be resistant to major changes in diet. However, the oral administration of NaCl tablets and/or protein supplements may be salutary.[19] Oral urea (available in the U.S. as a "medical food supplement") has been successfully used as therapy, but should be initiated in collaboration with a nephrologist or endocrinologist.[20] In addition to disease-specific management, incurable conditions (e.g., chronic CNS or pulmonary disease, CHF, or cirrhosis) may require lifelong fluid restriction (10 to 15 ml/kg/day), high-protein[21] and high-electrolyte diets as tolerated, periodic monitoring of the S_{Na} to reduce the risk of recurrent hyponatremia, and possible use of tolvaptan (albeit at a retail cost of $200 per day).

REFERRAL

- Referral to specialists in nephrology, endocrinology, and/or critical care medicine are recommended in cases of severe or symptomatic hyponatremia. Expertise is required to establish appropriate rates of correction of S_{Na} and monitor and adjust therapeutic regimens to achieve target S_{Na}.
- Outpatient referral to nephrology or endocrinology may be required to facilitate the treatment of patients with mild, chronic, or recurrent hyponatremia.

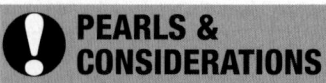

PREVENTION

Well-meaning family members, friends, news media, and health care providers often encourage patients who have chronic kidney disease or those who are prescribed diuretics to drink large amounts of water. When these patients consume more free water than they excrete, hyponatremia develops. Similarly, participants in marathons or other high-intensity endurance activities may ingest large volumes of water that more than offset losses, thereby self-inducing acute hyponatremia. Patients at risk for hyponatremia should have a specific fluid prescription that avoids both extremes. Conversely, patients with diarrheal losses or those who develop decreased ECFV from diuretics must be informed that intake of water or other hypotonic fluids alone will produce hyponatremia but will not effectively restore ECFV. Sodium, potassium, and water intake are all required for resolution of hyponatremia. Safe, outpatient correction of ECFV requires the consumption of electrolyte-containing tablets, powders, and solutions that are now widely promoted for adults. By contrast, originally available sports drinks have high sugar content but relatively low quantities of electrolytes and may be inadequate for electrolyte replacement.

REFERENCES

Available at eBooks.Health.Elsevier.com.

RELATED CONTENT

Syndrome of Inappropriate Antidiuresis (Related Key Topic)

AUTHOR: **MARK D. FABER, MD, MACM**

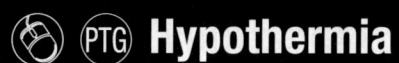
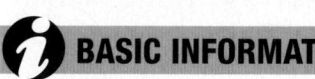 **BASIC INFORMATION**

DEFINITION

Hypothermia is a rectal temperature <35° C (95.8° F). "Accidental hypothermia" is an unintentionally induced decrease in core temperature in the absence of preoptic anterior hypothalamic conditions.

ICD-10CM CODES
R68.0	Hypothermia, not associated with low environmental temperature
T68	Hypothermia

EPIDEMIOLOGY & DEMOGRAPHICS

- Hypothermia occurs most frequently in the following groups: Alcoholics; homeless; learning-impaired; patients with cardiovascular, cerebrovascular, or pituitary disorders; those using sedatives or tranquilizers; and elderly patients.
- >700 persons in the U.S. die from hypothermia annually.

PHYSICAL FINDINGS & CLINICAL PRESENTATION

The clinical presentation varies with the severity of hypothermia. Shivering may be absent if body temperature is <33.3° C (92° F) or in patients taking phenothiazines.

Hypothermia may masquerade as cerebrovascular accident, ataxia, or slurred speech, or the patient may appear comatose or clinically dead. Signs of hypothermia are summarized in Box 1. The main physiologic effects of mild hypothermia are described in Table 1.

Physiologic stages of hypothermia (Table 2):
- Stage HT I: Mild hypothermia (typical core temperature 32.2° C to 35° C [90° F to 95° F]): Arrhythmias, ataxia
- Stage HT II: Moderate hypothermia (core temperature 28° C to 32.2° C [82.4° F to 90° F]):
  1. Progressive decrease of level of consciousness, pulse, cardiac output, and respiration
  2. Fibrillation, dysrhythmias (increased susceptibility to ventricular tachycardia)
  3. Elimination of shivering mechanism for thermogenesis
- Stage HT III: Severe hypothermia (core temperature ≤28° C to 24° C [82.4° F to 75° F]):
  1. Absence of reflexes or response to pain
  2. Decreased cerebral blood flow, decreased CO_2
  3. Increased risk of ventricular fibrillation or asystole
  4. Vital signs present
- Stage IV: No vital signs (core temperature <24° C [75° F])

ETIOLOGY

Exposure to cold temperatures for a prolonged period. Contributing factors include:
- Drugs: Ethanol, phenothiazines, sedative-hypnotics
- Skin disorders: Extensive burns, severe psoriasis, exfoliative dermatitis
- Metabolic disorders: Hypopituitarism, hypothyroidism, hypoadrenalism
- Neurologic abnormalities: Stroke, head trauma, acute spinal cord transection, impaired shivering
- Other: Lack of acclimatization, aggressive fluid resuscitation, sepsis, heat stroke treatment
- Table 3 summarizes factors predisposing to hypothermia

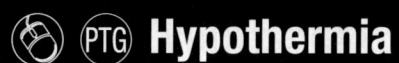 **DIAGNOSIS**

DIFFERENTIAL DIAGNOSIS

- It is crucial to determine an accurate core temperature measurement. Advantages and considerations of various methods to determine core temperature are summarized in Table 4. Core temperature is best monitored with an esophageal probe. Rectal and bladder temperature generally lag behind core temperatures during the rewarming process
- Cerebrovascular accident
- Myxedema coma
- Drug intoxication
- Hypoglycemia

LABORATORY TESTS

- Metabolic and respiratory acidosis are usually present.
  1. When blood cools, the arterial pH increases, oxygen tension (Po_2) increases, and the pCO_2 falls. Temperature correction factors for arterial blood gas specimens are summarized in Box 2.
  2. Blood gas analyzers warm the blood to 37° C (98.6° F), increasing the partial pressure of dissolved gases, resulting in higher oxygen and carbon dioxide levels and a lower pH than the patient's actual values. A decrease in K^+ initially, then an increase in K^+ with increasing hypothermia; extreme hyperkalemia indicates a poor prognosis.
- Hematocrit increases and can be perpetually high (caused by hemoconcentration and increased plasma volume), decreasing leukocytes and platelets (caused by splenic sequestration).
- Blood viscosity, increased clotting time.

BOX 1 Presenting Signs of Hypothermia

Head, Eye, Ear, Nose, Throat
- Mydriasis
- Decreased corneal reflexes
- Extraocular muscle abnormalities
- Erythropsia (altered color perception)
- Flushing
- Facial edema
- Epistaxis
- Rhinorrhea
- Strabismus

Cardiovascular
- Initial tachycardia
- Subsequent bradycardia
- Dysrhythmias
- Decreased heart tones
- Hepatojugular reflux
- Jugular venous distention
- Hypotension

Respiratory
- Initial tachypnea
- Adventitious sounds
- Bronchorrhea
- Progressive hypoventilation
- Apnea

Gastrointestinal
- Ileus
- Constipation
- Abdominal distention or rigidity
- Poor rectal tone
- Gastric dilation in neonates or in adults with myxedema

Genitourinary
- Anuria
- Oliguria
- Polyuria
- Testicular torsion

Neurologic
- Depressed level of consciousness
- Ataxia
- Hypesthesia
- Dysarthria
- Antinociception
- Amnesia
- Initial hyperreflexia
- Anesthesia
- Hyporeflexia
- Areflexia
- Central pontine myelinolysis

Psychiatric
- Impaired judgment
- Perseveration
- Mood changes
- Flat affect
- Altered mental status
- Paradoxic undressing
- Neuroses
- Psychoses
- Suicide
- Organic brain syndrome

Musculoskeletal
- Increased muscle tone
- Shivering
- Rigidity or pseudo–rigor mortis
- Paravertebral spasm
- Opisthotonos
- Compartment syndrome

Dermatologic
- Erythema
- Pernio
- Pallor
- Frostnip
- Cyanosis
- Frostbite
- Icterus
- Popsicle panniculitis (inflammation of the cheeks; also called "cold panniculitis")
- Sclerema (hardening of subcutaneous tissue)
- Cold urticaria
- Ecchymosis
- Necrosis
- Edema
- Gangrene

From Walls RM et al: *Rosen's emergency medicine, concepts and clinical practice,* ed 10, Philadelphia, 2023, Elsevier.

Diseases and Disorders

TABLE 1 Main Physiologic Effects of Mild Hypothermia

Physiologic Variables	Observed Effect
Cerebral metabolism	Decreased
Cerebral blood flow	Decreased
Fat metabolism	Increased
Lactate production	Increased
Oxygen consumption and carbon dioxide production	Decreased
Insulin secretion and sensitivity	Decreased
Inflammatory response	Decreased
Shivering	Increased
Cutaneous vasoconstriction	Increased
Renal electrolyte excretion (Mg, K, P)	Increased
Heart rate (if euvolemia)	Decreased
Myocardial contractility	Increased
Myocardial sensitivity to mechanical manipulation	Increased
Response to antiarrhythmic drugs	Decreased
Platelet function	Decreased
Drug clearance	Decreased
Bowel function	Decreased

From Vincent JL et al: *Textbook of critical care,* ed 8, Philadelphia, 2024, Elsevier.

TABLE 2 Hypothermia: Stages and Associated Clinical Manifestations

Stage	°F	°C	Clinical Manifestations
Normothermia	98.6	37.0	
Mild hypothermia	95.0	35.0	Cold diuresis, maximal shivering
	93.0	33.8	Ataxia, poor judgment, J wave
	91.0	32.7	Amnesia, blood pressure difficult to measure
Moderate hypothermia	89.0	31.6	Stupor, pupils dilated
	87.0	30.5	Shivering ceases
	85.0	30.0	Cardiac arrhythmias, insulin inactive
	82.0	27.8	Unconsciousness, ventricular fibrillation likely
	80.0	26.6	No muscle reflexes
Profound hypothermia	78.0	25.5	Acid-base disturbances, no response to pain
	75.0	23.8	Pulmonary edema, hypotension
	73.0	22.7	No corneal reflexes
	66.0	18.8	Heart standstill
	62.0	16.6	Isoelectric electrocardiogram
	57.6	14.2	Lowest infant survival from accidental hypothermia
	48.2	9.0	Lowest adult survival from accidental hypothermia

From Goldman L, Shafer AI: *Goldman-Cecil medicine,* ed 26, Philadelphia, 2019, Elsevier.

TABLE 3 Factors Predisposing to Cold Injury

Individual Factors

Inadequate clothing and shelter
Lean and low body fat
Low physical fitness
Prior exhaustive physical exercise
Advanced age
Young age
Black race (men and women)

Health Conditions

Burns
Diabetes mellitus
Hypoglycemia
Neurologic lesions
Dementia
Hypoadrenalism, hypopituitarism, hypothyroidism
Prior frostbite or trench foot
Raynaud phenomenon
Sickle cell trait
Trauma
Spinal cord injury

Drugs

Alcohol
Anesthetics
Antidepressants
Antithyroid agents
Sedatives and narcotics

Environmental Factors

Cold temperatures
High air motion
Rain and immersion
Skin contact with metal and fuels
Repeated cold exposure
Physical fatigue
Immobility
High-altitude and low-oxygen-tension environments

From Goldman L, Shafer AI: *Goldman-Cecil medicine,* ed 26, Philadelphia, 2019, Elsevier.

TABLE 4 Core Temperature Measurements

Type	Advantages	Considerations
Rectal	Convenient Continuous monitoring	Insert 15 cm (6 in) Lags during transition from cooling to rewarming Falsely elevated with peritoneal lavage Falsely low if probe is in cold feces or when lower extremities are frozen
Esophageal	Convenient Continuous monitoring	Insert 24 cm (9.5 in) below larynx Tracheal misplacement Aspiration Falsely elevated with heated inhalation
Tympanic	Approximates hypothalamic temperature via internal carotid artery	Probe: Tympanic membrane perforation; canal hemorrhage. Infrared: Unreliable; cerumen effect
Bladder	Convenient Continuous monitoring	Unreliable Falsely elevated with peritoneal lavage Falsely low with cold diuresis

From Auerbach P: *Wilderness medicine, expert consult premium edition—enhanced online features and print,* Philadelphia, 2012, Saunders.

BOX 2 Temperature Correction Factors for Arterial Blood Gas Specimens

ABG Component Correction Factor
pH $+ 0.015 (37 - T_c)$
$Pao_2 - 0.072 (37 - T_c) \times Pao_2$
$Paco_2 - 0.044 (37 - T_c) \times Paco_2$

Example
A patient presents with a core temperature of 32°C with the following ABG values: pH 7.12, $Paco_2$ 52 mm Hg, and Pao_2 52 mm Hg. Corrections for temperature are as follows:
pH $= 7.12 + [0.015 (37 - 32)] = 7.195$
$Pao_2 = 52 - [0.072 (37 - 32) \times 52] = 33.28$ mm Hg
$Paco_2 = 52 - [0.044 (37 - 32) \times 52] = 40.56$ mm Hg
These corrections also may be used for hyperthermia.*

*Arterial blood gas (ABG) values not corrected for temperature in significantly hypothermic patients yield falsely low pH and falsely elevated $Paco_2$ and Pao_2 values.
From Parrillo JE, Dellinger RP: *Critical care medicine, principles of diagnosis and management in the adult,* ed 5, Philadelphia, 2019, Elsevier.

IMAGING STUDIES

- Chest x-ray examination: Generally not helpful; may reveal evidence of aspiration (e.g., intoxicated patient with aspiration pneumonia).
- ECG: Prolonged PR, QT, and QRS segments, depressed ST segments, inverted T waves, atrioventricular block, and hypothermic J waves (Osborne waves) may appear at temperatures less than 33.0° C (91.4° F); characterized by notching of the junction of the QRS complex and ST segments (Fig. 1).

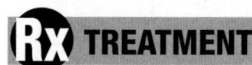 **TREATMENT**

NONPHARMACOLOGIC THERAPY

- The first critical step in management of accidental hypothermia is initiating passive external rewarming by removing wet clothing and covering the patient with insulating material.
- Specific treatment of hypothermia varies with the following:
  1. Degree of hypothermia
  2. Existence of concomitant diseases (e.g., cardiovascular insufficiency)
  3. Patient's age and medical condition (e.g., elderly; debilitated patients vs. young, healthy patients)
- General measures:
  1. Secure an airway before warming all unconscious patients; precede endotracheal intubation with oxygenation (if possible) to minimize the risk of arrhythmias during the procedure.
  2. Peripheral vasoconstriction may impede placement of a peripheral intravenous catheter; consider femoral venous access as an alternative to the jugular or subclavian sites to avoid ventricular stimulation.
  3. A Foley catheter should be inserted, and urinary output should be monitored and maintained >0.5 to 1 ml/kg/h with intravascular volume replacement.
  4. Box 3 summarizes measures for preparing hypothermic patients for transport.

ACUTE GENERAL Rx

- An emergency department rewarming protocol is described in Box 4.

- Continuous ECG monitoring of patients is recommended. Ventricular arrhythmias can be treated with bretylium; lidocaine is generally ineffective, and procainamide is associated with an increased incidence of ventricular fibrillation in hypothermic patients.
- Correct severe acidosis and electrolyte abnormalities.
- Hypothyroidism, if present, should be promptly treated (see "Myxedema Coma[A1]").
- If clinical evidence suggests adrenal insufficiency, administer IV methylprednisolone.

In patients unresponsive to verbal or noxious stimuli or with altered mental status, 100 mg of thiamine, 0.4 mg of naloxone, and 1 ampule of 50% dextrose may be given.

Warm (104° F to 113° F [40° C to 45° C]), humidified oxygen should also be given if available.

- Specific treatment:
  1. Mild hypothermia (rectal temperature <32.3° C [90° F]): Passive external rewarming is indicated. Place the patient in a warm room (temperature >21° C [69.8° F]), and cover with insulating material after gently removing wet clothing; recommended rewarming rates vary between 0.5° C/h and 20° C/h (32.9° F/h and 68° F/h) but should not exceed 0.55° C/h (32.99° F/h) in elderly persons. Therapeutic options to treat shivering during hypothermia are described in Table 5.
  2. Moderate to severe hypothermia:
     a. Active core rewarming
        (1) Delivery of heat by way of fluids: Warm GI irrigation (with saline enemas and by nasogastric tube); IV fluids (usually D_5NS without potassium) warmed to 104° F to 107.6° F (40° C to 42° C), peritoneal dialysis with dialysate heated to 40.5° C to 42.5° C (104.9° F/h to 108.5° F/h).

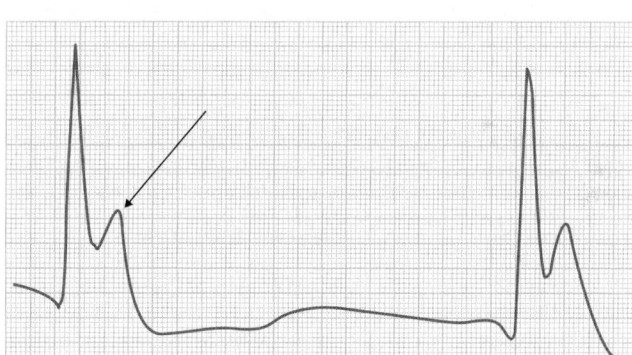

FIG. 1 **J (Osborne) wave.** (From Goldman L: *Goldman-Cecil medicine,* ed 26, Philadelphia, 2020, Elsevier.)

BOX 3 Preparing Hypothermic Patients for Transport

1. The patient must be dry. Gently remove or cut off wet clothing and replace it with dry clothing or a dry insulation system. Keep the patient horizontal, and do not allow exertion or massage of the extremities.
2. Stabilize injuries (i.e., the spine; place fractures in the correct anatomic position). Open wounds should be covered before packaging.
3. Initiate heated intravenous infusions (IVs) if feasible; bags can be placed under the patient's buttocks or in a compressor system. Administer a fluid challenge.
4. Active rewarming should be limited to heated inhalation and truncal heat. Insulate hot water bottles in stockings or mittens, and then place them in the patient's axillae and groin.
5. The patient should be wrapped. Begin building the wrap by placing a large plastic sheet on the available surface (floor, ground), and on it place an insulated sleeping pad. A layer of blankets, a sleeping bag, or bubble wrap insulating material is laid over the sleeping pad. The patient is then placed on the insulation. Heating bottles are put in place along with IVs, and the entire package is wrapped layer over layer, with the plastic as the final closure. The patient's face should be partially covered, but a tunnel should be created to allow access for breathing and monitoring.

From Auerbach P: *Wilderness medicine, expert consult premium edition—enhanced online features and print,* Philadelphia, 2012, Elsevier.

(2) Inhalation of heated, humidified oxygen (warmed to 40° C [104° F]) increases core temperature by 1° C (1.8° F) per h and decreases evaporative heat loss from respiration.

3. Active external rewarming: Immersion in a bath of warm water (40° C to 41° C [104° F to 105.8° F]); active external rewarming may produce shock because of excessive peripheral vasodilation. Ideal candidates are previously healthy, young patients with acute immersion hypothermia.
4. Extracorporeal blood warming with cardiopulmonary bypass appears to be an efficacious rewarming technique in young, otherwise healthy persons.
5. Patients with cardiac instability and those in cardiac arrest should be transported to a center capable of providing extracorporeal membrane oxygenation (ECMO) unless other conditions (e.g., trauma) require transport to a closer facility.

RELATED CONTENT

Hypothermia (Patient Information)

AUTHOR: **FRED F. FERRI, MD**

BOX 4 Emergency Department Rewarming Protocol

Prethaw
- Assess Doppler pulses and appearance.
- Protect part—no friction massage.
- Stabilize core temperature.
- Address medical and surgical conditions.
- Administer volume replacement as indicated.

Thaw
- Provide parenteral opiate analgesia as needed.
- Administer ibuprofen 400-600 mg (or aspirin, 325 mg).
- Immerse part in circulating water at 37°-39°C (98.6°-102.2°F), monitored by thermometer.
- Encourage gentle motion, but do not massage.

Postthaw
- Dry and elevate.
- Aspirate or débride clear vesicles.
- Débride broken vesicles and apply topical antibiotic or sterile aloe vera ointment every 6 h.
- Leave hemorrhagic vesicles intact.
- Administer tetanus prophylaxis if indicated.
- Provide streptococcal prophylaxis if high risk.
- Consider phenoxybenzamine in severe cases.
- Perform imaging, including angiography, if thrombolysis may be indicated.
- Carry out thrombolysis, if indicated and available.
- Obtain admission photographs.

From Walls RM et al: *Rosen's emergency medicine, concepts and clinical practice*, ed 10, Philadelphia, 2023, Elsevier.

TABLE 5 Therapeutic Options to Treat Shivering During Hypothermia (Not Exhaustive)

Drug or Strategy	Pros	Cons
Passive cutaneous counter-warming (i.e., blanket, room temperature)	Inexpensive, widely available	Unprecise, might require time to be effective
Active cutaneous counterwarming (i.e., heated forced-air blanket)	Relatively cheap, fast, evidence supported	Requires specific material
Selected cutaneous counterwarming (i.e., face, hands)	Fast; the patient remains accessible all the time	Unprecise, may be less effective than full-body surface counterwarming
Acetaminophen	Well tolerated, widely available	Liver toxicity; might mask fever. Limited usefulness to treat shivering
Magnesium sulfate (IV)	Well tolerated, efficient with surface cooling technique	Risks of hypermagnesemia
Serotonin modulators (i.e., buspirone, ondansetron)	Effective for shivering prevention	Often ineffective for moderate and severe shivering
Opioids (i.e., morphine, sufentanil, meperidine)	Widely available, often already part of the treatment in patients requiring TTM	Might increase the risk of seizures, respiratory depression, dependency
Alpha-agonists (i.e., dexmedetomidine, clonidine)	Fast acting, widely available, effective for mild and intermittent shivering	Bradycardia, hypotension
Ketamine	Effective as bolus to prevent and treat shivering	Hypertension, lack of evidence for continuous infusion, hallucinations
Sedatives (i.e., propofol, midazolam, thiopental)	Widely available, often part of the treatment in patients requiring TTM	Risk of hypotension and propofol-related infusion syndrome. Increased delirium incidence (midazolam). Long-lasting sedation (thiopental, midazolam)
Neuromuscular blockers	Effective for moderate and severe shivering, widely available	Increase necessity for sedation, prolonged ICU stay. Increase risk of ventilator-associated pneumonia

ICU, Intensive care unit; *IV*, intravenous; *TTM*, target temperature management.
From Vincent JL et al: *Textbook of critical care*, ed 8, Philadelphia, 2024, Elsevier.

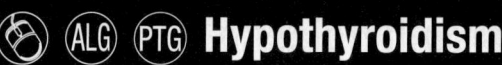

 BASIC INFORMATION

DEFINITION

Hypothyroidism is a disorder caused by the inadequate secretion of thyroid hormone.

SYNONYM

Myxedema

ICD-10CM CODES

E00.9	Congenital iodine-deficiency syndrome, unspecified
E02	Subclinical iodine-deficiency hypothyroidism
E03.0	Congenital hypothyroidism with diffuse goiter
E03.1	Congenital hypothyroidism without goiter
E03.2	Hypothyroidism due to medicaments and other exogenous substances
E03.3	Postinfectious hypothyroidism
E03.8	Other specified hypothyroidism
E03.9	Hypothyroidism, unspecified
E89.0	Postprocedural hypothyroidism

EPIDEMIOLOGY & DEMOGRAPHICS

INCIDENCE & PREVALENCE: 1.5% to 2% of women and 0.2% of men. Overall, about 1 in 300 persons in the U.S. has hypothyroidism.

PREDOMINANT AGE: Incidence of hypothyroidism increases with age; among persons older than 60 yr, 6% of women and 2.5% of men have laboratory evidence of hypothyroidism (thyroid-stimulating hormone [TSH] more than twice normal level).

PHYSICAL FINDINGS & CLINICAL PRESENTATION (BOX 1)

- Hypothyroid patients generally present with the following signs and symptoms: Fatigue, lethargy, weakness, constipation, weight gain, cold intolerance, muscle weakness, slow speech, slow cerebration with poor memory
- Skin: Dry, coarse, thick, cool, sallow (yellow color caused by carotenemia); nonpitting edema in skin of eyelids and hands (myxedema) secondary to infiltration of subcutaneous tissues by a hydrophilic mucopolysaccharide substance (Fig. E1, *A* and *B*)

BOX 1 Symptoms and Signs of Hypothyroidism

Vital Signs
- Systolic blood pressure, normal or low
- Diastolic blood pressure, normal or elevated
- Slow pulse to sinus bradycardia
- Respirations, normal or slow, shallow
- Temperature, normal, but prone to hypothermia with stress

Hypometabolic Complaints
- Cold intolerance
- Fatigue
- Weight gain, but decreased appetite

Cutaneous
- Coarse, brittle hair
- Alopecia
- Dry skin, decreased perspiration
- Pallor, cool hands and feet
- Coarse, rough skin
- Yellow tinge from carotenemia
- Thin, brittle nails
- Lateral thinning of the eyebrows

Neurologic
- Slow mentation and speech
- Impaired concentrating ability and attention span
- Lethargy
- Decreased short-term memory
- Agitation, psychosis
- Seizures
- Ataxia, dysmetria
- Mononeuropathy
- Carpal tunnel syndrome
- Sensorineural hearing loss
- Peripheral neuropathy, paresthesias

Muscular
- Proximal myopathy
- Pseudohypertrophy
- Delayed relaxation of reflexes (hung up or pseudomyotonic)

Cardiac
- Decreased exercise capacity
- Dyspnea on exertion
- Sinus bradycardia
- Long QT with increased ventricular arrhythmia
- Chest pain, accelerated coronary disease
- Diastolic heart failure (delayed ventricular relaxation)
- Pericardial effusion (asymptomatic)
- Peripheral edema

Respiratory
- Dyspnea on exertion
- Obstructive sleep apnea
- Primary pulmonary hypertension

Gastrointestinal
- Constipation
- Ileus
- Gastric atrophy

Reproductive
- Oligomenorrhea and amenorrhea
- Menorrhagia
- Decreased fertility
- Early abortions
- Decreased libido
- Erectile dysfunction

Rheumatic
- Polyarthralgias
- Joint effusions
- Acute gout or pseudogout

Head, Ear, Eyes, Nose, and Throat
- Hoarseness
- Deep husky voice
- Macroglossia
- Hearing loss
- Periorbital swelling
- Broad nose
- Swollen lips
- Goiter

- Hair: Brittle and coarse; loss of outer third of eyebrows
- Face: Dulled expression, thickened tongue, thick and slow-moving lips
- Thyroid gland: May or may not be palpable (depending on the cause of the hypothyroidism)
- Heart sounds: Distant, possible pericardial effusion
- Pulse: Bradycardia
- Neurologic: Delayed relaxation phase of the deep tendon reflexes, cerebellar ataxia, hearing impairment, poor memory, peripheral neuropathies with paresthesia
- Musculoskeletal: Carpal tunnel syndrome, muscular stiffness, weakness

ETIOLOGY (TABLE 1)

- Primary hypothyroidism (thyroid gland dysfunction): The cause of >90% of the cases of hypothyroidism
  1. Hashimoto thyroiditis is the most common cause of hypothyroidism after age 8 yr
  2. Idiopathic myxedema (nongoitrous form of Hashimoto thyroiditis)
  3. Previous treatment of hyperthyroidism (radioiodine therapy, subtotal thyroidectomy)
  4. Subacute thyroiditis
  5. Radiation therapy to the neck (usually for malignant disease)
  6. Iodine deficiency or excess
  7. Drugs (lithium, paraaminosalicylate, sulfonamides, phenylbutazone, amiodarone, thiourea). Box 2 summarizes medications that may cause iatrogenic hypothyroidism
  8. Congenital (approximately one case per 2000 to 4000 live births)
  9. Prolonged treatment with iodides
- Secondary hypothyroidism: Pituitary dysfunction, postpartum necrosis, neoplasm, infiltrative disease-causing deficiency of TSH
- Tertiary hypothyroidism: Hypothalamic disease (granuloma, neoplasm, or irradiation causing deficiency of thyrotropin-releasing hormone)
- Tissue resistance to thyroid hormone: Rare

Dx **DIAGNOSIS**

DIFFERENTIAL DIAGNOSIS

- Depression
- Dementia from other causes
- Systemic disorders (e.g., nephrotic syndrome, congestive heart failure, amyloidosis)

LABORATORY TESTS (TABLE 2)

- TSH, free T_4, thyroid peroxidase antibodies (TPOAB)
- Increased TSH: TSH may be normal if patient has secondary or tertiary hypothyroidism, is receiving dopamine or corticosteroids, or the level is obtained after severe illness
- Decreased free T_4 in hypothyroidism, normal free T_4 in subclinical hypothyroidism
- Other common laboratory abnormalities: Hyperlipidemia, hyponatremia, and anemia
- Increased antimicrosomal and antithyroglobulin antibody titers: Useful when autoimmune

From Walls RM et al: *Rosen's emergency medicine, concepts and clinical practice*, ed 10, Philadelphia, 2023, Elsevier.

TABLE 1 Causes of Hypothyroidism

Primary Hypothyroidism
- Chronic autoimmune thyroiditis (also known as Hashimoto thyroiditis)
- Iodine—severe iodine deficiency, mild and severe iodine excess
- Drugs—for example, amiodarone, lithium, tyrosine kinase inhibitors, interferon-α, thalidomide, monoclonal antibodies (e.g., ipilimumab and nivolumab), antiepileptic drugs (e.g., valproate), drugs for second-line treatment of multidrug-resistant tuberculosis
- Iatrogenic—radioiodine treatment (e.g., for Graves disease or toxic nodular disease), hemithyroidectomy, radiotherapy or surgery in the neck or head region
- Transient thyroiditis—viral (de Quervain syndrome), postpartum, silent thyroiditis, destructive thyroiditis
- Thyroid gland infiltration[a]—infectious (e.g., mycoplasma), malignant (e.g., thyroid malignancy, lymphoma, metastasis of malignancy elsewhere), autoimmune (e.g., sarcoidosis), inflammatory (e.g., Riedel thyroiditis)
- Genetic[a]—autoimmunity-related genes (e.g., *HLA* class 1 region, *PTPN22*, *SH2B3*, and *VAV3*), general and thyroid-specific genes (e.g., *FOXE1*, *ATXN2*, and *PDE86*)

Central Hypothyroidism
- Pituitary tumors (secreting or nonsecreting)
- Pituitary dysfunction (e.g., Sheehan syndrome)
- Hypothalamic dysfunction (e.g., posttraumatic)
- Resistance to thyroid-stimulating hormone (TSH) or thyrotropin-releasing hormone
- Drugs (e.g., dopamine, somatostatins, glucocorticosteroids, and retinoid X receptor-selective ligands)
- Increased TSH concentration because of leptin stimulation[b]

Peripheral (Extrathyroidal) Hypothyroidism
- Consumptive hypothyroidism
- Tissue-specific hypothyroidism owing to decreased sensitivity to thyroid hormone (e.g., mutations in *MCT8* [also known as *SLC16A2*], *SEQSBP2*, *TH RA*, *TH RB*)

[a]Rare cause of primary hypothyroidism.
[b]Evidence mainly from animal models.
From Chaker L et al: Hypothyroidism, *Lancet* 390:1550-1562, 2017. In Robertson RP et al: *DeGroot's endocrinology, basic science and clinical practice*, ed 8, Philadelphia, 2023, Elsevier.

BOX 2 Medications That May Cause Iatrogenic Hypothyroidism

Inhibition of Thyroid Hormone Synthesis or Secretion
- Aminoglutethimide
- Lithium
- Perchlorate
- Thalidomide
- Thionamides (methimazole, propylthiouracil)
- Iodine-containing medications
  1. Amiodarone
  2. Iodinated IV contrast
  3. Guaifenesin
  4. Kelp
  5. Potassium iodide
  6. Topical antiseptics

Immune Dysregulation
- Interferon alfa
- Interleukin-2
- Alemtuzumab
- Ipilimumab
- Nivolumab
- Pembrolizumab

TSH Suppression
- Dopamine

Destructive Thyroiditis
- Sunitinib

Increased Type 3 Deiodinase Activity
- Sorafenib

Increased T$_4$ Clearance and TSH Suppression
- Bexarotene

IV, Intravenous; *TSH,* thyroid-stimulating hormone.
From Townsend CM et al: *Sabiston textbook of surgery,* ed 21, St Louis, 2022, Elsevier.

TABLE 2 Laboratory Evaluation of Patients with Suspected Hypothyroidism or Thyroid Enlargement[a]

TSH, Free T$_4$	TPOAb	Diagnosis
TSH >10 mU/L		
Low	+	Primary hypothyroidism due to autoimmune thyroid disease
Low-normal	+	Primary "subclinical" hypothyroidism (autoimmune)
Low or low-normal	−	Recovery from systemic illness
		External irradiation, drug-induced, congenital hypothyroidism
		Iodine deficiency
		Seronegative autoimmune thyroid disease
		Rare thyroid disorders (amyloidosis, sarcoidosis, etc.)
		Recovery from subacute granulomatous thyroiditis
Normal	+, −	Consider TSH or T$_4$ assay artifacts
Elevated	−	Thyroid hormone resistance
		Blockade of T$_4$ to T$_3$ conversion (amiodarone) or a congenital 5′-deiodinase deficiency
		Consider assay artifacts
TSH 5-10 mU/L		
Low, low-normal	+	Early primary autoimmune hypothyroidism
Low, low-normal	−	Milder forms of nonautoimmune hypothyroidism (see earlier)
		Central hypothyroidism with impaired TSH bioactivity
Elevated	− (+)	Consider thyroid hormone resistance
		T$_4$ to T$_3$ conversion blockade (e.g., amiodarone)
TSH 0.5-5 mU/L		
Low, low-normal	− (+)	Central hypothyroidism
		Salicylate or phenytoin therapy
		Desiccated thyroid or T$_3$ replacement
TSH <0.5 μU/L		
Low, low-normal	− (+)	"Post-hyperthyroid" hypothyroidism (^{131}I or surgery)
		Central hypothyroidism
		T$_3$ or desiccated thyroid excess
		Following excess levothyroxine withdrawal

TgAb, Antithyroglobulin antibody; *TPOAb,* thyroid peroxidase autoantibody; *TSH,* thyroid-stimulating hormone (thyrotropin); +, present; −, not present.
[a]Initial tests: Serum TSH, serum free T$_4$, TPO, or TgAb.
From Melmed S et al: *Williams textbook of endocrinology,* ed 14, Philadelphia, 2019, Elsevier.

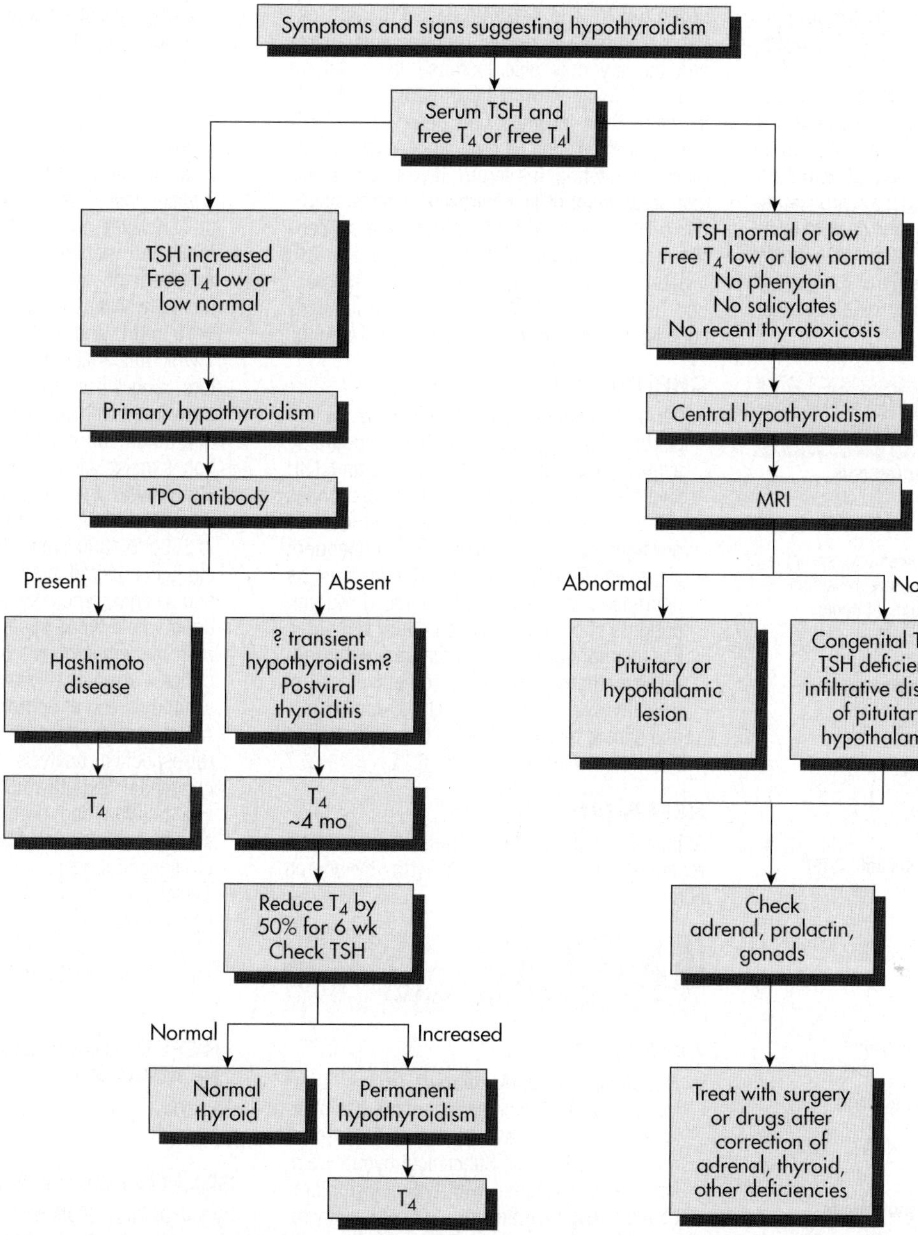

FIG. 2 Strategy for the laboratory evaluation of patients with suspected hypothyroidism.

```
                    Symptoms and signs suggesting hypothyroidism

                                   Serum TSH and
                                   free T₄ or free T₄I

        TSH increased                           TSH normal or low
        Free T₄ low or                          Free T₄ low or low normal
        low normal                              No phenytoin
                                                No salicylates
                                                No recent thyrotoxicosis

        Primary hypothyroidism                  Central hypothyroidism

        TPO antibody                            MRI

   Present        Absent                 Abnormal              Normal

  Hashimoto    ? transient          Pituitary or        Congenital TRH,
  disease      hypothyroidism?      hypothalamic        TSH deficiency
               Postviral           lesion              infiltrative disease
               thyroiditis                             of pituitary,
                                                       hypothalamus

     T₄           T₄
                  ~4 mo

                Reduce T₄ by                      Check
                50% for 6 wk                      adrenal, prolactin,
                Check TSH                         gonads

      Normal          Increased

   Normal      Permanent                         Treat with surgery
   thyroid     hypothyroidism                    or drugs after
                                                 correction of
                 T₄                              adrenal, thyroid,
                                                 other deficiencies
```

FIG. 2 Strategy for the laboratory evaluation of patients with suspected hypothyroidism. The principal differential diagnosis is between primary and central hypothyroidism. The serum thyrotropin *(TSH)* concentration is the critical laboratory determination that in general allows recognition of the cause of the disease. An exception is the individual with a recent history of thyrotoxicosis (and suppressed TSH) in whom a low free thyroxine *(T₄)* level may be associated with a reduced TSH level for several months after relief of the thyrotoxicosis. In patients with primary hypothyroidism, the absence of thyroid peroxidase *(TPO)* antibodies raises a possible diagnosis of transient hypothyroidism following an undiagnosed episode of subacute or postviral thyroiditis. In such patients, a trial of levothyroxine in reduced dosage after 4 mo may reveal recovery of thyroid function, thus avoiding permanent levothyroxine replacement. *MRI,* Magnetic resonance imaging; *TRH,* thyrotropin-releasing hormone; *T₄I,* thyroxine index. (From Melmed S et al: *Williams textbook of endocrinology,* ed 14, Philadelphia, 2019, Elsevier.)

thyroiditis is suspected as the cause of the hypothyroidism. The American Thyroid Association recommends treatment of pregnant patients with subclinical hypothyroidism and antithyroid peroxidase (anti-TPO) antibody positivity
- Fig. 2 describes a strategy for the laboratory evaluation of patients with suspected hypothyroidism

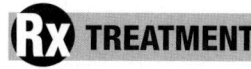 **TREATMENT**

NONPHARMACOLOGIC THERAPY
Patients should be educated regarding hypothyroidism and its possible complications. Patients should also be instructed about the need for lifelong treatment and monitoring of their thyroid abnormality. Patients should also be informed

about potential drug and food interactions. Levothyroxine is best taken with water on an empty stomach 60 min before breakfast or at bedtime 3 h after last meal.

ACUTE GENERAL Rx
Start replacement therapy with levothyroxine (L-thyroxine) 25 to 100 µg/day, depending on the patient's age and the severity of the disease.

Physiologic combinations of L-thyroxine plus liothyronine do not offer any objective advantage over L-thyroxine alone. The levothyroxine dose may be increased every 6 to 8 wk, depending on the clinical response and serum TSH level. Elderly patients and patients with coronary artery disease should be started with 12.5 to 25 µg/day (higher doses may precipitate angina). The average maintenance dose of levothyroxine is 1.7 µg/kg/day (100 to 150 µg/day in adults). The elderly may require <1 µg/kg/day, whereas children generally require higher

TABLE 3 Conditions That Alter Levothyroxine Requirements

Increased Levothyroxine Requirements

Pregnancy

Gastrointestinal Disorders

Mucosal diseases of the small bowel (e.g., sprue)
After jejunoileal bypass and small-bowel resection
Impaired gastric acid secretion (e.g., atrophic gastritis)
Diabetic diarrhea

Drugs That Interfere with Levothyroxine Absorption

Cholestyramine
Sucralfate
Aluminum hydroxide
Calcium carbonate
Ferrous sulfate

Drugs That Increase the Cytochrome P450 Enzyme (CYP 3A4) Activity

Rifampin
Carbamazepine
Estrogen
Phenytoin
Sertraline

Drugs That Block T_4-to-T_3 Conversion

Amiodarone

Conditions That May Block Deiodinase Synthesis

Selenium deficiency
Cirrhosis

Decreased Levothyroxine Requirements

Aging (≥65 yr)
Androgen therapy in women

T_3, Triiodothyronine; T_4, thyroxine.
From Melmed S et al: *Williams textbook of endocrinology,* ed 14, Philadelphia, 2019, Elsevier.

doses (up to 3 to 4 µg/kg/day). Pregnant patients also have increased requirements. Estrogen therapy may also increase the need for thyroxine. Women with hypothyroidism should increase their levothyroxine dose by approximately 30% as soon as pregnancy is confirmed. Close monitoring of serum thyrotropin levels and adjustment of levothyroxine dose to maintain a TSH level of a <2.5 mU/L before conception and during the first trimester and a TSH level of 4.0 mU/L as upper limit during the second and third trimester. Table 3 summarizes conditions that alter levothyroxine requirements.

CHRONIC Rx

- Periodic monitoring of TSH level is an essential part of treatment. Patients should be evaluated initially with office visit and TSH levels every 6 to 8 wk until the patient is clinically euthyroid and the TSH level is normalized. The frequency of subsequent visits and TSH measurement can then be decreased to every 6 to 12 mo. Pregnant patients should be checked every trimester.
- For monitoring therapy in patients with central hypothyroidism, measurement of serum free thyroxine (free T_4 level) is appropriate and should be maintained in the upper half of the normal range.

REFERRAL

Admission to the hospital intensive care unit is recommended in all patients with myxedema coma.

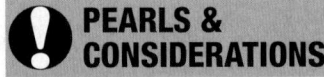

PEARLS & CONSIDERATIONS

COMMENTS

- ***Subclinical hypothyroidism*** occurs in as many as 20% of elderly patients and is characterized by an elevated serum TSH and a normal free T_4 level. Subclinical hypothyroidism is not associated with typical symptoms of overt hypothyroidism.[1] Subclinical hypothyroidism can progress to overt hypothyroidism, especially if antithyroid antibodies are present. It is associated with an increased risk of coronary heart disease events and

mortality, particularly in those with a TSH concentration of 10 mU/L or greater. Treatment is individualized and controversial. Some trials have shown that levothyroxine provides no apparent benefit in older persons (≥80 yr of age) with subclinical hypothyroidism. The management of subclinical hypothyroidism should be individualized on the basis of TSH level, comorbid conditions, risk factors, and patient preference. In general, replacement therapy is recommended by most physicians for patients with serum TSH >10 mU/L and with presence of goiter or thyroid autoantibodies or patient has risk factors. Subclinical thyroid dysfunction is not associated with cognitive decline or dementia and treatment of subclinical thyroid dysfunction is unlikely to improve cognitive function.[2]

- ***Congenital hypothyroidism*** is a pediatric disorder with an observed prevalence of one in 2000 to 4000 live births in the U.S. Screening is conducted in all newborns in all states and accomplished by measuring TSH from dried whole blood spots collected on a newborn by heel stick within the first 24 to 48 h of life. Currently 14 states perform a routine second screen at approximately 2 wk of age. A two-screen approach is preferred because retrospective analysis found that 20% of congenital hypothyroidism cases were in infants who had normal TSH on the first screen but elevated TSH concentrations on the second screen.
- Switching among FDA-approved generic levothyroxine preparations in patients with stable doses and normal TSH levels is safe and not associated with changes in TSH.[3]

REFERENCES & SUGGESTED READINGS

Available at eBooks.Health.Elsevier.com.

RELATED CONTENT

Hypothyroidism (Patient Information)
Myxedema Coma (Related Key Topic)

AUTHOR: **FRED F. FERRI, MD**

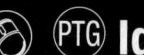

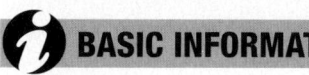 **BASIC INFORMATION**

DEFINITION

Idiopathic pulmonary fibrosis (IPF) is a specific form of chronic, progressive, fibrosing interstitial pneumonia with a histologic pattern of usual interstitial pneumonia (UIP) occurring in the absence of an identifiable cause of lung injury. Clinically, it is characterized by progressive parenchymal scarring and loss of pulmonary function.

SYNONYMS

Cryptogenic fibrosing alveolitis
IPF
Pulmonary fibrosis
Usual interstitial pneumonia

ICD-10CM CODE
J84.112   Idiopathic pulmonary fibrosis

EPIDEMIOLOGY & DEMOGRAPHICS

- Incidence: 7 to 16 cases/100,000 persons/yr in the U.S.
- Clinically IPF affects >50,000 people in the U.S. and accounts for 20% to 30% of interstitial lung diseases. It is the most common idiopathic interstitial pneumonia.
- Most commonly presents in sixth and seventh decades.
- More common in men than women.
- More common in current and past smokers.
- No distinct geographic distribution.
- No clear racial predilection.

GENETICS:
Familial forms account for 3% to 25% of cases. Genetic variants include mutations in surfactant protein C and telomerase as well as polymorphisms of the *MUC5B* gene.

PHYSICAL FINDINGS & CLINICAL PRESENTATION

- Most present with gradual onset (>6 mo) of exertional dyspnea and nonproductive cough. Progressive dyspnea is usually the most prominent symptom. Cough affects up to 80% of patients with IPF and is frequently disabling.
- Fine bibasilar inspiratory crackles, "Velcro-like crackles" in >80% of patients, with progression up the lung fields as disease advances.
- Clubbing is found in 25% to 50% of patients.
- Cyanosis and right heart failure (cor pulmonale) may occur late in the disease course.
- There are no extrapulmonary findings beyond clubbing and signs of right heart failure.
- Fever and wheezing are rare and suggest an alternative diagnosis.

ETIOLOGY

- Unknown. Fig. 1 illustrates a proposed pathogenetic sequence in IPF.
- Cigarette smoking, environmental exposures, gastroesophageal reflux, and microaspiration have been associated with IPF.
- Aberrant tissue repair and fibrosis are believed to play a greater role in the pathogenesis

than generalized inflammation. Immune system activation and increased vascular permeability contribute to the underlying pathology.

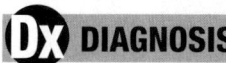 **DIAGNOSIS**

DIFFERENTIAL DIAGNOSIS

- Occupational exposures (e.g., asbestos) may cause pneumoconiosis with a UIP pattern
- Connective tissue diseases (e.g., rheumatoid arthritis [RA], systemic sclerosis) can cause a UIP pattern
- Chronic hypersensitivity pneumonitis (HP)
- Idiopathic fibrotic nonspecific interstitial pneumonia (NSIP)
- Drug-induced interstitial lung disease
- Desquamative interstitial pneumonia (DIP)
- Respiratory bronchitis–interstitial lung disease (RB-ILD)
- Pleuroparenchymal fibroelastosis
- NOTE: IPF is considered a diagnosis of exclusion

WORKUP

It is critical to establish a confident diagnosis to distinguish IPF from other diseases with better prognosis and different treatment. Multidisciplinary discussion with pulmonology, radiology, and pathology is encouraged as standard of care to decide if a surgical lung biopsy is necessary and to reach consensus on the diagnosis.[1]

- Laboratory tests: There are no specific laboratory tests for IPF; however, IPF requires excluding connective tissue disease-associated interstitial lung disease. Thus serologic testing is recommended. Antinuclear antibodies, rheumatoid factor, and anticyclic citrullinated

peptide are helpful to exclude RA, in which UIP is the most common pattern.[2]

IMAGING STUDIES

- Chest x-ray examination shows bilateral reticular opacities most prominent in the periphery and lower lobes. Fig. 2 is a chest x-ray examination showing diffuse bilateral lower lung predominant reticular opacities in a patient with IPF.
- High-resolution computed tomography scan (HRCT) of the chest (Fig. 3) is the most useful diagnostic test. HRCT can show one of four radiographic patterns.
  1. UIP: Lower lobe and peripheral predominant honeycombing, reticulation, and traction bronchiectasis. Mild ground-glass opacities (GGO) could be present in areas of fibrosis. It predicts histologic UIP and precludes the need for surgical lung biopsy.
  2. Probable UIP: Same as UIP, but without honeycombing. When the pretest probability is high—severe traction bronchiectasis in a patient of male sex, >60 yr —it predicts histologic UIP in >90% of cases.[3]
  3. Indeterminate for UIP: Lower lobe and peripheral predominant subtle reticulation, with or without mild GGO. The pattern does not suggest a specific etiology.
  4. Alternative diagnosis: Findings suggestive of another etiology such as mosaic attenuation, air trapping, predominant GGO, consolidation, nodules, cysts, a peribronchovascular, perilymphatic, or upper/mid lung predominant distribution, pleural plaques, etc.
- Surgical lung biopsy: Obtained by video-assisted thoracoscopy or open thoracotomy in carefully selected patients when the

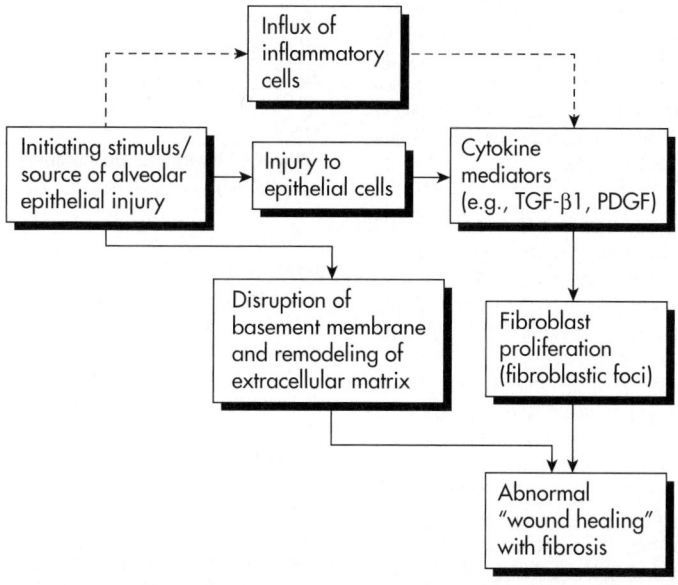

FIG. 1 Proposed pathogenetic sequence in idiopathic pulmonary fibrosis. *Dotted lines* indicate that although there is an influx of inflammatory cells, this is not thought to be a primary component of pathogenesis. *PDGF,* Platelet-derived growth factor; *TGF-β1,* transforming growth factor-β1. (From Weinberger SE: *Principles of pulmonary medicine,* ed 7, Philadelphia, 2019, Elsevier.)

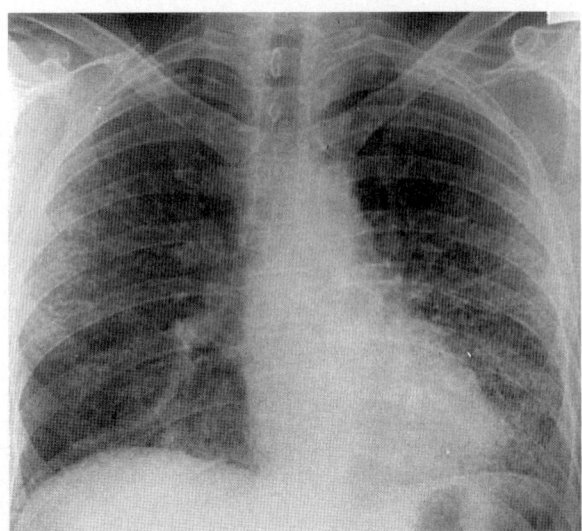

FIG. 2 Chest radiograph shows diffuse bilateral lower lung predominant reticular opacities in a patient with idiopathic pulmonary fibrosis. (From Mason RJ: *Murray & Nadel's textbook of respiratory medicine,* ed 5, Philadelphia, 2010, Saunders.)

Establishes IPF diagnosis in combination with a radiographic UIP pattern.

4. Alternative diagnosis: Features of other diseases. Excludes IPF. Table 1 summarizes histologic findings for immunologic diseases.

- Transbronchial lung biopsy with a molecular classifier (Envisia) has a specificity of 88% and sensitivity of 70% compared to diagnosis from pathology review, with 84% positive and 77% negative predictive value for UIP.[4] Its use could be considered when avoiding the risk of surgical lung biopsy is preferred.
- Pulmonary function tests show a restrictive pattern and reduced diffusing capacity.
- Six-min walk test may show reduced exercise tolerance and/or exertional hypoxia.

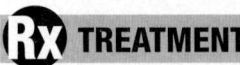 **TREATMENT**

- Two FDA-approved oral medications have similar proven efficacy in slowing disease progression, but neither restores normal lung parenchyma nor improves quality of life.

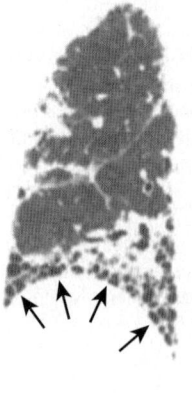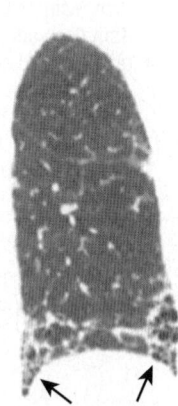

FIG. 3 Pulmonary fibrosis, honeycombing, and a usual interstitial pneumonia (UIP) pattern in idiopathic pulmonary fibrosis (IPF). Coronal high-resolution computed tomography reconstruction shows honeycombing *(arrows)* with a basal and subpleural predominance. This is typical of a UIP pattern. (From Webb WR et al: *Fundamentals of body CT,* ed 4, Philadelphia, 2015, Saunders.)

radiographic pattern is indeterminate for UIP, and the diagnosis remains unclear. It can show one of four patterns.

1. UIP: Normal lung with patchy, mostly subpleural or paraseptal, areas of dense fibrosis with distortion (e.g., microscopic honeycombing), fibroblastic foci, and no features to suggest other diagnosis. Establishes IPF diagnosis in the absence of a radiographic alternative diagnosis.
2. Probable UIP: Same as UIP but the extent is insufficient to exclude other diagnoses. Establishes IPF diagnosis in combination with radiographic probable UIP.
3. Indeterminate for UIP: Some features of UIP but with features suggesting another cause of UIP or an alternative diagnosis.

TABLE 1 Summary of Histologic Findings for Immunologic Lung Diseases

Disease	Histology
Granulomatous	
Foreign body, inorganic dust	Simple granuloma
Hypersensitivity pneumonitis	Poorly formed granulomas, peribronchiolar lymphoplasma-cytic infiltrate, organizing pneumonia
Infections	
Tuberculosis	Caseating granulomas
Sarcoidosis	Noncaseating granulomas in a lymphangitic pattern
Granulomatous Vasculitides	
Wegener granulomatosis	Necrotizing granulomas involving vasculature
Churg-Strauss syndrome	Necrotizing granulomas involving vasculature
Eosinophilic pneumonias	Granulomas with eosinophilic predominance; interstitial edema
Histiocytosis X	Granulomas with Langerhans cells
Alveolitic	
Drug-associated injury	Interstitial edema with inflammatory cells
Goodpasture syndrome	Linear staining of basement membrane with anti-IgG antibodies typically seen on renal biopsy; interstitial edema with inflammatory cells
Idiopathic Interstitial Pneumonias	
Idiopathic pulmonary fibrosis	Peripheral lobular fibrosis with less involvement of the centrilobular region, and fibroblastic foci in the interface of both
Desquamative interstitial pneumonia	Accumulation of macrophages in the alveolar spaces
Idiopathic nonspecific interstitial pneumonia	Alveolar septa diffusely thickened with inflammation and fibrosis. Preserved architecture
Acute interstitial pneumonia	Diffuse alveolar damage with thickened fibrotic interstitium; proliferating fibroblasts
Respiratory bronchiolitis–associated interstitial lung disease	Macrophages infiltrating distal bronchioles
Organizing pneumonia	Alveolar filling with polypoid plugs of granulation tissue that can contain inflammatory cells.
Lymphocytic interstitial pneumonia	Diffuse thickening of alveolar septa with lymphocytes forming lymphoid aggregates with germinal centers
Idiopathic pleuroparenchymal fibroelastosis	Diffuse alveolar damage with fibrosis

Modified from Sellke FW et al: *Sabiston & Spencer surgery of the chest,* ed 9, Philadelphia, 2016, Elsevier; and Jones et al: Histopathologic approach to the surgical lung biopsy in interstitial lung disease. In Collard HR, Richeldi L (eds): *Interstitial lung disease,* Philadelphia, 2018, Elsevier, pp. 141-155.

BOX 1 Guidelines for Lung Transplantation for Interstitial Lung Disease

Timing of Referral
Referral should be made at time of diagnosis, even if a patient is being initiated on therapy, for histopathologic UIP or radiographic evidence of a probable or definite UIP pattern.
Abnormal lung function: FVC <80% predicted or DLCO <40% predicted.
Any form of pulmonary fibrosis with one of the following in the past 2 yr:
- Relative decline in FVC 10%
- Relative decline in DLCO 15%
- Relative decline in FVC 5% in combination with worsening of respiratory symptoms or radiographic progression

Supplemental oxygen requirement either at rest or on exertion.
For inflammatory ILDs, progression of disease (either on imaging or pulmonary function) despite treatment.
For patients with connective tissue disease or familial pulmonary fibrosis, early referral is recommended as extrapulmonary manifestations may require special consideration.

Timing of Listing
Any form of pulmonary fibrosis with one of the following in the past 6 mo despite appropriate treatment:
- Absolute decline in FVC >10%
- Absolute decline in DLCO >10%
- Absolute decline in FVC >5% with radiographic progression.

Desaturation to <88% on 6-min walk test or >50 m decline in 6-min walk test distance in the past 6 mo.
Pulmonary hypertension on right heart catheterization or two-dimensional echocardiography (in the absence of diastolic dysfunction).
Hospitalization because of respiratory decline, pneumothorax, or acute exacerbation.

DLCO, Diffusion of carbon monoxide; *FVC,* Forced vital capacity; *ILDs,* interstitial lung diseases; *UIP,* usual interstitial pneumonia.
From Leard LE et al: Consensus document for the selection of lung transplant candidates: an update from the International Society for Heart and Lung Transplantation, *J Heart Lung Transpl* 40(11):1349-1379, 2021.

Both are associated with substantial side effects.[5]
1. Pirfenidone is an antifibrotic medication without a known mechanism of action. It is taken three times a day with food. Its major side effects are nausea, abdominal discomfort, and photosensitivity. Liver function tests (LFTs) must be monitored.[6]
2. Nintedanib is a tyrosine kinase inhibitor taken twice daily. Its major side effect is diarrhea, which often resolves. LFTs also need to be followed.[7]
- Additional new therapies are being investigated and are in phase I, II, and III trials.
- The food supplement epigallocatechin gallate (EGCG) blocks collagen cross-linking, suppressing TGFβ1-induced matrix production, and is associated with decrease in fibroblast-derived serum biomarkers.[8] Its efficacy in the treatment of IPF is currently being assessed in a randomized controlled trial.
- The combination of prednisone, azathioprine, and *N*-acetylcysteine was associated with increased mortality in a randomized clinical trial and is contraindicated.
- Treatment includes supportive care (pulmonary rehabilitation, supplemental oxygen, influenza and pneumococcal vaccination), referral for lung transplant consideration, and palliative care.[9]

- Gabapentin (up to 1800 mg/day) acts on airway nerves and is effective for cough, though side effects of sedation and fatigue may limit its use.[10] Other options include benzonatate, guaifenesin with codeine, and menthol lozenges. If postnasal drip or gastroesophageal reflux could be contributing to cough, it is reasonable to treat them.
- Treatment of asymptomatic gastroesophageal reflux may be reasonable given association between pulmonary fibrosis and reflux or microaspiration.
- Lung transplantation is the only therapy shown to prolong survival in IPF. Guidelines for transplantation in patients with interstitial lung disease, including IPF, are summarized in Box 1.[11] Posttransplant 5-yr survival for IPF patients is approximately 50% to 60%. Median survival time is longer after bilateral lung transplantation than single lung transplantation but is associated with more complications during the first yr.[12]
- Acute exacerbation of IPF, defined as worsening dyspnea (<1 mo), the presence of new opacities on chest imaging, and the lack of evidence of infection, has a yearly incidence of 7% to 32%. Progressive respiratory failure may require mechanical ventilation; however, a palliative care approach is often chosen

instead. Treatment for exacerbations typically includes high-dose corticosteroids and broad-spectrum antibiotics, although the efficacy of this approach is unproven and questionable.[13]

DISPOSITION
- Spontaneous remissions do not occur, although long periods of stability can occur.
- Natural history includes progressive loss of pulmonary function. Predictors of poor outcome include older age, male gender, moderately to severely reduced forced vital capacity (FVC) and diffusion of carbon monoxide (DLCO), and development of pulmonary hypertension.
- There is an increased risk of lung cancer.
- Mean survival after the diagnosis of biopsy-confirmed IPF is 3 to 5 yr, although with new therapies available, survival is less defined.
- Lung transplantation is the only therapy shown to prolong survival.
- Respiratory failure is the most common cause of death.

REFERRAL
- To pulmonologist, with review in multidisciplinary discussion to establish confident diagnosis.
- Referral for participation in clinical trials.
- Early referral to a lung transplant center for evaluation.
- Late-stage management should include palliative care referral.

! PEARLS & CONSIDERATIONS

- The course is progressive, with a high mortality. The most common cause of death in IPF is respiratory failure.
- Critical to differentiate IPF from other interstitial lung diseases because prognosis and treatment approaches differ.
- Two oral therapies have been shown to slow disease progression are available. Additional novel treatments are being investigated.
- Patients with IPF should be referred early for consideration of lung transplantation.

REFERENCES
Available at eBooks.Health.Elsevier.com.

RELATED CONTENT
Idiopathic Pulmonary Fibrosis (Patient Information)
Interstitial Lung Disease (Related Key Topic)

AUTHOR: **AIDA VENADO, MD, MAS**

BASIC INFORMATION

DEFINITION

Immune thrombocytopenic purpura (ITP) is an autoimmune disorder in which antibody-coated or immune complex–coated platelets are destroyed prematurely, resulting in peripheral thrombocytopenia.[1] The autoantibodies may also affect megakaryocytes and impair platelet production. In primary ITP, the thrombocytopenia is isolated, whereas in secondary ITP, the condition is associated with other disorders (e.g., systemic lupus erythematosus [SLE], HIV, chronic lymphocytic leukemia [CLL], lymphoma). Distinguishing ITP from other causes of thrombocytopenia is very important because ITP requires a different approach to treatment rather than addressing the underlying causes of other types of thrombocytopenia.

SYNONYMS

ITP
Immune thrombocytopenia

ICD-10CM CODE
D69.3   Immune thrombocytopenic purpura

EPIDEMIOLOGY & DEMOGRAPHICS

INCIDENCE: Primary ITP occurs in 1 to 6/100,000 adults/yr.[2]
PREVALENCE: In the U.S., 8/100,000 in children and 12/100,000 in adults.[3] Since ITP is often a chronic condition, prevalence significantly exceeds incidence.
PREDOMINANT SEX: 72% of patients >10 yr old are female; males are more commonly affected among children.[2]
PREDOMINANT AGE: Children aged 1 to 6 yr and women of childbearing age (70% are <40 yr).[4] New onset of ITP after age 60 yr is uncommon; comprehensive workup for secondary ITP may be required.

PHYSICAL FINDINGS & CLINICAL PRESENTATION

The presentation of ITP is different in children and adults:
- Children generally present with sudden onset of bruising and petechiae from severe thrombocytopenia.
- In adults, the presentation is insidious; a history of prolonged purpura may be present. Many patients are diagnosed incidentally based on automated laboratory tests that now routinely include platelet counts. Bleeding may be present in up to two thirds of patients.
- Fatigue is a common symptom and often correlates with platelet count.
- The physical examination may be entirely normal.
- Patients with severe thrombocytopenia may have petechiae, purpura, epistaxis, or heme-positive stool from gastrointestinal bleeding. Life-threatening bleeding is uncommon and generally confined to patients with platelets <10,000/mm³.

- Splenomegaly is unusual; its presence should alert to the possibility of other etiologies of thrombocytopenia.
- The presence of dysmorphic features (skeletal anomalies, auditory abnormalities) may indicate a congenital disorder as the cause of the thrombocytopenia.

ETIOLOGY

Increased platelet destruction is caused by autoantibody targets to platelet-membrane antigens, particularly antibodies against platelet GPIIb/IIIa or GPIb/IX.[5] The spleen has a major role in ITP by producing autoantibodies in the white pulp and removing autoantibody-coated platelets in the red pulp. Production of antibodies could be triggered either by the immunogenicity of membrane glycoproteins (GPs) on the platelet surface or by external factors such as infections or medications. Reduced platelet lifespan due to clearance is the predominant cause of thrombocytopenia.

DIAGNOSIS

DIFFERENTIAL DIAGNOSIS

- ITP is a diagnosis of exclusion.
- Falsely low platelet count due to aggregation (resulting from ethylenediaminetetraacetic acid [EDTA]-dependent or cold-dependent agglutinins). Platelet count is corrected by using a heparin or citrate anticoagulated tube.
- Variety of infections, including viral infections (e.g., HIV, hepatitis C, Epstein-Barr virus causing mononucleosis, cytomegalovirus, *H. pylori*, SARS-CoV-2, rubella).
- Drugs commonly implicated are heparin (heparin-induced thrombocytopenia [HIT]), quinidine, antibiotics (linezolid, vancomycin, sulfonamides, rifampin), platelet inhibitors (tirofiban, abciximab, eptifibatide), cimetidine, NSAIDs, thiazide diuretics, antirheumatic agents (gold salts, penicillamine), and many chemotherapeutic agents (cyclosporine, fludarabine, carboplatin, oxaliplatin).
- Hypersplenism resulting from liver disease.
- Myelodysplastic and lymphoproliferative disorders.
- Pregnancy.
- Hypothyroidism.
- SLE, rheumatoid arthritis, antiphospholipid syndrome.
- Microangiopathic processes include thrombotic thrombocytopenic purpura (TTP), hemolytic-uremic syndrome (HUS), and disseminated intravascular coagulation (DIC).
- Congenital thrombocytopenia (e.g., Fanconi syndrome, May-Hegglin anomaly, Bernard-Soulier syndrome).
- Evans syndrome is a rare autoimmune disorder characterized by autoimmune hemolytic anemia (AIHA) and immune thrombocytopenia (ITP).

LABORATORY TESTS

- CBC, platelet count, and peripheral smear: Platelets are decreased. The peripheral smear should show large platelets and no

schistocytes (Fig. E1). Red blood cells and white blood cells have a normal morphology. The hemoglobin level should be normal unless the patient has been bleeding.
- Reticulated platelets (RPs) are the youngest circulating platelets, analogous to the relationship between reticulocytes and mature red blood cells. RPs can be quantified by flow cytometry or with an automated measurement called the "immature platelet fraction" (IPF), which can diagnose ITP if the clinical picture is unclear.[6] The IPF is typically elevated in thrombocytopenia caused by peripheral consumption/destruction (e.g., ITP), and it is usually normal in production defects such as bone marrow failure syndromes.
- Additional tests may be ordered to exclude other causes of the thrombocytopenia when clinically indicated (e.g., HIV screening test, antinuclear antibody [ANA], thyroid-stimulating hormone [TSH] [hypothyroidism and hyperthyroidism can cause thrombocytopenia], liver enzymes, hepatitis C Ab, coagulation tests [PT, aPTT] to rule out other possible factors including DIC [moderate to severe bleeding] or vitamin K deficiency, *H. pylori* testing especially in endemic regions, and nutritional testing [vitamin B₁₂, folate]).
- Direct assay of platelet-bound antibodies has an estimated positive predictive value of only 80% to 83%. A negative test cannot be used to rule out the diagnosis.
- Bone marrow aspiration and biopsy are recommended in adults older than >60 yr if there is evidence of immature cells on peripheral smear or persistent neutropenia. Biopsy in an ITP patient shows normal cellularity and increased megakaryocytes; other hemopoietic lineages are normal.

IMAGING STUDIES

Computed tomography (CT) scan of abdomen/pelvis in patients with splenomegaly to exclude other disorders causing thrombocytopenia

TREATMENT

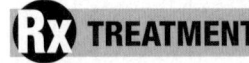

NONPHARMACOLOGIC THERAPY

- Minimize activity to prevent injury or bruising (e.g., contact sports should be avoided).
- Stop any potentially offending drugs (see "Etiology"). Avoid medications that increase the risk of bleeding (e.g., aspirin and other NSAIDs).

ACUTE GENERAL Rx

- Treatment varies with the platelet count, patient's age, and bleeding status. It is important to recognize secondary ITP as management would include treatment of the underlying cause, if possible. Therapy aims to provide a safe platelet count to prevent clinically significant bleeding. For newly diagnosed patients with minimal bleeding, treatment consists of corticosteroids vs. observation when platelet counts are <30,000 /mm³ and hospital admission when platelet counts are <20,000 /mm³ (Fig. E2).

- Outpatient observation and frequent platelet count monitoring is needed in asymptomatic established ITP patients with platelet counts >20,000/mm³.
- The most common initial regimen is oral prednisone 1 mg/kg/day for 1 to 2 wk, followed by a gradual taper. Prolonged courses (>6 wk) of prednisone are not recommended. Response rates range from 50% to 75%, and most responses occur within the first 3 wk.[7]
- IV methylprednisolone: 30 mg/kg/day (maximum dose of 1 g/day for 2 or 3 days) infused over 20 to 30 min plus IVIG (1 g/kg/day for 2 or 3 days).
- Pulse-dose oral dexamethasone: Given at a dose of 40 mg/day for 4 consecutive days when given for three to four cycles every 4 wk results in a high response rate (80% to 85%) and has been shown to have fewer side effects when compared to longer courses of prednisone.[8] A meta-analysis of nine randomized trials revealed no significant increase in efficacy but confirmed less toxicity and faster increases in platelet counts using high-dose dexamethasone.[9]
- Continuation of corticosteroids is limited by long-term complications associated with its use (osteoporosis, weight gain, hyperglycemia, facial swelling, opportunistic infections, emotional lability, and avascular necrosis).
- Infusion of platelets should only be given to patients with life-threatening bleeding or those undergoing emergent surgery.
- IVIG (typically 1 to 2 g/kg in divided doses) is used in two settings: Corticosteroid-refractory and pregnant patients. It rapidly increases platelet count in nearly 80% of patients, but its effect is transient, usually lasting only 3 to 4 wk.
- Anti-D immunoglobulin, a pooled IgG product derived from the plasma of Rh(D)-negative donors, is also effective. It can be given only to patients who are Rh(D) positive with hemoglobin >8 mg/dl; the usual dose is 50 to 75 mcg/kg.
- Rituximab, a monoclonal antibody directed against the CD20 antigen, is a second-line agent. The usual dose is 375 mg/m² weekly ×4 wk. All patients receiving rituximab should be screened for hepatitis B virus infection to avoid reactivation.
- Splenectomy is considered a subsequent option in case of rituximab failure. Previously, it

was considered in adults with platelet count <20,000/mm³ after 6 wk of medical treatment or after 6 mo if more than 10 to 20 mg/day of prednisone is still required to maintain a platelet count >30,000/mm³. In children, splenectomy is generally reserved for persistent thrombocytopenia (>1 yr) and clinically significant bleeding. Appropriate immunizations (pneumococcal vaccine in adults and children, *Haemophilus influenzae* vaccine, meningococcal vaccine in children) should be administered earlier than 2 wk before planned splenectomy. Postsplenectomy vaccinations should be performed in all cases.
- Additional second-line agents are thrombopoietin receptor agonists (TPO-RA), azathioprine, cyclosporin A, cyclophosphamide, danazol, dapsone, mycophenolate mofetil, and *Vinca* alkaloids. A recent trial of mycophenolate mofetil addition to a glucocorticoid for first-line ITP treatment yielded a greater response and a lower risk of refractory or relapsed ITP but with somewhat decreased quality of life.[10]
- TPO-RAs such as romiplostim (Nplate), a subcutaneously administered recombinant fusion protein, and the oral nonpeptide molecules eltrombopag or avatrombopag are effective in increasing the platelet count in adult patients with chronic ITP refractory to corticosteroids and/or splenectomy.[11] They are titrated to achieve platelet count in a safe range.
- Fostamatinib is an inhibitor of the enzyme spleen tyrosine kinase (Syk). Syk plays an important role in phagocytosis of FcγR-mediated signal transduction and inflammatory propagation.[12] It received FDA approval for chronic ITP in adults who had an insufficient response to previous treatment, including corticosteroids, intravenous immunoglobulin (IVIG), splenectomy, and/or a TPO-RA (10). The recommended initial dose is 100 mg PO twice daily. It can be increased to 150 mg twice daily if the platelet count has not responded to at least 50,000/mm³ at 1 mo.
- Preliminary trials with rilzabrutinib, an oral, reversible covalent inhibitor of Bruton's tyrosine kinase (BTK), have shown that it may increase platelet counts in patients with ITP through a dual mechanism of action: Decreased macrophage-mediated platelet destruction and reduced production of pathogenic autoantibodies.[12,13]

- Other investigational drugs include FcRn inhibitors (efgartigimod and rozanolixizumab), which are currently undergoing phase III studies, are postulated to work by decreasing the levels of antiplatelet IgG levels, leading to less platelet destruction.[14,15] Studies on complement pathway inhibitors are also ongoing.
- A combination of various agents rather than a single agent is helpful in specific cases with severe or symptomatic thrombocytopenia refractory to the single drug to achieve more effective and durable responses.[16]
- Adjunctive therapies, including aminocaproic acid or tranexamic acid, are also suggested. They do not necessarily affect platelet levels but help control local bleeding by inhibiting fibrinolysis.

PREGNANCY Rx

- No treatment of ITP in pregnancy has been approved by regulatory agencies.[4]
- No treatment is required when platelet count is >30,000/mm³ or higher until 36 wk gestation or earlier in case of premature labor.
- When needed, prednisone is given at the lowest effective dose, usually with an initial dose of 10 to 20 mg daily. Dexamethasone is likely to effect the fetus, whereas prednisone is almost completely inactivated by the placenta. IVIG, at a dose of 400 mg/kg of body weight per day given for up to 5 d may be added.[4]
- Refractory ITP may require splenectomy in the second trimester.

DISPOSITION

- More than 80% of children have a complete remission within 8 wk.
- In adults, the course of the disease is chronic; only 5% of adults have spontaneous remission. However, most adults will reach a stable, safe platelet count.
- The principal cause of death from ITP is intracranial hemorrhage (1% of children and 5% of adults).

REFERENCES
Available at eBooks.Health.Elsevier.com.

RELATED KEY CONTENT
Immune Thrombocytopenic Purpura (Patient Information)

AUTHORS: **TARUNA AURORA, MD** and **PATAN GULTAWATVICHAI, MD**

Diseases and Disorders

I

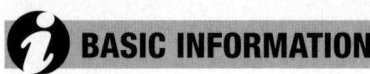 **BASIC INFORMATION**

DEFINITION

Urinary incontinence is the involuntary leakage of urine.

ICD-10CM CODES
N39.3	Stress incontinence (female) (male)
N39.41	Urgency urinary incontinence
N39.46	Mixed incontinence
N39.49	Disorder of urinary system, unspecified
R32	Unspecified urinary incontinence
R39.81	Functional urinary incontinence

EPIDEMIOLOGY & DEMOGRAPHICS

PREVALENCE: In the general population between the ages of 15 and 64, 1.5% to 5% of men and 25% to 57% of women have urinary incontinence (UI).[1] The prevalence of UI among young women is 25%;[2] in middle-aged and postmenopausal women it was found to be 44% to 57%;[1] and in a study of over 96,000 nursing home residents with a mean age of 82, prevalence was 75%.[3] The Women's Preventive Services Initiative (WPSI) recommends screening women for urinary incontinence annually.

CLINICAL, PSYCHOLOGIC, & SOCIAL IMPACT

Fewer than 50% of women living with incontinence in the U.S. consult health care professionals for care, resulting in significant physical and psychologic limitations.[4] Many women choose to turn to home remedies, commercially available absorbent materials, and supportive aids. As the incontinence worsens, many women become depressed, limit social interaction, refrain from sexual intimacy, and become homebound. It is estimated that $19.5 billion in direct costs is spent annually on incontinence in the U.S.[5] Urinary incontinence contributes to approximately 6% of nursing home admissions in the older population, leading to a cost of $3 billion per yr.

MAJOR TYPES OF INCONTINENCE

The continence mechanisms are complex and include multiple levels of control: Central and peripheral nervous systems (Fig. E1), the detrusor muscle, the urethra, and pelvic floor muscles. Dysfunction at any of these levels can lead to incontinence. Transient causes of urinary incontinence in the elderly are described in Table 1.

- **Stress urinary incontinence (SUI)** is the involuntary loss of urine with effort or physical exertion, or with any activity that increases intraabdominal pressure (sneezing, coughing, etc.) (Fig E2). The pathophysiology behind SUI is an inability of the urethral closing pressure to remain higher than intraabdominal, and thus intravesical, pressure. Continence during activities that increase intravesical pressure is afforded by adequate supportive tissue tone via levator ani muscles and connective tissue strength, and many factors can lead to inadequate support and stress incontinence. The most common risk factors are parity and obesity. Table 2 summarizes typical symptom differences in stress and urge incontinence. SUI may be demonstrated with a simple cough stress test during examination.

- **Intrinsic sphincter deficiency (ISD)** is the most severe form of SUI and indicates a urethra that cannot remain closed even at rest. On urodynamic testing, this is diagnosed with a maximal urethral closure pressure <20 cm H_2O and leak point pressure <60 cm H_2O.

- **Urgency urinary incontinence (UUI)** is the involuntary loss of urine associated with urgency, a sudden compelling desire to pass urine that is difficult to defer. The diagnosis is often made clinically based on patient's report of symptoms but may also be associated with involuntary detrusor contractions on urodynamic investigation. May be idiopathic or neurogenic.

- **Overactive bladder (OAB)** is a related condition described as a constellation of symptoms, including urgency, with or without urgency urinary incontinence, usually with urinary frequency and nocturia. It should be distinguished from excessive fluid intake and must exclude urinary tract infection. Can occur in up to 27% of men and up to 43% of women.

- **Mixed urinary incontinence** is the involuntary leakage of urine associated with urgency and with physical exertion, effort, sneezing, or coughing.

- **Overflow incontinence** is the leakage of urine resulting from urinary retention with resultant overflow or spilling of the urine. Causes include hypotonic bladder resulting from age, neurologic conditions such as diabetes or spinal cord injury, prior surgery, drug effects (e.g., intravesical Botox), or fecal impaction. It may also be caused by obstruction at the bladder neck and urethra, such as from prior antiincontinence surgery, pelvic organ prolapse, urethral stenosis, or detrusor-sphincter dyssynergia.

- **Functional urinary incontinence** is the involuntary leakage of urine resulting from chronic cognitive, functional, or mobility impairments. This is a diagnosis of exclusion and may be cured by improving the patient's functional status, treating comorbidities, changing medications, and reducing environmental barriers.

- **Extraurethral urinary incontinence** is leakage that bypasses the urethral meatus (i.e., vesicovaginal fistula or ectopic ureter).

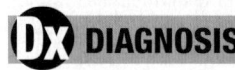 **DIAGNOSIS**

HISTORY

Because many women are hesitant to bring up symptoms of incontinence, these symptoms should be elicited through simple screening (Tables 3 and 4). Lower urinary tract symptoms are summarized in Table 5. A thorough history should include current symptom course, psychosocial factors, congenital disorders, access issues for those with mobility issues, neurologic disorders, and medication use or coexistent disorders that may affect the urinary tract. Urinary incontinence may be characterized by

TABLE 1 Transient Causes of Urinary Incontinence (DIAPPERS)

D	Delirium/AMS state
I	Infection, urinary (symptomatic)
A	Atrophic urethritis/vaginitis
P	Pharmaceuticals (diuretics, etc.)
P	Psychological, especially depression
E	Endocrine (hypercalcemia, hypokalemia, glycosuria)
R	Restricted mobility
S	Stool impaction

AMS, Altered mental status.
From Floege J et al: *Comprehensive clinical nephrology,* ed 4, Philadelphia, 2010, Saunders.

TABLE 2 Typical Symptom Differences in Stress and Urge Incontinence

Symptom	Stress Incontinence	Urge Incontinence
Leakage with exertion, cough, sneeze, activity	Yes	No
Leakage with sensation or urgency	No	Yes
Frequency, nocturia	No	Yes
Large volume urine loss	No	Yes
Leakage with running water, key in the door	No	Yes
Leakage with position change from sitting to standing	Possible	Yes
Leakage while recumbent	No	Possible
History of childhood bedwetting	No	Yes

From Gershenson DM et al: *Comprehensive gynecology,* ed 8, Philadelphia, 2022, Elsevier.

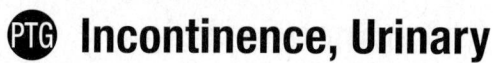

TABLE 3 Recommendations for Urinary Incontinence (UI) Screening

Organization	Target Population	Recommendation	Level of Evidence/Grade of Recommendation/Rationale
USPSTF	All older adults	Screen for UI as part of an overall prevention recommendation for older adults	Not provided
Women's Preventive Services Initiative	All women	Screen annually for UI	Weak; detect UI before it significantly affects women's lives
World Health Organization	All older persons	Routinely check for UI in older women and men	Rationale: At least half of women with UI do not report this issue to their general practitioner
ACOVE	All persons age ≥75 yr	1. During an initial evaluation, all persons should have documentation of the presence or absence of UI 2. During annual evaluations, all persons should have documentation of the presence or absence of UI	N/A

ACOVE, Assessing Care of Vulnerable Elderly; *USPSTF,* US Preventive Services Task Force.
From Warshaw G et al: *Ham's primary care geriatrics,* ed 7, Philadelphia, 2022, Elsevier.

TABLE 4 Screening Questions for Incontinence

Type of Incontinence	Question	Psychometrics
Any	"Have you had any problems with bladder or urine control?" "Do you ever leak urine when you don't want to?"	Kappa 0.8 (95% CI, 0.3-0.9) Percentage agreement 90% (95% CI, 84%-95%)
Stress incontinence	"Do you ever leak urine coughing, sneezing, lifting, walking, or running?"	Positive LR 2.2 (95% CI, 1.6-3.2) Negative LR 0.39 (95% CI, 0.25-0.61) Sensitivity 0.86 (95% CI, 0.79-0.90) Specificity 0.60 (95% CI, 0.51-0.68) Posttest probability decreases with age (from 87%-42%)
Urge incontinence	"Do you experience such a strong and sudden urge to void that you leak before reaching the toilet?"	Positive LR 4.2 (95% CI, 2.3-7.6) Negative LR 0.48 (95% CI, 0.36-0.62) Sensitivity 0.75 (95% CI, 0.68-0.81) Specificity 0.77 (95% CI, 0.69-0.84) Posttest probability increases with age (from 52%-91%)

CI, Confidence interval; *LR,* likelihood ratio (likelihood that a given test result would be expected in a patient with the target disorder compared with the likelihood that the same result would be expected in a patient without the target disorder).
From Warshaw G et al: *Ham's primary care geriatrics,* ed 7, Philadelphia, 2022, Elsevier.

TABLE 5 Lower Urinary Tract Symptoms

Symptom	Description
Urgency	Compelling, often sudden need to void that is difficult to defer.
Urge incontinence	Leakage preceded by/associated with urgency. Common precipitants include running water, hand washing, going out in the cold, even the sight of the garage or trying to unlock the door when returning home. The need to "rush to the toilet" and length of time one can forestall an urgency episode are less useful symptoms because they reflect cognition, mobility, toilet availability, and sphincter control, as well as bladder function.
Stress incontinence	Leakage with effort, exertion, sneezing, or coughing. Leakage may be provoked by minimal or no activity when there is severe sphincter damage. Leakage coincident with cough, laugh, sneeze, or physical activity suggests failure of sphincter mechanisms. Leakage that occurs seconds after the activity, especially if difficult to stop, suggests a cough-induced uninhibited detrusor contraction.
Mixed incontinence	Presence of both urgency and stress UI symptoms. Patients vary in the predominance, severity, and/or bother of urge versus stress leakage.
Overactive bladder	Symptom syndrome (not a specific pathologic condition) consisting of urgency, frequency, and nocturia, with or without urge incontinence.
Frequency	Complaint of needing to void too often during the day, as defined by the patient.
Nocturia	Complaint of waking at night one or more times to void. If these voids are associated with UI, the term *nocturnal enuresis* may be used.
Slow (weak) stream	Perception of reduced urine flow, usually compared with previous performance.
Hesitancy	Difficulty in initiating voiding, resulting in a delay in the onset of voiding after the individual feels ready to pass urine.
Straining	Muscular effort either to initiate, maintain, or improve the urinary stream.
Intermittent stream	Sensation that the bladder is not empty after voiding.
Postvoid dribbling	Small amounts/drops of urine after voiding has stopped. More common in men.

UI, Urinary incontinence.
From Warshaw GA et al: *Ham's primary care geriatrics,* ed 7, Philadelphia 2022, Elsevier.

frequency of incontinence episodes, severity, and extent of bother. A voiding diary can help assess total voided volume, frequency of micturition, mean volume voided, largest single volume, diurnal distribution, and nature and severity of incontinence. Assessments of the severity of symptoms and goals for treatment are important parts of the history.

PHYSICAL EXAMINATION

GENERAL PHYSICAL EXAMINATION: Performing a thorough general physical examination can highlight confounding conditions, including mobility issues. The examination should include a gait assessment to assess for neuromuscular deficits. Comorbid conditions that can cause or contribute to urinary incontinence in elderly patients are summarized in Table 6. Table 7 describes medications that can cause or contribute to urinary incontinence.

PELVIC EXAMINATION: The pelvic examination should include assessment for a number of related conditions as well as any findings that may be contributing to incontinence, including:
- Concurrent pelvic organ prolapse (POP)
- Vaginal discharge
- Estrogen status
- Pelvic floor strength assessment
- Neurologic examination to assess sacral nerves with anal wink and bulbocavernosus reflex
- Rectal examination to assess sphincter tone and stool impaction
- Cough stress test
- Urethral hypermobility via cotton swab test (performed by inserting the soft end of a cotton swab in the urethra to the urethrovesical junction and assessing angle change between the urethra at rest and with Valsalva maneuver; angle change or a resting angle of >30° suggests hypermobility)
- Postvoid residual with bladder scan or catheter to exclude retention

LABORATORY TESTS

It is important to rule out urinary tract infection and microscopic hematuria with urinalysis and/or culture prior to more invasive testing for other causes for incontinence.

TABLE 6 Comorbid Conditions That Can Cause or Contribute to Urinary Incontinence in Frail Older Adults

Conditions	Comments	Implications for Management
Comorbid Medical Illnesses		
Diabetes mellitus	Poor control can cause polyuria and precipitate or exacerbate incontinence; also associated with increased likelihood of urgency incontinence and diabetic neuropathic bladder	Better control of diabetes can reduce osmotic diuresis and associated polyuria, improve incontinence
Degenerative joint disease	Can impair mobility and precipitate urgency UI	Optimal pharmacologic and nonpharmacologic pain management can improve mobility, toileting ability
Chronic pulmonary disease	Associated cough can worsen stress UI	Cough suppression can reduce stress incontinence and cough-induced urgency UI
Congestive heart failure Lower extremity venous insufficiency	Increased nighttime urine production can contribute to nocturia and UI	Optimizing pharmacologic management of congestive heart failure, sodium restriction, support stockings, leg elevation, and late afternoon dose of rapid-acting diuretic may reduce nocturnal polyuria, associated nocturia, nighttime UI
Sleep apnea	May increase nighttime urine production by increasing production of atrial natriuretic peptide	Diagnosis and treatment of sleep apnea, usually with continuous positive airway pressure devices, may relieve UI, reduce nocturnal polyuria and associated nocturia
Severe constipation and fecal impaction	Associated with "double" incontinence (urine and fecal)	Appropriate use of stool softeners Adequate fluid intake and exercise Disimpaction if necessary
Neurologic and Psychiatric Conditions		
Stroke	Can precipitate urgency UI and, less often, urinary retention; also impairs mobility	UI after acute stroke often resolves with rehabilitation; persistent UI should be further evaluated. Regular toileting assistance essential for those with persistent mobility impairment
Parkinson disease	Associated with urgency UI; also causes impaired mobility and cognition in late stages	Optimizing management may improve mobility, improve UI. Regular toileting assistance essential for those with mobility and cognitive impairment in late stages
Normal-pressure hydrocephalus	Presents with UI, along with gait and cognitive impairments	Patients presenting with all three symptoms should be considered for brain imaging to rule out this condition; may improve with a ventricular-peritoneal shunt
Dementia (Alzheimer, multiinfarct, others)	Associated with urgency UI; impaired cognition and apraxia interfere with toileting and hygiene	Regular toileting assistance essential for those with mobility and cognitive impairment in late stages
Depression	May impair motivation to be continent; may also be a consequence of incontinence	Optimizing pharmacologic and nonpharmacologic management of depression may improve UI Discontinuation or modification of drug regimen
Medications		
Functional Impairments		
Impaired mobility, impaired cognition	Impaired cognition and/or mobility due to a variety of conditions (listed above) and others can interfere with ability to toilet independently and can precipitate UI	Regular toileting assistance essential for those with severe mobility and/or cognitive impairment
Environmental Factors		
Inaccessible toilets Unsafe toilet facilities No contrasting color between toilet and seat Caregivers unavailable for toileting assistance	Frail, functionally impaired persons require accessible and safe toilet facilities and, in many cases, human assistance to be continent	Environmental alterations may be helpful; supportive measures such as pads may be necessary if caregiver assistance not regularly available

UI, Urinary incontinence.
From Fillit HM: *Brocklehurst's textbook of geriatric medicine and gerontology*, ed 8, Philadelphia, 2017, Elsevier.

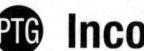

TABLE 7 Medications That Can Cause or Contribute to Urinary Incontinence in Frail Older Adults

Medications	Effects on Continence
α-Adrenergic agonists	Increased smooth muscle tone in urethra and prostatic capsule may precipitate obstruction, urinary retention, related symptoms
α-Adrenergic antagonists	Decreased smooth muscle tone in urethra may precipitate stress urinary incontinence in women
Angiotensin-converting enzyme inhibitors	Cause cough that can exacerbate UI
Anticholinergics	May cause impaired emptying, urinary retention, and constipation, which can contribute to UI; may cause cognitive impairment, reduce effective toileting ability
Calcium channel blockers	May cause impaired emptying, urinary retention, and constipation, which can contribute to UI; may cause dependent edema, which can contribute to nocturnal polyuria
Cholinesterase inhibitors	Increase bladder contractility, may precipitate urgency UI
Diuretics	Cause diuresis and precipitate UI
Lithium	Polyuria due to diabetes insipidus
Opioid analgesics	May cause urinary retention, constipation, confusion, immobility, all of which can contribute to UI
Psychotropic drugs Sedatives Hypnotics Antipsychotics Histamine-1 receptor antagonists	May cause confusion and impaired mobility and precipitate UI; anticholinergic effects; confusion
Selective serotonin reuptake inhibitors	Increase cholinergic transmission, may lead to urinary UI
Others—gabapentin, glitazones, nonsteroidal antiinflammatory drugs	Can cause edema, which can lead to nocturnal polyuria and cause nocturia and nighttime UI

UI, Urinary incontinence.
From Fillit HM: *Brocklehurst's textbook of geriatric medicine and gerontology,* ed 8, Philadelphia, 2017, Elsevier.

SPECIALIZED STUDIES

- **Urodynamic testing** measures different facets of urine storage and evacuation; usually necessary only if basic office evaluation does not elicit the cause of incontinence, if incontinence is persistent despite treatments, or if there are confounding contributors to incontinence including prior surgery.
  1. Uroflowmetry and pressure-flow studies: Measure the mechanisms of bladder emptying and rate of urine flow; can also measure detrusor pressure during voiding
  2. Simple cystometrogram: Graph of bladder and abdominal pressures related to fluid volume during filling/storage/voiding to assess sensation and capacity; also assesses presence of detrusor contractions and whether they are voluntary or involuntary
  3. Urethral pressure profile: Measures maximum urethral closure pressure (MUCP) and can aid in the diagnosis of intrinsic sphincter deficiency
  4. Electromyography studies the neuromuscular activity of pelvic muscles and striated urethral sphincter during filling and micturition
- **A cystourethroscopy** is a procedure that can be done in the office or the operating room. An endoscope is inserted into the urethra to view the inside of the bladder and urethra. This procedure is not routinely used to evaluate incontinence unless hematuria is present or prior pelvic surgery is noted on history.

IMAGING STUDIES

Imaging is usually ordered only if history and/or physical findings suggest other, less common, causes of incontinence (i.e., genitourinary fistula) or if microscopic hematuria is present.

- Renal ultrasound: Can assess for hydronephrosis
- CT urogram: Can assess for upper urinary tract abnormalities, congenital anomalies, genitourinary fistula, and microscopic hematuria etiologies

Rx TREATMENT

CONSERVATIVE/NONSURGICAL TREATMENT

The recommended approach to urinary incontinence is a stepwise care plan first offering noninvasive behavioral modifications such as bladder training, weight loss, and fluid management, before escalating to medications and/or surgical procedures. Treatment for urinary retention and overflow incontinence specifically focuses on reversal of modifiable factors and drainage of urine from the bladder via clean intermittent self-catheterization.

- **Pelvic floor muscle training (PFMT),** including Kegel exercises, often augmented with biofeedback or electrical stimulation, is an important component of first-line therapy for stress, urge, and mixed incontinence. Women should perform 45 to 50 exercises per day to achieve good results. One systematic review from the Agency for Healthcare

Research and Quality showed that PFMT is effective alone or in combination with other modalities such as medications or weight loss in improving continence for patients.[6]

- **Local estrogen** may have some benefit in decreasing urinary incontinence, especially in women who have some degree of atrophy.[7] Systemic estrogen therapy does not appear to be effective in treatment or prevention of incontinence.
- **Continence devices** are available as a nonsurgical option for women who experience primarily stress incontinence and can be used as a bridge to a surgical option. Continence pessaries help increase urethral resistance during increased intraabdominal pressure. Over-the-counter vaginal or urethral inserts are disposable devices used to support the urethra. They have been shown to reduce leakage episodes by about 50%[8] and may be a good option for women with situational stress incontinence (i.e., only when exercising).
- **Pharmacotherapy** is usually reserved for urgency urinary incontinence (Table 8). There are a number of medications that can be used alone or in combination with other treatment modalities to achieve the best symptom control for patients. The combination of anticholinergic drug and a β3 agonist may be more effective than either drug alone in patients who do not respond to monotherapy.
  1. Antimuscarinic (anticholinergic) medications: Block parasympathetic muscarinic receptors (detrusor M2/M3 receptors) to inhibit involuntary detrusor contractions
     a. Agents: Darifenacin, fesoterodine, oxybutynin (available orally and as a transdermal patch), solifenacin, tolterodine, and trospium
     b. Efficacy: Shown to improve symptoms and continence but only modestly compared with placebo
     c. Side effects: High rates of discontinuation due to side effects, most often dry mouth and constipation. May also exacerbate urinary retention, blurred vision, dyspepsia, and impaired cognitive function, with some studies now showing an association with dementia if used for >2 yr; contraindicated in narrow-angle glaucoma
     d. Of note, trospium may have a lower risk of cognitive impairment given the size of the molecule as it is less likely to cross the blood-brain barrier
  2. β-agonists: Stimulate β3-adrenergic receptor in the detrusor muscle to cause relaxation and increase bladder capacity
     a. Agents available: Mirabegron, vibegron
     b. Efficacy: Significant reductions in urgency incontinence in randomized trials
     c. Side effects:
        (1) Mirabegron: Tachycardia, hypertension, headache, and diarrhea (similar to placebo); not recommended in uncontrolled hypertension
        (2) Vibegron: most common side effects are headaches and nasopharyngitis; not associated with hypertension

Diseases and Disorders

I

TABLE 8 Pharmacologic Treatment for Urgency Urinary Incontinence

Indication(s)	Agent	Comments
Urgency UI OAB Urgency predominant–stress UI	All agents	With baseline average UI episodes/day of 1.6 to 5.3, mean reduction in episodes/day with placebo 1.08 (95% CI, 0.86-1.30); vs. IR formulations 1.46 (1.28, 1.64), and ER formulations 1.78 (1.61, 1.94). Head-to-head comparison trials of agents of limited quality
Antimuscarinics	Oxybutynin Immediate release (IR) 2.5-5 mg three to four times daily Extended release (ER, Ditropan XL) 5-20 mg once daily Topical patch (Oxytrol) 3.9-mg patch applied twice weekly Topical gel (Gelnique) 3% (84 mg, pump) and 10% (100 mg, sachet) once daily	Highest rate of dry mouth with immediate release, lowest with topical forms Application site rash in ~15% with patch
	Tolterodine	
	IR (Detrol) 1-2 mg one tab twice daily	
	ER (Detrol LA) 2-4 mg once daily	
	Fesoterodine (Toviaz) 4-8 mg once daily	Prodrug of tolterodine
	Darifenacin (Enablex) 7.5-15 mg once daily	Constipation
	Solifenacin (VESIcare) 5-10 mg once daily	
	Trospium IR (Sanctura) 20 mg once to twice daily ER (Sanctura XR) 60 mg daily β-3 agonist	Must be given on empty stomach
Urgency UI OAB	Mirabegron (Myrbetriq) 25-50 mg once daily	ADEs include hypertension; use with caution in patients with hypertension. Use with caution with metoprolol and digoxin

ADEs, Adverse drug effects; *OAB,* overactive bladder; *UI,* urinary incontinence.
From Warshaw G et al: *Ham's primary care geriatrics,* ed 7, Philadelphia, 2022, Elsevier.

TABLE 9 Minimally Invasive Treatment for Refractory Urge Urinary Incontinence

Treatment	Method	Efficacy/Level of Evidence	Comments
Botulinum toxin	Injection in detrusor during cystoscopy	Can reduce UI with a slightly higher cure compared with antimuscarinics, although with a greater risk of urinary retention (Level of Evidence = B)	Patients must be willing to do self-catheterization because of the risk of urinary retention Optimal dosing for specific patient groups such as older women is uncertain
Sacral nerve modulation	Percutaneous implantation of a trial electrode at the S3 sacral root, which is connected to an external stimulator. Patients responding to the trial have a permanent lead with a pacemaker-like energy source implanted		Anticipated newer MRI-compatible models will end need to explant stimulators before imaging
Percutaneous tibial nerve stimulation		Very small trials only	Patients unlikely to see efficacy before 6 wk of treatment Limited coverage by insurance

MRI, Magnetic resonance imaging; *UI,* urinary incontinence.
From Warshaw G et al: *Ham's primary care geriatrics,* ed 7, Philadelphia, 2022, Elsevier.

MINIMALLY INVASIVE TREATMENT OPTIONS

For urgency urinary incontinence specifically, there are multiple minimally invasive treatment options that can provide relief for patients whose symptoms do not respond to conservative measures and allow them to avoid surgery (Table 9).

- **OnabotulinumtoxinA (Botox A)** inhibits the presynaptic release of acetylcholine from motor neurons at the neuromuscular junction to paralyze the muscle and is administered via cystoscopic intravesical injection every 6 to 12 mo. It shows similar rates of improvement compared with antimuscarinic medications, but more women report complete resolution of urgency urinary incontinence with Botox A. It is considered a third-line treatment due to adverse effects, including urinary retention or incomplete

bladder emptying (5% requiring catheterization) and urinary tract infections (33%).[9]
- **Peripheral tibial nerve stimulation** has a pooled success rate of 60% compared with placebo in a guideline published by American Urological Association. Patients receive 30 min sessions of tibial nerve stimulation once per wk for 12 wk followed by a customized maintenance plan to treat OAB. Fewer adverse events were noted when compared with antimuscarinic medication.
- **Sacral neuromodulation** refers to the stimulation of the bladder and pelvic floor nerves to treat OAB, UUI, and idiopathic urinary retention via a currently unknown mechanism. It consists of a two-stage procedure: An electrode is placed near S3 and connected to an external generator that can be adjusted to maximize symptom control. If symptoms are improved

by 50%, planning to implant the pulse generator can begin. Evidence suggests 70% of women experience significant improvement in their symptoms with sacral neuromodulation.

SURGERY

Surgical options for treatment of stress urinary incontinence are outlined in Table 10. These are indicated for women who have not achieved symptom control with conservative management or as a first-line treatment in appropriately counseled women who decline more conservative treatment.

- Synthetic slings are the most common primary surgical treatment for SUI. Cure rates of 62% to 98% have been reported in a recent systematic review:
  1. Transvaginal/retropubic: Trocars are passed through the retropubic space from the midurethra to the abdomen (or vice versa).

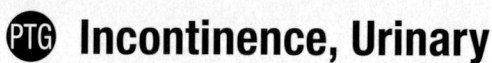

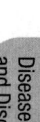

TABLE 10 Surgical Treatment of Stress Incontinence

Abdominal retropubic urethropexy (suspension)
Marshall-Marchetti-Krantz
Burch operation
Sling procedure:
  Pubovaginal (bladder neck) sling
Autologous:
  Rectus abdominis fascia
  Tensor fascia lata
  Anterior vaginal wall sling
  Allograft (cadaveric fascia lata fascia)
Xenograft:
  Porcine dermis
  Small intestinal submucosa
  Synthetic mesh (polypropylene)
Tension-free midurethral sling (polypropylene):
  Retropubic
  Transobturator
  Single incision
Urethral-bulking agents:
  Carbon-coated zirconium beads
  Calcium hydroxyapatite
  Cross-linked polydimethylsiloxane

From Lipshultz LI et al: *Urology and the primary care practitioner*, ed 3, Philadelphia, 2008, Elsevier.

Short-term cure rates range from 73% to 82%, according to a 2009 Cochrane meta-analysis, with de novo urgency in approximately 6% of patients

2. Transobturator: Trocars are passed from the vagina behind the ischium (or vice versa), with similar cure rates as the retropubic slings
3. Single-incision slings: Only one vaginal incision is needed beneath the urethra; ends of the sling are secured in the internal obturator muscle. A trial comparing mini-slings with midurethral slings revealed that single-incision mini-slings were noninferior to standard midurethral slings with respect to patient-recorded success at 15 mo, and the percentage of patients reporting success remained similar in the two groups at the 36-mo follow-up[10]

- Autologous fascial slings: Usually considered second line after the failure of synthetic slings due to length and morbidity of the operation. Cure rates estimated to be 50% to 75% depending on definition of cure
- Cadaveric slings: Usually second line; use has declined more recently because of concerns with early failure and declining success rate over time. Cure rates of 74% at 12 to 23 mo and 80% at 48 mo or greater

- Retropubic urethropexy (i.e., Burch procedure [open abdominal or laparoscopic]): A large meta-analysis estimated cure rates to be 82% at 12 to 23 mo and 73% at 48 mo or longer for open procedures
- **Bulking agents** injected into the urethra are used for the treatment of stress incontinence without hypermobility or in poor surgical candidates. Available agents include carbon-coated zirconium beads, calcium hydroxyapatite, and cross-linked polydimethylsiloxane. This option is relatively noninvasive but less effective than surgical intervention. The cure rate at 1 yr is 63% to 80%
  1. Fig. E3 illustrates a treatment algorithm for stress, urge, and mixed incontinence.
  2. Fig. E4 summarizes the diagnosis and treatment of overactive bladder.

REFERENCES & SUGGESTED READINGS
Available at eBooks.Health.Elsevier.com.

RELATED CONTENT
Urinary Incontinence (Patient Information)
Pelvic Organ Prolapse (Related Key Topic)

AUTHORS: **SAMANTHA BARTA, DO** and **ANTHONY SCISCIONE, DO**

 BASIC INFORMATION

DEFINITION

Inflammatory anemia, also known as anemia of chronic disease (ACD), refers to the impaired production of erythrocytes associated with chronic inflammatory states, such as cancer, chronic infection, or autoimmune diseases. Recent data have connected inflammatory anemia with severe, acute inflammation, such as critical illness, or with milder but persistent inflammatory signals that occur in obesity, aging, and kidney failure.[1] It is a disorder of iron homeostasis (Table 1) promoted by hepcidin-25 in response to an inflammatory condition.

SYNONYMS

Anemia of chronic disease
ACD
Anemia, inflammatory

ICD-10CM CODES

D63.8	Anemia in chronic diseases classified elsewhere
D63.0	Anemia in neoplastic disease
D64.8	Anemia, unspecified

EPIDEMIOLOGY & DEMOGRAPHICS

PREVALENCE:
- Second-most prevalent anemia after iron deficiency anemia:
  1. Around 11% of men and 10% of women ages 65 to 85 yr
  2. >20% of adults older than 85 yr

PATHOPHYSIOLOGY (FIG. 1)

Iron is carried in the bloodstream shelled by a hollow protein called transferrin (<0.2% of total iron body content) or at the core of hemoglobin in red blood cells (RBCs; 60% of total iron body content). It is mainly stored (15% to 30% of total iron body content) inside the liver, spleen, and skeletal muscle as ferritin and in lysosomes as hemosiderin. The rest of the body iron content is trapped in skeletal muscle myoglobin and mitochondrial cytochromes. In clinical practice, ferritin is a surrogate for iron stores, and total iron binding capacity (TIBC) is a surrogate for transferrin and iron carrying capacity.

Cells involved in the response to inflammation cause the release of cytokines, such as interleukin 6 (IL-6), which stimulates hepatic release of hepcidin. Hepcidin is a circulating protein that blocks ferroportin, an iron channel responsible for the exit of iron from enterocytes

TABLE 1 Suspected Causes of Anemia of Chronic Disease

Shortened erythrocyte survival

Block in reuse of iron by erythrocyte

Direct inhibition of erythropoiesis

Relative deficiency of erythropoietin

From Hoffman R et al: *Hematology, basic principles and practice,* ed 7, Philadelphia, 2018, Elsevier.

(and thus gastrointestinal absorption) and macrophages (which accumulate iron from engulfed senescent blood cells). IL-1 and tumor necrosis factor (TNF)-alpha stimulate interferon-gamma release by marrow stromal cells, which in turn suppress the erythroid response to erythropoietin (EPO). In chronic kidney disease, ACD is a consequence of decreased production of EPO and decreased renal clearance of hepcidin. The low availability of serum iron causes iron deficiency in the bone marrow compartment and decreased reticulocyte levels.

PHYSICAL FINDINGS & CLINICAL PRESENTATION

- Generalized symptoms include fatigue, shortness of breath, and weakness.
- It is important to consider other complaints if the underlying diagnosis is unknown, such as weight loss (malignancy, chronic infections, connective tissue diseases), anorexia, nausea, paresthesias, pleuritic chest pain, weight gain (chronic kidney disease [CKD]), diarrhea, bloody stools, abdominal pain, oral ulcers (inflammatory bowel disease [IBD]), and fevers (HIV, chronic infections).
- Physical findings may include pallor, lymphadenopathy, signs of connective tissue diseases (malar rash, sclerodactyly), palpable or visible masses, and localized findings for infection or malignancy.

ETIOLOGY

- Malignancy
- CKD (patients with CKD stage IV [glomerular filtration rate {GFR} <30 ml/min] should be screened for ACD)
- Congestive heart failure (CHF; ACD is the main cause of anemia in CHF patients)
- Chronic infections
- Anemia of critical illness (develops within days)
- Connective tissue diseases

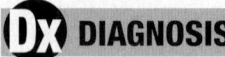 DIAGNOSIS

Isolated ACD:
- CBC with differential: Normocytic, normochromic, moderate (Hb rarely <8 g/dl) anemia
- Hypoproliferative anemia (low reticulocyte index; corrected reticulocyte count <2%)

Iron studies:
- Low iron concentration as in IDA (iron deficiency anemia)
- Normal/high ferritin (>35 mg/dl) in ACD as it is an acute phase reactant (Fig. 2)
- Low/normal TIBC (as opposed to IDA) and low transferrin saturation (as in IDA)
- Normal soluble transferrin receptor (sTfR, high in IDA)

Combined ACD/IDA:
- If normal to high ferritin, sTfR/log ferritin ratio <1 defines isolated ACD, and ratio >2 defines combined IDA/ACD

DIFFERENTIAL DIAGNOSIS

- Liver injury (increases ferritin):
  1. Iron deficiency anemia:
     a. Other causes of normocytic anemia or microcytic anemia (Table 2)
     b. Red blood cell loss or destruction:
        (1) Acute blood loss
        (2) Hypersplenism
        (3) Hemolysis
     c. Decreased red blood cell production:
        (1) Primary causes:
            (a) Bone marrow hypoplasia or aplasia
            (b) Myeloproliferative disease
            (c) Pure red blood cell aplasia
     d. Secondary causes:
        (1) Chronic renal failure
        (2) Liver disease
        (3) Endocrine deficiency states
        (4) Sideroblastic anemia

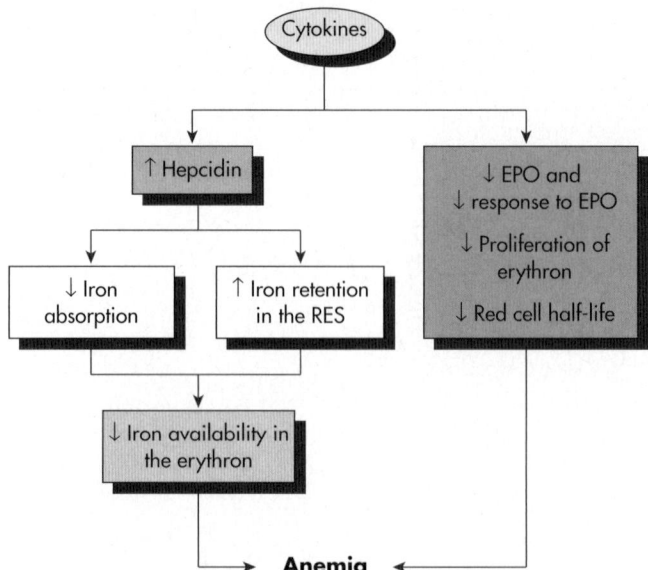

FIG. 1 Pathophysiologic factors associated with the development of anemia of chronic disease. *EPO,* Erythropoietin; *RES,* reticuloendothelial system. (From Hoffman R et al: *Hematology, basic principles and practice,* ed 7, Philadelphia, 2018, Elsevier.)

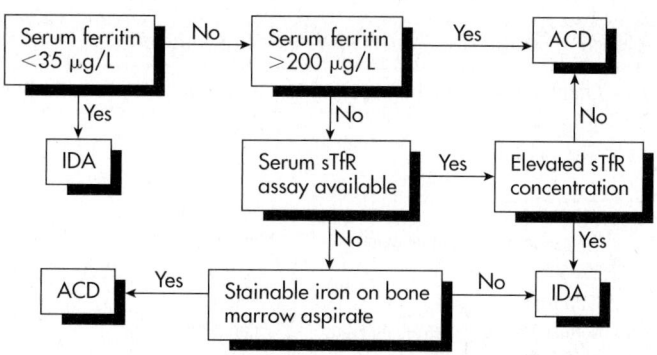

FIG. 2 Differential diagnosis of anemia with low serum iron. *ACD,* Anemia of chronic disease; *IDA,* iron deficiency anemia; *sTfR,* soluble transferrin receptor.

TABLE 2 Laboratory Features in Microcytic Hypochromic Anemias

| | Serum Iron | Serum TIBC | % Saturation | MARROW | | Serum Ferritin | ZPP | Hb A₂ | Hb F |
				% Sideroblasts	Iron Stores				
Iron deficiency	↓	↑	↓	↓	↓	↓	↑	N-↓	N
β-Thalassemia trait	N (↑)	N	N	N	N-↑	N-↑	N	↑	N-↑
ACD	↓	N-↓	↓	↓	N-↑	N-↑	↑	N	N
Sideroblastic anemia	↑	↓	↑	↑	↑	↑	↑ (↓)	N	N-↑

ACD, Anemia of chronic disease; *Hb,* hemoglobin; *N,* normal; *TIBC,* total iron-binding capacity; *ZPP,* zinc protoporphyrins; ↓, decreased; ↑, increased.
From McPherson RA, Pincus MR: *Henry's clinical diagnosis and management by laboratory methods,* ed 23, Philadelphia, 2017, Elsevier.

WORKUP

CBC, reticulocyte count, peripheral smear (Fig. E3), iron level, ferritin, TIBC. Table 3 summarizes characteristic findings in inflammatory anemia. Characteristic bone marrow findings of increased iron stores in stromal histiocytes and impaired erythroid iron incorporation are shown in Fig. E4.

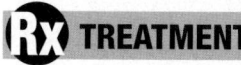 **TREATMENT**

Treat the underlying disorder/disease.

ACUTE GENERAL Rx

- The treatment of inflammatory anemia is directed primarily at treatment of underlying conditions, which can improve symptoms and facilitate hemoglobin recovery.
- Packed RBC (PRBC) transfusion is usually reserved for severe anemia (with Hb level <7 g/dl or <8 g/dl in patients with cardiac disease), especially if complicated with ongoing bleeding.

CHRONIC Rx

- Erythropoiesis-stimulating agents (ESA) (epoetin alfa and darbepoetin alfa) are FDA approved for use in patients with anemia resulting from:
  1. Chronic kidney disease
  2. Chemotherapy

- A 1998 study, the Normal Hematocrit Cardiac Trial (NHCT), showed a nonsignificant increase in the combined endpoint death and nonfatal myocardial infarction in patients with goal hematocrit of 33% versus 27%. Subsequent studies (CHOIR, CREATE, and TREAT) showed that higher doses and higher hematocrit targets were associated with increased cardiovascular events.
- ESA dose should be individualized for each patient, and the lowest sufficient dose to reduce PRBC transfusions should be used.[2] A hemoglobin target of ~10 g% is widely accepted. Iron deficiency should be ruled out before ESA is started. After starting ESA therapy, ASH/ASCO guidelines recommend periodic monitoring of iron status. When there is no or suboptimal response to oral therapy, parenteral iron therapy should be considered before concluding that a patient is nonresponsive to iron therapy.
- The hepcidin–ferroportin axis is the target of development of novel agents of which the most promising are hypoxia-induced factor modulators. Hypoxia-inducible factor (HIF) is a transcription factor that promotes expression of erythropoietin. HIF is upregulated by inhibition of PHD. Small molecule inhibitors of prolyl hydroxylase domain dioxygenases (HIF-PHI [prolyl hydroxylase inhibitor]) stimulate the production of endogenous erythropoietin and improve iron metabolism.[3] The clinical development of three oral agents targeting this axis—daprodustat, roxadustat, and vadadustat—has now completed randomized clinical development.

- Among patients with CKD undergoing dialysis, the oral hypoxia-inducible factor prolyl hydroxylase inhibitors (HIF-PHI) daprodustat was noninferior to ESAs regarding the change in the hemoglobin level from baseline and cardiovascular outcomes.
- Additionally, among patients with CKD and anemia who were not undergoing dialysis, daprodustat was noninferior to darbepoetin alfa with respect to the change in the hemoglobin level from baseline and with respect to cardiovascular outcomes.

AUTHOR: **DONNY V. HUYNH, MD**

REFERENCES

Available at eBooks.Health.Elsevier.com.

TABLE 3 Laboratory Characteristics of ACD, IDA, and IDA with Inflammation

	Anemia of Chronic Disease (ACD)	Iron Deficiency Anemia (IDA)	IDA With Inflammation
Mean corpuscular volume (MCV)	72-100 fl	<85 fl	<100 fl
Mean corpuscular hemoglobin concentration (MCHC)	<36 g/dl	<32 g/dl	<32 g/dl
Serum iron	Decreased	Decreased	Decreased
Serum total iron-binding capacity (TIBC)	Typical below midnormal range	Elevated	Less than upper limit of normal range
Transferrin saturation*	2%-20%	<15% (usually <10%)	<15%
Serum ferritin	>35 μg/L	<35 μg/L	>35 μg/L, <200 μg/L
Serum soluble transferrin receptor concentration (sTfR)	Normal (may be increased if serum ferritin >200 μg/L)	Increased	Increased
TfR index (sTfR/log ferritin)	<1	>2	>2
Hepcidin	High	Low	Normal
Stainable iron in bone marrow	Present	Absent	Absent

*Serum Iron concentration ÷ TIBC x 100.

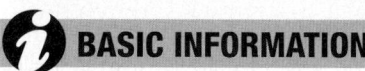

BASIC INFORMATION

DEFINITION

Inflammatory myopathies are idiopathic diseases of muscle characterized clinically by muscle weakness and pathologically by inflammation and muscle fiber breakdown. They may be further classified as dermatomyositis (DM), immune-mediated necrotizing myopathy, polymyositis (PM), antisynthetase syndrome, and inclusion body myositis (IBM).[1] See separate topics on "Inclusion Body Myositis" and "Necrotizing Autoimmune Myopathy" for details regarding these topics.

SYNONYMS

Immune-mediated myopathies
Idiopathic inflammatory myopathies
Myositis syndromes
Polymyositis
Dermatomyositis
IMM

ICD-10CM CODES

M33.02	Juvenile dermatopolymyositis with myopathy
M33.12	Other dermatopolymyositis with myopathy
M33.20	Polymyositis, organ involvement unspecified
M33.22	Polymyositis with myopathy
M33.90	Dermatopolymyositis, unspecified, organ involvement unspecified
M33.92	Dermatopolymyositis, unspecified with myopathy

EPIDEMIOLOGY & DEMOGRAPHICS

Inflammatory myopathies are the largest group of potentially treatable myopathies in children and adults.
DM:
- Occurs in children and in adults (bimodal age peak)
- Average age at diagnosis is 40 to 60 yr in adults, 4 to 14 yr in children[2]
- More common in females than in males (2:1)[2]
- Incidence: 9.54 to 32.74:100,000[2]
- Dermatomyositis is associated with a higher risk of cancer, especially in those older than age 50 yr[3]
PM:
- Occurs mostly in adults, very rarely in children[4]
- Average age at diagnosis is over 20 yr[4]
- More common in females[4]
- Least common inflammatory myopathy[4]
- Exact incidence unknown
Antisynthetase syndrome:
- Associated with antibodies against aminoacyl transfer RNA synthetases[5]
- More common in women[5]
- Average age at diagnosis is 48 yr[5]

PHYSICAL FINDINGS & CLINICAL PRESENTATION

- Most patients have a subacute onset over weeks to months.

- Pattern is typically symmetric proximal muscle weakness involving the proximal limbs (shoulder and pelvic girdles).
- Weakness of neck flexion and extension is common.
- Difficulty getting up from a chair, climbing stairs, reaching for objects above head, or combing hair.
- Distal muscle involvement and ocular involvement are uncommon.
- Sensation is preserved.
- Reflexes may be preserved or diminished.
- Dysphagia and dysphonia result from involvement of striated muscle of the pharynx and proximal esophagus.
- Esophageal dysmotility is common in DM.
- Respiratory failure from associated pulmonary fibrosis.
- Cardiac conduction abnormalities can be seen with DM.
- Systemic autoimmune disease occurs frequently in PM and rarely in DM.
- Skin findings in DM:
  1. Heliotrope rash on the upper eyelids
  2. Erythematous rash on the face
  3. May also involve the back and shoulders (shawl sign), neck and chest (V-shape), knees (Fig. E1), and elbows
  4. Photosensitivity
  5. Gottron papules (violaceous papules overlying dorsal interphalangeal or metacarpophalangeal areas, elbow or knee joints)
  6. Nail cracking, thickening, and irregularity (Fig. E2) with periungual telangiectasia
  7. Associated with increased risk of interstitial lung disease
- Antisynthetase syndrome is associated with:
  1. Interstitial lung disease[5]
  2. Arthritis[5]
  3. Raynaud phenomenon[5]
  4. Mechanic's hands (dry, cracked skin on hands)[5]

ETIOLOGY

Mechanisms of muscle fiber damage in myositis are illustrated in Fig. E3.
- DM: Complex, immune-mediated microangiopathy. Adaptive immune response via humorally mediated complement attack
- PM: Unknown:
  1. Cell-mediated immune major histocompatibility-I (MHC-1) process directed against muscle fibers is likely, given biopsy features.

DIAGNOSIS

- The diagnosis of each subtype of inflammatory myopathy is based on clinical history, pattern of muscle involvement, electromyographic findings, muscle biopsy (Table E1), and presence of certain antibodies.
  1. Myopathic pattern of muscle weakness
  2. Characteristic rash in DM
  3. Electromyography (EMG) shows myopathic (small-amplitude, short-duration, polyphasic) motor potentials with early recruitment

4. Majority of patients have "irritable" features (fibrillations and positive sharp waves) on EMG
5. See "Laboratory Tests"
6. Biopsy is required for diagnosis and should confirm inflammation before treatment is started. Table 2 describes histologic features of idiopathic inflammatory myopathies. In idiopathic inflammatory myopathies, myopathic features (variation in fiber size, fiber splitting, fatty replacement of muscle tissue, and increased endomysial connective tissue) should be seen in addition to:
   a. DM: Perifascicular atrophy, membrane attack complex (MAC) deposition along capillaries
   b. PM: Endomysial infiltrates composed of CD8+ T cells and macrophages invading nonnecrotic muscle fibers that express MHC-I antigen

DIFFERENTIAL DIAGNOSIS (TABLE E3)

- IBM
- Muscular dystrophies
- Amyloid myoneuropathy
- Amyotrophic lateral sclerosis
- Myasthenia gravis
- Eaton-Lambert syndrome
- Drug-induced myopathies (e.g., quinidine, NSAIDs, penicillamine, HMG-CoA-reductase inhibitors)
- Diabetic amyotrophy
- Guillain-Barré syndrome
- Hyperthyroidism or hypothyroidism
- Lichen planus
- Amyopathic DM (rash without weakness)
- DM sine rash (weakness with characteristic biopsy, but no rash)
- Systemic lupus erythematosus (SLE)
- Contact atopic or seborrheic dermatitis
- Psoriasis

LABORATORY TESTS

- Creatine kinase (CK) is the most sensitive muscle enzyme test for muscle breakdown.
- CK is typically elevated (5 to $50\times$ normal) in active PM.
- CK may be normal or only slightly elevated in DM.
- Aldolase, aspartate aminotransferase, alanine aminotransferase, alkaline phosphatase, and lactate dehydrogenase (LDH) may be elevated.
- Anti-Jo-1 antibodies are seen in myositis with associated interstitial lung disease but are not specific for either DM or PM.
- Myositis-specific and myositis-associated autoantibodies in adult polymyositis and dermatomyositis and juvenile dermatomyositis are summarized in Table E4.
- DM: Anti-MDA-5, anti-Mi-2, anti-TIF-1, and anti-NXP2 (implicated in cancer-associated dermatomyositis).
- PM: Antisynthetase antibodies associated with interstitial lung disease, arthritis, fever, and "mechanic's hands."

Diseases and Disorders

I

TABLE 2 Histologic Features of Idiopathic Inflammatory Myopathies

Feature	Dermatomyositis	Polymyositis	Inclusion Body Myositis
Necrosis of muscle fibers	+	+	+
Variation in fiber diameter	+	+	+
Regeneration of muscle fibers	+	+	+
Proliferation of connective tissue	+	+	+
Infiltration of mononuclear cells*	+	+	+
Perivascular and perimysial inflammation	+	−/+	−/+
Endomysial inflammation	−/+	+	+
Perifascicular atrophy	+	−	−
Abnormally dilated capillaries	+	−/+	−
Reduced capillary density	+	−/+	−
Deposition of complement on vessel walls	+	−/+	−
Microinfarcts	+	−	−
Invasion of nonnecrotic fibers by cytotoxic T lymphocytes and macrophages	−	+	+
Expression of major histocompatibility complex class I on muscle fibers	−/+	+	+
Rimmed vacuoles with amyloid deposits and tubulofilaments†	−	−	+
Angulated or atrophic and hypertrophic fibers	−	−	+
Ragged red or cytochrome oxidase–negative fibers	−	−	+

*Inflammation is absent in a small proportion of polymyositis and dermatomyositis biopsies.
†Also seen in chronic neurogenic conditions and distal myopathies.
From Firestein GS et al: *Firestein & Kelley's textbook of rheumatology,* ed 9, Philadelphia, 2013, Saunders.

- Electrolytes, thyroid-stimulating hormone, Ca, and Mg should be evaluated to exclude other causes of weakness.
- Check ECG for cardiac involvement.

IMAGING STUDIES

- Chest x-ray is used to rule out pulmonary involvement. If suspicious for pulmonary interstitial disease, a high-resolution computed tomography scan of the chest may be helpful.
- Radiography is an efficient means of identifying and characterizing soft-tissue calcinosis (Fig. E4).
- Although MRI arguably has greater diagnostic value than electromyography or serum enzyme measurements in cases of suspected idiopathic inflammatory myopathy, MRI findings have not been formalized as a diagnostic criterion for idiopathic inflammatory myopathy. The acceptance of MRI as a diagnostic tool in myositis may be inhibited by the high cost and the need for more reliable and validated methods of summarizing the findings of MRI. MRI evaluation before biopsy, however, has become routine at many tertiary care centers. Fascial disease is manifested on MRI by fascial or perifascial hyperintensity on fluid-sensitive sequences. The edema-like signal in the deep subcutis may accompany fasciitis and can indicate associated panniculitis.
- Video fluoroscopy or barium swallow study to look for upper esophageal dysfunction in patients with dysphagia and DM.
- Table E5 summarizes affected organs and their evaluation in inflammatory muscle disease.

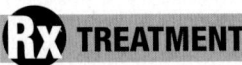 TREATMENT

Goal: Maintain function, minimize disease/iatrogenic sequelae

NONPHARMACOLOGIC THERAPY

- Sun-blocking agents with SPF 15 or greater for skin protection in patients with DM
- Physical therapy beneficial for gait training and increasing muscle tone and strength
- Occupational therapy assists with activities of daily living
- Speech therapy to monitor patients with swallowing dysfunction

ACUTE GENERAL Rx

- Corticosteroids are the mainstay of therapy. Start prednisone 0.7 to 1 mg/kg per day, up to a maximum dose of 60 mg/day. If severe disease, can give methylprednisolone 1 g intravenous (IV) daily for 3 to 5 days before starting prednisone. Continue until muscle strength improves. Begin tapering by 5 to 10 mg/mo. Consider every-other-day prednisone treatment at same dose (may decrease side effects).[6]
- Consider IV immunoglobulin (IVIG) if patient fails to improve on prednisone, or muscle enzymes begin rising when tapering off prednisone. See "Chronic Rx" for specific dosage.
- Hydroxychloroquine can be used to treat the cutaneous lesions of DM.
- A treatment algorithm for adult patients with inflammatory myopathies is illustrated in Fig. 5.

CHRONIC Rx

- Chronic prednisone therapy may be needed for years, but other immunosuppressive ("steroid-sparing") agents may be added early to decrease long-term steroid side effects.
- Azathioprine starting with 50 g daily, titrating to 100 mg/day after 1 wk to goal of 2 mg/kg/day.[6]
- Methotrexate 5 to 7.5 mg weekly, increased by 2.5 mg/wk to total of 25 mg/wk; consider intramuscular dosing if PO is ineffective. Use cautiously in patients with interstitial lung disease due to possible pulmonary fibrosis.
- IV immunoglobulin 2 g/kg total dose over 2 to 5 days.
- IV cyclophosphamide 0.5 to 1 g/m^2 monthly for 6 mo is preferred to oral dosing for refractory cases. However, oral dosing of cyclophosphamide is 1 to 2 mg/kg per day PO or 2 to 4 mg/kg per day in conjunction with prednisone.[6]
- Cyclosporine A: Initial dose 2.0 to 2.5 mg/kg bid; long-term maintenance is lowest effective dose.
- Mycophenolate mofetil 500 mg PO bid, titrate to 1500 mg PO bid over 1 to 2 mo.[6]

DISPOSITION

- 20% to 30% of patients achieve clinical remission with treatment.[6]
- In patients with residual weakness, deficits typically remain stable over long-term follow-up.
- 10% experience recurrent disease.
- Serum CK often returns to normal before symptoms improve.
- During exacerbations, enzymes may rise before clinical symptoms appear.
- Poor prognostic indicators include delay in diagnosis, older age, recalcitrant disease, malignancy, interstitial pulmonary fibrosis, dysphagia, leukocytosis, fever, and anorexia.
- Infection, malignancy, and cardiac and pulmonary dysfunction are the most common causes of death.

REFERRAL

Neurology or rheumatology referral should be made to help establish the diagnosis and implement treatment.

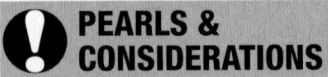 PEARLS & CONSIDERATIONS

- Do not implement treatment before muscle biopsy.
- When assessing response to treatment, clinical muscle strength is more important than muscle enzyme tests.
- The concern for malignancies (ovary, lung, breast, GI) associated with DM is legitimate and merits screening in patients older than age 40 at time of diagnosis and every 2 to 3 yr thereafter.
- No association exists between juvenile DM and malignancy.
- Overlap syndrome refers to patients with DM who also meet criteria for a connective tissue disorder (e.g., rheumatoid arthritis, scleroderma, SLE).

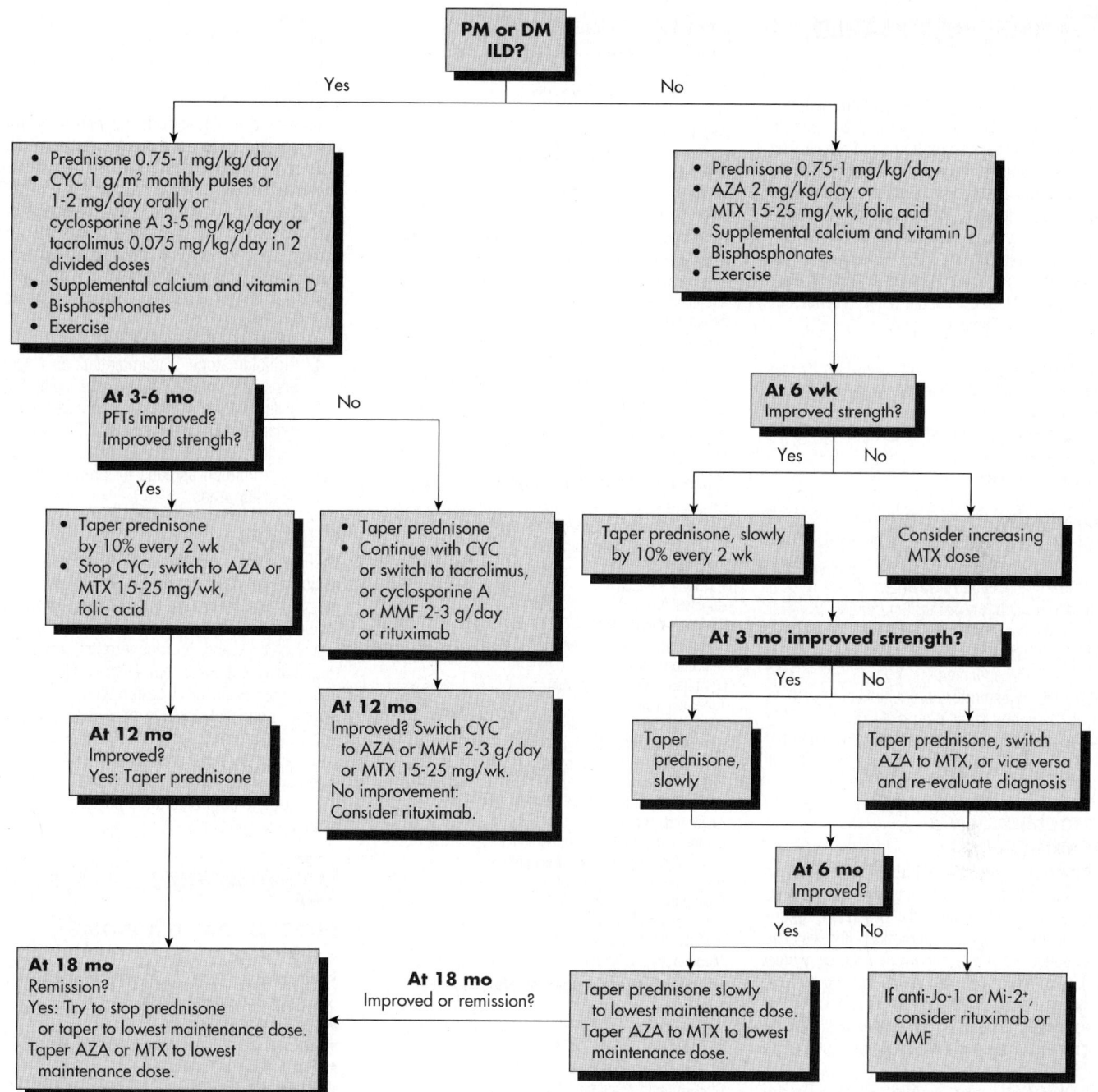

FIG. 5 Treatment algorithm for adult patients with polymyositis *(PM)* or dermatomyositis *(DM)*. *AZA,* Azathioprine; *CYC,* cyclophosphamide; *ILD,* interstitial lung disease; *MMF,* mycophenolate mofetil; *MTX,* methotrexate; *PFT,* pulmonary function test; *SC,* subcutaneous. (From Firestein GS et al: *Firestein & Kelley's textbook of rheumatology,* ed 11, Philadelphia, 2021, Elsevier.)

- In any patient taking steroids, closely monitor for:
  1. Diabetes or glucose intolerance (2-h oral glucose tolerance test)
  2. Osteopenia/osteoporosis (DEXA scan q6mo)
  3. Cataracts (yearly ophthalmologic appointment)
  4. Hypertension
  5. Psychiatric side effects including depression or psychosis
  6. Poor sleep
  7. Peptic ulcer disease (prescribe H₂ antagonist or proton pump inhibitor)
- Clinical and immune response features can be used for categorizing heterogeneous myositis syndromes and mutually exclusive and stable phenotypes and are useful for predicting clinical signs and symptoms, associated environmental and genetic risk factors, and responses to therapy and prognosis.

REFERENCES

Available at eBooks.Health.Elsevier.com.

RELATED CONTENT

Dermatomyositis and Polymyositis (Patient Information)
Inclusion Body Myositis (Related Key Topic)
Necrotizing Autoimmune Myopathy (Related Key Topic)

AUTHORS: **NAOMI R. KASS BA** and **LYDIA SHARP, MD**

Diseases and Disorders

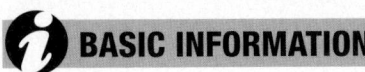 **BASIC INFORMATION**

DEFINITION

Interstitial lung disease (ILD) is a heterogenous group of disorders, characterized by varying patterns of lung inflammation and fibrosis. The term "ILD" arises from the histologic appearance that the interstitium is abnormal, although the alveoli, airways, blood vessels, lymphatic vessels, and pleura are often altered as well.[1] ILDs are classified as either arising from an identified cause or idiopathic.[2] A clinical classification of the interstitial lung diseases is summarized in Table 1.

SYNONYMS

Interstitial pulmonary disease
ILD
Diffuse parenchymal lung disease (DPLD)
Interstitial pneumonia
Pulmonary fibrosis

ICD-10CM CODES

J84.17	Other interstitial pulmonary diseases with fibrosis in diseases classified elsewhere
J84.89	Other specified interstitial pulmonary diseases
J84.9	Interstitial pulmonary disease, unspecified
J84.115	Respiratory bronchiolitis interstitial lung disease
J84.848	Other interstitial lung diseases of childhood

EPIDEMIOLOGY & DEMOGRAPHICS

INCIDENCE & PREVALENCE: Incidence varies widely with type of ILD. The most common ILDs are sarcoidosis, cryptogenic organizing pneumonia, and idiopathic pulmonary fibrosis. The prevalence of these syndromes varies widely across different populations as defined by age, gender, and race. The overall prevalence of ILD is estimated to be up to 76.0 cases per 100,000 people in Europe and 74.3 cases per 100,000 in the U.S.[3]

PREDOMINANT SEX & AGE: Some ILDs are more common in women, such as those resulting from autoimmune diseases, also known as connective tissue disorders.[4] Lymphangioleiomyomatosis (LAM) occurs almost exclusively in premenopausal women. ILDs caused by occupational exposures are more common in men. Most ILDs occur in people >50 yr; however, sarcoidosis most often presents in younger populations.

RISK FACTORS: Common identifiable risk factors include environmental exposures such as down, mold, silicone, and asbestos; reactions to drugs such as chemotherapeutic agents, tyrosine kinase inhibitors, amiodarone, and nitrofurantoin; radiation therapy; connective tissue disease including rheumatoid arthritis, scleroderma, and myosis; and pathologic acid reflux. Both tobacco and drug use can cause ILD. Some individuals have increased genetic

TABLE 1 Clinical Classification of the Interstitial Lung Diseases

Connective Tissue Diseases

Scleroderma
Polymyositis-dermatomyositis
Systemic lupus erythematosus
Rheumatoid arthritis
Mixed connective tissue disease
Ankylosing spondylitis

Treatment-Related or Drug-Induced Diseases

Antibiotics (nitrofurantoin, sulfasalazine)
Antiarrhythmics (amiodarone, tocainide, propranolol)
Antiinflammatories (gold, penicillamine)
Anticonvulsants (Dilantin)
Chemotherapeutic agents (mitomycin C, bleomycin, busulfan, cyclophosphamide, chlorambucil, methotrexate, azathioprine, BCNU [carmustine], procarbazine)
Therapeutic radiation
Oxygen toxicity
Narcotics

Primary and Idiopathic Diseases

Sarcoidosis
Primary pulmonary Langerhans cell histiocytosis (eosinophilic granuloma)
Amyloidosis
Pulmonary vasculitis
Gaucher disease
Niemann-Pick disease
Hermansky-Pudlak syndrome
Neurofibromatosis
Lymphangioleiomyomatosis
Tuberous sclerosis
Idiopathic pulmonary fibrosis
Nonspecific interstitial pneumonia
Cryptogenic organizing pneumonia
Respiratory bronchiolitis ILD or desquamative interstitial pneumonia
Acute interstitial pneumonia
Lymphocytic interstitial pneumonia
Pleuroparenchymal fibroelastosis
Bone marrow transplantation
Eosinophilic pneumonia
Alveolar proteinosis
Alveolar microlithiasis
Metastatic calcification

Occupational and Environmental Diseases

Inorganic
Silicosis
Asbestosis
Hard-metal pneumoconiosis
Coal worker's pneumoconiosis
Berylliosis
Talc pneumoconiosis
Siderosis (arc welder)
Stannosis (tin)

Organic (hypersensitivity pneumonitis)

Bird breeder's lung
Farmer's lung

ILD, Interstitial lung disease.
Modified from Mason RJ: *Murray & Nadel's textbook of respiratory medicine,* ed 5, Philadelphia, 2010, Saunders.

susceptibility to developing ILD from impaired cellular repair mechanisms, such as telomere shortening.

PHYSICAL FINDINGS & CLINICAL PRESENTATION

- Shortness of breath (especially with exertion)
- Cough (dry)
- Tachypnea
- Bibasilar end-inspiratory dry crackles
- Pulmonary hypertension
- Cyanosis
- Clubbing

Hallmarks of ILD include restriction of lung volumes and reduced diffusing capacity. The restrictive process can result from different abnormalities depending on the type of ILD including acute and subacute inflammatory changes, which are potentially reversible, and fibrosis, which is largely irreversible. Diffusion abnormalities can result from loss of functional capillaries from fibrosis, emphysema, or pulmonary hypertension.

- Specific changes may be seen:
  1. Granulomatous: Accumulation of T lymphocytes, macrophages, and epithelioid cells into granulomas in lung parenchyma
  2. Inflammation and fibrosis: Injury to epithelium causes inflammation; if chronic, inflammation spreads to interstitium and vascular areas

ETIOLOGY

The lungs are constantly exposed to potentially noxious stimuli from environmental and occupational exposures, smoking, drugs, radiation, autoimmune disease, pathologic acid reflux, etc. Lung injury leads to regeneration, repair, or remodeling responses that can result in restoration of normal tissue, inflammation, or fibrosis. Alveolar epithelial damage from repeated injuries promotes migration of inflammatory cells into the lungs. If regeneration or repair of the epithelium fails, remodeling occurs.[5] A fibrotic milieu promotes proliferation of fibroblasts and collagen deposition.

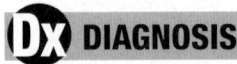 **DIAGNOSIS**

DIFFERENTIAL DIAGNOSIS

- Heart failure
- Pneumonia: Viral, bacterial, mycobacterial, fungal, and pneumocystis
- Pulmonary embolism
- Chronic obstructive pulmonary disease
- Pulmonary hypertension
- Vasculitis
- Metastatic malignancy manifesting as lymphangitic carcinomatosis
- Conditions associated with nonspecific interstitial pneumonitis pattern are summarized in Table 2

WORKUP

- Establishing a confident ILD diagnosis, as well as the type of ILD, which has treatment and prognostic implications, requires identifying clinical, radiographic, and histologic patterns of lung injury.
- Multidisciplinary discussion (MDD), which is considered the standard of care to diagnose ILD, includes a pulmonologist, radiologist, and pathologist. Detailed exposure history, exam findings, pulmonary function tests (PFT), laboratory tests, and high-resolution computed tomography (HRCT) scan of the chest are

I

TABLE 2 Conditions Associated with Nonspecific Interstitial Pneumonitis Pattern

Autoimmune connective tissue diseases
Chronic hypersensitivity pneumonitis
Infection (e.g., viral or atypical bacterial)
Inherited or acquired immunodeficiency
Drug toxicity
Idiopathic

From Broaddus VC et al: *Murray & Nadel's textbook of respiratory medicine,* ed 7, Philadelphia, 2022, Elsevier.

reviewed. If a confident diagnosis remains unclear, surgical lung biopsy should be considered and then reviewed in MDD. Fig. 1 illustrates the approach to ILD diagnosis.

- PFTs most often show restriction, characterized by decreased total lung capacity (TLC) and forced vital capacity (FVC) due to reduced lung compliance caused by alveolar wall thickening or filling of alveolar spaces as a result of inflammation and fibrosis. Inflammation, fibrosis, emphysema, and pulmonary vascular alterations can lead to impaired gas exchange, measured by the diffusing capacity of carbon monoxide (DLCO). FEV_1/FVC is usually normal or increased because lung stiffness keeps small airways open, although some conditions (e.g., sarcoidosis, hypersensitivity pneumonitis) may cause small airway obstruction and air trapping.
- Bronchoscopy with bronchoalveolar lavage (BAL) can show increased lymphocytes in chronic hypersensitivity pneumonitis and sarcoidosis, increased eosinophils in eosinophilic pneumonia, and can exclude infection.
- Bronchoscopic transbronchial biopsy is of limited utility. Cryobiopsy may yield sufficient tissue when done by experienced operators. Surgical lung biopsy provides sufficient tissue for diagnosis in >90% of cases. Histologic patterns of lung injury and their ILD associations are summarized in Tables 3 and 4 and illustrated in Figs. E2 and E3.

LABORATORY TESTS

- Arterial blood gases may be normal or show respiratory alkalosis and widened Aa gradient.
- Serologic tests can identify autoimmune features and connective tissue diseases: Antinuclear antibodies, rheumatoid factor, anticyclic citrullinated peptide, SS-A, SS-B, Scl-70, RNA pol III, RNP, myositis panel, creatinine kinase, aldolase. Antineutrophil cytoplasmic antibodies or antibasement membrane antibodies should be obtained if vasculitis is suspected.
- Serum precipitins are of limited utility to investigate exposures associated with hypersensitivity pneumonitis.
- ACE testing (ACE levels) in sarcoidosis is of unclear value.
- Laboratory findings in the interstitial lung diseases are summarized in Table 5.

IMAGING STUDIES

- Chest x-ray examination may appear normal or show opacities, often in a reticular pattern.

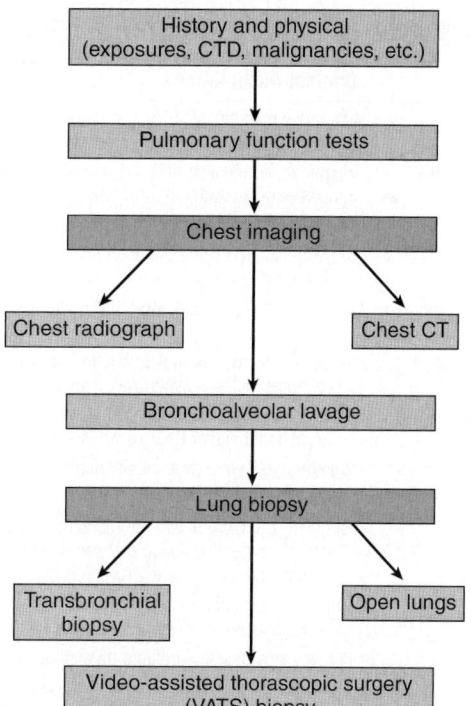

FIG. 1 Algorithm for the approach to a patient with interstitial lung disease. *CT,* Computed tomography; *CTD,* connective tissue disease. (From Sellke FW et al: *Sabiston and Spencer surgery of the chest,* ed 9, Philadelphia, 2016, Elsevier.)

- Chest computed tomography (CT) scan (Fig. E4) : High resolution CT (HRCT) is necessary to evaluate the radiographic pattern of lung injury. It can demonstrate consolidation, ground glass opacity, reticulation, traction bronchiectasis, fibrosis, air trapping, and cysts. It also may identify pulmonary artery enlargement in patients with pulmonary hypertension. Table 6 summarizes radiographic features of ILDs.
- Echocardiography is useful to evaluate cardiac size and function, and to screen for pulmonary hypertension, which can complicate advanced ILD.

Rx TREATMENT

NONPHARMACOLOGIC THERAPY

- Avoidance of tobacco and occupational exposures
- The mainstay of therapy is to identify the cause of the lung injury and completely avoid it, e.g., discontinue offending drugs or remove environmental exposures. Avoidance alone may be sufficient to reverse acute and subacute inflammation.

ACUTE GENERAL Rx

- Pharmacologic treatment varies significantly depending on the type of ILD; thus it is essential to try to correctly classify the type of ILD. Steroids and other immunosuppressants are beneficial for inflammatory conditions, such as hypersensitivity pneumonitis and connective tissue disease, but should be avoided in idiopathic pulmonary fibrosis. Please see specific

chapters on Asbestosis, Cryptogenic Organizing Pneumonia, Eosinophilic Granulomatosis with Polyangiitis, Eosinophilic Pneumonia, Hypersensitivity Pneumonitis, and Idiopathic Pulmonary Fibrosis that discuss specific treatment regimens.

- For patients with acute or subacute inflammation demonstrated by consolidation or ground glass opacity in HRCT, immunosuppression with steroids or steroid-sparing agents, such as mofetil mycophenolate and azathioprine, could expedite improvement. While steroids often cause rapid improvement, their multiple side effects may limit their prolonged use. Patients should be closely monitored with PFTs to assess the ILD trajectory. If there is improvement or stabilization after 4 to 12 wk of steroids, the dose should be tapered. If the patient's condition declines as steroids are weaned, starting mofetil mycophenolate or azathioprine for maintenance may allow steroid tapering. If patients are at high risk for steroid-induced side effects, mofetil mycophenolate or azathioprine monotherapy could be considered from the beginning.
- For patients with scleroderma-associated ILD and those with other progressive fibrosing ILDs, nintedanib added to immunosuppression or monotherapy should be considered. Nintedanib is a tyrosine kinase inhibitor with antifibrotic and antiinflammatory properties that lowers the annual rate of FVC decline compared to placebo.[6,7]

CHRONIC GENERAL Rx

- Supplemental oxygen in patients with hypoxemia is beneficial to support physical activity

TABLE 3 Histologic Patterns in the Interstitial Lung Diseases and Their Disease Associations

Histologic Patterns	Clinical Associations
Usual interstitial pneumonia	Idiopathic pulmonary fibrosis; connective tissue diseases (uncommon); asbestosis; chronic hypersensitivity pneumonitis; chronic aspiration pneumonia; chronic radiation pneumonitis; Hermansky-Pudlak syndrome
Nonspecific interstitial pneumonia	Idiopathic; connective tissue diseases; drugs; AIDS
Diffuse alveolar damage	Acute interstitial pneumonia (Hamman-Rich syndrome); acute respiratory distress syndrome (ARDS); drugs (cytotoxic agents, heroin, paraquat, ethchlorvynol, aspirin); toxic gas inhalation; radiation therapy; oxygen toxicity; connective tissue disease; infections
Organizing pneumonia	Cryptogenic organizing pneumonia; organizing stage of diffuse alveolar damage; drugs (amiodarone, cocaine); infections; connective tissue diseases
Desquamative interstitial pneumonia/ respiratory bronchiolitis	Cigarette smoking; idiopathic DIP of childhood
Lymphocytic interstitial pneumonia	Idiopathic; hypogammaglobulinemia; autoimmune diseases, including Hashimoto thyroiditis, lupus erythematosus, primary biliary cirrhosis, Sjögren syndrome, myasthenia gravis, chronic active hepatitis; AIDS; allogeneic bone marrow transplantation
Eosinophilic pneumonia	Idiopathic acute and chronic; tropical filarial eosinophilia; parasitic infections; allergic bronchopulmonary aspergillosis; allergic granulomatosis of Churg and Strauss; hypereosinophilic syndrome; AIDS
Alveolar proteinosis	Pulmonary alveolar proteinosis; acute silicosis; aluminum dust; AIDS; myeloproliferative disorder
Diffuse alveolar hemorrhage	
with capillaritis	Wegener granulomatosis; microscopic polyangiitis; systemic lupus erythematosus; polymyositis; scleroderma; rheumatoid arthritis; mixed connective tissue disease; lung transplantation; drugs (retinoic acid, propylthiouracil, Dilantin); Behçet disease; cryoglobulinemia; Henoch-Schönlein purpura; pauci-immune glomerulonephritis; immune complex glomerulonephritis
without capillaritis	Idiopathic pulmonary hemosiderosis; systemic lupus erythematosus; Goodpasture syndrome; diffuse alveolar damage; pulmonary venoocclusive disease; mitral stenosis; lymphangioleiomyomatosis
Amyloid deposition	Primary amyloidosis; multiple myeloma; lymphocytic interstitial pneumonia
Granuloma	Sarcoidosis; hypersensitivity pneumonitis; pulmonary Langerhans cell histiocytosis; silicosis; intravenous talcosis; berylliosis; lymphocytic interstitial pneumonia; infections

AIDS, Acquired immunodeficiency syndrome; *DIP,* desquamative interstitial pneumonia.
Modified from Broaddus VC et al: *Murray & Nadel's textbook of respiratory medicine,* ed 7, Philadelphia, 2022, Elsevier.

TABLE 4 Histologic Patterns of Interstitial Lung Disease

Acute lung injury
1. Diffuse alveolar damage
2. Organizing pneumonia
3. Acute fibrinous and organizing pneumonia
Consolidation of alveolar spaces
1. Eosinophilic pneumonia
2. Desquamative interstitial pneumonia
3. Pulmonary alveolar proteinosis
Interstitial fibrosis
1. Usual interstitial pneumonia
2. Nonspecific interstitial pneumonia (fibrosing NSIP)
Interstitial inflammation
1. Nonspecific interstitial pneumonia (cellular NSIP)
2. Lymphocytic interstitial pneumonia
3. Hypersensitivity pneumonitis

From Broaddus VC et al: *Murray & Nadel's textbook of respiratory medicine,* ed 7, Philadelphia, 2022, Elsevier.

and prevent development of pulmonary hypertension. Patients with interstitial disease should receive long-term oxygen therapy for severe resting hypoxemia and ambulatory oxygen for severe exertional desaturation.[8]
- Pulmonary rehabilitation improves exercise tolerance and strength in patients with ILD.[9]

- Lung transplant should be considered in appropriate patients.[10]

DISPOSITION
The prognosis is highly variable and depends on the cause, severity of illness, and initial response to treatment.

REFERRAL
- Pulmonary referral for workup and management
- Surgical referral for biopsy
- Referral for lung transplant evaluation

! PEARLS & CONSIDERATIONS

COMMENTS
- In ILD evaluation, it is important to obtain a thorough history of tobacco and drug use, prior medications, workplace and environmental exposures, and pets, as well as to conduct a complete review of systems, including signs and symptoms that might suggest an underlying connective tissue disease.
- Establishing the specific type of ILD is essential for both management and prognosis.

PREVENTION
- Proper industrial hygiene, including use of necessary respiratory protective equipment, is important, as well as close monitoring of patients receiving medications with known pulmonary toxicity.
- Symptoms of an ILD in the setting of an autoimmune condition need to be evaluated thoroughly.

REFERENCES
Available at eBooks.Health.Elsevier.com.

RELATED CONTENT
Asbestosis (Related Key Topic)
Cryptogenic Organizing Pneumonia (Related Key Topic)
Eosinophilic Granulomatosis with Polyangiitis (Related Key Topic)
Eosinophilic Pneumonia (Related Key Topic)
Hypersensitivity Pneumonitis (Related Key Topic)
Idiopathic Pulmonary Fibrosis (Related Key Topic)
Interstitial Pulmonary Disease (Patient Information)
Sarcoidosis (Related Key Topic)

AUTHOR: **AIDA VENADO, MD, MAS**

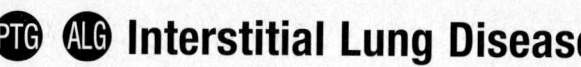

TABLE 5 Radiographic Features of the Interstitial Lung Diseases

Feature	Diseases
Upper zone–predominant disease	Radiation pneumonitis; neurofibromatosis; chronic sarcoidosis; pulmonary Langerhans cell histiocytosis; silicosis; chronic hypersensitivity pneumonitis; chronic eosinophilic pneumonia; ankylosing spondylitis; nodular rheumatoid arthritis; berylliosis; drug induced (amiodarone, gold, BCNU [carmustine]); radiation
Increased lung volumes	Lymphangioleiomyomatosis; chronic sarcoidosis; chronic pulmonary Langerhans cell histiocytosis; tuberous sclerosis; neurofibromatosis
Radiographic honeycomb lung	Idiopathic pulmonary fibrosis; connective tissue disease; asbestosis; drug induced; lymphocytic interstitial pneumonia; chronic aspiration pneumonia; hemosiderosis; Hermansky-Pudlak syndrome; alveolar proteinosis
Pneumothorax	Pulmonary Langerhans cell histiocytosis; lymphangioleiomyomatosis; tuberous sclerosis; neurofibromatosis, IPF
Kerley B lines	Lymphangitic carcinomatosis; lymphangioleiomyomatosis; left atrial hypertension (mitral valve disease, venoocclusive disease); lymphoma; amyloidosis
Lymphadenopathy	Sarcoidosis; lymphoma; lymphangitic carcinomatosis; lymphoid interstitial pneumonia; berylliosis; amyloidosis; Gaucher disease
Pleural disease	Lymphangitic carcinomatosis; connective tissue disease; asbestosis (pleural calcification); lymphangioleiomyomatosis (chylous effusion); drug induced (nitrofurantoin, radiation); sarcoidosis
Eggshell calcification of lymph nodes	Silicosis; sarcoidosis; radiation

IPF, Idiopathic pulmonary fibrosis.
From Mason RJ: *Murray & Nadel's textbook of respiratory medicine,* ed 5, Philadelphia, 2010, Saunders.

TABLE 6 Laboratory Findings in the Interstitial Lung Diseases

Finding	Diseases
Leukopenia	Sarcoidosis; connective tissue disease; lymphoma; drug induced
Leukocytosis	Systemic vasculitis; hypersensitivity pneumonitis; lymphoma
Eosinophilia	Eosinophilic pneumonia; sarcoidosis; systemic vasculitis; drug induced (sulfa, methotrexate)
Thrombocytopenia	Sarcoidosis; connective tissue disease; drug induced; Gaucher disease; idiopathic pulmonary fibrosis
Hemolytic anemia	Connective tissue disease; sarcoidosis; lymphoma; drug induced; idiopathic pulmonary fibrosis
Normocytic anemia	Diffuse alveolar hemorrhage syndromes; connective tissue disease; lymphangitic carcinomatosis
Urinary sediment abnormalities	Connective tissue disease; systemic vasculitis; drug induced
Hypogammaglobulinemia	Lymphocytic interstitial pneumonia
Hypergammaglobulinemia	Connective tissue disease; sarcoidosis; systemic vasculitis; idiopathic pulmonary fibrosis; asbestosis; silicosis; lymphocytic interstitial pneumonia; lymphoma
Serum autoantibodies	Rheumatoid arthritis, scleroderma, inflammatory myopathies (dermatomyositis, polymyositis, immune-mediated necrotizing myopathy), mixed connective tissue disease, Sjogren syndrome, systemic lupus erythematosus
Serum immune complexes	Idiopathic pulmonary fibrosis; lymphocytic interstitial pneumonia; systemic vasculitis; connective tissue disease; pulmonary Langerhans cell histiocytosis
Serum angiotensin-converting enzyme	Sarcoidosis; hypersensitivity pneumonitis; silicosis; acute respiratory distress syndrome; Gaucher disease
Antibasement membrane antibody	Goodpasture syndrome
Antineutrophil cytoplasmic antibody	Systemic vasculitis

Adapted from Mason RJ: *Murray & Nadel's textbook of respiratory medicine,* ed 5, Philadelphia, 2010, Saunders.

Diseases and Disorders

I

BASIC INFORMATION

DEFINITION

Classified into two broad categories:
- Acute interstitial nephritis (AIN):
  1. Decrease in kidney function resulting from delayed hypersensitivity immune-mediated injury; most often drug-induced
  2. Characterized on kidney biopsy by edema and leukocyte infiltration of the renal interstitium and tubules (tubulitis), which classically spares glomeruli and blood vessels
- Chronic interstitial nephritis:
  1. Final common pathway of many chronic kidney diseases (CKD) including diabetic kidney disease, hypertensive kidney disease, unresolved AIN, chronic obstruction, high-grade vesicoureteral reflux, and chronic bacterial infections
  2. Characterized on renal biopsy by interstitial fibrosis with mononuclear leukocyte infiltration and tubular atrophy

SYNONYMS

Acute tubulo-interstitial nephritis
Contracted kidney
Cirrhosis of the kidney
Granular kidney
Renal sclerosis

ICD-10CM CODES
N05.8	Unspecified nephritic syndrome with other morphologic changes
N05.9	Unspecified nephritic syndrome with unspecified morphologic changes
N10	Acute tubulo-interstitial nephritis
N11	Chronic tubulo-interstitial nephritis
N11.8	Other chronic tubulo-interstitial nephritis
N11.9	Chronic tubulo-interstitial nephritis, unspecified
N12	Tubulo-interstitial nephritis, not specified as acute or chronic
N14	Drug- and heavy metal-induced tubulo-interstitial and tubular conditions
N15	Other renal tubulo-interstitial diseases
N16	Renal tubulo-interstitial disorders in diseases classified elsewhere
N17.8	Other acute kidney failure

EPIDEMIOLOGY & DEMOGRAPHICS

PREVALENCE:
- Prevalence of AIN is significantly underestimated.
- AIN is found in 0.5% to 2.6% of all kidney biopsies, but prevalence may be as high as 12.9% to 18.6% in patients who have had biopsy for acute kidney injury (AKI) of unknown etiology.

PREDOMINANT AGE:
- Increased incidence in older adults attributed to reduced glomerular filtration rate (GFR), immune-mediated dysfunction, increasing medication use, and comorbidities.[1]
- Median age at presentation is 65 yr.

RISK FACTORS:
- Advanced age (>65 yr)
- Volume depletion
- Underlying kidney disease
- Congestive heart failure
- Diabetes
- HIV infection

PHYSICAL FINDINGS & CLINICAL PRESENTATION[2-4]

SIGNS & SYMPTOMS:
- For AIN, the most common presentation is an asymptomatic elevation of serum creatinine and blood urea nitrogen (BUN) levels. When advanced, AIN is associated with nonspecific symptoms of AKI from any cause:
  1. Malaise
  2. Anorexia
  3. Nausea and vomiting
  4. Oliguria or polyuria
  5. Hematuria
  6. Flank pain
- Classic triad (fever, maculopapular rash, and eosinophilia) is present in only 5% to 10% of cases:[1-3]
  1. If present, the rash is usually a truncal maculopapular morbilliform eruption.
  2. Triad is characteristic of methicillin-related AIN; this antibiotic has not been prescribed in the U.S. for 4 decades.
- A small minority present with tubulo-interstitial nephritis and uveitis (TINU) syndrome. The uveitis may be symptomatic or subclinical and may develop before, during, or after kidney injury. Adolescent females are most often affected by TINU.[1]
- For chronic interstitial nephritis, there may be a subacute to protracted rise in serum creatinine without obvious symptomatology that is classified as unspecified CKD.

ETIOLOGY

ACUTE INTERSTITIAL NEPHRITIS:
- **Drug-induced:** Accounts for 70% of cases, and more than 150 agents have been implicated.[4] AKI usually develops 10 to 14 days after exposure to the drug but may develop earlier when there has been prior drug exposure.
  1. Antibiotics (beta-lactams, sulfonamides, rifampin, fluoroquinolones)
  2. NSAIDs, including selective cyclooxygenase-2 (COX-2) inhibitors
  3. Proton pump inhibitors and H$_2$ blockers (primarily cimetidine)
  4. Loop diuretics (furosemide, bumetanide) and thiazide diuretics
  5. Antineoplastic agents
  6. Anticonvulsants
  7. Allopurinol (particularly common cause of drug rash or reaction with eosinophilia and systemic symptoms [DRESS] with AIN)
  8. Immunotherapy with checkpoint pathway inhibitors
  9. 5-aminosalicylates (mesalamine)
- **Infection** (10% to 15%): Systemic or localized to genitourinary system.

  1. Bacteria: Streptococci, *Corynebacterium diphtheriae,* legionellae, Yersinia, *Mycobacteria* spp., Mycoplasma, rickettsiae, *E. coli*
  2. Viruses: Cytomegalovirus, Epstein-Barr virus, Orthohantavirus, hepatitis C virus, herpes simplex virus-1 and -2, human immunodeficiency virus-1, rubulavirus (mumps), human polyomavirus-1 (BK) and -2 (JC), influenza A virus
  3. Other: *Treponema pallidum, Toxoplasma gondii, Babesia* species
- **Other Causes** (15% to 20%):[1,2]
  1. Idiopathic (10%)
- Immune disorders: Systemic lupus erythematosus, Sjögren syndrome, small-vessel vasculitides, autoimmune pancreatitis
- Neoplastic disorders (multiple myeloma)
- DRESS syndrome
- Immunoglobulin G4 (IgG4)-related disease
- Hypocomplementemic tubulointerstitial nephritis

CHRONIC INTERSTITIAL NEPHRITIS:
- Metabolic diseases (urate nephropathy, hypercalcemic nephropathy, hypokalemic nephropathy, oxalate nephropathy)
- Sarcoidosis
- Heavy metals
- Chronic urinary tract obstruction
- Aristolochic acid
- Diabetic kidney disease
- Hypertensive kidney disease
- Chronic pyelonephritis
- Drugs: Indinavir, cisplatin, tacrolimus, cyclosporine, lithium

OVERLAP OF ACUTE & CHRONIC INTERSTITIAL NEPHRITIS: Some metabolic processes and autoimmune disorders can present either as acute or chronic interstitial nephritis. For example, oxalate nephropathy can present as acute interstitial nephropathy in the setting of ethylene glycol ingestion or chronic interstitial nephritis in cases of bariatric surgery and high oxalate-containing diet.

DX DIAGNOSIS

DIFFERENTIAL DIAGNOSIS

Other causes of AKI or CKD include acute tubular necrosis, atheroembolic disease, glomerulonephritis, hypertensive nephrosclerosis, prerenal azotemia, obstructive nephropathy, and renal vascular disease.

WORKUP
- Diagnosis is typically recognized by the temporal relationship between onset and resolution of AKI with use and discontinuation of a known or suspected culprit drug.
- Gold standard for diagnosis is kidney biopsy. This procedure is reserved for clinical situations with an unclear diagnosis, when removal of the offending agent does not result in improvement or influences medical care, or when steroid initiation is being considered.

LABORATORY TESTS
- No single laboratory test has sufficient positive or negative predictive value to diagnose interstitial nephritis.

- Diagnosis is based on clinical history, urine and serum abnormalities, and clinical course.[3,5]

URINE TESTS:

- Urine eosinophils: Historical marker of AIN. Eosinophiluria is not sensitive or specific enough to establish AIN and occurs more frequently in noninterstitial kidney disorders.[6]
- Urinalysis: Sterile pyuria, microhematuria, glucosuria, and proteinuria usually <300 mg/dl.
  1. Urine protein < 1 g in 24 h
  2. Microscopic hematuria (less than 50%)
  3. FeNa > 1%
- Nephrogenic diabetes insipidus, especially in chronic tubulointerstitial disease.
- Urine sediment analysis: Leukocytes, leukocyte casts, red cells, and tubular epithelial cells (Fig. E1). However, a bland urine sediment can also be seen in interstitial nephritis, especially if chronic. A lack of pyuria does not exclude AIN. Additionally, granular casts may be noted when tubulitis is present.[3]

BLOOD TESTS:

- Serum chemistry profile: Elevated BUN, elevated creatinine, low serum phosphorus, and low serum urate concentrations may be present.
- CBC with differential findings include the following:
  1. Eosinophilia: Not sensitive; if present, this finding greatly increases clinical suspicion for a systemic drug reaction. Eosinophilia may also occur in other causes of AKI including cholesterol emboli, vasculitis, and hematologic or solid organ malignancy.
- Hemoglobin level that is disproportionately low compared to degree of AKI, attributed to loss of interstitial erythropoietin-producing cells.
- If drug-related AIN is not suspected, laboratory testing for infection, vasculitis, and autoimmune disorders is warranted depending on the clinical context.
- Low complements and elevated serum total IgG and/or IgG4 levels or hypergammaglobulinemia in patients with immunoglobulin G4 (IgG4)-related disease or hypocomplementemic interstitial nephritis.

IMAGING STUDIES

Gallium scintigraphy (gallium-67 scan), positron emission tomography, and computed tomography have been used to evaluate AIN in patients. These tests may distinguish between AIN and other forms of AKI in patients who are not candidates for kidney biopsy.[3]

KIDNEY BIOPSY[3,7]

Critical to diagnosis of interstitial nephritis in patients with broad differential diagnosis of AKI. Biopsy findings include the following (Fig. E2):

- Predominant lymphocytic and monocytic infiltrate
- Eosinophils suggestive of drug-induced AIN
- Tubulitis (renal tubular invasion by inflammatory cells) compatible with AIN
- Early inflammation with edema may transition to fibrosis with tubular atrophy as disorder becomes chronic
- Granuloma formation implies infectious origin of AIN, especially in regions where the infectious etiologies described earlier are endemic. Necrotizing granulomas typically seen in fungal infections and tuberculosis

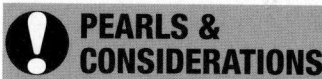

TREATMENT

NONPHARMACOLOGIC THERAPY

Largely supportive; removal of offending agent, if known, will resolve 60% of cases.

ACUTE GENERAL Rx

- Maintain adequate volume status and urine output.
- Identify and treat infection(s).
- Avoid nephrotoxins and medications that impair renal blood flow.
- Uveitis in TINU syndrome may be asymptomatic. An ophthalmologic exam is recommended in idiopathic AIN.
- Retrospective studies and anecdotal literature have shown that steroid treatment initiated within 7 days of diagnosis may reduce the requirement for long-term dialysis in patients with drug-induced AIN who have not responded to drug withdrawal alone. A retrospective, multicenter study of 61 patients with biopsy-proven AIN showed that among treated patients, those who started glucocorticoids within 7 days of withdrawal of the offending drug were more likely to recover kidney function compared with those who started later.[8] Steroids are the basis of treatment in idiopathic AIN, AIN associated with systemic disease, and TINU. Regimens vary. Some include an initial steroid pulse of methylprednisolone, 250 to 500 mg for 3 consecutive days, followed by prednisone 1 mg/kg.[8] Alternative regimen: Prednisone 1 mg/kg with no intravenous steroid pulse, with tapering over 4 to 6 wk; prolonged steroid tapering does not improve outcomes. Steroids are not administered to patients with significant kidney fibrosis on histologic examination.
- Cyclophosphamide, cyclosporine, and mycophenolate mofetil are anecdotal therapies for steroid-resistant disease. Mycophenolate mofetil has the most evidence for use as a steroid-sparing agent if AKI recurs when

steroids are tapered or discontinued, or when adverse effects from steroid therapy occur.

CHRONIC Rx

- Limit exposure to known nephrotoxic agents
- Medication dosage adjustments by glomerular filtration rate
- Rigorous control of blood pressure, diabetes, and cholesterol
- Treat causes of chronic obstructive uropathy

DISPOSITION

With AIN:

- Complete recovery with return to baseline creatinine occurs in 60% to 65% of cases.[4]
- Partial recovery is seen in 10% to 20%.[4]
- Irreversible damage in 5% to 10%.[4]
- Relapse is common with repeated exposure to offending agents.

REFERRAL

Renal consultation is often required when diagnosis is unclear, biopsy is required, or there is treatment-resistant disease.

⊘ PEARLS & CONSIDERATIONS

COMMENTS

Drug-induced AIN occurs primarily when the offending agent is initiated within the preceding 30 days of diagnosis. The most common drug classes are beta-lactam antibiotics, NSAIDs, and proton pump inhibitors. In contrast to acute tubular necrosis, which is often associated with oliguria, early AIN may be associated with polyuria. Therefore a high index of suspicion in this clinical setting is critical for establishing early diagnosis.

PREVENTION

Use known offending agents with care, especially in older adults and persons with known underlying kidney disease.

PATIENT & FAMILY EDUCATION

https://www.nlm.nih.gov/medlineplus/ency/article/000464.htm.

REFERENCES

Available at eBooks.Health.Elsevier.com.

RELATED CONTENT

Interstitial Nephritis (Patient Information)

AUTHORS: **SANDEEP SOMAN, MD, FNKF, FAMIA** and **HAMMOOD AHMED, MD**

Diseases and Disorders

I

Iron Deficiency Anemia

BASIC INFORMATION

DEFINITION

Anemia is defined as a hemoglobin level 2 standard deviations below normal for age and sex. Iron deficiency anemia is anemia resulting from inadequate iron supplementation or excessive blood loss.

SYNONYMS

Anemia Iron deficiency

ICD-10CM CODES

D50.0	Iron deficiency anemia secondary to blood loss (chronic)
D50.8	Other iron deficiency anemias
D50.9	Iron deficiency anemia, unspecified
O99.019	Anemia complicating pregnancy, unspecified trimester

EPIDEMIOLOGY & DEMOGRAPHICS

- Dietary iron deficiency occurs often in infants as a result of unsupplemented milk diets. It is also commonly seen in women during their reproductive years, as a result of heavy menstrual periods, and during pregnancy (increased demand).
- Iron deficiency is the most common nutritional deficiency worldwide.
- The prevalence of iron deficiency is greatest among toddlers ages 1 to 2 yr (7%) from inadequate intake and female individuals ages 12 to 49 yr (9% to 16%) from menstrual losses.
- The prevalence of iron deficiency is 2% in adult men, 9% to 12% in non-Hispanic White women, and 20% in Black and Mexican American women.
- GI cancer is diagnosed in 10% of elderly patients with iron deficiency anemia.

PHYSICAL FINDINGS & CLINICAL PRESENTATION

- Most patients have normal examination results.
- Skin pallor and conjunctival pallor may be present.
- Signs and symptoms specific for iron deficiency are koilonychias, pica, pagophagia, blue sclera, glossitis, and angular stomatitis (Fig. E1).
- Patients with severe anemia can have palpitations, headache, weakness, dizziness, and easy fatigability.

ETIOLOGY

- Blood loss from GI or menstrual bleeding (genitourinary blood loss less often the cause)
- Dietary iron deficiency (rare in adults)
- Poor iron absorption in patients with gastric or small-bowel surgery
- Repeated phlebotomy
- Increased requirements (e.g., during pregnancy)
- Other: Traumatic hemolysis (abnormally functioning cardiac valves), idiopathic pulmonary hemosiderosis (iron sequestration in pulmonary macrophages), paroxysmal nocturnal hemoglobinuria (intravascular hemolysis)
- The most common cause worldwide is hookworm infection

DIAGNOSIS

DIFFERENTIAL DIAGNOSIS

- Anemia of chronic disease
- Sideroblastic anemia
- Thalassemia trait
- Lead poisoning

WORKUP

Diagnostic workup consists primarily of laboratory evaluation. Table 1 describes laboratory studies differentiating the most common microcytic anemias. Most patients with iron deficiency anemia are asymptomatic in the early stages. With progressive anemia, the major symptoms are fatigue, dizziness, exertional dyspnea, pagophagia (ice eating), and pica. Patient history may also suggest GI blood loss (melena, hematochezia, hemoptysis).

LABORATORY TESTS

- Laboratory results vary with the stage of deficiency.
- Absent iron marrow stores and decreased serum ferritin are the initial abnormalities.
- Decreased serum iron and increased total iron-binding capacity (TIBC) are the next abnormalities.
- Hypochromic microcytic anemia is present with significant iron deficiency.
- Peripheral smear in patients with iron deficiency generally reveals microcytic hypochromic red blood cells (Fig. E2) with a wide area of central pallor, anisocytosis, and poikilocytosis when severe.
- Laboratory abnormalities consistent with iron deficiency are low serum ferritin level, increased red blood cell (RBC) distribution width with values generally >15, low mean corpuscular volume, low mean corpuscular hemoglobin, increased TIBC, and low serum iron.
- In patients diagnosed with iron deficiency anemia, a GI workup including an upper endoscopy and colonoscopy is recommended to look for source of iron loss.

TREATMENT

The goal of therapy is to supply sufficient iron to correct the low hemoglobin and replenish iron stores.

NONPHARMACOLOGIC THERAPY

Patients should be instructed to consume foods that contain large amounts of iron, such as liver, red meat, and legumes.

ACUTE GENERAL Rx

- Iron supplementation will result in reticulocytosis and will generally increase hemoglobin levels by 0.5 to 1 g per wk.
- Treatment consists of ferrous sulfate 325 mg PO daily for 3 to 6 mo. Doses higher than 325 mg/day are poorly tolerated. Calcium supplements can decrease iron absorption; therefore these medications should be staggered. Supplemental vitamin C can increase oral absorption.
- Parenteral iron therapy is reserved for patients with poor tolerance, noncompliance with oral preparations, or malabsorption. Indications for intravenous iron therapy are summarized in Table 2.
- Transfusion of packed RBCs is indicated in patients with severe symptomatic anemia.

CHRONIC Rx

Patients should be instructed to continue their iron supplements for at least 6 mo or longer to correct depleted body iron stores.

DISPOSITION

- Most patients respond rapidly to iron supplementation with improvement in CBC and

---

TABLE 1 Laboratory Studies Differentiating the Most Common Microcytic Anemias

Study	Iron Deficiency Anemia	α or β Thalassemia	Anemia of Chronic Disease
Hemoglobin	Decreased	Decreased	Decreased
MCV	Decreased	Decreased	Normal-decreased
RDW	Increased	Normal	Normal-increased
RBC	Decreased	Normal-increased	Normal-decreased
Serum ferritin	Decreased	Normal	Increased
Total Fe binding capacity	Increased	Normal	Decreased
Transferrin saturation	Decreased	Normal	Decreased
FEP	Increased	Normal	Increased
Transferrin receptor	Increased	Normal	Increased
Reticulocyte hemoglobin concentration	Decreased	Normal	Normal-decreased

Fe, Ferritin; *FEP,* free erythrocyte protoporphyrin; *MCV,* mean corpuscular volume; *RBC,* red blood cell; *RDW,* red cell distribution width.
From Kliegman RM: *Nelson textbook of pediatrics,* ed 21, Philadelphia, 2020, Elsevier.

TABLE 2   Indications for Intravenous Iron Therapy

Accepted Indications

- Oral iron intolerance
- Oral iron refractoriness, including iron refractory iron deficiency anemia (IRIDA)
- Need for a quick recovery, e.g., severe anemia of pregnancy
- Chronic bleeding not manageable with oral iron
- Concurrently with erythropoiesis-stimulating agents in chronic kidney disease
- Gastrointestinal disorders (inflammatory bowel disease, acute flares)
- Substitution for blood transfusions when not accepted by patient

Novel Proposed Indications

- Iron deficiency in chronic heart failure
- Perioperative anemia (transfusion sparing strategy)
- Anemia of chronic kidney disease before treatment with erythropoiesis-stimulating agents
- Persistent anemia after erythropoiesis-stimulating agents in cancer patients on chemotherapy

From Goldman L, Shafer AI: *Goldman-Cecil medicine,* ed 26, Philadelphia, 2019, Elsevier.

TABLE 3   Responses to Iron Therapy in Iron Deficiency Anemia

Time After Iron Administration	Response
12-24 h	Replacement of intracellular iron enzymes; subjective improvement; decreased irritability; increased appetite
36-48 h	Initial bone marrow response; erythroid hyperplasia
48-72 h	Reticulocytosis, peaking at 5-7 days
4-30 days	Increase in hemoglobin level
1-3 mo	Repletion of stores

From Kliegman RM: *Nelson textbook of pediatrics,* ed 21, Philadelphia, 2020, Elsevier.

TABLE 4   Differential Diagnosis of Microcytic Anemia That Fails to Respond to Oral Iron

Poor compliance (true intolerance of iron is uncommon)
Incorrect dose or medication
Malabsorption of administered iron
Ongoing blood loss including gastrointestinal, menstrual, and pulmonary
Concurrent infection or inflammatory disorder inhibiting the response to iron
Concurrent vitamin B_{12} or folate deficiency
Diagnosis other than iron deficiency:

- Thalassemias
- Hemoglobin C and E disorders
- Anemia of chronic disease
- Lead poisoning
- Sickle thalassemias, hemoglobin SC disease
- Rare microcytic anemias

SC, Sickle cell.
From Kliegman RM: *Nelson textbook of pediatrics,* ed 21, Philadelphia, 2020, Elsevier.

general well-being (Table 3). GI side effects from oral iron therapy are common and may require decreased dosage to once every other day or to change to parenteral iron.

- A differential diagnosis of microcytic anemia that fails to respond to oral iron is described in Table 4.

REFERRAL

GI referral for evaluation of GI malignancy is recommended in all patients with iron deficiency and suspected GI blood loss.

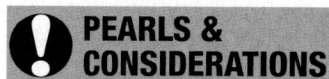 **PEARLS & CONSIDERATIONS**

COMMENTS

- Iron deficiency may impair aerobic performance and worsen symptoms in patients with heart failure. Treatment with intravenous iron in patients with chronic heart failure and iron deficiency has been shown to improve symptoms, quality of life, and functional capacity.
- If the diagnosis of iron deficiency anemia is made, locating the suspected site of iron loss is mandatory.

RELATED CONTENT

Algorithm for Diagnosis of Anemias (Algorithm in Section III)
Anemia (Patient Information)

AUTHOR: **FRED F. FERRI, MD**

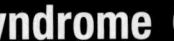

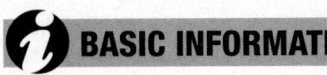

BASIC INFORMATION

DEFINITION

Irritable bowel syndrome (IBS) is a chronic functional disorder manifested by alteration in bowel habits and recurrent abdominal pain and bloating. IBS is a symptom complex influenced by a variety of physiologic determinants from gut to brain and back. The ROME IV criteria for diagnosis of IBS are:

- Patient has recurrent abdominal pain ≥1 day per wk, on average, in the previous 3 mo, with an onset ≥6 mo before diagnosis.
- Abdominal pain is associated with at least two of the following three symptoms:
  1. Pain related to defecation
  2. Change in frequency of stool
  3. Change in form (appearance) of stool
- Patient has none of the following warning signs:
  1. Age ≥50 yr, no previous colon cancer screening, and presence of symptoms
  2. Recent change in bowel habit
  3. Evidence of overt GI bleeding (e.g., melena or hematochezia)
  4. Nocturnal pain or passage of stool
  5. Unintentional weight loss
  6. Family history of colorectal cancer or inflammatory bowel disease
  7. Palpable abdominal mass or lymphadenopathy
  8. Evidence of iron deficiency anemia on blood testing
  9. Positive test for fecal occult blood
- The criteria must be fulfilled for at least the past 3 mo with symptom onset at least 6 mo before the diagnosis.
- Table 1 subtypes IBS by predominant stool pattern.

SYNONYMS

Irritable colon
Spastic colon
IBS

ICD-10CM CODES
K58	Irritable bowel syndrome
K58.9	Irritable bowel syndrome without diarrhea
K58.0	Irritable bowel syndrome with diarrhea

EPIDEMIOLOGY & DEMOGRAPHICS

- IBS is the most common functional bowel disorder. An estimated 15 million people in the U.S. have IBS.
- IBS occurs in 7% to 21% of the general population of industrialized countries and is responsible for >50% of GI referrals. Worldwide adult prevalence is 12%. Incidence increases during adolescence and peaks in third and fourth decades of life.
- Female:male ratio is 2:1. Peak prevalence is from 20 to 39 yr of age.
- Nearly 50% of patients have psychiatric abnormalities, with anxiety disorders being most common.

PHYSICAL FINDINGS & CLINICAL PRESENTATION

- The clinical presentation of IBS consists of abdominal pain and abnormalities of defecation, which may include loose stools, usually after meals and in the morning, alternating with episodes of constipation.
- Physical examination is generally normal.
- Nonspecific abdominal tenderness and distention may be present.

ETIOLOGY

- Unknown, believed to be multifactorial. Fig. 1 illustrates a biopsychologic model of IBS pathophysiology.
- Associated pathophysiology includes altered GI motility, alteration in gut flora, and increased gut sensitivity.
- Risk factors: Anxiety, depression, personality disorders, history of childhood sexual abuse, and domestic abuse in women.

DIAGNOSIS

DIFFERENTIAL DIAGNOSIS

- Inflammatory bowel disease (IBD)
- Diverticulitis
- Colon malignancy
- Endometriosis
- Peptic ulcer disease
- Biliary liver disease
- Chronic pancreatitis
- Constipation caused by medications (opiates, calcium channel blockers, anticholinergics)
- Diarrhea caused by medications (metformin, colchicine, proton pump inhibitors, antacids, antibiotics)
- Small-bowel overgrowth
- Celiac disease
- Parasites
- Lymphoma of GI tract
- Pelvic floor dyssynergia

TABLE 1 Subtyping Irritable Bowel Syndrome by Predominant Stool Pattern

- IBS with constipation (IBS-C)—hard or lumpy stools* ≥25% and loose (mushy) or watery stools† ≥25% of bowel movements‡
- IBS with diarrhea (IBS-D)—loose (mushy) or watery stools† ≥25% and hard or lumpy stool* ≥25% of bowel movements‡
- Mixed IBS—hard or lumpy stools* ≥25% and loose (mushy) or watery stools† ≥25% of bowel movements‡
- Unsubtyped IBS (IBS unclassified)—insufficient abnormality of stool consistency to meet criteria for IBS with constipation, diarrhea, or mixed‡

IBS, Irritable bowel syndrome.
*Bristol Stool Form Scale 1-2 (separate hard lumps like nuts [difficult to pass] or sausage-shaped but lumpy).
†Bristol Stool Form Scale 6-7 (fluffy pieces with ragged edges, a mushy stool or watery, no solid pieces, entirely liquid).
‡In the absence of use of antidiarrheals or laxatives.
Adapted from Sayuk GS, Gyawali CP: Irritable bowel syndrome: modern concepts and management options, *Am J Med* 128(8):817-827, 2015.

WORKUP

Diagnostic workup (Table 2) is aimed primarily at excluding the conditions listed in the differential diagnoses. A step-wise approach is critical. It is important to identify red flags of other diseases, such as weight loss, rectal bleeding, onset in patients >50 yr, fever, nocturnal pain, and family history of malignancy or IBD. Additional red flags include abnormal examination (e.g., mass, enlarged lymph nodes, stool positive for occult blood, muscle wasting) and abnormal laboratory values (anemia, leukocytosis, abnormal chemistry).

LABORATORY TESTS

- Blood work is generally normal. CBC is reasonable to evaluate for anemia. The presence of anemia should alert to the possibility of a colonic malignancy or IBD.
- Other reasonable tests include C-reactive protein, tissue transglutaminase antibody (rule out celiac disease), and thyroid-stimulating hormone (TSH; rule out thyroid abnormalities).
- Fecal calprotectin level is useful to differentiate IBS from inflammatory bowel disease in patients who have IBS with diarrhea or with both diarrhea and constipation. Fecal calprotectin levels less than 40 mcg/g exclude IBD in patients with IBS.
- Testing of stool for ova and parasites should be considered only in patients with chronic diarrhea. Evaluation of stool for *C. difficile* may be helpful in patients with predominant diarrhea symptoms who have recently taken antibiotics.

IMAGING STUDIES

- Imaging studies (e.g., flat and upright abdominal radiograph, small-bowel series, sonogram or computed tomography [CT] of abdomen and pelvis) are normal and not necessary for diagnosis.
- Lower endoscopy is generally normal except for the presence of some spasms. Colonoscopic imaging should be performed only in persons who have alarm features to rule out organic disease and in persons older than 50 yr to screen for colorectal cancer.

TREATMENT

NONPHARMACOLOGIC THERAPY

- The patient should be encouraged to maintain an adequate fiber intake and to eliminate foods that aggravate symptoms. Avoidance of caffeine, dairy products, fatty foods, and dietary excesses is also helpful. Several clinical trials have shown that a diet low in fermentable oligosaccharides, disaccharides, monosaccharides, and polyols (FODMAPs) improves symptoms in nearly 70% of patients with IBS.[1]
- Cognitive-behavioral therapy is also recommended, particularly in younger patients, because psychosocial stressors are important triggers of IBS. Reassurance that the disorder is benign and education about trigger avoidance and stress management are important.

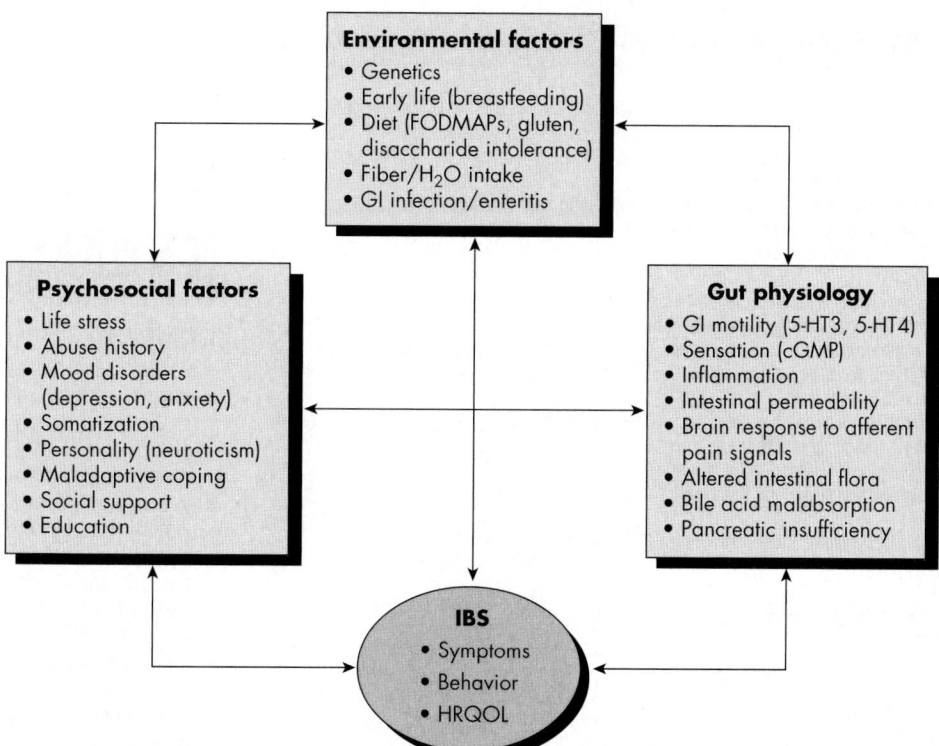

FIG. 1 A biopsychosocial model of irritable bowel syndrome pathophysiology. Irritable bowel syndrome is thought to be a multifactorial disorder, deriving from a potential multitude of etiopathogenic factors, including environmental, psychologic, and physiologic factors. This model highlights the complex, often bidirectional interplay of these factors in the experience of irritable bowel syndrome symptoms. *cGMP,* Cyclic guanosine monophosphate; *5-HT3,* serotonin type 3; *5-HT4,* serotonin type 4; *FODMAPS,* fermentable oligosaccharides, disaccharides, monosaccharides, and polyols; *GI,* gastrointestinal; *H₂0,* water; *HRQOL,* health-related quality of life; *IBS,* irritable bowel syndrome. (Modified from Sayuk GS, Gyawali CP: Irritable bowel syndrome: modern concepts and management options, *Am J Med* 128[8]:817-827, 2015.)

- Importance of regular exercise and adequate fluid intake should be stressed.
- Fig. E2 illustrates the management of IBS.

GENERAL Rx

- The mainstay of treatment of IBS is diet. A FODMAP diet has been proven effective. Fiber is helpful for relief of constipation but not for relief of pain. Because symptoms are chronic, the use of laxatives should generally be avoided.
- Soluble fiber (psyllium) is more effective in symptom relief than insoluble fiber (bran). Fiber supplementation with psyllium 1 tbsp bid or calcium polycarbophil (FiberCon) 2 tablets one to four times daily followed by 8 oz of water may be necessary in some patients.
- Patients should be instructed that there might be some increased bloating on initiation of fiber supplementation, which should resolve within 2 to 3 wk. It is important that patients take these fiber products on a regular basis and not only as needed. Fiber is not effective in patients with diarrhea-predominant IBS and may worsen symptoms in these patients.
- Patients who appear anxious can benefit from use of sedatives or selective serotonin reuptake inhibitors (SSRIs). Tricyclic antidepressants in low doses are also effective in some patients with diarrhea-predominant IBS.

- C-2 chloride channel activators: Lubiprostone (Amitiza) is a chloride channel activator that stimulates chloride-rich intestinal fluid secretion and accelerates small intestine and colonic transmit time. It may be effective in chronic constipation-predominant IBS unresponsive to conventional treatment. Usual dose is 8 to 24 mcg bid with food. Side effects include headache and nausea.
- Linaclotide (Linzess) is a guanylate cyclase-C (GC-C) agonist FDA approved for IBS with constipation. It stimulates secretion of chloride and bicarbonate into the intestinal lumen, mainly through activation of the CFTR ion channel, resulting in increased intestinal fluid and accelerated transit. Usual dose for IBS is 290 mcg 30 min before eating. The most common adverse effects are diarrhea, abdominal pain, flatulence, and abdominal distension.
- Tenapanor (Ibsrela) is an FDA-approved sodium/hydrogen exchanger 3 (NHE3) for twice daily oral treatment of IBS with constipation in adults. Its mechanism of action involves decreasing absorption of sodium, increasing osmotic secretion of water into the gut, shortening intestinal transit time, and softening stool consistency.[2]
- Loperamide is effective for diarrhea. Alosetron, a serotonin type-3 receptor antagonist previously withdrawn because of severe constipation and ischemic colitis, has been reintroduced with limited availability. It is

indicated only for women with severe chronic diarrhea-predominant IBS unresponsive to conventional therapy and not caused by anatomic or metabolic abnormality. Starting dose is 1 mg qd.
- Eluxadoline (Viberzi) is an FDA-approved μ-opioid receptor agonist and Δ-opioid receptor antagonist for IBS with diarrhea. It decreases muscle contractility, inhibits water and electrolyte secretion, and increases rectal sphincter tone. Usual dose is 100 mg PO bid taken with food.
- Alterations in gut flora have been identified as potentially contributing to IBS (84% of IBS patients have an abnormal lactulose breath test, suggesting small-intestinal bacterial overgrowth). Rifaximin, a gut-selective antibiotic, has been used in recent trials to eradicate bacterial overgrowth (70% eradication rate). A dose of 400 mg tid for 10 days was reported effective in improving IBS symptoms up to 10 wk after discontinuation of therapy. Until additional evidence is available, use of rifaximin or other antibiotics in IBS should be reserved for patients with proven bacterial overgrowth.
- Antispasmodics-anticholinergics (e.g., dicyclomine, hyoscyamine) are often used, but efficacy data from clinical trials are inconclusive.
- Probiotics: Bifidobacteria and some combinations of probiotics have shown some limited efficacy. Lactobacilli do not appear to be

---

TABLE 2 Irritable Bowel Syndrome Treatment Strategy: A Way Forward

- Evaluation
  1. Consider conditions that mimic IBS (e.g., celiac disease, microscopic colitis, bile acid diarrhea, pancreatic insufficiency, carbohydrate intolerances, medication side effects, postsurgical neoanatomy)
  2. Assess for the presence of alarm symptoms
  3. Evaluate for symptom triggers (e.g., stressors, diet)
  4. Explore presence of other functional GI (e.g., functional dyspepsia) and non-GI disorders (e.g., fibromyalgia), psychiatric comorbidity, and drug intolerances
  5. Understand previous IBS treatment experiences
- Selection of treatment approach
  1. Predicated on symptom severity and dominant symptoms
  2. Symptom severity (intensity, bother, effects on quality of life)
     a. Mild symptoms, intermittent symptoms, low symptom burden: Symptomatic or peripheral therapy
     b. Moderate symptoms: Centrally acting neuromodulators, especially if symptomatic therapy does not provide adequate benefit
     c. Severe symptoms and those with comorbidities (non-GI functional disorders, psychiatric): Both centrally acting neuromodulators and peripheral therapy
        (1) Concurrent affective disorders need to be managed
        (2) Other central therapies (cognitive and behavioral therapy, hypnosis, stress reduction) may need to be considered
  3. Dominant symptoms (diarrhea, constipation, pain, other GI symptoms)
     a. Constipation predominant
        (1) Laxatives, fiber
        (2) Novel agents (linaclotide, lubiprostone)
     b. Diarrhea predominant
        (1) Antidiarrheals
        (2) Alosetron
        (3) Address dysbiosis (rifaximin, probiotics)
        (4) Diet (low FODMAP)
        (5) Bile binders (cholestyramine, colesevelam)
        (6) Disaccharidases (lactase)
     c. Pain predominant
        (1) Antidepressants (TCAs and SNRIs preferred)
        (2) Linaclotide when constipation present
        (3) Avoid narcotics
- Education and therapeutic alliance
  1. Inform patient about etiopathogenesis
  2. Reaffirm legitimacy of diagnosis; allay concerns about organic disease
  3. Provide information about support organizations (International Foundation for Functional Gastrointestinal Disorders)

FODMAP, Fermentable oligosaccharides, disaccharides, monosaccharides, and polyols; *GI,* gastrointestinal; *IBS,* irritable bowel syndrome; *SNRI,* serotonin-norepinephrine reuptake inhibitor; *TCA,* tricyclic antidepressant.

---

effective for the treatment of IBS. Additional data showing efficacy is needed before probiotics can be endorsed for treatment of IBS.
- Antidepressants: SSRIs are more effective than placebo for relief of global IBS symptoms.

DISPOSITION

More than 60% of patients respond successfully to treatment over the initial 12 mo; however, IBS is a chronic, relapsing condition and requires prolonged therapy.

REFERRAL

GI referral is recommended in patients with rectal bleeding, fever, nocturnal diarrhea, anemia, weight loss, or onset of symptoms >40 yr. Consultation is also necessary if specialized diagnostic procedures such as endoscopy are necessary.

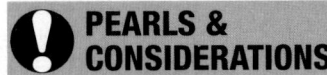

PEARLS & CONSIDERATIONS

COMMENTS

- Patients should be educated regarding maintenance of a high-fiber diet and elimination of stressors, which can precipitate attacks of IBS. They should be reassured that their condition does not lead to cancer.
- Recent drug efforts (alosetron, tegaserod) are aimed at serotonergic receptors in the gut because most of the serotonin in the body is found in the GI tract and is believed to be involved in the mediation of visceral sensation and motility.
- Cognitive-behavioral therapy is effective in the treatment of patients with IBS and should be considered as part of the armamentarium against this disorder.
- Some patients with IBS but without celiac disease show symptom improvement on a wheat-free diet. A 2- to 3-wk trial of wheat avoidance may be reasonable in patients with treatment-resistant IBS.
- Fecal microbiota transplantation (FMT) delivered via upper endoscopy seems to be efficacious in improving symptoms in all IBS subtypes in some clinical trials.

REFERENCES & SUGGESTED READINGS

Available at eBooks.Health.Elsevier.com.

RELATED CONTENT

Irritable Bowel Syndrome (Patient Information)

AUTHOR: **FRED F. FERRI, MD**

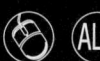 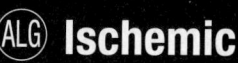

I

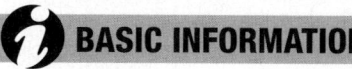 **BASIC INFORMATION**

DEFINITION

Ischemic colitis (IC) is tissue damage and inflammation of the large intestine due to a reduction in blood flow.

SYNONYMS

Intestinal ischemia
Colonic ischemia
IC

ICD-10CM CODES

K51.50	Left-sided colitis without complications
K51.51	Left-sided colitis with complications
K51.511	Left-sided colitis with rectal bleeding
K51.512	Left-sided colitis with intestinal obstruction
K51.513	Left-sided colitis with fistula
K51.514	Left-sided colitis with abscess
K51.518	Left-sided colitis with other complication
K51.519	Left-sided colitis with unspecified complications
K52.3	Indeterminate colitis
K55.0	Acute vascular disorders of intestine
K55.031	Focal (segmental) acute (reversible) ischemia of large intestine
K55.032	Diffuse acute (reversible) ischemia of large intestine
K55.039	Acute (reversible) ischemia of large intestine, extent unspecified
K55.9	Vascular disorder of intestine, unspecified

EPIDEMIOLOGY & DEMOGRAPHICS

INCIDENCE: IC is the most common type of intestinal ischemia, with an overall age- and sex-adjusted annual incidence of 15.6 to 17.7 per 100,000 person-yr. Those under 40 yr had an incidence of 1.1 per 100,000, while those over 80 yr had incidence rates of 107 per 100,000.[1]

PREDOMINANT SEX & AGE:
- More common among older patients (60s to 70s)
- Female predominance

RISK FACTORS:
- Older age
- Atherosclerotic disease, with associated disease processes such as diabetes, hypertension, and hyperlipidemia
- Abdominal Aortic Aneurysm Repair: There is an overall higher incidence IC after AAA repair, and it was higher in open repair compared to endovascular repair
- Atrial fibrillation
- Chronic constipation: Possible mechanism is increased intraluminal pressure resulting in decreased blood flow to the mucosa, thus resulting in ischemic attacks
- Hypercoagulable state (factor V leiden)
- Sickle cell disease, vasculitis, and lupus
- Hypoalbuminemia

- Shock and hypotension
- Heavy exercise
- Infection (cytomegalovirus [CMV], E. coli)
- Surgeries involving the heart, vasculature (aorta), digestive, or gynecologic systems
- Iatrogenic: Prescription drugs include oral contraceptives, migraine medications, antibiotics, Pseudoephedrine, opioids, some medications for irritable bowel syndrome, chemotherapeutic medications, bowel preparation for colonoscopy, and vasopressors[2]
- Lifestyle: Illicit drug use, such as cocaine or methamphetamine use, can result in IC, with most changes on the right side.[2] A total of 27% recreational triathletes, 20% marathon runners, and 87% ultramarathon runners tested positive for fecal occult blood, with accounts of IC developing in high endurance runners[3]

PHYSICAL FINDINGS & CLINICAL PRESENTATION

Classic presentation of IC is of an elderly patient presenting with sudden crampy abdominal pain and hematochezia within the first 24 h. Pain secondary to large bowel ischemia is often not as severe as pain associated with small bowel ischemia. Associated symptoms include the urge to defecate (tenesmus) accompanying the developing abdominal pain.[2]

The initial physical exam of the abdomen may be normal. However, the patient may also have peritoneal signs in severe illness or bowel perforation, with associated hypotension and tachycardia. Rectal exam will demonstrate guaiac positive stool.

ETIOLOGY

GENERAL:
- A reduction in blood flow, usually sudden, to a segment of the bowel causes inadequate oxygenation for normal cellular metabolism.
- Overall, the superior mesenteric artery provides blood flow from the duodenum to the mid transverse colon, while the inferior mesenteric artery supplies blood to the remaining part of the colon and superior rectum. Particularly affected are the watershed regions of the colon (Fig. E1), which have limited collateral circulation (splenic flexure aka Grifith point and sigmoid colon aka Sudeck point).
- Medical and surgical conditions associated with ischemic colitis are summarized in Box 1.

SPECIFIC:
- Nonocclusive disease (20%):
  1. Hypoperfusion: Cardiac failure, septic shock, hemorrhagic shock, hemodialysis, or any other condition that can cause hypotension
  2. Iatrogenic: Drugs (especially constipation-inducing). Medications associated with ischemic colitis are summarized in Box 2
  3. Colonic obstruction: Colon cancer, constipation, volvulus, bowel obstruction
  4. Long-distance running or other endurance sports

BOX 1 Medical and Surgical Conditions Associated with Ischemic Colitis

Cardiovascular/Pulmonary
Atherosclerosis*
Atrial fibrillation
Chronic obstructive pulmonary disease
Hypertension

Gastrointestinal
Constipation
Diarrhea
Irritable bowel syndrome

Low Flow State
Septic shock
Congestive heart failure
Hemorrhagic shock
Hypotension

Surgery
Abdominal surgery
Aortic surgery
Cardiovascular surgery

Invasive Interventions
Post Endovascular abdominal manipulations (e.g., chemoembolization)
Postcolonoscopy

Metabolic/Rheumatoid
Diabetes mellitus
Dyslipidemia
Rheumatoid arthritis
Systemic lupus erythematosus

Miscellaneous
Hypercoagulable states[†]
Sickle cell disease
Long-distance running*[†]

*For example, ischemic heart disease, cerebrovascular disease, peripheral vascular disease.
[†]Antiphospholipid syndrome, factor V Leiden deficiency, protein C and S deficiency.
From Cameron JL, Cameron AM: *Current surgical therapy*, ed 12, Philadelphia, 2017, Elsevier.

BOX 2 Drugs Associated with Ischemic Colitis

Constipation-inducing drugs (opioids and nonopioids)
Immunomodulator drugs (anti-TwNFα, type 1 interferon-α, type 1 interferon-β)
Chemotherapeutic drugs (e.g., Taxanes)
Cocaine and methamphetamines
Female hormones
Oral contraceptive medications
Antibiotics
Pseudoephedrine
Serotonergic (e.g., Alosetron, Sumatriptan)
Diuretics

- Occlusive disease (80%):
  1. Arterial: Thrombus/emboli (Fig. E2), cholesterol emboli, small vessel disease (atherosclerosis, diabetes, vasculitis, rheumatoid arthritis, radiation, amyloidosis), trauma
  2. Surgical: Aortic aneurysm repair, cardiac catheterization, cardiopulmonary bypass, colectomy, endoscopy, renal transplant
  3. Venous: Mesenteric venous thrombosis, hypercoagulable state, sickle cell disease, pancreatitis, portal hypertension, lymphocytic phlebitis

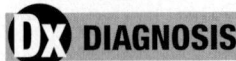 **DIAGNOSIS**

DIFFERENTIAL DIAGNOSIS

- Infectious colitis (e.g., *Clostridium difficile*, *Salmonella*, *Shigella*)
- Inflammatory bowel disease, inflammatory bowel syndrome, celiac disease
- Small bowel ischemia
- Constipation
- Diverticulitis
- Bowel obstruction
- Pancreatitis
- Appendicitis
- Malignancy
- Radiation enteritis

WORKUP

The clinical presentation is often vague and can be variable from patient to patient. A high index of suspicion must be maintained in any patient presenting with abdominal pain and bloody stool, especially if they are elderly or have risk factors. In addition to the physical exam, the following are key to confirming the diagnosis:
- Laboratory studies
- Computed tomography (CT)
- Lower endoscopy

LABORATORY TESTS

- General:
  1. CBC: Leukocytosis
  2. Comprehensive metabolic panel
  3. Liver function panel
- Specific markers: There are no specific laboratory tests for ischemic colitis. However, elevated levels of certain markers suggest inadequate global perfusion:
  1. Lactate
  2. Lactate dehydrogenase
  3. Creatine kinase (CK)
  4. Amylase
  5. Promising biomarkers: Intestinal fatty acid binding protein (I-FABP), a-glutathione S-transferase (a-GST), D-dimer, L- and D- lactate, citrulline, ischemia modified albumin, procalcitonin (PCT)5
- Infectious workup: Stool studies, parasite testing, virus panel
- Coagulation studies
- Type and screen

IMAGING STUDIES

- Abdominal CT with contrast: Although findings can be nonspecific, the value of CT is in distinguishing ischemic colitis from nonischemic causes of abdominal pain. It also assesses the degree of ischemia and gauges the need for surgical intervention, and may identify arterial emboli or venous obstruction. Specific findings suggestive of ischemic colitis include, but are not limited to, intestinal wall thickening, thumbprinting, pericolonic stranding, and peritoneal free fluid or free air. Pneumatosis (the presence of gas in the colonic wall), portal venous gas, and the presence of megacolon usually indicate severe disease requiring immediate surgical intervention.

- Abdominal radiograph: Should be used in critical patients who are too unstable for a CT scan to look for gas formation in the bowel wall or free air in the abdomen suggestive of perforation.
- Lower endoscopy: This is the gold standard for confirming diagnosis of ischemic colitis in the stable patient. In the absence of peritoneal signs, colonoscopy is the test of choice on an unprepared colon to evaluate the degree of ischemia. If ischemia is suspected, lower endoscopy should be performed within the first 24 to 48 h. In most cases, visual inspection of the colonic wall will confirm the diagnosis and dictate the need for conservative versus surgical management. However, endoscopy should not be performed in patients with acute peritonitis or evidence of irreversible ischemic damage on CT. There is a risk of perforation.[2]

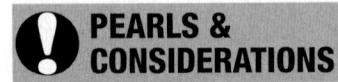 **TREATMENT**

- Treatment depends on disease severity and the specific etiology of colonic ischemia. The mainstay of therapy consists of optimizing blood flow to ischemic regions of bowel and removing any potential exacerbating factors. Initial care consists of aggressive intravenous (IV) crystalloid resuscitation, bowel rest, and broad-spectrum antibiotics with aerobic and anaerobic coverage. A treatment algorithm is illustrated in Fig. 3.
- **In patients with mild disease who are hemodynamically stable and without peritoneal signs**, colonoscopy should be performed. Patients with nonviable bowel seen on endoscopy require immediate operative intervention. **The remainder of patients** should be managed medically. Consider the use of a nasogastric tube in patients with abdominal distention, signs of ileus or bowel obstruction, with parenteral nutrition for those requiring prolonged bowel rest. Avoid vasoconstrictive medications, as they can exacerbate colonic hypoperfusion. Monitor the adequacy of end organ perfusion (e.g., mental status, abdominal pain, urine output). Management of underlying causes (e.g., heart failure, vascular disease, sepsis) should also be addressed.
- **In severe cases unresponsive to supportive therapy,** and in patients exhibiting peritonitis, sepsis, hypotension, and pain out of proportion to exam, surgical abdominal exploration is immediately warranted. Resection of gangrenous segments of bowel may be necessary. Colonoscopy should be avoided in these patients.[2,4]

NONPHARMACOLOGIC THERAPY

- Open or laparoscopic abdominal exploration to identify necrotic bowel. Box 3 summarizes indications for surgical intervention in patients with ischemic colitis.
  1. Bowel prep should not be given due to risk of perforation or toxic dilation[4]
  2. Bowel resection may be indicated in severe colitis

  3. Repeat surgical exploration normally is performed within 12 to 24 h, especially after colonic resection, to assess the viability of colonic tissue and state of the anastomosis. Intraoperative infrared angiography based on IV injection of indocyanine green (Fig. E4) may be used to determine the margins and the integrity of the intestinal anastomoses
  4. Primary anastomosis after colonic resection is contraindicated in certain cases (e.g., presence of aortic or iliac grafts; or when tissue is too friable for stable anastomosis).
- Nasogastric tube placement for bowel decompression is warranted for ileus or obstruction, with subsequent bowel rest and the possible need for parenteral nutrition.

ACUTE GENERAL Rx

- Supportive care:
  1. IV fluids
  2. Bowel rest
  3. Broad-spectrum antibiotics (aerobic and anaerobic coverage)
  4. Pain control
- Anticoagulation (not indicated in nonocclusive ischemia but may be considered in proven arterial occlusion or mesenteric vein thrombosis)

CHRONIC Rx

- Avoid overly aggressive hypertension treatment.
- Avoid dehydration.
- Avoid extreme exercise.

DISPOSITION

- Overall prognosis for ischemic colitis is dependent upon location of disease, comorbidities, and whether surgery was required.
- Most cases of acute ischemic colitis are nongangrenous and resolve completely with medical care in 1 to 2 days.
- The need for surgery in more severe cases portends a worse prognosis and is associated with increased morbidity and mortality. Any risk factors for ischemic colitis should be identified and mitigated as much as possible.
- Follow-up colonoscopy or imaging should be used to evaluate for structure or resolution of the colitis.

REFERRAL

Prompt general surgery consultation is indicated in patients with the following:
- Hemodynamic instability and peritoneal signs on examination
- CT showing signs of bowel infarction or perforation
- Endoscopy showing nonviable bowel or peritoneal signs

PEARLS & CONSIDERATIONS

- Ischemic colitis typically occurs in older patients who have multiple comorbidities.

Algorithm for the management of patients suspected of having colon ischemia

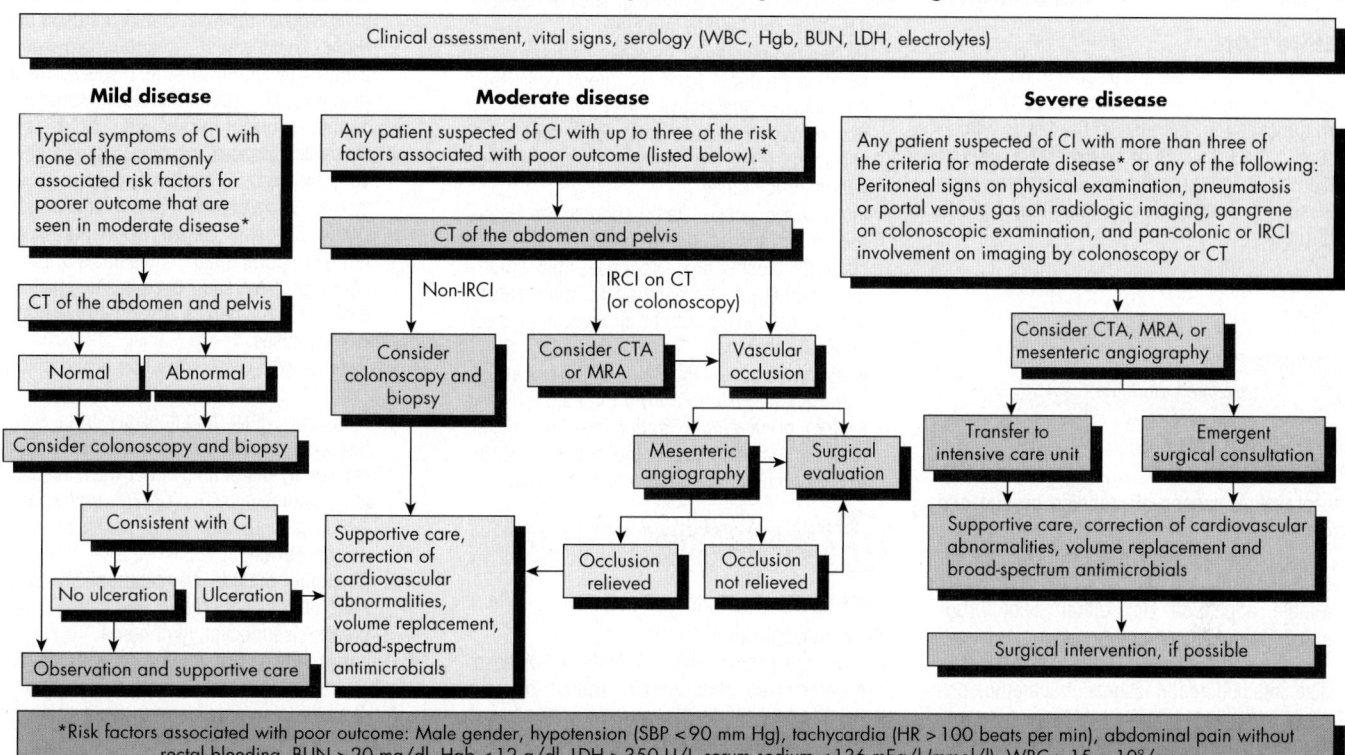

FIG. 3 Colon ischemia algorithm. Diagnosis and treatment of colon ischemia *(CI)* based upon disease severity. *BUN,* Blood urea nitrogen; *CT,* computed tomography; *CTA,* computed tomography angiography; *Hgb,* hemoglobin; *IRCI,* isolated right-colon ischemia; *LDH,* lactate dehydrogenase; *MRA,* magnetic resonance angiography; *MRI,* magnetic resonance imaging; *WBC,* white blood cell count. (From Brandt LJ et al: ACG clinical guideline: epidemiology, risk factors, patterns of presentation, diagnosis, and management of colon ischemia [CI], *Am J Gastroenterol* 110:18-44, 2015. In Goldman L, Shafer AI: *Goldman-Cecil medicine,* ed 26, Philadelphia, 2019, Elsevier.)

BOX 3   Indications for Surgical Intervention in Patients with Ischemic Colitis

Acute
Peritonitis
Bowel perforation
Bowel necrosis
Fulminant colitis
Massive hemorrhage
Sepsis

Chronic
Intractable symptoms (abdominal pain, bloody diarrhea, etc.) lasting >2 wk
Recurrent sepsis
Chronic colitis
Ischemic stricture
Malnutrition from protein-losing enteropathy

From Cameron JL, Cameron AM: *Current surgical therapy,* ed 12, Philadelphia, 2017, Elsevier.

- A high index of suspicion should be maintained for patients with recent endovascular procedures. These patients require close outpatient follow-up and management by a primary care provider.
- Avoid overly aggressive hypertension treatment, dehydration, and extreme exercise.

REFERENCES & SUGGESTED READINGS

Available at eBooks.Health.Elsevier.com.

RELATED CONTENT

Mesenteric Venous Thrombosis (Related Key Topic)
Acute Mesenteric Ischemia (Related Key Topic)

AUTHORS: **DIANA X. ZHOU, MD** and
TRACY LEIGH LEGROS, MD, PhD

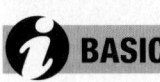 **BASIC INFORMATION**

DEFINITION

Jaundice is a yellowish discoloration of the sclera, skin, and mucous membranes resulting from deposition of bilirubin in the tissue, which occurs in the presence of an excessive amount of bilirubin in the bloodstream. Clinically detectable jaundice in adults is a serum bilirubin of 2.5 to 3 mg/dl.

SYNONYM

Icterus

ICD-10CM CODE
R17   Unspecified jaundice

EPIDEMIOLOGY & DEMOGRAPHICS

The prevalent causes of jaundice by age and sex:
- Young adulthood (for either sex): Viral hepatitis, Gilbert disease
- Middle adulthood (for either sex): Drug-induced hepatitis and cirrhosis
- Middle-aged and older men: Alcoholic liver disease, pancreatic cancer, hepatoma, primary hemochromatosis
- Women: Primary biliary cirrhosis, chronic active hepatitis, choledocholithiasis, carcinoma of the gallbladder

PHYSICAL FINDINGS & CLINICAL PRESENTATION

Presentation can vary from an incidental finding to acute and life-threatening. History and physical examination give important clues to the underlying condition.
Key history of present illness findings:
- Duration of jaundice
- Associated symptoms: Abdominal pain, fever, nausea, malaise, pruritus, chills, changes in urine and stool color (acholic stools), arthralgias, myalgias, rash, anorexia and/or weight loss
Key social history/exposure findings:
- Alcohol use, injection of illicit drugs, tattoos, use of hepatotoxic medication or herbal products, blood transfusions, unprotected sex, ingestion of shellfish, travel, occupational exposure to toxins
Key medical history findings:
- Prior abdominal/biliary surgery, prior episodes of jaundice, prior diagnosis of hepatitis B or C, inflammatory bowel disease
Key physical findings:
- Vital sign abnormalities: Fever, hypotension, tachycardia
- Signs of acute disease: Abdominal tenderness, splenomegaly, abdominal mass, encephalopathy, Murphy sign
- Signs of chronic liver disease: Palmar erythema, spider angiomas/nevi, bruising, gynecomastia, testicular atrophy, ascites, weight loss, Kayser-Fleischer rings (Wilson), caput medusa, internal hemorrhoids, scleral icterus, hepatic hydrothorax, Dupuytren contractures, muscle wasting

ETIOLOGY

Disruption in any of the three phases of bilirubin metabolism can lead to jaundice:
- Prehepatic phase: An increase in heme degradation products from red blood cell (RBC) catabolism, ineffective erythropoiesis, or breakdown of muscle myoglobin and cytochromes; leads to indirect (unconjugated) hyperbilirubinemia
- Intrahepatic phase: Destruction of the hepatocytes or disruption of either of the two separate biochemical processes that conjugate bilirubin in the hepatocyte; may lead to indirect (unconjugated) or direct (conjugated) hyperbilirubinemia
- Posthepatic phase: Blockage of the release of water-soluble bilirubin from the hepatobiliary system, preventing excretion into the stool or urine or recycling within the gut flora; leads to direct (conjugated) hyperbilirubinemia

 DIAGNOSIS

DIFFERENTIAL DIAGNOSIS

Prehepatic causes:
- Hemolytic processes (e.g., sickle cell disease, spherocytosis, thalassemia, G6PD, immune hemolysis, hemolytic uremic syndrome [HUS], microangiopathic hemolytic anemia [MAHA], paroxysmal nocturnal hemoglobinuria [PNH]), sepsis (hypoxia, hypotension with shock liver), heart failure, ineffective erythropoiesis (e.g., thalassemia, folate, severe iron deficiency), or large hematoma reabsorption
Intrahepatic causes:
- If unconjugated hyperbilirubinemia: Enzyme metabolism disorders (Gilbert disease, Crigler-Najjar syndrome), drugs that alter the enzymatic pathways such as rifampin, isoniazid, and probenecid
- If conjugated hyperbilirubinemia: Intrahepatic cholestasis caused by:
  1. Viruses: Hepatitis A, B, and C; Epstein-Barr (EBV), hemorrhagic viruses (yellow fever, Ebola)
  2. Other infections: Bacteria (leptospirosis, MAI), parasites (schistosomiasis, malaria, amebiasis), fungal (*Blastomyces, Histoplasma*)
  3. Alcohol: Alcoholic hepatitis, alcoholic cirrhosis
  4. Autoimmune: Primary biliary cirrhosis, primary sclerosing cholangitis, autoimmune hepatitis
  5. Hepatotoxic drug-induced: Acetaminophen (most common), antibiotics (amoxicillin-clavulanate [most common], sulfamethoxazole-trimethoprim, ciprofloxacin, isoniazid [INH]), cardiovascular drugs (statins, amiodarone), central nervous system agents (valproate, phenytoin, chlorpromazine), antineoplastic drugs (tyrosine kinase inhibitors, tumor necrosis factor inhibitors, methotrexate), tumor necrosis factor inhibitors, steroids (estrogenic or anabolic), NSAIDs, valproic acid, some herbals such as kava, ma huang, and off-market weight-loss supplements

6. Hereditary/metabolic: Sickle cell disease and other RBC dyscrasias, hemochromatosis, Wilson disease, Dubin-Johnson and Rotor syndromes, α-antitrypsin deficiency, glycogen storage disease, NASH (nonalcoholic steatohepatitis), porphyria, benign recurrent intrahepatic cholestasis
7. Systemic diseases invading liver: Sarcoidosis, amyloidosis, hemochromatosis, tuberculosis, *Mycobacterium avium intracellulare*
8. Other: Cirrhosis, sepsis, total parenteral nutrition, intrahepatic cholestasis of pregnancy, graft-versus-host disease, environmental toxins, benign postoperative state
Posthepatic causes:
- Intrinsic or extrinsic obstruction of the biliary system:
  1. Blockage within hepatobiliary tree: Strictures, cholangiocarcinoma, gallbladder cancer, carcinoma of ampulla of Vater, infection (e.g., cytomegalovirus [CMV], *Cryptosporidium* in patients with AIDS, parasites), choledocholithiasis
  2. Blockage outside of hepatobiliary tree: Pancreatitis, pancreatic carcinoma, pancreatic pseudocyst, lymphoma
- Pseudojaundice: Not related to bilirubin but rather resulting from excessive ingestion of foods containing beta carotene (e.g., carrots, melons, squash)

WORKUP

- History, physical examination, and first-line lab tests can often clarify diagnosis. Figs. 1 and 2 describes a clinical approach to jaundice.
Table 1 summarizes the differential diagnosis of critical and emergent diagnoses in patients with jaundice.

LABORATORY TESTS

- First-line tests:
  1. Serum total and direct bilirubin
  2. Urinalysis
  3. Liver function tests (aspartate aminotransferase [AST], alanine transaminase [ALT], gamma-glutamyl transpeptidase [GGTP], alkaline phosphatase), CBC, liver synthetic function (albumin, prothrombin time [PT], partial thromboplastin time [PTT]), pancreatic function (amylase, lipase)
- If serum total bilirubin and direct bilirubin are elevated and urine is positive for bilirubin, consider intrahepatic or posthepatic process. If serum total bilirubin is elevated but direct bilirubin is normal (unconjugated hyperbilirubinemia) and urine is negative for bilirubin, consider prehepatic or intrahepatic processes
Additional tests if diagnosis unclear:
- Screen for hepatitis A, B, and C; if still unclear, then consider following options based on history and physical
- Other viruses: EBV, CMV, COVID 19
- Autoimmune disorders: Antimitochondrial antibody (elevated in primary biliary cirrhosis); antismooth muscle antibody, antinuclear antibodies (ANA; elevated in autoimmune hepatitis); antinuclear cytoplasmic antibody (elevated in primary sclerosing cholangitis)

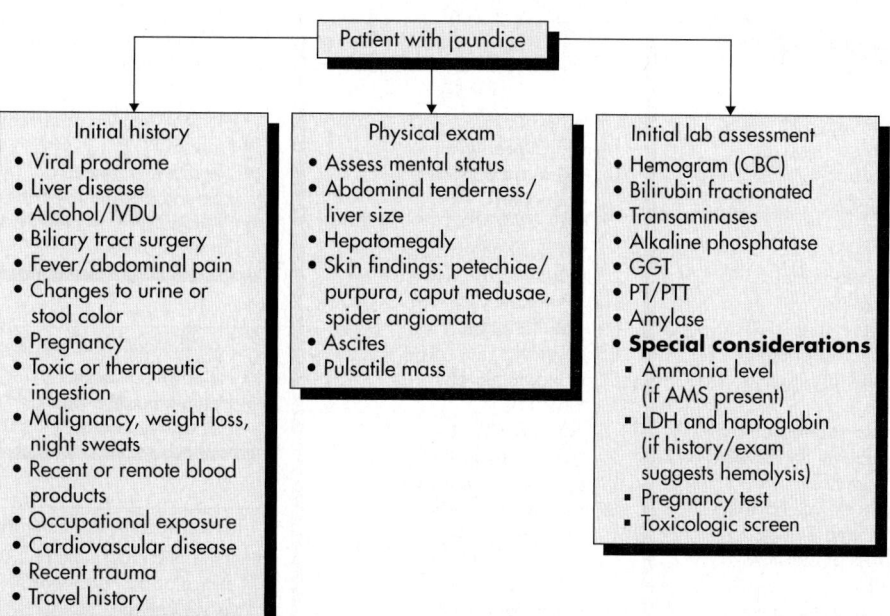

FIG. 1 Initial approach to the patient with jaundice. *AMS,* Altered mental status; *CBC,* complete blood count; *GGT,* gamma-glutamyl transferase; *IVDU,* intravenous drug use; *LDH,* lactate dehydrogenase; *PT,* prothrombin time; *PTT,* partial thromboplastin time. (From Walls RM et al: *Rosen's emergency medicine, concepts and clinical practice,* ed 10, Philadelphia, 2023, Elsevier.)

- Ceruloplasmin (elevated in Wilson disease)
- Alpha-1 antitrypsin deficiency (elevated in cirrhosis and emphysema)
- Ferritin, Fe saturation (elevated in hemochromatosis)
- Blood smear (RBC dyscrasias)
- Diagnosis of exclusion: Gilbert syndrome
- Liver biopsy: Essential in diagnosis of chronic hepatitis. Can be used for diagnosis of liver masses but carries a substantial risk

IMAGING STUDIES

- Abdominal ultrasound: First-line study (Figs. 3 and 4) may be completed bedside, most sensitive for proximal biliary tract disease; presence of dilated ducts hints at an extrahepatic process.
- Abdominal computed tomography (CT): Often necessary to elucidate more information on liver, pancreas, and distal biliary system.
- Endoscopic retrograde cholangiopancreatography: Rarely necessary for diagnostics. Refer to GI consultant.
- Percutaneous transhepatic cholangiography: Rarely necessary for diagnostics. Refer to GI or surgical consultant.
- Magnetic resonance cholangiopancreatography: Noninvasive visualization of bile and pancreatic ducts. Refer to GI consultant.
- Endoscopic ultrasound: Used for characterization and, if needed, biopsy of any focal lesions found within biliary tree and/or pancreas. Refer to GI consultant.

- Liver elastography: Can be done via ultrasound, CT, and MRI to predict the stage of hepatic fibrosis.

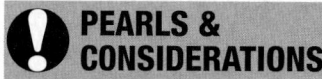

Rx TREATMENT

NONPHARMACOLOGIC THERAPY

Depends on underlying cause of the jaundice and clinical stability of the patient. Generally, obstructive causes require surgical treatment, while nonobstructive causes require medical treatment.

ACUTE GENERAL Rx

Acute, life-threatening illness (e.g., cholecystitis or ascending cholangitis) requires prompt diagnosis with basic labs and bedside diagnostics, with early surgical and GI consultation in conjunction. Suspicious medications should be stopped. Initiate medical management of symptoms with analgesia, intravenous (IV) fluids, correction of coagulopathies, and consideration of antibiotics. *N*-Acetylcysteine can be given for acetaminophen overdose.

CHRONIC Rx

Reversible causes must be ruled out first—suspicious medications and EtOH must be discontinued. Consider GI consult for management of many intrahepatic diseases, such as treatment of hepatitis B or C, Wilson disease with penicillamine, hemochromatosis with

phlebotomy, or for stent insertion with ERCP for posthepatic obstruction. Consider surgical consult for resection of pancreatic masses, cholecystectomy, etc.

Symptomatic pruritus may be treated with cholestyramine for bilirubin binding or with antihistamines to decrease the itch reflex. Ursodiol may be used to treat primary biliary cirrhosis and for gallstone prevention/dissolution.

! PEARLS & CONSIDERATIONS

COMMENTS

- Heed the warning of unstable vital signs to diagnose life-threatening illness; early collaboration with surgical and gastroenterology colleagues is helpful in complex patient care scenarios.
- Careful history and physical examination, basic labs, and prompt bedside imaging frequently lead to accurate diagnosis.
- Very high serum bilirubin (>15 mg/dl) is most likely to be seen in cirrhosis. Watch for hepatorenal syndrome in these patients.

RELATED CONTENT

Jaundice (Patient Information)

AUTHORS: **ALLA GOLDBURT, MD,** **PAOLO G. PACE, MASC, MD,** and **MINTA PATEL, MD**

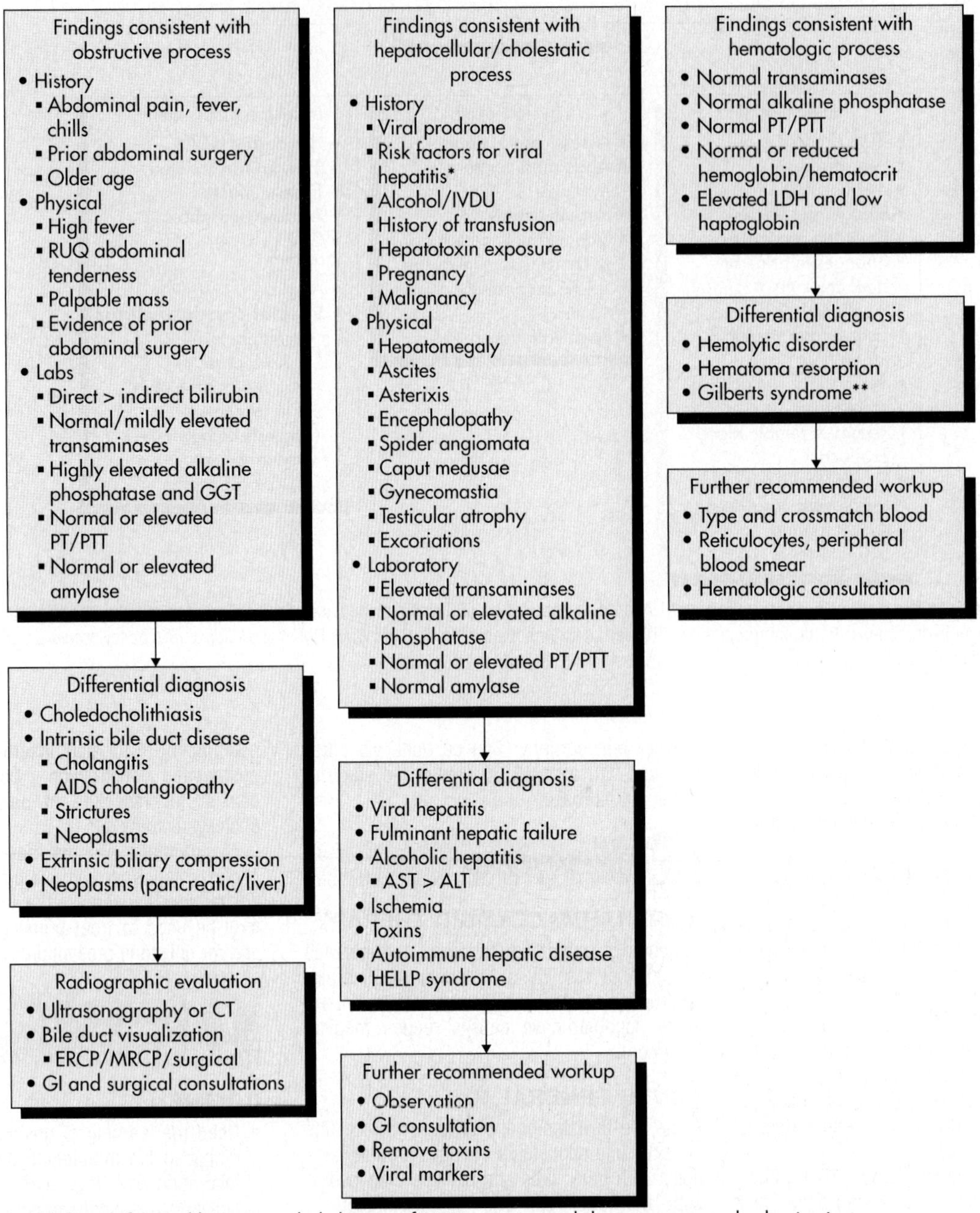

Findings consistent with obstructive process
- History
  - Abdominal pain, fever, chills
  - Prior abdominal surgery
  - Older age
- Physical
  - High fever
  - RUQ abdominal tenderness
  - Palpable mass
  - Evidence of prior abdominal surgery
- Labs
  - Direct > indirect bilirubin
  - Normal/mildly elevated transaminases
  - Highly elevated alkaline phosphatase and GGT
  - Normal or elevated PT/PTT
  - Normal or elevated amylase

Findings consistent with hepatocellular/cholestatic process
- History
  - Viral prodrome
  - Risk factors for viral hepatitis*
  - Alcohol/IVDU
  - History of transfusion
  - Hepatotoxin exposure
  - Pregnancy
  - Malignancy
- Physical
  - Hepatomegaly
  - Ascites
  - Asterixis
  - Encephalopathy
  - Spider angiomata
  - Caput medusae
  - Gynecomastia
  - Testicular atrophy
  - Excoriations
- Laboratory
  - Elevated transaminases
  - Normal or elevated alkaline phosphatase
  - Normal or elevated PT/PTT
  - Normal amylase

Findings consistent with hematologic process
- Normal transaminases
- Normal alkaline phosphatase
- Normal PT/PTT
- Normal or reduced hemoglobin/hematocrit
- Elevated LDH and low haptoglobin

Differential diagnosis
- Hemolytic disorder
- Hematoma resorption
- Gilberts syndrome**

Further recommended workup
- Type and crossmatch blood
- Reticulocytes, peripheral blood smear
- Hematologic consultation

Differential diagnosis
- Choledocholithiasis
- Intrinsic bile duct disease
  - Cholangitis
  - AIDS cholangiopathy
  - Strictures
  - Neoplasms
- Extrinsic biliary compression
- Neoplasms (pancreatic/liver)

Differential diagnosis
- Viral hepatitis
- Fulminant hepatic failure
- Alcoholic hepatitis
  - AST > ALT
- Ischemia
- Toxins
- Autoimmune hepatic disease
- HELLP syndrome

Radiographic evaluation
- Ultrasonography or CT
- Bile duct visualization
  - ERCP/MRCP/surgical
- GI and surgical consultations

Further recommended workup
- Observation
- GI consultation
- Remove toxins
- Viral markers

*Risk factors for viral hepatitis include history of IVDU or intranasal drug use, tattoos, body piercings, blood transfusions, high risk sexual conduct or men who have sex with men, birth in HBV endemic area, known human immunodeficiency virus infection, birth between 1945 and 1965 (hepatitis C), dialysis patients (hepatitis B), recent travel (hepatitis A).

**A benign hereditary condition characterized by hyperbilirubinemia and jaundice due to inadequate hepatic conjugation of bilirubin.

FIG. 2 Differentiation and further evaluation of the jaundiced patient. *AIDS,* Acquired immunodeficiency syndrome; *ALT,* alanine aminotransferase; *AST,* aspartate aminotransferase; *CT,* computed tomography; *ERCP,* endoscopic retrograde cholangiopancreatography; *GGT,* gamma-glutamyl transferase; *GI,* gastrointestinal; *HELLP,* hemolysis, elevated liver enzymes, low platelet count; *IVDU,* intravenous drug use; *LDH,* lactate dehydrogenase; *MRCP,* magnetic resonance cholangiopancreatography; *PT,* prothrombin time; *PTT,* partial thromboplastin time; *RUQ,* right upper quadrant. (From Walls RM et al: *Rosen's emergency medicine, concepts and clinical practice,* ed 10, Philadelphia, 2023, Elsevier.)

TABLE 1 Jaundice: Differential Diagnosis of Critical and Emergent Diagnoses

System	Critical	Emergent	Nonemergent
Hepatic	Fulminant hepatic failure (toxin, virus, alcohol, ischemic insult, Reye syndrome)	Hepatitis of any cause with confusion, bleeding, or coagulopathy	Hepatitis with normal mental status, normal vital signs, and no active bleeding
		Wilson disease	
		Primary biliary cirrhosis	
		Autoimmune hepatitis	
		Liver transplant rejection	
		Infiltrative liver disease	
		Drug induced (isoniazid, phenytoin, acetaminophen, ritonavir, halothane, sulfonamides)	
		Toxin ingestion or exposure	
Biliary	Cholangitis	Bile duct obstruction (stone, inflammation, stricture, neoplasm)	
Systemic	Sepsis	Sarcoidosis	Posttraumatic hematoma resorption
	Heatstroke	Amyloidosis	Total parenteral nutrition
		Graft-versus-host disease	
Cardiovascular	Obstructing AAA	Right-sided congestive heart failure	
	Budd-Chiari syndrome	Veno-occlusive disease	
	Severe congestive heart failure		
Hematologic-oncologic	Transfusion reaction	Hemolytic anemia	Gilbert syndrome
		Massive malignant infiltration	Physiologic neonatal jaundice
		Inborn error of metabolism	
		Pancreatic head tumor	
		Metastatic disease	
Reproductive	Preeclampsia or HELLP syndrome	Hyperemesis gravidarum	
	Acute fatty liver of pregnancy		Cholestasis of pregnancy

AAA, Abdominal aortic aneurysm; *HELLP,* hemolysis, elevated liver enzymes, low platelets.
From Walls RM et al: *Rosen's emergency medicine, concepts and clinical practice,* ed 10, Philadelphia, 2023, Elsevier.

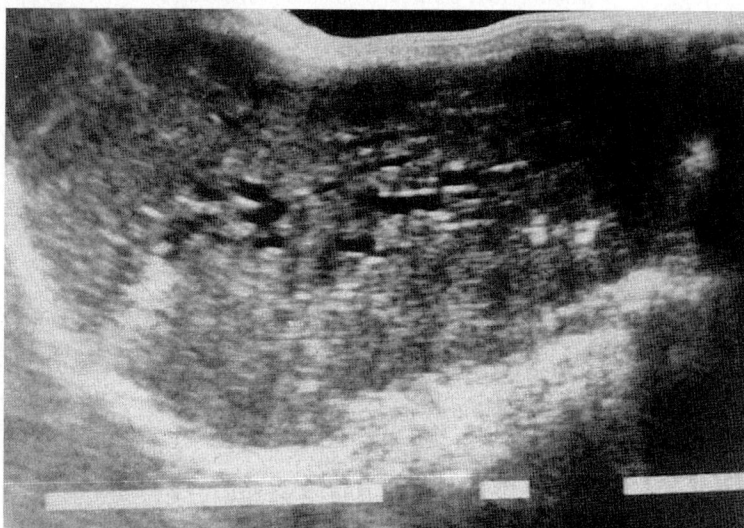

FIG. 3 Ultrasound showing a large calculus in the extrahepatic biliary tree. Dilated bile ducts can be seen to the left. (Courtesy Dr. MC Collins. From Forbes A et al [eds]: *Atlas of clinical gastroenterology,* ed 3, St Louis, 2005, Mosby.)

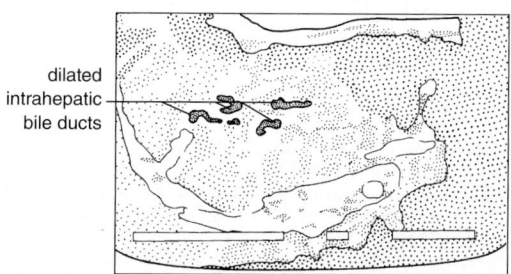

dilated intrahepatic bile ducts

FIG. 4 Schematic representation of ultrasound abnormality seen in Fig. 3. (From Forbes A et al [eds]: *Atlas of clinical gastroenterology,* ed 3, St Louis, 2005, Mosby.)

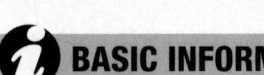 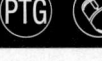 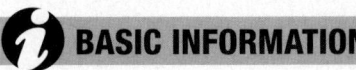
BASIC INFORMATION

DEFINITION

Labyrinthitis is an acute vestibular syndrome resulting from inflammation of the membranous labyrinth of the inner ear.[1] Symptoms include acute onset of dizziness with either hearing loss or tinnitus in association with nausea or vomiting, gait instability, nystagmus, and head-motion intolerance that lasts days or weeks.[2] Vestibular neuritis or neuronitis is often used interchangeably with labyrinthitis because the clinical presentation is so similar. However, vestibular neuritis does not result in hearing loss and is due to inflammation of the vestibular nerve without membranous labyrinth involvement.

SYNONYMS

Acute labyrinthitis
Acute vestibular neuronopathy
Vestibular neuronitis
Vestibular neuritis
Viral neurolabyrinthitis

ICD-10CM CODES	
H81.23	Vestibular neuronitis, bilateral
H83.01	Labyrinthitis, right ear
H83.02	Labyrinthitis, left ear
H83.03	Labyrinthitis, bilateral
H83.09	Labyrinthitis, unspecified ear

EPIDEMIOLOGY & DEMOGRAPHICS

INCIDENCE (IN U.S.): Incidence of labyrinthitis specifically (as opposed to vestibular neuritis) is not known
PREDOMINANT AGE: Any

PHYSICAL FINDINGS & CLINICAL PRESENTATION

CLINICAL PRESENTATION:

- Acute-onset dizziness with hearing loss or tinnitus
- Nausea or vomiting
- Gait instability
- Nystagmus
- Head-motion intolerance
- Duration of symptoms: Days to weeks
- During the first day, the patient usually has difficulty focusing the eyes because of spontaneous nystagmus
- Usually has benign course with complete recovery within 1 to 3 mo, although older patients may have intractable dizziness that persists for many months

PHYSICAL FINDINGS:

- Nystagmus: Spontaneous unidirectional horizontal-torsional nystagmus that attenuates with fixation and whose fast phase beats away from the affected side and intensifies when looking in the direction of the fast phase and diminishes when looking away[3]
- No skew deviation on Alternate Cover Test. The presence of skew deviation is a very specific finding for a brain stem lesion rather than a peripheral cause of acute vestibulopathy
- Corrective saccade on head impulse test (HIT)
- Nausea
- Vomiting
- Vertigo worsening with head movement
- Abnormal caloric electronystagmography (ENG) tests
- Hearing loss in the affected ear or ears
- Normal otoscopic examination typically
- Normal elemental neurologic examination aside from elements related to vestibulopathy such as nystagmus and a positive head thrust test

ETIOLOGY

Symptoms often preceded for 1 to 2 wk by a viral-like illness. Labyrinthitis may be either bacterial or viral and may be either tympanogenic (i.e., resulting from spread of infection into the inner ear from the middle ear, antrum, or petrous apex), meningogenic, or hematogenic from encephalitis or brain abscess. The round window membrane is considered the most likely pathway of inflammatory mediators from the middle to the inner ear that subsequently give rise to labyrinthitis.

Dx DIAGNOSIS

DIFFERENTIAL DIAGNOSIS (TABLE 1)

- Acute labyrinthine ischemia (ischemic stroke of the labyrinthine artery)
- Labyrinthine fistula
- Benign paroxysmal positional vertigo
- Ménière disease
- Cholesteatoma
- Drug-induced vestibulocochlear nerve damage
- Vestibulocochlear nerve (cranial nerve VIII) tumor
- Head trauma
- Vertebrobasilar stroke
- Dehiscence of the superior semicircular canal

WORKUP

Physical examination should include the following elements:[3]
- Otoscopic examination
- HINTS Plus Exam to distinguish patients with an acute vestibular syndrome due to peripheral cause from those with brain stem stroke:
  1. Head Impulse Test: A test of the vestibuloocular reflex (VOR) performed as follows: "Standing in front of the patient, the examiner holds the patient's head by each side, instructs the patient to maintain focus on the examiner's nose and to keep the head and neck loose. Then the examiner quickly turns the patient's head approximately 10 to 20 degrees, using a lateral to center motion. The normal (individuals with normal vestibular function) response is that the patient's focus stays locked on the examiner's nose. The presence of a corrective saccade (the eyes move with the head, then snap back in a fast corrective movement to the examiner's nose) is a positive test (abnormal VOR), which generally indicates a peripheral process, usually vestibular neuritis. The absence of a corrective saccade in an acute vestibular syndrome is consistent with a stroke. If an acutely dizzy patient with an acute vestibular syndrome does not have nystagmus, it is unlikely to be vestibular and, therefore, the HIT should not be used."[3]
  2. Nystagmus: Spontaneous unidirectional horizontal-torsional nystagmus that attenuates with fixation indicates a peripheral lesion. Direction-changing gaze-evoked nystagmus or nystagmus that is pure torsional or vertical should be considered central in origin.[3]
  3. Test of skew deviation with Alternative Cover Test: "With the patient looking directly at the examiner's nose, the examiner alternately covers the right eye, then the left eye, and continues alternating back and forth, approximately every 2 sec. In patients with skew deviation, each time the covered eye is uncovered, there is a slight

TABLE 1 Acute Vestibular Syndrome Oculomotor Physical Findings

Oculomotor Examination Component	Peripheral (Usually Vestibular Neuritis)	Central (Usually Posterior Circulation Stroke)
Nystagmus (neural gaze and gaze to the right and left)	Dominantly horizontal, direction-fixed, beating away from the affected side	Direction-changing horizontal or dominantly vertical and/or torsional, then central[a] (often mimics peripheral)
Test of skew (alternate cover test)	Normal vertical eye alignment (i.e., no skew deviation)	Often mimics peripheral, but if skew deviation is present then central[b]
HIT	Unilaterally abnormal toward the affected side (presence of a corrective saccade)	Usually bilaterally normal (no corrective saccade)

NOTE: Strokes in the AICA territory may produce a unilaterally HIT that mimics vestibular neuritis, but hearing loss is usually present as a clue. If a patient has bilaterally abnormal HIT, this is also suspicious for a central lesion if nystagmus is present (AICA stroke or Wernicke's syndrome).
[a]Inferior branch vestibular neuritis presents with down-beat-torsional nystagmus in a patient with an AVS should be considered to be central (a stroke).
[b]Skew deviation evident by bedside alternate cover testing is rare in peripheral vestibular cases; its presence should be considered to be central (a stroke, often in the brain stem).
From Edlow JA. A new approach to the diagnosis of acute dizziness in adult patients, *Emerg Med Clin North Am* 34(4):717-742, 2016.

vertical correction. One side corrects upward and the other corrects downward. The amplitude of correction is small—1 to 2 mm; therefore, it is key for the examiner to focus on one eye (either one), rather than following the uncovered eye. A normal response is no vertical correction, and an abnormal response should be considered a stroke in patients with an acute vestibular syndrome."[2]

4. Test of hearing (the Plus): Loss of hearing could indicate either labyrinthitis (if the rest of the examination is consistent with a peripheral etiology) or can be part of an anterior inferior cerebellar artery (AICA) stroke syndrome (if the rest of the examination suggests a central etiology).

- General neurologic examination, focusing on cranial nerves, including hearing, cerebellar testing, and long-tract signs. Because a lateral medullary stroke (Wallenberg syndrome) can present with an acute vertigo (with accompanying dysarthria, dysphagia, or hoarseness and may have a Horner's syndrome and decreased ipsilateral facial pain and temperature sensation and contralateral decreased body pain and temperature sensation without any weakness or loss of light touch sensation), it is important to test the cranial nerves carefully.

- Gait testing: Patients who cannot walk independently are unsafe for discharge and are more likely to have a stroke as a cause of their acute vestibular syndrome. Patient with cerebellar dysfunction may have truncal ataxia without abnormalities on finger to nose or rapid alternating movement testing. Patients too symptomatic to walk can be assessed for truncal ataxia by asking them to sit upright on the stretcher without holding onto the side rails.[2]

LABORATORY TESTS

- Routine laboratory tests are generally not helpful.
- If there is a history of significant emesis, check electrolytes, blood urea nitrogen, and creatinine.

IMAGING STUDIES

- Imaging studies are usually not useful but are relied on to evaluate for stroke as a cause of acute vestibular syndrome.
  1. Computed tomography (CT) is a poor test for posterior circulation stroke.
  2. MRI with diffusion-weighted imaging, misses 10% to 20% of strokes in the first 24 to 48 h of an acute vestibular syndrome patient.
- Therefore, in patients with an acute vestibular syndrome, the physical examination leads to a correct diagnosis more frequently than imaging.
- MRI of the brain with and without contrast with fine cuts through the internal auditory canal is indicated if there is an abnormal cranial nerve examination, headache, concern for stroke, or suspicion of cranial nerve VIII nerve tumor.
- Head CT with fine cuts through temporal bones is indicated if there is a history of trauma or suspicion of cholesteatoma.

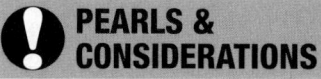

TREATMENT

NONPHARMACOLOGIC THERAPY

- Reassurance
- Initial bed rest, then encourage increase in activity as tolerated
- Vestibular rehabilitation

ACUTE GENERAL Rx

- Treatment options include antiemetics such as promethazine or ondansetron; vestibular suppressants such as the antihistamines meclizine or diphenhydramine; the anticholinergic scopolamine; and the benzodiazepines diazepam or lorazepam. These medications should be continued for only a few days during the acute phase. These medications should be used with caution in the elderly. Methylprednisolone 100 mg/day for 3 days, with slow taper is sometimes used but has not shown benefit in hastening recovery.

- Valacyclovir has not been shown to be helpful.

CHRONIC Rx

- No specific pharmacologic chronic therapy. Meclizine should not be used chronically.
- Vestibular rehabilitation is useful for patients with persistent symptoms.

DISPOSITION

Usually does not require hospital admission unless the patient is unable to tolerate oral intake of liquids

REFERRAL

- Refer if symptoms persist or neurologic abnormalities are present.
- Consider vestibular rehabilitation.

❗ PEARLS & CONSIDERATIONS

COMMENTS

Labyrinthitis is a term that usually implies peripheral vestibulopathy associated with hearing loss. The term *vestibular neuronitis* is typically used when hearing is not affected. Despite this technical distinction, many physicians use these terms interchangeably.

The HINTS Plus Exam is useful in patients with an acute vestibular syndrome to determine whether the lesion is peripheral or possibility due to a stroke.

REFERENCES

Available at eBooks.Health.Elsevier.com.

RELATED CONTENT

Labyrinthitis (Patient Information)
Benign Paroxysmal Positional Vertigo (Related Key Topic)
Vestibular Neuronitis (Related Key Topic)

AUTHOR: **JOSEPH S. KASS, MD, JD, FAAN**

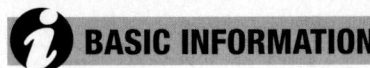
BASIC INFORMATION

DEFINITION

Lactose intolerance is the insufficient concentration of lactase enzyme, leading to fermentation of malabsorbed lactose by intestinal bacteria with subsequent production of intestinal gas and various organic acids, manifesting clinically with diarrhea, abdominal pain, flatulence, or bloating after lactose intake. Lactose malabsorption occurs when a substantial amount of lactose is not absorbed in the intestine. Lactase deficiency is defined as brush-border lactase activity that is markedly reduced relative to the activity observed in infants.

SYNONYMS

Lactose malabsorption
Lactase deficiency
Milk intolerance
Carbohydrate malabsorption

ICD-10CM CODES	
E73.9	Lactose intolerance, unspecified
E73.8	Other lactose intolerance

EPIDEMIOLOGY & DEMOGRAPHICS

- Nearly 50 million people in the U.S. have partial or complete lactose intolerance. There are racial differences, with <25% of White adults being lactose intolerant but >85% of Asian Americans and >60% of African Americans having some form of lactose intolerance.
- There are geographic variations: Highest in Asians (up to 90%), lowest in northern Europeans (approximately 10%), intermediate in southern Europeans and Middle Eastern populations (up to 40%).

PHYSICAL FINDINGS & CLINICAL PRESENTATION

- The main symptoms of lactose intolerance are bloating, abdominal cramps, increased flatus, and diarrhea. Development of bloating and abdominal cramps is presumably associated with increased perception of luminal distention by gas, because no clear relation has been observed between the amount of lactose ingested and the severity of symptoms.
- Physical examination: May be entirely within normal limits.

ETIOLOGY[1]

- Deficiency of the intestinal brush border enzyme lactase can lead to lactose malabsorption. Ingestion of as little as 3 g of lactose may induce symptoms in persons with lactose malabsorption. The pathophysiologic mechanisms resulting in lactose intolerance are currently unclear and may be related to milk protein allergy or fat intolerance on ingestion of nonlactose sugars with the lactose or to functional GI disorders.
- Acquired primary lactase deficiency (adult-type hypolactasia, OMIM #223100) is the most common form of lactase deficiency worldwide. Most populations lose considerable lactase activity in adulthood, which explains why adult mammals are unable to digest lactose and most refuse to drink milk. This decline in lactase activity is a multifactorial process that is regulated at the gene transcription level and leads to decreased biosynthesis, retardation of intracellular transport, or maturation of the enzyme lactase-phlorizin hydrolase. In Whites, an SNP—13910 T/C upstream of the gene that codes for the *LPH* gene has been found to be involved in regulation of the enzyme. The CC genotype of the SNP—13910 T/C upstream of the *LPH* gene is associated with adult-type hypolactasia; TC and TT genotypes are linked with lactase persistence, and, hence, the ability to consume lactose without adverse effect. In other populations (e.g., some African and sub-Saharan African populations), the SNP—13910*T polymorphism is not associated with lactase persistence. Because it is present in most of the adult human population, this form of lactase deficiency has to be considered normal rather than abnormal.
- Congenital lactase deficiency: Common in premature infants; rare in term infants and generally inherited as a chromosomal recessive trait.
- Secondary lactose intolerance: Usually a result of injury of the intestinal mucosa (Crohn disease, viral gastroenteritis, AIDS enteropathy, cryptosporidiosis, Whipple disease, sprue).

DIAGNOSIS

DIFFERENTIAL DIAGNOSIS

- Inflammatory bowel disease
- Irritable bowel syndrome
- Pancreatic insufficiency
- Nontropical and tropical sprue
- Cystic fibrosis
- Diverticular disease
- Bowel neoplasm
- Laxative abuse
- Celiac disease
- Parasitic disease (e.g., giardiasis)
- Viral or bacterial infections

WORKUP

- In patients with lactose malabsorption, it may be unclear whether the condition results from acquired primary lactase deficiency or is a consequence of another small intestinal disorder. Therefore, in the individual patient who demonstrates lactose malabsorption, especially if there is an ethnic background associated with a low prevalence of acquired primary lactase deficiency, it may be necessary to exclude other malabsorptive disorders such as celiac disease. GI symptoms, including diarrhea, have been shown to be more severe in adults with shorter small intestinal transit time, but no such relation between intestinal transit and symptoms is observed in children. Also, in pregnant women and in thyrotoxic patients with Graves disease, changes in intestinal motility play a role in the clinical manifestation of lactose malabsorption. To make a diagnosis of lactose intolerance, and in view of the poor correlation between lactose malabsorption and lactose intolerance, it is very important to monitor symptoms during a lactose HBTest and to confirm that any symptoms experienced by the patient during the test are truly those the patient complains of and that they are associated with a significant increase in breath hydrogen levels.
- Diagnostic workup may include confirming the diagnosis with hydrogen breath test and excluding other conditions listed in the differential diagnosis that may also coexist with lactase deficiency.

LABORATORY TESTS

- Malabsorption of lactose can be diagnosed by the measurement of hydrogen and methane excretion in the breath after a provocative testing dose of lactose. For this purpose, 25 to 50 g of lactose have been used in the past, with the current suggestions leaning toward a testing dose of 25 g. Sampling every 30 min for up to 4 h has been suggested, and a rise in hydrogen of greater than 20 ppm or of methane of greater than 10 ppm is considered positive.[1] This test is positive in 90% of patients with lactose malabsorption. Common causes of false-negative results are recent use of oral antibiotics or recent high colonic enema. Fig. 1 illustrates the role of symptoms in determining the clinical importance of lactose malabsorption.
- The lactose tolerance test is an older and less accurate testing modality (20% rate of false-positive and false-negative results). The patient is administered an oral dose of 1 to 1.5 g of lactose/kg body weight. Serial measurement of blood glucose level on an hourly basis for 3 h is then performed. The test is considered positive if the patient develops intestinal symptoms and the blood glucose level rises <20 mg/dl above the fasting baseline level.
- Diarrhea associated with lactase deficiency is osmotic in nature with an osmotic gap and a pH <6.5.
- Laboratory evaluation may not be necessary in patients with significant history.

IMAGING STUDIES

Imaging studies are generally not indicated. A small bowel series may be useful in patients with significant malabsorption.

TREATMENT

NONPHARMACOLOGIC THERAPY

Management consists of reducing lactose exposure by avoiding milk and milk-containing products or using milk in which the lactose has been prehydrolyzed with lactase. A lactose-free diet generally results in prompt resolution of symptoms. Lactose is primarily found in dairy products

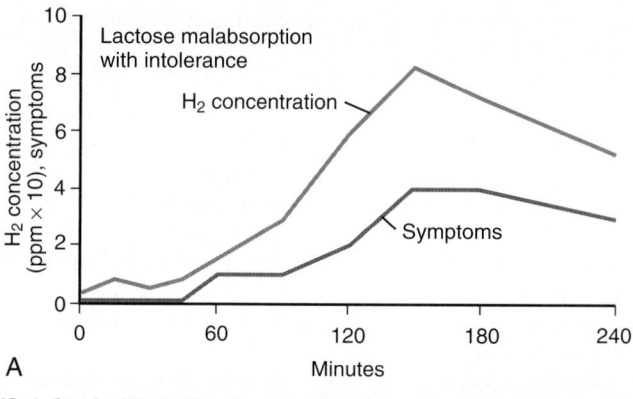
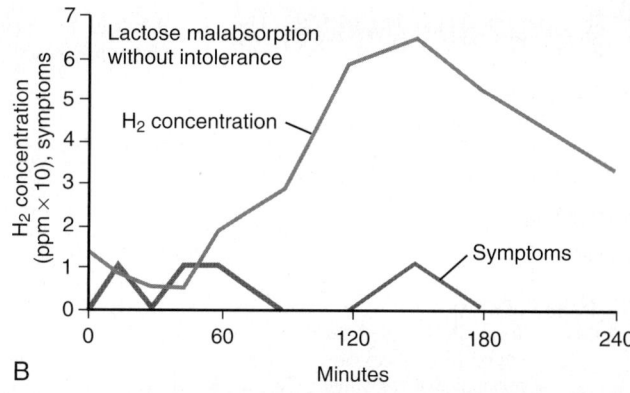

FIG. 1 Graphs illustrating the role of symptoms in determining the clinical importance of lactose malabsorption. Assessment of the clinical relevance of an abnormal lactose hydrogen breath test is made by monitoring abdominal symptoms (bloating, cramps, pain) during the test. Breath hydrogen concentration in parts per million (ppm) and GI symptoms using an arbitrary scoring system for two different patients are plotted on the graphs. **A,** The patient has symptoms associated with an increase in breath hydrogen concentration and therefore can be considered to have lactose intolerance. **B,** The patient has no increase in symptoms, although the breath hydrogen concentration increases considerably, so the patient has lactose malabsorption without lactose intolerance. (From Feldman M et al: *Sleisenger and Fordtran's gastrointestinal and liver disease,* ed 11, Philadelphia, 2021, Elsevier.)

but may be present as an ingredient or component of common foods and beverages. Possible sources of lactose include breads, candies, cold cuts, dessert mixes, cream soups, bologna, commercial sauces and gravies, chocolate, drink mixes, salad dressings, and medications. Labels should be read carefully to identify sources of lactose.

ACUTE GENERAL Rx

- Patients in whom a clear association can be established between symptoms and lactose ingestion (with or without proven lactose malabsorption) should be educated about lactose-reduced or lactose-free diets. Patients should be informed that the commonly ingested doses of lactose (e.g., up to a cup of milk) usually do not cause symptoms when ingested with a meal. Dietary instructions may help the large majority of lactose-intolerant subjects. Daily consumption of lactose-containing food may be better tolerated than intermittent consumption. Yogurt may be tolerated by such patients and provides a good source of calcium. Consuming whole milk or chocolate milk rather than skim milk and drinking milk with meals can reduce symptoms of lactose intolerance, presumably as a result of prolonged gastric emptying.

Alternatively, supplementation of dairy products with lactase of microbiologic origin can be suggested. The results of controlled studies on the use of lactose-reduced products or lactase capsules are inconsistent. Furthermore, because many carbohydrates other than lactose are incompletely absorbed by the normal small intestine and because dietary fiber also may be metabolized by colonic bacteria, persistence of some symptoms while the patient is on a lactose-free diet is not uncommon. It must also be kept in mind that symptoms arising after ingestion of dairy products may be from milk protein allergy or fat intolerance rather than lactose intolerance.[1]

- Addition of lactase enzyme supplement (Lactaid tablets, Dairy Ease) before the ingestion of milk products may prevent symptoms in some patients. However, it is not effective for all lactose-intolerant patients.

CHRONIC Rx

Lactose-intolerant patients must ensure adequate calcium intake. Calcium supplementation is recommended to prevent osteoporosis.

DISPOSITION

Clinical improvement with restriction or elimination of milk products

REFERRAL

GI referral for endoscopic procedures if concomitant GI disorders are suspected

❗ PEARLS & CONSIDERATIONS

COMMENTS

- There is great variability in signs and symptoms in patients with lactose intolerance depending on the degree of lactase deficiency. Most individuals with presumed lactose malabsorption can tolerate 12 to 15 g of lactose or up to 12 oz of milk daily without symptoms.
- Nondairy synthetic drinks (e.g., Coffee-Mate) and use of rice milk are generally well tolerated.

REFERENCE

Available at eBooks.Health.Elsevier.com.

RELATED CONTENT

Lactose Intolerance (Patient Information)

AUTHOR: **FRED F. FERRI, MD**

Lead Poisoning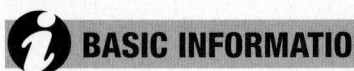

BASIC INFORMATION

DEFINITION
Lead is a potent, pervasive neurotoxicant. Lead poisoning refers to multisystem abnormalities resulting from excessive lead exposure.

SYNONYM
Plumbism

ICD-10CM CODES
T56.0X1A	Toxic effect of lead and its compounds, accidental (unintentional), initial encounter
T56.0X1D	Toxic effect of lead and its compounds, accidental (unintentional), subsequent encounter
T56.0X1S	Toxic effect of lead and its compounds, accidental (unintentional), sequela
T56.0X2A	Toxic effect of lead and its compounds, intentional self-harm, initial encounter
T56.0X2D	Toxic effect of lead and its compounds, intentional self-harm, subsequent encounter
T56.0X2S	Toxic effect of lead and its compounds, intentional self-harm, sequela
T56.0X3A	Toxic effect of lead and its compounds, assault, initial encounter
T56.0X3D	Toxic effect of lead and its compounds, assault, subsequent encounter
T56.0X3S	Toxic effect of lead and its compounds, assault, sequela
T56.0X4A	Toxic effect of lead and its compounds, undetermined, initial encounter
T56.0X4D	Toxic effect of lead and its compounds, undetermined, subsequent encounter
T56.0X4S	Toxic effect of lead and its compounds, undetermined, sequela

EPIDEMIOLOGY & DEMOGRAPHICS
- Lead poisoning is most common in children ages 1 to 5 yr (17,000 cases/100,000 persons). The highest rates are among Blacks, those with low income, and urban children.
- In 1991 the Centers for Disease Control and Prevention (CDC) lowered the definition of a safe blood lead level to <10 mcg/dl of whole blood (a blood lead level of 25 mcg/dl was considered acceptable before 1991).
- It is estimated that >15% of preschoolers in the U.S. have a blood lead level >15 mcg/dl.

PHYSICAL FINDINGS & CLINICAL PRESENTATION
- Findings vary with the degree of toxicity (Table 1). Examination may be normal in patients with mild toxicity.
- Myalgias, irritability, headache, and general fatigue may be present initially.
- Abdominal cramping, constipation, weight loss, tremor, paresthesias and peripheral neuritis, seizures, and coma may occur with severe toxicity.
- Motor neuropathy is common in children with lead poisoning; learning disorders are also frequent.

ETIOLOGY
Chronic, repeated exposure to paint containing lead, plumbing, storage of batteries, pottery, or lead soldering. Concentration of lead is generally highest in lead-based paint on exterior surfaces. Among interior surfaces, windows are most likely to have the highest lead content. Table 2 summarizes common sources of lead.

DIAGNOSIS

DIFFERENTIAL DIAGNOSIS
- Polyneuropathies from other sources
- Anxiety disorder, attention deficit disorder
- Malabsorption, acute abdomen
- Iron deficiency anemia

WORKUP
Laboratory screening: All U.S. children should be considered to be at risk for lead poisoning and should be screened routinely starting at age 1 yr for low-risk children and age 6 mo for high-risk children. Lead poisoning risk assessment questions to be asked between 6 mo and 6 yr are summarized in Table 3.

LABORATORY TESTS
- Venous blood lead level: Normal level, <5 mcg/dl; levels of 50 to 70 mcg/dl, indicative of moderate toxicity; levels >70 mcg/dl, associated with severe poisoning
- Mild anemia with basophilic stippling on peripheral smear
- Elevated zinc protoporphyrin levels or free erythrocyte protoporphyrin level

- An increased body burden of lead with previous high-level exposure in patients with occupational lead poisoning can be demonstrated by measuring the excretion of lead in urine after premedication with calcium ethylenediaminetetraacetic acid (EDTA) or another chelating agent

IMAGING STUDIES
- Imaging studies are generally not necessary.
- A plain abdominal film can visualize lead particles in the gut.
- "Lead lines" may be noted on x-ray films of long bones.

TABLE 1 Typical Blood Lead Levels and Correlative Signs and Symptoms in Children and Adults

Level (μg/dl)	SYMPTOMS Adults	Children
10	None	Decreased IQ
		Decreased hearing
		Decreased growth
20	Increased protoporphyrin	Decreased nerve conduction velocity
	No symptoms	Increased protoporphyrin
30	Increased blood pressure	Decreased vitamin D metabolism
	Decreased hearing	
40	Peripheral neuropathies	Decreased hemoglobin synthesis
	Nephropathy	
	Infertility (men)	
50	Decreased hemoglobin synthesis	Lead colic
70	Anemia	Anemia
		Encephalopathy
		Nephropathy
100	Encephalopathy	Death

IQ, Intelligence quotient.
From Walls RM et al: *Rosen's emergency medicine, concepts and clinical practice*, ed 10, Philadelphia, 2023, Elsevier.

TABLE 2 Sources of Lead

Paint chips
Dust
Soil
Parent's or older child's occupational exposure (auto repair, smelting, construction, remodeling, plumbing, gun/bullet exposure, painting, e-scrap)
Glazed ceramics
Herbal remedies (e.g., Ayurvedic medications)
Home remedies including antiperspirants, deodorants (litargirio)
Jewelry (toys or parents')
Stored battery casings (or living near a battery smelter)
Lead-based gasoline
Moonshine alcohol
Mexican candies; Ecuadorian chocolates
Indoor firing ranges
Retained bullet fragments
Imported spices (svanuri marili, zafron, kuzhambu)
Lead-based cosmetics (kohl, surma)
Lead plumbing (water)
Imported foods in lead-containing cans
Imported toys
Home renovations
Antique toys or furniture

From Kliegman RM: *Nelson's textbook of pediatrics*, ed 21, Philadelphia, 2020, Elsevier.

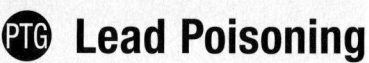
TABLE 3 Lead Poisoning Risk Assessment Questions to Be Asked Between 6 Mo and 6 Yr

Does the child live in or regularly visit a home built before 1950?

Does the child spend any time in a building built before 1978 with recent or ongoing painting, repair work, remodeling, or damage?

Is there a brother, sister, housemate, playmate, or community member being followed or treated (or even rumored to be) for lead poisoning?

Does the child live with an adult whose job or hobby involves exposure to lead (e.g., lead smelting and automotive radiator repair)?

Does the child live near an active lead smelter, battery recycling plant, or other industry likely to release lead?

Does the family use home remedies or pottery from another country?

From Marcdante KJ et al: *Nelson essentials of pediatrics,* ed 9, Philadelphia, 2023, Elsevier.

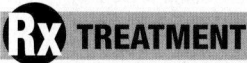 **TREATMENT**

NONPHARMACOLOGIC THERAPY

- Provide adequate amounts of calcium, iron, zinc, and protein in patient's diet.
- Family education on sources of lead exposure and potential adverse health effects.

ACUTE GENERAL Rx

- The use of chelation in cases of acute lead poisoning is guided by the patient's clinical status and the blood lead level. For children with blood levels of 10 to 19 mcg/dl, the CDC recommends nonpharmacologic interventions (see "Nonpharmacologic Therapy").
- For children with blood levels between 20 and 44 mcg/dl, the CDC recommendations include case management by a qualified social worker, clinical management, environmental assessment, and lead hazard control. Chelation therapy should be considered in children with refractory blood lead levels.
- Chelation therapy (Table 4) is indicated in children with blood lead levels >45 mcg/dl.
- Succimer (DMSA) 10 mg/kg PO q8h for 5 days then q12h for 2 wk can be used in patients with levels between 45 and 70 mcg/dl.
- Edetate calcium disodium (EDTA) and dimercaprol (BAL) are effective in patients with severe toxicity.
- Use of both EDTA and DMSA is indicated in children with blood levels >70 mcg/dl.
- D-Penicillamine (Cuprimine) also can be used for lead poisoning, but it is not FDA approved for this condition.

CHRONIC Rx

- Reduce exposure, remove any potential lead sources.
- Correct iron deficiency and any other nutritional deficiencies.
- Recheck blood lead level 7 to 21 days after chelation therapy.

DISPOSITION

Patients with mild to moderate toxicity generally improve without any residual deficits. The presence of encephalopathy at diagnosis is a poor prognostic sign. Residual neurologic deficits may persist in these patients. Chelation therapy seems to slow the progression of renal insufficiency in patients with mildly elevated body lead burden.

REFERRAL

If exposure to lead is work related, it should be reported to the Office of the United States Occupational Safety and Health Administration (OSHA). Follow-up testing is mandatory in all patients after an abnormal screening blood lead level.

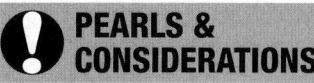 **PEARLS & CONSIDERATIONS**

COMMENTS

- Even blood lead concentrations as low as 5 to 10 mcg/dl are inversely associated with children's IQ scores at age 3 and 5 yr. A recent study evaluating long-term ramifications of childhood lead exposure revealed that childhood lead exposure was associated with lower cognitive function and socioeconomic status at age 38 yr, with declines in IQ, and downward social mobility.
- Screening of household members of affected individuals is recommended.
- In children with blood lead levels of >45 mg/dl, treatment with succimer does not improve scores on tests of cognition, behavior, or neuropsychologic function.
- Lead toxicity may delay growth and pubertal development in girls.
- Low-level environmental lead exposure may accelerate progressive renal insufficiency in patients without diabetes who have chronic renal disease. Repeated chelation therapy may improve renal function and slow the progression of renal failure.

RELATED CONTENT

Lead Poisoning (Patient Information)

AUTHOR: **FRED F. FERRI, MD**

TABLE 4 Chelators*

Chelator	Dose	Indications	Contraindications
Deferoxamine	15 mg/kg/h up to 24 h (titrate up slowly because of hypotension)	Iron level >500 g/dl or systemic symptoms	
Dimercaprol (British anti-Lewisite [BAL])	Lead encephalopathy: 75 mg/m² deep IM injection every 4 h for 5 days in children or 4 mg/kg every 4 h for adults Arsenic (severe): No established regimen; consider 3 mg/kg IM every 4 h for 48 h; then twice daily for 7-10 days Mercury: 5 mg/kg IM first; then 2.5 mg/kg every 12-24 h	Lead level >70 g/dl or encephalopathy Arsenic: Symptomatic patient with known exposure Mercury: Inorganic	Peanut allergy Organic mercury poisoning
CaNa₂EDTA	1500 mg/m²/day continuous IV infusion 50 mg/kg/day or 1000 mg/m²/day in 2-4 divided doses for up to 5 days if less severe symptoms	Lead: Given after first dose of BAL for blood lead level above 70 g/dl or encephalopathy	
Succimer (DMSA)	10 mg/kg q8h × 5 days; then q12h for 14 days	Lead level of 45-69 g/dl Arsenic: If tolerated orally for subacute and chronic toxicity Mercury: Acute and chronic	
D-Penicillamine	25 mg/kg q6h × 5 days	Lead level of 45-69 g/dl, succimer not tolerated Arsenic: Only if BAL and DMSA are unavailable Mercury: If BAL and DMSA are unavailable or not tolerated	Penicillin allergy
DMPS (investigational)	5 mg/kg/dose IM q6-8h day 1, q8-12h day 2, q12-24h day 3 and until 24-h urine is <50 µg/L	Lead (chronic) Arsenic Mercury	

DMPS, 2,3-Dimercapto-1-propanesulfonic acid; *EDTA,* edetate calcium disodium; *IM,* intramuscular; *IV,* intravenous; *q,* every.

*Indications for chelation and dosing regimens may change. Consult with a toxicologist or poison control center for the most up-to-date recommendations.

From Walls RM et al: *Rosen's emergency medicine, concepts and clinical practice,* ed 10, Philadelphia, 2023, Elsevier.

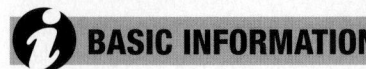

BASIC INFORMATION

DEFINITION

Liver abscess is a necrotic infection of the liver usually classified as pyogenic or amebic.

SYNONYMS

Pyogenic hepatic abscess
Amebic hepatic abscess

ICD-10CM CODE
K75.0   Abscess of liver

EPIDEMIOLOGY & DEMOGRAPHICS

INCIDENCE: Incidence of pyogenic liver abscess is 2.3 cases/100,000 population.
PREVALENCE (WORLDWIDE): Amebic liver abscess is more common than pyogenic liver abscess.
PREVALENCE (IN U.S.): Pyogenic liver abscess is more common than amebic liver abscess.
PREDOMINANT SEX & AGE: More common in men than women; male:female ratio of 2:1; most common in fourth to sixth decades of life.

PHYSICAL FINDINGS & CLINICAL PRESENTATION

- Fever, chills, and sweats
- Weakness/malaise
- Anorexia with weight loss
- Nausea, vomiting, and diarrhea
- Cough with pleuritic chest pain
- Right upper quadrant abdominal pain
- Hepatomegaly
- Splenomegaly
- Jaundice
- Pleural effusions, rales, and friction rubs may be present
- Most abscesses occur on the right lobe of the liver

ETIOLOGY

- Pyogenic liver abscess is usually polymicrobial (*Klebsiella pneumoniae* [43%], *Escherichia coli* [33%], *Streptococcus* spp. [37%], *Pseudomonas aeruginosa*, *Proteus* spp., *Bacteroides* spp. [24%], *Fusobacterium* spp., *Actinomyces* spp., gram-positive anaerobes, and *Staphylococcus aureus*).
- Pyogenic liver abscess occurs from:
  1. Biliary disease with cholangitis (accounts for approximately 40% to 60%)
  2. Gallbladder disease with contiguous spread to the liver
  3. Diverticulitis or appendicitis with spread via the portal circulation
  4. Hematogenous spread via the hepatic artery, though uncommon; if a solitary organism is isolated, a distant source of hematogenous seeding should be sought
  5. Penetrating wounds
  6. Cryptogenic
  7. Infection by way of portal system (portal pyemia)
  8. No causes found in approximately half of cases
  9. Incidence increased in patients with diabetes and metastatic cancer
  10. Table 1 summarizes underlying etiology and bacteriology of liver abscesses
- Amebic hepatic abscess is caused by the parasite *Entamoeba histolytica*. Amebiasis is usually due to fecal-oral contamination and invades the intestinal mucosa, gaining entry into the portal system to reach the liver. Amebic abscess occurs in 3% to 7% of patients with amebiasis.
- A comparison of pyogenic and amebic liver abscess is summarized in Table 2.

Box 1 describes pearls for amebic liver abscesses. The abscess is usually solitary (85%) and in the right lobe (72%).

DIAGNOSIS

The diagnosis of liver abscess requires a high index of suspicion after a detailed history and physical examination. Imaging studies and microbiologic, serologic, and percutaneous techniques (e.g., aspiration) confirm the presence of a liver abscess.

TABLE 1   Underlying Etiology and Bacteriology

Etiology	Bacteriology
Biliary, benign	*Escherichia coli* *Klebsiella* spp. *Enterococcus*
Biliary, malignant	*Pseudomonas* spp. Multiply resistant GN aerobes VRE Yeast
Diverticulitis/appendicitis	GN aerobes *Bacteroides fragilis*
Severe cholecystitis	See "Biliary, benign" *Clostridium perfringens Bacteroides* spp.
Subcutaneous abscess	*Staphylococcus* spp. MRSA
Endocarditis	*Enterococcus* spp. *Staphylococcus* spp.
Cryptogenic	Anaerobes

GN, Gram-negative; *MRSA*, methicillin-resistant *Staphylococcus aureus*; *VRE*, vancomycin-resistant *Enterococcus*.
From Cameron JL, Cameron AM: *Current surgical therapy*, ed 10, Philadelphia, 2011, Saunders.

TABLE 2   Features of Bacterial and Amebic Abscesses

	Demographics	Risk Factors	Symptoms	Laboratory Findings	Radiographic Features	Diagnosis	Treatment
Bacterial liver abscess	50-70 yr Male = female	Recent bacterial infection, biliary obstruction, diabetes mellitus	Fevers, chills, malaise, anorexia, diarrhea, cough, pleuritic chest pain, RUQ pain	Leukocytosis, anemia, elevated alkaline phosphatase and bilirubin, low albumin, positive blood cultures (50%)	Multifocal (50%), usually right lobe, irregular margins	Aspirate (70%-80% positive)	Percutaneous drainage and antibiotics
Amebic liver abscess	18-50 yr Male > female	Alcohol intake, HLA-DR3, oral and anal sex, contaminated enema apparatus, travel to or living in an endemic area	Fever, RUQ pain, hepatic tenderness, anorexia, weight loss, uncommon to have colitis	Leukocytosis, no eosinophilia, mild anemia, elevated alkaline phosphatase, elevated ESR, positive serology	Single abscess (80%), usually right lobe, wall enhancement seen on CT scan with IV contrast	Aspirate (trophozoites rarely seen) can rule out superimposed bacterial infection, positive serology and risk factors	Metronidazole and iodoquinol

CT, Computed tomography; *ESR*, erythrocyte sedimentation rate; *HLA*, human leukocyte antigen; *IV*, intravenous; *RUQ*, right upper quadrant.
From Goldman L, Schafer AI: *Goldman-Cecil medicine*, ed 26, Philadelphia, 2019, Elsevier.

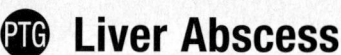

BOX 1 Pearls for Amebic Liver Abscesses

- Only 10%-20% of patients with amebic liver abscess have a history of diarrhea.
- Treat the intestinal infection to prevent relapse of amebic liver abscess. Failure to use luminal amebicidal agents after metronidazole in cases of amebic abscess results in a 10% relapse rate.
- Failure to show response to antiamebic medication requires evaluation for polymicrobial infection with bacteria.
- Amebic abscess usually responds clinically to antimicrobial therapy in 3-7 days, although imaging takes several months to show resolution.
- Percutaneous drainage is rarely required.

From Cameron JL, Cameron AM: *Current surgical therapy,* ed 10, Philadelphia, 2011, Saunders.

DIFFERENTIAL DIAGNOSIS

- Cholangitis
- Cholecystitis
- Diverticulitis
- Appendicitis
- Perforated viscus
- Mesentery ischemia
- Pulmonary embolism
- Pancreatitis

WORKUP

- The workup of a liver abscess should focus on differentiating between amebic and pyogenic causes.
- Features suggesting an amebic cause include travel to an endemic area, single abscess rather than multiple abscesses, subacute onset of symptoms, and absence of conditions predisposing to pyogenic liver abscess, as highlighted under "Etiology."
- Laboratory studies are not specific but are useful as adjunctive tests.
- Imaging studies cannot differentiate between the two, and bacteriologic cultures may be sterile in 50% of the cases.

LABORATORY TESTS

- CBC: Leukocytosis
- Liver function tests: Alkaline phosphatase is most commonly elevated (95% to 100%); aspartate transaminase (AST) and alanine transaminase (ALT) elevated in 50% of cases; elevated bilirubin (28% to 30%); decreased albumin
- Prothrombin time (INR): Prolonged (70%)
- Blood cultures: Positive in 50% of cases
- Aspiration (50% sterile)
- Stool samples for *E. histolytica* trophozoites (positive in 10% to 15% of amebic liver abscess cases)
- Serologic testing for *E. histolytica* should be done on all patients, but it is important to remember that it does not differentiate acute from old infections

IMAGING STUDIES

- Ultrasound (80% to 100% sensitivity in detecting abscesses) shows round or oval hypoechogenic mass (Fig. E1, *A*).
- Computed tomography (CT) scan is more sensitive in detecting hepatic abscesses and contiguous organ extension and is the imaging study of choice (see Fig. E1, *B*, and Fig. E2).

- Chest x-ray: Abnormal in 50% of the cases, may reveal elevated right hemidiaphragm, subdiaphragmatic air-fluid levels, pleural effusions, and consolidating infiltrates.
- Most liver abscesses are single; however, multiple liver abscesses can occur with systemic bacteremia.

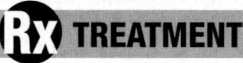 TREATMENT

NONPHARMACOLOGIC THERAPY

- The management of pyogenic liver abscess differs from that of amebic liver abscess.
- Medical management is the cornerstone of therapy in amebic liver abscess, whereas early intervention in the form of surgical therapy or catheter drainage and parenteral antibiotics is the rule in pyogenic liver abscess greater than 3 cm. Smaller abscesses (<3 cm) can generally be treated with broad-spectrum antibiotics.

ACUTE GENERAL Rx

- Percutaneous drainage under CT or ultrasound guidance is essential in the treatment of pyogenic liver abscesses.
- Aspiration of hepatic amebic abscesses is not required unless there is no response to treatment or a pyogenic cause is being considered.
- Empiric broad-spectrum antibiotics are recommended initially until culture results are available. Common choices include:
  1. Metronidazole (500 mg intravenous [IV] q8h) plus ceftriaxone or levofloxacin.
  2. Monotherapy with a beta-lactam/beta-lactamase inhibitor, such as piperacillin/tazobactam (4.5 g q6h), ticarcillin-clavulanate (3.1 g q4h), or ampicillin-sulbactam (3 g q6h).
  3. Monotherapy with a carbapenem, such as imipenem (500 mg IV q6h), meropenem (1 g q8h), or ertapenem (1 g daily).
  4. Duration of antibiotic treatment is usually 4 to 6 wk with IV antibiotics used for the first 1 to 2 wk or until a favorable clinical response, followed thereafter with oral antibiotics (e.g., metronidazole 500 mg PO q8h plus ciprofloxacin 500 mg PO q12h).
  5. Third-generation cephalosporins should not be used as single agents for empiric therapy because of risk of the emergence of beta-lactamase–producing bacteria.

- Antibiotic coverage for amebic liver abscesses includes:
  1. Metronidazole 750 mg PO tid for 10 days or tinidazole
  2. Eradication of the coexistent intestinal infection with paromomycin for 10 days

CHRONIC Rx

- If fever persists for 2 wk despite percutaneous drainage and antibiotic therapy as outlined under "Acute General Rx," or if there is failure of aspiration or failure of percutaneous drainage, surgery is indicated.
- In patients not responding to IV antibiotics and percutaneous drainage, hepatic artery antibiotic infusion can be considered.
- In patients with evidence of metastatic disease that is causing biliary obstruction, a gastroenterology consultation for endoscopic retrograde cholangiopancreatography and stenting should be considered.

DISPOSITION

- Most patients with pyogenic liver abscesses defervesce within 2 wk of treatment with antibiotics and drainage.
- No randomized controlled studies have evaluated the optimal duration of antibiotic therapy for pyogenic liver abscess. Typical duration of antibiotic therapy is at least 4 to 6 wk.
- Pyogenic liver abscess cure rates using percutaneous drainage and antibiotics have been reported to be between 88% and 100%.
- Mortality rate of untreated pyogenic liver abscess is nearly 100%.
- Most patients with amebic liver abscesses defervesce within 4 to 5 days of treatment.
- Amebic liver abscess mortality rate is <1% unless complications occur (see "Comments").
- Follow-up imaging should be used to monitor response to therapy; continue treatment until CT scan shows complete or near-complete resolution of cavity.

REFERRAL

Infectious disease, gastroenterology, interventional radiology, and general surgical consultations are recommended in any patient with hepatic abscess.

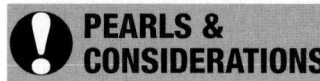 PEARLS & CONSIDERATIONS

COMMENTS

- Complications of pyogenic and amebic liver abscesses include:
  1. Pleuropulmonary extension, resulting in empyema, abscess, and fistula formation
  2. Peritonitis
  3. Purulent pericarditis
  4. Sepsis
- Amebic liver abscesses complicate amebic colitis in nearly 10% of cases.

RELATED CONTENT

Liver Abscess (Patient Information)
Amebiasis (Related Key Topic)

AUTHOR: **FRED F. FERRI, MD**

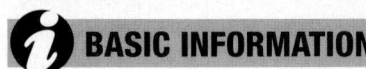
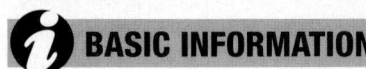

BASIC INFORMATION

DEFINITION
A lung abscess is an infection of the lung parenchyma resulting in necrosis and cavity formation.

SYNONYMS
Pulmonary abscess
Abscess, lung

ICD-10CM CODES	
A06.5	Amebic lung abscess
J85.1	Abscess of lung with pneumonia
J85.2	Abscess of lung without pneumonia

EPIDEMIOLOGY & DEMOGRAPHICS
INCIDENCE:
- The exact incidence is unknown; however, it has significantly decreased with the advent of antibiotics.
- Lung abscess is more common in the elderly because of an increased risk of periodontal disease and dysphagia.
RISK FACTORS (TABLE 1):
- Alcohol use disorder
- Seizure disorders
- Cerebrovascular disorders with dysphagia
- Head trauma
- Substance use disorders
- General anesthesia
- Esophageal disorders (e.g., scleroderma, esophageal carcinoma)
- Poor oral hygiene
- Poor cough reflex
- Obstructive lung neoplasm
- Bronchiectasis
- Obstructive foreign body

PHYSICAL FINDINGS & CLINICAL PRESENTATION
Symptoms are generally insidious, occurring over weeks to months:
- Fever
- Cough
- Sputum production (purulent with foul odor)
- Pleuritic chest pain
- Hemoptysis
- Dyspnea
- Malaise, fatigue, and weakness
Physical examination findings:
- Tachycardia and tachypnea
- Poor dentition
- Dullness to percussion, whispered pectoriloquy, and bronchophony
- Amphoric breath sounds (low-pitched sound of air moving across a large open cavity)

ETIOLOGY
- Aspiration is the most common cause of lung abscess, with periodontal disease being a major predisposing factor.[1]
- Septic emboli, superinfection of a pulmonary infarct, or extension from an adjacent mediastinal or subphrenic abscess could result in lung abscess formation.
- Lung abscesses are most often caused by anaerobic microorganisms (Peptostreptococcus, Bacteroides species, Fusobacterium, Prevotella) and microaerophilic streptococci such as Streptococcus milleri, Streptococcus anginosus, and Streptococcus mitis.[2]
- They frequently are polymicrobial with an anaerobic infection mixed with aerobic or facultative anaerobic organisms (S. aureus, E. coli, K. pneumoniae, P. aeruginosa).
- Nonbacterial pathogens include parasitic organisms (Paragonimus westermani, Entamoeba histolytica) and fungi (Aspergillus, Cryptococcus, Histoplasma, Blastomyces, and Coccidioides spp.)
- Lung abscesses in immunocompromised hosts are commonly due to Gram-negative bacilli but can include many organisms including Nocardia, Legionella micdade, Rhodococcus equi, mycobacteria, and fungi.
- Lung necrosis caused by community strains (USA 300 strain) of methicillin-resistant Staphylococcus aureus (MRSA) in adolescents and young adults following an acute influenza infection can be quite fulminant.
- Multidrug-resistant Klebsiella pneumoniae has been isolated from lung abscesses in Taiwan.[3]

DIAGNOSIS

Lung abscess may be classified as primary or secondary.[1]
- Primary lung abscess refers to abscess formation in immunocompetent hosts; usually a result of aspiration.
- Secondary lung abscess refers to abscess formation in individuals with immunodeficiency or those with a preexisting pulmonary condition (e.g., lung cancer, bronchiectasis).

Lung abscess may be defined as acute or chronic.
- Acute lung abscess denotes symptoms being present for <4 wk.
- Chronic lung abscess denotes symptoms being present for >4 wk.

DIFFERENTIAL DIAGNOSIS
The differential diagnosis for cavitary lung lesions can be separated into infectious and noninfectious causes.
INFECTIOUS:
- Bacterial (anaerobic, aerobic, facultative anaerobes, mycobacteria)
- Fungal (histoplasmosis, coccidioidomycosis, blastomycosis, aspergillosis, cryptococcosis, mucormycosis)
- Parasitic (amebiasis, echinococcosis)
NONINFECTIOUS:
- Malignancy (primary lung carcinoma, metastatic lung disease, lymphoma)
- Vasculitis (granulomatosis with polyangiitis)
- Septic emboli
- Bronchiectasis
- Obstructive mass or foreign body

WORKUP
- The workup of a patient with lung abscess attempts to elicit a primary or secondary cause.
- Routine blood tests are not specific in diagnosing lung abscesses.
- Most diagnoses are made from imaging studies.
- Bacteriologic, fungal, and parasitic studies are necessary to diagnose a specific pathogen.

LABORATORY TESTS
- CBC with leukocytosis
- Bacteriologic studies:
  1. Sputum Gram stain and culture (commonly contaminated by oral flora).
  2. Fiberoptic bronchoscopy with bronchial brushings and/or bronchial washings is commonly performed in those who have failed standard therapy and in immunocompromised individuals to rule out opportunistic infections. Of note, caution should be taken when performing bronchoalveolar lavage or biopsies of the cavity as this could cause spillage of abscess material.[2]
  3. Percutaneous transthoracic aspiration may also be used to identify an organism, especially when located adjacent to the pleura.
  4. Blood cultures in those with sepsis or septic shock.
If a pleural effusion is present, performing a thoracentesis may provide an uncontaminated specimen to isolate the causative organism of the neighboring abscess.

IMAGING STUDIES
- The diagnosis of lung abscess can be made by chest x-ray demonstrating a cavitary lesion with an air-fluid level.
- Lung abscesses are most commonly found in the posterior segment of the right upper

---

TABLE 1 Risk Factors for Aspiration Pneumonia and Lung Abscess

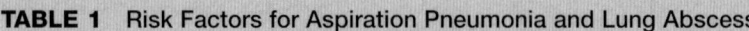

Increased bacterial inoculum	Periodontal disease, gingivitis, tonsillar or dental abscess, drugs that decrease gastric acidity
Impairment of consciousness	Drugs, alcohol, general anesthesia, metabolic encephalopathy, coma, shock, cerebrovascular accident, cardiopulmonary arrest, seizures, surgery, trauma
Impairment of cough and gag reflexes	Vocal cord paralysis, intratracheal anesthesia, endotracheal tube, tracheostomy, myopathy, myelopathy, other neurologic disorders
Impairment of esophageal function	Diverticula, achalasia, strictures, disorders of GI motility, neoplasm, tracheoesophageal fistula, pseudobulbar palsy
Emesis	Nasogastric tube, gastric dilation, ileus, intestinal obstruction

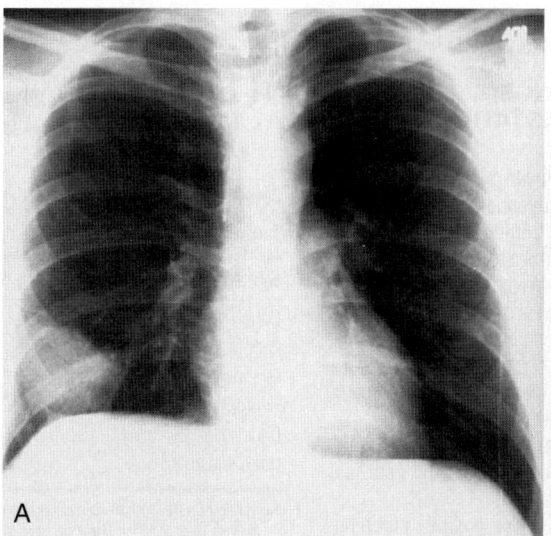
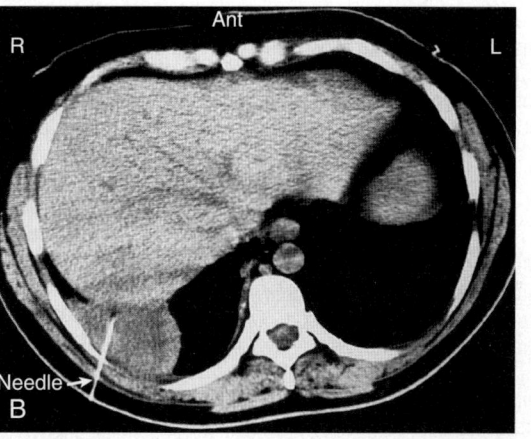
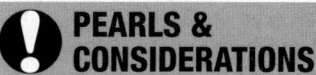

FIG. 1 Lung abscess. On a chest radiograph, a lung abscess may look to be a solid, rounded lesion **(A)**, or, if it has a connection with the bronchus, there may be an air-fluid level in a thick-walled cavitary lesion. CT scanning **(B)** can be used to localize the lesion and to place a needle for drainage and aspiration of contents for culture. (From Mettler FA [ed]: *Primary care radiology*, Philadelphia, 2000, Saunders.)

lobe or the superior segment of the lower lobes (the dependent regions of the lung when supine).
- Chest computed tomography (CT) scan can help to localize and size the lesion. In addition, it can assist in differentiating lung abscesses from other pathologic processes (e.g., tumor, empyema, infected bulla) (Fig. 1).
- Transthoracic echocardiogram may be indicated to rule out vegetations/endocarditis if imaging is suggestive of septic emboli.

Rx TREATMENT

NONPHARMACOLOGIC THERAPY
- Oxygen therapy.
- The efficacy of airway clearance maneuvers including postural drainage and chest percussion is less established and holds a risk of abscess rupture.

ACUTE GENERAL Rx
Antibiotics are the mainstay of treatment and are largely empiric due to the difficulty in isolating anaerobes on culture. Regimens should include combination of a beta-lactam/beta-lactamase inhibitor or a carbapenem.[2]
- Piperacillin/tazobactam 3.375 g intravenous (IV) q6h in aspiration pneumonia with lung abscess.
- Ceftriaxone 1 to 2 g IV q24h plus metronidazole 500 mg IV q8h.
- Clindamycin can be used and is more effective for anaerobic lung abscess than penicillin alone. Dose: 900 mg IV q8h until improved, then 300 to 600 mg PO q6h. (However, other regimens are often preferred to decrease risk of *Clostridioides difficile*.)
- Penicillin 1 to 2 million units IV q4h until improvement (afebrile, decreased phlegm production), followed by penicillin VK 500 mg PO q6h for 2 to 3 wk but often up to 6 to 8 wk

and can be given with metronidazole doses of 7.5 mg/kg IV q6h, followed by PO 500 mg bid to 4×per day dosing as an alternative to clindamycin.
- Penicillin should not be used alone because many mouth flora anaerobes now produce penicillinase enzymes.
- Metronidazole should not be used alone because it is not active against microaerophilic streptococci and some anaerobic cocci.
- Other alternatives are ampicillin/sulbactam and carbapenems such as imipenem and meropenem.

Duration of antibiotic therapy ranges from weeks to months. This largely depends on clinical and radiographic improvement.

CHRONIC Rx
- Bronchoscopy to assist with drainage and/or diagnosis is indicated in patients who fail to respond to antibiotics. Evaluating the airways is important if there is concern for an underlying malignancy or foreign body obstruction.
- Surgery is indicated in rare cases (~10%) in patients with complications of lung abscess (see "Comments").[1]

DISPOSITION
- Majority of patients fully recover with the use of antibiotics alone.
- Complications of lung abscesses include:
  1. Empyema
  2. Massive hemoptysis
  3. Pneumothorax
  4. Bronchopleural fistula
  5. Hepatobronchial fistula
  6. Pleurocutaneous fistula
  7. Brain abscess
  8. Bronchiectasis
- Mortality from lung abscess is approximately 15% to 20%.[4]
- Despite appropriate therapy, mortality may be as high as 75% in immunocompromised

patients, those with bronchial obstruction, or those with large abscesses (>6 cm).

REFERRAL
- Pulmonary and infectious disease consultation is recommended if a lung abscess is present.
- An interventional radiologist may be able to perform drainage and obtain cultures if indicated.

⚠ PEARLS & CONSIDERATIONS

COMMENTS
- It is essential to choose antibiotics with good anaerobic coverage.
- Cases refractory to antibiotics are usually the result of:
  1. Large cavity size (>6 cm)
  2. Recurrent aspiration
  3. Thick-walled cavities
  4. Obstructive lesion (e.g., lung mass or foreign body)
  5. Empyema formation
  6. Resistant organisms or other organisms such as mycobacterium, fungi, or parasites that are not covered by current therapy
- Percutaneous transthoracic tube drainage, endoscopic drainage or surgery may be indicated if the patient is not improving with antibiotic therapy.[5,6]

REFERENCES
Available at eBooks.Health.Elsevier.com.

RELATED CONTENT
Lung Abscess (Patient Information)
Aspiration Pneumonia (Related Key Topic)

AUTHOR: **NISHA H. GIDWANI, MD**

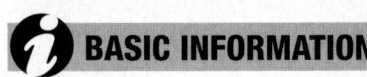 **BASIC INFORMATION**

DEFINITION

Primary lung neoplasms are malignancies arising from lung tissue and comprise of two different major subtypes: Non–small cell lung cancer (NSCLC, 85% of all lung cancers) and small cell lung cancer (SCLC, 15% of all lung cancers).

SYNONYM

Lung cancer

ICD-10CM CODES

C34.10	Malignant neoplasm of upper lobe, unspecified bronchus or lung
C34.11	Malignant neoplasm of upper lobe, right bronchus or lung
C34.12	Malignant neoplasm of upper lobe, left bronchus or lung
C34.2	Malignant neoplasm of middle lobe, bronchus or lung
C34.30	Malignant neoplasm of lower lobe, unspecified bronchus or lung
C34.31	Malignant neoplasm of lower lobe, right bronchus or lung
C34.32	Malignant neoplasm of lower lobe, left bronchus or lung
C34.80	Malignant neoplasm of overlapping sites of unspecified bronchus and lung
C34.81	Malignant neoplasm of overlapping sites of right bronchus and lung
C34.82	Malignant neoplasm of overlapping sites of left bronchus and lung
C34.90	Malignant neoplasm of unspecified part of unspecified bronchus or lung
C34.91	Malignant neoplasm of unspecified part of right bronchus or lung
C34.92	Malignant neoplasm of unspecified part of left bronchus or lung

EPIDEMIOLOGY & DEMOGRAPHICS

- Lung cancer causes >30% of male cancer deaths and >25% of female cancer deaths. Globally, it is the second-most common cancer (behind breast cancer) and is the leading cause of cancer-related death.
- Tobacco smoke is implicated in 90% of cases with secondhand smoke responsible for ~20% of cases.
- In the U.S., there were an estimated 238,340 new cases of lung cancer and 127,070 deaths from lung cancer in 2023.[1] Worldwide, the estimated number of new cases and deaths in 2020 was 2.2 million and 1.8 million, respectively.
- From 1990 through 2013 the percentage of patients with non–small cell lung cancer who never smoked rose from 8% to 16%, raising concerns about environmental carcinogens.
- Coincident with the decrease in smoking rates and the introduction of lung cancer low-dose computed tomography (CT) screening, as well as the introduction of newer immunotherapy treatments, the mortality from lung cancer in the U.S. continues to decrease.[2]

However, death rates among African Americans continue to be disproportionately higher.

PHYSICAL FINDINGS & CLINICAL PRESENTATION (TABLES 1 & 2)

- Weight loss, fatigue, fever, anorexia, dysphagia
- Cough, hemoptysis, dyspnea, wheezing
- Chest, shoulder, and bone pain
- Paraneoplastic syndromes (see Table 3):
  1. Lambert-Eaton myasthenic syndrome: Myopathy involving proximal muscle groups
  2. Endocrine manifestations: Hypercalcemia, ectopic adrenocorticotropic hormone secretion, syndrome of inappropriate excretion of adrenocorticotropic hormone (SIADH)
  3. Neurologic: Subacute cerebellar degeneration, peripheral neuropathy, cortical degeneration
  4. Musculoskeletal: Polymyositis, clubbing, hypertrophic pulmonary osteoarthropathy
  5. Hematologic or vascular: Migratory thrombophlebitis, marantic thrombosis, anemia, thrombocytosis, or thrombocytopenia
  6. Cutaneous: Acanthosis nigricans, dermatomyositis
- Pleural effusion (10% of patients), recurrent pneumonias (from obstruction), localized wheezing
- *Superior vena cava syndrome:* Obstruction of venous return of the superior vena cava is most commonly caused by bronchogenic carcinoma or metastasis to paratracheal nodes.
  1. The patient usually reports headache, nausea, dizziness, visual changes, syncope, and respiratory distress.
  2. Physical examination reveals distention of thoracic and neck veins, edema of face and upper extremities, facial plethora, and cyanosis.
     - *Horner syndrome:* Constricted pupil, ptosis, facial anhidrosis caused by spinal cord damage between C8 and T1 because of a superior sulcus tumor (bronchogenic carcinoma of the extreme lung apex).
     - *Pancoast tumor:* A superior sulcus tumor associated with ipsilateral Horner syndrome and shoulder pain.

TABLE 1 Presenting Symptoms with Bronchogenic Carcinoma

Symptoms	Patients (%)
Cough	45-75
Weight loss	8-68
Dyspnea	37-58
Hemoptysis	27-57
Chest pain	27-49
Hoarseness	2-18

From Midthun DE, Jett JR: Clinical presentation of lung cancer. In Pass HI et al (eds): *Lung cancer: principles and practice,* Philadelphia, 1996, Lippincott-Raven, p. 422.

TABLE 2 Expanded Clinical Evaluation

Symptoms Elicited In History

Constitutional—weight loss >10 lb
Musculoskeletal—focal skeletal pain
Neurologic—headaches, syncope, seizures, extremity weakness, recent change in mental status

Signs Found on Physical Examination

Lymphadenopathy (>1 cm)
Hoarseness
Superior vena cava syndrome
Bone tenderness
Hepatomegaly (>13 cm span)
Focal neurologic signs, papilledema
Soft tissue mass

Routine Laboratory Tests

Hematocrit <40% in males
Hematocrit <35% in females
Elevated alkaline phosphatase, γ-glutamyl transferase, aspartate aminotransferase, calcium

From Broaddus VC et al: *Murray & Nadel's textbook of respiratory medicine,* ed 7, Philadelphia, 2022, Elsevier.

TABLE 3 Paraneoplastic Syndromes Associated with Bronchogenic Carcinoma

Syndrome	Cell Type	Mechanism
Hypertrophic pulmonary osteoarthropathy and clubbing	All types	Unknown
Hyponatremia	SCLC most common; may be any type	SIADH, ectopic antidiuretic hormone production by tumor
Hypercalcemia	Usually squamous cell	Bone metastases, osteoclast-activating factor, parathyroid hormone–like hormone, prostaglandins
Cushing syndrome	Usually SCLC	Ectopic ACTH production
Lambert-Eaton myasthenic syndrome	Usually SCLC	Voltage-sensitive calcium channel antibodies in >75%; affects presynaptic neuronal calcium channel activity
Other neuromyopathic disorders	SCLC most common; may be any type	Antineuronal nuclear antibodies, also known as anti-Hu; others unknown
Thrombophlebitis	All types	Unknown

ACTH, Adrenocorticotropic hormone; *SCLC,* small cell lung cancer; *SIADH,* syndrome of inappropriate secretion of antidiuretic hormone.
Adapted from Andreoli TE et al: *Andreoli and Carpenter's Cecil essentials of medicine,* ed 8, Philadelphia, 2010, Saunders.

Phases of Molecular Carcinogenesis, Lung

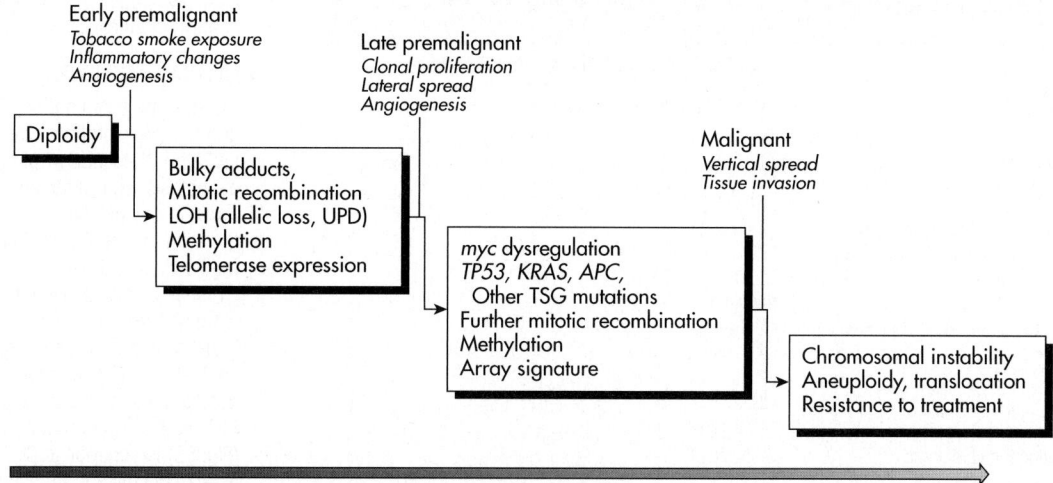

FIG. 1 The molecular pathology of smoking-related lung cancer begins with the direct interaction between metabolites of carcinogenic polyaromatic hydrocarbons in cigarette smoke with host DNA. This creates bulky adducts that affect DNA repair and create transcription errors. The result is a wide range of genomic losses, gains, translocations, and point mutations that account for the high degree of molecular heterogeneity in lung tumors with diverse physiologic effects. *LOH,* Loss of heterozygosity; *TSG,* tumor suppressor gene; *UPD,* uniparental disomy. (From Niederhuber JE: *Abeloff's clinical oncology,* ed 6, Philadelphia, 2020, Elsevier.)

ETIOLOGY & PATHOLOGY

- Tobacco abuse: The molecular pathology of smoking-related lung cancer is illustrated in Fig. 1. The chance of developing lung cancer for a 40-pack-yr persistent smoker is 20 times that of someone who never smoked.
- Environmental agents (e.g., radon) and industrial agents (e.g., ionizing radiation, asbestos, nickel, uranium, vinyl chloride, chromium, arsenic, coal dust).
- Lung cancer susceptibility and risk increased in inherited cancer syndromes caused by germline mutations in p53, retinoblastoma, and epidermal growth factor receptor *(EGFR)* genes.
- Adenocarcinoma: Represents 35% to 40% of lung carcinomas; frequently located in mid-lung and periphery; initial metastases are to lymphatics; frequently associated with peripheral scars; adenocarcinoma is described as preinvasive, minimally invasive, or invasive.
- Squamous cell: Represents 20% to 30% of lung cancers; central location; metastasis by local invasion; frequent cavitation and obstructive phenomena.
- Small cell: Represents 15% of lung carcinomas; central location; metastasis through lymphatics; associated with lesion of the short arm of chromosome 3; high cavitation rate.
- Large cell: Represents 10% to 15% of lung carcinomas; frequently located in the periphery; metastasis to central nervous system and mediastinum; rapid growth rate with early metastasis.
- Lepidic-predominant pattern (bronchoalveolar): Represents 5% of lung carcinomas; frequently located in the periphery; may be bilateral; initial metastasis through lymphatic, hematogenous, and local invasion;

no correlation with cigarette smoking; cavitation rare.
Fig. E2 illustrates the multistep cellular carcinogenesis in lung cancer.

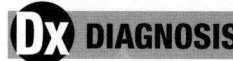 **DIAGNOSIS**

DIFFERENTIAL DIAGNOSIS

- Pneumonia
- Tuberculosis (TB)
- Metastatic carcinoma to the lung
- Lung abscess
- Granulomatous disease
- Carcinoid tumor
- Sarcoidosis
- Benign lesions that simulate thoracic malignancy:
  1. Lobar atelectasis: Pneumonia, chronic inflammatory disease, allergic bronchopulmonary aspergillosis
  2. Multiple pulmonary nodules: Septic emboli, Wegener granulomatosis, sarcoidosis, rheumatoid nodules, fungal disease, multiple pulmonary atrioventricular fistulas
  3. Mediastinal adenopathy: Sarcoidosis, lymphoma, primary TB, fungal disease, silicosis, pneumoconiosis, drug-induced (e.g., phenytoin, trimethadione)
  4. Pleural effusion: Congestive heart failure, pneumonia with parapneumonic effusion, TB, viral pneumonitis, ascites, pancreatitis, collagen-vascular disease

WORKUP

- The workup generally includes chest CT, PET scan, and tissue biopsy. Molecular testing for treatable oncogenic alterations should be performed to further classify NSCLC. Common immunohistochemical markers used in the diagnosis of lung tumors are summarized

in Table 4. Table 5 describes common molecular alterations in lung tumors.
- Additional laboratory tests include CBC, serum chemistry studies.
- Diagnosis and staging of lung cancer should be performed simultaneously to minimize invasive testing.

LABORATORY TESTS

Various modalities are available to obtain a tissue diagnosis:

- Biopsy of any suspicious lymph nodes (e.g., supraclavicular or mediastinal node).
- Flexible fiberoptic bronchoscopy: Brush and biopsy specimens are obtained from any visualized endobronchial lesions. The use of a gene-expression classifier has a high sensitivity across different lesion sizes, locations, stages, and cell type of lung cancer. The combination of the classifier plus bronchoscopy has a sensitivity of >85%. In intermediate-risk patients with a nondiagnostic bronchoscopic examination, a negative classifier score provides support for a more conservative diagnostic approach.
- Transbronchial needle aspiration: Done with a special needle passed through the bronchoscope; this technique is useful to sample mediastinal masses or paratracheal lymph nodes.
- Transthoracic fine-needle aspiration biopsy with fluoroscopic or CT scan guidance to evaluate peripheral pulmonary nodules.
- Endobronchial ultrasound (EBUS) guided biopsy and staging is now routinely used to evaluate suspected mediastinal and hilar nodes.
- Mediastinoscopy and anteromedial sternotomy in suspected tumor involvement of the mediastinum.
- Pleural biopsy in patients with pleural effusion.

TABLE 4 Common Immunohistochemical Markers Used in the Diagnosis of Lung Tumors

Diagnosis	Positive Immunohistochemical Markers
Squamous cell carcinoma	Cytokeratin (CK) cocktail (e.g., AE1/AE3) p63 p40 CK5/6 CK7 in up to 30%
Adenocarcinoma, including adenocarcinoma in situ or minimally invasive adenocarcinoma, nonmucinous	CK cocktail CK7 TTF-1 Napsin A
In situ and invasive mucinous adenocarcinoma	CK cocktail CK7 CK20 cdx-2 TTF-1 rare
Large cell neuroendocrine carcinoma	CK cocktail TTF-1 CD56 Chromogranin A Synaptophysin
Carcinoid tumor	CK cocktail TTF-1 (weaker than in high-grade neuroendocrine tumors) CD56 Chromogranin A Synaptophysin
Atypical carcinoid tumor	CK cocktail (tends to be patchy) TTF-1 (weaker than in high-grade neuroendocrine tumors) CD56 Chromogranin A Synaptophysin
Common differential diagnoses: • Colonic adenocarcinoma • Lung, breast, pancreatobiliary, upper GI adenocarcinoma • Urothelial carcinoma • Prostatic adenocarcinoma • Mesothelioma • Malignant melanoma	 CK20+/CK7− CK7+/CK20− CK7+/CK20+ CK7−/CK20− Calretinin, WT1, CK5/6 S-100, HMB-45, Melan-A

GI, Gastrointestinal.
From Niederhuber JE: *Abeloff's clinical oncology,* ed 6, Philadelphia, 2020, Elsevier.

TABLE 5 Examples of Common Molecular Alterations in Lung Tumors

Diagnosis	Common Molecular Alterations
Squamous preneoplasia	LOH—3p, 9p21, 8p21–23, aneuploidy, methylation
Atypical adenomatous hyperplasia	LOH—3p, 9p, aneuploidy K-ras codon 12 mutation
Adenocarcinoma	p53 mutation p16 mutation/inactivation K-Ras (42%); smokers more common EGFR overexpression (40%) EGFR mutation Her2/neu, COX-2 overexpression
Squamous cell carcinoma	p53 mutation p16 inactivation Allelic loss 3p EGFR overexpression (80%)
Large cell carcinoma	K-Ras, p53, loss p16
Large cell neuroendocrine carcinoma	p53 bcl-2 overexpression Rb mutation 3p21, FHIT, 3p22-24, 5q21,9p21
Small cell carcinoma	Rb mutation (80+%) p53 mutation 50%-80% BCL-2 expression 3p21, FHIT, 3p22-24, 5q21,9p21

COX-2, Cyclooxygenase 2; *EGFR,* epidermal growth factor receptor; *LOH,* loss of heterozygosity.
From Niederhuber JE: *Abeloff's clinical oncology,* ed 6, Philadelphia, 2020, Elsevier.

• Thoracentesis of pleural effusion and cytologic evaluation of the obtained fluid may confirm diagnosis.

IMAGING STUDIES

• Chest x-ray examination (Fig. 3): The radiographic presentation often varies with the cell type. Presence of pleural effusion, lobar atelectasis, and mediastinal adenopathy can occur in any cell type.
• CT scan of the chest (Fig. 4) can evaluate mediastinal and pleural extension. The chest CT should include liver and adrenal glands (common sites of metastases). CT or MRI of brain should be considered in a patient presenting with neurologic symptoms (e.g., headaches, vision disturbances).
• PET with ^{18}F-fluorodeoxyglucose (^{18}F-FDG) (Fig. E5) is superior to CT in detecting mediastinal and distant metastases in NSCLC. It is useful for preoperative staging of NSCLC.
• The use of PET-CT (Fig. E6) for preoperative staging of NSCLC reduces both the total number of thoracotomies and the number of futile thoracotomies.

STAGING

After confirmation of diagnosis, patients should undergo staging:
• In NSCLC, the TNM staging system is used (Table 6). Both stage I (no lymph node involvement) and stage II (ipsilateral bronchopulmonary/hilar lymph nodes or T_3 tumor) include localized tumors for which surgical resection is the preferred treatment. Stage III is subdivided into III$_A$ (potentially resectable) and III$_B$/III$_C$ (unresectable). Stage IV indicates metastatic disease with stage IV$_A$ referring to intrathoracic metastases or pleural involvement or single extrathoracic metastasis. Stage IV$_B$ includes tumors with multiple extrathoracic metastases.
• In SCLC, the staging system developed by the Veterans Administration Lung Cancer Study Group is used. It contains two stages:
  1. Limited-stage disease: Confined to the regional lymph nodes and to one hemithorax (excluding pleural surfaces), which can be included in a single radiation portal
  2. Extensive-stage disease: Spread beyond the confines of limited-stage disease
• Pretreatment staging procedures for lung cancer patients, in addition to complete history and physical examination, generally include the following tests:
  1. Laboratory evaluation: CBC, complete metabolic panel; arterial blood gases and pulse oximetry in selected cases
  2. Biopsy of any accessible suspect lesions
  3. Pulmonary function studies
  4. CT scan of chest and PET scan: There is a reduction in futile thoracotomies for patients undergoing preoperative PET assessment in addition to conventional workup
  5. Mediastinoscopy or anterior mediastinotomy in patients being considered for curative lung resection. Newer staging technologies include endoscopic bronchial ultrasonography (EBUS) and esophageal ultrasonography (EUS) to guide biopsies
  6. MRI brain to assess for metastases

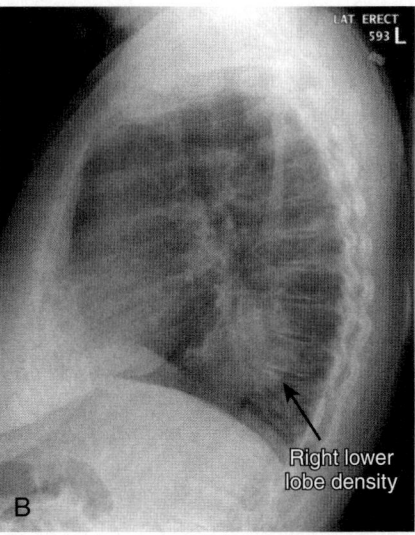

FIG. 3 Lung neoplasm, primary. Lung mass presenting with hemoptysis. **A,** Posterior-anterior (PA) chest x-ray examination. **B,** Lateral chest x-ray examination. This 83-yr-old woman presented with hemoptysis of a quarter-sized clot. Her PA chest x-ray film shows a rounded right lower lobe density. On the lateral view, this is visible in the retrocardiac space. This density measures 7.6 cm in diameter. Pneumonia, neoplasm, or abscess could have this appearance on chest x-ray examination. Computed tomography was performed to further delineate the pathology (see Fig. 5). (From Broder JS: *Diagnostic imaging for the emergency physician*, Philadelphia, 2011, Saunders.)

TABLE 6 TNM Stage Groups for Non–Small Cell Lung Cancer

Stage	T	N	M
Stage 0	T_{is}	N_0	M_0
Stage I_{A1}	T_{mi} or T_{1a}	N_0	M_0
Stage I_{A2}	T_{1b}	N_0	M_0
Stage I_{A3}	T_{1c}	N_0	M_0
Stage I_B	T_{2a}	N_0	M_0
Stage II_A	T_{2b}	N_0	M_0
Stage II_B	T_{1a-c}	N_1	M_0
	T_{2a-b}	N_1	M_0
	T_3	N_0	M_0
Stage III_A	T_{1a-c}	N_2	M_0
	T_{2a-b}	N_2	M_0
	T_3	N_1	M_0
	T_4	N_{0-1}	M_0
Stage III_B	T_{1a-c}	N_3	M_0
	T_{2a-b}	N_3	M_0
	T_{3-4}	N_2	M_0
Stage III_C	T_{3-4}	N_3	M_0
Stage IV_A	Any T	Any N	M_{1a-1b}
Stage IV_B	Any T	Any N	M_{1c}

TNM, Tumor, node, metastases.

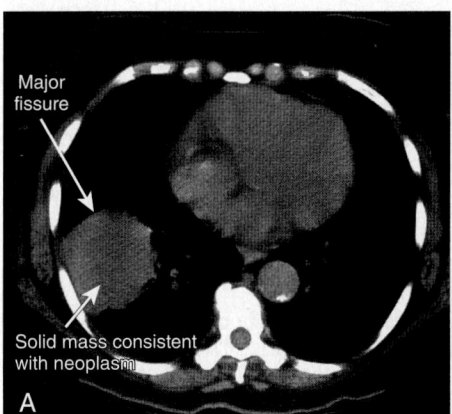
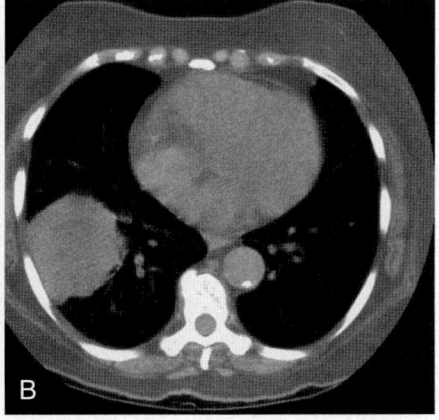

FIG. 4 Lung neoplasm, primary. Lung mass presenting with hemoptysis. Same patient as in Fig. 3. Noncontrast computed tomography was performed (contrast was withheld as a consequence of the patient's renal dysfunction) and shows a 6 × 6 cm round lesion abutting the oblique fissure (also called the major fissure) and lateral chest wall. **A,** Soft tissue windows. **B,** Lung windows. On soft tissue windows the center appears slightly darker, indicating lower density that may represent central necrosis. If intravenous contrast had been given, an area of necrosis would have failed to enhance. Infection or infarction is technically possible, but a pulmonary neoplasm is the most likely explanation for this lesion. Biopsy showed this to be a moderately differentiated squamous cell carcinoma. (From Broder JS: *Diagnostic imaging for the emergency physician*, Philadelphia, 2011, Saunders.)

Rx TREATMENT

NONPHARMACOLOGIC THERAPY

- Nutritional support
- Supplemental oxygen

ACUTE GENERAL Rx

Non–small cell carcinoma (Tables 7 and 8):
- Surgical resection is standard in patients with operable NSCLC (stage I or II) who are surgical candidates. This represents approximately 15% to 30% of cases. Lobectomy is the traditional standard surgical approach. Lesser resections including sublobar resections are now deemed equivalent in appropriate cases with smaller or peripheral tumors or in patients with marginal pulmonary reserve.[3] A recent trial[4] revealed that in patients with NSCLC with tumor sizes of ≤2 cm and pathologically confirmed negative hilar and mediastinal lymph nodes, the use of sublobar resection was not inferior to lobectomy with respect to disease-free interval.
- Stereotactic ablative radiotherapy is a reasonable option for patients with localized NSCLC who are not surgical candidates.[5] Multimodality treatment guidelines are summarized in Table 9.
- Preoperative evaluation includes cardiac status and pulmonary function assessment. Pneumonectomy is feasible if the patient has a preoperative FEV_1 = 2 L or if the maximal voluntary ventilation is >50% of predicted capacity. Individuals with FEV_1 >1.5 L are suitable for lobectomy without further evaluation unless there is evidence of interstitial lung disease or undue dyspnea on exertion. In that case, carbon dioxide diffusion in the lung (DLCO) should be measured. If the DLCO is <80% predicted normal, the individual may not be clearly operable.
- Conventional radiotherapy fails to durably control the primary lung tumor in nearly 70% of patients and 2-yr survival is less than 40%. Stereotactic body radiation (SBRT) uses several highly focused radiation beams to deliver total higher doses of radiotherapy (in high doses in 3 to 5 fractions) and is more effective than conventional radiotherapy with local control rates equivalent to that with surgery in inoperable early-stage lung cancer.
- Preoperative chemotherapy plus immunotherapy in resectable stage IB-IIIA NSCLC patients and has demonstrated improved pathological complete response rates, and both event-free survival and overall survival in recent trials with the use of neoadjuvant nivolumab, pembrolizumab, or durvalumab plus chemotherapy in comparison to chemotherapy alone.[6-8] Importantly, the addition of

TABLE 7 Summary of Current Treatment Strategies for Non–Small Cell Lung Cancer

Stage	Surgery	Chemotherapy	Radiotherapy	Chemoradiotherapy	Comments
IA and IB	First line	Adjuvant—tumors ≥4 cm	First line[a]	No	Role of adjuvant chemotherapy for stage IB not clearly defined but should be considered in tumors ≥4 cm in size and/or high-risk features (vascular invasion, visceral pleural involvement)
IIA and IIB	First line	Adjuvant	No	No	5-yr survival improvement with adjuvant chemotherapy about 5%
T3 due to multiple tumor nodules same lobe	Lobectomy to resect primary and satellite nodules				
T3 due to chest wall invasion	En bloc resection				
Superior sulcus tumors					Neoadjuvant chemoradiotherapy improves survival in this subset of stage IIB
IIIA	First line for N0-1	Adjuvant treatment in completely resected IIIA	Neoadjuvant or adjuvant in the setting of N2 nodes	First line for unresectable N2 disease. Followed by consolidation immunotherapy	Combined chemotherapy ± radiotherapy followed by surgery is feasible in select N2 disease, but more data are needed to recommend routinely
IIIB and IIIC	No	No	No	First line. Followed by consolidation immunotherapy	
IV	No	First line: Systemic therapy[b]: • Chemotherapy • Targeted therapy • Immunotherapy • Chemotherapy and immunotherapy	Radiotherapy is used for palliation only	No	All stage IV adenocarcinomas should have mutational analysis, including *EGFR*, *ALK*-fusion, *ROS1,* and *KRAS*. All stage IV NSCLC should be tested for PD-L1

[a]SBRT for patients who are medically unfit or who refuse surgery.
[b]First-line therapy in stage IV NSCLC is selected based on (1) histology: Pemetrexed for nonsquamous cell, gemcitabine for squamous cell, and bevacizumab is approved as an adjunct to chemotherapy in the first-line setting in patients with nonsquamous histology and no other contraindications; (2) presence of molecular target guides first-line therapy; (3) PD-L1 expression >50% used to select patients eligible for first-line pembrolizumab.
From Broaddus VC et al: *Murray & Nadel's textbook of respiratory medicine,* ed 7, Philadelphia, 2022, Elsevier.

TABLE 8 Targeted Therapy for Metastatic NSCLC with Molecular Target

Biomarker	First-Line Therapy	Second-Line Therapy	Promising Therapies
EGFR mutations	Erlotinib Gefitinib Afatinib Osimertinib	Osimertinib (after first- or second-generation TKI if T790M)	
ALK-fusion	Crizotinib Alectinib Ceritinib	Lorlatinib Brigatinib	
ROS1	Crizotinib Entrectinib		Repotrectinib
BRAF		Dabrafenib/trametinib	
RET-fusions			LOXO-292 BLU-667
MET exon 14 mutation		Crizotinib	Capmatinib Savolitinib Tepotinib
HER2 dysregulation			Trastuzumab[a] Ado-trastuzumab[a]
*KRAS*G12C mutation			AMG510 MRTX849

[a]Off-label use.
From Broaddus VC et al: *Murray & Nadel's textbook of respiratory medicine,* ed 7, Philadelphia, 2022, Elsevier.

immunotherapy to chemotherapy did not increase the incidence of adverse events or impede the feasibility of surgery. Early results from a similar second trial, evaluating pembrolizumab with chemotherapy in resectable NSCLC has also demonstrated improved pathologic complete response rates and event-free survival. Consequently, neoadjuvant chemoimmunotherapy is now an acceptable option in selected cases.
• Postoperative adjuvant chemotherapy with doublet regimens significantly increases 5-yr survival (69% vs. 54%) in patients with completely resected stage II-IIIA NSCLC. Some stage I NSCLC patients (tumors >4 cm) potentially benefit from adjuvant chemotherapy. In addition, postoperative adjuvant immunotherapy followed by 1 yr of checkpoint inhibitor therapy (atezolizumab, pembrolizumab) has shown improvement in survival over chemotherapy alone. An algorithm for selecting patients with stage I NSCLC for postoperative adjuvant chemotherapy is outlined in Fig. 7.
• Postoperative adjuvant targeted therapy with EGFR inhibitor osimertinib in patients with EGFR-mutated, resected stage IB-IIIA NSCLC conveys a major survival benefit

TABLE 9 Summary of Multimodality Guidelines

Stage	Surgery	Adjuvant Therapy	Radiation	Chemotherapy	Level of Evidence
I	Yes	No	No	No	1B—Surgical resection 1B—Against postoperative chemotherapy 1A—Against postoperative radiation therapy
II	Yes	Yes	No	Yes	1B—Surgical resection 1A—Postoperative chemotherapy 2A—Against postoperative radiation therapy
IIIA (N2-occult)	Yes	Yes	May be considered	Yes	1A—Adjuvant chemo 2C—Adjuvant radiation
(N2-discrete)	Yes	No	Yes (Definitive or induction recommended)	Yes	1A—Definite or induction followed by surgery 1C—Against primary resection followed by adjuvant therapy
IIIB (N2, N3)	No	No	Yes (Definitive concurrent)	Yes	1A—Definitive concurrent 1A—Against induction followed by surgery

From Sellke FW et al: *Sabiston & Spencer surgery of the chest,* ed 9, Philadelphia, 2016, Elsevier.

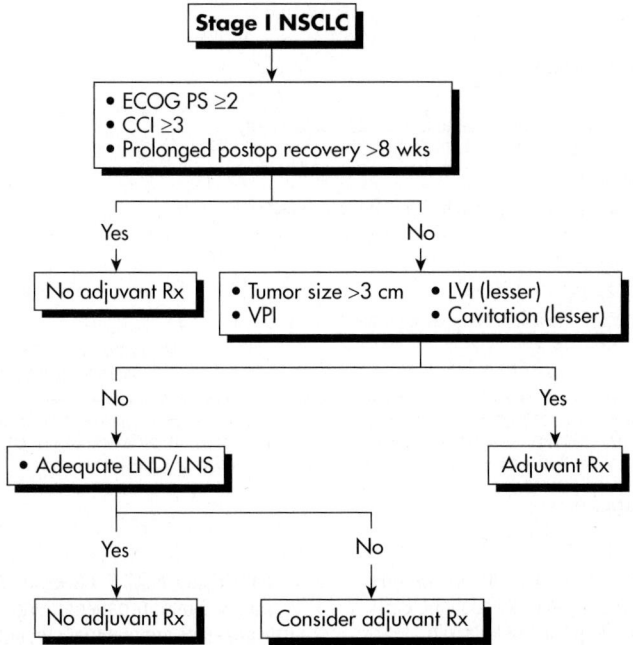

FIG. 7 Algorithm for selecting patients with stage I non–small cell lung cancer *(NSCLC)* for postoperative adjuvant chemotherapy. *CCI,* Charlson Comorbidity Index; *ECOG PS,* Eastern Cooperative Oncology Group Performance Status; *LND,* mediastinal lymph node dissection; *LNS,* systematic mediastinal lymph node sampling; *LVI,* lymphovascular invasion; *Rx,* treatment; *VPI,* visceral pleural invasion. (From Niederhuber JE: *Abeloff's clinical oncology,* ed 6, Philadelphia, 2020, Elsevier.)

when administered with or without chemotherapy use.

Treatment of unresectable NSCLC:
- Radiotherapy alone can be used primarily for treatment of central nervous system metastases, skeletal metastases, and superior vena cava syndrome.
- In unresectable stage 3 disease, concurrent chemotherapy and thoracic radiotherapy, followed by maintenance immunotherapy with checkpoint inhibitor durvalumab (in responding patients), is the standard therapeutic approach with a 5-yr survival rate of 43%.
- Chemotherapy, targeted therapy, and immune checkpoint inhibitor therapy are the mainstays of treatment for relapsed or metastatic NSCLC. Initial stratification is done based on pathology (squamous vs. nonsquamous cancers), presence of driver mutations (e.g., *EGFR, ALK, ROS1, BRAF, MET, RET, KRASC-G12C,* and *NTRK* mutations in adenocarcinomas), and expression of programmed death receptor ligand-1 (PD-L1). A recent phase 3 trial involving first-line treatment with osimertinib chemotherapy has also shown significantly longer progression-free survival than osimertinib monotherapy among patients with *EGFR*-mutated advanced NSCLC.[9] Table 10 summarizes selected NSCLC oncogenes and targeted therapy.
- The current approach in advanced NSCLC without driver mutations relies on using the PD-L1 score to generate recommendations for immunotherapy alone (PD-L1 score >50%), combination chemotherapy and immunotherapy (PD-L1 score 1% to 49%). For patients with undetectable PD-L1 (score 0%) options include chemotherapy plus anti-VEGF therapy or chemotherapy plus dual immunotherapy combinations.
- Platinum-based chemotherapy doublet regimens are recommended for fit patients including platinum plus pemetrexed for nonsquamous cancers, whereas for squamous cancers taxane plus carboplatin, cisplatin plus vinorelbine, and gemcitabine plus cisplatin are utilized with none being clearly superior to the others. The addition of bevacizumab to chemotherapy results in significant survival benefit in nonsquamous cancers.
- Single-agent immune checkpoint inhibitors approved for first-line use in patients with PD-L1 score >50% include pembrolizumab, atezolizumab, and cemiplimab.[10] Inhibitors approved for use in combination with doublet chemotherapy include pembrolizumab, cemiplimab, and atezolizumab. The dual immunotherapy combinations of ipilimumab and nivolumab in combination with short-course chemotherapy[11] or the combination of chemotherapy plus durvalumab and tremelimumab immunotherapy[12] have both been shown to improve survival in metastatic NSCLC patients.

TABLE 10 Selected Non–Small Cell Lung Cancer Oncogenes and Targeted Therapy

Oncogene Alteration	Incidence (%)	Clinical Relevance	Treatment
BRAF			
Mutation	1-3	V600E mutation: Most common, equal association with smokers and nonsmokers May be mechanism of acquired EGFR TKI resistance	Dabrafenib plus trametinib
EGFR (ErbB1, HER1)			
Mutation	13-50	Exon 19 deletion and exon 21-point mutation are the most common Predominantly adenocarcinoma and nonsmokers; up to 50% frequency in Asians	TKI: Gefitinib, erlotinib, afatinib, osimertinib
EML4-ALK			
Fusion	3-7	Most frequent in adenocarcinomas, nonsmokers, men, and younger patients	Nonspecific TKI: Crizotinib, ceritinib, alectinib, brigatinib
Her2/neu (ErbB2)			No approved therapy
Mutation	2-6	Mostly adenocarcinomas and nonsmokers	
Amplification	23	Mechanism of resistance to EGFR TKI	
KRAS			
Mutation	5-30	Mostly adenocarcinomas and smokers May contribute to resistance to ALF, BRAF, and PI3K inhibitors	No approved therapy
MET			No approved therapy
Mutation	<5		
Amplification	21	Mechanism of resistance to EGFR TKI	
PIK3CA			No approved therapy
Mutation	<10	Frequently occurs in association with other mutations; more common in squamous cell	
Amplification	5-43	Mechanism of resistance to EGFR TKI	
PTEN			
Mutation	1.7-10	Associated with PI3K activation, resistance to EGFR TKI, and sensitivity to PI3K inhibitors More frequent in squamous cell	
Loss of function	4-21	Associated with PI3K activation, resistance to EGFR TKI, and sensitivity to PI3K inhibitors More frequent in squamous cell	
RET fusion gene	1-2	Mostly adenocarcinomas and nonsmokers	No approved therapy
ROS1 fusion gene	2	Mostly adenocarcinomas, nonsmokers, and younger patients	TKI: Crizotinib
VEGF			Monoclonal antibodies: Bevacizumab VEGFR TKI

BRAF, v-Raf murine sarcoma viral oncogene homolog B1; *EGFR*, epidermal growth factor receptor; *EML4-ALK*, echinoderm microtubule-associated protein-like 4 anaplastic lymphoma kinase; *ERBB*, avian erythroblastosis oncogene B; *Her2*, human epidermal growth factor receptor 2; *KRAS*, Kirsten Rat sarcoma viral oncogene homolog; *MET*, mesenchymal-epithelial transition; *PIK3CA*, phosphoinositide-3-kinase catalytic alpha polypeptide; *PTEN*, phosphatase and tensin homolog; *RET*, rearranged during transfection; *ROS1*, reactive oxygen species 1; *TKI*, tyrosine kinase inhibitor; *VEGF*, vascular endothelial growth factor; *VEGFR*, vascular endothelial growth factor receptor.
From Sellke FW et al: *Sabiston & Spencer surgery of the chest*, ed 9, Philadelphia, 2016, Elsevier.

- Tyrosine kinase inhibitors that target activating driver mutations are used as initial and/or subsequent therapy in patients whose adenocarcinomas that harbor such mutations:
  1. EGFR mutations (20% to 25% cases) are more commonly detected in never or light smokers and in Asian patients. Gefitinib, erlotinib, afatinib, osimertinib, and dacomitinib are oral EGFR inhibitors that have showed impressive response rates and median overall survival in the range of 30 mo. Currently, first-line therapy with the oral inhibitor osimertinib is the preferred option based on updated data demonstrating median overall survival of 36 mo.[13] EGFR exon 20 insertion mutations (which do not respond to oral EGFR inhibitors) can now be treated with the recently approved bispecific EGFR/c-met antibody amivantamab.
  2. Oncogenic fusion genes consisting of *EML4* and anaplastic lymphoma kinase (ALK) are present in 4% to 5% of cases and can be treated with oral inhibitors crizotinib, ceritinib, alectinib, brigatinib, or lorlatinib.
  3. ~2% of adenocarcinomas have genetic rearrangements involving the ROS1 proto-oncogenic receptor tyrosine kinase (ROS1), and these patients can be treated with the oral inhibitors crizotinib and ceritinib.
  4. ~2% of adenocarcinomas harbor the BRAF V600E mutation, and these patients can be treated with the combination of oral BRAF/MEK inhibitor (dabrafenib plus trametinib) therapy.
  5. Mutations leading to MET exon 14 skipping are found in 3% to 4% of patients with advanced non–small cell lung cancer. The FDA has approved the oral inhibitors capmatinib and tepotinib for the treatment of adult patients with NSCLC harboring this specific MET mutation.
  6. RET (rearranged during transfection) rearrangements occur in 1% to 2% of unselected NSCLC cases and are commonly found in patients who have never smoked or are minimal smokers. The oral inhibitors selpercatinib and pralsetinib are now approved in patients with RET fusion-positive NSCLC who were previously treated with platinum-based chemotherapy and who had never undergone treatment.
  7. *NTRK* fusions are clinically targetable and have been identified to be the predominant drivers of growth in <1% of advanced lung cancers. The treatment of patients with NTRK fusion-positive cancers with a first-generation TRK inhibitor, such as larotrectinib or entrectinib, is associated with high response rates but eventual development of resistance.
  8. *KRAS G12C* mutations occur in 13% of patients with advanced NSCLC. The FDA approved the oral inhibitors sotorasib and adagrasib in previously treated patients

who had received chemotherapy and/or immunotherapy.[14]

9. Early initiation of palliative care focusing on management of symptoms, psychosocial support, and assistance with decision making in patients with metastatic NSCLC leads to improved quality of life, longer survival, and less use of aggressive end-of-life care.

Small cell lung cancer:

- Limited-stage disease: Standard treatments include thoracic radiotherapy and chemotherapy (cisplatin and etoposide).
- Extensive-stage disease: Standard combination chemotherapy regimens include platinum plus etoposide or platinum plus irinotecan. The addition of the PD-1 antibody atezolizumab or durvalumab to standard first-line chemotherapy has been proven to improve overall survival and is considered a standard approach in current practice.
- Prophylactic cranial irradiation for patients in complete remission to decrease the risk of central nervous system metastasis.
- Despite high initial response rates, most patients eventually relapse. Topotecan or irinotecan may be an option for these patients. Immune checkpoint inhibitors have demonstrated survival benefit in SCLC patients who have failed standard therapies. Lurbinectedin, a selective inhibitor of oncogenic transcription, is now approved for

patients who developed disease progression after first-line therapy.[15]

DISPOSITION

- The 5-yr survival of patients with resectable NSCLC (stages I-III) is ~30%. The 5-yr survival for stage 4 patients is increasing, with survival rates in the 25% range reported in current trials with the use of targeted therapy and immunotherapy.
- Median survival time in patients with limited-stage disease SCLC is 15 mo; in patients with extensive-stage SCLC, it is in the range of 12 mo.
- Among patients with metastatic NSCLC, early palliative care results in longer survival and significant improvements in both quality of life and mood.
- Population-level mortality from NSCLC in the United States fell sharply from 2013 to 2016, and survival after diagnosis improved substantially. Reduction in incidence along with modern treatment advances are likely explanations for the reduction in mortality observed.

 PEARLS & CONSIDERATIONS

Screening with use of low-dose CT (LDCT) for detection of lung cancer among persons with a

heavy history of smoking increases the percentage of lung cancer cases that are diagnosed in stage 1 and reduces mortality from lung cancer. The National Lung Screening Trial (NLST) showed that lung cancer screening with LDCT resulted in a 20% reduction in lung cancer mortality.[16] New guidelines (Table 11 and Fig. 8) recommend annual LDCT for those who are current or former smokers ages 50 to 77 yr with a smoking history threshold of 20 pack-yr. Screening should be discontinued once a person has not smoked for 15 yr or develops a health problem that substantially limits life expectancy or the ability or willingness to have curative lung surgery.

REFERENCES

Available at eBooks.Health.Elsevier.com.

RELATED CONTENT

Lung Cancer (Patient Information)
Lung Cancer Screening (Patient Information)
Horner Syndrome (Related Key Topic)
Lambert-Eaton Myasthenic Syndrome (Related Key Topic)
Paraneoplastic Syndromes (Related Key Topic)
Superior Vena Cava Syndrome (Related Key Topic)

AUTHOR: **RITESH RATHORE, MD**

TABLE 11 Lung Cancer Screening Recommendations

Asymptomatic patients age 55-77 yr	>30 pack-yr	Current smoker or quit <15 yr	Annual screening with low-dose CT
Asymptomatic patients >77 yr	<30 pack-yr	Quit smoking >15 yr ago	Low-dose CT screening should not be performed
Patients with comorbidities that adversely influence their ability to tolerate treatment of early-stage screen-detected lung cancer or that substantially limit their life expectancy			Low-dose CT screening should not be performed

CT, Computed tomography.
From Warshaw G et al: *Ham's primary care geriatrics*, ed 7, Philadelphia, 2022, Elsevier.

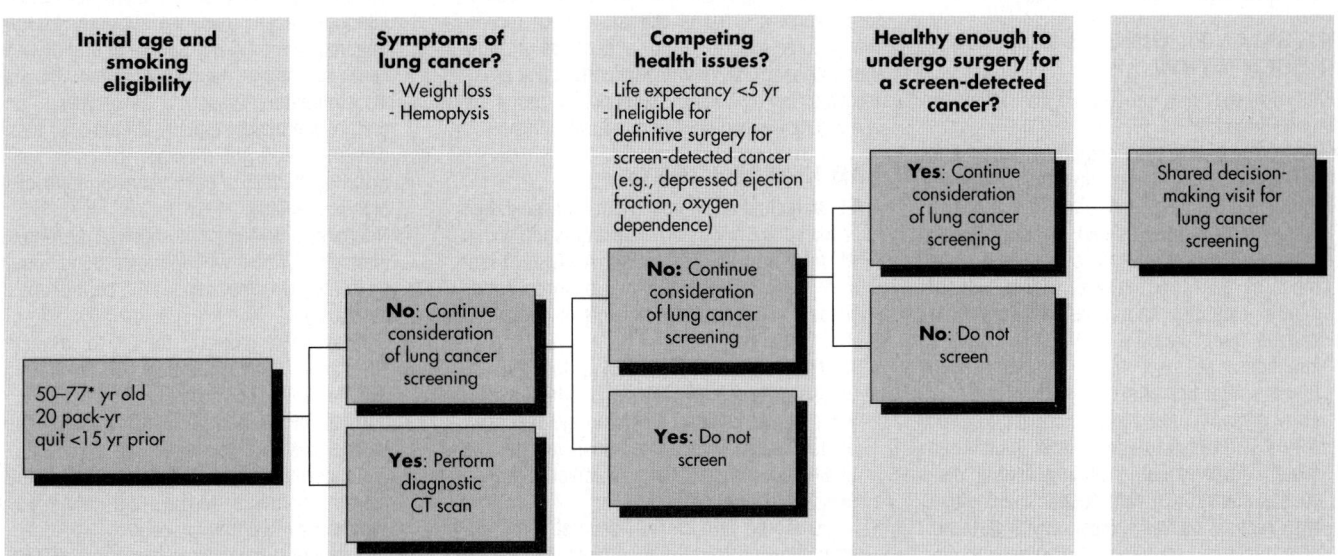

FIG 8 Algorithm for considering patient eligibility for lung cancer. *Centers for Medicare and Medicaid Services eligibility criteria. *CT*, Computed tomography. (Modified from Broaddus VC et al: *Murray & Nadel's textbook of respiratory medicine*, ed 7, Philadelphia, 2022, Elsevier.)

BASIC INFORMATION

DEFINITION

Lyme disease is a multisystem inflammatory disorder caused by the transmission of a spirochete, *Borrelia burgdorferi,* via the bite of infected *Ixodes* ticks, taking 36 to 48 h for a tick to take a blood meal and transmit the infecting organism to the host. Table E1 summarizes the Centers for Disease Control and Prevention (CDC) Lyme disease surveillance case definition.

SYNONYMS

Bannwarth syndrome (Europe)
Acrodermatitis chronica atrophicans

ICD-10CM CODES	
A69.20	Lyme disease, unspecified
A69.21	Meningitis due to Lyme disease
A69.22	Other neurologic disorders in Lyme disease
A69.23	Arthritis due to Lyme disease
A69.29	Other conditions associated with Lyme disease

EPIDEMIOLOGY & DEMOGRAPHICS

INCIDENCE (IN U.S.): In the U.S., 4.4 cases/100,000 persons; it is the most common vector-borne infection in the U.S., with more than 30,000 new cases reported each year. 90% of cases are found in Massachusetts, Connecticut, Rhode Island, New York, New Jersey, Pennsylvania, Minnesota, Wisconsin, and California. The area of transmission in the U.S. is expanding farther into the South and upper Northeast. The disease also occurs in Europe and Asia with a different *Ixodes* tick vector. Table E2 summarizes principal vector ticks and spirochetes associated with Lyme borreliosis.
PREDOMINANT SEX: Male = female
PREDOMINANT AGE: Median age of 28 yr
PEAK INCIDENCE: May to November

PHYSICAL FINDINGS & CLINICAL PRESENTATION

Lyme disease may present in the following stages (Table E3):
- *Early localized stage (incubation period 3 to 30 days):* Early Lyme disease, erythema migrans (EM); skin rash, often at site of tick bite (the CDC has defined EM rash as an expanding red macule or papule that must reach at least 5 cm in size, with or without central clearing); target lesions from ECM can be found in 60% to 80% of localized infections; possible fever, myalgias 3 to 32 days after tick bite
- *Early disseminated stage (incubation period 3 to 6 wk):* Days to weeks later; multiorgan system involvement, including central nervous system (CNS) with aseptic meningitis–type picture or Bell's palsy, joints (arthritis or arthralgias), cardiac including varying degrees of heart block; related to dissemination of spirochete

- *Late stage (incubation period month to year):* Month to year after tick exposure; affects central and peripheral nervous system, cardiac, joints

Common presenting signs and symptoms include:
- EM (Fig. E1). Most patients with EM (about 80%) have a single lesion, but the bacteria can disseminate hematogenously to other sites in the skin and result in often smaller erythema migrans lesions (Figs. E2 and E3).
- Lymphadenopathy, neck pains, pharyngeal erythema, myalgias, hepatosplenomegaly.
- Patients will complain of malaise, fatigue, lethargy, headache, fever/chills, neck pain, myalgias, back pain.

ETIOLOGY

B. burgdorferi transmitted from bite of an *Ixodes* tick (Fig. E4) (mostly in the nymph stage but also can be from adult ticks). Human infection occurs through inoculation of spirochetes in infected saliva and usually requires tick attachment for more than 36 h.

DIAGNOSIS

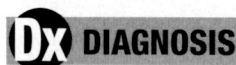

Clinical presentation, exposure to ticks in endemic area, and diagnostic testing for antibody response to *B. burgdorferi* (Fig. E5). Serologic testing at early stages is usually negative; therefore, in early stage, documentation of erythema migrans lesion with a compatible epidemiologic history is sufficient for diagnosis, and laboratory testing is not indicated.

DIFFERENTIAL DIAGNOSIS

- Chronic fatigue/fibromyalgia
- Acute viral illnesses
- Babesiosis
- Human granulocytic anaplasmosis
- Ehrlichiosis
- STARI: Southern tick-associated rash illness

WORKUP

Serologic testing is the principal means of laboratory diagnosis of Lyme disease. Current recommendations include using a sensitive enzyme immunoassay (EIA) or immunofluorescence assay, followed by a Western immunoblot assay for specimens yielding positive or equivocal results.

LABORATORY TESTS

- ELISA testing and if positive or equivocal then followed by a Western blot immunoglobulin M (IgM) and IgG (Table E4). A Western blot IgM assay is positive if two of three bands present. The Western blot IgG is positive if 5 of 10 bands present.
- An alternative serologic test is the VlsE C6 ELISA (enzyme-linked immunosorbent assay) (C6 peptide), which detects an IgG response earlier and may be more sensitive than the ELISA, but its specificity is lower than the two-tier testing method.
- In 2019, the FDA cleared several Lyme assays allowing for an EIA serology test rather than the western blot assay as the second test in the Lyme disease testing algorithm.

- Early disease often is difficult to diagnose serologically, secondary to slow immune response.
- Culturing of skin lesions (EM) and polymerase chain reaction (PCR) of synovial fluid or cerebrospinal fluid can also give the diagnosis of active infection.
- Fig. 6 is an algorithm for the diagnosis and treatment of arthritis associated with Lyme disease.

IMAGING STUDIES

- ECG
- Echocardiogram if conduction abnormalities are present with cardiac involvement
- CT, MRI of brain in patients with CNS involvement

TREATMENT (TABLE E5)

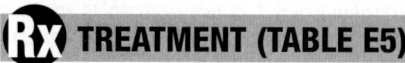

Early localized Lyme disease:
- Doxycycline 100 mg bid in adults (children: 2 mg/kg bid if ≥8 yr) for 10 to 14 days or amoxicillin 500 mg tid for adults (children: 50 mg/kg per day in three divided doses) for 14 to 21 days. Doxycycline offers the advantage of treating possible coinfection with the bacterial agents of ehrlichiosis.
- Alternative treatments for pregnancy and children ≤8 yr: Cefuroxime axetil 500 mg bid for 14 to 21 days (children: 30 mg/kg per day in two divided doses), azithromycin 500 mg PO for 7 to 10 days but should **not** be used as a first-line agent, as it is less effective than doxycycline and amoxicillin. NOTE: The American Academy of Pediatrics (AAP Red Book) now considers doxycycline safe regardless of age for up to 21 days.
- A single dose of 200 mg doxycycline given within 72 h of removing an engorged *Ixodes* tick can significantly reduce the risk of development of Lyme disease in endemic areas and is reasonable prophylaxis in nonpregnant adults and children ≥8 yr old.

Early disseminated and late persistent infection:
- 28 days of treatment is often prescribed, although recent evidence supports treating patients with a 14-day course of oral doxycycline for early neurologic Lyme disease in ambulatory patients. Doxycycline and ceftriaxone appear equally effective for acute disseminated Lyme disease.
- Arthritis: 28 days of doxycycline or amoxicillin plus probenecid.
- Neurologic involvement requires parenteral antibiotics. Those who fail to respond should be treated with intravenous (IV) ceftriaxone or cefotaxime.
- Ceftriaxone 2 g/day IV for 21 to 28 days; alternative: Cefotaxime 2 g q8h IV; alternative: Penicillin G 5 million U qid.
- Cardiac involvement: IV ceftriaxone or cefotaxime plus cardiac monitoring.
- Prolonged treatment with IV or PO antibiotic therapy for up to 90 days did not improve symptoms more than placebo.

Posttreatment Lyme disease syndrome (PTLDS):
- Presence of disabling symptoms such as fatigue, malaise, diffuse pains, and poor

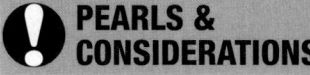
DIAGNOSIS AND TREATMENT OF LYME ARTHRITIS

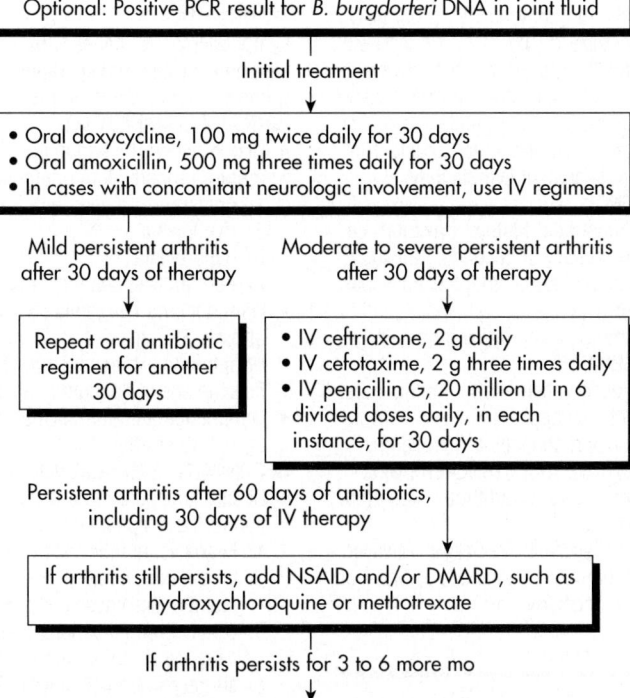

FIG. 6 Algorithm for the diagnosis and treatment of arthritis associated with Lyme disease. *DMARD*, Disease-modifying antirheumatic drug; *DNA*, deoxyribonucleic acid; *ELISA*, enzyme-linked immunosorbent assay; *Ig*, immunoglobulin; *IV*, intravenous; *NSAID*, nonsteroidal antiinflammatory drug; *PCR*, polymerase chain reaction. (From Hochberg MC: *Rheumatology*, ed 7, Philadelphia, 2019, Elsevier.)

concentration, which may be due to an exuberant host inflammatory response even in patients who have received proper antibiotic treatment.

- Antibiotics are not indicated. Antibiotic treatment of patients with persistent unexplained symptoms despite previous antibiotic treatment of Lyme disease provides little, if any, benefit and carries significant risk.
- Treatment of PTLDS is supportive care.

DISPOSITION

- The patient often needs careful follow-up and supportive care for the arthralgia-neuritis symptoms.

- 10% to 20% of treated patients may have lingering symptoms of fatigue, disrupted sleep, and musculoskeletal complaints. Repeat episodes of EM in appropriately treated patients are due to reinfection and not to relapse.

REFERRAL

- To a neurologist if significant neurologic complications (meningitis, myelitis, ophthalmoplegia, Bell palsy)
- To a cardiologist if the patient develops evidence of cardiac conduction disturbances or pericarditis

PEARLS & CONSIDERATIONS

- A physician diagnosis of classic EM in an endemic region of Lyme disease is sufficient to make a definitive diagnosis.
- In some patients with Lyme disease, nonspecific complaints such as headache, fatigue, and arthralgia may persist for months after appropriate (and ultimately successful) antibiotic treatment. Long-term antibiotic treatment does not provide additional beneficial effects.
- There is no evidence of current or previous *Borrelia burgdorferi* infection in most patients evaluated at university-based Lyme disease referral centers. Psychiatric comorbidity and other psychologic factors are prominent in the presentation and outcome of some patients who inaccurately ascribe long-standing symptoms to "chronic Lyme disease."
- It is important to realize that one tick bite can transmit Lyme disease *and* the bacterial agents of either ehrlichiosis or babesiosis (protozoan parasite), or even both, and these latter agents require separate serologic testing and possibly therapy. *Ehrlichiosis* is treated with doxycycline, but *Babesia* would require a different therapy. Powassan virus can also be transmitted by the *Ixodes* tick bite and causes an encephalitis seen in eastern Canada and northcentral, northeastern, and upper midwestern United States. Cases have been increasing.
- Tick bite protection: EPA-registered insect repellents containing DEET, picaridin, IR3535, oil of lemon eucalyptus (OLE), para-menthane-3, 8-diol (PMD), or 2-undecanone can prevent ticks from attaching when applied and can last for several hours. OLE and PMD products cannot be used on children under 3 yr of age.

SUGGESTED READINGS

Available at eBooks.Health.Elsevier.com.

RELATED CONTENT

Lyme Disease (Patient Information)

AUTHOR: **GLENN G. FORT, MD, MPH**

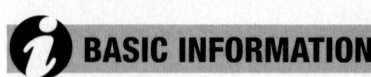 **BASIC INFORMATION**

DEFINITION

A primary role of the lymphatic system is to transport proteins from the interstitium to the heart. When the transport capacity of the lymphatic system is reduced, proteins accumulate in the interstitium. Accumulated proteins attract water, which creates a high protein swelling in the subcutaneous tissues called lymphedema. Lymphedema can be classified as primary or secondary (Box 1).

SYNONYM

Elephantiasis

ICD-10CM CODES
I89.0	Lymphedema, not elsewhere classified
I97.2	Postmastectomy lymphedema syndrome
Q82.0	Hereditary lymphedema

EPIDEMIOLOGY & DEMOGRAPHICS

PRIMARY LYMPHEDEMA:
- Found in 1.1/100,000 people aged <20 yr
- Females outnumber males 3.5:1
- Incidence peaks between ages 12 and 16 (puberty)

SECONDARY LYMPHEDEMA: See "Etiology"

PHYSICAL FINDINGS & CLINICAL PRESENTATION

Lymphedema is a slow-onset, progressive disease characterized by an asymmetric, inflammatory swelling, traveling distal to proximal, that can affect any body part including limbs, trunk, head/neck, and genitals (Fig. E1). Box 2 summarizes lymphedema staging from the International Society of Lymphology.

STAGE 0: LATENCY:
- Decreased lymphatic system transport capacity due to primary or secondary etiology
- Subjective complaints of affected body part feeling heavy or achy
- No objective findings, no apparent swelling

STAGE I: REVERSIBLE:
- Edema is observable, soft, pitting, and reversible with elevation.
- No secondary skin changes are present.

STAGE II: SPONTANEOUSLY IRREVERSIBLE:
- Skin becomes more firm/fibrotic, therefore less pitting.
- Edema does not reverse to normal with elevation.
- Possibility of infections (cellulitis), wounds, or weeping (lymphorrhea).

STAGE III: ELEPHANTIASIS:
- Skin becomes very firm/fibrotic, therefore nonpitting.
- Evidence of substantial skin changes (e.g., papillomas, lobules, "peau d' orange").

ETIOLOGY

Lymphedema is caused by a reduction in lymphatic system transport and is classified into primary and secondary forms.

PRIMARY LYMPHEDEMA:
- Occurs when the lymphatic system does not mature properly during fetal development
  1. Aplasia
  2. Hypoplasia
  3. Hyperplasia
- Can be familial, genetic, or hereditary
- Lymphedema congenital: Symptoms present at birth (Fig. 2)
- Lymphedema praecox: Symptoms onset before the age of 35 (commonly during puberty)
- Lymphedema tardum: Symptoms onset at the age of 35 or after

SECONDARY LYMPHEDEMA:
- Occurs secondary to a disruption or obstruction of the lymphatic system caused by:
  1. Filariasis (number one cause worldwide)
  2. Lymph node surgery/radiation due to cancer (number one cause in the U.S.)
  3. Other: Chronic venous insufficiency (CVI), deep vein thrombosis (DVT), infection, surgery/trauma, lipedema, and obesity

Dx DIAGNOSIS

- Lymphedema is primarily a clinical diagnosis made on the basis of past medical history and objective findings that distinguish it from other causes of chronic edema.
- A Stemmer sign is often used to identify lymphedema (inability to pick up or pinch a fold of skin at the base of the second toe or finger).

BOX 1 Classification of Lymphedema

Primary Lymphedema
- Congenital lymphedema (Milroy disease)
- Lymphedema praecox
- Lymphedema tarda

Syndromes Associated With Primary Lymphedema
- Yellow nail syndrome
- Turner syndrome
- Noonan syndrome
- Pes cavus
- Phakomatosis pigmentovascularis
- Distichiasis-lymphedema
- Emberger syndrome
- WILD syndrome
- Hypotrichosis-telangiectasia-lymphedema syndrome

Cutaneous Disorders Sometimes Associated With Primary Lymphedema
- Yellow nails
- Hemangiomas
- Xanthomatosis and chylous lymphedema
- Congenital absence of nails

Secondary Lymphedema
- Postmastectomy lymphedema
- Melphalan isolated limb perfusion
- Malignant occlusion with obstruction
- Extrinsic pressure
- Factitial lymphedema
- Postradiation therapy
- Following recurrent lymphangitis/cellulitis
- Lymphedema of upper limb in recurrent eczema
- Granulomatous disease
- Rosaceous lymphedema
- Primary amyloidosis

Complications of Lymphedema
- Cellulitis of lymphedema
- Elephantiasis nostra verrucosa
- Ulceration
- Lymphangiosarcoma

From James WD et al: *Andrews' diseases of the skin,* ed 12, Philadelphia, 2016, Elsevier.

BOX 2 Lymphedema Staging

Stage 0: Latent
- Impaired lymphatic function
- No evident edema; subclinical
- May last months or years before progression

Stage I: Spontaneously Reversible
- Early accumulation of protein-rich fluid
- Pitting edema
- Subsides with elevation

Stage II: Spontaneously Irreversible
- Accumulation of protein-rich fluid
- Pitting edema progresses to fibrosis
- Does not resolve with elevation alone

Stage III: Lymphostatic Elephantiasis
- Nonpitting
- Significant fibrosis
- Trophic skin changes

From International Society of Lymphology: The diagnosis and treatment of peripheral edema: 2009 consensus document of the International Society of Lymphology, *Lymphology* 42(2):51-60, 2009.

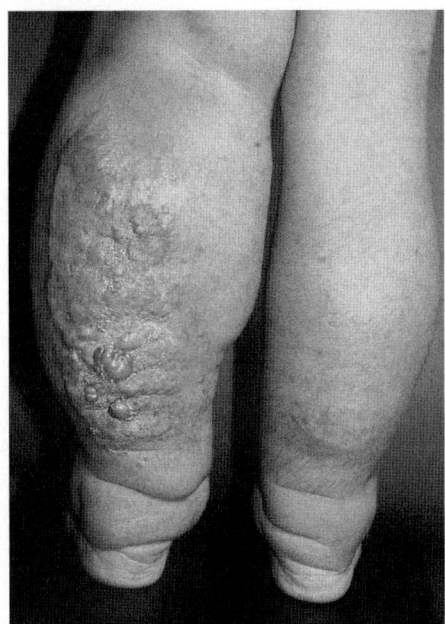

FIG. 2 Milroy disease.

- When physical examination is inconclusive, other available imaging tests can help make the diagnosis (see "Imaging Studies").

DIFFERENTIAL DIAGNOSIS

Other causes of edema that should be ruled out before treatment for lymphedema include cardiac, renal, hepatic, and thyroid dysfunction.

WORKUP

A detailed history and physical examination should help exclude most of the differential diagnoses.

LABORATORY TESTS

- Blood urea nitrogen, creatinine, liver function tests, albumin, urine analysis, and thyroid function tests are obtained to exclude possible systemic causes of edema.
- Genetic testing may be practical in defining a specific hereditary syndrome with a discrete gene mutation such as lymphedema distichiasis *(FOXC2)*, Milroy disease *(VEGFR-3)*, Meige disease, or Klippel-Trenaunay-Weber syndrome.

IMAGING STUDIES

- Lymphoscintigraphy: Diagnostic image of choice for lymphedema (if needed)
- Indocyanine green (ICG) fluorescent lymphography: Can now be used to identify sentinel nodes, to demonstrate superficial lymph channels and functional lymphatics, to indicate treatment pathways, and to confirm the effectiveness of therapeutic techniques
- MRI: Primarily used in tumor diagnosis
- Duplex ultrasound: Determines venous involvement in the edema
- Computed axial tomography (CAT): Distinguishes between fatty tissue and accumulations of protein-rich fluids

- Lymphography: Phased out in favor of less invasive techniques

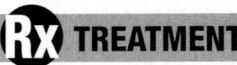 **TREATMENT**

NONPHARMACOLOGIC THERAPY

- Complete decongestive therapy (CDT) is backed by long-standing research and experience as the primary treatment of choice for lymphedema in both children and adults (Fig. E3). It should be delivered by a certified lymphedema therapist (CLT). CDT involves a two-phase treatment program:
  1. Phase 1—Reduce tissue congestion of affected body part with daily treatments:
     a. Manual lymph drainage
     b. Skin care
     c. Compression wrapping of limb
     d. Decongestive exercises
  2. Phase 2—Maintain decongestion with home maintenance program:
     a. Daily use of elastic and inelastic compression garments that are properly fitted according to circumference and length to prevent lymphedema from returning.
     b. Compression is graduated; most of the compression is distal with decreasing compression in the stocking proximally.
     c. Different knits and compression classes are available for different stages of lymphedema.
     d. Choices of garments include below-the-knee stockings, thigh-high stockings, pantyhose, sleeves, bras, and truncal garments.
- Massage (or any modality that increases blood flow) can have negative effects on

lymphedema by increasing vasodilation. Therefore it is contraindicated on the lymphedematous quadrants.
- Compression pumps have not been found to be effective in removing proteins from lymphedematous quadrants.
- Nutritional therapy (reducing the amount of proteins ingested) is ineffective in the treatment of lymphedema.

PHARMACOLOGIC THERAPY

No drugs have been shown to be beneficial in the treatment of lymphedema. Diuretics in particular have not been found to be effective in removing proteins from lymphedematous quadrants and may promote the development of volume depletion.

SURGERY

Surgery for lymphedema has been proven largely unsuccessful and should not be considered before CDT. Surgical procedures are divided into two types:
- Physiologic procedures: Those performed to improve lymph node drainage (e.g., anastomoses of the lymph system with the venous system, lymph node transplant).
- Excisional or debulking procedures: Those performed to excise the subcutaneous tissue (e.g., Charles procedure [Fig. E4], Thompson procedure, the modified Homans procedure [Fig. E5], and liposuction). Liposuction-circumferential suction-assisted lipectomy represents a newly proposed method to reduce morbidity involved in the traditional excisional techniques.

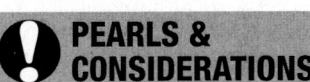 **PEARLS & CONSIDERATIONS**

- Lymphedema is a chronic, generally incurable but very manageable condition that requires lifelong care and attention along with psychosocial support.
- Children and adolescents (along with parents and adults) should be encouraged to pursue a normal life, participating in school activities and sports (preferably noncontact, such as swimming).
- Infections such as cellulitis should be treated promptly.
- If the etiology is filariasis caused by the parasites *Wuchereria bancrofti* or *Brugia malayi*, treatment is diethylcarbamazine citrate 5 mg/kg in divided doses for 3 wk.
- Patients with lymphedema commonly manifest psychiatric comorbidities as a result of their disease, such as anxiety; depression; adjustment problems; and difficulty in vocational, domestic, or social domains.
- Lymphedema can be complicated in rare cases by development of lymphangiosarcomata or other cutaneous malignancies. Chronic upper extremity lymphedema after mastectomy increases the risk for cutaneous angiosarcoma of the affected limb and lower extremity lymphadoma is associated with excess risk for nonmelanoma skin cancer.[1]

- Gene therapy to develop new lymphangiosis in the affected body parts is a potential clinical remedy in the future.

REFERENCE & SUGGESTED READING
Available at eBooks.Health.Elsevier.com.

RELATED CONTENT
Lymphedema (Patient Information)

AUTHORS: **FRANK G. FORT, MD, FACS, RPHS** and **KATHRYN MARIE TAYLOR, PT, DPT, CLT-LANA**

BASIC INFORMATION

DEFINITION

Malabsorption is the diminished intestinal absorption of dietary nutrients. The majority of malabsorption is due to either congenital or acquired defects in the membrane transport system, absorption, and brush border processing in the intestinal epithelium.

SYNONYM

Maldigestion

ICD-10CM CODES
K90.4	Malabsorption due to intolerance, not elsewhere classified
K90.89	Other intestinal malabsorption
K90.9	Intestinal malabsorption, unspecified
K91.2	Postsurgical malabsorption, not elsewhere classified

EPIDEMIOLOGY & DEMOGRAPHICS

PREDOMINANT SEX & AGE:
More common in females, with a mean age of 40

RISK FACTORS:
- Excessive alcohol consumption
- History of celiac disease
- History of irritable bowel disease
- Intestinal surgery

GENETICS: HLA-DQ2 present in 95% of celiac disease

PHYSICAL FINDINGS & CLINICAL PRESENTATION
- Most commonly nonspecific symptoms such as abdominal flatulence and distention are seen.
- Due to the osmotic load from maldigestion/malabsorption, watery diarrhea may be present. In the case of fat digestive disorder, steatorrhea ensues.
- Weight loss is very common, but many patients are able to compensate by increased caloric load. Diffuse disease often has much more pronounced weight loss.
- Chronic protein malabsorption can cause hypoalbuminemia, leading to edema and ascites.
- Both microcytic and macrocytic anemia can result from micronutrient deficiency (iron/B_{12}). These patients can be pale and present with fatigue.
- Bleeding disorders from vitamin K deficiency can lead to ecchymosis, melena, and hematuria.
- Vitamin D deficiency can lead to bone disorders. Secondary hyperparathyroidism can be a presenting feature.
- Electrolyte and vitamin deficiency can lead to neurologic disorders such as ataxia, weakness, and neuropathy, and may have positive Chvostek or Trousseau sign.
- Autoimmune disease-specific dermatologic findings such as alopecia, pellagra, erythema nodosum, pyoderma gangrenosum, cheilosis, glossitis, and aphthous ulcers may be present.
- Cardinal clinical features of specific malabsorptive disorders are summarized in Table 1.

ETIOLOGY
- Can be congenital or acquired.
- Disease-specific etiology. Mechanisms of malabsorption, malabsorbed substrates, and representative causes are summarized in Table 2.

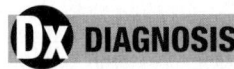 DIAGNOSIS

DIFFERENTIAL DIAGNOSIS
- Crohn disease
- Celiac disease
- Hartnup disease

TABLE 1 Cardinal Clinical Features of Specific Malabsorptive Disorders

Disorder	Cardinal Clinical Features
Adrenal insufficiency	Skin darkening, hyponatremia, hyperkalemia
Amyloidosis	Renal disease, nephrotic syndrome, cardiomyopathy, neuropathy, carpal tunnel syndrome, macroglossia, hepatosplenomegaly
Bile acid deficiency	Ileal resection or disease, liver disease
Carcinoid syndrome	Flushing, cardiac murmur
Celiac disease	Variable symptoms: Dermatitis herpetiformis, alopecia, aphthous mouth ulcers, arthropathy, neurologic symptoms, and (life-threatening) malnutrition; elevated liver biochemical test levels, mild iron deficiency
Crohn disease	Arthritis, aphthous mouth ulcers, episcleritis, uveitis, pyoderma gangrenosum, erythema nodosum, abdominal mass, fistulas, perianal fistulae, primary sclerosing cholangitis (PSC), laboratory signs of inflammation
CF	Chronic sinopulmonary disease, meconium ileus, distal intestinal obstruction syndrome (DIOS), elevated sweat chloride
Cystinuria, Hartnup disease	Kidney stones, dermatosis
Diabetes mellitus	Long history of diabetes and diabetic complications
Disaccharidase deficiency	Bloating and cramping, intermittent diarrhea
GI fistulas	Previous intestinal surgery or trauma, Crohn disease
Glucagonoma	Migratory necrolytic erythema, enlarged gallbladder
Hyperthyroidism, hypothyroidism	Symptoms and signs of thyroid disease
Hypogammaglobulinemia	Recurrent infections
Intestinal ischemia	Other ischemic organ manifestations; abdominal pain with eating (chronic mesenteric ischemia)
Lymphoma	Enlarged mesenteric or retroperitoneal lymph nodes, abdominal mass, abdominal pain, fever
Mastocytosis	Urticaria pigmentosum, peptic ulcer
Mycobacterium avium complex infection	AIDS
Pancreatic insufficiency	History of pancreatitis, abdominal pain, or alcoholism; large-volume fatty, oily stools; passage of orange oil
Parasitic infection	History of travel to endemic areas
PBC	Jaundice, itching
Scleroderma	Dysphagia, inability to open the mouth widely, Raynaud phenomenon, skin tightening
SIBO	Previous intestinal surgery, motility disorder (scleroderma, pseudo-obstruction), small intestinal diverticula, strictures
Tropical sprue	History of travel to endemic area
Tuberculosis	Specific history of exposure, living in or travel to endemic area, immunosuppression, abdominal mass or intestinal obstruction, ascites
Whipple disease	Lymphadenopathy, fever, arthritis, cerebral symptoms, heart murmur (pulmonary valve), oculomasticatory myorhythmia
ZES	Peptic ulcers, diarrhea

AIDS, Acquired immunodeficiency syndrome; *CF,* cystic fibrosis; *GI,* gastrointestinal; *PBC,* primary biliary cholangitis; *SIBO,* small intestinal bacterial overgrowth; *ZES,* Zollinger-Ellison syndrome.
From Feldman M et al: *Sleisenger and Fordtran's gastrointestinal and liver disease,* ed 11, Philadelphia, 2021, Elsevier.

Diseases and Disorders

TABLE 2 Mechanisms of Malabsorption, Malabsorbed Substrates, and Representative Causes

Pathophysiologic Mechanism	Malabsorbed Substrate(s)	Representative Causes
Maldigestion		
Conjugated bile acid deficiency	Fat Fat-soluble vitamins Calcium Magnesium	Hepatic parenchymal disease Biliary obstruction SIBO with bile acid deconjugation Ileal bile acid malabsorption CCK deficiency
Pancreatic insufficiency	Fat Protein Carbohydrate Fat-soluble vitamins Vitamin B_{12} (cobalamin)	Congenital defects Chronic pancreatitis Pancreatic tumors Inactivation of pancreatic enzymes (e.g., ZES)
Reduced mucosal digestion	Carbohydrate Protein	Congenital defects Acquired lactase deficiency Generalized mucosal disease (e.g., celiac disease, Crohn disease)
Intraluminal consumption of nutrients	Vitamin B_{12} (cobalamin)	SIBO Helminthic infections (e.g., *Diphyllobothrium latum* infection)
Malabsorption		
Reduced mucosal absorption	Fat Protein Carbohydrate Vitamins Minerals	Congenital transport defects Generalized mucosal diseases (e.g., celiac disease, Crohn disease) Previous intestinal resection or bypass Infections Intestinal lymphoma
Decreased transport from the intestine	Fat Protein	Intestinal lymphangiectasia Primary Secondary (e.g., solid tumors, Whipple disease, lymphomas) Venous stasis (e.g., from heart failure)
Other Mechanisms		
Decreased gastric acid and/or intrinsic factor secretion	Vitamin B_{12}	Pernicious anemia Atrophic gastritis Previous gastric resection
Decreased gastric mixing and/or rapid gastric emptying	Fat Calcium Protein	Previous gastric resection Autonomic neuropathy
Rapid intestinal transit	Fat	Autonomic neuropathy Hyperthyroidism

CCK, Cholecystokinin; *SIBO*, small intestinal bacterial overgrowth; *ZES*, Zollinger-Ellison syndrome.
Modified from Feldman M et al: *Sleisenger and Fordtran's gastrointestinal and liver disease*, ed 11, Philadelphia, 2021, Elsevier.

- Chronic pancreatitis
- Pancreatic insufficiency
- Cystic fibrosis
- Short bowel syndrome
- Neoplasm
- Abetalipoproteinemia
- Lactose intolerance
- Small intestine bacterial overgrowth
- Chronic atrophic gastritis
- Zollinger-Ellison syndrome
- Chronic cholestasis
- Cirrhosis

WORKUP
- A detailed history including alcohol consumption and surgical history as well as autoimmune disease can help diagnose the underlying disease. It is important to screen for anemia and electrolyte abnormalities due to malabsorption.
- Table E3 summarizes malabsorptive diseases or conditions in which noninvasive tests can establish malabsorption or provide a diagnosis.

LABORATORY TESTS
- CBC, serum iron, vitamin B_{12}, and folate to detect for anemia.
- **Prothrombin time:** Elevated prothrombin time can suggest vitamin K deficiency.
- **Fat malabsorption:** The gold standard is the 72-h stool elastase or fat collection. More than 6/g day in the stool is pathologic. This test can be cumbersome, so other options are available. Sudan III stain and acid steatocrit tests are qualitative measures of steatorrhea. Serologic testing for celiac disease should be considered as well.
- **Carbohydrate malabsorption:** Carbohydrate malabsorption leads to fermentation of the undigested carbohydrates by intestinal bacteria.
- The urinary D-xylose test for carbohydrate absorption in the small intestine. After loading with D-xylose, urinary D-xylose levels are measured. Low levels suggest intestinal malabsorption.

- Lactose intolerance can be tested by the lactose tolerance test or the breath test. The lactose tolerance test measures blood glucose after lactose administration. Development of symptoms or inadequate increase in blood sugar is indicative of lactose intolerance. H_2/CO_2 breath tests using specific forms of carbohydrates can detect malabsorption as well.
- **Protein malabsorption:** Protein malabsorption is likely due to small intestinal bacterial overgrowth or protein gastroenteropathies. Alpha-1 antitrypsin clearance or 99mTc-albumin gamma camera scintigraphy may aid in this diagnosis.
- **Pancreatic insufficiency:** Fecal elastase and chymotrypsin levels can distinguish from pancreatic and intestinal causes.
- **Vitamin deficiency:** It is important to assess serum vitamin B_{12} and methylmalonic acid levels. Schilling test is rarely used but can be useful in some cases.
- **Bile acid malabsorption:** Quantitative stool bile acid measurement is the preferred method of diagnosis. SeHCAT test (selenium homocholic acid taurine test) is another option but less likely used.
- **Bacterial overgrowth:** This can be detected with endoscopic jejunal aspirate culture or a less invasive hydrogen breath test.

Table 4 summarizes useful laboratory tests for evaluating patients with suspected malabsorption and for establishing possible nutrient deficiencies.

IMAGING STUDIES
- Abdominal ultrasound can identify thickened small bowel wall
- Endoscopy for visualization and biopsy
- Small bowel follow through
- Abdominal computed tomography (CT)/MRI
- Endoscopic retrograde cholangiopancreatography/magnetic resonance cholangiopancreatography/endoscopic ultrasound for identification of pancreatic abnormalities
- Capsule endoscopy

Rx TREATMENT

Involves identification and treatment of the underlying illness, treatment of diarrhea, and nutritional repletion

NONPHARMACOLOGIC THERAPY
- A gluten-free diet in patients with celiac disease. Avoidance of lactose-containing product in lactose intolerance.
- Avoidance of caffeine and high sugar containing compounds has been found to decrease diarrhea in some cases.

ACUTE GENERAL Rx
- Control of the underlying disease should be primary goal.
- It is also essential to control any volume and electrolyte abnormalities that might exist.

CHRONIC Rx
- Control of chronic diarrhea with loperamide should be one of the goals in a chronic malabsorptive state.

TABLE 4 Useful Laboratory Tests for Patients With Suspected Malabsorption and for Establishing Possible Nutrient Deficiencies

Test	Comment(s)
Blood Cell Count	
Hematocrit, hemoglobin	Decreased in iron, vitamin B_{12}, and folate malabsorption or with blood loss
Mean corpuscular hemoglobin or mean corpuscular volume	Decreased in iron malabsorption; increased in folate and vitamin B_{12} malabsorption
White blood cells, differential	Decreased in vitamin B_{12} and folate malabsorption; low lymphocyte count in lymphangiectasia
Biochemical Tests (Serum)	
TGs	Decreased in severe fat malabsorption
Cholesterol	Decreased in bile acid malabsorption or severe fat malabsorption
Albumin	Decreased in severe malnutrition, lymphangiectasia, protein-losing enteropathy
Alkaline phosphatase	Increased in calcium and vitamin D malabsorption (severe steatorrhea); decreased in zinc deficiency
Calcium, phosphorus, magnesium	Decreased in extensive small intestinal mucosal disease, after extensive intestinal resection, or in vitamin D deficiency
Zinc	Decreased in extensive small intestinal mucosal disease or intestinal resection
Iron, ferritin	Decreased in celiac disease, in other extensive small intestinal mucosal diseases, and with chronic blood loss
Other Serum Tests	
Prothrombin time	Prolonged in vitamin K malabsorption
β-Carotene	Decreased in fat malabsorption from hepatobiliary or intestinal diseases
Immunoglobulins	Decreased in lymphangiectasia, diffuse lymphoma
Folic acid	Decreased in extensive small intestinal mucosal diseases, with anticonvulsant use, in pregnancy; may be increased in SIBO
Vitamin B_{12}	Decreased after gastrectomy, in pernicious anemia, terminal ileal disease, SIBO, and infection with *Diphyllobothrium latum*
Methylmalonic acid	Markedly elevated in vitamin B_{12} deficiency
Homocysteine	Markedly elevated in vitamin B_{12} or folate deficiency
Citrulline	May be decreased in destructive small intestinal mucosal disease or intestinal resection
Stool Tests	
Fat	Qualitative or quantitative increase in fat malabsorption
Elastase, chymotrypsin	Decreased concentrations and output in exocrine pancreatic insufficiency
pH	Less than 5.5 in carbohydrate malabsorption

SIBO, Small intestinal bacterial overgrowth; *TGs,* thyroglobulins.
From Feldman M et al: *Sleisenger and Fordtran's gastrointestinal and liver disease,* ed 11, Philadelphia, 2021, Elsevier.

- Correction of volume and electrolyte disturbance with oral rehydration therapy should be made a priority.
- Bile acid conjugates can decrease steatorrhea in some cases.
- Pancreatic insufficiency is typically treated with a low-fat diet and exogenous pancreatic enzymes.
- Teduglutide-homolog of GLP-2 has been shown to increase absorptive surface area in short bowel syndrome.
- Periodic DEXA scans are indicated in chronic malabsorption in the setting of vitamin D deficiency.
- Oral supplementation with vitamins and minerals is important, sometimes requiring parenteral therapy.

REFERRAL
- Gastroenterology consultation can help in diagnosis when initial laboratory testing is unclear.
- Nutrition consultation can help patients with diet modification to alleviate symptoms.

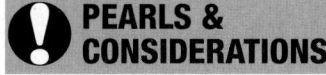 **PEARLS & CONSIDERATIONS**

COMMENTS
- Malabsorption should be considered a sign of an underlying disease.
- Treatment should focus on treating the underlying disorder.

- Nutrient and volume repletion should be priority in any treatment plan of malabsorption.

RELATED CONTENT
Celiac Disease (Related Key Topic)
Crohn Disease (Related Key Topic)
Cystic Fibrosis (Related Key Topic)
Irritable Bowel Syndrome (Related Key Topic)
Lactose Intolerance (Related Key Topic)
Chronic Pancreatitis (Related Key Topic)
Short Bowel Syndrome (Related Key Topic)
Small Bowel Intestinal Bacterial Overgrowth (Related Key Topic)
Ulcerative Colitis (Related Key Topic)

AUTHOR: **FRED F. FERRI, MD**

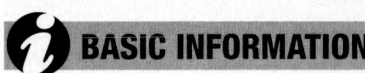
BASIC INFORMATION

DEFINITION

Mastitis is local painful inflammation of the breast that may or may not be accompanied by infection, flulike symptoms, and abscess formation.

ICD-10CM CODES	
N61	Inflammatory disorders of breast
O91.12	Abscess of breast associated with the puerperium
O91.22	Non-purulent mastitis associated with the puerperium

EPIDEMIOLOGY & DEMOGRAPHICS

- Mastitis is the most common cause of inflammatory breast disease, and most cases are related to lactation (puerperal mastitis).
  1. Nonpuerperal cases of mastitis can affect either the periareolar (periductal) region or peripheral breast tissue.
  2. Periductal mastitis (PM, also known as duct ectasia) is most common in younger, reproductive-age women. The majority of those affected are active smokers.
- In lactating mothers, mastitis typically occurs in the first 3 mo of the postpartum period (74 to 95% of cases).
- When severe, mastitis can lead to a breast abscess (5% to 11%) or septicemia.
- Delayed diagnosis and treatment of lactational mastitis can lead to discontinuation of breast-feeding, breast tissue damage, or recurrence.
- In younger nonlactating women, infection often presents as periductal mastitis and is caused by inflamed milk ducts near the nipple.
- Granulomatous mastitis (GM) is a rarer form of benign inflammation of the breast and also most commonly occurs in reproductive-age women. It generally affects the peripheral breast tissue.
- Mastitis also can occur in infancy when there is breast hypertrophy from maternal hormones, called neonatal mastitis (NM). ~50% of neonates with mastitis will develop an abscess.

PREVALENCE: Lactational mastitis occurs in up to 33% of mothers.
PREDOMINANT SEX & AGE: Females of reproductive age
RISK FACTORS:
- Previous mastitis
- Milk stasis and missed feedings, or extended periods between feedings such as when an infant begins to sleep through the night
- Milk oversupply
- Cracked, fissured, or sore nipples
- Primiparity and infant attachment difficulties
- Cleft lip or palate or short frenulum in infant
- Use of manual breast pump
- Foreign material: Breast implants, nipple piercings
- Rapid weaning
- Smoking (PM)
- Obesity (PM)
- Conditions that impair immunity (peripheral or granulomatous mastitis): Diabetes, steroid use, rheumatoid arthritis

PHYSICAL FINDINGS & CLINICAL PRESENTATION

- Warmth, redness, noncyclic tenderness in breast
- Unilateral or bilateral
- Flulike symptoms: Malaise, myalgias, fevers, chills, nausea
- Decreased milk output
- Breast is hard and swollen in a wedge-shaped area
- Lactational mastitis tends to be found in the breast periphery, whereas nonlactational mastitis tends to be peri- or sub-areolar
- In PM, there is often a breast mass near the nipple with retraction or discharge, and it can manifest simultaneously with abscess or even mammary duct fistula
- In GM, enlarged axillary lymph nodes or sinus tract formation

ETIOLOGY

- In lactational mastitis, infection occurs as a result of milk stasis and irritation of the milk ducts as a result of local immune response to milk proteins.
- Breaks in the skin also increase bacterial infection risk of subcutaneous tissues.
- Most common pathogen: *Staphylococcus aureus*
- Less common pathogens: *S. epidermidis,* group A beta-hemolytic streptococci, *S. pneumoniae, Escherichia coli, Candida albicans, Mycobacterium tuberculosis.*
- Up to 40% are polymicrobial.
- GM results from inflammation with epithelioid histiocytes and multinucleated giant cells and can be caused by etiologies like tuberculosis, sarcoidosis, foreign body reaction, parasitic and mycotic infections, or idiopathic.
- Periductal mastitis occurs after inflammation around nondilated subareolar ducts and often can progress to abscess formation. Peripheral abscesses can result from trauma, usually in the setting of comorbid conditions impairing immunity such as diabetes or use of immunosuppressive medications.
- Neonatal mastitis is most often caused by *S. aureus* or gram-negative enteric bacteria.

DIAGNOSIS

DIFFERENTIAL DIAGNOSIS

- Engorgement, plugged duct (Table 1)
- Breast abscess
- Inflammatory or other breast cancer (3% of women diagnosed with breast cancer are lactating)

- Paget disease of breast
- Hyperprolactinemia or galactorrhea
- GM can be manifestation of systemic disease (sarcoidosis, Wegener granulomatosis, giant cell arteritis [GCA], polyarteritis nodosa, tuberculosis [TB], syphilis)

WORKUP

- History and clinical examination with thorough breast examination are generally sufficient for diagnosis.
  1. Be sure to address time, course, and duration of symptoms as well as breast history, including lactation, recent trauma, and prior treatment
  2. Physical examination should include special attention to inflammatory changes and their location, skin changes, assessment of nipple for skin changes and discharge, axillary or supraclavicular adenopathy, and presence or absence of breast mass
  3. Assess for signs of systemic infection, such as fever, white blood cell count, tachycardia
- Recurrent mastitis should include workup for underlying breast disease.

LABORATORY TESTS

- Simple lactational mastitis requires no milk culture or laboratory studies.
- Obtain midstream sample of milk for culture and sensitivities in refractory mastitis or in methicillin-resistant *S. aureus*-suspected cases.
- CBC and blood cultures in toxic-appearing patients.
- In abscess formation, consider culture of drainage or aspirate fluid.
- Inpatient intravenous antibiotics may be necessary in severe cases or those recalcitrant to outpatient treatment.
- Gram stain and culture should be obtained in infant mastitis.

IMAGING STUDIES

- Not necessary unless refractory mastitis or abscess suspected.
- An abscess generally presents as a hypoechoic mass on ultrasound.
- In the context of a discrete mass on exam, age-appropriate breast imaging starting with ultrasound (US) (Fig. E1) is recommended to exclude carcinoma.

TABLE 1 Comparison of Findings of Engorgement, Plugged Duct, and Mastitis

Characteristics	Engorgement	Plugged Duct	Mastitis
Onset	Gradual, immediately	Gradual, after feedings	Sudden, after 10 days postpartum
Site	Bilateral	Unilateral	Usually unilateral
Swelling and heat	Generalized	May shift/little or no heat	Localized red, hot, and swollen
Body temperature	<38.4°C; 101.1°F	<38.4°C; 101.1°F	>38.4°C; 101.1°F
Systemic symptoms	Feels well	Feels well	Flulike symptoms

From Lawrence RA, Lawrence RM: *Breastfeeding: a guide for the medical profession,* ed 5, St Louis, 1999, Mosby.

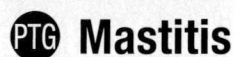

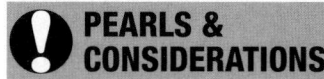

NONPHARMACOLOGIC THERAPY

- Mainstay of therapy is effective milk removal through continued breastfeeding or pumping. Patient should be encouraged to continue breastfeeding infant(s) throughout treatment unless otherwise indicated.
- Consider referral to a certified lactation consultant to improve breastfeeding technique.
  1. Positioning the infant with its chin pointed toward the affected area can help to drain the affected area.
- Encourage warm compresses, increased fluid intake, good nutrition, and rest.
- If abscess is present, surgical drainage or needle aspiration is necessary, followed by antibiotic therapy based on sensitivities of culture.
- In PM, aspiration or incision and drainage of abscesses should be performed, followed by culture of aspirate to guide antibiotic selection. If applicable, smoking cessation should be encouraged.

ACUTE GENERAL Rx

- NSAIDs and analgesics (e.g., acetaminophen, ibuprofen). There is insufficient evidence to support or refute the effectiveness of antibiotic therapy.
- Patients should be asked about history of penicillin allergy and history of methicillin-resistant *S. aureus* infection, either in herself or members of her household. Common antibiotic regimens include:
  1. No history of MRSA (methicillin-resistant *S. aureus*):
     a. Penicillinase-resistant antibiotic: Dicloxacillin 250 mg 4×/day for 7 days
     b. Cephalexin 500 mg 4×/day for 10 to 14 days
     c. Inpatient: Nafcillin or oxacillin 2 g intravenous (IV) q4h
     d. Erythromycin may be used in patients allergic to penicillin
  2. Suspected MRSA or high-risk penicillin allergy:
     a. Trimethoprim/sulfamethoxazole 160 mg/800 mg 2×/day for 10 to 14 days; should not be used when breastfeeding healthy infants <2 mo or compromised infants
     b. Clindamycin 300 mg 4×/day for 10 to 14 days
     c. Inpatient: Vancomycin 1 g IV q12h
- Women should be reassured that antibiotics and antiinflammatory medicines are safe for her infant(s).
- If no clinical response to antibiotics, MRSA or abscess should be considered. Again, if abscess is suspected or symptoms do not resolve with empiric antibiotic treatment, imaging should be performed to exclude other pathology. A biopsy should be performed based on imaging results.
- Antibiotic treatment in patients with abscesses should continue for up to 10 days following aspiration or incision and drainage, and antibiotic choice should be guided by culture results.
- Oxytocin nasal spray can be used if letdown reflex is disturbed.
- Consider treatment for candida infection if *bilateral* symptoms and/or infant with thrush. Both infant and mother will require treatment.
  1. Topical clotrimazole for mother and oral nystatin for infant, with careful washing of all pacifiers and nipples
  2. If resistant to topical treatment, can consider oral fluconazole; however, data in breastfeeding are limited
  3. Onset of candida infection can follow antibiotic treatment for presumed mastitis
- Infant mastitis typically is treated in an inpatient setting with parenteral antibiotics based on results of Gram stain.
- Most PM cases are treated adequately with a combination of antibiotics including anaerobic coverage (supported by culture results if available), needle aspiration/incision, and drainage. In recurrent cases, surgical removal of diseased ducts may be needed, which may necessitate referral to an experienced breast surgeon.
- If antibiotic and NSAID treatment for GM fails, immunosuppressive drugs (steroids, methotrexate) can be used. Surgical management is not recommended due to associated slow wound healing.

CHRONIC Rx

- No evidence proving benefit of prophylactic antibiotics to prevent lactational mastitis.
- In GM, systemic corticosteroids or wide surgical resection are recommended.

DISPOSITION

- Most women with mastitis can be treated with antibiotics on an outpatient basis.
- Criteria for admission include:
  1. Signs of sepsis, systemic infection, or hemodynamic instability
  2. Rapidly progressing infection
  3. Immunocompromised status
- If admission is necessary, the infant should be admitted with her to allow for continued breastfeeding.

COMPLEMENTARY & ALTERNATIVE MEDICINE

- Complementary therapies not assessed in prospective studies: *Belladonna, Phytolacca,* *Chamomilla,* sulfur, *Bellis perennis,* mupirocin, fucidic acid ointment, antisecretory factor, nisin.
- Several strains of lactobacilli have shown promise as probiotic agents that might be useful in treating mastitis, including *L. fermentum* and *L. salivarius.* These results should be replicated before this approach is adopted widely.

REFERRAL

Refer to breast surgeon for severe PM or significant lactational abscesses that do not resolve with conservative measures

PEARLS & CONSIDERATIONS

COMMENTS

- Early recognition and treatment is important to prevent complications such as breast abscesses, sepsis, and early weening. Mothers should be encouraged to continue breastfeeding throughout treatment.
- 25% of breastfeeding mothers with one episode of mastitis stop breastfeeding.
- Patients may experience a temporary decrease in milk supply that should improve once she begins to recover and as long as she continues to breastfeed or adequately express.
- Increasing incidence of MRSA mastitis.
- Lactational mastitis is a risk factor for vertical transmission of infections (i.e., HIV-1, cytomegalovirus, measles, hepatitis B and C).
- When reassessing refractory nonlactational mastitis, the most important consideration is the possibility of cancer.
- Nonlactational mastitis can be a manifestation of systemic disease.
- GM mimics breast cancer both clinically and radiologically (>50% of reported cases are initially mistaken for carcinoma). This includes FNA, which is sometimes interpreted as malignant.

RELATED CONTENT

Lactational Mastitis (Patient Information)
Mastitis (Patient Information)
Breast Abscess (Related Key Topic)
Fibrocystic Breast Disease (Related Key Topic)

AUTHORS: **ANTHONY SCISCIONE, DO** and **ERIN BISHOP, MD**

M

Diseases and Disorders

I

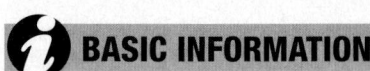
BASIC INFORMATION

DEFINITION

Medical marijuana or medical cannabis refers to the use of the unprocessed *Cannabis sativa* plant, part of the plant, or extracts from the plant as medical therapy to treat disease or alleviate symptoms.

SYNONYMS

Medical cannabis

Cannabinoids—biologically active compounds that activate the cannabinoid receptors. They may be derived from the plant or be synthetic.

CBD—cannabinol

THC—Δ^9-tetrahydrocannabinol

ICD-10CM CODES

F12.9	Cannabis use, unspecified
Z02.79	Encounter for issue of other medical certificate
Z79.899	Other long-term (current) drug therapy

BACKGROUND

- Medical use of marijuana has been restricted since classification as a Schedule I substance by the Controlled Substance Act in 1970.[1]
- First medical marijuana law (MML) was enacted in California in 1996, allowing for use of medical cannabis despite lack of FDA testing for safety and efficacy.[1]
- As of April 24, 2023, medical use of marijuana is permitted at the state level for 38 states, 3 territories, and the District of Columbia.[1]
- Cannabis is the second most commonly used recreational drug worldwide after alcohol.[2]
  1. In 2021, 52.5 million Americans >12 yr old (18.7% of the U.S. population) reported any marijuana use at least once in the past year.[3]
  2. In 2018, 2% of the U.S. population reported medical marijuana use.
  3. Of 2014 marijuana smokers, 6.2% used medical marijuana only, and 3.6% used medical and recreational marijuana.[4]
  4. Residents of medical marijuana states were 1.3 times more likely to use medical marijuana in 2015 compared to 2013.[5]

MECHANISM OF ACTION

- Cannabinoids elicit their effects by interacting with cannabinoid receptors in various central nervous system (CNS) locations, eliciting diverse CNS and peripheral nervous system (PNS) effects (Box 1).
- Primarily bind to CB1 G-protein-coupled receptors in the basal ganglia, hippocampus, cortex, and cerebellum, eliciting antinociception, locomotor, and psychoactive effects.
- Marijuana contains >400 plant-derived compounds, >60 classified as cannabinoids, with the major phytocannabinoids being cannabidiol (CBD) and Δ^9-tetrahydrocannabinol (THC).

FORMULATIONS

Research has demonstrated a wide range of THC and CBD concentrations in various formulations, with frequent inaccurate labelling.

- Cigarettes
- Tinctures
- Capsules
- Vaporization cartridges
- Purified cannabinoids butane hash oil (BHO)
- Supercritical fluid extracts (SFEs or "dabs")
- Buccal sprays
- Edibles
- Lozenges
- Transdermal patches

INDICATIONS

- Variable evidence for treatment of:
  1. Chronic pain
  2. Chemotherapy-induced nausea/vomiting
  3. HIV-related anorexia
  4. Glaucoma
  5. Anxiety
  6. Multiple sclerosis (MS)
  7. Seizures
- Marijuana has not been FDA approved as safe and effective for any indication and remains a Schedule I drug.
- However, there are phytocannabinoids and synthetic phytocannabinoid analogs that have received FDA approval.
  1. Dronabinol and Nabilone (synthetic THC analogs) are schedule II FDA approved medications for AIDS-associated anorexia and chemotherapy-induced nausea, respectively.[6]
  2. Purified cannabidiol oral solution (Epidiolex) is FDA approved for seizures associated with Dravet or Lennox-Gastaut syndrome.
- Qualifying diagnoses for certification for prescription medical marijuana vary by state, but typically include:
  1. Cancer
  2. Glaucoma
  3. HIV/AIDS
  4. Hepatitis C
  5. Cachexia
  6. Severe, debilitating, chronic pain
  7. Severe nausea
  8. Seizures
  9. Severe muscle spasms
  10. Crohn disease
  11. Alzheimer disease
  12. Posttraumatic stress disorder (PTSD)
  13. Sickle cell disease

EFFICACY

- There is published evidence demonstrating that marijuana improves noncancer-related pain, chemotherapy-induced nausea and vomiting, and spasticity in multiple sclerosis.[6,7]
  1. A 2011 systematic review of randomized controlled trials (RCTs) demonstrated statistically significant improvement in pain scores for noncancer-related chronic pain in 15 of 18 trials with no serious adverse effects.[7]
  2. A 2015 systematic review and meta-analysis showed improved response in nausea and vomiting compared to placebo (odds ratio 3.82).[8]
  3. A 2018 systematic review demonstrated a decrease in nausea and vomiting following chemotherapy (relative risk [RR] 3.60 compared to placebo), improved spasticity with MS (RR 1.45 compared to placebo), and a modest benefit with primarily neuropathic pain (RR 1.37 compared to placebo) with frequent adverse effects including psychosis, "feeling high," and somnolence (number needed to harm = 5 to 8).[9]
     a. No statistically significant improvement was noted in acute pain.
  4. A Cochrane review in 2013 found no statistically significant weight gain with dronabinol in HIV/AIDS patients, and multiple RCTs have identified megestrol acetate as superior to dronabinol for weight gain in cancer patients.[10]
  5. A 2020 systematic review and meta-analysis showed extremely limited evidence for benefits for Crohn disease and ulcerative colitis, with only three RCTs all showing no improvement of marijuana over placebo.[11]
  6. In 2019, a systematic review determined that there was sufficient evidence from

---

BOX 1 Acute Effects of Marijuana

Relaxation, euphoria, jocularity
Jitteriness, anxiety, paranoia, panic
Depersonalization, subjective time-slowing
Dizziness, sensation of floating
Impaired coordination and balance
Impaired memory and judgment
Conjunctival injection, decreased salivation
Urinary frequency
Tachycardia
Systolic hypertension and postural hypotension
Bradycardia, hypotension
Increased appetite and thirst
Decreased intraocular pressure
Analgesia
Auditory and visual illusions or hallucinations
Psychosis

From Jankovic J et al: *Bradley and Daroff's neurology in clinical practice*, ed 8, Philadelphia, 2022, Elsevier.

five reviews that cannabinoids may be effective for multiple sclerosis symptoms of pain and/or spasticity.[8,12]

7. In a study of 54,000 adults in 37 states with medical cannabis access, more than half reported that cannabis use led to less use of other analgesics both opioid and nonopioid and one quarter to one third reported that cannabis use led to less use of physical therapy or cognitive-behavioral therapy.[13]

RISKS OF USE

- Marijuana use has been demonstrated to impair short-term memory consolidation, reaction time, and concept formation, and to increase incidence of road traffic accidents, ataxia, euphoria, disorientation, dry mouth, somnolence, and, at high doses, psychosis, panic, and paranoia.
- Marijuana has been shown to worsen preexisting anxiety, depression, and schizophrenia. It should be used with caution, particularly in combination with other drugs with similar effects.[14]
- Meta-analyses demonstrate increased respiratory symptoms of cough, sputum production, and wheeze with smoking marijuana; however, there was no statistical difference in pulmonary function.
- Medical marijuana does have drug–drug interactions, and adverse effects can be potentiated by other medications. In particular, concomitant use of other medications such as opiates and benzodiazepines should be avoided as it could lead to somnolence and respiratory suppression.[14]
- Cannabinoid hyperemesis syndrome, a form of cyclic vomiting syndrome that is often accompanied by abdominal pain, occurs during or within 48 h after frequent and heavy cannabis use.[15]
- In utero exposure is associated with increased risk among newborns of having low birth weight, being small for gestational age, and being admitted to the neonatal intensive care unit.[15]
- Acute marijuana intoxication is associated with reversible changes in P and T waves and ST segments (pseudo-Wellens syndrome).
- Medical marijuana should be stored away from children given the risk of toxic ingestion.

PRESCRIBING

- Marijuana remains classified as a schedule I drug under the Controlled Substance Act of 1970.
- However, the Justice Department declared it would not prosecute any physician who recommends medical marijuana for a legitimate medical indication in a state where it has been legalized.[1]
- Medical marijuana card (MMC)
  1. MMC allows a patient to possess a certain amount of marijuana for medical use

and not be prosecuted for possession of marijuana.
  2. To obtain an MMC, a patient must obtain physician certification confirming a clinical indication for medical marijuana.
  3. With an MMC, the patient can go to a licensed medical marijuana compassion center (dispensary), which will dispense a dose and formulation of medical marijuana appropriate for the patient's medical condition.
  4. Physicians do not prescribe the dose or formulation of medical marijuana.
- To certify a patient for a medical marijuana card, physicians must
  1. Complete a Department of Health certification form.
  2. Forms vary by state, but typically consist of a single-page form indicating a qualifying diagnosis that is to be signed by the physician. Complete and document a full medical history and physical exam.
  3. Explain the risks, benefits, and side effects of medical marijuana.
  4. Continue an ongoing role on the patient's health care team.
  5. Maintain accurate medical records and documentation of the patient's clinical indication for medical marijuana.
- Some states require additional physician training and registration with the state medical marijuana program prior to being able to certify patients.
- Physicians are under no obligation to issue medical marijuana certifications.

ⓘ PEARLS & CONSIDERATIONS

- Medical marijuana has been shown to improve noncancer-related pain, chemotherapy-induced nausea and vomiting, and spasticity in multiple sclerosis.
  1. Qualifying diagnoses (may vary from state to state) for a medical marijuana card include
    a. Cancer
    b. Glaucoma
    c. HIV/AIDS
    d. Hepatitis C
    e. Cachexia
    f. Debilitating chronic pain
    g. Severe nausea
    h. Seizures
    i. Severe muscle spasms
    j. Crohn disease
    k. Alzheimer disease
    l. PTSD
    m. Sickle cell disease
  2. Adverse effects include increased incidence of road traffic accidents and pulmonary

and cognitive side effects. At high doses, psychosis, panic, and paranoia can occur. Hospitals may also have specific restrictions and policies regarding medical marijuana for inpatient stays.

- Medical marijuana laws and regulations permit patients to use medical marijuana if certified by a physician but vary by state.
  1. Physician certification involves documentation that a patient has a qualifying clinical condition.
  2. A medical marijuana card entitles a patient or designated caregiver to possess a given amount of marijuana and therefore will not be prosecuted for possession of marijuana.
  3. Medical marijuana can be obtained at state regulated medical marijuana compassion centers (dispensaries). Compassion centers obtain marijuana from licensed cultivators and offer a variety of formulations that are regulated by the state.
  4. There is no FDA oversight of the compassion centers.
- Physicians do not prescribe the dose or formulation of medical marijuana.
- Physicians are under no obligation to issue medical marijuana certifications.
- Emergency department (ED) visits attributable to inhaled cannabis are more frequent than those attributable to edible cannabis, although the latter is associated with more acute psychiatric visits and more ED visits than expected.

PATIENT & FAMILY EDUCATION

- Patients must possess a valid state-issued ID and apply for a state medical marijuana card.
- Patients can obtain medical marijuana from compassion centers without a medical marijuana card but could then be prosecuted for possession of marijuana.
- Patients should be aware that concomitant use of other medications such as opiates and benzodiazepines should be avoided as it could lead to somnolence and respiratory suppression.
- Patients should store medical marijuana away from children given the risk of toxic ingestions.

REFERENCES

Available at eBooks.Health.Elsevier.com.

RELATED CONTENT

Pain Management in Chronic Pain (Related Key Topic)
Chemotherapy-Induced Nausea and Vomiting (Related Key Topic)

AUTHOR: **SETH CLARK, MD, MPH, FASAM**

🛈 BASIC INFORMATION

DEFINITION

Melanoma is a skin neoplasm arising from the malignant degeneration of melanocytes, a pigment-producing cell found in the epidermal skin layer

It is classically subdivided in four histopathologic subtypes (Table 1):
- Superficial spreading melanoma (SMM)
- Nodular melanoma (NM)
- Lentigo maligna melanoma (LMM)
- Acral lentiginous melanoma (ALM)

SYNONYMS

Malignant melanoma
Cutaneous malignant melanoma

ICD-10CM CODES

C43.30	Malignant melanoma of unspecified part of face
C43.31	Malignant melanoma of nose
C43.4	Malignant melanoma of scalp and neck
C43.51	Malignant melanoma of anal skin
C43.52	Malignant melanoma of skin of breast
C43.59	Malignant melanoma of other part of trunk
C43.8	Malignant melanoma of overlapping sites of skin
C43.9	Malignant melanoma of skin, unspecified
D03.8	Melanoma in situ of other sites
D03.9	Melanoma in situ, unspecified

EPIDEMIOLOGY & DEMOGRAPHICS

Melanoma accounts for 1% of all skin cancers. The predicted estimate of new cases for 2023 is 97,610 with approximately 7990 deaths.
- Melanoma is more common in men than women, between the ages of 65 to 74.
- Melanoma is the fourth most common cancer in men and the fifth most common in women.
- It is the leading cause of death from all skin cancers.
- Melanoma is much more common in Whites (17.2 per 100,000 White men) than in African Americans (1 per 100,000 African American men). Increased risk of developing melanomas is found in patients with fair skin, red hair, light eyes, abundance of freckles, atypical moles, or

---

TABLE 1 Histologic Subtypes of Cutaneous Melanoma

	Frequency	Location	Characteristics	Morphology
Superficial spreading melanoma 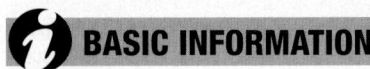	70% Women > men	Lower extremities	Slow radial growth phase	Flat during early phase, macule or papule
Nodular melanoma	15%-30%	Trunk, head	Rapid vertical growth	Papule or nodule
Lentigo maligna 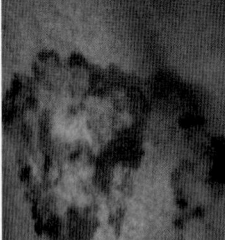	10%-15% More common in the elderly	Face, neck, arms Chronically sun-damaged skin	Slow radial growth, confirmed to the epidermis for many years	Large macule, arises in a preexisting nevus
Acral lentiginous 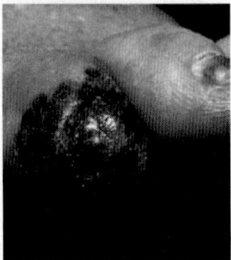	<5% More common in Asians and African Americans	Soles, palms Beneath nail beds (subungual)	Slow radial growth phase with vertical phase later on	Large dark patch, arising in a preexisting lesion

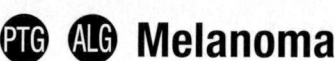

large congenital nevi. A personal or family history of melanoma also increases the risk.

- Individuals with high recreational/intermittent sun exposure, history of blistery sunburns in childhood or adolescence, and exposure to artificial ultraviolet radiation from use of tanning beds have a higher risk for developing melanoma.
- Superficial spreading melanoma occurs most often in young adults on sun-exposed areas.
- Acral lentiginous melanoma is most often found in Asian Americans and African Americans and is unrelated to sun exposure.
- 8% to 10% of melanomas arise in people with a family history of the disease.

PHYSICAL FINDINGS & CLINICAL PRESENTATION

Variable depending on the subtype of melanoma:

- Superficial spreading melanoma is most often found on the lower legs, arms, and upper back. It may have a combination of many colors or may be uniformly brown or black.
- Nodular melanoma can be found anywhere on the body, but it most frequently occurs on the trunk on sun-exposed areas. It has a dark-brown or red-brown appearance and can be dome shaped (or pedunculated). Lesions are frequently misdiagnosed because they may resemble a blood blister or hemangioma (Fig. E1) and may also be amelanotic.
- Lentigo maligna melanoma is generally found in older adults in areas continually exposed to the sun and frequently arising from lentigo maligna (Hutchinson freckle) or melanoma in situ. It might have a complex pattern and variable shape; color is more uniform than in superficial spreading melanoma.
- Acral lentiginous melanoma frequently occurs on soles, subungual mucous membranes, and palms (sole of the foot is the most prevalent site). Unlike other types of melanoma, it has a similar incidence in all ethnic groups.
- The warning signs that the lesion may be a melanoma can be summarized with the ABCDE mnemonic (Table E2):
  1. **A:** Asymmetry (e.g., lesion is bisected and halves are not identical)
  2. **B:** Border irregularity (uneven, ragged border) (Fig. E2)
  3. **C:** Color variegation (presence of various shades of pigmentation)
  4. **D:** Diameter enlargement (>6 mm)
  5. **E:** Evolving (mole changing in size, shape, or color, or mole that differs visibly from surrounding moles ["ugly duckling" sign])

ETIOLOGY

- Ultraviolet light is the most important cause of malignant melanoma.
- There is a modest increase in melanoma risk in patients with small nondysplastic nevi and a much greater risk in those with dysplastic lesions.
- The *CDKN2A* gene, residing at the 9p21 locus, is often deleted in patients with familial melanoma.

- A mutated signal transduction molecule, v-raf murine sarcoma viral oncogene homolog B *(BRAF),* has been identified in 40% to 60% of patients with melanoma.

Dx DIAGNOSIS

DIFFERENTIAL DIAGNOSIS

- Dysplastic nevi
- Solar lentigo
- Vascular lesions
- Blue nevus
- Basal cell carcinoma
- Seborrheic keratosis

WORKUP

- Dermoscopy (use of an instrument that shines polarized light on skin surfaces and magnifies skin lesions) can increase the accuracy in diagnosing melanoma by 10% to 27%.
- Any suspicious lesion should be biopsied. Perform excisional biopsy with elliptical excision that includes 1 to 2 mm of normal skin surrounding the lesion and extends to the subcutaneous tissue; incisional punch biopsy is sometimes necessary in surgically sensitive areas (e.g., digits, nose). It is essential that the size of the specimen be adequate to determine the histologic depth of penetration, which is known as the Breslow depth.
- Sentinel lymph node excision (SLNE) is the most important staging and potentially prognostic procedure for patients with melanoma. It should be considered at the time of excision as it provides important information regarding a patient's subclinical lymph node status with minimal morbidity. The National Comprehensive Cancer Network (NCCN) recommends that SLNE be discussed with and offered to patients classified as stage IB or II, and should be considered for patients with stage IA melanoma with high risk features such as ulceration. SLNE involves the use of radiologic lymphoscintigraphy to map lymphatic drainage from the site of the primary melanoma to the first sentinel lymph node in the region. When properly performed, if the sentinel node is negative, the remaining lymph nodes in the region will not have metastases in more than 98% of cases. A positive sentinel node biopsy provides important prognostic information and identifies patients who are eligible for adjuvant therapy.
- The staging system for melanoma adapted by the American Joint Committee on Cancer (AJCC) can be found in Table 3.

LABORATORY TESTS

The pathology report should indicate the following:
- Tumor thickness (Breslow microstage).
- Tumor depth: The depth of invasion is the most important histologic prognostic parameter in evaluating the primary tumor.
- Mitotic rate: Tabulated as mitoses per square millimeter in the dermal part of the tumor in which most mitoses are identified.
- Radial growth rates vs. vertical growth rate: Radial growth phase describes the growth of

melanoma within the epidermis and along the dermal-epidermal junction.
- Tumor infiltrating lymphocytes have a strong predictive value in vertical growth phase melanomas and are defined as brisk, non-brisk, or absent.
- Histologic regression: Characterized by the absence of melanoma in the epidermis and dermis flanked on one or both sides by melanoma.
- Reverse-transcription polymerase chain reaction assay for tyrosine messenger RNA is a useful marker for the presence of melanoma cells. It is performed on sentinel lymph node biopsy and is useful for detection of submicroscopic metastases.

Rx TREATMENT (FIG. 3)

- Initial excision of the melanoma
- Wide local excision is the primary treatment of localized melanomas.
- The margin is determined based on tumor thickness.

Tumor Thickness	Surgical Margin
1. Melanoma in situ	0.5-1.0 cm
2. <1.0 mm	1.0 1.0 cm
3. 1.01-2.00 mm	1.0-2.0 cm
4. 2.01-4.00 mm	2.0 cm
5. >4.00 mm	2.0 cm

- Sentinel lymph node excision is recommended in all patients with melanoma greater than 1 mm in depth or ulcerated melanomas of 0.8 to 1.0 mm depth
- Complete lymph node dissection is not recommended for microscopic nodal involvement and has not shown benefit when compared to surveillance with clinical exams and imaging of the lymph node basin.
- Complete lymph node dissection is recommended for patients who present with palpable lymph nodes at the time of diagnosis.
- Adjuvant therapy: Offered to eliminate potential micrometastatic disease.
- Approved for high risk stage IIB (tumor 2 to 4 mm in depth with ulceration or >4 mm without ulceration) stage IIC (melanoma with a thickness greater than 4 mm with ulceration) and stage III melanomas (melanoma spread to regional Lymph nodes)
- Adjuvant therapy decreases the risk of melanoma recurrence by 40% to 50%
  1. Immune checkpoint PD-1 (programmed death receptor-1) antibodies, nivolumab and pembrolizumab, have demonstrated superiority to ipilimumab (Anti CTLA-4) in patients with resected high-risk stage III melanoma and are considered the standard of care.
  2. Pembrolizumab (Anti PD-1) is the only immune checkpoint inhibitor approved to date for stage IIB,IIC melanoma.
  3. The combination regimen of BRAF inhibitor and MEK inhibitor (dabrafenib plus trametinib) has shown improved relapse-free survival in resected BRAF V600E/

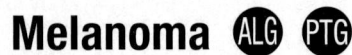

TABLE 3 The TNM Classification for Melanoma Adapted by the American Joint Committee on Cancer (AJCC, 8th edition)

T Classification	Thickness	Ulceration Status/Mitoses
T_{is} (in situ)	n/a	n/a
T_1	<1.0 mm	Unknown or unspecified
T_{1a}	<0.8 mm	Without ulceration
T_{1b}	0.8-1.0 mm	With/without ulceration
T_2	>1.0-2.0 mm	Unknown or unspecified
T_{2a}	>1.0-2.0 mm	Without ulceration
T_{2b}	>1.0-2.0 mm	With ulceration
T_3	>2.0-4.0 mm	Unknown or unspecified
T_{3a}	>2.0-4.0 mm	Without ulceration
T_{3b}	>2.0-4.0 mm	With ulceration
T_4	>4.0 mm	Unknown or unspecified
T_{4a}	>4.0 mm	Without ulceration
T_{4b}	>4.0 mm	With ulceration

Regional Nodes (N)	Number of Nodes	Presence of In-Transit, Satellite, and/or Microsatellite Metastases
N_0	0	None
N_1	One tumor-involved node or any number of in-transit, satellite, and/or microsatellite metastases with no tumor-involved nodes	
N_{1a}	One clinically occult (sentinel biopsy detected)	No
N_{1b}	One clinically detected	No
N_{1c}	No regional node	Yes
N_2	Two or three tumor-involved nodes or any number of in-transit, satellite, and/or microsatellite metastases with one tumor-involved node	
N_{2a}	Two or three clinically occult (sentinel biopsy detected)	No
N_{2b}	Two or three, at least one clinically detected	No
N_{2c}	One clinically occult or clinically detected	Yes
N_3	Four or more tumor-involved nodes or any number of in-transit, satellite, and/or microsatellite metastases with two or more tumor-involved nodes, or any number of matted nodes without or with in-transit, satellite, and/or microsatellite metastases	
N_{3a}	Four or more clinically occult (sentinel biopsy detected)	No
N_{3b}	Four or more, at least one of which was clinically detected, or the presence of any number of matted nodes	No
N_{3c}	Two or more clinically occult or clinically detected and/or presence of any number of matted nodes	Yes

M Category	Anatomic Site	LDH Level
M_0	No distant metastases	n/a
M_1	Evidence of distant metastases	
M_{1a}	Distant metastasis to skin, soft tissue including muscle, and/or nonregional lymph node	$M_{1a}(0)$: Normal $M_{1a}(1)$: Elevated
M_{1b}	Distant metastasis to lung with or without M_{1a} sites of disease	$M_{1b}(0)$: Normal $M_{1b}(1)$: Elevated
M_{1c}	Distant metastasis to non-CNS visceral sites with or without M_{1a} or M_{1b} sites of disease	$M_{1c}(0)$: Normal $M_{1c}(1)$: Elevated
M_{1d}	Distant metastasis to CNS with or without M_{1a}, M_{1b}, or M_{1c} sites of disease	$M_{1d}(0)$: Normal $M_{1d}(1)$: Elevated

CNS, Central nervous system; *LDH,* lactic dehydrogenase; *TNM,* tumor, nodes, metastases.

K-mutant stage III melanoma and is another option for these patients.

- Advanced or metastatic disease:
  1. The use of immune checkpoint inhibitors has improved overall survival in patients with previously treated or untreated metastatic melanoma irrespective of BRAF mutation status. Monotherapy with the PD-1 inhibitors nivolumab or pembrolizumab has been approved for the treatment of metastatic melanoma in treatment-naïve patients with a 5 yr OS of 40%.
  2. Combination immunotherapy of nivolumab (anti PD-1) and ipilimumab (anti CTLA-4) in previously untreated patients with unresectable or metastatic melanoma and those with brain metastasis has shown to improve survival compared to monotherapy with either ipilimumab or nivolumab. It is the most effective first-line therapy to date.
  3. Common immune-mediated toxicity seen with the use of the combination includes dermatitis, colitis, hepatitis, hypothyroidism, and hypophysitis. High-grade toxicity with treatment discontinuation is seen in 50% of patients. In patients who carry the V600E *BRAF* mutation, the combination of oral BRAF inhibitors and oral MEK inhibitors improves overall survival in patients with previously untreated melanoma. Three such combination regimens (vemurafenib plus cobimetinib; dabrafenib plus trametinib; and encorafenib plus binimetinib) are approved by the FDA for use in this setting. Targeted therapy is useful in patients with rapidly growing melanoma with *BRAF* mutations, but resistance appears in almost all patients, with a median progression-free survival of 15 to 18 mo. High-risk patients with brain metastases appear to have response rates of 40% to 50%.
  4. The combination of atezolizumab (PD-L1 checkpoint inhibitor), cobimetinib (MEK inhibitor), and vemurafenib (BRAF inhibitor) has been shown to improve progression-free survival compared with placebo in patients with *BRAF* mutated advanced melanoma and is likely to be another option in this setting.
  5. Relatlimab, a LAG-3 inhibitor, is approved in combination with Nivolumab for unresectable or metastatic melanoma. This combination is associated with longer progression-free survival compared to Nivolumab monotherapy (10.1 vs 4.2 mo).
  6. Adaptive cell therapy with tumor-infiltrating lymphocytes (TILs) have shown promising responses. In a recent phase 3 trial[1] in patients with advanced melanoma progression-free survival was significantly longer among those who received TIL therapy then among those who received ipilimumab.

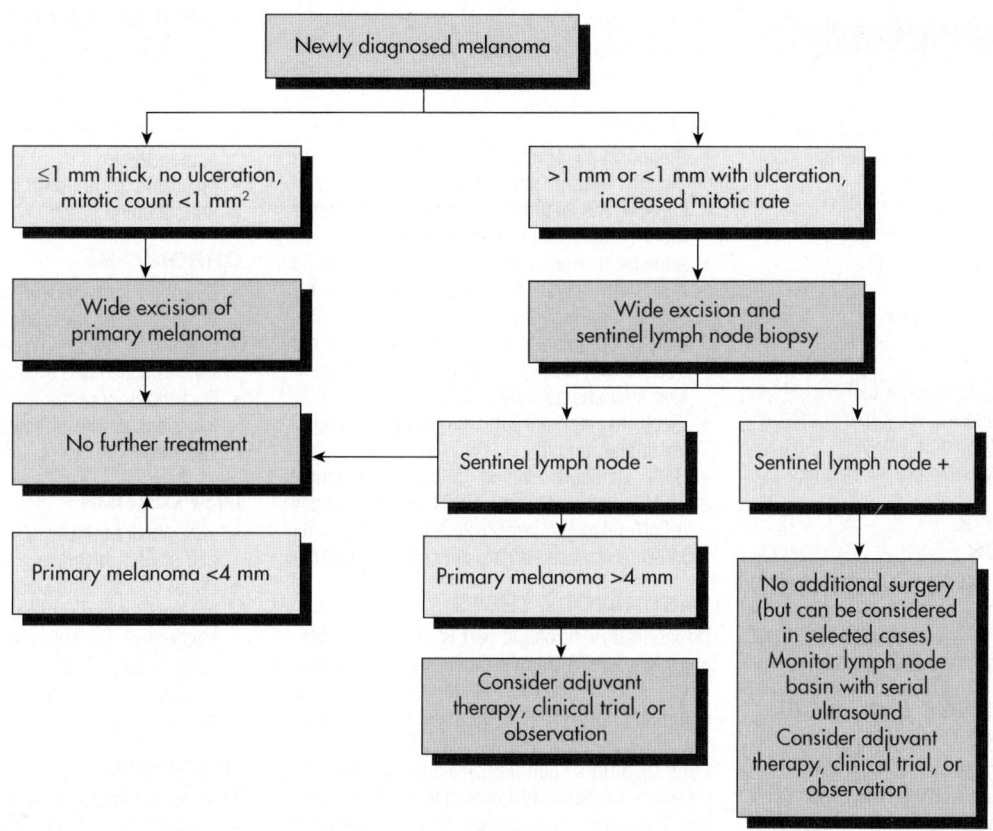

FIG. 3 Treatment algorithm for newly diagnosed melanoma. (From Goldman L, Schafer AI: *Goldman-Cecil medicine,* ed 26, Philadelphia, 2019, Elsevier.)

- All patients with a history of resected melanomas should be followed up with skin examinations every 3t to 6 mo.
- Patients with high-risk melanoma need clinical assessments that consist of medical history, physical examination, laboratory values, and computed tomography or PET imaging.

DISPOSITION

- Prognosis varies with the stage of the melanoma. The 5-yr survival varies depending on the melanoma thickness, the presence or absence of ulceration, and the number of involved lymph nodes.

- The 5-yr survival in patients with distant metastasis was historically <10% but has improved to 50%.[2]
- Treatment of advanced disease consists of immunotherapy and targeted therapy (BRAFI/MEKI). Brain metastasis is seen commonly in metastatic melanoma, and Nivolumab combined with ipilimumab has shown clinically meaningful activity in this setting. Chemotherapy has limited benefit for patients with advanced melanoma. Radiation therapy can be used for symptom palliation such as pain or vasogenic edema.

REFERENCES & SUGGESTED READINGS

Available at eBooks.Health.Elsevier.com.

RELATED CONTENT

Melanoma (Patient Information)

AUTHOR: **MARIA CONSTANTINOU, MD**

Diseases
and Disorders

I

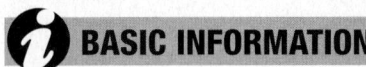

BASIC INFORMATION

DEFINITION
Ménière disease is a syndrome characterized by recurrent vertigo with fluctuating hearing loss, tinnitus, and fullness in the ear.

SYNONYMS
Endolymphatic hydrops
Lermoyez syndrome
Idiopathic endolymphatic hydrops

ICD-10CM CODES
H81.01 Ménière disease, right ear
H81.02 Ménière disease, left ear
H81.03 Ménière disease, bilateral
H81.09 Ménière disease, unspecified ear

EPIDEMIOLOGY & DEMOGRAPHICS
INCIDENCE (IN U.S.): Approximately 190/100,000 persons
PREDOMINANT SEX: Female:male ratio of 1.3:1
PEAK INCIDENCE: Fourth to sixth decade of life

PHYSICAL FINDINGS & CLINICAL PRESENTATION
- Hearing may be unilaterally decreased.
- Pallor, sweating, and nausea may occur during a severe attack.
- Usually the patient develops a sensation of fullness and pressure along with decreased hearing and tinnitus in a single ear.
- The patient typically experiences severe vertigo, which peaks within minutes, then slowly subsides over hours.
- May see spontaneous nystagmus on examination.
- Persistent sense of disequilibrium for days is typical after an acute episode.
- May have vestibulopathy demonstrable with a positive head thrust test.

ETIOLOGY
- Unknown; viral, autoimmune, and genetic causes have been suggested.
- Endolymphatic hydrops is the postmortem histologic hallmark. Endolymphatic hydrops may create cytochemical changes that disturb endolymphatic fluid homeostasis, leading to spiral ganglion cell death.

DIAGNOSIS

Proposed guidelines by the American Academy of Otolaryngology-Head and Neck Surgery (AAO-HNS) for diagnosis and severity of Ménière disease (Box E1).

DIFFERENTIAL DIAGNOSIS
- Acoustic neuroma
- Migrainous vertigo
- Multiple sclerosis
- Autoimmune inner ear syndrome
- Otitis media
- Vertebrobasilar disease
- Labyrinthitis

WORKUP
- Diagnosis is primarily made by history, although further diagnostic tests may help support the diagnosis. Guidelines to define Ménière disease are described in Table 1.
- Audiogram may show sensorineural hearing loss with lower frequencies primarily affected. Hearing loss may recover either partially or completely after an attack. Recurrent attacks may lead to a persistent and progressive sensorineural hearing loss.
- Electronystagmography may show peripheral vestibular deficit.
- Both vestibular-evoked myogenic potential (VEMP) studies and electrocochleography (ECoG) have low sensitivity and specificity for Ménière disease and are not clinically useful.

LABORATORY TESTS
No laboratory serologic test is specific for Ménière disease. A thyroid panel, glucose, hemoglobin A1C, antinuclear antibodies, urinalysis, chemistry panel, RPR, Lyme disease antibodies, and allergy testing can be ordered to screen for other disorders such as thyroid or autoimmune diseases, diabetes, otorenal syndrome, syphilis, Lyme disease, and allergy-mediated Ménière disease.

IMAGING STUDIES
- MRI to rule out acoustic neuroma or other retrocochlear lesion, especially if cerebellar or central nervous system dysfunction is present.
- Recent efforts have shown a role for MRI with intratympanic gadolinium.

TREATMENT

NONPHARMACOLOGIC THERAPY
Limit activity during attacks.

ACUTE GENERAL Rx
- Prochlorperazine 5 to 10 mg PO q6h or 25 mg PO bid
- Promethazine 12.5 to 25 mg PO q4 to 6h
- Diazepam 5 to 10 mg intravenous PO for acute attack
- Meclizine 25 mg q6h
- Scopolamine patch

CHRONIC Rx
- Diuretics such as furosemide, hydrochlorothiazide, or acetazolamide.
- Lifestyle modification recommendations include salt restriction and avoidance of caffeine.
- For refractory cases, intratympanic gentamicin injections to the affected ear; endolymphatic sac surgery.

DISPOSITION
- Patients are usually followed by an neurotologist or ENT specialist.
- Usual course of disease consists of alternating attacks and remissions.
- Majority of patients can be managed medically. Of all patients, 10% to 30% will undergo surgical intervention for persistent incapacitating vertigo.

REFERRAL
To an otolaryngologist for surgical intervention if attacks persist despite medical therapy

REFERENCES
Available at eBooks.Health.Elsevier.com.

RELATED CONTENT
Ménière Disease (Patient Information)

AUTHOR: **JOSEPH S. KASS, MD, JD, FAAN**

TABLE 1 Guidelines to Define Ménière Disease

Definition	Symptoms
Certain Ménière disease	Histopathologic confirmation
Definite Ménière disease	≥2 definitive spontaneous episodes of vertigo 20 min to 12 h
	Audiometrically documented low- to medium-frequency sensorineural hearing loss in one ear, defining the affected ear on at least one occasion before, during, or after one of the episodes of vertigo
	Fluctuating aural symptoms (hearing, tinnitus, or fullness) in the affected ear
	Not better accounted for by another vestibular diagnosis
Probable Ménière disease	One definite episode of vertigo
	Audiometrically documented hearing loss on at least one occasion
	Tinnitus or aural fullness in the treated ear
	Other causes excluded
Possible Ménière disease	Episodic vertigo without documented hearing loss, or sensorineural hearing loss (SNHL) fluctuating or fixed, with disequilibrium but nonepisodic
	Other causes excluded

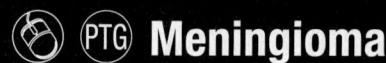

M

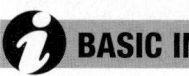 BASIC INFORMATION

DEFINITION
Meningiomas are generally slow-growing tumors arising from arachnoid cells of the arachnoid villi; 90% are benign.

ICD-10CM CODE
D32.0   Benign neoplasm of cerebral meninges

EPIDEMIOLOGY & DEMOGRAPHICS
INCIDENCE: 7.92/100,000 persons/yr but increases with age. Most common primary type of central nervous system tumor, and most common nonmalignant primary central nervous system tumor.[1]

PREDOMINANT SEX & AGE: Female:male ratio of almost 3:1 (in ages 35 to 54) in the brain and up to 6:1 in the spinal cord; 1:1 in childhood.[1]

PEAK INCIDENCE: Males: Sixth decade, females: Seventh decade, incidence increases with age, dramatic increase in incidence after age 65; rare in childhood.[1]

RISK FACTORS: Ionizing radiation results in increased incidence and a shorter latency period. Neurofibromatosis type 2 (NF2) is an autosomal dominant genetic disorder that predisposes to multiple intracranial tumors. Approximately half of all individuals with NF2 have meningiomas, most of which are intracranial.[2] Studies have suggested a link between hormonal factors and development of meningioma, specifically estrogen exposure. Multiple prospective cohort studies have also found an association between higher body mass index and meningioma, possibly relating to increased levels of circulating estrogen through increased adipose tissue. At present, there is no conclusive evidence to support a causal relationship with cell phone usage and subsequent development of meningioma.[1]

GENETICS: Meningiomas may be isolated or found in association with other genetic diseases, such as NF2 and familial meningioma. Other genetic conditions associated with increased incidence of meningioma include BAP1 tumor predisposition syndrome, Rubinstein-Taybi syndrome, multiple endocrine neoplasia, type 1, Gorlin syndrome, Cowden syndrome 1, Werner syndrome, and familial meningiomatosis. Approximately half of meningiomas have allelic losses involving the NF2 and DAL-1 genes. Allelic losses of chromosomes 1p, 2p, 6q, 9q, 10q, 14q, 17p, and 18q may be associated with histologic progression. Genome-wide association studies (GWAS) have discovered two genomic variants associated with increased meningioma risk in genes for MLLT10 and possibly RIC8A. Further, GWAS analysis also demonstrates an association between longer telomere length and increased risk of meningiomas.[3]

PHYSICAL FINDINGS & CLINICAL PRESENTATION
- Neurologic symptoms vary with location and size (Table 1); meningiomas can arise from the dura at any site, although they most commonly occur within the skull and at sites of dural reflection (i.e., the cerebral convexities and the falx). Other less common locations include the sphenoid wing, olfactory groove, and optic nerve sheath.[4]
- The presence of focal symptoms such as vision loss, hearing loss, or mental status change depend on the site of origin and the time course of growth.
- Most common presentation is with a focal or generalized seizure or gradually worsening neurologic deficit. Seizures are present preoperatively in 30% to 40%.[5]
- Typically slow growing and asymptomatic; many meningiomas are asymptomatic and/or discovered incidentally on a neuroimaging study or at autopsy.

ETIOLOGY
- Meningiomas are thought to arise from a multistep progression of genetic changes.
- Mutations of the NF2 gene on chromosome 22 are found in patients with neurofibromatosis type 2 and >50% of sporadic meningiomas. This gene is thought to act as a tumor suppressor gene; the protein product, merlin, is also involved in cytoskeletal organization.[2]
- DAL-1, located on chromosome 18p, is another tumor suppressor gene that has been identified in a subset of the approximately 40% of sporadic meningiomas with neither the NF2 gene mutations nor allelic loss of chromosome 22q.[2-3]
- Cranial radiation may be responsible for some cases following an appropriate latency period from 10 to 20 yr. Meningiomas that result from radiation are generally more aggressive.[5]
- The link with steroid hormones and their receptors is suggested by the increase in growth rate and/or development of meningiomas during pregnancy, increased incidence in women who use postmenopausal hormones, and in association with breast carcinomas.[4]

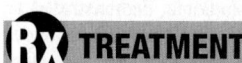 DIAGNOSIS

DIFFERENTIAL DIAGNOSIS
Other well-circumscribed intracranial tumors that involve the dura or subdural space:
- Acoustic schwannoma (typically at the pontocerebellar junction)
- Ependymoma, lipoma, and metastases within spinal cord
- Metastatic disease from lymphoma/adenocarcinoma
- Inflammatory disease such as sarcoidosis and Wegener granulomatosis
- Infections such as tuberculosis

WORKUP
Imaging studies with computed tomography (CT) or MRI, followed by surgical removal with histologic confirmation

LABORATORY TESTS
According to the World Health Organization (WHO) classification, there are nine benign histologic variants (accounting for 90% of all meningiomas) and four variants associated with increased recurrence and rates of metastasis. 80% of meningiomas are classified as benign meningiomas or WHO grade I.[6]

IMAGING STUDIES
- Cranial CT scanning or MRI can detect and determine the extent of meningiomas (Fig. 1). CT can show hyperostosis and/or intratumoral calcifications. MRI with contrast (Fig. 2) is the imaging modality of choice to demonstrate the dural origin of the tumor in most cases, with the characteristic "tail" sign that tracks along the dura outside brain parenchyma.[7]
- On nonenhanced scans, meningiomas are typically isodense or slightly hyperdense to brain and are homogeneous in appearance. They show homogeneous contrast enhancement; gadolinium can facilitate imaging of smaller additional lesions that are missed on unenhanced images.[7]
- Indistinct margins, marked edema, mushroom-like projections from tumor, brain parenchymal infiltration, and heterogeneous enhancement are suggestive of more aggressive behavior.[7]
- PET scan may help in predicting the aggressiveness of the tumor and the potential for recurrence, but it is not used routinely.[7]

Rx TREATMENT

Primary management depends on signs or symptoms, age of patient, and location and size of tumor. Observation may be appropriate if tumors are discovered incidentally and/or if growth is indolent and unlikely to cause symptoms.[8]

TABLE 1   Locations and Presentations of Meningiomas

Location	Presenting Manifestation
Parasagittal	Urinary incontinence, dementia, gradual paraparesis, seizures
Lateral convexity	Variable depending on structures compressed, including slow hemiparesis, speech abnormalities
Olfactory groove	Anosmia, visual disturbance, dementia, Foster-Kennedy syndrome
Suprasellar	Hormonal failure, bitemporal hemianopsia, optic atrophy
Sphenoid ridge	Extraocular nerve paresis, exostoses, proptosis, seizures

From Goetz CG, Pappert EJ: *Textbook of clinical neurology*, Philadelphia, 1999, Saunders.

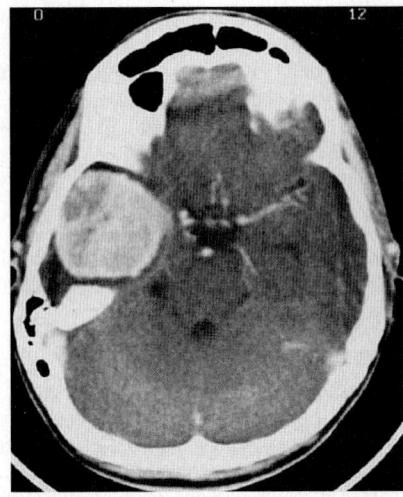

FIG. 1 Contrast-enhanced computed tomography scan demonstrates a large contrast-enhancing right sphenoid wing meningioma.

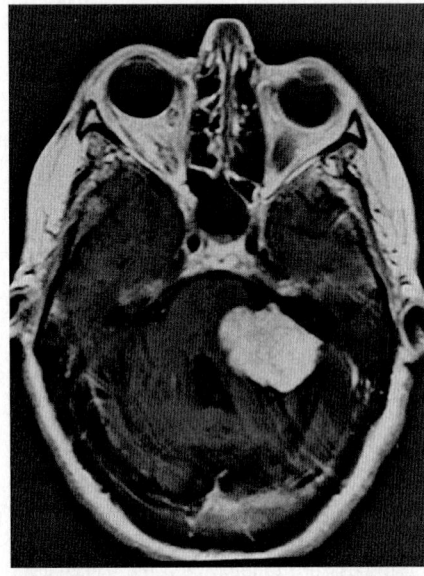

FIG. 2 Magnetic resonance imaging picture of a posterior fossa meningioma, demonstrated an extra-axial homogeneously contrast-enhanced mass arising from the tentorium and compressing the cerebellar hemisphere. (From Goetz CG, Pappert EJ: *Textbook of clinical neurology*, Philadelphia, 1999, Saunders.)

PHARMACOLOGIC THERAPY

- Although a variety of chemotherapeutic agents have been studied, there is no established effective systemic therapy.[8]
- In 2020, the CEVOREM trial in France, a phase 2 trial, demonstrated efficacy in treating recurrent meningioma with everolimus (an mTOR inhibitor) and octreotide (a somatostatin agonist).[9]
- Inhibition of hormone receptors, such as progesterone, estrogen, and androgen, has failed to demonstrate clinical benefit.[8]
- Treatment with molecularly targeted approaches, such as angiogenesis inhibition, is currently under study. Most recently, interim results from the ALLIANCE trial show promise for utilization of FAK inhibitors for patients with an NF2 mutation. However, the studied agent is currently not available for use and other FAK inhibitors are pending testing.[10]

NONPHARMACOLOGIC THERAPY

- The mainstay of treatment for meningiomas remains surgical removal. Complete resection is usually attempted when feasible. After total excision, recurrence rates of 0% to 20% have been observed, while 20% to 50% of patients recur within 5 yr of a subtotal resection.[8]
- Active surveillance to monitor for tumor recurrence is important in higher grade tumors.
- Radiation therapy is the only validated form of adjuvant therapy and may be beneficial in patients with incomplete resections or inoperable tumors. Stereotactic radiosurgery can provide local control with more limited toxicity.[8]

ACUTE GENERAL Rx

- For lesions that cause significant mass effect, steroids are sometimes used to decrease brain edema.
- Anticonvulsants are used if the patient presents with seizures.

CHRONIC Rx

- Prophylactic use of anticonvulsants is not recommended in patients without a history of seizures.
- There are limited data on the efficacy of traditional chemotherapy, and the evidence is largely anecdotal. The most extensively evaluated agents are hydroxyurea, mifepristone (RU486), and interferon alfa-2b. Recently, somatostatin analogs and mTOR inhibitors have been evaluated in multicenter clinical trials, primarily in malignant recurrent meningiomas.[8]

DISPOSITION

- Estimated surgical mortality is 7%. Significant morbidity and mortality can be observed in meningiomas with otherwise favorable pathology secondary to unfavorable location (e.g., skull base). 10-yr relative survival is 80.4% in the cerebral meninges vs. 93.2% in spinal meninges.[11,12]
- Long-term outcome varies based on pathology, tumor grade, location, and completeness of resection. 10-yr relative survival for nonmalignant meningioma is 81.5%, with highest survivability in the youngest age group. 10-yr relative survival for malignant meningioma is 53.5%, with similar age-based effects.[7]
- Most incidentally discovered meningiomas remain asymptomatic and have a slow rate of growth. Calcified tumors may be less likely to progress than noncalcified ones.
- Meningiomas may recur after surgical resection or progress to a higher grade. Risk factors for recurrence include multiple allelic chromosomal losses, local brain invasion, high rate of mitosis, and highly anaplastic features.[13]

REFERRAL

- Neurosurgical consultation for all cases
- Neurology, radiation oncology, and oncology consults depending on presence of other sequelae or in the setting of recurrence

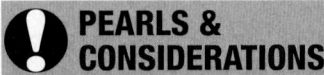

! PEARLS & CONSIDERATIONS

COMMENTS

- Many meningiomas are discovered incidentally; most are benign and remain asymptomatic. A first follow-up MRI should be performed 3 to 6 mo after the tumor is identified to rule out an atypical meningioma with rapid growth.
- "Dural tail," which is the thickening of the dura adjacent to the mass, is a classic finding on neuroimaging studies.
- Individuals with neurofibromatosis type 2 are at high risk to develop meningiomas.

PATIENT & FAMILY EDUCATION

- Meningioma Mommas: https://meningioma-mommas.com
- Meningioma Support and Patient Information Group
- National Brain Tumor Society
- Meningioma Online Support Group: https://braintrust.org/meningioma.html

REFERENCES

Available at eBooks.Health.Elsevier.com.

RELATED CONTENT

Meningioma (Patient Information)

AUTHOR: **LILY C. PHAM, MD**

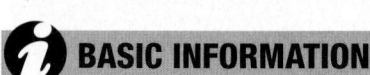
BASIC INFORMATION

DEFINITION
Bacterial meningitis is an inflammation of meninges with increased intracranial pressure and pleocytosis or increased WBCs in cerebrospinal fluid (CSF) secondary to bacteria in the pia-subarachnoid space and ventricles, leading to neurologic sequelae and abnormalities.

SYNONYMS
Spinal meningitis
Bacterial meningitis

ICD-10CM CODES
G00.9	Bacterial meningitis, unspecified
G00.8	Other bacterial meningitis
G01	Meningitis in bacterial diseases classified elsewhere

EPIDEMIOLOGY & DEMOGRAPHICS
INCIDENCE (IN U.S.): There are around 0.9 cases per 100,000 in the U.S. (about 2600 cases) and high-income nations yearly; 80 per 100,000 in low-income nations. About 1.2 million cases per yr in the world; 135,000 deaths annually worldwide. The rate of bacterial meningitis declined dramatically in the U.S. starting in the early 1990s with the introduction of the *Haemophilus influenzae* type b (Hib) vaccine and in 2000 with the introduction of the conjugate pneumococcal vaccine.
PREDOMINANT SEX: Male = female
PREDOMINANT AGE: All ages, neonate to geriatric

PHYSICAL FINDINGS & CLINICAL PRESENTATION
- Fever
- Headache
- Neck stiffness, nuchal rigidity, meningismus
- Altered mental state, lethargy
- Vomiting, nausea
- Photophobia
- Seizures
- Coma; lethargy, stupor
- Rash: Petechial and purpuric lesions (Fig. E1) associated with meningococcal infection, purpura fulminans
- Myalgia
- Cranial nerve abnormality (unilateral)

- Papilledema
- Dilated, nonreactive pupil(s)
- Posturing: Decorticate/decerebrate
- Physical examination findings of Kernig sign and Brudzinski sign (Fig. E2) in adults with meningitis are often seen later in the course of disease and may not be helpful in determining early meningeal inflammation

ETIOLOGY
The bacterial etiology of meningitis depends on the age of the patient (Table 1). *Neisseria meningitidis* is now more common than *Haemophilus influenzae* as a cause of bacterial meningitis in children as well as adults, and *Streptococcus pneumoniae* accounts for 72% of cases in persons older than 16.
- Neonates: Group B *Streptococcus*, gram-negative rods such as *E. coli, Listeria monocytogenes*
- Infants ≥1 mo and <3 mo: Group B streptococci (40%), gram-negative rods (30%), *Streptococcus pneumoniae* (14%), and *Neisseria meningitidis* (12%)
- Infants ≥3 mo and <3 yr:
  1. *S. pneumoniae* (45%)
  2. *N. meningitidis* (34%)
  3. *S. agalactiae* (group B streptococci) (11%)
  4. *H. influenzae*
  5. *E. coli*
- Ages ≥3 yr and <10 yr:
  1. *S. pneumoniae* (47%)
  2. *N. meningitidis* (32%)
- Ages ≥10 yr and <19 yr
  1. *N. meningitidis* (55%)
  2. *S. pneumoniae*
- Adults: *S. pneumoniae* (72% of cases), *N. meningitidis* (11% of cases), and *Streptococcus agalactiae* (third most common cause in adults)
- *Listeria monocytogenes* is uncommon in the general population but is often seen in older adults and in those with cell-mediated immune deficiencies
- People with HIV/AIDS are at increased risk for invasive meningococcal disease (IMD)

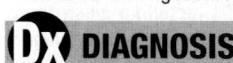 DIAGNOSIS

An algorithm for early management of suspected bacterial meningitis is illustrated in Fig. 3. Lumbar puncture should be performed as soon as possible. Key elements to diagnosis are

CSF evaluation and computed tomography (CT) scan or MRI if the patient is in a coma or has focal neurologic deficits, pupillary abnormalities, or papilledema. Tables 2 and 3 describe tests of CSF in patients with suspected CNS infection.

DIFFERENTIAL DIAGNOSIS (BOX E1)
- Endocarditis, bacteremia
- Intracranial tumor
- Lyme disease
- Brain abscess
- Partially treated bacterial meningitis
- Medications
- SLE
- Seizures
- Acute mononucleosis
- Other infectious meningitides
- Neuroleptic malignant syndrome
- Subdural empyema
- Subarachnoid hemorrhage (Table 4)
- Rocky Mountain spotted fever

WORKUP
CSF examination (Table 5):
- Opening pressure >100 to 200 mm Hg
- WBC usually >1000/mm³
- Neutrophilic predominance: >80%
- Gram stain of CSF: Positive in 60% to 90% of patients
- CSF protein: >50 mg/dl
- CSF glucose: <40 mg/dl
- Culture: Positive in 65% to 90% of cases
- Multiplex PCR assay for detection of *S. pneumoniae, H. influenza, N. meningitidis,* and *L. monocytogenes* offer 100% sensitivity and 98% specificity

LABORATORY TESTS
Blood culturing, WBC with differential, and CSF examination (see "Workup")

IMAGING STUDIES
- Guidelines from the Infectious Society of America recommend CT of brain before lumbar puncture in patients presenting with:
  1. A high clinical suspicion for subarachnoid hemorrhage
  2. New focal neurologic deficit
  3. Papilledema
  4. Seizures within a week
  5. Altered mental status

TABLE 1 Relationship Between Common Bacterial Pathogens and Factors Predisposing to Meningitis

Predisposing Factor	Bacterial Pathogens
Age	
<1 mo	*Streptococcus agalactiae, Escherichia coli, Listeria monocytogenes*
1-23 mo	*S. agalactiae, E. coli, Haemophilus influenzae, Streptococcus pneumoniae, Neisseria meningitidis*
2-50 yr	*S. pneumoniae, N. meningitidis*
>50 yr	*S. pneumoniae, N. meningitidis, L. monocytogenes,* aerobic gram-negative bacilli
Immunocompromised state	*S. pneumoniae, N. meningitidis, L. monocytogenes,* aerobic gram-negative bacilli (including *Pseudomonas aeruginosa*)
Basilar skull fracture	*S. pneumoniae; H. influenzae;* group A streptococci
Head trauma; after neurosurgery	*Staphylococcus aureus,* coagulase-negative staphylococci (especially *Staphylococcus epidermidis*), aerobic gram-negative bacilli (including *P. aeruginosa*)

From Bennett JE et al: *Mandell, Douglas, and Bennett's principles and practice of infectious diseases,* ed 9, Philadelphia, 2020, Elsevier.

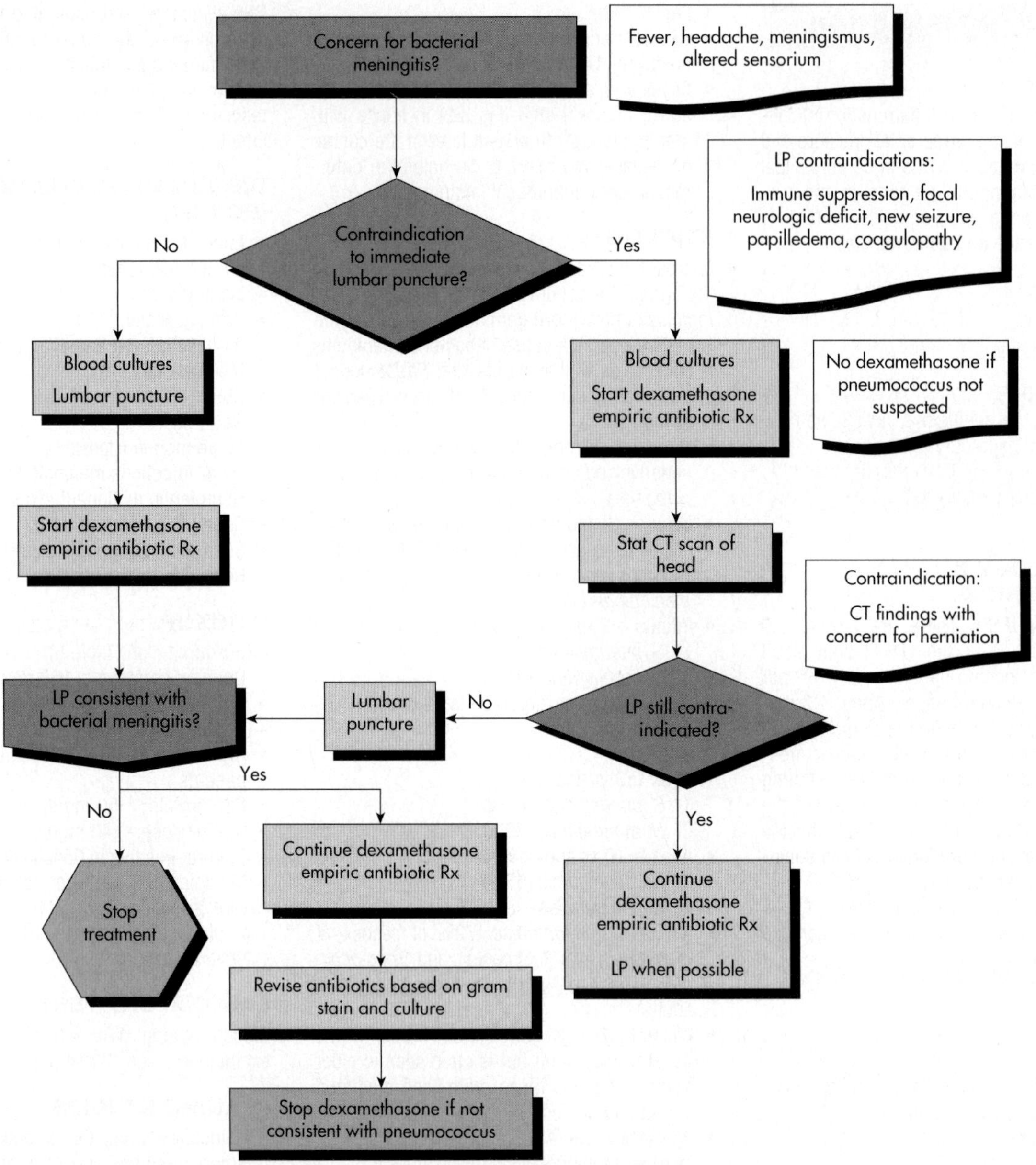

FIG. 3 Algorithm for early management of suspected bacterial meningitis including when to suspect the diagnosis, when imaging prior to lumbar puncture is appropriate, and when to initiate and discontinue empiric antibiotics and adjuvant dexamethasone. *CT,* Computed tomography; *LP,* lumbar puncture; *Rx,* treatment. (Based on Tunkel AR et al: Practice guidelines for the management of bacterial meningitis, *Clin Infect Dis* 39:1267-1284, 2004; and additional information from Hasbun R et al: Computed tomography of the head before lumbar puncture in adults with suspected meningitis, *N Engl J Med* 345:1727-1733, 2001; Glimåker M et al: Adult bacterial meningitis: earlier treatment and improved outcome following guideline revision promoting prompt lumbar puncture, *Clin Infect Dis* 60:1162-1169, 2015; and Brouwer MC et al: Corticosteroids for acute bacterial meningitis, *Cochrane Database Syst Rev* 12(9):CD004405, 2015.)

6. History of central nervous system disease (e.g., tumor, stroke)
7. Immunodeficiency
8. Age 60 or older

Rx TREATMENT

Empiric therapy (Table 6) is necessary with intravenous (IV) antibiotic treatment if patient has purulent CSF fluid at time of lumbar puncture, is asplenic, or has signs of DIC/sepsis pending Gram stain and culture results. Try to obtain blood and CSF cultures before starting antimicrobial therapy, but do not delay therapy if obtaining them is not possible. If CT scan is indicated (see "Imaging Studies" for indications) it should not delay empiric antibiotic therapy. Therapy after Gram stain pending cultures is recommended for the following:

- Neonates: Ampicillin: 200 to 400 mg/kg per day divided q6 to 8 h plus ceftazidime with or without gentamicin: 7.5 mg/kg IV in three divided doses
- 1 to 23 mo: Vancomycin: 60 mg/kg per day IV (maximum up to 4 g/day) divided in four doses plus third-generation cephalosporin: Ceftriaxone: 100 mg/kg (maximum dose 4 g/day) in one or two divided doses or cefotaxime: 300 mg/kg per day IV (maximum dose of 12 g/day) in three or four divided doses

- Children: Vancomycin: 60 mg/kg per day IV (maximum dose 4 g/day) in four divided doses plus third-generation cephalosporin: Ceftriaxone 100 mg/kg per day IV (maximum 4 g/day) or cefotaxime: 300 mg/kg IV (maximum dose of 12 g/day) in three or four divided doses
- Adults: Vancomycin: 15 to 20 mg/kg IV every 8 to 12 h plus third-generation cephalosporin: Ceftriaxone: 2 g IV q12h or cefotaxime: 2 g IV q4 to 6 h. For adults over 50 yr of age also add ampicillin 2 g IV every 4 h to cover *Listeria*
- Immunocompromised patients: Vancomycin *plus* ampicillin *plus* either cefepime 2 g IV every 8 h to cover *Pseudomonas* or meropenem 2 g IV q8h for adults, which also covers *Pseudomonas*

TABLE 2 Tests of Cerebrospinal Fluid in Patients with Suspected Central Nervous System Infection

Routine Tests

White blood cell count with differential

Red blood cell count[a]

Glucose concentration[b]

Protein concentration

Gram stain

Bacterial culture

Selected Specific Tests Based on Clinical Suspicion

Viral culture[c]

Smears and culture for acid-fast bacilli

Venereal Disease Research Laboratory (VDRL)

India ink preparation

Cryptococcal polysaccharide antigen

Fungal culture

Antibody tests (IgM or IgG, or both)[d]

Nucleic acid amplification tests (e.g., polymerase chain reaction)[e]

Cytology[f]

Flow cytometry

[a]Should be checked in the first and last tubes; in patients with a traumatic tap, there should be a decrease in the number of red blood cells with continued flow of cerebrospinal fluid (CSF). See text for the formula for determining whether the numbers of CSF red blood cells and white blood cells are consistent with a traumatic tap.
[b]Compare with serum glucose drawn just before lumbar puncture.
[c]Yield of viral culture may be low.
[d]May be useful for specific causes of meningitis and encephalitis.
[e]Most useful for specific viral causes of encephalitis and causes of chronic meningitis.
[f]In patients with suspected malignancy.

From Bennett JE et al: *Mandell, Douglas, and Bennett's principles and practice of infectious diseases*, ed 8, Philadelphia, 2015, Saunders.

Use of corticosteroids in adults:
• Dexamethasone 0.15 mg/kg q6h for first 4 days of therapy should be used for adults in developed countries with known or suspected bacterial meningitis. Decreased mortality and neurologic sequelae (hearing loss, etc.) are seen with adjunct therapy in patients with pneumococcal meningitis but not other pathogens. The benefit of dexamethasone is less clear in developing countries with high HIV prevalence and malnutrition or with delayed clinical presentations.
• Dexamethasone also benefits children with Hib meningitis if given at the same time or before the first dose of the antibiotic: 0.15 mg/kg per dose q6h for 2 to 4 days. The use and benefit of corticosteroids in children with suspected or pneumococcal or meningococcal meningitis to prevent neurologic sequelae is not as clear and should be individualized after analysis of risk and benefits.

DISPOSITION

Bacterial meningitis is a reportable disease that needs to be reported to local health authorities. Droplet precautions should be used for first 24 h of therapy for suspected or confirmed *N. meningitidis* infection.

REFERRAL

• To a neurologist if persistent neurologic sequelae develop after bacterial meningitis
• To an infectious disease consultant if a patient has recurrent bacterial meningitis; such patients deserve a workup for an anatomic (CSF dural leak) or immunologic defect (complement defect, hyposplenism, immunoglobulin deficiency)

PEARLS & CONSIDERATIONS

COMMENTS

• Patients with bacterial meningitis often require ICU care either to manage complications evident on presentation or for monitoring for any complications that may subsequently develop during their course. Criteria for admission to an ICU are summarized in Table 7.
• Nosocomial bacterial meningitis may result from invasive procedures (e.g., placement of ventricular catheters, lumbar puncture, craniotomy, spinal anesthesia). Treatment of this different spectrum of microorganisms requires empirical antimicrobial therapy with vancomycin plus either cefepime, ceftazidime, or meropenem. In cases of basilar skull fracture, effective empirical antimicrobial therapy consists of vancomycin plus a third-generation cephalosporin.
• False-positive elevations of CSF where blood cell counts can be found after traumatic lumbar puncture or in patients with intracerebral or subarachnoid hemorrhage in which RBCs and WBCs are introduced into the subarachnoid space. In those instances, the following formula should be used as a correction factor for the true WBC count in the presence of CSF RBCs:

$$\text{Adjusted WBC in CSF} = \text{Actual WBC in CSF} - \frac{\text{WBC in blood} \times \text{RBC in CSF blood}}{\text{RBC in blood}}$$

In the previous equation, the amount being subtracted is the predicted CSF WBC that would occur if all the CSF WBCs were the result of blood contamination.

TABLE 3 Bacterial Meningeal Pathogens and Their Diagnostic Tests

Organism	Blood	Cerebrospinal Fluid
Streptococcus pneumoniae	Culture	Gram stain: Gram-positive diplococci in pairs Culture Meningitis/encephalitis panel
Listeria monocytogenes	Culture	Gram stain: Gram-positive rods Culture Meningitis/encephalitis panel
Neisseria meningitides	Culture	Gram stain: Gram-negative diplococcus Culture
Haemophilus influenzae type b	Culture	Gram stain: Gram-negative coccobacillus Culture Meningitis/encephalitis panel
Mycobacterium tuberculosis		20-30 ml for AFB stain and culture; PCR
Treponema pallidum	RPR/VDRL; MHA-TPA; FTA-ABS; TPPA	VDRL (nontraumatic tap)
Coxiella burnetii	Acute and convalescent serologies	
Brucella spp.	Culture: Acute and convalescent serologies	Gram stain: Gram-negative coccobacillus Culture
Borrelia spp.	ELISA→if equivocal or +, then IgG and IgM WB (follow CDC guidelines for + WB)	Antibody index: Anti-*Borrelia* IgG in CSF/anti-*Borrelia* IgG in serum to total IgG in CSF/total IgG in serum
Leptospira spp.	Acute and convalescent serologies (MAT only done in reference labs, ELISA and lateral flow dipstick less sensitive and specific) Culture: Special media; may need to keep for 8-12 wk	Culture: Special media, fastidious

AFB, Acid-fast bacilli; *CDC,* Centers for Disease Control and Prevention; *CSF,* cerebrospinal fluid; *ELISA,* enzyme-linked immunosorbent assay; *FTA-ABS,* fluorescent treponemal antibody absorbed; *Ig,* immunoglobulin; *MAT,* microscopic agglutination test; *MHA-TPA,* microhemagglutination assay–*Treponema* antibody absorption test; *PCR,* polymerase chain reaction; *RPR,* rapid plasma reagin test; *TPPA, Treponema pallidum* particle agglutination; *VDRL,* Venereal Disease Research Laboratory test; *WB,* Western blot test.
From Jankovic J et al: *Bradley and Daroff's neurology in clinical practice*, ed 8, Philadelphia, 2022, Elsevier.

TABLE 4 Acute Bacterial Meningitis and Subarachnoid Hemorrhage

Finding	Frequency (%)
Acute Bacterial Meningitis	
Neck stiffness	84
Fever	66-97
Altered mental status	55-95
Kernig or Brudzinski sign	61
Focal neurologic signs	9-37
Seizures	5-28
Petechial rash	3-52
Subarachnoid Hemorrhage	
Neck stiffness	21-86
Seizures	7-32
Altered mental status	29-64
Focal neurologic findings	10-36
Fever	6
Preretinal hemorrhage	4

Diagnostic standard: For *meningitis,* cerebrospinal fluid pleocytosis and microbiologic or postmortem data supporting bacterial meningitis; for *subarachnoid hemorrhage,* computed tomography or lumbar puncture.

From McGee S: *Evidence-based physical diagnosis,* ed 4, Philadelphia, 2018, Elsevier.

PREVENTION

- Prevention of meningitis can be achieved through chemoprophylaxis of close contacts (household members and anyone exposed to oral secretions).
- Effective medications are rifampin 10 mg/kg PO bid for 2 days or ceftriaxone 250 mg intramuscularly (IM) single dose in patients older than age 12; 125 mg IM if age 12 or younger.
- Ciprofloxacin 500 mg for prevention of *Neisseria* meningitis can be given to patients older than 18 yr who cannot tolerate rifampin to eradicate pharyngeal colonization.
- Menactra: A protein-conjugate vaccine against serogroup A, C, Y, W-135 capsular polysaccharides is available for adults (up to 55 yr) and children older than 2 yr.
- Two vaccines are now available for *Neisseria* meningitis serogroup B (MenB): Bexsero and Trumenba. The FDA has also recently licensed MenQuadfi, a quadrivalent polysaccharide conjugate vaccine that uses tetanus toxoid as a protein carrier for prevention of *Neisseria meningitidis* serogroups A, C, W, and Y in persons >2 yr old.
- Children with cochlear implants are at increased risk of developing bacterial meningitis.
- Patients on eculizumab (Soliris) are at high risk for invasive meningococcal disease and should receive Menactra and a MenB vaccine and may need lifelong antibiotic prophylaxis as well.

SUGGESTED READINGS

Available at eBooks.Health.Elsevier.com.

RELATED CONTENT

Meningitis (Patient Information)
Meningitis, viral (Related Key Topic)
Meningitis, fungal (Related Key Topic)

AUTHOR: **GLENN G. FORT, MD, MPH**

TABLE 5 Cerebrospinal Fluid Findings in Various Central Nervous System Disorders

Condition	Pressure (CM H2O)	Leukocytes (Cells/μL)	Protein (mg/dl)/ Glucose (mg/dl)	Comments
Normal	10-20	<5; 60-70% lymphocytes, 30-40% monocytes, 1-3% neutrophils	20-45/>50% of serum glucose	WBC up to 10-20 cells/μL can be normal in neonates
Acute bacterial meningitis	Usually elevated (>25)	>100; usually thousands; PMNs predominate	100-500/usually <40 or <40% of serum glucose	Organisms may be seen on Gram stain and recovered by culture
Partially treated bacterial meningitis	Normal or elevated	1-10,000; PMNs usual but mononuclear cells may predominate if pretreated for extended period	>100/depressed or normal	Pretreatment may render CSF sterile, but bacteria may be detected by PCR
Tuberculous meningitis	Usually elevated; may be low because of CSF block in advanced stages	10-500; PMNs early but lymphocytes and monocytes predominate later	100-500; may be higher in presence of CSF block/ usually <50	Acid-fast smear and culture or mycobacteria PCR may be positive. Adenine deaminase can be used to aid in the diagnosis
Fungal	Usually elevated	10-500; PMNs early; mononuclear cells predominate later	20-500/usually <50	Organisms may be seen on smear, in culture, or by India ink preparation, and antigen may be positive in cryptococcal disease
Viral meningitis or meningoencephalitis	Normal or slightly elevated	10-1,000; PMNs early; mononuclear cells predominate later	<50/normal or depressed	Viruses may be detected by PCR
Abscess (parameningeal infection)	Normal or elevated	0-100 PMNs unless rupture into CSF	20-200/normal	Profile may be completely normal

CSF, Cerebrospinal fluid; *PCR,* polymerase chain reaction; *PMNs,* polymorphonuclear leukocytes.
From Marcdante KJ et al: *Nelson essentials of pediatrics,* ed 9, Philadelphia 2023, Elsevier.

M

Diseases
and Disorders

I

TABLE 6 Empiric Treatment of Suspected Bacterial Meningitis in Adults[a,1,2,3,4]

Host Factors to Consider			
Age >50 yr? Risk for *Listeria monocytogenes* and aerobic gram-negative rods			
Immune suppression? Includes host defects (e.g., HIV, alcoholism, lymphoma) and treatment-related (e.g., posttransplant, corticosteroids)			
Health care–associated? Includes trauma, postneurosurgical, shunt- or ventriculostomy-related			
Life-threatening penicillin/β-lactam allergy? Aztreonam or fluoroquinolone alternatives for gram-negative rods; trimethoprim-sulfamethoxazole an alternative for *L. monocytogenes*			

Host	Likely Pathogens	Empiric Therapy	Additional Considerations
Age 15-50 yr without Immune Suppression	*Streptococcus pneumoniae, Neisseria meningitidis,* group B β-hemolytic streptococci	Vancomycin + third-generation cephalosporin[b]	Adjuvant dexamethasone Consider rifampin if high rates of cephalosporin-resistant *S. pneumoniae*
Age ≥50 yr without Immune Suppression	*S. pneumoniae, N. meningitidis,* group B β-hemolytic streptococci, *L. monocytogenes,* aerobic gram-negative rods	Vancomycin + ampicillin + third-generation cephalosporin[b]	Adjuvant dexamethasone Consider rifampin if high rates of cephalosporin-resistant *S. pneumoniae*
Immune Suppression	*S. pneumoniae, N. meningitidis,* group B β-hemolytic streptococci, *L. monocytogenes, Staphylococcus aureus,* aerobic gram-negative rods including *Pseudomonas aeruginosa*	Vancomycin + ampicillin + cefepime or meropenum[c]	Adjuvant dexamethasone Consider rifampin if high rates of cephalosporin-resistant *S. pneumoniae*
Health Care–Associated: Trauma, Postneurosurgical, or Shunt-Associated[c]	*S. aureus,* coagulase-negative staphylococci, aerobic gram-negative rods including *P. aeruginosa*	Vancomycin + ceftazidime or cefepime or meropenem[c]	Dexamethasone not indicated Consider rifampin for staphylococci Consider intrathecal therapy for shunt-/ventriculostomy-associated infection
Health Care–Associated: Basilar Skull Fracture	*S. pneumoniae, Haemophilus influenzae,* group A β-hemolytic streptococci	Vancomycin + third-generation cephalosporin[b]	Adjuvant dexamethasone Consider rifampin if high rates of cephalosporin-resistant *S. pneumoniae*

HIV, Human immunodeficiency virus.

[a]Age older than 15 yr.

[b]Third-generation cephalosporin: Ceftriaxone 2 g q12h or cefotaxime 2 g q4-6h.

[c]Dosing of other agents (modified for renal insufficiency): Vancomycin targeted to vancomycin trough levels of 15-20 µg/ml; ampicillin 2 g q4h; ceftazidime 2 g q8h; cefepime 2 g q8h; meropenem 2 g q8h.

[1]van de Beek D et al: Community-acquired bacterial meningitis, *Nat Rev Dis Primers* 2, 16074, 1-20, 2016.

[2]Thigpen MC et al for the Emerging Infections Programs Network: Bacterial meningitis in the United States, 1998-2007, *N Engl J Med* 364(21):2016-2025, 2011.

[3]Tunkel AR et al: Practice guidelines for the management of bacterial meningitis, *Clin Infect Dis* 39(9):1267-1284, 2004.

[4]Tunkel AR et al: 2017 Infectious Diseases Society of America's clinical practice guidelines for health care-associated ventriculitis and meningitis, *Clin Infect Dis* 64(6):e34-e65, 2017.

From Parrillo JE, Dellinger RP: *Critical care medicine, principles of diagnosis and management in the adult,* ed 5, Philadelphia, 2019, Elsevier.

TABLE 7 Major Complications of Bacterial Meningitis Requiring ICU Level of Care for Monitoring and Management[1,2,3,4,5]

Type of Complication	Etiologies, Prevalence	Management Strategies
Neurologic Complications		
Increasing intracranial pressure	Brain edema, 6%-10%	Strategies: Osmotic diuresis, intracranial pressure monitoring, head of bed elevation, prophylactic lumbar drain Glycerol and hypothermia not beneficial and may result in higher mortality
Hydrocephalus	Communicating hydrocephalus, 3%-8% Obstructive hydrocephalus uncommon	Repeated lumbar puncture, lumbar drain, ventriculostomy
Focal neurologic deficits	Arterial infarct or vasculitis, 10%-15% Venous infarction, 3%-5% Hearing loss, 14%-30% Cranial nerve deficits, especially eighth nerve, 15%-30% Hemorrhage, <1% Brain abscess, subdural empyema <1%	Radiographic studies to look for focal intracranial complications Administer dexamethasone for suspected pneumococcal meningitis to decreases risk of hearing loss
Seizures	Multiple etiologies, 14%-33%	Continuous EEG monitoring, antiepileptic agents Prophylactic antiepileptic agents not routinely recommended
Agitation	Common	Careful sedation
Other Complications		
Hyponatremia	Up to 25%-30%	? Hypertonic saline solution Presence of hyponatremia did not affect outcome
Sepsis and cardiorespiratory failure	38%	Hemodynamic support, mechanical ventilation
Pneumonia	17%, most often with *Streptococcus pneumoniae*	Ventilatory support

EEG, Electroencephalographic.

[1]van de Beek D et al: Community-acquired bacterial meningitis, *Nat Rev Dis Primers* 2(16074):1-20, 2016.

[2]Bijlsma MW et al: Community-acquired bacterial meningitis in adults in the Netherlands, 2006-2014: a prospective cohort study, *Lancet Infect Dis* 16(3):339-347, 2016.

[3]Durand ML et al: Acute bacterial meningitis in adults: review of 493 episodes, *N Engl J Med* 328(1):21-28, 1993.

[4]Tunkel AR et al: Practice guidelines for the management of bacterial meningitis, *Clin Infect Dis* 39(9):1267-1284, 2004.

[5]Brouwer MC et al: What's new in bacterial meningitis, *Intensive Care Med* 42(3):415-417, 2016.

From Parrillo JE, Dellinger RP: *Critical care medicine, principles of diagnosis and management in the adult,* ed 5, Philadelphia, 2019, Elsevier.

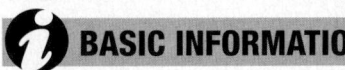

BASIC INFORMATION

DEFINITION

Viral meningitis is an acute febrile illness with signs and symptoms of meningeal irritation, usually with a lymphocytic pleocytosis of the cerebrospinal fluid (CSF) and negative CSF bacterial stains and cultures.

SYNONYMS

Aseptic meningitis
Viral meningitis

ICD-10CM CODES
A87.8	Other viral meningitis
A87.9	Viral meningitis, unspecified

EPIDEMIOLOGY & DEMOGRAPHICS (TABLE 1)

INCIDENCE (IN U.S.): 11 cases/100,000 persons; leads to 26,000 to 42,000 hospitalizations per yr
PREDOMINANT SEX: Male = female
GENETICS: Those with abnormal humoral immunity and agammaglobulinemia have associated difficulty with viral clearance

PHYSICAL FINDINGS & CLINICAL PRESENTATION

- Fever
- Headache
- Nuchal rigidity
- Photophobia
- Myalgias
- Vomiting
- Rash

ETIOLOGY

- Enterovirus: 85% to 95% of all cases. Most common are coxsackieviruses and echoviruses
- Parechoviruses
- Mumps virus
- Measles
- Arboviruses from mosquitoes: Eastern equine encephalitis (EEE), West Nile, St. Louis
- Herpes: HSV-1, HSV-2, VZV, HHV-6, and HHV-7
- Acute HIV
- Lymphocytic choriomeningitis virus
- Adenovirus
- Cytomegalovirus (CMV) and Epstein-Barr virus (EBV)
- Other arthropod-borne viruses: Powassan virus
- Influenza A and B virus
- Coronaviruses
- Box E1 summarizes etiologic agents, factors, and diseases associated with aseptic meningitis

DIAGNOSIS

The diagnostic approach is similar to that for bacterial meningitis (see "Meningitis, Bacterial"); the foremost need is to rule out bacterial meningitis with CSF evaluation (Table 2). Presentation may be similar to that of meningitis with bacterial involvement.

DIFFERENTIAL DIAGNOSIS

- Bacterial meningitis
- Meningitis secondary to Lyme disease, tuberculosis (TB), syphilis, amebiasis, leptospirosis
- Rickettsial illnesses: Rocky Mountain spotted fever
- Migraine headache
- Medications
- Systemic lupus erythematosus (SLE)
- Acute mononucleosis/EBV
- Seizures
- Carcinomatous meningitis

WORKUP

CSF examination:
- Usually shows pleocytosis
- Lymphocytic predominance (neutrophils in early stages)
- Opening pressure: 200 to 250 mm Hg H_2O ($\leq$250 mm/H_2O)
- WBC: 100 to 1000 mm^3
- Increased CSF protein (<200 mg/dl)
- Slightly decreased or normal CSF glucose (>45 mg/dl)
- Negative Gram stain, cultures, CIE, latex agglutination
- Viral cultures or serologic testing may be diagnostic
- Polymerase chain reaction (PCR) for HSV or enterovirus (which could shorten duration of antibiotic treatment and hospitalization if bacterial meningitis was suspected); multiplex or panel-based PCR tests that test for multiple viruses and bacteria at the same time in a single CSF sample are available. CSF PCR diagnosis of viral nervous system disease is summarized in Table 3
- Antibody detection in CSF for diagnosis of West Nile virus meningitis

LABORATORY TESTS

CBC with differential, blood culturing, and CSF examination (see "Workup")

IMAGING STUDIES

CT scan or MRI: If cerebral edema, focal neurologic findings develop

TREATMENT

- No specific antiviral therapy for most viruses. Treatment is supportive unless herpes simplex virus (HSV) is detected, which would be treated with IV acyclovir: 10 to 12.5 mg/kg q8h in adults for 14 to 21 days. Pediatric dose: 10 to 15 mg/kg q8h in children <12 yr and 20 mg/kg q8h in neonatal herpes.
- Empiric antibiotics may be given until CSF cultures exclude bacterial meningitis.

DISPOSITION

Viral meningitis is almost always an uncomplicated illness that will resolve; however, relapsing headache, myalgia, and weakness may occur for 2 to 3 wk after onset of symptoms.

PEARLS & CONSIDERATIONS

- Enteroviruses are the most common cause of viral meningitis and are transmitted by fecal-oral route and less commonly by the respiratory route. They are more common in summer and fall mos. Currently the most common serotypes are Group B coxsackie virus serotypes 2 through 5 and echoviruses 4, 6, 9, 11, 16, and 30. Aseptic meningitis is most commonly associated with echovirus 30.
- Herpes simplex type 2 (HSV-2) can be a cause of a primary episode of meningitis and also be a cause of recurrent episodes of

---

TABLE 1 Epidemiology of Acute Viral Meningitis

			EPIDEMIOLOGIC FACTORS*	
Season	Patient's Age (yr)	Patient's Sex	Risk Factor	Suggested Viral Agent
Summer-fall	Infant	—	Infected mother	Coxsackievirus B
	1-15	—	Swimming pools, closed communities	Enteroviruses
			Geographic area: California, southeastern U.S.	California serogroup virus
Winter	1-15	—	School exposure	Varicella virus, measles virus
		Male:female 3:1		Mumps virus
	16-21	—	College exposure	Measles virus
		Male:female 3:1		Mumps virus
				Epstein-Barr virus (mononucleosis)
	Any	—	Mice, rats, hamsters	Lymphocytic choriomeningitis virus
	Adults	—	Varicella-zoster	Varicella-zoster virus
Any	Any	—	Immunocompromise	Adenovirus
		—	Acquired immunodeficiency syndrome	Human immunodeficiency virus

*Epidemiologic factors are suggestive but should not be used to exclude diagnoses in individual cases.
From Gorbach SI: *Infectious diseases*, ed 2, Philadelphia, 1998, Saunders.

TABLE 2 Typical CSF Findings for Various Etiologies of Meningitis and Encephalitis

	Normal	Bacterial	Viral	Fungal/TB
Pressure (cm H$_2$O)	5-20	>30	Normal or increased	Increased
Protein (mg/dL)	18-45	Increased	Normal or increased	Normal or increased
Glucose	2/3 serum glucose	Decreased	Normal	Normal or decreased
Gram stain	Negative	60%-90% positive	Negative	Negative
White blood cells	<5	Usually >1000	100-1000	50-500
WBC differential predominance	None	Neutrophils	Lymphocytes	Lymphocytes or monocytes

From Walls RM et al: *Rosen's emergency medicine, concepts and clinical practice,* ed 10, Philadelphia, 2023, Elsevier.

TABLE 3 CSF PCR Diagnosis of Viral Nervous System Disease

Virus	Sensitivity	Specificity
Adenovirus	Unknown	
Dengue	Unknown	
Enterovirus	>95% (meningitis), <10% for AFM with EV-D68 or <25% with neuroinvasive EV-A71	>95%
Herpesviruses		
HCMV	100% in immunocompromised	High
	>60% in congenital CMV infection	High
EBV	98.5% as tumor marker in HIV patients with primary CNS lymphoma	Unknown
HSV-1 and -2	>95%	>95%
HHV-6	Unknown	Unknown
VZV	>95%	>95%
HIV	HIV RNA present at all stages	High
HTLV I and II	75%	98.5%
Influenza	Unknown but > culture	Unknown
Japanese encephalitis virus	Unknown (higher early)	High
JC virus	50%-90% in PML, lower copy # in more immunocompetent pts	98%
LCMV	Unknown	Unknown
Mumps	Unknown	High
Measles	Unknown	High
Parvovirus B-19	80%	Unknown
Rabies	90%	High
WNV	70% (higher early)	High
SARS-CoV2	Unknown, likely low (nasopharyngeal RT-PCR high acutely)	High
ZIKV	Unknown (congenital ZIKV syndrome)	High

AFM, Acute flaccid myelitis; *CNS,* central nervous system; *CSF,* cerebral spinal fluid; *EBV,* Epstein-Barr virus; *HCMV,* human cytomegalovirus; *HHV,* human herpesvirus; *HSV,* herpes simplex virus; *HTLV,* human T-cell lymphotropic virus; *LCMV,* lymphocytic choriomeningitis virus; *PCR,* polymerase chain reaction; *PML,* progressive multifocal leukoencephalopathy; *RT-PCR,* reverse transcription polymerase chain reaction; *VZV,* varicella-zoster virus; *WNV,* West Nile virus; *ZIKV,* Zika virus.
From Jankovic J et al: *Bradley and Daroff's neurology in clinical practice,* ed 8, Philadelphia 2022, Elsevier.

lymphocytic meningitis. HSV-2 meningitis presents most often without a history of genital herpes or genital symptoms. Recurrent aseptic meningitis, also known as Mollaret disease, is predominantly caused by HSV-2 infection.

SUGGESTED READING
Available at eBooks.Health.Elsevier.com.

RELATED CONTENT
Meningitis (Patient Information)
Meningitis, Bacterial (Related Key Topic)
Meningitis, Fungal (Related Key Topic)

AUTHOR: **GLENN G. FORT, MD, MPH**

M

Diseases and Disorders

I

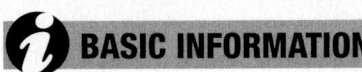
BASIC INFORMATION

DEFINITION

Menopause is the permanent cessation of menstrual periods for 1 yr or permanent cessation of ovulation after lost ovarian activity without any other obvious pathologic or physiologic cause. It is the reproductive stage of life marked by waxing and waning estrogen levels followed by decreasing ovarian function. Primary ovarian insufficiency (previously also referred to as premature ovarian failure) and no menstrual periods may also occur because of depletion of ovarian follicles before the age of 40 yr and is considered to be abnormal.

SYNONYMS

Change of life
Climacteric ovarian failure

ICD-10CM CODES
E28.310	Symptomatic premature menopause
E28.319	Asymptomatic premature menopause
N95.1	Menopausal and female climacteric states
N95.8	Other specified menopausal and perimenopausal disorders
Z78.0	Asymptomatic menopausal state

EPIDEMIOLOGY & DEMOGRAPHICS

- Average age of menopause in the U.S. is 51 yr.
- Age at which menopause occurs is primarily genetically determined.
- Smokers experience menopause an average of 1.5 yr earlier than nonsmokers.
- The menopausal transition, or perimenopause, begins on average 4 yr before the last menstrual period, which is usually in a woman's mid- to late-40s.
- Approximately 70% of middle-aged women experience vasomotor symptoms (hot flashes, night sweats, or both).

PHYSICAL FINDINGS & CLINICAL PRESENTATION

- Menopausal vasomotor symptoms (VMS, hot flashes, flushes): Night sweats, cardiovascular disease, coronary artery disease, atherosclerosis, headaches, tiredness, and lethargy; vasomotor symptoms typically begin around entry into the menopausal transition and tend to continue well after the final menstrual period. The median duration of hot flashes has been reported as 4 yr in some studies and in others, 10.2 yr, but the length of hot flashes was largely dictated by how early they began in the perimenopause. Variations in duration of hot flashes also may vary between racial/ethnic groups.
- Either complete cessation of menses or a period of irregular cycles and diminished or heavier bleeding

- Atrophic vaginitis, which can cause burning, itching, bleeding, dyspareunia
- Osteoporosis
- Osteopenia
- Psychological dysfunction:
  1. Anxiety
  2. Depression
  3. Insomnia
  4. Nervousness
  5. Irritability
  6. Inability to concentrate
  7. Sleep disturbance
- Sexual changes, decreased libido, dyspareunia
- Urinary incontinence

ETIOLOGY

- The most common etiology: Physiologic, caused by depleted granulosa and theca cells that fail to react to endogenous gonadotropins, producing less estrogen; decreased negative feedback in the hypothalamic pituitary access, increased follicle-stimulating hormone (FSH), and increased luteinizing hormone (LH), which leads to stromal cells that continue to produce androgens as a result of the LH stimulation.
- Surgical castration.
- Other factors that contribute to menopause (Table 1) can be family history of early menopause, cigarette smoking, blindness, abnormal chromosomal karyotype (Turner syndrome, gonadal dysgenesis), precocious puberty, and left-handedness.

DIAGNOSIS

DIFFERENTIAL DIAGNOSIS

- Primary ovarian insufficiency
- Asherman syndrome
- Hypothalamic dysfunction

TABLE 1 Etiologic Factors in Early Menopause

Race/ethnicity

Parity

Prior oral contraceptive use

Socioeconomic status

Lower educational attainment

Marital status

Stress

Familial/genetic factors

Blepharophimosis gene

POF 1/POF 2 gene

Fragile X syndrome

PVU II polymorphic allele

Environmental toxins

Smoking

Chemotherapy

Irradiation

Galactose consumption

Body mass index (BMI)

Depression

From Robertson RP et al: *DeGroot's endocrinology, basic science and clinical practice*, ed 8, Philadelphia, 2023, Elsevier.

- Hyper or hypothyroidism
- Pituitary tumors
- Adrenal abnormalities
- Ovarian abnormalities
- Polycystic ovarian syndrome
- Pregnancy
- Ovarian neoplasm
- Tuberculosis of the endometrium

WORKUP

- Physical examination, height, weight, blood pressure, breast examination, and pelvic examination are needed.
- If the clinical picture is highly suggestive of menopause, reassurance or hormone replacement therapy such as estrogen can be prescribed to help with menopausal symptoms (after appropriate counseling). If all symptoms resolve, then a diagnosis essentially has been made. Before estrogen is prescribed, however, a complete history and physical examination are needed. If a patient has an estrogen-dependent malignancy, unexplained abnormal uterine bleeding, a history of thrombophlebitis, or acute liver disease, estrogen therapy is contraindicated.
- Progesterone challenge test: Medroxyprogesterone 10 to 20 mg PO or progesterone 100 mg intramuscularly (IM) to induce withdrawal bleeding. If no withdrawal bleeding is obtained, a hypoestrogenic state is assumed to be present.
- Assess risk for coronary artery disease, osteoporosis, cigarette smoking, personal history, history of breast cancer, liver disease, active coagulation disorder, or any unexplained vaginal bleeding.

LABORATORY TESTS

- No laboratory tests may be indicated if the patient fulfills clinical criteria of menopause at an anticipated average age.
- The possibility of pregnancy must always be excluded in a woman with new onset amenorrhea by a serum hCG.
- FSH, LH, and estrogen levels: Markedly elevated FSH and markedly depressed estrogen level constitute laboratory diagnosis of ovarian failure; LH only if polycystic ovarian disease is to be ruled out in a younger patient. It is not necessary to obtain an FSH if the patient fulfills the clinical criteria for menopause. Similarly, since estradiol levels vary during the menstrual cycle, estradiol levels are rarely necessary or informative.
- Anti-Müllerian hormone (produced by the granulosa cells) will demonstrate a decrease.
- TSH to rule out thyroid dysfunction and prolactin level if patient has symptoms of galactorrhea and if suspicion of pituitary adenoma exists.
- A general chemistry profile to check for any systemic diseases.
- Pap smear per standard guidelines, endometrial biopsy, or dilation and curettage in patients who have had irregular periods or intermenstrual or postmenopausal bleeding.
- Mammogram as recommended by American Congress of Obstetricians and Gynecologists for preventive care.

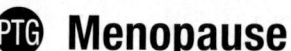

- For women under the age of 40, a complete evaluation for abnormal uterine bleeding is suggested.

IMAGING STUDIES

- Per standard protocols, computed tomography (CT) scan or MRI of sella if pituitary tumor is suspected
- Bone density studies if high-risk condition for osteoporosis exists
- Pelvic ultrasound to check endometrial stripe as determined by clinical history (i.e., in the setting of postmenopausal bleeding)

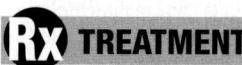 **TREATMENT**

NONPHARMACOLOGIC THERAPY

- A balanced diet: Low in fat, with total fat intake being <30% of calories; total calories sufficient to maintain body weight or produce weight loss if that is desired
- Avoidance of smoking, excessive alcohol or caffeine intake, and spicy foods (if they trigger hot flashes)
- Exercise: Weight-bearing exercise for osteoporosis prevention
- Kegel exercises for strengthening the pelvic floor
- Adequate calcium intake: 1200 mg of calcium daily (total diet plus supplement) and 800 IU of vitamin D daily in patients with osteoporosis. Many patients, however, do not need additional supplementation if getting adequate calcium and vitamin D from dietary intake and sun exposure
- Change in the ambient temperature (may ameliorate hot flashes and reduce night sweats)
- Vitamin E
- Vaginal lubricants to help with the dyspareunia attributable to vaginal dryness (e.g., Replens, K-Y Jelly, or Gyne-Moistrin cream)

ACUTE GENERAL Rx

Vasomotor symptoms are best managed with systemic hormone therapy given in the lowest dose and for the shortest period possible. Estrogen replacement in symptomatic patients can be administered in a variety of forms, including oral estrogen and transdermal estrogen patch. The lowest effective dose should be prescribed.

- Examples of oral estrogen include:
  1. Conjugated estrogens: Start with 0.3 mg daily and increase to 1.25 mg daily depending on symptoms.
  2. Estradiol: Start with 0.5 mg daily and increase up to 2 mg daily.
  3. Esterified estrogens: Start with 0.3 to 1.25 mg daily.
  4. Estropipate: Start with 0.75 to 3.0 mg daily.
  5. Esterified estrogen/testosterone combination: Give 1.25 mg and methyltestosterone 2.5 mg (Estratest) and esterified estrogen 0.625 mg and methyltestosterone 1.25 mg (Estratest HS [half-strength]). May improve sexual enjoyment and libido.
- If the patient has had a hysterectomy for benign disease, estrogen alone is sufficient. In patients who have an intact uterus, progestin

is critical to prevent endometrial hyperplasia associated with unopposed estrogen, which is protective against endometrial cancer. Progestins can be prescribed as continual daily dose or cyclic fashion. Most commonly prescribed progestins include medroxyprogesterone acetate 2.5 mg, 5 mg, and 10 mg; Prometrium 100 mg, 200 mg, and 400 mg; and Aygestin 5 mg. Continuous hormone replacement therapy is preferred because after time the patient should be amenorrheic. Patients should be counseled that they may experience some irregular spotting for the first 6 to 9 mo after starting hormone replacement therapy. Cyclic therapy will cause withdrawal bleeding.

- Combination oral preparations Femhrt, Prefest, Prempro, Activella, Premphase are commonly used. However, the U.S. Preventive Services Task Force recommends against the use of combined estrogen and progestin for the prevention of chronic conditions such as cardiovascular disease in postmenopausal women.
- The combination of conjugated estrogen and bazedoxifene is approved for the treatment of moderate to severe vasomotor symptoms associated with menopause and also for prevention of postmenopausal osteoporosis in women with an intact uterus.
- Transdermal patches can be either estradiol (Estraderm, Vivelle, FemPatch) 0.025 to 0.1 mg applied twice weekly or Climara 0.025 to 0.1 mg used once per wk. With these preparations, progesterone should be used in a similar fashion. Apply CombiPatch twice weekly (combination estrogen and progesterone) or Climara Pro once per wk (one patch).
- Vaginal estrogen creams can be used; these should be reserved for local therapy of atrophic vaginitis. Minimal systemic absorption does occur; however, blood levels are unpredictable. Usual dose 0.5 to 2 g intravaginally daily, cyclically 3 wk on and 1 wk off. When symptoms improve, once to twice weekly is adequate maintenance.
- Vagifem estradiol vaginal tablets. Initial dosage: One Vagifem tablet, inserted vaginally, daily for 2 wk. Maintenance dose: One Vagifem tablet, inserted vaginally, twice weekly.
- Femring vaginal ring delivering the equivalent of 0.5 mg/day inserted every 3 mo or Estring 0.0075 mg/day.
- EstroGel 0.06% (estradiol gel). One pump (1.25 g/day) applied to one arm from wrist to shoulder.
- The FDA contraindications to menopause hormone therapy include the following diseases and disorders: Active liver disease; current, past, or suspected breast cancer; active or recent anterior thromboembolic disease; cardiac disease (angina, myocardial infarction); known or suspected estrogen-sensitive malignant conditions; known hypersensitivity to the active substance of the therapy or to any of the excipients; porphyria cutanea tarda; previous idiopathic or current venous thromboembolism; undiagnosed genital bleeding; untreated hypertension; untreated endometrial hyperplasia.

- For women in whom estrogen is contraindicated or for those who do not wish to take estrogen, the following regimens can be used:
  1. Serotonin reuptake inhibitors, especially in women with menopausal mood disorders
  2. Depo-Provera 150 mg IM every month (may be helpful in alleviating hot flashes)
  3. Clonidine 0.05 to 0.15 mg PO daily (questionable efficacy) or transdermal clonidine patch
  4. Bellergal-S (questionable efficacy)
  5. Nonhormonal therapies for vasomotor symptoms are summarized in Box 1
- Tibolone significantly improves vasomotor symptoms, libido, and vaginal lubrication. Not available in the U.S.

CHRONIC Rx

Hormone replacement therapy should be used only for the short term unless benefits outweigh the risks of long-term use. Following the results of the Women's Health Initiative (WHI), the FDA has instituted a "black box" warning on postmenopausal hormone replacement products, suggesting that the lowest dose should be used for the shortest period of time. This necessitates a considered counseling session with patients contemplating hormone replacement prior to the initiation of therapy and then on a periodic basis after that, usually at least on a yearly basis.

DISPOSITION

If treated, the patient should have resolution of her symptoms and reduced incidence of osteoporosis. Hormonal and osteoporosis treatments available and approved for use in postmenopausal women are summarized in Box 2.

Lifelong medical supervision is necessary to monitor adequacy of treatment and prevention of complications. This should include regular Pap smears in accordance with the American Society for Colposcopy and Cervical Pathology (ASCCP) guidelines until the age of 65, pelvic examinations, breast examinations, mammography, and endometrial sampling of any type of abnormal bleeding. If untreated, the vasomotor symptoms will eventually dissipate; however, this may take several years in a small percentage of women. Some women who are in their 80s have experienced hot flashes. Urogenital atrophy will continue to worsen. Osteoporosis and coronary artery disease risks will increase with every passing year.

BOX 1 Nonhormonal Therapies for Vasomotor Symptoms

Antidepressants (SSRIs/SNRIs)
Gabapentin
Clonidine
Isoflavones, red clover, black cohosh
Cognitive behavior therapy
Acupuncture
Stellate ganglion block

From Gershenson DM et al: *Comprehensive gynecology*, ed 8, Philadelphia, 2022, Elsevier.

BOX 2 Hormonal and Osteoporosis Treatments: Available and Approved for Use in Postmenopausal Women

Estrogens

Oral
CEE, 0.3, 0.45, 0.625, 0.9, 1.25, and 2.5 mg
Piperazine estrone sulfate, equivalent of 0.625, 1.25, and 2.5 mg
Esterified, 0.3, 0.625, 0.9, 1.25, and 2.5 mg
Micronized estradiol, 0.5, 1, and 2 mg

Transdermal
Estradiol patches, 0.014, 0.025, 0.0375, 0.05, 0.75, and 0.10 mg/day
Estradiol gels, 0.25 to 1.5 mg/day various brands
Estradiol spray, 1.53 mg/day

Vaginal
Cream, CEE (0.0625%), estradiol (0.01%)
Estradiol ring, 2 mg: Release for atrophy 7.5 μg/day for 3 mo
Estradiol acetate ring for vasomotor symptoms: 50 to 100 μg/day for 3 mo
Estradiol hemihydrate (tablet) 10 μg: 1 tablet per day for 2 wk, then twice/wk
Estradiol soft gel inset, 4 μg and 10 μg: Daily use for 2 wk, then twice/wk

Parenteral
Intramuscular injections should be avoided

Progestins

Oral
Medroxyprogesterone acetate, 2.5, 5, and 10 mg
Norethindrone acetate, 5 mg
Micronized progesterone, 100 and 200 mg

Vaginal
Micronized progesterone, 100 mg
Progesterone gel, 4% and 8%

Combinations

Oral
CEE + MPA (0.625 mg) + MPA (2.5 or 5 mg)
CEE + MPA (0.3 mg + MPA, 1.5 mg)
Micronized estradiol (1 mg) + norethindrone, acetate (0.5 mg); or 0.5 mg with 0.1 orethindrone acetate
Micronized estradiol (1 mg) + 0.5 mg drospirenone; or 0.5 mg estradiol and 0.25 mg drospirenone
Ethinyl estradiol (5 μg), norethindrone acetate (1 mg or 2.5 μg), and 0.5 mg norethindrone acetate
CEE + bazedoxifene (SERM), 0.45 + 20 mg/day
Micronized estradiol (1 mg) + micronized progesterone (100 mg) in single tablet

Transdermal
Patch, 0.05 mg estradiol with 140 μg or 250 μg norethindrone acetate
Patch, 0.045 mg estradiol with levonorgestrel 0.015 mg

Androgens

Oral
Esterified estrogen and methyl testosterone (0.625/1.25 mg and 1.25/2.5 mg)

Transdermal
Patch, 150 μg/300 μg, approved outside the United States

Other Nonhormonal Products
Ospemifene (SERM), 60 mg/day for vulvovaginal atrophy
Paroxetine (SSRI), 7.5 mg/day for vasomotor symptoms

Medications for Osteoporosis

Bisphosphonates
Alendronate, 5 and 10 mg daily; 35 and 70 mg weekly
Risedronate, 5 mg; 35 mg weekly
Ibandronate, 150 mg monthly and 3l mg IV every 3 mo
Zoledronic acid 5 mg once yearly
Etidronate, 200 mg (intermittent)

Selective Estrogen Receptor Modulators (SERMs)
Raloxifene, 60 mg

Others for Osteoporosis
Tibolone, 2.5 mg (not approved in the United States)
Denosumab, 60 mg subcutaneously every 6 mo
Human parathyroid hormone 1-34; 20 μg subcutaneously daily
Romosozumab 105 mg × 2 (prefilled syringes) subcutaneously once/mo

From Gershenson DM et al: *Comprehensive gynecology*, ed 8, Philadelphia, 2022, Elsevier.

REFERRAL

Most menopausal women are managed by their gynecologists. However, this condition can be managed adequately by a primary care physician who has an interest in treating menopausal women.

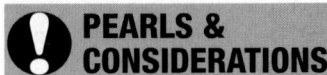 **PEARLS & CONSIDERATIONS**

COMMENTS

- Short-term risks of hormone replacement therapy (HT) include an eighteenfold increased rise for cholecystitis, three-and-a-half-fold risk of a thrombo-cardiac event in the first year, and possible increased risk of stroke and myocardial infarction.
- Results of the WHI study found that for every 10,000 women taking HT (combination of both estrogen and progesterone) for 1 yr (10,000 person-yr), seven more would have coronary events, eight would have more strokes, eight would have more pulmonary emboli, and eight would have earlier breast cancer than would 10,000 women taking a placebo. Benefits of HT were six fewer cases of colorectal cancer and five fewer hip fractures per 10,000 women.
- HT should not be initiated or continued for the primary or secondary prevention of coronary heart disease.
- Estrogen-replacement therapy should only be prescribed for patients with sufficient menopausal symptoms that impact the patient's quality of life.
- Interestingly, women who start hormone therapy early in menopause may have cardiac and other benefits. A recent trial showed that oral estradiol therapy was associated with less progression of subclinical atherosclerosis (measured as change in carotid-artery intima media thickness [CIMT]) than with placebo when therapy was initiated within 6 yr after menopause but not when it was initiated 10 or more yr after menopause. Estradiol had no significant effect on cardiac CT measures of atherosclerosis in either postmenopausal stratum.

SUGGESTED READINGS
Available at eBooks.Health.Elsevier.com.

RELATED CONTENT
Menopause (Patient Information)
Hot Flashes (Related Key Topic)
Osteoporosis (Related Key Topic)

AUTHORS: **SHANICE AKOTO, MD, MPH** and **RACHEL WRIGHT HEINLE, MD, FACOG**

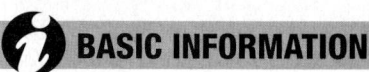 **BASIC INFORMATION**

DEFINITION

Malignant mesothelioma is a neoplasm originating from the mesothelial surfaces of the pleura, peritoneum, or pericardium with 80% cases occurring in the pleural cavity. The three major histologic subtypes are epithelial (commonest), sarcomatous, and mixed (epithelial/sarcomatous).

SYNONYM

Malignant mesothelioma

ICD-10CM CODES
C45.0	Mesothelioma of pleura
C45.1	Mesothelioma of peritoneum
C45.2	Mesothelioma of pericardium
C45.7	Mesothelioma of other sites
C45.9	Mesothelioma, unspecified

EPIDEMIOLOGY & DEMOGRAPHICS

- Associated with asbestos exposure with a latency of 20 to 50 yr.
- About 2500 new cases annually are diagnosed in the U.S. with an incidence of <1 case per 100,000 population.
- More common in men (5:1).
- Incidence of mesothelioma increases with age; median age at presentation is >70 yr.
- More than 8 million persons in the U.S. are at risk due to prior asbestos exposure.
- Family members of exposed workers have a higher risk due to cleaning of contaminated clothes, but incidence in the U.S. has leveled off due to regulation of asbestos use.

PHYSICAL FINDINGS & CLINICAL PRESENTATION

- Dyspnea
- Nonpleuritic chest pain
- Fever, weight loss, sweats, fatigue, loss of appetite
- Dysphagia, superior vena cava syndrome, Horner syndrome in advanced stages
- Auscultation may reveal unilateral loss of breath sounds
- Dullness on percussion may be present

ETIOLOGY

- Asbestos exposure (>70% of patients).
- Other reported potentially causal factors include prior radiation therapy and extravasated Thorotrast, zeolite, and erionite fibers.
- Mutations of BRCA1-associated protein 1 (BAP1) cyclin-dependent kinase inhibitor 2A gene *(CDKN2A)* have been causally linked to development of mesothelioma.

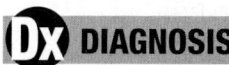 **DIAGNOSIS**

DIFFERENTIAL DIAGNOSIS

Metastatic adenocarcinomas (from lung, breast, ovary, kidney, stomach, prostate)

WORKUP

- Contrast-enhanced computed tomography (CT) of the chest and upper abdomen is recommended as the initial method of investigation.[1]
- Staging evaluation (Box 1) includes complete history (including occupational history), physical examination, and testing to determine potential operability (CT, bone scan, pulmonary function tests [PFTs]).
- Thoracoscopy, pleuroscopy, and open-lung biopsy are useful in obtaining adequate tissue samples for diagnosis.
- Pulmonary function tests.
- PET-CT scan (Figs. E1 and E2) is performed only in patients considered candidates for surgery to determine resectability.
- Staging: The tumor, node, metastasis (TNM) system categorizes mesothelioma in stages I to IV similar to that used for non–small cell lung cancer.

LABORATORY TESTS

- Diagnostic thoracentesis is generally insufficient for diagnosis because pleural effusions may only reveal atypical mesothelial cells.
- Immunohistochemistry can distinguish adenocarcinoma from malignant mesothelioma (mesotheliomas are carcinoembryonic antigen negative and cytokeratin positive).
- Thrombocytosis and anemia may be found on initial laboratory evaluation.
- Soluble mesothelin levels have been demonstrated to track with ongoing systemic therapy, but its clinical utility has not been validated.
- Serum osteopontin levels (when available) can also be used to distinguish persons with

---

BOX 1 International Mesothelioma Interest Group (IMIG) Staging System

T: Primary Tumor and Extent

T_1:
1. Tumor limited to ipsilateral parietal pleura, including mediastinal and diaphragmatic pleura; no involvement of the visceral pleura
2. Tumor involving the ipsilateral parietal pleura, including mediastinal and diaphragmatic pleura; scattered foci or tumor also involving the visceral pleura

T_2 Tumor involving each of the ipsilateral pleural surfaces (parietal, mediastinal, diaphragmatic pleura); scattered foci or tumor also involving the visceral pleura:
1. Involvement of diaphragmatic muscle
2. Confluent visceral pleura (including the fissures) or extension of tumor from visceral pleura into the underlying pulmonary parenchyma

T_3 Locally advanced but potentially resectable tumor; tumor involving all the ipsilateral pleural surfaces (parietal, mediastinal, diaphragmatic, and visceral pleura) with at least one of the following features:
1. Involvement of the endothoracic fascia
2. Extension into mediastinal fat
3. Solitary, complete resectable focus or tumor extending into the soft tissues of the chest wall
4. Nontransmural involvement of the pericardium

T_4 Locally advanced, technically nonresectable tumor; tumor involving all the ipsilateral pleural surfaces (parietal, mediastinal, diaphragmatic, and visceral pleura) with at least one of the following features:
1. Diffuse extension or multifocal mass of tumor in the chest wall, with or without associated rib destruction
2. Direct transdiaphragmatic extension of the tumor to the peritoneum
3. Direct extension of tumor to the contralateral pleura
4. Direct extension of tumor to one or more mediastinal organs
5. Direct extension of tumor into the spine
6. Tumor extending through the internal surface of the pericardium with or without a pericardial effusion or tumor involving the myocardium

N: Lymph Nodes

N_x Regional lymph nodes cannot be assessed
N_0 No regional lymph node metastases
N_1 Metastases in ipsilateral bronchopulmonary or hilar lymph nodes
N_2 Metastases in the subcarinal or the ipsilateral mediastinal lymph nodes, including the ipsilateral internal mammary nodes
N_3 Metastases in contralateral mediastinal, contralateral internal mammary, ipsilateral, or contralateral supraclavicular scalene lymph nodes

M: Metastases

M_x Presence of distant metastases cannot be assessed
M_0 No (known) metastasis
M_1 Distant metastasis present

Stage Grouping

I.
   a. $T_{1a}N_0M_0$
   b. $T_{1b}N_0M_0$
II. $T_2N_0M_0$
III. Any T_3M_0, any N_1M_0, any N_2M_0
IV. Any T_4, any N_3, any M_1

From Sellke FW et al: *Sabiston & Spencer surgery of the chest,* ed 9, Philadelphia, 2016, Elsevier.

Diseases and Disorders

I

BOX 2   Therapeutic Options for Malignant Pleural Mesothelioma

Single-Modality Therapy
- Debulking surgery (pleurectomy/decortication or extrapleural pneumonectomy)
- Radiation (external beam, brachytherapy)
- Chemotherapy (single- or double-agent approach: Doxorubicin, cyclophosphamide, cisplatinum; gemcitabine, pemetrexed, and cisplatin)

Multimodality Therapy
- Surgery and adjuvant radiation
- Surgery and adjuvant chemotherapy
- Surgery and adjuvant chemoradiotherapy

Innovative Therapies Under Investigation
- Intracavitary lavage with hyperthermic chemotherapy
- Photodynamic therapy
- Gene therapy
- Angiogenesis
- Immunogenic therapy

From Sellke FW et al: *Sabiston & Spencer surgery of the chest,* ed 9, Philadelphia, 2016, Elsevier.

exposure to asbestos who do not have cancer from those with exposure to asbestos who have pleural mesothelioma. Higher levels are correlated with a poorer prognosis.

IMAGING STUDIES
- Chest radiographs may reveal pleural plaques (Fig. E3) or calcifications in the diaphragm.
- CT scans of the chest and abdomen, bone scan, and PET scan are used to assess the stage of disease.

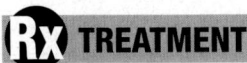 **TREATMENT**

GENERAL Rx
- Treatment is guided by staging, histologic subtype, and the patient's functional status.[1,2]
- Box 2 summarizes therapeutic options for malignant pleural mesothelioma.
- Operable patient (epithelial type, no positive nodes, confined to pleura, adequate PFTs): The two surgical techniques for therapeutic intervention are:
  1. Decortication (pleurectomy).
  2. Extrapleural pneumonectomy (EPP).
  3. With EPP, patients are eligible to be treated with either preoperative or postoperative radiation therapy to improve local control.
  4. Postoperative chemotherapy with cisplatin and pemetrexed and subsequent external-beam radiation are used with limited success.
- Inoperable patient (elderly patient, extensive disease, sarcomatous or mixed histology type, poor PFTs):
  1. Systemic therapy is administered to improve survival; supportive care is a standard option.
  2. Combined modality therapies (radiotherapy, chemotherapy, and biologic therapy) are used to reduce both local and distant recurrences.
  3. First-line chemotherapy options include the combination of cisplatin and pemetrexed with or without bevacizumab (anti-angiogenic agent).[3]

4. Dual immunotherapy with ipilimumab and nivolumab as first-line therapy in advanced mesothelioma results in a 14% improvement in 2-yr overall survival and a 4-mo improvement in median overall survival.[4]
5. The FDA has approved a device called NovoTTF-100L for first-line treatment for malignant pleural mesothelioma patients. This is based on the delivery of specific electric frequencies (tumor treating fields [TTFs]) in combination with chemotherapy, to interfere with cancer cell proliferation. The reported median overall survival was 18.2 mo with no increase in systemic toxicity with this approach.[5]
6. Improvement in survival has been shown with use of immune checkpoint inhibitors targeting the programmed death-1 (PD-1) pathway (pembrolizumab, durvalumab, nivolumab with or without ipilimumab) in patients previously treated with chemotherapy alone.
7. Patients with progressive cancer after initial chemotherapy can also be treated with single-agent chemotherapy (gemcitabine or vinorelbine).
8. Intrapleural instillation of cisplatin or biologics (e.g., interferons, interleukin-2) is generally limited to very early disease because it can penetrate to only a very limited depth of the tumor and there is a propensity of the pleural space to become progressively obliterated with advancing disease.
9. Among nonmetastatic patients who underwent nonradical lung-sparing surgery and chemotherapy, the use of radical hemithoracic radiotherapy (RHR) to the involved pleural cavity is associated with a 2-yr survivor of 58% vs. 28% in patients receiving palliative radiotherapy.[6] However, there is a major increase in pulmonary toxicity with the use of RHR.
10. ONCOS-102, an oncolytic adenovirus expressing granulocyte-macrophage colony-stimulating factor, can alter the tumor microenvironment to an immunostimulatory

state and is being evaluated in combination with chemotherapy. ONCOS-102 is well tolerated by patients, promotes a proinflammatory environment, including T-cell infiltration, and may potentially impact survival.[7]
- In advanced stages, radiation therapy is often used for palliation of local chest pain.
- Obliteration of the pleural space (pleurodesis) with instillation of talc or tetracycline into the pleural cavity is done in the treatment of recurrent symptomatic pleural effusions.
- Several biomarkers have been evaluated extensively in mesothelioma management.[8]
  1. Serum mesothelin is not sensitive or specific for diagnostic purposes, but serial measurements during chemotherapy can be useful as a monitoring tool.
  2. Recent data reveal that plasma fibulin-3 levels can distinguish healthy persons with exposure to asbestos from patients with mesothelioma. In conjunction with effusion fibulin-3 levels, plasma fibulin-3 levels can further differentiate mesothelioma effusions from other malignant and benign effusions.

DISPOSITION
- The overall prognosis of malignant mesothelioma is dismal, with a median survival of 8 mo. The 5-yr overall survival is better for patients with lower stages: Localized (20%), regional (12%), and distant (8%).
- Patients who receive trimodality therapy (surgery, radiation therapy, systemic therapy) have improved survivals of ~18 mo; however, less than 10% of cases fit in this category.
- In the U.S., age-adjusted mortality has been reduced from almost 14 deaths per 1 million persons in 2000 to 11 deaths per 1 million in 2015.[1]

! PEARLS & CONSIDERATIONS

- Patients with early disease should be referred to treatment centers specializing in multidisciplinary therapy before attempts are made to obliterate the pleural space with pleurodesis.
- Patients with advanced or resected disease should be treated with appropriate combination chemotherapy as listed previously.

REFERENCES
Available at eBooks.Health.Elsevier.com.

RELATED CONTENT
Mesothelioma (Patient Information)
Asbestosis (Related Key Topic)

AUTHOR: **BHARTI RATHORE, MD**

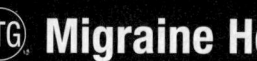

M

BASIC INFORMATION

DEFINITION

Migraine headaches are recurrent severe headaches that either are preceded by a focal neurologic symptom (migraine with aura), occur independently without preceding focal neurologic symptoms (migraine without aura), or have atypical presentations (migraine variants). The migraine aura (Box 1) typically is characterized by visual or sensory symptoms that develop over 5 to 60 min. If the aura includes unilateral motor weakness, the migraine is referred to as hemiplegic. In migraine with and without aura, the headache is typically moderate to severe, unilateral, pulsatile, made worse with head movement, and associated with nausea and vomiting, photophobia, and phonophobia. Migraines that occur $\geq$15 days every mo for $\geq$3 mo are known as chronic; otherwise, they are referred to as episodic. *Status migrainosus* (SM) is a complication of migraine with debilitating pain and associated symptoms lasting for more than 72 h. The most common triggers are stress and sleep disruption.[1]

ICD-10CM CODES
G43.909	Migraine, unspecified, not intractable, without status migrainosus
G43.1	Migraine with aura (classical migraine)
G43.0	Migraine without aura (common migraine)
G43.2	Status migrainosus
G43.3	Complicated migraine

EPIDEMIOLOGY & DEMOGRAPHICS

INCIDENCE: Increases from infancy, peaks during the third decade of life, then decreases. It is the second leading cause of years lived with disability worldwide for all ages and the leading cause in woman aged 16 to 49 yr.[2]

PREVALENCE (IN U.S.): Migraine is the third most prevalent disease in the world. Globally, it is estimated to affect 1 billion people, and it has an estimated 1-yr prevalence of approximately 12% in the general population.[3] It affects approximately 39 million people in the U.S.[4-5]

BOX 1 Auras of Migraine

Sensory phenomena
- Special senses
  1. Visual, olfactory, auditory, gustatory
- Paresthesias, especially lips and hand
Motor deficits
- Hemiparesis, hemiplegic
Neuropsychologic changes
Aphasia
Perceptual impairment, especially for size, shape, and time
Emotional and behavioral
- Anxiety, depression, irritability, (rarely) hyperactivity

From Kaufman DM et al: Kaufman's clinical neurology for psychiatrists, ed 9, Philadelphia, 2023, Elsevier.

PREDOMINANT SEX: Female:male ratio of about 3:1.[5]

PREDOMINANT AGE: Peak prevalence between ages of 18 and 49.

GENETICS: Familial predisposition: More than 50% of migraine sufferers have an affected family member.[3]
- Autosomal-dominant transmission for some rare migraine variants (familial hemiplegic migraine, cerebral autosomal-dominant arteriopathy with subcortical infarcts and leukoencephalopathy [CADASIL]); familial hemiplegic migraines have been associated with calcium channelopathy, sodium channelopathy, and Na^+/K^+-ATPase dysfunction.

PHYSICAL FINDINGS & CLINICAL PRESENTATION
- Normal exam between episodes
- Normal exam for migraine without aura
- Focal motor or sensory abnormalities (Fig. E1) possible for migraine with aura or migraine variants
- Common aura types include scintillating scotoma, bright zigzags (fortifications), and other visual distortions (Fig. E2) such as macropsia or micropsia (enlargement or shrinkage of objects) that often cross visual fields. Homonymous visual disturbance, sensory phenomena such as hemibody paresthesia, speech disturbances, or hemiparesis (familial or sporadic hemiplegic migraine) also can occur independently or associated with visual symptoms

ETIOLOGY

The pathophysiology of migraines is not clearly understood, although the primary neuronal event results in a trigeminovascular reflex causing neurogenic inflammation. Calcitonin-gene related peptide (CGRP) is released by the trigeminal ganglion and binds receptors around meningeal vessels leading to inflammation. Serotonin, substance P, and nitric oxide also play a role, but the exact mechanism is unknown. Cortical spreading depressions are likely responsible for the aura.[6]

DIAGNOSIS

Migraine without aura:[7]
- Five attacks fulfilling criteria
- Headache attacks lasting 4 to 72 h
- Headache has at least two of the following characteristics:
  1. Unilateral location
  2. Pulsating quality
  3. Moderate or severe pain intensity
  4. Aggravation or causing avoidance of routine physical activity
- At least one of the following during headache:
  1. Nausea and/or vomiting
  2. Photophobia and phonophobia
Migraine with typical aura:[7]
- At least two attacks
- Aura consisting of at least one of the following, but no motor weakness:
  1. Fully reversible visual symptoms, including positive and/or negative features
  2. Fully reversible sensory symptoms, including positive and/or negative features

3. Fully reversible dysphasic speech disturbance
- At least two of the following:
  1. Homonymous visual symptoms and/or unilateral sensory symptoms
  2. At least one aura symptom develops gradually over >5 min and/or different aura symptoms occur in succession over >5 min
  3. Each symptom lasts between 5 and 60 min
- A migraine occurring during or within 60 min of the aura

DIFFERENTIAL DIAGNOSIS
- A diagnosis of migraine is possible only after five recurrent episodes.
- The first or the worst headache should always be investigated, and the differential includes headaches from all secondary causes.
- Headache red flags can be remembered by the mnemonic SSNOOP5:
  1. S: Systemic symptoms of fever, weight loss
  2. S: Secondary risk factors of immunosuppression from any cause, cancer
  3. N: Neurologic deficits, altered consciousness
  4. O: Onset is sudden, abrupt, split second thunderclap
  5. O: Older, age >50 for new-onset headache should be worked up for giant cell arteritis
  6. P: Pattern: Change in headache pattern
  7. P: Pregnancy
  8. P: Positional or postural
  9. P: Papilledema
  10. P: Precipitation with Valsalva maneuver or exertion
- Table 1 compares tension-type and migraine headaches.
- Useful mnemonic for migraine is POUND: Pulsatile, One day in duration, Unilateral, Nausea/vomiting, Disabling.

WORKUP
- In general, no additional investigation is needed with recurrent, typical attacks with usual age of onset, family history, and a normal physical examination.
- Fundus examination is important to evaluate for the possibility of optic disk edema, which would suggest a secondary cause of headache such as idiopathic intracranial hypertension (IIH).
- If there is an unusual presentation, headache with red flags, and/or unexpected findings on examination, investigation for other causes is required including imaging.

LABORATORY TESTS

Lumbar puncture for history of abrupt-onset headaches and uncertain diagnosis of migraine

IMAGING STUDIES
- Imaging should be done in patients with any of the red flags for secondary headache, such as described by the SSNOOP5 mnemonic (see "Differential Diagnosis" above).
- MRI brain with and without contrast is the imaging modality of choice for almost all headache types, although computed tomography head without contrast may be used in the acute setting to evaluate for subarachnoid

Diseases and Disorders

I

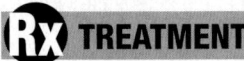

TABLE 1 Comparison of Tension-Type and Migraine Headaches

	Tension-Type	Migraine
Location	Bilateral	Hemicranial*
Nature	Dull ache	Throbbing*
Severity	Slight–moderate	Moderate–severe
Associated symptoms	None	Nausea, hyperacusis, photophobia
Behavior	Continues working	Seeks seclusion
Effect of alcohol	Reduces headache	Worsens headache

*In approximately half of patients, at least at onset.
From Kaufman DM et al: *Kaufman's clinical neurology for psychiatrists*, ed 9, Philadelphia 2023, Elsevier.

hemorrhage or other causes of acute intracranial hemorrhage.

Rx TREATMENT

Consider the use of a headache log/diary to identify triggers of headaches, record efficacy of treatments, and track history of headaches.

NONPHARMACOLOGIC THERAPY

- Avoid any identifiable provoking factors: Caffeine, tobacco, and alcohol may trigger attacks, as may dietary or other environmental precipitants (less common).
- Avoid emotional stressors and minimize variations in daily routine with regular sleep, meals, and exercise.
- Relaxation training, behavioral therapy, and biofeedback. Trials have shown that among young persons with chronic migraine, the use of cognitive-behavioral therapy (CBT) plus amitriptyline results in greater reductions in days with headaches and migraine-related disability compared with use of headache education plus amitriptyline;[8] however, overall evidence is mixed.[9]
- Trials in patients with migraine without aura have shown that acupuncture may be associated with long-term reduction in migraine recurrence.[10]

ACUTE ANALGESIC Rx (TABLE 2)

- Many oral agents are ineffective because of poor absorption from migraine-induced gastric stasis. Nonoral route of administration should be selected in patients with severe nausea or vomiting.
- An oral nonopioid analgesic is often sufficient for acute treatment of mild to moderate migrane pain without severe nausea or vomiting. NSAIDs such as ketorolac, ibuprofen, and naproxen, or combination analgesics, may be used first line for mild migraine headaches.[3,11]
- Barbiturate-containing compounds should be avoided because they are potentially addictive and promote medication overuse headaches.
- Opioids are not effective for treating patients with migraine headaches and should not be used.

ACUTE ABORTIVE Rx

- Triptans (subcutaneous [SC], PO, and intranasal) are the drug class of choice for abortive therapy. Meta-analysis suggests that 10 mg rizatriptan, 40 mg eletriptan, and 12.5 mg almotriptan are most effective. Sumatriptan may also be given, especially in combination with an NSAID, like naproxen. Early administration improves effectiveness. Triptans are relatively contraindicated in heart disease, cerebrovascular disease, and hemiplegic migraine.[2,3,11]
- Gepants (rimegepant, ubrogepant, and zavegepant): Small-molecule CGRP antagonists newly approved for acute migraine abortive therapy, especially when triptans are ineffective or contraindicated.[2,3]
- Ditans (lasmiditan): 5HT1-F agonist newly approved for acute migraine abortive therapy, especially when triptans are ineffective or contraindicated. There have been no clear cardiac risks with this class. Patients should not drive for 8 h after taking due to concern for somnolence.[2,3,12]
- Intravenous (IV) antiemetics (prochlorperazine, metoclopramide, chlorpromazine) may be used in addition to triptans. Acute dystonic reactions, QT prolongation, and akathisia are rare side effects. These are generally not used as monotherapy.
- Ergotamine, ergotamine combinations (PO/PR), and dihydroergotamine (DHE 45) (SC, IV, intramuscular [IM], intranasal) have well-documented efficacy against migraines. DHE is usually administered in combination with an antiemetic drug but cannot be given within 24 h of a triptan.
- IV dexamethasone may be used to prevent recurrence but should not be used frequently due to risk for toxicity.
- Greater and lesser occipital nerve blocks (Fig. 3) may also be performed to alleviate pain in the acute setting. These injections may be combined with auriculotemporal, supraorbital, and supratrochlear nerve block to achieve anesthesia in the area of perceived pain.

PROPHYLAXIS Rx

- Prophylactic treatment is generally indicated when headaches are disabling more than 6 days of the month, less than 5 days per mo but significantly disabling, or when symptomatic treatments are contraindicated or not effective. The goal of these medications are to reduce the frequency and intensity of the migraine attacks. All prophylaxes should be taken daily at an adequate dose for at least 3 mo before deeming the medication a failure.[13]
- Well-established options for prophylactic treatment include β-blockers (propranolol, timolol, atenolol, metoprolol), tricyclic antidepressants (amitriptyline, nortriptyline), and the antiepileptic drugs topiramate and sodium divalproate (valproic acid).[13]

- CGRP monoclonal antibodies: A new class of injectable drugs that target the CGRP molecule or its receptor.[14] There are currently four FDA-approved drugs in this class, erenumab (Aimovig, once-a-mo injection), fremanezumab (Ajovy, once-a-mo or quarterly injection), galcanezumab (Emgality, once-a-mo injection), and eptinezumab[15] (Vyepti, quarterly infusion), with more under study. These drugs can be used first line for episodic and chronic migraine but are usually used after failure of oral prophylactic treatment.[3,14]
- Gepants (rimegepant and atogepant): Small-molecule CGRP antagonist newly approved for acute migraine abortive therapy as well as prophylaxis.
- Less-established options include calcium channel blockers, selective norepinephrine serotonin reuptake inhibitors, memantine, and other antiepileptic medications.
- Supraorbital transcutaneous electrical stimulation has been approved by the FDA for prophylaxis of episodic migraine and is widely available with a prescription in Europe and North America.[16]
- For prevention of headaches in adult patients with chronic migraines only (≥15 headache days/mo for ≥3 mo), onabotulinum toxin A (Botox) injections are the only approved therapy.[17] However, prophylaxis for episodic migraine also have efficacy including topiramate as well as the CGRP injectable or oral agents.[18]

DISPOSITION

With advancing age, many patients will have sustained reduction in frequency of migraine headaches.

REFERRAL

To neurologist if uncertain about diagnosis or treatment not effective

! PEARLS & CONSIDERATIONS

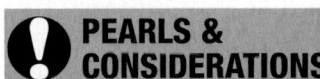

- Migraines that change in character or headaches that are different from the patient's typical ones need to be reevaluated.
- Long-term and frequent use of analgesic medications can result in medication overuse or rebound headaches. Early initiation of prophylactic medication is key.
- Avoid use of narcotics, barbiturates, and benzodiazepines because they are habit forming. Narcotics and barbiturates also promote medication overuse headaches.
- Migraine with aura is associated with an increase in stroke and thromboembolism risk and is a relative contraindication to the use of combined oral contraceptives in women.

REFERENCES

Available at eBooks.Health.Elsevier.com.

RELATED CONTENT

Migraine Headache (Patient Information)

AUTHOR: **ANJALI SUNDARAMOORTHY, DO**

TABLE 2 Selected Medications for Acute Migraine Attacks

Medication	Dosage and Route Administered	Comments
Oral Medication		
Ibuprofen	400 mg PO	Gastrointestinal upset
Naproxen sodium	500 mg PO	Gastrointestinal upset
Acetaminophen + metoclopramide	650 mg + 10 mg PO	Combination therapy has better efficacy than acetaminophen alone
Sumatriptan	50-100 mg PO	Use cautiously in patients with cardiovascular risk factors
Eletriptan	40 mg PO	Use cautiously in patients with cardiovascular risk factors
Ubrogepant	50-100 mg	May cause transaminitis
First-Line Parenteral Medication		
Prochlorperazine	10 mg IV	Sedation and dystonic reaction
Metoclopramide	10 mg IV	Dystonic reaction
Droperidol	2.5 mg IV	QT prolongation; dystonic reaction
Ketorolac	15 mg IV or 15 mg IM	Gastrointestinal upset; avoid this medication in elderly patients and in patients with renal insufficiency
Sumatriptan	6 mg SC	Chest pain, throat tightness, flushing
		Contraindicated with hypertension, coronary artery disease, peripheral vascular disease, and pregnancy
		Cannot be used within 24 h of ergot use
Second-Line Parenteral medication:		
Dihydroergotamine (DHE)	1 mg IV or IM; may be repeated in 1 h	Nausea (pretreat with antiemetic)
		Often causes chest pain
		Caution in inhibitors of enzyme CYP450 3A4
Magnesium sulfate	2 g IV	More efficacious in migraine with aura
Procedures		
Greater occipital nerve block	6 ml of bupivacaine 0.5% injected bilaterally	Can also target lesser occipital nerve
To Prevent Headache Recurrence After Emergency Department Discharge		
Dexamethasone	10 mg IV	Use cautiously in diabetics

IM, Intramuscular; *IV*, intravenous; *PO*, per os (by mouth); *SC*, subcutaneous.
From Walls RM et al: *Rosen's emergency medicine, concepts and clinical practice,* ed 10, Philadelphia, 2023, Elsevier.

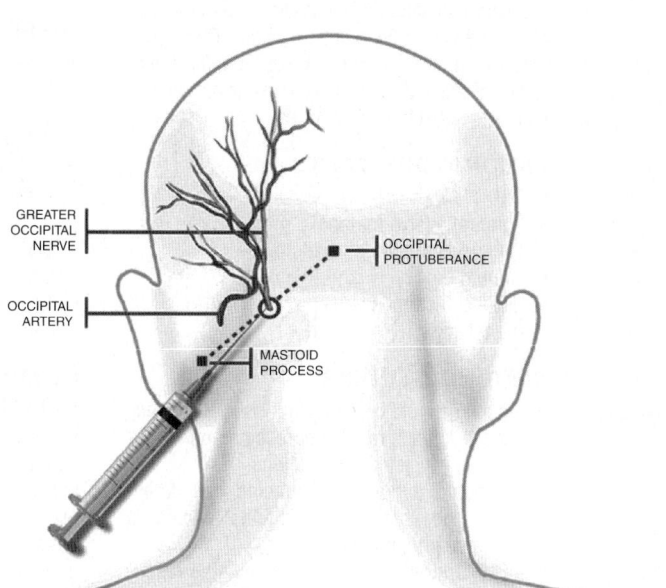

FIG. 3 Technique of greater occipital nerve block. The injector identified the appropriate location using landmarks on the patient's head. The medial landmark was the occipital protuberance. The lateral landmark was the mastoid process. Using these landmarks to form a line, the injector identified the correct location, which was one third of the distance from the occipital protuberance along this line (two thirds of the distance away from the mastoid process). The injector felt for pulsation of the occipital artery and attempted to elicit pain or paresthesia in the distribution of the GON by pressing slightly. The injector then used a fan technique, placing 1 mm of anesthetic at the correct spot, 1 mm slightly medial of the correct spot, and 1 mm slightly lateral to the correct spot. (From Walls RM et al: *Rosen's emergency medicine, concepts and clinical practice,* ed 10, Philadelphia, 2023, Elsevier.)

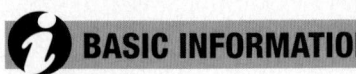 **BASIC INFORMATION**

DEFINITION

Significant cognitive impairment in the absence of dementia with preserved activities of daily living (ADLs). Mild cognitive impairment (MCI) is an intermediate state between normal cognitive function and dementia. The main distinctions between MCI and mild dementia are that in the latter, more than one cognitive domain is invariably involved and substantial interference with daily life is evident.

SYNONYMS

Mild neurocognitive disorder
MCI

ICD-10CM CODE
G31.84   Mild cognitive impairment, so stated

EPIDEMIOLOGY & DEMOGRAPHICS

INCIDENCE:
- 12 to 15 cases per 1000 person/yr age $\geq$65
- 51 to 77 cases per 1000 person/yr age $\geq$75

PREVALENCE: 15% to 25% in those older than age 70

PREDOMINANT SEX & AGE: Male, age $\geq$75

PEAK INCIDENCE: In the elderly

RISK FACTORS: Male sex, age, lower socioeconomic status, lower educational level, vascular risks (diabetes, obesity, cerebrovascular attack [CVA], myocardial infarction [MI], hypertension [HTN]), obstructive sleep apnea, depression, sedentary lifestyle.

GENETICS: *APOE4* genotype
- Various pathways result in amyloid accumulation and deposition in pre-Alzheimer presenting as MCI.

CLINICAL PRESENTATION

- Subjective memory problems, preferably corroborated by another person.
- Preserved functional status (ADLs).
- Normal general thinking and reasoning skills.
- Subtypes of MCI include amnestic (mainly involves memory loss) vs. nonamnestic with involvement of other cognitive domains (single domain vs. multiple domains).
- Domains affected in MCI include memory, visuospatial skills, learning, language, attention, and executive function.
- Olfactory dysfunction may be associated with amnestic MCI and progression to Alzheimer dementia.

ETIOLOGY

Neurodegenerative, vascular, or traumatic

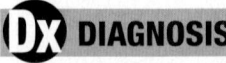 **DIAGNOSIS**

DIFFERENTIAL DIAGNOSIS

- Age-associated memory impairment (AAMI)
- Delirium
- Dementia
- Depression

- "Reversible" cognitive impairment:
  1. Medication related (anticholinergics)
  2. Hypothyroidism
  3. Vitamin B$_{12}$ deficiency
- Reversible central nervous system (CNS) conditions:
  1. Subdural hematoma
  2. Normal pressure hydrocephalus

WORKUP

HISTORY:
- Focus on specific cognitive deficits and impairment with emphasis on time course of deficits.
- Review all medications that may impact cognition (i.e., anticholinergics).
- Rule out depression and delirium.
- Perform functional assessment.
- Additional history from family members or caregivers is important.
- Assess vascular risks.
- Evaluate sleep issues and pain.
- Assess how cognitive concerns affect day to day life.

PHYSICAL EXAM:
- Check blood pressure
- Neurologic exam to rule out reversible CNS causes of cognitive impairment
- Gait and balance assessment
- Cardiovascular exam

COGNITIVE FUNCTION TESTING: Mental status testing using brief cognitive assessment tool (MOCA [Montreal Cognitive Assessment] or SLUMS [St. Louis University Mental Status] or others) followed by neuropsychologic testing if appropriate for quantifying specific deficits in cognitive domains. MOCA may be a better tool in identifying and following MCI with higher sensitivity to monitor cognitive decline in longitudinal monitoring. Neuropsychologic testing longitudinally for the first couple of years can help to determine stability vs. progression. It can establish a baseline for future testing of cognition and can help to rule out concurrent factors that impact cognition.

LABORATORY TESTS

- CBC
- Comprehensive metabolic profile
- Thyroid-stimulating hormone
- Vitamin B$_{12}$
- Syphilis testing
- HIV testing

IMAGING STUDIES

- Imaging should be performed with focal neurologic deficits, rapid progression and symptoms, or atypical presentations.
- Computed tomography imaging can detect most reversible CNS conditions leading to cognitive impairment.
- MRI is preferred and further evaluates vascular, infectious, neoplastic, and inflammatory conditions.

Rx **TREATMENT**

- There is insufficient evidence to recommend use of cholinesterase inhibitors for MCI. They

are not approved for treating MCI, have shown little efficacy in altering progression to dementia, and can have significant side effects.
- Consider treatment with these medications only if memory complaints appear to be significantly affecting day-to-day quality of life in individual patients or in amnestic subtypes of MCI after risk-vs.-benefit discussion with patient and family.
- Newer agents targeting cerebral amyloid can be considered if MCI is worked up and found to be due to pre-Alzheimer's.

NONPHARMACOLOGIC THERAPY

- Role of cognitive rehabilitation to target specific deficits.
- Regular dental exams and good dental hygiene should be encouraged. Significant periodontal disease is associated with MCI.
- Caregiver education and counseling.
- Multicomponent physical and mental exercises to maintain cognition should be recommended. Daily physical activity, at least 30 min on most days, has been shown to be beneficial in maintaining cognition. Reading and group discussion can also be beneficial.
- Address and correct hearing loss and visual impairment as best possible.
- Cognition can improve in those with obstructive sleep apnea who become compliant with continuous positive airway pressure (CPAP).
- Alcohol consumption in excess can worsen cognition.
- Aids and strategies for memory impairment are summarized in Box 1.

DISPOSITION

- Progression to Alzheimer at the rate of 5% to 15% per yr.
  1. Risk factors for progression to dementia include presence of vascular risk factors, significant cognitive impairment, depression, hearing loss, loss of smell, and presence of extrapyramidal signs.
- Mortality of those with MCI is twice that of those without MCI.
- Two- to threefold increase in risk of nursing home placement in those with MCI.

COMPLEMENTARY & ALTERNATIVE MEDICINE

No clear indications for antioxidants, and studies in humans are inconclusive. Over-the-counter herbs and supplements for memory should be discouraged, since they do not have any good evidence to prove efficacy and can have interactions and significant side effects. These agents are not FDA approved for MCI.

REFERRAL

Consider referral to a memory specialist if more than just memory is involved or for further evaluation of specific deficits.

BOX 1 Aids and Strategies for Memory Impairment

External

Reminders by Others
Tape recorder or portable voice organizer
Notes written by hand or entered into smartphone calendar

Time Reminders
Alarm clock, phone call, smartphone app
Personal organizer or diary
Calendar or wall planner
Orientation board

Place Reminders
Labels
Codes (colors, symbols)

Person Reminders
Name tags
Clothes that offer a cue

Organizers
Lists
Personal organizer or diary
Numbered series of reminders
Items grouped for use
Calendar and event alarm on smartphone or tablet

Internal
Mental retracing of events
Visual imagery
Alphabet searching
Associations to what is already recalled
Rehearsal
First-letter mnemonics
Chunking or grouping of items

From Jankovic J et al: *Bradley and Daroff's neurology in clinical practice,* ed 8, Philadelphia, 2022, Elsevier.

PREVENTION

Patients with MCI should be counseled on strategies to prevent progression to dementia. They should remain physically and mentally active, have a well-balanced diet, continue activities that are socially engaging, reduce stress in their lives, and aggressively pursue treatment of vascular risk factors.

PATIENT & FAMILY EDUCATION

- Patients with MCI typically have poor retention and rapid loss of newly learned information.
- For additional information for patients, families, and clinicians: Alzheimer's Association (https://www.alzheimers.org).

AUTHOR: **BIRJU B. PATEL, MD**

PEARLS & CONSIDERATIONS

COMMENTS

- Patients with MCI usually report short-term memory concerns such as misplacing things, not remembering names of people, word-finding difficulties, forgetting day-to-day tasks, not being able to read a book, or not being able to follow a conversation.
- Women with MCI are higher risk for progression to dementia than men.
- MCI becomes clinically relevant when quality of life is affected such as problems making financial decisions and problems with personal day-to-day interactions.
- Depression should be ruled out prior to making a diagnosis of MCI since it is highly prevalent in the elderly.
- Anticholinergic medication use should be evaluated carefully prior to making a diagnosis of MCI.

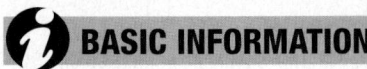

DEFINITION

Mitral regurgitation (MR) is retrograde blood flow into the left atrium resulting from any part of an incompetent mitral valve apparatus. This condition may cause left ventricular (LV) failure, as well as increased left atrial and pulmonary pressures leading to pulmonary hypertension and right-sided heart failure.

SYNONYMS

Mitral insufficiency
MR

ICD-10CM CODES	
I34.0	Nonrheumatic mitral (valve) insufficiency
I05.1	Rheumatic mitral insufficiency
I05.9	Mitral valve disease, unspecified
I05.2	Rheumatic mitral stenosis with insufficiency
Q23.3	Congenital mitral insufficiency

EPIDEMIOLOGY & DEMOGRAPHICS

Mitral regurgitation is a common valvular abnormality occurring in about 10% of the total population. The incidence of MR has increased over that past few decades. However, this may be due to increasing availability of echocardiography leading to MR diagnosis rather than to an actual increase in the prevalence of this condition.

PHYSICAL FINDINGS & CLINICAL PRESENTATION

Heart sounds:
- Diminished S1 as valve leaflets fail to coapt properly
- Widely split S2 as A2 occurs earlier because of decreased LV ejection time
- Presence of an S3 as a result of increased flow into a dilated LV caused by severe MR with systolic impairment

Heart murmurs:
- Holosystolic, high-pitched, "blowing" murmur is most easily audible at apex with radiation to base, left axilla, or back. There is a poor correlation between the intensity of the systolic murmur and the degree of regurgitation. However, an early diastolic to mid-diastolic rumble (pseudomitral stenosis) suggests severe MR. The murmur of acute MR may be short and unimpressive. This is because the sudden volume overload increases left atrial and pulmonary venous pressures leading to pulmonary congestion and hypoxia, whereas decreased blood delivery to the tissues with concomitant decrease in LV systolic pressure limits the pressure gradient driving MR to early systole.
- Hyperdynamic apex, sometimes with palpable LV lift and apical thrill.
- Symptomatic patients with MR generally present with the following:
  1. Symptoms suggestive of heart failure (fatigue, dyspnea, orthopnea, paroxysmal nocturnal dyspnea, edema)

2. Hemoptysis (caused by pulmonary hypertension)
3. Atrial fibrillation

ETIOLOGY (FIG. E1)

Primary MR:
- Idiopathic myxomatous degeneration of the mitral valve, mitral valve prolapse (most common cause of MR in industrialized countries)[1]
- Papillary muscle dysfunction or rupture (typically as a result of an inferior wall myocardial infarction)
- Ruptured chordae tendineae
- Infective endocarditis
- Calcified mitral valve annulus
- Rheumatic valvulitis (may be combined with mitral stenosis; common in developing countries)
- Systemic lupus erythematosus (Libman-Sacks endocarditis)
- Drugs: Fenfluramine, dexfenfluramine, pergolide, cabergoline
- Congenital cleft valve
- Radiation heart disease
- Ischemic MR due to papillary muscle dysfunction from multivessel coronary artery disease (CAD)

Secondary MR:
- Hypertrophic cardiomyopathy
- LV dilation (e.g., secondary to dilated cardiomyopathy)

DIAGNOSIS

DIFFERENTIAL DIAGNOSIS

- Hypertrophic cardiomyopathy
- Tricuspid regurgitation
- Aortic stenosis
- Aortic sclerosis
- Ventricular septal defect
- Atrial septal defect

WORKUP

- Diagnostic workup consists of echocardiography, ECG, and chest radiograph; cardiovascular magnetic resonance (CMR) and cardiac catheterization are sometimes needed to confirm severity of the disease.
- Brain natriuretic peptide (BNP) level may be used as a complementary tool in addition to echocardiography to identify patients who may need surgical management rather than conservative treatment. Recent studies suggest that in patients with severe asymptomatic MR, normal LV function and elevations of BNP >105 pg/ml have an independent and additive prognostic value that may identify high-risk patients and aid in the selection of patients for early surgery. However, cutoff value for BNP has not been clearly established.[2]

IMAGING STUDIES

- Echocardiography (Fig. E2): Transthoracic echocardiography (TTE) is the initial imaging modality of choice, with TEE performed if insufficient or discordant information is

obtained from TTE[3]. Findings include dilated left atrium, hyperdynamic left ventricle, erratic motion of the leaflet in patients with ruptured chordae tendineae, and color flow Doppler with evidence of MR. The most important aspect of the echocardiographic examination is the quantification of the severity of MR. A vena contracta width ≥ 0.7 cm, a regurgitant volume ≥ 60 ml, regurgitant orifice area ≥ 0.40 cm^2 by proximal isovelocity surface area (PISA), and systolic pulmonary vein flow reversal are all echocardiographic criteria of severe MR.
- Chest x-ray examination:
  1. Left atrial enlargement, LV enlargement
  2. Possible pulmonary congestion, although most often normal
- ECG:
  1. Left atrial enlargement
  2. LV hypertrophy
  3. Atrial fibrillation
- Cardiac catheterization: To confirm severity of MR, or to rule out presence of coronary artery disease in patients being evaluated for surgical replacement. Can also be considered in cases where there is discrepancy between symptomatic status and other noninvasive testing.[3]
- CMR imaging: Can be considered in cases where echocardiography is limited or LV function/dimensions are borderline, or when clinical condition and echocardiographic findings are discordant.[3]

TREATMENT[3]

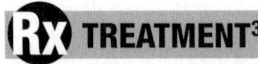

Treatments can vary depending on chronicity and the severity of MR. In chronic MR, distinguishing between primary and secondary MR is pertinent for management.

NONPHARMACOLOGIC THERAPY

- Salt restriction
- Surgical repair or replacement (see "Acute General Rx" and "Chronic Rx")

ACUTE GENERAL Rx

ACUTE MR:
- Medical Therapy:
  1. In acute MR, intravenous vasodilators (such as sodium nitroprusside or nicardipine) has shown some utility. However, the use of vasodilators is limited by hypotension with decreased peripheral resistance.
  2. Afterload reduction can also be achieved by intraaortic balloon counter pulsation. Use of percutaneous circulatory assist device can be used to establish hemodynamic stability before procedure.
- Surgical Intervention: For acute severe MR, mitral valve surgery, preferably mitral valve repair, is critical. Most patients, especially those with severe MR due to complete papillary muscle rupture, require early surgical intervention for correction of hemodynamic status and symptoms (Class I recommendation).

CHRONIC Rx

CHRONIC PRIMARY MR:

- Medical Therapy: While useful in acute severe MR, there is no evidence of vasodilator reducing severity in chronic primary MR. Guideline-directed medical therapy (GDMT) can be helpful in patients who are unable to undergo surgery to treat LV dysfunction. Stages of chronic primary mitral regurgitation are outlined in Table E1. Fig. 3 and Table E2 illustrate management strategy for intervention for primary MR.
- Surgical Intervention: Surgery is the only definitive treatment for MR. Although no randomized trial of mitral valve repair vs. replacement exists, repair is favored over replacement[4] in degenerative mitral valve disease due to its lower perioperative risk, improved event-free survival, freedom from complications of prosthetic valves, and better postoperative LV function.
- Surgery is a class I recommendation in patients with the following diagnoses:
  1. Symptomatic patients with severe primary MR irrespective of LV systolic function.
  2. Asymptomatic patients with severe primary MR and LV systolic dysfunction (left ventricular ejection fraction [LVEF] ≤60%) or progressive dilation (left ventricular end-systolic diameter [LVESD] ≥40 mm).
- Surgery is a class IIa recommendation in:
  1. Asymptomatic severe MR with normal LV systolic function (LVEF ≥60% and LVESD ≤40 mm) in whom the likelihood of successful repair without residual MR is >95% and operative mortality is <1%.
  2. Severely symptomatic patients (New York Heart Association [NYHA] class III/IV) with primary severe MR and high surgical risk, transcatheter edge to edge repair is reasonable if patient life expectancy is at least 1 yr.
- Surgery is a class IIb recommendation in:
  1. Asymptomatic patients with severe primary MR and normal LV systolic function but with progressive increase in LV size or decrease in ejection fraction (EF) on three or more serial imaging studies.
  2. Symptomatic patients with severe primary MR due to rheumatic valve disease, mitral valve repair may be considered if surgical treatment is indicated and successful repair is likely.

CHRONIC SECONDARY MR:

- Medical Therapy: Because secondary MR usually develops due to LV systolic dysfunction, GDMT is mainstay of therapy. It is often responsive to GDMT and reduces the severity of secondary MR. Coronary revascularization or cardiac revascularization can be considered. Stages of chronic secondary mitral regurgitation are outlined in Table E3. Table E4 and Fig. E4 illustrate management strategy for intervention for secondary MR.
- Surgical Intervention: In chronic secondary MR, appropriate and proper trial with GDMT is crucial before determining necessity for surgical or transcatheter interventions.
- Surgery is a class IIa recommendation in:
  1. Chronic severe secondary MR related to LV systolic dysfunction of EF <50% with persistent symptoms (NYHA class II/III/IV) while on optimal GDMT for HF. If mitral anatomy is favorable on TEE, transcatheter edge-to-edge repair (TEER) is reasonable.
  2. Severe secondary MR when coronary artery bypass graft (CABG) was undertaken for myocardial ischemia.
- Surgery is a class IIb (reasonable) recommendation in:
  1. Chronic severe secondary MR from atrial annular dilation with EF ≥50% with severe persistent symptoms (NYHA class III/IV)

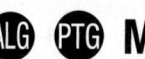

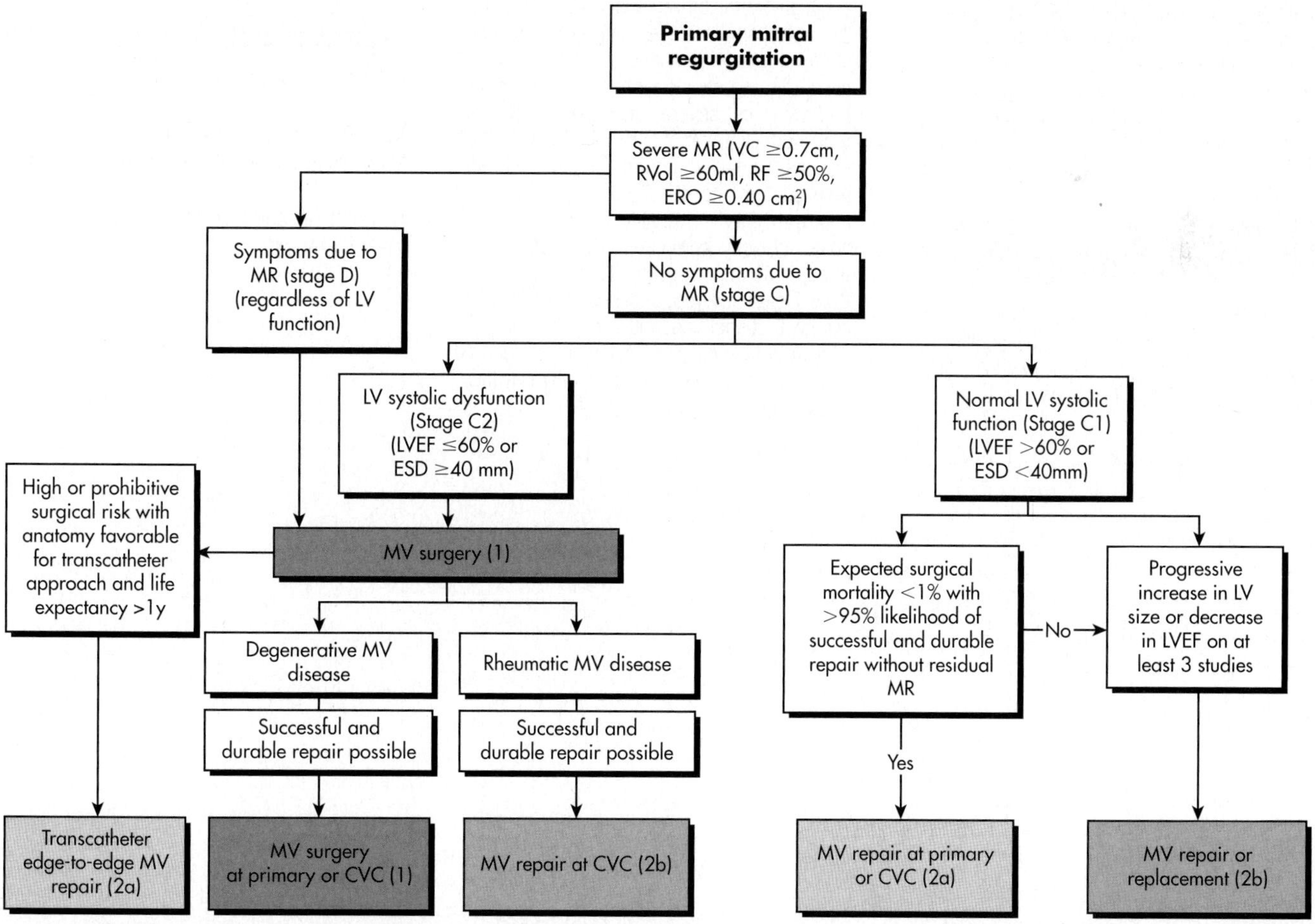

FIG. 3 Management strategy for intervention for primary mitral regurgitation. Colors correspond to Table E2. *CVC,* Comprehensive valve center; *ERO,* effective regurgitant orifice; *ESD,* end-systolic dimension; *LVEF,* ejection fraction; *MR,* mitral regurgitation; *MV,* mitral valve; *MVR,* mitral valve replacement; *RF,* regurgitant fraction; *RVol,* regurgitant volume; *VC,* vena contracta. (From Otto CM et al: 2020 AHA/ACC guideline for the management of patients with valvular heart disease: a report of the American College of Cardiology/American Heart Association Task Force on Practice Guidelines, *J Am Coll Cardiol* 77:e25-e197, 2021. In Libby P et al: *Braunwald's heart disease, a textbook of cardiovascular medicine,* ed 12, Philadelphia, 2022, Elsevier.)

despite therapy for heart failure (HF), atrial fibrillation (AF), or other comorbidities.

2. Chronic severe secondary MR with LEVF<50% and persistent severe symptoms (NYHA class III/IV) on optimal GDMT. In these patients with CAD, chordal sparing MV replacement may be reasonable over downsized annuloplasty repair.

DISPOSITION

Prognosis is generally good unless there is significant impairment of LV function or significantly elevated pulmonary artery pressures. Most patients remain asymptomatic for many years (average interval from diagnosis to onset of symptoms is 16 yr). In patients with chronic severe MR, MR is commonly progressive, with onset of other symptoms or LV dysfunction within 6 to 10 yr. However, surgery should be advised well before the onset of symptoms in case of worsening LVEF and LV systolic dimensions and presence of pulmonary hypertension or atrial fibrillation, all of which are poor prognostic signs.

REFERRAL

- Surgical referral in selected patients (see "Acute General Rx" and "Chronic Rx").
- Emergency surgery is usually necessary in patients with acute MR caused by ruptured papillary muscle or chordae tendineae after myocardial infarction.
- Mitral valve repair can also be accomplished with percutaneous implantation of a MitraClip device in patients who are too high risk for surgery.

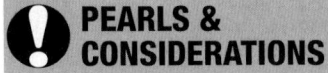

PEARLS & CONSIDERATIONS

- Medical therapy toward etiology or complications should be assessed (e.g., atrial fibrillation, ischemic heart disease, infective endocarditis, hypertension, and heart failure).

1. Control ventricular response in atrial fibrillation when rapid ventricular response is present. Use anticoagulants if atrial fibrillation occurs. Note that current guidelines do not consider atrial fibrillation in patients with MR "valvular" and nonvitamin K anticoagulation agents may be used for stroke prophylaxis.

2. Diuresis and achieving a euvolemic state may significantly decrease the degree of functional MR caused by volume overload and heart failure.

- Quantitative grading of MR is a powerful predictor of the clinical outcome of asymptomatic MR. In general, patients with regurgitant orifice areas of ≥ 40 mm^2 should be considered for prompt surgery, whereas those with orifices between 20 and 39 mm^2 can be followed closely.

- Percutaneous mitral valve repair methods are continually being investigated. The MitraClip is a catheter-delivered clip that grasps and approximates the edges of the mitral leaflets at the origin of the regurgitant jet. This device is FDA approved for use in patients with significant symptomatic degenerative or primary MR ($>3+$) who are too high risk for surgery. Transcatheter edge-to-edge repair in severely symptomatic patients with primary severe MR and high or prohibitive surgical risk has a class IIa indication. In 2019, the FDA expanded approval for symptomatic secondary or functional MR. In patients with HF and moderate-to-severe or severe secondary MR who remained symptomatic despite GDMT, TEER was safe, provided a durable reduction in MR, reduced the rate of HF hospitalizations, and improved survival, quality of life, and functional capacity compared with GDMT alone through 36 mo.[5] Secondary analysis of the COAPT data showed presence of moderate to severe tricuspid regurgitation (TR) worsened clinical outcomes and should be considered when selected patients for this minimally invasive therapy vs. surgical repair.[6]

- In 2023, follow-up of patients with HF on GDMT and severe secondary MR who underwent transcatheter edge to edge repair in the COAPT trial, continued to have lower rate of hospitalization for HF and lower all-cause mortality through 5-yr follow-up. Symptomatic improvement was also noted throughout the period with only 1.4% of the device group having device specific complications. However, adverse events continued, involving 73.6% of the device group and 91.5% of the control group either dying or being hospitalized for HF.[7]

COMMENTS

- Although vasodilators and other agents should be used to treat hypertension in patients with severe MR, there is no evidence that they will delay the need for eventual valve surgery, which is the definitive treatment for severe MR.

- In 2007, the American Heart Association guidelines for prevention of infectious endocarditis were revised, and routine antibiotic prophylaxis to undergo dental or other invasive procedures is no longer recommended, unless the patient has had prior endocarditis.

REFERENCES

Available at eBooks.Health.Elsevier.com.

RELATED CONTENT

Mitral Regurgitation (Patient Information)

AUTHORS: **HEESUNG MOON, MD** and **UYEN T. LAM, MD**

BASIC INFORMATION

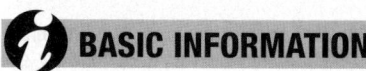

DEFINITION

Mitral stenosis (MS) is a narrowing of the mitral valve orifice that prevents proper opening during diastole and obstruction of blood flow from the left atrium to the left ventricle. Due to thickening of the leaflets, there is restricted movement. This obstruction leads to increased pressure in the left atrium, pulmonary vasculature, and the right side of the heart. The cross section of a normal orifice measures 4 to 6 cm^2. Symptoms usually develop with exercise when the orifice measures <2.5 cm^2, and symptoms may develop at rest when the orifice is <1.5 cm^2.

SYNONYM

MS

ICD-10CM CODES
I05.0	Rheumatic mitral stenosis
I05.2	Rheumatic mitral stenosis with insufficiency
I34.2	Nonrheumatic mitral (valve) stenosis
Q23.2	Congenital mitral stenosis

EPIDEMIOLOGY & DEMOGRAPHICS

- The predominant cause of mitral stenosis is rheumatic heart disease; however, the occurrence of mitral valve stenosis has decreased worldwide over the past 30 yr (particularly in developed countries) as a result of declining incidence of rheumatic fever due to appropriate antibiotic use.
- However, rheumatic heart disease remains endemic in many low and middle income countries, particularly in Africa, South Asia, East Asia, and South-East Asia.[2]
- Rheumatic heart disease has a predilection for the mitral valve, aortic valve, and to some extent the tricuspid valve.
- The incidence of MS is higher in women (2:1 female:male ratio).
- Outbreaks of rheumatic fever in the United States are due to increased virulence of a streptococcal strain or enhanced immigration from where rheumatic heart disease is prevalent.

PHYSICAL FINDINGS & CLINICAL PRESENTATION

PHYSICAL FINDINGS: "Mitral facies" that are pinkish-purple patches on the cheek due to low cardiac output and vasoconstriction usually indicate severe MS. Loud first heart sound (S1) caused by delayed valve closure preceded by an opening snap and rapid rising left ventricular (LV) pressure. A low-pitched rumbling diastolic murmur is heard best at the apex. The intensity of the murmur is not related to the severity of the stenosis, but the duration is holodiastolic in severe MS. An opening snap (OS) caused by tensing of the valve leaflets after the cusps have opened completely. The OS follows S2 by 0.03 to 0.14 sec, and the shorter the S2 to OS interval, the more severe the MS, due to the increasing left atrial pressures. A diastolic thrill may be palpable at the apex, especially with the patient in the left lateral recumbent position. A left parasternal heave secondary to right ventricular (RV) hypertrophy and pulmonary hypertension. An accentuated P2 and/or a soft, early diastolic decrescendo murmur (Graham Steell murmur) caused by pulmonary regurgitation may be present in patients with pulmonary hypertension (not specific for mitral stenosis).

SYMPTOMS & PRESENTATION:

- Dyspnea is the most common symptom, along with fatigue and decreased exercise capacity. These symptoms occur due to an inability to increase cardiac output, especially with exercise, and elevated pulmonary capillary wedge pressures, with resultant increase in pulmonary artery pressures. The stages of mitral stenosis are summarized in Table 1.
- Pregnancy in females with advanced MS may be poorly tolerated due to the 50% increase in cardiac output that occurs in pregnancy. This can often be the initial presentation of symptoms in a previously asymptomatic patient.
- Acute pulmonary edema may occur after an increase in flow across the mitral valve secondary to an increase in cardiac output or heart rate (exertion, tachyarrhythmias, fever, anemia, pregnancy etc.).
- Paroxysmal nocturnal dyspnea (PND) and orthopnea secondary to elevated left atrial pressure may occur.
- Hemoptysis can be present secondary to rupture of thin-walled dilated bronchial veins due to an abrupt increase in left atrial pressure.
- Chest pain can be caused by RV pressure overload and/or concomitant coronary artery disease in up to 15% of patients.
- Hoarseness can occur due to enlargement of the left atrium leading to compression of the recurrent laryngeal nerve.

COMPLICATIONS

- Pulmonary hypertension that results from chronically elevated pulmonary capillary wedge pressures can lead to RV dysfunction and signs and symptoms of right heart failure (hepatomegaly, pulsatile liver, peripheral edema, ascites). This is sometimes referred to the "second stenosis" of mitral stenosis.

TABLE 1 Stages of Mitral Stenosis (MS)

Stage	Definition	Valve Anatomy	Valve Hemodynamics*	Hemodynamic Consequences	Symptoms
A	At risk for MS	Mild valve doming during diastole	Normal transmitral flow velocity	None	None
B	Progressive MS	Rheumatic valve changes with commissural fusion and diastolic doming of mitral valve leaflets Planimetered MVA >1.5 cm^2	Increased transmitral flow velocities MVA >1.5 cm^2 Diastolic pressure half-time <150 msec	Mild to moderate LA enlargement Normal pulmonary pressure at rest	None
C	Asymptomatic severe MS	Rheumatic valve changes with commissural fusion and diastolic doming of mitral valve leaflets Planimetered MVA ≤1.5 cm^2	MVA ≤1.5 cm^2 Diastolic pressure half-time ≥150 msec	Severe LA enlargement Elevated PASP >50 mm Hg	None
D	Symptomatic severe MS	Rheumatic valve changes with commissural fusion and diastolic doming of mitral valve leaflets Planimetered MVA ≤1.5 cm^2	MVA ≤1.5 cm^2 Diastolic pressure half-time ≥150 msec	Severe LA enlargement Elevated PASP >50 mm Hg	Decreased exercise tolerance Exertional dyspnea

LA, Left atrial; *MVA*, mitral valve area; *PASP*, pulmonary artery systolic pressure.
*The transmitral mean pressure gradient should be obtained to determine the full hemodynamic effect of the MS and usually is greater than 5 to 10 mm Hg in severe MS; however, because of the variability of the mean pressure gradient with heart rate and forward flow, it has not been included in the criteria for severity.
From Otto CM et al: 2020 AHA/ACC guideline for the management of patients with valvular heart disease: a report of the American College of Cardiology/American Heart Association Task Force on Practice Guidelines, *J Am Coll Cardiol* 77:e25-197, 2021. In Libby P et al: *Braunwald's heart Disease, a textbook of cardiovascular medicine*, ed 12, Philadelphia, 2022, Elsevier.

- Atrial fibrillation is more prevalent in patients with more severe MS, increasing age, and other valvular abnormalities. This is classified as "valvular Afib," and current guidelines recommend anticoagulation with warfarin.
- The left ventricle is typically "protected" in mitral stenosis and exists in a low-pressure state; however, rheumatic MS often coexists with mitral regurgitation and occasionally with aortic valve dysfunction, both of which can cause LV dysfunction.
- Systemic embolic events are caused by left atrial thrombi. These are associated with atrial fibrillation 80% of the time, since mitral stenosis leads to left atrial enlargement, which is a predisposing factor for atrial arrhythmias.

RADIOGRAPHIC & HEMODYNAMIC FINDINGS

- Prominent A wave on the pulmonary capillary wedge pressure tracing. This is analogous to the prominent A wave seen in systemic venous pressure tracings with tricuspid stenosis.
- Straightening of the left heart border seen on chest radiography indicative of left atrial enlargement.
- Fig. E1 shows schematic representations of LV, aortic, and left atrial pressures, showing normal relationships and alterations with mild and severe MS.

ETIOLOGY

- Rheumatic fever (RF) is the predominant cause of MS. RF causes thickening of the leaflet tips, commissure fusion, and chordal shortening and fusion. This leads to the classic doming of the leaflets in diastole due to fusion of the leaflet tips at the commissures. Rheumatic fever involves the leaflet tips first with progression toward the annulus. This is opposite of mitral annular calcification, which typically starts in the annulus and proceeds out to the leaflet tips, leading to mitral stenosis in severe cases.
- An atrial septal defect associated with rheumatic mitral stenosis is termed *Lutembacher syndrome*. This can classically lead to right ventricular overload and right-sided heart failure.
- Parachute valve, a congenital defect, has the usual two mitral leaflets, but the chordae, instead of diverging to insert into two papillary muscles, converge into one major papillary muscle, which allows little mobility of the leaflets, as in cor triatriatum (heart with three atria), in which there is a thin membrane that obstructs the pulmonary vein flow and simulates mitral stenosis.
- Less common causes are severe mitral annular calcification usually seen in end-stage renal disease patients, endomyocardial fibroelastosis, malignant carcinoid syndrome, systemic lupus erythematosus, Whipple disease, Fabry disease, rheumatoid arthritis, 3,4-methylenedioxy-methamphetamine (MDMA) use, and significant age-related changes.

- Medications: Ergot alkaloids (methysergide and ergotamine).

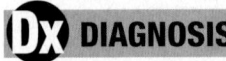

DIFFERENTIAL DIAGNOSIS

Causing similar symptoms of LV inflow obstruction
- Left atrial myxoma
- Ball valve thrombus
- Other valvular abnormalities (e.g., tricuspid stenosis, mitral regurgitation)
- Atrial septal defect

IMAGING STUDIES

- Echocardiography (Fig. E2):
  1. Two-dimensional echocardiogram can be used to measure valve area by direct planimetry or calculate it by the Doppler pressure half-time method (this may be inaccurate in patients with concomitant diastolic dysfunction, atrial septal defects, or aortic insufficiency, and those who recently have undergone mitral valvuloplasty), or the continuity equation can be used to calculate the valve area. It also can be measured using the proximal isovelocity surface area method. A valve area ≤ 1.5 cm^2 is consistent with moderate MS (and ≤ 1.0 cm^2 with severe MS). The transmitral gradient can also be calculated. A mean gradient of >10 mm Hg indicates severe MS, a gradient of 5 to 10 mm Hg is consistent with moderate MS, and 0 to 5 mm Hg is consistent with mild MS or no MS.
  2. M-Mode echocardiography will also show a markedly diminished E-to-F slope of the anterior mitral valve leaflet during diastole. There can be loss of the "A-wave" due to increased left atrial pressure or the presence of associated atrial fibrillation. There is also fusion of the commissures, resulting in "doming" of the leaflets during diastole.
  3. Grading of leaflet thickness, mobility, calcification, and subvalvular thickening (Wilkins score) with a score of 0 to 4 for each characteristic can predict hemodynamic results and outcome of balloon mitral valvuloplasty (a low score of less than 8 is favorable for balloon valvuloplasty and a high score is unfavorable). A score above 8 would favor a surgical approach. In addition, mitral regurgitation that is greater than mild would preclude a balloon mitral valvuloplasty procedure.
  4. Doppler echocardiography can be used to assess for pulmonary hypertension and to give an estimate of the pulmonary artery systolic pressure at rest and with exercise.
  5. Patients with known mitral stenosis: A follow-up echocardiography is recommended to assess for pulmonary artery pressures and valve gradient, and to determine the optimal timing of surgical or percutaneous intervention. According to the 2020 American Heart Association/American College of Cardiology (AHA/ACC)

focused valve guideline, echocardiogram is recommended every year for very severe MS with mitral valve area <1.0 cm^2, every 1 to 2 yr with severe MS with mitral valve area ≤ 1.5 cm^2, and every 3 to 5 yr with progressive MS with mitral valve area >1.5 cm^2.[1]
- Chest x-ray examination:
  1. Straightening of the left cardiac border caused by enlarged left atrium
  2. Left atrial enlargement on lateral chest x-ray examination
  3. Prominence of pulmonary arteries that indicates pulmonary hypertension
  4. Possible pulmonary congestion and edema (Kerley B lines)
- ECG:
  1. RV hypertrophy; right axis deviation caused by pulmonary hypertension
  2. Left atrial enlargement (broad, biphasic P waves in lead V1 and duration of P-waves >0.11 sec in lead II); this is termed "P-mitrale"
  3. Atrial fibrillation
- Cardiac catheterization:
  1. Measurement of pulmonary artery pressure and transmitral pressure gradients at rest or with exercise (supine biking or raising weights with arms while lying supine)
  2. Measurement of transmitral flow and calculation of the valve area
  3. Is not routinely recommended for the evaluation of MS but is useful when the echocardiographic findings are nondiagnostic or discrepant with the clinical scenario
  4. Cardiac catheterization in addition to echocardiography can be used to monitor the hemodynamics during a balloon mitral valvuloplasty procedure

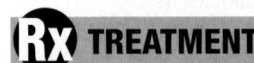

NONPHARMACOLOGIC THERAPY

Decrease level of activity in symptomatic patients, and salt restriction if pulmonary congestion is present.

ACUTE GENERAL Rx (FIG. 3)

- Medical:
  1. Anticoagulation for the prevention of systemic embolic events in patients with MS and:
     a. Atrial fibrillation: In patients with atrial fibrillation and rheumatic mitral stenosis, anticoagulation with a vitamin K antagonist with a goal international normalized ratio (INR) of 2.5 is indicated. Vitamin K antagonists remain superior to direct oral anticoagulants (DOACS) in this setting.[3]
     b. Prior embolic event.
  2. Documented left atrial thrombus or left atrial appendage thrombus.
  3. Ventricular rate control (to increase diastolic filling period) with β-blockers, non-dihydropyridine calcium channel blockers, or digitalis and aggressive treatment of tachyarrhythmias.

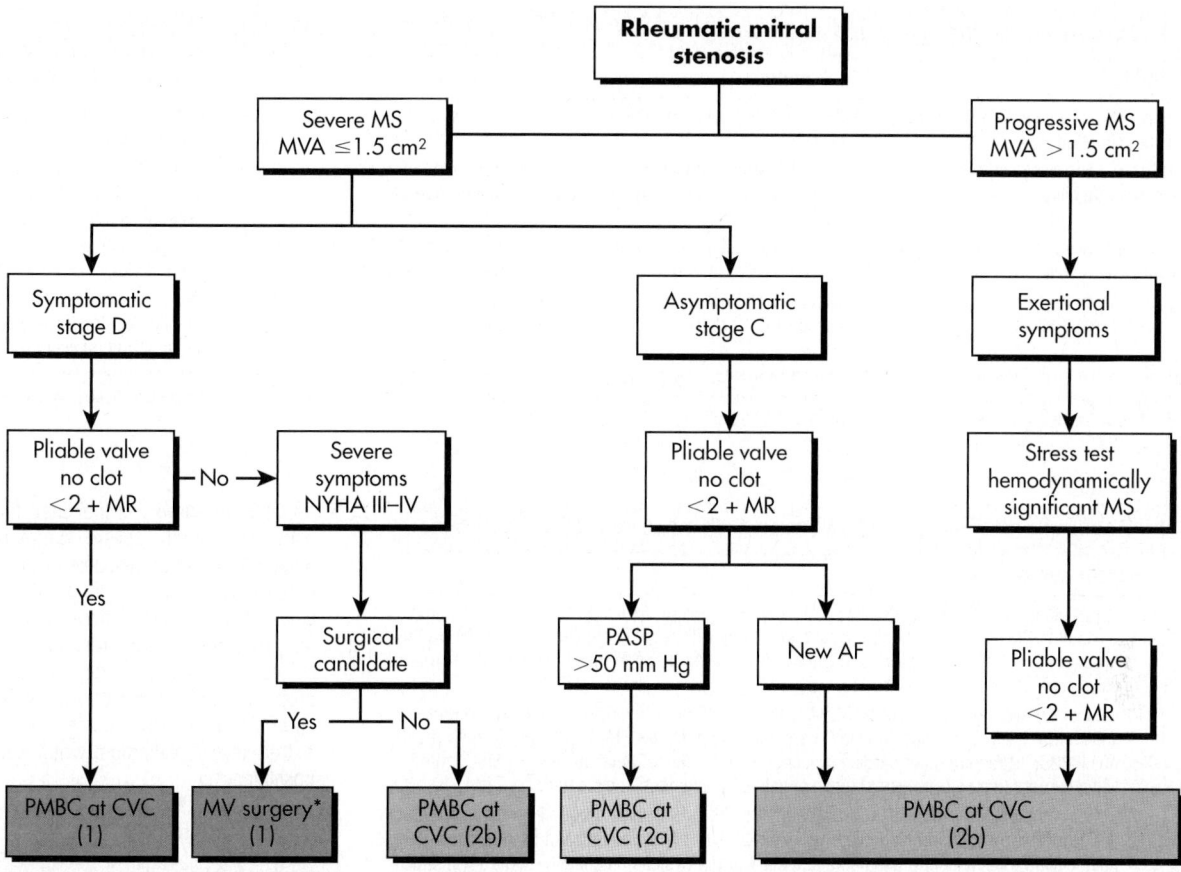

FIG. 3 **Management strategy for rheumatic mitral stenosis.** *MV surgery could be repair, commissurotomy, or valve replacement. *AF,* Atrial fibrillation; *CVC,* comprehensive valve center; *MR,* mitral regurgitation; *MS,* mitral stenosis; *MV,* mitral valve; *MVA,* mitral valve area; *NYHA,* New York Heart Association; *PASP,* pulmonary artery systolic pressure; *PMBC,* percutaneous mitral balloon commissurotomy. (From Otto CM et al: 2020 AHA/ACC guideline for the management of patients with valvular heart disease: a report of the American College of Cardiology/American Heart Association Task Force on Practice Guidelines, *J Am Coll Cardiol* 77:e25-197, 2021. In Libby P et al: *Braunwald's heart disease, a textbook of cardiovascular medicine,* ed 12, Philadelphia, 2022, Elsevier.)

4. Treat congestive heart failure with loop diuretics and sodium restriction.
5. Antibiotic prophylaxis to prevent recurrent rheumatic fever is usually not indicated unless there is presence of high-risk features such as prior endocarditis, prosthetic heart valves, valvulopathy of the transplanted heart, and certain cases of cyanotic congenital heart disease.
6. Physical activity and exercise. Patients with mild MS in sinus rhythm with a peak pulmonary artery pressure <50 mm Hg can participate in all competitive sports. Patients with moderate MS and in sinus rhythm or atrial fibrillation with a peak pulmonary artery pressure of <50 mm Hg can participate in low to moderate static and dynamic sports. Patients in sinus rhythm with severe MS should not participate in any competitive sports. Patients in atrial fibrillation with any degree of MS and on anticoagulation should avoid all competitive sports.
7. Mild to moderate MS may be tolerated in pregnancy with medical therapy alone.
• Table 2 summarizes approaches to mechanical relief of mitral stenosis.

TABLE 2 Approaches to Mechanical Relief of Mitral Stenosis

Approach	Advantages	Disadvantages
Closed surgical valvotomy	Inexpensive Relatively simple Good hemodynamic results in selected patients Good long-term outcome	No direct visualization of valve Only feasible with flexible, noncalcified valves Contraindicated with MR grade higher than 2+ Surgical procedure with general anesthesia
Open surgical valvotomy	Visualization of valve allows directed valvotomy Concurrent annuloplasty for MR is feasible	Best results with flexible, noncalcified valves Surgical procedure with general anesthesia
Valve replacement	Feasible in all patients regardless of extent of valve calcification or severity of MR	Surgical procedure with general anesthesia Effect of loss of annular-papillary muscle continuity on LV function Prosthetic valve Chronic anticoagulation
Balloon mitral valvotomy	Percutaneous approach Local anesthesia Good hemodynamic results in selected patients Good long-term outcome	No direct visualization of valve Only feasible with flexible noncalcified valves Contraindicated with MR grade higher than 2+

LV, Left ventricular; *MR,* mitral regurgitation.
From Zipes DP et al [eds]: *Braunwald's heart disease, a textbook of cardiovascular medicine,* ed 11, Philadelphia, 2019, Elsevier.

TABLE 3 Wilkins Score for Assessing Appropriateness of Percutaneous Balloon Mitral Commissurotomy

Grade	Mobility	Thickening	Calcification	Subvalvular Thickening
1	Highly mobile valve with only leaflet tips restricted	Leaflets near normal in thickness (4-5 mm)	A single area of increased echocardiographic brightness	Minimal thickening just below the mitral leaflets
2	Leaflet mid and base portions have normal mobility	Midleaflets normal, considerable thickening of margins (5-8 mm)	Scattered areas of brightness confined to leaflet margins	Thickening of chordal structures extending to one-third of the chordal length
3	Valve continues to move forward in diastole, mainly from the base	Thickening extending through the entire leaflet (5-8 mm)	Brightness extending into the midportions of the leaflets	Thickening extended to distal third of the chords
4	No or minimal forward movement of the leaflets in diastole	Considerable thickening of all leaflet tissue (>8-10 mm)	Extensive brightness throughout much of the leaflet tissue	Extensive thickening and shortening of all chordal structures extending down to the papillary muscles

Sum of the four items ranges between 4 and 16. With a score of 8 or less, percutaneous balloon mitral valvuloplasty is likely to be successful. If the score is more than 8, surgery is recommended.
From Townsend CM et al: *Sabiston textbook of surgery*, ed 21, St Louis, 2022, Elsevier.

TABLE 4 Recommendations for Intervention for Rheumatic Mitral Stenosis

COR	LOE	Recommendations
1	A	1. In symptomatic patients (NYHA Class II, III, or IV) with severe rheumatic MS (mitral valve area ≤1.5 cm², Stage D) and favorable valve morphology with less than moderate (2+) MR* in the absence of LA thrombus. PMBC is recommended if it can be performed at a comprehensive valve center.
	B-NR	2. In severely symptomatic patients (NYHA Class III or IV) with severe rheumatic MS (mitral valve area ≤1.5 cm², Stage D) who (1) are not candidates for PMBC, (2) have failed a previous PMBC, (3) require other cardiac procedures, or (4) do not have access to PMBC, mitral valve surgery (repair, commissurotomy, or valve replacement) is indicated.
2a	B-NR	3. In asymptomatic patients with severe rheumatic MS (mitral valve area ≤1.5 cm², Stage C) and favorable valve morphology with less than 2 + MR in the absence of LA thrombus who have elevated pulmonary pressures (pulmonary artery systolic pressure >50 mm Hg), PMBC is reasonable if it can be performed at a comprehensive valve center.
2b	C-LD	4. In asymptomatic patients with severe rheumatic MS (mitral valve area ≤1.5 cm², Stage C) and favorable valve morphology with less than 2f/ MR* in the absence of LA thrombus who have new onset of AF, PMBC may be considered if it can be performed at a comprehensive valve center.
	C-LD	5. In symptomatic patients (NYHA Class II, III, or IV) with rheumatic MS and a mitral valve area >1.5 cm², if there is evidence of hemodynamically significant rheumatic MS on the basis of a pulmonary artery wedge pressure >25 mm Hg or a mean mitral valve gradient >15 mm Hg during exercise, PMBC may be considered if it can be performed at a comprehensive valve center.
	B-NR	6. In severely symptomatic patients (NYHA Class III or IV) with severe rheumatic MS (mitral valve area ≤1.5 cm², Stage D) who have a suboptimal valve anatomy and who are not candidates for surgery or are at high risk for surgery, PMBC may be considered if it can be performed at a comprehensive valve center.

PMBC, Percutaneous mitral balloon commissurotomy.
*2+ on a 0 to 4+ scale according to Sellar's criteria or less than moderate by Doppler echocardiography.
From Otto CM et al: 2020 AHA/ACC guideline for the management of patients with valvular heart disease: a report of the American College of Cardiology/American Heart Association Task Force on Practice Guidelines, *J Am Coll Cardiol* 77:e25-197, 2021. In Libby P et al: *Braunwald's heart disease, a textbook of cardiovascular medicine*, ed 12, Philadelphia, 2022, Elsevier.

- Mitral valve surgery is indicated for patients with moderate to severe symptomatic MS when PMBC is not available or is contraindicated (valvuloplasty score ≤8) or the valve is calcified, when MR is more than mild, when left atrial thrombus is present, and when the surgical risk is acceptable. The surgical approaches include closed mitral valvotomy, open valvotomy and repair (preferred), and mitral valve replacement when repair is not possible.
- Table 4 summarizes guidelines for intervention for mitral stenosis.

PROGNOSIS

- Prognosis is generally good except in patients with chronic pulmonary hypertension.
- Operative mortality rates for mitral valve replacement are 1% to 5% at most institutions.

RELATED CONTENT

Mitral Stenosis (Patient Information)

AUTHORS: **VISHNU KADIYALA, MD** and **ARAVIND RAO KOKKIRALA, MD, FACC**

REFERENCES

Available at eBooks.Health.Elsevier.com.

- Percutaneous mitral balloon commissurotomy (PMBC) is the therapy of choice for symptomatic patients with severe MS (valve area ≤1.5 cm²) with a favorable valvuloplasty score (Table 3), minimal or no mitral regurgitation, and no left atrial thrombus. PMBC is reasonable for asymptomatic patients with very severe MS (mitral valve area ≤1.0 cm²) and favorable valve morphology in the absence of left atrial thrombus or moderate to severe MR (class IIa indication). PMBC is also considered the procedure of choice in pregnant women with rheumatic MS and in New York Heart Association (NYHA) class III to IV heart failure and/or unresponsive to adequate medical treatment. In addition, it may be considered for severely symptomatic (NYHA class III/IV) patients with very severe MS (mitral valve area ≤1.5 cm²) who are not candidates for surgery or are at high risk for surgery, even if they have suboptimal valve anatomy (class IIb indication). Regular follow-up is needed after PMBC because restenosis may occur. Repeat intervention can be performed as long as valve anatomy remains favorable; however, there is usually more fibrosis and deformation of the valve with subsequent procedures. The approximate frequency of repeat intervention is 10% at 7 yr.

ℹ️ BASIC INFORMATION

DEFINITION

Mitral valve prolapse (MVP) is the bulging of one or both of the mitral valve leaflets ≥2 mm above the annular plane into the left atrium during systole. MVP syndrome refers to a constellation of MVP and associated symptoms (e.g., autonomic dysfunction, palpitations) or other physical abnormalities (e.g., pectus excavatum).

SYNONYMS

MVP
Mitral click murmur syndrome
Barlow syndrome

ICD-10CM CODES
I34.1 Nonrheumatic mitral (valve) prolapse
I34.0 Nonrheumatic mitral (valve) insufficiency

EPIDEMIOLOGY & DEMOGRAPHICS[1]

- MVP is the leading cause of organic mitral regurgitation (MR). It is the most common cause of chronic primary MR in high-income countries.
- MVP can be found by echocardiogram in 2.4% of the general population with some studies suggesting that it is more common in women than in men and some studies suggesting approximately equal distribution.
- Increased incidence is seen with autoimmune thyroid disorders, Ehlers-Danlos syndrome, Marfan syndrome, osteogenesis imperfecta, pseudoxanthoma elasticum, pectus excavatum, anorexia nervosa, and bulimia.
- Compared to men, women with MVP have less posterior prolapse (22% vs. 31%), less flail (2% vs. 8%), more leaflet thickening (32% vs. 28%), and less frequent severe MR (10% vs. 23%).
- Although MVP is more common in women than men, men more often develop severe regurgitation requiring surgical intervention.

PHYSICAL FINDINGS & CLINICAL PRESENTATION

- The most common auscultatory finding in cardiac examination is a nonejection mid to late systolic click best heard at the apex. When the valve prolapses, it gets caught by the subvalvular structures, causing an abrupt halt that creates the click. It is caused by degeneration of the valve resulting in an abnormal ratio between the length of the mitral apparatus and left ventricle (LV) during contraction.
- If regurgitation is present, a crescendo mid to late systolic murmur may be heard that worsens with standing and Valsalva maneuver.
- Timing of click within the cardiac cycle varies with loading conditions within the left ventricle (i.e., may occur earlier with standing or Valsalva and later with squatting or expiration).

- May be associated with small anteroposterior chest diameter, scoliosis, pectus excavatum, or low body mass index.
- Most patients with MVP are asymptomatic; symptoms, if present, consist primarily of chest pain, palpitations, fatigue, dyspnea, and anxiety.
- Neurologic abnormalities (e.g., transient ischemic attack [TIA] or stroke) are rare.
- A spectrum of arrhythmias, mainly paroxysmal supraventricular tachycardia and atrial and ventricular premature beats, etc., is also observed with mitral valve prolapse. There is also an increased association with Wolff-Parkinson-White syndrome and QT prolongation.

ETIOLOGY[1]

- Myxomatous degeneration of connective tissue within mitral valve, usually involving multiple leaflet segments (e.g., Barlow disease). In contrast, fibroelastic deficiency of single leaflet segment (usually the middle scallop of the posterior leaflet) develops in elderly patients.
- Congenital deformity of mitral valve and supportive structures.
- Secondary to other disorders of connective tissue such as Ehlers-Danlos, Marfan, or pseudoxanthoma elasticum. Association with other connective tissue disorders suggests that MVP results from defective embryogenesis in cells of mesenchymal origin.

🔬 DIAGNOSIS

DIFFERENTIAL DIAGNOSIS

- Other valvular abnormalities (especially MR)
- Anxiety or panic disorders
- Pulmonary embolism
- Atypical chest pain

WORKUP

- Medical history and physical examination with increased suspicion in patients with other findings of connective tissue disorder.
- 2D or 3D echocardiography in patients with a systolic click or murmur on careful auscultation. 2D echocardiography is the gold standard for diagnosis of MVP.
- Cardiac MRI is an emerging tool for the evaluation and diagnosis of MVP but has not been widely used. It can identify MVP with sensitivity and specificity of 100%.[1] MRI should be considered because it may be helpful in accurately quantifying the amount of mitral regurgitation when present. ECG is most often normal but may show nonspecific ST-T wave changes, prolonged QT interval, prominent Q waves, or early repolarization with J-point elevation in young patients.

IMAGING STUDIES

Echocardiography (Fig. 1) shows one or more leaflets prolapsing >2 mm into the left atrium during systole in a long axis view. Mitral leaflets may be thickened (>5 mm) with myxomatous degeneration. MR is typically present but may only occur during late systole or with exertion. If

moderate or severe MR is present, findings of dilated left atrium, LV dilation and/or dysfunction, and elevated estimated RV systolic pressure may also be present. There is an increased incidence of secundum-type atrial septal defects (ASDs) in patients with MVP are readily identified by echocardiography.

℞ TREATMENT[2]

NONPHARMACOLOGIC THERAPY

Avoidance of stimulants (e.g., caffeine, nicotine) in patients with palpitations. Sometimes reassurance is sufficient to reduce the severity of symptoms in many patients.

ACUTE GENERAL Rx

Beta-blockers may be used in symptomatic patients (e.g., palpitations, chest pain) to decrease the heart rate and contractility, thus potentially decreasing the stretch on the prolapsing valve leaflets.

CHRONIC Rx

Monitoring for complications:
- MR (most common complication); on rare occasion may occur acutely due to rupture of chordae tendineae.
- Routine echocardiographic monitoring is indicated at the following intervals with patients with evidence of mitral regurgitation.

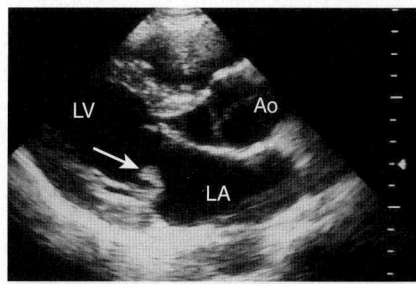
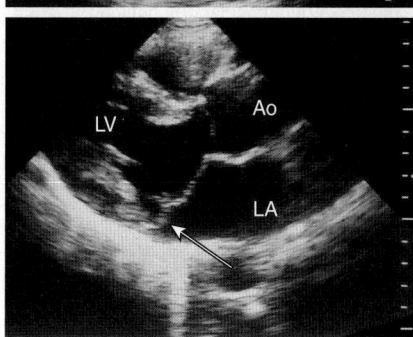

FIG. 1 Mitral valve prolapse. Parasternal long-axis view in diastole *(top)* and systole *(bottom)* in a patient with mitral valve prolapse and myxomatous changes. In the *upper panel,* note the open mitral valve and the diffuse thickening of the posterior mitral valve leaflet *(arrow).* The lower panel was recorded in systole. Note that both leaflets prolapse behind the plane of the mitral valve annulus. The prolapse of the posterior leaflet is somewhat more prominent *(arrow). Ao,* Aorta; *LA,* left atrium; *LV,* left ventricle. (From Zipes DP et al [eds]: *Braunwald's heart disease,* ed 7, Philadelphia, 2005, Saunders.)

TABLE 1   Predictors of Clinical Outcome in Mitral Valve Prolapse

Predictor	Survival	Valve Surgery	Arrhythmias or Sudden Death	Endocarditis
Age	+++	+++	−	−
Gender	++	++	−	−
Leaflet thickness or redundancy	+++	+++	++++	++++
Severity of mitral regurgitation	++++	++++	++++	++++
Systolic click	+	−	−	−
Left ventricular dilation	+	++++	++	−
Left atrial dilation	−	++	+	−

Symbols indicate the relative predictive value of each variable for the listed clinical outcomes on a scale of no predictive value (−) to strongly predictive (++++).
From Bonow RO et al: *Braunwald's heart disease, a textbook of cardiovascular medicine,* ed 12, Philadelphia, 2012, Saunders.

In addition, if there are new symptoms or change in physical examination, repeat echo may be necessary:

1. Stage B with mild regurgitation: Every 3 to 5 yr. Follow-up interval can be extended for patients who show no progression over a 10 to 15 yr period.
2. Stage B with moderate regurgitation: Every 1 to 2 yr.
3. Stage C1 (asymptomatic severe MR without LV dysfunction): Every 6 to 12 mo.
4. Stage C2 and D diseases are candidates for intervention.

- Bacterial endocarditis (risk is three to eight times that of the general population); higher risk in patients with concomitant regurgitation. However, routine antibiotic prophylaxis is not recommended.[3]
- TIA or stroke caused by embolic phenomena (from fibrin and platelet thrombi) in patients with thickened leaflets; risk in young patients is <0.05% per yr. If present, aspirin (75 to 325 mg) is indicated for secondary prevention.
- Cardiac arrhythmias with the vast majority being supraventricular and benign.
- Sudden death (rare); most often associated with acute flail leaflets or caused by ventricular arrhythmias especially ventricular fibrillation associated with other structural heart disease. There are studies suggesting that it predominantly affects young females.[4]
- The incidence of complications of MVP is very low (<1% per yr). Table 1 lists variables that are predictors of favorable clinical outcome in mitral valve prolapse.

Major predictors of outcomes were moderate or severe MR and depressed ejection fraction (EF); minor predictors were LA diameter 40 mm or greater, flail leaflet, atrial fibrillation, and age 50 yr or older.

REFERRAL

Surgical referral may be necessary in patients who develop progressive MR with surgical indications as per guidelines for valvular heart disease (see topic on "Mitral Regurgitation").

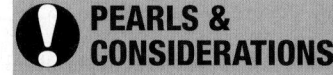 **PEARLS & CONSIDERATIONS**

COMMENTS

- Recent studies suggest that the prevalence of MVP and its propensity to cause symptoms and serious complications have been overestimated in the past.
- MVP is the most common cause of severe MR requiring surgery with 0.2% to 3.5% of patients with MVP requiring surgery at some point in their life. Less invasive percutaneous catheter procedures are now available for patients who are not candidates for surgery. It has been shown to improve quality of life and decrease rehospitalization, although survival at 1 yr did not improve.[3]
- The relationship between MVP syndrome and sudden cardiac death is unclear. The best evidence suggests that there is only a slight risk in subsets of patients with MVP who have severe MR, severe valvular deformity, complex ventricular arrhythmias, QT prolongation, and a history of syncope.
- Asymptomatic patients with MVP and mild or no MR can be evaluated clinically every 3 to 5 yr. High-risk patients (those with symptoms, arrhythmias, or significant regurgitation) should undergo a follow-up examination once a year.
- In 2007, the AHA guidelines for prevention of infectious endocarditis were revised, and prophylactic antibiotics are no longer recommended for patients with MVP without previous endocarditis.

PATIENT & FAMILY EDUCATION

https://www.themitralvalve.org

REFERENCES

Available at eBooks.Health.Elsevier.com.

RELATED CONTENT

Mitral Valve Prolapse (Patient Information)

AUTHORS: **HEESUNG MOON, MD** and **UYEN T. LAM, MD**

BASIC INFORMATION

DEFINITION

Molluscum contagiosum (MC) is a DNA poxvirus characterized by discrete skin lesions with central umbilication. It predominantly affects children.

SYNONYM

MC

ICD-10CM CODE
B08.1 Molluscum contagiosum

EPIDEMIOLOGY & DEMOGRAPHICS

- Peak occurrence ranges from 2 to 5 yr, with an estimated overall prevalence of 2.8% among children.
- The disease tends to occur in epidemics, characteristically targeting child care centers, swimming pools, and schools.
- Molluscum contagiosum spreads by autoinoculation, scratching, or touching a lesion.
- It usually occurs in young children. It is also common in sexually active adults and patients with HIV infection.
- Incubation period varies between 4 and 8 wk.
- Spontaneous resolution in immunocompetent patients can occur after several months.

PHYSICAL FINDINGS & CLINICAL PRESENTATION

- The characteristic lesions appear as flesh-colored, domed papules with central umbilication that may present anywhere on the body surface, including the genitalia in sexually active individuals. The individual lesion appears initially as a small (2 to 3 mm), flesh-colored, firm, smooth-surfaced papule with subsequent central umbilication. Lesions are frequently grouped (Fig. 1). The size of each lesion generally varies from 2 to 6 mm in diameter.
- Typical distribution in children involves the face, extremities, and trunk. Mucous membranes are spared.

- Distribution in adults generally involves pubic and genital areas (Figs. E2 and E3).
- Severe, diffuse involvement may be seen in patients with immunosuppression, including HIV infection.
- Erythema and scaling at the periphery of the lesions may be present as a result of scratching or hypersensitivity reaction.
- Lesions are not present on the palms and soles.

ETIOLOGY

Viral infection of epithelial cells caused by a poxvirus, molluscum contagiosum

DIAGNOSIS

Diagnosis is usually established by the clinical appearance of the lesions (distribution and central umbilication). A magnifying lens can be used to observe the central umbilication. If necessary, the diagnosis can be confirmed by removing a typical lesion with a curette and examining the content on a slide after adding potassium hydroxide and gentle heating. Staining with toluidine blue will identify viral inclusions.

DIFFERENTIAL DIAGNOSIS

- Verruca plana (flat warts): No central umbilication, not dome shaped, irregular surface, can involve palms and soles
- Herpes simplex: Lesions become rapidly umbilicated
- Varicella: Blisters and vesicles are present
- Folliculitis: No central umbilication, presence of hair piercing the pustule or papule
- Cutaneous cryptococcosis in AIDS patients: Budding yeasts will be present on cytologic examination of the lesions
- Basal cell carcinoma: Multiple lesions are absent
- Cellulitis

WORKUP

Careful examination of the papules

LABORATORY TESTS

Generally not indicated in children.
- Dermoscopy to confirm the presence of the characteristic amorphous, lobular, yellow central umbilication
- Methylene blue smear preparation to identify molluscum bodies
- Histopathology to identify eosinophilic intracellular inclusion bodies (Henderson–Paterson bodies)

These investigations are required only when the diagnosis is in doubt.

Screening for other sexually transmitted diseases is recommended in all cases of genital molluscum contagiosum.

TREATMENT

GENERAL Rx

- Therapy is individualized depending on number of lesions, immune status, and patient's age and preference.
- Observation for spontaneous resolution is reasonable in patients with few, small, nonirritated, and nonspreading lesions. In patients with limited disease, MC frequently resolves in months without scarring.
- Genital lesions should be treated in all sexually active patients.
- Liquid nitrogen cryotherapy.
- Carbon dioxide laser.
- Curettage after pretreatment of the area with combination prilocaine 2.5% with lidocaine 2.5% cream (EMLA) for anesthesia is useful for treatment of a few lesions. Curettage should be avoided in cosmetically sensitive areas because scarring may develop.
- Treatments with liquid nitrogen therapy in combination with curettage are effective in older patients who do not object to some discomfort.
- Application of cantharidin 0.7% to individual lesions covered with clear tape will result in blistering over 24 h and possible clearing without scarring. This medication should be avoided on facial lesions.
- Other treatment measures include use of imiquimod cream or tretinoin 0.025% gel or 0.1% cream at bedtime, daily use of salicylic acid (Occlusal) at bedtime, and use of laser therapy.
- Trichloroacetic acid peel generally repeated every 2 wk for several wk is useful in immunocompromised patients with extensive lesions.

PEARLS & CONSIDERATIONS

COMMENTS

Genital molluscum contagiosum in children may be indicative of sexual abuse.

RELATED CONTENT

Molluscum Contagiosum (Patient Information)

AUTHOR: **FRED F. FERRI, MD**

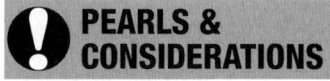

FIG. 1 Grouped molluscum. (From Kliegman, RM: *Nelson textbook of pediatrics*, ed 21, Philadelphia, 2020, Elsevier.)

Monoclonal Gammopathy of Undetermined Significance (MGUS)

BASIC INFORMATION

DEFINITION

MGUS is a premalignant disorder characterized by clonal expansion of plasma cells or lymphoplasmacytic cells. It is defined by the presence of <3 g/dl serum monoclonal (M) protein and <10% clonal plasma cells in the bone marrow.[1] In addition, there should be no end-organ damage such as hypercalcemia, renal insufficiency, anemia, or bony lesions demonstrated by skeletal surveys (Table 1).

SYNONYMS

MGUS
Light chain MGUS
Monoclonal gammopathy of unknown significance

ICD-10CM CODE
D47.2 Monoclonal gammopathy of undetermined significance (MGUS)

EPIDEMIOLOGY & DEMOGRAPHICS

INCIDENCE: In the U.S., the estimated age-adjusted incidence of MGUS is higher in men than in women. The annual incidence of MGUS in men is 120 per 100,000 at age 50 yr and increases to 530 per 100,000 at age 80 yr, whereas the incidence for women is 60 per 100,000 at age 50 yr and 370 per 100,000 at age 80 yr.[2]

PREVALENCE: MGUS is associated with increasing age; approximately 3.2% of persons older than 50 yr and 5.3% of persons older than 70 yr have an elevated M protein level without end organ dysfunction.[3] At clinical diagnosis, MGUS is most likely to have been present undetected for a median duration of >10 yr. The prevalence of MGUS is also higher in African Americans, with a twofold to threefold increase in prevalence compared with the Caucasian population.

PREDOMINANT SEX & AGE: Median age at diagnosis is about 70 yr, and the prevalence is higher in men than in women.

RISK FACTORS: Race (African American), older age, male sex, obesity, pesticide exposure, and family history of MGUS or other plasma cell disorders confer a higher risk of MGUS with a cumulative risk of progression into multiple myeloma or related disorders of approximately 1% per yr.[4] A variety of disorders (Table 2) are also associated with monoclonal gammopathy.

PHYSICAL FINDINGS & CLINICAL PRESENTATION

- MGUS typically is detected after a routine blood test reveals an elevated total protein concentration.
- Patients are mostly asymptomatic.
- Physical exam is normal.
- Increased osteoporosis and risk for fractures (relative risk of approximately 2.5).[5]
- Absolute prevalence of peripheral neuropathy <5% most commonly in IgM-MGUS.[5] A decision-making pathway in the diagnosis and management of peripheral neuropathy with MGUS is illustrated in Fig. E1.
- A twofold to threefold increased risk in bacterial and viral infections compared to normal population, which confers increased mortality.[5]
- Some patients can develop monoclonal gammopathy of renal (MGRS) or neurologic significance (MGNS), and treatment sometimes is indicated in these cases.[6,7]
  1. MGRS is typically associated with non-IgM MGUS and should be proven by a kidney biopsy. Treatment should follow myeloma or amyloidosis-targeted regimens.
  2. MGNS is associated with IgM MGUS and can be sensory, bilateral, symmetric, and length dependent. Nerve conductions studies should show demyelination, and anti-MAG antibodies can be positive in 50% of the cases. Treatment should follow Waldenström macroglobulinemia–targeted regimens.

ETIOLOGY

- The mechanism is unknown, and most cases are sporadic. The causes of malignant transformation of MGUS into multiple myeloma is still not well understood. Genetic predisposition, cytokine release, and bone marrow angiogenesis may play a role in the progression of MGUS into multiple myeloma.
- Characterized by a rearrangement of immunoglobulin (Ig) genes resulting in the production of a monoclonal protein.

DIAGNOSIS

DIFFERENTIAL DIAGNOSIS

- Smoldering myeloma (Table E3)
- Multiple myeloma
- Waldenström agammaglobulinemia
- Secondary monoclonal gammopathies
  1. Chronic liver disease
  2. Rheumatologic diseases
  3. Chronic myelomonocytic leukemia
  4. Chronic neutrophilic leukemia
  5. Lichen myxedematosus
- Pyoderma gangrenosum
- AL amyloidosis
- Idiopathic Bence Jones proteinuria

LABORATORY TESTS

- Protein studies with serum free light chain assay
- Serum protein electrophoresis (Fig. E2): IgG most common, followed by IgM and IgA
- 24-h urine protein excretion and urine electrophoresis
- Serum and urine immunofixation
- Determination of serum free light chain ratio (kappa and lambda free light chains)
- Hemoglobin
- Serum calcium and creatinine
- Bone marrow examination is unnecessary in low-risk MGUS patients (no end-organ damage, Ig gammopathy less than 1.5 g/dl, normal serum free light chain ratio)

IMAGING STUDIES

- Skeletal survey
- Bone mineral density at baseline (MGUS is associated with increased risk of osteoporosis)

TREATMENT

- Risk stratification per International Myeloma Working Group (IMWG) consensus:[8]
  1. Low risk: Serum M protein <1.5 g/dl, IgG subtype, normal genetics, free light chain ratio between 0.26 and 1.65. Absolute risk of progression (ARP) at 20 yr is 5%.
  2. Low-intermediate risk: Any 1 factor abnormal. ARP at 20 yr is 21%.
  3. High-intermediate risk: Any 2 factors abnormal. ARP at 20 yr is 37%.
  4. High risk: More than 3 factors abnormal. ARP at 20 yr is 58%.
- Follow-up by risk category: Patients should be retested within 4 to 6 mo in order to exclude evolving multiple myeloma. Low-risk MGUS patients can be followed every 1 to 2 yr, whereas those with intermediate- or high-risk MGUS need at least annual follow-up or until they develop a life expectancy–threatening condition.
- Reevaluation consists of:
  1. Serum protein electrophoresis with immunofixation
  2. 24-h urine protein excretion
  3. Serum free light chain assessment:
     a. CBC
     b. Serum creatinine and calcium
     c. Careful history and physical examination for signs and symptoms known to evolve from MGUS

DISPOSITION

- Annual risk of progression to malignancy depends on type of M protein:[9,10]
  1. Non-IgM MGUS: 1% per yr
  2. IgM MGUS: 1.5% per yr
  3. Light-chain MGUS: 0.3% per yr
- Non-IgM and light-chain MGUS tend to progress to myeloma or amyloidosis
- IgM MGUS tends to progress to Waldenström macroglobulinemia

REFERRAL

To hematologist/oncologist for evaluation

PEARLS & CONSIDERATIONS

- Approximately 55% of 70-yr-old patients diagnosed with MGUS have had the condition for more than 10 yr.
- Most patients with MGUS should be monitored every 6 to 12 mo for signs and symptoms of progression to a malignancy.
- There is no indicated treatment for asymptomatic MGUS.

REFERENCES

Available at eBooks.Health.Elsevier.com.

AUTHOR: **BHARTI RATHORE, MD**

TABLE 1 Disease Definitions for the Monoclonal Gammopathies: MGUS and Related Disorders

Type of Monoclonal Gammopathy	Premalignancy with a Low Risk of Progression (1%-2% per yr)	Premalignancy with a High Risk of Progression (10% per yr)	Malignancy
IgG and IgA (non-IgM) monoclonal gammopathies*	**Non-IgM MGUS** All 3 criteria must be met: Serum monoclonal protein <3 g/dl Clonal bone marrow plasma cells <10%, and absence of end-organ damage such as hypercalcemia, renal insufficiency, anemia, and bone lesions (CRAB) that can be attributed to the plasma cell proliferative disorder	**Smoldering multiple myeloma** Both criteria must be met: Serum monoclonal protein (IgG or IgA) ≥3 g/dl and/or clonal bone marrow plasma cells ≥10%, and absence of end-organ damage such as lytic bone lesions, anemia, hypercalcemia, or renal failure that can be attributed to a plasma cell proliferative disorder	**Multiple myeloma** All 3 criteria must be met except as noted: Clonal bone marrow plasma cells ≥10% Presence of serum and/or urinary monoclonal protein (except in patients with true nonsecretory multiple myeloma), and evidence of end-organ damage that can be attributed to the underlying plasma cell proliferative disorder, specifically Hypercalcemia: Serum calcium >11.5 mg/dl or renal insufficiency: Serum creatinine >2 mg/dl or estimated creatinine clearance <40 ml/min Anemia: Normochromic, normocytic with a hemoglobin value of >2 g/dl below the lower limit of normal or a hemoglobin value <10 g/dl Bone lesions: Lytic lesions or severe osteopenia attributed to a plasma cell proliferative disorder or pathologic fractures
IgM monoclonal gammopathies	**IgM MGUS[†]** All 3 criteria must be met: Serum IgM monoclonal protein of any level Normal bone marrow and absence of end-organ damage such as anemia, constitutional symptoms, hyperviscosity, lymphadenopathy, or hepatosplenomegaly that can be attributed to the underlying lymphoproliferative disorder	**Smoldering Waldenström macroglobulinemia** Both criteria must be met: Serum IgM monoclonal protein of any level and/or bone marrow lymphoplasmacytic infiltration of any level, and no evidence of anemia, constitutional symptoms, hyperviscosity, lymphadenopathy, or hepatosplenomegaly that can be attributed to the underlying lymphoproliferative disorder	**Waldenström macroglobulinemia** All criteria must be met: IgM monoclonal gammopathy of any level, and any level of bone marrow lymphoplasmacytic infiltration (usually intratrabecular) by small lymphocytes that exhibit plasmacytoid or plasma cell differentiation and a typical immunophenotype (e.g., surface IgM+, CD5±, CD10−, CD19+, CD20+, CD23−) that satisfactorily excludes other lymphoproliferative disorders, including chronic lymphocytic leukemia and mantle cell lymphoma Evidence of anemia, constitutional symptoms, hyperviscosity, lymphadenopathy, or hepatosplenomegaly that can be attributed to the underlying lymphoproliferative disorder. Presence of the *MYD88* L265P mutation **IgM myeloma** All criteria must be met: Symptomatic monoclonal plasma cell proliferative disorder characterized by a serum IgM monoclonal protein regardless of size Presence of 10% plasma cells on bone marrow biopsy Presence of lytic bone lesions related to the underlying plasma cell disorder and/or translocation t(11;14) on fluorescence in situ hybridization
Light-chain monoclonal gammopathies	**Light-chain MGUS** All criteria must be met: Abnormal FLC ratio (<0.26 or >1.65) Increased level of the appropriate involved light-chain (increased kappa FLC in patients with ratio >1.65 and increased lambda FLC in patients with ratio <0.26) No immunoglobulin heavy-chain expression on immunofixation Clonal bone marrow plasma cells <10%, and absence of end-organ damage such as hypercalcemia, renal insufficiency, anemia, and bone lesions (CRAB) that can be attributed to the plasma cell proliferative disorder	**Idiopathic Bence Jones proteinuria** All criteria must be met: Urinary monoclonal protein on urine protein electrophoresis ≥500 mg/24 h and/or clonal bone marrow plasma cells ≥10% No immunoglobulin heavy-chain expression on immunofixation Absence of end-organ damage such as hypercalcemia, renal insufficiency, anemia, and bone lesions (CRAB) that can be attributed to the plasma cell proliferative disorder	**Light-chain multiple myeloma[†]** Same as multiple myeloma except no evidence of immunoglobulin heavy-chain expression

*Occasionally patients with IgD and IgE monoclonal gammopathies have been described and will be part of this category as well.
†Note that conventionally IgM MGUS is considered a subtype of MGUS, and similarly light-chain multiple myeloma is considered as a subtype of multiple myeloma. Unless specifically distinguished, when the terms MGUS and multiple myeloma are used in general, they include IgM MGUS and light-chain multiple myeloma, respectively.
CRAB, Hypercalcemia, renal failure, anemia, and bone disease; *FLC*, free light chain; *Ig*, immunoglobulin; *MGUS*, monoclonal gammopathy of undetermined significance.
Modified from Rajkumar SV et al: Advances in the diagnosis, classification, risk stratification, and management of monoclonal gammopathy of undetermined significance: implications for recategorizing disease entities in the presence of evolving scientific evidence, *Mayo Clin Proc* 85:945-948, 2010.

Diseases and Disorders

I

TABLE 2 Diseases Associated with Monoclonal Gammopathy

Plasma cell and related disorders	MGUS Solitary plasmacytoma: Bone Soft tissue Multiple myeloma Waldenström macroglobulinemia Primary amyloidosis	
Lymphoid disorders	Non-Hodgkin lymphoma	Monoclonal protein observed in CLL (>20% of cases with IgM, ≈50% with IgG, light chains also observed), extranodal marginal zone lymphomas (>30% of cases and correlated with BM involvement), follicular, mantle cell, and diffuse large B-cell lymphomas also reported with serum M proteins as has AITL
	Hodgkin lymphoma	Rare but reported
	Castleman disease	<2% with monoclonal gammopathy
Other hematologic disorders	Acquired von Willebrand disease	IVIG more effective than factor concentrate in increasing factor VIII coagulant and VWF levels
	Gaucher disease	Observed in 25% in one study; M protein declined after splenectomy
	Pernicious anemia, pure RBC aplasia, hereditary spherocytosis, MPD, MDS	
Connective tissue disorders	SLE	IgG, IgM, and IgA have been observed, no difference in disease activity or outcome
	Inclusion body myositis	80% with IgG M protein
	Polymyositis, RA, scleroderma	
Neurologic disorders	POEMS syndrome	Most have M-protein of λ light chain
	Peripheral neuropathy	Most common is IgM In half, IgM protein binds to myelin-associated glycoprotein Size of M protein not correlated with severity of neuropathy Treatment with Waldenström macroglobulinemia regimens
	Myasthenia gravis, ALS, Alzheimer disease	
Dermatologic disorders	Schnitzler syndrome	Neutrophilic urticarial dermatitis, monoclonal IgM protein, and two of: Lymphadenopathy, fever, hepatosplenomegaly, joint pain, increased ESR, increased neutrophils, or abnormal bone imaging
	Scleredema	
	Pyoderma gangrenosum	Frequently an IgA protein
Infections	HIV	Both IgG and IgM M proteins observed
	HCV	M protein present in up to 10% of patients
Immunosuppression	Renal transplant	In children CMV infection associated with M protein
	Liver and heart transplant	Most patients with posttransplant lymphoproliferative disorders have M proteins
	BM transplant	Observed in both autologous and allogeneic transplants Appearance of M protein correlated with GVHD
Renal dysfunction	AL amyloidosis Monoclonal fibrillary glomerulonephritis Immunotactoid glomerulonephritis Cryoglobulinemic glomerulonephritis Light-chain proximal tubulopathy Crystal storing histiocytosis Crystal globulin glomerulonephritis Monoclonal immunoglobulin deposition disease Proliferative glomerulonephritis and monoclonal immunoglobulin deposition	Biopsy advised if acute kidney injury (AKI) stage 3, estimated glomerular filtration rate (eGFR) <60 ml/min and >2 ml/min/yr decline, proteinuria >1 g/24 h, albumin/creatinine ratio >30, Fanconi syndrome Consider biopsy if AKI stage 1 or 2, eGFR <60 ml/min and <2 ml/min/yr decline, albumin/creatinine ratio 3:30 and eGFR >60 ml/min, hematuria, and eGFR <60 ml/min, evidence of light chain proteinuria Defer biopsy if stable eGFR, bland urinalysis, no evidence of light chain proteinuria

AITL, Angioimmunoblastic T-cell lymphoma; *ALS,* amyotrophic lateral sclerosis; *BM,* bone marrow; *CLL,* chronic lymphocytic leukemia; *CMV,* cytomegalovirus; *ESR,* erythrocyte sedimentation rate; *GVHD,* graft-versus-host disease; *HCV,* hepatitis C virus; *HIV,* human immunodeficiency virus; *Ig,* immunoglobulin; *IVIG,* intravenous immunoglobulin; *MDS,* myelodysplastic syndrome; *MGUS,* monoclonal gammopathy of uncertain significance; *MPD,* myeloproliferative disorder; *POEMS,* polyneuropathy, organomegaly, endocrinopathy, monoclonal gammopathy, and skin changes; *RA,* rheumatoid arthritis; *RBC,* red blood cell; *SLE,* systemic lupus erythematosus; *VWF,* von Willebrand factor.
From Hoffman R et al: *Hematology, basic principles and practice,* ed 8, Philadelphia, 2023, Elsevier.

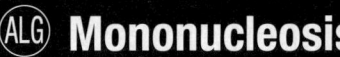
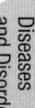

BASIC INFORMATION

DEFINITION

Infectious mononucleosis (IM) is a symptomatic infection most commonly caused by Epstein-Barr virus (EBV) and characterized by a classic triad of fever, tonsillar pharyngitis, and lymphadenopathy (predominantly cervical).[1] Fatigue is also a very common finding. IM was first coined in 1920 to describe a syndrome characterized as an acute infectious process accompanied by atypical large peripheral blood lymphocytes.

SYNONYMS

Mononucleosis
EBV
Kissing disease

ICD-10CM CODES
B27	Infectious mononucleosis
B27.0	Gamma herpesviral mononucleosis
B27.1	Cytomegaloviral mononucleosis
B27.8	Other infectious mononucleosis
B27.9	Infectious mononucleosis

EPIDEMIOLOGY & DEMOGRAPHICS

INCIDENCE (IN U.S.): 500 cases/100,000 persons/yr; worldwide, approximately 90% lifetime prevalence by age 30 yr.
PREDOMINANT SEX: Incidence is the same but occurs earlier in females.
PREDOMINANT AGE: Symptomatic infection most common between the ages of 15 and 24 yr. The age at which primary EBV infection is acquired is potentially increasing in developed countries.[2]

Young children rarely develop clinical signs of IM. Infection during childhood is more common in lower socioeconomic groups and may vary by geographic location or social factors, such as crowding, sharing a bedroom, maternal education, day care attendance, and school catchment area.

PHYSICAL FINDINGS & CLINICAL PRESENTATION

- Following an incubation period of 4 to 7 wk, there are two common presentations.[1-3] The first presentation represents the prodromal period with gradual onset of fever, chills, malaise, and anorexia for several days. This is followed by the second presentation of the classic triad of pharyngitis, fever, and lymphadenopathy. These patients often report the worst sore throat of their life. Pharyngitis (Fig. E1) is typically the most severe symptom and is characterized by white tonsillar exudates that may spread to the tongue. Up to half of patients may have palatal petechiae.
- Lymphadenopathy (nonnecrotic) can be diffuse, but most commonly occurs in both the anterior and posterior triangles of the neck.
- Splenomegaly may be palpable, most commonly during the second wk of illness. Most patients have some degree of splenomegaly on ultrasound assessment. Hepatomegaly

with some degree of hepatitis is also common. In 75% of cases there is some increase in alanine aminotransferase (ALT).[3]
- Rash (Fig. E2) is uncommon but will occur in nearly all patients who receive ampicillin or amoxicillin due to a transient penicillin hypersensitivity.
- IM is usually a self-limited illness (2 to 4 wk), but symptoms of malaise and fatigue may last months before resolving.[1]
- At times, IM can present as fever and adenopathy without pharyngitis.
- Although acute complications may be severe, they are uncommon and tend to resolve completely. Reported complications include cholestatic liver disease, chronic hepatitis, or even liver failure; hemolytic anemia; splenic rupture; or airway compromise.[3,4]
- Splenic rupture is rare, with an incidence rate <1%, but it is the most feared.[4] It should be suspected in anyone with confirmed or suspected IM who presents with acute abdominal or chest pain. Most cases occur in the first 3 wk of symptoms.
- Airway compromise, as evidenced by stridor, cyanosis, and/or tachypnea, is reported in 1% to 3% of cases and is an indication for hospitalization.
- Systemic corticosteroids are indicated for treating those at risk or with impending airway

obstruction, and usually lead to improvement in 12 to 36 h. Acute tonsillectomy may be pursued if steroids are not sufficient to mitigate the risk for obstruction.[5]
- Late complications may include lymphoproliferative cancers (Burkitt lymphoma and Hodgkin lymphoma), multiple sclerosis, rheumatoid arthritis, and chronic active EBV infection (CAEBV).[3]
- EBV may also cause hemophagocytic disease, alternatively referred to as EBV-associated hemophagocytic lymphohistiocytosis (EBV-HLH), characterized by fever, splenomegaly, and cytopenias with high ferritin and soluble CD25.
- Box 1 and Table 1 summarize the features of IM in immunocompetent patients.

ETIOLOGY

The most common cause of IM (90%) is primary infection with EBV.[1] Cytomegalovirus (CMV) is the most common cause of the other 10% of IM, but CMV infection often occurs in infancy or early childhood and is minimally symptomatic. Other causes include human herpes virus-6, herpes simplex virus-1, and HIV. Primary EBV infection during childhood also often causes few or no symptoms; persistent fatigue and recurrent/persistent fevers are the most common reasons parents bring symptomatic children to medical care.

BOX 1 Summary of Features of Infectious Mononucleosis (IM) in Immunocompetent Patients

Epstein-Barr virus (human herpesvirus-4)

Pathophysiology
- Virus enters through oropharyngeal epithelial and lymphoid cells.
- Virus attaches to CD21 on B cells.
- Viral antigens—viral capsid antigen (VCA), early antigen (EA), Epstein-Barr nuclear antigen (EBNA)—are produced and elicit antibody production.

Humoral Immune Response
- Immunoglobulin (Ig)M against VCA rises during incubation and prodrome, falls over few weeks to months.
- IgG against VCA rises during incubation, decreases during convalescence, remains detectable for life.
- Antibodies to EA rise 2-3 wk after onset of illness, then fall.
- Antibodies to EBNA rise during convalescence, detectable for life.

Cellular Immune Response
- T cells activated during second week of illness.
- CD8-positive cytotoxic T cells kill infected B cells.
- Natural killer cells kill infected B cells.
- Some resting memory B cells remain latently infected.

Clinical Features
- 4- to 7-wk incubation period
- Vague onset of symptoms
- Fever, sore throat, lymphadenopathy
- Adolescents, young adults more often symptomatic than younger children

Laboratory Features
- Leukocytosis with absolute lymphocytosis and atypical lymphocytes
- Transient monocytosis
- Relative and absolute neutropenia early on
- Mild thrombocytopenia in half of cases
- Hemolytic anemia in 1%-3% of cases, often with anti-I specificity
- Elevated transaminases in 85%-100% of cases, but clinical jaundice rare
- Spot test is simple, rapid, specific, based on agglutination of horse red blood cells (RBCs)
- Heterophil antibody (HA) test is based on differential absorption of IM-specific HA by beef RBC stroma and guinea pig kidney

From McPherson RA, Pincus MR: *Henry's clinical diagnosis and management by laboratory methods,* ed 23, Philadelphia, 2017, Elsevier.

TABLE 1 Clinical Manifestations of Infectious Mononucleosis in Children and Adults

Sign or Symptom	FREQUENCY (%)		
	Age <4 yr	Age 4-16 yr	Adults (Range)
Lymphadenopathy	94	95	93-100
Fever	92	100	63-100
Sore throat or tonsillopharyngitis	67	75	70-91
Exudative tonsillopharyngitis	45	59	40-74
Splenomegaly	82	53	32-51
Hepatomegaly	63	30	6-24
Cough or rhinitis	51	15	5-31
Rash	34	17	0-15
Abdominal pain or discomfort	17	0	2-14

From Hoffman R et al: *Hematology, basic principles and practice*, ed 7, Philadelphia, 2018, Elsevier.

EBV infects epithelial cells and resting B cells of the oropharynx. It is then found in saliva, making it transmittable through coughing, sharing drink/food, and kissing; thus the pseudonym "kissing disease." IM is more prevalent during adolescence when these types of close contact increase. How it is transmitted in younger children is less clear.

EBV levels peak during the active phase of infection but can persist in the oropharynx for up to 18 mo. Transmission may also occur sexually because EBV can be isolated in cervical epithelial cells and male seminal fluid. It has also been shown to be transmitted by blood transfusion, solid organ transplantation, or hematopoietic cell transplantation.

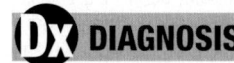 **DIAGNOSIS**

DIFFERENTIAL DIAGNOSIS
- Heterophile-negative IM caused by CMV
- Bacterial and viral causes of pharyngitis
- Toxoplasmosis
- Acute retroviral syndrome of HIV, lymphoma

WORKUP[2]

Initial testing consists of heterophile antibody (monospot) and CBC with differential. Fig. 3 illustrates the serologic evaluation of patients with clinical symptoms of acute IM and atypical lymphocytosis.

LABORATORY TESTS
- About 85% of patients with EBV-related IM will have a positive heterophile antibody test, making it the best initial test for diagnosis of EBV infection (sensitivity of 71% to 90% for diagnosing IM). However, the test has a 25% false-negative rate in the first wk of illness because the amount of heterophile antibody may not be above the limit for detection early in the disease. A negative test should be repeated if clinical suspicion is high; negative results are common in patients symptomatic for <2 wk and children <4 yr. False-positive heterophile antibody tests have been reported in other acute infections, autoimmune diseases, and cancer.
- About 10% of patients will have a persistently negative heterophile antibody test. In this event, further testing may be pursued with EBV viral capsid antigen (VCA) IgG and IgM antibody testing, as well as EBV nuclear antigen (EBNA) antibodies for staging of infection. Early diagnosis in monospot-negative cases may be made by isolating IgM to the VCA, which is usually positive during the acute illness and disappears after 4 to 6 wk. If the monospot test remains negative (without evidence of acute infection with antibody testing) for 8 wk, alternative diagnoses should be considered. The monospot usually remains positive for 3 to 6 mo but can last >1 yr.
- Increased white blood count (WBC) is common, with a relative lymphocytosis and neutropenia. Atypical lymphocytes (Fig. E4) are the hallmark of IM but are not pathognomonic. Mild thrombocytopenia is common. A falling hematocrit

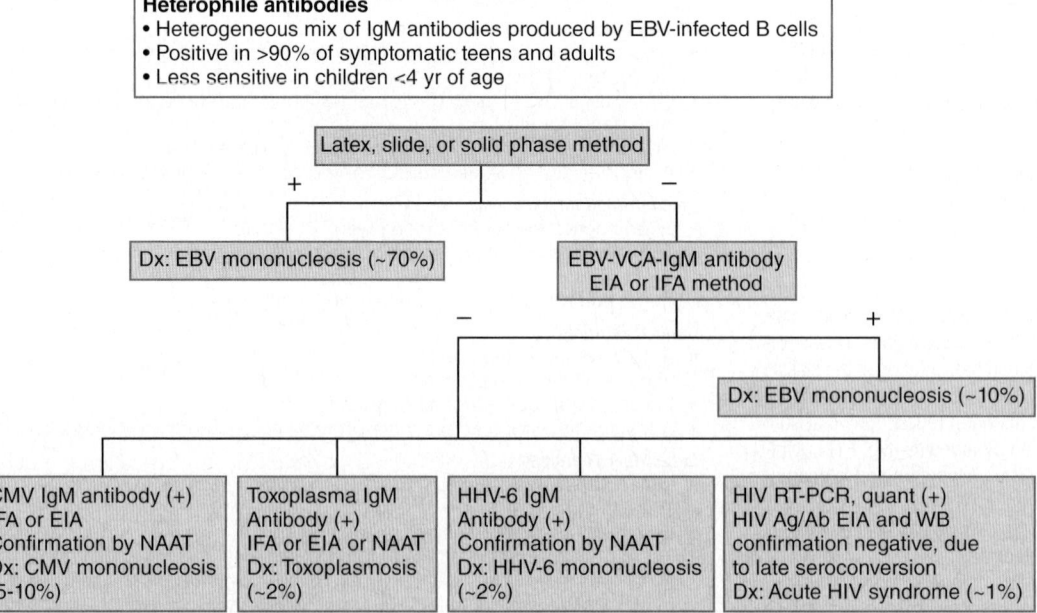

FIG. 3 Serologic evaluation of patients with clinical symptoms of acute infectious mononucleosis and atypical lymphocytosis. *Ab,* Antibody; *Ag,* antigen; *CMV,* cytomegalovirus; *Dx,* diagnosis; *EBV,* Epstein-Barr virus; *EIA,* enzyme immunoassay; *HHV-6,* human herpesvirus 6; *HIV,* human immunodeficiency virus; *IFA,* immunofluorescent assay; *IgM,* immunoglobulin M; *NAAT,* nucleic acid amplification testing; *quant,* quantitative; *RT-PCR,* reverse transcriptase polymerase chain reaction; *VCA,* viral capsid antigen; *WB,* Western blot. (From McPherson RA, Pincus MR: *Henry's clinical diagnosis and management by laboratory methods,* ed 23, Philadelphia, 2017, Elsevier.)

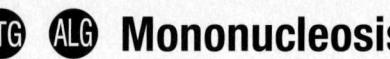

may signal splenic rupture or severe immune-mediated hemolytic anemia. Elevated hepatocellular enzymes and cryoglobulins occur in many cases.

IMAGING STUDIES

Chest x-ray examination may rarely show infiltrates. An elevated left hemidiaphragm may occur in cases of splenic rupture.

Rx TREATMENT

NONPHARMACOLOGIC THERAPY

- No specific treatment exists; focus is on supportive care and symptomatic relief with analgesics, antipyretics, and hydration. Supportive rest is advocated by some, but the effect on outcome is not clear. Prolonged rest may result in deconditioning, which may contribute to further fatigue.
- Splenectomy if rupture occurs; transfusions for severe anemia or thrombocytopenia.

GENERAL Rx

There is no role for antiviral agents such as acyclovir in the management of IM.

CHRONIC Rx

CAEBV is treated with hematopoietic cell transplantation.

DISPOSITION

Eventual resolution of all symptoms is the rule.

! PEARLS & CONSIDERATIONS

COMMENTS

- Contact sports should be avoided during the first month of illness because splenic rupture can occur during this time, even in the absence of clinically detectable splenomegaly.[3]
- Between 30% and 75% of college freshmen are seronegative for EBV. Each year nearly 20% of susceptible persons become infected, and up to 50% of these persons develop IM.
- Pharmacologic therapy, including corticosteroids, is not indicated in mild illness or for symptomatic relief. Use of corticosteroids is controversial because they may impair clearance of the viral load.
- The use of steroids, however (Fig. 5), should be considered in patients who have severe acute complications, such as thrombocytopenia, hemolytic anemia, or impending airway obstruction.

REFERENCES

Available at eBooks.Health.Elsevier.com.

RELATED CONTENT

Mononucleosis (Patient Information)
Epstein-Barr Virus Infection (Related Key Topic)

AUTHOR: **RUSSELL J. MCCULLOH, MD**

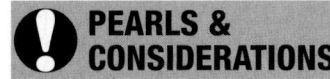

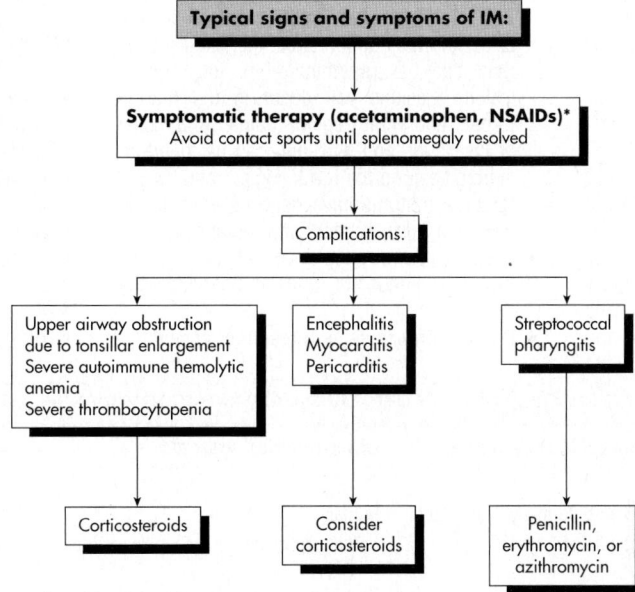

FIG. 5 Algorithm for management of infectious mononucleosis. *IM,* Infectious mononucleosis; *NSAID,* nonsteroidal antiinflammatory drug. *Consider corticosteroids in moderate/severe cases.

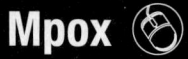

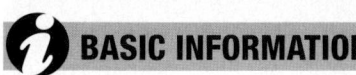 BASIC INFORMATION

DEFINITION

Mpox is a linear double-strand DNA virus approximately 250 kb in size and is of the family *Poxviridae*, subfamily *Cordopoxvirinae,* genus *Orthopoxvirus,* and species *mpox* (Table 1). The virus is considered a zoonotic disease first identified in laboratory monkeys in the 1950s. The natural hosts of mpox virus include rope squirrels, tree squirrels, Gambian pouched rats, and African dormice. In the U.S. it is commonly found in prairie dogs. There are two main clades of mpox that have been identified: Clade I (formerly Central African clade) and clade II (formerly West African clade), with the latter being the more severe form of the virus. In addition, clade II consists of two subclades, clade IIa and IIb.

SYNONYMS

MPX
MPXV
Monkeypox (former name)
Monkeypox virus (former name of virus)

ICD 10-CM CODE	
B04	Mpox

EPIDEMIOLOGY & DEMOGRAPHICS

INCIDENCE: The first case in the current outbreak was diagnosed in a[1] traveler to the U.K. from Nigeria in May 2022.
PREVALENCE: The Centers for Disease Control and Prevention (CDC) indicates a total of 30,671 cases, 46 deaths in the U.S. with 89,385 cases documented globally since the start of the current outbreak. In the U.S., more than 30,000 cases of Mpox occurred as of March 1, 2023 in an outbreak disproportionately affecting transgender, gay, and bisexual persons and other men who have sex with men.[2]
PREDOMINANT SEX & AGE: Males: Can affect any age group but typically seen in sexually active individuals
RISK FACTORS: Men who have sex with men (MSM), multiple sex partners, anonymous sex, LGBTQ+ community, close intimate contact with someone who has confirmed mpox, or coming into contact with bedding, towels, clothing, etc., that has been in contact with an infected person
GENETICS: Uncertain, but viral tropism appears to occur downstream of virus binding and entry into the cell.

PHYSICAL FINDINGS & CLINICAL PRESENTATION

- Patients can be asymptomatic during the incubation period, which can last from 3 to 17 days, and the illness typically lasts from 2 to 4 wk.
- Lesions can be firm, rubbery, deep-seated, with an umbilication at the center, and are purulent-filled. The outbreak that started in 2022 has demonstrated variations in the classical mpox appearance, including rashes that[3] can be disseminated or localized to lesions. Lesions can occur in the mouth, throat, anorectal region, palms and soles of the hands and feet, and can be found on extremities and the trunk (Figs. 1 and 2).
- Rectal symptoms have been noted, such as bloody or purulent stool and rectal pain.
- Patients can develop fever, chills, malaise, myalgias, headache, and lymphadenopathy (Fig. E3).
- Rashes sometimes are present or absent.
- Respiratory symptoms have been described, including sore throat, congestion, and cough.
- The lesions usually evolve together and progress through four stages, which include macular, papular, vesicular, and pustular before scabbing, and lesions are considered healed and noncontagious when scabs fall off and a new layer of skin has replaced the lesion.

ETIOLOGY

- Caused by the mpox virus and by coming into contact with individuals who have active mpox lesions or their bedding, towels, and clothing.
- Other modes of transmission include coming into contact with infected wildlife (Fig. E4).
- The virus gains access to the body by entering through the oropharynx, nasopharynx, or intradermal routes. Once entry is gained, the virus replicates at the site of inoculation and makes copies of itself within the cell cytoplasm upon hijacking cellular machinery; it does not enter the cell nucleus. The virus then spreads to lymph nodes and other bodily organs (Fig. E5).

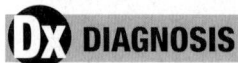 DIAGNOSIS

DIFFERENTIAL DIAGNOSIS (TABLE 2)

- Smallpox
- Syphilis (primary and secondary)
- Bacterial skin infection (cellulitis, impetigo, etc.)
- Herpes simplex virus
- Varicella
- Molluscum contagiosum
- Disseminated cryptococcal infection
- Disseminated gonococcal infection
- Scabies
- Drug eruptions

TABLE 1   Genera and Species of the Family Poxviridae, Subfamily Chordopoxvirinae, That Affect Humans

Genus and Species	Geographic Distribution	Other Infected Animals	Reservoir
Orthopoxvirus			
Variola	Eradicated (formerly worldwide)	Humans	None
Mpox	Africa (United States)*	Humans, primates, zoo animals, prairie dogs	Squirrels, dormice, Gambian giant rat, hedgehog, jerboa, opossum, woodchuck
Cowpox	Western Eurasia	Humans, cats, cows, elephants, gerbils, rats, okapi, zoo animals	Rodents (bank voles, long-tailed field mouse)
Vaccinia	Worldwide	Humans, cows, buffalo, rabbits, pigs	Most likely rodents
Parapoxvirus			
Bovine papular stomatitis	Worldwide	Humans, cows	Unknown (cows?)
Orf (contagious ecthyma, contagious pustular dermatitis)	Worldwide	Humans, sheep, goat, Artiodactyla, other ruminants	Unknown (sheep? goats?)
Pseudo-cowpox (paravaccinia, milker's nodule)	Worldwide	Humans, cows	Unknown (cows?)
Parapoxvirus of seals	Worldwide	Humans, seals	Unknown (seals?)
Parapoxvirus of reindeer	Finland	Humans, reindeer	Unknown
Molluscipoxvirus			
Molluscum contagiosum	Worldwide	Humans	Humans
Yatapoxvirus			
Tanapox	Africa	Humans, rodents	Mosquitoes(?), rodents(?)
Yabapox	Africa	Humans, primates	Unknown (primates?)
Yaba monkey tumor	Africa	Primates	Unknown

*Import of mpox to the United States with Gambian giant rats.
Adapted from Damon IK: Poxviruses. In Knipe DM, Howley PM (eds): *Field's virology*, Philadelphia, 2007, Lippincott Williams & Wilkins, pp. 2948-2975; Essbauer S et al: Zoonotic poxviruses, *Vet Microbiol* 229-236, 2009; and Breman JG: Poxviruses. In Strickland GT (ed): *Hunter's tropical medicine*, ed 8, Philadelphia, 2000, Saunders, pp. 207-210.

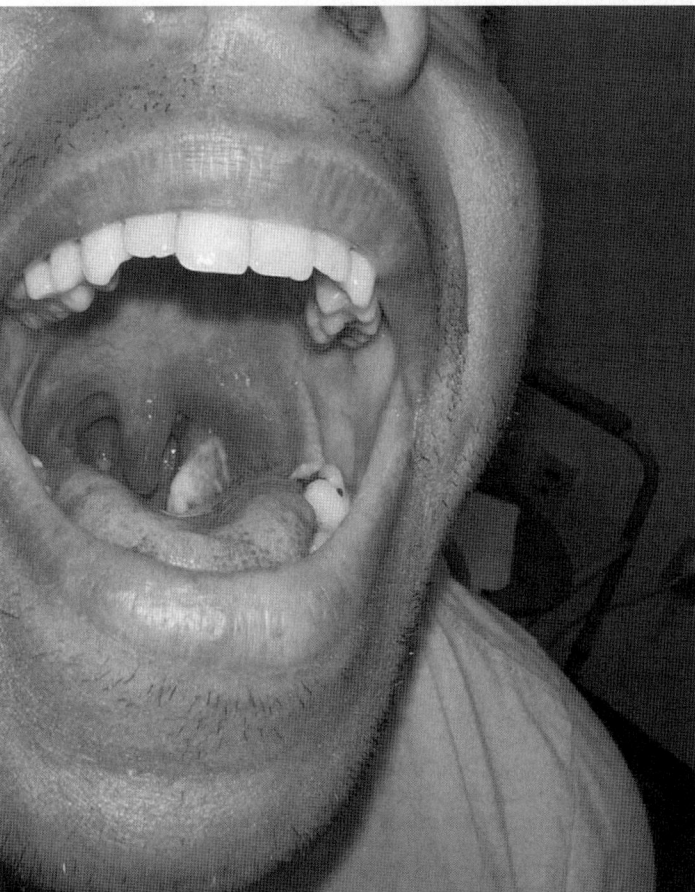

FIG. 1 Left and right tonsils with overlying purulent exudates. The left tonsil has extensive purulence, and the right tonsil has early development of lesions. (Image courtesy of Glenn Fort, MD, MPH and Frank Sanchez, MD, MBA.)

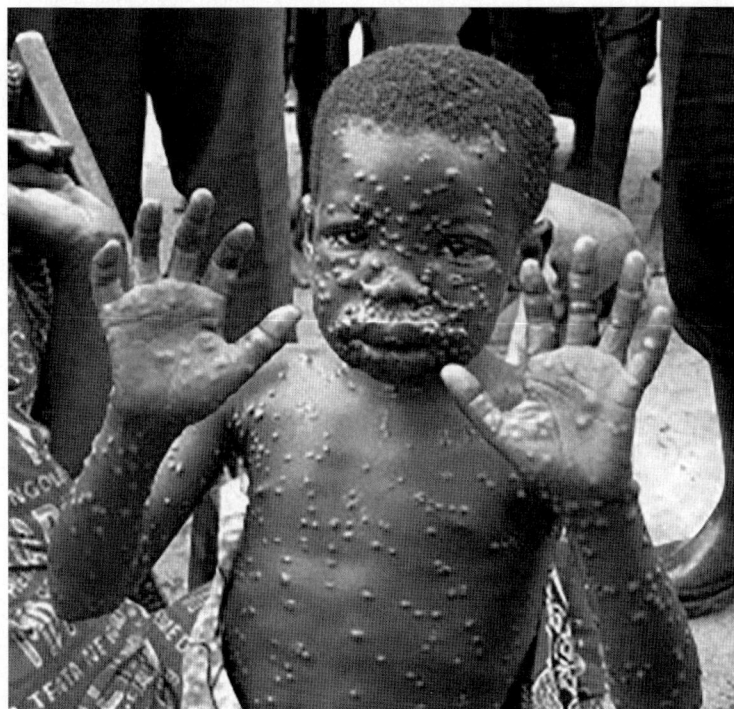

FIG. 2 Mpox. Patient with pox during a mpox outbreak in the Democratic Republic of the Congo. (From Jahrling PB. Smallpox and related orthopoxviral infections. In: Guerrant RL, et al [eds]: *Tropical infectious diseases: principles, pathogens and practice,* ed 3, Philadelphia, 2011, Saunders Elsevier, pp. 369-377.)

- Contact dermatitis/atopic dermatitis
- Measles

WORKUP

- The CDC has established case definitions for mpox to guide clinicians encountering suspected patients (Table 3).
- This includes suspecting a case in a patient who has developed a new rash or had contact with someone who had similar symptoms, is part of a high-risk population (MSM, LGBTQ+, sex worker), or has traveled to an endemic region and developed symptoms within 21 days.
- If there is high clinical suspicion of a mpox diagnosis given the above information, it is advised that individuals undergo testing and receive treatment.

LABORATORY TESTS

- Detection of *Orthopoxvirus* DNA by polymerase chain reaction testing of a clinical specimen
- Detection of *Orthopoxvirus* using immunohistochemical or electron microscopy testing methods
- Detection of mpox virus DNA by polymerase chain reaction testing or next-generation sequencing of a clinical specimen
- Isolation of mpox virus in culture from a clinical specimen
- Demonstration of detectable levels of anti *Orthopoxvirus* immunoglobin M (IgM) antibody 4 to 56 days after rash onset
- If superimposed bacterial infection is suspected, blood cultures and CBC can help determine if sepsis is occurring

IMAGING STUDIES

- Computed tomography (CT) scan head if encephalitis suspected, although this is a rare complication. Lymphadenopathy can be a prominent but nonspecific feature detected. Cutaneous lesions may be seen.
- MRI can show mpox encephalitis, with findings being diffuse edema with increased fluid-attenuated inversion recovery (FLAIR) signal in the thalamus, parietal cortex, and meningeal enhancement may be present. Other sites can be visualized as well, including the internal rectal wall.

Rx TREATMENT

ACUTE GENERAL Rx

- Typically, mpox infection is a self-limiting disease.
- Tecovirimat, aka "Tpoxx," antiviral medication
  1. 600 mg PO q12h for 14 days, 200 mg intravenous (IV) q12h treatment can be shorter depending on clinical course
- Pre-/postexposure prophylaxis
  1. Vaccination can either be given as preexposure prophylaxis or postexposure prophylaxis; if it is given as postexposure prophylaxis, it is recommended to be given with 4 to 14 days of exposure to lessen disease severity and duration.

TABLE 2 Differential Diagnosis of Mpox, Smallpox, and Chickenpox

Variable	Mpox	Smallpox	Chickenpox
Incubation period, days	7-17	7-17	12-14
Prodrome period, days	1-4	2-4	0-2
Symptom			
Fever, severity	Moderate	Severe	Mild or none
Malaise, severity	Moderate	Moderate	Mild
Headache, severity	Moderate	Severe	Mild
Lymphadenopathy, severity	Moderate	None	None
Lesions			
Depth (diameter in mm)	Superficial to deep (4-6)	Deep (4-6)	Superficial (2-4)
Distribution	Centrifugal (mainly)	Centrifugal	Centripetal
Evaluation	Homogeneous rash	Homogeneous rash	Heterogeneous rash
Time to desquamation, days	14-21	14-21	6-14
Frequency of lesions on palms or soles of feet	Common	Common	Rare

From Nalca A, et al: Reemergence of monkeypox: prevalence, diagnostics, and countermeasures, *Clin Infect Dis* 41:1765-1771, 2005.

2. Two vaccines are available in the U.S: Jynneos and ACAM2000.
3. ACAM200 is a live replication competent smallpox vaccine used only in a select group of patients and is associated with more adverse effects. Use of this vaccine is contraindicated in immunosuppressed populations.
4. Modified Vaccinia Ankara (MVA) Jynneos is a live, attenuated nonreplicating vaccinia virus given in two doses that are spaced 28 days apart and injected into the triceps of the arm. Recently, the CDC has recommended switching the site of injection to intradermally in the forearm to allow for a much lower volume injected than the subcutaneous route, in order to provide more vaccine to the population.
5. Tpoxx can be used for postexposure prophylaxis in patients unable to receive vaccination.
6. Trifluridine Ophthalmic Solution (Viroptic): Q4h for 7 to 10 days has been used off-label for ocular complications due to mpox.

DISPOSITION

Patients usually have a self-limiting course, and recover completely without any long-term sequelae. Scarring has been noted following some lesions. Mortality has been estimated to be 1% to 4% with common causes of death being bacterial superinfection of lesions.

REFERRAL

- To the local/state Department of Health with suspected cases and vaccination
- Infectious diseases consultant for guidance on oral therapy and vaccination

! PEARLS & CONSIDERATIONS

COMMENTS

- Be sure to inquire about sexual and travel history, as this information will help significantly in guiding the clinician to the correct diagnosis.

- Be aware that there is considerable overlap with common rashes and sexually transmitted infections, such as syphilis.
- There are now cases that have involved children, likely through skin-to-skin contact with infected individuals.
- In November 2022, the World Health Organization (WHO) renamed monkeypox to Mpox citing racist stigma that came with name monkeypox. The WHO anticipated phasing out the original name in 1 yr.

INFECTION PREVENTION & CONTROL

- Individuals with mpox should quarantine from others until all lesions have scabbed and fallen off and a new layer of skin has grown over the lesion(s); this can be anywhere from 2 to 4 wk.
- Vaccination with the Jynneos vaccine is recommended for all men who have sex with men.
- The WHO recommends consistent condom use during any sexual activity for 12 wk following recovery.
- Individuals with mpox should also quarantine from their pets as there have been recent reports of pets becoming infected with mpox from their owners.
- Standard precautions are advised when interacting with infected patients, which includes gowns, gloves, and protective eyewear.
- Infected patients who are hospitalized should be placed in a single room with a private restroom.

PATIENT & FAMILY EDUCATION

- Avoid close intimate contact with individuals suspected of mpox infection and their clothing, bed coverings, and surfaces that have been exposed to their lesions.
- Patients with multiple sex partners and individuals of the LGBTQ+ community appear to be affected in higher proportions than other individuals (over 90% of cases in the 2022 outbreak); however, this is a disease that can affect all populations.
- The role of sexual transmission of mpox virus is still being evaluated.

TABLE 3 2022 Centers for Disease Control and Prevention Case Definition for Mpox

Clinical Criteria

A person presenting with new onset of:
- Clinically compatible rash lesions*; OR
- Lymphadenopathy or fever**

Laboratory Criteria

Confirmatory laboratory evidence:
- Detection of mpox virus nucleic acid by molecular testing in a clinical specimen; OR
- Detection of mpox virus by genomic sequencing in a clinical specimen.

Presumptive laboratory evidence:
- Detection of orthopoxvirus nucleic acid by molecular testing in a clinical specimen AND no laboratory evidence of infection with another non-variola orthopoxvirus; OR
- Detection of presence of orthopoxvirus by immunohistochemistry in tissue; OR
- Detection of orthopoxvirus by genomic sequencing in a clinical specimen; OR
- Detection of anti-orthopoxvirus Immunoglobulin M (IgM) antibody using a validated assay on a serum sample drawn 4-56 days after rash onset, with no recent history (last 60 days) of vaccination***.

Supportive laboratory evidence:
N/A

Epidemiologic Linkage

Epidemiologic risk factors within 21 days of illness onset:
- Higher Risk Epidemiologic Linkages
  1. Contact, without the use of appropriate personal protective equipment (PPE)‡, with a person or animal with a known orthopoxvirus or mpox virus infection; OR
  2. Contact, without the use of appropriate PPE‡ or Biosafety Level (BSL) protocols‡, with laboratory specimens or other items that could serve as fomites that have been in contact with a person or animal with a known orthopoxvirus or mpox virus infection; OR
  3. Member of an exposed cohort as defined by public health authorities experiencing an outbreak (e.g., participated in activities associated with risk of transmission in a setting where multiple cases occurred).
- Lower Risk Epidemiologic Linkages
  1. Member of a cohort as defined by public health authorities experiencing mpox activity; OR
  2. Contact with a dead or live wild or exotic pet animal of an African species, or used or consumed a product derived from such an animal (e.g., game meat, powders, etc.); OR
  3. Residence in or travel to a country where mpox is endemic.

Criteria to Distinguish a New Case from an Existing Case

For surveillance purposes, a new case of mpox virus infection meets the following criteria:
- Healthy tissue has replaced the site of all previous lesions after they have scabbed and fallen off; AND
- New lesions are present which have tested positive for orthopoxvirus or mpox virus DNA by molecular methods or genomic sequencing.

Case Classification

Suspect
- Meets clinical criteria AND epidemiologic criteria^ AND no evidence of a negative test for either non-variola orthopoxvirus or mpox virus

Probable
- Meets presumptive laboratory criteria

Confirmed
- Meets confirmatory laboratory criteria

*The presence of clinically compatible rash lesions should be combined with either a higher or lower epidemiologic linkage criterion for case classification.

**A person presenting with lymphadenopathy or fever without any clinically compatible rash lesions must meet a higher epidemiologic risk criterion for case classification.

***Recent administration of ACAM2000 and JYNNEOS vaccines need to be considered when interpreting an antibody titer. RABORAL V-RG, an oral rabies vaccine product for wildlife, is a recombinant vaccinia virus, and could lead to an antibody response in an individual exposed to the liquid vaccine; this is expected to be an extremely rare occurrence.

Note: The categorical labels used here to stratify laboratory evidence are intended to support the standardization of case classifications for public health surveillance. The categorical labels should not be used to interpret the utility or validity of any laboratory test methodology.

‡The language "without the use of appropriate PPE or Biosafety Level (BSL) protocols" includes breaches in the recommended PPE and deviations from appropriate BSL protocols.

^The presence of clinically compatible rash lesions should be combined with either a higher or lower epidemiologic linkage criterion for case classification. A person presenting with lymphadenopathy or fever without any clinically compatible rash lesions must meet a higher risk epidemiologic risk criterion for case classification.

From Centers for Disease Control and Prevention: Mpox Virus Infection 2022 Case Definition. Available at https://ndc.services.cdc.gov/case-definitions/monkeypox-virus-infection/.

REFERENCES & SUGGESTED READINGS

Available at eBooks.Health.Elsevier.com.

AUTHORS: **FRANK A. SANCHEZ, MD, MBA** and **GLENN G. FORT, MD, MPH**

Diseases and Disorders

I

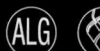
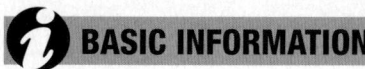 **BASIC INFORMATION**

DEFINITION

Multifocal atrial tachycardia (MAT) is a supraventricular tachyarrhythmia (rate greater than 100 beats per minute) with organized atrial activity, showing P waves having at least three or more different morphologies and irregular P-P, P-R, and R-R intervals. MAT is differentiated from atrial fibrillation by discrete P wave depolarizations and an isoelectric baseline between P waves.

SYNONYMS

MAT
Chaotic atrial rhythm
Multiform atrial rhythm
Chronic atrial tachycardia
Repetitive multifocal paroxysmal atrial tachycardia
Multifocal ectopic atrial tachycardia
The term *wandering pacemaker* or multifocal atrial rhythm is used for a similar arrhythmia associated with heart rates less than 100 bpm.

ICD-10CM CODE	
I47.1	Supraventricular tachycardia

EPIDEMIOLOGY & DEMOGRAPHICS

Estimated prevalence in hospitalized patients is 0.05% to 0.37%.[1] Right atrial hypertension and distention (from secondary pulmonary hypertension from advanced chronic obstructive pulmonary disease [COPD] or left ventricular dysfunction) potentially cause MAT.[2] The average age of onset is 70 yr of age.

The entity is usually associated with underlying pulmonary disease with right atrial electromechanical delay (60% of cases);[1] the arrhythmia has been identified in up to 20% of patients hospitalized for acute respiratory failure.[3] COPD is present in approximately 55% of patients with MAT, and significant lung disease is associated in roughly 60% of cases, including pneumonia, pulmonary embolism, hypoxia, hypercapnia, and acidosis.

MAT may also be seen in patients with heart failure, valvular heart disease, pulmonary hypertension, and hypomagnesemia. These patients are in general quite ill and have an in-hospital mortality rate of 40% to 60% from pulmonary, cardiac, and/or other serious diseases.

MAT has been identified in patients with coronavirus disease 2019; however, it was not associated with increased mortality.[4]

PHYSICAL FINDINGS & CLINICAL PRESENTATION

Symptoms:
- Palpitations
- Light-headedness
- Presyncope and/or syncope are rare
- Symptoms of the underlying pulmonary disease, if applicable

- Physical findings associated with the underlying pulmonary disease, if applicable
- Most episodes do not cause hemodynamic compromise; however, it can lead to decompensation if there is coexisting advanced cardiac disease (i.e., severe multivessel obstructive coronary artery disease or decompensated heart failure)
- High heart rates associated with MAT can sometimes worsen systemic oxygenation or exacerbate heart disease if there is coexisting pulmonary or cardiac disease, respectively

ETIOLOGY

- Exact mechanism is unknown; however, there are two leading theories:
  1. Atrial pacemaker activity arises from different atrial locations. This is supported by variable P waves and PR intervals.
  2. A single focus with different exit pathways or abnormalities in intraatrial conduction.
- MAT has been associated with abnormal intraatrial, atrionodal, and atrioventricular nodal conduction.
- Potentially caused by right atrial hypertension and distention such as that found in pulmonary hypertension (from advanced COPD) or left ventricular dysfunction.
- Also seen in other circumstances; therefore atrial distention may not be a universal mechanism.
- Exacerbated by underlying pulmonary disease COPD, hypoxia, pulmonary embolism, pneumonia), cardiac disease, hypercarbia, acidosis, electrolyte disturbances (hypokalemia and hypomagnesemia).
- Other associations:
  1. Drugs like isoproterenol, aminophylline, and theophylline
  2. Chronic renal failure (15% of patients with MAT has chronic renal failure)
  3. Sepsis and recent surgery

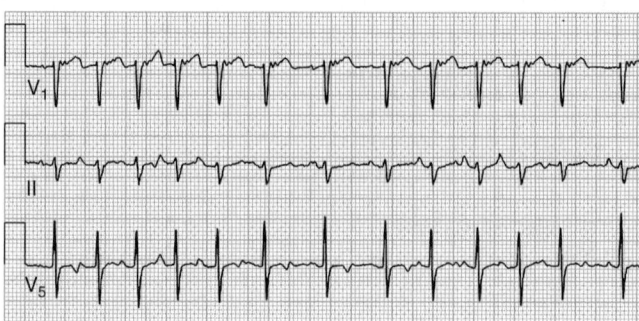 **DIAGNOSIS**

DIFFERENTIAL DIAGNOSIS

- Atrial fibrillation (no discernable P waves; up to 55% of patients with MAT will develop

atrial fibrillation, MAT can degenerate into atrial fibrillation)
- Atrial flutter with variable atrioventricular conduction (regular P-P intervals; MAT has variable P-P intervals)
- Sinus tachycardia with frequent premature atrial contractions (PACs) or ventricular premature beats (regular P-P intervals)
- Paroxysmal atrial tachycardia

WORKUP

- ECG (Fig. 1)
- Chest x-ray examination
- Pulmonary function tests
- Electrolytes
- Arterial blood gases

TREATMENT

- Correction and/or improvement in the underlying pulmonary or metabolic dysfunction if possible (e.g., electrolyte repletion if associated with hypomagnesemia and/or hypokalemia).[5]
- Correction of oxygenation and acid-base disorders, if present.
- Avoid drugs such as theophylline, isoproterenol, etc.
- Intravenous magnesium infusion may occasionally be helpful even in patients with normal magnesium levels.
- Calcium channel blockers: Verapamil may be effective acutely and chronically and is often used as first line in patients with preserved left ventricular function *if there are symptoms related to tachycardia.*
- β-Blockers (metoprolol is relatively cardioselective) can be used if not contraindicated by obstructive lung disease, acute heart failure, hypotension, hypersensitivity, heart block, or sinus node dysfunction.
- If the arrhythmia is asymptomatic, it can be left untreated.
- Direct current cardioversion is ineffective, therefore there is no role for cardioversion.
- Antiarrhythmics are ineffective.
- Anticoagulation is currently not indicated, although some recent studies have linked

FIG. 1 Multifocal atrial tachycardia (MAT). This three-lead rhythm strip (leads II, V₁, and V₅) shows an irregularly irregular narrow QRS complex rhythm. However, unlike in atrial fibrillation, each QRS complex is preceded by discrete, conducted P waves. There are at least three different P wave morphologies and PR intervals, consistent with MAT. (From Olshansky B et al: *Arrhythmia essentials,* ed 2, Philadelphia, 2017, Elsevier.)

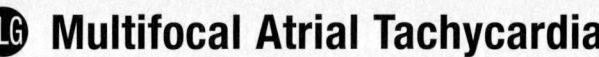
frequent atrial ectopy on ambulatory monitoring with stroke risk
- No significant role for catheter ablation; however, in extreme cases of refractory MAT in symptomatic patients who cannot tolerate medical therapy or in MAT resistant

to medical therapy, atrioventricular nodal ablation with pacemaker implantation has been performed.
- Table 1 summarizes the treatment of multifocal atrial tachycardia.

REFERENCES
Available at eBooks.Health.Elsevier.com.

AUTHOR: **VYBHAV JETTY, MD, MHA**

TABLE 1	Multifocal Atrial Tachycardia Therapy
Acute therapy, stable and unstable	• Treat underlying condition. Aggressive treatment of COPD exacerbation usually treats arrhythmia, but MAT may persist for hours to days after management of the underlying condition is effective. Treatment of the MAT itself does not affect the course or prognosis of the medical illness. • Avoid digoxin, as AV block and slowing of ventricular rate is unlikely to occur. • Cardioversion is of no benefit for MAT. However, AF may be confused with MAT; if the diagnosis is uncertain and the patient is hemodynamically unstable, cardioversion can be considered in selected cases. Hemodynamic instability generally results from the underlying medical condition and not from the rhythm or rapid rate per se. • Lower the dose of sympathomimetics and methylxanthines, as tolerated, if applicable. • Maintain K^+ and $Mg2^+$ within normal limits, ideally $K^+ \geq 4.0$ mEq/L and $Mg2^+ \geq 2.0$ mEq/L. • Drugs to control ventricular rate (data on effectiveness are inconclusive): Preferred: Calcium blocker (IV or PO diltiazem). Verapamil can cause substantial hypotension in patients with COPD but may be effective. Ventricular rate control is difficult due to excess catecholamines. β-Adrenergic blockers rarely can be given due to concurrent bronchospastic pulmonary disease. • Magnesium sulfate, IV bolus of 2- to 4-g, may terminate the episodes and help control the ventricular rate, but success is limited and unpredictable. • Potassium chloride, 20-60 mEq per day if hypokalemic. • Digoxin may worsen MAT and is unlikely to control the ventricular response. • Amiodarone can be considered to control ventricular rate and suppress the arrhythmia, but there are no data to support its use.
Chronic prevention	• Options include calcium channel blockers (e.g., oral diltiazem) for ventricular rate control or possibly amiodarone to prevent recurrences; drug therapy without aggressive treatment of the underlying condition is often futile. • Treat pulmonary disease; maintain $K^+ \geq 4.0$ mEq/L and $Mg2^+ \geq 2.0$ mEq/L, if possible.
MI	• Rapid rate and ineffective atrial kick (PR interval ≤0.14 s) can worsen ischemia and CHF. Rate control is often required. A calcium channel blocker such as diltiazem is the first-line therapy, unless β-adrenergic blockers can be tolerated.

AF, Atrial fibrillation; *AV,* atrioventricular; *CHF,* congestive heart failure; *COPD,* chronic obstructive pulmonary disease; *DCC,* direct current cardioversion; *IV,* intravenous; *MAT,* multifocal atrial tachycardia; *MI,* myocardial infarction; *PO,* oral.
Modified from Olshansky B et al: *Arrhythmia essentials,* ed 2, Philadelphia, 2017, Elsevier.

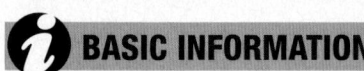 BASIC INFORMATION

DEFINITION

Multiple endocrine neoplasia (MEN) refers to a group of heritable genetic syndromes characterized by the development of specific groups of tumors of the endocrine glands.

SYNONYMS

MEN I: Wermer syndrome
MEN IIA: Sipple syndrome

ICD-10CM CODES

E31.2	Multiple endocrine neoplasia [MEN] syndromes
E31.20	Multiple en docrine neoplasia [MEN] syndrome, unspecified
E31.21	Multiple endocrine neoplasia [MEN] syndrome type I
E31.22	Multiple endocrine neoplasia [MEN] syndrome type IIA
E31.23	Multiple endocrine neoplasia [MEN] syndrome type IIB

EPIDEMIOLOGY & DEMOGRAPHICS[1,2]

INCIDENCE:
- MEN I: 25 in 10,000
- MEN II: 1 in 30,000

PREVALENCE:
- MEN I: 1/30,000
- MEN II: 1/35,000 (predominantly MEN IIA)

RISK FACTORS: Family history of MEN syndrome, although it can also occur sporadically

GENETICS:
- MEN I: Autosomal-dominant mutation in MEN1 tumor-suppressor gene[1]
- MEN IIA and MEN IIB: Autosomal-dominant mutations in RET protooncogene[2]

PHYSICAL FINDINGS & CLINICAL PRESENTATION

- Patients may present due to screening or may present with a MEN-associated tumor. Tumors are found incidentally due to biochemical abnormalities or to symptoms.
- MEN I (PPP [pituitary, pancreas, parathyroid])[3,4]
- Diagnostic criteria generally include two MEN-associated tumors, one tumor in a patient with a family history, or positive genetic testing.
- Primary hyperparathyroidism (parathyroid adenoma or hyperplasia) is the most common manifestation and can cause hypercalcemia (urolithiasis, GI disturbance, bone pain, neuropsychiatric disturbances) and also affect bone density.
- Pancreatic neuroendocrine tumors cause symptoms related to their secretory properties or metastases.
  1. Gastrinoma: Peptic ulcers, diarrhea, esophageal symptoms (see "Gastrinoma")
  2. Insulinoma: Hypoglycemic symptoms upon fasting and after exercise (see "Insulinoma")
  3. Glucagonoma: Necrolytic migratory erythema (a blistering skin lesion), diabetes/glucose intolerance, weight loss

4. VIPoma: Diarrhea, hypokalemia, decreased gastric acid
5. Somatostatinoma: Hyperglycemia, cholelithiasis, diarrhea, abdominal pain, weight loss
6. Nonfunctioning tumors can metastasize (frequently to the liver), a frequent cause of death in MEN I
- Pituitary tumors may cause compressive symptoms, such as visual field defects or hypopituitarism (see "Pituitary Adenoma"). Hormonal secretion may also cause symptoms.
  1. Prolactinoma (most common pituitary tumor in MEN I): Menstrual irregularities, hypogonadism, gynecomastia, and/or galactorrhea (see "Prolactinoma")
  2. Somatotroph adenomas (producing growth hormone): Gigantism or acromegaly (frontal bossing, increased shoe/hat size, hyperglycemia, hyperhidrosis) depending on patient age (see "Acromegaly")
  3. Corticotroph adenomas (producing adrenocorticotropic hormone): Cushingoid features such as weight gain, moon facies, hyperglycemia, bone loss, proximal muscle weakness, hypertension, hypokalemia (see "Cushing Disease and Syndrome")
  4. Nonfunctioning (nonsecretory) tumors
- Other manifestations: Carcinoid tumors, collagenomas, angiofibromas, meningiomas, lipomas
- MEN IIA:[5,6]
  1. Medullary thyroid carcinoma (MTC) is a tumor of the thyroid's calcitonin-secreting C cells. It can present with a neck mass, as well as flushing and diarrhea due to elevated calcitonin levels.
  2. Primary hyperparathyroidism: See "Physical Findings & Clinical Presentation, MEN I." Less aggressive in "MEN IIA."
  3. Pheochromocytoma is an adrenal tumor producing catecholamines, which can lead to life-threatening hypertensive crises.
- MEN IIB:[5,6]
  1. MTC
  2. Pheochromocytoma
  3. Oral mucosal neuromas

ETIOLOGY

Tumor development facilitated by the previously described genetic mutations (Table E1).

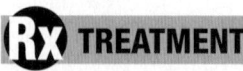 DIAGNOSIS

DIFFERENTIAL DIAGNOSIS

Tumors associated with MEN may occur sporadically.

WORKUP

- MEN I: Note that opinions vary regarding the aggressiveness and frequency of screening for MEN-associated tumors. Fig. E1 illustrates an algorithm for screening and management of MEN1 syndromes.
  1. Genetic testing: Offered to patients meeting MEN I clinical criteria or to patients in whom there is high suspicion, as well as to first-degree relatives of MEN I patients.

2. Hyperparathyroidism screening: Parathyroid hormone (PTH) and calcium annually.
3. Pancreatic tumor screening: Annual pancreas imaging (endoscopic ultrasonography, computed tomography [CT], or MRI) and annual biochemical testing (glucose, gastrin, vasoactive intestinal peptide [VIP], glucagon, insulin, pancreatic polypeptide, chromogranin A). Notably, Gallium-68 DOTATATE PET-CT is an exciting new tool for neuroendocrine tumor localization, though it is not typically utilized in screening at this time.
4. Pituitary tumor screening: Insulin-like growth factor 1 (IGF-1) and prolactin annually and pituitary MRI every 3 to 5 yr.
5. Carcinoid tumor screening: Chest CT or MRI every 2 yr.
- MEN IIA:
  1. Genetic testing: At-risk members of families with known RET mutations should undergo screening for the specific mutation. Patients with MTC should have genetic testing of the tumor and genetic testing based on results. Cutaneous lichen amyloidosis (a skin finding) should prompt testing; Hirschsprung disease may also prompt testing.[2]
  2. Hyperparathyroidism screening: PTH and calcium annually.
  3. Pheochromocytoma: Plasma catecholamines and metanephrines annually for screening, age to begin depending on specific mutation; CT and MRI may localize; I-123 and PET (possibly including gallium-68 DOTATATE PET-CT) also helpful for localization.[7]
  4. MTC screening: Depends on risk category; physical exam, neck ultrasound, and calcitonin level yearly; carcinoembryonic antigen may also be indicated.[5,6]
- MEN IIB:
  1. Genetic testing: See "Workup, MEN IIA"
  2. Pheochromocytoma: See "Workup, MEN IIA"
  3. MTC screening: Although there may be a role for monitoring, prophylactic thyroidectomy is typically performed early

LABORATORY TESTS

See "Workup."

IMAGING STUDIES

See "Workup."

TREATMENT

No therapy available at this time to reverse the underlying genetic cause. Treatment (both medical and surgical) focuses on tumor prevention and management.

NONPHARMACOLOGIC THERAPY

- MEN I:[3,4]
  1. For hyperparathyroidism, surgical parathyroidectomy is indicated in patients with significant hypercalcemia, osteoporosis, renal disease, or nephrolithiasis or found

to be at high risk for nephrolithiasis. Hyperparathyroidism may be treated surgically with parathyroidectomy.

2. Pituitary tumors may be surgically excised via transsphenoidal approach; notably, medical therapy is first line for prolactinoma.

3. Pancreatic tumor treatment is extremely variable. Gastrinoma is frequently complicated by duodenal metastases, which are difficult to treat surgically, so treatment choice varies between centers. Ulcers caused by gastrinoma may require endoscopic or surgical management. Surgery is preferred for insulinoma, VIPoma, and glucagonoma. Nonfunctioning tumors may be treated surgically depending on tumor size and location. Conservative management for insulinoma may involve frequent carbohydrate intake. Cytotoxic chemotherapy and tyrosine kinase inhibitors are options for patients with metastatic disease. Peptide receptor radionucleotide therapy (PRRT) is an emerging and exciting therapeutic modality for metastatic disease.

- **MEN IIA:**
  1. MTC is generally treated surgically. Prophylactic thyroidectomy is considered based on genetic mutation. Almost all children with MEN IIA will require thyroidectomy (screening as previously described). Patients should undergo ultrasound and total thyroidectomy with cervical lymph node dissection. Extent of further neck dissection depends on metastases and may be guided by calcitonin levels. A more palliative surgical approach is considered in the setting of advanced disease.[5,6]
  2. Hyperparathyroidism: Resection of only enlarged glands with intraoperative PTH monitoring is preferred.
  3. Pheochromocytoma is treated surgically. Unilateral adrenalectomy is preferred, although many patients will develop a contralateral pheochromocytoma. Preoperative blood pressure control with alpha blockade is key. If present, pheochromocytoma must be removed before thyroidectomy.[7]

- **MEN IIB:**
  1. MTC: Prophylactic thyroidectomy offered in childhood.[5,6]
  2. Pheochromocytoma: See "Nonpharmacologic Therapy, MEN IIA."

ACUTE GENERAL Rx

- **MEN I:[3,4]**
  1. Hyperparathyroidism causes hypercalcemia that may be treated with intravenous (IV) hydration, diuretics, and bisphosphonates. Early vitamin D repletion prevents bone destruction postoperatively due to the "hungry bone syndrome."

2. Gastrinoma may lead to peptic ulcers requiring IV proton pump inhibitor (PPI).
3. Supportive care (glucose for hypoglycemia caused by insulinoma; fluids and electrolytes for hypovolemia caused by diarrhea from VIPoma or gastrinoma) is required.

- **MEN IIA:**
  1. Hyperparathyroidism: See "Acute General Rx, MEN I."
  2. Pheochromocytoma: Preoperative blood pressure control is key; alpha blockers are first line. Phenoxybenzamine irreversibly blocks alpha adrenergic receptors; doxazosin may also be helpful. Calcium channel blockers can be utilized. There is concern that unopposed beta blockade may allow for alpha-medicated vasoconstriction.[7]

- **MEN IIB:**
  1. Pheochromocytoma: See "Acute General Rx, MEN IIA."

CHRONIC Rx

- **MEN I:[3,4]**
  1. Hyperparathyroidism may be amenable to agonists of the calcium-sensing receptor (cinacalcet), although surgery is preferred in patients who meet surgical criteria and are operative candidates.
  2. Pancreatic tumors may benefit from medical therapy.
     a. Gastrinoma: PPI or H2 antagonists, somatostatin agonists (such as octreotide)
     b. Insulinoma: Diazoxide or somatostatin agonists
     c. Glucagonoma and VIPoma: Somatostatin agonists
  1. Adjunctive medical therapy can be considered for pituitary tumors, although surgical treatment is first-line with the exception of prolactinoma (for which dopamine agonists are first line). Radiation therapy and/or medical therapy are considered in cases of incomplete resection or regrowth.
     a. Prolactinoma: Dopamine agonists (bromocriptine or cabergoline). Temozolomide is a chemotherapeutic agent for refractory cases.
     b. Somatotroph adenoma: Somatostatin or dopamine agonists, growth hormone receptor antagonist
     c. Corticotroph adenoma: Antiadrenal agents, adrenal enzyme blocker (such as ketoconazole), somatostatin or dopamine agonists, glucocorticoid receptor blockers

- **MEN II A:**
  1. Hyperparathyroidism: See "Chronic Rx, MEN I."
  2. MTC: Tyrosine kinase inhibitors and chemotherapy may help treat metastatic disease. After thyroidectomy, levothyroxine is

indicated (thyroid-stimulating hormone suppression not required).[5,6]

- **MEN IIB:**
  1. MTC: See "Chronic Rx, MEN II A."

DISPOSITION

Most workup can be done as an outpatient (multidisciplinary team); inpatient stays may be required due to acute complications or for surgical procedures.

COMPLEMENTARY & ALTERNATIVE MEDICINE

MEN is unlikely to be amenable to this.

REFERRAL

Patients with MEN should be followed by a multispecialty team, including endocrinologists, endocrine surgeons, and genetic counselors.

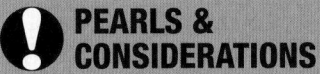

COMMENTS

MEN is a group of genetic syndromes that requires close monitoring and intervention to prevent and treat tumor development, as well as genetic counseling of patients and family members.

PREVENTION

Prevention focuses on screening for MEN in persons at risk and early identification of MEN-associated tumors.

PATIENT & FAMILY EDUCATION

- American Multiple Endocrine Neoplasia Support: https://www.amensupport.org/
- Association for Multiple Endocrine Neoplasia Disorders: https://www.amend.org.uk/

REFERENCES

Available at eBooks.Health.Elsevier.com.

RELATED CONTENT

Acromegaly (Related Key Topic)
Cushing Disease and Syndrome (Related Key Topic)
Gastrinoma (Related Key Topic)
Hyperparathyroidism (Related Key Topic)
Insulinoma (Related Key Topic)
Pheochromocytoma (Related Key Topic)
Pituitary Adenoma (Related Key Topic)
Prolactinoma (Related Key Topic)
Thyroid Carcinoma (Related Key Topic)

AUTHORS: **HARIKRASHNA B. BHATT, MD** and **RUSSELL E. BRATMAN, MD**

M

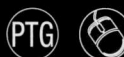

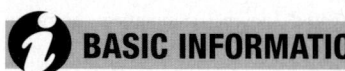 **BASIC INFORMATION**

DEFINITION

Multiple sclerosis (MS) is a chronic, predominantly autoimmune demyelinating disease of the central nervous system (CNS), characterized by subacute neurologic deficits correlating with CNS lesions (typical for MS in location, shape, and orientation) separated in time (typically at least 1 mo) and space, and excluding other possible disease.[1-3]

An MS relapse is defined as an acute to subacute (peaking over hours to days) onset of neurologic dysfunction (typically focal) lasting at least 24 h, and caused by inflammatory CNS demyelination. Relapses can be symptomatic or asymptomatic, the latter of which are represented by new enhancing MRI lesions without correlating symptoms.

Active subtypes include:

- **Relapsing-remitting MS (RRMS)** (85%): Relapses followed by complete or near-complete recovery over weeks to months (rarely beyond 6 mo), 50% to 85% of which later evolve to secondary progressive MS.[2-3]
- **Primary progressive MS (PPMS)** (10% to 15%): Progressive worsening of neurologic disability from the onset, with rare distinct relapses.[2-3]
- **Secondary progressive MS (SPMS):** Progressive worsening of neurologic disability over at least 1 yr with few or no distinct relapses, from a prior course consistent with RRMS.
  1. Progressive-relapsing or relapsing-progressive courses can be incorporated into definitions of PPMS or SPMS, respectively.
- **Clinically isolated syndrome (CIS):** An initial, isolated clinical event lasting at least 24 h and typical for MS relapse, but not yet meeting criteria for dissemination in time and space. Correlating demyelinating lesions on MRI arc associated with 60% to 80% risk of developing a second relapse (and therefore, MS) within several years, vs. 20% without the presence of typical MS lesions on MRI.[2] Factors associated with conversion to clinically definite MS (CDMS) include additional T2 lesions on MRI, younger age, and CSF-specific oligoclonal bands (OCBs).[4] The definition for RRMS is met when another distinct relapse occurs or when MRI demonstrates new lesions typical for MS.[2,5]
- **Radiologically isolated syndrome (RIS):** The presence of CNS lesions on MRI that meet the diagnostic imaging criteria for MS found incidentally without correlating symptoms or symptoms typical for MS. Approximately 50% develop MS within 10 yr.[1,2] Factors associated with increased risk of conversion to MS include younger age, male sex, spinal cord lesions, CSF-specific OCBs, and gadolinium-enhancing lesions on MRI.[6]
- **Solitary sclerosis:** Characterized by isolated or minimal CNS demyelinating lesion(s) with associated progressive neurologic morbidity similar to that in progressive MS, without any

clinical or radiologic evidence of new MS-type lesions.[2]

Rare MS variants include:

- **Marburg variant:** Characterized by acute onset and a fulminant, often malignant course (severe disability or death can occur within a year of initial symptoms). MRI reveals tumefactive (tumor-like) demyelinating lesion(s) with extensive edema. Pathology shows severe inflammation with extensive necrosis. May also involve the peripheral nerves.[7]
- **Baló's concentric sclerosis:** Has a monophasic and rapidly progressive course. Neuroimaging and pathology show alternating rings of high- and low-signal intensity (on MRI) representing demyelination and intact myelination, resembling an onion bulb.[7] More common in those of Chinese and Filipino descents.
- **Schilder's disease (myelinoclastic diffuse sclerosis):** Onset is typically in childhood with 1 to 2 large, confluent lesions. Usually progresses to involve widespread, bilateral regions of the CNS, and has variable course and prognosis.[8] Etiology is unclear but may have a possible association with preceding infectious illness.

SYNONYMS

MS
Disseminated sclerosis

ICD-10CM CODE	
G35	Multiple sclerosis

EPIDEMIOLOGY & DEMOGRAPHICS

PREVALENCE: More common in people raised in northern latitudes and in certain genetic clusters.[1] Global prevalence of MS is estimated to be around 36 per 100,000 people (~3 million people).[9] There are currently nearly 1 million people living with MS in the United States.[10]

PREDOMINANT SEX & AGE: Female:male ratio is approximately 3:1.[1]

PEAK INCIDENCE: Most common permanently disabling disorder of the central nervous system in young adults.[1] Two thirds of patients have incidence between 20 and 40 yr; mean age of onset is 30 yr. Ranges from infancy to 70 yr.[11]

RACE: Although more common in White people of Northern European descent, MS has been demonstrated to occur across most races and ethnic backgrounds. Recent studies suggest up to 47% higher risk of MS in Black vs. White women in the United States. Social determinants of health probably contribute to this risk. Hispanic, Asian, and Native American populations have demonstrated lower incidence of MS thus far, compared to White and Black populations. Features of MS that have been more commonly associated with Black patients (compared to White patients) include transverse myelitis, vision loss from optic neuritis, earlier progression to disability, and higher lesion burden. Hispanic patients may also more frequently have optic neuritis and transverse myelitis, as

well as younger age of disease onset and more severe disease course. Asian patients may have higher rates of optic nerve and spinal cord involvement.

GENETICS: Frequency of MS in dizygotic twins and siblings is 3% to 5%, and 30% to 50% in monozygotic twins. ~200 genes have been identified that contribute to the risk of developing MS.[1] Most common associations include human leukocyte antigen classes I and II (*DRB1*1501, DQA1*0102, DQB1*0602*), (*DRB1*0405-DQA1*0301-DQB1*0302* in the Mediterranean population). A notable epigenetic interaction between vitamin D and the main MS-linked *HLA-DRB1*1501* allele has been elucidated. Conversely, *HLA-A*02* has been associated with a reduced odds of developing MS.[12]

PHYSICAL FINDINGS & CLINICAL PRESENTATION

Findings depend on the location of the CNS lesion(s) and may include the following:

- Common: Nonspecific complaints such as fatigue (most common, with 80% lifetime prevalence), blurred vision, diplopia, vertigo, falls, hemiparesis, paraparesis, monoparesis, numbness, paresthesias, ataxia, cognitive impairment, depression, anxiety, pseudobulbar affect (involuntary crying or laughing out of context), sexual dysfunction, and bowel/bladder dysfunction
- Visual abnormalities: Horizontal nystagmus, visual field deficits, Marcus Gunn pupil (i.e., relative afferent papillary defect—normal consensual light reflex; however, when swinging a flashlight from the unaffected eye to the affected eye, direct light causes paradoxical pupillary dilation in the affected eye), sixth nerve palsy, internuclear ophthalmoplegia (paresis of the adducting eye on conjugate lateral gaze with simultaneous horizontal nystagmus of the abducting eye) (Fig. 1)
- Corticospinal tract(s) involvement: Transverse myelitis, upper motor neuron signs such as spasticity (particularly leg spasms at night or after prolonged immobility), hyperreflexia,

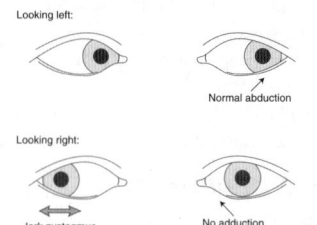

FIG. 1 Internuclear ophthalmoplegia. When the patient in the figure looks to the left *(top row)*, both eyes move normally, but when the patient looks to the right *(bottom row)*, the left eye fails to adduct ("weak" medial rectus) and the contralateral eye develops a jerk nystagmus. The finding is named for the side with weak adduction (i.e., in this example, a *left* internuclear ophthalmoplegia), and the lesion is in the *ipsilateral* medial longitudinal fasciculus (i.e., *left* medial longitudinal fasciculus in this example). See the text. (From McGee S: *Evidence-based physical diagnosis*, ed 4, Philadelphia, 2018, Elsevier.)

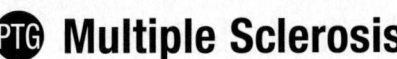

clonus, extensor plantar responses, tonic spasms, upper motor neuron pattern of weakness
- Sensory involvement: May include partial or full dermatomal loss of pain and temperature, loss of vibration (common) and position sense, temperature dysregulation, thoracic band of pressure or squeezing sensation ("MS hug"), paresthesias, trigeminal neuralgia
- Ataxia: Intention tremor, dysmetria, dysdiado-chokinesis, titubation, inability to tandem gait
- Bladder dysfunction: Detrusor hyperreflexia (urge incontinence), urinary frequency, flaccidity (neurogenic bladder), and dyssynergia (bladder contracts against a closed sphincter)
- **Lhermitte sign:** Flexion of the neck elicits an electrical sensation extending down the spine and occasionally into the extremities, due to involvement of the posterior cervical spinal cord[1-2]
- **Uhthoff phenomenon:** Transient recurrence or worsening of preexisting neurologic deficits with small elevations in core body temperature (e.g., during exercise or warm bathing)[2]

ETIOLOGY

Likely multifactorial, with evidence for autoimmunity (autoreactive T and B lymphocytes), environmental factors (low sunlight exposure, vitamin D deficiency, smoking, obesity, shift work), and genetics (Mendelian and epigenetic). Environmental risk factors during childhood include exposure to certain viruses (e.g., Epstein-Barr virus and human herpes virus 6), low ultraviolet light exposure, and month of birth (higher in spring).[1,13]

Dx DIAGNOSIS

- **MS:** Based on the revised 2017 McDonald criteria[2] (Table 1)
- **RRMS:** See Table 1
- **PPMS:** Insidious progression of neurologic disability for at least 1 yr, independent of disability associated with clinical relapse(s), with at least two of the following: (1) evidence of positive cerebrospinal fluid (CSF)-specific oligoclonal bands (OCBs), and (2) MRI evidence of at least one brain or (3) at least two spinal cord MS-like lesions[2]
- **MRI diagnostic criteria for dissemination in space:** At least one T_2-hyperintense lesion in at least two of the following regions: Periventricular, cortical or juxtacortical, infratentorial, spinal cord[2]
- **MRI and CSF diagnostic criteria for dissemination in time:** (1) Presence of both gadolinium-enhancing and nonenhancing lesions on a single MRI; (2) presence of new T_2-hyperintense or enhancing lesion(s) on a subsequent MRI; (3) at least two CSF-specific OCBs[2]

DIFFERENTIAL DIAGNOSIS[14] (TABLE 2)

- **Autoimmune:** Acute disseminated encephalomyelitis (ADEM), postvaccination encephalomyelitis, neuromyelitis optica spectrum disorder (NMOSD), myelin oligodendrocyte glycoprotein antibody disease (MOGAD), antiphospholipid antibody syndrome, autoimmune glial fibrillary acidic protein (GFAP) astrocytopathy
- **Degenerative:** Amyotrophic lateral sclerosis, primary lateral sclerosis, cerebral autosomal dominant arteriopathy with subcortical infarcts and leukoencephalopathy (CADASIL), multisystem atrophy
- **Genetic:** Fabry disease, Wilson disease, spinocerebellar ataxia, hereditary spastic paraparesis
- **Hematologic:** Lymphoma, histiocytosis, thrombotic thrombocytopenic purpura
- **Infectious:** Lyme disease, neurosyphilis, HIV, tropical spastic paraparesis (human T-lymphotropic virus type 1 or HTLV-1), progressive multifocal leukoencephalopathy (PML, caused by the JC virus), Listeria, Whipple disease (*Tropheryma whipplei*), acute flaccid myelitis, chronic meningitis, CNS tuberculosis, or fungal disease
- **Inflammatory:** Systemic lupus erythematosus, vasculitis, neurosarcoidosis, Sjögren syndrome, Guillain-Barré syndrome, Behçet disease, celiac disease

TABLE 1 Summary of Revised 2017 McDonald Criteria for Diagnosis of Multiple Sclerosis

RRMS/Clinical Attacks	Clinical Lesions	Paraclinical Testing Needed
2	2	None
2	1	MRI dissemination in space *or* a second clinical attack at a different CNS site
1	2	MRI dissemination in time *or* CSF-specific oligoclonal bands
1	1	Additional clinical attack at a different CNS site or MRI dissemination in space
		MRI dissemination in time *or* CSF-specific oligoclonal bands

Evidence of clinical lesions by physical examination or evoked potentials.
CNS, Central nervous system; *CSF,* cerebrospinal fluid; *MRI dissemination in space,* ≥1 T2 lesions in 2 of the 4 typical areas for MS lesions—periventricular, juxtacortical, infratentorial, or spinal cord; *MRI dissemination in time,* a new lesion at follow-up MRI at any time, or presence of both an enhancing and nonenhancing lesion at any time; *RRMS,* relapsing-remitting multiple sclerosis.

TABLE 2 Conditions That Can Be Mistaken for Multiple Sclerosis and Other Diseases of Myelin

Vascular Disease
Small-vessel cerebrovascular disease
Vasculitis
CADASIL
Antiphospholipid antibody syndrome

Structural Lesions
Craniocervical junction, posterior fossa, or spinal tumors
Cervical spondylosis or disc herniation
Chiari malformation or syrinx

Degenerative Diseases
Hereditary myelopathy
Spinocerebellar degeneration

Infections
HTLV-1 infection
HIV myelopathy or HIV-related cerebritis
Neuroborreliosis (e.g., Lyme disease)
JC virus/progressive multifocal leukoencephalopathy
Neurosyphilis

Other Inflammatory Conditions
Systemic lupus erythematosus
Sjögren syndrome

Sarcoidosis

Monofocal or Monophasic Demyelinating Syndromes
Neuromyelitis optica spectrum disorder
Acute disseminated encephalomyelitis

Other Conditions
Hashimoto thyroiditis with or without encephalopathy
Nonspecific MRI abnormalities related to migraine, aging, or trauma

CADASIL, Cerebral autosomal dominant arteriopathy with subcortical infarcts and leukoencephalopathy; *HIV,* human immunodeficiency virus; *HTLV,* human T-cell lymphotropic virus; *JC,* John Cunningham; *MRI,* magnetic resonance imaging.
From Goldman L, Schafer AI: *Goldman's Cecil medicine,* ed 24, Philadelphia, 2012, Saunders.

TABLE 3 Comparison of Sensitivity of Laboratory Testing in Multiple Sclerosis

	VER	BAER	SSEP	OCB	MRI
Clinically definite multiple sclerosis	80%-85%*	50%-65%	65%-80%	85%-95%	90%-97%

*Numbers show the percentage of patients with abnormal study results.
BAER, Brain stem auditory evoked response; *MRI,* magnetic resonance imaging; *OCB,* oligoclonal band; *SSEP,* somatosensory evoked potential; *VER,* visual evoked response.
From Jankovic J et al: *Bradley and Daroff's neurology in clinical practice,* ed 8, Philadelphia, 2022, Elsevier.

- **Toxic/Nutritional/Metabolic:** Vitamin B_{12} deficiency, copper deficiency, nitrous oxide toxicity, inherited leukodystrophies, central pontine myelinolysis
- **Mitochondrial:** Leber hereditary optic neuropathy; mitochondrial encephalopathy, lactic acidosis, and stroke-like episodes (MELAS)
- **Neoplasms:** CNS lymphoma, metastases, paraneoplastic disease, gliomatosis cerebri
- **Vascular:** Susac syndrome, subcortical infarcts, Binswanger disease, amyloid angiopathy, cavernous or arteriovenous malformation, cerebral venous sinus thrombosis

DIAGNOSTIC STUDIES (TABLE 3)

- Lumbar puncture to evaluate for presence of CSF-specific OCBs (Fig. 2), for cases that are atypical, and to evaluate for mimics of MS.[15] Typical CSF abnormalities (Table 4) may include elevated protein (>100 mg/dl), mild pleocytosis, and elevated CSF-specific immunoglobulin G (IgG) index and synthesis rate. >75% of clinically definite MS (CDMS) demonstrate elevated CSF-specific IgG synthesis and >90% demonstrate CSF-specific OCBs[2] (serum protein electrophoresis should be sent to the lab simultaneously with CSF for

TABLE 4 Cerebrospinal Fluid Abnormalities in Multiple Sclerosis

	Albumin	IgG/TP	IgG/Albumin	IgG Index	Oligoclonal Banding of Ig
Clinically definite multiple sclerosis	23%	67%	60%-73%	70%-90%	85%-95%
Normal controls	3%	—	36%	3%	7%*

*Other neurologic disease.
IgG/TP, Immunoglobulin G value/total protein.
From Jankovic J et al: *Bradley and Daroff's neurology in clinical practice,* ed 8, Philadelphia, 2022, Elsevier.

both of these tests). CSF kappa free light chain may have similar sensitivity and specificity for MS to OCBs.[16]
- Serum: CBC with differential, comprehensive metabolic panel, liver function tests (LFTs), vitamin B_{12}, copper, 25-OH vitamin D_3.
- Consider in the appropriate clinical setting:[14] CT angiogram and/or venogram of brain and carotids with and without contrast, AQP4-IgG and MOG-IgG (by cell based assay), antinuclear antibody (ANA), double-stranded DNA antibody, antineutrophil cytoplasmic antibodies, antiphospholipid antibodies, CSF soluble interleukin-2 receptor, CSF cytology and flow cytometry, Sjögren antibodies, thyroid-stimulating hormone (TSH), thyroglobulin antibody, peripheral blood smear, very-long-chain fatty acids, arylsulfatase A, lactate, pyruvate, urine organic acids, plasma amino acids, HIV serology, Lyme western blot, syphilis serology, quantiferon TB Gold
- Consider optical coherence tomography (OCT) or evoked potentials (visual, somatosensory, and brain stem auditory evoked response).
- In the evaluation of atypical cases of possible MS, myelin oligodendrocyte glycoprotein and aquabrim antibodies should be considered.

IMAGING

MRI of the brain with and without gadolinium contrast Fig. 3 is recommended in all cases. MRI with and without contrast of the cervical (Fig. E4) and thoracic spines should also be performed to screen for spinal cord lesions. MRI assesses for both acute and chronic lesions, as well as for atrophy, and should be repeated at least annually for disease surveillance and monitoring of disease-modifying therapy (DMT) efficacy. A normal MRI of the brain does not definitively exclude early MS but makes it extremely unlikely.[5]

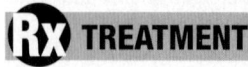 **℞ TREATMENT**

NONPHARMACOLOGIC THERAPY

Patient education regarding disease characteristics, treatment options, risks and benefits of

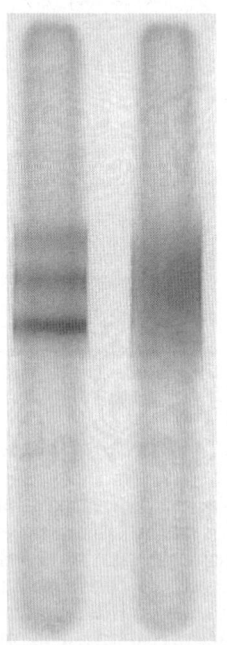

FIG. 2 Electrophoresis of cerebral spinal fluid (CSF) of a patient with multiple sclerosis *(left),* compared to the CSF of someone with no central nervous system inflammatory disease *(right),* shows three distinct, horizontal oligoclonal bands. (From Kaufman DM et al: *Kaufman's clinical neurology for psychiatrists,* ed 9, Philadelphia, 2023, Elsevier.)

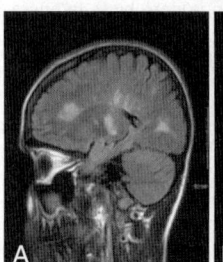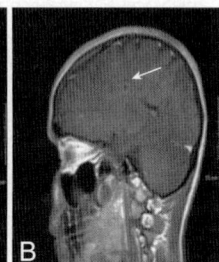

FIG. 3 Multiple sclerosis. A, Sagittal fluid-attenuated inversion recovery image magnetic resonance scan shows multiple lesions in corpus callosum, "Dawson fingers" (periventricular fingerlike lesions oriented toward the ventricles), along with ovoid and punctuate lesions in the deep white matter. **B,** Gadolinium-enhanced scan shows an enhancing lesion *(arrow).*

treatment, and prognosis. Often, patients need to incorporate intermittent rest periods on a daily basis and when physically active (for energy conservation), and avoid or limit exposure to heat (using cooling aids), which typically exacerbates symptoms.

Recommend physical therapy for new or worsening weakness, incoordination, or spasticity. Please see "Chronic Rx, Symptomatic therapy."

ACUTE GENERAL Rx (TABLE 5)

For relapses: High-dose intravenous (IV) or oral methylprednisolone (1 g/day for 3 to 5 days).[17] A proton pump inhibitor and insulin sliding scale should be simultaneously administered to prevent GI ulcers and treat steroid-induced hyperglycemia.

The Optic Neuritis Treatment Trial showed worse outcomes in optic neuritis after oral methylprednisolone compared with intravenous.[17] However, the COPOUSEP trial published in 2015 demonstrated nearly equivalent efficacy in improvement of symptoms and/or full recovery between 1000 mg daily for 3 days of oral and IV methylprednisolone in all types of relapses. High-dose corticosteroids do not alter

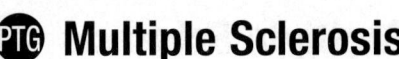

TABLE 5 Some Selected Approved Medications for Multiple Sclerosis

Generic (Brand Name: Mode of Administration)	Indications(s)	Side Effects	Chemical Structure
Glatiramer acetate (Copaxone: daily SQ)	To reduce relapse frequency in patients with relapsing-remitting multiple sclerosis (MS) and patients who have experienced a first clinical episode and have MRI features consistent with MS	Injection site reactions, lipoatrophy with prolonged use	Synthetic polymer
IFN-β-1a, (Avonex: weekly IM, Plegridy: q2wk IM, Rebif: TIW SQ)	To slow accumulation of physical disability and decrease frequency of clinical exacerbations in patients with relapsing forms of MS and patients who have experienced a first clinical episode and have MRI features consistent with MS	Flulike symptoms, injection site reactions, neutropenia, anemia, liver function test abnormalities	Interferon beta-1 alpha
IFN-β-1b (Betaseron: Every other day SQ injections)	To reduce the frequency of clinical exacerbations in patients with relapsing forms of MS and patients who have experienced a first clinical episode and have MRI features consistent with MS	Flulike symptoms, injection site reactions, neutropenia, anemia, liver function test abnormalities	Interferon beta-1-beta
Ofatumumab (Kesimpta: SQ monthly)	To reduce the frequency of clinical exacerbations in patients with relapsing forms of MS	Injection site reactions, headache, HBV reactivation, increased risk infections	B cell antibody
Natalizumab (Tysabri: Monthly IV infusions)	As monotherapy for relapsing forms of MS; to delay accumulation of physical disability and reduce frequency of clinical exacerbations	PML brain infection (risk 1:1,000)	α4-integrin adhesion molecule blocker
Ocrelizumab (Ocrevus: Every-6-mo infusion)	To reduce frequency of relapses in relapsing-remitting MS; slows progression in primary progressive MS	Infusion reactions; risk of infection	B-cell antibody
Teriflunomide (Aubagio: daily oral t)	To reduce frequency of relapses in relapsing-remitting MS	Hepatotoxicity, bone marrow suppression, peripheral neuropathy	Pyrimidine synthesis inhibitor
Dimethyl fumarate (Tecfidera), diroximel fumarate (Vumerity), monomethyl fumarate (Bafiertam): Twice daily capsules	To reduce frequency of relapses in relapsing-remitting MS	Flushing, gastrointestinal side effects, lymphopenia	Inhibits transcription of nuclear factor
Cladribine 2 wk of oral pills/yr	To reduce frequency of relapses in relapsing-remitting MS	Potential cancer risk; risk of infection	Purine synthesis modulator
Mitoxantrone (Novantrone: IV chemotherapy)	To reduce neurologic disability and/or the frequency of clinical relapses in secondary (chronic) progressive, progressive relapsing, or worsening relapsing-remitting MS	Cardiomyopathy, increased risk of secondary lymphoid malignancies (now used less commonly due to risks)	Cytotoxic chemotherapy; synthetic antineoplastic anthracenedione

HBV, hepatitis B virus; *IFN,* interferon; *IM,* intramuscular; *IV,* intravenous; *MRI,* magnetic resonance imaging; *PML,* progressive multifocal leukoencephalopathy; *SQ,* subcutaneous; *TIW,* three times a week.
Adopted from Jankovic J et al: *Bradley and Daroff's neurology in clinical practice,* ed 8, Philadelphia, 2022, Elsevier.

long-term outcomes of the disease, but instead accelerate recovery from symptoms of the current relapse.[18-19]

Plasma exchange can be considered for steroid-refractory cases.[20]

CHRONIC Rx

- Most FDA-approved disease-modifying therapies (DMTs) are only approved for use in relapsing forms of MS (which include CIS, RRMS, and active SPMS—or SPMS with relapses). Ocrelizumab and mitoxantrone are the first FDA-approved DMTs for use in PPMS and SPMS, respectively.
- **Injectable DMTs:** These medications include the first generation of MS drugs (interferons and glatiramer acetate), which have a low risk of side effects but modest efficacy in preventing future relapses. Ofatumumab is a newer injectable DMT with high efficacy but higher risk of side effects than the older injectable's DMTs.
  1. **Interferons:** Include interferon beta-1a (intramuscular injection [IM Avonex, dose of 30 mcg once per wk; IM Plegridy, starting dose of 63 mcg uptitrated over 1 mo to 125 mcg every 2 wk; subcutaneous (SC) Rebif, dose of 22 or 44 mcg three times per wk]) and **interferon beta-1b** (SC Betaseron, SC Extavia; doses of 0.25 mg every other day). Involve a complex and multifactorial mechanism of action, including increased expression of antiinflammatory mediators and downregulated expression of proinflammatory cytokines. Side effects can include fatigue, flulike symptoms, injection site reactions such as skin necrosis, depression, hepatotoxicity, seizures, anemia, leukopenia, thrombocytopenia, and thrombotic microangiopathy. CBC with differential, LFTs, and thyroid function tests should be obtained before initiating and regularly monitored during treatment (initially every 3 mo for 6 mo, then annually).
  2. **Glatiramer acetate** (SC Copaxone, SC Glatopa; doses of 20 mg daily or 40 mg three times per wk): Synthetic protein that simulates myelin basic protein and shifts T cells from the proinflammatory Th1 to regulatory Th2 profile. Common side effects include injection site reactions (such as lipoatrophy and skin necrosis) and brief postinjection reactions such as flushing, chest tightness, tachycardia, and dyspnea; no laboratory monitoring is needed.
  3. **Ofatumumab** (SC Kesimpta; dose of 20 mg weekly for 3 wk, no injection for 1 wk, then 20 mg per mo):[21] Anti-CD20 monoclonal antibody injectable. Side effects can include injection site reactions, headache, hepatitis B virus (HBV) reactivation, low immunoglobulins, and increased risk of infections (especially upper respiratory tract infections [URIs]). Before initiating and during treatment, obtain CBC with differential (including lymphocyte subsets), LFTs, immunoglobulins, TB, and HBV and JC virus antibodies. Live or live-attenuated vaccinations should be administered at least 1 mo before starting treatment.
- **Oral DMTs:** These medications are newer and more efficacious than the initial injectable DMTs in preventing MS relapses, but carry a higher risk of serious side effects and infections. Review the patient's general risk of infections before starting any oral DMT.
  1. Fingolimod (Gilenya; dose of 0.5 mg daily)[22], siponimod (Mayzent; starting dose of 0.25 mg daily, titrated up to 1 to 2 mg daily over 4 to 5 days), ozanimod (Zeposia;

starting dose of 0.23 mg uptitrated over 1 wk to 0.92 mg daily), or ponesimod (Ponvory; starting dose of 2 mg uptitrated over 2 wk to 20 mg daily): Mechanism of action involves sphingosine-1-phosphate receptor modulation and lymphocyte sequestration. Side effects can include diarrhea, headache, back pain, abdominal pain, cough, hepatotoxicity, bradycardia with the first dose (requiring cardiac monitoring and ECG for at least 8 h after administration), arrhythmia, orthostatic hypotension, hypertension, pancytopenia, macular edema (requiring ophthalmologic exam at baseline, at 3 mo, and annually thereafter for those with history of diabetes or uveitis), increased risk of infections (including PML, cryptococcal meningitis, herpes simplex virus [HSV] encephalitis, disseminated VZV), posterior reversible encephalopathy syndrome (PRES), increased risk of skin cancers (requiring regular skin examinations), and reduced pulmonary function. Before initiating treatment, obtain baseline HSV, TB, JC virus, and VZV serologies, CBC with differential, LFTs, macular OCT, and possibly CYP2C9 genotype (if considering siponimod); monitor CBC with differential and LFTs every 3 to 6 mo during treatment. Live or live-attenuated vaccinations should be administered at least 1 mo before starting treatment.

2. **Teriflunomide** (Aubagio; dose of 14 mg daily):[23] Reversible inhibitor of pyrimidine synthesis (enzyme dihydroorotate dehydrogenase). Side effects can include headache, nausea, diarrhea, hypertension, alopecia, peripheral neuropathy, paresthesias, severe hepatotoxicity, hypersensitivity reactions (anaphylaxis, angioedema, Stevens-Johnson syndrome, toxic epidermal necrolysis, drug reaction with eosinophilia and systemic symptoms [DRESS]), and interstitial lung disease. Patients should avoid becoming pregnant while on teriflunomide (pregnancy category X). Serum levels can be measured, and the drug can be eliminated by a course of activated charcoal or cholestyramine. Before initiating treatment, check baseline blood pressure, CBC with differential, LFTs, and TB test; monitor monthly LFTs for the first 6 mo, and CBC and LFTs every 3 to 6 mo during treatment.

3. **Dimethyl fumarate** (Tecfidera; starting dose of 120 mg twice daily for 2 wk, then 240 mg twice daily), **diroximel fumarate** (Vumerity; starting dose of 231 mg twice daily for 1 wk, then 462 mg twice daily), or **monomethyl fumarate** (Bafiertam; starting dose of 95 mg twice daily for 1 wk, then 190 mg twice daily): Inhibit transcription of nuclear factor-κB (NF-κB; in the nuclear factor erythroid 2–related factor 2 [Nrf-2] pathway). Side effects can include nausea, abdominal discomfort (can be reduced with use of H2 blockers or proton pump inhibitors), pruritus, and flushing (can be reduced with concurrent use of aspirin and taking with food)—especially

during the first mo—and rarely, lymphopenia, with increased risk of infections such as PML. Before initiating treatment, check CBC with differential, LFTs, TB, VZV and JC virus antibodies; monitor CBC with differential and LFTs every 3 to 6 mo during treatment.

4. **Cladribine** (Mavenclad; total dose of 3.5 mg/kg administered orally in two short courses 1 yr apart): A purine antimetabolite that inhibits DNA synthesis and depletes both T and B lymphocytes. FDA-approved for use in relapsing forms of MS, except for CIS. Side effects can include hematologic toxicity, alopecia, increased risk of infections, increased risk of malignancy, weight loss, and hepatic injury. Pregnancy should be avoided during treatment and for at least 6 mo after the last dose, and breastfeeding is contraindicated during treatment days and for 10 days after the last dose. Cladribine is also contraindicated in patients who are immunocompromised, have active chronic infections, or have cancer. CBC with differential, TB, and viral serologies (e.g., HIV, VZV, HSV, hepatitis B and C, JC virus) should be checked before initiating treatment and monitored regularly during treatment. Live or live-attenuated vaccinations should be administered at least 1 mo before starting treatment.

- **IV DMTs:** These are generally the newest and most efficacious for preventing MS relapses. They consequently also carry a higher risk of serious side effects and infections. Live or live-attenuated vaccinations should be administered at least 1 mo before starting treatment with any of these.

1. **Ocrelizumab** (Ocrevus; dose of 600 mg every 6 mo, with the first dose divided as 300 mg given 2 wk apart):[24] Humanized monoclonal antibody to CD20+ B cells. FDA-approved for use in PPMS as well as all relapsing forms of MS. Side effects can include leukopenia, low immunoglobulins, infusion reactions, increased risk of infections (upper and lower respiratory tract infections, UTI, HSV, skin infections), HBV reactivation, and possibly an increased risk of breast cancer. Before starting treatment, obtain baseline CBC with differential, immunoglobulins, TB test, and viral serologies, including HBV, HCV, VZV, HSV, HIV, and JC virus. Monitor CBC with differential, T and B lymphocyte counts, immunoglobulins, TB, HBV, and JC virus antibodies 1 to 2 times per year. This medication is contraindicated in patients with history of active HBV infection.

2. **Ublituximab** (Briumvi; dose of 450 mg every 6 mo, with first dose at 150 mg and second dose at 450 mg given 2 wk after first dose): Chimeric monoclonal antibody to CD20+ B cells (binding to a different epitope than other anti-CD20 therapies). Has enhanced affinity to CD16a variants, therefore activating natural killer-cell function. FDA approved for use in all

relapsing forms of MS. Second and subsequent doses are administered over 1 h (more rapid than standard ocrelizumab infusion rate). Side effects, risks, and required screening and monitoring tests are similar to those of ocrelizumab.

3. **Natalizumab** (Tysabri; dose of 300 mg monthly): A humanized monoclonal antibody that binds to the lymphocyte surface protein α4-integrin, which inhibits binding to VCAM-1 and, therefore, movement of lymphocytes across the bloodstream. It has been associated with a *higher* risk of PML than other immunomodulatory therapies. Testing for JC virus antibody (along with CBC with differential and LFTs) should be done every 6 mo because conversion to a positive antibody occurs at increased frequency while on this drug. If positive, PML is still rare, but the risk increases with increased length of therapy (>2 yr), history of chemotherapy or prior immunosuppression, and high level of JC virus antibodies. Other potential serious side effects can include infusion reactions, HSV and other infections, hepatotoxicity, and thrombocytopenia. Stopping natalizumab has increased risk of rebound relapse.

4. **Alemtuzumab** (Lemtrada; dose of 12 mg daily for 5 days, then 12 mg daily for 3 days 1 yr later): Anti-CD52 humanized monoclonal antibody and second-line therapy for patients who have failed at least two FDA-approved MS therapies. FDA-approved for use in relapsing forms of MS, except for CIS. Side effects can include the development of autoimmune conditions (34% developed autoimmune thyroid disorders), cytopenias, hepatotoxicity, infusion reactions, stroke, arterial dissection, hemophagocytic lymphohistiocytosis (HLH), bleeding or clotting disorders such as immune thrombocytopenic purpura (ITP) and TTP, pneumonitis, Goodpasture disease, increased risk of certain cancers, and increased risk of infections including PML. Only available through a restricted access program. It is contraindicated in patients who are immunocompromised or have chronic active infections. Requires monthly monitoring of CBC with differential (including lymphocyte subsets), LFTs, TSH, renal function tests, and urinalysis until at least 4 yr after the last course, and HSV prophylaxis for at least 2 mo after each dose.

5. **Mitoxantrone** (Novantrone; 12 mg/m² every 3 mo for 2 yr): An antineoplastic anthracenedione (DNA-reactive agent) that inhibits B-cell, T-cell, and macrophage proliferation and impairs antigen presentation. FDA-approved for use in SPMS, progressive-relapsing MS, and worsening RRMS; however, now used very infrequently. Potential serious side effects include secondary acute myeloid leukemia, neutropenia, and cardiotoxicity (CHF). Is contraindicated if baseline neutrophil

count <1,500 cells/mm^3 and hepatic impairment (due to reduced clearance). Requires initial evaluation and regular monitoring (prior to each dose) of CBC with differential, LFTs, ECG, echocardiogram (for left ventricular ejection fraction), and pregnancy test if relevant (pregnancy category D).

- Symptomatic therapy:
  1. **Gait dysfunction:** Initial management should be referral to physical therapy, use of ankle-foot orthoses (for footdrop), and/or mobility aids. Dalfampridine (Ampyra) is a potassium channel blocker that is FDA-approved to improve walking speed (objectively measured by a timed 25-ft walk test) in patients with MS; contraindicated in patients with epilepsy.
  2. **Spasticity:** Initial management should be twice-daily stretching exercises and referral to physical therapy. Can next consider baclofen (starting dose of 10 mg twice daily) or tizanidine (starting dose of 2 mg nightly; requires monitoring of liver enzymes). For severe spasticity not responsive to these medications, dantrolene (starting dose of 25 mg daily; requires monitoring of liver enzymes) or diazepam (average daily dose of 15 mg) may be tried. Onabotulinum toxin type A injection can be used for focal intractable spasticity. Intrathecal baclofen pump can be used for generalized intractable spasticity. Acute worsening of spasticity may be caused by infections such as UTI, injury, recent surgery, or colder temperatures.[25]
  3. **Urge incontinence and retention:** Obtain urinalysis and post-void residual bladder ultrasound. Recommend fluid restriction at night, scheduled voiding, and avoidance of caffeine and alcohol. Incontinence can be initially treated with anticholinergic/muscarinic therapy such as oxybutynin, trospium, tolterodine, or solifenacin. Mirabegron is a beta-3 agonist indicated for treatment of neurogenic detrusor overactivity (overactive or neurogenic bladder). Urinary retention can be treated with tamsulosin. In both cases, UTI or bladder infection should be ruled out. Intermittent catheterization, intradetrusor onabotulinum toxin A injections, and neuromodulation (tibial nerve stimulation) are more advanced options for severe neurogenic bladder symptoms and require management by a urologist.[26]
  4. **Dysesthesias:** Can treat with carbamazepine (200 mg twice daily), oxcarbazepine (starting dose of 300 mg daily), gabapentin (starting dose of 300 mg daily), pregabalin (starting dose of 50 mg daily), or duloxetine (starting dose 30 mg daily; can treat comorbid depression and anxiety).
  5. **Fatigue:** Initial management should involve medication review, depression screening, evaluating for underlying sleep disorder (e.g., obstructive sleep apnea), energy conservation strategies, exercise program, and weight loss for obesity. Can next consider medical management with amantadine (100 mg twice daily), modafinil (starting dose of 100 mg daily), or a stimulant such as methylphenidate.
  6. **Tremor:** Can treat with clonazepam (starting dose of 0.5 mg daily), propranolol (starting dose of 20 to 40 mg twice daily), or gabapentin (starting dose of 300 mg daily).
  7. **Cognitive impairment:** Can objectively screen with the Symbol Digit Modalities Test, if available. Assess for other causes of cognitive impairment, such as neurodegenerative disease, depression, fatigue, disordered sleep, and polypharmacy. Recommend conservative strategies, such as the use of checklists, reminders, diaries, and calendars, and regular physical exercise and social activity.
  8. **Depression and anxiety:** Refer for cognitive-behavioral therapy. Consider starting a selective serotonin reuptake inhibitor (SSRI) or serotonin norepinephrine reuptake inhibitor (SNRI). Distinguish between depression and pseudobulbar affect, which is treated with dextromethorphan/quinidine (Nuedexta).

DISPOSITION

Most patients have complete or near-complete recovery weeks to months after a relapse, even without acute treatment with high-dose steroids. Typically, two relapses occur in RRMS patient not on DMT per yr (75% will have >1 relapse). Although the rate of disease progression is highly variable, there is higher risk of greater long-term disability with higher relapse rate during the first 2 to 5 yr, poor recovery from initial relapses, older age of onset, involvement of multiple systems, male sex, African American, and primary progressive disease.

The development of higher-efficacy DMTs, since the introduction of the first DMT (interferon 1-b) approved for treatment of RRMS in 1993, has significantly improved the prognosis of patients newly diagnosed with MS. The current treatment goal for these patients is no relapses and no disease progression on imaging.

REFERRAL

- Referral to a neurologist is necessary. Referral to an MS specialist is recommended for all patients based on availability and especially for those with questionable diagnosis, poor response to initial therapy, high relapse rate, progressive MS, and concern about monitoring/managing complications of therapies.
- Referrals for physical, speech, and occupational therapy for motor, sensory, and speech symptoms.
- Referral to a mental health provider and/or psychiatrist for depression/anxiety.
- Referral to neuropsychology and cognitive rehabilitation for cognitive impairment symptoms.
- Referral to urology if bladder-sphincter dyssynergia is possible, if symptoms are not responsive to first-line medications, or in case of complications such as recurrent UTI, hematuria, renal impairment, hydronephrosis, or stress incontinence.
- Referral to ophthalmology (or neuroophthalmology, if available) for optic neuritis (with optical coherence tomography for measurement of retinal nerve fiber layer and ganglion cell layer thickness).

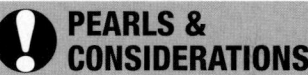

PEARLS & CONSIDERATIONS

- Pseudorelapse or pseudoexacerbation or recrudescence, terms used to describe recurrence of symptoms from a prior relapse (either symptomatic or asymptomatic) without new inflammation may occur with heat, exercise, fatigue, fever, or infections (urinary tract infections are common in patients with MS). Symptoms should subside within 24 h after elimination of the trigger; if symptoms persist, consider obtaining MRI to rule out a new symptomatic relapse.
- Pseudoprogression is the insidious progression of neurologic disability due to factors unrelated to MS pathogenesis, typically that of other comorbidities (degenerative joint disease, neurodegenerative disease, etc.).
- Headache, fever, altered mental status, marked CSF pleocytosis, or recurrent relapses over days to weeks raises concern for CNS infection or ADEM.

REFERENCES & SUGGESTED READING

Available at eBooks.Health.Elsevier.com.

RELATED CONTENT

Multiple Sclerosis (Patient Information)
Neuromyelitis Optica Spectrum Disorder (Related Key Topic)
Optic Neuritis (Related Key Topic)

AUTHORS: **NATASHA CHOUDHURY, MD** and **ROUMEN BALABANOV, MD**

BASIC INFORMATION

DEFINITION

Myasthenia gravis (MG) is an autoimmune disorder affecting postsynaptic neuromuscular transmission, most commonly mediated by antibodies directed against the nicotinic acetylcholine receptor (AChR) of the neuromuscular junction. Anti-AChR antibodies cause a decrease in functional postsynaptic ACh receptors, resulting in fatigable weakness. A small percentage of MG patients lack AChR antibodies, and a subset of these patients possess antibodies against muscle-specific tyrosine kinase (MuSK) or low-density lipoprotein receptor–related protein 4 (LRP4), which both affect pre- and postsynaptic function of the neuromuscular junction.[1,2] Finally, a portion of AChR antibody-negative myasthenia patients do not possess any detectable antibodies, and this group of patients is appropriately termed "seronegative." A classification of MG is described in Table 1.

SYNONYM

MG

ICD-10CM CODES

G70.00	Myasthenia gravis without (acute) exacerbation
G70.01	Myasthenia gravis with (acute) exacerbation
P94.0	Transient neonatal myasthenia gravis

EPIDEMIOLOGY & DEMOGRAPHICS

INCIDENCE (IN U.S.): 8 to 10 cases annually per 1 million persons. It is the most common disorder of neuromuscular junction transmission.
PREVALENCE (IN U.S.): 150 to 250 cases per 1 million persons.
PREDOMINANT SEX: Females are affected more often than males (3:2) in adults; they are equally affected in the elderly.
PEAK INCIDENCE: Female, second to third decades; male, sixth to eighth decades.
GENETICS: Increased frequency of HLA-B8, DR3.[3]

PHYSICAL FINDINGS & CLINICAL PRESENTATION

- The hallmark of MG is weakness worsened with exercise and improved with rest.[4]
- Generalized weakness involving proximal muscles, the diaphragm, and neck extensors is common.
- Weakness is confined to eyelids and extraocular muscles in approximately 15% of patients (Figs. E1, E2, E3, and Box 1). This is referred to as ocular myasthenia gravis.
- Bulbar symptoms of ptosis, diplopia, dysarthria, and dysphagia are common.
- Reflexes, sensation, and coordination remain normal.

ETIOLOGY

An antibody-mediated decrease in nicotinic AChRs in the postsynaptic neuromuscular junction results in defective neuromuscular transmission and subsequent muscle weakness and fatigue. Early-onset MG is associated with *HLA-B8.1*, whereas late-onset MG is associated with *HLA-DQB1, HLA-DQA1,* and *HLA-DRB1*.[3]

Some myasthenia gravis patients present with MuSK or LRP4 antibodies instead of AChR antibodies. The MuSK antibody is present in about 40% to 50% of the subset of individuals who lack the AChR antibody, and the LRP4 antibody is present in a fraction of the remainder.[1] Both MuSK and LRP4 antibodies interrupt the process of AChR aggregation at the neuromuscular junction. Anti-MuSK patients can have a similar syndrome to AChR MG, although they may have fewer ocular symptoms, more bulbar weakness, facial tongue and proximal muscle atrophy, and either lack of or paradoxic response to pyridostigmine. Anti-LRP4 patients generally have milder symptoms that favor ocular findings. However, serious cases can still yield severe clinical symptoms.[1] Both MuSK and LRP4 antibody MG have not been shown to have any association with thymoma.[4]

Less than 10% of myasthenia gravis patients are seronegative for AChR, MuSK, and LRP4 antibodies. This syndrome is termed *seronegative myasthenia gravis* and presents with a higher proportion of entirely ocular symptoms. Generally, this group of patients responds well to classic MG therapies, including pyridostigmine, steroids, immunosuppression, and thymectomy.

Serologic and clinical presentation of myasthenia gravis subgroups are summarized in Table 2.

Dx DIAGNOSIS

DIFFERENTIAL DIAGNOSIS

Lambert-Eaton myasthenic syndrome, botulism, medication-induced myasthenia, chronic progressive external ophthalmoplegia, congenital myasthenic syndromes, thyroid disease, basilar meningitis, intracranial mass lesion with cranial neuropathy, Miller-Fisher variant of Guillain-Barré syndrome

WORKUP

- Edrophonium (Tensilon) test (Fig. E4): Useful in MG patients with ocular symptoms, although uncommonly used now. Cardiac

TABLE 1 Osserman Classification Used by the Myasthenia Gravis Foundation of America to Standardize Clinical Symptoms[a]

Class I	Any ocular muscle weakness
Class II	Ocular muscle weakness of any severity, MILD limb weakness
Class IIa	Predominantly limb and/or axial muscle weakness
Class IIb	Predominantly bulbar and/or respiratory muscle weakness
Class III	Ocular muscle weakness of any severity, MODERATE weakness of other muscles
Class IIIa	Predominantly limb and/or axial muscle weakness
Class IIIb	Predominantly bulbar and/or respiratory muscle weakness
Class IV	Ocular muscle weakness of any severity, SEVERE weakness of other muscles
Class IVa	Predominantly limb and/or axial muscle weakness
Class IVb	Predominantly bulbar and/or respiratory muscle weakness
Class V	Intubation with or without mechanical ventilation

[a]Jaretzki A et al: Myasthenia gravis: recommendations for clinical research standards. Task Force of the Medical Scientific Advisory Board of the Myasthenia Gravis Foundation of America, *Neurology* 55:16-23, 2000.
From Parrillo JE, Dellinger RP: *Critical care medicine: principles of diagnosis and management in the adult,* ed 5, Philadelphia, 2019, Elsevier.

BOX 1 Ocular Findings in Myasthenia Gravis (MG)

1. Weakness usually involves one or more ocular muscles without overt pupillary abnormality.
2. Weakness is typically variable, fluctuating, and fatigable.
3. Ptosis that shifts from one eye to the other is virtually pathognomonic of MG.
4. With limited ocular excursion, saccades are superfast, producing ocular "quiver."
5. After downgaze, upgaze produces lid overshoot ("lid twitch")
6. Pseudo-internuclear ophthalmoplegia—limited adduction, with nystagmoid jerks in abducting eye.
7. In asymmetric ptosis, covering the ptotic eye may relieve contraction of the opposite frontalis.
8. Passively lifting a ptotic lid may cause the opposite lid to fall: "Enhanced ptosis" or "curtain sign."
9. Edrophonium may improve only some of several weak ocular muscles; others may actually become weaker.
10. Edrophonium may relieve asymmetric ptosis and produce retraction of the opposite lid from frontalis contraction.
11. The opposite lid may droop further as the more involved lid improves after edrophonium.
12. Cold applied to the eye may improve lid ptosis: "Ice-pack test" (see Fig. E5).

From Jankovic J et al: *Bradley and Daroff's neurology in clinical practice,* ed 8, Philadelphia, 2022, Elsevier.

M

I

TABLE 2 Serologic and Clinical Presentation of Myasthenia Gravis Subgroups[a-h]

	AChR Antibody	MuSK Antibody	LRP4 Antibody	Striated Muscle Antigens Titin Antibody RyR Antibody	Age at Onset Sex	Clinical Findings	Response to Therapy	Response to Thymectomy	Prognosis
Ocular MG	50%-75%	None	None	None	Older Male	Ocular	Good	Good	Good (but 50% can develop generalized MG in 2 yr)
Early-onset generalized MG	80%-85% (high titer)	None	None	None-rare	<50 yr	General	Rarely needs immunosuppression	Good	Less severe Low mortality
Late-onset generalized MG	None-rare	None	None	50% 54% titin 33% RyR	≥50 yr	General	Often requires immunosuppression	Poor	Severe
Thymomatous-associated MG	Positive, nearly 100% (low titer)	None	None	95% 50% titin 47% RyR	Ranges: Older but <40 yr if RyR	General If RyR: Ocular, bulbar, respiratory weakness	Often requires immunosuppression	Fair	RyR: Invasive, malignant thymoma Severe Higher mortality
Generalized MG MuSK positive	None	100%	None	None	Younger female	Facial, bulbar, neck, respiratory weakness paraspinal, esophageal muscles	Poor response to AChE inhibitors	Poor (no thymic changes)	Severe, progressive course
Generalized MG LRP4 positive	None	None	100%	None	Younger female	General	Good	Not enough data	Fair
MG with thymic hyperplasia	89%	None	None	None	Younger female	General	Good	Good	Good
ACh antibody negative	Negative	Negative	Negative	Present	Younger female	General	Poor		Fair

ACh, Acetylcholine; *AChE*, acetylcholinesterase; *AChR*, acetylcholine receptor; *MG*, myasthenia gravis; *MuSK*, muscle-specific tyrosine kinase; *LRP4*, low-density lipoprotein receptor-related protein 4; *RyR*, ryanodine receptor.

[a]Romi F et al: Myasthenia gravis patients with ryanodine receptor antibodies have distinctive clinical features, *Eur J Neurol* 14:617-620, 2007.
[b]Romi F et al: Myasthenia gravis: clinical, immunological, and therapeutic advances, *Acta Neurol Scand* 111:134-141, 2005.
[c]Akaishi T et al: Response to treatment of myasthenia gravis according to clinical subtype, *BMC Neurol* 16:225, 2016.
[d]Gilhus NE, Verschuuren JJ: Myasthenia gravis: subgroup classification and therapeutic strategies, *Lancet Neurol* 14:1023-1036, 2015.
[e]Hong Y et al: Autoantibody profile and clinical characteristics in a cohort of Chinese adult myasthenia gravis patients, *J Neuroimmunol* 298:51-57, 2016.
[f]Gilhus NE et al: Myasthenia gravis-autoantibody characteristics and their implications for therapy, *Nat Rev Neurol* 12:259-268, 2016.
[g]Roberts PF et al: Thymectomy in the treatment of ocular myasthenia gravis, *J Thorac Cardiovasc Surg* 122:562-568, 2001.
[h]Rivner MH et al: Clinical features of LRP4/agrin-antibody-positive myasthenia gravis: a multicenter study, *Muscle Nerve* 62(3):333-343, 2020. https://doi.org/10.1002/mus.26985.
From Parrillo JE, Dellinger RP: *Critical care medicine: principles of diagnosis and management in the adult*, ed 5, Philadelphia, 2019, Elsevier.

monitoring and atropine ready at the bedside are essential.
- Patients with MG may also have a positive ice-pack test (Fig. E5).
- Repetitive nerve stimulation: Successive stimulation shows decrement of muscle action potential in clinically weak muscle; may be negative in up to 50%.
- Single-fiber electromyography: Highly sensitive; abnormal in up to 95% of patients.
- Serum AChR antibodies MuSK and/or LRP4 antibodies.

LABORATORY TESTS

- Forced vital capacity (FVC) is the most useful test for assessing neuromuscular respiratory status. Patients with an FVC of <20 ml/kg are at high risk of respiratory failure and should be monitored in an ICU setting. Although the decision of when to intubate is a clinical one, FVC falling below 10 to 15 ml/kg generally requires intubation.
- Computed tomography scan with contrast of anterior chest to look for thymoma (about 10% of patients) or thymic hyperplasia (about 80% of patients). Prevalence increases with age.
- Thyroid-stimulating hormone and free T$_4$ to rule out thyroid disease.

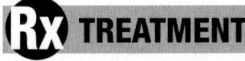 **TREATMENT**

NONPHARMACOLOGIC THERAPY

- Patient education to facilitate recognition of worsening symptoms and impress need for medical evaluation at onset of clinical deterioration
- Avoidance of selected drugs (Table 3) known to provoke exacerbations of MG (β-blockers, aminoglycoside and quinolone antibiotics, penicillamine, interferons, class I antiarrhythmics [procainamide, quinidine, etc.])
- Prompt treatment of infections, diet modification, and speech evaluation with dysphagia

ACUTE THERAPY

- The initial step in managing the myasthenic patient in crisis is stabilization of the airway and supporting ventilation. Respiratory failure ensues from muscle weakness, not inadequate oxygenation; therefore, supplemental oxygenation does not address the problem, and mechanical ventilation is indicated. Endotracheal intubation may be necessary, but biphasic positive airway pressure (BiPAP) support may be sufficient if the patient is otherwise able to protect their airway. Capnometry monitoring can be useful in detecting respiratory fatigue well in advance of

TABLE 3 Medications to Avoid in Myasthenia Gravis[a]

Medications to Avoid	Examples	Recommendation for Avoidance	Mechanism of Weakness
Antibiotics			
Aminoglycosides	Gentamycin Streptomycin Tobramycin Amikacin	Contraindicated Less likely problematic	Blocks ACh receptor, prevents release of ACh
Antimalarials	Quinine Chloroquine	Contraindicated	Presynaptic blockage of voltage-dependent sodium channels and postsynaptic potentiation of depolarization
Macrolides	Erythromycin, Tetracycline Azithromycin	Relative	Affects presynaptic transmission
Fluoroquinolones	Moxifloxacin Ciprofloxacin Levofloxacin Ofloxacin	FDA black box warning	Unknown
Ketolide	Telithromycin	FDA black box warning	Unknown
	Polymyxins	Contraindicated	Presynaptic and postsynaptic effects
Cardiovascular			
Antiarrhythmics	Procainamide Propafenone	Contraindicated	Decreases the release of AChSodium influx blocker
β-Blockers	Propranolol Atenolol Ophthalmic timolol	Relative	Unclear—may be at the neuromuscular junction or muscle membrane
Calcium channel blocker	Verapamil Amlodipine	Relative	Presynaptic and postsynaptic blockade of L-type calcium channels
Anticonvulsants			
	Phenytoin	Relative	Depressed postsynaptic response to ACh; inhibition of calcium channel; increase in muscle membrane threshold
	Carbamazepine	Relative	Triggers immune response
	Gabapentin	Relative	Binds voltage-gated calcium channel
Chemotherapeutic Agents			
	Doxorubicin Etoposide Cisplatin	Relative	Unknown
Others			
	Interferon	Relative	Autoantibody production
Neuromuscular blocking agents	Atracurium Cisatracurium Vecuronium	Relative	Blocks ACh receptors
Statins		Relative	Unknown
Corticosteroids		Relative	Direct blocking of ACh receptor through ionic channels
Botulinum toxin		Contraindicated	Impairs synaptic transmission
Magnesium		Relative	Impairs synaptic transmission
Penicillamine		Contraindicated	Binds the ACh receptor; induces antibodies to receptor

ACh, Acetylcholine; *FDA,* Food and Drug Administration.

[a]Ahmed A, Simmons Z: Drugs which may exacerbate or induce myasthenia gravis: a clinician's guide, *Internet J Neurol* 10:1-8, 2008.

From Parrillo JE, Dellinger RP: *Critical care medicine: principles of diagnosis and management in the adult,* ed 5, Philadelphia, 2019, Elsevier.

oxyhemoglobin desaturation and obvious clinical findings of respiratory distress.[5] Consider elective intubation if forced vital capacity is <10 to 15 ml/kg.

- Plasmapheresis and intravenous immunoglobulin (IVIG) are short-term options for immunotherapy during an exacerbation. There is no significant difference in efficacy between IVIG and plasmapheresis.[6]
- Fig. E6 illustrates a flowchart for the management of myasthenic crisis.

CHRONIC Rx (TABLE E4)

- Symptomatic treatment with acetylcholinesterase inhibitors:
  1. Pyridostigmine 30 to 60 mg PO q4 to 6h initially; onset of effect is 30 min, duration 4 h. May be titrated up to 120 mg every 4 h. GI upset is common with higher doses and may respond to hyoscyamine. Patients with MUSK+ disease often do not respond to pyridostigmine.
- Long-term immunosuppressive treatment with corticosteroids is first-line treatment; however, patients are often transitioned to a nonsteroidal immunosuppressive agent such as azathioprine or mycophenolate to avoid the significant side effects of long-term steroid use:
  1. Prednisone initiated at 10 to 20 mg daily titrated by 5-mg increments to effect or dose of 1 mg/kg/day with improvement in 2 to 4 wk and maximal response by 3 to 6 mo.
  2. Azathioprine initiated at 50 mg daily titrated to 2 to 3 mg/kg/day with clinical effect in 6 to 12 mo. Steroid-sparing agent. Azathioprine is not recommended in patients with no thiopurine methyltransferase activity.
  3. Mycophenolate mofetil 500 mg twice a day titrated to 2 g/day with clinical effect in 3 to 6 mo, but can be up to 12 mo. Steroid-sparing agent.
  4. Cyclosporine initiated at 5 mg/kg/day with clinical effect within 1 to 2 mo. Steroid sparing agent. Note a faster onset of effect than azathioprine or mycophenolate, but also a less tolerable side-effect profile due to concerns for renal toxicity and drug interactions.
  5. Tacrolimus initiated at 0.1 mg/kg/day divided into two doses then titrated to

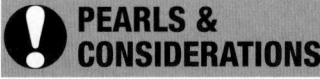
plasma concentration of 7 to 8 ng/ml with clinical effect within 6 to 12 mo. Steroid sparing agent. This drug is better tolerated than cyclosporine but still has potential for serious side effects.

- Targeted immunotherapy for myasthenia gravis allows quicker and more effective treatment with fewer side effects. Multiple new therapies are currently being researched and/or in clinical trials, including Fc receptor inhibitors, complement inhibitors, interlukin-6 inhibitors, chimeric antigen receptor (CAR) and chimeric autoantibody receptor (CAAR) T cell therapy, and hematopoietic stem cell transplantation.[7] A current list of some alternative agents is below:

1. Efgartigimod alfa given at 10 mg/kg for 4 wk in weekly infusions with clinical effect within 1 mo. This drug is an Fc receptor inhibitor that promotes IgG degradation and was approved by the FDA in 2021. Further research is needed to determine the long term benefit of this drug, but it can be considered as a glucocorticoid-sparing bridge until slower-acting agents such as azathioprine and mycophenolate take effect.[8]

2. Ravulizumab initiated as IV infusion at 2.4 to 3 g (weight based) followed by 3 to 3.6 g (weight based) 2 wk after loading dose, followed by every 8 wk afterwards. This drug is a human monoclonal antibody that binds complement C5 similar to eculizumab but with a more convenient dosing schedule. It was FDA approved for AChR antibody positive patients in 2022.[9]

3. Eculizumab initiated at 900 mg IV weekly for four doses, then 1200 mg on the fifth wk and every 2 wk afterwards. Like ravulizumab, this drug is a complement inhibitor approved for adult patients who are acetylcholine-antibody positive and have severe symptoms despite current immunotherapy use.[7]

4. Rozanolixizumab initiated at 420 to 840 mg SQ weekly for 6 wk depending on body weight. With a similar target to efgartigimod, it is a monoclonal antibody that binds to the Fc receptor to promote lysosomal degradation of IgG autoantibodies and is approved for AChR+ and MUSK+ myasthenia gravis.

5. Rituximab initiated at 1 g every 2 wk for two doses, OR 375 mg/m² weekly for four doses. Generally used in refractory MG or earlier in MuSK antibody MG. Redosing interval varies per protocol and by clinical response of the patient.[7]

SURGICAL Rx

- In thymomatous MG, thymectomy is indicated in all patients. If the tumor cannot be surgically resected, chemotherapy can be considered for prevention of local invasion and symptom relief.
- For nonthymomatous AChR-antibody positive MG, thymectomy improves clinical outcomes and reduces the need for steroids sustained over at least a 5-yr period. Surgical referral should be considered in patients <60 yr old without significant medical comorbidities even if no frank thymic tissue is seen on imaging, especially if they are refractory to therapy.[10,11]
- MuSK and LRP4 myasthenia are not associated with thymic pathology and generally thymectomy is not beneficial for these patients.[12]

DISPOSITION

Course of disease is highly variable. Mortality rate has decreased from 75% to 4.5% over the past four decades.

REFERRAL

- Referral to a general neurologist or neuromuscular specialist is appropriate.

- Surgical referral for thymectomy in selected cases (see "Surgical Rx").

⚠ PEARLS & CONSIDERATIONS

- Sustained upward or lateral gaze and arm abduction for 120 sec may be necessary to elicit subtle signs on examination.
- Myasthenic patients can worsen rapidly and warrant careful observation during an exacerbation or when ill.
- Cholinergic crisis, caused by excessive ACh activity related to acetylcholinesterase inhibitor therapy, is rarely seen, particularly with close management of pyridostigmine dosing. It may occur when patients deliberately or inadvertently take pyridostigmine in excess of the recommended dose. Cholinergic crisis is manifest by excessive cholinergic activity, which may include bradycardia, diarrhea and abdominal cramping, increased secretions, and muscle weakness, which might mimic a myasthenic crisis (Table 5).[1]

REFERENCES

Available at eBooks.Health.Elsevier.com.

RELATED CONTENT

Myasthenia Gravis (Patient Information)

AUTHOR: **LYDIA SHARP, MD**

TABLE 5 Notable Differences between Myasthenic Crisis and Cholinergic Crisis Pertaining to Myasthenia Gravis Patients

Myasthenic Crisis	Cholinergic Crisis
Generally minimal abdominal symptoms	Presence of abdominal pain, nausea and vomiting
Increased HR and BP	Decreased heart rate and blood pressure
Normal secretions	Increased secretions
Mydriasis	Miosis
Caused by undermedication of myasthenia gravis treatment	Caused by overmedication of myasthenia gravis treatment
Treat with cholinergic agent (edrophonium)	Treat with anticholinergic agent (atropine)

BP, Blood pressure; *HR,* heart rate.
From Walls RM et al: *Rosen's Emergency Medicine, concepts and clinical practice,* ed 10, Philadelphia, 2023, Elsevier.

BASIC INFORMATION

DEFINITION

Myocardial infarction (MI) is a clinical syndrome characterized by symptoms of myocardial ischemia, persistent electrocardiographic (ECG) changes, and release of biomarkers of myocardial necrosis resulting from an insufficient supply of oxygenated blood to an area of the heart. MI may be classified as ST-segment elevation MI (STEMI) and non–ST-segment elevation MI (NSTEMI) depending on the ECG findings on MI presentation. Acute coronary syndrome (ACS) refers to acute myocardial ischemia without myocardial necrosis (unstable angina) and myocardial necrosis and infarction (NSTEMI or STEMI). According to the European Society of Cardiology/American College of Cardiology guidelines, the following criteria for acute evolving or recent MI (NSTEMI and STEMI) satisfies the diagnosis:

- Detection of the rise and/or fall of cardiac biomarker values (preferably cardiac troponin [cTn]) with at least one value above the 99th percentile upper reference limit and with at least one of the following:
  1. Symptoms of ischemia
  2. Development of pathologic Q waves in the ECG
  3. Imaging evidence of new loss of viable myocardium or a new regional wall motion abnormality
  4. Identification of an intracoronary thrombus by angiography or autopsy pathologic findings of acute MI.
- ECG criteria:
  1. STEMI:
     a. New, or presumed new, significant ST-T changes or new left bundle branch block (LBBB) in appropriate clinical setting.
     b. New ST elevation at the J-point in at least 2 contiguous leads of >2 mm (0.2 mV) in men or ≥1.5 mm (0.15 mV) in women in leads V2 to V3 and/or of ≥1 mm (0.1 mV) in another contiguous chest leads or the upper limb leads
  2. NSTEMI:
     c. New ST-segment depression ≥0.5 mV (0.5 mm) and T-wave abnormalities
     d. New generation troponin assays are extremely sensitive to small changes in serum troponin levels at the cost of diagnostic specificity for MI related to plaque rupture or erosion.

Universal classification of acute MI:
- Type 1: Spontaneous MI related to ischemia due to a primary coronary event such as plaque erosion and/or rupture, fissuring, or dissection.
- Type 2: MI secondary to ischemia, other than coronary artery disease, due to either increased oxygen demand or decreased supply (e.g., coronary endothelial dysfunction, coronary artery spasm, coronary embolism, anemia, arrhythmias, respiratory failure, hypertension with/without left ventricular hypertrophy [LVH], or hypotension). Also, in critically ill patients or in patients undergoing major noncardiac surgery, elevated values of cardiac biomarkers may appear due to the direct toxic effects of endogenous or exogenous high circulating catecholamine levels.

- Type 3: Sudden unexpected cardiac death, including cardiac arrest, often with symptoms suggestive of myocardial ischemia, accompanied by presumed new ST elevation, new left bundle branch block, or evidence of fresh thrombus in a coronary artery by angiography and/or at autopsy, or death occurring before blood samples could be obtained or at a time before the appearance of cardiac biomarkers in the blood.
- Type 4a: MI associated with percutaneous coronary intervention. Elevation of cTn >5× percentile of upper reference limit (URL) in patients with normal baseline value, or a rise of cTn >20% if the baseline values are stable and are stable or falling. In addition to either symptoms of ischemia, new ischemic ECG changes or new LBBB, or angiographic loss of a patent coronary artery, persistent slow or no-flow, or embolization, or imaging of new wall motion abnormality.
- Type 4b: MI associated with stent thrombosis as documented by angiography or at autopsy in the setting of myocardial ischemia and with a rise/fall of cardiac biomarker values.
- Type 5: MI associated with coronary artery bypass grafting. Elevation of cardiac biomarker values >10× 99% URL in patients with normal baseline cTn values, in addition to either new pathologic Q waves or new LBBB, or new native coronary artery occlusion or imaging of new abnormal wall motion abnormality.
- Myocardial Infarction With Nonobstructive Coronary Arteries (MINOCA): It is defined as acute myocardial infarction in the absence of obstructive coronary artery disease. Conditions like Takotsubo cardiomyopathy, spontaneous coronary artery dissection, coronary artery spasm, microvascular dysfunction, and pulmonary embolism come under this novel category.

SYNONYMS

MI
ST-elevation MI
Heart attack
Acute myocardial infarction
AMI
Coronary thrombosis
Coronary occlusion

EPIDEMIOLOGY & DEMOGRAPHICS

INCIDENCE & PREVALENCE (IN U.S.)

- According to data from National Health and Nutrition Examination Survey (NHANES) 2013 to 2016 (National Heart, Lung, and Blood Institute [NHLBI] tabulation), cardiovascular disease prevalence excluding hypertension was 9% (24.3 million in 2016).
- In 2013 in the U.S., coronary heart disease alone caused 1 of every 7 deaths. In 2013, 370,213 Americans died of coronary heart disease. Each year, an estimated 660,000 Americans have a new coronary attack (defined as first hospitalized myocardial infarction or coronary heart disease death), and 305,000 have a recurrent attack. It is estimated that an additional 160,000 silent myocardial infarctions occur each year. Approximately every 34 sec, one American has a coronary event, and approximately every 1 min 24 sec, an American will die of one.[1]
- Community incidence rates as well as mortality rates from STEMI have declined over the past decade, whereas those for NSTEMI have increased. At present, STEMI comprises approximately 30% to 40% of MI presentations. In-hospital mortality (approximately 5% to 6%) and 1-yr mortality (approximately 7% to 18%). The most common cause of death in adults over the age of 40 is myocardial infarction. A heart attack takes the life of >1,500,000 people each year in the U.S.
- Modifiable risk factors such as hypertension, diabetes, and cigarette smoking have recently declined, although hyperlipidemia has shown no significant change, and obesity has steadily increased.
- Tobacco use remains the second-leading cause of total deaths and disability. The percentage of adults who reported current cigarette use declined from 24.1% in 1998 to 15.5% in 2016. Still, almost one third of coronary heart disease deaths are attributable to smoking and exposure to secondhand smoke.

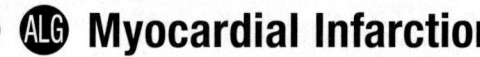

Patients with first acute MI were found to have an almost threefold increase in cigarette smoking from 2002 to 2009. Cigarette smoking is associated with endothelial dysfunction, prothrombotic defects, and increased oxidative stress.

- It is more prevalent in males between the ages of 45 and 65 yr old; there is no predominant sex differential after the age of 65.
- Women comprised 30% of STEMI patients. They experience more lethal and severe first acute MIs than men regardless of comorbidity, previous angina, or age. Studies have suggested that women are less likely to receive reperfusion therapy, have longer reperfusion times, are often given the standard of care treatment within 24 h of presentation, and have higher risk of bleeding with antithrombotic therapy.
- At least one fourth of all MIs are clinically unrecognized. Approximately 23% of patients with STEMI in the U.S. have diabetes mellitus, and three quarters of all deaths among patients with diabetes mellitus are related to coronary artery disease. Diabetes mellitus is associated with higher short- and long-term mortality after STEMI. In the CRUSADE (Can Rapid risk stratification of Unstable angina patients Suppress Adverse outcomes with Early implementation of the ACC/AHA guidelines) trial, 7% of eligible patients did not receive reperfusion therapy. The most important factor for not providing reperfusion therapy in eligible patients was increasing age.
- 6% to 15% of MIs are not associated with obstructive coronary disease or angiography.[1]

PHYSICAL FINDINGS & CLINICAL PRESENTATION

The clinical presentation of myocardial infarction is usually based on a history of substernal pressure–type chest pain radiated to the neck, lower jaw, left arm, or mid-back lasting 20 min or more that is not completely relieved by sublingual nitroglycerin. The pain may not be severe. Some patients may present with atypical symptoms such as nausea/vomiting, shortness of breath, fatigue, palpitations, and diaphoresis. The elderly may present with dizziness or syncope. The patients who tend to present with atypical symptoms are more likely to be women, diabetic patients, or elderly patients and less frequently receive reperfusion therapy and other evidence-based therapies than patients with a typical chest pain presentation. Records show that up to 30% of patients with STEMI present with atypical symptoms.

Physical findings:
- Skin may be diaphoretic and exhibit pallor (because of decreased oxygen).
- Rales may be present at the bases of lungs (indicative of heart failure [HF]).
- Cardiac auscultation may reveal an apical systolic murmur caused by mitral regurgitation from papillary muscle dysfunction; S3 or S4 may also be present.
- Up to 10% of patients may present with acute pulmonary edema and/or cardiogenic shock.

- Physical examination may be completely normal.

ETIOLOGY

- Coronary atherosclerosis and plaque rupture
- Coronary artery spasm
- Coronary embolism (caused by infective endocarditis, rheumatic heart disease, intracavitary thrombus, atrial fibrillation)
- Periarteritis and other coronary artery inflammatory diseases
- Dissection into coronary arteries (aneurysmal or iatrogenic or spontaneous)
- Anomalous origin of coronary artery, especially interarterial (aorta and pulmonary artery) course of coronary artery
- MI with normal coronaries: More frequent in younger patients and cocaine addicts. The risk of acute MI is increased by a factor of 24 during the 60 min after the use of cocaine in persons who are otherwise at relatively low risk. Most patients with cocaine-related MI are young, non-White, male cigarette smokers without other risk factors for coronary heart disease and who have a history of repeated cocaine use. Blood and urine toxicology screen for cocaine is recommended in all young patients who present with acute MI.
- Hypercoagulable states, increased blood viscosity (polycythemia vera and autoimmune diseases such as systemic lupus, antiphospholipid syndrome)

DX DIAGNOSIS

DIFFERENTIAL DIAGNOSIS

The various causes of myocardial ischemia are described along with the differential diagnosis of chest pain.

LABORATORY TESTS

- ECG (Fig. 1): A 12-lead ECG should be performed and shown to an experienced emergency physician within 10 min of emergency department (ED) arrival for all patients with chest discomfort (or anginal equivalent) or other symptoms suggestive of MI. Table 1 and Table 2 describe ECG findings in myocardial infarction. If the initial ECG is not diagnostic for MI but the patient remains symptomatic and there is a high clinical suspicion for MI, serial ECGs at 5- to 10-min intervals or continuous 12-lead ST-segment monitoring should be performed to detect the potential development of ST deviation. In patients with inferior STEMI, right-sided ECG leads should be obtained to look for ST elevation suggestive of right ventricular (RV) infarction. The joint ESC/ACCF/AHA committee for the definition of MI established the definition for the diagnosis of ST-elevation MI, which is considered to be present when there is an ST-segment elevation in two contiguous leads, ≥2 mm for men and ≥1.5 mm for women in precordial leads and/or ≥1 mm in limb leads. ST-segment elevation is measured at 0.08 sec after the J point (the junction between the end of the QRS and the

beginning of the ST segment). In addition, ST depression in >2 precordial leads (V1 to V4) may indicate transmural posterior injury; ST depression in multiple leads with coexistent ST elevation in lead aVR has been described in patients with left main or proximal left anterior descending artery involvement.
- New or presumably new LBBB at presentation occurs infrequently, may interfere with ST-elevation analysis. Thus consider MI only if clinically appropriate.
- Diagnosing new STEMI in patients with old left bundle branch block could be challenging. Sgarbossa and colleagues emphasized that concordant 1 mm ST-segment elevation in any lead with a positive QRS deflection or discordant ST-segment elevation >5 mm in any lead with negative QRS deflection suggest STEMI.
- New ST-segment depression ≥0.5 mV (0.5 mm) and T-wave abnormalities suggest NSTEMI. ECG findings alone, without laboratory results, are sufficient to diagnose STEMI; therefore treatment should not be delayed until biomarkers are available.
- Cardiac troponin levels: Cardiac-specific troponin T (cTnT) and cardiac-specific troponin I (cTnI) are generally indicative of myocardial injury with increases in serum levels of >99th percentile of a normal reference population. Detection of a rise and fall pattern of the measurements is essential to the diagnosis of AMI. The rise may occur relatively early after muscle damage (3 to 6 h), peak at 12 to 16 h, and may be present for several days after MI (up to 7 days for cTnI and more than 14 days for cTnT). Earlier peaking and rapid decline of cardiac enzymes may present in light of successful revascularization (Fig. 2). cTnT or cTnI tests can be falsely positive for myocardial infarction in patients with renal failure, heart failure, myocarditis, aortic dissection, and pulmonary embolism. Recently, highly sensitive troponin assays (hs-cTnI, hs-cTnT) have also been developed to facilitate an early diagnosis of AMI. Most patients can be diagnosed with AMI within the first 2 to 3 h of presentation. However, an initial negative high-sensitivity troponin at the time of presentation is not sensitive enough to completely rule out AMI. MI can be excluded in most patients by 6 h of presentation, and guidelines suggest serial samples be obtained every 3 to 6 h after an initial sample if there is a high degree of suspicion for AMI.[1,2]
- Troponin is the preferred marker for the diagnosis of myocardial necrosis. A single high-sensitivity assay for cardiac troponin (hs-cTnT) concentration below the limit of detection in combination with a nonischemic ECG may successfully rule out an MI in patients presenting to EDs with possible emergency acute coronary syndrome.[2] Because troponins need 7 to 14 days to be cleared by the kidneys, they are not sensitive enough to detect a recurrent MI within days from the initial MI. CK-MB isoenzyme can be useful in such circumstances (see Fig. 2).
- CK-MB isoenzyme is also a useful marker for MI if troponin levels are not available. It is

M

Diseases and Disorders

I

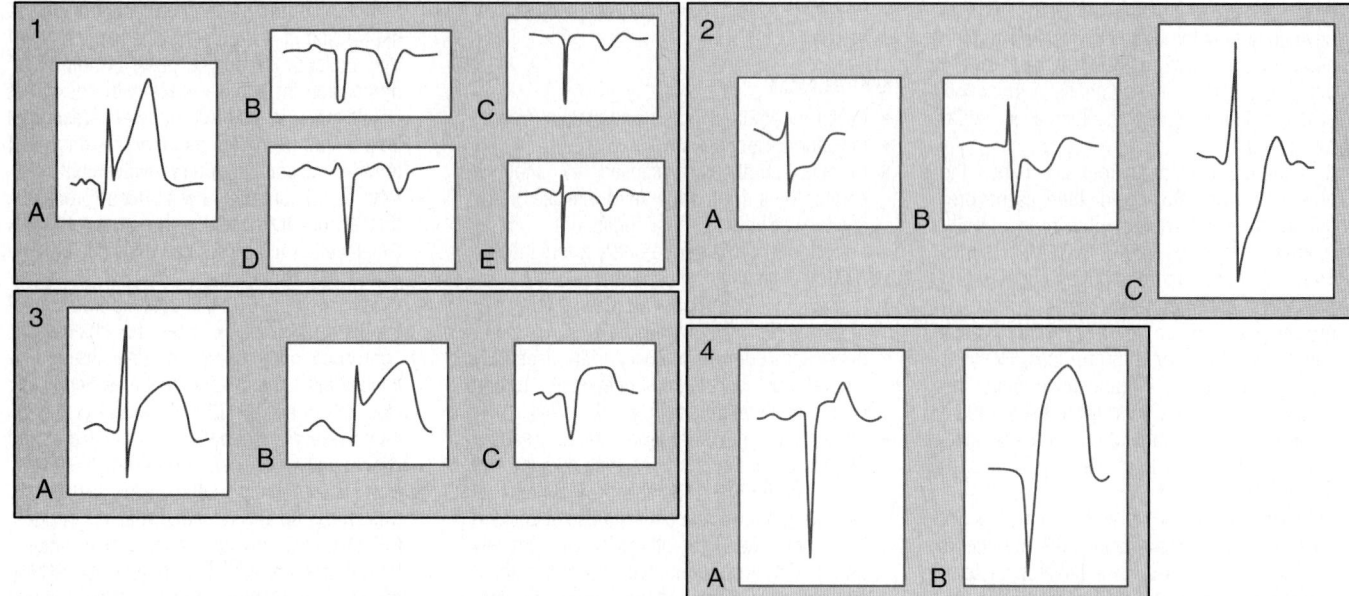

FIG. 1 Electrocardiographic findings of acute myocardial infarction (AMI). (1) T-wave abnormalities of AMI. *A,* Prominent "hyperacute" T wave. *B* through *E,* T-wave inversions of non–ST-segment elevation MI (NSTEMI). (2) ST-segment depression. *A,* Flat. *B,* Downsloping. *C,* Upsloping. (3) ST-segment elevation. *A,* Convex ST-segment elevation. *B,* Obliquely straight ST-segment elevation. *C,* Convex ST-segment elevation. (4) Pathologic Q waves. *A,* Pathologic Q wave of completed myocardial infarction. *B,* Simultaneous ST-segment elevation with pathologic Q wave 2 h into the course of ST-segment elevation MI (STEMI). (From Vincent JL et al: *Textbook of critical care,* ed 6, Philadelphia, 2011, Saunders.)

TABLE 1 Leads Showing Abnormal Electrocardiographic Findings in Myocardial Infarction

	Limb Leads	Precordial Leads
Lateral	I, aVL	V5, V6
Anterior		V1, V2, V3
Anterolateral	I, aVL	V2-V6
Diaphragmatic	II, III, aVF	
Posterior		V1-V3*

aVF, Augmented vector foot; *aVL,* augmented vector left.

*None of the leads is oriented toward the posterior surface of the heart. Therefore in posterior infarction, changes that would have been present in the posterior surface leads will be seen in the anterior leads as a mirror image (e.g., tall and slightly wide R waves in V1 and V2, comparable to abnormal Q waves, and tall and wide, symmetric T waves in V1 and V2).

From Park MK: *Park's pediatric cardiology for practitioners,* ed 6, Philadelphia, 2014, Elsevier.

released in the circulation in amounts that correlate with the size of the infarct. An increased CK-MB value for the diagnosis of MI is defined as a measurement above the 99th percentile of the upper reference limit. CK-MB can be detected within 3 to 8 h of the onset of chest pain, peak at 12 to 24 h, and return to baseline levels within 24 to 48 h.

IMAGING STUDIES

Imaging studies such as a high-quality portable chest x-ray examination, transthoracic echocardiography, and a contrast chest computed tomography (CT) scan should be used to differentiate MI from aortic dissection, pulmonary embolism, and other intrathoracic causes of chest pain

(i.e., pneumonia and pneumothorax) in patients for whom this distinction is initially unclear, or to assess for complications of AMI such as pulmonary edema. Transthoracic echocardiography may provide evidence of focal wall motion abnormalities and facilitate triage in patients with ECG findings that are difficult to interpret.

RISK ASSESSMENT

For STEMI patients, TIMI (Thrombolysis in Myocardial Infarction) risk index, TIMI risk score (30-day outcomes), and GRACE (Global Registry of Acute Coronary Events) risk score (6-mo outcomes) are commonly available risk assessment models. In the TIMI risk score for STEMI, the mean 30-day mortality was 6.7%. It is composed of eight baseline variables. The risk score showed a >fortyfold graded increase in mortality, with scores ranging from 0 to >8 ($P < 0.0001$); 30-day mortality was 0.1% among patients with a score of 0, 2.25 with a score of 5, and >8.8% among patients with a score of 8 or greater. The higher the score, the higher the 30-day mortality rate. The variables are divided between historic, exam, and presentation:
History:
• Age 65 to 74 (2 points), >75 (3 points)
• Diabetes/HTN or angina (1 point)
Exam:
• Systolic blood pressure (SBP) <100 mm Hg (3 points)
• Heart rate >100 bpm (2 points)
• Killip 2 to 4 (2 points)
• Weight <67 kg (1 point)
Presentation:
• Anterior ST elevation or LBBB (1 point)
• Time to reperfusion >4 h (1 point)
For NSTEMI patients, TIMI risk score (14-day outcomes) and GRACE (Global Registry of Acute

Coronary Events) risk score (in hospital outcomes) are available. See variables for TIMI risk score below.[3,4]
• Age ≥65 yr
• Presence of ≥3 risk factors for CAD
• Known CAD (coronary artery stenosis ≥50%)
• Aspirin use in the past 7 days
• ≥2 episodes of angina within 24 h
• ST changes ≥0.05 mV
• Positive cardiac enzymes
In TIMI score for the NSTEMI patients, each variable scores one point. The risk score of 6 to 7 carries an estimated major acute coronary event (MACE) rate of 41% during 14 days of post-MI. Risk assessment is a continuous process that should be repeated throughout hospitalization and at time of discharge.

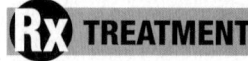 **TREATMENT**

NONPHARMACOLOGIC THERAPY

• Limit patient's activity: Bed rest with bedside commode for the initial 12 to 24 h. If the patient remains stable, it gradually increases.
• Diet: Nothing by mouth until stable, then clear liquids as tolerated to advance gradually to a diet tailored to the patient's comorbidities (i.e., diabetes, hypertension, heart failure, hyperlipidemia, renal failure, chronic obstructive pulmonary disease [COPD], etc.). The Mediterranean diet is recommended for the long term.
• Patient education to decrease the risk of subsequent cardiac events, counseling on smoking cessation, dietary restrictions, regular exercise, and medication compliance should be initiated when the patient is medically stable.

TABLE 2 Electrocardiographic Manifestations of Myocardial Infarction

ST Elevation

Electrocardiographic Manifestations of Acute Myocardial Ischemia (in the Absence of Left Bundle Branch Block)

New ST elevation at the J point in two contiguous leads with the following cut points:
- ≥0.1 mV in all leads (except V2-V3)
- In leads V2-V3 the following cut points apply:
  1. ≥0.2 mV in men ≥40 yr
  2. ≥0.25 mV in men <40 yr
  3. ≥0.15 mV in women

ST Depression and T Wave Changes
- New horizontal or downsloping ST depression ≥0.05 mV in two contiguous leads
- T-wave inversion ≥0.1 mV in two contiguous leads with a prominent R wave or R/S ratio >1

Electrocardiographic Manifestations of Ischemia in the Setting of Left Bundle Branch Block

Electrocardiographic Criterion	Points
ST-segment elevation ≥1 mm and concordant with the QRS complex	5
ST-segment depression ≥1 mm in lead V1, V2, or V3	3
ST-segment elevation ≥5 mm and discordant with the QRS complex	2
A score of ≥3 had a specificity of 98% for acute MI	

Electrocardiographic Changes Associated with Previous Myocardial Infarction (in the Absence of Left Ventricular Hypertrophy and Left Bundle Block)

Any Q wave in leads V2-V3 ≥0.02 sec or a QS complex in leads V2 and V3

Q wave ≥0.03 sec and ≥0.1-mV deep or QS complex in leads I, II, aVL, aVF, or V4-V6 in any 2 leads of a contiguous lead grouping (I, aVL; V1-V6; II, III, aVF)

R wave ≥0.04 sec in V1-V2 and R/S ≥1 with a concordant positive T wave in absence of a conductions defect.

aVF, Augmented vector foot; *aVL,* augmented vector left; *MI,* myocardial infarction.

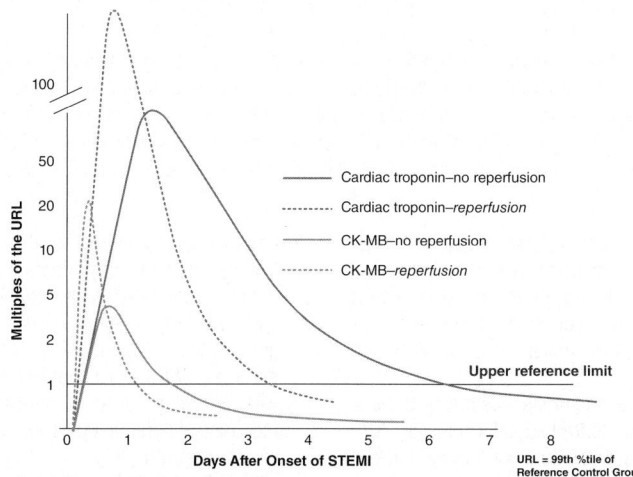

FIG. 2 Trends of troponin and CK-MB following revascularization in MI. *CK-MB,* Creatine kinase-MB; *MI,* myocardial infarction; *STEMI,* ST-segment elevation myocardial infarction; *URL,* upper reference limit. (Modified from Shapiro BP, Jaffe AS: Cardio biomarkers. In Murphy JG, Lloyd MA [eds]: *Mayo Clinic cardiology: concise textbook,* ed 3, Rochester, MN, 2007, Mayo Clinic Scientific Press, and New York, 2007, Informa Healthcare USA. Used with permission of Mayo Foundation for Medical Education and Research.)

- Cardiac rehabilitation prevents future major adverse cardiac events and increases medication compliance.

ACUTE GENERAL Rx

- Fig. 3 shows a treatment algorithm for STEMI. Assessment and treatment algorithm for non–ST-segment MI is described in Fig. 4. Rationale of the treatment of a patient with STEMI is based on "time is muscle." Therefore all communities should create and maintain a regional system of STEMI care that includes assessment and continuous quality improvement of emergency medical services (EMS) and hospital-based activities. A 12-lead ECG must be done by EMS personnel at the site of first medical contact (FMC).
- Reperfusion therapy should be administered to all eligible patients with STEMI with symptom onset within 12 h. Indications for primary angioplasty and comparison with fibrinolytic therapy are described in Table 3. Primary percutaneous coronary intervention (PCI) is the recommended method of reperfusion when it can be performed in a timely fashion by experienced operators with an ideal FMC-to-device time system goal of 90 min or less.
- In the absence of contraindications, fibrinolytic therapy (Table 4) should be administered to patients with STEMI at non–PCI-capable hospitals when the anticipated FMC-to-device time at a PCI-capable hospital exceeds 120 min because of unavoidable delays. Door-in door-out time (DIDO) for fibrinolytic therapy should be less than 30 min. If there is more than 30 min delay, transfer the patient to a PCI-capable hospital.
- Among STEMI patients who were treated with fibrinolytics, patients with >50% ST-segment resolution on ECG were at much lower risk for cardiac-related mortality compared with those with <50% resolution at 30 days.
- PCI is superior to thrombolytic therapy and is the standard of care. It is effective and generally results in more favorable outcomes than thrombolytic therapy.
- Primary PCI should be performed in patients with STEMI and persistent ischemic symptoms and who have contraindications to fibrinolytic therapy, irrespective of the time delay from FMC, or in patients with cardiogenic shock or acute severe HF irrespective of time delay from MI onset, first medical contact to balloon time is <90 min or door to balloon/door to needle time is <1 h, symptoms onset was >3 h ago and when diagnosis of STEMI in doubt. Coronary stents (drug-eluting or bare-metal) are useful in patients with STEMI.[5-8]
- The question of culprit vessel vs. complete revascularization during PCI has been brought up since the stent technology was applied to the management of STEMI. The most recent clinical trials (CuLPRIT, PRAMI, and DANAMI3-PRIMULTI [FFR-driven revascularization]) appear to favor complete revascularization in the setting of acute coronary syndrome. However, CULPRIT-SHOCK trial showed culprit vessel only PCI associated with 9.5% absolute reduction in the rate of death or renal replacement therapy at 30 days compared to multivessel PCI in acute MI patients with cardiogenic shock. One-yr outcomes did not show significant difference in mortality between two groups. Korea Acute Myocardial Infarction-National Institutes of Health (KAMIR-NIH) Registry data showed better outcomes with multivessel PCI in cardiogenic shock patients compared to culprit vessel-only PCI. Thus multivessel PCI should be reserved for a few selective patients.[6,7]
- For patients presenting to a non–PCI-capable hospital, rapid assessment should be done of (1) the time from onset of symptoms, (2) the risk of complications related to STEMI, (3) the risk of bleeding with fibrinolysis, (4) the presence of shock or severe HF, and (5) the time required for transfer to a PCI-capable hospital and a decision about administration of fibrinolytic therapy reached. Because the effectiveness of thrombolytics is time dependent, these agents should ideally be administered either in the field or within 30 min of the patient's arrival to the emergency department (door-to-needle time).

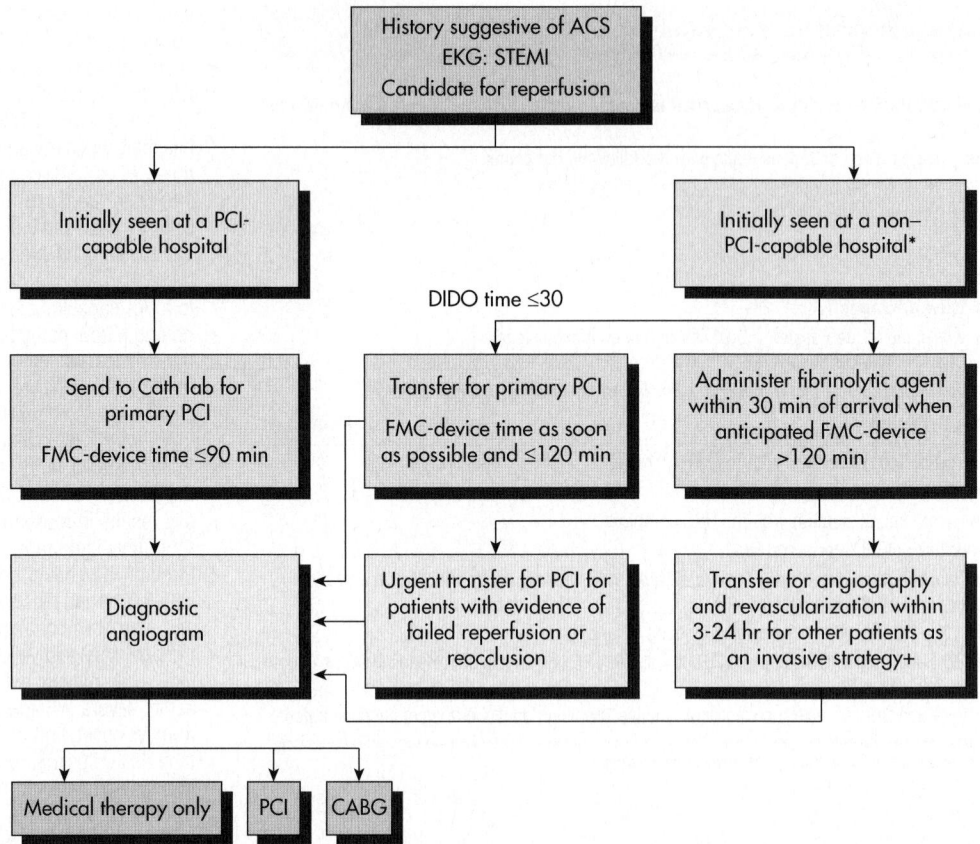

FIG. 3 Reperfusion therapy for patients with STEMI. *Patients with cardiogenic shock or severe heart failure initially seen at a non–PCI-capable hospital should be transferred for cardiac catheterization and revascularization as soon as possible, irrespective of time delay from MI onset. +Angiography and revascularization should not be performed within the first 2 to 3 h after administration of fibrinolytic therapy. *ACS,* Acute coronary syndrome; *CABG,* coronary artery bypass graft; *Cath,* catheterization; *DIDO,* door-in to door-out; *EKG,* electrocardiogram; *FMC,* first medical contact; *MI,* myocardial infarction; *PCI,* percutaneous coronary intervention; *STEMI,* ST-elevation myocardial infarction. (Modified from O'Gara PT et al: 2013 ACCF/AHA guideline for the management of ST-elevation myocardial infarction, *JACC* 61(4):e78-e140, 2013.)

- Fibrinolytic therapy: If tissue plasminogen activator (t PA) or reteplase is used, anticoagulants, such as heparin, are given to increase the likelihood of patency in the infarct-related artery for 48 h and preferably for the duration of the index hospitalization, up to 8 days. In patients receiving fibrinolysis for STEMI, treatment with enoxaparin is superior to treatment with unfractionated heparin for 48 h but is associated with an increase in major bleeding episodes. In patients receiving streptokinase or APSAC, heparin after thrombolysis is not indicated because it does not offer any additional benefit and can result in increased bleeding complications. Tenecteplase and reteplase are comparable with accelerated infusion recombinant t-PA in terms of efficacy and safety but are more convenient because they are administered by bolus injection. Lanoplase and heparin bolus plus infusion are as effective as tPA with regard to mortality rate, but the rate of intracranial hemorrhage is significantly higher.
- Absolute contraindications to thrombolytic therapy (Table 5) include history of intracranial hemorrhage, known intracranial malignant neoplasm or arteriovenous malformation, ischemic stroke within 3 mo (except acute ischemic stroke within 4.5 h), suspected aortic dissection, active bleeding or bleeding diathesis (except

menses), significant closed head or facial trauma within 3 mo, intracranial or intraspinal surgery within 2 mo, or severe uncontrolled hypertension (unresponsive to therapy). For streptokinase, this applies to prior treatment within 6 mo.
- Relative contraindications: History of chronic severe, poorly controlled hypertension, SBP >180 mm Hg, diastolic blood pressure (DBP) >110 mm Hg, history of prior ischemic stroke more than 3 mo, dementia, known intracranial pathology, traumatic or prolonged cardiopulmonary resuscitation (CPR) (>10 min), major surgery <3 wk, recent internal bleeding within 2 to 4 wk, noncompressible vascular punctures, pregnancy, active peptic ulcer, oral anticoagulant therapy. After the administration of thrombolytics, immediate transfer to a PCI-capable facility is advisable without waiting for lytic results.
- Transfer to a PCI-capable hospital: Immediate transfer for STEMI patients who develop cardiogenic shock or acute severe HF, irrespective of the time delay from MI onset. Urgent transfer if the patient demonstrates evidence of failed reperfusion or reocclusion after fibrinolytic therapy.
- Coronary angiography should not be performed within the first 2 to 3 h after administration of fibrinolytic therapy.

- Coronary artery bypass graft (CABG): Urgent CABG is indicated in patients with STEMI and coronary anatomy not amenable to PCI who have ongoing or recurrent ischemia, cardiogenic shock, severe HF, or other high-risk features. CABG is recommended in patients with STEMI at time of operative repair of mechanical defects. Box 1 summarizes CABG in patients with MI.[8]
- Therapeutic hypothermia should be started as soon as possible in comatose patients with STEMI and out-of-hospital cardiac arrest caused by ventricular fibrillation (VF) or pulseless ventricular tachycardia, including patients who undergo primary PCI.
- Immediate angiography and PCI when indicated should be performed in resuscitated out-of-hospital patients.
- The use of mechanical circulatory support is reasonable in patients with STEMI who are hemodynamically unstable and require urgent CABG.
- For NSTEMI patients, immediate invasive strategy (within 2 h) recommended in patients with refractory angina, signs, or symptoms of congestive heart failure or new or worsening ischemic mitral regurgitation, hemodynamic instability, recurrent angina or ischemia at rest or with low level activities despite intensive medical therapy and

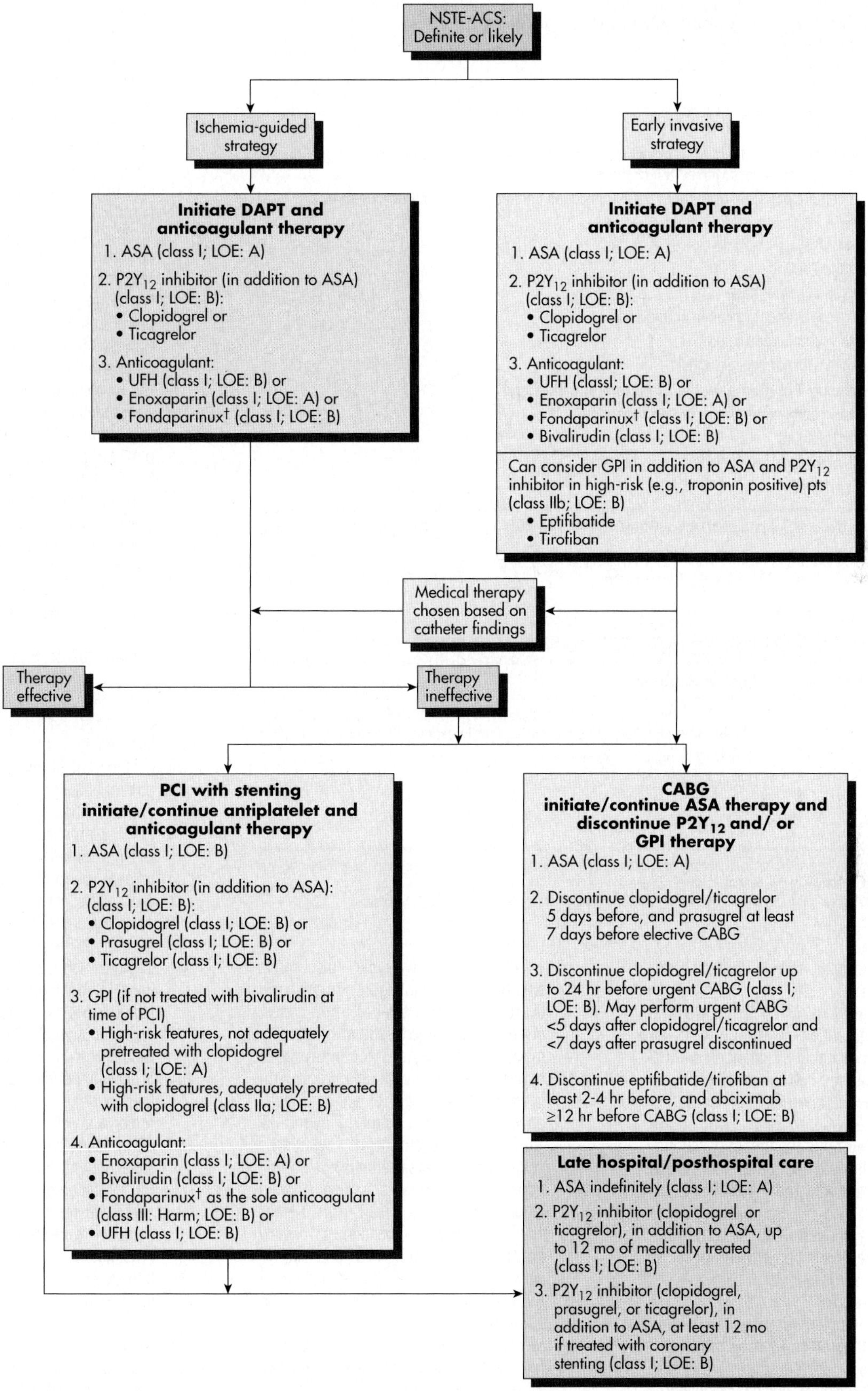

NSTE-ACS:
Definite or likely

Ischemia-guided
strategy

Early invasive
strategy

**Initiate DAPT and
anticoagulant therapy**

1. ASA (class I; LOE: A)

2. P2Y$_{12}$ inhibitor (in addition to ASA)
(class I; LOE: B):
• Clopidogrel or
• Ticagrelor

3. Anticoagulant:
• UFH (class I; LOE: B) or
• Enoxaparin (class I; LOE: A) or
• Fondaparinux† (class I; LOE: B)

**Initiate DAPT and
anticoagulant therapy**

1. ASA (class I; LOE: A)

2. P2Y$_{12}$ inhibitor (in addition to ASA)
(class I; LOE: B):
• Clopidogrel or
• Ticagrelor

3. Anticoagulant:
• UFH (classI; LOE: B) or
• Enoxaparin (class I; LOE: A) or
• Fondaparinux† (class I; LOE: B) or
• Bivalirudin (class I; LOE: B)

Can consider GPI in addition to ASA and P2Y$_{12}$
inhibitor in high-risk (e.g., troponin positive) pts
(class IIb; LOE: B)
• Eptifibatide
• Tirofiban

Medical therapy
chosen based on
catheter findings

Therapy
effective

Therapy
ineffective

**PCI with stenting
initiate/continue antiplatelet and
anticoagulant therapy**

1. ASA (class I; LOE: B)

2. P2Y$_{12}$ inhibitor (in addition to ASA):
(class I; LOE: B):
• Clopidogrel (class I; LOE: B) or
• Prasugrel (class I; LOE: B) or
• Ticagrelor (class I; LOE: B)

3. GPI (if not treated with bivalirudin at
time of PCI)
• High-risk features, not adequately
pretreated with clopidogrel
(class I; LOE: A)
• High-risk features, adequately pretreated
with clopidogrel (class IIa; LOE: B)

4. Anticoagulant:
• Enoxaparin (class I; LOE: A) or
• Bivalirudin (class I; LOE: B) or
• Fondaparinux† as the sole anticoagulant
(class III: Harm; LOE: B) or
• UFH (class I; LOE: B)

**CABG
initiate/continue ASA therapy and
discontinue P2Y$_{12}$ and/ or
GPI therapy**

1. ASA (class I; LOE: A)

2. Discontinue clopidogrel/ticagrelor
5 days before, and prasugrel at least
7 days before elective CABG

3. Discontinue clopidogrel/ticagrelor up
to 24 hr before urgent CABG (class I;
LOE: B). May perform urgent CABG
<5 days after clopidogrel/ticagrelor and
<7 days after prasugrel discontinued

4. Discontinue eptifibatide/tirofiban at
least 2-4 hr before, and abciximab
≥12 hr before CABG (class I; LOE: B)

Late hospital/posthospital care

1. ASA indefinitely (class I; LOE: A)

2. P2Y$_{12}$ inhibitor (clopidogrel or
ticagrelor), in addition to ASA, up
to 12 mo of medically treated
(class I; LOE: B)

3. P2Y$_{12}$ inhibitor (clopidogrel,
prasugrel, or ticagrelor), in
addition to ASA, at least 12 mo
if treated with coronary
stenting (class I; LOE: B)

FIG. 4 Algorithm for management of patients with definite or likely non–ST-elevation acute coronary syndromes (NSTE-ACS). †In patients who have been treated with fondaparinux (as upfront therapy) who undergo percutaneous coronary intervention (PCI), an additional anticoagulant with anti-IIa activity should be administered at the time of PCI because of the risk of catheter thrombosis. ASA, Acetylsalicylic acid (aspirin); CABG, coronary artery bypass grafting; DAPT, dual-antiplatelet therapy; GPI, glycoprotein inhibitor; LOE, level of evidence; pts, patients; UFH, unfractionated heparin. (From Amsterdam EA et al: 2014 AHA/ACC guideline for the management of patients with non–ST-elevation acute coronary syndromes: a report of the American College of Cardiology/American Heart Association Task Force on Practice Guidelines, J Am Coll Cardiol 64:e139-228, 2014. In Zipes DP et al [eds]: Braunwald's heart disease, a textbook of cardiovascular medicine, ed 11, Philadelphia, 2019, Elsevier.)

TABLE 3 Indications for Primary Angioplasty and Comparison with Fibrinolytic Therapy

Indications

Alternative recanalization strategy for ST segment elevation or LBBB acute MI within 12 h of symptom onset (or >12 h if symptoms persist)

Cardiogenic shock developing within 36 h of ST segment elevation/Q wave acute MI or LBBB acute MI in patients >75 yr old who can be revascularized within 18 h of shock onset

Recommended only at centers performing >200 PCI/yr with backup cardiac surgery and for operators performing <75 PCI/yr

Advantages of Primary PCI

Higher initial recanalization rates

Reduced risk of intracerebral hemorrhage

Less residual stenosis; less recurrent ischemia or infarction

Usefulness when fibrinolysis contraindicated

Improvement in outcomes with cardiogenic shock

Disadvantages of Primary PCI (Compared with Fibrinolytic Therapy)

Access, advantages restricted to high-volume centers, operators

Longer average time to treatment

Greater dependence on operators for results

Higher system complexity, costs

LBBB, Left bundle branch block; *MI,* myocardial infarction; *PCI,* percutaneous coronary intervention (includes balloon angioplasty, stenting).
From Goldman L, Schafer AI: *Goldman's Cecil medicine,* ed 24, Philadelphia, 2012, Saunders.

TABLE 4 Dosing Regimens of Commonly Used Thrombolytic Agents

Thrombolytic Agents	Dosing Regimen
t-PA (alteplase)	15 mg bolus IV, followed by 0.75 mg/kg body weight (not to exceed 50 mg) over 30 min, followed by 0.5 mg/kg (not to exceed 35 mg) over 60 min
r-PA (reteplase)	Two 10-U IV boluses, given 30 min apart
TNK–t-PA (tenecteplase)	Single bolus IV 0.5 mg/kg (dose rounded to the nearest 5 mg, ranging from 30 to 50 mg)
Streptokinase	1.5 million U IV over 60 min

IV, Intravenous; *PA,* plasminogen activator; *r-PA,* recombinant plasminogen activator; *TNK–t-PA,* tenecteplase tissue plasminogen activator; *t-PA,* tissue plasminogen activator; *U,* units.
From Andreoli TE et al: *Andreoli and Carpenter's Cecil essentials of medicine,* ed 8, Philadelphia, 2010, Saunders.

sustained ventricular tachycardia or ventricular fibrillation.

- Early invasive strategy (<24 h) for NSTEMI patients recommended if GRACE risk for more than 140, dynamic ST changes on ECG and temporal change in troponin levels.
- NSTEMI patient with low-risk TIMI score (0 or 1) and/or low GRACE score (<109) and/or troponin-negative female patients can benefit from ischemia-guided strategy. Fibrinolytic therapy is contraindicated in NSTEMI patients.
- Medical therapy should be initiated immediately in the emergency department for all MI patients. This includes:
  1. Routine measures
     a. Oxygen: Supplemental oxygen should be administered to patients with arterial oxygen desaturation (SaO$_2$ less than 90%). No benefit has been demonstrated to supplemental oxygen in patients with normal SaO$_2$.
     b. Nitroglycerin: Increase oxygen supply by reducing coronary vasospasm and decrease oxygen consumption by reducing ventricular preload. Patients with ongoing ischemic discomfort should receive sublingual nitroglycerin every 5 min for a total of three doses, after which an assessment should be made about the need for intravenous nitroglycerin. Intravenous nitroglycerin is indicated for relief of ongoing ischemic discomfort, control of hypertension, or management of pulmonary congestion. Nitrates should not be administered to patients whose systolic blood pressure is <90 mm Hg or ≥30 mm Hg below baseline or severe bradycardia (<50 beats/min), tachycardia (>100 beats/min), or suspected RV infarction. Nitrates should not be administered to patients who have received a phosphodiesterase inhibitor for erectile dysfunction within the last 24 h (48 h for tadalafil).
     c. Adequate analgesia: Morphine sulfate 2 to 4 mg intravenous (IV) initially with increments of 2 to 8 mg IV at 5- to 10-min intervals can be given for severe pain unrelieved by nitroglycerin. Morphine can reduce the catecholamine surge caused by anxiety and pain, particularly in patients with anterior myocardial infarctions, which in turn can reduce heart rate and pulmonary capillary wedge pressure (PCWP), the increased cardiac workload and oxygen demand, leading to decreased ischemia and pulmonary congestion. Hypotension from morphine can be treated with careful IV hydration with saline solution. If sinus bradycardia accompanies hypotension, use atropine (0.5 to 1.0 mg IV q5min prn to a total dose of 2.5 mg). Respiratory depression caused by morphine can be reversed with naloxone 0.8 mg. Morphine sulfate and nitroglycerine should be avoided in patients with RV involvement who usually present with bradycardia and hypotension. Pain management in these cases should be provided preferentially with meperidine 25 to 50 mg intravenously q4h, in combination with Phenergan 12.5 mg to prevent nausea and/or vomiting. Blood pressure support with normal saline solution is of critical importance to maintain adequate hemodynamics until optimal revascularization is accomplished.
     d. Aspirin 162 to 325 mg PO should be crushed and chewed to enhance drug absorption and delivery. It should be given as soon as possible and continued indefinitely at 81 mg daily.[5] Depending on the clinical and ECG findings, if the patient is suspected to have a coronary anatomy that needs CABG rather than PCI, aspirin should be continued. P2Y12 receptor antagonists should be avoided (except cangrelor) because they increase the perioperative bleeding risk; on-pump surgery should be deferred for at least 24 h after clopidogrel and ticagrelor. Off-pump surgery might be considered within 24 h of clopidogrel or ticagrelor if the benefits of revascularization outweigh the risk of bleeding. However, if the coronary artery disease is likely to benefit from PCI alone, then a loading dose of clopidogrel 600 or 300 mg or ticagrelor 180 mg PO or prasugrel 60 mg should be given as early as possible and no later than 1 h after PCI. P2Y12 receptor antagonist should be continued for at least 1 yr after acute coronary syndrome or after primary PCI. Prasugrel showed significant net clinical benefit (MACE vs. bleeding complications) only in patients with MI who underwent revascularization. It shouldn't be given to non-revascularized patients. Ticagrelor or clopidogrel can be given to patients with MI with or without catheter-based revascularization. Cangrelor is the newest direct-acting P2Y12 platelet receptor inhibitor. It has a similar chemical structure to ATP, with a half-life of 3 to 6 min. It is given IV as a bolus plus 120 min of infusion at the time of primary

TABLE 5 Contraindications to and Cautions in the Use of Fibrinolytics for Treating ST-Elevation Myocardial Infarction*

Absolute Contraindications

Any previous intracranial hemorrhage
Known structural cerebral vascular lesion (e.g., arteriovenous malformation)
Known malignant intracranial neoplasm (primary or metastatic)
Ischemic stroke within 3 mo *except* acute ischemic stroke within 4.5 h
Suspected aortic dissection
Active bleeding or bleeding diathesis (excluding menses)
Significant closed-head or facial trauma within 3 mo
Intracranial or intraspinal surgery within 2 mo
Severe uncontrolled hypertension (unresponsive to emergency therapy)
For streptokinase, previous treatment within the previous 6 mo

Relative Contraindications

History of chronic, severe, poorly controlled hypertension
Significant hypertension at initial evaluation (SBP >180 mm Hg or DBP >110 mm Hg)[†]
History of previous ischemic stroke >3 mo
Dementia
Known intracranial pathology not covered in Absolute Contraindications
Traumatic or prolonged (>10 min) cardiopulmonary resuscitation
Major surgery (<3 wk)
Recent (within 2 to 4 wk) internal bleeding
Noncompressible vascular punctures
Pregnancy
Active peptic ulcer
Oral anticoagulant therapy

DBP, Diastolic blood pressure; *MI,* myocardial infarction; *SBP,* systolic blood pressure.
*Viewed as advisory for clinical decision making and may not be all-inclusive or definitive.
[†]Could be an absolute contraindication in low-risk patients with MI.
From O'Gara PT et al: 2013 ACCF/AHA guideline for the management of ST-elevation myocardial infarction: a report of the American College of Cardiology Foundation/American Heart Association task force on practice guidelines, *J Am Coll Cardiol* 61:e78, 2013. In Libby P et al: *Braunwald's heart disease, a textbook of cardiovascular medicine,* ed 12, Philadelphia, 2022, Elsevier.

BOX 1 CABG in Patients with Acute MI

Class I
1. Emergency CABG is recommended in patients with acute MI in whom (1) primary PCI has failed or cannot be performed, (2) coronary anatomy is suitable for CABG, and (3) persistent ischemia of a significant area of myocardium at rest or hemodynamic instability refractory to nonsurgical therapy is present.
2. Emergency CABG is recommended in patients undergoing surgical repair of a postinfarction mechanical complication of MI, such as ventricular septal rupture, mitral valve insufficiency because of papillary muscle infarction or rupture, or free wall rupture.
3. Emergency CABG is recommended in patients with cardiogenic shock and who are suitable for CABG irrespective of the time interval from MI to onset of shock and time from MI to CABG.
4. Emergency CABG is recommended in patients with life-threatening ventricular arrhythmias (believed ischemic in origin) in the presence of left main stenosis greater than or equal to 50% or three-vessel CAD.

Class IIa
1. The use of CABG is reasonable as a revascularization strategy in patients with multivessel CAD with recurrent angina or MI within the first 48 h of STEMI presentation as an alternative to a more delayed strategy.
2. Early revascularization with PCI or CABG is reasonable for selected patients older than 75 yr of age with ST-segment elevation or left bundle branch block who are suitable for revascularization irrespective of the time interval from MI to onset of shock.

Class III
1. Emergency CABG should not be performed in patients with persistent angina and a small area of viable myocardium who are stable hemodynamically.
2. Emergency CABG should not be performed in patients with no reflow (successful epicardial reperfusion with unsuccessful microvascular reperfusion).

CABG, Coronary artery bypass grafting; *CAD,* coronary artery disease; *MI,* myocardial infarction; *PCI,* percutaneous coronary intervention; *STEMI,* ST-segment elevation MI.
From Hillis LD et al: 2011 ACCF/AHA guideline for coronary artery bypass graft surgery: a report of the American College of Cardiology Foundation/American Heart Association task force on practice guidelines, *J Am Coll Cardiol* 58:e123-e210, 2011. In Parrillo JE et al: *Critical care medicine, principles of diagnosis and management in the adult,* ed 5, Philadelphia, 2019, Elsevier.

PCI in patients who are naïve to P2Y12 receptor antagonists. It was approved by the FDA in 2015 after the CHAMPION PHOENIX trial. Clopidogrel and prasugrel should be started after its infusion is finished. The ticagrelor loading dose can be given during the infusion. Considering rapid onset action and clearance, cangrelor can be started in the emergency room at the time of high-risk acute myocardial infarction diagnosis irrespective surgical or catheter-based revascularization.

2. In patients receiving fibrinolytics only or balloon angioplasty without stent, P2Y12 antagonists can be given for as little as 14 days. Clopidogrel is recommended for post fibrinolytic patients.

3. Unfractionated heparin (UFH) is recommended in all patients with NSTEMI and STEMI (fibrinolysis or invasive revascularization). UFH infusion should not exceed more than 48 h after PCI or fibrinolysis in the absence of an ongoing indication due to risk of heparin-induced thrombocytopenia. NSTEMI patients who underwent ischemia-guided therapy, low-molecular-weight heparin (LMWH) showed better MACE outcomes compared with UFH. The benefit was not significant in revascularized patients. Bivalirudin was associated with lower MACE and bleeding events in STEMI patients compared with UFH. However, it increased the risk of stent thrombosis. In NSTEMI patients who are undergoing PCI, LMWH, bivalirudin, and UFH are acceptable.

4. Beta-adrenergic blocking agents should generally be given to all patients who do not exhibit evidence of shock. Table 6 summarizes recommendations for β-blocker therapy for STEMI. β-blockers are useful to reduce myocardial oxygen consumption and prevent tachyarrhythmias. Early IV beta blockage (in the initial 24 h) followed by institution of an oral maintenance regimen is also effective in reducing recurrent infarction and ischemia. Oral β-blockers should be initiated in the first 24 h in patients with MI who do not have any of the following: Signs of HF, evidence of a low-output state, sinus tachycardia, increased risk for cardiogenic shock, or other contraindications for its use (bradycardia, PR interval more than 0.24 sec, second- or third-degree heart block, active asthma, or reactive airways disease).

5. They should be continued during and after hospitalization for all patients with MI and with no contraindications to their use for at least 2 yr. Patients with initial contraindications to the use of β-blockers in the first 24 h after MI should be reevaluated to determine their subsequent eligibility. It is reasonable to administer intravenous β-blockers at the time of presentation to patients with MI and no

M

Diseases and Disorders

I

TABLE 6 Recommendations for β-Blocker Therapy for ST-Elevation Myocardial Infarction (STEMI)

Recommendation	COR	LOE
Oral β-blockers should be initiated in the first 24 h in patients with STEMI who do not have any of the following:	I	B
Signs of heart failure or evidence of a low-output state		
Increased risk for cardiogenic shock*:		
• Age >70 yr		
• Systolic blood pressure <120 mm Hg		
• Sinus tachycardia >110 beats/min or heart rate <60 beats/min		
• Increased time since the onset of symptoms of STEMI		
Other relative contraindications to use of oral β-blockers:		
• PR interval longer than 0.24 sec		
• Second- or third-degree heart block		
• Active asthma or reactive airways disease		
β-blockers should be continued during and after hospitalization for all patients with STEMI and no contraindications to their use.	I	B
Patients with initial contraindications to the use of β-blockers in the first 24 h after STEMI should be reevaluated to determine their subsequent eligibility.	I	C
It is reasonable to administer IV β-blockers at initial encounter to patients with STEMI and no contraindications to their use who are hypertensive or have ongoing ischemia.	IIa	B

COR, Class of recommendation; *IV*, intravenous; *LOE*, level of evidence.
*The greater the number of risk factors present, the higher the risk for development of cardiogenic shock.
Modified from O'Gara PT et al: 2013 ACCF/AHA guideline for the management of ST-elevation myocardial infarction: a report of the American College of Cardiology Foundation/American Heart Association task force on practice guidelines, *J Am Coll Cardiol* 61:e78, 2013. In Libby P et al: *Braunwald's heart disease, a textbook of cardiovascular medicine*, ed 12, Philadelphia, 2022, Elsevier.

contraindications to their use who are hypertensive or have ongoing ischemia.

6. In patients with acute MI, treatment with drug-eluting stents is associated with decreased mortality rates and a reduction in the need for repeated revascularization procedures compared with treatment including bare-metal stents.

7. Gp IIb/IIIa inhibitors in the era of DAPT therapy and primary PCI have failed to show benefit with "upstream" treatment. Abciximab might be useful in the presence of large thrombus burden during primary PCI. For patients receiving bivalirudin as the primary anticoagulant, routine adjunctive use of GP IIb/IIIa inhibitors is not recommended but may be considered as adjunctive or "bail-out" therapy in selected cases. In patients with acute coronary syndrome with high-risk features and not adequately pretreated with P2Y12 inhibitors, it is useful to administer GP IIb/IIIa inhibitors at the time of PCI.

CHRONIC Rx
- Discharge medications in all patients with MI (unless contraindicated) should include antiischemic medications (e.g., nitroglycerin, β-blocker), lipid-lowering agents, and antiplatelet therapy (aspirin and/or P2Y12 antagonists).
- Aspirin, 81 mg PO daily, but should be continued indefinitely unless not tolerated (e.g., GI bleed). In MI patients, clopidogrel 75 mg PO daily; ticagrelor, 90 mg bid, or prasugrel, 10 mg PO daily, can be combined with aspirin and should be continued without interruption

for a minimum of 12 mo after drug-eluting stent placement; however, aspirin should be continued indefinitely. In cases of high bleeding risk or significant overt bleeding, consider discontinuation of P2Y12 inhibitor after 6 mo (Fig. 5). Combining P2Y12 antagonists with aspirin reduces the risk for repeat myocardial infarction and stent thrombosis. If there is an elective surgical intervention pending, it is recommended to defer the surgery until completion of the full course of the P2Y12 antagonist treatment. Duration dual antiplatelet therapy in high-bleeding-risk (HBR) patients is debatable. Many randomized controlled trials support single antiplatelet therapy 1 or 3 mo after PCI in HBR acute coronary syndrome populations.

- ACE inhibitors (ACEIs) should be started within the first 24 h of MI to all patients having MI with anterior infarction, pulmonary congestion, or LV EF <40%, in the absence of hypotension. They reduce LV dysfunction and dilation and slow the progression to HF during and after acute MI. Angiotensin receptor blockers (ARBs) should be given to patients who have indication but are intolerant of ACEIs. IV formulations of ACEIs should not be given within the first 24 h of STEMI due to risk of hypotension. ARBs offer no advantage over ACEIs and should be considered only in patients who are intolerant to ACEIs.
  1. ACEIs may be stopped in patients without complications and no evidence of LV dysfunction after 6 to 8 wk.
  2. ACEIs should be continued indefinitely in patients with impaired LV function (EF <40%) or clinical HF.

3. ARNI (angiotensin receptor and neprilysin inhibitor) showed more benefit compared to ARB in preventing major adverse cardiovascular events in heart failure patients.

- Long-term aldosterone antagonist therapy should be prescribed for post-MI patients without significant renal dysfunction (creatinine ≤2.5 mg/dl in men and ≤2.0 mg/dl in women) or hyperkalemia who are already taking an ACEI, a β-blocker, and have LV EF <40% with symptomatic HF or diabetes.

- In late 2018, American College of Cardiology (ACC) recommended LDL goal of <70 mg/dl for secondary prevention of atherosclerotic cardiovascular disease. The goal should further be reduced to <55mg/dl in patients with existing atherosclerotic vascular disease and familial hypercholesterolemia. High-intensity statins (atorvastatin 40 to 80 mg or rosuvastatin 20 to 40 mg) should be started as early as possible in all patients with MI regardless of lipid panel, not only for their lipid-lowering effects, but also their antiinflammatory properties (JUPITER trial), which can stabilize the ruptured plaque. Atorvastatin 80 mg can be used (PROVE IT-TIMI 22 and MIRACL trials). IMPROVE-IT trial showed adding ezetimibe to statin treatment could decrease recurrent MI and ischemic stroke in MI patients. FDA also approved two PCSK9 (proprotein convertase subtilisin/kexin type 9) inhibitors (alirocumab and evolocumab) for heterozygous familial hypercholesterolemia patients who are receiving maximally tolerated statins or patients with clinical atherosclerotic cardiovascular disease who require lowering LDL levels. Newer 2018 lipid guidelines suggested starting PCSK9 inhibitor in very high-risk atherosclerotic cardiovascular disease patients who did not meet the LDL goal on high intensity statin and ezetimibe. One should always consider adding ezetimibe to high intensity statin prior to initiation of PCSK9 inhibitor due to cost issues. A fasting lipid panel should be checked during the first 24 h of hospital course, and the intensive therapy can be stepped down if appropriate. Inclisiran, Evinacumab, and Bempedoic acid are excellent non–statin therapy alternatives in patients who are unable to tolerate statin and reach target LDL levels.

- In diabetic patients, HbA1c goal should be aimed at below or around 7.0% to reduce micro- and macrovascular complications. Oral hypoglycemic agents GLP1 (glucagon-like peptide) agonist (liraglutide) and SGLT2 (sodium-glucose cotransporter) inhibitor (empagliflozin) showed significant mortality benefit in type 2 diabetic patients with history of CAD.

- ACC/AHA 2017 hypertension guidelines recommend initiation of blood pressure (BP)-lowering medications in patients with clinical cardiovascular disease and an average SBP ≥130 mm Hg or a DBP ≥80 mm Hg for goal BP of <130/80.

COMPLICATIONS OF MI
- Cardiogenic shock: Emergent revascularization with either PCI or CABG is the recommended treatment.

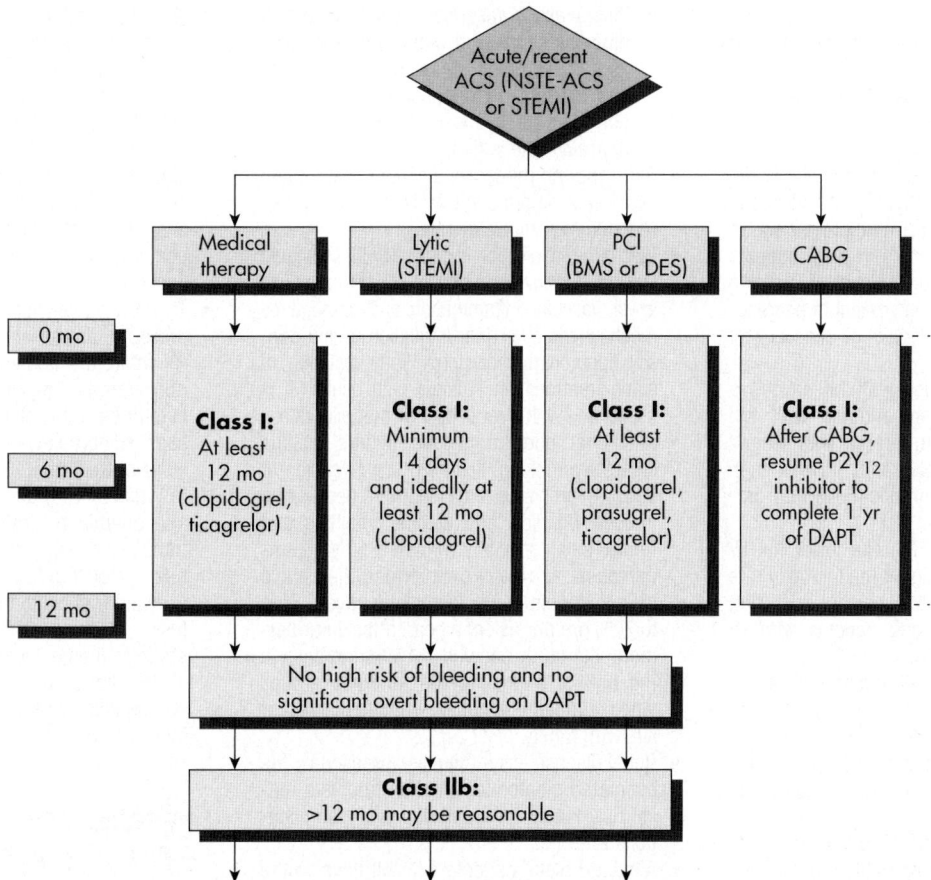

FIG. 5 ACC/AHA guideline recommendation for duration and choice of antiplatelet agent in patients with recent acute coronary syndrome (ACS), including STEMI aspirin therapy is generally continued indefinitely post-ACS. In patients treated with dual-antiplatelet therapy (DAPT) after DES implantation who have a high risk of bleeding (e.g., use of oral anticoagulant therapy, major intracranial surgery) or develop significant overt bleeding, discontinuation of P2Y12 inhibitor therapy after 6 mo for ACS may be reasonable. The optimal duration of prolonged DAPT is not established. *BMS,* Bare-metal stent; *CABG,* coronary artery bypass grafting; *DES,* drug-eluting stent; *lytic,* fibrinolytic therapy; *NSTE-ACS,* non–ST-elevation acute coronary syndrome; *PCI,* percutaneous coronary intervention; *STEMI,* ST-elevation myocardial infarction. (Modified from Levine GN et al: 2016 ACC/AHA guideline focused update on duration of dual antiplatelet therapy in patients with coronary artery disease, *J Am Coll Cardiol* 68(10):1082-115, 2016. In Zipes DP: *Braunwald's heart disease, a textbook of cardiovascular medicine,* ed 11, Philadelphia, 2019, Elsevier.)

- Sustained ventricular tachycardia: Implantable cardioverter-defibrillator therapy (ICD) is indicated before discharge in patients who develop sustained ventricular tachycardia/ventricular fibrillation more than 48 h after STEMI, provided the arrhythmia is not due to transient or reversible ischemia, reinfarction, or metabolic abnormalities.
- Pacing in MI: Temporary pacing is indicated for symptomatic bradyarrhythmias unresponsive to medical treatment and after revascularization. AV block and bradyarrhythmia in the setting of inferior wall MI are usually transient, will not require long-term pacing, and usually resolve within 2 to 4 wk of the event. On the contrary, AV block and bradyarrhythmia or new LBBB in the presence of anterior wall MI is usually a sign of severe disruption of the bundle of His and often requires a permanent pacemaker.
- Pericarditis after MI: Post-MI pericarditis can occur early after MI. Dressler syndrome is an autoimmune inflammatory reaction to myocardial antigen after myocardial infarction. Symptoms of pericarditis usually occur 2 to 3 wk after myocardial infarction. Aspirin is recommended for treatment of pericarditis

after MI. Glucocorticoids and NSAIDs are potentially harmful for treatment of pericarditis after STEMI.
- Severe mitral regurgitation from papillary muscle rupture (1%), interventricular septum rupture (0.2%), and free wall rupture (1% to 3%) are the three major mechanical complications that can occur after acute myocardial infarction. Echocardiogram is helpful in diagnosing papillary muscle rupture, ventricular septal rupture, and free wall rupture. Right heart catheterization is needed to show "step-up" in oxygen saturation at the level of right ventricle. Emergent surgical repair is the treatment of choice for ventricular free wall rupture, intraventricular septum rupture, and papillary muscle rupture.

EVALUATION OF POST-MI PATIENTS

- Noninvasive testing for ischemia should be performed before discharge to assess the presence and extent of inducible ischemia in patients with STEMI who have not had coronary angiography and do not have high-risk clinical features for which coronary angiography would be warranted. It might be

considered before discharge to evaluate the functional significance of a non-infarct artery stenosis previously identified at angiography and/or before discharge to guide the postdischarge exercise prescription.
- Assessment of LV function: LV ejection fraction should be measured in all patients with STEMI. Echocardiography to rule out presence of mural thrombi in patients suspected of having an extensive infarction (more common with anterior wall MI); contrast echocardiography is added if mural thrombus is suspected.
- Assessment of risk for sudden cardiac death: Patients with an initially reduced LV ejection fraction, <40%, who are possible candidates for implantable cardioverter-defibrillator therapy should undergo reevaluation of LV ejection fraction at 90 days (or 42 days if no revascularization was performed). ICD is recommended when LVEF remains <35% in the presence of NYHA class II or III heart failure, or in patients with LVEF <30% regardless of symptoms, if the life expectancy is >1 yr.
- Cardiac rehabilitation/secondary prevention programs are recommended for patients with STEMI.

DISPOSITION

The prognosis after MI depends on multiple factors:

- New bundle branch block, Mobitz II second-degree block, and third-degree heart block adversely affect outcome.
- Size of infarct: The larger it is, the higher the post-MI mortality rate. Significant myocardial stunning with subsequent improvement of ventricular function occurs in most patients after anterior MI. A lower level of creatine kinase, an estimate of the extent of necrosis, is independently predictive of recovery of function.
- Site of infarct: Inferior wall MI carries a better prognosis than anterior wall MI; however, patients with inferior wall MI and right ventricular involvement have a high risk for arrhythmic complications and cardiogenic shock.
- Ejection fraction after MI: The lower the LV ejection fraction, the higher the mortality rate after MI. The risk of death is higher in the first 30 days after MI among patients with LV dysfunction, HF, or both.
- The presence of post-MI angina indicates a high mortality rate.
- Performance on low-level exercise test: The presence of ST-segment changes during the test is a predictor of high mortality rate during the first yr.
- The presence of pericarditis during the acute phase of MI increases mortality rate at 1 yr.
- The Killip classification is an independent predictor of all-cause 30-day mortality:
  1. Killip class I include individuals with no clinical signs of HF. Mortality rate is 6%.
  2. Killip class II includes individuals with rales or crackles in the lungs, S3 gallop, and elevated jugular venous pressure. Mortality rate is 17%.
  3. Killip class III describes individuals with frank acute pulmonary edema. Mortality rate is 38%.

4. Killip class IV describes individuals in cardiogenic shock or hypotension (measured as systolic blood pressure <90 mm Hg) and evidence of peripheral vasoconstriction (oliguria, cyanosis, or sweating). The mortality rate is 67%.

- Self-reported moderate alcohol consumption in the year before acute MI is associated with reduced 1-yr mortality rate.
- Discharge medication in patients with MI should include lipid-lowering agents. Statins may also lower vascular inflammation and damage by mechanisms other than reduction of low-density lipoprotein cholesterol. Early initiation of statin treatment in patients with acute MI is associated with a reduced 1-yr mortality rate.
- Additional poor prognostic factors include cigarette smoking, history of hypertension or prior MI, presence of ST-segment depression in acute MI, older age, diabetes mellitus, and female sex (especially women >50 yr). Lammintausta and Fonarow reported that single men and women who live alone have a 60% to 70% greater risk of a heart attack. Furthermore, the study showed >160% increase in the risk of sudden death in these groups when compared to people who are married or live with family.
- Renal disease, even mild, as assessed by the estimated glomerular filtration rate, is a major risk factor for cardiovascular complications after MI.
- Although black patients with MI have worse outcomes than their white counterparts, these differences did not persist after adjustment for patient factors and site of care.

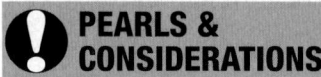

COMMENTS

- Approximately 1.5 million patients undergo PCI in the U.S. each year. Depending on local practices and the diagnostic criteria used, 5% to 30% of these patients have evidence of a periprocedural MI.
- The 12-lead ECG has low sensitivity for the detection of MI if the culprit lesion is in the left circumflex artery (LCX). If the initial 12-lead ECG is not diagnostic and high clinical suspicion for acute coronary syndrome exists, it is reasonable to obtain additional posterior chest leads (V7 to V9) to detect LCX occlusion.
- Triad of hypotension, elevated jugular venous pressure, and clear lungs are suggestive of RV infarction in patients with inferior AMI. Administration of nitroglycerin is contraindicated due to hypotension. IV fluids, inotropic support, and early reperfusion are the mainstays of treatment.
- In patients with acute myocardial infarction and anemia a strategy of administering a transfusion only when the hemoglobin falls below 7 or 8 g/dL has been widely adapted. A recent trial comparing the restrictive transfusion strategy versus a liberal transfusion strategy (hemoglobin cut off <10 g/dL) revealed that a liberal transfusion strategy did not significantly reduce the risk of recurrent MI or death at 30 d.[9]

REFERENCES

Available at eBooks.Health.Elsevier.com

RELATED CONTENT

Heart Attack (Patient Information)
Acute Coronary Syndrome (Related Key Topic)
Angina Pectoris (Related Key Topic)
Coronary Artery Disease (Related Key Topic)

AUTHOR: **MAHESWARA SATYA GANGADHARA RAO GOLLA, MD**

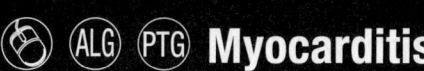

BASIC INFORMATION

DEFINITION

Myocarditis broadly refers to inflammatory disease of the heart muscle (myocardium). Disease severity may range from benign and self-limiting illness to severe, acute decompensation requiring intensive care. Myocarditis may result from exposure to a variety of infectious (Table E1) and noninfectious (Table E2) triggers.

ICD-10CM CODES

I40.0	Infective myocarditis
I40.1	Isolated myocarditis
I40.8	Other acute myocarditis
I40.9	Acute myocarditis, unspecified
A39.52	Meningococcal myocarditis
B26.82	Mumps myocarditis
B33.22	Viral myocarditis
B58.81	Toxoplasma myocarditis
D86.85	Sarcoid myocarditis
I01.2	Acute rheumatic myocarditis
I09.0	Rheumatic myocarditis
I41	Myocarditis in diseases classified elsewhere
I51.4	Myocarditis, unspecified

EPIDEMIOLOGY & DEMOGRAPHICS

- Myocarditis is often underdiagnosed.
- The incidence of focal myocarditis reported at autopsy is 1% to 9% in asymptomatic patients and 50% in patients infected with HIV.
- Myocarditis is the third leading cause of sudden unexpected death (as high as 8% to 9%), especially in competitive athletes. Approximately 1% to 5% of patients who test positive for viral infections may develop myocarditis.

PHYSICAL FINDINGS & CLINICAL PRESENTATION

- Clinical symptoms are heterogeneous, ranging from asymptomatic to severe forms resulting in cardiogenic shock and arrhythmias.
- The most common presentations in patients are new-onset heart failure (HF) (<6 mo), chest pain, and arrhythmias, which include sinus tachycardia as well as atrial and ventricular tachyarrhythmias.
- Chest pain, especially pleuritic and positional, presents when the pericardium is involved.
- Persistent tachycardia may be present, out of proportion to fever.
- Bradyarrhythmia and new-onset unexplained heart block may also occur both in infectious (e.g., Lyme disease) and in immune-mediated forms of myocarditis.
- Faint S_1, S_3, and S_4 gallops on auscultation are important signs of impaired ventricular function.
- Murmur of functional mitral regurgitation and functional tricuspid regurgitation caused by severe left ventricular and right ventricular dilation.
- Pericardial friction rub if associated with pericarditis as in the clinical syndrome of myopericarditis.

- Patients may present with a history of a recent flu-like syndrome or nonspecific viral prodrome (fever, arthralgias, malaise, fatigue). Children often have a more fulminant presentation than adults. Difficulty breathing is the most common presentation of pediatric myocarditis.
- Congestive heart failure (CHF) symptoms that usually manifest with fatigue and decreased exercise capacity and appetite.
- Signs of biventricular failure (hypotension, hepatomegaly, peripheral edema, distention of neck veins, S_3 sounds, and pulmonary edema).
- Presyncope or syncope can occur secondary to ventricular arrhythmias.
- Sudden cardiac death from ventricular tachycardia/ventricular fibrillation mediated by inflammation and/or a scar, which sets up a reentry-mediated pathway for ventricular arrhythmias.
- Acute coronary syndrome, which can occur as a result of local coronary spasm and inflammation and can present on ECG as acute injury pattern or ischemic changes.

ETIOLOGY

- Infection:
  1. Viral (adenovirus, parvovirus B19, hepatitis C virus [HCV], Coxsackie B virus, cytomegalovirus, enterovirus, poliovirus, mumps, HIV, and Epstein-Barr virus, etc.). Viruses are the most common cause of myocarditis in developed countries. In the 1980s and 1990s, enteroviruses and adenoviruses were frequently associated with myocarditis and dilated cardiomyopathy (DCM). In the past 20 yr, however, other viruses such as HCV, parvovirus B19, herpesvirus 6 (HH6), HIV, and COVID-19, have emerged as the significant pathogens
  2. Bacterial (*Staphylococcus aureus, Clostridium perfringens,* diphtheria, mycoplasma, *Mycobacterium tuberculosis,* and any severe bacterial infection)
  3. Mycotic (*Candida, Mucor, Aspergillus, Blastomyces, Histoplasma*)
  4. Parasitic (*Trypanosoma cruzi*—most common worldwide, *Trichinella, Echinococcus, Amoeba, Toxoplasma*)
  5. *Rickettsia rickettsii*
  6. Spirochetal (*Borrelia burgdorferi*—Lyme carditis)
- Rheumatic fever
- Systemic lupus erythematosus
- Granulomatosis with polyangiitis
- Giant cell arteritis and Takayasu arteritis
- Drugs and medications (e.g., cocaine, emetine, doxorubicin, sulfonamides, isoniazid, methyldopa, amphotericin B, tetracycline, phenylbutazone, lithium, 5-fluorouracil, phenothiazines, interferon-alfa, nivolumab, ipilimumab, tricyclic antidepressants, cyclophosphamides, smallpox vaccination)
- Toxins (carbon monoxide, ethanol, diphtheria toxin, lead, arsenicals)
- Systemic and collagen-vascular disease (scleroderma, sarcoidosis, celiac disease, Sjögren syndrome, Kawasaki syndrome, etc.)

- Celiac disease: Two reports from Italy suggest that celiac disease, which is often clinically unsuspected, accounts for as many as 5% of patients with autoimmune myocarditis or idiopathic DCM
- Radiation
- Postpartum status
- Post–stem cell transplantation
- Hypersensitivity reactions from insect bites, such as bee and wasp bites; from snake bites; and from tetanus toxoid
- Vaccine-associated myocarditis

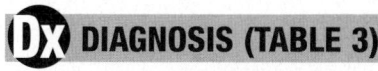 DIAGNOSIS (TABLE 3)

DIFFERENTIAL DIAGNOSIS

- Ischemic cardiomyopathy and nonischemic cardiomyopathies, including dilated idiopathic cardiomyopathy
- Acute coronary syndrome
- Valvular heart disease
- Infiltrative diseases of the myocardium, such as sarcoidosis, amyloidosis, hemochromatosis, and Chagas disease

The differential diagnosis of chest pain is described in Section II.

WORKUP

- Medical history: The clinical presentation of myocarditis is nonspecific and can consist of fatigue, palpitations, dyspnea, precordial discomfort, and myalgias.
- Diagnostic workup includes chest x-ray examination, ECG, laboratory evaluation, echocardiogram, cardiac catheterization, cardiac MRI, and endomyocardial biopsy (in selected patients on the basis of the likelihood of finding specific treatable disorders such as giant cell myocarditis). Of note, endomyocardial biopsy has a sensitivity of only 10% to 35% using standard histologic criteria. This is due to variability in interpretation and sampling error.
- A three-tiered clinical classification for diagnosis of myocarditis by level of diagnostic certainty is summarized in Table 4.

LABORATORY TESTS

- Elevated cardiac troponin is suggestive of myocarditis in patients with clinically suspected myocarditis. Troponin I specificity is 89%; sensitivity is 34% to 53%.[265] Elevated troponin aids in diagnosis but does not confer a prognostic value. A normal level does not rule out the diagnosis.
- Increased creatine kinase (CK) (with elevated MB fraction, lactate dehydrogenase), and aspartate aminotransferase from myocardial necrosis.
- Elevation of cardiac troponin I or T is more common than CK-MB elevation in patients with biopsy-proven myocarditis.
- The elevations of cardiac troponin I were correlated with a short duration (typically <1 mo) of CHF symptoms, indicating that the majority of myocardial necrosis occurs early in the disease course.
- Persistent elevations of cardiac biomarkers are indicative of ongoing myocardial necrosis.

TABLE 3 Expanded Criteria for Diagnosis of Myocarditis

Suggestive of Myocarditis	2 Positive Categories
Compatible with myocarditis:	3 positive categories
High probability of being myocarditis:	all 4 categories positive

(Any matching feature in category = positive for category)

Category I: Clinical Symptoms
- Clinical heart failure
- Fever
- Viral prodrome
- Fatigue
- Dyspnea on exertion
- Chest pain
- Palpitations
- Presyncope or syncope

Category II: Evidence of Cardiac Structural or Functional Perturbation *in the Absence* of Regional Coronary Ischemia
- Echocardiography evidence
- Regional wall motion abnormalities
- Cardiac dilation
- Regional cardiac hypertrophy
- Troponin release
- High sensitivity (>0.1 ng/ml)
- Positive indium-111 antimyosin scintigraphy
- Normal coronary angiography *or*
- Absence of reversible ischemia by coronary distribution on perfusion scan

Category III: Cardiac Magnetic Resonance Imaging
- Increased myocardial T2 signal on inversion recovery sequence
- Delayed contrast enhancement after gadolinium-DTPA infusion

Category IV: Myocardial Biopsy—Pathologic or Molecular Analysis
- Pathology findings compatible with Dallas criteria
- Presence of viral genome by polymerase chain reaction or in situ hybridization

DTPA, Diethylenetriamine penta-acetic acid.
From Bonow RO et al: *Heart disease,* ed 9, Philadelphia, 2012, Saunders.

TABLE 4 Three-Tiered Clinical Classification for Diagnosis of Myocarditis by Level of Diagnostic Certainty

Diagnostic Category	Criteria	Histologic Confirmation	Biomarker, ECG, or Imaging Abnormalities Consistent with Myocarditis	Treatment Needed
Possible subclinical acute myocarditis	In the clinical context of possible myocardial injury *without* cardiovascular symptoms but with at least one of the following: Biomarkers of cardiac injury raised ECG findings suggestive of cardiac injury Abnormal cardiac function on echocardiogram or CMR	Absent	Required	Not known
Probable acute myocarditis	In clinical context of possible myocardial injury *with* cardiovascular symptoms and at least one of the following: Biomarkers of cardiac injury raised ECG findings suggestive of cardiac injury Abnormal cardiac function on echocardiogram or CMR	Absent	Required	Per clinical syndrome
Definite myocarditis	Histologic or immunohistologic evidence of myocarditis	Present	Not required	Tailored to specific cause

CMR, Cardiac magnetic resonance imaging; *ECG,* electrocardiogram.

- Brain natriuretic peptide (BNP) or N terminal (NT)-proBNP is recommended if patient has HF symptoms.
- Increased erythrocyte sedimentation rate and C-reactive protein (nonspecific but may be of value in following the progress of the disease and the response to therapy).
- Increased white blood cell count (also nonspecific). An increase in eosinophils can be seen with parasitic infections.
- Viral titers (acute and convalescent).
- Cold agglutinin titer, antistreptolysin O titer, blood cultures when appropriate.
- Lyme disease antibody titer.
- Rapid plasma reagin, Venereal Disease Research Laboratory.
- Histology on endomyocardial biopsy (Fig. E1) may reveal histiocytic and mononuclear cellular infiltrates, fulfilling the Dallas criteria, which were developed by a panel of cardiac pathologists as a working standard to define the disease; active myocarditis is defined as "an inflammatory infiltrate of the myocardium with necrosis and/or degeneration of adjacent myocytes not typical of the ischemic damage associated with coronary artery disease."
- Based on the European Society of Cardiology Working Group on Myocardial and Pericardial Diseases, immunohistochemical criteria of myocarditis are abnormal inflammatory infiltrates defined as >14 leukocytes/mm^2 including up to 4 monocytes/mm^2 with the presence of >7 CD^3 positive T lymphocytes/mm^2.
- A novel microRNA (the human homologue hsa-mir-Chr8:96) has been reported useful to distinguish patients with myocarditis from those with myocardial infarction.[266]

IMAGING STUDIES

- Chest x-ray examination: Enlargement of cardiac silhouette with or without pulmonary congestion may be present.
- ECG: May be normal or show nonspecific findings. Sinus tachycardia with nonspecific ST-T wave changes unless there is concomitant pericarditis in which the ECG changes are more specific; intraventricular conduction defects and bundle branch blocks are uncommon in typical viral myocarditis but are common manifestations in cardiac sarcoid and idiopathic giant cell myocarditis. The presence of Q waves or left bundle branch block was associated with higher rates of death or transplantation in some patients.
- Lyme disease and diphtheria can cause varying degrees of heart block.
- Changes mimicking acute myocardial infarction (regional ST elevations and Q waves) can occur with focal necrosis from myocarditis.
- Echocardiogram:
  1. The most useful test in detecting decreased ventricular function in suspected myocarditis even when subclinical.
  2. Acute severe myocarditis is associated with left ventricular systolic dysfunction with decreased ejection fraction.
  3. The systolic dysfunction is generally global but may be regional or segmental as in the case of focal myocarditis.

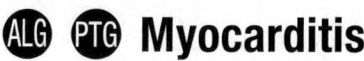

4. Exercise-induced wall motion abnormalities may also be seen. This is usually due to microvascular dysfunction.
5. Abnormal tissue Doppler signal can provide additional evidence for the presence of myocarditis.
6. The echocardiogram can also be helpful with diagnosing coexisting pericardial involvement (e.g., with the presence of a pericardial effusion).
7. The spheroid dysfunctional ventricle in acute myocarditis tends to remodel to the more normal elliptical shape over several months.
- Cardiac catheterization and angiography:
1. To rule out coronary artery disease. Coronary angiography is most commonly normal with evidence of minimal or no coronary artery disease.
- Endomyocardial biopsy.
1. A right ventricular endomyocardial biopsy can confirm the diagnosis, although a negative biopsy result does not exclude myocarditis owing to the low sensitivity of this test. Recent studies have shown that myocardial biopsy may be unnecessary because immunosuppression therapy based on biopsy results is generally ineffective. However, if idiopathic giant cell myocarditis is suspected, biopsy can confirm this diagnosis, and aggressive immunosuppression therapy is indicated in this patient cohort.
- Cardiac MRI (Fig. E2):
1. Can be used to detect myocardial edema and myocyte injury in myocarditis.
2. Increased focal or global signal intensity can be used to calculate an edema ratio. Edema in the absence of necrosis or scar represents reversible injury and thus can predict functional recovery.
3. Late gadolinium enhancement (LGE) and the presence of increased focal and global myocardial contrast enhancement relative to skeletal muscle.
4. Any combination of two of the above has a sensitivity and specificity of 76% and 96%, with 85% diagnostic accuracy, and is the gold standard for diagnosis of myocarditis, as opposed to routine biopsy.
5. Cardiac MRI has demonstrated that myocarditis tends to start as a focal process and becomes a more global process over time, with the extent of myocardial enhancement correlating with clinical status and left ventricular function.
6. The pattern of LGE is different from that in ischemic cardiomyopathy. LGE in myocarditis tends to involve the epicardium with variable extension into the mid myocardium and sparing of the endocardium. This is in contrast to ischemic injury, which involves endocardium first with extension outward.
- Indium-111–labeled antimyosin antibody scintigraphy is positive in myocarditis with a sensitivity of up to 65%.

Rx TREATMENT

NONPHARMACOLOGIC THERAPY
- Supportive care is the first line of therapy for patients with myocarditis.
- Restrict physical activity (to decrease cardiac work). Bed rest is advisable during viremia.
- Avoid heavy use of alcohol.
- NSAIDs should be avoided in patients with HF generally, given the risk of HF exacerbation and possible risk of increased mortality. NSAIDs in the lowest required dose are reserved for patients with perimyocarditis in whom left ventricular function is normal and who have prominent chest pain from pericarditis.

ACUTE GENERAL Rx
- Treat the underlying cause (e.g., use specific antibiotics for bacterial infection, management of autoimmune disease).
- Treat CHF with diuretics, ACE inhibitors, and salt restriction. A beta-blocker may be added once clinical stability has been achieved. In patients with myocarditis associated with severe left ventricular dysfunction, major treatment decisions such as referral for heart transplant, left ventricular assist device, and with implantable cardioverter-defibrillator (ICD) implantation should be deferred for 3 to 6 mo when feasible to allow for improvement with optimal medical therapy.
- Patients who are left with an LVEF ≤35% despite optimal medical therapy for 3 to 6 mo, and who have good functional status with prognosis >1 yr, may benefit from primary prevention therapy with ICD implantation as in patients with ischemic cardiomyopathy and other nonischemic cardiomyopathies.
- Antiarrhythmics if needed for ventricular arrhythmias. When antiarrhythmic therapy is necessary, options include amiodarone, dofetilide, and, in patients without class IV HF, cautious use of beta-blockers or calcium channel blockers. ICD implantation for secondary prevention in patients who have life-threatening ventricular arrhythmias and have good functional status with prognosis >1 yr.
- Complete heart block and/or symptomatic bradycardia are indications for pacing during the acute phase of myocarditis but are usually transient. Permanent pacing is typically not required.
- Management of HF with reduced ejection fraction follows the AHA/ACC guidelines in order to decrease mortality. (See "Heart Failure")
- Anticoagulation is indicated in patients with evidence of systemic embolism or presence of acute left ventricular thrombus. Standard criteria for anticoagulation for atrial fibrillation should also be applied.
- Mechanical assist devices such as intraaortic balloon pumps, Impella device, and left ventricular assist device (LVAD) if low output HF or cardiogenic shock persists despite medical therapy.

- Cardiac transplantation in patients with chronic or acute fulminant myocarditis with intractable cardiomyopathy and persistent CHF.
- Corticosteroid use is contraindicated in early infectious myocarditis. It is the treatment of choice in patients with immune-checkpoint inhibitor related myocarditis. Steroids also may be indicated in select patients with intractable CHF, severe systemic toxicity, severe life-threatening arrhythmias, and when it is the treatment for the underlying etiology as later.
- Immunosuppressive drugs (prednisone with cyclosporine/Cytoxan or azathioprine) do not have any significant effect on the prognosis of myocarditis and should not be used in the routine treatment of patients with myocarditis. Immunosuppression may have a role in the treatment of myocarditis from systemic autoimmune disease (e.g., lupus, scleroderma); in idiopathic giant cell myocarditis, sarcoidosis, or myocarditis caused by hypersensitivity reactions; or in severe hemodynamic compromise.
- Observational data suggest that patients with giant cell myocarditis treated with certain immunosuppressive regimens have improved survival compared with patients who do not receive immunosuppressive treatment.
- In patients with ongoing viral genomic expression, preliminary data suggest that treatment with interferons may improve both symptoms and left ventricular function when compared with standard HF therapy.
- Intravenous (IV) immunoglobulins have been studied, but because of lack of efficacy data, at present there is no indication for their use except in some pediatric cases or those refractory to immunosuppressive therapy.
- Improved cardiac function and arrhythmias have been reported in patients with celiac disease and myocarditis or DCM following a gluten-free diet with or without immunosuppressive therapy, but controlled data are lacking.
- In patients who develop myocarditis following the first dose of a COVID-19 mRNA vaccine, we suggest that the second dose be deferred in most cases; it is reasonable for such individuals to choose to receive a second dose once the episode has completely resolved if the risk of severe COVID-19 is high. Individuals with a history of resolved myocarditis or pericarditis unrelated to COVID-19 vaccination can receive an mRNA vaccine. Of note, myocarditis secondary to COVID-19 vaccine is typically mild in severity with a trend toward normalization of left ventricular systolic function within 6 mo in preliminary observational studies.[267,268]
- A treatment algorithm for patients with myocarditis is described in Fig. 3.

DISPOSITION
- The natural history of myocarditis is illustrated in Fig. E4. Most patients with acute myocarditis and mild cardiac involvement have a partial or a full clinical recovery. In some cases, however, the process may continue subclinically with eventual progression

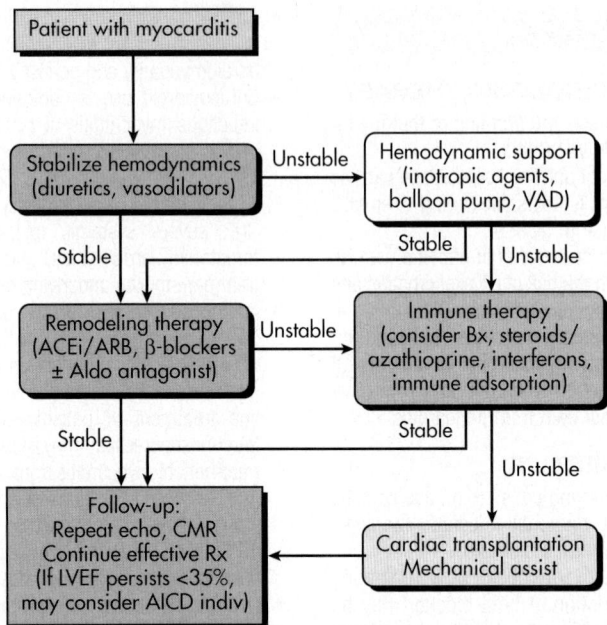

FIG. 3 Treatment algorithms for patients with myocarditis, depending on hemodynamic stability and response to general supportive and remodeling treatment regimen at each step. All patients require aggressive support and appropriate follow-up. Immune therapy at present is still indicated mainly to support those who have failed to improve spontaneously. *ACEi,* Angiotensin-converting enzyme inhibitor; *AICD,* automatic implantable cardioverter-defibrillator; *Aldo,* aldosterone; *ARB,* angiotensin receptor blocker; *Bx,* biopsy; *CMR,* cardiac magnetic resonance; *echo,* echocardiography; *indiv,* based on individual assessment of risk vs. benefit; *LVEF,* left ventricular ejection fraction; *VAD,* ventricular assist device. (From Libby P: *Braunwald's heart disease, a textbook of cardiovascular medicine,* ed 12, Philadelphia, 2022, Elsevier.)

to a cardiomyopathy. Therefore all patients with myocarditis should be followed up at least initially at intervals of 1 to 3 mo, depending on their initial severity of illness. Of those with advanced cardiac dysfunction, 33% will have residual cardiac dysfunction, and 25% may progress to cardiac transplantation or death.

- Prognosis is best for patients with fulminant lymphocytic myocarditis (severe hemodynamic compromise, rapid onset of symptoms, or high fever). These patients tend to have complete recovery with total resolution of myocarditis on repeat biopsy.
- In contrast, patients with giant cell myocarditis have an extremely poor prognosis with a median survival of <6 mo, and most require cardiac transplantation.
- In patients with immune-checkpoint inhibitor related myocarditis, regardless of the severity of presentation, the patient should not be rechallenged with immunotherapy.
- The American Heart Association recommends 3 to 6 mo abstinence from competitive sports after myocarditis.[269]

REFERRAL

Consider heart transplant if intractable CHF develops.

REFERENCES

Available at eBooks.Health.Elsevier.com.

RELATED CONTENT

Myocarditis (Patient Information)

AUTHORS: **VISHNU KADIYALA, MD** and **ARAVIND RAO KOKKIRALA, MD, FACC**

BASIC INFORMATION

DEFINITION

Nasopharyngeal carcinoma (NPC) is an epithelial carcinoma originating in the nasopharynx that has a distinct clinical behavior in comparison to other head and neck carcinomas.

SYNONYMS

Nasopharynx cancer
NPC

ICD-10CM CODE
C11.9   Malignant neoplasm of
               nasopharynx, unspecified

EPIDEMIOLOGY & DEMOGRAPHICS

- NPC is an uncommon cancer that is endemic to east and southeast Asia (70% of cases). In 2020, there were an estimated 133,354 new cases and 80,008 deaths globally.[1]
- The incidence rate is 3 per 100,000 population in China and is <1 per 100,000 in the United States. Its incidence is decreasing steadily in the endemic regions in Asia.
- Incidence is higher in males (2.5 times higher than females).

RISK FACTORS:
- Epstein-Barr virus (EBV) infection
- Tobacco smoking
- Alcohol consumption
- Family history
- Consumption of preserved foods
- Poor oral hygiene

GENETICS:
- Human leukocyte antigen (HLA) genes residing at the major histocompatibility complex (MHC) region on chromosome 6p21 have been widely recognized as major risk loci conferring nasopharyngeal carcinoma risk.
- Genomic changes involved in the development of NPC include: Multiple loss-of-function mutations in the NFkB–negative regulators, recurrent genetic lesions such as loss of the CDKN2A/CDKN2B locus, CCND1 amplification, TP53 mutation, and mutations in the PI3K/MAPK signaling pathways.[2]

PHYSICAL FINDINGS & CLINICAL PRESENTATION

- Chronically blocked or stuffy nose
- Recurrent epistaxis and bloody rhinorrhea
- Hearing impairment and tinnitus
- Headache
- Ear pain
- Palpable neck adenopathy
- Cranial nerve palsies

ETIOLOGY

- Pathologic subtypes of squamous NPC are keratinizing, nonkeratinizing, and basaloid types. The keratinizing subtype accounts for less than 20% of cases worldwide and is seen in nonendemic areas. The nonkeratinizing subtype constitutes most cases in endemic areas (>95%) and is predominantly associated with Epstein-Barr virus (EBV) infection.

- Persistent EBV infection in genetically mutated epithelial cells and the proliferation of infected cells lead to tumorigenic transformation.[3,4] Chronic exposure of the nasopharyngeal mucosa to environmental carcinogens increases DNA damage and leads to somatic genetic changes in the nasopharyngeal epithelial cells. EBV infection in turn facilitates inactivation of a variety of cancer-related genes. During tumor development, acquired mutations of regulatory factors in the NF-κB signaling pathway alter the activity of additional cancer-related genes. Mutations in the MHC class I genes, PI3K/MAPK pathways as well as somatic mutations of TP53 and RAS genes may be at play in the development of tumor recurrence and metastasis.

DIAGNOSIS

DIFFERENTIAL DIAGNOSIS

- Nasal polyps
- Nasopharyngeal lymphoma
- Nasopharyngeal sarcoma

WORKUP

Direct nasopharyngoscopy by ear, nose, throat (ENT) physician followed by biopsy (Fig. E1) and imaging studies (Fig. E2)

LABORATORY TESTS

- Complete blood count (CBC)
- Comprehensive chemistry panel
- Circulating cell-free EBV DNA is a biomarker for nasopharyngeal carcinoma. Pretreatment plasma EBV-DNA levels may add to the prognostic value of conventional Tumor, Node, Metastasis (TNM) staging systems (Table E1)

IMAGING STUDIES

- Computed tomography (CT) or MRI of the head and neck; MRI is better than CT for soft-tissue extent assessment and retropharyngeal nodal detection.
- PET/CT is used to assess for detection of distant metastasis and for detection of residual cancer after completion of therapy.

TREATMENT

The mainstay of therapy is concurrent chemotherapy and radiation therapy. Both adjuvant chemotherapy and to a lesser extent neoadjuvant chemotherapy are routinely utilized after and before chemoradiotherapy in the clinical setting.[5]

NONPHARMACOLOGIC THERAPY

- Surgery is utilized for diagnostic biopsies and for neck dissection in the setting of residual neck lymphadenopathy after completion of definitive chemoradiotherapy.
- Supportive care with gastrostomy tube nutrition is often required to maintain nutritional and hydration status during treatment.

ACUTE GENERAL Rx

- Intensity modulated radiotherapy (IMRT) is the definitive treatment for NPC. It is typically administered with concurrent every 3-wk

cycles of cisplatin and 5-fluorouracil chemotherapy in patients with locoregionally advanced NPC. Weekly cisplatin resulted in similar survival benefit as triweekly cisplatin but with higher hematological toxicity. Adjuvant chemotherapy with cisplatin and gemcitabine is routinely administered with improved overall survival through reduction of distant metastases.

- Induction multiagent chemotherapy prior to definitive chemoradiotherapy has been shown to improve survival but with increased hematologic and gastrointestinal toxicity in a recent meta-analysis of seven randomized controlled trials involving 2311 patients.[6]
- In recurrent or metastatic disease, the addition of immune checkpoint inhibitor camrelizumab to chemotherapy demonstrated improved progression-free survival and has the potential to change standard practice on maturity of data.[7]
- Systemic chemotherapy and antiepidermal growth factor receptor inhibitor (EGFR) approaches improve survival in these patients. Additionally, single-agent immune checkpoint inhibitors (pembrolizumab, nivolumab, camrelizumab) have demonstrated significant antitumor efficacy and improved safety profile in patients with recurrent or metastatic disease.[8]
- Significant supportive care with nutrition, hydration, and mucositis management (especially pain control) is required.
- Posttherapy rehabilitation with swallowing therapy, dental care, endocrinology care, and lymphedema care are often required.

DISPOSITION

Early-stage disease patients typically have a good outcome (5-yr survival 60% to 75%), whereas stage 4 patients have a poor outcome (5-yr survival <40%).

REFERRAL

Referrals include to medical oncology, radiation oncology, dietitian, and gastroenterology.

PEARLS & CONSIDERATIONS

- Analysis of EBV DNA in plasma samples has been found to be useful in screening for early asymptomatic cases. NPC was detected significantly earlier and outcomes were better in participants who were identified by screening compared to those in a historical cohort.[3]
- Higher pretreatment, mid-treatment, and posttreatment EBV DNA levels have been significantly correlated with poor outcomes for patients afflicted with NPC.[4]

REFERENCES
Available at eBooks.Health.Elsevier.com.

RELATED CONTENT
Head and Neck Squamous Cell Carcinoma (Related Key Topic)

AUTHOR: RITESH RATHORE, MD

Diseases and Disorders

N

I

BASIC INFORMATION

DEFINITION

Nephrotic syndrome is not a specific disease, but rather an umbrella term characterized by heavy proteinuria (usually defined as >3.5 g/24 h), hypoalbuminemia, hyperlipidemia, lipiduria, and edema. Nephrotic-range proteinuria involves urine protein excretion of >3.5 g/24 h without other features of the nephrotic syndrome. Proteinuria, primarily in the form of albuminuria, can have many causes that share a common mechanism of glomerular injury, the most common being diabetes, focal segmental glomerulosclerosis, membranous nephropathy, minimal change disease, and amyloidosis. Though less common, disorders that are classically categorized under the nephritic syndrome may also lead to nephrotic-range proteinuria.[1]

ICD-10CM CODES

N04.9 Nephrotic syndrome with unspecified morphologic changes
N04.0 Nephrotic syndrome with minor glomerular abnormality
N04.1 Nephrotic syndrome with focal and segmental glomerular lesions
N04.2 Nephrotic syndrome with diffuse membranous glomerulonephritis
N04.3 Nephrotic syndrome with diffuse mesangial proliferative glomerulonephritis
N04.4 Nephrotic syndrome with diffuse endocapillary proliferative glomerulonephritis
N04.5 Nephrotic syndrome with diffuse mesangiocapillary glomerulonephritis
N04.6 Nephrotic syndrome with dense deposit disease
N04.7 Nephrotic syndrome with diffuse crescentic glomerulonephritis
N04.8 Nephrotic syndrome with other morphologic changes

EPIDEMIOLOGY & DEMOGRAPHICS

- Among children (especially <6 yr), the most common causes of nephrotic syndrome (NS) are the following: Minimal change disease (MCD) (75% of pediatric cases) and primary focal and segmental glomerulosclerosis (FSGS) (7% to 20% of cases).[2] Variation in incidence of NS depending on country of origin, or ethnicity, with proportions ranging from 1.15 to 16.9 per 100,000 children. Incidence is highest among children of south Asian ancestry.[1]
- In adults, diabetes mellitus is the most frequent cause of nephrotic syndrome, followed by membranous nephropathy and FSGS. FSGS is also the most common primary (nonsystemic) cause of nephrotic-range proteinuria and is more common in persons of African ancestry, especially in patients with high-risk APOL1 genotypes.[1,3,4]
- Membranous nephropathy is the second most common primary cause of nephrotic syndrome in adults.
- Membranous nephropathy can be found in all racial and ethnic groups.

PHYSICAL FINDINGS & CLINICAL PRESENTATION[1,2]

- Peripheral edema, periorbital edema, ascites, anasarca, and weight gain
- Hypercoagulability is a potential clinical manifestation, especially with serum albumin less than 2 g/dl
- Patients are at higher risk for infections due to urinary immunoglobulin loss even without being on systemic immunosuppression.

ETIOLOGY

Disorders that exclusively affect the basement membrane or podocyte generally have a noninflammatory pathology and lead to proteinuria as primarily albuminuria, the hallmark of glomerular disease.[1-3,5]

Traditionally, the clinical approach to this pathologic schema has been a subdivision of patients into those with a nephrotic vs. those with a nephritic presentation. Nephritic disorders classically have subnephrotic proteinuria, low glomerular filtration rates, and hematuria whereas nephrotic (or nonnephrotic) disorders have greater proteinuria, often normal glomerular filtration rates, and lack hematuria. While generally true, this schema may cause diagnostic confusion because nephritic disease may present with nephrotic-range proteinuria, especially earlier in the disease course before glomerular filtration is substantially reduced. It is better to categorize these disorders as nephrotic, with a noninflammatory urine sediment (i.e., proteinuria without casts or cellular elements) vs. nephritic, with an inflammatory sediment (i.e., proteinuria plus red blood cell [RBC] casts and/or dysmorphic RBCs), regardless of the amount of proteinuria.[2]

Fig. E1 details the clinical breakdown. In this chapter, we focus on primary diseases that present with a noninflammatory sediment (MCD, FSGS, membranous nephropathy, and amyloidosis) and on primary disorders with inflammatory sediment that are often with nephrotic-range proteinuria, such as membranoproliferative glomerulonephritis (MPGN). The evaluation of nephritic syndrome is noted by worsening glomerular filtration in the setting of proteinuria and hematuria. Important points regarding the most common etiologies of nephrotic syndrome are detailed in the following text (Table 1).

- MCD has a bland urine sediment with abrupt onset of disease and abrupt remission. Thought to be secondary to antibodies targeting nephrin, present in podocytes.
  1. Proteinuria may exceed 20 g daily.
  2. Acute kidney injury may occur in severe NS associated with MCD.
  3. NSAID use, chronic lithium ingestion, viral infections, and lymphomas are associated with secondary forms of MCD.
- FSGS, primary and secondary: Primary FSGS, possibly caused by an autoimmune triggered circulating permeability factor, typically manifests with full nephrotic syndrome and requires immunosuppressive therapy.
  1. FSGS is more prevalent in persons of African ancestry.[5,6]
  2. Secondary FSGS is caused by a known etiology, including heroin use, sickle cell disease, scarring of any kind from prior injury, obesity, low nephron mass, HIV, etc. Most cases of secondary FSGS are associated with lower levels of proteinuria (often subnephrotic), higher serum albumin levels, and less edema. HIV-associated nephropathy is an important exception and is associated with heavy proteinuria and rapid progression if untreated. Distinguishing between primary and secondary FSGS is important therapeutically as secondary FSGS should be treated by managing the underlying disease rather than with immunosuppression. Many forms of glomerular injury can produce morphologic features of FSGS, and worsening proteinuria attributable to secondary FSGS generally portends worse outcomes.[5,6]
- Membranous nephropathy may be primary or secondary. Primary membranous nephropathy is due to in situ deposition of antibodies directed against a glomerular antigen. In 70% or more cases, the epitope is identified as phospholipase A2 receptor. Less common epitopes are neural epidermal growth-factor like 1 (NELL1), exostosin 1/exostosin 2 (EXT1/2), and thrombospondin type-1 domain-containing 7A (THSD7A). Secondary membranous nephropathy is often due to infection (e.g., hepatitis B, malaria, schistosomiasis, syphilis), autoimmune disease (e.g., systemic lupus erythematosus [SLE]), medications (e.g., D-penicillamine, gold), and malignancies. Distinguishing between the two subtypes is important for management.[4,7,8]
- Kidney amyloidosis is frequently due to aberrantly folded immunoglobulin light chains (AL amyloid) or serum amyloid A protein (AA amyloid associated with chronic inflammation), and other less common amyloid-types. Kidney size is often enlarged, and proteinuria may be massive. On histology, Congo red staining detects amyloid proteins.[9]
- Diabetic nephropathy occurs most commonly in diabetics with longstanding and/or uncontrolled diabetes. The correlation between retinopathy, proteinuria, and diabetic nephropathy is well established in patients with type 1 diabetes. The relationship is less well established in type 2 diabetes, and absence of retinopathy does not preclude a diagnosis of diabetic nephropathy.
- MPGN usually has immune complex deposition with complement or alternate complement system activation without immune complex formation (e.g., C3 glomerulopathy). The prior classification of types 1, 2, and 3 MPGN is obsolete, and a pathophysiologic scheme is used now. Common causes are infections (e.g., hepatitis C), autoimmune disorders (e.g., SLE), disorders of the alternative complement pathway (C3 glomerulopathy), or dysproteinemias (e.g., monoclonal gammopathies). Distinguishing between these

TABLE 1 Important Clinical, Serologic, and Pathologic Features of Selected Diseases Causing Nephrotic Syndrome

Disease	Important Clinical Features	Serologic Features	Pathologic Features
Minimal change disease	Rapid onset with heavy proteinuria and rapid remission with therapy. True steroid resistance is rare and should prompt repeat biopsy to rule out FSGS.	Complements are normal.	Light microscopy (LM) shows completely normal kidney architecture. Immunofluorescence microscopy: Normal. Electron microscopy (EM): Diffuse podocyte effacement.
Primary FSGS	Often heavier proteinuria and low serum albumin and edema. Tip lesion subtype and collapsing FSGS often have more explosive onset. Sediment usually bland, but RBCs can be seen. Usually no cellular casts.	Complements are normal.	LM: Only one glomerulus need show features of FSGS to make diagnosis. Immunofluorescence microscopy: Often devoid of immunoglobulin, although IgM can be seen. EM: Often has diffuse podocyte effacement.
Secondary FSGS	Proteinuria is often subnephrotic, or if nephrotic, serum albumin levels are maintained. Minimal edema.	HIV and parvovirus infection can cause phenotype identical to idiopathic collapsing FSGS.	LM: Often shows evidence of glomerulomegaly. EM: Foot process effacement is less diffuse.
Primary membranous nephropathy	Often seen in older White patients. More likely than other forms of nephrotic syndrome to be associated with thrombotic complications. Sediment: Bland. RBCs can be found, although RBC casts are usually found.	Serum antiphospholipase A2 receptor antibodies are found in 70% of patients with idiopathic primary membranous nephropathy. Antineutral endopeptidase antibodies are found in a minority of others.	LM: Characterized by thickening of the GBM; "spikes" can be seen on silver stain. Immunofluorescence microscopy: C3 and IgG noted in granular pattern. Newer techniques stain for antiphospholipase A2 receptor antibody in situ. EM: Associated with subepithelial deposits.
Secondary membranous nephropathy	Associated with malignancy, lupus, syphilis, hepatitis B and C, medications (gold, captopril, penicillamine, etc.).	Notable for the absence of antiphospholipase A2 antibodies. ANA, hepatitis B, HCV serologies are helpful. RPR can be sent in context of appropriate history.	Morphology is exactly the same except when examined by EM. On high power, one sees both subendothelial and mesangial deposits in addition to classic subepithelial deposits.
Amyloidosis	Often found with massive proteinuria. Kidney size is enlarged. Bland sediment.	UPEP, SPEP, serum free light chains may be positive. The UPEP will show glomerular proteinuria, which can help differentiate from myeloma kidney.	LM: Often notable for nodular pattern. Diagnosis can be made by staining using Congo red or thioflavin T. Immunofluorescence microscopy: Antibody use can differentiate AA from AL amyloid. EM: Shows characteristic random 10-nm fibrils.
Diabetes	Often associated with nephrotic-range proteinuria in the setting of retinopathy. Kidney sizes are preserved.	No specific serologic tests are positive.	LM: Nodular pattern often seen, thickened GBM.
MPGN	Often associated with nephrotic-range proteinuria with a "nephritic" sediment. RBC casts often seen along with dysmorphic RBC.	C3 and C4 are often low in immune complex MPGN. Immune complex GN warrants checking SPEP and UPEP, as gammopathy is associated with MPGN. Hepatitis B, HCV, ANA, and cryoglobulins are also warranted. C3 alone is low in dense deposit disease and C3 glomerulonephritis, which may prompt specific tests for complement dysregulation.	The key point here is to look at the IF. If immunofluorescence shows both immunoglobulin and complement deposition, the diagnosis is immune complex MGPN. If only complement, the diagnosis is most likely C3 glomerulopathy (either dense deposit disease or C3 glomerulonephritis).

ANA, Antinuclear antibody; *C3*, complement component 3; *FSGS*, focal and segmental glomerulosclerosis; *GBM*, glomerular basement membrane; *GN*, glomerulonephritis; *HCV*, hepatitis C virus; *Ig*, immunoglobulin; *MPGN*, membranoproliferative glomerulonephritis; *RBC*, red blood cell; *RPR*, rapid plasma reagin; *SPEP*, serum protein electrophoresis; *UPEP*, urine protein electrophoresis.

possibilities guides therapy. Urinary sediment often contains dysmorphic erythrocytes and erythrocyte casts and is also associated with heavy proteinuria.[10]

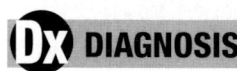 **DIAGNOSIS**

DIFFERENTIAL DIAGNOSIS
- Other conditions that present with edema (congestive heart failure, cirrhosis, protein-losing enteropathy, severe malnutrition)
- Glomerulonephritis from disorders commonly associated with inflammatory urinary sediment and glomerular inflammation

WORKUP
Initial workup includes serum creatinine, blood urea nitrogen, 24-h urine protein collection and urinary sediment examination.[1,11] Abnormalities in any of the these tests should prompt nephrology consultation.
- Testing may include urine and serum electrophoresis, serum-free light chains, and serologic testing for HIV, hepatitis B surface antigen, hepatitis C virus (HCV) antibody, and antinuclear antibody (ANA). As urinary sediment examination is not 100% sensitive in ruling out an inflammatory process, C3 and C4 can be checked, as complement levels are often low in many inflammatory

glomerulonephritides and often low in MPGN.
1. Depending on practice patterns, these tests are used selectively before or, in some cases, after biopsy to better define an etiology.
- Antiphospholipase A2 receptor antibody (anti-PLA2R) titer. Elevated titers are found in primary membranous nephropathy and less commonly in secondary membranous nephropathy. With treatment, patients may develop immunologic remission (decreasing anti-PLA2R titers) prior to a clinical remission based on urine proteinuria. Monitoring titers during the treatment course may guide treatment

duration and limit toxic side effects of therapy.[3,4,11,12]

- Kidney biopsy is performed in most instances unless there is a contraindication to biopsy or the disease is diagnosed through serologic testing (i.e., anti-PLA2R antibody in nondiabetic patients with preserved kidney function) or other organ biopsy (i.e., fat pad or bone marrow in amyloidosis).

Rx TREATMENT

NONIMMUNOSUPPRESSIVE THERAPY

- Control of proteinuria is key to treating progressive kidney disease. Nearly all trials of nondiabetic chronic kidney disease demonstrate that reducing proteinuria improves renal survival. ACE inhibitors (ACEIs) or angiotensin II type 1 receptor blockers (ARBs) should be used at maximally tolerated doses.[1,11] SGLT2 inhibitors are also likely to be beneficial in these patients given their antiproteinuric effects.[12]
  1. Nondihydropyridine calcium channel blockers (verapamil, diltiazem) can be used in lieu of ACEIs or ARBs when these agents are contraindicated.
- For proteinuria >1 g per day, the target blood pressure is <125/75 mm Hg.
- With the exception of MCD, patients with nephrotic-range proteinuria and hyperlipidemia should be treated with HMG-CoA synthetase inhibitors (statins).
- Although some patients with nephrotic syndrome are hypercoagulable (particularly those with membranous nephropathy), the role of prophylactic anticoagulation is controversial and not well defined. For patients with membranous nephropathy and serum albumin levels <2.0 g/dl, anticoagulation should be considered if bleeding risk is low.[2,11] An online calculator is available (https://www.med.unc.edu/gntools/) to help decide about prophylactic anticoagulation for membranous nephropathy.[13]
- Low sodium diet (<2 g daily) with diuretics.
- Diuretic resistance is common due to gut wall edema and hypoalbuminemia. More bioavailable diuretics (bumetanide, torsemide) may better increase urine output compared to furosemide. Thiazide diuretics can be added to loop agents to augment diuresis.
- Loop diuretics should be dosed at least on a twice-daily basis.

IMMUNOSUPPRESSIVE THERAPY

Important terms in dealing with the management of nephrotic-range proteinuria due to primary glomerular diseases are listed in Table E2. First-line therapies for each disease are highlighted in the following.[11]

- MCD: First-line therapy in adults is prednisone (1 mg/kg per day to a maximum of 80 mg per day) for a minimum of 4 wk and maximum of 16 wk. Steroids are tapered over 6 mo for favorable responses. Second-line options include cyclophosphamide and/or calcineurin inhibitors. Newer, randomized controlled trial data from studies of children reveal efficacy of rituximab in steroid-dependent patients with recurrent relapsing MCD. Consequently, rituximab may become a reasonable option for patients who do not respond to conventional therapy.[12]
- FSGS: Primary FSGS is often treated with high-dose prednisone (maximum, 80 mg daily in adults) tapered over 6 mo. Alternative regimens include low-dose prednisone with cyclosporine. Mycophenolate mofetil (MMF) has also been used in primary FSGS. Treatment of secondary FSGS is based on arresting the underlying cause and nonspecific therapy with an ACEI or ARB, blood pressure control, weight loss, and dietary protein restriction. Immunosuppression is avoided.[11]
- Membranous nephropathy: Acceptable treatments include alternating months of cyclophosphamide and steroids, calcineurin inhibitors with low-dose steroids or without steroids, and rituximab. Therapy for secondary membranous nephropathy is directed at treating the underlying cause (malignancy, SLE, etc.).[11]
- Amyloidosis, diabetes, and immune complex MPGN: Treatment is specific for the underlying disorder. In rapidly progressive HCV-related MPGN, immunosuppressive therapy with rituximab or glucocorticoids and cyclophosphamide can be administered during direct-acting antiviral therapy.[11]
- MPGN: A reclassification of MPGN highlights alternative complement cascade activation (C3 glomerulonephritis) as etiologic. MPGN is considered immune complex mediated or complement mediated by immunofluorescent microscopy. Treatment may now involve agents (e.g., eculizumab) that inhibit the complement cascade. Prior nontargeted approaches (e.g., steroids) for MPGN have been largely unsuccessful, except in selected pediatric cases.[11,14]

REFERRAL

Nephrology consultation is recommended for all cases of nephrotic syndrome.

! PEARLS & CONSIDERATIONS

- Albuminuria generally implies that glomerular disease is present. The urine protein electrophoresis defines the type(s) of proteins excreted: Albumin, immunoglobulins, and/or tubular.
- Massive proteinuria (>20 g daily) is rarely encountered with inflammatory glomerulonephritis and generally indicates MCD, FSGS, membranous nephropathy, or amyloidosis.
- Partial remissions and steroid resistance are rarely seen in primary minimal change disease. These circumstances require repeat kidney biopsy because FSGS is often revealed.
- Proteinuria is quantitated by a 24-h urine collection with evaluation of urinary creatinine excretion to document adequacy of collection. Spot collections have not been validated for heavy proteinuria or patients with rapidly changing creatinine values. A spot urine protein:creatinine ratio directly obtained from the 24-h collection defines the relationship between spot and true ratios for therapeutic monitoring.
- Most noninflammatory processes progress slowly. If a sediment without RBC casts is detected with a rapidly increasing serum creatinine and heavy proteinuria, the differential is relatively narrow:
  1. MCD with acute tubular necrosis or acute interstitial nephritis that may occur with NSAID administration[7]
  2. Any form of nephrotic syndrome associated with acute tubular necrosis
  3. Bilateral renal vein thrombosis superimposed on nephrotic syndrome
  4. Myeloma cast nephropathy
  5. Collapsing FSGS from lupus, HIV infection, bisphosphonate therapy, or thrombotic microangiopathy[5,6]

REFERENCES & SUGGESTED READING

Available at eBooks.Health.Elseviver.com.

RELATED CONTENT

Nephrotic Syndrome (Patient Information)

AUTHORS: **NATHANIEL HOCKER, MD** and **RUPALI AVASARE, MD**

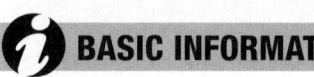

BASIC INFORMATION

DEFINITION

Neuropathic pain is defined as a persistent pain with neuropathic features (burning, tingling, prickling, etc.), resulting from abnormal discharges of impaired or injured neural structures in either the peripheral or central nervous system (CNS). Neuropathic pain is not itself a disease but rather a symptom associated with multiple different diseases and localizations within the nervous system. Thus it is not enough to define its presence without searching for a cause.

SYNONYMS

Neuralgia
Neuropathy

ICD-10CM CODES

B02.29	Postherpetic neuralgia
G50.0	Trigeminal neuralgia
G58.0	Intercostal neuropathy
G58.7	Mononeuritis multiplex
G58.8	Other specified mononeuropathies
G58.9	Mononeuropathy, unspecified
G61.9	Inflammatory polyneuropathy, unspecified
G62.0	Drug-induced polyneuropathy
G62.1	Alcoholic polyneuropathy
G62.9	Polyneuropathy, unspecified
G63.2	Diabetic polyneuropathy
G63.5	Polyneuropathy in systemic connective tissue disease
G63.8	Polyneuropathy in other diseases classified elsewhere
G79.2	Neuralgia and neuritis
G89.0	Central pain syndrome
M79.2	Neuralgia and neuritis, unspecified

EPIDEMIOLOGY & DEMOGRAPHICS

- Estimates of the prevalence of neuropathic pain in the general population range from 1.6% to 8.2%,[1] affecting up to 20 million Americans.[2]
- Overall, neuropathic pain affects women more commonly than men (8% compared to 5.7%) and patients >50 yr;[3] however, demographics vary widely with etiology:
  1. Postherpetic neuralgia: Affects almost 100% of cases, mainly elderly
  2. AIDS: 30% of patients affected
  3. Diabetes mellitus: 20% to 24% affected, with higher prevalence among those with longer disease duration; diabetic neuropathy is typically painless, but given the high diabetes prevalence, diabetic neuropathy is a common etiology of neuropathic pain
  4. Fabry disease: Affects mostly children, pain in 81% to 90% of patients
  5. Cryptogenic sensory polyneuropathy: At least 25% of neuropathies are idiopathic and likely genetic, with 70% to 80% of these being painful
  6. Chemotherapy: Affects 20% to 50% of patients with cancer[4]

PATHOGENESIS

- Neuropathies often preferentially affect different categories of axons that can be subdivided based on the diameter of the impaired axon:
  1. Large myelinated axons: Motor axons and sensory axons responsible for proprioception, vibration, and light touch.
  2. Thinly myelinated axons: Sensory fibers responsible for light touch, pain, temperature, and preganglionic autonomic functions.
  3. Small unmyelinated fibers: convey pain, temperature, and postganglionic autonomic functions.
- Neuropathic pain typically occurs in neuropathies with prominent involvement of the small thinly myelinated (Aδ) and unmyelinated (C) nerve fibers.
- Hyperexcitability and lack of inhibition of Aδ and C nerve fibers by descending central pathways leading to ectopic firing and central sensitization is considered the main mechanism of neuropathic pain.[5]
- Axonal and neuronal ion channels (particularly voltage-gated sodium channels) play an important role in facilitating hyperexcitability in painful neuropathies.[6]

PHYSICAL FINDINGS & CLINICAL PRESENTATION

- History is important for localization and diagnosis.[1,7] Characterization and localization of neuropathic pain can help identify the underlying etiology and inform management.
- Quality: Burning, lancinating, stinging, stabbing, electrical, tingling, hot or cold, "pins and needles" or "icy hot."
- Patients may also report the following:
  1. Allodynia: Pain provoked by a non-noxious stimulus (wind, clothing, etc.).
  2. Hyperesthesia: Increased pain provoked by a non-noxious stimulus (e.g., light touch).
  3. Hyperalgesia: Increased pain provoked by a noxious stimulus (e.g., pinprick).
  4. Hyperpathia: Increased and delayed response to a noxious stimulus.
  5. Paresthesia: Spontaneous or provoked nonpainful, abnormal sensations, typically "tingling" or "prickling."
  6. Dysesthesia: Spontaneous or provoked unpleasant sensation.
- Pain may be accompanied by deficits in large-fiber function (e.g., tactile sensibility, position sense, and vibration perception) and/or small-fiber function (e.g., pain and temperature perception).
- Distribution of symptoms may aid in localization (i.e., "stocking-glove" symptoms in generalized neuropathy, numbness in a peripheral nerve territory in focal neuropathy or dermatomal involvement in radiculopathy).
- Generalized small-fiber neuropathy: Dysesthesias without numbness common, but many etiologies (e.g., diabetes) cause both small- and large-fiber dysfunction.
- Large-fiber neuropathy (LFPN): Coexisting numbness, hyporeflexia, or weakness may be seen, usually worse distally.
  1. Nerve root: Coexisting neck or low back pain that radiates along a specific dermatome; most common cause is structural compression.
  2. Spinal cord symptoms: Coexisting spasticity, bowel or bladder involvement, sensory level.
  3. History of thalamic stroke in central thalamic pain syndrome (Dejerine-Roussy syndrome).
- Family history may suggest a genetic cause.
- Examination: See Table 1. Table 2 describes joint involvement in neuropathic arthropathy. Fig. 1 illustrates a diagnostic approach to neuropathy pain. Fig. E2 shows a neuropathic ankle.

ETIOLOGY

- Metabolic: Diabetes mellitus, nutritional deficiencies (vitamin B_{12}, vitamin B_6, vitamin E, thiamine, copper), malnutrition, alcoholism, porphyria, Fabry disease.
- Vascular: Prior stroke usually in the thalamus, peripheral nerve vasculitis.

TABLE 1   Examination

Examination Finding	Localization
Pinprick/temperature loss alone	Small fibers only
Pinprick/temperature loss + vibratory/proprioceptive loss	Small and large fibers
Sensory loss and motor dysfunction worse distally than proximal	Large-fiber neuropathy
Sensory loss and motor dysfunction along single nerve distribution	Single nerve
Sensory loss and motor dysfunction along multiple single nerves	Multiple mononeuropathies (i.e., mononeuropathy multiplex)
Motor and sensory loss involving multiple nerves belonging to specific region of brachial or lumbar plexus	Plexopathy
Sensory loss along dermatome with multiple myotomal muscles affected	Nerve root lesion
Asymmetric sensory loss without weakness and pseudoathetosis	Dorsal root ganglion
Vibratory/proprioceptive loss without pinprick/temperature loss	Dorsal column dysfunction (from compressive lesion, B_{12} deficiency, or tabes dorsalis from neurosyphilis)
Sensory level with weakness below the level of lesion and long tract signs (spasticity/Babinski sign)	Spinal cord lesion
Hemisensory hyperalgesia	Contralateral thalamus

TABLE 2 Joint Involvement in Neuropathic Arthropathy

Disease	Site of Involvement
Diabetes mellitus	Midtarsal, metatarsophalangeal, tarsometatarsal
Syringomyelia	Shoulder, elbow, wrist
Amyloidosis	Knee, ankle
Congenital sensory neuropathy	Knee, ankle, intertarsal, metatarsophalangeal
Tabes dorsalis	Knee, hip, ankle
Leprosy	Tarsal, tarsometatarsal

From Hochberg MC et al: *Rheumatology,* ed 8, Philadelphia, 2023, Elsevier.

- Inflammatory: Autoimmune diseases (systemic vasculitides, systemic lupus erythematosus, Sjögren syndrome, etc.), acute inflammatory demyelinating polyneuropathy (classically manifests with ascending weakness without numbness, although pain is also a common feature), chronic inflammatory demyelinating polyneuropathy, sarcoidosis, multiple sclerosis.
- Infiltrative: Amyloidosis, paraproteinemias (e.g., monoclonal gammopathy of uncertain significance [MGUS] associated neuropathy).
- Hematologic: Plasma cell disorders (multiple myeloma, POEMS syndrome, light chain amyloidosis, Waldenström macroglobulinemia, cryoglobulinemia), myeloproliferative disorders (polycythemia vera).
- Infectious: Postviral (brachial neuritis), HIV/AIDS, herpes simplex virus (HSV), varicella-zoster virus (VZV; postherpetic neuralgia), Lyme disease, leprosy (thickened nerves and skin lesions), syphilis.
- Neoplastic and paraneoplastic-carcinomatous infiltration of nerve/nerve root, anti-Hu.
- Drugs/toxins: Chemotherapeutic agents (paclitaxel, vincristine), antimicrobials (isoniazid, metronidazole, fluoroquinolones), amiodarone, colchicine, or heavy metals (thallium, arsenic).
- Genetic/idiopathic: Many neuropathies are cryptogenic and/or genetic and are often painful. Sodium channel mutations are thought to account for many of these.
- Peripheral neuropathies frequently associated with pain are summarized in Box E1
- See Table 3 for the typical clinical presentation and laboratory and electrophysiologic study findings of the common etiologies of neuropathic pain.

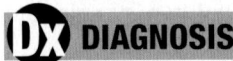 **DIAGNOSIS**

DIFFERENTIAL DIAGNOSIS

- Nociceptive pain: Results from tissue damage by inflammatory, ischemic, infectious, or mechanical/compressive injury; dissipates as the affected body part recovers. It occurs due to nociceptive signals from external stimuli, as opposed to neuropathic pain, which arises as a result of damage mediated directly to sensory nerves.

- Complex regional pain syndrome (CPRS): Patients present with spontaneous, asymmetric, regional, extremity pain, allodynia, and/or hyperalgesia following trauma affecting the distal part of an extremity (type II). In some patients, injury to a major peripheral nerve and associated focal deficits also may be present (type II). Both types may also manifest with autonomic abnormalities (e.g., swelling, sweating, change in skin blood flow), trophic signs (e.g., abnormal nail growth, increased or decreased hair growth, fibrosis, thin glossy skin, and osteoporosis), and weakness of all muscles.

LABORATORY TESTS (SEE TABLE 3)

- Selective use of blood tests may provide a specific diagnosis in patients presenting with neuropathic pain:
  1. Fasting blood glucose
  2. 2-h oral glucose tolerance test (OGTT)
  3. Vitamin B_{12} level
  4. Serum methylmalonic acid and homocysteine levels (if B_{12} level normal)
  5. Serum erythrocyte sedimentation rate (ESR), antinuclear antibodies (ANA), Sjögren syndrome (SS)-A and SS-B, c-ANCA, p-ANCA
  6. Rapid plasma reagin or fluorescent treponemal antibody absorption (FTA-ABS)
  7. Serum ACE level (sarcoidosis)
  8. HIV antibody
- Serum protein electrophoresis (SPEP), urine protein electrophoresis (UPEP), immunofixation
- Urine and stool protoporphyrin, if porphyria is suspected clinically
- Hu antibody: Can be seen in both small cell and non–small cell lung cancers and may be positive without evidence of lung cancer

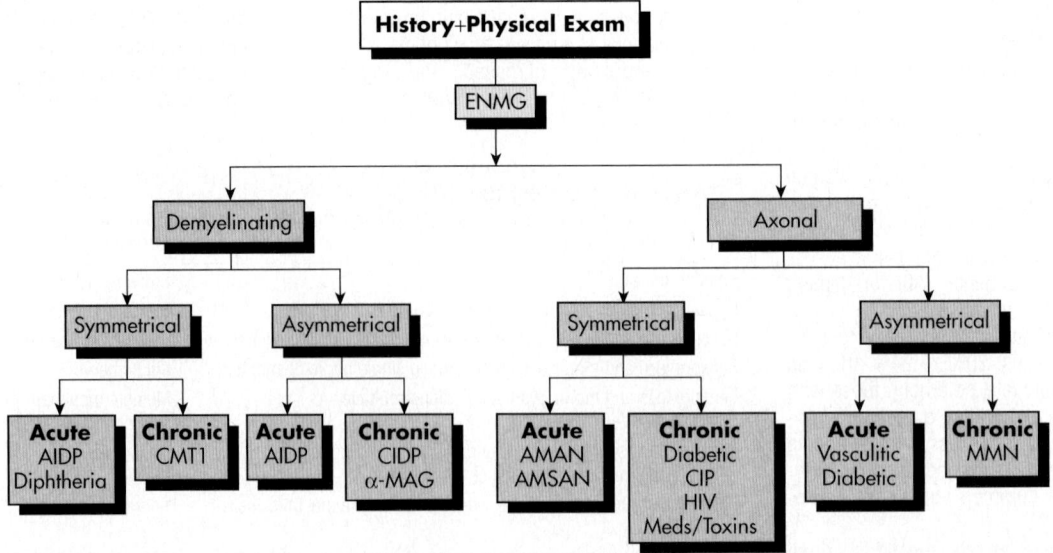

FIG. 1 A systematic approach to evaluate neuropathy. The diseases listed are examples of neuropathies associated with specific neurophysiologic and clinical findings. Diabetic distal, predominantly sensory neuropathies are manifested as chronic axonal neuropathies; acute asymmetric neuropathies can also occur with diabetes. Most neuropathies caused by toxins or by side effects of medication are chronic, symmetric axonal neuropathies. AIDP, AMAN, and AMSAN are subtypes of Guillain-Barré syndrome. These and other examples are discussed in more detail in the text. *AIDP,* Acute inflammatory demyelinating polyradiculoneuropathy; *AMAN,* acute motor axonal neuropathy; *AMSAN,* acute motor and sensory axonal neuropathy; *CIDP,* chronic inflammatory polyradiculoneuropathy; *CIP,* chronic illness polyneuropathy; *CMT1,* Charcot-Marie-Tooth disease type 1, a genetic disorder; *ENMG,* electroneuromyography; *HIV,* human immunodeficiency virus–related neuropathy; α-*MAG,* alpha-myelin-associated glycoprotein; *MMN,* multifocal motor neuropathy. (From Goldman L, Schafer AI: *Goldman's Cecil medicine,* ed 24, Philadelphia, 2012, Saunders.)

TABLE 3 Clinical Presentation and Laboratory Findings

Neuropathy Type	Predisposition	Examination Findings	EMG/NCS	Laboratory Analysis
Idiopathic small-fiber PN	Age >50	Strength: Normal Reflexes: Normal Pos/vib: Normal Pain/temp: Decreased distally	Normal	Serum studies: Normal Skin biopsy: Abnormal Sudomotor studies: Abnormal
Diabetic PN	Long-standing disease, family history	Strength normal to reduced, sensation reduced distally	Abnormal	Abnormal glucose tolerance: High fasting glucose
Inherited PN	Family history	Pes cavus, hammer toes, reduced reflexes, sensation reduced distally	Abnormal	Genetic studies may be abnormal, other studies normal
Familial amyloid PN	Family history	Pain/temp loss, reduced reflexes, orthostasis	Abnormal if large fibers affected; also carpal tunnel syndrome	Transthyretin genetic study
Acquired amyloid PN	Monoclonal gammopathy	Pain/temp loss, reduced reflexes, orthostasis	Abnormal if large fibers affected; also carpal tunnel syndrome	SPEP, UPEP, immunofixation abnormal
Fabry disease	Age, renal failure, strokes	Normal; possible reduced pain/temp sensation	Normal	α-Galactosidase levels in cultured fibroblasts
PN + mixed connective tissue disease	History of lupus, rheumatoid arthritis, Sjögren syndrome	Reduced reflexes and distal sensation	Abnormal	ANA, RF, SS-A/SS-B may be abnormal
Peripheral nerve vasculitis	Asymmetric disease	Multiple peripheral nerves involved	Abnormal	ANA, RF, SS-A/SS-B, ANCA, cryoglobulins may be abnormal
Paraneoplastic neuropathy	Lung cancer risk factors, chemical exposures	Asymmetric sensory loss, pseudoathetosis, relatively preserved strength	Abnormal	Anti-Hu
Sarcoidosis	Pulmonary sarcoid	Multiple mononeuropathies	Abnormal	Abnormal biopsy, elevated serum ACE, CXR abnormal
Arsenic	Pesticides, copper smelting	Reduced reflexes and distal sensation	Abnormal	Elevated arsenic in plasma, urine, and hair
HIV	Multiple partners, unprotected sex, IV drug abuse, blood transfusion	Variable, but most often reduced reflexes and distal sensation	Abnormal if large fibers involved	HIV antibody

ACE, Angiotensin-converting enzyme; *ANA*, antibody to nuclear antigens; *ANCA*, antineutrophil cytoplasmic antibodies; *CXR*, chest x-ray; *EMG*, electromyography; *HIV*, human immunodeficiency virus; *IV*, intravenous; *NCS*, nerve conduction studies; *PN*, polyneuropathy; *Pos*, position sensation; *RF*, rheumatoid factor; *SPEP*, serum protein electrophoresis; *SS-A*, Sjögren syndrome A; *SS-B*, Sjögren syndrome B; *Temp*, temperature sensation; *UPEP*, urine protein electrophoresis; *Vib*, vibration sensation.
Adapted from Mendell JR, Sahenk Z: Painful sensory neuropathy, *N Engl J Med* 348(13):1243, 2003.

- Lumbar puncture: Protein elevation, oligoclonal bands, cerebrospinal fluid (CSF)/serum IgG index

ELECTROPHYSIOLOGY STUDIES (SEE TABLE 3)

- Painful peripheral neuropathies preferentially involve the small unmyelinated or lightly myelinated Aδ and C.
- Electrophysiologic testing (electromyography with nerve conduction studies): May be normal in small-fiber neuropathies or CNS lesions, but is often abnormal in large-fiber neuropathies.
- Quantitative sensory testing: Abnormal in small- and large-fiber neuropathy.
- Evoked potentials (only if suspicion for spinal cord lesion).
- Autonomic testing: Assesses sympathetic cholinergic function; abnormal in small-fiber neuropathy.

PATHOLOGY STUDIES

- Nerve biopsy is occasionally useful in selected cases, particularly when vasculitides, sarcoidosis, or amyloid neuropathy are in the differential.
- Skin biopsy for intraepidermal nerve fiber (IENF) density may be useful for small-fiber neuropathy when other studies are normal.

- Rectal or abdominal fat pad biopsy sample may show amyloid deposition in systemic amyloidosis.

IMAGING STUDIES

Based on localization:
- MRI (with and without contrast):
  1. Brain: Evaluated for thalamic pathology if symptoms and signs are consistent with thalamic lesion (hemibody pain)
  2. Spinal cord and nerve roots: Evaluates for structural, inflammatory, neoplastic, or infectious causes if localization is consistent with spinal cord
  3. Lumbar spine: Evaluates for arachnoiditis
- If MRI cannot be performed, consider:
  1. CT of the brain for thalamic pathology
  2. CT myelography of the spinal cord to evaluate for structural/neoplastic disease, but only if clinical signs of spinal or nerve root compression are present

Rx TREATMENT

NONPHARMACOLOGIC THERAPY

- Counseling should be initiated at the beginning of therapy to address psychologic issues exacerbating physiologic pain and set realistic expectations for pain management as complete pain relief is typically not possible.[8]

- Moderate aerobic exercise (30 min daily) in addition to strength training improves pain and objective parameters of neuropathy.[9]
- Tai chi, yoga, and massage therapy, may help in cases of chronic neck and low back pain but have not been specifically studied in neuropathic pain.[10,11]
- Optimization of glucose control.
- Cognitive-behavioral therapy.
- Percutaneous electrical nerve stimulation (TENS unit).
- Dorsal column spinal cord stimulation is FDA-approved for treatment of painful diabetic neuropathy given demonstration of short-term benefit.[12] However, cost is relatively high and not all patients benefit long term.[13]

ACUTE GENERAL Rx

- Treatment of the underlying cause, if possible, will help slow or prevent worsening.
- Medications may reduce or alleviate pain but do not affect numbness.
- Overall, tricyclic antidepressants (TCAs), serotonin-norepinephrine reuptake inhibitors (SNRIs), gabapentinoids, and/or sodium channel blockers show equivalent efficacy in treating diabetic neuropathic pain and are used by extension in most types of neuropathic pain. The decision of which to use depends on side effects, comorbidities, and

patient preferences. If one category is not effective, a different category should be tried or added.[8]

- Gabapentinoids:[8,14-16]
  1. Pregabalin has the best level of evidence: Begin 50 mg PO tid, increase slowly to 100 to 200 mg PO tid.
  2. Gabapentin: Begin 300 mg PO qd, advance to 300 mg PO tid by the end of the first wk. Effective dose: >1600 mg/day. Max daily dose: 1200 mg PO tid. Gabapentin and pregabalin have similar efficacy, but patients may differ in response and/or tolerance.
- TCAs and SNRIs:[8,14-16]
  1. TCAs: Nortriptyline preferred over amitriptyline (fewer anticholinergic side effects). Begin 25 mg PO qd in adults or 10 mg qd in elderly. Increase dose by 25 mg every week as tolerated until usual maximal effective dose of 150 mg/day.
  2. Duloxetine: Begin 30 mg PO qd, advance to 30 to 60 mg bid. Duloxetine is effective in diabetic neuropathy, postherpetic neuropathy, and chemotherapy-induced painful peripheral neuropathy.
  3. Venlafaxine and desvenlafaxine: Begin 37.5 mg PO qd, advance to 225 mg/day in two to three divided doses once higher than 37.5 mg/day.
- Sodium-channel blockers—less commonly used first-line:[8,14]
  1. Topiramate: Begin 25 mg PO qd daily then increase by 25- to 50-mg increments at intervals ≥1 wk up to 100 mg PO bid
  2. Oxcarbazepine: Begin 300 mg PO bid, then titrate to pain relief by 300 mg every 3 days to a maximum daily dose of 900 mg bid
  3. Lamotrigine: Begin 25 mg PO qd then increase as needed at weekly intervals by 50 mg/day in one to two divided doses to a maximum of 400 mg/day in one to two divided doses
  4. Lacosamide: Begin 50 to 100 mg PO bid, then increase as needed at weekly intervals by 50 mg bid. Typical maintenance dose is 150 to 200 mg PO bid

- Lidocaine (5%) patch: Apply to area of pain, max three patches every 12 h. Most useful in postherpetic neuralgia because pain is localized; less useful when the neuropathy progresses and becomes more proximal and diffuse.
- Capsaicin cream and patches are inconsistent in their ability to relieve pain and may exacerbate it. A capsaicin 8% patch is approved specifically for postherpetic neuralgia and is applied for 60 minutes under medical supervision.
- Opioids (including tramadol): Overall not recommended for neuropathic pain. Only use when first- and second-line agents are ineffective and patients have severe and refractory symptoms that have not responded to all other options.[8]
- Procedural/surgical: This option is considered mostly when the patient suffers from pain secondary to spinal cord or cauda equina injury. Procedures should be considered only when all other therapeutic modalities have failed. In addition, the patient should be cautioned that surgical procedures may not result in pain relief and may be associated with significant morbidity and even mortality.
  1. Dorsal root rhizotomy
  2. Nerve blocks
  3. Spinal cord stimulator[12,13]

DISPOSITION

Prognosis depends on multiple factors, including:
- Etiology of pain
- Treatment of any underlying condition
- Initiation of appropriate (often multiple) therapeutic modalities
- Patient compliance with prescribed regimen

Most care is accomplished in the outpatient setting, except when surgery is required.

REFERRAL

- Pain clinic
- Neurology
- Psychiatry
- Psychology
- Physiatry
- Anesthesiology (nerve blocks)
- Neurosurgery (surgical management)

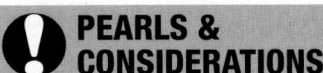

PEARLS & CONSIDERATIONS

- Factitious disorder and malingering frequently manifest with pain complaints. These are diagnoses of exclusion and require negative evaluation for organic etiologies before diagnosis is made.
- Peripheral neuropathy in patients with diabetes increases the risk of foot ulceration by seven-fold. Abnormal results in monofilament testing and vibratory perception (alone or in combination with the appearance of the feet, ulceration, and ankle reflexes) are the most helpful sign for the detection of LFPN.

REFERENCES

Available at eBooks.Health.Elsevier.com.

RELATED CONTENT

Trigeminal neuralgia (Related Key Topic)

AUTHORS: **OMAIR SHAKIL, MD, MPH** and **COREY ELAM GOLDSMITH, MD, FAAN**

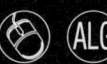
BASIC INFORMATION

DEFINITION

- Nonalcoholic *fatty liver disease* (NAFLD) is a spectrum of diseases based on histopathologic findings and representing a morphologic rather than a clinical diagnosis (Fig. 1). It is liver disease occurring in patients who do not abuse alcohol and manifesting histologically by mononuclear cells and/or polymorphonuclear cells, hepatocyte ballooning, and spotty necrosis. Nonalcoholic steatohepatitis (NASH) is a subset of NAFLD. Patients with NASH have progressive disease that can result in fibrosis and cirrhosis. A diagnosis of NAFLD is contingent on the following factors:
  1. Alcohol consumption in amounts less than those considered hepatotoxic.
  2. Absence of serologic evidence of other hepatic diseases or disorders.
  3. Liver biopsy showing predominant macrovesicular steatosis or steatohepatitis.
- NAFL is defined as ≥5% hepatic steatosis without evidence of hepatocellular injury or fibrosis.
- NASH is ≥5% hepatic fibrosis with inflammation and hepatocellular injury with or without fibrosis.
- *NASH cirrhosis* is the presence of cirrhosis with current or past evidence of steatosis.

SYNONYMS

Nonalcoholic steatohepatitis (NASH)
NAFLD
Fatty liver hepatitis
Diabetes hepatitis
Alcohol-like liver disease
Laënnec disease

ICD-10CM CODE
K76.0 Fatty (change of) liver, not elsewhere classified

EPIDEMIOLOGY & DEMOGRAPHICS

- NAFLD affects 30% of the adult general population in the U.S.
- Increased prevalence in obese persons (57% to 74%), type 2 diabetes mellitus, and hyperlipidemia (primarily hypertriglyceridemia).
- Most common cause of abnormal liver test results in adults in the U.S. (accounts for up to 90% of cases of asymptomatic alanine aminotransferase [ALT] elevations).
- NAFLD is more prevalent in men than women.
- NAFLD is more prevalent in the Hispanic population.
- ~20% of patients with NAFLD have NASH, and 10% to 30% of patients with NASH have NASH cirrhosis.

PHYSICAL FINDINGS & CLINICAL PRESENTATION

- Most patients are asymptomatic.
- Patients may report a sensation of fullness or discomfort on the right side of the upper abdomen.
- Nonspecific complaints of fatigue or malaise may be reported.
- Hepatomegaly (Table 1) is generally the only positive finding on physical examination.
- Acanthosis nigricans may be found in children.

ETIOLOGY

- Metabolic syndrome and insulin resistance are the most reproducible factors in the development of NAFLD and accumulation of triglycerides within the liver. High baseline and continuously increasing fasting insulin levels are independent determinants for future development of NAFLD. The transition from NAFLD to NASH is poorly understood; there may be a genetic component. The presence of the I48M variant of PNPLA3 increases risk for and severity of NAFLD. Genetic polymorphism (TM6SF2) also increases NAFLD risk.
- Risk factors are obesity (especially truncal obesity), diabetes mellitus, hyperlipidemia.

DIAGNOSIS

DIFFERENTIAL DIAGNOSIS

- Alcohol-induced liver disease (a daily alcohol intake of 20 g in females and 30 g in males [three 12-oz beers or 12 oz of wine] may be enough to cause alcohol-induced liver disease)
- Viral hepatitis
- Autoimmune hepatitis
- Toxin- or drug-induced liver disease
- Box 1 summarizes the various causes of fatty liver disease

WORKUP

Diagnosis is usually suspected on the basis of hepatomegaly, asymptomatic elevations of transaminases, or "fatty liver" on sonogram of abdomen in obese patients with little or no alcohol use. Fig. 2 illustrates an algorithm for the diagnostic approach to NAFLD. Transient elastography is a noninvasive imaging modality that can be used to screen for the development of hepatic fibrosis (Fig 3). In obese patients newer "XL" FibroScan machines are more accurate. Liver biopsy can confirm diagnosis

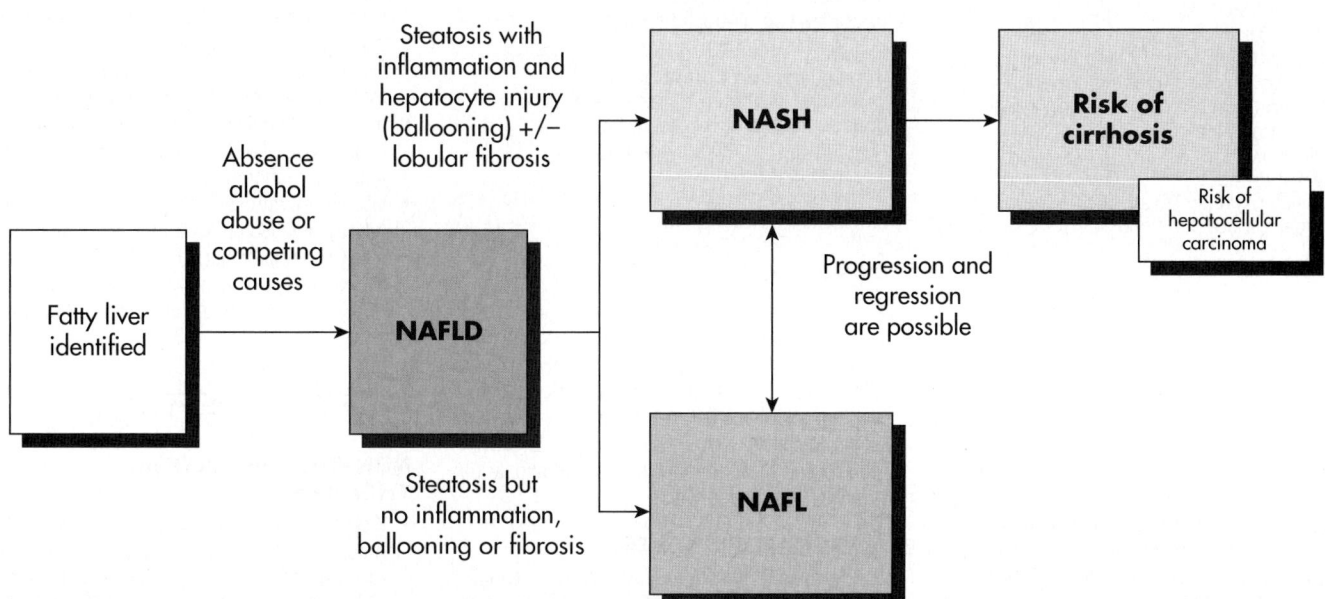

FIG. 1 Relationship between fatty liver, NAFLD, NAFL, and NASH. *NAFL,* Nonalcoholic fatty liver; *NAFLD,* nonalcoholic fatty liver disease; *NASH,* nonalcoholic steatohepatitis. (From Budd J, Cusi K: Nonalcoholic fatty liver disease: what does the primary care physician need to know? *Am J Med* 133:536-543, 2020.)

TABLE 1 Symptoms, Signs, and Laboratory Features of Nonalcoholic Fatty Liver Disease

Symptoms	Signs	Laboratory Features
Common		
None (48%-100% of patients)	Hepatomegaly	2- to 4-fold elevation of serum ALT and AST levelsAST/ALT ratio <1 in most patients
		Serum alkaline phosphatase level slightly elevated in one third of patients
		Normal serum bilirubin, serum albumin, and prothrombin time
		Elevated serum ferritin level
Uncommon		
Vague right upper quadrant pain	Splenomegaly	Low-titer (<1:320) antinuclear antibodies
Fatigue	Spider telangiectasias	
Malaise	Palmar erythema	
	Ascites	

ALT, Alanine aminotransferase; *AST,* aspartate aminotransferase.
From Feldman M et al: *Sleisenger and Fordtran's gastrointestinal and liver disease,* ed 11, Philadelphia, 2021, Elsevier.

BOX 1 Causes of Fatty Liver Disease

Acquired Metabolic Disorders
Diabetes mellitus
Dyslipidemia
Kwashiorkor and marasmus
Obesity
Rapid weight loss
Starvation

Cytotoxic and Cytostatic Drugs
L-Asparaginase
Azacitidine
Bleomycin
Cisplatin
5-Fluorouracil
Methotrexate
Tetracyclines (inhibit mitochondrial beta oxidation)

Other Drugs and Toxins
Amiodarone
Camphor
Chloroform
Cocaine
Ethanol
Ethyl bromide
Estrogens
Glucocorticoids
Griseofulvin
Highly active antiretroviral therapy (zidovudine, stavudine, didanosine)
Lycopodium serratum (*Jin Bu Huan,* an herbal supplement)
Nifedipine
Nitrofurantoin
Nonsteroidal antiinflammatory drugs (piroxicam, ibuprofen, indomethacin, sulindac)

Tamoxifen
Valproic acid

Metals
Antimony
Barium salts
Chromates
Mercury
Phosphorus
Rare earth metals of low atomic number
Thallium compounds
Uranium compounds

Inborn Errors of Metabolism
Abetalipoproteinemia
Familial hepatosteatosis
Galactosemia
Glycogen storage disease
Hereditary fructose intolerance
Homocystinuria
Systemic carnitine deficiency
Tyrosinemia
Weber-Christian syndrome
Wilson disease

Surgical Procedures
Biliopancreatic diversion
Extensive small bowel resection
Jejunoileal bypass

Miscellaneous Conditions
Industrial exposure to petrochemicals
Inflammatory bowel disease
Jejunal diverticulosis with bacterial overgrowth
Partial lipodystrophy
Total parenteral nutrition

From Feldman M et al: *Sleisenger and Fordtran's gastrointestinal and liver disease,* ed 11, Philadelphia, 2021, Elsevier.

and provide prognostic information. It should be considered in patients with suspected advanced liver fibrosis (presence of obesity or type 2 diabetes, aspartate aminotransferase [AST]:ALT ratio 1, age 45 yr). NAFLD activity score on liver biopsy is described in Table 2. The FIB-4 score can screen noninvasively for clinically significant fibrosis. It is derived from AGG, ALT, and AST levels and platelet count and can be obtained using online calculators. Patients with low-risk FIB-4 scores (<1.3) can be followed routinely in primary care. Patients

with FIB-4 scores between 1.3 and 2.67 are considered to be at intermediate risk for fibrosis and should undergo transient elastography scan. Patients with FIB-4 scores >2.67 are considered high risk for fibrosis and should be referred to a hepatologist.[1]

LABORATORY TESTS
- Elevated ALT, AST: AST:ALT ratio is usually <1, but can increase as fibrosis advances. In advanced fibrosis AST to ALT ratio is >1 and platelet count is low.

- Negative serology for infectious hepatitis; generally normal gamma-glutamyl transpeptidase and serum alkaline phosphatase.
- Hyperlipidemia (primarily hypertriglyceridemia) may be present.
- Elevated glucose levels may be present.
- Prolonged prothrombin time, hypoalbuminemia, and elevated bilirubin may be present in advanced stages.
- Elevated serum ferritin and increased transferrin saturation may be found in up to 10% of patients; however, hepatic iron index and hepatic iron level are normal.
- Antismooth muscle antibodies and antinuclear antibodies at low titer are not uncommon.

IMAGING STUDIES
- Ultrasound generally reveals diffuse increase in echogenicity however standard B-mode ultrasound is not recommended as a tool to identify hepatic steatosis due to los sensitivity; computed tomography (CT) scan reveals diffuse low-density hepatic parenchyma. The sensitivity of CT scan for detection of fat in liver is higher (over 70%) if hepatic steatosis exceeds 33%.
- Occasionally patients may have focal rather than diffuse steatosis, which may be misinterpreted as a liver mass on ultrasound or CT (Fig. 4); use of MRI in these cases will identify focal fatty infiltration.
- Vibration-controlled transient elastography (VCTE) can also be used to evaluate noninvasively for hepatic fibrosis and to further stratify patients and is more cost effective than MRI.[2] VCTE should be considered for patients with FIB-4 scores >1-3.[3]

(Rx) **TREATMENT**

NONPHARMACOLOGIC THERAPY
- Weight reduction in all obese patients. The American Gastroenterological Association recommends that the initial target weight loss be 10% of baseline weight at a rate of 1 to 2 lb (0.45 to 0.90 kg) per wk. The Mediterranean diet reduces fat intake and enables

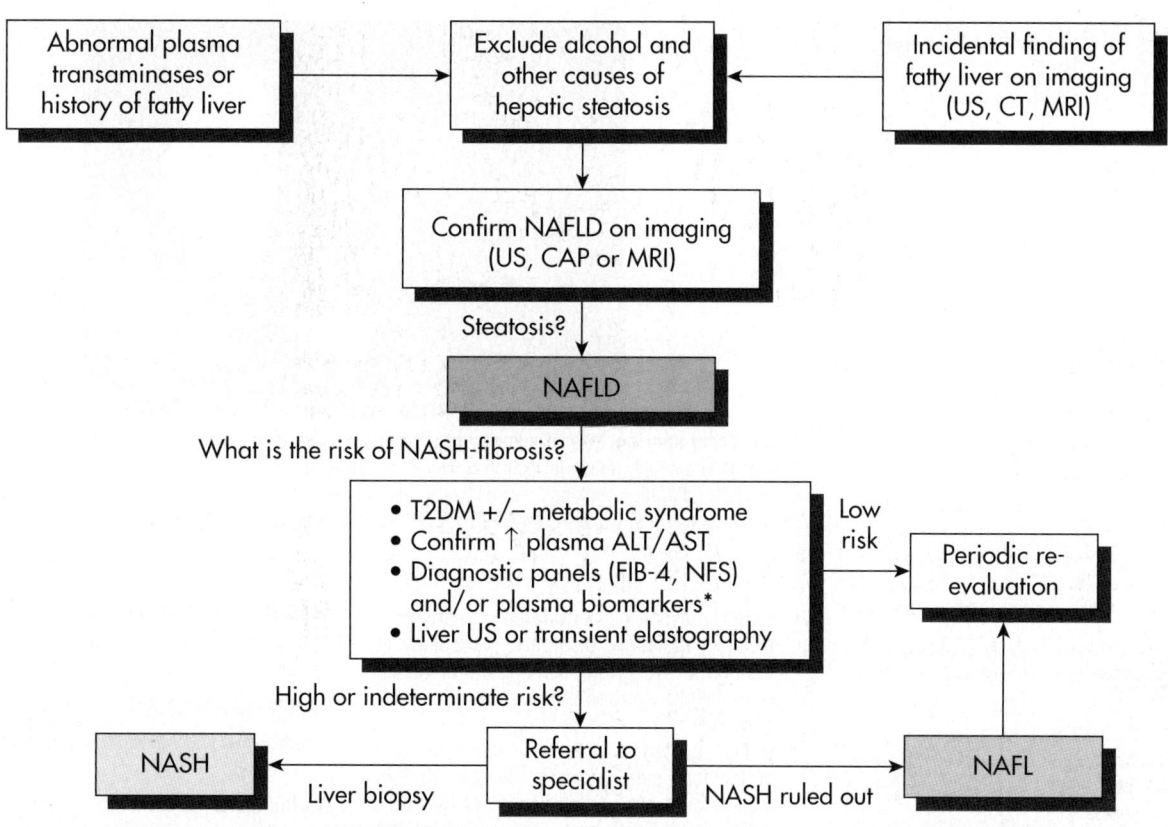

FIG. 2 Diagnosis of NAFLD, NAFL, and NASH. *ALT,* Alanine aminotransferase; *AST,* aspartate aminotransferase; *CAP,* controlled attenuation parameter; *CT,* computed tomography; *MRI,* magnetic resonance imaging (used largely in research settings); *NAFL,* nonalcoholic fatty liver; *NAFLD,* nonalcoholic fatty liver disease; *NASH,* nonalcoholic steatohepatitis; *NFS,* NAFLD fibrosis score; *T2DM,* type 2 diabetes mellitus; *US,* liver ultrasound. *Plasma biomarkers: several commercial ones are available and others are in development.[6-13] (From Budd J, Cusi K: Nonalcoholic fatty liver disease: what does the primary care physician need to know? *Am J Med* 133:536-543, 2020.)

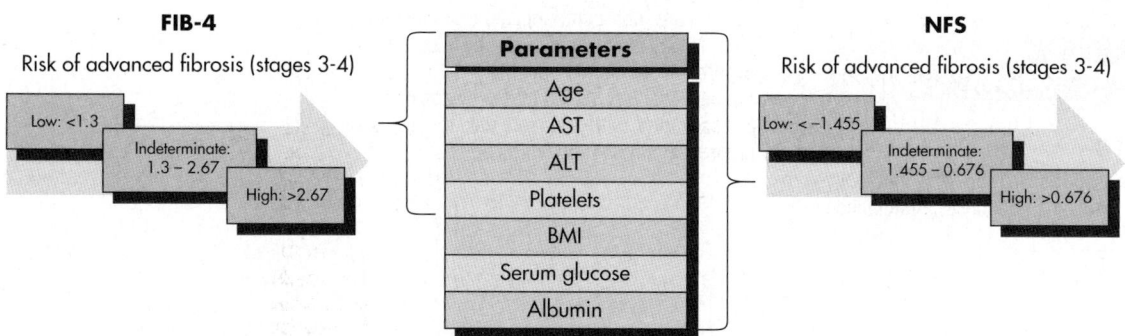

FIG. 3 Parameters and interpretation of FIB-4 and NFS for establishing the risk of advanced fibrosis (stages 3-4). *ALT,* Alanine aminotransferase; *AST,* aspartate aminotransferase; *BMI,* body mass index; *FIB-4,* fibrosis-4 score; *NFS,* NAFLD fibrosis score. (From Budd J, Cusi K: Nonalcoholic fatty liver disease: what does the primary care physician need to know? *Am J Med* 133:536-543, 2020.)

weight loss. A diet with fish may slow fatty liver disease progression in patients who also consume meat.[4] Fresh fish consumption is associated with increases in short-chain fatty acids, unconjugated bile acids, and increases in intestinal faecalibacterium which may improve hepatic steatosis.[5]

- Increase physical activity. Vigorous and moderate exercise are equally effective in reducing intrahepatic triglyceride content, the effect being largely mediated by weight loss.
- Alcohol has a deleterious effect on NAFLD and should be avoided.

ACUTE GENERAL Rx

- There are no drugs currently approved by FDA for NAFLD. Medications to control hyperlipidemia (e.g., fenofibrates for elevated triglycerides) and hyperglycemia (e.g., pioglitazone, insulin, metformin) can lead to improvement in abnormal liver test results.
- A 3-yr trial with pioglitazone (30 mg/day), an insulin-sensitizing thiazolidinedione, revealed that pioglitazone treatment was associated with long-term metabolic and histologic improvement in patients with prediabetes or type 2 diabetes mellitus and NASH. These

results suggest that NASH progression may be halted, and the natural history of the disease may be modified with the use of pioglitazone in patients with prediabetes or type 2 diabetes mellitus.[1] Glucagon-like peptide-1 receptor agonists (GLP-1RA) like liraglutide have shown modest improvement in reduction of plasma aminotransferase and steatosis.

DISPOSITION

- Patients with pure steatosis on liver biopsy generally have a relatively benign course.

TABLE 2	NAFLD Activity Score on a Liver Biopsy Specimen
Steatosis	
5%	1
5%-33%	2
33%-66%	3
Ballooning	
None	0
Few	1
Many	2
Lobular Inflammation	
Mild	1
Moderate	2
Severe	3
Total Score	
0-2	Likely not NASH
3-4	Intermediate
5-8	Likely NASH

NAFLD, Nonalcoholic fatty liver disease; *NASH,* nonalcoholic steatohepatitis.
From Feldman M et al: *Sleisenger and Fordtran's gastrointestinal and liver disease,* ed 11, Philadelphia, 2021, Elsevier.

- The presence of steatohepatitis or advanced fibrosis on liver biopsy is associated with a worse prognosis.

REFERRAL

Liver transplantation should be considered in patients with decompensated, end-stage disease; however, in these patients there may be a recurrence of NAFLD posttransplantation.

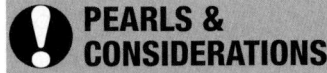

PEARLS & CONSIDERATIONS

COMMENTS

- NAFLD is closely associated with metabolic disorders, even in nonobese, nondiabetic

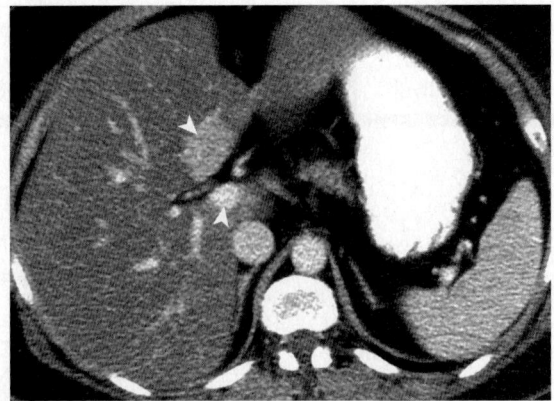

FIG. 4 Focal sparing. Two islands of normal parenchyma *(arrowheads)* in segment IVb and the caudate lobe (segment 1) simulate mass lesions in a liver with extensive fatty infiltration. Most of the liver parenchyma shows fatty infiltration, making these islands of normal parenchyma appear of high attenuation by comparison. (From Webb WR et al: *Fundamentals of body CT,* ed 4, Philadelphia, 2015, Saunders.)

subjects. It can be considered an early predictor of metabolic disorders, particularly in the normal-weight population. The presence of metabolic syndrome is a strong predictor of NAFLD.
- NAFLD is associated with an increased risk of incident cardiovascular disease that is independent of the risk conferred by traditional risk factors and components of the metabolic syndrome.
- 10% of patients with NASH have progression to advanced fibrosis. Most common in patients older than 50, ALT > twice normal, body mass index >28, triglycerides >150 mg/dl.
- Statins are not contraindicated in patients with NASH and should be considered in hypercholesterolemic patients.
- A recent trial has shown that daily aspirin use is associated with reduced risk for fibrosis progression in patients with NAFLD.[1]

RELATED CONTENT

Fatty Liver (Patient Information)

REFERENCES

Available at eBooks.Health.Elsevier.com.

AUTHOR: **FRED F. FERRI, MD**

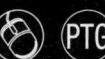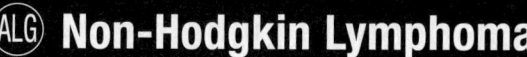

N

Diseases and Disorders

I

 BASIC INFORMATION

DEFINITION

Non-Hodgkin lymphoma (NHL) is a heterogeneous group of malignancies of the lymphoreticular system. There are ~60 different NHL subtypes.[1] The WHO classification of lymphomas is summarized in Fig. 1.

SYNONYM

NHL

ICD-10CM CODES

C85.90	Non-Hodgkin lymphoma, unspecified, unspecified site
C85.91	Non-Hodgkin lymphoma, unspecified, lymph nodes of head, face, and neck
C85.92	Non-Hodgkin lymphoma, unspecified, intrathoracic lymph nodes
C85.93	Non-Hodgkin lymphoma, unspecified, intra-abdominal lymph nodes
C85.94	Non-Hodgkin lymphoma, unspecified, lymph nodes of axilla and upper limb
C85.95	Non-Hodgkin lymphoma, unspecified, lymph nodes of inguinal region and lower limb
C85.96	Non-Hodgkin lymphoma, unspecified, intrapelvic lymph nodes
C85.97	Non-Hodgkin lymphoma, unspecified, spleen
C85.98	Non-Hodgkin lymphoma, unspecified, lymph nodes of multiple sites
C85.99	Non-Hodgkin lymphoma, unspecified, extranodal and solid organ sites

EPIDEMIOLOGY

- Seventh most common neoplasm in the U.S. (>80,000 new cases annually).[2] Incidence increases with age; majority of patients are >60 yr of age (median 66 yr).
- In the U.S. and Europe, diffuse large B-cell lymphoma (DLBCL) is the most common subtype (30% of the cases), and follicular lymphoma (FL) is the second most common subtype (25% of cases).[3]
- In patients with HIV, NHL is the most common tumor (followed by Kaposi sarcoma). DLBCL accounts for 80% to 90% of the cases.[4]
- Factors associated with an increased risk of NHL are summarized in Box 1.

PHYSICAL FINDINGS & CLINICAL PRESENTATION

- Patients often present with lymphadenopathy.
- Approximately one third of the NHL involve extranodal sites, which can result in unusual presentations (e.g., GI tract involvement can simulate peptic ulcer disease).
- Presence of B symptoms like unexplained weight loss, fever, fatigue, and night sweats are seen typically in aggressive lymphomas.

- Aggressive lymphomas have acute or subacute presentation with increasing size of the mass and B symptoms.
- Indolent lymphomas have a more chronic course, with asymptomatic lymphadenopathy and/or slowly progressive cytopenias.
- Hepatomegaly and splenomegaly may be present.
- Cough, dyspnea can occur with bulky mediastinal involvement.

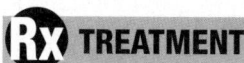 **DIAGNOSIS**

DIFFERENTIAL DIAGNOSIS

- Hodgkin lymphoma
- Viral infections (e.g., mononucleosis)
- Metastatic carcinoma
- Autoimmune conditions
- Sarcoidosis

WORKUP

Initial laboratory evaluation may be entirely normal. Elevated serum lactate dehydrogenase (LDH) may be seen in aggressive lymphoma or in indolent lymphoma with high disease burden. In cases of highly aggressive NHL (e.g., Burkitt lymphoma [BL]), spontaneous tumor lysis syndrome (TLS) may be seen, characterized by hyperkalemia, hyperuricemia, hypocalcemia, hyperphosphatemia, and acidosis. TLS can be life threatening and is considered a medical emergency. Acute management includes aggressive intravenous (IV) fluid repletion and/or rasburicase. Nephrology consult is recommended. Proper staging of NHL includes the following:

- A thorough history and physical examination.
- Excisional or incisional surgical biopsy is preferred. Image-guided core needle biopsies may be acceptable in patients without peripheral adenopathy. Fine needle aspirates are not adequate for precise lymphoma subclassification. Laparoscopic lymph node biopsy or mediastinoscopy can be used on an outpatient basis for most patients with intraabdominal or mediastinal lymphoma, respectively.
- Tissue biopsy with histologic, immunophenotypic, and genetic studies interpretation. Major molecular alterations in NHLs are summarized in Table 1.
- Routine laboratory evaluation (CBC, flow cytometry in selected circumstances, urinalysis, serum LDH, blood urea nitrogen, creatinine, serum calcium, uric acid, liver function tests, serum protein electrophoresis).
- HIV and hepatitis B testing. Human T-lymphotrophic virus (HTLV-1) testing is encouraged in peripheral T-cell lymphomas (especially in patients of Japanese, Caribbean, and South American descendants).[5,6]
- Bone marrow evaluation (aspirate and biopsy) in selected patients (Fig. E2).
- Fluorine-18 fluorodeoxyglucose (FDG) PET integrated with computed tomography (CT) (Fig. E3) has emerged as a tool for staging, response evaluation, and posttreatment surveillance in patients with aggressive subtypes of NHL.

- CT scan of chest, abdomen, and pelvis with IV contrast in selected patients.
- Depending on the histopathology, the results of the previous studies, and the planned therapy, some other tests may be performed (e.g., next generation sequencing, T-cell receptor rearrangement).
- Lumbar puncture is needed in some patients with aggressive NHL (e.g. BL), and most patients with HIV-associated NHL, to evaluate for CNS involvement by lymphoma.
- The evaluation of a new patient with NHL is summarized in Table 2.

CLASSIFICATION

For clinical approach, NHL is subdivided into indolent, aggressive, and highly aggressive disease.

STAGING

The Ann Arbor staging system that was initially developed for Hodgkin lymphoma (HL) was revised as the Lugano criteria and remains the current standard; but unlike HL, NHL does not spread predictably via lymphatic channels to contiguous nodal regions, so stage is only one of multiple contributors to prognosis (Table 3). Disease subtype has greater therapeutic implications in NHL than in HL. Fig. 4 illustrates a diagnostic algorithm outlining the steps in classification of B-cell lymphomas composed of cells of small to intermediate size.

 TREATMENT

ACUTE GENERAL Rx

The therapeutic regimen varies with specific lymphoma subtype and pathologic stage. Following are the commonly used therapeutic modalities:

INDOLENT NHL:

- The GELF criteria remains the tool to categorize patients in need of immediate therapy vs. those who would be candidates for a watch-and-wait strategy.[7]
- Deferment of therapy and careful observation in asymptomatic patients with low volume (burden) disease.
- Local radiotherapy for stage I disease, depending on location of disease.
- Rituximab, an anti-CD20 monoclonal antibody, with or without chemotherapy is used in patients with symptomatic, high volume (burden) or progressive disease.
- The addition of rituximab to chemotherapy is generally well tolerated and has increased response and survival rates in NHL patients. Patients who received rituximab, cyclophosphamide, doxorubicin, vincristine, and prednisone (R-CHOP) had higher response rates (96% vs. 90%) with a better 2-yr overall survival rate (95% vs. 90%) than patients who received CHOP without rituximab.[8] Similarly, patients who received rituximab, cyclophosphamide, vincristine, and prednisone (R-CVP) had higher response rates (81% vs. 57%) and better overall survival at 4 yr (83% vs. 77%) than patients who were treated with CVP without rituximab.[9]

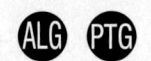

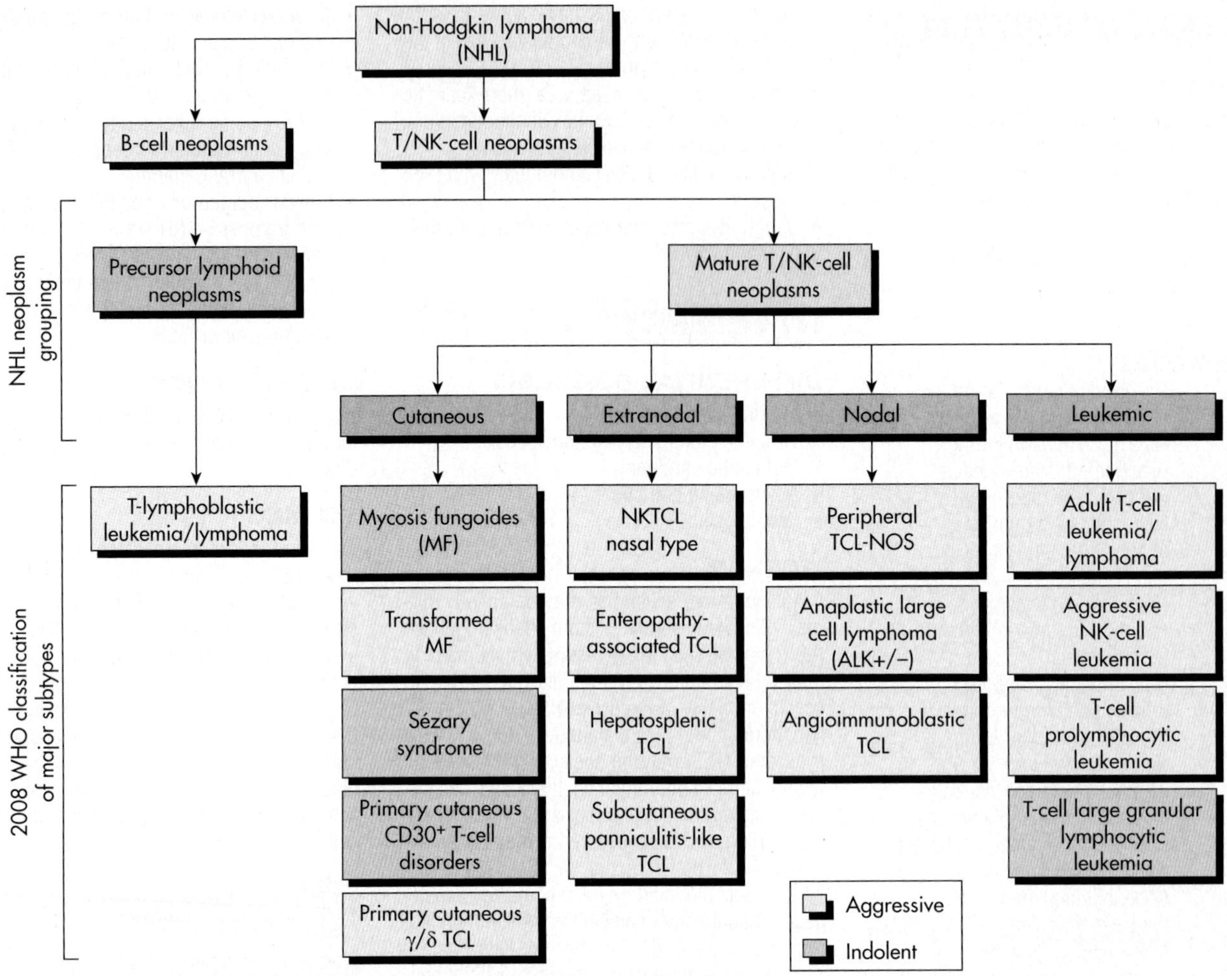

FIG. 1 World Health Organization (WHO) classification of the mature T-cell neoplasms. *NK,* Natural killer; *NKTCL,* nasal NK/T-cell lymphoma; *NOS,* not otherwise specified; *TCL,* T-cell lymphoma; *WHO,* World Health Organization. (From Hoffman R et al: *Hematology: basic principles and practice,* ed 7, Philadelphia, 2018, Elsevier.)

BOX 1 Factors Associated with an Increased Risk of Non-Hodgkin Lymphoma

Immunosuppression, acquired
  After solid-organ or hematopoietic stem cell transplantation
  HIV/AIDS
Congenital immunodeficiency syndromes
Increasing age (waning immunity)
Previous history of HL or NHL
Family history of NHL
Drugs
  Methotrexate
  TNF-α inhibitors
Occupational exposures
  Herbicides, pesticides, wood dust, epoxy glue, organic solvents
  Farming, forestry, painting, carpentry, tanning

HL, Hodgkin lymphoma; *NHL,* non-Hodgkin lymphoma; *TNF,* tumor necrosis factor.
From Niederhuber JE: *Abeloff's clinical oncology,* ed 6, Philadelphia, 2020, Elsevier.

- In a phase III noninferiority study, the combination of bendamustine and rituximab was associated with better progression-free survival rates than R-CHOP (70 vs. 31 mo) with fewer toxic effects.[10] Subset analyses showed better progression-free survival in patients with FL, mantle cell lymphoma, and lymphoplasmacytic lymphoma.
- The combination of obinutuzumab and chemotherapy followed by obinutuzumab maintenance was approved by the FDA in previously untreated patients with FL based on a randomized study, in which obinutuzumab and chemotherapy were associated with longer median progression-free survival than rituximab and chemotherapy.[11]
- Combination regimens containing cytarabine such as R-CHOP alternating with R-DHAP or the NORDIC regimen are used for the frontline treatment of aggressive mantle cell lymphoma.[12] Bendamustine and rituximab, R-CHOP, and lenalidomide and

rituximab are less aggressive regimens for mantle cell lymphoma.[10,13,14] Mantle cell lymphoma can have indolent or aggressive clinical behavior.
- Maintenance rituximab after rituximab-containing regimens has been associated with better progression-free survival rates than observation in follicular and mantle cell lymphoma.[15] However, its practice has been impacted by the COVID-19 pandemic given the association between rituximab use and the development of severe COVID-19 infection and decreased responses to vaccination.
- *H. pylori*–associated gastric marginal zone lymphoma can be treated with a course of antibiotics. For persistent cases after eradication or for *H. pylori*–negative cases, radiotherapy is highly effective.
- Splenic marginal zone lymphoma is typically treated with rituximab. Splenectomy can be performed for symptomatic splenomegaly.

TABLE 1 Major Molecular Alterations in Non-Hodgkin Lymphomas

NHL Histologic Type	Alteration	Cases Affected (%)	Proto-oncogene Involved	Mechanism of Proto-oncogene Activation	Proto-oncogene Function
Lymphoplasmacytic lymphoma	MYD88 L265P mutation	95	MYD88	Activation	B-cell signaling
Follicular lymphoma	t(14;18)(q32;q21)	90	BCL-2	Transcription deregulation	Negative regulator of apoptosis
Mantle cell lymphoma	t(11;14)(q13;q32)	70	BCL-1/cyclin D1	Transcription deregulation	Cell cycle regulator
MALT lymphoma	t(11;18)(q21;q21)	50	API$_2$/MLT	Fusion protein	API$_2$ has antiapoptotic activity
	t(1;14)(p22;q32)		BCL-10	Transcription deregulation	Antiapoptosis
Diffuse large B-cell lymphoma	der(3)(q27)	35	BCL-6	Transcription deregulation	Transcriptional repressor required for GC formation
	t(14;18)(q32;q21)	15	BCL-2	Transcription deregulation	Negative regulator of apoptosis
	t(8;14)(q24;q32)	10	MYC	Transcription deregulation	Transcription factor regulating cell proliferation and growth
Burkitt lymphoma	t(8;14)(q24;q32)	80	MYC	Transcription deregulation	Transcription factor regulating cell proliferation and growth
	t(2;8)(p11;q24)	15	MYC		
	t(8;22)(q24;q11)	5	MYC		
Anaplastic large T-cell lymphoma	t(2;5)(p23;q35)	60	NPM/ALK	Fusion protein	ALK is a tyrosine kinase
	Locus 6p25.3	30	DUSP22/IRF4	Tumor suppressor	Inhibit T-cell lymphomagenesis in ALK negative ALCL
	inv(3)(q26q28)	8	TBL1XR1/TP63	Inhibit apoptosis	Inhibit apoptosis in ALK negative ALCL

GC, Gastric cancer; *MALT,* mucosa-associated lymphoid tissue; *NHL,* non-Hodgkin lymphoma.
From Niederhuber JE: *Abeloff's clinical oncology,* ed 6, Philadelphia, 2020, Elsevier.

TABLE 2 Evaluation of a New Patient with Non-Hodgkin Lymphoma

Evaluation	Mandatory	As Indicated
Confirm diagnosis	Adequate biopsy reviewed by experienced hematopathologists	Immunophenotyping with immunohistochemistry ± flow cytometry Cytogenetics/molecular studies
General overview and risks of therapy	History and physical examination CBC Chemistry screen (including liver and renal function studies) HIV serology Hepatitis B serologies	Blood coagulation studies EBV serology and PCR assay Hepatitis C serology HTLV-1 serology Serum electrolytes, uric acid Assessment of cardiac ejection fraction Pregnancy testing in women Discussion of fertility issues
Prognostic categorization	Serum lactate dehydrogenase Serum albumin	Erythrocyte sedimentation rate Serum β$_2$-microglobulin
Anatomic disease	Chest, abdominal, and pelvic CT with contrast enhancement	Ultrasonography FDG-PET/CTMRI
Occult sites of involvement		Unilateral bone marrow biopsy with aspirate Lumbar puncture with flow cytometry of CSF Biopsy of suspicious sites Blood flow cytometry

CBC, Complete blood count; *CSF,* cerebrospinal fluid; *CT,* computed tomography; *EBV,* Epstein-Barr virus; *FDG-PET,* fluorodeoxy-glucose-18–labeled positron emission tomography; *HIV,* human immunodeficiency virus; *MRI,* magnetic resonance imaging; *PCR,* polymerase chain reaction.
From Niederhuber JE: *Abeloff's clinical oncology,* ed 6, Philadelphia, 2020, Elsevier.

- Rituximab or chemoimmunotherapy regimens can be used in patients with advanced stage extranodal, splenic, or nodal marginal zone lymphoma.[16]
- The oral BTK inhibitor ibrutinib is FDA-approved for the treatment of patients with lymphoplasmacytic lymphoma. It was previously approved for mantle cell lymphoma and marginal zone lymphoma.[17-19] In April 2023, the U.S. indications for ibrutinib in patients with mantle cell lymphoma and marginal zone lymphoma were voluntarily withdrawn after the Phase III SHINE study failed to demonstrate overall survival benefit but increased adverse reactions compared to the placebo-controlled arm (although it met its primary endpoint of progression-free survival benefit), and the Phase III SELENE study did not meet its primary endpoint of progression-free survival in patients with relapsed/refractory FL or marginal zone lymphoma.[20,21]
- Acalabrutinib and zanubrutinib, second-generation BTK inhibitors, have been approved for relapsed mantle cell lymphoma.[22,23] Zanubrutinib has been approved for lymphoplasmacytic lymphoma and marginal zone lymphoma.[24,25]
- The oral PI3K inhibitors idelalisib and copanlisib and the EZH2 inhibitor tazemetostat have been FDA-approved for the treatment of relapsed FL.[26-28]
- The PI3K inhibitor umbralisib had its FDA approval withdrawn in June 2022 due to safety concerns. It was formerly approved for use in previously treated marginal zone lymphoma (at least one prior therapy) and FL (at least three prior therapies).
- The proteasome inhibitor bortezomib and the immunomodulating agent lenalidomide are FDA-approved for the treatment of relapsed mantle cell lymphoma but are less preferred than BTK inhibitors.
- CAR T-cell therapy has been approved for relapsed or refractory FL (axicabtagene ciloleucel and tisagenlecleucel)[29,30] and mantle cell lymphoma (brexucabtagene autoleucel).[31]

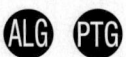

TABLE 3	Non-Hodgkin Lymphoma: Lugano Staging Classification
Stage	**Features**
I	Involvement of a single lymph node region or lymphoid structure (e.g., spleen, thymus, Waldeyer ring), or a single extranodal location without nodal involvement (IE)
II	Involvement of two or more lymph node regions on the same side of the diaphragm or limited nodal disease with limited contiguous extranodal involvement (IIE)
III	Involvement of lymph node regions or structures on both sides of the diaphragm
IV	Involvement of diffuse or noncontiguous extranodal site(s)

From Niederhuber JE: *Abeloff's clinical oncology,* ed 6, Philadelphia, 2020, Elsevier.

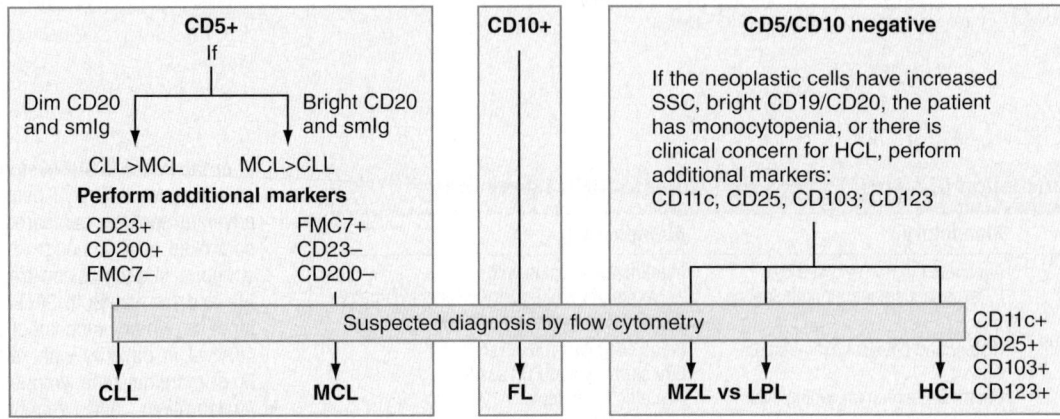

FIG. 4 This diagnostic algorithm outlines the steps in classification of B-cell lymphomas composed of cells of small to intermediate size. *BL,* Burkitt lymphoma; *CLL,* chronic lymphocytic leukemia; *FL,* follicular lymphoma; *HCL,* hairy cell leukemia; *IgM,* immunoglobulin M; *IHC,* immunohistochemistry; *LPL,* lymphoplasmacytic lymphoma; *MBL,* monoclonal B-cell lymphocytosis; *MCL,* mantle cell lymphoma; *MZL,* marginal zone lymphoma; *SmIg,* surface immunoglobulin; *SSC,* scleroderma and systemic sclerosis. (From McPherson RA, Pincus MR: *Henry's clinical diagnosis and management by laboratory methods,* ed 23, Philadelphia, 2017, Elsevier.)

- Stem cell transplantation (autologous or allogeneic) may confer long-term disease control in multiple relapsed or refractory disease.
- Table 4 summarizes chemotherapy regimens in indolent lymphomas.

AGGRESSIVE NHL: The most common aggressive NHL is DLBCL. The 5-yr overall survival rate is 60%. The addition of rituximab against CD20 B-cell lymphoma to the CHOP regimen (R-CHOP) increased the complete response rate and prolonged overall survival in patients with DLBCL, based on randomized controlled trials, without clinically significant increase in toxicity.[32-34] R-CHOP has shown to be safe and effective in patients with HIV-associated NHL.[35]

Most common regimens used in DLBCL include:

- Three to four cycles of R-CHOP followed by involved-field radiotherapy, or four to six cycles of R-CHOP alone are appropriate approaches in patients with localized DLBCL, even if high grade B cell lymphoma (e.g., double hit lymphoma; DLBCL NOS).[36-38]

- Six cycles of R-CHOP are appropriate in patients with advanced-stage DLBCL.
- The antibody-drug conjugate targeting CD79b polatuzumab vedotin, in combination with R-CHP, has emerged as an option for the treatment of previously untreated DLBCL and received FDA approval in April 2023.[39] Subgroup analysis and a subsequent publication shown greater benefit in those >60 yr, ABC phenotype, and IPI score of >2.[40]
- For patients with double-hit (defined as harboring rearrangement of MYC, BCL-2, and/or BCL-6), HIV-associated and primary mediastinal large cell lymphoma, R-EPOCH (infusional etoposide, doxorubicin, and vincristine, along with cyclophosphamide, prednisone, and rituximab) is preferred over R-CHOP.[41]
- Granulocyte-colony stimulating factor (e.g., filgrastim) may be effective in reducing the risk of febrile neutropenia in patients over 65 yr with aggressive lymphoma undergoing chemotherapy.
- Treatment with high-dose chemotherapy and autologous bone marrow transplant: Compared with conventional chemotherapy, increases overall survival in patients with chemotherapy-sensitive relapsed DLBCL (if relapse happens >1 yr post first-line).
- Chimeric antigen receptor T-cell therapy agents (axicabtagene ciloleucel, tisagenlecleucel, and lisocabtagene maraleucel) have been FDA approved for patients with relapsed (<1 yr) or refractory DLBCL after two prior lines of chemotherapy.[42-44]
- Axicabtagene ciloleucel and lisocabtagene maraleucel have been FDA-approved for patients with relapsed or refractory DLBCL within 12 mo of first-line chemoimmunotherapy or relapse after first-line chemoimmunotherapy and are not eligible for hematopoietic stem cell transplant due to comorbidities or age.[45,46]
- Two global phase 3 studies are evaluating the efficacy of axicabtagene ciloleucel as first-line therapy in patients with high-risk (IPI 4-5) large B-cell lymphoma, and in patients with relapsed/refractory FL that relapsed within 24 mo after first line or after ≥2 lines of systemic therapy.[47,48]
- The anti-CD79 antibody drug conjugate polatuzumab vedotin in combination with bendamustine and rituximab[49]; the selective inhibitor of nuclear export selinexor[50]; the anti-CD19 monoclonal antibody tafasitamab in combination with lenalidomide[51]; and loncastuximab tesirine[52] have been FDA approved for the treatment of relapsed and/or refractory DLBCL.
- Results of the randomized, phase II GUIDANCE-01 trial establishes the basis for combination of targeted agents with R-CHOP based on genetic subtyping for newly diagnosed, intermediate- or high-risk DLBCL.[53]

HIGHLY AGGRESSIVE NHL: The most common high-grade NHL subtype is BL. BL affects younger patients than DLBCL and is common in HIV-infected individuals. Regimens more intensive than R-CHOP are needed to cure patients with high-grade NHL. The most used multi-agent regimens include hyper-CVAD, CODOX-M/IVAC, and dose-adjusted EPOCH, usually in combination with rituximab.[54-56] The 5-yr survival approximates 75%. Regimens with high central nervous system (CNS) penetrance are recommended for patients with high risk for CNS recurrence (e.g., HIV infection, poor performance status, ≥2 extranodal sites, LDH level >3 times the upper limit of normal, and bone marrow involvement).[57] Relapsed/refractory BL has a dismal outcome with median survival of <4 mo.[58] The use of blinatumomab and polatuzumab-based therapy has been reported with varied responses in relapsed/refractory BL.[59,60] CAR-T cell therapy does not seem to improve outcomes in relapsed/refractory BL patients.[61]

DISPOSITION

- Patients with indolent NHL in the rituximab era experience long survival despite the lack of curative potential of chemoimmunotherapy.

TABLE 4 Chemotherapy Regimens in Lymphomas

BR (Every 28 Days)

- Bendamustine 90 mg/m² on days 1 and 2
- Rituximab 375 mg/m² IV on day 1

CVP-R (Every 21 Days)

- Cyclophosphamide 750 mg/m² IV on day 1
- Vincristine 1.4 mg/m², up to a maximal dose of 2 mg IV, on day 1
- Prednisone 40 mg/m² daily PO on days 1-5
- Rituximab 375 mg/m² IV day 1

R-CHOP (Every 21 Days)

- Cyclophosphamide 750 mg/m² IV on day 1
- Doxorubicin 50 mg/m² IV on day 1
- Vincristine 1.4 mg/m², up to a maximal dose of 2 mg IV, on day 1
- Prednisone 100 mg daily PO on days 1-5
- Rituximab 375 mg/m² IV on day 1

R-EPOCH (Every 21 Days)

- Rituximab 375 mg/m² IV on day 0 or 1 of each therapy cycle
- Doxorubicin 10 mg/m² IV per day on days 1-4
- Vincristine 0.4 mg/m² IV per day on days 1-4 (dose not capped)
- Etoposide 50 mg/m² IV per day on days 1-4
- Cyclophosphamide 750 mg/m² IV on day 5
- Prednisone 60 mg/m² PO twice daily on days 1-5

R-Hyper-CVAD (Every 21 Days)[36]

Cycles 1, 3, 5, and 7

- Rituximab 375 mg/m² IV on day 1
- Cyclophosphamide (with mesna) 300 mg/m² IV over 3 h every 12 h on days 2-4 (total six doses)
- Vincristine 1.4 mg/m² (maximum 2 mg) IV on days 5 and 12
- Doxorubicin 16.6 mg/m² IV by continuous infusion on days 5-7
- Dexamethasone 40 mg/day PO/IV on days 2-5 and days 12-15

Cycles 2, 4, 6, and 8

- Rituximab 375 mg/m² IV on day 1
- Methotrexate 200 mg/m² IV over 2 h, followed by 800 mg/m² IV continuous infusion over 22 h on day 2
- Leucovorin 50 mg PO starting 12 h after completion of methotrexate infusion, followed by 15 mg PO every 6 h for eight doses until the methotrexate level is <0.1 μM/L
- Cytarabine 3000 mg/m² IV over 2 h every 12 h on days 3 and 4 (four doses total)

Rituximab Monotherapy

- Rituximab 375 mg/m² weekly for 4 wk

R2 (Every 28 Days)

- Rituximab 375 mg/m² weekly for 4 wk, then every 28 days until cycle 5 (eight doses total)
- Lenalidomide 20 mg PO daily, 21 days on and 7 days off, for 12 cycles

From Hoffman R et al: *Hematology: basic principles and practice*, ed 7, Philadelphia, 2018, Elsevier.

N

Diseases and Disorders

I

Patients with aggressive NHL may achieve a cure with chemoimmunotherapy. Chimeric antigen receptor T-cell therapy agents have emerged as a novel therapeutic option for relapsed and refractory indolent and aggressive B-cell NHL.

- Prognostic factors include the lymphoma subtype, age of patient, and extent of disease. Table 5 describes the International Prognostic Index (IPI) for aggressive lymphomas.[62] Studies of the IPI in the modern era incorporating the anti-CD20 monoclonal antibody rituximab show an overall improved prognosis with 33% of the highest-risk patients alive 5 yr from diagnosis and 96% in the lowest risk.

- Patients who present with HIV-related NHL and low CD4$^+$ cell count have a poor prognosis (median duration of survival is 15 to 34 mo). Despite therapeutic advances, the management of HIV-associated lymphomas is challenging due to potential pharmacologic interactions and increased risk of infectious complications. It is important to optimize the CD4 cell count during treatment. Referral to an HIV specialist is recommended.

REFERENCES

Available at eBooks.Health.Elsevier.com.

RELATED CONTENT

Non-Hodgkin Lymphoma (Patient Information)

AUTHORS: **LUIS MALPICA, MD** and
JORGE J. CASTILLO, MD

TABLE 5 Clinical Prognostic Indexes

International Prognostic Index (IPI) for Aggressive Lymphomas[a]

Risk Group	IPI Score*	CR Rate (%)	5-Yr OS Rate (%)
Low	0, 1	87	73
Low intermediate	2	67	51
High intermediate	3	55	43
High	4, 5	44	26

Follicular International Prognostic Index (FLIPI)[b]

Risk Group	FLIPI Score†	Distribution (%)	5-Yr OS Rate (%)
Low	0-1	36	90.6
Intermediate	1-2	37	77.6
Poor	≥3	27	52.5

Mantle Cell International Prognostic Index (MIPI)[c]

Risk Group	MIPI Score‡	Distribution (%)	Median Survival Rate
Low	0-3	44	Not reached
Intermediate	4-5	35	51 mo
High	6-11	21	29 mo

CR, Complete response; *OS*, overall survival.

*One point is given for the presence of each of the following characteristics: Age >60 yr, elevated serum lactate dehydrogenase (LDH) level, Eastern Cooperative Oncology Group performance status ≥2, Ann Arbor stage III or IV, and more than two extranodal sites.

†One point is given for the presence of each of the following characteristics: Age >60 yr, elevated serum LDH level, hemoglobin level <12 g/dl, Ann Arbor stage III or IV, and number of nodal sites ≥5.

‡Points are based on age, ECOG performance status, white blood cell count, and serum LDH level.

[a]The International Non-Hodgkin's Lymphoma Prognostic Factors Project: A predictive model for aggressive non-Hodgkin's lymphoma, *N Engl J Med* 329:987-994, 1993.

[b]Solal-Celigny P et al: Follicular lymphoma international prognostic index, *Blood* 104:1258-1265, 2004.

[c]Hoster E et al: A new prognostic index (MIPI) for patients with advanced-stage mantle cell lymphoma, *Blood* 111:558-565, 2008.

From Niederhuber JE: *Abeloff's clinical oncology,* ed 6, Philadelphia, 2020, Elsevier.

ℹ BASIC INFORMATION

DEFINITION

Normal pressure hydrocephalus (NPH) is a syndrome of symptomatic communicating hydrocephalus in the setting of normal cerebrospinal fluid (CSF) pressure. Ventricular expansion results in compression of brain parenchyma and stretching of the corticospinal and other tracts of the internal capsule (Fig. E1). The classic clinical triad of NPH includes gait disturbance, cognitive decline, and incontinence.

SYNONYMS

Hydrocephalus, normal pressure
NPH
Occult hydrocephalus
Extraventricular obstructive hydrocephalus
Chronic hydrocephalus

ICD-10CM CODES
G91.2　Normal pressure hydrocephalus
G91.8　Other hydrocephalus

EPIDEMIOLOGY & DEMOGRAPHICS

INCIDENCE: The exact incidence is not known. In one study the incidence was found to be 5.5/100,000, but it may account for up to 5% of dementia in the U.S. Hospital discharge data suggest ~11,500 new cases diagnosed annually (may be overestimated). The prevalence of NPH was found to be 21.9/100,000 (~0.22%) in one study but also may be as high as 14% among extended-care facility patients.
PREDOMINANT SEX: Males = females
PREDOMINANT AGE: NPH is more common with increasing age. In one study of 1238 patients who had undergone a head computed tomography (CT) scan and neuropsychiatric evaluation, 0.2% of patients between 70 and 79 had probable NPH, and 5.9% of those ≥80 yr had probable NPH.[1]

PHYSICAL FINDINGS & CLINICAL PRESENTATION[2]

- Gait difficulty (Fig. E2): A "magnetic" gait, in which patients have difficulty initiating ambulation. The gait may be broad-based and shuffling, with the appearance that the feet are stuck to the floor. Difficulty with turns may also be seen.
- Cognitive decline: Mental slowing, forgetfulness, and inattention, typically without agnosia, aphasia, or other cortical disturbances. The main cognitive feature is executive dysfunction.
- Incontinence: Initially may have urinary urgency; incontinence later develops. Fecal incontinence also occurs. In one prospective study of 55 consecutive patients with idiopathic NPH, nocturia was the most common symptom, urge incontinence was the most bothersome, and 100% had detrusor overactivity on urodynamic studies.[3]
- *Gegenhalten* (paratonia or involuntary resistance with passive movement) or other frontal lobe signs may be seen.

ETIOLOGY

- ~50% of cases are idiopathic; the prevailing thought is that these cases are due to either increased CSF production or reduced absorption.
- The remaining cases are secondary to a variety of causes, including prior subarachnoid hemorrhage, meningitis, head trauma, or intracranial surgery.
- Symptoms are presumed to result from stretching of cortical, limbic, and thalamocortical fibers that lie near the ventricles as dilation occurs.

Dx DIAGNOSIS

DIFFERENTIAL DIAGNOSIS

- Vascular dementia
- Alzheimer disease with extrapyramidal features
- Cognitive impairment in the setting of Parkinson disease or parkinsonism-plus syndromes
- Dementia with Lewy bodies
- Frontotemporal dementia
- Cervical spondylosis with cord compromise in the setting of degenerative dementia
- HIV-associated dementia
- Chronic bifrontal subdural hematomas
- Table E1 differentiates MRI findings between hydrocephalus and atrophy

WORKUP

Alternative causes of cognitive complaints, gait abnormalities, and urinary complaints are very common, and workup should include investigation for alternative explanations. Gait problems occur in 20% of individuals >75 yr and is associated with the development of dementia.[4]

Large-volume lumbar puncture should be performed with assessment of improvement in gait.[2] Speed of walking 30 ft and number of steps when turning should be evaluated. Improvement in gait after a high-volume lumbar puncture is highly correlated with shunt responsiveness.[5]

Measurement of CSF outflow resistance by an infusion test or CSF pressure monitoring is sometimes used to help predict surgical outcome. External lumbar drainage (ELD) is being used more commonly and can be done over a period of 1 to 3 days at special centers that specialize in evaluating patients with adult hydrocephalus.

LABORATORY TESTS

- CSF should be sent for routine fluid analysis to exclude other pathologies.
- CSF biomarkers may be useful in excluding Alzheimer disease (e.g., Tau/A-beta 42). However, there may be overlap with patients with comorbid other neurodegenerative diseases.

IMAGING STUDIES

- CT scan or MRI (Fig. 3) can be used to document ventriculomegaly. The distinguishing feature of NPH is ventricular enlargement out of proportion to sulcal atrophy (Fig. E4), and typically the frontal horn ratio (Evans index) exceeds 0.30.[2,6] An algorithm for evaluation of patients with enlarged ventricles is described in Fig. 5.
- MRI has advantages over CT, including better ability to visualize structures in the posterior fossa, visualize transependymal CSF flow (seen as periventricular T2 FLAIR hyperintensity), and document extent of white matter lesions. On MRI a flow void in the aqueduct and third ventricle ("jet sign"), thinning and elevation of the corpus callosum on sagittal images, rounding of the frontal horns, and a pattern known as *disproportionately enlarged subarachnoid space hydrocephalus* (DESH) may be seen. DESH is characterized by narrow CSF space at the high convexity/midline areas and enlarged sylvian fissures and is associated with a good response to CSF shunting.[7] MRI time-resolved 2D phase contrast imaging with velocity encoding also can be used to visualize CSF flow.
- Isotope cisternography and dynamic MRI studies have not been shown to be superior in predicting shunt outcome.

Rx TREATMENT

- There is no evidence that NPH can be effectively treated with medications. CSF diversion via a ventriculoperitoneal (VP) vs. less commonly ventriculoatrial or lumboperitoneal shunt is a definitive treatment.[8,9] Fig. 6 illustrates an algorithm for selection of patients for VP shunt.

NONPHARMACOLOGIC THERAPY

Response to VP shunting is variable ranging from 90% to much less. Patient selection is key. Effectiveness of shunting has never been demonstrated in a randomized controlled trial. Based on a metanalysis, in appropriately chosen patients, gait improvement was observed in 75%, cognitive function improvement in 60%, and improvement of incontinence in 55% of patients.[9]

- Factors that may predict positive outcome with surgery:[8]
  1. NPH caused by prior trauma, subarachnoid hemorrhage, or meningitis
  2. History of mild impairment in cognition <2 yr duration
  3. Presence of gait abnormality
  4. Onset of gait abnormality before cognitive decline
  5. Imaging demonstrates hydrocephalus without sulcal enlargement, including normal-size sylvian fissures and cortical sulci, and absent or mild white matter lesions
  6. Transependymal CSF flow visualized on MRI
  7. Large-volume tap or ELD produces dramatic but temporary relief of symptoms
  8. High *normal* opening pressure
- Factors that may predict negative outcome with surgery:
  1. Extensive white matter lesions or diffuse cerebral atrophy on MRI
  2. Moderate to severe cognitive impairment
  3. Onset of cognitive impairment before gait disorder
  4. History of alcohol abuse

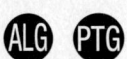
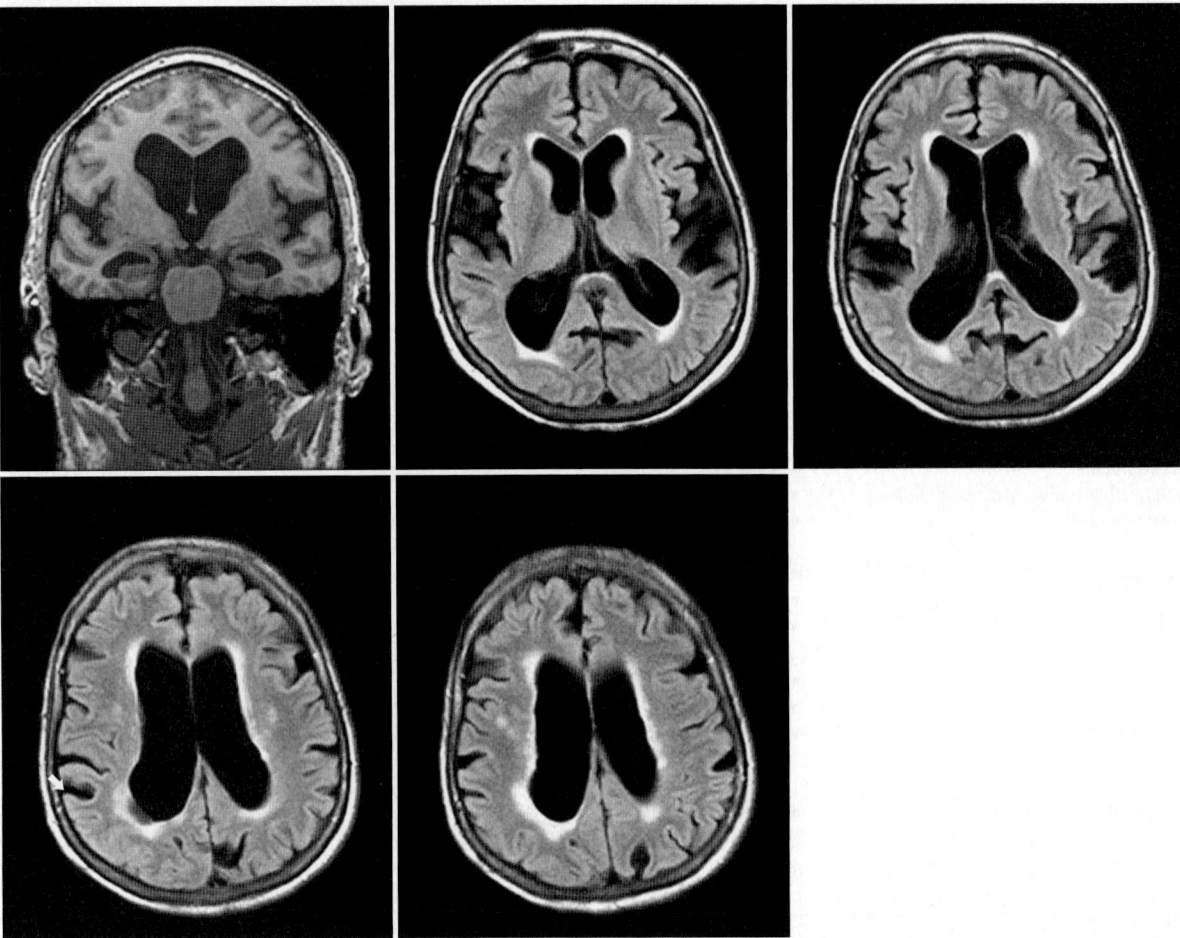

FIG. 3 *Top row: Left image* reveals enlargement of the sylvian fissures and crowding at the apex consistent with disproportionately enlarged subarachnoid space hydrocephalus. *Middle and right images* demonstrate ventricular enlargement and transependymal flow seen in normal pressure hydrocephalus (NPH). *Bottom row:* Entrapped sulci seen in NPH *(white arrow).* (From Jankovic J et al: *Bradley and Daroff's neurology in clinical practice,* ed 8, Philadelphia, 2022, Elsevier.)

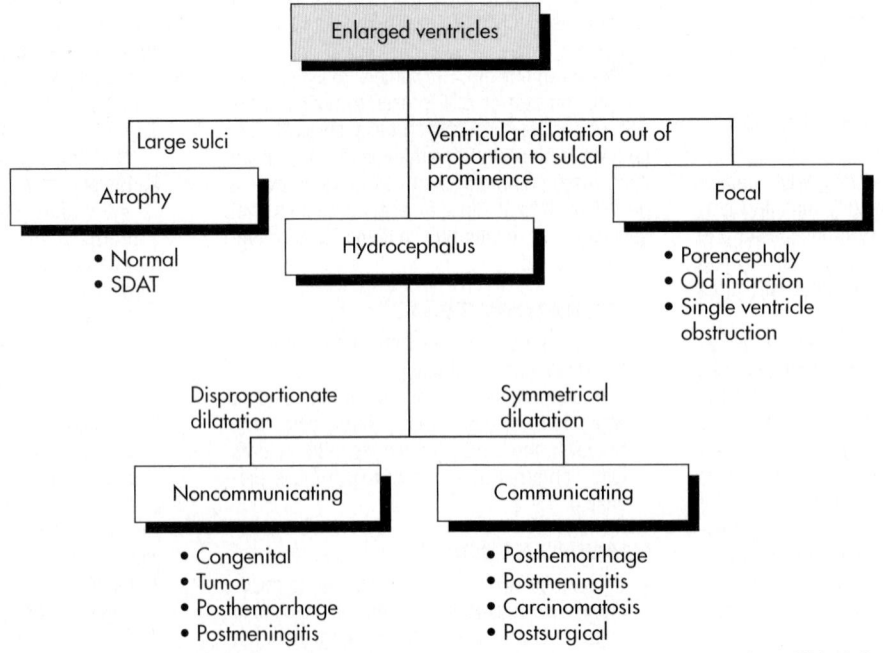

FIG. 5 Radiographic differential diagnosis of enlarged ventricles. *SDAT,* Senile dementia of the Alzheimer type. (From Weissleder R et al: *Primer of diagnostic imaging,* ed 5, St Louis, 2011, Mosby.)

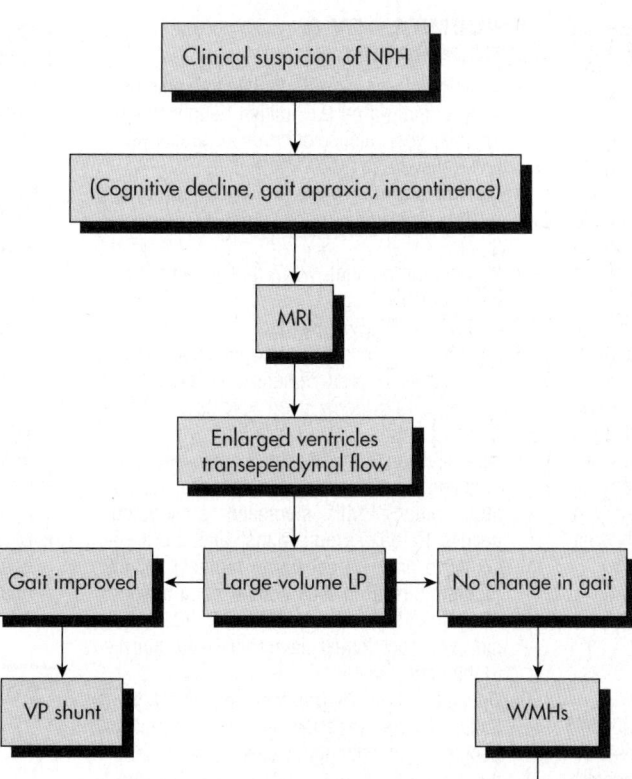

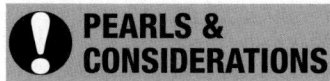

FIG. 6 An algorithm for selection of patients for ventriculoperitoneal (VP) shunt. Patients with the clinical triad undergo FLAIR MRI. If communicating hydrocephalus is found without excessive atrophy and with transependymal absorption, then a large volume of cerebrospinal fluid is removed, and the changes in the gait observed over several days. In those with improvement in gait, a VP shunt is done. Patients with white-matter changes in the deep white matter probably have lacunar state. Those with white matter changes compatible with microvascular disease most likely have lacunar state or parkinsonism. *FLAIR,* Fluid-attenuated inversion recovery; *LP,* lumbar puncture; *MRI,* magnetic resonance imaging; *NPH,* normal-pressure hydrocephalus; *WMHs,* white matter hyperintensities. (From Jankovic J et al: *Bradley and Daroff's neurology in clinical practice,* ed 8, Philadelphia, 2022, Elsevier.)

ACUTE GENERAL Rx
Shunting in selected patients

DISPOSITION
Symptoms of NPH may progress over time. Prompt diagnosis may improve chances for treatment success.

REFERRAL
Patients should be referred to a neurologist with experience in evaluating NPH followed by a neurosurgeon for shunting in appropriate patients.

❗ PEARLS & CONSIDERATIONS

Each of the cardinal symptoms of NPH is commonly seen in the elderly and occurs in multiple disease processes; therefore, differential diagnoses should always be considered carefully.

REFERENCES
Available at eBooks.Health.Elsevier.com.

RELATED CONTENT
Normal Pressure Hydrocephalus (Patient Information)

AUTHOR: **COREY ELAM GOLDSMITH, MD, FAAN**

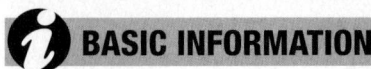

BASIC INFORMATION

DEFINITION

Opioid use disorder (OUD) is defined as a cluster of cognitive, behavioral, and physiologic symptoms in which the individual continues use of opioids despite significant drug use–associated problems. OUD is a chronic, relapsing disorder characterized by repeated self-administration of opioids that commonly results in emergence of tolerance/dependence with chronic use, as well as withdrawal with abrupt drug discontinuation. Tolerance occurs as opioid receptors become less responsive to stimulation over time and is associated with the need to increase the dose to achieve the same effect. Dependence may occur with or without the physiologic symptoms of tolerance and withdrawal and is associated with physiologically unpleasant reactions with drug discontinuation.

SYNONYMS

OUD
Opioid addiction
Substance use disorder

Historically, terms including "opioid abuse" and "opioid dependence" were used to describe various aspects of OUD. Similarly "addict" was a term commonly used to describe patients using various substances, including opioids. These terms are perceived as stigmatizing and should be avoided. Furthermore, drug abuse/dependence both are no longer valid diagnostic categories in *Diagnostic and Statistical Manual of Mental Disorders,* Fifth Edition, Text Revision (DSM-5-TR). As apparent in the following text, unfortunately the language remains common in the medical setting, including in the ICD-10M codes outlined here.

ICD-10CM CODES

F11.10	Opioid abuse, uncomplicated
F11.120	Opioid abuse with intoxication, uncomplicated
F11.121	Opioid abuse with intoxication delirium
F11.122	Opioid abuse with intoxication with perceptual disturbance
F11.129	Opioid abuse with intoxication, unspecified
F11.14	Opioid abuse with opioid-induced mood disorder
F11.150	Opioid abuse with opioid-induced psychotic disorder with delusions
F11.151	Opioid abuse with opioid-induced psychotic disorder with hallucinations
F11.159	Opioid abuse with opioid-induced psychotic disorder, unspecified
F11.181	Opioid abuse with opioid-induced sexual dysfunction
F11.182	Opioid abuse with opioid-induced sleep disorder
F11.188	Opioid abuse with other opioid-induced disorder
F11.19	Opioid abuse with unspecified opioid-induced disorder

EPIDEMIOLOGY & DEMOGRAPHICS

- There has been a dramatic rise in opioid use, with an estimated 9.5 million people reporting past-year misuse of heroin or prescription pain relievers in 2020.[1]
- Opioids were involved in ~15% of drug-related emergency department (ED) visits in 2021.[2]
- It is estimated that >2.7 million Americans have an OUD.[3]

INCIDENCE & PREVALENCE:

- Each year, U.S. retail pharmacies dispense >170 million prescriptions for opioid pain relievers. Commonly used opioids are summarized in Box 1.
- Opioid-associated fatalities have been increasing over the past two decades, associated initially with increased prescribing/access to pain medications, and more recently to growing access to fentanyl (illicitly manufactured) in vulnerable communities. After briefly plateauing in 2018 to 2019, opioid overdose deaths have increased sharply in the past 3 yr.[5]
- Opioid (e.g., heroin, prescription pain medications) use was reported by 3.4% (9.5 million people), with patients disclosing to prescription pain reliever misuse (9.3 million people).[1]
- Fentanyl is a synthetic opioid 50 to 100 times more potent than morphine and approved for the management of surgical/postoperative pain, severe chronic pain, and breakthrough cancer pain. The Drug Enforcement Administration and Centers for Disease Control and Prevention have issued nationwide alerts identifying fentanyl, particularly illicitly manufactured fentanyl, as a threat to public health and safety.

Incidence of chronic pain in the U.S. population is estimated at close to 20%. In 2019, some 22.1% of U.S. adults with chronic pain used a prescription opioid, with the highest prevalence noted among adults aged 45 to 64 (25.9%). Sex (24.3% women vs. 19.4% men), employment status (27.8% unemployed vs. 15.2% employed adults), and financial insecurity were all associated with higher rates of opioid prescribing. High rates of opioid prescriptions for chronic pain remain despite inadequate evidence of long-term benefits and growing evidence of harm.

PREDOMINANT SEX & AGE: Rates of opioid use and OUD are higher in men compared to women. Adults aged 35 to 44 show some of the highest rates of OUD-associated complications, including overdose/death.[4]

PEAK INCIDENCE: The majority of new opioid users are <26 yr. The majority of opioid-related complications, including overdoses, are in individuals aged 35 to 44 yr.[4]

RISK FACTORS:

- Family history
- History of substance use
- Psychiatric disorders

GENETICS:

- Similar to other substance use disorders, genetic epidemiologic studies suggest a high degree of heritable vulnerability for OUD.
- Gene polymorphism for dopamine receptor/transporters, opioid receptors, serotonin receptors/transporters, proenkephalin, and catechol-*O*-methyltransferase all appear to be associated with vulnerability to OUD.

PHYSICAL FINDINGS & CLINICAL PRESENTATION

- Acute opioid intoxication: Physical examination is often notable for miosis. Progressive sedation and reduced respiratory rate may be present with significant use. Respiratory compromise, coma, and death can all occur with overdose. Acute opioid intoxication: Behaviorally, acute intoxication is marked by euphoria and sense of well-being. Irritability can occur, and, as noted, progressive sedation is hallmark of significant use. Acute effects of opioid agonists are summarized in Box 2.
- Chronic opioid use can cause distal esophageal spasm and esophagogastric outflow obstruction.[6]

BOX 1   Commonly Used Opioids

Agonist
    Camphorated tincture of opium (paregoric)
    Morphine
    Meperidine (Demerol)
    Methadone
    Fentanyl
    Hydromorphone (Dilaudid)
    Oxycodone
    Hydrocodone
    Propoxyphene (Darvon)
    Heroin
Antagonist
    Naloxone (Narcan)
    Naltrexone
Mixed Agonist–Antagonist
    Pentazocine (Talwin)
    Butorphanol (Stadol)
    Buprenorphine (Buprenex, Subutex, Belbuca, and others)

From Jankovic J et al: Bradley and Daroff's neurology in clinical practice, ed 8, Philadelphia, 2022, Elsevier.

BOX 2   Acute Effects of Opioid Agonists

"Rush"
Euphoria or dysphoria
Drowsiness, "nodding"
Analgesia
Nausea, vomiting
Miosis
Dryness of the mouth
Sweating
Pruritus
Cough suppression
Respiratory depression
Hypothermia
Postural hypotension
Constipation
Biliary tract spasm
Urinary retention

From Jankovic J et al: Bradley and Daroff's neurology in clinical practice, ed 8, Philadelphia, 2022, Elsevier.

- Scars or track marks from chronic intravenous (IV) use may be visible over the veins of the arms, hands, ankles, neck, and breasts. Inflamed nasal mucosa and/or respiratory wheezing may be apparent in patients who are insufflating opioids.
- Opioid withdrawal: Patients in withdrawal generally do not show significant vital sign abnormalities. Physical examination may evidence piloerection (goose flesh), mydriasis, lacrimation, rhinorrhea, sweating, and repeated yawning. Box 3 summarizes symptoms and signs of opioid withdrawal.
- Opioid withdrawal: Though uncommonly life-threatening, opioid withdrawal is markedly uncomfortable. Patients will commonly describe significant irritability, physical discomfort, cramps (abdominal), nausea/vomiting, and diarrhea.
- Given the high risk for complications associated with IV drug use (IVDU), in an appropriate clinical setting consider additional causes of GI discomfort as gastroenteritis, pancreatitis, peptic ulcer disease, and intestinal obstruction. In patients with significant vital sign changes and fever, consider potential occult infectious causes.
- The history may provide relevant information in making the diagnosis. Significant findings may include:
  1. A long history of opioid self-administration, typically by the IV or intranasal route but sometimes through smoking as well.
  2. Use of multiple substances. Intoxication by drugs other than opioids is common and should be ruled out because it may have an impact on risk stratification and treatment.
     a. A high incidence of non–opioid-related psychiatric disorders (>80%).
     b. History of problems at work, at school, or in relationships associated with drug use.
     c. History of interpersonal violence and trauma.
     d. History of adverse childhood experiences.
     e. History of drug use–associated infectious complications, including cellulitis/abscesses, phlebitis, and endocarditis. History of liver diseases attributable to acute drug-related toxicity, coingestion of other substances (e.g., acetaminophen in Vicodin/Percocet) or viral hepatitis. Hepatitis C is the most prevalent blood-borne pathogen in patients with IVDU. ~72% of hepatitis C cases reported to the Centers for Disease Control and Prevention (CDC) in 2018 were associated with IVDU. HIV is likewise strongly associated with IVDU and OUD.

ETIOLOGY

OUD is a biopsychosocial disorder. Pharmacologic, social, genetic, and psychodynamic factors interact to influence use behaviors. Pharmacologic factors are especially prominent in OUD. With initial use, opioids can be strongly reinforcing because of their analgesic, euphoric, and anxiolytic effects. With chronic exposure, compensatory changes in the reward circuits result in emergence of emotion/context-based cuing (triggers/cravings to use) and reduced ability to effectively resist drug use–associated behaviors (even if associated with reduced reward or punishment).

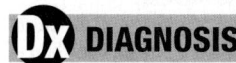 **DIAGNOSIS**

DIFFERENTIAL DIAGNOSIS

- Psychiatric disorders (e.g., anxiety, depression, bipolar disorder, posttraumatic stress disorder).
- Acute medical illness (e.g., hypoglycemia, seizure disorder, sepsis, renal or hepatic insufficiency) may mimic opioid withdrawal symptoms.
- Pseudo-addiction: Patients with chronic opioid exposure may exhibit both tolerance and withdrawal associated with chronic use. Rarely, these patients may apparently engage in behavioral patterns that raise concern for addiction (e.g., frequent emergency room visits, access to multiple prescriptions or providers), but their behavior may reflect maladaptive coping associated with chronic opioid exposure (and potentially anxiety regarding said medications being tampered with) rather than OUD.

WORKUP

The history is the most important part of the workup. A single question screening test ("How many times in the past year have you used a street drug or a prescription medication for non-medical reasons?") should be incorporated in the medical history. Useful screening tools for OUD are the CAGE-AID (Table 1), the DAST 10 (Table 2), and the CRAFFT (Table 3). The CAGE-AID has a sensitivity of 70% and a specificity of 85% when two questions are answered in the affirmative.[7] The DAST 10 can discriminate between current users and former users. The CRAFFT is a useful screening tool for adolescents. A CRAFFT score of ≥2 is optimal for identifying any problem (sensitivity 76%, specificity 94%), disorder (sensitivity 80%, specificity 86%), and drug dependence (sensitivity 92%, specificity 80%).[8] COWS (Clinical Opioid Withdrawal Scale) is used to assess the severity of opioid withdrawal.

- Observation of opioid withdrawal is indicative of opioid dependence, but does not necessarily confirm the presence of OUD (e.g., patients

---

BOX 3 Symptoms and Signs of Opioid Withdrawal

Drug craving
Anxiety, irritability
Lacrimation
Rhinorrhea
Yawning
Sweating
Mydriasis
Myalgia, muscle spasms
Piloerection
Anorexia, nausea, vomiting
Diarrhea
Abdominal cramps
Productive coughing
Hot flashes
Fever
Tachycardia
Tachypnea
Hypertension
Erection, orgasm

From Jankovic J et al: *Bradley and Daroff's neurology in clinical practice,* ed 8, Philadelphia, 2022, Elsevier.

TABLE 1 CAGE-AID

1. Have you ever tried to **C**ut down on your alcohol or drug use?
2. Do you get **A**nnoyed when people comment about your drinking or drug use?
3. Do you feel **G**uilty about things you have done while drinking or using drugs?
4. Do you need an **E**ye-opener to get started in the morning?
   Two or more questions answered in the affirmative require further assessment.

AID, Adapted to include drugs.
From Bowman S et al: Reducing the health consequences of opioid addiction in primary care, *Am J Med* 126:565-571, 2013.

TABLE 2 Drug Abuse Screening Test (DAST-10)

1. Have you used drugs other than those required for medical reasons?
2. Do you abuse more than one drug at a time?
3. Are you unable to stop using drugs when you want to?
4. Have you ever had blackouts or flashbacks as a result of drug use?
5. Do you ever feel bad or guilty about your drug use?
6. Does your spouse (or parents) ever complain about your involvement with drugs?
7. Have you neglected your family because of your use of drugs?
8. Have you engaged in illegal activities in order to obtain drugs?
9. Have you ever experienced withdrawal symptoms (felt sick) when you stopped taking drugs?
10. Have you had medical problems as a result of your drug use (e.g., memory loss, hepatitis, convulsions, bleeding)?
    Two or more questions answered in the affirmative require further assessment.

From Bowman S et al: Reducing the health consequences of opioid addiction in primary care, *Am J Med* 126:565-571, 2013.

From Bowman S et al: Reducing the health consequences of opioid addiction in primary care, *Am J Med* 126:565-571, 2013.

TABLE 3 CRAFFT Screening Tool for Adolescents

1. Have you ever ridden in a **C**ar driven by someone (including yourself) who was high or had been using alcohol or drugs?
2. Do you ever use alcohol or drugs to **R**elax, feel better about yourself, or fit in?
3. Do you ever use alcohol or drugs while you are by yourself **A**lone?
4. Do you ever **F**orget things you did while using alcohol or drugs?
5. Do your **F**amily or Friends ever tell you that you should cut down on your drinking or drug use?
6. Have you ever gotten into **T**rouble while you were using alcohol or drugs?
   Two or more questions answered in the affirmative require further assessment.

with chronic pain, patients on methadone or Suboxone).

- Observation of purposeful behaviors such as complaints and manipulations directed at getting more drugs is potentially concerning for malingering, though it can also reflect undertreated pain (see "Differential Diagnosis") or withdrawal needs.
- Screen urine for opioid metabolites. If feasible, consider buccal screens preferentially, as harder to tamper with. Be familiar with common false positive/negatives, and have low threshold to reach out to toxicology laboratories if unexpected findings.
- Screen for communicable diseases: HIV, hepatitis B and hepatitis C, tuberculosis. Discuss safe needle use practices with patients as a harm reduction approach.
- Screen for endocarditis in patients with newly diagnosed murmurs.

LABORATORY TESTS

- Urine and serum toxicology screen
- CBC
- Chemistries (alanine aminotransferase, aspartate aminotransferase, serum creatinine): Elevated liver function test (LFT) results may be from viral hepatitis or acetaminophen toxicity
- Hepatitis screen: If hepatitis C antibody positive, follow up with hepatitis C polymerase chain reaction (viral load) even in patients with normal LFTs
- HIV
- Purified protein derivative

IMAGING STUDIES

Generally, not helpful in routine diagnosis and treatment. Consider echocardiography in patients with heart murmurs and liver sonography or computed tomography scan in patients with elevated LFTs or who are positive for hepatitis C or B (increased risk of hepatocellular carcinoma).

Ⓡⓧ TREATMENT

NONPHARMACOLOGIC THERAPY

- Brief counseling interventions during a visit with their primary care physician or OB/GYN have proved efficacious in motivating patients for treatment.
- Treatment with either full agonist (methadone) or partial agonist (buprenorphine) is the standard of care and should ALWAYS be discussed with patient. Naltrexone intramuscularly (IM) is likewise an option, though less effective

overall. Please note that although all of the later-noted nonpharmacologic options are worth considering, none have shown superiority to pharmacologic methods for OUD. Nonpharmacologic options should never be forced on the patient (because they have been repeatedly shown to be ineffective).

- For patients with housing instability or significant community-associated triggers to use, consider referral to therapeutic communities (residential, CSS/TSS).
- Peer support should likewise be considered, including recovery coaching (if access), as well as 12-step or other self-help groups (e.g., Alcoholics Anonymous, Narcotics Anonymous). Note that considerable variability exists across NA/AA groups regarding acceptance of methadone/Suboxone; routinely screen and counsel patients about this. Alternative self-help and peer groups include SMART Recovery, Dharma Recovery, and Refuge Recovery.
- Relapse prevention counseling can be of considerable benefit if the patient is willing to engage, in particular if incorporating aspects of motivational interviewing (MI) into therapeutic practice.
- Opioid prevention education (Table 4).
- Nonpharmacologic strategies have the greatest documented efficacy: Education, feedback, goal setting, problem solving, and additional contacts for further assistance.

- Consider psychiatry referrals to address co-occurring psychiatric conditions, as well as social work and case management referrals to address common psychosocial barriers to recovery (e.g., access to safe housing).

ACUTE GENERAL Rx

- The majority of intoxicated patients will do adequately with supportive care alone.
- This noted, opioid overdose is an acute medical emergency that requires immediate attention to the maintenance of airway, breathing, and circulation (i.e., ABCs of resuscitation). If severe, opioid-induced respiratory depression can be treated with 0.4 mg/ml of IV or IM naloxone, which can be repeated every 2 min, as needed (up to a total dose of 2 mg). If no response after 20 min, or if partial response noted, strongly consider combined drug overdose or other contributors (e.g., infection). Naloxone is also available as an intranasal formulation. The FDA has also approved an intranasal formulation of the opioid antagonist nalmefene for emergency treatment of known or suspected opioid overdose in persons ≥12 yr old.
- CDC guidelines advise naloxone co-prescription to patients with active OUD and specifically for patients with a history of overdose, concurrent benzodiazepine use, and for all patients using high doses of opioids (≥50 mg of morphine [or equivalent] per day).
- Treatment of opioid overdose is summarized in Box 4.
- Acute management of opioid withdrawal should always include consideration of a potential opioid agent (typically buprenorphine or methadone). Opioid withdrawal using "comfort medications" alone (commonly clonidine, dicyclomine, and NSAIDs) should always be avoided because it is associated with limited patient compliance and considerable discomfort (despite the name).

TABLE 4 Basic Components of Opioid Overdose Prevention Education Curriculum

1. Know the signs of an opioid overdose (e.g., unresponsive, limp, slow, shallow breathing, pale or clammy, fingernails or lips turning blue, gurgling).
2. Call 911.
3. Administer rescue breathing.
4. Administer naloxone if no response and Emergency Medical Services has not yet arrived.
5. Stay with the person until help arrives.

From Bowman S et al: Reducing the health consequences of opioid addiction in primary care, *Am J Med* 126:565-571, 2013.

BOX 4 Treatment of Opioid Overdose

Respiratory support
If hypotension does not respond promptly to ventilation, IV fluids (pressors rarely needed)
Consider prophylactic intubation
If respiratory depression, naloxone, 2 mg IV, IM, or SC, and then 2-4 mg repeated as needed up to 20 mg. If no respiratory depression, naloxone 0.4-0.8 mg IV, IM, or SC, and if no response, 2 mg repeated as needed
Hospitalization and close observation, with additional naloxone as needed
Consider additional drug overdose, such as, alcohol or cocaine

IM, Intramuscular; *IV,* intravenous; *SC,* subcutaneous.

From Jankovic J et al: *Bradley and Daroff's neurology in clinical practice,* ed 8, Philadelphia, 2022, Elsevier.

- Acute management of opioid withdrawal without consideration of long-term treatment should be avoided because it is associated with increased risk of overdose/death and new infectious disease (e.g., HIV) after detoxification.
  1. If detoxification is considered, either buprenorphine (partial agonist) or methadone (agonist) can be initiated in tapering doses. Before starting buprenorphine, patients must be tapered off all opioids and start experiencing mild-moderate withdrawal (COWS >12) to avoid precipitating worsened acute withdrawal.
  2. If considering methadone, most patients will note some benefit regarding acute withdrawal with methadone dose of 30 to 45 mg/day (usually divided into three doses to minimize risk of oversedation), though cravings may not abate until higher doses (≥60 mg/day). QTc prolongation is a common concern with methadone administration, though it is uncommon at lower doses.
- In addition to methadone or Suboxone, always consider adjunct agents, including clonidine (e.g., 0.1 mg three times daily for aniety, insomnia, and autonomic symptoms), NSAIDs for body/muscle aches, and dicyclomine for GI hyperactivity.
- Nonbenzodiazepine sedatives, including low-dose atypical antipsychotics (e.g., quetiapine), are effective for promoting adequate sleep. Opioid agonist treatment:
- As noted, strongly recommend considering methadone or buprenorphine/naloxone as the preferred first-line treatment for OUD. They are largely equivalent in efficacy, though patient-specific factors may influence choice of treatment (see "Patient Selection for Buprenorphine or Methadone").
- Buprenorphine: After induction, most patients can be maintained on buprenorphine 16 to 24 mg/day (either as a single daily dose or divided twice or three times daily). Because of the ceiling effect seen with partial opioid agonists, there are limited pharmacologic benefits from buprenorphine doses >32 mg/day
- Buprenorphine initiation: As noted, ensure patient is in moderate opioid withdrawal before offering buprenorphine (COWS >12); otherwise, there is risk for precipitating withdrawal. Most patients with short-acting opioid use will be able to take Suboxone 10 to 12 h after last use, though this may prove considerably longer in patients with exposure to chronic agents (e.g., methadone). For most OUD patients, first-day buprenorphine dose is 8 to 12 mg (commonly divided into two or three 4-mg doses), and most patients will stabilize on buprenorphine 16 mg (either as single daily dose or twice daily) by treatment day 2. Buprenorphine is now also FDA approved as a subcutaneously inserted, extended-release formulation (brixadi) for once-weekly or once-monthly treatment of moderate to severe opioid use disorder.
- Sublocade is an injectable, long-term buprenorphine that provides sufficient mediation maintenance up to 4 wk. Sublocade has been found to be effective at reducing opioid use.[9]

- Methadone is likewise an effective treatment for OUD. It involves administration of once-daily methadone in a controlled setting by methadone clinics. Though methadone is an effective analgesic at doses of 5 mg three times daily in opioid-naïve patients, patients with OUD show considerable tolerance. For most patients, the starting dose of methadone is 30 to 40 mg/day. Though beneficial for withdrawal management, cravings to use usually do not abate until higher doses are reached. Most patients on methadone will stabilize at doses between 80 and 120 mg/day.
- Methadone is associated with risk for QTc prolongation (at higher doses), oversedation (especially if used in conjunction with other sedatives), and drug-drug interactions (e.g., rifampin).
- Although all physicians can prescribe methadone for pain management, outpatient treatment with methadone for OUD can be dispensed only through specific federally mandated facilities (i.e., clinics).
- NOTE: Buprenorphine and methadone are both metabolized by the cytochrome P-450 3a4 and 2d6 I isoenzyme pathways. Prescribers should be aware of multiple possible drug interactions, especially with methadone.
- Naltrexone: Full and reversible antagonist at the opioid receptor. Naltrexone treatment is generally associated with less optimal outcomes (when compared to methadone/Suboxone), which appears driven primarily by low compliance. If considering naltrexone for OUD, note that the IM formulation carries FDA approval and the PO formulation should not be used (given aforementioned low adherence rates)
- In a patient with active OUD, administration of naltrexone can precipitate withdrawal if offered too soon after last use; therefore, it is recommended to wait 7 to 14 days after last opioid use before administering IM naltrexone. This is often a considerable challenge for patients in early sobriety and may prove difficult to achieve outside of sober therapeutic setting (e.g., detox or residential). Always consider PO naltrexone challenge before administering IM naltrexone.
- Naltrexone (oral or injectable) also may be used for maintenance in opioid dependence treatment, though evidence of effectiveness is limited. In a patient with opioid dependence, naltrexone can precipitate withdrawal if it is given too soon after an agonist; therefore, it is best to wait 7 to 14 days after last opioid use to prevent patient discomfort.
- Always combine pharmacotherapy with counseling. There is good evidence that this combination improves outcome.
- Treatment of comorbid psychiatric disorders improves outcomes.

PATIENT SELECTION FOR BUPRENORPHINE OR METHADONE

- Appropriate patients for buprenorphine office-based treatment:
  1. Patients interested (motivated) in treatment

  2. Have no major contraindications (see following)
  3. Can be expected to be reasonably compliant with treatment
  4. Understand the benefits and risks of buprenorphine treatment
  5. Willing to follow safety precautions
- Less likely to be appropriate for office-based treatment:
  1. Have comorbid use of benzodiazepines or other CNS depressants (including alcohol), though buprenorphine is still safer here than alternatives.
  2. Have multiple previous failed treatment attempts with buprenorphine, including frequent relapses
  3. Have active treatment with an opioid agonist (e.g., chronic pain) and are unwilling to consider tapering off said agent
  4. Have significant prior concerns for buprenorphine diversion
- Methadone maintenance: Narcotic treatment program (clinic setting) indications:
  1. Evidence of opioid addiction >1 yr
  2. Two failed previous treatment attempts
  3. Patients not appropriate for office-based treatment
  4. Eligible without active "use" if prior methadone maintenance patient within previous 2 mo
  5. Pregnancy

DISPOSITION

- OUD is a chronic, relapsing disease.
- High rate of relapse after detox alone.
- Relapse potential after medically supervised withdrawal from methadone:
  1. 90% after 1 yr stable in treatment
  2. 80% after 3 yr stable in treatment
  3. 70% after 5 yr stable in treatment

REFERRAL

Refer to addiction medicine specialist or narcotic treatment program when the neurobiologic disease of opioid addiction is identified.

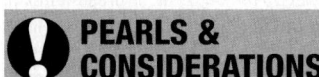

PEARLS & CONSIDERATIONS

COMMENTS

- Detoxification is contraindicated during pregnancy given risks to the fetus; always consider methadone or Suboxone initiation. Methadone maintenance has been the gold standard for pregnant patients with OUD regardless of the duration of the OUD or prior treatment attempts. The use of buprenorphine in pregnancy is associated with a lower risk of neonatal complications compared to methadone and may be easier to implement given the ease of access to buprenorphine by office-based treatment; the risk of adverse maternal outcomes is similar among patients who receive buprenorphine and those who receive methadone.[10]
- Breastfeeding is encouraged in pregnant people on methadone maintenance. The American Academy of Pediatrics statement

regarding "Transfer of Drugs and Other Chemicals into Human Milk" has placed methadone into the "usually compatible with breastfeeding" group based on the assumption that maternal urine is monitored to detect use of illicit drugs. The U.S. Department of Health and Human Services also recommends that mothers on methadone be encouraged to breastfeed.

- When a physician identifies a patient as "drug seeking," it is imperative that the physician avoid abruptly stopping the opioid prescription because this will often result in the patient buying the drugs illegally. These patients should be counseled and referred for treatment.
- Patients on methadone who have pain resulting from an acute injury will need pain medication in addition to their daily dose of methadone. They will require higher than usual doses of pain medications because of tolerance resulting from chronic exposure to methadone.
- Patients with chronic opioid use have a likewise lower pain threshold resulting from hyperalgesia related to long-term use of opioids.
- Patients on buprenorphine requiring acute opioid pain management should reduce their buprenorphine dose to 4 mg twice daily at this dose, sufficient buprenorphine is present to avoid withdrawal emergence and also to provide baseline analgesia, yet sufficient receptors are available for conventional short-acting opioid agents to provide acute pain control.
- In 2017, the federal government declared the opioid epidemic a national public health emergency within the U.S. Since then, attention (in treatment and funding) has focused mainly on White suburban and rural communities. Between 2015 and 2016 the rate of increase of drug overdose deaths was 40% in Black/African Americans compared with 21% in the overall population.[11] Systems of stigma, negative societal representations, health care inequity, and historical injustices (e.g., the "War on Drugs") have led to discrimination and harsh (often criminal) punishment for Black/African Americans with substance use disorder instead of compassionate medical treatment and recovery services. Even for those seeking recovery, unequal access exists (e.g., Black/African Americans and Latino low-income individuals are more likely to be in treatment with methadone compared with high-income patients who are more likely to be in treatment with Suboxone). Using community-informed and culturally appropriate strategies in addition to expanding access to Suboxone will be key to addressing opioid (and other substance) use disorder within the Black/African American and Latino low-income populations.
- Another group in which there exist disparities in substance use care is among sexual minorities (SMs). Data show that there are higher rates of substance use and substance use disorders among SMs than in heterosexual individuals.[12] There are high levels of unmet mental health needs among this group, particularly among SM women. There exist different patterns of substance use within the various sexual identity groups (e.g., abuse of cocaine and OxyContin is more common among lesbian and bisexual individuals); thus, understanding this heterogeneity and applying treatment models that address the unique challenges of the various SM groups will be key to delivering equitable substance use care to this population.[12]

PREVENTION

Education is the hallmark of prevention:
- School drug prevention education programs.
- Educate children about their family medical history, including diseases of addiction.
- Address childhood psychiatric disorders and adverse childhood experiences to prevent self-medicating.

- Educate patients on nonopioid analgesics for pain management.

PATIENT & FAMILY EDUCATION

- Stigma of substance use and treatment often interferes with good treatment.
- Family needs to be educated so they can support the patient's efforts.
- Encourage family meeting with substance use specialist, counselor.
- Recommend support groups for family members. Table 5 identifies organizations providing referral information for patients. Recommendations for integrating risk reduction strategies for addressing opioid misuse in the primary care setting are summarized in Table E6.
- Physicians should offer reliant immunizations to people with OUD, including hepatitis A and B and TDAP, and consider referral to syringe service programs.[1]

REFERENCES

Available at eBooks.Health.Elsevier.com.

RELATED CONTENT

Drug Use Disorder (Patient Information)
Opioid Overdose (Related Key Topic)

AUTHORS: **MOLLIE C. MARR, MD, PHD** and **MLADEN NISAVIC, MD**

TABLE 5 Organizations Providing Referral Information for Patients

Organization	Resources/Website
Substance Abuse and Mental Health Services Administration (SAMHSA)	Opioid treatment program directory: https://dpt2.samhsa.gov/treatment/directory.aspx.
Physicians who provide buprenorphine	Buprenorphine physician and treatment program locator: https://www.samhsa.gov/medication-assisted-treatment/treatment/buprenorphine.
Pain Action	Chronic pain management materials for patients: https://www.painaction.com/.
Substance abuse treatment facilities	https://findtreatment.gov/.
Harm Reduction Coalition	Local risk reduction resources and programs, overdose prevention education, and naloxone prescribing information: https://www.harmreduction.org/.
Narcotics Anonymous (NA)	General information and meeting information for NA, a 12-step program modeled after Alcoholics Anonymous: https://www.na.org/.

From Bowman S et al: Reducing the health consequences of opioid addiction in primary care, *Am J Med* 126:565-571, 2013.

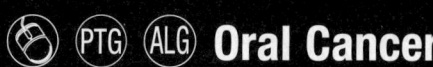

BASIC INFORMATION

DEFINITION

Oral cancers refer to the malignant transformation of the oral tissues through sequential dysplastic changes leading to the development of squamous carcinoma. Oral squamous cell cancers (OSCCs) include oral cavity cancers (lip, floor of mouth, buccal mucosa, anterior tongue, gingivae, hard palate, retromolar trigone), oropharynx cancers (base of tongue, tonsils, soft palate, pharyngeal walls), and hypopharynx cancers (pyriform sinus, postcricoid area, posterior pharyngeal wall).

SYNONYMS

Head and neck cancer
Oral malignant neoplasm
OSCC

ICD-10CM CODES

C01	Malignant neoplasm of base of tongue
C03	Malignant neoplasm of gum
C04	Malignant neoplasm of floor of mouth
C05	Malignant neoplasm of palate
C06	Malignant neoplasm of other and unspecified parts of mouth
C09	Malignant neoplasm of tonsil
C10	Malignant neoplasm of oropharynx
C11	Malignant neoplasm of nasopharynx
C12	Malignant neoplasm of piriform sinus
C13	Malignant neoplasm of hypopharynx
C14	Malignant neoplasm of other and ill-defined sites of lip, oral cavity, and larynx
C14.0	Malignant neoplasm of pharynx, unspecified
C14.2	Malignant neoplasm of Waldeyer ring
C14.8	Malignant neoplasm of overlapping sites of lip, oral cavity, and pharynx

EPIDEMIOLOGY & DEMOGRAPHICS

INCIDENCE & PREVALENCE:

- In 2023, there were an estimated 54,540 new cases and 11,580 deaths in the U.S.[1]
- The incidence of oral cancers linked to alcohol and tobacco use has declined in developed countries, while those linked to the human papillomavirus (HPV), primarily HPV type 16, primarily cancers in the tonsils and base of tongue.[2] Differences between the traditional nonhuman papillomavirus–associated vs. HPV-associated oropharyngeal squamous cell carcinoma are summarized in Table 1.
- In Asian countries where chewing betel nut is customary, oral cancer accounts for up to 40% of cancers in some regions.

PREDOMINANT SEX & AGE:

- The ratio of oral cancer in males:females is 2.5:1 in the U.S.
- Black males have a higher early incidence in the 50-yr to 60-yr age group, but with increasing age, White men predominate.

RISK FACTORS (FIG. 1): The following factors are implicated in the development of oral cancer:

- Tobacco use
- HPV infection (primarily types 16 and 18)
- Alcohol
- Immune deficiency
- Radiation
- Betel nut consumption
- Solar radiation

GENETICS: The genes that are critically altered in OSCC include *TP53,* the retinoblastoma family, *p16* and cyclin *D1.* The *TP53, CCND1,* and *CDKN2A* genes are established cancer genes in HPV-negative cancers.[3] *TP53* and the genes encoding the Rb family are established cancer genes in HPV-positive cancers. Signaling pathways that are involved in the pathogenesis of oral cancers include that of the human epidermal receptor (HER) family, vascular endothelial growth factor (VEGF) receptor, and signal transducer and activator of transcription 3 (STAT 3). The tumor suppressor gene *TP53* is frequently mutated in HPV-negative tumors.

PHYSICAL FINDINGS & CLINICAL PRESENTATION

- Specific patient complaints may include the following: Oral ulcers or mass, choking,

TABLE 1 Differences between the Traditional Nonhuman Papillomavirus–Associated Versus Human Papillomavirus–Associated Oropharyngeal Squamous Cell Carcinoma

Variables	Traditional Non–HPV-Associated OPSCC	HPV-Associated OPSCC
Demographics	Older (age ≥60 yr); male:female = 3:2	Younger (age 40-60 yr); male:female = 3:1, Whites
Risk profile	Tobacco, alcohol	Minimal/no addiction habit, epidemiologic correlation with sexual history
Molecular biology	p16 inactivation, p53 mutation, higher mutation rates and genetic instability	p16 overexpression, wild-type p53, lower mutation rates
Pathology	Keratinizing SCC, well to moderate to poorly differentiated	Nonkeratinizing SCC, poorly differentiated
Clinical presentation	Less bulky nodes	Small/unknown primary with bulky, cystic, or multiple nodes
Prognosis	Guarded, 5-yr survivals ~40%-60%	Good, 5-yr survivals ~80%-90%
Prognostic variables	T- and N-category, margin, ENE, smoking	T-category, five or more metastatic nodes, margins (?)
Mode of recurrence	Locoregional recurrence more frequent	Locoregional recurrence infrequent, distant metastasis predominant mode

ENE, Extracapsular extension; *HPV,* human papillomavirus; *OPSCC,* oropharyngeal squamous cell carcinoma; *SCC,* squamous cell carcinoma.
From Flint PW et al: *Cummings otolaryngology, head and neck surgery,* ed 7, Philadelphia, 2021, Elsevier.

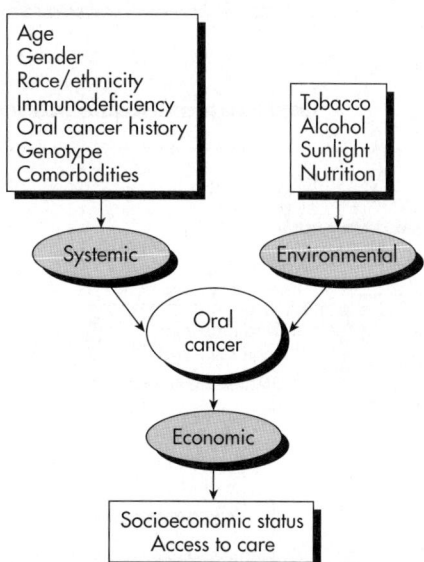

FIG. 1 Risk model for oral cancer. Oral cancer is a multifactorial disease process that includes systemic, environmental, and economic effects. The interplay of these variables ultimately leads to the incidence of this disease. The multifactorial nature of oral cancer should be addressed in the assessment of a patient's risk. (From Jones DL, Rankin KV: Oral cancer and associated risk factors. In Cappelli D, Mobley C [eds]: *Prevention in clinical oral health care,* St Louis, 2008, Elsevier, pp. 68-77.)

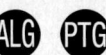

difficulty breathing, dysphagia, odynophagia, voice hoarseness, globus sensation, otalgia, ear or nose stuffiness, hemoptysis, trismus, neck mass, and pain in the head/neck region.
- Generalized symptoms and signs may include weight loss, fatigue, anorexia, altered mood, and sleep.
- Clinically, oral cancers can present as:
  1. Erythroplakia (flat red patch); can mimic inflammatory or traumatic lesions
  2. Leukoplakia (white patch; Fig. E2)
  3. Raised lesion
  4. Ulcerated lesion
  5. Warty lesion or growth

Dx DIAGNOSIS

DIFFERENTIAL DIAGNOSIS
- Oral leukoplakia
- Invasive fungal infections
- Chancre of early syphilis and gumma of tertiary syphilis
- Chronic ulcer

- Metastatic or locally invading cancers from sinuses or other sites of the body

WORKUP
- Primary workup includes either biopsy or fine-needle aspiration (FNA) of the presenting lesion or suspected neck lymph node for histopathologic analysis. HPV assessment with p16 immunohistochemical staining and confirmatory in situ hybridization (ISH) testing is performed when indicated for oropharynx primary tumors.
- Detailed examination of the oral cavity, pharynx, larynx, neck, ears, nose, and cranial nerves should be performed.
- Laryngoscopy and examination under anesthesia are commonly performed.
- Pretreatment evaluation of tumor size, the extent of invasion, and the presence or absence of regional lymph node metastases is critical for planning treatment.
- Laboratory workup can include CBC, complete chemistry panel, and thyroid function.

- Staging workup includes computed tomography (CT) or MRI imaging of the head and neck and a chest X-ray examination. If locoregional or advanced disease is a consideration, a PET scan is typically completed.
- The tumor, node, and metastasis (TNM) system is used for staging of OSCC and is subdivided according to primary tumor sites: (1) lip and oral cavity, (2) pharynx.

Rx TREATMENT

- Fig. 3 illustrates a management algorithm for squamous cell carcinoma of the oropharynx.
- Surgery, radiation therapy, and chemotherapy are treatment modalities involved in the treatment plan for OSCC.
- The use of supportive and special therapeutic modalities such as nutritional therapy including feeding gastrostomy, speech and swallowing therapy, reconstructive surgery, and speech prosthesis is required often.
- For treatment purposes OSCC are classified as early (T1 or T2 lesions), locoregional (T3 to T4

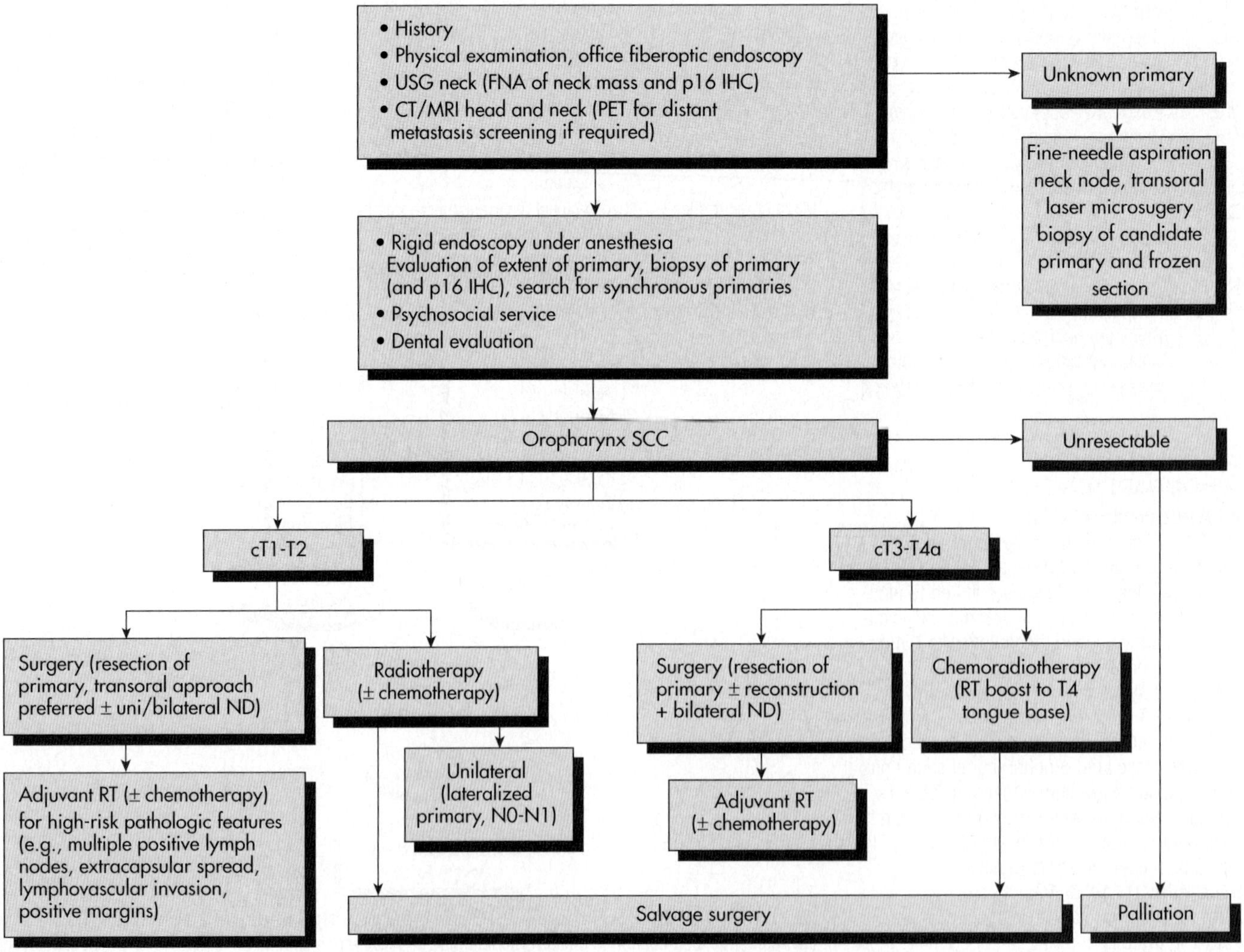

```
• History
• Physical examination, office fiberoptic endoscopy
• USG neck (FNA of neck mass and p16 IHC)
• CT/MRI head and neck (PET for distant
  metastasis screening if required)
                    │                              ──────────→  Unknown primary
                    ▼                                                   │
                                                                        ▼
• Rigid endoscopy under anesthesia                        Fine-needle aspiration
  Evaluation of extent of primary, biopsy of primary       neck node, transoral
  (and p16 IHC), search for synchronous primaries           laser microsugery
• Psychosocial service                                    biopsy of candidate
• Dental evaluation                                         primary and frozen
                    │                                             section
                    ▼
        Oropharynx SCC  ──────────────────→  Unresectable
         │                        │
         ▼                        ▼
      cT1-T2                   cT3-T4a
      │      │                 │        │
      ▼      ▼                 ▼        ▼
Surgery (resection of  Radiotherapy  Surgery (resection of  Chemoradiotherapy
primary, transoral     (± chemo-     primary ± reconstruction  (RT boost to T4
approach preferred ±   therapy)      + bilateral ND)          tongue base)
uni/bilateral ND)         │                 │
      │                   ▼                 ▼
Adjuvant RT (± chemo-  Unilateral      Adjuvant RT
therapy) for high-risk  (lateralized   (± chemotherapy)
pathologic features     primary, N0-N1)
(e.g., multiple positive lymph
nodes, extracapsular spread,
lymphovascular invasion,
positive margins)
                 Salvage surgery                          Palliation
```

FIG. 3 Management algorithm for squamous cell carcinoma *(SCC)* of the oropharynx. *CT,* Computed tomography; *cT#,* clinical tumor stage; *FNA,* fine-needle aspiration; *IHC,* immunohistochemistry; *MRI,* magnetic resonance imaging; *ND,* neck dissection; *PET,* positron emission tomography; *RT,* radiotherapy; *USG,* ultrasonography. (From Flint PW et al: *Cummings otolaryngology, head and neck surgery,* ed 7, Philadelphia, 2021, Elsevier.)

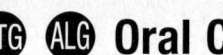
O

or any N), or metastatic (M1) stages. Site-specific TNM staging is done as per the primary tumor site (e.g., oral cavity, oropharynx, hypopharynx, etc.).

- After staging completion, the initial treatment considerations include:[4,5]
  1. Determination of primary tumor resectability
  2. Management of neck nodes
  3. Intent of radiation therapy (curative vs. palliative)
  4. Need for organ preservation
  5. Need for reconstructive surgery
  6. Need for chemotherapy
  7. HPV status of tumor
- Localized tumors (stage I or II) can be approached by initial surgical resection or definitive radiotherapy. Resectable locoregionally advanced tumors (stage III and localized IV) are typically approached by upfront surgery followed by adjuvant radiation and/or chemotherapy. Unresectable patients are treated with definitive chemotherapy and radiotherapy. Patients with distant metastatic disease are treated with systemic chemotherapy and immunotherapy, while locally recurrent tumors can be approached with either surgery or systemic therapy or both.
- Surgery is typically associated with less long-term morbidity than radiation therapy. Surgical therapy traditionally involved wide-exposure approaches (mandibulotomy, transpharyngeal access). Newer surgical techniques allow tumor resection through the mouth. Recently, transoral robotic surgery (TORS) has been developed to improve access to oropharyngeal squamous cell carcinomas with excellent oncologic outcomes.[6]
  1. Acute surgical complications can include infection, bleeding, aspiration, wound breakdown, fistula, and flap loss.
  2. Surgical procedures can cause functional deficits in speech and swallowing, but these adverse effects can be minimized by appropriate reconstruction and prostheses.
  3. Recent randomized trial data results have demonstrated equivalent results with sentinel lymph node biopsy vs. neck dissection in early (T1 to T2) oral cancer cases.
  4. Newer approaches with the goal of toxicity reduction include dysphagia-optimised intensity modulated radiotherapy (DO-IMRT) and deescalated radiotherapy. Results from a randomized trial have demonstrated that DO-IMRT significantly improves patient-reported swallowing function compared with standard IMRT.[7] Among patients with HPV-positive OSCC, early data about deescalated radiotherapy dosing has been associated with encouraging survival and toxicity outcomes.[8]

- Definitive radiation therapy is reserved for patients who cannot tolerate surgery or when surgical resection would result in severe functional impairment.
  1. Radiation therapy options include external beam radiation and brachytherapy.
  2. Side effects include mucositis, radiation dermatitis, dysgeusia, dysphagia, dental caries and decay, and xerostomia.
  3. Late complications can include skin/soft tissue atrophy and fibrosis, hypothyroidism, osteoradionecrosis, and trismus.
- Systemic chemotherapy can be administered alone or in combination with radiotherapy, depending on the disease stage. Agents typically used include cisplatin, carboplatin, 5-fluorouracil, taxanes, and the epidermal growth factor receptor (EGFR) antibody cetuximab.
- For locally advanced OSCC, the combination of cisplatin and radiotherapy is the regimen of choice. Recent reports have demonstrated similar outcomes with every-3-wk administered standard-dose cisplatin and once-weekly administered low-dose cisplatin, but with lower toxicity rates.[7] Cetuximab was demonstrated to be inferior to cisplatin when used concurrently with radiotherapy in patients with locally advanced HPV-positive oral cancers. In selected patients with large primary tumors or bulky nodal disease, neoadjuvant TPF chemotherapy (docetaxel, cisplatin, and 5-FU) may be used before chemoradiotherapy administration.
- Patients who have metastatic cancers or unresectable locoregional recurrences usually are treated with systemic therapy.
- Chemoimmunotherapy consisting of platinum plus 5-FU chemotherapy in combination with pembrolizumab has superior survival outcomes in patients with recurrent or metastatic head and neck cancer.[8] Alternatively, doublet chemotherapy regimens (platinum plus either 5-fluorouracil or platinum plus taxane) can be combined with the EGFR–targeting antibody cetuximab in this setting.

- In patients who have not received checkpoint inhibitor therapy previously, nivolumab and pembrolizumab have been shown to improve survival outcomes after failure of first-line chemotherapy.
- The negative predictive value of posttreatment PET imaging in patients with locally advanced cancer who have been treated with chemoradiotherapy is 98% to 99%.

DISPOSITION

- Prognosis depends on the staging and resectability of the primary tumor as well as on patient performance status.
- Tumor HPV status is a strong and independent prognostic factor for survival among patients with base of tongue and oropharyngeal cancer.

REFERRAL

Referral to multidisciplinary head and neck cancer team consisting of ENT or head/neck surgeon, radiation oncologist, medical oncologist, speech therapy, and dietitian.

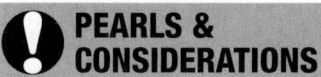 **PEARLS & CONSIDERATIONS**

COMMENTS

- Oral cavity cancer is the sixth most common cancer globally.
- Biopsy with HPV-status assessment is the key for accurate diagnosis.
- Posttreatment rehabilitation and surveillance is important.

PREVENTION

- Encourage patients to stop using any type of tobacco and drinking alcohol.
- Examine oral cavities at annual checkups and work up suspicious lesions.

REFERENCES & SUGGESTED READINGS

Available at eBooks.Health.Elsevier.com.

RELATED CONTENT

Mouth Cancer (Patient Information)

AUTHOR: **RITESH RATHORE, MD**

ⓘ BASIC INFORMATION

DEFINITION
Oral hairy leukoplakia (OHL) is a painless, white, nonremovable, plaque-like lesion typically located on the lateral aspect of the tongue.

SYNONYMS
Oral hairy leukoplakia
OHL

ICD-10CM CODE
K13.3   Hairy leukoplakia

EPIDEMIOLOGY & DEMOGRAPHICS
INCIDENCE & PREVALENCE: Epstein-Barr virus (EBV) is implicated in the etiology of OHL, and the incidence of EBV seroprevalence is high in individuals who are HIV seropositive. OHL may also occur in other immunosuppressed individuals, for example, organ transplant recipients, as well as individuals receiving systemic or inhaled steroids.[1]
RISK FACTORS: OHL is usually found in HIV-seropositive individuals but may also be identified in smokers and other immunocompromised patients, such as transplant recipients (particularly renal and bone marrow transplants) and patients taking steroids.[2] Diagnosis of OHL is an indication to test for HIV.

PHYSICAL FINDINGS & CLINICAL PRESENTATION
- Varying morphology and appearance (Fig. E1), which may change daily.
- May be unilateral or bilateral.
- White plaques can be small with fine, vertical corrugations on the lateral margin of the tongue (Fig. 2). The plaques from OHL are adherent to the tongue surface (in contrast to candidal plaques, which may be easily scraped off).
- Irregular surface; may have prominent folds or projection, occasionally markedly resembling hairs.

- May spread to cover the entire dorsal surface or spread onto the ventral surface of the tongue where the lesions usually appear flat.
- Rarely, lesions can manifest on the soft palate, buccal mucosa, or posterior oropharynx.
- Usually asymptomatic, but some patients have mouth pain, soreness, or a burning sensation; impaired taste, or difficulty eating; others complain of its unsightly appearance.[3]

ETIOLOGY
EBV is implicated in the etiology of OHL. It likely results from unchecked lytic replication of EBV in the epithelium of keratinized cells. OHL differs from most EBV-related diseases in that infection is predominantly lytic rather than latent, with abundant virus production resulting in cell lysis.

OHL should be differentiated from oral leukoplakia, which is a potentially premalignant condition.

Ⓓ DIAGNOSIS

DIFFERENTIAL DIAGNOSIS
- Oral homogenous/nonhomogeneous leukoplakia
- *Candida albicans*
- Lichen planus
- Idiopathic leukoplakia
- White sponge nevus
- Dysplasia
- Squamous cell carcinoma

WORKUP
Requires physical examination and testing for HIV

LABORATORY TESTS
The *provisional* diagnosis is clinical and based on:
- Visual inspection
- Inability to scrape the lesion off the tongue with a blade
- Failure to respond to antifungal therapy
The *presumptive* diagnosis requires biopsy and histologic demonstration of:
- Epithelial hyperplasia with hairs
- Absence of inflammatory cell infiltrate

The *definitive* diagnosis requires:
- In situ hybridization of histologic or cytologic specimens revealing EBV DNA *or*
- Electron microscopy of specimens revealing herpes-like particles
- Measurement of the DNA content in cells of oral leukoplakia may be used to predict the risk of oral carcinoma
- NOTE: Specimens obtained from lesions may demonstrate hyphae of *Candida albicans,* which may coexist and potentiate EBV-induced OHL[3]

℞ TREATMENT

NONPHARMACOLOGIC THERAPY
OHL is usually asymptomatic and requires no specific therapy. It may resolve spontaneously and is generally benign in HIV-seropositive patients.

ACUTE GENERAL Rx
- Antiretroviral therapy (ART) has considerably decreased the frequency of oral lesions caused by opportunistic infections in HIV-seropositive individuals.
- Topical retinoids (0.1% vitamin A) may improve the appearance of OHL-affected oral surfaces through their dekeratinizing and immunomodulation effects; however, they are expensive, and prolonged use may result in a burning sensation over the treated area.
- Topical podophyllin resin 25% solution has been reported to induce resolution.
- Surgical excision and cryotherapy may help, but the lesions may recur.
- High-dose acyclovir 800 mg five times per day, valacyclovir 1000 mg three times daily, famciclovir 500 mg three times daily, ganciclovir 1000 mg three times daily, or foscarnet 40 mg/kg intravenous three times daily will cause lesions to resolve but only temporarily.[3]

REFERRAL
Referral to ear, nose, throat (ENT) or oral surgeon for biopsy of tongue to confirm diagnosis

❗ PEARLS & CONSIDERATIONS

- OHL may be the presenting sign of patients infected with HIV who are unaware of their status.
- The incidence of OHL has decreased significantly in the era of antiretroviral therapy.

REFERENCES
Available at eBooks.Health.Elsevier.com.

RELATED CONTENT
Acquired Immunodeficiency Syndrome (Related Key Topic)
Oral Hairy Leukoplakia (Patient Information)
Epstein-Barr Virus Infection (Related Key Topic)
Human Immunodeficiency Virus (Related Key Topic)

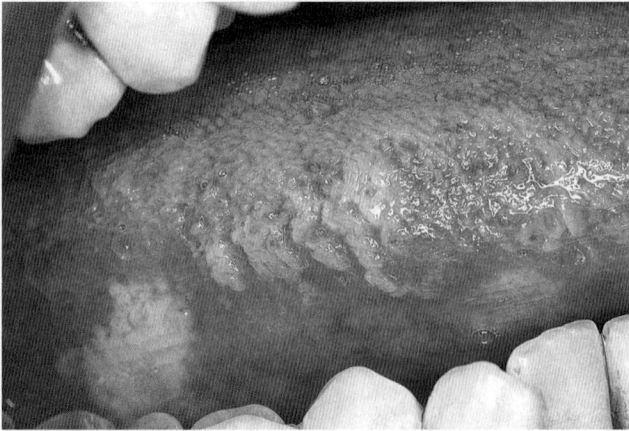

FIG. 2 Oral hairy leukoplakia along the lateral tongue margin is characterized by vertically corrugated keratotic ridges. (From Flint PW et al: *Cummings otolaryngology, head and neck surgery,* ed 7, Philadelphia, 2021, Elsevier.)

AUTHORS: **SAJEEV HANDA, MD, SFHM** and **ANNA HARDESTY, MD**

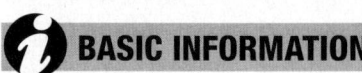

BASIC INFORMATION

DEFINITION

Orthostatic hypotension (OH) is defined as the presence of at least one of the following:
- Decrease in systolic blood pressure by ≥20 mm Hg *or*
- Decrease in diastolic blood pressure by ≥10 mm Hg, within 3 min of standing
  It is a physical sign that requires further investigation to discern its underlying etiology.
  Recent studies have shown that blood pressure measurements within 1 min might be more useful in predicting fractures, falls, and other adverse events and that for most patients, assessment within 1 min of standing rather than waiting for 3 min may be sufficient.[1]

SYNONYMS

Postural hypotension
OH

ICD-10CM CODE

I95.1   Orthostatic hypotension

EPIDEMIOLOGY & DEMOGRAPHICS

- The incidence of OH is increased in older people. Surveys have shown OH to be present in approximately 20% of adults over 65 yr of age.
- Also, higher incidence noted in those with diseases associated with autonomic dysfunction (e.g., Parkinson disease, diabetes mellitus).
- OH may cause up to 30% of all syncopal events in the elderly, and OH is associated with an increased risk of heart failure among those aged 45 to 55 yr and an increased risk of cardiovascular disease and all-cause mortality among those aged 55 yr and older.
- OH can be a common cause and/or a contributor to hospitalization in older adult patients.[2]
- There is an association between OH and cognitive dysfunction among older adults.

PHYSICAL FINDINGS & CLINICAL PRESENTATION

- Symptoms may include dizziness, lightheadedness, syncope, visual and auditory disturbances, weakness, diaphoresis, pallor, and nausea.
- OH may be asymptomatic, especially in older hypertensive patients with autonomic dysfunction. These patients tend to have systolic hypertension when seated or supine.
- Associated with increased autonomic activity during meals (from increased splanchnic blood flow), exercise, prolonged standing, and hot weather.
- Supine and nocturnal hypertension in patients with OH may indicate an underlying autonomic dysfunction.

ETIOLOGY

- There are two main mechanisms for OH: Autonomic dysfunction and volume depletion.

- Normal response: Assumption of an upright posture results in the pooling of ∼500 ml of blood in the lower extremities as a result of gravity and decreased venous return, decreased cardiac output, and decreased arterial pressure. The consequent increase in sympathetic tone due to increased carotid baroreceptor activity causes arterial and venous constriction as well as positive inotropic and chronotropic effects, thereby limiting the fall in upright blood pressure. Peripheral vasoconstriction is also mediated by increased activity of the renin-angiotensin system and decreased activity of atrial natriuretic factor.
- Autonomic dysfunction: Impairment of the baroreceptor reflex, as in central (e.g., Parkinson disease) or peripheral autonomic dysfunction (such as diabetes) and aging, may cause OH because decreased blood pressure cannot be counteracted by the aforementioned regulatory mechanisms.
- Volume depletion: May be caused by diuretics, vomiting, hemorrhage, and hyperglycemia. Mechanism of OH in these patients is similar to what is described earlier, with failure of the regulatory mechanisms kicking in.

DIAGNOSIS

DIFFERENTIAL DIAGNOSIS (BOX 1)

Common:
- Medications: Antihypertensives, antidepressants (tricyclics), antipsychotics (phenothiazines), alcohol, narcotics, barbiturates, insulin, nitrates, PDE-5 inhibitors, alpha-adrenergic antagonists
- Reduced intravascular volume (hemorrhage, dehydration, hyperglycemia, hypoalbuminemia)
- Postprandial effect (especially in the elderly)
- Vasovagal syncope
- Deconditioning
- Central autonomic dysfunction (Parkinson disease)
- Peripheral autonomic dysfunction (diabetes mellitus, Guillain-Barré syndrome)

Uncommon:
- Central autonomic dysfunction (Shy-Drager syndrome)
- Postganglionic autonomic dysfunction: Impaired norepinephrine release
- Autoimmune autonomic dysfunction: Nicotinic acetylcholine receptor autoantibodies
- Paraneoplastic autonomic dysfunction: Anti-Hu antibodies (in small-cell lung cancer)
- Postural tachycardia syndrome (POTS): Usually occurs in young women; an abnormally large increase in heart rate is observed in the upright position, caused by increased venous pooling from autonomic dysfunction of the lower extremities, but blood pressure is not affected because of an excess of plasma norepinephrine
- Impaired cardiac output (myocardial infarction, aortic stenosis, arrhythmias)
- Cerebrovascular accident
- Adrenal insufficiency
- Deconditioning
- Carotid sinus hypersensitivity

- Anxiety, panic attacks
- Seizures
- Sepsis
- Idiopathic

WORKUP

- Obtain a detailed history including medication list, recent history of potential volume loss, medical history of congestive heart failure, malignancy, diabetes and alcoholism, evidence on history and physical examination of parkinsonism, ataxia, peripheral neuropathy, or dysautonomia.[3]
- In assessing patients for OH, blood pressure measurement changes going from supine to standing are more sensitive than going from sitting to standing.[4]
- Measure supine blood pressure after the patient has been resting comfortably. The duration of time that the patient should spend supine and standing when measuring OH is controversial. Limited evidence supports having the patient remain supine for 5 to 10 min before obtaining the supine blood pressure, followed by blood pressure measurement

---

BOX 1 Differential Diagnosis of Orthostatic Hypotension

Autonomic Disorders
Pure autonomic failure
Multiple system atrophy
Familial dysautonomia
Dopamine β-hydroxylase deficiency
Baroreflex failure
Secondary autonomic neuropathies

Hypovolemia Disorders
Hemorrhage or plasma loss
Overdiuresis
Overdialysis
Idiopathic hypovolemia

Endocrinologic Disorders
Addison disease
Hypoaldosteronism
Pheochromocytoma
Renovascular hypertension

Vascular Insufficiency
Varicose veins
Absent venous valves
Arteriovenous malformations

Vasodilator Excess
Mastocytosis (histamine, prostaglandin D_2)
Hyperbradykininism (bradykinin)
Carcinoid (bradykinin)
Hypermagnesemia

Paroxysmal Autonomic Syncope
Glossopharyngeal syncope
Micturition syncope
Carotid sinus syncope
Swallow syncope
Cough syncope
Bezold-Jarisch reflex activation

Miscellaneous
Drugs and toxins
Stokes-Adams attacks
Gastrectomy
Hypokinesia, weightlessness, bed rest

From Jankovic J et al: *Bradley and Daroff's neurology in clinical practice*, ed 8, Philadelphia, 2022, Elsevier.

within 1 min of standing and again after 3 min of standing. The blood pressure cuff must be held at the level of the right atrium; holding the cuff below this level will result in a 5 to 10 mm Hg underestimation of blood pressure.
- Thorough neurologic examination should be performed.

LABORATORY TESTS
- Hemoglobin and hematocrit
- Consider blood urea nitrogen/creatinine if suspecting dehydration as the cause
- ECG if suspecting underlying cardiac cause
- Consider when treatable causes of OH have been ruled out:
  1. Blood pressure and heart rate monitoring with a tilt-table test
  2. Plasma norepinephrine measurements (to distinguish postganglionic from preganglionic autonomic dysfunction)
  3. Other methods, which use the Valsalva maneuver or measure sweating as indirect means of evaluating the autonomic nervous system

IMAGING STUDIES
None

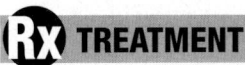 **TREATMENT**

NONPHARMACOLOGIC THERAPY[4]
- Patient education (leg crossing, prolonged sitting before first standing in the morning, avoid excessive straining and hot baths)
- High-salt diet (e.g., bouillon cubes); caution if history of heart failure
- Liberal fluid intake
- Take needed antihypertensive medications at different times of the day
- Raise the head of the bed at night
- Compression stockings (to include splanchnic circulation)
- Multiple low-carbohydrate meals to avoid postprandial OH
- Avoid large carbohydrate loads and excess alcohol consumption

ACUTE GENERAL Rx
- Correction of volume status and impairment of cerebral perfusion.
- Review medication list and attempt to eliminate those potentially contributing to OH.

CHRONIC Rx
- Fludrocortisone: 0.1 mg/day (may combine with an alpha-1 agonist to lower the dose of

each); monitor for electrolyte disturbances and supine hypertension
- Midodrine (alpha-1 agonist): 10 mg three times a day; monitor for supine hypertension
- Erythropoietin (consider if anemic)
- Caffeine (for postprandial hypotension)
- Table 1 summarizes management of OH in older adults

OTHER TREATMENTS
- Pyridostigmine (enhances renal sodium reabsorption): 0.2 to 0.6 mg/day (not FDA approved for this indication)
- Octreotide: 300 to 600 mg/day (not FDA approved for this indication)
- Indomethacin (prostaglandin inhibitor)
- DDAVP (experimental)
- Droxidopa (used for patients with autonomic dysfunction to increase the availability of norepinephrine) has been FDA approved for treatment of adults with symptomatic neurogenic OH caused by primary autonomic failure or nondiabetic autonomic neuropathy

⚠ PEARLS & CONSIDERATIONS

COMMENTS
- The presence of OH should always trigger a search for an underlying etiology.
- OH is diagnosed by observing changes in blood pressure, not heart rate.
- Volume depletion should cause an increased heart rate on standing; a lack of heart rate response in this setting suggests autonomic dysfunction.
- Pharmacotherapy with mineralocorticoids may require concomitant potassium replenishment and monitoring for hypertension.
- Evidence to support the efficacy of pharmacologic interventions to treat OH, including midodrine, is limited.
- The etiology of OH is often multifactorial in older patients, but increased susceptibility to volume depletion due to decreased baroreceptor reflexes frequently contributes. Chronic vitamin D deficiency is associated with the development of OH.
- Intensive blood pressure control did not increase injurious falls compared with controls among community-dwelling older adults participating in the Systolic Blood Pressure Intervention Trial (SPRINT).
- The physical examination of patients with dizziness, gait disturbance, and/or falls should include an assessment for OH. OH is

TABLE 1 Management of Orthostatic Hypotension in Older Adults

Identify and treat correctable causes.

Reduce or eliminate drugs causing orthostatic hypotension.

Avoid situations that may exacerbate orthostatic hypotension.
- Standing motionless
- Prolonged recumbency
- Large meals
- Hot weather
- Hot showers
- Straining at stool or with voiding
- Isometric exercise
- Ingesting alcohol
- Hyperventilation
- Dehydration

Raise the head of the bed to a 5- to 20-degree angle.

Wear waist-high, custom-fitted, elastic stockings and an abdominal binder.

Participate in physical conditioning exercises.

Participate in controlled postural exercises using the tilt table.

Avoid diuretics and eat salt-containing fluids (unless congestive heart failure is present).

Drug therapy:
- Caffeine
- Fludrocortisone
- Midodrine
- Desmopressin
- Erythropoietin

From Fillit HM: *Brocklehurst's textbook of geriatric medicine and gerontology,* ed 8, Philadelphia, 2017, Elsevier.

an independent predictor of unexplained falls in older adults.
- Because OH may be asymptomatic, physical examination of those at risk must include assessment of blood pressure in both the supine and upright positions.

REFERENCES
Available at eBooks.Health.Elsevier.com.

AUTHOR: **HUSSAIN R. KHAWAJA, MD, FACP**

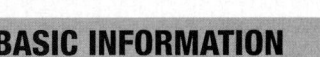 BASIC INFORMATION

DEFINITION

Osteomyelitis is an acute or chronic infection of the bone secondary to the hematogenous or contiguous source of infection or direct traumatic inoculation, which is usually bacterial.

SYNONYM

Bone infection

ICD-10CM CODES
M86	Osteomyelitis
M86.0	Acute hematogenous osteomyelitis
M86.1	Other acute osteomyelitis
M86.2	Subacute osteomyelitis
M86.3	Chronic multifocal osteomyelitis
M86.6	Other chronic osteomyelitis
M86.9	Osteomyelitis, unspecified

EPIDEMIOLOGY & DEMOGRAPHICS

PREDOMINANT SEX: Male > female
PREDOMINANT AGE: All ages

PHYSICAL FINDINGS & CLINICAL PRESENTATION

HEMATOGENOUS OSTEOMYELITIS:
- Usually occurs in tibia/fibula (children)
- Localized inflammation: Often secondary to trauma with accompanying hematoma or cellulitis
- Abrupt fever
- Lethargy
- Irritability
- Pain in involved bone

VERTEBRAL OSTEOMYELITIS:
- Usually hematogenous
- Fever: 50%
- Localized pain/tenderness. Back pain is the most common initial symptom (86% of cases)
- Neurologic defects: Motor/sensory (sensory loss, weakness, radiculopathy)

CONTIGUOUS OSTEOMYELITIS:
- Direct inoculation
- Associated with trauma, fractures, surgical fixation
- Chronic infection of skin/soft tissue
- Fever, drainage from surgical site

CHRONIC OSTEOMYELITIS:
- Bone pain
- Sinus tract drainage, nonhealing ulcer
- Chronic low-grade fever
- Chronic localized pain

ETIOLOGY

- MSSA: Methicillin-sensitive *Staphylococcus aureus*
- MRSA: Methicillin-resistant *S. aureus*
- *Pseudomonas aeruginosa*
- *Enterobacteriaceae*
- *Streptococcus pyogenes*
- *Enterococcus*
- Mycobacteria
- Fungi
- Coagulase-negative staphylococci
- *Salmonella* (in sickle cell disease)

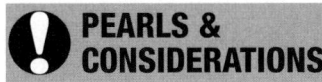 DIAGNOSIS

DIFFERENTIAL DIAGNOSIS

- Gaucher disease
- Bone infarction
- Charcot joint
- Fracture

WORKUP

- Erythrocyte sedimentation rate (ESR), C-reactive protein: Nondiagnostic but if significantly elevated they increase the pretest probability of osteomyelitis and can be useful in monitoring therapeutic response.
- Blood culturing, CBC with differential.
- Bone culture. A culture of a biopsy specimen has a significantly higher overall diagnostic yield than does a blood culture. Bone samples should be cultured for aerobic and anaerobic bacteria and for fungi.
- Pathologic evaluation of bone biopsy for acute/chronic changes consistent with necrosis or acute inflammation.
- Polymerase chain reaction (PCR) analysis of specimens obtained by means of biopsy or puncture may be useful for organisms that are difficult to identify (anaerobic bacteria, *Bartonella* sp., *Kingella kingae*); however, broad-range PCR has suboptimal sensitivity and specificity due to contamination and may not provide sufficient information on the susceptibility of the microorganisms to antibiotics.
- Probe to bone to detect osteomyelitis in diabetic feet: The theory is that if a probe can reach to bone, then so can bacteria. The probe is a sterile, metal surgical probe into diabetic foot ulcer and is positive if a hard gritty surface is felt inside. A systematic review concluded that the probe to bone test can accurately rule in diabetic foot osteomyelitis in high-risk patients and rule out osteomyelitis in low-risk patients.[1]

IMAGING STUDIES

- Bone radiograph examination (Fig. E1): Initial study but not sensitive in early osteomyelitis as may not show changes for as much as 2 wk
- MRI with and without contrast (Fig. E2): Most accurate imaging study. Computed tomography (CT) only if patient has contraindication to MRI
- Triple-phase technetium-99m bone scan (Fig. E3) when MRI is unavailable or contraindicated. Typically positive within a few days after onset of symptoms but accuracy is lower than that of MRI
- Positron emission tomography (PET) scanning with ^{18}F-fluorodeoxyglucose has high accuracy (similar to MRI) and is useful in patients with metallic implants
- Gallium scan (Ga-67) scintigraphy with single-photon emission CT (SPECT) has higher accuracy than bone scan but is less sensitive for detection of epidural abscess in vertebral osteomyelitis. Useful when MRI is contraindicated or unavailable
- Indium-111–labeled leukocyte scintigraphy scan; low sensitivity (<20%) for vertebral osteomyelitis

- Table 1 summarizes imaging findings in osteomyelitis

⟨Rx⟩ TREATMENT

- Surgical debridement in biopsy-positive cases will guide direction for antibiotic therapy. This will vary with type of osteomyelitis. Duration of therapy is usually 4 to 6 wk for acute osteomyelitis; chronic osteomyelitis may need a longer course of medication
- Orthopedic hardware should be removed if possible
- *S. aureus* (MSSA): Cefazolin IV, nafcillin IV, vancomycin IV (in patient allergic to penicillin)
- *S. aureus* (MRSA): Vancomycin IV, linezolid IV or PO, daptomycin IV
- *Streptococcus* spp: Ceftriaxone, IV penicillin G in sensitive species
- *P. aeruginosa:* Cefepime, imipenem/cilastatin, or meropenem
- *Enterobacteriaceae:* Ceftriaxone or ertapenem
- Anaerobes: Clindamycin, piperacillin-tazobactam, cefotetan, or metronidazole
- In general, higher doses of antibiotics are necessary in order to achieve optimal bone penetration
- Table 2 summarizes antimicrobial therapy for selected microorganisms in osteomyelitis. A retrospective analysis revealed that in diabetic foot osteomyelitis adjunctive rifampin is associated with improved amputation-free survival
- Hyperbaric oxygen therapy: May be useful in chronic osteomyelitis
- Wound-assisted vacuum device may help closure of wound
- Surgical debridement of all devitalized bone and tissue
- Immobilization of affected bone (plaster, traction) if bone is unstable
- Recommended antibiotic therapy for osteomyelitis in children is summarized in Table E3

DISPOSITION

Acute hematogenous osteomyelitis usually resolves without recurrence or long-term complications, but contiguous focus osteomyelitis, bone infections from open fractures, or osteomyelitis frequently recurs.

REFERRAL

- To an orthopedic surgeon if chronic osteomyelitis with need for bone debridement, bone grafting, or stabilization of infected tissue adjacent to a bone fracture
- To an infectious disease specialist for appropriate treatment for difficult-to-treat or recalcitrant infections
- To a hyperbaric oxygen chamber service for nonhealing, chronic osteomyelitis

ⓘ PEARLS & CONSIDERATIONS

- Chronic osteomyelitis is one of the most challenging infections to treat; the high failure rate is a consequence of poor vascular supply, nondistensible bone tissue, and limited penetration of bone tissue.

TABLE 1 Imaging Findings in Osteomyelitis

	Plain Radiograph	CT	MRI	NM
Acute	Minimal findings Soft-tissue swelling may be seen	Not useful	Bone marrow edema can occur as early as 24-48 h, seen as low T1 and high T2 signal	May show increased uptake, but takes a few days
Subacute	Lucent or sclerotic lesion, periosteal reaction, soft-tissue swelling	Cortical and marrow abnormalities including abscess, periosteal reaction, soft-tissue edema, and abscess	Bone marrow changes, cortical abnormalities seen as thickening, bone abscess, periosteal reaction, increased T2 signal in soft tissues, abscess formation. Postgadolinium T1W sequences outline abscess cavities clearly	Three-phase bone scintigram, indium-111 WBC scan and combined studies are useful, especially to assess multifocal involvement. PET-CT generally not used in this context, but may be useful in exceptional circumstances
Chronic	Bone sclerosis, cortical thickening, sequestrum and cloaca, bone destruction, resorption, and deformities	Much better than plain radiographs to demonstrate cloaca and sequestrum, periosteal new bone formation, and abscess	Better soft-tissue and bone marrow resolution to demonstrate medullary and cortical changes, sequestra and cloaca well demonstrated, useful to outline soft-tissue abscess, and sinus tracts	Generally useful if there is a problem with diagnosis. Combined WBC and bone marrow scintigram is useful. May highlight multiple sites of involvement

CT, Computed tomography; *MRI,* magnetic resonance imaging; *NM,* nuclear medicine; *PET,* positron emission tomography; *WBC,* white blood cell.
From Grant LA: *Grainger & Allison's diagnostic radiology essentials,* ed 2, Philadelphia, 2019, Elsevier.

TABLE 2 Antimicrobial Therapy for Selected Microorganisms in Chronic Osteomyelitis in Adults

Microorganism	First Choice*	Alternative Choice
Methicillin/oxacillin/nafcillin-sensitive staphylococci	Nafcillin sodium or oxacillin sodium 1.5-2 g IV q4h for 4-6 wk *or* cefazolin 1-2 g IV q8h for 4-6 wk	Vancomycin 15 mg/kg IV q12h for 4-6 wk
Methicillin/oxacillin/nafcillin-resistant staphylococci (MRSA)	Vancomycin[†] 15 mg/kg IV q12h for 4-6 wk *or* daptomycin 6 mg/kg IV q24h	Linezolid 600 mg PO/IV q12h *or* levofloxacin[†] 500-750 mg PO/IV daily, plus rifampin 600-900 mg PO for 6 wk if susceptible to both drugs
Penicillin-sensitive streptococci	Aqueous penicillin G 20 epto[6] U/24 h IV either continuously or in six equally divided daily doses *or* ceftriaxone 1-2 g IV q24h *or* cefazolin 1-2 g IV q8h for 4-6 wk	Vancomycin 15 mg/kg IV q12h for 4-6 wk
Enterococci	Aqueous crystalline penicillin G 20 × 10[6] U/24 h IV either continuously or in six equally divided daily doses *or* ampicillin sodium 12 g/24 h IV either continuously or in six equally divided daily doses; the addition of gentamicin sulfate 1 mg/kg IV or IM q8h for 1-2 wk is *optional*	Vancomycin[†] 15 mg/kg IV q12h; the addition of gentamicin sulfate 1 mg/kg IV or IM q8h for 1-2 wk is *optional*
Enterobacteriaceae	Ceftriaxone 1-2 g IV q24h for 4-6 wk or ertapenem 1 g IV q24h	Ciprofloxacin 500-750 mg PO q12h for 4-6 wk or levofloxacin 500-750 mg PO q24h
Pseudomonas aeruginosa	Cefepime 2 g IV q12h, meropenem 1 g IV q8h, or imipenem 500 mg IV q6h for 4-6 wk	Ciprofloxacin 750 mg PO q12h for 4-6 wk or ceftazidime 2 g IV q8h

IM, Intramuscular; *IV,* intravenous; *MRSA,* methicillin-resistant *Staphylococcus aureus; PO,* by mouth.
*Antimicrobial selection should be based on in vitro sensitivity data, as well as allergies, intolerances, and drug interactions in individual patients.
[†]Doses shown are based on normal renal and hepatic function and may need to be adjusted or serum levels monitored (vancomycin).

- Parenteral antibiotics are usually chosen initially, but oral fluoroquinolones have good bone penetration and may be used in stable patients. A recent trial comparing oral versus IV antibiotics for bone and joint infections found that oral antibiotic therapy is not inferior to IV antibiotic therapy when used during the first 6 wk for complex orthopedic infections.

- The optimal duration of therapy for vertebral osteomyelitis is unclear. Trials comparing 6 wk to 12 wk of antibiotic treatment in pyogenic vertebral osteomyelitis showed similar cure rates (91%) in both groups.

REFERENCE

Available at eBooks.Health.Elsevier.com.

RELATED CONTENT

Osteomyelitis (Patient Information)

AUTHOR: **GLENN G. FORT, MD, MPH**

BASIC INFORMATION

DEFINITION

Osteoporosis is a skeletal disorder characterized by a progressive loss of bone mass and a decline in bone density and quality that results in increased bone fragility and a higher fracture risk. Poor bone mass acquisition during adolescence and bone loss during the sixth decade of life are the main processes responsible for osteoporosis. The various types are as follows:

PRIMARY OSTEOPOROSIS: Primary osteoporosis is the loss of bone mass due to aging and decreased gonadal function, not to any other chronic illness.

- Idiopathic osteoporosis: Unknown pathogenesis; may occur in children and young adults.
- Type I osteoporosis (postmenopausal women): Occurs after menopause due to an abrupt decline in estrogen production. It is characterized by accelerated and disproportionate trabecular bone loss and is associated with fractures of the spine, hip, and wrist.
- Type II osteoporosis (involutional): Occurs in both men and women aged >70 yr due to the progressively negative balance between bone formation and resorption. It is characterized by both trabecular and cortical bone loss and associated with fractures of the spine, long bones, and hip.

SECONDARY OSTEOPOROSIS: Secondary osteoporosis is bone loss due to another chronic condition such as thyroxine excess, hyperparathyroidism, malignancies, gastrointestinal disease, medications, renal failure, and connective tissue diseases (see "Differential Diagnosis").

ICD-10CM CODES
M81.0	Age-related osteoporosis without current pathological fracture
M81.4	Drug-induced osteoporosis
M81.5	Idiopathic osteoporosis
M81.6	Localized osteoporosis

EPIDEMIOLOGY & DEMOGRAPHICS

PREVALENCE (IN U.S.):
- Affects more than 10 million people in the U.S.
- Annual incidence of osteoporotic fractures exceeds 1.5 million in the U.S. (70% women)
- Twice as common in women than in men
- Health care costs in excess of $17 billion annually
- Health inequities in screening and treatment: Black women are less likely to be screened for osteoporosis and receive fewer prescriptions for osteoporosis treatment after diagnosis when compared with white women

RISK FACTORS:
- Female sex
- Postmenopausal state
- Advanced age
- Small body frame, low body weight (<58 kg)
- White or Hispanic ancestry
- Sedentary lifestyle
- Nulliparity
- Calcium deficiency
- Previous low-trauma fracture
- Parental history of hip fracture
- Tobacco use
- Excess alcohol use (>3 drinks per day)
- Long-term glucocorticoid use
- Chronic disease states; e.g., primary ovarian insufficiency, diabetes mellitus, androgen deficiency, inflammatory bowel disease, hyperthyroidism, hypercortisolism
Conditions and drugs associated with osteoporosis are summarized in Table 1.

PHYSICAL FINDINGS & CLINICAL PRESENTATION
- Most commonly asymptomatic.
- Insidious and progressive development of dorsal kyphosis *(dowager's hump)*, loss of height, and skeletal pain typically associated with fracture; reduced gait speed or grip strength; other physical findings related to other conditions with associated increased risk for osteoporosis such as nodular thyroid, hepatic enlargement, jaundice, cushingoid features (see "Risk Factors" and Boxes 1 and 2).

ETIOLOGY

Normal bone turnover involves balance between process of bone resorption and bone formation. Osteoclasts resorb bone, and osteoblasts secrete bone matrix for building bone. In postmenopausal women, rate of bone turnover increases after loss of ovarian function, leading to progressive bone loss.

Several fracture risk calculation tools have been developed. Clinical risk factors used in the World Health Organization Fracture Risk Assessment Tool (WHO FRAX) 10-yr fracture risk calculator are summarized in Box 3.

DIAGNOSIS

DIFFERENTIAL DIAGNOSIS
- Malignancy (multiple myeloma, lymphoma, leukemia, metastatic carcinoma)
- Primary hyperparathyroidism
- Osteomalacia
- Paget disease
- Osteogenesis imperfecta: Types I, III, and IV

SCREENING
- History and physical examination with appropriate evaluation for risk factors and secondary causes. Medications associated with osteoporosis are summarized in Table 2. Investigations for secondary osteoporosis are summarized in Box 4.
- WHO guidelines for the diagnosis of osteoporosis are based on bone mineral density (BMD) measurements of the hip or spine in g/cm^2 and are reported as a T score.
- Dual-energy x-ray absorptiometry (DEXA) is the gold standard for screening and monitoring changes in BMD due to excellent precision, widespread availability, low cost, and minimal radiation exposure.
- DEXA (Fig. 1) is indicated in all women 65 yr and older and in postmenopausal women younger than 65 yr of age who are at risk for fracture (e.g., weight <127 lb, parental history of hip fracture, use of medications that cause bone loss, current smoking, excessive alcohol use, rheumatoid arthritis, or presence of diseases that cause bone loss). Clinical indications for bone densitometry are summarized in Table 3. Causes of erroneous bone mineral density measures by DEXA in the lumbar spine are summarized in Table 4.

Diseases and Disorders

I

TABLE 1 Conditions and Drugs Associated with Osteoporosis

Inflammatory Disorders
- Rheumatoid arthritis
- Inflammatory bowel disease
- Cystic fibrosis

Bone Marrow Disorders
- Multiple myeloma
- Mastocytosis
- Leukemia

Hypogonadism
- Athletic amenorrhoea
- Hemochromatosis
- Turner syndrome
- Klinefelter syndrome
- Postchemotherapy
- Hypopituitarism

Malabsorption
- Celiac disease
- Gastrectomy
- Bariatric surgery
- Liver disease
- Total parenteral nutrition

Endocrine Disorders
- Cushing syndrome
- Diabetes
- Thyrotoxicosis
- Hyperparathyroidism

Low Body Weight
- Anorexia nervosa
- Human immunodeficiency virus infection

Immobilization
- Parkinson disease
- Poliomyelitis
- Cerebral palsy
- Paraplegia

Defective Synthesis of Connective Tissue
- Osteogenesis imperfecta
- Marfan syndrome
- Homocystinuria

Miscellaneous
- Chronic obstructive lung disease
- Congestive heart failure
- Pregnancy/lactation
- Ankylosing spondylitis
- Hypercalciuric nephrolithiasis
- Depression

Drugs
- Glucocorticoids, alcohol
- Medroxyprogesterone acetate
- Anticonvulsants, methotrexate
- Heparin, cyclosporin, omeprazole
- Aromatase inhibitors, glitazones
- Androgen deprivation therapy

From Robertson RP et al: *DeGroot's endocrinology, basic science and clinical practice*, ed 8, Philadelphia, 2023, Elsevier.

- Fracture risk calculators: The relationships among clinical risk factors, BMD, and fracture incidence are complex. As such, several fracture risk calculators have been developed to facilitate the assessment of fracture risk. There are major differences in the variables that have been incorporated into the commonly used calculators, partly because different variables were available in the cohorts on which these calculators were based (Table 5). Both the FRAX and Garvan calculators can be used with or without entering BMD. For FRAX, inclusion of BMD makes surprisingly little difference to its predictive efficacy.[1]

BOX 1 Major Clinical Risk Factors for Osteoporotic Fracture

- Age
- Gender
- Previous fragility fracture
- Glucocorticoid therapy
- History of falls
- Family history of hip fracture
- Other causes of secondary osteoporosis
- Low body mass index
- Smoking
- High alcohol intake

From Hochberg MC: *Rheumatology,* ed 7, Philadelphia, 2019, Elsevier.

BOX 2 Causes of Secondary Osteoporosis

Endocrine
- Hypogonadism in either sex, including untreated, premature menopause and treatment with aromatase inhibitors or androgen deprivation therapy
- Hyperthyroidism
- Hyperprolactinemia
- Cushing disease
- Diabetes

Gastrointestinal
- Celiac disease
- Inflammatory bowel disease
- Chronic liver disease
- Chronic pancreatitis
- Other causes of malabsorption

Rheumatologic
- Rheumatoid arthritis
- Other inflammatory arthropathies

Hematologic
- Multiple myeloma
- Hemoglobinopathies
- Systemic mastocytosis
- Chronic heparin treatment

Respiratory
- Cystic fibrosis
- Chronic obstructive pulmonary disease

Metabolic
- Homocystinuria

Chronic Renal Disease

Immobility

From Hochberg MC: *Rheumatology,* ed 7, Philadelphia, 2019, Elsevier.

BOX 3 Clinical Risk Factors Included in the FRAX Case-Finding Algorithm

- Age (50-90 yr)
- Sex
- Weight (in kilograms) and height (in centimeters). Body mass index is automatically computed from height and weight
- Previous fragility fracture (yes/no)
- Parental history of hip fracture (yes/no)
- Current tobacco smoking (yes/no)
- Long-term use of oral glucocorticoids (over 3 mo) (yes/no)
- Rheumatoid arthritis (yes/no)
- Alcohol consumption of 3 or more units daily (yes/no)
- Other causes of secondary osteoporosis (yes/no): Includes type 1 diabetes, osteogenesis imperfecta, longstanding untreated hyperthyroidism, hypogonadism or premature menopause (<45 yr), chronic malnutrition, malabsorption, chronic liver disease

From World Health Organization: WHO risk fracture assessment tool. www.sheffield.ac.uk/FRAX/. From Hochberg MC: *Rheumatology,* ed 7, Philadelphia, 2019, Elsevier.

TABLE 2 Medications Associated with Osteoporosis

System	Medication
Endocrine	Aromatase inhibitors (e.g., anastrozole)
	Excess thyroxine replacement
	Glucocorticoids
	Gonadotropin-releasing hormone agonists
	Ovarian-suppressing drugs (e.g., medroxyprogesterone acetate)
	Thiazolidinediones
	SGLT2 inhibitors
Gastrointestinal	Proton pump inhibitors
Hematologic	Heparin
	Warfarin
Infectious disease	Antiretroviral therapy
Immunosuppressant	Cyclosporine
	Cytotoxic drugs
	Tacrolimus
Neurologic	Anticonvulsants—phenytoin, phenobarbital, carbamazepine
Psychiatric	Selective serotonin reuptake inhibitors
Renal	Loop diuretics (e.g., furosemide)

From Hochberg MC et al: *Rheumatology,* ed 8, Philadelphia, 2023, Elsevier.

BOX 4 Investigations for Secondary Osteoporosis in Older People with Low-Trauma Fractures or Low Bone Mineral Density

- CBC
- ESR or CRP
- Biochemical profile: Including renal function, adjusted serum calcium, and alkaline phosphatase
- Thyroid function tests
- Serum testosterone, sex hormone–binding globulin, LH, FSH (men)
- Serum and urine electrophoresis (vertebral fractures)
- Serum 25OHD and PTH

From Fillit HM: *Brocklehurst's textbook of geriatric medicine and gerontology,* ed 8, Philadelphia, 2017, Elsevier.

- FRAX questionnaire (Fig. 2): Use of FRAX calculator (www.sheffield.ac.uk/FRAX/) is proposed by the U.S. Preventive Services Task Force (USPSTF) to determine the need for screening in women between the ages of 50 and 64. If the FRAX 10-yr major osteoporotic risk is greater than or equal to 9.3%, the USPSTF recommends screening with DEXA scan.
- Currently, routine testing in men for osteoporosis is not recommended unless there are clinical manifestations of low bone mass.
- Recommendations as to when to repeat bone density testing should be based on initial T scores (Fig. 3). Data from the Study of Osteoporotic Fractures indicates that in women with normal bone density or mild osteopenia, repeat testing might not be necessary for another 10 to 15 yr. For women with moderate osteopenia, a screening interval of 3 to 5 yr may be appropriate. For women with advanced bone loss/osteoporosis, testing every 1 to 2 yr is recommended.

LABORATORY TESTS (BOX 5)
- Comprehensive metabolic panel
- Complete blood count

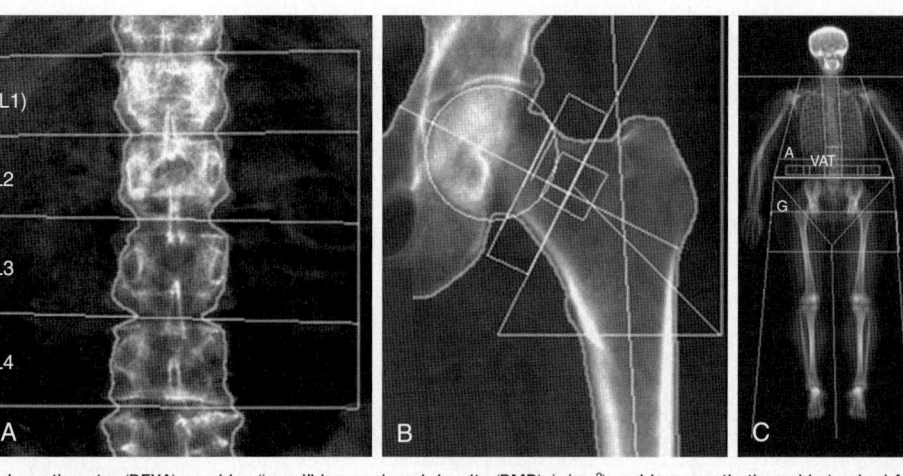

FIG. 1 Dual-energy x-ray absorptiometry (DEXA) provides "areal" bone mineral density (BMD) (g/cm²) and is currently the gold standard for diagnosis of osteoporosis by bone densitometry (World Health Organization definition T score −2.5 or below) in **(A)** posteroanterior lumbar spine (L1 through L4) or **(B)** hip (femoral neck or total). **C,** DEXA of the whole body can provide information on total and regional BMD and body composition (fat and muscle mass). Recent additional parameters measured are android A/gynoid G ratio and visceral adipose tissue (VAT). (From Pope TL et al: *Musculoskeletal imaging,* ed 2, Philadelphia, 2015, Saunders.)

TABLE 3 Clinical Indications for Bone Densitometry

All postmenopausal women <65 yr who have one or more additional risk factors for osteoporosis (besides menopause)
All women >65 yr regardless of additional risk factors
To document reduced bone density in patients with vertebral abnormalities or osteopenia on radiographs
Estrogen-deficient women at risk for low bone density who are considering use of estrogen or an alternative therapy, if bone density would influence the decision
Women who have been receiving estrogen replacement therapy for prolonged periods or to monitor the efficacy of a therapeutic intervention or interventions for osteoporosis
To diagnose low bone mass in people treated with glucocorticoids
To document low bone density in people with asymptomatic primary or secondary hyperparathyroidism

From Firestein GS et al: *Firestein & Kelley's textbook of rheumatology,* ed 11, Philadelphia, 2021, Elsevier.

TABLE 4 Causes of Erroneous Bone Mineral Density Measures by DEXA in the Lumbar Spine

Overestimation of Bone Mineral Density

Extraneous calcification (lymph nodes, aorta)
Degenerative disk and spine disease (osteophytes)
Ankylosing spondylitis
Vertebral fracture
Sclerotic metastases
Vertebral hemangioma
Overlying metal artifacts (navel rings)
Surgical interventions (metallic rods, spinal fusion)
Vertebroplasty
Paget disease
Treatment with strontium ranelate

Underestimation of Bone Mineral Density

Laminectomy

DEXA, Dual-energy x-ray absorptiometry.
From Pope TL et al: *Musculoskeletal imaging,* ed 2, Philadelphia, 2015, Saunders.

- Thyroid-stimulating hormone
- 24-h urinary calcium levels and 26-hydroxy-vitamin D level may be helpful in evaluating for secondary causes of osteoporosis
- Consider celiac panel and serum protein electrophoresis
- Biochemical markers of bone remodeling may be useful to predict rate of bone loss and/or follow therapy response. Specific biochemical markers (listed below) are followed to document response to therapy
  1. High-turnover osteoporosis: High levels of resorption markers (lysyl pyridinoline, deoxy lysyl pyridinoline, n-telopeptide of collagen cross-links, C-telopeptide of collagen cross-links) and formation markers (osteocalcin and bone-specific alkaline phosphatase); indicates accelerated bone loss responding best to antiresorptive therapy
  2. Low or normal-turnover osteoporosis: Normal or low levels of the markers of resorption and formation (see "high-turnover osteoporosis" listed previously); no accelerated bone loss; responds best to drugs that enhance bone formation

IMAGING STUDIES

- Bone mineral density (BMD) determination (see "Workup") should be performed on all women with determined risk factors and/or associated secondary causes. Criteria for the diagnosis of osteoporosis based on measurement of bone density and T score are summarized in Table 6.
  1. Normal: BMD <1 standard deviation (SD) below the young adult reference mean
  2. Osteopenia: BMD 1 to 2.5 SD below the young adult reference mean
  3. Osteoporosis: BMD >2.5 SD below the young adult reference mean
- For patients undergoing treatment: The frequency of BMD monitoring is controversial, and many experts recommend that clinicians should not monitor BMD during the initial 5-yr drug treatment period because no studies have proven that such monitoring improves fracture outcomes.

TABLE 5 Characteristics of Two Widely Used Fracture Risk Calculators

	FRAX	Garvan
Clinical risk factors	Age (40-90 yr) Sex Weight Height Previous fracture in adulthood (yes or no) Parent fractured hip Current smoking Glucocorticoid use Rheumatoid arthritis Secondary osteoporosis Alcohol Bone mineral density (optional) Country ± ethnicity	Age (50-96 yr) Sex Fractures since age of 50 yr (up to three) Falls over last 12 mo (up to three) Bone mineral density or weight
Competing risk of death	Allowed for	Not allowed for
Fracture risk outputs	10-yr risk of hip fracture or of a major osteoporotic fracture (i.e., hip, clinical spine, humerus, or forearm)	5- or 10-yr risk of hip or any fragility fracture

From Robertson RP et al: *DeGroot's endocrinology, basic science and clinical practice,* ed 8, Philadelphia, 2023, Elsevier.

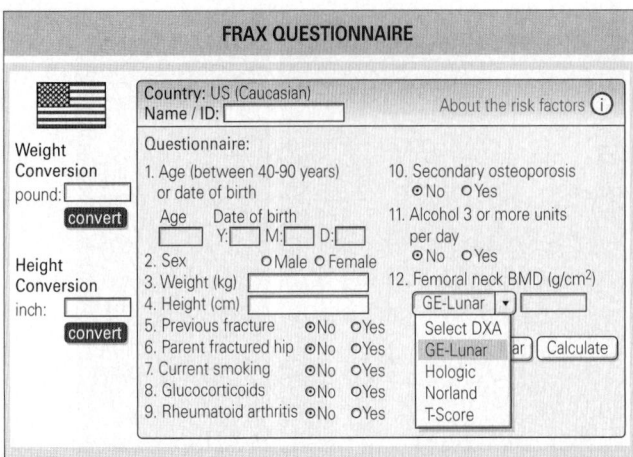

FIG. 2 FRAX questionnaire. (From Hochberg MC et al: *Rheumatology*, ed 8, Philadelphia, 2023, Elsevier.)

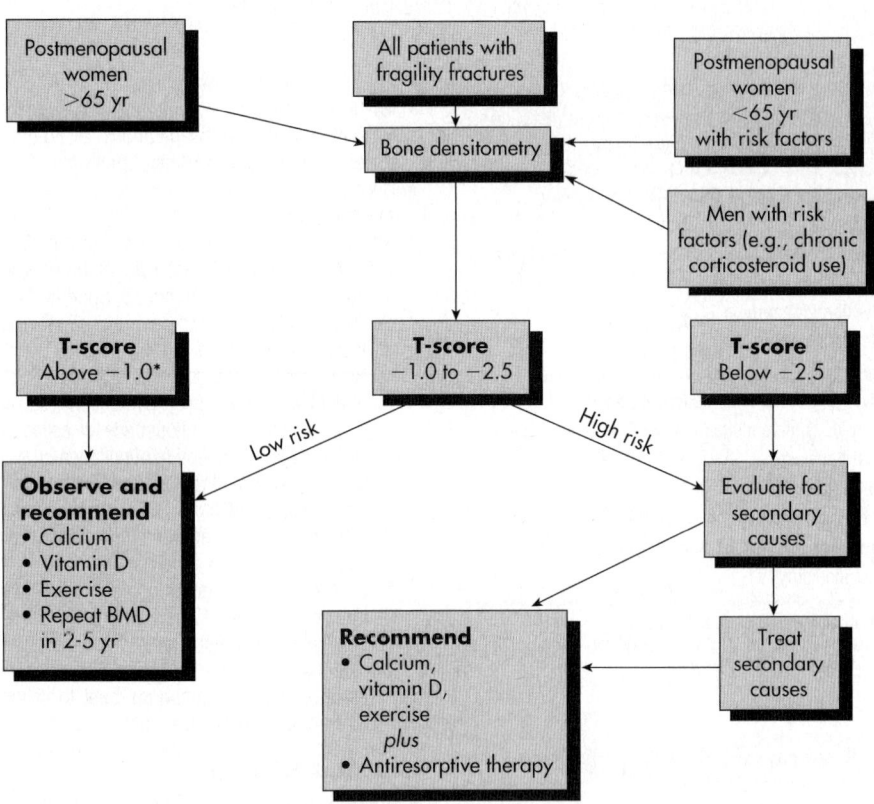

*Patients with fragility fractures and a T-score above −1.0 should be evaluated for other causes of pathologic fracture.

FIG. 3 Diagnosis and management of osteoporosis.

1. X-ray exam of appropriate part of skeleton (Figs. 4 and 5) is indicated to evaluate clinical osteoporotic fracture only.

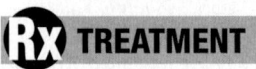 **TREATMENT**

When to treat:
- Osteoporosis criteria met based on DEXA measurements of BMD
- History of hip or vertebral fracture
- Osteopenia on DEXA + 10-yr FRAX score of greater than or equal to 3% at hip or greater than or equal to 20% of major osteoporotic fracture

NONPHARMACOLOGIC THERAPY

Prevention:
- Identification and minimization of risk factors
- Appropriate diagnosis and treatment of secondary causes
- Behavioral modification: Proper nutrition, physical activity (specifically weight-bearing activity), fracture prevention strategies, fall risk reduction

---

BOX 5   Recommended Laboratory Investigations for Individuals with Osteoporosis

Recommended Screening in All Patients
- Serum calcium, albumin, phosphorus*, †, ‡, §
- Serum creatinine*, †, ‡, §
- Liver function tests*
- Bicarbonate*
- Complete blood count*
- 24-h urinary calcium level*, †, ‡, §
- 25-hydroxyvitamin D level*, †, ‡, §
- Thyroid-stimulating hormone level*, †, ‡, §

Other Testing, if Appropriate
- Biochemical markers of bone turnover*, †, ‡, §
- Cortisol levels*, ‡
- Protein electrophoresis*, †, §
- Parathyroid hormone level*, §

*American Association of Clinical Endocrinologists guidelines.
‡U.S. Surgeon General's report.
†National Osteoporosis Foundation Physician's Guide.
§American College of Obstetricians and Gynecologists.
From Hochberg MC: *Rheumatology,* ed 7, Philadelphia, 2019, Elsevier.

ACUTE GENERAL Rx

- Vitamin D supplement: 600 IU/day for persons 19 to 70 yr of age and 800 IU/day for persons 71 yr and older. Recommended supplementation of calcium and vitamin D is summarized in Table 6.
- Calcium supplement: The recommended dietary intake of calcium for women 19 to 50 yr of age and men 19 to 70 yr of age is 1000 mg/day; women older than age 50 and men older than age 70 require 1200 mg/day. Calcium intake above 2500 mg/day (2000 mg/day in persons >50 yr of age) should be avoided. Consumption of calcium-rich foods and beverages is the preferred approach to ensuring adequate calcium intake.[2]
- Bisphosphonates have been used in osteoporosis and remain the most widely used agents, being joined more recently by denosumab (Table 7). Oral bisphosphonates (alendronate, risedronate): Decrease bone resorption by attenuating osteoclast activity. They are first-line therapy for the treatment of most patients with osteoporosis, with proven efficacy to reduce fracture risk. The bisphosphonates differ in binding affinity, dose frequency, and route of administration. To facilitate absorption, most oral bisphosphonates are taken on an empty stomach with a full glass of water. Patients are instructed to remain in a sitting or standing position for 30 to 60 min. Contraindications include esophageal disorders, inability to remain standing for 30 to 60 min after taking the medication, chronic kidney disease, and Roux-en-Y gastric bypass procedures. Adverse side effects include gastroesophageal reflux disease, esophagitis, transient hypocalcemia, musculoskeletal pain, renal impairment, ocular side effects, jaw necrosis, and atypical femur fracture.

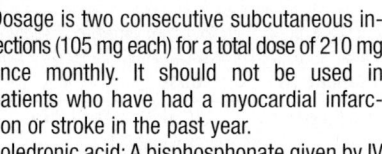

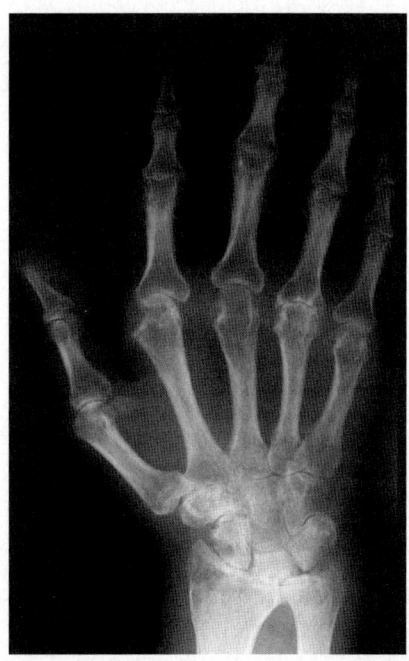

FIG. 4 Regional osteoporosis. Hand radiograph in early rheumatoid arthritis (RA) shows periarticular osteopenia at the metacarpophalangeal and interphalangeal joints, with joint space narrowing and juxtaarticular erosions. The periarticular osteopenia is the earliest radiographic feature of RA and is related to hyperemia, synovial inflammation, and local cytokines that stimulate osteoclastic bone resorption. (From Pope TL et al: *Musculoskeletal imaging*, ed 2, Philadelphia, 2015, Saunders.)

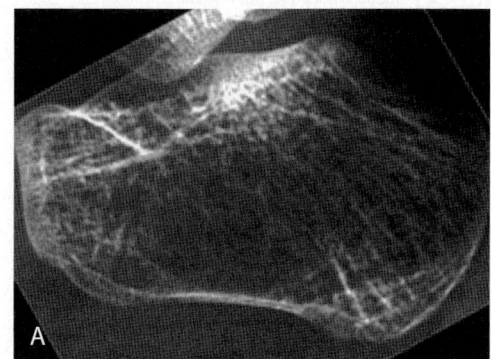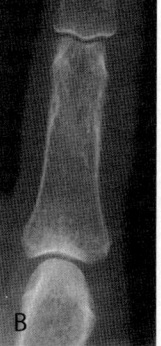

FIG. 5 General osteoporosis. Radiographic features include reduced radiographic density (osteopenia) with reduction in the number of trabeculae, which may be destroyed completely, and the bone cortex becomes thinned as evident in the lateral radiograph of the calcaneus **(A)** and radiograph of the phalanx **(B)**. When these features are present, bone densitometry using dual-energy x-ray absorptiometry (DEXA) should be suggested. (From Pope TL et al: *Musculoskeletal imaging*, ed 2, Philadelphia, 2015, Saunders.)

TABLE 6 Diagnostic Categories for Osteoporosis Based on World Health Organization Criteria

Category	Definition
Normal	BMD not more than 1 SD below the young adult mean value
Low bone mass (osteopenia)	BMD lying between 1 and 2.5 SD below the young adult mean value
Osteoporosis	BMD more than 2.5 SD below the young adult mean value

BMD, Bone mineral density; *SD*, standard deviation.
From World Health Organization data, 1994. Hochberg MC et al: *Rheumatology*, ed 8, Philadelphia, 2023, Elsevier.

Dosage is two consecutive subcutaneous injections (105 mg each) for a total dose of 210 mg once monthly. It should not be used in patients who have had a myocardial infarction or stroke in the past year.
- Zoledronic acid: A bisphosphonate given by IV infusion over at least 15 min, 5 mg once per yr may be used in patients who are unable to tolerate oral bisphosphonates. It is contraindicated in patients with acute renal failure.
- Teriparatide is a recombinant human parathyroid hormone used for postmenopausal women with osteoporosis who are at high risk for fracture, especially vertebral fractures. It is also used in men with primary or hypogonadal osteoporosis who are at high risk of fracture. It is administered by injection 20 mcg daily, subcutaneously into the thigh or abdominal wall. Use for more than 2 yr is not recommended. It stimulates bone formation and reduces the risk of fracture but may increase the risk of stroke in older women with osteoporosis. Common side effects include headaches, myalgia, hypercalcemia, and hypercalciuria. Trials involving abaloparatide, a selective activator of the parathyroid hormone type 1 receptor, have also shown reduced risk of new vertebral and nonvertebral fractures in postmenopausal women with osteoporosis. Use of teriparatide is followed by a biphosphonate upon its discontinuation in females with primary osteoporosis and a very high risk of fractures.[3]
- Estrogen prescription drugs or raloxifene should not be prescribed to treat women with osteoporosis.

- Biologic agents: Denosumab is a human monoclonal antibody that inhibits osteoclast formation and prevents resorption for treatment of postmenopausal osteoporosis. It is used as a second-line pharmacologic treatment to reduce the risk of fractures in postmenopausal females diagnosed with primary osteoporosis who have contraindications to or experience adverse effects of biphosphonates.[3] Dosage is 60 mg subcutaneously every 6 mo. Romosozumab is a monoclonal antibody that increases bone formation and decreases bone resorption by binding to sclerostin. It may be considered for patients who are at high risk for fracture and cannot tolerate any other osteoporotic therapies.

CHRONIC Rx
- Lifelong attention to behavior modification (nutrition, physical activity, fracture prevention strategies) and compliance with pharmacologic intervention. Recommendations include weight-bearing and muscle-strengthening exercises, smoking cessation, reduced alcohol intake, and adoption of fall prevention strategies.
- There is little evidence to guide physicians about long-term bisphosphonate therapy. The decision to continue drug therapy beyond 5 yr should reflect reassessment of risk and benefit. The risks of atypical fracture of the femur and osteonecrosis of the jaw (ONJ)[3] increase after 5 yr of bisphosphonate use. It is reasonable to consider a drug holiday in postmenopausal women who are not at high fracture risk after 3 yr (IV) to 5 yr (oral) of bisphosphonate therapy. Continued treatment may be advisable in those at highest risk.
- Continuing need to eliminate high-risk factors when possible and to optimally manage secondary causes of osteoporosis.

DISPOSITION

Goals for diagnosis and treatment include identification of women at risk; initiation of lifelong preventive measures for all women; institution of treatment modalities that will result in a decrease in fracture risk; and reduction of morbidity,

---

TABLE 7 Principal Medications for Management of Osteoporosis

Medication	Dose	Indications	Dosing Instructions	Comments
Alendronate	70 mg/wk PO 10 mg/d PO	Treatment of postmenopausal, male and glucocorticoid osteoporosis	Take fasting with a glass of water while sitting or standing. Remain upright and fasting for 30 min	
	35 mg/wk PO 5 mg/d PO	Prevention of postmenopausal osteoporosis		
Risedronate	5 mg/d, 35 mg/wk, 75 mg ×2 per mo, 150 mg/mo, all PO	Treatment or prevention of postmenopausal osteoporosis; treatment of male and glucocorticoid osteoporosis		
Ibandronate	150 mg/mo PO	Treatment or prevention of postmenopausal osteoporosis	As above, but remain upright and fasting for 60 min	
	3 mg/3 mo IV	Treatment of postmenopausal osteoporosis	Inject over 15-30 sec	
Zoledronate or zoledronic acid	5 mg/yr IV	Treatment of postmenopausal, male, and glucocorticoid osteoporosis, fracture prevention after hip fracture	IV infusion in 100 ml over at least 15 min	
	5 mg every 2 yr	Prevention of postmenopausal osteoporosis		
Raloxifene	60 mg/d PO	Prevention and treatment of postmenopausal osteoporosis		
Denosumab	60 mg every 6 mo SC	Treatment of postmenopausal, male, and glucocorticoid osteoporosis patients at high fracture risk		
Teriparatide	20 μg/d SC for 18-24 mo	Treatment of postmenopausal, male, and glucocorticoid osteoporosis patients at high fracture risk	Follow with antiresorptive agent	FDA recommends considering >2 yr of cumulative use during a patient's lifetime only if fracture risk remains high
Abaloparatide	80 μg/d SC for 18-24 mo	Treatment of postmenopausal osteoporosis patients at high fracture risk	Inject into the periumbilical region. Administer initial doses where the patient can lie down if orthostatic hypotension occurs Follow with antiresorptive agent	See above Declined registration in Europe
Romosozumab	210 mg/mo SC for 12 mo	Treatment of postmenopausal osteoporosis at high fracture risk or patients who have failed or are intolerant to other available osteoporosis therapy	Follow with antiresorptive agent	

FDA, U.S. Food and Drug Administration; *IV,* intravenously; *PO,* by mouth; *SC,* subcutaneously.
From Robertson RP et al: *DeGroot's endocrinology, basic science and clinical practice,* ed 8, Philadelphia, 2023, Elsevier.

TABLE 8 Effect of Major Treatment Options on the Risk of Vertebral, Nonvertebral, and Hip Fractures

	Vertebral Fractures	Nonvertebral Fractures	Hip Fractures
Alendronate	A	A	A
Etidronate	A	ND	ND
Risedronate	A	A	A
Raloxifene	A	ND	ND
Strontium ranelate	A	A	(A)
Teriparatide	A	A	ND
Denosumab	A	A	A
Zoledronate*	A	A	A
Ibandronate*	A	(A)	ND
Calcium and vitamin D*	ND	A	A

A indicates evidence from randomized, controlled trials and/or meta-analysis; *(A)* reflects that a beneficial effect on fracture risk was found only in post hoc subgroup analysis; *ND* indicates that fracture reduction has not been demonstrated.
From Fillit HM: *Brocklehurst's textbook of geriatric medicine and gerontology,* ed 8, Philadelphia, 2017, Elsevier.

mortality, and unnecessary institutionalization, thereby improving quality of independent life and productivity. Table 8 summarizes the effect of major treatment options on the risk of vertebral, nonvertebral, and hip fractures.

REFERENCES & SUGGESTED READING

Available at eBooks.Health.Elsevier.com

AUTHORS: **SYDNEY FORD, MD, MPH** and **RACHEL WRIGHT HEINLE, MD, FACOG**

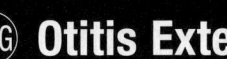

O

 BASIC INFORMATION

DEFINITION

Otitis externa refers to a variety of conditions causing inflammation and/or infection of the external auditory canal (and/or auricle and tympanic membrane).[1] There are six subgroups of otitis externa:

- Acute localized otitis externa (furunculosis)
- Acute diffuse bacterial otitis externa (i.e., "swimmer ear")
- Chronic otitis externa
- Eczematous otitis externa
- Fungal otitis externa (otomycosis)
- Invasive or necrotizing (malignant) otitis externa

SYNONYM

See "Definition."

ICD-10CM CODES
H60.90	Unspecified otitis externa, unspecified ear
H60.2	Malignant otitis externa
H60.3	Other infective otitis externa
H60.5	Acute otitis externa, non-infective
H60.8	Other otitis externa

EPIDEMIOLOGY & DEMOGRAPHICS[2]

INCIDENCE (IN U.S.):
- Among the most common disorders
- An estimated 10% of people develop external otitis during their lifetime
- Affects 3% to 10% of patients seeking otologic care

PREVALENCE (IN U.S.):
- Diffuse otitis externa is most often seen in swimmers and in hot, humid climates, conditions that lead to water retention in the ear canal. In the U.S., 44% of AOE-related health care visits occur June to August[1]
- Necrotizing otitis externa is more common in elderly, diabetics, and immunocompromised patients[3]

PREDOMINANT SEX: None
PREDOMINANT AGE:
- Occurs at all ages; however, incidence is highest during childhood and decreases with age[1]
- Necrotizing otitis externa: Typically occurs in elderly; mean age >65 yr[3]

PHYSICAL FINDINGS & CLINICAL PRESENTATION

The two most common symptoms are otalgia, ranging from pruritus to severe pain exacerbated by motion (e.g., chewing), and otorrhea. Patients may also experience aural fullness and hearing loss due to swelling and occlusion of the canal. More intense symptoms may occur with bacterial otitis externa, with or without fever, and lymphadenopathy (anterior to tragus).[1] Findings unique to specific forms of the infection include:

- Acute localized otitis externa (furunculosis):[1]
  1. Occurs from infected hair follicles, usually in the outer third of the ear canal, forming pustules and furuncles

  2. Furuncles are superficial and pointing or deep and diffuse
- Impetigo:[1]
  1. In contrast to furunculosis, this is a superficial spreading infection of the ear canal that may also involve the concha and the auricle
  2. Begins as a small blister that ruptures, releasing straw-colored fluid that dries as a golden crust
- Erysipelas:[1]
  1. Caused by group A streptococcus (Streptococcus pyogenes [GAS])
  2. May involve the concha and canal
  3. May involve the dermis and deeper tissues
  4. Area of cellulitis, often with severe pain
  5. Fever, chills, malaise
  6. Regional adenopathy
- Eczematous or seborrheic otitis externa:[1]
  1. Stems from a variety of dermatologic problems that can involve the external auditory canal
  2. Severe itching, erythema, scaling, crusting (Fig.E1), and fissuring possible
- Acute diffuse otitis externa (swimmer ear):[1]
  1. Begins with itching and a feeling of pressure and fullness in the ear that becomes increasingly tender and painful
  2. Mild erythema and edema of the external auditory canal, which may cause narrowing and occlusion of the canal (Fig. E2), leading to hearing loss
  3. Minimal serous secretions, which may become profuse and purulent
  4. Tympanic membrane may appear dull and infected
  5. Usually absence of systemic symptoms such as fever, chills
- Otomycosis:[1]
  1. Chronic superficial infection of the ear canal and tympanic membrane
  2. In primary fungal infection, major symptom is intense itching
  3. In secondary infection (fungal infection superimposed on bacterial infection), major symptom is pain
  4. Fungal growth of variety of colors
- Chronic otitis externa:[1]
  1. Dry and atrophic canal
  2. Typically lack of cerumen
  3. Itching, often severe, and mild discomfort rather than pain
  4. Occasionally mucopurulent discharge
  5. With time, thickening of the walls of the canal, causing narrowing of the lumen
- Necrotizing otitis externa (also known as malignant otitis externa). Typically seen in older patients with diabetes or in patients who are immunocompromised[3]
  1. Redness, swelling, and tenderness of the ear canal
  2. Classic finding of granulation tissue on the floor of the canal and the bone–cartilage junction
  3. Small ulceration of necrotic soft tissue at bone–cartilage junction
  4. Most common symptoms: Pain (often severe) and otorrhea
  5. Lessening of purulent drainage as infection advances

  6. As the infection advances, osteomyelitis of the base of the skull and temporomandibular joint osteomyelitis can develop
  7. Facial nerve palsy often the first and only cranial nerve defect
  8. Possible involvement of other cranial nerves

ETIOLOGY[1]

- Box 1 summarizes common pathogens in otitis externa
- Acute localized otitis externa: *Staphylococcus aureus*
- Impetigo:
  1. *S. aureus* including MRSA
  2. *Streptococcus pyogenes* (GAS)
- Erysipelas: GAS
- Eczematous otitis externa:
  1. Seborrheic dermatitis
  2. Atopic dermatitis
  3. Psoriasis
  4. Neurodermatitis
  5. Lupus erythematosus
- Acute diffuse otitis externa:
  1. Swimming
  2. Hot, humid climates
  3. Tightly fitting hearing aids
  4. Use of ear plugs
  5. *Pseudomonas aeruginosa*
  6. *S. aureus* including MRSA
- Otomycosis:
  1. Prolonged use of topical antibiotics and steroid preparations
  2. Uncontrolled diabetes mellitus can contribute to risk
  3. *Aspergillus* (80% to 90%)
  4. *Candida*
- Chronic otitis externa: Persistent low-grade infection and inflammation
- Necrotizing otitis externa (NOE):[3]
  1. Complication of persistent otitis externa
  2. Typically starts in the external auditory canal and spreads to the stylomastoid foramen, then to the mastoid tip and the jugular foramen. Finally, it extends to the petrous apex and the middle cranial fossa
  3. *P. aeruginosa*
  4. High index of suspicion for atypical organisms (MRSA) in patients without diabetes

---

BOX 1 Common Pathogens in Otitis Externa

Gram-Negative Organisms
- *Pseudomonas aeruginosa*
- *Pseudomonas* spp. Nov. "otitidis"
- *Proteus mirabilis*
- *Serratia marcescens*

Gram-Positive Organisms
- *Staphylococcus aureus*
- *Staphylococcus epidermidis*
- *Corynebacterium auris*
- *Enterococcus faecalis*

Fungi and Yeasts
- *Aspergillus fumigatus*
- *Candida albicans*
- *Candida parapsilosis*

From Cherry JD et al: *Feigin and Cherry's pediatric infectious diseases*, ed 8, Philadelphia, 2019, Elsevier.

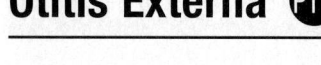

Dx DIAGNOSIS

DIFFERENTIAL DIAGNOSIS

- Acute otitis media
- Bullous myringitis
- Mastoiditis
- Foreign bodies
- Neoplasms
- Contact dermatitis
- Eczema
- Ramsey-Hunt syndrome
- Seborrhea
- Otomycosis
- Referred pain
- Table 1 describes the differential diagnosis of painful external ear and auditory canal disorders

WORKUP

Thorough history and physical examination, including pneumatic otoscopy if available

LABORATORY TESTS

- Cultures from the canal are usually not necessary unless the condition does not respond to treatment.
- Leukocyte count normal or mildly elevated.
- Erythrocyte sedimentation rate is often quite elevated in malignant otitis externa.

IMAGING STUDIES

- Computed tomography scan (Fig. E3) is the best technique for defining bone involvement and extent of disease in malignant otitis externa.
- MRI is slightly more sensitive in evaluation of soft tissue changes and intracranial extension of infection.
- Gallium scans are more specific than bone scans in diagnosing NOE.
- Follow-up scans are helpful in determining efficacy of treatment. NOTE: Expert opinion supports history and physical examination as the best means of diagnosis. Persistent pain that is constant and severe should raise the question of NOE (particularly in the elderly, diabetics, and immunocompromised patients).

Rx TREATMENT

NONPHARMACOLOGIC THERAPY

- Cleansing and debridement of the ear canal with cotton swabs and hydrogen peroxide or other antiseptic solution allows a more thorough examination of the ear.
- If the canal lumen is edematous and too narrow to allow adequate cleansing, a cotton wick or gauze strip inserted into the canal serves as a conduit for topical medications to be drawn into the canal. Usually remove wick after 2 days.
- Local heat is useful in treating deep furunculosis.
- Incision and drainage are indicated in treatment of superficial pointing furunculosis.

ACUTE GENERAL Rx

Topical medications:
- An acidifying agent such as 2% acetic acid (Vosol) inhibits growth of bacteria and fungi.

- Topical antibiotics (in the form of otic or ophthalmic solutions) or antifungals, often in combination with an acidifying agent and a steroid preparation. Direct application of topical agents to the infected site is a key element in the treatment of external otitis regardless of severity. Proper installation of eardrops entails tilting the head toward the opposite shoulder, pulling the superior aspect of the auricle upward, and filling the ear canal with drops. In young children, the earlobe should be pulled downward to fill the canal.
- The ideal antibiotic regimen should have coverage against the most common pathogens, S. aureus and P. aeruginosa.
- Side effect profile can also influence choice of treatment. Ototoxicity is the most important concern with aminoglycoside drugs, including neomycin, tobramycin, and gentamicin. Aminoglycosides are a significant potential source for iatrogenic hearing loss and balance dysfunction, particularly in the presence of tympanic membrane perforation. Allergic contact dermatitis is commonly associated with neomycin when used for prolonged courses. Topical fluoroquinolones can cause local irritation.
- The following are some of the available preparations:
  1. Neomycin otic solutions and suspensions:
     a. With polymyxin-B-hydrocortisone (Cortisporin)
     b. With hydrocortisone-thonzonium (Coly-Mycin S)
  3. Polymyxin-B-hydrocortisone (Otobiotic)
  4. Quinolone otic solutions:
     a. Ofloxacin 0.3% solution (Floxin Otic)
     b. Ciprofloxacin 0.3% with hydrocortisone (Cipro HC)
  5. Quinolone ophthalmic solutions:
     a. Ofloxacin 0.3% (Ocuflox)
     b. Ciprofloxacin 0.3% (Ciloxan)
  6. Aminoglycoside ophthalmic solutions:
     a. Gentamicin sulfate 0.3% (Garamycin)
     b. Tobramycin sulfate 0.3% (Tobrex)
     c. Tobramycin 0.3% and dexamethasone 0.1% (TobraDex)
  7. Chloramphenicol 0.5% otic solution or 0.25% ophthalmic solution (Chloromycetin)
  8. Gentian violet (methylrosaniline chloride 1%, 2%)
  9. Antifungals:
     a. Amphotericin B 3% (Fungizone lotion)
     b. Clotrimazole 1% solution (Lotrimin)
     c. Tolnaftate 1% (Tinactin)
- Topical preparations should be applied qid (bid for quinolones, antifungals), generally for 3 days after cessation of symptoms (average 10-14 days total).

Systemic antibiotics:
- Reserved for when the infection has spread beyond the ear canal.
- Treatment usually for 10 days with ciprofloxacin 750 mg q12h or ofloxacin 400 mg q12h, or with antistaphylococcal agent (e.g., dicloxacillin or cephalexin 500 mg q6h). Use Bactrim or clindamycin when MRSA suspected or cultured at one DS twice a day instead of cephalexin or dicloxacillin. For

TABLE 1	Differential Diagnosis of Painful External Ear and Auditory Canal Disorders
Disorder	**Clinical Features**
Acute otitis externa	Diffuse redness, swelling, and pain of the canal with greenish to whitish exudate; often very tender pinna
Malignant otitis externa	Rapidly progressive, severe swelling and redness of pinna, which may be laterally displaced
Dermatitis	
Eczema	History of atopy, presence of lesions elsewhere; lesions are scaly, red, pruritic, and weeping
Contact	History of cosmetic use or irritant exposure; lesions are scaly, red, pruritic, and weeping
Seborrhea	Scaly, red, papular dermatitis; scalp may have thick, yellow scales
Psoriasis	History or presence of psoriasis elsewhere; erythematous papules that coalesce into thick, white plaques
Cellulitis	Diffuse redness, tenderness, and swelling of the pinna
Furuncles	Red, tender papules in areas with hair follicles (distal third of the ear canal)
Infected periauricular cyst	Discrete, palpable lesions; history of previous swelling at same site; cellulitis may develop, obscuring cystic structure
Insect bites	History of exposure; lesions are red, tender papules
Herpes zoster	Painful, vesicular lesions in the ear canal and tympanic membrane in the distribution of cranial nerves V and VII
Perichondritis	Inflammation of the cartilage, usually secondary to cellulitis
Tumors	Palpable mass, destruction of surrounding structures
Foreign body	Foreign body may cause secondary trauma to the ear canal or become a nidus for an infection of the ear canal
Trauma	Bruising and swelling of external ear; there may be signs of basilar skull fracture (cerebrospinal fluid otorrhea, hemotympanum)

From Kliegman RM: *Nelson textbook of pediatrics*, ed 21, Philadelphia, 2020, Elsevier.

malignant otitis externa (due to *Pseudomonas aeruginosa* in >90% of cases), effective agents are meropenem 1 g intravenous (IV) q8h or ciprofloxacin 400 mg IV q12h or 750 mg PO q12h or cefepime 2 g q12h.

Treatment for NOE:
- Combined oral quinolones with topical quinolones for 4 to 6 wk may be sufficient for initial therapy.[3]
- IV antipseudomonals with or without aminoglycosides are appropriate in refractory cases.[3]
- Local debridement.

Pain control:
- May require NSAIDs or opioids
- Topical corticosteroids to reduce swelling and inflammation

CHRONIC Rx
- Patients prone to recurrent infections should try to identify and avoid precipitants to infection.
- Swimmers should try tight-fitting ear plugs or tight-fitting bathing caps and remove all excess water from the ears after swimming.

- Treat underlying systemic diseases and dermatologic conditions that predispose to infection.
- Hearing aids should be removed nightly and regularly cleaned.

DISPOSITION
- Inadequate treatment of otitis externa may lead to NOE and mastoiditis.
- Considerations if acute otitis externa fails to respond to initial ototopical therapy are summarized in Box 2.
- Complications of acute and chronic otitis externa are summarized in Table 2.

REFERRAL
To an otolaryngologist:
- NOE
- Treatment failure
- Severe pain

BOX 2 Considerations if Acute Otitis Externa Fails to Respond to Initial Ototopical Therapy

- Self-instrumentation trauma
- Malignant external otitis
- Contact dermatitis
- Failure to adhere to preventive measures (such as avoidance of water exposure)
- Improper administration of ototopical therapy
- Immunosuppression: Diabetes, prior radiotherapy
- Inadequate penetration of ototopical therapy due to copious debris or thickened canal skin
- Misdiagnosis: Canal cholesteatoma or keratosis obturans, autoimmune condition, mycobacterial infection, malignancy
- Resistance of involved organism to ototopical therapy choice

From Flint PW et al: *Cummings otolaryngology, head and neck surgery,* ed 7, Philadelphia, 2021, Elsevier.

TABLE 2 Complications of Acute and Chronic Otitis Externa

Complication	Description	Treatment
Cellulitis/perichondritis/chondritis	Extension of infection into soft tissues and cartilage of the auricle	Oral administration of antibiotics with adequate coverage of *Pseudomonas* species
Malignant otitis externa	Extension of infection beyond the EAC into soft tissue, mastoid and skull base; can evolve into temporal bone osteomyelitis	Underlying metabolic or immune abnormality to be addressed; culture-directed antibiotic therapy; typically requires a prolonged (6-wk) course of antipseudomonal antibiotic
Medial canal fibrosis	Fibrous scar of the medial EAC; a sequela of COE	Surgical treatment with canalplasty vs. lateral graft tympanoplasty; bone-anchored hearing device if surgery is not indicated
Perforation of the tympanic membrane	Often seen in the setting of fungal OE	Elimination of infection; tympanoplasty if spontaneous repair does not occur

COE, Chronic otitis externa; *EAC,* external auditory canal; *OE,* otitis externa.
From Flint PW et al: *Cummings otolaryngology, head and neck surgery,* ed 7, Philadelphia, 2021, Elsevier.

! PEARLS & CONSIDERATIONS

Otitis externa varies in severity from a mild irritation of the external acoustic canal (swimmer ear) that resolves spontaneously by simply removing the offending agent (stay out of freshwater or wear ear plugs when swimming) to a life-threatening infection with the risk of intracranial extension, gram-negative bacterial meningitis, and severe neurologic impairment with multiple cranial neuropathy. Do not miss severe malignant otitis externa in patients who are diabetic, elderly, or immunocompromised.

REFERENCES
Available at eBooks.Health.Elsevier.com

RELATED CONTENT
Otitis Externa (Patient Information)

AUTHOR: **LYNN C. FULLENKAMP, MD, JD**

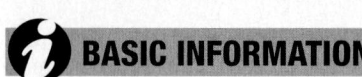
BASIC INFORMATION

DEFINITION

Acute otitis media (AOM) is defined by infected middle ear fluid resulting in moderate to severe bulging of the tympanic membrane (TM) or new onset of otorrhea not due to acute otitis externa. Table 1 summarizes otitis media definitions and terminology. Care should be taken to differentiate AOM from serous otitis media, which involves noninfected middle ear fluid that does not result in bulging of the TM. Serous otitis media does not require antibiotic treatment.[1,2]

SYNONYMS

Acute suppurative otitis media
Purulent otitis media
Acute otitis media
AOM

ICD-10CM CODES

H65.3	Chronic mucoid otitis media
H66.0	Acute suppurative otitis media
H66.4	Suppurative otitis media, unspecified
H66.9	Otitis media, unspecified
H66.1	Chronic tubotympanic suppurative otitis media
H66.2	Chronic atticoantral suppurative otitis media

EPIDEMIOLOGY & DEMOGRAPHICS

INCIDENCE (IN U.S.):

- Affects patients of all ages but is largely a disease of infants and young children
- Affects approximately 80% of all children by age 5 yr
- Occurs three or more times in one third of all children by age 3 yr
- Costs associated with otitis media exceed $5 billion, with 40% of the costs occurring from patients ages 1 to 3 yr

- One of the most common indications for antibiotic prescription among children

PEAK INCIDENCE:

- AOM occurs at all ages but is most prevalent between 6 and 24 mo of age.
- A second peak in incidence occurs between 4 and 6 yr of age.
- AOM is most frequent in the fall, winter, and early spring (coincident with peak respiratory virus prevalence in the community).
- Incidence of infection declines with age; AOM is seen infrequently in adults.

RISK FACTORS:

- Daycare attendance
- Limited or no breastfeeding
- Tobacco smoke exposure
- Pacifier use
- Craniofacial anomalies
- Immune globulin G (IgG) or subclass deficiencies

PHYSICAL FINDINGS & CLINICAL PRESENTATION[3]

- Moderate to severe bulging of the TM.
- Fluid in the middle ear along with signs and symptoms of local inflammation.
  1. Erythema with diminished light reflex (Fig. E1)
- As infection progresses, middle ear exudation occurs (exudative phase); the exudate rapidly changes from serous to purulent (suppurative phase).
- Retraction and poor mobility of the TM ensues, and the TM begins to bulge.
- At any time during the suppurative phase, the TM may rupture, releasing the middle ear contents (otorrhea).
- Erythema of the TM without other abnormalities is not a diagnostic criterion for acute otitis media (AOM) because it may occur with any inflammation of the upper respiratory tract, crying, or nose blowing.
- Symptoms:[1]

1. Rapid- or recent-onset otalgia, ranging from slight discomfort to severe, is the most common presenting symptom.
2. Hearing loss while middle ear fluid is present.
3. Otorrhea (if TM has ruptured).
4. Systemic symptoms such as fever, listlessness, irritability, decreased appetite, vomiting, and diarrhea are common. Although vertigo, facial swelling, nystagmus, tinnitus, lethargy, and facial nerve palsies can occur as rare complications of AOM; these symptoms should prompt consideration of an alternate diagnosis.
5. Table 2 summarizes symptom scoring systems designed to aid in diagnosis.
- After an episode of AOM:
  1. Persistence of effusion for weeks or months (called secretory, serous, or nonsuppurative otitis media)
  2. Fever and otalgia usually absent
  3. Hearing loss possible (10 to 50 dB, with predominant involvement of the low frequencies)
  4. Manifestations of the sequelae and complications of otitis media are summarized in Table E3

ETIOLOGY

- Most common etiology is a viral upper respiratory tract infection, which causes inflammation and dysfunction of the eustachian tube and transient aspiration of nasopharyngeal secretions into the middle ear (Fig. 2). Bacterial colonization from the nasopharynx in conjunction with eustachian tube dysfunction leads to infection.
- May occasionally develop as a result of hematogenous spread or by direct invasion from the nasopharynx.
- Conjugated pneumococcal vaccination of children has resulted in decreases in *Streptococcus pneumoniae* causing AOM.

TABLE 1 Otitis Media Definitions and Terminology

Preferred Term	Definition	Comment
Otitis media (OM)	Inflammation of the middle ear without reference to etiology or pathogenesis	Nonspecific umbrella term for any condition associated with middle ear inflammation
Acute otitis media (AOM)	Rapid onset of signs and symptoms of inflammation in the middle ear	Diagnosed when there is moderate to severe bulging of the ear drum; mild bulging of the ear drum and recent (<48 h) onset of ear pain or intense erythema of the ear drum; or acute ear discharge unrelated to otitis externa (inflammation of the external ear canal)*
Recurrent AOM (rAOM)	≥3 well-documented and separate AOM episodes in the preceding 6 mo or ≥4 episodes in the preceding 12 mo with >1 episode in the past 6 mo	Children without persistent MEE tend to have a good prognosis and often improve spontaneously; children with persistent MEE have a poorer prognosis and might benefit from ventilation tubes
Otitis media with effusion (OME)	Fluid in the middle ear without signs or symptoms of acute ear infection	Diagnosed by one or more of the following: Reduced ear drum mobility on pneumatic otoscopy, reduced ear drum mobility on tympanometry, opaque ear drum or a visible air-fluid interface behind the ear drum on otoscopy
Chronic OME	OME persisting for ≥3 mo from date of onset (if known) or from date of diagnosis (if onset is unknown)	Chronic OME has much lower rates of spontaneous resolution compared to OME of new onset or following an episode of AOM
Chronic suppurative otitis media (CSOM)	Chronic inflammation of the middle ear and mastoid mucosa with a nonintact ear drum (perforation or ventilation tube) and persistent ear discharge	No consensus on duration of ear discharge needed for diagnosis, with recommendations ranging from 2 wk to at least 3 mo
Middle ear effusion (MEE)	Fluid in the middle ear from any cause	MEE is present with both OME and AOM and might persist for weeks or months after the signs and symptoms of AOM resolve

*The degree of bulging does not reflect AOM severity. Severe AOM is defined as having moderate-to-severe ear pain, ear pain for at least 48 h, or temperature 39°C or higher.
From Flint PW et al: *Cummings otolaryngology, head and neck surgery,* ed 7, Philadelphia, 2021, Elsevier.

TABLE 2 Acute Otitis Media Symptom Scoring Systems Designed to Aid in Diagnosis

3-Item Otitis Media Score (OM-3)	Ear Treatment Group Symptom Questionnaire (ETG-5)	Acute Otitis Media Faces Scale (AOM-FS)	Otoscopic Severity Scale (OS-8)	Acute Otitis Media Severity of Symptom Scale (AOM-SOS)	Otitis Media Clinical Severity Index (OM-CSI) 30-Point Scale[a]	Otitis Media Clinical Severity Index (OM-CSI) 10-Point Scale[a]
Physical suffering	Ear pain	Seven facial expressions ranging from no problem to extreme problem	Eight categories of TM inflammation[b]	Ear pain	Ear pain	Ear pain
Emotional distress	Fever			Ear tugging	Fever	Fever
Limitation of activities	Irritability			Irritability	Irritability	Irritability
	Appetite			Decreased play	Fever at examination	Fever at examination
	Sleep quality			Decreased appetite	TM erythema	TM erythema
				Difficulty sleeping	TM mobility	TM mobility
				Fever	TM position	TM position
					Effusion color	Effusion color
					Otorrhea	Otorrhea

TM, Tympanic membrane.

[a] The 30-point scale used a 2- to 5-point Likert scale, and the 10-point scale used a 2- to 3-point Likert scale.

[b] 0 = normal; 1 = erythema only; 2 = erythema, air-fluid level, clear fluid; 3 = erythema, complete effusion, no opacification; 4 = erythema, opacification with air-fluid level or air bubbles, no bulging; 5 = erythema, complete effusion, opacification, no bulging; 6 = erythema, bulging rounded doughnut appearance of the tympanic membrane; 7 = erythema, bulging, complete effusion and opacification with bulla formation.

From Cherry JD et al: *Feigin and Cherry's pediatric infectious diseases,* ed 8, Philadelphia, 2019, Elsevier.

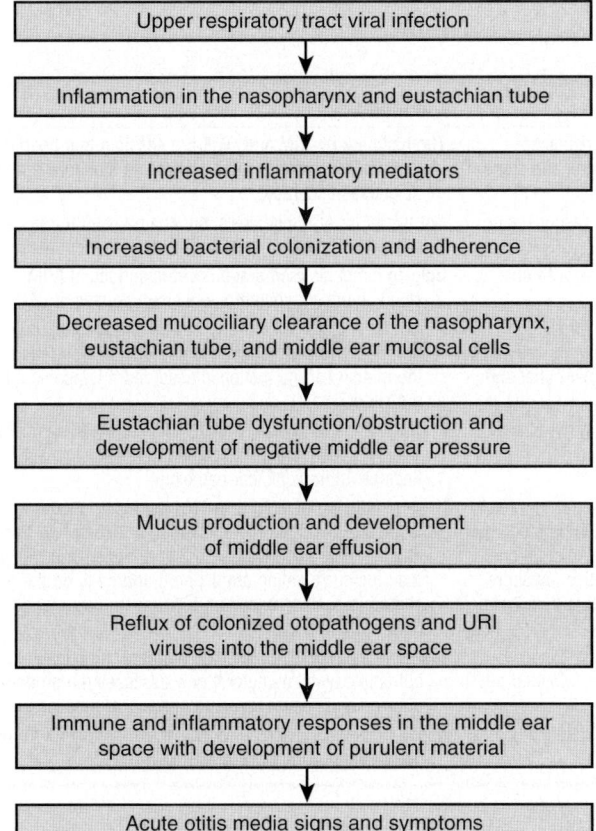

FIG. 2 Pathogenesis of virus-induced acute otitis media. *URI,* Upper respiratory infection. (From Cherry JD et al: *Feigin and Cherry's pediatric infectious diseases,* ed 8, Philadelphia, 2019, Elsevier.)

- Most common bacterial pathogens:[4,5]
  1. *Haemophilus influenzae* is now the most common causative pathogen of AOM in children.
  2. *S. pneumoniae* causes up to half of cases and is the least likely of the major pathogens to resolve without treatment.
  3. *Moraxella catarrhalis.*

- Of increasing importance, infection caused by penicillin-nonsusceptible *S. pneumoniae* (MIC >0.1 mg/ml), ranging from 8% to 34%. About 50% of PNSSP isolates are penicillin-intermediate (MIC 0.1 to 2.0 mg/ml).
- Group A streptococci is associated with higher rates of TM perforation than AOM caused by other pathogens.

- Viral pathogens:
  1. Respiratory syncytial virus (RSV)
  2. Rhinovirus
  3. Adenovirus
  4. Influenza
- Others:
  1. *Mycoplasma pneumoniae*
  2. *Chlamydia trachomatis*
  3. *Streptococcus pyogenes* (Latin America)

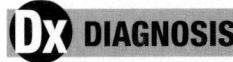 **DIAGNOSIS**

DIFFERENTIAL DIAGNOSIS
- Otitis externa
- Otitis media with effusion (OME): An algorithm for distinguishing between acute otitis media and otitis media with effusion is illustrated in Fig. 3
- Referred pain from mouth, nasopharynx, or throat
- Section II describes the differential diagnosis of earache

WORKUP (TABLE 4)
Thorough otoscopic examination. AOM is a visual diagnosis based on viewing the tympanic membrane. Adequate visualization of the tympanic membrane may require removal of cerumen and debris from the external ear canal.
- Tympanometry
  1. Measures compliance of the tympanic membrane and middle ear pressure
  2. Detects the presence of fluid, but cannot determine whether the fluid is infected
- Acoustic reflectometry
  1. Measures sound waves reflected from the middle ear
  2. Is useful in infants >3 mo
  3. Increased reflected sound correlated with the presence of effusion, but cannot determine whether the fluid is infected

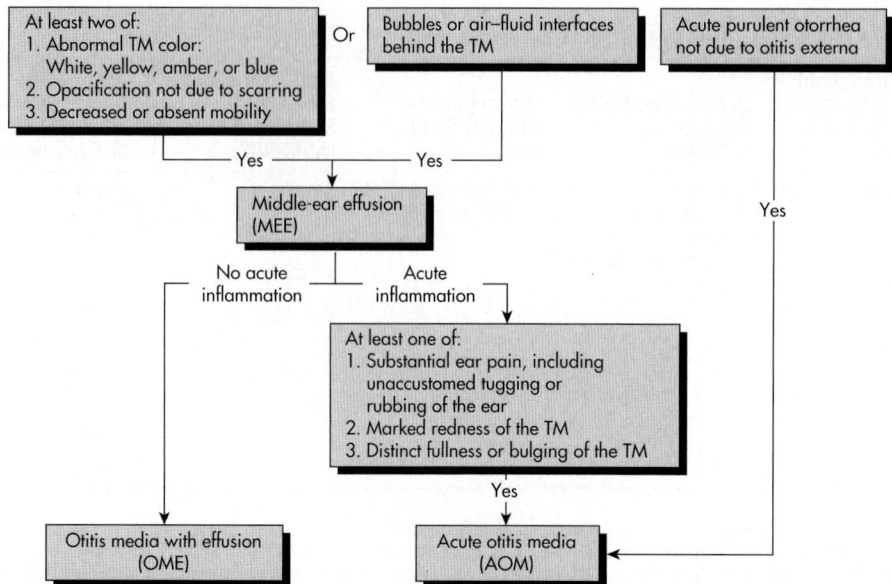

FIG. 3 **Algorithm for distinguishing between acute otitis media and otitis media with effusion.** *TM,* tympanic membrane. (From Kliegman RM: *Nelson textbook of pediatrics,* ed 21, Philadelphia, 2020, Elsevier.)

TABLE 4 Diagnostic Modalities for Otitis Media

Modality	Description	Comment
Signs and symptoms (obtained by history)	Includes ear-specific symptoms (ear pain, hearing loss), nonspecific symptoms (nausea, irritability, sleep disturbance, anorexia), and signs (fever, vomiting)	The hallmark of AOM and OME are ear pain and hearing loss, respectively, but signs and symptoms alone have poor diagnostic accuracy
Symptom severity scales	Parent-reported measures of AOM severity using categoric responses or a faces scale	Not useful for AOM diagnosis, but can be used to rate severity, follow the course of disease, and assess outcomes
Otoscopy	Visual examination of the ear canal and tympanic membrane with an otoscope	Bulging tympanic membrane is characteristic of AOM; opaque or cloudy tympanic membrane is characteristic of OME
Pneumatic otoscopy	Examination of the middle ear using an otoscope to create an air-tight (hermetic) seal in the ear canal and then gently squeezing (or releasing) the attached rubber bulb to change the pressure in the ear canal and observe the tympanic membrane	A normal tympanic membrane moves briskly with applied pressure, but the movement is minimal or sluggish when there is fluid in the middle ear; no motion is observed if tympanic membrane is not intact
Otomicroscopy	Examination of the ear canal and tympanic membrane using the binocular, otologic microscope to obtain a magnified view with good depth perception	Primary use is to assess tympanic membrane abnormalities (atrophy, sclerosis, retraction pockets) and to help distinguish surface findings from middle ear pathology
Tympanometry	An objective measure of middle ear function that requires an air-tight seal in the ear canal. Tympanometry provides a graph showing how energy admitted to the ear canal is reflected back to an internal microphone while the canal pressure is varied from negative to positive (pressure admittance function) and can be performed with a portable (handheld) unit or a desktop machine	If the middle ear is filled with fluid, tympanic membrane vibration is impaired and the result is a flat, or nearly flat, tracing. If the middle ear is filled with air but at a higher or lower pressure than the surrounding atmosphere, the peak on the graph will be shifted in position based on the pressure (to the left if negative, to the right if positive)
Acoustic reflectometry	Uses a transducer and microphone at the entrance of the ear canal, without an air-tight seal, to measure how much sound is reflected off the tympanic membrane	Higher reflectivity levels indicate a greater probability of effusion, but unlike tympanometry it only assesses the probability of effusion and cannot measure middle ear function
Computed tomography	An imaging procedure, using ionizing radiation, to create a detailed scan of the temporal bone	Useful in surgical planning for CSOM but not useful for primary diagnosis of AOM, OME, or CSOM

AOM, Acute otitis media; *CSOM,* chronic suppurative otitis media; *OME,* otitis media with effusion.
From Flint PW et al: *Cummings otolaryngology, head and neck surgery,* ed 7, Philadelphia, 2021, Elsevier.

LABORATORY TESTS
- Tympanocentesis.
  1. Not necessary in most cases because the microbiology of middle ear effusions has been shown to be extremely consistent
  2. May be indicated in:
     a. Patients who do not respond to treatment in 72 h or those who experience multiple treatment failures
     b. Immunocompromised patients

- Cultures of the nasopharynx are not helpful.
- Blood counts (generally unnecessary) usually reveal leukocytosis with polymorphonuclear elevation.
- Plain mastoid radiographs (generally unnecessary) reveal haziness in the periantral cells that may extend to entire mastoid.
- Computed tomography (CT) or MRI may be indicated if serious complications are suspected (meningitis, brain abscess, severe mastoiditis).

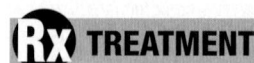 **TREATMENT**

ACUTE GENERAL Rx
- Hydration, avoidance of irritants (e.g., tobacco smoke, air pollution, bottle feeding), nasal decongestants, cool mist humidifier, and oral ibuprofen or acetaminophen. Topical procaine or lidocaine preparations (if available) are an alternative to oral analgesics for children ≥2 yr

but should not be used in children with tympanic membrane perforation.[3]
- Antibiotics: See "Complementary & Alternative Medicine."

SURGICAL Rx

- There is no evidence to support the routine use of myringotomy, but in severe cases it provides prompt pain relief and accelerates resolution of infection.
- Purulent secretions retained in the middle ear can lead to increased pressure that may lead to spread of infection to contiguous areas. Myringotomy to decompress the middle ear is sometimes necessary to avoid complications such as mastoiditis, facial nerve paralysis, labyrinthitis, meningitis, and brain abscess.

CHRONIC Rx

- Among children 6 to 35 mo of age with recurrent acute otitis media, the rate of episodes of acute otitis media during a 2-yr period is not significantly lower with tympanostomy-tube placement than with medical management, however myringotomy and tympanostomy tube placement for persistent or recurrent middle ear effusion unresponsive to medical therapy can be considered if fluid has persisted for ≥3 mo if bilateral or ≥6 mo if unilateral.
- Adenoidectomy, with or without tonsillectomy, often is advocated for treatment of recurrent otitis media, although evidence for this procedure is controversial.
- Long-term complications include tympanic membrane perforations, cholesteatoma, tympanosclerosis, ossicular necrosis, toxic or suppurative labyrinthitis, hearing loss, and intracranial suppuration.

DISPOSITION

Patients can be treated at home as outpatients with the rare exception of patients with evidence of local suppurative complications (e.g., meningitis, acute mastoiditis, brain abscess, cavernous sinus, or lateral sinus thrombosis).

COMPLEMENTARY & ALTERNATIVE MEDICINE[6]

- Xylitol and vitamin intake may help prevent further otitis media.[7]
- Biologically based therapies such as botanical extracts can be used if there is no perforation (all prepared in an olive oil base) and can be a reasonable complement during observation period or with the wait-and-see approach.
  1. Calendula
  2. Hypericum perforatum homeopathic preparation—can help with pain[7]
  3. Lavendar
  4. Vitamin E oil
- Manipulative methods have also been used by those properly trained in osteopathic manipulation and chiropractic techniques. Osteopathy requires weekly treatment for 3 wk and is an adjunct to other treatment modalities. Chiropractic techniques: Little is published, and there are currently no randomized controlled trials on PubMed.
- Chinese medicine has shown promising results but demands further research.[7]

Antimicrobials:
- NOTE: Most uncomplicated cases of AOM resolve spontaneously, without complications. Studies have demonstrated limited therapeutic benefit from antibiotic therapy. Watchful waiting is appropriate for children who look well, can be comforted with supportive care, and are old enough to easily evaluate. Children <24 mo with bilateral AOM should receive antibiotic therapy. Children with severe signs or symptoms (moderate or severe otalgia or otalgia for ≥48 h or temperature ≥39° C) should also receive antibiotic therapy. Fig. E4 illustrates an algorithm for management of acute otitis media in pediatric populations.

When opting to use antibiotic therapy:[2,4,8-10]
- Amoxicillin has been used for years as first line treatment of AOM but because of increased prevalence of AOM caused by beta-lactamase strains of *H. influenzae* and *M. catarrhalis,* some expert clinicians now recommend amoxicillin-clavulanate for initial treatment.
- Treatment failure is defined by lack of clinical improvement of signs or symptoms after 3 days (72 h or greater) of therapy.
- With treatment failure (if using amoxicillin), in the absence of an identified etiologic pathogen, therapy should be redirected to cover:
  1. Drug-resistant *S. pneumoniae*
  2. β-lactamase–producing strains of *H. influenzae* and *M. catarrhalis*
- Agents fulfilling these criteria include amoxicillin-clavulanate, second-generation (e.g., cefuroxime axetil, cefaclor) or third-generation (e.g., oral cefdinir or cefpodoxime or IM ceftriaxone) cephalosporins. Cefaclor, cefixime, loracarbef, and ceftibuten should be avoided given their limited activity against pneumococci.
- Cross-resistance between TMP/SMX and macrolides and the β-lactams exists; therefore patients who do not respond to amoxicillin are more likely to have infections resistant to TMP/SMX and macrolides.
- Fluoroquinolones are not indicated as first- or second-line therapy for AOM and should be avoided in young children due to risks of

musculoskeletal effects and limited dosing guidance and limited availability of oral suspension compounds or compounding pharmacies.
- Treatment should be modified according to cultures and sensitivities when available.
- Treatment course is 10 days for children <2 yr and those with severe symptoms, 7 days for children age 2 to 5 yr, and 5 to 7 days for children ≥6 yr.
- Follow-up should be tailored to clinical improvement and concern for neurocognitive developmental delays in at-risk children. Standard follow-up of all cases is no longer recommended.
- Antibiotic prophylaxis to reduce the frequency of AOM episodes in children with recurrent AOM is not recommended.
- Table E5 summarizes suggested antibiotics for treatment of otitis media and for patients who have failed first-line antibiotic treatment.

REFERRAL

- To otorhinolaryngologist in cases of:
  1. Medical treatment failure
  2. An uncertain diagnosis; adults with one or more episodes of AOM should be referred for evaluation to rule out an underlying process (e.g., malignancy)
  3. Any of the above-mentioned acute and chronic complications

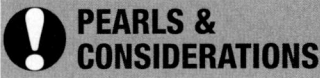

PEARLS & CONSIDERATIONS

COMMENTS

- Otoscopic findings are critical for accurate AOM diagnosis.[11]
- AOM microbiology has changed with use of pneumococcal conjugate vaccine (PCV13).
- Antibiotics are modestly more effective than no treatment but cause adverse effects in 4% to 10% of children.
- Most antibiotics have comparable clinical success.

PREVENTION

- Vaccinate against common pathogens.
- Breastfeed and bottle-feed infants in an upright position.
- Avoid irritants (e.g., tobacco smoke).

REFERENCES

Available at eBooks.Health.Elsevier.com

AUTHOR: **KATHERINE ELIZABETH MCGRAW, MD**

Diseases and Disorders

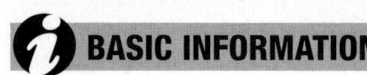

BASIC INFORMATION

DEFINITION

Ovarian cancer is not one disease but a constellation of distinct cancer subtypes classified according to their tissue of origin. About 90% of tumors are epithelial ovarian cancers, 5% are germ cell tumors, and 5% are sex cord-stromal tumors. A classification of ovarian epithelial tumors is summarized in Table E1.

SYNONYMS

Epithelial ovarian cancer
Germ cell tumor
Sex cord stromal tumor
Ovarian tumor of low malignant potential
Ovarian malignancy

ICD-10CM CODES
C56.9   Malignant neoplasm of unspecified ovary
C56.1   Malignant neoplasm of right ovary
C56.2   Malignant neoplasm of left ovary

EPIDEMIOLOGY & DEMOGRAPHICS

INCIDENCE: Ovarian cancer ranks fifth in cancer deaths among biologic females and is the leading cause of gynecologic cancer–related deaths. There are 10.6 cases/100,000 persons and ~19,880 new cases annually. Lifetime risk for developing ovarian cancer is 1.1%. The rate of diagnosis of ovarian cancer has been slowly declining over the past 20 yr.[1]
PREVALENCE: Median age at time of diagnosis: 63 yr
RISK FACTORS:
- Low parity
- Delayed childbearing
- Smoking
- Polycystic ovary syndrome
- Endometriosis
- High-fat diet
- Lynch II syndrome (nonpolyposis colon cancer, endometrial cancer, breast cancer, and ovarian cancer clusters in first- and second-degree relatives)
- Breast-ovarian familial cancer syndrome
- Site-specific familial ovarian cancer
- The **strongest** risk factors are advancing age and family history of ovarian and breast cancer
- Factors that **decrease** the risk of ovarian cancer include previous pregnancy, oral contraceptive pill use, hysterectomy, tubal ligation, or salpingectomy
- Table 2 summarizes risk and protective factors for ovarian cancer
GENETICS: The greatest risk factors of ovarian cancer are a family history and associated genetic syndromes. More than 90% of inherited ovarian malignancies are associated with *BRCA1* and *BRCA2* mutations. *BRCA* mutations interact with and affect DNA repair proteins. The estimated lifetime risk of ovarian cancer for patients with either of these mutations is 65% to 74%.
Genetic counseling is recommended for certain patients, including those with:

- Epithelial ovarian cancer at any age
- Breast cancer diagnosed at age 45 yr or younger
- Breast cancer with two distinct and sequential primaries, the first one diagnosed at age 50 yr or younger
- Breast cancer that is triple-negative and diagnosed at age 60 yr or younger
- Breast cancer at any age, with at least one close relative diagnosed at age 50 yr or younger
- Breast cancer diagnosed at any age, with two or more close relatives with breast cancer; one close relative with epithelial ovarian cancer; or two close relatives with pancreatic cancer or aggressive prostate cancer
- Breast cancer, with a close male relative at any age who has breast cancer
- Breast cancer and Ashkenazi Jewish ancestry
- A family with a known deleterious *BRCA1* or *BRCA2* mutation

PHYSICAL FINDINGS & CLINICAL PRESENTATION

- Patients with ovarian cancer commonly present with nonspecific symptoms. A recent study revealed that at the time of diagnosis 72% of women had at least one symptom and 32% had two or more symptoms (Table 3). The most common presenting symptoms were abdominal or pelvic pain (31%) and bloating or a sensation of abdominal fullness (26%)[2]
- 60% present with advanced disease
- Abdominal fullness, early satiety, dyspepsia
- Pelvic pain, back pain, constipation

TABLE 2   Risk and Protective Factors for Ovarian Cancer

Increased Risk	Protective
Lifestyle and diet factors	Lifestyle and diet factors
Aging	Soy intake
Obesity	Flavonoids
Tall stature	High calcium
Animal fat intake	Sun exposure
α-linolenic acid	Adequate sleep
Dairy foods	Metformin
Lactose product	
Cigarette use	
Diabetes mellitus	
Reproductive factors	Reproductive factors
Menopausal hormone therapy	Oral contraceptive
Menopausal age	Breastfeeding
Infertility	Tubal sterilization
Polycystic ovarian syndrome	Salpingectomy
Endometriosis	Hysterectomy
Pelvic inflammatory disease	Parity
Genetic factors	

From Niederhuber JE: *Abeloff's clinical oncology,* ed 6, Philadelphia, 2020, Elsevier.

- Pelvic or abdominal mass (Table 4)
- Lymphadenopathy (inguinal)
- Sister Mary Joseph nodule (umbilical mass)

ETIOLOGY

- Can be inherited as site-specific familial ovarian cancer (two or more first-degree relatives have ovarian cancer)
- Breast-ovarian cancer syndrome (clusters of breast and ovarian cancer among first- and second-degree relatives)
- Lynch syndrome
- There is no contributory family history and an unknown etiology in the majority of ovarian cancer cases

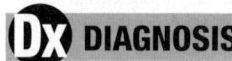 DIAGNOSIS

DIFFERENTIAL DIAGNOSIS

- Primary peritoneal cancer mesothelioma
- Benign ovarian tumor
- Functional ovarian cyst
- Endometriosis
- Ovarian torsion
- Pelvic kidney
- Pedunculated uterine fibroid
- Primary cancer from breast, gastrointestinal tract, or other pelvic organ metastasized to the ovary

TABLE 3   Symptoms in Ovarian Cancer

Symptom	% of patients
Pain (late symptom)	50-60
Abdominal swelling (persistent bloating)	50-65
Anorexia	20
Nausea and vomiting	20
Weight loss	15
Abnormal vaginal bleeding	15
Frequency	10
Malaise	5
Change in bowel habit	5
Virilization	Rare
Precocious puberty	Rare

From Magowan BA: *Clinical obstetrics & gynecology,* ed 4, London, 2019, Elsevier.

TABLE 4   Signs of Ovarian Cancer

Sign	% of patients
Pelvic mass	70-80
Abdominal mass	60-70
Ascites	30-40
Pleural effusion	10-15
Hepatomegaly	<5
Cervical lymphadenopathy	<5

From Magowan BA: *Clinical obstetrics & gynecology,* ed 4, London, 2019, Elsevier.

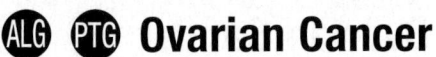

WORKUP

- Definitive diagnosis made at laparotomy; epithelial ovarian cancer most common type of ovarian cancer (90% of ovarian cancer cases)
- Careful physical and history, including family history
- Exclusion of nongynecologic etiologies
- Observation of small cystic masses in premenopausal women for regression for 2 mo
- FIGO classification of ovarian carcinoma is described in Table 5
- Referral to specialists who have extensive training and experience in treating ovarian cancer significantly increases survival after an ovarian cancer diagnosis

LABORATORY TESTS

- Complete blood count.
- Chemistry profile including liver tests and calcium (to evaluate for paraneoplastic syndrome).
- CA-125 or lysophosphatidic acid level. Use of these tests for annual screening is controversial, and most experts warn against universal screening with this marker. Only about 50% of early-stage ovarian cancers will be associated with elevated CA-125. Additionally, false elevations may occur with uterine leiomyoma, endometriosis, pregnancy, and intraabdominal infections. The PLCO cancer screening trial revealed that annual screening based on CA-125 and vaginal ultrasound is ineffective,

and diagnostic follow-up of false positives resulted in a 15% serious complication rate.
- Consider the following laboratory tests: Human chorionic gonadotropin, inhibin, alpha-fetoprotein, neuron-specific enolase, and lactate dehydrogenase.
- A panel of three serum biomarkers (apolipoprotein A-1 [ApoA-1], transthyretin [TTR], and transferrin [TF]) has been reported useful in distinguishing normal samples from early-stage ovarian cancer with a sensitivity of 84% and normal samples from late-stage ovarian cancer with a sensitivity of 97%.
- *BRCA1/2* testing is recommended for all women with ovarian cancer.

IMAGING STUDIES

- Ultrasound
- Chest x-ray examination
- Computed tomography or MRI of abdomen and pelvis help evaluate extent of disease (Fig. E1)
- Mammogram

Rx TREATMENT

NONPHARMACOLOGIC THERAPY

Virtually all cases of ovarian cancer involve surgical exploration. This includes:
- Abdominal cytology
- Total abdominal hysterectomy and bilateral salpingo-oophorectomy (except when fertility

preservation is desired and the disease is in the early stage)
- Omentectomy
- Diaphragm sampling
- Selective lymphadenectomy (pelvic and para-aortic nodes)
- Primary cytoreduction with a goal of residual tumor diameter <2 cm
- Bowel surgery, splenectomy if needed to obtain optimal (<2 cm) cytoreduction
- Conventional treatment includes surgical debulking (cytoreduction) followed by chemotherapy. However, patients with low-grade, well-differentiated stage I ovarian cancer do not benefit from adjuvant chemotherapy

ACUTE GENERAL Rx

- Optimal cytoreduction (debulking) is generally followed by chemotherapy (except in some early-stage disease [stage I without high-risk features is treated with surgery alone]).
- Cisplatin-based combination chemotherapy is used for stage II or greater, 6-mo treatment. Compared with IV paclitaxel plus cisplatin, IV paclitaxel plus intraperitoneal cisplatin and paclitaxel improves survival rates in patients with optimally debulked stage III ovarian cancer.
- Chemotherapy regimens continue to change as research continues. Bevacizumab, a humanized antivascular endothelial growth factor monoclonal antibody, has been shown to be effective in improving progression-free survival in women with ovarian cancer. Trials using bevacizumab during and up to 10 mo after carboplatin and paclitaxel chemotherapy have shown prolongation of the median progression-free survival by about 4 mo in patients with advanced epithelial ovarian cancer.
- Antibody drug conjugates in conjunction with VEG-F inhibitors such as bevacizumab are a promising new area of study that is currently under investigation for treatment of patients who are resistant to platinum-based chemotherapy. This area remains under investigation.[3]
- Mirvetuximab soravtansine-gynx (MIRV), a first-in-class antibody-drug conjugate targeting folate receptor alpha (FRα) is approved for treatment of platinum-resistant ovarian cancer in the U.S. and recent phase 3 trials have shown a significant benefit over chemotherapy with respect to progression-free and overall survival and objective response.[4]
- PARP inhibitors are up-and-coming chemotherapeutic agents that have been used for maintenance therapy and have been shown to improve progression-free survival among patients with platinum-sensitive high-grade serous cancers. PARP inhibitors work by pharmacologically inhibiting the enzyme poly (ADP-ribose) polymerase. Three PARP inhibitors are currently U.S. Food and Drug Administration approved for different indications. Olaparib, an oral polymerase inhibitor, was approved in 2014 and has shown antitumor activity in patients with high-grade serous ovarian cancer with or without *BRCA1* and *BRCA2* germline

TABLE 5 Staging of Ovarian Carcinomas*

Stage	Characteristics
I	Tumor confined to the ovaries
IA	Growth limited to one ovary (capsule intact); no tumor on ovarian surface; no malignant cells in the ascites or peritoneal washings
IB	Tumor limited to both ovaries (capsule intact); no tumor on ovarian surface; no malignant cells in the ascites or peritoneal washings
IC	Tumor limited to one or both ovaries
1C1	Surgical spill
1C2	Capsule ruptured before surgery or tumor on ovarian surface
1C3	Malignant cells in the ascites or peritoneal washings
II	Tumor involves one or both ovaries with pelvic extension
IIA	Extension or metastases to the uterus or fallopian tubes
IIB	Extension to other pelvic intraperitoneal tissues
III	Tumor involving one or both ovaries with cytologically or histologically confirmed spread to the peritoneum outside the pelvis or metastasis to the retroperitoneal lymph nodes
IIIA1	Positive retroperitoneal lymph nodes only (cytologically or histologically proved)
IIIA1 (i)	Metastasis up to 10 mm in greatest dimension
IIIA1 (ii)	Metastasis more than 10 mm in greatest dimension
IIIA2	Microscopic extrapelvic (above the pelvic brim) peritoneal involvement with or without positive retroperitoneal lymph nodes
IIIB	Macroscopic peritoneal metastasis beyond the pelvis up to 2 cm in greatest dimension, with or without metastasis to the retroperitoneal lymph nodes
IIIC	Macroscopic peritoneal metastasis beyond the pelvis more than 2 cm in greatest dimension, with or without metastasis to the retroperitoneal lymph nodes (includes extension of tumor to capsule of liver and spleen without parenchymal involvement of either organ)
IV	Distant metastases excluding peritoneal metastases
IVA	Pleural effusion with positive cytology
IVB	Parenchymal metastases and metastases to extraabdominal organs (including inguinal lymph nodes and lymph nodes outside of the abdominal cavity)

*According to the International Federation of Gynecology and Obstetrics (FIGO), 2014.
From Berek JS et al: Cancer of the ovary, fallopian tube, and peritoneum: 2021 update, *Int J Gynecol Obstet* 155(Suppl 1):61-85, 2021. https://doi.org/10.1002/ijgo.13878.

mutations. Rucaparib was approved in 2016 to treat high-grade serous cancers with *BRCA1* and *BRCA2* germline or somatic mutations. Last, niraparib was approved in 2017 for use in high-grade serous cancers with or without *BRCA1* and *BRCA2* mutations.

- Second-look surgery when chemotherapy is complete generally is no longer recommended because this has not been shown to improve survival.
- In most cases, neoadjuvant (presurgical) chemotherapy has no advantage over postsurgical initiation of chemotherapy. However, some trials have shown that neoadjuvant chemotherapy followed by interval debulking surgery is not inferior to debulking surgery followed by chemotherapy as a treatment option for patients with bulky stage IIIC or IV ovarian carcinoma. Complete resection of all macroscopic disease, whether performed as primary treatment or after neoadjuvant chemotherapy, remains the objective whenever cytoreductive surgery is performed.

CHRONIC Rx

- If CA-125 is increasing, this may indicate recurrent disease. However, routine monitoring of CA-125 at every visit does not improve survival and should be reserved for addressing specific clinical concerns.
- Physical and pelvic examinations recommended every 2 to 4 mo for 2 yr, every 3 to 6 mo during third yr, then annually after 5 yr.
- Annual Pap smear.
- A treatment approach algorithm for recurrent ovarian cancer is illustrated in Fig. 2.
- A recent randomized trial of cytoreductive surgery for relapsed ovarian cancer revealed that in women with recurrent ovarian cancer, cytoreductive surgery followed by chemotherapy results in longer overall survival than chemotherapy alone. Secondly, cytoreductive surgery should be considered an appropriate option in properly selected patients if it can be performed by experienced surgeons in centers of excellence.[5]

DISPOSITION

- Overall 5-yr survival rates remain low because of the preponderance of late-stage disease:
  1. Stage I and II: 80% to 100%
  2. Stage III: 15% to 20%
  3. Stage IV: 5%
- Younger patients (<50 yr) in all stages have a considerably better 5-yr survival than older patients (40% vs. 15%).
- Among women with high-grade serous ovarian cancer, *BRCA2* mutation, but not *BRCA1* deficiency, is associated with improved survival, improved chemotherapy response, and genome instability compared with *BRCA* wild-type.
- Among patients with invasive epithelial ovarian cancer (EOC), having a germline mutation in *BRCA1* or *BRCA2* is associated with improved 5-yr overall survival. *BRCA2* carriers have the best prognosis.

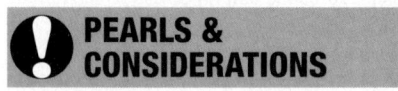 **PEARLS & CONSIDERATIONS**

COMMENTS

- The U.S. Preventive Services Task Force has concluded that current evidence does not show any mortality benefit to routine screening for ovarian cancer with transvaginal ultrasonography or single-threshold serum CA-125 testing and that the harms of such screening are at least moderate. This recommendation applies to asymptomatic women who are not known to have a high-risk hereditary cancer syndrome.
- Oral contraceptives reduce the risk of ovarian cancer by 40% to 50%. The greatest risk reduction is present after ≥15 yr of oral contraceptive use.
- Patients at high risk for developing ovarian cancer (*BRCA1/BRCA2* gene mutation, hereditary nonpolyposis colorectal cancer syndrome) should consider prophylactic salpingo-oophorectomy after childbearing is complete. Prophylactic bilateral salpingo-oophorectomy reduces ovarian cancer by 80%. It is recommended by age 35 to 40 yr for *BRCA1* carriers and by age 45 for *BRCA2* carriers. If surgery is declined, the National Comprehensive Cancer network guidelines recommend intensive surveillance with pelvic and abdominal sonogram and serum CA-125 every 6 mo starting at age 35 or 10 yr earlier than cancer diagnosis in family member.

REFERENCES

Available at eBooks.Health.Elsevier.com.

RELATED CONTENT

Ovarian Cancer (Patient Information)
Ovarian Neoplasm, Benign (Related Key Topic)

AUTHORS: **LAUREN DAVIS RIVERA, MD, MSED** and **SUDESHNA CHATTERJEE-PAER, MD**

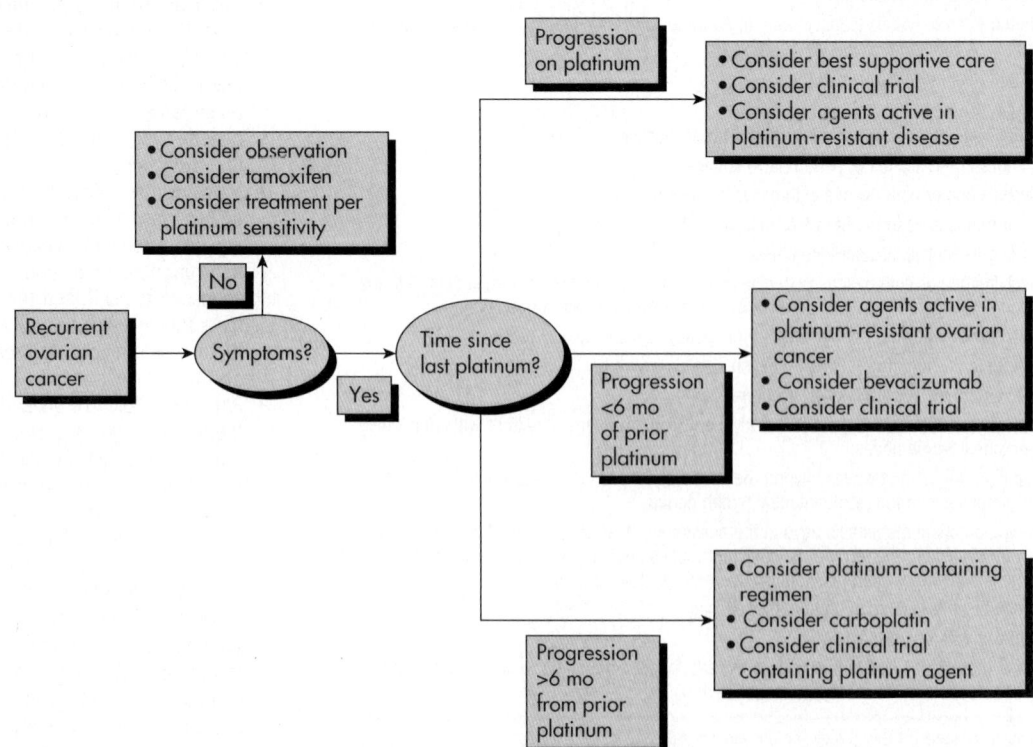

FIG. 2 Treatment approach algorithm for recurrent ovarian cancer. (From Niederhuber JE: *Abeloff's clinical oncology,* ed 6, Philadelphia, 2020, Elsevier.)

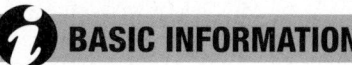

DEFINITION

Paget disease of bone is a nonmalignant focal disorder of chaotic bone remodeling with increased osteoblastic and osteoclastic activity that results in a disorganized mosaic pattern of woven and lamellar bone (Fig. E1) in one or more skeletal sites.[1] This disordered remodeling results in enlarged, hypervascular bone susceptible to deformation and fracture.

SYNONYM

Osteitis deformans

ICD-10CM CODES
M88.9	Osteitis deformans of unspecified bone
M88.0	Osteitis deformans of skull
M88.1	Osteitis deformans of vertebrae
M88.869	Osteitis deformans of unspecified lower leg
M88.89	Osteitis deformans of multiple sites
M90.60	Osteitis deformans in neoplastic diseases, unspecified site
M90.679	Osteitis deformans in neoplastic diseases, unspecified ankle and foot
M90.68	Osteitis deformans in neoplastic diseases, other site
M90.69	Osteitis deformans in neoplastic diseases, multiple sites

EPIDEMIOLOGY & DEMOGRAPHICS

Epidemiologic data suggest Paget disease originated in Great Britain, and English colonists spread the disease to other areas beginning in the seventeenth century. Highest prevalence occurs in Eastern and Western Europe and in those of European descent who have emigrated to New Zealand, Australia, South Africa, and North America. Paget disease is rarely seen in Scandinavians, Japanese, Chinese, Asian Indians, sub-Saharan Africans, and Middle Eastern Arabs.[1,2]

- Most common diagnosis is above the age of 50 yr and rare before the age of 40 yr.
- Prevalence estimates suggest up to 3% of population ages >50 yr and up to 10% in those ages >90 yr.

INCIDENCE: Family history positive in up to 40% of cases[3]

PREDOMINANT SEX: Variable preponderance of males[2]

PREDOMINANT AGE: Presentation is rare before the age of 55 yr, with prevalence of Paget disease increasing with age.[2,3]

PHYSICAL FINDINGS & CLINICAL PRESENTATION

- Most common sites of involvement: Pelvis (70%), lumbar spine (53%), sacrum, femur (55%), skull (42%), tibia (30%) (Fig. E2), humerus, scapula.[3]

- Uncommon sites of involvement: Hand, foot, fibula.[1,3]
- Lesions can occur in one (monostotic) or more bones/locations (polyostotic).[1,2]
- Gradual progression of disease in affected bone(s) with a rare appearance at new site(s).
- Many patients are asymptomatic, but up to 40% of patients who come to medical attention present with bone pain.[3]
- Symptoms and signs include bone and articular pain often related to secondary arthritis, bone deformities and enlargement, increased warmth over pagetic bone, skull enlargement, nerve entrapment or compression syndromes, cranial nerve deficits, especially deafness (Fig. E3), spinal cord compression, vascular steal syndromes, fissure fractures, fractures, and neoplastic degeneration.[3]

ETIOLOGY

Fig. E4 illustrates the pathophysiology of Paget disease. Extensive epidemiologic and laboratory data are in keeping with potential role of paramyxoviral infection of osteoclasts in a genetically susceptible individual with or without documented genetic mutations.[4]

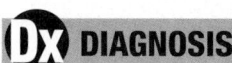

Diagnosis is often suspected in asymptomatic patients with isolated elevation of alkaline phosphatase without evidence of liver disease. The use of imaging studies is effective in determining the extent of disease.[1]

DIFFERENTIAL DIAGNOSIS[1]

- Osteosclerosis
- Hyperphosphatasia
- Familial expansile osteolysis
- Fibrous dysplasia
- Skeletal neoplasm (primary or metastatic)
- Osteomalacia with secondary hyperparathyroidism

LABORATORY TESTS[1]

- Isolated increase in serum alkaline phosphatase is highly indicative of Paget disease.[1,3]
- Assessing bone-specific alkaline phosphatase or procollagen type I N-terminal propeptide can be helpful in patients with coexisting liver disease.[3]
- Increase in urine N-terminal telopeptide/creatinine ratio or plasma C-terminal telopeptide.
- Bone biopsy is rarely needed but can be necessary in selected cases to rule out sarcomatous degeneration or metastatic disease.

IMAGING STUDIES

Bone scintigraphy (Fig. E5) is the most sensitive test for delineating the extent and site of pagetic lesions; however, it lacks specificity, as areas of uptake may be related to arthritis or metastatic lesions. Radiographs (Fig. E6) will further delineate characteristic pagetic changes (thickening of cortical bone, coarsened trabecular markings, distortion, and expansion of involved bone). Magnetic resonance imaging or computing tomography are

TABLE 1 Indications for Treatment of Paget Disease of Bone

Pain
Hypercalcemia
Fractures
High-output cardiac failure (rare)
Skull involvement
Neurologic compromise
Periarticular disease
Prevention of progression of Paget disease

From Firestein GS et al: *Firestein & Kelley's textbook of rheumatology,* ed 11, Philadelphia, 2021, Elsevier.

not recommended for diagnosis but are effective in assessing disease complications.[1]

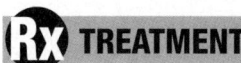

Indications for therapy (Table 1) include extensive or symptomatic disease; neurologic complications; involvement of weight-bearing bones, skull, vertebrae, and other areas of critical involvement (e.g., in proximity to joints); prevention of excess bleeding from an orthopedic procedure on pagetic bone; and if serum alkaline phosphatase is more than four times the upper limit of normal.[1]

NONPHARMACOLOGIC THERAPY

- Optimization of calcium and vitamin D intake and appropriate guidance regarding ambulatory needs.[1]
- Orthopedic stabilization may be required for patients with pseudofractures.[3]
- In the setting of acute unstable fractures, orthopedic preoperative planning and instrument selection should account for abnormal, hardened bone quality.

SPECIFIC THERAPY

Osteoclast inhibitors reduce the elevated rates of bone turnover that occur in active disease.[1] Bisphosphonates are the mainstay of therapy and include oral alendronate or risedronate and intravenous pamidronate or zoledronic acid. A one-time dose of zoledronic acid (5 mg intravenously) may be effective in controlling symptoms for over 3 yr.[5]

- Salmon calcitonin (SC) when bisphosphonates are not tolerated or are contraindicated as in those with glomerular filtration rate (GFR) of <35 ml/min
- Acetaminophen, aspirin, and nonsteroidal drugs for relief of pain

DISPOSITION

- Without treatment, progression of disease is common.
- With treatment, remissions of varying duration in most patients. For most patients with Paget disease, a single infusion of zoledronic acid will provide a prolonged suppression of pagetic activity and for many elderly patients a possible lifelong remission. Careful and regular clinical and biochemical follow-up at 3- to 6-mo intervals with necessity of retreatment in patients with continued pagetic activity or reactivation.[1]

- With first-ever intravenous dose of pamidronate or zoledronic acid, patients may experience a flulike syndrome that may be prevented with acetaminophen.
- A rare but serious complication of Paget disease is osteosarcoma (0.3% of patients).[1]
- Bisphosphonate therapy has been effective in reducing markers of bone turnover and total alkaline phosphatase values.[1-3]

REFERENCES

Available at eBooks.Health.Elsevier.com.

RELATED CONTENT

Paget Disease of Bone (Patient Information)

AUTHORS: **NISHANT JAYACHANDRAN, BA, SURYA KHATRI, BA,** and **JONATHAN LIU, MD**

ℹ BASIC INFORMATION

DEFINITION

Pancreatic cancer is an adenocarcinoma derived from pancreatic duct epithelium. Pancreatic intraepithelial neoplasia (PIN) refers to microscopic premalignant pancreatic ductal lesions that accumulate genetic alterations and undergo stepwise progression from low grade to high grade. Intraductal papillary mucinous neoplasms (IPMN) are precursors to pancreatic cancer with a 25% overall risk of invasive cancer especially in lesions arising from the main pancreatic duct.

ICD-10CM CODES
C25.9	Malignant neoplasm of pancreas, unspecified
C25.0	Malignant neoplasm of head of pancreas
C25.1	Malignant neoplasm of body of pancreas
C25.2	Malignant neoplasm of tail of pancreas
C25.3	Malignant neoplasm of pancreatic duct

EPIDEMIOLOGY & DEMOGRAPHICS

INCIDENCE:
- In 2023, it is estimated that there were 64,050 new cases and 49,830 deaths in the U.S.[1] It is the third-leading cause of cancer-related death in the U.S.
- Majority of patients present with advanced disease, and <20% patients present with potentially resectable tumors. At diagnosis, 35% have stage III disease, and 50% of patients have stage IV disease.[2]

PREDOMINANT SEX: The male:female ratio is 2:1.
PREDOMINANT AGE: Median age at diagnosis is 71 yr.

PHYSICAL FINDINGS & CLINICAL PRESENTATION

Presenting symptoms are generally related to primary tumor location:[3]
- Jaundice (60% to 70% of pancreatic cancers are located in the head of the pancreas)
- Dull abdominal pain or vague abdominal discomfort
- Weight loss
- Anorexia/change in taste, asthenia
- Nausea
- Uncommonly: Depression, gastrointestinal bleeding, acute pancreatitis (due to pancreatic duct obstruction), severe back pain (celiac axis involvement)
- Trousseau syndrome may be the initial presentation in some patients
- Table 1 summarizes demographic features and presenting symptoms in pancreatic cancer patients

PHYSICAL FINDINGS:
- Icterus
- Excoriations from scratching pruritic skin
- Cachexia and temporal wasting
- Ascites
- Hepatomegaly

ETIOLOGY

Unknown, but several conditions have been associated with pancreatic cancer:[3]
- Smoking
- Alcoholism
- Genetics: Up to 20% of patients have a family history of the disease
- Genetic syndromes and associated genes: Hereditary pancreatitis (*PRSS1, SPINK1*), Peutz-Jeghers syndrome (*STK11[LKB1]*), familial atypical multiple mole and melanoma syndrome (*p16*), hereditary breast and ovarian cancer syndromes (*BRCA1, BRCA2, PALB2*), ataxia telangiectasia (*ATM*), and Li-Fraumeni syndrome (*P53*)
- Gallstones
- Diabetes mellitus (present in at least 50% of patients with pancreatic cancer): New-onset diabetes after age 50 yr confers a six- to eightfold increased risk for pancreatic ductal adenocarcinoma[2]
- Chronic pancreatitis
- Diet rich in animal fat
- Occupational exposure: Oil refining, paper manufacturing, chemical industry
- Overweight or obesity during early adulthood is associated with a greater risk of pancreatic cancer and a younger age of disease onset. Obesity at an older age is associated with a lower overall survival in patients with pancreatic cancer
- There are four major driver genes for pancreatic cancer: *KRAS, CDKN2A, TP53*, and *SMAD4. KRAS* mutation and alterations in *CDKN2A* are early events in pancreatic cancer tumorigenesis
- Table 2 summarizes nongenetic and genetic risk factors for pancreatic cancer

Dx DIAGNOSIS

DIFFERENTIAL DIAGNOSIS
- Common duct cholelithiasis
- Cholangiocarcinoma
- Common duct stricture
- Sclerosing cholangitis
- Primary biliary cirrhosis
- Autoimmune pancreatitis
- Drug-induced cholestasis (e.g., phenothiazines)
- Other pancreatic tumors (islet cell tumor, cystadenocarcinoma, epidermoid carcinoma, sarcomas, lymphomas)

WORKUP
- Initial laboratory testing includes complete blood count, comprehensive chemistry panel.
- The bile duct antigen CA 19-9 is not useful for screening but is utilized for risk assessment after surgical resection, detecting recurrence, and therapeutic monitoring in patients undergoing systemic therapy.[4]
- All patients diagnosed with pancreatic cancer should undergo risk assessment for underlying cancer-associated hereditary syndromes. Germline genetic testing for cancer susceptibility should be considered even if family history is unremarkable.

Routine Laboratory Tests	% Abnormal
Alkaline phosphatase	80
Bilirubin	55
Total protein	15
Amylase	15
Hemoglobin	60

IMAGING STUDIES
- Multidetector helical computed tomography (CT) (Fig. E1) with intravenous administration of contrast is the imaging procedure of choice for initial evaluation.
- Endoscopic ultrasonography (Fig. E2) is useful when the diagnosis is strongly suspected and tissue is required for diagnostic purposes. Fine-needle aspiration biopsy combined with endoscopic ultrasonography is the preferred modality for evaluation of cystic or mass lesions to determine malignancy.

TABLE 1 Demographic Features and Presenting Symptoms and Signs in Patients with Unresectable (Palliated) and Resectable (Resected) Pancreatic Cancer

	Palliated (*N* = 256)	Resected (*N* = 512)
Demographic Features		
Age, average (yr)	64.0	65.8
Men/women	57%/43%	55%/45%
Race	91% white	91% white
Symptoms and Signs (%)		
Abdominal pain	64	36*
Jaundice	57	72*
Weight loss	48	43
Nausea/vomiting	30	18*
Back pain	26	2*

*P = 0.001 vs. palliated group.
Modified from Sohn T et al: Surgical palliation of unresectable periampullary adenocarcinoma in the 1990s, *J Am Coll Surg* 188:658-666, 1999. In Feldman M et al: *Sleisenger and Fordtran's gastrointestinal and liver disease*, ed 11, Philadelphia, 2021, Elsevier.

TABLE 2 Nongenetic and Genetic Risk Factors for Pancreatic Cancer

Variable	Risk Increase
Nongenetic Risk Factors	
Chronic pancreatitis	13.3
New-onset type 2 diabetes	7.9
Long-standing diabetes mellitus	2.0
Obesity	2.0
Smoking	1.8
Alcohol abuse	1.2
Non-O blood group	1.3
Genetic Syndrome and Associated Genes	
Familial pancreatic cancer (unknown gene)	
One first-degree relative	9
Three first-degree relatives	32
Familial adenomatous polyposis (APC)	4.5-6
Breast and ovarian cancer syndrome (BRCA1, BRCA2, PALB2)	2-3.5
Peutz-Jeghers syndrome (STK11/LKB1)	132
Hereditary pancreatitis (PRSS1, SPINK1)	69
Familial atypical multiple mole melanoma pancreatic carcinoma syndrome (P16INK4A/CDKN2A)	47
Lynch syndrome (MLH1, MSH2, MSH6, PMS2, EPCAM)	8.6
Cystic fibrosis (CFTR)	3.5
Ataxia-telangiectasia (ATM)	Unknown
Genetic Polymorphisms	
ABO	1.3
NR5A2	1.3
TERT	1.2
PDX1	1.2
BCAR1, CTRB1, CTRB2	1.5
ZNRF3	1.2
LINC00673	1.3
ETAA1	1.1
TP63	1.1
SUGCT	1.1

From Niederhuber JE: *Abeloff's clinical oncology*, ed 6, Philadelphia, 2020, Elsevier.

- Endoscopic retrograde cholangiopancreatography (ERCP, Fig. E3) is useful in patients with jaundice needing an endoscopic stent to relieve obstruction.
- PET scans are of limited value in pancreatic cancer and are not part of standard management.

Noninvasive Imaging	% Abnormal
Abdominal ultrasonography	60
Abdominal CT scan (with contrast) (Fig. E4)	90
Abdominal MRI scan	90
Invasive Imaging	**% Abnormal**
ERCP	90
CT scan or ultrasonography-guided needle aspiration cytology	90-95

STAGING

2018 AJCC eighth edition of staging system for pancreatic cancer:

PRIMARY TUMOR (T):

T_X	Primary tumor cannot be assessed
T_0	No evidence of primary tumor
T_1	Tumor <2 cm
T_2	Tumor >2 cm and <4 cm
T_3	Tumor >4 cm
T_4	Tumor involves celiac axis or superior mesenteric artery (unresectable primary)

LYMPH NODES (N):

N_0	No regional lymph nodes
N_1	Metastasis in 1-3 regional lymph nodes
N_2	Metastasis in >4 regional lymph nodes

DISTANT METASTASES (M):

M_X	Presence of distant metastasis cannot be assessed
M_0	No distant metastasis
M_1	Distant metastasis

STAGING GROUPS:

I_A	T_1, N_0, M_0
I_B	T_2, N_0, M_0
II_A	T_3, N_0, M_0
II_B	T_{1-3}, N_1, M_0
III	$T_{1-3}, N_2, M_0 T_4$, any N, M_0
IV	Any T, any N, M_1

Rx TREATMENT

Treatment sequencing strategies are summarized in Fig. 5 and Table 3.
- The overall treatment strategy is guided by the tumor resectability status and the patient's functional status. Pancreatic cancer (exocrine) is initially classified as resectable, borderline resectable, unresectable, and metastatic.[3]
- Palliative therapeutic ERCP with metal or plastic stents is performed for biliary decompression.

RESECTABLE DISEASE

Surgery:
- Classification of resectability of pancreatic cancer per the National Comprehensive Cancer Network and Surgical Oncology Expert Consensus Statement is summarized in Table 4.
- Curative pancreaticoduodenectomy (Whipple procedure) for pancreatic head and neck tumors is feasible in only 10% to 20% of patients (solitary lesion <5 cm, no locoregional invasion). Surgical mortality rate can be up to 5%. Distal pancreatectomy (+/- splenectomy) is used for pancreatic body or tail tumors.
- Due to the complexity of surgery and risk for significant morbidity and mortality, current guidelines recommend that pancreatic resections be carried out in centers that perform at least 15 to 20 cases annually. High-volume institutions are associated with higher negative-margin status and higher 5-yr survival rates, and that patients are more likely to receive multimodality therapy at these centers.[5]

ADJUVANT THERAPY

- Adjuvant chemotherapy improves postoperative survival and is considered the standard of care in patients with resected cancers.
- In older patients or those with borderline performance status, single-agent chemotherapy with either 5-fluorouracil (5-FU) or gemcitabine is used and results in median overall survival in the 20-mo range. The combination chemotherapy consisting of gemcitabine and capecitabine (GEMCAP) results in median overall survival of 28-mo range.
- In patients with maintained performance status (ECOG 0-1), the use of the modified FOLFIRINOX (5-FU, oxaliplatin, and irinotecan) chemotherapy regimen is the standard of care and results in striking outcomes with reported median overall survival of 54 mo.[6] Adjuvant use of gemcitabine and nab-paclitaxel is potentially useful, but a clear survival benefit has not been demonstrated.

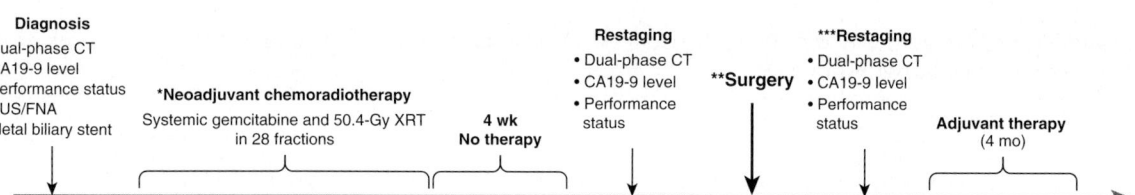

*Systemic therapy alone (FOLFIRINOX, gem-nab) is being considered by many clinicians because of the efficacy of these regimens in advanced disease and the challenges of delivering FOLFIRINOX in the adjuvant setting after such a large operation.
**Surgery is typically performed in the fifth week after the completion of XRT.
***Patients are restaged during postop week six if their recovery has been uncomplicated; however, there is no need to restage if recovery is complicated and the patient is not a suitable candidate to receive further systemic therapy.

A

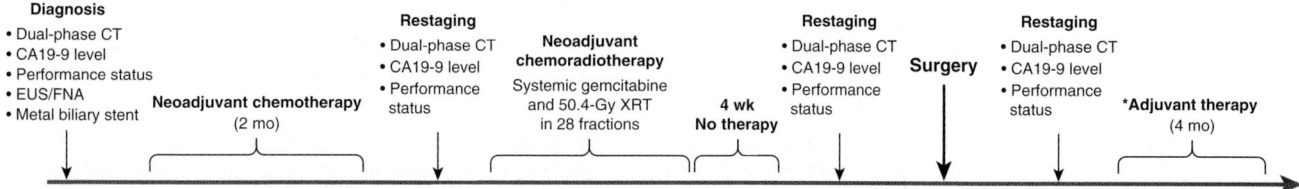

*The benefit of further postoperative/adjuvant systemic therapy after a more prolonged induction phase is being questioned, especially in those patients of advanced age or when postoperative recovery is slow.

B

FIG. 5 Schematic representation of treatment sequencing in **(A)** resectable and **(B)** borderline resectable pancreatic cancer (PC). *CA 19-9*, Cancer antigen 19-9; *CT*, computed tomography; *EUS*, endoscopic ultrasound scan; *FNA*, fine-needle aspiration; *FOLFIRINOX*, 5-fluorouracil, leucovorin, irinotecan, and oxaliplatin; *gem-nab*, gemcitabine/nab-paclitaxel; *XRT*, external radiotherapy. (From Cameron JL, Cameron AM: *Current surgical therapy*, ed 12, Philadelphia, 2017, Elsevier.)

TABLE 3 Comparison of Treatment Sequencing Strategies for Patients with Pancreatic Cancer (Outside of a Clinical Trial)

Stage	NCCN	MCW
Resectable	• Surgery • Restaging • Adjuvant therapy (+/− chemoradiotherapy; 6 mo)	• Neoadjuvant chemoradiotherapy (5.5 wk)* • Restaging • Surgery • Restaging • Adjuvant therapy (4 mo)
Borderline resectable	• Neoadjuvant therapy (regimen not specified) • Restaging • Surgery • Restaging • Consider adjuvant therapy	• Neoadjuvant chemotherapy (2 mo) • Restaging • Neoadjuvant chemoradiotherapy (5.5 wk) • Restaging • Surgery • Restaging • Adjuvant therapy (4 mo)
Locally advanced	• Chemotherapy • Restaging • Chemoradiotherapy in selected patients	• Chemotherapy (minimum 4 mo) • Restaging • Chemoradiotherapy • Restaging • Surgery in highly selected patients
Metastatic	• Systemic therapy • Clinical trial	• Systemic therapy • Clinical trial

NOTE: Clinical trials are preferred in all patients with pancreatic cancer (regardless of stage of disease) who have a performance status acceptable for treatment.
FOLFIRINOX, 5-fluorouracil, leucovorin, irinotecan, and oxaliplatin; *gem-nab*, gemcitabine/nab-paclitaxel; *MCW*, Medical College of Wisconsin; *NCCN*, National Comprehensive Cancer Network.
*Systemic therapy alone (FOLFIRINOX, gem-nab) is being considered by many clinicians because of the efficacy of these regimens in advanced disease and the challenges of delivering FOLFIRINOX in the adjuvant setting after such a large operation.
From Cameron JL, Cameron AM: *Current surgical therapy*, ed 12, Philadelphia, 2017, Elsevier.

• Adjuvant radiotherapy is controversial and is best limited to patients with poor risk features, margin-positive status, multiple involved nodes, or extranodal extension.

NEOADJUVANT THERAPY

• In patients with resectable and borderline-resectable pancreatic cancer, the use of upfront combination chemotherapy and concurrent radiotherapy modestly improved median overall survival but significantly improved the 5-yr overall survival rate from 6.5% to 20% while also significantly improving the complete resection rates.[7]

• Neoadjuvant chemotherapy alone followed by resection is also performed, and both FOLFIRINOX and gemcitabine-based regimens are routinely used in this setting.

RECURRENT/METASTATIC DISEASE

• In patients with metastatic disease, accepted upfront chemotherapy treatment approaches have demonstrated improvement in survival outcomes. Acceptable chemotherapy regimens for locally advanced and metastatic disease are summarized in Table 5.

• Options can include gemcitabine alone, combination regimen consisting of 5-fluorouracil, leucovorin, irinotecan, and oxaliplatin (FOLFIRINOX), or the combination of nab-paclitaxel plus gemcitabine. Multiagent regimens have an improved survival outcome compared with single-agent therapy.

• Liposomal irinotecan in combination with infusional 5-fluorouracil is now also approved in the setting of progressive disease after failure of first-line chemotherapy. Recent results have also demonstrated the superiority of first-line use of liposomal irinotecan containing chemotherapy (NALIRIFOX) regimen.

• Maintenance therapy with the PARP inhibitor olaparib (after systemic chemotherapy) in germline *BRCA* mutated pancreatic cancer improves progression-free survival.[8]

• Poor survival outcomes are seen in patients with poor performance status, significant weight loss, and with liver metastases.

• Combined chemoradiotherapy can be utilized in the case of patients with locally advanced but unresectable cases and confers a modest improvement in median overall survival.

DISPOSITION

Adjuvant postoperative chemotherapy has a significant survival benefit in patients with resected pancreatic cancer.

Diseases and Disorders

I

TABLE 4 Classification of Resectability of Pancreatic Cancer per the National Comprehensive Cancer Network and Surgical Oncology Expert Consensus Statement

Resectability Status	Criteria
Resectable	• No distant metastases • No radiographic evidence of SMV and portal vein abutment, distortion, tumor thrombus, or venous encasement • Clear fat planes around the celiac axis, hepatic artery, and SMA
Borderline resectable	• For tumors of the head or uncinate process: 　1. Solid tumor contact with the SMV or portal vein of >180 degrees with contour irregularity of the vein or thrombosis of the vein but with suitable vessel proximal and distal to the site of involvement, allowing for safe and complete resection and vein reconstruction 　2. Solid tumor contact with the IVC 　3. Solid tumor contact with the common hepatic artery without extension to the celiac axis or hepatic artery bifurcation, allowing for safe and complete resection and reconstruction 　4. Solid tumor contact with the SMA ≤180 degrees 　5. Solid tumor contact with variable anatomy (e.g., accessory right hepatic artery, replaced right hepatic artery, replaced common hepatic artery, and the origin of replaced or accessory artery), and the presence and degree of tumor contact should be noted if present, as it may affect surgical planning • For tumors of the body or tail: 　1. Solid tumor contact with the celiac axis of ≤180 degrees 　2. Solid tumor contact with the celiac axis >180 degrees without involvement of the aorta and with an intact and uninvolved gastroduodenal artery, thereby permitting a modified Appleby procedure (although some members of the consensus committee preferred this criterion to be in the unresectable category)
Unresectable/locally advanced	• Head of pancreas or uncinate lesions: 　1. Solid tumor contact with the SMA >180 degrees 　2. Solid tumor contact with the celiac axis >180 degrees 　3. Solid tumor contact with the first jejunal SMA branch 　4. Unreconstructable SMV or portal vein because of tumor involvement or occlusion (can be because of tumor or bland thrombus) 　5. Contact with the most proximal draining jejunal branch into the SMV • Body and tail lesions: 　1. Solid tumor contact of >180 degrees with the SMA or celiac axis 　2. Solid tumor contact with the celiac axis and aortic involvement 　3. Unreconstructable SMV or portal vein because of tumor involvement or occlusion (can be because of tumor or bland thrombus) • For all sites: 　1. Distant metastases 　2. Metastases to lymph nodes beyond the field of resection
Metastatic	• Any presence of distant metastases

IVC, Inferior vena cava; *SMA,* spinal muscular atrophy; *SMV,* superior mesenteric vein.
From Niederhuber JE: *Abeloff's clinical oncology,* ed 6, Philadelphia, 2020, Elsevier.

TABLE 5 Acceptable Chemotherapy Regimens for Locally Advanced and Metastatic Disease[a]

Locally Advanced or Unresectable	Metastatic Disease
Options for patients with good performance status: • FOLFIRINOX • Gemcitabine + albumin bound-paclitaxel • Gemcitabine + erlotinib • Gemcitabine + capecitabine • Gemcitabine + cisplatin (especially in patients with *BRCA1/2* mutation and/or family history) • Capecitabine single agent • CI 5-FU • Fixed-dose gemcitabine/docetaxel/capecitabine (GTX regimen) • Fluoropyrimidine + oxaliplatin • Chemotherapy (any of above) followed by chemoradiation or SBRT • Chemoradiation or SBRT	Options for patients with good performance status: • FOLFIRINOX (category 1) • Gemcitabine + albumin bound-paclitaxel (category 1) • Gemcitabine + erlotinib (category 1) • Gemcitabine (category 1) • Gemcitabine + capecitabine • Gemcitabine + cisplatin (especially in patients with *BRCA1/2* mutation and/or family history) • Fixed-dose gemcitabine/docetaxel/capecitabine (GTX regimen) (category 2B) • Fluoropyrimidine + oxaliplatin (category 2B)
Options for patients with poor performance status: • Gemcitabine • Capecitabine • CI 5-FU	Options for patients with poor performance status: • Gemcitabine (category 1) • Capecitabine (category 2B) • CI 5-FU (category 2B)

CI, Continuous infusion; *FOLFIRINOX,* 5-FU, irinotecan, oxaliplatin; *5-FU,* 5-fluorouracil; *GTX,* gemcitabine, docetaxel, capecitabine; *SBRT,* stereotactic body radiation therapy.
[a]Level of recommendation is based on National Comprehensive Cancer Network (NCCN) Guidelines. Category 1 is based on high-level evidence with uniform NCCN consensus that the intervention is appropriate. Category 2B is based on lower level evidence with NCCN consensus that the intervention is appropriate.
From Niederhuber JE: *Abeloff's clinical oncology,* ed 6, Philadelphia, 2020, Elsevier.

- Adjuvant chemotherapy with FOLFIRINOX regimen significantly delays the development of recurrence and results in median survival of approximately 54 mo.
- The role of radiotherapy in the adjuvant setting is best restricted to patients who have a high risk for locoregional recurrence.

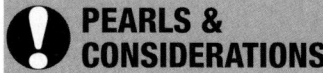

PEARLS & CONSIDERATIONS

COMMENTS

- Risk factors for pancreatic cancer and recommendations for screening of individuals at risk are summarized in Tables 6 and 7. New-onset diabetes (NOD) after age 50 yr confers a sixfold to eightfold increased risk for sporadic (nonfamilial) pancreatic ductal adenocarcinoma (PDAC) in the 3 yr after diagnosis. About 20% of patients with PDAC have NOD, and about 1% of patients with NOD will be diagnosed with PDAC in the 3 yr after NOD.[9]
- The U.S. Preventive Services Task Force (USPSTF) recommends against routine screening for pancreatic cancer in asymptomatic adults since it found no evidence that screening is effective in reducing mortality rates. There is potential for significant harm because of the low prevalence of pancreatic cancer, limited accuracy of available screening tests, invasive nature of diagnostic tests, and poor outcome of treatment.
- Alcohol consumption, specifically liquor consumption of more than three drinks per day, increases pancreatic cancer mortality independent of smoking.
- Patients should be referred for pancreatic cancer surgery to high-volume medical centers that perform at least 15 to 20 cases per yr.

REFERENCES

Available at eBooks.Health.Elsevier.com.

RELATED CONTENT

Pancreatic Cancer (Patient Information)

AUTHOR: **RITESH RATHORE, MD**

TABLE 6 Risk Factors for Pancreatic Cancer

Risk Factor	Relative Increase in Risk
High Risk (>10-fold)	
FAMMM	13- to 47-fold
Hereditary pancreatitis	50- to 83-fold
Peutz-Jeghers syndrome	132-fold
Three or more first-degree relatives with PC	14- to 32-fold
Moderate Risk (5- to 10-fold)	
Two first-degree relatives with PC	4- to 6.4-fold
Cystic fibrosis	5.3-fold
Chronic pancreatitis	2- to 19-fold
BRCA2 mutation carrier	3.5- to 10-fold
PALB2 mutation carrier	6-fold
Low Risk (<5-fold)	
Cigarette smoking	1.5- to 3-fold
Alcohol consumption	None to 1.2-fold
Obesity	None to 1.7-fold
Diabetes mellitus	1.3- to 2.6-fold
One first-degree relative with PC	3-fold
BRCA1 mutation carrier	None to 2-fold
Familial adenomatous polyposis	4-fold
Li-Fraumeni syndrome	2-fold
Lynch syndrome	2- to 8-fold

FAMMM, Familial atypical multiple-mole melanoma; *PC,* pancreatic cancer.
From Niederhuber JE: *Abeloff's clinical oncology,* ed 6, Philadelphia, 2020, Elsevier.

TABLE 7 Recommendations for Screening

HRIs to Consider for Screening

FAMMM patients with *CDKN2A*
Patients with hereditary pancreatitis
Patients with hereditary PJS
Three or more first-, second-, or third-degree relatives with PC with at least one being a first-degree relative
Two or more first-degree relatives with PC
BRCA1, BRCA2, or *PALB2* mutation carriers with at least one first- or second-degree relative with PC

Age to Start Screening

Age 45-50 yr *or* 15 yr before age of earliest occurrence of PC in the family (whichever is earliest)
Consider age 30 yr for patients with PJS

FAMMM, Familial atypical multiple-mole melanoma; *HRI,* high-risk individual; *PC,* pancreatic cancer; *PJS,* Peutz-Jeghers syndrome.
From Niederhuber JE: *Abeloff's clinical oncology,* ed 6, Philadelphia, 2020, Elsevier.

BASIC INFORMATION

DEFINITION

- Acute pancreatitis is an inflammatory process of the pancreas with intrapancreatic activation of enzymes that may also involve peripancreatic tissue and/or remote organ systems. The diagnosis of acute pancreatitis requires at least two of the following criteria: Serum amylase or lipase ≥3 times normal, abdominal pain consistent with pancreatitis, and radiographic findings (computed tomography [CT] or MRI) of acute pancreatitis.
- Severity scoring systems: Table 1 summarizes commonly used severity scoring systems.
- The **Revised Atlanta Criteria** (Box 1) uses early prognostic signs, organ failure, and local complications to define disease severity:
  1. **Mild pancreatitis:** No organ failure, no local or systemic complications, pancreatitis typically resolves in first wk
  2. **Moderate pancreatitis:** Transient organ failure (≤48 h) *or* local complications (e.g., pancreatic necrosis, peripancreatic fluid collections, peripancreatic necrosis) *or* exacerbation of comorbid disease
  3. **Severe pancreatitis:** Persistent organ failure (>48 h)
- The **BALI Score** evaluates only four variables:
  1. BUN ≥25 mg/dl
  2. Age ≥65 yr
  3. LDH ≥300 U/L
  4. Interleukin-6 level ≥300 pg/ml
- These measurements are taken at admission and at 48 h. Mortality is >25% for a score of 3 and exceeds 50% with a score of 4.

- **Severe acute pancreatitis (SAP)** is diagnosed by the presence of any of the following four criteria:
  1. Organ failure with one or more of the following: Shock (systolic blood pressure <90 mm Hg), pulmonary insufficiency (PaO$_2$ ≤60 mm Hg), renal failure (serum creatinine >2 mg/dl after rehydration), and gastrointestinal bleeding (>500 ml/24 h)
  2. Local complications such as necrosis, pseudocyst, or abscess
  3. At least three of the Ranson criteria (Boxes 2 and 3) *or*
  4. At least eight of the Acute Physiology and Chronic Health Evaluation II (APACHE II) criteria

ICD-10CM CODES

K85.0	Idiopathic acute pancreatitis
K85.1	Biliary acute pancreatitis
K85.2	Alcohol-induced acute pancreatitis
K 85.3	Drug-induced pancreatitis
K85.6	Other acute pancreatitis
K85.9	Acute pancreatitis, unspecified

EPIDEMIOLOGY & DEMOGRAPHICS

- The incidence of pancreatitis is increasing in the U.S. Admissions for acute pancreatitis have increased dramatically, and acute pancreatitis was the number-one GI-related cause for admission across U.S. hospitals in 2012. There are >270,000 cases of acute pancreatitis reported annually in the U.S., with 40%+ resulting from gallstone disease (most common cause) and 30% caused by alcohol consumption.

- Incidence in urban areas is twice that of rural areas (20/100,000 persons in urban areas).
- 20% of patients have necrotizing pancreatitis; the remainder have interstitial, or edematous, pancreatitis.
- Drugs are responsible for less than 5% of all cases of acute pancreatitis.

BOX 1 Atlanta Criteria for Acute Pancreatitis

Organ Failure, as Defined by
- Shock (systolic blood pressure <90 mm Hg)
- Pulmonary insufficiency (PaO$_2$ <60 mm Hg)
- Renal failure (creatinine level >2 mg/dl after fluid resuscitation)
- Gastrointestinal bleeding (>500 ml/24 h)

Systemic Complications
- Disseminated intravascular coagulation (platelet count ≤100,000)
- Fibrinogen <1 g/L
- Fibrin split products >80 µg/dl
- Metabolic disturbance (calcium level ≤7.5 mg/dl)

Local Complications
- Necrosis
- Abscess
- Pseudocyst
- Severe pancreatitis is defined by the presence of any evidence of organ failure or a local complication

From Townsend CM et al: *Sabiston textbook of surgery,* ed 21, St Louis, 2022, Elsevier.

TABLE 1 Summary of Severity Scoring Systems

Ranson Criteria	APACHE II Variables	Modified CTSI	BISAP
At admission	Age	**Pancreatic inflammation**	BUN > 25 mg/dl
Age >55 yr	Temperature	0: Normal pancreas	Impaired mental status
WBC >16,000/mm³	Mean arterial pressure	2: Intrinsic pancreatic abnormalities ± inflammatory	(disorientation, lethargy,
Glucose >200 mg/dl	Heart rate	changes in peripancreatic fat	somnolence, coma)
AST >250 IU/L	Respiratory rate	4: Pancreatic or peripancreatic fluid collection or	≥ SIRS criteria
LDH >350 IU/L	PaO$_2$ pH or HCO$_3$	peripancreatic fat necrosis	Age >60 yr
At admission (if biliary cause)	Serum sodium	**Pancreatic necrosis**	Pleural effusion present
Age >70 yr	Serum potassium	0: None	
WBC >18,000/mm³	Serum creatinine	2: 30% or less	
Glucose >220 mg/dl	Hematocrit	4: More than 30%	
AST >250 IU/L	WBC count	**Extrapancreatic complications**	
LDH >400 IU/L	Glasgow Coma Scale	2: One or more of pleural effusion, ascites, vascular	
At 48 h	Chronic health problems:	complications, parenchymal complications, and/or	
Hematocrit drop >10%	• Cirrhosis of the liver confirmed by	gastrointestinal involvement	
BUN rise >5 mg/dl	biopsy		
Calcium <8 mg/dl	• New York Heart Association Class IV		
PaO$_2$ <60 mm Hg	• Severe COPD		
Base deficit >4 mEq/L	1. Hypercapnia, home O$_2$ use, or		
Fluid needs >6 L	pulmonary hypertension		
At 48 h (if biliary cause)	• On regular dialysis		
Hematocrit drop >10%	• Immunocompromised		
BUN rise >2 mg/dl			
Calcium <8 mg/dl			
Base deficit >5 mEq/L			
Fluid needs >4 L			

APACHE, Acute Physiology and Chronic Health Evaluation; *AST,* aspartate transaminase; *BISAP,* Bedside Index of Severity in Acute Pancreatitis; *BUN,* blood urea nitrogen; *CTSI,* computed tomography severity index; *COPD,* chronic obstructive pulmonary disease; *LDH,* lactate dehydrogenase; *PaO₂,* partial pressure of oxygen; *SIRS,* systemic inflammatory response syndrome; *WBC,* white blood cell.
From Walls RM et al: *Rosen's emergency medicine, concepts and clinical practice,* ed 10, Philadelphia, 2023, Elsevier.

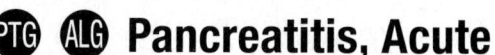
BOX 2   Ranson Prognostic Criteria for Nongallstone Pancreatitis

- At presentation
  1. Age >55 yr
  2. Blood glucose level >200 mg/dl
  3. White blood cell count >16,000 cells/mm^3
  4. Lactate dehydrogenase level >350 IU/L
  5. Aspartate aminotransferase level >250 IU/L
- After 48 h of admission
  1. Hematocrit*: Decrease >10%
  2. Serum calcium level <8 mg/dl
  3. Base deficit >4 mEq/L
  4. Blood urea nitrogen level: Increase >5 mg/dl
  5. Fluid requirement >6 L
  6. Pao$_2$ <60 mm Hg
- Ranson score ≥3 defines severe pancreatitis

*Compared with admission value.
From Townsend CM et al: *Sabiston textbook of surgery,* ed 21, St Louis, 2022, Elsevier.

BOX 3   Ranson Prognostic Criteria for Gallstone Pancreatitis

- At presentation
  1. Age >70 yr
  2. Blood glucose level >220 mg/dl
  3. White blood cell count >18,000 cells/mm^3
  4. Lactate dehydrogenase level >400 IU/L
  5. Aspartate aminotransferase level >250 IU/L
- After 48 h of admission
  1. Hematocrit*: Decrease >10%
  2. Serum calcium level <8 mg/dl
  3. Base deficit >5 mEq/L
  4. Blood urea nitrogen level: Increase >2 mg/dl
  5. Fluid requirement >4 L
  6. Pao$_2$: Not available
- Ranson score ≥3 defines severe pancreatitis

*Compared with admission value.
From Townsend CM et al: *Sabiston textbook of surgery,* ed 21, St Louis, 2022, Elsevier.

PHYSICAL FINDINGS & CLINICAL PRESENTATION

- Epigastric tenderness and guarding, often radiating to the back; pain usually developing suddenly, reaching peak intensity within 10 to 30 min, severe and lasting several hours without relief. Rarely, some patients can have painless severe pancreatitis
- Nausea and vomiting (up to 90% of cases)
- Hypoactive bowel sounds (from ileus)
- Tachycardia, shock (from decreased intravascular volume)
- Confusion (from metabolic disturbances)
- Fever (SIRS response or infection when pancreatic necrosis is present)
- Decreased breath sounds (pleural effusions) or rales (atelectasis, acute respiratory distress syndrome [ARDS])
- Jaundice (from obstruction or compression of biliary tract)
- Ascites (from tear in pancreatic duct, leaking pseudocyst)
- Palpable abdominal mass (pseudocyst, phlegmon, abscess, carcinoma)
- Evidence of hypocalcemia (Chvostek sign, Trousseau sign)
- Evidence of retroperitoneal bleeding (hemorrhagic pancreatitis):
  1. Ecchymosis around the umbilicus **(Cullen sign)**
  2. Ecchymosis involving the flanks **(Grey Turner sign)**
- Tender subcutaneous nodules (caused by subcutaneous fat necrosis)

ETIOLOGY

- The most common causes of acute pancreatitis are gallstones (40% of cases) and excessive alcohol consumption (30% of cases). Alcohol-related pancreatitis is most common after long term (>10 yr of heavy drinking). The pathophysiology of severe acute pancreatitis is illustrated in Fig. 1
- Hypertriglyceridemia (usually >1000 mg/dl) from any cause
- Drugs (e.g., thiazides, furosemide, corticosteroids, tetracycline, estrogens, valproic acid, metronidazole, azathioprine, methyldopa, pentamidine, ethacrynic acid, procainamide, amiodarone, sulindac, nitrofurantoin, ACE inhibitors, danazol, cimetidine, piroxicam, gold, ranitidine, sulfasalazine, isoniazid, acetaminophen, cisplatin, didanosine, opiates, erythromycin, metformin, GLP-1 receptor agonists, incretin mimetics)
- Abdominal trauma
- Surgery
- Endoscopic retrograde cholangiopancreatography (ERCP), especially with manipulation of the pancreatic duct
- Infections (predominantly viral)
- Peptic ulcer (penetrating duodenal ulcer)
- Pancreas divisum (congenital failure to fuse of dorsal or ventral pancreas)
- Idiopathic
- Pregnancy
- Vascular (vasculitis, ischemic)
- Hypercalcemia
- Pancreatic carcinoma (primary or metastatic)
- Renal failure
- Hereditary pancreatitis, such as in patients with cystic fibrosis
- Immunoglobulin G subclass 4 (IgG4) disease
- Occupational exposure to chemicals: Methanol, cobalt, zinc, mercuric chloride, creosol, lead, organophosphates, chlorinated naphthalenes
- Others: Scorpion venom, obstruction at ampulla region (neoplasm, duodenal diverticula, Crohn disease, rarely celiac disease), hypotensive shock, autoimmune pancreatitis

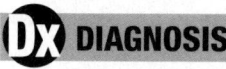 **DIAGNOSIS**

DIFFERENTIAL DIAGNOSIS

- Peptic ulcer disease
- Acute cholangitis, biliary colic
- High intestinal obstruction
- Early acute appendicitis
- Diabetic ketoacidosis
- Pneumonia (basilar)
- Myocardial infarction (inferior wall)
- Renal colic
- Ruptured or dissecting aortic aneurysm
- Mesenteric ischemia

LABORATORY TESTS

Pancreatic enzymes:
- Amylase is increased, usually elevated in the initial 3 to 5 days of acute pancreatitis. Isoamylase determinations (separation of pancreatic cell isoenzyme components of amylase) are useful in excluding occasional cases of salivary hyperamylasemia. The use of isoamylase rather than total serum amylase reduces the risk of erroneously diagnosing pancreatitis and is preferred by some as initial biochemical test in patients suspected of having acute pancreatitis.
- Urinary amylase determinations are useful to diagnose acute pancreatitis in patients with lipemic serum, to rule out elevated serum amylase caused by macroamylasemia, and to diagnose acute pancreatitis in patients whose serum amylase is normal.
- Serum lipase levels are elevated in acute pancreatitis; the elevation is less transient than serum amylase and more sensitive in patients with alcoholic pancreatitis. Concomitant evaluation of serum amylase and lipase does not improve diagnostic accuracy of acute pancreatitis. Serial measurements have limited usefulness because levels are not predictors of severity. Elevated serum trypsin levels are diagnostic of pancreatitis (in absence of renal failure).
- Serum C-reactive protein is an excellent laboratory marker of severity; a level >150 mg/dl at 48 h is associated with severe pancreatitis.

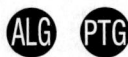

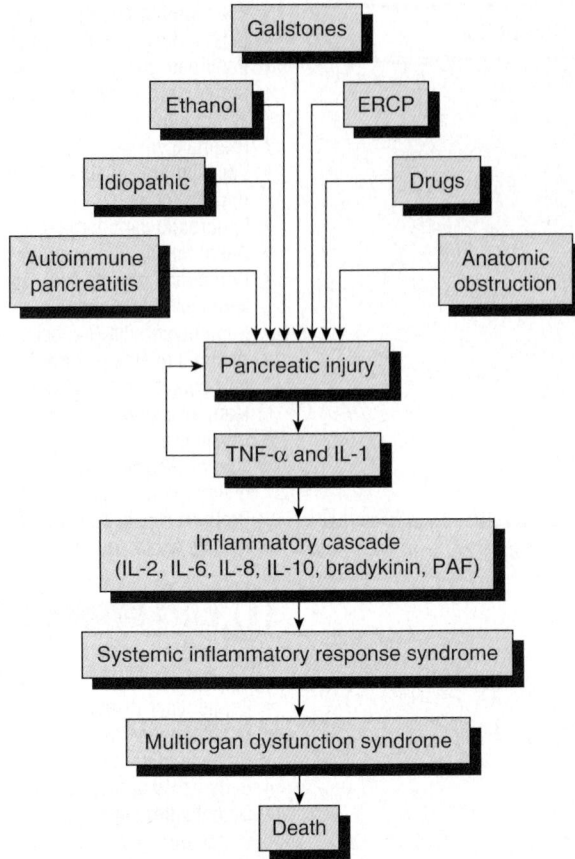

FIG. 1 Pathophysiology of severe acute pancreatitis. The local injury induces the release of tumor necrosis factor-alpha (TNF-α) and interleukin-1 (IL-1). Both cytokines produce further pancreatic injury and amplify the inflammatory response by inducing the release of other inflammatory mediators, which cause distant organ injury. This abnormal inflammatory response is responsible for the mortality seen during the early phase of acute pancreatitis. *ERCP*, Endoscopic retrograde cholangiopancreatography; *PAF*, platelet-activating factor. (From Townsend CM et al: *Sabiston textbook of surgery,* ed 21, St Louis, 2022, Elsevier.)

- Rapid measurement of urinary trypsinogen-2 (if available) is useful in the emergency department as a screening test for acute pancreatitis in patients with abdominal pain; a negative dipstick test for urinary trypsinogen-2 rules out acute pancreatitis with a high degree of probability, whereas a positive test indicates need for further evaluation.
- Interleukin-6 level: Worse prognosis with level ≥300 pg/ml.

Additional tests:
- CBC: Reveals leukocytosis; hematocrit (Hct) may be initially increased as a result of hemoconcentration; decreased Hct may indicate hemorrhage or hemolysis.
- Blood urea nitrogen (BUN) is increased because of dehydration. Serial BUN measurements are the most valuable lab test for predicting mortality during the initial 48 h.
- Elevation of serum glucose in a previously normal patient correlates with the degree of pancreatic malfunction and may be related to increased release of glycogen, catecholamines, and glucocorticoid release and decreased insulin release.
- Liver profile: Aspartate aminotransferase (AST) and lactate dehydrogenase (LDH) are increased as a result of tissue necrosis; bilirubin and alkaline phosphatase may be increased from common bile duct obstruction. A threefold or greater rise in serum alanine aminotransferase concentrations is an excellent indicator (95% probability) of biliary pancreatitis.
- Serum calcium is decreased because of saponification, precipitation, and decreased parathyroid hormone response.
- Arterial blood gases: Pao$_2$ may be decreased as a result of ARDS, pleural effusion(s); pH may be decreased as a result of lactic acidosis, respiratory acidosis, and renal insufficiency.
- Serum electrolytes: Potassium may be increased from acidosis or renal insufficiency; sodium may be increased from dehydration.

IMAGING STUDIES
- Abdominal plain films are useful initially to distinguish other conditions that may mimic pancreatitis (perforated viscus). They may reveal localized ileus (sentinel loop), pancreatic calcifications (chronic pancreatitis), blurring of left psoas shadow, dilation of transverse colon, calcified gallstones.
- Chest x-ray may reveal elevation of one or both diaphragms, pleural effusions, basilar infiltrates, or platelike atelectasis.

- Abdominal ultrasonography is useful in detecting gallstones (sensitivity of 60% to 70% for detecting stones associated with pancreatitis). Its availability and noninvasive nature make it the initial imaging study of choice; its major limitation is the presence of distended bowel loops overlying the pancreas.
- CT scan (Fig. 2) is less sensitive than ultrasound in identifying gallstones and exposes the patient to risk of contrast-induced nephropathy. It is, however, superior to ultrasonography in identifying pancreatitis and defining its extent, and it also plays a role in diagnosing pseudocysts (they appear as a well-defined area surrounded by a high-density capsule); gastrointestinal fistulization or infection of a pseudocyst can also be identified by the presence of gas within the pseudocyst. Sequential contrast-enhanced CT is useful for detection of pancreatic necrosis. The severity of pancreatitis can also be graded by CT scan (Table 2). (A = normal pancreas, B = enlarged pancreas [1 point], C = pancreatic and/or peripancreatic inflammation [2 points], D = single peripancreatic collection [3 points], E = at least two peripancreatic collections and/or retroperitoneal air [4 points]. Percentage of pancreatic necrosis <30% [2 points], 30% to 50% [4 points], >50% [6 points]. The CT severity index is calculated by adding grade points to points assigned for percentage of necrosis.)
- Magnetic resonance cholangiopancreatography (MRCP) has >90% sensitivity for choledocholithiasis and can identify other anatomic abnormalities.
- Endoscopic ultrasonography (EUS) is a minimally invasive test that provides high-resolution imaging of the pancreas. It is useful to identify anatomic abnormalities of the pancreas and has good sensitivity and specificity for small gallstones (≤5 mm).
- ERCP indications: Useful to perform biliary sphincterotomy and stone removal in the presence of a retained bile duct stone seen on imaging. The role and timing of ERCP in patients with acute biliary pancreatitis has been controversial. Guidelines from the American College of Gastroenterology suggest that urgent ERCP (within 24 h of admission) is indicated in patients with biliary pancreatitis who have concurrent acute cholangitis, but it is not needed in most patients who do not have evidence of ongoing biliary obstruction.

Ⓡ TREATMENT

NONPHARMACOLOGIC THERAPY
- Bowel rest with avoidance of liquids or solids during the acute illness. Limited data suggest that early feeding in patients with acute pancreatitis does not seem to increase adverse events and, for patients with mild to moderate pancreatitis, may reduce length of hospital stay.
- Avoidance of alcohol and any drugs associated with pancreatitis.

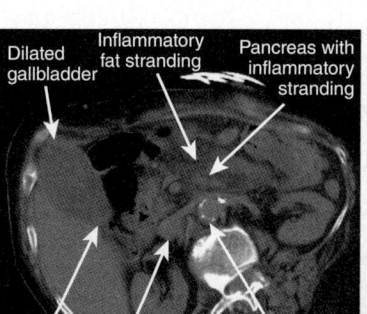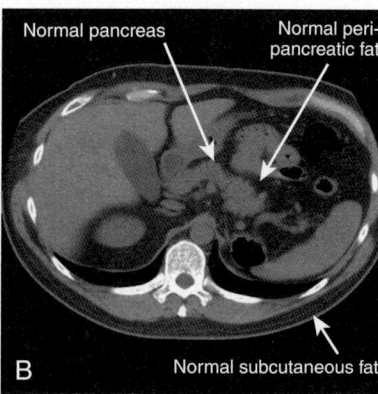

FIG. 2 Gallstone pancreatitis and normal pancreas for comparison, axial computed tomography without contrast. A, Gallstone pancreatitis CT. A dilated gallbladder is visible with a hyperdense dependent lesion consistent with a gallstone. The region of the pancreas shows significant inflammatory stranding. In this patient the pancreas lies just anterior to the left renal vein, which can be seen crossing anterior to the aorta and entering the inferior vena cava. **B,** A normal pancreas is visible. This pancreas is surrounded by uninflamed fat, which is dark (nearly black). Compare this normal fat with normal subcutaneous fat. (From Broder JS: *Diagnostic imaging for the emergency physician,* Philadelphia, 2011, Saunders.)

TABLE 2 Computed Tomography (CT) Severity Index Score for Pancreatitis*

Grade[†]	CT Findings	Score
A	Normal pancreas	0
B	Focal or diffuse enlargement of the pancreas, contour irregularities, heterogeneous attenuation, no peripancreatic inflammation	1
C	Grade B plus peripancreatic inflammation	2
D	Grade C plus a single fluid collection	3
E	Grade C plus multiple fluid collections or gas	4
Percent Necrosis Present on CT		
0		
<33		
33-50		
>50		

*Severity Index Score = Grade score + Percent necrosis score. Maximum score = 10; severe disease = 6 or higher.
[†]Severity of the acute inflammatory process.
From Adams JG et al: *Emergency medicine: clinical essentials,* ed 2, Philadelphia, 2013, Elsevier.

ACUTE GENERAL Rx

GENERAL MEASURES:

- Assess severity of pancreatitis.
- An algorithm for the management of acute pancreatitis is described in Fig. 3.
- Maintain adequate intravascular volume with intravenous (IV) hydration. The ideal quantity of fluid resuscitation has been controversial. Traditionally aggressive fluid resuscitation (250 to 500 ml/h) with isotonic crystalloids was regarded as critical in managing acute pancreatitis, unless cardiac or renal disease precluded it. Recent trials have shown that moderate fluid resuscitation results in similar clinical outcomes as did aggressive resuscitation with less fluid overload.[1]
- Patient should remain NPO (nothing by mouth) until clinically improved, stable, and hungry. Enteral feedings are preferred over total parenteral nutrition if supplemental nutrition is necessary. Enteral nutrition reduces mortality, multiple organ failure, systemic infections, and operative interventions more than total parenteral nutrition does in patients with acute pancreatitis. Parenteral nutrition may be necessary in patients who do not tolerate enteral feeding or in whom an adequate infusion rate cannot be reached within 2 to 4 days. The American Gastroenterological Association recommends that oral feedings be started within 24 h of admission in patients with mild to moderate pancreatitis. A recent trial revealed that patients started on a low-fat diet on admission were discharged about 5 days earlier than patients in whom feeding was delayed.
- Nasogastric suction is useful only in severe pancreatitis to decompress the abdomen in patients with ileus.
- Control pain: IV hydromorphone or fentanyl. Meperidine and morphine are also commonly used narcotics for pain control, although morphine has been shown to increase sphincter of Oddi pressure and has delayed metabolite clearance in patients with concomitant renal failure.

- Correct metabolic abnormalities (e.g., replace calcium and magnesium as necessary).
- Prophylactic antibiotics are not recommended, regardless of the severity or presence of pancreatic necrosis.
- An algorithm for the management of acute pancreatitis at various stages is described in Fig. 3.

SPECIFIC MEASURES:

- Pancreatic or peripancreatic infection develops in 30% of patients with pancreatic necrosis. The use of antibiotics is justified if the patient has evidence of septicemia, pancreatic abscess, or pancreatitis caused by biliary calculi with concomitant cholangitis. Their use should generally be limited to 5 to 7 days to prevent development of fungal superinfection. Appropriate empiric antibiotic therapy should penetrate pancreatic necrosis. Options include a carbapenem alone (due to anaerobic coverage) or a quinolone, ceftazidime, or cefepime, combined with an enteric anaerobic agent such as metronidazole. CT-guided fine-needle aspiration (FNA) can be performed to culture the infected necrosis and tailor antibiotic therapy. If sampling of infected necrosis occurs and is sterile, antibiotics should be discontinued
- Surgical therapy has a limited role in acute pancreatitis; it is indicated in the following:
  1. Gallstone-induced pancreatitis: Cholecystectomy when acute pancreatitis subsides. However, randomized trials have shown that patients with mild gallstone pancreatitis can undergo cholecystectomy safely during the first 48 h of hospitalization.
  2. Perforated peptic ulcer.
  3. Necrotizing pancreatitis with infected necrotic tissue is associated with an elevated rate of complications and increased risk of death. Traditional treatment has been open necrosectomy; surgical necrosectomy induces a proinflammatory response and is associated with a high complication rate. Recent trials have shown that a step-up approach consisting of percutaneous drainage followed, if necessary, by minimally invasive retroperitoneal necrosectomy may have a lower rate of complications and death. A recent trial did not show superiority of immediate drainage over postponed drainage with regard to complications in infected necrotizing pancreatitis. Endoscopic transgastric necrosectomy, a form of natural orifice transluminal endoscopic surgery, has been shown in recent trials to be effective in reducing the proinflammatory response as well as reducing complications.
- Identification and treatment of complications:
  1. **Pseudocyst:** Round or spheroid collection of fluid, tissue, pancreatic enzymes, and blood.
     a. Diagnosed by CT scan or sonography.
     b. Treatment: Pancreatic pseudocysts can be drained surgically or endoscopically. The endoscopic approach is preferable when the patient's anatomy is suitable and an experienced endoscopist is

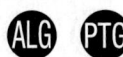
Early course: 0-72 h
Is there organ failure?

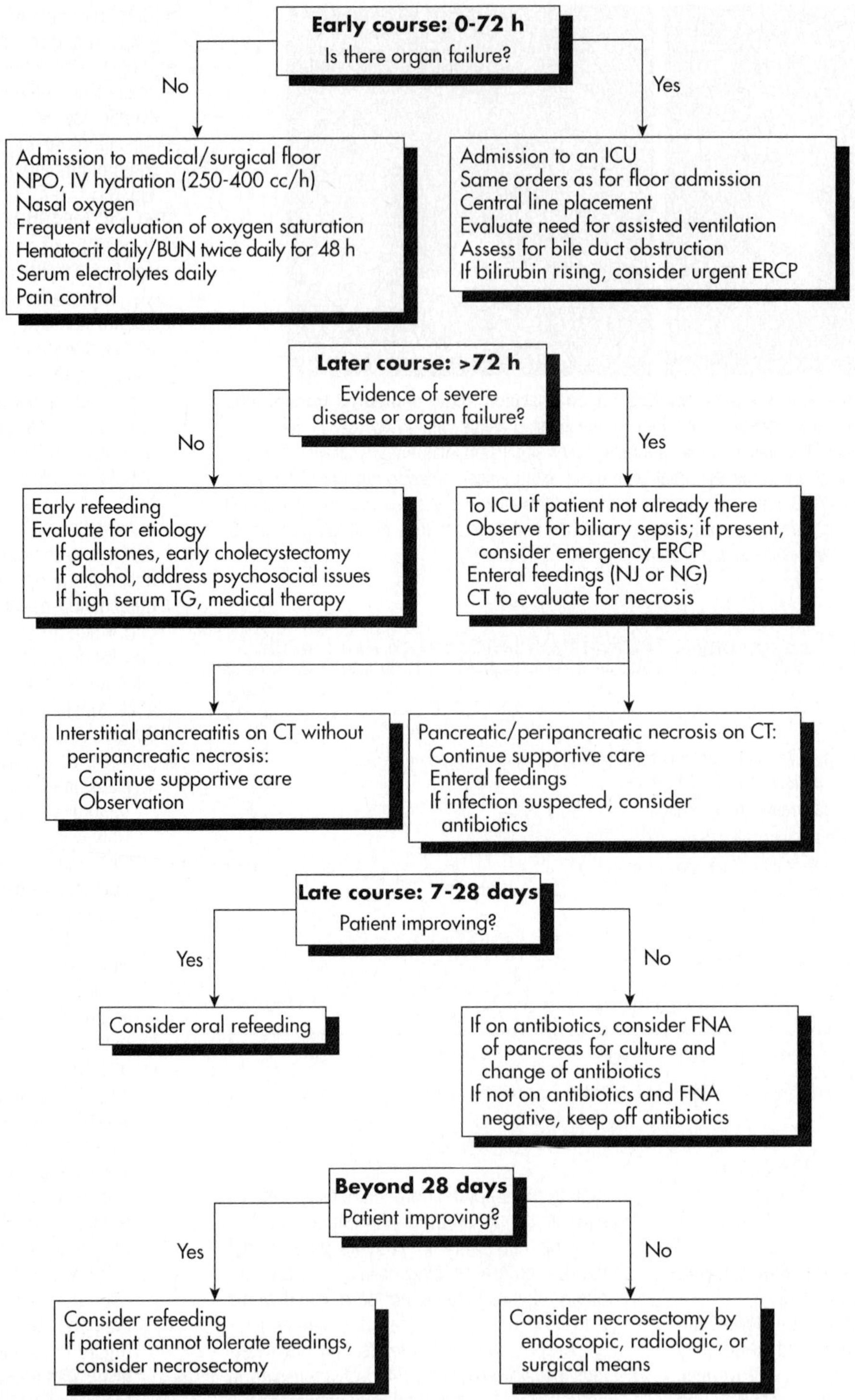

No →

Admission to medical/surgical floor
NPO, IV hydration (250-400 cc/h)
Nasal oxygen
Frequent evaluation of oxygen saturation
Hematocrit daily/BUN twice daily for 48 h
Serum electrolytes daily
Pain control

Yes →

Admission to an ICU
Same orders as for floor admission
Central line placement
Evaluate need for assisted ventilation
Assess for bile duct obstruction
If bilirubin rising, consider urgent ERCP

Later course: >72 h
Evidence of severe
disease or organ failure?

No →

Early refeeding
Evaluate for etiology
　If gallstones, early cholecystectomy
　If alcohol, address psychosocial issues
　If high serum TG, medical therapy

Yes →

To ICU if patient not already there
Observe for biliary sepsis; if present,
　consider emergency ERCP
Enteral feedings (NJ or NG)
CT to evaluate for necrosis

Interstitial pancreatitis on CT without
peripancreatic necrosis:
　Continue supportive care
　Observation

Pancreatic/peripancreatic necrosis on CT:
　Continue supportive care
　Enteral feedings
　If infection suspected, consider
　　antibiotics

Late course: 7-28 days
Patient improving?

Yes →

Consider oral refeeding

No →

If on antibiotics, consider FNA
　of pancreas for culture and
　change of antibiotics
If not on antibiotics and FNA
　negative, keep off antibiotics

Beyond 28 days
Patient improving?

Yes →

Consider refeeding
If patient cannot tolerate feedings,
consider necrosectomy

No →

Consider necrosectomy by
endoscopic, radiologic, or
surgical means

FIG. 3 Algorithm for the management of acute pancreatitis at various stages in its course. *NJ,* Nasojejunal. (From Feldman M et al: *Sleisenger and Fordtran's gastrointestinal and liver disease,* ed 11, Philadelphia, 2021, Elsevier.)

available. CT scan or ultrasound-guided percutaneous drainage (with a pigtail catheter left in place for continuous drainage) can be used, but the recurrence rate is high; the conservative approach is to reevaluate the pseudocyst (with CT scan or sonography) after 6 to 7 wk and surgically drain it if the pseudocyst has not decreased in size.

　c. Generally, pseudocysts <5 cm in diameter are reabsorbed without intervention, whereas those >5 cm require surgical intervention after the wall has matured.
2. **Phlegmon:** Represents pancreatic edema. It can be diagnosed by CT scan or sonography. Treatment is supportive as it usually resolves spontaneously.
3. **Pancreatic abscess:** Diagnosed by CT scan (presence of air in the retroperitoneum);

Gram staining and cultures of fluid obtained from guided percutaneous aspiration usually identify bacterial organism. Therapy is surgical (or catheter) drainage and IV antibiotics (carbapenem is the drug of choice).
4. **Pancreatic ascites:** Usually caused by leaking of pseudocyst or tear in pancreatic duct. Paracentesis reveals very high amylase and lipase levels in the pancreatic fluid; ERCP may demonstrate the lesion.

P

TABLE 3 Features of Type 1 and Type 2 Autoimmune Pancreatitis

Feature	Type 1	Type 2
Histology	Lymphoplasmacytic infiltration Dense periductal infiltrate without damage to ductal epithelium Storiform fibrosis Obliterative phlebitis Abundant (>10 cells/HPF) IgG4-positive cells Fibroinflammatory process may extend to peripancreatic region	Periductal lymphoplasmacytic and neutrophilic infiltration Destruction of the duct epithelium by neutrophils (granulocytic epithelial lesion [GEL]) Obliterative phlebitis is rare No IgG4-positive cells
Average age at presentation	60-70 yr	40-50, but may present in young adults and even children
Gender predominance	Male	Equal
Usual clinical presentations	Obstructive jaundice (75%) Acute pancreatitis (15%)	Obstructive jaundice (50%) Acute pancreatitis (33%)
Pancreatic imaging	Diffuse pancreatic enlargement (40%) Focal pancreatic enlargement (60%)	Diffuse pancreatic enlargement (15%) Focal pancreatic enlargement (85%)
IgG4	Level elevated in serum (~⅔ of patients) Positive in staining of involved tissues	Not associated
Other organ involvement	Biliary strictures Pseudotumors Kidney Lung Others Retroperitoneal fibrosis Sialoadenitis	Not associated
Associated diseases	See above (other organ involvement)	IBD
Long-term outcome	Frequent relapses	Rare or no relapse

HPF, High power field; *IBD,* inflammatory bowel disease; *IgG4,* immunoglobulin G, subclass 4.
From Feldman M et al: *Sleisenger and Fordtran's gastrointestinal and liver disease,* ed 11, Philadelphia, 2021, Elsevier.

Treatment is surgical correction if exudative ascites from severe pancreatitis does not resolve spontaneously.

- **Abdominal compartment syndrome:** Caused by intraabdominal leakage of fluids from volume resuscitation or ascites. Diagnosed with sustained intraabdominal pressure >20 mm Hg with new-onset organ failure
- **Gastrointestinal bleeding:** Caused by alcoholic gastritis, bleeding varices, stress ulceration, or disseminated intravascular coagulation (DIC)
- **Renal failure:** Caused by hypovolemia, resulting in oliguria or anuria, cortical or tubular necrosis (shock, DIC), or thrombosis of renal artery or vein
- **Hypoxia:** Caused by ARDS, pleural effusion, or atelectasis
- **Vascular:** Splenic, portal, or superior mesenteric vein thrombosis; pseudoaneurysm

THERAPY OF UNCOMMON FORMS OF PANCREATITIS

- **Autoimmune pancreatitis (AIP):** Fibroinflammatory disease characterized by an IgG4 lymphoplasmacytic infiltrate. It is a variant of chronic pancreatitis and has been associated with other autoimmune disorders (e.g., primary sclerosing cholangitis, Sjögren syndrome). The inflammatory process is generally responsive to corticosteroid therapy. Older men aged 60 to 70 yr are primarily affected. Patients present with abdominal pain, weight loss, anorexia, and obstructive jaundice. IgG4

levels are elevated. Radiographically on CT, the pancreas is diffusely enlarged, with a characteristic smooth, capsulelike rim ("sausage pancreas"). Features of type 1 and type 2 autoimmune pancreatitis are summarized in Table 3. Type II autoimmune hepatitis (idiopathic duct-centric chronic pancreatitis) is associated with inflammatory bowel disease and not related to IgG4 cell deposition.

- **Hypertriglyceridemic pancreatitis (HTGP):** IV insulin therapy is the cornerstone of immediate treatment, with supplemental IV glucose infusion if the serum glucose levels are not elevated. IV heparin was previously used as well, but its effectiveness has come into question. Antihyperlipidemic agents (fibrates) should be initiated as adjuvant therapy as soon as possible for long-term control. Beneficial results have been reported with early (within 48 h) initiation of apheresis with therapeutic plasma exchange when there is concomitant hypocalcemia, lactic acidosis, or other signs of organ dysfunction.

DISPOSITION

Prognosis varies with the severity of pancreatitis; overall mortality rate in acute pancreatitis is 5% to 10%. Prognostic criteria for acute pancreatitis are described in Table 4.

REFERRAL

- Hospitalization is indicated in moderate to severe cases of pancreatitis.

- Surgical consultation is needed in suspected gallstone pancreatitis, perforated peptic ulcer, or presence of necrotic or infected foci. Acute pancreatitis can generally be attributed to gallstones when patients have both abnormal liver enzymes and gallstones (or sludge) on imaging. Such patients should consider cholecystectomy before discharge to prevent recurrent pancreatitis.
- Gastroenterology consultation in severe or recurrent pancreatitis, when ERCP is needed for gallstone pancreatitis, or when the cause of pancreatitis is unclear.
- Consider intensive care unit transfer for patients who require aggressive fluid resuscitation and are at risk of volume overload from cardiac or renal causes. Similarly, consider transfer for patients with developing ARDS, patients with abdominal compartment syndrome (with surgical consultation), and those who require apheresis.

! PEARLS & CONSIDERATIONS

- Acute pancreatitis is the most common major complication of ERCP. NSAIDs are potent inhibitors of phospholipase A_2, cyclooxygenase, and neutrophil-endothelial interactions, which play an important role in the pathogenesis of acute pancreatitis. Preliminary trials show that among patients at high risk for

TABLE 4 Prognostic Criteria for Acute Pancreatitis

Ranson Criteria*	Simplified Glasgow Criteria†	Computed Tomography Criteria‡
On admission: Age >55 yr	*Within 48 h of admission:* Age >55 yr	Normal
WBC >16,000/μL	WBC >15,000/μL	Enlargement
AST >250 U/L LDH >350 U/L	LDH >600 U/L	Pancreatic inflammation
Glucose >200 mg/dl	Glucose >180 mg/dl	Single fluid collection
48 h after admission:	Albumin <3.2 g/dl	Multiple fluid collection
Hematocrit decrease by >10	$Ca^{2}+$ <8 mg/dl	
BUN increase by >5 mg/dl	Arterial Po_2 <60 mm Hg	
$Ca^{2}+$ <8 mg/dl	BUN >45 mg/dl	
Arterial Po_2 <60 mm Hg		
Base deficit >4 mEq/L		
Fluid sequestration >6 L		

AST, Aspartate aminotransferase; *BUN,* blood urea nitrogen; *LDH,* lactate dehydrogenase; *WBC,* white blood cells.

*Three or more Ranson criteria predict a complicated clinical course. Data from Ranson JH et al: Prognostic signs and nonoperative peritoneal lavage in acute pancreatitis, *Surg Gynecol Obstet* 143:209-219, 1976.

†Data from Blamey SL et al: Prognostic factors in acute pancreatitis, *Gut* 25:1340, 1984.

‡Grades A and B represent mild disease with no risk of infection or death. Grade C represents moderately severe disease with a minimal likelihood of infection and essentially no risk of mortality. Grades D and E represent severe pancreatitis with an infection rate of 30% to 50% and mortality rate of 15%. Data from Balthazar EJ et al: Acute pancreatitis value of CT in establishing prognosis, *Radiology* 174:331, 1990.

From Goldman L, Ausiello D (eds): *Cecil textbook of medicine,* ed 24, Philadelphia, 2012, Saunders.

post-ERCP pancreatitis, rectal indomethacin (given as two 50-mg indomethacin suppositories administered immediately after ERCP) significantly reduced the incidence of post-ERCP pancreatitis.
- Pancreatic stent placement decreases the risk of post-ERCP pancreatitis.
- Statins reduce risk for pancreatitis in adults. Fibrates do not affect risk for pancreatitis other than in patients with hypertriglyceridemia-induced pancreatitis.
- Diabetes mellitus may develop from extensive pancreatic necrosis.

REFERENCE & SUGGESTED READINGS

Available at eBooks.Health.Elsevier.com.

RELATED CONTENT

Acute Pancreatitis (Patient Information)
Chronic Pancreatitis (Related Key Topic)

AUTHOR: **DAVID J. LUCIER JR., MD, MBA, MPH**

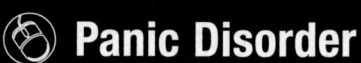

P

BASIC INFORMATION

DEFINITION

A **panic attack** is a relatively brief, sudden episode of intense fear or apprehension, often associated with a sense of impending doom and various uncomfortable and disquieting physical and/or cognitive symptoms. Panic attacks may be unexpected ("out of the blue") or expected (i.e., triggered by a particular object or situation). They can happen in a calm or an anxious state; their rapid peak intensity differentiates them from continuous anxiety. Panic attacks may be present in a variety of different anxiety-related disorders (e.g., phobias, social anxiety, obsessive-compulsive disorder) and other mental disorders (e.g., depression, substance use, PTSD, and psychosis).

Panic disorder is diagnosed after at least one uncued panic attacks have occurred followed by at least 1 mo (or more) of significant concern about future attacks, worry about their implications, or a major change in behavior related to these attacks.

According to the *Diagnostic and Statistical Manual of Mental Disorders,* Fifth Edition, Text Revision (DSM-5-TR), key criteria for panic disorder include recurrent, unexpected panic attacks, accompanied by 1 mo or more of persistent worry and changes in behavior related to the panic attacks.[1]

SYNONYMS

Anxiety attacks
Fear attacks
Ataque de nervios (Latin America), "soul loss" (Cambodia), "hit by the wind" (Vietnam)
Fearful spells

ICD-10-CM CODES	
F41.0	Panic disorder
DSM-5-TR CODES	
300.01	Panic disorder

EPIDEMIOLOGY & DEMOGRAPHICS

PREVALENCE:
- There is a 12% to 28% estimated lifetime prevalence of one or more panic attacks.[2,3]
- Panic disorder is much less common, with a lifetime prevalence of 3.8%; the chronicity of panic disorder is reflected in a similar 1-yr prevalence rate of 2.4%.[2]

PREDOMINANT SEX & AGE:
- Panic disorder is reported 2× more in women.[2]
- Median age of onset is 20 to 24 yr in the U.S.[2]
- Onset after age 60 yr is rare and should raise suspicion of different etiology.[2,4]

PEAK INCIDENCE:
- Bimodal incidence peaks noted, with the first peak between ages 15 and 24 yr and second peak between ages 35 and 44 yr.[5]

RISK FACTORS:
- Environmental triggers: Adverse childhood, recent separation and loss, long-lasting stressful events; smoking.

- Temperamental: Negative affect, anxiety sensitivity, and harm avoidance. Severe separation anxiety in childhood may precede the panic disorder.

GENETICS:
- Risk of developing panic disorder in first-degree relatives of individuals with panic disorder is four to seven times that of general population.[6]
- Findings in twin studies: Heritability estimates for panic disorder range from 24% to 55%.[6,7]
- It is thought that multiple genes may contribute to susceptibility; however, reported effect sizes have been small.[8]

PHYSICAL FINDINGS & CLINICAL PRESENTATION
- May present either with a panic attack or worries related to anticipation of a future panic attack or its implications.
- Physical findings may include but are not limited to sweating, tremulousness, hyperventilation, tachycardia, and nausea.
- 10% of patients with comorbid panic attacks and noncardiac chest pain may develop panic disorder.[9]
- Given overlapping physical symptoms and the often unexpected and untriggered nature of panic attacks, patients may present to the emergency department or primary care physician with concerns of heart attack, stroke, death, passing out, losing control, or losing one's mind.

ETIOLOGY
The exact etiology is not yet known. Hypotheses include:
- Central dysregulation of autonomic arousal (typically localized to the locus ceruleus); similar symptoms may be chemically induced with yohimbine, caffeine, or cholecystokinin[10]
- Cognitive overreaction (i.e., "catastrophic misinterpretation") to relatively mild or benign physiologic cues that then triggers a genuine autonomic[10] cascade and further misinterpretations[10]
- Dysfunction of a central suffocation alarm mechanism; some signs of compensated respiratory alkalosis. Can be experimentally induced with sodium lactate or carbon dioxide[10]
(NOTE: The above models are not mutually exclusive.)

DIAGNOSIS

DIFFERENTIAL DIAGNOSIS
Medical conditions:
- Endocrinopathies:
  1. Hyperthyroidism
  2. Hyperparathyroidism
  3. Pheochromocytoma
  4. Carcinoid tumor
- Cardiac and respiratory diseases:
  1. Arrhythmias
  2. Myocardial infarction
  3. Chronic obstructive pulmonary disease
  4. Asthma

  5. Mitral valve prolapse
  6. Pulmonary embolism
- Metabolic:
  1. Hypoglycemia
  2. Electrolyte imbalances
  3. Porphyria
- Seizure disorders: Ictal fear happens with simple partial seizures of meso-temporal lobe origin and lasts for seconds to minutes. May evolve to a focal seizure with impaired awareness
- Substance- or medication-induced anxiety disorder: Therapeutic (theophylline, steroids), intoxication (cocaine, amphetamine, caffeine, diet pills, cannabis) or withdrawal (alcohol, barbiturates, benzodiazepines)
- Psychiatric disorders (Note: Panic attacks are common in a variety of psychiatric disorders. Panic disorder could be conceptualized as a phobia of the somatic sensations or situations that have become paired with panic attacks.):
  1. Phobias (e.g., specific phobia or social phobia). Note that fear of going on a plane because of crashing would be a specific phobia, whereas fear of going on a plane because one is then trapped and worries about panic is more suggestive of panic disorder with comorbid agoraphobia
  2. Obsessive-compulsive disorder (cued by exposure to the object of the obsession)
  3. Posttraumatic stress disorder (cued by recall of a trauma)
  4. Generalized anxiety disorder (cued by excessive worry)
  5. Somatic symptom disorder (cued by more persistent anxiety and somatic symptoms)

WORKUP
- Emergency presentation: Cardiac, respiratory, or neurologic symptoms
- History and physical examination to rule out a concomitant medical or substance-related condition
NOTE: Panic disorder is not a diagnosis of exclusion, but exclusion of other conditions is usually required.

LABORATORY TESTS
- Thyroid profile
- Electrolyte measures, including calcium
- Human chorionic gonadotropin (hCG)
- Toxicology screen
- ECG
- Acute cases: Possible monitoring and cardiac enzymes to rule out arrhythmia or ischemia

IMAGING STUDIES
- Imaging studies can be considered based on the differential diagnosis and clinical suspicion
- For temporal lobe dysfunction (e.g., temporal lesions or as ictal or interictal manifestation of temporal lobe focal seizures): Brain CT scan or MRI or an electroencephalogram in some patients
- Holter monitor to rule out occult or episodic arrhythmias
- Chest x-ray, arterial blood gases, or pulmonary function tests if respiratory compromise suspected

TREATMENT

NONPHARMACOLOGIC THERAPY

- Recent systematic review of randomized controlled clinical trials demonstrate that cognitive-behavioral therapy (CBT) and short-term psychodynamic therapy are reliable first-line psychotherapies.[11]
- Cognitive-behavioral therapy (CBT), in particular panic control treatment (PCT), is generally very effective, with strongest results for cognitive restructuring (i.e., challenging catastrophic misinterpretations of somatic symptoms), in vivo or imaginal exposures (i.e., exposure to panic triggers in a controlled graded hierarchical fashion from least to most difficult with the goal of habituation and extinction of the fear response), and interoceptive exposures (i.e., repeated recreation and management of feared somatic sensations via activities such as chair spinning, straw breathing, and hyperventilation).[12,13]
- CBT effect sizes are equal to or larger than for pharmacotherapy, attrition rates are lower, and relapse rates are lower. Treatment may take several sessions spread over weeks and may require referral to a behavioral specialist. CBT has been shown to be the most effective intervention for panic disorder with or without agoraphobia across treatment sites. CBT may also be effectively delivered online (e.g., iCBT).[14]
- A recent dismantling study of cognitive-behavioral therapy components for panic disorder suggests that interoceptive exposure and a face-to-face setting were associated with better treatment efficacy whereas muscle relaxation and virtual reality exposure were associated with significantly lower efficacy.[11]

ACUTE GENERAL Rx

- Benzodiazepines, particularly clonazepam and alprazolam: Highly effective in the acute setting, although long-term use is not recommended for effective outcome and due to addictive potential.
- Low-dose clonazepam for patients with rare panic attacks and asymptomatic periods (0.25 to 0.5 mg PO or sublingually PRN).
- Start patient on selective serotonin reuptake inhibitor (SSRI) or similar agent and taper patient off benzodiazepine by wk 2 to 3.

CHRONIC Rx

- Preferred pharmacologic agents: Antidepressants with a significant serotonin reuptake inhibitory action, usually SSRIs. Generally, start at low dose and titrate upward. Minimum treatment duration is 6 to 8 mo, but many patients need to take medications indefinitely. These medications should not be discontinued abruptly; they should be tapered due to withdrawal effects including rebound anxiety.
    1. SSRIs: Sertraline (50 to 200 mg/day), citalopram (20 to 60 mg/day), escitalopram (5 to 30 mg/day), fluoxetine (5 to 60 mg/day), fluvoxamine (50 to 300 mg/day) and paroxetine (10 to 60 mg/day)
    2. Imipramine (100 to 300 mg/day)
    3. Serotonin-norepinephrine reuptake inhibitors (SNRIs): Venlafaxine (37.5 to 225 mg/day), duloxetine (30 to 120 mg/day)
- Combination CBT plus SSRI has shown good long-term effects and is somewhat better than antidepressants or CBT alone. Combination CBT plus benzodiazepine does not provide any added benefit and may undermine CBT (interoceptive and in vivo exposures may be less effective if the benzodiazepine is completely controlling the anxiety).

DISPOSITION

- Typical course is chronic but with significant waxing and waning (common to have long periods of remission).
- Presence of agoraphobia associated with a more chronic course.

Findings with long-term follow-up studies: 6 to 10 yr after treatment some 30% are in remission, 40% to 50% have improved with residual symptoms, and the remainder are either unchanged or worse.[11,15]

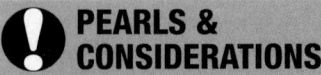

PEARLS & CONSIDERATIONS

- Panic disorder is not a diagnosis of exclusion, but exclusion of other conditions is usually required.
- Patient and family education is an important first step in the management of panic disorder. Psychoeducation provides more adaptive explanations for the benign somatic sensations paired with panic. Presentation of genetic information and explanation of the non-threatening nature of the physiology of each of the symptoms the patient experiences serve as a good start to allay fears and reduce stigma. It may also ensure compliance with treatment.
- Combination CBT plus SSRI has shown good long-term effects and is somewhat better than antidepressants or CBT alone.

REFERENCES
Available at eBooks.Health.Elsevier.com.

RELATED CONTENT

Agoraphobia (Related Key Topic)
Generalized Anxiety Disorder (Related Key Topic)

AUTHORS: **ERIKA KASKE, MD, RILEY LONGTAIN, MD, PERLA M. ROMERO GÓMEZ, MD,** and **JOHN W. DENNINGER, MD, PhD**

Diseases and Disorders

(i) BASIC INFORMATION

DEFINITION

Idiopathic Parkinson disease (PD) is a progressive neurodegenerative synucleinopathy defined by bradykinesia plus either resting tremor or rigidity.

SYNONYMS

PD
Paralysis agitans

ICD-10CM CODES

G20	Parkinson disease
G21.1	Other drug-induced secondary parkinsonism
G21.11	Neuroleptic-induced parkinsonism
G21.2	Secondary parkinsonism due to other external agents
G21.3	Postencephalitic parkinsonism
G21.4	Vascular parkinsonism
G21.8	Other secondary parkinsonism
G21.9	Secondary parkinsonism, unspecified

EPIDEMIOLOGY & DEMOGRAPHICS

PREVELANCE:

- It is the second most common neurodegenerative disease worldwide and is found in every country.[1]
- Affects more than 1 million people in North America at 0.3% of the population and 1% of people over the age of 60. Prevalence increases with age.
- In those aged >70 yr, 700/100,000 are affected.
- Lifetime risk of PD is 2% in men and 1.3% in women.

PHYSICAL FINDINGS & CLINICAL PRESENTATION

- Prodromal symptoms during 3 yr before patients receive a diagnosis of PD include problems with working, lifting heavy objects, and balance.[2]
- Tremor (Fig. 1 and Fig. 2): Typically a resting tremor with a frequency of 4 to 6 Hz that is often first noted in the hand as a pill-rolling tremor (thumb and forefinger). Can also involve the leg and lip. Tremor improves with purposeful movement. Usually starts asymmetrically.
- Rigidity (Fig. 3): Increased muscle tone that persists throughout the range of passive movement of a joint. Rigidity, like resting tremor, is usually asymmetric at onset.
- Akinesia/bradykinesia (Fig. E4 and Fig. 5): Slowness in initiating movement and decrement with repeated movements.
- Postural instability: Tested by "pull test." Ask patient to stand in place with back to examiner. Examiner pulls patient back by the shoulders, and proper response would be to take no steps back or very few steps back without falling. Retropulsion is a positive test,

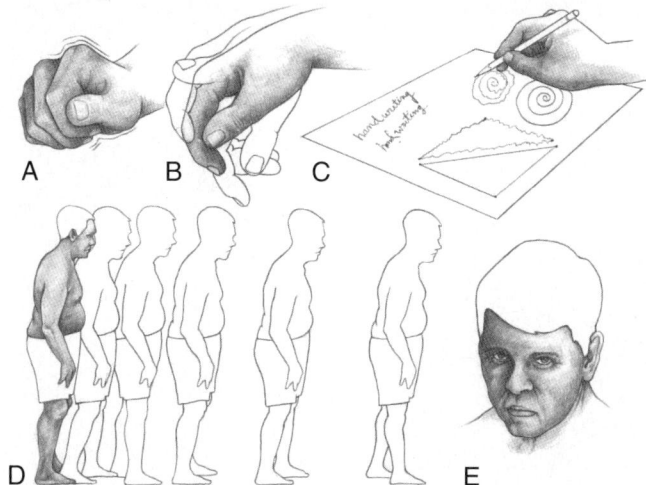

FIG. 1 The parkinsonian syndrome. A, The "pill-rolling" tremor. **B,** Tremor that can worsen with emotional stress. **C,** Handwriting abnormalities, including micrographia. **D,** Typical posture and gait, which becomes faster (festination). **E,** Lack of facial expression as well as "stare" from decreased blinking.

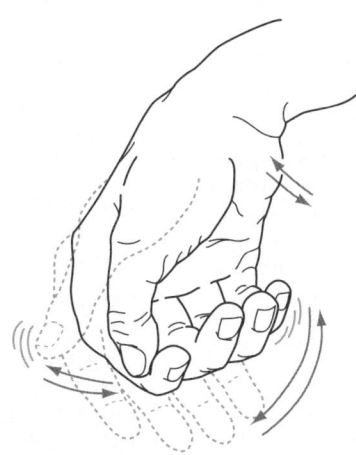

FIG. 2 Resting tremor. *Resting tremor*—a cardinal feature of Parkinson disease—consists of a relatively slow (4 to 6 Hz) to-and-fro flexion movement of the wrist, hand, thumb, and fingers most apparent when patients sit comfortably. Its similarity to rolling a pill or a coin between the thumb and index finger gave rise to the description "pill-rolling" tremor. The tremor is exaggerated or sometimes apparent only when patients are anxious. (From Kaufman DM et al: *Kaufman's clinical neurology for psychiatrists,* ed 9, Philadelphia, 2023, Elsevier.)

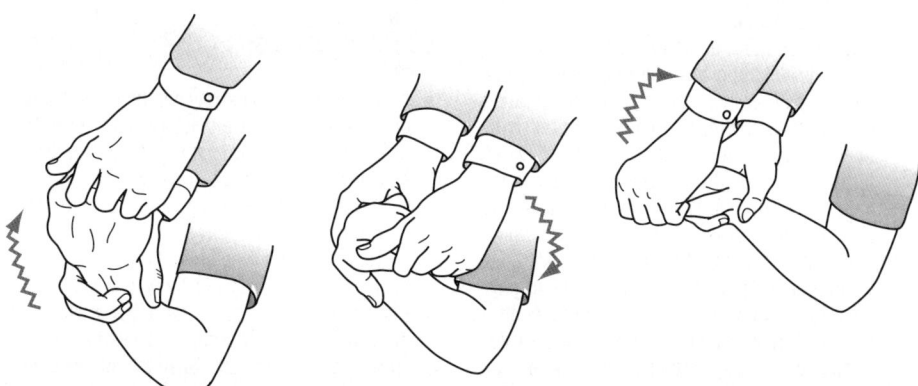

FIG. 3 Neurologists describe resistance to passive movement of the patient's limbs as rigidity. A superimposed tremor creates ratchet-like *cogwheel rigidity*. (From Kaufman DM et al: *Kaufman's clinical neurology for psychiatrists,* ed 9, Philadelphia, 2023, Elsevier.)

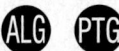
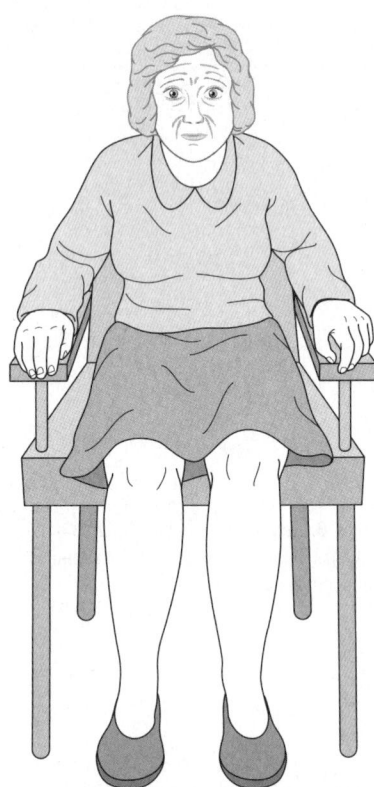

FIG. 5 Parkinson disease patients typically sit motionless with their legs uncrossed and their feet flat. Their arms remain on the chair or in their lap and rarely participate in normal gestures or re-positioning movements. They do not shift their weight from one hip to another or make any unnecessary movements. (From Kaufman DM et al: *Kaufman's clinical neurology for psychiatrists,* ed 9, Philadelphia, 2023, Elsevier.)

as is falling straight back. Postural instability is usually mild early in the disease course but can be significant in later stages. If falls and postural reflexes are greatly impaired early on, then consider other disorders, such as progressive supranuclear palsy (PSP).
- Masked facies (hypomimia) (Fig. 6): Face seems expressionless, giving the appearance of depression. Decreased blink; often there is excess drooling.
- Gait disturbance.
- Stooped posture, decreased arm swing.
- Difficulty initiating the first step; small shuffling steps that increase in speed (festinating gait) (Fig. E7). Steps become progressively faster and shorter while the trunk inclines further forward. Other complaints and findings early on include handwriting becoming smaller (micrographia) and voice becoming softer and often "gruffer" (hypophonia).
- Nonmotor symptoms in PD include neuropsychiatric (depression, apathy, impulse control disorders, hallucinations), cognitive, dysautonomia (especially orthostatic hypotension, sexual dysfunction, and anosmia), and sensory abnormalities. These symptoms also may be subject to fluctuations during "on" vs. "off" states.

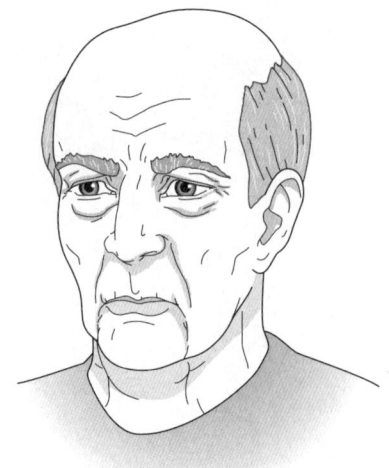

FIG. 6 Compared to normal individuals of the same age, Parkinson disease patients blink less frequently, show less facial expression, and move their head less frequently. Neurologists have called patients' facial appearance a "stare" or "masked facies" (Latin, face or countenance). Even when subtle, the masked face gives the appearance of apathy or depression. (From Kaufman DM et al: *Kaufman's clinical neurology for psychiatrists,* ed 9, Philadelphia, 2023, Elsevier.)

- Common premotor symptoms of PD include constipation, anosmia, depression, and REM sleep behavior disorder (Table 1).

ETIOLOGY

- Most cases are sporadic. Age is the most common risk factor, although a combination of both environmental and genetic factors likely contributes to disease expression.
- Both pesticides and drinking well water are factors correlated with a higher incidence of PD.
- 10% to 15% have a genetic etiology. Several different genes have been identified; these include the parkin gene (a significant cause of early-onset autosomal recessive PD), *LRRK2* (the most common cause of familial and sporadic parkinsonism associated with later onset of PD), and *PINK1* (associated with early-onset PD).[1]

Dx DIAGNOSIS

- A clinical diagnosis usually can be made based on a comprehensive history and physical examination. The cardinal signs used to diagnose PD are (mnemonic = ART):
  1. **A**kinesia/bradykinesia: Slowing and decrement of movement
  2. **R**igidity, of the cogwheel type
  3. **T**remor (resting, typically 4 to 6 Hz)
- Diagnostic criteria require bradykinesia plus either resting tremor or rigidity plus at least two supporting criteria and absence of absolute exclusion criteria and absence of red flags.[3]
  1. Supporting criteria: Clear benefit of dopaminergic therapy, presence of levodopa-induced dyskinesia, rest tremor, presence

of hyposmia, or cardiac sympathetic denervation on MIBG scintigraphy.
  2. Absolute exclusion criteria: No response to high-dose levodopa therapy, cerebellar abnormalities, downward vertical supranuclear gaze palsy, frontotemporal dementia symptoms early in the disease process, only lower limb involvement >3 yr, cortical sensory loss, progressive aphasia, or alternative diagnosis. These findings would suggest another diagnosis.
  3. Red flags: Severe autonomic failure or rapid progression of gait impairment in the first 5 yr, early bulbar involvement, inspiratory respiratory dysfunction, early recurrent falls, contractures, or bilateral symmetric parkinsonism. These findings would suggest another diagnosis.

DIFFERENTIAL DIAGNOSIS
Other diseases that cause parkinsonism:
- Multiple system atrophy (MSA): Distinguishing features include early autonomic dysfunction (including urinary incontinence, orthostatic hypotension, and erectile dysfunction), parkinsonism, cerebellar signs, and normal cognition.
- Dementia with Lewy bodies (DLB): Parkinsonism with concomitant dementia; patients often have early hallucinations and fluctuations in level of alertness and mental status.
- Corticobasal syndrome (CBD): Often begins asymmetrically with apraxia, cortical sensory loss in one limb, and, sometimes, alien limb phenomenon.
- Progressive supranuclear palsy (PSP): Tends to have axial rigidity greater than appendicular (limb) rigidity. These patients have early and severe postural instability. Hallmark is supranuclear gaze palsy that usually involves vertical gaze (especially downward) before horizontal.
- Essential tremor: Bilateral postural and action tremor.
- Secondary (acquired) parkinsonism (Box 1):
  1. Iatrogenic: Many, including any of the neuroleptics and antipsychotics. The high-potency D_2-blocker neuroleptics are most likely to cause parkinsonism. Metoclopramide can also cause parkinsonism. Abuse of methamphetamine has been linked to risk of PD
  2. Postinfectious parkinsonism: Von Economo encephalitis
  3. Chronic traumatic encephalopathy (dementia pugilistica): Parkinsonism and dementia after repeated head trauma
  4. Toxins (e.g., MPTP, manganese, carbon monoxide)
  5. Cerebrovascular disease: "Vascular parkinsonism" (basal ganglia infarcts); often lower limbs (especially gait) affected more than upper extremities
  6. Red flags suggesting a diagnosis other than PD are summarized in Box 2

WORKUP
- Identification of clinical signs and symptoms associated with PD (see "Physical Findings &

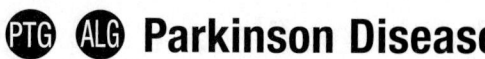

P

TABLE 1 Sleep and Night Problems in Parkinson Disease and Suggested Management

Problem	Potential Diagnosis	Proposed Management
Frequent Nocturia (± Two Episodes/Night)		
Normal volumes	Sleep apnea syndrome	Check for sleep apnea and treat appropriately
Small volumes, poor stream	Prostatism	Refer to urologist
Small volumes, good stream	Parkinsonism: associated nocturia	Intranasal desmopressin, oral amitriptyline, or transdermal rotigotine patch; if detrusor instability: oxybutynin, tolterodine, Myrbetriq
		Decrease evening fluid intake; empty bladder before bed; avoid evening dosing with diuretics, antihypertensives, or vasodilators; have a urinal at the bedside table
Difficulty Initiating Sleep		
Early in the evening	Too early lights-off	Switch off lights later
	Anxiety or behavioral insomnia	Sleep hygiene; treat anxiety
		Evening melatonin, eszopiclone, doxepin
With restlessness	Restless legs syndrome	Check for low ferritin; remove antidepressant drugs; if the diagnosis is uncertain, consider polysomnography with leg monitoring; try gabapentin, pregabalin or opiates, such as tramadol, if not confused
Late in the night	Altered circadian cycle	Sleep hygiene; decrease levodopa/dopamine agonists in the evening
		Melatonin 1-2 h before the desired bedtime
Late in night, hypomanic	Assess for impulse control disorder	Decrease dopamine agonists; keep on levodopa monotherapy; close neuropsychologic follow-up
Difficulty Resuming Sleep		
With cramps, muscle pain, slowness	Nocturnal bradykinesia	Immediate-release levodopa with a glass of water during awakenings
		Continuous drug delivery (ropinirole transdermal patch; pramipexole or extended-release ropinirole; apomorphine infusion; intrajejunal levodopa-carbidopa infusion)
		Satin bed sheets to aid movement in bed
With restlessness	Restless legs syndrome	Similar to nocturnal bradykinesia treatment
With anxiety	Anxious disorder	Evening antidepressants (mirtazapine, doxepin, paroxetine)
With low mood	Depressive disorder	Treat the depression
Nightmares, Agitation		
Confused at night when awake	Hallucinations, psychosis, confusion	Remove or reduce the evening dose of dopamine agonist or antidepressant; assess for sleep apnea
		Antipsychotics (quetiapine, clozapine)
Kicks, shouts, slaps	REM sleep behavior disorders	Secure the bed environment; discontinue antidepressant; assess likelihood of sleep apnea (video-PSG before treating)
		Melatonin, 3-9 mg in the evening, clonazepam, 0.5-2 mg in the evening
Daytime Sleepiness		
Falls asleep unexpectedly	Sleep attack	Check for possible sedating drugs (e.g., dopamine agonists) and remove or change them; warn patient not to drive
Falls asleep more often than before		Consider the Epworth Sleepiness Score; ask about associated hallucinations; consider PSG and MSLT
		Treat sleep apnea if severe
		Decrease/stop the dopamine agonist during daytime, and other sedative drugs
		Caffeine, modafinil, methylphenidate

MSLT, Multiple Sleep Latency Test; *PSG,* polysomnography; *REM,* rapid eye movement.
From Kryger M et al: *Principles and practice of sleep medicine,* ed 7, Philadelphia, 2023, Elsevier.

I

Clinical Presentation"), and elimination of conditions that may mimic it with a comprehensive history and physical examination.
- Routine genetic testing is not recommended.
- Can evaluate for response to carbidopa/levodopa (C/L) to differentiate PD from other causes of parkinsonism such as PSP, MSA, CBD.

IMAGING STUDIES

- MRI of the head may sometimes distinguish between idiopathic PD and other conditions that present with signs of parkinsonism (see "Differential Diagnosis").

- Dopamine transporter imaging (DaTscan with [¹²³I]β-CIT SPECT) evaluates the level of dopamine in the striatum and can be used to confirm parkinsonism in atypical cases. Normally there is dopamine reuptake in the caudate and putamen that can light up to look like a comma. If there is poor reuptake in the putamen as seen in PD, only the caudate lights up, similar to a period on imaging. DaTscan is approved to distinguish essential tremor from parkinsonism but cannot distinguish between different causes of parkinsonism.[3] Interpretation can be tricky, and routine use is not recommended at this time.

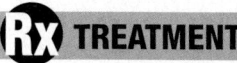 **TREATMENT**

NONPHARMACOLOGIC THERAPY

- Physical therapy (to help with exercise and help in evaluation of safe equipment to use), speech therapy, swallow evaluation. A safe, practical, and reasonable exercise regimen should be encouraged.[4,5]
- Avoidance of drugs that can induce or worsen parkinsonism: Neuroleptics (especially high potency), certain antiemetics (prochlorperazine, trimethobenzamide), metoclopramide, nonselective MAO inhibitors (MAO-Is) (may induce hypertensive crisis), reserpine, methyldopa.

BOX 1   Causes of Parkinsonism

Primary Parkinsonism
- Parkinson disease (idiopathic/sporadic parkinsonism)

Secondary Parkinsonism
- Drug-induced parkinsonism
  1. Neuroleptic drugs
  2. Calcium blocker cinnarizine
- Vascular parkinsonism (pseudoparkinsonism)
  1. Multiinfarct states
  2. Single basal ganglia/thalamic infarct
  3. Binswanger disease
- Multisystem degenerative diseases
  1. Progressive supranuclear palsy
  2. Multiple system atrophy (striatonigral type)
  3. Corticobasal degeneration
  4. Alzheimer disease
  5. Wilson disease (young-onset parkinsonism)
  6. Dementia with Lewy bodies
  7. Neurofibrillary tangle parkinsonism
- Toxins
  1. MPTP
  2. Manganese
- Familial parkinsonism
- Postinfectious parkinsonism
  1. Creutzfeldt-Jakob disease
  2. AIDS
  3. Postencephalitis (encephalitis lethargica)
- Miscellaneous causes
  1. Hydrocephalus
  2. Posttraumatic
  3. Tumors
- Metabolic causes (postanoxic)

From Fillit HM: *Brocklehurst's textbook of geriatric medicine and gerontology,* ed 8, Philadelphia, 2017, Elsevier.

BOX 2   "Red Flags" Suggesting a Diagnosis Other Than Parkinson Disease

- Early or prominent dementia
- Symmetric signs
- Bulbar dysfunction
- Early gait disorder
- Falls within the first yr
- Wheelchair dependence within 5 yr
- Early autonomic failure
- Sleep apnea
- Inspiratory stridor
- Apraxia
- Alien limb
- Cortical sensory loss

From Jankovic J et al: *Bradley and Daroff's neurology in clinical practice,* ed 8, Philadelphia, 2022, Elsevier.

ACUTE GENERAL Rx

- Levodopa is the gold standard, but patients <65 can be started on agonists if preferred.[6]
- It is appropriate to initiate pharmacotherapy when required by symptoms. Fig. 8 describes treatment of motor symptoms in patients with parkinsonism.
- Motor complications do develop during the course of the disease and likely reflect the combination of disease progression and the side effects of dopaminergic medications.

CHRONIC Rx

- Levodopa therapy:
  1. The gold standard is levodopa with a peripheral dopa decarboxylase inhibitor (carbidopa) to minimize side effects (nausea, light-headedness, postural hypotension).[6,7] The combination of the two drugs is marketed under the trade name Sinemet. Levodopa therapy has been found to reduce morbidity and mortality in PD patients.
  2. Usual starting dose is 25/100 mg (C/L) tid 1 h before (or after) meals. Typically better effect before meals, but lower side effects when taken with protein-rich meals.
  3. Controlled-release (Sinemet CR), extended-release (Rytary), infusion (Duopa), and inhaled (Inbrija) preparations are also available, but their use should be supervised by a neurologist.
  4. Stalevo (combination Sinemet and entacapone, a COMT inhibitor). Useful for patients with motor fluctuations (wearing off); has no role in treating patients with early PD.
  5. Duopa (C/L), administered by a 16-h infusion to the jejunum through either a nasojejunal tube (short-term) or PEG-J tube (long-term), is used for treating motor fluctuations in patients with advanced PD.
  6. Inbrija (levodopa inhalation powder) is used to treat "off" periods in patients taking C/L, but does not replace taking regular C/L. It works quickly and is easy to carry. It cannot be used if an MAO-I was used in the past 2 wk.
  7. Treatment of levodopa-related motor complications in PD are summarized in Fig. 9.
- Dopamine receptor agonists (ropinirole, pramipexole, rotigotine) are not as potent as levodopa, but they are often used as initial treatment in younger patients in an attempt to delay the onset of complications (dyskinesias, motor fluctuations) associated with levodopa therapy.[6,7] In general, they cause more side effects than levodopa, including nausea, vomiting, light-headedness, peripheral edema, confusion, and somnolence. They can also cause impulse control behaviors such as hypersexuality, binge eating, and compulsive shopping and gambling. Presence of these must be assessed at each visit as the appearance of these side effects is often underreported and their consequences can be severe. Dopamine agonists also can be associated with a prolonged withdrawal syndrome.
  1. Ropinirole: Initial dose is 0.25 mg tid but must be titrated over the course of 4 wk to 1 mg tid and then may be increased by 1.5 mg/wk to a maximum of 24 mg/day. An extended-release formulation is also available.
  2. Pramipexole: Initial dose is 0.125 mg tid but must be titrated over the course of weeks to 1.5 to 4.5 mg/day in three doses. An extended-release formulation is also available.
  3. Rotigotine: 2 mg to 6 mg/24 h as transdermal patch.
  4. Apomorphine: A dopamine agonist used for acute, intermittent treatment of unpredictable "off" episodes with advanced Parkinson disease.
- COMT inhibitors (entacapone, opicapone, and tolcapone) are used as adjunct to levodopa therapy to treat end-of-dose wearing off.
- MAO-B inhibitors can be used as monotherapy early in the disease or as adjunctive therapy in later stages; they have been shown to have milder symptomatic benefit than dopamine agonists or levodopa.[6,7] They are well tolerated and easy to titrate. Concurrent use of stimulants and sympathomimetics should be avoided. Certain food restrictions may apply.
  1. Rasagiline: Initial dose is 0.5 mg/day, then 1 mg/day. The ADAGIO study suggests that 1 mg rasagiline may have disease-modifying benefits, but results must be interpreted with caution.
  2. Selegiline: Usual dose, 5 mg bid with breakfast and lunch. Has amphetamine by-product, so has mild stimulant-like effects, which can be beneficial in some patients.
  3. Safinamide: FDA approved as add-on therapy for C/L that reduces "off time" and increases "on time" with fewer dyskinesias. Starting dose is 50 mg/day for 2 wk, which can be increased if needed to 100 mg/day.
- Istradefylline is the first FDA-approved adenosine A 2A receptor agonist for use as an adjunct to C/L in adults with PD experiencing "off" episodes.
- Amantadine (unclear mechanism of action, but reported to modulate the dopamine and glutamate systems in the CNS) can be used alone early in the disease. Later in the disease, it is especially useful in the treatment of dyskinesias. Dosage is 100 mg tid (titrate weekly from 100 mg daily). Must adjust for elderly and renal impairment. The most notable side effect, especially in the elderly, is confusion. Extended-release amantadine (Gocovri) may have fewer side effects.
- Anticholinergic agents are only helpful in treating tremor but may be more effective than levodopa for tremor in some circumstances. They can also be used to treat drooling in patients with PD. Potential side effects include constipation, urinary retention, memory impairment, and hallucinations. They should be avoided in the elderly.
  1. Trihexyphenidyl: Initial dose, 1 mg PO tid
  2. Benztropine: Usual dose, 0.5 to 1 mg daily or bid
- Treatment of nonmotor symptoms:[4] Nonmotor symptoms such as depression, anxiety, irritability, dementia, psychosis, constipation, urinary and sexual dysfunction, sleep disturbances such as REM behavior disorder, decreased sense of smell, and impulsive behavior, among others, often cause a great deal of distress for patients and caretakers alike. Treatable symptoms should be addressed pharmacologically using medications appropriate for elderly patients sensitive to antidopaminergic medications.

Treatment of motor symptoms of Parkinson disease

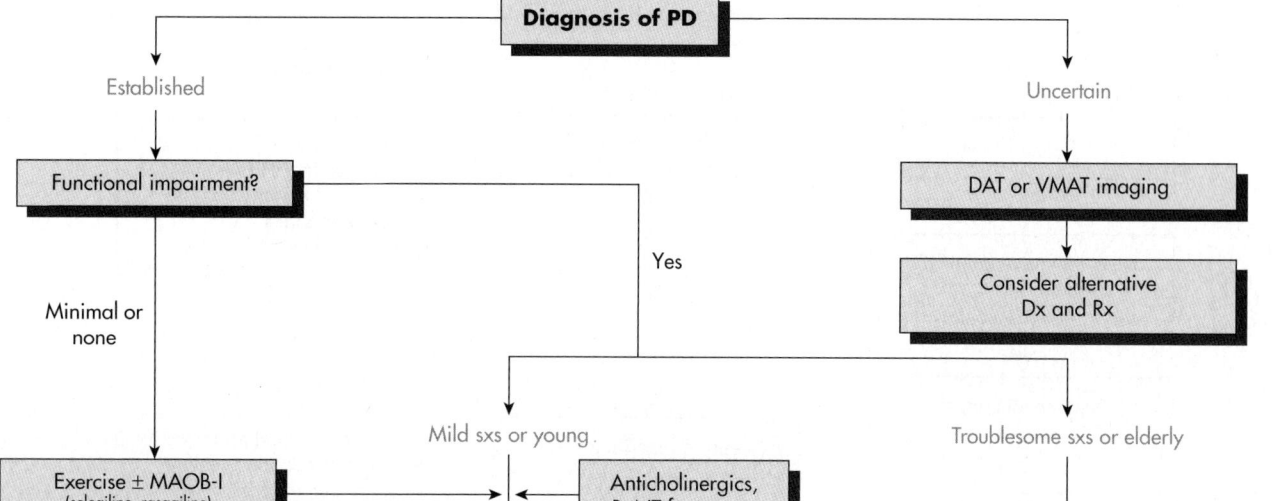

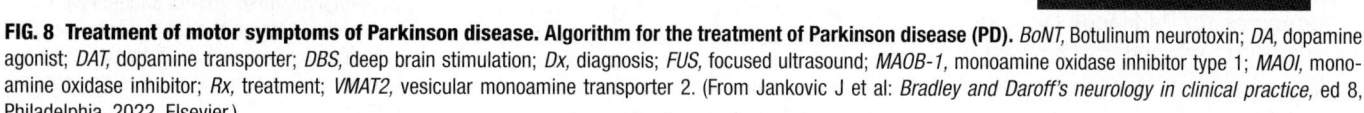

FIG. 8 Treatment of motor symptoms of Parkinson disease. Algorithm for the treatment of Parkinson disease (PD). *BoNT,* Botulinum neurotoxin; *DA,* dopamine agonist; *DAT,* dopamine transporter; *DBS,* deep brain stimulation; *Dx,* diagnosis; *FUS,* focused ultrasound; *MAOB-1,* monoamine oxidase inhibitor type 1; *MAOI,* monoamine oxidase inhibitor; *Rx,* treatment; *VMAT2,* vesicular monoamine transporter 2. (From Jankovic J et al: *Bradley and Daroff's neurology in clinical practice,* ed 8, Philadelphia, 2022, Elsevier.)

- Psychosis: Dopamine agonists and anticholinergics can cause hallucinations, so adjustment of these medications should be the first step. Pimavanserin (Nuplazid) is FDA approved for the treatment of PD psychosis and has been shown effective for the treatment of hallucinations and delusions associated with PD psychosis. The medication is an inverse agonist of 5-HT$_{2A}$ and 5-HT$_{2C}$ receptors without any evidence of dopamine blockade.
- PD dementia: Rivastigmine (Exelon), a cholinesterase inhibitor available both orally and transdermally as a patch (with few GI side effects), is approved to treat not only Alzheimer disease but also PD dementia.
- There are monoclonal antibody therapies against alpha synuclein in the pipeline to help with treatment of motor symptoms and cognitive symptoms in PD; however, thus far trials have been unsuccessful.

SURGICAL OPTIONS (BOX 3)

- Pallidal (globus pallidus interna) and subthalamic deep-brain stimulation (subthalamic nucleus) are currently the surgical options of choice for patients with advanced PD; similar improvement in motor function and adverse effects have been reported after either procedure.[8-10] Subthalamic targets have the benefit of possible medication lowering compared to pallidal targets. Compared with ablative procedures, DBS has the advantage of being reversible and adjustable. Thalamic DBS may be useful for refractory tremor. It improves the cardinal motor symptoms, extends medication "on" time, and reduces motor fluctuations during the day. In general, patients are likely to benefit from this therapy if they show a clear response to levodopa. Therefore, when considering DBS, patients should be evaluated for motor response to levodopa by stopping

levodopa overnight and evaluating motor response before and after a dose of levodopa.
- Focused ultrasound (FUS) is an imaging-guided method for creating therapeutic lesions in dead-brain structures, including the subthalamic nucleus. FUS subthalamotomy in one hemisphere improved motor features of PD in selected patients with asymmetric signs.[11] At 3 mo, patients who were most likely to benefit were younger, had lower motor severity scores, or had higher dyskinesia scores.[12] Longer and larger trials are required to determine the effect and safety of FUS in persons with Parkinson disease. DBS is currently favored over FUS as it can be continually reprogrammed to account for worsening disease and does not cause a permanent lesion.
- Surgery is often limited to patients with disabling, medically refractory problems, and patients must still have a good response to

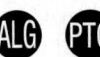
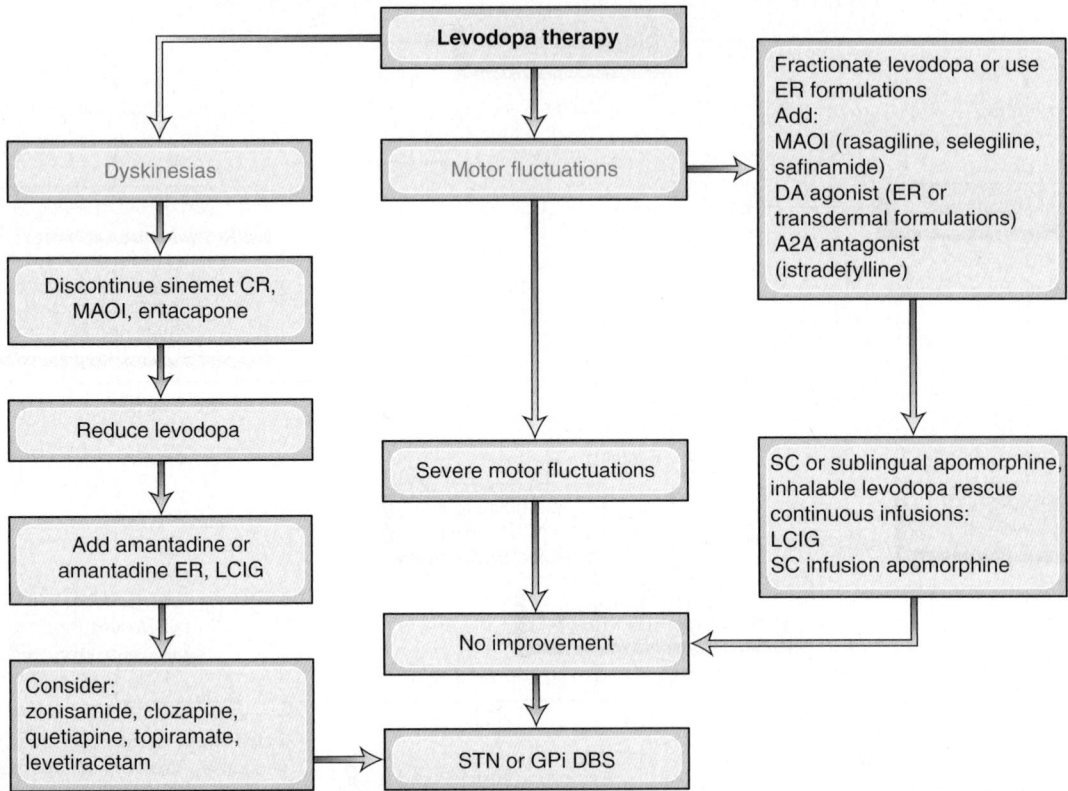

FIG. 9 Treatment of levodopa-related motor complications in Parkinson disease. *A2A,* Adenosine A2A receptor; *COMTI,* catechol-o-methyl-transferase inhibitor; *CR,* controlled release; *DA,* dopamine agonist; *DBS,* deep brain stimulation; *ER,* extended release; *GPi,* globus pallidus interna; *LCIG,* levodopa-carbidopa infusion gel; *MAOI,* monoamine oxidase inhibitor; *SC,* subcutaneous; *STN,* subthalamic nucleus. (From Jankovic J et al: *Bradley and Daroff's neurology in clinical practice,* ed 8, Philadelphia, 2022, Elsevier.)

BOX 3 Ablative and Stimulation Procedures for Parkinson Disease

- Ablative procedures
- Thalamotomy
- Pallidotomy
- Subthalamotomy
- Deep brain stimulation (DBS) procedures
- Thalamus (Vim nucleus)
- Globus pallidus pars interna (Gpi)
- Subthalamic nucleus (STN)
- Restorative procedures

From Warshaw G et al: *Ham's primary care geriatrics,* ed 7, Philadelphia, 2022, Elsevier.

L-dopa to undergo surgery. Yet for many patients, earlier stimulation might provide an improved motor benefit before disability from other symptoms has occurred and should be considered at an earlier stage of PD. DBS results in decreased dyskinesias, fluctuations, rigidity, and tremor.

DISPOSITION

PD usually follows a slowly progressive course leading to disability over the course of several years. However, every patient will progress individually, and patients should be reassured that this diagnosis does not, by definition, result in being either wheelchair or bed bound.

REFERRAL

- Neurology consultation is recommended at initial diagnosis of PD.
- Exercise is important for all patients with PD.
- Participation in outpatient physical and speech therapy program is recommended for patients with moderate to advanced disease.
- Neuropsychiatry in patients considering DBS.

 **PEARLS & CONSIDERATIONS**

- Asymmetry of symptoms at onset is typical of PD and therefore very useful in distinguishing PD from other causes of parkinsonism.

- Although resting tremor is a common presenting symptom, up to 25% of patients with idiopathic PD do not have classic resting tremor.
- PD patients can have mouth tremor, but head tremors are commonly seen with essential tremor.

REFERENCES

Available at eBooks.Health.Elsevier.com.

RELATED CONTENT

Parkinson Disease (Patient Information)

AUTHOR: **COREY ELAM GOLDSMITH, MD, FAAN**

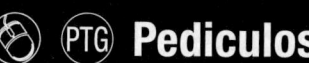
 BASIC INFORMATION

DEFINITION

Pediculosis is lice infestation. Humans can be infested with three kinds of lice: *Pediculus capitis* (head louse), *Pediculus corporis* (body louse), and *Phthirus pubis* (pubic, or crab, louse).[1] Lice inject saliva into the skin and feed on human blood, causing local inflammation and pruritis.[2] They deposit eggs (nits) on hair shafts (head lice and pubic lice) and along the seams of clothing (body lice). Nits remain firmly attached and hatch within 7 to 10 days. Lice are obligate human parasites and cannot survive away from their hosts for longer than 7 to 10 days.

SYNONYM

Lice

ICD-10CM CODES
B85.0	Pediculosis due to *Pediculus humanus capitis*
B85.1	Pediculosis due to *Pediculus humanus corporis*
B85.2	Pediculosis, unspecified
B85.3	Phthiriasis
B85.4	Mixed pediculosis and phthiriasis
Z11.8	Screening for head lice
Z20.7	Exposure to head lice
Z83.1	Family history of lice
Z86.19	History of lice

EPIDEMIOLOGY & DEMOGRAPHICS

- There are 6 to 12 million cases of head lice in the U.S. annually in children between ages 3 and 11, with infection more common in females.[1]
- Head lice affect children of all socioeconomic levels. Risk factors include sharing hair care items and attending day care. Frequency of hair washing, brushing, and hair length do not modify risk of infestation.[3]
- Risk factors for body lice include poor hygiene, homelessness, and crowded living conditions. Unlike head and pubic lice, body lice can transmit disease.[1]
- Pubic lice in a child, including infestation of the eyelashes, may indicate sexual abuse.[1,3]
- Pubic lice are usually spread during sexual intercourse, are most common in adolescents and young adults, and diagnosis should prompt additional evaluation for sexually transmitted infections.[1,3]
- Pets are not implicated in the transmission of lice.

PHYSICAL FINDINGS & CLINICAL PRESENTATION

- Infections may be asymptomatic. However, pruritis is the most common symptom, caused by hypersensitivity to lice saliva and fecal material. Secondary bacterial infections may develop from excoriation sores from scratching (Fig. E1).[3]
- Nits can be identified by examining hair shafts (Fig. E2) in cases of head and pubic

lice or on clothing (Fig. E3) in instances of body lice.[1-3]
- Head lice are most frequently found on the nape of the neck and behind the ears.[2]
- Lymphadenopathy may be present (cervical adenopathy with head lice, inguinal lymphadenopathy with pubic lice).[3]
- Pubic lice may affect the hair around the anus.[1]
- Nits found more than 1 cm away from the scalp are not likely to be viable.

ETIOLOGY

Lice are most commonly transmitted by close personal contact and less commonly by use of contaminated objects (e.g., combs, clothing, bed linen, hats). Lice cannot jump or fly.[1-3]

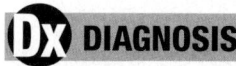 **DIAGNOSIS**

DIFFERENTIAL DIAGNOSIS

- Seborrheic dermatitis
- Scabies
- Eczema
- Other: Pilar casts, trichonodosis (knotted hair), monilethrix (beaded hair), dandruff
- Table 1 describes the differential diagnosis of nits

WORKUP

Diagnosis is made by seeing live, adult lice (Fig. 4), which are typically 2 to 3 mm in length, and have six legs. Nits alone may be hatched or nonviable. Using bright light, a magnifying glass, and a fine-toothed comb can aid in diagnosis.

LABORATORY TESTS

Wood's light examination is useful to screen a large number of children: Live nits fluoresce, empty nits have a gray fluorescence, and nits with unborn lice reveal white fluorescence.

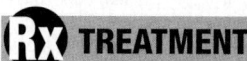 **TREATMENT**

ACUTE GENERAL Rx (TABLE 2)

The following products are available for treatment of head and pubic lice. Generally, body lice can be treated with nonpharmacologic therapies. Because head and pubic lice present minimal health risk, only children with proven or highly suspected active infestation should be

treated, and therapy should prioritize safety and cost. Side effects of topical therapy include pruritus, erythema, and mild burning. These side effects do not indicate treatment failure and do not necessitate retreatment. Additionally, clinicians should heed local resistance patterns, and if patients fail standard therapy, consultation with an infectious disease specialist may be beneficial.

- Permethrin is available over the counter (1% permethrin [Nix]) or by prescription (5% permethrin [Elimite]). It should be applied to damp hair and rinsed out after 10 min. Hair should not be shampooed for 1 to 2 days after application. Repeat application is generally not necessary in patients with head lice, but if required, it is most efficacious when performed 9 days after first treatment. Permethrin is nontoxic and FDA approved for use in children >2 mo old. Resistance to permethrin is widespread.[2,3] Permethrin or pyrethrin-piperonyl butoxide are first-line treatments for head lice.[2]
- Pyrethrin with piperonyl butoxide applied to dry hair and washed off after 10 min, for use in children 24 mo and older. Hair should not be washed for 1 to 2 days after application. Repeat application in 9 to 10 days is recommended. Resistance is widespread.
- Malathion (Ovide), an organophosphate, is effective in head lice, but is available by prescription only. It is applied to dry hair but is not commonly used due to its malodor, risk of flammability, and prolonged application time (8 to 12 h). Hair should not be washed for 1 to 2 days after application. It is not indicated for use in children <6 yr old. Most children do not require a second treatment.
- Ivermectin 0.5% lotion is FDA approved and now available OTC as a single-use topical treatment for head lice in patients >6 mo, but it may be cost prohibitive.[2,3] Ivermectin can also be applied to dried hair and rinsed after 10 min. Only one application is needed. Ivermectin is given as an oral dose of 200 to 400 mcg/kg of body weight. A second dose in 7 to 10 days may be needed for cases of persistent head lice. Ivermectin should not be used in children <15 kg given risk of neurotoxicity.
- Spinosad is a topical suspension applied to dry hair for 10 min, then rinsed out. The hair should not be washed for 1 to 2 days after

TABLE 1 Differential Diagnosis of Nits

Diagnosis	Comment
Nits	Firmly adherent to hair shaft; not easily removed with fingers
Seborrheic dermatitis (dandruff)	Diffuse scalp scaling; scales occasionally adhere to hair but easy to remove; scalp erythema may be present
Hair casts	Keratin protein that encircles hair shaft; easily removed
Piedra	Fungal infection of hair; firm nodules attached to hair shafts, white or black in color
Psoriasis	Thick silvery scales, often present overlying red plaques on the scalp
Hair products	Hairspray, mousse, gel

From Paller AS, Mancini AJ: *Hurwitz clinical pediatric dermatology, a textbook of skin disorders of childhood and adolescence,* ed 5, Philadelphia, 2016, Elsevier.

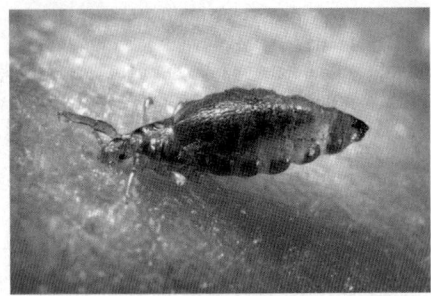

FIG. 4 Body louse, *Pediculus humanus* var. *corporis*, as it was obtaining a blood meal from human host. (Courtesy Public Health Image Library, Centers for Disease Control and Prevention. From Vincent JL et al: *Textbook of critical care,* ed 6, Philadelphia, 2011, Saunders.)

application. Its application may be repeated 7 days later if live lice are seen. It is more effective than permethrin, but more expensive. It is safe for use in pregnant persons (category B—no evidence of risk in humans) and in children >6 mo old.[2-3]
- Eyelash infestation can be treated with the application of ophthalmic-grade, prescription petroleum jelly rubbed into the eyelashes two to four times a day for 10 days.

COMPLEMENTARY & ALTERNATIVE MEDICINE
- Wet combing is a widely recommended but unproven adjunctive therapy.
- Personal items such as combs and brushes should be soaked in hot water for 15 to 30 min. Clothing, towels, and bed linens used in the 48 h prior to treatment should be washed in hot water (>130 °F [>54.4 °C]), and then dried for 10 min at the hottest setting. Items that cannot be washed should be sealed in a plastic bag for 2 wk.
- Vacuuming floors and furniture is recommended, but excessive, costly household cleaning is not needed.
- Gaseous pesticides are toxic and should not be used.

ⓘ PEARLS & CONSIDERATIONS

COMMENTS
- Given the low risk of classroom transmission, the American Academy of Pediatrics does not support exclusion from school because of head lice. Parents should be notified of the child's condition with recommendation for prompt treatment.[2]

- Close contacts and household members should also be examined for the presence of lice and treated if lice or nits within 1 cm of the scalp are identified.[2]
- Patients with pubic lice should notify their sexual contacts. Sexual partners within the last month should be treated.
- Finding nits without live, adult lice, especially >0.25 inches from the scalp, suggests past infection.
- Lice-removal companies may be helpful for some families, but no studies exist comparing efficacy of professional vs. home removal.

RELATED CONTENT
Lice (Patient Information)

REFERENCES
Available at eBooks.Health.Elsevier.com.

AUTHOR: **CINDY W. CHRISTIAN, MD**

TABLE 2 Recommended Pediculicide Treatments for Pediculosis Capitis[a]

Pediculicide	Tradenames	Therapeutic Efficacy (Ovicidal, Pediculicidal)	Safety Profile	Contraindications
0.33% Pyrethrins + 4% piperonyl butoxide shampoo	A-200 (OTC) RID (OTC)	95% ovicidal; no residual activity; increasing drug resistance	Excellent	Chrysanthemum and daisy (plant family *Compositae*) allergies possible contraindications
1%-5% Permethrin cream rinse	Acticin (OTC, Rx) Nix (OTC)	2-wk residual activity; increasing drug resistance	Excellent	Prior allergic reactions
0.5% Malathion lotion, 1% malathion shampoo	Ovide (Rx)	95% ovicidal; rapid (5-min) killing; good residual activity; increasing drug resistance, but not in the U.S.	Flammable 78% isopropyl alcohol vehicle stings eyes, skin, mucosa; increasing drug resistance; organophosphate poisoning risks with overapplication and ingestion	Infants and children <6 mo of age; pregnancy; breastfeeding
1% Lindane lotion and shampoo	Generic (Rx)	95% ovicidal; no residual activity; increasing drug resistance	Potential for CNS toxicity from organochlorine poisoning, usually manifesting as seizures, with overapplication and ingestion	Preexisting seizure disorder; infants and children <6 mo of age; pregnancy; breastfeeding; not recommended for use due to toxicity
0.9% Spinosad suspension	Natroba (Rx)	New to market; no reports of resistance; not ovicidal	Excellent	Infants and children age 4 yr and younger; presumed safe in pregnancy based on animal studies
5% Benzyl alcohol lotion	Ulesfia (Rx)	No resistance reported; not ovicidal	Excellent	Infants and children age 6 mo and younger; presumed safe in pregnancy based on animal studies
0.5% Ivermectin lotion	Sklice (Rx)	No resistance; single 10-min application; not ovicidal but nymphs die when they emerge from nits	Excellent	Infants and children age 6 mo and younger; safety in pregnancy uncertain
Ivermectin, 200-400 µg/kg tablet	Stromectol (Rx)	Excellent; not ovicidal; single PO dose, second dose in 7-10 days recommended	Excellent, but not in widespread use; nausea and vomiting possible; take on empty stomach with water only	Safety in pregnancy uncertain; not recommended for children weighing <5 kg

CNS, Central nervous system; *FDA,* US Food and Drug Administration; *OTC,* over-the-counter availability; *Rx,* available by prescription only.
[a]Carbaryl (Sevin), a carbamate pesticide, is not currently approved or available as a human topical preparation for use for pediculosis in the U.S. Carbaryl is, however, prescribed for pediculosis in Europe and elsewhere. Ectoparasite resistance to carbaryl has not been reported.
From Bennett JE et al: *Mandell, Douglas, and Bennett's principles and practice of infectious diseases,* ed 9, Philadelphia, 2020, Elsevier.

P

BASIC INFORMATION

DEFINITION

Pelvic abscess is an acute or chronic infection, most commonly involving the pelvic viscera. Treatment requires directed therapy including broad-spectrum antimicrobials and, if medical therapy fails, surgical intervention. There are four categories based on etiologic factors:

- Ascending infection, spreading from cervix through endometrial cavity to adnexa, forming a tuboovarian complex
- Infection occurring in the puerperium, which spreads to the adnexa from the endometrium or myometrium by a hematogenous or lymphatic route
- Abscess complicating pelvic surgery
- Involvement of the pelvic viscera as a result of spread from contiguous organs, such as appendicitis or diverticulitis

SYNONYMS

Tuboovarian abscess (TOA)
Vaginal cuff abscess

ICD-10CM CODES
K63.0	Abscess of intestine
K65.1	Peritoneal abscess
K68.11	Postprocedural retroperitoneal abscess
K68.12	Psoas muscle abscess
K68.19	Other retroperitoneal abscess
N70.93	Salpingitis and oophoritis, unspecified
N70.0	Acute salpingitis and oophoritis
N70.1	Chronic salpingitis and oophoritis

EPIDEMIOLOGY & DEMOGRAPHICS
INCIDENCE:
- 34% of hospitalized patients with pelvic inflammatory disease
- <1% of patients undergoing hysterectomy for benign gynecologic disease, most frequently with vaginal approach[1]
- Peak incidence between 15 and 40 yr

RISK FACTORS: Same risk factors as for pelvic inflammatory disease, although in 30% to 50% of patients there is no prior history of salpingitis before abscess forms.
- Untreated pelvic inflammatory disease
- Bacterial vaginosis
- Endometrioma
- Hydrosalpinx
- Prior laparotomy
- Anatomic anomalies
- Renal comorbidities
- Abdominal hysterectomy (vs. laparoscopic approach)
- Prolonged operative time (>3 h)
- Diabetes
- Smoking
- Respiratory disease
- Overweight or obesity
- Postoperative hematoma[1]

PHYSICAL FINDINGS & CLINICAL PRESENTATION
- Abdominal or pelvic pain (90%)
- Fever or chills (50%)
- Abnormal bleeding (21%)
- Vaginal discharge (28%)
- Nausea (26%)
- Up to 60% to 80% present without fever or leukocytosis; absence of these findings should not exclude diagnosis

ETIOLOGY
- Mixed flora of anaerobes, aerobes, and facultative anaerobes, such as *Escherichia coli*, *Bacteroides fragilis*, *Prevotella* spp., aerobic streptococci, and *Peptococcus* and *Peptostreptococcus* spp.
- *Neisseria gonorrhoeae* and *Chlamydia* are the major etiologic bacteria in cervicitis and salpingitis but are rarely found in abscess cavity cultures.
- After cesarean delivery, the most common site is the broad ligament, followed by the posterior cul-de-sac and retropubic space.[2]
- After vaginal delivery or hysterectomy, the most common site is the apex of the vagina or the adnexa.[2]
- In elderly patients, consider diverticular disease.

DIAGNOSIS

DIFFERENTIAL DIAGNOSIS
- Pelvic neoplasms, such as ovarian tumors and leiomyomas
- Ovarian torsion
- Inflammatory masses involving adjacent bowel or omentum, such as ruptured appendicitis or diverticulitis
- Pelvic hematomas, as may occur after cesarean section or hysterectomy
- Ectopic pregnancy
- Nephrolithiasis
- Urinary tract infection

LABORATORY TESTS
- CBC with differential
- Aerobic as well as anaerobic cultures of cervix, blood, urine, sputum, peritoneal cavity (if entered), and abscess cavity before starting antibiotics
- Pregnancy test in patients of reproductive age

IMAGING STUDIES
- Sonogram: Noninvasive, inexpensive study to confirm diagnosis, estimate size of abscess, and monitor response to therapy; sensitivity >90%
- Computed tomography (CT) scan: Used for both diagnosis and therapy (CT-guided drainage) (Fig. 1)
  1. Useful where sonogram provides insufficient information, as with intraabdominal abscesses
  2. Success rate with CT-guided abscess drainage: Unilocular, 90%; multilocular, 40%

TREATMENT

Major concerns:
- Desire for future fertility
- Likelihood of rupture of abscess, with resulting peritonitis, septic shock, and morbid sequelae

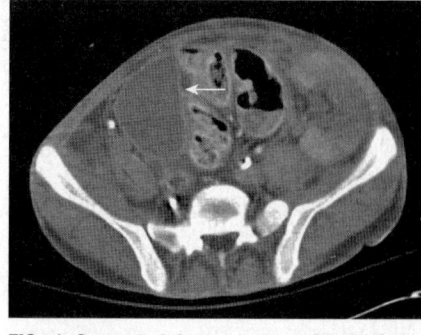
FIG. 1 Computed tomography with oral and intravenous contrast in a patient with a large pelvic abscess amenable to percutaneous drainage. There is classic "rim enhancement" of the abscess cavity (arrow). (From Vincent JL et al: *Textbook of critical care*, ed 8, Philadelphia, 2024, Elsevier.)

ACUTE GENERAL Rx
- Clinical quandary is whether patient requires immediate surgical intervention (uncertain diagnosis or suspicion of rupture) or management with intravenous (IV) antibiotics, reserving surgery for those with inadequate clinical response (e.g., 48 to 72 h of therapy, with persistent fever or leukocytosis, increasing size of mass, or suspicion of rupture). Laparoscopic surgery should be reserved for experienced surgeons and in cases of unruptured pelvic abscess.
- Surgery indicated in poor response to medical therapy. Early surgery may be needed in those with large adnexal masses (>8 cm), or in immunocompromised patients.
- 60% of patients with abscesses ≥10 cm will require surgical intervention.[1]
- Antibiotic combinations:
  1. Cefotetan 2 g IV q12h or cefoxitin 2 g IV q6h or ampicillin-sulbactam 3 g IV q6h plus doxycycline 100 mg PO or IV q12h
  2. For penicillin allergic patients: Clindamycin 900 mg IV q8h plus gentamicin either 3 to 5 mg/kg q24h or loading dose 2 mg/kg IV/IM loading dose plus maintenance dose 1.5 mg/kg q8h
- During medical management, high index of suspicion for acute rupture, such as acute worsening of abdominal pain or new-onset tachycardia and hypotension, mandating immediate surgical intervention after patient stabilization.
- Surgical options:
  1. Laparoscopy with drainage and irrigation
  2. CT-guided drainage (interventional radiology)
  3. Transvaginal colpotomy (abscess must be midline, dissect rectovaginal septum, and be adherent to vaginal fornix)
  4. Laparotomy, including total abdominal hysterectomy with bilateral salpingo-oophorectomy or unilateral salpingo-oophorectomy
  5. Evidence of ruptured tuboovarian abscess is a surgical emergency
  6. Antibiotics should be continued during and after surgery[2]

Diseases and Disorders

I

DISPOSITION

- Of patients treated with medical therapy alone, pregnancy rate is 25%. Of patients treated with both medical and laparoscopic surgical management, pregnancy rate is between 32% and 63%. Pregnancy rate decreases with recurrent episodes.
- No response in 30% to 40%; can be treated with either CT-guided drainage or surgical intervention, keeping in mind that unilateral adnexectomy may give equal chance of cure versus hysterectomy, yet preserve reproductive potential.

REFERRAL

If patient has a tuboovarian abscess, refer to gynecologist.

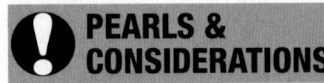

COMMENTS

- If *Actinomyces* species is isolated from culture, treatment with penicillin is required for an extended period (6 wk to 3 mo).
- Most common cause of preventable death: Physician delay in diagnosis.

REFERENCES

Available at eBooks.Health.Elsevier.com.

RELATED CONTENT

Pelvic Abscess (Patient Information)
Pelvic Inflammatory Disease (Related Key Topic)

AUTHORS: **ALEXANDRA MULLIKEN, MD,** **ELLA STERN, MD,** and **MARWAN MA'AYEH, MD**

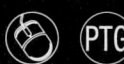 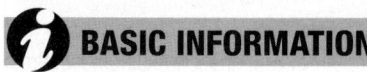
Diseases and Disorders

I

BASIC INFORMATION

DEFINITION

Pelvic inflammatory disease (PID) is infection and inflammation of the female upper genital tract (including uterus, fallopian tubes, ovaries, and/or pelvic peritoneum) unrelated to pregnancy or surgical intervention. PID can be classified as acute (≤30 days' duration), subclinical, or chronic (>30 days' duration).

SYNONYMS

PID
Endometritis
Salpingitis
Oophoritis
Adnexitis
Pelvic peritonitis
Pyosalpinx
Tuboovarian abscess
TOA

ICD-10CM CODES

A18.17	Tuberculous female pelvic inflammatory disease
A52.76	Syphilitic pelvic inflammatory disease
A54.2*	Gonococcal pelviperitonitis and other gonococcal genitourinary infections
A54.24	Gonococcal female pelvic inflammatory disease
A56.1*	Chlamydial infection of pelviperitoneum and other genitourinary organs
A56.11	Chlamydial female pelvic inflammatory disease
A56.19	Other chlamydial genitourinary infection
N70*	Salpingitis and oophoritis
N70.0*	Acute salpingitis and oophoritis
N70.01	Acute salpingitis
N70.02	Acute oophoritis
N70.03	Acute salpingitis and oophoritis
N70.1*	Chronic salpingitis and oophoritis
N70.11	Chronic salpingitis
N70.12	Chronic oophoritis
N70.13	Chronic salpingitis and oophoritis
N70.9*	Salpingitis and oophoritis, unspecified
N70.91	Salpingitis, unspecified
N70.92	Oophoritis, unspecified
N70.93	Salpingitis and oophoritis, unspecified
N71*	Inflammatory disease of uterus, except cervix
N71.0	Acute inflammatory disease of uterus
N71.1	Chronic inflammatory disease of uterus
N71.9	Inflammatory disease of uterus, unspecified
N72	Inflammatory disease of cervix uteri
N73*	Other female pelvic inflammatory diseases
N73.0	Acute parametritis and pelvic cellulitis
N73.1	Chronic parametritis and pelvic cellulitis
N73.2	Unspecified parametritis and pelvic cellulitis
N73.3	Female acute pelvic peritonitis
N73.4	Female chronic pelvic peritonitis
N73.5	Female pelvic peritonitis, unspecified
N73.6	Female pelvic peritoneal adhesions (postinfective)
N73.8	Other specified female pelvic inflammatory diseases
N73.9	Female pelvic inflammatory disease, unspecified
N74	Female pelvic inflammatory disorders in diseases classified elsewhere

*Indicates nonbillable codes.

EPIDEMIOLOGY & DEMOGRAPHICS

INCIDENCE & PREVALENCE: Pelvic inflammatory disease is most often diagnosed in young, sexually active women. The incidence of PID is difficult to ascertain given its broad diagnostic criteria, its propensity to be missed as a diagnosis, and the challenges with follow-up due to patients seeking urgent or emergent care for this condition. The Centers for Disease Control and Prevention (CDC) estimates 1 million new cases of PID are diagnosed yearly. The incidence may be rising given recent sharp increases in sexually transmitted diseases (STDs) associated with PID in the United States. PID has long-term health risks for women, including recurrent infection, chronic pelvic pain, pelvic adhesive disease, and tubal disease resulting in ectopic pregnancy and infertility.

RISK FACTORS:

- Sexually active adolescent and young women
- History of PID
- Prior chlamydial or gonorrheal infection
- Multiple or new sexual partners within past 12 mo
- Sexual partner diagnosed with sexually transmitted infection (STI)
- Lack of barrier contraception use

PHYSICAL FINDINGS & CLINICAL PRESENTATION

- Pelvic or lower abdominal pain
- Abnormal vaginal discharge
- Abnormal uterine bleeding
- Postcoital bleeding
- Dysuria
- Dyspareunia
- Fever
- Nausea and vomiting (suggestive of peritonitis)
- Cervical friability
- Cervical motion tenderness
- Uterine tenderness
- Adnexal tenderness
- Adnexal mass
- Right upper quadrant tenderness (perihepatitis, Fitz-Hugh-Curtis syndrome [Fig. E1]): 5% to 10% of PID cases may develop right upper quadrant pain, pleuritic pain, and tenderness in the right upper quadrant when the liver is palpated. The pain may radiate to the shoulder or into the back. Liver transaminase levels may be elevated.

NOTE: Women with PID may be asymptomatic and/or have a benign physical examination.

ETIOLOGY

PID occurs as a result of ascending infection from the lower genital tract. Infections are often polymicrobial, and although gonorrheal and chlamydial infections are commonly implicated in the development of PID, fewer than 50% of women test positive for these organisms. This is likely due in part to increased STI screening efforts. PID may also arise in the setting of organisms associated with normal vaginal flora such as:

- Bacteroides fragilis
- Escherichia coli and other enteric gram-negative rods
- Gardnerella vaginalis
- Haemophilus influenzae
- Streptococcus agalactiae

Less common infectious causes include the following: *Trichomonas vaginalis*, *Mycoplasma hominis*, *Ureaplasma urealyticum*, *Mycoplasma genitalium* (a concern because of antibiotic resistance), *Mycobacterium tuberculosis* (an important cause in developing countries), and cytomegalovirus (CMV).

DIAGNOSIS

Diagnosis of PID is made when a sexually active female has clinical or pathologic evidence of upper genital tract infection and inflammation, which includes any cervical motion tenderness, uterine tenderness, or adnexal tenderness. Box 1 summarizes the CDC criteria for diagnosing PID. Although no single test or measure reliably diagnoses the spectrum of disorders that comprise PID, a clinical diagnosis of symptomatic PID has a positive predictive value of 65% to 90%:

- Providers should maintain a low threshold for diagnosis and treatment of PID given significant long-term health risks associated with the disease, especially if untreated.
- The CDC suggests that women with risk factors, abdominal or pelvic pain, and any pelvic tenderness (cervical, uterine, and/or adnexal) be treated for PID.
- Definitive criteria for diagnosis of PID include:
  1. Laparoscopic abnormalities consistent with PID
  2. Histopathologic evidence of endometritis in women with clinical suspicion for PID
  3. Transvaginal sonography or other imaging techniques showing thickened, fluid-filled tubes with or without free pelvic fluid, tuboovarian complex, or Doppler studies indicative of pelvic infection such as tubal hyperemia

However, requiring the aforementioned criteria before empiric treatment would not only lead to underdiagnosis and treatment but also delay treatment and lead to unnecessary morbidity.

- Supportive criteria for that enhance diagnostic specificity of PID include:
  1. Oral temperature >38.3° C (>101° F)
  2. Abnormal cervical mucopurulent discharge or cervical friability
  3. Predominance of white blood cells (WBCs) on saline microscopy of vaginal fluid
  4. Elevated acute inflammatory markers (erythrocyte sedimentation rate [ESR] or C-reactive protein)
  5. Neisseria gonorrhoeae or Chlamydia trachomatis infection

DIFFERENTIAL DIAGNOSIS

- Appendicitis
- Ectopic pregnancy
- Intrauterine/other pregnancy
- Ovarian cyst
- Adnexal torsion
- Endometriosis
- Urinary tract infection (cystitis or pyelonephritis)
- Diverticulitis

WORKUP

- History: See "Risk Factors" and "Physical Findings & Clinical Presentation"
- Physical examination: See "Physical Findings & Clinical Presentation"

LABORATORY TESTS

- Wet mount: Clue cells, increased WBCs
- Gram stain of endocervical exudate: >30 polymorphonuclear cells per high-power field correlates with chlamydial or gonococcal infection
- Endocervical cultures for *N. gonorrhoeae* and *C. trachomatis*
- CBC: Leukocytosis
- Human chorionic gonadotropin to rule out intrauterine or ectopic pregnancy
- Elevated acute phase reactants: ESR >15 mm/h, C-reactive protein
- HIV and rapid plasma reagin, with consideration for other STI screening such as hepatitis B surface antigen, hepatitis C Ab (HIV increases incidence of tuboovarian abscess [TOA])
- Fallopian tube aspirate or peritoneal exudate culture if laparoscopy or drainage of TOA performed
- Endometritis on endometrial biopsy if performed

IMAGING STUDIES

Ultrasonography is commonly used to assess for PID and can be used to determine inpatient vs. outpatient treatment by presence or absence of TOA. Ultrasonographic findings include:

- Thick-walled adnexal mass with heterogenous or cystic contents suggestive of abscess
- Dilated fallopian tubes (note that normal fallopian tubes are rarely identified on ultrasonography)
- "Cogwheel sign" indicating thickened fallopian tube walls
- Heterogenous fluid within the endometrium

Computed tomography or MRI scan may be useful to better characterize adnexal masses and/or rule out other pathology, such as appendicitis or renal calculus. Choice of imaging modality will depend on clinical suspicion, logistic access, and associated cost.

PROCEDURES

Endometrial biopsy that reveals endometritis may support a diagnosis of PID. Laparoscopy has been utilized as a gold standard for diagnosing PID, but due to the invasive nature of this procedure and the risks and costs associated, it is rarely indicated as a diagnostic tool.

℞ TREATMENT (TABLE 1)

Primary management of PID is medical, with broad-spectrum antibiotics administered in an outpatient setting. Inpatient treatment should be initiated when:

- Surgical emergency is not excluded (such as acute appendicitis, ruptured ectopic pregnancy, or ovarian torsion)
- Severe illness, nausea or vomiting, or temperature >38.5° C (>101.3° F)
- TOA (Fig. E2) is present
- Patient is unable or unwilling to complete outpatient treatment (including medication regimen and clinical follow-up)
- Outpatient treatment fails to improve symptoms in 48 to 72 h
- Pregnancy, immunodeficiency, or other complicating medical condition exists

The following are evidence-based guidelines recommended by the CDC for acute PID.

INPATIENT REGIMENS

Recommended parenteral regimens:

- Ceftriaxone 1 g intravenous (IV) q24h *PLUS* doxycycline 100 mg oral (PO) or IV q12h *PLUS* metronidazole 500 mg IV q12h *OR*
- Cefotetan 2 g IV q12h *PLUS* doxycycline 100 mg PO or IV q12h *OR*
- Cefoxitin 2 g IV q6h *PLUS* doxycycline 100 mg PO or IV q12h *OR*

Alternative parenteral regimen:

- Ampicillin/sulbactam 3 g IV q6h *PLUS* doxycycline 100 mg PO or IV q12h.
- Clindamycin 900 mg IV q8h *PLUS* gentamicin loading dose IV or intramuscular (IM) (2 mg/kg of body weight), followed by a maintenance dose (1.5 mg/kg) q8h. Single daily dosing (3 to 5 mg/kg) can be substituted.
- When clinical improvement is apparent based on symptoms, physical exam, and laboratory criteria, antibiotics may be transitioned from IV to PO with doxycycline PO and metronidazole PO or clindamycin PO (depending on the regimen selected) administered to complete 14 days of total antibiotic therapy. If a patient does not improve despite use of a recommended antibiotic regimen, further workup and potential procedural intervention are warranted.

OUTPATIENT REGIMENS

Recommended IM/PO regimens:

- Ceftriaxone 500 mg IM in a single dose *PLUS* *doxycycline* 100 mg PO bid for 14 days *PLUS* metronidazole 500 mg PO bid for 14 days *OR*
- Cefoxitin 2 g IM in a single dose and probenecid 1 g PO administered concurrently in a single dose *PLUS* doxycycline 100 mg PO bid for 14 days *PLUS* metronidazole 500 mg PO bid for 14 days *OR*

TABLE 1 Recommended Treatment of Acute Pelvic Inflammatory Disease

Hospitalized Patients

Regimen A

- Cefotetan, 2 g IV q12h, or cefoxitin, 2 g IV q6h

plus

- Doxycycline, 100 mg IV or PO q12h
- Continue both drugs IV for 24 h after the patient substantially improves, then continue doxycycline, 100 mg PO bid, to complete 14 days total therapy. Either clindamycin or metronidazole may be added to the oral regimen if tuboovarian abscess is suspected.

or

Regimen B

- Clindamycin, 900 mg IV q8h

plus

- Gentamicin, 2 mg/kg IV once, followed by 1.5 mg/kg q8h[a]
- Continue both drugs IV for 24 h after the patient substantially improves, then continue doxycycline, 100 mg PO twice daily, or clindamycin, 450 mg PO four times daily, to complete 14 days total therapy. Clindamycin may be preferable when tuboovarian abscess is suspected.

Outpatients

- Single-dose cefoxitin, 2 g IM, plus probenecid, 1 g PO; or ceftriaxone, 250 mg IM; or other parenteral third-generation cephalosporin (e.g., ceftizoxime or cefotaxime)

plus

- Doxycycline, 100 mg PO bid for 14 days

with or without

- Metronidazole, 500 mg PO bid for 14 days

bid, Twice daily; *IM,* intramuscular; *IV,* intravenous; *PO,* by mouth (per os).
[a]Single daily dosing may be substituted.
Modified from Centers for Disease Control and Prevention: Sexually transmitted diseases treatment guidelines, 2015, *MMWR Morb Mortal Wkly Rep* 64:60-68, 2015; and www.cdc.gov/std/treatment.

- Other third-generation cephalosporin (ceftizoxime or cefotaxime) *PLUS* doxycycline 100 mg PO bid for 14 days *PLUS* metronidazole 500 mg PO bid for 14 days

Alternative intramuscular/oral regimen if the patient has a cephalosporin allergy:

- Levofloxacin 500 mg PO daily *PLUS* metronidazole 500 mg PO bid for 14 days
- Moxifloxacin 400 mg PO daily for 14 days (preferred if *M. genitalium*)
- Azithromycin 500 mg IV daily for 1 to 2 doses followed by 250 mg PO daily for 7 days or in combination with metronidazole 500 mg PO tid for 12 to 14 days

Due to quinolone-resistant *N. gonorrhoeae,* antimicrobial susceptibility testing should be performed if a culture is positive for gonorrhea in a patient with a cephalosporin allergy. If the isolate is quinolone-resistant, consultation with an infectious disease specialist is recommended.

TREATMENT CONSIDERATIONS

- Antimicrobials should include coverage against *N. gonorrhoeae* and *C. trachomatis* even if these organisms are not identified on culture.
- Women should avoid sexual activity until they and their sexual partners have been adequately treated and symptoms have resolved.
- TOA may require drainage, which may be accomplished by interventional radiology via aspiration or placement of a drain, or by a gynecologist via vaginal or laparoscopic means. Recurrent/persistent TOAs may be managed by total hysterectomy with bilateral salpingo-oophorectomy after acute treatment of infection.
- Treatment of PID in women with intrauterine devices (IUDs) does not include/require removal of the device unless there is no clinical improvement after 48 to 72 h of treatment with an

approved regimen. IUDs rarely serve as a source for PID, especially >3 wk after insertion.
- Sexual partners of patients diagnosed with PID or other STIs should be evaluated and treated appropriately. In the setting of PID, treat all sexual partners within 60 days of onset of symptoms. Some states allow for expedited partner therapy (EPT), such that a woman's provider is able to supply her with enough medication to treat herself and her partner(s).
- Treatment of chronic PID may be aimed at a different spectrum of microbes and should be tailored appropriately.

DISPOSITION

- Given the risk of reinfection, all women should be retested for gonorrhea and chlamydia 3 mo after treatment.
- Follow-up includes confirmation of partner treatment, education on use of barrier contraception, and risks of PID and long-term sequelae, including:
  1. Recurrent PID
  2. Chronic pelvic pain
  3. Fallopian tube damage that leads to infertility and/or ectopic pregnancy
  4. Fitz-Hugh-Curtis syndrome
  5. Potential risk for cancer: Limited studies have suggested a small association between PID and ovarian, endometrial, and colon cancer

⚠ PEARLS & CONSIDERATIONS

COMMENTS

- Maintain a low threshold for the diagnosis and treatment of PID given the risks for progression to severe infection and to significant and chronic medical and reproductive complications.

- Most patients are candidates for outpatient therapy, but inpatient hospitalization is recommended in select cases.
- Use only CDC-recommended treatment regimens unless contraindicated due to severe patient allergy; in such cases, check local susceptibilities of suspected pathogen.
- Offer HIV and other STI screening to all women with suspected or diagnosed PID.
- IUDs may be retained unless women have failed to improve with 48 to 72 h of treatment.
- Treat sexual partners of women with PID, with EPT if possible.
- Counsel patients on abstinence until they and their partners have completed treatment.
- Test for reinfection with gonorrhea and chlamydia 3 mo after treatment.

PREVENTION

Women aged <25 yr and/or participating in high-risk sexual behavior should be screened annually for gonorrhea and chlamydia; studies have shown such screening to reduce cases of PID by >50%. The importance of minimizing partner exposures and using barrier contraception (either alone or in conjunction with another method) should also be emphasized.

SUGGESTED READINGS

Available at eBooks.Health.Elsevier.com.

RELATED CONTENT

Pelvic Inflammatory Disease (Patient Information)
Chlamydia Genital Infections (Related Key Topic)
Gonorrhea (Related Key Topic)
Pelvic Abscess (Related Key Topic)

AUTHOR: **COURTNEY PFEUTI, MD**

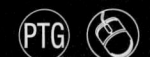
 BASIC INFORMATION

DEFINITION

Peptic ulcer disease (PUD) is an ulceration in the stomach (Table 1) or duodenum resulting from an imbalance between mucosal protective factors and various mucosal damaging mechanisms (see "Etiology").

SYNONYMS

PUD
Duodenal ulcer (DU)
Gastric ulcer (GU)

ICD-10CM CODES

K25.3	Acute gastric ulcer without hemorrhage or perforation
K25.7	Chronic gastric ulcer without hemorrhage or perforation
K26.3	Acute duodenal ulcer without hemorrhage or perforation
K26.7	Chronic duodenal ulcer without hemorrhage or perforation
K27.0	Acute peptic ulcer, site unspecified, with hemorrhage
K27.1	Acute peptic ulcer, site unspecified, with perforation
K27.2	Acute peptic ulcer, site unspecified, with both hemorrhage and perforation
K27.3	Acute peptic ulcer, site unspecified, without hemorrhage or perforation
K27.4	Chronic or unspecified peptic ulcer, site unspecified, with hemorrhage
K27.5	Chronic or unspecified peptic ulcer, site unspecified, with perforation
K27.6	Chronic or unspecified peptic ulcer, site unspecified, with both hemorrhage and perforation
K27.7	Chronic peptic ulcer, site unspecificd, without hemorrhage or perforation
K27.9	Peptic ulcer, site unspecified, unspecified as acute or chronic, without hemorrhage or perforation
P78.82	Peptic ulcer of newborn
Z87.11	Personal history of peptic ulcer disease

TABLE 1 Gastric Ulcer Types

Type	Location	Acid Level
I	Lesser curve at incisura	Low to normal
II	Gastric body with duodenal ulcer	Increased
III	Prepyloric	Increased
IV	High on lesser curve	Normal
V	Anywhere	Normal, NSAID-induced

NSAID, Nonsteroidal antiinflammatory drug.
From Townsend CM et al: *Sabiston textbook of surgery,* ed 21, St Louis, 2022, Elsevier.

BOX 1 Key Symptoms and Signs of Peptic Ulcer

Uncomplicated Ulcer
No symptoms ("silent ulcer" in up to 40% of cases)
Epigastric pain
Pain may radiate to the back, thorax, other parts of abdomen (cephalad most likely, caudad least likely)
Pain may be nocturnal (most specific),"painful hunger" relieved by food, or continuous (least specific)
Nausea
Vomiting
Heartburn (mimics or associated with gastroesophageal reflux)

Complicated Ulcer
Acute perforation
Severe abdominal pain
Shock
Abdominal board-like rigidity (and rebound and other signs of peritoneal irritation)
Free intraperitoneal air
Hemorrhage
Hematemesis and/or melena
Hemodynamic changes, anemia
Previous history of ulcer symptoms (80%)
Gastric outlet obstruction
Satiation, inability to ingest food, eructation
Nausea, vomiting (and related disturbances)
Weight loss

From Goldman L, Schafer AI: *Goldman's Cecil medicine,* ed 24, Philadelphia, 2012, Saunders.

EPIDEMIOLOGY & DEMOGRAPHICS

INCIDENCE:
• 250,000 to 500,000 (200,000 to 400,000 duodenal; 50,000 to 100,000 gastric) annually; duodenal ulcer/gastric ulcer ratio is 4:1.

ANATOMIC LOCATION:
• <90% of duodenal ulcers occur in the first portion of the duodenum; gastric ulcers occur most frequently in the lesser curvature near the incisura angularis.

PHYSICAL FINDINGS & CLINICAL PRESENTATION

• Box 1 describes key symptoms and signs of peptic ulcer.
• Epigastric pain is the most frequently reported symptom of PUD. The pain is typically improved with food or antacids and worsened by fasting.
• Physical examination is often unremarkable.
• Patient may have epigastric tenderness, tachycardia, pallor, hypotension (from acute or chronic blood loss), nausea and vomiting (if pyloric channel is obstructed), board-like abdomen and rebound tenderness (if perforated, Fig. E1), and hematemesis or melena (with a bleeding ulcer).

ETIOLOGY

Often multifactorial. The following are common mucosal damaging factors:
• *Helicobacter pylori* infection. *H. pylori* is the major cause of PUD. It is found in more than 70% of patients with duodenal ulcers and gastric ulcers in the U.S. Rates are much higher (>90%) in other parts of the world. Eradication of *H. pylori* markedly reduces peptic ulcer recurrence
• Medications (NSAIDs, glucocorticoids). Risk factors for development of NSAID-related ulcers are described in Box 2

BOX 2 Risk Factors for Development of NSAID-Related Ulcers

Definite
Advanced age
History of ulcer
Concomitant corticosteroid therapy
Concomitant anticoagulation therapy
High doses of NSAIDs
Serious systemic disorders

Possible
Concomitant infection with *Helicobacter pylori*
Cigarette smoking
Consumption of alcohol

NSAIDs, Nonsteroidal antiinflammatory drugs.
From Andreoli TE et al: *Andreoli and Carpenter's Cecil essentials of medicine,* ed 8, Philadelphia, 2010, Saunders.

• Incompetent pylorus or lower esophageal sphincter
• Bile acids
• Impaired proximal duodenal bicarbonate secretion
• Decreased blood flow to gastric mucosa
• Acid secreted by parietal cells and pepsin secreted as pepsinogen by chief cells
• Cigarette smoking
• Alcohol

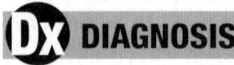 **DIAGNOSIS**

DIFFERENTIAL DIAGNOSIS

• Gastroesophageal reflux disease
• Cholelithiasis syndrome
• Pancreatitis
• Gastritis
• Nonulcer dyspepsia

- Neoplasm (gastric carcinoma, lymphoma, pancreatic carcinoma)
- Angina pectoris, myocardial infarction, pericarditis
- Dissecting aneurysm
- Other: High small-bowel obstruction, pneumonia, subphrenic abscess, early appendicitis

WORKUP

Comprehensive history and physical exam to exclude other diagnoses. Diagnostic modalities include endoscopy or upper GI series. Endoscopy is preferred and remains the gold standard for diagnosis of PUD. The presence of a mucosal break ≥5 mm in the stomach or duodenum confirms the diagnosis. An algorithm for evaluation, treatment, and surveillance of a patient with gastric ulcer is illustrated in Fig. 2.

LABORATORY TESTS

- Routine laboratory evaluation is usually unremarkable.
- Anemia may be present in patients with significant GI bleeding.
- *H. pylori* testing by endoscopic biopsy, urea breath test, or stool antigen test (*H. pylori* stool antigen) is recommended:
  1. The urea breath test documents active infection (sensitivity and specificity >90%). The patient ingests a small amount of urea labeled with carbon 13 or carbon 14. If urease is present (produced by the organism), the urea is hydrolyzed and the patient exhales labeled carbon dioxide that is then collected and measured. Use of proton pump inhibitors (PPIs) within 2 wk of the urea breath test may interfere with test results.
  2. Stool antigen test is an ELISA that identifies *H. pylori* antigen in a stool specimen through a polyclonal anti–*H. pylori* antibody. It is as accurate as the urea breath test for diagnosis of active infection and follow-up evaluation of patients treated for *H. pylori*. A negative result on the stool antigen test 6 wk after completion of therapy identifies patients in whom eradication of *H. pylori* was successful.
  3. Serologic testing for antibodies to *H. pylori* is easy and inexpensive; however, the presence of antibodies demonstrates previous but not necessarily current infection. Antibodies to *H. pylori* can remain elevated for months to years after infection has cleared; therefore antibody levels must be interpreted in light of the patient's symptoms and other test results (e.g., PUD seen on upper GI series).
  4. Histologic evaluation of endoscopic biopsy samples is considered by many the gold standard for accurate diagnosis of *H. pylori* infection. However, detection of *H. pylori* depends on the site and number of biopsy samples, the method of staining, and experience of the pathologist.
- Additional laboratory evaluation is indicated only in specific cases (e.g., amylase

level in suspected pancreatitis, serum gastrin level in suspected Zollinger-Ellison [ZE] syndrome).

IMAGING STUDIES

- Conventional upper GI barium studies (rarely performed) identify ~70% to 80% of PUD; accuracy can be increased to ~90% by using double contrast.
- Abdominal CT is helpful when suspecting perforating PUD (sensitivity >95%).

RX TREATMENT

NONPHARMACOLOGIC THERAPY

- Stop smoking; smoking increases the risk of PUD, decreases the healing rate, and increases the frequency of recurrence.
- Avoid NSAIDs and alcohol.
- Special diets have been proved unrelated to ulcer development and healing; however, avoid foods that cause symptoms.
- It is recommended that patients with acute upper gastrointestinal bleeding undergo endoscopy within 24 h after GI consultation. The rate of endoscopy within time frames shorter than 24 h is not clearly defined but a recent trial[1] revealed that endoscopy performed within 6 h after GI consultation is not associated with lower 30-day mortality than

endoscopy performed between 6 and 24 hr after consultation.

ACUTE GENERAL Rx

Eradication of *H. pylori*, when present, can be accomplished with various regimens (see "*Helicobacter pylori* Infection").

PUD patients testing negative for *H. pylori* should be treated with antisecretory agents:

- H₂-Receptor antagonists (H₂RAs): Famotidine and nizatidine are effective; they are usually given in split dose or at nighttime.
- PPIs: Can also induce rapid healing; they are usually given 30 min before meals.

Antacids and sucralfate are also effective agents for the treatment and prevention of PUD.

- Glycopyrrolate, an anticholinergic drug, is available as a generic 2-mg tablet and as an oral disintegrating tablet (ODT) to reduce symptoms of peptic ulcer by decreasing volume and acidity of gastric secretions. Formulary and cost are limiting factors of the oral disintegrating tablet.

CHRONIC Rx

Maintenance therapy in peptic ulcer patients is indicated in the following situations:

- Persistent smokers
- Recurrent ulcerations
- Long-term treatment with NSAIDs, glucocorticoids

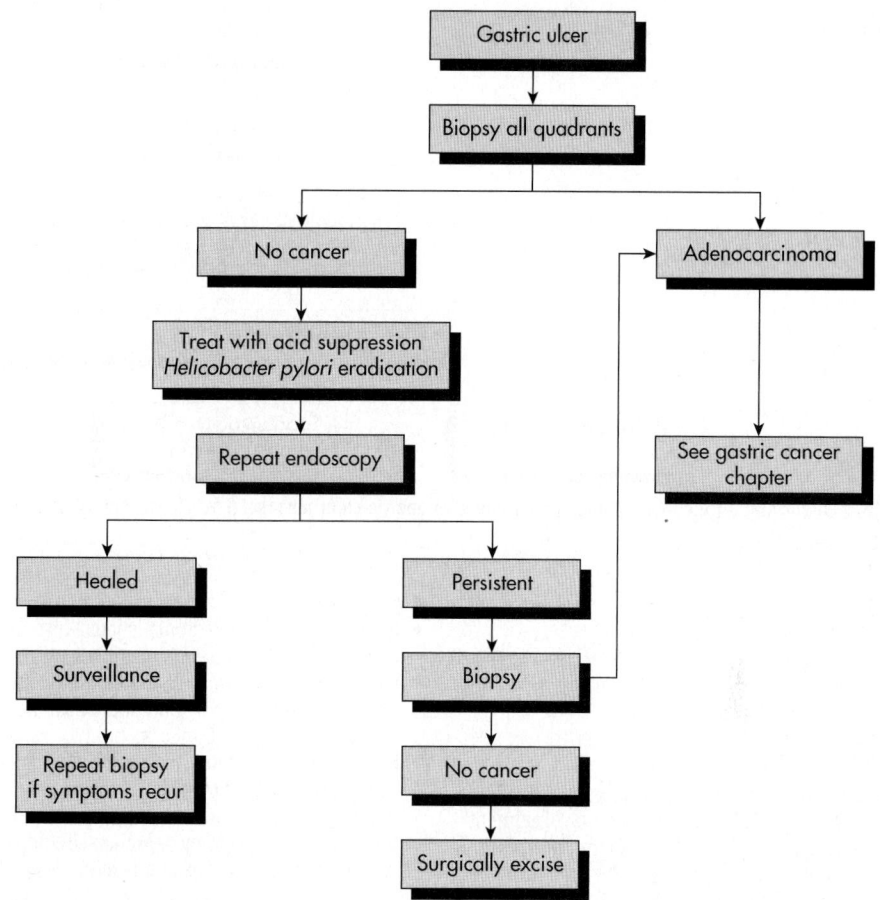

FIG. 2 Algorithm for evaluation, treatment, and surveillance of a patient with a gastric ulcer. (From Townsend CM et al: *Sabiston textbook of surgery,* ed 21, St Louis, 2022, Elsevier.)

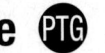

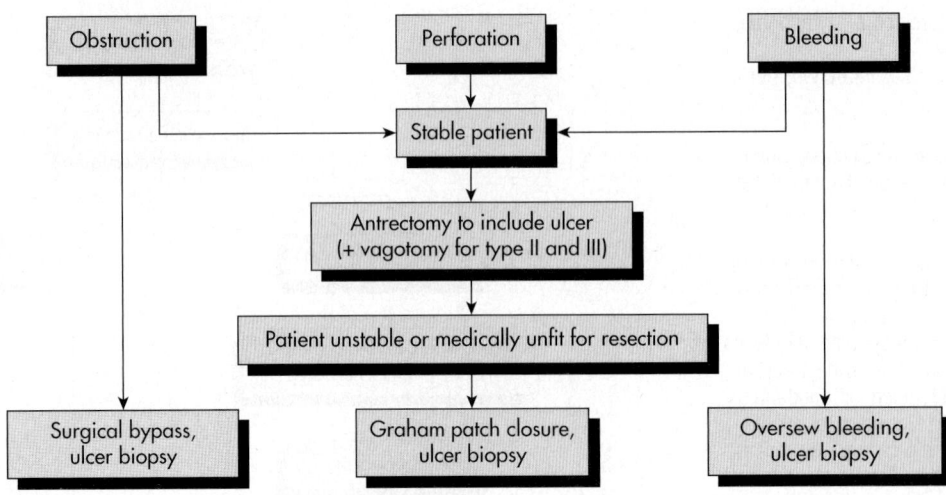

FIG. 3 Algorithm for the management of complicated gastric ulcer disease. (From Townsend CM et al: *Sabiston textbook of surgery,* ed 21, St Louis, 2022, Elsevier.)

- Elderly or debilitated patients
- Aggressive or complicated ulcer disease (e.g., perforation, hemorrhage)
- Asymptomatic bleeders

DISPOSITION

- The recurrence rate for untreated PUD is ~60% (>70% in smokers). Treatment decreases the recurrence rate by nearly 30%.
- Patients with recurrent ulcers should be retreated for an additional 8 wk and then placed on maintenance therapy with H$_2$RAs, PPIs, sucralfate, or antacids.
- An ulcer is considered refractory to treatment if healing is not evident after 8 wk for duodenal ulcers and 12 wk for gastric ulcers. In these patients, maximum acid inhibition (e.g., esomeprazole 40 mg bid) is preferred over continued therapy with standard antiulcer therapy.
- An algorithm for the management of complicated gastric ulcer disease is illustrated in Fig. 3.
- Eradication of *H. pylori* (when present) is indicated in all patients. A negative stool antigen test for *H. pylori* 6 wk after treatment accurately confirms cure of *H. pylori* infection with reasonable sensitivity in initially seropositive healthy subjects.

- Screening for ZE syndrome should also be considered in patients with multiple recurrent ulcers; in patients with ZE, the serum gastrin level is >1000 pg/ml and the basal acid output is usually >15 mEq/h.
- Surgery for refractory ulcers is now only rarely performed; it consists of highly selective vagotomy for duodenal ulcers or ulcer removal with antrectomy or hemigastrectomy without vagotomy for gastric ulcers.

REFERRAL

- GI referral for patients requiring endoscopy
- Surgical referral for patients with nonhealing ulcers despite appropriate medical therapy

PEARLS & CONSIDERATIONS

COMMENTS

- Patients with gastric ulcers should generally have repeat endoscopy after 8 to 12 wk of antisecretory therapy to document healing and test exfoliative cytology for gastric carcinoma. Patients with duodenal ulcers and those with low-risk gastric ulcers, such as young patients on NSAIDs, generally do not require endoscopic surveillance.

- After endoscopic treatment of bleeding peptic ulcers, bleeding recurs in up to 20% of patients. PPI administration intravenously by continuous infusion substantially reduces the risk of recurrent bleeding. High-dose intravenous (IV) esomeprazole (80 mg IV bolus followed by 8 mg/h infusion over 72 h) given after successful endoscopic therapy to patients with high-risk peptic ulcer bleeding has been reported to reduce recurrent bleeding at 72 h and to maintain sustained clinical benefits for up to 30 days.
- Among low-dose aspirin recipients who had peptic ulcer bleeding, continuous aspirin therapy may increase the risk for recurrent bleeding.

REFERENCE

Available at eBooks.Health.Elsevier.com.

RELATED CONTENT

Peptic Ulcer (Patient Information)
Helicobacter pylori Infection (Related Key Topic)

AUTHOR: **FRED F. FERRI, MD**

REFERENCE

1. Lau JYW et al: Timing of endoscopy for acute upper gastrointestinal bleeding, *N Engl J Med* 382(14):1299-1308, 2020.

P

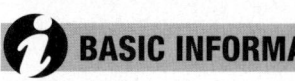 **BASIC INFORMATION**

DEFINITION

Performance-enhancing drugs (PEDs) are substances used by individuals, typically recreational and professional athletes, to improve body aesthetics and potentially their performance. Commonly used agents include hormones with anabolic properties (Table 1), such as insulin, insulin-like growth factor-1 (IGF-1), growth hormone (GH), erythropoietin, diuretics, levothyroxine, aromatase inhibitors, clomiphene, selective estrogen receptor modulators (SERMs), gamma-hydroxybutyrate, and stimulants.[1,2] The focus of this chapter will be the hormonal PEDs, particularly androgenic-anabolic steroids (AAS), the most frequently used class of PEDs among weightlifters and athletes, GH, and insulin.[3]

SYNONYM

PED Anabolic steroids

ICD-10CM CODES
F55.3	Abuse of steroids or hormones
F55.0	Abuse of nonpsychoactive substances
F55.8	Abuse of other nonpsychoactive substances
F15.10	Other stimulant abuse, uncomplicated

EPIDEMIOLOGY & DEMOGRAPHICS

INCIDENCE: The CDC reported that 3.2% of high school students had taken AAS at least once without a doctor's prescription.[4]

PREVALENCE: A global meta-analysis of AAS demonstrated a lifetime prevalence of 3.3%, with a higher prevalence in men than women (6.4% vs. 1.6%), with a higher rate among recreational athletes (18.4%) than professional athletes (13.3%).[5]

Field et al found that 12% of adolescent boys and 8% of girls reported use of some type of

TABLE 1 Performance-Enhancing Hormones

Anabolic Androgenic Steroids

17β-Esters of testosterone (cypionate, enanthate, heptylate, propionate, undecanoate, buciclate)
17α-Alkyl derivatives of testosterone (methyltestosterone, fluoxymesterone, oxandrolone, stanozolol)
19-Nortestosterone (nandrolone)
17β-Esters of 19-nortestosterone (decanoate, phenpropionate)
19-Norandrostenedione
19-Norandrostenediol
Tetrahydrogestrinone
Peptide hormones
Growth hormone
Insulin-like growth factor 1
Insulin
Erythropoietin

From Melmed S et al: *Williams textbook of endocrinology*, ed 14, Philadelphia, 2019, Elsevier.

product to improve strength, gain muscle mass, or improve appearance.[6] About 5% of high school athletes and 24% of community gym members report using GH and 12% of male weightlifters use GH or IGF-1.[7]

PREDOMINANT SEX & AGE: The average age of onset of androgen use appears to be in the early 20s,[3] although use is common among teenagers.[6] The ratio of use in men to women is >50:1.[8,9]

RISK FACTORS: Adolescents and teenagers are at increased risk for use of PED because of their nature of risk-taking behaviors, experimentation, and lack of insight into long-term complications.[10] Athletes in certain sports such as football, baseball, basketball, wrestling, gymnastics, and weight training are at increased risk.[11] No significant difference has been seen in racial/ethnic prevalence of AAS use.[8] Substance abuse and mental health disorders are more common in those with AAS dependence. In a study of 223 men entering a drug treatment program, it was found that men using opioids used AAS more than men using other drugs (25% vs. 5%).[12] In another study, 50% of users dependent on AAS met *Diagnostic and Statistical Manual of Mental Disorders-IV* (DSM-IV) criteria for lifetime history of opioid dependence or abuse.[12] AAS use also has been linked to alcohol use.[13] In an online survey of 492 male bodybuilders, AAS use was associated with higher odds of psychopathic traits.[14]

PHYSICAL FINDINGS & CLINICAL PRESENTATION

AAS abuse may be suspected in men who present with gynecomastia, decreased testicular size, hair loss, sexual dysfunction, acne, infertility, and a muscular appearance. Women who have AAS abuse may present with a muscular appearance, male-pattern baldness, menstrual irregularity, decreased voice pitch, and acne. GH results in increased fat mass with abdominal obesity and decreased lean body mass, and patients may have decreased aerobic capacity.[3] Athletes abusing insulin may present with increased weight, despite physical training, or hypoglycemic events.

ADVERSE EFFECTS

- AAS abuse can affect multiple organ systems (Table 2, Fig. E1), which include the following:[3]
  1. Cardiovascular: Dyslipidemia, cardiomyopathy, conduction abnormalities, hypertension
  2. Neuroendocrine: Hypothalamic-pituitary suppression leading to hypogonadism, gynecomastia
  3. Neuropsychiatric: Major mood disorders (mania or hypomania, depression), aggression, AAS dependence
  4. Hematologic: Coagulation abnormalities, polycythemia
  5. Hepatic: Inflammatory and cholestatic effects
  6. Renal: Renal failure secondary to rhabdomyolysis, focal segmental glomerulosclerosis
  7. Other reported effects include premature epiphyseal closure, tendon rupture, acne,

and striae. Infectious complications can occur with use of contaminated needles or products obtained on the black market.
- GH abuse can lead to systemic adverse effects such as edema, cardiomyopathy, glucose intolerance or diabetes mellitus, excessive sweating, myalgias, arthralgias, and carpal tunnel syndrome.[3]
- Use of insulin may result in hypoglycemia, which can lead to coma and death if left untreated.
- Erythropoietin increases plasma viscosity and red cell mass and thereby results in increased risk of thromboembolic events, cardiovascular events, hypertension, stroke, and death.[3]

TABLE 2 Side Effects of Anabolic Androgenic Steroids

Cardiovascular

Cardiomyopathy
Lipid disorders (decreased HDL, increased LDL)
Increased platelet aggregation
Increased hematocrit
Elevated blood pressure

Cosmetic

Gynecomastia
Acne
Hair loss
Cutaneous striae

Reproductive-Endocrine

Libido changes
Subfertility

In Males

Testicular atrophy
Impaired spermatogenesis
Erectile dysfunction
Prostate diseases

In Females

Hirsutism
Breast atrophy
Voice deepening
Virilization (clitoromegaly)
Menstrual disturbances

Hepatic

Cholestasis
Steatosis
Tumors
Hepatocellular adenoma and carcinoma
Hepatic angiosarcoma and cholangiocarcinoma

Psychologic

Aggression
Mood swings
Anxiety
Psychosis
Irritability
Dependence
Withdrawal
Depression

Injection Related

Infection
Bruising
Fibrosis
Injection site pain

HDL, High-density lipoprotein; *LDL*, low-density lipoprotein.
From Melmed S et al: *Williams textbook of endocrinology*, ed 14, Philadelphia, 2019, Elsevier.

ETIOLOGY

AAS:

- AAS are synthesized from structural modifications of the testosterone molecule. The synthetic derivatives differ in their affinity for the androgen receptor, metabolism and duration of action, and anabolic effects.[3]
- Drugs used in direct and indirect doping are summarized in Table 3. The commonly used AAS are testosterone, dihydrotestosterone, boldenone, trenbolone, parenteral 19-nortestosterone derivatives such as nandrolone, and oral 17-α-alkylated androgens such as stanozolol.[3,15]
- Testosterone increases muscle mass and maximal voluntary strength, increases net oxygen delivery to the tissue by increasing red cell mass and tissue capillarity, and improves neuromuscular transmission.[3]
- Testosterone derivatives promote increase in nitrogen concentration in muscle, which results in an anabolic state, preserve muscle mass, and prohibit muscle breakdown by inhibiting the binding of glucocorticoids to muscle.[10]
- Testosterone effects on mood and aggression promote more intense training in athletes.[10]

GH:

- GH, or somatotropin, is an amino acid protein involved in skeletal and organ growth, lipolysis, and regulation of lean body mass.[16]
- Use of GH in GH-deficient individuals stimulates lipolysis and fatty acid oxidation to provide energy during the fasting state, spares protein oxidation, increases lean body mass, and decreases fat mass.[3]
- A meta-analysis of 11 studies showed improvement in body composition including increased lean body mass and decreased fat mass but no significant change in muscle strength or aerobic exercise capacity in healthy young subjects who administered GH.[17]
- There is little evidence that the use of supraphysiologic GH improves physical performance.[3,16]

Insulin:

- Insulin, with glucose, as a PED is primarily anecdotal but is possible because of its wide availability and affordability.
- It is thought to be used to enhance recovery after a heavy workout through increasing glucose and amino acid transport into human muscles[3] and thus stimulating protein synthesis to promote muscle anabolism.[18]
- It can also help endurance athletes through lipogenesis and inhibiting the release of free fatty acids, which are muscle fuel.[3]

Erythropoietin:

- Erythropoietin is a glycoprotein hormone that binds to red cell progenitor receptors to activate the JAK-2 signaling pathway, promote red cell production, and increase red cell mass.[3]
- Erythropoietin-stimulating agents (ESAs) increase oxygen delivery to the muscle.
- ESAs are most often used in endurance sports, such as cycling, triathlons, long-distance running, and cross-country skiing.[19]

Dx DIAGNOSIS

DIFFERENTIAL DIAGNOSIS

- Hyperprolactinemia: Elevated prolactin resulting in hypogonadism
- Acromegaly: GH-secreting pituitary adenoma
- Insulinoma: Rare tumor secreting insulin

WORKUP

Use of the biologic passport has recently been adapted in the detection of AAS use. The biologic passport is based on the concept that an individual's serum and urine hormones do not change significantly over time.[20] Baseline and follow-up laboratory testing are done to monitor the hormonal levels. Effect of different doping strategies on serum hormone concentrations are summarized in Table 4. Use of athlete biologic passport has also been studied for use in detection of GH.[21]

LABORATORY TESTS

AAS

- Hemoglobin and hematocrit: Increased
- Serum total and free testosterone: Suppressed
- Serum luteinizing hormone and follicular-stimulating hormone: Suppressed
- Sperm count: Low
- Urinary ratio of testosterone glucuronide to epitestosterone glucuronide (>4:1)[10]
- The ratio of carbon 13 (13C) to carbon 12 (12C) in urinary metabolites of testosterone using isotope ratio mass spectrometry[22]

TABLE 3 Drugs Used in Direct and Indirect Doping

Direct Doping	Indirect Doping
Naturally Occurring	**Testosterone Precursors**
Anabolic Steroids	DHEA
Testosterone	Androstenedione
Epitestosterone	**Selective Estrogen**
Dihydrotestosterone	**Receptor Modulators**
Nandrolone	Clomiphene
Boldenone	Droloxifene
Synthetic Anabolic Steroids	Raloxifene
Clostebol	Tamoxifen
Danazol	Toremifene
Drostanolone	**Gonadotropins**
Ethylestrenol	Human chorionic gonadotropin
Fluoxymesterone	Recombinant human LH
Gestrinone	**Aromatase inhibitors**
Methandienone	Anastrozole
Methenolone	Letrozole
Methyltestosterone	Vorozole
Norethandrolone	Atamestane
Oxandrolone	Exemestane
Oxymetholone	Testolactone
Stanozolol	**Selective Estrogen**
Tibolone	**Receptor Degraders**
Trenbolone	Fulvestrant
Designer Steroids	
Boldione (precursor to boldenone)	
Dimethazine	
Mentabolan	
Methasteron	
Methoxygonadiene	
Methylclostebol	
Methylepistiostanol	
Methylstenbone	
Methylstenbolone	
Prostanozolol (precursor to stanozolol)	
Selective Androgen Receptor Modulators	
GTx-024	
LGD-4033	
RAD140	
S-4	
S-23	
YK11	

TABLE 4 Effect of Different Doping Strategies on Serum Hormone Concentrations

	LH and FSH	Testosterone	Estradiol
Indirect Doping			
SERMs	↑	↑	↑
Aromatase inhibitors	↑	↑	↓
hCG	↓	↑	↑
Testosterone precursors	↓	↑	↑
Direct Doping			
Testosterone	↓	↑	↑
Nontestosterone AAS	↓	↓	↓

From Robertson RP et al: *DeGroot's endocrinology, basic science and clinical practice,* ed 8, Philadelphia, 2023, Elsevier.

GH
- Measurement of the variants of GH (isoforms) secreted by the pituitary gland: Increase in the ratio of recombinant/pituitary 22-kDA isoforms. Test must be done within 12 to 24 h of the last dose.[23]
- Measurement of the downstream products: IGF-1 and procollagen type III amino-terminal propeptide (P-III-NP). Test can be done up to 7 days.[23]

Insulin
- Insulin: Increased
- C-peptide: Decreased
- Glucose
- Erythropoietin-stimulating agents
- Total hemoglobin mass and hematocrit
- Reticulocyte count
- Urine electrophoresis to detect recombinant erythropoietin[3]

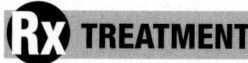 **TREATMENT**

NONPHARMACOLOGIC THERAPY
- Management of AAS abuse is based on the patient's willingness to quit. If the patient is not willing or ready to quit, the patient should be informed of the side effects of continued use.
- For those who use AAS for less than 1 yr, many have spontaneous recovery of the hypothalamic-pituitary axis in 1 to 3 mo and normalization of sperm concentrations within 12 to 16 mo after cessation.[24]

ACUTE GENERAL Rx
- For increased hematocrit and hemoglobin caused by erythropoietin or AAS abuse, therapeutic phlebotomy can be used along with cessation of use of the abused substance.
- Hypoglycemia caused by insulin abuse can be treated with oral or intravenous glucose or administration of glucagon intramuscularly.

CHRONIC Rx
- Prescription of intramuscular testosterone at dosage of up to twice the usual replacement dosage with taper to a physiologic dosage over several months has been done to convince men to quit AAS use and avoid severe AAS withdrawal in the process.[15]
- A trial of clomiphene or human chorionic gonadotropin (hCG) therapy to increase testosterone concentrations and spermatogenesis may be considered for those who desire fertility, especially for men who use AAS for more than 1 yr.[25,26]

REFERRAL
- Referral for treatment of users with associated mood disorder and alcohol or illicit drug use.[15]
- Individuals with AAS dependence may have "muscle dysmorphia" or depression related to AAS withdrawal, which may require psychotherapy interventions such as cognitive behavioral therapy.[26]
- Peer-led programs such as ATLAS (Adolescents Training and Learning to Avoid Steroids) for male athletes and ATHENA (Athletes Targeting Healthy Exercise & Nutrition Alternatives) for female athletes.[16]

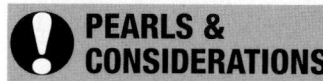 **PEARLS & CONSIDERATIONS**

PREVENTION
- Early education and discussion with youth and athletes.
- Educational programs such as ATLAS and ATHENA have been shown effective in preventing substance abuse.[16]

PATIENT & FAMILY EDUCATION
- Maintaining an open dialogue and understanding the motive behind the use of PED are a few suggestions to address PED use.[10]
- Educating the athletes against the use of PEDs and discussing the side effects of PEDS also have been suggested.[10]

REFERENCES
Available at eBooks.Health.Elsevier.com.

AUTHORS: **LAKSHMI RAVINDRA, MD** and **VICKY CHENG, MD**

P

Diseases and Disorders

I

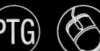

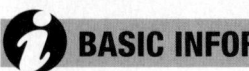

BASIC INFORMATION

DEFINITION

Acute pericarditis is the inflammation (or infiltration) of the pericardium. The pericardium is a rigid, avascular fibrous sac with both visceral and richly innervated parietal layers where fluid resides for lubrication. It is characterized by at least two of the following four criteria:[1] (1) Chest pain, (2) specific electrocardiographic changes, (3) pericardial friction rub, and (4) new or worsening pericardial effusion.

ICD-10CM CODES

I30.0	Acute nonspecific idiopathic pericarditis
I30.1	Infectious pericarditis
I30.8	Other forms of acute pericarditis
I30.9	Acute pericarditis, unspecified
I31.0	Chronic adhesive pericarditis
I31.1	Chronic constrictive pericarditis
I31.3	Pericardial effusion (noninflammatory)
I31.9	Diseases of pericardium, unspecified (tamponade)
I31.2	Hemopericardium

EPIDEMIOLOGY & DEMOGRAPHICS

- Most common form of pericardial disease worldwide
- Observed in 0.1% to 0.2% of hospitalized patients and accounts for 5% of emergency room admissions for chest pain[2]
- Recurrence rate as high as 20% to 30% of cases, while 50% of recurrent pericarditis cases persist
- Four definitions: Acute (<4 to 6 wk), incessant (>4 to 6 wk), recurrent (after symptom-free interval), and chronic (>3 mo)

PHYSICAL FINDINGS & CLINICAL PRESENTATION (TABLE 1)

- Chest pain: Characteristically sharp, pleuritic, positional (improved by sitting up and leaning forward).
- Pericardial rub: A triphasic (ventricular systole, early diastole, atrial contraction), scratchy sound best heard at the lower left sternal border is pathognomonic. Unlike pleural friction rub, the rub of pericarditis is not affected by respiration.
- Pericardial effusion: Beck triad (hypotension, elevated jugular venous pressure, and muffled heart sounds) suggests pericardial tamponade.

ETIOLOGY (TABLE 2)

- In developed countries, viral and idiopathic etiologies are the most common.[3]
- Viral causes can include common gastrointestinal or respiratory flulike illnesses, whereas Parvovirus B19, Epstein-Barr, and HIV are also quite common precipitants.[4]
- The novel coronavirus SARS-CoV-2, as well as its vaccines, have been rarely associated with pericarditis.

- Tuberculosis accounts for 80% to 90% of pericarditis in developing countries, with a high prevalence in HIV-positive patients.
- Neoplastic etiologies (7% to 13%) are typically of lung, breast, esophageal, hematologic, and melanoma origin.
- Autoimmune syndromes (3% to 4%) include systemic lupus erythematosus and rheumatoid arthritis, Sjögren syndrome, sarcoidosis, scleroderma.
- Drug-induced: Procainamide, hydralazine, phenytoin, isoniazid, rifampin, doxorubicin, mesalamine, adalimumab, immune checkpoint inhibitors.
- Radiation-induced pericarditis prevalence is improving, with better radioprotective techniques. Morbidity is closely related to the radiation dose due to damage of capillary endothelial cells, lymphatic stenosis or occlusion.
- Metabolic: Uremia, myxedema, anorexia nervosa.
- Postcardiac injury syndrome: Postpericardiotomy, postpacemaker lead placement, postcatheter ablation, post-CPR, post-PCI, perimyocardial infarction, or Dressler syndrome.

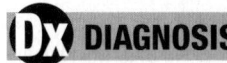

DIAGNOSIS

DIFFERENTIAL DIAGNOSIS

- Angina pectoris and acute coronary syndrome
- Myopericarditis, perimyocarditis, Takotsubo stress cardiomyopathy syndrome

TABLE 1 Manifestations of Pericarditis

Symptoms

Chest pain (worsened if lying down or with inspiration)
Dyspnea
Malaise
Patient assumes sitting position

Signs

Nonconstrictive

Fever
Tachycardia
Friction rub (accentuated by inspiration, body position)
Enlarged heart by percussion and x-ray examination
Distant heart sounds

Tamponade

As above, plus:
Distended neck veins
Hepatomegaly
Pulsus paradoxus (>10 mm Hg with inspiration)
Narrow pulse pressure
Weak pulse, poor peripheral perfusion

Constrictive

Distended neck veins
Kussmaul sign (inspiratory increase in jugular venous pressure)
Distant heart sounds
Pericardial knock
Hepatomegaly
Ascites
Edema
Tachycardia

From Marcdante KJ et al: *Nelson essentials of pediatrics,* ed 9, Philadelphia, 2023, Elsevier.

TABLE 2 Etiology of Pericarditis and Pericardial Effusion

Idiopathic (Presumed Viral) Infectious Agents

Bacterial

Group A streptococci
Staphylococcus aureus
Pneumococcus, meningococcus*
Haemophilus influenzae*
Mycobacterium tuberculosis

Viral[†]

Coxsackievirus (group A, B)
Echovirus
Mumps
Influenza
Epstein-Barr
Cytomegalovirus

Fungal

Histoplasma capsulatum
Coccidioides immitis
Blastomyces dermatitidis
Candida

Collagen Vascular-Inflammatory and Granulomatous Diseases

Rheumatic fever
Systemic lupus erythematosus (idiopathic and drug-induced)
Rheumatoid arthritis
Kawasaki disease
Scleroderma
Mixed connective tissue disease
Inflammatory bowel disease
Sarcoidosis
Vasculitis

Traumatic

Cardiac contusion (blunt trauma)
Penetrating trauma
Postpericardiotomy syndrome
Radiation

Contiguous Spread

Pleural disease
Pneumonia
Aortic aneurysm (dissecting)

Metabolic

Hypothyroidism
Uremia
Chylopericardium

Neoplastic

Primary
Contiguous (lymphoma)
Metastatic
Infiltrative (leukemia)

Other Etiologic Disorders/Factors

Drug reaction
Pancreatitis
After myocardial infarction
Thalassemia
Central venous catheter perforation
Heart failure
Hemorrhage (coagulopathy)

*Infectious or immune complex.
[†]Common (viral pericarditis or myopericarditis is probably the most common cause of acute pericarditis in a previously normal host).
From Kliegman RM et al (eds): *Practical strategies in pediatric diagnosis and therapy,* ed 2, Philadelphia, 2004, Saunders. In Marcdante KJ et al: *Nelson essentials of pediatrics,* ed 9, Philadelphia, 2023, Elsevier.

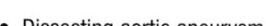

P

- Dissecting aortic aneurysm
- Pulmonary and thoracic causes: Thromboembolism, infarction, pneumothorax, pneumonia with pleurisy, costochondritis
- Gastrointestinal causes: Hepatitis, cholecystitis, gastroesophageal reflux disease, esophageal spasm or rupture
- Box 1 summarizes the differential diagnosis of pericardial effusion by etiology

WORKUP (TABLE 3)

Table 4 summarizes an initial approach to acute pericarditis. Diagnosis of pericarditis requires at least two of the four following clinical criteria:
- Typical pleuritic chest pain
- Pericardial friction rub
- Suggestive ECG changes (diffuse concave ST segment elevation, PR depression in all leads except for AVR where there is elevation)
- New or worsening pericardial effusion

LABORATORY TESTS

Initial laboratory tests may determine severity of inflammation and acuity of patient's condition, while also guiding workup and treatment timeline:[5]
- Inflammatory markers: Erythrocyte sedimentation rate, (high-sensitivity) C-reactive protein (CRP), and complete blood count with differential
- Cardiac biomarkers (troponin T and I) suggest myocardial involvement
- Basic metabolic profile

Additional lab studies:
- HIV
- PPD/QuantiFERON-TB Gold
- Antinuclear antibody, rheumatoid factor
- Thyroid-stimulating hormone
- Routine viral studies are not indicated since they are low yield

PERICARDIAL FLUID & TISSUE SAMPLING

Indications for pericardiocentesis are:
- Tamponade physiology
- Moderate to large pericardial effusion with symptoms, or refractory to medical therapy
- Suspicion of a neoplastic, bacterial, or tuberculous process
- Evidence of constrictive or effusive-constrictive pericarditis
- Pericardiocentesis is for diagnostic and therapeutic purposes. The pericardial fluid should be analyzed for RBC, WBC, Gram

---

BOX 1 Major Differential Diagnosis of Pericardial Effusion by Etiology

Noninfectious
- Malignancy (usually metastatic)
- Myocardial infarction associated (Dressler syndrome)
- Uremia
- Myxedema (rare cause of tamponade physiology)
- Trauma (penetrating or nonpenetrating)
- Chylopericardium
- Acute idiopathic
- Rheumatic fever
- Collagen vascular disease (systemic lupus erythematosus, rheumatoid arthritis, scleroderma, Wegener granulomatosis)
- Postsurgical (cardiac and intrathoracic)
- Drug induced (procainamide, hydralazine, phenytoin, doxorubicin, isoniazid)

Infectious
- Viral (coxsackievirus, echovirus, mumps, adenovirus, hepatitis, human immunodeficiency virus)
- Bacterial (pneumococcus, *Streptococcus*, *Staphylococcus*)
- Tuberculous
- Fungal (histoplasmosis, coccidiomycosis, *Candida*, particularly in immunosuppressed patients)

From Niederhuber JE: *Abeloff's clinical oncology*, ed 6, Philadelphia, 2020, Elsevier.

TABLE 3 Diagnostic Pathway and Sequence of Performance in Acute Pericarditis

Diagnostic Measure	Characteristic Findings
Obligatory	
Auscultation	Pericardial rub (monophasic, biphasic, or triphasic)
ECG*	*Stage I:* Anterior and inferior concave ST segment elevation. PR segment deviations opposite to P wave polarity
	Early stage II: All ST junctions return to the baseline. PR segments deviated
	Late stage II: T waves progressively flatten and invert
	Stage III: Generalized T-wave inversions in most or all leads
	Stage IV: ECG returns to prepericarditis state
Echocardiography	Effusion types B to D (Horowitz)
	Signs of tamponade
Blood analyses	Erythrocyte sedimentation rate, C-reactive protein, lactate dehydrogenase, leukocytes (inflammation markers)
	Troponin I,† CK-MB (markers of myocardial involvement)
Chest radiograph	Ranging from normal to "water bottle" shape of the heart shadow
	Performed primarily to reveal pulmonary or mediastinal pathology
Mandatory in Tamponade, Optional in Large/Recurrent Effusions or if Previous Tests Inconclusive in Small Effusions	
Pericardiocentesis/drainage	Polymerase chain reaction and histochemistry for etiopathogenetic classification of infection or neoplasia
Optional or if Previous Tests Inconclusive	
CT	Effusions, pericardium, and epicardium
MRI	Effusions, pericardium, and epicardium
Pericardioscopy, pericardial/epicardial biopsy	Establishing the specific etiology

CK-MB, Creatine kinase-MB; *CT*, computed tomography; *ECG*, electrocardiogram; *MRI*, magnetic resonance imaging.

*Typical lead involvement: I, II, aVL, aVF, and V3-V6. The ST segment is always depressed in aVR, frequently in V1, and occasionally in V2. Stage IV may not occur, and there are permanent T-wave inversions and flattenings. If an ECG is first recorded in stage III, pericarditis cannot be differentiated by ECG from diffuse myocardial injury, "biventricular strain," or myocarditis. ECG in early repolarization is very similar to stage I. Unlike stage I, this ECG does not acutely evolve, and J-point elevations are usually accompanied by a slur, oscillation, or notch at the end of the QRS just before and including the J point (best seen with tall R and T waves—large in an early repolarization pattern). Pericarditis is likely if, in lead V6, the J point is greater than 25% of the height of the T-wave apex (using the PR segment as a baseline).

†A rise in cardiac muscle troponin I (cTnI) is detected in 32.2% of patients, more frequently in younger, male patients, with ST segment elevation and pericardial effusion at presentation. An increase beyond 1.5 ng/ml is uncommon (7.6%) and associated with CK-MB elevation. cTnI increase and is not a negative prognostic marker for the incidence of recurrences, constrictive pericarditis, cardiac tamponade, or residual left ventricular dysfunction.

From Vincent JL et al: *Textbook of critical care*, ed 8, Philadelphia, 2024, Elsevier.

TABLE 4 Initial Approach to the Patient With Definite or Suspected Acute Pericarditis

1. If the diagnosis is suspected but not certain, listen often for pericardial rub and obtain ECGs frequently to check for diagnostic findings.
2. If the diagnosis is suspected or certain, obtain the following tests to help confirm the diagnosis (if necessary) and determine whether a specific causative diagnosis and/or significant associated conditions and/or complications are present:
   a. Hemogram hsCRP
   b. Troponin I
   c. Chest radiograph
   d. Echocardiogram
   e. Consider additional testing on the basis of clinical suspicion of a specific etiology
3. If the diagnosis is likely or certain, initiate therapy with an NSAID plus colchicine.

From Libby P et al: *Braunwald's heart disease, a textbook of cardiovascular medicine,* ed 12, Philadelphia, 2022, Elsevier.

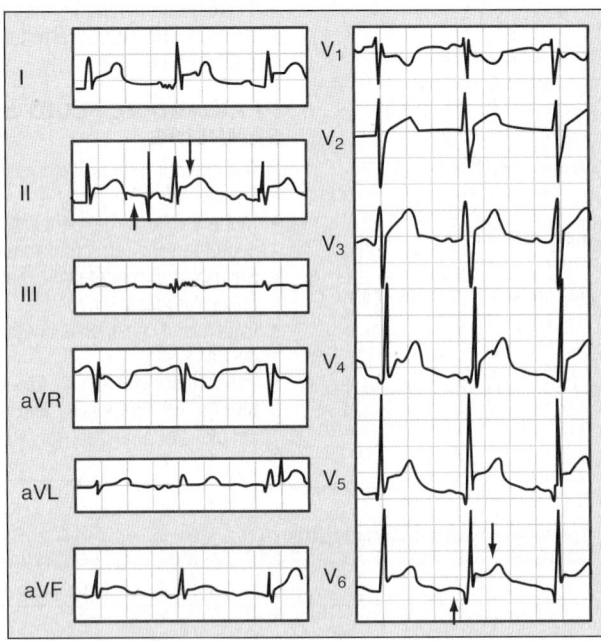

FIG. 1 Typical electrocardiographic changes in acute pericarditis: PR depression *(small arrow)* and concave ST-segment elevation *(large arrow)*. *aVF,* Augmented vector foot; *aVL,* augmented vector left; *aVR,* augmented vector right. (From Vincent JL et al: *Textbook of critical care,* ed 8, Philadelphia, 2024, Elsevier.)

stain, culture, cytology, glucose, pH, lactate dehydrogenase, and protein. In select cases, consider checking triglyceride for chylopericardium, adenosine deaminase, or polymerase chain reaction for tuberculosis
• Pericardial biopsy can be performed for cases of recurrent pericardial effusion when pericardial fluid analysis does not reveal etiology, and especially if malignancy or tuberculosis is suspected

IMAGING STUDIES

• ECG (Fig. 1): Changes in the ECG reflect inflammation of the epicardium, because the parietal pericardium is electrically inert. The ECG changes are staged as follows:
   1. Stage I (Acute phase): Hours to few days. PR-segment depression in all leads except aVR (where PR elevation is seen) and diffuse concave ST-segment elevations
   2. Stage II (Intermediate phase): Seen in first week with return of PR and ST segments to baseline
   3. Stage III (Intermediate): T-wave inversion in leads previously showing ST-segment elevation
   4. Stage IV (Late phase): Normalization of the ECG or indefinite persistence of T-wave inversions
• Echocardiogram is used to evaluate for pericardial effusion (present in 50% to 60% of patients) (Fig. E2). Echocardiogram can help exclude STEMI (through absent wall motion abnormality) and support the diagnosis of constrictive pericarditis or tamponade. Echocardiogram is also recommended for guidance for pericardiocentesis.
• Chest x-ray: Performed to rule out abnormalities of the mediastinum or lung fields. Cardiac silhouette may appear enlarged when pericardial effusion accumulates over ≥200 ml of fluid (Fig. E3). Calcifications around the heart may be seen with chronic constrictive pericarditis.
• Computed tomography: Evaluation of associated pleuropulmonary and extra thoracic diseases and pericardial calcifications.

• Cardiac MRI (Fig. E4) is recommended in patients with elevated troponin I or T and can also be helpful in cases of chronic constrictive pericarditis and malignancy.

℞ TREATMENT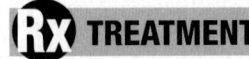

NONPHARMACOLOGIC THERAPY

• Physical activity should be restricted until pain resolves, and inflammatory markers, ECG, and echocardiogram normalize.
• Athletes should avoid competitive activity for 3 mo at a minimum. Exercise intensity, heart rate >100 bpm, and shear stress on pericardium are thought to worsen inflammation. With myocardial involvement (positive troponin), athletic activity must be avoided for at least 6 mo.
• Patient education should be provided of potential warning signs of complications such as cardiac tamponade, recurrent pericarditis (which can occur in up to one third of patients), and chronic constrictive pericarditis.

ACUTE GENERAL Rx

• High-dose aspirin (750 to 1000 mg tid) or NSAIDs (e.g., ibuprofen 600 to 800 mg tid, indomethacin 50 mg tid) for 1 to 2 wk. Proton pump inhibitor should be provided for gastric protection. NSAIDs should be avoided in patients with recent myocardial infarction, congestive heart failure, acute renal failure, and upper GI bleed.
• Colchicine 0.5 to 0.6 mg once daily (<70 kg) or bid (>70 kg) for 3 mo. Current evidence (COPE, CORE, CORP, ICAP, CORP-2 trials)[6] supports the effectiveness of colchicine in symptomatic relief and prevention of recurrent pericarditis.
• Corticosteroids are prescribed for refractory recurrent pericarditis, or in the setting of established rheumatologic disease, renal failure, or other contraindications to NSAID or colchicine therapies. They can be associated with severe adverse effects, more hospitalizations, and high rate of recurrence.
• In tuberculous pericarditis, adjunctive corticosteroids can prevent development of constriction with tapering dose of 120 mg prednisolone over 6 wk in patients without HIV. Because of increased risk of malignancy, corticosteroids should be avoided in persons with combined tuberculosis and HIV infection.
• When corticosteroids are indicated, recommended dosing is as follows: Low- to moderate-dose (0.25 to 0.5 mg/kg/day) systemic steroid therapy for 1 mo, followed by a long taper (6 to 12 wk).
• Azathioprine, intravenous immunoglobulins, and anti–interleukin-1 therapies (e.g., anakinra) can be considered for patients with refractory recurrent pericarditis.[7] In addition, a phase 3 trial demonstrated reduction of recurrent pericarditis with interleukin 1-α/1-β inhibition (rilonacept).[8]
• For acute pericarditis in pregnancy, NSAIDs are the cornerstone for management in the first and second trimesters. Ibuprofen is

preferred due to reduced cross-placental transfer and shorter half-life. Low-dose ASA and glucocorticoids (ideally <20 mg/day to limit trans-placental passage) are considered safe as well. Azathioprine and IVIG are considered safe although evidence is limited.

- Pericardiectomy and pericardiotomy at specialized centers are a last-resort procedure reserved for recurrent cardiac tamponade, refractory pericarditis, and hemodynamically significant constrictive pericarditis.
- Avoidance of anticoagulants (increased risk of hemopericardium).

TREATMENT OF UNDERLYING CAUSE

- Purulent bacterial pericarditis: Systemic antibiotics and drainage of pericardium
- Collagen vascular disease: Corticosteroid therapy (prednisone)
- Tuberculous pericarditis: Rifampicin, isoniazid, pyrazinamide, and ethambutol for 2 mo, then isoniazid and rifampicin for 6 mo. Isoniazid is the most effective agent in penetrating the pericardial space
- Thyroid-related pericardial effusion: Thyroid replacement therapy
- Uremic: Dialysis
- Malignant pericardial effusion: Fig. 5

POTENTIAL COMPLICATIONS FROM PERICARDITIS

- **Chronic constrictive pericarditis:** Occurs in <1% of patients with acute idiopathic pericarditis. New awareness of subset of patients with "transient constrictive pericarditis" who have an initial hyperacute stage of inflammation that must be identified before progression to fibrosis and calcification of the pericardium.
  1. Physical examination: Signs of right heart failure—hepatomegaly, splenomegaly, ascites, pedal edema, scrotal edema, possible anasarca, jugular venous pressure, Kussmaul sign (paradoxic increase in jugular venous pressure during inspiration), pericardial knock (early diastolic filling sound heard 0.06 to 0.1 sec after S2), and clear lungs.

2. ECG: Low QRS voltage, nonspecific ST-segment changes, biatrial enlargement.
3. Chest radiograph: Mild alveolar edema, pleural effusions, biatrial enlargement, pericardial calcification (seen in tuberculous pericarditis).
4. Echocardiography: May show thickened pericardium (>4 mm), >25% mitral and >50% tricuspid valve inflow variation with respiration, interventricular septal bounce; and mitral annulus reversus (medial e' velocity > lateral e' velocity) suggests constrictive pericarditis.
5. Hemodynamics (Fig. E6): Elevation of right-sided filling pressures, equalization of diastolic pressures, as well as prominent "x" and rapid "y" descent in the atrial tracing are seen in constrictive pericarditis. Right ventricular pressure tracing typically shows a "dip and plateau" (square root sign) that is a result of the unimpeded early filling of the RV with an abrupt halt to the late diastolic filling by the stiff pericardium. Discordance of right ventricular and left ventricular systolic pressures during respiration is also suggestive of constrictive pericarditis.
6. Therapy: Complex surgical stripping or removal of both layers of the constricting pericardium improves the functional class in majority of late survivors, but has high operative mortality.
- **Cardiac tamponade:** Occurs in 5% to 15% of patients with idiopathic pericarditis, but in up to 60% of those with neoplastic, tuberculous, or purulent pericarditis.
  1. Signs and symptoms: Dyspnea, orthopnea, chest pain, fatigue.
  2. Physical examination: Beck triad (distended neck veins, distant heart sounds, hypotension), reduced apical impulse, diaphoresis, tachypnea, tachycardia, narrowed pulse pressure, or pulsus paradoxus (decrease in systolic blood pressure ≥10 mm Hg during inspiration; most specific sign).
  3. ECG: Decreased amplitude of the QRS complex, electrical alternans (occurs more frequently with large neoplastic effusions).

4. Chest x-ray: Cardiomegaly ("water-bottle" configuration of the cardiac silhouette may be seen) with clear lungs.
5. Echocardiography (Table 5): Pericardial effusion, >30% mitral and >60% tricuspid valve inflow variation with respiration, paradoxic motion of interventricular septum, diastolic right or left atrium collapse, diastolic right ventricular collapse (pathognomonic).[9]
6. Hemodynamics: Equalization of diastolic pressures within chambers of the heart, elevation of right atrial pressure with a prominent "x" but blunted "y" descent. Table 6 summarizes hemodynamics in cardiac tamponade and constrictive pericarditis.
7. Therapy: Cardiac tamponade is a life-threatening condition usually requiring emergent pericardiocentesis. Avoid drugs (diuretics, nitrates) or therapies (high PEEP) that reduce the preload. Fluid resuscitation can temporize hemodynamics while awaiting pericardiocentesis. In patients with recurrent effusions (e.g., neoplasms), placement of a percutaneous drainage catheter or pericardial window may be necessary.
- **Effusive-constrictive pericarditis:** Uncommon syndrome characterized by concomitant tamponade caused by tense pericardial effusion and constriction caused by the visceral pericardium.
  1. Signs and symptoms of both tamponade and/or constriction. Pulsus paradoxus is present, but Kussmaul sign and pericardial knock are typically absent.
  2. Echocardiography: Low sensitivity to distinguish effusive-constrictive pericarditis from other types.
  3. Cardiac catheterization: Before drainage, "y" descent is usually less prominent than expected, and right atrial "v" wave persists. After drainage, may continue to have elevated right atrial and pulmonary wedge pressures.
  4. Therapy: Extensive epicardiectomy (with disruption of the visceral layer of pericardium) is the procedure of choice in symptomatic patients.
- **Myopericarditis:** Defined by an elevated cardiac biomarker. Myocarditis and pericarditis may coexist in 20% to 30% of patients presenting with pericarditis. Hospitalization and cardiac MRI are favored in these patients. Overall, myopericarditis has a good prognosis with appropriate guideline medical therapies and has very low rates of morbidity, mortality, and heart failure.

DISPOSITION

- Complete resolution of pain and other signs and symptoms during the initial 3 wk of therapy occurs in 70% to 90% of cases.
- Admission is highly recommended if any of the following high risk and poor prognostic features exist: Fever >38° C (>100.4° F) during tamponade, failure to respond to 1 wk of outpatient treatment.

FIG. 5 Treatment approach algorithm to malignant pericardial effusions. (From Niederhuber JE: *Abeloff's clinical oncology,* ed 6, Philadelphia, 2020, Elsevier.)

TABLE 5 Hemodynamic and Echocardiographic Features of Constrictive Pericarditis Compared With Restrictive Cardiomyopathy

	Constriction	Restriction
Prominent y descent in venous pressure	Present	Variable
Paradoxic pulse	~1/3 cases	Absent
Pericardial knock	Present	Absent
Equal right- and left-sided filling pressures	Present	Left at least 3-5 mm Hg higher than right
Filling pressures >25 mm Hg	Rare	Common
Pulmonary artery systolic pressure >60 mm Hg	No	Common
"Square root" sign	Present	Variable
Respiratory variation in left-sided and right-sided pressures/flows	Exaggerated	Normal
Ventricular wall thickness	Normal	Usually increased
Pericardial thickness	Increased	Normal
Atrial size	Possible LA enlargement	Biatrial enlargement
Septal bounce	Present	Absent
Tissue Doppler E' velocity	Increased	Reduced
Speckle tracking	Normal longitudinal, decreased circumferential restoration	Decreased longitudinal, normal circumferential restoration

From Libby P et al: *Braunwald's heart disease, a textbook of cardiovascular medicine*, ed 12, Philadelphia, 2022, Elsevier.

TABLE 6 Hemodynamics in Cardiac Tamponade and Constrictive Pericarditis

	Tamponade	Constriction
Paradoxic pulse	Usually present	Present in ~1/3
Equal left-/right-sided filling pressure	Present	Present
Systemic venous wave morphology	Absent y descent	Prominent y descent (M or W shape)
Inspiratory change in systemic venous pressure	Decrease (normal)	Increase or no change (Kussmaul sign)
"Square root" sign in ventricular pressure	Absent	Present

From Mann DL et al: *Braunwald's heart disease, a textbook of cardiovascular medicine*, ed 10, Philadelphia, 2015, Elsevier.

- The following are considered moderate risk factors but should also prompt admission: Myopericarditis, trauma, immunosuppression, oral anticoagulant therapy.
- Recurrent pericarditis occurs after a symptom-free interval (4 to 6 wk) following the initial episode of pericarditis. Incidence is reported as 10% to 15% and increases to 50% in patients who are not on colchicine. Standard first line treatment for recurring pericarditis is colchicine plus an NSAID. Colchicine plus low dose prednisone can be used for second-line treatment. Rilonacept, an interleukin-1 antagonist was FDA approved in 2021 for treatment of recurrent pericarditis and prevention of further recurrences in patients greater than or equal to 12 yr old. Its use should be reserved for patients with recurrences refractory to colchicine-based regimens.
- Incessant pericarditis is defined as pericarditis lasting for >4 to 6 wk but <3 mo without remission, while chronic pericarditis is pericarditis lasting for >3 mo.
- In patients with pericardial effusion after cardiac surgery, use of NSAIDs are not recommended because they have not been shown to reduce the size of the effusions or prevent late cardiac tamponade. The COPPS trial suggested that prophylactic colchicine may reduce the risk of developing a post-pericardiotomy pericarditis.[10]

REFERENCES & SUGGESTED READING

Available at eBooks.Health.Elsevier.com.

RELATED CONTENT

Pericarditis (Patient Information)
Cardiac Tamponade (Related Key Topic)

AUTHORS: **PERSEY BEDIAKO, MD** and **MAXWELL EYRAM AFARI, MD**

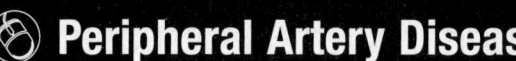

 BASIC INFORMATION

DEFINITION

Peripheral artery disease (PAD) refers to atherosclerotic, inflammatory, occlusive, and aneurysmal diseases that lead to acute or chronic obstruction of the arteries involving the noncerebral and noncoronary arteries. (This topic focuses on lower-extremity PAD.)

SYNONYMS

PAD
Peripheral vascular disease (PVD)
Arteriosclerosis obliterans
Atherosclerotic occlusive disease
Atherosclerosis of the extremities
Peripheral arterial stenosis
Vasoocclusive disease of the legs
Critical limb ischemia (CLI)
Chronic limb threatening ischemia (CTLI)
Acute limb ischemia (ALI)
Intermittent claudication (IC)

ICD-10CM CODES

I70	Atherosclerosis
I70.2	Atherosclerosis of native arteries of the extremities
I70.21	Atherosclerosis of native arteries of extremities with intermittent claudication
I70.22	Atherosclerosis of native arteries of extremities with rest pain
I70.23	Atherosclerosis of native arteries of right leg w/ulceration
I70.24	Atherosclerosis of native arteries of left leg w/ulceration
I70.25	Atherosclerosis of native arteries of other extremities w/ulceration
I70.26	Atherosclerosis of native arteries of extremities with gangrene
I70.29	Other atherosclerosis of native arteries of extremities
I73	Other specified peripheral vascular diseases
I70.3	Atherosclerosis of unspecified type of bypass graft(s) of the extremities
I70.31	Atherosclerosis of unspec. type of bypass graft(s) of extremities w/intermittent claudication
I70.32	Atherosclerosis of unspec. type of bypass graft(s) of extremities w/rest pain
I70.33	Atherosclerosis of unspec. type of bypass graft(s) of right leg w/ulceration
I70.34	Atherosclerosis of unspec. type of bypass graft(s) of left leg w/ulceration
I70.35	Atherosclerosis of unspec. type of bypass graft(s) of other extremity w/ulceration
I70.4	Atherosclerosis of autologous vein bypass graft(s) of the extremities
I70.5	Atherosclerosis of non-autologous biological bypass graft(s) of the extremities
I70.6	Atherosclerosis of non-biological bypass graft(s) of the extremities
I70.7	Atherosclerosis of other type of bypass graft(s) of the extremities
I73.8	Other specified peripheral vascular diseases
I73.9	Peripheral vascular disease, unspecified
I79	Disorders of arteries, arterioles, and capillaries in diseases classified elsewhere

EPIDEMIOLOGY & DEMOGRAPHICS

- There are more than 200 million patients afflicted with PAD globally (ankle-brachial index [ABI] ≤0.9); it affects approximately 8 to 12 million Americans.[1]
- The prevalence is nearly equal in men and women. It increases with age, from roughly 6% in those aged 40 to 49 yr to 15% to 20% in those aged 70 to 79 yr. However, symptoms of claudication are more likely to be present in males with PAD (50%) vs. in women with PAD (25%).[2]
- Risk factors for PAD include:
  1. Smoking
  2. Diabetes
  3. Hypertension
  4. Hypercholesterolemia
  5. Chronic kidney disease
  6. C-reactive protein
- As per the PARTNERS study, the prevalence of PAD in patients 50 to 69 yr or >70 yr with history of smoking or diabetes was 29%.[3]
- Smoking is three times more likely to lead to PAD than coronary artery disease (CAD). Conversely, the association of hypertension (HTN) and hyperlipidemia with PAD is lower than that with CAD and cerebrovascular disease.[3]
- Patients at increased risk of PAD include those >65 yr, those aged 50 to 64 yr with risk factors of atherosclerosis, those <50 yr with diabetes and an additional risk factor, as well as those individuals with known atherosclerotic disease in another vascular bed.[2]
- Black race and female sex are particularly sensitive to aggregate effects of multiple risk factors (HTN, diabetes, hypercholesterolemia, smoking, kidney disease). With one of these risk factors, the odds ratio (OR) of developing PAD was found to be 4.9 in Blacks and 2.8 in females. For >3 of these risk factors, the OR was 14.7 in Blacks and 18.6 in females.[4]
- Patients with newly diagnosed PAD are six times more likely to die within the next 10 yr when compared with patients without PAD.[4]
- Patients with heart failure and PAD have increased risk of mortality (hazard ratio 1.36), increased risk of myocardial infarction (MI), and less improvement in a structural physical exercise program.[4]
- Concomitant renal failure (Cr >2) is associated with worse overall cardiovascular (CV) prognosis in addition to lower rates of amputation-free survival to the point that the *European Journal of Vascular Medicine* guidelines recommend a special attention to be paid to atherosclerosis in lower extremities in these patients.[4]
- The total annual costs associated with the hospitalization of patients with PAD in the U.S. exceed $21 billion and account for ~13% of all Medicare Part A and B expenditures.[5]
- Those with PAD had average annual expenditures of $11,553 compared with only $4219 in matched cohort without PAD.[5]

PHYSICAL FINDINGS & CLINICAL PRESENTATION

- PAD may present in a variety of ways:
  1. 20% to 50%: Asymptomatic (estimated three times more than symptomatic patients)
  2. 10% to 35%: Intermittent claudication (IC), defined as aching pain, cramping, weakness, numbness, or heaviness of the leg induced by exercise, particularly walking, and relieved by rest; up to 75% of people experiencing intermittent claudication will not develop further progression of disease throughout life
  3. 1% to 2%: Critical limb ischemia (CLI), defined as chronic (>2 wk) rest pain, or tissue loss with nonhealing ulceration, necrosis, or gangrene (Fig. E1)
  4. 40% to 50%: Atypical symptoms involving the calf, thigh, or buttock do not restrict the ability to walk and not relieved in 10 min on activity cessation
  5. Acute limb ischemia (ALI) will be present in 14 per 100,000 individuals in the general population. It is defined as acute (<2 wk) onset of symptoms due to severe poor perfusion of the extremities, and further categorized into the following:
     a. Viable: No sensory or muscle weakness with audible Doppler pulses
     b. Threatened: Mild to moderate sensory or motor loss; inaudible arterial Doppler
     c. Irreversible: Severe sensory loss and muscle weakness; inaudible arterial Doppler
        (1) Claudication can be categorized using the Rutherford and Fontaine classification symptoms.
- Physical findings include:
  1. Diminished pulses and/or cool skin temperature of lower extremities
  2. Bruits heard over the distal aorta, iliac, or femoral arteries (femoral bruit is an independent marker for ischemic cardiac events)
  3. Change in skin color:
     a. Dependent rubor in CLI
     b. Livedo reticularis, or a mottled reticulated vascular pattern that appears lacelike
     c. Severe limb ischemia may also have petechiae, persistent cyanosis or pallor, pedal edema, skin fissures, ulceration, or gangrene
  4. Trophic changes of hair loss, thickened and brittle toenails, smooth and shiny skin, and muscle atrophy

P

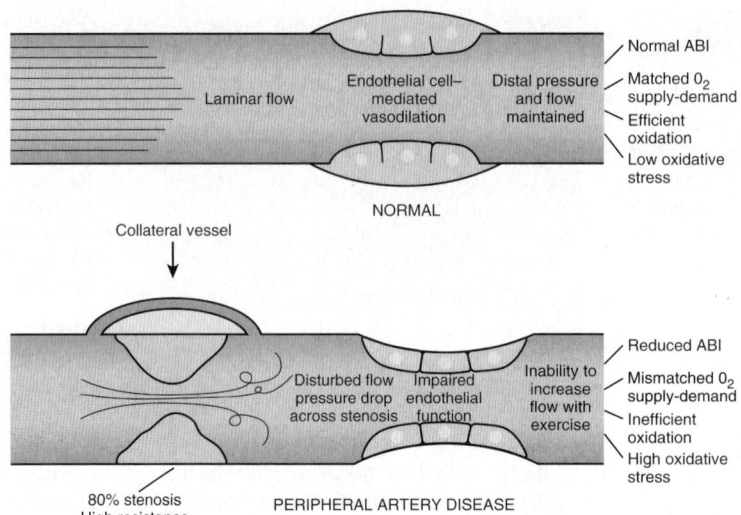

FIG. 2 Pathophysiology of intermittent claudication. In healthy arteries *(top)*, flow is laminar and endothelial function is normal; therefore blood flow and oxygen delivery match muscle metabolic demand at rest and during exercise. Muscle metabolism is efficient and results in low oxidative stress. In contrast, in peripheral artery disease *(PAD) (bottom)*, arterial stenosis results in disturbed flow, and the loss of kinetic energy results in a drop in pressure across the stenosis. Collateral vessels have high resistance and only partially compensate for the arterial stenosis. In addition, endothelial function is impaired, thereby resulting in further loss of vascular function. These changes limit the blood flow response to exercise and result in a mismatch of oxygen delivery to muscle metabolic demand. Changes in skeletal muscle metabolism further compromise the efficient generation of high-energy phosphates. Oxidant stress, the result of inefficient oxidation, further impairs endothelial function and muscle metabolism. *ABI*, Ankle-brachial index. (From the text *Anatomie, physiologie, pathologie des vaisseaux lymphatiques* by PC Sappey [1874], courtesy Harvard Medical Library, Francis A. Countway Library of Medicine. In Hiatt WR, Brass EP: Pathophysiology of intermittent claudication. In Creager MA et al [eds]: *Vascular medicine: a companion to Braunwald's heart disease*, ed 2, Philadelphia, 2013, Elsevier.)

ETIOLOGY

- PAD is primarily the result of atherosclerotic narrowing of the arterial lumen that results in impaired blood flow to the lower-extremity tissues and an oxygen supply-demand mismatch. Fig. 2 illustrates the pathophysiology of IC, from which symptoms initially manifest with exercise as metabolic demands increase.
- The mechanism of oxygen supply-demand mismatch is multifactorial, including stenosis-related turbulent flow and loss of kinetic energy with subsequent pressure loss across a stenosis, endothelial dysfunction, abnormal skeletal muscle metabolism, and increased oxidant stress.
- CLI may develop gradually from progressive atherosclerosis or in a subacute fashion from multisegmented atherothrombosis or atheroembolism, such that blood supply at rest cannot sufficiently supply the nutritional needs of the affected limb, leading to rest pain and tissue loss.
- ALI is marked by a sudden onset of symptoms (<2 wk) due to arterial occlusion and reduced blow flow to the affected extremity.

DX DIAGNOSIS

DIFFERENTIAL DIAGNOSIS

- Vascular etiologies
  1. Thrombus or embolism
  2. Vasculitis, such as thromboangiitis obliterans, giant cell arteritis, and Takayasu arteritis
  3. Fibromuscular dysplasia
  4. Aortopathy, including coarctation of the aorta
  5. Raynaud phenomenon

  6. Irradiation-related vascular fibrosis or injury
  7. Extravascular compression, such as compartment syndrome or popliteal artery entrapment
  8. Direct vascular injury
  9. Deep venous thrombosis
- Nonvascular etiologies
  1. Musculoskeletal disorder, such as arthritis or myositis
  2. Spinal stenosis or nerve root compression (neurogenic or pseudoclaudication)
  3. Peripheral neuropathy
  4. Reflex sympathetic dystrophy

WORKUP

- Thorough history, including identifying walking distance, speed, and incline to qualitatively assess for claudication, presence of ischemic rest pain, or presence of nonhealing wounds in patients ≥70 yr or those ≥50 yr with a history of smoking and/or diabetes.
- Careful physical examination includes:
  1. Measurement of blood pressure in both arms; pressure difference of >15 to 20 mm Hg is abnormal and suggestive of subclavian artery stenosis (marker of vascular disease risk and death)
  2. Palpation and recording of carotid pulses, upstroke, amplitude, and presence of bruits
  3. Auscultation and palpation of abdomen for bruits, aortic pulsation, and diameter
  4. Palpation of brachial, radial, ulnar, femoral, popliteal, dorsalis pedis, and posterior tibial pulses. Pulse intensity should be recorded as follows: 0, absent; 1+, diminished; 2+, normal; 3+, bounding
  5. Auscultation of femoral arteries for the presence of bruits

  6. Extremities should be inspected for color, temperature, integrity of the skin, hair loss, and hypertrophic nails
- Categorization of the clinical symptoms helps to identify risk and types of therapeutic intervention. One such classification is the Fontaine staging system (Table 1) for PAD:
  1. I: Asymptomatic
  2. II: Intermittent claudication
  3. IIa: Claudication walking >200 m (mild)
  4. IIb: Claudication walking <200 m (moderate)
  5. III: Nocturnal or rest pain
  6. IV: Evidence of tissue lost with ulceration, gangrene, or necrosis
- Segmental pressure measurement, where pneumatic cuffs are placed on multiple portions of the upper and lower extremity, is a simple tool that can identify the presence and severity of stenosis in the peripheral arteries.
- Resting ABI, a simplified form of segmental pressure measurement, is a first-line noninvasive test to establish a diagnosis of PAD in individuals with symptoms or signs suggestive

TABLE 1 Fontaine Classification of Peripheral Artery Disease

Stage	Symptoms
I	Asymptomatic
II	Intermittent claudication
IIa	Pain free, claudication walking >200 m
IIb	Pain free, claudication walking <200 m
III	Rest and nocturnal pain
IV	Necrosis, gangrene

From Libby P et al: *Braunwald's heart disease, a textbook of cardiovascular medicine*, ed 12, Philadelphia, 2022, Elsevier.

of disease (individuals with one or more of the following exertional leg symptoms: Nonhealing wounds, age >65 yr, or age >50 yr with smoking or diabetes history).

- ABI of each leg is calculated by dividing the highest dorsalis pedis or posterior tibial systolic blood pressure by the highest systolic brachial pressure obtained from either the right or left arm.
  1. Noncompressible/calcified: >1.40
  2. Normal: 1.00 to 1.40 at rest
  3. Borderline: 0.91 to 0.99 at rest
  4. Abnormal: ≤0.90
     a. ABI <0.5 severe PAD
     b. 0.5 <ABI <0.75 moderate PAD
     c. 0.75 <ABI <0.9 mild PAD
- ABI should be measured in both legs in all new patients (Fig. 3).
- Exercise ABI is recommended if resting ABI is borderline or normal (>0.9) and symptoms of claudication are present; a 25% or greater decrease in ABI after exercise is considered diagnostic.
- Toe-brachial index (TBI) should be used in patients suspected of PAD with an ABI of >1.40. A TBI of <0.70 is abnormal and diagnostic of PAD. TBI may be used to assess perfusion in patients with suspected CLI.
- Routine screening for lower-extremity PAD in the absence of risk factors, history, signs, or symptoms is not recommended.
- PAD is recognized as a risk factor for abdominal aortic aneurysm (AAA), and in observational studies the prevalence of AAA was higher in patients with symptomatic PAD.

LABORATORY TESTS

Laboratory tests can help identify risk factors or other potential causative etiologies. These include lipid profile, hemoglobin A_{1C}, D-dimer, and C-reactive protein/erythrocyte sedimentation rate.

ADDITIONAL PHYSIOLOGIC TESTING & IMAGING STUDIES

- Rest or exercise pulse volume recordings (PVR) are also useful, depicting the volume of limb flow per pulse in different segments of the limb (e.g., thigh, calf, ankle, metatarsal, and toes). Segmental analysis of the pulse wave may identify the location and severity of a lesion and assess the integrity of blood flow in noncompressible vessels.
- Duplex ultrasound incorporates anatomic and physiologic evaluation by combining 2D ultrasound to visualize arterial segments and pulse wave Doppler to sample blood flow velocities at specific locations in the arterial lumen.
- Transcutaneous oxygen pressure (TcPO2) measurement can quantify skin oxygenation and is useful in evaluating the severity of limb ischemia or predicting wound healing after amputation.
- Computed tomography angiography (CTA) with intravenous radiocontrast administration is a highly sensitive and specific imaging modality that provides a detailed view of lower limb vasculature, and it is the preferred testing for treatment planning and disease assessment in CLI patients.
- Magnetic resonance angiography (MRA) is a useful alternative to CTA with the benefit of not requiring iodinated contrast or radiation. However, gadolinium used in MRA can increase the risk of nephrogenic systemic fibrosis in patients with renal failure.
- Contrast-enhanced digital subtraction angiography (DSA) allows for real-time visualization of the arteries, which involves taking a series of x-rays while injecting a radioopaque contrast media. While it remains the gold standard for diagnosis of PAD, duplex ultrasonography, CTA and MRA have largely replaced catheter-based angiography in anatomic assessment for revascularization. DSA (Fig. E4) is now reserved for patients with PAD who are being considered for endovascular revascularization. It allows assessment of translesional pressure gradients before percutaneous intervention.

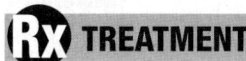

TREATMENT

The treatment goal in patients with PAD is to focus on CV risk factor reduction to decrease morbidity and mortality as well as to improve limb-related symptoms. There are also medical and surgical approaches to management of limb-related symptoms to improve blood supply and preserve limb viability. Fig. 5 illustrates an approach to a patient with PAD. 2016 American College of Cardiology Foundation/American Heart Association (ACCF/AHA) guidelines for medical management of patients with PAD are summarized in Table 2.

MEDICAL THERAPY (TABLE 3)
LOWERING CV RISK FACTORS, MORBIDITY, AND MORTALITY:
- Smoking cessation or avoidance of secondhand smoke should be emphasized in patients with PAD at each visit with assistance of behavioral and pharmacologic treatment (Class I).[6]
- E-cigarettes may be considered as an interim activity to reduce habituation and to make smoking cessation possible.
- Control of blood sugar in diabetic patients with PAD is recommended (hemoglobin A_{1C} goal <6.5), although studies have failed to demonstrate a beneficial effect on intensive insulin therapy in lowering risk of PAD.
- In all patients with diabetes and lower-extremity PAD, proper foot care, including use of appropriate footwear, chiropody/podiatric medicine, daily foot inspection, skin cleansing, and use of topical moisturizing creams, should be encouraged, and skin lesions and ulcerations should be addressed urgently (Class I).
- A foot infection should be suspected in patients presenting with local pain, periwound erythema, edema, or discharge; these patients should undergo prompt diagnosis and treatment with an interdisciplinary care team to avoid amputation.
- Antihypertensive therapy also provides reduced CV risk in patients with PAD, and while data regarding specific targets for blood pressure goal and types of agents to be used are mixed, standard therapy per the AHA/ACC guidelines should be utilized (Class I).[7]
- Antiplatelet therapy is indicated to reduce risk of MI, stroke, and vascular death in individuals with symptomatic PAD with either aspirin (75 to 325 mg) or clopidogrel (75 mg) (Class I) and in asymptomatic patients (Class

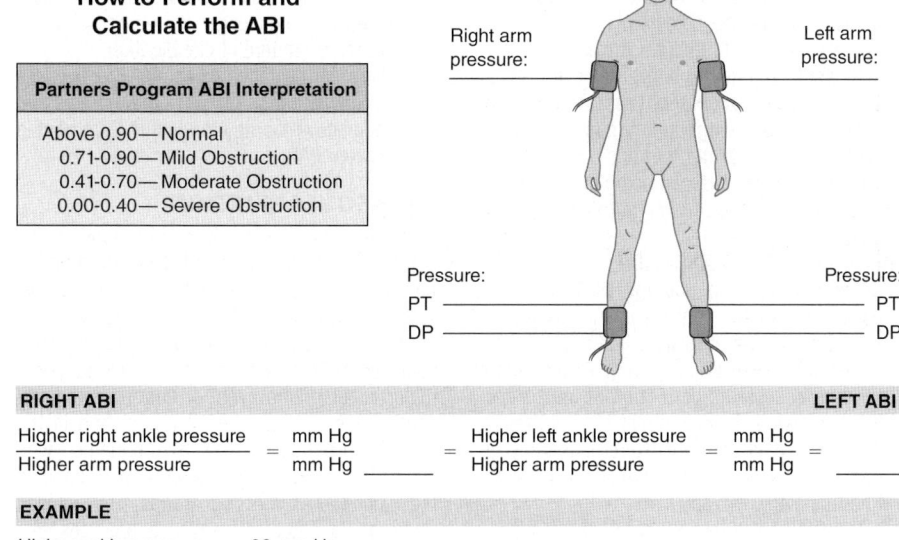

FIG. 3 Performing pressure measurements and calculating the ankle-brachial index (ABI). To calculate the ABI, systolic pressures are determined in both arms and both ankles with the use of a handheld Doppler instrument. The highest readings for the dorsalis pedis (DP) and posterior tibial (PT) arteries are used to calculate the index. (From Goldman L, Schafer AI: Goldman's Cecil medicine, ed 24, Philadelphia, 2012, Saunders.)

How to Perform and Calculate the ABI

Partners Program ABI Interpretation

Above 0.90— Normal
0.71-0.90— Mild Obstruction
0.41-0.70— Moderate Obstruction
0.00-0.40— Severe Obstruction

RIGHT ABI   **LEFT ABI**

$$\frac{\text{Higher right ankle pressure}}{\text{Higher arm pressure}} = \frac{\text{mm Hg}}{\text{mm Hg}} \_\_\_\_ = \frac{\text{Higher left ankle pressure}}{\text{Higher arm pressure}} = \frac{\text{mm Hg}}{\text{mm Hg}} \_\_\_\_$$

EXAMPLE

$$\frac{\text{Higher ankle pressure}}{\text{Higher arm pressure}} = \frac{92 \text{ mm Hg}}{164 \text{ mm Hg}} = 0.56 \qquad \text{See ABI Chart}$$

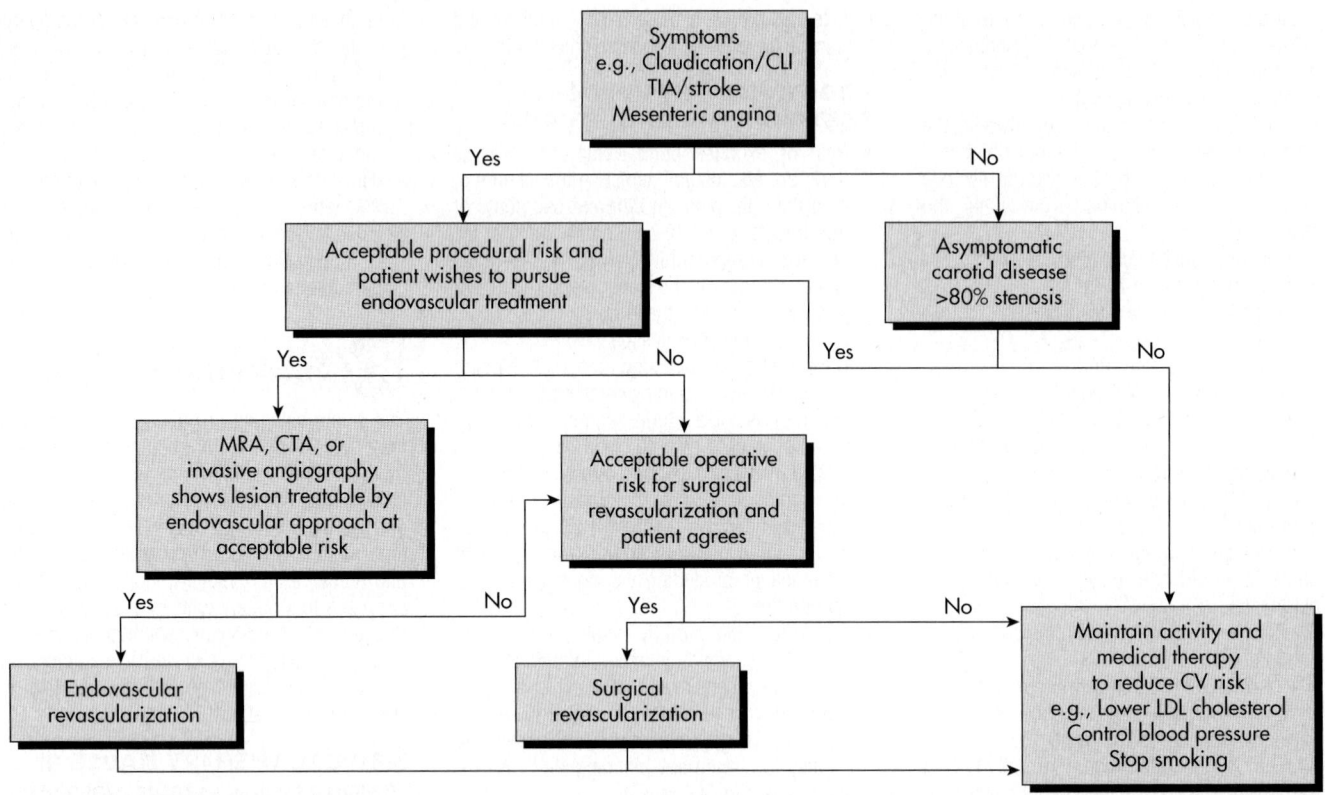

FIG. 5 Approach to a patient with peripheral artery disease. This strategy is based on assessment of the risk for adverse events with and without treatment by taking into consideration procedural or operative risks and the patient's informed decision to proceed with revascularization. *CLI,* Critical limb ischemia; *CTA,* computed tomographic angiography; *CV,* cardiovascular; *LDL,* low-density lipoprotein; *MRA,* magnetic resonance angiography; *TIA,* transient ischemic attack. (From Libby P et al: *Braunwald's heart disease, a textbook of cardiovascular medicine,* ed 12, Philadelphia, 2022, Elsevier.)

IIa). Uncertain benefit has been observed with combination aspirin and clopidogrel therapy (Class IIb). There are limited data on the use of newer P2Y12 receptor antagonists in PAD. In the EUCLID trial, ticagrelor was not shown to be superior to clopidogrel for the reduction of CV events, with major bleeding being similar in the two groups.[8] There is uncertain benefit with vorapaxar (Class IIb).

- Anticoagulation with low-dose (2.5 mg twice daily) rivaroxaban (Xarelto) plus aspirin 100 mg daily showed significant reductions in both major CV and limb events, including amputations, in patients with PAD in the COMPASS trial. (Class IIa—Level B per 2019 *European Journal of Vascular Medicine* PAD guidelines.)[9]
- Similarly, the VOYAGER PAD trial studied patients who had undergone lower-extremity revascularization with therapy with rivaroxaban 2.5 mg twice daily plus aspirin or aspirin alone. The rivaroxaban/aspirin group had significantly lower incidence of the composite outcome of ALI, major amputation for vascular causes, MI, ischemic stroke, or death from CV causes.[10]
- Lipid-lowering therapy in patients with lower limb PAD has been shown to help slow disease progression, alleviate symptoms, and improve walking distance. The 2018 ACC/AHA Guideline on the Treatment of Blood Cholesterol recommends that patients with

atherosclerotic PAD receive high-intensity statin therapy to lower risk of CV events regardless of baseline cholesterol values (Class I). In patients who are judged to be at very high risk and considered for PCSK9 inhibitor therapy, maximally tolerated low-density lipoprotein–cholesterol (LDL-C) lowering therapy should include maximally tolerated statin therapy and ezetimibe (Class I). 2019 *European Journal of Vascular* Medicine PAD guidelines also recommends addition of ezetimibe to get better tolerance of the statin medication (with reduced dose) or to achieve target level of LDL <70 mg/dl or >50% decrease.[11,12]

TREATMENT OF CLAUDICATION:
- Supervised exercise therapy (SET) may be as beneficial as stent revascularization in symptomatic improvement. Patients should be prescribed exercise for a minimum of 30 to 45 min, in sessions performed at least three times per wk for a minimum of 12 wk (Class I). ACCF/AHA guidelines for exercise therapy in patients with PAD are summarized in Table 4.
- Pharmacologic therapy:
  1. Cilostazol (100 mg PO twice daily) is indicated as effective therapy for enabling pain-free and maximal walking distance (Class 1). It is a phosphodiesterase (PDE-3) inhibitor that enables vasodilation and also inhibits thromboxane A2–mediated platelet aggregation. It may have an added

benefit of reducing restenosis and repeat revascularization following endovascular therapy. Cilostazol is contraindicated in patients with systolic heart failure.
  2. Pentoxifylline, prostanoids, L-arginine, buflomedil, ginkgo biloba, and chelation therapy are no longer considered effective in the treatment of claudication.
  3. No clear evidence exists for effectiveness of hyperbaric oxygen therapy as an adjunctive therapy for wound treatment in severe PAD.

REVASCULARIZATION

In general, there is no clear consensus on the use of open versus endovascular revascularization. A recent trial[13] in patients with chronic limb-threatening ischemia (CLTI) who had adequate great saphenous vein for surgical revascularization revealed that the incidence of a major adverse limb event or death was significantly lower in the surgical group than in the endovascular group. Among patients who lacked an adequate saphenous vein conduit, the outcomes in the two groups were similar. However, in other retrospective analyses, the endovascular approach was associated with improved amputation-free survival compared to open repair in the short (at 30 days) and long term (at 4 yr), with additional data reporting lower complication rates, shorter hospital stays, and lower amputation and mortality rates with

TABLE 2 ACCF/AHA Guidelines for Medical Therapy for Patients With Peripheral Artery Disease

COR	Indication	LOE
I	Antiplatelet therapy with aspirin alone (range, 75-325 mg/day) or clopidogrel alone (75 mg/day) is recommended to reduce MI, stroke, and vascular death in patients with symptomatic PAD.	A
	Treatment with a statin medication is indicated for all patients with PAD.	A
	Antihypertensive therapy should be administered to patients with hypertension and PAD to reduce the risk of MI, stroke, heart failure, and CV death.	A
	Patients with PAD who smoke cigarettes or use other forms of tobacco should be advised at every visit to quit.	A
	Patients with PAD who smoke cigarettes should be assisted in developing a plan for quitting that includes pharmacotherapy (varenicline, bupropion, and/or nicotine replacement therapy) and/or referral to a smoking cessation program.	A
	Patients with PAD should avoid exposure to environmental tobacco smoke at work, at home, and in public places.	B-NR
	Management of diabetes mellitus in the patient with PAD should be coordinated between members of the health care team.	C-EO
	Cilostazol is an effective therapy to improve symptoms and increase walking distance in patients with claudication.	A
	Patients with PAD should have an annual influenza vaccination.	C-EO
IIa	In asymptomatic patients with PAD (ABI ≤0.90), antiplatelet therapy is reasonable to reduce the risk of MI, stroke, or vascular death.	C-EO
	The use of angiotensin-converting enzyme inhibitors or angiotensin receptor blockers can be effective to reduce the risk of CV ischemic events in patients with PAD.	A
	Glycemic control can be beneficial for patients with CLI to reduce limb-related outcomes.	B-NR
IIb	In asymptomatic patients with borderline ABI (0.91-0.99), the usefulness of antiplatelet therapy to reduce the risk of MI, stroke, or vascular death is uncertain.	B-R
	The effectiveness of dual-antiplatelet therapy (aspirin and clopidogrel) to reduce the risk of CV ischemic events in patients with symptomatic PAD is not well established.	B-R
	Dual-antiplatelet therapy (aspirin and clopidogrel) may be reasonable to reduce the risk of limb-related events in patients with symptomatic PAD after lower extremity revascularization.	C-LD
	The overall clinical benefit of vorapaxar added to existing antiplatelet therapy in patients with symptomatic PAD is uncertain.	B-R
	The usefulness of anticoagulation to improve patency after lower extremity autogenous vein or prosthetic bypass is uncertain.	B-R
III	Anticoagulation should not be used to reduce the risk of CV ischemic events in patients with PAD.	A
	Pentoxifylline is not effective for treatment of claudication.	B-R
	Chelation therapy (e.g., ethylenediaminetetraacetic acid) is not beneficial for treatment of claudication.	B-R
	B-complex vitamin supplementation to lower homocysteine levels for prevention of CV events in patients with PAD is not recommended.	B-R

ABI, Ankle-brachial index; *ACCF,* American College of Cardiology Foundation; *AHA,* American Heart Association; *CLI,* critical limb ischemia; *COR,* class of recommendation; *CV,* cardiovascular; *LOE,* level of evidence; *MI,* myocardial infarction; *PAD,* peripheral artery disease.
From Libby P et al: *Braunwald's heart disease, a textbook of cardiovascular medicine,* ed 12, Philadelphia, 2022, Elsevier.

the endovascular approach compared to the open surgical approach.[14,15]

- The 2016 ACCF/AHA guidelines on PAD (Table 5) have recommended revascularization as a reasonable treatment option for the patient with lifestyle-limiting claudication with inadequate response to guideline-directed medical therapy. A multidisciplinary approach by vascular specialists in all chronic limb ischemia patients for management of pain, risk factors, and comorbidities is appropriate. ACC/AHA guidelines for wound healing therapies for patients with CLI are summarized in Table 6.
- The following approach is discussed:
  1. Considerations in percutaneous/endovascular treatment:
     a. In patients with a vocational- or lifestyle-limiting disability due to claudication or limb ischemia from either significant aortoiliac or femoropopliteal disease despite optimal medical therapy when clinical features suggest a reasonable likelihood of symptomatic improvement with endovascular intervention.
     b. Endovascular intervention is not indicated as prophylactic therapy in an asymptomatic patient with lower-extremity PAD.
     c. Durability of endovascular intervention is greater in aortoiliac disease than in the femoropopliteal segment.
  2. Considerations in surgical revascularization:
     a. Individuals with claudication symptoms that have a vocational- or lifestyle-limiting disability. These patients need to also be unresponsive to exercise or pharmacotherapy and should have a reasonable likelihood of symptomatic improvement with an acceptable surgical risk and technical factors favoring surgical versus endovascular approach.
     b. Autogenous vein graft is superior to prosthetic graft if surgical revascularization is performed (Class I).
     c. Iliac or femoropopliteal disease with long segments; multifocal segments; long segment occlusions; and eccentric, calcified stenosis, which are less amenable to percutaneous interventions.
     d. Surgical intervention is not indicated to prevent progression to limb-threatening ischemia in patients with IC as generally claudication does not progress to severe ischemia.
  3. Revascularization for ALI (Table 7):
     a. Management approach is dependent on whether affected limb is viable, threatened, or irreversible. Initial management will depend on the absence of sensation and movement. If absent, then urgent surgery should be considered.
     b. Heparin should be given to all patients with ALI; direct thrombin inhibitor is used if patient has history of HIT.
     c. Catheter-based thrombolysis is effective in ALI with salvageable limb.
     d. Amputation should be performed in patients with irreversible damage.
     e. Rivaroxaban 2.5 mg PO bid is now FDA approved to reduce the risk of major thrombotic vascular events in patients with PAD, including those who have recently undergone a lower extremity revascularization procedure for symptomatic PAD.

DISPOSITION

Risk factors for atherosclerosis should be assessed, and appropriate modification instituted. Focus should be placed on smoking cessation, dietary adjustment, and pharmacotherapy for dyslipidemia, hyperglycemia, and hypertension. All patients with PAD should receive aspirin therapy unless contraindicated. Revascularization should be considered for refractory lifestyle-limiting symptoms.

More than one in six patients with peripheral arterial disease who undergo peripheral arterial revascularization have unplanned readmission within 30 days with high associated mortality risks and costs. Procedure- and patient-related factors were the primary reasons for readmission.[16]

TABLE 3 Approved Medical Therapies for Patients With Peripheral Artery Disease

			INDICATIONS			
Therapy	**Mechanism of Action**	**Key Clinical Trials**	**European Medicines Agency**	**European Society of Cardiology**	**FDA**	**ACC/AHA**
Statin (Class effect)	Cholesterol-lowering HMG-CoA reductase inhibitor	Heart Protection Study 3% RRR with simvastatin 40 mg/day vs. placebo in all-cause mortality, 18% RRR in coronary heart death Approval for PAD based on subgroup of 6748 patients, 2700 had PAD and no CHD	Reduction in MACE and mortality	Class I for lipid lowering with LDL <2.5 mmol/L, optimally <1.8 mmol/L	Reduction in MACE and mortality	Class I, LOE A
ACEI or ARB (Class effect)	Blood pressure lowering and other vascular effects Renin-angiotensin system inhibition	HOPE 22% RRR with ramipril 10 mg daily vs. placebo for composite of MI, stroke, or CV death Approval for PAD based on subgroup of 4051 patients, 1725 with "clinical PAD"	Reduction in MACE	Class I for blood pressure lowering to ≤40/90 mm Hg	Reduction in MACE	Class I, LOE A for antihypertensive therapy Class IIa, LOE A for ACEI/ARB specifically
Clopidogrel	Antiplatelet P2Y$_{12}$ inhibitor	CAPRIE 8.7% RRR vs. aspirin for composite of ischemic stroke, MI, or vascular death Approval for PAD based on subgroup of 6452 patients	As monotherapy Reduction in MACE	Class I monotherapy for risk reduction Class I added to ASA after lower-extremity stenting	As monotherapy Reduction in MACE	Class I, LOE A for monotherapy Class IIb, LOE B-R, C-LD, when added to aspirin as DAPT
Vorapaxar	Antiplatelet PAR-1 antagonist	TRA2P-TIMI 50 20% RRR vs. placebo for composite of MI, stroke, or CV death Approval for PAD based on subgroup of 3787 patients	Added to aspirin or clopidogrel Reduction in MACE, limb benefits mentioned	Approved after most recent guidelines	Added to aspirin and/or clopidogrel Reduction in MACE	Class IIb, LOE B-R added to aspirin and/or clopidogrel
Pentoxifylline	Decreases blood viscosity Mechanism not fully understood	Meta-analysis of six studies including 788 patients who showed minimal increase in maximal walking distance with (+59 m)	Improve function and symptoms in patients with intermittent claudication	Described but no clear recommendation	Improve function and symptoms in patients with intermittent claudication	Class III, LOE B-R
Cilostazol	Antiplatelet and vasodilator Mechanism not fully understood	50 mg bid (n = 303), 100 mg bid (n = 998), and placebo (n = 973) Improvement in maximal walking distance with 100 mg bid, expressed as the percent mean change from baseline, 28%-100% vs. placebo, which were 0%-41%	Reduction of symptoms of intermittent claudication, as indicated by an increased walking distance	Class I for symptoms	Reduction of symptoms of intermittent claudication, as indicated by an increased walking distance	Class I, LOE A

ACC/AHA, American College of Cardiology/American Heart Association; *ACEI,* angiotensin-converting enzyme inhibitor; *ARB,* angiotensin receptor blocker; *bid,* twice daily; *ASA,* acetylsalicylic acid; *CAPRIE,* Clopidogrel versus Aspirin in Patients at Risk of Ischaemic Events; *CHD,* coronary heart disease; *CV,* cardiovascular; *DAPT,* dual-antiplatelet therapy; *FDA,* U.S. Food and Drug Administration; *HOPE,* Heart Outcomes Prevention Evaluation; *LDL,* low-density lipoprotein; *LOE,* level of evidence (*B-R,* moderate-quality evidence from one or more randomized clinical trials; *C-LD,* randomized or nonrandomized observational/registry studies or a meta-analysis); *MACE,* major adverse cardiovascular events; *MI,* myocardial infarction; *PAR-1,* protease-activated receptor 1; *RRR,* relative risk reduction; *TRA2P-TIMI 50,* Thrombin Receptor Antagonist in Secondary Prevention of Atherothrombotic Ischemic Events–Thrombolysis in Myocardial Infarction.
From Zipes DP et al (eds): *Braunwald's heart disease, a textbook of cardiovascular medicine,* ed 11, Philadelphia, 2019, Elsevier.

TABLE 4 ACCF/AHA Guidelines for Exercise Therapy in Patients With Peripheral Artery Disease

COR	Indication	LOE
I	In patients with claudication, a supervised exercise program is recommended to improve functional status and quality of life and to reduce leg symptoms.	A
	A supervised exercise program should be discussed as a treatment option for claudication before possible revascularization.	B-R
IIa	In patients with PAD, a structured community- or home-based exercise program with behavioral change techniques can be beneficial to improve walking ability and functional status.	A
	In patients with claudication, alternative strategies of exercise therapy, including upper-body ergometry, cycling, and pain-free or low-intensity walking that avoids moderate to maximum claudication while walking, can be beneficial to improve walking ability and functional status.	A

COR, Class of recommendation; *LOE,* level of evidence; *PAD,* peripheral artery disease.
From Libby P et al: *Braunwald's heart disease, a textbook of cardiovascular medicine,* ed 12, Philadelphia, 2022, Elsevier.

TABLE 5 ACCF/AHA Guidelines for Revascularization of Patients With Peripheral Artery Disease

COR	Indication	LOE
I	In patients with CLI, revascularization should be performed when possible to minimize tissue loss.	B-NR
	An evaluation for revascularization options should be performed by an interdisciplinary care team before amputation in the patient with CLI.	C-EO
	Endovascular procedures are recommended to establish in-line blood flow to the foot in patients with nonhealing wounds or gangrene.	B-R
	Surgical procedures are recommended to establish in-line blood flow to the foot in patients with nonhealing wounds or gangrene.	C-LD
	When surgery is performed for CLI, bypass to the popliteal or infrapopliteal arteries (i.e., tibial, pedal) should be constructed with suitable autogenous vein.	A
	Endovascular procedures are effective as a revascularization option for patients with lifestyle-limiting claudication and hemodynamically significant aortoiliac occlusive disease.	A
	When surgical revascularization is performed, bypass to the popliteal artery with autogenous vein is recommended in preference to prosthetic graft material.	A
IIa	Revascularization is a reasonable treatment option for the patient with lifestyle-limiting claudication with an inadequate response to GDMT.	A
	Endovascular procedures are reasonable as a revascularization option for patients with lifestyle-limiting claudication and hemodynamically significant femoropopliteal disease.	B-R
	Surgical procedures are reasonable as a revascularization option for patients with lifestyle-limiting claudication with inadequate response to GDMT, acceptable perioperative risk, and technical factors suggesting advantages over endovascular procedures.	B-NR
	A staged approach to endovascular procedures is reasonable in patients with ischemic rest pain.	C-LD
	Evaluation of lesion characteristics can be useful in selecting the endovascular approach for CLI.	B-R
	In patients with CLI for whom endovascular revascularization has failed and a suitable autogenous vein is not available, prosthetic material can be effective for bypass to the below-knee popliteal and tibial arteries.	B-NR
	A staged approach to surgical procedures is reasonable in patients with ischemic rest pain.	C-LD
IIb	The usefulness of endovascular procedures as a revascularization option for patients with claudication due to isolated infrapopliteal artery disease is unknown.	C-LD
	Use of angiosome-directed endovascular therapy may be reasonable for patients with CLI and nonhealing wounds or gangrene.	B-NR
III	Endovascular procedures should *not* be performed in patients with PAD solely to prevent progression to CLI.	B-NR
	Surgical procedures should not be performed in patients with PAD solely to prevent progression to CLI.	B-NR
	Femoral-tibial artery bypasses with prosthetic graft material should not be used for the treatment of claudication.	B-R

CLI, Critical limb ischemia; *COR,* class of recommendation; *GDMT,* guideline-directed medical therapy; *LOE,* level of evidence; *PAD,* peripheral artery disease.
From Libby P et al: *Braunwald's heart disease, a textbook of cardiovascular medicine,* ed 12, Philadelphia, 2022, Elsevier.

TABLE 6 ACCF/AHA Guidelines for Wound Healing Therapies for Patients With Critical Limb Ischemia

COR	Indication	LOE
I	An interdisciplinary care team should evaluate and provide comprehensive care for patients with CLI and tissue loss to achieve complete wound healing and a functional foot.	B-NR
	In patients with CLI, wound care after revascularization should be performed with the goal of complete wound healing.	C-LD
IIb	In patients with CLI, intermittent pneumatic compression (arterial pump) devices may be considered to augment wound healing and/or ameliorate severe ischemic rest pain.	B-NR
	In patients with CLI, the effectiveness of hyperbaric oxygen therapy for wound healing is unknown.	C-LD
III	Prostanoids are not indicated in patients with CLI.	B-R

CLI, Critical limb ischemia; *COR,* class of recommendation; *LOE,* level of evidence.
From Libby P et al: *Braunwald's heart disease, a textbook of cardiovascular medicine,* ed 12, Philadelphia, 2022, Elsevier.

TABLE 7 ACCF/AHA Guidelines for Management of Patients With Acute Limb Ischemia

COR	Indication	LOE
I	Patients with ALI should be emergently evaluated by a clinician with sufficient experience to assess limb viability and implement appropriate therapy.	C-EO
	In patients with suspected ALI, initial clinical evaluation should rapidly assess limb viability and potential for salvage and does not require imaging.	C-LD
	In patients with ALI, systemic anticoagulation with heparin should be administered unless contraindicated.	C-EO
	In patients with ALI, the revascularization strategy should be determined by local resources and patient factors (e.g., etiology, degree of ischemia).	C-LD
	Catheter-based thrombolysis is effective for patients with ALI and a salvageable limb.	A
	Amputation should be performed as the first procedure in patients with a nonsalvageable limb.	C-LD
	Patients with ALI should be monitored and treated (e.g., fasciotomy) for compartment syndrome after revascularization.	C-LD
	In the patient with ALI, a comprehensive history should be obtained to determine the cause of thrombosis and/or embolization.	C-EO
IIa	In patients with ALI with a salvageable limb, percutaneous mechanical thrombectomy can be useful as adjunctive therapy to thrombolysis.	B-NR
	In patients with ALI due to embolism and with a salvageable limb, surgical thromboembolectomy can be effective.	C-LD
	In the patient with a history of ALI, testing for a cardiovascular cause of thromboembolism can be useful.	C-EO
IIb	The usefulness of ultrasound-accelerated catheter-based thrombolysis for patients with ALI with a salvageable limb is unknown.	C-LD

ACCF, American College of Cardiology Foundation; *AHA*, American Heart Association; *ALI*, acute limb ischemia; *COR*, class of recommendation; *LOE*, level of evidence.
From Libby P et al: *Braunwald's heart disease, a textbook of cardiovascular medicine*, ed 12, Philadelphia, 2022, Elsevier.

REFERRAL

Consultation with vascular medicine, vascular surgery, interventional cardiology, or other physicians with expertise in PAD is recommended in patients with rest pain, functional disability from pain, ABI <0.90 at rest, or any physical signs of limb ischemia or gangrene.

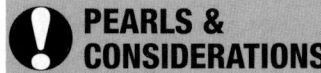

PEARLS & CONSIDERATIONS

COMMENTS

- PAD is a highly prevalent disease process that remains underdiagnosed and undertreated.
- Patients with PAD are at markedly higher risk of future coronary, cerebrovascular, and other vascular events.
- Medical treatment is aimed mainly at cardiovascular risk factor modification, except for cilostazol, which treats IC.
- Studies of the natural history of claudication show the relative safety of initial conservative treatment of PAD in the absence of CLI.

- When PAD limits a patient's ability to walk and exercise, revascularization should be considered.
- Exercise training is an important and often neglected treatment strategy that has proven beneficial in improving functional status, reducing symptoms, and improving quality of life. Exercise capacity alone is the strongest predictor of mortality in patients with PAD.
- Surgical intervention should be considered in patients who meet the criteria for intervention but have lesions that are not amenable to PTA/stenting or in older patients with a low surgical risk. Advances in endovascular therapy have broadened the range of revascularization options for refractory claudication and critical ischemia and ALI in patients with multiple comorbidities.
- Among patients with chronic limb-threatening ischemia (CLTI) and infrapopliteal artery disease, angioplasty has been associated with frequent reintervention and adverse limb outcomes from restenosis. The use of an everolimus-eluting resorbable scaffold

was found to be superior to angioplasty with respect to freedom from major adverse limb events at 6 mo in a recent multicenter trial.[17]

PREVENTION

CV disease is the major cause of death in patients with IC. Therefore, the treatment of claudication is directed not only at improving walking distance but also at reducing CV risk.

PATIENT & FAMILY EDUCATION

The following organization offers more information about PAD:
- American College of Cardiology (http://www.acc.org/)

REFERENCES

Available at eBooks.Health.Elsevier.com.

RELATED CONTENT

Claudication (Related Key Topic)

AUTHORS: **MURTAZA BHARMAL, MD** and **PRANAV M. PATEL, MD, FACC, FAHA, FSCAI**

P

I

BASIC INFORMATION

DEFINITION

A perirectal abscess is a localized inflammatory process that can be associated with infections of soft tissue and anal glands based on anatomic location. Perianal and perirectal abscesses may be simple or complex, causing suppuration. Infections in these spaces may be classified as superficial perianal or perirectal with involvement in the following anatomic spaces: Ischiorectal, intersphincteric, perianal, and supralevator (Table 1). The Parks classification of anorectal abscess is subdivided into intersphincteric, transsphincteric, suprasphincteric, and extrasphincteric abscess (Fig. E1).

SYNONYMS

Rectal abscess
Perianal abscess
Anorectal abscess

ICD-10CM CODES
K61.0   Anal abscess
K61.1   Rectal abscess

EPIDEMIOLOGY & DEMOGRAPHICS

INCIDENCE (IN U.S.): Commonly encountered
PREDOMINANT SEX: Male > female
PREDOMINANT AGE: All ages
PEAK INCIDENCE: Not seasonal; common
GENETICS: None known

PHYSICAL FINDINGS & CLINICAL PRESENTATION

- Localized perirectal or anal pain—often worsened with movement or straining
- Perirectal erythema or cellulitis
- Perirectal mass by inspection or palpation
- Fever and signs of sepsis with deep abscess
- Urinary retention

ETIOLOGY

- Polymicrobial aerobic and anaerobic bacteria involving one of the anatomic spaces (see "Definition"), often associated with localized trauma
- Microbiology: Most infections are polymicrobial, mixed enteric, and skin flora
- Predominant anaerobic bacteria:
  1. *Bacteroides fragilis*
  2. *Peptostreptococcus* spp.
  3. *Prevotella* spp.
  4. *Porphyromonas* spp.
  5. *Clostridioides* spp.
  6. *Fusobacterium* spp.
- Predominant aerobic bacteria:
  1. *Staphylococcus aureus*
  2. *Streptococcus* spp.
  3. *Escherichia coli*
  4. *Enterococcus* spp.

DIAGNOSIS

Many patients will have predisposing underlying conditions including:
- Malignancy or leukemia
- Immune deficiency
- Diabetes mellitus
- Recent surgery
- Steroid therapy

DIFFERENTIAL DIAGNOSIS

- Neutropenic enterocolitis
- Crohn disease (inflammatory bowel disease)
- Pilonidal disease
- Hidradenitis suppurativa
- Tuberculosis or actinomycosis; Chagas disease
- Cancerous lesions
- Chronic anal fistula
- Rectovaginal fistula
- Proctitis—often sexually transmitted disease–associated, including syphilis, gonococcal, chlamydia, chancroid, condylomata acuminata
- AIDS-associated: Kaposi sarcoma, lymphoma, cytomegalovirus

WORKUP

- Examination of rectal, perirectal/perineal areas
- Rule out necrotic process and crepitance suggesting deep tissue involvement
- Local aerobic and anaerobic culture
- Blood cultures if toxic, febrile, or compromised
- Possible sigmoidoscopy

IMAGING STUDIES

Usually not indicated unless extensive disease is suspected. Computed tomography (CT) has a sensitivity of 77% and is relatively poor in detecting a perirectal abscess in immunocompromised patients.

TREATMENT

ACUTE GENERAL Rx

- Incision and drainage of abscess
- Debridement of necrotic tissue
- Rule out need for fistulectomy
- Local wound care—packing
- Sitz baths
- Antibiotic treatment: Directed toward coverage for mixed skin and enteric flora

OUTPATIENT—ORAL:
- Trimethoprim/sulfamethoxazole DS bid or ciprofloxacin 500 mg bid or levofloxacin 500 mg q24h plus metronidazole 500 mg q8h × 7 to 10 days
- Amoxicillin/clavulanic acid 875 to 1000 mg 1 tabs bid
- Clindamycin 150 to 300 mg PO q6 to 8h, for its anaerobic coverage

INPATIENT—INTRAVENOUS:
- Piperacillin/tazobactam 3.375 g intravenous (IV) q6 to 8h
- Ampicillin/sulbactam 1.5 to 3 g IV q6h
- Cefotetan 1 to 2 g IV q8h
- Imipenem or meropenem 500 to 1000 mg IV q8h

DISPOSITION

Follow-up with a general surgeon or infectious disease physician is often warranted.

REFERRAL

- General surgeon or colorectal surgeon for drainage.
- AIDS specialist may be needed for perirectal complications of HIV infection.
- Gastroenterologist follow-up may be warranted in Crohn disease with perirectal fistula and other complications.
- Endoscopic ultrasound–guided perirectal abscess drainage is a recently described promising alternative treatment.

PEARLS & CONSIDERATIONS

Perirectal abscess may be a presenting manifestation of type 2 diabetes mellitus in older adults. Check the blood sugar or hemoglobin A1C in patients to exclude the possibility of undiagnosed diabetes mellitus.

SUGGESTED READINGS
Available at eBooks.Health.Elsevier.com.

RELATED CONTENT
Perirectal Abscess (Patient Information)

AUTHOR: **GLENN G. FORT, MD, MPH**

TABLE 1 Types of Abscesses of the Anorectum

Feature	Perianal	Ischiorectal	Intersphincteric	Supralevator	Postanal
Incidence	40%-45%	20%-25%	20%-25%	<5%	5%-10%
Location	Outside and verge	Buttocks	Lower rectum	Above levator ani	Deep to external sphincter
Symptoms	Painful perianal mass	Buttock pain	Rectal fullness	Perianal and buttock pain	Rectal fullness, pain near coccyx
Fever, ↑ WBCs	−	±	±	+	+
Associated fistula	++	+	+++	+++	−
ED incision and drainage	+	±	−	−	−

ED, Emergency department; *WBCs*, white blood cells; −, does not occur; ±, occurs sometimes; ++, occurs often; +++, usually occurs.
From Walls RM et al: *Rosen's emergency medicine, concepts and clinical practice*, ed 10, Philadelphia, 2023, Elsevier.

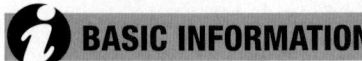 **BASIC INFORMATION**

DEFINITION

Peritonitis refers to the acute onset of severe abdominal pain caused by peritoneal inflammation.

Secondary peritonitis is peritonitis stemming from another condition; commonly a defect in an abdominal viscus.

SYNONYMS

Acute abdomen
Surgical abdomen

ICD-10CM CODES	
K65.0	Generalized (acute) peritonitis
K65.8	Other peritonitis
K65.9	Peritonitis, unspecified
A18.31	Tuberculous peritonitis
A54.85	Gonococcal peritonitis
A74.81	Chlamydial peritonitis
K35.2	Acute appendicitis with generalized peritonitis
K35.3	Acute appendicitis with localized peritonitis
K65.2	Spontaneous bacterial peritonitis
N73.3	Female acute pelvic peritonitis
N73.4	Female chronic pelvic peritonitis
N73.5	Female pelvic peritonitis, unspecified
P78.1	Other neonatal peritonitis

EPIDEMIOLOGY & DEMOGRAPHICS

Common presentation as a result of diverse etiologies; for example, 5% to 10% of the population has acute appendicitis at some point in their lives.

PHYSICAL FINDINGS & CLINICAL PRESENTATION

- Acute abdominal pain
- Abdominal distention and ascites
- Abdominal rigidity, rebound, and guarding
- Altered mental status
- Fever, chills
- Exacerbation with movement
- Anorexia, nausea, and vomiting
- Constipation or diarrhea
- Decreased bowel sounds
- Hypotension and tachycardia
- Tachypnea, dyspnea

ETIOLOGY

- One of the early steps is disturbance in gut flora with overgrowth and extraintestinal organismal overtake. Most common are gram-negative bacteria *(Escherichia coli, Enterobacter, Klebsiella, Proteus)*, gram-positive bacteria (enterococci, streptococci, staphylococci), anaerobic bacteria *(Bacteroides, Clostridioides),* and fungi

- Perforation peritonitis: Gastrointestinal perforation, intestinal ischemia, pelvic peritonitis, and other forms
- Postoperative peritonitis: Anastomotic leak, accidental perforation, and devascularization
- Posttraumatic peritonitis: After blunt or penetrating abdominal trauma

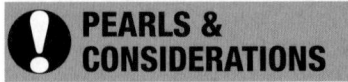 **DIAGNOSIS**

DIFFERENTIAL DIAGNOSIS

- Postoperative: Abscess, sepsis, bowel obstruction, injury to internal organs
- Gastrointestinal: Perforated viscus, appendicitis, inflammatory bowel disease, infectious colitis, diverticulitis, acute cholecystitis, peptic ulcer perforation, pancreatitis, bowel obstruction
- Gynecologic: Ruptured ectopic pregnancy, pelvic inflammatory disease, ruptured hemorrhagic ovarian cyst, ovarian torsion, degenerating leiomyoma
- Urologic: Nephrolithiasis, interstitial cystitis
- Miscellaneous: Abdominal trauma, penetrating wounds, infections caused by intraperitoneal dialysis

WORKUP

- Acute peritonitis is mainly a clinical diagnosis based on patient history and physical examination.
- Laboratory and imaging studies assist in determining the need for and type of intervention. Typical pretreatment peritoneal fluid and blood culture results in peritonitis are summarized in Table E1.
- If patient is hemodynamically unstable, immediate diagnostic laparotomy should be performed in lieu of adjuvant diagnostic studies.

LABORATORY TESTS

- Ascitic fluid testing
  1. Anaerobic and aerobic cultures
  2. Cell count and differential
  3. Albumin, protein, amylase, bilirubin
  4. Glucose
  5. Lactate dehydrogenase (LDH)
- CBC: Leukocytosis, left shift, anemia
- SMA7: Electrolyte imbalances, kidney dysfunction
- Liver function tests: Indicative of cirrhosis as ascites from liver disease, cholelithiasis
- Amylase: Pancreatitis
- Blood cultures: Bacteremia, sepsis
- Blood gas: Respiratory versus metabolic acidosis
- Urinalysis and culture: Urinary tract infection
- Cervical cultures for gonorrhea and *Chlamydia*
- Urine/serum human chorionic gonadotropin

IMAGING STUDIES

- Abdominal series: Free air from perforation, small or large bowel dilation from obstruction, identification of fecalith

- Chest x-ray examination: Elevated diaphragm, pneumonia
- Pelvic/abdominal ultrasound: Abscess formation, abdominal mass, intrauterine versus ectopic pregnancy, identify free fluid suggestive of hemorrhage or ascites
- Computed tomography (CT): Mass, ascites

TREATMENT

NONPHARMACOLOGIC THERAPY

- Intravenous (IV) hydration to correct dehydration, hypovolemia
- Blood transfusion to correct anemia from hemorrhage
- Nasogastric decompression, especially if obstruction is present
- Oxygen: Intubation if necessary
- Bed rest

ACUTE GENERAL Rx

- Surgery to correct underlying pathology, such as controlling hemorrhage, correcting perforation, and draining abscess
- Broad-spectrum antibiotics to cover both gram-negative aerobic and gram-negative anaerobic bacteria:
  1. Mild-moderate disease: Piperacillin-tazobactam 3.375 g IV q6h or 4.5 g IV q8h *or* ticarcillin-clavulanate 3.1 g IV q6h. Alternative agents are ciprofloxacin 400 mg IV q12h or levofloxacin 750 mg IV q24h *plus* metronidazole 1 g IV q12h.
  2. Severe life-threatening disease: Imipenem 500 mg IV q6h or meropenem 1 g IV q8h. Alternative agents are ampicillin *plus* metronidazole *plus* ciprofloxacin.
  3. Antibiotic therapy should be tailored to culture results and sensitivities.
- Pain control: Morphine or meperidine as needed (hold until diagnosis confirmed)

DISPOSITION

Depends on etiology of peritonitis, age of patient, coexisting medical disease, and duration of process before presentation.

REFERRAL

Surgical consultation is required in all cases of acute peritonitis.

PEARLS & CONSIDERATIONS

CT scan guides therapeutic approach and should be considered as the primary imaging study if available. As with forms of sepsis, early administration of broad-spectrum antibiotics, fluid resuscitation, and rapidly obtaining anatomic source control (when appropriate) will lead to improved outcomes.

AUTHOR: **GHAMAR BITAR, MD**

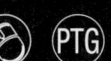 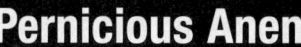
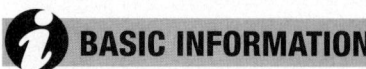 BASIC INFORMATION

DEFINITION

Pernicious anemia (PA) is an autoimmune disease resulting from antibodies against gastric intrinsic factor and gastric parietal cells that results in vitamin B_{12} deficiency due to decreased absorption and leading to megaloblastic anemia. Pernicious anemia also manifests with neurologic symptoms.

SYNONYMS

Megaloblastic anemia resulting from vitamin B_{12} deficiency
Addison-Biermer anemia
Anemia, pernicious

ICD-10CM CODES
D51.0	Vitamin B_{12} deficiency anemia due to intrinsic factor deficiency
D51.8	Other vitamin B_{12} deficiency anemias
D51.9	Vitamin B_{12} deficiency anemia, unspecified
D51.1	Vitamin B_{12} deficiency anemia due to selective vitamin B_{12} malabsorption with proteinuria

EPIDEMIOLOGY & DEMOGRAPHICS

- Increased incidence in females and older adults (40 to 70 yr)
- More frequent in patients of northern European ancestry
- Overall prevalence of undiagnosed PA after age 60 yr is 1.9%
- Prevalence is higher in women (2.7%), particularly in Black women (4.3%)
- Associated with other autoimmune diseases (e.g., type 1 diabetes mellitus, Graves disease, Addison disease), along with possible *Helicobacter pylori* association

PHYSICAL FINDINGS & CLINICAL PRESENTATION[1,2]

- Mucosal pallor and/or glossitis ("beefy red tongue")
- Angular cheilosis
- Mild jaundice (representative of intramedullary hemolysis of megaloblastic cells); "lemon yellow" skin due to pallor and jaundice
- Peripheral sensory neuropathy with paresthesia initially and absent reflexes in advanced disease
- Delirium or dementia
- Worsening weakness and possible subacute combined degeneration of spinal cord (Fig. E1)
- Loss of proprioception and an unsteady gait
- GI symptoms including anorexia, pyrosis, nausea, and vomiting
- Possible splenomegaly and mild hepatomegaly

ETIOLOGY[3,4]

- Parietal cell antibodies are present in >70% of patients, while intrinsic factor antibodies are noted in >50% of patients.

- Atrophic gastric mucosa (Fig. E2) with achlorhydria.
- Inborn errors of cobalamin-cofactor synthesis are rare. Fig. E3 illustrates the components and mechanism of cobalamin absorption. An etiopathophysiologic classification of cobalamin deficiency is described in Section II.

DX DIAGNOSIS

DIFFERENTIAL DIAGNOSIS

- Nutritional vitamin B_{12} deficiency
- Malabsorption (e.g., celiac disease)
- Chronic alcoholism (multifactorial)
- Chronic gastritis related to *H. pylori* infection
- Folic acid deficiency
- Myelodysplasia
- Thyroid abnormalities
- Atrophic gastritis
- Paraproteinemias
- Gastrectomy or use of H2 blockers
- Insufficient pancreatic enzymes (Zollinger-Ellison syndrome, chronic pancreatitis, post-Whipple procedure)

WORKUP

- The clinical presentation of PA varies with the stage. Initially, patients may be asymptomatic. In advanced stages, patients may have impaired memory, depression, gait disturbances, paresthesias, and generalized weakness.
- Investigation consists primarily of laboratory evaluation. Table 1 describes a step-wise approach to the diagnosis of cobalamin and folate deficiency.

- Endoscopy and biopsy for atrophic gastritis may be performed in selected cases.
- Diagnosis is crucial because failure to treat may result in irreversible neurologic deficits.

LABORATORY TESTS

- CBC generally reveals macrocytic anemia, thrombocytopenia, and mild leukopenia with hypersegmented neutrophils (Fig. E4).
- Mean corpuscular volume (MCV) is significantly elevated in advanced stages.
- Reticulocyte count is low to normal.
- False low serum cobalamin levels can occur in patients who are pregnant or taking oral contraceptives, have multiple myeloma, have transcobalamin I (TCI) deficiency, have severe folic acid deficiency, or are taking large doses of ascorbic acid. False high normal levels in patients with cobalamin deficiency can occur in several conditions including hepatomas, severe liver disease, or monoblastic leukemias (Table 2).
- The absence of anemia or macrocytosis does not exclude the diagnosis of cobalamin deficiency. Anemia is absent in 20% of patients with cobalamin deficiency, and macrocytosis is absent in >30% of patients at the time of diagnosis. Macrocytosis can be masked by concurrent iron deficiency, anemia of chronic disease, or thalassemia trait.
- Laboratory tests used for detecting cobalamin deficiency in patients with normal vitamin B_{12} levels include serum and urinary methylmalonic acid (MMA) level (elevated), total homocysteine level (elevated), and

TABLE 1 Stepwise Approach to the Diagnosis of Cobalamin and Folate Deficiency

Megaloblastic Anemia or Neurologic-Psychiatric Manifestations Consistent with Cobalamin Deficiency *Plus* Test Results on Serum Cobalamin and Serum Folate

Cobalamin[a] (pg/ml)	Folate[b] (ng/ml)	Provisional Diagnosis	Proceed With Metabolites?[c]
>300	>4	Cobalamin or folate deficiency is unlikely	No
<200	>4	Consistent with cobalamin deficiency	No
200-300	>4	Rule out cobalamin deficiency	Yes
>300	<2	Consistent with folate deficiency	No
<200	<2	Consistent with (1) combined cobalamin plus folate deficiency or (2) isolated folate deficiency	Yes
>300	2-4	Consistent with (1) folate deficiency or (2) an anemia unrelated to vitamin deficiency	Yes

Test Results on Metabolites: Serum Methylmalonic Acid and Total Homocysteine

Methylmalonic Acid (Normal, 70-270 nM)	Total Homocysteine (Normal, 5-14 μM)	Diagnosis
Increased	Increased	Cobalamin deficiency confirmed; folate deficiency still possible (i.e., combined cobalamin plus folate deficiency possible)
Normal	Increased	Folate deficiency is likely
Normal	Normal	Cobalamin and folate deficiency is excluded

[a]Serum cobalamin levels: Abnormally low, <200 pg/ml; clinically relevant low-normal range, 200-300 pg/ml.
[b]Serum folate levels: Abnormally low, <2 ng/ml; clinically relevant low-normal range, 2-4 ng/ml.
[c]Any frozen-over sample from serum folate/cobalamin determination can be subjected to metabolite tests.
From Hoffman R et al: *Hematology, basic principles and practice*, ed 8, Philadelphia, 2023, Elsevier.

TABLE 2 Serum Cobalamin: False-Positive and False-Negative Test Results

Falsely Low Serum Cobalamin in the Absence of True Cobalamin Deficiency

- Folate deficiency (one third of patients)
- Multiple myeloma
- TCI deficiency
- Megadose vitamin C therapy
- Pregnancy
- Oral contraceptives

Falsely Raised Cobalamin Levels in the Presence of a True Deficiency[a]

- Cobalamin binders (TCI and II) increased (e.g., myeloproliferative states, hepatomas, and fibrolamellar hepatic tumors)
- TCII-producing macrophages are activated (e.g., autoimmune diseases, monoblastic leukemias and lymphomas)
- Release of cobalamin from hepatocytes (e.g., active liver disease)
- High serum anti-IF antibody titer

IF, Intrinsic factor; *TC,* transcobalamin.

[a]Although a low serum cobalamin level is not synonymous with cobalamin deficiency, 5% of patients with true cobalamin deficiency have low-normal cobalamin levels, a potentially serious problem because the patient's underlying cobalamin deficiency will progress if uncorrected.

From Hoffman R et al: *Hematology, basic principles and practice,* ed 8, Philadelphia, 2023, Elsevier.

intrinsic factor antibody (positive). Cobalamin is a cofactor for the enzymes L-methylmalonyl coenzyme A mutase and methionine synthase. Inadequate levels of cobalamin will thus result in increased MMA and homocysteine levels. Plasma MMA levels can also be used to differentiate cobalamin deficiency from folate deficiency because patients with folate deficiency have normal or mild elevations of MMA levels.

- An increased concentration of plasma MMA does not predict clinical manifestations of vitamin B_{12} deficiency and should not be used as the only marker for diagnosis of B_{12} deficiency.
- Additional laboratory abnormalities can include elevated lactate dehydrogenase, direct hyperbilirubinemia, and decreased haptoglobin, due to rapid destruction of red blood cells.
- Bone marrow aspirate is not necessary to diagnose cobalamin deficiency. It may show giant C-shaped neutrophil bands and megaloblastic normoblasts (Fig. E5).
- Schilling test: No longer used or available. It was historically used to identify the locus of cobalamin malabsorption and the cause of cobalamin deficiency.

Rx TREATMENT[5-7]

NONPHARMACOLOGIC THERAPY

Avoid folic acid supplementation without proper vitamin B_{12} supplementation. Folic acid supplementation alone may result in hematologic remission in patients with vitamin B_{12} deficiency but will not treat or prevent neurologic manifestations.

ACUTE GENERAL Rx

Traditional therapy of cobalamin deficiency consists of intramuscular (IM) or deep subcutaneous (SC) injections of vitamin B_{12} 1000 mcg/day for 1 wk followed by a weekly administration for 1 to 2 mo and then monthly lifelong. Monitor response and increase dosing if serum B_{12} levels decline.

CHRONIC Rx

- Parenteral vitamin B_{12} 1000 mcg/mo or intranasal cyanocobalamin 500 mcg/wk for the remainder of life.
- In patients who have no nervous system involvement, intranasal cyanocobalamin may be used in place of parenteral cyanocobalamin after hematologic parameters have returned to normal range. Macrocytosis correction can be noted during the first mo of treatment. The initial dose of intranasal cyanocobalamin is 1 spray (500 mcg) in one nostril once per wk. Nasal cyanocobalamin is expensive.
- Oral cobalamin (1000 to 2000 mcg/day) is also being effective in mild cases of pernicious anemia because approximately 1% of an oral dose is absorbed by passive diffusion, a pathway that does not require intrinsic factor. Cost for 1 mo of therapy is approximately $5. Consider returning to IM vitamin B_{12} supplementation if decline recurs.

DISPOSITION

Anemia generally resolves with appropriate cobalamin replacement therapy. Neurologic deficits, on the other hand, may be corrected only if treated early on.

REFERRAL

Gastroenterology referral for endoscopy on diagnosis of PA followed by periodic surveillance endoscopies to rule out gastric adenocarcinoma or carcinoid tumors.

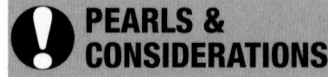

! PEARLS & CONSIDERATIONS

COMMENTS

- Early manifestations of negative cobalamin balance are increased serum methylmalonic

TABLE 3 Causes of Megaloblastosis Not Responding to Therapy with Cobalamin or Folate

Wrong Diagnosis

Combined folate and cobalamin deficiencies being treated with only one vitamin

Associated iron deficiency

Associated hemoglobinopathy (e.g., sickle cell disease, thalassemia)

Associated anemia of chronic disease

Associated hypothyroidism

From Hoffman R et al: *Hematology, basic principles and practice,* ed 8, Philadelphia, 2023, Elsevier.

acid and total homocysteine levels. This occurs when the total cobalamin in serum is still in the low-normal range.

- Vitamin B_{12} deficiency that is allowed to progress for longer than 3 mo may produce permanent degenerative lesions of the spinal cord (e.g., subacute combined degeneration of spinal cord).
- Vitamin B_{12} deficiency may suppress signs of polycythemia vera; treatment of B_{12} deficiency may unmask this disorder.
- Blunted or impeded therapeutic response to vitamin B_{12} may be due to concurrent iron or folic acid deficiency, uremia, infections, or use of drugs with bone marrow suppressant properties. Causes of megaloblastosis not responding to therapy with cobalamin or folate are summarized in Table 3.
- Drugs that interfere with B_{12} absorption include metformin, colchicine, neomycin, and aminosalicylic acid.
- Patients must understand that cobalamin replacement therapy is lifelong.
- Self-injection of vitamin B_{12} may be taught in selected patients. Cost of monthly injections is less than $10.
- Patients who have had bariatric surgery should receive 1 mg of oral vitamin B_{12} per day indefinitely.

REFERENCES

Available at eBooks.Health.Elsevier.com.

RELATED CONTENT

Pernicious Anemia (Patient Information)

AUTHOR: **SHIVA KUMAR R. MUKKAMALLA, MD, MPH**

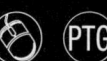 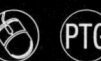
Diseases
and Disorders

I

BASIC INFORMATION

DEFINITION

Sore throat may represent pain or soreness in the pharynx or surrounding anatomy. Pharyngitis specifically refers to inflammation of the pharynx. Tonsillitis refers to inflammation of the tonsils, which are situated in the rear of the pharynx. Either pharyngitis or tonsillitis may present with pain, erythema, edema, exudates or enanthems (e.g., ulcers, vesicles).[1]

SYNONYMS

Sore throat
Acute pharyngitis
Pharyngitis
Tonsillitis
Group A *Streptococcus* (GAS)
Strep throat
Group A beta-hemolytic *Streptococcus* (GABHS)

ICD-10CM CODES
J02.0	Streptococcal pharyngitis
J02.8	Acute pharyngitis due to other specified organisms
J02.9	Acute pharyngitis, unspecified
J03.0	Streptococcal tonsillitis
J03.8	Acute tonsillitis due to other specified organisms
J03.9	Acute tonsillitis, unspecified

EPIDEMIOLOGY & DEMOGRAPHICS

Acute pharyngitis accounts for 1% to 2% of all ambulatory care visits and 12 million outpatient visits each year in the U.S.[2]

PREDOMINANT SEX: Females = males
PREDOMINANT AGE:
- All ages are affected (children <3 yr have atypical symptoms and rarely complain of sore throat).
- Incidence peaks in childhood and adolescence, with 50% of cases before age 18 yr.
- Streptococcal pharyngitis is most common among school-age children (ages 5 to 15 yr). GAS infections are responsible for 5% to 15% of cases of pharyngitis in adults and 35% to 40% of cases in children (ages 5 to 15 yr).

PEAK INCIDENCE:
- Late winter/early spring (GAS infections)[3]

PHYSICAL FINDINGS & CLINICAL PRESENTATION

- Pharynx:
  1. May appear normal to severely erythematous (Fig. E1).
  2. Tonsillar hypertrophy and exudates are commonly seen but do not confirm etiology.
- Common associated viral symptoms:
  1. Coryza
  2. Conjunctivitis
  3. Cough
  4. Cervical lymphadenopathy
  5. Findings associated with specific viral etiology
     a. Herpes simplex or enterovirus infection: Exudates and vesicles

  b. Severe acute respiratory syndrome coronavirus 2 (SARS-CoV-2): Fever, cough, diarrhea, and vomiting
  c. Epstein-Barr virus (EBV): Malaise, cervical node enlargement, exudates
  6. Rhinorrhea
- Common symptoms of candida:
  1. Pseudomembranous white plaques on buccal mucosa, palate, tongue
- Common bacterial symptoms, especially for GAS:
  1. Fever >38° C (100.4° F)
  2. Tonsillar exudate
  3. Scarlatiniform rash
  4. Strawberry tongue
  5. Systemic signs of infection
- Rare complications associated with GAS infection:
  1. Scarlet fever
  2. Rheumatic fever
  3. Acute glomerulonephritis
  4. Streptococcal toxic shock syndrome
  5. Pediatric autoimmune neuropsychiatric disorders associated with streptococcal infections (PANDAS) syndrome
- Extension of infection (Fig. E2): Tonsillar, parapharyngeal, or retropharyngeal abscess presenting with severe pain, high fever, trismus, respiratory distress, difficulty swallowing, and drooling.
- Streptococcal tonsillitis is manifested as acute onset of fever, headache, neck pain, dysphagia, odynophagia, sore throat, otalgia, red tongue with enlargement of papillae, sore throat, red swollen uvula, palatal petechiae, and tender anterior cervical adenitis.
- Peritonsillar abscess (accumulation of pus between the tonsil and its capsule) is the most common complication of acute tonsillitis. Clinical signs include dysphagia, odynophagia, drooling, neck stiffness, deformed posterior pharynx, displacement of the uvula, trismus, muffled voice (hot-potato voice), and respiratory distress.
- Lingual tonsillitis is a rarely diagnosed cause of pharyngitis that predominantly occurs in patients who have had their palatine tonsils removed. The lingual tonsils are located below the inferior pole of the palatine tonsils and anterior to the vallecula at the base of the tongue. The lymphoid tissue may enlarge after tonsillectomy and repeated infections. Patients have a sore throat that worsens with movement of the tongue. Physical findings often include a normal-appearing pharynx because the lingual tonsils cannot be visualized on routine oral examination. Lateral soft tissue neck films reveal an obliterated vallecular space and a thick-appearing epiglottis (Fig. E3).[4]
- Box 1 describes seven danger signs in patients with sore throat.

ETIOLOGY

- Viruses:
  1. Adenovirus
  2. Coronavirus, including SARS-CoV-2
  3. Cytomegalovirus
  4. Enterovirus

  5. Epstein-Barr virus
  6. Herpes simplex virus
  7. Human metapneumovirus
  8. Influenza
  9. Parainfluenza
  10. Respiratory syncytial virus
  11. Rhinovirus
  12. HIV
- Bacteria:
  1. GAS: The most common cause of acute tonsillitis
  2. *Fusobacterium necrophorum* (10% of pharyngitis): Highest incidence in patients ages 15 to 30 yr
  3. *Haemophilus influenzae* B
  4. *Neisseria gonorrhoeae*
  5. *Peptostreptococcus*
  6. *Prevotella*
  7. Mixed anaerobes: Associated with Vincent angina
- Other organisms:
  1. Arcanobacterium haemolyticum
  2. Candida albicans
  3. Chlamydophila pneumoniae
  4. Chlamydia trachomatis
  5. Mycoplasma pneumoniae
  6. Corynebacterium diphtheriae
  7. Francisella tularensis
  8. Yersinia pestis
  9. Yersinia enterocolitica

DIAGNOSIS

DIFFERENTIAL DIAGNOSIS

- Infectious: Viral, bacterial, fungal, peritonsillar abscess, Lemierre syndrome, epiglottitis, tracheitis, croup, lateral or retropharyngeal abscess, uvulitis. Table 1 summarizes characteristics of viral and bacterial pharyngitis
- Allergic/inflammatory: Allergic rhinitis/sinusitis, gastroesophageal reflux disease, Kawasaki disease, periodic fever with aphthous stomatitis, Stevens-Johnson syndrome, Behçet syndrome, angioedema, anaphylaxis, sore throat associated with granulocytopenia, thyroiditis
- Environmental exposure: Foreign body ingestion, chemical exposure (e.g., smoke), irritative pharyngitis, trauma
- Referred pain: Psychogenic pharyngitis, referred pain from dental abscess, otitis media, cervical adenitis

---

BOX 1 Seven Danger Signs in Patients with Sore Throat

1. Persistence of symptoms longer than 1 wk without improvement
2. Respiratory difficulty, particularly stridor
3. Difficulty in handling secretions
4. Difficulty in swallowing
5. Severe pain in the absence of erythema
6. A palpable mass
7. Blood, even in small amounts, in the pharynx or ear

From Andreoli TE et al: *Andreoli and Carpenter's Cecil essentials of medicine,* ed 8, Philadelphia, 2010, Saunders.

TABLE 1 Characteristics of Viral and Bacterial Pharyngitis

	Viral Pharyngitis	Infectious Mononucleosis	Group A Streptococcal Pharyngitis	Diphtheria
Population	*Any*	*Older Children*	*Peak 5-6 Yr Old*	*Unimmunized*
Onset	Slow	Variable	Rapid	Rapid
Associated symptoms	Rhinorrhea, congestion, hoarseness, oral ulcers	General malaise, headache	Headache, otalgia, nausea, abdominal pain	None
Fever	None or low-grade	High	High	High
Sore throat severity	Mild to moderate	Moderate to severe	Severe	Severe
Dysphagia	Possible	Yes	Yes	Yes
Odynophagia	None	Yes	Yes	Yes
Toxic appearance	No	Sometimes airway obstruction	No	Yes, severe upper airway obstruction
PE findings	Pharyngeal erythema; no exudate; ± tonsil hypertrophy	Palatal petechiae ± tonsil hypertrophy ± exudate; large tender cervical lymphadenopathy; splenomegaly; hepatomegaly	Palatal petechiae, pharyngeal erythema, tonsil hypertrophy ± exudate; large tender cervical lymphadenopathy; scalariform rash; strawberry tongue	Thick exudate, pharyngeal membrane
Diagnostic testing	None	Heterophile or EBV titers	Rapid strep or strep culture	Culture on tellurite media
Treatment	Supportive	Supportive, ibuprofen, steroids, rare airway obstruction	Penicillin or amoxicillin	Antitoxin, penicillin G, amoxicillin

EBV, Epstein-Barr virus; *PE,* Physical examination.
From Flint PW et al: *Cummings otolaryngology, head and neck surgery,* ed 7, Philadelphia, 2021, Elsevier.

BOX 2 Centor Score (Modified/McIsaac) for Determining Group A Beta-Hemolytic Streptococcal Pharyngitis

- Age
- Tonsillar exudate or swelling
- Tender/swollen anterior lymphadenopathy or lymphadenitis
- Absence of cough
- History of fever 38° C (100.4° F) or higher

- Oncologic: Tonsillar hypertrophy associated with lymphoma, lymphangioma, or hemangioma of airway
- Section II describes the differential diagnosis of sore throat

WORKUP

The Centor criteria identify patients at risk for GAS and consist of (1) fever subjective or measured >38° C (100.5° F), (2) absence of cough, (3) tonsillar exudates, and (4) tender anterior cervical lymphadenopathy. The McIsaac criteria add 1 point for ages 3 to 14 and subtract 1 point for ages ≥45 yr (Box 2 and Table 2). Patients with ≤1 criteria are at low risk and do not need additional testing. Indications for screening for GABHS carrier state are summarized in Table 3.

- Rapid antigen detection test (RADT) (culture should be performed if RADT negative)
- Gold standard: Throat swab for culture

LABORATORY TESTS

- Testing for bacteria other than GAS is performed infrequently.
- Reserved for patients with persistent signs or symptoms suggestive of a specific non-GAS bacteria.
- For example, gonococcal testing in a sexually active patient. In a patient with suspected EBV,

TABLE 2 Centor Criteria (Modified/McIsaac) Scoring for Determining Testing and Treatment for Group A Beta-Hemolytic Streptococcal Pharyngitis

Centor Score	Testing and Treatment
0-1	No further testing or antibiotics
2	Optional rapid strep testing and/or culture
3	Consider rapid strep testing and/or culture
4	Consider rapid strep testing and/or culture. Empiric antibiotics may be appropriate depending on the specific scenario

TABLE 3 Screening for Group A β-Hemolytic *Streptococcus* Carrier State

Screening for GABHS carrier state is not indicated except:
1. In patients with a history or family history of rheumatic fever
2. During a community outbreak of rheumatic fever, poststreptococcal glomerulonephritis, or invasive GABHS infection
3. When tonsillectomy is being considered
4. When symptomatic GABHS spreads among household members

Although both have positive throat culture results, true infections are distinguished from the carrier state by the addition of:
1. A rise in the antistreptolysin-O titer of ≥0.2 log₁₀ between the acute and convalescent phase (2-4 wk after presentation)
2. Relevant history of symptoms and signs during episode

Documented response to antibiotics

GABHS, Group A β-hemolytic *Streptococcus.*
From Flint PW et al: *Cummings otolaryngology, head and neck surgery,* ed 7, Philadelphia, 2021, Elsevier.

a CBC may show atypical lymphocytes or a mononucleosis slide agglutination test (Monospot) may confirm clinical diagnosis of EBV. When indicated based on population prevalence and supply availability, a nasal swab for a general respiratory viral panel or specifically SARS-CoV-2 will help indicate a viral etiology.

IMAGING STUDIES

- Seldom indicated.
- Imaging is not necessary to make the diagnosis of a peritonsillar abscess.

- If there is concern for parapharyngeal or retropharyngeal space infection, computed tomography (CT) or MRI is preferred over plain radiographs.[5]

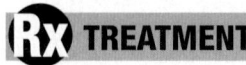 **TREATMENT**

NONPHARMACOLOGIC THERAPY

- Rest
- Soft diet
- Hydration

- Warm saltwater gargles
- Warm beverages with honey or lemon (avoid honey in children <12 mo of age due to risk of infantile botulism)
- Cold beverages/ice chips
- Anesthetic spray/lozenges (Avoid lozenges in children <4 yr due to choking hazard. Avoid benzocaine-containing sprays in children <2 due to risk of methemoglobinemia)

ACUTE GENERAL Rx

- Analgesics: Acetaminophen (adults and children) or ibuprofen (adults and children ≥6 mo of age).
- Systemic glucocorticoids are not recommended in uncomplicated pharyngitis/tonsillitis because of increased risk of adverse events; analgesics are effective for pain. However, low-dose corticosteroids can be considered in patients >3 yr.
- The primary benefit and intent of antibiotic treatment in GAS pharyngitis is the prevention of acute rheumatic fever.[6]
- If streptococcal infection is proven or suspected:
  1. Amoxicillin Immediate Release Tablets: 50 mg/kg/day PO once daily or divided every 12 h for 7 to 10 days. Maximum daily dose: 1000 mg/day.
  2. Amoxicillin Extended Release (≥12 yr old): 775 mg PO once daily for 7 to 10 days.
  3. Penicillin V (≤27 kg) 250 mg PO every 8 to 12 h for 7 to 10 days or (>27 kg) 500 mg PO every 8 to 12 h for 7 to 10 days.
  4. Benzathine penicillin (≤27 kg) 600,000 U intramuscularly (IM) once or (>27 kg) 1.2 million U IM once. Consider in noncompliant patients with history of acute rheumatic fever.
  5. If avoiding penicillin, cephalexin 40 mg/kg/day PO divided every 12 h for 7 to 10 days. Maximum 500 mg/dose.
  6. If anaphylactically sensitive to penicillin, clindamycin 7 mg/kg PO (max. 300 mg/dose) every 8 h for 7 to 10 days.
- If uncomplicated gonococcal pharyngitis infection:[7]
  1. <150 kg: Ceftriaxone 500 mg IM once; ≥150 kg: Ceftriaxone 1g IM once.
  2. Unless chlamydia is excluded via microbiologic testing: Doxycycline 100 mg PO twice a day for 7 days. If pregnant: Azithromycin 1g PO once.

3. Consult infectious disease specialist for alternative regimen if anaphylaxis or severe allergic reaction to ceftriaxone.
- Treatment of peritonsillar abscess is drainage through needle or incision.

CHRONIC Rx

- Recurrent streptococcal infections are common and may represent chronic carrier status, reinfection before antibody development, new infection to a different GAS M subtype, poor compliance to antibiotic, or rarely, an immune disorder.
- Recurrence in children is defined as seven or more infections in 1 yr, five or more infections in 2 yr, or three or more infections in 3 yr.
- Chronic carrier: Oral treatment options include clindamycin, amoxicillin-clavulanate, and penicillin plus rifampin.
- In adults, tonsillectomy is rarely indicated for patients with recurrent GAS.
- In children, tonsillectomy may lower the incidence for recurrent pharyngitis.
- In both children and adults, each individual case is reviewed based on patient age, frequency or severity of infections, history of antibiotic use, and patient preferences.
- Indications for tonsillectomy in treatment of recurrent streptococcal tonsillitis are summarized in Box 3.

DISPOSITION

- Tonsillopharyngitis is generally managed in an outpatient setting with follow-up arranged in 1 to 2 wk.

BOX 3 Indications for Tonsillectomy in Treatment of Recurrent Strep Tonsillitis

Well-documented clinical features for each episode:
- Sore throat associated with fever >38.3° C (>100.9° F)
- Cervical lymphadenopathy, tonsillar exudate, or GABHS positive testing
- Frequency of seven episodes or more in the preceding year, five or more episodes in each of the preceding 2 yr, or three or more episodes in each of the preceding 3 yr

Other factors that inform decision making about surgical intervention:
- How well infections have responded to medical therapy
- Quality-of-life issues (e.g., days of work/school missed)
- Children who have multiple antibiotic allergies or intolerance
- Periodic fever with aphthous stomatitis, pharyngitis, and adenitis
- History of peritonsillar abscess

From Flint PW et al: *Cummings otolaryngology, head and neck surgery*, ed 7, Philadelphia, 2021, Elsevier.

- Admission to the hospital is indicated for local suppurative complications (peritonsillar abscess; lateral pharyngeal, posterior, or retropharyngeal abscess; concern for impending airway closure or respiratory distress; or inability to swallow food, medications, or water).

REFERRAL

- To otolaryngologist:
  1. If peritonsillar or other abscess is suspected
  2. If tonsillar hypertrophy persists

PREVENTION

- Hand hygiene.
- Antimicrobial prophylaxis is only recommended in patients with a history of acute rheumatic fever and is based on the risk of recurrence and severity of disease.
- Influenza vaccine for children ≥6 mo.[8] COVID-19 vaccine for children ≥6 mo.[9]

REFERENCES

Available at eBooks.Health.Elsevier.com.

RELATED CONTENT

Sore Throat (Patient Information)
Strep Throat (Patient Information)
Tonsillitis (Patient Information)

AUTHORS: **VIKNESH S. KASTHURI, AB** and **MARK F. BRADY, MD, MPH, MMSc**

BASIC INFORMATION

DEFINITION

Enterobius vermicularis is a small (5 to 13 mm) helminth of the nematode (roundworm) family that can cause noninvasive infestation of the large intestine.[1] Female worms have a notably long, pointed tail that is similar in appearance to a pin; therefore *E. vermicularis* is also referred to as pinworms. Other species such as *Enterobius gregorii* and *Syphacia obvelata* have been described to cause pinworms; however, *E. vermicularis* is the most frequent culprit.[2]

SYNONYMS

Pinworms
Enterobiasis
Oxyuriasis
Seatworms
Threadworms
Roundworms

ICD-10CM CODE
B80   Enterobiasis

EPIDEMIOLOGY & DEMOGRAPHICS

- *E. vermicularis* is the most prevalent helminth infection in the U.S., with an estimated prevalence of 20 to 40 million infected individuals.[3,4]
- *E. vermicularis* is found worldwide, although most commonly in temperate climates and tropical regions.[4]
- Close proximity and poor hand hygiene raise the risk of infection.[2]
- Pinworms are easily spread in day care settings, institutions, within homes, and in other environments with overcrowded living conditions.[3]
- Preschool/early grade school age children and their caretakers, as well as institutionalized persons, have the highest risk of infection.[2]

PHYSICAL FINDINGS & CLINICAL PRESENTATION

- Many individuals (30% to 50%) with pinworms are asymptomatic.[3]
- The most common symptom is perianal pruritus, often worse at night, and resulting in nocturnal restlessness. Itching can lead to excoriations and secondary bacterial infection.[2]
- Symptomatic individuals may display insomnia, enuresis, and teeth-grinding, secondary to constant scratching in attempts to relieve irritation. Anorexia secondary to pinworms has been reported.[4]
- Abdominal pain and nausea/vomiting may occur in individuals with high worm burden.[1]
- While pinworms live primarily in the cecum of the large intestine, infestations are not just limited to the gastrointestinal tract; pinworms can also infest the urethra and vulva, presenting as urethritis and vaginitis, respectively. Though rare, salpingitis and oophoritis have been reported.[3]
- Although rare, complications occur including appendicitis, resulting from a high worm burden obstructing the lumen of the appendix, eosinophilic enteritis, and urinary tract infection.[1]

ETIOLOGY & PATHOGENESIS

- Humans are the definitive host for *E. vermicularis*.[2]
- *E. vermicularis* has a fecal-oral transmission pattern. It is spread directly via hand-to-mouth contact, indirectly via fomites, through person-to-person contact, and through ingestion of contaminated food.[4]
- In rare cases, pinworm eggs can become airborne and subsequently inhaled.[3]
- *E. vermicularis* may be transmitted between sexual partners, especially those engaging in oral-anal sex.[5]
- The pinworm species that infect humans and animals are different from each other and do not spread between species.[2]
- Upon ingestion of embryonated eggs, larvae hatch in the small intestine and then migrate to the large intestine once matured (1 to 2 mo). Gravid females tend to occupy distal aspects of the large intestine and migrate to the perianal region at night to release approximately 10,000 eggs.[2]
- The larvae within the eggs mature and become infectious within 4 to 6 h of deposition. Eggs may survive and remain infectious for up to 2 to 3 wk in an indoor environment.[2]
- Embryonated eggs are pruritic, and when the host scratches the perianal region, the eggs are retained under the fingernails. This can lead to autoinfection via hand-to-mouth contact or infection of others via the fecal-oral route.[2]
- Retroinfection, when newly hatched larvae migrate from the perianal region into the rectum, can occur but is not thought to be common.[5]
- In the absence of autoinfection, *Enterobius* infestation lasts only 4 to 6 wk.[1]

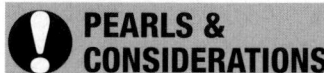 **DIAGNOSIS**

DIFFERENTIAL DIAGNOSIS

- Perianal itching related to poor hygiene. Section II describes the causes of pruritus ani, which include infectious (e.g., group A strep, *Mycoplasma pneumoniae*) and inflammatory (e.g., lichen sclerosis) pathologies
- Perineal yeast/fungal infection
- Sexually transmitted infections
- Hemorrhoids and anal fissures

WORKUP

Direct visualization of the adult worm or microscopic examination of eggs confirms the diagnosis; however, only up to 5% of infected patients will have eggs in their stool.[1] *E. vermicularis* ova are 50 by 30 microns with one flattened side and surrounded by a thick, smooth, and colorless shell (Fig. E1).[4] The eggs are best identified via the cellophane (Scotch) tape test in which transparent tape (Fig. E2) is placed on the perianal skin and viewed under the microscope.[6] The test is most effective on awakening prior to bathing.[4] A single examination detects 50% of infections, three examinations detect 90%, and five examinations detect 99%.[4] Examinations should be performed on different days. Five consecutive negative tests effectively rule out the diagnosis. Pinworm paddles are clear plastic paddles that can be used in place of transparent tape. No serologic testing for *E. vermicularis* is available. Given that *E. vermicularis* does not cause invasive disease, there is no associated peripheral eosinophilia.

Rx **TREATMENT**

- It is reasonable to empirically treat patients with anal pruritus.
- Treatment options include either a single dose of mebendazole (100 mg), albendazole (400 mg), or pyrantel pamoate (11 mg/kg up to 1g) followed by a repeat dose in 2 wk. Mebendazole and albendazole are expensive and require a prescription whereas pyrantel pamoate is available over the counter.[2,4,5]
- It can be difficult to eradicate infestations due to reinfection and autoinfection.[5] Retreatment at 2 wk targets newly hatched pinworms before they can lay eggs.[2,5]
- Other infected family members and asymptomatic close contacts and sexual contacts should be treated.[4,5]
- Clothing and bedding should be cleaned to prevent reinfection.[4]

! **PEARLS & CONSIDERATIONS**

PREVENTION

- Good compliance with basic hand hygiene is the most effective method of prevention.[2-4]
- Control of *E. vermicularis* infection and prevention of recurrence and autoinfection require both antihelminthic treatment of all close contacts (including sexual partners) and household members as well as decontamination of the environment (mopping or using a wet disinfectant is preferred to sweeping or dusting) and frequent changing of clothing and bedding.[2]

PATIENT & FAMILY EDUCATION

- Fingernails should be cut short and scrubbed frequently as pinworm eggs can reside beneath the nails.[2,3]
- Morning showering to clear the eggs deposited on the skin overnight helps to prevent recurrent autoinfection.[2]
- Showering is preferred over taking baths to limit the risk of ingesting pinworms from contaminated bath water; infected individuals should not cobathe with others while infected.[2]

REFERENCES
Available at eBooks.Health.Elsevier.com.

RELATED CONTENT
Pinworms (Patient Information)

AUTHORS: **CAROLINE LEAHY, MD** and **JEREMY MICHEL, MD, MHS**

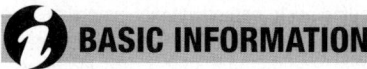

DEFINITION

The diagnosis of placenta previa is based on sonography and requires the identification of echogenic homogeneous placental tissue over the internal cervical os. When the placental edge is <2 cm from the internal os, the placenta is called "low-lying." The historic terms "marginal" and "partial" for characterizing a placenta previa are no longer used. A classification of placenta previa in "major" or "minor" is described in Table 1 and illustrated in Fig. 1.

One hypothesis is that the lower uterine cavity contains more vascularized decidua, which promotes implantation of trophoblast toward the cervical os. Another hypothesis is that a particularly large placental surface area increases the probability that the placenta will implant over the cervical os.

ICD-10CM CODES

O44	Placenta previa
O44.0	Complete placenta previa NOS or without hemorrhage
O44.1	Complete placenta previa with hemorrhage
O44.2	Partial placenta previa without hemorrhage
O44.3	Partial placenta previa with hemorrhage
O44.4	Low-lying placenta NOS or without hemorrhage
O44.5	Low-lying placenta with hemorrhage

TABLE 1 Classification of Placenta Previa

Minor	I	Encroaches the lower uterine segment
	II	Reaches internal os of the cervix (marginal)
Major	III	Covers part of internal os (partial)
	IV	Completely covers the internal os (complete)

From Magowan BA: *Clinical obstetrics and gynecology,* ed 4, London, 2019, Elsevier.

EPIDEMIOLOGY & DEMOGRAPHICS

INCIDENCE: The pooled prevalence of major placenta previa was 4.3 cases/1000 pregnancies. Prevalence was highest among Asian studies (12.2/1000) and lower among studies from Europe (3.6/1000), North America (2.9/1000), and sub-Saharan Africa (2.7/1000).

RISK FACTORS:
- Previous placenta previa (recurs in 4% to 8% of subsequent pregnancies)
- Previous cesarean delivery (increases incidence by 47% to 60%)
- Multiparity
- Multiple gestation (increases prevalence by 40%)
- Smoking and cocaine use
- Previous intrauterine surgical procedure or Asherman syndrome
- Abnormal or large placenta

PHYSICAL FINDINGS & CLINICAL PRESENTATION

The classic presentation of placenta previa is painless vaginal bleeding, usually in the second or third trimester. 10% to 20% of women present with uterine contractions, pain, and bleeding. On physical examination, the uterus is soft and pain free. The fetus is often in breech, transverse lie, or high. Fetal distress is usually not present.

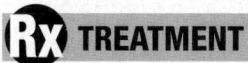

DIFFERENTIAL DIAGNOSIS

- Morbidly adherent placenta (accreta, increta, percreta)
- Vasa previa
- Abruptio placentae
- Vaginal or cervical trauma
- Labor
- Local malignancy

WORKUP

- Do *not* perform a digital vaginal examination.
- Perform a speculum examination in a hospital setting to exclude any local bleeding.
- Perform a transvaginal ultrasonography to assess for placental location.

- Exclude the presence of placenta previa-accreta in patients with a history of cesarean deliveries. The frequency of placenta accreta increases with an increasing number of cesarean deliveries.

LABORATORY TESTS

- A CBC can be used to monitor hemoglobin and hematocrit.
- A Kleihauer-Betke preparation of maternal blood in all Rh-negative women and Rh-immune globulin when indicated.

IMAGING STUDIES

- The simplest and safest method of placental localization is transabdominal sonography with confirmatory imaging by transvaginal ultrasonography (TVUS). Transabdominal ultrasonography alone is inaccurate in the diagnosis of placenta previa and should be used only as a screening tool. TVUS (Fig. 2) has become the gold standard for the diagnosis of placenta previa. It is safe even in the presence of active bleeding.
- MRI has also been effective in detecting placenta previa, although sonography remains the preferred method due to lower cost, widespread availability, and well-established accuracy.

Rx TREATMENT

MANAGEMENT OF ASYMPTOMATIC PLACENTA PREVIA

- Avoid sexual activity, digital exams, and extraneous exercise.
- Review bleeding precautions and anticipatory guidance, including the need for cesarean delivery and the risk for hysterectomy early in pregnancy.

Sequential assessment of placental location:
- At 32 wk, follow-up is indicated:
  1. If the placental edge is ≥2 cm from the internal os, placenta previa has resolved, and no further assessment is required.
  2. If the placental edge is over or <2 cm from the internal os, placenta previa persists, and repeat at 36 wk is indicated.

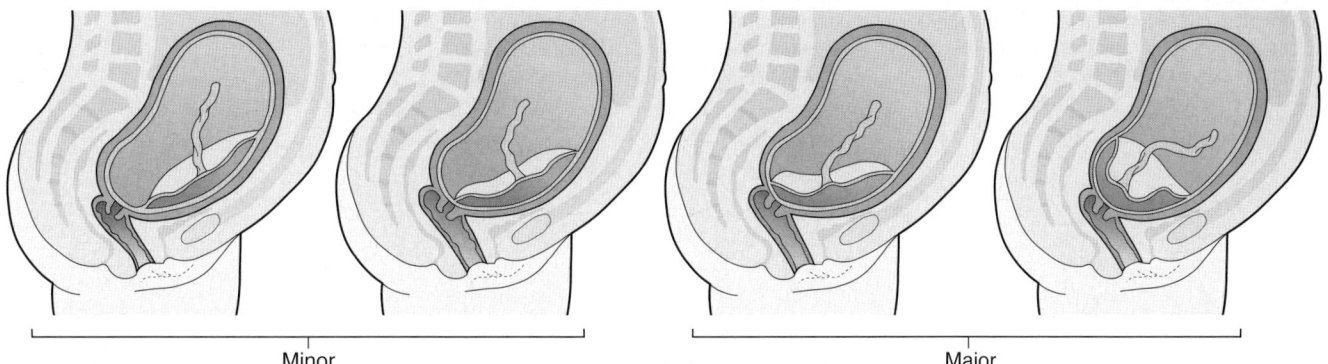

Minor   Major

FIG. 1 Classification into "major" and "minor" placenta previa depends on the distance of the placenta from the internal os of the cervix. In the presence of a cesarean delivery scar, an anterior placenta previa may result in abnormal invasion (morbidly adherent placenta, placenta accreta). (From Magowan BA: *Clinical obstetrics and gynecology,* ed 4, London, 2019, Elsevier.)

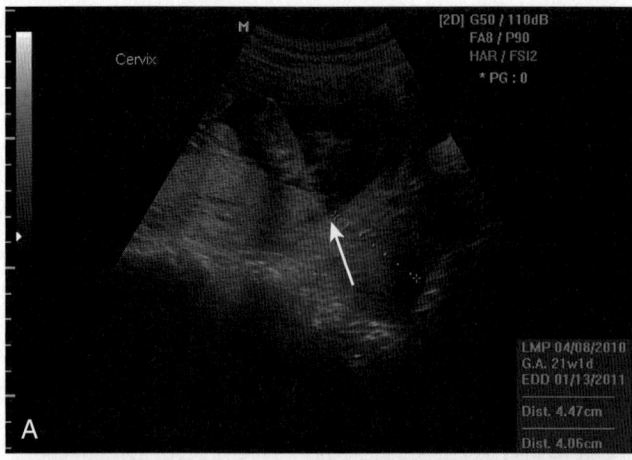

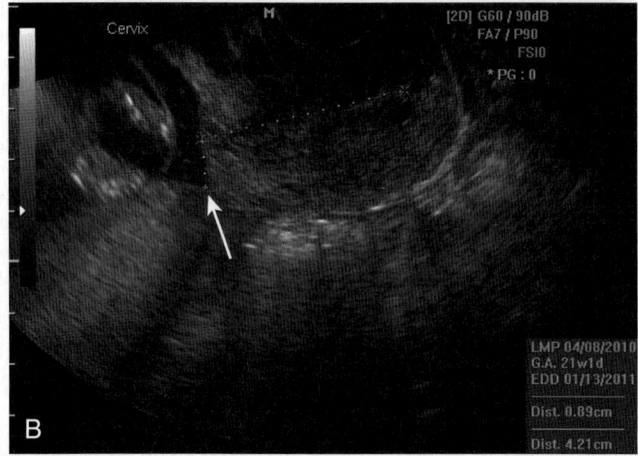

FIG. 2 Transabdominal ultrasonography and transvaginal ultrasonography of marginal placenta previa. *Arrows* identify placental edge. (Courtesy K. Francois. From Gabbe SG: *Obstetrics,* ed 6, Philadelphia, 2012, Saunders.)

- At 36 wk:
  1. If the placental edge is ≥2 cm, the patient is consented for vaginal delivery.
  2. If the placental edge is over the internal os, cesarean delivery is scheduled.

Timing of delivery:
- Cesarean delivery at 36+0 to 37+6 wk in pregnancies with uncomplicated placenta previa

MANAGEMENT OF SYMPTOMATIC PLACENTA PREVIA

- Initial assessment for signs of maternal hemodynamic compromise or hemorrhagic shock; large-bore intravenous (IV) access with crystalloid fluid resuscitation.
- Assess fetal status and gestational age by sonogram and continuous fetal heart rate monitoring.
- Cross-matched blood should be made available during bleeding episodes.
- Tocolytic therapy should not be administered in an actively bleeding patient.
- Magnesium sulfate therapy for fetal neuroprotection should be considered in those with symptomatic preterm (<32 wk) placenta previa if the decision has been made to likely deliver the patient within 24 h. Emergent delivery should not be delayed to administer magnesium.
- Cesarean delivery is indicated for active labor, nonreassuring fetal heart rate tracing, active bleeding with hemodynamic instability, and significant bleeding after 34 wk gestation.

Expectant management after a resolved bleed:
- Antenatal corticosteroid should be administered to symptomatic women between 23+0 and 36+6 wk gestation to enhance fetal pulmonary maturity.
- Correct anemia.
- Administer anti-D immune globulin to D-negative women.

DISPOSITION

Inpatient vs. outpatient: Consider discharge for women whose bleeding has stopped for 24 h and live in close proximity to the hospital, demonstrate compliance with medical management, can maintain bed rest, understand bleeding precautions, and have an adult companion available for transport 24 h a day.

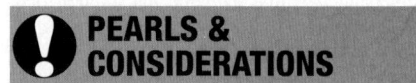

COMMENTS

- Placenta previa is diagnosed by TVUS, with repeat assessment at 32 and 36 wk when indicated.
- Asymptomatic placenta previa can be managed expectantly with a planned cesarean delivery at 36+0 to 37+6 wk.
- Symptomatic placenta previa is managed by assessing hemodynamic stability, considering steroids for fetal lung maturity, magnesium sulfate for fetal neuroprotection when indicated, and cesarean delivery.

RELATED CONTENT

Placenta Previa (Patient Information)
Vaginal Bleeding During Pregnancy (Related Key Topic)

AUTHORS: **HELEN B. GOMEZ SLAGLE, MD** and **ANTHONY SCISCIONE, DO**

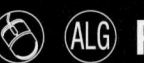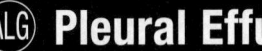

P

BASIC INFORMATION

DEFINITION

A pleural effusion is the pathologic accumulation of fluid in the pleural space, stemming from a wide range of etiologies.

SYNONYMS

Exudates
Transudates
Hydrothorax
Hemothorax
Chylothorax
Empyema

ICD-10CM CODES
J90   Pleural effusion, not elsewhere classified
J91.8 Pleural effusion in other conditions classified elsewhere

PHYSICAL FINDINGS & CLINICAL PRESENTATION

- Subjective symptoms largely depend on the underlying etiology and may include dyspnea, cough, fatigue, fever, chest pain.
- Box 1 summarizes signs and symptoms of pleural effusion.
- Physical examination findings include asymmetric chest wall expansion, dullness to percussion, decreased tactile fremitus, and decreased breath sounds.

ETIOLOGY

A pleural effusion may be caused by increased fluid entry into the pleural space; this can occur in the setting of increased capillary permeability, increased vascular hydrostatic pressure or decreased vascular oncotic pressure. Decreased exit of the fluid from the pleural space in the setting of inflammation of the pleura, traumatic/iatrogenic causes, and/or obstruction of normal pleural fluid efflux can also lead to effusion formation. Box 2 summarizes causes of pleural effusion.[1]

BOX 1   Signs and Symptoms of Effusion

Dyspnea
Cough (dry, nonproductive)
Chest pain (pleuritic or nonpleuritic)
Chest wall discomfort
Decreased breath sounds
Dullness to percussion
Egophony, decreased tactile fremitus
Pleural friction rub
Asymmetric chest wall excursion

Disease-Specific Signs and Symptoms may Include:
Orthopnea
Paroxysmal nocturnal dyspnea
Fever
Night sweats

From Adams JG et al: *Emergency medicine: clinical essentials,* ed 2, Philadelphia, 2013, Elsevier.

BOX 2   Causes of Pleural Effusions

Transudates
Atelectasis (early)
Congestive heart failure
Central venous occlusion
Glomerulonephritis
Hepatic hydrothorax
Hypoalbuminemia
Myxedema
Nephrotic syndrome
Peritoneal dialysis
Pulmonary embolism
Veno-occlusive disease

Exudates
Infectious
Bacterial infection
Fungal infection
Lung abscess
Parasitic infection
Traumatic hemothorax
Tuberculosis
Viral illness

Malignancies
Lymphoma
Mesothelioma
Primary lung cancer
Pulmonary metastasis

Connective Tissue Disease
Eosinophilic granulomatosis
Granulomatosis with polyangiitis
Rheumatoid arthritis
Systemic lupus erythematosus
Sjögren syndrome

Abdominal/Gastrointestinal
Esophageal rupture
Pancreatic disorders
Subphrenic abscess

Other
Asbestos
Atelectasis (chronic)
Chylothorax
Cerebrospinal fluid leak or ventriculopleural shunt
Drug reactions (amiodarone, nitrofurantoin)
Hemothorax
Meigs syndrome
Myxedema
Postpartum state
Postsurgical (abdominal, cardiac bypass)
Pulmonary infarction or embolism
Thoracic endometriosis
Uremia
Superior vena cava syndrome
Yellow nail syndrome

From Adams JG et al: *Emergency medicine: clinical essentials,* ed 2, Philadelphia, 2013, Elsevier.

DIAGNOSIS

DIFFERENTIAL DIAGNOSIS

Differential diagnosis for causes of pleural effusion includes:

- **Transudate:** Effusions that stem from hydrostatic and oncotic imbalances; characterized by pleural: serum lactate dehydrogenase (LDH) ratio ≤0.6, pleural: serum protein ratio ≤0.5, and pleural LDH ratio ≤⅔ upper limit of normal serum LDH.[2] Possible causes of transudative pleural effusions include:
  1. Heart failure
  2. Cirrhosis (hepatic hydrothorax)
  3. Chronic renal insufficiency (nephrotic syndrome or peritoneal dialysis)
  4. Hypoalbuminemia
  5. Myxedema
  6. Pericardial disease
  7. Urinothorax
- **Exudate:** Effusions that stem from an infiltrative or inflammatory process; characterized by pleural to serum LDH ratio >0.6 or total protein ratio >0.5 or pleural to upper limit of normal for serum LDH ratio >2:3. Box 3 describes cellular differential of pleural effusions. Possible causes of exudative pleural effusions include:
  1. Malignancy: metastatic cancer or primary (e.g., mesothelioma)
  2. Infection (Table E1)
     a. Parapneumonic effusion (simple = pH >7.2, complicated = ≤7.2 or glucose <60)[3]
     b. Empyema (pus in the pleural space, positive pleural fluid cultures or Gram stain from pleural fluid; see chapter on "Empyema")
     c. Fungal
     d. Tuberculous effusion
     e. Viral

BOX 3   Cellular Differential of Pleural Effusions

Neutrophilia (>50%)
- Bacterial pneumonia (parapneumonic effusion)
- Pulmonary infarction
- Pancreatitis
- Subphrenic abscess
- Early tuberculosis
- Transudates (>10%)

Lymphocytosis (>50%)
- Tuberculosis
- Viral infection
- Malignancy (lymphoma, other neoplasms)
- True chylothorax
- Rheumatoid pleuritis
- Systemic lupus erythematosus
- Uremic effusions
- Transudates (≈30%)

Eosinophilia (>10%)
- Pneumothorax (air in pleural space)
- Trauma
- Pulmonary infarction
- Congestive heart failure
- Infection (especially parasitic, fungal)
- Hypersensitivity syndromes
- Drug reaction
- Rheumatologic diseases
- Hodgkin disease
- Idiopathic
- Iatrogenic (repeat taps introducing blood/air)

From McPherson RA, Pincus MR: *Henry's clinical diagnosis and management by laboratory methods,* ed 23, St Louis, 2017, Elsevier.

3. Pulmonary embolism (rarely can present as transudate)
4. Hemothorax
5. Chylothorax
6. Esophageal perforation
7. Pleuropancreatic fistula
8. Biliothorax
9. Collagen vascular disease (e.g., rheumatoid arthritis, systemic lupus erythematosus, eosinophilic granulomatosis, granulomatosis with polyangiitis [Table E2])
10. Asbestos
11. Meigs syndrome (association of pleural effusion with ascites and ovarian fibroma)

WORKUP

After a careful history and physical exam, thoracentesis can help to establish the etiology of a pleural effusion. The Light criteria should be used for classification of the pleural effusion (summarized in Box 4). Fig. 1 illustrates a diagnostic algorithm for pleural effusions. A thorough history and physical examination can avoid unnecessary instrumentation, as it is important to remember that not all pleural effusions need to be immediately sampled (e.g., clear history of heart failure).[1,4] Fig. E2 illustrates an approach to malignant pleural effusions.

LABORATORY TESTS

See Table 3.

IMAGING STUDIES

- **Chest x-ray examination** (Fig. 3): Blunting of the costophrenic angle, ipsilateral atelectasis, contralateral shift of the mediastinum with large effusions, elevated hemidiaphragm with subpulmonic effusions, "spine sign" on lateral chest x-ray examination, may be free-flowing or fixed on lateral decubitus film depending on etiology.
- **Ultrasonography** (Fig. E4): Bedside transthoracic ultrasound can be helpful to identify characteristics of pleural effusions, including:
  1. Size, location, and laterality
  2. Echogenicity of pleural fluid, presence of loculations, pleural adhesions, or pleural implants
  3. Procedure planning (e.g., thoracentesis, chest tube)
  4. Underlying lung parenchymal pathology (e.g., pulmonary edema, consolidation, pneumothorax)
  5. Signs of other pathologies (e.g., ascites, B lines)
  6. Diaphragmatic excursion
- **Computed tomography** (Fig. E5): Useful to identify loculated effusions and to assess underlying lung parenchyma to aid in establishing a diagnosis. In empyema, can demonstrate heterogeneity and gas bubbles. (See chapter on "Empyema.")

(Rx) TREATMENT

- Table 4 summarizes treatment options for pleural effusions.
- Table 5 summarizes options for control of symptomatic malignant effusions. Fig. 6 describes a treatment approach to malignant pleural effusions.

REFERRAL

Negative diagnostic workup after initial pleural fluid sampling should be followed by referral to a pulmonologist for further evaluation (including consideration for thoracoscopy for pleural biopsy).

(!) PEARLS & CONSIDERATIONS

- One-time drainage of a pleural effusion is seldom a definitive therapy.
- Early identification of the underlying etiology of new effusions should be pursued. Pleural biopsy should be considered when the underlying etiology is uncertain.[4]
- Pleural drainage with a catheter should be considered when the pleural infection is suspected.[4]
- Managing patients with malignant pleural effusion can be challenging and should be tailored to the patient on a case-by-case basis. In patients near the end of life with malignant pleural effusions that are slow to reaccumulate fluid, repeat thoracentesis, as needed, is a reasonable strategy.[4]
- Tunneled indwelling pleural catheters have gained favor for ambulatory management of malignant pleural effusions[5] and are increasingly utilized for the management of refractory noncancerous pleural effusions.[6]
- The LENT score is a validated prognostic score (incorporating LDH in pleural fluid, ECOG score, neutrophil to lymphocyte ratio in serum, and tumor type) that can be used to predict survival in malignant pleural effusions and to help inform treatment decisions in patients.[7]
- Pleurodesis should also be considered when feasible. A recent trial showed that, among patients with malignant pleural effusion, outpatient administration of talc via an indwelling tunneled pleural catheter resulted in a higher rate of pleurodesis and catheter removal than placement of a tunneled catheter alone.[8]

BOX 4 Light Criteria for Classification of Pleural Effusions

In 1972, Light et al. developed the currently accepted benchmark for classifying pleural fluid, as follows:
Pleural fluid protein to serum protein ratio >0.5:1
Pleural fluid lactate dehydrogenase (LDH) to serum LDH ratio >0.6:1
Pleural fluid LDH greater than two thirds the upper limit of normal for serum LDH (a cutoff value of 200 IU/L was used previously)
Pleural fluid is classified as an exudate if it meets any of the aforementioned criteria. Conversely, if all three characteristics are absent, the fluid is classified as a transudate. These researchers achieved a diagnostic sensitivity of 99% and a specificity of 98% for classification of an exudate.

From Adams JG etal: *Emergency medicine: clinical essentials*, ed 2, Philadelphia, 2013, Elsevier.

REFERENCES

Available at eBooks.Health.Elsevier.com.

RELATED CONTENT

Empyema (Related Key Topic)
Heart Failure (Related Key Topic)
Lung Neoplasms, Primary (Related Key Topic)

AUTHORS: **ILANA KRUMM, MD** and **YARON B. GESTHALTER, MD**

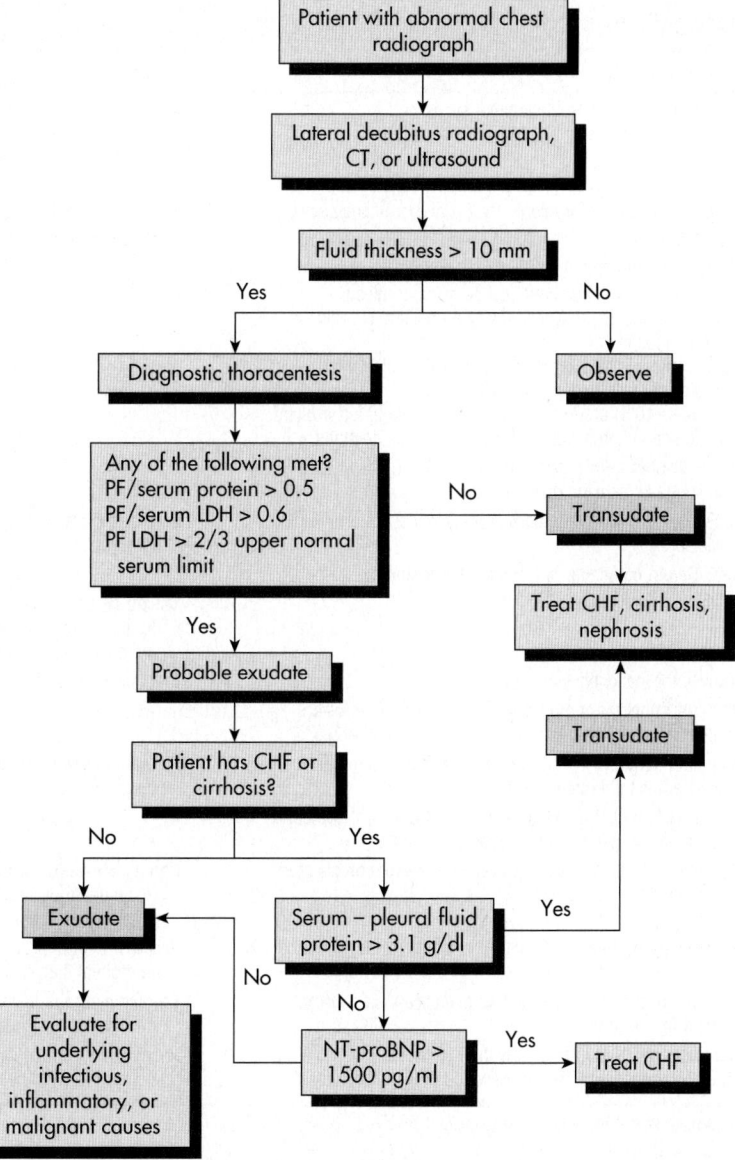

FIG. 1 Algorithm for distinguishing transudative from exudative pleural effusions. With the results of the initial thoracentesis, one can usually determine whether the effusion is an exudate or a transudate. If a transudate, the treatment can be directed to the likely causes—*congestive heart failure* (CHF), liver disease, or kidney disease. If the protein and *lactate dehydrogenase* (LDH) results are borderline exudative and there is also CHF or cirrhosis present, there is a possibility that the effusion is still transudative. To determine this, one can measure the difference between the serum and pleural fluid protein concentrations; when greater than 3.1 g/dl, one can assume that the effusion is transudative. The serum and pleural albumin gradient can also be used to identify transudates in cases of pseudoexudates (e.g., diuresed patients) using a cutoff of 1.2 g/dl. If not, one can test the pleural or serum *N-terminal pro–brain natriuretic peptide* (NT-proBNP); if greater than 1500 pg/ml, one can conclude that CHF is at least one of the causes of the effusion. Once the effusion is determined to be exudative, one can focus on further evaluation of the underlying inflammatory, infectious, or malignant cause. *CT*, Computed tomography; *PF*, Pleural fluid. (From Broaddus VC et al: *Murray & Nadel's textbook of respiratory medicine,* ed 7, Philadelphia, 2022, Elsevier.)

TABLE 3 Selected Laboratory Tests Used to Diagnose Pleural Effusion

Test	Diagnostic Utility	Comments
Adenosine deaminase (ADA)	<40 IU/L excludes tuberculous pleurisy	Values >72 IU/L highly specific for tuberculosis, with improved yield with pleural biopsy and PCR, can also be elevated in lymphoma and parapneumonic effusions. Can be falsely low in elderly patients.
Albumin	Pleural Serum albumin gradient >1.2 g/dl more consistent with transudate	Can be used to corroborate mixed findings from LDH and protein ratios
Amylase	Esophageal perforation, pancreatitis, malignancy	
Cell count	Lymphocyte predominance suggestive of tuberculosis, lymphoma, malignancy, pulmonary embolism, chronic pleural effusion Neutrophil predominant effusions seen with bacterial infection, occasionally with malignancy (20%) Eosinophil (>10%) predominance is suggestive of air or blood, can be seen in drug reactions or helminthic infections	Helpful in distinguishing causes of exudative effusions
Cholesterol	A pleural level of >45 mg/dl correlates with Light's criteria and suggests an exudative effusion	
Chylomicrons	Positive finding adds to specificity of triglycerides for establishing chylothorax	Consider thoracic duct defect (due to malignancy, trauma or iatrogenic)
Creatinine	Pleural: Serum creatinine >1 suggests urinothorax	
Culture	Positive findings used to narrow therapy	Should be sent from every suspected parapneumonic effusion to guide antimicrobial selection. Use of blood culture bottles increase culture yield
Cytology	Sensitivity for malignancy of ~65%	Diagnostic yield increases with two serial samples (~90%)
Glucose	<60 mg/dl suggests complicated parapneumonic effusion, malignancy, tuberculous pleurisy, or rheumatoid effusion	
Hematocrit	Pleural fluid hematocrit >50% peripheral blood hematocrit consistent with hemothorax	Pleural fluid with relatively low hematocrit can appear bloody on gross exam, does not necessarily represent hemothorax
Lactate dehydrogenase (LDH)	Pleural to serum LDH ratio >0.6 or pleural LDH >⅔ the upper limit of normal serum LDH suggests exudate	
pH	≤7.2 with clinical suspicion highly suggestive of complicated parapneumonic effusion	Can also have low pH with malignant pleural effusions and esophageal perforation. Measurement of pH can be temperamental, and subject to change based on collection methods
Protein	Pleural to serum protein ratio >0.5 suggests exudate	Very low pleural protein (<0.5g/dl) suggests urinothorax or peritoneal dialysis associated effusion
NT-proBNP	>1500 pg/ml suggests heart failure even if effusion meets criteria for exudate	Chronic pleural effusions related to heart failure in patients on diuretic therapy may appear exudative
Triglycerides	Triglycerides >110 mg/dl seen with chylothorax <50 mg/dl argues against the presence of a chylothorax	Absent triglycerides with high suspicion for chylothorax can be confirmed with pleural chylomicrons

NT-proBNP, N-terminal pro b-type natriuretic peptide; *PCR,* polymerase chain reaction.

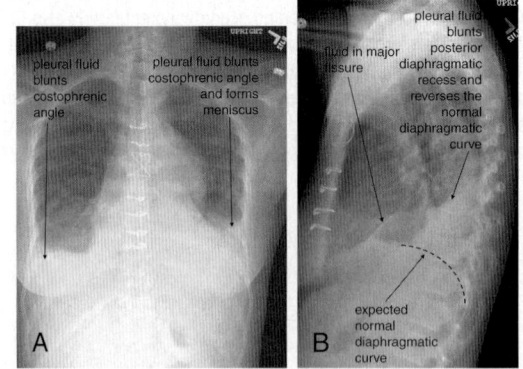

FIG. 3 Pleural effusions. **A,** Posterior-anterior upright view in which a pleural effusion is most evident on this patient's left side. Both costophrenic angles are blunted. The pleural effusion forms a meniscus against the left lateral chest wall. **B,** Lateral upright view shows two meniscus densities, suggesting bilateral pleural effusions. The posterior diaphragmatic recess is filled with pleural fluid, which forms a meniscus with the posterior chest wall. (From Broder JS: *Diagnostic imaging for the emergency physician,* Philadelphia, 2011, Saunders.)

TABLE 4 Treatment Options for Pleural Effusion

Thoracentesis	Site selection should be guided by ultrasonography whenever possible; evacuation of pleural fluid can be limited when the lung cannot fully re-expand, including central airway obstruction, chronic atelectasis, and the presence of extensive pleural adhesions or pleural thickening; aspiration in these circumstances can lead to pneumothorax ex vacuo
Tube thoracostomy	Consider when ongoing drainage will be needed, especially for empyema or hemothorax
Indwelling tunneled pleural catheter	A cuffed pleural drainage catheter tunneled through subcutaneous tissue, drained regularly on an outpatient basis, most commonly used to manage malignant pleural effusions
Pleurodesis	Instillation of a chemical irritant under direct thoracoscopic visualization (e.g., talc poudrage) or via tube thoracostomy to adhere the visceral and parietal pleurae, can also be done with mechanical pleurodesis via video-assisted thoracic surgery
Pharmacotherapy	Based on underlying etiology (e.g., diuretics, antimicrobials, chemotherapy)

TABLE 5 Options for Control of Symptomatic Malignant Effusions

Option	Patient Eligibility and Considerations
Chemotherapy, targeted therapy	Responsive tumor
Therapeutic thoracentesis	Slowly recurring effusion
	Used for patients with very short life expectancy
Pleurodesis	
Via chest tube	Lung able to reinflate
Via thoracoscopy	Can free up lung tacked down by adhesions, obtain biopsies
	Thoracoscopy must be available
Indwelling pleural catheter	Can be used as first line and coupled with talc pleurodesis if suitable
	Good outpatient situation
	Good for trapped lung
Pleuroperitoneal shunt	Patient able to operate pump
	Good for the non-expandable lung
	Good for chylothorax (provided there is no concurrent ascites)
Pleurectomy	
Via thoracoscopy	When other less-invasive options have failed
Via thoracotomy	Good patient status and life expectancy

From Broaddus VC et al: *Murray & Nadel's textbook of respiratory medicine,* ed 7, Philadelphia, 2022, Elsevier.

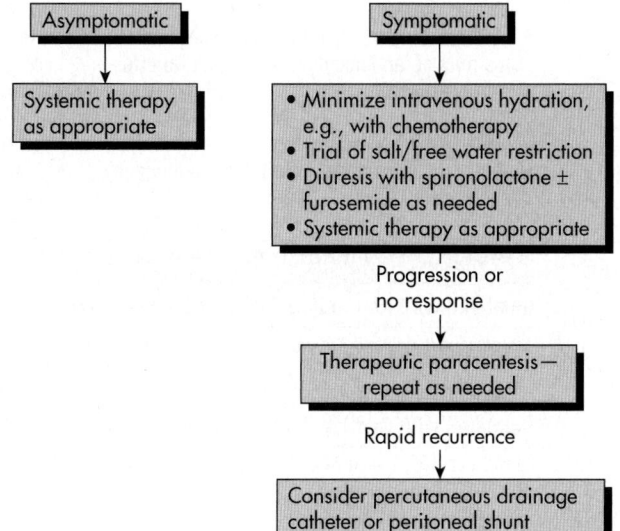

FIG. 6 Treatment approach algorithm to malignant pleural effusions. (From Niederhuber JE: *Abeloff's clinical oncology,* ed 6, Philadelphia, 2020, Elsevier.)

Diseases and Disorders

BASIC INFORMATION

DEFINITION

Pneumonia is defined as inflammation of the pulmonary parenchyma caused by an infectious agent (in this case, bacteria). It can be further categorized as community-acquired or hospital-acquired pneumonia. Community-acquired pneumonia (CAP), traditionally referred to as alveolar infection that develops in the outpatient setting or within 48 h of admission, now also includes patients previously categorized as having health care-associated pneumonia (HCAP) since the microbiology and treatment are similar. Hospital-acquired pneumonia (HAP) is pneumonia occurring ≥48 h after hospital admission and not incubating at the time of admission.[1]

SYNONYMS

Community-acquired pneumonia
CAP
Health care-associated pneumonia
Hospital-acquired pneumonia

ICD-10CM CODES
J15.9	Unspecified bacterial pneumonia
J13	Pneumonia due to *Streptococcus pneumoniae*
J15.1	Pneumonia due to *Pseudomonas*
J15.20	Pneumonia due to staphylococcus, unspecified
J15.0	Pneumonia due to *Klebsiella pneumoniae*
J14	Pneumonia due to *Haemophilus influenzae*
J15.211	Pneumonia due to methicillin-susceptible *Staphylococcus aureus*
J15.212	Pneumonia due to methicillin-resistant *Staphylococcus aureus*
J15.6	Pneumonia due to other aerobic gram-negative bacteria
J15.7	Pneumonia due to *Mycoplasma pneumoniae*

EPIDEMIOLOGY & DEMOGRAPHICS

- The annual incidence of pneumonia in the U.S. is 24.8 cases per 10,000 adults, with the highest rates among adults between 65 to 79 yr of age (63 cases per 10,000 adults) and those >80 yr old (164.3 cases per 10,000 adults). Health care expenditures for CAP exceed $10 billion annually.
- Hospitalization rate for pneumonia is 15% to 20%. Incidence is highest among the oldest adults.
- In 2017, the tenth leading cause of mortality in the U.S. reported by the National Center for Health Statistics was influenza and pneumonia together. Deaths per 100,000 population: 15.1.
- Globally, *Streptococcus pneumoniae* (pneumococcus) is the most common pathogen causing community-acquired pneumonia.

PHYSICAL FINDINGS & CLINICAL PRESENTATION

- Fever, tachypnea, chills, tachycardia, cough, and sometimes pleuritic chest pain (especially if a pleural effusion is present)
- Presentation varies with the cause of pneumonia, the patient's age, and the clinical situation:
  1. Patients with streptococcal pneumonia usually present with high fever, chills, atypical chest pain, cough, and copious production of rusty-appearing purulent sputum. Pleurisy in the setting of parapneumonic effusions can also occur. Potential complications include bacteremia, empyema, and distant infections (e.g., meningitis).
  2. *Mycoplasma pneumoniae:* Insidious onset; headache; dry, paroxysmal cough that is worse at night; myalgias; malaise; sore throat; extrapulmonary manifestations (e.g., erythema multiforme, aseptic meningitis, urticaria, erythema nodosum) may be present. (See chapter on "*Mycoplasma* Pneumonia".)
  3. *Chlamydia pneumoniae:* Persistent, nonproductive cough, low-grade fever, headache, sore throat.
  4. *Legionella pneumophila:* High fever, mild cough, mental status change, myalgias, diarrhea, respiratory failure. (See chapter on "Legionnaires Disease.")
  5. MRSA pneumonia: Often preceded by influenza, may present with shock and respiratory failure.
  6. Elderly or immunocompromised hosts with pneumonia may initially present with only minimal symptoms (e.g., low-grade fever, confusion); respiratory and nonrespiratory symptoms are less commonly reported by older patients with pneumonia.
- In general, auscultation of lungs in patients with pneumonia reveals crackles/rhonchi and diminished breath sounds. Egophany may also be present.
- Dullness on percussion or decreased fremitus may be an indication that a pleural effusion is present.

ETIOLOGY[2]

- Table 1 summarizes common pathogens causing CAP

- *Streptococcus pneumoniae* (5% to 15% of hospitalized CAP cases): Incidence has been declining due to widespread use of pneumococcal vaccination and reduced rate of cigarette smoking
- *Haemophilus influenzae* (Fig. E1) (3% to 10% of CAP cases)
- *L. pneumophila* (1% to 5% of adult pneumonias) (2% to 8% of CAP cases)
- *Klebsiella pneumoniae* (Fig. E2), *Pseudomonas aeruginosa, Escherichia coli*
- *Staphylococcus aureus* (Fig. E3) (3% to 5% of CAP cases)
- Atypical organisms such as *Mycoplasma pneumoniae, Chlamydia pneumoniae,* and *Legionella pneumophila* implicated in up to 40% of cases of CAP
- Gram-negative organisms cause >80% of nosocomial pneumonias
- Predisposing factors (Table 2 and Table 3):
  1. Influenza infection is one of the important predisposing factors to *S. pneumoniae* and *S. aureus* pneumonia
  2. Chronic obstructive pulmonary disease: *H. influenzae, S. pneumoniae, Legionella, Moraxella catarrhalis*
  3. Seizures: Aspiration pneumonia
  4. Compromised hosts: *Legionella,* gram-negative organisms
  5. Alcoholism: *K. pneumoniae, S. pneumoniae, H. influenzae*
  6. HIV: *S. pneumoniae*
  7. Intravenous (IV) drug users with right-sided bacterial endocarditis: *S. aureus*
  8. Older patient with comorbid diseases: *C. pneumoniae*

DIAGNOSIS

DIFFERENTIAL DIAGNOSIS

- Viral pneumonias (see chapter on "Viral Pneumonia")
- Aspiration pneumonia (see chapter on "Aspiration Pneumonia")
- Exacerbation of chronic bronchitis
- Pulmonary embolism or infarction (see chapter on "Pulmonary Embolism")
- Lung neoplasm
- Bronchiolitis

TABLE 1 Common Pathogens Causing Community-Acquired Pneumonia

Inpatient, with No Cardiopulmonary Disease or Modifying Factors

Streptococcus pneumoniae, Haemophilus influenzae, Mycoplasma pneumoniae, Chlamydophila pneumoniae, mixed infection (bacteria plus atypical pathogen), viruses (including influenza), *Legionella* spp., and others (*Mycobacterium tuberculosis,* endemic fungi, *Pneumocystis jirovecii*)

Inpatient, with Cardiopulmonary Disease and/or Modifying Factors

All of the above, but drug-resistant *S. pneumoniae* (DRSP) and enteric gram-negative organisms are more of a concern

Severe Community-Acquired Pneumonia, with No Risks for *Pseudomonas Aeruginosa*

S. pneumoniae (including DRSP), *Legionella* spp., *H. influenzae,* enteric gram-negative bacilli, *Staphylococcus aureus* (including methicillin-resistant *S. aureus*), *M. pneumoniae,* respiratory viruses (including influenza), others (*C. pneumoniae, M. tuberculosis,* endemic fungi)

Severe CAP, with Risks for *P. Aeruginosa*

All of the pathogens above plus *P. aeruginosa*

From Vincent JL et al: *Textbook of critical care,* ed 8, Philadelphia, 2024, Elsevier.

TABLE 2 Risk Factors for Developing Severe Community-Acquired Pneumonia

Advanced age

Comorbid illness (e.g., chronic respiratory illness, cardiovascular disease, diabetes mellitus, neurologic illness, renal insufficiency, malignancy)

Cigarette smoking

Alcohol abuse

Absence of antibiotic therapy before hospitalization

Failure to contain infection to its initial site of entry

Immune suppression

Genetic polymorphisms in the immune response

From Vincent JL et al: *Textbook of critical care*, ed 8, Philadelphia, 2024, Elsevier.

TABLE 3 Clinical Associations with Specific Pathogens

Condition	Commonly Encountered Pathogens
Alcoholism	*Streptococcus pneumoniae* (including penicillin-resistant), anaerobes, gram-negative bacilli (possibly *Klebsiella pneumoniae*), tuberculosis
Chronic obstructive pulmonary disease/current or former smoker	*S. pneumoniae, Haemophilus influenzae, Moraxella catarrhalis*
Residence in nursing home	*S. pneumoniae*, gram-negative bacilli, *H. influenzae, Staphylococcus aureus, Chlamydophila pneumoniae;* consider *M. tuberculosis.* Consider anaerobes, but these are less common
Poor dental hygiene	Anaerobes
Bat exposure	*Histoplasma capsulatum*
Bird exposure	*Chlamydophila psittaci, Cryptococcus neoformans, H. capsulatum*
Rabbit exposure	*Francisella tularensis*
Travel to southwestern United States	*Coccidioidomycosis;* hantavirus in selected areas
Exposure to farm animals or parturient cats	*Coxiella burnetii* (Q fever)
Postinfluenza pneumonia	*S. pneumoniae, S. aureus* (including the community-acquired strain of methicillin-resistant *S. aureus*), *H. influenzae*
Structural disease of the lung (e.g., bronchiectasis, cystic fibrosis)	*Pseudomonas aeruginosa, Pseudomonas cepacia,* or *S. aureus*
Sickle cell disease, asplenia	Pneumococcus, *H. influenzae*
Suspected bioterrorism	Anthrax, tularemia, plague
Travel to Asia	Severe acute respiratory syndrome, tuberculosis, melioidosis

From Vincent JL et al: *Textbook of critical care*, ed 8, Philadelphia, 2024, Elsevier.

- Sarcoidosis (see chapter on "Sarcoidosis")
- Hypersensitivity pneumonitis (see chapter on "Hypersensitivity Pneumonitis")
- Pulmonary edema
- Drug-induced lung injury
- Fungal pneumonias
- Parasitic pneumonias
- Atypical pneumonia
- Tuberculosis
- Cryptogenic organizing pneumonia

WORKUP

Diagnostic testing for CAP is summarized in Table 4. Useful tools for assessing severity of illness are the *CURB-65* (see "Disposition") and *Pneumonia Severity Index* (Fig. 4 and Box 1). Poor prognostic indicators are hypotension (SBP <90 or DBP <60), respiratory rate >30/min, fever (>40° C; 104° F), or hypothermia (<35° C; 95° F). None of these indices is as valuable as clinical judgment.[3]

LABORATORY TESTS

- Complete blood count with differential; white blood cell count is elevated, usually with left shift or the presence of bandemia.
- Sputum culture should be obtained, ideally prior to initiation of antibiotics, in hospitalized patients or if drug-resistant or unusual pathogen is suspected.
- Blood cultures (hospitalized patients only): Positive in approximately 20% of cases of pneumococcal pneumonia.
- Pneumococcal urinary antigen test can be used to detect the C-polysaccharide antigen of *S. pneumoniae* (70% sensitivity). It is a useful tool in the treatment of hospitalized adult patients with CAP.[4]
- When suspecting *Legionella,* a respiratory specimen culture on special media and/or a urinary antigen should be requested.

TABLE 4 Diagnostic Testing for Community-Acquired Pneumonia

Test	Sensitivity	Specificity	Comment
Chest radiograph	65%-85%	85%-95%	Computed tomography is more sensitive to infiltrates. Recommended for all patients.
Computed tomography	Gold standard	Not infection specific	Should not be performed routinely but helpful to identify cavitation and loculated pleural fluid. Recommended in the evaluation of nonresponding patients.
Blood cultures	10%-20%	High when positive	Usually shows pneumococcus (in 50%-80% of positive samples) and defines antibiotic susceptibility. Recommended in patients with severe CAP, particularly if not on antibiotic therapy at the time of testing.
Sputum Gram stain	40%-100% depending on criteria	0%-100% depending on criteria	Can correlate with sputum culture to define predominant organism and can be used to identify unsuspected pathogens. Recommended if sputum culture is obtained. May not be able to narrow empiric therapy choices.
Sputum culture			Use if suspect drug-resistant or unusual pathogen, but a positive result cannot differentiate colonization from infection. Obtain via tracheal aspirate in all intubated patients.
Oximetry or arterial blood gas			Define both severity of infection and need for oxygen; if hypercarbia is suspected, a blood gas sample is needed. Recommended in severe community-acquired pneumonia.
Serologic testing for *Legionella, Chlamydophila pneumoniae, Mycobacterium pneumoniae,* viruses			Accurate, but usually requires acute and convalescent titers collected 4 to 6 wk apart. Not routinely recommended.
Legionella urinary antigen	50%-80%		Specific to serogroup 1, but the best acute diagnostic test for *Legionella.*
Pneumococcal urinary antigen	70%-100%	80%	False positives if recent pneumococcal infection. Can increase sensitivity with concentrated urine.
Serum procalcitonin			Not a routine test, but if performed, should be measured with the highly sensitive Kryptor assay. May help guide duration of therapy and need for ICU admission.

From Vincent JL et al: *Textbook of critical care*, ed 8, Philadelphia, 2024, Elsevier.

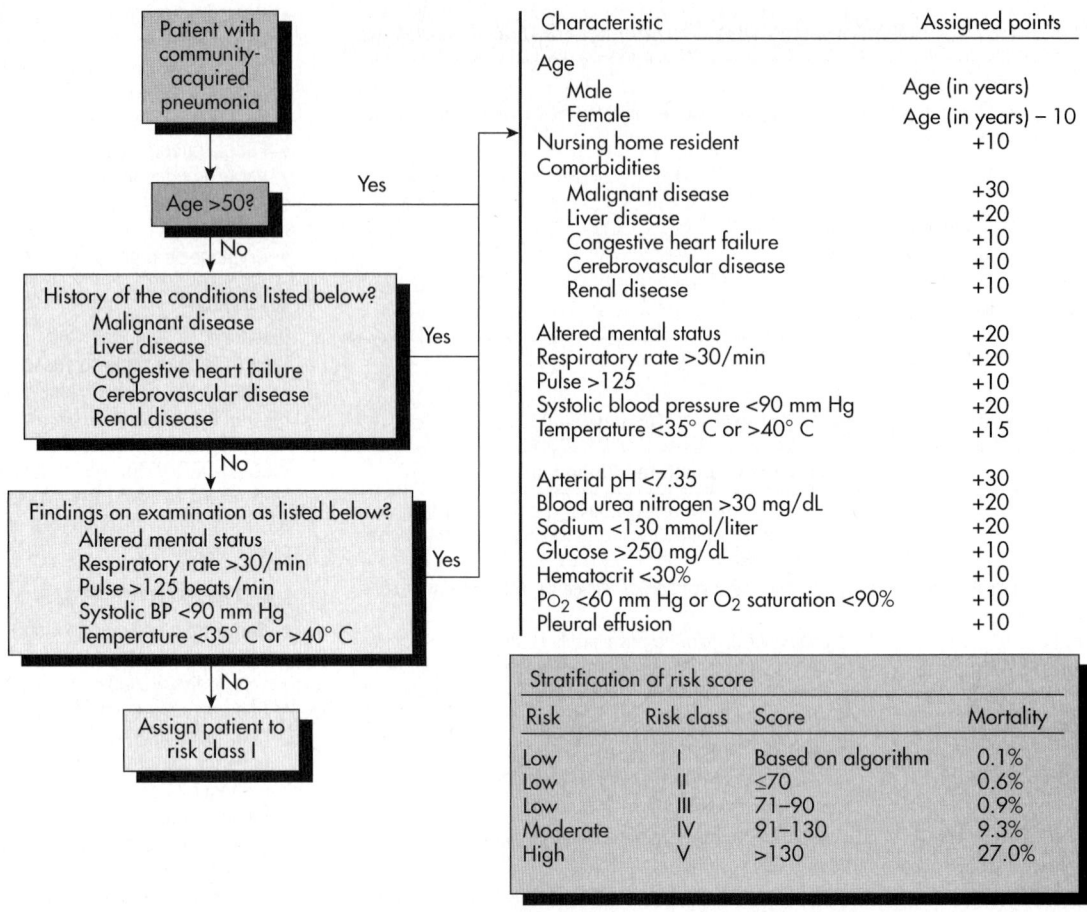

FIG. 4 The pneumonia severity index. *BP,* Blood pressure; *O₂,* oxygen; *Po₂,* partial pressure of oxygen. (From Sellke FW et al: *Sabiston & Spencer surgery of the chest,* ed 9, Philadelphia, 2016, Elsevier.)

BOX 1 Severe Pneumonia: Diagnostic Criteria*

Major Criteria
Invasive mechanical ventilation
Use of vasopressors to maintain blood pressure

Minor Criteria
Respiratory rate ≥30 breaths/min
Multilobar infiltrates
New-onset confusion/disorientation
Uremia (BUN >20 mg/dl)
Leukopenia (WBC count <4000 cells/μL)
Pao₂/Fio₂ ratio ≥250
Thrombocytopenia (platelet count <100,000 cells/μL)
Hypothermia (core temperature <36° C; 96.8° F)
Hypotension requiring aggressive fluid resuscitation*

*According to ATS/IDSA 2007 guidelines.
From Parrillo JE, Dellinger RP: *Critical care medicine: principles of diagnosis and management in the adult,* ed 4, Philadelphia, 2014, Saunders.

- Serologic testing for HIV in selected patients.
- Serum electrolytes (hyponatremia in suspected *Legionella* pneumonia), blood urea nitrogen (BUN), creatinine.
- Nasopharyngeal swab for rapid and polymerase chain reaction testing for influenza.
- Testing for SARS-COVID19.

- Serum procalcitonin level: Often used to distinguish pneumonia from heart failure in patients presenting to the emergency department with acute dyspnea. The procalcitonin level is significantly higher in patients with pneumonia than in those without. However, serum procalcitonin should not be used to determine initiation or duration of antibiotic therapy in patients with radiographically confirmed CAP unless antibiotic therapy is being extended beyond 5 to 7 days. Recent trials regarding procalcitonin-guided use of antibiotics for lower respiratory tract infections did not result in less use of antibiotics than did usual care among patients with suspected lower respiratory tract infection.[5]
- Pulse oximetry or arterial blood gases: Hypoxemia with partial pressure of oxygen <60 mm Hg while the patient is breathing room air, a standard criterion for hospital admission.
- Table 5 summarizes recommended microbiologic evaluation in patients with community acquired pneumonia.
- Fig. 5 illustrates an algorithm for the diagnosis and treatment of nosocomial pneumonia.
- Ventilator-associated pneumonia: Table 6 and Fig. E6 summarize a proposed strategy for managing antimicrobial therapy in patients with ventilator-associated pneumonia.

IMAGING STUDIES

Chest x-ray (PA and lateral) (Fig. 7): Findings vary with the stage and type of pneumonia and the hydration of the patient:
- Classically, pneumococcal pneumonia presents with a segmental lobe infiltrate (Fig. E8).
- Diffuse infiltrates on chest x-ray can be seen with *L. pneumophila* (Fig. 9), *M. pneumoniae,* viral pneumonias, *P. jirovecii (carinii),* miliary tuberculosis, aspiration, aspergillosis.
- An initial chest x-ray is also useful to rule out the presence of complications (pneumothorax, empyema, abscesses).

Rx TREATMENT

NONPHARMACOLOGIC THERAPY

- Avoidance of tobacco use
- Oxygen to maintain partial oxygen pressure in arterial blood >60 mm Hg or oxygen saturation >88% in COPD patients and >92% in non-COPD patients
- IV hydration, correction of dehydration
- Assisted ventilation in patients with significant respiratory failure

ACUTE GENERAL Rx

- Antibiotic therapy should be based on clinical, radiographic, and laboratory evaluation.[6-8]

TABLE 5 Recommended Microbiologic Evaluation in Patients with Community-Acquired Pneumonia

Patients Who Do Not Require Hospitalization

None*

Patients Who Require Hospitalization

Two sets of blood cultures (obtained prior to antibiotics) in selected patients

Gram stain and culture of a valid sputum sample in selected patients

Urinary antigen test for detection of *Legionella pneumophila* (in endemic areas or during outbreaks)

Stain for acid-fast bacilli and culture of sputum (if tuberculosis is suggested by clinical history or radiologic findings)

Fungal stain and culture of sputum, and fungal serologies (if infection by an endemic fungus is suggested by the clinical history or radiologic findings)

Sputum examination for *Pneumocystis jirovecii* (if suggested by clinical history, HIV infection, or radiologic findings)

Nucleic acid amplification tests for *Mycoplasma pneumoniae, Chlamydophila pneumoniae, Chlamydophila psittaci, Coxiella burnetii, Legionella* species, respiratory viruses (in endemic areas or during outbreaks) and other agents (e.g., *Streptococcus pneumoniae*) if available

Culture and microscopic evaluation of pleural fluid (if significant fluid is present)

Additional Tests for Patients Who Require Treatment in an ICU

Gram stain and culture of endotracheal aspirate or bronchoscopically obtained specimens using a protected specimen brush or BAL

BAL, Bronchoalveolar lavage; *ICU,* intensive care unit.
*Gram stain and culture should be strongly considered in patients with risk factors for infection by an antimicrobial-resistant organism or unusual pathogen.
From Broaddus VC et al: *Murray & Nadel's textbook of respiratory medicine,* ed 7, Philadelphia, 2022, Elsevier.

Empiric therapy regimens for community-acquired pneumonia are summarized in Tables 7 and 8.

- Macrolides (azithromycin or clarithromycin) or doxycycline can be used for empiric outpatient treatment of CAP as long as the patient has not received antibiotics within the past 3 mo and does not reside in a community in which the prevalence of macrolide resistance is high.[9] Updated guidelines from the American Thoracic Society and Infectious Diseases Society of America have added amoxicillin as a first-line agent for healthy adult outpatients with CAP.[10] The treatment of choice in suspected *Legionella* pneumonia is either a quinolone (e.g., moxifloxacin) or a macrolide (e.g., azithromycin) antibiotic. A beta-lactam antibiotic is usually added to macrolides.
- In the hospital setting, patients not requiring intensive care unit (ICU) care can be treated empirically with a second- or third-generation cephalosporin (ceftriaxone, cefotaxime, or cefuroxime) plus a macrolide (azithromycin or clarithromycin) or doxycycline. An antipseudomonal quinolone (levofloxacin or moxifloxacin) can be substituted in place of the macrolide or doxycycline.[11]
- Empiric therapy in ICU patients: IV beta-lactam (ceftriaxone, cefotaxime, ampicillin-sulbactam) plus an IV quinolone (levofloxacin, moxifloxacin) or IV azithromycin.
- In hospitalized patients at risk for *P. aeruginosa* infection, empiric treatment should consist of an antipseudomonal beta-lactam (meropenem, doripenem, imipenem, or piperacillin-tazobactam) with or without a second antipseudomonal agent such as an aminoglycoside or an antipseudomonal quinolone.
- In patients with suspected methicillin-resistant *S. aureus,* vancomycin or linezolid is effective.
- Corticosteroids: Clinical trials evaluating adjunctive use of corticosteroids in severe CAP have produced mixed results. There is no

evidence that adjunctive use of corticosteroids improves outcomes in mild to moderate CAP. Guidelines advise against adjunctive treatment of CAP with corticosteroids except in patients with septic shock that is refractory to fluid resuscitation and vasopressor support.[12-14] A recent trial revealed that among patients with severe community-acquired pneumonia being treated in the ICU, those who received hydrocortisone (200 mg daily for either 4 or 8 days) had a lower risk of death by day 28 than those who received placebo.[15]

- Duration of antibiotic treatment ranges from 5 to 14 days. Trials have shown that in adults hospitalized with CAP, stopping antibiotic treatment after 5 days in clinically stable patients is reasonable and noninferior to usual care.[8,16] Hematogenous *Staphylococcus* infection, abscesses, and cavitary lesions might require prolonged antibiotic therapy, sometimes until radiologic resolution is documented.

CHRONIC Rx

Parapneumonic effusion and empyema can be managed with chest tube placement for drainage. (See chapters on "Pleural Effusion" and "Empyema.")

DISPOSITION

Risk factors for a poor outcome from CAP are summarized in Table 9. Indications for hospital admission are:
- Hypoxemia (oxygen saturation <90% while patient is breathing room air)
- Hemodynamic instability
- Inability to tolerate medications
- Active coexisting condition requiring hospitalization. A criterion often used to determine hospital admission is known as the **"CURB-65": C**onfusion, B**UN >19.6 mg/dl, **R**espiratory rate >30 breaths/min, systolic **B**P <90 mg Hg, and diastolic BP ≤60 mm Hg, age ≥**65.** Patients are generally admitted to the hospital if they fulfill two or more criteria and to the ICU if they have three or more criteria[17]

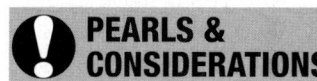

PEARLS & CONSIDERATIONS

COMMENTS

- "Recurrent pneumonia": Table 10 summarizes the differential diagnosis of recurrent pneumonia.
- Causes of slowly resolving or nonresolving pneumonia:
  1. Difficult to treat infections: Viral pneumonia, *Legionella,* pneumococci or staphylococci with impaired host response, tuberculosis, atypical mycobacteria, nocardia, or fungi
  2. Neoplasm: Lung, lymphoma, metastasis
  3. Congestive heart failure
  4. Pulmonary embolism
  5. Immunologic or idiopathic: Cryptogenic organizing pneumonia, eosinophilic pneumonia, granulomatosis with polyangiitis
  6. Drug toxicity (e.g., amiodarone, methotrexate)
- Repeat imaging: If patients with pneumonia are not improving, repeat thoracic imaging should be done promptly. In those with complete clinical recovery, it is reasonable to wait 6 to 8 wk before repeating the imaging study to document clearing of the infiltrate. However, the latest guidelines (2019 ATS/IDSA) do not recommend follow-up imaging.[10]

Patients may be eligible for lung cancer screening, which should be performed as clinically indicated.

PREVENTION

- Four pneumococcal vaccines are currently available: The 23-valent pneumococcal polysaccharides vaccine (PPSV23), the pneumococcal conjugated vaccine (PCV13), a new 15 valent PVC (PVC-15), and a 20-valent PVC-20 (Prevnar). The Centers for Disease Control and Prevention (CDC) recommends giving the PCV13 to all children. PPSV20 is recommended as a single dose for all adults >65 yr and any other individual with risk factors (including smoking; alcoholism; diabetes

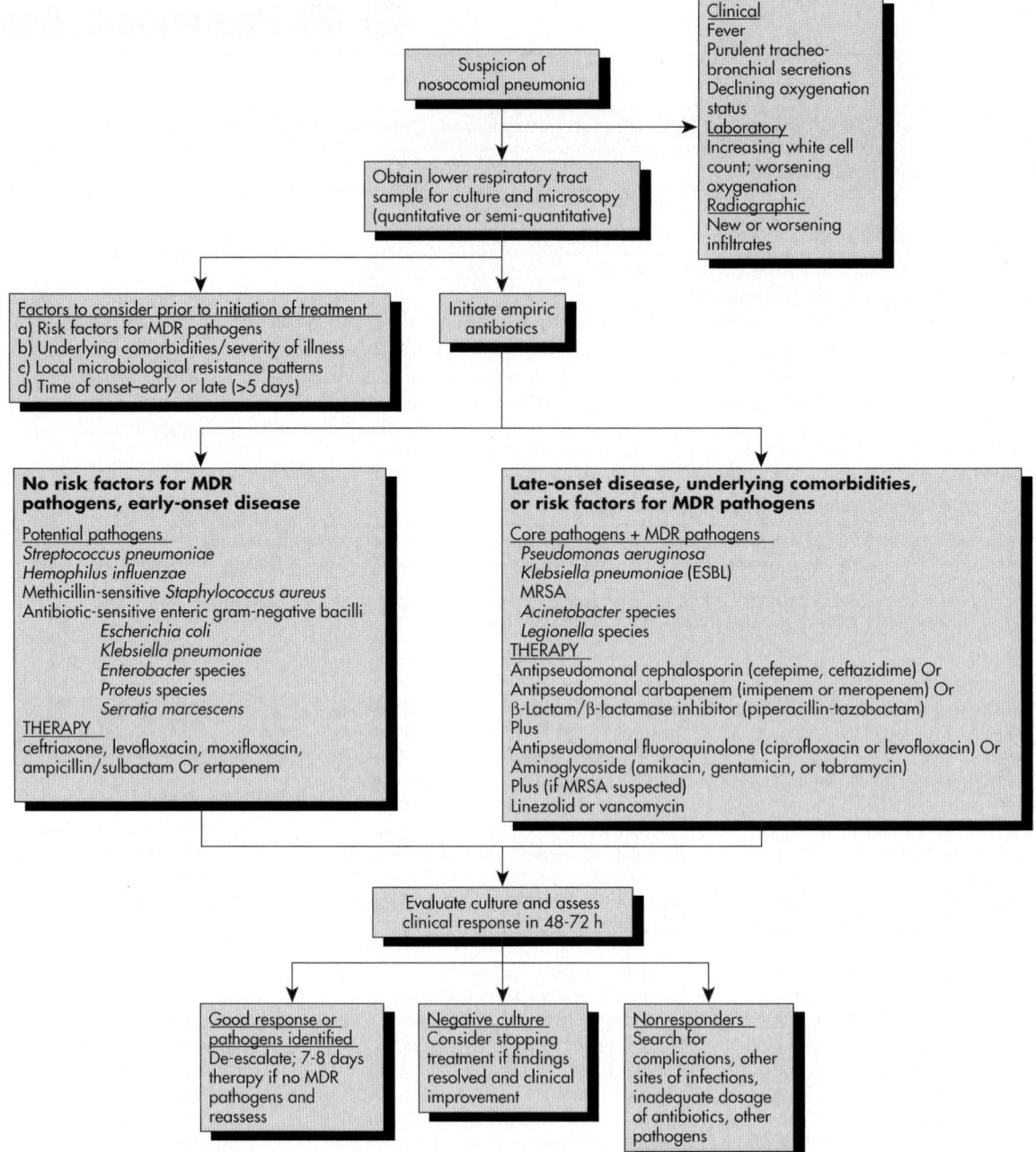

FIG. 5 A suggested algorithm for the diagnosis and treatment of nosocomial pneumonia. (From Parrillo JE, Dellinger RP: *Critical care medicine, principles of diagnosis and management in the adult*, ed 4, Philadelphia, 2014, Elsevier.)

TABLE 6	Proposed Strategy for Managing Antimicrobial Therapy in Patients with Ventilator-Associated Pneumonia

Proposed Strategy	Rationale
Step 1: Start therapy using broad-spectrum antibiotics	Due to the emergence of multiresistant GNB, such as *P. aeruginosa* and ESBL-producing GNB, and the increasing role of MRSA, empirical treatment with broad-spectrum antibiotics is justified in most patients with a clinical suspicion of VAP.
Step 2: Stop therapy if the diagnosis of infection becomes unlikely	The goal is to ensure that ICU patients with true bacterial infection receive immediate appropriate treatment. However, this can result in more patients receiving antimicrobial therapy than necessary because clinical signs of infection are nonspecific.
Step 3: Use narrower spectrum antibiotics once the etiologic agent is identified	For many patients with VAP, including those with late-onset infection, therapy can be narrowed once the results of respiratory tract and blood cultures are available, either because an anticipated organism (e.g., *P. aeruginosa* and *Acinetobacter* spp. or MRSA) was not recovered, or because the organism isolated is sensitive to a more narrow-spectrum antibiotic than used in the initial regimen.
Step 4: Use pharmacokinetic-pharmacodynamic data to optimize treatment	Clinical and bacteriologic outcomes can be improved by optimizing the therapeutic regimen according to pharmacokinetic and pharmacodynamic properties of the agents selected for treatment.
Step 5: Switch to monotherapy on days 3 to 5	There are no clinical benefits to using a regimen combining two antibiotics for more than days 3 to 5, provided that initial therapy was appropriate, the clinical course appears favorable, and microbiologic data do not point to a very difficult-to-treat microorganism.
Step 6: Shorten the duration of therapy	Reducing duration of therapy in patients with VAP has led to good outcomes with less antibiotic use. Prolonged therapy leads to colonization with antibiotic-resistant bacteria, which may precede a recurrent episode of VAP.

ESBL, Extended-spectrum β-lactamase; *GNB*, gram-negative bacteria; *ICU*, intensive care unit; *MRSA*, methicillin-resistant *Staphylococcus aureus*; *VAP*, ventilator-associated pneumonia.
From Broaddus VC et al: *Murray & Nadel's textbook of respiratory medicine*, ed 7, Philadelphia, 2022, Elsevier.

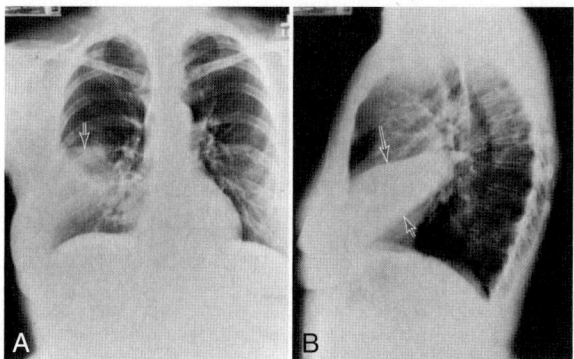

FIG. 7 Posteroanterior **(A)** and lateral **(B)** chest radiographs show lobar pneumonia (probably caused by *Streptococcus pneumoniae*) affecting the right middle lobe. In **(A)** the *arrow* points to a minor fissure, which defines the upper border of the middle lobe. In **(B)** the *long arrow* points to a minor fissure, and the *short arrow* points to a major fissure. (From Weinberger SE: *Principles of pulmonary medicine,* ed 7, Philadelphia, 2019, Elsevier.)

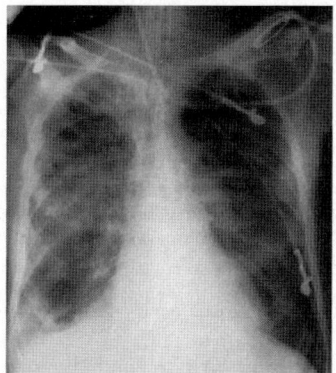

FIG. 9 Chest radiograph of a patient with extensive gram-negative pneumonia. Note the patchy infiltrates throughout both lungs, which are more prominent on the right. (From Weinberger SE: *Principles of pulmonary medicine,* ed 7, Philadelphia, 2019, Elsevier.)

TABLE 7 Guidelines for Empirical Oral Outpatient Treatment of Immunocompetent Adults with Community-Acquired Pneumonia

ATS/IDSA

No modifying factors[a]: Amoxicillin,[b] doxycycline or advanced macrolide if *S. pneumoniae* macrolide resistance <25%[c,d]
Comorbidities[a]: Beta-lactam,[e] macrolide[f] or doxycycline,[d] or fluoroquinolone[g] alone

BTS

Primary: Amoxicillin
Alternatives: Clarithromycin or doxycycline

ERS/ESCMID

Amoxicillin or doxycycline with macrolide as alternative if low levels of resistance

DRSPTWG

Primary: Amoxicillin, amoxicillin-clavulanate, cefuroxime, doxycycline, macrolide (if low rate of resistance)
Alternative: Fluoroquinolone[h]

ATS/IDSA, American Thoracic Society/Infectious Diseases Society of America; *BTS,* British Thoracic Society; *DRSPTWG,* Drug-Resistant *Streptococcus pneumoniae* Therapeutic Working Group; *ERS/ESCMID,* European Respiratory Society and European Society for Clinical Microbiology and Infectious Diseases.
[a]American Thoracic Society/Infectious Diseases Society of America comorbidities (modifying factors) include chronic heart, lung, liver or kidney disease; diabetes; asplenia; alcoholism; and malignancy.
[b]Amoxicillin 1 g q8h, doxycycline 100 mg q12h, azithromycin 500 mg on first day then 250 mg/day, clarithromycin 500 mg q8h, or clarithromycin extended release 1000 mg/day.
[c]Advanced macrolides are azithromycin and clarithromycin.
[d]Second-choice agent.
[e]Amoxicillin-clavulanate (500 mg amoxicillin plus 125 mg clavulanate q8h, 875 mg amoxicillin plus 125 mg clavulanate q12h or 2 g amoxicillin plus 125 mg clavulanic acid q12h), cefpodoxime, cefprozil, or cefuroxime.
[f]Because of increasing macrolide resistance, erythromycin cannot be relied upon to ensure coverage of beta-lactamase–producing *Haemophilus influenzae.* A combination of a beta-lactam/beta-lactamase inhibitor is preferred.
[g]Antipneumococcal fluoroquinolones include levofloxacin, and moxifloxacin.
[h]Levofloxacin or moxifloxacin.
From Broaddus VC et al: *Murray & Nadel's textbook of respiratory medicine,* ed 7, Philadelphia, 2022, Elsevier.

mellitus; or chronic heart, lung, or liver disease). It is administered as a single dose. Eligible adults who have received only PPSV23 may receive either PVC-20 or PVC-15 1 yr later. Eligible adults who have received PVC-13 alone should receive a chaser dose of PPSV23 at 1 yr later. During the influenza season, patients should also receive influenza vaccination.
• COVID-19 vaccination should be recommended.[18]

REFERENCES

Available at eBooks.Health.Elsevier.com.

RELATED CONTENT

Bacterial Pneumonia (Patient Information)
Aspiration Pneumonia (Related Key Topic)
Legionnaires disease (Related Key Topic)
Pneumonia, Mycoplasma (Related Key Topic)

AUTHOR: **JORGE MERCADO, MD**

TABLE 8 Guidelines for Empirical Parenteral Inpatient Treatment of Immunocompetent Adults with Community-Acquired Pneumonia

Mild to Moderate Disease

ATS/IDSA

- Primary:[c] Ampicillin and sulbactam, cefotaxime, ceftriaxone, or ceftaroline with azithromycin or clarithromycin
- Alternative: Fluoroquinolone[a] alone or, if history of prior respiratory isolation of MRSA[d] or *Pseudomonas aeruginosa*,[e] treatment to cover these agents

BTS

- Mild: Oral amoxicillin. Alternatives parenteral amoxicillin or benzylpenicillin or clarithromycin
- Moderate: Oral amoxicillin and clarithromycin (can consider clarithromycin monotherapy if prior therapy with amoxicillin)
- Alternative if unable to take oral medication: Parenteral amoxicillin or benzylpenicillin plus clarithromycin (if intolerant of penicillin but able to take a cephalosporin parenteral second- or third-generation cephalosporin plus clarithromycin)
- Alternative: If unable to take penicillin or macrolide,[b] oral doxycycline, or if not able to take any of these, a respiratory fluoroquinolone[a]

ERS/ESCMID

- Aminopenicillin, aminopenicillin with beta-lactamase inhibitor, penicillin, cefotaxime, ceftriaxone with or without macrolide[b]
- Respiratory fluoroquinolone alone[a]

DRSPTWG

- Primary: Cefuroxime, cefotaxime, ceftriaxone, or ampicillin-sulbactam; macrolide[b]
- Alternative: Fluoroquinolone[a]

Severe Disease

ATS/IDSA

- Primary[c]: Ampicillin and sulbactam, cefotaxime, ceftriaxone, or ceftaroline with azithromycin or clarithromycin
- Alternative: Broad-spectrum β-lactam as for primary with fluoroquinolone[a] or, if history of prior respiratory isolation or prior hospitalization with parenteral antimicrobials within 90 days in setting of locally validated risk factors for MRSA[d] or *P. aeruginosa*,[e] treatment to cover these agents

BTS

- Primary: Amoxicillin/clavulanate (or if penicillin intolerant cefuroxime, cefotaxime, or ceftriaxone) plus macrolide[b]

ERS/ESCMID

- Cefotaxime or ceftriaxone plus macrolide or respiratory fluoroquinolone
- Alternative: Respiratory fluoroquinolone alone if no sepsis
- Alternative if risk factors for *P. aeruginosa*: Piperacillin/tazobactam, antipseudomonal cephalosporin (ceftazidime[f] or cefepime) plus ciprofloxacin or plus macrolide[b] and aminoglycoside[g]

DRSPTWG

- Primary: Ceftriaxone or cefotaxime, macrolide;[b] or ceftriaxone or cefotaxime, fluoroquinolone[a]
- Alternative (with caution): Fluoroquinolone[a]

ATS/IDSA, American Thoracic Society/Infectious Diseases Society of America; *BTS*, British Thoracic Society; *DRSPTWG*, Drug-Resistant *Streptococcus pneumoniae* Therapeutic Working Group; *ERS/ESCMID*, European Respiratory Society and European Society for Clinical Microbiology and Infectious Diseases.
[a]Antipneumococcal fluoroquinolones include levofloxacin 750 mg/day and moxifloxacin 400 mg/day.
[b]Advanced macrolides are azithromycin and clarithromycin.
[c]Ampicillin and sulbactam 1.5-3 g q6h, cefotaxime 1-2 g q8h, ceftriaxone 1-2 g/day, or ceftaroline 600 mg q12h and azithromycin 500 mg/day or 500 mg on day 1 and 250 mg once a day thereafter for mild disease or clarithromycin 500 mg bid.
[d]Antistaphylococcal treatments include vancomycin (15 mg/kg q12h, adjust based on levels) or linezolid (600 mg q12h).
[e]Antipseudomonal β-lactams include piperacillin-tazobactam (4.5 g q6h), cefepime (2 g q8h), ceftazidime (2 g q8h), imipenem (500 mg q6h), meropenem (1 g q8h), or aztreonam (2 g q8h).
[f]If ceftazidime used should be combined with penicillin to ensure coverage of pneumococci per ERS/ESCMID guideline.
[g]Recommendation to double cover *P. aeruginosa* with both a β-lactam and either ciprofloxacin or an aminoglycoside per ERS/ESCMID guideline.
From Broaddus VC et al: *Murray & Nadel's textbook of respiratory medicine,* ed 7, Philadelphia, 2022, Elsevier.

TABLE 9 Risk Factors for a Poor Outcome from Community-Acquired Pneumonia

Patient-Related Factors

Male sex
Absence of pleuritic chest pain
Nonclassic clinical presentation
Neoplastic illness
Neurologic illness
Age >65 yr old
Family history of severe pneumonia or death from sepsis

Abnormal Physical Findings

Respiratory rate >30 breaths/min on admission
Systolic (<90 mm Hg) or diastolic (<60 mm Hg) hypotension
Tachycardia (>125 beats/min)
High fever (>40° C; 104° F) or afebrile
Confusion

Continued

TABLE 9 Risk Factors for a Poor Outcome from Community-Acquired Pneumonia—cont'd

Laboratory Abnormalities

Blood urea nitrogen >19.6 mg/dl

Leukocytosis or leukopenia (<4000/mm^3)

Multilobar radiographic abnormalities

Rapidly progressive radiographic abnormalities during therapy

Bacteremia

Hyponatremia (<130 mmol/L)

Multiple organ failure

Respiratory failure

Hypoalbuminemia

Thrombocytopenia (<100,000/mm^3) or thrombocytosis (>400,000/mm^3)

Arterial pH <7.35

Pleural effusion

Pathogen-Related Factors

High-risk organisms

Type III pneumococcus, *Staphylococcus aureus,* gram-negative bacilli (including *Pseudomonas aeruginosa*), aspiration organisms, severe acute respiratory syndrome

Possibly high levels of penicillin resistance (minimal inhibitory concentration of at least 4 mg/L) in pneumococcus

Therapy-Related Factors

Delay in initial antibiotic therapy (more than 4 h)

Initial therapy with inappropriate antibiotic therapy

Failure to have a clinical response to empiric therapy within 72 h

From Vincent JL et al: *Textbook of critical care,* ed 8, Philadelphia, 2024, Elsevier.

TABLE 10 Differential Diagnosis of Recurrent Pneumonia

Hereditary Disorders

Cystic fibrosis

Sickle cell disease

Disorders of Immunity

AIDS

Bruton agammaglobulinemia

Complement deficiency

Selective IgG subclass deficiencies

Common variable immunodeficiency syndrome

Severe combined immunodeficiency syndrome

Disorders of Leukocytes

Chronic granulomatous disease

Hyperimmunoglobulin E syndrome (Job syndrome)

Leukocyte adhesion defect

Disorders of Cilia

Primary ciliary dyskinesia

Kartagener syndrome

Anatomic Disorders

Sequestration

Lobar emphysema

Foreign body

Tracheoesophageal fistula (H type)

Congenital pulmonary airway malformation (cystic adenomatoid malformation)

Gastroesophageal reflux

Bronchiectasis

Aspiration (oropharyngeal incoordination)

Noninfectious Mimics of Pneumonia

Autoimmune diseases (e.g., granulomatosis with polyangiitis)

Hypersensitivity pneumonitis

From Marcdante KJ et al: *Nelson essentials of pediatrics,* ed 9, Philadelphia, 2023, Elsevier.

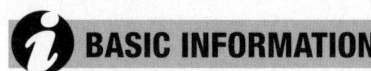

BASIC INFORMATION

DEFINITION

Viral pneumonia is a lung infection caused by any of a large number of viral pathogens. Some of the most important viruses are discussed in this chapter.

SYNONYMS

Viral pneumonia
Nonbacterial pneumonia

ICD-10CM CODES
J12.9	Viral pneumonia, unspecified
J12.89	Other viral pneumonia

EPIDEMIOLOGY & DEMOGRAPHICS

INCIDENCE (IN U.S.):

- COVID-19 (SARS-CoV-2 virus):
  1. The novel coronavirus disease (COVID-19) was first detected in December 2019 and became a worldwide pandemic in 2020. (See "COVID-19 Disease" and "COVID-19 Cardiac Effects" chapters for further information.)
  2. There has been a decline of 47% in the age adjusted COVID-19 death in 2022 compared to 2021.[1]
- Influenza virus:
  1. The CDC estimated ~27 million illnesses, ~12 million medical visits, 300,000 hospitalizations, and ~19,000 deaths caused by influenza in the 2022 to 2023 influenza season.[2]
  2. Secondary bacterial pneumonia develops in a small percentage of infected persons.
- Incidence of other important viral pathogens can vary widely depending on setting, geography, and testing modalities. With the more widespread use of rapid molecular testing of respiratory secretions, an increase in the detection of viral pathogens has been observed. However, determining causality of the identified virus to the suspected pneumonia remains challenging because respiratory viruses remain detectable for several weeks after initial infection, and the pneumonia may be due to secondary bacterial infection.

PREVALENCE (IN U.S.):

- Often related to immune status of the population or presence of an epidemic/pandemic.
- Normal hosts (estimates):
  1. Viral pneumonia requiring children's hospitalization accounts for ~66% cases.
  2. Viruses have been detected in ~23% of adults with clinical pneumonia.

PREDOMINANT SEX:

- Equal predominance.
- Male sex may predispose to more severe respiratory disease in respiratory syncytial virus (RSV) infection.
- Case fatality ratio of COVID-19 is greater among men than among women.

PREDOMINANT AGE:

- COVID-19:
  1. Hospitalizations and deaths increase with age
  2. More prevalent in adults >30 yr

- Influenza:
  1. Overall incidence greatest in children <5 yr
  2. In general, lower incidence with increasing age
  3. Hospitalizations are greatest in infants and children aged <5 yr and adults aged >64 yr
  4. Mortality is greater in adults >64 yr
- RSV and parainfluenza virus:
  1. Young children (as the major cause of pneumonia)
  2. Occurs throughout life
- Human metapneumovirus:
  1. Children: Peak incidence 11 mo
  2. Increasingly detected in adults (bronchitis, chronic obstructive pulmonary disease [COPD] exacerbation, pneumonia)
  3. Frequent cause of lower respiratory tract infection (LRTI) in lung transplant recipients
- Adenoviruses:
  1. Young children
  2. Adults, primarily military recruits
- Varicella:
  1. Approximately 16% of adults (not infected in childhood) who contract varicella develop pneumonia
  2. Acute varicella during pregnancy is more likely to be complicated by severe pneumonia
  3. 90% of reported varicella pneumonia cases are in adults (highest incidence ages 20 to 60 yr)
- Measles:
  1. Young adults and older children who only received a single vaccination (5% failure rate)
  2. Currently most cases are seen in unvaccinated individuals
  3. Measles during pregnancy more likely to be complicated by pneumonia
  4. Underlying cardiopulmonary diseases and immunosuppression predispose to serious pneumonia
  5. Before availability of measles vaccine, 90% of pneumonias in those <10 yr
  6. ~6% of measles cases are complicated by pneumonia
- Cytomegalovirus (CMV):
  1. Neonatal through adult
  2. Immunosuppression is key predisposing factor
  3. Hematopoietic stem cell transplant recipients are at highest risk

PEAK INCIDENCE:

- COVID-19:
  1. Onset in December 2019 without clear seasonal variation
- Influenza:
  1. Winter months for influenza A
  2. Year-round for influenza B
  3. Peak of pneumonia seen weeks into the outbreak of infection
- RSV and parainfluenza virus: Winter and spring
- Human metapneumovirus: Winter months
- Adenovirus: Endemic (military)
- Varicella: Spring in temperate zones
- Measles: Year-round
- Cytomegalovirus (CMV): Year-round

GENETICS: Familial disposition:

- Close contact, not genetics, is important in acquisition
- Congenital anomalies and immunosuppression worsen course of RSV pneumonia

Congenital infection:

- CMV is the most common intrauterine infection in the U.S.
- Pneumonia occurs occasionally in infants with symptomatic congenital infection

Neonatal infection:

- Severe RSV pneumonia
- Adenovirus pneumonia
  1. 5% to 20% mortality rate
  2. Can lead to residual restrictive or obstructive functional abnormalities
- "Varicella neonatorum"
  1. Disseminated visceral disease including pneumonia
  2. May develop in neonates whose mothers develop peripartum chickenpox
- CMV pneumonia:
  1. Generally fatal
  2. Associated with severe cerebral damage in this population

PHYSICAL FINDINGS & CLINICAL PRESENTATION

- COVID-19: Wide range, from mild symptoms to severe illness
  1. Fever, chills, fatigue, myalgias, headache
  2. Cough, shortness of breath, sore throat, congestion, rhinorrhea
  3. Loss of taste or smell
  4. Nausea, vomiting, diarrhea
- Influenza:
  1. Fever, cough, or sore throat (referred to as influenza-like illness [ILI])
  2. Uncomfortable or lethargic appearance
  3. Prominent dry cough (rarely hemoptysis)
  4. Flushed skin and erythematous mucous membranes
  5. Rales or rhonchi
- RSV, parainfluenza, and human metapneumovirus:
  1. Fever
  2. Tachypnea
  3. Prolonged expiration
  4. Wheezes and rales
  5. Diarrhea[3]
- Adenoviruses:
  1. Hoarseness, pharyngitis
  2. Conjunctivitis
  3. Tachypnea
  4. Cervical adenitis
  5. Diarrhea, nausea, vomiting
- Measles:
  1. Conjunctivitis
  2. Rhinorrhea
  3. Koplik spots (white lesions on the buccal mucosa)
  4. Exanthem (maculopapular rash that starts on the head, then moves down to rest of body)
  5. Pneumonitis (coincident with rash, may also develop after apparent recovery from measles)
  6. Fever
  7. Dry cough

- Varicella:
  1. Fever
  2. Maculopapular or vesicular rash (all lesions at the same stage) becomes encrusted
  3. Pneumonia typically 1 to 6 days after rash appears. Pneumonia (Fig. E1) may be accompanied by cough and occasionally hemoptysis
  4. Few auscultatory abnormalities noted on examination of the lungs
- CMV:
  1. Fever
  2. Paroxysmal cough
  3. Occasional hemoptysis
  4. Diffuse adenopathy when pneumonia occurs after transfusion
  5. Severe immunosuppression associated with symptomatic CMV pneumonia (may be reactivation of latent infection or in previously seronegative recipients from the donor)

ETIOLOGY

Viral infection can lead to pneumonia in both immunocompetent and immunocompromised hosts.

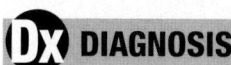

DIAGNOSIS

DIFFERENTIAL DIAGNOSIS

- Bacterial pneumonia; primary bacterial, secondary bacterial infection, or bacterial coinfection
- Other causes of atypical pneumonia:
  1. *Mycoplasma* spp.
  2. *Chlamydia* spp.
  3. *Coxiella* spp.
  4. Legionnaires disease.
  5. In certain patient populations (e.g., immunocompromised) consider fungal infections, pneumocystis, tuberculosis, or atypical mycobacterium.
- Acute respiratory distress syndrome (ARDS)
- Pulmonary emboli

WORKUP

- Information about the current prevalent strain of influenza virus or local prevalence of COVID-19 can be obtained from local health departments or from the Centers for Disease Control and Prevention (CDC).
- Influenza and other viruses may be cultured from respiratory secretions during the initial few days of the illness (special media and techniques necessary).
- Respiratory viral panels that use polymerase chain reaction (PCR)-based assays from nasopharyngeal or bronchoalveolar lavage samples to test for a variety of viruses are extremely sensitive and are becoming the test of choice.
- Rapid flu tests have a 50% to 70% sensitivity in diagnosing influenza (a negative test does not mean the patient does not have influenza).
- Measles and adenovirus pneumonia are usually diagnosed clinically and can be confirmed with serology.
- CMV may be grown in culture or PCR amplified from bronchoalveolar lavage samples.

- An algorithm for the workup and management of suspected severe influenza pneumonia in the critical care unit is described in Fig. E2.
- COVID-19 can be assessed by nasopharyngeal or tracheal aspirate PCR tests for diagnostic workup. Rapid antigen tests are also available and provide results more quickly; however, a single negative test does not rule out an infection, especially in those who are asymptomatic. Antibody serology testing is not generally useful for acute diagnosis.

LABORATORY TESTS

- COVID-19, influenza, RSV, and several other respiratory viruses can be assessed by nasopharyngeal or tracheal aspirate PCR tests for diagnostic workup.
- Sputum Gram stain (usually produced in scanty amounts) typically shows few polymorphonuclear leukocytes and few bacteria.
- White blood cell (WBC) count may vary from leukopenia to modest elevation, usually without a leftward shift. COVID-19 is particularly characterized by leukopenia with predominant lymphopenia.
- Disseminated intravascular coagulation occasionally complicates adenovirus type 7 pneumonia.
- Multinucleated giant cells on Tzanck preparation of an unroofed vesicular lesion are useful in diagnosing varicella (also found in herpes simplex).
- CMV PCR can detect CMV virus but may be negative even with organ involvement in immunosuppressed patients.
- Cultures (blood, sputum, or bronchoalveolar lavage) may be helpful in identifying superinfecting bacterial pathogens.

IMAGING STUDIES

- Chest x-rays may demonstrate a spectrum of findings from ill-defined, patchy, or generalized interstitial opacities (see Fig E1), which can be associated with ARDS.
- Chest CT most commonly demonstrates ground glass opacities, which are usually patchy and peripheral in COVID-19.
- A localized dense alveolar opacification suggests a superimposed bacterial pneumonia.
- Small, calcified nodules may develop as a radiographic residual of varicella pneumonia.

TREATMENT

NONPHARMACOLOGIC THERAPY

General:
- Measures to diminish person-to-person transmission
- Maintenance of adequate hydration
- Possible ventilation support for severe pneumonia or ARDS

COVID-19:
- Facial coverings, social distancing, and quarantine are important in limiting spread of disease.
- COVID-19 vaccines became available in the United States in December 2020. The

messenger RNA vaccines (Pfizer and Moderna) require two doses and a booster. The Janssen vaccine requires a single dose and can be given as a booster, but the CDC generally recommends Pfizer or Moderna for both primary series and booster.[4] Vaccines have been proven to be effective in reducing severity of illness in COVID-19 pneumonia.

Influenza:
- Yearly prophylactic strain-specific influenza vaccination can be given to prevent infection.

RSV:
- Isolation techniques are important in limiting spread of RSV infections.
- Immunoglobulins with a high RSV-neutralizing antibody titer are beneficial in treatment.

Adenoviruses:
- Intestinal inoculation of respiratory adenoviruses has been used to successfully immunize military recruits.
- Although they produce no disease in recipients, the viruses may be shed chronically and may infect others at a later date.
- These vaccines are not available for civilian populations.

Varicella:
- Live, attenuated varicella vaccine has been successfully used in clinical trials.
- Varicella-zoster immune globulin should be administered within 4 days of exposure to prevent or modify the disease in susceptible persons.
- Nonimmunized persons exposed to varicella are potentially infectious between 10 and 21 days after exposure.

Measles:
- Effective measles vaccine (MMR) is available.
  1. The vaccine should be administered at age 15 mo.
  2. A second dose should be administered at the time of school entry.
- Live, attenuated vaccine or gammaglobulin can prevent measles in unvaccinated persons if administered early after exposure.
- Vitamin A given PO for 2 days reduces morbidity and mortality rates from measles in exposed children.

ACUTE GENERAL Rx

- General: Administer antibiotics for bacterial superinfections when appropriate.
- COVID-19:
  1. Supportive care is the mainstay of treatment in outpatient and inpatient cases.
  2. Remdesivir has been shown to shorten the time to recovery in adults hospitalized with COVID-19 with lower respiratory tract infection.
  3. Dexamethasone decreases 28-day mortality in patients requiring respiratory support.
  4. Paxlovid has been shown to reduce the risk of hospitalization and death when used in the outpatient setting in patients who are at high risk for progression to severe disease. It should be initiated within 5 days of symptom onset. Individuals considered at high risk include age >50 yr

and unvaccinated status, >65 yr, immunocompromised individuals, and those with multiple medical comorbidities.[5]

5. In cases where Paxlovid cannot be used, a 3-day course of remdesivir is the preferred alternate treatment in qualifying individuals.

6. In situations when Paxlovid and remdesivir are not available or cannot be administered, molnupiravir can be used.[5]

- Influenza:
  1. Oseltamivir is recommended in patients of any age suspected or confirmed to have influenza.
  2. Oseltamivir is recommended in outpatients with complicated disease or exacerbation of preexisting conditions with suspected or confirmed influenza.
  3. Antiviral treatment should be initiated as soon as possible in hospitalized patients, those with severe illness, or at higher risk for complications. [6]
  4. In individuals who are not high risk, antiviral treatment can be initiated if within 48 h of illness onset.[6]
  5. Baloxavir, oseltamivir, peramivir, or zanamivir may be used in uncomplicated outpatients suspected or confirmed to have influenza.
  6. Amantadine and rimantadine are not recommended for treatment in the United States due to high resistance.
- RSV and parainfluenza:
  1. Ribavirin aerosol may be effective for severe RSV pneumonia.
  2. No approved antiviral therapy for parainfluenza virus pneumonia.
- Human metapneumovirus: No specific antiviral treatment is available.
- Adenoviruses: No approved antiviral therapy for adenovirus; cidofovir has been used in severe cases.

- Varicella:
  1. Patients over age 12 yr who develop chickenpox should be treated with acyclovir or valacyclovir, which may prevent the development of pneumonia.
  2. Varicella pneumonia can be treated with intravenous (IV) acyclovir.
- Measles:
  1. No effective antiviral agent.
  2. Vitamin A should be given to children with measles.
- CMV:
  1. Acyclovir, ganciclovir, and valganciclovir are used to prevent CMV infection in transplant recipients.
  2. Ganciclovir and foscarnet, with or without CMV hyperimmune globulin, are used to treat CMV infection, including pneumonia.

DISPOSITION

- Supportive therapy is useful.
- Death is possible during acute illness.
- Residual functional abnormalities may be persistent or develop into or predispose to chronic respiratory diseases later in life.
- Morbidity and mortality rates after most viral pneumonias are increased by bacterial superinfection.

REFERRAL

- To infectious disease specialist and/or pulmonologist if uncertainty about the diagnosis.
- If symptoms or findings are progressive, with severe respiratory compromise, diffuse infiltrates, or the development of ARDS, referral for supportive care on extracorporeal life support could be considered in select patients.

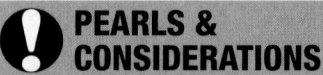

COMMENTS

- Facial coverings, social distancing, and quarantine are important in reduction of COVID-19 transmission, which is spread by droplets and aerosols.
- Influenza spreads through close contact and by small droplets transmitted by cough.
- RSV is effectively transmitted by fomites and by direct contact (little by aerosol).
- Varicella is transmitted by direct contact or by aerosol.
- Of the three major forms of parainfluenza viruses (types 1 to 3), type 3 is the most common cause of viral pneumonia; types 1 and 2 primarily cause laryngotracheitis.
- Human metapneumovirus is a common cause of upper respiratory infections and pneumonia.

REFERENCES

Available at eBooks.Health.Elsevier.com.

RELATED CONTENT

Viral Pneumonia (Patient Information)
Cytomegalovirus Infection (Related Key Topic)
Influenza (Related Key Topic)
Varicella (Related Key Topic)
COVID-19 Disease (Related Key Topic)

AUTHORS: **BETELHEM KIFLE, MD** and **LEKSHMI SANTHOSH, MD, MAED**

Diseases and Disorders

I

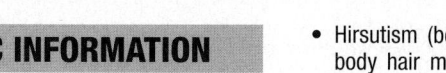 BASIC INFORMATION

DEFINITION

Polycystic ovary syndrome (PCOS) is characterized by an accumulation of incompletely developed follicles in the ovaries due to anovulation and associated with an excess of ovarian androgen production. In its complete form, it is associated with polycystic ovaries, amenorrhea, hirsutism, and obesity. However, a woman with polycystic ovaries but no clinical symptoms does not meet criteria for PCOS. Table 1 describes criteria for a diagnosis of PCOS.

SYNONYMS

Polycystic ovarian syndrome
Polycystic ovary disease
Stein-Leventhal syndrome
PCOS

ICD-10CM CODE
E28.2   Polycystic ovarian syndrome

EPIDEMIOLOGY & DEMOGRAPHICS

- 6% to 21% of reproductive-age women depending on region and diagnostic criteria applied (most common endocrine disorder in this population)[1,2]
- Symptoms usually begin around the time of menarche, and the diagnosis is often made during adolescence or young adulthood.
- Increased risk of endometrial and ovarian cancers due to unopposed estrogen by anovulation (therefore prompt recognition is crucial).
- PCOS is the most common cause of anovulatory infertility.
- Pregnant women with PCOS have higher rates of gestational diabetes and perinatal mortality.

PHYSICAL FINDINGS & CLINICAL PRESENTATION

- Oligomenorrhea or amenorrhea
- Dysfunctional uterine bleeding
- Infertility
- Hirsutism (because the definition of normal body hair may vary depending on patient's race and ethnicity, providers may use the Ferriman-Gallwey scoring system to evaluate hirsutism)[3]
- Acne
- Androgenic alopecia
- Acanthosis nigricans (Fig. E1)
- Obesity (40% only), predominantly abdominal obesity
- Insulin resistance/type 2 diabetes mellitus (may be present in both obese and non-obese women)
- Hypertension
- Dyslipidemia
- Depression
- Nonalcoholic steatohepatitis
- Sleep apnea

ETIOLOGY & PATHOGENESIS

Elevated serum luteinizing hormone (LH) concentrations and an increased serum LH/follicle-stimulating hormone (FSH) ratio result either from an abnormal pulsatile gonadotropin-releasing hormone hypothalamic secretion or, less likely, from a primary pituitary abnormality. This results in increased intraovarian androgen production by theca cells and subsequent dysregulation of androgen secretion, the effect of which in the ovary is follicular atresia, maturation arrest, polycystic ovaries, and anovulation. Hyperandrogenism further exacerbates abnormal GnRH pulsation and subsequent FSH and LH secretion. Anti-Mullerian hormone secretion by follicles accumulated in the ovaries also abnormally affects GnRH pulsation and ovarian environment of follicles. Hyperinsulinemia is a contributing factor to ovarian hyperandrogenism, independent of LH excess, as it activates androgen secretion by theca cells, and additionally inhibits the production of sex hormone-binding globulin in the liver which increases circulating testosterone. A role for insulin growth factor (IGF) receptors has been postulated for the association of PCOS and diabetes. Although there is likely a genetic basis to PCOS, there is currently no recommended genetic screening testing.[4] Iatrogenic causes of PCOS include the antiepileptic medication Valproic Acid.[5] Fig. E2 illustrates the pathologic mechanisms in PCOS.

Dx DIAGNOSIS

The diagnosis of PCOS excludes secondary causes (androgen-producing neoplasm, hyperprolactinemia, adult-onset congenital adrenal hyperplasia).
    Clinical:
- The symptoms, signs, and biochemical features of PCOS vary greatly among women and may change over time.
- There are various diagnostic schemes (Table 1). However, generally the presence of oligomenorrhea, hirsutism, obesity, and documented polycystic ovaries establishes the diagnosis.
- PCOS is the most common cause of chronic anovulation with estrogen present. A positive progesterone withdrawal test establishes the presence of estrogen. Medroxyprogesterone (Provera) 10 mg qd is administered for 5 days and bleeding occurs if estrogen is present.

DIFFERENTIAL DIAGNOSIS

Causes of amenorrhea:
- Primary (unusual in PCOS):
  1. Genetic disorder (Turner syndrome)
  2. Anatomic abnormality (e.g., imperforate hymen)
- Secondary:
  1. Pregnancy
  2. Functional (cause unknown, anorexia nervosa, stress, excessive exercise, hyperthyroidism, hypothyroidism, adrenal dysfunction, pituitary dysfunction, severe systemic illness, drugs such as oral contraceptives, estrogens, or dopamine agonists)
  3. Abnormalities of the genital tract (uterine tumor, endometrial scarring, ovarian tumor)

LABORATORY TESTS

- Glucose tolerance test at the initial presentation and every 2 yr thereafter (rule out diabetes mellitus). Impaired glucose tolerance is very common, occurring in approximately 30% of women with PCOS
- Fasting lipid panel (rule out dyslipidemia)
- Alanine aminotransferase, aspartate aminotransferase (rule out hepatic steatosis)
- Elevated LH/FSH ratio >2.5
- Prolactin level elevation in 25% (rule out hyperprolactinemia)

TABLE 1   Criteria for Diagnosis of Polycystic Ovary Syndrome

Study*	Criteria
National Institute of Child Health and Human Development 1990	Menstrual irregularity
	Hyperandrogenism (clinical or biochemical)
ESHRE-ASRM 2003 Rotterdam criteria	Menstrual irregularity
	Hyperandrogenism (clinical or biochemical)
	Polycystic ovaries on ultrasound (two of three required)
AEPCOS Society 2006	Hyperandrogenism (clinical or biochemical) and menstrual irregularity
	Polycystic ovaries on ultrasound (either or both of the latter two)
NIH Workshop 2012	Endorsement of Rotterdam criteria, acknowledging its limitations, and suggesting the name "PCOS" should be changed

AEPCOS, Androgen Excess and PCOS; *ASRM*, American Society for Reproductive Medicine; *ESHRE*, European Society of Human Reproduction and Embryology; *NIH*, National Institutes of Health; *PCOS*, polycystic ovary syndrome.
*All required the exclusion of other underlying hormonal disorders or tumors.
From Gershenson DM et al: *Comprehensive gynecology*, ed 8, Philadelphia, 2022, Elsevier.

TABLE 2   Laboratory Testing to Exclude Other Causes of Ovulatory Dysfunction and Hyperandrogenism

Lab	Evaluation for:	Comment
Total and/or bioavailable testosterone	Androgen-secreting tumor	Measure if there are symptoms concerning for an androgen-secreting tumor or if biochemical evidence of hyperandrogenism is needed to make the diagnosis of polycystic ovary syndrome. Rapid progression or a total testosterone >200 ng/dl should prompt a workup for an androgen-secreting tumor.
Dehydroepiandrosterone sulfate	Androgen-secreting tumor	Measure if there are symptoms concerning for an androgen-secreting tumor. Although modest elevations in dehydroepiandrosterone sulfate can be seen in polycystic ovary syndrome, rapid progression or greater elevations should prompt a workup for an adrenal androgen-secreting tumor.
Morning 17-hydroxyprogesterone	Late-onset congenital adrenal hyperplasia	This disorder is caused by a partial adrenal enzyme defect that leads to impaired cortisol production, compensatory elevation in adrenocorticotropic hormone, and subsequent excess androgen production. Symptoms may mimic polycystic ovary syndrome. Normal values <200 ng/dl. If higher than this, adrenocorticotropic hormone stimulation test recommended.
24-h urine for cortisol and creatinine; dexamethasone suppression test; salivary cortisol	Cushing syndrome	Consider ruling out Cushing syndrome in women with an abrupt change in menstrual pattern, later-onset hirsutism, or other evidence of cortisol excess such as hypertension, facial plethora, supraclavicular fullness, hyperpigmented striae, and fragile skin.
Prolactin	Hyperprolactinemia	May be accompanied by galactorrhea. Consider ruling this out in all women with irregular menstrual cycles.
Thyroid function studies	Hyperthyroidism or hypothyroidism	Consider ruling out thyroid dysfunction in all women with irregular menstrual cycles.

From Setji TL, Brown AJ: Polycystic ovary syndrome: update on diagnosis and treatment, *Am J Med* 127:912-919, 2014.

- Elevated androgens (testosterone [free and total levels], DHEA-S) and sex hormone-binding globulin (rule in biochemical hyperandrogenemia or rule out androgen-secreting tumor)
- Other: Thyroid-stimulating hormone (rule out hypothyroidism), 17-hydroxyprogesterone (rule out congenital adrenal hyperplasia), 24-h urine for cortisol and creatinine (rule out Cushing syndrome)
- Table 2 summarizes laboratory testing to exclude other causes of ovulatory dysfunction and hyperandrogenism

IMAGING STUDIES

Pelvic ultrasound (Fig. E3) reveals the presence of twofold to fivefold ovarian enlargement with a thickened tunica albuginea, thecal hyperplasia, and 20 or more subcapsular follicles from 1 to 15 mm in diameter. It is important to note that having polycystic ovaries alone does not make the diagnosis of PCOS because 20% of women with polycystic ovaries have no symptoms.

🆁🆇 TREATMENT (TABLE 3)

Clinical practice guidelines for PCOS vary greatly; however, the general goal is to interrupt the self-perpetuating abnormal hormone cycle:[6,7]
- Weight reduction for all obese women with PCOS via exercise and diet as loss of abdominal fat seems to be crucial to restore ovulation. A recent study showed that a short-term ketogenic diet may reduce hormonal imbalances in PCOS.[8]
- Reduction of ovarian androgen secretion by using oral contraceptives or LH-releasing hormone (LHRH) analogs.
- Letrozole (aromatase inhibitor) or FSH stimulation with Clomiphene HMG
- If letrozole or clomiphene fail, pulsatile GnRH and reduction of ovarian androgen secretion

TABLE 3   Treatment for Women with Polycystic Ovary Syndrome

Complaint	Treatment Options
Infertility	Letrozole, clomiphene, with or without metformin, gonadotropins, ovarian cautery ("drilling")
Skin manifestations	Oral contraceptive + antiandrogen (spironolactone, finasteride), GnRH agonists
Abnormal bleeding	Cyclic progestogen, oral contraceptives
Weight, metabolic concerns	Diet/lifestyle management, metformin

From Gershenson DM et al: *Comprehensive gynecology*, ed 8, Philadelphia, 2022, Elsevier.

by laparoscopic ovarian wedge resection may induce ovulation. Laparoscopic ovarian surgery (laparoscopic ovarian drilling [LOD]) is a useful alternative that does not trigger ovarian hyperstimulation.
- Urofollitropin (pure FSH) administration.
- Metformin improves ovulation, insulin sensitivity, and possibly hyperandrogenemia.

Choice of treatment:[6,7]
- Medical methods may improve hirsutism, however are mainly palliative and not curative. Management includes oral contraceptives with or without spironolactone (antiandrogen), topical eflornithine, finasteride, flutamide, shaving or laser hair removal (with eflornithine).
- The management of androgen-related acne includes oral contraceptives, spironolactone, topic treatments (benzoyl peroxide), or oral antibiotics.
- The management of androgen-related alopecia includes oral contraceptives, finasteride, topical minoxidil, or hair transplantation.
- Pregnancy can be achieved with letrozole as the primary ovulation-induction agent. Alternatively, with clomiphene (alone or with glucocorticoids, human chorionic gonadotropin, or bromocriptine), HMG, urofollitropin, pulsatile GnRH, or ovarian wedge resection. Metformin may also induce ovulation. If weight loss,

ovulation induction, and wedge resection are unsuccessful, consider in vitro fertilization (IVF). Of note, recent data suggests that frozen-embryo transfer is associated with a higher rate of live birth and a lower risk of the ovarian hyperstimulation syndrome, however also a higher risk of preeclampsia, when compared to fresh-embryo transfer.[9]
- Psychologic screening and management for depression is recommended as women with PCOS are fourfold more likely to have abnormal depression scores.

DISPOSITION

Table 4 summarizes metabolic complications in PCOS. Cardiovascular risk factors associated with PCOS are described in Table 5.

REFERENCES

Available at eBooks.Health.Elsevier.com.

RELATED CONTENT

Polycystic Ovarian Syndrome (Patient Information)
Amenorrhea (Related Key Topic)
Abnormal Uterine Bleeding (Related Key Topic)

AUTHORS: **FRED F. FERRI, MD** and **MARCELA OSORIO, BA**

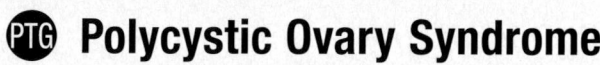

TABLE 4 Metabolic Complications in Polycystic Ovary Syndrome

Abnormal glucose tolerance (impaired glucose tolerance or type 2 diabetes)	30% of obese polycystic ovary syndrome women have impaired glucose tolerance, and 10% have type 2 diabetes by age 40. In thin women with polycystic ovary syndrome, 10% have impaired glucose tolerance, and 1.5% have type 2 diabetes.
Obesity	Prevalence of obesity varies considerably in women with polycystic ovary syndrome. Previously, prevalence rates of obesity were estimated based on populations of women with polycystic ovary syndrome seeking care. A recent study comparing patients presenting for care in a polycystic ovary syndrome clinic with an unselected population evaluated during a preemployment physical suggests that obesity and overweight may not be more common in polycystic ovary syndrome. In that study, 63.7% of polycystic ovary syndrome clinic patients were obese, compared with 28% of unselected women with polycystic ovary syndrome identified during screening, and 28% of nonpolycystic ovary syndrome controls. Polycystic ovary syndrome symptoms, including hyperandrogenism and oligo-ovulation, are exacerbated by obesity.
Metabolic syndrome	33%-50% of U.S. women with polycystic ovary syndrome have metabolic syndrome compared to only 12% in a similarly aged National Health and Nutrition Examination Survey population. In contrast, only 8.2% of women with polycystic ovary syndrome in Italy met criteria for metabolic syndrome. Thus, metabolic syndrome varies by geographic location, a finding likely related to different body mass index, though other causes including genetics and diet could also be playing a part.
High blood pressure	Data have been conflicting, but a large Kaiser Permanente study demonstrated that hypertension or elevated blood pressure was more than twice as common in women with polycystic ovary syndrome (27% vs. 12%).
Dyslipidemia	Dyslipidemia is more prevalent in women with polycystic ovary syndrome compared to controls (15% vs. 6%). In a meta-analysis, triglyceride values were 26 mg/dl higher (95% CI 17-35), low-density lipoprotein cholesterol was 12 mg/dl higher (95% CI 10-16), and high-density lipoprotein-cholesterol was 6 mg/dl lower (95% CI 4-9) in women with polycystic ovary syndrome compared with controls. Women with polycystic ovary syndrome also have higher concentrations and proportions of small, dense low-density lipoprotein cholesterol.
Nonalcoholic fatty liver disease and nonalcoholic steatohepatitis	Nonalcoholic fatty liver disease and nonalcoholic steatohepatitis have recently been recognized as a potential complication in women with polycystic ovary syndrome. Prevalence of fatty liver disease in polycystic ovary syndrome women has been estimated to be 15%-55%, depending on the diagnostic parameter used (level of serum alanine aminotransferase or ultrasound). Individuals that may be at higher risk of nonalcoholic fatty liver disease including nonalcoholic steatohepatitis include those with metabolic syndrome, insulin resistance, and possibly hyperandrogenemia.
Cardiovascular disease	Many studies demonstrate abnormal surrogate markers of cardiovascular disease in women with polycystic ovary syndrome. However, data regarding cardiovascular disease risk are conflicting with some studies suggesting an increased risk in women with polycystic ovary syndrome, whereas other studies have not found this difference in cardiovascular risk. While it is important to recognize and treat cardiovascular risk factors in this population, further research of cardiovascular risk and complications is still needed to clarify the long-term risk.

CI, Confidence interval.
From Setji TL, Brown AJ: Polycystic ovary syndrome: update on diagnosis and treatment, *Am J Med* 127:912-919, 2014.

TABLE 5 Cardiovascular Risk Factors in Polycystic Ovary Syndrome

Risk Factor	Features
Traditional risk factors	Obesity, insulin resistance, dyslipidemia, abnormal homocysteine, C-reactive protein, plasminogen activator inhibitor-1, increase in inflammatory adipocytokines such as TNF-α, decrease in adiponectin; higher prevalence of diabetes, hypertension
Atherosclerosis	Coronary catheterization studies, increase in carotid intima-media thickness, coronary calcium
Endothelial dysfunction by blood flow studies	All increased in classic PCOS; less of a concern with milder phenotypes using Rotterdam criteria

PCOS, Polycystic ovary syndrome; *TNF-α,* tumor necrosis factor alpha.
From Gershenson DM et al: *Comprehensive gynecology,* ed 8, Philadelphia, 2022, Elsevier.

BASIC INFORMATION

DEFINITION

Polymyalgia rheumatica (PMR) is an inflammatory condition characterized by muscle pain and stiffness of the shoulders and hips. PMR primarily affects the elderly and can occur alone or in conjunction with giant cell arteritis (GCA).[1]

SYNONYMS

PMR
Anarthritic rheumatoid syndrome

ICD-10CM CODES
M31.5   Polymyalgia rheumatica with giant cell arteritis
M35.3   Polymyalgia rheumatica

EPIDEMIOLOGY & DEMOGRAPHICS

- PMR almost exclusively occurs above age 50 with peak incidence between ages 70 and 79. Women are 2 to 3 times more likely to be affected by PMR compared to men.[1,2] Only behind rheumatoid arthritis, PMR is the second most common inflammatory rheumatic disease in the US among the elderly population.[3]
- In the U.S., incidence is 52.5 cases per 100,000, increasing with advancing age, with a prevalence of 0.5% to 0.7%. A recent literature review showed the global epidemiology of PMR is more limited with a greater variation in prevalence and estimates. Of note, PMR is higher in Scandinavian countries and populations of Northern European ancestry.[1,2] In Olmsted Country, MN, where there the population is predominantly of Scandinavian and Northern European descent, the incidence of PMR was 63.9 per 100,00 inhabitants aged 50 yr or older.[4]
- PMR is often associated with giant cell arteritis (GCA); approximately 50% of patients with GCA also have PMR.[2,5] Genetic links in PMR are not as clear as in GCA; HLA-DRB1 alleles have been linked with GCA development repeatedly, but that link has not been established with PMR.[5] There is evidence suggesting proinflammatory cytokines such as interleukin (IL)-1α, IL-6, and IL-8 and T-helper lymphocytes may be important in the pathogenesis of PMR.[6]

PHYSICAL FINDINGS & CLINICAL PRESENTATION

- Patients with PMR often have symptoms for 1 to 3 mo before a diagnosis is made.
- Onset of symmetric muscle pain and stiffness, which is worse in the morning (similar to other inflammatory disorders) and recurs with periods of inactivity.[7]
- Neck, shoulders, lower back, hips, thighs, and occasionally trunk and arms are involved. Shoulders are usually affected first. Pain distribution in PMR is illustrated in Fig. E1.
- Constitutional symptoms of fatigue, malaise, weight loss, loss of appetite, and low-grade fever may accompany pain and stiffness.

- Physical exam may reveal limited range of motion of shoulder (most common), cervical spine, and hips. May have subdeltoid and subacromial bursitis and peripheral joint synovitis. Motor exam is normal, although can be limited by pain.
- High-spiking fevers, night sweats, visual disturbances, headaches, or jaw claudication should raise suspicion of giant cell arteritis and be further evaluated promptly.[3]

ETIOLOGY

The cause is unknown, but both PMR and GCA are associated with HLA-DRB1 haplotype. With both conditions, also see elevated Th17 cells and decreased regulatory T cells.[7]

Dx **DIAGNOSIS**

DIFFERENTIAL DIAGNOSIS

See Box 1.

WORKUP

- Initial laboratory evaluation: Erythrocyte sedimentation rate (ESR), C-reactive protein (CRP), CBC, creatine phosphokinase (CPK).[8]
- ESR >30 mm/h in majority of patients. CRP elevation may be more common than high ESR.
- CBC may show a normocytic anemia and thrombocytosis.
- CPK is normal. Antibodies (antinuclear antibody, rheumatoid factor, cyclic citrullinated peptide) are typically negative.
- An algorithm for diagnosing polymyalgia rheumatica without giant cell arteritis (GCA) is described in Fig. E2, and Tables 1 and 2 describe various classification criteria for PMR.
- Ultrasonography, MRI, and PET may identify bursitis or tenosynovitis, (features of the 2012 PMR classification of criteria), which increase sensitivity and specificity.[9]

BOX 1   Differential Diagnosis of Polymyalgia Rheumatica

- Rheumatoid arthritis
- Rotator cuff syndrome
- Osteoarthritis of shoulder and hip joints
- Fibromyalgia
- Polymyositis/dermatomyositis
- Spondyloarthritis
- Systemic lupus erythematosus
- Vasculitides
- Paraneoplastic myalgias
- Infection-associated myalgias
- RS3PE (remitting seronegative symmetric synovitis and pitting edema)
- Parkinson disease
- Hypothyroidism
- There has been a report of a case of polymyalgia rheumatica being an adverse event after administration of a COVID-19 vaccine, but this is uncommon[11]

Rx **TREATMENT**

- Start prednisone 12.5 to 25 mg/day. Dramatic improvement usually occurs within 3 days.
- Dosage should be tailored to patient's weight, symptom severity, and comorbidities (e.g., diabetes, hypertension, or heart failure). If nighttime side effects are experienced, can divide prednisone dose. If symptoms persist after 1 wk, increase dose by 5 mg. Ongoing symptoms require consideration of alternative diagnosis.
- Initial prednisone dose should be maintained for 4 to 8 wk. Steroid dose is then tapered every 2 to 4 wk as tolerated to minimum amount required to remain symptom free. When dose reaches 10 mg/day, taper slowly, usually by 1 mg/mo.
- Flares are typical during tapering, can manage by increasing prednisone 10% to 20%. Most require treatment for 1 to 2 yr with steroids; others are unable to taper off fully.
- Monitor both clinical response and ESR and CRP intermittently.
- Gastroprotection should be considered. Start calcium and vitamin D supplementation for bone health. Start prophylactic bisphosphonates if indicated.
- More than half of patients cannot successfully taper glucocorticoid therapy. Adjunctive treatments including methotrexate have been investigated without clear demonstration of benefit.[10]
- Sarilumab, a human monoclonal antibody that binds interleukin-6 receptor alpha has showed significant efficacy in achieving sustained remission and reducing the cumulative glucocorticoid dose in patients with a relapse of PMR during glucocorticoid tapering.[10] Sarilumab (kevzara) is now FDA approved for PMR patients who have responded inadequately to corticosteroid or who cannot tolerate corticosteroid taper. Cost and formulary are major barriers to its use.

! **PEARLS & CONSIDERATIONS**

Patients with PMR should be monitored closely for the development of GCA. Patients who have incomplete response to prednisone or have an evolving pattern of pain and swelling should be reevaluated for the possibility of a different diagnosis such as rheumatoid arthritis.

REFERENCES
Available at eBooks.Health.Elsevier.com.

RELATED CONTENT

Polymyalgia Rheumatica (PMR) (Patient Information)
Giant Cell Arteritis (Related Key Topic)
Vasculitis, Systemic (Related Key Topic)

AUTHORS: **RISHUBH JAIN, BA** and **MANUEL F. DASILVA, MD**

TABLE 1 2012 European League Against Rheumatism/American College of Rheumatology Classification Criteria for Polymyalgia Rheumatica*

Criteria	Points with Ultrasonography	Points without Ultrasonography
Morning stiffness duration >45 min	2	2
Hip pain or limited range of movement	1	1
Absence of rheumatoid factor or anticitrullinated protein antibody	2	2
Absence of other joint involvement	1	1
≥1 shoulder with subdeltoid bursitis and/or biceps tenosynovitis and/or glenohumeral synovitis (either posterior or axillary) and ≥1 hip with synovitis and/or trochanteric bursitis	1	Not applicable
Both shoulders with subdeltoid bursitis, biceps tenosynovitis, or glenohumeral synovitis	1	Not applicable

*Score ≥4 without ultrasonography or ≥5 with ultrasonography is categorized as polymyalgia rheumatica.

TABLE 2 Classification Criteria for Polymyalgia Rheumatica

Chuang Criteria
1. Patients aged 50 yr or older
2. Bilateral aching and stiffness persisting for 1 mo or more involving two of the following areas: Neck or torso, shoulders or proximal regions of the arms, and hips or proximal aspects of the thighs
3. ESR >40 mm/h
4. Exclusion of other diagnoses except GCA
The presence of all these criteria defines diagnosis of PMR.

Healey Criteria (22)
1. Persistent pain (for at least 1 mo) involving two of the following areas: Neck, shoulders, and pelvic girdle
2. Morning stiffness lasting >1 h
3. Rapid response to prednisone (≤20 mg/day)
4. Absence of other diseases capable of causing the musculoskeletal symptoms
5. Age >50 yr
6. ESR >40 mm/h
The diagnosis of PMR is made if all the above criteria are satisfied.

Bird Criteria (23)*
1. Bilateral shoulder pain and/or stiffness
2. Onset of illness within 2 wk
3. Initial ESR >40 mm/h
4. Morning stiffness >1 h
5. Age >65 yr
6. Depression or loss of weight
7. Bilateral upper arm tenderness

ESR, Erythrocyte sedimentation rate; *GCA*, giant cell arteritis.
*A diagnosis of probable polymyalgia rheumatica (PMR) is made if any three or more of these criteria are fulfilled. The presence of any three or more criteria yields a sensitivity of 92% and a specificity of 80%.
From Hochberg MC et al: *Rheumatology*, ed 8, Philadelphia, 2023, Elsevier.

P

Diseases
and Disorders

I

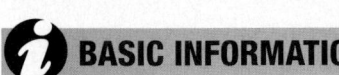

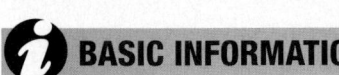 BASIC INFORMATION

DEFINITION
Clinically significant portal hypertension is defined as a portal vein pressure >10 mm Hg, most commonly attributable to liver disease.

ICD-10CM CODE	
K76.6	Portal hypertension

EPIDEMIOLOGY & DEMOGRAPHICS
- Incidence of portal hypertension is not known.
- Cirrhosis is the most common cause of portal hypertension in the U.S.
- Portal hypertension is developed by >90% of patients with cirrhosis.
- Alcoholic and viral liver diseases are the most common causes of cirrhosis and portal hypertension in the U.S.
- Schistosomiasis is the main cause of portal hypertension outside the U.S.
- Esophageal varices may appear when portal vein pressure rises to >10 mm Hg.
- Variceal hemorrhage is the most serious complication of portal hypertension and may occur when portal pressures rise >12 mm Hg.

PHYSICAL FINDINGS & CLINICAL PRESENTATION
- Jaundice
- Ascites (Fig. 1)
- Spider angiomata
- Testicular atrophy
- Gynecomastia
- Palmar erythema
- Dupuytren contracture
- Asterixis (with advanced liver failure)
- Irritability, encephalopathy

- Splenomegaly
- Dilated veins in the anterior abdominal wall
- Venous pattern on the flanks
- Caput medusae (tortuous collateral veins around the umbilicus)
- Hemorrhoids
- Hematemesis
- Melena
- Pruritus

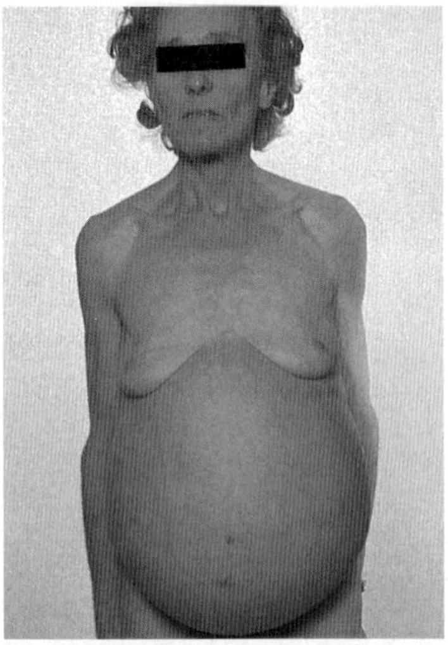

ETIOLOGY
Pathophysiologically caused by:
- Conditions resulting in an increased resistance to flow:
  1. **Prehepatic** (e.g., portal vein thrombosis, splenic vein thrombosis, congenital stenosis)
  2. **Hepatic** (e.g., cirrhosis, alcoholic liver disease, primary biliary cirrhosis, schistosomiasis)
  3. **Posthepatic** (e.g., Budd-Chiari syndrome, constrictive pericarditis, inferior vena cava obstruction, cor pulmonale, tricuspid regurgitation)
- Conditions leading to increase in portal blood flow:
  1. Splanchnic arterial vasodilation accompanying portal hypertension, mediated by local release of nitric oxide
  2. Arterial-portal venous fistulae

Table 1 describes the pathophysiologic changes in portal hypertension, and Table 2 summarizes the etiologies of portal hypertension.

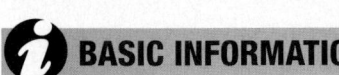 DIAGNOSIS

- The diagnosis of portal hypertension is made on clinical grounds after a comprehensive history and physical examination.
- Noninvasive and invasive procedures confirm diagnosis and determine the severity of portal hypertension.

DIFFERENTIAL DIAGNOSIS
- Ascites from infection, neoplasm, or other inflammatory processes
- Obesity
- Abdominal organomegaly

WORKUP
The workup of portal hypertension includes blood tests and noninvasive imaging studies to determine if the cause of portal hypertension is prehepatic, hepatic, or posthepatic. Ascitic fluid analysis is a key part of the diagnosis.

LABORATORY TESTS
- Complete blood count with platelets
- Liver function tests with serum albumin
- Prothrombin and partial thromboplastin times
- Hepatitis B surface antigen and antibody
- Hepatitis C antibody
- In selected cases: Iron, total iron-binding capacity, and ferritin; antinuclear antibody, anti–smooth muscle antibodies, antimitochondrial antibody, ceruloplasmin, alpha-1 antitrypsin
- Ascitic fluid analysis: A serum-ascites albumin gradient ≥1.1 mg/dl suggests portal hypertension. Polymorphonuclear cells ≥250 cells/ml or positive Gram stain or culture suggest complicating spontaneous bacterial peritonitis (SBP)

IMAGING STUDIES
- Duplex-Doppler ultrasound is effective in screening for portal hypertension.
- Less commonly, CT/MRI/MRA scanning (Figs. E2 and E3) or liver-spleen nuclear medicine scanning can be used if the results from ultrasound are equivocal.
- Upper endoscopy is the most reliable test documenting the presence of esophageal varices.

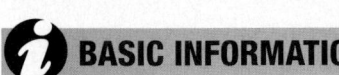

FIG. 1 Ascites secondary to portal hypertension. Note the dilated collateral vein running up the right side of the abdomen. (From Forbes A et al [eds]: *Atlas of clinical gastroenterology,* ed 3, Oxford, 2005, Mosby.)

TABLE 1 Pathophysiologic Changes in Portal Hypertension

Pathophysiologic Change	Specifics
Hepatic resistance	Passive, mechanical component: 60%-70%
	Active, dynamic component: 30%-40%
Portal hypertension	
Shunts	
Splanchnic vasodilation	
Increased portal inflow	
Decrease in effective circulating volume; redistribution total blood volume	
Increase in endogenous vasopressors (RAA, SNS, VP)	
	Increase in endothelin-1
	Angiotensin II
	Norepinephrine
	Vasopressin
	PGF-2 alpha
Decrease in NO, CO	

CO, Carbon monoxide; *NO,* nitrogen monoxide; *PGF,* prostaglandin; *RAA,* renin-angiotensin-aldosterone; *SNS,* sympathetic nervous system; *VP,* vasopressin.
From Vincent JL et al: *Textbook of critical care,* ed 7, Philadelphia, 2017, Elsevier.

TABLE 2 Etiology of Portal Hypertension Grouped by Location of Insult

Site of Increased Resistance	Condition	FHVP	WHVP	HVGP	SPP
Presinusoidal (extrahepatic)	Extrahepatic portal, splenic, or mesenteric vein thrombosis	Normal	Normal	Normal	Increased
Presinusoidal (intrahepatic)	Early primary biliary cirrhosis	Normal	Normal/raised (?)	Normal/raised (?)	Increased
Presinusoidal (intrahepatic)	PSC	Normal	Normal/raised (?)	Normal/raised (?)	Increased
Presinusoidal (intrahepatic)	Sarcoid	Normal	Normal/raised (?)	Normal/raised (?)	Increased
Presinusoidal (intrahepatic)	Schistosomiasis	Normal	Normal/raised (?)	Normal/raised (?)	Increased
Presinusoidal (intrahepatic)	Congestive heart failure	Normal	Normal/raised (?)	Normal/raised (?)	Increased
Presinusoidal (intrahepatic)	Noncirrhotic portal fibrosis	Normal	Normal/raised (?)	Normal/raised (?)	Increased
Intrahepatic sinusoidal	Cirrhosis (any etiology)	Normal	Increased	Increased	Increased
Intrahepatic sinusoidal	Alcoholic hepatitis	Normal	Increased	Increased	Increased
Intrahepatic sinusoidal	Fulminant liver failure (any etiology)	Normal	Increased	Increased	Increased
Extrahepatic postsinusoidal hypertension	Budd-Chiari syndrome	Increased	Increased	Normal	Increased
Extrahepatic postsinusoidal hypertension	Constrictive pericarditis	Increased	Increased	Normal	Increased
Extrahepatic postsinusoidal hypertension	Inferior vena cava obstruction	Increased	Increased	Normal	Increased
Extrahepatic postsinusoidal hypertension	Congenital inferior vena cava web	Increased	Increased	Normal	Increased
Extrahepatic postsinusoidal hypertension	Right heart failure	Increased	Increased	Normal	Increased

FHVP, Free hepatic venous pressure; *HVGP,* hepatic venous pressure gradient; *PSC,* primary sclerosing cholangitis; *SPP,* systolic pulse pressure; *WHVP,* wedged hepatic venous pressure.
From Vincent JL et al: *Textbook of critical care,* ed 7, Philadelphia, 2017, Elsevier.

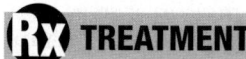 **TREATMENT**

The treatment of portal hypertension is complex and involves measures to reduce the hypertension directly, minimize volume overload, correct underlying disorders, and prevent complications (most notably SBP and variceal bleeding).

NONPHARMACOLOGIC THERAPY
Dietary sodium restriction to generally 2000 mg/day forms the basis of therapy to limit fluid overload.

ACUTE GENERAL Rx
- For tense ascites, serial large-volume paracentesis (LVP) is generally recommended. The use of albumin infusion (8 to 10 g/L of ascites fluid removed) during LVP >5 L has been shown to reduce the incidence of postparacentesis circulatory dysfunction, although its use remains somewhat controversial.
- Intravenous (IV) diuretics, typically furosemide and spironolactone, are used to achieve natriuresis and net negative salt and water balance. Renal function and serum electrolytes are monitored frequently, with transition to an oral regimen for long-term therapy.
- SBP is treated with IV antibiotics directed against enteric bacteria.
- Acute variceal hemorrhage is treated with crystalloid and blood product resuscitation, IV octreotide, terlipressin/vasopressin or somatostatin, and urgent upper endoscopy, often with sclerotherapy or band ligation. Patients with acute variceal hemorrhage should receive empiric antibiotic therapy for SBP.
- Traditionally, a transjugular intrahepatic portosystemic shunt (TIPS) or surgical shunt placement may be considered in patients not responding to above measures. However, recent data show *early* TIPS placement improved outcomes in acute variceal hemorrhage. Table 3 summarizes indications, contraindications, and complications of the TIPS procedure.
- Table 4 compares treatment modalities for portal hypertension.

CHRONIC Rx
- Dietary sodium restriction in combination with diuretics: The typical ratio of furosemide 40 mg to spironolactone 100 mg retains normal serum potassium levels in most patients.
- Nonselective beta-blockers (propranolol and nadolol) in dosages sufficient to reduce the resting heart rate by 25% have been shown to be effective in primary prophylaxis for first-time variceal bleeding and for preventing recurrent variceal bleeding. Dosages are usually given bid and decreased if heart rate falls to <55 beats/min or systolic blood pressure drops to <90 mm Hg. The addition of a long-acting nitrate (e.g., isosorbide-5-mononitrate)

TABLE 3 Indications, Contraindications, and Complications of the TIPS Procedure

Indications	Relative Contraindications	Contraindications	Acute Complications	Chronic Complications
Upper GI bleeding	Pulmonary hypertension	Right-sided heart failure	Neck hematoma	Congestive heart failure
Ascites	Severe liver failure	Biliary tract obstruction	Arrhythmia	Portal vein thrombosis
Hepatic hydrothorax	Portal vein thrombosis	Uncontrolled infection	Stent displacement	Progressive liver failure
	Multiple hepatic cysts	Chronic recurrent disabling hepatic encephalopathy	Hemolysis	Chronic recurrent encephalopathy
		Hepatocellular carcinoma involving hepatic veins	Bilhemia	Stent dysfunction
			Hepatic vein obstruction	TIPSitis
			Shunt thrombosis	
			Hemoperitoneum	
			Hemobilia	
			Liver ischemia	
			Cardiac failure	
			Sepsis	

GI, Gastrointestinal; *TIPS,* transjugular intrahepatic portosystemic shunt.
From Vincent JL et al: *Textbook of critical care,* ed 7, Philadelphia, 2017, Elsevier.

TABLE 4 Comparison of Treatment Modalities

Treatment Modality	No (%), N = 77	Age, Yr (Mean)	Female %	Initial Meld (Mean, Range)	Child-Pugh Score (N = 74)	Ascites Size	Death (No, %) (N = 44)	Days from Presentation until Death or End of Study
Medical management	64/77 (83%)	52	23/64 (36%)	16 (4-46)	A = 1 B = 31	None: 6 Small: 34 Moderate: 16 Large: 8	40/64 (63%)	321 ± 463
TIPS	8/77 (10%)	56	5/8 (63%)	12 (7-28)	A = 0 B = 5 C = 2	None: 1 Small: 3 Moderate: 3 Large: 1	4/8 (50%)	845 ± 407
Transplant	5/77 (7%)	54	0	21 (10-40)	A = 1 B = 1 C = 1	Large: 1	0	1896 ± 1752

TIPS, Transjugular intrahepatic portosystemic shunt.
From Vincent JL et al: *Textbook of critical care,* ed 7, Philadelphia, 2017, Elsevier.

has been shown to improve portal hemodynamics. Findings of a prospective trial of beta-blockers to prevent the formation of varices were negative. The combination of beta-blockade plus endoscopic esophageal variceal banding is superior to either intervention alone.

- Intermittent LVP may be needed in "diuretic-resistant" patients.
- Patients with prior SBP merit lifelong antibiotics for secondary prevention.
- Abstinence from alcohol or treatment for hepatitis B or hepatitis C. Vaccination for hepatitis A and B as appropriate.
- Hepatic transplantation is an option in selected patients.

DISPOSITION

- The most common complication associated with portal hypertension is variceal bleeding. The risk of bleeding from varices is approximately 15% at 1 yr.

- Development of the hepatorenal syndrome (HRS) is associated with high near-term mortality. In particular, HRS may complicate SBP, which emphasizes the importance of making the diagnosis of SBP and instituting appropriate prophylaxis.

REFERRAL

Consultation with a gastroenterologist is recommended in all patients with portal hypertension to screen for esophageal varices.

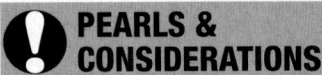 **PEARLS & CONSIDERATIONS**

Splanchnic arterial vasodilation is increasingly recognized as an important component of the pathophysiology of portal hypertension and ascites. There may be vasodilation in other capillary beds as well; of note, pulmonary arteriolar vasodilation can create a significant shunt fraction and resultant hypoxemia in the absence of chest radiograph or CT chest evidence of parenchymal disease. The diagnosis is suspected when otherwise unexplained hypoxia arises in a patient with cirrhosis, along with platypnea (dyspnea worse when sitting upright) and orthodeoxia (desaturation with upright posture). The diagnosis is confirmed by echocardiography with agitated saline, in which there is delayed appearance of bubbles in the left heart after injection into a peripheral vein.

COMMENTS

Portal hypertension and its complications carry significant morbidity and mortality rates. Emphasize ethanol abstinence, provide vaccinations and prophylactic therapy where indicated, and consider early referral to a specialist for assistance with management and consideration for hepatic transplantation.

AUTHOR: **FRED F. FERRI, MD**

BASIC INFORMATION

DEFINITION

Postconcussion syndrome (PCS) refers to nonspecific neurologic, cognitive, and psychologic symptoms that result from traumatic brain injury (TBI) and persist beyond the expected recovery period, usually greater than 3 mo. Concussion is an acute trauma-induced alteration of mental function lasting <24 h, with or without preceding loss of consciousness. Approximately 90% of concussion symptoms resolve within 10 to 14 days, but some may linger.[1] The extent and severity of lingering symptoms are highly dependent on the testing and reporting used. PCS can also follow moderate and severe brain injury, although it is more commonly associated with mild brain injury or concussion often without loss of consciousness.

SYNONYMS

PCS
Postconcussive syndrome
Posttraumatic nervous instability or brain injury
Postcontusion syndrome or encephalopathy

ICD-10CM CODE
F07.81   Postconcussional syndrome

EPIDEMIOLOGY & DEMOGRAPHICS

- Incidence is approximately 27 cases per 100,000 persons/yr.
- From 30% to 80% of patients with mild to moderate brain injury will experience some symptoms of PCS, though this is variable.[1]
- Risk factors for prolonged symptoms include children, female sex, low socioeconomic status, anxiety sensitivity, previous TBI, severe bodily injury from TBI, headaches, and unsettled litigation.[2]
- Recurrent TBI, especially when symptoms of previous injuries still exist, significantly increases the risk and severity of future postconcussive syndrome.
- Acute postinjury symptoms such as headache, dizziness, photophobia, diplopia, or tinnitus are associated with development of persistent symptoms.[1]

PHYSICAL FINDINGS & CLINICAL PRESENTATION

- Symptoms start within a few days to weeks after the head injury, and greater than 30% of patients still have some symptoms 3 mo after injury; 15% of patients or more will have persistent symptoms 1 yr later.[2]
- At least three of the following symptoms after TBI are required to meet ICD-10 criteria:[3]
  1. Headache (usually of frontooccipital location and showing characteristics of tension or migraine headache)—occurring in 25% to 78% of persons after mild TBI
  2. Fatigue
  3. Dizziness and/or vertigo—occurring in approximately 50%. Associated with risk for prolonged recovery

  4. Impaired memory
  5. Difficulty in concentrating
  6. Insomnia—occurring in approximately 33% acutely and 25% more chronically
  7. Irritability/frustration
  8. Lowered tolerance of stress, emotion, or alcohol
- Other associated symptoms: Noise sensitivity, neck pain, nondermatomal paresthesias, interference with social role functioning.
- Detailed neurologic exam is required focusing on orthostatic intolerance, cognitive function, vestibular function, extraocular movements, gait, balance, and coordination. Abnormalities are often subtle.[3-5]
- May need to test for impaired saccades or vestibulo-ocular reflex abnormalities, cervical motion abnormalities, and impairment on tandem gait forward and backward.[5]

ETIOLOGY

- The inciting TBI may occur as a result of events such as falls, motor vehicle accidents, military injuries, and contact sports.
- The primary injury triggers a slew of pathophysiological changes at the cellular level secondary to the axonal stretching and injury, leading to alterations in membrane and intracellular physiology, thereby affecting neurotransmission. These changes are believed to be a factor in determining whether the outcome will be an apparent normal recovery or persistent postconcussion symptoms.
- Postmortem findings reveal diffuse axonal injury as the primary pathologic finding, along with small petechial hemorrhages and local edema.
- Prior history of anxiety is a strong risk factor for occurrence of PCS.

Dx DIAGNOSIS

A careful history will usually establish the diagnosis and rule out other etiologies.

DIFFERENTIAL DIAGNOSIS

- Headache (dissection of the vertebral artery, occipital neuralgia)
- Epidural hematoma
- Subdural hematoma
- Skull fracture
- Cervical spine disk disease
- Whiplash
- Cerebrovascular accident
- Benign paroxysmal positional vertigo—common after head injury
- Depression
- Anxiety
- Posttraumatic stress disorder

WORKUP

- Neuropsychologic testing, which often reveals difficulties in concentration, memory, language, and executive function
- To exclude other causes of neurologic symptoms after TBI:
  1. Normal results of electroencephalography
  2. Normal evoked potentials

LABORATORY TESTS

Various biomarkers in blood and cerebrospinal fluid and genetic testing have been proposed and studied in patients with TBI, but these tests are not specific and are not routinely used in clinical practice.

Chronically, if not improving, consider growth factor and other neuroendocrine markers.[5]

IMAGING STUDIES

- There is no imaging modality to diagnose PCS. PCS is primarily a clinical diagnosis. The American College of Emergency Physicians' clinical policy regarding neuroimaging in adults with mild traumatic brain injury is summarized in Box 1.
- 10% of computed tomography (CT) scans of the head following mild TBI are abnormal, showing mild subarachnoid hemorrhage, subdural hemorrhage, or contusions.[1,2]
- MRI of the head after a mild traumatic brain injury (mTBI) is abnormal in 30% of patients with normal CT scans and may show irregular brain contours or cerebral contusions.
- More advanced imaging modalities, including diffuse tensor imaging (DTI) and susceptibility weighted imaging (SWI) in MRI, functional MRI (fMRI), and metabolic imaging such as magnetic resonance spectroscopy (MRS), positron emission tomography (PET), and single-photon emission computed tomography (SPECT) imaging, can show acute and chronic changes even after one mTBI, although they have not found a major role in clinical practice yet.[3-4]
- None of the imaging modalities have been able to predict the occurrence of PCS in patients with mild TBI.[3-4]

Rx TREATMENT

PCS must be recognized as a physiologic and psychologic problem and treated accordingly. Treatment should be individualized to target the patient's particular symptoms and is typically completed on an outpatient basis. Some symptoms may be refractory to treatment.

NONPHARMACOLOGIC THERAPY

- Early reassurance and patient education are major components of treatment. Explanation of symptoms and expectations, combined with early follow-up with reassurance, may hasten resolution of symptoms.
- Early and graduated physical activity is preferred over prolonged cognitive and physical rest. Light aerobic activity that avoids risk for reinjury has been shown beneficial in mitigating refractory concussion symptoms. Physical and occupational therapy may be beneficial.[3-4]
- Cognitive behavioral therapy may be effective in treating symptoms.
- Avoidance of alcohol, narcotics, and sleep deprivation.

PHARMACOLOGIC THERAPY

- Supportive symptomatic care may include the use of non-narcotic analgesics and antiemetics.

BOX 1   American College of Emergency Physicians' Clinical Policy Regarding Neuroimaging in Adults with Mild Traumatic Brain Injury

A noncontrast head CT is indicated (level one recommendation) in adults with altered LOC or posttraumatic amnesia only if at least one of the following is present:
- Headache
- Vomiting
- Age older than 60 yr
- Drug or alcohol intoxication
- Deficits in short-term memory
- Physical evidence of trauma above the clavicle
- Posttraumatic seizure
- GCS score below 15
- Focal neurologic deficit
- Coagulopathy

A noncontrast head CT should be considered (level two recommendation) in head trauma patients with no altered LOC or posttraumatic amnesia if any of the following is present:
- Focal neurologic deficit
- Vomiting
- Severe headache
- Age 65 yr or older
- Physical signs of a basilar skull fracture
- GCS score below 15
- Coagulopathy
- A dangerous mechanism (e.g., ejection from motor vehicle, pedestrian struck, fall of more than 3 feet or 5 stairs)

CT, Computed tomography; *GCS,* Glasgow coma scale; *LOC,* level of consciousness.
From Marx J et al: *Rosen's emergency medicine, concepts and clinical practice,* ed 7, Philadelphia, 2010, Mosby.

- Early treatment of symptoms may improve outcomes and improve quality of life.
- Amitriptyline has been widely used for posttraumatic tension-type headaches as well as for nonspecific symptoms such as irritability, dizziness, insomnia, and depression.[2-3] Amantadine is also a consideration.
- Posttraumatic migraine-type headaches can be treated with a trial of propranolol or amitriptyline alone or in combination.
- Depression can be treated with selective serotonin reuptake inhibitors but may not respond as well when compared with patients without PCS who have depression.
- If symptoms are not improving, consider testing for hypopituitarism since complete or partial hypopituitarism (most commonly growth factor) can be a sequelae of mild TBI and has overlapping symptoms with postconcussion syndrome.[6]

DISPOSITION

- Most patients improve after mild TBI without any residual deficits within 3 mo, though the cognitive and emotional symptoms resolve more slowly.
- Although good improvement is typically seen within the first 6 mo, patients can continue to show improvement for up to 12 to 18 mo.
- Patients with very severe brain injuries (low Glasgow Coma Scale [GCS] score) and prolonged anterograde amnesia are at increased risk of development of some degree of permanent cognitive and personality disturbance.

- Predictors for the development of persistent PCS (symptoms greater than 3 mo) include:
  1. Female sex
  2. Ongoing litigation (conflicting studies)
  3. Low socioeconomic status
  4. Prior headaches
  5. Prior TBI
  6. Prior psychiatric illnesses, particularly anxiety

REFERRAL

Early consultations with psychologists, psychiatrists, neurologists, and rehabilitation specialists in an outpatient setting may be beneficial.

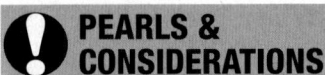

❗ PEARLS & CONSIDERATIONS

- Recognizing depression and treating pain symptoms early in the course may help prevent the development of persistent PCS (>3 mo).
- The severity of the trauma does not clearly predict the risk of PCS, and symptoms do not cluster in a predictable manner.
- The severity of brain injury is usually documented by initial GCS score, duration of loss of consciousness, and duration of amnesia; however, there is a move toward tests of function, such as neuropsychologic testing or fMRI.
- Engaging in physical activity within 2 days after concussion is associated with a lower rate of persistent postconcussive symptoms.

REFERENCES

Available at eBooks.Health.Elsevier.com.

RELATED CONTENT

Postconcussion Syndrome (Patient Information)
Concussion (Related Key Topic)
Traumatic Brain Injury (Related Key Topic)

AUTHOR: **COREY ELAM GOLDSMITH, MD, FAAN**

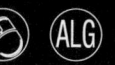

BASIC INFORMATION

DEFINITION

Postherpetic neuralgia (PHN) is a pain syndrome that results as a complication of herpes zoster (HZ). HZ, also known as shingles, is a painful vesicular eruption in a dermatomal distribution. HZ is caused by the reactivation of varicella zoster virus (VZV) in someone with a known history of varicella. PHN is pain and/or dysesthesia that persist for 3 or more mo at the site of resolved HZ.[1]

SYNONYMS

PHN
Shingles neuropathy

ICD-10CM CODE
B02.29   Other postherpetic nervous system involvement

EPIDEMIOLOGY & DEMOGRAPHICS

INCIDENCE: PHN occurs in up to 12.8% of HZ patients. It is the most frequent chronic complication of HZ and the most common neuropathic pain disorder resulting from infection.[2] From 1994 through 2018, the overall incidence of PHN increased across all ages, races/ethnicities, and sexes.[2] The median age of patients with PHN was 65.9 yr old, nearly 10 yr older than the median age of patients with HZ, indicating its predominance in the elderly.[2] In one study, approximately 60% of patients with HZ developed PHN at age 60 yr, and 75% developed PHN at age 70 yr. In another study, the incidence of PHN at 9 yr post-HZ eruption was 21%.[3]

PREDOMINANT SEX & AGE:
- PHN occurs equally in males and females.
- The likelihood of developing PHN significantly increases with advancing age.

PEAK INCIDENCE: Unknown

RISK FACTORS:
- Advanced age
- Greater severity of HZ prodromal pain
- Greater severity of pain during acute HZ eruption
- Location—specifically ophthalmic (V1) location and brachial plexus
- Severe immunosuppression
- Severe rash[4]

GENETICS: Family history of HZ is considered a risk factor for HZ, with higher risk if multiple family members have had HZ.[5]

PHYSICAL FINDINGS & CLINICAL PRESENTATION

- HZ typically presents as a painful vesicular eruption in a dermatomal distribution. Rarely, HZ can occur subclinically with dermatomal pain in the absence of a rash (zoster sine herpete).[6]
- PHN is pain that continues for 3 mo at the dermatomal site of the resolved HZ. The pain may be described as burning, stabbing, shooting, or shocklike.
- Patients may note an amplified response to stimuli at the site of PHN, with increased pain

response (hyperalgesia), pain to typically nonnoxious stimuli (allodynia), or focal changes in autonomic function (e.g., increased sweating).
- Physical examination should include a comparison of sensory function in the affected dermatome with that on the contralateral side.

ETIOLOGY

PHN is associated with damage and scarring to the dorsal root ganglion secondary to inflammation related to active herpes zoster infection.[6]

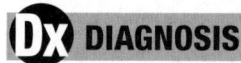

DIAGNOSIS

DIFFERENTIAL DIAGNOSIS

Zoster sine herpete (subclinical HZ without skin eruption)

TREATMENT

ACUTE GENERAL Rx

- Administration of acyclovir or valacyclovir within 72 h of HZ onset is thought to help reduce the likelihood of developing PNH. However, one Cochrane review paper found no difference with acyclovir administration.[7]
- A single published study supports the use of amitriptyline (25 mg daily) as an adjunct to an antiviral agent in acute HZ to decrease the incidence of PHN and the pain associated with subsequent PHN.[8]
- A suggestive noncontrolled study with co-administration of valacyclovir and gabapentin during acute HZ reduced the incidence of PHN as well.[9]
- Corticosteroids do NOT prevent PHN.[10]

CHRONIC Rx (TABLE E1)[11-15]
TOPICAL TREATMENTS:
- Lidocaine 5% patches may be used for mild pain.
- Capsaicin 0.075% cream (although little reported efficacy)[16] 5 times per day.
- Capsaicin 8% patch has greater efficacy,[16] but overall analgesia may be minimal at best, with one third of patients unable to tolerate the agent due to burning, stinging, and erythema. However, a single 60-min treatment with high concentration capsaicin patch was found in one study to reduce PHN for up to 12 wk regardless of concomitant systemic neuropathic pain medication use.[17]

ORAL TREATMENTS: First line:
- Gabapentinoids (gabapentin, pregabalin) are the only FDA-approved oral therapy for PHN and are some of the most used first-line therapies for chronic PHN pain.[18] Gabapentin may be administered in the immediate-release or extended-release formulation. Dosing includes gabapentin 300 mg 3 times a day (titrating up to max 3600 mg/day) and pregabalin 75 mg nightly (titrating up to 300 mg twice daily).
- Tricyclic antidepressants such as amitriptyline (25 mg/day, increased by 25 mg every night to

a maximum of 75 mg/night), desipramine (10 to 25 mg/day, increased by 25 mg/day every 3 days as needed to a maximum of 150 mg/day), and nortriptyline (10 to 25 mg/day, increased by 25 mg/day weekly as needed to maximum of 75 mg day) are other first-line treatments.[19] These medications have a delayed onset of action and may not work as well in patients with certain types of pain, such as burning pain or allodynia. They have a considerable side effect profile. Their use in elderly patients should be carefully considered. A randomized controlled crossover study showed the combination of gabapentin and nortriptyline was more efficacious than either drug as monotherapy for neuropathic pain.[20]
Second line:
- Opiates (e.g., controlled-release oxycodone):[21] Side effects, the possibility of misuse, and the potential for abuse must be weighed.
Other modalities:
- Dorsal root entry zone (DREZ) lesioning has been used with an improvement rate of up to 45% in long-term studies.[22]
- For recalcitrant cases, epidural corticosteroids[23] and nerve blocks,[24] botulinum toxin,[25,26] cryotherapy,[27] and pulsed radiofrequency.[28]
- Fig. 1 describes a treatment algorithm for HZ and PHN.

COMPLEMENTARY & ALTERNATIVE MEDICINE

Acupuncture: Studies on acupuncture and PHN pain have had varying results. A recent systematic review and meta-analysis of seven randomized, controlled studies showed superior pain reduction in the acupuncture arm compared with pharmacologic therapy, although their effects on improving the global impression or life quality were similar.[29]

REFERRAL

For complicated cases, dermatology, neurology, and/or pain management input can be helpful.

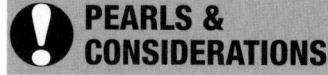

PEARLS & CONSIDERATIONS

COMMENTS

- Careful consideration of treatment side effects and drug interactions is needed.
- The natural history of PHN is slow resolution, and most individuals respond to medical therapy. However, a subtype of patients may develop severe, long-lasting pain that is recalcitrant to medical therapy.
- In a questionnaire study of 385 adults age >65 yr with persistent acute pain, the mean duration of PHN was 3.3 yr.[30]
- Only consider topical capsaicin on intact skin.[31]

PREVENTION

- Vaccination:
  1. A non-live VZV vaccine (Shingrix®) is approved by the FDA for individuals age 50 and older. It is administered as two shots spaced 2 mo apart and is 97% effective against shingles in people ages 50 to 69,[32]

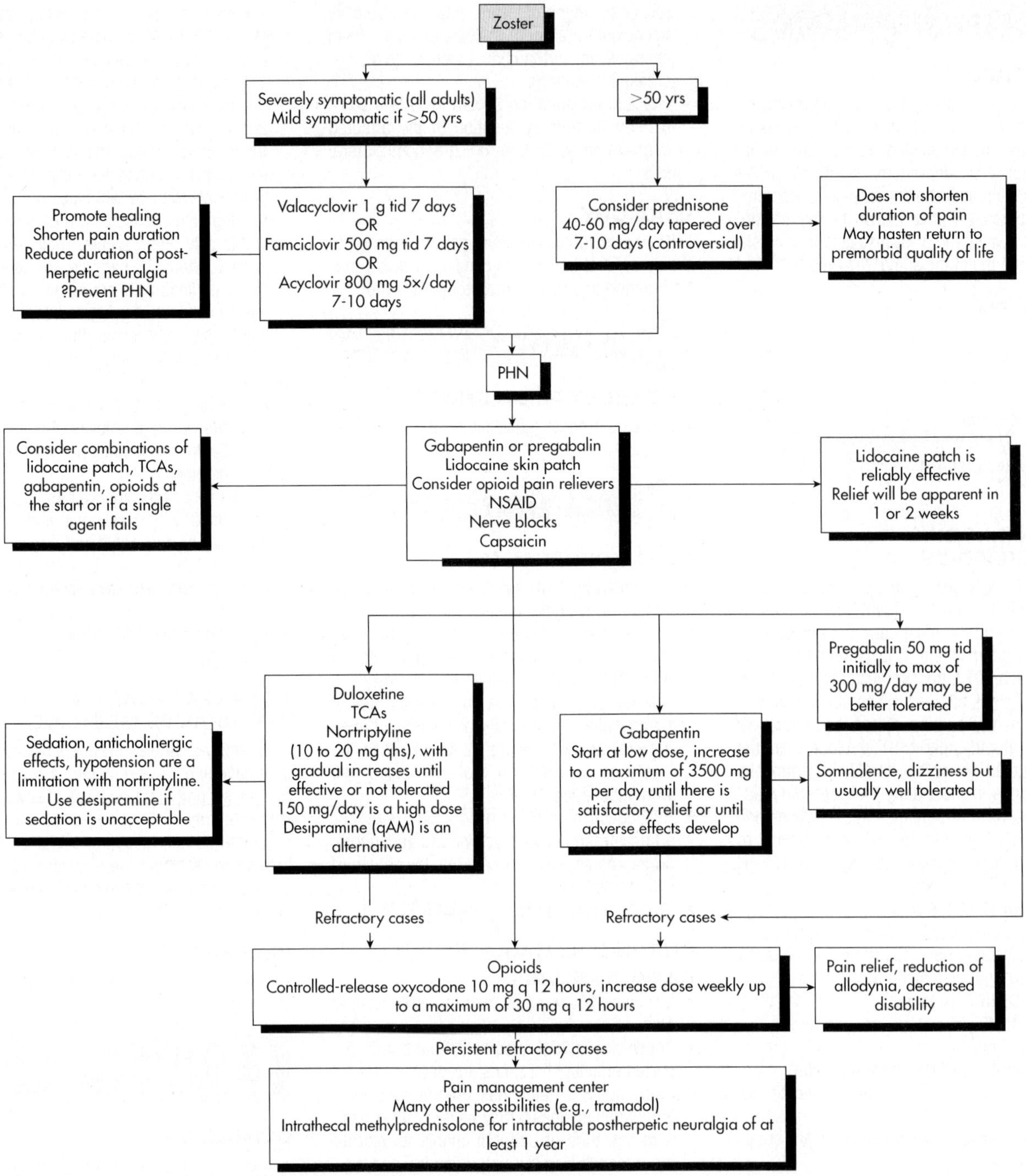

FIG. 1 Treatment of herpes zoster and postherpetic neuralgia. *NSAID,* Nonsteroidal antiinflammatory drug; *PHN,* postherpetic neuralgia; *TCA,* Tricyclic antidepressants. (Modified from Habif TA: *Clinical dermatology,* ed 6, St Louis, 2016, Elsevier.)

and 91% effective against PHN in people 50 and older.[33] It is more effective than the live attenuated VZV vaccine (Zostavax).[34]

2. The Centers for Disease Control and Prevention (CDC) recommends that those who received Zostavax be revaccinated with Shingrix.[35]

3. Those who have had HZ should still receive the vaccine.[36]

4. All immunosuppressed individuals, regardless of age, should receive VZV vaccine.[36]

- Combination therapies can be effective in preventing PHN. Continuous epidural blocks with local anesthetics, antiviral agents with intracutaneous or subcutaneous injection with local anesthetics and steroid, and paravertebral block combined with antiviral antiepileptic agents have shown efficacy in preventing PHN.[37]

PATIENT & FAMILY EDUCATION

- The only well-documented means of preventing PHN is the prevention of herpes zoster through vaccination.
- Patients should understand both the benefits and the potential adverse effects of treatment.
  1. They should be informed that pain relief will likely not be immediate.
  2. Frequent reassessment may be needed, and drug doses should be increased as necessary.

REFERENCES
Available at eBooks.Health.Elsevier.com.

RELATED CONTENT
Herpes Zoster (Related Key Topic)

AUTHOR: **LISA PAPPAS-TAFFER, MD**

BASIC INFORMATION

DEFINITION

Postpartum hemorrhage (PPH) is defined, for both vaginal and cesarean deliveries, as an estimated blood loss ≥1000 ml OR blood loss resulting in signs/symptoms of hypovolemia within 24 h following delivery. PPH is further categorized into primary or secondary.[1,2] Primary PPH occurs within the first 24 h after delivery. Secondary PPH occurs more than 24 h after delivery but within 12 wk following delivery.

SYNONYMS

Obstetric hemorrhage
Maternal hemorrhage
PPH

ICD-10CM CODES
072.0	Third stage hemorrhage
072.1	Other immediate postpartum hemorrhage
072.2	Delayed and secondary postpartum hemorrhage
072.3	Postpartum coagulation defects

EPIDEMIOLOGY & DEMOGRAPHICS

INCIDENCE: Depending on definitions used and scope considered, anywhere from 1% to 6% of obstetric patients will experience postpartum hemorrhage. Postpartum hemorrhage is the leading cause of maternal mortality worldwide and is implicated in >11% of maternal deaths in the United States and 20% of maternal deaths in developing nations.[2]
PREDOMINANT SEX & AGE: Female of reproductive age
RISK FACTORS:
- Antepartum factors: History of PPH, primiparity or high parity, fetal macrosomia, multiple gestation, polyhydramnios, uterine fibroids, prior uterine surgery, abnormal placentation, bleeding disorder[1,2]
- Intrapartum factors: Prolonged labor, augmented labor, rapid labor, preeclampsia, chorioamnionitis, operative delivery, episiotomy, lacerations, retained products, placental abruption, fetal demise[1,2]

PHYSICAL FINDINGS & CLINICAL PRESENTATION (TABLE 1)

- Bleeding is generally brisk at time of delivery.
- Examination findings can include a boggy uterus with continued passage of clot or blood with fundal pressure[1]
- Objective findings can also include hypotension, tachycardia, and oliguria with substantial blood loss[1]

ETIOLOGY

- Primary: Uterine atony (70% to 80%), retained placenta, lacerations, and coagulopathies[1]
- Secondary: Subinvolution of placental site, retained products (includes abnormal placentation), infection, and coagulopathies[1]

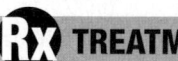 DIAGNOSIS

WORKUP

- Bimanual examination to evaluate for atony; remove clots; massage if it is present
- Bladder should be emptied
- Examination to verify that placenta is intact
- Ensure adequate intravenous (IV) access
- Consider ultrasonography at bedside to evaluate for retained tissue or clot
- Examination to verify that no lacerations are present, including cervical examination with necessary lighting and retractors (may require examination in OR for adequate exposure)

LABORATORY TESTS

Significant hemorrhage can lead to disseminated intravascular coagulation (DIC). If DIC is suspected, CBC and coagulation panels should be ordered. Similarly, if coagulopathy is suspected, evaluation of clotting factors should be ordered. Thromboelastography (TEG) is a useful test to guide product replacement in association with coagulation cascade dysfunction.

IMAGING STUDIES

Ultrasonography can be used to scan for retained products, including clot or placenta. It can be performed to assess the need for more invasive measures, such as instrumentation or a manual sweep.

Rx TREATMENT

The most effective strategy for the prevention of postpartum hemorrhage is active management of the third stage of labor (AMTSL). Medical management with uterotonics is generally the first line of treatment. None of the following medications has been demonstrated to be superior in treating PPH compared with the others.[1,3]
- Oxytocin (IV, 10 to 40 units diluted into IV solution, or 10 units intramuscularly [IM]); often given prophylactically immediately after delivery to minimize EBL with delivery of placenta
- Methylergonovine (IM, 0.2 mg): Contraindicated in hypertensive patient
- Carboprost (IM, 0.25 mg): Contraindicated in patient with history of asthma
- Misoprostol (400 to 800 mcg sublingually, buccally, or rectally)
Other medical management:
- Tranexamic acid (IV, 1 g): Trials[4] have shown that among women who undergo cesarean delivery, tranexamic acid treatment results in significantly longer incidents of blood loss greater than 1000 ml or red-cell transfusion by day 2 than placebo, but it does not result in lower incidence of hemorrhage-related secondary clinical outcomes (use of additional uterotonic agents, provider-assessed clinically significant postpartum hemorrhage). Recent investigation showed that prophylactic use of tranexamic acid for cesarean delivery when compared to placebo did not significantly lower the risk of maternal death or decrease the risk for blood transfusion.[5]

NONPHARMACOLOGIC THERAPY[1,2]

- Active management of third stage of labor: Controlled cord traction (Brandt-Andrews maneuver) and uterine massage after delivery of placenta (in addition to Pitocin)
- Uterine tamponade (Fig. E1): Packing with gauze, Foley catheter, or tamponade balloon (Bakri)
- Intrauterine negative pressure system (Jada system)
- Uterine curettage for suspected retained products
- Uterine artery embolization
- Surgical management with laparotomy:
  1. Hypogastric artery ligation
  2. Bilateral uterine artery ligation (O'Leary sutures)
  3. B-lynch sutures
  4. Hysterectomy

ACUTE GENERAL Rx

- Uterotonics, surgical management, embolization, blood transfusion. Fig. E2 outlines the management of postpartum hemorrhage.
- Table 2 describes therapeutic response to initial fluid resuscitation. Dosing regimen for oxytocic drugs is summarized in Table 3. Blood product replacement is described in Box 1.

CHRONIC Rx

For anemia (Hb <10 g/dl): Ferrous sulfate and ascorbic acid supplementation to support new red blood cell production. Can also consider IV iron replacement.[1]

DISPOSITION

- The patient should be closely watched for at least 24 h after a postpartum hemorrhage. Vital signs should be monitored for evidence of hemodynamic stability and appropriate response to anemia. Serial laboratory tests

TABLE 1 Presentation of Symptoms in Postpartum Hemorrhage

% Blood Loss (ml)	Systolic Blood Pressure (mm Hg)	Signs and Symptoms
10-15 (500-1000)	Normal	Tachycardia, palpitations, dizziness
15-25 (1000-1500)	Low-normal	Tachycardia, weakness, diaphoresis
25-35 (1500-2000)	70-80	Restlessness, pallor, oliguria
35-45 (2000-3000)	50-70	Collapse, air hunger, anuria

From Vincent JL et al: *Textbook of critical care*, ed 8, Philadelphia, 2024, Elsevier.

TABLE 2 Therapeutic Response to Initial Fluid Resuscitation

Response	Description	Follow-Up Treatment
Rapid response	<20% of blood volume lost	No additional fluids or blood are needed
Transient response	20%-40% of blood volume lost; responds to initial fluid bolus but later has worsening vital signs	Continue fluids and consider blood transfusions
Minimal or no response	Ongoing severe hemorrhage with >40% blood volume lost	Continue aggressive fluid and blood product replacements

From Vincent JL et al: *Textbook of critical care*, ed 8, Philadelphia, 2024, Elsevier.

TABLE 3 Dosing Regimens for Oxytocic Drugs

Drugs	Regimens
Oxytocin (Pitocin)	5-unit IV bolus
	Add 20-40 units oxytocin to 1 L of fluids for continuous infusion
	10 units intramyometrially
Methylergonovine (Methergine)	0.2 mg IM every 2-4 h
Ergonovine maleate (Ergotrate)	100-125 μg IM or intramyometrially every 2-4 h
	200-250 μg IM
	Total dose 1.25 mg
Carboprost (Hemabate)	250 μg IM or intramyometrially every 15-90 min
	Total dose 2 mg (8 doses maximum)
Misoprostol	800-1000 μg PR, oral, or sublingual

IM, Intramuscular; *IV,* intravenous; *PR,* per rectum.
From Vincent JL et al: *Textbook of critical care*, ed 8, Philadelphia, 2024, Elsevier.

BOX 1 Blood Product Replacement

Crossmatched blood
Type-specific or "saline crossmatched" blood
Compatible ABO and Rh blood types
Rh-negative blood is preferable
Warm the blood, if possible, especially if the rate of infusion is >100 ml/min or if the total volume transfused is high; cold blood is associated with an increased incidence of arrhythmias and paradoxic hypotension
Administer calcium if blood is transfused rapidly at >100 ml/min because of binding of calcium by anticoagulants in banked blood
Give 6-10 units fresh frozen plasma (FFP) for every 10 units of packed red blood cell (PRBC) transfusions
Give 10-12 units of platelets if the platelet count decreases to <50 × 10⁹/L
Cryoprecipitate can be given to replace fibrinogen in addition to the FFP
Consider 60-120 μg/kg intravenous bolus injection of recombinant activated factor VII (rFVIIa)

From Vincent JL et al: *Textbook of critical care,* ed 7, Philadelphia, 2017, Elsevier.

can be performed in the setting of concern for ongoing bleeding.
- Morbidity can include: Shock, acute respiratory distress syndrome, Sheehan syndrome, thromboembolic disease, and loss of fertility.[1]
- For cases with large blood loss (e.g., >2 L) and hemodynamic instability, surgical intensive care unit admission may be warranted.

REFERRAL

During the course of a postpartum hemorrhage, the anesthesiology department, blood bank, and OR staff should be notified, and adequate nursing should be available.[1] Early considerations should be made to notify obstetricians. If bleeding is brisk or estimated blood loss is considerable, preparation should be made for transfusion of blood products, including notification of the blood bank to facilitate type and crossmatching blood products.

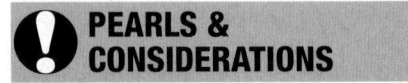

PEARLS & CONSIDERATIONS

PREVENTION
- Active management of third stage of labor
- Implementation of institution-specific PPH risk assessment tools effective for identifying patients at increased risk, though clinical suspicion should be maintained in all patients

REFERENCES
Available at eBooks.Health.Elsevier.com.

AUTHOR: **JESSICA C. FIELDS, MD**

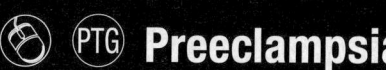

BASIC INFORMATION

DEFINITION

Hypertensive disorders of pregnancy represent a spectrum of disease ranging from gestational hypertension to severe preeclampsia. Preeclampsia is defined as new-onset hypertension (systolic blood pressure ≥140 or diastolic ≥90) after 20 wk gestation or up to 6 wk postpartum in the presence of proteinuria or evidence of end-organ injury.[1] In the absence of proteinuria, other criteria, including thrombocytopenia, acute kidney injury, impaired liver function, pulmonary edema, and new-onset neurologic symptoms, can be used for diagnosis. In 2013, the American College of Obstetricians and Gynecologists (ACOG) Task Force on Hypertension in Pregnancy revised the criteria, making the presence of proteinuria unnecessary to make the diagnosis.[2] The task force reinforced the importance of hypertension as a necessary condition and deemphasized proteinuria. Hypertensive disorders of pregnancy can be categorized as follows:[1]

- Gestational hypertension: Hypertension in pregnancy after 20 wk without proteinuria or evidence of end-organ injury
- Preeclampsia: Hypertension in pregnancy after 20 wk, with proteinuria but without evidence of end-organ injury
- Preeclampsia with severe features (Table 1)
- Chronic hypertension: Hypertension pre-dating pregnancy or present at <20 wk gestation
- Chronic hypertension with superimposed preeclampsia: The presence of chronic hypertension with elevation in blood pressure from baseline often requiring increasing antihypertensives or with development of new onset of signs or symptoms meeting criteria for severe preeclampsia (Table 1)
- Hemolysis, elevated liver enzymes, and low platelet count (HELLP) syndrome: A severe form of preeclampsia defined by lactate dehydrogenase (LDH) greater than 600 IU/L, liver enzymes (aspartate aminotransferase [AST], alanine transaminase [ALT]) greater than twice the upper limit of normal, and a platelet count less than 100 × 10⁹/L

SYNONYMS

Pregnancy-induced hypertension (PIH)
Hypertensive disorders of pregnancy (HDP)
Severe gestational hypertension

ICD-10CM CODES

O11.1	Pre-existing hypertension with pre-eclampsia, first trimester
O11.2	Pre-existing hypertension with pre-eclampsia, second trimester
O11.3	Pre-existing hypertension with pre-eclampsia, third trimester
O11.9	Pre-existing hypertension with pre-eclampsia, unspecified trimester
O14.00	Mild to moderate pre-eclampsia, unspecified trimester
O14.02	Mild to moderate pre-eclampsia, second trimester
O14.03	Mild to moderate pre-eclampsia, third trimester
O14.10	Severe pre-eclampsia, unspecified trimester
O14.12	Severe pre-eclampsia, second trimester
O14.13	Severe pre-eclampsia, third trimester
O14.90	Unspecified pre-eclampsia, unspecified trimester
O14.92	Unspecified pre-eclampsia, second trimester
O14.93	Unspecified pre-eclampsia, third trimester

EPIDEMIOLOGY & DEMOGRAPHICS

INCIDENCE: Hypertensive disorders of pregnancy are recognized as the second leading cause of maternal mortality (after hemorrhage) and are attributed to 18% of maternal mortality globally. The global incidence of preeclampsia is estimated to be 2% to 4% with significant regional variation.[3,4] The disease burden is borne disproportionately by women in low- and middle-income countries or who are otherwise disadvantaged.[5]

RISK FACTORS: See Table 2. Recently, SARS-COV-2 infection has been associated with a twofold increased risk of preeclampsia. Vaccination has been shown to be safe in pregnancy and reduce the likelihood of infection.[6,7]

GENETICS: Preeclampsia is a complex genetic disorder that is not yet well understood.[8] However, large studies describing the epigenetics of maternal hypertension have implicated alterations of the fetal FLT1 locus in the development of preeclampsia.[9] There are both fetal and maternal genetic factors influencing the risk of developing preeclampsia. The maternal genetic contribution has been estimated at 30% to 35% and the fetal contribution at 20%.[10]

PATHOGENESIS

The underlying causes of preeclampsia have been studied extensively for over a century; however, many uncertainties remain.[11]

PHYSICAL FINDINGS & CLINICAL PRESENTATION

Headache that persists despite treatment with acetaminophen is one of the classic neurologic symptoms of preeclampsia. **Visual changes** associated with preeclampsia, including scotoma, blurred vision, or aura.[1,12] Classic neurologic exam findings of preeclampsia include hyperreflexia, clonus, or cranial nerve VI palsy.[13]

Endothelial dysfunction and elevated perfusion pressure accompanied by cerebral edema are considered the underlying cause of cerebral injury, including posterior reversible encephalopathy syndrome (PRES), in patients with preeclampsia. PRES is characterized by cerebral edema classically affecting the occipital and parietal lobes. Patients with PRES may manifest headache, visual loss or disturbance, altered sensorium, or altered consciousness.[13] Severe cases of PRES may result in seizure or coma. PRES is also associated with increased risk of hemorrhagic and ischemic cerebrovascular accident. Importantly, patients with hypertensive disorders of pregnancy have a fivefold increased risk for occurrence of hemorrhagic or ischemic stroke.[13]

Patients with persistent neurologic symptoms are at highest risk for developing PRES. Management of PRES includes controlling hypertension, possible antiepileptic therapy, and indicated follow-up care.

Shortness of breath is often an indicator of underlying pulmonary edema from elevated pulmonary perfusion pressure accompanied by endothelial dysfunction. Rales may be auscultated, and a chest x-ray examination may be useful in confirming the presence of edema. Management includes fluid restriction and use of diuretics as clinically indicated.[1]

TABLE 2 Risk Factors for Preeclampsia

Nulliparity
Multifetal gestations
Preeclampsia in a previous pregnancy
Chronic hypertension
Pregestational diabetes
Gestational diabetes
Thrombophilia
Systemic lupus erythematosus
Prepregnancy body mass index greater than 30
Antiphospholipid antibody syndrome
Maternal age 35 yr or older
Kidney disease
Assisted reproductive technology
Obstructive sleep apnea

From American College of Obstetricians and Gynecologists: Gestational hypertension and preeclampsia: ACOG Practice Bulletin No. 222, *Obstet Gynecol* 135:e237-e260, 2020.

TABLE 1 Criteria for the Diagnosis of Preeclampsia with Severe Features

In patients with preeclampsia, **severe features** can be diagnosed if any one of the following criteria is present:
Blood pressure ≥160 mm Hg systolic or ≥110 mm Hg diastolic on two separate occasions at least 4 h apart (unless antihypertensive therapy is initiated before this time)
Serum creatinine >1.1 mg/dl or a doubling of the serum creatinine
New onset of visual disturbances
New-onset headache unresponsive to medication and not accounted for by alternative diagnoses
Pulmonary edema
Hepatocellular injury (serum transaminases at least twice the upper limit of normal) or severe persistent right upper quadrant or epigastric pain unresponsive to medications
Thrombocytopenia (platelet count <100 × 10⁹/L)

Dependent edema, which may affect the lower extremities, vulva, or back, is also frequently seen. It occurs due to increased vascular permeability and sodium retention related to renal injury and abnormal RAAS activation. It can be managed with compression and diuretics. Physiologic edema of pregnancy can sometimes be distinguished from pathologic edema by timing of onset. Rapidly progressing edema >4 to 5 lbs of weight gain per wk and facial edema are not typical of healthy pregnancy.[1]

The **right upper quadrant** or **epigastric pain** classically associated with preeclampsia is thought to be the result of periportal and parenchymal necrosis, with hepatocellular edema sometimes resulting in distension of the Glisson capsule. However, no strong correlation between symptoms and laboratory abnormalities exists.[14]

Oliguria in preeclampsia is due to decreased intravascular volume as a result of vascular endothelial dysfunction and RAAS activation.[1,12]

1% of patients with preeclampsia and 3% of patients with severe preeclampsia will develop placental abruption. **Vaginal bleeding** in a preeclamptic patient should prompt a workup for abruption.[1]

It is important to remember that patients can be asymptomatic with elevated blood pressures and high risk. Rarely, HELLP or eclampsia may present in a normotensive patient. It is important to maintain a high level of suspicion for preeclampsia in patients at increased risk.

Dx DIAGNOSIS

DIFFERENTIAL DIAGNOSIS

- Acute fatty liver of pregnancy
- Appendicitis
- Autoimmune hepatitis
- Chronic hypertension
- Chronic kidney disease
- Diabetic ketoacidosis
- Gallbladder disease
- Gastroenteritis
- Glomerulonephritis
- Hemolytic-uremic syndrome
- Idiopathic thrombocytopenia
- Thrombotic thrombocytopenic purpura
- Pancreatitis
- Peptic ulcer disease
- Secondary hypertension
- Systemic lupus erythematosus
- Viral hepatitis
- Medications or medication withdrawal
- Migraine headache

WORKUP

Hypertension:
- Two blood pressure measurements at least 4 h apart, with a systolic BP of 140 mm Hg or more or a diastolic blood pressure of 90 mm Hg or more.
- Severe hypertension with systolic BP of 160 mm Hg or more or a diastolic blood pressure of 110 mm Hg or more.
- Severe hypertension can be confirmed in a brief period to allow for immediate treatment of severe range blood pressure.

Proteinuria:
- ≥300 mg per 24-h urine collection
- Protein/creatinine ratio ≥0.3
- 2+ on dipstick (only if other methods not available)

Other diagnostic labs:
- See Table 1

LABORATORY TESTS

- Generally, the recommended laboratory testing is consistent with labs that can be used to identify end-organ dysfunction.
- **CBC** to assess for anemia or thrombocytopenia.
- **Liver function tests** (aspartate aminotransferase, alanine aminotransferase) are useful in determining the presence of hepatic injury and are also useful in excluding HELLP syndrome.
- Serum creatinine (and uric acid).
- Prothrombin time, partial thromboplastin time, and fibrinogen can be checked to rule out disseminated intravascular coagulation, if clinically appropriate.

IMAGING STUDIES

- Computed tomography or MRI scan of head if persistent headache or neurologic symptoms raising concern for PRES or stroke
- Chest x-ray examination if there is concern for pulmonary edema
- Sonogram of fetus to evaluate for intrauterine growth restriction, amniotic fluid level, placental location
- Sonogram of maternal liver if subcapsular hematoma suspected

Rx TREATMENT

ACUTE GENERAL Rx[1,2,15]

Delivery is the treatment of choice and the only cure for the disease. This must be taken in the context of the gestational age of the fetus and severity of the preeclampsia.

- For preeclampsia with severe features, administer magnesium sulfate 4 to 6 g intravenous (IV) loading dose, with 2 g/h maintenance (adjust dosage for renal insufficiency). If there is a contraindication to magnesium sulfate, such as myasthenia gravis, then use phenytoin at 10 to 15 mg/kg loading dose, then 200 mg IV q8h starting 12 h after loading dose.
- Treat blood pressure (BP) >160 mm Hg systolic or >110 mm Hg diastolic either with hydralazine 5 to 10 mg IV, then 10 mg, every 20 min to a max dose of 20 mg; or with labetalol hydrochloride 20, 40, 60, 80 mg IV, escalating dosage every 10 min to a max dose of 300 mg IV; or with nifedipine 10 to 20 mg orally every 20 min to a max dose of 180 mg/day for acute blood pressure control. If maximum dose of one medication is reached, add an additional medication to reach goal of BP 140 to 150/90 to 100 mm Hg.
- Continuous fetal monitoring.
- Epidural is anesthesia of choice for pain management in labor or cesarean delivery.
- All patients undergoing induction of labor or cesarean delivery should receive antiseizure medications (magnesium sulfate) if disease with severe features, for delivery and 12 to 24 h postpartum.

CHRONIC Rx[1,2,15]

Preeclampsia without severe features: If <37 wk, close observation for worsening maternal or fetal condition with delivery at 37 wk. If 24 to 36 wk, consider antenatal corticosteroids. If severe features develop or there is evidence of fetal compromise, earlier delivery is appropriate.

Preeclampsia with severe features: Delivery in the presence of maternal or fetal compromise, labor, or 34 wk. From 24 to 34 wk consider steroids with close monitoring, and at <24 wk offer termination of pregnancy (Fig. 1). Risks of expectant management include severe worsening of disease, eclampsia, abruptio placenta, stillbirth, HELLP syndrome, and intensive care unit (ICU) admission. Contraindications to expectant management include eclampsia, HELLP syndrome, pulmonary edema, disseminated intravascular coagulation, abruptio placenta, uncontrollable severe hypertension, fetal demise, and nonreassuring fetal status. Labetalol, hydralazine, and nifedipine are the drugs of choice for long-term blood-pressure control during pregnancy.

DISPOSITION

- Preeclampsia is a progressive and unpredictable disease process; a course of expectancy should be managed with caution. Up to 20% of patients who have seizures are normotensive.
- The reoccurrence rate for preeclampsia in a subsequent pregnancy is approximately 20%, and higher in cases with a second trimester presentation or complications. This risk may be decreased with the use of daily low-dose aspirin.
- For high-risk patients, baseline assessment of renal function (24-h urine collection for total protein and creatinine clearance or protein:creatinine ratio), CBC, serum creatinine, liver function tests (LFTs), and uric acid should be obtained at the first prenatal visit.

REFERRAL

Obstetric management with input from maternal-fetal subspecialists in severe cases. Transfer of care to facilities with appropriate level of care for all cases <34 wk.

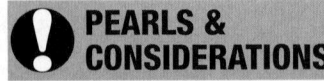 PEARLS & CONSIDERATIONS

COMMENTS

- Low-dose aspirin exposure during the early stages of placentation decreases the risk of preeclampsia, preterm birth, and intrauterine growth restriction in women who are at high risk of preeclampsia. The ACOG and the U.S. Preventive Services Task Force (USPSTF) recommend the use of low-dose aspirin as

P

Diseases
and Disorders

I

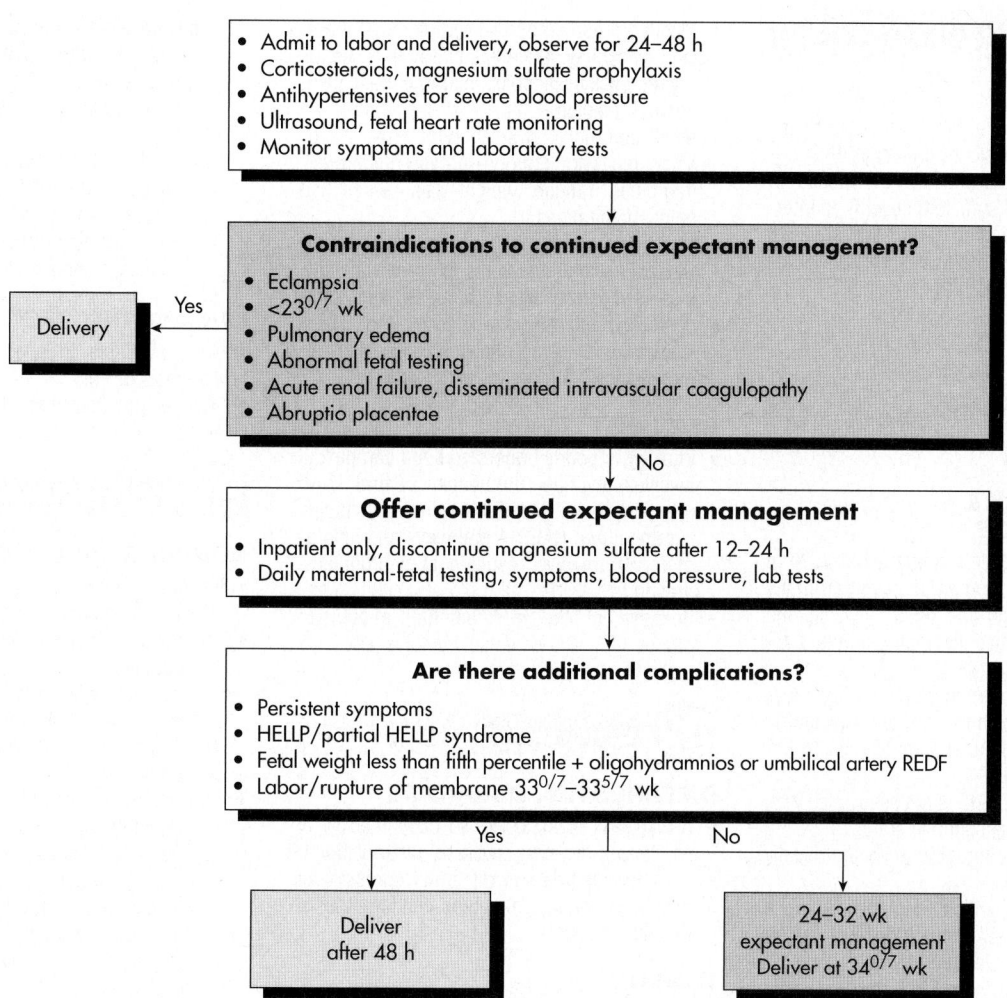

- Admit to labor and delivery, observe for 24–48 h
- Corticosteroids, magnesium sulfate prophylaxis
- Antihypertensives for severe blood pressure
- Ultrasound, fetal heart rate monitoring
- Monitor symptoms and laboratory tests

Contraindications to continued expectant management?

- Eclampsia
- $<23^{0/7}$ wk
- Pulmonary edema
- Abnormal fetal testing
- Acute renal failure, disseminated intravascular coagulopathy
- Abruptio placentae

Yes → Delivery

No

Offer continued expectant management

- Inpatient only, discontinue magnesium sulfate after 12–24 h
- Daily maternal-fetal testing, symptoms, blood pressure, lab tests

Are there additional complications?

- Persistent symptoms
- HELLP/partial HELLP syndrome
- Fetal weight less than fifth percentile + oligohydramnios or umbilical artery REDF
- Labor/rupture of membrane $33^{0/7}$–$33^{5/7}$ wk

Yes → Deliver after 48 h

No → 24–32 wk expectant management Deliver at $34^{0/7}$ wk

FIG. 1 Management plan for patients with preeclampsia with severe features before 34 wk gestation. *HELLP,* Hemolysis, elevated liver enzymes, and low platelets; *REDF,* reversed end-diastolic flow. (From Gabbe SG et al: *Obstetrics: normal and problem pregnancies,* ed 7, Philadelphia, 2017, Elsevier.)

preventive medication starting after 12 wk of gestation (ideally before 16 wk) in women who are at high risk for preeclampsia.[16,17]

- The development of preeclampsia may be one of the earliest identifiable risk markers for potential future cardiovascular disease in women. Women with a history of

preeclampsia are at increased risk for cardiovascular disease, and appropriate follow-up should be encouraged.

REFERENCES

Available at eBooks.Health.Elsevier.com.

RELATED CONTENT

Preeclampsia (Patient Information)
Eclampsia (Related Key Topic)
Hypertension (Related Key Topic)

AUTHORS: **BETHANY K. SEDERDAHL, MPH, MD** and **PHILIP A. SHLOSSMAN, MD**

BASIC INFORMATION

DEFINITION

Premenstrual syndrome (PMS) consists of various somatic and physical complaints that develop during the luteal phase of the menstrual cycle and that are of sufficient severity to interfere with daily functioning and/or interpersonal relationships. The symptoms resolve shortly after the onset of menses.[1]

SYNONYM

PMS

ICD-10CM CODE
N94.3   Premenstrual tension syndrome

EPIDEMIOLOGY & DEMOGRAPHICS

- Premenstrual disorders affect about 12% of reproductive-age women, although as many as 80% of women will report at least one somatic or affective symptom during their luteal phase (Table 1).[2]
- Severe cases of premenstrual dysphoric disorder (PMDD), which is more of a psychiatric diagnosis, occur in approximately 3% to 8% of women in the U.S.[3]
- The prevalence of PMS is not associated with age, race, or socioeconomic status.
- Those seeking treatment for PMS are usually in their 30s or 40s.
- Based on some identical twinning studies, a genetic component is thought to exist, but no genes have been identified.[4]
- The natural history of PMS has not been clearly elucidated.

PHYSICAL FINDINGS & CLINICAL PRESENTATION

- Diverse and potentially disabling symptoms. Table 1 summarizes common symptoms of PMS[2]
- Associated with multiple psychologic, physical, and behavioral symptoms
- Most frequent reason for seeking treatment: Emotional symptoms

- Most common emotional symptoms: Depression, irritability, anxiety, labile moods, anger, crying easily, sadness, extreme sensitivity, nervous tension
- Most common physical symptoms: Headache, bloating, cramps, breast tenderness, migraines, fatigue, weight gain, aches and pains, palpitations
- Most common behavior symptom: Food cravings
- Other behavioral symptoms: Increased appetite, increased alcohol intake, decreased motivation, decreased efficiency, avoidance of activities, staying home, sleep changes, libido changes, forgetfulness, decreased concentration

ETIOLOGY

- Etiology is poorly understood and complex. It involves ovarian hormones, central neurotransmitters, and neurosteroids including serotonin and GABS-A pathways and inflammatory pathways resulting in neuroinflammation.[1,3,5]
- Because of the multifactorial, multiorgan nature of PMS, a single etiologic cause is unlikely.

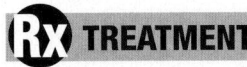 **DIAGNOSIS**

DIFFERENTIAL DIAGNOSIS

- A diagnosis of exclusion, so other medical or psychologic disorders should be ruled out (Box 1)
- Common disorders to rule out: Depression or anxiety, anemia, migraines, endometriosis, thyroid disease

WORKUP

- History
- Physical examination
- Laboratory studies to rule out alternative diagnosis
- If no alternative diagnosis, confirm by either history of regular menses, basal body temperature charting, or elevated luteal progesterone that patient is ovulatory
  1. If she is not ovulating, it is not PMS.
  2. A prospective questionnaire given over two menstrual cycles has been found to

be the most accurate way to assess the presence of PMS or PMDD.[1] If symptoms are not occurring only in the luteal phase, it is not PMS, and further investigation is needed.
  a. If symptoms occur in the follicular phase, patient has premenstrual exacerbation of another condition.
  b. If symptoms do not occur in the follicular phase, diagnosis of PMS is confirmed.

LABORATORY TESTS

- None available to specifically confirm the diagnosis of PMS
- Thyroid function tests to rule out thyroid disease

Rx **TREATMENT**

NONPHARMACOLOGIC THERAPY

- Individualization of the treatment plan to maximize therapeutic response
- Psychosocial intervention:
  1. Education
  2. Stress management
  3. Environmental changes
  4. Adequate rest and sleep
  5. Regular exercise
- Nutritional recommendations:
  1. Regularly eaten, well-balanced meals
  2. Adequate amounts of protein, fiber, and complex carbohydrates; low fat
  3. Avoidance of foods that are high in salt and simple sugars; may promote water retention, weight gain, and physical discomfort
  4. Avoidance of alcohol and illicit drugs; may worsen emotional lability
  5. Calcium supplementation (1000 mg/day for women 19 to 50 yr, 1300 mg/day for girls 14 to 18 yr) to reduce the physical and emotional symptoms[2]
  6. The data are mixed regarding the benefits of vitamin D supplementation in reducing PMS symptoms, so more studies are needed

---

BOX 1   Considerations in the Differential Diagnosis of Premenstrual Dysphoric Disorder

Premenstrual syndrome
Endometriosis
Dysmenorrhea
Physical disorders with premenstrual exacerbations
Autoimmune disorders
Diabetes mellitus
Anemia
Hypothyroidism
Psychiatric disorders with luteal phase exacerbation
Depression
Anxiety
Dysthymic disorder
Bipolar disorder

From Gershenson DM et al: *Comprehensive gynecology,* ed 8, Philadelphia, 2022, Elsevier.

TABLE 1   Common Symptoms of Cyclic Premenstrual Syndrome

Somatic Symptoms

Abdominal bloating	Constipation or diarrhea
Acne	Headache
Alcohol intolerance	Peripheral edema
Breast engorgement and tenderness	Weight gain
Clumsiness	

Emotional and Mental Symptoms

Anxiety	Insomnia
Change in libido	Irritability
Depression	Lethargy
Fatigue	Mood swings
Food cravings (especially salt and sugar)	Panic attacks
Hostility	Paranoia
Inability to concentrate	Violence toward self and others
Increased appetite	Withdrawal from others

From Goldman L, Schafer AI: *Goldman's Cecil medicine,* ed 24, Philadelphia, 2012, Saunders.

TABLE 2 SSRIs for Premenstrual Dysphoric Disorder

SSRI	Effective Doses
Fluoxetine hydrochloride*	20 mg/day
Sertraline hydrochloride	50-150 mg/day
Paroxetine hydrochloride*	20-30 mg/day
Paroxetine controlled release (CR)	25 mg/day
Citalopram	20-30 mg/day
Escitalopram	10-20 mg/day
SNRI	
Venlafaxine	37.5-112.5 mg/day

PMDD, Premenstrual dysphoric disorder; *SNRI*, selective norepinephrine reuptake inhibitor; *SSRI*, selective serotonin reuptake inhibitor.
*Only fluoxetine and paroxetine are approved for PMDD.
From Gershenson DM et al: *Comprehensive gynecology*, ed 8, Philadelphia, 2022, Elsevier.

7. Pyridoxine (vitamin B$_6$) 80 mg qd to improve depression, fatigue, and irritability has been suggested in small studies

ACUTE GENERAL Rx

Suppression of ovulation:
- Oral contraceptives: One pill per day; continuous use of a combinaton pill with drospirenone is associated with better treatment effect[3]
- Progestin-only oral contraceptive: One pill per day
- Oral micronized progesterone: 100 mg every morning and 200 mg every evening on days 17 through 28 of menstrual cycle
- Progestin suppository: 200 to 400 mg bid on days 17 through 28 of menstrual cycle
- Medroxyprogesterone: 150 mg intramuscularly q3mo
- Levonorgestrel implants: Surgical insertion every 5 yr
- Transdermal estradiol: One or two 100-μg patches every 3 days
- Danazol: 100 to 200 mg/day by mouth (ovulation not suppressed at this dose); has significant side-effect profile and is not commonly utilized
- Gonadotropin-releasing hormone (GnRH) agonists: Daily by intranasal spray or monthly by depot injection; profound hypoestrogenism, concerns for osteoporosis and vasomotor symptoms

Suppression of physical symptoms:
- Spironolactone: 25 to 50 mg PO bid on days 14 through 28 of menstrual cycle—need a reliable form of birth control
- Mefenamic acid
  1. For fluid retention: 250 mg PO tid on days 24 through 28 of cycle
  2. For pain: 500 mg PO tid on days 19 through 28 of cycle
- Bromocriptine: 5 mg/day by mouth on days 10 through 26 of cycle
- Naproxen: 550 mg PO bid on days 17 through 28 of cycle; Naprosyn: 500 mg PO bid on days 17 through 28 of cycle

Suppression of psychologic symptoms (Table 2):
- SSRIs, or serotonergic antidepressants, are first-line treatment for PMS/PMDD, treating mostly the psychologic aspects but also some physical aspects[2,4,5]
- Sertraline, paroxetine, fluoxetine, citalopram, escitalopram are most commonly used[4,5]
- In 2013 the *Cochrane Reviews* reported a statistically significant benefit over placebo when taken either continuously or in the luteal phase[4]
- Serotonin-norepinephrine reuptake inhibitors (SNRIs) such as venlafaxine; use is off-label, but onset of action is quick and has been found to be helpful[2]

- Seroquel: Smaller studies[2]
- Wellbutrin: Not as effective as the other options
- Ulipristal acetate is a second-generation selective progesterone receptor modulator (SPRM) that shows promise at low doses (5 mg/day) in ameliorating symptoms of PMDD[6]
- Off-label use of dutasteride to increase local allopregnanolone levels and ameliorate physical and psychologic symptoms of PMDD[3]

CHRONIC Rx

- Therapy is largely trial and error, with the goal of providing effective treatment with the safest therapy. Provider should initially attempt to ameliorate the most pronounced symptom(s).
- Limited evidence exists that acupuncture and/or acupressure may ameliorate some symptoms associated with PMS and improve quality of life.[1,6] More studies are needed to determine if this option is as good as or better than conventional therapies such as treatment with an SSRI.
- Newer pharmacologic therapies that target neurotransmitter systems in the brain through the action of allopregnanolone on the GABA receptor show promise.[3,7]
- For severe intractable PMS bilateral oophorectomy has been considered but should be last resort after a trial of GnRH agonists have been shown to resolve symptoms.[1] This course of action should be exceedingly rare.

DISPOSITION

Improved symptoms in 90% of women over time

REFERENCES

Available at eBooks.Health.Elsevier.com.

RELATED CONTENT

Premenstrual Syndrome (Patient Information)
Dysmenorrhea (Related Key Topic)
Premenstrual Dysphoric Disorder (Related Key Topic)

AUTHOR: **ADRIENNE B. NEITHARDT, MD**

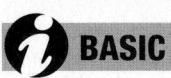
BASIC INFORMATION

DEFINITION

Preterm labor is defined as regular contractions that result in cervical dilation or effacement prior to 37 wk gestation. Preterm birth is one that occurs after 20 wk gestation and before the completion of 37 wk gestational age and is further classified as early preterm birth (before 34 wk, 0 days of gestation) and late preterm birth (between 34 wk 0 days and 36 wk 6 days of gestation).[1]

SYNONYM

Premature labor

ICD-10CM CODES
O60.0	Preterm labor without delivery
O60.1	Preterm spontaneous labor with preterm delivery
O60.2	Preterm spontaneous labor with term delivery

EPIDEMIOLOGY & DEMOGRAPHICS

INCIDENCE: The incidence of preterm births in the U.S. increased from 9.5% in 1981 to 12.8% in 2006 before falling gradually between 2007 and 2014. It is now is increasing with the 2019 preterm birth rate of 10.2%.[2-4] The increase over time is attributed to improvements in pregnancy dating by ultrasound, increased use of assisted reproductive technology, and increased preterm induction or preterm operative delivery for maternal or fetal indications with a particular rise in late preterm deliveries. Between 40% and 45% of these births follow spontaneous preterm labor; either the remaining preterm births result from preterm premature rupture of membranes (PPROM), or they occur secondary to intentional delivery for maternal or fetal indications.[5]

PREDOMINANT SEX & AGE & RACIAL DIFFERENCES: Pregnant women at the extremes of reproductive age (<17 yr and >35 yr) are at greatest risk. Non-Hispanic Black race is one of the most significant risk factors with the rate of preterm birth being 14.4% in 2019 compared to 9.3% in White women and 10% in Hispanic women.[4] The disparity between African American and other ethnic American races persists after adjusting for income, education, and other medical risk factors.

RISK FACTORS: Risk factors for premature labor include a prior preterm delivery, intrauterine infection, systemic or genital tract infections, periodontal disease, short interpregnancy interval (<18 mo), short cervical length (<25 to 30 mm), low prepregnancy body mass index (BMI) (<18.5 kg/m²), age (<17 yr or >35 yr), a history of elective pregnancy termination, history of prior stillbirth, African-American race, vaginal bleeding, polyhydramnios or oligohydramnios, multiple gestation, structural abnormalities of the uterus, history of cervical cone biopsy or loop electrocautery excision, in vitro fertilization or ovulation induction, tobacco use, heavy alcohol consumption, cocaine use, heroin use, and psychologic or social stress. The strongest historic risk factor for preterm birth is a previous birth between 16 and 36 wk gestation.[1]

GENETICS: A genetic component has been suggested. Women with sisters who have had preterm births and women with grandparents who were born preterm may be at increased risk for having preterm deliveries themselves. Gene variants have recently been found to be associated with gestational duration and preterm birth.[6]

PHYSICAL FINDINGS & CLINICAL PRESENTATION

Presenting symptoms include increased pelvic pressure, abdominal cramping or contractions, increased vaginal discharge, vaginal bleeding or spotting, or leakage of fluid.

ETIOLOGY

Causes of premature labor are varied and often difficult to determine. Premature labor may be secondary to infection, systemic illness, trauma, anatomic abnormalities (i.e., uterine anomaly), or a combination of factors.[1] It is thought that cervical ripening is the most common first step to premature labor or delivery. Subsequently, decidual-membrane activation occurs followed by contractions (Box 1).

DIAGNOSIS

DIFFERENTIAL DIAGNOSIS

The differential diagnosis for preterm labor should include preterm rupture of membranes, preterm contractions (contractions before 37 wk gestation that do not result in cervical change), and abdominal pain or cramping secondary to other medical conditions. There are many medical conditions that may cause preterm contractions or premature labor. Treating some of these underlying conditions may improve the prognosis for stopping the preterm labor.
Possible medical conditions include:
- Infection
  1. Intraamniotic infection
  2. Genital tract infections, including bacterial vaginosis, gonorrhea, chlamydia
  3. Urinary tract infections, including pyelonephritis, cystitis, or asymptomatic bacteriuria
  4. Gastroenteritis
- Trauma
- Placental abruption
- Illicit drug use
- Preterm premature rupture of membranes
- Appendicitis
- Nephrolithiasis
- Pancreatitis
- Cholelithiasis
- Uterine fibroids

WORKUP

- History and physical exam to rule out trauma, abuse, other causes of abdominal pain, and infection
- Fetal heart rate monitoring and tocometry to determine fetal status and contraction frequency
- Speculum exam to visually assess the cervix and assess for rupture of membranes, bleeding, infection, or advanced cervical dilation
  1. If the patient is <35 wk gestation, a Fetal Fibronectin (FFN) test should be collected prior to performing a digital exam or transvaginal ultrasound. A FFN test can help predict preterm delivery.
- Digital exam in the unruptured patient with normal placentation to determine cervical dilation and effacement, and fetal station

---

BOX 1 Factors Linked to Preterm Labor

Demographic and Psychosocial
- Extremes of age (>40 yr, teenagers)
- Lower socioeconomic status
- Tobacco use
- Cocaine abuse
- Prolonged standing (occupation)
- Psychosocial stressors

Reproductive and Gynecologic
- Prior preterm delivery
- Diethylstilbestrol exposure
- Multiple gestations
- Anatomic endometrial cavity anomalies
- Cervical incompetence
- Low pregnancy weight gain
- First-trimester vaginal bleeding
- Placental abruption or previa

Surgical
- Prior reproductive organ surgery
- Prior paraendometrial surgery other than genitourinary (appendectomy)

Infectious
- Urinary tract infections
- Nonuterine infections
- Genital tract infections (bacterial vaginosis)

From Walls RM et al: *Rosen's emergency medicine, concepts and clinical practice*, ed 10, Philadelphia, 2023, Elsevier.

LABORATORY TESTS

- CBC
- Urine analysis and culture
- Urine toxicology screen
- Collect tests for GBS, gonorrhea, and *Chlamydia*
- Perform a wet prep for yeast, bacterial vaginosis, and *Trichomonas*
- Fetal fibronectin swab as described earlier
- Consider PT, PTT, INR, CMP, amylase, and lipase
- Amniocentesis may be performed if an intraamniotic infection is suspected

IMAGING STUDIES

- A formal ultrasound is indicated to determine estimated fetal weight, fetal presentation, amniotic fluid volume, placental location and appearance, and cervical length.

The diagnosis of preterm labor is confirmed in the presence of regular contractions with subsequent cervical change. Suspicion for preterm labor may be heightened if FFN is positive.

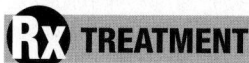 **TREATMENT**

Patients with premature labor should be delivered promptly when an intraamniotic infection is suspected or when they have advanced cervical dilation >5 cm, a persistently nonreassuring fetal heart rate tracing, an intrauterine fetal demise, or significant vaginal bleeding concerning for placental abruption having maternal or neonatal implications.[7]

NONPHARMACOLOGIC THERAPY

- Bedrest, activity restriction, and pelvic rest are often recommended by clinicians, but there are insufficient data to support this practice, and it is currently not recommended.[7]

ACUTE GENERAL Rx

- Antenatal administration of corticosteroids between 24 wk and 33 6/7 wk gestation is recommended for women at risk of preterm delivery to prevent neonatal respiratory distress syndrome and decrease the incidence

---

BOX 2   Commonly Used Tocolytic Agents

Magnesium sulfate
- 4-6 g IV bolus over 20 min
- 1-2 g/h IV infusion

Terbutaline
- 5-10 mg PO q4-6h
- 0.25 mg SC q20 min
- 2.5-5 mcg/min increased every 20 min to max 25 mcg/min

Ritodrine[a]
- 10 mg PO q2-4 h
- 10 mg IM q3-8 h
- 0.05-0.35 mg/min IV infusion

Isoxsuprine
- 20 mg PO q6h
- 0.2-0.5 mg/min IV infusion

IM, Intramuscular; *IV,* intravenous; *PO,* by mouth (per os); *SC,* subcutaneous.
[a]Ritodrine and Isoxsuprine have been discontinued in the United States.
From Walls RM et al: *Rosen's emergency medicine, concepts and clinical practice,* ed 10, Philadelphia, 2023, Elsevier.

---

of intraventricular hemorrhage and necrotizing enterocolitis.[7] It is also recommended between 34.0 and 36.6 wk gestation if there is no prior steroid exposure.[8]

- Numerous tocolytic agents have been used in an attempt to inhibit contractions (Box 2). Although efficacy is unclear, they can be utilized during an observation period in an effort to prolong gestation for administration and exposure of steroids or to transfer the mother to a facility capable of caring for preterm infants. This, of course, assumes there are no maternal or fetal medical contraindications to use of tocolytic drugs and no indications for rapid delivery. The most commonly used tocolytics are beta-mimetics (terbutaline), intravenous magnesium sulfate, calcium channel blockers (nifedipine), or prostaglandin synthetase inhibitors (indomethacin, ketorolac, sulindac). Table E1 summarizes side effect profiles of tocolytic agents.

- Routine antibiotic use has failed to show benefit in the absence of a known infection, but all mothers in preterm labor (without a documented negative group B strep culture) should be given antibiotics to prevent neonatal GBS infection.[7]
- Intravenous magnesium sulfate has been shown to decrease cerebral palsy in children exposed antenatally with premature labor or premature rupture of the membranes at less than 32 wk gestation.[7,9]

PROPHYLACTIC OR CHRONIC Rx

- Patients with a history of prior spontaneous preterm birth may benefit from transvaginal cervical length screening in pregnancy to monitor for short cervix. Prophylactic use of 17 alpha-hydroxyprogesterone caproate is no longer recommended for the prevention of preterm birth in patients with a history of spontaneous preterm birth.[10]
- Patients with a history of preterm birth and short cervix may also be candidates for prophylactic or rescue cerclage.[7]
- Patients with a short cervix may be candidates for vaginal progesterone for prevention.[7]
- There is no evidence supporting the use of maintenance tocolytic therapy.[7,11]

REFERRAL

- Women who present in preterm labor should be referred to an obstetrician and transferred to a facility with a neonatal intensive care unit.
- For women who present for prenatal care with a history of preterm delivery, early referral to an obstetrician is also recommended.

REFERENCES

Available at eBooks.Health.Elsevier.com.

RELATED CONTENT

Abruptio Placentae (Related Key Topic)
Breech Birth (Related Key Topic)

AUTHOR: **JESSICA C. FIELDS, MD**

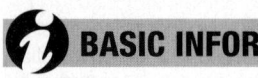 **BASIC INFORMATION**

DEFINITION

Primary biliary cholangitis (PBC), previously known as primary biliary cirrhosis, is a chronic, variably progressive immune-mediated cholestatic liver disease manifested by fatigue and pruritus. Most often diagnosed in middle-aged women, this condition is characterized by autoimmune destruction of small intralobular bile ducts leading to portal inflammation, hepatic cell necrosis, fibrosis, and, if left untreated, cirrhosis, liver failure, and death.[1]

SYNONYMS

PBC
Primary biliary cirrhosis
Biliary cirrhosis
Nonsuppurative destructive cholangitis
Autoimmune cholangiopathy (AIC)

ICD-10CM CODE
K74.3   Primary biliary cholangitis

EPIDEMIOLOGY & DEMOGRAPHICS

INCIDENCE:
- Most recent annual incidence rate in European countries is 1.87 new cases per 100,000 patients.[1]
- Most recent annual incidence rate in the Asia-Pacific region is 0.86 new cases per 100,000 patients.[2]
- Most recent annual incidence rate in North America is 2.75 new cases per 100,000 patients.[3]
- Pooled global annual incidence is estimated at 1.76 new cases per 100,000 patients.[3]

PREVALENCE: Prevalence is greatest in North America and Northern Europe and varies tremendously by time and geographic areas, but most recent data show an incidence of 22.27 cases per 100,000 patients in European countries, 11.88 cases per 100,000 patients in the Asia-Pacific region, and 21.81 per 100,000 patients in North America.[1,3] Pooled global prevalence is estimated at 14.60 per 100,000 patients. Disease incidence and prevalence appear to be increasing worldwide, particularly in North America.[3,4] However, a recent study showed a decrease in incidence and in the female:male ratio of those with PBC in a Taiwanese population from 2002 to 2015.[5]

PREDOMINANT SEX: While a female:male ratio of 9:1 is often described, recent studies suggest that PBC may be more common in men than previously understood with a female:male ratio of 4 or 5:1.[6,7] Men with PBC typically present with more advance disease at the time of diagnosis, and those with well-compensated cirrhosis have been reported to have a higher risk of death and liver-related death or transplantation.[7]

PREDOMINANT AGE: Onset typically occurs between the ages of 30 and 65 yr of age

PREDOMINANT RACE: Most often described in Caucasians, but PBC affects all races.

GENETICS:
- Pathogenesis is unknown, but it is thought to be in the setting of environmental influences and genetic predisposition.[8]
- There is a clear familial occurrence. At least one genetic locus has been identified that is likely associated with increased risk of PBC.[9] However, there is no genetic testing currently available for clinical practice.
- Up to 73% of patients with PBC have at least one other extrahepatic autoimmune disorder such as thyroiditis, Sjögren syndrome, rheumatoid arthritis, cutaneous scleroderma (including CREST syndrome), systemic lupus erythematosus, pernicious anemia, celiac disease, inflammatory bowel disease, autoimmune thrombocytopenia purpura, autoimmune diabetes mellitus, and/or other autoimmune diseases.[10,11]
- A variant form of PBC exists as an overlap syndrome with autoimmune hepatitis (AIH).
- PBC is closely associated with a greater risk of hepatocellular carcinoma as well as an overall greater risk of cancer.

PHYSICAL FINDINGS & CLINICAL PRESENTATION

Clinical stages:
- Asymptomatic
- Symptomatic
- Cirrhotic
- Hepatic failure

Symptoms:
- 50% to 65% of patients may be asymptomatic at time of diagnosis; between 35% and 89% become symptomatic within 4.5 to 17.8 yr.[12]
- Fatigue (50% to 78% of patients) and pruritus (20% to 70% of patients) are the usual presenting symptoms and are independent of disease severity.[12]
- Fatigue can be chronic and correlate with daytime somnolence and autonomic dysfunction.
- Pruritus is present predominantly on the palm and soles, is worse at night and with constricting garments, and is worse with dry skin and humid weather. The cause is unknown but elevated histamine, bile salt concentration, endogenous opioids, lysophosphatidic acid, and female steroid hormones and their metabolites have been discussed as potential causes. Pruritus may first occur during pregnancy but is distinguished from pruritus of pregnancy because it persists into the postpartum period and beyond.
- Symptoms include jaundice, unexplained right upper quadrant pain, manifestations of portal hypertension, dyslipidemia, xanthomas, and osteoporosis, and may be associated with Sjögren syndrome, rheumatoid arthritis, systemic lupus erythematosus, celiac disease, and thyroid disorders (with the most common being Hashimoto thyroiditis).
- Other symptoms can include steatorrhea, osteopenia, fat-soluble vitamin deficiencies, and anemia.

Physical examination:
- Variable: Findings depend on stage of disease at time of presentation; patients at the early stage may be completely unaffected.

- Excoriations may be present due to extensive scratching from pruritus and can be severe enough to cause bleeding.
- Hepatomegaly is more common with disease progression but can be seen even in asymptomatic patients. Splenomegaly can worsen with disease progression and is often a sign of portal hypertension.
- Xanthomas and jaundice generally appear in advanced disease. Kayser-Fleischer rings are rare and result from copper retention. Hyperpigmentation of the skin due to melanin deposition can occur.
- Late physical findings mirror those of cirrhosis: Spider nevi, caput medusae, temporal and proximal limb wasting, ascites, palmar erythema, digital clubbing, gynecomastia, and edema.

ETIOLOGY
- Although the cause of PBC remains unknown, it is believed to require both a genetic susceptibility as well as an environmental trigger, ultimately leading to the modification of mitochondrial proteins triggering a persistent T lymphocyte–mediated attack on intrahepatic biliary epithelial cells.
- Antimitochondrial antibodies are present in the majority of patients with PBC. PBC is otherwise associated most strongly with HLA alleles DRA, DRB1, DPB1, DQB1, BTNL2, and c6orf10. PBC is also associated with ORMDL3, CD80, STAT1/STAT4, IL12A, NF-κB, and RPL3/SYNGR1. Positive ANA is also common. However, there is significant variation across ethnic groups.
- Possible environmental triggers include infectious agents, cigarette smoking, environmental pollutants, radiation, urinary tract infections, reproductive hormone replacement, prior pregnancy, toxic waste sites (particularly exposure to halogenated hydrocarbons), electrophilic drugs, and xenobiotics found in food additives and cosmetics.
- The enzyme complex subunit PDC-E2 is an autoantigen that plays a major role in the early pathogenesis of PBC. Patients with PBC have a tenfold increased concentration of PDC-E2-specific cytotoxic CD8$^+$ lymphocytes in their livers compared to their blood, and antimitochondrial antibodies (AMAs), which are the serologic hallmark of this disease, react to the PDC-E2 subunit leading to a strong inflammatory response. In addition, biliary epithelial cells handle PDC-E2 in a unique way that exposes them to immune-mediated attack. Future therapies may be specific immunomodulation directed at these peptides.
- Damage to bile ducts results in bile leaking into liver parenchyma resulting in hepatocyte necrosis, which can lead to fibrosis and eventual cirrhosis.

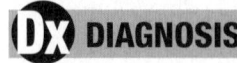 **DIAGNOSIS**

The diagnosis of PBC can be established when two of the following three criteria are met in the absence of extrahepatic biliary obstruction.

- Positive serum AMA (titer >1:40) or PBC-specific antibodies to sp100 or gp210 in AMA-negative patients[12]
- Biochemical evidence of cholestasis (mainly alkaline phosphatase elevation [ALP] ≥1.5 times the upper limit of normal [ULN])
- Characteristic liver histology demonstrating nonsuppurative destruction of small to medium-sized interlobular biliary ducts
- Recent guidelines suggest that the above criteria may lead to a delay in diagnosis, so clinical judgment and expert referral should be considered[5]

DIFFERENTIAL DIAGNOSIS

- Drug-induced cholestasis (common medications: Phenothiazines, anabolic steroids, diclofenac, some antibiotics as TMP-SMX, oxacillin, and ampicillin)
- PBC-AIH overlap syndrome; reported in 1% to 14.2% of patients initially diagnosed with PBC. Transition from stable PBC to AIH and vice versa also seen
- Other etiologies of chronic liver disease and cirrhosis, such as alcoholic cirrhosis, chronic viral hepatitis, primary sclerosing cholangitis, AIH, sarcoidosis, hepatic amyloidosis, chemical/toxin-induced cirrhosis, other hereditary or familial disorders (e.g., cystic fibrosis, α-1-antitrypsin deficiency)
- Biliary obstruction
- Secondary biliary cirrhosis or secondary sclerosing cholangitis

WORKUP

History, physical examination, laboratory evaluation, liver biopsy

LABORATORY TESTS

- AMAs are found in 90% to 95% of patients with PBC and are 98% specific, although ANA-negative PBC is possible.[9] ANA is also found in about 30% to 50% of patients.[13] Most patients have ANA or AMAs, or both.
- Cholestatic pattern of liver biochemical markers; markedly increased ALP (of hepatic origin). ALP levels below 1.5× ULN are associated with more favorable prognosis.
- γ-Glutamyl transpeptidase is increased and may be indicative of biliary origin of ALP elevation.
- Serum immunoglobulin M (IgM) levels are increased (lower in AMA-negative PBC).
- Bilirubin level is normal early on and increases with disease progression (direct and indirect). Increased serum bilirubin level is generally regarded as a poor prognostic indicator.
- Rising serum hyaluronate levels correlate with the serum bilirubin and histologic worsening of the disease.
- Aminotransferase level may be normal and, if increased, is rarely more than 5× ULN.
- Bile acid levels are strikingly elevated, and this accumulation is thought to cause foamy degeneration of hepatocytes due to toxic effects.
- Serum ceruloplasmin may also be elevated.
- Markedly increased serum lipids is largely due to increased lipoprotein X (LpX). Total cholesterol may surpass 1000 mg/dl (with

increased xanthomas rather than xanthelasmas). In the early stages of PBC, patients can have relatively higher high-density lipoprotein (HDL) in comparison to low-density lipoprotein (LDL) and very (V)-LDL. This rise in HDL might explain the lack of increased risk for cardiovascular disease. However, cardiovascular risk may still exist due to other risk factors (e.g., family history and metabolic syndrome).

- Percutaneous liver biopsy is helpful to rule out or confirm PBC in patients with superimposed NASH or AIH overlap syndrome but is not always necessary for diagnosis.[14] Biopsy is also helpful for disease staging.
- Histology is not uniform, so histologic stage is based on the most advanced lesion present.
  1. Stage I: Nonsuppurative cholangitis indicated by lymphocytic infiltration of small bile ducts with or without epithelioid granulomas or plasma cells, limited to portal areas
  2. Stage II: Extension of inflammatory cells to periportal parenchyma, ductular proliferation
  3. Stage III: Bridging necrosis or fibrous septa linking portal triads
  4. Stage IV: Frank cirrhosis with regenerative nodules

IMAGING STUDIES

If history, physical examination, blood tests, and liver biopsy are all consistent with PBC, neither imaging nor cholangiography (Fig. E1) is necessary. MRI or transient elastography (TE) is important for determination of degree of cirrhosis if present and may be indicated for monitoring of disease progression. Notably, the cutoffs for transient elastography are different from those established for other diseases, such as hepatitis C.

PROGNOSIS

- There is widespread variation in progression between phases of PBC. Some patients advance rapidly to cirrhosis and require transplant whereas others remain asymptomatic for decades.
- Median time to development of extensive fibrosis in untreated patients is 2 yr.[12]
- Median survival is 7.5 yr in untreated patients and 16 yr in asymptomatic patients; however, this has improved with earlier diagnosis and initiation of treatment.[12] Table 1 summarizes time course of histologic progression to a higher stage in patients with PBC.

TABLE 1 Rate of Histologic Progression to a Higher Stage in Patients with PBC

Rate of Progression (%) at	INITIAL HISTOLOGIC STAGE		
	1	2	3
1 yr	41	43	35
2 yr	62	62	50

From Feldman M et al: *Sleisenger and Fordtran's gastrointestinal and liver disease*, ed 11, Philadelphia, 2021, Elsevier.

- Neither presence nor total titer level of AMAs predicts survival, disease progression, or response to therapy. As such, AMA should not be serially measured.
- Serum bilirubin is the best predictor of survival and the most heavily weighted factor in prognostic models. Box E1 summarizes independent predictors of survival in patients with PBC.[1]
- Serum ALP >1.5× ULN has been shown to be a risk factor for a more progressive course of PBC including cirrhosis.[14]
- Response to ursodeoxycholic acid (UDCA) therapy can be prognostic, with approximately 40% of patients failing to respond. There are multiple biochemical response criteria that, if met after 1 yr of treatment with UDCA, are associated with improved clinical outcomes. Three of these criteria are Barcelona (decrease in ALP level of at least 40% or to the reference range), Paris I (ALP <3× ULN, AST <2× ULN and bilirubin within normal limits), and Paris II (ALP <1.5× ULN, ALT <1.5× ULN and bilirubin within normal limits).[15-17]
- Nonresponse to UDCA is also associated with increased HCC risk compared to UDCA-responsive PBC.
- Similarly, the Mayo Risk score, a predictor of short-term survival probability in nontransplanted patients (www.mayoclinic.org/medical-professionals/transplant-medicine/the-updated-natural-histo/the-updated-natural-history-model-for-primary-biliary-cirrhosis/itt-20434724), can also reliably predict life expectancy when calculated after 6 mo of UDCA therapy.[18]
- Several predictive models based upon laboratory and clinical data have been proposed, and two such models (GLOBE score and UK-PBC score) are based on multicenter studies including large cohorts of patients with PBC.
  1. GLOBE score: Includes the following five variables: Serum bilirubin, albumin, serum ALP, platelet count after 1 yr of UDCA treatment, and age at start of therapy. It estimates the duration of transplant-free survival.[19]
  2. UK-PBC score: Includes serum ALP, aminotransferases, and bilirubin after 12 mo of UDCA therapy, in addition to baseline albumin and platelet count. This model estimates the risk of liver transplantation or liver-related death.[20]
- Transient elastography is a valuable noninvasive means of determining prognosis, treatment response, and fibrosis staging and to rule out cirrhosis in clinical practice.[21] It has been reported to be significantly superior to biochemical markers and risk scores (APRI, FIB-4, Mayo risk score) in predicting fibrosis and cirrhosis in PBC. In a prospective study of PBC patients treated with UDCA, noncirrhotic PBC patients (F0 to F3 stages) were found to have either limited or no significant progression of liver stiffness whereas cirrhotic PBC patients developed significant increases in liver stiffness. Increasing liver stiffness (>2.1 kPa/yr) has been associated with an 8.4-fold increased risk of decompensation, liver transplantation, or death.[22]

- Poorer prognosis is associated with jaundice, advanced histologic stage, elevated bilirubin or ALP, low albumin, hepatocellular carcinoma, nonresponse to UDCA, and esophageal varices.

Rx TREATMENT

- Treatment is guided by the clinical stage of the disease.
- Asymptomatic stage:
  1. Follow liver function tests every 3 mo.
  2. Once ALP is elevated up to 1.5× ULN, begin UDCA at 13 to 15 mg/kg/day in two to four divided doses regardless of histologic stage.
  3. Side effects may include headaches, dizziness, diarrhea or constipation, dyspepsia, nausea, weight gain, back pain, and upper respiratory infections.
  4. Watch for interactions with fibric acid derivatives, bile acid sequestrants, estrogen derivatives, and aluminum hydroxide, which may interfere with the therapeutic effect or serum concentration of UDCA.
  5. Efficacy is best if started during stage I or II disease but should be started at any stage of disease. Lifelong therapy is currently recommended.
- Treatment also includes treatment of associated conditions such as fatigue, pruritus, osteoporosis, hypercholesterolemia, malabsorption, fat-soluble vitamin deficiencies, anemia, hypothyroidism, and any complications of cirrhosis.

ACUTE GENERAL Rx

- Symptomatic stage: Goals of treatment are resolution of symptoms such as pruritus, treatment of chronic cholestatic complications, and delay of liver failure.
- Obeticholic acid (OCA), a farnesoid X receptor agonist, has been approved as a second-line treatment for PBC and is indicated in patients who are nonresponders to UDCA as evidenced by persistently elevated ALP, lack of normalization of bilirubin, high risk on predictive models, and/or evidence of fibrosis by any modality.[4]
  1. It is initially dosed at 5 mg once daily and can be increased to 10 mg once daily after 3 mo if there has been an inadequate decrease in bilirubin and/or ALP.
  2. OCA may be given as adjunctive therapy along with UDCA, or as an alternative in patients intolerant of UDCA.
  3. The most common adverse event noted is pruritus, and therefore this drug may not be ideal for patients with that symptom.
  4. OCA has been associated with severe liver injury and close monitoring of liver function is warranted. OCA use is contraindicated in those with advanced cirrhosis with current or prior decompensation and/or portal hypertension. It should be used with caution and with frequent monitoring in those with cirrhosis that is not advanced.[23]
  5. A recent trial showed that patients with inadequate response to UDCA who were then also treated with OCA had significantly greater transplant-free survival as compared to patients who did not receive OCA.[24]
- Fibrates can be considered as off-label alternatives for patients with inadequate response to UDCA, although they should not be used in patients with decompensated liver disease.[23]
- For the pruritus, cholestyramine resin (4 to 16 g/day) reduces pruritus in most patients but must be given at least 4 h before UDCA to avoid reducing the efficacy of that drug. Antihistamines at bedtime help nighttime symptoms. Rifampin (150 to 300 mg bid), oral opiate antagonists such as naltrexone (12.5 to 50 mg daily), and sertraline (75 to 100 mg daily) can be used for pruritus refractory to bile acid sequestrants. Table E2 summarizes treatment recommendations for pruritus in PBC. Intractable pruritus can be an indication for liver transplantation.
- Newer agents that are being investigated for pruritus include ileal bile acid transporter inhibitors such as Linerixibat and fibrates such as bezafibrate.[25-27]
- Fibrates may be used in those with inadequate response to UDCA but should be avoided in those with decompensated liver disease.[23]
- A selective peroxisome proliferator-activated receptor-δ (PPAR) agonist, seladelpar, is currently being investigated as a means to improve biochemical markers of cholestasis and inflammation in patients with PBC at risk of disease progression.[28,29]
- Prednisone, azathioprine, colchicine, methotrexate, penicillamine, cyclosporine, silymarin, and mycophenolate mofetil are no longer used because of limited efficacy and/or significant toxicity.

CHRONIC Rx

- Liver function tests should be checked every 3 to 6 mo.
- Management of chronic liver disease: Immunization against hepatitis A and B, minimizing ETOH consumption, monitoring for HCC via alpha fetoprotein and ultrasound every 6 mo, and monitoring for varices via EGD every 1 to 3 yr in patients with cirrhosis or Mayo risk score >4.1.
- Management of sicca syndrome: Artificial tears can be used initially for dry eyes. Saliva substitutes can be used for xerostomia and dysphagia; pilocarpine or cevimeline can be used for refractory cases. Moisturizers can be given for vaginal dryness.
- Treatment/prevention of osteopenia/osteoporosis: Patients with PBC should be given 1000 to 1200 mg calcium daily in divided doses and 1000 IU of vitamin D daily in the diet and as supplements if needed. Weight-bearing exercises are also recommended. Bone densitometry should be done at time of diagnosis, after a fragility fracture, in patients with cirrhosis, prior to transplant, or in patients receiving steroids more than 3 mo. It should then be performed every 2 to 4 yr. Alendronate (70 mg weekly) or other bisphosphonates should be considered if patients have osteopenia in the absence of acid reflux or known varices.
- Hyperlipidemia is common in patients with PBC. However, there is no elevated risk of cardiovascular disease. Statins are safe and effective in patients who may need treatment even if liver chemistry is abnormal.
- Vitamin A, K, E, and D deficiencies can be clinically important in advanced cases and respond to oral replacement. Consider annual vitamin K and vitamin D levels, and prothrombin time.
- Liver transplantation is the only effective treatment for patients with liver failure, and approximately 25% of PBC patients ultimately need a liver transplant. Indications for transplantation include hepatic decompensation (encephalopathy, recurrent variceal bleeding, intractable ascites and spontaneous bacterial peritonitis), hepatocellular carcinoma fulfilling Milan criteria (see "Hepatocellular Carcinoma"), and intractable pruritus. Liver transplant should also be considered with a Mayo risk score >7.8, MELD score >12, and bilirubin ≥6 mg/dl.
- The outcome of liver transplantation for patients with PBC is more favorable than that of nearly all other liver disease categories. The survival rates at 1 yr are now up to 90% to 95%. Although recurrent disease may develop in about one third of patients after liver transplantation, patient and graft survival is usually not affected.

DISPOSITION

Definitive treatment requires liver transplantation. Patients treated with UDCA have been reported to have transplant-free survival of 90%, 78%, and 66% at 5, 10, and 15 yr, respectively. Among untreated patients, transplant-free survival is 79%, 59%, and 32% at 5, 10, and 15 yr, respectively.[30,31]

REFERRAL

Refer to gastroenterology and/or hepatology for treatment, evaluation for liver transplantation, and management of portal hypertension.

REFERENCES & SUGGESTED READING

Available at eBooks.Health.Elsevier.com.

RELATED CONTENT

Primary Biliary Cirrhosis (PBC) (Patient Information)

AUTHORS: **KIRSTEN LOSCALZO, MD** and **JEANETTE G. SMITH, MD**

BASIC INFORMATION

DEFINITION

Primary sclerosing cholangitis (PSC) is a chronic, cholestatic, immune-mediated liver disease characterized by progressive inflammation and fibrosis of the intrahepatic and extrahepatic bile ducts. PSC has a strong association with inflammatory bowel disease (IBD) and may be complicated by recurrent cholangitis, colorectal and hepatobiliary malignancies, and cirrhosis.[1]

SYNONYMS

PSC
Chronic obliterative cholangitis
Fibrosing cholangitis
Stenosing cholangitis

ICD-10CM CODES
K83.0	Cholangitis
K83.9	Disease of biliary tract, unspecified

EPIDEMIOLOGY & DEMOGRAPHICS

- The incidence and prevalence of PSC are 1 case/100,000 persons per yr and 6 to 16 cases/100,000 persons, respectively.[2]
- About 60% of patients with PSC are men.
- PSC can present at any age. The median age of diagnosis is 36 to 39 yr.[3,4]
- Over 70% of patients with PSC also have IBD, most commonly with an ulcerative colitis (UC) phenotype. Approximately 5% to 10% of patients with IBD will develop PSC. Eight percent to 9% of adults and 15% of children with IBD were found to have PSC after undergoing universal screening with liver biopsy or cholangiography.[5] PSC-IBD may represent a phenotypic entity on its own and typically presents with right-sided colitis, "backwash" ileitis, and rectal sparing.[6]
- PSC is an independent risk factor for developing colorectal cancer in patients with IBD. PSC-IBD is associated with a fourfold increased risk of colorectal cancer compared to IBD alone.[7]
- Patients with PSC are at increased risk of gallbladder cancer. Review of cholecystectomy specimens with gallbladder cancer varies from 18% to 56%.[8]
- Patients with PSC are at increased risk of hepatobiliary cancers, most commonly cholangiocarcinoma (CCA). CCA is present in 2.5% of PSC patients at diagnosis. PSC should be considered a premalignant disease with a lifetime risk of developing CCA between 5% and 10%.[9]
- PSC can coexist with other autoimmune liver diseases. PSC–autoimmune hepatitis (AIH) overlap syndrome is more common in young adults and children.[10]
- Box 1 summarizes a classification of diseases associated with sclerosing cholangitis.
- The median survival from time of diagnosis is 10 to 15 yr without liver transplantation.[11] While deaths from end-stage liver disease have decreased, deaths from cholangiocarcinoma have remained unchanged.[12]

PHYSICAL FINDINGS & CLINICAL PRESENTATION

- Up to 50% of patients are asymptomatic at the time of diagnosis, with normal physical examination findings. Abnormal liver tests and a known diagnosis of IBD are often the only signs at diagnosis.
- The most common symptoms on presentation include right upper quadrant abdominal pain, fever, pruritus, and fatigue. Additional symptoms include abdominal distention, confusion, jaundice, recurrent cholangitis, or other symptoms related to portal hypertension. On physical exam, patients may have jaundice, skin excoriation and hyperpigmentation from scratching, hepatosplenomegaly, and xanthelasmas.

ETIOLOGY

- The cause of PSC is unknown. Like other autoimmune diseases, the most likely mechanism is immunologic priming in a genetically susceptible patient causing phenotypic expression of the disease.[2]
- Genetic and immunologic factors are supported by reports of familial occurrence of this disorder and increased frequency of human leukocyte antigen (HLA) B8 and DR3. Genome-wide association studies have discovered novel loci associated with PSC, but the functional aspects of these genes are still unknown.
- Portosystemic inflammation caused by translocation of the gut microbiota is an increasing area of research. The close association with UC and PSC may be secondary to gut-activated T lymphocytes in IBD causing portal inflammation because of overlapping adhesion molecules in the gut and liver. Furthermore, intestinal dysbiosis and impaired gut barrier in PSC have also been seen and remain an area of ongoing research.
- Dysregulated inflammatory cytokine production by cholangiocytes is also more recently suggested to be playing a role in the pathogenesis of PSC.

DIAGNOSIS

DIFFERENTIAL DIAGNOSIS

- Immunoglobulin G4 (IgG4)-associated cholangitis (IAC)
- Surgical biliary trauma
- Ischemic cholangitis, recurrent pyogenic cholangitis, recurrent pancreatitis
- Choledocholithiasis, cholangiocarcinoma
- Intraarterial chemotherapy (5-FU/floxuridine)
- Diffuse intrahepatic metastasis, sarcoidosis, or amyloidosis
- AIDS-related, eosinophilic, or mast cell cholangiopathy
- Histiocytosis X, graft-versus-host disease
- Hepatic inflammatory pseudotumor, portal hypertensive biliopathy
- Primary biliary cholangitis (Table 1)

WORKUP

Diagnosis is based on characteristic (1) laboratory findings, (2) cholangiographic findings, and (3) the exclusion of secondary cholangitis. Though liver biopsy is now rarely used to diagnose PSC, it may be indicated in patients with normal cholangiograms and a high suspicion of small-duct PSC, or if PSC-AIH overlap is being considered. Table 2 describes the staging of PSC.

LABORATORY TESTS

- A persistent elevated serum alkaline phosphatase is characteristic of PSC.
- Also, patients frequently have elevated serum aminotransferase levels, and this may suggest an overlap syndrome, such as PSC-AIH.
- However, liver enzymes fluctuate as part of the natural history of PSC, and some patients may have normal liver enzymes.
- Serum bilirubin is usually normal at the time of diagnosis unless the patient has advanced stricturing disease or advanced liver disease. Initial elevation of bilirubin at diagnosis may be related to a worse prognosis.[9]
- A wide range of autoantibodies can be detected in patients with PSC, including anti-neutrophil cytoplasmic antibodies (ANCAs; 26% to 96% of PSC patients), antinuclear antibody (ANA; 8% to 77% of PSC patients), and anti–smooth muscle antibody (ASMA; 83% of PSC patients).[13] These antibodies are not specific for PSC and do not reflect prognosis.
  1. Antimitochondrial antibody (AMA), which is characteristic of primary biliary cholangitis (PBC), is NOT found in PSC and can be helpful in excluding PSC.
  2. Serum IgG levels are useful in the diagnosis of PSC-AIH overlap syndrome (more common in pediatric patients) and IAC with autoimmune pancreatitis.
  3. In particular, elevated levels of IgG4 are found in 10% to 20% of PSC patients, with a subset of these patients displaying features of autoimmune pancreatitis. PSC patients with elevated IgG4 tend to have worse outcomes and seem to respond to corticosteroid therapy; hence, IgG4 levels should be checked at least once in all patients with PSC.

IMAGING STUDIES

- Cholangiography with magnetic resonance cholangiopancreatography (MRCP), endoscopic retrograde cholangiopancreatography (ERCP), and percutaneous transhepatic cholangiography (PTC) are considered to be the gold standard for the diagnosis of PSC. Characteristic findings reveal segmental fibrosis of bile ducts with saccular dilation of normal intervening areas resulting in a "beads-on-a-string" appearance (Fig. 1).
- MRCP has largely supplanted ERCP and PTC as the diagnostic study of choice because it is noninvasive, less expensive.
- In a meta-analysis of six studies, the sensitivity and specificity of MRCP for diagnosing PSC were 86% and 94%, respectively.[14]
- MRCP, however, does not allow sampling of strictures for brush cytology or biopsy, nor does it allow therapeutic interventions if a

BOX 1 Classification of and Diseases Associated with Sclerosing Cholangitis

Primary sclerosing cholangitis
Principal disease associations
Inflammatory bowel disease:
- Crohn colitis or ileocolitis
- Ulcerative colitis

Other disease associations
Systemic diseases with fibrosis:
- Inflammatory pseudotumor
- Mediastinal fibrosis
- Peyronie disease
- Pseudotumor of the orbit
- Retroperitoneal fibrosis
- Riedel thyroiditis

Autoimmune or collagen vascular disorders:
- Autoimmune hemolytic anemia
- Celiac disease
- Chronic sclerosing sialadenitis
- Membranous nephropathy
- Progressive systemic sclerosis
- Rapidly progressive glomerulonephritis
- Rheumatoid arthritis
- Sjögren syndrome
- Systemic lupus erythematosus
- Type 1 diabetes mellitus

Alloimmune diseases:
- Hepatic allograft rejection
- Hepatic graft-versus-host disease after bone marrow transplantation

Infiltrative diseases:
- Hypereosinophilic syndrome
- Histiocytosis X
- Sarcoidosis
- Systemic mastocytosis

Immunodeficiency:
- Congenital immunodeficiency
  1. Combined immunodeficiency
  2. Dysgammaglobulinemia
  3. X-lined agammaglobulinemia
- Acquired immunodeficiency:
  1. AIDS
  2. Angioimmunoblastic lymphadenopathy
  3. Opportunistic infections (e.g., cryptosporidiosis, cytomegalovirus, microsporidiosis)
  4. Selective IgA deficiency

Secondary sclerosing cholangitis
Obstructive
- Autoimmune pancreatitis
- Chronic pancreatitis
- Caroli disease
- Choledocholithiasis
- Intrahepatic lithiasis
- Portal hypertension biliopathy
- Surgical stricture

Congenital abnormalities:
  1. Cystic fibrosis
  2. Choledochal cyst
- Infectious
- HIV
- Recurrent pyogenic cholangitis
- Parasitic
- Hydatid
- Echinococcus
- Fluke
- Ascariasis
- Schistosomiasis
- Fascioliasis
- Autoimmune
- Eosinophilic cholangitis
- Hepatic inflammatory pseudotumor
- IgG4 associated cholangitis
- Mast cell cholangiopathy
- Sarcoidosis
- Immunotherapy-associated (checkpoint inhibitor)

Toxic
- Intraarterial floxuridine (FUDR)
- Intraductal formaldehyde or hypertonic saline (echinococcal cyst treatment)

Ischemic
- Hepatic arterial thrombosis
- Hereditary hemorrhagic telangiectasis
- Paroxysmal nocturnal hemoglobinuria
- Toxic vasculitis (FUDR)
- Vascular trauma

Neoplastic
- Cholangiocarcinoma
- Hepatocellular carcinoma
- Lymphoma
- Metastatic cancer

Modified from Feldman M et al: *Sleisenger and Fordtran's gastrointestinal and liver disease*, ed 11, Philadelphia, 2021, Elsevier.

mechanical reason for obstruction is found such as stone, stricture, or tumor.[7]
- Noninvasive measurements of liver elastography including MR elastography are promising methods for evaluating for cirrhosis but have not yet been validated in this patient cohort.[15]

Rx TREATMENT

- No medical therapy has been established to be effective in treating PSC. Management of PSC patients is aimed at symptom relief and management of complications from PSC (i.e., obstruction/strictures, portal hypertension).[16]
- Ursodeoxycholic acid (UDCA) has shown to be associated with improvement in ALP, and significant reductions in ALP have been shown to result in better outcomes. However, because ALP and GGT can spontaneously normalize, the American Association for Liver Diseases recommends observing for 6 mo and only initiating UDCA if ALP remains elevated. High-dose UDCA is not recommended as it has been associated with increased adverse outcomes.[17]
- Bile acid–based therapy options being tested in clinical trials include 24-norursodeoxycholic acid (norUDCA), steroidal and nonsteroidal bile acid receptor/farnesoid X receptor (FXR) agonists (e.g., obeticholic acid, cilofexor), and the FXR-downstream target fibroblast growth factor-19 (FGF19; nontumorigenic recombinant FGF19/NGM-282 [aldafermin]).[18]
- The use of corticosteroids and other immunosuppressive agents is not recommended in patients with PSC alone; however, it is recommended in patients with PSC-AIH overlap syndrome or elevated IgG4.[2] Randomized control trials are ongoing exploring the use of immune modulators and have shown some promise in reducing ALP levels, especially in patients with worse disease.[19]

- Manipulation of the microbiome is an exciting area being explored as a future treatment for PSC. This is being tried with antibiotics (e.g., vancomycin), fecal microbiota transplantation (FMT), and bacteriophage-based therapy.
  1. Oral vancomycin may show clinical and biochemical response in pediatric patients, but no randomized clinical trial has been performed.[3]
  2. Recent studies have shown that FMT in PSC is safe, improves liver biochemistries, and improves microbiome diversity. This is a rapidly expanding area of gastroenterology that shows promise. However, larger studies are needed to determine if such treatments can affect mortality or reduce liver transplantation.[20]

ACUTE GENERAL Rx

- For mild pruritus, cooling gels (e.g., menthol gels), skin emollients, antihistamines, and

TABLE 1 Primary Sclerosing Cholangitis (PSC) Versus Primary Biliary Cholangitis (PBC)

Feature	PSC	PBC
Age	Young	Middle-aged and elderly
Sex	Typically men (70%)	Typically women (90%)
Clinical	Pain Cholangitis Hepatosplenomegaly ALP elevated	Pruritus Xanthomas, xanthelasma Hyperpigmentation Hepatosplenomegaly ALP elevated
Liver function tests	Bilirubin fluctuates	
Antimitochondrial antibody	Negative	Positive in 90% (also elevated in chronic hepatitis, connective tissue disease)
pANCA	Positive (up to 80%)	Negative
MRCP	Irregular and beaded ducts	Pruned ducts
Associated diseases	Ulcerative colitis (70%) Crohn disease (rare) Sjögren syndrome (rare) Thyroiditis (rare) Hypothyroidism (rare) Pancreatitis (rare) Retroorbital and retroperitoneal fibrosis (rare)	CREST syndrome Sjögren syndrome Thyroiditis Renal tubular acidosis
Complications	Portal hypertension Liver failure Bile duct carcinoma	Osteomalacia Steatorrhea (due to bile acid deficiency, associated pancreatic insufficiency, or coexisting celiac disease) Portal hypertension, liver failure (late)
Treatment	Ursodeoxycholic acid Liver transplant	Liver transplant

ALP, Serum alkaline phosphatase; *CREST*, calcinosis, Raynaud syndrome, esophageal dysmotility, sclerodactyly, and telangiectasia; *MRCP*, magnetic resonance cholangiopancreatography; *pANCA*, perinuclear antineutrophil cytoplasmic antibody.
From Talley NJ et al: *Essentials of internal medicine,* ed 4, Chatswood, NSW, 2021, Elsevier Australia.

TABLE 2 Staging of Primary Sclerosing Cholangitis

Stage	Description
I—Portal	Portal edema, inflammation, ductal proliferation; abnormalities do not extend beyond the limiting plate
II—Periportal	Periportal fibrosis with or without inflammation extending beyond the limiting plate
III—Septal	Septal fibrosis, bridging necrosis, or both
IV—Cirrhotic	Biliary cirrhosis

From Cameron JL, Cameron AM: *Current surgical therapy,* ed 10, Philadelphia, 2011, Saunders.

cholestyramine are recommended as the first-line treatment.[9,17]

- For moderate or severe pruritus, bezafibrate and rifampicin are now recommended first-line agents.[18] Alternative agents include naltrexone, sertraline, phenobarbital, and phototherapy.[17,21]
- Patients who present with increasing serum bilirubin, worsening pruritus, progressive bile duct dilation on imaging studies, or cholangitis should be evaluated for dominant strictures with imaging. A dominant stricture is a stenosis <1.5 mm in the common bile duct or <1 mm in the hepatic duct.[9]

- ERCP with brushings, cytology, and fluorescent in situ hybridization (FISH) is recommended to evaluate dominant strictures for CCA, which is found in 15% to 20% of cases. Once malignancy is excluded, balloon dilation with or without stenting is recommended to treat symptomatic patients. Routine stenting is not required, but short-term stenting may be helpful in patients with severe stricture. If ERCP is unsuccessful, percutaneous cholangiopancreatography with stenting should be considered.[9]
- Probe–based confocal laser endomicroscopy (pCLE) can visualize the gut epithelium at ultra-high magnification (1000×) and resolution (<10 microns) and allows targeted biopsy. pCLE enhances standard imaging by offering in vivo histopathology and visualization of vasculature and architecture using fluorescein dye.
- Recent literature has shown that the combination of ERCP and pCLE was more accurate than ERCP and tissue sampling (90% vs. 73%, $P = .001$).[22,23]
- In noncirrhotic patients with dominant strictures refractory to endoscopic or percutaneous management, surgery should be considered, although this may complicate future liver transplantation.[9]
- Antibiotic usage is recommended in patients with dominant strictures/obstructions both acutely and for long-term prophylaxis in patients with recurrent cholangitis.[9]

CHRONIC Rx

- Alcohol avoidance and vaccination against hepatitis A and B are advised.
- Patients with PSC are at risk for osteoporosis and osteopenia; therefore DEXA scan should be performed at diagnosis and repeated every 2 to 4 yr. The pathophysiology of osteopathy in PSC is not well understood but has been hypothesized to be related to decreased absorption of fat-soluble vitamins and impairment of osteoblasts by bilirubin.[9]
- With advanced disease, fat-soluble vitamin deficiencies such as A, E, and D should be assessed and replaced as needed.
- Patients with newly diagnosed PSC should undergo colonoscopy with biopsies to exclude concurrent IBD and for surveillance of colorectal cancer. In patients with PSC and IBD, continued surveillance colonoscopy with biopsies, or chromoendoscopy, at 1- to 2-yr intervals is recommended. In patients without IBD, a 3- to 5-yr surveillance interval has been recommended due to an increased risk of colorectal cancer.[9]
- Screening for CCA and gallbladder cancer should be performed at least yearly with ultrasound and/or MRI/MRCP, with or without serum CA 19-9 regardless of disease stage. CCA screening is not indicated in PSC patients <18 yr of age or in those who have small duct PSC. ERCP with brush cytology or cholangioscopy should be performed in patients who have biochemical or symptomatic deterioration or dominant stricture to rule out CCA.[9,17]
- Annual transabdominal ultrasound is recommended due to the increased risk of gallbladder malignancy, even in patients who are not cirrhotic. The AASLD and the American College of Gastroenterology (ACG) recommend cholecystectomy for polyps >8 mm.[9,17]
- Patients with PSC and cirrhosis are recommended to have hepatocellular carcinoma (HCC) surveillance with ultrasound, with or without α-fetoprotein, every 6 mo and gastroesophageal variceal surveillance at regular intervals.[24]
- In patients with HCC and CCA, resection versus liver transplantation may be indicated depending on the extent of disease.[9]

DISPOSITION

Liver transplantation is the only effective treatment for patients with decompensated cirrhosis, liver failure, intractable pruritus, and recurrent bacterial cholangitis. Survival is excellent, with 90% and 80% survival rates at 1 and 5 yr, respectively. The recurrence of PSC after transplant is reportedly 5% to 20%, with IBD and younger age at transplant being important risk factors.[2] Transplant referral is warranted in patients with MELD score ≥15, refractory cholangitis, and early-stage HCC/CCA7.[4]

REFERRAL

All patients with suspected PSC should be referred to a gastroenterologist or hepatologist for formal diagnosis, management of complications, surveillance of associated malignancies, and evaluation for liver transplantation.

P

Diseases and Disorders

I

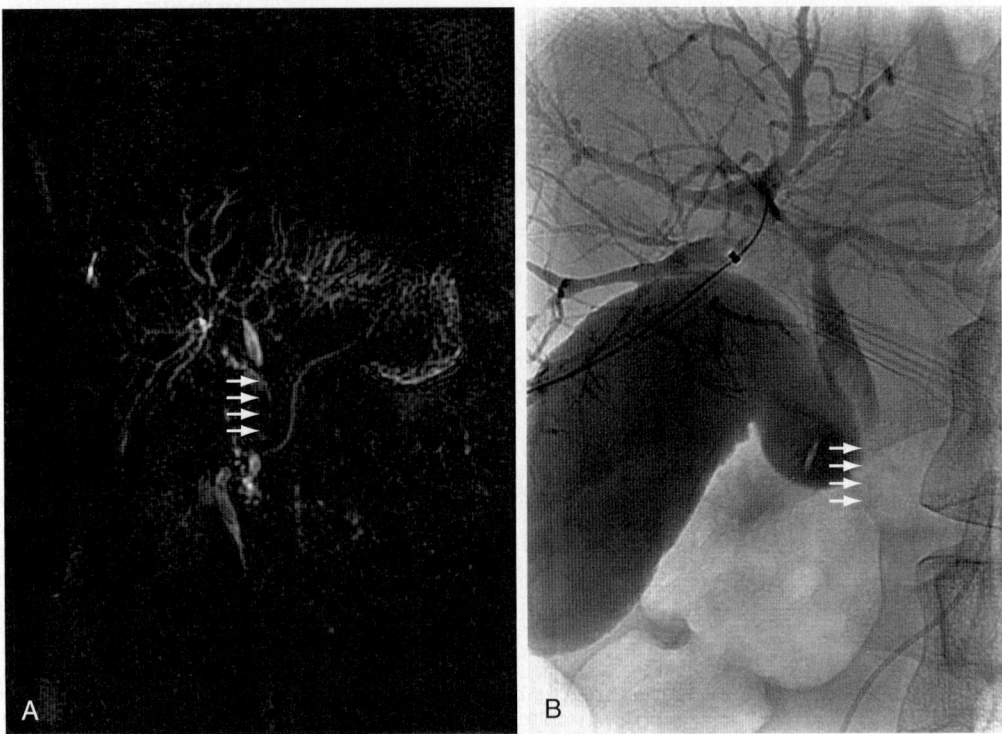

FIG. 1 A, Reconstructed magnetic resonance cholangiopancreatography images in a patient with primary sclerosing cholangitis. The intrahepatic biliary radicles are diffusely abnormal and characterized by pruning and a beaded appearance. There is a dominant stricture at the level of the distal bile duct *(arrows)* indicated by a signal void on magnetic resonance image. **B,** A percutaneous cholangiogram in the same patient. Note the high-grade, dominant, distal bile duct stenosis *(arrows)* with a markedly enlarged gallbladder, suggesting that the stricture involves the insertion of the cystic duct. Similar findings could be seen in a patient with a distal cholangiocarcinoma. (From Feldman M et al: *Sleisenger and Fordtran's gastrointestinal and liver disease*, ed 11, Philadelphia, 2021, Elsevier.)

ⓘ PEARLS & CONSIDERATIONS

- Diagnosis of PSC is made by a combination of clinical presentation, cholestatic liver function tests, cholangiographic evidence of multifocal biliary strictures, and the exclusion of secondary cholangitis.
- There is currently no effective medical treatment of PSC. Management of PSC targets symptom relief, complications of PSC, cirrhosis, early hepatobiliary and colorectal cancer detection, and timely referral for liver transplantation. Liver transplant remains the only definitive therapy for complications of PSC.
- Patients are at increased risk for the development of colorectal cancer, gallbladder cancer, and cholangiocarcinoma and need surveillance.
- In patients with cirrhosis, surveillance for gastroesophageal varices and HCC is recommended.

REFERENCES

Available at eBooks.Health.Elsevier.com.

RELATED CONTENT

Ulcerative Colitis (Related Key Topic)

AUTHOR: **LI WANG, MD, MHA**

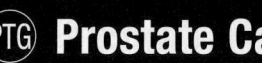
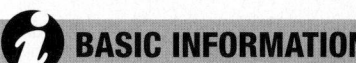

BASIC INFORMATION

DEFINITION & CLASSIFICATION

Prostate cancer is a neoplasm involving the prostate. Various classifications have been developed to evaluate malignancy potential and prognosis.

- The degree of malignancy varies with the stage:
  1. Stage A: Confined to the prostate, no nodule palpable
  2. Stage B: Palpable nodule confined to the gland
  3. Stage C: Local extension
  4. Stage D: Regional lymph nodes or distant metastases
- In the Gleason classification (Box 1 and Fig. E1), two histologic patterns are independently assigned numbers 1 to 5 (best to least differentiated). These numbers are added to give a total tumor score between 2 and 10. Prognosis is best for highly differentiated tumors (e.g., Gleason score 2 to 6) compared with most poorly differentiated tumors (Gleason score 7 to 10).
- Another commonly used classification is the Tumor-Node-Metastasis (TNM) classification of prostate cancer (Table 1).
- Table 2 summarizes the definition of risk groups and biopsy criteria.

ICD-10CM CODES
C61   Malignant neoplasm of prostate
D07.5   Carcinoma in situ of prostate

EPIDEMIOLOGY & DEMOGRAPHICS

- Prostate cancer has surpassed lung cancer as the most common nonskin cancer in men.
- In the United States, more than 220,000 new cases are diagnosed yearly, and nearly 30,000 males die from prostate cancer each year (second leading cause of death from cancer in U.S. men).
- Incidence of prostate cancer increases with age: Uncommon <50 yr; 80% of new cases are diagnosed in patients aged ≥65 yr. Widespread prostate-specific antigen (PSA) testing has doubled the incidence of prostate cancer and the lifetime risk for prostate cancer to approximately 16%. Prostate cancer is also diagnosed earlier, and the incidence of clinically "silent" T_1 tumors has increased from 17% in 1989 to 48% in 2001 since the advent of PSA screening. Currently, approximately 80% of prostate cancer cases are diagnosed as localized disease and only 4% as metastatic disease. The incidence of metastatic prostate cancer for middle-aged men was stable from 2004 to 2010 and then increased from 12 to 17 cases/100,000 from 2010 to 2018.[1] It is unclear if this increase was due to U.S. Preventive Services Task Force (USPSTF) recommendations against PSA screening in 2008 and 2012 or to more aggressive diagnostic strategies.
- Prostate cancer is found at autopsy in more than half of U.S. men older than 50 yr but is the cause of death in only 3%.
- Average age at time of diagnosis is 72 yr.
- Blacks in the U.S. have the highest incidence of prostate cancer in the world (one in every nine males).
- Incidence is low in Asians.
- Approximately 9% of all prostate cancers may be familial. Obesity is a risk factor for prostate cancer. High-fat, low-fiber diet increases risk. High insulin levels may also increase the risk of prostate cancer. Dietary supplementation with vitamin E has been reported to significantly increase the risk of prostate cancer among healthy men. Linkage studies have implicated chromosome 17p21-22 as a possible location of a prostate-cancer susceptibility gene. Germline mutations in *HOXB13* are associated with a significantly increased risk of hereditary prostate cancer.
- Mortality rates of prostate cancer have declined substantially in the past 15 yr from 34% in 1990 to <20% currently.

PHYSICAL FINDINGS & CLINICAL PRESENTATION

- Generally silent disease until it reaches advanced stages.
- Bone pain and pathologic fractures may be initial symptoms of prostate cancer.
- Local growth can cause symptoms of outflow obstruction.
- Digital rectal examination (DRE) may reveal an area of increased firmness; 10% of patients will have a negative DRE.
- Prostate may be hard, fixed, with extension of tumor to the seminal vesicles in advanced stages.

DIAGNOSIS

DIFFERENTIAL DIAGNOSIS

- Benign prostatic hypertrophy
- Prostatitis
- Prostate stones

LABORATORY TESTS

- Measurement of PSA is controversial in early diagnosis of prostate cancer. Main benefits and harms of PSA testing are summarized in Box 2. PSA screening is associated with psychological harm, and its potential benefits remain uncertain. In asymptomatic men with no history of prostate cancer, screening using PSA does not reduce all-cause mortality or death from prostate cancer. Normal PSA is found in >20% of patients with prostate cancer, whereas only 20% of men with PSA levels between 4 ng/ml and 10 ng/ml have prostate cancer. Most guidelines encourage a shared decision-making approach between patient and physician regarding PSA testing. Available evidence favors clinician discussion of the pros and cons of PSA screening with average-risk men aged 65 to 69 yr. Only men who express a definite preference for screening should have PSA testing. Rather than widespread annual PSA screening, a reasonable approach may be to focus on high-risk men (those with PSA levels ≥2 ng/ml at age 60). The American Cancer Society recommends offering the PSA test and DRE yearly to men aged ≥50 yr who have a life expectancy of at least 10 yr. Earlier testing, starting at age 40 to 45 yr, is recommended for men at high risk (e.g., blacks, men with family history of prostate cancer). An isolated elevation in PSA level should be confirmed several weeks later before proceeding with further testing, including prostate biopsy. Screening for prostate cancer in men aged ≥75 yr is controversial and generally not recommended. The American College of Physicians (ACP) recommends that clinicians should not screen for prostate cancer using the PSA in average-risk men

---

BOX 1   2005 International Society of Urological Pathology Modified Gleason System

Pattern 1
Circumscribed nodule of closely packed but separate, uniform, rounded to oval, medium-sized acini (larger glands than pattern 3)

Pattern 2
Like pattern 1, fairly circumscribed, yet at the edge of the tumor nodule there may be minimal infiltration
Glands are more loosely arranged and not quite as uniform as Gleason pattern 1

Pattern 3
Discrete glandular units
Typically smaller glands than seen in Gleason pattern 1 or 2
Infiltrates in and among nonneoplastic prostate acini
Marked variation in size and shape

Pattern 4
Fused microacinar glands
Ill-defined glands with poorly formed glandular lumens
Large cribriform glands
Cribriform glands
Hypernephromatoid

Pattern 5
Essentially no glandular differentiation, composed of solid sheets, cords, or single cells
Comedocarcinoma with central necrosis surrounded by papillary, cribriform, or solid masses

From Wein AJ et al: *Campbell-Walsh urology,* ed 11, Philadelphia, 2016, Elsevier.

under age 50, men over age 69, or men with a life expectancy of <10 to 15 yr. The U.S. Preventive Services Task Force (USPSTF) recommends against PSA-based screening for prostate cancer in all age groups. According to the USPSTF:

1. The magnitude of harms from screening (e.g., falsely high PSA levels, psychological effects, unnecessary biopsies, overdiagnosis of indolent tumors) is "at least small."
2. The magnitude of treatment-associated harms (i.e., adverse effects of surgery, radiation, and hormonal therapy) is "at least moderate."
3. The 10-yr mortality benefit of PSA-based prostate cancer screening is "small to none."
4. The overall balance of benefits and harms results in "moderate certainty that PSA-based screening has no net benefit."

- The USPSTF currently recommends individualized screening decisions for men between ages 55 and 69 and advises against screening for older men.
- Free PSA: The use of serum free PSA for prostate screening has been proposed by some urologists as a means to decrease unwarranted biopsies without missing a significant number of prostate cancers. This approach is based on the higher free PSA in men with benign prostatic hyperplasia and the higher protein-bound PSA levels in men with prostate cancer. For example, in men with total PSA levels of 4 to 10 ng/ml, the cancer probability is 0.25, but if the percentage of free PSA is ≤17%, the probability of cancer increases to 0.45.
- PSA velocity: The rate of increase of serum PSA over time (PSA velocity) can aid in the diagnosis of prostate cancer. A yearly PSA velocity >0.75 ng/ml increases the likelihood of later malignancy when total PSA is still within normal range. Proper interpretation of PSA velocity requires at least three PSA measurements over an 18-mo period because most PSA variations are physiologic. Recent trials have cast a doubt on the value of PSA velocity by showing that adding PSA velocity as a trigger for biopsy did not improve predictive accuracy beyond that of using PSA threshold values alone. Retrospective studies[2] have also shown that PSA velocity threshold is different in black and non-Hispanic white men treated for low-risk prostate cancer with active surveillance. PSA velocity associated significantly with grade progression was 0.44 mg/ml/yr in black patients and 1.18 mg/ml/yr in non-Hispanic whites. The optimal PSA velocity threshold for development of metastases was 1.77 mg/ml/yr.

TABLE 1 Prostate Cancer

T Stage		
T_x		Primary tumor is not assessable
T_0		There is no evidence of primary tumor
T_1		Tumor is not clinically palpable or detected with imaging
	T_{1a}	*An incidental histologic finding in ≤5% of resected tissue (e.g., TURP)*
	T_{1b}	*An incidental histologic finding in >5% of resected tissue (e.g., TURP)*
	T_{1c}	*Tumor is identified by needle biopsy*
T_2		Prostate-confined tumor that is clinically palpable or detected with imaging
	T_{2a}	*Tumor involves ≤1/2 of one prostate lobe*
	T_{2b}	*Tumor involves >1/2 of one prostate lobe (but not both lobes)*
	T_{2c}	*Tumor involves both lobes*
T_3		There is tumor extension through the prostate capsule
	T_{3a}	*Unilateral or bilateral tumor extension through the prostate capsule*
	T_{3b}	*Seminal vesical involvement*
T_4		Tumor invades structures other than the seminal vesicles (e.g., the bladder neck, rectum, or pelvic wall)
N Stage		
N_x		The lymph nodes are not assessable
N_0		There is no tumor spread
N_1		There is tumor spread to one or more regional pelvic nodes
M Stage		
M_0		There is no tumor spread beyond the regional pelvic nodes
M_1		There is tumor spread beyond the regional pelvic nodes
	M_{1a}	*Tumor spread to nodes outside of the pelvis*
	M_{1b}	*Tumor spread to bones*
	M_{1c}	*Tumor spread to other organs (e.g., lung, liver and brain) ± bone involvement*

From Grant LA: *Grainger & Allison's diagnostic radiology essentials*, ed 2, Philadelphia, 2019, Elsevier.

TABLE 2 Definition of Risk Groups

Risk Group	Clinical Stage	PSA (ng/ml)	Gleason Score	Biopsy Criteria
Low	T_{1a} or T_{1c}	<10	2-6	Unilateral or <50% of core involved
Intermediate	T_{1b}, T_{1c}, or T_{2a}	<10	3 + 4 = 7	Bilateral
High	T_{1b}, T_{1c}, T_{2b}, or T_3	10-20	4 + 3 = 7	>50% of core involved or perineural invasion or ductal differentiation
Very high	T_4	>20	8-10	Lymphovascular invasion or neuroendocrine differentiation

From Wein AJ et al: *Campbell-Walsh urology*, ed 11, Philadelphia, 2016, Elsevier.

BOX 2 Main Benefits and Harms of PSA Testing

Benefits	Limitations
Increased detection of prostate cancer earlier in disease course.	False-positive PSA tests lead to unnecessary biopsies, which have potential complications including urinary incontinence, erectile dysfunction, and bowel disturbance.
Reduction in prostate cancer mortality.	The advent of new risk stratification scores may help to avoid unnecessary biopsies following positive PSAs.
	May identify cancers that would not have become clinically relevant in a man's lifetime.

From Robertson RP et al: *DeGroot's endocrinology, basic science and clinical practice*, ed 8, Philadelphia, 2023, Elsevier.

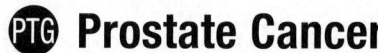
- Age-adjusted PSA: There is evidence that the current threshold of 4.0 ng/ml is inadequate for younger men, because in a recent study 22% of men with PSA levels between 2.6 and 4.0 were found to have prostate cancer. The concept of age-related cutoffs remains controversial. Lowering the upper limit of normal for PSA would improve sensitivity but decrease specificity.
- Prostatic acid phosphatase can be used for evaluation of nonlocalized disease.
- Prostate cancer gene 3 *(PCA3)* is overexpressed in prostate cancer cell, and high levels are suggestive of prostate cancer. Measurement of *PCA3* in urine specimens collected after digital exams is helpful to make decisions about prostate biopsy in men with elevated PSA.
- Ultrasound-guided transrectal biopsy and fine-needle aspiration of prostate can confirm the diagnosis. Indications for biopsy include an abnormal PSA level, an abnormal DRE, or a previous biopsy specimen that showed prostatic intraepithelial neoplasia or prostatic atypia. The number of cores taken is patient specific, typically including a minimum of 10 cores. Prostate volume negatively affects cancer detection rate (23% in glands >50 cm³, 38% in glands <50 cm³). MRI-targeted biopsy identifies clinically significant prostate cancers more accurately than conventional systematic biopsy in men with suspected localized prostate cancer but misses one in five clinically significant cancers.[3]

IMAGING STUDIES (FIGS. E2 TO E5)

- MRI can be used to guide decisions on whether to perform biopsies in men with elevated PSA levels on prostate cancer screening. MRI also facilitates targeted biopsy or suspicious areas.[4] However the avoidance of systematic biopsy in favor of MRI-directed targeted biopsy for screening and early detection in persons with elevated PSA levels reduces the risk of over-diagnosis by half at the cost of delaying detection of intermediate-risk tumors in a small proportion of patients.[5]
- Bone scan is useful to evaluate bone metastasis (present or eventually develops in almost 80% of patients). However, according to the American Urological Association (AUA), the routine use of bone scanning is not required for staging of prostate cancer in asymptomatic men with clinically localized cancer if the PSA level is ≤20 ng/ml.
- Computed tomography (CT) scan, MRI, and transrectal ultrasonography may be useful in selected patients to assess extent of prostate cancer. High-resolution has been used for the detection of small and otherwise undetectable lymph node metastases in patients with prostate cancer. However, according to the AUA, transrectal ultrasonography adds little to the combination of PSA and DRE. Similarly, CT and MRI imaging are generally not indicated for cancer staging in men with clinically localized cancer and PSA <25 ng/ml. With regard to pelvic lymph node dissection in staging, the AUA states that it may not be required in patients with PSA levels <10 ng/ml and when PSA level is <20 ng/ml and the Gleason score is <6.

Rx TREATMENT

NONPHARMACOLOGIC THERAPY
Localized prostate cancer management is summarized in Box 3. Active surveillance is reasonable in selected patients with early-stage (T_{1a}) and projected life expectancy <10 yr or in patients with focal and moderately differentiated carcinoma.

ACUTE GENERAL Rx
- Therapeutic approach varies with the following:
  1. Stage of the tumor
  2. Patient's life expectancy
  3. General medical condition
  4. Patient's treatment preference (e.g., patient may be opposed to orchiectomy)
- The optimal treatment of clinically localized prostate cancer is unclear. It is important to remember that all forms of treatment have potential adverse effects. Management requires careful consideration of the potential benefits and harms of intervention and the patient's age, health status, and individual preferences. A treatment algorithm for prostate cancer is described in Fig. 6. Table 3 summarizes recommended treatment based on risk group and life expectancy.
  1. Radical prostatectomy is generally performed in patients with localized prostate cancer and life expectancy >10 yr. Radical prostatectomy reduces disease-specific mortality, overall mortality, and the risks of metastasis and local progression. The absolute reduction in the risk of death after 10 yr is small, but the reductions in the risks of metastasis and local tumor progression are substantial. A 29-yr follow-up comparing radical prostatectomy with watchful waiting showed that men with clinically detected, localized prostate cancer and a long life expectancy benefited from radical prostatectomy with a mean 2.9 yr of life gained. A trial[6] comparing surgery with radiation therapy for high-risk localized prostate cancer showed that prostate cancer-specific mortality at 5 yr was significantly lower with surgery than with external beam radiation therapy (2.3% vs 4.1% PS 0.001). Postoperative complications of radical prostatectomy include urinary incontinence (10% to 20% depending on degree of neurovascular bundle and urethral preservation, patient age, and correct mucosal apposition) and erectile dysfunction (percentage >50% and varies with patient age, preoperative erectile dysfunction, stage of tumor at time of surgery, and preservation of neurovascular bundle). Lower complication rates occur in hospitals that perform a large number of prostatectomies. Fewer men will have postsurgical erectile dysfunction after unilateral or bilateral nerve-sparing surgery. In men undergoing prostatectomy, robotic-assisted laparoscopic surgery represents an alternative to open retropubic radical prostatectomy. Box 4 compares robotic surgery to open radical prostatectomy. Trials have shown that prostatectomy is preferred over active surveillance in patients with localized prostate cancer detected by PSA if the PSA level is >10 ng/ml. In this subgroup, the 10-yr mortality is 48.4% with prostatectomy versus 61.6% with active surveillance. In men who have low-risk disease (PSA level <10 mcg/L, stage <T_{2a}, Gleason score ≤3 + 3), and <6% risk for prostate cancer–specific death at 15 yr, active surveillance is a reasonable and underutilized option.
  2. Radiation therapy (external-beam irradiation or brachytherapy with implantation of radioactive pellets [iodine-125 or palladium-103 seeds] into the prostate

---

BOX 3   Localized Prostate Cancer Management

Active Surveillance
Includes
- Regular PSA assessment (3 to 6 monthly)
- Multiparametric MRI (1 to 3 yearly)
- Repeat biopsies (1 to 3 yearly) with treatment reserved for those patients who demonstrate disease progression
- *For low- or intermediate-risk localized prostate cancer*

Radical Prostatectomy (RP)
- Removal of prostate with adjoining seminal vesicles, with a vesicourethral anastomosis +/− pelvic lymph node dissection
- *For low-, intermediate-, or high-risk localized prostate cancer*

Radiotherapy
- Radical external beam radiotherapy
- Low-dose rate or high-dose brachytherapy
- *For low-, intermediate-, or high-risk localized prostate cancer*
- *Can be administered with or without neoadjuvant/adjuvant androgen deprivation therapy*

Androgen Receptor–Signaling Inhibitors (ARSIs) or Chemotherapy with Docetaxel
Can be considered in those with high-risk, localized prostate cancer

From Robertson RP et al: *DeGroot's endocrinology, basic science and clinical practice*, ed 8, Philadelphia, 2023, Elsevier.

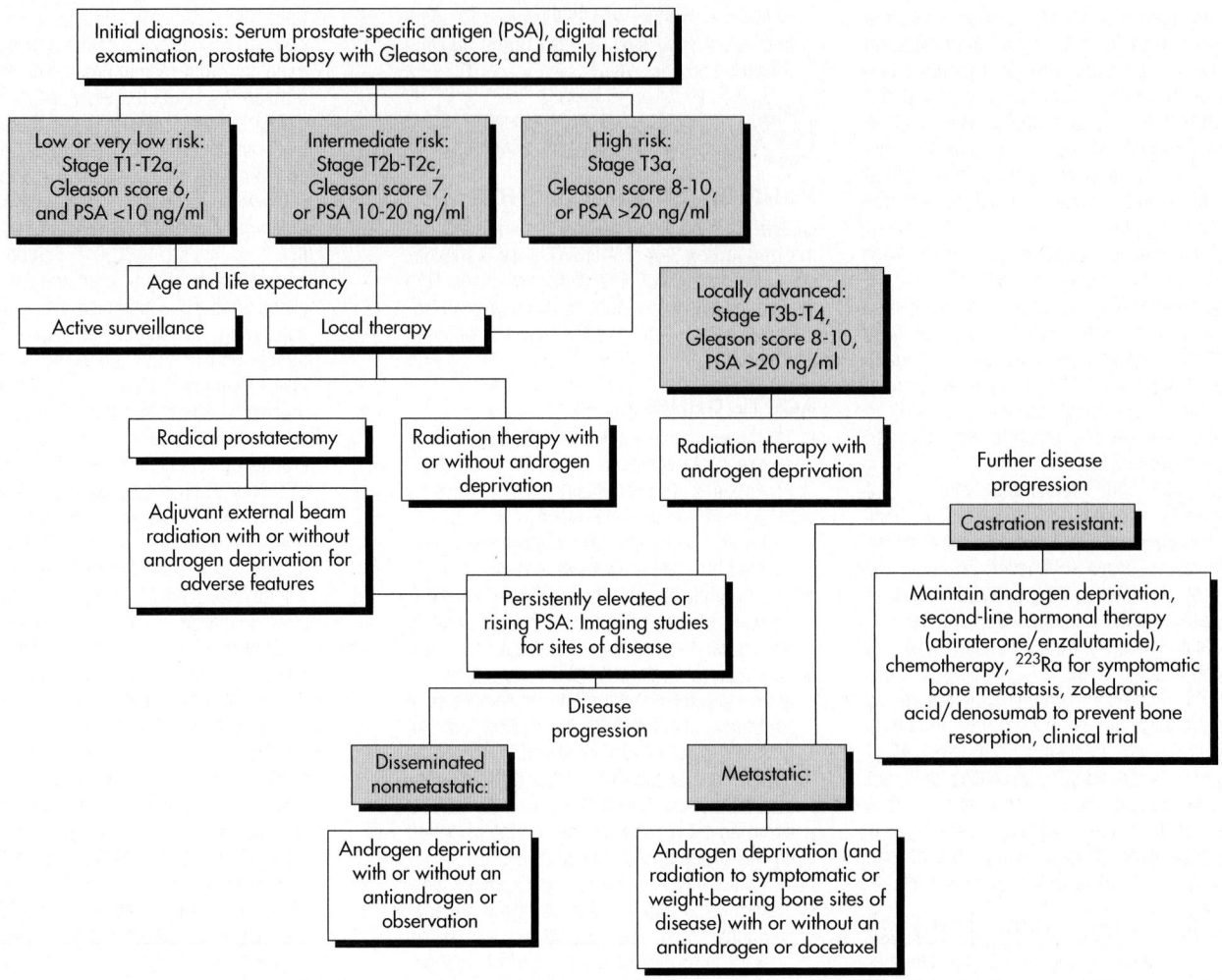

FIG. 6 Treatment algorithm. ^{223}Ra, Radium-223. (From Niederhuber JE: *Abeloff's clinical oncology,* ed 6, Philadelphia, 2020, Elsevier.)

TABLE 3 Recommended Treatment

Risk Group	Life Expectancy (Yr)	Recommended Treatment
Low	0-5	AS, HT
	5-10	AS, RT, HT, O
	>10	RP, RT, AS, O
Intermediate*	0-5	AS, HT, RT, O
	5-10	RT, HT, RP, O
	>10	RP, RT, O, HT
High*	0-5	AS, RT + HT, O
	5-10	RT + HT, HT, RP, O
	>10	RT + HT, RP + RT + HT, HT
Very high*	0-5	AS, RT + HT, O
	5-10	H, RT + HT, ST
	>10	RT + HT, RP + RT + HT, HT, ST, IT

AS, Active surveillance; *HT,* hormone therapy; *IT,* investigational multimodal therapy; *O,* others; *RP,* radical prostatectomy; *RT,* radiation therapy; *ST,* systemic therapy.
*If there is more than a 20% probability of positive lymph nodes, AS, HT, ST + HT.
From Wein AJ et al: *Campbell-Walsh urology,* ed 11, Philadelphia, 2016, Elsevier.

BOX 4 Robotic Surgery vs Open Radical Prostatectomy

Small but significant advantage of robotic over open surgery, with regard to erectile dysfunction (68 vs 74%).
No difference identified in:
- Incontinence
- Sexual dysfunction
- Positive surgical margins
- Oncological outcomes

From Robertson RP et al: *DeGroot's endocrinology, basic science and clinical practice,* ed 8, Philadelphia, 2023, Elsevier.

gland) represents an alternative in patients with localized prostate cancer, especially poor surgical candidates or patients with a high-grade malignancy. The efficacy of brachytherapy is comparable to external radiation and radical prostatectomy. In patients receiving external-beam radiation, a total dose of 79.2 Gy (high dose) compared with a total dose of 70.2 Gy (conventional dose) has been reported to lower the risk of recurrence without increased risk of morbidity and mortality. Newer radiation treatments such as intensity-modulated radiation therapy (IMRT) and proton therapy are becoming increasingly popular and replacing the older technique of conformal radiation therapy over the past 10 yr. Trials have shown that among patients with nonmetastatic prostate cancer, the use of

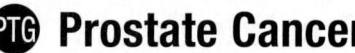

IMRT compared with conformal therapy is associated with less GI morbidity and fewer hip fractures but more erectile dysfunction; IMRT compared with proton therapy is associated with less GI morbidity. Patients with localized prostate cancer and high risk for extraprostatic disease and disease recurrence (e.g., Gleason score ≤ 7 with multiple positive biopsy cores and clinical stage T_{1b}-T_{2b}) may benefit (increased overall survival) with the addition of 6 mo of androgen suppression therapy to radiation therapy. High-intensity focused ultrasound (HIFU) is a newer treatment option for patients with prostate cancer. It ablates localized areas of the prostate with the goal of sparing patients the morbidity of whole-gland therapy. Longer-term studies comparing HIFU with standard therapy are needed. Hemigland cryoablation is another newer treatment modality for intermediate-risk prostate cancer. Longer studies are needed before drawing conclusions.

3. Active surveillance is reasonable in patients who are too old or too ill to survive longer than 10 yr. Conservative management is also reasonable for patients with Gleason score of 2 to 4 because these patients do not have a shortened life expectancy and treatment is associated with long-term side effects. Active surveillance also appears to be safe in older men with less-aggressive disease. Individual preferences play a central role in the decision whether to treat or to pursue active surveillance. If the cancer progresses to the point at which it becomes symptomatic, palliation can be attempted with several methods..

- Patients with advanced disease and projected life expectancy <10 yr are candidates for radiation therapy and hormonal therapy (diethylstilbestrol, luteinizing hormone–releasing hormone analogues, antiandrogens, bilateral orchiectomy). Box 5 summarizes advanced prostate cancer management.
- Recommended treatment of patients with regional metastatic prostate cancer with projected life expectancy ≥ 10 yr includes radiation therapy and hormonal therapy.
- Prostate cancer is an androgen receptor–dependent disease, and the blocking of androgen-receptor signaling is an effective treatment modality. Table E4 summarizes major circulating androgens. Androgen deprivation therapy (ADT) is the mainstay of treatment for metastatic prostate cancer. Adverse effects of ADT include decreased libido, impotence, hot flashes, osteopenia with increased fracture risk, metabolic alterations, and changes in mood and cognition. Adjuvant treatment with luteinizing hormone-releasing hormone (LHRH) agonists (goserelin, leuprolide, or triptorelin) plus antiandrogens (flutamide, bicalutamide, or nilutamide), when started simultaneously with external-beam radiation, improves local control and survival in patients with locally advanced prostate cancer. Pamidronate

inhibits osteoclast-mediated bone resorption and prevents bone loss in the hip and lumbar spine in men receiving treatment for prostate cancer. Gonadotropin-releasing hormone (GnRH) receptor antagonists can be used for rapid medical castration of men with advanced prostate cancer. Degarelix is an injectable GnRH agonist useful to suppress testosterone in patients with prostate cancer who are not good candidates for LHRH agonists and refuse surgical castration. Assessment of bone density and treatment with once-weekly oral alendronate can prevent and improve the bone loss that occurs in men receiving ADT for prostate cancer.

- Docetaxel plus prednisone or docetaxel plus estramustine can be used in metastatic hormone–refractory prostate cancer. Newer treatments for hormone–refractory prostate cancer (castration-resistant cancer) include immunotherapy with sipuleucel and cabazitaxel, a microtubule inhibitor that interferes with cell mitosis and replication. Both agents can prolong survival but adverse effects can be severe, and both agents are very expensive. Abiraterone is an oral agent that blocks biosynthesis of androgens by inhibiting CYP17, an enzyme required for androgen biosynthesis. It has been FDA approved for oral treatment, in combination with prednisone, of metastatic castration-resistant prostate cancer in patients previously treated with docetaxel. Darolutamide is an androgen-receptor inhibitor approved for the treatment of nonmetastatic castration-resistant prostate cancer. The addition of darolutamide to androgen-deprivation therapy and docetaxel has also been shown to prolong survival in patients with metastatic, hormone-sensitive prostate cancer.[7]
- Enzalutamide is a newer nonsteroidal antiandrogen. Trials have shown it to be highly effective in extending survival in patients with metastatic castration-resistant prostate cancer. It can be used sequentially with other agents such as docetaxel, abiraterone, cabazitaxel, and immunotherapy.

- Radium-223, an alpha emitter, selectively targets bone metastases and has been found effective in improving survival in men with castration-resistant prostate cancer and bone metastases.
- The polyadenosine diphosphate [ADP]-ribose) polymerase (PARP) inhibitor olaparib has shown a high response rate in trials in patients whose prostate cancers were no longer responding to standard treatments with enzalutamide or abiraterone and who had defects in DNA-repair genes.

CHRONIC Rx

- Patients should be monitored at 3- to 6-mo intervals with clinical examination and PSA for the first year, then every 6 mo for the second year, then yearly if stable. For patients who have undergone radical prostatectomy, a rising PSA level suggests evidence of residual or recurrent prostate cancer. A recent study revealed that if the PSA level remains undetectable 3 to 5 yr after radical prostatectomy, the probability of biochemical recurrence is extremely low, and it is reasonable to stop PSA monitoring. Salvage radiotherapy may potentially cure patients with disease recurrence after radical prostatectomy. Recent trials have shown that addition of 24 mo of antiandrogen therapy with daily bicalutamide to salvage radiation therapy results in significantly higher rates of long-term overall survival and lower incidences of metastatic prostate cancer and death from prostate cancer than radiation therapy plus placebo.
- Chest radiography and bone scan should be performed yearly or sooner if patient develops symptoms.

DISPOSITION

- Prognosis varies with the stage of the disease and the Gleason classification (see "Definition"). For patients between ages 65 and 69 yr at diagnosis and a Gleason score of 2 to 4, the probability of dying from prostate cancer 15 yr after diagnosis is 0.06 and that of dying from other causes is 0.56. If the Gleason

---

BOX 5 Advanced Prostate Cancer Management

Androgen Deprivation Therapy
- Gonadotropin-releasing hormone (GnRH) agonists (goserelin, leuprorelin, diphereline)
- GnRH antagonists are also available (degarelix, relugolix)
- *Most men initially respond to ADT, but inevitably, patients develop castration-resistant prostate cancer (CRPC).*

Androgen Receptor–Signaling Inhibitors (ARSIs)
- Abiraterone, enzalutamide, apalutamide, and darolutamide
- *Improve survival in men with CRPC and recently shown to improve survival in high-risk, castrate sensitive prostate cancer (CSPC)*

Chemotherapy
Taxane chemotherapy
Docetaxel—*Improves overall survival* in CRPC and CSPC
Cabazitaxel—*Used subsequent to docetaxel and ARSIs*
Personalized therapy
Treatment based upon genomic abnormalities within a particular tumor
Poly-ADP ribose polymerase (PARP) inhibitors—*Olaparib*
AKT-signaling inhibitors—*Ipatasertib*

From Robertson RP et al: *DeGroot's endocrinology, basic science and clinical practice*, ed 8, Philadelphia, 2023, Elsevier.

Diseases and Disorders

P

I

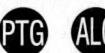

score is 7 to 10, the probability of dying from prostate cancer increases to 0.72 and from other causes varies from 0.25 to 0.36.

- The ploidy of the tumor also has prognostic value; prognosis is better with diploid tumor cells and worse with aneuploid tumor cells.
- For grade 1 tumors, the extended 10-yr, disease-specific survival is similar for patients with prostatectomy (94%), radiotherapy (90%), and conservative management (93%); survival rate is better with surgery than with radiotherapy or conservative management in patients with grade 2 or 3 localized prostate cancer.
- Expression of the gene *EZH2* has been identified as an important factor in the determination of the aggressiveness of prostate cancer. A recent study revealed that expression of the *EZH2* gene may be a better predictor of clinical failure than Gleason score, tumor stage, or surgical margin status. Testing for *EZH2* protein in prostate cancer tissue may be useful to determine prognosis and direct treatment.
- Preoperative PSA level and PSA velocity have prognostic significance. Men whose PSA level increases by >2.0 mcg/ml during the year before the diagnosis of cancer may have a relatively high risk of death from

prostate cancer despite undergoing radical prostatectomy.

- Extraprostatic disease is detected at radical prostatectomy in 38% to 52% of patients and is associated with a risk of disease recurrence, progression, and death. In these patients, adjuvant radiotherapy results in significantly reduced risk of PSA relapse and disease recurrence; however, the improvements in metastases-free survival and overall survival are not statistically significant. Table 5 summarizes common pain syndromes in metastatic castration-resistant prostate cancer.
- The Prostate Cancer Prevention trial revealed that the use of 5-alpha-reductase inhibitors lowers the incidence of prostate cancer but also increases the incidence of high-grade tumors (Gleason score >7). It is possible that these agents delay diagnosis of prostate cancer by lowering PSA levels and decreasing prostate size. The trade-off inherent in using 5-alpha-reductase inhibitors for prostate cancer prevention is risk of one additional high-grade cancer in order to avert three or four lower-grade cancers. Based on these results, the FDA's Oncologic Drugs Advisory Committee concluded that finasteride

and dutasteride do not have a favorable risk-benefit profile for chemoprevention of prostate cancer in healthy men.

- Patients undergoing prostatectomy are more likely to have urinary incontinence than those undergoing radiotherapy at 2 yr and 5 yr. However, at 15 yr there are no significant relative differences in disease-specific functional outcomes among men undergoing prostatectomy or radiotherapy.
- Bone health is a significant concern in men with prostate cancer. Trials involving bisphosphonates and denosumab reveal that both improve bone mineral density (BMD) in men with nonmetastatic prostate cancer receiving androgen deprivation therapy. Denosumab has also been shown to reduce the risk of vertebral fractures.

REFERENCES

Available at eBooks.Health.Elsevier.com.

RELATED CONTENT

Prostate Cancer (Patient Information)

AUTHOR: **FRED F. FERRI, MD**

TABLE 5 Common Pain Syndromes in Metastatic Castration-Resistant Prostate Cancer

Pain Syndrome	Initial Management	Other Therapeutic Alternatives
Localized bone pain	Pharmacologic pain management	Surgical stabilization of pathologic fractures or extensive bone erosions
	Localized radiotherapy (special attention to weight-bearing areas, lytic metastasis, and extremities)	Epidural metastasis and cord compression should be evaluated in all patients with focal back pain
		Radiopharmaceuticals should be considered if local radiation therapy fails
Diffuse bone pain	Pharmacologic pain management	Corticosteroids
	"Multispot" or wide-field radiotherapy	Bisphosphonates or RANK ligand inhibitors
	Radiopharmaceuticals	Calcitonin
		Chemotherapy
Epidural metastasis and cord compression	High-dose corticosteroids	Pharmacologic pain management
	Radiation therapy	Physical therapy for recovery of neurologic function
	Surgical decompression and stabilization are indicated in high-grade epidural compressions, extensive bone involvement, or recurrence after irradiation	
Nerve plexopathies caused by direct tumor extension or previous therapy (rare)	Pharmacologic pain management	Tricyclic antidepressants (amitriptyline)
	Radiation therapy (if not previously used)	Anticonvulsants (gabapentin, pregabalin)
	Neurolytic procedures (nerve blocks)	
Miscellaneous neurogenic causes: Postherpetic neuralgia, peripheral neuropathies	Complete neurologic evaluation	Tricyclic antidepressants (amitriptyline)
	Pharmacologic pain management	Anticonvulsants (gabapentin, pregabalin)
	Discontinuation of neurotoxic drugs: Docetaxel, platinum compounds	
Other uncommon pain syndromes: Extensive skull metastasis with cranial nerve/skull base involvement, extensive painful liver metastasis, or pelvic masses	Radiation therapy	Chemotherapy
	Pharmacologic pain management	Intrathecal chemotherapy may ameliorate symptoms of meningeal involvement
	Corticosteroids (cranial nerve involvement)	

From Wein AJ et al: *Campbell-Walsh urology*, ed 11, Philadelphia, 2016, Elsevier.
RANK, Receptor activator of nuclear factor-κB.

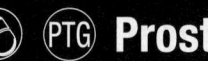

 BASIC INFORMATION

DEFINITION

Prostatitis refers to inflammation of the prostate gland. There are four major categories (Table 1):
- Acute bacterial prostatitis (type I)
- Chronic bacterial prostatitis (type II)
- Chronic prostatitis/pelvic pain syndrome (CP/CPPS) (type III): Subdivided into type IIIA (inflammatory) and IIIB (noninflammatory)
- Asymptomatic inflammatory prostatitis (type IV)

ICD-10CM CODES
N41.0   Acute prostatitis
N41.1   Chronic prostatitis

EPIDEMIOLOGY & DEMOGRAPHICS

- 50% of men will have symptoms of prostatitis in their lifetime.
- Prostatitis accounts for >8% of visits to urologists and 1% of visits to primary care physicians.
- The prevalence of chronic bacterial prostatitis is 5% to 10%.
- CP/CPPS is the most common of the clinically defined prostatitis syndromes, with prevalence ranging from 9% to 12% of men.
- Acute bacterial prostatitis accounts for 10% of all cases of prostatitis.

PHYSICAL FINDINGS & CLINICAL PRESENTATION

- Acute bacterial prostatitis:
  1. Sudden or rapidly progressive onset of:
     a. Dysuria
     b. Frequency
     c. Urgency
     d. Nocturia
     e. Perineal pain that may radiate to the back, rectum, or penis
  2. Hematuria or a purulent urethral discharge may occur.
  3. Occasionally urinary retention complicates the course.
  4. Fever, chills, and signs of sepsis can also be part of the clinical picture.
  5. On rectal examination the prostate is typically tender.
- Chronic bacterial prostatitis:
  1. Characterized by positive culture of expressed prostatic secretions. May cause symptoms such as suprapubic, low back, or perineal pain; mild urgency, frequency, and dysuria with urination; and possibly recurrent urinary tract infections.
  2. May be asymptomatic when the infection is confined to the prostate.
  3. May present as an increase in severity of baseline symptoms of benign prostatic hypertrophy (BPH).
  4. When cystitis is also present, urinary frequency, urgency, and burning may be reported.
  5. Hematuria may be a presenting complaint.

6. In elderly men, new onset of urinary incontinence may be noted.
- CP/CPPS:
  1. Presents similarly with pain in the pelvic region lasting >3 mo. Symptoms also can include pain in the suprapubic region, low back, penis, testes, or scrotum.
  2. The symptoms can be of variable severity and may include lower urinary tract symptoms, sexual dysfunction, and reduced quality of life.

ETIOLOGY

- Acute bacterial prostatitis:
  1. Acute, usually gram-negative infection of the prostate gland. *Escherichia coli* is the most commonly isolated organism.
  2. Generally associated with cystitis.
  3. Results from the ascent of bacteria into the urethra.
  4. Occasionally the route of infection is hematogenous or a lymphatogenous spread of rectal bacteria.
  5. Consider *Neisseria gonorrhoeae* or *Chlamydia trachomatis* in young patients (age <35 yr) with risk of sexually transmitted disease (STD).
- Chronic bacterial prostatitis:
  1. Often asymptomatic. *E. coli* is the most commonly isolated organism.
  2. Exacerbation of symptoms of BPH caused by the same mechanism as in acute bacterial prostatitis.
- CP/CPPS:
  1. Type IIIA: Refers to symptoms of prostatic inflammation associated with the presence of white blood cells in prostatic secretions with no identifiable bacterial organism.
  2. *Chlamydia* infection may be etiologically implicated in some cases.
  3. Type IIIB: Refers to symptoms of prostatic inflammation with no or few white blood cells in the prostatic secretion. Its cause is multifactorial (Fig. 1).

DX DIAGNOSIS

DIFFERENTIAL DIAGNOSIS

- BPH with lower urinary tract symptoms
- Prostate cancer
- Interstitial cystitis/bladder pain syndrome
- Pelvic floor dysfunction
- Bladder cancer
- Urolithiasis
- Urinary tract infection
- Proctitis

WORKUP

- Rectal examination:
  1. Tender prostate most suggestive of acute bacterial prostatitis
  2. Enlarged prostate common in chronic bacterial prostatitis
  3. Normal prostate is consistent with chronic bacterial prostatitis and CP/CPPS
- Expression of prostatic secretions by prostate massage is contraindicated in acute bacterial prostatitis but is appropriate in the other three situations.

LABORATORY TESTS

- Urinalysis
- Urine culture and sensitivity
- Bacterial localization studies can be performed but are cumbersome and impractical in most clinical settings
- Cell count and culture of expressed prostatic secretions
- Prostate-specific antigen (PSA) is not used to diagnose prostatitis and is not recommended unless a nodule is present on digital examination. A rapid rise over baseline should raise the possibility of prostatitis even in the absence of symptoms. In such cases, a follow-up PSA after treatment of prostatitis is appropriate
- CBC and blood cultures if fever, chills, or signs of sepsis exist

TABLE 1   Classification System for the Prostatitis Syndromes

Traditional	National Institutes of Health	Description
Acute bacterial prostatitis	Category I	Acute infection of the prostate gland
Chronic bacterial prostatitis	Category II	Chronic infection of the prostate gland
N/A	Category III Chronic pelvic pain syndrome (CPPS)	Chronic genitourinary pain in the absence of uropathogenic bacteria localized to the prostate gland employing standard methodology
Nonbacterial prostatitis	Category IIIA Inflammatory CPPS	Significant number of white blood cells in expressed prostatic secretions, postprostatic massage urine sediment (VB3), or semen
Prostatodynia	Category IIIB Noninflammatory CPPS	Insignificant number of white blood cells in expressed prostatic secretions, postprostatic massage urine sediment (VB3), or semen
N/A	Category IV Asymptomatic inflammatory prostatitis (AIP)	White blood cells (and/or bacteria) in expressed prostatic secretions, postprostatic massage urine sediment (VB3), semen, or histologic specimens of prostate gland

From Wein AJ et al: *Campbell-Walsh urology*, ed 11, Philadelphia, 2016, Elsevier.

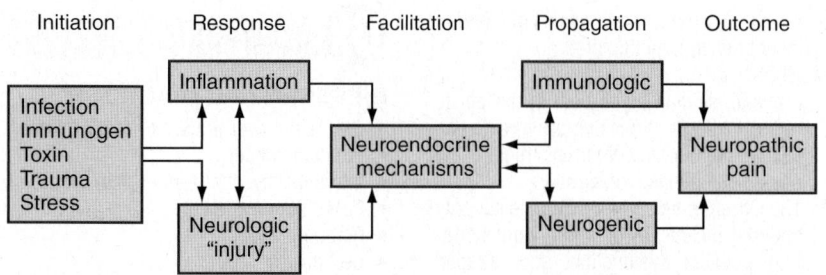

FIG. 1 The cause and pathogenesis of chronic prostatitis/chronic pelvic pain syndrome (category III chronic pelvic pain syndrome) appear to involve a pluricausal, multifactorial mechanism. An initiating stimulus, such as infection, reflux of some toxic or immunogenic urine substance, or perineal or pelvic trauma, starts a cascade of events in an anatomically or genetically susceptible man, resulting in a local response of inflammation or neurogenic injury or both. Further interrelated immunologic, neuropathic, endocrinologic, and psychologic mechanisms propagate or sustain the chronicity of the initial (or ongoing) event. The final outcome is the clinical manifestation of chronic perineal or pelvic pain and associated symptoms with local and central neuropathic mechanisms involving areas outside the prostate or pelvic area. (From Wein AJ et al: *Campbell-Walsh urology*, ed 11, Philadelphia, 2016, Elsevier.)

BOX 1 Suggested Therapies for Chronic Prostatitis and Chronic Pelvic Pain Syndrome (National Institutes of Health Category III)

Recommended
1. α-Blocker therapy as part of a multimodal treatment strategy for newly diagnosed, α-blocker–naive patients who have voiding symptoms
2. Antimicrobial therapy trial for selected newly diagnosed, antimicrobial-naive patients
3. Selected phytotherapies: Cernilton and quercetin
4. Multimodal therapy directed by clinical phenotype
5. Directed physiotherapy. Although level 1 evidence is not available, evidence from multiple weak trials and vast clinical experience strongly suggests benefit for selected patients

Not Recommended
1. α-Blocker monotherapy, particularly in patients previously treated with α-blockers
2. Antiinflammatory monotherapy
3. Antimicrobial therapy as primary therapy, particularly for patients in whom treatment with antibiotics has previously failed
4. 5α-Reductase inhibitor monotherapy; can be considered in older patients with coexisting benign prostatic hyperplasia
5. Most minimally invasive therapies such as transurethral needle ablation (TUNA), laser therapies
6. Invasive surgical therapies such as transurethral resection of the prostate (TURP) and radical prostatectomy

Requiring Further Evaluation
1. Low-intensity shock wave treatment
2. Acupuncture
3. Biofeedback
4. Invasive neuromodulation (e.g., pudendal nerve modulation)
5. Electromagnetic stimulation
6. Botulinum toxin A injection
7. Medical therapies including mepartricin, muscle relaxants, neuromodulators, and immunomodulators

Modified from Nickel JC et al: Male chronic pelvic pain syndrome (CPPS). In Chapple C, Abrams P (eds): *Male lower urinary tract symptoms (LUTS): an international consultation on male LUTS, Fukuoka, Japan, Sept 30-Oct 4, 2012,* Montreal, 2013, Société Internationale d'Urologie. From Wein AJ et al: *Campbell-Walsh urology*, ed 11, Philadelphia, 2016, Elsevier.

(Rx) TREATMENT

- Acute bacterial prostatitis:
  1. Uncomplicated (with risk of STD, age <35 yr): Ceftriaxone 250 mg intramuscular (IM) × 1 dose *or* cefixime 400 mg PO × 1, *then* doxycycline 100 mg bid × 10 days
  2. Uncomplicated with low risk of STD: Levofloxacin 500 mg qid or ciprofloxacin 500 mg bid × 10 to 14 days
- Chronic bacterial prostatitis:
  1. First-line choice is a quinolone (ciprofloxacin or levofloxacin) for 4 wk.
  2. Trimethoprim-sulfamethoxazole (TMP-SMX) is second-line choice for 1 to 3 mo if the organism is sensitive. Tissue penetration for TMP-SMX is not as good as quinolones, and there is evidence of increasing uropathogenic resistance.
- CP/CPPS:
  1. Suggested therapies for CP/CPPS are summarized in Box 1.

RELATED CONTENT

Prostatitis (Patient Information)

AUTHOR: **FRED F. FERRI, MD**

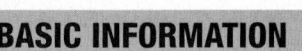

BASIC INFORMATION

DEFINITION

Psoriasis is a chronic skin disorder characterized by excessive proliferation of keratinocytes, resulting in the formation of thickened scaly plaques, itching, and inflammatory changes of the epidermis and dermis. Psoriasis is also associated with cardiovascular, metabolic, and neuropsychiatric effects. The various forms of psoriasis include plaque (most common), guttate, erythrodermic, pustular, inverse, and arthritis variants.

ICD-10CM CODES
L40	Psoriasis
L40.0	Psoriasis vulgaris
L40.1	Generalized pustular psoriasis
L40.4	Guttate psoriasis
L40.8	Other psoriasis
L40.9	Psoriasis unspecified
L40.54	Psoriatic juvenile arthropathy

EPIDEMIOLOGY & DEMOGRAPHICS

- Psoriasis affects 2% to 4% of the world's population. Most patients have limited psoriasis involving <5% of their body surface.
- There is a strong association between psoriasis and human leukocyte antigens (HLAs) B13, B17, and B27 (pustular psoriasis).
- Peak age of onset is bimodal (age 30 to 39 yr and at age 60 yr). Mean age at diagnosis is 34 yr.
- Men and women are affected equally. Approximately 20% of patients with psoriasis also have psoriatic arthritis. Median time from development of joint symptoms to diagnosis of psoriatic arthritis is 5 yr. Nail psoriasis affects over 50% of patients with psoriasis and can occur with any of the subtypes.

PHYSICAL FINDINGS & CLINICAL PRESENTATION

- Approximately 67% of patients with psoriasis have mild-to-moderate disease.
- The primary psoriatic lesion is an erythematous papule topped by a loosely adherent scale. Scraping the scale results in several bleeding points *(Auspitz sign)*.
- Chronic plaque psoriasis generally manifests with symmetric, sharply demarcated, erythematous, silver-scaled patches affecting primarily the intergluteal folds, elbows, scalp, fingernails, toenails, and knees (Figs. 1 and 2). This form accounts for 80% of psoriasis cases. Psoriasis may also involve the forehead, particularly contiguous to the scalp (Fig. E3).
- Psoriasis can also develop at the site of any physical trauma (sunburn, scratching). This is known as *Koebner phenomenon.*
- Nail involvement is common (pitting of the nail plate), resulting in hyperkeratosis, onychodystrophy with onycholysis (Fig. E4).
- Pruritus is variable; soreness and bleeding may occur.
- Joint involvement can result in sacroiliitis and spondylitis.

- Guttate psoriasis is generally preceded by streptococcal pharyngitis and manifests with multiple droplike lesions on the extremities and the trunk.
- Erythrodermic psoriasis is characterized by widespread cutaneous erythema and scaling.
- Pustular psoriasis manifests with widespread pustules. Localized forms may affect palms and soles.
- Inverse psoriasis is characterized by red and sharply demarcated thinner patches involving intertriginous areas (axillae, inguinal areas).
- Adverse effect on psychological and social functioning, with affected persons often feeling stigmatized.

ETIOLOGY

- Unknown, but there is a strong genetic component and high heritability. There are at least nine chromosomal loci with linkage to psoriasis. These loci are called psoriasis susceptibility 1 through 9 (PSORS1-PSORS9). PSORS1 locus in the major histocompatibility complex (MHC) region on chromosome 6 is considered the most important susceptibility locus and is believed to account for 35% to 50% of the heritability of the disease.
- Familial clustering (genetic transmission with a dominant mode with variable penetrants).
- One third of persons affected have a positive family history.
- A high prevalence of celiac disease has been noted in patients with psoriasis.

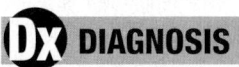

DIAGNOSIS

DIFFERENTIAL DIAGNOSIS
- Contact dermatitis
- Atopic dermatitis
- Stasis dermatitis
- Tinea
- Nummular dermatitis
- Candidiasis
- Mycosis fungoides, Sezary syndrome
- Cutaneous systemic lupus erythematosus
- Secondary and tertiary syphilis
- Drug eruption

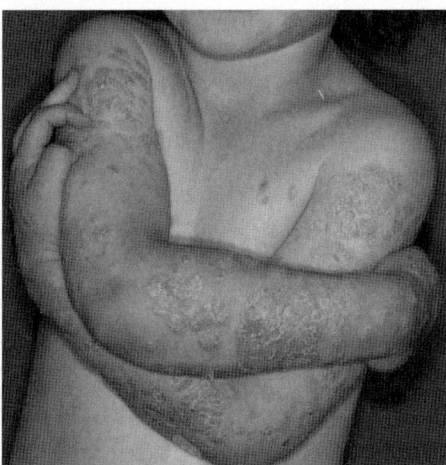

FIG. 1 Psoriasis. Variably sized erythematous plaques with moderately thick overlying scale. (From Paller AS, Mancini AJ: *Hurwitz clinical pediatric dermatology: a textbook of skin disorders of childhood and adolescence,* ed 5, Philadelphia, 2016, Elsevier.)

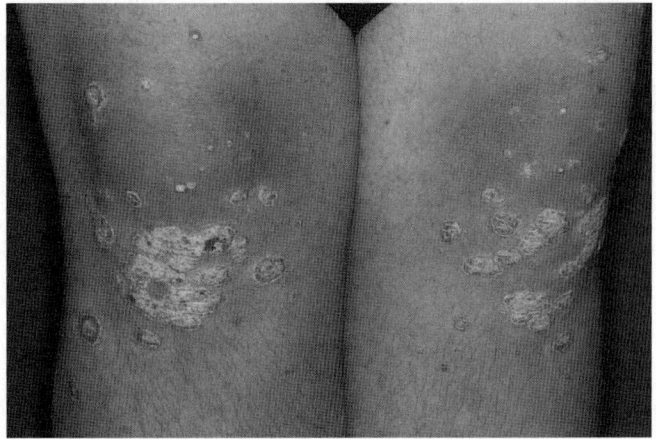

FIG. 2 Typical plaques of psoriasis with thick, micaceous scale overlying erythema. (From Paller AS, Mancini AJ: *Hurwitz clinical pediatric dermatology: a textbook of skin disorders of childhood and adolescence,* ed 5, Philadelphia, 2016, Elsevier.)

- Dermatomyositis (DM)
- Lupus erythematosus (LE)
- Seborrheic dermatitis
- Pityriasis rosea
- Lichen planus
- Pityriasis rubra pilaris

WORKUP

- Diagnosis is clinical. Blood work is rarely needed. A rapid plasma reagin test is useful when ruling out syphilis. Antinuclear antibody (ANA) and anti-Ro and anti-La antibodies are helpful in ruling out subacute cutaneous lupus.
- Skin biopsy is rarely necessary.

LABORATORY TESTS

Generally not necessary for diagnosis.

- Skin biopsy (only if the clinical diagnosis of psoriasis is uncertain)
- Serum electrolytes and calcium for patients with generalized pustular psoriasis (GPP)
- Antistreptolysin O or bacterial cultures for patients with guttate psoriasis
- Appropriate drug-related monitoring for patients on systemic therapies including annual tuberculosis testing except for acitretin and apremilast

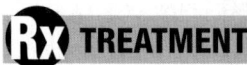 **TREATMENT**

NONPHARMACOLOGIC THERAPY

- Sunbathing generally leads to improvement.
- Eliminate triggering factors (e.g., stress, certain medications [e.g., lithium, β-blockers, antimalarials]). Severe emotional stress tends to aggravate psoriasis.
- Patients with psoriasis benefit from a daily bath in warm water followed by application of a cream or ointment moisturizer. Regular use of an emollient moisturizer limits evaporation of water from the skin and allows the stratum corneum to rehydrate itself.
- Psoralen and ultraviolet A (PUVA) therapy (see "General Rx").
- Local hyperthermia has been used successfully to clear psoriatic plaques, but relapse is common.
- Occlusive treatment with surgical tape or dressings is effective as monotherapy or in combination with topical medications.
- Avoidance of tobacco. Smoking tobacco may worsen psoriasis.

GENERAL Rx

Therapeutic options vary according to the extent of disease and comorbidities. Topical therapies remain the cornerstone for treating mild psoriasis. Approximately 70% to 80% of all patients can be treated adequately with topical therapy.

- Patients with limited disease (<20% of the body) can be treated with the following:
  1. Topical steroids: Disadvantages are brief remissions, expense, and decreased effect with continued use. Salicylic acid can be compounded by pharmacist in concentrations of 2% to 10% and used in combination with a corticosteroid to decrease the amount of scale.

2. Calcipotriene: A vitamin D analogue effective for moderate plaque psoriasis. Adults should comb the hair, apply solution to the lesions, and rub it in, avoiding uninvolved skin. Disadvantages include its cost and potential burning and skin irritation. It should not be used concurrently with salicylic acid because calcipotriene is inactivated by the acidic nature of salicylic acid. Taclonex ointment and Enstilar aerosol foam formulation are a combination of calcipotriene and the high-potency corticosteroid betamethasone dipropionate. They are well tolerated and more effective than either agent used alone but also much more expensive.
3. Tar products (Estar, liquor carbonis detergens [LCD], Psorigel) can be used overnight and are most effective when combined with ultraviolet B (UVB) light (Goeckerman regimen).
4. Anthralin: Useful for chronic plaques; can result in purple-brown staining; best used with UVB light.
5. Retinoids, such as tazarotene 0.05%, 0.1% cream or gel, are effective in thinning plaques but are expensive and can cause skin irritation.
6. Other useful measures include tape or occlusive dressing, UVB and lubricating agents, and interlesional steroids.

- Therapeutic options for persons with generalized disease (affecting >20% of the body) and for those with inadequate response to topical agents:
  1. UVB light exposure three times a wk: This therapy does not require administration of a systemic drug (unlike psoralen plus ultraviolet A [PUVA]), but to be effective, it requires removal of scale with keratolytic agents and emollients.
  2. Oral PUVA administered two to three times weekly is effective for generalized disease. It is often considered in patients for whom narrow-band UVB therapy is ineffective. However, many PUVA treatments are required, necessitating frequent office visits, and it may be associated with phototoxicity, such as erythema and blistering, and increased risk of skin cancer.
- Systemic treatments include methotrexate 25 mg/wk for severe psoriasis. Etretinate (a synthetic retinoid) is most effective for palmar-plantar pustular psoriasis. Dose is 0.5 to 1 mg/kg/day. It can cause liver enzyme and lipid abnormalities and is teratogenic.
- Apremilast is a phosphodiesterase type-4 inhibitor used in moderate to severe plaque psoriasis. Side effects include diarrhea, nausea, headache, and worsening depression. Cost and formulary are limiting factors.
- Cyclosporine is also effective in severe psoriasis; however, relapses are common.
- Chronic plaque psoriasis may be treated with alefacept, a recombinant protein that selectively targets T lymphocytes. Treatment with alefacept for 12 wk (0.025, 0.075, or 0.150 mg/kg of body weight intravenous [IV] weekly) may result in significant improvement. Some

patients also demonstrate a sustained clinical response after the cessation of treatment. Cost and formulary are limiting factors.

- Tapinarof (Vtama), 1% cream formulation, has been FDA approved for treatment of adults with plaque psoriasis.
- Biologic therapies are now routinely used when traditional systemic agents are ineffective or poorly tolerated. Screening for tuberculosis is necessary before initiating treatment with these agents. Active, serious infection is a contraindication to the use of biologics.
- Tumor necrosis factor (TNF) inhibitors (adalimumab [Humira], etanercept [Enbrel], infliximab [Remicade]) are effective in reducing severity of plaque psoriasis. Efalizumab, a humanized monoclonal antibody that inhibits the activation of T cells, has also been reported to produce significant improvement in plaque psoriasis treatment period.
- Newer biologic agents in patients with moderate to severe plaque psoriasis are ustekinumab (Stelara; an interleukin-12 and interleukin-23 blocker); brodalumab (SILIQ); ixekizumab (Taltz); secukinumab (Cosentyx) antiinterleukin-17 receptor antagonists; and guselkumab (Tremfya), risankizumab (Skyrizi), and tildrakizumab (ILUMYA) interleukin-23 blockers. The injectable interleukin (IL)-17A/17F antagonist bimekizumab-BKZX is now FDA approved for moderate to severe plaque psoriasis. Cost and formulary are limiting factors with all these agents.
- The topical PDE4 inhibitor roflumilast has been approved for plaque psoriasis.
- Deucravacitinib, an oral tyrosine kinase 2 (TYK2), is FDA approved for moderate to severe plaque psoriasis.
- The multiple newer agents offer nonsteroidal options for treatment of psoriasis, but older, less expensive drugs should be tried first.

DISPOSITION

The course of psoriasis is chronic, and the disease may be refractory to treatment.

REFERRAL

- Dermatology referral is recommended in all patients with generalized disease.
- Hospital admission may be necessary for severe diffuse or poorly responsive psoriasis. The Goeckerman regimen combines daily application of tar with UVB exposure and can result in prolonged remissions.

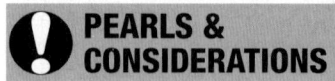 **PEARLS & CONSIDERATIONS**

COMMENTS

Psoriasis is more emotionally than physically disabling for most patients. Counseling may be indicated, particularly when it affects younger patients.

RELATED CONTENT

Psoriasis (Patient Information)
Psoriatic Arthritis (Related Key Topic)

AUTHOR: **FRED F. FERRI, MD**

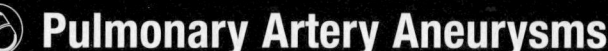

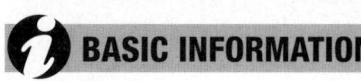 **BASIC INFORMATION**

DEFINITION

Pulmonary artery (PA) aneurysms (PAAs) are a rare diagnosis.[1] PAA is defined as focal dilation of PA including all three layers, that is, tunica intima, media, and adventitia. Several studies have different cutoff values of upper limit of normal for PA diameter, ranging from 29 to 40 mm.[2,3]

SYNONYM

Pulmonary artery dilation

ICD 10-CM CODE
I28.1   Aneurysm of pulmonary artery

EPIDEMIOLOGY & DEMOGRAPHICS

Approximately 50% of PAAs have been reported in the congenital heart disease (CHD) population. There is an equal gender distribution.
INCIDENCE: PAA is an extremely rare abnormality with an incidence of approximately 1 in 14,000 based on an autopsy study conducted by the Mayo Clinic.[1] During the index study, out of 109,571 autopsies, 8 were found to have PAAs.
PREDOMINANT SEX & AGE: There is an equal gender distribution in reported cases.[1]
RISK FACTORS: CHD remains the most prevalent risk factor in this population. More than 50% of known cases of PAAs had concomitant CHD, including persistent ductus arteriosus, ventricular septal defect (VSD), atrial septal defect (ASD), and bicuspid aortic valve, in decreasing order.[4,5] Infectious causes such as untreated tuberculosis[6] and syphilis and vasculitis remain other prominent risk factors. Iatrogenic pseudoaneurysms were reported in several cases due to trauma from Swan-Ganz catheter.
GENETICS: PAAs are a topic of great interest because they are a complex genetic mechanism involving connective tissue disease. Fig. 1 describes the relationship of increased extracellular matrix and increased cell proliferation in PAA formation.

PHYSICAL FINDINGS & CLINICAL PRESENTATION

Clinical presentation ranges from asymptomatic patients to debilitating dyspnea, hoarseness of voice, chest pain, and syncopal episodes. Compression of bronchus by large PAA has been reported with cough, increasing dyspnea, pneumonia, and bronchiectasis. Exertional chest pain can be a rare presentation of PAA due to compression of left main coronary artery. Hemoptysis, when present, can be worrisome for impending rupture.[7] On physical exam, S1 may be combined with a diastolic murmur.

ETIOLOGY

Focal dilation secondary to increased pressure in PA remains the key mechanism for PAAs due to CHD.

In acquired cases, tissue inflammation and destruction due to vasculitis or untreated tuberculosis and syphilis causes dilation of the PA. Trauma from procedures such as Swan-Ganz catheterization resulted in 10 out of 18 reported cases of postprocedure pseudoaneurysm formation.

DX **DIAGNOSIS**

DIFFERENTIAL DIAGNOSIS

Differential diagnoses of PAAs include pulmonary arterial hypertension (PAH), pulmonary hypertension (PH), pulmonary venous hypertension, heart failure with preserved ejection fraction, and coronary artery disease.

LABORATORY TESTS

Lab tests are nonspecific for PAAs.

IMAGING STUDIES

- ECG can show right heart strain pattern.
- Chest x-ray usually reveals hilar lymphadenopathy or dilation.
- Echocardiography with Doppler technique can provide a noninvasive assessment of right ventricular function, estimated PA pressures, and congenital abnormalities, particularly patent ductus arteriosus (PDA), VSDs, ASDs, pulmonary valve regurgitation, stenosis or absence, and bicuspid aortic valve.
- Computed tomography (CT) chest with contrast can accurately assess diameter of the PA, as well as screening for congenital abnormalities. Bronchoscopy can be done to evaluate for the compression of the bronchus and for anatomic assessment of hemoptysis. A PA angiogram is the most sensitive and specific test to evaluate for PAA and its treatment with coil embolization if needed. One of the major limitations of pulmonary angiogram is its inability to show surrounding structures. Therefore CT scan remains an essential tool in procedural planning as well as assessment of PAAs. MRI can be utilized alternatively in patients where a CT scan with contrast is contraindicated.

Rx **TREATMENT**

Due to rarity of PAAs, there are no guidelines for the treatment of PAAs.

NONPHARMACOLOGIC THERAPY

Surgical or interventional treatment is recommended by experts for symptomatic large PAAs (>5.5 cm in diameter)[8] with impending rupture, increase of 0.5 cm in 6 mo, compression of adjacent structures, thrombus formation, or for valvular pathologies and shunt flow. Aneurysmectomy and repair or replacement of right ventricular outflow tract (RVOT) are surgical procedures of choice for large symptomatic PAAs.[9] When feasible, endovascular repair with coils has been performed with success in case reports. An Amplatzer plug has been utilized as well for PAAs.

Medical management of symptomatic PAAs with PAH include reducing PA pressures with diuretic therapy, vasodilators (calcium channel blockers as well as use of endothelin receptor antagonists), phosphodiesterase inhibitors, and prostacyclin analogs. Asymptomatic benign PAAs do not warrant treatment without associated PAH. Periodic assessment for increase in size should be performed.

REFERRAL

Patient should follow up with a pulmonologist and a cardiologist. Appropriate referral to a cardiothoracic surgeon should be made in select cases of large and symptomatic PAAs.

REFERENCES
Available at eBooks.Health.Elsevier.com.

RELATED CONTENT

Pulmonary hypertension (PH) (Related Key Topic)
Patent ductus arteriosus (PDA) (Related Key Topic)

AUTHOR: **TAYEBAH MUMTAZ, MD**

P

Diseases and Disorders

I

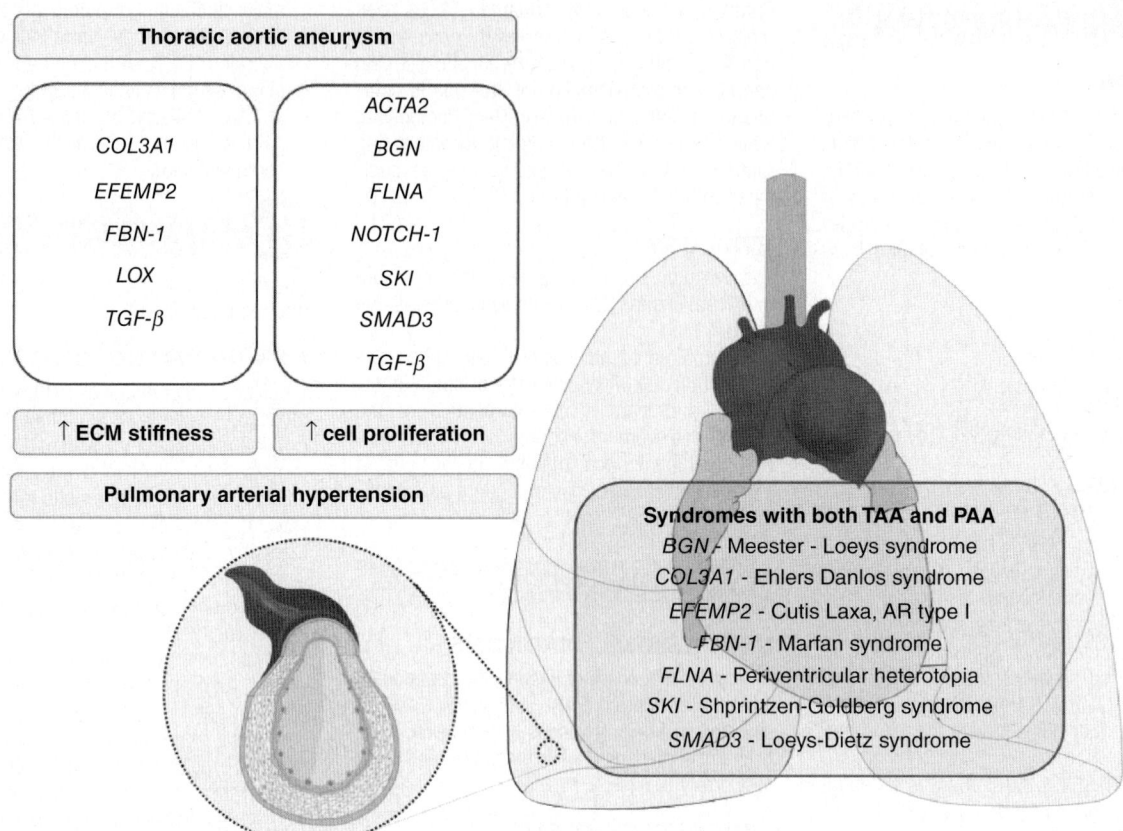

FIG. 1 Interplay of genetic pathways related to thoracic aortic aneurysms (TAA) and potentially contributing to pulmonary artery aneurysms (PAAs) and resultant pulmonary arterial hypertension (PAH). Extracellular matrix stiffness and increased cell proliferation may play a role in PAA formation. (From Nuche J et al: Potential molecular pathways related to pulmonary artery aneurysm development: lessons to learn from the aorta, *Int J Mol Sci* 21:2509, 2020. https://doi.org/10.3390/ijms21072509.)

🛈 BASIC INFORMATION

DEFINITION

Acute cardiogenic pulmonary edema (ACPE) arises from an increased leakage of fluid into the interstitial space and/or alveolar spaces within the pulmonary vasculature. This leads to a combination of clinical signs and symptoms resulting from compromised gaseous exchange.[1]

SYNONYMS

ACPE
ADHF
CPE
Cardiogenic pulmonary edema (CPE)
Acute cardiogenic pulmonary edema (ACPE)
Acute decompensated heart failure (ADHF) with pulmonary edema
Acute diastolic heart failure with pulmonary edema
Acute systolic heart failure with pulmonary edema
Acute combined heart failure with pulmonary edema

ICD-10CM CODES
J81.0	Acute pulmonary edema
J81.1	Chronic pulmonary edema
I50.1	Left ventricular failure
J68.1	Pulmonary edema due to chemicals, gases, fumes and vapors

EPIDEMIOLOGY & DEMOGRAPHICS

- **Prevalence of Heart Failure (HF):** Affects approximately 6.5 million individuals in the U.S. and 23 million globally. In the U.S. this number is expected to rise to 8 million by 2030.[2]
- **Healthcare Utilization:** In 2012, there were 1.7 million HF-related visits to U.S. physician offices and half a million emergency department visits reported.
- **Age-Related Impact:** About 20% of all-cause admissions among individuals over the age of 65 are linked to HF.
- **Readmission Rates:** Within 30 days of discharge, 25% to 30% of these patients are readmitted due to recurrent ADHF.
- **Mortality Rates:** The in-hospital mortality rate for HF ranges from 10% to 20%, particularly when HF is associated with acute myocardial infarction (MI).

PHYSICAL FINDINGS & CLINICAL PRESENTATION

Signs (physical findings):
- Hypertension (in cardiogenic shock, could be hypotensive)
- Tachycardia
- Elevated jugular venous pressure with hepatojugular reflex
- Bilateral pulmonary rales/decreased breath sounds/pleural effusions
- S3 gallop/S4 and/or laterally displaced apex
- Abdominal distention/ascites
- Peripheral edema
- Cold and clammy skin
- Perioral and peripheral cyanosis
- Pink, frothy sputum

Symptoms (clinical presentations):
- Weight gain
- Altered mental status
- Dyspnea (exertional or at rest, paroxysmal nocturnal dyspnea, orthopnea)
- Cough and wheezing (cardiac asthma)
- Diaphoresis

ETIOLOGY

Common causes of acute pulmonary edema include:
Cardiac causes:
- Acute MI
- Atrial and ventricular arrhythmias
- Valvular heart disease (mitral, aortic, tricuspid, and pulmonary valve disease)
- Peripartum cardiomyopathy/HF of pregnancy
- Infections (myopericarditis, endocarditis, HIV, Chagas)
- Uncontrolled hypertension
- Structural heart disease (ventricular septal defect, infiltrative heart disease, hypertrophic cardiomyopathy)
- Postcardioversion syndrome
Noncardiac causes:
- Poor dietary compliance or medication nonadherence
- Renal and liver disease
- Endocrine (thyrotoxicosis, obesity, metabolic syndrome, diabetes)
- Toxin mediated (cocaine, alcohol, chemotherapy agents, ephedra)
- Pulmonary embolism
Box 1 summarizes common causes of cardiogenic and noncardiogenic pulmonary edema.

🔷 DIAGNOSIS

DIFFERENTIAL DIAGNOSIS
- Noncardiogenic pulmonary edema (Fig. 1 and Table 1)
- Viral pneumonitis including COVID 19[3] and other pulmonary infections.
- Pulmonary embolism
- Exacerbation of asthma/chronic obstructive pulmonary disease
- High-altitude pulmonary edema (HAPE)
- Sarcoidosis
- Pulmonary fibrosis
- Lymphangitic carcinomatosis

LABORATORY TESTS
- Arterial blood gases (ABGs): Respiratory and metabolic acidosis, decreased PaO_2, increased $PaCO_2$, low pH. (NOTE: The patient may initially show respiratory alkalosis because of hyperventilation in attempts to maintain PaO_2.)
- B-type natriuretic peptide (BNP) and NT-pro BNP add diagnostic value to the history and physical examination as evidenced in the Breathing Not Properly (BNP) study.
- Cardiac biomarkers: Troponin T or I if suspicion for acute coronary syndrome.
- Basic metabolic profile: Assess for electrolyte abnormalities and kidney function.
- Elevated liver function tests (LFTs) are indicative of congestive hepatopathy or shock liver.

- Serology for suspected inciting agents, including HIV, Chagas, adenovirus, enterovirus, parvovirus, herpes virus, and more recently the novel Coronavirus disease (COVID-19).[3]
- CBC: Anemia can trigger acute pulmonary edema.
- Glucose, HgbA1c, fasting lipid profile, thyroid-stimulating hormone (TSH) for risk stratification.
- Urinalysis and urine toxicology if indicated.
- Genetic testing for unexplained cardiomyopathies.[4]

IMAGING STUDIES
NONINVASIVE IMAGING:
- ECG: May elucidate the etiology of pulmonary edema. Causes may include ischemia/infarct, arrhythmias, left ventricular (LV) hypertrophy, and atrial enlargement.
- Chest x-ray (Fig. 2):
  1. Bilateral interstitial and alveolar infiltrates
  2. Cephalization of the pulmonary vessels
  3. Kerley B lines; fluffy perihilar infiltrates
  4. Pleural effusions
  5. Enlarged cardiac silhouette
- Echocardiogram:
  1. Assess left and right ventricular systolic/diastolic function.
  2. Structural abnormalities (VSD, LV rupture).
  3. Evaluate valvular abnormalities including endocarditis.
  4. Engorged inferior vena cava (IVC) and IVC plethora, based on bedside ultrasound, suggests elevated filling pressures.
- Computed tomography (CT) of the chest: May differentiate between cardiogenic and noncardiogenic pulmonary edema.
- Lung ultrasound (LUS) has emerged as a tool to diagnose pulmonary edema. It is easy to use, accessible, and noninvasive, and has a

---

BOX 1 Common Causes of Cardiogenic and Noncardiogenic Pulmonary Edema

Cardiogenic Pulmonary Edema
- Acute exacerbation of heart failure
- Acute valve dysfunction (e.g., mitral valve chordae tendineae rupture)
- Arrhythmia/myocardial infarction
- Hypertensive crisis
- Fluid overload following aggressive volume resuscitation (e.g., postoperative)
- Ventricular septal rupture
- Pericardial tamponade

Noncardiogenic Pulmonary Edema
- Direct lung injury
  1. Pneumonia
  2. Gastric aspiration
  3. Toxic inhalation
  4. Negative pressure related (e.g., strangulation)
- Indirect causes of lung injury
  1. Sepsis
  2. Trauma
  3. Pancreatitis
  4. Multiple blood transfusions
  5. Burn injury

From Vincent JL et al: *Textbook of critical care*, ed 8, Philadelphia, 2024, Elsevier.

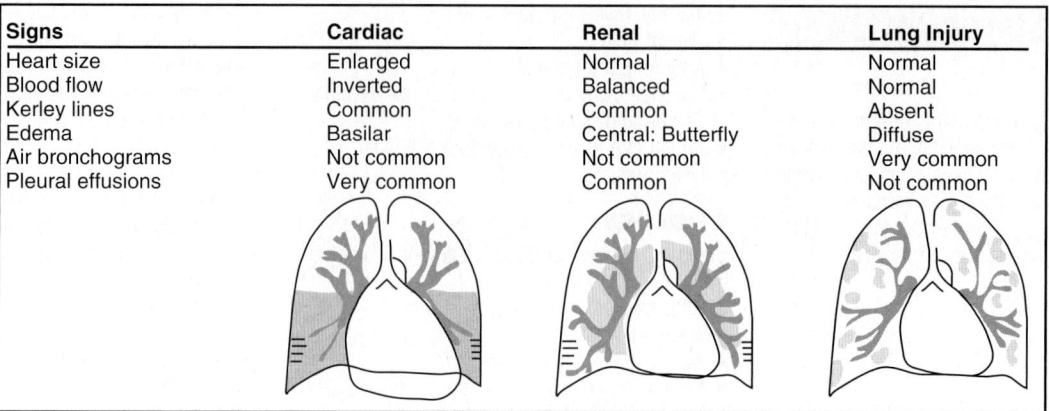

Signs	Cardiac	Renal	Lung Injury
Heart size	Enlarged	Normal	Normal
Blood flow	Inverted	Balanced	Normal
Kerley lines	Common	Common	Absent
Edema	Basilar	Central: Butterfly	Diffuse
Air bronchograms	Not common	Not common	Very common
Pleural effusions	Very common	Common	Not common

FIG. 1 Types of pulmonary edema. (From Weissleder R et al: *Primer of diagnostic imaging,* ed 4, St Louis, 2007, Mosby.)

TABLE 1 Distinguishing Cardiogenic and Noncardiogenic Pulmonary Edema

	History	Exam	Labs	Imaging	Pulmonary Artery Catheter
Cardiogenic	Heart disease Renal disease Uncontrolled HTN Edema Orthopnea Recent administration of IV fluids or blood products	Heart failure exam findings: Distended neck veins S3 heart sound Dependent edema Elevated blood pressure Cool extremities	↑BNP >1200 pg/ml ↑Creatinine (in setting of volume overload) ↑Troponin	CXR: CMG pleural effusions Kerley B lines TEE: ↓LVEF Diastolic filling defect Severe mitral or aortic valvular disease Pericardial effusion with tamponade VSD	PCWP >18 mm Hg Prominent V-waves (mitral regurgitation) Elevation and equilibration of right atrial pressure, pulmonary artery diastolic and PCWP (tamponade physiology) CVP >12 mm Hg
Noncardiogenic	Sepsis Aspiration event Trauma (long bone fractures) Burn injury Pancreatitis Multiple transfusions	Signs of active infection Extensive burn injury Evidence of trauma (absence of heart failure exam findings)	↑WBC BNP <200 pg/ml	CXR: Diffuse central and peripheral infiltrates Normal heart size No or minimal pleural effusions TEE: Normal LV and valvular function No evidence of volume overload	PCWP <18 mm Hg CVP <12 mm Hg

BNP, Brain natriuretic peptide; *CVP,* central venous pressure; *CXR,* chest x-ray; *HTN,* hypertension; *IV,* intravenous; *LVEF,* left ventricle ejection fraction; *PCWP,* pulmonary capillary wedge pressure; *S3,* third heart sound; *TFF,* transesophageal echocardiogram; *VSD,* ventricular septal defect; *WBC,* white blood count.
From Vincent JL et al: *Textbook of critical care,* ed 8, Philadelphia, 2024, Elsevier.

high negative predictive value. Positive predictive value for LUS is slightly lower, but LUS remains a versatile, easily accessible and reliable tool at points of triage.[1] Kerley B lines and pleural effusions are highly suggestive of pulmonary edema.[5-7]

INVASIVE IMAGING:
- Right heart catheterization (RHC): Obtain estimated filling pressures, assess cardiac output, differentiate between different shocks, and use to guide tailored inotropic and pressor therapy. Despite the widespread availability of Swan-Ganz catheters the ESCAPE trial failed to demonstrate the utility of pulmonary artery catheters in acute decompensated HF.
- Coronary angiogram: Rule out acute MI/progressive coronary artery disease.
- Left heart catheterization (LHC): Measure left ventricular end-diastolic pressure (LVEDP) to estimate left-sided filling pressure.

- CardioMEMS (St. Jude Medical) is an invasive pulmonary artery pressure monitoring device that can provide remote monitoring capability and aid in reduction of frequency of HF hospitalizations.[2]

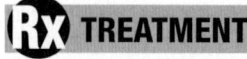 **TREATMENT**

ACUTE GENERAL Rx (FIG. 3)
Nonpharmacologic treatment:
- Sodium restriction in American College of Cardiology (ACC)/American Heart Association (AHA) class C and D HF patients has conflicting data
- Restrict 1.5 to 2 L of free water in the setting of hyponatremia
- Risk factor modification (blood pressure [BP] and glucose control, dietary modifications)
- Oxygen supplementation if signs of hypoxia are present

- Noninvasive ventilation (continuous positive airway pressure [CPAP]) or bilevel noninvasive positive-pressure ventilation (NPPV) reduces dyspnea and may reduce the need for endotracheal intubation. Positive pressure ventilation (invasive or noninvasive) decreases preload and afterload and reduces the work of breathing, while positive end expiratory pressure improves oxygenation
- HF teaching

Pharmacologic treatment:
- Loop diuretics such as furosemide, torsemide, bumetanide, and ethacrynic acid are the cornerstones of the treatment of volume overload. Intravenous treatment might be required in acute pulmonary edema due to coexistent gut edema that is a barrier to effective GI absorption. There is no difference in symptoms or kidney function whether the diuretic is given as a bolus or continuous

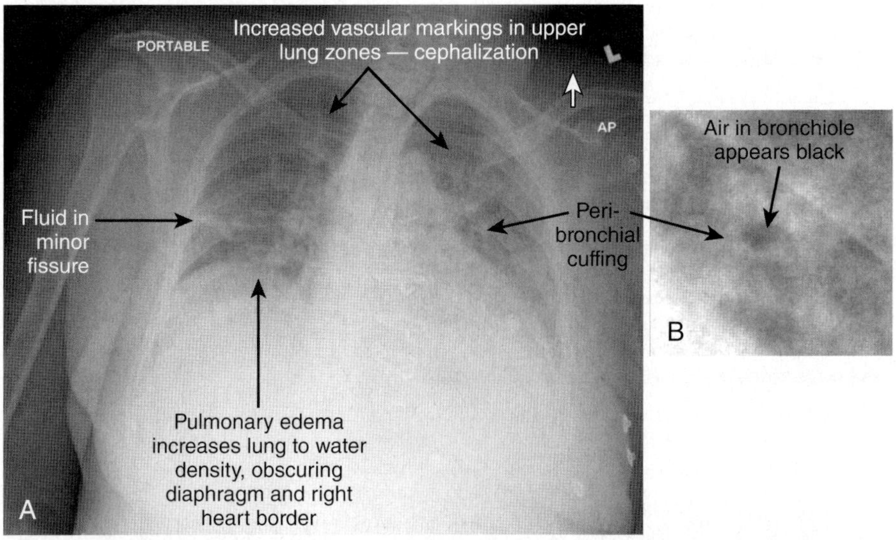

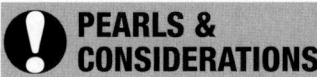

FIG. 2 **Pulmonary edema. A,** Anterior-posterior chest x-ray. **B,** Close-up from **A.** This 53-yr-old woman with end-stage renal disease missed dialysis and presented to the emergency department. Her examination demonstrated bilateral rales. Her x-ray shows mild cardiomegaly, bilateral interstitial opacities, and cephalization of the pulmonary vascular markings. The minor fissure appears thickened. These findings are consistent with pulmonary edema. In addition, peribronchial cuffing is present. As discussed elsewhere, this is a nonspecific thickening of the bronchial wall that can occur from edema in the setting of heart failure, asthma, viral illness, or even infections such as pertussis. The thickened wall appears white, whereas the air-filled bronchiole appears black and has a circular short-axis cross section. (From Broder JS: *Diagnostic imaging for the emergency physician,* Philadelphia, 2011, Saunders.)

infusion (DOSE trial; New England Journal of Medicine, March 3, 2011).[8]

- Nitrates: Particularly useful if the patient has concomitant chest pain or is hypertensive.
  1. Nitroglycerin: 0.4 to 0.8 mg sublingual (SL) or nitroglycerin spray may be given immediately on arrival and repeated every 5 min up to three times if the patient remains symptomatic and BP remains stable.
  2. 2% nitroglycerin ointment: 1 to 3 inches out of the tube applied continuously; absorption may be erratic.
  3. IV nitroglycerin for refractory chest pain and hypertension: Start at 0.2 to 0.4 mcg/kg/min.
- Nitroprusside is useful for afterload reduction in severe hypertension, acute mitral regurgitation, or acute aortic regurgitation.
  1. Start at low-dose 0.5 μg/kg/min with an arterial line in place.
  2. Monitor for cyanide toxicity.
- ACE inhibitors, angiotensin II receptor blockers, aldosterone antagonist, and angiotensin receptor–neprilysin inhibitors are vasodilators with long-term mortality benefit in patients with HF with reduced ejection fraction.[4,9,10]
- In patients with HF with reduced ejection fraction, with and without type 2 diabetes, SGLT2 inhibitors decrease frequency of hospitalization for HF, an urgent visit resulting in intravenous therapy for HF, or death from cardiovascular causes (EMPA-REG OUTCOME,

DAPA HF trial). They can be initiated before discharge during acute hospitalizations for ADHF.
- Ultrafiltration/aquapheresis if diuretic resistant.
- Morphine was previously thought to be beneficial in patients with ACPE, but recent data suggested that it can be detrimental with increase in rates of in hospital mortality, increased need for invasive and noninvasive ventilation, and increased need for pressors/inotropes.[11]

Pharmacologic-vasopressors:
- Patients with profound hypotension benefit from vasopressors.
  1. Norepinephrine: Powerful vasoconstrictor with small inotropic effect.[12]
  2. Dopamine: Low doses (0.5 to 3 μg/kg/min) increase blood flow to coronary, renal, and cerebral beds. Intermediate doses (3 to 10 μg/kg/min) increase cardiac contractility while high doses (10 to 20 μg/kg/min) have a pressor effect.

Pharmacologic-inotropes:
- Dobutamine: Potent inotrope, mild chronotropic effects. Dose ranges from 2.5 to 20 mcg/kg/min.
- Phosphodiesterase inhibitors (amrinone, milrinone, and enoximone [not available in U.S.]) may be useful in refractory cases.

Mechanical support:
- Intra-aortic balloon pump (IABP): Decreases afterload, increases coronary blood flow.

- Impella: Axial-flow pump on a pigtail catheter that crosses the aortic valve and unloads the left ventricle.
- Tandem heart device: Oxygenated blood is pumped from the left atrium into the femoral artery. It can provide 3.5 to 4.5 L/min of cardiac output.
- Extracorporeal membrane oxygenation (ECMO) as a bridge to heart transplant or recovery.
- Durable mechanical circulatory support such as left ventricular assist device can be considered for those in cardiogenic shock refractory to medical therapy.

DISPOSITION
Admit to intensive care unit (ICU)/critical care unit (CCU) if:
- Need for intubation
- Signs and symptoms of hypoperfusion/shock
- SpO_2 <90% despite supplemental oxygen
- Use of accessory muscles/respiratory rate (RR) >25/min
- Heart rate <40 or >130, systolic BP <90

PEARLS & CONSIDERATIONS

- ACPE is the outcome of decompensation of mechanical function of the heart due to variable etiologies.
- Accurate identification of etiology and prompt steps in management concurrent to management of pulmonary edema itself can improve outcomes.
- Use of bedside LUS or other easily accessible noninvasive and reliable methods to be used in rapid diagnosis to facilitate early initiation of therapy.
- Choice of pharmacologic agents on case-by-case basis depending on etiology. Early use of mechanical support in addition if indicated.
- Emphasis to be placed on patient education and utilization of quality metrics after discharge as well as continued follow-up in the outpatient setting.

COMMENTS
Accumulated evidence still favors the use of noninvasive ventilation, especially CPAP, in patients with ACPE, especially as this therapy reduces dyspnea and helps correct metabolic abnormalities more rapidly than standard oxygen therapy. The role of morphine in the treatment of ACPE has come into question.

REFERENCES
Available at eBooks.Health.Elsevier.com.

RELATED CONTENT
Heart Failure (Related Key Topic)

AUTHOR: **SAEED ABUGHAZALEH, MD**

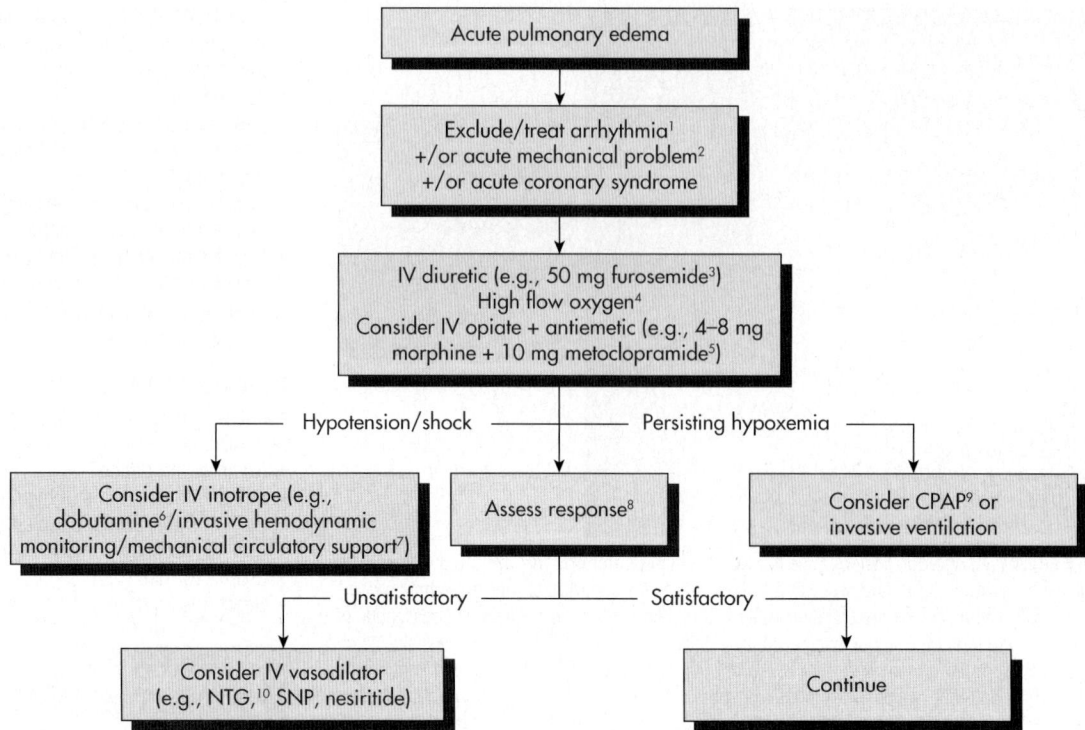

¹ Casual arrhythmia (e.g., ventricular tachycardia). It can be difficult to determine whether atrial fibrillation is a primary cause of acute pulmonary edema or secondary to it. An ECG is an essential investigation.

² Acute mechanical problems include ventricular septal rupture and mitral valve papillary muscle rupture. Mechanical support (e.g., an intraaortic balloon pump) and urgent surgery should be considered. An echocardiogram should be performed as soon as possible, especially in a patient without a prior diagnosis of heart failure/other relevant heart disease (e.g., prior myocardial infarction or valve disease).

³ Dose of diuretic depends on prior diuretic use and renal function—a lower dose may suffice if preserved renal function and no prior diuretic use.

⁴ Oxygen causes an increase in systemic vascular resistance and a reduction in heart rate and cardiac output and should only be administered to patients with hypoxemia.

⁵ Consider if patient is agitated/distressed/in pain; may cause respiratory depression and dose should be reduced in very elderly.

⁶ An intravenous infusion of dobutamine may be started at a dose of 2.5 μg/kg/min, doubling every 15 minutes according to response and tolerability (dose titration usually limited by excessive tachycardia, arrhythmias, or ischemia). A dose above 20 μg/kg/min is rarely needed.

⁷ E.g., an intraaortic balloon pump

⁸ Improvement in symptoms and peripheral perfusion and adequate urine output—patient should be monitored closely, and usually a response will occur within 30 minutes. Bladder catheterization may help in monitoring urine output.

⁹ Continuous positive airways pressure (CPAP) is valuable in severe pulmonary edema, especially if associated with hypoxemia. Endotracheal intubation and invasive mechanical ventilation should be considered in patients with persisting hypoxemia and physical ventilatory exhaustion.

¹⁰ If systolic blood pressure is adequate (>100 mm Hg), an intravenous infusion of nitroglycerin (NTG) can be considered. Start at a dose of 10 μg/min and double every 10 minutes according to response and tolerability (usually dose up-titration is limited by hypotension). A dose of more than 100 μg/min is rarely needed.

FIG. 3 Approach to the patient with acute pulmonary edema. *IV,* Intravenous; *SNP,* sodium nitroprusside. (From Goldman L, Shafer AI: *Goldman-Cecil medicine,* ed 26, Philadelphia, 2019, Elsevier.)

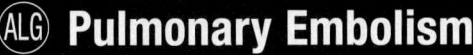

BASIC INFORMATION

DEFINITION

Pulmonary embolism (PE) refers to the lodging of a thrombus or other embolic material from a distant site in the pulmonary circulation. A classification of acute PE is described in Table 1.

SYNONYMS

PE
Pulmonary thromboembolism

ICD-10CM CODES	
I26	Pulmonary embolism
I26.01	Septic pulmonary embolism with acute cor pulmonale
I26.09	Other pulmonary embolism with acute cor pulmonale
I26.90	Septic pulmonary embolism without acute cor pulmonale
I26.99	Other pulmonary embolism without acute cor pulmonale
I27.82	Chronic pulmonary embolism
Z86.711	Personal history of pulmonary embolism

EPIDEMIOLOGY & DEMOGRAPHICS

- Approximately 650,000 cases of PE occur in the U.S. each year (increased incidence in women and with advanced age); annually, as many as 100,000 people in the U.S. die from acute PE, and the diagnosis is often not made until after autopsy. The incidence of PE is increasing with the increasing use of spiral computed tomography (CT) scans, with a lower severity of illness and lower mortality, suggesting that the increase is the result of earlier diagnosis.
- More than 90% of PEs originate in the deep venous system of the lower extremities. (See chapter "Deep Vein Thrombosis".)
- Pulmonary thromboembolism is associated with >200,000 hospitalizations per yr.
- Up to 8% to 10% of victims of PE die within the first h.
- Although nearly 20% of patients who are treated for PE die within 90 days, PE is not commonly the cause of death because it frequently coexists with other serious conditions, such as cancer, sepsis, or illness leading to hospitalization. The true mortality associated with undiagnosed PE is estimated to be less than 5%.[1]

PHYSICAL FINDINGS & CLINICAL PRESENTATION

- Most common symptom: Dyspnea (82% to 85%)
- Tachypnea (30% to 60%)
- Cough (30% to 40%)
- Wheezing (20%)
- Chest pain: May be nonpleuritic or pleuritic (infarction) (40% to 49%); angina may reflect right ventricle (RV) ischemia
- Syncope (massive PE) (10% to 14%)
- Fever, diaphoresis, apprehension
- Hemoptysis (2%)
- Evidence of deep vein thrombosis (DVT) may be present (e.g., swelling and tenderness of extremities)
- Cardiac examination may reveal: Tachycardia (23%), increased pulmonic component of S2, murmur of tricuspid insufficiency, right ventricular heave, right-sided S3
- Pulmonary examination: May demonstrate rales, localized wheezing, friction rub

ETIOLOGY

- Thrombus, fat, air, tumor, or other foreign material
- Major transient risk factors for PE:
  1. Postoperative state, major surgery including hip or knee replacement
  2. Trauma to lower extremities, immobilizer, or cast
  3. Prolonged immobilization, reduced mobility
  4. Central venous catheter
  5. Pregnancy and early puerperium
- Minor transient risk factors for PE:
  1. Estrogen-containing birth control pills, hormone replacement therapy, estrogen-modulators (e.g., raloxifene, tamoxifen)
  2. Prolonged air travel
  3. Acute medical illness (e.g., infection, disseminated intravascular coagulation)
- Persistent risk factors for PE:
  1. History of DVT or PE
  2. Heart failure

3. Visceral cancer (lung, pancreas, alimentary and genitourinary tracts)
4. Spinal cord injury
5. Advanced age
6. Obesity
7. Hematologic disease (e.g., factor V Leiden mutation, antithrombin III deficiency, protein C deficiency, protein S deficiency, lupus anticoagulant, polycythemia vera, dysfibrinogenemia, paroxysmal nocturnal hemoglobinuria, acquired protein C resistance without factor V Leiden, G20210A prothrombin mutation)
8. Chronic obstructive pulmonary disease (COPD)
9. Diabetes mellitus
10. Autoimmune diseases (systemic lupus erythematosus, inflammatory bowel disease, rheumatoid arthritis)

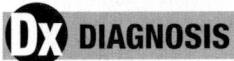 DIAGNOSIS

DIFFERENTIAL DIAGNOSIS

- Myocardial infarction
- Pericarditis
- Pneumonia
- Pneumothorax
- Chest wall pain
- GI abnormalities (e.g., peptic ulcer, esophageal rupture, gastritis)
- Heart failure
- Pleuritis
- Anxiety disorder with hyperventilation
- Pericardial tamponade
- Dissection of aorta
- Asthma or COPD exacerbation
- Chronic thromboembolic pulmonary hypertension (CTEPH)

WORKUP

- Guidelines from the Clinical Guidelines Committee of the American College of Physicians for the Evaluation of Patients with Suspected Acute Pulmonary Embolism recommend the following:
  1. Use of validated clinical prediction rules to estimate pretest probability in patients in whom acute PE is being considered.

TABLE 1 Classification of Acute Pulmonary Embolism

European Society of Cardiology (esc, 2019)	American Heart Association (AHA, 2011)	Hemodynamic Status	Pe Severity Index (Pesi) (or Simplified Pesi)	Evidence of Dysfunction	Treatment
High risk	Massive	Unstable	High	Typically abnormal RV on imaging, elevated troponin, OR both	Anticoagulation and advanced therapy
Intermediate-high risk	Submassive	Stable	High	Abnormal RV on imaging, AND elevated troponin	Anticoagulation with advanced therapy if clinical deterioration
Intermediate-low risk			High	May have abnormal RV on imaging OR elevated troponin BUT not both	Anticoagulation
Low risk	Low risk	Stable	Low	None	Anticoagulation with home therapy in subset with reliable follow-up

From Libby P et al: *Braunwald's heart disease, a textbook of cardiovascular medicine*, ed 12, Philadelphia, 2022, Elsevier.

2. Not obtaining a D-dimer measurement or imaging studies in patients with low pretest probability of PE and who meet all PE rule-out criteria.

3. Obtaining a high-sensitivity D-dimer measurement as the initial diagnostic test in patients who have an intermediate pretest probability of PE or in patients with low pretest probability of PE who do not meet all PE rule-out criteria. Clinicians should not use imaging studies as the initial test in patients who have a low or intermediate pretest probability of PE.

4. Use of age-adjusted D-dimer thresholds (age $\times$ 10 ng/ml rather than a generic 500 ng/ml) in patients >50 yr to determine whether imaging is warranted.

5. Clinicians should not obtain any imaging studies in patients with a D-dimer level below the age-adjusted cutoff.

6. CT pulmonary angiography (CTPA) should be obtained in patients with high pretest probability of PE. Ventilation-perfusion (V/Q) scans should be reserved for patients who have a contraindication to CTPA or if CTPA is not available.

7. A D-dimer measurement should not be obtained in patients with a high pretest probability of PE.

- Clinical assessment alone is insufficient to diagnose or rule out PE. It is also important to remember that no single noninvasive test has both high sensitivity and high specificity for PE. Consequently, in addition to clinical assessment, most patients require an imaging test to diagnose PE. An integrated diagnostic approach to PE is illustrated in Fig. 1. Prediction models for PE are summarized in Table 2.
- CTPA (Fig. E2) is an excellent diagnostic modality (83% sensitivity and 96% specificity).

- V/Q scan is reserved for patients with clinically significant contrast allergies or renal insufficiency, or when CTPA is not available.
- Pulmonary angiogram (gold standard) can confirm the diagnosis in equivocal cases, but is rarely used.
- Serial compressive duplex ultrasonography of lower extremities can be used in patients with "low-probability" V/Q scans and high clinical suspicion (see "Imaging Studies"). It is useful if positive; negative results do not exclude PE.

LABORATORY TESTS
- Arterial blood gas may reveal hypoxemia and respiratory alkalosis (decreased PaO_2 and $PaCO_2$ and increased pH); normal results do not rule out PE.
- Alveolar-arteriolar (A-a) oxygen gradient, a measure of the difference in oxygen concentration between alveoli and arterial blood,

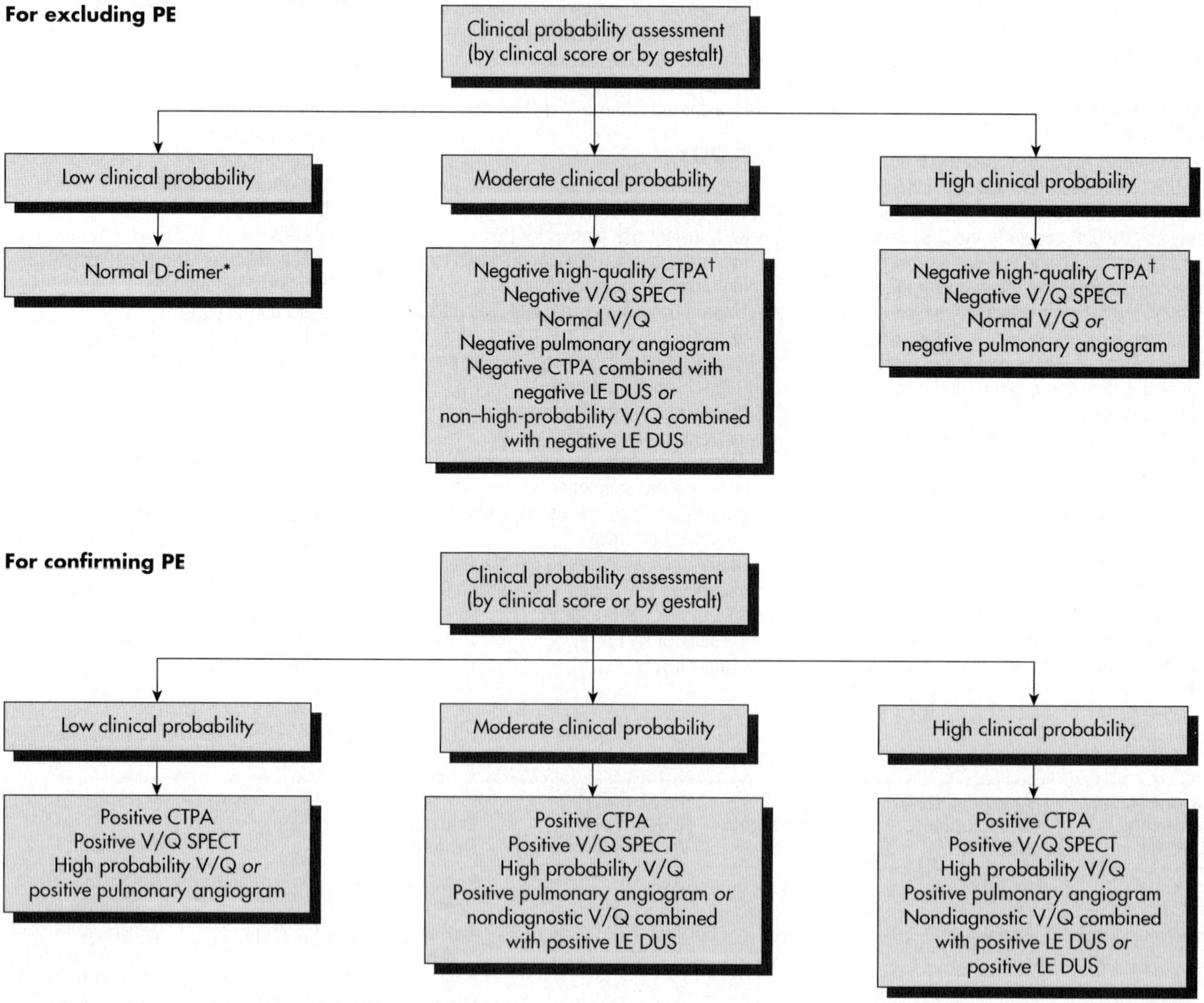

For excluding PE

Clinical probability assessment (by clinical score or by gestalt)

Low clinical probability → Normal D-dimer*

Moderate clinical probability → Negative high-quality CTPA† / Negative V/Q SPECT / Normal V/Q / Negative pulmonary angiogram / Negative CTPA combined with negative LE DUS *or* non–high-probability V/Q combined with negative LE DUS

High clinical probability → Negative high-quality CTPA† / Negative V/Q SPECT / Normal V/Q *or* negative pulmonary angiogram

For confirming PE

Clinical probability assessment (by clinical score or by gestalt)

Low clinical probability → Positive CTPA / Positive V/Q SPECT / High probability V/Q *or* positive pulmonary angiogram

Moderate clinical probability → Positive CTPA / Positive V/Q SPECT / High probability V/Q / Positive pulmonary angiogram *or* nondiagnostic V/Q combined with positive LE DUS

High clinical probability → Positive CTPA / Positive V/Q SPECT / High probability V/Q / Positive pulmonary angiogram / Nondiagnostic V/Q combined with positive LE DUS *or* positive LE DUS

FIG. 1 Diagnostic strategies capable of excluding or confirming the diagnosis of pulmonary embolism. Depending on the assessed clinical probability, the tests and their results can be used either to exclude or to confirm a diagnosis of pulmonary embolism. *CTPA,* Computed tomographic pulmonary angiography; *DUS,* Doppler ultrasound; *LE,* lower extremity; *V/Q,* ventilation-perfusion scan; *V/Q SPECT,* ventilation-perfusion scan performed with a SPECT (single-photon emission computerized tomography) protocol. *The limits of normal for D-dimer are best appreciated when the patient's age is taken into account. †Artifacts may interfere with the sensitivity of CTPA, especially in scanners with four or fewer detectors. (From Broaddus VC et al: *Murray & Nadel's textbook of respiratory medicine,* ed 7, Philadelphia, 2022, Elsevier.)

TABLE 2 Prediction Models for Pulmonary Embolism

Clinical Variable	Wells Clinical Model	Revised Geneva	PERC	YEARS**
	SCORING MODEL			
Patient population in which clinical rule was validated	ED patients suspected of having PE	ED patients suspected of having PE	ED patients at low or very low risk of PE	Outpatients and inpatients suspected of having PE
Clinical signs/symptoms of deep venous thrombosis	3	4	1	1
PE is most likely or as likely as alternative diagnosis	3			1
Heart rate:				
75-94 beats/min		3		
≥95 beats/min		5		
≥100 beats/min	1.5		1	
Immobilization, surgery or trauma in the previous 4 wk requiring hospitalization or fracture of the lower limb within 1 mo (Geneva)	1.5	2	1	
Prior DVT or PE	1.5	3	1	
Hemoptysis	1	2	1	1
Malignancy (on treatment, treated in last 6 mo, cured <1 yr or palliative)	1	2		
SaO₂ <95% on room air			1	
Unilateral lower limb pain		3		
Exogenous estrogen use			1	
Age:				
≥50 yr			1	
≥65 yr		1		
Clinical Assessment Probability:				
Low probability	<2 points	0-3 total	0 points*	0 points†
Intermediate probability	2-6 points	4-10 total		
High probability	>6 points	≥11 total		
Dichotomous Wells Score With D-Dimer				
Pulmonary embolism "unlikely"		≤4 points		D-dimer <500 ng/ml: PE excluded; D-dimer >500 ng/ml, consider CTPA
Pulmonary embolism "likely"		>4 points		PE not excluded, consider additional testing with CTPA

Age-Adjusted D-Dimer Cutoff for VTE:

Formula for use in patients ≥50 yr of age in whom clinical suspicion for PE is low or intermediate

Units	*Age-Adjusted D-Dimer*	*Interpretation/Recommendation*
FEU (fibrinogen equivalent units)‡	Age × 10 μg/L	Above age-adjusted cutoff: VTE *likely*, consider confirmatory testing
DDU (D-dimer units)‡	Age × 5 μg/L	Below age-adjusted cutoff: VTE *unlikely*, consider alternative diagnosis

CTPA, Computed tomography pulmonary angiography; *DVT*, deep venous thrombosis; *ED*, emergency department; *PE*, pulmonary embolism; *PERC*, Pulmonary Embolism Rule out Criteria; *SaO₂*, arterial saturation of oxygen; *VTE*, venous thromboembolism.

*If no criteria are positive and the clinician's pretest probability of PE <15%, PERC criteria is satisfied, and there is <2% chance of PE.

†In patients with no YEARS items and D-dimer <1000 ng/ml, PE is excluded. In patients with one or more YEARS items, PE is excluded if D-dimer is <500 ng/ml. If PE is not excluded, CTPA is recommended.

‡Must check laboratory closely to ensure correct use of units.

** Years algorithm is a modification of the Wells Clinical Decision Rule. It combines an evaluation of three characteristics (clinical signs of DVT, hemoptysis, and whether PE is the most likely diagnosis) with a differential analysis of D-dimer concentrations.

From Broaddus VC et al: *Murray & Nadel's textbook of respiratory medicine*, ed 7, Philadelphia, 2022, Elsevier.

may be elevated. However, a normal A-a gradient does not rule out PE.

- High-sensitivity plasma D-dimer measurement: D-dimer assays by enzyme-linked assay detect the presence of plasmin-mediated degradation products of fibrin that contain cross-linked D fragments in the whole blood or plasma. A normal plasma D-dimer level is useful to exclude PE in patients with a low pretest probability of PE. However, it cannot be used to "rule in" the diagnosis because it increases with many other disorders (e.g., metastatic cancer, trauma, sepsis, postoperative state). Plasma D-dimer can also be used in conjunction with lower-extremity compression ultrasonography in patients with indeterminate V/Q and spiral CT scans. Absence of DVT and presence of a normal D-dimer level in these settings generally rule out clinically significant PE.

- Elevated cardiac troponin levels also occur in patients with PE because of RV dilation and myocardial injury; therefore, PE should be considered in the differential diagnosis of all patients presenting with chest pain or dyspnea and elevated cardiac troponin levels.

- Elevated serum BNP levels in patients with acute PE may reflect RV overload. The pathophysiology of RV dysfunction in PE is illustrated in Fig. 3.

- ECG is abnormal in 85% of patients with acute PE. Frequent abnormalities are sinus tachycardia; nonspecific ST-segment or T-wave changes; S-1, Q-3, T-3 pattern (10% of patients); S-1, S-2, S-3 pattern; T-wave inversion in V₁ to V₆ acute RBBB; new-onset atrial fibrillation; ST segment depression in lead II; RV strain. An RV strain pattern on ECG in patients with PE and normal blood pressure is associated with adverse short-term outcome and adds incremental prognostic value to echocardiographic evidence of RV function.

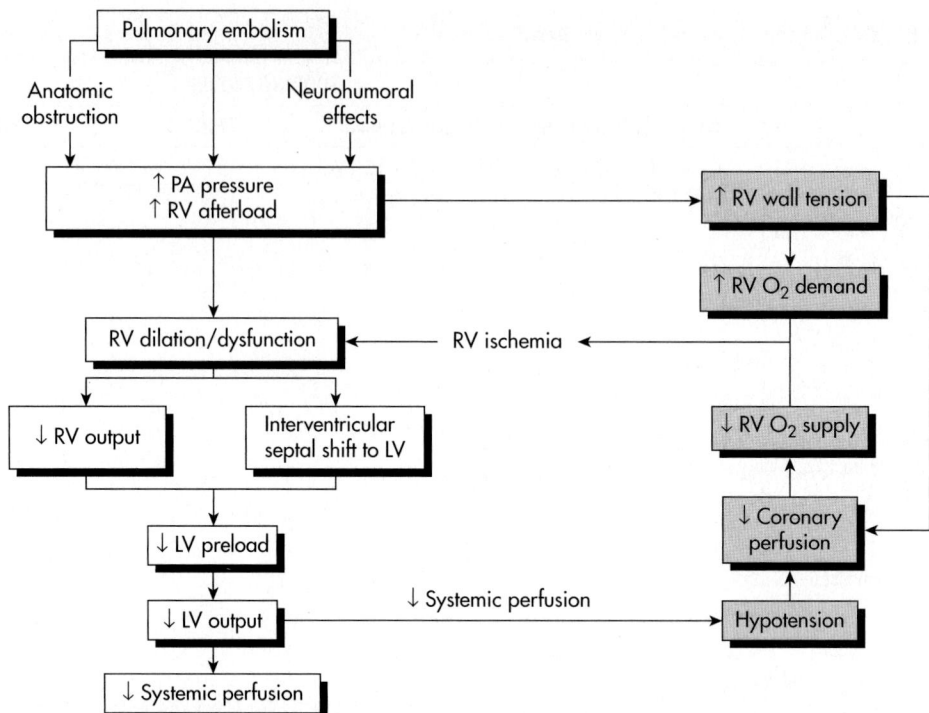

FIG. 3 Pathophysiology of right ventricular dysfunction and its deleterious effects of causing decreased systemic arterial pressure, decreased coronary perfusion, and deteriorating ventricular function. *LV,* Left ventricle/ventricular; *PA,* pulmonary artery; *RV,* right ventricle/ventricular. (From Libby P et al: *Braunwald's heart disease, a textbook of cardiovascular medicine,* ed 12, Philadelphia, 2022, Elsevier.)

IMAGING STUDIES

- Chest x-ray can be normal but is typically abnormal (Fig. E4); suggestive findings include elevated diaphragm, pleural effusion, dilation of pulmonary artery, infiltrate or consolidation, abrupt vessel cut-off, oligemia distal to the PE *(Westermark sign),* or atelectasis. A wedge-shaped consolidation in the middle and lower lobes is suggestive of a pulmonary infarction and is known as a *Hampton hump.*
- CT pulmonary angiography (CTPA) is an accurate, noninvasive tool in the diagnosis of PE (Fig. E5) at the main, lobar, and segmental pulmonary artery levels. A major advantage of CTPA over standard pulmonary angiography is its ability to diagnose intrathoracic disease other than PE that may account for the patient's clinical picture. It is also less invasive, less costly, and more widely available. Its major shortcoming is its poor sensitivity for subsegmental emboli. It is important to recognize signs of chronic clot on CT scan. These signs include eccentric thrombus, intraluminal webs/bands, mosaic attenuation of lung fields, and presence of bronchial artery collaterals, which may suggest chronic rather than acute PE, warranting a different treatment approach (see Fig. E2).
- V/Q lung scan (in patient with normal chest x-ray examination): This test must be interpreted within the pretest probability of having a PE.
  1. A normal lung scan rules out PE.
  2. A V/Q mismatch is suggestive of PE, and a lung scan interpretation of high probability is confirmatory (Fig. E6).

3. If the clinical suspicion of PE is high and the V/Q lung scan is interpreted as low probability, moderate probability, or indeterminate, a pulmonary angiogram is diagnostic. A positive angiogram confirms diagnosis. A positive compressive duplex ultrasonography for DVT obviates the need for an angiogram, because treatment with anticoagulants is indicated in these patients. The overall sensitivity of compressive ultrasonography for DVT in patients with PE is 29% with a specificity of 97%. Adding ultrasonography in patients with a nondiagnostic lung scan prevents 9% of angiographies; however, this improvement in efficacy is achieved at the cost of unnecessary anticoagulant therapy in 26% of patients who have false-positive ultrasonography results.

- Pulmonary angiography is the historic gold standard; however, it is invasive, expensive, and not readily available in some clinical settings. False-positive pulmonary angiograms may result from mediastinal disorders such as radiation fibrosis and tumors.
- Echocardiography is useful for identifying patients with PE who are high risk for poor outcomes. Moderate or severe RV hypokinesis, persistent pulmonary hypertension, patent foramen ovale, and free-floating right heart thrombus are markers of increased risk of death or recurrent thrombosis. RV pressure overload may be inferred from a RV:LV ratio ≥1.0 and predicts higher rates of in-hospital death or clinical deterioration. McConnell's sign, akinesia of mid-free wall with normal

motion at apex, is 77% sensitive and 94% specific for acute PE.
- Gadolinium-enhanced magnetic resonance angiography (MRA/MRV) of the pulmonary arteries has a moderate sensitivity and high specificity for the diagnosis of PE at experienced centers, but obtaining acceptable images is technically challenging and should only be performed if other imaging tests are contraindicated.

Rx TREATMENT

NONPHARMACOLOGIC THERAPY
Modification of risk factors (see "Etiology") to prevent future PE.

ACUTE GENERAL Rx
Patients with acute PE should be initially stratified according to risk (see Table 1) so that higher-risk therapies (e.g., thrombolysis, embolectomy) are offered to patients with the greatest chance of benefit. Many tertiary and quaternary care centers deploy a multidisciplinary Pulmonary Embolism Response Team (PERT) to determine the optimal course of treatment for patients with intermediate- and high-risk PE, given the highly variable mortality risk in the intermediate-risk group.

Anticoagulation is recommended as initial therapy in all patients with small to moderate PE without a contraindication. Fig. 7 illustrates the treatment of PE in hemodynamically stable patients. Anticoagulant treatments for acute PE are summarized in Table 3.

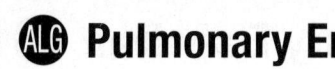

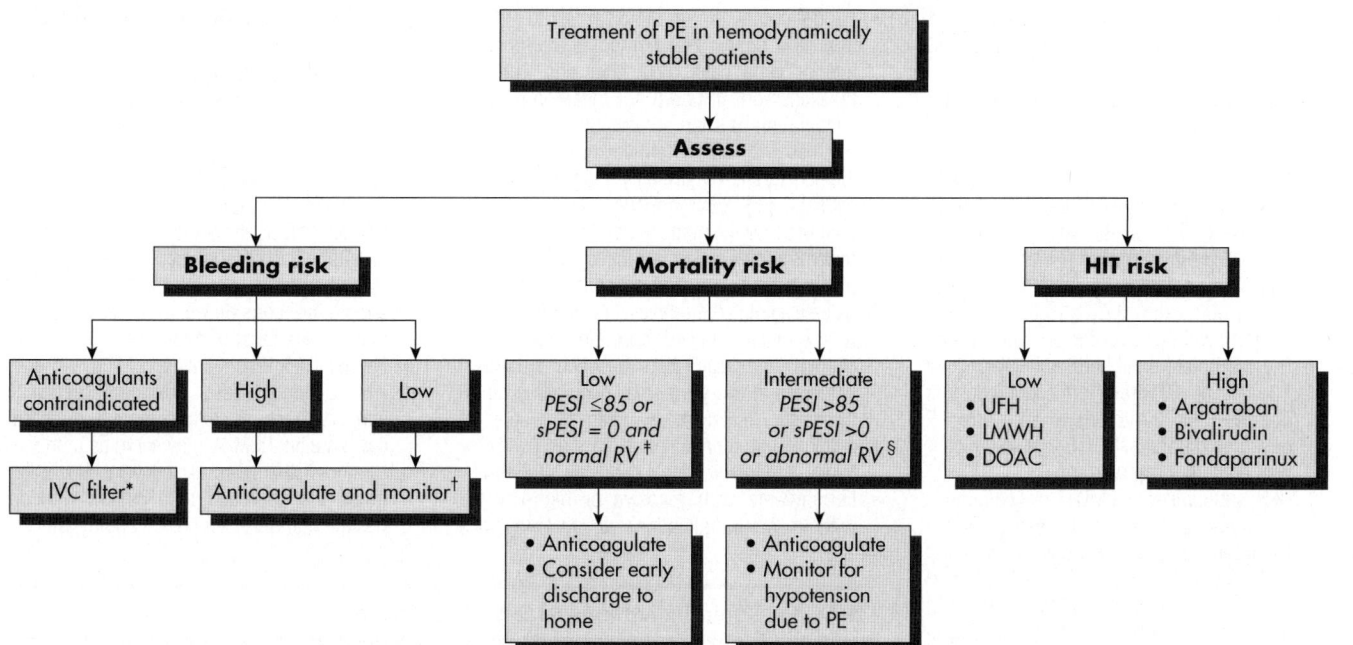

FIG. 7 Treatment of pulmonary embolism (PE) in hemodynamically stable patients. Decisions require assessment of bleeding risk, mortality risk, and risk of *heparin-induced thrombocytopenia* (HIT). *DOAC,* Direct oral anticoagulant; *LMWH,* low-molecular-weight heparin; *PESI,* pulmonary embolism severity index; *sPESI,* simplified PESI; *UFH,* unfractionated heparin. *Consider echocardiography to rule out pulmonary embolism in transit (if not already done) before *inferior vena cava* (IVC) filter placement. †See Table 3 for assessment of bleeding risk and recommendations for anticoagulation in patients at high risk for major bleeding. ‡No abnormality of the *right ventricle* (RV) is detected on initial diagnostic testing (e.g., computed tomography pulmonary angiography, echocardiography, troponin). §Obtain an echocardiogram and biomarker test (e.g., troponin or natriuretic peptides) if not done previously. (From Broaddus VC et al: *Murray & Nadel's textbook of respiratory medicine,* ed 7, Philadelphia, 2022, Elsevier.)

TABLE 3   Anticoagulant Treatments for Acute Pulmonary Embolism

Clinical	Initial*	Long-Term*	Extended*
Unstable	UFH† (5+ days)	DOAC or warfarin‡	DOAC or warfarin‡
High risk for bleed§	UFH† (5+ days)	DOAC or warfarin‡	DOAC or warfarin‡
Stable, cancer	Dalteparin 200 IU/kg/day‖ (1 mo)	Dalteparin 150 IU/kg/day	Dalteparin 150 IU/kg/day
Stable, cancer	Enoxaparin 1 mg/kg/bid‖	Enoxaparin 1 mg/kg/bid	Enoxaparin 1 mg/kg/bid
Stable, cancer	Enoxaparin 1 mg/kg bid (7 days)	Edoxaban 60 mg/day¶	Edoxaban 60 mg/day¶
Stable, no cancer	Apixaban 10 mg bid (7 days)	Apixaban 5 mg bid	Apixaban 2.5 mg bid
Stable, no cancer	Rivaroxaban 15 mg bid (21 days)	Rivaroxaban 20 mg qd	Rivaroxaban 20 mg qd
Stable, no cancer	Enoxaparin 1 mg/kg bid (5-7 days)	Dabigatran 150 mg bid	Dabigatran 150 mg bid

aPTT, Activated partial thromboplastin time; *bid,* twice daily; *DOAC,* direct oral anticoagulant; *HIT,* heparin-induced thrombocytopenia; *INR,* international normalized ratio; *LMWH,* low-molecular-weight heparin; *PE,* pulmonary embolism; *qd,* once daily; *UFH,* unfractionated heparin.
*Initial anticoagulant period from day 1 to day 5 to 7 of treatment, followed by long-term anticoagulation from day 5 to 7 to 3 mo, with anticoagulation extended beyond 3 mo when the risk of recurrent PE exceeds the risk of major bleeding.
†UFH dosed according to a standardized protocol; monitor for HIT.
‡If oral vitamin K antagonist (e.g., warfarin) treatment is planned, begin with 4 to 5 mg once daily and transition entirely to warfarin after all the following criteria are satisfied: (1) at least 5 days of UFH or LMWH; (2) INR >2.0 for two determinations; (3) PE symptoms and PE-related hypoxemia significantly improved, then monitor INR; and (4) adjust dose to maintain INR in range of 2.0 to 3.0.
§High risk for bleeding as defined by Kearon and colleagues. Some experts advise intravenous UFH 400 U/h without a bolus and observe for bleeding/hemostasis. After 6 h with hemostasis, increase to 600 U/h with continued observation. Keep aPTT <50 sec and anti–factor Xa level <0.5 U/ml. If hemostasis is maintained, then slowly increase UFH dose over 24 h to 800 U/h.
‖LMWHs accumulate with renal dysfunction. Titrate doses to produce anti–factor Xa levels of 0.4 to 0.85 U/ml and monitor for HIT.
¶Edoxaban 30 mg once daily for creatinine clearance 15 to 50 ml/min or body weight <60 kg.
From Broaddus VC et al: *Murray & Nadel's textbook of respiratory medicine,* ed 7, Philadelphia, 2022, Elsevier.

- For patients with low-risk or intermediate-low–risk PE, anticoagulation can be initiated right away with the direct oral anticoagulant (DOAC) rivaroxaban or apixaban (Table E4); subcutaneous low-molecular-weight heparin (LMWH) or fondaparinux; or IV unfractionated heparin (UFH). When oral anticoagulation is initiated, a DOAC is recommended over a vitamin K antagonist. Reversal agents for DOAC in patients with significant bleeding are summarized in Table E5.
  1. Oral rivaroxaban, a factor Xa inhibitor (15 mg bid for 3 wk, then 20 mg/day), has been studied as a treatment for DVT and PE, without prior parenteral therapy. For both DVT and PE, treatment with rivaroxaban alone was noninferior to treatment with LMWH followed by a vitamin K antagonist with the endpoint of recurrent venous thromboembolism (VTE). Use of rivaroxaban should be avoided in patients with severe renal failure.
  2. Apixaban, a factor Xa inhibitor (10 mg bid for a wk, followed by 5 mg bid), is approved for the treatment of acute PE based on the data in the AMPLIFY and AMPLIFY-EXT trials, in which apixaban

met its noninferiority mark in terms of efficacy and improved safety compared to warfarin.

3. Dabigatran, a direct thrombin inhibitor (150 mg bid following 5 to 10 days of parenteral anticoagulation), is approved for treatment of DVT and PE in patients with CrCl >30 ml/min based on data in the RE-COVER and RE-COVER II trials, in which it was noninferior to warfarin.

4. Edoxaban, a factor Xa inhibitor (60 mg/day, or 30 mg/day if CrCl 15 to 50 ml/min or body weight ≤60 kg or if on certain P-glycoprotein inhibitors, following 5 to 10 days of parenteral anticoagulation) is approved for treatment of DVT and PE based on the Hokusai VTE trial, in which it was noninferior to warfarin.

5. UFH, subcutaneous LMWH, or subcutaneous fondaparinux can be used for initial treatment for at least 5 days when used with warfarin, dabigatran, or edoxaban. If IV UFH is used, a bolus dose (80 U/kg) followed by a weight-based (18 U/kg/h) continuous infusion to achieve therapeutic anti–factor Xa (or aPTT) levels should be used. LMWH and fondaparinux should be avoided in patients with severe renal failure.

- For patients with intermediate-high risk or high-risk PE, anticoagulation with LMWH or IV UFH (if LMWH is contraindicated due to renal failure or bleeding concerns) is recommended and can be transitioned to an oral agent prior to hospital discharge.

- For patients with contraindications to anticoagulation, consider placement of a *temporary* inferior vena cava (IVC) filter and frequent reassessment of safety for initiation of anticoagulation as soon as possible.

- For patients with intermediate-high risk PE (demonstrating RV strain by imaging and myocardial injury with positive biomarkers), attempts should be made to risk stratify individual patients as this cohort may have multiple therapeutic options including anticoagulation alone, catheter-directed therapies, or systemic thrombolysis at a reduced dose. In high-volume centers, the distinction between treatment strategies in this group may occur via a multidisciplinary PERT team, often consisting of pulmonary and critical care, cardiology, hematology, and interventional radiology specialists.

- For patients with massive or high-risk PE without contraindications to thrombolytics (Box 1), thrombolytic agents (urokinase, tPA, streptokinase) provide rapid resolution of clots with some increased risk of major bleeding (up to 3% incidence of intracranial hemorrhage with systemic thrombolytic administration). The standard dosing for systemic thrombolytic is 100 mg of alteplase (synthetic tPA), administered over 2 h.

- In high-risk patients with absolute contraindications to thrombolytics, catheter-directed thrombectomy or surgical embolectomy should be considered at centers with the appropriate level of expertise.

- For high-risk PE patients in refractory shock or with cardiac arrest, additional mechanical support, such as extracorporeal membrane oxygenation (ECMO), may serve as a bridge to advanced therapies or recovery. Fig. 8 illustrates the approach to a patient with suspected pulmonary embolism and hypotension.

BOX 1 Contraindications to Systemic Thrombolysis

Absolute Contraindication to Systemic Thrombolytics TPA:
(Prior intracranial hemorrhage, known structural intracranial cerebrovascular disease, known malignant intracranial neoplasm, ischemic CVA within 3 mo, suspected aortic dissection, active bleeding, recent surgery encroaching on spinal canal or brain, recent significant closed head or facial trauma)

Relative Contraindication to Systemic Thrombolytics
(Age >75, current use of anticoagulation, pregnancy, noncompressible vascular punctures, CPR >10 min, recent internal bleeding, dementia, remote history of CVA [<3 mo], major surgery within 3 wk)

Modified from Parrillo JE, Dellinger RP: *Critical care medicine, principles of diagnosis and management in the adult,* ed 5, Philadelphia, 2019, Elsevier.

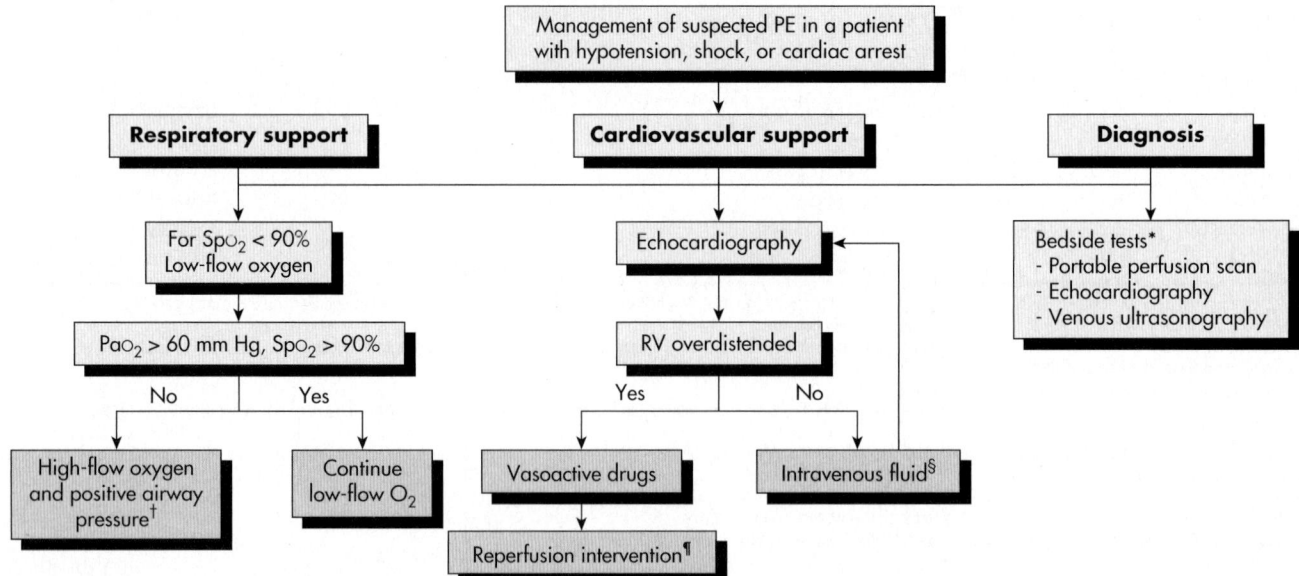

FIG. 8 Management of a patient with suspected pulmonary embolism and hypotension. Hypotension (defined by systolic blood pressure <90 mm Hg), shock, and cardiac arrest represent a life-threatening spectrum of hemodynamic compromise, and these conditions often limit diagnostic options. At times, thrombolysis must be tried even though the diagnosis of pulmonary embolism (PE) is unproven. *Pao₂*, arterial partial pressure of oxygen; *Spo₂*, oxygen saturation as measured by pulse oximetry. *A bedside echocardiogram can support the diagnosis of acute pulmonary embolism (e.g., McConnell's sign) or can provide another diagnosis (e.g., pericardial tamponade), and venous ultrasonography can show deep venous thrombosis. ¶Reperfusion interventions include thrombolysis, surgical embolectomy, and catheter-based treatment. The choice of reperfusion strategy depends on patient-related factors (e.g., bleeding risk and hemodynamic stability) and the institutional resources that can be mobilized (e.g., cardiovascular surgical team). †Suspect right-to-left shunting of venous blood when low-flow oxygen is insufficient. Provide high-flow oxygen. Assess the location of shunting (e.g., atelectasis and/or shunt through the foramen ovale). Provide positive airway pressure with mask ventilation and avoid intubation, if possible, for intrapulmonary shunt, and monitor and manage adverse effects of positive airway pressure on cardiac output. §Intravenous fluids should be titrated carefully to avoid overdistention of the right ventricle (RV). (From Broaddus VC et al: *Murray & Nadel's textbook of respiratory medicine,* ed 7, Philadelphia, 2022, Elsevier.)

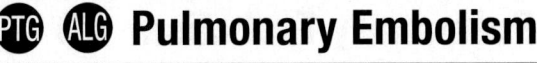

- Long-term treatment for PE not associated with malignancy can be carried out with a DOAC, LMWH, or warfarin.
- For PE associated with malignancy, DOACs or LMWH is recommended for long-term therapy.
- If thrombolytics and anticoagulants are contraindicated (e.g., GI bleeding, recent CNS surgery, recent trauma) or if the patient continues to have recurrent PE despite anticoagulation therapy, an IVC filter is recommended.
- In older adults, IVC filters are associated with higher 30-day and 1-yr mortality (11.6% and 20.5%, respectively, versus 9.3% and 13.4% in those who do not undergo filters); however, these patients tended to be sicker. An IVC filter is not advised for patients with recurrent VTE, unless risk for cardiopulmonary deterioration outweighs risk for IVC filter replacement.
- For PE occurring in the setting of pregnancy, LMWH is the treatment of choice. Dosing is based on early pregnancy weight. Planned delivery should be strongly considered to avoid complications with anticoagulation and spinal anesthesia. For a patient with a recent PE, LMWH should be switched to UFH approximately 36 h prior to planned delivery and the drip should be stopped 4 to 6 h prior to delivery, with a normal partial thromboplastin time (PTT) at the time of spinal anesthesia initiation. LMWH should be restarted as soon as it is deemed safe by the obstetrician. Duration of anticoagulation should be at least 3 mo total with at least 6 wk of anticoagulation after delivery. Breastfeeding mothers can be prescribed either LMWH or warfarin. Thrombolytic therapy should only be used for life-threatening PE during pregnancy due to the high risk of peri-partum and post-partum bleeding.
- For patients with antiphospholipid syndrome, Warfarin is recommended over DOAC therapy.[2]
- For patients with isolated subsegmental PE, rule proximal DVT out. If risk of recurrent venous thromboembolism (VTE) is low, surveillance is recommended over anticoagulation. If risk for recurrent VTE is high, anticoagulation is recommended.[2] However, a recent study revealed that overall, patients with subsegmental PE who did not have proximal DVT had a higher-than-expected rate of recurrent VTE.[3]

CHRONIC Rx
- Elimination of risk factors (see "Etiology").
- Duration of anticoagulation:
  1. Patients with PE attributed to a major transient risk factor that is no longer present should complete at least 3 mo of therapeutic anticoagulation.
  2. Patients with PE occurring in the setting of a minor transient risk factor should complete at least 6 mo of therapeutic anticoagulation. If bleeding risk is low and patient is tolerating therapy well, consider low-dose extended DOAC (apixaban 2.5 mg PO bid or rivaroxaban 10 mg/day) indefinitely.
  3. Patients with PE occurring in the setting of persistent risk factors such as hematologic thrombotic disorders, antiphospholipid syndrome, and ongoing active malignancy, therapeutic anticoagulation should continue during the presence of the persistent risk factor.
  4. For unprovoked PE, lifelong anticoagulation should be considered, as long as bleeding risk is low. If bleeding risk is moderate or high after a single unprovoked PE, stopping anticoagulation can be considered. Indefinite long-term anticoagulation should be used in patients with recurrent unprovoked PE.
  5. Recurrence risk calculators help inform the risk/benefit discussion with patients interested in avoiding indefinite anticoagulation. Such calculators include the modified Vienna prediction model, the HERDOO-2 score, the DASH model, and the Louzada score.
- Patients with unprovoked DVT/PE have a high rate of recurrent VTE. Longer durations of chronic anticoagulation after unprovoked DVT/PE result in lower rates of recurrent DVT/PE while on anticoagulation, but benefits are lost once anticoagulation is halted. The use of indefinite anticoagulation in select individuals with apparently unprovoked DVT/PE must be weighed against ongoing bleeding risk and other factors.
- Aspirin (100 mg/day) is superior to placebo in preventing recurrence of VTE in patients with a first-ever unprovoked VTE who completed 6 to 18 mo of oral anticoagulation. This suggests that aspirin could be offered as an alternative to oral anticoagulants for prevention of recurrent VTE in patients who refuse to or cannot continue oral anticoagulant therapy but who have a high risk of recurrent VTE.

DISPOSITION
- Mortality can be reduced to <10% by rapid and effective treatment. Stratification of risk of death associated with PE and severity-adjusted treatment is described in Table 6. Indicators of poor prognosis include hemodynamic instability/hypotension, signs of RV dysfunction, elevated BNP, elevated troponin, thrombus burden, coexisting DVT, and RV thrombus. The Pulmonary Embolism Severity Index (PESI) is summarized in Table 7.
- Risk stratification tools may be used to identify select low-risk patients who may be considered for home treatment.
- Mortality from recurrent PE is 8% with effective treatment and >30% in patients with untreated PE.

OUTPATIENT FOLLOW-UP
- Monitor for recurrent, persistent, or progressive symptoms after PE.
- Determine appropriate plan for type, dosing, duration, and monitoring of anticoagulation.
- Ensure appropriate evaluation of underlying factors contributing to the development of the

TABLE 6 Stratification of Risk of Death Associated With Pulmonary Embolism and Severity-Adjusted Treatment*

		RISK FACTOR		
Early Risk of Death	Shock or Hypotension (on Clinical Examination)	Right Ventricular Dysfunction (on Echocardiography or Multidetector CT)	Myocardial Injury (on Cardiac Troponin Testing)	Recommended Treatment
High	Present	Present[†]	NA[‡]	LMWH or unfractionated heparin plus thrombolysis or embolectomy
Intermediate-high	Absent	Both present		LMWH, fondaparinux, or UFH; consideration of reperfusion therapy
Intermediate-low	Absent	Only one present		LMWH, fondaparinux, or UFH; avoid early thrombolysis; monitor clinical status and right ventricular function
Low	Absent	Absent	Absent	DOAC, LMWH, fondaparinux, or UFH; consider outpatient treatment

CT, Computed tomography; *DOAC,* direct oral anticoagulant; *LMWH,* low-molecular-weight heparin; *RV,* right ventricle; *UFH,* unfractionated heparin.
*Adapted with modifications from the 2019 Guidelines on the Diagnosis and Management of Acute Pulmonary Embolism of the European Society of Cardiology. NA denotes not applicable.
[†]If RV function is normal on echocardiography, or if a CT scan shows no RV dilation in a patient with hemodynamic compromise and clinically suspected pulmonary embolism, an alternative diagnosis should be sought.
[‡]Troponin test results do not influence risk assessment or treatment in hemodynamically compromised patients with acute pulmonary embolism.
From Konstantinides S: Acute pulmonary embolism, *N Engl J Med* 359:2804-2813, 2008.

TABLE 7 Original and Simplified Pulmonary Embolism Severity Index (PESI)

Variable	Original PESI	Simplified PESI
Age	Age, in yr	1 (if age >80 yr)
Male sex	+10	—
History of cancer	+30	1
History of heart failure	+10	1 for either or both of these items
History of chronic lung disease	+10	
Pulse >110 beats/min	+20	1
Systolic blood pressure <100 mm Hg	+30	1
Respiratory rate >30 breaths/min	+20	—
Temperature <36° C	+20	—
Altered mental status	+60	—
Arterial oxyhemoglobin saturation (Sa O_2) <90%	+20	1

30-Day Mortality Risk Strata (Based on the Sum of Points)

Low-Risk Pesi	*Low-Risk Spesi*
Class I: <65 Points	0 Points
(event rate 95% CI, 0-1.6)	(event rate 95% CI, 0-2.1)
Class II: 66-85 Points	
(event rate 95% CI, 1.7-3.5)	

High-Risk Pesi	*High-Risk Spesi*
Class III: 86-105 Points	≥1 Point
(event rate 95% CI, 3.2-7.1)	(event rate 95% CI, 8.5-13.2)
Class IV: 106-125 Points	
(event rate 95% CI, 4.0-11.4)	
Class V: >125 Points	
(event rate 95% CI, 10.0-24.5)	

CI, Confidence interval; *PESI*, Pulmonary Embolism Severity Index; *sPESI*, simplified P.
From Vincent JL et al: *Textbook of critical care,* ed 7, Philadelphia, 2017, Elsevier.

PE, including hypercoagulable workup and age-appropriate cancer screening.
- Facilitate appropriate and expeditious removal of temporary IVC filters.
- Monitor for sequelae of PE, such as post-PE syndrome (functional and exercise limitation 1 yr post PE), chronic thromboembolic disease (CTED), and chronic thromboembolic pulmonary hypertension (CTEPH). Between 0.1% and 9% of patients who experience PE develop CTEPH, which can be a life-threatening disease if not identified and treated in a timely fashion.

REFERENCES

Available at eBooks.Health.Elsevier.com.

AUTHORS: **ALEXANDER SHERMAN, MD** and **SONIA JASUJA, MD**

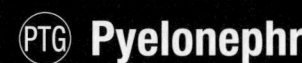

P

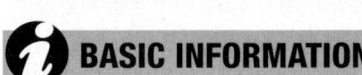 **BASIC INFORMATION**

DEFINITION

Pyelonephritis is an ascending infection of a bacterial pathogen that infects the renal pelvis and kidney. It primarily presents as a urinary tract infection (UTI) characterized by painful urination (dysuria) with associated flank pain/tenderness, nausea, vomiting, and/or fever. Older adults may also present with failure-to-thrive, unexplained anorexia, other organ system decompensation, or generalized deterioration.
Consists of two groups:

- *Uncomplicated:* Can be treated as an outpatient with oral (PO) antibiotics.
- *Complicated:* Inpatient treatment with intravenous (IV) antibiotics is required. Hospitalization is indicated for persistent vomiting, progression of uncomplicated UTI, suspected sepsis, immunosuppression, or urinary tract obstruction. This is a potentially life-threatening infection that can lead to renal parenchymal damage. Timely diagnosis and management can significantly impact patient outcomes.

SYNONYMS

Acute pyelonephritis
Pyonephrosis
Renal carbuncle
Lobar nephronia
Acute bacterial nephritis

ICD-10CM CODES	
N10	Acute pyelonephritis
N11	Chronic tubulo-interstitial nephritis
N11.0	Nonobstructive reflux-associated chronic pyelonephritis
N11.1	Chronic obstructive pyelonephritis
N11.8	Other chronic tubulo-interstitial nephritis
N11.9	Chronic tubulo-interstitial nephritis, unspecified
N12	Tubulo-interstitial nephritis, not specified as acute or chronic
N20.9	Calculus pyelonephritis

Use additional code (B95-B97) to identify infectious agent.

EPIDEMIOLOGY & DEMOGRAPHICS

INCIDENCE: Pyelonephritis is common in the U.S. with overall rates of 15 to 17 cases/10,000 women and 3 to 4 cases/10,000 men.[1] Pyelonephritis accounts for 9.1% to 31% of severe sepsis cases annually, depending on geographic area. Average annual mortality is 16.1%, ranging from 5% for patients <25 yr to 43% for ages >64 yr.

PREDOMINANT SEX: Women are 5 times more likely to be hospitalized than men until the age of 65 yr. In men beyond the age of 65 yr, the difference in prevalence narrows. Risk factors associated with pyelonephritis in healthy women are sexual intercourse (≥3 times wk over the previous 30 days), a new sex partner in the past year, use of spermicide, UTI during the

past 12 mo, mother with a history of UTI, diabetes mellitus, and urinary incontinence. Urinary tract obstruction is the most important risk factor for a complicated UTI.

PREDOMINANT AGE: Trimodal distribution described in female patients:
- Girls, ages 0 to 4 yr
- Women, ages 15 to 35 yr, especially if sexually active
- Gradual increase in frequency after age 50 yr, with peak incidence at 80 yr

Bimodal distribution in male patients:
- Boys, ages 0 to 4 yr
- Gradual increase in prevalence after age 35 yr, with peak incidence at 85 yr

GENETICS: Congenital urologic structural disorders associated with vesicoureteral reflux predispose individuals to infections at an early age (<5 yr) and produce renal scarring in most male and some female patients. Pyelonephritis may produce an Ask-Upmark kidney (segmental renal hypoplasia) that is found more often in young female patients with severe hypertension.

PHYSICAL FINDINGS & CLINICAL PRESENTATION

Diagnosis established by clinical presentation, history, and physical examination.

Pyelonephritis is suspected in cases of lower urinary tract symptoms (e.g., urinary frequency, urgency, and dysuria) and frequently accompanied by any of the following:[2]
- Fever, rigors, chills (fever may not be present in older adults or the immunosuppressed)
- Flank pain
- Hematuria: Gross hematuria occurs rarely in acute pyelonephritis and raises suspicion for acute cystitis, papillary necrosis, or lower genitourinary malignancy
- Toxic appearance
- Nausea and vomiting
- Headache
- Diarrhea

Physical examination may elicit costovertebral angle tenderness with flank pain, a nearly universal finding. Its absence suggests an alternative diagnosis. Patients presenting with nephrolithiasis/ureterolithiasis usually do not present with costovertebral angle tenderness. Usually, abdominal or suprapubic tenderness is present.[2]

ETIOLOGY

Ascending infections from intestinal bacteria that colonize the perineum and vulvae in women account for most infections. Less commonly, bacteria, viruses, or fungal pathogens may produce hematogenously induced pyelonephritis.
- Gram-negative bacilli cause >80% of cases (e.g., *Escherichia coli* and *Klebsiella* species).[3]
- Less common gram-negative bacteria may produce infection, particularly after urinary tract instrumentation (e.g., *Proteus mirabilis, Enterobacter, Serratia,* and *Pseudomonas* species).
- Resistant gram-negative organisms or fungi such as *Candida* may colonize indwelling catheters.

- Gram-positive organisms such as enterococci and rarely *Staphylococcus saprophyticus.*
- *Staphylococcus aureus* indicates hematogenous spread to the kidneys.
- Viruses generally are limited to the lower urinary tract.
- Urea-splitting organisms generate alkaline urine that fosters production of staghorn calculi. These stones may grow to large size and cause infection, obstruction, or both.

In older adults, *E. coli* is less common (60%). Patients with diabetes develop infections from *Klebsiella* species, *Enterobacteriaceae, Clostridioides* species, or *Candida* species.

During the past decade, community-acquired bacteria (particularly *E. coli*) that produce extended-spectrum beta-lactamases have emerged as a cause of acute pyelonephritis worldwide. The most common risk factors for these uropathogens include frequent visits to health care centers, recent use of antimicrobials (e.g., cephalosporins and fluoroquinolones), older age, immunosuppression, recurrent pyelonephritis, nephrolithiasis, and comorbid conditions such as diabetes mellitus and recurrent UTIs.

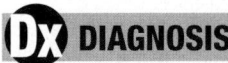 **DIAGNOSIS**

DIFFERENTIAL DIAGNOSIS

Differential diagnosis includes the following:
- Abdominal abscess
- Acute abdomen
- Appendicitis
- Basilar pleural process
- Diverticulitis
- Endometriosis
- Herpes zoster
- Lower rib fracture
- Metastatic disease
- Musculoskeletal disorders
- Nephrolithiasis
- Pancreatitis
- Papillary necrosis
- Pelvic inflammatory disease
- Prostatitis
- Pulmonary infarctions
- Renal corticomedullary necrosis
- Renal vein thrombosis
- Retroperitoneal hemorrhage or abscess
- Splenic abscess or infarct
- Urinary tract obstruction
- Vascular pathology

WORKUP

URINALYSIS: Obtained from and conducted on a clean-catch voided or catheterized specimen, if unable to void or cooperate. Dipstick and microscopic examination must be performed on a fresh specimen for preservation of formed elements (e.g., cells, casts, and microorganisms). Most cases demonstrate pyuria in association with a positive blood reaction and microhematuria. Leukocyte casts are generally of kidney origin but may be absent.

URINE CULTURE: Historically, clean, midstream cultures are obtained from all patients suspected of having acute pyelonephritis to guide antibiotic therapy. However, a clean-catch specimen may not be necessary. Recent evidence demonstrates no significant difference in the number of contaminated or unreliable culture results when urine is collected with or without preparatory cleansing. Obtain a catheterized urine sample if the patient is unable to void, uncooperative, or has an altered mental status. There is no difference in colony counts or organisms between catheterized and midstream voiding samples.

More than 95% of acute pyelonephritis cases exhibit $>10^5$ colony forming units of a single bacterium per milliliter of urine. However, it is important to obtain an accurate history regarding the timing of culture acquisition and prior antibiotic administration. A negative culture with classic clinical and radiologic findings does not rule out acute pyelonephritis, as shown by a prospective study, in which only 23.5% of 196 patients with clinical and radiologic evidence of acute pyelonephritis had demonstrated positive urine cultures.[4] A urine Gram stain may aid in the choice of empiric antimicrobial therapy pending urine culture. If gram-positive cocci are seen, consider *Enterococcus* species or *S. saprophyticus* as causative.

Posttreatment urinalysis and culture are unnecessary if symptomatic improvement occurs, but these studies should be obtained when symptomatic improvement does not occur after 2 or 3 days of antibiotic treatment, or if symptoms recur within 2 wk of treatment. Urinary tract imaging is recommended in such cases.

BLOOD CULTURES: Cultures are obtained from hospitalized patients but may not be routinely required in uncomplicated cases. Approximately 15% to 30% of patients with acute pyelonephritis are bacteremic.[1] Older adults and individuals with complicated acute pyelonephritis are more likely to develop bacteremia and sepsis.

Urine cultures yield a causative organism in nearly all cases of acute pyelonephritis. Therefore, a positive blood culture may be diagnostically redundant. However, in unclear cases, or when an alternative diagnosis to acute pyelonephritis is considered, blood cultures should be obtained.

IMAGING STUDIES

The primary imaging modalities used in patients with pyelonephritis are computed tomography (CT), MRI, and ultrasound.[5] Most uncomplicated cases of acute pyelonephritis do not require imaging studies unless symptoms do not improve, recurrence occurs, or if the patient has prolonged fever (>72 h) or persistent bacteremia. Abdominal radiographs (i.e., kidney, ureter, and bladder x-ray [KUB]) are of limited utility in acute pyelonephritis, unless staghorn calculi are present. Retrograde or antegrade pyelography may be helpful in severe obstruction that is not evident after noninvasive evaluations. Voiding cystourethrography demonstrates vesicoureteral reflux and generally is conducted routinely only in children.

Recommendations for radiologic tests:
- Healthy patients with uncomplicated pyelonephritis typically do not require radiologic

evaluation when therapeutic responses occur within 72 h of antibiotic therapy.
- If no response to therapy occurs within 72 h, abdominal CT is the study of choice.
- Patients with diabetes and immunocompromised patients should undergo precontrast and postcontrast abdominal and pelvic CT scans (Fig. E1) within 24 h of diagnosis when response to therapy is not prompt.
- Ultrasound (Fig. E2) is reserved for patients in whom exposure to contrast or radiation is considered hazardous. There is a high false-negative rate for renal abscess with ultrasound. In a prospective study of acute pyelonephritis that included 213 patients who had a CT/nuclear magnetic resonance (NMR) study done, 50 patients (23.5%) had a renal abscess, yet only 2 were detected by ultrasound.
- All other adults with complicated cases (i.e., history of stones or other urologic conditions, prior urologic surgery, repeated episodes of pyelonephritis) should be evaluated early by CT.
- Helical CT detects calculi with high sensitivity.
- Urologic imaging studies should be conducted in all young men and boys.

Although the risk of contrast-induced nephropathy has declined substantially, exert caution during contrast administration in patients with chronic kidney disease or for those taking metformin. When evaluating kidney function, diagnostic decision-making must include estimated glomerular filtration rate trends, not serum creatinine levels, especially in older adults with reduced muscle mass. Patients with acute pyelonephritis and acutely elevated baseline serum creatinine concentrations may warrant CT imaging to rule out obstruction. If the risk of radiocontrast media administration outweighs its benefits, consider MRI or retrograde or antegrade pyelography.

The purpose of imaging is to identify underlying structural abnormalities such as occult obstruction from a stone or abscess and serious complications such as emphysematous pyelonephritis (EPN). In a prospective study of 213 patients with acute pyelonephritis, there were no differences in frequency of fever, leukocytosis, C-reactive protein, pyuria, urine cultures, and duration of symptoms before hospitalization for positive or negative CT.[4] Accordingly, systematic CT or MRI is not required to exclude an anatomic abnormality. Such abnormalities cannot be predicted based on clinical, biochemical, or culture parameters.

EPN is a necrotizing infection that produces intraparenchymal kidney gas visualized by renal imaging. This disorder is associated with high mortality. Risk factors include diabetes mellitus and/or urinary tract obstruction. Gas-forming bacteria, most commonly *E. coli*, produce gas typically restricted within the Gerota fascia. Studies suggest an overall EPN mortality rate of 19%, reporting significant treatment success rates with percutaneous drainage and antibiotics (66%) and with nephrectomy (90%).[6] EPN must be differentiated from a renal abscess, which can also be associated with a gas collection. With drainage and antibiotic treatment, a renal abscess has a favorable prognosis.

LABORATORY TESTS

A basic metabolic profile and CBC with differential count are required to estimate kidney function in patients with suspected acute pyelonephritis. If the diagnosis is in doubt, other laboratory tests may be appropriate to clarify the differential diagnosis (e.g., lipase, transaminase, and β-hCG levels).

🆁🅇 TREATMENT

ACUTE GENERAL Rx

UNCOMPLICATED ACUTE PYELONEPHRITIS: Close outpatient follow-up is possible for patients with minimal GI symptoms and the ability to maintain fluid intake and oral medications. Prompt antibiotic therapy prevents progression of infection and must be initiated following acquisition of appropriate cultures. Begin empiric therapy based on risk of adverse effects, local community bacterial profiles, and resistance rates. Antibiotics are revised after urine culture results are available.

The concept of requiring long-term treatment for acute pyelonephritis has been questioned. Women with acute pyelonephritis were randomized to PO treatment with ciprofloxacin 500 mg bid for 7 days or 14 days, and 27% of these patients experienced bacteremia from *E. coli*. No differences in the cure rates were found (87% and 96%, respectively).[7]

Outpatient regimens:[8]
- Fluoroquinolones are preferred in communities where the local prevalence of resistant *E. coli* is ≤10%.
- Ciprofloxacin 500 mg PO bid or a single, 1000-mg/day PO dose in the extended-release form for 7 days.
- Levofloxacin 750 mg/day PO for 5 to 7 days.
- The initial dose may be administered intravenously (ciprofloxacin 400 mg or levofloxacin 500 mg).
- When a fluoroquinolone is contraindicated, alternative treatment with trimethoprim-sulfamethoxazole (TMP-SMX) 160/800 mg PO bid for 10 to 14 days may be administered if the pathogen is susceptible.
- Antibiotic options for acute uncomplicated pyelonephritis are summarized in Table 1.

Because of the high prevalence of resistance to PO beta-lactam antibiotics and TMP-SMX, these agents usually are reserved for cases in which susceptibility results are known. Additional factors (e.g., allergy history, potential drug–drug interactions, drug availability) may require empiric treatment with these agents before susceptibility testing results are known. In this circumstance, a long-acting, broad-spectrum parenteral drug (e.g., ceftriaxone 1 g or gentamicin 5 mg/kg) may be administered as a one-time dose or longer, until sensitivities of the organism are known. If the local prevalence of fluoroquinolone resistance to *E. coli* exceeds 10%, an initial IV dose of ceftriaxone or gentamicin is recommended, followed by an oral fluoroquinolone regimen.

Significant clinical improvement during appropriate empiric antibiotic therapy should occur within 48 to 72 h. If improvement does not occur, a complication of acute pyelonephritis or an alternative diagnosis such as an abscess, EPN, or an obstructing calculus should be considered. Any unexpected change in the clinical picture warrants immediate investigation with a CT scan.

COMPLICATED ACUTE PYELONEPHRITIS: Hospitalization is indicated for the following reasons:

- Toxic patients
- Complicated infections
- Diabetes or otherwise immunosuppressed
- Suspected bacteremia

Inpatient care includes supportive care, monitoring of culture results, adjustment of antibiotic regimen, and IV volume repletion as required. IV antibiotics are continued until defervescence occurs and clinical improvement occurs. Next, there is conversion to a PO antibiotic regimen for a total duration of 10 to 14 days.

- IV antibiotic options for more toxic patients pending cultures include[8] IV ceftriaxone (once daily), IV ciprofloxacin (400 mg bid), IV levofloxacin (500 mg/day), piperacillin/tazobactam (3.375 g IV qid), or carbapenems such as meropenem (500 mg IV tid).
- Ceftazidime 1 to 2 g IV tid, piperacillin/tazobactam, or carbapenems are optimal choices for *Pseudomonas* because of increasing ciprofloxacin resistance.
- Aminoglycosides are potentially nephrotoxic. These agents should be used only if no better alternative exists.
- Vancomycin 1 g IV bid, linezolid 600 mg IV or PO bid, or daptomycin 4 to 6 mg/kg/day IV for gram-positive cocci (e.g., enterococci, staphylococci).
- Ampicillin 1 to 2 g IV every 4 to 6 h for ampicillin-sensitive enterococci with aminoglycoside for synergy. Urinary obstruction is promptly drained by nephrostomy tube. Surgical drainage of abscess formation(s).

- Pregnant women with acute pyelonephritis are hospitalized and treated initially with a second- or third-generation cephalosporin.
- Antibiotic options for complicated pyelonephritis are summarized in Table 2.

RENAL ABSCESSES (RENAL CARBUNCLES): Cortical abscesses historically required surgical drainage; however, using current antibiotics is commonly sufficient for cure.[9]

- Semisynthetic penicillin, cephalosporin, fluoroquinolone, or vancomycin with guidance from culture and sensitivity results.
  1. Parenteral therapy for 10 to 14 days followed by PO therapy for 2 to 4 wk.
  2. Fever should resolve in 5 to 6 days and pain within 24 h.
  3. If no clinical response occurs within 48 h, percutaneous (preferred) or open drainage should be considered. More extreme measures are occasionally required, including enucleation or nephrectomy.

CORTICOMEDULLARY ABSCESSES:

- Parenteral therapy for at least 48 h is generally successful.
- May require incision and drainage and possibly, nephrectomy.
- If defervescence occurs, IV antibiotic treatment may be switched to complete a 2-wk course of PO antibiotic therapy.

PERINEPHRIC ABSCESSES:

- Serious complication with mortality in the 25% to 50% range.
- Lesions require early recognition, surgical drainage, and parenteral antibiotics (not adequate alone) to reduce mortality.
- Initial antibiotic therapy may include piperacillin-tazobactam, cefepime, or meropenem.
- Empiric therapy in the setting of *S. aureus* bacteremia includes nafcillin, oxacillin, cefazolin, or vancomycin (when methicillin-resistant *Staphylococcus aureus* is suspected).

- Tuberculosis and fungi are rare reported causes.
- Deterioration despite aggressive therapy.

CALCULI-RELATED INFECTIONS: Chronic pyelonephritis may lead to formation of struvite stones (magnesium ammonium phosphate stones). Formation requires infection with a urease-producing organism such as *Proteus* or *Klebsiella*. Symptoms directly attributable to struvite stones are uncommon. Typically, patients will present with symptoms of a UTI, mild flank pain, or hematuria. The stone may grow rapidly over a period of weeks to months if treatment is inadequate. Medical treatment for struvite stones is often ineffective and only indicated when surgery is not an option. The most common surgical intervention is percutaneous nephrolithotomy. Open surgery, once the gold standard, is now rarely used.

Surgical intervention is generally recommended in patients with newly discovered stones or in patients with a solitary kidney or two equally functioning kidneys. Nephrectomy is a reasonable option in patients with a nonfunctional kidney, particularly when chronic infection is present.

RENAL PAPILLARY NECROSIS:

- Admission for parenteral antibiotics:
  1. Initial therapy should cover *E. coli, Enterobacter, Proteus,* and *Klebsiella* species, pending culture results.
  2. For more serious infections, *Pseudomonas* and *Enterococcus* should also be covered.
  3. Empiric therapy agent options include the following:
     a. Aminoglycosides
     b. Cefotaxime
     c. Ceftriaxone
     d. Ceftazidime
     e. Cefepime
     f. Piperacillin-tazobactam
     g. Imipenem-cilastatin
     h. Meropenem
     i. Ciprofloxacin
  4. Continue parenteral therapy until fever and clinical symptoms improve.

Xanthogranulomatous pyelonephritis (XGP) is a rare variant of chronic pyelonephritis with destruction of renal parenchyma.

- Generally unilateral
- Affects women more than men from newborn to advanced age
- Usually in individuals with obstructing stones
- Presents with flank or abdominal pain, lower urinary tract symptoms, fever, palpable mass, gross hematuria, or weight loss
- Urine cultures commonly demonstrate *E. coli* or *Proteus mirabilis*
- CT is the diagnostic modality of choice and provides staging information
- Can be confused with malignancy
- Treatment is surgical nephrectomy

Chronic nephrolithiasis, especially in high-risk populations such as patients with diabetes or immunosuppressed patients, can predispose individuals and promote complicated infections leading to XGP and ENP. These are very rare disorders that are difficult to diagnose, and an unrecognized renal tumor can be hidden behind a suspected diagnosis of XGP and ENP.

TABLE 1   Antibiotic Options for Acute Uncomplicated Pyelonephritis

Antimicrobial	Dose (Oral)	Duration	Common Side Effects
Ciprofloxacin	500 mg bid	7 days	Gastrointestinal disturbance, headache, dizziness, tremors, restlessness, confusion, rash, *Candida* infections
Levofloxacin	750 mg once daily	5 days	Same as for ciprofloxacin
Trimethoprim-sulfamethoxazole	160/800 mg bid	10-14 days	Nausea, vomiting, anorexia, hypersensitivity reactions

From Walls RM et al: *Rosen's emergency medicine, concepts and clinical practice*, ed 10, Philadelphia, 2023, Elsevier.

TABLE 2   Antibiotic Options for Complicated Pyelonephritis

Antimicrobial	Dose (IV)	Common Side Effects
Cefepime	1-2 g every 8 h	Abdominal pain, muscle cramps, nausea, vomiting
Ceftriaxone	1 g every 24 h	Fever, cough, sore throat, fatigue
Piperacillin-tazobactam	3.375 g every 6 h	Diarrhea, nausea, vomiting, rash
Aztreonam	1 g every 8-12 h	Cough, abdominal pain, nausea, vomiting
Ciprofloxacin	400 mg every 12 h	GI disturbance, headache, dizziness, tremors, restlessness, confusion, rash, *Candida* infections
Levofloxacin	500 mg every 24 h	Same as for ciprofloxacin

From Walls RM et al: *Rosen's emergency medicine, concepts and clinical practice*, ed 10, Philadelphia, 2023, Elsevier.

CHRONIC Rx

- Repair underlying structural problems, especially when kidney function is compromised.
  1. Reflux
  2. Obstruction
  3. Suspect nephrolithiasis
- Avoid urinary catheters.

DISPOSITION

- If pyelonephritis is uncomplicated with no significant GI symptoms, treatment may be initiated on an outpatient basis with close monitoring of therapeutic response(s) in 48 to 72 h.
- If pyelonephritis is complicated and symptoms persist for >48 to 72 h, admission is recommended for any of the following: Significant GI symptoms that preclude PO therapy, pregnancy, urinary tract obstruction, suspected renal or perinephric abscess, bacterial sepsis, diabetes or other immuno-compromised states, recurrent or refractory pyelonephritis, or infection with unusual or antibiotic-resistant microorganisms.
- If sepsis is present, consider intensive care unit hospitalization.
- Acute pyelonephritis may be fatal when complications develop such as EPN (mortality rate, 20% to 80%), perinephric abscess (mortality rate, 20% to 50%), or sepsis syndrome (>25% overall mortality rate).
- Acute deterioration or nonresponse to conventional therapy may be due to a complication, resistant organism, or unrecognized comorbidity.
- Patients with diabetes and acute pyelonephritis are prone to bacteremia, longer hospital stays, and greater mortality. Those with diabetes should be considered to have complicated status.
- Patients older than 65 yr have greater mortality, septic shock, bedridden status, and immunosuppression. In men, mortality is also increased with the use of antibiotics in the previous month.

REFERRAL

- General surgery or urology for suspected abscess
- Infectious disease for resistant organisms and poor response to routine antibiotic therapy as outlined
- Urology to correct underlying urologic problems (e.g., reflux and hydronephrosis)
- Nephrology consult for renal dysfunction or nephrolithiasis evaluation
- Critical care monitoring, if intensive care unit admission is required

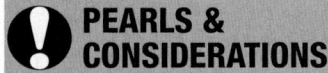

PEARLS & CONSIDERATIONS

- Consider acute pyelonephritis in patients with urinary symptoms, flank pain, and fever.
- Obtain a urinalysis and culture before starting empiric antibiotic therapy. Adjust treatment pending antibiotic sensitivity testing.
- Evaluate clinical response in 48 to 72 h during outpatient therapy. If there is no or delayed improvement, continue evaluation to rule out urinary tract obstruction.
- Pursue urology consultation in all cases of urinary tract obstruction or detection of urinary tract gas (e.g., emphysematous pyelonephritis).
- Treat all patients who have diabetes as having complicated acute pyelonephritis.

REFERENCES

Available at eBooks.Health.Elsevier.com.

RELATED CONTENT

Pyelonephritis (Patient Information)

AUTHORS: **JAMES P. REICHART, MD** and **NELSON KOPYT, DO**

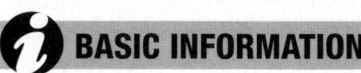 **BASIC INFORMATION**

DEFINITION

Raynaud phenomenon (RP) is a vasospastic disorder that causes an exaggerated response to cold temperatures and/or emotional stress, resulting in episodic digital ischemia. It presents as a cold-induced, symmetric, sharply demarcated white or blue discoloration of the distal fingers or toes, followed by erythema at a variable time after rewarming.

SYNONYMS

Primary Raynaud phenomenon or Raynaud disease
Secondary Raynaud phenomenon
RP

ICD-10CM CODES
I73.0	Raynaud syndrome
I73.00	Raynaud syndrome without gangrene
I73.01	Raynaud syndrome with gangrene

EPIDEMIOLOGY & DEMOGRAPHICS

- RP is classified clinically into primary or secondary forms and affects ~3% to 5% of the general population, 15% of children <12 yr, and <1% of adults >60 yr.
- Occurs more commonly in colder climates.
- Primary RP usually occurs between the ages of 12 and 25 yr.
- It is more likely to affect more women than men (4:1).
- 5% to 15% of patients with primary RP develop a secondary cause later in the course of the disease (mostly a connective tissue disorder).
- Secondary RP tends to begin after age 35 to 40 yr.
- Secondary RP occurs in >90% of patients with scleroderma and in ~30% of patients with systemic lupus erythematosus or Sjögren syndrome.

PHYSICAL FINDINGS & CLINICAL PRESENTATION

- The typical manifestation of RP is the biphasic color response of the digits to cold exposure and rewarming, which may or may not be accompanied by pain. RP most often affects the hand (Fig. E1).
  1. White (pallor) or blue (cyanotic) discoloration of the digit(s) resulting from vasospasm on cold or vibration exposure.
  2. Red (rubor) with or without pain and paresthesia when vasospasm resolves and blood returns to the digit.
- Color changes can sometimes be induced by placing the hand in an ice bath, although this is not recommended as a diagnostic maneuver because responses may be inconsistent even in patients with definite RP.
- Color changes are well delineated, symmetric, and usually bilateral, involving the fingers and toes. The index, middle, and ring fingers are commonly involved and the thumb infrequently;

however, if the thumb is involved, that suggests secondary causes of RP.
- Fingertips are most often involved, but feet, ears, nose, tongue, and nipples can also be affected.
- Patients with RP may exhibit a violaceous or reticular pattern of skin of arms and legs, sometimes with regular, unbroken circles (livedo reticularis).
- Duration of attacks can range from seconds to hours and averages 15 to 20 min.
- Chronic skin changes resulting from repeated attacks may include skin thickening and brittle nails. Ulcerations and, rarely, gangrene may occur.
- Physical examination should also include examination for symptoms associated with autoimmune disease, such as fever, rash, arthritis, dry eyes, dry mouth, myalgias, or cardiopulmonary abnormalities.

ETIOLOGY

- Primary RP also can be called idiopathic RP, primary Raynaud syndrome, or Raynaud disease. It occurs in the absence of any associated disease.
- With primary RP, the possibility that another first-degree family member is affected is reported as ~25%.
- Secondary RP is associated with an underlying pathologic condition or disorder, use of certain drugs, or related occupation. Secondary causes of RP are summarized in Box 1.

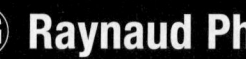 **DIAGNOSIS**

Clinical criteria:
- Definite RP: Repeated episodes of biphasic color change on cold exposure
- Possible RP: Uniphasic color changes plus numbness or paresthesia on cold exposure
- No RP: No color change on cold exposure
The suggested criteria for primary RP are:
- Symmetric attacks
- Absence of tissue necrosis, ulceration, gangrene, or peripheral vascular disease
- Absence of a secondary cause on the basis of a patient's history and general physical examination
- Negative nail-fold capillary examination
- Negative test for antinuclear antibody (ANA)
- Normal erythrocyte sedimentation rate (ESR)
Secondary RP is suggested by the following findings:
- Onset of symptoms after age 30 yr
- Male sex
- Episodes that are painful, asymmetric, or associated with ischemic skin lesions
- Clinical features suggestive of a connective-tissue disease
- Elevated specific autoantibody tests and ESR
- Evidence of microvascular disease on microscopy of nail-fold capillaries
- It is critical to differentiate primary and secondary RP because management is significantly different for the two conditions. Table 1 summarizes characteristics of primary and secondary RP

BOX 1 Secondary Causes of Raynaud Phenomenon

Rheumatologic
Systemic sclerosis (CREST syndrome)
Sjögren syndrome
Systemic lupus erythematosus
Ehlers-Danlos syndrome
Rheumatoid arthritis
Dermatomyositis
Polymyositis
Mixed connective tissue disease

Autoimmune
Reiter syndrome
Vasculitis (polyarteritis nodosa, Henoch-Schönlein purpura)
Antiphospholipid syndrome
Primary pulmonary hypertension

Endocrine
Hypothyroidism
Pheochromocytoma
Carcinoid

Infectious
Hepatitis B and C infection
Mycoplasma pneumonia

Medications
Cyclosporine
Ergotamine
Beta-blockers
Cytotoxic (bleomycin, cisplatin, vinblastine)
Bromocriptine
Nicotine
Cocaine
Sulfasalazine
Interferon-alpha and interferon-beta
Clonidine
Sympathomimetics
Estrogen in oral contraceptives
Caffeine

Occlusive Vascular
Arteriosclerosis
Vascular trauma (hypothenar hammer syndrome)
Buerger disease
Thoracic outlet syndrome
Thromboembolism

Hematologic Proliferative
Leukemia
Lymphoma
Polycythemia vera
Multiple myeloma
Disseminated intravascular coagulation
Cryoglobulinemia
Cold agglutinin disease

Neurologic
Migraines
Carpal tunnel syndrome
Polyneuropathy

Environmental
Emotional stress
Frostbite
Repetitive trauma or injuries to hand

Malignancy
Lung, stomach, small bowel
Paraneoplastic syndrome
Neurofibromatosis

From Cameron JL, Cameron AM: *Current surgical therapy,* ed 12, Philadelphia, 2017, Elsevier.

TABLE 1 Characteristics of Primary and Secondary Raynaud Phenomenon

Characteristic	Primary	Secondary
Age	Younger (<30 yr)	Older (>30 yr)
Gender preference	Female	Male (depending on secondary cause)
Incidence	Most common	Less common
Familial predisposition	Yes	Yes
Combination with other disease	No, idiopathic	Associated with systemic disease
Vascular defect	Functional dysregulation of autonomic nervous system	Structural changes in connective tissue or vessels
Associated signs	None	Arthritis, sclerodactyly, cardiopulmonary abnormality, rash
Frequency	Precipitated by stimuli	Periodic and stimuli trigger
Severity of symptoms	Long history of mild attacks	Severe and disabling pain
Distribution	Symmetric	Asymmetric
Duration	Self-limited	Need for additional treatment (pharmacologic, surgery)
Critical complications	None	Ischemia and ulcers
Capillaroscopy	Normal (symmetric, thin, and uniform)	Abnormal (dilated, irregular, elongated, and tortuous vessel)
Vascular examination	Normal pulses	Abnormal pulses
Erythrocyte sedimentation rate	Normal	Elevated
Serologic studies	Negative	Antinuclear antibody, autoantibodies
C-reactive protein	Normal	Elevated

From Cameron JL, Cameron AM: *Current surgical therapy*, ed 12, Philadelphia, 2017, Elsevier.

DIFFERENTIAL DIAGNOSIS

- Neurogenic thoracic outlet syndrome or carpal tunnel syndrome
- Frostbite or cold weather injury
- Medication reaction (ergotamine, chemotherapeutic agents)
- Atherosclerosis, thromboembolic disease
- Buerger disease, embolic disease
- Acrocyanosis
- Livedo reticularis
- Injury from repetitive motion

WORKUP

- An algorithm for the evaluation of RP is illustrated in Fig. 2.
- Once the diagnosis of RP is established, differentiating primary from secondary is helpful in treatment and prognosis.
- Patients who are younger when their symptoms occur, have a normal history and physical examination and normal nail-fold capillaries, and have no history of digital ischemic lesions can be considered as having primary RP. These patients can be monitored clinically without any further testing.
- If a secondary cause of RP is suspected, appropriate laboratory testing is recommended (see "Laboratory Tests"). Secondary RP has associated abnormal nail-fold microscopy.

LABORATORY TESTS

- CBC, serum electrolytes, blood urea nitrogen, creatinine, ESR, ANAs, venereal disease research laboratory (VDRL) antibody test, rheumatoid factor, and urinalysis should be included in the initial evaluation.
- If the history, physical examination, and initial laboratory tests suggest a possible secondary cause, specific serologic testing (e.g., anticentromere antibodies, anti-Scl 70, cryoglobulins, complement testing, and serum protein electrophoresis) may be indicated.
- Noninvasive vascular testing includes finger systolic blood pressures, segmental blood pressure measurements, cold recovery time (measure vasoconstrictor and vasodilator responses of finger to cold), fingertip thermography, and laser Doppler with thermal challenge (measures relative change in skin blood flow with ambient warming).

IMAGING STUDIES

- The diagnosis of RP should not be made on the basis of laboratory tests, and imaging studies should not replace a good history and physical examination.
- Duplex ultrasound can image the palmar arch and digital arteries for patency.
- Magnetic resonance angiography is useful for imaging larger arteries.
- Contrast angiography is the gold standard for arterial imaging.
- Nail-fold capillary microscopy can differentiate primary from secondary RP.
- Videomicroscopy and thermography are also useful for diagnosis of RP.

Rx TREATMENT

NONPHARMACOLOGIC THERAPY

- Avoid drugs that may precipitate RP (see "Etiology").
- Avoid cold exposure and sudden temperature shifts. Use warm gloves, hats, and garments during the winter months or before going into cold environments (e.g., air-conditioned rooms).
- Avoid stressful situations, and use relaxation techniques in preventing RP attacks.

ACUTE GENERAL Rx

- Acute measures to terminate an attack include rotating the arms in a windmill pattern, placing the hands under warm water or in a warm body fold such as the axilla, and the swing-arm maneuver.
- Medications are indicated in the treatment of RP if there are signs of critical ischemia or if the quality of life of the patient is affected to the degree that activities of normal living are no longer possible and preventive techniques do not work. Fig. 3 illustrates an approach to drug treatment of RP. Table 2 summarizes drugs commonly used in RP.

CHRONIC Rx

- Dihydropyridine calcium channel blockers (e.g., nifedipine, amlodipine, felodipine, nisoldipine, isradipine) are the most effective pharmacologic treatment for RP and are the drugs of choice. Amlodipine or nifedipine are commonly used.
- Amlodipine dosage ranges from 2.5 to 10 mg/day. Nifedipine is most often prescribed at a dose of 10 to 20 mg 30 min before cold exposure. If symptoms occur with long duration, nifedipine XL 30 to 180 mg PO qd is often effective.
- When calcium channel blockers do not appropriately control symptoms, phosphodiesterase inhibitors (cilostazol, pentoxifylline, and sildenafil) can be added or substituted. Sildenafil can be started at a dosage of 20 mg/day. Angiotensin 2 receptor antagonists (losartan), and selective serotonin reuptake inhibitors (fluoxetine) have also been used with some limited success.
- Some potential therapeutic options include direct vasodilators such as nitroprusside, hydralazine, papaverine, minoxidil, niacin, and griseofulvin. Topical 1% nitroglycerin or topical l-arginine, ethyl nicotinate, hexyl nicotinate, thurfyl salicylate may also be useful, particularly if low blood pressure is a concern.
- Alpha receptor antagonists such as prazosin and phenoxybenzamine have also shown some effectiveness in treating RP.
- The prostaglandins, including inhaled iloprost, intravenous (IV) epoprostenol, alprostadil, and tadalafil, may be promising in severe RP. However, additional experience and controlled studies are needed.
- Antioxidants like zinc gluconate have been used to decrease tissue damage.
- *N*-Acetylcysteine and probucol have been shown to lead to improvement in RP.
- Anticoagulation with IV unfractionated heparin or subcutaneous low–molecular-weight heparin and addition of aspirin can be considered during the acute phase of a severe ischemic event. Aspirin (81 mg/day) therapy can be considered in all patients with secondary RP with a history of ischemic ulcers or thrombotic events; however, caution should

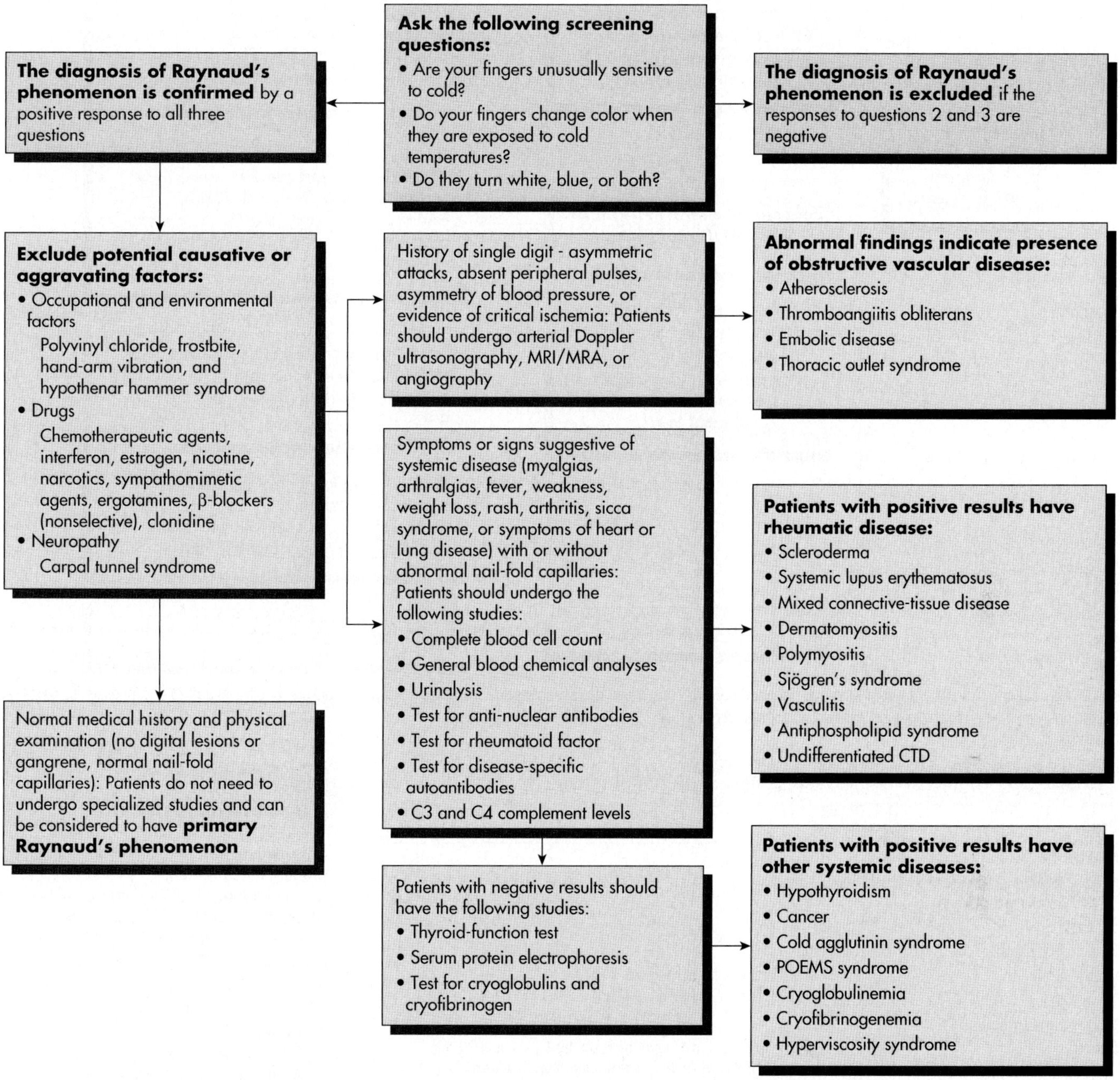

Diseases
and Disorders

I

The diagnosis of Raynaud's phenomenon is confirmed by a positive response to all three questions	**Ask the following screening questions:** • Are your fingers unusually sensitive to cold? • Do your fingers change color when they are exposed to cold temperatures? • Do they turn white, blue, or both?	**The diagnosis of Raynaud's phenomenon is excluded** if the responses to questions 2 and 3 are negative

Exclude potential causative or aggravating factors:
• Occupational and environmental factors
  Polyvinyl chloride, frostbite, hand-arm vibration, and hypothenar hammer syndrome
• Drugs
  Chemotherapeutic agents, interferon, estrogen, nicotine, narcotics, sympathomimetic agents, ergotamines, β-blockers (nonselective), clonidine
• Neuropathy
  Carpal tunnel syndrome

History of single digit - asymmetric attacks, absent peripheral pulses, asymmetry of blood pressure, or evidence of critical ischemia: Patients should undergo arterial Doppler ultrasonography, MRI/MRA, or angiography

Abnormal findings indicate presence of obstructive vascular disease:
• Atherosclerosis
• Thromboangiitis obliterans
• Embolic disease
• Thoracic outlet syndrome

Symptoms or signs suggestive of systemic disease (myalgias, arthralgias, fever, weakness, weight loss, rash, arthritis, sicca syndrome, or symptoms of heart or lung disease) with or without abnormal nail-fold capillaries: Patients should undergo the following studies:
• Complete blood cell count
• General blood chemical analyses
• Urinalysis
• Test for anti-nuclear antibodies
• Test for rheumatoid factor
• Test for disease-specific autoantibodies
• C3 and C4 complement levels

Patients with positive results have rheumatic disease:
• Scleroderma
• Systemic lupus erythematosus
• Mixed connective-tissue disease
• Dermatomyositis
• Polymyositis
• Sjögren's syndrome
• Vasculitis
• Antiphospholipid syndrome
• Undifferentiated CTD

Normal medical history and physical examination (no digital lesions or gangrene, normal nail-fold capillaries): Patients do not need to undergo specialized studies and can be considered to have **primary Raynaud's phenomenon**

Patients with negative results should have the following studies:
• Thyroid-function test
• Serum protein electrophoresis
• Test for cryoglobulins and cryofibrinogen

Patients with positive results have other systemic diseases:
• Hypothyroidism
• Cancer
• Cold agglutinin syndrome
• POEMS syndrome
• Cryoglobulinemia
• Cryofibrinogenemia
• Hyperviscosity syndrome

FIG. 2 Approach to diagnosis of Raynaud phenomenon. *CTD,* Connective tissue disease; *MRA,* magnetic resonance angiography; *POEMS,* polyneuropathy, organomegaly, endocrinopathy, monoclonal gammopathy, and skin changes. (From Firestein GS et al: *Firestein & Kelley's textbook of rheumatology,* ed 11, Philadelphia, 2021, Elsevier.)

be exercised because aspirin can theoretically worsen vasospasm by the inhibition of prostacyclin. Long-term anticoagulation with heparin or warfarin is not recommended unless there is evidence of a hypercoagulable state.
• Bypass surgery can be performed for severe RP associated with reconstructible arterial occlusive disease.
• Sympathectomy is available for unreconstructible occlusive disease or pure vasospastic disease refractory to medical treatment.
• Microsurgical revascularization of the hand and digital reconstruction may improve digital vascular perfusion and heal digital ulcers

when proximal arterial occlusion is associated with digital vasospasm.
• Ischemic digital lesions should be treated with topical antibiotics and daily cleansing with soap and water. Digits that progress to dry gangrene should be permitted to undergo autoamputation. Surgical amputation is limited for intractable pain or deep tissue infection.

DISPOSITION
The prognosis of patients with RP depends on the etiology.
• Primary RP is fairly benign, usually remaining stable and controlled with nonpharmacologic medical treatment.

• Remission of primary RP can occur spontaneously.
• Patients with secondary RP, specifically those with scleroderma, CREST syndrome, or thromboangiitis obliterans, may develop severe ischemic digits with ulceration, gangrene, and autoamputation.
• Box E2 summarizes features suggestive of progression of Raynaud phenomenon.

REFERRAL
• Rheumatology consult is indicated if secondary collagen vascular disease is diagnosed.
• Vascular surgery consult is indicated if ulcers, gangrene, or threatened digit loss is noted.

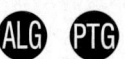

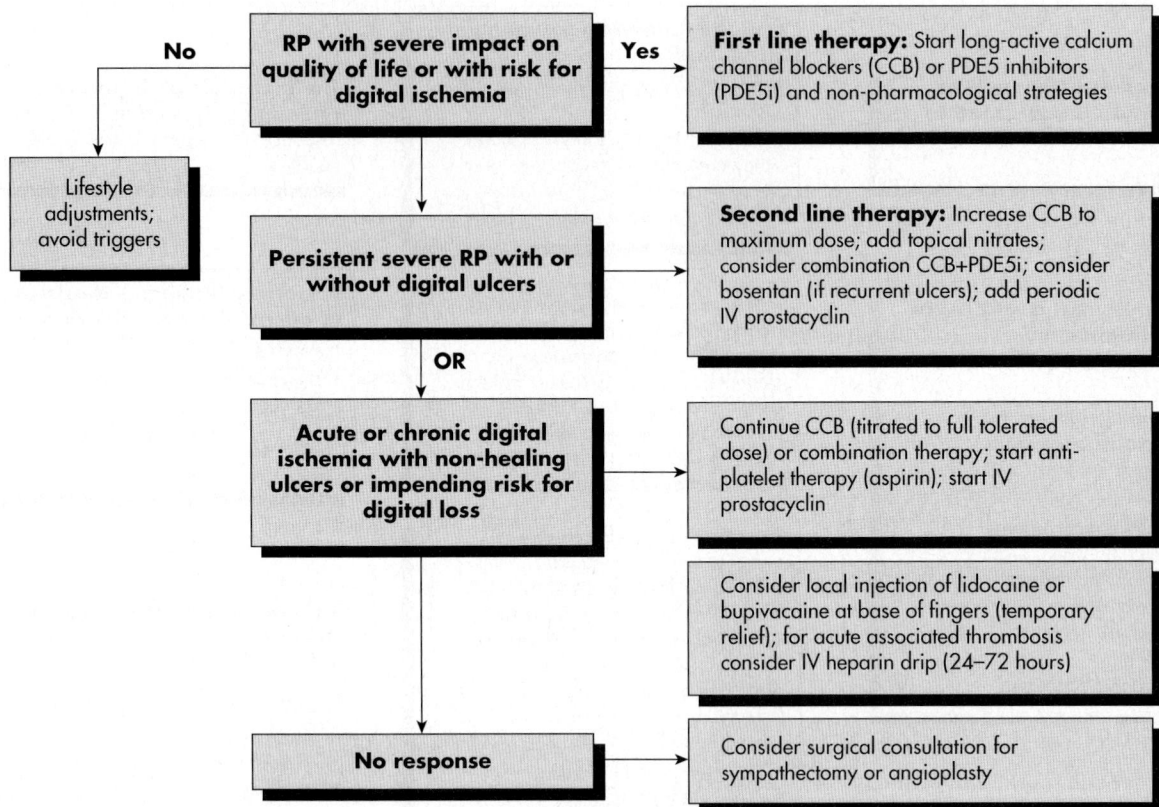

FIG. 3 Approach to drug treatment of Raynaud phenomenon (RP) and acute digital ischemia. *CCB,* Calcium channel blockers; *IV,* intravenous; *PDE-5,* phosphodiesterase-5. (From Firestein GS et al: *Firestein & Kelley's textbook of rheumatology,* ed 11, Philadelphia, 2021, Elsevier.)

TABLE 2	Drugs Commonly Used in Raynaud Phenomenon

Drug	Dosage
Oral	
Nifedipine (or other long-acting calcium channel blocker)	10-20 mg bid or tid
Sildenafil	25-50 mg tid
Naftidrofuryl oxalate	100-200 mg tid
Inositol nicotinate	1 g tid or inositol nicotinate forte 1.5 g bid
Thymoxamine	40-80 mg qid (stop after 2 wk if no response)
Intravenous Infusion	
Iloprost	Start infusion (peripheral line) at 1 μg/h; increase by 1 μg every 30 min until reach maximum tolerable dose (maximum dose should not be greater than 3 μg/h). Infusions are given over 6 h each day for 3-7 days on each occasion
Prostaglandin E_1	60 μg in 250-ml physiologic infusion over 3 h daily for 5-6 days. This could be repeated every 6 wk to cover the cold weather in severe cases, especially if associated with critical ischemia or digital ulceration, and should be given via a central line

bid, Twice a day; *qid,* four times a day; *tid,* three times a day.
From Hochberg MC et al: *Rheumatology,* ed 8, Philadelphia, 2023, Elsevier.

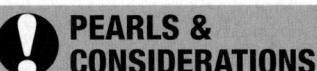 **PEARLS & CONSIDERATIONS**

- Most patients with RP can be managed by a primary care provider.
- It is important to differentiate primary from secondary forms. Secondary forms may become manifest as far out as 10 yr from the diagnosis of RP. It is important to take immediate action during an attack, and patients are encouraged to:
  1. Keep warm
  2. Not use tobacco products
  3. Avoid aggravating medications
  4. Control stress
  5. Exercise
  6. Follow up with a physician

RELATED CONTENT

Raynaud Phenomenon (Patient Information)
Clinical

AUTHOR: **FRED F. FERRI, MD**

R

I

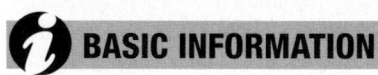 **BASIC INFORMATION**

DEFINITION

Renal cell carcinoma (RCC) is a primary carcinoma originating in the renal parenchyma from the malignant transformation of proximal renal tubular epithelial cells. The majority of renal cell cancers are of clear cell type; 15% are papillary tumors, and 10% are chromophobe cancers.

SYNONYMS

RCC
Hypernephroma
Renal cell adenocarcinoma

ICD-10CM CODES
C64.9	Malignant neoplasm of kidney, except renal pelvis
C64.1	Malignant neoplasm of right kidney, except renal pelvis
C64.2	Malignant neoplasm of left kidney, except renal pelvis
C64.9	Malignant neoplasm of unspecified kidney, except renal pelvis
C65.9	Malignant neoplasm of renal pelvis

EPIDEMIOLOGY & DEMOGRAPHICS

INCIDENCE: In 2023, there were an estimated 81,800 new cases and 14,890 deaths in the U.S.[1] Two percent of cases of renal cancer are associated with inherited syndromes.
PREDOMINANT SEX: Male:female ratio is ~2:1.
PREDOMINANT AGE: Peak incidence is at age 50 to 70 yr.
RISK FACTORS:
- Cigarette smoking
- Obesity
- Phenacetin-containing analgesics
- Asbestos, lead, Thorotrast, and chromium exposure
- Gasoline and other petroleum products
- Role of the *VHL* gene on chromosome 3

PHYSICAL FINDINGS & CLINICAL PRESENTATION

- Patients are often asymptomatic until they have advanced disease.
- Paraneoplastic syndromes such as hypercalcemia, erythrocytosis, anemia, and hepatic dysfunction (Stauffer syndrome) may occur with RCC.
- The classic triad of flank pain, hematuria, and a palpable abdominal mass currently represents an unusual presentation.
- Current manifesting findings in RCC include:

Hematuria	50%-60%
Elevated erythrocyte sedimentation rate	50%-60%
Abdominal mass	25%-45%
Anemia	20%-40%
Flank pain	35%-40%
Hypertension	20%-40%
Weight loss	30%-35%

Fever	5%-15%
Hepatic dysfunction	10%-15%
Classic triad (hematuria, abdominal mass, flank pain)	5%-10%
Hypercalcemia	3%-6%
Erythrocytosis	3%-4%
Varicocele	2%-3%

ETIOLOGY

Hereditary forms:
- Familial renal carcinoma
- Renal carcinoma associated with von Hippel-Lindau disease
- Hereditary papillary RCC

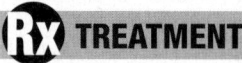 **DIAGNOSIS**

DIFFERENTIAL DIAGNOSIS

- Transitional cell carcinomas of the renal pelvis (8% of all renal cancers)
- Wilms tumor
- Other primary renal carcinomas and sarcomas
- Renal cysts
- Retroperitoneal tumors

WORKUP

LABORATORY TESTS:
- Urinalysis: Hematuria
- CBC: Anemia or erythrocytosis
- Chemistry panel: Renal failure and electrolyte issues, including hypercalcemia
- Liver function tests: Hepatic dysfunction with elevated alkaline phosphatase, prolonged prothrombin time, and hypoalbuminemia

IMAGING STUDIES

Nearly 50% of renal cancers are now detected because a renal mass is incidentally detected on radiographic evaluation.
- Renal ultrasound
- Abdominal computed tomography (CT) scan with contrast (Fig. E1)
- CT-guided biopsy is generally not necessary for diagnosis of solid masses >4 cm (high likelihood of cancer)
- MRI
- Renal arteriogram
- Intravenous pyelography

STAGING

See Table 1.

TREATMENT

NONMETASTATIC CANCERS

- Surgery:
  1. Surgical nephrectomy (open and laparoscopic approaches) is the only effective management for stages I, II, and some stage III tumors. Although radical nephrectomy had been a standard treatment, partial nephrectomy is associated with improved survival and is appropriate for patients with neoplasms <4 cm that are not adjacent to the renal pelvis or invading the vena cava.[2]
  2. Laparoscopic robotic-assisted nephrectomy has been adopted in multiple centers, primarily for nephron-sparing surgery in the case of tumors <4 cm. Advantages

TABLE 1 TNM Staging of Renal Cell Carcinomas as per the AJCC Eighth Edition

T Stage	Description
T_x	Tumor cannot be assessed
T_1: Tumor ≤7 cm, limited to kidney	T_{1a}: Tumor <4 cmT_{1b}: Tumor ≥4 cm to ≤7 cm
T_2: Tumor >7 cm, limited to kidney	T_{2a}: Tumor >7 cm but ≤10 cm T_{2b}: Tumor >10 cm
T_3: Tumor extending into major veins or perinephric tissue but not into ipsilateral adrenal gland or beyond Gerota fascia	T_{3a}: Tumor extends to renal vein/branches or invades perirenal and/or renal sinus fatT_{3b}: Tumor extends into IVC below diaphragmT_{3c}: Tumor extends into IVC above diaphragm or wall of IVC
T_4	Tumor invades beyond Gerota fascia (including contiguous extension into ipsilateral adrenal gland)
N stage	Description
N_x	Regional nodes cannot be assessed
N_1	No regional nodes involved
N_2	Metastasis in regional node(s)
M stage	Description
M_0	No distant metastases
M_1	Distant metastasis present
Stage	TNM grouping
I	$T_1N_0M_0$
II	$T_2N_0M_0$
III	$T_3N_0M_0$ or $T_{1-3}N_1M_0$
IV	$T_4N_{any}M_{any}$ or $T_{any}N_{any}M_1$

AJCC, American Joint Committee on Cancer; *IVC*, intravenous cholangiography; *TNM*, tumor, node, metastases.

include less blood loss, minimal effects on renal function, and similar oncologic outcomes. Disadvantages include increased costs and limitations in tumor size and locations eligible for robotic surgery.

3. Various forms of partial nephrectomy may be available for patients with bilateral cancers or with a solitary kidney.

- Systemic therapy:
  1. Adjuvant targeted therapy with the tyrosine kinase inhibitor sunitinib modestly improves survival in resected high-risk cases but has not been readily adopted into clinical practice.
  2. Adjuvant immunotherapy with pembrolizumab after resection in high-risk patients has demonstrated improvement in disease-free survival and overall survival.[3] Adjuvant nivolumab has also demonstrated a benefit in disease-free survival in this setting.

METASTATIC CANCERS

- Surgery:
  1. Cytoreductive nephrectomy in patients with metastatic RCC in the preimmunotherapy era improved survival in patients compared to cytokine therapy alone based on randomized trials data. However, recent results from the randomized Clinical Trial to Assess the Importance of Nephrectomy (CARMENA) demonstrated no benefit for intermediate- and poor-risk patients in the setting of modern tyrosine kinase inhibitor (sunitinib) therapy. Additional trial data are awaited to assess the role of nephrectomy in favorable-risk patients and with the use of neoadjuvant tyrosine kinase inhibitor therapy.
- Angioinfarction, cryoablation, or radiotherapy (for palliation).
- Systemic therapy:
  1. Risk stratification using the International mRCC Database Consortium Prognostic Model (IMDC score) is the initial step in planning systemic therapy.[4] Patients are categorized into favorable risk (no risk factors), intermediate risk (one or two risk factors), or poor risk (three or more risk factors) status according to the following risk factors:
     a. Karnofsky performance status <80%
     b. Time from diagnosis to treatment <1 yr
     c. Hemoglobin concentration < lower limit of normal
     d. Serum calcium > upper limit of normal
     e. Neutrophil count > upper limit of normal
     f. Platelet count > upper limit of normal

2. Until recently, monotherapy with multitargeted kinase inhibitors was the initial treatment option for metastatic cancers followed by the use of second-line therapy with mTOR inhibitors. However, the use of immunotherapy (including dual immunotherapy combinations) or immunotherapy/targeted therapy combinations is now established as initial therapy in this setting:[5]
   a. Immune checkpoint inhibitors: These have demonstrated efficacy in both treatment-naïve and previously treated patients. Dual immunotherapy with ipilimumab plus nivolumab has superior efficacy in treatment-naïve patients with IMDC intermediate- and poor-risk status.
   b. Combination tyrosine kinase inhibitors and immune checkpoint inhibitors: The upfront use of combination regimens (axitinib plus pembrolizumab, axitinib plus avelumab, cabozantinib plus nivolumab, lenvatinib plus pembrolizumab, atezolizumab plus cabozantinib) all have demonstrated superiority compared to monotherapy with tyrosine kinase inhibitors.
   c. Tyrosine kinase inhibitors: In patients with advanced disease, therapy with the multitargeted inhibitors (axitinib, sunitinib, pazopanib, cabozantinib, lenvatinib, tivozanib, and sorafenib) followed by mTOR kinase inhibitors (everolimus and temsirolimus) can be used as sequential therapeutic options. The combination of lenvatinib plus everolimus also has been approved in second-line therapy after demonstrating improved outcomes compared to single-agent everolimus use. Most responses with these agents are typically partial or stable disease, and relapse is the norm.
   d. With a view to improve outcomes further among patients with previously untreated, advanced RCC with intermediate or poor prognostic risk, treatment with triplet combination of cabozantinib plus nivolumab and ipilimumab results in significantly longer progression-free survival than treatment with dual immunotherapy alone.[6] However, severe adverse events were more common in the triple therapy group while overall survival results are awaited.

- Cytokine therapy: High-dose interleukin-2 (IL-2) therapy has a 10% to 15% response

rate, which is often durable and associated with long-term survival in highly selected patients with excellent performance status. Severe toxicities associated with this therapy have limited the use of this approach.

PROGNOSIS

The 5-yr overall survival rate among patients with kidney cancer has increased from 57% in 1987 to 76% in 2015. According to a SEER database report, the outcomes of surgically treated patients is shown in the following table though it does not reflect gains made in the immunotherapy era:

Stage	5-Yr Survival (%)
Localized	90-95
Regional	70
Distant	13
Total	76

REFERRAL

- To urologist for staging and surgery
- To medical oncologist if metastatic disease is present

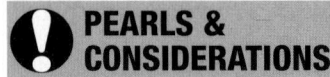

PEARLS & CONSIDERATIONS

- Patients should be considered for nephron-sparing surgery in case of smaller tumors (<4 cm).
- Laparoscopic robotic-assisted surgery is used for standard nephron-sparing surgery routinely; it is used for central tumors and tumors >4 cm in some experienced centers.
- Adjuvant use of tyrosine kinase inhibitors has showed mixed results and is not approved in this setting. An intergroup study showed no survival benefit, whereas a smaller study limited to high-risk patients showed a progression-free survival benefit.

REFERENCES

Available at eBooks.Health.Elsevier.com.

RELATED CONTENT

Kidney Cancer (Patient Information)

AUTHOR: **BHARTI RATHORE, MD**

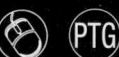

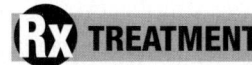 BASIC INFORMATION

DEFINITION

Restless legs syndrome (RLS) is an awake phenomenon consisting of an urge to move legs, usually associated with feeling of discomfort in legs. Symptoms typically are present only at rest and at least partially improve with movement. Additionally, symptoms are usually worse at night. RLS can result in sleep disturbance with associated executive dysfunction and depression.

CLASSIFICATION

- Primary RLS is without any obvious cause, with no associated disorder.
- Secondary RLS results from other medical conditions.

SYNONYMS

RLS
Wittmaack-Ekbom syndrome

ICD-10CM CODE
G25.81 Restless legs syndrome

EPIDEMIOLOGY & DEMOGRAPHICS

PREVALENCE: Average prevalence rate is 1% to 29%. Prevalence estimates in Europe are around 10%, and 0.1% to 12% in East Asian population.[1-3]

PREDOMINANT SEX: Early-onset RLS is more common in females, with female:male ratio of 2:1.[1-5]

PREDOMINANT AGE: Prevalence of RLS increases with age, and it is more commonly seen in the elderly population[2] but can occur in children.

PEAK PREVALENCE: 10% in persons aged 30 to 79 and 19% in persons aged 80 or above.[1-5]

RISK FACTORS:
- Iron deficiency anemia (IDA): 25% to 35%
- Pregnancy: Increases in severity and prevalence with each passing trimester
- End-stage renal disease (ESRD) requiring hemodialysis: Improves with transplant but not dialysis
- Peripheral neuropathy: 5% to 54% of patients with peripheral neuropathy also have symptoms of RLS[6]
- Many other neurologic diseases such as Parkinson disease, multiple sclerosis, and myelopathy increase risk as do mood disorders, other inflammatory disease, and cardiovascular disease
- Medications: Antidepressants (mirtazapine, venlafaxine), dopamine antagonists (neuroleptics and antinausea agents), and antihistamines[2]

GENETICS: Genetic basis of RLS has been reported, particularly in early-onset RLS.
- Autosomal dominant disorder
- Common among first-degree relatives
- RLS associated with certain sequences in chromosomes 6p, 12q, 14q, 9p, 20p, 2p, 16p
- These include polymorphisms in the genes *BTBD9, MEIS1,* and *MAP2K5/SKOR1*[2]

PHYSICAL FINDINGS & CLINICAL PRESENTATION

- Wide spectrum of severity of clinical manifestations has been reported in RLS.[1,2]
- Most common symptom is unpleasant sensations in legs ("dysesthesias"), reported as discomfort or "creepy-crawling" sensations, mostly bilateral. Arms are occasionally involved.
- There is an extreme urge to move legs, and relief is sustained as long as the movement continues.
- Symptoms are worse at night or evening. Best sleep is usually early in the morning.

ETIOLOGY

The exact etiology remains unknown. Pharmacologic, pathologic, physiologic, and imaging studies have implicated dopaminergic pathways, brain iron metabolism, and endogenous opioid pathways. Drugs that may be associated with RLS are summarized in Table E1.

DIAGNOSIS

DIFFERENTIAL DIAGNOSIS

- Periodic limb movement disorder
- Nocturnal leg cramps
- Leg ischemia/pain
- Leg arthritis
- Painful peripheral neuropathy
- Akathisia
- Positional discomfort
- Volitional movements, foot tapping, leg rocking

WORKUP

- Diagnosis of RLS is based on established clinical criteria (Table 2) and normal neurologic examination.
- Testing is done to determine possible cause of secondary RLS. All patients with RLS should be screened for iron deficiency because iron supplementation in patients with iron deficiency may resolve the symptoms.[1,2]
- Polysomnography with leg activity monitors to determine limb movements during sleep, which occur in 80% of people with RLS but are also common in the general population and not necessary for diagnosis.[2]
- Nerve conduction studies and electromyography for associated peripheral neuropathy given the high prevalence.[5]

LABORATORY TESTS

- Iron status: Serum ferritin, total iron binding capacity, percent saturation
- CBC for anemia in case of iron deficiency
- Metabolic panel: Blood urea nitrogen and serum creatinine for renal insufficiency

IMAGING STUDIES

No imaging studies are required for diagnosis of RLS.

TREATMENT

NONPHARMACOLOGIC THERAPY[5]

- Avoid caffeine, alcohol, and nicotine, which can exacerbate RLS.

- Review and adjust medications that may exacerbate or cause RLS (selective serotonin reuptake inhibitors, dopamine blocking agents, stimulants).
- Physical and mental activity.
- Good sleep hygiene.
- Monitoring for depression as RLS has an elevated suicide risk. Bupropion may be the best agent for depression in RLS due to lack of dopamine effects.
- Mild symptoms are associated with resolution or quick response to treatment.[7]

CHRONIC Rx

Once the diagnosis of RLS is considered based on clinical criteria as mentioned in Table 2 and causes impairment of quality of life, an anticonvulsant (gabapentin, enacarbil, or pregabalin) or dopamine agonist (bromocriptine, pramipexole, or ropinirole) should be started at low dose and then gradually tapered depending on tolerance.

Treatment options (Table 3) for RLS include:
- Anticonvulsants, such as gabapentin, have been shown to be effective in multiple studies. Gabapentin, enacarbil, and pregabalin are now considered first-line agents in the treatment of RLS. These agents do not cause iatrogenic worsening (augmentation) of RLS with long-term treatment. Carbamazepine and valproic acid likely are efficacious.[8]
- Dopaminergic agents such as levodopa and dopamine agonists help to ameliorate RLS symptoms, decrease periodic limb movements, and improve sleep. Dopamine agonists, pramipexole and ropinirole, can be first-line agents in the treatment of RLS but often cause augmentation of RLS with long-term treatment.
- Rotigotine patch (Neupro) is also effective and FDA approved for moderate to severe RLS.[8]
- Opiates, mostly methadone, are generally reserved as last line of treatment.[9]
- Iron replacement with vitamin C should be started concurrently in case of iron deficiency. Iron supplements are indicated even with low-normal ferritin levels (<75 ng/ml).[8,9] Sometimes intravenous iron replacement is used especially if no symptom improvement on oral supplementation or severe symptoms.

REFERRAL

Refer to neurologist if diagnosis is uncertain or an underlying disorder is suspected.

REFERENCES

Available at eBooks.Health.Elsevier.com.

RELATED CONTENT

Restless Legs Syndrome (Patient Information)

AUTHOR: **COREY ELAM GOLDSMITH, MD, FAAN**

TABLE 2 Diagnostic Criteria for Restless Legs Syndrome

Minimal Criteria
- Desire to move the legs usually associated with paresthesias
- Motor restlessness, as characterized by floor pacing, leg rubbing, stretching, and flexing
- Worse at rest, with relief by activity
- Worse at night

Additional Criteria
- Sleep disturbances, as difficulty in sleep onset and maintaining sleep, daytime fatigue, or somnolence
- Involuntary movements, as periodic limb or leg movements in sleep and periodic or aperiodic limb movements while awake
- Neurologic examination is normal in idiopathic restless legs syndrome
- Clinical course may begin at any age but most severe in middle and older age
- Family history suggests autosomal dominant mode of inheritance in one third of the cases

From Stiasny K et al: Clinical symptomatology and treatment of restless legs syndrome and periodic limb movement disorder, *Sleep Med Rev* 6(4):253-265, 2002.

TABLE 3 Management of Restless Legs Syndrome

Agent and Daily Dosage	Side Effects	Countermeasures
Step 1: $\alpha2\delta$ Agents		
First-line treatment, particularly if sleep disturbance, pain, or anxiety is present		
Gabapentin enacarbil, 300-600 mg Pregabalin, 50-450 mg[a] Gabapentin, 100-1800 mg[a]	Dizziness	Reduce dose and add alternative medication class as needed. If fall risk, then discontinue and change to alternative medication class.
	Somnolence, daytime fatigue	Reduce dose and add alternative medication class as needed. If significant, discontinue and change to alternative medication class.
	Tolerance	Discontinue, take drug holiday with return to medication. Switch to alternate medication class.
	Weight gain	Reduce dose and add alternative medication class as needed. If significant, discontinue and change to alternative medication class.
Step 2: Dopamine Agonists		
Alternative first-line treatment if depression is present and dose kept low.		
Pramipexole, 0.125-0.5 mg[a] (0.75 mg in Europe)	Nausea and orthostatic hypotension	Slowly increase dosage or use domperidone if available (10-30 mg).
Ropinirole, 0.5-4.0 mg[a] Rotigotine, 1-3 mg/24 h	Insomnia	Add or switch to $\alpha2\delta$ agent. Use a small dose of benzodiazepines in association with dopamine agonists.
	Daytime fatigue and somnolence	Reduce dosage or discontinue dopamine agonists.
	Compulsive or impulsive behavior	Reduce dose and add alternative medication class as needed. If significant, discontinue and change to alternative medication class.
	Tolerance	Discontinue and switch to longer-acting dopamine agonist or alternative medication class.
	Augmentation	Discontinue and switch to alternative medication class or longer-acting dopamine agonist.
Step 3: Dopamine Precursors		
Useful for intermittent treatment, such as twice a week		
Levodopa-benserazide or levodopa-carbidopa (regular or slow release), 100/25 or 200/50 mg[b]	Same as for dopamine agonists	See "Countermeasures" for dopamine agonists.
	Morning rebound or augmentation of restless legs syndrome in early evening	Use small extra dose of levodopa during daytime or reduce dosage or combine levodopa with dopamine agonists or benzodiazepines or discontinue levodopa (if severe and persistent).
	Augmentation	Do not use daily. Discontinue and switch to dopamine agonists or a nondopamine medication.
Benzodiazepines		
Useful for sleep promotion		
Clonazepam, 0.5-2.0 mg[c]	Daytime somnolence	Reduce dosage.
Temazepam, 15-30 mg[c] Nitrazepam, 5-10 mg[a]	Tolerance	Take drug holiday for 2 wk then return to lower dosage.
Opiates		
Second-line treatment		
Oxycodone-naloxone, 10/5 to 40/20 mg/day	Constipation	Use for symptom treatment.
Methadone, 2.5-20 mg Oxycodone, 5-40 mg	Dependency	Take a drug holiday. Discontinue and switch to alternative medication.
Oral Iron		
Always consider if serum iron ≤75 mcg/L *or* transferrin saturation ≤17%		
Ferrous sulfate, 650 mg (325 mg with vitamin C, 100 mg twice a day)	Constipation, stomach upset and pain	Reduce dose, discontinue, take with food.
	Diarrhea, nausea, vomiting	Reduce dose, discontinue, take with food.

[a]One hour before onset of symptoms in the evening or 1-2 h before bedtime if symptoms are not present in the evening.
[b]Considered most appropriate for prn dosing not more than 3×/wk rather than daily use.
[c]Before bedtime usually to promote sleep with restless legs syndrome.
From Kryger M et al: *Principles and practice of sleep medicine*, ed 6, Philadelphia, 2017, Elsevier.

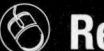

BASIC INFORMATION

DEFINITION

- Retinal vein occlusions (RVOs) are defined as retinal vascular disorders caused by complete or partial obstruction of a retinal vein characterized by tortuosity and dilation of the retinal veins with secondary intraretinal hemorrhages, macular edema, and retinal ischemia (including cotton-wool spots and retinal neovascularization).
- Central retinal vein occlusion (CRVO) is defined by obstruction at or posterior to the optic nerve head.
- Branch retinal vein occlusion (BRVO) is defined by partial or complete obstruction at a tributary or branch of the central retinal vein.

SYNONYMS

RVO
CRVO
BRVO

ICD 10-CM CODES

H34.819	Central retinal vein occlusion, unspecified eye
H34.811	Central retinal vein occlusion, right eye
H34.812	Central retinal vein occlusion, left eye
H34.813	Central retinal vein occlusion, bilateral
H34.8130	Central retinal vein occlusion, bilateral, with macular edema
H34.8131	Central retinal vein occlusion, bilateral, with retinal neovascularization
H34.831	Tributary (branch) retinal vein occlusion, right eye
H34.832	Tributary (branch) retinal vein occlusion, left eye
H34.8190	Central retinal vein occlusion, unspecified eye, with macular edema
H34.8111	Central retinal vein occlusion, right eye, with retinal neovascularization
H34.8121	Central retinal vein occlusion, left eye, with retinal neovascularization
H348191	Central retinal vein occlusion, unspecified eye, with retinal neovascularization
H34.833	Tributary (branch) retinal vein occlusion, bilateral
H34.8311	Tributary (branch) retinal vein occlusion, right eye, with retinal neovascularization
H34.8321	Tributary (branch) retinal vein occlusion, left eye, with retinal neovascularization
H34.8331	Tributary (branch) retinal vein occlusion, bilateral, with retinal neovascularization
H34.8391	Tributary (branch) retinal vein occlusion, unspecified eye, with retinal neovascularization
H34.8330	Tributary (branch) retinal vein occlusion, bilateral, with macular edema
H34.8390	Tributary (branch) retinal vein occlusion, unspecified eye, with macular edema
H34.8392	Tributary (branch) retinal vein occlusion, unspecified eye, stable
H34.9	Unspecified retinal vascular occlusion
H34.8110	Central retinal vein occlusion, right eye, with macular edema
H34.233	Retinal artery branch occlusion, bilateral Bilateral branch retinal artery occlusion; Occlusion of bilateral branch retinal arteries
H34.8310	Tributary (branch) retinal vein occlusion, right eye, with macular edema
H34.8320	Tributary (branch) retinal vein occlusion, left eye, with macular edema

EPIDEMIOLOGY & DEMOGRAPHICS

INCIDENCE: BRVO is 6 to 7 times more prevalent than CRVO.
PREDOMINANT SEX & AGE:
- Over 50% of cases occur in patients older than 65.
- Population-based studies report the prevalence of CRVO at <0.1% to 0.4%.

PEAK INCIDENCE: 0.7% incidence for patients ages 49 to 60 yr and 4.6% incidence for those older than 80 yr.
RISK FACTORS:
- Risk factors for BRVO and CRVO differ.
- A prior RVO is a risk for RVO in the other eye.
- Age: Most important factor for both BRVO and CRVO; majority of cases occur in elderly patients.
- Glaucoma: Open-angle glaucoma is the most common ocular factor predisposing to CRVO.
Systemic conditions that impair vascular health:
- Hypertension: A common finding is recently diagnosed or uncontrolled hypertension. This major risk factor is more prevalent in patients with BRVO than in those with CRVO. More than 64% of RVO patients in the age group over 50 yr are hypertensive, and it is a predominant finding in recurrent RVO (88%).
- Diabetes mellitus: Diabetes mellitus is significantly associated with CRVO.
- Hyperlipidemia: This is the predominant risk factor for RVO in patients under 50 yr old. It is also found in up to 50% of older patients.
- Coagulation defects:
  1. Consider workup only in atypical situations such as patients with family history of clotting at a young age (deep venous thrombosis, pulmonary emboli, or multiple spontaneous abortions), personal history of clotting, or bilateral simultaneous RVO.
  2. Thrombophilia: Factor V Leiden mutation increases the risk of RVO by about 50% to 60%, whereas other prothrombotic

defects (i.e., prothrombin G21201A and deficiencies of antithrombin and of protein C or S) are not associated with RVO.
- The role of lupus anticoagulant and anticardiolipin antibodies in RVO is uncertain. The relationship between fibrinolysis and RVO is not strong. Since RVO occurs at arteriovenous crossings, where the blood flow is locally turbulent, changes in platelet reactivity due to polymorphisms in the platelet receptors may be important.
- Hyperhomocysteinemia.
- High body mass index (BMI) and smoking have also been implicated in RVO, but these associations are less consistent.
- High plasma viscosity (e.g., leukemia or multiple myeloma).
- Waldenström macroglobulinemia.
- Myelofibrosis.
- Systemic inflammatory conditions (Behçet disease, polyarteritis nodosa, sarcoidosis, granulomatosis with polyangiitis, Goodpasture syndrome).

PHYSICAL FINDINGS & CLINICAL PRESENTATION

Visual acuity (VA) is reduced compared with unaffected eye, but it varies by occlusion severity and site. Ischemic central retinal vein and branch retinal vein occlusions are associated with worse visual acuity (20/400 or worse) than nonischemic central and branch retinal vein occlusions (better than 20/200). In BRVO, visual function and recovery of vision are correlated with thickness of the central macula, and that is correlated with the integrity of the inner and outer segments of the photoreceptors in the fovea.

Pupillary reflexes may be affected. Patients may or may not show relative afferent pupillary defect (Marcus Gunn pupil), depending on severity.
- Fundoscopic exam may reveal:
  1. Optic disc edema (Fig. E1) in central retinal vein occlusion (may or may not be present in branch retinal vein occlusion) and macular edema
  2. Increased dilation and tortuosity of retinal veins
  3. Central retinal vein occlusion: All retinal veins are dilated and tortuous
  4. Branch retinal vein occlusion: Only affected branch is dilated and tortuous
  5. Widespread deep and superficial hemorrhages (dot-and-blot and flame shaped)
  6. Cotton-wool spots
  7. Neovascularization in advanced cases
- Findings outside fundus may include neovascularization of iris (rubeosis iridis) and/or anterior chamber (iridocorneal) angle (in advanced cases)
Presentation of retinal vein occlusion is variable:
- Clinically ischemic CRVO is generally painless and may present with unilateral loss of vision on awakening.
- Nonischemic central retinal vein occlusion may be asymptomatic and be discovered on routine ophthalmic examination. It most commonly presents with gradual development of

central visual blurring that is usually worse on awakening in the morning with a variable degree of improvement after a few hours or in the afternoon. VA is impaired to a variable degree dependent on severity; eyes with initially good VA tend to have a good prognosis and vice versa; initial VA in the middle range (6/30 to 6/60) is an unreliable predictor of outcome. VA worse than 6/60 commonly indicates that substantial ischemia is present. In cases that do not become ischemic, vision returns to normal or near normal in about 50%.

- In some instances, patients may complain of transient visual blurring before a constant diminution of vision followed by permanent central scotoma.
- Branch retinal vein occlusion usually presents with a sudden painless decrease in visual acuity or a visual field defect. It may also be asymptomatic and discovered on routine ophthalmic examination.

ETIOLOGY
- Compression of retinal vein wall or obstruction by thrombosis.
- In BRVO, arteriolosclerotic thickening of a branch retinal arteriole is associated with compression of a venule at an arteriovenous crossing point, exacerbated by sharing an adventitial sheath. This leads to secondary changes that include endothelial cell loss, turbulent flow, and thrombus formation. Similarly, the central retinal vein and artery possess a common sheath at crossing points posterior to the lamina cribrosa so that atherosclerotic changes of the artery may precipitate CRVO. Hematologic prothrombotic factors are thought to be important in a minority, amplifying an atherosclerotic anatomic predisposition. Once venous occlusion has occurred, elevation of venous and capillary pressure with stagnation of blood flow ensues, resulting in retinal hypoxia, which in turn results in damage to the capillary endothelial cells, extravasation of blood constituents, and liberation of mediators such as vascular endothelial growth factor (VEGF).

Dx DIAGNOSIS

DIFFERENTIAL DIAGNOSIS (IN ORDER OF IMPORTANCE)
- Ocular ischemic syndrome
- Diabetic retinopathy
- Chronic hypertensive retinopathy
- Papilledema

WORKUP
- History and physical examination, including direct funduscopy and measurement of visual acuity by Snellen chart; both eyes are examined
- Slit-lamp biomicroscopy (directed or performed by ophthalmologist): Indicated in all cases when history and physical examination findings lead to suspicion of retinal vein occlusion
- Ophthalmologist-performed assessment

- Evaluation for afferent pupillary defect that corresponds with level of ischemia and risk of neovascular complications
- Measure intraocular pressure before dilated indirect funduscopic examination
- Careful slit-lamp iris examination for neovascularization before dilation
- Dilated binocular funduscopic examination
- Visual field findings may help differentiate vein occlusion findings from ischemic optic neuropathy
- Optical coherence tomography (OCT): Indicated to detect presence and quantify severity of macular edema
- OCT angiography may help in quantifying capillary nonperfusion and foveal ischemia
- Fluorescein angiography (Figs. E2 and E3):
  1. Valuable to help determine location and extent of venous occlusion and to differentiate ischemic from nonischemic retinal vein occlusion, as well as extent of macular edema
  2. Also helps differentiate neovascularization from collateral vessels that form with chronicity
  3. May help guide laser treatment
- Electroretinography: May be used to differentiate ischemic from nonischemic retinal vein occlusion but not used widely

LABORATORY TESTS
In general, there are no clear guidelines for systemic testing in these patients unless the RVO is bilateral, in a person younger than age 40 yr, or there is medical history and/or systemic symptoms to warrant a workup.
- CBC, sedimentation rate, C-reactive protein
- FBS, HBA1c
- Lipid panel
- Evaluation for hypercoagulable state when suspecting thrombotic occlusion: Factor V Leyden, lupus anticoagulant, antithrombin II, international normalization ratio, activated partial thromboplastin time, anticardiolipin antibodies, anti–beta 2-glycoprotein-I antibodies
- Plasma homocysteine level
- Antinuclear antibody test

IMAGING STUDIES
- Optical coherence tomography: Provides visualization of central macula to detect edema and to measure macular thickness
- Fluorescein angiography: Indicated for suspected retinal vein occlusion to determine site of occlusion, perfusion status of retina, presence of neovascularization, and presence of macular edema

Rx TREATMENT

NONPHARMACOLOGIC THERAPY
- Control of systemic risk factors: Investigating major systemic risk factors is essential as patients with RVO are at increased risk of cardiovascular disease, cerebrovascular accidents, and all-cause mortality. Addressing these as appropriate is critical, and as well as conferring systemic benefit this may also

reduce the risk of the recurrence of retinal vein occlusion.
  1. Lifestyle changes to correct hypertension, hyperglycemia, hyperlipidemia, hyperhomocysteinemia
  2. Avoidance of tobacco products
  3. Reduction of obesity to maintain normal BMI

ACUTE GENERAL Rx
VEGF-A plays a major role in the ocular complications of retinal vein occlusions and therefore treatment with intravitreal antivascular endothelial growth factor agents is very effective and has become the standard of care for reducing macular edema and ocular neovascularization.

MEDICATIONS:
- Vascular endothelial growth factor inhibitors
  1. Ranibizumab
  2. Aflibercept
  3. Bevacizumab
  4. Injected monthly but interval may be extended in some patients; over 50% will have persistent macular edema and require ongoing injections more than 5 yr after onset
- Corticosteroids
  1. Typically a second- or third-line treatment after exhaustion of all anti-VEGF drugs
  2. Reduce pro–permeability factors that cause macular edema in RVO
  3. Glaucoma may influence risk-benefit assessment of intravitreal steroids, as corticosteroids can produce a rise in intraocular pressure
  4. Promotes cataract so more commonly used in pseudophakic eyes
- Intravitreal dexamethasone: Dexamethasone intraocular implant; sustained delivery formulation (containing 0.7 mg dexamethasone in a solid polymer delivery system) approved for injection every 6 mo
- Intravitreal triamcinolone: Triamcinolone acetonide suspension for injection; adults: 1 to 4 mg (100 μL of 40 mg/ml suspension) injected into the vitreous cavity

PROCEDURES: LASER PHOTOCOAGULATION:
- Two types of laser treatment may be performed: Focal macular laser photocoagulation to treat macular edema when the edema is noncentral (more common in BRVO) and panretinal photocoagulation to ischemic peripheral retina to manage neovascular complications, particularly iris neovascularization (more common in CRVO).
- Peripheral scatter photocoagulation is indicated for BRVO with retinal or disc neovascularization to lessen the risk of vitreous hemorrhage.
- The 2019 guidelines from the European Society of Retina Specialists suggest that focal laser photocoagulation should be considered only as a second-line treatment of macular edema secondary to BRVO. Intravitreal anti-VEGF injections remain the standard of care for center-involving macular edema for any RVO.

CHRONIC Rx
Monitor monthly during initial therapy using slit-lamp examination to detect neovascularization

and to assess iris and anterior chamber (iridocorneal) angle.

- Subsequent follow-up plan depends on degree of ischemia found:
  1. In patients with significant ischemia (i.e., more than 10 disc areas of retinal capillary nonperfusion), evaluate every 3 mo for 1 yr; then continue monitoring for another year, with frequency determined by the treatment given and any complications experienced.
  2. In patients without significant ischemia, evaluate at 3 mo and at 6 mo, and then as determined by the treatment given and any complications experienced.
  3. In patients receiving injection therapy for macular edema, follow up more frequently (e.g., every 4 wk).

DISPOSITION

- In patients with nonischemic (well-perfused) CRVO and good visual acuity on presentation (better than 20/40, corrected), prognosis is favorable; however, 30% of eyes with initially nonischemic CRVO may convert to ischemic subtype.
- According to the Central Vein Occlusion Study:
  1. 20% of eyes with visual acuity at presentation of 20/50 to 20/200 improve spontaneously to 20/50
  2. 80% of patients with initial visual acuity worse than 20/200 have no improvement or have deterioration
- The ischemic form accounts for 20% of all cases of CRVO. The most concerning complication of CRVO is neovascular glaucoma, occurring in approximately 50% of ischemic cases.
- Prognosis is guarded in cases that have progressed to macular ischemia as demonstrated by fluorescein angiography.
- In BRVO with perfused periphery and normal visual acuity, prognosis is favorable, even with monitoring alone and no therapy.
- Because visual disturbance is often mild to moderate at first but progresses with no treatment, prognosis is generally improved with early diagnosis and treatment.
- CRVO is usually a unilateral disease; however, the annual risk of developing a CRVO in the other eye is approximately 1% per yr, and it is estimated that up to 7% of persons with CRVO may develop CRVO in the other eye within 5 yr of onset in the first eye.

REFERRAL

Urgent referral to an ophthalmologist (retina specialist if available)

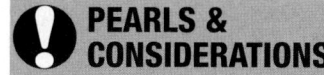

PEARLS & CONSIDERATIONS

PREVENTION

- Appropriate management of chronic systemic diseases associated with the development of vascular disease (e.g., hypertension, diabetes mellitus, hyperlipidemia, coagulation disorders, systemic inflammatory conditions) is important for prevention of RVO.
- Smoking cessation reduces risk of developing RVO.
- Appropriate management of glaucoma may also reduce risk of RVO because open-angle glaucoma is the most common ocular factor predisposing to RVO.

SUGGESTED READINGS

Available at eBooks.Health.Elsevier.com.

RELATED CONTENT

Glaucoma, Open Angle (Related Key Topic)
Diabetes Mellitus (Related Key Topic)
Hypertension (Related Key Topic)

AUTHORS: **ROBERT H. JANIGIAN JR., MD** and **FRED F. FERRI, MD**

Diseases
and Disorders

BASIC INFORMATION

DEFINITION

Rhabdomyolysis is a syndrome characterized by striated muscle lysis with resulting muscle damage and leakage of intracellular contents into the circulation. The presentation may range from an asymptomatic elevation of creatine kinase (CK), also known as creatine phosphokinase (CPK), to severe muscle injury with irreversible kidney failure. In general, a five- to tenfold elevation of CK levels, muscle pain, and myoglobinuria in an appropriate clinical setting (see below) are sufficient criteria for the diagnosis of rhabdomyolysis. Acute kidney injury (AKI), which is not a diagnostic criterion of rhabdomyolysis, typically results from multiple factors, including volume depletion, tubular obstruction, direct heme pigment–induced proximal tubular cell injury, and renal vasoconstriction.

ICD-10CM CODES
M62.82	Rhabdomyolysis (idiopathic)
T79.6	Traumatic ischemia of muscle
M62.89	Other specified disorders of muscle

EPIDEMIOLOGY & DEMOGRAPHICS[1-3]

- Incidence is approximately 1 per 10,000 persons in the U.S.
- Rare in children, increased risk with age, i.e., >80 yr.
- Reported incidence of AKI with rhabdomyolysis is 10% to 55%.
- 7% to 10% of cases of AKI are due to rhabdomyolysis.

MORTALITY RATE: 5% to 8%, with better prognosis when AKI is absent.

ONSET:

- Evidence is limited regarding the onset of physical exertion–induced rhabdomyolysis. Exercise levels that exceed an individual's usual exercise tolerance level can induce rhabdomyolysis. Extracellular volume depletion and vasoconstriction are common predisposing features (Fig. E1). Patients with risk factors (e.g., metabolic myopathies, advanced age) develop symptoms associated with rhabdomyolysis within 2 to 6 h after activity. Concurrent electrolyte abnormalities such as hypokalemia, hyponatremia, hypernatremia, hypomagnesemia, hypophosphatemia, and hypocalcemia increase the risk for rhabdomyolysis. Patients without risk factors generally become symptomatic 12 to 36 h after muscle injury.
- CK levels increase within 2 to 12 h of the onset of muscle injury, generally peak after 24 to 72 h, and decline 3 to 5 days after cessation of muscle injury. Peak CK levels may predict development of AKI.
- Rhabdomyolysis from cholesterol-lowering therapy by HMG-CoA reductase inhibitors (statins) requires hospitalization in less than 0.1% of cases. The mechanism of damage is multifactorial: Bioavailability, lipophilicity, efficiency of uptake of transport proteins in hepatocytes, blood level of statins, and level of extrahepatic inhibition of mitochondrial

respiration, bioavailability, and lipophilicity. Among the statins, pravastatin has a lower risk for induction of rhabdomyolysis than other statins, presumably due to lower lipid solubility. The average duration of statin therapy before onset of myopathy is 6 mo. Symptom resolution with normalization of serum CK concentrations occurs in days to weeks following drug discontinuation. The average time for onset of rhabdomyolysis after the addition of a fibrate to statin therapy is 32 days. Rare genetic variants are associated with statin-induced myopathy.

PHYSICAL FINDINGS & CLINICAL PRESENTATION

- Classic triad of muscle pain, weakness, and dark urine from myoglobinuria
- Muscle tenderness is present in half of cases
- Muscle swelling occurs after intravenous fluid repletion
- Muscular rigidity
- Fever
- In rhabdomyolysis secondary to long-term statin administration, fatigue (74%) is nearly as common as muscle pain (88%)
- Oliguria or anuria with AKI

ETIOLOGY[1-4]

Causes can be divided into three categories:
- Traumatic or muscle compression
  1. High-current electrical injury
  2. Crush injury and compartment syndrome
  3. Tourniquet and limb ischemia
  4. Reperfusion after revascularization procedures for ischemia
  5. Extensive surgical (spinal) dissection, bariatric surgery
- Nontraumatic exertional
  1. Exercise: More than 10 genetically predisposing gene sequence variants are associated with exertional rhabdomyolysis
  2. Sickle cell trait, rarely: Usually additional predisposing factors are involved (e.g., body mass index [BMI] >30 kg/m², tobacco use, statin use, antipsychotic use, high altitude)
  3. Heat stroke
  4. Metabolic myopathies
  5. Malignant hyperthermia and neuroleptic malignant syndrome
  6. Seizure activity
- Nontraumatic, nonexertional
  1. Drug-induced (statins alone, combinations of statins with fibrates or erythromycin, simvastatin and amiodarone, amphetamines, haloperidol, levofloxacin, macrolide antibiotics)
  2. Chronic ethanol ingestion
  3. Hypothyroidism
  4. Infectious and inflammatory myositis

Table 1 summarizes various causes of rhabdomyolysis.

DIAGNOSIS

DIFFERENTIAL DIAGNOSIS

"Creatine Kinase Elevation" in Section IV describes a clinical algorithm for the evaluation of CK elevation.

LABORATORY TESTS[1-3]

- Creatine kinase: Usually CK is 5 to 10 times the upper limit of the normal range and typically peaks 24 to 72 h after the initial insult (Fig. 2). Levels >15,000 IU/L are more likely associated with AKI. However, in patients with concomitant risk factors such as hypokalemia or volume depletion, CK levels as low as 5000 U/L may be associated with AKI.
- Myoglobin: Filtration into urine produces a "port wine" color at concentrations of 100 to 300 mg/dl. Myoglobinuria can be suspected by a positive urine dipstick test for blood within urine or by light microscopy detection of red blood cells. Due to its rapid hepatic metabolism, myoglobin lacks sensitivity for detection and diagnosis of rhabdomyolysis. Therefore serum and/or urine myoglobin measurement is not recommended to establish the diagnosis of rhabdomyolysis. Blood urea nitrogen and plasma creatinine concentrations are used to monitor severity of AKI.
- Potassium, calcium, phosphorus, and uric acid are released from damaged muscle, and levels should be monitored. Hyperkalemia is less common in nontraumatic rhabdomyolysis.
- Calcium: Hypocalcemia from deposition of calcium phosphate complexes in damaged muscle tissue. Hypercalcemia may follow resolution of rhabdomyolysis from liberation of calcium from damaged muscle into the circulation and increased gut calcium absorption from enhanced vitamin D production.
- Anion gap metabolic acidosis may occur from release of organic acids and phosphates from damaged muscle. Metabolic acidosis is less common in nontraumatic rhabdomyolysis.
- Urinalysis: Myoglobin is detected as blood on dipstick, but red blood cells are absent on

---

TABLE 1 Causes of Rhabdomyolysis

Muscle injury/ ischemia	Trauma, pressure necrosis, electric shock, burns, acute vascular disease
Myofiber exhaustion	Seizures, excessive exercise, heat exhaustion
Toxins	Alcohol, cocaine, heroin, amphetamines, ecstasy, phencyclidine, snakebite
Drugs	Statins, fibrates, zidovudine, neuroleptic malignant syndrome, azathioprine, theophylline, lithium, diuretics, colchicine
Electrolyte disorders	Hypophosphatemia, hypokalemia, hyperosmolar states
Infections	Viral (influenza, HIV, coxsackievirus, Epstein-Barr virus, COVID-19), bacterial *(Legionella, Francisella, Streptococcus pneumoniae, Salmonella, Staphylococcus aureus)*
Familial	McArdle disease, carnitine palmitoyl transferase deficiency, malignant hyperthermia
Other	Hypothyroidism, polymyositis, dermatomyositis

From Johnson RJ et al: *Comprehensive clinical nephrology*, ed 7, Philadelphia, 2024, Elsevier.

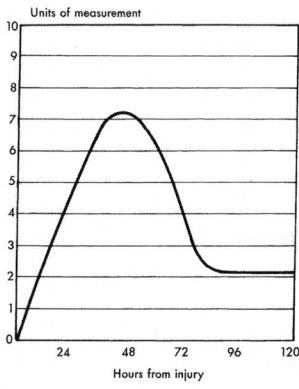

FIG. 2 Typical creatine kinase elimination curve.

microscopy. Microscopic identification of pigmented tubular casts establishes acute tubular necrosis.

- Rhabdomyolysis-induced acute tubular necrosis may occur with a low fractional excretion of sodium (FE_{Na} <1%).
- Box 1 summarizes laboratory abnormalities observed with rhabdomyolysis.

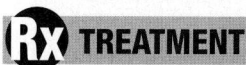 **TREATMENT**

ACUTE GENERAL Rx[1-3]

- Identify precipitating factor(s) and discontinue potentially contributory drugs or toxins.
- Early, aggressive, high-volume intravenous fluid replacement with normal saline. Extracellular fluid volume-loading and diuresis reduce the risk for renal damage by elimination of urate and phosphate that can precipitate in the kidneys. Fig. 3 describes a treatment algorithm for rhabdomyolysis.
- Fasciotomy is indicated in compartment syndrome for preservation of muscle and nerve function.
- Initiate volume repletion with normal saline at a rate of 200 to 1000 ml/h, depending on clinical circumstances and severity of muscle damage. Titrate the infusion rate to maintain a urine output of at least 200 ml/h. Consider treatment with mannitol (up to 200 g per day with cumulative dose up to 800 g) to enhance urine flow rate. Typically, a 20% mannitol infusion at a dose of 0.5 g/kg is given over a 15-min interval followed by an infusion at 0.1 gram/kg per h. Discontinue mannitol and volume resuscitation if a diuresis threshold of >20 ml/h is not established. Maintain volume repletion until myoglobinuria stops (negative urine dipstick blood test) or plasma CK levels decrease to <5000 U/L.
- Correct hypocalcemia if symptomatic or hyperkalemia that produces electrocardiographic changes.
- Treatment of all electrolyte imbalances.
- Urine alkalinization: Maintain urine pH at 6 to 7 and plasma pH at ~7.50. This recommendation is controversial. Early volume resuscitation and expansion are the most important treatments.
- Initiation of renal replacement therapy is determined by severity of kidney injury and/or

---

BOX 1   Laboratory Abnormalities Observed with Rhabdomyolysis

Potassium
Elevated
Risk for acute kidney injury

Bicarbonate
Decreased (20 mEq/L)
Metabolic acidosis

Uric Acid
Elevated (>7 mg/dl)
Marker of acute renal failure

Sodium
Usually normal
Can decrease with mannitol therapy
Use serum osmolality values as a guide

Phosphate
Elevated
Risk for precipitation of calcium phosphate
May need phosphate binders if phosphate >7 mg/dl

Creatine Kinase
Elevated
Associated with creatine kinase level of 15 to 75,000

Blood Urea Nitrogen
Elevated (>20 mg/dl)

Creatinine
Elevated

Calcium
Initially low
Rebound phase may demonstrate hypercalcemia

Liver Function Tests
Occasionally elevated
Serum aspartate transaminase, lactate dehydrogenase, aldolase, muscle enzyme levels elevated

Troponin
Normal
Suspect myocardial damage as a cause (or effect) if elevated
7% false-positive rate for troponin I

Anion Gap
Sometimes elevated
May predict acute kidney injury

Prothrombin Time, Partial Thromboplastin Time, D-Dimer
Disseminated intravascular coagulation in up to 30% of severe cases
Associated with greater mortality

From Adams JG et al: *Emergency medicine, clinical essentials,* ed 2, Philadelphia, 2013, Elsevier.

---

electrolyte imbalances. Continuous renal replacement therapy and specialized hemodialysis membranes to enhance myoglobin clearance have not been systematically studied or proven superior to intermittent hemodialysis.

DISPOSITION

Early diagnosis and management are required to prevent AKI.

REFERRAL

Renal consultation and surgical consultation if compartment syndrome develops

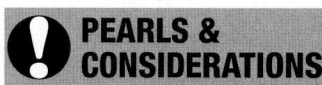 **PEARLS & CONSIDERATIONS**

COMMENTS

- Statin-induced rhabdomyolysis occurs 12 times more frequently when statins are combined with fibrates than when used alone.

- Short-term, high-dose glucocorticoid steroid administration (500 to 1000 mg methylprednisolone) has been used for treatment of alcohol-induced rhabdomyolysis that is refractory to volume repletion. This treatment may be efficacious in cases of severe rhabdomyolysis by reducing secondary leukocyte inflammatory muscle injury. Watch for potential rebound hypercalcemia in the recovery phase of rhabdomyolysis.

REFERENCES

Available at eBooks.Health.Elsevier.com.

RELATED CONTENT

Rhabdomyolysis (Patient Information)
Statin-Induced Muscle Syndrome (Related Key Topic)

AUTHOR: **HESHAM SHABAN, MD**

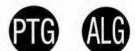

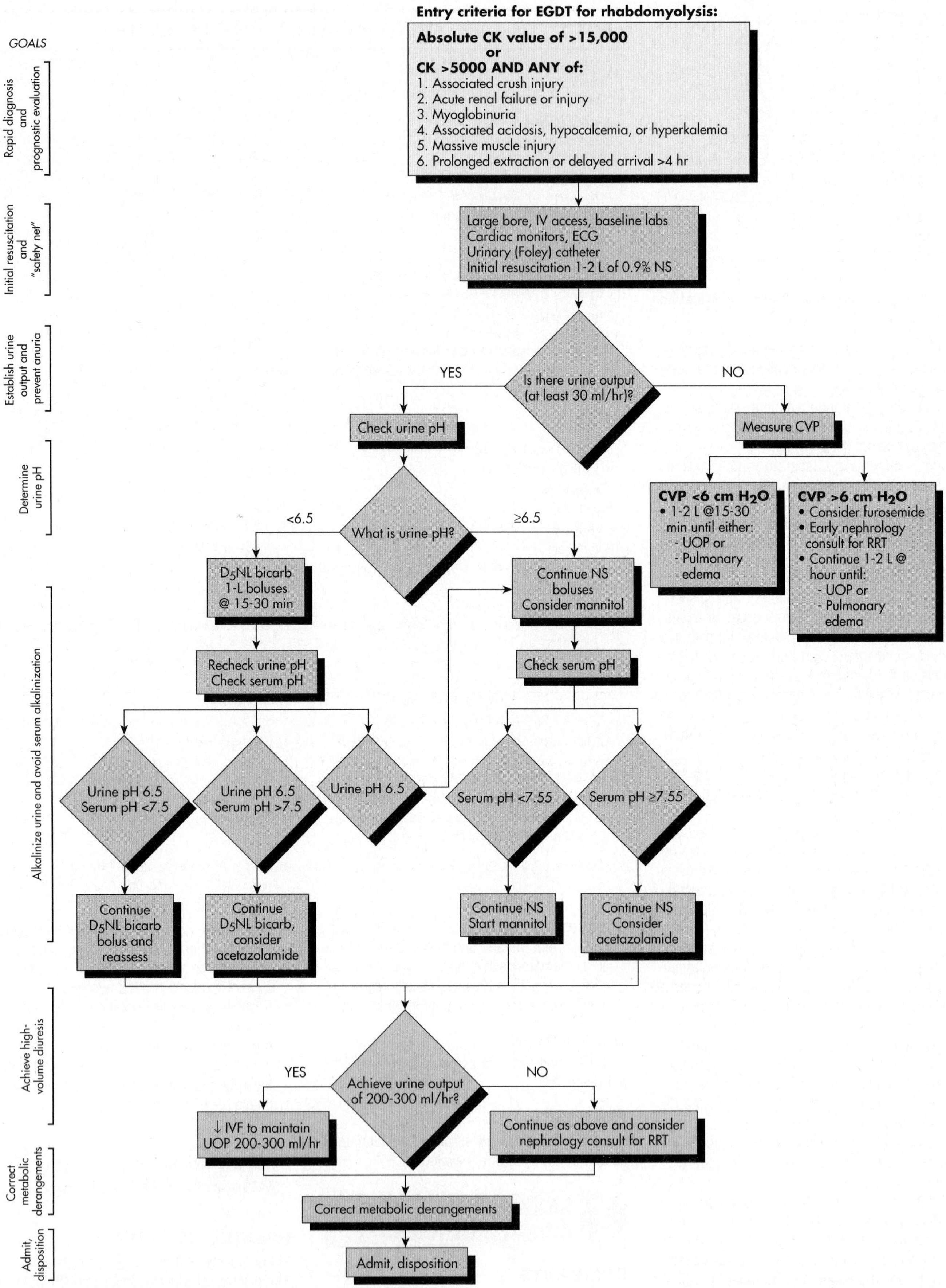

GOALS

Rapid diagnosis and prognostic evaluation

Entry criteria for EGDT for rhabdomyolysis:

Absolute CK value of >15,000
or
CK >5000 AND ANY of:
1. Associated crush injury
2. Acute renal failure or injury
3. Myoglobinuria
4. Associated acidosis, hypocalcemia, or hyperkalemia
5. Massive muscle injury
6. Prolonged extraction or delayed arrival >4 hr

Initial resuscitation and "safety net"

Large bore, IV access, baseline labs
Cardiac monitors, ECG
Urinary (Foley) catheter
Initial resuscitation 1-2 L of 0.9% NS

Establish urine output and prevent anuria

Is there urine output (at least 30 ml/hr)?

YES → Check urine pH

NO → Measure CVP

Determine urine pH

What is urine pH?

<6.5 → D₅NL bicarb 1-L boluses @ 15-30 min

≥6.5 → Continue NS boluses Consider mannitol

CVP <6 cm H₂O
- 1-2 L @15-30 min until either:
  - UOP or
  - Pulmonary edema

CVP >6 cm H₂O
- Consider furosemide
- Early nephrology consult for RRT
- Continue 1-2 L @ hour until:
  - UOP or
  - Pulmonary edema

Alkalinize urine and avoid serum alkalinization

Recheck urine pH
Check serum pH

Check serum pH

Urine pH 6.5
Serum pH <7.5

Urine pH 6.5
Serum pH >7.5

Urine pH 6.5

Serum pH <7.55

Serum pH ≥7.55

Continue D₅NL bicarb bolus and reassess

Continue D₅NL bicarb, consider acetazolamide

Continue NS Start mannitol

Continue NS Consider acetazolamide

Achieve high-volume diuresis

Achieve urine output of 200-300 ml/hr?

YES → ↓ IVF to maintain UOP 200-300 ml/hr

NO → Continue as above and consider nephrology consult for RRT

Correct metabolic derangements

Correct metabolic derangements

Admit, disposition

Admit, disposition

FIG. 3 Early goal-directed therapy for rhabdomyolysis. *CK,* Creatine kinase; *CVP,* central venous pressure; *D5NL bicarb,* 5% dextrose in normal sodium bicarbonate solution; *EGDT,* early goal-directed therapy; *IV,* intravenous; *IVF,* intravenous fluid; *NS,* normal saline; *RRT,* renal replacement therapy; *UOP,* urinary output. (From Adams JG et al: *Emergency medicine, clinical essentials,* ed 2, Philadelphia, 2013, Elsevier.)

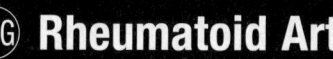
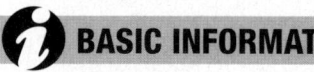

DEFINITION

Rheumatoid arthritis (RA) is a systemic autoimmune disease characterized by inflammatory polyarthritis that affects peripheral joints, especially the small joints of the hands and feet.[1] It is a chronic, progressive disease in which untreated inflammation may lead to cartilage and bone erosions and joint destruction resulting in functional impairment.[1]

SYNONYM

RA

ICD-10CM CODES

M06.9	Rheumatoid arthritis, unspecified
M05.10	Rheumatoid lung disease with rheumatoid arthritis of unspecified site
M05.20	Rheumatoid vasculitis with rheumatoid arthritis of unspecified site
M05.39	Rheumatoid heart disease with rheumatoid arthritis of multiple sites
M05.49	Rheumatoid myopathy with rheumatoid arthritis of multiple sites
M05.59	Rheumatoid polyneuropathy with rheumatoid arthritis of multiple sites
M05.69	Rheumatoid arthritis of multiple sites with involvement of other organs and systems
M05.79	Rheumatoid arthritis with rheumatoid factor of multiple sites without organ or systems involvement
M05.80	Other rheumatoid arthritis with rheumatoid factor of unspecified site

EPIDEMIOLOGY & DEMOGRAPHICS

INCIDENCE: Annual incidence of 12 to 1200 per 100,000[2]

PREVALENCE: 0.5% to 1.0% of the worldwide population, with different rates in different ethnic groups[2]

PREDOMINANT SEX: Females are at higher risk of developing RA than males (2 to 3:1)[3]

PREDOMINANT AGE: Diagnosis usually between age 30 and 50.[4] Steadily increases with age until the mid-70s

RISK FACTORS: Female sex, age, tobacco use, silica exposure, obesity, and family history. Smoking has an additive detrimental effect in RA patients (twofold excess mortality risk).[2]

PHYSICAL FINDINGS & CLINICAL PRESENTATION

Initial presentation:
- Pain, swelling, warmth in one or more peripheral joints, frequently with symmetric small joint involvement, often associated with >1 h of morning stiffness and constitutional symptoms such as fatigue, malaise, low-grade fevers, and weight loss occurring over a period of weeks to months.[4] A subset of patients can also present with acute-onset polyarthritis instead of insidious symptoms.[2]
- Most common joints involved include the metacarpophalangeal (MCP) joints, proximal interphalangeal (PIP) joints (Fig. E1), and metatarsophalangeal (MTP) joints (Fig. E2), as well as the wrists.[4]
- Other affected joints involved include the elbows, shoulders, hips, knees, and ankles.[4]
- Distal interphalangeal (DIP) joints are spared.[1]
- Sacroiliac and vertebral joints are spared, except for the C1 and C2 articulations.[4]

Chronic longstanding disease:
- "Swan-neck" (DIP flexion and PIP hyperextension) (Fig. E3), "boutonniere" (DIP hyperextension and PIP flexion), "Z-thumb" (MCP flexion and IP hyperextension) deformities (Fig. 4), ulnar deviation of the fingers, radial deviation of the wrists, and subluxation of the MCP joints.
- C1 to C2 (atlantoaxial) inflammation can lead to odontoid erosion and transverse ligament laxity/rupture, resulting in atlantoaxial subluxation (Fig. E5) and cord compression.[5]
- Joint damage to wrists, elbows, shoulders, hips, and knees can lead to severe secondary osteoarthritis, necessitating joint surgery and/or replacement.[4]

Extraarticular manifestations:
- Secondary Sjögren syndrome (~35%): Immune-mediated inflammation of lacrimal and salivary glands, resulting in dry mouth (xerostomia) and eyes (keratoconjunctivitis sicca).[6]
- Rheumatoid nodules (25%): Nontender, firm nodules on extensor surfaces and pressure points, usually in rheumatoid factor positive (RF+) disease.[6] Histopathology demonstrates palisading histiocytes surrounding a central area of fibrinoid necrosis.[7]
- Felty syndrome: RA with splenomegaly and leukopenia.[4] Most patients are positive for HLA-DR4 and RF.

Pulmonary disease:
- Pleural disease (exudative effusions, pleuritis)[4]
- Interstitial lung disease (up to 10% clinically significant)[4]
- Bronchiolitis obliterans[4]
- Cryptogenic organizing pneumonia[4]
- Pulmonary nodules: A combination of RA and pneumoconiosis is called Caplan syndrome (rheumatoid pneumoconiosis)[4]

Neuromuscular:
- Entrapment neuropathy (carpal tunnel, tarsal tunnel, and cubital tunnel are most commonly affected)[4,8,9]
- Mononeuritis multiplex[4]
- Peripheral neuropathy[9]
- Cervical myelopathy and cord compression secondary to atlantoaxial subluxation[4]
- Pachymeningitis (rare)[10]
- Vasculitis[4]

Cardiac disease:
- Pericarditis (most common)[4]
- Myocarditis[11]
- Valvular nodules[11]
- There is an increased risk of cardiovascular disease compared to the general population, thought to be secondary to accelerated atherosclerosis from systemic inflammation[11]

Ocular disease:
- Keratoconjunctivitis sicca (dry eye, without dry mouth) (10%)[4]
- Episcleritis, scleritis, scleral thinning, scleromalacia perforans, ulcerative keratitis[4]

Other conditions:
- Amyloidosis: Occurs in longstanding, poorly controlled RA. Usually presents as nephrotic syndrome. Organs affected include the heart, kidney, liver, spleen, intestines, and skin[4]
- Osteoporosis[12]

ETIOLOGY

The exact cause of RA remains unknown despite extensive research. It is likely that a combination of genetic, hormonal, and environmental factors leads to aberrant immune activation and inflammatory response within joints. Genetic factors have been found to be involved in susceptibility to disease, as twins and first-degree relatives of RA patients are at an increased risk of developing the disease compared to the general population.[13] Patients with HLA-DR4, DR1, and DR14 alleles have increased susceptibility to RA; in particular, one amino acid sequence in the DR β

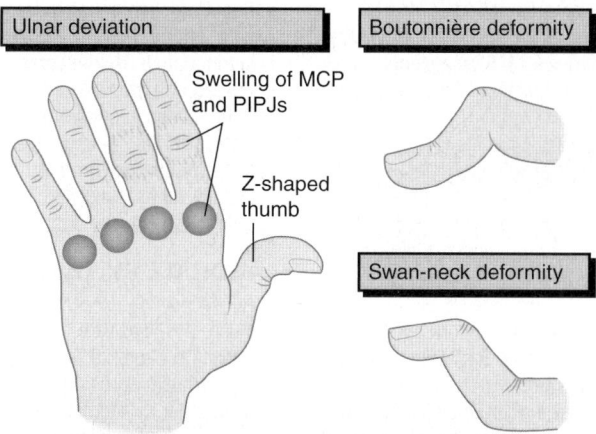

FIG. 4 Characteristic hand deformities in rheumatoid arthritis. *MCP,* Metacarpophalanges; *PIPJs,* proximal interphalangeal joints. (From Ballinger A: *Kumar & Clark's essentials of clinical medicine,* ed 6, Edinburgh, 2012, Saunders.)

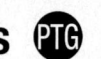

chain, known as the shared epitope, is overrepresented in these patients.[13] Other identified genetic associations include polymorphisms in *PTPN22, PADI4, CTLA4, TRAF1-C5, STAT4, TNFAIP3*.[13] Epigenetic factors are also likely to be involved.[13] Multiple environmental factors have been implicated as potential etiologic factors, including cigarette smoking, silica exposure, and low socioeconomic class.[13] Infectious agents such as *P. gingivalis*, Epstein-Barr virus, and parvovirus B19 have also been reported as potential triggers.[13]

Stages of disease development presumably include:

- Initiation of the innate immune response through toll-like receptor (TLR) activation by a stimulating signal.[13] The preclinical stages of seropositive rheumatoid arthritis are characterized by disordered immunity, often associated with mucosal surfaces, including the oral cavity, lungs, and GI tract, in addition to local and systemic generation of anti-citrullinated protein antibodies (ACPAs). These autoantibodies can be detected in the blood a median of 4.5 yr before the onset of symptomatic arthritis.[14]
- Perpetuation of inflammatory responses through activation of the adaptive immune system. There is migration of inflammatory cells (autoreactive B and T cells, monocytes) into the joint space, activation of macrophage-like and fibroblast-like synoviocytes, and development of a "synovial pannus," a thickened synovial membrane.[15]
- The pannus releases proinflammatory cytokines (tumor necrosis factor alpha [TNF-α], interleukin [IL]-1, IL-6, IL-15, IL-17, IL-18) as well as proteases, which erode cartilage and bone.[15] Bone erosions are caused mainly by osteoclasts, which express the receptor activator of NF-κB (RANK).[13] TNF-α, IL-1, IL-6, and IL-17 promote the expression of RANK ligand (RANKL) on T cells and fibroblast-like synoviocytes, thus creating a positive feedback loop.[13] IL-6 and TNF-α act synergistically to increase vascular endothelial growth factor levels, which in turn stimulate angiogenesis, thereby maintaining pannus formation. IL-6 also promotes B-cell differentiation and production of autoantibodies.[13]
- Many of the new "biologic" disease-modifying antirheumatic drugs (DMARDs) are engineered to target these cytokines (see "Treatment" section).[16]

Dx DIAGNOSIS

The American College of Rheumatology (ACR) and the European League Against Rheumatism (EULAR) developed new classification criteria for RA in 2010 (Table 1). These are based on a point system where patients with score ≥6/10 are considered to have "definite RA." Four variables constitute the new criteria:

- The number and size of involved joints (0 to 5 points, with higher scores for a larger number of small joints affected)
- Levels of rheumatoid factor (RF) and anti-cyclic citrullinated peptide (anti-CCP) antibody

(0 to 3 points, with a higher score for a high-titer positive RF or anti-CCP)
- Elevated erythrocyte sedimentation rate (ESR) or C-reactive protein (CRP) (1 point)
- Symptom duration ≥6 wk (1 point)

DIFFERENTIAL DIAGNOSIS

- Infectious causes: Parvovirus B19, hepatitis B, hepatitis C, poststreptococcal reactive arthritis, acute rheumatic fever[4]
- Connective tissue diseases: Systemic lupus erythematosus, scleroderma, mixed connective tissue disease, Sjögren syndrome[4]
- Seronegative spondyloarthropathies[4]
- Calcium pyrophosphate deposition (CPPD or "pseudo-RA")[4]
- Polyarticular gout[4]
- Polymyalgia rheumatica[4]
- Remitting seronegative symmetric synovitis with pitting edema (RS3PE) can resemble seronegative RA in elderly patients[17]
- Hemochromatosis[18]
- Paraneoplastic syndromes
- Osteoarthritis, a degenerative arthritis that lacks prolonged morning stiffness and that usually lacks synovitis, should not be confused with RA (see Table 2)

LABORATORY TESTS

- RF (sensitivity ~60%; specificity ~80%): False positives are seen with hepatitis C, subacute bacterial endocarditis, primary biliary cirrhosis, sarcoidosis, malignancy, Sjögren syndrome, systemic lupus erythematosus (SLE), and increasing age.[4]
- Anti-CCP antibodies: Sensitivity is similar to RF, but it is more specific for RA than RF (up to 95% to 98%).[19]

- The presence of either RF or anti-CCP ("seropositive RA") is associated with more severe disease, more extraarticular manifestations, and worse prognosis.[19]
- Elevated ESR and/or CRP: These markers decline with treatment; thus they can be used to monitor disease activity along with physical examination and clinical presentation.[19]
- CBC with differential: RA may lead to anemia of chronic disease (through upregulation of the iron-regulating hormone, hepcidin) and thrombocytosis.[19]
- Hypoalbuminemia and hypergammaglobulinemia.
- Antinuclear antibody (ANA) is present in 20% to 30% of patients. However, complement will usually be normal or increased, in contrast to patients with systemic lupus erythematosus. Many patients will have secondary Sjögren syndrome (positive ANA with negative SSA and SSB).[19]
- Inflammatory synovial fluid with >2,000 polymorphonuclear neutrophils (PMNs): Of note, patients with RA have an increased risk of developing septic arthritis.[20] Hence, synovial fluid with white blood cells >50,000 cells/mm^3 is concerning for an infectious process and must always be ruled out.[20]

IMAGING STUDIES

Recommendations for the use of imaging in the clinical management of rheumatoid arthritis are summarized in Table 3.

Plain radiography (Table E4):
- Early changes include soft tissue swelling, symmetric joint space narrowing, and periarticular osteopenia.

TABLE 1 The 2010 American College of Rheumatology/European League Against Rheumatism Classification Criteria for Rheumatoid Arthritis[a]

Criteria	Score
Joint involvement	
2-10 large joints	1
1-3 small joints (with or without involvement of large joints)	2
4-10 small joints (with or without involvement of large joints)	3
>10 joints (with at least one small joint)	5
Serology (at least one test result is needed for classification)	
Negative RF and negative ACPA	0
Low-positive RF or low-positive ACPA	2
High-positive RF or high-positive ACPA	3
Acute-phase reactants	
Normal CRP and normal ESR	0
Abnormal CRP or abnormal ESR	1
Duration of symptoms	
<6 wk	0
≥6 wk	1

A score of ≥6 is needed for classification of a patient as having definite rheumatoid arthritis.
If incontrovertible radiographic evidence of rheumatoid arthritis exists, the diagnosis can be made even if the criteria provided are not fulfilled.
If a patient has previously fulfilled the criteria for rheumatoid arthritis, the diagnosis is maintained even if the criteria are not fulfilled on current reexamination.
ACPA, Anticitrullinated protein antibodies; *CRP*, C-reactive protein; *ESR*, erythrocyte sedimentation rate; *RF*, rheumatoid factor.
[a]Target population (patients who can be evaluated using these criteria): Those who have *at least one joint with definite clinical synovitis* (swelling), with the synovitis not better explained by another disease.
From Firestein GS et al: *Firestein & Kelley's textbook of rheumatology*, ed 11, Philadelphia, 2021, Elsevier.

TABLE 2 Factors Useful for Differentiating Early Rheumatoid Arthritis from Osteoarthritis

	Rheumatoid Arthritis	Osteoarthritis
Age at onset	Across age spectrum, peak incidence in 50s	Increases with age
Predisposing factors	Susceptibility epitopes (HLA-DRB1*01, HLA-DRB1*04)	Trauma, overuse
	PTPN22, PADI4 polymorphisms; RF and ACPA positivity	Congenital abnormalities (e.g., shallow acetabulum)
	Smoking	
Early symptoms	Morning stiffness and gelling phenomenon, pain improves with activity	Pain increases through the day and with use
Joints involved	Proximal interphalangeal joints, metacarpophalangeal joints, wrists most often; distal interphalangeal joints almost never	Distal interphalangeal joints (Heberden's nodes), proximal interphalangeal joints (Bouchard's nodes), knees, lumbar spine
Physical findings	Soft tissue swelling, warmth	Bony osteophytes, minimal soft tissue swelling early
Radiographic findings	Periarticular osteopenia, marginal erosions, symmetric joint space narrowing in large joints	Subchondral sclerosis, osteophytes, asymmetric joint space loss in large joints
Laboratory findings	Increased C-reactive protein, positive RF, positive ACPA, anemia, thrombocytosis	Normal

ACPA, Anticitrullinated protein antibody; *HLA*, human leukocyte antigen; *RF*, rheumatoid factor.
From Firestein GS et al: *Firestein & Kelley's textbook of rheumatology*, ed 11, Philadelphia, 2021, Elsevier.

TABLE 3 EULAR Recommendations for the Use of Imaging in the Clinical Management of Rheumatoid Arthritis[a]

When there is diagnostic doubt, conventional radiography, ultrasonography, or MRI can be used to improve the certainty of a diagnosis of RA in addition to clinical criteria alone.[b]

The presence of inflammation seen with ultrasonography or MRI can be used to predict the progression to clinical RA from undifferentiated inflammatory arthritis.

Ultrasonography and MRI are superior to clinical examination in the detection of joint inflammation; these techniques should be considered for more accurate assessment of inflammation. Conventional radiography of the hands and feet should be used as the initial imaging technique to detect damage. However, ultrasonography and/or MRI should be considered if conventional radiographs do not show damage and may be used to detect damage at an earlier time point (especially in early-stage RA).

MRI bone edema is a strong independent predictor of subsequent radiographic progression in early RA, and should be considered as a prognostic indicator. Joint inflammation (synovitis) detected by MRI or ultrasonography as well as joint damage detected by conventional radiographs, MRI, or ultrasonography can also be considered for the prediction of further joint damage.

Inflammation seen on imaging may be more predictive of a therapeutic response than clinical features of disease activity; imaging may be used to predict response to treatment.

Given the superior detection of inflammation by MRI and ultrasonography versus clinical examination, they may be useful in monitoring disease activity.

The periodic evaluation of joint damage, usually by radiographs of the hands and feet, should be considered. MRI (and possibly ultrasonography) is more responsive to change in joint damage and can be used to monitor disease progression.

Monitoring of functional instability of the cervical spine by lateral radiography obtained in flexion and neutral positions should be performed in patients with clinical suspicion of cervical involvement. When radiography is positive or specific neurologic symptoms and signs are present, MRI should be performed.

MRI and ultrasonography can detect inflammation that predicts subsequent joint damage, even when clinical remission is present and can be used to assess persistent inflammation.

EULAR, European League Against Rheumatism; *MRI*, magnetic resonance imaging; *RA*, rheumatoid arthritis.
[a]Recommendations are based on data from imaging studies that have mainly focused on the hands (particularly wrists, metacarpophalangeal, and proximal interphalangeal joints). There are few data with specific guidance on which joints to image.[8]
[b]In patients with at least one joint with definite clinical synovitis, which is not better explained by another disease.
From Firestein GS et al: *Firestein & Kelley's textbook of rheumatology*, ed 11, Philadelphia, 2021, Elsevier.

- Later changes include periarticular erosions and deformities. This reflects cartilage and bone destruction secondary to pannus formation (Fig. E6).
- Radiographs of hands and feet should be obtained at disease onset and repeated to monitor disease progression and to ensure that adequate treatment is achieved.

MRI and musculoskeletal ultrasound:
- More sensitive for detecting erosive disease and joint effusions/synovitis.

Rx TREATMENT

- Early identification and treatment of RA with DMARDs is crucial.[21] More than half of patients have radiographic joint damage within 2 yr of disease onset, but early aggressive treatment with DMARDs and/or biologic agents is associated with decreased progression of synovitis and bone erosions, and with decreased disability.[22]
- There are several tools to measure disease activity (Table 5) and define remission in rheumatoid arthritis, including (but not limited to) Clinical Disease Activity Index (CDAI), Simplified Disease Activity Index (SDAI), Disease Activity Score (DAS) 28, Routine Assessment of Patient Index Data 3 (RAPID3), Stanford Health Assessment Questionnaire (HAQ), and Patient Activity Scale (PAS).

ACUTE GENERAL Rx

- NSAIDs: Can be used initially to relieve pain and mild inflammation or used later in the disease course for additional control of mild pain.[4] NSAIDs are not disease modifying.
- Corticosteroids: Oral or intraarticular, frequently used initially to rapidly reduce inflammation until oral DMARD treatments take effect.[4] They may also be used during acute flares or in low doses for additional control of inflammation.[4] The use of corticosteroids at the lowest dose and shortest duration possible is recommended.[4] Corticosteroids have many side effects, including but not limited to weight gain, increased risk of diabetes, osteoporosis, cataract formation, peptic ulcer disease (especially when used in combination with NSAIDs), and avascular necrosis.

CHRONIC Rx

- DMARDs: Can be classified into "nonbiologic" and "biologic" treatments (Table 6).
  1. Nonbiologic DMARDs: Most commonly used agents are methotrexate (MTX), hydroxychloroquine (HCQ), sulfasalazine (SSZ), and leflunomide (LEF).[4] Most of these are associated with potential toxicity and require close monitoring. They are also slow-acting drugs that generally require >8 wk to start taking effect.
  2. MTX is the most commonly used DMARD worldwide for the treatment of RA.[4] It is effective as monotherapy in about 30% of patients with RA.
  3. "Triple therapy"—MTX, HCQ, and SSZ—has been shown to be superior to MTX alone.[21]
- Biologic DMARDs: Newer biologically engineered therapies, which target cytokines and cells involved in the RA inflammatory response.[4] Major side effects include an increased risk of infections and potential reactivation of latent tuberculosis.[4] A negative purified protein derivative (PPD) or interferon γ-release assay is a prerequisite to initiate therapy.[4] Biologic DMARDs are most effective when used in combination with a nonbiologic DMARD, usually MTX.[4]
- The five approved tumor necrosis factor α inhibitors (TNFI) include infliximab, etanercept, adalimumab, certolizumab pegol, and golimumab.[4]

TABLE 5 Instruments Used to Measure Rheumatoid Arthritis Disease Activity

Instrument	Score Range	Remission	THRESHOLDS OF DISEASE ACTIVITY		
			Low	Moderate	High
Disease Activity Score in 28 joints (DAS28)	0-9.4	≤2.6	≤3.2	>3.2 and ≤5.1	>5.1
Simplified Disease Activity Index (SDAI)	0.1-86.0	≤3.3	≤11	>11 and ≤26	>26
Clinical Disease Activity Index (CDAI)	0-76.0	≤2.8	≤10	>10 and ≤22	>22
Rheumatoid Arthritis Disease Activity Index (RADAI)	0-10	≤1.4	<2.2	2.2 and ≤4.9	>4.9
Patient Activity Scale (PAS or PASII)	0-10	≤1.25	<1.9	≥1.9 and ≤5.3	>5.3
Routine Assessment Patient Index Data (RAPID)	0-30	≤1	<6	≥6 and ≤12	>12

From Firestein GS et al: *Firestein & Kelley's textbook of rheumatology*, ed 11, Philadelphia, 2021, Elsevier.

TABLE 6 Disease-Modifying Drugs and Biologics for Rheumatoid Arthritis

Drugs	Usual Dose	Side Effects and Cautions
DMARDs		
Methotrexate	7.5-25 mg/wk in a single dose orally or SQ. Start low and increase by 5 mg every 1-2 mo until desired effects are achieved	Myelosuppression, hepatotoxicity, hepatic fibrosis, cirrhosis, pulmonary infiltrates or fibrosis, mouth sores (daily folic acid can prevent this), nausea, hair loss
Sulfasalazine (Azulfidine, Azulfidine EC)	500-3000 mg/day in 2-4 divided doses orally	Myelosuppression, hepatotoxicity, nausea
Hydroxychloroquine sulfate (Plaquenil)	200-400 mg per day in 2 divided doses orally Not to exceed 6.5 mg/kg of actual body weight	Retinal toxicity, rash
Leflunomide (Arava)	10-20 mg per day in a single dose orally	Myelosuppression, hepatotoxicity, cirrhosis, diarrhea, hair loss
Azathioprine (Imuran)	50-150 mg per day in 1-3 divided doses orally	Myelosuppression, hepatotoxicity, lymphoproliferative disorders, nausea, hair loss; check TPMT before initiation
BIOLOGICS		Must check T-SPOT and hepatitis B and C serology before starting all biologics; discuss updating vaccinations before initiation
TNF blockers:	40 mg SQ once a wk or every 2 wk	Increased risk of infections, tuberculosis, histoplasmosis, or others
Adalimumab (Humira)	25 mg SQ twice a wk, or 50 mg SQ once a wk	
Etanercept (Enbrel)	3-10 mg/kg IV. Given at 0, 2, 6 wk then every 8 wk (usually taken with methotrexate)	Injection site or infusion reaction
Infliximab (Remicade)		Congestive heart failure
Golimumab (Simponi)	50 mg SQ once a mo	
Certolizumab (Cimzia)	400 mg SQ loading at 0, 2, 4 then 200 mg every 2 wk vs. 400 mg q 4 wk	
T-cell costimulation blocker: Abatacept (Orencia)	500-1000 mg IV 0, 2, 4 wk then every 4 wk or 500-1000 mg IV one time, then 125 mg SQ weekly	Increased risk of infections; injection site or infusion reaction; COPD exacerbation
IL-6 blocker: Tocilizumab (Actemra)	4-8 mg/kg IV every 4 wk; 162 mg SQ once every other wk or every wk	Increased risk of infections; myelosuppression; hepatotoxicity; hyperlipidemia
B-cell depletion: Rituximab	1000 mg IV 0, 2 wk and again when arthritis becomes active; on average every 6 mo	Increased risk of infection; progressive multifocal leukoencephalopathy (PML); tumor lysis syndrome
IL-1 blocker: Anakinra	100 mg SQ daily, 100 mg SQ every other day in severe kidney disease	Increased risk of infections; injection site reaction

COPD, Chronic obstructive pulmonary disease; *DMARDs*, disease-modifying antirheumatic drugs; *IL*, interleukin; *SQ*, subcutaneously; *TNF*, tumor necrosis factor; *TPMT*, thiopurine S-methyltransferase.
From Warshaw G et al: *Ham's primary care geriatrics*, ed 7, Philadelphia, 2022, Elsevier.

- Abatacept (CTLA-4Ig) is a recombinant protein that prevents costimulatory binding of antigen presenting cell to T cell, preventing T-cell activation.[4]
- Tocilizumab (anti–IL-6) is a monoclonal antibody against the IL-6 receptor.[4]
- Sarilumab is another IL-6 inhibitor monoclonal antibody, approved by the FDA in 2017 for treatment of RA, and can be used as monotherapy or in combination with MTX or other conventional DMARDs.[23]
- Tofacitinib (JAK1/2/3 inhibitor) inhibits the JAK-STAT intracellular signaling pathway, thus preventing the production of inflammatory mediators.[13] The first oral biologic DMARD, it can be used as monotherapy or in combination with MTX. Baricitinib, an oral, once-daily Janus kinase (JAK1 and JAK2) inhibitor, was approved by the FDA in May 2018 for treatment of moderate to severe RA in patients who did not respond adequately to one or more TNFIs.[24] A dose of 2 mg was approved, with concerns that higher doses had increased adverse events. Upadacitinib (JAK1 > JAK2/3 inhibitor) was approved in 2019 at 15 mg once daily for moderate to severely active RA resistant or intolerant to MTX, or in combination with MTX with other nonbiologic DMARDs.[24]
- Rituximab (anti-CD20) is a monoclonal antibody against the CD20 antigen on B lymphocytes.[4]
- Biosimilars are beginning to be available.[25] These molecules are highly similar, but not identical, to the original drugs. Legal disputes have delayed the widespread adoption of these drugs in the U.S., but they are likely to be of increasing prevalence in the future.
- Treatment recommendations in RA patient with high-risk comorbidities:
  1. TNFI should be avoided in patients with congestive heart failure, as it can worsen the condition.[26]
  2. In patients with hepatitis B, immunosuppressive therapy can be safely prescribed along with concomitant antiviral therapy.[4]
  3. Treatment of hepatitis C patients with RA should be done following standard guidelines in collaboration with gastroenterology/hepatology.[4] Immunosuppressive therapy can be used safely in conjunction with

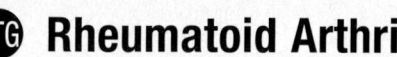
TABLE 7	Factors Associated with Poorer Prognosis in Rheumatoid Arthritis

Presence of rheumatoid factor and titer
Presence of antibodies to CCP and titer
Presence of shared epitope and number of alleles
Presence of erosive disease at presentation
Disease activity at presentation
Magnitude of ESR or CRP elevations
Presence of nodules or extraarticular features
Female sex
Smoking currently and in the past
Obesity

CCP, Cyclic citrullinated peptide; *CRP,* C-reactive protein; *ESR,* erythrocyte sedimentation rate.
From Firestein GS et al: *Firestein & Kelley's textbook of rheumatology,* ed 11, Philadelphia, 2021, Elsevier.

antiviral therapy; avoidance of DMARDs such as MTX and LEF should be taken into consideration.[16]

4. In patients with a history of skin cancer, DMARDs are recommended over the use of biologics.[27] For patients with previously treated lymphoproliferative disorders, use of rituximab should be considered first, as well as combination DMARDs and non-TNF biologics.[28] One should avoid TNFI, as there is an increased risk of lymphoma with these agents. Recommendations for treatment of patients with previously treated solid organ malignancy are the same as for patients without the condition.

Rx in pregnancy:[29]

- Patients with active rheumatoid arthritis should be tested for anti-Ro/SSA and anti-La/SSB antibodies once before or early in pregnancy, due to their associated increased in risk for neonatal lupus and congenital heart block.[30]
- Fluorinated glucocorticoids (e.g., betamethasone and dexamethasone) cross the placenta at higher concentrations without significant metabolism and can hasten lung maturity. These should not be used routinely for the management of active RA during pregnancy.[31] Glucocorticoids (e.g., prednisone, prednisolone, and methylprednisolone) should be maintained at the lowest dose possible.[32]

- Hydroxychloroquine (HCQ) has been shown to cross the placenta. However, most studies have not described fetal toxicity with HCQ doses used for the treatment of rheumatic diseases.[33]
- Methotrexate (MTX) should be stopped 1 to 3 mo before conception because of its teratogenic risks. If conception occurs while a woman is taking MTX, the medication should be stopped immediately and folic acid 5 mg/day taken for the remainder of the pregnancy.[34]
- Leflunomide (LEF) should be avoided in pregnancy due to its teratogenic effects. Conception should be delayed until LEF is undetectable in the serum (<0.02 mg/L), typically 2 yr after discontinuation. An enhanced drug elimination procedure using cholestyramine can be used for faster results.[33]
- TNF-α inhibitors, DMARDs, and other biologics can be continued throughout pregnancy. Most professional societies recommend discontinuing these medications in the third trimester. Noteworthy exception is certolizumab, which is pegylated and does not cross the placenta in significant amounts and can be continued throughout the pregnancy.[35]

Immunization, cardiovascular disease prevention (smoking cessation, blood pressure control, cholesterol control), and osteoporosis prevention (calcium and vitamin D supplementation, bisphosphonate therapy) should be addressed in all RA patients.

DISPOSITION

- Remissions and exacerbations are common, but RA is chronically progressive in the majority of cases.
- Joint degeneration and deformity often lead to disability. Joint replacement is indicated for patients with severe joint damage whose symptoms are poorly controlled by medical management. The ACR published guidelines in 2017 concerning the perioperative management of antirheumatic medications in patients undergoing elective total hip or total knee arthroplasty.[36]
- Early and aggressive diagnosis and treatment are crucial in preventing or slowing joint destruction.
- Factors associated with a poorer prognosis in RA are summarized in Table 7.

REFERRAL

- Early referral to a rheumatologist
- Orthopedic consultation for corrective surgery

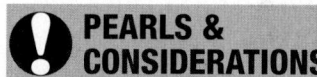 **PEARLS & CONSIDERATIONS**

RA sometimes develops acutely in the postpartum patient; conversely, as high as 75% of pregnant RA patients will experience remission during pregnancy.

REFERENCES

Available at eBooks.Health.Elsevier.com.

RELATED CONTENT

Rheumatoid Arthritis (Patient Information)

AUTHORS: **OSCAR COVARRUBIAS, BS** and **MANUEL F. DASILVA, MD**

R

Diseases and Disorders

I

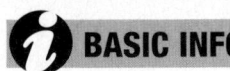
BASIC INFORMATION

DEFINITION

Sarcoidosis is a chronic multisystem granulomatous disease of unknown cause characterized histologically by the presence of noncaseating granulomas and manifesting with a wide range of clinical disturbances.

SYNONYM

Boeck sarcoid

ICD-10CM CODES
D86	Sarcoidosis
D86.0	Sarcoidosis of lung
D86.1	Sarcoidosis of lymph nodes
D86.2	Sarcoidosis of lung with sarcoidosis of lymph nodes
D86.3	Sarcoidosis of skin
D86.8	Sarcoidosis of other and combined sites
D86.9	Sarcoidosis, unspecified

EPIDEMIOLOGY & DEMOGRAPHICS

INCIDENCE (IN U.S.): Incidence is 11 in 100,000 in Whites and 35 in 100,000 in Blacks; presents most commonly in the winter and early spring. (The adjusted annual incidence among Black Americans is roughly 3 times higher than among white Americans [35.5 cases/100,000, as compared with 10.9/100,000] and is likely more chronic and fatal in Black Americans.)
PREDOMINANT SEX: Increased incidence in females.
PREDOMINANT AGE: 20 to 50 yr, second peak after 60 yr[1]
GENETICS: Familial clustering has been described. Having a first-degree relative with sarcoidosis increases the risk for disease fivefold.[2] There have been reports of association between sarcoidosis and gene products, specifically human leukocyte antigen (HLA) class II antigens, encoded by HLA-DRB1 and DQB1 alleles.[3]

PHYSICAL FINDINGS & CLINICAL PRESENTATION

- Clinical manifestations often vary with the stage of the disease and degree of organ involvement. Patients may be asymptomatic, but a chest radiograph may demonstrate findings consistent with sarcoidosis (see "Imaging Studies"). Nearly 50% of patients with sarcoidosis are diagnosed by incidental findings on chest radiograph. Lung involvement occurs in >90% of patients with sarcoidosis.
- Frequent manifestations:
  1. Pulmonary manifestations: Dry, nonproductive cough; dyspnea; chest discomfort. Pleural effusion is an uncommon manifestation but can occur in stage II or III of pulmonary involvement.
  2. Constitutional symptoms: Fatigue, weight loss, anorexia, malaise, night sweats.
  3. Visual disturbances: Blurred vision, ocular discomfort, conjunctivitis, iritis, uveitis (65% of patients).

4. Dermatologic manifestations (30% of patients): Erythema nodosum (10% of patients), macules, papules, subcutaneous nodules, hyperpigmentation, lupus pernio (indurated violaceous lesions on the nose, lips, ears, and cheeks that can erode into underlying cartilage and bone) (Fig. E1).
5. Myocardial disturbances, arrhythmias, cardiomyopathy, various conduction abnormalities, and pericardial effusion. Cardiac sarcoidosis is much more common than clinically appreciated and is found in up to 25% of patients in the U.S.
6. Splenomegaly, hepatomegaly, and rarely, can involve the pancreas.
7. Rheumatologic manifestations: Arthralgias have been reported in up to 40% of patients. It typically affects the ankles but can also involve the knees, wrists, and small joints of the hands and feet.
8. **Löfgren syndrome,** consisting of the triad of arthritis, erythema nodosum, and bilateral hilar adenopathy, occurs in 9% to 34% of patients. Fever is frequently present.
9. Neurologic and other manifestations: Cranial nerve palsies, diabetes insipidus, meningeal involvement, parotid enlargement, hypothalamic and pituitary lesions, peripheral adenopathy. Neurosarcoidosis is detected in up to 25% of patients and can occur in the absence of apparent disease elsewhere. Cranial nerve dysfunction is the most common neurologic complication of sarcoidosis. Basilar granulomatous meningitis is the usual cause (Fig. E2), but the facial nerve may also be involved when parotitis is present.
10. The presence of anterior uveitis, parotiditis, fevers, and facial nerve palsy is known as **Heerfordt syndrome.**
11. Renal involvement in 7% to 22% in multisystem disease. Epididymis and the testis can be involved in male patients. Initial presentation can be of hydronephrosis due to external compression by retroperitoneal lymph nodes.
12. Hypercalcemia is seen in about 10% to 13% of patients with multisystem involvement. Abnormal production of 1-alpha-hydroxylase and PTHrp is thought to contribute to the hypercalcemia in some patients with sarcoidosis. Hypercalciuria is also common.

ETIOLOGY & PATHOGENESIS

A cardinal feature of sarcoidosis is the presence of CD4+ T cells that interact with antigen-presenting cells to initiate the formation and maintenance of granulomas (Fig. E3). Multiple lines of evidence suggest that sarcoidosis may result from the interaction of multiple genes with environmental exposures or infection.
GENETIC PREDISPOSITION TO SARCOIDOSIS: Various HLA antigens have been implicated in diverse patient populations. Familial predisposition has been reported dating back to 1923,

with a wide percentage of variability of affected relatives (0.4% to 21%) and heterogeneity based on genetic background. A more recent study was published by the ACCESS (A Case Controlled Etiologic Survey of Sarcoidosis) study group, which confirmed increased risk for family members with an odds ratio of 4.6 for all relatives. Absolute risk, however, for a family member to be affected was less than 1%. This study also showed a higher risk in white versus black American siblings and parents.
IMMUNOPATHOGENESIS OF SARCOIDOSIS: Numerous chemokines and cytokines have been implicated in the development and/or resolution of the disease. In sarcoidosis, the alveolitis seen at disease presentation represents an increase in primarily lymphocytic cellularity, predominated by CD4 cells. Presence of increased neutrophils in the bronchoalveolar lavage of patients with sarcoidosis has been associated with persistence of disease, with spontaneous remission noted in 36% of patients with elevated neutrophil counts.

DIAGNOSIS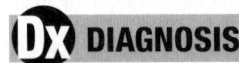

DIFFERENTIAL DIAGNOSIS

- Infection:
  1. Tuberculosis
  2. Fungal infection (e.g., *Coccidioides*, histoplasmosis, blastomycosis)
  3. Infectious mononucleosis
- Malignancies:
  1. Lymphoma
  2. Metastatic cancer
  3. Lymphangitic carcinomatosis
- Pneumoconioses including berylliosis and silicosis
- Other interstitial lung diseases (e.g., hypersensitivity pneumonitis)
- Vascular abnormalities (e.g., enlarged pulmonary arteries)
- Parasitic infection
- Other diseases such as amyloidosis

WORKUP

- No pathognomonic diagnostic test exists for sarcoidosis, so the diagnosis remains one of exclusion. The presence of noncaseating granulomas does not establish the diagnosis, because conditions such as tuberculosis and malignancies, among others, can cause granulomas.
- Workup is aimed at excluding critical organ involvement, determining extent and severity of disease, and excluding other disease. A complete neurologic and ophthalmologic examination is mandatory.
- A complete occupational and environmental exposure history is recommended.
- In patients with a history of beryllium exposure, beryllium lymphocyte proliferation testing should be obtained to assess for berylliosis.
- Initial laboratory evaluation should include complete blood count, serum chemistries (alanine aminotransferase, aspartate aminotransferase, alkaline phosphatase, electrolytes, blood urea nitrogen, creatinine, serum calcium), urinalysis, 24-h urinary excretion of

calcium, C-reactive protein (CRP), erythrocyte sedimentation rate (ESR), and tuberculin skin test or QuantiFERON gold test for tuberculosis. Routine vitamin D screening is generally not recommended; if done, it should measure both 25-hydroxyvitamin D and 1,25-dihydroxyvitamin D because sarcoidosis increases conversion of the former to the latter.[4]

- Chest x-ray and ECG should also be obtained in all patients suspected to have sarcoidosis.
- Pulmonary function testing: Spirometry, diffusion capacity of carbon monoxide.
- Biopsy (Fig. 4) in symptomatic patients should be done on accessible tissues suspected of sarcoid involvement (conjunctiva, skin, lymph nodes); bronchoscopy with transbronchial biopsy (85% diagnostic yield) is often performed in patients without any readily accessible site. Among patients with suspected Stage I/II pulmonary sarcoidosis undergoing tissue confirmation, the addition of endobronchial ultrasound (EBUS) transbronchial needle aspiration (TBNA) resulted in greater diagnostic yield. EBUS-TBNA of lymph nodes has a diagnostic yield of approximately 87%. Although in some studies, mediastinoscopy may have a higher diagnostic yield than EBUS-guided lymph node biopsy (98% and 87%, respectively), EBUS-TBNA is less invasive and has become the standard diagnostic modality for patients with mediastinal adenopathy with high clinical suspicion for sarcoidosis.

LABORATORY TESTS

The following laboratory abnormalities are often present in sarcoidosis:

- Hypergammaglobulinemia, anemia, leukopenia may be present.
- Liver function test abnormalities are common, e.g., elevated alkaline phosphatase.
- Hypercalcemia (11% of patients), hypercalciuria (40% of patients; attributable to increased gastrointestinal absorption, abnormal vitamin D metabolism, and increased calcitriol production by sarcoid granuloma).
- Angiotensin-converting enzyme: Elevated in approximately 75% of patients with untreated sarcoidosis; nonspecific and poor sensitivity; generally not useful as a diagnostic tool or in following the course of the disease.
- Serum adenosine deaminase (ADA), serum amyloid A (SAA) elevated but nonspecific.

IMAGING STUDIES

- Chest x-ray (Fig. 5): Pulmonary sarcoidosis is classified based on radiographic pattern. Adenopathy of the hilar and paratracheal nodes is a frequent finding. Parenchymal changes may also be present, depending on the stage of the disease (stage 0, normal radiograph; stage I, bilateral hilar adenopathy; stage II, stage I plus pulmonary infiltrate; stage III, pulmonary infiltrate without adenopathy; stage IV, advanced fibrosis with evidence of "honeycombing," hilar retraction, bullae, cysts, and emphysema).
- Computed tomography (CT) imaging: High-resolution CT may help detect early

parenchymal abnormalities. A chest CT scan with contrast can better define mediastinal adenopathy.

- For patients without apparent lung involvement, ^{18}F-fluorodeoxyglucose positron emission tomography (FDG-PET) (Fig. E6) is useful in identifying sites for diagnostic biopsy.

- FDG-PET and cardiac MRI (Fig. E7) with gadolinium are useful in patients with suspected cardiac and neurologic involvement.
- Gallium-67 scan: Represents an older testing modality. It will localize in areas of granulomatous infiltrates; however, it is not specific and not necessary. The "panda" sign (localization in the lacrimal and salivary glands, giving a

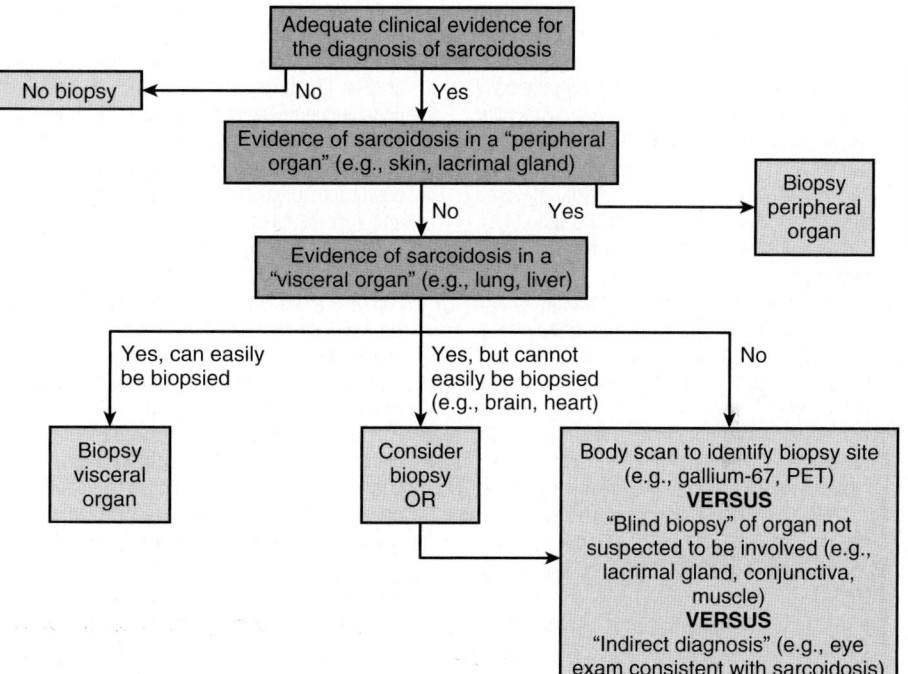

FIG. 4 Diagnostic approach to selecting a biopsy site for pathologic confirmation of granulomatous inflammation consistent with sarcoidosis. This approach emphasizes selection of a relatively noninvasive biopsy site when possible, biopsy of a site suspected to be clinically involved unless the biopsy would be highly invasive, and various approaches when no obvious organ involvement is demonstrated or only organs requiring very invasive biopsies demonstrate potential involvement. *PET,* Positron emission tomography. (From Broaddus VC et al: *Murray & Nadel's textbook of respiratory medicine,* ed 7, Philadelphia 2022, Elsevier.)

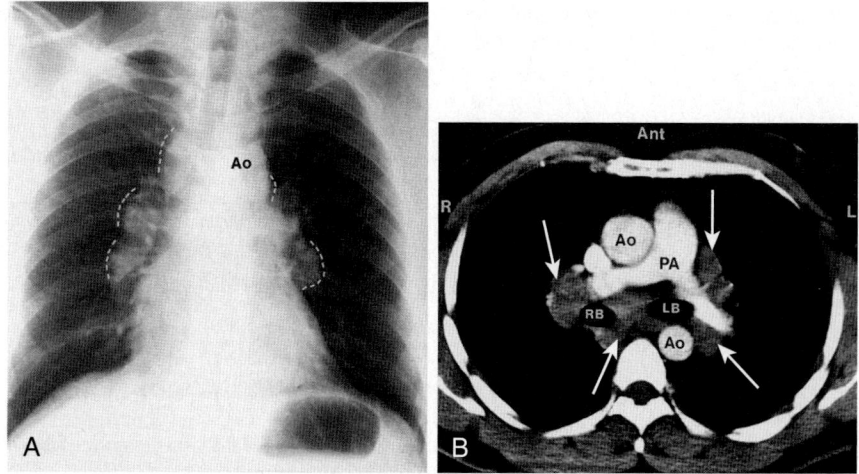

FIG. 5 Sarcoid. Marked lymphadenopathy *(dotted lines)* is seen in the region of both hila in the right paratracheal region **(A).** The transverse contrast-enhanced computed tomography (CT) scan of the upper chest **(B)** clearly shows the ascending and descending aorta *(Ao)* as well as the pulmonary artery *(PA)* and superior vena cava. The right and left mainstem bronchus area is also seen. The *arrows* indicate the extensive lymphadenopathy. *LB,* Left bronchus; *RB,* right bronchus. (From Mettler FA [ed]: *Primary care radiology,* Philadelphia, 2000, Saunders.)

"panda" appearance to the face) is suggestive of sarcoidosis.

Additional diagnostic tests:

- Pulmonary function tests (spirometry, lung volumes, and diffusing capacity for carbon monoxide): May be normal; may reveal a restrictive ventilatory defect with reduced forced vital capacity and/or reduced DLCO; may reveal an obstructive pattern; or may reveal a combination.
- Bronchoscopy: Flexible bronchoscopy and bronchoalveolar lavage (BAL) with transbronchial biopsy (showing noncaseating granulomas) are traditional methods for the minimally invasive diagnosis of sarcoidosis. With hilar adenopathy, EBUS-TBNA is the preferred method for lymph node sampling. BAL may show predominantly lymphocytosis, elevated ADA levels, and elevated CD4:CD8 ratio (4:1).
- Mediastinoscopy: Now rarely used for lymph node sampling and diagnosis.
- Routine eye examination is recommended, even for patients without ocular symptoms.
- For patients with extracardiac sarcoidosis or suspected cardiac involvement, cardiac MRI is indicated.
- Echocardiogram is indicated in patients with suspected pulmonary hypertension. If suggested by transthoracic echocardiogram, right heart catheterization should be done.

(Rx) TREATMENT

- Many patients with sarcoidosis will not require any treatment, and the disease resolves spontaneously.
- Multisystem sarcoidosis is best treated with a multidisciplinary approach that may include a pulmonologist, rheumatologist, cardiologist, and thoracic radiologist.
- Treatment should be instituted when organ function is threatened.
- Corticosteroids (Table 1) are the mainstay of therapy when treatment is required (e.g., prednisone 40 mg daily for 8 to 12 wk with gradual tapering of the dose to 10 mg every other day over 8 to 12 mo). Corticosteroids

should be considered in patients with severe symptoms (e.g., dyspnea, chest pain); hypercalcemia; ocular, central nervous system, or cardiac involvement; or progressive pulmonary disease. Patients with interstitial lung disease benefit from oral steroid therapy for 6 to 24 mo. A lack of response to steroid therapy may be due to the presence of irreversible fibrotic disease.

- Methotrexate: Patients with progressive disease refractory to corticosteroids or in patients unable to locate corticosteroids may be treated with methotrexate 7.5 to 15 mg once per wk or another immunosuppressant such as azathioprine, leflunomide, or mycophenolate mofetil.
- The antimalarial agent hydroxychloroquine is also a corticosteroid sparing agent particularly useful for cutaneous disease, hypercalcemia, and in some cases of neurosarcoidosis.[1]
- Immunomodulators: Represent third line alternatives. Adalimumab and infliximab may be considered. Infliximab has been used with some benefits in cutaneous, pulmonary, and neurologic disease.
- NSAIDs are useful for musculoskeletal symptoms and erythema nodosum.
- Pulmonary rehabilitation is recommended for patients with significant respiratory impairment.
- Lung transplantation should be considered in patients with advanced lung disease, unresponsive to medical therapy.

DISPOSITION

- The majority of patients with sarcoidosis have spontaneous remission within 2 yr and do not require treatment. Their course can be followed by periodic clinical evaluation, chest CT scans, and pulmonary function tests.
- Blacks have increased rates of pulmonary involvement, a worse long-term prognosis, and more frequent relapses.
- Up to one third of patients have unrelenting disease, leading to clinically significant organ impairment. Adverse prognostic factors in sarcoidosis include age of onset >40 yr, cardiac involvement, neurosarcoidosis, progressive pulmonary fibrosis, chronic hypercalcemia,

chronic uveitis, involvement of nasal mucosa, nephrocalcinosis, and presence of cystic bone lesions and lupus pernio.

- Prognosis for Loeffler syndrome is good with remittance within 16 wk in most patients. Symptoms can generally be controlled with NSAIDs. Low-dose glucocorticoids, hydroxychloroquine, and colchicine are also effective.
- Pulmonary hypertension is a poor prognostic sign and warrants consideration of referral for lung transplant evaluation. Transplantation for sarcoidosis is performed in 3% to 5% of patients and posttransplant survival rate is approximately 70% at 5 yr. The main factors associated with worse survival are older age and extensive preoperative lung fibrosis.[1]

REFERRAL

- Patients with progressive pulmonary disease or development of pulmonary hypertension despite therapy should be referred for consideration of lung transplant candidacy.
- Ophthalmologic examination is indicated in all patients with suspected sarcoidosis because ocular findings (iridocyclitis, uveitis, conjunctivitis, and keratopathy) are found in ≥25% of documented cases.
- Dermatology consultation for possible biopsy is indicated for patients with possible skin manifestations.
- Patients with suspected cardiac involvement should be referred to cardiology and those with CNS involvement referred to neurology.

❶ PEARLS & CONSIDERATIONS

COMMENTS

- Serial spirometry and measurement of DLCO can be useful in following response to therapy and disease progression.
- Approximately 15% to 20% of patients with lung involvement advance to irreversible lung impairment (bronchiectasis, cavitation, progressive fibrosis, pneumothorax, and respiratory failure). Death from pulmonary failure occurs in 5% to 7% of patients with sarcoidosis.
- Newer treatment approaches are aimed at targeting mechanisms involving CD4 type 1 helper T cells.
- The diagnosis of sarcoidosis should be reconsidered in the presence of atypical manifestations or persistent/progressive disease despite appropriate therapy.
- Diagnostic biopsy may not be necessary in most patients presenting with asymptomatic bilateral lymphadenopathy (with no other evidence of malignancy), in those with Lofgren syndrome, or in those with Heerfordt syndrome.

REFERENCES

Available at eBooks.Health.Elsevier.com.

RELATED CONTENT

Sarcoidosis (Patient Information)

TABLE 1 Indications for Use of Corticosteroids in Sarcoidosis

Disorder	Treatment
Iridocyclitis	Corticosteroid eye drops; local subconjunctival deposit of cortisone
Posterior uveitis	Oral prednisone
Pulmonary involvement	Steroids rarely recommended for stage I; typically used if infiltrate remains static or worsens over 3-mo period or the patient is symptomatic
Upper airway obstruction	Rare indication for intravenous steroids
Lupus pernio	Oral prednisone shrinks the disfiguring lesions
Hypercalcemia	Responds well to corticosteroids
Cardiac involvement	Corticosteroids usually recommended if patient has arrhythmias or conduction disturbances
Central nervous system involvement	Response is best in patients with acute symptoms
Lacrimal/salivary gland involvement	Corticosteroids recommended for disordered function, not gland swelling
Bone cysts	Corticosteroids recommended if symptomatic

From Andreoli TE (ed): *Cecil essentials of medicine*, ed 8, Philadelphia, 2010, Saunders.

AUTHOR: **IMRANA QAWI, MD**

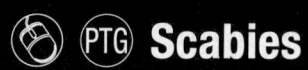
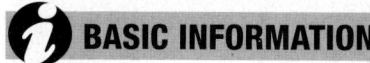 **BASIC INFORMATION**

DEFINITION

Scabies is a parasitic skin infestation caused by the mite *Sarcoptes scabiei*.

ICD-10CM CODE
B86   Scabies

EPIDEMIOLOGY & DEMOGRAPHICS

- Scabies is generally acquired by prolonged direct skin-to-skin contact with an infected individual.
- Scabies is endemic in many developing countries; however, it can affect individuals of any age and socioeconomic status.
- Prevalence is 100 to 200 million people worldwide,[1] with more than 200,000 U.S. cases/yr.
- Risk factors include living in crowded conditions (homes, shelters, nursing homes, extended care facilities, and prisons). More common in resource-limited areas and in tropical climates.[1]

PHYSICAL FINDINGS & CLINICAL PRESENTATION

- Primary lesions are caused when the microscopic mite burrows into the upper layer of the skin, laying eggs within the tract she leaves behind; burrows (linear or serpiginous tracts, see Fig. E1) end with a minute papule or vesicle.
- The distribution of primary lesions (Fig. E2) is usually widespread, and lesions are most commonly found in the web spaces of the hands, flexor aspects of wrists, buttocks, genitalia, breasts, axillae, and knees. In children <2 yr, they can also involve the head, neck, face, palms of the hands, and soles of the feet.[2] They are often confused with eczema (Fig. E3).
- Secondary lesions result from repeatedly scratching or secondary staphylococcal or streptococcal infections.
- Intense itching, especially at night, is the hallmark of this condition; it is caused by a delayed hypersensitivity to the mite or fecal pellets and is usually noted 2 to 6 wk after the primary infestation.
- Examination of the skin may reveal burrows, tiny vesicles, excoriations, or inflammatory papules.[2]
- Widespread hyperkeratotic crusted lesions (Norwegian or crusted scabies) may be seen in the elderly, in immunocompromised patients, or in patients who do not have the ability to scratch (Fig. E4). Pruritus may be mild or absent due to impaired host immune response.

Table 1 summarizes the different presenting forms of scabies.

ETIOLOGY

- Human scabies is caused by the mite *Sarcoptes scabiei* var. *hominis* (Fig. 5). After impregnation on the skin surface, the gravid female burrows in the stratum corneum and gradually extends the tract along the boundary with the stratum granulosum laying two to three eggs per day for 4 to 6 wk.[3] The eggs hatch in 3 to 4 days, and larvae move to the skin surface and mature in 2 to 3 wk, resuming the cycle.
- Transmission is usually due to prolonged skin-to-skin contact. In some cases minimal contact with crusted scabies can result in transmission due to mites from large exfoliative scales, because they can survive off a host for 24 to 36 h.
- Clinical manifestations result from a delayed type IV hypersensitivity reaction to the mite, eggs, saliva, or scybala (fecal pellets).
- Infestation from house pets and other animals is uncommon.

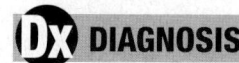 **DIAGNOSIS**

DIFFERENTIAL DIAGNOSIS

- Pediculosis
- Atopic dermatitis
- Flea bites
- Seborrheic dermatitis
- Dermatitis herpetiformis
- Contact dermatitis
- Nummular eczema
- Infantile acropustulosis
- Langerhans cell histiocytosis
- Arthropod bites

WORKUP

Diagnosis is made based on the clinical appearance of the rash and burrows and should be suspected if the patient presents with intense itching out of proportion to skin findings or there is a history of other family members with similar symptoms. Diagnosis can be confirmed by microscopic detection of mites, eggs, or mite feces from scrapings of burrows or intact papules.

LABORATORY TESTS

- Microscopic demonstration of the mites, feces, or eggs: A drop of mineral oil may be placed over the suspected lesion before removal (Box 1); the scrapings are transferred directly to a glass

TABLE 1	Different Presenting Forms of Scabies		
Presenting Forms of Scabies	**Specific High-Risk Populations**	**Clinical Manifestations**	**Limited Differential Diagnoses**
Classic scabies (scabies vulgaris)	Infants and children; sexually active adults; men who have sex with men	Intense generalized pruritus, worse at night; inflammatory pruritic papules localized to finger webs, flexor aspects of wrists, elbows, axillae, buttocks, genitalia, female breasts; lesions and pruritus spare the face, head, and neck; secondary lesions include eczematization, excoriation, impetigo	Dermatitis herpetiformis, drug reactions, eczema, pediculosis corporis, lichen planus, pityriasis rosea
Scalp scabies	Infants and children; institutionalized older adults; AIDS patients; patients with preexisting crusted scabies	Atypical crusted papular lesions of the scalp, face, palms, and soles	Dermatomyositis, ringworm, seborrheic dermatitis
Crusted scabies (Norwegian scabies, scabies norvegica, scabies crustosa)	Institutionalized older adults; institutionalized developmentally disabled (Down syndrome); homeless, especially HIV-positive; all immunocompromised patients, particularly those with AIDS or positive for HIV or HTLV-1; transplant recipients; patients on prolonged systemic corticosteroids and chemotherapy	Psoriasiform hyperkeratotic papular lesions of the scalp, face, neck, hands, feet, with extensive nail involvement; eczematization and impetigo common	Contact dermatitis, drug reactions, eczema, erythroderma, ichthyosis, psoriasis
Nodular scabies	Sexually active adults; men who have sex with men; HIV-positive men > HIV-positive women	Violaceous pruritic nodules localized to male genitalia, groin, axillae, representing hypersensitivity reaction to mite antigens	Acropustulosis, atopic dermatitis, Darier disease, lupus erythematosus, lymphomatoid papulosis, papular urticaria, necrotizing vasculitis, secondary syphilis

AIDS, Acquired immunodeficiency syndrome; *HIV,* human immunodeficiency virus; *HTLV-1,* human T-cell lymphotropic virus type 1.
From Bennett JE et al: *Mandell, Douglas, and Bennett's principles and practice of infectious diseases,* ed 9, Philadelphia, 2020, Elsevier.

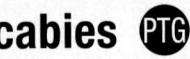
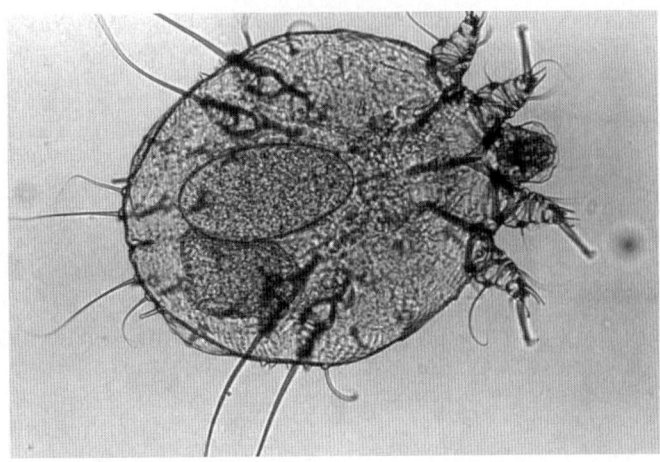

FIG. 5 Scabies mite. Note the eggs within the body of the mite. (Live scabies mite, ×40 magnification.) (From Paller AS, Mancini AJ: *Hurwitz clinical pediatric dermatology: a textbook of skin disorders of childhood and adolescence,* ed 5, Philadelphia, 2016, Elsevier.)

BOX 1   Performing a Mineral-Oil Examination for Scabies

---

1. Apply a drop of mineral oil to the lesion(s) to be scrapped.
2. Scrape through the lesion with a no. 15 scalpel blade (a small amount of bleeding is expected with appropriately deep scrapings).
3. Smear contents of scraping on a clean glass slide.
4. Add a few more drops of mineral oil.
5. Place cover slip over oil and examine under microscope at low power.

Criteria for a positive mineral oil examination:
Scabies mite
or
Ova (eggs)
or
Scybala (feces)

From Paller AS, Mancini AJ: *Hurwitz clinical pediatric dermatology: a textbook of skin disorders of childhood and adolescence,* ed 5, Philadelphia, 2016, Elsevier.

slide; a drop of potassium hydroxide is added, and a cover slip is applied.[3]
- Skin biopsy is rarely necessary to make the diagnosis.

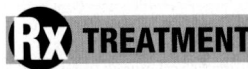 TREATMENT

NONPHARMACOLOGIC THERAPY

Clothing, underwear, bedding, and towels used 72 h before treatment must be washed in hot water and put in a dryer or sealed in a plastic bag for at least 72 h. Scabies mites generally do not survive more than 2 to 3 days away from human skin.

ACUTE GENERAL Rx

- Permethrin 5% cream is usually effective with one treatment; it should be massaged into the skin from head to soles of feet and applied under fingernails and toenails. Cream should be applied overnight and then washed off after 8 to 14 h. In children, cream should also be applied to the scalp and face. May need a second application in 1 to 2 wk. Permethrin is safe for children >2 mo old.[4]
- A single dose of ivermectin (200 μg/kg), an antiparasitic agent, can be used as initial therapy or for those who have failed topical treatment. Repeat doses, along with topical therapy, are recommended for Norwegian (crusted) scabies.[4]
- Pruritus generally abates 24 to 48 h after treatment but can last up to 2 wk; oral antihistamines can be effective. Retreatment may be necessary if pruritus is persistent for 2 to 4 wk or if new burrows or rash appears.
- Any sores that become infected should be treated with appropriate antibiotics if needed.
- It is essential that all close contacts and household members are treated at the same time whether symptomatic or not. If the patient is a resident of an extended care facility, it is important to educate the patients, staff, family, and frequent visitors about scabies and the need to have full cooperation with treatment.
- Table 2 summarizes currently recommended treatment for scabies.

DISPOSITION

Treatment failure is often result of poor adherence to treatment regimen or reinfestation. Scabies infection can be complicated by *Streptococcus pyogenes* and *Staphylococcus aureus* impetigo.[3] Refractory cases are usually only seen with immunocompromised hosts or patients with underlying skin diseases. ***Norwegian scabies (crusted scabies)*** refers to a highly contagious, severe variant often found in institutions caring for the elderly or physically and mentally disabled individuals.[5]

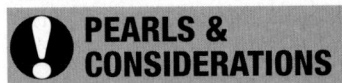 PEARLS & CONSIDERATIONS

COMMENTS

- Symptoms can take 4 to 6 wk to develop; however, individuals can still spread scabies before symptoms arise.
- Sexual partners and household members should be notified and treated simultaneously.
- It is important to decontaminate all bedding, clothing, and towels used by infested persons.

REFERENCES

Available at eBooks.Health.Elsevier.com.

RELATED CONTENT

Scabies (Patient Information)

AUTHOR: **MARY E. BOVE, MD**

TABLE 2   Currently Recommended Treatment for Scabies

Scabicides	FDA Approved?	Pregnancy Category[a]	Dosing Schedule	Safety Profile	Contraindications
5% Permethrin cream (Actin, Nix, Elimite)	Yes	B	Apply from neck down; wash off after 8-14 h; good residual activity, but second application recommended after 1 wk	Excellent; itching and stinging on application	Prior allergic reactions; infants <2 mo of age; breastfeeding
1% Lindane lotion or cream	Yes	B	Apply 30-60 ml from neck down; wash off after 8-12 h; no residual activity; increasing drug resistance	Potential for central nervous system toxicity from organochloride poisoning, usually manifesting as seizures, with overapplication and ingestions	Preexisting seizure disorder; infants and children <6 mo of age; pregnancy; breastfeeding
10% Crotamiton cream or lotion (Eurax)	Yes	C	Apply from neck down on two consecutive nights; wash off 24 h after second application	Excellent; not very effective; exacerbates pruritus	None
2%-10% Sulfur in petrolatum ointments	No	C	Apply for 2-3 days, then wash	Excellent; not very effective	Preexisting sulfur allergy
10%-25% Benzoyl benzoate lotion	No	None	Two applications for 24 h with 1-day to 1-wk interval	Irritant; exacerbates pruritus; can induce contact irritant dermatitis and pruritic cutaneous xerosis	Preexisting eczema
0.5% Malathion lotion (Ovide), 1% malathion shampoo (unavailable in the U.S.)	No	B	95% ovicidal; rapid (5 min) killing; good residual activity; increasing drug resistance	Flammable 78% isopropyl alcohol vehicle stings eyes, skin, mucosa; increasing drug resistance; organophosphate poisoning risk with overapplication and ingestions	Infants and children <6 mo of age; pregnancy; breastfeeding
Ivermectin (Stromectol)	Yes	C	200 μg/kg single PO dose, may be repeated in 14-15 days; not ovicidal, second dose on day 14 or 15 highly recommended; recommended for endemic or epidemic scabies in institutions and refugee camps	Excellent; may cause nausea and vomiting; take on empty stomach with water	Safety in pregnancy uncertain; probably safe during breastfeeding; not recommended for children <5 yr of age or weighing <15 kg

FDA, U.S. Food and Drug Administration; *PO,* by mouth.
[a]U.S. Food and Drug Administration (FDA) safety in pregnancy categories: A, safety established; B, presumed safe; C, uncertain safety; D, unsafe; X, highly unsafe.
From Bennett JE et al: *Mandell, Douglas, and Bennett's principles and practice of infectious diseases,* ed 8, Philadelphia, 2015, Saunders.

BASIC INFORMATION

DEFINITION

Tonic clonic seizures are characterized by sudden loss of consciousness, muscle contraction (tonic phase), followed by rhythmic jerking activity (clonic phase).

SYNONYMS

Bilateral tonic-clonic seizures
Convulsive seizures
Grand mal seizures
Generalized tonic clonic seizures

ICD-10CM CODES
G40.6   Grand mal seizures, unspecified
G41.0   Grand mal status epilepticus

EPIDEMIOLOGY & DEMOGRAPHICS

INCIDENCE: 40 to 70 cases per 100,000 person-yr (epilepsy incidence)[1]
PREVALENCE: 4 to 12 cases/1000 persons (epilepsy prevalence)[1]
PREDOMINANT SEX & AGE: No gender preference
PEAK INCIDENCE: Not applicable

PHYSICAL FINDINGS & CLINICAL PRESENTATION

- Patients with unprovoked tonic clonic seizures usually have normal physical and neurologic examinations.[2]
- A generalized seizure may start without warning and can typically last from 1 to 3 min, during which the patient will be unconscious and may have increased rigidity and/or jerking of the whole body, or staring spells. Cyanosis (especially of the lips and face) can result from temporary airway compromise due to muscle spasms. Patients are usually unaware of the seizure afterwards. A post-ictal state characterized by confusion, lethargy, headaches, or drowsiness may result and can last from minutes to hours depending on the severity of the seizure (Fig. 1).
- Tonic clonic seizures can cause injuries, bladder incontinence, and tongue biting.[3]
- Any warning or aura before onset of the seizure or focal post-ictal weakness (Todd paralysis) may point toward a focal cortical lesion.[2]

ETIOLOGY

- Seizures are a cardinal sign of cortical neurologic injury. Generalized seizures include both hemispheres of the brain at onset. However, seizures can start focally and then rapidly spread and generalize across both hemispheres of the brain, and this progression can make them appear very similar to primary generalized seizures. Any warning or aura symptoms before the generalized seizure starts would point to a focal onset.
- Acute symptomatic generalized seizures can be due to systemic causes (e.g., systemic infections, meningitis, encephalitis,

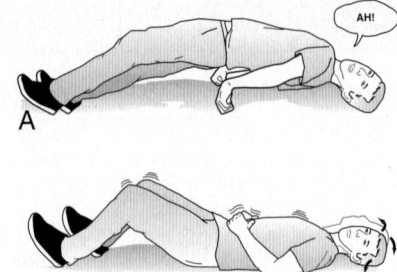

FIG. 1 A, This man in the tonic phase of a tonic-clonic seizure arches his torso and extends his arms and legs. He assumes this position because of the relatively greater strength of the extensor muscles compared to the flexor muscles. Simultaneous diaphragm, chest wall, and laryngeal muscle contractions force air through his tightened larynx to produce the shrill "epileptic cry." During this phase, he may also bite his tongue and lose control of his urine. **B,** In the clonic phase, his head, neck, and legs contract symmetrically and forcefully for about 10 to 20 sec. Saliva, aerated and often blood-tinged from tongue lacerations, froths from his mouth. His pupils dilate, and he sweats profusely. Finally, his muscular contractions lose strength. The seizure usually ends with stertorous breathing. In the immediate post-ictal period, he remains unresponsive. Before regaining consciousness, he may pass through a state of confusion and agitation. (From Kaufman DM et al: *Kaufman's clinical neurology for psychiatrists*, ed 9, Philadelphia, 2023, Elsevier.)

electrolyte abnormalities, hypoglycemia, malignant hypertension, eclampsia, drug intoxication or withdrawal).[4]
- Generalized seizures are seen in many epilepsy syndromes with genetic causes.[3]

DIAGNOSIS

DIFFERENTIAL DIAGNOSIS

- Convulsive syncope
- Psychogenic nonepileptic spells, conversion disorder, somatic symptom disorder, dissociative disorder, functional neurologic disorder
- Focal seizure with secondary generalization
- Factitious disorder
- Malingering
- Myoclonus (from metabolic disturbance)

WORKUP

- Electroencephalogram (EEG) (Fig. 2): An EEG can help confirm the presence of epilepsy but cannot be used to exclude the diagnosis.[5]
- Ambulatory EEG and/or video EEG recommended for patients with diagnostic uncertainty.[5]

LABORATORY TESTS

- Routine blood workup (CBC, comprehensive metabolic panel, glucose, electrolytes)[2]
- Urine drug screen[2]
- Lumbar puncture is recommended in patients with suspicion of encephalitis

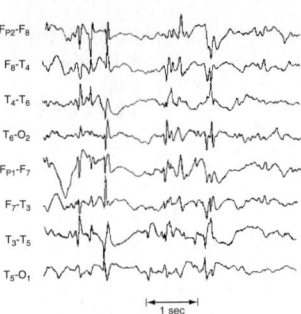

FIG. 2 Electroencephalogram (EEG). During a tonic-clonic seizure, the EEG ideally shows paroxysms of spikes, polyspikes, and occasional slow waves in all channels; however, muscle artifact can obscure this pattern. Even during interictal periods, the EEG contains multiple bursts of generalized spikes in the background. In contrast to occasional temporal lobe spikes, this pattern confirms a diagnosis of epilepsy in patients with seizures. (From Kaufman DM et al: *Kaufman's clinical neurology for psychiatrists*, ed 9, Philadelphia, 2023, Elsevier.)

IMAGING STUDIES

- Neurodiagnostic imaging studies such as computed tomography (CT) of the head or, preferably, MRI of the brain should be performed in all patients with first unprovoked seizure.[2]
- CT scans of the head should be avoided in children due to unnecessary exposure to radiation and the low yield of the test.[6] CT scans of the head are reserved for neurologic emergencies and are adjusted for weight in children.

TREATMENT

ACUTE Rx

- The immediate management of a seizure focuses on stabilization of the patient with focus on the airway and vital signs and rapid identification and correction of reversible causes.
- Seizures lasting >5 min or multiple seizures without return to baseline in between should be treated as status epilepticus.[7]
- Treatment is based on the type and etiology of seizures (i.e., metabolic disturbance, infectious, etc.).[2]
- Provoked seizures due to metabolic derangements, infections, fever, alcohol, or drug withdrawal are typically generalized and likely do not need long-term treatment.[2]
- Multiple antiseizure medication choices are available. Choice depends on side effect profile as well as whether the seizure started focally or is secondary to an idiopathic generalized epilepsy syndrome.[2]

NONPHARMACOLOGIC THERAPY

Not applicable

GENERAL Rx

- Patients with a first unprovoked seizure who have a normal EEG, imaging, lab values, and physical exam do not require treatment with antiseizure medications but may be offered therapy because the use of an antiseizure medication after a first unprovoked seizure in an adult reduces the absolute risk of seizure recurrence at 2 yr by 35%. However, there is no difference at 3 yr. This decision should be made in conjunction with the patient and should take into consideration the patient's job, risks of medications, and individual preferences.[2]

- Patients with two or more unprovoked seizures, or those with one seizure and an abnormal workup consistent with epilepsy findings, should be started or continued on antiseizure medications. Patients on antiseizure therapy with negative workup may be considered for weaning off antiseizure medication if seizure-free after 2 yr.[2]
- Primary generalized epilepsies:
  1. Levetiracetam (Keppra): Initial dose of 250 to 500 bid, maximum dose 2000 mg bid
  2. Lamotrigine (Lamictal): Initial dose of 25 mg daily and increase slowly to goal dose 200 to 300 mg daily (depends on combination of other medications)
  3. Topiramate (Topamax): Initial dose of 25 mg bid and increase to usual dose of 100 to 400 mg bid
  4. Perampanel (Fycompa): Initial dose of 2 mg once daily at bedtime, increments of 2 mg once daily at weekly intervals to a recommended maintenance dose of 4 to 8 mg (adjunctive treatment in patients with epilepsy 12 yr of age and older)
  5. Valproic acid (Depakote): Initial dose of 10 to 15 mg/kg/day (divided bid), maximum dose 60 mg/kg/day. Valproic acid should

be avoided in girls and women with childbearing potential due to the risk of teratogenicity[4]

- Focal epilepsies with secondary generalization: Almost all antiseizure medications are approved for focal seizures, either in monotherapy or in adjunct. Carbamazepine, oxcarbazepine, eslicarbazepine, lamotrigine, levetiracetam, lacosamide, or perampanel are all possibilities, among others.
- Patients who continue to have seizures despite adequate trials on at least two antiseizure medications should be referred to a tertiary care epilepsy center for evaluation of surgical treatment of epilepsy.

DISPOSITION

- Patients should avoid situations that may cause injuries or accidents in the event of a seizure, such as climbing ladders, using heavy machinery, swimming unsupervised, or taking baths (rather than showers).
- No driving until seizure-free in accordance with local laws and regulations.

REFERRAL

Patients with epilepsy and seizures should be referred for a consultation by a neurologist.

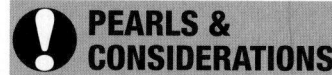 **PEARLS & CONSIDERATIONS**

COMMENTS

- It is crucial to understand that tonic-clonic seizures can occur in a variety of acute neurologic diseases.

- Successful treatment depends on the correct choice of antiseizure medications based on the type (focal onset vs. generalized onset) and etiology of the seizures.
- All women of childbearing age taking antiseizure medications should take folic acid supplementation (1 to 4 mg/day) for the prevention of neural tube defects.
- Many antiseizure medications also affect vitamin D absorption or metabolism, prompting attention to patients' bone health.

PREVENTION

Sleep deprivation and alcohol consumption should be avoided.

PATIENT & FAMILY EDUCATION

Patients with ongoing seizures are forbidden to drive; check your state regulations and laws regarding driving and epilepsy.

REFERENCES

Available at eBooks.Health.Elsevier.com.

RELATED CONTENT

Generalized Tonic-Clonic Seizures (Patient Information)
Status Epilepticus (Related Key Topic)

AUTHOR: **PEDRO BALAGUERA, MD**

S

Diseases and Disorders

I

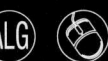
 BASIC INFORMATION

DEFINITION

An unprovoked seizure is a seizure that occurs without triggers or precipitating factors. In contrast, an acute symptomatic seizure occurs in the setting of an insult to the brain (infectious, toxic, etc.).[1,2] The presentation of a new seizure can vary greatly depending on the type (focal or generalized), progression, and severity.

Epilepsy is a disorder of the brain characterized by an enduring predisposition to generate seizures. For epidemiologic and, commonly, for clinical purposes, epilepsy is considered present when two or more unprovoked seizures occur in a time frame of longer than 24 h or after a single event that occurs in a person who is considered to have a high risk of recurrence (>60% risk in a 10-yr period).[3,4] A classification of seizure descriptions is summarized in Box 1.

SYNONYM

Convulsions

ICD-10CM CODES

G40.001	Localization-related (focal) (partial) idiopathic epilepsy and epileptic syndromes with seizures of localized onset, not intractable, with status epilepticus
G40.009	Localization-related (focal) (partial) idiopathic epilepsy and epileptic syndromes with seizures of localized onset, not intractable, without status epilepticus
G40.10	Localization-related (focal) (partial) symptomatic epilepsy and epileptic syndromes with simple partial seizures, not intractable
G40.101	Localization-related (focal) (partial) symptomatic epilepsy and epileptic syndromes with simple partial seizures, not intractable, with status epilepticus
G40.109	Localization-related (focal) (partial) symptomatic epilepsy and epileptic syndromes with simple partial seizures, not intractable, without status epilepticus
G40.201	Localization-related (focal) (partial) symptomatic epilepsy and epileptic syndromes with complex partial seizures, not intractable, with status epilepticus
G40.209	Localization-related (focal) (partial) symptomatic epilepsy and epileptic syndromes with complex partial seizures, not intractable, without status epilepticus
G40.301	Generalized idiopathic epilepsy and epileptic syndromes, not intractable, with status epilepticus
G40.309	Generalized idiopathic epilepsy and epileptic syndromes, not intractable, without status epilepticus
G40.A01	Absence epileptic syndrome, not intractable, with status epilepticus
G40.A09	Absence epileptic syndrome, not intractable, without status epilepticus
G40.4	Other generalized epilepsy and epileptic syndromes
G40.401	Other generalized epilepsy and epileptic syndromes, not intractable, with status epilepticus
G40.409	Other generalized epilepsy and epileptic syndromes, not intractable, without status epilepticus
G40.501	Epileptic seizures related to external causes, not intractable, with status epilepticus
G40.509	Epileptic seizures related to external causes, not intractable, without status epilepticus
G40.909	Epilepsy, unspecified, not intractable, without status epilepticus

EPIDEMIOLOGY & DEMOGRAPHICS

INCIDENCE: 29 to 39 per 100,000 per yr for acute symptomatic seizures. 23 to 61 per 100,000 person-yr for unprovoked seizures.[1] Approximately 8% to 10% of the population will experience a seizure during their lifetime; however, less than 3% go on to develop epilepsy

PREVALENCE: 5 to 8.4 cases per 1000 persons

PREDOMINANT SEX & AGE: Males younger than 12 mo and older than 65 yr[1]

RISK FACTORS:[1]
- Age of onset
- Family history of epilepsy
- Excessive sleep deprivation, use of alcohol, or illicit drugs
- History of head trauma, diseases of the brain, brain surgeries, and strokes

---

BOX 1   Classification of Seizure Descriptions (International League Against Epilepsy, 2017 Revision, Modified)

Focal onset
Aware vs. impaired awareness (formerly called complex partial)
Motor onset vs. nonmotor onset (autonomic, behavior arrest, cognitive, emotional, sensory)
Focal to bilateral tonic-clonic (formerly called secondarily generalized)

Generalized onset
Motor
Tonic-clonic (formerly called grand mal)
Other motor: Myoclonic, tonic, clonic, atonic, epileptic spasms
Nonmotor: Absence

Unknown onset
Motor: Tonic-clonic, epileptic spasms
Nonmotor: Behavior arrest

Unclassified

Modified from Kaufman DM et al: *Kaufman's clinical neurology for psychiatrists*, ed 9, Philadelphia, 2023, Elsevier.

- History of congenital cerebral anomalies or developmental delay

GENETICS: Although some new onset seizures are related to specific genes, most are not.

PHYSICAL FINDINGS & CLINICAL PRESENTATION

- Patients with generalized seizures will typically have normal physical exams. Patients with focal seizures due to persistent structural central nervous system damage may have exam findings consistent with the location of the lesion.
- A generalized seizure may start without warning[5] and can typically last from 30 to 120 sec, during which the patient will be unconscious and may have increased rigidity and/or jerking of the whole body, or staring spells. Cyanosis (especially of the lips and face) can result from temporary airway compromise due to muscle spasms. Tonic-clonic seizures can cause injuries, tongue biting, and bladder incontinence. Patients are usually unaware of the seizure afterwards. A post-ictal state characterized by confusion, lethargy, headaches, or drowsiness may result and can last from minutes to hours depending on the severity of the seizure.
- During a focal seizure, a patient may be aware (focal aware seizure) or have impaired consciousness (focal impaired awareness seizures).[6] A focal impaired awareness seizure may be associated with an aura (itself a focal aware seizure) and lasts between 30 and 120 sec. Motor or nonmotor symptoms may predominate in focal seizures, including jerking of one limb, automatisms, head turning, auditory hallucinations, or feelings of derealization. A focal seizure may progress to a generalized seizure, which usually involves the head and eyes turning to one side. Postictal weakness may result after focal seizures and can last for hours but usually resolves within 1 day. Patients with associated focal neurologic deficits, fever, persistent headache, cognitive changes, or a recent history of head trauma should be investigated.

ETIOLOGY (TABLE 1)

- New, unprovoked seizures are often idiopathic.
- Acute symptomatic seizures can be due to cerebral abnormalities (e.g., infections/abscesses, subarachnoid hemorrhages, ischemic strokes, tumors, vascular malformations) or systemic causes (e.g., systemic infections, electrolyte abnormalities, hypoglycemia, malignant hypertension, drug intoxication or withdrawal).[2]

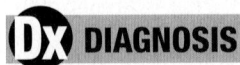 **DIAGNOSIS**

DIFFERENTIAL DIAGNOSIS[5,7]

- Syncope
- Transient ischemic attacks
- Migraines
- Sleep disorders
- Paroxysmal movement disorders
- Panic attacks, hallucinations, and other psychiatric disorders

TABLE 1 Causes of Seizures

Etiology	Examples
Infection and inflammation	Infective (meningo)encephalitis Chronic CNS infection (e.g., neurocysticercosis) Autoimmune limbic encephalitis (may present bizarrely) Cerebral lupus
Neoplasia	Gliomas and other primary CNS neoplasms Metastases Lymphoma
Vascular	Stroke* Subarachnoid hemorrhage* Subdural hematoma Eclampsia Hypertensive encephalopathy
Metabolic	Hyponatremia Hypoglycemia Hypocalcemia Uremia Porphyria
Trauma	Head injury* Neurosurgery*
Drugs and withdrawal	Alcohol Amphetamines, MDMA Pethidine Benzodiazepine or barbiturate withdrawal Many others
Neurodegeneration	Alzheimer disease Creutzfeldt-Jakob disease
Epilepsy	Multiple causes
Psychiatric	Psychogenic nonepileptic seizures

CNS, Central nervous system; *MDMA*, ecstasy.
*May occur at the time of the insult or may occur up to years later.
From Talley NJ et al: *Essentials of internal medicine*, ed 4, Chatswood, NSW, 2021, Elsevier Australia.

WORKUP

- Ambulatory 30-min electroencephalogram (EEG) if patient fully recovers after seizure within 30 to 60 min. May be delayed if treatment does not depend on EEG result.[5]
- Consider inpatient continuous EEG if patient does not fully recover within 60 min or for recurrent seizures.
- ECG.
- Fig. 1 illustrates the initial approach to patients with suspected seizures. The approach to a child with a suspected convulsive disorder is outlined in Fig. E2.
- Critical and emergent diagnoses to consider in a patient with seizures are summarized in Box 2.

LABORATORY TESTS

Comprehensive metabolic panel and urine drug screen[5]

IMAGING STUDIES

- Acutely, computed tomography (CT) of the head with and without contrast to evaluate for hemorrhage and space-occupying lesions
- Brain MRI with and without contrast with epilepsy protocol in patients with no clear provoking cause of a seizure, in consultation with a neurologist[5]

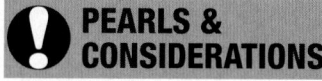 **TREATMENT**

ACUTE Rx

- The immediate management of a seizure focuses on stabilization of the patient with focus on the airway and vital signs and rapid identification and correction of reversible causes.[8]
- Seizures lasting >5 min or multiple seizures without return to baseline in between should be treated as status epilepticus.[7]
- Treatment is based on the type and etiology of seizures (i.e., metabolic disturbance, infectious, unprovoked, etc.).[5]

CHRONIC Rx

- Provoked seizures do not need long-term treatment.[5]
- Patients with a first unprovoked seizure who have a normal EEG, imaging, lab values, and physical exam do not require treatment with antiseizure medications but may be offered therapy because the use of an antiseizure medication after a first unprovoked seizure in an adult reduces the absolute risk of seizure recurrence at 2 yr by 35%. However, there is no difference at 3 yr.[8] This decision should be made in conjunction with the patient and should take into consideration the patient's job, risks of medications, and individual preferences.
- Patients with two or more unprovoked seizures, or those with one seizure and an abnormal workup consistent with epilepsy findings, should be started or continued on antiseizure medications. Patients on antiseizure therapy with negative workup may be considered for weaning off antiseizure medication if seizure-free after 2 yr.[5]
- The choice of treatment depends largely on seizure type and etiology (Table 2). Antiseizure medications may be thought of as narrow- or wide-spectrum drugs. Treatment with wide-spectrum antiseizure medications is advisable in generalized seizures or those of unknown type, whereas partial seizures are better controlled with narrow-spectrum antiseizure medications.[5]
- Narrow-spectrum drugs include carbamazepine, oxcarbazepine, eslicarbazepine, gabapentin, lacosamide, and phenytoin. Wide-spectrum drugs include valproate, topiramate, zonisamide, lamotrigine, and levetiracetam.[5]
- In patients with significant comorbidities, the use of antiseizure medications with limited drug interactions is advised (lamotrigine, levetiracetam, lacosamide).[5]
- Older patients may benefit from lamotrigine, levetiracetam, or gabapentin due to a lower risk of adverse events.[5]
- Some patients may benefit from having a seizure rescue medication that could be used if they have a prolonged seizure or cluster of seizures.

DISPOSITION

- Patients should avoid swimming unobserved, bathing alone, working at heights, using heavy machinery, or other activities that may be high-risk in the event of a seizure.[5]
- Discontinue driving until seizures are well controlled and in accordance with state laws.[5]

REFERRAL

Patients should be referred to a neurologist, especially if they experience recurrent unprovoked seizures.[5]

⚠ PEARLS & CONSIDERATIONS

COMMENTS

- Driving: Physicians should be aware of the law in their jurisdiction about driving after a seizure. Although a few U.S. states require physicians to notify the state government authority that issues driver's licenses, most do not impose such an obligation on physicians. However, states do require patients to self-report and abstain from driving until seizure-free for a specified period of time, depending on the state.[5]
- Recurrence risk: After a first unprovoked seizure, the overall risk of recurrence may be as high as 60% and is highest within the first 2 yr. Greatest recurrence risk in an adult with a first unprovoked seizure is within the first 2 yr and is between 21% and 45%. The recurrence risk is lower in patients treated with an antiseizure medication and higher in patients with a brain MRI abnormality causing the seizure or an EEG showing epileptiform activity.[8]

PREVENTION

Patients with recurrent seizures should be extensively counseled on avoiding seizure triggers such as sleep deprivation, alcohol or drug use, stress, and exposure to excessive flashing lights. Such patients may need dose titration of antiseizure medication and referral to a neurologist.[5]

PATIENT & FAMILY EDUCATION

- Physicians should inform patients with first-time seizures that they are subject to state law restrictions on driving after a seizure. Physicians should also counsel patients with epilepsy about not swimming unattended, not climbing heights, and taking showers rather than baths (because of the risk of drowning in a bathtub during a generalized seizure).[5] Physicians should counsel women of childbearing potential about effects of antiseizure medications on both oral contraceptive efficacy and on a developing fetus.[5] They should recommend supplemental folic acid for such women if they are taking antiseizure medications. They should also recommend that women plan pregnancy if they are on antiseizure medications to minimize adverse effects on the pregnancy. All such counseling should be documented in the medical record.
- Patients must be informed of the potential risks of recurrent seizures, including aspiration, status epilepticus, and sudden unexpected death in epilepsy (SUDEP).

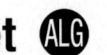

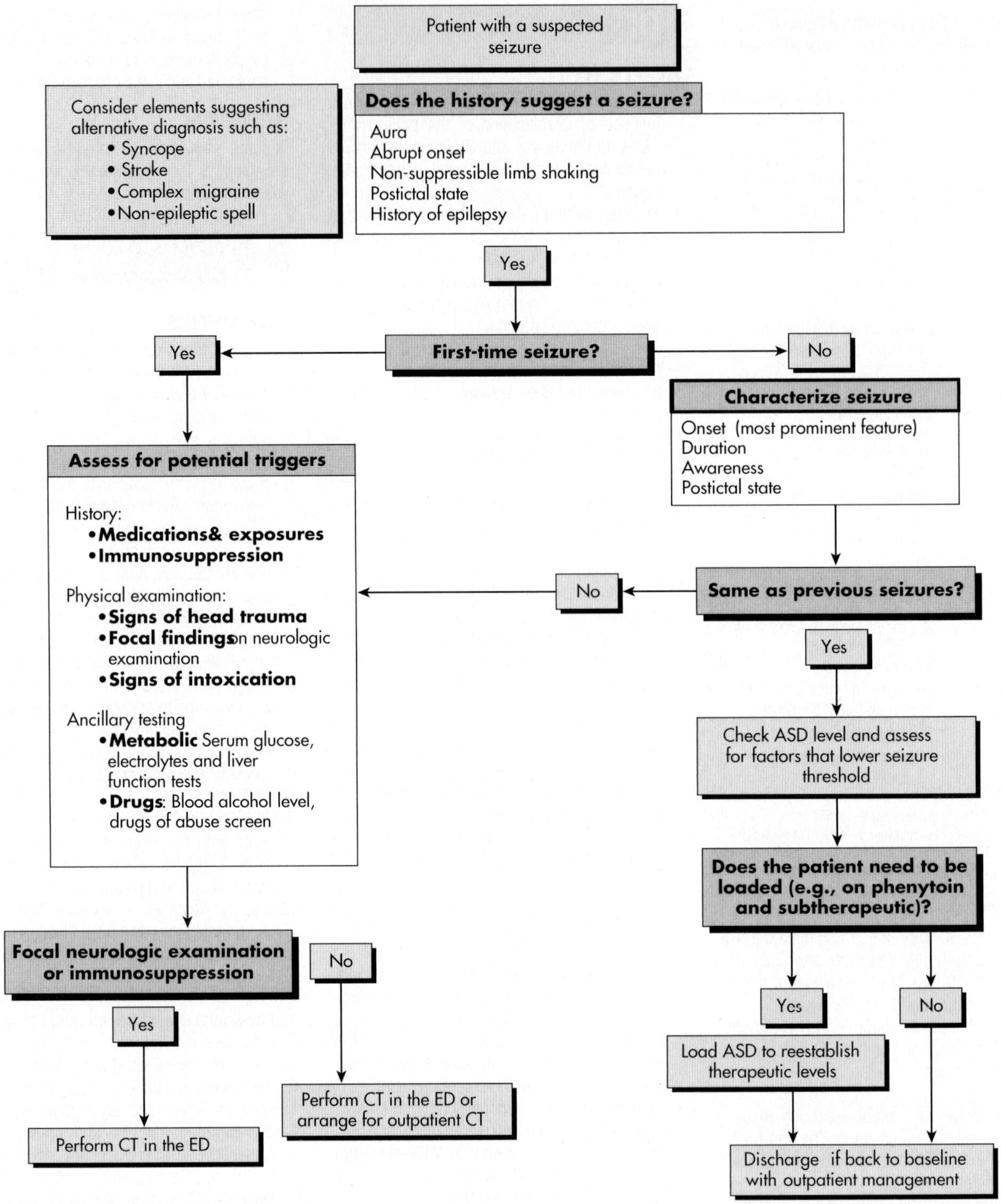

Patient with a suspected seizure

Consider elements suggesting alternative diagnosis such as:
- Syncope
- Stroke
- Complex migraine
- Non-epileptic spell

Does the history suggest a seizure?
Aura
Abrupt onset
Non-suppressible limb shaking
Postictal state
History of epilepsy

Yes

First-time seizure?

Yes ← First-time seizure? → No

Characterize seizure
Onset (most prominent feature)
Duration
Awareness
Postictal state

Assess for potential triggers

History:
- **Medications& exposures**
- **Immunosuppression**

Physical examination:
- **Signs of head trauma**
- **Focal findings** on neurologic examination
- **Signs of intoxication**

Ancillary testing
- **Metabolic** Serum glucose, electrolytes and liver function tests
- **Drugs**: Blood alcohol level, drugs of abuse screen

No ← **Same as previous seizures?**

Yes

Check ASD level and assess for factors that lower seizure threshold

Does the patient need to be loaded (e.g., on phenytoin and subtherapeutic)?

Focal neurologic examination or immunosuppression

No

Yes

Perform CT in the ED or arrange for outpatient CT

Perform CT in the ED

Yes

Load ASD to reestablish therapeutic levels

No

Discharge if back to baseline with outpatient management

FIG. 1 Initial approach to patients with suspected seizure. *ASD,* Antiseizure drug; *CT,* computed tomography; *ED,* emergency department. (From Walls RM et al: *Rosen's emergency medicine, concepts and clinical practice,* ed 10, Philadelphia, 2023, Elsevier.)

BOX 2 Critical and Emergent Diagnoses to Consider in a Patient with Seizures

Critical Diagnoses

Status epilepticus, convulsive and non-convulsive, regardless of cause

Seizures with specialized treatments
- Eclampsia
- Toxic ingestion (e.g., isoniazid, lithium, tricyclic antidepressants)
- Hypoglycemia
- Hyponatremia, hypocalcemia
- Increased intracranial pressure

Emergent Diagnoses

Infection

Acute brain injury: ischemic or hemorrhagic strokes, traumatic brain injury, cerebral venous thrombosis

Serious mimics of seizure activity (e.g., cardiogenic syncope)

From Walls RM et al: *Rosen's emergency medicine, concepts and clinical practice*, ed 10, Philadelphia, 2023, Elsevier.

- A diagnosis of epilepsy has significant medical, social, and emotional consequences. Patient information on seizures and locating support groups can be found at the Epilepsy Foundation website: https://www.epilepsy.com.

REFERENCES

Available at eBooks.Health.Elsevier.com.

RELATED CONTENT

Absence Seizures (Related Key Topic)
Febrile Seizures (Related Key Topic)
Seizures, Generalized Tonic-Clonic (Related Key Topic)
Focal Seizures (Related Key Topic)
Status Epilepticus (Related Key Topic)

AUTHOR: **PEDRO BALAGUERA, MD**

TABLE 2 A Selection of Antiseizure Medication

Drug	Mechanism of Action	Uses	Side Effects
Carbamazepine	Sodium-channel blocking agent	Focal seizures	May worsen generalized seizures Nausea, ataxia, elevated hepatic enzymes, drowsiness, rash Potential for Stevens-Johnson syndrome in Han Chinese ethnicity, so must be avoided Agranulocytosis, which is usually reversible
Sodium valproate	Multiple, including sodium-channel blockade, and increasing cerebral GABA	Multiple actions Broad-spectrum anticonvulsant First-line therapy in generalized epilepsies	Weight gain, tremor, thrombocytopenia, LFT dysfunction Rarely but importantly, hyperammonemic encephalopathy Teratogenic, in particular neural tube defects Interacts with lamotrigine
Lamotrigine	Sodium-channel blocker	Broad-spectrum anticonvulsant Focal epilepsies Useful in generalized epilepsies Second-line therapy in JME	CNS side effects Stevens-Johnson syndrome
Topiramate	Enhances central GABA activity, and antagonizes AMPA and kainate glutamate receptors	Broad-spectrum anticonvulsant Migraine prophylaxis	Cognitive blunting and speech disturbance Acral paresthesias Kidney stones Mood disturbance
Levetiracetam and brivaracetam (less neuropsychiatric events)	Not fully known	Broad-spectrum anticonvulsant Renally excreted with minimal interactions	Lethargy Possible neuropsychiatric disturbance with mood change and irritability
Clonazepam + clobazam	Benzodiazepines	Broad-spectrum effect on seizures Predominantly used in the short-term control of epilepsy while titrating other medication	Longer-term use should be limited to intractable epilepsies due to tolerance, difficulty with withdrawal, and the potential for abuse
Phenobarbitone + primidone	Barbiturates	Less commonly used now, but some patients have been on these drugs for many years	Sedation Narrow therapeutic index Withdrawal seizures
Lacosamide	Slow inactivation of sodium channels	Narrow spectrum, usually as add-on therapy Few interactions	Dizziness, diplopia, and visual disturbance Nausea and headache
Perampanel	Inhibition of AMPA glutamate excitatory channels	Broad spectrum with uses in generalized and focal epilepsy; less helpful in absences	Somnolence, dizziness, and behavioral disturbance may occur
Phenytoin	Sodium-channel blocking agent	Status epilepticus (due to availability for IV infusion)	Ataxia, drowsiness, nausea, encephalopathy Multiple drug interactions Gum hypertrophy or cerebellar degeneration possible with long-term use

AMPA, Alpha-amino-3-hydroxy-5-methyl-4-isoxazolepropionic acid; *CNS,* central nervous system; *GABA,* gamma-aminobutyric acid; *IV,* intravenous; *JME,* juvenile monoclonic epilepsy; *LFT,* liver function test.

From Talley NJ et al: *Essentials of internal medicine*, ed 4, Chatswood, NSW 2021, Elsevier Australia.

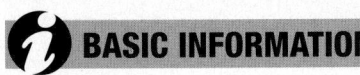

BASIC INFORMATION

DEFINITION

Sepsis is an exaggerated inflammatory response to an infectious stimulus. It is usually caused by generalized bacterial or fungal infection and characterized by evidence of infection, fever or hypothermia, hypotension, and evidence of end-organ compromise. The Sepsis Definitions Task Force in 2016 updated definitions for sepsis and septic shock (Table 1). A major change in the definitions is the elimination of mention of SIRS.* According to the new definitions, sepsis is now defined as evidence of infection plus life-threatening organ dysfunction, clinically codified by an acute change in 2 points or greater in the SOFA score (Table 2). The new clinical criteria for septic shock include sepsis with fluid, unresponsive hypotension, serum lactate level greater than 2 mmol/L, and the need for vasopressors to maintain mean arterial pressure of 65 mm Hg or greater.*

SYNONYMS

Septicemia
Sepsis syndrome
Severe sepsis
Systemic inflammatory response syndrome
Septic shock

ICD-10CM CODES
A41.9   Sepsis, unspecified organism
A41.50   Gram-negative sepsis, unspecified

*SIRS (Systemic Inflammatory Response Syndrome): Variables in SIRS criteria include respiratory rate (breaths/min), white blood cell count (109/L), hands (%), heart rate (beats/min), temperature (° C), and arterial carbon dioxide tension (mm Hg). Score range is 0 to 4.

A41.2	Sepsis due to unspecified *Staphylococcus*
A41.4	Sepsis due to anaerobes
A41.51	Sepsis due to *Escherichia coli* [E. Coli]
A41.52	Sepsis due to Pseudomonas
A54.86	Gonococcal sepsis
B37.7	Candidal sepsis
A32.7	Listerial sepsis
A40.0	Sepsis due to streptococcus, group A
A40.1	Sepsis due to streptococcus, group B
A40.3	Sepsis due to Streptococcus pneumoniae
A40.8	Other streptococcal sepsis
A40.9	Streptococcal sepsis, unspecified
A41.01	Sepsis due to Methicillin susceptible *Staphylococcus aureus*
A41.02	Sepsis due to Methicillin resistant *Staphylococcus aureus*

EPIDEMIOLOGY & DEMOGRAPHICS

INCIDENCE (IN U.S.):
- Sepsis occurs in 6% of hospitalized patients; approximately half require intensive care unit (ICU) admission.
- More than 1.7 million cases of sepsis occur each year in the U.S. and cases have been increasing annually. It leads to 250,000 deaths per yr and is the leading cause of death in noncardiac ICUs.
- The most common sources of sepsis leading to ICU admissions include lungs (64%), abdomen (20%), bloodstream (15%), and urinary tract (14%).
- The most common isolated organisms causing sepsis are Gram-negative bacteria (62%), Gram-positive bacteria (47%), and fungi (19%).[1]

PREDOMINANT SEX: Males are slightly more commonly affected than females.

PREDOMINANT AGE:
- Neonatal period.
- Patients >65 yr of age account for 60% of all cases of sepsis.

GENETICS:
- Familial disposition: A great variety of congenital immunodeficiency states and other inherited disorders may predispose to septicemia.
- Neonatal infection: Incidence is high in neonatal period.

PHYSICAL FINDINGS & CLINICAL PRESENTATION
- Fever or hypothermia
- Hypotension
- Tachycardia
- Tachypnea
- Altered mental status
- Bleeding diathesis
- Skin rashes
- Symptoms that reflect primary site of infection: Urinary tract, GI tract, central nervous system (CNS), respiratory tract
- Table 3 describes some clinical signs and symptoms of sepsis

ETIOLOGY
- Disseminated infection with a great variety of bacteria:
  1. Gram-negative bacteria:
     a. *Escherichia coli*
     b. *Klebsiella* spp.
     c. *Pseudomonas aeruginosa*
     d. *Proteus* spp.
     e. *Neisseria meningitides*
  2. Gram-positive bacteria:
     a. *Staphylococcus aureus* (including MRSA)
     b. *Streptococcus* spp.
     c. *Enterococcus* spp.

TABLE 1   Proposed New Definitions of Sepsis

Term	Definition	Criteria	Notes
Sepsis[a] (previously severe sepsis)	Life-threatening organ dysfunction caused by a dysregulated host response to infection	Organ dysfunction is identified as an acute change in the SOFA score, ≥2 points from the baseline consequent to the infection.	qSOFA (quick Sequential Organ Failure Assessment) Prolonged ICU stay or in-hospital mortality can be identified at the bedside with qSOFA 1. Respiratory rate ≥22 breaths/min 2. Acute mental status change 3. Systolic blood pressure ≤100 mm Hg 4. An increase in SOFA of ≥2 predicts a 10% mortality in the general hospital population. Presume a baseline SOFA of 0 unless the patient has known (acute or chronic) organ dysfunction before the onset of infection
Septic shock	It is a subset of sepsis in which the underlying circulatory and cellular/metabolic abnormalities are profound enough to substantially increase mortality	A clinical construct of sepsis with persisting hypotension requiring vasopressors to maintain MAP ≥65 mm Hg and having a serum lactate level ≥2 mmol/L despite adequate volume resuscitation	Septic shock portends hospital mortality in excess of 40%

MAP, Mean arterial pressure.
[a]Note that the proposed new definitions abandon the previous term "severe sepsis" to describe infection-induced organ dysfunction and now use "sepsis" in its place. The previous condition called "sepsis" is now just called "infection," and when infection is not associated with organ dysfunction, there is no differentiation between infection with or without systemic manifestations.
From Parrillo JE, Dellinger RP: *Critical care medicine, principles of diagnosis and management in the adult,* ed 5, Philadelphia, 2019, Elsevier.

TABLE 2 The Sequential Organ Failure Assessment (SOFA) Score

Score	0	1	2	3	4
Respiration					
PaO$_2$/FiO$_2$, mm Hg	>400	≤400	≤300	≤200 With respiratory support	≤100
Coagulation					
Platelets × 10^3/mm^3	>150	≤150	≤100	≤50	≤20
Liver					
Bilirubin, mg/dl (μmol/L)	<1.2 (<20)	1.2-1.9 (20-32)	2.0-5.9 (33-101)	6.0-11.9 (102-204)	>12.0 (>204)
Cardiovascular					
Hypotension	No hypotension	MAP <70 mm Hg	Dopamine ≤5 or dobutamine (any dose)*	Dopamine >5 or epinephrine ≤0.1 or norepinephrine ≤0.1*	Dopamine >15 or epinephrine >0.1 or norepinephrine >0.1*
Central Nervous System					
Glasgow coma score	15	13-14	10-12	6-9	<6
Renal					
Creatinine, mg/dl (μmol/L) OR urine output	<1.2 (<110)	1.2-1.9 (110- 170)	2.0-3.4 (171-299)	3.5-4.9 (300-440) <500 ml/d	>5.0 (>440) <200 ml/d

*Adrenergic agents administered for at least 1 h (doses given are in mcg/kg per min).
From Ronco C et al: *Critical care nephrology,* ed 3, Philadelphia, 2019, Elsevier.

TABLE 3 Clinical Signs and Symptoms of Sepsis

Infection	General	Inflammatory	Hemodynamic	Tissue Perfusion
Documented or suspected	Temperature >38° C (100.4° F) or <36° C (96.8° F) Heart rate >90 beats/min Respiratory rate ≥20 breaths/min Altered mental status Hyperglycemia Third spacing of fluid	WBC count <4000 or >12,000 cells/μL or ≥10% bands	Hypotension: Systolic blood pressure <90 mm Hg MAP <70 mm Hg SVo$_2$ >70 CI >3.5 L/min/m^2	Hypoxemia: (Pao$_2$/Fio$_2$ <300) Acute oliguria (urine output <0.5 ml/kg/h) Coagulopathy Abnormal liver function tests Platelet count <100,000 cells/μL Lactic acidosis Skin mottling

CI, Cardiac index; *MAP,* mean arterial pressure; *SVo$_2$,* mixed venous oxygen saturation; *WBC,* white blood cell.
From Cameron JL, Cameron AM: *Current surgical therapy,* ed 10, Philadelphia, 2011, Saunders.

- Less common infections:
  1. Fungal
  2. Viral
  3. Rickettsial
  4. Parasitic
- Sepsis is a complex dysregulation of both inflammation and coagulation (Fig. E1). There is activation of coagulation, inflammatory cytokines, complement, and kinin cascades with release of a variety of vasoactive endogenous mediators. The innate immune system recognizes pathogens by means of pattern-recognition receptors (toll-like receptors [TLRs], Table 4). TLRs bind to structures on microorganisms and, based on the composite information gained, generate a tailored response to the invading pathogen.
- Predisposing host factors (Table 5):
  1. General medical condition
  2. Extremes of age
  3. Immunosuppressive therapy
  4. Recent surgery
  5. Granulocytopenia
  6. Hyposplenism
  7. Diabetes
  8. Instrumentation

PATHOGENESIS

Patients with sepsis show signs of both hyper-inflammation and immunosuppression, two seemingly opposite reactions that involve partially different cell types and organ systems (Fig. E2). Likely, this disturbed immune response is not only the result of persistent stimulation by pathogens and their virulence factors but also the release of damage-associated molecular patterns (DAMPs), or alarmins, which are molecules derived from host cells released into the extracellular environment on injury. Sepsis is associated with a strong activation of coagulation, which, together with an impairment of endogenous anticoagulant mechanisms, results in a net procoagulant state and a tendency toward microvascular thrombosis (Fig. E3). The most severe manifestation of coagulopathy in sepsis is DIC, which clinically can be associated with both microvascular thrombosis and hemorrhage, owing to widespread fibrin depositions and consumption of clotting factors and platelets, respectively.

🄳🅇 **DIAGNOSIS**

DIFFERENTIAL DIAGNOSIS

- Cardiogenic shock
- Acute pancreatitis
- Pulmonary embolism
- Systemic vasculitis
- Toxic ingestion
- Exposure-induced hypothermia
- Fulminant hepatic failure
- Collagen-vascular diseases

WORKUP

- Evaluation should focus on identifying a specific pathogen and localizing the site of primary infection. Box 1 summarizes a general approach to shock.
- Hemodynamic, metabolic, coagulation disorders should be carefully characterized.
- Intensive monitoring.

LABORATORY TESTS

- Cultures of blood and examination and culture of sputum, urine, wound drainage, stool, and cerebrospinal fluid (CSF), depending on the presenting signs and symptoms for each patient
- CBC with differential, coagulation profile
- Routine chemistries, liver function tests (LFTs)
- Arterial blood gases (ABGs), lactic acid level
- Procalcitonin can be useful as a serum marker of bacterial infection as a cause of the sepsis, and has been shown to improve survival and facilitate earlier discontinuation of antibiotics
- Urinalysis

TABLE 4	Toll-Like Receptors
Toll-Like Receptor	**Pathogen or Disease State**
TLR1	Lyme disease
	Neisseria meningitidis
TLR2	*Mycobacterium tuberculosis*
	Chagas disease
	Leptospirosis
	Fungal sepsis
	CMV viremia
TLR3	Many
TLR4	Gram-negative bacteria
	Septic shock
	Chlamydia trachomatis
	Chlamydia pneumoniae
	Certain viruses
	Mycobacterium tuberculosis
TLR5	Flagellated bacteria (e.g., *Salmonella*)
TLR7	Viral infections
TLR8	Viral infections
TLR9	Bacterial and viral infections
TLR10	Unknown

CMV, Cytomegalovirus; *TLR,* toll-like receptor.
From Parrillo JE, Dellinger RP: *Critical care medicine, principles of diagnosis and management in the adult,* ed 5, Philadelphia, 2019, Elsevier.

TABLE 5	Risk Factors for Sepsis

Demographic Factors

Older age (>65 yr old)
Male sex
Black race
Nutrition
Vaccination status
Genetic polymorphisms

Environmental Factors

Poor socioeconomic status
Seasonal variation and contacts
Disease outbreaks
Travel

Comorbidities

Diabetes
Chronic obstructive pulmonary disease
Cancer
Chronic renal disease
Chronic liver disease
Human immunodeficiency virus
Use of immunosuppressive agents

Hospital Factors

Duration of hospitalization
Antibiotic resistance
Catheters (e.g., urine catheters, intravenous lines)
Complications of surgery (wound infection, emergency vs. elective surgery)

Bennett JE et al: *Mandell, Douglas, and Bennett's principles and practice of infectious diseases,* ed 9, Philadelphia, 2020, Saunders.

IMAGING STUDIES

- Chest x-ray
- Other radiographic and radioisotope procedures according to suspected site of primary infection

---

BOX 1 General Approach to Shock: Initial Diagnosis and Evaluation

Clinical (primary diagnosis)
- Tachycardia, hypotension (systolic blood pressure <90 mm Hg) tachypnea, oliguria, encephalopathy (confusion), peripheral hypoperfusion (mottled extremities), cyanosis

Laboratory (confirmatory)
- Hemoglobin, WBC, platelets

Prothrombin time/partial thromboplastin time
- Electrolytes, arterial blood gases, Ca, Mg, BUN, creatinine, serum lactate
- ECG

Monitoring (continuous ECG and respiratory monitors)
- Pulse oximetry
- Urinary catheter (urine output)
- Point-of-care ultrasonography (heart, lung, abdominal, and major vessels)
- Arterial pressure catheter
- Central venous pressure monitor (uncomplicated shock)
- Pulmonary artery flotation catheter
  1. Cardiac output
  2. Pulmonary artery occlusion pressure
  3. Central and/or mixed venous oxygen saturation (intermittent or continuous)
- Oximetry

Imaging
- Chest x-ray
- X-ray views of abdomen
- Computed tomographic scan: Abdomen or chest
- Formal transthoracic and/or transesophageal echocardiogram

From Parrillo JE, Dellinger RP: *Critical care medicine, principles of diagnosis and management in the adult,* ed 5, Philadelphia, 2019, Elsevier.

Rx TREATMENT (FIG. 4)

NONPHARMACOLOGIC THERAPY

- Tissue oxygenation: Mixed venous oxygen saturation maintained >70% if possible; early mechanical ventilation with low tidal volume (6 ml/kg predicted body weight) to protect lung parenchyma from overstretching and "volutrauma." Recommended plateau pressure for sepsis-related acute respiratory distress syndrome (ARDS) is ≤30 cm H_2O.
- Focal infection should be drained if possible, and potentially infected catheters should be removed.

ACUTE GENERAL Rx

- Blood pressure support, intravenous (IV) fluid resuscitation and vasopressors (Table 6), if needed, with the goal of reestablishing a mean arterial blood pressure >65 mm Hg; reduction in blood lactate and improved mixed venous oxygen saturation >70% within 6 h of recognition of septic shock is associated with improved survival. If possible, measure vena cava oxygen saturation ($ScvO_2$) to assess adequacy of resuscitation. If the $ScvO_2$ is <70%, consider packed red blood cell transfusion to achieve Hct >30%. Start inotropic agents if $ScvO_2$ is <70% despite transfusion and adequate fluid resuscitation.
  1. IV hydration; patients receiving balanced crystalloids as resuscitation fluids appear to have a lower 30-day mortality compared with patients who received saline (26% versus 31%) in a recent trial. Use of the fluid challenge technique to evaluate the effect (and safety) of fluid administration

has been downgraded from a strong recommendation to a weak one in recent guidelines.[2] For sepsis-induced hypoperfusion, give 30 ml/kg of IV crystalloids within 3 h, with additional fluid based on frequent reassessment using dynamic variables (e.g., passive leg raise test or pulse or stroke volume variations induced by mechanical ventilation) rather than previous guidelines using target-specific values of central venous pressure. Fluid administration should be discontinued when the response to fluids is no longer beneficial. Most patients need 4 to 6 L of fluid in the first 6 h. Trials have shown that resuscitation with balanced crystalloids or albumin compared with other fluids seems to be associated with reduced mortality, and that albumin replacement in addition to crystalloids alone does not improve the rate of survival at 28 and 90 days. There is considerable debate about how much fluid is enough fluid before initiating vasopressors. A recent trial comparing a restrictive fluid strategy (prioritizing vasopressors and lower intravenous fluid volumes) with a liberal fluid strategy (prioritizing higher intravenous fluids before vasopressor use) for a 24-h period did not result in significantly lower liberal fluid strategy.[3]

2. Therapy with vasopressors if mean arterial blood pressure of >65 mm Hg cannot be maintained by hydration alone. Use norepinephrine as a first-choice vasopressor and target a mean arterial pressure (MAP) of 65 mm Hg. Administration of vasopressors should be initiated via peripheral access, as opposed

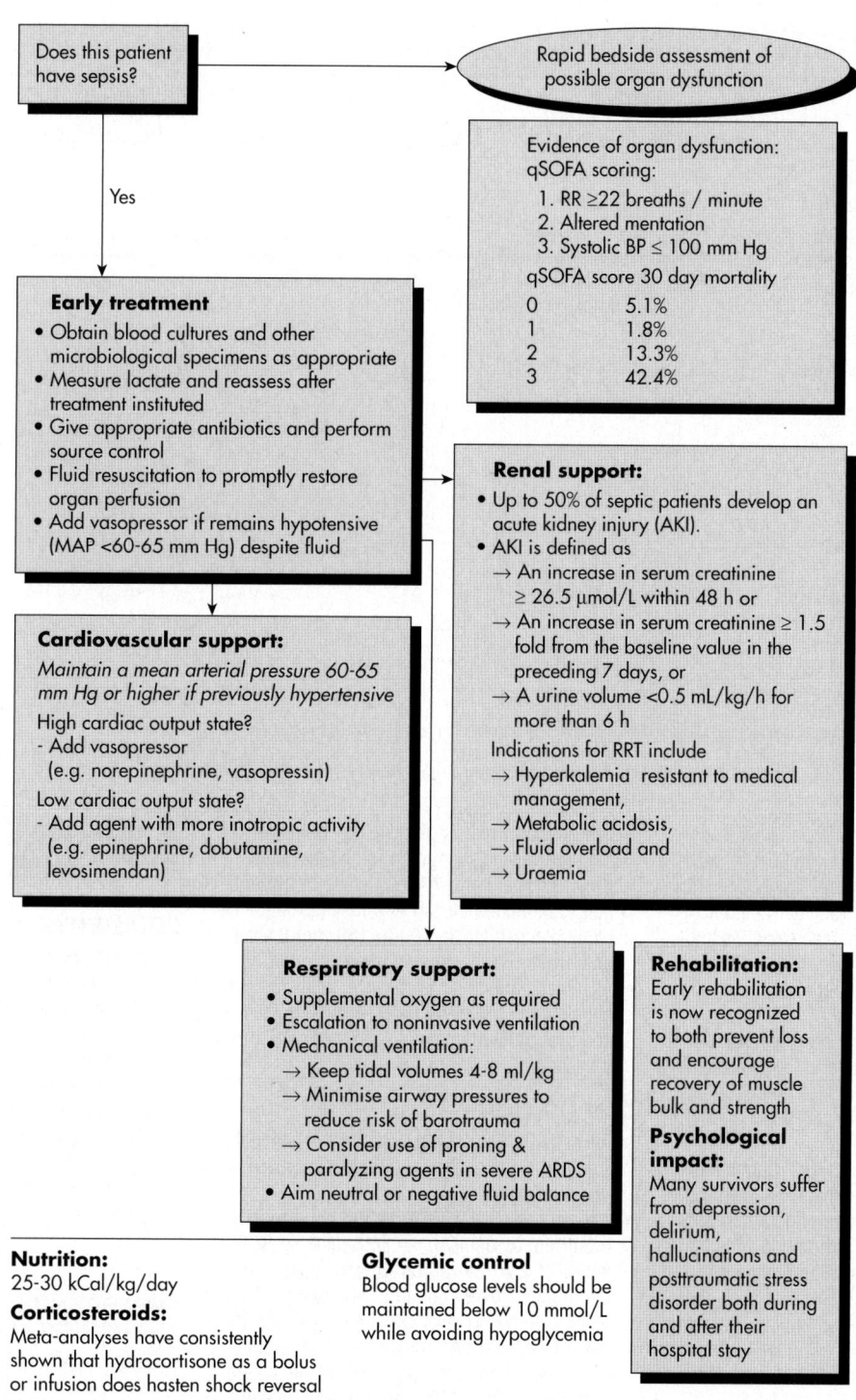

FIG. 4 Flow diagram for the management of sepsis and septic shock. Starting with rapid recognition of the septic patient, early initiation of appropriate antibiotics, and fluid resuscitation with supportive management. *ARDS,* Acute respiratory distress syndrome; *BP,* blood pressure; *MAP,* mean arterial pressure; *RR,* respiratory rate. (From Newman M et al: *Perioperative medicine,* ed 2, Philadelphia, 2022, Elsevier.)

to waiting for placement of central venous access.[2]
- Correction of acidosis by improving the tissue perfusion, not by giving bicarbonate.
- Mechanical ventilation as needed.
- Antibiotics:
  1. Directed at the most likely sources of infection. Table 7 describes initial antibiotic recommendations for septic patients.

2. Should generally provide broad coverage of gram-positive and gram-negative bacteria (or fungi if clinically indicated).
3. Antibiotics should be administered within 1 h of the diagnosis of septic shock—this is a medical emergency.
4. Antimicrobial therapy should be narrowed based on culture results and clinical improvement (antibiotic stewardship). Serial

procalcitonin levels (PCT) can help guide length of therapy.
- Updated guidelines[2] recommend that patients with ongoing vasopressor requirements should receive IV corticosteroids. Patients with relative adrenal insufficiency may benefit from low-dose therapy with hydrocortisone (200 mg IV by continuous infusion for 7 days). Current evidence and guidelines support limiting the

TABLE 6 Relative Potency of Intravenously Administered Vasopressors/Inotropes Used in Shock[a]

Drug	Dose	CARDIAC		PERIPHERAL VASCULATURE			Typical Clinical Use
		Heart Rate	Contractility	Vasoconstriction	Vasodilation	Dopaminergic	
Dopamine	1-4 μg/kg/min	1+	1-2+	0	1+	4+	All shock
	5-10 μg/kg/min	2+	2+	1-2+	1+	4+	
	11-20 μg/kg/min	2+	2+	2-3+	1+	4+	
Norepinephrine	0.01-0.3 μg/kg/min	2+	2+	4+	0	0	Refractory shock
Dobutamine	1-20 μg/kg/min	1-2+	3+	1+	2+	0	CHF; cardiogenic, obstructive and septic shock
Dopexamine[b]	0.5-6 μg/kg/min	2+	1+	0	3-4+	4+	CHF; cardiogenic shock
Epinephrine	0.05-0.2 μg/kg/min	4+	4+	4+	3+	0	Refractory or anaphylactic shock
Phenylephrine	0.1-1 μg/kg/min	0	1+	4+	0	0	Neurogenic or septic shock
Isoproterenol	1-8 μg/min	4+	4+	0	4+	0	Cardiogenic shock (bradyarrhythmia), torsades de pointes, ventricular tachycardia
Vasopressin	0.02-0.04 U/min	0	0	4+	0	0	Vasodilatory (e.g., septic) shock
Milrinone	37.5-75 μg/kg bolus over 10 min; 0.375-0.75 μg/kg/min infusion	1+	3+	0	2+	0	CHF; cardiogenic shock

CHF, Congestive heart failure.
[a]The 1 to 4+ scoring system represents an arbitrary quantitation of the comparative potency of different vasopressors/inotropes.
[b]Not clinically released in the U.S.
From Parrillo JE, Dellinger RP: *Critical care medicine, principles of diagnosis and management in the adult,* ed 5, Philadelphia, 2019, Elsevier.

use of IV hydrocortisone for patients with septic shock to these instances with fluid resuscitation and vasopressor therapy are inadequate to restore hemodynamic stability. The corticotropin (ACTH) stimulation test is not helpful and should not be used to determine the need for corticosteroid in these patients. During the COVID-19 pandemic, the RECOVERY trial provided evidence that treatment with dexamethasone in hospitalized patients at a dose of 6 mg once a day (IV or oral) for up to 10 days reduced 28-day mortality in patients with COVID-19.

- Blood transfusion: A lower hemoglobin threshold is preferred. Trials have shown that among patients with septic shock, mortality at 90 days and rates of ischemic events and use of life support is similar among those assigned to blood transfusion at a higher hemoglobin threshold (hemoglobin level of 9 g/dl or less) and those assigned to blood transfusion at a lower threshold (hemoglobin level of 7 g/dl or less).

CHRONIC Rx

- Adjust antibiotic therapy on the basis of culture results.
- In general, continue antibiotic therapy for a minimum of 7 to 10 days.

- Infection source control (e.g., removal of catheter/device suspected to be infected).
- If hyperglycemia develops during treatment, start continuous insulin IV infusion, maintain blood glucose in the 110 to 180 mg/dl level, and avoid insulin-induced hypoglycemia.
- All adult patients who survive to discharge should have follow-up for physical, cognitive, and emotional problems associated with their admission.[2]

DISPOSITION

- All patients with sepsis should be hospitalized and given access to intensive monitoring and nursing care.
- Among adults with suspected infection admitted to an ICU, an increase in SOFA score of 2 or more has greater prognostic accuracy for in-hospital mortality than SIRS criteria or the qSOFA score (quick SOFA). The qSOFA can be done at bedside and consists of increased respiratory rate ≥22/min, altered mentation and systolic blood pressure (BP) ≤100 mm Hg with each allocated 1 point.

REFERRAL

- To infectious diseases expert
- To physician experienced in critical care

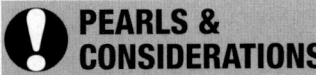 **PEARLS & CONSIDERATIONS**

COMMENTS

- Mortality rises quickly if antibiotic therapy is not instituted promptly (preferably within 1 h of onset of shock) and metabolic derangements are not treated aggressively.
- Early, goal-directed therapy (EGDT) does not result in better outcomes than usual care and is associated with higher hospitalization costs across a broad range of patient and hospital characteristics.
- Use of vitamin C is not recommended for sepsis.[2]

REFERENCES & SUGGESTED READINGS

Available at eBooks.Health.Elsevier.com.

AUTHORS: **GLENN G. FORT, MD, MPH,** and **FRED F. FERRI, MD**

TABLE 7 Empiric Antibiotic Options for Patients With Severe Sepsis or Septic Shock

	SUSPECTED SOURCE				
	Lung	**Abdomen**	**Skin/Soft Tissue**	**Urinary Tract**	**Source Uncertain**
Major Community-Acquired Pathogens	*Streptococcus pneumoniae* *Haemophilus influenzae* *Legionella* *Chlamydia pneumoniae*	*Escherichia coli* *Bacteroides fragilis*	*Streptococcus pyogenes* *Staphylococcus aureus* Polymicrobial	*E. Coli* *Klebsiella spp.* *Enterobacter spp.* *Proteus spp.* *Enterococci*	
Empirical Antibiotic Therapy	Moxifloxacin or levofloxacin *or* azithromycin *plus* cefotaxime *or* ceftazidime *or* cefepime *or* piperacillin-tazobactam	Imipenem *or* meropenem *or* doripenem *or* Piperacillin-tazobactam ± aminoglycoside. If biliary source: Piperacillin-tazobactam, ampicillin-sulbactam, *or* ceftriaxone with metronidazole	Vancomycin or daptomycin *plus* either imipenem *or* meropenem *or* piperacillin-tazobactam; ± clindamycin (see text)	Ciprofloxacin *or* levofloxacin (if gram-positive cocci, use ampicillin *or* vancomycin ± gentamicin)	Vancomycin plus either doripenem *or* ertapenem *or* imipenem *or* meropenem
Major Commensal or Nosocomial Microorganisms	Aerobic gram-negative bacilli	Aerobic gram-negative rods Anaerobes *Candida* spp.	*Staphylococcus aureus* (? MRSA) Aerobic gram-negative rods	Aerobic gram-negative rods *Enterococci*	Consider MDRO if in area of high prevalence. Consider echinocandin if neutropenic or indwelling intravascular catheter
Empirical Antibiotic Therapy	Imipenem *or* meropenem *or* doripenem *or* cefepime (if *Acinetobacter baumannii* or carbapenem-resistant *Klebsiella* in ICU, add colistin)	Imipenem *or* meropenem ± aminoglycoside (consider echinocandin)	Vancomycin or daptomycin *plus* imipenem-cilastatin *or* meropenem *or* cefepime, ± clindamycin	Vancomycin plus imipenem or meropenem or cefepime	Cefepime plus vancomycin ± caspofungin

Dosages for intravenous administration (normal renal function):
- Imipenem-cilastatin, 0.5-1.0 g q6-8h
- Meropenem, 1-2 g q8h
- Doripenem, 0.5 g q8h
- Piperacillin-tazobactam, 3.375 g q4h or 4.5 g q6h
- Vancomycin, load 25-30 mg/kg, then 15-20 mg/kg q8-12h
- Cefepime, 1-2 g q8h
- Levofloxacin, 750 mg q24h
- Ciprofloxacin, 400 mg q8-12h
- Moxifloxacin, 400 mg daily
- Ceftriaxone, 2 g q24h
- Caspofungin, 70 mg, followed by 50 mg q24h
- Colistin: Loading dose = 5 mg/kg body weight

ICU, Intensive care unit; *MDRO,* multidrug-resistant organisms; *MRSA,* methicillin-resistant Staphylococcus aureus. For *MDRO,* resistance usually includes carbapenems. Carbapenems are less susceptible to extended-spectrum β-lactamases; base choice on local resistance pattern.

From Bennett JE et al: *Mandell, Douglas, and Bennett's principles and practice of infectious diseases,* ed 8, Philadelphia, 2015, Saunders.

BASIC INFORMATION

DEFINITION

Sinus node dysfunction is a group of cardiac rhythm disturbances characterized by abnormalities of the sinus node leading to the inability of the sinoatrial (SA) node to react to heart rate changes and physiologic demands. This entity includes (1) sinus bradycardia (sinus rate <50 beats per min); (2) ectopic atrial bradycardia; (3) sinus pauses or arrest; (4) sinoatrial exit block; (5) chronotropic incompetence; (6) alternating sinus bradycardia with paroxysmal supraventricular tachyarrhythmias (frequently atrial fibrillation), known as tachycardia-bradycardia syndrome; and (7) isorhythmic dissociation. When sinus node dysfunction is associated with symptoms, it is called sick sinus syndrome (SSS). The term *chronotropic incompetence* represents the inability to augment heart rates appropriately in response to exercise or activities of daily living.

SYNONYMS

Sinus pause
Sinus arrest
Inappropriate persistent sinus bradycardia
Tachycardia-bradycardia syndrome
Bradycardia-tachycardia syndrome
Sinoatrial exit block
SSS

ICD-10CM CODE

I49.5   Sick sinus syndrome

EPIDEMIOLOGY & DEMOGRAPHICS

- In children: Associated with genetic, congenital, and acquired heart disease, particularly after cardiac surgery.
- In adults: It is primarily a disease of the elderly secondary to progressive idiopathic degenerative disease. A modern population study has suggested that White race, increased body mass index, prolonged baseline QRS or right bundle branch block, elevated N-terminal pro-B-type natriuretic peptide, hypertension, or other cardiovascular diseases are associated with increased incidence of sick sinus syndrome. With an aging population, the annual incidence of SSS is projected to increase significantly.

PHYSICAL FINDINGS & CLINICAL PRESENTATION

- Fatigue, light-headedness, syncope, presyncope, palpitations. Other manifestations include dyspnea on exertion and chest pain. Usually symptoms are progressive; however, abrupt symptoms can occur (i.e., syncope).
- Physical examination may be normal or reveal abnormalities (e.g., irregular heart rhythm, signs of congestive heart failure, heart murmurs or gallop sounds) associated with the underlying heart disease.

ETIOLOGY

- Sinus node fibrosis is the primary etiology, which may also affect the atrioventricular node, the His bundle, or its branches.
- Polypharmacy should be considered and obtaining an accurate medicine list is essential. Common medications include β-blockers, nondihydropyridine calcium channel blockers, digoxin, and antiarrhythmic medications.
- Additional etiologies include acute coronary syndromes, diseases of the SA nodal artery, inflammatory and infiltrative diseases (hemochromatosis, amyloidosis, sarcoidosis), collagen vascular diseases (systemic lupus erythematosus and scleroderma), epicardial and pericardial diseases, trauma following cardiac surgery, hypothyroidism, hypothermia, hypoxia, sepsis, muscular dystrophies (e.g., myotonic dystrophy, Friedreich ataxia), infectious etiologies such as Lyme disease and increased intracranial pressure.
- Note that the sinus node artery arises from right coronary artery in 60% of people and the left circumflex artery in 40%.

DIAGNOSIS

DIFFERENTIAL DIAGNOSIS

- Atrioventricular block
- Medication toxicity
- Carotid sinus hypersensitivity
- Metabolic abnormality (e.g., hyperkalemia in acute kidney injury)
- Normal physiologic response (e.g., increased vagal tone)

WORKUP

- ECG (Fig. E1)
- Ambulatory cardiac rhythm monitoring with diary to correlate symptoms to findings. Event recorders, wearable ECG devices, or an implantable loop recorder can be used if symptoms are less frequent. Note that establishment of diagnosis is more effective with longer-term recording (at least 2 to 4 wk) compared with 24-h ambulatory ECG
- Exercise stress testing to evaluate the severity of chronotropic incompetence
- If possible, discontinue or down-titrate medications associated with bradycardia
- Electrophysiologic testing, including sinus node recovery time and sinoatrial conduction time

TREATMENT

- Permanent pacemaker placement is primarily indicated if bradycardic patient is symptomatic and a reversible etiology is not identified. Indications for permanent pacemaker in sinus node dysfunction are described in Table 1.[1]
- In tachycardia-bradycardia syndrome, drug treatment or ablation is often indicated for tachycardia after placement of a permanent pacemaker for bradycardia.

REFERENCE

Available at eBooks.Health.Elsevier.com.

AUTHORS: **DANIEL R. FRISCH, MD,** and **EITAN S. FRANKEL, MD**

TABLE 1	Indications for Permanent Pacing in Chronic Sinus Node Dysfunction
Class	**Indications**
I	• In patients who are symptomatic due to sinus node dysfunction, permanent pacing is indicated to increase heart rate and improve symptoms. • In patients with symptomatic sinus bradycardia as a consequence of necessary therapy for which there is no alternative treatment, permanent pacing is recommended to increase heart rate and improve symptoms.
IIa	• For patients with tachy-brady syndrome and symptomatic bradycardia, permanent pacing is reasonable to increase heart rate and reduce symptoms attributable to hypoperfusion. • In patients with symptomatic chronotropic incompetence, permanent pacing with rate-responsiveness is reasonable to improve symptoms and increase exertional heart rates.
IIb	• In patients with symptoms that are likely attributable to SND, a trial of oral theophylline may be considered to increase heart rate, improve symptoms, and help determine the potential benefits of permanent pacing.
III	• In asymptomatic patients with sinus bradycardia or sinus pauses that are secondary to physiologically elevated parasympathetic tone, permanent pacing should not be performed. • In patients with sleep-related sinus bradycardia or transient sinus pauses occurring during sleep, permanent pacing should not be performed in the absence of other indications for pacing. • In patients with asymptomatic SND, or in those in whom the symptoms have been documented to occur in the absence of bradycardia or chronotropic incompetence, permanent pacing is not indicated.

ACC, American College of Cardiology; *AHA,* American Heart Association; *HRS,* Heart Rhythm Society; *SND,* sinus node dysfunction. Adapted from Kusumoto FM et al: 2018 ACC/AHA/HRS guideline on the evaluation and management of patients with bradycardia and cardiac conduction delay: a report of the American College of Cardiology/American Heart Association Task Force on Clinical Practice Guidelines and the Heart Rhythm Society [published correction appears in *J Am Coll Cardiol* 74(7):1016-1018, 2019] *J Am Coll Cardiol* 74(7):e51-e156, 2019. doi:10.1016/j.jacc.2018.10.044.

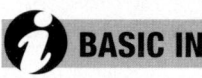

i BASIC INFORMATION

DEFINITION

Sickle cell disease (SCD) is a hemoglobin synthesis disorder arising from the substitution of valine for glutamic acid at position six of the beta-globin chain thus yielding a variant hemoglobin S. In its deoxygenated form, hemoglobin S (deoxy HgbS) polymerizes into long strands, deforming red blood cells (RBCs) into a characteristic sickle shape. Chronic membrane damage from this process locks RBCs into an abnormal sickle shape that along with an abnormal adherence to vascular endothelium leads to microcirculatory obstruction and the hallmark painful crises of this disease.

SCD patients include those who are homozygous for sickle cell hemoglobin (HbS) and those with one sickle hemoglobin gene inherited with other hemoglobin abnormalities, notably beta thalassemia (Hgb S/β⁰ or Hgb S/β⁺ thalassemia) and hemoglobin C (HbSC). A comparison of sickle cell syndromes is summarized in Table 1.

SYNONYMS

Sickle cell anemia
SCD
Hemoglobin S disease

ICD-10CM CODES
D57.1	Sickle-cell disease without crisis
D57.20	Sickle-cell/Hb-C disease without crisis
D57.211	Sickle-cell/Hb-C disease with acute chest syndrome
D57.212	Sickle-cell/Hb-C disease with splenic sequestration
D57.219	Sickle-cell/Hb-C disease with crisis, unspecified
D57.3	Sickle-cell trait
D57.40	Sickle-cell thalassemia without crisis
D57.411	Sickle-cell thalassemia with acute chest syndrome
D57.412	Sickle-cell thalassemia with splenic sequestration
D57.419	Sickle-cell thalassemia with crisis, unspecified
D57.80	Other sickle-cell disorders without crisis
D57.811	Other sickle-cell disorders with acute chest syndrome
D57.812	Other sickle-cell disorders with splenic sequestration
D57.819	Other sickle-cell disorders with crisis, unspecified

EPIDEMIOLOGY & DEMOGRAPHICS

- SCD is an autosomal-recessive disorder that affects approximately 100,000 Americans. One in 13 African American children has sickle cell trait, and approximately 1 in 365 Black children born in the U.S. has sickle cell anemia. Among children born to Hispanic Americans, the incidence of SCD is 1 in 16,300 live births.[1]
- Sickle cell trait occurs in approximately 300 million people worldwide, with the highest prevalence of approximately 30% to 40% in sub-Saharan Africa, but also in the southern Mediterranean region (usually as Hgb S/β⁰ or Hgb S/β⁺), parts of the Middle East, and India. In the U.S., it is found in nearly 10% of African Americans.
- An estimated 2000 babies are born with sickle cell disease in the U.S. each yr, and worldwide 275,000 infants are born with the disease annually.
- There is no predominant sex.

PHYSICAL FINDINGS & CLINICAL PRESENTATION

- Physical examination is variable depending on the degree of anemia and presence of acute vasoocclusive syndromes, as well as acute pulmonary, neurologic, cardiovascular, genitourinary, and musculoskeletal complications. Clinical manifestations of sickle cell disease are described in Table 2. Table 3 summarizes organ damage seen in sickle cell disease. Table 4 summarizes acute problems in sickle cell disease.
- A study of the prevalence of pain in sickle cell patients found that they complained of pain on 55% of days surveyed. Chronic pain may be due to avascular necrosis of joints and is sometimes poorly explained.
- There is no clinical laboratory finding that is pathognomonic of an episode of painful SCD crisis. The diagnosis is made solely on the basis of the medical history and physical examination. Elevated total bilirubin, reticulocytosis, and lactate dehydrogenase (LDH) can be seen due to increased hemolysis. However, hemolytic anemia is typical for sickle cell disease at baseline. "Aplastic crisis" refers to crisis presenting with severe anemia and low reticulocyte count, usually caused by B19 parvovirus infection.
- Bones are the most common site of pain. Dactylitis, or hand-foot syndrome (acute, painful swelling of the hands and feet), is the first manifestation of sickle cell disease in many infants. Irritability and refusal to walk are other common symptoms. After infancy, musculoskeletal pain can be symmetric, asymmetric, or migratory, and it may or may not be associated with swelling, low-grade fever, redness, or warmth.
- In both children and adults, sickle vasoocclusive episodes are difficult to distinguish from osteomyelitis, septic arthritis, synovitis, rheumatic fever, or gout.
- Cholecystitis presents with abdominal pain in patients with chronic hemolysis.
- In general, localizing symptoms for infections should be evaluated because these can trigger sickle crisis. Infections, particularly involving *Salmonella, Staphylococcus aureus, Mycoplasma,* and *Streptococcus,* are relatively common. Catheter-associated bacteremia should be considered if a vascular access device is present; these may present without fever.
- Severe splenomegaly as a result of sequestration often occurs in children before splenic atrophy. Adult patients with severe SCD have splenic atrophy, whereas patients with milder disease (e.g., Hgb S/C) may have splenic infarct-related pain.
- Acute chest syndrome is a potentially life-threatening complication that manifests with chest pain, fever, wheezing, tachypnea,

TABLE 1 Comparison of Sickle Cell Syndromes

Genotype	Clinical Condition	PERCENT HEMOGLOBIN					Other Finding(S)
		HB A	HB S	HB A₂	HB F	HB C	
SA	Sickle cell trait	55-60	40-45	2-3	–	–	Usually asymptomatic
SS	Sickle cell anemia	0	85-95	2-3	5-15	–	Clinically severe anemia; Hb F heterogeneous in distribution
S-β⁰ thalassemia	Sickle cell β⁰-thalassemia	0	70-80	3-5	10-20	–	Moderately severe anemia; splenomegaly in 50%; smear: hypochromic, microcytic anemia
S-β⁺ thalassemia	Sickle cell β⁺-thalassemia	10-20	60-75	3-5	10-20	–	Hb F distributed heterogeneously; mild microcytic anemia
SC	Hb SC disease	0	45-50	–	–	45-50	Moderately severe anemia; splenomegaly; retinopathy; target cells
S-HPFH	Sickle-hereditary persistence of Hb F	0	70-80	1-2	20-30	–	Often asymptomatic; Hb F is uniformly distributed

From Andreoli T et al: *Cecil essentials of medicine,* ed 7, Philadelphia, 2007, Saunders. In Marcdante KJ et al: *Nelson essentials of pediatrics,* ed 9, Philadelphia, 2023, Elsevier.

TABLE 2   Clinical Manifestations of Sickle Cell Disease*

Manifestation	Comments
Anemia	Chronic, onset 3-4 mo of age; hemoglobin usually 6-10 g/dl
Aplastic crisis	Parvovirus infection, reticulocytopenia; acute and reversible; may need transfusion
Sequestration crisis	Massive splenomegaly (may involve liver), shock; treat with transfusion
Hemolytic crisis	May be associated with G6PD deficiency
Dactylitis	Hand-foot swelling in early infancy
Pain	Microvascular painful vasoocclusive infarcts of muscle, bone, bone marrow, lung, intestines; chronic pain (nervous system sensitization)
Cerebrovascular accidents (overt and silent)	Large and small vessel occlusion → thrombosis/bleeding (stroke); requires chronic transfusion; neurocognitive deficits
Acute chest syndrome	Infection, asthma, atelectasis, infarction, fat emboli, severe hypoxemia, infiltrate, dyspnea, absent breath sounds; treated with transfusions, antibiotics, oxygen, bronchodilators
Chronic lung disease	Pulmonary fibrosis, restrictive lung disease, cor pulmonale, pulmonary hypertension
Priapism	Causes eventual impotence; treated with transfusion, oxygen, or corpora cavernosa-to-spongiosa shunt
Ocular	Retinopathy
Gallbladder disease	Bilirubin stones; cholecystitis
Renal	Hematuria, papillary necrosis, renal concentrating defect; nephropathy
Cardiomyopathy	Heart failure
Skeletal	Osteonecrosis (avascular) of femoral or humeral head
Leg ulceration	Seen in older patients
Infections	Functional asplenia, defects in properdin system; pneumococcal bacteremia, meningitis, and arthritis; deafness from meningitis; *Salmonella* and *Staphylococcus aureus* osteomyelitis; severe *Mycoplasma* pneumonia
Growth failure, delayed puberty	May respond to nutritional supplements
Psychosocial issues	Depression, anxiety, attention deficit hyperactivity disorder (ADHD)

G6PD, Glucose-6-phosphate dehydrogenase.
*Clinical manifestations with sickle cell trait are unusual but include renal papillary necrosis (hematuria), sudden death on exertion, intraocular hyphema extension, and sickling in unpressurized airplanes.
From Marcdante KJ et al: *Nelson essentials of pediatrics*, ed 9, Philadelphia, 2023, Elsevier.

TABLE 3   Organ Damage Seen in Sickle Cell Disease

Organ or System	Injury
Skin	Stasis ulcer
Central nervous system	Cerebrovascular accident
Eye	Retinal hemorrhage, retinopathy
Cardiac	Congestive heart failure
Pulmonary	Intrapulmonary shunting, embolism, infarct, infection
Vascular	Occlusive phenomenon at any site
Liver	Hepatic infarct, hepatitis resulting from transfusion, hepatic sequestration, intrahepatic cholestasis
Gallbladder	Increased incidence of bilirubin gallstones caused by hemolysis
Spleen	Acute sequestration
Urinary	Hyposthenuria, hematuria
Genital	Decreased fertility, impotence, priapism
Skeletal	Bone infarcts, osteomyelitis, aseptic necrosis
Placenta	Insufficiency with fetal wastage
Leukocytes	Relative immunodeficiency
Erythrocytes	Chronic hemolysis

From Walls RM et al: *Rosen's emergency medicine, concepts and clinical practice*, ed 10, Philadelphia, 2023, Elsevier.

and cough and pulmonary infiltrates on imaging. Causes include infection (*Mycoplasma, Chlamydia,* viruses), infarction, and fat embolism; Fig. E1 illustrates the pathogenesis of the acute chest syndrome.

- Musculoskeletal and skin abnormalities include leg ulcers (particularly on the malleoli) and limb-girdle deformities caused by avascular necrosis of the femoral and humeral heads. Osteonecrosis of the heads of the femur and humerus is found in nearly 50% of adults with Hgb S/S disease.
- Endocrine abnormalities include delayed sexual maturation and late physical maturation, especially evident in boys.
- Neurologic abnormalities on examination may include seizures and altered mental status. Strokes occur in about 10% of children and adults with sickle cell anemia and approximately 35% of children with sickle cell anemia have cerebrovascular disease.

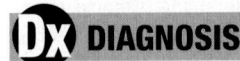 **DIAGNOSIS**

DIFFERENTIAL DIAGNOSIS

- Thalassemia
- Other hemolytic anemias
- The differential diagnosis of patients presenting with a painful crisis is discussed in "Physical Findings"

WORKUP (TABLE 5)

- Screening of all U.S. newborns regardless of racial background is performed with approaches such as the sodium metabisulfite reduction test (Sickledex test).
- Hemoglobin electrophoresis is confirmatory and identifies hemoglobin variants such as fetal hemoglobin and hemoglobin C.
- Patients will have evidence of hemolysis (elevated reticulocyte count, low haptoglobin, variable elevation of LDH and total bilirubin).
- Chest x-ray examination often reveals typical vertebral body changes ("fish mouth" vertebrae) caused by chronic vasoocclusive injury to vertebral bodies.
- For prenatal diagnosis, initial step is identification of parenteral globin gene mutation by DNA-based testing. If positive, then DNA-based testing of chorionic villus sampling or amniotic fluid cells is performed.

LABORATORY TESTS

- Anemia (from chronic hemolysis), reticulocytosis, leukocytosis, and thrombocytosis are common. Hgb S/β⁰ and Hgb S/β⁺ thalassemia will have microcytosis; Hgb S/C is also typically microcytic. Hgb S/C may have normal or near-normal hematocrit but will have characteristic changes on peripheral smear (target cells).
- Elevations of bilirubin, lactate dehydrogenase, and low haptoglobin are consistent with chronic hemolysis.
- Peripheral blood smear may reveal sickle cells, target cells, poikilocytosis, and hypochromia (Fig. 2).
- Elevated blood urea nitrogen and creatinine may be present in patients presenting acutely with dehydration or chronically with progressive renal insufficiency.
- Urinalysis may reveal hematuria and proteinuria. Patients with SCD should be screened for microalbuminuria and proteinuria with spot urine testing by 10 yr of age.

IMAGING STUDIES (FIGS. E3 & E4)

- Chest x-ray examination or noncontrast chest computed tomography (CT) scan to evaluate acute and chronic lung changes is helpful.

TABLE 4 Acute Problems in Sickle Cell Disease

Dactylitis. Typically the bones of the hands and feet are affected, with fever and leukocytosis. It is often the first event in young children and can occur multiple times until the age 3 yr.

Painful crises. Typically occurs after the first few years in bones or occasionally abdominal viscera. Pain is caused by ischemia and can be very severe. Crises are associated with low-grade fever and mild leukocytosis compared with osteomyelitis, in which fever and leukocytosis are more pronounced. Pain relief with paracetamol, nonsteroidal antiinflammatory drugs, or opioids, as appropriate, should be instigated immediately. Supportive measures such as hydration, intravenously if necessary, and oxygen also help to reduce the duration of the pain crisis. Any precipitating cause such as infection should be treated.

Central nervous system events. Strokes occur in up to 17% of children and young adults. The pathogenesis is unclear, but angiography often shows occlusions or stenosis. Recurrence is likely unless a long-term transfusion program is initiated.

Acute chest syndrome. This is a common cause of death presenting with fever, tachypnea, chest pain, and leukocytosis, often with a sudden drop in hemoglobin. It can be difficult to differentiate among infection, infarction, and embolism. Common precipitating causes are pulmonary fat embolism and infections. Treatment is with transfusion (simple or exchange), antibiotics, and aggressive treatment of hypoxia.

Splenic sequestration. This occurs in children between ages 6 mo and 2 yr. It is caused by sudden trapping of red cells within the spleen, producing a sudden drop in hemoglobin and rapidly enlarging spleen, eventually leading to hypovolemic shock and death. Management includes early detection of the rapidly enlarging spleen and blood transfusion.

Priapism. Engorgement of the penis can be short-lived and self-terminating, or it can last in excess of 24 h and may lead to impotence. Initial management is with fluids and analgesia, but persistent priapism (>12 h) may need partial exchange transfusion and corporal aspiration.

Infections. Overwhelming infection with *Streptococcus pneumoniae* is the most common cause of death in children. Other common causes of infections in sickle cell disease include *Haemophilus influenzae* and *Salmonella*. A significant reduction in the number of deaths from sepsis has resulted from the routine use of vaccinations against these organisms and antibiotic prophylaxis. Malaria prophylaxis should be considered in endemic areas.

From Ryan ET et al: *Hunter's tropical medicine and emerging infectious diseases*, ed 10, Philadelphia, 2019, Elsevier.

TABLE 5 Baseline Evaluations to Consider

	Tests
Blood tests	CBC with differential
	Reticulocyte count
	Hemoglobin HPLC or electrophoresis
	LDH
	Renal function tests
	Liver function tests
	Mineral panel
	Serum iron, ferritin, TIBC
	Vitamin D level
	Hepatitis B sAg
	Hepatitis C antibody
	RBC alloantibody screen
	RBC typing
	D-dimer[a]
	C-reactive protein[a]
	Brain natriuretic peptide
Urine and kidney tests	Urinalysis
	Renal ultrasonography[b]
Radiology	MRI or MRA brain (adults)[c] or transcranial Doppler ultrasonography starting at age 2 yr (children)
	Chest radiography[d]
	Hip or shoulder radiograph or MRI (or both)[c]
	Bone density in teenagers and adults
Cardiology and pulmonary	Echocardiogram
Neurocognitive	Neurocognitive testing[d]

CBC, Complete blood count; *HPLC,* high-performance liquid chromatography; *LDH,* lactate dehydrogenase; *MRA,* magnetic resonance angiography; *MRI,* magnetic resonance imaging; *RBC,* red blood cell; *sAg,* surface antigen; *TIBC,* total iron-binding capacity.
[a]Consider following as surrogate markers after initiation of disease-modifying intervention.
[b]If hematuria with red blood cells in urine.
[c]As clinically indicated.
[d]If the patient has poor school performance, an abnormal memory, or abnormal MRI findings.
From Hoffman R et al: *Hematology, basic principles and practice*, ed 8, Philadelphia, 2023, Elsevier.

- Routine skeletal imaging is rarely helpful in acute crisis and should usually be reserved for pain that is not consistent with transient acute crisis.
- MRI or bone scan is useful to address chronic avascular necrosis or, in the acute setting, osteomyelitis.
- CT or MRI scan of brain is not indicated in asymptomatic adults and children with SCD but is often needed in patients with neurologic complications, such as transient ischemic attack, cerebrovascular accident, seizures, or altered mental status.
- Transcranial Doppler ultrasonography (TCD) can identify children with sickle cell anemia who are at risk for stroke. There should be an annual screening starting at age 2 until age 16. Patients determined to be at risk (transcranial Doppler velocity ≥200 cm/s) should be enrolled in long-term transfusion programs. These approaches reduce the risk of stroke by >90%.[2] In adults, magnetic resonance angiography (MRA) can be used to identify those at risk for stroke.
- Doppler echocardiography should be performed in patients with unexplained respiratory symptoms to evaluate for pulmonary hypertension (Fig. E5), with right heart catheterization performed if abnormal. Screening for vasculopathy is done by estimating the tricuspid regurgitant jet velocity (TRV). Elevated values are predictive of early mortality. The prevalence of pulmonary hypertension when right heart catheterization is performed is approximately 6% in adults with sickle cell disease.

TREATMENT

NONPHARMACOLOGIC THERAPY

- Patients are instructed to avoid conditions that precipitate sickling crisis, such as extremes of cold and heat and dehydration.
- Maintain adequate hydration (by mouth [PO] or intravenous [IV]).
- Correct hypoxia when present.

ACUTE GENERAL Rx

- Initiate aggressive IV and oral hydration; most patients in crisis are dehydrated. Use hypo-osmolar fluids, such as lactated Ringer or 0.45 normal saline, for IV hydration during acute crisis in the hospitalized patient. Normal saline has adverse biochemical effects on sickled cells and may lead to increase pain.
- L-arginine 1000 mg/kg PO tid, decreases narcotic use by approximately 54% in the hospitalized patient during a vasoocclusive crisis.[3]
- Aggressively diagnose and treat suspected urinary, respiratory, or catheter-associated infections. Table 6 summarizes bacteria and viruses that most frequently cause serious infection in patients with sickle cell disease.
- Provide pain relief during the vasoocclusive crisis (Table 7). Most patients will have a treatment history that can guide dosing. Opiate management is complicated by high levels of tolerance in patients often treated over many years. Patient-controlled analgesic pumps are often helpful; caution should

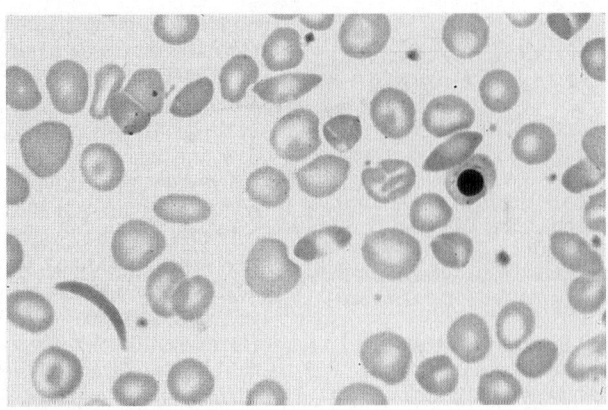

FIG. 2 Photomicrograph of a blood film. Sickle cell anemia (homozygosity for hemoglobin S). Shown are a sickle cell, boat-shaped cells, a nucleated red cell, and target cells. (From Bain BJ et al: *Dacie and Lewis practical haematology,* ed 12, Philadelphia, 2017, Elsevier.)

TABLE 6 Bacteria and Viruses That Most Frequently Cause Serious Infection in Patients with Sickle Cell Disease

Microorganism	Type of Infection	Comments
Streptococcus pneumoniae	Septicemia	Common despite prophylactic penicillin and pneumococcal vaccine
	Meningitis	Less frequent than in years past
	Pneumonia	Rarely documented except in infants and young children
	Septic arthritis	Uncommon
Haemophilus influenzae type b	Septicemia	
Meningitis		
Pneumonia	Much less common in recent years because of immunization with conjugate vaccine	
Salmonella species	Osteomyelitis	
Septicemia	Most common cause of bone and joint infection	
Escherichia coli and other gram-negative enteric pathogens	Septicemia	
Urinary Tract Infection		
Osteomyelitis	Focus sometimes not apparent	
Staphylococcus aureus	Osteomyelitis	Uncommon
Mycoplasma pneumoniae	Pneumonia	Pleural effusions; multilobe involvement
Chlamydia pneumoniae	Pneumonia	
Parvovirus B19	Bone marrow suppression (aplastic crisis)	High fever common; rash and other organ involvement infrequent
Hepatitis viruses (A, B, and C)	Hepatitis	Marked hyperbilirubinemia

Data from Buchanan GR, Glader BE: Benign course of extreme hyperbilirubinemia in sickle cell anemia: analysis of six cases, *J Pediatr* 91:21, 1977. From Hoffman R et al: *Hematology, basic principles and practice,* ed 8, Philadelphia, 2023, Elsevier.

be used when employing continuous infusions, which are usually not necessary or helpful. Morphine and hydromorphone are most commonly used. Meperidine is rarely used now and generally discouraged because of neurologic side effects, although some patients state a preference for it.
- Oral diphenhydramine is used to control pruritus, which is commonly associated with opiate analgesics.
- Tables 8 and 9 summarize overall strategies for the management of acute chest syndrome.

- Follow oxygenation in patients presenting with chest pain or respiratory symptoms; assess for evolving acute chest syndrome if oxygenation deteriorates.
- Urology evaluation for priapism.

CHRONIC Rx
- Hydroxyurea increases hemoglobin F levels, reduces the incidence of vasoocclusive complications, and improves survival especially in patients with Hgb S/S and S/β⁰ thalassemia with uncertain benefit in other variants.[4] Hydroxyurea therapy in children ages 9 mo and older decreases the frequency of vasoocclusive crises and acute chest syndrome. It is also strongly recommended for adults with three or more crises during any 12-mo period, with SCD pain or chronic anemia interfering with daily activities, or with severe or recurrent episodes of acute chest syndrome. It should be stopped in pregnancy, and contraception counseling should be given to all patients.
- Recommended starting doses for hydroxyurea are 15 mg/kg/day PO in adults and 5 to 10 mg/kg/day PO in patients with renal disease. Recent data has shown markedly superior efficacy with a dose escalation up to 30 mg/kg/day compared with 20 mg/kg/day.[5]
- Pharmaceutical grade L-glutamine can decrease crisis symptoms in patients with Hgb S/S and Hgb S/β⁰ thalassemia; benefits include decrease in acute crisis episodes, reduced hospitalization, and decrease in episodes of acute chest syndrome.[6] Dosing is 5 g to 15 g PO thrice daily, taken with food or cold or room-temperature fluid. Constipation, nausea, headache, and abdominal discomfort are occur commonly in 15% to 20% of patients. It may work with or without concomitant use of hydroxyurea. Caution may be warranted in prescribing L-glutamine to patients with significant renal or hepatic dysfunction.
- Replace folic acid (1 mg PO daily) to replace increased utilization of folic acid stores from chronic hemolysis. Patients also have mineral and vitamin deficiencies (calcium; zinc; and vitamins A, C, D, and E) and may need oral supplementation.
- Chronic pain management represents an enduring challenge, made more difficult by the current opiate addiction and overdose epidemic. Review of guidelines for safe opiate prescribing is strongly recommended and management with pain management specialists is also strongly recommended.
- Indications for packed red blood cell (PRBC) transfusion in SCD are described in Table 10. Urgent exchange transfusion for acute chest syndrome with progressive hypoxia (arterial oxygen saturation <90%) or multiorgan failure may be lifesaving. Simple transfusion may be adequate in milder cases with a target Hgb of 10 g/dl. Transfusion therapy is appropriate for patients with stroke or at high risk by transcranial Doppler study (see "Imaging Studies") if possible. Transfusion has shown to be beneficial in children with silent infarcts by MRI in preventing progression. Transfusion to Hgb 10 g/dl is recommended in anemic patients undergoing general anesthesia to reduce crisis and respiratory complications after surgery. Patients on chronic transfusion therapy should receive RBC matched at C, E, and K antigens to avoid alloimmunization.
- Serum ferritin level should be monitored quarterly. Iron overload due to blood transfusions (transfusional hemosiderosis) can be treated with chelating agents (deferoxamine [subcutaneous infusion], deferasirox [PO], and deferiprone [PO]).

TABLE 7 Recommended Dose and Interval of Analgesics Necessary to Obtain Adequate Pain Control in Patients with Sickle Cell Disease

	Dose/Rate	Comments
Severe to Moderate Pain		
Morphine	Parenteral: 0.1-0.15 mg/kg every 3-4 h Recommended maximum single dose, 10 mg PO: 0.3-0.6 mg/kg every 4 h	Drug of choice for pain; lower doses in elderly adults and infants and in patients with liver failure or impaired ventilation
Meperidine	Parenteral: 0.75-1.5 mg/kg every 2-4 h Recommended maximum dose, 100 mg PO: 1.5 mg/kg every 4 h	Increased incidence of seizures; avoid in patients with renal or neurologic disease and those who receive MAOIs
Hydromorphone	Parenteral: 0.01-0.02 mg/kg every 3-4 h PO: 0.04-0.06 mg/kg every 4 h	
Oxycodone	PO: 0.15 mg/kg/dose every 4 h	
Ketorolac	IM: Adults: 30 or 60 mg initial dose followed by 15-30 mg; children: 1 mg/kg load followed by 0.5 mg/kg every 6 h	Equal efficacy to 6 mg MS; helps narcotic-sparing effect; not to exceed 5 days; maximum, 150 mg first day, 120 mg maximum on subsequent days; may cause gastric irritation
Butorphanol	Parenteral: Adults: 2 mg every 3-4 h	Agonist–antagonist; can precipitate withdrawal if given to patients who are being treated with agonists
Mild Pain		
Codeine	PO: 0.5-1 mg/kg every 4 h Maximum dose, 60 mg	Mild to moderate pain not relieved by aspirin or acetaminophen; can cause nausea and vomiting
Aspirin	PO: Adults: 0.3-6 mg every 4-6 h; children: 10 mg/kg every 4 h	Often given with a narcotic to enhance analgesia; can cause gastric irritation; avoid in febrile children
Acetaminophen	PO: Adults: 0.3-0.6 g every 4 h; children: 10 mg/kg	Often given with a narcotic to enhance analgesia
Ibuprofen	PO: Adults: 300-400 mg every 4 h; children: 5-10 mg/kg every 6-8 h	Can cause gastric irritation
Naproxen	PO: Adults: 500 mg/dose initially and then 250 every 8-12 h; children: 10 mg/kg/day (5 mg/kg every 12 h)	Long duration of action; can cause gastric irritation
Indomethacin	PO: Adults: 25 mg every 8 h; children: 1-3 mg/kg/day given 3 or 4 times	Contraindicated in psychiatric, neurologic, renal diseases; high incidence of gastric irritation; useful in gout

IM, Intramuscular; *MAOI,* monoamine oxidase inhibitor; *MS,* morphine sulphate; *PO,* oral.
Adapted from Charache S et al: Effect of hydroxyurea on the frequency of painful crises in sickle cell anemia: investigators of the multicenter study of hydroxyurea in sickle cell anemia, *N Engl J Med* 332:1317, 1995. From Hoffman R et al: *Hematology, basic principles and practice,* ed 8, Philadelphia, 2023, Elsevier.

TABLE 8 Overall Strategies for the Management of Acute Chest Syndrome

Prevention

Incentive spirometry and periodic ambulation in patients admitted for sickle cell pain, surgery, or febrile episodes
Watchful waiting in any hospitalized child or adult with sickle cell disease (pulse oximetry monitoring and frequent respiratory assessments)
Cautious use of intravenous fluids
Intense education and optimum care of patients who have sickle cell anemia and asthma

Diagnostic Testing and Laboratory Monitoring

Blood cultures, if febrile
Nasopharyngeal samples for viral culture (respiratory syncytial virus, influenza), depending on clinical setting
Complete blood counts every day and appropriate chemistries
Continuous pulse oximetry
Chest radiographs for persistent or progressive illness

Treatment

Blood transfusion (simple or exchange) depending on clinical features; consider maintaining an active type and crossmatch
Supplemental O_2 for drop in pulse oximetry by 4% over baseline, or values <90%
Empirical antibiotics (third-generation cephalosporin and macrolide)
Continued respiratory therapy (incentive spirometry and chest physiotherapy as necessary)
Bronchodilators and corticosteroids for patients with asthma
Optimum pain control and fluid management

From Kliegman RM: *Nelson textbook of pediatrics,* ed 21, Philadelphia, 2020, Elsevier.

- Annual screening for proteinuria is recommended. ACE inhibitor therapy should be started for microalbuminuria in adults with SCD to prevent progression of renal injury. Progressive renal injury may cause worsening anemia and responds to erythropoietin.
- Annual retinopathy screening should be performed beginning at age 10, especially for patients with Hgb S/C variant, in whom proliferative retinopathy occurs in about 30% to 50%. It is less common in Hgb S/S and other variants.
- Gene therapy for SCD patients represents a novel approach. Clinical trials with lentiviral vector-mediated addition of an antisickling β-globin gene into autologous hematopoi-etic stem cells are ongoing with encouraging early results in terms of reduction of sickle cell crises and correction of the biologic hallmarks of the disease.[7] A level of erythrocyte fetal hemoglobin (HbF) comprising alpha and gamma globins may ameliorate the hemolytic anemia of sickle cell disease by mitigating sickle hemoglobin polymerization and erythrocyte sickling. BCL11A is a repressor of gamma-globin expression and HbF production in adult erythrocytes. Its downregulation is a promising therapeutic strategy for induction of HbF. Gene therapy trials with the use of LentiGlobin have shown sustained production of HbA^{T87Q} in most red cells, leading to reduced hemolysis and complete resolution of severe vasoocclusive events.[1] Two cell-based gene therapies exagamglogene autotemcel (casgevy-vertex) and lovotibeglogene autotemcel (lyfgenia-bluebird bio) have been FDA approved for treatment of sickle cell disease in patients ≥12 years old with recurrent venoocclusive crises. Cost is a major barrier to their use.

- Allogeneic stem cell transplantation can be curative in young patients with symptomatic SCD.
- Crizanlizumab, an antibody against the adhesion molecule p-selectin, has a significantly lower rate of sickle cell–related pain crisis than placebo and was associated with a low incidence of adverse events in a recent study.[8] It has been approved for the prevention of

TABLE 9 Treatment of the Acute Chest Syndrome

Oxygen therapy to maintain arterial hemoglobin oxygen saturation >92%

Pain control and incentive spirometry to reduce chest wall splinting and pulmonary atelectasis

Close clinical observation
- Monitor Po2/Fio2 ratio
- Particular attention to worsening respiratory function

Asthma therapy if indicated

Empirical antibiotics
- Cover typical and atypical respiratory pathogens
- Consider regional and seasonal risk of methicillin-resistant *Staphylococcus aureus*
- Anticipate influenza A or B infections and treat/prevent accordingly

Transfusion therapy
- Main indication for transfusion therapy in ACS is worsening respiratory function
- Simple transfusion is as effective as erythrocytapheresis in the usual patient
- Patients with high initial hemoglobin concentrations (≥9 g/dl) or patients with more severe disease should receive erythrocytapheresis
- Transfused blood should be matched to Rh, C, E, and Kell antigens, and transfusion records documenting history of prior alloantibodies should be obtained

ACS, Acute chest syndrome; *Fio2,* fractional concentration of oxygen in inspired gas; *Po2,* partial pressure of oxygen.
From Broaddus VC et al: *Murray & Nadel's textbook of respiratory medicine,* ed 7, Philadelphia, 2022, Elsevier.

TABLE 10 Indications for Transfusion in Sickle Cell Disease

	Duration	Consensus	Method	Goal*
Stroke, acute	Single	+	Ex	HbS <30%
Stroke, ongoing care	Chronic	+	Either	HbS <30%
High-velocity transcranial Doppler	Chronic	+	Either	HbS <30%
ACS, initial episode	Single	+	Dir > Ex	Hgb 10
ACS, recurrent	6-12 mo	+	Either	
Pulmonary hypertension	Chronic	+	Either	
Multiorgan failure	Single	+	Ex	
Major surgery	Single	+	Dir	Hgb 10
Acute anemia	Single	+	Dir	
Recurrent spleen sequestration	Chronic	+		
Sepsis/meningitis	Single	+	Dir	
Severe chronic pain	6-12 mo	+		
Congestive heart failure	Chronic	+		
Silent infarct with abnormal neuropsychology	Chronic	−		
Pregnancy		−		
Anemia/renal failure	Chronic	−		
Leg ulcers	6-12 mo	−		
Severe growth delay		−		
Severe eye disease		−		
Priapism		−		

ACS, Acute chest syndrome; *Dir,* direct; *Ex,* exchange; *Hb,* hemoglobin type; *Hgb,* hemoglobin concentration; +, consensus reached; −, consensus not reached.
*Goal of transfusion if a consensus has been reached.
From Fuhrman BP et al: *Pediatric critical care,* ed 4, Philadelphia, 2011, Saunders.

vasoocclusive crises in adults and pediatric patients ages 16 yr and older.
- Voxelotor, an inhibitor of sickle hemoglobin (HbS) polymerization, significantly increases hemoglobin levels and reduces markers of hemolysis and is approved for the therapy of adults and children over age 12 yr.[9]
- Penicillin V 125 mg PO bid should be administered by age 2 mo and increased to 250 mg bid by age 3 yr. Penicillin prophylaxis can be discontinued after age 5 yr, except in children who have had splenectomy.

- Table 11 summarizes disease-modifying treatments to consider.

REFERRAL
- Hospitalization for pain crisis unresponsive to oral analgesics, or involving fever, respiratory symptoms, or vomiting and diarrhea
- Optimal management requires coordination with hematology, blood banking, pain management, and psychosocial counseling and support
- Referral for patients with organ-specific complications, notably pulmonary hypertension, acute/chronic kidney disease, and ophthalmologic complications
- Referral to an ophthalmologist for an annual dilated retinal examination beginning at 10 yr of age

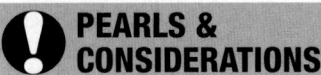

PEARLS & CONSIDERATIONS

COMMENTS
- The average life span of individuals with sickle cell trait is similar to that of the general population. Chronic pain and acute pain are not typical of sickle cell trait. Chronic problems in sickle cell disease are summarized in Table 12.
- Regular immunizations, especially pneumococcal vaccination, are recommended. The prophylactic administration of penicillin soon after birth and the timely administration of pneumococcal and *Haemophilus influenzae* type b vaccines have resulted in a significant decline in the incidence of these infections. The heptavalent conjugated pneumococcal vaccine (Prevnar) should be administered from 2 mo of age. The 23-valent unconjugated pneumococcal vaccine (Pneumovax) is given from age 2 yr and can be boosted once 3 yr later. Influenza vaccination can be given after 6 mo of age.
- In patients with SCD presenting with acute crisis, IV hydration with hypotonic saline is favored over normal saline. Normal saline can have adverse biochemical effects on sickle cell and possibly lead to increased pain.
- Pulmonary hypertension due to chronic hemolysis is associated with a high risk of death. It can be detected by Doppler echocardiography in >30% of adult patients with sickle cell disease. Cardiac catheterization will confirm the diagnosis. It is resistant to hydroxyurea therapy.
- Malnutrition can lead to poor clinical outcomes in patients with SCD. Identifying patients at risk might improve outcomes.
- Vitamin D deficiency is common and should be treated to prevent adverse skeletal outcomes.
- Metformin increases fetal hemoglobin (HbF) levels in patients with SCD. A recent study revealed that metformin use in SCD patients with diabetes is associated with fewer episodes of consequential SCD complications and with lower health care utilization.[10]
- Exposure to systemic corticosteroids is associated with a fourfold excess risk for hospitalization for a vasoocclusive episode (VOE).

REFERENCES
Available at eBooks.Health.Elsevier.com.

RELATED CONTENT
Sickle Cell Anemia (Patient Information)

AUTHOR: **RELINDIS AZENWI FRU, MD**

TABLE 11 Disease-Modifying Treatments to Consider[a]

Robust Clinical Data	Penicillin prophylaxis
	Streptococcus pneumoniae vaccination
	Hydroxyurea
	Chronic exchange transfusion
	Iron chelation for chronic iron overload[b]
Limited Clinical Data	Daily multivitamin without iron or folate supplementation *and* vitamin D replacement[c]
	Haemophilus influenzae vaccination
	Influenza vaccination
	Erythropoietin
	Phlebotomy
Experimental	Hb F reactivation with decitabine, histone deacetylase inhibitors, or imids
	Erythropoietin for chronic relative reticulocytopenia
	Nutritional supplements and antioxidants (e.g., glutamine, zinc, multivitamins)
	N-acetylcysteine

Hb F, Fetal hemoglobin.
[a]See text for specific indications and limitations.
[b]Best data from thalassemia patient experience.
[c]Risks minimal; therefore it is generally done.
From Hoffman R et al: *Hematology, basic principles and practice,* ed 8, Philadelphia, 2023, Elsevier.

TABLE 12 Chronic Problems in Sickle Cell Disease

Growth and development	Reduced height and weight
	Pubertal delay
	Cognitive impairment (recurrent small strokes)
Locomotor	Osteonecrosis of humeral and femoral heads
	Chronic leg ulcers
Cardiovascular	Myocardial infarction
	Left and right ventricular dilatation
Pulmonary	Pulmonary fibrosis
	Pulmonary hypertension
	Cor pulmonale
Genitourinary	Renal papillary necrosis hematuria and tubular defects
	Chronic renal failure
	Frequent urinary tract infections in women
	Impotence (secondary to priapism)
Ocular	Proliferative retinopathy (30% of patients)
	Blindness (especially in SC disease)
	Retinal detachment

SC, Sickle cell.
From Ryan ET et al: *Hunter's tropical medicine and emerging infectious diseases,* ed 10, Philadelphia, 2019, Elsevier.

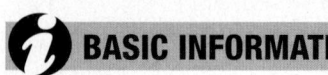
BASIC INFORMATION

DEFINITION

Silicosis is a spectrum of chronic fibrotic lung disease caused by inhalation of crystalline silica.

SYNONYMS

Pneumoconiosis caused by silica
Silicoproteinosis
Progressive massive fibrosis

ICD-10CM CODE

J62.8   Pneumoconiosis due to other dust containing silica

EPIDEMIOLOGY & DEMOGRAPHICS

- Occupational lung disease impacting workers exposed to respirable crystalline silica across a number of professions. Jobs associated with an increased risk of silicosis are described in Box 1.
- According to the Occupational Safety and Health Administration (OSHA), approximately 2.3 million Americans are exposed to respirable crystalline silica at work.[1]
- Within the U.S., age-adjusted death rates due to silicosis have decreased over time.[2] However, the quality of mortality data is limited. New outbreaks of silicosis have been described worldwide among engineered stone fabricators.[3]

PHYSICAL FINDINGS & CLINICAL PRESENTATION

There are three classic patterns of silicosis: Acute silicoproteinosis, simple chronic silicosis, and progressive massive fibrosis.[4]

- Acute silicosis is also known as silicoproteinosis.

BOX 1   Occupational Exposures Associated with Silicosis

Mining: Surface or underground mining (tunneling)
Milling: Ground silica for abrasives and filler
Quarrying
Sandblasting (e.g., of buildings, preparing steel for painting)
Pottery; ceramic or clay work
Grinding, polishing using silica wheels
Engineered stone fabrication: Cutting, grinding engineered stone products
Foundry work: Grinding, molding, chipping
Refractory brick work
Glass making: To polish and as an abrasive
Boiler work: Cleaning boilers
Manufacture of abrasives
Hydraulic fracturing

Adapted from Goldman L, Schafer AI: *Goldman's Cecil medicine*, ed 24, Philadelphia, 2012, Saunders.

---

1. Develops within days to weeks of a high level respirable crystalline silica exposure.
2. Presents with rapid onset acute hypoxic respiratory failure, cough, and fatigue.
- Chronic silicosis is the most common clinical presentation, and onset occurs after years of repeated exposure. It has two types:
  1. Simple silicosis, which may be asymptomatic, with the only manifestation being an abnormal chest x-ray examination. Latency period is 10 to 20 yr. Over time, patients may develop increasing dyspnea and cough.
  2. Progressive massive fibrosis characterized by x-ray progression and resulting fibrosis. Patients report dyspnea, cough, and pleuritic chest pain and may be hypoxic on examination.
- Patients with chronic silicosis may develop an accelerated form of disease, with rapid progression to progressive massive fibrosis (less than 10 yr after first exposure). Patients with recurrent, high-level exposures have a greater risk of developing accelerated disease.

ETIOLOGY

- Inhaled respirable crystalline silica becomes lodged in the terminal bronchioles
- Engulfed by alveolar macrophages, which release interleukin-1 (IL-1) and tumor necrosis factor alpha (TNF-alpha) triggering the inflammatory cascade
- Persistent inflammatory cytokine release recruits type 2 pneumocytes and fibroblasts
- Collagen deposition in the interstitium, leading to fibrosis (Fig. E1)

DIAGNOSIS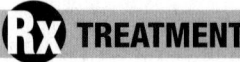

DIFFERENTIAL DIAGNOSIS

- Other pneumoconiosis (coal workers' pneumoconiosis, siderosis, talcosis)
- Sarcoidosis
- Fungal infection (blastomycosis, coccidioidomycosis, histoplasmosis)
- Tuberculosis
- Interstitial lung disease
- Lung cancer
- Amyloidosis

WORKUP

- Occupational and exposure history
- Chest x-ray examination (Fig. E2)
- High resolution computed tomography (CT) imaging (Fig. E3)
- Pulmonary function testing
- Lung biopsy (not required if history and imaging are suggestive)

Acute silicosis:
- Chest x-ray examination demonstrates typical pattern of perihilar or basilar opacities.
- Chest CT demonstrates diffuse nodular and ground glass opacities with enlargement of hilar lymph nodes.

- Bronchoscopy: Milky and lipoproteinaceous effluent is seen on bronchoalveolar lavage (BAL).
- Lung biopsy is not necessary in the setting of a definite exposure history.
- Exclusion of other causes like pulmonary edema, alveolar hemorrhage, and pulmonary alveolar proteinosis is necessary.

Chronic silicosis:
- Chest x-ray examination demonstrates multiple small, rounded opacities (<1 cm in diameter) distributed in the upper lung zones. Eggshell calcification of the hilar lymph nodes may be noted.
- Conglomerate masses >1 cm in diameter with an upper lobe predominance are characteristic of progressive massive fibrosis (PMF) (Fig. E4).
- Pulmonary function tests (PFT) show mixed obstructive and restrictive defect.
- Bronchoscopy and lung biopsies have limited diagnostic role unless atypical imaging features are noted.[4]

Accelerated silicosis:
- Chest x-ray examination pattern initially suggestive of simple silicosis, with rapid (less than 10 yr) progression to changes characteristic of PMF.

TREATMENT

- Treatment is symptomatic (supplemental O_2 for hypoxemia, bronchodilators, antibiotics for infections)
- Prevention (industrial hygiene)
- Smoking cessation
- Pulmonary rehabilitation
- Vaccination against influenza and pneumococcus
- Treatment of associated tuberculosis if present
- Screening for secondary complications of silica exposure
- Consider lung transplant for patients who develop chronic respiratory failure

ASSOCIATED COMPLICATIONS

Silica exposure/silicosis is associated with an increased risk of the following:
- Lung and renal cancer[5]
- Acute kidney injury[6]
- Mycobacterial and chronic fungal infections[5]
- Rheumatologic disease, particularly rheumatoid arthritis and scleroderma[5]

REFERENCES

Available at eBooks.Health.Elsevier.com.

RELATED CONTENT

Interstitial Lung Disease (Related Key Topic)
Silicosis (Patient Information)

AUTHOR: **MAEVE G. MACMURDO, MBCHB, MPH**

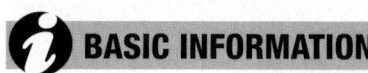

BASIC INFORMATION

DEFINITION

Sinus venous thrombosis (SVT) is an uncommon form of stroke due to thrombosis of one of the intracranial veins or sinuses resulting in increased intracranial pressure and possibly venous infarction or hemorrhage.

SYNONYMS

SVT
Intracranial venous sinus thrombosis or thrombophlebitis
Dural sinus thrombosis
Cerebral venous thrombosis
Venous sinus thrombosis

ICD-10CM CODES

I67.6	Nonpyogenic thrombosis of intracranial venous system
O87.3	Cerebral venous thrombosis in the puerperium

EPIDEMIOLOGY & DEMOGRAPHICS

INCIDENCE:
- 5 to 12 per million people annually[1,2]
- SVT represents 0.5% to 1% of all strokes but a large percentage of strokes in young women and during pregnancy
- 78% in people <50 yr old[1-3]
- 3:1 female-to-male ratio mainly due to the higher incidence during pregnancy and the postpartum period

RISK FACTORS:[3-5]
- Prior prothrombotic medical conditions including thrombophilias, inflammatory bowel disease, nephrotic syndrome, iron deficiency anemia, polycythemia, antiphospholipid syndrome, antithrombin III deficiency, protein C deficiency, protein S deficiency, factor V Leiden gene mutation, coronavirus (COVID-19) vaccines,[5] hyperhomocysteinemia, and cancers
- Transient conditions causing a prothrombotic state including pregnancy and the postpartum period, dehydration
- Infections (usually parameningeal—ear, sinus, mouth, face, neck, or meningeal, but also COVID-19)
- Medications including oral contraceptives and cytotoxic medications
- Mechanical factors such as head trauma, lumbar puncture, and neurosurgical procedures

PHYSICAL FINDINGS & CLINICAL PRESENTATION

- Symptom onset occurs acutely within 48 h in 37% and chronically over more than 30 days in up to 10%.[3]
- Headache, although not specific, is the most common presenting symptom in up to 90% of patients. It is often diffuse and progressive over days and weeks, although it may present more acutely. Up to 25% present with only headache without other focal neurologic symptoms.[2-3]
- Papilledema and/or isolated cranial VI nerve palsies as a manifestation of increased cerebral pressure.
- Seizures occur in ~40%.[2,3]
- Bilateral involvement and symptoms are frequent and progressive.
- The physical findings and presentation depend on the venous sinus involved.[1]
  1. Superior sagittal sinus (62%): Headache, papilledema, focal motor weakness
  2. Lateral sinus thrombosis (41% to 45%): Hemianopia, contralateral weakness, aphasia
  3. Cavernous sinus—ptosis, vision loss, ophthalmoplegia, hypoesthesia or hyperesthesia of V1 and V2, chemosis, periorbital edema, and proptosis due to involvement of cranial nerves III to VI, as well as impaired venous drainage from the orbit and eye (Table 1)
  4. Deep cerebral veins (internal cerebral vein, vein of Galen, straight sinus)—alteration in consciousness due to bilateral thalamic or basal ganglia infarction

ETIOLOGY

- 34% had an inherited or acquired prothrombotic condition.[2-4]
- 25% of patients had more than one risk factor.
- Infective sinus venous thrombosis, usually in the cavernous sinus, most commonly results from contiguous spread of an infection from either the sinuses (sphenoid, ethmoid, or frontal) or the medial third of the face (areas around the eyes and nose that drain to the ophthalmic vein). Hematogenous spread can also occur.

DIAGNOSIS

The diagnosis of SVT is made by clinical suspicion and confirmed by appropriate imaging studies.

DIFFERENTIAL DIAGNOSIS

- Idiopathic intracranial hypertension
- Arterial ischemic infarction
- Primary intracerebral hemorrhage
- Migraine headache
- Meningitis
- Epidural and subdural infections
- Epidural and subdural hematoma
- Subarachnoid hemorrhage
- Trauma

WORKUP

SVT is a clinical diagnosis, with laboratory tests and imaging studies confirming the clinical impression.

LABORATORY TESTS

- CBC, complete metabolic panel (CMP), prothrombin time/partial thromboplastin time (PT/PTT).
- Screening of potential prothrombotic conditions included infections, underlying inflammatory disease, or inherited/acquired prothrombotic conditions.
- Anti-PF4 antibodies and platelet activation assay if heparin-induced thrombocytopenia (HIT) or vaccine-induced immune thrombotic thrombocytopenia (VITT), often after a COVID-19 vaccine, is suspected.[5]
- A normal D-dimer assay may make the diagnosis of SVT very unlikely except in the setting of isolated headache.[1]
- Lumbar puncture (LP) is not often necessary except in cases of infection where it may help distinguish from more localized processes (e.g., sinusitis, orbital cellulitis). Elevated opening pressure is a common finding and may be a clue to consider SVT in patients presenting with isolated headache.[2] Elevated cell counts and protein are often but not always present. In the setting of an infection, the cerebrospinal fluid profile is typical for a parameningeal focus (high white blood cells with polymorphonuclear and/or mononuclear cells, normal glucose, normal protein, culture negative), and in one third may be similar to that of bacterial meningitis.

IMAGING STUDIES

- Computed tomography (CT) scan of head without contrast: 30% to 40% present with intracerebral hemorrhage (ICH). Bilateral ICH or lobar ICH of unclear etiology should raise a strong suspicion for SVT. However, head CT without contrast by itself is often normal, with only one third of cases showing a hyperdense sinus. Head CT with contrast may sometimes show enhancement of the dural lining of the sinus with an associated filling defect like the "empty delta sign."
- MRI with gadolinium, including magnetic resonance angiography and magnetic resonance venogram (Fig. 1), is more sensitive than CT scan and is the imaging study of choice to diagnose SVT. Findings may include an obvious signal hyperintensity within thrombosed vascular sinuses, focal edema, and/or hemorrhage in a nonarterial or bilateral distribution or associated with a venous sinus.

If high level of suspicion (such as when there are multiple intraparenchymal hemorrhages or bilateral thalamic or basal ganglia ischemic infarctions) but no thrombosis is visualized, CT

TABLE 1 Cavernous Venous Thrombosis Clinical Syndromes

Clinical Syndrome	Features
Intracranial hypertension	Persistent headache, decreased visual acuity, papilledema
Focal neurologic deficits	Motor weakness, aphasia
Seizures	Focal, generalized, status epilepticus
Encephalopathy	Altered mental status, coma

From Walls RM et al: *Rosen's emergency medicine, concepts and clinical practice,* ed 10, Philadelphia, 2023, Elsevier.

Diseases and Disorders

S

I

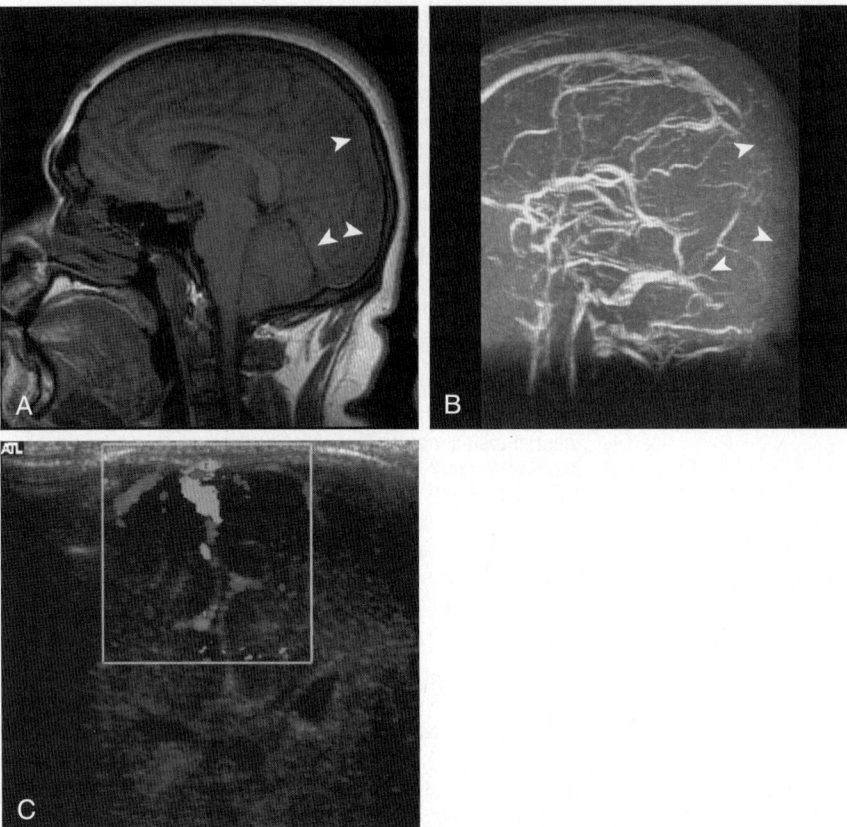

FIG. 1 Superior sagittal sinus (SSS) thrombosis on magnetic resonance venogram (MRV). Sagittal T1 magnetic resonance imaging **(A)** shows intermediate signal intensity in sagittal and straight sinuses *(arrowheads)*. No flow is seen on MRV **(B)** in these vessels *(arrowheads)*, which is consistent with thrombosis. Color Doppler evacuation **(C)** of the SSS in another 6-mo-old patient with suspected thrombosis demonstrated a patent SSS with normal draining cortical veins. (From Fuhrman BP et al: *Pediatric critical care,* ed 4, Philadelphia, 2011, Saunders.)

or magnetic resonance venogram may demonstrate the thrombosis.

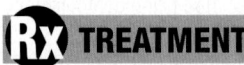 **TREATMENT**

ACUTE GENERAL Rx

- Acute treatment with anticoagulation, even in the setting of already present intracerebral hemorrhage, is necessary to prevent thrombus growth, facilitate recanalization, and prevent deep vein thrombosis or pulmonary embolism.[2]
  1. Cerebral hemorrhage on presentation is associated with adverse outcomes, but anticoagulation does not result in further worsening outcomes.
- Low molecular weight heparin (LMWH) is preferred to unfractionated heparin when medically indicated.[6]
- If the venous sinus thrombosis occurs in the setting of VITT, treatment involves intravenous immunoglobulin (IVIG) and nonheparin anticoagulation.[5]
- Anticoagulation alone is sometimes not sufficient to dissolve a large and extensive thrombus. In the setting of clinical deterioration, direct catheter thrombolysis, mechanical thrombectomy, or surgical thrombectomy could be considered.[2]

- If concern for infection due to local invasion (from otitis, mastoiditis) or systemic (meningitis), broad-spectrum intravenous (IV) antibiotics are used as empiric therapy until a definite pathogen is found, considering the source.
- Treatment of intracranial pressure, seizures, and hydrocephalus if and when required may be necessary.[2] Acetazolamide treatment can be helpful.

CHRONIC Rx

- Overall 6.5% annual risk of any type of recurrent thrombosis; however, venous thromboembolism is more common than recurrent SVT.[2]
- In patients with provoked SVT associated with a transient risk factor, treatment with warfarin or a direct oral anticoagulant (DOAC) for 3 to 6 mo is recommended. If the SVT occurred in the setting of pregnancy, LMWH should be continued for at least 6 wk postpartum.
- In patients with an unprovoked SVT, warfarin or a DOAC should be continued for 6 to 12 mo.[2,7]
- Testing for prothrombotic conditions, including protein C, protein S, antithrombin deficiency, antiphospholipid syndrome, prothrombin G20210A mutation, and factor V Leiden is recommended 2 to 4 wk after completion of

anticoagulation. If positive, indefinite anticoagulation should be considered.[2]
- In patients with antiphospholipid antibody syndrome, coumadin is preferred over DOACs.[2]
- In women with a history of SVT, prophylaxis with LMWH during future pregnancies and the postpartum period is recommended.[2]
- Patients with infected SVT are usually treated with prolonged courses (3 to 4 wk) of IV antibiotics. If there is evidence of complications, such as intracranial suppuration, 6 to 8 wk of total therapy may be warranted.
- Headache is common chronically and often is not related to recurrent SVT, although this may need to be investigated.[2]
- SVT of the cavernous, lateral, or sagittal sinus can induce dural arteriovenous fistula formation.[2]

DISPOSITION

- SVT can be life-threatening or more indolent, but generally has a favorable outcome. Mortality ranges from 8% to 10% with complete recovery in 79% of patients.
- Risk factors for long-term poor outcome include central nervous system infection, malignancy, thrombosis of deep venous system, intracranial hemorrhage on admission, Glasgow Coma Scale <9, mental status disturbance, age >37, and male sex.[3]

- Complications of untreated SVT include extension of thrombus to other dural sinuses, carotid thrombosis with concomitant strokes, subdural empyema, brain abscess, or meningitis. Septic embolization may also occur.
- Long-term complications of treated SVT include epilepsy and chronic headaches.[5]

REFERRAL

If suspected, SVT should be considered a medical emergency.

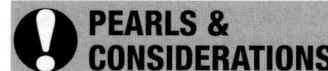

PEARLS & CONSIDERATIONS

COMMENTS

Sinus venous thrombosis can present with isolated headache and papilledema mimicking idiopathic intracranial hypertension. In a patient with possible intracranial hypertension, evaluation of the cerebral venous sinuses is required to rule out a secondary cause.

Delays in diagnosis of SVT are common, and a high level of suspicion is necessary.

REFERENCES

Available at eBooks.Health.Elsevier.com.

RELATED CONTENT

Idiopathic Intracranial Hypertension (Related Key Topic)

AUTHOR: **COREY ELAM GOLDSMITH, MD, FAAN**

S

Diseases and Disorders

I

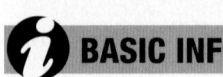
BASIC INFORMATION

DEFINITION

Sinusitis is inflammation of the mucous membranes lining one or more of the paranasal sinuses. The various presentations are:

- Acute sinusitis: Infection lasting <4 wk, with complete resolution of symptoms.
- Subacute infection: Lasts from 4 to 12 wk, with complete resolution of symptoms.
- Recurrent acute infection: Episodes of acute infection lasting <30 days, with resolution of symptoms, which recur at intervals at least 10 days apart.
- Chronic sinusitis: Inflammation of the paranasal sinuses and nasal cavities lasting >12 wk, with persistent upper respiratory symptoms. It accounts for 1% to 2% of total physician encounters.
- Acute bacterial sinusitis superimposed on chronic sinusitis: New symptoms that occur in patients with residual symptoms from prior infection(s). With treatment, the new symptoms resolve, but the residual ones do not.

SYNONYM

Rhinosinusitis: Sinusitis is almost always accompanied by inflammation of the nasal mucosa; thus it is now the preferred term.

ICD-10CM CODES

J32.9	Chronic sinusitis, unspecified
J01.90	Acute sinusitis, unspecified
J01.00	Acute maxillary sinusitis, unspecified
J01.01	Acute recurrent maxillary sinusitis
J01.10	Acute frontal sinusitis, unspecified
J01.11	Acute recurrent frontal sinusitis
J01.20	Acute ethmoidal sinusitis, unspecified
J01.21	Acute recurrent ethmoidal sinusitis
J01.30	Acute sphenoidal sinusitis, unspecified
J01.31	Acute recurrent sphenoidal sinusitis
J01.80	Other acute sinusitis
J01.81	Other acute recurrent sinusitis
J01.91	Acute recurrent sinusitis, unspecified
J32.0	Chronic maxillary sinusitis
J32.1	Chronic frontal sinusitis
J32.2	Chronic ethmoidal sinusitis
J32.3	Chronic sphenoidal sinusitis
J32.8	Other chronic sinusitis

EPIDEMIOLOGY & DEMOGRAPHICS

INCIDENCE (IN U.S.): Seems to correlate with the incidence of upper respiratory tract infections and higher in women than men; 30 million cases per yr in the U.S.

PEAK INCIDENCE:

- Fall, winter, spring: September through March
- In adults: Greatest incidence between 45 and 74 yr of age
- Approximately 6% to 7% of children presenting with respiratory symptoms have acute sinusitis

PHYSICAL FINDINGS & CLINICAL PRESENTATION

- Patients often give a history of a recent upper respiratory illness with some improvement, then a relapse.
- Mucopurulent secretions in the nasal passage:
  1. Purulent nasal and postnasal discharge lasting 7 to 10 days
  2. Facial tightness, pressure, or pain
  3. Nasal obstruction
  4. Headache
  5. Decreased sense of smell
  6. Purulent pharyngeal secretions, brought up with cough, often worse at night
- Erythema, swelling, and tenderness over the infected sinus in a small proportion of patients:
  1. Diagnosis cannot be excluded by the absence of such findings.
  2. These findings are not common, and do not correlate with number of positive sinus aspirates.
- Intermittent low-grade fever in about half of adults with acute bacterial sinusitis.
- Toothache is a common complaint when the maxillary sinus is involved.
- Periorbital cellulitis and excessive tearing with ethmoid sinusitis:
  1. Orbital extension of infection: Chemosis, proptosis, impaired extraocular movements
- Characteristics of acute sinusitis in children with upper respiratory tract infections:
  1. Persistence of symptoms
  2. Cough
  3. Bad breath
- Symptoms of chronic sinusitis (may or may not be present):
  1. Nasal or postnasal discharge
  2. Fever
  3. Facial pain or pressure
  4. Headache
- Nosocomial sinusitis is typically seen in patients with nasogastric tubes or nasotracheal intubation.

ETIOLOGY

- Each of the four paranasal sinuses is connected to the nasal cavity by narrow tubes (ostia), 1 to 3 mm in diameter; these drain directly into the nose through the turbinates. The sinuses are lined with a ciliated mucous membrane (mucoperiosteum).
- Acute viral infection:
  1. Infection with the common cold or influenza
  2. Mucosal edema and sinus inflammation

3. Decreased drainage of thick secretions/obstruction of the sinus ostia
4. Subsequent entrapment of bacteria
   a. Multiplication of bacteria
   b. Secondary bacterial infection
- Other predisposing factors:
  1. Tumors
  2. Polyps
  3. Foreign bodies
  4. Congenital choanal atresia
  5. Other entities that cause obstruction of sinus drainage
  6. Allergies
  7. Asthma
- Dental infections lead to maxillary sinusitis.
- Viruses recovered alone or in combination with bacteria (in 16% of cases):
  1. Rhinovirus
  2. Coronavirus
  3. Adenovirus
  4. Parainfluenza virus
  5. Respiratory syncytial virus
- The principal bacterial pathogens in sinusitis are *Streptococcus pneumoniae,* nontypable *Haemophilus influenzae,* and *Moraxella catarrhalis* (Table 1).
- In the remainder of cases *Streptococcus pyogenes, Staphylococcus aureus,* beta-hemolytic streptococci, and mixed anaerobic infections (*Peptostreptococcus, Fusobacterium, Bacteroides,* and *Prevotella* spp.) are found.
- Infection is polymicrobial in about one third of cases.
- Anaerobic infections are seen more often in cases of chronic sinusitis and in cases associated with dental infection; anaerobes are unlikely pathogens in sinusitis in children.
- Fungal pathogens are isolated with increasing frequency in immunocompromised patients but remain uncommon pathogens in the paranasal sinuses. Fungal pathogens include *Phaeohyphomycosis, Aspergillus, Pseudallescheria, Sporothrix,* and *Zygomycetes* spp.
- Nosocomial infections: Occur in patients with nasogastric tubes, nasotracheal intubation, cystic fibrosis, and immunocompromised state.
  1. *S. aureus* (including methicillin-resistant *Staphylococcus aureus* [MRSA])
  2. *Pseudomonas aeruginosa*
  3. *Klebsiella pneumoniae*
  4. *Enterobacter* spp.
  5. *Proteus mirabilis*
- Organisms typically isolated in chronic sinusitis:
  1. *S. aureus*
  2. *S. pneumoniae*

TABLE 1   Microbiology of Acute Bacterial Rhinosinusitis in Adults

Organism	Range of Prevalence (%)
Streptococcus pneumoniae	20-43
Haemophilus influenzae	22-35
Streptococcus spp	3-9
Anaerobes	0-9
Moraxella catarrhalis	2-10
Staphylococcus aureus	0-8
Other	4

From Broaddus VC et al: *Murray & Nadel's textbook of respiratory medicine,* ed 7, Philadelphia, 2022, Elsevier.

3. *H. influenzae*
4. *P. aeruginosa*
5. Anaerobes

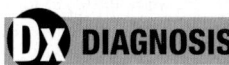 **DIAGNOSIS**

DIFFERENTIAL DIAGNOSIS
- Temporomandibular joint disease
- Migraine headache
- Cluster headache
- Dental infection
- Trigeminal neuralgia
- Allergic rhinitis
- Drugs (cocaine, decongestant overuse)
- Gastroesophageal reflux disease
- Wegener granulomatosis
- Cystic fibrosis

WORKUP
- The diagnosis is generally based on clinical signs and symptoms (purulent rhinorrhea and facial pain). Radiologic tests and cultures are not recommended initially and should be considered only when treatment is ineffective, and sinusitis persists.
- In the normal healthy host, the paranasal sinuses should be sterile. Although the contiguous structures are colonized with bacteria and likely contaminate the sinuses, the mucociliary lining functions to remove these bacteria.
- Gold standard for diagnosis: Recovery of bacteria in high-density $\geq 10^4$ colony-forming units/ml from a paranasal sinus, in the setting of a patient with history of upper respiratory infection and symptoms persisting for 7 to 10 days. Sinus aspiration is the best method for obtaining cultures; however, it must be performed by an otorhinolaryngologist and is not practical for the primary care practitioner. Therefore, most diagnoses are based on the clinical history and presentation, possibly supported by radiologic evaluations.
  1. Overall, standard radiographs are of limited use in diagnosis, although negative films are strong evidence against the diagnosis
  2. Computed tomography (CT) scans (Figs. E1 and E2):
     a. Much more sensitive than plain x-rays in detecting acute changes and disease in the sinuses
     b. Recommended for patients requiring surgical intervention, including sinus aspiration; it is a useful adjunct to guide therapy
  3. Transillumination:
     a. Used for diagnosis of frontal and maxillary sinusitis
     b. Absence of light transmission indicates that sinus is filled with fluid
     c. Dullness (decreased light transmission) is less helpful in diagnosing infection
  4. Endoscopy:
     a. Used to visualize secretions coming from the ostia of infected sinuses
     b. Culture collection via endoscopy often contaminated by nasal flora; not nearly as good as sinus puncture

- Sinus puncture:
  1. Gold standard for collecting sinus cultures
  2. Generally reserved for treatment failures, suspected intracranial extension, and nosocomial sinusitis

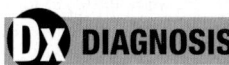 **TREATMENT**

NONPHARMACOLOGIC THERAPY
To help promote sinus drainage:
- Air humidification with vaporizers (for steam) or humidifiers (for a cool mist)
- Application of hot, wet towel over the face
- Sipping hot beverages
- Hydration

ACUTE GENERAL Rx
- Sinus drainage:
  1. Nasal vasoconstrictors, such as phenylephrine nose drops, 0.25% or 0.5%.
  2. Topical decongestants should not be used for more than a few days because of the risk of rebound congestion.
  3. Systemic decongestants.
  4. Corticosteroids: Nasal or systemic corticosteroids, such as nasal beclomethasone. Oral corticosteroids combined with antibiotics may be associated with modest benefit for short-term relief of symptoms in adults with severe symptoms of acute sinusitis compared with antibiotics alone. Oral corticosteroids as monotherapy are not associated with improved clinical outcomes in adults with clinically diagnosed acute sinusitis.
  5. Nasal irrigation, with hypertonic or normal saline (saline may act as a mild vasoconstrictor of nasal blood flow).
  6. Use of antihistamines has no proven benefit, and the drying effect on the mucous membranes may cause crusting, which blocks the ostia, thus interfering with sinus drainage.
- Analgesics, antipyretics
Antimicrobial therapy:
- Most cases of acute sinusitis have a viral cause and will resolve within 2 wk without antibiotics.
- Current treatment recommendations favor symptomatic treatment for those with mild symptoms. 85% of persons have a reduction or resolution of symptoms within 7 to 15 days

without antibiotic therapy. Physicians grossly overprescribe antibiotics for presumed bacterial sinusitis despite a much higher prevalence of viral infections.
- Antibiotics should not be prescribed for mild to moderate sinusitis within the first wk of illness. They should be reserved for those with persistent symptoms for more than 10 days, high fever and purulent nasal discharge or facial pain lasting for at least 3 consecutive days, or worsening symptoms after a typical viral illness lasting >5 days that had initially improved ("double sickening").
- Antibiotic therapy (Tables 2 and 3) is usually empiric, targeting the common pathogens:
  1. First-line antibiotics in children include amoxicillin or amoxicillin/clavulanate. For adults, amoxicillin/clavulanate or doxycycline is first-line agent, with quinolones (levofloxacin or moxifloxacin) reserved as second-line agents unless patient is penicillin allergic.
  2. Second-line antibiotics include the newer macrolides: Clarithromycin and oral cephalosporins: Cefuroxime axetil, cefprozil, cefaclor, loracarbef, but high rate of resistance of *S. pneumoniae* is a concern with these agents as is *H. influenzae* resistance with TMP-SMX and azithromycin such that they should no longer be used as first-line agents.
  3. For patients with uncomplicated acute sinusitis, the less expensive first-line agents appear to be as effective as the costlier second-line agents.
  4. During the COVID-19 pandemic, symptoms on presentation could be those of a sinus infection; however, although a loss of smell is common in COVID-19 infection, it is generally not seen in bacterial sinusitis or other viral sinus infections.
- Hospitalization and intravenous (IV) antibiotics may be required for more severe infection and those with suspected intracranial complications. Broader-spectrum antibiotic coverage may be indicated in severe cases, to cover for MRSA, *Pseudomonas*, and fungal pathogens.
- Duration of therapy generally 5 to 7 days in adults rather than 10 to 14 days as recommended in the past.
  1. Optimal duration of treatment in children varies from 10 to 28 days.

TABLE 2 Comparison of Two Major Guidelines for the Diagnosis and Treatment of Acute Bacterial Sinusitis

	Diagnosis	Treat	Antimicrobial of Choice	Amoxicillin Dose
IDSA	Clinical	All patients	Amoxicillin/clavulanate	40-45 mg/kg/day 80-90 mg/kg/day or 2 g/day for high risk[a]
AAP	Clinical	All severe patients Treat or wait 3 days for mild-moderate	Amoxicillin with or without clavulanate	40-45 mg/kg/day 80-90 mg/kg/day or 2 g/day for high risk[a]

AAP, American Academy of Pediatrics; *IDSA,* Infectious Diseases Society of America.
[a]High risk: ≥10% nonsusceptible pneumococci, severe infection, attend day care, age <2 yr or >65 yr, recent hospitalization, antibiotics in the past month.
From Bennett JE et al: *Mandell, Douglas, and Bennett's principles and practice of infectious diseases,* ed 9, Philadelphia, 2020, Elsevier.

TABLE 3 Oral Antimicrobial Agents for Acute Bacterial Sinusitis

Antimicrobial	Adult Dosage	Pediatric Dosage
Amoxicillin	500-875 mg q12h	40-80 mg/kg/day divided q12h
Amoxicillin/clavulanate[a]	875 or 2000 mg 12h	40-80 mg/kg/day divided q12h
Cefpodoxime proxetil	200 mg 12h	10 mg/kg/day divided 12h
Cefixime[b]	400 mg q12-24h	8 mg/kg/day divided q12-24h
Cefdinir	300 mg q12h or 600 mg q24h	14 mg/kg/day divided 12-24h
Azithromycin[c]	500 mg daily for 3 days	10 mg/kg daily for 3 days
Clarithromycin[c]	500 mg q12h for 14 days 1000 mg daily for 14 days	15 mg/kg/day divided q12h
Levofloxacin	500 mg daily	16-20 mg/kg/day divided every 12h[b]
Moxifloxacin	400 mg daily	400 mg daily for adolescents[b]

[a]Dosages specify amoxicillin component.
[b]Not U.S. Food and Drug Administration approved for this indication.
[c]Macrolides not preferred because of poor activity against *Haemophilus influenzae*.
From Bennett JE et al: *Mandell, Douglas, and Bennett's principles and practice of infectious diseases*, ed 9, Philadelphia, 2020, Elsevier.

Surgery:
- Surgical drainage indicated
  1. If intracranial or orbital complications suspected
  2. Many cases of frontal and sphenoid sinusitis
  3. Chronic sinusitis recalcitrant to medical therapy
- Surgical debridement imperative in the treatment of fungal sinusitis

Complications:
- Untreated, sinusitis may lead to a number of serious, life-threatening complications.
- Intracranial complications include meningitis, brain abscess, and epidural and subdural empyema.
- Intracranial sequelae are more common with frontal and ethmoid infections.
- Extracranial complications include orbital cellulitis, blindness, orbital abscess, osteomyelitis.
- Extracranial sequelae are more commonly seen with ethmoid sinusitis.

CHRONIC Rx

- Chronic sinusitis: Evidence supports daily high-volume saline irrigation with topical corticosteroid therapy as a first-line therapy for chronic sinusitis. A short course of systemic corticosteroids (1 to 3 wk), short course of doxycycline (3 wk), or a leukotriene antagonist may be considered in patients with nasal polyps. A prolonged course (3 mo) of macrolide antibiotic may be considered for patients without polyps. A clinical algorithm for the management of chronic rhinosinusitis in children is illustrated in Fig. E3.
- Dupilumab (Dupixent), a monoclonal antibody that targets interleukin -4 and -13, was FDA approved in 2017 for chronic rhinosinusitis with nasal polyps (CRSwNP). Cost is a limiting factor.
- Surgical intervention may be necessary in nonresponders.

REFERRAL

- To infectious disease specialist if failure to respond to initial therapy
- To otorhinolaryngologist for:
  1. Failure to respond to therapy
  2. Suspected fungal infection
  3. Suspected intracranial or orbital complications

SUGGESTED READINGS

Available at eBook.Health.Elsevier.com.

RELATED CONTENT

Sinusitis (Patient Information)

AUTHOR: **GLENN G. FORT, MD, MPH**

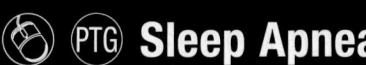
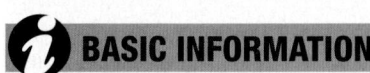 BASIC INFORMATION

DEFINITION

Sleep apnea refers to repetitive episodes of reduction or cessation of inspiratory airflow during sleep, usually associated with episodes of hypoxemia or physiologic arousal. Inspiratory airflow limitation is due to some combination of upper airway collapse and loss or instability of ventilatory drive. When sleep apnea is primarily due to upper airway collapse, it is referred to as obstructive sleep apnea (OSA); when it is predominantly due to loss of ventilatory drive, it is referred to as central sleep apnea (CSA; Fig. 1). This chapter will focus on OSA.

OSA is clinically defined and classified using the apnea-hypopnea index (AHI), the number of apneas or hypopneas occurring per h of sleep (Table 1).

SYNONYMS

Sleep-disordered breathing

Sleep-disordered breathing refers to a broader category of sleep breathing problems that includes OSA, CSA, elevated AHI regardless of symptoms, hypoventilation syndromes, and the interaction of these with other respiratory conditions such as chronic obstructive pulmonary disease (COPD).

Obstructive sleep apnea syndrome (OSAS)

The concept of sleep apnea syndrome refers to an elevated AHI in the presence of symptoms such as excessive daytime sleepiness or nocturnal choking and gasping. OSA is diagnosed with AHI ≥15 regardless of symptoms.

Obstructive sleep apnea–hypopnea syndrome (OSAHS)

ICD-10CM CODES
G47.30	Sleep apnea, unspecified
G47.31	Primary central sleep apnea
G47.33	Obstructive sleep apnea (adult) (pediatric)
G47.37	Central sleep apnea in conditions classified elsewhere
G47.39	Other sleep apnea
P28.3	Primary sleep apnea of newborn

EPIDEMIOLOGY & DEMOGRAPHICS

- OSA is an increasingly common disease worldwide, rising in prevalence in conjunction with obesity.
- Latest estimates suggest nearly one third of U.S. adults ages 30 to 69 yr have some degree of sleep-disordered breathing, and nearly 15% have moderate or severe OSA.[1]
- Risk of OSA increases with age, male sex, postmenopausal status, and obesity and other features of the metabolic syndrome. Age and obesity appear to have a powerful interaction.
- Due to the very high prevalence in the general population, clinicians should retain a high index of suspicion for OSA in patients

who may not fit the stereotype of the OSA patient. Factors such as chronic nasal congestion, tonsillar hypertrophy, conditions affecting upper airway tone, and unfavorable craniofacial and upper airway anatomy can predispose patients of any weight or sex to OSA. Family history may give an indication that some of these risk factors are present.

- OSA in pregnant patients is less common than in the general population but is not rare; one recent meta-analysis estimated prevalence (AHI ≥5) at 15%.[2] OSA prevalence in pregnancy increases with gestational age and is also higher in older mothers. In premenopausal women, obesity is the most significant risk factor for OSA.
- Prevalence in the general pediatric population is estimated to be 1% to 6%, but may be higher in obese adolescents.[3]

PHYSICAL FINDINGS & CLINICAL PRESENTATION

The clinical presentation of sleep apnea varies by etiology and subtype (Table 2). Cardinal symptoms of OSA include loud snoring, nocturnal choking or gasping, frequent awakenings from sleep, and feeling unrestored or excessively sleepy during the day, even if sleeping an adequate amount of time.

Some patients may have no symptoms at all, even with severe OSA, or symptoms only noted by the bed partner. Often, the patient may not associate systemic symptoms with sleep symptoms.

NOCTURNAL SYMPTOMS:
- Snoring (especially when loud, habitual, and bothersome to others, most sensitive symptom)[4]
- Witnessed apneas (often interrupting snoring and end with a snort)

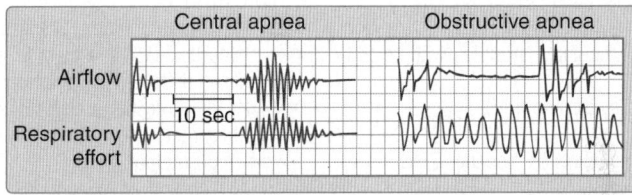

FIG. 1 Central and obstructive sleep apnea. The relationship between airflow and respiratory effort in central and obstructive apnea. During central apnea, cessation of airflow occurs without associated ventilatory effort. Respiratory effort is present during an obstructive apnea. (From Wellman A, White DP: Central sleep apnea and periodic breathing. In Kryger M, Dement W [eds]: *Principles and practice of sleep medicine,* ed 5, Philadelphia, 2011, Saunders, pp. 1140-1152.)

TABLE 1 Definitions

Apnea
- An event lasting ≥10 sec characterized by ≥90% reduction from pre-event baseline in oronasal thermistor airflow. An apnea is scored as:
  1. Obstructive, if there is continued or increasing respiratory effort throughout the event
  2. Central, if respiratory effort is absent throughout the entire event
  3. Mixed, if effort is initially absent, then resumes in the latter part of the event
- There is no minimum desaturation or microarousal requirement for scoring of an apnea.

Hypopnea
- An event lasting ≥10 sec characterized by a ≥30% reduction from pre-event baseline in peak nasal pressure inspiratory airflow that is associated with:
  1. Definition 1A*: Either a ≥3% reduction in arterial SpO_2 pre-event baseline *or* an arousal on EEG (recommended definition by the AASM and most commonly used in U.S. sleep labs for non-Medicare patients)
  2. Definition 1B*: A ≥4% reduction in arterial SpO_2 from pre-event baseline value (definition required by Medicare)

Respiratory Event–Related Arousal (RERA)
- A sequence of breaths lasting ≥10 sec that does not meet criteria for apnea or hypopnea, which is characterized by increasing respiratory effort or inspiratory flattening of the nasal pressure flow signal leading to a microarousal.

Hypoventilation
- An increase in arterial Pco_2 to >55 mm Hg for ≥10 min or an increase in arterial Pco_2 ≥10 mm Hg above awake supine values to >50 mm Hg for ≥10 min

Metrics of Severity
- *Apnea-Hypopnea Index:* Average number of apneas plus hypopneas per h of sleep.
- *Respiratory Disturbance Index:* Average number of apneas plus hypopneas plus RERAs per h of sleep.

Consensus Definitions of Severity in Adults
- Normal: <5 episodes/h
- Mild sleep apnea: ≥5 and <15 episodes/h
- Moderate sleep apnea: ≥15 and <30 episodes/h
- Severe sleep apnea: ≥30 episodes/h

---

*The choice of which definition to use for any given patient is at the discretion of each individual sleep lab and may vary by insurer. This can have diagnostic implications, as definition 1A is more sensitive.

Adapted from Broaddus C et al: *Murray and Nadel's textbook of respiratory medicine,* ed 7, Philadelphia, 2022, Saunders.

TABLE 2 Clinical Characteristics of Patients with Sleep Apnea

CENTRAL		
Nonhypercapnic	**Hypercapnic**	**Obstructive**
Insomnia	Daytime sleepiness Morning headache	Daytime sleepiness
Mild intermittent snoring	Snoring	Prominent snoring
Awakenings (choking/dyspnea)	Respiratory failure	Witnessed apneas/gasping
Normal body habitus	Normal or obese	Commonly obese
	Polycythemia	Upper airway narrowing
	Cor pulmonale	

From Kryger M et al: *Principles and practice of sleep medicine*, ed 7, Philadelphia, 2023, Elsevier.

- Awakening with gasping, choking, or smothering sensations (most specific indicator)[4]
- Restless sleep
- Frequent awakenings
- Nightmares
- Insomnia (particularly trouble with sleep maintenance)
- Restless legs syndrome (RLS)
- Nocturia
- Gastroesophageal reflux disease (GERD)
- Night sweats

DAYTIME SYMPTOMS:
- Excessive daytime sleepiness (a commonly used instrument is the Epworth Sleepiness Scale; a score ≥10 suggests abnormal sleepiness)
- Unrefreshing sleep regardless of duration
- Daytime fatigue
- Morning headache (improving within a few hours of waking, fairly specific for OSA)[4]
- Dry mouth or throat on awakening
- Mental fog, or problems with memory, concentration, and cognitive function
- Depressed mood
- Anxiety, irritability, or short temper
- Chronic pain or fibromyalgia-like symptoms
- Inattentiveness or, in children, attention-deficit/hyperactivity disorder (ADHD) symptoms
- Decreased libido, or erectile dysfunction in men

HISTORICAL FINDINGS & ASSOCIATED CONDITIONS:
- Weight gain (in one study, a 10% increase in weight over 4 yr predicts a sixfold increase in the likelihood of developing an AHI ≥15)[5]

- Chronic nasal congestion (often with allergic triad in children)
- Cardiovascular, cerebrovascular, and metabolic disease
  1. In pregnant women, this includes history of hypertensive diseases of pregnancy, gestational diabetes, and advanced maternal age
- Motor vehicle accidents or occupational accidents
- Posttraumatic stress disorder, particularly with nightmares
- Family history of OSA (odds increase with each additional close family member)
- Conditions affecting shape or compensatory tone of the airway:
  1. Neuromuscular disorders (e.g., demyelinating diseases, amyotrophic lateral sclerosis [ALS], muscular dystrophy, severe cervical spondylosis)
  2. Hypermobility syndromes (e.g., Marfan, Ehlers-Danlos)
  3. Disorders affecting craniofacial development (cleft palate, Down syndrome)
  4. OSA should always be suspected in patients with Down syndrome

OSA may cause or exacerbate comorbid sleep disorders, most commonly insomnia, but also RLS, nightmares, or parasomnias. The latter may be the presenting complaints.

OBJECTIVE FINDINGS:
- Obesity
- Neck circumference of ≥43 cm (17 in) in men and ≥38 cm (15 in) in women[6]
  1. OSA is more likely at lower body mass index (BMI) and neck circumference in Asian populations

- Tonsillar hypertrophy: In many pediatric patients and the occasional adult patient, identification of enlarged tonsils can prompt referral for curative tonsillectomy
- Low-hanging soft palate (i.e., a high Mallampati classification; Fig. 2)
- Signs of nasal congestion (e.g., turbinate hypertrophy, severely deviated nasal septum)
- Retrognathia or micrognathia (often associated with dental crowding and overbite/overjet; Fig. E3)
- Scalloping of the edge of the tongue (evidence of tongue too large for oral cavity; see Fig. E3)

The STOP-BANG Questionnaire (Fig. 4) and the Berlin Questionnaire are widely used and well-validated screening instruments that summarize some of the most common signs, symptoms, and associated conditions. These can be helpful in developing a clinic protocol for referral.

ETIOLOGY

OSA is characterized by upper airway collapse. Several features of sleep make it a vulnerable time for breathing: Postural changes alter upper airway mechanics and lung volumes, the wakefulness drive to breathe is absent, and upper airway dilator reflexes attenuate. Ventilatory instability is most classically illustrated by Cheyne-Stokes respirations (CSR), but a similar tendency to hyperventilate after an obstructive apnea can also contribute to perpetuation of obstructive events in a repetitive fashion. A low arousal threshold (tendency to awaken easily) also contributes to OSA and unstable breathing.
- Mechanical loads resulting in narrowing of upper airway (Fig. E5)
  1. Obesity (likely mediated by lingual fat deposition)
  2. Size and position of maxilla, mandible, palate, and other craniofacial properties
  3. Adenotonsillar hypertrophy
  4. Fluid overload
  5. Inflammation (e.g., allergies, GERD, local tissue trauma from snoring)
- Impairment of compensatory neuromuscular or central nervous system activity
  1. Neuromuscular disorders or metabolic disorders
  2. Diminished airway muscle activity/reflexes (may be exacerbated by local trauma due to snoring and reflux)

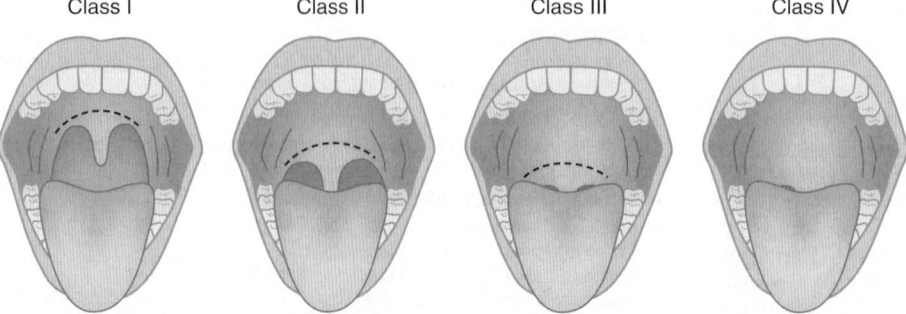

FIG. 2 Mallampati classification. Visualized with the patient in the sitting position, head held in a neutral position, mouth wide open, tongue protruding to the maximum, without phonation. Class I is characterized by direct visualization of the soft palate, uvula, palatine tonsils, and pillars. Classification increases until only the hard palate is visible (class IV). (From Mallampati SR et al: A clinical sign to predict difficult tracheal intubation: a prospective study, *Can Anaesth Soc J* 32:429-434, 1985.)

The STOP-BANG Questionnaire

Snoring	Do you snore loudly (louder than talking or loud enough to be heard through closed doors)?
Tired	Do you often feel tired, fatigued, or sleepy during the daytime?
Observed	Has anyone observed you stop breathing during your sleep?
Blood pressure	Do you have or are you being treated for high blood pressure?
BMI	Body mass index >35?
Age	Age over 50 yr old?
Neck circumference	Neck circumference greater than 40 cm?
Gender	Gender male?

FIG. 4 The STOP-BANG Questionnaire. High risk of obstructive sleep apnea is indicated by answering YES to ≥5 questions OR answering YES to ≥2 more of the STOP questions (the first 4 questions) plus YES to at least one of the following: Male gender, body mass index *(BMI)* ≥35, neck circumference ≥40 cm (16 inches). Intermediate risk is YES to ≥3 questions. (Adapted from Kryger M et al: *Atlas of clinical sleep medicine,* ed 2, Philadelphia, 2014, Saunders.)

3. Instability or impairment of ventilatory drive
4. Low arousal threshold

Dx DIAGNOSIS

DIFFERENTIAL DIAGNOSIS

Consider other causes of sleepiness, fatigue, or paroxysmal awakenings. A systematic approach can involve considering other sleep disorders and then considering non–sleep-related causes. Other etiologies that should not be missed:
- Decompensated heart failure or arrhythmia, or cardiac ischemia presenting with paroxysmal nocturnal dyspnea
- Decompensated COPD or asthma presenting as above or with nocturnal cough
- If reports of sleepiness, fatigue, or exertional intolerance are relatively abrupt, consider an undetected cardiac or pulmonary event

Sleep disorders likely to mimic OSA:
- Primary snoring
- Central sleep apnea (especially in patients with heart failure or on opioids)
- Obesity hypoventilation syndrome (OHS, 90% of cases coexist with OSA, but 10% of cases can be seen in absence of OSA, risk increases with BMI, particularly ≥40)

Sleep disorders likely to cause sleepiness and fatigue (often comorbid with OSA, but can independently explain sleepiness as well):
- Insufficient sleep
- Insomnia

- RLS (exacerbated by untreated OSA)
- Circadian rhythm disorder
- Shift work sleep disorder

Less common sleep disorders that may cause sleepiness:
- Narcolepsy (but OSA must be ruled out or treated prior to diagnosis)
- Idiopathic hypersomnia
- Parasomnias (includes sleep walking, sleep eating, REM behavior disorder)
- Periodic limb movement disorder

Non–sleep-related disorders likely to cause nocturnal symptoms or abrupt awakening:
- Alcohol use, particularly heavy or close to bed time
- Nocturnal gastroesophageal reflux
- Asthma
- Anxiety or panic disorder
- Benign prostatic hyperplasia
- Nocturnal seizures (not common, but important to consider)

Non–sleep-related disorders likely to cause fatigue or sleepiness:
- Medication side effects (particularly when several centrally acting agents are combined, consider over-the-counter sleep aids also)
- Iron deficiency (even in absence of anemia or RLS)
- Mood disorders (antidepressants, antipsychotics, anxiolytics can also cause hypersomnia)
- Hypothyroidism
- Anemia
- Traumatic brain injury

- Neurologic conditions (e.g., Parkinson disease, multiple sclerosis, dementia)
- Connective tissue diseases or chronic pain
- Other advanced systemic illness or malignancy

WORKUP
SAFETY:
- All patients with suspected OSA should be screened for drowsiness while driving, recent motor vehicle accidents, or "close calls" while driving.
- An occupational history focused on professional operation of vehicles or other modes of transportation, long commute times, operation of heavy machinery, or other occupations where falling asleep on the job might have catastrophic effects is essential.[7]
- A thorough review of prescribed and recreational substances should be performed, including alcohol, opioids, muscle relaxants, other sedatives, and centrally acting medications.

DIAGNOSTIC EVALUATION (FIG. 6):
- OSA is confirmed by nocturnal polysomnography (PSG), which is the gold standard for diagnosis, or home sleep apnea testing (HSAT). Particularly in the wake of the COVID-19 pandemic, HSAT has become a more reasonable option in many circumstances.
- PSG is recommended for occupational screening (e.g., pilots, train operators, commercial drivers).
- In most settings, PSG is optimal for suspected mild OSA (e.g., a young adult patient

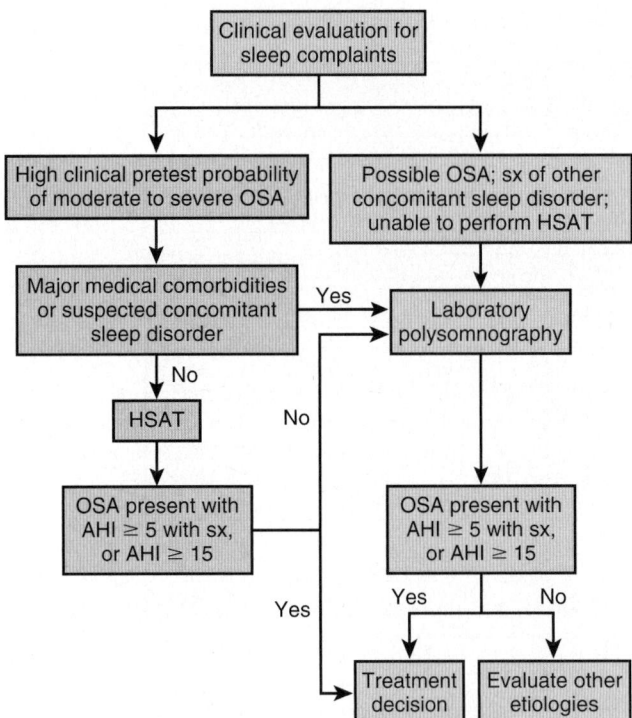

FIG. 6 Approach to the diagnosis of obstructive sleep apnea (OSA). An ambulatory pathway for patients with symptomatic moderate to severe OSA without other major comorbidities is shown in *blue*. Patients with a lower pretest probability of OSA or who are suspected of having another sleep disorder are recommended for evaluation in the laboratory-based pathway in *orange*. *AHI,* Apnea-hypopnea index; *HSAT,* home sleep apnea testing. (From Broaddus C et al: *Murray and Nadel's textbook of respiratory medicine,* ed 7, Philadelphia, 2022, Saunders.)

without other comorbidities) because it may detect more subtle respiratory events than HSAT and can accurately quantify total sleep time (rather than simply time in bed).

- HSAT is best used as an alternative to PSG in cases where clinical suspicion is high for moderate or severe OSA and there are no comorbidities that might influence sleep testing. Referral to a sleep specialist or PSG should be considered when there is comorbid COPD, heart failure, neuromuscular weakness, or a suspected hypoventilation syndrome, or if there is concern for another nonrespiratory sleep disorder requiring PSG (e.g., narcolepsy, severe insomnia, or parasomnias).
- HSAT is not recommended for pediatric use.
- Diagnosis of OSA in adults is made using a combination of AHI and symptoms:
  1. Mild: ≥5 to <15 respiratory events per h (with symptoms or comorbidities)
  2. Moderate: ≥15 to <30 respiratory events per h
  3. Severe: ≥ 30 respiratory events per h
- Note that formal diagnosis of mild OSA requires the presence of symptoms (including those noted by the bed partner) or presence of a comorbidity such as hypertension, excessive daytime sleepiness, heart attack, heart failure, stroke, mood disorders or insomnia, or impaired cognition.
- The respiratory disturbance index (RDI) includes additional respiratory events (RERAs; see Table 1) that are not captured in the AHI.

Using the more sensitive RDI for diagnosis instead of the AHI may be most appropriate in sleepy, symptomatic patients.
- Diagnostic AHI thresholds are lower in children.

LABORATORY TESTS

- CBC to look for anemia or erythrocytosis
- Ferritin and iron panel if RLS or anemia (or other relevant CBC abnormality) is present
- Thyroid studies if thyroid dysfunction is suspected
- Bicarbonate level on basic metabolic panel can serve as a surrogate marker for chronic hypercapnia and can be used to stratify risk for OHS as an alternative or additional diagnosis; bicarbonate <27 in a patient with BMI <35 has high negative predictive value for OHS
- Arterial blood gas testing if hypercapnia needs to be ruled out
- Cardiac and pulmonary testing as guided by history and symptomatology

🆁🆇 TREATMENT

ACUTE GENERAL Rx

- Avoid alcohol for 4 to 6 h before bedtime.
- Avoid narcotics, muscle relaxants, and sedating medications.
- Treat nasal congestion.
- Consider side sleeping and/or elevating head of bed.

CHRONIC Rx

- Weight loss
  1. Most patients with OSA will benefit from weight loss. Weight loss by any modality is effective for reducing the severity of OSA, and sufficient weight loss can be curative in some patients.[8,9]
  2. Exercise without weight loss may improve OSA,[5] and lifestyle interventions reduce OSA in proportion to weight loss.[8]
  3. Medication-assisted weight loss should be considered.[8,10,11] Many patients with OSA who are overweight or obese will have comorbidities that can guide selection of a weight loss agent.
  4. Bariatric surgery leads to improvement or resolution of OSA for most patients, in addition to improvements in metabolic syndrome outcomes.
- Positive airway pressure (PAP)
  1. Continuous positive airway pressure (CPAP) is the first-line and most effective therapy for OSA (Fig. 7). It delivers a constant airway pressure that serves as a pneumatic splint relieving upper airway obstruction.[12] Most new devices sold today can be in autotitrating CPAP mode (auto-CPAP or APAP), which increases or decreases the level of pressure in response to change in airflow, vibratory snoring, or changes in circuit pressure. This allows for prescription of APAP immediately after diagnostic PSG or HSAT, with titration of pressures done at home.
  2. Other methods of delivering positive pressure include bilevel positive airway pressure (BPAP).[12] In addition to delivering expiratory positive airway pressure (EPAP, equivalent to CPAP), BPAP also delivers a higher inspiratory positive airway pressure (IPAP). BPAP may be used for certain patients with hypoventilation syndromes, or occasionally in the treatment of OSA where CPAP is not well-tolerated.
- Oral appliance
  1. Mandibular advancement devices fit over the teeth like a mouthguard while engaging the maxillary and mandibular dental arches, inducing protrusion of the mandible and more favorable positioning of the tongue and other airway structures. They are most effective for the treatment of mild to moderate OSA and tend to work better in those with retrognathia, supine OSA, and lower BMI. They can be considered for severe OSA if CPAP is absolutely not tolerated. Although CPAP is more efficacious, this advantage may be offset by inferior compliance relative to oral appliance, resulting in similar effectiveness. There is no overall difference between oral appliances and CPAP with respect to improvement in blood pressure, daytime sleepiness, or quality of life.[13] Severely hypoxemic patients or patients requiring rapid treatment should be treated with CPAP.
- Surgical treatment (Box 1):
  1. Presurgical planning may involve several visits to identify specific anatomic areas of

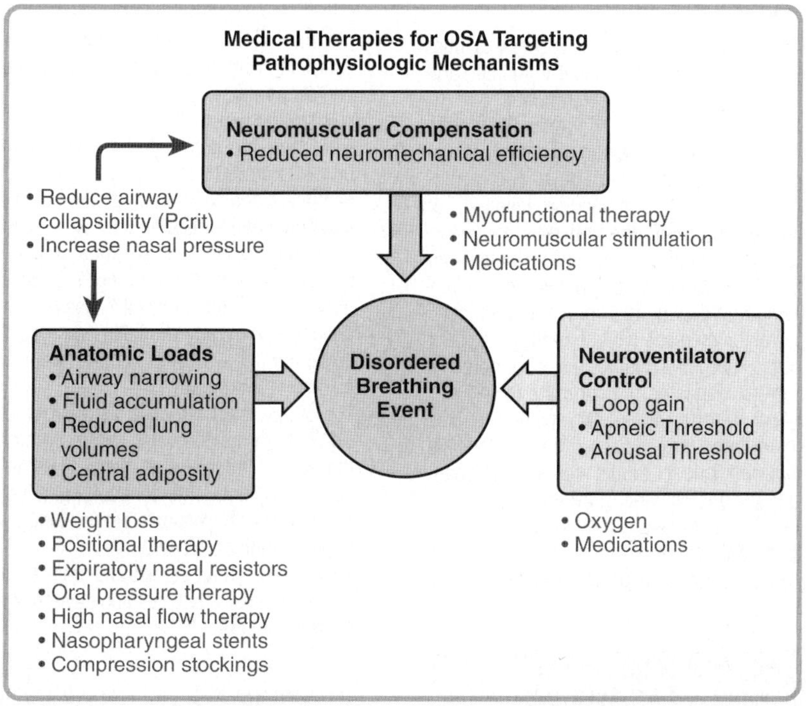

Medical Therapies for OSA Targeting Pathophysiologic Mechanisms

Neuromuscular Compensation
• Reduced neuromechanical efficiency

• Reduce airway collapsibility (Pcrit)
• Increase nasal pressure

• Myofunctional therapy
• Neuromuscular stimulation
• Medications

Anatomic Loads
• Airway narrowing
• Fluid accumulation
• Reduced lung volumes
• Central adiposity

Disordered Breathing Event

Neuroventilatory Control
• Loop gain
• Apneic Threshold
• Arousal Threshold

• Weight loss
• Positional therapy
• Expiratory nasal resistors
• Oral pressure therapy
• High nasal flow therapy
• Nasopharyngeal stents
• Compression stockings

• Oxygen
• Medications

FIG. 7 Therapies for obstructive sleep apnea (OSA) stratified by mechanism. Traditional therapies such as continuous positive airway pressure (CPAP) use nasal pressure to overcome anatomic loads. By contrast, upper airway surgery and weight loss reduce anatomic loads (measured as airway collapsibility, *Pcrit*). Therapeutic strategies that address impairments in neuromuscular function and neuroventilatory control are less well established, but include myofunctional therapies, neuromuscular stimulation, use of medications to modulate tone or increase arousal threshold, and supplemental oxygen. (Adapted from Kryger M et al: *Principles and practice of sleep medicine,* ed 6, Philadelphia, 2017, Elsevier.)

BOX 1 Surgical Treatment Options

Nasal Surgery
• Nasal septoplasty
• Inferior turbinate reduction
• Adenoidectomy
• Nasal tumor or polyp resection
• Nasal valve reconstruction

Palatal Surgery
• Palatal radiofrequency ablation
• Pillar implants
• Injection snoreplasty
• Tonsillectomy
• Uvulopalatopharyngoplasty/Z-palatoplasty
• Transpalatal advancement pharyngoplasty

Hypopharyngeal Surgery
• Lingual tonsillectomy
• Partial midline glossectomy
• Tongue base radiofrequency ablation
• Mandibular osteotomy and genioglossal advancement
• Hyoid myotomy and suspension
• Tongue-suspension suture
• Maxillomandibular osteotomy and advancement

From Flint PW et al: *Cummings otolaryngology, head and neck surgery,* ed 7, Philadelphia, 2021, Elsevier.

narrowing (nasal, pharyngeal, tongue base, hypopharynx) and select the appropriate surgery. See details that are listed below. Sometimes, these surgeries may be performed in combination or in sequence.
2. Adenotonsillectomy is often curative for children with OSA, and for select adults with tonsillar hypertrophy.

3. Uvulopalatopharyngoplasty, which involves resection of the uvula and soft palate.
4. Maxillomandibular advancement surgery involves osteotomies of the maxilla and mandible to allow the entire lower face to be projected forward, creating a more favorable configuration for the soft tissues and dilators of the oropharynx.[14]

5. Hypoglossal nerve stimulation (HGNS) involves surgical placement of an implant in the upper chest, connected to the hypoglossal nerve, which helps recruit lingual muscles, reducing pharyngeal collapsibility and decreasing upper airway resistance. Operation of the device requires nightly activation by the patient with a remote control.
6. Palatal implant surgery and maxillary expansion for high-arched palates are other surgical options.
7. Nasal septoplasty/turbinectomy could be considered for patients with severe anatomic deformities or chronic nasal congestion refractory to medical therapy.
• Other treatments: These treatments are generally best used as adjunctive strategies or used in mild cases with patients seeking to avoid devices and surgery.
  1. Optimal treatment of allergic rhinitis, including nasal irrigation, nasal steroids, antihistamines, and modifications to environment.
  2. Side sleeping will reduce OSA in many patients. In well-selected patients, guided by PSG or HSAT results, positional therapy may even be a first-line choice. Body pillows, wedge pillows, physical or electronic position trainers, or other devices can be helpful.
  3. Nasal EPAP devices are one-way expiratory valves worn over the nose. Resistance to exhalation at the nose generates positive airway pressure, reducing apneas.
  4. Myofunctional therapy, a set of upper airway exercises to reduce snoring and apneas, can be suggested to motivated patients as an adjunctive therapy.
  5. Orthodontic treatment (palatal expansion) may be an option in children.

DISPOSITION
• Patients should be counseled on risks of untreated sleepiness, particularly when it comes to driving. Short-term prognosis for excessive daytime sleepiness and snoring is good with regular use of CPAP.
• Problems with tolerance of CPAP at initiation are common but surmountable. Scheduled follow-up to assess CPAP usage and to address problems proactively is necessary.
• Mask fit, claustrophobia, nasal congestion, and the habitual nature of the therapy are common barriers to care.
• CPAP machines provide daily usage reports logging hours of use and estimated AHI (Fig. E8). In most U.S. practice settings, the durable medical equipment company supplying the CPAP device can provide these reports on request and provide assistance with troubleshooting issues related to CPAP comfort or equipment malfunction.
• Residual excessive sleepiness (RES) despite adequate treatment of OSA should prompt consideration of alternative causes. Modafinil or armodafinil can be considered for treatment once other causes are ruled out and are first-line medications for RES. Solriamfetol is

a dopamine and norepinephrine reuptake inhibitor FDA approved for RES, although it may be limited by formulary.

- If central sleep apnea is diagnosed, evaluate for underlying heart failure or opioid use, and treat underlying heart failure as appropriate or reduce opioid use to the extent possible. Consult sleep medicine to determine if PAP therapy is indicated.
- Although evidence on the matter is not entirely straightforward, patients should be counseled on likely long-term risks of untreated OSA, which may include increased risks of hypertension, stroke, heart failure, arrhythmia, cognitive impairment, and others (Fig. E9).
  1. Observational studies show strong association between increasing OSA severity, vascular events, and early mortality. These studies have long follow-up times, on the order of 10 yr or longer, and inflection points in mortality curves do not appear until late into the observation period.[15]
  2. Randomized controlled trials (RCTs) have failed to show that CPAP reduces incident cardiovascular events in those with moderate to severe OSA.[15] Critiques of these studies include low adherence to CPAP (3 h/night), the necessity of excluding excessively sleepy patients for ethical reasons, selection of composite outcomes (obscuring effectiveness in preventing stroke), and insufficient follow-up time (follow-up times on the order of 3 to 5 yr).
  3. RCT evidence supports improvement in mood and quality of life with CPAP.

REFERRAL

- HSAT and APAP can lower barriers to care and for some patients enable diagnosis and treatment initiation entirely at home.
- Referral to sleep medicine may be helpful when ruling out other sleep disorders, evaluating SDB in the setting of advanced cardiopulmonary or neuromuscular disease, or when seeking CPAP alternatives.
- Sleep psychologists can be consulted for CPAP desensitization or motivational interviewing approaches to improve adherence.
- Referral to medical weight management or bariatric surgery should be considered if weight is suspected to contribute to OSA.
- Surgical referral to otolaryngology should be considered for children with adenotonsillar hypertrophy and for adults who are unresponsive to weight loss and CPAP therapy.
- Referral to a qualified dentist for treatment with an oral appliance is a good alternative to CPAP for those with uncomplicated mild to moderate OSA.

❗ PEARLS & CONSIDERATIONS

- OSA is a common disorder that is highly prevalent. OSA should be considered in patients of every age, gender, and weight status. Prevalence is particularly high in patients with the metabolic syndrome.
- An atypical presentation of a common disorder will still be common. Symptoms such as mental fog, nocturia, night sweats, insomnia, nightmares, and mood disturbances can be useful in prompting diagnostic evaluation.
- An occupational and driving history is a key component of the sleep history. In most situations, the greatest short-term morbidity from untreated OSA is due to excessive daytime sleepiness leading to motor vehicle and occupational accidents.
- Allow the presence or absence of significant symptoms to guide treatment recommendations in borderline and mild cases.
- Weight loss by any modality can lead to improvement of OSA and should be discussed as part of treatment.
- The single most effective therapy for OSA is CPAP, with quieter and more comfortable masks and machines developed over the last decade. Adjustments to equipment settings and behavioral therapies can be employed to improve patient acceptance.
- There are effective alternatives to CPAP, including oral appliances and several surgical options for OSA.

REFERENCES
Available at eBooks.Health.Elsevier.com.

RELATED CONTENT
Sleep Apnea (Patient Information)

AUTHORS: **DAVID CLAMAN, MD** and **ALEXANDER GOMEZ, MD**

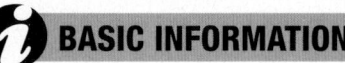 **BASIC INFORMATION**

DEFINITION

- Small bowel obstruction (SBO) can be **functional** (as a result of intrinsic abnormal intestinal pathology; dysfunction peristalsis, also called "ileus") or **mechanical** (which may occur acutely or may be chronic).
- SBO is due to intraluminal or extraluminal mechanical compression.
- Mechanical obstruction means the blockage of the intestinal lumen, preventing the passage of luminal contents through the gut tube. Intraabdominal adhesion disease is the most common cause of mechanical SBO in developed countries.
- Mechanical obstruction may be either:
  1. **Simple obstruction:** In which the lumen may be *partially* or *completely blocked* but with intact intestinal blood flow OR
  2. **Strangulated obstruction:**
     a. This is a surgical emergency.
     b. Usually the obstruction is complete; blood flow to the obstructed segment is cut off; and tissue necrosis, gangrene, and perforation may occur.

ICD-10CM CODES	
K56	Paralytic ileus and intestinal obstruction
K56.1	Intussusception
K56.2	Volvulus
K56.3	Gallstone ileus
K56.4	Other impaction of intestine
K56.5	Intestinal adhesions (bands) with obstruction
K56.6	Other and unspecified intestinal obstruction
K56.9	Ileus, unspecified

EPIDEMIOLOGY & DEMOGRAPHICS

- An estimated 300,000 laparotomies are performed yearly in the U.S. for SBO.
- The most frequently encountered surgical disorder of the small intestines is mechanical SBO. This is a common surgical emergency accounting for 2% to 4% of emergency room visits and 15% of hospital admissions.
- 75% of all cases of SBO result from intraabdominal adhesion related to prior abdominal surgery, such as appendectomy, colorectal surgery, and gynecologic procedures.

PREDOMINANT SEX & AGE: Incidence is similar for males and females.

RISK FACTORS:
- Previous abdominal or pelvic surgery—most important risk factor for mechanical SBO in the U.S.
- Hernia (abdominal wall or groin)
- Prior abdominal irradiation
- Bowel neoplasm
- Foreign-body ingestion
- Parasitic infestation
- Gallstones
- Inflammatory/ischemic stricture

PHYSICAL FINDINGS & CLINICAL PRESENTATION

PHYSICAL FINDINGS: These may include:
- Dehydration (manifested by tachycardia, decreased urine output, orthostatic hypotension, dry mucous membrane)
- Abdominal distention may suggest an abnormal accumulation of air or fluid
- Hyperactive bowel sounds (an early occurrence)
- Tympany to abdominal percussion over a distended abdomen may indicate the presence of air
- Percussion dullness over a distended abdomen may indicate fluid
- High-pitched "tinkling" sound on auscultation of the abdomen
- Hypoactive bowel sounds (late finding)
- Hernia

Rectal examination may reveal:
- Blood (suggestive of neoplasm or strangulation or mucosal ischemia)
- Masses (may suggest obturator hernia)
- Fecal impaction

CLINICAL PRESENTATION: There are four key symptoms: Abdominal pain, vomiting, distention, and constipation.
- Abdominal pain (abrupt onset):
  1. Intermittent, crampy, or colicky
  2. Constant pain (that is, change in pain's character) signifies serious complication
- Abdominal distention: Indicates abnormal accumulation of air or fluid
- Nausea
- Vomiting (bilious vomiting seen in proximal obstructions)
- Diarrhea (early finding)
- Constipation (a late finding)
- Obstipation (inability to pass gas or stool)
- Hypotension, fever, tachycardia, leukocytosis, and peritoneal signs (these late findings may be seen with strangulation or intestinal ischemia) should compel urgency toward operative management
- It is important to perform serial abdominal examinations to detect changes early

ETIOLOGY
- Postoperative adhesions, especially prior abdominopelvic operations (may cause acute obstruction usually within 1 mo of surgery; or chronic obstructions can occur years later)
- Incarcerated inguinal hernia
- Malignant tumor
- Inflammatory bowel disease
- Gallstone ileus
- Stool impaction
- Stricture
- Cystic fibrosis
- Volvulus
- In children consider pyloric stenosis, intussusception, congenital atresia

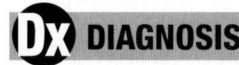 **DIAGNOSIS**

DIFFERENTIAL DIAGNOSIS
- Paralytic ileus
- Pseudoobstruction

- Acute cholangitis
- Cholecystitis
- Gastroenteritis
- Inflammatory bowel disease
- Diverticulitis
- Endometriosis
- Mesenteric ischemia
- Pancreatitis
- Dysmenorrhea
- Ovarian torsion

WORKUP (FIG. 1)

All patients diagnosed with acute SBO should be admitted to the hospital, as they need immediate surgical evaluation. During the initial evaluation, the primary objectives are to gauge the degree of metabolic derangement and volume depletion, and to assess the need for GI decompression with nasogastric (NG) tube and expediency of surgery. It is also important to exclude sepsis, perforation, and bowel ischemia. As with many surgical conditions, determining the correct diagnosis and management strategy hinges on a focused, yet thorough history and physical examination.

LABORATORY TESTS

- Laboratory abnormalities are not diagnostic of bowel obstruction but instead may indicate complications of obstruction. Essential laboratory tests include:
  1. Basic metabolic panel (hyponatremia, hypokalemia)
  2. CBC: Hemoconcentration, leukocytosis
  3. Urinalysis
  4. Serum amylase: May be elevated
  5. Lactate dehydrogenase
  6. Hepatic panel
  7. Check serum lactate, blood cultures, arterial blood gas in patients with signs such as fever, hypotension, or change in mental status
  8. Type and cross-match (in anticipation of possible surgical intervention)

IMAGING STUDIES

- Image to confirm diagnosis, identify the location of the obstruction, and access the type of obstruction.
- Imaging also helps identify complications (perforation, necrosis, etc.) and possible cause of the obstruction.
- Initial radiographic evaluation begins with plain x-ray films of the abdomen (supine and upright) and an upright chest radiograph. An upright chest radiograph is of paramount importance to inspect for pneumoperitoneum and also for evidence of aspiration in a patient with a history of vomiting. A supine and upright plain abdominal x-ray in patients with suspected SBO may show:
  1. Ladderlike pattern of dilated small bowel loops with air-fluid levels (Fig. 2) indicating SBO
  2. Accumulation of air and fluid proximal and clearance of fluid and air distal to the point of obstruction
  3. Proximal small bowel dilation with distal loop collapse

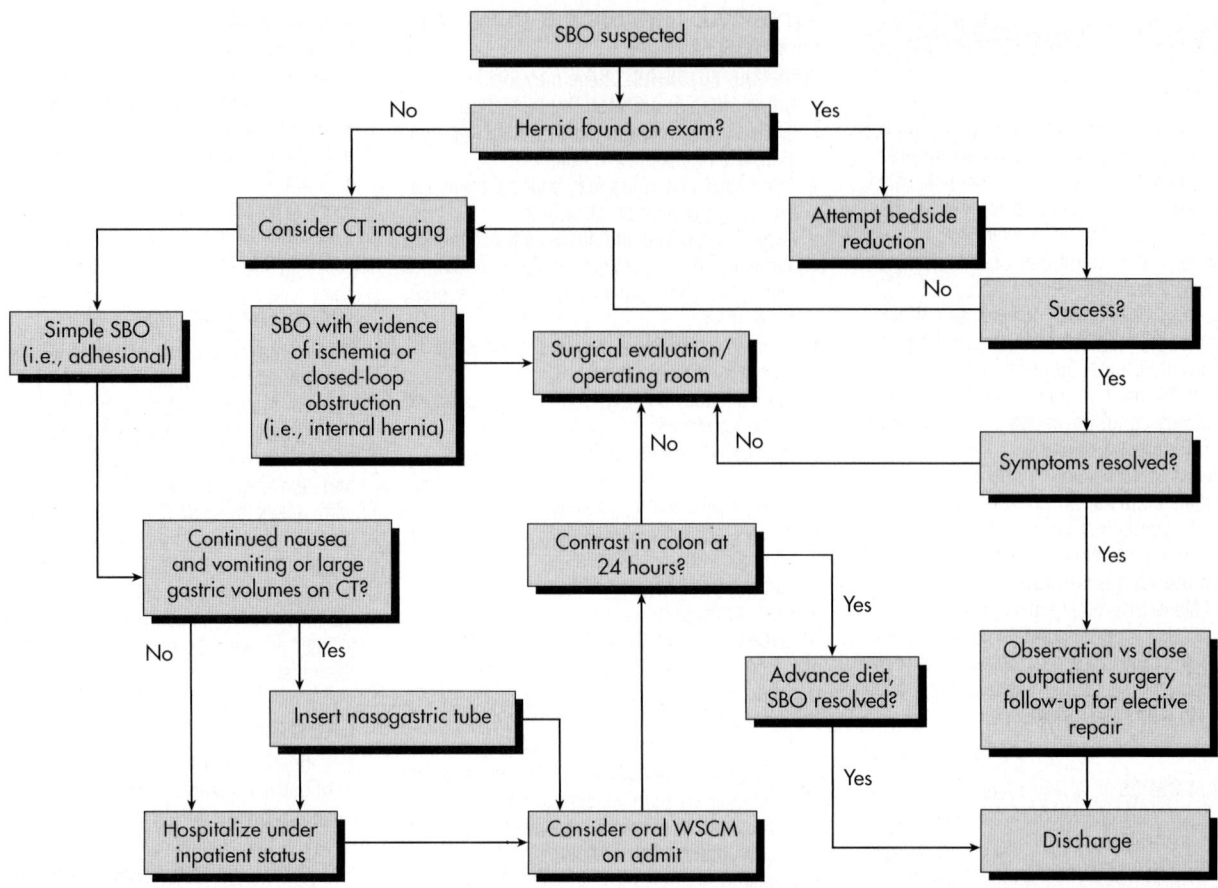

FIG. 1 **Management algorithm of small bowel obstruction** *(SBO)*. *CT,* Computed tomography; *WSCM,* water-soluble contrast medium. (From Walls RM et al: *Rosen's emergency medicine, concepts and clinical practice,* ed 10, Philadelphia, 2023, Elsevier.)

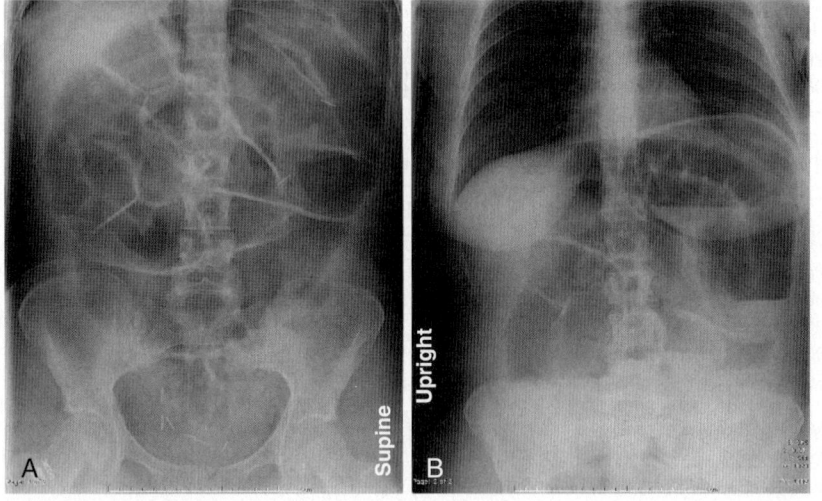

FIG. 2 A, Supine film showing dilated loops of small bowel in a patient with small bowel obstruction. **B,** Upright abdominal film revealing multiple air-fluid levels and small bowel dilation, consistent with a diagnosis of small bowel obstruction. (From Walls RM et al: *Rosen's emergency medicine, concepts and clinical practice,* ed 10, Philadelphia, 2023, Elsevier.)

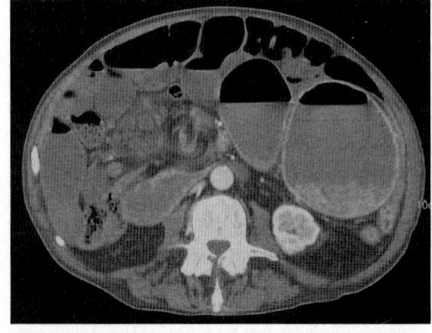

FIG. 3 Computed tomography scan of small bowel volvulus with notable mesenteric torsion. (From Cameron JL, Cameron AM: *Current surgical therapy,* ed 10, Philadelphia, 2011, Saunders.)

- Enteroclysis (a fluoroscopic x-ray of the small intestine) is useful in detecting obstruction and can distinguish partial from complete blockage and adhesions from metastases.
- Computed tomography (CT) scan of the abdomen and pelvis with contrast is the gold standard imaging modality.

- CT scan is the study of choice if the patient has fever, tachycardia, abdominal pain, and leukocytosis. It can reveal the etiology of the obstruction: Abscess, inflammatory process, extraluminal pathology, and/or metastases.
- CT can elucidate the cause, such as the presence of a mass (Fig. 3) or a hernia with subsequent obstruction (Fig. 4). In addition, CT has high sensitivity for detecting strangulation and pneumoperitoneum indicative of a perforation and is particularly useful in the early postoperative setting to rule out ischemia, intraabdominal abscess, or morbidity as the underlying cause. It is also useful in patients with a history of malignancy to differentiate potentially recurrent disease from adhesions (Fig. 5).
- CT enterography, in which intraluminal distention is achieved with administration of large volumes of oral contrast such as

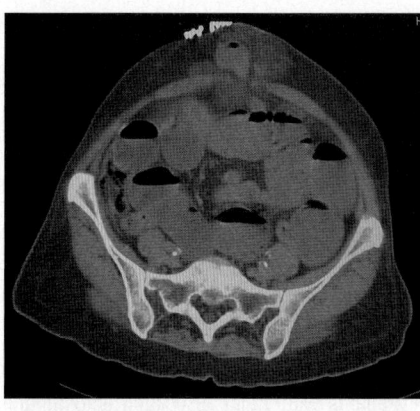

FIG. 4 Computed tomography scan of complete small bowel obstruction due to incisional hernia. (From Cameron IL, Cameron AM: *Current surgical therapy,* ed 10, Philadelphia, 2011, Saunders.)

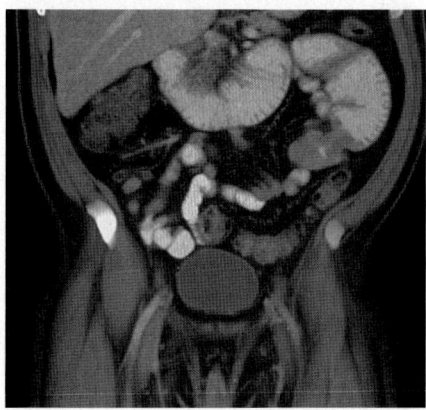

FIG. 5 Coronal image of computed tomography scan showing mass in proximal small bowel with decompressed loops of small bowel distal to obstruction. (From Cameron JL, Cameron AM: *Current surgical therapy,* ed 10, Philadelphia, 2011, Saunders.)

water-methylcellulose solution, can be useful. This modality is most often used to diagnose patients with Crohn disease–related strictures, and its benefit is high-resolution imaging of the bowel wall; however, it is impractical in the patient with GI distress who is nauseated and vomiting.

℞ TREATMENT

- Immediate admission to the hospital if acute SBO is suspected.
- Prompt surgical consultation to determine if surgical intervention is needed.

EMERGENCY DEPARTMENT CARE

- Vigorous fluid resuscitation and correction of electrolyte disorders underpin the initial therapeutic goals of both nonoperative and preoperative management strategies. Placing a Foley catheter to measure urinary output, establishing adequate intravenous access, and reassessing hemodynamic and electrolyte status are all essential in the initial management.
- Initial treatment:
  1. Designate the patient nothing by mouth; *nil per os* ("NPO")
  2. Fluid resuscitation (with isotonic Ringer or normal saline solution)
  3. Bowel decompression (via nasogastric [NG] tube placement): A standard NG tube provides symptomatic relief, prevents added gas and fluid accumulation proximally, and enables the serial assessment of antegrade fluid movement
  4. Correction of metabolic and electrolyte abnormalities
  5. Pain management
  6. Antiemetic administration
  7. Surgical consultation: Must be done early
  8. Antibiotic administration

NONSURGICAL INPATIENT CARE

General principles:
- Bowel rest
- Continue NG suction for decompression
- Serial abdominal examination (q4 to 6h)
- Check labs, for example, CBC, basic metabolic panel, lactic acid q6h
- Provide adequate fluid

Patients with low-grade partial SBOs are prone to spontaneous resolution with conservative interventions such as bowel rest, NG decompression, and appropriate fluid resuscitation. For partial or simple obstructions resolution usually occurs within 72 h.

SURGICAL CARE

More than 25% of inpatients admitted because of SBO will require an operation. Patients with complete or high-grade partial SBO are most likely to need surgery, with less than 20% successfully managed nonoperatively. Surgery is indicated in:
- Strangulated obstruction (which is a surgical emergency)
- Patients with clinical signs including fever, tachycardia, and peritonitis
- Patients with radiologic signs of ischemia/necrosis or perforation (require prompt surgery)
- Simple complete obstruction: After failed nonoperative care

AUTHOR: **FRED F. FERRI, MD**

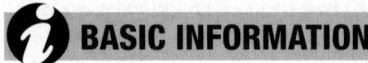 **BASIC INFORMATION**

DEFINITION

Statin-induced muscle syndromes (SIMS) include myopathy, myalgia, myositis, and rhabdomyolysis. Definitions for these syndromes are inconsistent in the medical literature.

- Myopathy: A general term defined as any disease of muscles
- Myalgia: Muscle weakness or pain without serum creatinine kinase elevation
- Myositis: Muscle weakness or pain with an increased serum creatinine kinase level
- Rhabdomyolysis: Muscle weakness or pain and a marked serum creatinine kinase level usually greater than 10× the upper limit of normal and serum creatinine elevation as well as signs of brown urine and elevated urine myoglobin. A rare **immune-mediated necrotizing myopathy (IMNM)**, also known as **statin-associated autoimmune myopathy**, has also been associated with the use of statins with symptoms persisting after discontinuation of the drug. This condition presents with symmetric proximal arm and leg weakness and severe elevations of muscle enzymes

SYNONYMS

SIMS
Statin-induced myopathies
Statin-induced myositis
Statin-induced myalgias
Statin-induced rhabdomyolysis
Statin-associated autoimmune myopathy

ICD-10CM CODES	
M60.9	Myositis, unspecified
M62.82	Rhabdomyolysis
G72.2	Myopathy due to other toxic agents
G72.9	Myopathy, unspecified
G72.81	Critical illness myopathy
G72.89	Other specified myopathies
M60.89	Other myositis, multiple sites

EPIDEMIOLOGY & DEMOGRAPHICS

INCIDENCE: Risk of statin-induced rhabdomyolysis is 1.2 per 10,000 persons/yr. Rhabdomyolysis risk of death is 0.15 deaths per 1 million prescriptions. SIMS most commonly occur in people aged 51 to 75, which may reflect the pattern of statin use. Statin-associated autoimmune myopathy occurs in an estimated 2 or 3 of every 100,000 patients treated with statins.
PREVALENCE: The prevalence of statin-induced myalgias is about 1% to 5%, similar to placebo in clinical trials, although observational studies have suggested a prevalence of 10% or higher. Statins may cause elevated transaminases (alanine transaminase [ALT], aspartate aminotransferase [AST]) at a prevalence of 0.5% to 2.0% and rhabdomyolysis ~0.08%.
PREDOMINANT SEX & AGE: The mean age of hospitalized patients with statin-induced myopathy or rhabdomyolysis was 64 yr old and was slightly more common in women (56%).
PEAK INCIDENCE: Patients on high-dose statins have a 0.9% incidence of statin-induced rhabdomyolysis.
RISK FACTORS: Small body frame; age over 80 yr; women, particularly frail elderly women; patients taking multiple drugs, especially gemfibrozil, niacin, colchicine, cyclosporine, itraconazole, ketoconazole, erythromycin, clarithromycin, verapamil, amiodarone; renal or liver impairment; pharmacogenetic variability; hypothyroidism; excessive alcohol intake; vigorous exercise; severe infections; excessive grapefruit juice ingestion; low vitamin D levels; inherited defects of muscle metabolism such as carnitine palmityl transferase II deficiency, McArdle disease, and myoadenylate deaminase deficiency; acquired myopathies such as postpoliomyelitis syndrome; lipophilic statins (simvastatin, atorvastatin, lovastatin); multiple conditions such as diabetes; renal impairment, and prior elevated creatine kinase (CK) and drugs of abuse (amphetamines, heroin, cocaine, phencyclidine).
GENETICS: Interpatient variability exists in the activity of the *CYP3A4* gene for the metabolism of simvastatin, atorvastatin, and lovastatin. Homozygous carriers of *CYP2D6* (poor metabolizers) had a higher rate of discontinuation of simvastatin due to muscle syndromes compared with the *CYP2D6* wild-type genotype; patients taking atorvastatin and having a muscle event were more likely to have the CYP2D6*4 allele. *SLCO1B1* polymorphisms encode for the organic anion transport of statins into the liver cells. The variant C allele may increase the risk of the *SLCO1B1* statin–induced myopathy in patients taking simvastatin and atorvastatin. Simvastatin-induced myopathy is more likely to be associated with *SLO1B1* genotype and not *ABCB1* genotype. However, a statin-associated autoimmune myopathy has shown a link to class II HLA allele DRB1*11:01 in the development of anti-HMG CoA reductase antibodies, leading to an increase in expression of the antibodies in the muscles of patients exposed to statins. Deficiencies in ubiquinone (coenzyme Q10) may exist in patients with a mutation in the *COQ2* gene. The *EYS* gene can affect neuromuscular tissue and may have a role. In addition, *RYR1* and *CACNA1S* genetic variants may be associated with statin-induced muscle syndromes and elevated CK levels.

PHYSICAL FINDINGS & CLINICAL PRESENTATION

- Myopathy can occur at any time, although it is more common within the first 4 wk of therapy; statin-associated necrotizing myopathy may occur after months of using statins
- Proximal generalized muscle aches, body aches, and pains, and may be mild or severe
- Dark-colored urine
- Muscle cramps, spasms, tenderness, proximal muscle weakness, or stiffness
- Unusually tired or weak
- Nocturnal cramping
- Tendon pain

ETIOLOGY

- History of current statin use.
- May be explained by one of three deficiencies of end products of the 3-hydroxy-3-methyl-glutaryl-coA reductase pathway: Cell signaling and apoptosis, mitochondrial function and ubiquinone concentrations, and cholesterol concentrations and cell membrane integrity.
- The risk may be enhanced by drug interactions that interfere with hepatic metabolism and gut wall transport of interacting medications and by pharmacodynamic effects.
- Underlying metabolic muscle disorder may predispose a patient to develop myopathy.
- Patients with statin-associated autoimmune myopathy have been found to have anti–HMG-CoA reductase antibodies even prior to exposure to statin therapy.

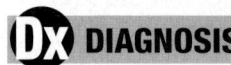 **DIAGNOSIS**

DIFFERENTIAL DIAGNOSIS

Bursitis, tendinitis, radiculopathy, osteoarthritis, muscle strain, myofascial pain, hypothyroidism, proton pump inhibitor–induced polymyositis, viral illness, polymyositis, idiopathic inflammatory myositis, and polymyalgia rheumatica

WORKUP

Workup consists of a thorough history, including exercise history, urine color, medication history, and physical exam to palpate tenderness and obtain blood tests to evaluate muscle and kidney damage.

LABORATORY TESTS

If severe myopathy or rhabdomyolysis is suspected:

- Elevated CK, positive serum myoglobin, elevated blood urea nitrogen (BUN), serum creatinine, AST, ALT, lactate dehydrogenase, and potassium
- Urine creatinine, positive casts, and hemoglobin in urine with absence of red blood cells
- Anti-3-hydroxy-3-methylglutaryl-coenzyme A (anti–HMG-CoA) antibody
- Consider electrocardiogram and assessment of calcium, phosphate, and uric acid

If mild to moderate myopathy is suspected:

- Monitor thyroid-stimulating hormone (TSH) and CK levels; CK may only be elevated when sudden severe myopathy occurs.
- If the patient has brown or dark urine or elevated CK monitor BUN and serum creatinine.
- In statin-associated autoimmune myopathy, the CK level is usually ≥10 times the upper limit of normal. In these patients, muscle biopsy specimens will be positive for autoantibodies against HMG-CoA reductase and may have necrosis.

IMAGING STUDIES

- Not recommended.
- In statin-associated autoimmune myopathy, electromyography shows small-amplitude motor-unit potentials with increased spontaneous activity characteristic of an active myopathic process. Muscle edema is evident on MRI.

- Statin Intolerance Tool:
  1. The American College of Cardiology (ACC) has created a tool to assess statin muscle symptoms and to guide clinicians that can be of value: http://tools.acc.org/statinintolerance/#!/

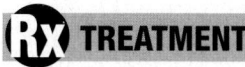 TREATMENT

NONPHARMACOLOGIC THERAPY

Treatment of rhabdomyolysis is generally supportive in nature (see "Rhabdomyolysis" topic).

ACUTE GENERAL Rx

- Stop statin therapy immediately if muscle symptoms occur. Check history, potential drug-drug interactions, CK, TSH, renal function, hepatic function, and urinalysis.
- If patients have suspected rhabdomyolysis, they should be hospitalized and treated with supportive therapy and monitoring of complications.
- If CK <10× the upper limit of normal without symptoms, continue statin therapy at the same or lower dosage.
- If CK <10× the upper limit of normal with intolerable symptoms, discontinue statin.
- If CK >10× the upper limit of normal, discontinue statin.
  Box E1 describes recommendations of the National Lipid Association Statin Safety Assessment Task Force regarding statin and muscle safety.

CHRONIC Rx

- After stopping the statin and symptom or CK resolution, which may take up to 4 mo, consider the same statin at a lower dosage or a different statin at an equivalent or lower dosage.
- When restarting therapy, consider statins such as low-dose rosuvastatin; pravastatin; and alternate-day dosing of rosuvastatin or atorvastatin.
- If patient had rhabdomyolysis secondary to statin therapy, consider nonstatin treatments.
- If the patient develops myopathy after a second trial of therapy, statin treatment should be permanently discontinued and nonstatin cholesterol-lowering therapy initiated.
- A nocebo effect of statin-induced myopathy has been demonstrated in some patients.
- Bempedoic acid may offer a safe and effective lipid-lowering therapeutic option for patients unable to tolerate statins.
- For IMNM (statin-associated autoimmune myopathy and idiopathic inflammatory myositis), immunosuppressive therapy with prednisone

(1 mg per kg of body weight per day) and at least one agent (methotrexate, azathioprine, or mycophenolate mofetil) have been used. In resistant cases, IV immune globulin or another agent such as rituximab may be added.

INTEGRATIVE MEDICINE

- The effect of coenzyme Q10 on reducing or preventing SIMS remains controversial; although it may be effective in reducing muscle pain, weakness, cramps, and tiredness, it has no effect on lowering CK levels. Given its safety, coenzyme Q10 can be recommended if the actions listed under "Chronic Rx" are insufficient to continue the use of the statin and if the muscle symptoms have been limited to myalgias. Use coenzyme Q10 with caution in patients taking warfarin, as its anticoagulant effect may be decreased.
- A 2015 meta-analysis of observational studies reported that vitamin D levels were lower in patients with statin-induced myalgias than in individuals who did not have these symptoms.
- A more recent trial[1] comparing statin users who took vitamin D supplements to those who took placebo revealed that both had the same incidence of muscle symptoms. The mean 25 hydroxyvitamin D level at baseline was 30 mg/ml. Vitamin D did not prevent symptoms in subgroups with baseline levels less than 30 mg/ml or <20 mg/ml.

DISPOSITION

- Usually resolves within 1 wk up to 4 mo after discontinuing statin therapy.
- Once the patient has a full recovery, an alternative statin can be tried.
- Statins should not be restarted in IMNM or idiopathic inflammatory myositis.

REFERRAL

If rhabdomyolysis is suspected, immediate referral for hospitalization is suggested.

⚠ PEARLS & CONSIDERATIONS

COMMENTS

- SIMS are usually mild and will resolve within a few wk after discontinuing statin therapy. However, such syndromes may progress to rhabdomyolysis.
- A recent meta-analysis[2] revealed that among participants taking statins 27.1% reported muscle symptoms compared with 26.6% in the placebo group for a 3% small increase

during a median of 4 yr which is considered barely significant. All excess risk occurred in the first yr of therapy.

PREVENTION

- Follow the 2013 American Heart Association (AHA)/ACC treatment guidelines and the 2017 ACC focused update on nonstatin therapies for low-density lipoprotein (LDL) cholesterol and limit the concomitant use of fibrates with statins.
- Discontinue statin therapy prior to and during surgical procedures.
- If patient requires a short-term therapy with an interacting medication such as an azole antifungal, temporarily discontinue statin until interacting therapy is completed.
- If statin–fibric acid therapy is warranted, fenofibrate is preferred over gemfibrozil to decrease risk of myopathy.
- Baseline liver function testing before initiation of statin therapy and only if clinically indicated thereafter.

PATIENT & FAMILY EDUCATION

- Inform patients to promptly report muscle weakness, unexpected muscle pain, or brownish urine.
- Providers should be cautious of the impact of media coverage of statin-induced side effects, which may include the nocebo effect.
- Ensure that the pharmacist and/or primary care physician checks for drug-drug interactions with every new prescription, including those from dentists and physicians from other specialties.
- Coenzyme Q10 may lessen milder muscle symptoms from statins, but patients should inform their physician and pharmacist if they decide to use this supplement.
- A recent clinical trial comparing lipid-lowering efficacy for two nonstatin therapies, ezetimibe and evolocumab, among patients with statin intolerance revealed that evolocumab resulted in a significantly greater reduction in LDL-C levels after 24 wk. Further studies are needed to assess long-term efficacy and safety.

REFERENCES & SUGGESTED READINGS

Available at eBooks.Health.Elsevier.com.

RELATED CONTENT

Rhabdomyolysis (Related Key Topic)

AUTHORS: **LISA COHEN, PHARMD** and **ANNE L. HUME, PHARMD**

Diseases
and Disorders

I

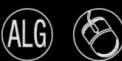

 BASIC INFORMATION

DEFINITIONS

Status epilepticus is a medical neurologic emergency. It is historically defined as 30 min of continuous seizure activity or two or more seizures without full recovery of consciousness between seizures. However, in practice, a continuous seizure that lasts >5 min is treated as status epilepticus.[1]

Refractory status epilepticus: Status epilepticus persisting despite administration of at least two appropriately selected and dosed parenteral medications including a benzodiazepine. No specific seizure duration is required.[2]

Super-refractory status epilepticus exists if status epilepticus continues for 24 h or longer after anesthesia is administered.[2]

SYNONYMS

Convulsive status epilepticus
Nonconvulsive status epilepticus

ICD-10CM CODES
G41	Status epilepticus
G40.301	Generalized idiopathic epilepsy and epileptic syndromes, not intractable, with status epilepticus

EPIDEMIOLOGY & DEMOGRAPHICS

INCIDENCE: 18.3 to 41 per 100,000 people per yr in the U.S.[3]

PREDOMINANT SEX & AGE: From population-based studies, it seems that status epilepticus is more common in Black males and in either young children or older adults.[4]

PEAK INCIDENCE: The highest incidences occur in young children and in those aged 60 and above. The incidence in the elderly is about 3 to 10 times that of younger adults.[4]

PHYSICAL FINDINGS & CLINICAL PRESENTATION

- Patients can present with repetitive tonic-clonic movements of the body (convulsive status epilepticus); other patients are comatose and nonresponsive (nonconvulsive status epilepticus).[5]
- Patients may also present with lethargy, intermittent confusion, and involuntary movements.

ETIOLOGY

- Status epilepticus can be the result of an acute neurologic injury, such as stroke, meningitis, brain tumor.[6] Table 1 summarizes causes of status epilepticus in adults presenting in the community.
- In patients with epilepsy, low antiseizure medication levels can result in status.[2]

Dx **DIAGNOSIS**

DIFFERENTIAL DIAGNOSIS

- Encephalopathies: Metabolic, infectious, toxic, cerebral hypoperfusion, etc.
- Nonepileptic psychogenic events

WORKUP

- Airway, breathing, circulation (ABCs)
- Intensive care unit (ICU) admission
- Emergent electroencephalogram (EEG), especially if the patient does not start returning to baseline[2]
- Continuous EEG in refractory cases[2]
Table 2 describes a suggested timetable for emergency diagnosis and treatment of status.

TABLE 1 Causes of Status Epilepticus in Adults Presenting From the Community

Previous Seizures	No Previous Seizures
Common	
Subtherapeutic anticonvulsant	Ethanol-related
Ethanol-related	Drug toxicity
Intractable epilepsy	CNS infection
	Head trauma
	CNS tumor
Less Common	
CNS infection	Metabolic aberration
Metabolic aberration	Stroke
Drug toxicity	
Stroke	
CNS tumor	
Head trauma	

CNS, Central nervous system.
From Vincent JL et al: *Textbook of critical care*, ed 8, Philadelphia, 2024, Elsevier.

epilepticus. A treatment approach is summarized in Table 3 and Fig. 1.

LABORATORY TESTS

- Routine blood workup (CBC, comprehensive metabolic panel [CMP], glucose, electrolytes)
- Urine drug screen
- Lumbar puncture and cerebrospinal fluid (CSF) analysis in patients with suspected infectious meningitis or encephalitis or suspected autoimmune or paraneoplastic encephalitis

IMAGING STUDIES

- Immediate computed tomography (CT) scan of the head.
- MRI of the brain with and without contrast should be performed once the patient is in a stable condition.[2,6]

Rx **TREATMENT**

- The longer a patient is in status epilepticus, the harder it is to treat and the more likely permanent damage is done.[2]
- Patients with continuous seizure activity over 5 min should be given intravenous lorazepam 0.1 mg/kg/dose, max: 4 mg/dose, may repeat dose once (or diazepam 0.15 to 0.2 mg/kg/dose, max 10 mg/dose, may repeat dose once only when lorazepam is not available).[2,7]
- In the absence of intravenous access, intramuscular administration of midazolam 10 mg in an adult is a superior alternative.[2,7]
- It is not uncommon for patients in convulsive status epilepticus to transition to nonconvulsive

TABLE 2 Suggested Timetable for Emergency Diagnosis and Treatment of Status Epilepticus

Time	Exam/Intervention	Testing
Initial presentation: 0 min	Airway, breathing, circulation, IV access, monitoring	Glucose, oxygenation via pulse oximetry ± blood gas analysis
Primary survey: 5 min	Neurologic exam Administer antiseizure medications Lorazepam, 0.1 mg/kg IV Phenobarbital, 20 mg/kg IV Normal saline maintenance IV Reduce fever	Electrolytes, renal and liver function, ammonia, anticonvulsant levels, toxicology, complete blood cell count, urinalysis
Secondary survey: 15-30 min	Evaluate treatment results Second-line antiseizure medication if seizure persists Fosphenytoin, 20 mg/kg IV; or phenytoin, 20 mg/kg IV	Patient-specific: Cranial imaging (CT vs. MRI), lumbar puncture, EEG, ECG
Status epilepticus: >30 min	Intubation and mechanical ventilation	
Refractory status epilepticus: >60 min	Titrate antiseizure medications to burst suppression Pentobarbital, 10 mg/kg IV given over 30 min, then 5 mg/kg every h for 3 doses, then 1 mg/kg/h; titrate to effect Midazolam, 0.15 mg/kg IV, then 1-2 μg/kg/min, titrate to effect Phenobarbital, 5-10 mg/kg IV every 20 min to achieve burst suppression, then every 12 h Evaluate need for vasopressors	Continuous EEG Neurologic consultation Consider anesthesia consultation for treatment with inhaled anesthetic

CT, Computed tomography; *ECG,* electrocardiogram; *EEG,* electroencephalogram; *IV,* intravenous; *MRI,* magnetic resonance imaging.
From Vincent JL et al: *Textbook of critical care*, ed 7, Philadelphia, 2017, Elsevier.

TABLE 3 Treatment Approach to Status Epilepticus

1. Appropriate critical care treatment should be provided as soon as possible and simultaneously with emergent initial therapy for seizures. Treatment should be escalated quickly until seizures are controlled.
2. Critical care treatment (dictated by clinical circumstances):
   a. Intubation for airway protection and mechanical ventilation
   b. Vital sign monitoring
   c. Peripheral IV access
   d. Treatment of hypotension with vasopressors
   e. Finger stick blood glucose
   f. Nutrient resuscitation (thiamine before dextrose)
   g. Hypertension may be related to ongoing seizure activity, and termination of status epilepticus often substantially corrects it. Additionally, many agents used to terminate status epilepticus can produce hypotension
3. Emergent initial therapy with benzodiazepines:
   a. Lorazepam 0.1 mg/kg up to 4 mg per dose, may repeat after 5-10 min
   b. Midazolam 0.2 mg/kg IM/IV up to 10 mg
   c. Diazepam 0.15 mg/kg up to 10 mg per dose, may repeat after 5 min
4. Urgent control therapy—antiseizure drugs available in IV formulations:
   a. Fosphenytoin/phenytoin 20 mg PE/kg IV, may repeat bolus of 5 mg/kg IV
   b. Valproic acid 20-40 mg/kg IV, may repeat bolus of 20 mg/kg IV
   c. Levetiracetam 1000-3000 mg IV
   d. Phenobarbital 20 mg/kg IV, may repeat bolus of 5-10 mg/kg
   e. Lacosamide 200-400 mg IV
   f. Midazolam bolus 0.2 mg/kg IV, followed by 0.05-2 mg/kg/h continuous infusion
5. Refractory therapy–continuous infusion of antiseizure drugs, titrated to either seizure cessation, suppression-burst, or complete suppression on EEG:
   a. Midazolam bolus 0.2 mg/kg IV, followed by 0.05-2 mg/kg/h continuous infusion
   b. Propofol bolus 1-2 mg/kg, followed by 20 mcg/kg/min continuous infusion, titrate up to 30-200 mcg/kg/min
   c. Pentobarbital 5-15 mg/kg, may repeat bolus of 5-10 mg/kg, followed by 0.5-5 mg/kg/h continuous infusion
6. Treat complications
7. Complications of status epilepticus are numerous and can involve multiple organ systems. In particular, convulsive status epilepticus is associated with cardiac complications such as hypertension and tachycardia, as well as rhabdomyolysis and hyperthermia. Respiratory complications, including respiratory failure, hypoxia, and neurogenic pulmonary edema, may be seen. Status epilepticus is associated with neuronal damage and cerebral edema with increased intracranial pressure, which may require intracranial pressure monitoring and aggressive treatment with hypertonic agents

IV, Intravenous.
From Vincent JL et al: *Textbook of critical care,* ed 8, Philadelphia, 2024, Elsevier.

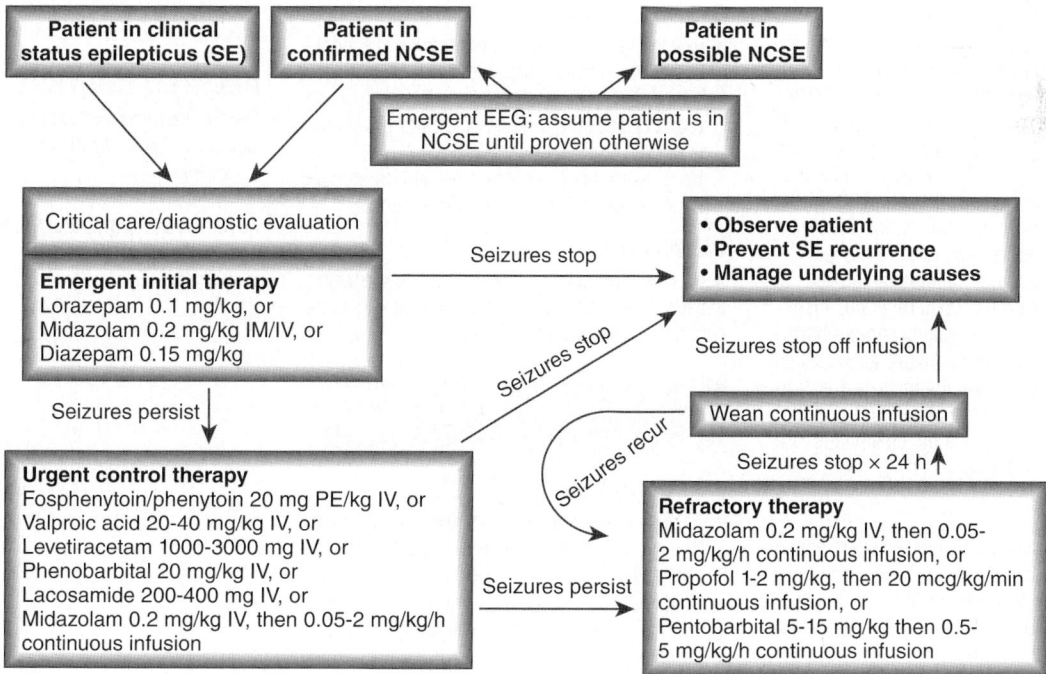

FIG. 1 Management algorithm for status epilepticus. *EEG,* Electroencephalogram; *IM,* intramuscular; *IV,* intravenous; *NCSE,* nonconvulsive status epilepticus; *SE,* status epilepticus. (From Vincent JL et al: *Textbook of critical care,* ed 8, Philadelphia, 2024, Elsevier.)

TABLE 4 Treatment Alternatives for Refractory and Super-Refractory Status Epilepticus

	Comments	Adverse Events
Thiopental	Metabolized to pentobarbital	Hypotension Respiratory depression Cardiac depression
Ketamine	Mechanism of action particularly well-suited to treat refractory and super-refractory SE (NMDA receptor antagonist)	High intracranial pressure Hypotension Hallucinations
Inhaled anesthetics	High rate of complications Needs closed system (gas recovery)	Hypotension Infection Paralytic ileus
Ketogenic diet	Relatively safe (no respiratory and cardiocirculatory instability) Slow onset of action Requires skilled dietitian	Gastroesophageal reflux Constipation Acidosis Hypertriglyceridemia
Lidocaine	Minor respiratory depression compared with other drugs	Cardiocirculatory instability Possible induction of seizures
Hypothermia	Only transitory control (cannot be a prolonged therapy)	Hypotension Cardiovascular instability Impaired coagulation (bleeding risks)
Resective surgery	Long-term treatment of seizures Not all patients are eligible	Surgical risks

NMDA, N-methyl-D-aspartate; *SE,* status epilepticus.
From Swaiman KF et al: *Swaiman's pediatric neurology, principles and practice,* ed 6, Philadelphia, 2017, Elsevier. See original table for references.

status epilepticus with time or with benzodiazepine treatment. If a patient does not start improving or has any subtle signs (subtle jerks, gaze deviation, or hippus) of ongoing seizures, consider nonconvulsive status epilepticus.

- Failure of response to lorazepam or midazolam is referred to as established status epilepticus and should be followed by second-line therapy of intravenous (IV) fosphenytoin 20 mg/kg (PE) at a rate not greater than 150 mg/min, phenytoin 20 mg/kg IV at up to 50 mg/min as tolerated, intravenous valproic acid 40 mg/kg IV (max: 300 mg/dose), or intravenous levetiracetam 60 mg/kg IV (max: 4500 mg/dose). Vital signs should be monitored during the infusion.[2,7]
- If seizures continue, an additional infusion of intravenous valproate; levetiracetam; lacosamide; or continuous infusions of pentobarbital, midazolam, and propofol are alternatives. Superiority of any one agent is not established.[2,6] Treatment alternatives for refractory and super-refractory status epilepticus are summarized in Table 4.

GENERAL Rx

It is important to find out the etiology of the status epilepticus (e.g., metabolic disturbance, infection). The appropriate treatment/understanding of the underlying cause of the status epilepticus will impact successful treatment.

CHRONIC Rx

- Chronic treatment of status epilepticus depends on underlying etiology.
- Patient with status epilepticus due to epilepsy will need chronic treatment.

DISPOSITION

- Response to treatment depends on the etiology of the status epilepticus.
- When there is no CNS injury as a cause or result of the status epilepticus, the prognosis is good.
- No driving until seizure freedom in accordance with local laws and regulations.

REFERRAL

Status epilepticus is a neurologic emergency; therefore immediate inpatient neurologic consultation is warranted.

ⓘ PEARLS & CONSIDERATIONS

COMMENTS

- Status epilepticus is a medical emergency that carries a high risk of mortality. Mortality among patients who present in status epilepticus approaches 20%. Among those who survive, functional ability will decline in 25% of cases.[5]

- Continuous video EEG is crucial in the treatment of these patients because some of them may not be clinically seizing (convulsing) but electrographically they may still have subclinical repetitive seizures or subclinical status epilepticus.[2]
- In the context of benzodiazepine-refractory convulsive status epilepticus, the anticonvulsant drugs levetiracetam, fosphenytoin, and valproate each led to seizure cessation and improved alertness by 60 min in approximately half the patients, and the three drugs were associated with similar incidences of adverse events.[8]

PREVENTION

Medication compliance is crucial in patients with epilepsy.

PATIENT & FAMILY EDUCATION

- Patients with epilepsy have normal lives.
- The goal of treatment is no seizures and no side effects to medications.
- Patient education and information can be obtained at the Epilepsy Foundation: www.epilepsyfoundation.org.
- Pregnant women with epilepsy should visit the Antiepileptic Drug Pregnancy Registry website for information and assistance: www.aedpregnancyregistry.org.
- Patients with ongoing seizures are forbidden from driving; check state regulations and laws regarding driving and epilepsy.

REFERENCES

Available at eBooks.Health.Elsevier.com.

RELATED CONTENT

Febrile Seizures (Related Key Topic)
Seizures, Generalized Tonic-Clonic (Related Key Topic)

AUTHOR: **PEDRO BALAGUERA, MD**

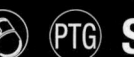
Diseases and Disorders

I

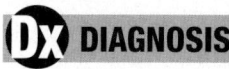 BASIC INFORMATION

DEFINITION
Ischemic stroke is the sudden onset of a focal neurologic deficit due to cerebral ischemia resulting in cell death.[1] The purpose of this chapter is to help the provider make decisions about the management of the acute stroke patient within the first several hours of symptoms—this is the crucial time for definitive treatment interventions.

SYNONYMS
Stroke
Cerebral infarction
Brain attack
Cerebrovascular accident

ICD-10CM CODES
I63	Cerebral infarction
I63.3	Cerebral infarction due to thrombosis of cerebral arteries
I63.4	Cerebral infarction due to embolism of cerebral arteries
I63.5	Cerebral infarction due to unspecified occlusion or stenosis of cerebral arteries
I63.6	Cerebral infarction due to cerebral venous thrombosis, nonpyogenic
I63.8	Other cerebral infarction
I63.9	Cerebral infarction, unspecified
I67.89	Other cerebrovascular disease

EPIDEMIOLOGY & DEMOGRAPHICS
INCIDENCE:
- ~795,000 new or recurrent strokes occur each year in the U.S.[2]
- Stroke is the fifth leading cause of death (~160,000 deaths/yr) and the leading cause of long-term disability in the U.S.[2]

PREVALENCE:
- There are ~9.4 million stroke survivors in the U.S., two thirds of whom are currently disabled.[2]
- Stroke prevalence in the U.S in adults is 2.8%.[2]

RISK FACTORS: Hypertension, dyslipidemia, diabetes mellitus, and smoking are the four major modifiable risk factors. Other risk factors include age, gender, atrial fibrillation (most common cause of cardioembolic stroke), mechanical heart valve, patent foramen ovale, recent myocardial infarction, metabolic syndrome, carotid artery stenosis, vertebral artery stenosis, intracranial artery stenosis, hypercoagulable states, subclinical atrial tachyarrhythmias without clinical atrial fibrillation, sickle cell disease, and obesity.[3] Inherited and miscellaneous disorders causing cerebral infarction are summarized in Box 1.

GENETICS: Multifactorial

PHYSICAL FINDINGS & CLINICAL PRESENTATION
When a patient presents with an acute ischemic stroke acutely, the most important considerations are determination of the time the patient

was last known normal, to rule out a hemorrhagic stroke, and the severity, because these aspects will determine acute treatment. The time last known normal was when the patient was last witnessed to be normal (by themselves or by someone else). If they awoke with the deficits, the time last seen normal was when they went to bed.[4]

Clinical presentation varies with the artery and region of the central nervous system (CNS) affected. Clinical presentation cannot reliably distinguish between hemorrhagic and ischemic causes, and so imaging must be done. Following is a noncomprehensive list of common stroke syndrome presentations based on the cerebral vascular territory affected. Please note that this list is not comprehensive and that all findings for a particular syndrome may not be listed here.[4]
- Large- to medium-sized arteries:
  1. Dominant middle cerebral artery (MCA) (left in 90% of people): Right face and arm > leg weakness and sensory loss with aphasia (expressive, receptive, or both); possible hemianopia.
  2. Nondominant MCA: Contralateral face and arm > leg weakness and sensory loss with hemineglect; possible hemianopia.
  3. Anterior cerebral artery (ACA): Contralateral leg weakness and sensory loss.
  4. Internal carotid artery: Combination of contralateral MCA and ACA.
  5. Basilar artery: Typically, acute loss of consciousness preceded by vertigo, nausea, vomiting, and diplopia; quadriparesis or quadriplegia may be seen, including "locked-in" syndrome.
  6. Posterior cerebral artery: Unilateral hemianopia; blindness with anosognosia if bilateral (Anton syndrome).
  7. Posterior inferior cerebellar artery: Lateral medullary (Wallenberg) syndrome—ipsilesional loss of pinprick and temperature on the face and contralateral loss of pinprick and temperature on the body; ipsilesional Horner syndrome and ipsilesional palatal weakness with resulting dysphagia, dysarthria. Also with vertigo, nystagmus, ataxia.

- Small arteries: Lacunar syndromes; no cortical signs are present in lacunar syndromes.[5]
  1. Pure motor hemiparesis: Typically, due to an ischemic lesion in either the internal capsule or pons.
  2. Pure hemisensory loss: Typically, due to an ischemic lesion of the thalamus.
  3. Ataxic hemiparesis: Ataxia out of proportion to the hemiparesis; typically due to an ischemic lesion of either the internal capsule or pons.
  4. Sensorimotor stroke: Typically, due to ischemic lesion involving both the thalamus and internal capsule.
  5. Dysarthria–clumsy hand syndrome: Multiple localizations possible but typically the pons; facial weakness, dysarthria, and mild clumsiness and weakness of the hand.

ETIOLOGY
Etiologies include large artery atherosclerosis, artery-to-artery embolism, cardioembolism, small-vessel lipohyalinosis, arterial dissection, and vasospasm.[6]

DX DIAGNOSIS

DIFFERENTIAL DIAGNOSIS
The differential diagnosis of acute ischemic stroke includes hemorrhagic stroke (intracerebral hemorrhage), subarachnoid or subdural hemorrhage, seizure with postictal paralysis, migraine with hemiparesis or other aura, syncope, hypoglycemia, hypertensive encephalopathy, and conversion disorder.[7]

LABORATORY TESTS
- Immediate (Box 2): Complete blood count, metabolic panel that includes blood glucose and renal function, prothrombin time/international normalized ratio (PT/INR), activated partial thromboplastin time (aPTT), troponin I, and urinalysis. Blood glucose is the only test required before initiation of intravenous (IV) thrombolysis (alteplase or tenecteplase). Although it is desirable to know the results of

---

BOX 1   Inherited and Miscellaneous Disorders Causing Cerebral Infarction

- Homocystinuria
- Fabry disease
- Marfan syndrome
- Ehlers-Danlos syndrome
- Pseudoxanthoma elasticum
- Sneddon syndrome
- Hereditary hemorrhagic telangiectasia
- Neoplastic angioendotheliomatosis
- Susac syndrome
- Eales disease
- Reversible cerebral segmental vasoconstriction syndrome
- Hypereosinophilic syndrome
- Cerebral amyloid angiopathy
- Coils and kinks
- Arterial dolichoectasia
- Complications of coarctation of the aorta
- Air, fat, amniotic fluid, bone marrow, and foreign particle embolism

From Jankovic J et al: *Bradley and Daroff's neurology in clinical practice*, ed 8, Philadelphia, 2022, Elsevier.

BOX 2   Immediate Diagnostic Studies: Evaluation of a Patient with Suspected Acute Ischemic Stroke

All Patients
- Noncontrast brain computed tomographic scan (magnetic resonance imaging, if immediately available, preferred at the institution, and only DWI/ADC sequence)
- Blood glucose level
- Serum electrolyte and renal function tests
- Electrocardiography
- Markers of cardiac ischemia
- Complete blood count, including platelet count
- Prothrombin time/international normalized ratio
- Activated partial thromboplastin time
- Oxygen saturation

Selected Patients
- CT angiogram head and neck or MR angiogram head and neck
- CT or MR perfusion
- Hepatic function tests
- Toxicology screen
- Blood alcohol level
- Pregnancy test
- Arterial blood gas tests (if hypoxia is suspected)
- Chest radiography (if lung disease is suspected)
- Lumbar puncture (if subarachnoid hemorrhage is suspected and computed tomography scan is negative for blood)
- Electroencephalogram (if seizures are suspected)

ADC, Apparent diffusion coefficient; *CT,* computed tomography; *DWI,* diffusion-weighted imaging; *MR,* magnetic resonance.
From Christensen H et al: Abnormalities on ECG and telemetry predict stroke outcome at 3 months, *J Neurol Sci* 234:99-103, 2005.

BOX 3   Specialized Laboratory Tests for Thrombophilia

- Antithrombin activity
- Protein C
- Protein S (total and free antigen levels)
- Activated protein C resistance
- Factor V Leiden
- Prothrombin gene (G20210 A) mutation
- Cardiolipin (IgG, IgM) antibodies
- β_2-Glycoprotein 1 (IgG, IgM) antibodies
- Lupus anticoagulant
- Fibrinogen
- Plasminogen
- Plasminogen activator inhibitor
- Plasmin functional activity
- Factors V, VII, VIII, IX, X, XI, and XIII levels
- Hemoglobin electrophoresis
- Plasma homocysteine

Ig, Immunoglobulin.
From Jankovic J et al: *Bradley and Daroff's neurology in clinical practice,* ed 8, Philadelphia, 2022, Elsevier.

CBC and PT/INR/aPTT before giving a patient thrombolytics, this should not be delayed while awaiting the results unless, there is clinical suspicion of a bleeding abnormality or thrombocytopenia, the patient has received heparin or warfarin, or the patient's use of anticoagulants is uncertain.[8]
- Specialized laboratory tests for thrombophilia are summarized in Box 3.
- National Institutes of Health Stroke Scale (NIHSS) (Table 1): A brief, focused neurologic examination aimed at providing a numeric estimate of the severity of stroke; can be performed by any health care provider trained in its use.[8]
- ECG and telemetry monitoring.
- Echocardiogram to look for potential cardiogenic source of embolism, infective endocarditis, and intracardiac shunts.[9]

IMAGING STUDIES
- Immediate (Fig. 1): Computed tomography (CT) of the head without contrast to rule out hemorrhage, required before initiation of IV thrombolytics.[10]
- CT angiogram of the head and neck is necessary acutely in selected patients if deficits are severe to assess whether there is a thrombus that is amenable to intervention as well as CT head perfusion to assess for the degree of salvageable tissue (Table 2).[10]
- MRI of the brain with stroke protocol to assess the extent of stroke (higher sensitivity and specificity compared to CT) but it is rarely needed in the hyperacute setting to determine appropriateness of reperfusion strategy.[10]

See "Transient Ischemic Attack" for general workup, which is identical to that for ischemic stroke.

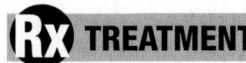 **TREATMENT**

NONPHARMACOLOGIC THERAPY
GENERAL CONSIDERATIONS:
- Airway, breathing, and circulation should be maintained.
- Supplemental oxygen should be provided to keep the oxygen saturation $\geq$92%.
- Pneumatic compression devices or pharmacologic means should be applied to help prevent deep venous thrombosis.
- Avoid oral intake until swallowing is evaluated and found to be unimpaired; this helps to avoid aspiration pneumonia.
- Early mobilization for rehabilitation is desirable.
- Consider neurosurgical intervention for craniectomy in select cases. Typical cases in which craniectomy may be performed include cerebellar ischemia with compression of the brain stem and/or the fourth ventricle as well as large middle cerebral artery ischemia. Available evidence suggests that it may be better to perform early hemicraniectomy (<48 h) to achieve better outcomes in malignant hemispheric strokes. Decompressive hemicraniectomy has shown good benefit in terms of mortality and morbidity.[11]

ACUTE GENERAL Rx (TABLE 3)
INTRAVENOUS THROMBOLYSIS:
- IV t-PA, or alteplase, is currently the only medical therapy approved by the U.S. FDA[12-15] for the treatment of acute ischemic stroke; however, tenecteplase, a recombinant DNA–derived version of alteplase, has been recently shown to be noninferior and is used as an alternative in some centers.[16] The most recent American Heart Association/American Stroke Association (AHA/ASA) guidelines include it as a reasonable option for thrombolysis in patients who are also eligible for endovascular thrombectomy.[12]
- The time window for administration of thrombolysis is generally accepted to be within 4.5 h of symptom onset, although the FDA indication is still within 3 h. The AHA/ASA guidelines recommend thrombolysis administration window of up to 4.5 h with certain additional exclusion criteria when compared to the 3-h administration.[12] Time goals for evaluation and treatment of patients with acute ischemic stroke are summarized in Table 4.[17]
- There are strict criteria for the administration of IV thrombolysis[12,18] (Tables 5 and 6).
- Alteplase protocol is weight based, at a dose of 0.9. mg/kg (90 mg maximum) with the initial 10% given as a bolus and the rest as a 1-h infusion.
- Tenecteplase is administered as a single bolus of 0.25 mg/kg (maximum 25 mg) with comparable risk of bleeding to alteplase.
- The risk of brain hemorrhage with IV t-PA is about 6% in stroke patients. The management

TABLE 1 National Institutes of Health Stroke Scale

1A. Level of Consciousness (LOC)	1B. LOC Questions	1C. LOC Commands
0 = Alert 1 = Not alert, but arousable 2 = Not alert, obtunded 3 = Coma	Ask the month and his/her age. 0 = Answers both correctly 1 = Answers one correctly 2 = Answers neither correctly	Open and close the eyes. Open and close the nonparetic hand. 0 = Performs both tasks correctly 1 = Performs one task correctly 2 = Performs neither task correctly

2. Best Gaze (Horizontal)	3. Visual Fields	4. Facial Palsy
0 = Normal 1 = Partial gaze palsy 2 = Forced deviation or total gaze paresis	0 = No visual loss 1 = Partial hemianopia 2 = Complete hemianopia 3 = Bilateral hemianopia	0 = Normal 1 = Minor paralysis 2 = Partial paralysis (total or near total paralysis of lower face) 3 = Complete paralysis of upper and lower face

5. Motor Arm	6. Motor Leg	7. Limb Ataxia
Arm extended with palms down 90 degrees (if sitting) or 45 degrees (if supine) for 10 sec 0 = No drift 1 = Drift; limb drifts down from position and does not hit bed or support in 10 sec 2 = Some effort against gravity 3 = No effort against gravity 4 = No movement	Leg extended at 30 degrees, always tested supine for 5 sec 0 = No drift 1 = Drift; limb drifts down from position and does not hit bed or support in 5 sec 2 = Some effort against gravity 3 = No effort against gravity 4 = No movement	The finger-nose-finger and heel-shin tests 0 = Absent 1 = Present in one limb 2 = Present in two limbs

8. Sensory	9. Best Language	10. Dysarthria
To Pinprick or Noxious Stimuli 0 = Normal 1 = Mild to moderate sensory loss 2 = Severe to total sensory loss	0 = No aphasia, normal 1 = Mild-to-moderate aphasia 2 = Severe aphasia 3 = Mute, global aphasia, coma	0 = Normal 1 = Mild-to-moderate 2 = Severe (including mute/anarthric due to aphasia) Do not score if intubated.

11. Extinction and Inattention		Total Score:
0 = No abnormality 1 = Present 2 = Profound (two modalities)		

From Vincent JL et al: *Textbook of critical care*, ed 8, Philadelphia, 2024, Elsevier.

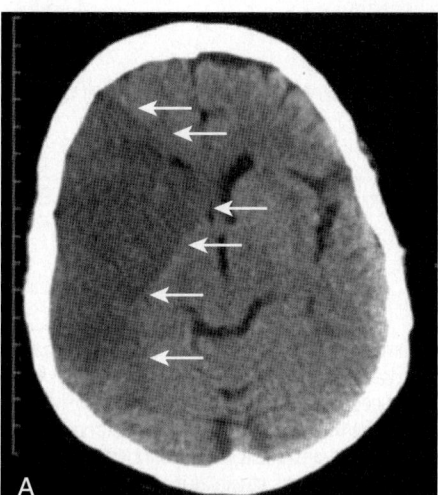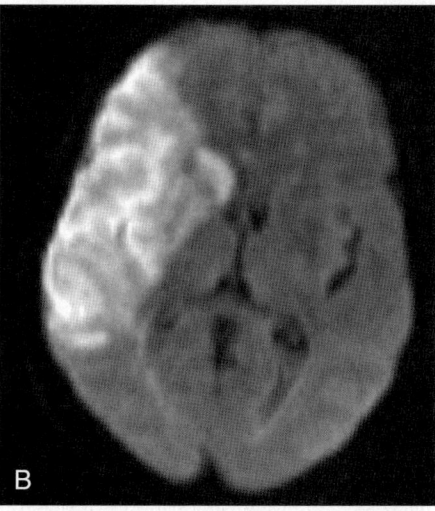

FIG. 1 Large right middle cerebral artery infarct on an unenhanced computed tomographic scan **(A)** and a diffusion-weighted magnetic resonance image **(B)**. There is a mass effect, and this patient is at risk for cerebral herniation syndromes.

of suspected intracranial hemorrhage after use of t-PA is summarized in Box 4.[19]

- Endovascular intervention is useful only for large, accessible thrombi. Therefore if a stroke patient is a candidate for IV thrombolysis, treatment with IV alteplase/tenecteplase should be started and then the patient should be assessed for possible endovascular therapy.[12] Table 7 summarizes AHA/ASA recommendations for endovascular therapy in patients with acute ischemic stroke.

IMMEDIATE CATHETER CEREBRAL ANGIOGRAPHY FOR ENDOVASCULAR INTERVENTION: Methods available (Figs. 2 and 3):

- The AHA/ASA 2018 guidelines with an update in 2019 recommend endovascular thrombectomy with a stent-retriever device for highly selected patients who present with large vessel occlusion (LVO) up to 16 h after last known normal and suggest that it is reasonable up to 24 h.[12,20,21]
  1. IV thrombolysis should be administered in this group if eligible.
  2. All patients should be assessed with CT angiogram head and neck or MRA head and neck for possible LVO if they have an NIHSS of ≥6 or suspicion of a large vessel stroke.
  3. In selected patients with acute ischemic stroke within 6 to 24 h of last known normal who have LVO on noninvasive angiogram, obtaining a CT perfusion, diffusion weighted–MRI, or perfusion is recommended to aid in patient selection for endovascular thrombectomy.[20,21]

- Adult patients should receive endovascular thrombectomy with a stent retriever if they present within 6 h of last known normal with a causative LVO (especially of the internal carotid artery or MCA segment 1 [M1] but reasonable in the setting of a causative MCA segment 2 or 3 [M2/3] or other large vessel cerebral artery) if they were relatively independent before the stroke and have an NIHSS score of ≥6 and an ASPECTS score of ≥6.[22-27]

- Patients should receive endovascular thrombectomy with a stent retriever if treatment can be initiated within 16 h (and up to 24 h) of last known normal with a large anterior circulation LVO and they meet the DAWN[21] or DEFUSE-3[20] criteria (a defined mismatch between clinical severity and/or infarct volume compared to the penumbra [tissue at risk]). The number needed to treat to improve functional outcomes is only 2.8, and so patients should be aggressively evaluated for possible treatment.

- Complications can ensue from the endovascular procedure itself, including an intracerebral hemorrhage rate that is similar to that associated with thrombolysis. A meta-analysis revealed that among patients with acute ischemic stroke, endovascular therapy with endovascular thrombectomy + medical therapy versus standard medical care with t-PA alone was associated with improved functional outcomes and higher rates of angiographic revascularization, but no significant difference in

TABLE 2 Imaging Modalities for Stroke

Imaging Modality	Advantages	Disadvantages
Cerebral catheter angiography	• Allows for the definitive assessment of cerebral circulation (gold standard) • Allows for the deployment of intraarterial thrombolysis and thrombectomy devices if a thrombus is found • Allows for the assessment of collateral circulation	• Invasive (significant risks) • High cost • Not available at all facilities
Doppler studies	• Noninvasive • May be performed at the patient's bedside	• Can be limited by the patient's body habitus • Operator dependent
Magnetic resonance angiography	• Excellent view of the large arteries of the neck and brain • No contrast material needed	• Cannot be performed in patients who are critically ill, who are unable to tolerate supine positioning, who have a pacemaker or other ferromagnetic hardware, or who are claustrophobic
Magnetic resonance perfusion	• Assesses cerebral hemodynamics • May show ischemic penumbra (i.e., the area of the brain that may be saved by timely intervention)	• Not commonly available • Not well standardized
CT angiography	• Excellent view of the large arteries of the neck and brain • Similar to magnetic resonance angiography with regard to resolution	• Requires intravenous contrast
CT perfusion	• Assesses cerebral hemodynamics • May show ischemic penumbra (i.e., the area of the brain that may be saved by timely intervention)	• Challenging to interpret in some cases • Not routinely available at many facilities • Requires intravenous contrast

CT, Computed tomography.

TABLE 3 Treatment Options for Acute Ischemic Stroke

Time Window	Treatment Options
0-3 h	IV thrombolysis with alteplase Mechanical thrombectomy (terminal ICA or M1 occlusion)
3-4.5 h	IV thrombolysis with alteplase (relative contraindications) Mechanical thrombectomy (terminal ICA or M1 occlusion)
4.5-6 h	Mechanical thrombectomy (terminal ICA or M1 occlusion)

6-24 h	• Mechanical thrombectomy (large vessel occlusion + favorable perfusion imaging) 6-16 h (DEFUSE 3 Criteria):
	  1. Occlusion of terminal ICA or MCA - M1
	  2. Clinical imaging mismatch
	• Infarct core volume <70 ml
	• Mismatch volume >15 ml
	• Mismatch ratio (penumbra/core) >1.8
	• 16-24 h (DAWN Criteria):
	  1. Occlusion of terminal ICA or MCA - M1
	  2. Clinical imaging mismatch:
	• ≥80 yr, NIHSS ≥10 + core <21 ml
	• <80 yr, NIHSS ≥10 + core <31 ml
	• <80 yr, NIHSS ≥20 + core <51 ml

Wake-up stroke	• Age 18-80 yr old • Stroke symptoms at awakening or could not report symptom onset • MRI brain including DWI, FLAIR, a sequence sensitive to hemorrhage, and time-of-flight magnetic resonance angiography of circle of Willis • Patients are eligible for thrombolysis if: 1. Abnormal signal in DWI + no signal change in FLAIR

DWI, Diffusion-weighted imaging; *FLAIR,* fluid-attenuated inversion recovery; *ICA,* internal carotid artery; *MCA,* middle cerebral artery; *MRI,* magnetic resonance imaging; *NIHSS,* National Institutes of Health stroke scale.
From Warshaw G et al: *Ham's primary care geriatrics,* ed 7, Philadelphia, 2022, Elsevier.

symptomatic intracranial hemorrhage or all-cause mortality at 90 days.[28]
- More recently, at least six randomized controlled trials are examining the benefit of extending endovascular thrombectomy to patients with a large infarct core volume and ASPECTS ≥6. These trials have yielded mixed results, with improvement in functional outcome, but with an increased risk of vascular complications.[29] A comprehensive review of these randomized controlled trials is beyond the scope of this chapter.
- Endovascular intervention is typically available only at comprehensive stroke centers.

HYPERTENSION: Elevated blood pressure is common during acute stroke, and it often subsides without specific therapy. In general, hypertension is not treated acutely unless it is extremely high (e.g., >220 mm Hg systolic blood pressure), there is evidence of hypertension-induced organ damage, or thrombolysis is being considered, in which case the blood pressure needs to be reduced (if it can be safely accomplished) to <185/110 mm Hg. It is risky to decrease blood pressure dramatically and quickly in the presence of acute ischemic stroke as it can cause an extension of the infarction into the ischemic penumbra. A gradual 15% to 25% decrease over the first 24 h is recommended when more acute lowering is not required. Blood pressure goals and treatment

TABLE 4 Time Goals for Evaluation and Treatment of Patients with Acute Ischemic Stroke

Time after Emergency Department Arrival	Goals
10 min	Assess ABCs, vital signs
	Provide oxygen if hypoxemic
	Obtain intravenous access
	Obtain laboratory studies
	CBC, coagulation, electrolytes
	Check glucose level, treat if indicated
	Perform screening neurologic assessment
	Activate stroke team
	Order "stroke code" brain CT or MRI
	Obtain 12-lead ECG
25 min	Review history
	Establish time at onset or last known normal
	Perform neurologic examination
	NIH Stroke Scale
45 min	Review laboratory studies
	Review brain CT or MRI results
	Evaluate inclusion and exclusion criteria (see Table 4)
60 min	Review risks and benefits
	Obtain consent
	Begin infusion

ABCs, Airway, breathing, circulation; *CBC*, complete blood count; *CT*, computed tomography; *ECG*, electrocardiogram; *MRI*, magnetic resonance imaging; *NIH*, National Institutes of Health.
From Goldman L, Schafer AI: *Goldman-Cecil medicine*, ed 26, Philadelphia, 2019, Elsevier.

TABLE 5 Eligibility Criteria for Thrombolysis in Acute Ischemic Stroke

Eligibility Criteria
- Diagnosis of ischemic stroke causing measurable and "disabling" neurologic deficit
- The neurologic signs should not be minor and isolated. Caution should be exercised in treating a patient with major deficits
- Onset of symptoms <4.5 h before beginning treatment
- The neurologic signs should not be clearing spontaneously
- The symptoms of stroke should not be suggestive of subarachnoid hemorrhage
- The patient or family members should understand the potential risks and benefits from treatment

Contraindications for Thrombolysis
- Evidence of intracranial hemorrhage on CT
- Head trauma or prior stroke in previous 3 mo
- Myocardial infarction in the previous 3 mo
- Gastrointestinal or urinary tract hemorrhage in previous 21 days
- Arterial puncture at a noncompressible site in the previous 7 days
- Major surgery in the previous 14 days
- History of previous intracranial hemorrhage
- Elevated blood pressure (systolic >185 mm Hg and diastolic >110 mm Hg)
- Evidence of active bleeding or acute trauma (fracture) on examination
- Taking an oral anticoagulant or, if taking anticoagulant, INR ≥1.7 is a contraindication
- If receiving heparin in previous 48 h, aPTT must be in normal range
- Platelet count ≤100,000 mm^3
- Blood glucose concentration ≥50 mg/dl (2.7 mmol/L)
- Seizure with postictal residual neurologic impairments
- CT shows a multilobar infarction (hypodensity >⅓ cerebral hemisphere)

aPTT, Activated partial thromboplastin time; *CT*, computed tomography; *INR*, international normalized ratio.
From Hoffman R et al: *Hematology, basic principles and practice*, ed 8, Philadelphia, 2023, Elsevier.

options in acute ischemic stroke are summarized in Box 5.[30]

HYPOTENSION: The presence of systemic hypotension in acute ischemic stroke portends a poor outcome. The cause should be sought, and volume depletion should be corrected with normal saline. Cardiac arrhythmias should be treated. Induced hypertension with vasopressor agents may be useful for select cases with an ischemic penumbra that is at risk, but caution is strongly advised.[12]

HYPOGLYCEMIA: Hypoglycemia can mimic stroke. Prompt assessment of serum glucose level and replacement as necessary are important.[12]

HYPERGLYCEMIA: Hyperglycemia should be treated with sliding scale insulin, taking into consideration the patient's oral intake. The presence of hyperglycemia worsens ischemic stroke outcomes, but recent evidence has not shown that aggressive treatment with an insulin pump improves outcomes and in-hospital goals of <180 mg/dl are considered adequate.[31]

FEVER: Fever is harmful during acute stroke. Ascertaining and addressing the cause while lowering an elevated temperature is strongly advised.

ELEVATED INTERCRANIAL PRESSURE: Traditional treatment of increased intracranial pressure associated with acute ischemic stroke is shown in Box 6.

ANTIPLATELET THERAPY: Oral, rectal, or feeding tube administration of aspirin (81 to 325 mg/day) within 48 h of stroke onset is advised to decrease the likelihood of a repeat ischemic stroke. Other oral antiplatelet regimens including dual antiplatelet therapy may be indicated.[32] Please see further discussion in Stroke, Secondary Prevention. Patients who have received thrombolysis should not be given antithrombotic or anticoagu[n]tion agents within the first 24 h after administration.

ANTICOAGLUATION THERAPY: In patients with acute ischemic stroke presumed secondary to embolism and atrial fibrillation, full-dose anticoagulation with heparin infusion or low-molecular-weight heparin is seldom indicated in the acute setting due to the relatively high risk of hemorrhagic conversion and little evidence to suggest any benefit except in very select circumstances. However, chronic anticoagulation is indicated and is usually started 2 to 14 days after the acute ischemic stroke, depending on the size.[33] In some circumstances, such as a cardiac thrombus or mechanical valves, anticoagulation may need to be started more quickly.

DISPOSITION

Patients with acute ischemic stroke should be cared for in a stroke unit or an intensive care unit. Nurses with skills in stroke care and telemetry monitoring should be routine. Once the patient is stable and the workup is complete, rehabilitation should be arranged.[5,34]

REFERRAL

Patients with acute ischemic stroke should be transported to a hospital in which providers are skilled in stroke care. Depending on the severity and duration of symptoms, the patient may qualify for immediate endovascular intervention at a comprehensive stroke center, even if he or she is not a candidate for thrombolysis. If complications from brain edema develop, further evaluation by a neurosurgeon may be helpful during the acute phase.[12]

❗ PEARLS & CONSIDERATIONS

PREVENTION
- The prevention of acute ischemic stroke depends on the aggressive management of risk factors in individual patients.
- Paroxysmal atrial fibrillation is common in patients with cryptogenic stroke. Ambulatory

TABLE 6 Administration of rtPA for Acute Ischemic Stroke

Infuse 0.9 mg/kg (maximum dose 90 mg) over 60 min, with 10% of the dose given as a bolus over 1 min.

Admit the patient to an intensive care or stroke unit for monitoring.

If the patient develops severe headache, acute hypertension, nausea, or vomiting or has a worsening neurologic examination, discontinue the infusion (if IV rtPA is being administered) and obtain emergent CT scan.

Measure blood pressure and perform neurologic assessments every 15 min during and after IV rtPA infusion for 2 h, then every 30 min for 6 h, then hourly until 24 h after IV rtPA treatment.

Increase the frequency of blood pressure measurements if systolic blood pressure is >180 mm Hg or if diastolic blood pressure is >105 mm Hg; administer antihypertensive medications to maintain blood pressure at or below these levels.

Delay placement of nasogastric tubes, indwelling bladder catheters, or intraarterial pressure catheters if the patient can be safely managed without them.

Obtain a follow-up CT or MRI scan at 24 h after IV rtPA before starting anticoagulants or antiplatelet agents.

CT, Computed tomography; *IV,* intravenous; *MRI,* magnetic resonance imaging; *rtPA,* recombinant tissue plasminogen activator.
From Powers WJ et al: Guidelines for the early management of patients with acute ischemic stroke: 2019 update to the 2018 guidelines for the early management of acute ischemic stroke: a guideline for healthcare professionals from the American Heart Association/American Stroke Association, *Stroke* 50:e344-e418, 2019.

BOX 4 Management of Suspected Intracerebral Hemorrhage after Use of Tissue Plasminogen Activator

- Discontinue the t-PA infusion if it remains in progress.
- Obtain noncontrast CT scan of the head stat.
- Order PT, PTT, platelet count, fibrinogen level, type and cross-match stat.
- In event of hemorrhage, consult hematology and neurosurgery.
- Give 6 to 8 units of cryoprecipitate, then 6 to 8 units of platelets.
- Administer aminocaproic acid 4 to 5 g IV over 1 h, followed by 1 g PO or IV per h.
- Check fibrinogen every 4 h and give cryoprecipitate to keep fibrinogen >150 mg/dl.
- Monitor blood pressure every 15 min.
- Periodically repeat CBC, PT, PTT.
- Consider repeat head CT.

CBC, Complete blood count; *CT,* computed tomography; *IV,* intravenous; *PO,* by mouth (per os); *PT,* prothrombin time; *PTT,* partial thromboplastin time; *t-PA,* tissue plasminogen activators.
From Parrillo JE, Dellinger RP: *Critical care medicine: principles of diagnosis and management in the adult,* ed 5, Philadelphia, 2019, Elsevier.

TABLE 7 AHA Recommendations for Endovascular Therapy in Patients with Acute Ischemic Stroke

Patients should receive endovascular therapy with a stent retriever if they meet all of the following criteria (class I; level of evidence, A):

- Prestroke modified Rankin score 0 to 1 (functionally independent)
- Acute ischemic stroke receiving intravenous recombinant tissue plasminogen activator within 4.5 h of onset according to guidelines from professional medical societies
- Causative occlusion of the internal carotid artery or proximal middle cerebral artery
- Age 18 yr or older
- National Institutes of Health Stroke Scale (NIHSS) score of 6 or greater
- Alberta Stroke Program Early CT Score (ASPECTS) of 6 or greater
- Treatment can be initiated (groin puncture) within 6 h of symptom onset

CT, Computed tomography.
From Zipes DP et al: *Braunwald's heart disease, a textbook of cardiovascular medicine,* ed 11, Philadelphia, 2019, Elsevier.

ECG monitoring with a loop recorder or other device for 30 days or more significantly improved the detection of atrial fibrillation by a factor of >5 and nearly doubled the rate of anticoagulant treatment compared to the standard practice of short-duration ECG monitoring.[35]

PATIENT & FAMILY EDUCATION

Patients and families need to be taught about ways to reduce the risk for recurrent stroke, including lifestyle modifications. Education about rehabilitation goals, when appropriate, should also be accomplished.

REFERENCES

Available at eBooks.Health.Elsevier.com.

RELATED CONTENT

Stroke (Patient Information)
Stroke, Secondary Prevention (Related Key Topic)
Transient Ischemic Attack (Related Key Topic)
Atrial Fibrillation (Related Key Topic)

AUTHORS: **CÉSAR E. ESCAMILLA-OCAÑAS, MD** and **COREY ELAM GOLDSMITH, MD, FAAN**

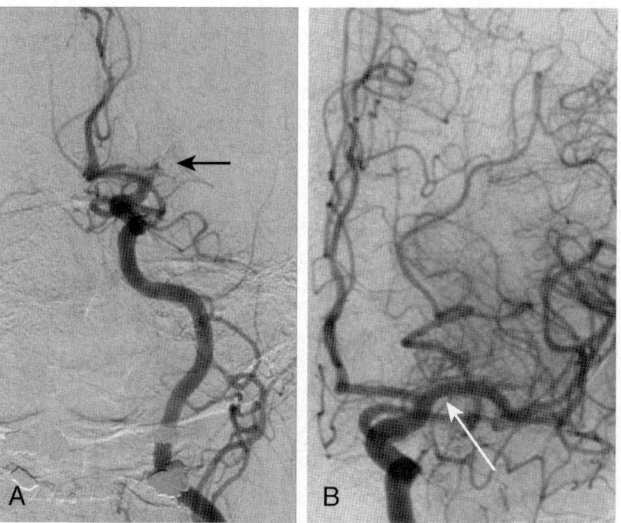

FIG. 2 A, A catheter angiogram showing left middle cerebral artery occlusion, which caused severe stroke symptoms for several hours. **B,** The artery was opened with the Merci clot retrieval system, and this resulted in normal flow.

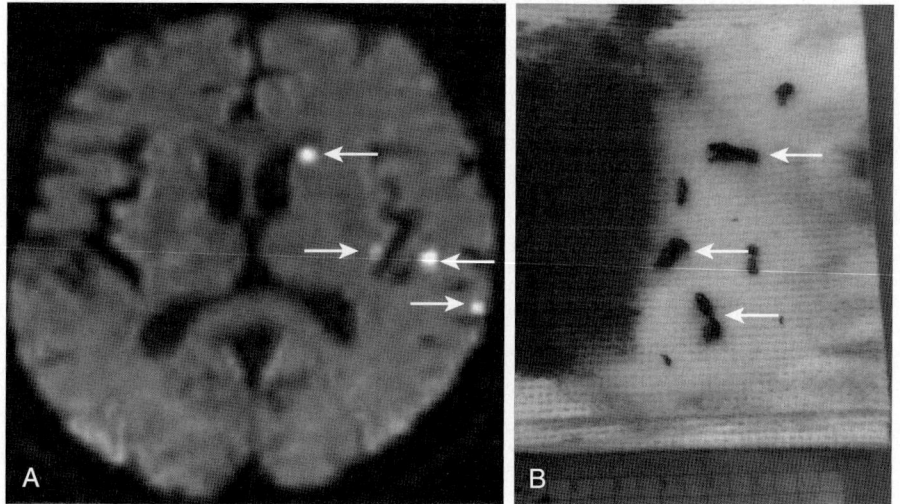

FIG. 3 A, A diffusion-weighted magnetic resonance image of the same patient as shown in previous figure, this time showing only mild left cerebral ischemia after intervention. The patient was clinically normal. **B,** Thrombi removed from the middle cerebral artery using the Merci clot retrieval system.

BOX 5 Blood Pressure Goals in Acute Ischemic Stroke

- If not a candidate for thrombolysis: <220/120 mm Hg
- If candidate for thrombolysis: <185/110 mm Hg
- After thrombolysis: <180/105 mm Hg
- After revascularization: <140/80 mm Hg

From Warshaw G et al: *Ham's primary care geriatrics,* ed 7, Philadelphia, 2022, Elsevier.

BOX 6 Medical Management Guidelines for Elevated Intracranial Pressure in Patients with Acute Ischemic Stroke

Correction of Factors Exacerbating Increased Intracranial Pressure
- Hypercarbia
- Hypoxia
- Hyperthermia
- Acidosis
- Hypotension
- Hypovolemia

Positional
- Avoidance of head and neck positions compressing jugular veins
- Avoidance of flat supine position; elevation of head of bed 15 degrees

Medical Therapy
- Endotracheal intubation and mechanical ventilation if Glasgow Coma Scale score ≤8
- Hyperventilation to a $PaCO_2$ of 35 ± 3 mm Hg (if herniating)
- Hyperosmolar therapy with mannitol or hypertonic saline

Fluid Management
- Maintenance of euvolemia with isotonic solutions using normal saline; avoidance of glucose-containing solutions because hyperglycemia is associated with worse prognosis for stroke; replacement of urinary losses with normal saline in patients receiving mannitol

From Jankovic J et al: *Bradley and Daroff's neurology in clinical practice,* ed 8, Philadelphia, 2022, Elsevier.

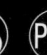
BASIC INFORMATION

DEFINITION

Hemorrhagic stroke is the sudden onset of a focal neurologic deficit caused by hemorrhage into (intracerebral hemorrhage) or around (subarachnoid hemorrhage) the brain. Etiologically, hemorrhage in the brain can be traumatic or nontraumatic.

Subarachnoid hemorrhage commonly occurs as a result of a ruptured aneurysm. Please see "Subarachnoid Hemorrhage" for additional information. This section will discuss nontraumatic intracerebral hemorrhage only.

Intracerebral hemorrhage (ICH) can have associated intraventricular extension/hemorrhage (IVH).

SYNONYMS

Intracerebral hemorrhage
Intracranial hemorrhage
Cerebrovascular attack (this is a nonspecific term and should not be used)

ICD-10CM CODES
I61	Intracerebral hemorrhage
I61.0	Intracerebral hemorrhage in hemisphere, subcortical
I61.1	Intracerebral hemorrhage in hemisphere, cortical
I61.2	Intracerebral hemorrhage in hemisphere, unspecified
I61.3	Intracerebral hemorrhage in brainstem
I61.4	Intracerebral hemorrhage in cerebellum
I61.5	Intracerebral hemorrhage, intraventricular
I61.6	Intracerebral hemorrhage, multiple localized
I61.9	Nontraumatic intracerebral hemorrhage, unspecified

EPIDEMIOLOGY & DEMOGRAPHICS

INCIDENCE: There are approximately 795,000 new or recurrent strokes per yr in the U.S., of which approximately 10% are hemorrhagic.[1,2] Risk increases sharply with age. Intracerebral hemorrhage has a mortality rate of 30% to 40%.[3]

RISK FACTORS:
- Increased age
- Hypertension
- Cerebral amyloid angiopathy
- Anticoagulant use
- Antithrombotic medication
- Sympathomimetic drugs (e.g., cocaine, heroin, amphetamine, ephedrine)
- Alcoholism
- African American race
- Low cholesterol, low-density lipoprotein, and triglycerides
- Minuscule increase in absolute risk from antiplatelet therapy

GENETICS: Multifactorial

PHYSICAL FINDINGS & CLINICAL PRESENTATION

Patients with intracerebral hemorrhage present with focal neurologic signs that are abrupt in onset. The evolution is typically over minutes and may be associated with headache, nausea, or vomiting and, in many cases, a depressed level of consciousness.[3,4] The presentation varies with the region of the brain that is affected. Table 1 summarizes clinical features of anatomic forms of intracerebral hemorrhage. There is no exact clinical way to distinguish between a primary cerebral hemorrhage and an ischemic stroke; therefore imaging is required. Imaging can also help determine if the diagnosis is ischemic stroke with hemorrhagic conversion versus primary hemorrhage.[3-5]

The following are common locations for hypertensive hemorrhage:
- Basal ganglia
- Cerebellum
- Pons
  Lobar hemorrhage in an older adult is likely due to amyloid angiopathy.

A systematic, detailed examination is necessary when approaching a comatose patient (Box 1). The ICH score is a widely used grading scale to estimate mortality based on computed tomography (CT) scan results. Parameters used to calculate the ICH score include Glasgow Coma Scale (GCS) (0 to 2 points) at presentation, patient age ≥80 (1 point), ICH volume ≥30 ml (1 point), presence of intraventricular blood (1 point), and infratentorial origin of blood (1 point). Scores range from 0 to 6, with a score of 0 conferring 0% mortality and a score of 6 with estimated 100% mortality.[5] This score, however, should not be used as the sole prognostic indicator or decision maker for discontinuing aggressive care. Accuracy of prognosis, especially early after ICH onset, is difficult, and aggressive treatment is recommended for at least the first 48 h before discussing prognosis.[3]

ETIOLOGY
- Arteriolosclerosis
- Amyloid angiopathy
- Aneurysm
- Arteriovenous malformation
- Brain tumor
  Nonhypertensive causes of intracerebral hemorrhage are summarized in Box 2.

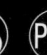 DIAGNOSIS

DIFFERENTIAL DIAGNOSIS
- Ischemic stroke, possibly with hemorrhagic conversion
- Seizure with postictal paralysis
- Syncope
- Migraine with hemiparesis
- Conversion disorder

LABORATORY TESTS
- CBC, metabolic panel including blood glucose, renal and liver function, prothrombin time/international normalized ratio, activated partial thromboplastin time, urinalysis, cardiac troponin, and toxicology screens[3]
- ECG and telemetry monitoring

IMAGING STUDIES
- Immediate: CT scan of the head without contrast is highly sensitive for hemorrhage (Fig. E1).
- Intraventricular extension of ICH occurs in 30% to 50% of patients with ICH and predisposes to the development of hydrocephalus in approximately half of patients. IVH predicts a worse prognosis.
- CT or magnetic resonance angiogram to rule out an underlying vascular malformation. CT spot sign on the CT angiography has been shown to be a reliable early predictor of hematoma expansion.[6]
- MRI of the brain with a gradient echo sequence is also highly sensitive for hemorrhage, including intracerebral microhemorrhages that may not be visible with computed tomography scanning. While CT and MRI are equivalent for detecting acute ICH, MRI is more accurate to detect chronic ICH.[3] MRI may also help to identify underlying brain tumors or vascular malformations, especially if the bleeding occurs at atypical sites. In the acute setting the MRI may show only the hematoma, but repeat MRI approximately 6 wk after initial hemorrhage may help exclude these other etiologies.

℞ TREATMENT

NONPHARMACOLOGIC THERAPY
- Urgent neurosurgical evaluation is needed in many cases either for evacuation of the hematoma or for relieving raised intracranial pressure by procedures such as external ventricular drain (EVD) placement or decompressive surgeries.
- Surgery should be performed promptly for cases of cerebellar hemorrhage of >3 cm when the patient is deteriorating clinically, showing brain stem edema or hydrocephalus.[4]
- Surgery for evacuation of lobar or deep brain clots may be considered for select cases, although the level of evidence for efficacy is not high. Surgery is often considered in lobar hemorrhages close to the surface and/or when the patient is neurologically deteriorating.[3]
- Minimally invasive surgery for hematoma evacuation in ICH >20 to 30 ml can be effective in improving mortality.[3]
- In patients with ICH <30 ml and IVH, the addition of thrombolytic irrigation with alteplase or urokinase with the EVD placement hastens intraventricular clot removal and results in further mortality reduction.[3]

ACUTE GENERAL Rx

The cornerstones of medical management of acute intracerebral hemorrhage (Table 2) include:
- Control of hypertension
- Correction of coagulopathy
- Management of elevated intracranial pressure
- Treatment of seizures

HYPERTENSION: Blood pressure should be quickly lowered in most patients to ensure continuous and sustained control of blood pressure in the systolic blood pressure range of

TABLE 1 Clinical Features of Anatomic Forms of Intracerebral Hemorrhage

Type of Intracerebral Hemorrhage	Hemiplegia	Hemisensory Syndrome	Aphasia	Homonymous Visual Defects	GAZE PALSY		Brainstem Signs
					Horizontal	Vertical	
Putaminal	Generally dense	Frequent	Global > motor > conduction	In large hematomas	Contralateral	No	No (only present with herniation)
Caudate	Absent or mild, transient	Absent	Transcortical motor (in dominant hemisphere hematomas)	No	Generally absent	No	No
Thalamic	Generally dense	Frequent, prominent	Occasional, thalamic variety	In large hematomas	Contralateral, occasionally ipsilateral	Yes, upward	Skew deviation, Horner syndrome, Parinaud syndrome
Lobar	Prominent in frontoparietal location	Prominent in frontoparietal location	In dominant temporoparietal location	In occipital hematomas	Contralateral in frontal hematomas	No	No (only present with herniation)
Cerebellar	Absent	Absent	No	No	Ipsilateral	No	Ipsilateral fifth through seventh nerve palsy, Horner syndrome
Pontine	Variable, usually bilateral	Variable, usually bilateral	No	No	Bilateral	No	Pinpoint reactive pupils, ocular "bobbing," decerebrate rigidity, respiratory rhythm abnormalities
Mesencephalic	Variable, usually present	Rare	No	No	No	Occasional, upward	Unilateral or bilateral third nerve palsy
Medullary	Generally absent	Occasional	No	No	No	No	Nystagmus, ataxia, hiccups, facial hypesthesia, dysarthria, dysphagia, 12th nerve palsy, Horner syndrome
Intraventricular	Generally absent	Rare	No	No	Occasional	Occasional	Rare (decerebrate rigidity)

From Jankovic J et al: *Bradley and Daroff's neurology in clinical practice*, ed 8, Philadelphia, 2022, Elsevier.

BOX 1 Neurologic Profile: A Modified Glasgow Coma Scale

Verbal Response
- Oriented speech
- Confused conversation
- Inappropriate speech
- Incomprehensible speech
- No speech

Eye Opening
- Spontaneous
- Response to verbal stimuli
- Response to noxious stimuli
- None

Motor Response
- Obeys
- Localizes
- Withdraws (flexion)
- Abnormal flexion
- None

Pupillary Reaction
- Present
- Absent

Spontaneous Eye Movement
- Orienting
- Roving conjugate
- Roving disconjugate
- Miscellaneous abnormal movements
- None

Oculocephalic Response
- Normal (unpredictable)
- Full
- Minimal
- None

Oculovestibular Response
- Normal (nystagmus)
- Tonic conjugate
- Minimal or disconjugate
- None

Deep Tendon Reflexes
- Normal
- Increased
- Absent

From Parrillo JE, Dellinger RP: *Critical care medicine: principles of diagnosis and management in the adult*, ed 4, Philadelphia, 2014, Elsevier.

BOX 2 Nonhypertensive Causes of Intracerebral Hemorrhage

- Vascular malformations (saccular or mycotic aneurysms, arteriovenous malformations, cavernous angiomas)
- Intracranial tumors
- Bleeding disorders, anticoagulant and fibrinolytic treatment
- Cerebral amyloid angiopathy
- Granulomatous angiitis of the central nervous system and other vasculitides, such as polyarteritis nodosa
- Sympathomimetic agents (including amphetamine and cocaine)
- Hemorrhagic infarction
- Head trauma
- Miscellaneous: Other vasculopathies (e.g., moyamoya disease, reversible cerebral vasoconstriction syndrome, cerebral autosomal dominant arteriopathy with subcortical infarcts and leukoencephalopathy [rarely]), and septic emboli/arteritis in the setting of infective endocarditis (all discussed elsewhere)

From Jankovic J et al: *Bradley and Daroff's neurology in clinical practice*, ed 8, Philadelphia, 2022, Elsevier.

---

150 to 130 mm Hg and avoiding hypotension or significant blood pressure variability. More aggressive control of systolic blood pressure (SBP) to 140 or less in the acute setting has been shown to be safe in clinical trials (Intensive Blood Pressure Reduction in Acute Cerebral Hemorrhage Trial 2 [INTERACT2]) with nonsignificant improvement in outcomes compared to less aggressive BP control (target SBP <180 mm Hg).[7] Antihypertensive Treatment of Acute Cerebral Hemorrhage II (ATACH 2) studied aggressive blood pressure lowering in patients randomized within 4.5 h of symptom onset. Patients were randomized to aggressive blood pressure lowering to a target SBP of 110 to 139 mm Hg compared to standard blood pressure lowering to target SBP of 179 to 140 mm Hg. The trial was stopped early because there was no difference in neurologic outcome or death, but patients in the aggressive blood pressure lowering arm suffered more kidney injury.[8] More recent analysis has failed to demonstrate functional outcome improvement but found it to be safe.[9]

The most recent guidelines state that for ICH patients presenting with SBP between 150 and 220 mm Hg and without contraindication to acute BP treatment, acute lowering of SBP to a target range of 150 to 130 mm Hg is safe and can be effective for improving functional outcome. For ICH patients presenting with SBP >220 mm Hg, it may be reasonable to consider aggressive reduction of BP with a continuous intravenous infusion and frequent BP monitoring but not to 150 mm Hg.[3]

CORRECTION OF COAGULOPATHY:
- Anticoagulation-associated ICH accounts for about 20% of all cases. Early hematoma expansion has been associated with poor outcome. Rapid reversal of coagulopathy should be performed as soon as possible after diagnosis of ICH to improve outcome.[3]
- Protamine sulfate is used to treat cases of heparin-induced intracerebral hemorrhage. Protamine dosage is 1 mg intravenous (IV) for every 100 units of heparin administered in the previous 2 to 3 h (maximum dose is 50 mg).

- Prothrombin concentrate complex (PCC) is recommended for reversal of warfarin-associated ICH in INR >2 and may be reasonable in INR 1.9 to 1.3 at a lower dose. FFP may be used instead if PCC not available but showed slower reversal of coagulopathy and was associated with more hematoma expansion compared to PCC. Vitamin K should be administered IV along with PCC for sustained effects. Routine use of recombinant factor VII concentrates is not recommended due to insufficient evidence and concern for increased risk of thromboembolic events.[3,10]
- Idarucizumab (Praxbind) is a humanized monoclonal antibody fragment that can be used for urgent reversal of the anticoagulant effect of the direct thrombin inhibitor dabigatran (Pradaxa). PCC infusion is also recommended if idarucizumab is not available.[3,10]
- Andexanet alfa, a recombinant modified human factor X2 decoy protein, has been effective for reversion of the anticoagulant effect of apixaban (Eliquis), rivaroxaban (Xarelto), and edoxaban (Savaysa), though it requires continuous infusion. PCC infusion is also recommended if andexanet alfa is not available.[3,10]
- Recommendations for thrombolytic-associated intracerebral hemorrhage treatment include the consideration of the infusion of platelets and cryoprecipitate.
- Platelet transfusion for patients experiencing ICH while on aspirin appears to result in worse outcomes than no platelet transfusion according to the Platelet Transfusion in Cerebral Hemorrhage (PATCH) trial is not recommended unless the patient requires emergency neurosurgery.[3,11]

ELEVATED INTRACRANIAL PRESSURE: This condition should be treated with a graded approach, which may include the elevation of the head of the bed, analgesia/sedation, hyperventilation, and osmotic therapy. In patients clinically suspected to have elevated ICP or with GCS <8, invasive monitoring of the ICP may be required. If conservative treatment fails to control ICP, EVD placement or other decompressive procedures like craniotomy should be pursued.[3]

SEIZURES: If seizures occur, they should be treated aggressively, including with intravenous medications, if needed. Although widely practiced, routine use of prophylactic antiepileptic medications is not recommended and, if used, should be stopped after 7 days if no evidence of seizures. Continuous EEG monitoring should be employed in patients with suspected seizures or unexplained low levels of consciousness.[3]

SUPPORTIVE TREATMENT:[3]
- Hyperglycemia: A high blood glucose level predicts a worse outcome. Markedly elevated glucose levels should be lowered to <180 mg/dl.
- Antipyretics should be administered for fever in addition to searching for a cause of the fever.

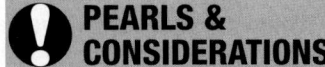
TABLE 2 Medical Management Protocol for Acute Intracranial Hemorrhage

Blood pressure	• Maintain mean arterial pressure <140 mm Hg with continuous infusion labetalol (2-10 mg/min), nicardipine (5-15 mg/h), or clevidipine (2-6 mg/h) • If stuporous or comatose, measure ICP and maintain CPP >70 mm Hg.

Reversal of anticoagulation	• For elevated INR: Vitamin K 10 mg IV push and 4F-PCC
	  1. INR 1.3-1.9: consider 10-20 units/kg
	  2. INR 2 to <4: 25 units/kg; not to exceed 2500 units
	  3. INR 4-6: 35 units/kg; not to exceed 3500 units
	  4. INR >6: 50 units/kg; not to exceed 5000 units
	• For heparin: Protamine sulfate 10 to 50 mg slow IV push (1 mg reverses approximately 100 units of heparin)
	• For dabigatran: Idarucizumab 5g IV (Praxbind)
	• For the factor Xa inhibitors (rivaroxaban, apixaban, and edoxaban): Andexanet-alpha IV. Low dose (≤10 mg rivaroxaban or ≤5 mg apixaban per dose): 400 mg IV bolus, followed by 4 mg/kg for 2 h. High dose (higher doses given within 8 h): 800 mg bolus, followed by 8 mg/kg for 2 h.
	• For thrombocytopenia or platelet dysfunction: Desmopressin 0.3 μg/kg intravenous push. Platelet transfusion is reasonable in the setting of thrombocytopenia but is not effective and may be harmful when given to patients on NSAIDs or other antiplatelet agents.
	• Expedited INR reversal for life-saving neurosurgical intervention: Recombinant activated factor VII 40-80 μg/kg (approximately 3.0-6.0 mg) intravenous push

Intracranial hypertension	• Elevate head of bed to 30 degrees • Hyperventilate to pCO$_2$ of 30 mm Hg • EVD placement • Mannitol 1.0-1.5 g IV prn to surgery
Fluids and nutrition	• Normal (0.9%) saline at 1.0 ml/kg/h • Begin enteral feeding via nasoduodenal tube within 24 h
Seizure	• For coma, start continuous EEG monitoring. • If clinical or electrographic seizures, treat with phenytoin or levetiracetam
Physiologic homeostasis	• Cooling blankets to maintain temperature ≤37.5° C • Insulin as needed to maintain glucose 120-180 mg/dl

CPP, Cerebral perfusion pressure; *EEG*, electroencephalogram; *EVD*, external ventricular drain; *FEIBA*, factor VIII inhibitor bypass activity; *4F-PCC*, four factor prothrombin complex concentrate, containing factors II, VII, IX, and X; *INR*, international normalization ratio; *IV*, intravenous; *NSAIDs*, nonsteroidal antiinflammatory drugs; *prn*, as needed.
From Goldman L, Schafer AI: *Goldman-Cecil medicine,* ed 26, Philadelphia, 2019, Elsevier.

• Care should be taken to avoid hypoxia. Airway and ventilatory management should happen early and concurrently with the primary management of ICH.
• Pneumatic compression devices should be applied from the start of hospitalization to help prevent deep venous thrombosis. Chemical deep venous thrombosis prophylaxis can be started after 24 to 48 h in most situations once the bleed has been determined to be stable.
• Early mobilization for rehabilitation is desirable in the first 24 to 48 h.

DISPOSITION

For large hemorrhages or unstable patients, immediate referral to a stroke center

REFERRAL

Patients with hemorrhagic stroke should be transported to a hospital where providers are skilled in the treatment of stroke and cerebrovascular diseases including the availability of neurosurgery services and neurocritical care. Depending on the severity and duration of symptoms, the patient may require neurosurgical intervention.

PEARLS & CONSIDERATIONS

Outcomes are inversely correlated with hemorrhage size; however, accuracy of prognosis, especially early after ICH onset, is difficult.

PREVENTION

• Prevention depends on the aggressive management of risk factors in individual patients, including hypertension, smoking, alcohol use, and cocaine use.
• Uncontrolled hypertension accounts for more than 70% of the attributable risk for ICH. Patients with prior ICH attributable to hypertension should have a blood pressure goal of <130/80 mm Hg.[3]
• Patients with prior ICH are at higher risk for ischemic strokes than recurrent hemorrhagic strokes.[12] Therefore initiation or resumption of antiplatelets is safe if indicated.[13]
• Direct oral anticoagulants (DOACs) dabigatran, apixaban, rivaroxaban, and edoxaban are uniformly associated with an overall reduced risk of iatrogenic ICH when used for stroke prevention in atrial fibrillation when compared to warfarin. Any of the currently available DOACs can be considered first line for patients at high risk for ICH if anticoagulation is indicated.

PATIENT & FAMILY EDUCATION

Patients and families need to understand that most patients will not soon achieve functional independence and that rehabilitation will be a long process. Education about avoiding antithrombotic agents should be stressed as appropriate for individual circumstances.

REFERENCES

Available at eBooks.Health.Elsevier.com.

RELATED CONTENT

Stroke (Patient Information)
Stroke, Secondary Prevention (Related Key Topic)

AUTHOR: **COREY ELAM GOLDSMITH, MD, FAAN**

BASIC INFORMATION

DEFINITION

Subarachnoid hemorrhage (SAH) is defined as hemorrhage into the subarachnoid space surrounding the brain. This can be either nontraumatic or traumatic in nature. Cerebral aneurysms are the most common cause of nontraumatic SAH (up to 85%) and have the most devastating consequences. Other causes include venous bleed, which have less severe sequelae. Here we will focus on aneurysmal nontraumatic subarachnoid hemorrhage.

SYNONYMS

Subarachnoid bleed
SAH

ICD-10CM CODES

I60	Subarachnoid hemorrhage
I60.1	Subarachnoid hemorrhage from middle cerebral artery
I60.2	Subarachnoid hemorrhage from anterior communicating artery
I60.3	Subarachnoid hemorrhage from posterior communicating artery
I60.4	Subarachnoid hemorrhage from basilar artery
I60.5	Subarachnoid hemorrhage from vertebral artery
I60.7	Subarachnoid hemorrhage from intracranial artery, unspecified

EPIDEMIOLOGY & DEMOGRAPHICS

INCIDENCE: Aneurysmal SAH: 6.1/100,000 persons worldwide and varies from 0.5 to 27.9 per 100,000 persons depending on geography. Annual incidence estimated at 500,000 cases worldwide.[1, 2]

PREDOMINANT SEX & AGE: Women in the fifth and sixth decades of life.[3]

PEAK INCIDENCE: Most aneurysmal SAH occurs in people who are between the ages of 55 and 60 yr.

RISK FACTORS: Although genetics seem to play a factor in aneurysm formation, age and lifestyle factors are more important for determining overall risk of rupture. These risk factors include smoking, hypertension, oral contraception, pregnancy, and sympathomimetic use.

GENETICS:

- Several genes and medical conditions such as collagen vascular disease and autosomal dominant polycystic kidney disease have been associated with aneurysm formation, but their association with SAH remains controversial.[4,5]
- Current guidelines recommend screening for aneurysms only if 2 or more first-degree relatives have a history of SAH or cerebral aneurysms.
- Genetic screening is not recommended for patients with SAH.[5]

PHYSICAL FINDINGS & CLINICAL PRESENTATION

- The primary symptom is a sudden, severe headache in >90% of cases. About 50% have a headache that is classically described as the "worst headache of my life" and reaches maximal intensity within 1 min—a "thunderclap" headache. This headache may be associated with nausea/vomiting, neck pain, seizure, or complete loss of consciousness.
- 10% to 45% of patients report a history of headaches during the weeks preceding the actual hemorrhage event. These are most likely sentinel bleeds that represent microhemorrhages.[6]
- A posterior communicating artery aneurysm may present as oculomotor (cranial nerve III) palsy, typically involving the pupillary fibers, even in a nonruptured setting.
- The World Federation of Neurosurgeons (WFNS) score and the Hunt and Hess score are clinical scores that correlate with mortality (higher numbers indicating higher mortality) (Table 1).

ETIOLOGY

- Trauma.
- About 85% of nontraumatic SAHs are caused by a ruptured berry aneurysm, whereas 10% do not reveal a bleeding source despite modern imaging techniques. About 5% are due to other causes, which include arteriovenous malformations (AVMs), tumors, vasculitis, reversible cerebrovascular vasoconstriction syndrome, cerebral sinus venous thrombosis, and coagulopathies.
- Table 2 summarizes nonaneurysmal causes of subarachnoid hemorrhage.

DIAGNOSIS

DIFFERENTIAL DIAGNOSIS

Other headache syndromes: Thunderclap headaches due to reversible cerebral vasoconstriction syndrome (often with recurrent thunderclap headaches), migraine headache, sexual headache, cough headache, exertional headache, secondary causes including, but not limited to, pituitary apoplexy or acute hydrocephalus.

WORKUP

IMAGING STUDIES:

- The Ottawa SAH Rule can assist in selecting patients who require further neuroimaging and workup (Fig. 1).

TABLE 1 Most Commonly Used Clinical Grading Scales for Subarachnoid Hemorrhage

Hunt and Hess Scale

- Grade 0: Asymptomatic
- Grade 1: Mild headache and mild nuchal rigidity, no neurologic deficit
- Grade 2: Moderate to severe headache but no neurologic deficit other than cranial nerve palsy
- Grade 3: Drowsy, confused, or mild focal deficit
- Grade 4: Stupor, moderate to severe hemiparesis, and early decerebrate posturing
- Grade 5: Deep comatose, decerebrate posturing

World Federation of Neurological Surgeons Scale

	Glasgow Coma Scale	Motor Deficit
Grade 0	15	Absent
Grade 1	15	Absent
Grade 2	13-14	Absent
Grade 3	13-14	Present
Grade 4	7-12	Present or absent
Grade 5	3-6	Present or absent

From Jankovic J et al: *Bradley and Daroff's neurology in clinical practice,* ed 8, Philadelphia, 2022, Elsevier.

TABLE 2 Nonaneurysmal Causes of Subarachnoid Hemorrhage

Trauma

Idiopathic perimesencephalic subarachnoid hemorrhage

Arteriovenous malformation

Intracranial arterial dissection

Cocaine and amphetamine use

Mycotic aneurysm

Pituitary apoplexy

Moyamoya disease

Central nervous system vasculitis

Sickle cell disease

Coagulation disorders

Primary or metastatic neoplasm

Causes are listed in approximate order of frequency.
From Goldman L, Shafer AI: *Goldman-Cecil medicine,* ed 26, Philadelphia, 2019, Elsevier.

OTTAWA SUBARACHNOID HEMORRHAGE RULE*

Patients who are ≥15 yr old and have a new severe atraumatic headache with maximum intensity within 1 h.

↓

Patient characteristics

Age ≥40 yr
Neck pain or stiffness
Witnessed loss of consciousness
Onset during exertion
Thunderclap headache (peaking pain within 1 sec)
Limited neck flexion on examination

All no
Probability of subarachnoid hemorrhage = 0

Any yes
An evaluation for subarachnoid hemorrhage (see text) should be undertaken in a patient with one or more criteria

*Should not be used in patients with new neurologic deficits, a prior aneurysm, prior subarachnoid hemorrhage, known brain tumors, or chronic recurrent headaches.

FIG. 1 The Ottawa Subarachnoid Hemorrhage Rule. (From Goldman L, Shafer AI: *Goldman-Cecil medicine,* ed 26, Philadelphia, 2019, Elsevier.)

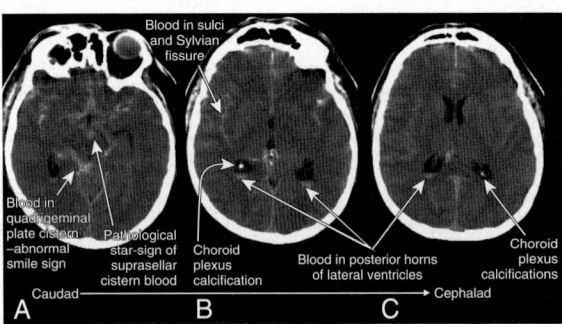

FIG. 2 Subarachnoid hemorrhage (SAH), noncontrast computed tomography (CT), brain windows. Acute SAH appears white on noncontrast CT brain windows. **A** through **C,** Nonconsecutive axial slices, progressing from caudad to cephalad. In this case of diffuse SAH, note the presence of subarachnoid blood filling the sulci, as well as extending into the cisterns, Sylvian fissures, and even lateral ventricles. In **A,** blood *(white)* fills the suprasellar cistern. This star-shaped structure is normally filled with cerebrospinal fluid (CSF) *(black).* The quadrigeminal plate cistern is normally a smile-shaped black crescent, filled with CSF, but in this case it is filled with blood. Extremely bright calcifications in the choroid plexus of the posterior horns of the lateral ventricles are common, normal findings—do not mistake these for hemorrhage. Note their similarity in density to bone of the calvarium. (From Broder JS: *Diagnostic imaging for the emergency physician,* Philadelphia, 2011, Saunders.)

- Computed tomography (CT) of the brain without contrast (Fig. 2) shows hemorrhage in around 95% of cases, especially during the acute phase (i.e., 24 to 48 h) after the onset of bleeding. Box 1 describes a CT scan classification of subarachnoid hemorrhage. About 3% to 5% of SAH may be missed on initial CT of the head. MRI brain, specifically FLAIR sequence, is helpful in detecting subarachnoid blood if clinically suspected.
- Lumbar puncture should be performed in all cases of suspected SAH with "normal CT of the head," especially when clinical suspicion is high and the patient presents beyond 6 h from symptom onset. The following suggest SAH:
  1. An RBC count of more than 100,000/m^3 in tubes 1 AND 4. This is to differentiate from a traumatic tap in which there will be a drop in RBC count from tube 1 to 4.
  2. Presence of xanthochromia or bilirubin in the cerebrospinal fluid.
  3. SAH can also be excluded by the following two criteria: CSF RBC count <2000 × 10^6/L and no xanthochromia.
- CT angiogram of the brain (Fig. E3 and Fig. E4).
- Digital subtraction angiography with 3D processing when indicated is the gold standard for diagnosis of etiology in subarachnoid hemorrhage.
- ECG may reveal diffuse repolarization abnormalities in precordial leads (Fig. E5).[7]

BOX 1   Computed Tomography Scan Classification of Subarachnoid Hemorrhage (Fisher Scale)

Group 1: No blood detected
Group 2: Diffuse deposition or thin layer of blood, with all vertical layers of blood (interhemispheric fissure, insular cistern, ambient cistern) <1 mm thick
Group 3: Localized clots or vertical layers of blood 1 mm or greater in thickness
Group 4: Diffuse or no subarachnoid hemorrhage but with intraparenchymal or intraventricular clots

From Jankovic J et al: *Bradley and Daroff's neurology in clinical practice,* ed 8, Philadelphia, 2022, Elsevier.

LABORATORY TESTS

- Basic laboratory values, including CBC, chemistry panel, prothrombin time, partial thromboplastin time, and platelet count.
- Serum troponin to evaluate for severe cardiac stress; elevated troponins indicate cardiac damage secondary to a catecholamine surge and can be associated with poor outcomes.
- Patients with SAH are prone to developing cerebral salt wasting, resulting in hyponatremia. Sodium levels should be monitored frequently.

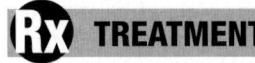 **TREATMENT**

NONPHARMACOLOGIC THERAPY

- Airway, breathing, and circulation.
- Once stabilized, good neurologic exam.
- Cerebrospinal fluid (CSF) drainage may be required for patients who develop hydrocephalus and increased intracranial pressure. It is also recommended for patients with Hunt and Hess grade 3 or higher. CSF drainage can be achieved through an extra ventricular drain or a lumbar drain.
- Recent data suggest that prophylactic lumbar drainage may reduce the burden of secondary infarction and decrease the rate of unfavorable outcomes.[8]

ACUTE GENERAL Rx

- Critical care management: Initial management strategies are geared toward stabilizing the patient and preventing re-hemorrhage and hydrocephalus. Re-hemorrhage occurs within 72 h in up to 23% and is associated with very high mortality rates.
- Blood pressure control: Tight blood pressure control is paramount before securing the aneurysm to protect against re-rupture. Blood pressure control can be achieved with the use of antihypertensive infusions such as intravenous nicardipine. A systolic blood pressure of less than 160 mm Hg is recommended. Placement of arterial line is recommended.

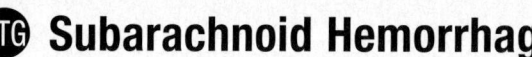

After securing the aneurysm, liberalization of blood pressure parameters is the standard. Hypotension should be avoided as it may worsen outcomes.

- Intracranial pressure control: Raised intracranial pressure occurs in more than 50% of patients with subarachnoid hemorrhage secondary to hydrocephalus, cerebral edema, cerebral infarction or other causes. Insertion of a ventricular catheter to treat acute hydrocephalus and maintain intracranial pressure <20 mm Hg can be lifesaving. Patients who are unable to be weaned may require permanent CSF diversion.
- In cases of aneurysmal SAH, treatment focuses on occlusion/exclusion of the aneurysm to prevent rebleeding. Most aneurysms currently are treated endovascularly. The most common treatment methods are:
  1. Microsurgical clipping: Performed through a craniotomy by placing a clip around the neck of the aneurysm
  2. Endovascular coiling (Fig. E6): Performed via digital subtraction angiography; it consists of deploying platinum coils inside the aneurysm (Fig. E7) or stents in the parent artery to cause thrombosis of the aneurysmal sac.
  3. Flow diverters and the Woven EndoBridge (WEB) device are also treatment options.
- Vasospasm: Cerebral vasospasm is a morbid complication leading to cerebral ischemia, disability, and death after SAH. It typically develops between day 4 and 14 (but may occur up to day 21) after the hemorrhage, and it reaches a peak on day 6 to 8. Treatment strategies include:
  1. Induced hypertension with typical mean arterial pressure goals of 90 to 100 (after aneurysm is secured) and with euvolemia instead of hypervolemia, as the latter was found to lead to significant cardiopulmonary and hemodynamic complications. "Triple H" therapy—*H*ypertension, *H*ypervolemia, and *H*emodilution—was originally employed to maintain cerebral perfusion, but it has fallen out of favor due to its many complications.
  2. Nimodipine (60 mg q4h or 30 mg q2h if blood pressure is low) has been shown to improve outcomes if it is administered

between days 4 and 21 after the hemorrhage. Nimodipine has not been shown to reduce the incidence of vasospasm but does have a mortality benefit, likely acting as a neuroprotective agent.
  3. Intraarterial therapies such as intraarterial calcium channel blockers and balloon angioplasty may be employed as needed for symptomatic vasospasm.
- Seizures occur in about 3% of patients during the acute phase.
- Use of prophylactic antiseizure medications is generally not recommended but can be considered in high-risk patients such as those with high-grade SAH, MCA aneurysm, or cortical stroke. Phenytoin should be avoided as it can worsen long-term cognitive outcomes.
- Pain control: Use short-acting and less-sedating medications (e.g., codeine, low-dose morphine).
- Monitor and treat for cerebral salt wasting and any other electrolyte abnormalities or anemia.
- Maintain normothermia.
- Avoid hyperglycemia or hypoglycemia.
- Management of SAH is complex and requires a multidisciplinary approach that includes expertise from neurology, critical care, neurosurgery, neuro-interventionalists, cardiologists, and endocrinologists, to name a few. A brief summary of the management is outlined above, but a detailed discussion is outside the scope of this text. The authors recommend supplementing this material with society guidelines such as those laid out by the Neurocritical Care Society.[5,9]

CHRONIC Rx

- Management of reversible risk factors mentioned earlier (smoking, hypertension, drug use)
- Management of neurologic disability through physical therapy and rehabilitation

DISPOSITION

- Outcomes after SAH have been improving over the years, with a 17% to 50% decrease in case fatality. The prehospital and 30-day mortality rates are still reported at around 15% to 33%.

- Almost half of those who survive hospitalization have cognitive impairments or disability that affect their lifestyles.[10]

REFERRAL

All patients should be managed at high-volume SAH centers, which are defined as having a case volume of more than 35 SAHs per yr. Patients who present to alternative facilities should be transferred to a high-volume SAH center as soon as possible.

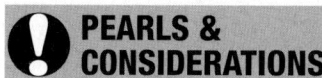 **PEARLS & CONSIDERATIONS**

COMMENTS

- "Thunderclap" headaches should be considered SAH until proven otherwise and evaluated by CT of the head with/without LP. MRI FLAIR sequence is also a helpful modality.
- All SAH should be managed in a critical care setting (preferably neurocritical care unit) with neurosurgical care available.
- Measures to prevent rebleeding include adequate control of blood pressure and aneurysm treatment with the use of coiling or clipping.

PREVENTION

Controlling some of the modifiable risk factors, especially smoking and blood pressure, may help to decrease the risk of aneurysmal rupture.

PATIENT & FAMILY EDUCATION

- SAH is a devastating condition, with most survivors developing significant neurologic or cognitive deficits. A good support system and an adequate physical and cognitive rehabilitation program may prove useful to survivors.
- Screening may be useful for patients with two or more first-degree relatives with SAH.

REFERENCES
Available at eBooks.Health.Elsevier.com.

RELATED CONTENT
Subarachnoid Hemorrhage (Patient Information)

AUTHORS: **KHWAJA A. SIDDIQUI, MD** and **EMERY STEELE, MD**

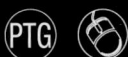

 BASIC INFORMATION

DEFINITION
A subdural hematoma (SDH) is a collection of blood or blood products between the brain and dura mater. Subdural hematomas can be acute (ASDH) or chronic (CSDH) and vary significantly in presentation and treatment.

SYNONYMS
Acute subdural hematoma
ASDH
Chronic subdural hematoma
CSDH
Subdural hemorrhage

ICD-10CM CODES	
I62.01	Acute subdural hematoma
I62.03	Chronic subdural hematoma
S06.5	Traumatic subdural hemorrhage

EPIDEMIOLOGY & DEMOGRAPHICS
INCIDENCE:
- ASDH: The exact incidence of ASDH is unknown, but it is commonly seen in patients with head injuries.
- CSDH: It is most common in the elderly with an estimated incidence of 1.72 to 20.6 per 100,000.[1]
- Recurrent CSDH: Between 10% and 20% of cases will experience reaccumulation of CSDH after evacuation.[1]

PREVALENCE: Unknown
PREDOMINANT SEX & AGE:
- CSDH has a peak incidence in the eighth decade of life and is notably higher in males.
- ASDH usually presents with trauma and can happen in all age groups. In particular, shaken baby syndrome can be associated with SDH in the infant population.[1]

RISK FACTORS: Factors such as antithrombotic therapy, coagulopathy, thrombocytopenia, early childhood, advanced age, brain atrophy, and chronic alcoholism can increase the risk of bleeding.[2,3] Intracranial hypotension associated with cerebral spinal fluid (CSF) shunts or leaks is uncommon but can result in acute or chronic SDH.[2,4]

PHYSICAL FINDINGS & CLINICAL PRESENTATION
- Symptoms vary on the basis of acuity, size, and location. Acute traumatic SDHs are often seen in traumatic brain injury patients, and their Glasgow Coma Scale may vary according to the extent of brain injury, size of hematoma, and associated compression. When associated with a midline shift (i.e., >5 mm), they can cause signs of cerebral herniation (e.g., ipsilateral pupil dilation, contralateral weakness) requiring prompt surgical evacuation.[5]
- Patients with CSDH may present with diverse nonspecific symptoms such as headaches, confusion, gait disturbance, incontinence, aphasia, hemiparesis, transient ischemic at-tacklike symptoms, and seizures.

ETIOLOGY
ASDH is usually the result of shearing and tearing of bridging veins between the brain parenchyma and the dura mater. Other causes of bleeding into the subdural space include traumatic contusion and extension of parenchymal hemorrhage. In the setting of spontaneous SDH, vascular abnormalities, such as arteriovenous (AV) malformation, aneurysm, and dural AV fistula, should be considered.[5]

For CSDH, it has been proposed that initial minor trauma splits the inner dural cell layer, leading to a self-perpetuating inflammatory cascade that causes membrane formation and neovascularization in the subdural space through the release of procollagen, fibrinolytic, and angiogenic factors. The resulting weak and rigid blood vessels and ongoing fibrinolysis lead to recurrent accumulation of blood in the subdural space.[1]

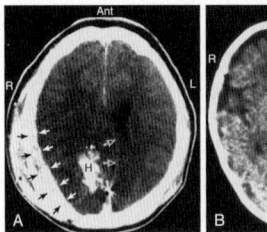 **DIAGNOSIS**

DIFFERENTIAL DIAGNOSIS
CSF hygromas, abscesses, and tumor infiltrations

WORKUP
- Clinical assessment: Patient history screening for provoking factors, including medications, specifically anticoagulants/antiplatelets; alcohol abuse; recent trauma; cancer; and recent bacterial infections
- Neurologic examination: Glasgow Coma Scale, cranial nerves, motor, and sensory exam

LABORATORY TESTS
Assessment of the patient's coagulation status including CBC with platelet count, prothrombin time, partial thromboplastin time, and liver function test (especially with a history of alcoholism or liver failure)

IMAGING STUDIES
CT of the head (Fig. 1) demonstrates the classic crescentic collection between the brain and

FIG. 1 A, Noncontrast computed tomography scan of an acute subdural hematoma shows a crescentic area of increased density in the right posterior parietal region between the brain and the skull *(black and white arrows)*. An area of intraparenchymal hemorrhage (*H*) is also seen. **B,** A chronic subdural hematoma for a different patient is shown. There is an area of decreased density in the left frontoparietal region *(arrows)* that effaces the sulci, compresses the anterior horn of the left lateral ventricle, and shifts the midline somewhat to the right. (From Mettler FA [ed]: *Primary care radiology,* Philadelphia, 2000, Saunders.)

inner table. For comatose and trauma patients, include a cervical spine CT scan. ASDH is usually hyperdense, whereas a CSDH is usually hypodense on noncontrast CT. Contrast is only needed if there are concerns about tumor or infection.

Rx TREATMENT

- Admission for monitoring in the setting of ASDH.
- Correction of underlying coagulopathy, if present (e.g., warfarin/direct oral anticoagulants [DOAC]/ acetylsalicylic acid [ASA]/clopidogrel reversal).
- The majority of SDH can be managed without surgery in awake patients with normal neurologic examinations.
- Atorvastatin and tranexamic acid have shown promising results in reducing the reaccumulation of CSDH, although results from larger randomized controlled trials are still awaited, and these drugs are not used in routine clinical practice.[6-8]
- Corticosteroids have not demonstrated any clinical benefit and may be associated with more adverse events in two randomized controlled trials.[9,10]
- The irritative effects of blood products on the brain can contribute to seizures, in both acute and chronic subdural hematomas. If seizures occur, aggressive treatment with antiepileptic drugs should be undertaken. Nonclinical seizures should be considered in cases with depressed or fluctuating mental status, and video EEG monitoring should be instituted in such cases. In traumatic ASDH, seizure prophylaxis with phenytoin or levetiracetam for 7 days can be considered as there is underlying injury to the brain parenchyma.[11,12]

NONPHARMACOLOGIC THERAPY
Surgical treatment is indicated in:
- ASDHs measuring >10 mm in thickness with a midline shift >5 mm on CT scan and a compromised neurologic status (Glasgow Coma Scale <9, pupillary asymmetry or fixation) should be immediately evacuated.[5]
- In CSDH with a mass effect, a clear change in the neurologic examination from baseline, and/or enlargement of the hematoma size, evacuation (Fig. 2) via craniotomy or burr hole should be considered.
- In cases of recurrent CSDHs or otherwise high-risk patients such as those who need antiplatelet or anticoagulant therapies for other medical indications, middle meningeal artery embolization has emerged as an effective treatment option.[13]

DISPOSITION
Depending on the size and location of the SDH and the examination of the patient, disposition can range from the ICU to outpatient management. When observation of the patient is considered, clinical examinations should be serially performed. Patient baseline and follow-up clinical examinations are more important than CT scan findings.

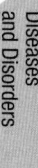

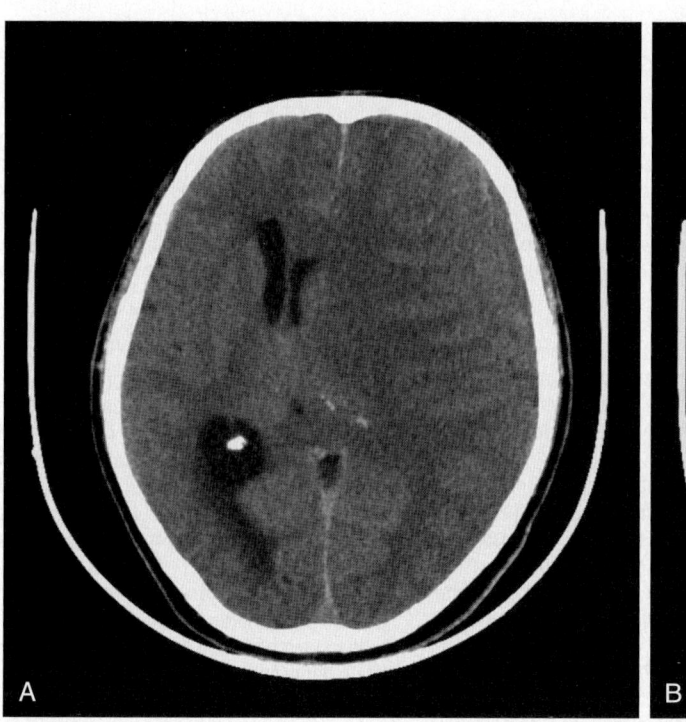

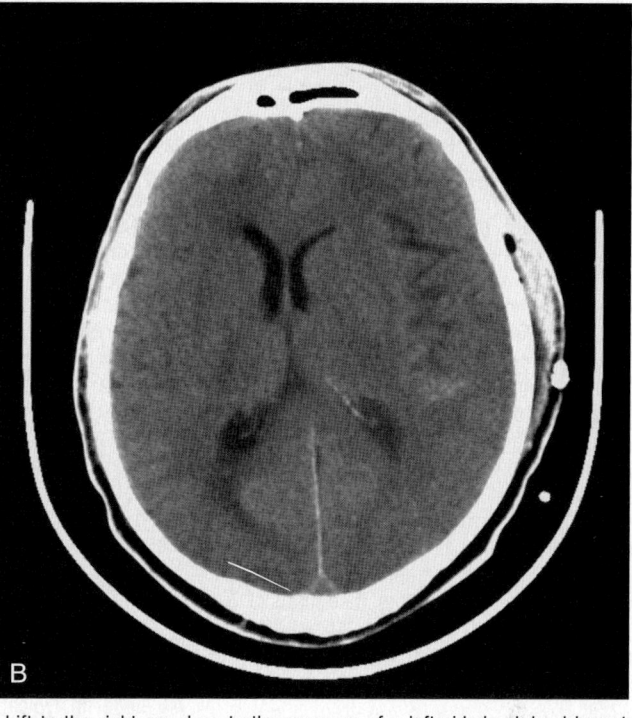

FIG. 2 An isodense subdural hematoma. A, Sulcal effacement and a midline shift to the right are clues to the presence of a left-sided subdural hematoma. **B,** Reexpansion of the left Sylvian fissure and a reduction in midline shift after evacuation. (From Soto JA, Lucey BC: *Emergency radiology, the requisites,* ed 2, Philadelphia, 2017, Elsevier.)

REFERRAL

Neurosurgical and operative consultation should be made available.

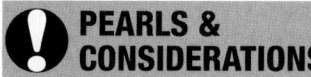

PEARLS & CONSIDERATIONS

COMMENTS

- Traumatic acute subdural hematomas frequently warrant surgical evaluation by means of a craniotomy (bone flap replaced) or decompressive craniectomy (bone flap not replaced). A trial comparing the two found that disability and quality of life outcomes were similar with the two approaches.[1] Additional surgery was performed in a higher proportion of the craniotomy group, but more wound complications occurred in the craniectomy group.[14]
- Many elderly patients have small CSDHs or hygromas. Unless these are associated with seizures or clinical or radiographic progression, they are usually not emergent and usually do not require neurosurgical intervention.
- SDHs in elderly patients can have a mixed hyperdense and hypodense appearance on noncontrast CT scan; this finding is suggestive of subdural membranes and chronic components.

PATIENT & FAMILY EDUCATION

Individuals with SDHs are at higher risk for seizure, so surveillance is important.

REFERENCES

Available at eBooks.Health.Elsevier.com.

RELATED CONTENT

Subdural Hematoma (Patient Information)

AUTHOR: **MUHAMMAD UBAID HAFEEZ, MD**

BASIC INFORMATION

DEFINITION

Supraventricular tachycardia (SVT) refers to a group of rapid regular tachyarrhythmia. There are three major categories of SVT:

- Atrial tachycardia (AT): An arrhythmia that originates from the atrium and does not involve the AV node. This is usually a focal arrhythmia. In some cases, the underlying mechanism may be a reentry circuit, either a small circuit (micro-reentry) or a large circuit (macro-reentry)
- AV nodal reentrant tachycardia (AVNRT)
- AV reentrant tachycardia (AVRT) (Fig. 1)

The latter two are reentrant arrhythmia that always involve the AV node as part of the circuit (see Fig. 1).

Other forms of arrhythmia that involve the atria, such as atrial fibrillation and atrial flutter, have distinct electrocardiographic features and are covered in separate chapters. Rare forms of SVT such as inappropriate sinus tachycardia, sinus mode reentry tachycardia, and junctional tachycardia are beyond the scope of this chapter.

SYNONYMS

SVT
Paroxysmal supraventricular tachycardia
PSVT

ICD-10CM CODE
I47.1   Supraventricular tachycardia

EPIDEMIOLOGY & DEMOGRAPHICS

The exact epidemiology of SVT is difficult to estimate because there is poor differentiation between SVT and atrial fibrillation/flutter in the literature. According to older reports from the U.S., the estimated prevalence of SVT was 225/100,000 persons and estimated incidence was 35/100,000 persons/yr.[1] Yet, most contemporary data suggest a remarkable rise in the prevalence and incidence of SVT in the U.S., which were estimated at 332.9/100,000 people and 57.8/100,000 people/yr, respectively.[2] SVT is most commonly diagnosed between the second and fourth decades of life and mostly in patients without prior cardiac conditions.[3] AVNRT is the most common type of SVT in both genders and in all ages, but is most common among young women.[4] AVRT is the second most common SVT, and it is typically diagnosed in younger patients as compared to the age of patients with AVNRT.[4] AT is more commonly associated with structural heart disease.[4]

PHYSICAL FINDINGS & CLINICAL PRESENTATION

- Patients may be either symptomatic or asymptomatic.
- Patient may be aware of "fast" regular heartbeat (but sometimes complain of irregular heartbeat, palpitations); may complain of weakness, dyspnea, dizziness, chest pain, presyncope or, rarely, syncope.[5]

- Patients with AVNRT may complain of neck pounding during the episode due to simultaneous contraction of the atria and ventricles with closed AV valves causing a sharp increase in atrial and jugular venous pressure.[6]
- In some cases the episodes can be triggered by physical activity or psychological stress, but in others there may not be an obvious trigger.[5] In patients with AVNRT, sometimes the arrhythmia is reproducibly initiated when bending forward to pick up an item from the floor.[7]
- Hemodynamic status during the arrhythmia may vary and depend on the patient's comorbidities and presence of underlying structural heart disease. Usually, patients are hemodynamically stable.[7]
- Physical examination is most commonly normal and unrevealing, except rapid regular heart rate and occasionally hypotension. In patients with AVNRT, sharp tall jugular vein A waves may be seen when the right atrium contracts against a closed tricuspid valve.[6]

ETIOLOGY (SEE FIG. 1)

- AVNRT: Dual electrical pathways within the AV node. In typical AVNRT the anterograde limb conducts slowly (slow pathway), and the retrograde limb has fast conduction properties (fast pathway), and vice versa in atypical AVNRT.[3]
- AVRT is accessory pathway mediated, either orthodromic (antegrade through the AV node and retrograde through the accessory pathway) or, much less commonly, antidromic (antegrade through the accessory pathway and retrograde through the AV node). In the case of antidromic tachycardia, the QRS will be wide and fully preexcited. In some patients, the presence of accessory pathway is not evident on the baseline ECG (concealed accessory pathway), while in others it is

manifest in the baseline ECG, presenting the typical features of the Wolff-Parkinson-White (WPW) syndrome.
- Paroxysmal atrial tachycardia and multifocal atrial tachycardia: Abnormal automaticity of atrial tissue or triggered activity. In some cases (especially in patients who underwent previous cardiac surgery such as valve replacement or atrial septal defect [ASD] closure), the underlying mechanism is macroreentrant AT.[3]

DX DIAGNOSIS

The diagnosis of SVT relies principally on the 12-lead ECG. Every patient suspected of having an episode of SVT should have a 12-lead ECG done immediately. Typically, patients with SVT will present with a narrow complex QRS tachycardia with a ventricular rate faster than 100 beats per min (bpm) and typically faster than 130 to 150 bpm.[8]

P wave morphology can be useful in discriminating rhythms. P waves with a similar axis to the sinus node can be atrial tachycardias and sinus tachycardias. P waves with retrograde depolarization of the atria (seen as inverted in the inferior leads) can be seen in AVNRT, AVRT, and atrial tachycardia. Sawtooth P waves are indicative of atrial flutter, and an absence of P waves with irregular R-R intervals points to atrial fibrillation. Variable (>3) morphologies of P wave are suggestive of multifocal atrial tachycardia. Wide QRS complex (>0.12 sec) with initial slurring (delta wave) during sinus rhythm and short PR (<0.12 sec) is characteristic of Wolff-Parkinson-White syndrome.

In typical AVNRT, due to the small size of the circuit within the AV node and the fast retrograde conduction, there is simultaneous depolarization of the ventricles and atria, thus making the P wave "buried" in the QRS and therefore not visible or inscribed very close to

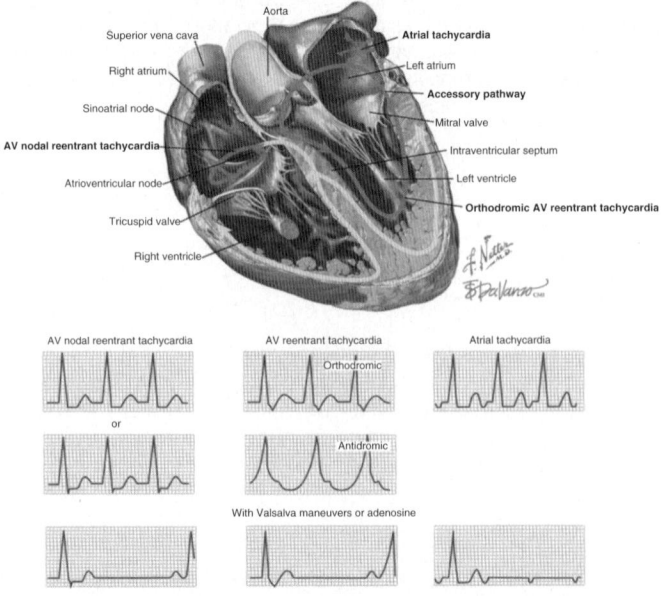

FIG. 1 Typical electrocardiographic recordings and anatomic representation of the common supraventricular tachycardias. (From Runge MS et al [eds]: *Netter's cardiology,* ed 2, Philadelphia, 2010, Saunders. Adapted from Delacretaz E: Clinical practice: supraventricular tachycardia, *N Engl J Med* 354:1039-1051, 2006.)

the QRS at the final part of the QRS complex, and sometimes creating a "pseudo terminal S wave" usually seen in leads II, III, and aVF and "pseudo terminal R waves" at the end of the QRS in V1 and avR[3,8] (see Fig. 1).

In orthodromic AVRT, the P wave is usually visible close after the QRS due to the rapid conduction properties of the accessory pathway (short RP tachycardia). In AT, the P wave is usually noticed farther away after the QRS (long RP tachycardia)[3,8] (see Fig. 1). A unique form of orthodromic AVRT termed *paroxysmal junctional reentrant tachycardia* (PJRT) involves a concealed accessory pathway, usually located in the posteroseptal region, and typically presents with deeply inverted retrograde P waves in leads II, III, and aVF, with a long RP interval.[9]

Other diagnostic maneuvers that may assist in the differential diagnosis are vagal maneuvers (such as carotid sinus massage) or giving intravenous AV nodal blocking agents (such as adenosine or verapamil) to produce AV nodal conduction block. This will terminate reentrant arrhythmia dependent on the AV node—AVNRT and AVRT—but not AT, which will continue, albeit with nonconducted P waves.[10,11]

Other arrhythmias that present with narrow complex tachycardia like PSVT are:
- Fascicular VT
- Junctional tachycardias
- Artifact such as with Parkinson disease

SVT can conduct with bundle branch block (BBB) and wide QRS either due to preexisting BBB on the baseline ECG or due to aberrant conduction (rapid rate–dependent BBB). When a patient presents with wide QRS tachycardia, VT must be excluded first.[12] Features to distinguish SVT from ventricular tachycardia are outlined in Table 1.

WORKUP

- Electrocardiography
- Echocardiography to exclude structural heart disease

- Thyroid function tests
- Complete blood count to exclude anemia or infection as an underlying trigger for the event
- In most cases the workup will be negative, with no underlying cardiac or systemic pathology and no clear triggers for an acute episode
- Holter or event monitor to document the arrhythmias if they are paroxysmal and not documented yet

Rx TREATMENT (FIG. 2)

NONPHARMACOLOGIC THERAPY

Acute termination: If the patient is hemodynamically unstable, prompt synchronized cardioversion with an external defibrillator using 50 to 100 J should be performed.[10,11]

If the patient is stable, Valsalva maneuver in the supine position is the most effective way to

terminate most types of SVT; carotid sinus massage (after excluding occlusive carotid disease and murmurs over the carotid arteries) is also commonly used to elicit vagal efferent impulses. These are effective in terminating AVRT, AVNRT, and may occasionally terminate some types of atrial tachycardia, but in the case of sinus tachycardia, atrial flutter, and atrial fibrillation, they only transiently slow down AV conduction without terminating the actual tachycardia.[10,11]

ACUTE TREATMENT

- Adenosine is useful to terminate acutely orthodromic AVRT and AVNRT and can uncover the underlying rhythm in paroxysmal atrial tachycardia (Fig. 3); it is the first choice of therapy for treatment of almost all episodes of SVT unresponsive to vagal maneuvers. The dose is 6 mg given as a rapid intravenous (IV) bolus; tachycardia is usually terminated

TABLE 1 Features That May Differentiate Ventricular Tachycardia from Supraventricular Tachycardia with Aberrancy

Helpful Features	Implications
Positive QRS concordance	Diagnostic of VT
Presence of AV dissociation, capture beats, or fusion beats	Diagnostic of VT
R to S interval >100 ms in any one precordial lead	Suggests VT
Atypical RBBB (monophasic R, QR, RS, or triphasic QRS in V_1; R:S ratio <1, QS or QR, monophasic R in V_6)	Suggests VT
Atypical LBBB (R >30 min or R to S [nadir or notch] >60 min in V_1 or V_2; R:S ratio <1, QS or QR in V_6)	Suggests VT
Shift of axis from baseline	Suggests VT
History of CAD	Suggests VT
QRS during tachycardia identical to QRS during sinus rhythm	Suggests SVT
Termination with adenosine	Suggests SVT

AV, Atrioventricular; *CAD*, coronary artery disease; *LBBB*, left bundle branch block; *RBBB*, right bundle branch block; *SVT*, supraventricular tachycardia; *VT*, ventricular tachycardia.
Adapted from Josep Brugada et al: 2019 ESC Guidelines for the management of patients with supraventricular tachycardia, *Euro Heart J* 41(5):655-720, 2020. https://doi.org/10.1093/eurheartj/ehz467.

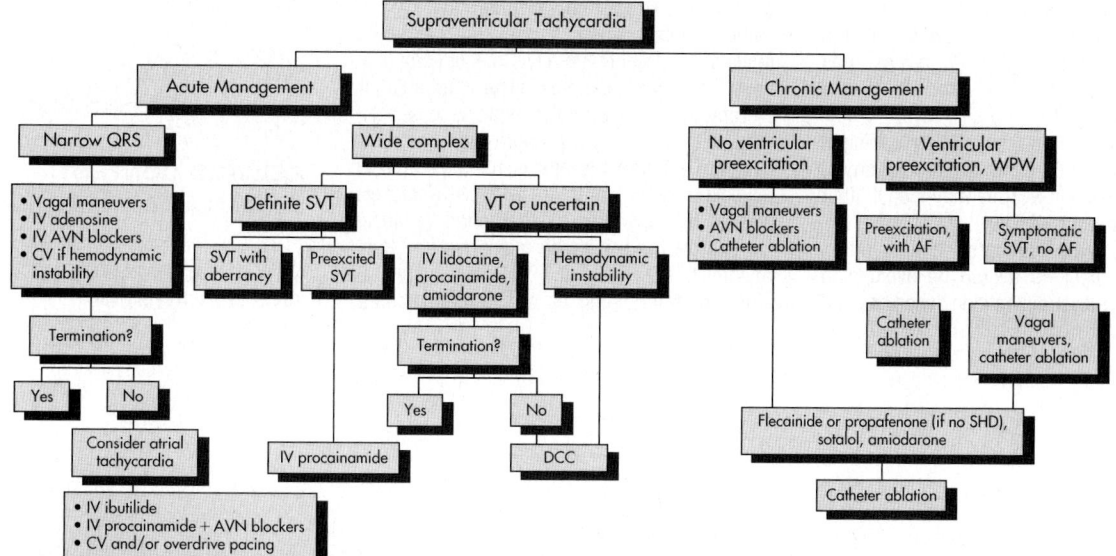

FIG. 2 Supraventricular tachycardia. *AF,* Atrial fibrillation; *AVN,* atrioventricular node; *CV,* cardioversion; *DCC,* direct current cardioversion; *IV,* intravenous; *SHD,* structural heart disease (no overt evidence of myocardial, valvular, congenital, or coronary heart disease); *SVT,* supraventricular tachycardia; *VT,* ventricular tachycardia; *WPW,* Wolff-Parkinson-White. (From Olshansky B et al: *Arrhythmia essentials,* ed 2, Philadelphia, 2017, Elsevier.)

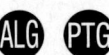

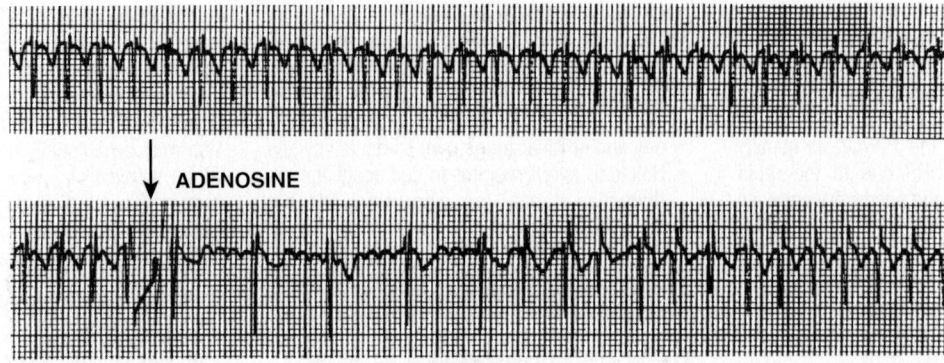

FIG. 3 Adenosine can uncover the mechanism of supraventricular tachycardia. A 3-mo-old infant developed an extremely fast narrow QRS complex tachycardia and a heart rate of 220 beats/min after insertion of a central line through a jugular vein. Adenosine produced a transient atrioventricular block and unmasked very rapid atrial fibrillation waves (570 beats/min). (From Park MK: *Park's pediatric cardiology for practitioners,* ed 6, Philadelphia, 2014, Elsevier.)

within a few seconds. If this fails, one may repeat with 12 mg IV bolus for up to two times. Contraindications are second- or third-degree atrioventricular block; WPW with atrial fibrillation; sick sinus syndrome; and chronic use of drugs such as dipyridamole, theophylline, or aminophylline; and heart transplant. Adenosine may cause broncho-spasm in asthmatics as well as chest dis-comfort, flushing, and shortness of breath, but these usually last for a very short time and serious adverse effects are extremely rare due to the drug's very short half-life.[10,11]

- Verapamil 5 to 10 mg IV is given over 5 min; if no effect, may repeat in 30 min.
  1. Verapamil should be used cautiously in patients with SVT associated with hypo-tension and should not be used in patients with heart failure with reduced ejection fraction or those who are under regular beta-blocker treatment.
  2. Slow injection of calcium chloride (10 ml of a 10% solution given over 5 to 8 min before verapamil administration) decreases the hypotensive effect without compromising its antiarrhythmic effect.[10,11]
- Metoprolol (IV 5 mg/2 min up to 15 mg) or esmolol (500 μg/kg IV bolus, then 50 μg/kg/min) may be effective in the treatment of SVT.[10,11]
  1. IV digoxin (0.75 to 1 mg slow IV loading in increments of 0.25 mg over several hours) is rarely used in SVT but may tried if other agents are not effective.
  2. Digoxin, beta-blockers, and calcium channel blockers should be avoided in patients with preexcitation syndrome and

antidromic AVRT or preexcited atrial fibril-lation to avoid increased conduction through the accessory pathway.
- Etripamil, a novel fast-acting intranasal calcium channel blocker, was recently shown to be effective in converting SVT to sinus rhythm acutely.[13] Etripamil (70 mg) may be nasally administered twice in a 10-min interval, depending on symptom persistence. In a randomized clinical trial, self-administered etripamil was shown to achieve a 64% return to sinus rhythm within 30 min compared with 31% with a placebo. No serious adverse events were associated with treatment, and most adverse events (~5%) were related to nasopharyngeal symptoms following the nasal drug admin-istration. This drug may be an essential self-administered treatment modality but is not yet approved for routine clinical use.

ONGOING MANAGEMENT

The main goal of treatment is the prevention of recurrent episodes and eliminating symptoms. Current guidelines recommend referring patients with recurrent, symptomatic SVT to catheter ablation, which is a highly effective mode of treatment with a low risk of complica-tions.[10,11] Recent studies show that ablation therapy is highly effective, safe, and associ-ated with a very low recurrence rate.[14] If catheter ablation therapy is not desirable or feasible, regular treatment with beta-blockers or nondihydropyridine calcium channel block-ers can be tried; if these fail, class Ic antiar-rhythmics are optional.[10,11] Rarely, when all other treatments fail or are contraindicated,

class III antiarrhythmics, such as amiodarone or sotalol, may be tried.[10,11] In patients with infrequent and minimally symptomatic episodes without preexcitation, it is optional to provide treatment only during acute episodes with a "pill-in-the-pocket" strategy with either beta-blockers or other antiarrhythmics.[10,11]

DISPOSITION

Most patients respond well with resolution of the SVT upon treatment (see "Acute General Rx"). Some patients may need chronic AV blocking agents for recurrence.

Radiofrequency ablation (RFA) is the proce-dure of choice in symptomatic patients with SVT and particularly in AVRT, AVNRT, and atrial flutter.[10,11] RFA has high efficacy rates (single procedure success is 93.2%), low all-cause mortality (0.1%), and low adverse events (2.9%). Recent technologic developments provided the ability to perform RFA with no to minimal radia-tion using advanced electroanatomic mapping systems and intracardiac echocardiography.[15] Despite high reported success rates and high safety profile, RFA appears to be underused in clinical practice.

REFERENCES

Available at eBooks.Health.Elsevier.com.

RELATED CONTENT

Supraventricular Tachycardia (Patient Information)

AUTHORS: **GAL TSABAN, MD, MPH** and **YUVAL KONSTANTINO, MD**

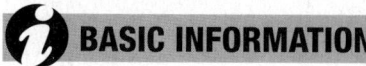
BASIC INFORMATION

DEFINITION

Syncope is a symptom that presents with an abrupt, transient, complete loss of consciousness, associated with inability to maintain postural tone, with rapid and spontaneous recovery. The presumed mechanism is cerebral hypoperfusion. There are three major types: Neurocardiogenic, orthostatic, and cardiac. Syncope is a symptom, and the goal is to distinguish lethal causes from benign causes of transient loss of consciousness.

ICD-10CM CODE
R55   Syncope and collapse

EPIDEMIOLOGY & DEMOGRAPHICS[1-3]

- Syncope accounts for 1% to 3% of emergency department visits and 6% of hospital admissions.
- 40% of the adult population will experience at least one syncopal episode during their lifetimes.
- Incidence of syncope is highest in elderly men and young women.
- 15% of children and adolescents experience syncope; fewer than 5% have cardiac causes.
- Older age (>60 yr), males, known ischemic or structural heart disease, previous arrhythmias, brief or absent prodrome, syncope during exertion or in the supine position, abnormal cardiac examination, family history of inheritable conditions or premature sudden cardiac death, and presence of known congenital heart disease are all associated with increased risk for cardiac etiology of syncope.

PHYSICAL FINDINGS & CLINICAL PRESENTATION

- Blood pressure: If low, consider orthostatic hypotension; if unequal in both arms (difference >20 mm Hg), consider subclavian steal or dissecting aneurysm. (NOTE: Blood pressure [BP] and heart rate [HR] should be recorded in the supine and standing positions, waiting at least 5 min between each position.) If there is a drop in BP but no change in HR, the patient may be taking a β-blocker or may have an autonomic neuropathy.
- Pulse: If patient has tachycardia, bradycardia, or irregular rhythm, consider arrhythmia.
- Heart: If there are murmurs present, consider syncope attributable to left ventricular outflow obstruction (aortic stenosis or idiopathic hypertrophic subaortic stenosis); if there are jugular venous distention and distal heart sounds, consider cardiac tamponade.
- Carotid sinus pressure: Can be diagnostic if it reproduces symptoms and other causes are excluded; a pause >3 sec or a systolic BP drop >50 mm Hg without symptoms or <30 mm Hg with symptoms when sinus pressure is applied separately on each side for <5 sec is considered abnormal. This test should be avoided in patients with carotid bruits or cerebrovascular disease. ECG monitoring, intravenous (IV) access, and bedside atropine should be available when carotid sinus pressure is applied.

ETIOLOGY

- Consider blood pressure equation: MAP − RAP = CO × resistance
  1. Where MAP = mean arterial pressure, RAP = right atrial pressure or central venous pressure, CO = cardiac output = heart rate × stroke volume
  2. Transient drop in heart rate, stroke volume, and/or resistance causes syncope
- Neurocardiogenic or neurally mediated syncope: Most common type, accounting for two thirds of cases. It includes vasovagal, situational, carotid hypersensitivity, and postexertional syncope (Box 1).
  1. Psychophysiologic (emotional upset, panic disorders, hysteria, hyperventilation)
  2. Visceral reflex (micturition, defecation, food ingestion, coughing, ventricular contraction, glossopharyngeal neuralgia)
  3. Carotid sinus pressure
  4. Reduction of venous return caused by Valsalva maneuver
  5. Postural tachycardia syndrome (POTS)

- Orthostatic hypotension (10% of cases):
  1. Hypovolemia
  2. Vasodilator medications
  3. Neurogenic orthostatic hypotension (primary autonomic failure, Parkinson disease, multiple system atrophy)
  4. Autonomic neuropathy (diabetes, amyloid)
  5. Pheochromocytoma
  6. Carcinoid syndrome
- Cardiac (10% to 20%):
  1. Reduced cardiac output—which should be transient, quickly reversible or compensated by increased resistance:
     a. Left ventricular obstruction (aortic stenosis, hypertrophic cardiomyopathy)
     b. Obstruction to pulmonary flow (pulmonary embolism, pulmonic stenosis, primary pulmonary hypertension); prevalence of pulmonary embolism in patients hospitalized for first episode of syncope up to 17% (mean age 76 yr)[4]
     c. Myocardial infarct with pump failure
     d. Cardiac tamponade
     e. Mitral stenosis
     f. Reduction of venous return (atrial myxoma, valve thrombus)
     g. Aortic dissection
     h. β-blocker therapy

BOX 1   Causes of Syncope

Reflex Syncopal Syndromes
- Vasovagal faint (common faint)
- Carotid sinus syncope
- Situational faint:
  1. Acute hemorrhage
  2. Cough, sneeze
  3. Gastrointestinal stimulation (swallow, defecation, visceral pain)
  4. Micturition (postmicturition)
  5. Postexercise
  6. Pain, anxiety
- Glossopharyngeal and trigeminal neuralgia

Orthostatic
- Aging
- Antihypertensives
- Autonomic failure:
  1. Primary autonomic failure syndromes (e.g., pure autonomic failure, multiple system atrophy, Parkinson disease with autonomic failure)
  2. Secondary autonomic failure syndromes (e.g., diabetic neuropathy, amyloid neuropathy)
- Medications
- Volume depletion:
  1. Hemorrhage, diarrhea, Addison disease, diuretics, febrile illness, hot weather

Cardiac Arrhythmias
- Sinus node dysfunction (including bradycardia-tachycardia syndrome)
- Atrioventricular conduction system disease
- Paroxysmal supraventricular and ventricular tachycardias
- Implanted device (pacemaker, implantable cardioverter defibrillator) malfunction
- Drug-induced proarrhythmias

Structural Cardiac or Cardiopulmonary Disease
- Cardiac valvular disease:
  1. Acute myocardial infarction, ischemia
  2. Obstructive cardiomyopathy
  3. Atrial myxoma
  4. Acute aortic dissection
  5. Pericardial disease, tamponade
  6. Pulmonary embolus, pulmonary hypertension

Cerebrovascular
- Vascular steal syndromes

Multifactorial

2. Arrhythmias or asystole:
   a. Extreme tachycardia (>160 to 180 beats/min)
   b. Severe bradycardia (<30 to 40 beats/min)
   c. Sick sinus syndrome
   d. Atrioventricular block (second or third degree)
   e. Ventricular tachycardia or fibrillation
   f. Long QT syndrome, with R-on-T leading to polymorphic ventricular tachycardia
   g. Pacemaker malfunction, leading to bradycardia
   h. Psychotropic medications and beta-blockers (Table 1)

TABLE 1 Drugs That Can Cause or Contribute to Syncope

Drug	Mechanism
Diuretics	Volume depletion
Vasodilators:	Reduction in systemic vascular resistance and venodilation
• Angiotensin-converting enzyme inhibitors	
• Calcium channel blockers	
• Hydralazine	
• Nitrates	
• α-Adrenergic blockers	
• Prazosin	
Other antihypertensive drugs:	Centrally acting antihypertensives
• α-Methyldopa	
• Clonidine	
• Guanethidine	
• Hexamethonium	
• Labetalol	
• Mecamylamine	
• Phenoxybenzamine	
Drugs associated with torsades de pointes:	Ventricular tachycardia associated with a prolonged QT interval
• Amiodarone	
• Disopyramide	
• Encainide	
• Flecainide	
• Quinidine	
• Procainamide	
• Sotalol	
Digoxin	Cardiac arrhythmias
Psychoactive drugs:	Central nervous system effects causing hypotension; cardiac arrhythmias
• Tricyclic antidepressants	
• Phenothiazines	
• Monoamine oxidase inhibitors	
• Barbiturates	
Alcohol	Central nervous system effects causing hypotension; cardiac arrhythmias

From Fillit IIM: *Brocklehurst's textbook of geriatric medicine and gerontology,* ed 8, Philadelphia, 2017, Elsevier.

(Dx) DIAGNOSIS

DIFFERENTIAL DIAGNOSIS

- Seizure (Table 2)
- Vertebrobasilar transient ischemic attack (TIA) usually manifests as diplopia, vertigo, or ataxia but not loss of consciousness. Isolated episodes of transient loss of consciousness (TLOC, Fig. 1) without accompanying neurologic symptoms are unlikely to be TIAs
- Recreational drugs or alcohol
- Functional causes such as somatoform disorders
- Sleep disorders, such as sleep attacks and narcolepsy, are also in the differential for TLOC
- Head trauma

WORKUP

The history is crucial to diagnosing the cause of syncope and may suggest a diagnosis that can be evaluated with directed testing. History is also important to determine other etiologies for TLOC, such as seizure.

- Sudden loss of consciousness (LOC): Consider cardiac arrhythmias (Boxes 2 and 3).
- Gradual LOC: Consider orthostatic hypotension, vasodepressor syncope, hypoglycemia.
- History of aura before LOC or prolonged confusion (>1 min), amnesia, or lethargy after LOC suggests seizure rather than syncope.
- Patient's activity at the time of syncope:
  1. Micturition, coughing, defecation: Consider syncope caused by decreased venous return.
  2. Turning head or while shaving: Consider carotid sinus syndrome.
  3. Physical exertion in a patient with murmur: Consider aortic stenosis or hypertrophic obstructive cardiomyopathy.
  4. Arm exercise: Consider subclavian steal syndrome.
  5. Assuming an upright position: Consider orthostatic hypotension.
- Associated events:
  1. Chest pain: Consider myocardial infarction, pulmonary embolism.

TABLE 2 Clinical Features That Help Distinguish a Generalized Tonic-Clonic Seizure From Syncope

	Seizure	Syncope
Clinical context and circumstances	Neurologic or systemic conditions that predispose to seizures, family history of seizures. Mental fatigue, sleep deprivation, alcohol use or withdrawal, systemic illness	Cardiovascular disorders, dehydration, anemia. Family history of syncope
Triggers	Usually none (unless reflex epilepsy)	Orthostatic hypotension, venipuncture, painful and noxious stimuli, emotional stress, micturition, Valsalva maneuver
Clinical features		
• Onset	No warning unless there is a warning symptom. Abrupt loss of consciousness, generalized stiffening, and fall. Occurs in any position	Tiredness, nausea, diaphoresis, tunneling of vision. Loss of consciousness over few seconds and fall. Occurs usually standing
• Course	Prominent tonic phase then clonic movements lasting about 1 min, cyanosis, labored breathing, may bite tongue or cheeks, sometimes urinary incontinence	Usually loss of tone, pallor, multifocal myoclonic jerks lasting <15 sec, sometimes urinary incontinence, usually no tongue or cheek biting
• Offset	Postictal sleepiness and confusion lasting up to hours, headache, myalgia	Rapid recovery over seconds to less than few minutes, no confusion, headache, or myalgia. May have fatigue

From Goldman L, Schafer AI: *Goldman-Cecil medicine,* ed 26, Philadelphia, 2019, Elsevier.

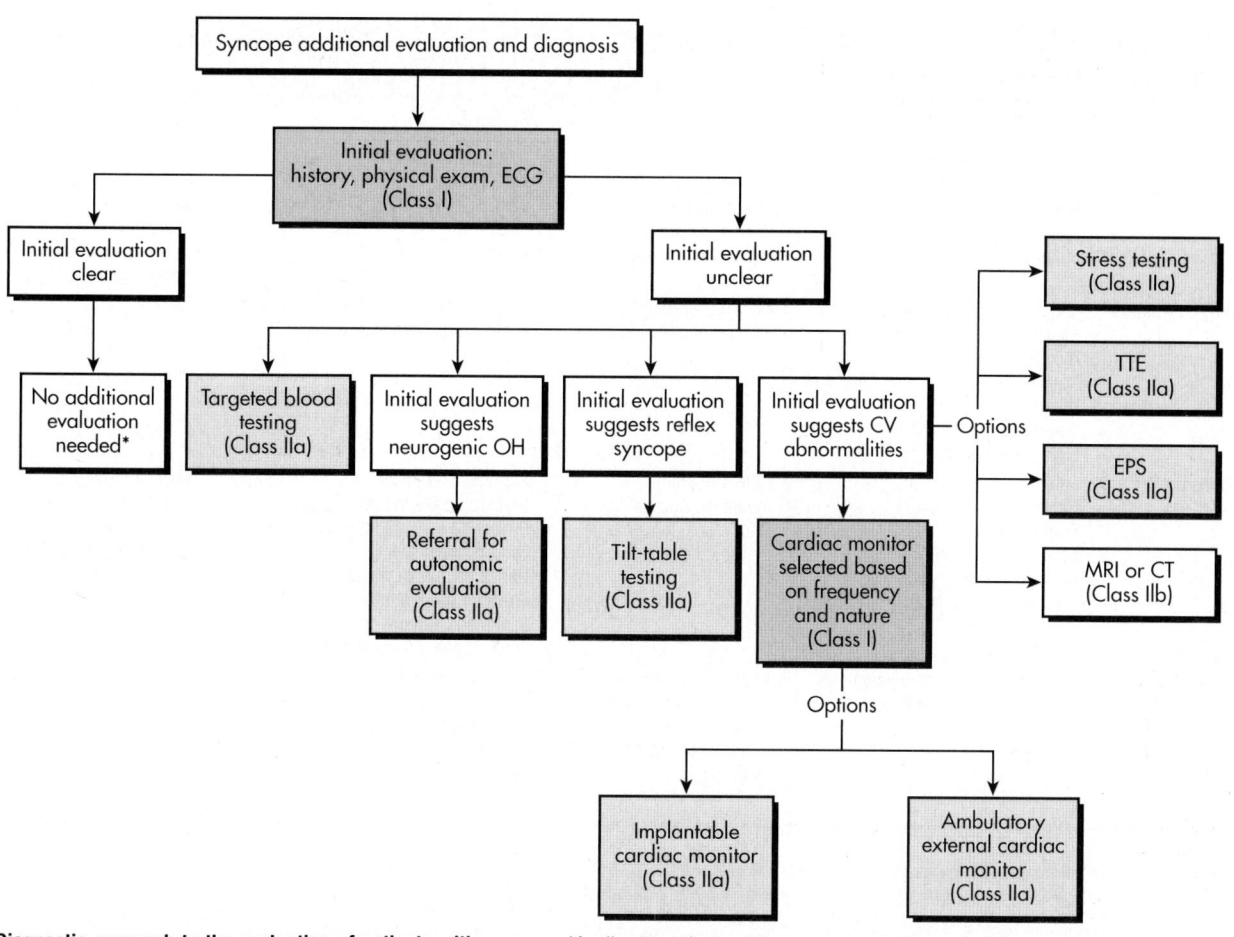

FIG. 1 Diagnostic approach to the evaluation of patients with syncope. *Applies to patients with a normal evaluation, no significant cardiovascular morbidity, or significant injuries with syncope. The recommendation in the *yellow boxes* are for selected patients; see text for details. (From Shen WK et al: 2017 ACC/AHA/HRS guideline for the evaluation and management of patients with syncope: a report of the American College of Cardiology/American Heart Association Task Force on Clinical Practice Guidelines and the Heart Rhythm Society, *J Am Coll Cardiol* 70(5):e39-110, 2017.)

BOX 2 Cardiac Diagnoses Associated with Syncope

- Dysrhythmias (see Boxes 3 and 4 for further detail):
  1. Tachydysrhythmias
  2. Bradydysrhythmias
- Structural causes:
  1. Hypertrophic cardiomyopathy
  2. Aortic stenosis
  3. Severe pulmonic stenosis
  4. Acute myocardial infarction/ischemia
  5. Cardiac masses (e.g., atrial myxoma)
  6. Pericardial tamponade
  7. Prosthetic valve dysfunction
  8. Ventricular assist device (VAD) dysfunction
- Cardiopulmonary causes:
  1. Acute aortic dissection
  2. Pulmonary embolism
  3. Pulmonary hypertension

From Walls RM et al: *Rosen's emergency medicine, concepts and clinical practice*, ed 10, Philadelphia, 2023, Elsevier.

BOX 3 Dysrhythmias Potentially Associated with Syncope

- Atrioventricular (AV) block
  1. Mobitz type II second degree
  2. Third degree (complete heart block)
- Sinus pause >3 sec
- Sick sinus syndrome
- Persistent sinus bradycardia (<40 beats/min)
- Ventricular tachyarrhythmias
  1. Monomorphic ventricular tachycardia
  2. Polymorphic ventricular tachycardia (i.e., Torsades de pointes)
  3. Ventricular fibrillation
- Supraventricular tachyarrhythmias
  1. Atrial flutter/fibrillation
  2. AV nodal reentry tachycardia
  3. AV reentry tachycardia
- Alternating left and right bundle branch block
- Pacemaker or automatic implantable cardioverter-defibrillator malfunction with cardiac pauses

From Walls RM et al: *Rosen's emergency medicine, concepts and clinical practice*, ed 10, Philadelphia, 2023, Elsevier.

2. Palpitations: Consider arrhythmias or POTS.
3. Incontinence (urine or fecal) and tongue biting are associated with seizure or syncope.
4. Brief, transient shaking after LOC may represent myoclonus from global cerebral hypoperfusion and not seizures. However, sustained tonic/clonic muscle action is more suggestive of seizure.
5. Focal neurologic symptoms or signs point to a neurologic event such as a seizure with residual deficits (e.g., Todd paralysis) or cerebral ischemic injury.
6. Psychologic stress: Syncope may be vasovagal.
7. Multiple nonspecific symptoms (fatigue, diffuse weakness, headache, "brain fog," exercise intolerance, "coat hanger sign") can be seen in POTS and neurogenic orthostatic hypotension.
- Review current medications, particularly antihypertensive and psychotropic drugs.
- Table 3 differentiates syncope caused by neutrally mediated hypotension, arrhythmias, seizures, and psychogenic causes.

TABLE 3 Differentiation of Syncope Caused by Neurally Mediated Hypotension, Arrhythmias, Seizures, and Psychogenic Causes

	Neurally Mediated Hypotension	Arrhythmias	Seizures	Psychogenic
Demographics and clinical setting	Female > male sex Younger age (<55 yr) More episodes (>2) Standing, warm room, emotional upset	Male > female sex Older age (>54 yr) Fewer episodes (<3) During exertion or supine Family history of sudden death	Younger age (<45 yr) Any setting	Female > male sex Occurs in presence of others Younger age (<40 yr) Many episodes (often many episodes in a day) No identifiable trigger
Premonitory symptoms	Longer duration (>5 sec) Palpitations Blurred vision Nausea Warmth Diaphoresis Light-headedness	Shorter duration (<6 sec) Palpitations less common	Sudden onset or brief aura (déjà vu, olfactory, gustatory, visual)	Usually absent
Observations during the event	Pallor Diaphoresis Dilated pupils Slow pulse, low BP Incontinence may occur Brief clonic movements may occur	Blue, not pale Incontinence may occur Brief clonic movements may occur	Blue face, no pallor Frothing at the mouth Prolonged syncope (duration > 5 min) Tongue biting Horizontal eye deviation Elevated pulse and BP Incontinence more likely* Tonic-clonic movements if grand mal	Normal color Not diaphoretic Eyes closed Normal pulse and BP No incontinence Prolonged duration (minutes) common
Residual symptoms	Residual symptoms common Prolonged fatigue common (>90%) Oriented	Residual symptoms uncommon (unless prolonged unconsciousness) Oriented	Residual symptoms common Aching muscles Disoriented Fatigue Headache Slow recovery	Residual symptoms uncommon Oriented

BP, Blood pressure.
*May be observed with any of these causes of syncope but more common with seizures.
From Libby P et al: *Braunwald's heart disease, a textbook of cardiovascular medicine,* ed 12, Philadelphia, 2022, Elsevier.

LABORATORY TESTS
Routine blood tests rarely yield diagnostically useful information and should be done only if they are specifically suggested by the results of the history and physical examination. The following are commonly ordered tests:
- Pregnancy test in women of childbearing age
- CBC to look for anemia and signs of infection
- Electrolytes, blood urea nitrogen, creatinine, magnesium, and calcium to look for electrolyte abnormalities and evaluate fluid status
- Serum glucose level
- Cardiac troponins, especially if the patient gives a history of chest pain before the syncopal episode
- Drug and alcohol levels with suspected toxicity

IMAGING STUDIES
- ECG to rule out arrhythmias in all patients; may be diagnostic in 5% to 10% of patients (Box 4).
- Echocardiography: Indicated in patients where initial evaluation suggests structural heart disease (based on physical exam and/or ECG) or have known heart disease.
- Exercise stress testing can be useful to establish the cause of syncope in selected patients who experience syncope or presyncope during exertion.

- If seizure is suspected, MRI of the brain and electroencephalogram may be useful.
- If head trauma or neurologic signs on examination, computed tomography (CT) or MRI may be helpful.
- If arrhythmias are suspected, a 24-h Holter monitor or admission to a telemetry unit in high risk patients is appropriate. In general, Holter monitoring is rarely useful, revealing a cause for syncope in <3% of cases. Loop recorders that can be activated after syncopal episode to retrieve information about the cardiac rhythm during the preceding 4 min add considerable diagnostic yield in patients with unexplained syncope.
- Implantable cardiac monitors that function as permanent loop recorders or implantable cardioverter-defibrillators, which are placed subcutaneously in the pectoral region with the patient under local anesthesia, are useful in patients with cardiac syncope.
- Electrophysiologic studies (EPS) may be indicated in patients with structural heart disease and/or recurrent syncope. The diagnostic yield of EPS was approximately 50% and 10% in patients with and without structural heart disease, respectively.

TILT-TABLE TESTING
- Useful to support a diagnosis of neurocardiogenic syncope. Patients age >50 yr should have stress testing before tilt-table testing. Positive results would preclude tilt-table testing.

BOX 4 ECG Abnormalities Potentially Associated with Syncope

- Signs of acute myocardial ischemia (e.g., ST elevation/depression, T-wave inversions, new bundle branch block, new abnormal Q waves)
- Pre-excitation suggestive of Wolff-Parkinson-White syndrome
- Long QT interval suggestive of congenital or acquired form of the long QT syndrome (e.g., Jervell and Lange-Nielsen syndrome.)
- Short QT interval suggestive of short QT syndrome
- Right bundle branch block pattern with ST elevation in leads V1-V3 suggestive of Brugada syndrome
- Inverted T waves in right precordial leads and epsilon waves suggestive of arrhythmogenic right ventricular cardiomyopathy
- Left ventricular hypertrophy, prominent abnormal Q waves, or deeply inverted T waves suggestive of hypertrophic cardiomyopathy
- Low voltages or electrical alternans suggestive of pericardial effusion
- Right ventricular strain pattern suggestive of pulmonary embolism

From Walls RM et al: *Rosen's emergency medicine, concepts and clinical practice,* ed 10, Philadelphia, 2023, Elsevier.

- Indicated in patients with recurrent episodes of unexplained syncope as well as patients in high-risk occupations (e.g., pilots, bus drivers). The test is also useful for identifying patients with prominent bradycardic response who may benefit from implantation of a permanent pacemaker. The test is contraindicated in patients with recent stroke, MI, and severe coronary or carotid disease.
- It is performed by keeping the patient strapped in an upright posture on a tilt table with footboard support. The angle of the tilt table varies from 60 to 80 degrees. The duration of upright posture during tilt-table testing varies from 25 to 45 min.
- The hallmark of neurocardiogenic syncope is severe hypotension associated with a paradoxical bradycardia triggered by a specific stimulus. The diagnosis of neurocardiogenic syncope is likely if upright tilt testing reproduces these hemodynamic changes in <15 min and causes presyncope or syncope.
- Postural orthostatic tachycardia syndrome is diagnosed if there is a sustained heart rate increase of not less than 30 beats/min (40 beats/min if age <18 yr old) and above 120 beats/min within 10 min of active standing or head-up tilt without associated orthostatic hypotension and with reproduction of symptoms.

PSYCHIATRIC EVALUATION

- May be indicated in young patients without heart disease who have frequently recurring transient loss of consciousness and other somatic symptoms.
- Generalized anxiety disorder, pain disorder, and major depression predispose patients to neurally mediated reactions and may result in syncope.

Rx TREATMENT[3,5]

NONPHARMACOLOGIC THERAPY

- Education about condition, avoidance of triggers, reassurance of benign nature of neurocardiogenic syncope.
- Ensure proper hydration; consider compression stockings and salt tablets in appropriate patients.
- Perform physical counter-pressure maneuvers if sufficient prodrome.
- Eliminate medications that may induce hypotension.
- Elevate the head of the bed by 10 to 30 degrees while sleeping.
- There is uncertainty in orthostatic training/exercise for sustained benefit.

ACUTE GENERAL Rx

- Varies with the underlying etiology of syncope (e.g., pacemaker in patients with syncope resulting from bradycardia or prolonged pauses). Clinical variables for identification of high-risk syncope patients who may benefit from hospitalization or an accelerated outpatient evaluation are summarized in Table 4.

TABLE 4 Clinical Variables for Identification of High-Risk Syncope Patients Who May Benefit from Hospitalization or an Accelerated Outpatient Evaluation

Severe structural heart disease (low ejection fraction, previous myocardial infarction, heart failure)
Clinical or ECG features suggesting arrhythmic syncope:
- Syncope during exertion or while supine
- Palpitations at the time of syncope
- Family history of sudden death
- Nonsustained ventricular tachycardia
- Bifascicular block or QRS >120 msec
- Severe sinus bradycardia (<50 beats/min) in the absence of medications or physical training
- Preexcitation
- Prolonged or very short QT interval
- Brugada ECG pattern (right bundle branch block with ST elevation in leads V1-V3)
- Arrhythmogenic right ventricular dysplasia ECG pattern (T wave inversion in leads V1-V3 with or without epsilon waves)
- ECG suggestive of hypertrophic dilated cardiomyopathy
- Clinical evidence or suspicion of a pulmonary embolus (clinical setting, sinus tachycardia, shortness of breath)
- Severe anemia

Important comorbid conditions:
- Significant electrolyte abnormalities
- Severe anemia

ECG, Electrocardiogram.
From Libby P et al: *Braunwald's heart disease, a textbook of cardiovascular medicine*, ed 12, Philadelphia, 2022, Elsevier.

- Treatment of neurally mediated and reflex-mediated syncope is summarized in Table 5.
- Syncope caused by orthostatic hypotension is treated with volume replacement in patients with intravascular volume depletion. Also consider midodrine to promote venous return by adrenergic-mediated vasoconstriction and fludrocortisone for its mineralocorticoid effects to increase intravascular volume, although these medications can cause supine hypertension. Droxidopa is approved for neurogenic orthostatic hypotension in pure autonomic failure or multiple system atrophy.
- The alpha-1 agonist midodrine (starting dose 2.5 mg twice a day and titrated as tolerated) is effective for the prevention of vasovagal syncope in young healthy patients with frequent vasovagal syncope.[6]
- Beta-blockers in older patients (>42 yr) and selective-serotonin reuptake inhibitors may be considered for recurrent neurocardiogenic syncope.
- Catheter-based cardioneural ablation may have a role in targeting atrial ganglionic plexi to treat refractory cases of neurocardiogenic syncope. The largest multicenter registry (n = 71, 13 sites) in the U.S. showed 82% free of syncope at 8.5-mo median follow-up after single ablation.

DISPOSITION

Prognosis varies with the age of the patient and the etiology of the syncope. In general:
- Benign prognosis (very low 1-yr morbidity rate) in patients:
  1. Age <30 yr and having noncardiac syncope
  2. Age <70 yr and having vasovagal or psychogenic syncope or syncope of unknown cause
- Poor prognosis (high mortality and morbidity rates) in patients with cardiac syncope, with presenting systolic BP <90 mm Hg
- Patients with the following risk factors have a higher 1-yr mortality rate: Abnormal ECG, history of ventricular arrhythmia, history of congestive heart failure

REFERRAL

Hospital admission in elderly patients without prior history of syncope or unknown etiology of their syncope and in any patients suspected of having cardiac syncope, with presenting systolic BP <90 mm Hg.

The Canadian Syncope Risk Score has been prospectively validated to identify very-low-risk and low-risk patients who can be discharged safely while improving health care efficiency.[7]

PEARLS & CONSIDERATIONS

COMMENTS

- The etiology of syncope is identified in <50% of cases during the initial evaluation.
- A thorough history and physical examination are the most productive means of establishing a diagnosis in patients with syncope.
- Driving restrictions vary based on state but consider restricting driving if syncope is frequent or unpredictable.

REFERENCES

Available at eBooks.Health.Elsevier.com.

RELATED CONTENT

Syncope (Patient Information)
Orthostatic Hypotension (Related Key Topic)

AUTHOR: **WILSON LAM, MD**

TABLE 5 Treatment of Neurally Mediated and Reflex-Mediated Syncope

Treatment	Class	Level of Evidence
Patient education on diagnosis and prognosis.	I	C-EO
Physical counterpressure maneuvers can be useful in patients with vasovagal syncope (VVS) who have a sufficiently long prodromal period.	IIa	B-R
Midodrine is reasonable in patients with recurrent VVS with no history of hypertension, heart failure, or urinary retention. Cardiac pacing should be considered with frequent recurrent reflex syncope, age >40 yr, and documented spontaneous cardioinhibitory response during monitoring of recurrent syncope.	IIa	B-R
The use of orthostatic training is uncertain in patients with frequent VVS. Midodrine may be indicated in patients with neurally mediated syncope refractory to conservative treatment approaches.	IIb	B-R
Dual-chamber pacing might be reasonable in a select population of patients age 40 or older with recurrent VVS and prolonged spontaneous pauses.	IIb	B-R
Fludrocortisone might be reasonable for patients with recurrent VVS and inadequate response to salt and fluid intake, unless contraindicated.	IIb	B-R
Beta-blockers might be reasonable in patients age 42 or older with recurrent VVS.	IIb	B-NR
Encouraging increased salt and fluid intake may be reasonable in select patients with VVS, unless contraindicated.	IIb	C-LD
In select patients with VVS, it may be reasonable to reduce or withdraw medications that can cause hypotension when appropriate.	IIb	C-LD
In select patients with VVS, a selective serotonin reuptake inhibitor might be considered.	IIb	C-LD
Beta-blockers are not indicated in pediatric patients with VVS.	IIb	C-LD

Modified from Shen WK et al: 2017 ACC/AHA/HRS guideline for the evaluation and management of patients with syncope: a report of the American College of Cardiology/American Heart Association Task Force on Clinical Practice Guidelines and the Heart Rhythm Society, *J Am Coll Cardiol* 70:e39-e11, 2017. In Libby P et al: *Braunwald's heart disease, a textbook of cardiovascular medicine*, ed 12, Philadelphia, 2022, Elsevier.

BASIC INFORMATION

DEFINITION

In healthy individuals, the expected physiologic response to serum hypotonicity is inhibition of the hypothalamic synthesis and posterior pituitary gland release of antidiuretic hormone/arginine vasopressin (ADH/AVP). Decreased binding to renal medullary collecting duct vasopressin receptors results in the increased excretion of urine that is dilute (low osmolality) and hypotonic (low sodium and potassium concentrations). The syndrome of inappropriate antidiuresis (SIAD) is defined by inappropriately concentrated urine in patients with hypotonic hyponatremia and normal extracellular fluid (ECF) volume. In the absence of an elevated serum glucose or exogenous osmole such as mannitol, the serum sodium concentration (S_{Na}) is essentially determined by the ratio of total body exchangeable sodium and potassium ($Na_e + K_e$) (mmol) to total body water (TBW) (L).[1]

Hyponatremia results from a reduction in total body exchangeable sodium and potassium ($Na_e + K_e$), increase in TBW, or both. The normal, appropriate renal response that corrects hyponatremia is excretion of urine with (Na + K) concentrations significantly less than serum sodium (S_{Na}). In SIAD, TBW is increased by retention of water due to reduced excretion of electrolyte-free water (EFW), which is water essentially devoid of Na and K. The severity of hyponatremia in SIAD is determined by the magnitude of solute intake, electrolyte-free fluid intake, and the urinary dilution defect (the patient's minimum urine osmolality). The definition of SIAD excludes hemodynamic stimuli that stimulate ADH, including reduced ECF volume (decreased total body sodium content), hypotension, and disorders characterized by decreased effective arterial blood volume. The latter group is characterized by increased ECF volume (edema or ascites) from increased total body sodium content. This group includes cardiac disease (e.g., congestive heart failure or chronic pericardial disease), nephrotic syndrome, and cirrhosis.

The term *syndrome of inappropriate antidiuretic hormone* (SIADH) has fallen into disfavor because 10% to 15% of so-called SIADH patients manifest suppressed or undetectable serum ADH concentrations. The group with suppressed ADH may have renal collecting duct cells with increased sensitivity to ADH, secretion of other ADH-like peptides, or altered renal hemodynamics that reduce sodium and water delivery to distal diluting sites, thereby preventing maximal urinary dilution. Establishing a diagnosis of SIAD does not require the measurement of ADH levels. Patients with adrenal insufficiency are excluded from the definition of SIAD. Hypothyroidism has been considered a cause of SIADH previously but is no longer because bioscientific evidence of thyroid hormone influencing water metabolism is lacking. Instead, hyponatremia may result from impaired cardiac output (heart failure) in severe cases of hypothyroidism (i.e., myxedema). SIAD should not be diagnosed in acute or chronic kidney disease.

SYNONYMS

SIADH
SIAD
Syndrome of inappropriate antidiuretic hormone secretion
Syndrome of inappropriate ADH release
Inappropriate secretion of antidiuretic hormone

ICD-10CM CODE
E22.2   Syndrome of inappropriate secretion of antidiuretic hormone

EPIDEMIOLOGY & DEMOGRAPHICS

INCIDENCE: Hyponatremia occurs in nearly 14% of hospitalized patients and represents an acquired disorder in the majority of cases and is the most common electrolyte abnormality. It affects approximately 5% of adults overall and 35% of hospitalized patients.[2] The adjusted odds ratio for in-hospital mortality in patients with hyponatremia at hospital admission is 1.47 (95% confidence interval, 1.33 to 1.62).

PHYSICAL FINDINGS & CLINICAL PRESENTATION

- SIAD is defined as an S_{Na} <130 mmol/L persisting for more than 48 h with normal ECF volume and concentrated urine (Uosm > 100 mOsm/kg) in the absence of the exclusion criteria noted earlier. Patients are hemodynamically stable with no evidence of edema, ascites, pleural effusion, or pulmonary congestion.
- Manifestations: Weakness, dizziness, headache, nausea, vomiting, muscle cramps[3]; confusion, vomiting, seizure, coma, ataxia, collapse, and dyspnea (severe EAH); fever and delirium after 3,4-methylenedioxy-methamphetamine (MDMA, ecstasy) administration; stigmata of alcoholism or malnutrition, fever and/or localizing symptoms related to pneumonia or other pulmonary disease, or headaches and visual field defects from an intracranial mass.
- If hyponatremia occurs rapidly (<24 to 48 h), delirium, lethargy, or seizures may occur. Diminished reflexes and extensor plantar responses may occur with severe hyponatremia or an S_{Na} <120 mmol/L.
- Neurologic abnormalities, including ataxia, mood changes, and proximal muscle weakness, are frequent in chronic hyponatremia. Abnormalities may be subtle despite severe hyponatremia.

ETIOLOGY

- Drugs: Thiazide diuretics[4] and selective serotonin reuptake inhibitor (SSRI) antidepressants are the two most common causes of drug-related hyponatremia. Narcotic analgesics, carbamazepine, phenothiazines, tricyclic antidepressants, methylenedioxymethamphetamine (MDMA; ecstasy), nicotine, clofibrate, haloperidol, nonsteroidal antiinflammatory drugs (NSAIDs), monoamine oxidase inhibitors, chlorpropamide, vasopressin, desmopressin, oxytocin, and chemotherapeutic agents (vincristine, cyclophosphamide), proton pump inhibitors represent additional etiologies
- Neoplasms: Lung, oropharynx, stomach, duodenum, pancreas, brain, thymus, bladder, prostate, endometrium, mesothelioma, lymphoma, and Ewing sarcoma
- Pulmonary disorders: Coronavirus disease (SARS-CoV-2, COVID-19),[5] pneumonia, aspergillosis, pulmonary abscess, tuberculosis, bronchiectasis, emphysema, cystic fibrosis, status asthmaticus, and respiratory failure associated with positive-pressure breathing
- Intracranial pathology: Trauma, neoplasms, infections (meningitis, encephalitis, brain abscess), hemorrhage, hydrocephalus, multiple sclerosis, and Guillain-Barré syndrome
- Postoperative period: Surgical stress, positive pressure ventilation, anesthetic agents, and pain
- Other: Acute intermittent porphyria, psychosis, delirium tremens, general anesthesia, and EAH (associated with extreme endurance exercise such as marathon running)
- Table 1 summarizes common etiologies of SIAD

DIFFERENTIAL DIAGNOSIS[6]

- Hyponatremia associated with subclinical hypovolemia
- Solute-limited water excretion (e.g., "tea-and-toast" diet, beer-drinker's potomania); an acquired disorder in which the renal capacity to excrete sufficient EFW is impaired from an insufficient osmolar intake (sodium and potassium) and/or metabolism (generation of urea from protein metabolism)
- Primary polydipsia or water intake that exceeds renal dilutional capability and is frequently accompanied by solute-limited water excretion and/or incomplete suppression of ADH
- Endocrine disorders, including hypothyroidism and adrenal insufficiency
- Severe hypokalemia produces hyponatremia because the exchangeable potassium pool is twice the size of the exchangeable sodium pool. When intracellular potassium is in severe deficit, the resulting decrease in intracellular osmolality shifts water from the intracellular to extracellular space. Additionally, sodium ions exit the plasma, enter cells, and cause hyponatremia
- Hypertonic hyponatremia (hyperglycemia, iatrogenic administration of mannitol, sorbitol, glycine)
- Hyponatremia from subclinical heart or liver disease
- Pseudohyponatremia caused by extreme hyperglobulinemia or hyperlipidemia
- Reset osmostat: ADH regulation occurs at a lower-than-normal osmotic threshold, with intact urinary dilution and concentration
- Cerebral salt wasting syndrome (CSWS) in critically ill neurologic patients (Table E2)

WORKUP

- Normal ECF volume by history and physical examination. No history of large-volume fluid losses. No generalized edema, ascites, pulmonary congestion, or large pleural effusions

TABLE 1 Common Etiologies of the Syndrome of Inappropriate Antidiuretic Hormone Secretion (SIADH)

Tumors

Pulmonary/mediastinal (bronchogenic carcinoma, mesothelioma, thymoma)

Extrapulmonary (duodenal carcinoma, pancreatic carcinoma, ureteral/prostate carcinoma, uterine carcinoma, nasopharyngeal carcinoma, leukemia)

Central Nervous System Disorders

Mass lesions (tumors, brain abscesses, subdural hematoma)

Inflammatory diseases (encephalitis, meningitis, systemic lupus erythematosus, acute intermittent porphyria, multiple sclerosis)

Degenerative/demyelinating diseases (Guillain-Barré syndrome, spinal cord lesions)

Miscellaneous (subarachnoid hemorrhage, head trauma, acute psychosis, delirium tremens, pituitary stalk section, transsphenoidal adenomectomy, hydrocephalus)

Drug-Related

Stimulated release of AVP (nicotine, phenothiazines, tricyclics)

Direct renal effects and/or potentiation of AVP antidiuretic effects (desmopressin, oxytocin, prostaglandin synthesis inhibitors)

Mixed or uncertain actions (ACE inhibitors, carbamazepine and oxcarbazepine, chlorpropamide, clofibrate, clozapine, cyclophosphamide, 3,4-methylenedioxy-methamphetamine [ecstasy], omeprazole; serotonin reuptake inhibitors [SSRIs], vincristine)

Pulmonary

Infections (tuberculosis, acute bacterial and viral pneumonia, aspergillosis, empyema)

Mechanical/ventilatory causes (acute respiratory failure, COPD, positive-pressure ventilation)

Other Causes

Acquired immunodeficiency syndrome (AIDS) and AIDS-related complex

Prolonged strenuous exercise (marathon, triathlon, ultramarathon, hot-weather hiking)

Senile atrophy

Idiopathic

ACE, Angiotensin-converting enzyme; *AVP,* arginine vasopressin; *COPD,* chronic obstructive pulmonary disease.
From Melmed S et al: *Williams textbook of endocrinology,* ed 12, Philadelphia, 2011, Saunders.

TABLE 3 Diagnostic Criteria for the Syndrome of Inappropriate Antidiuretic Hormone Secretion

Essential Diagnostic Criteria

Decreased extracellular fluid effective osmolality (<270 mOsm/kg H_2O)

Inappropriate urinary concentration (>100 mOsm/kg H_2O)

Clinical normovolemia

Elevated urinary sodium concentration under conditions of normal salt and water intake

Absence of adrenal, thyroid, or pituitary insufficiency

Absence of chronic kidney disease

Absence of diuretic use

Supplemental Criteria

Abnormal water loading test (inability to excrete at least 90% of a 20 ml/kg H_2O load in 4 h and/or failure to dilute urine osmolality to <100 mOsm/kg H_2O). Plasma vasopressin level inappropriately elevated relative to the plasma osmolality

No significant correction of S_{Na} with volume expansion, but improvement after fluid restriction

$S_{Na},$ Serum sodium.

Modified from Verbalis J: The syndrome of inappropriate antidiuretic hormone secretion and other hypo-osmolar disorders. In Schrier RW (ed): *Diseases of the kidney and urinary tract,* ed 9, Philadelphia, 2013, Lippincott Williams & Wilkins. In Johnson RJ et al: *Comprehensive clinical nephrology,* ed 6, Philadelphia, 2019, Elsevier.

- Laboratory evaluation (see "Laboratory Tests") is consistent with excessive ADH secretion or sensitivity in the absence of osmotic or hemodynamic stimuli for ADH secretion
- Normal thyroid, adrenal, and cardiac function
- No recent or concurrent use of loop diuretics
- Failure to correct hyponatremia after ECF volume repletion by isotonic 0.9% saline solution
- Correction of hyponatremia solely by fluid restriction is generally unsuccessful

Diagnostic criteria for SIADH are described in Table 3.

LABORATORY TESTS

- Normal or low blood urea nitrogen (BUN) and/or serum creatinine
- S_{Na} lower than the limit of the normal range
- Decreased serum osmolality (<270 mOsm/kg H_2O) corrected for serum glucose, BUN, and exogenous osmoles
- Decreased serum uric acid concentration
- Urine osmolality >100 mOsm/kg H_2O
- Urine Na concentration is generally >40 mmol/L with normal dietary salt intake

IMAGING STUDIES

Imaging is not routinely required for diagnosis. Imaging may facilitate the diagnosis of an associated underlying pulmonary or central nervous system (CNS) disease or rule out intracranial pathology.

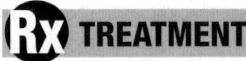 **TREATMENT**

NONPHARMACOLOGIC THERAPY

With mild SIAD, fluid restriction (10 to 15 ml/kg per day) combined with increased solute loads (diets high in protein, urea powder, sodium chloride, and potassium chloride) may normalize S_{Na}. The enhanced solute load produces an osmotic diuresis that increases EFW loss. Urea administration should be undertaken with a consulting nephrologist; it has been proven safe for decades[7] and is sold in the U.S. as a "medical food supplement."

ACUTE GENERAL Rx

RATE OF CORRECTION: In chronic hyponatremia, it is critical to avoid overly rapid correction of S_{Na} correction to prevent brain injury from osmotic demyelination syndrome.[8,9] Patients with moderate-to-severe hyponatremia should undergo serial monitoring of S_{Na} and serum potassium concentration (S_K), urine volumes, and urine chemistries (osmolality, K, and Na). Most SIAD patients have chronic hyponatremia (developing over more than 24 to 48 h) and mild symptoms. Target S_{Na} correction rates are 6 to 8 mmol/L per day in chronic hyponatremia. The S_{Na} should be actively lowered in patients who experience increases of >10 mmol/L during a 24-h period. The rate of S_{Na} change during conservative therapy or 0.9% infusion is often slow or flat because sodium is excreted while water

is mostly retained. However, administration of even limited volumes of isotonic saline (308 mOsm/L) may quickly lead to overcorrection of hyponatremia in misdiagnosed cases of inadequate generation/excretion of urinary solute (tea-and-toast diet or beer potomania) as administered osmoles are excreted in dilute urine. Correction of undiagnosed ECF volume depletion can also lead to overcorrection, but takes much longer times and larger volumes. Therefore close monitoring of serum and urine electrolytes, osmolality, and volume is always recommended. In addition, blind administration of isotonic saline prior to checking urine osmolality in hemodynamically stable euvolemic patients with hyponatremia is strongly discouraged.

ACUTE HYPONATREMIA: In patients with acute hyponatremia (duration <24 h), the goal of therapy is to increase S_{Na} sufficiently to prevent or reduce the severity of cerebral edema. S_{Na} should be increased by up to 3 to 6 mmol/L within the first 3 h if symptoms are mild to moderate and within the initial hour with severe symptoms (seizures, coma, obtundation).

Rapid correction of S_{Na} in acute hyponatremia may involve hypertonic saline therapy (3% saline, 513 mmol/L). As a general rule, 1 ml/kg body weight of 3% saline is expected to increase S_{Na} by 1 mmol/L, as shown in the following example:
- 80 kg male
- 80 ml 3% saline = .08 L × 513 mEq/L = 41 mEq
- TBW = 80 kg × 0.55 L/kg = 44 L
- Expected ΔS_{Na} = 41 mEq/ 44 L 1 mEq/L

S_{Na} correction rates may be greater than anticipated when unrecognized ECF volume depletion is concurrently corrected. The simultaneous delivery of the synthetic ADH analog desmopressin can mitigate S_{Na} overcorrection. Intravenous furosemide therapy may augment urinary EFW loss and prevent unintended ECF volume expansion during hypertonic saline therapy, which is contraindicated in individuals with heart failure.

CHRONIC HYPONATREMIA: The therapeutic goals of chronic hyponatremia from SIAD are normalization of TBW and restoration of Na and K stores to their respective normal levels. These goals may be achieved as follows.

- Choose a 24-h target S_{Na}, based on current S_{Na} and safe rates of correction (see "Rate of Correction").
- Estimate TBW and total body cation content. Estimation of current TBW should consider the patient's baseline TBW, volume of additional retained water, and changes in total body content of sodium and potassium (see example that follows).
- Account for all sources of EFW intake and loss (including insensible losses). Add/subtract this total volume to/from net target EFW to determine total EFW volume loss required to attain the target S_{Na}.
- Select a strategy that achieves target EFW volume loss: Collecting duct arginine vasopressin receptor-2 antagonist (e.g., tolvaptan), oral urea therapy, or loop diuretic combined with electrolyte replacement such as sodium chloride (salt) (17 mmol sodium per 1 g of NaCl) and potassium chloride tablets.

The following example demonstrates the method to determine the target TBW and EFW loss required to reach an appropriate S_{Na} target after 24 h of therapy in a patient with chronic hyponatremia.

- S_{Na} is 115 mmol/L in 75 kg, minimally symptomatic older woman who chronically takes an SSRI and hydrochlorothiazide.
  1. Step 1: Establish target S_{Na}:
     a. Target S_{Na} after 24 hr = Current S_{Na} + 6 = 121 mmol/L
  2. Step 2: Estimate current TBW and total body cations:
     a. Current weight = 75 kg
     b. Estimated TBW fraction = 0.55 (55%)
     c. Current TBW = 0.55 × 75 = 41.2 L
     d. Current total body (Na$_e$ + K$_e$) cation quantity = Current TBW × S_{Na} = 41.2 × 115 = 4743 mmol
  3. Step 3: Calculate target TBW:
     a. Target TBW (L) = Current [TBNa$_e$ + Total body potassium (TBK)$_e$]/Target S_{Na} = 4743 mmol/121 mmol/L = 39.2 L
  4. Step 4: Calculation of net EFW loss:
     a. Target net EFW loss after 24 h = Current TBW − Target TBW = 41.2 L − 39.2 L = 2 L

  5. Step 5: Calculate total urine EFW volume:
     a. Target total urine EFW excretion (estimate: 1 L oral fluid intake and 0.5 L net insensible loss) Urine EFW volume = 2 + (1 − 0.5) = 2.5 L
  6. Step 6: Choose therapeutic strategy
     a. Note that urinary EFW loss is calculated as Urine volume x [1 − (UNa + UK)/S_{Na}]
  7. Step 7: Implement strategy and monitor results frequently

LOOP DIURETIC PLUS SALINE STRATEGY: Before the advent of specific arginine vasopressin receptor-2 antagonists, SIAD was typically treated by increasing urine volume and EFW loss with a loop diuretic. In the earlier example a 24-h net EFW loss of 2.5 L is required. The urine cation (Na + K) concentration is approximately 75 mEq/L following loop diuretic administration. To maintain normal total body sodium and potassium, lost urine electrolytes need to be replaced.

Periodic monitoring of S_{Na}, S_K, urine volume, and urine chemistries (osmolality, sodium, and potassium) is recommended to prevent overly rapid correction of S_{Na}.

The use of hypertonic saline solutions should be guided by an expert. Urine potassium loss cannot be ignored, and these losses are corrected separately.

ARGININE VASOPRESSIN RECEPTOR ANTAGONISTS: Selective arginine vasopressin receptor antagonist therapy is straightforward and convenient for patients and medical personnel. Currently, two agents are available in the U.S: Intravenous (IV) conivaptan (20 mg IV once followed by continuous IV infusion of 20 to 40 mg/day for 2 to 4 days) and oral tolvaptan (15 to 90 mg/day, as needed). Tolvaptan must be initiated in-hospital, and conivaptan requires ICU monitoring. Urinary electrolyte losses are minimal, meaning that administration produces virtually electrolyte-free urines. In the earlier example, the dose would be titrated to produce a daily urine output of 2.5 L. Urine output in excess of this amount would require quantitative replacement with oral water or intravenously as D$_5$W until the effects of the AVP agonist wore off (in approximately 12 to 24 h in the case of tolvaptan).

CHRONIC Rx

- When SIAD is chronic, fluid restriction (<15 ml/kg per day) may be required indefinitely and combined with high dietary electrolyte and protein intake.
- NaCl tablets, electrolyte supplements, protein powders to generate urea production, and pharmaceutical-grade urea may be used to

correct hyponatremia.[10] Periodic monitoring of electrolytes is recommended in patients with chronic SIAD.

- Tolvaptan has been administered successfully in clinical trials. FDA labeling states that tolvaptan use is restricted to 30 days due to concerns regarding hepatotoxicity, which was detected during clinical trials for polycystic kidney disease. Additional contraindications include volume contraction and concomitant use of strong cytochrome P3A inhibitors. Patients undergoing tolvaptan therapy are not fluid-restricted.
- Demeclocycline variably increases urine EFW losses. This agent is contraindicated in hepatic disease and rarely used today.

DISPOSITION

- Mortality exceeding 40% has been reported in patients with S_{Na} <110 mmol/L.
- Hospital readmission rates are common in chronic SIAD when an underlying cause cannot be eliminated, especially if patients are unwilling or unable to restrict their fluid intake and follow dietary recommendations.
- Chronic, mild-to-moderate hyponatremia is associated with bone loss, falls, and increased fracture risk, particularly in older patients.

REFERRAL

Emergency department evaluation and hospital admission are appropriate for moderate-to-severe hyponatremia due to SIAD, especially when acute or symptomatic. Due to a high complication risk from overly aggressive or ineffective treatment, consultation by a nephrologist, endocrinologist, or critical care physician is recommended.

REFERENCES

Available at eBooks.Health.Elsevier.com.

RELATED CONTENT

Syndrome of Inappropriate Secretion of Antidiuretic Hormone (Patient Information)
Salt-Losing Nephropathy (Related Key Topic)

AUTHOR: **MARK D. FABER, MD, MACM**

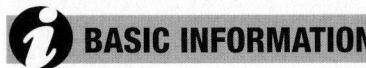
BASIC INFORMATION

DEFINITION

Syphilis is a systemic sexually transmitted infection caused by the spirochete *Treponema pallidum,* with acute and chronic manifestations, characterized by primary skin lesions; secondary eruption involving skin and mucous membranes; long periods of latency; and late lesions of the skin, bone, viscera, central nervous system, and cardiovascular system.[1]

ICD-10CM CODES
A50	Congenital syphilis
A51.0	Primary genital syphilis
A51.1	Primary anal syphilis
A51.2	Primary syphilis of other sites
A51.3	Secondary syphilis of skin and mucous membranes
A51.4	Other secondary syphilis
A51.5	Early syphilis, latent
A51.9	Early syphilis, unspecified
A52	Late syphilis
A52.0	Cardiovascular and cerebrovascular syphilis
A52.1	Symptomatic neurosyphilis
A52.2	Asymptomatic neurosyphilis
A52.3	Neurosyphilis, unspecified
A52.8	Late syphilis, latent
A52.9	Late syphilis, unspecified
A53.9	Syphilis, unspecified

EPIDEMIOLOGY & DEMOGRAPHICS

- Most diagnosed in people 20 to 30 yr old in urban areas and among people of lower socioeconomic status.
- Rates reached historic lows in the U.S. in 2000 but began increasing in 2001 with a continued increase observed. The number of cases reported to the U.S. Centers for Disease Control and Prevention (CDC) increased by 71% from 2014 to 2018, with men accounting for 85% of all cases. Additionally, rates are disproportionately higher among African American and Hispanic men and women, along with men who have sex with men (MSM). Rates of primary and secondary syphilis among women more than doubled between 2014 and 2018, and congenital syphilis rates are also increasing secondary to this.[2,3]
- Cases of congenital syphilis increased by 754.8% from 2012 to 2021. Currently 1 in every 1300 live births is affected.[4]

PHYSICAL FINDINGS & CLINICAL PRESENTATION

PRIMARY SYPHILIS:[1]
- Characteristic lesion is a painless chancre on genitalia, most commonly on the penis, cervix, or vagina (Figs. E1 and E2); mouth; or anus.
- May appear 3 days to 12 wk with median around 3 wk postexposure. May resolve without treatment within 6 wk.

SECONDARY SYPHILIS:[1]
- Bacteremia, also called spirochetemia, is associated with generalized lymphadenopathy and a characteristic maculopapular rash, including the palms, soles, trunk, and mucous membranes. Constitutional, flulike symptoms may also occur, as well as mild disturbances of multiple organ systems. Typically occurs 4 to 6 wk after appearance of chancre and can resolve within 1 wk to 12 mo even without treatment. Of note, there can be relapsing episodes up to 5 yr after the initial episode.
  - 60% to 80% have maculopapular lesions on palms and soles (Fig. E3).
  - 21% to 58% have mucocutaneous or mucosal lesions (pharyngitis, tonsillitis, "mucous patch" lesion on oral and genital mucosa).
  - Condylomata lata intertriginous papules (raised, gray-white lesions) form at areas of friction and moisture, such as the vulva (Fig. E4).

LATENT SYPHILIS—EARLY VS. LATE LATENT:[1]
- Generally asymptomatic, can occur between 1 and 30 yr after a primary infection. Early latent applies to relapses that occur within 1 yr, whereas late latent occurs more than 1 yr after acquisition.
- Seroreactivity is seen without other evidence of primary or secondary disease. Without treatment, one third will progress to tertiary syphilis.

TERTIARY SYPHILIS:[1]
- One half of patients with tertiary syphilis have late benign syphilis characterized by gummas (nodular, ulcerative lesions) that can involve the skin, mucous membranes, skeletal system, and viscera.
- One fourth of patients with tertiary syphilis will have manifestations of cardiovascular syphilis, including aortitis, aneurysm, or aortic regurgitation.
- Manifestations of the central nervous system (CNS); "neurosyphilis," which may be asymptomatic or symptomatic; tabes dorsalis; meningovascular syphilis; general paralysis; or insanity may occur.
- Manifestations of the eye, "ocular syphilis," which can affect any part of the eye, with posterior uveitis being the most common, iritis, choroidoretinitis, and leukoplakia may also occur. The Argyll Robertson pupil, a pupil that does not react to light but accommodates, is pathognomonic of tertiary syphilis.

ETIOLOGY

- Treponema pallidum, a spirochete
- Spread by sexual intercourse or by intrauterine transfer
- Congenital syphilis usually results from transplacental passage of *T. pallidum* to the fetus during disseminated maternal infection. Less frequently neonatal infection occurs through exposure to syphilitic genital lesions at the time of delivery.[4]

DIAGNOSIS

DIFFERENTIAL DIAGNOSIS

Other genitoulcerative diseases such as herpes or chancroid (Table 1)

WORKUP

Essentials of a proper sexual history are summarized in Table 2.
- Confirmation is primarily through laboratory diagnosis
- Culture of lesions
- Serologic testing (see "Laboratory Tests")
- Cerebrospinal fluid (CSF) testing

LABORATORY TESTS

- Dark-field microscopy of fluid from lesion to look for treponeme is the definitive method for diagnosis of early syphilis. Typically done if a chancre is cultured. It is then sent to the lab for dark-field microscopy.
- Serologic testing:
  1. Nontreponemal tests are sensitive to disease: Venereal Disease Research Laboratory (VDRL) or rapid plasma reagin (RPR).
  2. Treponemal tests are specific to disease: Fluorescent treponemal antibody absorbed (FTA-ABS) tests, the *T. pallidum* passive particle agglutination (TP-PA) assay, various enzyme immunoassays (EIAs), chemiluminescence immunoassays, immunoblots, or rapid treponemal assays.
  3. Antibody titers are used to assess for response to treatment and for reinfection in previously treated patients.
- Screening methods:
  1. Most traditional and most used include screening with nontreponemal tests (sensitive: VDRL, RPR), with confirmation using the treponemal tests (specific: FTA-ABS, TP-PA).
- Lumbar puncture (LP) is used for CSF-VDRL in patients with evidence of latent syphilis (good specificity, poor sensitivity). If negative with high suspicion, can also perform a CSF FTA-ABS (good sensitivity, less specificity). When reactive in the absence of substantial contamination of CSF with blood, it is considered diagnostic of neurosyphilis. The CDC indications for LP are not commonly used, but are needed in cases of neurologic symptoms, treatment failure, any eye or ear involvement, or evidence of active syphilis (aortitis, gumma, iritis).
- HIV testing in all patients.

TREATMENT[5] (BOX 1)

ACUTE GENERAL Rx

- Primary, secondary, early latent:
  1. Penicillin G benzathine 2.4 million U intramuscularly (IM) once.
  2. Infants and children: Benzathine penicillin G 50,000 units/kg IM, up to the adult dose of 2.4 million units in a single dose.
  3. Nonpregnant penicillin-allergic patients: Doxycycline 100 mg bid × 14 days. For pregnancy, patients are admitted as an inpatient and desensitized from penicillin allergy and then are treated with penicillin G once.
  4. Alternative regimens (contraindicated in MSM, persons with HIV, or pregnant women):
     a. Azithromycin 2 g by mouth (PO) × 1 dose

TABLE 1 Genital Ulcer Disease

Disease	Lesions	Lymphadenopathy	Systemic Symptoms
Primary syphilis	**Painless,** indurated, with a clean base, usually singular	Nontender, rubbery, nonsuppurative bilateral lymphadenopathy	None
Genital herpes	**Painful** vesicles, shallow, usually multiple	Tender, bilateral inguinal adenopathy	Present during primary infection
Chancroid	Tender papule, then **painful,** undermined purulent ulcer, single or multiple	Tender, regional, painful, suppurative nodes	None
Lymphogranuloma	Small, **painless** vesicle or papule progresses to an ulcer	Painful, matted, large nodes with fistulous tracts	Present after genital lesion heals

From Wein AJ et al: *Campbell-Walsh urology,* ed 11, Philadelphia, 2016, Elsevier.

TABLE 2 Essentials of the Sexual History

The Five Ps of the Sexual History	Essential Points to Cover
Partners	Last 3 mo who, how many, where from, risk factors in partners?
Practices	Is sexual contact vaginal, oral, anal and with whom? Are condoms used sometimes, always, never?
Protection	How is risk reduced (e.g., monogamy, condoms)?
Pregnancy	Plans around becoming or preventing pregnancy and details of contraception used
Past STIs	In patient and partners—what infections, when and how were they treated, how were they followed up? Screening since?

STIs, Sexually transmitted infections.
From Cameron P et al: *Textbook of adult emergency medicine,* ed 5, Edinburgh, 2019, Elsevier Australia.

b. Ceftriaxone 1 to 2 g IM or intravenous (IV) for 10 to 14 days
c. Tetracycline 500 mg PO qid for 14 days
d. Amoxicillin 3 g PO bid + probenecid 500 mg PO bid for 14 days

- Late latent syphilis, tertiary syphilis (not neurosyphilis):
  1. Penicillin G benzathine 2.4 million U IM weekly × 3 wk
  2. Infants and children: Benzathine penicillin G 50,000 units/kg IM, up to the adult dose of 2.4 million units in a single dose
  3. Nonpregnant penicillin-allergic patients: Doxycycline 100 mg PO bid × 4 wk
- Neurosyphilis:
  1. Aqueous crystalline penicillin G 18 to 24 million U/day, administered as 3 to 4 million U IV q4h or continuous infusion for 10 to 14 days
  2. Alternative regimen: Procaine penicillin 2.4 million U IM/day plus probenecid 500 mg PO qid, both for 10 to 14 days
- Congenital syphilis:
  1. Aqueous crystalline penicillin G 50,000 U/kg/dose IV q12h × first 7 days of life and q8h after that for a total of 10 days OR procaine penicillin G 50,000 U/kg/dose IM/day × 10 days.

BOX 1 Centers for Disease Control and Prevention Recommended Treatment of Syphilis (2014)

Early syphilis (primary, secondary, and early latent syphilis of less than 1 yr in duration)
Recommended regimen: Benzathine penicillin G, 2.4 million U IM, one dose
Alternative regimen (penicillin-allergic nonpregnant patients): Doxycycline, 100 mg orally bid for 2 wk *or* tetracycline, 500 mg orally qid for 2 wk

Late latent syphilis (>1 yr in duration, gummas, and cardiovascular syphilis)
Recommended regimen: Benzathine penicillin G, 7.2 million U total, administered as three doses of 2.4 million U IM at 1-wk intervals
Alternative regimen (penicillin-allergic nonpregnant patients): Doxycycline 100 mg orally 2 times a day for 2 wk if <1 yr, otherwise, for 4 wk; *or* tetracycline, 500 mg orally qid for 2 wk if <1 yr; otherwise, for 4 wk

Neurosyphilis
Recommended regimen: Aqueous crystalline penicillin G, 18-24 million U daily, administered as 3-4 million U IV every 4 h, for 10-14 days
Alternative regimen: Procaine penicillin, 2.4 million U IM daily, for 10-14 days plus probenecid, 500 mg PO qid for 10-14 days

Syphilis in pregnancy
Recommended regimen: Penicillin regimen appropriate for stage of syphilis. Some experts recommend additional therapy (e.g., second dose of benzathine penicillin, 2.4 million U IM) 1 wk after the initial dose for those who have primary, secondary, or early latent syphilis
Alternative regimen (penicillin allergy): Pregnant women with a history of penicillin allergy should be skin-tested and desensitized

Syphilis in HIV-infected patients
Primary and secondary syphilis: Benzathine penicillin G, 2.4 million U IM. Some experts recommend additional treatments, such as three weekly doses of benzathine penicillin G. Penicillin-allergic patients should be desensitized and treated with penicillin
Latent syphilis (normal CSF examination): Benzathine penicillin G, 7.2 million U as three weekly doses of 2.4 million U each

Data from Workowski KA, Bolan GA, Centers for Disease Control and Prevention: Sexually transmitted diseases treatment guidelines, 2015. *MMWR Recomm Rep.* 2015;64(RR-03):1-137. In Gershenson DM et al: *Comprehensive gynecology,* ed 8, Philadelphia, 2022, Elsevier.

2. An algorithm for evaluation and treatment of infants born to mothers with reactive serologic tests for syphilis is illustrated in Fig. E5.

DISPOSITION

Repeat quantitative nontreponemal tests at 6 and 12 mo to ensure adequate treatment. For HIV-infected patients, repeat testing at 3, 6, 9, 12, and 24 mo. Pregnancy requires monthly tests until delivery.
- Findings indicating need for retreatment of syphilis and additional testing for HIV:
  1. If a fourfold increase in titer occurs and is sustained over testing performed >2 wk apart
  2. If initial high titer fails to drop by fourfold within a year for early syphilis or 24 mo for late syphilis

3. If signs persist or patient develops new signs of infection
- Because treatment failure may be the result of unrecognized CNS infection, CSF examination can be considered in such situations. For retreatment, weekly infusions of benzathine penicillin G 2.4 million units IM for 3 wk is recommended, unless CSF examination indicates that neurosyphilis is present.
- Pregnant women without a fourfold drop in titer by 6 mo compared to pretreatment titer need to be retreated. Inadequate treatment is likely if patient delivers fewer than 30 days after treatment or if titers are fourfold higher than pretreatment at delivery. Titers should be repeated monthly during pregnancy for those infected.
- Cases should be reported to local or state health department for referral, follow-up, and partner notification.

REFERRAL

- Pregnant and possible congenital syphilis
- Pregnant and allergic to penicillin who need to be desensitized for treatment
- Late latent syphilis with serious central nervous system, cardiovascular, or other organ system compromise

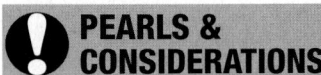

PEARLS & CONSIDERATIONS

- Jarisch-Herxheimer reaction (fever, myalgia, tachycardia, hypotension) may occur within 24 h of treatment.
- Fig. 6 illustrates the course of untreated syphilis. One third of untreated patients develop CNS and/or cardiovascular sequelae.
- Up to 80% of those treated during late stages remain seropositive indefinitely.
- Treponemal tests remain positive even after adequate therapy.
- Male circumcision does not decrease the incidence of syphilis (unlike HIV, herpes simplex virus 2 [HSV-2], and human papillomavirus [HPV] infection).
- Partner notification and treatment:
  1. Persons who are exposed within 90 days preceding the diagnosis of primary, secondary, or early latent syphilis in a sex partner might be infected even if seronegative; therefore, such persons should be treated presumptively.
  2. Persons who were exposed ≥90 days before the diagnosis of syphilis in a sex partner should be treated presumptively

if serologic test results are not available immediately and the opportunity for follow-up is uncertain.

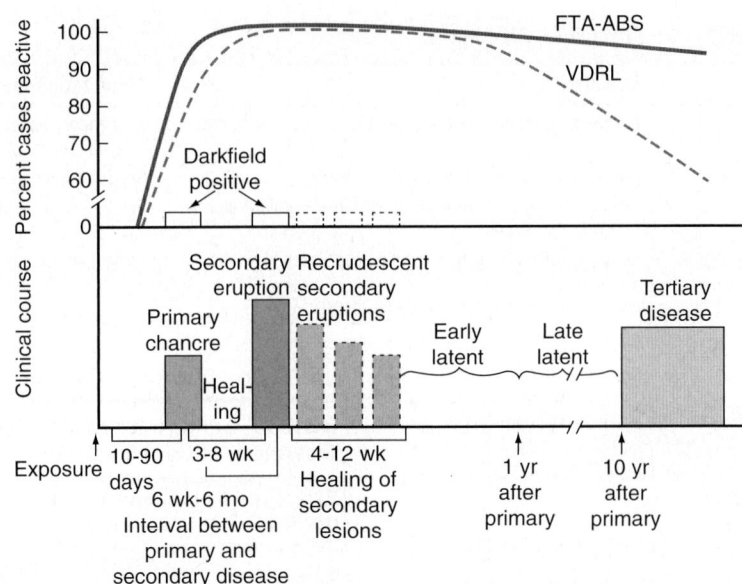

FIG. 6 The course of untreated syphilis. *FTA-ABS,* Fluorescent treponemal antibody absorption; *VDRL,* Venereal Disease Research Laboratory. (From Cherry JD et al: *Feigin and Cherry's textbook of pediatric infectious diseases,* ed 8, Philadelphia, 2019, Elsevier.)

REFERENCES

Available at eBooks.Health.Elsevier.com.

RELATED CONTENT

Syphilis (Patient Information)
Tabes Dorsalis (Related Key Topic)

AUTHORS: **LEAH SAYLOR, DO** and **STEVEN D. JOHNSON, MD**

BASIC INFORMATION

DEFINITION

Systemic lupus erythematosus (SLE) is a chronic inflammatory disorder characterized by autoantibody production responsible for antibody-mediated and immune complex deposition tissue damage. SLE involves multiple organ systems and has heterogeneous disease patterns. Relapses and remissions are a common feature.

SYNONYMS

SLE
Lupus

ICD-10CM CODES

M32	Systemic lupus erythematosus
M32.0	Drug-induced systemic lupus erythematosus
M32.8	Other forms of systemic lupus erythematosus
M32.9	Systemic lupus erythematosus, unspecified
M32.10	Systemic lupus erythematosus, organ or system involvement unspecified
M32.11	Endocarditis in systemic lupus erythematosus
M32.12	Pericarditis in systemic lupus erythematosus
M32.13	Lung involvement in systemic lupus erythematosus
M32.14	Glomerular disease in systemic lupus erythematosus
M32.15	Tubulo-interstitial nephropathy in systemic lupus erythematosus
M32.19	Other organ or system involvement in systemic lupus erythematosus

EPIDEMIOLOGY & DEMOGRAPHICS

INCIDENCE: Varies across gender, racial/ethnic groups, and geography, with a prevalence of 24 to 207 cases per 100,000 persons per yr. Prevalence is higher among African Americans, Asian Americans, and Hispanics. There are an estimated 350,000 people diagnosed with SLE in the U.S.[1,2]
PREDOMINANT SEX: Female:male ratio is 9:1. The ratio is highest in the reproductive age group, and about half of that in patients younger than 16 and older than 55.[3]
PREDOMINANT AGE: Mean age at diagnosis is 31.

PHYSICAL FINDINGS & CLINICAL PRESENTATION

- Constitutional: Unexplained fever, fatigue (80% to 100% patients), malaise (Table 1)
- Mucocutaneous lesions (more than 80% of patients):
  1. Acute (associated with + Ro antibody): Malar rash (Fig. E1) sparing nasolabial folds (acute cutaneous lupus); annular or papulosquamous rash (subacute cutaneous lupus)
  2. Chronic: Raised erythematous patches with subsequent edematous plaques and adherent scales (discoid cutaneous

lupus), lupus profundus, lupus tumidus; alopecia; photosensitivity; nasal or oropharyngeal ulcerations (classically painless, but discoid lesions [Fig. E2] may be painful); Raynaud phenomenon; leukocytoclastic vasculitis, chilblains; livedo reticularis or livedo racemosa (secondary to antiphospholipid antibody syndrome)
  3. Skin biopsy hallmark: Interface dermatitis
- Musculoskeletal (about 90% of lupus patients): Arthralgias are more common than true arthritis, but nonerosive deforming arthritis is not rare; myositis
- Cardiac: Pericardial rub (pericarditis) is most common; valvular heart disease (e.g., valve sclerosis, Libman-Sacks endocarditis); congestive heart failure, myocarditis, premature atherosclerotic heart disease
- Pulmonary: Pleuritis (most common), acute or chronic pneumonitis, diffuse alveolar hemorrhage, pulmonary hypertension
- Gastrointestinal: Dysphagia, mesenteric vasculitis, peritonitis, pancreatitis, hepatitis
- Neuropsychiatric: Headache, psychosis, seizure, acute confusion states, peripheral or cranial neuropathy, transverse myelitis, stroke (may be associated with antiphospholipid syndrome), cognitive dysfunction
- Hematologic (about 50% of lupus patients): Anemia (hemolytic, anemia of chronic disease, aplastic anemia), thrombocytopenia, leukopenia, lymphadenopathy, secondary antiphospholipid antibody syndrome
- Renal: Acute renal failure, proteinuria, nephritic syndrome, nephrotic syndrome

ETIOLOGY

Lupus may develop in genetically susceptible individuals, triggered by endogenous and exogenous factors. SLE susceptibility involves major histocompatibility complex (MHC) class II polymorphism with commonly observed association with *HLA-DR-2, DR3, DR4,* and *DR8.* SLE is also associated with inherited deficiencies of C1q, C2, C4a, and others. There is predilection for familial clustering of SLE with risk in monozygotic

twins—about 25% to 50%—and 5% in dizygotic twins. Environmental factors such as ultraviolet (UV) light, Epstein-Barr virus infection, and tobacco smoking may have a triggering role. Autoantibody production is the hallmark of disease development and diagnosis of SLE. Evidence supports the improper processing of nuclear proteins and nucleic acid from cell death. Impairments in neutrophil cell death via a process termed NET-osis (nuclear extracellular trap) contribute to the accumulation of nuclear debris. This, in turn, can lead to the presentation of self-nuclear material to plasmacytoid dendritic cells. Plasmacytoid dendritic cells propagate antibody and immune complex production via a type I interferon-dependent mechanism (Fig. E3).[4]

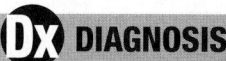 DIAGNOSIS

DIFFERENTIAL DIAGNOSIS

- Rheumatoid arthritis, mixed connective tissue disease, systemic vasculitis
- Neoplastic disorder
- Hematologic malignancy, paraneoplastic syndrome
- Systemic infection
- Other: Thrombotic thrombocytopenic purpura/hemolytic uremic syndrome, primary antiphospholipid antibody syndrome

EVALUATION

The diagnosis of SLE is clinical. The 2019 European League Against Rheumatism/American College of Rheumatology (ACR) classification criteria for SLE (Table 2) includes positive antinuclear antibody (ANA) at least once as obligatory entry criterion, followed by additive weighted criteria grouped in seven clinical (constitutional, hematologic, neuropsychiatric, mucocutaneous, serosal, musculoskeletal, renal), and three immunologic (antiphospholipid antibodies, complement proteins, SLE-specific antibodies) domains, and weighted from 2 to 10. Patients accumulating ≥10 points are classified

---

TABLE 1 Potential Clinical Manifestations of Systemic Lupus Erythematosus

Target Organ	Potential Clinical Manifestations
Constitutional	Fatigue, anorexia, weight loss, fever, lymphadenopathy
Musculoskeletal	Arthritis, myositis, arthralgias, myalgias, avascular necrosis, osteoporosis
Skin	Malar rash, discoid rash, photosensitive rash, cutaneous vasculitis, livedo reticularis, periungual capillary abnormalities, Raynaud phenomenon, alopecia, oral and nasal ulcers
Renal	Hypertension, proteinuria, hematuria, edema, nephrotic syndrome, renal failure
Cardiovascular	Pericarditis, myocarditis, conduction system abnormalities, Libman-Sacks endocarditis
Neurologic	Seizures, psychosis, cerebritis, stroke, transverse myelitis, depression, cognitive impairment, headaches, pseudotumor, peripheral neuropathy, chorea, optic neuritis, cranial nerve palsies
Pulmonary	Pleuritis, interstitial lung disease, pulmonary hemorrhage, pulmonary hypertension, pulmonary embolism
Hematologic	Immune-mediated cytopenias (hemolytic anemia, thrombocytopenia or leukopenia), anemia of chronic inflammation, hypercoagulability, thrombocytopenic thrombotic microangiopathy
Gastroenterology	Hepatosplenomegaly, pancreatitis, vasculitis affecting bowel, protein-losing enteropathy
Ocular	Retinal vasculitis, scleritis, episcleritis, papilledema

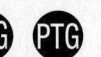

TABLE 2 The American College of Rheumatology/European League Against Rheumatism Classification Criteria for Systemic Lupus Erythematosus

Clinical			Immunologic		
Constitutional	Fever	2	aPL	aCL IgG or B2GP1 or LA	2
Cutaneous	Nonscarring alopecia	2	Complement	Low C3 or C4	3
	Oral ulcers	2		Low C3 + C4	4
	SCLE or discoid	4			
	ACLE	6			
Arthritis	Arthritis (synovitis in ≥2 joints or TTP and A.M. stiffness)	6	Antibodies	Anti-DNA	6
				Anti-Sm	6
Neurologic	Delirium	2			
	Psychosis	3			
	Seizure	5			
Serositis	Pleural/pericardial effusion	5			
	Acute pericarditis	6			
Hematologic	Leukopenia	3			
	Thrombocytopenia	4			
	AIHA	4			
Renal	UPCR >0.5	4			
	Class II or V	8			
	Class III or IV	10			

aCL, Anticardiolipin antibodies; *ACLE,* acute cutaneous lupus erythematosus; *AIHA,* autoimmune hemolytic anemia; *aPL,* antiphospholipid antibodies; *IgG,* immunoglobulin G; *SCLE,* subacute cutaneous lupus erythematosus; *Sm,* Smith; *TTP,* thrombotic thrombocytopenic purpura; *UPCR,* urine protein/creatinine ratio.
From Firestein GS et al: *Firestein & Kelley's textbook of rheumatology,* ed 11, Philadelphia, 2021, Elsevier.

as having systemic lupus. The new criteria has a sensitivity of 96.1% and specificity of 93.4%, compared with 82.8% sensitivity and 93.4% specificity of the ACR 1997 (see later) and 96.7% sensitivity and 83.7% specificity of the Systemic Lupus International Collaborating Clinics 2012 criteria.[5]
1997 ACR Criteria:
- Malar rash
- Discoid rash
- Photosensitivity (recurrence of unusual skin rash in sun-exposed areas)
- Oral or nasopharyngeal painless ulceration, observed by physician
- Arthritis (nonerosive)
- Serositis (pleuritis, pericarditis)
- Renal disorder (persistent proteinuria >0.5 g/day, or ≥3+ on dipstick if quantification not performed; cellular casts)
- Neurologic disorder (seizures, psychosis [in absence of offending drugs or metabolic derangement])
- Hematologic disorder:
  1. Hemolytic anemia with reticulocytosis
  2. Leukopenia (<4000/mm³ total on two or more occasions)
  3. Lymphopenia (<1500/mm³ on two or more occasions)
  4. Thrombocytopenia (<100,000/mm³ in the absence of offending drugs)
- Immunologic disorder:
  1. Anti–double-stranded DNA antibody (anti-dsDNA)
  2. Anti-Smith antibody (anti-Sm)
  3. Antiphospholipid antibodies (anticardiolipin immunoglobulin M [IgM] or IgG, lupus anticoagulant, antibeta-2 glycoprotein IgM or IgG, or false-positive fluorescent treponemal antibody absorption test or

Treponema pallidum immobilization for 6 mo)
- ANA: An abnormal titer of ANA by immunofluorescence or equivalent assay at any time in the absence of drugs known to be associated with drug-induced lupus syndrome
2012 SLICC Criteria: SLE can be diagnosed if:[6]
- Biopsy-proven nephritis with either ANA or anti-dsDNA antibodies *or*
- Patient satisfies four clinical criteria, requiring at least one clinical and at least one immunologic criterion
- Clinical criteria:
  1. Acute cutaneous lupus (malar rash, bullous lupus, toxic epidermal necrolysis, photosensitive lupus rash, maculopapular lupus, subacute cutaneous lupus)
  2. Chronic cutaneous lupus (discoid, hypertrophic verrucous, panniculitis, mucosal lupus, lupus tumidus, chilblains lupus, lichen planus)
  3. Oral ulcers or nasal ulcers
  4. Nonscarring alopecia
  5. Synovitis (more than two joints or inflammatory arthralgias of more than two joints)
  6. Serositis (pleurisy for more than 1 day, pericardial pain for more than 1 day)
  7. Renal (>500 mg proteinuria/24 h or red blood cell [RBC] casts)
  8. Neurologic (seizures, psychosis, mononeuritis multiplex, myelitis, peripheral or cranial neuropathy, acute confusion state)
  9. Hemolytic anemia
  10. Lymphopenia (<1000/mm³ at least once)
  11. Thrombocytopenia (<100,000/mm³ at least once)

- Immunologic criteria:
  1. ANA
  2. Anti-dsDNA (>2× laboratory reference range)
  3. Anti-Smith
  4. Antiphospholipid antibodies (lupus anticoagulant, rapid plasma reagin [RPR], anticardiolipin immunoglobulin [Ig]A, IgG, IgM, anti-β2 glycoprotein IgA, IgG, IgM)
  5. Low complement
  6. Direct Coombs test in the absence of hemolytic anemia
Definitions of SLE classification criteria are included in Table 3.

LABORATORY TESTS
Suggested initial laboratory evaluation of suspected SLE:
- ANA by immunofluorescence or similar high-quality method
  1. CBC with differential, blood urea nitrogen and serum creatinine, urinalysis, erythrocyte sedimentation rate (ESR), partial thromboplastin time (PTT), complements (C3, C4)
Consider additional laboratory testing in a patient with strong suspicion for systemic lupus:
- Anti-dsDNA, anti-Smith, anti-SSA, anti-SSB, anti-RNP antibodies. Table 4 summarizes autoantibodies and clinical significance in SLE
- Lupus anticoagulant, RPR, anticardiolipin antibodies, anti-beta-2 glycoprotein antibodies especially in patients with thrombotic events or recurrent miscarriages
- Urinalysis for RBC, cellular casts
- Random spot urine protein: Urine creatinine ratio, 24-h urine protein collection if proteinuria; >0.5 or >500 mg/24 h is abnormal, respectively. Evaluation of renal biopsy specimens in lupus nephritis (LN) is summarized in Table E5
- Direct Coombs test

IMAGING STUDIES
- Chest x-ray for evaluation of pulmonary involvement (pleural effusion, infiltrates)
- Electrocardiogram for chest pain
- Echocardiogram if murmur, evidence of new or unexplained congestive heart failure, or suspected pericarditis

℞ TREATMENT

NONPHARMACOLOGIC THERAPY
- Avoidance of sunlight and use of high-SPF sunscreen (>35)
- Screening and counseling for modifiable cardiovascular risk factors such as cigarette smoking, diet, exercise, cholesterol, and uncontrolled hypertension (HTN)
- Counseling for pregnancy planning for patients of childbearing age
- Calcium and vitamin D supplementation for prevention of early osteoporosis (see "Osteoporosis")[7]

TABLE 3 Definitions of SLE Classification Criteria 2019

Criteria	Definition
Antinuclear antibodies (ANA)	ANA at a titer of ≥1:80 on HEp-2 cells or an equivalent positive test at least once. Testing by immunofluorescence on HEp-2 cells or a solid-phase ANA screening immunoassay with at least equivalent performance is highly recommended.
Fever	Temperature >38.3° C (100.9° F)
Leukopenia	White blood cell count <4000/mm³
Thrombocytopenia	Platelet count <100,000/mm³
Autoimmune hemolysis	Evidence of hemolysis, such as reticulocytosis, low haptoglobin, elevated indirect bilirubin, elevated LDH, AND positive Coombs (direct antiglobulin) test
Delirium	Characterized by 1) change in consciousness or level of arousal with reduced ability to focus, 2) symptom development over hours to <2 days, 3) symptom fluctuation throughout the day, 4) either 4a) acute/subacute change in cognition (e.g., memory deficit or disorientation) or 4b) change in behavior, mood, or affect (e.g., restlessness, reversal of sleep/wake cycle)
Psychosis	Characterized by 1) delusions and/or hallucinations without insight and 2) absence of delirium
Seizure	Primary generalized seizure or partial/focal seizure
Nonscarring alopecia	Nonscarring alopecia observed by a clinician[†]
Oral ulcers	Oral ulcers observed by a clinician[†]
Subacute cutaneous OR discoid lupus	Subacute cutaneous lupus erythematosus observed by a clinician: [†]Annular or papulosquamous (psoriasiform) cutaneous eruption, usually photodistributed If skin biopsy is performed, typical changes must be present (interface vacuolar dermatitis consisting of a perivascular lymphohistiocytic infiltrate, often with dermal mucin noted) OR Discoid lupus erythematosus observed by a clinician:[†] Erythematous-violaceous cutaneous lesions with secondary changes of atrophic scarring, dyspigmentation, often follicular hyperkeratosis/plugging (scalp), leading to scarring alopecia on the scalp If skin biopsy is performed, typical changes must be present (interface vacuolar dermatitis consisting of a perivascular and/or lymphohistiocytic infiltrate of the appendages. In the scalp, follicular keratin plugs may be seen. In longstanding lesions, mucin deposition may be noted)
Acute cutaneous lupus	Malar rash or generalized maculopapular rash observed by a clinician.[†] If skin biopsy is performed, typical changes must be present (interface vacuolar dermatitis consisting of a perivascular lymphohistiocytic infiltrate, often with dermal mucin noted. Perivascular neutrophilic infiltrate may be present early in the course)
Pleural or pericardial effusion	Imaging evidence (such as ultrasound, x-ray, CT scan, MRI) of pleural or pericardial effusion, or both
Acute pericarditis	≥2 of 1) pericardial chest pain (typically sharp, worse with inspiration, improved by leaning forward), 2) pericardial rub, 3) EKG with new widespread ST elevation or PR depression, 4) new or worsened pericardial effusion on imaging (such as ultrasound, x-ray, CT scan, MRI)
Joint involvement	Either 1) synovitis involving two or more joints characterized by swelling or effusion, or 2) tenderness in two or more joints and at least 30 min of morning stiffness
Proteinuria >0.5 g/24 h	Proteinuria >0.5 g/24 h by 24-h urine or equivalent spot urine protein-to-creatinine ratio
Class II or V lupus nephritis on renal biopsy according to ISN/RPS 2003 classification	Class II: Mesangial proliferative lupus nephritis: Purely mesangial hypercellularity of any degree or mesangial matrix expansion by light microscopy, with mesangial immune deposit. A few isolated subepithelial or subendothelial deposits may be visible by immunofluorescence or electron microscopy, but not by light microscopy. Class V: Membranous lupus nephritis: Global or segmental subepithelial immune deposits or their morphologic sequelae by light microscopy and by immunofluorescence or electron microscopy, with or without mesangial alterations
Class III or IV lupus nephritis on renal biopsy according to ISN/RPS 2003 classification	Class III: Focal lupus nephritis: Active or inactive focal, segmental, or global endocapillary or extracapillary glomerulonephritis involving <50% of all glomeruli, typically with focal subendothelial immune deposits, with or without mesangial alterations Class IV: Diffuse lupus nephritis: Active or inactive diffuse, segmental, or global endocapillary or extracapillary glomerulonephritis involving ≥50% of all glomeruli, typically with diffuse subendothelial immune deposits, with or without mesangial alterations. This class includes cases with diffuse wire loop deposits but with little or no glomerular proliferation.
Positive antiphospholipid antibodies	Anticardiolipin antibodies (IgA, IgG, or IgM) at medium or high titer (>40 APL, GPL, or MPL, or >the 99th percentile) or positive anti-β₂GPI antibodies (IgA, IgG, or IgM) or positive lupus anticoagulant
Low C3 OR low C4	C3 OR C4 below the lower limit of normal
Low C3 AND low C4	Both C3 AND C4 below their lower limits of normal
Anti-dsDNA antibodies OR anti-Sm antibodies	Anti-dsDNA antibodies in an immunoassay with demonstrated ≥90% specificity for SLE against relevant disease controls OR anti-Sm antibodies

anti-β₂GPI, Anti-β₂-glycoprotein I; *anti-dsDNA*, anti-double-stranded DNA; *anti-Sm*, anti-Smith *CT*, computed tomography; *EKG*, electrocardiography; *Ig*, immunoglobulin; *ISN*, International Society of Nephrology; *LDH*, lactate dehydrogenase; *MRI*, magnetic resonance imaging; *RPS*, Renal Pathology Society; *SLE*, systemic lupus erythematosus.
[†]This may include physical examination or review of a photograph.

GENERAL Rx

- There are only four FDA-approved SLE medications: Aspirin, corticosteroids, hydroxychloroquine (1955), and belimumab (2011).
- Treatment should be targeted toward the involved organ(s). Recommended drugs for the treatment of SLE according to stratification of disease severity are described in Fig. 4. Indications for immunosuppressive therapy in SLE are summarized in Table 6.
- Limited and defined courses of corticosteroids are useful for a variety of SLE symptoms. Steroid therapy should be restricted to acute or subacute control of symptoms, due to the increased cardiovascular risk and increased organ damage associated with chronic steroid use. Recommended drug monitoring in SLE is summarized in Table 7.
- Consider checking G6PD in certain ethnic groups more predisposed to antimalarial-induced hemolytic anemia.
- Hydroxychloroquine has best evidence for reducing flares, organ damage, lipids,

TABLE 4 Autoantibodies and Clinical Significance in Systemic Lupus Erythematosus

Autoantibody	Prevalence in SLE (%)	Clinical Associations
Antinuclear Antibody		
Anti-dsDNA	60	95% specificity for SLE; fluctuates with disease activity; associated with glomerulonephritis
Anti-Smith	20-30	99% specificity for SLE; associated with anti-U1RNP antibodies
Anti-U1RNP	30	Antibody associated with mixed connective tissue disease and lower frequency of glomerulonephritis
Anti-Ro/SS-A	30	Associated with Sjögren syndrome, photosensitivity, SCLE, neonatal lupus, congenital heart block
Anti-La/SS-B	20	Associated with Sjögren syndrome, SCLE, neonatal lupus, congenital heart block, anti-Ro/SS-A
Antihistone	70	Also associated with drug-induced lupus
Antiphospholipid	30	Associated with arterial and venous thrombosis, pregnancy morbidity

SCLE, Subacute cutaneous lupus erythematosus; *SLE,* systemic lupus erythematosus.
From Firestein GS et al: *Firestein & Kelley's textbook of rheumatology,* ed 11, Philadelphia, 2021, Elsevier.

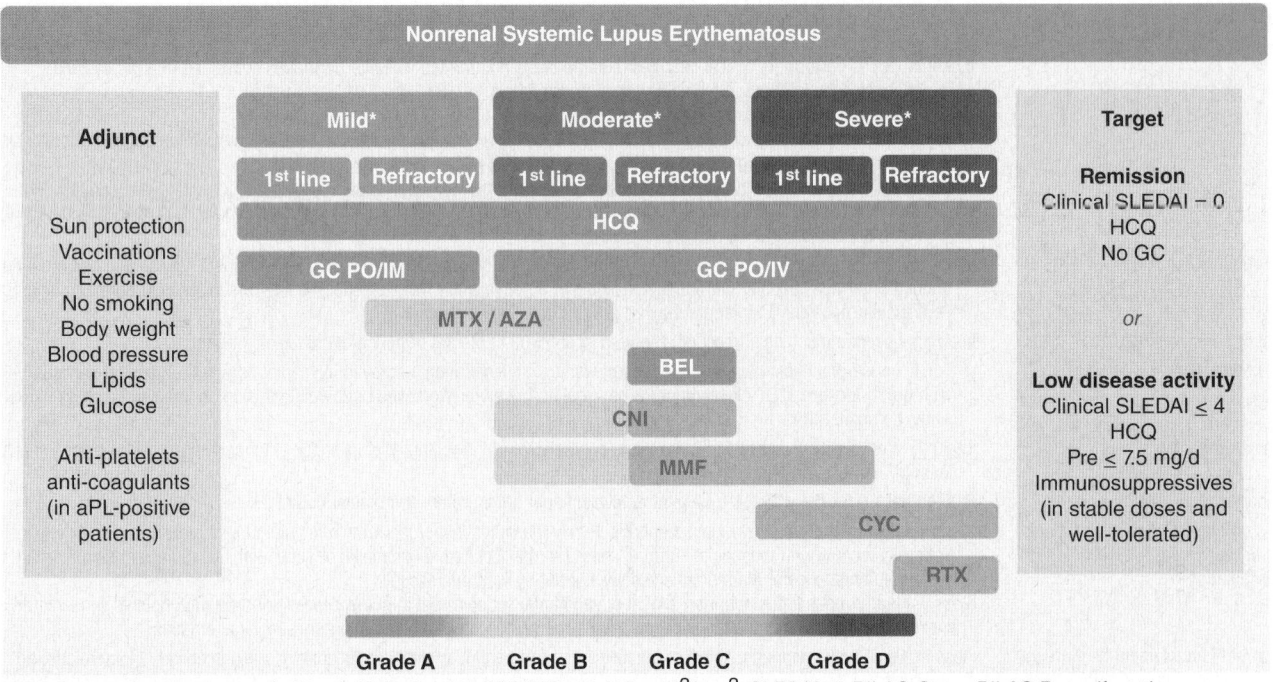

Mild: Constitutional symptoms/mild arthritis/rash $\leq$ 9% BSA/PLTs 50-100 $\times$ 10^3/mm^3; SLEDAI$\leq$6; BILAG C or $\leq$ BILAG B manifestation
Moderate: RA-like arthritis/rash 9-18% BSA/cutaneous vasculitis $\leq$ 18% BSA; PLTs 20-50$\times$10^3/mm^3/serositis; SLEDAI 7-12; $\geq$2 BILAG manifestations
Severe: major organ threatening disease (cerebritis, myelitis, pneumonitis, mesenteric vasculitis; thrombocytopenia with platelets <20$\times$10^3/mm^3; TTP-like disease or acute hemophagocytic syndrome; SLEDAI>12; $\geq$1 BILAG A manifestations)

FIG. 4 Recommended drugs for the treatment of SLE according to stratification of disease severity. The grading of recommendation/level of evidence refers to extrarenal manifestations. *aPL,* Antiphospholipid antibodies; *AZA,* azathioprine; *BEL,* belimumab; *CNI,* calcineurin inhibitors; *CYC,* cyclophosphamide; *GC,* glucocorticoids; *HCQ,* hydroxychloroquine; *IM,* intramuscular; *IV,* intravenous; *MMF,* mycophenolate mofetil; *MTX,* methotrexate; *PO,* per os; *Pre,* prednisone; *RTX,* rituximab; *SLEDAI,* Systemic Lupus Erythematosus Disease Activity Index. (From Firestein GS et al: *Firestein & Kelley's textbook of rheumatology,* ed 11, Philadelphia, 2021, Elsevier.)

thrombosis; improving survival; augmenting action of mycophenolate mofetil (MMF) in LN; and preventing seizures. Currently recommend not to exceed an oral dose of 5 mg/kg/day to decrease risk of retinal toxicity.[1]
• Methotrexate and azathioprine are used as steroid-sparing agents. Indications include cutaneous and joint involvement.[1]
• Joint pain and mild serositis are generally well controlled with NSAIDs or low-dose corticosteroids. Hydroxychloroquine and methotrexate are also effective for arthritis.

Belimumab does well for joint and cutaneous manifestations. Leflunomide and rituximab may be considered for refractory arthritis. Treatment approach for musculoskeletal features of SLE is summarized in Table 8.
• Cutaneous manifestations:
  1. Topical or intradermal corticosteroids are helpful for individual discoid lesions, especially in the scalp.
  2. Hydroxychloroquine alone or in combination with quinacrine and/or chloroquine can be considered for refractory skin disease.

3. Refractory cases may be treated with belimumab, MMF, dapsone, or combination treatment.[1,8]
4. Fig. 5 and Table E9 summarizes general management of cutaneous lesions in SLE.
• Hematologic manifestations:
  1. Corticosteroids are first-line therapy. Table E10 summarizes the treatment and main hematologic features of SLE.
  2. Azathioprine can be used for thrombocytopenia or hemolytic anemia. Check for TPMT genetic mutation before the first use.

TABLE 6 Indications for Immunosuppressive Therapy in Systemic Lupus Erythematosus

General Indications

Involvement of major organs or extensive involvement of non-major organs (skin) refractory to other agents, or both
Failure to respond to or inability to taper glucocorticoids to acceptable doses (<7.5 mg/day) for long-term use

Specific Organ Involvement

Renal

Proliferative or membranous nephritis, or mixed

Hematologic

Severe thrombocytopenia (platelets <20-30,000/mm³)
Thrombotic thrombocytopenic purpura-like syndrome
Severe autoimmune hemolytic or aplastic anemia (hemoglobin <8 g/dl) not responding to glucocorticoids

Pulmonary

Lupus pneumonitis and/or alveolar hemorrhage

Cardiac

Myocarditis with depressed left ventricular function, pericarditis with impending tamponade

Gastrointestinal

Abdominal vasculitis, peritonitis

Nervous System

Transverse myelitis, optic neuritis, psychosis refractory to glucocorticoids, mononeuritis multiplex, severe peripheral neuropathy, acute confusional state

From Firestein GS et al: *Firestein & Kelley's textbook of rheumatology*, ed 11, Philadelphia, 2021, Elsevier.

TABLE 7 Recommended Drug Monitoring in Systemic Lupus Erythematosus

Drug	Dosage	Dose Adjustment	Toxicities Requiring Monitoring	Baseline Evaluation	Laboratory Monitoring
Azathioprine	50-200 mg/day in 1-3 doses with food	↓ 25% if eGFR 10-30 ml/min; ↓ 50% if eGFR <10 ml/min	Myelosuppression, hepatotoxicity, lymphoproliferative diseases	CBC, platelets, Cr, AST or ALT	CBC and platelets every 2 wk, with changes in dosage; during monitoring every 1-3 mo
Mycophenolate mofetil	1-3 g/day in 2 divided doses with food	Maximum 1 g/day if eGFR <25 ml/min	Myelosuppression, hematotoxicity, infection	CBC, platelet, Cr, AST or ALT	CBCs and platelets every 1-2 wk with changes in dosage; during monitoring every 1-3 mo
Cyclophosphamide	50-150 mg/day in a single dose with breakfast. Increase fluid intake (at least 3 L water/day), empty bladder before bedtime	↓ 25% if eGFR 25-50 ml/min; ↓ 30%-50% if eGFR <25 ml/min; ↓ 25% if serum Bil 3.1-5 mg/dl or transaminases >3 times ULN	Myelosuppression, hemorrhagic cystitis, myeloproliferative disease, malignancies	CBC, platelet, Cr, AST or ALT, urinalysis	CBC with differential every 1-2 wk, with changes in dosage and then every 1-3 mo; keep WBC >4000/mm³ with dose adjustment; urinalysis for hematuria, AST or ALT every 3 mo; urinalysis for hematuria every 6-12 mo following cessation
Methotrexate	7.5-25 mg/wk in 1-3 doses with food or milk/water	↓ 50% if eGFR 10-50 ml/min; avoid use if eGFR <10 ml/min; avoid use in hepatic dysfunction (serum Bil 3.1-5 mg/dl or transaminases >3 times ULN)	Myelosuppression, hepatic fibrosis, pneumonitis	Chest radiograph, hepatitis B/C serology in high-risk patients, AST or ALT, Alb, ALP, Cr	CBC with platelet, AST, Alb, Cr every 1-3 mo
Cyclosporin A	100-400 mg/day in 2 doses at the same time every day with meal or between meals	Avoid in impaired renal function	Renal insufficiency, anemia, hypertension	CBC, Cr, uric acid, AST or ALT, Alb, ALP, blood pressure	Cr every 2 wk until dose is stable, then monthly; CBC, potassium, AST or ALT, Alb, and ALP every 1-3 mo; drug levels only with doses >3 mg/kg/day
Tacrolimus	1-4 mg/day in 2 doses at the same time every day	Cautious use in liver or renal insufficiency	Renal insufficiency, neurotoxicity, malignancy, infections, hyperkalemia	Cr, potassium, AST or ALT, glucose, blood pressure	Once a wk for the first 3-4 wk, then every 1-3 mo; monitor drug trough levels
Rituximab	1000 mg on day 1 and 15	None	HBV reactivation (rare)	CBC, Cr, AST or ALT, HBV serology (high-risk patients), TST	CBC and platelets

Note that placebo-controlled studies have failed to demonstrate efficacy in controlled clinical trials.

Alb, Serum albumin; *ALP,* alkaline phosphatase; *ALT,* alanine transaminase; *AST,* aspartate transaminase; *Bil,* bilirubin; *CBC,* complete blood cell count; *Cr,* serum creatinine; *eGFR,* estimated glomerular filtration rate; *HBV,* hepatitis B; *LFTs,* liver function tests; *MTX,* methotrexate; *TST,* tuberculin skin testing; *ULN,* upper limit of normal; *WBC,* white blood cell count.

From Firestein GS et al: *Firestein & Kelley's textbook of rheumatology*, ed 11, Philadelphia, 2021, Elsevier.

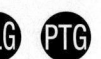

TABLE 8 Treatment Approach for Musculoskeletal Features of Systemic Lupus Erythematosus

	First-Line Therapy	Second-Line Therapy	Third-Line Therapy	Experimental Therapy
Arthritis	HCQ or CQ	MTX	Belimumab	Abatacept
	Low doses of glucocorticoids	Leflunomide	RTX	Sifalimumab
			Anti-TNF	
AVN	Avoid high doses of corticosteroid	Antiaggregation in aPL positivity	Core decompression	
			Percutaneous drilling	
			Arthroplasty	
Myositis	High-dose corticosteroid	MTX	IVIG	
		Azathioprine	RTX	

aPL, Antiphospholipid; *AVN,* avascular necrosis; *CQ,* chloroquine; *HCQ,* hydroxychloroquine; *IVIG,* intravenous immunoglobulin; *MTX,* methotrexate; *RTX,* rituximab; *TNF,* tumor necrosis factor.
From Hochberg MC et al: *Rheumatology,* ed 8, Philadelphia, 2023, Elsevier.

3. Intravenous immunoglobulin (IVIG) or rituximab may be considered for severe leukopenia, autoimmune hemolytic anemia, or autoimmune thrombocytopenia (Fig. E6).
- Central nervous system manifestations:
  1. Headaches are treated symptomatically. Most headaches will not be SLE-related and should be treated according to the underlying cause.
  2. Anticonvulsants and antipsychotics may be indicated.
  3. Standard therapy for other neuropsychiatric SLE symptoms is not established.
- Renal disease: The histologic classification of LN according to the International Society of Nephrology/Renal Pathology Society is summarized in Table E11. Severity of LN is described in Table E12. Treatment recommendations for LN are summarized in Table E13. (Class III, IV, or IV/V with cellular crescents LN; Table E14.) INDUCTION: 6-mo treatment.
  1. The typical treatment induction period is 6 mo. The use of intravenous cyclophosphamide (CYC) with corticosteroids given at monthly intervals is more effective in preserving renal function than is treatment with glucocorticoids alone. Low-dose "Euro-Lupus" protocol may be equally efficacious and less toxic for certain populations (e.g., Caucasians, Blacks) than high-dose regimen. MMF is considered equivalent to CYC based on high-quality studies, with better tolerability and fertility profile. MMF may be preferred in African Americans and Hispanics. MMF and azathioprine are good options for maintenance treatment.
  2. There is interest in and positive data for use of calcineurin inhibitors, such as tacrolimus, for treatment of LN. Newer and possibly less toxic voclosporin has entered phase III trial and when added to MMF showed better results in renal responses compared with MMF alone.[9]
- Severe nonrenal organ disease:
  1. Evidence from systematic randomized controlled trials for non-renal lupus treatment is comparatively limited.
  2. High-dose intravenous CYC is used as an induction treatment. Azathioprine or MMF may be used as maintenance.
  3. IVIG may be considered in severe disease especially when concomitant infection is present.
  4. Plasmapheresis or plasma exchange may be considered in critical situations: First-line therapy in Guillain-Barré syndrome, thrombotic thrombocytopenic purpura (TTP); second-line for SLE-related hemolytic anemia, cerebritis, and diffuse alveolar hemorrhage (DAH). Infectious complications are common.
- Fever/infection post-immunosuppressive therapy
  1. Immunosuppressive therapy can result in neutropenia and increased susceptibility to infection
  2. Fig. E7 illustrates an approach to SLE patients with fever and other signs of infection post-immunosuppressive therapy
- Therapy targeting B cells:
  1. Rituximab: Anti-CD20 monoclonal antibody. Randomized controlled trials for rituximab as an adjunct induction agent were negative in terms of both renal and nonrenal outcomes but were felt to be limited by study design. Some observational studies have shown efficacy in those who have failed other regimens.[1,10]
  2. Epratuzumab: An anti-CD22 agent. Studies initially showed positive data, but in July 2015 both phase III trials for SLE failed to meet their primary endpoint, and this medication is no longer studied.
  3. Belimumab: Decreases activation of B cells. When used in addition to standard therapy, patients on belimumab showed improvement in cutaneous and musculoskeletal disease. Belimumab-treated patients had decreased SLE activity, a reduced time to disease flare, and lower glucocorticoid exposure. Patients with central nervous system or serious kidney disease were excluded. There is interest in adding belimumab to standard LN regimen, but data from BLISS-LN are not yet available.[8,11]

4. Abatacept: Downregulates T-cell activation. Data are limited regarding improvement in arthritis, fatigue, sleep if added to routine therapy. Negative data as adjunct agent for lupus arthritis when added to MMF or CYC. Shows limited positive efficacy in patients refractory to other treatments.[1]
5. Interferon therapy: Interferon α (INFα) has been linked to increased disease activity in SLE. INFα blocking therapies are in phase II clinical trials. Sifalimumab, a monoclonal antibody against INFα, reduced moderate to severe mucocutaneous involvement in SLE and decreased active joint count and fatigue scores in preliminary data analysis. Development of sifalimumab has been terminated in favor of anifrolumab, a similar INFα blocking agent. The TULIP-1 study of that molecule did not meet response criteria based on score used in the BLISS trial. TULIP-2 used BICLA as a response measure and showed statistically significant improvement compared to placebo. The phase III trial is ongoing.[12,13]
6. There is continuous interest in studying B-cell and interferon-based treatment, but no FDA approved treatment, other than noted earlier, is currently used clinically.
7. Novel potential targeted treatment approaches may include blocking interleukin-17 (IL-17), IL-12/23, and JAK inhibitors (early data for 4-mg baricitinib showed positive results). Research remains very active and ongoing to find new therapeutic targets.[14,15]
- Recommended assessment and monitoring of patients with SLE with nonrenal, noncentral nervous system manifestations are summarized in Box 1.
- SLE in pregnancy (Table E15): Pregnancy in the setting of SLE is associated with a higher risk of complications compared to healthy women (preterm labor, unplanned cesarean delivery, fetal growth restriction, preeclampsia, and eclampsia). Ideally, conception should be attempted in a state of disease remission or stability. If pregnancy occurs during a period of disease relapse, medications need to be adjusted for maternal and fetal safety. Mothers with active SLE should be tested for anti-Ro/SSA and anti-La/SSB antibodies once before or early in pregnancy, due to their associated increase in risk for neonatal lupus and congenital heart block.[16]
  1. Recommended during pregnancy: Hydroxychloroquine, low-dose aspirin, antihypertensives (methyldopa, labetalol, nifedipine)
  2. Selective use allowed during pregnancy: NSAIDs, glucocorticoids, azathioprine, cyclosporine, tacrolimus, biologics
  3. Contraindicated: Cyclophosphamide, mycophenolate mofetil, methotrexate, leflunomide

DISPOSITION
- Most patients with SLE experience remissions and exacerbations.

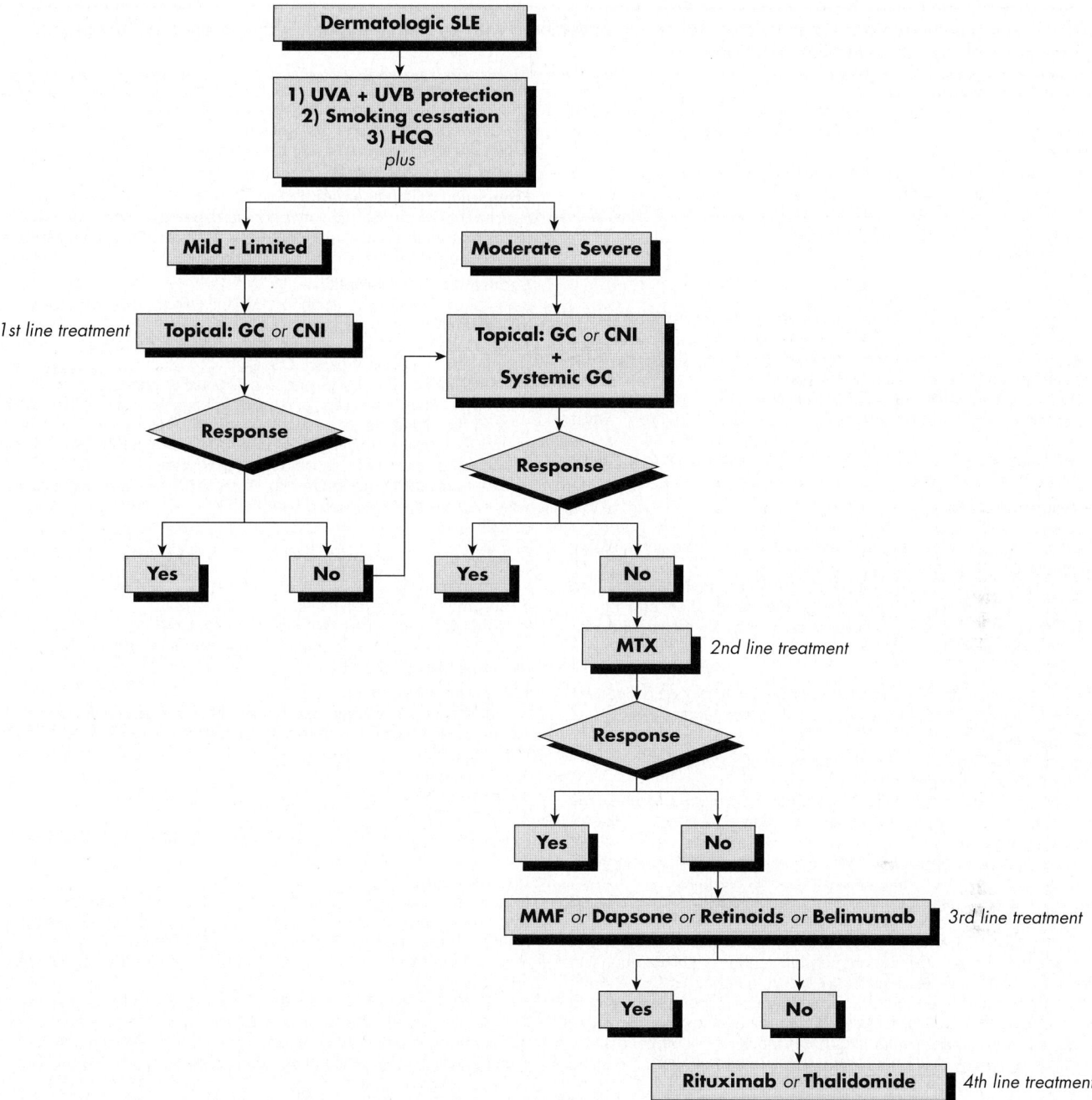

FIG. 5 Suggested algorithm for the management of cutaneous manifestations in systemic lupus erythematosus (SLE). *CNI,* Calcineurin inhibitors; *GC,* glucocorticoids; *HCQ,* hydroxychloroquine; *MMF,* mycophenolate mofetil; *MTX,* methotrexate; *UVA/UVB,* ultraviolet A/B. (From Firestein GS et al: *Firestein & Kelley's textbook of rheumatology,* ed 11, Philadelphia, 2021, Elsevier.)

- 5-yr survival rate has improved to more than 90% in patients with newly diagnosed SLE since the advent of potent immunosuppressive therapy. The 15-yr survival rate is now 85%.[3]
- Early death related to SLE activity and infections; late death due to cardiovascular disease.
- LN progression rate to end-stage renal disease (ESRD) is 10% to 30% within 15 yr.
- African Americans, Asian Americans, and Hispanic Americans in general have a worse prognosis. The leading cause of death in SLE patients in developed countries is premature atherosclerosis. The quality of life for many

SLE patients is poor due to fatigue, chronic pain, and cognitive impairment.[2]

REFERRAL
- Rheumatology consultation for all patients with SLE
- Hematology consultation for patients with significant hematologic abnormalities (e.g., severe hemolytic anemia or thrombocytopenia)
- Nephrology consultation in patients with proteinuria and/or suspected renal involvement
- Dermatology consultation for patients with unexplained or unusual skin rash

- Cardiology consultation for patients with lupus carditis, arrhythmias
- Ophthalmology referral for all patients on hydroxychloroquine and chloroquine

PEARLS & CONSIDERATIONS

- Arthritis in SLE often does not present with prolonged morning stiffness and is not erosive on x-rays; reversible joint deformities in lupus are termed Jaccoud arthropathy.

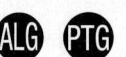
BOX 1 Recommended Assessment and Monitoring of Patients with Systemic Lupus Erythematosus With Nonrenal, Noncentral Nervous System Manifestations

Patient General Assessment
In addition to the standard care of patients without lupus of the same age and sex, the assessment of patients with SLE must include the evaluation of:
- Disease activity by a validated index at each visit
- Organ damage annually
- General quality of life by patient history and/or by a 0-10 VAS (patient global score) at each visit
- Comorbidities
- Drug toxicity

Cardiovascular Risk Factors
At baseline and during follow-up at least once a year:
- Assess smoking, vascular events (cerebral and cardiovascular), physical activity, oral contraceptives, hormonal therapies, and family history of cardiovascular disease
- Perform blood tests: Blood cholesterol, glucose
- Examine for blood pressure and BMI (and/or waist circumference)
- NB: Some patients may need more frequent follow-up (e.g., those taking glucocorticoids).

Osteoporosis Risk
All patients with SLE:
- Should be assessed for adequate calcium and vitamin D intake, regular exercise, and smoking habits
- Should be screened and followed for osteoporosis according to existing guidelines (1) for postmenopausal women and (2) for patients taking glucocorticoids or on any other medication that may reduce BMD

Cancer Risk
Cancer screening is recommended according to the guidelines for the general population, including cervical smear tests.

Infection Risk
Screening: Patients with SLE should be screened for:
- HIV based on the patient's risk factors
- HCV and HBV based on the patient's risk factors, particularly before immunosuppressive drugs including high-dose glucocorticoids are given
- Tuberculosis, according to local guidelines, especially before IS drugs including high-dose glucocorticoids are given
- CMV testing should be considered during treatment in selected patients.
Vaccination: Patients with SLE are at high risk of infections, and prevention should be recommended. The administration of inactivated vaccines (especially flu and pneumococcus), following CDC guidelines for patients who are immunosuppressed, should be encouraged strongly in patients with SLE who take IS drugs, preferably administered when the SLE is inactive. For other vaccinations, an individual risk–benefit analysis is recommended.

Monitoring: At follow-up visits, continuous assessment of the risk of infection by taking into consideration the presence of:
- Severe neutropenia (<500 cells/mm^3)
- Severe lymphopenia (<500 cells/mm^3)
- Low IgG (<500 mg/dl)

Frequency of Assessments
In patients with no activity, no damage, and no comorbidity, assessments are recommended every 6-12 mo. During these visits, preventive measures should be emphasized.

Laboratory Assessment
It is recommended to monitor the following autoantibodies and complement:
- At baseline: ANA, anti-dsDNA, anti-Ro, anti-La, anti-RNP, anti-Sm, antiphospholipid, C3, C4
- Reevaluation of aPLs in previously negative patients before pregnancy, surgery, transplant, and use of estrogen-containing treatments or in the presence of a new neurologic or vascular event; anti-Ro and anti-La antibodies before pregnancy; anti-dsDNA/C3 C4 may support evidence of disease activity or remission
Other laboratory assessments. At 6- to 12-mo intervals, patients with inactive disease should have:
- CBC
- ESR
- CRP
- Serum albumin
- Serum creatinine (or eGFR)
- Urinalysis and urine protein-to-creatinine ratio
NB: If a patient is on a specific drug treatment, monitoring for that drug is required as well

Mucocutaneous Involvement
Mucocutaneous lesions should be characterized, according to existing classification systems, as to whether they may be:
- LE specific
- LE nonspecific
- LE mimickers
- Drug-related
Lesions should be assessed for activity and damage using validated indices (e.g., CLASI).

Eye Assessment
In patients treated with glucocorticoids or antimalarials, a baseline eye examination is recommended according to standard guidelines. An eye examination during follow-up is recommended:
- In selected patients taking glucocorticoids (high risk of glaucoma or cataracts)
- In patients on antimalarial drugs. (Low risk: HCQ: No further testing is required until after 5 yr of baseline, and after the first 5 yr of treatment, eye assessment is recommended yearly; High risk: Eye assessment is recommended yearly, especially when using CQ.)

ANA, Antinuclear antibody; *anti-La,* anti-Sjögren syndrome type B (anti-SSB); *anti-RNP,* antinuclear ribonucleoprotein; *anti-Ro,* anti-Sjögren syndrome type A (SSA); *anti-Sm,* anti-Smith; *BMD,* bone mineral density; *BMI,* body mass index; *CBC,* complete blood count; *CDC,* Centers for Disease Control and Prevention; *CLASI,* cutaneous LE disease area and severity index; *CQ,* chloroquine; *CRP,* c-reactive protein; *dsDNA,* double-stranded deoxyribonucleic acid; *eGFR,* estimated glomerular filtration rate; *ESR,* erythrocyte sedimentation rate; *HBV,* hepatitis B virus; *HCQ,* hydroxychloroguine; *HCV,* hepatitis C vivrus; *HIV,* human immunodeficiency virus; *Ig,* immunoglobulin; *NB,* note well; *SLE,* systemic lupus erythematosus; *VAS,* visual analogue scale.
From Mosca M et al: European League Against Rheumatism recommendations for monitoring patients with systemic lupus erythematosus in clinical practice and in observational studies, *Ann Rheum Dis* 69:1269-1274, 2010. In Hochberg MC et al: *Rheumatology,* ed 8, Philadelphia, 2023, Elsevier.

- Myocardial infarction is 50 times more common in young female patients than in age-matched control groups.
- Prevent adverse effects of medications: Consider prophylaxis for infections and appropriate vaccinations, ensure yearly Pap and other cancer screening as clinically indicated; for patients taking CYC, intervention to preserve bladder and fertility should be considered; manage bone health.

- Based on small clinical data, a vitamin D level >40 may have modest reduction in disease activity; in addition, vitamin D may reduce risk of thrombosis, based on oncology research.[7]

REFERENCES
Available at eBooks.Health.Elsevier.com.

RELATED CONTENT
Systemic Lupus Erythematosus (Patient Information)
Discoid Lupus (Related Key Topic)
Renal Lupus (Related Key Topic)

AUTHOR: **VICTORIA KENT, BS**

BASIC INFORMATION

DEFINITION

Tardive dyskinesia (TD) is a medication-induced movement disorder associated with the prolonged use of dopamine receptor-blocking agents, including antipsychotic drugs and antiemetics. Patients exhibit involuntary rapid, repetitive, stereotypic movements that mostly involve the oral, lingual, trunk, and limb areas.

SYNONYMS

Orofacial dyskinesia
Tardive syndrome
TD

ICD-10CM CODE
G24.01 Drug induced subacute dyskinesia
DSM-5-TR CODE
333.85 Tardive dyskinesia

EPIDEMIOLOGY & DEMOGRAPHICS

- The disorder is caused by dopamine-blocking antipsychotics (e.g., haloperidol) and antiemetics (e.g., metoclopramide, prochlorperazine, and promethazine).
- The reported prevalence of TD can be variable; however, this is a serious clinical concern.[1]
- With first-generation antipsychotics, about 32% of patients are affected with TD, and ~5% are expected to develop TD with each year of antipsychotic treatment.[1,2]
- The incidence of TD with second-generation antipsychotics is about 21%. Thus, despite increasing use of these medications, TD remains a serious problem.[1,2]
- Risk increases with the duration of antipsychotic treatment, in female and in elderly patients, in patients with brain damage or dementia, with concurrent anticholinergic use, alcohol and substance use, comorbid diabetes, and in patients without schizophrenia spectrum diagnoses.[2]

PHYSICAL FINDINGS & CLINICAL PRESENTATION

- TD is classically described as a chronic condition of insidious onset, but symptoms are variable over time and may even improve despite continued antipsychotic therapy.
- TD classically involves uncontrollable stereotypic movements of the mouth and tongue, including lip smacking and puckering, tongue twisting and protrusion, and facial grimacing (Fig. 1).
- The involuntary mouth movements associated with TD may be suppressed by voluntary actions (e.g., putting food in the mouth, talking).
- TD may also involve slow, writhing movements of the trunk or choreoathetoid movements of the fingers and toes.
- Many patients may be unaware of or unbothered by the movements, but some find them disfiguring.
- A variant of the condition, named withdrawal TD or withdrawal dyskinesia, typically appears

with the reduction or withdrawal of the antipsychotic medications.
- Variants of TD with similar treatment include tardive dystonia (e.g., torticollis, blepharospasm), tardive myoclonus, tardive akathisia, and tardive tics.

ETIOLOGY

The pathophysiology of TD is not fully understood. The most commonly proposed mechanism suggests that exposure to dopamine receptor antagonists results in dopamine receptor hypersensitivity, upregulation, and/or an imbalance between dopamine type 1 (D1) and type 2 (D2) receptor-mediated effects in the basal ganglia. Damage to striatal cholinergic neurons and dysfunction of striatal GABAergic interneurons have also been implicated.

DIAGNOSIS

DIFFERENTIAL DIAGNOSIS

- Acute extrapyramidal symptoms (e.g., acute dystonic reaction, Parkinsonism, akathisia)
- Basal ganglia movement disorders (e.g., Huntington chorea, Tourette syndrome, levodopa-induced dyskinesia in Parkinson disease, Wilson disease, basal ganglia stroke and hemorrhage)
- Autoimmune diseases (Sydenham chorea, anti-N-methyl-D-aspartate [anti-NMDA] receptor encephalitis)
- Other causes of neurologic damage (e.g., lead or mercury toxicity, HIV, neurosyphilis, head injury, multiple sclerosis, neurodegeneration from illicit substances)
- Mannerisms associated with catatonia
- Hyperthyroidism-induced choreoathetosis
- Edentulous dyskinesias and improperly fitted dentures

- Rabbit syndrome (a rare variant of extrapyramidal symptoms with rapid vertical orofacial movements without tongue involvement); may respond to anticholinergic agents

WORKUP

TD is a clinical diagnosis of exclusion, based on complete neuropsychiatric and medication history showing the presence of typical dyskinetic involuntary movements, a history of at least 1 mo of ongoing or prior dopamine receptor-blocking agent exposure, and the exclusion of other causes. Abnormal Involuntary Movement Scale (AIMS) can be used to evaluate and monitor the severity of TD.

IMAGING STUDIES

Standard brain imaging is normal in patients with TD.

TREATMENT

ACUTE GENERAL Rx

- Treatment is predicated on prevention (Fig. 2): Limit the indications for antipsychotics; use the lowest effective dose; discontinue the drugs, when feasible; and monitor patients frequently. Anticholinergic medications may worsen symptoms.
- Switch to second-generation antipsychotics, if possible.

CHRONIC Rx

- If continued antipsychotic treatment is needed, switching to clozapine or quetiapine remains the preferred initial treatment if feasible, though evidence is insufficient.[3,4]
- Valbenazine and deutetrabenazine, inhibitors of the vesicular monoamine transporter 2 (VMAT2), are centrally acting synaptic dopamine

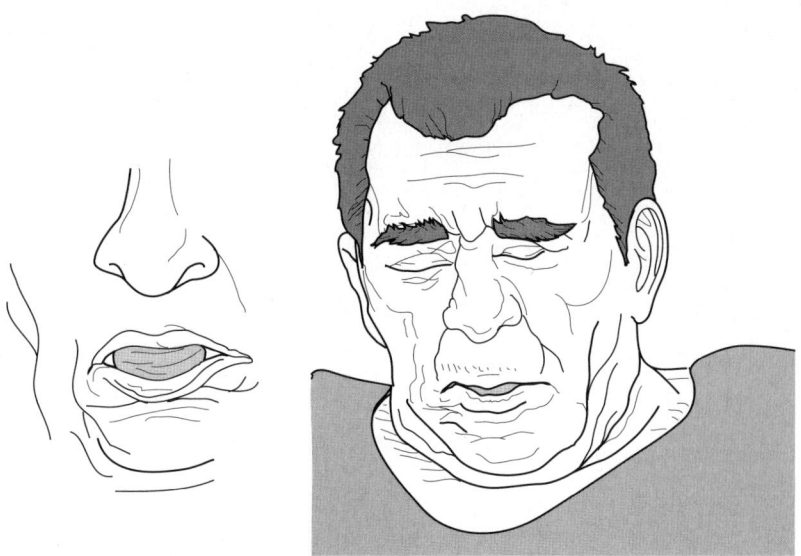

FIG. 1 The oral-buccal-lingual type of tardive dyskinesia consists of repetitive tongue darting, lip smacking, kissing, lip puckering, and chewing. Sometimes blepharospasm also is present. Tongue movements are not only prominent, but they may lead to tongue enlargement *(macroglossia)*. (From Kaufman DM et al: *Kaufman's clinical neurology for psychiatrists,* ed 9, Philadelphia, 2023, Elsevier.)

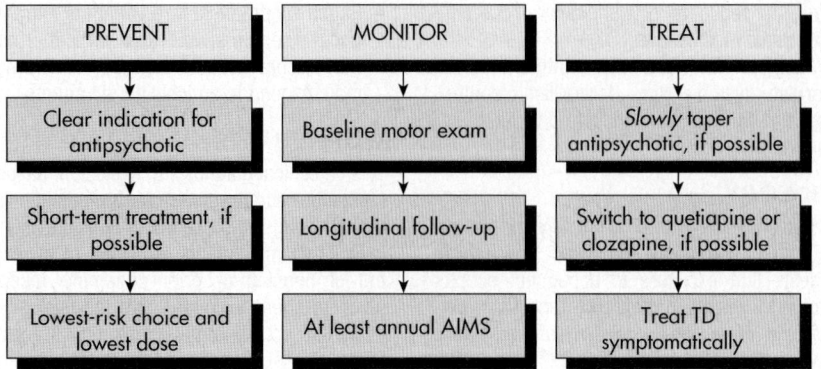

FIG. 2 Prevention and treatment of tardive dyskinesia *(TD)*. (From Stern TA: *Massachusetts General Hospital handbook of general hospital psychiatry,* ed 7, Philadelphia, 2018, Elsevier.)

depleters that are the first FDA-approved treatments for TD and are recommended as first-line treatment options when discontinuation of antipsychotic not indicated. An older VMAT2 inhibitor, tetrabenazine, may also improve TD and might be considered.[3-7]

- Clonazepam, vitamin E, vitamin B₆, botulinum toxin, amantadine, and ginkgo have limited evidence to improve TD.[3,4,8]
- For treatment-resistant, disabling TD, deep brain stimulation of internal globus pallidus seems to provide significant symptom reduction without exacerbation of psychiatric symptoms.[3]

- Using a higher dose of antipsychotic medication to mask TD is not considered a safe practice, as the risks might outweigh the benefits.[9]
- TD is potentially irreversible in nearly two thirds of patients; thus patients undergoing long-term treatment with dopamine receptor blocking agents require frequent monitoring and aggressive management at the onset of TD symptoms.

REFERRAL

Movement disorder specialist consultation if symptoms are severe

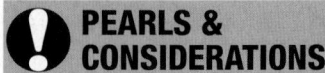 **PEARLS & CONSIDERATIONS**

- After removal of the causative medication, symptoms of tardive dyskinesia can take months to years to resolve or may become permanent (higher risk in elderly, female sex, prolonged use, and higher dose of causative medication).
- First-generation antipsychotics should be resumed to treat TD in the absence of active psychosis only as a last resort for persistent, disabling, and treatment-resistant TD.
- Avoid anticholinergic medications (e.g., benztropine) may exacerbate TD symptoms.
- Recent evidence suggests increased overall mortality among patients with TD, which highlights the need for referral for more aggressive specialized interventions.

REFERENCES

Available at eBooks.Health.Elsevier.com.

RELATED CONTENT

Tardive Dyskinesia (Patient Information)
Dyskinesia (Related Key Topic)

AUTHORS: **BAKTASH BABADI, MD, PhD** and **CAROL LIM, MD, MPH**

T

I

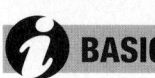 BASIC INFORMATION

DEFINITION

Tension-type headache (TTH) is a highly prevalent primary headache disorder. In contrast to migraine, it is not typically associated with nausea, vomiting, photophobia, or phonophobia.[1] Although previously thought to be caused by psychologic factors and muscle contraction, current thinking implicates neurobiologic mechanisms.

ICD-10CM CODES
G44.201 Tension-type headache, unspecified, intractable
G44.209 Tension-type headache, unspecified, not intractable

EPIDEMIOLOGY & DEMOGRAPHICS

Most common type of neurologic dysfunction and type of headache, representing 70% of all headaches presenting to primary care physicians. Yearly prevalence rates in the U.S. are more than 34,000 per 100,000 people. Women are slightly more affected than men.[2]

PHYSICAL FINDINGS & CLINICAL PRESENTATION

Headaches have an insidious progression, ranging from infrequent (<1 day per mo) to chronic (at least 180 days per yr).[1] Although considered a "featureless" headache disorder, either photophobia or phonophobia may still be present, but are typically more mild. Osmophobia, however, would not occur in tension headaches. In patients with migraine, some headaches may be less severe and suggestive of tension headaches.[3] Concurrent problems, such as anxiety, depression, and analgesic overuse, may aggravate the headaches. Patients may have pericranial tenderness to palpation on exam. The rest of the examination should be normal.

PATHOPHYSIOLOGY

- TTH is no longer thought to be due to either a psychologic problem or abnormal muscle contraction. Similar to migraine, TTH is likely a heterogeneous disorder with several possible pathophysiologic mechanisms, peripheral and central.[3]
- In episodic TTH, peripheral mechanisms may predominate, whereas in chronic TTH, central mechanisms are involved.

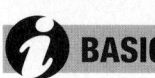 DIAGNOSIS

The International Headache Society criteria[1] for tension-type headache are as follows:
- At least 10 headaches
- Lasting from 30 min to 7 days
- Having at least two of the following features:
  1. Bilateral
  2. Pressure or tightening (nonpulsating) quality

  3. Mild or moderate intensity
  4. Not aggravated by routine physical activity such as walking or climbing stairs
- Both of the following:
  1. No nausea or vomiting
  2. No more than one of either photophobia or phonophobia
- Not better accounted for by another diagnosis

DIFFERENTIAL DIAGNOSIS[3]

- Migraine (would expect associated symptoms [i.e., nausea]; see Table 1 and "Migraine Headache" chapter)
- Cervicogenic headache
- Hypnic headache
- External compression headache
- Intracranial mass (may present with focal neurologic signs, seizures)
- Idiopathic intracranial hypertension (found more often in obese women of childbearing age)
- Medication overuse headache
- Secondary headache (e.g., obstructive sleep apnea, temporomandibular joint syndrome, hypo- or hyperthyroidism, systemic disease, drug side effects)
- Section II describes the differential diagnosis of headaches

WORKUP

- Routine testing is not needed; the diagnosis may be established clinically.
- Thorough history to identify any red flag features (see topic "Migraine Headache," SSNOOP5 mnemonic in "Differential Diagnosis") and physical examination (looking for papilledema) for all patients being evaluated for headache.
- Neuroimaging, preferably with contrast-enhanced MRI, should be performed only when red flag features are identified by history or unexplained neurologic findings are present on examination.
- Erythrocyte sedimentation rate and C-reactive protein in patients 50 yr of age and older to screen for giant cell arteritis.

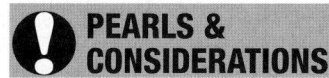 TREATMENT

Current evidence supports synergistic benefits of combined nonpharmacologic and pharmacologic

interventions. Nonpharmacologic therapy may include behavioral sleep modification, acupuncture, cognitive-behavioral therapy, relaxation training, and biofeedback.[4,5]

ACUTE Rx

- Simple analgesics (e.g., NSAID, acetaminophen).
- Combination analgesics containing caffeine may be used as second-line treatment, although use on more than 10 days per mo may lead to medication overuse headache.
- As with migraine headaches, narcotic- and barbiturate-containing analgesics should be avoided in tension-type headaches.

PREVENTIVE Rx

- Tricyclic antidepressants (e.g., amitriptyline 10 to 70 mg qhs) (first choice)
- Other options: Mirtazapine, selective serotonin reuptake inhibitors (SSRIs) or selective norepinephrine reuptake inhibitors (SNRIs) such as venlafaxine, and tizanidine[3]

DISPOSITION

For those with episodic or infrequent TTH, prognosis is generally favorable. Chronic TTH can be more difficult to treat as it is generally less responsive to therapeutic agents.[6]

REFERRAL

If red flags are present on history or exam or if the patient is not improving with treatment

PEARLS & CONSIDERATIONS

It is imperative to avoid overuse of caffeine as well as narcotic- and barbiturate-containing medications because of the risk of rebound headaches.

REFERENCES
Available at eBooks.Health.Elsevier.com.

RELATED CONTENT
Tension Headache (Patient Information)

AUTHOR: **ANJALI SUNDARAMOORTHY, DO**

TABLE 1 Comparison of Tension-Type and Migraine Headaches

	Tension-Type	Migraine
Location	Bilateral	Hemicranial*
Nature	Dull ache	Throbbing*
Severity	Slight–moderate	Moderate–severe
Associated symptoms	None	Nausea, hyperacusis, photophobia
Behavior	Continues working	Seeks seclusion
Effect of alcohol	Reduces headache	Worsens headache

*In approximately half of patients, at least at onset.
From Kaufman DM et al: *Kaufman's clinical neurology for psychiatrists*, ed 9, Philadelphia, 2023, Elsevier.

DEFINITION
Testicular cancers (TCs) are primordial germ cell cancers originating in the testis. They are the most common cancers in men between the ages of 15 and 39 yr.

SYNONYMS
TC
Testis tumor
Testicular neoplasms

ICD-10CM CODES
C62.00	Malignant neoplasm of unspecified undescended testis
C62.01	Malignant neoplasm of undescended right testis
C62.02	Malignant neoplasm of undescended left testis
C62.10	Malignant neoplasm of unspecified descended testis
C62.11	Malignant neoplasm of descended right testis
C62.12	Malignant neoplasm of descended left testis
D40.10	Neoplasm of uncertain behavior of unspecified testis
D40.11	Neoplasm of uncertain behavior of right testis
D40.12	Neoplasm of uncertain behavior of left testis

EPIDEMIOLOGY & DEMOGRAPHICS
INCIDENCE:
- There were an estimated 9190 new cases and 470 deaths associated with testicular cancer in the U.S. in 2023.[1]
- Globally, there were an estimated 74,400 new cases and 7300 deaths from testicular cancer in 2020.[2]
- In the U.S. the incidence is highest in non-Hispanic White men (7 per 100,000) followed by American Indians, Hispanics, Asian Americans, and least in African Americans (1.2 per 100,000).

PREVALENCE: TC accounts for 0.5% of all cancers in men.

RISK FACTORS:
- Cryptorchidism (undescended testes) is a major risk factor even if corrected by orchiopexy; however, treatment of undescended testis before puberty decreases the risk of testicular cancer from fivefold to twofold.
- Family history is an important risk factor (four to eight times as high in a brother of a person with testicular cancer and four to six times higher in sons of a father with testicular cancer).
- Other risk factors include genetic disorders (Down syndrome, testicular dysgenesis syndrome), Klinefelter syndrome, infertility, tobacco use, and White race (risk is highest among Whites and lowest among Blacks).

PHYSICAL FINDINGS & CLINICAL PRESENTATION
- TC typically presents as a painless testicular mass. Any mass within the testicle should be considered cancer until proven otherwise. It may be found by the patient on self-examination, or it may be found by a physician on a routine examination.
- Besides scrotal or testicular swelling, symptoms are typically absent unless the cancer has metastasized (10% of patients at diagnosis).[3,4] Occasionally a patient may report scrotal fullness or heaviness and approximately 10% of patients present with acute pain. Back pain secondary to enlarged retroperitoneal lymph nodes can occur. Gynecomastia from tumors that secrete beta-human chorionic gonadotropin (hCG) is found in 5% of men with testicular cancer.
- Testicular palpation should be performed with two hands. Transillumination may distinguish a solid mass (e.g., cancer) and a fluid-filled lesion (e.g., hydrocele or spermatocele). The mass is nontender; indeed, it is less sensitive than a normal testicle.

ETIOLOGY, CLASSIFICATION, & PATHOLOGY
CLASSIFICATION:
- TC can be classified as pure seminomas or nonseminomatous germ cell tumors (embryonal carcinoma, choriocarcinoma, yolk sac carcinoma, teratoma, or mixed germ cell tumors).
- Germ-cell neoplasia in situ (GCNIS) is a precursor lesion developing from gonocytes that have failed to mature. Approximately 90% of germ-cell tumors are associated with adjacent GCNIS, which carries a 50% risk of testicular cancer within 5 yr.[4] Table 1 summarizes germ cell tumors and serum markers.
- More than 80% of TC harbor an isochromosome of the short arm of chromosome 12, while the rest have amplification of 12p genetic material. Genes localized to the 12p region are associated with pluripotency, germ cell proliferation, and survival. After the development of GCNIS, subsequent steps occur that lead to malignant transformation, with a gain of 12p sequences possibly playing a major role.

- The incidence of various subtypes of TC is as below:

PATHOLOGY:

Cell Type	Frequency (%)
Seminoma	42
Embryonal cell carcinoma	26
Teratocarcinoma	26
Teratoma	5
Choriocarcinoma	1

- Other rare types:
  1. Yolk sac carcinoma
  2. Mixed germ cell tumors
  3. Carcinoid tumor
  4. Sertoli cell tumors
  5. Leydig cell tumors
  6. Lymphoma
  7. Metastatic cancer to the testes

STAGING
- The TNM staging system for TC is described in Table 2 and Table 3.
- The clinical stages consist of:
  1. Stage I, with tumor confined to the testis
  2. Stage II, with positive regional lymph nodes
  3. Stage III, with metastases
- Fig. 1 shows the clinical staging of TC.

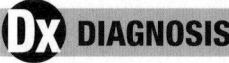 **DIAGNOSIS**

DIFFERENTIAL DIAGNOSIS
- Spermatocele
- Varicocele
- Hydrocele
- Epididymitis/orchitis
- Epidermoid cyst of the testicle
- Epididymis tumors
- Inguinal hernia
- Hematocele or testicular rupture
- Torsion of testicular appendage

WORKUP
Physical examination, laboratory tests, and imaging studies (Fig. 2). Immunohistochemical

---

TABLE 1 Germ Cell Tumors and Serum Markers

Histology	Marker Negative (%)	Elevated hCG Alone (%)	Elevated AFP Alone (%)
Seminoma	90	10 (usually <100 IU/ml)	0 (if +, by definition, NSGCT)
All NSGCTs	15	50-60	40
Embryonal		0	10-40
Yolk sac tumors		Rare	80-90 (alone or with elevated hCG)
Choriocarcinoma (or syncytiotrophoblast elements)		>90 (level can be very high)	0

AFP, α-Fetoprotein; *hCG*, human chorionic gonadotropin; *NSGCT*, nonseminoma germ cell tumor.
From Niederhuber JE: *Abeloff's clinical oncology*, ed 6, Philadelphia, 2020, Elsevier.

TABLE 2 TNM Staging for Testicular Cancer (AJCC 8th Edition Staging Cancer Manual)

pT Stage	Primary Tumor
pT$_X$	Primary tumor cannot be assessed
pT$_0$	No evidence of primary tumor
pT$_{is}$	Germ cell neoplasia in situ
pT$_1$	Tumor limited to testis (including rete testis invasion) without lymphovascular invasion pT$_{1a}$: Tumor smaller than 3 cm in size (seminoma only) pT$_{1b}$: Tumor 3 cm or larger in size (seminoma only)
pT$_2$	Tumor limited to testis (including rete testis invasion) with lymphovascular invasion OR tumor invading hilar soft tissue or epididymis or penetrating visceral mesothelial layer covering the external surface of tunica albuginea with or without lymphovascular invasion
pT$_3$	Tumor directly invades spermatic cord soft tissue with or without lymphovascular invasion
pT$_4$	Tumor invades scrotum with or without lymphovascular invasion
N Stage	**Regional Lymph Nodes**
N$_x$	Regional lymph nodes cannot be assessed
N$_0$	No regional lymph node metastasis
N$_1$	Metastasis with a lymph node mass 2 cm or smaller in greatest dimension OR multiple lymph nodes, none larger than 2 cm in greatest dimension
N$_2$	Metastasis with a lymph node mass larger than 2 cm but not larger than 5 cm in greatest dimension OR multiple lymph nodes, any one mass larger than 2 cm but not larger than 5 cm in greatest dimension
N$_3$	Metastasis with a lymph node mass larger than 5 cm in greatest dimension
M Stage	**Distant Metastasis**
M$_0$	No distant metastasis
M$_1$	Distant metastasis present M$_{1a}$: Nonretroperitoneal nodal or pulmonary metastases M$_{1b}$: Nonpulmonary visceral metastases
S	Serum Tumor Markers
S$_x$	Not available
S$_0$	Markers within normal levels
S$_1$	LDH $<1.5 \times$ N *and* hCG (mIU/ml) <5000 *and* AFP (ng/ml) <1000
S$_2$	LDH $1.5\text{-}10 \times$ N *or* hCG (mIU/ml) $5000\text{-}50,000$ *or* AFP (ng/ml) $1000\text{-}10,000$
S$_3$	LDH $>10 \times$ N *or* hCG (mIU/ml) $>50,000$ *or* AFP (ng/ml) $>10,000$

AJCC, American Joint Committee on Cancer; *TNM,* tumor, necrosis, metastases.

TABLE 3 AJCC Prognostic Stage Groupings

Stage	T	N	M	S
0	pT$_{is}$	N$_0$	M$_0$	S$_0$
I	pT$_{1-4}$	N$_0$	M$_0$	S$_X$
I$_A$	pT$_1$	N$_0$	M$_0$	S$_0$
I$_B$	pT$_{2-4}$	N$_0$	M$_0$	S$_0$
I$_S$	Any T	N$_0$	M$_0$	S$_{1-3}$
II	Any T	N$_{1-3}$	M$_0$	S$_X$
II$_A$	Any T	N$_1$	M$_0$	S$_0$-S$_1$
II$_B$	Any T	N$_2$	M$_0$	S$_0$-S$_1$
II$_C$	Any T	N$_3$	M$_0$	S$_0$-S$_1$
III	Any T	Any N	M$_1$	S$_X$
III$_A$	Any T	Any N	M$_{1a}$	S$_0$-S$_1$
III$_B$	Any T	Any N	M$_0$-M$_{1a}$	S$_2$
III$_C$	Any T	Any N	M$_0$-M$_{1a}$	S$_3$
	Any T	Any N	M$_{1b}$	Any S

AJCC, American Joint Committee on Cancer.

analysis of the testicular specimen is used to determine the histologic composition of the tumor. Staging involves computed tomography (CT) of chest, abdomen, and pelvis and measurement of beta subunit of human chorionic gonadotropins (β-hCG), alphafetoprotein (AFP), and lactate dehydrogenase (LDH).

LABORATORY TESTS

- Serum β-hCG is elevated in approximately 20% of patients with pure seminomas.
- Serum AFP is elevated in nonseminomas and never elevated in pure seminomas.
- One or both tumor markers will be elevated in 70% of cases of testicular cancer.
- Serum lactate LDH level is elevated with rapid turnover of malignant cells.
- Testicular biopsy is contraindicated.

IMAGING STUDIES

- Testicular ultrasound
- CT scan of chest, pelvis, and abdomen
- MRI of the brain in patients with neurologic symptoms
- PET scan is not recommended (frequent false positives)

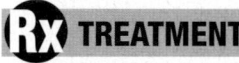 **TREATMENT**

- Fertility preservation is important but underutilized during the management of TC patients. Serum cryopreservation is the most cost-effective procedure for fertility preservation and should be offered to all patients before the start of therapy.
- The initial diagnostic procedure involves usually a radical inguinal orchiectomy, which is both diagnostic and therapeutic. Treatment recommendations are dependent on pathology (seminoma vs. nonseminoma), stage (I vs. II vs. III), and risk (good, intermediate, poor).
- Box E1 summarizes a treatment algorithm for TC.
- Seminoma:
  1. Stage I: Most patients (80% to 85%) are cured with orchiectomy. Adjuvant chemotherapy (one cycle of carboplatin) or radiation therapy (to the paraaortic lymph nodes) is standard and increases cure rates to >95%. Active post-orchiectomy surveillance is the routine approach in clinical practice in most cases. Recent randomized trials have shown that less intensive surveillance CT imaging strategies are noninferior to aggressive imaging strategies in this stage group. Long-term survival is the norm irrespective of the initial option chosen.
  2. Stage II$_A$ or II$_B$: Radiotherapy or combination chemotherapy (e.g., bleomycin, etoposide, and cisplatin [BEP] regimen).
  3. For stage II$_C$/III pure seminoma: Multiagent combination cisplatin-based chemotherapy for three to four cycles depending on risk stratification (low vs. intermediate). Residual disease post-chemotherapy is evaluated according to size and functional imaging (PET/CT scans) followed by options of resection.
- Nonseminoma:
  1. Stage I$_A$: Radical orchiectomy plus nerve-sparing retroperitoneal lymph node dissection (RPLND)

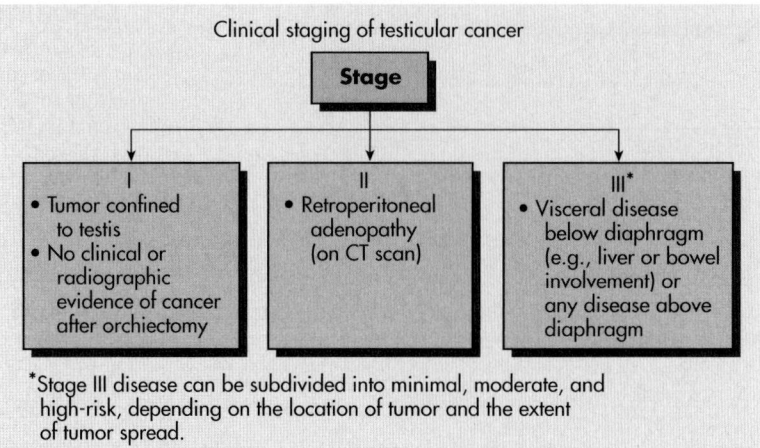

FIG. 1 **Clinical staging of testicular cancer.** The American Joint Committee on Cancer TNM staging system is less commonly used, because it is based upon histologic evaluation of the orchidectomy specimen and retroperitoneal periaortic lymph node dissection. Because the latter may not be performed in every patient, the clinical staging system is generally more practical. *CT,* Computed tomography; *TNM,* tumor, necrosis, metastases. (From Skarin AT: *Atlas of diagnostic oncology,* ed 4, St Louis, 2010, Mosby.)

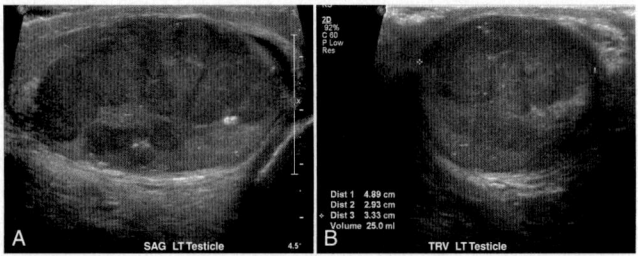

FIG. 2 **Seminoma in an 18-yr-old patient with painless left scrotal mass. A** and **B,** Sagittal and transverse sonograms of the left testis demonstrate a testicular volume of 25 ml, with a lobulated, heterogeneous, relatively hypoechoic mass occupying most of the testis with a thin rim of normal testis and a few tiny clusters of calcification, as well as multiple, tiny, brightly echoic speckles both inside and outside the mass. The tiny speckles represent microlithiasis. (From Rumack CM et al: *Diagnostic ultrasound,* ed 4, Philadelphia, 2011, Elsevier.)

2. Stage I$_B$: Same as stage I$_A$ plus two cycles of chemotherapy (bleomycin, etoposide, and cisplatin [BEP])
3. Stages II to III: Multiagent cisplatin-based chemotherapy regimens for three or four cycles depending on risk stratification (low/intermediate or high). RPLND is offered for residual lymph nodal disease after chemotherapy
- Relapsed disease:
  1. Salvage chemotherapy using multiagent regimens is offered. Active chemotherapy regimens include TIP (paclitaxel, ifosfamide, cisplatin) and VIP (vinblastine, ifosfamide, cisplatin) regimens.
  2. Chemotherapy-sensitive patients who have responded to salvage chemotherapy treatment are treated with high-dose chemotherapy followed by autologous stem cell transplantation (ASCT).
- Posttreatment surveillance for testicular cancer survivors (annually):
  1. Fertility assessment
  2. Physical examination and skin examination (increased risk of dysplastic nevi)

3. Testicular examination (3% to 4% risk of second testicular cancer)
4. Serum tumor markers (hCG, AFP)
5. Abdominal and pelvic CT every 3 to 4 mo for 2 yr, every 6 to 12 mo in third and fourth yr, and annually thereafter

DISPOSITION
- The overall cure rate for TC is >95% (80% for metastatic disease) with pure seminoma patients having a better prognosis. Prognosis can be determined by criteria established by the International Germ Cell Consensus Criteria (Table E4). Given these favorable outcomes, the U.S. Preventive Services Task Force recommends against screening asymptomatic men for testicular cancer.
- There is an increased risk for metabolic syndrome (insulin resistance, hypertension, dyslipidemia, abdominal obesity) after radiation or chemotherapy. Additionally, long-term effects on reproductive health, lower fertility, hearing impairment, neuropathy, and Raynaud phenomenon are long-term toxicities due to chemotherapy use.[5]

- Therapeutic radiation and chemotherapy are both risk factors for the development of solid and hematologic second malignant neoplasms (SMNs) in survivors. In a recent SEER analysis of 29,400 patients, the 30-yr cumulative incidences of solid-SMN after radiotherapy, chemotherapy, and surgery alone were 16.9%, 10.1%, and 8.8%, respectively.[6] Increased sevenfold excesses of acute myeloid leukemia were seen 1 to 10 yr after testicular cancer diagnosis. Risks for lymphoma and plasma cell dyscrasias were not elevated. Common reported cancers include those of the thyroid, kidney, pancreas, and stomach, as well as leukemia.

REFERENCES
Available at eBooks.Health.Elsevier.com.

RELATED CONTENT
Testicular Cancer (Patient Information)

AUTHOR: **BHARTI RATHORE, MD**

BASIC INFORMATION

DEFINITION[1-3]

Thoracic outlet syndrome (TOS) describes a condition producing upper extremity symptoms believed to result from neurovascular compression at the thoracic outlet (Fig. E1, Table 1). Three types are described on the basis of point of compression: (1) cervical rib and scalenus syndrome, in which abnormal scalene muscles or the presence of a cervical rib may cause compression; (2) costoclavicular syndrome, in which compression may occur under the clavicle; and (3) subcoracoid pectoralis minor syndrome, in which compression may occur in the subcoracoid area or retropectoralis minor area. The compression occurs in three anatomic structures: Arteries, veins, and nerves, and specific terminology is used to describe TOS depending on the predominantly affected structure: Arterial TOS, venous TOS, and neurogenic TOS.[1] TOS usually is caused by a combination of two factors: (1) having abnormal anatomy that creates compression in the thoracic outlet and (2) having some environmental factor such as injury at the thoracic outlet or excessive repetitive motion that predisposes to compression.

- Neurogenic TOS (nTOS): Caused by compression of brachial nerve plexus
- Arterial TOS (aTOS): Caused by subclavian artery compression and almost always associated with complete cervical rib or anomalous first rib
- Venous TOS (vTOS): Caused by compression of subclavian vein and may also occur in patients with chronic indwelling intravenous catheters

SYNONYM

TOS

ICD-10CM CODE
G54.0   Brachial plexus disorders

EPIDEMIOLOGY & DEMOGRAPHICS[2]

PREVALENCE: TOS is an uncommon disorder. Its prevalence varies from source to source, likely due to a lack of agreement on diagnostic criteria. Presence of cervical ribs occurs in 0.5% to 1% of the population (50% bilateral), but most are asymptomatic. Approximately 90% to 95% of all TOS disorders are neurogenic, and the remaining 5% to 10% are arterial or venous.

PREDOMINANT SEX: Females affected more often than males (ratio of 3.5:1).

PREDOMINANT AGE: TOS usually occurs in the third to fifth decades of life, although certain types occur in younger individuals.

PHYSICAL FINDINGS & CLINICAL PRESENTATION[2,4]

- Symptoms and signs are related to the degree of involvement of each of the various structures at the level of the first rib.
- True venous or arterial involvement is not common.
- Diagnosis is most often used in the consideration of neural pain affecting the arm, which suggests involvement of the brachial plexus.
  1. Arterial compression: Pallor, pain, paresthesias, diminished pulses, coolness, Raynaud phenomenon, digital gangrene, digital ischemia, supraclavicular bruit or mass, and stroke
  2. Venous compression: Edema, cyanosis and pain, thrombosis causing superficial venous dilation in the shoulder area
  3. Neurologic compression: Pain and/or paresthesia of neck, shoulder region, arm or hand, depending on the root involved; intrinsic weakness and diminished sensation on examination; occipital headache
  4. Possible supraclavicular tenderness
  5. Provocative tests:[5] Adson (Fig. E2), Wright (hyperabduction test where the strength of the radial pulse weakens as the arm is passively abducted and externally rotated), elevated arm stress test or EAST (Roos), upper limb tension test or ULTT (Elvey). May reproduce pain but are of disputed usefulness

ETIOLOGY[2,3]

- Congenital cervical rib or fibrous extension of cervical rib
- Abnormal scalene muscle insertion
- Drooping of shoulder girdle from generalized hypotonia or trauma
- Narrowed costoclavicular interval as a result of downward and backward pressure on shoulder (sometimes seen in individuals who carry heavy backpacks), poor posturing, pregnancy
- Acute venous thrombosis with exercise (effort thrombosis or Paget-Schroetter syndrome)
- Bony abnormalities of first rib
- Abnormal fibromuscular bands
- Malunion of clavicle fracture

DIAGNOSIS

DIFFERENTIAL DIAGNOSIS[5]

- Carpal tunnel syndrome
- Cervical radiculopathy
- Brachial neuritis
- Ulnar nerve compression (cubital tunnel syndrome)
- Complex regional pain syndrome
- Superior sulcus tumor
- Intrinsic shoulder dysfunction

WORKUP

Fig. E3 describes a diagnostic algorithm for thoracic outlet syndrome. Preliminary criteria for the clinical diagnosis of neurogenic thoracic outlet syndrome are summarized in Table 2. Except for venous or arterial pathology, no ancillary diagnostic tests are reliable for diagnostic confirmation.

IMAGING STUDIES[6]

- Electromyography and nerve conduction velocity studies to rule out carpal tunnel syndrome, cervical radiculopathy
- Doppler ultrasound for initial evaluation for arterial or venous thoracic outlet syndrome with provocative maneuvers
- Cervical spine radiographs to rule out cervical disk disease
- Chest x-ray examination to rule out lung tumor
- Computed tomography (CT) with intravenous (IV) contrast for detailed anatomic relationship of vascular structure to surrounding muscles and bones
- CT angiography or contrast-enhanced magnetic resonance angiography can be very useful in assessing vessel imaging while using provocative arm positions

---

TABLE 1 Sites and Structures Compressed in Thoracic Outlet Syndrome

Site	Description	Abnormalities	Structures Compressed
Sternal-costovertebral circle	This aperture can be narrowed by bony variations	• Cervical first rib • First rib • Long transverse process	• Subclavian artery • Subclavian vein • Brachial plexus
Scalene muscle triangle	The scalenus anterior and middle muscle insert on the first rib, creating a tunnel	• Scalenus anterior and middle	• Subclavian artery • Brachial plexus
First rib, clavicular space	The neurovascular structures lie above the rib and below the clavicle	• Costoclavicular ligament • Clavicle • First rib	• Subclavian vein • Subclavian artery • Brachial plexus
Behind the pectoralis minor muscle	The neurovascular structures travel to and from the arm behind this muscle	• Pectoralis minor • Costocoracoid ligament	• Subclavian vein • Subclavian artery • Brachial plexus

From Sellke FW et al: *Sabiston & Spencer surgery of the chest*, ed 9, Philadelphia, 2016, Elsevier.

TABLE 2 Preliminary Criteria for the Clinical Diagnosis of Neurogenic Thoracic Outlet Syndrome

Unilateral or bilateral upper extremity symptoms that:
- Extend beyond the distribution of a single cervical nerve root or peripheral nerve
- Have been present for at least 12 wk
- Have not been explained satisfactorily by another condition
- Meet at least one criterion in at least four of the following five categories:

1. Principal symptoms	1A. Pain in the neck, upper back, shoulder, arm, or hand
	1B. Numbness; paresthesias; or weakness in the arm, hand, or digits
2. Symptom characteristics	2A. Pain, paresthesias, or weakness exacerbated with elevated arm positions
	2B. Pain, paresthesias, or weakness exacerbated by prolonged or repetitive arm or hand use or by prolonged work on a keyboard or other repetitive strain
	2C. Pain or paresthesias radiate down the arm from the supraclavicular or infraclavicular space
3. Clinical history	3A. Symptoms began after occupational, recreational, or accidental injury of the head, neck, or upper extremity, including repetitive upper extremity strain or overuse activity
	3B. Previous clavicle or first rib fracture or known cervical rib(s)
	3C. Previous cervical spine or peripheral nerve surgery without sustained improvement
	3D. Previous conservative or surgical treatment for thoracic outlet syndrome
4. Physical examination	4A. Local tenderness on palpation over scalene triangle or subcoracoid space
	4B. Arm, hand, or digit paresthesias on palpation over scalene triangle or subcoracoid space
	4C. Weak handgrip, intrinsic muscles, or digit 5 or thenar or hypothenar atrophy
5. Provocative maneuvers	5A. Positive upper limb tension test (ULTT)
	5B. Positive 1- or 3-min elevated arm stress test (EAST)
	5C. Positive Adson test
	5D. Positive Wright test (or hyperabduction)

From Cameron JL, Cameron AM: *Current surgical therapy,* ed 12, Philadelphia, 2017, Elsevier.

- High-resolution ultrasound for visualization of ligaments in the thoracic outlet region that may lead to compression of neurovascular structures
- MRI with and without IV contrast for evaluation of neurogenic thoracic outlet syndrome
- Arteriography or venography (Fig. E4) can be used for dynamic studies while performing upper extremity maneuvers and also performing thrombolysis, if needed

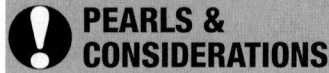 **TREATMENT**

ACUTE GENERAL Rx[2,3]
- Avoid weight gain
- Sling for pain relief
- Physical therapy modalities plus shoulder girdle–strengthening exercises

- Postural reeducation
- NSAIDs and other analgesics
- Muscle relaxants
- Muscle block with injection of local anesthetic agent or botulinum toxin A in anterior scalene (for diagnostic and therapeutic reasons, e.g., predicting response to surgical intervention)[7]

CHRONIC Rx[2,3]

Surgical treatment is indicated in the presence of the following:
- Symptomatic after failure of physical therapy
- With complications such as thrombosis, aneurysms
- With neurologic compressions
- With sympathetic cervical rib

Surgical options:
- Thoracic outlet decompression including cervical rib resection and anterior scalenectomy

- Thoracic sympathectomy
- Vascular reconstruction
- Catheter-directed thrombolysis or aspiration mechanical thrombectomy, with or without venous stenting, followed by thoracic outlet decompression and anticoagulation for deep vein thrombosis due to venous TOS

DISPOSITION[2,3,8]
- Nonsurgical treatment is often successful for patients with pain as the primary symptom.
- Nonsurgical management is initially recommended in neurogenic TOS. Operative management is often required in arterial TOS and venous TOS.
- Thoracic outlet decompression in neurogenic TOS can be effective in patients who fail conservative treatment.
- Complications of surgical treatment include transient dysesthesia, hematoma, pneumothorax, hemothorax, venous injury, arterial injuries, or brachial plexus injuries.

REFERRAL

For vascular surgery consultation when venous or arterial impairment is present

PEARLS & CONSIDERATIONS

COMMENTS
- True thoracic outlet syndrome is probably an uncommon condition with considerable disagreement regarding its frequency.
- Diagnosis is often used to describe a wide variety of clinical symptoms and should be modified by the affected structure such as nTOS, aTOS, and vTOS.

REFERENCES

Available at eBooks.Health.Elsevier.com.

RELATED CONTENT

Thoracic Outlet Syndrome (Patient Information)

AUTHORS: **ANNA ASTASHCHANKA, MD** and **PHILIPPE MONTGRAIN, MD**

Diseases and Disorders

I

BASIC INFORMATION

DEFINITION

Thrombocytosis is defined by an elevated platelet count (>450,000/ml) in peripheral blood. It is caused by overproduction of platelets (reactive thrombocytosis) or clonal expansion of megakaryocytes (clonal thrombocytosis). Reactive thrombocytosis is driven by excessive cytokines induced by various stimuli, such as trauma or inflammation. Clonal thrombocytosis is defined as chronic myeloproliferative neoplasms (MPNs), of which four subgroups are well characterized: Chronic myelogenous leukemia (CML), polycythemia vera (PV), primary myelofibrosis (PMF), and essential thrombocythemia (ET). In addition, platelet count can be spuriously elevated in some conditions (see "Differential Diagnosis"). Extreme thrombocytosis is defined as platelet count >1 million/ml. This chapter deals primarily with essential thrombocythemia.

SYNONYMS

Thrombocythemia
Essential thrombocythemia
ET

ICD-10CM CODES	
D47.3	Essential (hemorrhagic) thrombocythemia
D75.89	Other specified diseases of blood and blood-forming organs
D75.9	Disease of blood and blood-forming organs, unspecified
D77	Other disorders of blood and blood-forming organs in diseases classified elsewhere

EPIDEMIOLOGY & DEMOGRAPHICS

It has been estimated that about 88% to 97% of the cases of thrombocytosis are reactive rather than clonal proliferation.[1]

EPIDEMIOLOGY FOR ESSENTIAL THROMBOCYTHEMIA

INCIDENCE: 1 to 2 per 100,000 population/yr.[2]
PREVALENCE: Estimated at 38 to 57 cases/100,000 population.[3]
PREDOMINANT SEX & AGE: The median age at diagnosis is 65 to 70 yr. Female:male ratio is 2:1.[4]

PHYSICAL FINDINGS & CLINICAL PRESENTATION

- Regardless of the cause, a high platelet count may be associated with vasomotor symptoms such as headache, visual disturbances, dizziness, atypical chest pain, acral dysesthesia, and erythromelalgia.[1,4]
- Thrombotic and bleeding complications can occur. Thrombosis at unusual sites (hepatic vein, IVC, portal vein, splenic vein) are especially concerning.[1,4]
- Symptoms and complications are much more likely to occur in association with clonal thrombocytosis than reactive thrombocytosis.
- The degree of thrombocytosis does not predict the likelihood of clonal thrombocytosis

and does not generally correlate to the risk of thrombosis.[1]
- Splenomegaly is common with MPNs.[5]
- Coexistent leukocytosis and erythrocytosis are common with CML and PV.[5]
- Disease transformation from ET to PV, PMF, and acute myeloid leukemia (AML) is uncommon. In patients with ET, the 15-yr rate of leukemic transformation is estimated at 2% to 5%.[6]

ETIOLOGY

- Essential thrombocytosis, a myeloproliferative neoplasm, is a clonal disorder of a multipotent hematopoietic progenitor cell.[1]
- Abnormality in JAK2-STAT pathway (including *JAK2*, *CALR*, and *MPL* gene mutations) may play a role in pathogenesis of MPN.[1]

DIAGNOSIS

DIFFERENTIAL DIAGNOSIS

- Spurious thrombocytosis:
  1. Mixed cryoglobulinemia—precipitated cryoglobulin particles are counted as platelets by automatic counters; generally occurs at low temperatures
  2. Circulating cytoplasmic fragments miscounted as platelets—seen mainly in patients with leukemia, lymphoma, severe hemolysis, or burns
- Reactive thrombocytosis:
  1. Benign hematologic disorders
  2. Acute hemorrhage, iron deficiency anemia, hemolytic anemia
  3. Chronic infection, such as tuberculosis
  4. Acute and chronic inflammatory disorders
  5. Rheumatologic disorders
  6. Inflammatory bowel disease
  7. Celiac disease
  8. Functional and surgical asplenia
  9. Tissue damage
  10. Trauma, thermal burn

11. Myocardial infarction
12. Acute pancreatitis
13. Recent surgery
14. Renal failure, nephrotic syndrome
15. Exercise
16. Medications, such as vincristine, epinephrine
- Clonal thrombocytosis:
  1. CML
  2. PV
  3. PMF
  4. Myelodysplastic syndrome (5q- syndrome)
  5. AML with inv(3), t(3;3)
  6. Essential thrombocytosis (Box 1)

WORKUP

- Comprehensive history and physical examination to exclude many of the common causes of reactive thrombocytosis: History and physical examination suggestive of acute blood loss, iron deficiency, acute or chronic infection/inflammation, medication use, asplenia, malignancy, and trauma should be evaluated. Fig. E1 describes a diagnostic algorithm for thrombocytosis. The diagnosis of ET requires platelet counts >450 × 10³/ml on two separate occasions >4 wk apart, absence of BCR-ABL, and exclusion of secondary causes of thrombocytosis.
- Repeat CBC with peripheral blood smear and bone marrow biopsy (Figs. E2 and E3) to exclude spurious thrombocytosis.

LABORATORY TESTS

- CBC with peripheral blood smear: Howell-Jolly bodies and target cells are present in patients with asplenia; nucleated red blood cell (RBC), teardrop RBC and white blood cell (WBC) precursors in patients with PMF.
- Serum ferritin level: Low ferritin level suggests iron deficiency.
- Serum C-reactive protein, erythrocyte sedimentation rate, and plasma fibrinogen: Nonspecific markers of infection or inflammation.

BOX 1 World Health Organization Diagnostic Criteria for Essential Thrombocythemia

Diagnosis requires that all of the following criteria be met:
- Sustained platelet count ≥450 × 10⁹/L.*
- Bone marrow biopsy specimen showing proliferation mainly of the megakaryocytic lineage, with increased numbers of enlarged, mature megakaryocytes; no significant increase or left shift of neutrophil granulopoiesis or erythropoiesis.
- Failure to meet the WHO criteria for polycythemia vera,†† primary myelofibrosis,‡ BCR-ABL1–positive chronic myelogenous leukemia,§ myelodysplastic syndrome,¶ or other myeloid neoplasms.
- Demonstration of *JAK2 V617F* or other clonal marker; or, in the absence of *JAK2 V617F*, no evidence of reactive thrombocytosis.¶

*Sustained during the workup process.
‡Requires the absence of relevant reticulin fibrosis, collagen fibrosis, peripheral blood leukoerythroblastosis, or markedly hypercellular marrow accompanied by megakaryocyte morphology typical for primary myelofibrosis—small to large megakaryocytes with an aberrant nuclear-to-cytoplasmic ratio and hyperchromatic, bulbous, or irregularly folded nuclei and dense clustering.
†Requires the failure of iron replacement therapy to increase the hemoglobin level to the polycythemia vera range in the presence of decreased serum ferritin. Exclusion of polycythemia vera is based on hemoglobin and hematocrit levels; red cell mass measurement is not required.
§Requires the absence of BCR-ABL1.
¶Causes of reactive thrombocytosis include iron deficiency, splenectomy, surgery, infection, inflammation, connective tissue disease, metastatic cancer, and lymphoproliferative disorders. Requires the absence of dyserythropoiesis and dysgranulopoiesis. From Swerdlow SH et al (eds): *WHO classification of tumours of haematopoietic and lymphoid tissues*, Lyon, France, 2008, IARC Press.

- Philadelphia chromosome or BCR-ABL rearrangement: Positive in CML.
- Serum erythropoietin assay: Low to normal in PV and ET.
- *JAK2* mutation analysis: PV and ET; *JAK2* mutation is found in 95% of patients with PV and in 50% to 60% of patients with ET and PMF.[7]
- In ET, frequency of *MPL* and *CALR* mutations are estimated to be 5% and 27%, respectively.[8]
  1. These mutations are associated with differences in prognosis and risk of thrombosis.[8]
  2. *JAK2, CALR,* and *MPL* mutations are mutually exclusive. They are not confined to a particular myeloproliferative neoplasm, and their absence does not exclude any of the MPNs.[8]
  3. About 13% of patients with ET will be negative for *JAK2, CALR,* and *MPL* mutations.[8]
- Bone marrow chromosome analysis: 5q-syndrome and other myelodysplastic syndrome, CML.
- Bone marrow exam in ET may show clusters of abnormal megakaryocytes and increased reticulin fibrosis (see Fig. E3).

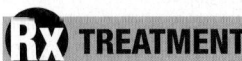

TREATMENT

No therapies are known to alter survival or leukemic transformation in ET. Reactive thrombocytosis has been rarely associated with thrombosis or bleeding and generally does not require specific therapy.

ACUTE GENERAL Rx

- Vasomotor symptoms easily manageable with low-dose aspirin (<100 mg/day).[5]
- Bleeding:
  1. Discontinue any platelet antiaggregating agent, such as aspirin or nonsteroidal anti inflammatory agents.
  2. Evaluate for disseminated intravascular coagulopathy and coagulation factor deficiency. Acquired factor V deficiency is occasionally present in association with clonal thrombocytosis. In that case, treat with fresh frozen plasma infusion.
  3. In case of extreme thrombocytosis (platelet count generally >1,000,000/microliter [1000 × 10⁹/L]), acquired von Willebrand disease may occur. Immediate definitive therapy with a platelet-lowering agent is essential in this instance. Platelet pheresis should be reserved for cases of acute thrombosis or bleeding.
- Thrombosis:
  1. Arterial or venous thrombosis occurs in 10% to 20% of patients.[8]
  2. If the platelet count is >800,000/ml, platelet apheresis coupled with a platelet-lowering agent should be considered with the goal of platelet count <400,000/mm³.
  3. Anticoagulant therapy for 3 mo to indefinite based on the presence or absence of additional thrombophilic defects.

CHRONIC Rx

Treatment strategies for ET are based on the presence or absence of risk factors for thrombosis. Objective risk stratification is done by calculating IPSET-thrombosis score with age, history of thrombosis, cardiac risk factor, and presence of JAK2 mutation. Smoking cessation and obesity management should be discussed with all patients with ET. In low-risk patients (age <60 yr, no history of thrombosis or hemorrhage, platelet count <1 million/ml), observation may be adequate. Treatment with low-dose aspirin is indicated in low-risk patients with vasomotor symptoms or with other indications for aspirin use. The cytoreductive therapy along with low-dose aspirin therapy is indicated in high-risk patients (age >60 yr and/or with previous history of thrombosis) regardless of vasomotor symptoms. Exception is if a high-risk patient has no history of arterial thrombosis but has history of venous thrombosis, in which case systemic anticoagulation instead of low-dose aspirin is recommended.[8]

- Low-dose aspirin (81 mg/day) may be safe and effective in preventing vascular events. It is also effective in preventing recurrent vascular events in high-risk patients and in treating the vasomotor symptoms.
- Cytoreductive therapy (Table 1):
  1. First-line therapy is hydroxyurea in majority of cases. Anagrelide and interferon (if not used previously) generally are considered second line.
  2. Hydroxyurea (HU) vs. anagrelide: A randomized trial comparing HU with aspirin and anagrelide with aspirin in patients with ET found that patients in the anagrelide group had increased rates of arterial thrombosis, serious hemorrhage, and transformation to myelofibrosis, but decreased rate of venous thrombosis.[9] However, another randomized trial found no difference between HU and anagrelide in terms of arterial and venous thrombosis and bleeding complications.[10] Current recommendation is to consider anagrelide after failure of other drug options, including HU, interferon, and busulfan.[8] Monitor liver function tests and the degree of neutropenia or anemia with HU therapy.

TABLE 1 Choice of Drugs for Treatment of Patients with High-Risk Essential Thrombocythemia

Age (yr)	Treatment of Choice	Second Line
<50	Interferon	Anagrelide
		Hydroxyurea
50-75	Hydroxyurea	Interferon
		Anagrelide
>75	Hydroxyurea	Anagrelide

From Hoffman R et al: *Hematology, basic principles and practice*, ed 8, Philadelphia, 2023, Elsevier.

3. The incidence of leukemic conversion in patients with ET treated with HU alone is reported as <1%. Interferon alpha may be effective for controlling platelet count in patients failing treatment with HU. A randomized control trial comparing HU with pegylated interferon (PEG) found no difference in complete response between the two treatments at 12 mo. However, PEG was associated with more Grade 3/4 adverse events compared to HU (46% vs. 28%).[11]
4. To date, there is no proven benefit to JAK2 inhibition with ruxolitinib compared to best available therapy in essential thrombocytosis with regard to platelet counts, thrombosis, hemorrhage, or transformation to AML.[12]

DISPOSITION

- Although long survival is expected in patients with ET, it is inferior to the sex- and age-matched U.S. population.
- An International Prognostic Score for Essential Thrombocythemia (IPSET) was proposed by International Working Group on Myelofibrosis Research and Treatment based on age, WDC count, and history of thromboembolism at diagnosis.

REFERRAL

Refer to hematologist/oncologist when platelet count is consistently elevated >450,000/mm³ without causes for reactive thrombocytosis.

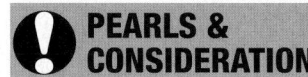

COMMENTS

- Some patients with clinically apparent ET have BCR-ABL rearrangement, even in the absence of other features of CML. It is suggested that it should be tested in all ET patients due to its potential therapeutic implications.
- The risk of bleeding with aspirin use in patients with ET paradoxically increases when the platelet count is >1 million/ml, likely due to acquired von Willebrand disease.

PATIENT & FAMILY EDUCATION

Smoking cessation is encouraged in both patients with ET and reactive thrombocytosis.

REFERENCES

Available at eBooks.Health.Elsevier.com.

AUTHORS: **SOVIJJA POU, MD** and **JOHN L. REAGAN, MD**

BASIC INFORMATION

DEFINITION

Superficial venous thrombophlebitis (SVT) is an inflammation of a vein with subsequent secondary thrombus formation. SVT most frequently involves superficial veins of the leg, but any superficial vein can be affected. SVT has been reported to occur in 125,000 people in the U.S. per yr; however, the actual incidence is likely far greater. SVT is not always a benign condition. SVT should be regarded as the superficial venous manifestation of a systemic process known as venous thromboembolism (deep vein thrombosis [DVT], pulmonary embolism [PE]).

SYNONYMS

SVT
Superficial phlebitis
Superficial suppurative thrombophlebitis
Suppurative thrombophlebitis

ICD-10CM CODES
I80.00	Phlebitis and thrombophlebitis of superficial vessels of unspecified lower extremity
I80.8	Phlebitis and thrombophlebitis of other sites
I80.9	Phlebitis and thrombophlebitis of unspecified site

EPIDEMIOLOGY & DEMOGRAPHICS

- Approximately 30% to 45% of patients diagnosed with SVT are men with an average age of 54 yr.
- Approximately 55% to 70% of patients diagnosed with SVT are women with an average age of 58 yr.
- The overall recurrence of SVT is 18% over an average observation period of 15 mo, equally involving varicose and nonvaricose veins.
- The lifetime incidence of SVT in those with untreated varicose veins has been estimated at 25% to 50%.

PHYSICAL FINDINGS & CLINICAL PRESENTATION

- Subcutaneous vein is palpable as a tender cord or "worm-like" mass with increased warmth and erythema.
- Induration, redness, and tenderness are localized along the course of the vein. This linear appearance (Fig. E1) rather than circular appearance is useful to distinguish thrombophlebitis from other conditions (cellulitis, erythema nodosum).
- There is some swelling of the overlying skin and subcutaneous tissue but without generalized edema of the limb.
- Low-grade fever may be present.

ETIOLOGY

- In the lower extremity, 70% of SVT occurs in patients with varicose veins, with the great saphenous vein being most commonly involved (60% to 80%)

- Intravenous catheters and infusion of caustic drugs are the most common cause of upper-extremity SVT
- Malignancy
- Pregnancy/puerperium
- Hypercoagulable states
- Previous DVT/SVT
- OCP (oral contraceptive pill)/HRT (hormone replacement therapy)

DIAGNOSIS

DIFFERENTIAL DIAGNOSIS

- Lymphangitis
- Cellulitis
- Erythema nodosum
- Panniculitis
- Acute lipodermatosclerosis

WORKUP

The clinical investigation includes not only the local findings but also the presence of varicose veins with or without the stigmata of chronic venous insufficiency. Today, duplex ultrasound is the most important additional diagnostic tool.

IMAGING STUDIES

- Duplex ultrasound offers the advantage of being inexpensive, noninvasive, and repeatable for follow-up examination.
- Ultrasonography confirms the diagnosis, shows the location of the thrombus and its location regarding the saphenofemoral and/or saphenopopliteal junctions.
- Ultrasound examination of patients with SVT has revealed that a concomitant DVT can exist in 15% to 20%.
- In up to 25% of these patients, the DVT may not be contiguous with the SVT and may be found in the contralateral leg.
- Therefore bilateral duplex exam is recommended in all cases of SVT that involve the main trunk of the great saphenous vein (GSV) or small saphenous vein (SSV).

TREATMENT

NONPHARMACOLOGIC THERAPY

- Warm, moist compresses
- Do not restrict activity. Immediate mobilization with walking exercises

ACUTE GENERAL Rx

- Treatment guidelines for SVT are not well established because of the lack of controlled clinical trials. In general, the primary goal of management should be to prevent thrombus extension and the risk of venous thromboembolism. All other therapy is directed at patient comfort with analgesics and NSAIDs (in patients not receiving anticoagulants).
- In patients with migratory SVT (Fig. E2), recurrent SVT, or SVT without varicose veins, the underlying condition should be investigated, and treatment directed accordingly.
- The most common cause of upper-extremity SVT is an intravenous catheter. Treatment starts with removal of the cannula and

application of warm compresses. The resultant lump may persist for months. No anticoagulant therapy is required.
- In patients with lower-extremity SVT in a varicose vein branch, control of pain with analgesics and the use of gradient compression stockings are usually sufficient. Patients are encouraged to continue their usual daily activities.
- Many investigators favor systemic anticoagulation when there is superficial thrombosis of 5 cm or more in length, the thrombus is within 1 cm of the saphenous junctions, or more than 5 cm of the saphenous trunk is involved, as shown by duplex ultrasonography. Anticoagulation is also reasonable for patients with SVT and cancer or previous DVT.
- The American College of Chest Physicians guidelines recommend anticoagulation for 45 days over no anticoagulation in patients with lower-extremity SVT within 1 cm of the saphenofemoral or saphenopopliteal junction.
- In the case of patients with varicose veins secondary to saphenous vein reflux, a catheter vein ablation procedure should be performed only after the acute SVT episode is over in order to avoid the thromboembolic complications induced by such procedures.

PEARLS & CONSIDERATIONS

SUPERFICIAL SUPPURATIVE THROMBOPHLEBITIS

- Superficial suppurative thrombophlebitis is associated with an intravenous catheter or multiple puncture sites secondary to intravenous (IV) drug abuse and is located primarily in the upper extremity.
- Clinical presentation is similar to that of nonsuppurative SVT but with associated fever, leukocytosis, and/or septicemia.
- Most cases of intravenous catheter sepsis are not complicated by suppurative thrombophlebitis; local IV catheter site infections occur in about 7% of cases and septicemia is found in only 1 of every 400 IV catheterizations.
- The incidence of peripheral vein suppurative thrombophlebitis is highest in patients with specific risk factors such as burns, steroids, and IV drug abuse.
- Treatment consists of antibiotics with adequate coverage of gram-negative rods and *Staphylococcus aureus,* including MRSA. Initial empirical treatment is with IV vancomycin 1 g q12h *plus* ceftriaxone 1 g IV q24h. Alternative regimen consists of daptomycin 6 mg/kg IV q12h *plus* ceftriaxone 1 g IV q24h.

RELATED CONTENT

Thrombophlebitis (Patient Information)
Deep Vein Thrombosis (Related Key Topic)

AUTHOR: **FRANK G. FORT, MD, FACS, RPHS**

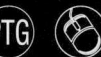
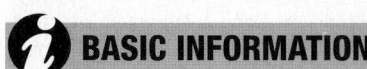 **BASIC INFORMATION**

DEFINITION

Thyroid carcinoma is a primary neoplasm of the thyroid and consists of four major subtypes: Papillary, follicular, anaplastic, and medullary. A classification of thyroid neoplasms is described in Table 1.

SYNONYMS

Papillary carcinoma of thyroid
Follicular carcinoma of thyroid
Anaplastic carcinoma of thyroid
Medullary carcinoma of thyroid

ICD-10CM CODES
C73	Malignant neoplasm of thyroid gland
D09.3	Carcinoma in situ of thyroid and other endocrine glands
D34	Benign neoplasm of thyroid gland
D44.0	Neoplasm of uncertain behavior of thyroid gland

EPIDEMIOLOGY & DEMOGRAPHICS

- Thyroid cancer is the most common endocrine cancer, with an estimated 43,720 new cases and 2120 deaths occurring in 2023 in the U.S.[1]
- Incidence is 13.9 per 100,000 people in the U.S. and increasing over last four decades.
- Female:male ratio is 3:1.
- Median age at diagnosis: 45 to 50 yr.
- Occult thyroid cancer is identified in 20% of autopsy specimens.

TABLE 1 Classification of Thyroid Neoplasms

Primary Epithelial Tumors
- Tumors of follicular cells
  1. Benign: Follicular adenoma
  2. Borderline follicular tumors
  3. Follicular tumor of uncertain malignancy potential
  4. Well-differentiated tumor of uncertain malignancy potential
  5. Noninvasive follicular neoplasm with papillary-like nuclear features (NIFTP)
  6. Malignant: Carcinoma
  7. Differentiated: Papillary, follicular, Hürthle cell, poorly differentiated
  8. Undifferentiated (anaplastic)
- Tumors of C cells
  1. Medullary carcinoma
- Tumors of follicular and C cells
- Mixed medullary-follicular carcinomas

Primary Nonepithelial Tumors
- Malignant lymphomas
- Sarcomas
- Others

Secondary Tumors

From Melmed S et al: *Williams textbook of endocrinology,* ed 14, Philadelphia, 2019, Elsevier.

PHYSICAL FINDINGS & CLINICAL PRESENTATION

- Thyroid cancer is often identified incidentally.
- Physical exam may reveal:
  1. Presence of thyroid nodule
  2. Hoarseness and cervical lymphadenopathy
  3. Painless swelling in the region of the thyroid

ETIOLOGY

- Risk factors: Prior neck irradiation.
- Multiple endocrine neoplasia II (medullary carcinoma).
- Inherited syndromes associated with thyroid cancer are described in Table 2.
- GLP-1 receptor agonists for the treatment of type 2 DM (e.g., exenatide, albiglutide) can increase the risk of medullary thyroid carcinoma (MTC).
- Papillary thyroid carcinoma is the commonest type of thyroid carcinoma of follicular origin and encompasses several tumor types that have mutually exclusive mutations that activate thyroid cell abnormal proliferation. BRAF V600E mutation accounts for 60% of these mutations; other mutations include *RAS* or *RET/PTC* rearrangements.[2,3]
- In follicular thyroid carcinoma, oncogenic drivers are primarily *RAS* alterations (40% to 50% of cases) and *PAX8/PPAR*γ rearrangements (30% to 40% of cases). Molecular alterations of the PI3K/Akt pathway and PTEN silencing by inactivating mutations or epigenetic changes also occur in some cases.[2,3]
- Poorly differentiated thyroid carcinomas are aggressive cancers with a high mutation rate. *RAS* and *BRAF* mutations are found in 20% to 50% and up to 35% of cases, respectively. Genetic alterations that characterize PDTC and are associated with tumor aggressiveness are *TERT* promoter (20% to 50%) mutations and *TP53* mutations (10% to 35%) that cooccur with *RAS* and *BRAF* mutations.[2,3]
- In anaplastic thyroid cancer, as many as 25% to 50% of cases harbor BRAFV600 mutations, which can be targeted with available BRAF/MEK inhibitor combination therapy. Other frequent mutations include *TERT* (75%), *TP53* (63%), and *RAS* (24%). Other actionable molecular drivers with available targeted therapies include *RET* rearrangements, *ALK* rearrangements, *NTRK* fusions, and *TSC2* mutations, suggesting the need for broad molecular profiling.[2,3]

TABLE 2 Inherited Syndromes Associated with Thyroid Cancer

Multiple endocrine neoplasia (MEN) 2A and 2B
Isolated familial medullary thyroid cancer
Gardner syndrome
Familial adenomatous polyposis
Carney complex
Cowden syndrome
Familial nonmedullary thyroid cancer

From Cameron JL, Cameron AM: *Current surgical therapy,* ed 10, Philadelphia, 2011, Saunders.

- Pathways in the development of thyroid cancer are depicted in Fig. E1.

DIAGNOSIS

DIFFERENTIAL DIAGNOSIS

- Multinodular goiter
- Lymphocytic thyroiditis
- Ectopic thyroid

WORKUP

The workup of thyroid carcinoma includes laboratory evaluation and diagnostic imaging. Key features of thyroid malignancies are summarized in Table 3. Diagnosis is confirmed with fine-needle aspiration or surgical biopsy. At diagnosis, the vast majority of thyroid cancers are well differentiated, with excellent prognosis. The characteristics of thyroid carcinoma vary with the type:

- Papillary carcinoma (80%):
  1. Most frequently occurs in women during second or third decades
  2. Histologically, psammoma bodies (calcific bodies present in papillary projections) are pathognomonic; found in 35% to 45% of papillary thyroid carcinomas
  3. Majority are not papillary lesions but mixed papillary follicular carcinomas
  4. Spread is by lymphatics and by local invasion
- Follicular carcinoma (10%):
  1. More aggressive than papillary carcinoma
  2. Incidence increases with age
  3. Tends to metastasize hematogenously to bone, producing pathologic fractures
  4. Tends to concentrate iodine (useful for radiation therapy)
- Poorly differentiated thyroid carcinoma (5% to 6%):
  1. Aggressive cancers with pathology characterized by high mitotic activity and tumor necrosis.
  2. Patients often develop vascular invasion, lymph node metastasis, extrathyroidal extension, and distant metastases.
  3. Associated with a mean survival of 3.2 yr.
  4. Radioiodine therapy is of limited benefit and most patients require systemic therapies.
- Anaplastic carcinoma (1%):
  1. Very aggressive neoplasm
  2. Two major histologic types: Small cell (less aggressive, 5-yr survival approximately 20%) and giant cell (death usually within 6 mo of diagnosis)
- MTC (4%):
  1. Unifocal lesion: Found sporadically in elderly patients
  2. Bilateral lesions: Associated with pheochromocytoma and hyperparathyroidism; this combination is known as MEN-II and is inherited as an autosomal-dominant disorder

LABORATORY TESTS

- Thyroid function studies are generally normal. Thyroid-stimulating hormone (TSH), T4, and

TABLE 3 Thyroid Malignancies—Key Features

	Description	Pattern of Spread
Papillary carcinoma (70%-80%)	Low-grade tumors with a good prognosis (histologically multicentric) ▶ Tumors concentrate radio-iodine	Early lymph node spread (metastatic lymph nodes may be normal in size, cystic, calcified, hemorrhagic, or contain colloid) ▶ Distant metastases are rare (and usually to the lungs)
Follicular carcinoma (10%-20%)	Slow growing ▶ Tumors concentrate radio-iodine	It rarely metastasizes to the regional lymph nodes ▶ The tendency is to spread via the bloodstream and disseminate to the lungs, bones, or liver
Anaplastic carcinoma (1%-2%)	Undifferentiated malignant tumors that do not concentrate radio-iodine ▶ There is a poor prognosis ▶ They tend to occur in older patients ▶ Punctate calcification and necrosis frequently are present	Lymphatic metastases occur in the majority of patients
Medullary carcinoma (5%-10%)	This originates from the parafollicular C cells ▶ It does not concentrate radio-iodine ▶ It may be sporadic or familial (and associated with the MEN type II syndrome or other endocrine neoplasms) ▶ It is usually a unilateral, solitary lesion ▶ Calcification is seen in 10% ▶ I¹²³-MIBG and somatostatin analogs (e.g., octreotide) can be used for evaluation ▶ Circulating calcitonin levels are usually elevated	It may invade locally, spread to the regional nodes, or demonstrate hematogenous spread to the lungs, bones, or liver
Lymphoma (10%)	It is usually a non-Hodgkin lymphoma ▶ It occurs in one third of patients with Hashimoto thyroiditis (a MALT-type lymphoma) ▶ It presents as a rapidly enlarging, solitary nodule (80%) or as multiple nodules (imaging cannot distinguish between a lymphoma and thyroiditis) ▶ Necrosis and calcification are uncommon	It can involve the nodes with spread to the GI tract
Metastases (<1%)	The most common primary is renal cell carcinoma	

¹²³-*MIBG,* Iodine-123 meta-iodobenzylguanidine; *GI,* gastrointestinal; *MALT,* mucosa associated lymphoid tissue; *MEN,* multiple endocrine neoplasia.
From Grant LA: *Grainger & Allison's diagnostic radiology essentials,* ed 2, Philadelphia, 2019, Elsevier.

TABLE 4 The Bethesda System for Thyroid Cytopathology

Category	Risk of Malignancy (%)	Recommended Management
Nondiagnostic or unsatisfactory	1-4	Repeat FNA with ultrasound guidance
Benign	0-3	Clinical follow-up
Atypia of undetermined significance (AUS) or follicular lesion of undetermined significance (FLUS)	5-15	Repeat FNA*
Follicular neoplasm or suspicious for follicular neoplasm	15-30	Lobectomy
Suspicious for malignancy	60-75	Lobectomy with or without frozen section or total thyroidectomy
Malignant	97-99	Total thyroidectomy

FNA, Fine-needle aspiration.
*Lobectomy also can be considered depending on clinical or sonographic characteristics.
From Niederhuber JE: *Abeloff's clinical oncology,* ed 6, Philadelphia, 2020, Elsevier.

serum thyroglobulin levels should be obtained before thyroidectomy in patients with confirmed thyroid carcinoma. Serum thyroglobulin levels can be useful postoperatively to monitor recurrence of thyroid carcinoma (Fig. E2).

- Increased plasma calcitonin assay in patients with medullary carcinoma (tumors produce thyrocalcitonin). RET proto-oncogene sequencing and measurement of plasma free metanephrine and normetanephrine levels to rule out coexistent pheochromocytoma are recommended in all patients with medullary thyroid cancer.
- Fine-needle aspiration biopsy is the best method to assess a thyroid nodule (see "Thyroid Nodule" in Section I). Table 4 describes the Bethesda system for thyroid cytopathology.

IMAGING STUDIES (FIG. E3)

- Thyroid ultrasound can detect solitary solid nodules that have a high risk of malignancy.

However, a negative ultrasound does not exclude diagnosis of thyroid carcinoma.
- Thyroid scanning with iodine-123 or technetium-99m can identify hypofunctioning (cold) nodules, which are more likely to be malignant. However, warm nodules can also be malignant.

STAGING (TABLE E5)

- Stage I: Thyroid cancer of any size without distal spread in patient <55 yr. In patients >55 yr, tumor size ≤4 cm without local invasion or positive cervical lymph nodes
- Stage II: Distal spread in patient <55 yr. In patients >55 yr, tumors >2 cm but <4 cm, spread to nearby lymph nodes, not spread to distant sites
- Stage III: Tumors >4 cm in patient >55 yr of age, not spread to distant sites
- Stage IV: Distal spread in patient >55 yr of age

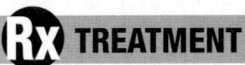 **TREATMENT**

ACUTE GENERAL Rx

- Papillary carcinoma:
  1. Total thyroidectomy is indicated if the patient has:
     a. Extrathyroid extension
     b. History of radiation exposure
     c. Poorly differentiated
     d. Cervical lymph node involvement
     e. Tumor >4 cm
     f. Known distant metastasis
  2. Lobectomy with isthmectomy may be considered in patients with intrathyroid papillary carcinoma <4 cm and no history of neck or head radiation; surgery should be followed with suppressive therapy with thyroid hormone because these tumors are TSH responsive. The accepted practice is to suppress serum TSH concentrations

---

TABLE 6 Indications for Iodine-131 Treatment in Patients with Papillary, Follicular, or Hürthle Cell Thyroid Carcinoma After Initial Definitive Near-Total Thyroidectomy

No Indication

Adult patients at very low risk for cause-specific mortality or relapse: Complete surgical resection, favorable histology, and limited extent of disease (e.g., PTC patients with MACIS scores <6; patients with tumor size <1 cm, N0, and M0)

Definite Indications

Distant metastasis at diagnosis

Incomplete tumor resection

Complete tumor resection but high risk for mortality or recurrence (e.g., PTC patients with MACIS scores ≥6 and pTNM stage II/III FTC or HCC)

Probable Indications

Incomplete surgery (less than near-total thyroidectomy, no lymph node dissection)

PTC or FTC in a child younger than 16 yr

If PTC, tall cell or columnar cell variant and diffuse sclerosing variant

If FTC, widely invasive or poorly differentiated tumor

Bulky nodal metastases

FTC, Follicular thyroid carcinoma; *HCC,* Hürthle cell carcinoma; *MACIS,* scoring system based on metastasis, age, completeness of resection, invasion, and size; *M0,* no distant cancer spread found; *N0,* no cancer in nearby lympnodes; *PTC,* papillary thyroid carcinoma; *pTNM,* pathologic tumor-node-metastasis classification.
From Melmed S et al (eds): *Williams textbook of endocrinology,* ed 12, Philadelphia, 2011, Saunders.

TABLE 7 Characteristics of Thyroid Cancers

Type of Cancer	Porcontago of Thyroid Cancers	Age of Onset (yr)	Treatment	Prognosis
Papillary	88	40-80	Thyroidectomy, followed by radioactive iodine ablation and TSH suppression	Good
Follicular	10	45-80	Thyroidectomy, followed by radioactive iodine ablation and TSH suppression	Fair to good
Medullary	3-4	20-50	Thyroidectomy and central compartment lymph node dissection and TSH suppression	Fair
Anaplastic	1	50-80	Isthmusectomy followed by palliative x-ray treatment	Poor
Lymphoma	<1	25-70	X-ray therapy and/or chemotherapy	Fair

From Andreoli TE et al: *Andreoli and Carpenter's Cecil essentials of medicine,* ed 8, Philadelphia, 2010, Saunders.

---

to <0.1 microunit/ml in patients with persistent disease, suppression to 0.1 to 0.5 microunit/ml in patients who are disease free but are at high risk of recurrence, and a goal TSH level of 0.3 to 2.0 microunits/ml in patients who are disease free and have a low risk of recurrence.

3. Radioiodine ablation reduces rates of death and recurrence (Table 6). Radioiodine is administered for stages III and IV disease.[4]

4. In cases that have progressed after radioiodine therapy, oral targeted inhibitors (lenvatinib, sorafenib) have significant survival benefit.[5,6]

5. Larotrectinib and entrectinib are both FDA approved for patients with NTRK gene fusion–positive advanced solid tumors.

6. If a patient is found to have a *BRAF* mutation, therapy with BRAF inhibitors vemurafenib or dabrafenib can be considered.[5,6]

- Follicular carcinoma:
  1. Total thyroidectomy followed by TSH suppression, as previously noted.
  2. Radiotherapy with iodine-131 followed by thyroid suppression therapy with triiodothyronine is useful in patients with metastasis (see Table 6).[4]
  3. In cases that have progressed after radioiodine therapy, oral targeted inhibitors

(lenvatinib, sorafenib) have significant survival benefit.

- Anaplastic carcinoma:
  1. At diagnosis, this neoplasm is rarely operable; palliative surgery is indicated for extremely large tumor compressing the trachea.
  2. Management is usually restricted to radiation therapy or chemotherapy (combination of doxorubicin, cisplatin, and other antineoplastic agents) (see Table 6); these measures rarely provide significant palliation.
  3. Patients with anaplastic thyroid cancer should have their tumors tested for *BRAF V600E* mutation and *NTRK* gene fusion. The FDA has approved dabrafenib 150 mg PO bid and trametinib 2 mg PO daily for patients who harbor the *BRAF* mutation.
  4. Larotrectinib or entrectinib can be offered to patients who have an *NTRK* gene mutation.

- Medullary carcinoma:
  1. Thyroidectomy should be performed, followed by TSH suppression.
  2. Vandetanib and cabozantinib are oral tyrosine kinase inhibitors that are FDA-approved for treatment of symptomatic or progressive, unresectable, locally advanced or metastatic medullary thyroid cancer.

3. Patients and their families should be screened for pheochromocytoma and hyperparathyroidism.

DISPOSITION

- Overall 5-yr survival rate is 98% and varies with the type of thyroid carcinoma: 5-yr survival is over 80% for follicular carcinoma and is approximately 5% with anaplastic carcinoma (Table 7).
- Factors used in prognostic classification systems are summarized in Table 8.
- Risk factors for aggressive behavior of well-differentiated thyroid carcinomas are described in Box 1.
- Box 2 summarizes risk stratification for thyroid cancer recurrence.

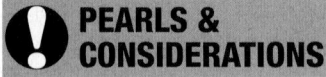 **PEARLS & CONSIDERATIONS**

COMMENTS

- Follow-up surveillance (Table 9) involves neck ultrasound 6 to 12 mo after initial treatment and periodically and lab evaluation with TSH, serum thyroglobulin (T8), and thyroglobulin antibody (T8 Ab).
- Family members of patients with medullary carcinoma should be screened; DNA analysis

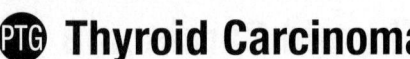

TABLE 8 Factors Used in Prognostic Classification Systems

	TNM	AMES	AGES	MACIS
Patient Factors				
Age	×	×	×	×
Gender	×	×		
Tumor Factors				
Size	×	×	×	×
Histologic grade		×		
Histologic type	×	×	*	*
Extrathyroid spread	×	×	×	×
Lymph node metastasis	×			
Distant metastasis	×	×	×	×
Incomplete resection				×

*AGES, A*ge at diagnosis, histologic tumor *g*rade, *e*xtent of disease at presentation, and tumor *s*ize; *AMES,* patient *a*ge, *m*etastases, *e*xtent of invasion, and tumor *s*ize; *MACIS, m*etastasis, *a*ge at diagnosis, completeness of surgical resection, extrathyroid *i*nvasion, and tumor *s*ize; *TNM,* tumor/node/metastasis.
*AGES/MACIS classifications for papillary carcinomas only.
From Flint PW et al: *Cummings otolaryngology, head and neck surgery,* ed 7, Philadelphia, 2021, Elsevier.

BOX 1 Risk Factors for Aggressive Behavior of Well-Differentiated Thyroid Carcinomas

Demographics
Age <20 yr
Men >55 yr
Women >55 yr
Male > female
History of radiation exposure/therapy
Family history of thyroid carcinoma

Physical Examination
Hard, fixed lesion
Rapid growth of mass
Pain
Lymphadenopathy
Vocal cord paralysis
Aerodigestive tract compromise
Dysphagia
Stridor

Histopathologic Factors (at Initial Presentation)
Size >4 cm
Extrathyroid spread
Vascular invasion
Lymph node metastasis
Distant metastasis
Histologic type
- Tall cell variant of papillary carcinoma
- Follicular carcinoma
- Hürthle cell carcinoma

From Flint PW et al: *Cummings otolaryngology, head and neck surgery*, ed 7, Philadelphia, 2021, Elsevier.

for the detection of mutations in the *RET* gene structure permits the identification of *MEN IIA* gene carriers.
- While there is little controversy regarding the benefit of radioactive iodine in iodine-avid advanced-stage well-differentiated thyroid cancer, the indications for radioactive iodine following total thyroidectomy in patients with very low risk disease is controversial. Proponents argue that its use may destroy microscopic metastases, while opponents counter that the risk of secondary cancer due to radioactive iodine is not warranted in patients whose prognosis is typically excellent.

- Metastatic thyroid cancers that are refractory to radioiodine (iodine-131) are associated with a poor prognosis.
- Small-molecule tyrosine kinase inhibitors, including vandetanib, cabozantinib, sorafenib, and lenvatinib, are now FDA-approved and have shown clinical benefit with improved survival in advanced differentiated and medullary thyroid cancer.[5,6]
- Targeted therapy with a combined regimen of BRAF/MEK inhibitors (dabrafenib plus trametinib) is efficacious and approved in patients with metastatic BRAFV600E-mutated anaplastic thyroid cancer.
- In a subset of patients with anaplastic thyroid cancer, the immune checkpoint inhibitor pembrolizumab may be an effective salvage therapy when added to kinase inhibitors at the time of progression on these drugs. In patients with advanced, differentiated thyroid cancer, pembrolizumab has a manageable safety profile and demonstrates evidence of antitumor activity in a minority of treated patients.
- Selpercatinib is approved for thyroid cancers with *RET* gene mutations.

REFERENCES
Available at eBooks.Health.Elsevier.com.

RELATED CONTENT
Thyroid Cancer (Patient Information)
Thyroid Nodule (Related Key Topic)
Multiple Endocrine Neoplasia (Related Key Topic)

AUTHOR: **BHARTI RATHORE, MD**

BOX 2   Risk Stratification for Thyroid Cancer Recurrence

High Risk
Gross extrathyroidal extension, incomplete tumor resection, distant metastases, or lymph node >3 cm

Intermediate Risk
Aggressive histology, minor extrathyroidal extension, vascular invasion, or >5 involved lymph nodes (0.2-3 cm)

Low Risk
Intrathyroidal DTC ≤5 LN micrometastases (<0.2 cm)

FTC, extensive vascular invasion (≈30%-55%)
pT4a gross ETE (≈30%-40%)
pN1 with extranodal extension, >3 LN involved (≈40%) PTC, >1 cm, TERT mutated ± BRAF mutated (≈40%) pN1, any LN >3 cm (≈30%)
PTC, extrathyroidal, BRAF mutated (≈10%-40%) PTC, vascular invasion (≈15%-30%)
Clinical N1 (≈20%)
pNl, >5 LN involved (≈20%)
Intrathyroidal PTC, <4 cm, BRAF mutated (≈10%) pT3 minor ETE (≈3%-8%)
pN1, all LN <0.2 cm (≈5%)
pN1 ≤5 LN involved (≈5%)
Intrathyroidal PTC, 2-4 cm (≈5%)
Multifocal PTMC (≈4%-6%)
pN1 without extranodal extension, ≤3 LN involved (2%)
Minimally invasive FTC (≈2%-3%)
Intrathyroidal, <4 cm, BRAF wild type (≈1%-2%)
 • Intrathyroidal unifocal PTMC, BRAF mutated, (≈1%-2%)
 • Intrathyroidal, encapsulated, FV-PTC (≈1%-2%)
Unifocal PTMC (≈1%-2%)

From Flint PW et al: *Cummings otolaryngology, head and neck surgery*, ed 7, Philadelphia, 2021, Elsevier.

TABLE 9   Overview of Plans for First Year of Follow-Up Following Initial Therapy

Initial Plan Based on ATA Risk for the First Year of Follow-Up	ATA Low Risk	ATA Intermediate Risk	ATA High Risk
Tg, TgAb, TFTs, every 3-6 mo	√	√	√
Neck US in 3-6 mo	–	√	√
Neck/chest CT with contrast in 6-12 mo	–	Consider[a]	√[b]
Cross-sectional imaging of other sites (brain, abdomen, pelvis)	–	–	Consider[c]
Routine surveillance diagnostic RAI scan	–	–	Consider
18FDG-PET scan	–	–	Consider
Dynamic risk assessment at each visit	√	√	√

ATA, American Thyroid Association; *CT*, computed tomography; *18FDG-PET*, fluorodeoxyglucose positron emission tomography; *RAI*, radioactive iodine; *Tg*, thyroglobulin; *TgAb*, antithyroglobulin antibodies; *TFTs*, thyroid function tests; *US*, ultrasound.
Note: Although most patients will return for physical examination and biochemical testing every 3-6 mo for the first yr, consideration for additional testing is based on ATA risk and on the dynamic risk assessment done at each follow-up visit.
[a]Considered for intermediate-risk patient status postresection clinical N1a or N1b disease.
[b]Depending on presenting features, CT of the neck/chest may need to be done as early as 2-3 mo after initial therapy.
[c]Depending on presenting features, functional imaging results, and serum Tg levels.
From Melmed S et al: *Williams textbook of endocrinology*, ed 14, Philadelphia, 2019, Elsevier.

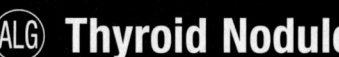
Diseases
and Disorders

I

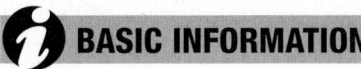 BASIC INFORMATION

DEFINITION

An abnormal growth of thyroid tissue detected on either physical examination or radiographic imaging, and ultimately confirmed by thyroid ultrasound.

ICD-10CM CODES

E04.1	Nontoxic single thyroid nodule or cyst
E04.9	Nontoxic goiter
E05.1	Thyrotoxicosis with toxic single thyroid nodule
E05.2	Thyrotoxicosis with toxic multinodular goiter
E05.11	Thyrotoxicosis with toxic single thyroid nodule with thyrotoxic crisis or storm

EPIDEMIOLOGY & DEMOGRAPHICS

- Thyroid nodules are present in up to 50% of the population.
- Only 5% of the population has a palpable nodule.
- Incidence of thyroid nodules increases after 45 yr. They are more common in women by a ratio of 4:1.
- The vast majority of nodules (approximately 95%), regardless of size, are benign.

PHYSICAL FINDINGS & CLINICAL PRESENTATION

- Anatomic: Characteristics of the nodule include size, firmness (ranges from soft to rock hard), mobility, presence of single or multiple nodules, and presence of enlarged cervical lymph nodes. Additional physical findings to look for include exophthalmos, which would suggest Graves disease, tracheal deviation, and hoarseness suggestive of recurrent laryngeal nerve dysfunction usually associated with advanced malignancy.
- Physiologic: Symptoms of thyrotoxicosis that can be seen with a toxic nodule or toxic multinodular goiter include palpitations, anxiety, insomnia, weight loss, and heat intolerance. The signs of thyrotoxicosis include tremor, lid lag, tachycardia, pressured speech, and restlessness.

ETIOLOGY

- Most nodules are benign. They can be solitary or multiple. Positive family history is common. Iodine deficiency is rarely a cause of nodule formation in developed countries, where salt is iodized.
- Malignancy risks include family history of thyroid cancer and prior head and neck irradiation. Indicators of malignancy: Nodule significantly increasing in size, regional lymphadenopathy, fixation to adjacent tissues, very young or very old age at onset, symptoms of local invasion (dysphagia, hoarseness, neck pain), male sex.
- Inherited syndromes: Multiple endocrine neoplasia (MEN) II predisposes to medullary thyroid cancer, and Cowden syndrome predisposes to follicular neoplasms. Other syndromic causes include Carney complex, Gardner syndrome, and familial adenomatous polyposis.

Dx DIAGNOSIS

DIFFERENTIAL DIAGNOSIS

- Benign functioning or nonfunctioning thyroid adenoma
- Benign thyroid cyst
- Thyroid carcinoma
- Multinodular goiter
- Thyroglossal duct cyst (midline neck mass at level of hyoid)
- Epidermoid cyst (subcutaneous firm mobile mass)
- Laryngocele (superior lateral neck mass)
- Nonthyroid neck neoplasm (lymphoma or lymph node metastases)
- Branchial cleft cyst (lateral neck mass, often with a draining fistula tract)

WORKUP (FIG. 1)

Physical exam is helpful if there are overt signs of hyperthyroidism or malignancy, but these are uncommon. Diagnosis usually relies on laboratory tests, radiographic studies, and cytology.[1]

LABORATORY TESTS

- Serum thyroid-stimulating hormone (TSH) required in all patients. If suppressed, obtain free T4 and free T3 and thyroid scan to screen for a "hot nodule," indicative of a hyperfunctioning adenoma (Fig. E2). If the TSH is normal or elevated, consider biopsy based on ultrasonographic characteristics.
- Serum calcitonin is only recommended when suspecting medullary carcinoma (MTC), such as a patient with a family history of MEN II or familial MTC, or history of pheochromocytoma or hyperparathyroidism.
- If the patient may have Hashimoto thyroiditis, check an antimicrosomal or antithyroid peroxidase antibody level to confirm (see "Thyroiditis"). These patients often have marked heterogeneity of the thyroid parenchyma on ultrasound, which can be mistaken for nodular disease.
- Molecular analysis of thyroid tissue is now commercially available, and it may be useful when fine needle aspiration (FNA) biopsy results are indeterminate.[2] Several companies offer the testing, and in general they are beneficial as rule-out tests. They can be used to identify a subpopulation of patients with a low likelihood of cancer, thereby avoiding unnecessary thyroid lobectomy in patients with indeterminate FNA. These tests have a high negative predictive value for cytologically indeterminate nodules (95% for an atypia or follicular lesion of undetermined significance, 94% for a follicular neoplasm). It is less common to find a gene that is highly predictive of cancer, such as *BRAF, RET/PTC,* and *PAX8-PPAR* gamma. The presence of *RAS* mutations is not as helpful, as it is commonly found in benign follicular adenomas, noninvasive follicular thyroid neoplasms with papillary-like nuclear features, and follicular cancers.

BIOPSY

- FNA biopsy is the best means of distinguishing benign from malignant nodules, but it requires the availability of an expert cytopathologist.
- Decision to perform ultrasound-guided biopsy is based on size and ultrasound features (Table 1). The American Thyroid Association guidelines for thyroid nodules tallies the number of benign or suspicious ultrasound features and then recommends biopsy or observation based on nodule size. The American College of Radiology (ACR) has published a thyroid nodule scoring system called Thyroid Imaging Reporting and Data System (TI-RADS [Table 2]), which is used in a similar way. If the likelihood of malignancy is low, a 1-yr follow-up ultrasound should be performed. The major limitation of ACR-TIRADS is the need to memorize a number of features and their associated scores. The attendant interobserver variability associated with each feature further constrains the reliability of this system for accurately characterizing malignancy risk. Another criticism of ACR-TIRADS is that using it can become time-consuming, particularly in the setting of having to categorize multiple nodules; assessing nodules with a pattern-based system is significantly quicker.[3]
- FNA is discouraged for thyroid nodules <1 cm in diameter unless there are highly concerning features, such as concern for tracheal or nerve involvement, or suspicion of metastatic disease.
- FNA biopsy is very low yield for thyroid cystic lesions because of a paucity of cellular material. Most asymptomatic simple cysts can be observed. Large compressive cysts, or those with a significant solid component, should be considered for resection.
- Previous endocrine, surgery, and radiology algorithms recommended biopsy of all solid thyroid nodules over 1 cm. Over the last 5 yr, there has been a marked shift toward risk stratifying nodules by their ultrasound characteristics using the TI-RADS scoring system or the American Thyroid Association risk assessment (Fig. 3).

IMAGING STUDIES

- Iodine uptake scanning (Fig. E4) is only indicated in patients with suppressed TSH levels to determine if the nodule is toxic or not. If it is hot, biopsy is not indicated.
- Ultrasonography is an inexpensive and effective modality to stratify malignancy risk. The ACR-TIRADS is illustrated in Fig. 3.[4]
- Ultrasound (Fig. E5) is useful to evaluate the size and number of nodules, as well as their characteristics. These include whether it is solid or cystic, echogenicity relative to normal thyroid tissue, irregular vs. smooth borders, presence of calcifications, shape, and vascularity. The three

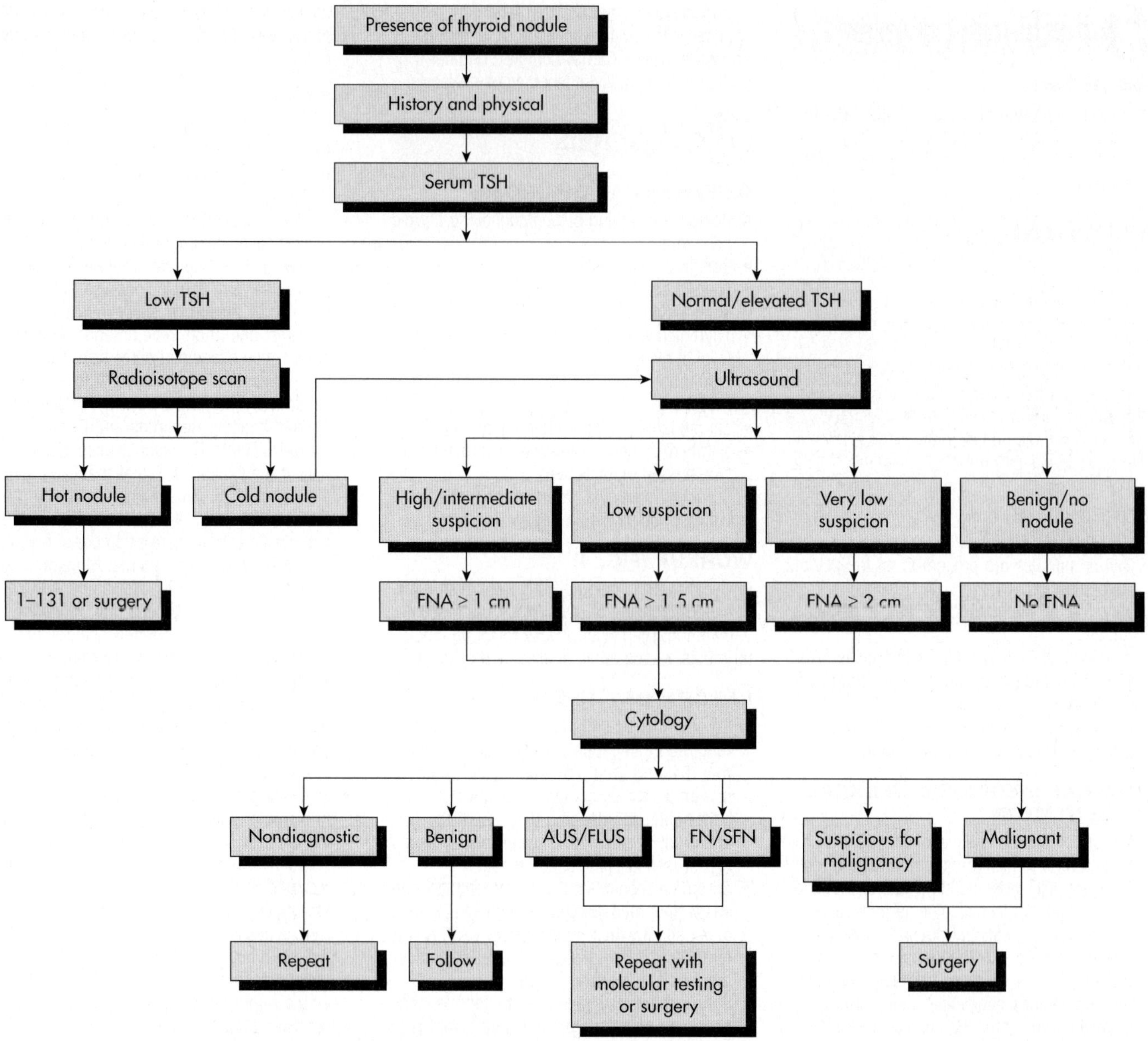

Presence of thyroid nodule

↓

History and physical

↓

Serum TSH

Low TSH

Normal/elevated TSH

Low TSH → Radioisotope scan

Normal/elevated TSH → Ultrasound

Radioisotope scan → Hot nodule / Cold nodule

Hot nodule → 1–131 or surgery

Ultrasound → High/intermediate suspicion / Low suspicion / Very low suspicion / Benign/no nodule

High/intermediate suspicion → FNA > 1 cm

Low suspicion → FNA > 1.5 cm

Very low suspicion → FNA > 2 cm

Benign/no nodule → No FNA

↓

Cytology

Cytology → Nondiagnostic / Benign / AUS/FLUS / FN/SFN / Suspicious for malignancy / Malignant

Nondiagnostic → Repeat

Benign → Follow

AUS/FLUS, FN/SFN → Repeat with molecular testing or surgery

Suspicious for malignancy, Malignant → Surgery

FIG. 1 Workup of a thyroid nodule. *AUS,* Atypia of undetermined significance; *FLUS,* follicular lesion of undetermined significance; *FN,* follicular neoplasm; *FNA,* fine-needle aspiration biopsy; *SFN,* suspicious for follicular neoplasm; *TSH,* thyroid-stimulating hormone. (Modified from Townsend CM et al: *Sabiston textbook of surgery,* ed 21, St Louis, 2022, Elsevier.)

ultrasound characteristics most predictive of malignancy in solid thyroid nodules are shape taller than wide, microcalcifications, and hypoechogenicity, in that order. The positive predictive value for malignancy steadily rises as the number of suspicious ultrasound findings mounts. However, FNA biopsy remains necessary for a definitive diagnosis. Very low risk ultrasound features include simple cystic lesions and spongiform nodules (sponge-like in appearance with layers of solid and cystic contents). Ultrasound follow-up is reasonable in such cases without biopsy, although it is acceptable to biopsy spongiform nodules over 2 cm based on practitioner and patient preference.

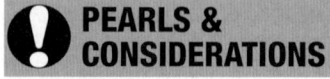 **TREATMENT**

GENERAL Rx
- Evaluation of results of FNA:
  1. The ACR recommendations based on FNA results are summarized in Table 3.
  2. Regardless of biopsy result, symptomatic compressive nodules, substernal nodules, and those causing tracheal deviation are all indications for thyroidectomy.

DISPOSITION

Variable with results of FNA biopsy. Once patients have had a benign biopsy and a 1-yr follow-up ultrasound shows no significant growth, they do *not* require annual thyroid ultrasound

exams. They can be followed with an annual neck exam. If growth is detected or symptoms develop, repeat ultrasound is indicated.

REFERRAL

Surgery or radiology referral for possible FNA biopsy if nodule is solid and over 1 cm

PEARLS & CONSIDERATIONS

COMMENTS
- Many solid, benign nodules grow; therefore, an increase in nodule volume alone is not a reliable predictor of malignancy.

TABLE 1 American Thyroid Association Risk Stratification System

Risk Category	Description	Malignancy Risk	Threshold for FNA
High	Solid hypoechoic nodule or solid hypoechoic component in partially cystic nodule with one or more suspicious features*	>70%-90%	≥1 cm
Intermediate	Hypoechoic solid nodule with smooth margins lacking suspicious features**	10%-20%	≥1 cm
Low	Isoechoic or hyperechoic solid or partially cystic with eccentric solid areas lacking suspicious features**	5%-10%	≥1.5 cm
Very low	Spongiform or partially cystic without suspicious features	<3%	Consider ≥2 cm or observe
Benign	Purely cystic (no solid component)	<1%	No FNA

FNA, Fine-needle aspiration.
*Irregular margins (infiltrative, microlobulated), microcalcifications, taller-than-wide shape, rim calcifications with small extrusive soft tissue component, evidence of extrathyroidal extension.
**Microcalcifications, extrathyroidal extension, or taller-than-wide shape.
From Robertson RP et al: *DeGroot's endocrinology, basic science and clinical practice,* ed 8, Philadelphia, 2023, Elsevier.

TABLE 2 American College of Radiology Thyroid Imaging Reporting and Data System

Nodule Features and Associated Points for Each Characteristic

Composition	Echogenicity	Shape	Margin	Echogenic Foci
Cystic 0	Anechoic 0	Wider than tall 0	Smooth 0	None 0
Spongiform 0	Hyper-/isoechoic 1	Taller than wide 3	Ill-defined 0	Comet tails 0
Mixed 1	Hypoechoic 2		Irregular 2	Macrocalcifications 1
Solid 2	Markedly hypoechoic 3		ETE 3	Peripheral/rim 2
				Punctate 3

ACR-TIRADS Scores and FNA Thresholds

Score	0	2	3	4-6	≥7
TIRADS Class	TR1	TR2	TR3	TR4	TR5
Description	Benign	Not suspicious	Mildly suspicious	Moderately suspicious	Highly suspicious
FNA Threshold	Not recommended	Not recommended	≥2.5 cm	≥1.5 cm	≥1 cm

ACR, American College of Radiology; *FNA*, Fine-needle aspiration; *TIRADS*, Thyroid Imaging Reporting and Data System.
From Robertson RP et al: *DeGroot's endocrinology, basic science and clinical practice,* ed 8, Philadelphia, 2023, Elsevier.

- Thyroid nodules incidentally identified as FDG avid on fluorodeoxyglucose-PET (FDG-PET) scan done for other disorders have a higher malignancy rate (25%).
- Highly suspicious nodules should be referred for surgical evaluation even if result of FNA is "benign."

- Most follicular neoplasms are benign, and patients should not be told they have a malignancy based on this cytology result.

REFERENCES

Available at eBooks.Health.Elsevier.com.

RELATED CONTENT

Thyroid Nodule (Patient Information)
Thyroiditis (Related Key Topic)
Thyroid Carcinoma (Related Key Topic)

AUTHORS: **PETER J. MAZZAGLIA, MD** and **FRED F. FERRI, MD**

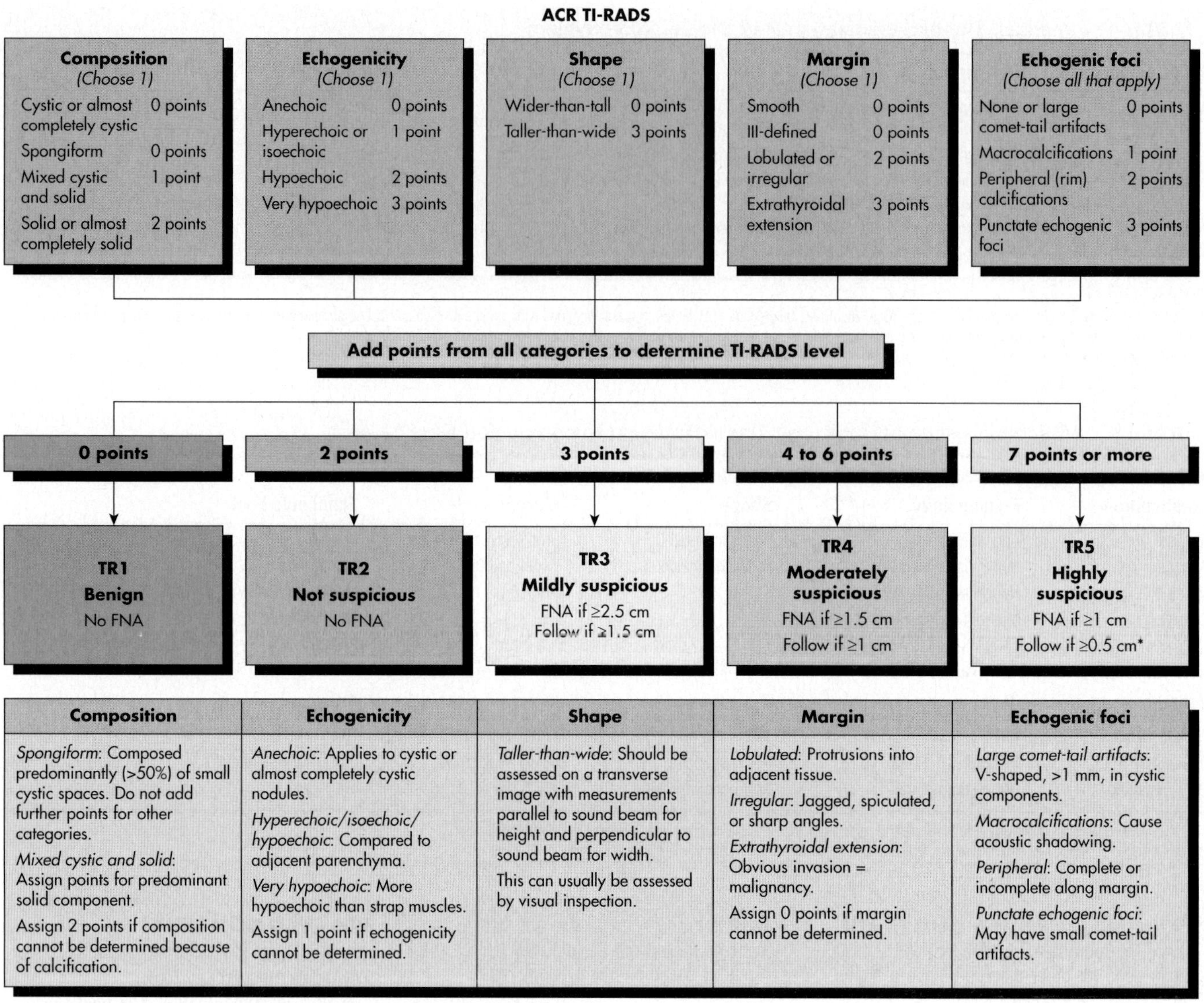

ACR TI-RADS

Composition (Choose 1)		Echogenicity (Choose 1)		Shape (Choose 1)		Margin (Choose 1)		Echogenic foci (Choose all that apply)	
Cystic or almost completely cystic	0 points	Anechoic	0 points	Wider-than-tall	0 points	Smooth	0 points	None or large comet-tail artifacts	0 points
Spongiform	0 points	Hyperechoic or isoechoic	1 point	Taller-than-wide	3 points	Ill-defined	0 points	Macrocalcifications	1 point
Mixed cystic and solid	1 point	Hypoechoic	2 points			Lobulated or irregular	2 points	Peripheral (rim) calcifications	2 points
Solid or almost completely solid	2 points	Very hypoechoic	3 points			Extrathyroidal extension	3 points	Punctate echogenic foci	3 points

Add points from all categories to determine TI-RADS level

0 points	2 points	3 points	4 to 6 points	7 points or more
TR1 Benign No FNA	**TR2** Not suspicious No FNA	**TR3** Mildly suspicious FNA if ≥2.5 cm Follow if ≥1.5 cm	**TR4** Moderately suspicious FNA if ≥1.5 cm Follow if ≥1 cm	**TR5** Highly suspicious FNA if ≥1 cm Follow if ≥0.5 cm*

Composition	Echogenicity	Shape	Margin	Echogenic foci
Spongiform: Composed predominantly (>50%) of small cystic spaces. Do not add further points for other categories. *Mixed cystic and solid:* Assign points for predominant solid component. Assign 2 points if composition cannot be determined because of calcification.	*Anechoic:* Applies to cystic or almost completely cystic nodules. *Hyperechoic/isoechoic/ hypoechoic:* Compared to adjacent parenchyma. *Very hypoechoic:* More hypoechoic than strap muscles. Assign 1 point if echogenicity cannot be determined.	*Taller-than-wide:* Should be assessed on a transverse image with measurements parallel to sound beam for height and perpendicular to sound beam for width. This can usually be assessed by visual inspection.	*Lobulated:* Protrusions into adjacent tissue. *Irregular:* Jagged, spiculated, or sharp angles. *Extrathyroidal extension:* Obvious invasion = malignancy. Assign 0 points if margin cannot be determined.	*Large comet-tail artifacts:* V-shaped, >1 mm, in cystic components. *Macrocalcifications:* Cause acoustic shadowing. *Peripheral:* Complete or incomplete along margin. *Punctate echogenic foci:* May have small comet-tail artifacts.

*Refer to discussion of papillary microcarcinomas for 5–9 mm TR5 nodules.

FIG. 3 The American College of Radiology (ACR) Thyroid Imaging, Reporting and Data System (TI-RADS) lexicon, TR levels, and criteria for fine-needle aspiration biopsy. (From Tessler FN et al: ACR Thyroid Imaging, Reporting and Data System [TI-RADS]: white paper of the ACR TI-RADS Committee, *J Am Coll Radiol* 14:587-595, 2017.)

TABLE 3 American College of Radiology Thyroid Nodule Scoring System: TI-RADS

Scoring and Classification	Recommendations
TR1: 0 points	TR1: No FNA required (0.3% risk)
TR2: 2 points	TR2: No FNA required (1.5% risk)
TR3: 3 points	TR3: ≥1.5 cm follow-up at 1, 3, 5 yr, ≥2.5 cm FNA (4.8% risk)
TR4: 4-6 points	TR4: ≥1.0 cm follow-up at 1, 2, 3, 5 yr ≥1.5 cm FNA (9.1% risk)
TR5: ≥7 points	TR5: ≥0.5 cm follow-up each year, ≥1.0 cm FNA (35% risk)

ACR TI-RADS is a reporting system for thyroid nodules on ultrasound proposed by the American College of Radiology (ACR) and is based on composition, echogenicity, shape, margin, and echogenic foci.

From Tessler FN et al: ACR Thyroid Imaging, Reporting and Data System (TI-RADS): white paper of the ACR TI-RADS committee, *J Am Coll Radiol* 14:587-595, 2017.

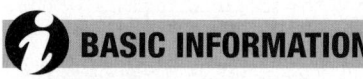
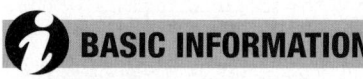 BASIC INFORMATION

DEFINITION

Thyroiditis is an inflammatory disease of the thyroid. It is a multifaceted disease with various etiologies, different clinical characteristics (depending on the stage), and distinct histopathology. Thyroiditis can be subdivided into three common types (Hashimoto, painful, and painless) and two rare forms (suppurative and Riedel). To add to the confusion, there are various synonyms for each form, and there is no internationally accepted classification of autoimmune thyroid disease. However, in general there is agreement on the use of several synonyms for equivalent entities (Table 1).

SYNONYMS

Hashimoto thyroiditis: Chronic lymphocytic thyroiditis, chronic autoimmune thyroiditis, lymphadenoid goiter

Painful subacute thyroiditis: Subacute thyroiditis, giant cell thyroiditis, de Quervain thyroiditis, subacute granulomatous thyroiditis, pseudogranulomatous thyroiditis

Painless postpartum thyroiditis: Subacute lymphocytic thyroiditis, postpartum thyroiditis

Painless sporadic thyroiditis: Silent sporadic thyroiditis, subacute lymphocytic thyroiditis

Infectious thyroiditis: Acute suppurative thyroiditis, bacterial thyroiditis, microbial inflammatory thyroiditis, pyogenic thyroiditis

Riedel thyroiditis: Fibrous thyroiditis

ICD-10CM CODES	
E06.3	Autoimmune thyroiditis
E06.1	Subacute thyroiditis
E06.9	Thyroiditis, unspecified
E06.0	Acute thyroiditis
E06.5	Other chronic thyroiditis

PHYSICAL FINDINGS & CLINICAL PRESENTATION

- Thyroiditis typically has three phases (Fig. 1): Thyrotoxic and hypothyroid (each lasting approximately 3 mo) and return to euthyroidism.
- Hashimoto: Patients may have signs of hyperthyroidism (tachycardia, diaphoresis, palpitations, weight loss) or hypothyroidism (fatigue, weight gain, delayed reflexes) depending on the stage of the disease. Usually there is diffuse, firm enlargement of the thyroid gland; the gland may also be of normal size (atrophic form with clinically manifested hypothyroidism).
- Painful subacute: Exquisitely tender, enlarged thyroid, fever; signs of hyperthyroidism are initially present; signs of hypothyroidism can subsequently develop.
- Painless thyroiditis: Clinical features are similar to subacute thyroiditis except for the absence of tenderness of the thyroid gland.
- Suppurative: Patient is febrile with severe neck pain, focal tenderness of the involved portion of the thyroid, erythema of the overlying skin.
- Riedel: Slowly enlarging hard mass in the anterior neck; often mistaken for thyroid cancer;

TABLE 1 Terminology for Thyroiditis

Type	Synonyms
Hashimoto thyroiditis	Chronic lymphocytic thyroiditis Chronic autoimmune thyroiditis Lymphadenoid goiter
Postpartum thyroiditis	Painless postpartum thyroiditis Subacute lymphocytic thyroiditis
Painless sporadic thyroiditis	Silent sporadic thyroiditis Subacute lymphocytic thyroiditis Lymphocytic thyroiditis with spontaneously resolving hyperthyroidism
Painful subacute thyroiditis	Subacute de Quervain thyroiditis Subacute nonsuppurative thyroiditis Giant-cell thyroiditis Subacute granulomatous thyroiditis Pseudogranulomatous thyroiditis
Suppurative thyroiditis	Infectious thyroiditis Acute suppurative thyroiditis Pyrogenic thyroiditis Bacterial thyroiditis
Drug-induced thyroiditis	Amiodarone, lithium, IFN-α, IL-2, tyrosine kinase inhibitors, checkpoint inhibitor immunotherapy
Radiation-induced thyroiditis	
Palpation- or trauma-induced thyroiditis	
Riedel's thyroiditis	Fibrous thyroiditis IgG4-induced thyroiditis

IFN, Interferon; *Ig,* immunoglobulin; *IL-2,* interleukin 2.
From Robertson RP et al: *DeGroot's endocrinology, basic science and clinical practice,* ed 8, Philadelphia, 2023, Elsevier.

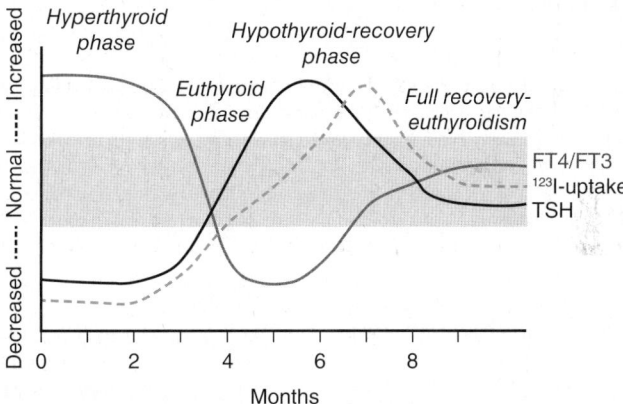

FIG. 1 Graphical representation of the typical clinical course of various forms of thyroiditis, mainly painful subacute thyroiditis, painless postpartum thyroiditis, and painless sporadic thyroiditis. Fluctuation is a frequent finding; patients with thyroiditis archetypally undergo an initial thyrotoxic phase, followed by hypothyroidism and eventual recovery. The horizontal axis represents time, and the vertical axis represents the quantity of thyroid-stimulating hormone *(green curve),* FT4/FT3 *(orange curve),* and ^{123}I uptake *(dotted blue curve).* The green area represents the normal range of values. *TSH,* Thyroid-stimulating hormone. (From Robertson RP et al: *DeGroot's endocrinology, basic science and clinical practice,* ed 8, Philadelphia, 2023, Elsevier.)

signs of hypothyroidism occur in advanced stages.

ETIOLOGY

- Fig. 2 illustrates the stages in the autoimmune process leading to thyroid dysfunction. The main differentiating characteristics between the different subtypes of thyroiditis are summarized in Table 2
- Hashimoto: Autoimmune disorder that begins with the activation of CD4 T-helper

lymphocytes specific for thyroid antigens. The etiologic factor for the activation of these cells is unknown. The natural history of Hashimoto thyroiditis is illustrated in Fig. E3
- Painful subacute: Possibly postviral; usually follows a respiratory illness not considered to be a form of autoimmune thyroiditis
- Painless thyroiditis: Frequently occurs postpartum
- Infectious (suppurative): Infectious etiology, generally bacterial, although fungi and parasites

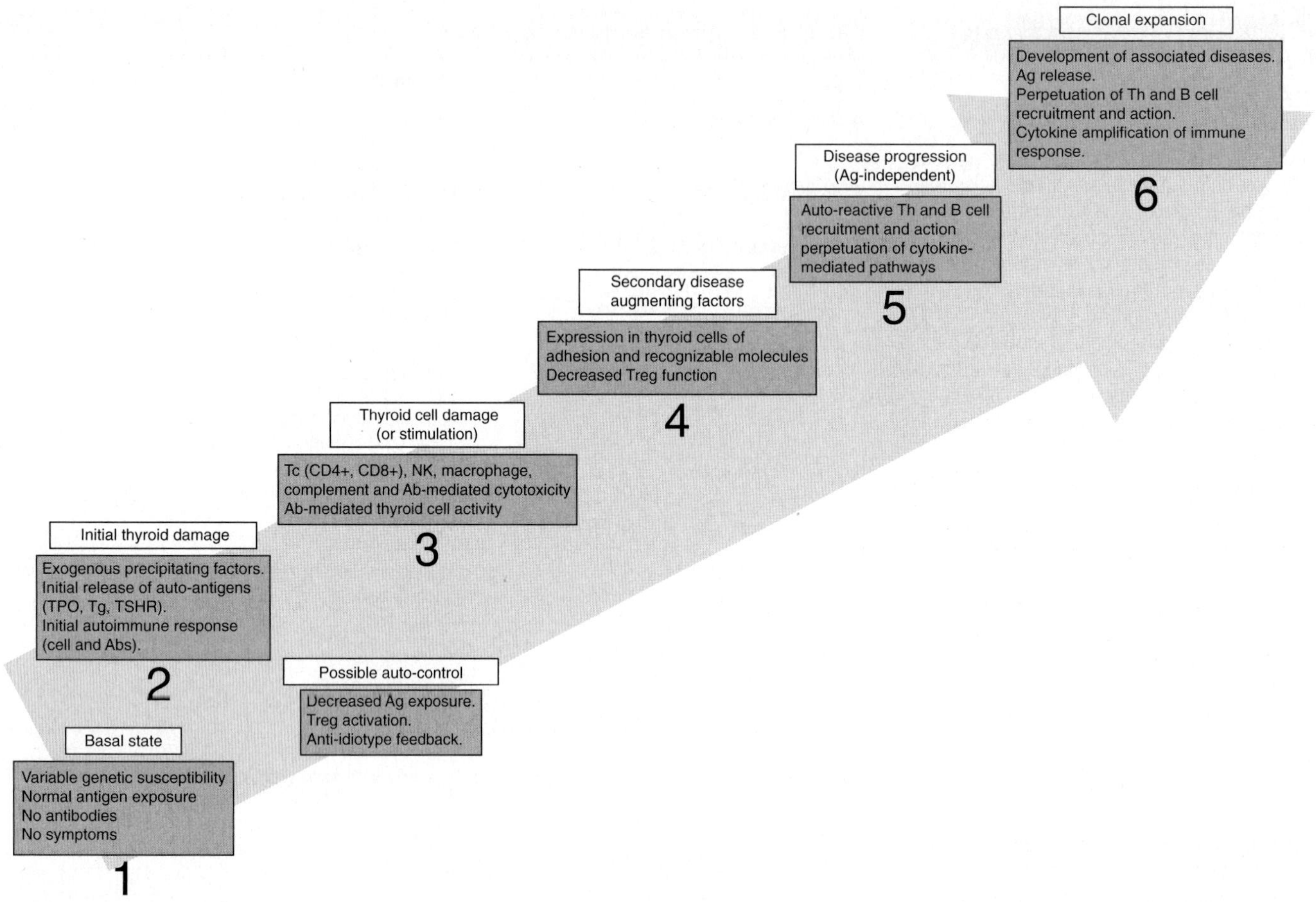

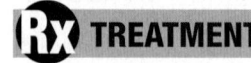

FIG. 2 Flow diagram to illustrate the stages in the autoimmune process leading to thyroid dysfunction. Starting at a first basal state, in which there is a variable genetic susceptibility, with normal antigen exposure, no antibodies, and no symptoms, exogenous precipitating factors may initiate the autoimmune response and thyroid damage. The possibility of autocontrol and returning point exists, but perpetuation of the autoimmune response will lead to secondary disease, augmenting factors, disease progression, and clonal expansion. *Ab,* Antibody; *Ag,* antigen; *NK,* natural killer cell; *Tc,* cytotoxic T cell; *Tg,* thyroglobulin; *Th,* T helper cell; *TPO,* thyroid peroxidase; *Treg,* regulatory T cell; *TSHR,* thyroid-stimulating hormone receptor. (From Robertson RP et al: *DeGroot's endocrinology, basic science and clinical practice,* ed 8, Philadelphia, 2023, Elsevier.)

have also been implicated; often occurs in immunocompromised hosts or after a penetrating neck injury
- Riedel: Fibrous infiltration of the thyroid; etiology unknown
- Drug induced: Typically painless due to lithium, interferon-alfa, amiodarone, interleukin-2
- Radiation thyroiditis: Occurs 5 to 10 days after treatment with radioactive iodine; it is painful and may result in transient exacerbation of hyperthyroidism

Dx DIAGNOSIS

DIFFERENTIAL DIAGNOSIS
- The hyperthyroid phase of Hashimoto, subacute, and silent thyroiditis can be mistaken for Graves disease.
- Riedel thyroiditis can be mistaken for carcinoma of the thyroid.
- Painful subacute thyroiditis can be mistaken for infections of the oropharynx and trachea or for suppurative thyroiditis.
- Factitious hyperthyroidism can mimic silent sporadic thyroiditis.

WORKUP
- The diagnostic workup includes laboratory and x-ray evaluation to rule out other conditions that may mimic thyroiditis (see "Differential Diagnosis") and differentiate the various forms of thyroiditis.
- The patient's medical history may be helpful in differentiating the various types of thyroiditis (e.g., presentation after childbirth is suggestive of silent [postpartum, painless] thyroiditis; occurrence after a viral respiratory infection suggests subacute thyroiditis; history of penetrating injury to the neck indicates suppurative thyroiditis).

LABORATORY TESTS
- Thyroid-stimulating hormone, free T4: May be normal or indicative of hypothyroidism or hyperthyroidism depending on the stage of the thyroiditis.
- White blood cell (WBC) with differential: Increased WBC with left shift occurs with subacute and suppurative thyroiditis.
- Antimicrosomal antibodies: Detected in >90% of patients with Hashimoto thyroiditis and 50% to 80% of patients with silent thyroiditis.

- Serum thyroglobulin levels are elevated in patients with subacute and silent thyroiditis; this test is nonspecific but may be useful in monitoring the course of subacute thyroiditis and distinguishing silent thyroiditis from factitious hyperthyroidism (low or absent serum thyroglobulin level).

IMAGING STUDIES (FIGS. E4 & E5)
24-h radioactive iodine uptake (RAIU) is useful to distinguish Graves disease (increased RAIU) from thyroiditis (normal or low RAIU). Table E3 summarizes factors that influence 24-h thyroid iodide uptake.

Rx TREATMENT

ACUTE GENERAL Rx
- The duration of the thyrotoxic phase of thyroiditis is usually 10 to 12 wk. This phase is followed by a hypothyroid phase typically lasting up to 12 wk.
- Treat hypothyroid phase in symptomatic patients somatic with levothyroxine 25 to

TABLE 2 Main Differentiating Characteristics between the Different Subtypes of Thyroiditis

	Etiology	Epidemiology	Clinical picture	Diagnosis	Treatment
Acute, suppurative	Infection (bacterial most frequent)	Prior upper respiratory infection No difference between sexes Children and 20-40 yr. Association to pyriform sinus fistula	Sudden, local symptoms (pain, swelling, dysphagia, etc.) Generalized symptoms (fever) Mild thyrotoxicosis very rare	↑ESR. ↑WBC. TSH/FT4 normal TPOAb and TgAb negative FNA (gram-positive staining) and culture	Antibiotics FNA and/or drainage
Painful, subacute (de Quervain)	Viral (almost)	Female predominance (5:1) 20-60 yr. Possible seasonal incidence related to prior viral infection. Associated with HLA-B35	Prodromal generalized symptoms (flulike) Local pain, extending to jaw and ears Initial hyperthyroid phase followed by hypothyroidism	↓TSH/↑FT4. ↑↑ESR, ↑CRP Negative TPOAb and TgAb. ↓RAIU FNA: inflammatory infiltrate (+ giant cells) Biopsy: inflammatory infiltrate (+ giant cells), granulomas > fibrosis	NSAID, especially aspirin 1-3 g/day. Glucocorticoids Beta-blockers
Painless, silent, subacute	Autoimmune Postpartum	Female predominance (2:1) All ages, peak 30-40 yr. Thyroid "aggressors" Potential progression to chronic	Initial hyperthyroid phase followed by hypothyroidism. No local symptoms	Abnormal TSH/FT4 ↑Thyroglobulin. (+) TPOAb and TgAb (persistent) (−) TSH-R–Ab. Normal inflammation reactants ↓RAIU	Expectant (observation) Beta-blockers for hyperthyroid symptoms L-T4 replacement therapy if needed
Chronic (Hashimoto)	Autoimmune	Middle-aged women Thyroid dysfunction precipitating factors	Goiter in the early phase Later hypothyroidism	Initial goiter and mild hyperthyroidism Then, ↑TSH/↓FT4. (++) TPOAb and TgAb Biopsy: inflammatory infiltrate + fibrosis + necrosis	L-T4 replacement therapy
Riedel	Fibrous, IgG4		Insidious compressive local symptoms Fibrosis in other extrathyroidal locations No signs of systemic inflammation Hypothyroidism	Biopsy: fibrosis	Glucocorticoids in the early phase Surgery for compressive symptoms and signs

↑ elevated; ↓: decreased; (+): positive; (−): negative.
CRP, C-reactive protein; *ESR,* Erythrocyte sedimentation rate; *FNA,* fine-needle aspiration; *FT4,* free T4; *L-T4,* levothyroxine; *NSAID,* nonsteroidal antiinflammatory drugs; *RAIU,* radioactive iodine uptake; *TgAb,* antithyroglobulin antibodies; *TPOAb,* antithyroperoxidase antibodies; *TSH,* thyroid-stimulating hormone; *WBC,* white blood cell.
From Robertson RP et al: *DeGroot's endocrinology, basic science and clinical practice,* ed 8, Philadelphia, 2023, Elsevier.

50 mcg/day initially and monitor serum thyroid-stimulating hormone initially every 6 to 8 wk.
- Control symptoms of hyperthyroidism with β-blockers (e.g., propranolol 20 to 40 mg PO q6h or atenolol).
- Control pain in patients with subacute thyroiditis with NSAIDs. Prednisone 20 to 40 mg daily may be used if nonsteroidals are insufficient, but it should be gradually tapered off over several weeks.
- Use intravenous antibiotics and drain abscess (if present) in patients with suppurative thyroiditis.

DISPOSITION

- Hashimoto thyroiditis: Long-term prognosis is favorable; most patients recover their thyroid function.

- Painful subacute thyroiditis: Permanent hypothyroidism occurs in 10% of patients.
- Painless thyroiditis: 6% of patients have permanent hypothyroidism.
- Infectious thyroiditis: There is usually full recovery after treatment.
- Riedel thyroiditis: Hypothyroidism occurs when fibrous infiltration involves the entire thyroid.

REFERRAL

- Surgical referral in patients with compression of adjacent neck structures and in some patients with infectious (suppurative) thyroiditis.
- Total thyroidectomy has been shown to improve symptoms in patients with Hashimoto thyroiditis who still have symptoms despite having normal thyroid gland function while receiving medical therapy.

RELATED CONTENT

Thyroiditis (Patient Information)
Hyperthyroidism (Related Key Topic)
Hypothyroidism (Related Key Topic)

AUTHOR: **FRED F. FERRI, MD**

BASIC INFORMATION

DEFINITION

Tinnitus is a perceived sound in the absence of acoustic stimulus external to the head. It may be unilateral, bilateral, or lateral dominant. It is commonly described as a ringing, buzzing, roaring, hissing, whistling, humming, cricket-like, or pulsing sound. It is frequently a symptom associated with hearing loss, Ménière disease, acoustic neuroma, drug toxicity, depression, or an autoimmune inner ear disease. The sound may be internal and perceived only by the patient, called subjective or tonal tinnitus, or it may be heard by both the patient and the examiner, called objective or nontonal tinnitus. Tinnitus can be subdivided into three key distinctions: Subjective versus objective, pulsatile versus nonpulsatile, and primary versus secondary. This early classification guides the history, physical examination, and subsequent diagnostic studies, thereby facilitating a simple and efficient approach to tinnitus management. Subjective tinnitus can only be heard by the patient, while objective tinnitus is also appreciated by the examiner. Objective tinnitus is rare: Even at an otolaryngology tertiary referral center, it represents only 1.5% of all tinnitus complaints. By definition, objective tinnitus implies an identifiable source for the acoustic stimulus, including joints, muscles, turbulent blood flow, or rarely, otoacoustic emissions. Objective tinnitus is usually pulsatile or rhythmic and can be auscultated in the periauricular region, ear canal, neck, or chest. Patient confirmation that the sound identified is identical to their perceived tinnitus is required for classifying the symptom as objective tinnitus.

Subjective nonpulsatile tinnitus is by far the most common type of tinnitus, representing an estimated 90% of all tinnitus referrals seen in an otolaryngology practice. Typically described as a "ringing," "hissing," "buzzing," or "roaring," nonpulsatile tinnitus is almost exclusively subjective. Conversely, pulsatile tinnitus, often described as rhythmic or pulse-like, can be either subjective or objective and may be altered by changes in position.

ICD-10CM CODES
H93.1	Tinnitus
H93.2	Other abnormal auditory perceptions
H93.11	Tinnitus, right ear
H93.12	Tinnitus, left ear
H93.13	Tinnitus, bilateral
H93.19	Tinnitus, unspecified ear

EPIDEMIOLOGY & DEMOGRAPHICS

PREVALENCE:
- The American Tinnitus Association reports 50 to 60 million Americans have tinnitus for >6 mo.
- Prevalence increases steadily with age, peaking for persons aged 60 to 69 yr.
- Prevalence in the U.S. based on National Health Interview Survey (NHIS) in 1996:
  1. 2.98% all ages
  2. 0.26% for persons <18 yr old
  3. 1.6% for persons aged 18 to 44 yr

4. 5.96% for persons aged 45 to 64 yr: 7.7% males, 4.3% females
5. 9.6% for persons aged 65 to 74 yr: 12% males, 7.7% females
6. 7.6% for persons >75 yr: 11.4% males, 5.3% females
7. 2:1 South/Northeast regions
- Up to 18% of people in industrialized societies are mildly affected by chronic tinnitus, and 0.5% report tinnitus having a severe effect on their daily life.
- Only 20% of patients with persistent tinnitus ever seek medical evaluation.

PREDOMINANT SEX & AGE: Persons most affected are male, Caucasian, elderly, persons with hearing impairment, persons living in southern U.S. For military veterans, tinnitus is the third most common service-related disability.

RISK FACTORS: Any condition causing hearing loss or damage to the auditory system can produce tinnitus. Cochlear damage from exposure to noise is the most common cause. Exposure to ototoxic drugs is also important.

PHYSICAL FINDINGS & CLINICAL PRESENTATION
- History should focus on exposure to loud noises, evidence of hearing loss, and ototoxic drugs.
- Patient should be screened for depression.
- Patient who complains of sound in ear may also complain of ear pain or fullness.
- Objective tinnitus is pulsatile and coincides with patient's pulse.
- Physical examination should focus on HEENT, neck, and neurologic exam.
- There may be no significant physical findings.

ETIOLOGY
- The mechanism behind tinnitus is poorly understood. It may originate at any point along the auditory pathway. Causes of tinnitus include injured cochlear hair cells, spontaneous activity in auditory nerve fibers, hyperactivity in the auditory nuclei in the brain stem, or a reduction in the suppressive activity of the central auditory cortex.
- Medications implicated in causing tinnitus include salicylates, NSAIDs, aminoglycosides, loop diuretics, valproate, quinine, chemotherapeutic agents, cisplatin, vincristine, and heavy metals such as lead.

DIAGNOSIS

DIFFERENTIAL DIAGNOSIS (TABLE 1, FIG.1)
- Subjective/tonal tinnitus:
  1. Otologic: Tympanic membrane disorder, inner ear disorder (hair cells, organ of Corti), Ménière disease. Sigmoid sinus diverticula (Fig. E2) may manifest as pulsatile venous tinnitus and account for approximately 20% of cases of pulsatile tinnitus
  2. Ototoxic medications
  3. Neurologic: Multiple sclerosis, head trauma, cochlear nerve lesion, acoustic schwannoma, neurofibroma, meningioma

4. Metabolic: Thyroid disorder, hyperlipidemia (leading to plaque formation), vitamin B_{12} deficiency
5. Psychogenic: Depression, anxiety, fibromyalgia
6. Infectious: Otitis media, Lyme disease, meningitis, syphilis
- Objective/nontonal tinnitus:
  1. Vascular: Arterial bruit, venous hum, arteriovenous malformation, vascular tumors
  2. Neurologic: Contraction of muscles of the eustachian tube, contraction of the stapedius muscle, contraction of the tensor tympani muscles, or a palatal myoclonus, glomus jugulare tumor
  3. Conductive: Patulous (wide-open) eustachian tube

WORKUP
- Audiometry.
- Tympanometry.
- Electronystagmography is used to evaluate for Ménière disease.
- An algorithm for tinnitus evaluation is described in Fig. 3.
- Targeted history in tinnitus and clinical significance are summarized in Table E2.

LABORATORY TESTS
Evaluate for metabolic abnormalities: Thyroid-stimulating hormone, CBC, B_{12}, and lipid panel.

IMAGING STUDIES (FIG. 4)
- Computed tomography (CT)/MRI: To evaluate for subjective tinnitus.
- MRI/Magnetic resonance angiography(MRA): To evaluate objective tinnitus.
- Imaging should not be part of routine management. Clinicians must distinguish patients with bothersome tinnitus from patients with nonbothersome tinnitus. For patients without persistent and bothersome tinnitus, audiometric testing is optional.

TREATMENT

NONPHARMACOLOGIC THERAPY
- It is best to avoid exposure to excessive noise, ototoxic agents, and to wear protective equipment in noisy environments, or mask the tinnitus through amplification of normal sounds with a hearing aid. Habituation techniques such as tinnitus retraining therapy may help. Cognitive-behavioral therapy helps patients cope with tinnitus distress through biofeedback.
- Recent trials involving brain stimulation in the form of repetitive transcranial magnetic stimulation (rTMS) have shown reduction in the perception or severity of tinnitus.

ACUTE GENERAL Rx
- If the tinnitus is severe enough to cause suicidal symptoms, immediate referral to a psychiatrist and an otolaryngologist is recommended to minimize the time to diagnosis and optimize treatment.

TABLE 1 Differential Diagnosis and Associated Conditions of Subjective Nonpulsatile Tinnitus

	Etiology or Associated Condition
Inner ear	Sensorineural hearing loss, Ménière disease, presbycusis, noise-induced hearing loss
Middle ear	Otosclerosis, ossicular or tympanic membrane abnormalities, cholesteatoma
External ear	Canal occlusion, cerumen impaction
Otologic infections	Otitis externa, otitis media, labyrinthitis, mastoiditis, herpes zoster oticus
Ototoxic medications	Antibiotics, antineoplastic drugs, corticosteroids, nonsteroidal antiinflammatory drugs, diuretics
Social habits	Alcohol, nicotine, and caffeine intake
Neurologic	Multiple sclerosis, Charcot-Marie-Tooth, epilepsy, migraine
Psychologic	Anxiety, depression
Autoimmune	Systemic lupus erythematosus, systemic sclerosis, rheumatoid arthritis
Musculoskeletal	Temporomandibular joint disorder
Endocrine	Diabetes mellitus, hyperinsulinemia, hypothyroidism, pregnancy

From Flint PW et al: *Cummings otolaryngology, head and neck surgery,* ed 7, Philadelphia, 2021, Elsevier.

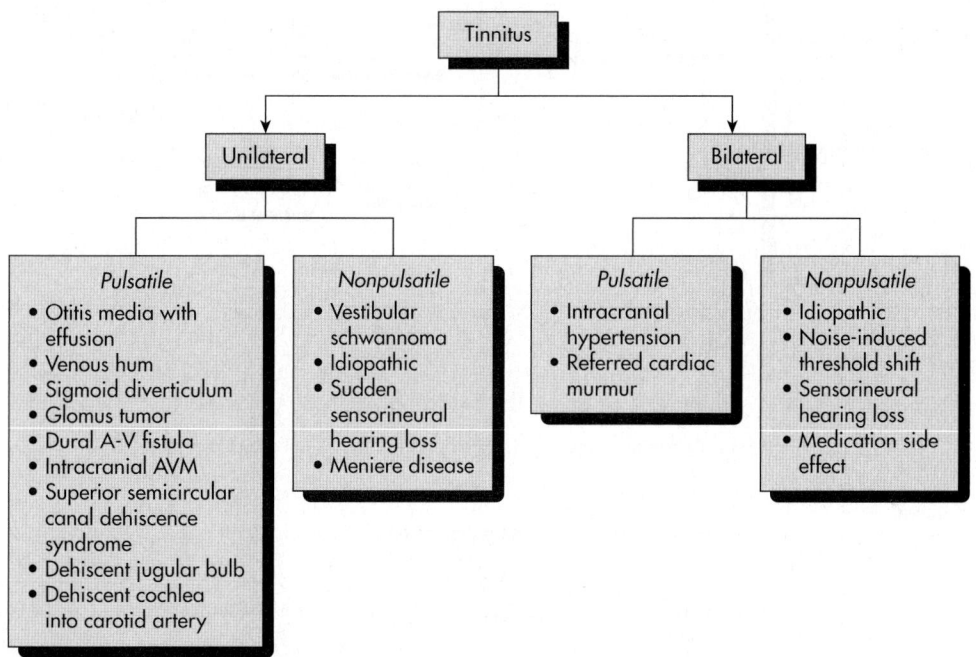

FIG. 1 Establishing a differential diagnosis with a chief complaint of hearing loss. This algorithm encourages the clinician to consider the patient complaint in categorical differential diagnosis families. It is not exhaustive. *SNHL,* Sensorineural hearing loss. (From Flint PW et al: *Cummings otolaryngology, head and neck surgery,* ed 7, Philadelphia, 2021, Elsevier.)

- Patients with persistent symptoms or tinnitus accompanied by visual changes or headache should be evaluated for tumors such as acoustic neuroma.
- Clinicians should not routinely recommend anxiolytics, anticonvulsants, or intratympanic medications.

CHRONIC Rx

There is insufficient evidence to support the use of any medication, vitamin, or nutritional supplement to treat tinnitus. Empirical use of over-the-counter supplements or prescription medications should be discouraged.

DISPOSITION

Clinical course is variable. About 20% to 25% of patients with chronic tinnitus consider it a significant problem. Individualized tinnitus management programs can be beneficial in most patients.

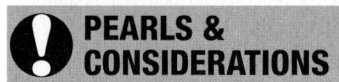 **PEARLS & CONSIDERATIONS**

PREVENTION

- Avoid loud, chronic noise and ototoxic drugs.
- Higher caffeine intake is associated with a lower risk of incidence of tinnitus in women.

RELATED CONTENT

Tinnitus (Patient Information)

AUTHOR: **FRED F. FERRI, MD**

T

Diseases and Disorders

I

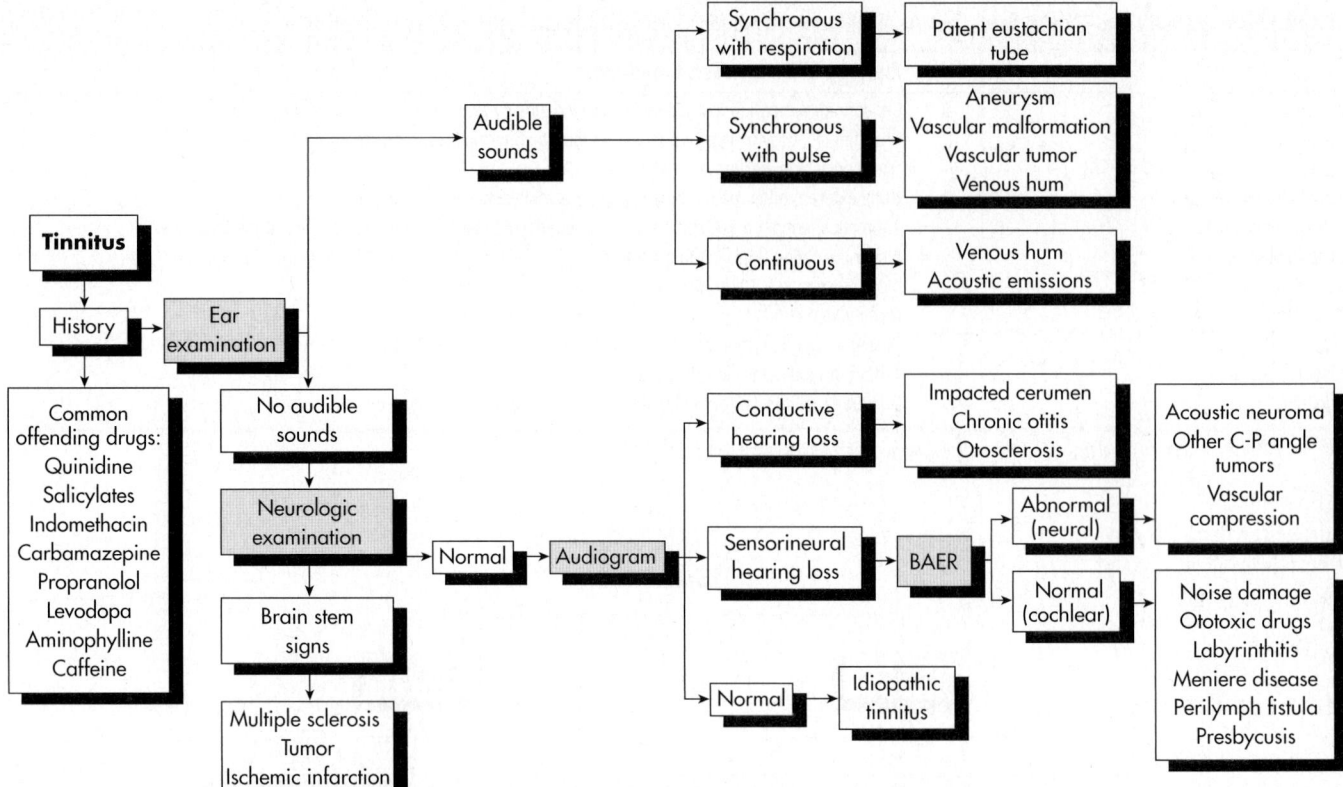

FIG. 3 Evaluation of tinnitus. *BAER,* Brain stem auditory evoked response; *C-P,* cerebellopontine. (From Goldman L, Schafer AI: *Goldman's Cecil medicine,* ed 24, Philadelphia, 2012, Saunders.)

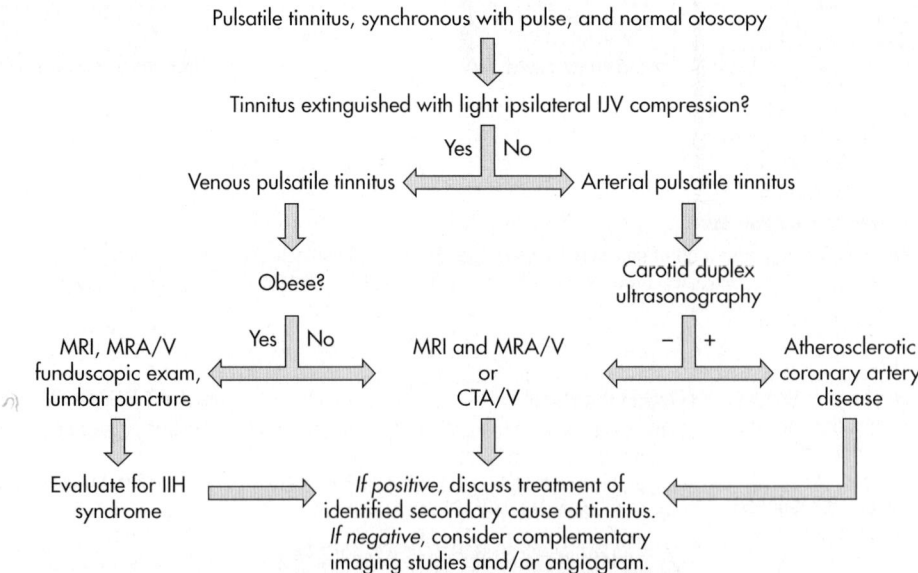

FIG. 4 Diagnostic imaging algorithm for pulsatile tinnitus. *CTA/V,* Computed tomography angiography/venography; *IIH,* idiopathic intracranial hypertension; *IJV,* internal jugular vein; *LP,* lumbar puncture; *MRA/V,* magnetic resonance angiography/venography; *MRI,* magnetic resonance imaging. (From Flint PW et al: *Cummings otolaryngology, head and neck surgery,* ed 7, Philadelphia, 2021, Elsevier.)

BASIC INFORMATION

DEFINITION

Tourette syndrome (TS) is an inherited neuropsychiatric disorder characterized by motor and phonic tics that wax and wane and change over time. Diagnosis requires onset of symptoms prior to age 18; however, symptom onset typically occurs in early childhood.

Tics are sudden, brief, patterned, repetitive, intermittent, movements (motor tics) or sounds (phonic tics) that may abruptly interrupt otherwise normal motor activity or speech.[1]

SYNONYMS

Gilles de la Tourette syndrome
TS
Tourette disorder

ICD-10CM CODE
F95.2 Combined vocal and multiple motor tic disorder [de la Tourette]

EPIDEMIOLOGY & DEMOGRAPHICS

PREVALENCE (IN U.S.): Estimates range from 0.3% to 3% in children.[2]
PREDOMINANT SEX: Approximate male:female ratio of 4:1.[2]
PREDOMINANT AGE: Typical age of onset is between 2 and 12 yr of age (most frequently between 3 and 8 yr).[3]

PHYSICAL FINDINGS & CLINICAL PRESENTATION

- Neurologic examination is normal.
- Phonic tics are characterized by simple meaningless sounds or noises (e.g., clearing of throat, sniffing, grunting, forceful exhales or inhales) or complex, which are semantically meaningful utterances (e.g., repetition of words or short phrases, swearing [coprolalia]).[3]
- Motor tics can be simple (e.g., blinking, grimacing, head jerking [Fig. E1]) or complex (e.g., gesturing [Fig. E2]). Tics wax, wane, change over time, and are often suppressible. Commonly, they are preceded by a premonitory urge that builds until the tic is performed, during which the urge is resolved and then later builds again.[4]
- TS is often associated with a variety of psychiatric conditions, most commonly attention-deficit/hyperactivity disorder (ADHD) and obsessive-compulsive disorder (OCD).[5]
- Diagnostic criteria of TS according to the *Diagnostic and Statistical Manual of Mental Disorders,* fifth edition (DSM-5), are as follows:
  1. Multiple motor tics and one or more phonic tics must be present for greater than 1 yr, although not necessarily concurrently.
  2. The tics may wax and wane in frequency but have persisted for more than 1 yr since onset.
  3. Age at onset is less than 18 yr.
  4. Disturbance is not attributable to the direct physiologic effects of a substance

(e.g., cocaine) or another medical condition (e.g., Huntington disease or post-viral encephalitis).

ETIOLOGY

The exact pathogenesis is unknown; however, current models describe inhibitory network dysfunction between the cortex, thalamus, and basal ganglia.[6,7] An alternative hypothesis is that tics may be habits that are reinforced by aberrant increased dopamine release, thus resulting in reinforced learning.[7] Genetic predisposition is likely, as there is a strong family history of OCD or TS in patients with tics, and twin studies provide evidence for the importance of genetic factors with a concordance rate of 77%.[8] Multiple genes have been explored as possible links to TS, but no causative gene has yet been identified.

DIAGNOSIS

DIFFERENTIAL DIAGNOSIS

- Autism spectrum disorder
- Carbon monoxide poisoning
- Sydenham chorea
- Brain tumor
- Drug intoxication: Many drugs are known to induce or exacerbate tic disorders, including cocaine and supratherapeutic levels of stimulants
- Postinfectious encephalitis
- Inherited disorders: Huntington disease, neurodegeneration with brain iron accumulation, and neuroacanthocytosis. These conditions should have other observed abnormalities on neurologic examination
- Functional neurologic symptom disorder

WORKUP

Clinical examination and history to confirm diagnosis

LABORATORY TESTS

No laboratory tests are required for the diagnosis.

IMAGING STUDIES

Computed tomography scan and MRI of brain are unremarkable in TS and unnecessary when the neurologic examination is within normal limits.

TREATMENT (FIG. 3)

NONPHARMACOLOGIC THERAPY

- Multidisciplinary: Education of patients, parents, teachers, psychologists, and school nurses is essential.
- Patients with tics require treatment only when movements and sounds are bothersome, impairing, or painful to the patient. If none of these characteristics are present, patient and caregiver education on the natural history of tics is appropriate. However, forceful motor tics involving the neck should be treated more aggressively (these often are bothersome and painful to the child), as these

may pose a risk of causing traumatic cervical myelopathy with associated spasticity, weakness, and eventual loss of mobility.[9]
- Cognitive-behavioral therapy, termed habit-reversal treatment or Comprehensive Behavioral Intervention for Tics (CBIT), is often recommended as first-line treatment.[10]
- Screening for comorbid psychiatric disorders such as ADHD, OCD, anxiety, and depression must be performed, as these symptoms often become more impairing than the tics.

ACUTE GENERAL Rx

In general, acute treatment of tics is not necessary unless tics are clearly self-injurious. In this case, one could consider short-term treatment with benzodiazepines until adequate doses of chronic anti-tic medications are achieved.[11]

CHRONIC Rx

Tics require treatment when movements and sounds are painful, bothersome, or impairing to the patient or if lack of treatment would cause imminent self-harm (e.g., forceful motor tics of the neck).[3]

Oral medications include alpha-2 agonists (clonidine, guanfacine), anticonvulsants (topiramate, clonazepam), dopamine-receptor blocking agents (haloperidol, pimozide, aripiprazole, fluphenazine), and vesicular monoamine transporter type 2 (VAMT2) inhibitors (tetrabenazine, valbenazine, deutetrabenazine).
TICS:
- Alpha-2 agonists (clonidine and guanfacine) can be used for treatment of mild motor and phonic tics; however, they may be limited by adverse effects.[12] They may also be beneficial for management of comorbid psychiatric conditions such as impulsivity.
- Haloperidol, aripiprazole, and pimozide are the only U.S. FDA–approved medications for the treatment of tics in TS; however, other dopamine receptor blocking agents may also be used such as fluphenazine or ziprasidone.[11,12] Dopamine receptor blocking medications carry a small but significant risk of tardive dyskinesia, especially in adults.
- Tetrabenazine, deutetrabenazine, and valbenazine are presynaptic dopamine-depleting agents that inhibit VMAT2 and have been found to provide meaningful benefit in treatment of tics and do not carry a risk of tardive dyskinesia.[13] However, large-scale randomized placebo-controlled trials have not shown the same benefit.[12]
- An antiepileptic (topiramate) has also been found to be helpful in reducing tics.[11,12]
- Botulinum neurotoxin injections are effective for simple motor tics and are particularly useful in forceful neck tics. Injections must be repeated every 3 mo.[14]
- In the case of tics that are refractory to treatments and are impairing, surgical treatment with deep brain stimulation can be considered.[15]

ADHD: Stimulants are the most common medications for the treatment of ADHD. Previous studies have reported exacerbations of tics in some patients; however, a meta-analysis

Treatment algorithm for Tourette syndrome

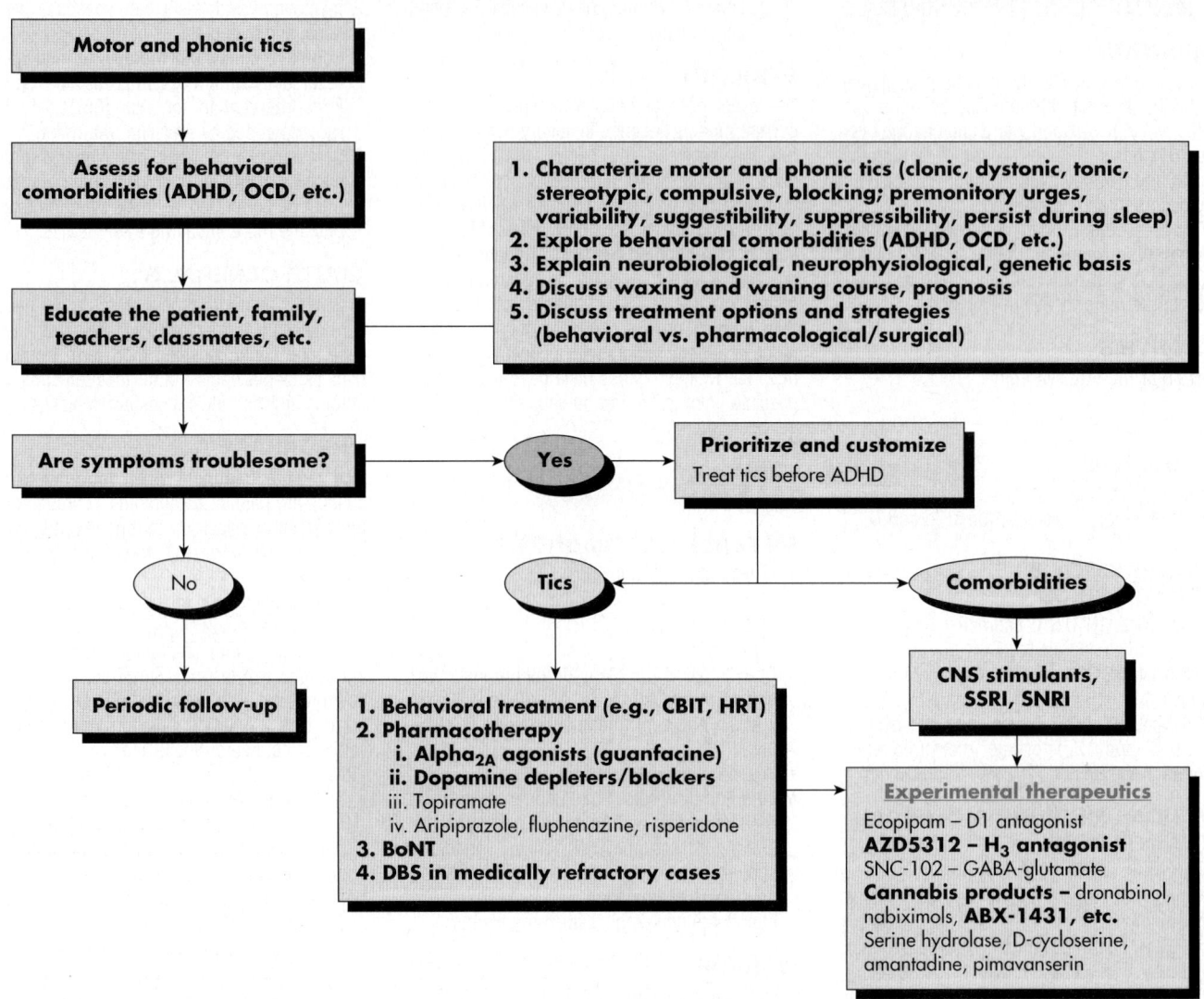

FIG. 3 Treatment algorithm for Tourette syndrome. *ADHD*, Attention-deficit/hyperactivity disorder; *CBIT*, comprehensive behavioral intervention for tics; *CNS*, central nervous system; *DBS*, deep brain stimulation; *GABA*, γ-aminobutyric acid; *HRT*, habit reversal training; *OCD*, obsessive compulsive disorder; *SNc*, substantia nigra pars compacta; *SNRI*, selective noradrenergic reuptake inhibitor; *SSRI*, selective serotonin reuptake inhibitor. (From Jankovic J et al: *Bradley and Daroff's neurology in clinical practice*, ed 8, Philadelphia, 2022, Elsevier.)

concluded that there was no concrete evidence that stimulants consistently worsened tic severity.[16] These medications should be used if impairing ADHD is present.

OCD: Selective serotonin reuptake inhibitors, such as fluoxetine, citalopram, escitalopram, or fluvoxamine, are the most effective medications for OCD.

DISPOSITION

- The intensity and frequency of tics often decrease in late adolescence and early adulthood.
- Approximately 75% of patients will have reduced severity of tics in adulthood; however, 90% will still have mild tics that are often not impairing as adults.[3]

REFERRAL

When tics do not require treatment, no referrals are necessary. The provider should educate the

patient and caregivers on the diagnosis and natural history of tics. However, referrals should be made to neurologists or subspecialty movement disorder neurologists if (1) the diagnosis is unclear, (2) treatment is required or has been refractory, or (3) there is risk of imminent self-harm when untreated. The latter should be expedited whenever possible.

If comorbid psychiatric disorders are bothersome or impairing, referral to a psychiatrist and/or psychologist should also be made.

❗ PEARLS & CONSIDERATIONS

- Tics require treatment when they are bothersome, impairing, or painful.
- An important part of treatment is appropriate evaluation and therapy of coexisting conditions (e.g., ADHD, OCD), as these conditions

often cause more disability than the tics themselves.
- Treatment of tics includes comprehensive behavioral intervention for tics, medications, botulinum neurotoxin injections, and deep brain stimulation.

COMMENTS

Patient education may be obtained from the Tourette Syndrome Association, 4240 Bell Blvd., Bayside, NY 11361-2864; 800-237-0717 or 718-224-2999; http://www.tsa-usa.org/.

REFERENCES

Available at eBooks.Health.Elsevier.com.

RELATED CONTENT

Tourette Syndrome (Patient Information)

AUTHOR: **MARIAM HULL, MD**

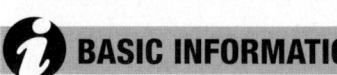

T

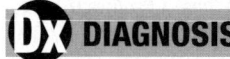 BASIC INFORMATION

DEFINITION

Transient ischemic attack (TIA) is a transient episode of neurologic dysfunction caused by focal brain, spinal cord, or retinal ischemia attributable to a vascular territory, without acute infarction on MRI.[1] TIA symptoms typically resolve within 60 min to 24 h. Despite complete symptom resolution, one third (20% to 50%) of patients clinically suspected to have suffered a TIA have evidence of acute tissue infarction on MRI and should be diagnosed with an ischemic stroke.[1-3]

SYNONYMS

TIA
Amaurosis fugax
Ophthalmologic TIA
"Mini-stroke"
Pre-stroke

ICD-10CM CODES	
G45.9	Transient cerebral ischemic attack, unspecified
G45.8	Other transient cerebral ischemic attacks and related syndromes
Z86.73	Personal history of transient ischemic attack (TIA), and cerebral infarction without residual deficits

EPIDEMIOLOGY & DEMOGRAPHICS

INCIDENCE: 240,000 persons annually[4]
PREVALENCE:
- 7.6 million persons in the U.S.
- Annual risk of stroke after either a TIA or minor stroke is approximately 3% to 4%.[3,4]

PREDOMINANT SEX & RACE: Males > females; African American > Caucasian
PEAK INCIDENCE: After age 60 yr[4]
RISK FACTORS: Same as for ischemic stroke (diabetes, hypertension, age, smoking, obesity, alcoholism, unhealthy diet, psychosocial stress, and lack of regular physical activity)

PHYSICAL FINDINGS & CLINICAL PRESENTATION

- TIAs often present with transient neurologic symptoms including ipsilateral transient monocular blindness (amaurosis fugax), contralateral numbness or weakness, contralateral homonymous hemianopsia, and/or aphasia.[1]
- Anatomy of carotid artery is illustrated in Fig. E1. Box 1 summarizes carotid artery TIAs.[5]
- Anatomy of vertebral arteries is illustrated in Fig. E2. Vertebrobasilar artery TIAs are described in Box 2.[5]

ETIOLOGY

Embolic (cardioembolism in 10% to 15%), large vessel atherothrombotic disease (20% to 25%), lacunar disease, hypoperfusion, hypercoagulable state, arteritis[6]

BOX 1 Carotid Artery Transient Ischemic Attacks (TIAs)

Symptoms
- Contralateral hemiparesis, hemianopsia, hemisensory loss
- Aphasia, if dominant hemisphere
- Neglect and hemi-inattention, if non-dominant hemisphere
- Ipsilateral amaurosis fugax

Associated Findings
- Carotid bruit
- Retinal artery emboli

Adapted from Kaufman DM et al: *Kaufman's clinical neurology for psychiatrists,* ed 9, Philadelphia, 2023, Elsevier.

BOX 2 Vertebrobasilar Artery Transient Ischemic Attacks (TIAs)

Symptoms
- Vertigo, vomiting, tinnitus
- Circumoral paresthesias or numbness
- Dysarthria, dysphasia
- Drop attacks

Associated Findings
- Nystagmus
- Ataxia
- Cranial nerve abnormalities

Adapted from Kaufman DM et al: *Kaufman's clinical neurology for psychiatrists,* ed 9, Philadelphia, 2023, Elsevier.

(Dx) DIAGNOSIS

DIFFERENTIAL DIAGNOSIS

Seizures, hypoglycemia, hemiplegic migraine, intracranial hemorrhage, mass lesion, vestibular disease, Bell palsy, meningitis, multiple sclerosis, subdural hematoma, brain abscess, cervical or lumbar spine disease, conversion disorder.[7]

WORKUP

Given the high risk of stroke within the first 48 h after TIA (up to 10%), hospital admission for workup is advised.[8] An outpatient workup can be considered if MRI and vascular neurology expertise can be arranged promptly (ideally <24 h).[9] Most of the immediate risk of stroke is secondary to carotid disease.

The American Heart Association recommends that the ABCD2 score be used in the evaluation of TIA.[8] It consists of 1 point for age ≥60 yr, 1 point for BP ≥140 mm Hg systolic or ≥90 mm Hg diastolic, clinical features (2 points for unilateral weakness, 1 point for speech impairment), duration of TIA (2 points for duration ≥60 min, 1 point for duration 10 to 59 min), presence of diabetes mellitus (1 point).[10,11] According to the guidelines, it is reasonable to hospitalize patients with TIA if they present within 72 h and have an ABCD2 score ≥3.[8,12] There is some debate about the usefulness of this scale because it fails to account for changes seen on echocardiogram, carotid Dopplers, or ECG that

---

may place the patient at more imminent risk of stroke (carotid stenosis, atrial fibrillation, cardiac thrombus, etc.). If patient cannot have outpatient evaluation, ideally within 48 h but no later than 1 wk after TIA, admission is also indicated. Alternatives to this scoring system are being investigated.[9,13]

LABORATORY TESTS

CBC, basic metabolic panel, prothrombin time, activated partial thromboplastin time, sedimentation rate, fasting lipid panel, serum glucose and hemoglobin A_{1c} (to detect latent diabetes mellitus), and thyroid-stimulating hormone.[8]

IMAGING STUDIES

- Computed tomography (CT) scan should be obtained to exclude hemorrhage; MRI with diffusion-weighted images if immediately available to determine whether infarction occurred.[8,9]
- Imaging of the vessels should be obtained via magnetic resonance angiography (MRA) head and neck, computed tomography angiography (CTA) head and neck, or, if CTA is not available, carotid Doppler/transcranial Doppler (CD/TCD). If symptoms are localizable to the posterior circulation, MRA or CTA should be obtained in lieu of CD/TCD.[14,15]
- Transthoracic echocardiogram should be obtained in all patients. A bubble study should be obtained in all patients younger than 50 yr with TIA symptoms to exclude patent formen ovale (PFO).[16]
- ECG should be obtained to exclude the presence of arrhythmias, namely atrial fibrillation.[17,18]
- At least 24 h of heart rhythm monitoring should be accomplished to screen for arrhythmia. Paroxysmal atrial fibrillation is common in patients with TIA and longer monitoring is encouraged.

Noninvasive ambulatory ECG monitoring for 30 days significantly improved the detection of atrial fibrillation by a factor of more than five and nearly doubled the rate of anticoagulant treatment as compared with the standard practice of short-duration ECG monitoring.[19]

Furthermore, a randomized study of insertable cardiac monitor vs. conventional follow-up in patients with cryptogenic stroke or TIA found that by 6 mo atrial fibrillation had been detected in 8.9% in the insertable cardiac monitor group vs. 1.4% in the control group.[20]

(Rx) TREATMENT

NONPHARMACOLOGIC THERAPY

- Carotid endarterectomy or carotid stenting should be considered for patients found to have carotid stenosis of ≥50% as the cause for TIA. Efficacy is greatest in the 2 wk immediately following a TIA or ischemic stroke.[21,22] Please refer to the "Carotid Artery Stenosis" chapter for more information.
- Intracranial angioplasty and stenting is only used in select patients, generally reserved for

ischemic stroke patients who fail maximal medical management with aggressive platelet inhibition, strict risk factor control such as hyperlipidemia, hypertension, diabetes mellitus, weight loss, treatment of sleep apnea, and smoking cessation, among others.[23-25]

ACUTE GENERAL Rx

- In the absence of contraindications, patients with atrial fibrillation should be considered for anticoagulation. Choices for anticoagulants include the direct oral anticoagulants (such as dabigatran, rivaroxaban, apixaban, edoxaban, betrixaban) and/or warfarin. In patients with TIA and some causes of embolism such as a cardiac thrombus, therapeutic anticoagulation should be achieved rapidly. Those who are not candidates for a direct oral anticoagulation and who will need chronic warfarin should first be started on either intravenous (IV) heparin or therapeutic anticoagulant doses of Lovenox, along with warfarin, until target international normalization ratio (INR) between 2.0 and 3.0 is achieved, at which point warfarin should be continued as monotherapy.[8]
- Patients with high-risk TIA (ABCD2 score >3) or minor stroke may be started on dual antiplatelet therapy (DAPT) of clopidogrel 300 to 600 mg on day 1 followed by clopidogrel 75 mg/day and aspirin for 21 to 30 days based on the CHANCE and POINT trials.[26,27] A study[28] examining whether starting DAPT for TIA can be beneficial beyond 24 h revealed that DAPT can be helpful when given as long as 72 h after high-risk TIA of presumed atherosclerotic origin.

CHRONIC Rx

- Please refer to the "Secondary Stroke Prevention" chapter for more complete discussion.
- Chronic therapy includes single antiplatelet (after 21 to 30 days) and modifying the four major risk factors: Hypertension, dyslipidemia, diabetes mellitus, and smoking cessation.
- If no evidence of atrial fibrillation, antiplatelet therapy alone should be used to reduce the risk of recurrent TIAs or subsequent stroke.[29,30] Antiplatelet agents commonly used in stroke prevention include aspirin, aspirin/dipyridamole, clopidogrel, and ticagrelor. All are reasonable choices, but practitioners should consider their individual patient's comorbidities when selecting an antiplatelet agent. Chronic long-term dual antiplatelet therapy is not recommended as this increases the risk of hemorrhagic complications.
- Warfarin (INR 2.0-3.0) or use of direct oral anticoagulants instead of an antiplatelet is indicated for prevention of future strokes in patients with atrial fibrillation.[8]

⚠ PEARLS & CONSIDERATIONS

- The 1-yr all-cause mortality rate is 25% in patients diagnosed with TIA.
- Approximately 20% to 30% of ischemic strokes are heralded by transient ischemic symptoms.
- Patients with nonclassic TIA symptoms (e.g., isolated symptoms of vertigo, ataxia, diplopia, dysarthria, bilateral decreased vision, numbness in one body segment) tend to wait longer before seeking medical attention and are more likely to have has a recurrent stroke before seeking attention (8% vs. 5%). Both classic and nonclassic symptoms of TIA confer similar 90-day stroke risk.[29]
- Previous studies conducted between 1987 and 2003 estimated the risk of stroke or an acute coronary syndrome was 12% to 20% during the first 3 mo after a TIA. New data estimate the 1-yr risk to be 6.2%. Multiple major risk factors: Hypertension, dyslipidemia, infarctions on brain imaging, large-artery atherosclerosis, and an ABCD score of 6 or 7 were each associated with more than a doubling of the risk of stroke.

PREVENTION

- A healthy lifestyle and management of cardiovascular risk factors should be encouraged.
- Antiplatelet therapy has not been proven efficacious in primary prevention of TIA or stroke but is very beneficial in secondary prevention.

PATIENT & FAMILY EDUCATION

Patients should be counseled on the early signs of stroke symptoms and instructed to promptly seek medical attention if they develop symptoms concerning for stroke. Patients should be encouraged to pursue a healthy lifestyle to include exercise and smoking cessation. In addition, patients should take an active role in controlling blood pressure and blood glucose. Further educational materials can be found online at https://www.stroke.org/.

REFERENCES & SUGGESTED READING

Available at eBooks.Health.Elsevier.com.

RELATED CONTENT

AUTHORS: **CÉSAR E. ESCAMILLA-OCAÑAS, MD** and **COREY ELAM GOLDSMITH, MD, FAAN**

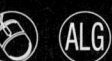
BASIC INFORMATION

DEFINITION

- Traumatic brain injury (TBI) is a broad term that encompasses multiple intracranial processes (including cerebral contusion, epidural hemorrhages, subdural hemorrhages, subarachnoid hemorrhages, skull fractures, diffuse axonal injury, and cerebral edema) that occur secondary to head trauma or if the head experiences a sudden deceleration injury without external trauma resulting in an injury to the brain.[1] An overview of classification of TBI is summarized in Table 1. These injuries result in varying levels of cellular and macroscopic changes, detected with clinical examination and supplemented by neuroimaging.
- Mild TBI is defined as loss of consciousness <30 min, a Glasgow Coma Scale (GCS) of 13 to 15, and normal imaging.
- Moderate TBI is defined as loss of consciousness for 30 min to 24 h with even longer alteration in consciousness, a GCS of 9 to 12, and may or may not have abnormal imaging.
- Severe TBI is defined as >24 h of loss of consciousness with a GCS of 3 to 8 and prolonged posttraumatic amnesia with normal or abnormal imaging.[1,2]

SYNONYMS

TBI
Head injury
Concussion
Intracranial contusion

ICD-10CM CODES

S06.9 X0A	Intracranial injury
S06.1X7A	Traumatic cerebral edema with loss of consciousness of any duration with death due to brain injury prior to regaining consciousness, initial encounter
S06.2X9A	Diffuse traumatic brain injury with loss of consciousness of unspecified duration, initial encounter
S06.300A	Unspecified focal traumatic brain injury without loss of consciousness, initial encounter
S06.305A	Unspecified focal traumatic brain injury with loss of consciousness greater than 24 h with return to preexisting conscious level, initial encounter
S06.309A	Unspecified focal traumatic brain injury with loss of consciousness of unspecified duration, initial encounter
S09.90	Unspecified injury of the head

EPIDEMIOLOGY & DEMOGRAPHICS

Traumatic brain injury (TBI) is a leading cause of mortality in the young and elderly worldwide. In the 2022 Centers for Disease Control and Prevention (CDC) surveillance report, suicide, unintentional falls, and motor vehicle crashes caused the majority of TBI-related deaths.[3]

INCIDENCE: Globally, more than 69 million people suffer from TBI each yr, with North America and Europe showing highest incidence and Southeast Asian and Western Pacific countries experiencing the greatest burden of disease. According to one estimate, up to 4.6 million individuals suffer from TBI in United States and Canada each yr.[4] In 2014, about 2.87 million emergency department visits, including deaths and hospitalizations, were associated with TBI. The financial burden of TBI has been estimated to be greater than $80 billion/yr in the United States and is approaching $400 billion worldwide in direct and indirect costs.[5]

PREVALENCE: In 2016, the global prevalence of TBI was estimated at 55.5 million. From 1990 to 2016, the age-standardized prevalence of TBI increased by 8.4%.[6] According to the CDC, there were 214,110 TBI-related hospitalizations in 2020 and 69,473 TBI-related deaths in 2021, an incidence that does not reflect people with TBI who were only treated in emergency departments or primary care or were untreated.[3]

PREDOMINANT SEX & AGE: TBI occurs more commonly in males and hospitalizations/deaths are the highest in adults >75 yr of age.[3]

RISK FACTORS:
- Falls
- Motor vehicle accidents
- Physical violence
- Sport injuries
- Ballistic injuries (gunshot wounds, blast injuries)

GENETICS: TBI and Apo E ∈4 synergistically are associated with a tenfold increased risk for Alzheimer disease. Apo E ∈4 is also associated with larger intracerebral hematomas and greater ischemia after TBI.[7]

PHYSICAL FINDINGS & CLINICAL PRESENTATION

TBI patients present with a spectrum of clinical symptoms including nausea, vomiting, headache, seizures, altered mental status, and/or coma. Stigmata of trauma, including bruises, scalp lacerations, and periorbital or mastoid ecchymosis suggesting skull base fractures, can be telltale signs of underlying traumatic brain injury. Box 1 describes risk stratification in patients with minor head trauma. The spectrum of TBI is most commonly assessed using the GCS (Table 2), which ranges from 3 to 15 and utilizes eye, motor, and verbal exams (Table 3). The reproducibility and the ease of administration across multiple specialties make the GCS scoring the ideal severity screening test.

ETIOLOGY

- Suicide, unintentional mechanical falls, motor vehicle accidents, and assaults resulting in direct or indirect head trauma are the most common etiologies, with suicides being the leading cause of TBI-related deaths in the U.S.[3] (Fig. E1, Fig. E2).
- Gunshot wounds are the most prevalent **penetrating injuries** (Fig. E3), accounting for 35% of deaths from TBI under the age of 45 yr in the United States. Self-inflicted injuries such as nail gun injuries can also lead to penetrating trauma (Fig. E4). Gunshot wounds are the most lethal type of brain injury, with 90% resulting in death.
- The most common mechanisms of pediatric TBI vary according to age. Falls are the leading cause of TBI in children under the age of 14 yr. Children younger than 4 yr of age are injured mainly by falls but are also affected by abusive injuries and motor vehicle accidents. Children 4 to 8 yr of age are injured in falls and motor vehicle accidents but also

TABLE 1 Overview of Classification of Traumatic Brain Injury

Mechanism	Blunt		High velocity (MVC)
			Low velocity (fall, assault)
	Penetrating		GSW
			Other (stab wounds, etc.)
	Blast		Explosive devices
Severity	Mild		GCS 14-15
	Moderate		GCS 9-13
	Severe		GCS 3-8
Morphology	Skull fracture	Vault	Linear versus stellate
			Depressed/nondepressed
			Open/closed
		Basilar	With/without CSF
			With/without CN palsy
	Intracranial lesions	Focal	Epidural
			Subdural
			Intracerebral
		Diffuse	Mild concussion
			Classic concussion
			Diffuse axonal injury

CN, Cranial nerve; *CSF,* cerebrospinal fluid; *GCS,* Glasgow Coma Scale; *GSW,* gunshot wound; *MVC,* motor vehicle collision.
Adapted from Jankovic J et al: *Bradley and Daroff's neurology in clinical practice,* ed 8, Philadelphia, 2022, Elsevier.

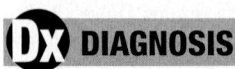

become more at risk for other transportation-related injuries such as bicycle-related incidents. Abusive head trauma (AHT) is particularly common in young infants less than 2 yr of age; approximately 30 of every 100,000 infants aged less than 1 yr were hospitalized for AHT.[8]

- Sports-related TBIs account for roughly one third of all causes of TBI, with higher incidence in males, adolescents, and young adults. Some common sports associated with TBI are football, horse riding, cycling, skateboarding, hockey, water sports, and snow sports.[9]

DIAGNOSIS

DIFFERENTIAL DIAGNOSIS

Differential diagnosis of TBI is quite limited; however, there are several considerations and diagnoses that should be considered. These are enumerated in the imaging section.

BOX 1 Risk Stratification in Patients with Minor Head Trauma

High Risk
- Focal neurologic findings
- Asymmetric pupils
- Skull fracture on clinical examination
- Multiple trauma
- Serious, painful, distracting injuries
- External signs of trauma above the clavicles
- Initial Glasgow Coma Scale score of 14 or 15
- Loss of consciousness
- Posttraumatic confusion or amnesia
- Progressively worsening headache
- Vomiting
- Posttraumatic seizure
- History of bleeding disorder or anticoagulation
- Recent ingestion of intoxicants
- Unreliable or unknown history of injury
- Previous neurologic diagnosis
- Previous epilepsy
- Suspected child abuse
- Age above 60 yr or below 2 yr

Medium Risk
- Initial Glasgow Coma Scale score of 15
- Brief loss of consciousness
- Posttraumatic amnesia
- Vomiting
- Headache
- Intoxication

Low Risk
- Currently asymptomatic
- No other injuries
- No focality on examination
- Normal pupils
- No change in consciousness
- Intact orientation and memory
- Initial Glasgow Coma Scale score of 15
- Accurate history
- Trivial mechanism
- Injury less than 24 h ago
- No or mild headache
- No vomiting
- No preexisting high-risk factors

TABLE 2 Glasgow Coma Scale

Response	Points
Speech	
Alert, oriented, and conversant	5
Confused, disoriented, but conversant	4
Intelligible words, not conversant	3
Unintelligible sounds	2
No verbalization, even with painful stimulus	1
Eye Opening	
Spontaneous	4
To verbal stimuli	3
To painful stimuli	2
None, even with painful stimuli	1
Motor	
Follows commands	6
Localizes painful stimulus	5
Withdraws from painful stimulus	4
Flexor posturing with central pain	3
Extensor posturing with central pain	2
No response to painful stimulus	1

Data from Teasdale G, Jennett B: Assessment of coma and impaired consciousness: a practical scale, *Lancet* 2:81-84, 1974. In Vincent JL et al: *Textbook of critical care*, ed 8, Philadelphia, 2024, Elsevier.

WORKUP

TBI workup is always a part of the advanced trauma life support (ATLS) protocol. Primary and secondary survey followed by imaging studies constitutes the standardized approach to TBI. Focused TBI workup includes:
- History: Including timing of injury, duration of loss of consciousness if applicable, events leading up to the injury, mechanism of injury,

seizures (if any), comorbidities, use of anticoagulants and antiplatelet agents (requires reversal in the event of intracranial blood on imaging).
- Neurologic examination: Glasgow Coma Scale, cranial nerves, motor/sensory exam. Assess for scalp lacerations, specifically overlying a skull fracture as well as cerebrospinal fluid (CSF) otorrhea or rhinorrhea.
- Computed tomography (CT) imaging of the head if there is a significant history of impact to the head, polytrauma, positive loss of consciousness, or stigmata of trauma to the head. Factors to consider regarding the need for CT imaging in head-injured patients are described in Table 4. The American College of Emergency Physicians Clinical Policy Regarding Neuroimaging in adults with mild TBI is summarized in Box 2.

LABORATORY TESTS

- Basic labs including CBC, basic metabolic panel, prothrombin time, activated partial thromboplastin time, urine drug screen, and ethanol blood level.
- Consider tests for platelet function analysis for unknown antiplatelet use.
- Consider cardiac evaluation (troponin, ECG, and echocardiography) in patients with history pointing to a cardiac event leading to TBI.
- No blood biomarker currently exists for TBI assessment (Fig. E5 and Fig. E6).

IMAGING STUDIES (TABLE 5)

CT scan is the cornerstone of imaging modalities for head trauma; however, it is not always necessary. Patients over the age of 16 with minimal head injury (i.e., no history of loss of

---

TABLE 3 Useful Criteria to Assess the Severity of Head Injury[a]

Quantifying the Degree of Head Injury	Glasgow Coma Scale (GCS)	Score
Moderate TBI (GCS 9-13)	**Eye Opening**	
Severe TBI (GCS <8)	Spontaneous	4
Significant head CT:	To speech	3
• Cerebral edema	To pain	2
• Midline shift	None	1
• Subdural/epidural bleeding	**Verbal Response**	
• Open head injury with intracranial air	Oriented	5
	Confused conversation	4
	Inappropriate words	3
	Incomprehensible sounds	2
	None	1
	Best Motor Response	
	Obeys commands	6
	Localizes pain	5
	Flexion withdrawal to pain	4
	Abnormal flexion (decorticate)	3
	Extension (decerebrate)	2
	None (flaccid)	1

TBI, Traumatic brain injury.
[a]Consultation with other specialists (i.e., neurosurgeon) may be valuable for the orthopedic surgeon unfamiliar with the process of "clearing" the patient's head injury for ischemic monomelic neuropathy (IMN) fixation.
From Browner B et al: *Skeletal trauma: basic science, management, and reconstruction*, ed 6, Philadelphia, 2019, Elsevier.

TABLE 4 Factors to Consider Regarding the Need for Computed Tomography in Head-Injured Patients

Indications for urgent CT include the following:
- Evidence of skull fracture—basal, depressed, or open
- Abnormal results of neurologic examination
- Seizure
- Vomiting more than once
- High-risk mechanism (e.g., ejection from vehicle; injury to pedestrian or cyclist vs. car occupant)
- Decreasing GCS score or persistently decreased GCS score below 15
- Indications for lower threshold for CT scan include the following:
  1. Age >60 yr
  2. Persistent anterograde amnesia
  3. Retrograde amnesia >30 min
  4. Coagulopathy
  5. Fall >5 stairs or >3 ft
  6. Intoxication (examination unreliable)
  7. LOC >30 min
  8. Mechanism and location of injury
  9. Social factors (e.g., abusive situation at home, language barriers precluding an accurate history)

CT, Computed tomography; *GCS*, Glasgow Coma Scale; *LOC*, loss of consciousness.
From Jankovic J et al: *Bradley and Daroff's neurology in clinical practice*, ed 8, Philadelphia, 2022, Elsevier.

BOX 2 American College of Emergency Physicians Clinical Policy Regarding Neuroimaging in Adults with Mild Traumatic Brain Injury

A noncontrast head computed tomography (CT) is indicated (level-1 recommendation) in adults with level of consciousness (LOC) or post-traumatic amnesia only if one or more of the following is present:
- Headache
- Vomiting
- Age >60 yr
- Drug or alcohol intoxication
- Deficits in short-term memory
- Physical evidence of trauma above the clavicle
- Posttraumatic seizure
- Glasgow Coma Scale (GCS) score <15
- Focal neurologic deficit
- Coagulopathy

A noncontrast head CT should be considered (level-2 recommendation) in head trauma patients with no LOC or posttraumatic amnesia if there is:
- Focal neurologic deficit
- Vomiting
- Severe headache
- Age ≥ 65 yr
- Physical signs of a basilar skull fracture
- GCS score <15
- Coagulopathy
- A dangerous mechanism (e.g., ejection from motor vehicle, pedestrian struck, fall of more than 3 feet or 5 stairs)

From Marx JA et al: *Rosen's emergency medicine*, ed 8, Philadelphia, 2014, Elsevier.

TABLE 5 Comparison of Head Imaging Modalities

	Computed Tomography Scans	**Magnetic Resonance Imaging**	**Angiography**	**Skull Radiography**
Advantages	Fast Patient accessible for monitoring Defines acute hemorrhages, mass effects, bone injuries, hydrocephalus, intraventricular blood, edema	Defines contusions and pericontusion edema, posttraumatic ischemic infarction, brainstem injuries	Helps localize acute traumatic lesions Defines vascular injuries, injuries to venous sinuses Detects mass effects	Readily available May help screen some patients for further imaging studies
Disadvantages	Artifacts arise from patient's movement, foreign bodies Streak artifacts may obscure brainstem or posterior fossa	Slow Patients not easily accessible for monitoring Does not define most acute hemorrhagic lesions Not useful for bone injuries	Does not define nature of acute lesion Does not detect infratentorial masses	Does not indicate presence or absence of intracranial injury
Indications	Acute severe head trauma Acute moderate head trauma Suspected depressed skull fracture High-risk minor head trauma Suspected child abuse in minor head trauma Deteriorating neurologic status	Persistent symptoms with postconcussive syndrome Suspected posttraumatic ischemic infarction Suspected contusions not seen on CT scan	Suspected vascular injury CT scan not available	CT scan may not be done Penetrating head trauma

CT, Computed tomography.
From Marx JA et al: *Rosen's emergency medicine, concepts and clinical practice*, ed 7, Philadelphia, 2010, Elsevier.

BOX 3 Clinical Decision Rules for Neuroimaging in Adults with Mild Traumatic Brain Injury Canadian Computed Tomography Head Rule (CCHR)

High-Risk Injury (May Require Neurologic Intervention)
- GCS score <15 at 2 h after injury
- Suspected open or depressed skull fracture
- Any sign of basal skull fracture (hemotympanum, raccoon eyes, CSF otorrhea or rhinorrhea, Battle sign)
- Vomiting >2 episodes
- Age >65 yr

Medium-Risk Injury (May Have Important Brain Injury on CT)
- Amnesia before impact ≤30 min
- Dangerous mechanism (pedestrian struck by vehicle, occupant ejected from vehicle, fall from elevation >3 feet [five stairs])

New Orleans Criteria (NOC)
- Headache
- Vomiting
- Age >60 yr
- Drug or alcohol intoxication
- Persistent anterograde amnesia
- Trauma above the clavicle
- Seizure

NEXUS II Criteria
- Evidence of significant skull fracture
- Scalp hematoma
- Neurologic deficit
- Altered level of alertness
- Abnormal behavior
- Coagulopathy
- Persistent vomiting
- Age >65 yr

CSF, Cerebrospinal fluid; *CT,* computed tomography; *GCS,* Glasgow Coma Scale.
From Walls RM et al: *Rosen's emergency medicine, concepts and clinical practice,* ed 10, Philadelphia, 2023, Elsevier.

consciousness, amnesia, and confusion), not on blood thinners, and without associated seizure generally do not need a CT scan. Canadian CT head rules (Box 3) for patients with GCS 13 to 15 who do have history of loss of consciousness, amnesia, and/or confusion are a useful guide in determining utility of obtaining a CT scan. If any of these risk factors are present, a CT scan of the head should be considered.

HIGH RISK:
- Failure to reach GCS of 15 within 2 h
- Suspected open or depressed skull fracture
- Any signs of basal skull fracture (hemotympanum, "raccoon" eyes, CSF otorrhea/rhinorrhea, Battle's sign)
- Two or more episodes of vomiting
- Age older than 65

MEDIUM RISK:
- Dangerous mechanism of injury or polytrauma
- Retrograde amnesia to the event >30 min

Usually, in addition to a plain CT of the head (Fig. E7), computed tomography angiography (CTA) head/neck or CT of the spine is helpful if arterial or C-spine injury is suspected, respectively. Other imaging modalities such as MRI can be helpful in certain situations but are typically adjuncts in the acute setting to CT-guided management.

Pathologies that can be identified with imaging are noted in the following:
- Primary extraaxial: Epidural, subdural, subarachnoid hemorrhage
- Primary intraaxial: Axonal injury, cortical contusion, intracerebral or intraventricular hemorrhage, encephalomalacia (from prior TBI or vascular insult)
- Skull fracture: Linear, depressed, open, involving frontal sinus or skull base
- Penetrating brain injury: Gunshot wounds, sharp objects resulting in parenchymal and vascular injury
- Vascular injury: Dissection, traumatic carotid-cavernous fistula (CCF), dural arteriovenous fistula (dAVF), pseudoaneurysm formation
- Secondary acute injury: Diffuse cerebral swelling/dysautoregulation (seen more commonly in children from posttraumatic hyperemia), infarction, infection from penetrating trauma, brain herniation from mass lesion or cerebral edema
- Secondary chronic injury: Hydrocephalus (posttraumatic due to disruption of normal CSF absorption pathways), encephalomalacia, CSF leak (from skull base fractures, manifests as otorrhea or rhinorrhea), leptomeningeal cyst (seen most commonly in infants, skull fracture resulting in underlying dural injury)

℞ TREATMENT (FIG. 8)

Prevention of secondary injury is the primary goal of prehospital and early in-hospital management. Most common mechanisms of secondary injury are either intracranial (increased intracranial pressure [ICP], hematoma) or systemic (hypoxia, hypovolemia, hypotension).

Early categorization of head trauma patients according to the severity (based on GCS) and transport to facilities equipped with personnel and technology to deal with issues pertaining to head trauma has improved the overall management of head injury patients and prevention of secondary injury.[10] Assessment and treatment recommendations for mild TBI are summarized in Table 6. Airway, breathing, and circulation remain the most important parameters to be stabilized, and both directly and indirectly affect GCS and overall outcome. Trauma guidelines suggest intubation should be performed in any patient with a GCS of 8 or less to prevent respiratory failure. Patients were previously hyperventilated to decrease pCO_2 in an effort to reduce ICP. Recent evidence suggests normoventilation for patients with severe TBI, with hyperventilation only being used as a temporary measure in patients with TBI and ICP crisis, until other methods of reducing ICP are employed.[11] Hypotension should also be avoided in patients with TBI, as it has been shown to increase mortality.[11] Transfer to and care in a Level 1 trauma center is associated with better outcomes. Monitoring and treatment recommendations for severe TBI are summarized in Table 7.

Details of in-hospital management including critical care and surgical intervention is beyond the scope of this text. Some important points are summarized below.
- Advanced trauma life support (ATLS) protocol (airway, breathing, circulation, disability, exposure).
- Ventilatory support.
- Optimization of oxygenation, ventilation, and fluid status. Goal-directed parameters for head injury are summarized in Table 8.
- CT head (Fig. E9) to evaluate for mass lesion (hematoma) or cerebral edema. These findings may necessitate either surgical intervention or ICP monitor placement. ATLS guidelines recommend a maximum of 30 minutes between initial assessment and CT head.
- In case of either a severe TBI (GCS 8 or less) or a moderate TBI (GCS 8 to 13) with an unreliable neurologic exam, patients should be admitted to the intensive care unit for frequent neurologic checks. TBI guidelines suggest ICP monitor placement for GCS 8 or less to monitor intracranial pressure closely.[11] Commonly used ICP monitors include intraparenchymal ICP monitors, subarachnoid bolt devices, epidural bolt devices, and external ventricular drains (EVDs). EVDs are considered gold standard, as they can provide diagnostic values and therapeutic management. Research has also supported the use of multimodality monitoring with brain tissue oxygen monitoring for severe TBI patients.[11]
- Surgical decompression may involve evacuation of hematoma (epidural, subdural, intraparenchymal, contusion) through craniotomy (replacement of bone after completion of operation) or decompressive craniectomy (complete removal of bone without replacement). Skull fractures are treated depending on the morphology and location of the fracture.

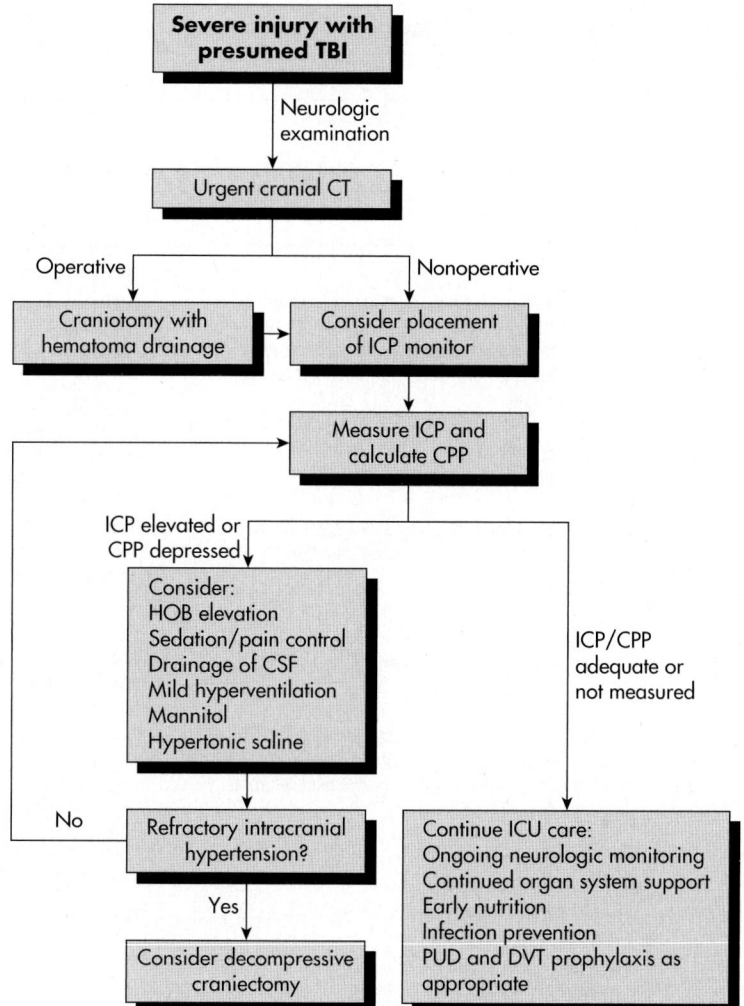

FIG. 8 Algorithm for the management of traumatic brain injury (TBI). *CPP,* Cerebral perfusion pressure; *CSF,* cerebrospinal fluid; *CT,* computed tomography; *DVT,* deep venous thrombosis; *HOB,* head of bed; *ICP,* intracranial pressure; *ICU,* intensive care unit; *PUD,* peptic ulcer disease. (From Townsend CM et al: *Sabiston textbook of surgery,* ed 21, St Louis, 2022, Elsevier.)

TABLE 6 Assessment and Treatment Recommendations for Mild Traumatic Brain Injury

Function	Assessment	Treatment
Overall recovery	Standardized symptom checklist	Physical rest 1-2 days[1] followed by subsymptomatic aerobic exercise[2]
Headache	Determine the type	HA persisting more than 3-4 days may require abortive treatment tailored to phenotype (migraine, tension-type, occipital neuralgia, etc.)
Vertigo	Romberg test, dynamic standing, tandem gait	If Hallpike Dix is normal, or if Epley maneuver does not relieve symptoms, consider physical therapy for vestibular rehabilitation
Eye movements	Examine cranial nerves 3, 4, 6 for tracking, saccades, diplopia, nystagmus	Physical therapy evaluation for vestibular rehabilitation
Near vision	Near-point accommodation and binocular convergence	Ophthalmologic evaluation for vision therapy
Cognitive function	Symptoms, cognitive testing, neuropsychologist evaluation	Sleep hygiene, neuropsychology evaluation for cognitive rehabilitation[3]

HA, Headache.

[1]Thomas DG et al: Benefits of strict rest after acute concussion: a randomized controlled trial, *Pediatrics* 135:213-223, 2015.
[2]Kurowski BG et al: Aerobic exercise for adolescents with prolonged symptoms after mild traumatic brain injury: an exploratory randomized clinical trial, *J Head Trauma Rehabil* 32:79-89, 2017.
[3]Cooper DB et al: Cognitive rehabilitation for military service members with mild traumatic brain injury: a randomized clinical trial, *J Head Trauma Rehabil* 32:E1-E15, 2017.
From Goldman L, Schafer AI: *Goldman-Cecil medicine,* ed 26, Philadelphia, 2019, Elsevier.

TABLE 7 Guidelines for the Management of Severe Traumatic Brain Injury

Topic	Level 1	Level 2	Level 3
Blood pressure and oxygenation	Insufficient data	Avoid systolic blood pressure <90 mm Hg	Avoid hypoxia (Pao_2 <60 mm Hg or O_2 saturation <90%)
Hyperosmolar therapy	Insufficient data	Mannitol is effective for control of raised ICP at doses of 0.25 g/kg to 1 g/kg body weight	Restrict mannitol use prior to ICP monitoring in patients with signs of transtentorial herniation
Prophylactic hypothermia	Insufficient data	Insufficient data	Pooled data indicate that prophylactic hypothermia is not significantly associated with decreased mortality as compared with normothermic controls
Infection prophylaxis	Insufficient data	Periprocedural antibiotics for intubation should be administered to reduce the incidence of pneumonia Early tracheostomy should be performed to reduce days on mechanical ventilation with pneumonia	To reduce infection, routine ventricular catheter exchange or prophylactic antibiotic use for ventricular catheter placement is not recommended
Deep venous thrombosis prophylaxis	Insufficient data	Insufficient data	Intermittent pneumatic compression stockings are recommended Low-molecular-weight heparin or low-dose unfractionated heparin should be used in combination with mechanical prophylaxis
Indications for ICP monitoring	Insufficient data	ICP should be monitored in all salvageable patients with a GCS score of 3-8 after resuscitation and an abnormal CT scan	ICP monitoring is indicated in patients with severe TBI with a normal CT scan if >40 yr of age with blood pressure <90 mm Hg
ICP pressure-monitoring technology	N/A	N/A	N/A
ICP thresholds	Insufficient data	Treatment should be initiated with ICP >20 mm Hg	A combination of ICP values and clinical and brain CT findings should be used to determine the need for treatment
Cerebral perfusion thresholds	Insufficient data	Aggressive attempts to maintain CPP above 70 mm Hg with fluids and pressors should be avoided because of the risk of adult respiratory distress syndrome	CPP of <50 mm Hg should be avoided The CPP value to target lies within the range of 50-70 mm Hg. Patients with intact pressure autoregulation tolerate higher CPP values. Ancillary monitoring of cerebral parameters that include blood flow, oxygenation, or metabolism facilitates CPP management
Brain oxygen monitoring and thresholds	Insufficient data	Insufficient data	Jugular venous saturation (<50%) or brain tissue oxygen tension (<15 mm Hg) are treatment thresholds
Anesthetics, analgesics, sedatives	Insufficient data	Prophylactic administration of barbiturates to induce burst suppression electroencephalogram is not recommended. High-dose barbiturate administration is recommended to control elevated ICP refractory to maximum standard medical and surgical treatment. Hemodynamic stability is essential before and during barbiturate therapy. Propofol is recommended for the control of ICP but not for improvement in mortality or 6-mo outcome	N/A
Nutrition	Insufficient data	Patients should be fed to attain full caloric replacement by day 7 postinjury	N/A
Antiseizure prophylaxis	Insufficient data	Anticonvulsants are indicated to decrease the incidence of early PTS (within 7 days of injury)	N/A
Hyperventilation	Insufficient data	Prophylactic hyperventilation ($Paco_2$ of 25 mm Hg or less) is not recommended	Hyperventilation is recommended as a temporizing measure for the reduction of ICP. Hyperventilation should be avoided during the first 24 h after injury, when cerebral blood flow is often critically reduced. If hyperventilation is used, jugular venous oxygen saturation (SjO_2) or brain-tissue oxygen tension ($PbtO_2$) measurements are recommended to monitor oxygen delivery
Steroids	The use of high-dose methylprednisolone is associated with increased mortality and is contraindicated	N/A	N/A

CT, Computed tomography; *CPP*, cerebral perfusion pressure; *ICP*, intracranial pressure; *GCS*, Glasgow Coma Scale; *PTS*, posttraumatic seizures; *TBI*, traumatic brain injury.
From Jankovic J et al: *Bradley and Daroff's neurology in clinical practice*, ed 8, Philadelphia, 2022, Elsevier.

Open, depressed fractures require surgical debridement and elevation in most cases, in addition to broad-spectrum antibiotics.

- Avoid electrolyte imbalance, especially hyponatremia and hyperglycemia, which may contribute to cerebral edema and increase intracranial pressure. A recent randomized controlled trial studied use of prophylactic continuous 20% hypertonic saline infusion in addition to standard therapy in patients with moderate to severe TBI (COBI trial) and did not improve neurologic status at 6 mo.[12]
- Elevation of head of bed to allow better venous drainage to reduce intracranial pressure.
- ICP management (Table 9), which may include the following: Drainage of cerebrospinal fluid via external ventricular drain, surgical hematoma evacuation, administration of hyperosmotic fluids to reduce edema, pharmacologic sedation and paralysis, pentobarbital-induced coma, and surgical decompression of the brain.[11]
- Decompressive craniectomy in patients with TBI and refractory intracranial hypertension may reduce intensive care unit (ICU) stay but does not clearly improve outcomes. DECRA[13] and RESCUEicp[14] are two randomized controlled trials that assessed decompressive craniectomy (DC) for reduction in ICP vs. medical management. Both trials were unable to provide definite evidence for or against DC, indicating that the decision to proceed with DC should be made on case-by-case basis, after assessment of individual risks and benefits.
- Normothermia: In patients with TBI, hypothermia can reduce intracranial hypertension, but recent trials in patients with an intracranial pressure of more than 20 mm Hg after TBI, therapeutichypothermia, plus standard care to reduce intracranial pressure did not result in outcomes better than those with standard care alone. The most recent TBI guidelines do not recommend hypothermia.[11]
- Prevention of seizures in the acute setting. Seizure prophylaxis can be considered for the first 7 days. Indications for acute seizure prophylaxis in severe head trauma are described in Box 4. Usually phenytoin or levetiracetam is used.[15] Seizure prophylaxis, however, has not been shown to prevent long-term development of traumatic epilepsy.
- Deep vein thrombosis (DVT) prophylaxis is recommended in almost all patients on hospital day 1 or 2 in addition to sequential compression devices (SCDs) for immobile or bedbound patients to prevent DVTs.[11]
- Early initiation of parenteral nutrition.
- Early tracheostomy for ventilator-dependent patients can be considered to reduce mechanical ventilation days and ventilator-dependent complications.[11]

CHRONIC Rx

- TBI can lead to short- and long-term emotional, physiologic, and cognitive sequelae. Patients suffering from TBI are shown to benefit from neurocognitive, occupational, and physical therapy. The Glasgow Outcome Scale is a comprehensive measure of severity and eventual outcome of brain injury. Posttraumatic amnesia, age, length of coma, GCS score within the first 24 h, and imaging study scales are some of the factors that impact long-term outcomes.
- Chronic treatment addresses several sequelae of TBI, including, but not limited to, the following: Dysautonomia, agitation, sleep disturbance, posttraumatic epilepsy, spasticity, dysphagia, syndrome of the trephined, posttraumatic hydrocephalus, apathy, fecal/urinary

---

TABLE 8 Goal-Directed Parameters for Head Injury

Pulse oximetry ≥95%	ICP 20-25 mm Hg	Serum sodium 135-145 mEq/L
PaO₂ ≥100 mm Hg	PbtO₂ ≥15 mm Hg	INR ≤1.4
PaCO₂ 35-45 mm Hg	CPP ≥60 mm Hg*	Platelets ≥75 × 10³/mm³
SBP ≥100 mm Hg	Temperature 36°-38°C	Hemoglobin ≥7 g/dl
pH 7.35-7.45	Glucose 80-180 mg/dl	

CPP, Cerebral perfusion pressure; *ICP*, intracranial pressure; *INR*, international normalized ratio; *PaCO₂*, partial pressure of carbon dioxide; *PaO₂*, partial pressure of oxygen; *PbtO₂*, brain tissue oxygen tension; *SBP*, systolic blood pressure.
*Depending on status of cerebral autoregulation.
From Vincent JL et al: *Textbook of critical care*, ed 8, Philadelphia, 2024, Elsevier.

TABLE 9 Elevated ICP Management

- Verify ICP
  1. Check if EVD is still patent
  2. Check to see if EVD waveform is present and adequate
  3. Check to see if EVD ICP correlates with intraparenchymal monitor if present
- Check for 30-degree head elevation
- Loosen cervical collar if in place
- Open EVD for ICP >20 mm Hg for 10 min and then close and transduce ICP
  1. Repeat once
  2. If ICP >20 mm Hg, keep open at 15 mm Hg above midbrain and proceed with ICP module
- Treat temperature >37.5°C with 650 mg of acetaminophen once
- Sedation
  1. Titrate propofol to a Ramsay score of 4
     a. Do not exceed 5 mg/kg/h for more than 24 h
  2. Check potassium, triglycerides, creatine kinase, and urinalysis for myoglobinuria q 8 h for 24 h
  3. If maximal dose of propofol is reached and ICP >20 mm Hg
  4. Start fentanyl drip at 0.8 µg/kg/h
  5. Apply bispectral index (BIS) monitor
  6. Titrate fentanyl drip to a bispectral index of 30 or to a maximum of 5 µg/kg/h
  7. Start chlorhexidine gluconate (Peridex) with a loading infusion of 1 µg/kg over 10 min
     a. Continue maintenance infusion of 0.2 to 0.7 µg/kg/h
- Hyperosmolar therapy
  1. 3% hypertonic saline bolus of 250 ml
  2. Before administering 3% hypertonic saline bolus, check if Na <130 mEq/L
  3. In emergency, administer mannitol 1-1.5 mg/kg bolus once
  4. Check sodium and serum osmolality q 4 h × 2 after every bolus
  5. Start 3% hypertonic saline drip at 0.5 ml/h or 250 ml 3% hypertensonic saline bolus q6h
  6. A central venous catheter will be needed for prolonged hypertonic saline administrations
  7. Check sodium and serum osmolality q3-6h while on drip
  8. If sodium >160 mEq/L or serum osmolality >320 sOsm/L, call physician
  9. If serum sodium has increased to >10 mEq/L within the last 24 h, call physician
  10. If CBF > 35 ml/min/100 g white matter or >80 ml/min/100 g gray matter refer to CBF module high flow
- If core body temperature ≥37.5°C, start normothermia protocol
- Hyperventilation
  1. Do not hyperventilate in the first 24 h (goal of Paco₂ of 35-40 mm Hg)
  2. If PbtO₂ is <20 mmHg, go to hypoxia module
  3. If CBF <18 ml/min/100 g white matter or <67 ml/min/100 g gray matter, go to CBF module
  4. If PbtO₂ and CBF are optimized, hyperventilate to 33-35 mm Hg
- Radiology
  1. Refractory ICP > 20 mm Hg despite intervention, obtain portable head CT without contrast immediately if no head CT since ICP is elevated despite maximal therapy
- Consider surgical decompression, if patient is a candidate
- Consider pentobarbital coma induction
  1. Only for diffuse nonoperative injuries
  2. Only with attending approval
  3. Order continuous EEG monitoring if not already in place
  4. Have norepinephrine drip ready at the bedside for MAP < 80 mm Hg/CPP < 60 mm Hg
  5. Pentobarbital bolus/loading: 10 mg/kg once over 60 min, then 5 mg/kg qh × 4 or until burst suppression
  6. Pentobarbital maintenance dose: 1 mg/kg/h titrated to burst suppression

CBF, Cerebral blood flow; *CPP*, cerebral perfusion pressure; *EEG*, electroencephalography; *EVD*, external ventricular drain; *ICP*, intracranial pressure; *MAP*, mean arterial pressure; *PbtO₂*, Brain tissue oxygen.
Modified from Jankovic J et al: *Bradley and Daroff's neurology in clinical practice*, ed 8, Philadelphia, 2022, Elsevier.

BOX 4 Indications for Acute Seizure Prophylaxis in Severe Head Trauma

- Depressed skull fracture
- Paralyzed and intubated patient
- Seizure at the time of injury
- Seizure at emergency department presentation
- Penetrating brain injury
- Severe head injury (Glasgow Coma Scale score ≤8)
- Acute subdural hematoma
- Acute epidural hematoma
- Acute intracranial hemorrhage
- Prior history of seizures

incontinence, headache, and neuropathic pain syndromes.
- Neurostimulants such as amantadine, modafinil, bromocriptine, amphetamine, and methylphenidate are used in the rehabilitation phase with anecdotal data, but good randomized controlled trials (RCTs) are lacking in this area.

DISPOSITION

- Patients may require admission to a rehabilitation facility or discharge to home with outpatient neurocognitive therapy depending on the severity of head injury.
- Despite individual clinical variability, several common neurobehavioral sequelae of moderate to severe TBI can be identified (Table 10). Cognitive recovery is protracted for moderate to severe TBIs, with most improvements occurring in the first yr but measurable recovery of cognitive functioning still occurring several yr after the injury. However, even after a prolonged length of time, individuals may not return to preinjury levels.

REFERRAL

Early transfer to a Level 1 Trauma Center with neurosurgical personnel if high-risk findings are noted on clinical exam or CT head, and is associated with better outcomes.[10]

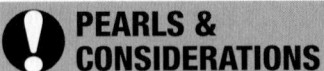

PEARLS & CONSIDERATIONS

TBI is a major health care issue. Guidelines (Table 11) have been developed to address TBI in a timely and effective fashion.[11] Clinical acumen and judgment, however, is irreplaceable and should be exercised for better patient care and outcomes. Early recognition of high-risk patients, early imaging, and early evaluation at a Level 1 Trauma Center by a specialist are associated with improved outcomes. The goal of health care providers in the field or in the community is to identify patients who need this attention.

PATIENT & FAMILY EDUCATION

Brain Injury Association of America: https://www.biausa.org/

TABLE 10 Common Neurocognitive Sequelae of Moderate to Severe Traumatic Brain Injury

Cognitive Domain	Clinical Manifestation of Impairment
Attention	Difficulty with sustained attention
	Poor concentration
	Psychomotor impersistence
Memory	Problems with acquiring and retaining new verbal or nonverbal information
	Problems in retrieving verbal and nonverbal memories
Speed of information processing	Slowed sensorimotor skills and information processing
Executive functioning	Problems in convergent and divergent reasoning
	Poor judgment
	Difficulty planning
	Problems in self-monitoring and self-correcting behavior
Awareness of symptoms	Difficulty recognizing deficits
	Unrealistic expectations concerning the recovery of functions
	Problems related to poor treatment compliance
Language and communication	Problems in word comprehension
	Impaired reading, spelling, and writing ability
	Tendency to become fragmented in free speech
Integrative functions	Problems in adequate or time-efficient execution of various perceptual-motor-spatial-sequential tasks

From Jankovic J et al: *Bradley and Daroff's neurology in clinical practice*, ed 8, Philadelphia, 2022, Elsevier.

TABLE 11 Brain Trauma Foundation Recommendations for Traumatic Brain Injury

Parameter	Guideline
Hyperosmolar therapy	Mannitol effective for control of raised ICP (0.25-1 g/kg)
Prophylactic hypothermia	Early (within 2.5 h), short term (48 h postinjury) hypothermia not recommended to improve outcomes in patients with diffuse injury
Infection prophylaxis	Routine external ventricular catheter exchange not recommended; oral care is not recommended to reduce ventilator-associated pneumonia; antimicrobial ventricular EVD catheters decrease infection
ICP monitoring	Indicated if GCS score = 3-8 on admission and abnormal CT. In severe traumatic brain injury and normal CT, indicated with two or more of the following: Age >40 yr, unilateral posturing, hypotension with SBP <90 mm Hg
CPP threshold	CPP <50 mm Hg should be avoided; aggressive interventions to maintain it above 70 mm Hg have a considerable risk of acute respiratory distress syndrome
Brain oxygen monitoring and thresholds	Jugular venous saturation (50%) or above
Blood pressure and oxygenation	Maintain SBP >100 mm Hg in patients 50-69 yr of age, >110 mm Hg in patients 15-49 and > 70 yr of age; hypoxia (saturation <90% or Po$_2$ <60 mm Hg) should be avoided
Nutrition	Should be initiated within at least by day 5 and at most day 7 postinjury
Sedatives	High-dose barbiturates recommended to control refractory ICP in the hemodynamically stable patient; propofol recommended for ICP control but does not improve mortality
Seizure prophylaxis	Decreases early posttraumatic seizures (<7 days after injury); insufficient evidence to recommend levetiracetam over phenytoin
Hyperventilation	Recommended as temporizing measure; Pco$_2$ below 25 mm Hg not recommended; avoid in first 24 h after injury
Steroids	Not recommended, contraindicated

CPP, Cerebral perfusion pressure; *CT,* computed tomography; *EVD,* external ventricular drain; *GCS,* Glasgow Coma Scale; *ICP,* intracranial pressure; *SBP,* systolic blood pressure.
From Townsend CM et al: *Sabiston textbook of surgery,* ed 21, St Louis, 2022, Elsevier.

Brain Injury Resource Center: https://www.headinjury.com/linktbisup.htm

REFERENCES

Available at eBooks.Health.Elsevier.com.

RELATED CONTENT

Concussion (Related Key Topic)
Postconcussion Syndrome (Related Key Topic)

AUTHOR: **LINTU RAMACHANDRAN, MD**

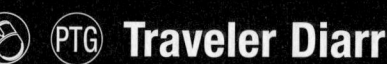
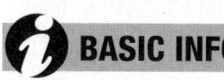 **BASIC INFORMATION**

DEFINITION

Traveler diarrhea (TD) is defined as three or more loose-to-watery stools, with or without associated fever, abdominal cramps, and vomiting, within a 24-h period. It develops during or within 10 days of traveling to developing areas of the world.

SYNONYMS

TD
Enterotoxigenic *Escherichia coli*
Enteroaggregative *E. coli*
Infectious diarrhea
Postinfectious irritable bowel syndrome

ICD-10CM CODE	
A09	Infectious diarrhea

EPIDEMIOLOGY & DEMOGRAPHICS

- TD is mostly caused by bacteria and other pathogens in food and water.
- At least one episode of diarrhea occurs in 40% to 50% of travelers during their stay abroad. Table 1 describes pathogens and epidemiologic features associated with TD.

INCIDENCE:

- **High risk (>20%):** South and Southeast Asia, Africa (except South Africa), South and Central America, and Mexico
- **Moderate risk (10% to 20%):** Caribbean Islands, South Africa, Central and East Asia (including Russia and China), Eastern Europe, and the Middle East, including Israel
- **Low risk (<10%):** Northern and Western Europe, Australia, New Zealand, U.S., Canada, Singapore, Japan

PREVALENCE: Acute and chronic diarrhea account for a third of medical visits by returned travelers as per the GeoSentinel database.

PREDOMINANT SEX & AGE:

- Travelers in their 30s are at highest risk, possibly secondary to more adventurous travel.
- Sex does not seem to influence the risk for TD.
- Infants and toddlers are more likely to have a more severe form of TD and are more likely to need hospitalization.

PEAK INCIDENCE:

- Peak incidence occurs during the first wk of travel and progressively declines after that.
- Seasonal variation does exist for TD, with lower rates in the winter months.

RISK FACTORS:

- Gastric acid protects against enteropathogens, so medications that reduce gastric acid secretion (i.e., proton pump inhibitor [PPI] or histamine-2 [H_2]-receptor blockers) are known to increase risk for TD by a factor of 12.
- Immunocompromised travelers such as those with HIV/AIDS are at higher risk for parasitic infections.
- Backpackers are at higher risk than those staying at a resort.
- Food bought from street vendors or prepared by persons not wearing gloves carries a higher risk.

GENETICS: Travelers with the O blood group are at higher risk for diarrhea caused by norovirus and *Shigella*.

PHYSICAL FINDINGS & CLINICAL PRESENTATION

- The clinical presentation does not allow determination of infectious cause.
- 90% of cases occur within 2 wk of stay.
- Acute watery diarrhea predominates in 90% of patients.
- Signs of invasive infection, including fever and bloody/mucoid diarrhea, occur in 3% to 30%.
- Most patients report three to five bowel movements a day, but in 20% a higher frequency of up to 20 daily bowel movements occurs.

- Nausea (10% to 70%), vomiting (4% to 36%), abdominal cramps/tenesmus (80%), urgency (90%).
- Other: Myalgia, arthralgia, headache.
- Average episode resolves in 3 to 5 days.
- Prolonged symptoms lasting more than 1 wk: 8% to 15%; chronic diarrhea >30 days: 1% to 3%.
- Severe episodes may result in electrolyte imbalance (K^+ loss).
- 50% of all travelers are incapacitated for at least 24 h, but up to 20% are ill in bed for 1 to 2 days.

ETIOLOGY

- *E. coli* (Table E2): Accounts for up to 60% of all cases of TD and is most prevalent in Central and South America, South Asia, and Africa. Table E3 summarizes etiology of TD in Latin America, Africa, and Asia
  1. Enterotoxigenic *E. coli* (ETEC): Produce heat labile and heat stable toxin and are the most common cause, accounting for 10% to 45% of cases. Frequently seen in Latin America, Africa, and South Asia
  2. Enteroaggregative *E. coli* (EAEC): More commonly seen in Latin America
  3. Other *E. coli* (enteropathogenic [EPEC], enteroinvasive [EIEC], enterohemorrhagic [EHEC]): Shiga toxin–producing or diffuse adhering *E. coli* are much less common
- *Campylobacter:* 2% to 32% of cases. More common in Southeast Asia, where it is more frequent than ETEC
- *Shigella:* 2% to 9%. More common in Africa
- *Salmonella:* <5% of cases except in Asia, where it is seen in up to 10% of cases
- Other bacteria: *Aeromonas, Arcobacter, Plesiomonas,* enterotoxigenic *Bacteroides fragilis, Vibrio cholera,* noncholera vibrios
- Viral pathogens:
  1. Norovirus: Up to 17% of cases from Caribbean and Africa
  2. Rotavirus: 4% to 7% of cases

TABLE 1 Pathogens and Epidemiologic Features Associated With Traveler Diarrhea

Organism	Approximate Percentage of Cases (%)	Epidemiologic Features
Enterotoxigenic *Escherichia coli*	15-50	Most important causative agent of traveler diarrhea overall; not diagnosed by routine microbiologic methods
Enteroaggregative *E. coli*	20-35	Not diagnosed by routine microbiologic methods
Shigella spp. and enteroinvasive *E. coli*	10-25	Most important causes of dysentery; enteroinvasive *E. coli* not diagnosed by routine microbiologic methods
Nontyphoidal *Salmonella* spp.	5-10	
Campylobacter jejuni	3-15	More common in Asia; antimicrobial resistance a concern
Aeromonas	5	
Plesiomonas	5	
Giardia lamblia	<2	Affects hikers and campers who drink from contaminated freshwater streams
Cryptosporidium hominis/parvum	<2	Occasional large-scale waterborne outbreaks
Cyclospora cayetanensis	<2	
Vibrio cholerae		Ongoing outbreaks in Haiti and Zimbabwe, and endemic in many countries in Asia; rare cause of disease in travelers
Norovirus		Outbreaks on cruise ships
Entamoeba histolytica		May cause liver abscess

From Bennett JE et al: *Mandell, Douglas, and Bennett's principles and practice of infectious diseases,* ed 8, Philadelphia, 2015, Saunders.

- Protozoans:
  1. *Entamoeba histolytica:* More common in South and Southeast Asia
  2. *Giardia lamblia:* More common in South and Southeast Asia, especially Nepal
  3. *Cryptosporidium, Cyclospora, Isospora*

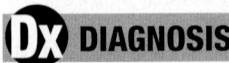

DIFFERENTIAL DIAGNOSIS

- Malaria
- Dengue fever
- Influenza
- Rocky Mountain spotted fever
- Irritable bowel syndrome
- Inflammatory bowel disease
- Shellfish poisoning
- Mushroom poisoning

WORKUP

- Most cases of TD are self-limiting, do not require workup, and are treated symptomatically without regard to etiologic agent.
- In patients with diarrhea, fever, and colitic symptoms (bloody stools, cramping), a stool culture should be obtained to look for specific bacterial pathogens.

LABORATORY TESTS

- Stool culture ×3 for bacterial pathogens.
- Stool for ova and parasites to help identify protozoans. Special stains such as modified acid-fast or trichrome stain may be necessary for *Cryptosporidium, Cyclospora,* and *Isospora.*
- Currently there are gastrointestinal multiplex panels that are based on nucleic acid amplification technologies that can detect bacteria, viruses, and parasites, all from one stool sample. They are highly sensitive and specific with fast turnaround times and can test for more than 20 pathogens at once. These panels are replacing stool cultures and ova and parasite testing in many hospitals.
- Blood cultures in patients with systemic illness to rule out *Salmonella* spp.

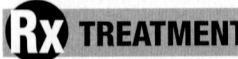

NONPHARMACOLOGIC THERAPY

- Fluid replacement to treat volume depletion of diarrhea is important.
- Mild cases: Alternate fluids that contain salts and fluids that contain sugars, such as broths or fruit juices. Pedialyte is effective as an over-the-counter product.
- Severe cases: Oral rehydration solution (ORS) packets are available in most pharmacies. They should be mixed with clean water to replace lost electrolytes and are used until patient is urinating regularly. An alternative home-based solution can be made with: ½ tsp of salt, ½ tsp of baking soda, and 4 tbsp of sugar in 1 L of clean water.

ACUTE GENERAL Rx

- Antisecretory agents may reduce symptoms but do not treat underlying cause:
  1. Bismuth subsalicylate: One dose of 525 mg (two tablets of Pepto-Bismol) by mouth (PO) every 30 min up to eight doses a day. Can reduce number of bowel movements by 50%. Dosages are available for children based on weight, and the product is available in liquid or chewable tablet form.
  2. Loperamide: 4 mg PO, then 2 mg after each loose bowel movement, not to exceed 16 mg/day. Use for up to 48 h. Has antisecretory and antimotility effect. Antimotility drugs should not be used in cases of bloody diarrhea or dysentery (increased risk of colitis and colonic perforation). When used, they should be given only in conjunction with antimicrobial therapy.
- Antibiotics are warranted only for moderate to severe diarrhea (i.e., more than four bowel movements a day; fever; or blood, pus, or mucus in stool. Antibiotics can reduce duration of diarrhea by 1 to 2 days.
  1. Azithromycin: The preferred antibiotic for empiric treatment of moderate to severe TD. It is also the preferred agent for children and pregnant women. Dose of 1 g PO is the single dose for women. Children: 10 mg/kg daily single dose or for 3 days. Particularly effective against quinolone-resistant *Campylobacter* infections in Southeast Asia. Another option for children: Ceftriaxone 50 mg/kg intravenous (IV) once daily ×3 days.
     a. Ciprofloxacin: 500 mg twice a day (bid) for 1 to 3 days
     b. Levaquin: 500 mg/day for 1 to 3 days
  2. Fluoroquinolones are also effective agents for bacterial causes of TD, but resistance to fluoroquinolones is increasing. Cannot be used in children under 15 and in pregnant women.
  3. Rifaximin: 200 mg PO three times a day (tid) for 3 days for children age >12 and adults is effective for afebrile, noncolitic diarrhea such as ETEC. Does not treat *Salmonella, Shigella,* or *Campylobacter.*
  4. Rifamycin is now FDA approved for TD caused by noninvasive strains of *E. coli.* It is not recommended for TD complicated by fever and/or bloody stools. Dosage is 388 mg (two tablets) bid ×3 days.
- Concerns of use of antibiotics:
  1. Widespread use of antibiotics has led to resistance. Tetracycline and sulfa agents such as trimethoprim-sulfamethoxazole (TMP-SMX; Bactrim) are no longer used due to widespread resistance.
  2. Antibiotic treatment may lead to prolonged colonization in infections with *Salmonella* and nontyphoid *Salmonella.*
  3. In cases of EHEC (Shiga toxin production) treatment with quinolones, but not rifaximin, may increase risk of complications such as hemolytic uremic syndrome.

  4. *Clostridium difficile* infection can occur with use of antibiotics.

PREVENTION BY ANTIBIOTICS & NONANTIBIOTIC AGENTS

- Antibiotic prophylaxis can be considered for certain groups, such as persons with underlying illness, athletes, and politicians for up to 2 to 3 wk. Ciprofloxacin 250 to 500 mg/day is effective in preventing 90% of TD. Rifaximin dosed daily has been shown to help prevent TD for U.S. travelers to Mexico, but not as effectively as ciprofloxacin.
- Bismuth subsalicylate can be used. It must be given 4× daily and can cause black tongue and stools. As it contains salicylates, it can interact with anticoagulants and lead to toxicity in patients on long-term salicylate therapy.
- Probiotics are being studied for their potential use but evidence of their effectiveness is limited.

REFERRAL

Infectious diseases physician for more difficult cases lasting more than 72 h

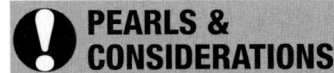

- Travelers on cruises have lower incidence of TD than land-based trips, but cruise ship passengers and staff are at higher risk of large outbreaks of norovirus that are difficult to contain. Norovirus infection needs only a low inoculum of virus to cause illness, and the virus is relatively resistant to cleaning.
- In up to 40% of cases of TD, no pathogen is identified.
- *Giardia* is the most frequent cause of long-lasting TD.

PREVENTION

- There are oral and injectable vaccines against *Salmonella typhi* available in the U.S.
- Dukoral is an oral vaccine available in some countries such as Canada and Australia and in Europe to help prevent cholera and ETEC.

PATIENT & FAMILY EDUCATION

Food hygiene education: Wash hands often, especially after going to bathroom and before eating. Avoid raw fruits and vegetables (unless peeled and washed in clean water). Avoid undercooked meats, fish, and seafood. Avoid tap water and ice. Choose beverages in factory-sealed containers (such as bottled water and carbonated soft drinks). Try to avoid buffet-style foods.

SUGGESTED READINGS
Available at eBooks.Health.Elsevier.com.

RELATED CONTENT
Traveler Diarrhea (Patient Information)

AUTHOR: **GLENN G. FORT, MD, MPH**

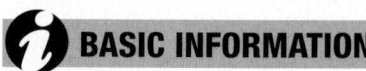
BASIC INFORMATION

DEFINITION
Ulcerative colitis (UC) is an idiopathic, remitting and relapsing, chronic inflammatory bowel disease (IBD) that starts in the rectum and extends proximally.

SYNONYMS
UC
Inflammatory bowel disease (IBD)
Idiopathic proctocolitis
Pancolitis

ICD-10CM CODES
K51.0	Ulcerative pancolitis
K51.2	Ulcerative proctitis
K51.3	Ulcerative rectosigmoiditis
K51.5	Left-sided colitis
K51.90	Ulcerative colitis, unspecified, without complications
K51.80	Other ulcerative colitis without complications
K51.811	Other ulcerative colitis with rectal bleeding
K51.812	Other ulcerative colitis with intestinal obstruction
K51.813	Other ulcerative colitis with fistula
K51.814	Other ulcerative colitis with abscess
K51.818	Other ulcerative colitis with other complication
K51.819	Other ulcerative colitis with unspecified complications
K51.911	Ulcerative colitis, unspecified with rectal bleeding
K51.912	Ulcerative colitis, unspecified with intestinal obstruction
K51.913	Ulcerative colitis, unspecified with fistula
K51.914	Ulcerative colitis, unspecified with abscess
K51.918	Ulcerative colitis, unspecified with other complication
K51.919	Ulcerative colitis, unspecified with unspecified complications

EPIDEMIOLOGY & DEMOGRAPHICS
INCIDENCE: The incidence of UC is 9 to 12 cases/100,000 persons per yr in the U.S.; worldwide, the estimated incidence ranges from 1.2 to 20.3 cases/100,000 person-yr, and its prevalence ranges from 7.6 to 246.0/100,000 persons. It is most common between ages 15 and 40 yr, with a second peak between 50 and 80 yr. The disease affects men and women at similar rates. Infection with nontyphoid *Salmonella* or *Campylobacter* is associated with an 8 to 10 times higher risk of developing UC in the following year. Worldwide, UC is more common than Crohn disease.
PREVALENCE: The prevalence of UC is 7.6 to 246.0 cases/100,000 per yr. Higher prevalence in Ashkenazi Jewish descendants.
GENETICS:
• Both specific and nonspecific gene variants are associated with UC.

• There are 47 loci associated with UC, of which 19 are specific for UC and 28 are shared with Crohn disease.
• Abnormalities in humoral and cellular adaptive immunity are also found in UC.
GEOGRAPHIC DISTRIBUTION: The highest incidence and prevalence of IBD are seen in northern Europe and North America, and the lowest in continental Asia.

PHYSICAL FINDINGS & CLINICAL PRESENTATION
• Patients with UC often present with acute onset of bloody diarrhea accompanied by tenesmus, fever, and dehydration. At presentation 40% of adults have proctitis, 40% have left-sided colitis, and 20% have pancolitis. Diarrhea is not always present in UC patients with proctosigmoiditis and proctitis, and patients may have constipation.
• Abdominal pain is not usually a prominent symptom. Abdominal distention and tenderness may indicate the presence of complications such as toxic megacolon.
• The onset of symptoms is typically acute and is generally followed by periods of spontaneous remission and frequent relapses.
• Fever, evidence of dehydration may be present during the acute flare-up.
• Evidence of extraintestinal manifestations may be present in nearly 25% of patients: Liver disease, sclerosing cholangitis, iritis, uveitis, episcleritis, arthritis, erythema nodosum, pyoderma gangrenosum, aphthous stomatitis. Box 1 summarizes common extraintestinal manifestations of UC.

ETIOLOGY & PATHOGENESIS
Accumulating evidence suggests that it may result from an inappropriate inflammatory response to environmental triggers and immune dysregulation involving CD4+ T-cell Th2 response in a genetically susceptible host.

DIAGNOSIS

DIFFERENTIAL DIAGNOSIS (TABLE 1, BOX 2)
• Crohn disease
• Bacterial infections:
  1. Acute: *Campylobacter, Yersinia, Salmonella, Shigella, Chlamydia, Escherichia coli, Clostridioides difficile,* gonococcal proctitis
  2. Chronic: Whipple disease, tuberculosis, enterocolitis
• Irritable bowel syndrome
• Protozoal and parasitic infections (amebiasis, giardiasis, cryptosporidiosis)
• Neoplasm (intestinal lymphoma, carcinoma of colon)
• Ischemic bowel disease
• Diverticulitis
• Celiac sprue, lymphocytic or collagenous colitis, radiation enteritis, endometriosis
• Solitary rectal ulcer
• Acute self-limited colitis
• Medication (NSAIDs, chemotherapy)

WORKUP
An accurate diagnosis of UC should define the extent and severity of inflammation. Diagnostic workup includes:
• Comprehensive history, physical examination
• Laboratory tests (see "Laboratory Tests")
• Colonoscopy to establish the presence of mucosal inflammation; typical endoscopic findings in UC are areas of continuous friable mucosa; diffuse, uniform erythema replacing the usual mucosal vascular pattern (Table 2); and pseudopolyps. The transition from abnormal to normal tissue tends to be abrupt. Rectal involvement is invariably present if the disease is active. Pathologic findings suggestive of UC include crypt abscesses and atrophy, mucin depletion, basal plasmacytosis, basal lymphoid aggregates, increased lamina propria cellularity, and Paneth cell metaplasia

LABORATORY TESTS
• Anemia and high erythrocyte sedimentation rate (in severe colitis) are common, but normal levels do not rule out the disorder.

BOX 1 Common Extraintestinal Manifestations of Ulcerative Colitis

Cutaneous/Oral
Angular stomatitis
Aphthous stomatitis
Erythema nodosum
Oral ulcerations
Psoriasis
Pyoderma gangrenosum
Pyostomatitis vegetans
Sweet syndrome (acute febrile neutrophilic dermatosis)

Ophthalmologic
Conjunctivitis
Episcleritis
Retinal vascular disease
Scleritis
Uveitis, iritis

Musculoskeletal
Ankylosing spondylitis
Osteomalacia
Osteonecrosis
Osteopenia
Osteoporosis
Peripheral arthropathy
Sacroiliitis

Hepatobiliary
Autoimmune hepatitis
Cholangiocarcinoma
Pericholangitis
Primary sclerosing cholangitis
Hepatic steatosis

Hematologic
Anemia of chronic disease
Autoimmune hemolytic anemia
Hypercoagulable state
Iron deficiency anemia
Leukocytosis or thrombocytosis
Leukopenia or thrombocytopenia

From Feldman M et al: *Sleisenger and Fordtran's gastrointestinal and liver disease,* ed 10, Philadelphia, 2016, Elsevier.

TABLE 1 Features that Distinguish Ulcerative Colitis from Other Diagnoses

Diagnosis	Clinical Features	Radiologic and Colonoscopic Features	Histologic Features
UC	Bloody diarrhea	Extends proximally from rectum; fine mucosal ulceration	Distortion of crypts; acute and chronic diffuse inflammatory cell infiltrate; goblet cell depletion; crypt abscesses; lymphoid aggregates
Crohn colitis	Perianal lesions are common; may be associated with ileitis; frank bleeding is less common than in UC	Segmental disease; rectal sparing; strictures, fissures, ulcers, fistulas; small bowel involvement	Focal inflammation; submucosal involvement; granulomas; goblet cell preservation; transmural inflammation; fissuring
Ischemic colitis	Occurs in older adults; sudden onset, often painful; usually resolves spontaneously in several days	Segmental splenic flexure and sigmoid involvement are most common, with thumb-printing early and ulceration after 24-72 h; rectal involvement is rare	Mucosal necrosis with ghost cells; congestion with red blood cells; hemosiderin-laden macrophages and fibrosis (when disease is chronic)
Microscopic colitis	Watery diarrhea; normal-appearing mucosa at colonoscopy	Usually normal	Chronic inflammatory infiltrate; increased intraepithelial lymphocytes (lymphocytic colitis) and/or subepithelial collagen band (collagenous colitis)
Infectious colitis	Sudden onset; identifiable source in some cases (e.g., *Salmonella* spp.); pain may predominate (e.g., *Campylobacter* spp.); pathogens are present in stool	Nonspecific findings	Crypt architecture is usually normal; edema, superficial neutrophilic infiltrate, crypt abscesses
Amebic colitis	History of travel to endemic area; amebae may be detected in a fresh stool specimen, but ELISA for amebic lectin antigen is the preferable diagnostic test	Discrete ulcers; ameboma or strictures	Similar to UC; amebae present in lamina propria or in flask-shaped ulcers, identified by periodic acid–Schiff stain
Gonococcal proctitis	Rectal pain; pus	Granular changes in rectum	Intense polymorphonuclear neutrophil infiltration; purulent exudate; gram-negative diplococci
Pseudomembranous colitis	Often a history of antibiotic use; characteristic pseudomembranes may be seen on sigmoidoscopy; *Clostridioides difficile* toxin is detectable in stools	Edematous; shaggy outline of colon; pseudomembranes may be identified radiologically or seen at colonoscopy	May resemble acute ischemic colitis; summit lesions of fibrinopurulent exudate

ELISA, Enzyme-linked immunosorbent assay; *UC,* ulcerative colitis.
From Feldman M et al: *Sleisenger and Fordtran's gastrointestinal and liver disease,* ed 10, Philadelphia, 2016, Elsevier.

- Potassium, magnesium, calcium, and albumin may be decreased.
- Antineutrophil cytoplasmic antibodies (ANCA) with a perinuclear staining pattern (pANCA) can be found in >45% of patients; there is an increased frequency in treatment-resistant left-sided colitis, suggesting a possible association between these antibodies and a relative resistance to medical therapy in patients with UC.
- Calprotectin is a protein that is measured in feces as a marker of intestinal mucosa leukocyte activity that may be useful for screening of patients with suspected IBD. Trials have shown that based on a pretest probability of IBD of 32% in adults, an abnormal fecal calprotectin test would increase the posttest probability to 91% and a normal result would reduce the probability to 3%.
- Fecal lactoferrin is also a sensitive marker of intestinal inflammation.
- Stool examinations for ova and parasites, stool culture, and testing for *C. difficile* toxin and *E. coli* O157:H7 may be useful to eliminate other causes of diarrhea in selected patients with risk factors.

IMAGING STUDIES

Image studies (plain radiography, CT scan [Fig. E1]) are generally reserved for suspected complications such as perforation of bowel or toxic megacolon.

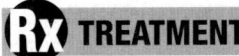 **TREATMENT**

NONPHARMACOLOGIC THERAPY

- Correct nutritional deficiencies; total parenteral nutrition with bowel rest may be necessary in severe cases. Folate supplementation may reduce the incidence of dysplasia and cancer in chronic UC.
- Avoid oral feedings during acute exacerbation to decrease colonic activity; a low-roughage diet may be helpful in early relapse.
- Psychotherapy is useful in most patients. Referral to self-help groups is also important because of the chronicity of the disease and the young age of the patients.

ACUTE GENERAL Rx

The therapeutic options (Table 3) vary with the degree of disease (mild, severe, fulminant) and areas of involvement (distal, extensive).

- Mild disease can be treated with 5-aminosalicylate agents (mesalamine, olsalazine, balsalazide, sulfasalazine). These agents can be used for both induction and maintenance of remission. Mesalamine can be administered as an enema (4 gm once daily at bedtime for 3 to 6 wk) or suppository (500 mg bid) for patients with distal colonic disease. Oral forms in which the 5-acetyl salicylic acid is in a slow-release or pH-dependent matrix (Pentasa 1 g qid, Asacol 800 mg PO tid) can deliver therapeutic concentrations to the more proximal small bowel or distal ileum. Olsalazine can be useful for maintenance of remission of UC in patients intolerant to sulfasalazine. Usual dose is 500 mg bid taken with food. Balsalazide is indicated for mild to moderately active UC. Usual dose is three 750-mg capsules tid. Probiotics may also be helpful in inducing remission in mild-to-moderate UC.
- Mild-to-moderate UC is often treated with a combination of rectal and oral 5-aminosalicylate. Refractory patients are candidates for oral glucocorticoids or immunosuppressive agents (e.g., cyclosporine).
- Severe disease usually responds to oral corticosteroids (e.g., prednisone 40 to 60 mg/day). In patients with moderately to severely active disease, a tumor necrosis factor (TNF) inhibitor (infliximab, adalimumab, golimumab), an integrin receptor antagonist (vedolizumab), or an interleukin (IL) 12-23 antagonist (ustekinumab) are useful for both induction and maintenance of remission. In patients with moderately to severely active ulcerative colitis who cannot tolerate or respond poorly to TNF inhibitors oral Janus kinase inhibitors (tofacitinib or upadacitinib) may be effective. The FDA has also approved ozanimod and etrasimod, oral sphingosine 1-phosphate (S1P) receptor modulators for treatment of adults with moderate to severe

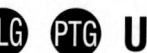 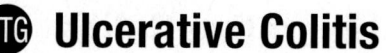
Diseases
and Disorders

I

BOX 2 Differential Diagnosis of Ulcerative Colitis

Infectious Causes
- *Aeromonas hydrophila*
- *Campylobacter jejuni*
- *Chlamydia* spp.
- *Clostridioides difficile*
- Cytomegalovirus
- *Entamoeba histolytica*
- *Escherichia coli* O157:H7, other EHEC
- Herpes simplex virus (HSV)
- *Listeria monocytogenes*
- *Neisseria gonorrhoeae*
- *Salmonella* spp.
- *Schistosomiasis*
- *Shigella* spp.
- *Yersinia enterocolitica*

Noninfectious Causes
- Acute self-limited colitis
- Behçet disease
- Crohn disease
- Diversion colitis
- Diverticulitis
- Drugs and toxins
  1. Chemotherapy
  2. Gold
  3. Penicillamine
- Eosinophilic colitis
- Graft-versus-host disease
- Ischemic colitis
- Microscopic colitis
  1. Collagenous
  2. Lymphocytic
- Neutropenic colitis (typhlitis)
- NSAIDs
- Radiation colitis
- Segmental colitis associated with diverticulosis
- Solitary rectal ulcer syndrome

From Feldman M et al: *Sleisenger and Fordtran's gastrointestinal and liver disease,* ed 10, Philadelphia, 2016, Elsevier.

TABLE 2 Endoscopic Differentiation of Ulcerative Colitis and Crohn Disease

Feature	Ulcerative Colitis	Crohn Disease
Distribution	Diffuse inflammation that extends proximally from the anorectal junction	Rectal sparing, frequent skip lesions
Inflammation	Diffuse erythema, early loss of vascular markings with mucosal granularity or friability	Focal and asymmetric, cobblestoning; granularity and friability less commonly seen
Ulceration	Small ulcers in a diffusely inflamed mucosa; deep, ragged ulcers in severe disease	Aphthoid ulcers, linear or serpiginous ulceration; intervening mucosa is often normal
Colonic lumen	Often narrowed in long-standing chronic disease; tubular colon; strictures are rare	Strictures are common

From Feldman M et al: *Sleisenger and Fordtran's gastrointestinal and liver disease,* ed 10, Philadelphia, 2016, Elsevier.

active ulcerative colitis who had an inadequate response to or would not tolerate other drugs.
- Fulminant disease generally requires hospital admission and parenteral corticosteroids (e.g., IV hydrocortisone 100 mg q6h). When bowel movements have returned to normal and the patient is able to eat normally, PO prednisone is resumed. IV cyclosporine can also be used in severe refractory cases; renal toxicity is a potential complication.
- Surgery is indicated in patients who do not respond to intensive medical therapy. Fig. 2 illustrates the surgical management of chronic UC.
- Proctocolectomy is usually curative in these patients and also eliminates the high risk of developing adenocarcinoma of the colon (10% to 20% of patients develop it after 10 yr with the disease). Total proctocolectomy with ileal pouch–anal anastomosis (IPAA) is the procedure of choice for most patients who require elective surgery, since it preserves anal sphincter function. Continent ileostomy is an alternative procedure.

CHRONIC Rx
- Colonoscopic surveillance and multiple biopsies should be instituted approximately 10 yr after diagnosis because of the increased risk of colon carcinoma.
- Erythropoietin is useful in patients with anemia refractory to treatment with iron and vitamins.
- In patients on long-term steroid therapy, periodic bone density scans are recommended to screen for glucocorticoid-induced osteoporosis.

DISPOSITION
- The natural history of the disease is one of remission and episodic flares.
- The clinical course is variable. ~66% of patients will achieve clinical remission with medical therapy, and nearly 80% of treatment-compliant patients maintain remission. 15% to 20% of patients eventually require colectomy. Pouchitis is the most common long-term complication of IPAA (up to 40% of patients). >75% of patients treated medically will experience relapse.

REFERRAL
- GI consultation for initial diagnostic sigmoidoscopy/colonoscopy in suspected cases.
- Surgical referral for patients with severe disease unresponsive to medical therapy. Indications for surgery in patients with UC are summarized in Box 3.

SUGGESTED READINGS
Available at eBooks.Health.Elsevier.com.

RELATED CONTENT
Ulcerative Colitis (Patient Information)

AUTHOR: **FRED F. FERRI, MD**

TABLE 3 Medical Therapy Used in Ulcerative Colitis

Drug	Release Site	Treatment of UC	Side Effects
Oral 5-aminosalicylates			
Sulfasalazine	Colon	Induce and maintain remission in mild-to-moderate UC	Sulfasalazine: Idiosyncratic (rash, hepatitis, aplastic anemia), dose-related (nausea, hemolytic anemia, inhibits folic acid transport), oligospermia (reversible)
Mesalamine (mesalazine)	Distal ileum, colon	Use in combination with topical mesalamine for distal colitis	
Mesalamine (mesalazine) (controlled-release)	Duodenum, jejunum, ileum, colon		
Olsalazine	Colon		
Balsalazide	Colon		
Topical 5-aminosalicylates			
Mesalamine (mesalazine) enema	Rectum, sigmoid	Induce and maintain remission in mild-to-moderate distal disease	
Mesalamine (mesalazine) suppository	Rectum	Combination therapy with oral aminosalicylates are superior to monotherapy	
Antibiotics			
Ciprofloxacin	Systemic	Antibiotics are not used for the treatment of UC but are used for pouchitis	Ciprofloxacin: Tendonitis and rupture
Metronidazole			Metronidazole: Neuropathy
Amoxicillin/clavulanic acid			Amoxicillin/clavulanic acid: Hepatitis
Rifaximin			
Corticosteroids			
Budesonide extended-release	Colon	Induce remission in mild-to-moderate UC Should not be used for maintenance	High first-pass metabolism More favorable side-effect profile than prednisone
Prednisone	Systemic	Induce remission in mild-to-moderate and some moderate-to-severe UC flares Not used for maintenance therapy	Infection, diabetes mellitus, osteoporosis, osteonecrosis, cataracts, glaucoma, and myopathy Increase risk of mortality
Methylprednisolone	Systemic	Induce remission in severe UC	As for prednisone
Immunomodulators			
6-Mercaptopurine	Systemic	Maintain remission in steroid-dependent, steroid-refractory, or steroid-induced-remission UC	Allergic reactions, pancreatitis, myelosuppression, nausea, infections, hepatotoxicity, and malignancy, in particular lymphoma
Azathioprine	Systemic	Not used to induce remission	
Cyclosporine	Systemic	Rescue therapy to induce remission in severe UC not responding to IV methylprednisolone	Infections, hypertension, renal insufficiency, tremor, headache, hepatotoxicity
Biologicals			
Infliximab	Systemic	Can be used to induce and maintain moderate-to-severe UC and are steroid-sparing	Infections (tuberculosis, fungal infections), autoantibody formation, psoriasis, drug-induced lupus
Adalimumab	Systemic	Infliximab is also used as a rescue therapy to induce remission in severe UC not responding to IV methylprednisolone	Infusion reactions (infliximab), injection-site reaction (adalimumab and golimumab), delayed hypersensitivity reaction (infliximab)
Golimumab	Systemic		Lymphoma (higher in combination therapy)
Vedolizumab	Systemic	Effective in the induction and maintenance of remission in moderate-to-severe UC	Headache, infections, abdominal pain, infusion reactions
Tofacitinib (small molecules)	Systemic	Effective in induction and maintenance	Infections (especially herpes zoster), lymphoma

UC, Ulcerative colitis.
From Talley NJ et al: *Essentials of internal medicine,* ed 4, Chatswood, NSW, 2021, Elsevier Australia.

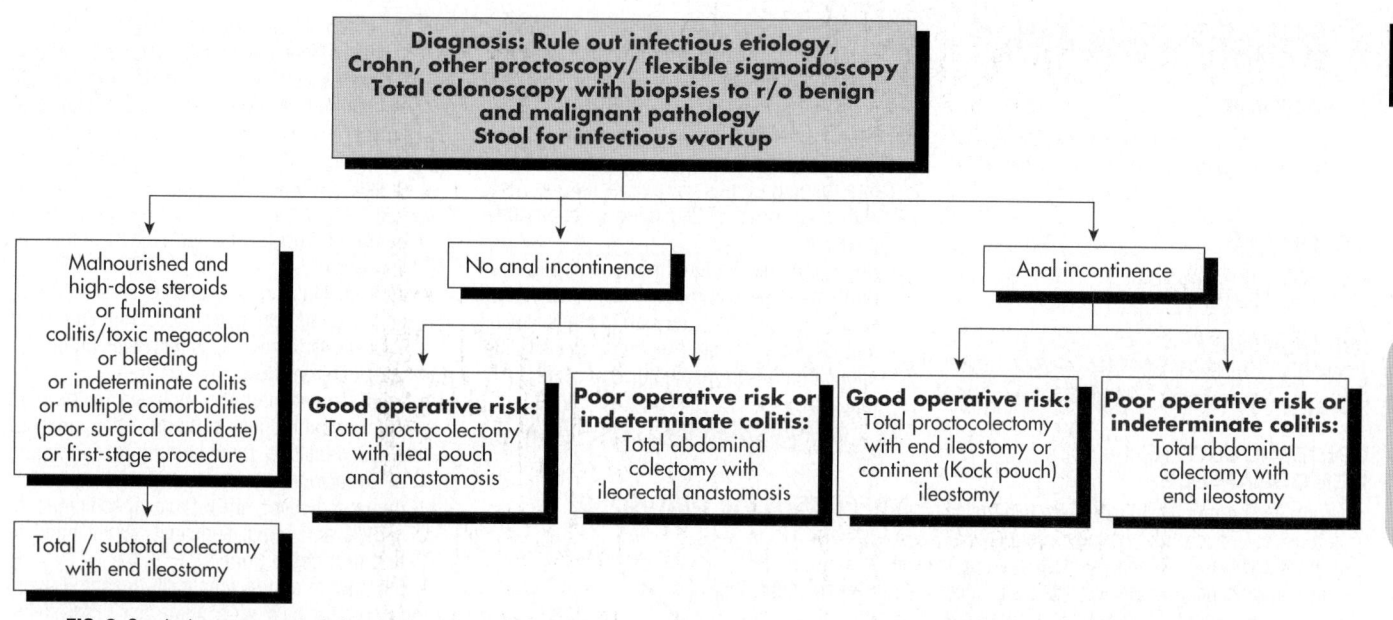

FIG. 2 Surgical management of chronic ulcerative colitis. (From Cameron JL, Cameron AM: *Current surgical therapy,* ed 12, Philadelphia, 2017, Elsevier.)

BOX 3 Indications for Surgery in Patients with Ulcerative Colitis

Colonic dysplasia or carcinoma
Colonic perforation
Growth retardation
Intolerable or unacceptable side effects
  of medical therapy
Medically refractory disease
Systemic complications that are recurrent
  or unmanageable
Toxic megacolon
Uncontrollable colonic hemorrhage

From Feldman M et al: *Sleisenger and Fordtran's gastrointestinal and liver disease,* ed 10, Philadelphia, 2016, Elsevier.

BASIC INFORMATION

DEFINITION

Urethritis is a well-defined clinical syndrome manifested by dysuria, a urethral discharge, or both.

SYNONYMS

Gonococcal urethritis
GCU

ICD-10CM CODE
A54.00 Gonococcal infection of lower genitourinary tract, unspecified

EPIDEMIOLOGY & DEMOGRAPHICS

- Urethritis commonly is divided into two major categories based on etiology: Gonococcal urethritis (GCU, *Neisseria gonorrhoeae* spp.) and nongonococcal urethritis (NGU, all other pathogens, most commonly *Chlamydia trachomatis* and *Mycoplasma genitalium*).[1]
- This differentiation is based historically on *N. gonorrhoeae*'s easy visualization on Gram stain as gram-negative, kidney-shaped diplococci.
- In the U.S., rates of gonorrheal urethritis are rising; however, the incidence varies greatly based on race and geography; the prevalence of GCU is disproportionately higher in the South and among Black, non-Hispanic men. The urethra is the most common site of infection in all men.

PHYSICAL FINDINGS & CLINICAL PRESENTATION

- Symptoms of GCU: Dysuria is the most common chief complaint in patients with GCU, which is often accompanied by discharge and pruritus. Acute-onset purulent discharge is a hallmark of this infection. Additionally, meatal edema and urethral tenderness to palpation may occur. Approximately 5% to 10% of patients with GCU remain asymptomatic.
- GCU may spread to other parts of the genitourinary system. Prostatic involvement can cause urinary frequency, urgency, and nocturia and may present with mucopurulent discharge. Epididymal involvement can result in unilateral testicular pain and edema.
- Time frame: The incubation period of GCU is variable but is commonly 4 to 7 days. Without treatment, urethritis will persist for 3 to 7 wk, with 95% of men becoming asymptomatic after 3 mo.
- Complications: Periurethritis leading to urethral stenosis can occur. Additionally, disseminated infection can lead to tenosynovitis and arthritis. Rarely, hepatitis, myocarditis, endocarditis, and meningitis can occur.

DIAGNOSIS

DIFFERENTIAL DIAGNOSIS (TABLE 1)

- NGU
- Herpes simplex virus

LABORATORY TESTS

- Urethritis is diagnosed when a symptomatic male has any of the following characteristics:
  1. Mucopurulent/purulent discharge on examination
  2. Urethral swab showing:
     a. ≥2 white blood cells (WBCs) per field in high-prevalence settings or ≥5 WBCs per field in lower prevalence settings
     b. Gram-negative diplococci seen within WBCs
- Urethritis can be diagnosed by culture or by NAATs.[2] The performance of NAATs with respect to overall sensitivity, specificity, and ease of specimen transport is better than that of any of the other tests available for the diagnosis of chlamydial and gonococcal infections. NAATs should be used as first line to detect chlamydia and gonorrhea, except in cases of child sexual assault, rectal and oropharyngeal infections in prepubescent girls, and when evaluating a potential gonorrhea treatment failure, in which case culture and susceptibility testing might be required.

- Of note, a presumptive diagnosis can be made without the earlier diagnostic criteria for males who are at high risk for sexually transmitted infections (i.e., more than one partner and >25 yr) and who are unlikely to return for follow-up. In these patients, empirical treatment to cover both gonococcal and nongonococcal infections can be given before the results of a nucleic acid amplification test (NAAT).
- If Gram staining is available, it is indicated and should be performed with modified Thayer-Martin media, as this helps differentiate GCU from NGU.
- NAATs have largely replaced culture in many health care settings. They are not more sensitive than culture for detecting *N. gonorrhoeae* in cervical or urethral specimens; however, they have specificities of >99% and retain sensitivity when used to test first-catch urine.
- For culture and susceptibility testing: Rayon, Dacron, or calcium alginate tips with plastic or wire shafts should be used (not cotton-tipped swabs, which are bactericidal). A swab of the urethra should be performed within 2 to 4 h after voiding to prevent bacterial washout with urination. Collect cultures of the pharynx and rectum when indicated for concomitant *Chlamydia* testing on all patients.
- Concomitant serologic testing for syphilis and HIV infections should be offered to all patients.

TREATMENT

Regimen for adults and adolescents weighing >45 kg with GCU:
- Ceftriaxone 500 mg intramuscular (IM) as a single dose for persons weighing <150 kg (300 lbs)
- For persons weighing ≥150 kg (300 lbs), 1 g of IM ceftriaxone should be administered.
- If chlamydial infection has not been excluded, providers should treat for chlamydia with doxycycline 100 mg orally (PO) twice daily for 7 days.

Alternative regimen for GCU if cephalosporin allergy:
- Gentamicin 240 mg IM as a single dose plus azithromycin 2 g PO as a single dose.

Alternative regimen for GCU if ceftriaxone not available or administration is not feasible:
- Cefixime 800 mg PO once. If chlamydial infection has not been excluded, providers should treat for chlamydia with doxycycline 100 mg PO twice daily for 7 days.

Regimen for infants and children weighing ≤45 kg:
- Ceftriaxone 25 to 50 mg/kg body weight intravenously (IV) or IM as a single dose, but not exceeding 250 mg IM[1]

FOLLOW-UP

It is imperative to appropriately counsel patients on the avoidance of intercourse or use of barrier protection until a cure has been obtained and sexual partners have been evaluated. Once treated, patients should be advised to abstain from sex for 7 days.

TABLE 1 Etiology of Urethritis	
Infectious	**Noninfectious**
Sexually Transmitted Infections	***Vasculitides***
Neisseria gonorrhoeae	Reiter syndrome
Chlamydia trachomatis	Erythema multiforme
Trichomonas vaginalis	Kawasaki disease
Herpes simplex virus type 2	
Mycoplasma spp.	
Nonsexually Transmitted Infections	***Mechanical***
Staphylococcus saprophyticus	Masturbation
Enterobacteriaceae	Foreign body
Gardnerella vaginalis	Trauma
Streptococcus spp.	Dysfunctional elimination
Enterobius vermicularis	***Chemical***
	Soaps
	Detergents
	Drugs

From Cherry JD: *Feigin and Cherry's pediatric infectious diseases*, ed 8, Philadelphia, 2019, Elsevier.

In cases of suspected cephalosporin treatment failure, clinicians should obtain relevant clinical specimens for culture and antimicrobial susceptibility testing, consult an infectious disease specialist or STD clinical expert (https://www.stdccn.org/) for guidance in clinical management, and report the case to the Centers for Disease Control and Prevention (CDC) through state and local public health authorities within 24 h. Health departments should prioritize notification and culture evaluation for the patient's sex partner(s) from the preceding 60 days for those with suspected cephalosporin treatment failure or persons whose gonococcal isolates demonstrate reduced susceptibility to cephalosporins.

A test of cure (repeat testing 1 to 3 wk after initial treatment) is unnecessary for persons with uncomplicated GCU treated with any of the recommended or alternative regimens. However, for persons with pharyngeal gonorrhea, a test of cure is recommended, using culture or NAATs 7 to 14 days after initial treatment, regardless of the treatment regimen.

Alternatively, repeat testing 3 mo after treatment is recommended for all persons diagnosed with GCU, regardless of treatment, because reinfections rates are so high: Reinfection within 12 mo ranges from 7% to 12% among persons previously treated for gonorrhea. If retesting at 3 mo is not possible, clinicians should retest within 12 mo after initial treatment.

CHRONIC INFECTION

- Reinfection is the most common cause of recurrence.
- Repeat swab and culture of the urethra, pharynx, and rectum (where applicable) are mandatory.
- Persistence of *N. gonorrhoeae* by smear or culture requires treatment for *N. gonorrhoeae*.
- Postgonococcal urethritis (PGU): Persistence of polymorphonuclear cells (PMNs) in the absence of gram-negative intracellular diplococci. This occurs when GCU is treated with a regimen that is ineffective against coincident nongonococcal infection; it represents NGU after GCU and should be treated as such.

PEARLS & CONSIDERATIONS

COMMENTS

- Partner notification: The names and contact information of sexual partners should be gathered at the time of diagnosis and referred to the health department, or the patient can notify the contact directly.
- Expedited partner treatment is recommended by the CDC and is approved in most states. This consists of giving prescriptions to the infected patient for their partner(s) who has not been evaluated by a physician and for whom health department partner-management strategies are impractical or unavailable.[1]
- On examination of the urethral smear, the presence of small numbers of PMNs provides objective evidence of urethritis. The complete absence of PMNs on a urethral smear argues against urethritis. If in addition to the PMNs there are gram-negative, intracellular diplococci, the diagnosis of gonorrhea is established.

REFERENCES & SUGGESTED READINGS

Available at eBooks.Health.Elsevier.com.

RELATED CONTENT

Gonococcal Urethritis (Patient Information)
Gonorrhea (Related Key Topic)

AUTHOR: **LAUREN C. ROBY, MD**

Diseases and Disorders

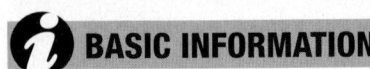

BASIC INFORMATION

DEFINITION

Nongonococcal urethritis (NGU) is urethral inflammation caused by any of several organisms (see "Etiology").

SYNONYMS

NGU
Nongonococcal urethritis

ICD-10CM CODES	
A56.0	Chlamydial infection of lower genitourinary tract
N34.1	Nonspecific urethritis

EPIDEMIOLOGY & DEMOGRAPHICS

- The occurrence is 50% in sexually transmitted disease clinics. *Chlamydia trachomatis* is the most common notifiable disease in the U.S., with >1.5 million infections reported to the Centers for Disease Control and Prevention (CDC) in 2016.
- NGU most commonly affects men in a higher socioeconomic class, affecting heterosexual men more frequently than men who have sex with men.
- NGU carries a greater morbidity rate than gonococcal urethritis (GCU).

PHYSICAL FINDINGS & CLINICAL PRESENTATION

- Incubation period: 2 to 35 days.
- Symptoms: Dysuria, whitish-clear urethral discharge, and urethral itching. The onset of symptoms in NGU is less acute than in GCU. The majority of persons with *C. trachomatis* infection are not aware of their infection because they do not have symptoms that would prompt them to seek medical care.
- Signs: Whitish-clear urethral discharge, meatal edema, and erythema. Infected women manifest pyuria, and the disease can present as acute urethral syndrome.

COMPLICATIONS

- Epididymitis in men may be linked to nonbacterial prostatitis, proctitis in men who have sex with men, or Reiter syndrome.
- Urethritis complications are more common in women and can be associated with ectopic pregnancy, pelvic inflammatory disease, or infertility.

ETIOLOGY

- Most common agent is *Chlamydia* spp., an obligate intracellular parasite possessing both DNA and RNA, which replicates by binary fission. It causes 20% to 50% of NGU cases. Two species exist:
  1. *Chlamydia psittaci*
  2. *Chlamydia trachomatis* with its 15 serotypes:
     a. Serotypes A through C cause hyperendemic-blinding trachoma.
     b. Serotypes D through K cause genital tract infection.
     c. Serotypes L1 through L3 cause lymphogranuloma venereum.
- Other causes of NGU: *Mycoplasma genitalium* (found in 44% of treatment failures with double infection with *C. trachomatis* in up to 15% of cases); *Ureaplasma urealyticum*, causing 15% to 30% of the cases of NGU; *Trichomonas vaginalis;* herpes simplex virus; and *Adenovirus*. However, the cause of up to 50% of the cases of NGU may not be identified.
- Asymptomatic infection occurs in 28% of the contacts of women with chlamydial cervical infection.

DIAGNOSIS

DIFFERENTIAL DIAGNOSIS

- Gonococcal urethritis
- Herpes simplex virus
- Trichomoniasis

LABORATORY TESTS

- Requires demonstration of urethritis and exclusion of infection with *N. gonorrhoeae*.
- Nucleic acid amplification tests (NAATs) have replaced culture where persons are screened for asymptomatic genital infection, and yields more sensitivity, specificity, and ease of specimen transport than any other tests available for the diagnosis of chlamydial and gonococcal infections. NAATs should be used to detect chlamydia and gonorrhea except in cases of child sexual assault, rectal and oropharyngeal infections in prepubescent girls, and when evaluating a potential gonorrhea treatment failure, in which case culture and susceptibility testing might be required.
- *Chlamydia* culture: The appearance of polymorphonuclear cells on urethral smear confirms the diagnosis of urethritis. Because *Chlamydia* is an intracellular parasite of the columnar epithelium, the best specimen for culture is an endourethral swab taken from an area 2 to 4 cm inside the urethra. For culture, a Dacron-tipped swab is used; avoid calcium alginate or cotton swabs. The organism can only be grown in tissue culture, which is expensive.

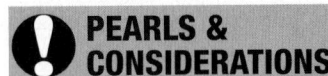 TREATMENT

- Because it is impossible to differentiate among the common causes of NGU, the condition is treated syndromically, including in the initial treatment regimen those drugs effective against the common causative agents.
- In patients with isolated uncomplicated NGU, the recommended regimen is doxycycline 100 mg twice daily for 7 days. An alternative regimen is azithromycin 1 g oral (PO) single dose or 500 mg PO in a single dose followed by 250 mg PO daily for 4 days.
- Recommended treatment for isolated uncomplicated NGU in pregnancy is azithromycin, 1 g PO as a single dose or amoxicillin 500 mg three times a day (tid) for 7 days.
- In patients with confirmed urethritis and unclear etiology, concurrent treatment for gonorrhea and *Chlamydia* is recommended. In these patients, uncomplicated infections of the urethra can be treated with combination of a single 1-g dose of oral azithromycin or 100 mg doxycycline bid for 7 days *plus* one dose of ceftriaxone 250 mg.
- In areas where *T. vaginitis* is prevalent, men who have sex with women and have persistent or recurrent urethritis should be presumably treated with metronidazole 2 g PO or a single dose of tinidazole 2 g PO.
- Patients with recurrent NGU should initially be assessed for compliance with treatment or reexposure; retreatment of initial therapy should be considered. Alternative retreatment regimens should take into consideration the original treatment. For patients initially treated with doxycycline, consider retreatment with a single dose of azithromycin 1 g. If azithromycin was used for initial treatment, consider retreatment with moxifloxacin 400 mg/day for 6 days.

! PEARLS & CONSIDERATIONS

COMMENTS

- Partner notification: The names and contact information of all sexual partners within preceding 60 days should be gathered at the time of the visit and referred to the health department, or the patient notifies the contacts directly. Expedited partner treatment is recommended by the CDC and approved in several states. This consists of giving prescriptions to the infected patient for their partner(s) who have not been evaluated by a physician and are unlikely to seek medical care.
- Patients should abstain from intercourse for 7 days after therapy completion.
- Test of cure for NGU in pregnancy should be performed 4 wk after therapy completion and patients should be rescreened 3 mo after treatment.

SUGGESTED READING

Available at eBooks.Health.Elsevier.com.

RELATED CONTENT

Nongonococcal Urethritis (Patient Information)
Cervicitis (Related Key Topic)
Chlamydia Genital Infections (Related Key Topic)

AUTHORS: **RACHEL WRIGHT HEINLE, MD, FACOG** and **CHRISTINE BURKE, MD**

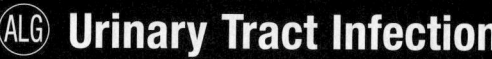
Diseases and Disorders

I

 BASIC INFORMATION

DEFINITION

Urinary tract infection (UTI) is a term that encompasses a broad range of clinical entities that have in common a positive urine culture. Most cases are caused by bacteria ascending from the urethra into the bladder. A conventional threshold is growth of >100,000 colony-forming units (CFUs)/ml from a midstream-catch urine sample with no more than two species of organisms and at least one sign or symptom of UTI (urgency, frequency, dysuria, suprapubic tenderness, fever >38.0°C [100.4°F]). In symptomatic patients, using a lower threshold of between 100 and 10,000 CFUs/ml increases diagnostic sensitivity without significantly compromising specificity.

CLASSIFICATION

- Uncomplicated UTI: Occurs in a normal urinary tract and resolves rapidly with conventional antimicrobials. These patients have a low risk of ascending infection.
- Complicated UTI: Occurs in patients with co-existing pathology (strictures, stones, comorbidities [diabetes mellitus, multiple sclerosis, spinal cord injuries]). These patients are considered at high risk for ascending infection.
- First infection: The first documented UTI; tends to be uncomplicated and is easily treated.
- Unresolved bacteriuria: UTI in which the urinary tract is not sterilized during therapy. Main causes are bacterial resistance, patient noncompliance with treatment, mixed bacterial infection, rapid reinfection, azotemia, infected stones, Munchausen syndrome, and papillary necrosis.
- Bacterial persistence: UTI in which the urine cultures become sterile during therapy, but a persistent source of infection gives rise to reinfection by the same organism. Causes include chronic bacterial prostatitis, atrophic infected kidney, vesicovaginal or enterovesical fistulas, obstructive uropathy, infected pyelocaliceal diverticula, infected ureteral stump after nephrectomy, infected necrotic papillae from papillary necrosis, infected urachal cysts, infected medullary sponge kidney, urethral diverticula, and foreign bodies.
- Reinfection: UTI in which a new infection occurs with new pathogens at variable intervals after a previous infection has been eradicated.
- Relapse: A less common form of recurrent infection; occurs within 2 wk of treatment when the same organism reappears in the same site as the previous infection. Relapsing infections of the urinary tract most commonly occur in pyelonephritis, kidney obstruction from a stone, foreign body, and prostatitis.

SYNONYM

UTI

ICD-10CM CODES

N39.0	Urinary tract infection, site not specified
N99.521	Infection of other external stoma of urinary tract
N99.531	Infection of other stoma of urinary tract
N30.00	Acute cystitis without hematuria
N30.30	Trigonitis without hematuria
N30.20	Other chronic cystitis without hematuria

EPIDEMIOLOGY & DEMOGRAPHICS

INCIDENCE:

- UTI is the most common bacterial infection encountered in the ambulatory care setting in the U.S. The self-reported annual incidence of UTI in women is 12%, and half of all women report having had at least one UTI by 32 yr of age.
- UTIs account for 8 million health care visits per yr and 15% of all outpatient prescriptions.
- Incidence by age group:
  1. In neonates: More common in boys as a result of anatomic abnormalities such as the posterior urethral valves.
  2. In preschool children: More common in girls than in boys (4.5% vs. 0.5%).
  3. In adulthood: More common in women, with a 1% to 3% prevalence in nonpregnant women. Table 1 describes risk factors for acute uncomplicated UTIs in women.
  4. In pregnancy: At 12 wk gestation, the incidence of asymptomatic bacteriuria is similar to that in nonpregnant women (2% to 10%). However, 25% to 30% of pregnant women with untreated asymptomatic bacteriuria develop acute pyelonephritis, especially in the second and third trimesters, and pregnant women have a pyelonephritic recurrence rate of 10%; therefore treatment of asymptomatic bacteriuria in pregnancy is recommended.
  5. In adults aged ≥65: At least 10% of men and 20% of women have bacteriuria.

PHYSICAL FINDINGS & CLINICAL PRESENTATION

- Typical symptoms of UTI include:
  1. Urinary frequency and/or urgency
  2. Dysuria
  3. Suprapubic pain
  4. Gross or microscopic hematuria

- The probability of cystitis is greater than 50% in women with any symptom of UTI and greater than 90% in women who have dysuria and frequency without vaginal symptoms.
- Clinical symptoms alone can be used to make the diagnosis of uncomplicated UTI in women without a urine culture.
- When negative cultures are associated with significant pyuria, vaginal discharge, or hematuria, infections with *Chlamydia trachomatis*, *Neisseria gonorrhoeae*, and *Trichomonas vaginalis* should be considered.
- Acute pyelonephritis presents with fever, flank or abdominal pain, chills, malaise, and vomiting. It is these systemic symptoms that distinguish pyelonephritis from cystitis. Complications of acute pyelonephritis are renal abscess, perinephric abscess, emphysematous pyelonephritis, and pyonephrosis.

ETIOLOGY & PATHOGENESIS

- Most UTIs are caused by fecal flora, which can colonize the vaginal and periurethral tissues and ascend into the bladder.
- Other risk factors include incomplete bladder emptying due to neurologic disease, bladder outlet obstruction or urethral stricture, renal failure, diabetes, vesicoureteral reflux, fistula, urinary diversion, advanced age, pregnancy, recent sexual activity, and instrumentation.
- Catheters: Patients who require a long-term Foley catheter will eventually develop significant levels of bacteriuria. Treatment is reserved for individuals who become symptomatic (fever, chills, malaise, loss of appetite, pain, etc.). Using prophylactic antibiotics to treat patients who have chronic catheters is not indicated because of the risk of acquiring bacteria resistant to antibiotic therapy.
- Once bacteria reach the urinary tract, three factors determine whether symptomatic infection occurs (Box 1). These factors also determine the anatomic level of the UTI:
  1. Virulence of the microorganism
  2. Inoculum size
  3. Adequacy of the host defense mechanisms
- Urinary pathogens: In 90% of UTIs the infecting organism is gram-negative bacilli. *Escherichia coli* is the most common pathogen, causing

---

TABLE 1 Factors Modulating Risk for Acute Uncomplicated Urinary Tract Infections in Women

Host Determinants	Uropathogen Determinants
Behavioral: Sexual intercourse, use of spermicidal products, recent antimicrobial use, suboptimal voiding habits	*Escherichia coli* virulence determinants: P, S, Dr, and type I fimbriae; hemolysin; aerobactin; serum resistance
Genetic: Innate and adaptive immune response, enhanced epithelial cell adherence, antibacterial factors in urine and bladder mucosa, nonsecretor of ABO blood group antigens, P_1 blood group phenotype, reduced *CXCR1* expression, previous history of recurrent cystitis	
Biologic: Estrogen deficiency in postmenopausal women, micturition	

From Johnson RJ et al: *Comprehensive clinical nephrology*, ed 6, Philadelphia, 2019, Elsevier.

BOX 1   Bacterial Factors

- The size of the inoculum
- The virulence of the infecting organism
  1. Virulence factors
     a. P-fimbriae facilitate the adherence of bacteria to biologic surfaces.
     b. K-antigens facilitate adherence and protect the organisms from the host-immune response.
     c. O-antigens are an important source of systemic reactions such as fever and shock that occur with bacterial infections.
     d. H-antigens are associated with flagella and are related to bacterial locomotion.
     e. Hemolysin may potentiate tissue damage and facilitate local bacterial growth.
     f. Urease alkalinizes the urine and facilitates stone formation, thus potentiating infection.
  2. Biofilms harbor bacteria on prosthetic devices and may be a source of recurrent infections.
  3. The presence of sialosyl galactosyl globoside on the surface of kidney cells. This compound is a highly powerful receptor for *Escherichia coli* bacteria.
  4. Women with a deficiency in human beta-defensin-1 are at greater risk for urinary tract infection.

85% of UTI cases (predominantly O, K, and H antigen serotypes). *Staphylococcus saprophyticus* causes 10% of infections, especially in young, sexually active women. Other less common urinary pathogens include *Klebsiella, Enterobacter, Serratia, Proteus,* and *Pseudomonas.*

- In contrast, the organisms that commonly colonize the distal urethra and skin of both men and women and the vagina of women are *Staphylococcus epidermidis,* diphtheroids, lactobacilli, *Gardnerella vaginalis,* and a variety of anaerobes that rarely cause UTIs. In general, the isolation of two or more bacterial species from a urine culture signifies a contaminated specimen unless the patient is being managed with an indwelling catheter or urinary diversion, or has a chronic complicated infection.
- Innate defense mechanisms against cystitis include low urine pH and high urine osmolarity, mucopolysaccharide glycosaminoglycan (GAG) protective layer, complete bladder emptying, and low vaginal pH due to the presence of estrogen and resulting colonization of the genital tract by lactobacillus. At the level of the kidney, uromodulin (also known as Tamm-Horsfall protein) is secreted by renal tubular epithelial cells to inhibit adherence of bacteria to urothelial cells.
- In uncomplicated, nonpregnant patients, cystitis rarely progresses to pyelonephritis or other serious infections such as bacteremia.

Dx DIAGNOSIS (FIG. 1)

DIFFERENTIAL DIAGNOSIS

- Vaginitis
- Urethritis (gonococcal, nongonococcal, *Trichomonas*)
- Interstitial cystitis (painful bladder syndrome)
- Pelvic inflammatory disease
- Nephrolithiasis
- Structural urethral abnormalities such as diverticulum or stricture

LABORATORY TESTS

- Microscopic urinalysis of clean-catch urine for bacteria and pyuria. The presence of ≥10 leukocytes/μl of unspun urine from a midstream catch indicates possible UTI. The absence of pyuria should call into question the diagnosis of UTI.
- Dipstick urinalysis with the presence of nitrites or leukocyte esterase is indicative of UTI. However, dipstick urinalysis may not be useful in symptomatic patients, as a negative dipstick urinalysis does not exclude the diagnosis of UTI. Additionally, dipsticks may be falsely positive when the urine is contaminated. Overall, a dipstick positive for nitrites and leukocyte esterase has a sensitivity of 75% and specificity of 82% in patients with >100,000 CFU/ml.
- Urine culture and sensitivity are useful in complicated UTIs and to help guide therapy in patients who fail initial therapy. They are generally not needed in uncomplicated UTIs.

IMAGING STUDIES

- Warranted only if renal infection or genitourinary abnormality is suspected
- Computed tomography (CT) urogram, voiding cystourethrogram, renal ultrasound, and intravenous pyelogram
- Specialty examination: Cystoscopy and retrograde pyelography to rule out obstructive uropathy, urethral diverticulum, mesh obstruction, or malignancy

Rx TREATMENT

SUPPORTIVE THERAPY

Urinary analgesics such as phenazopyridine and aggressive hydration

ACUTE GENERAL Rx

- First-line antimicrobials for uncomplicated UTI recommended by the Infectious Disease Society of North America, the American Urologic Society, and the American College of Obstetricians and Gynecologists include nitrofurantoin twice daily for 5 days, trimethoprim plus sulfamethoxazole (TMP-SMX) twice daily for 3 days, or fosfomycin 3-g sachet in a single dose.
- Antimicrobial stewardship and drug resistance needs to be considered when choosing antibiotic therapy. Nitrofurantoin continues to have the lowest rates of antimicrobial resistance. Empiric treatment with TMP-SMX is considered appropriate when resistance rates are below 20%. Beta-lactam antibiotics may be appropriate in cases of known patient intolerance or allergy to conventional first-line agents.
- Nitrofurantoin may have lower rates of bioavailability in patients >65 yr due to decline in renal function. If CrCl is <30 ml/min, nitrofurantoin should be avoided, as it may not reach therapeutic concentration in the urine.
- Many women with a history of UTIs are aware of symptom onset. Patient-initiated therapy, in which a patient is given a prescription for the treatment of an uncomplicated UTI and instructed to start therapy when symptoms develop, has been found to be safe, effective, and less costly.
- High rates of resistance and the potential for serious side effects should limit the use of fluoroquinolone antimicrobials. The U.S. FDA has warned against the use of fluoroquinolone antibiotics for routine infections when suitable alternatives are available.
- Pyelonephritis may be treated as an outpatient in stable, well-hydrated patients with close follow-up. Antimicrobial selection is ideally based on urine culture results. Empiric treatment with fluoroquinolone antimicrobials or TMP-SMX is acceptable. Initiation of treatment in the emergency room setting with a single parenteral dose of a long-acting beta-lactam or aminoglycoside antibiotic followed by oral treatment with fluoroquinolones or TMP-SMX is an acceptable regimen. Patients should be assessed for a proper response to treatment within 48 h. Nitrofurantoin and fosfomycin are not indicated for the treatment of pyelonephritis due to inadequate renal tissue levels.
- Inpatient management of pyelonephritis should begin with parenteral antimicrobials followed by transition to oral agents based on clinical response and culture results.
- Pyelonephritis may require a total duration of 10 to 14 days of therapy, although evidence exists that 7 to 10 days may be equally effective in low-risk patients (Table 2).

! PEARLS & CONSIDERATIONS

COMMENTS

- Asymptomatic bacteriuria occurs commonly in postmenopausal women. Treatment of asymptomatic bacteriuria with antimicrobials is discouraged because it can result in the development of drug-resistant organisms. Patients with cloudy or foul-smelling urine should be encouraged to aggressively hydrate to eliminate these symptoms. Postmenopausal

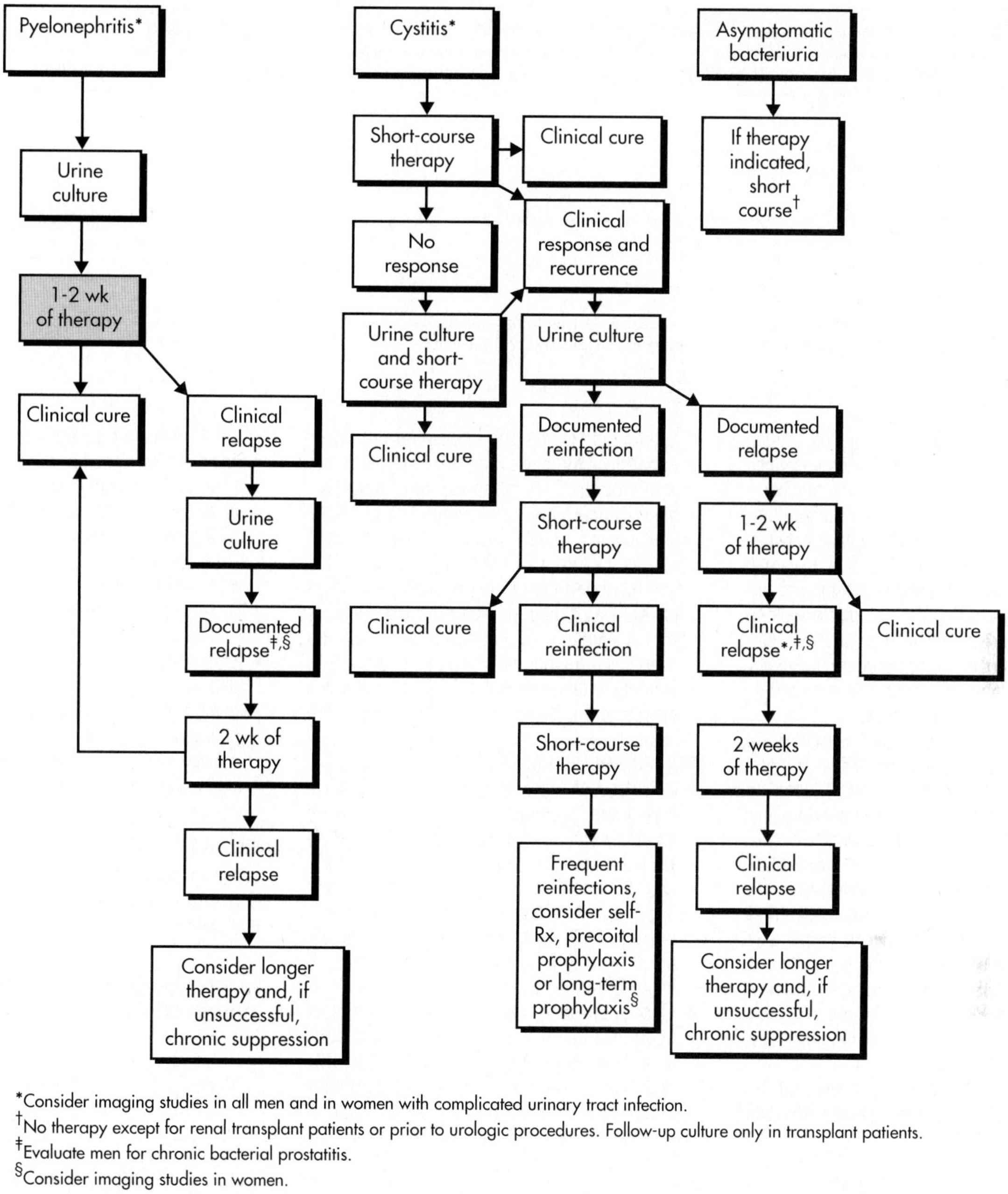
Pyelonephritis*
Urine culture
1-2 wk of therapy
Clinical cure
Clinical relapse
Urine culture
Documented relapse‡,§
2 wk of therapy
Clinical relapse
Consider longer therapy and, if unsuccessful, chronic suppression
Cystitis*
Short-course therapy
Clinical cure
No response
Clinical response and recurrence
Urine culture and short-course therapy
Urine culture
Clinical cure
Documented reinfection
Documented relapse
Short-course therapy
1-2 wk of therapy
Clinical cure
Clinical reinfection
Clinical relapse*,‡,§
Clinical cure
Short-course therapy
2 weeks of therapy
Frequent reinfections, consider self-Rx, precoital prophylaxis or long-term prophylaxis§
Clinical relapse
Consider longer therapy and, if unsuccessful, chronic suppression
Asymptomatic bacteriuria
If therapy indicated, short course†
*Consider imaging studies in all men and in women with complicated urinary tract infection.
†No therapy except for renal transplant patients or prior to urologic procedures. Follow-up culture only in transplant patients.
‡Evaluate men for chronic bacterial prostatitis.
§Consider imaging studies in women.

FIG. 1 Approach to the management of urinary tract infection in nonpregnant adults. (From Bennett JE et al: *Mandell, Douglas, and Bennett's principles and practice of infectious diseases*, ed 9, Philadelphia, 2020, Elsevier.)

TABLE 2 Dosage and Toxicity of Antibiotics Commonly Used to Treat Urinary Tract Infections

Drug	Oral Dose and Frequency	Minor Toxicity	Major Toxicity
Trimethoprim-sulfamethoxazole	160 mg/800 mg, q12h	Allergic	Serious skin reactions, blood dyscrasia
Nitrofurantoin macrocrystals	100 mg, q12h	GI upset	Peripheral neuropathy, pneumonitis
Ampicillin	250-500 mg, q6h	Allergic, candidal overgrowth	Allergic reactions, pseudomembranous colitis
Tetracycline	250-500 mg, q6h	GI upset, skin rash, candidal overgrowth	Hepatic dysfunction, nephrotoxicity
Cephalexin	250-500 mg, q6h	Allergic	Hepatic dysfunction
Ciprofloxacin	250 mg, q12h	Nausea, vomiting, diarrhea, abdominal pain, headache, skin rash	Arrhythmias, angina, convulsions, GI bleeding, nephritis

GI, Gastrointestinal.
From Walters M, Karram M: *Urogynecology and reconstructive pelvic surgery*, ed 4, Philadelphia, 2015, Elsevier.

TABLE 3 Spectrum of Antimicrobial Activity Against Common Lower Urinary Tract Pathogens

Organism	Nitrofurantoin	TMP-SMX	Ciprofloxacin	Levofloxacin	Cephalexin	Ampicillin	Fosfomycin
Escherichia coli	+	±	+	+	+	±	+
Pseudomonas	−	−	+	±	−	−	+
Klebsiella	−	±	+	+	+	−	+
Proteus	±	±	+	+	±	+	±
Enterobacter	±	±	+	+	−	−	±
Enterococcus	+	−	−	±	−	+	±
Staphylococcus	+	+	±	±	±	+	+
Serratia marcescens	−	±	+	+	−	−	±

From Walters M, Karram M: *Urogynecology and reconstructive pelvic surgery,* ed 4, Philadelphia, 2015, Elsevier.

women with vaginal atrophy can be treated with vaginal estrogen to reduce the incidence of bacteriuria. Exceptions include immunocompromised patients, patients with structural urinary tract abnormalities, and pregnant patients.

- Pregnancy: 25% to 30% of pregnant women with untreated asymptomatic bacteriuria develop pyelonephritis. All pregnant women should be screened for asymptomatic bacteriuria and treated. Nitrofurantoin, TMP-SMX, and beta-lactam antibiotics are appropriate first-line choices in pregnancy.
- Recurrent UTI: Two or more symptomatic UTIs over a 6-mo period or three or more episodes over a 12-mo period. Causes include unresolved infection, abnormal vaginal colonization by the originally infecting organism, or reinfection with a new strain. Management of recurrent UTI includes antibiotic prophylaxis for 6 mo or longer, intermittent self-treatment, and postcoital prophylaxis depending on the circumstances. Patients with recurrent UTIs can be considered for an anatomic evaluation including office cystoscopy and upper urinary tract imaging (renal ultrasound or CT urography).
- Nonantimicrobial strategies to prevent UTI have shown mixed results. Nonantimicrobial agents with antiseptic effects on the lower urinary tract include cranberry supplements with vitamin C, D-mannose, and methenamine. Studies demonstrating clinical effectiveness of these agents show modest effects with few side effects. Topical estrogen has been shown to normalize the vaginal flora and may increase the thickness of the urothelium over time and should be used as an adjunct in postmenopausal women with recurrent UTI. Oral probiotics may also be beneficial by decreasing the vaginal pH.

ANTIMICROBIAL RESISTANCE:
- Because of the overuse of antibiotics, organisms once sensitive to a number of antimicrobial agents are now increasingly resistant, making effective treatment of UTI and pyelonephritis more challenging. Most important has been the increasing resistance to TMP-SMX, the current primary care provider drug of choice for acute uncomplicated UTI in women.
- Fluoroquinolone use for the treatment of acute cystitis in women should be avoided when suitable alternatives exist. The U.S. FDA has changed the labeling of quinolone antibiotics to reflect this recommendation.

- When choosing a treatment regimen, physicians should consider such factors as:
  1. In vitro susceptibility
  2. Adverse effects on individual patients
  3. Adverse effects on the population (stewardship)
  4. Cost-effectiveness
  5. Resistance rates in their respective communities
- Meropenem (1 g intravenous [IV] q8h) or IV plazomicin (15 mg/kg body weight once daily) are effective for the treatment of complicated UTIs and acute pyelonephritis caused by *Enterobacteriaceae,* including multidrug-resistant strains (Table 3).

RELATED CONTENT

Urinary Tract Infection (Patient Information)
Urinary Tract Infection (Child) (Patient Information)
Pyelonephritis (Related Key Topic)

AUTHORS: **SYDNEY FORD, MD, MPH** and **ANTHONY SCISCIONE, DO**

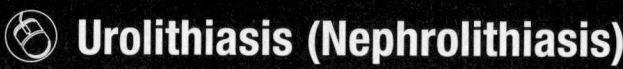
BASIC INFORMATION

DEFINITION

Urolithiasis is the presence of calculi (urinary stones) within the urinary tract. The five major types of urinary stones are calcium oxalate (60% to 70%), calcium phosphate (20%), uric acid (7%), struvite (7%), and cystine (1%) (Table 1).[1]

SYNONYMS

Kidney stones
Kidney calculi
Renal stones
Renal calculi
Ureteral stones
Ureteral calculi
Urinary stones
Nephrolithiasis
Ureterolithiasis

ICD-10CM CODES

N20.0	Calculus of kidney
N20.1	Calculus of ureter
N20.2	Calculus of kidney with calculus of ureter
N20.9	Urinary calculus, unspecified
N21.0	Calculus in bladder
N21.1	Calculus in urethra
N21.8	Other lower urinary tract calculus
N21.9	Calculus of lower urinary tract, unspecified

EPIDEMIOLOGY & DEMOGRAPHICS

INCIDENCE: Urinary stones affect approximately 1 in 11 persons in the United States.[2] It is estimated to cost over $5 billion on the U.S. health care system and accounts for approximately 1 million Emergency Department (ED) visits annually.

PREVALENCE: More commonly occurring in men than women, approximately 10% vs. 7%.[2] Recurrence rate of up to 50% within 5 yr of first stone episode.

PREDOMINANT SEX & AGE: Most common in men in their 30 to 50s.[2]

PEAK INCIDENCE: Fourth to sixth decade of life.[2]

RISK FACTORS: Dehydration, warm weather, prior stone episodes, metabolic syndrome, family history.

PHYSICAL FINDINGS & CLINICAL PRESENTATION

Obstructing ureteral stones, although asymptomatic at times, cause the following signs and symptoms:

- Renal colic: Acute, often severe flank pain
- Referred pain: Pain radiating from the flank downward to the lower back and abdomen and anteriorly to the groin and genitalia
- Inability to find a comfortable position
- Nausea and vomiting
- Hematuria, gross or microscopic
- Urinary urgency and frequency with distal ureteral stones mimicking a urinary tract infection
- Fever and chills accompanying acute renal colic from superimposed infection
- Older adult patients; children; and patients with diabetes mellitus, neurologic deficits, or kidney transplant may present with nonspecific and vague abdominal discomfort and pain

ETIOLOGY

- Low urine output
- Low or high urine pH, hypercalciuria, hypocitraturia, hyperoxaluria, and/or hyperuricosuria predispose patients to urinary stone formation[3]
- Diets high in sodium and animal protein, excessive oxalate content, and heavy intake of phosphoric acid can all increase the risk of urinary stone formation[2]
- Anatomic factors predisposing patients to urinary stasis: Malrotated, horseshoe, or ectopic kidney; ureteropelvic junction obstruction, bladder outlet obstruction, and urinary strictures affecting the urinary tract.[4,5]

DIAGNOSIS

DIFFERENTIAL DIAGNOSIS

- GI: Appendicitis, cholecystitis, constipation, diverticulitis, small bowel obstruction

- Genitourinary: Testicular torsion, ureteropelvic junction obstruction, urinary tract infection (cystitis and pyelonephritis)
- Obstetric-gynecologic: Dysmenorrhea, ectopic pregnancy, pelvic inflammatory disease, ovarian torsion
- Other: Malignancy (primary) urinary tract or retroperitoneal lymphadenopathy causing ureteral/kidney obstruction, musculoskeletal back pain, malingering or factitious disorder

WORKUP

- Vitals should be obtained to monitor for signs of sepsis (fever, tachycardia, hypotension) as an obstructing ureteral stone with superimposed urinary tract infection necessitates more urgent intervention.
- Imaging studies should be performed to determine the location of obstructing urinary stones. Urine and blood studies are obtained to assess the acuity of stone presentation and elucidate possible etiologies.

LABORATORY TESTS

- Blood work should include the following:
  1. A CBC should be obtained in anticipation of possible intervention associated with a significant bleeding risk or in those with bleeding disorders. Additionally, the presence of leukocytosis in the acute setting may influence the management approach.[4]
  2. A basic metabolic panel is appropriate in the acute setting. Patients undergoing a formal metabolic evaluation should have a comprehensive metabolic panel in addition to assessing levels of uric acid and parathyroid home.[2-5]
  3. A lactic acid should be obtained if there is concern for septic stone.
  4. Preprocedural tests as needed (coagulation profile, etc.) if procedure planned.
- Urine studies:
  1. A urinalysis (UA) should always be part of the workup for urolithiasis. Hematuria is often present, but the absence of hematuria does not exclude stones. Urine pH may help identify stone type, where pH >7.5 is associated with struvite stones, pH <5.5 is generally associated with uric acid stones, and low serum bicarbonate concentration with urine pH ≥6 is consistent with a renal tubular acidosis.[4,5]
  2. Urine culture and sensitivity should be obtained in patients suspected to have an underlying urinary tract infection or when surgery is planned.[4,5]
- A 24-h urine collection evaluates for urine chemistries. It is generally reserved for patients with recurrent stones, bilateral stones, large stone burden, young, and/or motivated first-time stone formers who are interested in preventive measures.[2,3,5]

IMAGING STUDIES

- Noncontrast computed tomography (CT) is the standard for diagnosing urolithiasis. It is rapid and accurate, has the greatest sensitivity (nearly 100%) and specificity (94% to

---

TABLE 1 Types of Urinary Tract Stones and Their Etiology

Composition	Etiological Factors	Percentage of All Stones
Calcium oxalate/calcium oxalate mixed with calcium phosphate	An underlying metabolic disorder (e.g., idiopathic hypercalciuria or hyperoxaluria) ► in 25% no metabolic abnormality is identified	75
Struvite or matrix calculi (composed of magnesium ammonium phosphate)	Renal infection	10-15
Uric acid	Hyperuricemia or hyperuricosuria ► it is idiopathic in 50%	6
Cysteine	A renal tubular defect	1-2

Other stones (e.g., xanthine stones, which may be related to a metabolic abnormality, or indinavir stones, which are drug related) are uncommon and account for <5% of all renal stones.
From Grant LA: *Grainger & Allison's diagnostic radiology essentials*, ed 2, Philadelphia, 2019, Elsevier.

96%), and can identify almost all stone types in essentially all locations. CT scan is the best test upon which to base stone treatment recommendations, evaluate stone persistence or passage, and plan for surgery.[4,6]

- Renal-bladder ultrasonography (RBUS) may be an adequate initial study to detect stone presence (i.e., hydronephrosis, absent ureteral jet), especially in patients known to have a history of stones and in patients where radiation should be avoided (e.g., pregnancy and children). RBUS is 50% to 70% sensitive in detecting stones within the kidneys and approximately 90% sensitive in detecting hydronephrosis. Initial RBUS may be associated with lower cumulative radiation exposure than initial CT, without significant differences in missing, serious, or alternative diagnoses; adverse events; pain scores; return emergency department visits; or hospitalizations.[4,6]
- A kidney-ureter-bladder x-ray (KUB) can identify radioopaque stones (e.g., calcium-containing) but not radiolucent stones (uric acid stones). However, the KUB has much lower detection rates than CT, with an estimated sensitivity of 44% and specificity of 77%.[5]

Rx TREATMENT

ACUTE GENERAL Rx

- NSAIDs are excellent for managing renal colic and are preferred first-line agents (e.g., ketorolac, ibuprofen). Opiates may be required for severe pain. Initial pain control with NSAIDs can reduce overall opiate dosing for renal colic.
- For patients who have a stone with a high probability of passage (i.e., small stone, especially in the distal ureter), medical expulsive therapy with alpha-blockers or calcium channel blockers (used less often due to side effects) may be helpful, particularly for stones in the distal ureter >5 mm in size.[5]
- Intravenous fluids and antiemetics may be required.
- Antibiotics are indicated if a urinary tract infection is present or suspected.

PREVENTION

Preventive measures for urolithiasis center around dietary measures, hydration, and lifestyle modifications.[2,5] Diets high in sodium and animal protein should be avoided in favor of those rich in vegetables and fiber and normal amounts of calcium. Fluid intake near 3 liters per day is advocated, with the goal of having a urine output of 2 liters or more on a daily basis. Furthermore, an active lifestyle with adequate physical activity is advocated in addition to maintaining a body mass index in the normal range. Despite popular belief, a diet of normal and high normal calcium intake has not been shown to increase the risk of stone formation. Pharmaceutical therapy may be necessary in those with recurrent urolithiasis despite following the aforementioned preventive measures.

- Thiazide diuretic agents are widely used for "prevention of recurrence of kidney stones," but a recent trial among patients with recurrent kidney stones revealed that the incidence of recurrence did not differ substantially among patients receiving hydrochlorothiazide once daily at a dose of 12.5 mg, 25 mg, or 50 mg or placebo daily.[7]

CHRONIC Rx

Pharmaceutical therapy may be indicated in patients with certain stone composition, specific metabolic abnormalities, and/or those with stone recurrence or stone growth despite preventive measures.[2,3] This includes allopurinol (normocalciuria with hyperuricosuria), potassium citrate (normocalciuria with hypocitraturia; normocalcemia with hypercalciuria; uric acid stone formers, cystinuria), thiazides (normocalcemia with hypercalciuria), calcium citrate (normocalciuria with hyperoxaluria), and tiopronin (cystine stone formers).[3]

DISPOSITION

- Patients with uncomplicated obstructing ureter stones may safely be observed. A 4- to 6-wk monitoring period is preferred, which may be paired with medical expulsion therapy.[4,5]
- Stone passage is influenced by size and location of stone. Smaller and more distal stones are more likely to pass spontaneously.[4,5] Stones less than <5 mm in size in the distal ureter have about an 80% to 90% chance of spontaneous passage.
- For high-risk patients, stone recurrence rates are estimated to be 50% at 10 yr compared to 10% to 20% in those with lower risk profile.[8]
- A formal metabolic evaluation should considered in those with stone recurrence, motivated first-time stone formers, and children after their first stone episode.

REFERRAL

- Urology referral is appropriate for any patient with urinary stones when a patient cannot be discharged from the emergency department; when a patient has an obstructing kidney stone and presumed or associated urinary tract infection; when there are large or recurrent stones; when patients have solitary kidneys or complex anatomy that may predispose them to stones; and when spontaneous passage is unlikely or does not occur despite an appropriate monitoring period.
- The mainstays of definitive treatment for obstructing ureteral stones that have failed a trial of passage are shockwave lithotripsy (SWL), ureteroscopy, and percutaneous nephrolithotomy (PCNL). Open procedures are relatively uncommon in the modern era.

! PEARLS & CONSIDERATIONS

COMMENTS

- Uncomplicated obstructing ureteral stones can safely be monitored for 4 to 6 wk.
- Medical expulsion therapy includes improved hydration, analgesics, and medications that may help with stone passage such as alpha-blockers (Tamsulosin) or calcium channel blockers.
- Consider NSAIDs as first-line therapy for pain control with kidney stones, unless there are contraindications (e.g., allergy or acute kidney injury).
- Imaging is key to diagnosing urolithiases. Ultrasound or KUB is a suitable screening test, while CT scan is most accurate and often determines treatment recommendations.
- Escalation of care is indicated if (1) spontaneous passage does not occur, (2) the patient is persistently symptomatic, (3) an underlying urinary tract infection is suspected, (4) significant acute kidney injury is present despite adequate hydration, and (5) concerns for systemic inflammatory response syndrome are present. Urology consultation is appropriate at this point to determine the need for prompt urinary tract drainage via insertion of a ureteral stent or percutaneous nephrostomy.
- The removal of small, asymptomatic kidney stones during surgery to remove ureteral or contralateral kidney stones is up to the urologist and the patient. Trials have shown that removal of small asymptomatic stones results in a lower incidence of relapse than nonremoval and in a similar number of emergency department visits related to the surgery.[9]

REFERENCES

Available at eBooks.Health.Elsevier.com.

AUTHORS: **MICHAEL CHIEN, MD** and **DAVID A. LEAVITT, MD**

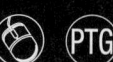 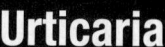

BASIC INFORMATION

DEFINITION

Urticaria is a pruritic rash involving the epidermis and the upper portions of the dermis caused by localized capillary vasodilation and the release of histamine and other vasoactive mediators. It is followed by transudation of protein-rich fluid in the surrounding tissue and manifests clinically with the presence of raised erythematous, circumscribed lesions with central pallor. Urticaria is classified according to its chronicity into acute (<6-wk duration) and chronic (≥6-wk duration). Chronic urticaria has been categorized on the basis of consensus criteria and guidelines as spontaneous urticaria (previously designated as chronic idiopathic urticarias) in which urticaria, angioedema, or both occur in unprompted fashion, or as inducible urticaria (previously designated as physical urticaria) in which urticaria, angioedema, or both are elicited by factors such as cold, heat, or pressure.[1]

SYNONYMS

Hives
Wheals

ICD-10CM CODES
L50.0	Allergic urticaria
L50.1	Idiopathic urticaria
L50.2	Urticaria due to cold and heat
L50.3	Dermatographic urticaria
L50.4	Vibratory urticaria
L50.5	Cholinergic urticaria
L50.6	Contact urticaria
L50.8	Other urticaria
L50.9	Urticaria, unspecified

EPIDEMIOLOGY & DEMOGRAPHICS

- Between 15% and 25% of the population will have at least one episode of urticaria during their lifetime.[2]
- The incidence of chronic urticaria (CU) is thought to be around 1.4% annually. It is more common in adults, with the average age of occurrence between the third and fifth decades of life. Females are twice as likely to be affected as males.[2,3]
- Incidence is increased in atopic patients.[2]

PHYSICAL FINDINGS & CLINICAL PRESENTATION

- Presence of elevated, erythematous, or white circumscribed lesions that change in size and shape over time (Fig. E1) in no specific distribution; they are characterized by extreme pruritus and are evanescent, with individual lesions generally lasting <24 h in duration and disappearing without scarring. If the patient has persistent symptoms, new lesions typically have a novel distribution.
- Stroking of the skin can lead to urticarial reaction (dermatographism) (Fig. E2).

- Angioedema occurs in approximately 40% of cases of urticaria and is caused by mast cell mediator release in the subcutaneous tissue and deep dermis.[3]
- Although not yet well understood, patients with CU may have a range of concurrent systemic symptoms such as fatigue, rhinorrhea, dyspnea, gastritis, joint pain, and hypertension. These patients also have higher rates of depression and anxiety.[3]

PATHOGENESIS

- Cellular mechanisms of acute and chronic urticaria are heterogenous and incompletely understood, but are known to involve pathologic activation of mast cells and basophils, which leads to the release of proinflammatory mediators, such as histamine, leukotrienes, and prostaglandins.[2]
- Autoimmunity plays a central role specifically in the pathogenesis of chronic spontaneous urticaria (CSU), with contributions from immunoglobulin G (IgG)- and IgE-specific autoantibodies (against interleukin-24 [IL-24] and FcεR1, the latter being found on the surface of dermal mast cells and basophils). CSU patients also tend to have higher levels of proinflammatory cytokines: IL-17, IL-31, and IL-33. The clinical significance of these antibodies and inflammatory markers is currently being studied and reviewed for potential therapeutic targets.[2,4]

ETIOLOGY

Acute urticaria (Table 1):
- Food allergies (e.g., shellfish [Fig. E3], tree nuts, legumes, milk, eggs)
- Medication allergies (e.g., penicillin, aspirin, sulfonamides, hormone therapy)
- Insect sting allergies (e.g., honey bee, *Hymenoptera,* fire ant)
- Systemic diseases (e.g., systemic lupus erythematosus, serum sickness, autoimmune thyroid disease, cutaneous mastocytosis, cryoglobulinemia)
- Infections (e.g., viral upper respiratory infections, hepatitis B and C, fungal infections, chronic bacterial infections, helminthic)
- Nonimmunologic contact urticaria (e.g., caterpillars, plants)
- Immunologic contact urticaria (e.g., natural rubber latex, nickel, parabens, benzoic acid, salicylic acid)
- Other: Pregnancy, hair bleaches, saliva, pemphigoid, emotional stress, malignancy (lymphomas, endocrine tumors)
- Idiopathic urticaria is diagnosed in ~50% of patients with acute urticaria

Chronic urticaria:
- CU is classified as either CSU or chronic inducible urticaria, depending on whether the skin lesions appear spontaneously or can be induced.
- Physical stimuli (e.g., pressure, cholinergic, solar, cold/heat, aquagenic, or vibration) are found in ~20% of patients.[3]

- Experts consider CSU to be autoimmune in nature but the exact mechanism remains unclear.[2]

DIAGNOSIS

DIFFERENTIAL DIAGNOSIS

- Erythema multiforme
- Erythema marginatum
- Erythema infectiosum
- Urticarial vasculitis
- Herpes gestationis
- Drug eruption
- Multiple insect bites
- Bullous pemphigoid
- Mastocytosis or other mast cell disease
- Viral exanthema
- Pityriasis rosea
- Atopic dermatitis
- Contact dermatitis
- Henoch-Schönlein purpura

WORKUP

- It is useful to determine whether hives are acute or chronic; a medical history focused on various etiologic factors is necessary before embarking on additional laboratory testing.
- Most cases of acute urticaria resolve spontaneously and diagnostic testing is not required. However, in patients with acute urticaria, it is crucial to consider anaphylaxis before further workup of urticaria because this may require urgent management.
- The cause of CU is often never determined.

LABORATORY TESTS

- Guidelines from the Academy of Allergy, Asthma & immunology (AAAAI) and the American College of Allergy, Asthma & Immunology (ACAAI) only recommend targeted laboratory testing based on clinical findings.[3] International guidelines, recommend CBC with differential, C-reactive protein and/or erythrocyte sedimentation rate (ESR), and, in special cases, total IgE and IgG anti-TPO.[5] Testing rarely leads to the identification of the cause of CU.
- If the history is consistent with allergen-induced contact urticaria, skin testing with allergen extracts and screening for dermatographism (i.e., by attempting to elicit a wheal after application of linear skin pressure) should be performed only after withholding antihistamines for 36 to 72 h to prevent false-negative results.[3]
- Measurement of C4, C1 inhibitor antigenic level and function, and C1q may be helpful in patients who present with angioedema alone. In these patients, C1-inhibitor deficiency should be considered.[3]
- Skin biopsy is helpful in patients with fever, arthralgias, and elevated ESR. Histologic evidence of leukocytoclasia (neutrophilic infiltration with fragmentation of nuclei) is indicative of urticarial vasculitis.[3]
- When food or contact allergy is suspected in acute urticaria, testing can be performed using skin prick or serum testing for allergen-specific IgE.[3]

TABLE 1 Some Causes of Urticaria*

Infections	Eggs[†]
Bacterial infections	Cheese
Dental abscess	Inhalants
Sinusitis	Animal dander
Otitis	Pollen
Pneumonitis	Contactants
Gastritis	Wool
Hepatitis	Silk
Cholecystitis	Occupational exposure
Cystitis	Potatoes
Vaginitis	Antibiotics
Fungal infections	Cosmetics
Dermatophytes	Dyes
Candida	Hairspray
Other Infections/Infestations	Nail polish
Scabies	Mouthwash
Helminth	Toothpaste
Protozoa	Perfumes
Trichomonas	Hand cream
Drugs and Chemicals	Soap
Salicylates	Insect repellent
Indomethacin and other, newer nonsteroidal antiinflammatory agents[†]	Physical stimuli
Opiates[†]	Light
Radiocontrast material[†]	Pressure
Penicillin (medication, milk, blue cheese)	Heat
Sulfonamides	Cold
Sodium benzoate	Water
Douches	Vibration
Ear drops or eye drops	Endocrinopathies
Insulin	Thyroid disease
Menthol (cigarettes, toothpaste, iced tea, hand cream, lozenges, candy)	Diabetes mellitus
Tartrazine (vitamins, birth control pills, antibiotics, FDC yellow #5)	Pregnancy
Foods	Menstruation
Nuts	Menopause
Berries[†]	Systemic diseases
Fish	Rheumatic fever
Seafood	Connective tissue diseases (lupus erythematosus, Sjögren syndrome, rheumatoid arthritis, Still disease, dermatomyositis, polymyositis, other)
Shellfish[†]	Leukemia
Bananas	Lymphoma
Grapes	Acquired immunodeficiency disease
Tomatoes	Ovarian tumors

*Partial list of most frequently described causes in each category.
[†]May be mediated by nonimmunologic mechanisms independent of immunoglobulin E.
From Callen JP et al: *Dermatological signs of systemic disease*, ed 5, Philadelphia, 2017, Elsevier.

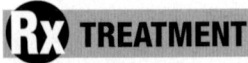

TREATMENT

NONPHARMACOLOGIC THERAPY

Remove all suspected etiologic agents (e.g., stop all nonessential drugs) and avoid any triggers that may have been observed to precipitate an attack (e.g., NSAIDs, alcohol, opiates, physical triggers, stress).[5,6]

ACUTE Rx

- Oral antihistamines: Use of second-generation H₁ antihistamines (e.g., cetirizine 10 mg/day, levocetirizine 5 mg/day, loratadine 10 mg/day, fexofenadine 180 mg/day) is preferred over first-generation sedating antihistamines (e.g., hydroxyzine, diphenhydramine). Higher doses of second-generation antihistamines up to four times the FDA-approved dose may be required to achieve adequate control of symptoms.[6]
- Leukotriene receptor antagonists (e.g., montelukast) can be added to H₁ antagonists in refractory cases, although the utility of this has not been consistently shown.[6]
- Oral corticosteroids should be reserved for refractory cases of acute urticaria and prescribed for a very limited course (e.g., prednisone 20 mg/day or 20 mg bid for 5 days).[6,7]

CHRONIC Rx

Stepwise approach for management of CU is described in Fig. E4.

- Step 1: Monotherapy with second-generation H₁ antihistamines.
- Step 2: If unresponsive, increase to up to 4× the daily recommended dose. Consider addition of leukotriene receptor antagonist (e.g., montelukast) or first-generation H₁ antihistamine (hydroxyzine or doxepin) to be taken at bedtime.[6]
- Step 3: Referral to an allergy specialist for evaluation and management. Consider addition of omalizumab (monoclonal anti-IgE antibody that downregulates surface IgE receptors) to antihistamine therapy.[6]
- Step 4: If adequate control is not reached, consider cyclosporine in addition to antihistamine therapy.[5]
- Refractory options available at specialty centers include antiinflammatory or immunosuppressive agents such as dapsone, hydroxychloroquine, sulfasalazine, methotrexate, cyclosporine A, mycophenolate, tacrolimus, sirolimus, interferon, TNFα, plasmapheresis, phototherapy, or intravenous immune globulin (IVIG).[5,6]
- Patients should be evaluated at each visit and, if symptoms are well managed, should be considered for step down in treatment.
- Numerous therapies are currently under investigation including BTK inhibitors, Anti-kit antibodies, vitamin D supplementation, Jak1/3 inhibition, tripterygium glycosides, IL-2 injections, and heparin and tranexamic acid.

DISPOSITION

- Most cases of urticaria resolve within 6 wk.[6]
- >50% of patients may not achieve satisfactory control of CU with antihistamines alone and may require additional therapies. The median duration of CU is between 3 and 5 yr, but it can often be present for much longer durations.

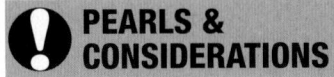

PEARLS & CONSIDERATIONS

COMMENTS

- Topical treatment (e.g., starch baths or oatmeal baths) may be temporarily soothing in selected patients; however, they are not recommended for long-term control of CU.
- If individual urticarial lesions leave residual ecchymoses, pigmentation, and/or lesions that typically last >24 h at a single location, consider skin biopsy to evaluate for urticarial vasculitis.
- Be judicious when prescribing NSAIDs in CU patients, as up to 30% of these patients will experience an exacerbation of urticaria and/or angioedema.

REFERENCES

Available at eBooks.Health.Elsevier.com.

RELATED CONTENT

Hives (Patient Information)
Chronic Urticaria (Related Key Topic)

AUTHORS: **JEFFREY YUNG, MD** and **SHYAM JOSHI, MD**

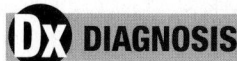 BASIC INFORMATION

DEFINITION

Trichomonas vulvovaginitis is inflammation of the vulva and vagina caused by the protozoan *Trichomonas vaginalis.*[1]

SYNONYMS

Trichomonas vaginalis
T. vaginalis
Trichomoniasis
Trich
TV
Vaginitis, trichomonas

ICD-10CM CODE
A59.01   Trichomonal vulvovaginitis

EPIDEMIOLOGY & DEMOGRAPHICS

- Epidemiologically, *T. vaginalis* infections are commonly associated with other sexually transmitted diseases (STDs) and are a marker of high-risk sexual behavior. Vertical transmission from mother to infant can occur rarely and cause genital infection or respiratory distress.
- *T. vaginalis* is the most common nonviral sexually transmitted infection in the U.S., caused by a parasitic protozoan.[2]
  1. Commonly transmitted male to female, female to male, and female to female
  2. Rarely transmitted male to male
- Overall prevalence is 2% in women 18 to 59; incidence increases with age.
- Diagnosed in:[3]
  1. 9.6% Black women, 1.4% Hispanic women, 0.8% non-Hispanic white women
  2. 14.6% to 27% women presenting to sexually transmitted infection (STI) clinics
  3. 9% to 32% incarcerated women
  4. Up to 70% of male partners of women with trichomonas

RISK FACTORS:[4]
- African descent
- Multiple sexual partners
- HIV infection
- IV drug use
- History of previous STIs
- History of incarceration
- Concurrent bacterial vaginosis (BV) infection
- Others: Less than a high school education, living below the national poverty level

PHYSICAL FINDINGS & CLINICAL PRESENTATION

These symptoms and physical findings (Table 1) may or may not be present depending on the case:[3,5]

- The discharge is classically described as "frothy," but it is actually frothy in only about 10% of patients (Fig. E1). The color of the discharge is variable. Yellow-green, malodorous vaginal discharge is common
- Vaginal and/or vulvar pruritus
- Dysuria

- Dyspareunia
- Intense erythema of the vaginal mucosa
- Cervical petechiae ("strawberry cervix")
- Infected men may have symptoms of urethritis, epididymitis, or prostatitis
- Asymptomatic in approximately 85% of women and 75% of men

ETIOLOGY

Single-cell protozoan *Trichomonas vaginalis*

DX DIAGNOSIS

DIFFERENTIAL DIAGNOSIS[5] (TABLE 2)
- Bacterial vaginosis
- Candida vulvovaginitis
- STI (gonorrhea or chlamydia)
- Others: Atrophic vulvovaginitis, contact dermatitis

WORKUP
- Pelvic examination
- Speculum examination
- Wet mount: Look for motile trichomonads on normal saline preparation (Fig. 2)
  1. 40% to 70% sensitivity[3]
  2. Evaluate within 10 min; sensitivity decreases over time
- Assess vaginal pH: *Trichomonas* is associated with elevated pH (>4.5)
- Laboratory testing (see "Laboratory Tests")
  1. NOTE: If wet mount negative, should evaluate with lab test if possible
- Recommend also screening for gonorrhea and chlamydia

LABORATORY TESTS
- Nucleic acid amplification tests (NAATs): Most sensitive and specific test (gold standard)[3]
  1. Can be collected as endocervical swab, vaginal swab, or urine
  2. Pros: More rapid turnaround time compared with culture
  3. Cons: More expensive, test results take 24 to 72 h
  4. Brands: Aptima, Amplicor, BD Max
- Rapid tests: Useful in areas with high prevalence of *Trichomonas*[3]
  1. Pros: Sensitivity 80% to 95%, specificity 97% to 100%; more accurate than wet mount
  2. Cons: More expensive
  3. Brands: OSOM *Trichomonas* Rapid Test (10 min), Affirm VP III (45 min)
- Culture: Was gold standard before polymerase chain reaction[3]
  1. Useful if negative wet mount or NAAT not available
  2. Pros: Sensitivity up to 93%, specificity up to 100%; can be used for antimicrobial susceptibility
  3. Cons: Not widely available, can take 3 to 7 days to get results
  4. Brands: InPouch
- Pap smear: Incidental finding of trichomonads is sometimes reported on Pap smear[5]
  1. Liquid-based cytology: High specificity, reasonable to treat if presence reported
  2. Conventional Pap smear: Lower specificity, recommend evaluating with diagnostic test, although still reasonable to treat if patient reports symptoms

TABLE 1 Sensitivity of Clinical and Laboratory Findings in Vaginal Trichomoniasis

	Clinical Manifestation	Percent Positive
Symptoms	None	9-56
	Discharge	50-75
	Malodorous	~10
	Irritating, pruritic	23-82
	Dyspareunia	10-50
	Dysuria	30-50
	Lower abdominal discomfort	5-12
Signs	None	~15
	Vulvar erythema	10-20
	Excessive discharge	50-75
	Yellow, green	5-20
	Frothy	10-50
	Vaginal wall inflammation	40-75
	Strawberry cervix (direct visualization)	1-2
	Colpitis macularis (colposcope)	45
Laboratory findings	pH >4.5	66-91
	Positive whiff test	~75
	Excess polymorphonuclear neutrophils on wet mount	~75

Data from Honigberg BM (ed): *Trichomonads parasitic in humans*, New York, 1990, Springer-Verlag. Bickley LS et al: Comparison of direct fluorescent antibody, acridine orange, wet mount, and culture for detection of *Trichomonas vaginalis* in women attending a public sexually transmitted disease clinic, *Sex Transm Dis* 16:127-131, 1989; and Rein MF: Uncertainties and controversies in trichomoniasis. In Sobel JD (ed): *Vulvovaginal infections: current concepts in diagnosis and therapy*, New York, 1990, Academy Professional Information Services, pp. 73-85.

TABLE 2 Features of Sexually Transmitted Infections Characterized by Vaginal Discharge

Feature	Physiologic Leukorrhea (Normal)	Trichomoniasis	Bacterial Vaginosis
Agent	Normal flora	*Trichomonas vaginalis*	Reduction in *Lactobacillus* and overgrowth organisms including *Gardnerella vaginalis*, *Bacteroides*, *Mobiluncus*, and *Peptostreptococcus*
Incubation	—	5-28 days	Not necessarily sexually transmitted
Predominant Symptoms			
Pruritus	None	Mild to moderate	None to mild
Discharge	Minimal	Moderate to severe	Mild to moderate
Pain	None	Mild	Uncommon
Vulvar inflammation	None	Common	Uncommon
Characteristics of Discharge			
Amount	Small	Profuse	Moderate
Color	Clear, milky	Yellow-green or gray	Gray
Consistency	Flocculent	Frothy	Homogeneous
Viscosity	Thin	Thin	Thin
Foul odor	None	Possible	Yes
Odor with KOH	None	Possible	Characteristic fishy odor (amine)
pH	<4.5	>5.0	>4.5
Diagnosis			
Saline drop	Squamous and few WBCs	WBC; motile flagellates, slightly larger than WBCs	Squamous cells studded with bacteria ("clue cells") and WBCs
Gram stain	Gram-positive and gram-negative rods and cocci	*Trichomonas*	Predominance of gram-negative rods and cocci with paucity of gram-positive rods
Culture	Mixed flora with *Lactobacillus* predominant	Culture generally not indicated; antibody and nucleic acid tests available	Culture not useful
Treatment	Reassurance	Metronidazole or tinidazole	Metronidazole or clindamycin

KOH, Potassium hydroxide; *WBCs*, white blood cells.
From Marcdante KJ et al: *Nelson essentials of pediatrics*, ed 9, Philadelphia, 2023, Elsevier.

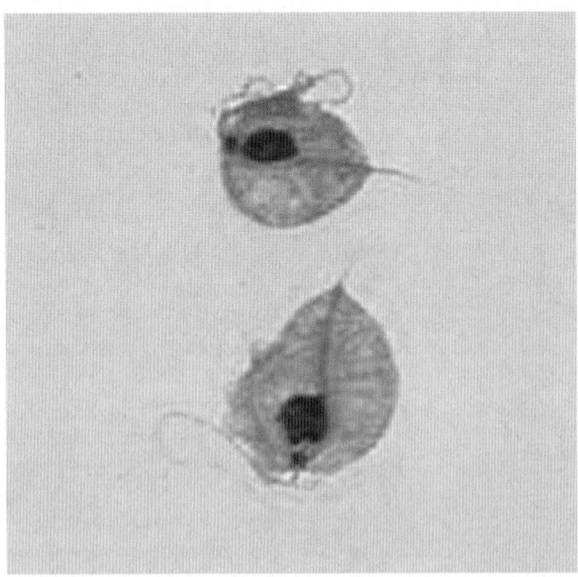

FIG. 2 *Trichomonas vaginalis.* (From Centers for Disease Control and Prevention, National Center for Infectious Diseases, Division of Parasitic Diseases.)

Rx TREATMENT

NONPHARMACOLOGIC THERAPY

- Barrier methods: Recommend using condoms, internal condoms, dental dams, or other barrier methods during all oral, anal, or vaginal intercourse.
- Hygiene: Recommend not sharing sex toys and cleaning after each use with a dedicated cleaner.
- Screening: Recommend regular STI screening if concern for a new partner or new exposure.

ACUTE GENERAL Rx

- Preferred initial treatment for women:[6] Metronidazole 500 mg by mouth (PO) twice a day (bid) × 7 days
  1. Second-line treatment for women:[6] Metronidazole, secnidazole, or tinidazole 2 g PO × 1 dose
- Preferred initial treatment for men:[3] Metronidazole 2 g PO × 1 dose
  1. Second-line treatment for men:[3] Tinidazole or secnidazole 2 g PO × 1 dose
- Special populations:
  1. Pregnancy:[3] Metronidazole only (either 500 mg PO bid × 7d or 2 g PO × 1 dose)
     a. Avoid tinidazole and secnidazole, minimal research has been done
     b. *Trichomonas* is associated with premature rupture of membranes, preterm delivery, and small-for-gestational-age infants; unclear if treatment improves outcomes

  2. Breastfeeding:[3] Consider deferring breastfeeding for 12 to 24 h after taking traditional dose of metronidazole
     a. Lowest concentration in breast milk: Metronidazole 400 mg PO tid × 7 days
  3. HIV:[3] Metronidazole 500 mg PO bid × 7 days
     a. Higher treatment failure with single-dose regimen
- Expedited partner therapy (EPT): Recommend sending Rx for sex partners and abstaining from sex for 7 days or until both partners are treated and symptoms resolved.[5]
- Centers for Disease Control and Prevention (CDC) recommends retesting sexually active women between 3 wk and 3 mo after completing treatment.[3]
- NOTE: Consider recommending avoidance of alcohol consumption during treatment with metronidazole (at least 24 h after completion of therapy) and tinidazole (at least 72 h after completion of therapy) to reduce the possibility of disulfiram-like reaction, although is likely unnecessary.[4]

CHRONIC Rx

- For persistent infections:[3] Repeat metronidazole 500 mg PO bid × 7 days
- If treatment is still unsuccessful:[3] Metronidazole or tinidazole 2 g PO daily × 7 days
- If still unsuccessful:[3]
  1. Option 1: Tinidazole 2 g PO daily PLUS intravaginal tinidazole 500 mg bid × 14 days
  2. Option 2: Tinidazole 1 g PO three times a day (tid) PLUS intravaginal paromomycin 4 g nightly (6.25% cream) × 14 days
  3. Option 3: Culture and susceptibility testing per the CDC (404-718-4141)
- Allergy, intolerance, or adverse reactions: Alternatives to metronidazole or tinidazole are not recommended. Patients who are allergic to nitroimidazoles can be managed by desensitization.[3,5]

DISPOSITION

- *Trichomonas* is considered an STI and treatment of sex partners is recommended.
- If diagnosed with *Trichomonas*, testing for other STIs is recommended, including HIV, syphilis, and gonorrhea/chlamydia.
- *Trichomonas* is associated with 1.5- to 2-fold increased risk for HIV acquisition.
- *Trichomonas* in pregnancy is associated with premature rupture of membranes, preterm birth, and delivery of low-birth-weight infants.

REFERRAL

To obstetrician/gynecologist for recurrent infection or pregnancy

REFERENCES

Available at eBooks.Health.Elsevier.com.

RELATED CONTENT

Trichomoniasis (Patient Information)
Pruritus Vulvae (Related Key Topic)

AUTHORS: **ALEXANDRA H. SMICK, MD** and **STEVEN D. JOHNSON, MD**

BASIC INFORMATION

DEFINITION

Bacterial vaginosis (BV) is a condition marked by alteration of the normal microbiome of the vagina due to overgrowth of facultative anaerobic bacteria in replacement of hydrogen peroxide-producing lactobacilli. The shift in vaginal flora causes a rise in vaginal pH and can produce symptoms such as thin, gray, and malodorous vaginal discharge.

SYNONYMS

Bacterial vaginosis
BV
Nonspecific vaginitis
Gardnerella vaginalis vaginitis

ICD-10CM CODES
N76.0   Acute vaginitis
N77.1   Vaginitis, vulvitis and vulvovaginitis in diseases classified elsewhere

EPIDEMIOLOGY & DEMOGRAPHICS

Most common cause of vaginal discharge in women of reproductive age.

- Commonly associated organisms include *Gardnerella vaginalis, Prevotella* species, *Porphyromonas* species, *Bacteroides* species, *Peptostreptococcus* species, *Mobiluncus* species, *Fusobacterium* species, *Mycoplasma hominis, Ureaplasma urealyticum,* and *Atopobium vaginae* (now renamed *Fannyhessea vaginae*).
- Women with BV are at increased risk for acquiring other sexually transmitted diseases (STDs) such as HIV, *N. gonorrhoeae, C. trachomatis,* and herpes simplex virus type 2 (HSV-2). BV may also contribute to persistent human papillomavirus (HPV) infection.
- May be associated with pelvic inflammatory disease (PID) and complications after gynecologic surgery. Preoperative evaluation and treatment before planned hysterectomy or abortion decreases the infection complication rate.
- May be associated with low birth weight, premature rupture of membranes (PROM), and prematurity in the obstetric setting.
- BV may recur in 30% of cases within the first 3 mo after treatment, which may be due to:
  1. Persistence of pathogenic bacteria
  2. Reinfection from exogenous sources including sexual partners
  3. Failure of the normal lactobacillus-dominant flora to reestablish

RISK FACTORS:
- Multiple female or male sexual partners
- Infection with sexually transmitted infections
- Douching
- Tobacco use
- Lack of condom use
- Lack of vaginal lactobacilli

PHYSICAL FINDINGS & CLINICAL PRESENTATION

- Asymptomatic: 50% to 70% of patients
- Symptomatic:
  1. A thin, dull, and gray homogeneous discharge (Fig. 1)
  2. Characterized by a "fishy" odor from the vagina
- BV alone does not typically cause dysuria, dyspareunia, burning, or vaginal inflammation (edema, erythema). Presence of these symptoms suggest concomitant infection with another pathogen.
- Vaginal pH >4.5
- Clue cells on microscopic examination (Fig. 2)

ETIOLOGY

- *Gardnerella vaginalis* is detected in 40% to 50% of vaginal secretions.
- Increase in vaginal pH secondary to decrease in hydrogen peroxide producing lactobacilli allows predominance of anaerobes that produce large amounts of proteolytic carboxylase enzymes. These enzymes break down vaginal peptides into amines, which are malodorous and associated with increased vaginal transudation and epithelial cell exfoliation, resulting in malodorous discharge.
- It is unclear how the vaginal floral imbalance occurs and the role sexual activity plays in the pathogenesis of BV.
- *G. vaginalis* may be important in epithelial biofilm formation, which may in turn become a scaffold to which other species adhere.
- Ethnicity and age may contribute to the vaginal microbial environment.

DIAGNOSIS

WORKUP

- At least three of the Amsel clinical diagnostic criteria must be present for diagnosis (sensitivity of 92% and specificity of 77%):
  1. Thin, gray, and homogeneous, malodorous discharge that adheres to the vaginal walls
  2. Vaginal pH >4.5
  3. Positive whiff-amine test
     a. Conducted by placing wet mount specimen and adding 10% potassium hydroxide, which creates a fishy odor.
  4. More than 20% of the epithelial cells on microscopy are clue cells

Clinical laboratory tests: Increasingly used due to greater sensitivity and specificity compared with pH testing and microscopy (>90%), ability to identify fastidious bacteria, ease of use, and ability to test for multiple infections from the same swab (*candidiasis, trichomonas, chlamydia, gonorrhea*):

- Nucleic acid amplification tests (NAATs): Exponentially multiply nucleic acid sequences through polymerase chain reactions to identify various vaginal pathogens.
  1. Aptima BV (Hologic): Measurement of lactobacillus, *G. vaginalis,* and *A. vaginae.* Sensitivity 95.0%, specificity 89.6%.
  2. BD Max vaginal panel (Cecton Dickinson): Measurement of *G. vaginalis, A. vaginae,* Megasphaera-1, BV-associated bacteria 2, *L. crispatus, L. jensenii,* and a proprietary algorithm to provide a positive/negative assessment for presence of BV. Sensitivity 90.5%, specificity 85.8%.
- Point of care tests: Used in conjunction with physical exam, vaginal pH, and whiff-amine tests. These are less commonly used since development of NAATs.
  1. Affirm VPIII (Becton Dickinson, Sparks, MD), a DNA-hybridization probe test of high concentrations of *G. vaginalis*
  2. OSOM BV Blue test (Sekisui Diagnostics, Framingham, MA), which detects vaginal fluid sialidase activity
- Gram staining: Considered the gold-standard for diagnosis of BV, but requires more time, resources, and expertise than Amsel's criteria or NAAT tests. Determines the concentration of lactobacilli, gram-negative, and gram-positive bacteria.
- Cultures are unnecessary.
- Pap smear is not a reliable test for BV.
- Rule out other causes such as vulvar diseases, STDs, and atrophic vaginitis.

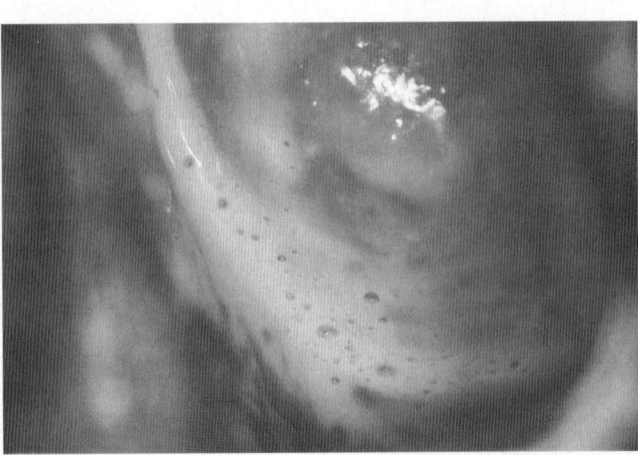

FIG. 1 Bacterial vaginosis. The gray, homogeneous discharge that coats the tissues is characteristic. (From Bennett JE et al: *Mandell, Douglas, and Bennett's principles and practice of infectious diseases,* ed 9, Philadelphia, 2020, Elsevier.)

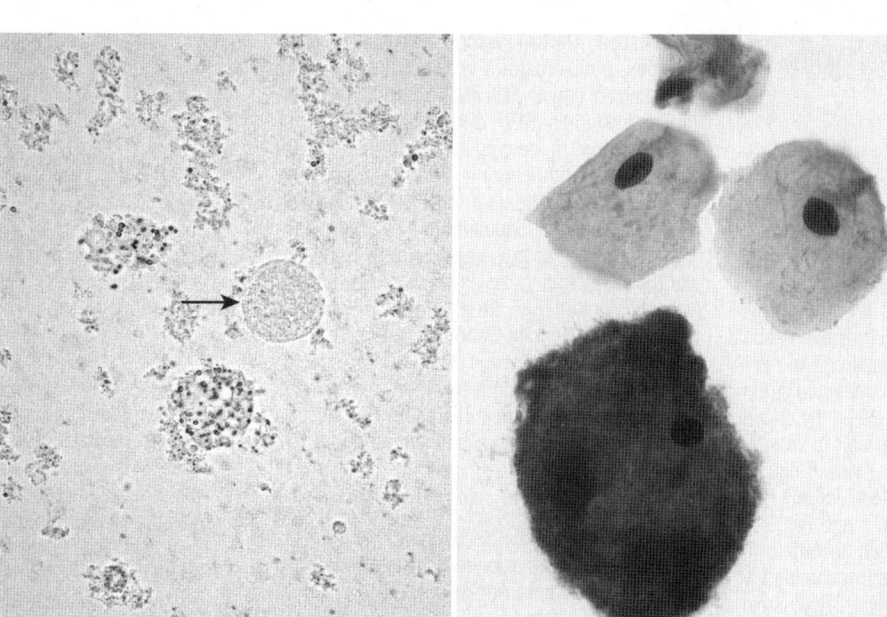

FIG. 2 Bacterial vaginosis, seen as dense, evenly distributed collections of rod-like bacteria forms in squamous cells as seen on a wet prep **(A)** or Papanicolaou stain (clue cells; **B**). (From Crum CP et al: *Diagnostic gynecologic and obstetric pathology,* ed 3, Philadelphia, 2018, Elsevier.)

Rx TREATMENT

ACUTE GENERAL Rx

- Recommended regimens (similar efficacy):
  1. Metronidazole 500 mg PO bid for 7 days *or*
  2. Metronidazole 0.75% gel, one full applicator (5 g of gel contains 37.5 mg of metronidazole) intravaginally daily for 5 days *or*
  3. Clindamycin 2% cream, one full applicator (5 g of cream contains 100 mg of clindamycin) intravaginally at bedtime for 7 days
- Alternative regimens:
  1. Clindamycin 300 mg PO bid for 7 days or
  2. Clindamycin 100 mg ovules (vaginal suppositories) intravaginally once at bedtime for 3 days
  3. May be associated with antimicrobial resistance
- Tinidazole 1g orally once daily for 5 days
  1. Longer half-life than metronidazole (~12 to 14 h vs. ~6 to 7 h)
- Secnidazole 2 g packet once orally
  1. Longer half-life than metronidazole (~17 h vs. ~8 h).
  2. Superior to placebo in phase 3 trial, and at least as effective as metronidazole 500 mg PO bid in noninferiority trial.
  3. Single 1-g oral dose appears to be effective as well.
  4. Improved compliance with single dose regimen, however, more expensive than metronidazole.
- Manufacturer packaging of metronidazole recommends abstinence from alcohol consumption during treatment and for 24 h after

treatment due to potential risk of disulfiram-type reactions.
- Sexual partners: It is not necessary to treat male partners of affected females; however, females who partner with females need to be aware of the signs and symptoms of BV, and treatment is indicated in this population if symptoms occur.
- Follow-up visits after treatment and resolution of symptoms are unnecessary, but patients are advised to return if symptoms recur.
- Not enough evidence for or against probiotic use for treatment and prevention.
- Clindamycin cream may weaken latex condoms if used together. Avoid treatment of asymptomatic patients.
- Treatment in pregnancy:
  1. Symptomatic pregnant patients with BV should be treated to relieve bothersome symptoms.
  2. Insufficient evidence to recommend routine screening for BV in asymptomatic pregnant women at high or low risk of preterm delivery.
  3. Can use oral or topical therapy for symptomatic pregnant women with same regimen as nonpregnant women.
  4. There is no evidence that metronidazole or clindamycin have any teratogenic effect during pregnancy. Tinidazole should be avoided in pregnancy.
- Recurrent BV:
  1. Condom use may help reduce the risk of recurrence.
  2. Chronic suppressive therapy with vaginal metronidazole gel has been proven to reduce the development or recurrence of BV.

3. Vaginal boric acid followed by the option for suppressive treatment with vaginal metronidazole gel may treat recurrent BV.
4. Hormonal contraception may help prevent BV recurrence based on observational data, but it is not a treatment.

! PEARLS & CONSIDERATIONS

BV is the most common cause of vaginitis in reproductive women.

- BV has been associated with pelvic inflammatory disease (PID), postprocedural gynecologic complications including postabortal infection and posthysterectomy vaginal cuff cellulitis, preterm delivery, plasma cell endometritis, and increased risk acquisition of sexually transmitted infections. It is reasonable to treat asymptomatic women who are to undergo gynecologic surgery and screen for other STDs.
- American College of Obstetricians and Gynecologists, U.S. Preventive Services Task Force (USPSFT), and Centers for Disease Control and Prevention all agree to not routinely screen and treat all pregnant women with asymptomatic BV to prevent preterm birth.

RELATED CONTENT

Bacterial Vaginal Infections (Patient Information)

AUTHORS: **LAUREN BURTON, MD** and **EMILY SAKS, MD, MSCE**

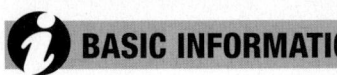

BASIC INFORMATION

DEFINITION

Vasculitis refers generically to inflammation occurring within the walls of blood vessels. Blood vessel inflammation can result in either perforation of affected vessels with hemorrhage into adjacent structures or thrombosis with subsequent ischemia and infarction of supplied tissues. Vasculitis can occur as a primary process or secondary to another connective tissue disease, infection, or drug exposure. The systemic vasculitides are a heterogeneous group of disorders (Table 1) characterized by blood vessel inflammation affecting vessels of varying size and location resulting in a wide range of clinical manifestations dictated largely by which vessels are affected (Fig. 1 and Fig. E2). Vasculitis is traditionally classified according to the size of the blood vessels predominantly affected (Table 2). Antineutrophilic cytoplasmic autoantibody (ANCA)–associated vasculitis (AAV) includes granulomatosis with polyangiitis (GPA); microscopic polyangiitis (MPA), including renal-limited vasculitis (RLV); and eosinophilic granulomatosis with polyangiitis (EGPA). All are associated with ANCA and have similar features on renal histology (e.g., a focal necrotizing, and often crescentic, pauciimmune glomerulonephritis). Several of these are covered in individual topics, including topics on ANCA-associated vasculitis, giant cell arteritis (GCA), Takayasu arteritis, and Henoch-Schönlein purpura (HSP). Severity varies between and within specific vasculitides from a relatively benign, self-limited process to severe, life-threatening multisystem organ involvement with significant morbidity and mortality.

ICD-10CM CODES
M30.0	Polyarteritis nodosa
M30.3	Mucocutaneous lymph node syndrome [Kawasaki]
M31.30 31	Wegener granulomatosis without renal involvement
M31.5	Giant cell arteritis with polymyalgia rheumatica
M31.6	Other giant cell arteritis
M31.4	Aortic arch syndrome [Takayasu]
D 69.0	Allergic purpura
L95.9	Vasculitis limited to the skin, unspecified

EPIDEMIOLOGY & DEMOGRAPHICS

- The epidemiology and demographics of the various vasculitides vary by the individual disease and, where applicable, are covered under the relevant vasculitis disease chapters.
- The most common form of systemic vasculitis in the U.S. is giant cell arteritis, with an approximate incidence of 170 cases/1 million per yr in individuals older than 50 yr.

TABLE 1 Comparing the Vasculitides

Disease	Pathophysiology	Classic Features	Testing	Treatment
Giant cell arteritis	Mononuclear cell infiltration and giant cell formation	Headache, scalp tenderness, visual disturbance	ESR, CRP biopsy	Prednisone and aspirin, may need tocilizumab or sarilumab
Takayasu arteritis	Mononuclear cell infiltration and giant cell formation	Visual disturbance, chest pain, abdominal pain, differences in extremity blood pressure and pulses	Angiography	Prednisone Surgical or angiographic intervention
Polyarteritis nodosa	Polymorphonuclear infiltration	Fever, hypertension, myalgias, abdominal pain, hematuria, CHF, GI bleeding, orchitis	ESR, CRP biopsy Angiography	Prednisone (mild disease) plus cyclophosphamide (moderate-severe disease) Antiviral therapy if concurrent hepatitis B or C Azathioprine or methotrexate for maintenance of remission
Kawasaki disease	Polymorphonuclear infiltration	5-day fever, conjunctivitis, oral lesions, rash, red palms and soles, edema, cervical lymphadenopathy	ESR, CRP leukocytosis Thrombocytosis Echocardiography	Aspirin plus IV gamma globulin
Granulomatosis with polyangiitis (Wegener granulomatosis)	Granuloma formation secondary to aggregating neutrophils	Upper and lower respiratory symptoms, renal insufficiency, skin lesions, visual disturbance	ESR, CRP c-ANCA/PR3	Prednisone and methotrexate (mild disease) Cyclophosphamide or rituximab plus prednisone (moderate to severe disease)
Eosinophilic granulomatosis with polyangiitis (Churg-Strauss syndrome)	Eosinophilic infiltration Allergic granulomas	Allergic rhinitis, nasal polyps, asthma	Leukocytosis Eosinophilia ESR, CRP biopsy	Prednisone with or without cyclophosphamide, mepolizumab
Henoch-Schönlein purpura	IgA complex deposition	Palpable purpura, arthralgias, GI disturbances, glomerulonephritis	Leukocytosis Eosinophilia Ig A elevation, skin biopsy	Usually self-limited NSAIDs Prednisone if necessary Rituximab (refractory cases)
Cryoglobulinemic vasculitis	Cold precipitable monoclonal or polyclonal immunoglobulins	Palpable purpura, glomerulonephritis, myalgias, weakness, peripheral neuropathy	Low complement levels, hepatitis C Renal biopsy	Rituximab with or without prednisone Peg interferon plus ribavirin (HCV infection)
Cutaneous leukocytoclastic vasculitis	Neutrophilic infiltration Mononuclear and eosinophilic infiltration	Palpable purpura, macules, vesicles, bullae, urticaria	Skin biopsy	Prednisone Colchicine Dapsone
Behçet syndrome	Polymorphonuclear infiltration	Recurrent oral aphthous ulcers, genital ulcers, skin lesions, visual disturbance	ESR, CRP leukocytosis Oral mucosa autoantibodies	Topical corticosteroids Prednisone with azathioprine (end-organ disease) Colchicine (aphthous ulcer and arthritis) Apremilast Infliximab (refractory disease)

c-ANCA, Cytoplasmic antineutrophil cytoplasmic antibody; *CHF,* congestive heart failure; *CRP,* C-reactive protein; *ESR,* erythrocyte sedimentation rate; *GI,* gastrointestinal; *HCV,* hepatitis C virus; *IgA,* immunoglobulin A; *IV,* intravenous.
From Adams JG et al: *Emergency medicine: clinical essentials,* ed 2, Philadelphia, 2013, Elsevier.

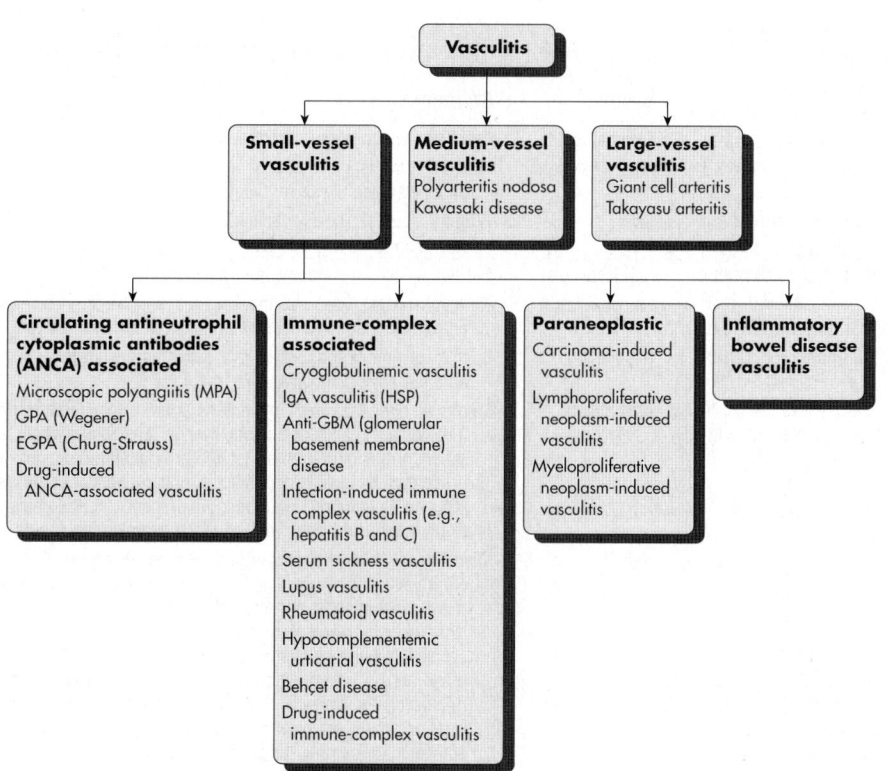

FIG. 1 Major categories of noninfectious vasculitis. Not included are vasculitides that are known to be caused by direct invasion of vessel walls by infectious pathogens, such as rickettsial vasculitis and neisserial vasculitis. *ANCA,* Antineutrophil cytoplasmic antibodies; *EGPA,* eosinophilic granulomatous polyangiitis; *GPA,* granulomatous polyangiitis; *HSP,* Henoch-Schönlein purpura; *IgA,* immunoglobulin A. (From Freehally J et al: *Comprehensive clinical nephrology,* ed 6, Philadelphia, 2019, Saunders.)

TABLE 2   Names and Definitions of Small Vessel Vasculitides as Presented by the 2012 Chapel Hill Consensus Conference

Name	Definition and Comments
Small-vessel vasculitis	Vasculitis predominantly affecting small vessels, defined as small intraparenchymal arteries, arterioles, capillaries, and venules. Medium-sized arteries and veins may be affected.
ANCA-associated vasculitis	Necrotizing vasculitis with few or no immune deposits predominantly affecting small vessels (i.e., capillaries, venules, arterioles, and small arteries), associated with MPO ANCA or PR3 ANCA. Not all patients have ANCA. Add a prefix indicating ANCA reactivity (e.g., MPO-ANCA, PR3-ANCA, ANCA-negative).
Granulomatosis with polyangiitis	Necrotizing granulomatous inflammation usually involving the upper and lower respiratory tract, and necrotizing vasculitis affecting predominantly small- to medium-sized vessels (e.g., capillaries, venules, arterioles, arteries, and veins). Necrotizing glomerulonephritis is common.
Microscopic polyangiitis	Necrotizing vasculitis with few or no immune deposits predominantly affecting small vessels (i.e., capillaries, venules, or arterioles). Necrotizing arteritis involving small- and medium-sized arteries may be present. Necrotizing glomerulonephritis is very common. Pulmonary capillaritis often occurs. Granulomatous inflammation is absent.
Eosinophilic granulomatosis with polyangiitis (Churg-Strauss syndrome)	Eosinophil-rich and necrotizing granulomatous inflammation often involving the respiratory tract, and necrotizing vasculitis predominantly affecting small- to medium-sized vessels, and associated with asthma and eosinophilia. ANCA is more frequent when glomerulonephritis is present.
Immune complex vasculitis	Vasculitis with moderate to marked vessel wall deposits of Ig and/or complement components predominantly affecting small vessels (i.e., capillaries, venules, arterioles, and small arteries). Glomerulonephritis is frequent.
Anti–glomerular basement membrane disease	Vasculitis affecting glomerular capillaries, pulmonary capillaries, or both, with GBM deposition of anti-GBM autoantibodies. Lung involvement causes pulmonary hemorrhage, and renal involvement causes glomerulonephritis with necrosis and crescents.
Cryoglobulinemic vasculitis	Vasculitis with cryoglobulin immune deposits affecting small vessels (predominantly capillaries, venules, or arterioles) and associated with serum cryoglobulins. Skin, glomeruli, and peripheral nerves are often involved.
IgA vasculitis (Henoch-Schönlein purpura)	Vasculitis, with IgA1-dominant immune deposits, affecting small vessels (predominantly capillaries, venules, or arterioles). Often involves skin and GI tract, and frequently causes arthritis. Glomerulonephritis indistinguishable from IgA nephropathy may occur.
Hypocomplementemic urticarial vasculitis (anti-C1q vasculitis)	Vasculitis accompanied by urticaria and hypocomplementemia affecting small vessels (i.e., capillaries, venules, or arterioles), and associated with anti-C1q antibodies. Glomerulonephritis, arthritis, obstructive pulmonary disease, and ocular inflammation are common.

ANCA, Anti-neutrophil cytoplasmic antibody; *GBM,* glomerular basement membrane; *GI,* gastrointestinal; *MPO,* myeloperoxidase; *PR3,* proteinase 3.
From Firestein GS et al: *Firestein & Kelley's textbook of rheumatology,* ed 11, Philadelphia, 2021, Elsevier.

- ANCA-associated vasculitis is significantly less common with aggregate incidence estimated at ~20 per million in the U.S.
- Polyarteritis nodosa (PAN) has an annual incidence of 1/100,000 persons but has a higher incidence in patients with existing hepatitis B or C infections.
- Age distribution can demonstrate significant variability between the vasculitides as shown by the fact that GCA generally does not occur before age 50, whereas 90% of cases of HSP occur in the pediatric population, and 80% of patients with Kawasaki disease are under age 5.
- Although genetic factors clearly play a role in disease susceptibility, familial cases of vasculitis are rare.

PHYSICAL FINDINGS & CLINICAL PRESENTATION

- Clinical presentation often includes nonspecific constitutional symptoms including fever, malaise, headache, and weight loss.
- Signs and symptoms are generally dictated by the tropism of involved vessels.
- Skin manifestations of vasculitis include petechiae, palpable purpura (Fig. E3), subcutaneous nodules, livedo reticularis, ulcerations, and digital ischemia.
- Kidney involvement of medium-sized and large vessel vasculitis is often in the form of renovascular hypertension. Glomerulonephritis may be seen in small vessel vasculitis.
- Pulmonary small vessel involvement can cause alveolar hemorrhage, which can present with cough, dyspnea, and alveolar hemorrhage.
- Organ involvement in polyarteritis nodosa is summarized in Table 3.
- Mononeuritis multiplex is the characteristic finding of vasculitis affecting the vasa nervorum of the peripheral nervous system.
- GI involvement of the mesenteric vasculature can cause postprandial pain, bleeding, and perforation.
- Testicular pain or tenderness can be seen with hepatitis B infection in PAN.
- Cardiac involvement can include chest pain secondary to ischemic infarcts in the coronary arteries, pericarditis, cardiomyopathy, and arrhythmias.
- Arthritis, while nonspecific, can be present.
- Significant clinical variability exists between the various vasculitides, although overlapping symptoms may be seen.

ETIOLOGY

Most forms of systemic vasculitis are of unknown etiology. Cryoglobulinemia vasculitis is often secondary to hepatitis C infection, and cutaneous leukocytoclastic vasculitis is often related to a drug exposure.

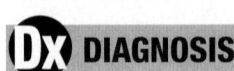 **DIAGNOSIS**

DIFFERENTIAL DIAGNOSIS

- Infective endocarditis
- Atrial myxoma

TABLE 3	Organ Involvement in Polyarteritis Nodosa	
System	**Comment**	**Frequency**
Constitutional	Fever and weight loss (current and previous)	>90%
Musculoskeletal	Arthritis, arthralgia, myalgia, or weakness; when muscle is involved, it provides a useful site for biopsy	24%-80%
Skin	Purpura, nodules, livedo reticularis, ulcers, bullous or vesicular eruptions, and segmental skin edema	44%-50%
Cardiovascular	Cardiac ischemia, cardiomyopathy, hypertension	35%
Ear, nose, and throat	No involvement; nasal crusting, sinusitis, and hearing loss suggest an alternative diagnosis such as granulomatosis with polyangiitis	None
Respiratory	Lung involvement not seen in PAN; abnormal respiratory findings suggest an alternative diagnosis	None
Abdominal	Pain is an early feature of mesenteric artery involvement; progressive involvement may cause bowel, liver, or splenic infarction, bowel perforation, or bleeding from a ruptured arterial aneurysm; less common presentations include appendicitis, pancreatitis, or cholecystitis as a result of ischemia or infarction; the presence of abdominal tenderness or peritonitis and blood loss on rectal examination should be assessed	33%-36%
Renal	Vasculitis involving the renal arteries is present in many cases but does not commonly give rise to clinical features; it can present with renal impairment, renal infarcts, or rupture of renal arterial aneurysms; glomerular ischemia may result in mild proteinuria or hematuria, but red cell casts are absent because glomerular inflammation is not a feature; if evidence of glomerular inflammation exists, then an alternative diagnosis such as microscopic polyangiitis or granulomatosis with polyangiitis must be considered; hypertension is a manifestation of renal ischemia causing activation of the renin-angiotensin system	11%-66%
Nervous system	Mononeuritis multiplex, with sensory symptoms preceding motor deficits; CNS involvement is a less frequent finding and can present with encephalopathy, seizures, and stroke	55%-79%
Ocular	Visual impairment, retinal hemorrhage, and optic ischemia	Rare
Other	Breast or uterine involvement is rare; testicular pain from ischemic orchitis is a characteristic feature, albeit an uncommon presentation	Rare

PAN, Polyarteritis nodosa.
From Firestein GS et al: *Firestein & Kelley's textbook of rheumatology*, ed 11, Philadelphia, 2021, Elsevier.

- Cholesterol emboli
- Malignancy
- Hypercoagulopathy
- Congenital collagen vascular disorder

WORKUP

- The diagnosis of most forms of systemic vasculitis relies on the history and physical examination as well as supportive laboratory testing. Table 4 describes differential diagnostic features of selected forms of small vessel vasculitis.
- Tissue biopsy is important in establishing an accurate diagnosis; biopsy sites should target affected tissues.
- Electromyography and nerve conduction studies can evaluate for site of nerve or muscle involvement before biopsy in patients with neuropathy or myopathy.
- Imaging such as mesenteric angiography can be supportive and may obviate the need for tissue biopsy.

LABORATORY TESTS

- Laboratory markers of systemic inflammation include elevated erythrocyte sedimentation rate (ESR), C-reactive protein (CRP), and anemia of chronic disease.
- ANCA targeting myeloperoxidase (MPO) and proteinase 3 (PR3) are frequently found in

several small vessel vasculitides, including GPA (Wegener), microscopic polyangiitis (MPA), and EGPA (Churg-Strauss).
- Hepatitis C antibodies and rheumatoid factor are often present in cryoglobulinemic vasculitis.
- Positive hepatitis B serologies are commonly found in PAN.
- Urinalysis in patients with glomerulonephritis due to small vessel ANCA-associated vasculitis will generally demonstrate hematuria with active urinary sediment, with red blood cell casts and proteinuria.

IMAGING STUDIES

- Computed tomography (CT) angiography, magnetic resonance angiography, and angiography can demonstrate vascular narrowing and aneurysm formation in suspected medium-size and large-vessel vasculitis.
- Pulmonary and sinus CT scans can demonstrate active pulmonary and upper airway disease in ANCA-associated vasculitis.

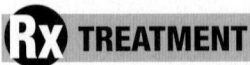 **TREATMENT**

Treatment of vasculitis depends on the specific type of vasculitis and is tailored to the severity of disease activity. Novel treatments are covered under the relevant vasculitis disease chapters.

TABLE 4 Differential Diagnostic Features of Selected Forms of Small Vessel Vasculitis

Features	Microscopic Polyangiitis (MPA)	Granulomatosis with Polyangiitis (GPA)	Eosinophilic Granulomatosis with Polyangiitis	Henoch-Schönlein Purpura (HSP)	Cryoglobulinemic Vasculitis
Vasculitic signs and symptoms	+	+	+	+	+
Immunoglobulin A–dominant immune deposits	–	–	–	+	–
Cryoglobulins in blood and vessels	–	–	–	–	+
Antineutrophil cytoplasmic antibodies in blood	+	+	+	–	–
Necrotizing granulomas	–	+	+	–	–
Asthma and eosinophils	–	–	+	–	–

From Freehally J et al: *Comprehensive clinical nephrology,* ed 6, Philadelphia, 2019, Saunders.

ACUTE GENERAL Rx

- Systemic corticosteroids are generally required to gain initial control of active vasculitis, although mild cases of drug-induced cutaneous leukocytoclastic vasculitis often require cessation of the offending medication and at times, low-dose corticosteroid use.
- HSP and vasculitis limited to the skin, including cutaneous PAN, can often be managed without further immunosuppression.
- Major organ-threatening disease in systemic vasculitis has traditionally required pulse steroids and oral or intravenous cyclophosphamide for induction of remission.
- Studies have demonstrated noninferiority of rituximab compared to cyclophosphamide in ANCA-associated vasculitis with major organ involvement, and it is approved for this use.
- Rituximab with prednisone has also been shown to be effective in the treatment of relapsing flares of disease activity in ANCA-associated vasculitis.
- Less severe disease such as GPA limited to the upper airways can be managed with methotrexate rather than cyclophosphamide.
- Trimethoprim-sulfamethoxazole should be used to prevent *Pneumocystis jirovecii* infection with concurrent immunosuppressive therapy.
- The goal of acute therapy is to induce remission of disease activity and is generally continued for 1 to 2 mo once this is achieved, at which point chronic therapy is used.

CHRONIC Rx

- The goal of chronic therapy is to prevent disease relapse and minimize medication side effects.
- Steroids are gradually tapered as allowed by disease activity.
- Immunomodulatory agents such as methotrexate or azathioprine are commonly used for maintenance therapy in place of cyclophosphamide to reduce side effects.
- Methotrexate and tocilizumab can be used as adjunctive therapy in refractory or relapsing cases of GCA and Takayasu's arteritis to help to reduce the toxicity of glucocorticoids.
- Cryoglobulinemic vasculitis due to chronic hepatitis C virus infection will often improve with treatment of the underlying viral infection.
- Rituximab is shown to be effective in the treatment of cryoglobulinemic vasculitis, and in severe disease it can be used in combination with cyclophosphamide.
- Belimumab can be considered in rituximab-refractory cases of cryoglobulinemic vasculitis as an add-on therapy.
- In PAN with concurrent hepatitis B infection, appropriate antiviral treatment (interferon alpha-2b or lamivudine with or without plasma exchange) is indicated.
- Rituximab may also be an appropriate remission maintenance agent in ANCA-associated vasculitis. For GPA or MPA, scheduled redosing of rituximab every 4 to 6 mo is conditionally recommended over redosing based on ANCA titers or CD19 B-cell counts.

DISPOSITION

Varies widely among the various vasculitides

REFERRAL

Systemic vasculitis care is generally coordinated by a rheumatologist. Renal, pulmonary, neurology, and GI consultations are often needed when vasculitis involves these organ systems. Isolated cutaneous leukocytoclastic vasculitis is often managed by dermatology.

RELATED CONTENT

Cogan Syndrome (Related Key Topic)
Cryoglobulinemia (Related Key Topic)
Giant Cell Arteritis (Related Key Topic)
ANCA-Associated Vasculitis (Related Key Topic)
IgA Vasculitis (Related Key Topic)
Kawasaki Disease (Related Key Topic)
Takayasu Arteritis (Related Key Topic)

AUTHORS: **SHADI JAFARI-ESFAHANI, MD** and **ANTHONY M. REGINATO, MD, PhD**

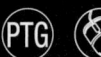
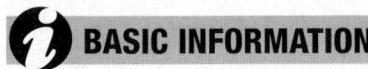 BASIC INFORMATION

DEFINITION

The spectrum of chronic venous disease (CVD) ranges from varicose veins to leg edema and skin manifestations consisting of hyperpigmentation, eczema, lipodermatosclerosis, and venous ulcer. These latter venous-specific skin changes constitute an advanced form of CVD known as chronic venous insufficiency (CVI).

SYNONYMS

Stasis dermatitis
Postthrombotic syndrome (PTS)
Chronic venous disease

ICD-10CM CODES
I87.2	Venous insufficiency (chronic) (peripheral)
I87.8	Other specified disorders of veins
I87.9	Disorder of vein, unspecified
I83.10	Varicose veins of unspecified lower extremity with inflammation

EPIDEMIOLOGY & DEMOGRAPHICS

- From 10% to 35% of adults in the U.S. have some form of CVI.
- Venous ulcers are the complication of CVI that results in the greatest morbidity and affects 4% of people over the age of 65.
- The population-based costs to the U.S. government for CVI treatment and venous ulcer care have been estimated at >$1 billion/yr.
- In addition, 4.6 million workdays/yr are lost to chronic venous-related diseases.

PHYSICAL FINDINGS & CLINICAL PRESENTATION

The manifestations of CVI can be viewed using the internationally accepted classification system, CEAP (clinical, etiology, anatomy, and pathophysiology) (Table E1). The spectrum of cutaneous changes of CVI in the affected leg include:

- Varicose eczema: The most common and earliest sign, this involves the skin above the medial ankle and consists of pruritic, red, and scaly eczematous patches and plaques.
- Hyperpigmentation: Caused by the breakdown of red blood cells and leads to hemosiderin deposition and dark staining of the skin (Fig. 1).
- Atrophie blanche: Usually presents as hypopigmented white patches with focal red punctate dots or telangiectasia surrounded by hyperpigmentation. Skin in this condition is avascular and prone to ulceration (Fig. 2).
- Lipodermatosclerosis: A chronic, brawny induration of the skin and underlying fat that usually involves the skin from medial malleolus up to the lower border of the calf. Progression of the disease leads to an "inverted champagne bottle" appearance. The induration and lack of perfusion of the skin in this area make it susceptible to ulcer formation.

ETIOLOGY

- CVI occurs as a result of sustained venous hypertension in the leg, which can be caused by the following:
  1. Primary: Vein valve failure with reflux in the superficial venous system or perforating veins (most common cause of CVI)
  2. Secondary: Postthrombotic syndrome in which a deep vein thrombosis causes outflow obstruction *or*
  3. Combination of the two previous processes
- This sustained elevation in venous pressure or venous hypertension results in pathologic effects in the skin and subcutaneous tissues such as edema, eczema, hyperpigmentation, fibrosis, and ultimately venous ulceration.

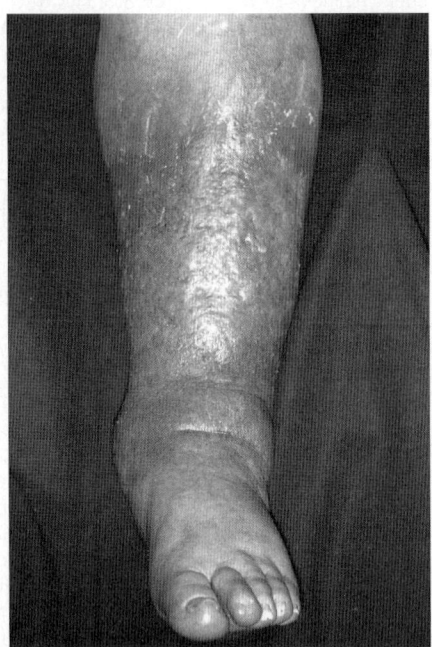 DIAGNOSIS

The diagnosis and evaluation of CVI are directed primarily by a detailed history and physical examination.

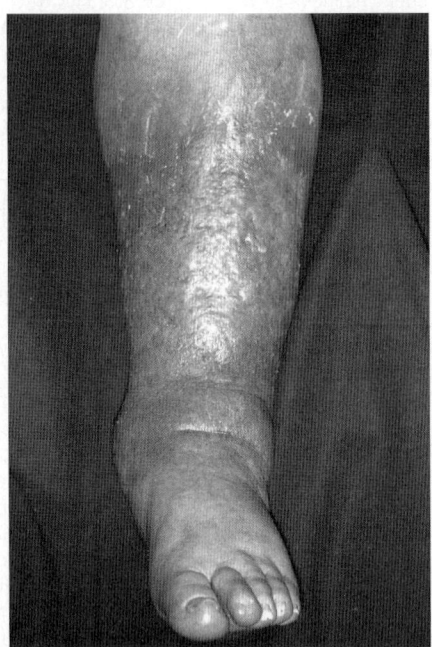

FIG. 1 Stasis dermatitis, venous insufficiency. (From James WD et al: *Andrews' diseases of the skin,* ed 12, Philadelphia, 2016, Elsevier.)

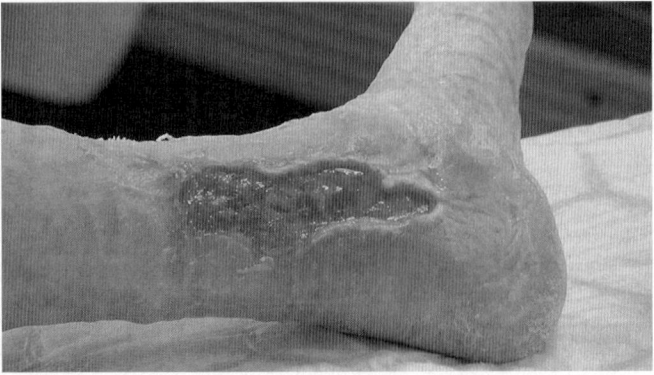

FIG. 2 Chronic venous ulcer likely to be resistant to treatment as it involves the space behind the medial malleolus, which is difficult to compress. (From Fillit HM: *Brocklehurst's textbook of geriatric medicine and gerontology,* ed 8, London, 2017, Elsevier.)

DIFFERENTIAL DIAGNOSIS

- Contact dermatitis
- Atopic dermatitis
- Cellulitis
- Dermatophyte infection
- Pretibial myxedema
- Nummular eczema
- Xerosis
- Asteatotic eczema

WORKUP

The primary goal is to identify the cause of sustained venous hypertension.

LABORATORY TESTS

Generally not indicated

IMAGING STUDIES

- Evaluation of the patient is performed in the standing position with duplex ultrasonography to identify reflux in the superficial, deep, and perforating veins as well as obstruction of the deep veins.

- No exam of a leg with CVI is complete without palpation of pulses and/or determination of ankle-brachial index (ABI).

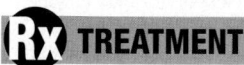 **TREATMENT**

NONPHARMACOLOGIC THERAPY

- Leg elevation above heart level for 30 min three to four times a day
- Weight reduction because obesity is a risk factor for deep vein thrombosis and CVI
- Walking exercises to improve calf function
- Physical therapy to improve ankle joint mobility
- For weeping skin lesions, wet-to-dry dressing changes

ACUTE GENERAL Rx

- The fundamental role of compression in the treatment of CVI is well recognized and has been validated by randomized controlled trials.
- The beneficial effects of gradient compression stockings (decrease in edema and control of discomfort) are due to their effect on microvascular hemodynamics and Starling forces.
- Below-knee compression stocking with a gradient of at least 20 to 30 mm Hg will control edema, alleviate pain, and improve the quality of life in CVI patients.
- Compression stockings are contraindicated in patients with an ABI of <0.6.
- Some patients (acute lipodermatosclerosis) may benefit from nonelastic compression with the unna gel paste gauze boot to alleviate their

symptoms and acute increase in their swelling. The Unna boot is changed once a week.
- Topical corticosteroid creams or ointments (e.g., triamcinolone 0.12% bid) may be used to help reduce inflammation and itching. Steroids should never be applied to ulcer.
- Antibiotics should only be used when treating a clinically apparent, culture-proved infection. Most secondary infections are the result of *Staphylococcus* or *Streptococcus* organisms.
- Diuretics have no role in the treatment of CVI-related edema.

CHRONIC Rx

- Although conservative care is fundamental, patients with CVI should be considered for correction of their underlying venous hypertension.
- The majority of patients with CVI have superficial vein or perforator vein reflux as their underlying pathology and would benefit from the newer vein ablation procedures listed below.
  1. Endovenous ablation of superficial (saphenous) or perforator vein reflux
  2. Radiofrequency ablation with VNUS closure
  3. Endovenous laser therapy (EVLT)
  4. Ultrasound-guided foam sclerotherapy

COMPLEMENTARY & ALTERNATIVE MEDICINE

Several groups of drugs have been evaluated in the treatment of CVI, including coumarins, flavonoids, and saponosides (horse chestnut extracts). These drugs have venoactive properties and are

widely used in Europe but are not approved for use in the U.S. The precise mechanism of action is not known. Horse chestnut seed extract has been found, in the short term, to be as effective as compression stockings in reducing pain and edema, but long-term efficacy has not been established.

REFERRAL

- Phlebology
- Vascular surgery
- Indications for referral:
  1. Skin and subcutaneous changes consistent with CVI
  2. Associated peripheral arterial insufficiency (peripheral artery disease)
  3. Long-standing varicose vein disease
  4. Consideration for vein ablation procedure

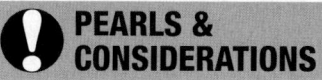 **PEARLS & CONSIDERATIONS**

COMMENTS

- Inflammatory skin changes from CVI are irreversible. The goal of therapy is to eliminate venous hypertension and prevent progression.
- Venous ulcers are often an end-stage manifestation of CVI. Refer to "Venous Ulcers" for more information.

RELATED CONTENT

Stasis Dermatitis (Patient Information)
Varicose Veins (Related Key Topic)
Venous Ulcers (Related Key Topic)

AUTHOR: **FRANK G. FORT, MD, FACS, RPHS**

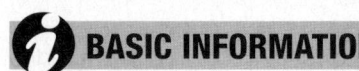 **BASIC INFORMATION**

DEFINITION

Venous ulcers are defined as chronic defects of the skin that fail to heal spontaneously and persist for longer than 4 wk. Venous ulcers account for about 70% of all lower-extremity ulcerations. They are usually located in the "gaiter" region and can be accompanied by varicose veins, edema, hyperpigmentation, and lipodermatosclerosis. Venous ulceration develops in patients as a result of sustained venous hypertension.

SYNONYM

Stasis ulcers

ICD-10CM CODES
I87.2	Venous insufficiency (chronic) (peripheral)
L97.909	Non-pressure chronic ulcer of unspecified part of unspecified lower leg with unspecified severity

EPIDEMIOLOGY & DEMOGRAPHICS

In industrialized nations, up to 1.5% of the population will suffer from venous ulcers. In patients ≥65 yr, the incidence increases to 4%. In the U.S., >500,000 people suffer from stasis ulcers.
RISK FACTORS:
- Obesity
- Increasing age
- Family history of chronic venous insufficiency
- History of deep venous thromboembolism

PHYSICAL FINDINGS & CLINICAL PRESENTATION

Venous ulcers are most commonly located in the lower leg just above the ankle (gaiter region). They are a partial-thickness, irregularly shaped wound with well-defined borders with granulation tissue and fibrin present in the ulcer base (Figs. E1 and E2). Venous ulcers are relatively painless and are surrounded by brown-stained skin and/or dry, itchy, and reddened skin. In about 50% of patients, there are visible varicose veins in an aching, swollen leg.

ETIOLOGY

The exact mechanism of the role of venous hypertension in the etiology of venous ulcers is not certain. Hemodynamic forces such as venous hypertension, circulatory stasis, and modified conditions of shear stress appear to play an important role in an inflammatory reaction accompanied by leukocyte activation that clinically leads to fibrosclerotic remodeling of the skin and then to ulceration.

DIAGNOSIS

DIFFERENTIAL DIAGNOSIS
- Arterial ulcer
- Neurotrophic ulcers (located predominantly in the foot)

- Vasculitis
- Pyoderma gangrenosum
- Ulcerated skin tumors like basal cell or squamous cell carcinoma (Marjolin ulcer)
- Rheumatoid arthritis

WORKUP
- The history and clinical signs and symptoms of leg ulcers are often misleading and may not differentiate venous ulcers from other leg ulcers; about 30% of leg ulcers are not of venous origin.
- Measurement of the ankle-brachial index (ABI) is essential in excluding peripheral arterial disease, which can be present in 20% of patients and is required before starting compression therapy. Arterial insufficiency is suggested by an ABI <0.9.
- Patients with lower-extremity ulcers should also be evaluated for diabetes.
- Coagulation defects have been found in 40% of patients with leg ulcers. This finding suggests that many patients with leg ulcers have a known or suspected history of deep venous thrombosis and a thrombophilia workup is indicated.
- If vasculitis is suspected, a biopsy of the edge of the ulcer can confirm the diagnosis.
- Any wound that has failed to improve after therapy of 4 wk should have a biopsy to rule out malignancy.

IMAGING STUDIES
- Evaluation of patients with venous leg ulcer should include duplex sonography to identify reflux in the superficial, deep, and perforating veins as well as possible obstruction of the deep veins.
- If the ulcer appears to be infected, consider tissue for culture, plain x-ray films, and bone scan to evaluate for osteomyelitis.

TREATMENT

NONPHARMACOLOGIC THERAPY
- Fig. 3 describes an algorithm for the treatment of venous ulcers.
- Surgical debridement to remove all nonviable material can be accomplished in the office setting with the use of a topical xylocaine gel. Debridement produces the release of growth factors that allow the development of healthy granulation tissue and the initiation of the healing process.
- The first-line treatment of ulcers includes below-knee compression stockings to improve venous return to the heart, thereby decreasing edema, inflammation, and tissue ischemia (used only if the ABI is between 0.6 and 0.85 because compression can cause limb ischemia).
- There is Level A evidence that graduated compression stockings alone can lead to healing of a venous ulcer. The stockings should be worn during the day and removed at night.
- Regular, brisk walking 30 min a day, five times a wk is recommended.

- Elevate leg above heart level and raise the foot of bed with 3-in blocks to reduce edema.
- Role of surgery: In a randomized controlled trial, endovenous catheter ablation of superficial reflux showed no improvement in the healing rate of ulcers but did demonstrate a reduction of ulcer recurrence from 28% to 12% at 12 mo. Longer term follow-up (median 3 to 5 yr) also confirmed that abrasive procedures lowered incidence of recurrent ulcers.

ACUTE GENERAL Rx
- Dressings are used under compression stockings to provide a clean, moist environment to promote healing.
- Modern, more complex dressings have been developed and include occlusive and semiocclusive dressings, classified according to their physical composition and ability to control wound drainage.
- Semiocclusive dressings have varying ability to absorb wound drainage. Some examples of this type are hydrocolloids (DuoDERM), hydrogels (DuoDERM hydrogel), foam dressings (Allevyn), and alginates.
- Biologic wound dressings (Apligraf) and tissue-engineered products (Oasis) have been developed, and these products can either directly provide growth factors or indirectly stimulate growth factors in the ulcer bed.
- Pentoxifylline (800 mg PO tid) has been shown to be an effective adjuvant to compression therapy as reported in a meta-analysis of nine clinical trials.
- Skin grafting should be considered for large or refractory ulcers as long as the wound is clean and there is healthy granulation tissue.
- Published randomized clinical trials on the value of the different types of dressings in the management of leg ulcers have not shown effects on ulcer healing. Despite the lack of evidence to support their use, modern dressings remain a part of the standard of care. Decisions regarding their use should be based on local cost of the dressings and the physician's clinical experience.
- Trials have shown that endovenous ablation of superficial veins lowers the probability of long-term recurrent venous ulcers.[1]
- Trials involving the use of weekly, low-dose, high-frequency ultrasound for hard-to-heal venous leg ulcers do not support adding therapeutic ultrasound to standard care for venous leg ulcers.

DISPOSITION

The overall prognosis for this condition is poor; the healing rate depends on the initial size of the ulcer. Although 65% to 70% of venous ulcers are healed within 6 mo, the 5-yr recurrence rate of healed venous ulcers can be as high as 40%. Maintenance of lifelong compression therapy is recommended.

REFERRAL

All patients should be evaluated weekly during the first month of therapy. Nonhealing ulcers with little to no improvement should also be referred to a wound care clinic.

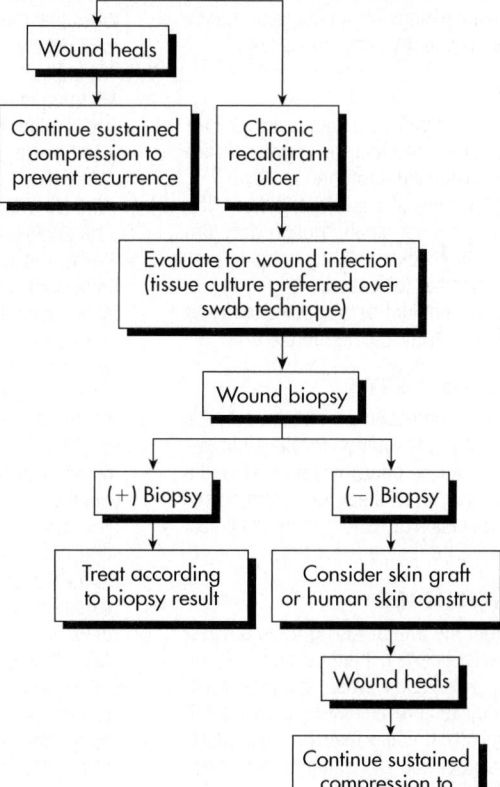

REFERENCE

Available at eBooks.Health.Elsevier.com.

AUTHOR: **FRANK G. FORT, MD, FACS, RPHS**

FIG. 3 Algorithm for the care of a patient with a venous leg ulcer. *ABI,* Ankle brachial index; *ASA,* acetylsalicylic acid.

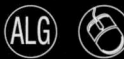

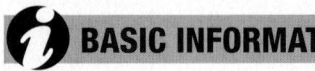 **BASIC INFORMATION**

DEFINITION

Vertebral compression fractures (VCFs) are defined as fractures of spinal vertebrae in which a bony surface is driven toward another bony surface. These fractures are classified as radiographic reductions in vertebral body height of more than 15%.

SYNONYMS

Thoracolumbar vertebral compression fractures
Osteoporotic fractures
VCF

ICD-10CM CODES

M80.0	Post-menopausal osteoporosis with pathologic fracture
M80.4	Drug-induced osteoporosis with pathological fracture
M80.5	Idiopathic osteoporosis with pathological fracture
M80.8	Other osteoporosis with pathological fracture
M80.9	Unspecified osteoporosis with pathological fracture
S32.009A	Unspecified fracture of unspecified lumbar vertebra, initial encounter for closed fracture
S22.009A	Unspecified fracture of unspecified thoracic vertebra, initial encounter for closed fracture

EPIDEMIOLOGY & DEMOGRAPHICS

Approximately 700,000 VCFs occur in the United States each yr, and they affect up to 25% of postmenopausal women. They are the most common complication of osteoporosis. The prevalence increases with age, reaching a peak of 40% to 50% among women aged >80 yr. Compression fractures are also a major concern among men, although their rates of VCF are lower.

RISK FACTORS:
- Modifiable: Tobacco or alcohol use, osteoporosis, estrogen deficiency (i.e., early menopause, bilateral oophorectomy, premenopausal amenorrhea for >1 yr), frailty, impaired vision, abusive situations, inadequate physical activity, low body mass index, and deficiency of vitamin D or calcium.
- Nonmodifiable: Advanced age, female gender, dementia, Caucasian descent, history of fractures in adulthood and among first-degree relatives, and falls.

PHYSICAL FINDINGS & CLINICAL PRESENTATION

- Asymptomatic: Most VCFs are asymptomatic, except for height loss or kyphosis (i.e., dowager's hump [Fig. E1]), which is often a sign of multiple VCFs, and height loss of >6 cm has a sensitivity/specificity of 94% and 30%, respectively, for VCF.
- Symptomatic: When symptomatic, VCFs usually present as acute back pain after activity (e.g., bending, lifting) or coughing; neck strain and radicular rib pain may also be present.

ETIOLOGY

- VCFs take place when the combination of bending and the axial load on the spine exceed the strength of the vertebral body.
- The primary etiology of VCF is osteoporosis, though a pathologic fracture from an underlying malignancy, typically metastatic disease, must be ruled out.

Dx **DIAGNOSIS**

DIFFERENTIAL DIAGNOSIS

- Osteoporosis
- Malignancy, most often metastases
- Hyperparathyroidism
- Osteomalacia
- Granulomatous diseases (e.g., tuberculosis)
- Hematologic/oncologic diseases (e.g., multiple myeloma, primary bone malignancy)

WORKUP

- Only one third of VCFs are diagnosed. Guidelines for patient selection for vertebral fractural assessment are described in Box E1.
- VCFs can be clinically suspected from the history and physical alone, though they are often diagnosed incidentally by imaging performed for another indication.
- There may or may not be a specific injury or a remembered event that led to the VCF.

LABORATORY TESTS

Tests to rule out infection or cancer may be helpful, such as a CBC, an erythrocyte sedimentation rate, an alkaline phosphatase level, and a C-reactive protein level; these tests can be reserved for individuals for whom there is clinical suspicion.

IMAGING STUDIES

- Plain frontal and lateral radiographs (x-rays) are the initial imaging method and may be sufficient, particularly when no neurologic abnormalities are present. MRI and computed tomography (CT) scans may be uncomfortable or painful for the patient, especially during the acute phase.
- Although CT scans are not routinely necessary for the diagnosis, they can be helpful for visualizing fractures that are not seen on plain films, for evaluating the integrity of the posterior vertebral wall, for ruling out other causes of back pain, for detecting spinal canal narrowing, and for assessing instability.
- MRI may be useful when spinal cord compression is suspected, if neurologic symptoms are present, or to distinguish malignancy from osteoporosis (e.g., in patients <55 yr with VCF after minimal or no trauma).
- Bone density studies may be helpful to determine the severity of osteoporosis, which is a key risk factor for future fractures.

Rx **TREATMENT (FIG. 2)**

NONPHARMACOLOGIC THERAPY

- Physical therapy
- External back braces: Frequently recommended to relieve pain and improve mobility; however, controlled trials have not shown any effect in patients with vertebral compression fractures
- Exercise programs: Getting active as soon as possible is extremely important for both short- and long-term recovery

ACUTE GENERAL Rx

- Analgesics are first line for pain control, including acetaminophen and opioids (oral or parenteral), and pain can be expected to diminish over 4 to 6 wk.
- NSAIDs are helpful but must be used with caution among elderly patients or when contraindicated.
- Muscle relaxants should be used judiciously because they have significant side effects, particularly in the elderly.
- Intranasal calcitonin (200 units once daily, alternating nostrils) has been shown in some small trials to hasten relief from pain when used as an adjunct to oral analgesics, and a 2- to 4-wk course may be useful for patients who do not achieve adequate control with oral analgesics alone.
- Early mobilization with physical therapy is important for recovery and prevention of subsequent fractures.
- The efficacy of vertebroplasty vs. kyphoplasty vs. conservative treatment remains controversial.
- Percutaneous vertebroplasty (Fig. E3) involves the injection of acrylic bone cement into the affected vertebral body in an effort to stabilize the fracture and reduce pain, whereas in kyphoplasty, a high-pressure inflatable bone tamp or balloon is expanded within the body of the affected vertebra to restore prefracture vertebral height before the injection of bone cement. These two procedures were thought to be helpful in patients who did not respond to conservative therapy; however, further studies showed them to be no more effective than sham procedures. Nonetheless, Klazen et al (2010)[1] demonstrated in an open-label prospective randomized trial that for the subgroup of patients with acute osteoporotic VCFs and persistent pain, percutaneous vertebroplasty may provide immediate pain relief, sustained for at least a yr, which may be significantly greater than that achieved with conservative treatment. Zampini (2010)[2] showed in a nonrandomized cohort study that elderly patients who underwent kyphoplasty were more likely to be discharged home. Analysis of Medicare claims of patients with VCF treated with kyphoplasty or vertebroplasty compared with medical management revealed no difference in mortality or major medical outcomes but decreased health care utilization in the conservatively managed

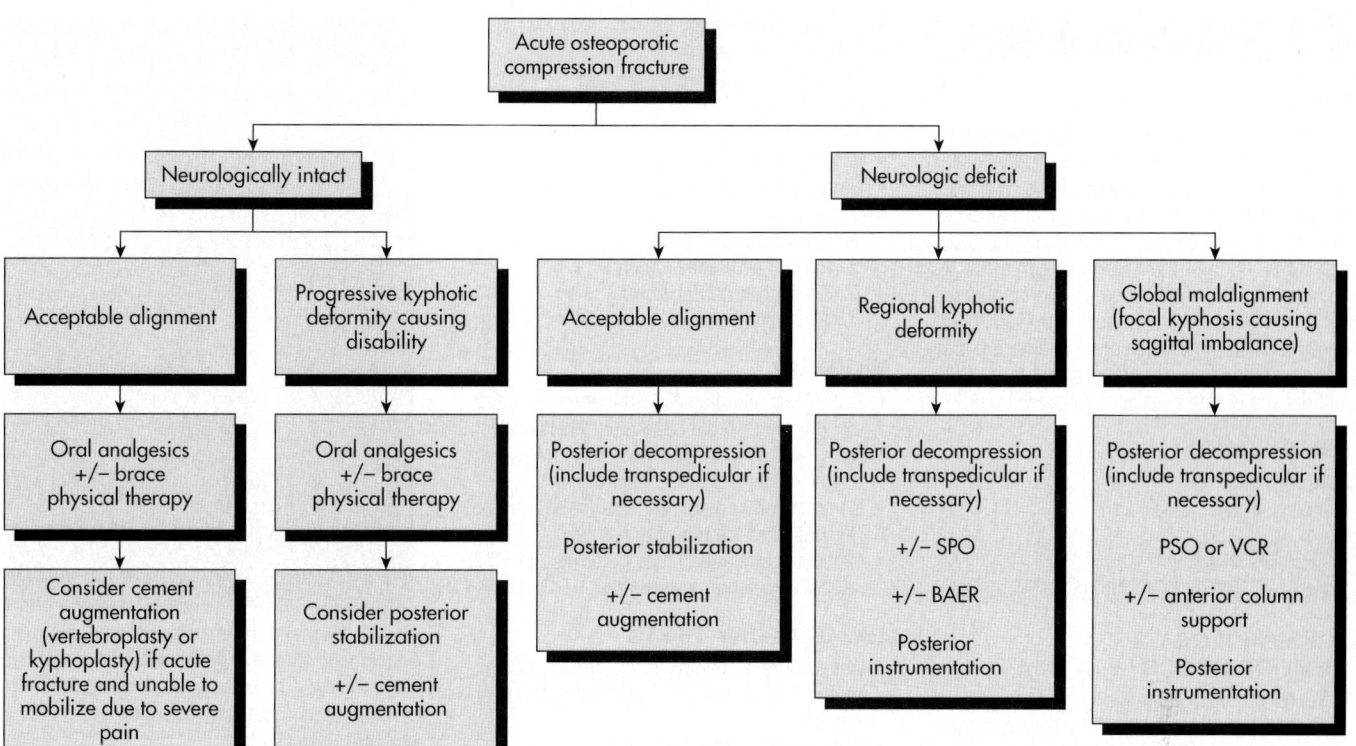

FIG. 2 A generalized treatment algorithm for osteoporotic spine fractures. *BAER,* Balloon-assisted endplate reduction; *PSO,* pedicle subtraction osteotomy; *SPO,* Smith–Petersen osteotomy; *VCR,* vertebral column resection. (From Browner BD et al: *Skeletal trauma: basic science, management, and reconstruction,* ed 6, Philadelphia, 2020, Elsevier.)

group. These procedures are still in their infancy, and more answers should be forthcoming as to their efficacy, as well as questions regarding the amount of time that conservative therapy alone should be pursued and which procedure, if any, should be advised. Most current guidelines recommend 4 to 6 wk of medical therapy before pursuing surgical intervention in neurologically intact VCF.

CHRONIC Rx
Osteoporosis should be treated with the reduction of risk factors (e.g., smoking, alcohol), diet, exercise, calcium and vitamin D supplements, and with medications used to treat osteoporosis (e.g., bisphosphonates).

REFERRAL
Referral is indicated for neurologic abnormalities, unremitting pain, instability, continued disability, or when the investigation of the cause of the fracture reveals serious underlying pathology.

ⓘ PEARLS & CONSIDERATIONS

Prevention of osteoporosis and conservative therapy remain the mainstay of treatment.

COMMENTS
- VCFs should be suspected in anyone aged >50 yr with the acute onset of low back pain. There are many opportunities for diagnosis and treatment that are easy to miss, especially for males.
- Solitary vertebral fractures higher than T7 are unusual and should raise suspicion for other pathologic causes.
- Diagnosing and treating osteoporosis reduce the incidence of VCFs.
- Getting people with VCF physically active as soon as possible will be efficacious both acutely and in the long term.
- In general, VCF will be best managed through a partnership of the patient, the primary care physician, an orthopedist, a physical therapist, a dietitian, and a social worker.
- Concerns that vertebroplasty and kyphoplasty increased risk for a new "secondary" fracture in adjacent vertebrae have not been confirmed in retrospective studies.[3]

PREVENTION
Reducing the effects of modifiable risk factors is key.

REFERENCES
Available at eBooks.Health.Elsevier.com.

AUTHOR: **FRED F. FERRI, MD**

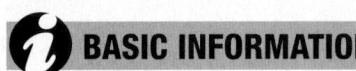 **BASIC INFORMATION**

DEFINITION

Vestibular schwannoma is a benign proliferation of the Schwann cells that cover the vestibular branch of the eighth cranial nerve (CN VIII). Symptoms are commonly a result of compression of the acoustic branch of CN VIII, the facial nerve (CN VII), and the trigeminal nerve (CN V). The glossopharyngeal nerve (CN IX) and vagus nerve (CN X) are less commonly involved. In extreme cases, compression of the brain stem may lead to obstruction of cerebrospinal fluid (CSF) outflow and elevated intracranial pressure (ICP).[1]

SYNONYMS

Acoustic neuroma
Acoustic schwannoma

ICD-10CM CODE
D33.3   Benign neoplasm of cranial nerves

EPIDEMIOLOGY & DEMOGRAPHICS

- Vestibular schwannomas account for 8% of all intracranial tumors and are the most common neoplasm of the cerebellopontine angle in adults.[2]
- Overall incidence is approximately 1 in 100,000 person-yr in the U.S., with a higher incidence in patients with neurofibromatosis type 2 (NF2). About 3000 new cases of acoustic neuroma are diagnosed each yr. The tumor most commonly presents in the fifth and sixth decades.[3]

PHYSICAL FINDINGS & CLINICAL PRESENTATION

- Most frequently unilateral hearing loss and/or tinnitus. Also balance problems, vertigo, facial pain (trigeminal neuralgia) and weakness, difficulty swallowing, fullness or pain of the involved ear. Headache may occur.[4]
- With elevated ICP, patients may also have vomiting, fever, and visual changes.
- Hearing loss is the most common presenting complaint and is usually high frequency.

ETIOLOGY

The etiology is incompletely understood, but long-term exposure to acoustic trauma has been implicated.[5] Bilateral acoustic neuromas may be inherited in an autosomal-dominant manner as part of NF2. This disease is associated with a defect on chromosome 22q1.[6] Childhood exposure to low-dose radiation for benign head and neck conditions may increase risk for acoustic neuromas.[7] There is inconclusive evidence to link chronic exposure to radiofrequency radiation from cellular telephone use and the risk for developing brain tumors.[8]

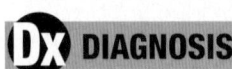 **DIAGNOSIS**

DIFFERENTIAL DIAGNOSIS

- Benign positional vertigo
- Ménière disease

- Trigeminal neuralgia
- Cerebellar disease
- Normal-pressure hydrocephalus
- Presbycusis
- Glomus tumors
- Vertebrobasilar insufficiency
- Ototoxicity from medications
- Other tumors:
  1. Meningioma, glioma
  2. Facial nerve schwannoma
  3. Cavernous hemangioma
  4. Metastatic tumors

WORKUP

- A detailed neurologic examination with special attention to the cranial nerves is crucial.
- Rinne and Weber tests help determine conductive or sensorineural hearing loss.
- Common office balance tests (i.e., Romberg, Dix-Hallpike) are typically normal.
- Otoscopic evaluation may help rule out other causes of hearing loss.[9,10]

LABORATORY TESTS

- Audiometry is useful, often showing asymmetric, sensorineural, high-frequency hearing loss.
- CSF protein may be elevated.

IMAGING STUDIES

- MRI with gadolinium (Fig. 1, Fig. 2, and Fig. 3) is the preferred test. It can detect tumors as small as 2 mm in diameter.[9]
- High-resolution computed tomography scan with and without contrast can detect tumors 1 cm in diameter or larger.
- Treatment decisions should be based on the size of the tumor, rate of growth (older patients tend to have slower-growing tumors), degree of neurologic deficit, desire to preserve hearing, life expectancy, age of the patient, and surgical risk. A combination of treatments can also be used.[10]

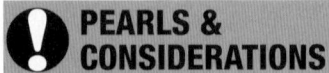 **TREATMENT**

NONPHARMACOLOGIC THERAPY

- Surgery is the definitive treatment. Choice of approach (middle cranial fossa, translabyrinthine, or retromastoid suboccipital) may vary depending on the size of the tumor, amount of residual hearing desired, and degree of surgical risk that can be tolerated. Partial resection is sometimes undertaken to minimize the risk of injury to nearby structures. Intraoperative facial nerve monitoring is recommended.[10]
- Radiation therapy (stereotactic radiotherapy, stereotactic radiosurgery, or proton beam radiotherapy) is useful for tumors <3 cm in diameter or for those in whom surgery is not an option. Radiotherapy after partial resection has also been used to minimize complications.[11,12]
- Age alone is not a contraindication to surgery.

GENERAL Rx

- Bevacizumab, an antivascular endothelial growth factor monoclonal antibody, has been shown to improve hearing and reduce the

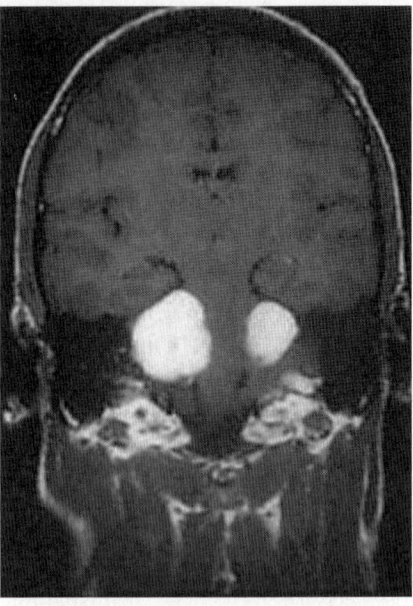

FIG. 1 Magnetic resonance imaging with enhancement shows bilateral acoustic neuromas. Coronal view. (From Kanski JJ, Bowling B: *Clinical ophthalmology, a systematic approach*, ed 7, Philadelphia, 2011, Saunders.)

volume of growing acoustic neuromas in some neurofibromatosis type 2 patients.[9]
- New therapeutic strategies being investigated include gene therapy and molecular targeted therapy.[13]
- Observation with MRI every 6 to 12 mo may be appropriate for frail patients with small tumors, but risk of unrecoverable hearing loss may increase if surgery is delayed. Also, progressive hearing loss may occur despite absence of growth on subsequent imaging.[9,10]

DISPOSITION

Hearing can be preserved at near-preoperative levels in more than two thirds of patients with small- to medium-sized tumors. Occurrence of secondary radiation-related tumors following radiosurgery is rare. There are no standard posttreatment follow-up recommendations. Therefore an individualized approach to follow-up imaging and audiometry is recommended.[3,9,10]

REFERRAL

Prompt referral to an otolaryngologist or neurosurgeon who is facile with all three surgical approaches is recommended.

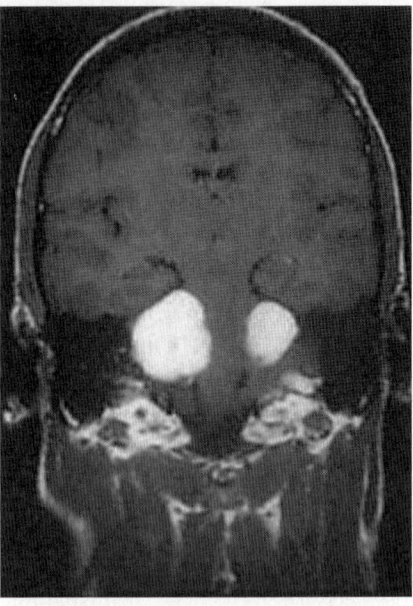 **PEARLS & CONSIDERATIONS**

COMMENTS

- Presents most commonly as unilateral, sensorineural hearing loss.
- Treatment outcomes are excellent, with surgical cure rates greater than 95%.
- Of those who are managed with observation only, approximately half have continued enlargement, and approximately one fifth eventually have a surgical intervention.

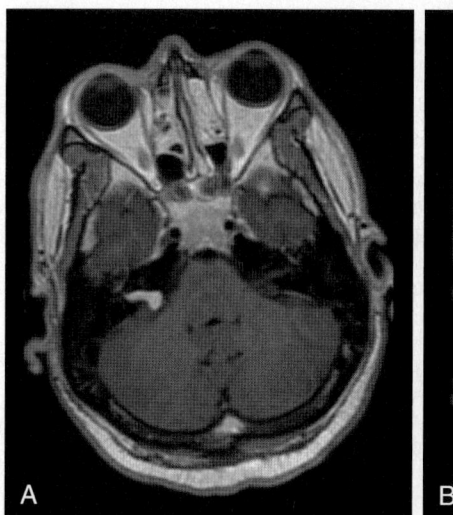
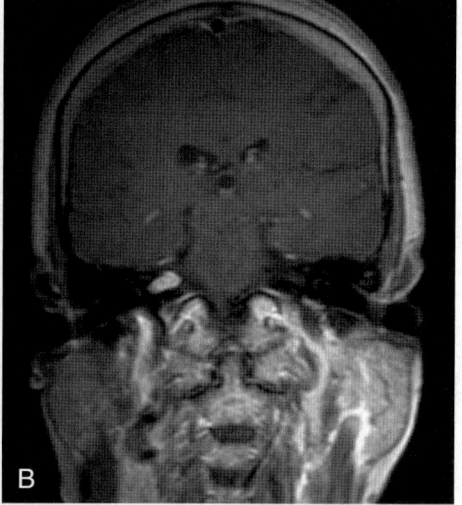

FIG. 2 T1-weighted postgadolinium contrast magnetic resonance image demonstrating a unilateral right enhancing mass within the internal auditory canal and cerebellopontine angle consistent on axial **(A)** and coronal **(B)** images consistent with a vestibular schwannoma. (From Flint PW et al: *Cummings otolaryngology, head and neck surgery,* ed 7, Philadelphia, 2021, Elsevier.)

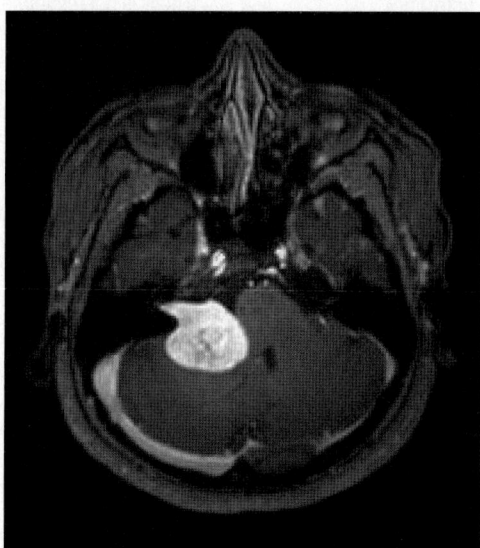

FIG. 3 A large acoustic neuroma, originating from the right cerebellopontine angle, compresses the pons and shifts the fourth ventricle. Patients with neurofibromatosis type 2, because they tend to develop bilateral acoustic neuromas, routinely undergo MRI with views of the internal auditory canals. (From Kaufman DM et al: *Kaufman's clinical neurology for psychiatrists, clinical atlas*, ed 9, Philadelphia, 2023, Elsevier.)

PATIENT & FAMILY EDUCATION
Acoustic Neuroma Association: www.anausa.org/

REFERENCES
Available at eBooks.Health.Elsevier.com.

RELATED CONTENT
Acoustic Neuroma (Patient Information)
Tinnitus (Related Key Topic)

AUTHOR: **COURTNEY CLARK BILODEAU, MD, FACP**

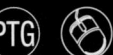

 BASIC INFORMATION

- Vitamin D is a hormone and a steroid and, by definition, not a vitamin. There are two forms of vitamin D: Vitamin D_2 and vitamin D_3.
- Vitamin D_2 (ergocalciferol) is mainly found in some plant foods.
- Vitamin D_3 (cholecalciferol) is produced in skin exposed to ultraviolet (UV) B radiation from sunlight (Fig. E1).
- The major functions of vitamin D include:
  1. Increasing calcium, magnesium, and phosphorus absorption from the small intestines
  2. Promoting the maturation of osteoclast to resorb calcium from bones

DEFINITION

Vitamin D deficiency is characterized by hypocalcemia and/or hypophosphatemia leading to impaired bone mineralization. It is classified as a serum 25-hydroxyvitamin D (25[OH]D) level of <20 ng/ml (50 nmol/L). This standard definition of vitamin D deficiency has been recently challenged, and some endocrinologists recommend a cutoff of 12 mg/ml for vitamin D deficiency. Vitamin D insufficiency is defined as a 25(OH)D between 12 and 20 ng/ml.

The consequences of vitamin D deficiency include:
- Bone disease (rickets, osteoporosis, low bone mass)
- May impair reproductive success
- Decrease the ability to combat infection (especially tuberculosis, influenza, viral infection)
- May induce or worsen autoimmune disorders
- May increase the incidence of death due to heart disease, inflammatory bowel disease, fracture, and cancer of the breast, colon, and prostate
- Subclinical vitamin D deficiency may occur in developed countries and be associated with increased fall risk and osteoporosis

SYNONYMS

The sunshine vitamin
The antirachitic factor
Cholecalciferol

ICD-10CM CODE
E55.9   Vitamin D deficiency, unspecified

EPIDEMIOLOGY & DEMOGRAPHICS

INCIDENCE:
- Vitamin D insufficiency is very high among older adults and hospitalized and institutionalized people.
- Worldwide deficiency and insufficiency affect about 1 billion people.
- Children and young adults: 40% to 50% of preadolescent Caucasian girls, and Hispanic and African American adolescents, are vitamin D deficient.

PREVALENCE: 41.6% of adults (at least 20 yr old) have 25(OH)D levels <20 ng/dl.

PREDOMINANT SEX & AGE:
- Decreased skin production of vitamin D with age
- Increased prevalence among darker-skinned individuals

PEAK INCIDENCE:
- In the U.S., 40% to 100% of the elderly are vitamin D deficient.
- Sixty percent of nursing home residents may be vitamin D deficient.

RISK FACTORS:
- Age (due to decreased ability to produce D_3)
- Sunshine-deficient areas (geographic location, living in higher latitudes)
- Dark-skinned individuals (melanin competes with vitamin D_3 precursors for UV photons and thus decreases pre-D_3 formation)
- Obese individuals
- Institutionalized individuals
- Pregnant and lactating women
- Use of sunscreen (sun radiation that causes skin cancer also produces pre-vitamin D_3 in skin)
- Patients on certain medications that antagonize vitamin D action (phenobarbital, phenytoin)
- Intestinal resection
- Severe chronic liver diseases (such as cirrhosis)
- Kidney disease (e.g., nephritic syndrome)
- Sarcoidosis and lymphomas (increased catabolism of 25[OH]D to 1,25[OH]2D)
- Intestinal malabsorption disease (caused by celiac sprue, cystic fibrosis, Whipple disease)

PHYSICAL FINDINGS & CLINICAL PRESENTATION

- Clinical presentation of vitamin D deficiency is dependent on the duration and severity of deficiency
- Most patients with mild to moderate vitamin D deficiency are asymptomatic
- Severe deficiency may lead to rickets (in children), osteomalacia (in adults), bone demineralization, hypokalemia, and phosphaturia
- Mild deficiency can lead to hypocalcemia and hyperparathyroidism
- Rickets: Seen in children; caused by defective mineralization in the skeleton (Fig. E2)
  1. Bowing of the legs
  2. Leg bone pain
  3. Delayed growth
  4. Seizure due to hypocalcemia
- Osteomalacia: Seen in adults with severe and prolonged vitamin D deficiency
  1. Periosteal bone pain (best detected by putting firm pressure on tibia or sternal bones)
  2. Proximal muscle weakness
  3. Chronic muscle aches/pain
- Fracture with very minimal trauma (brittle and easily broken bones)
- Severe hypocalcemia: Especially in late vitamin D deficiency leading to seizure tetany
- Hypophosphatemia
- Paresthesia
- Tetany
- Muscle cramps

ETIOLOGY

- Inadequate exposure to sunlight, such as:
  1. During winter
  2. In nursing home and health care institution residents
  3. With excessive use of sunscreen
- Medications: Individuals on certain medications, such as phenobarbital, phenytoin, and rifampin (antagonize vitamin D action/increase vitamin D catabolism)
- Diseases and disease states:
  1. Diseases causing vitamin D malabsorption:
     a. Cystic fibrosis
     b. Whipple disease
     c. Celiac sprue
  2. Diseases increasing vitamin D catabolism:
     a. Lymphoma
     b. Sarcoidosis
  3. Intestinal resection
  4. Decreased 25(OH)D production:
     a. Kidney disease
     b. Liver cirrhosis

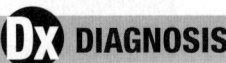 **DIAGNOSIS**

DIFFERENTIAL DIAGNOSIS
- Arthritis
- Fibromyalgia

WORKUP
- Population-wide screening for vitamin D deficiency is not recommended because evidence to support this practice is lacking. Appropriate to screen high-risk individuals.
- Screening is needed for individuals at risk (osteoporosis, history of falls, obese persons, pregnant and lactating women, diseases causing vitamin D malabsorption, African Americans). Workup involves blood and urine tests as well as radiography, as outlined in the next section.

LABORATORY TESTS (TABLE 1)
- Serum 25(OH)D: This is the best test to determine vitamin D status.
- Parathyroid hormone (PTH): Increased levels in vitamin D insufficiency. It is a marker of vitamin D insufficiency.
- Increased (serum or bone) alkaline phosphatase.
- Decreased 24-h urine calcium (patient should not be on a thiazide).
- In patients at risk for osteomalacia [s-25(OH)D is less than 10 ng/ml], check calcium, Ph, alkaline phosphatase, PTH, basic metabolic panel, and tissue transglutaminase antibodies.

IMAGING STUDIES
- Radiographs may show:
  1. Pseudofractures of the pelvis, femur, metatarsals
  2. Nontraumatic fractures
- Bone density:
  1. Decreased bone mineral density (osteopenia or osteoporosis). Note that bone mineral density is not routinely performed in patients whose only risk factor is decreased Vitamin D levels.

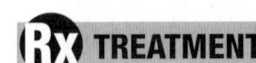 **TREATMENT**

NONPHARMACOLOGIC THERAPY
- Natural sources of vitamin D. These include:
  1. Exposure to sunlight. A mild sunburn is equivalent to consuming 10,000 to 25,000 IU of dietary vitamin D.

TABLE 1 Laboratory Tests

	SERUM			URINE
	Calcium	Phosphorus	Alkaline Phosphatase	Calcium
Osteoporosis	N	N	N	N
Hyperparathyroidism				
Primary	↑		N or ↑	N or ↑
Secondary	N or ↑	↑	↑	↓
Tertiary	↑	N or ↓	N or ↑	N or ↑
Hypoparathyroidism	↓	↑	N	↓
Pseudohypoparathyroidism	↓	↑	N	↓
Rickets/osteomalacia				
Vit D deficient	↓	↓	↑	
Vit D refractory	N	↓	↑	↓
Hypophosphatasia	N or ↑	N	↓	N or ↑

Vit, Vitamin.
From Grant LA: *Grainger & Allison's diagnostic radiology essentials,* ed 2, Philadelphia, 2019, Elsevier.

2. Dietary sources are not enough to meet daily requirements. Oily fish such as salmon, cod, and mackerel are rich sources of vitamin D_3.
- Foods fortified with vitamin D
  1. Mainly fortified dairy products
  2. Fortified orange juice

ACUTE GENERAL Rx
- Treating deficiency (general population): Cholecalciferol (vitamin D_3), when available, is preferred for vitamin D supplementation
  1. 50,000 IU (1250 mg) of vitamin D every wk for 8 wk, *or*
  2. 5000 IU (125 mg) daily to achieve a serum level of 25(OH)D of at least 30 ng/ml
- Maintenance measures after treatment (general population): 1500 to 2000 IU daily
- Treating deficiency (obese patients, patients with malabsorption syndromes, or those taking certain medications, as indicated earlier)
  1. 10,000 IU daily maintenance dose is recommended once s-25(OH)D level exceeds 30 ng/ml.
  2. After treating deficiency, recheck 25(OH)D in 12 to 16 wk.
  3. Maintenance measures after treatment (obese patients, patients with malabsorption syndromes, or those taking certain medications, as indicated earlier): 3000 to 6000 IU daily.
  4. If deficiency persists after several attempts at treatment, try UV B light therapy.

REFERRAL
Referral to an endocrinologist is recommended if there is no response to treatment.

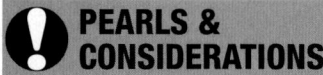

PEARLS & CONSIDERATIONS

- In the U.S., vitamin D supplements are available by prescription as vitamin D_2 (ergocalciferol) or over the counter as vitamin D_3 (cholecalciferol, usually in 400- to 1000-IU doses). Both vitamin D_2 and vitamin D_3 are acceptable as supplements. On average, oral vitamin D_3 raises blood levels more than does vitamin D_2.
- Upper limit of maintenance tolerability in healthy adults is 4000 IU a day. More than 4000 IU of vitamin D daily in nondeficient individuals increases the risk of harm. High-level supplements (>10,000 IU daily) are associated with kidney and tissue damage.
- Vitamin D supplementation is often recommended for fall prevention; however, trials have revealed that Vitamin D supplementation at doses of 1000 IU daily or higher did not prevent falls in older adults, and fall risk increased with higher doses.[1] A recent study[2] showed that vitamin D supplementation did not result in a significant lower risk of fractures.
- Prescribing more than the recommended daily amount to improve quality of life or prevent cardiovascular disease or death is not advised.
- Trials have shown that low vitamin D levels are associated with depressive symptoms, especially in persons with a history of depression. These findings suggest that measuring vitamin D levels may be useful in patients with a history of depression.
- Recent data suggest that vitamin D deficiency is associated with the risk of developing certain cancers (including breast, colon, and prostate).
- A randomized trial has shown that 5 yr of routing vitamin D supplementation does not lower 6 yr mortality in older adults.[3]
- Vitamin D deficiency is associated with some autoimmune diseases (types 1 and 2 diabetes, metabolic syndrome, multiple sclerosis). Daily vitamin D supplementation was found to be beneficial in preventing some new autoimmune diseases in older adults.[4]
- Serum vitamin D concentrations are affected by multiple variables (Tables E2 and E3).

Excessive supplementation can lead to vitamin D toxicity (Box E1).

PREVENTION
- Food fortification with vitamin D_2 or vitamin D_3
- Adequate sun exposure, for example, exposure in the middle of the day (between 10:00 A.M. and 3:00 P.M.)
- Use vitamin D_3 for supplementation when available
- Vitamin D supplementation (per the Endocrine Society):
  1. Infants (age range 1 to 12 mo) require at least 400 IU/day of vitamin D
  2. Children (age range 1 to 18 yr) require 600 IU/day of vitamin D
  3. Adult supplementation (adults 19 to 70 yr): 600 IU of vitamin D daily
  4. Adult supplementation (persons ≥70 yr): 800 IU of vitamin D daily
  5. Exceptions: Pregnant or lactating women, obese persons, and patients on antiseizure medications, steroids, antifungals, and AIDS medications should be given 2× to 3× more vitamin D
  6. To reduce the risk of fracture and falls, the American Geriatric Society recommends a daily intake of at least 1000 IU and the National Osteoporosis Foundation 800 to 1000 IU in adults 65 yr or older

SCREENING
Routine screening for low-risk adults is not recommended. Screening is recommended only for individuals at high risk for vitamin D deficiency such as Blacks and Hispanics, obese individuals (body mass index >30 kg/m²), patients with osteoporosis, the elderly, and patients with certain chronic diseases (see "Risk Factors"). According to the U.S. Preventive Services Task Force, current evidence is insufficient to assess the balance of benefits and harms of screening for vitamin D deficiency in asymptomatic adults.

REFERENCES
Available at eBooks.Health.Elsevier.com.

RELATED CONTENT
Vitamin D Deficiency (Patient Information)
Osteomalacia and Rickets (Related Key Topic)
Vitamin Deficiency (Related Key Topic)

AUTHOR: **FRED F. FERRI, MD**

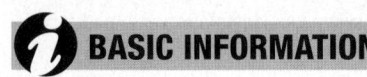 **BASIC INFORMATION**

DEFINITION

Vitamins are organic compounds that cannot be synthesized by humans but are required as nutrients in minute amounts for normal metabolism. Vitamins have several different functions: They may regulate cell growth and differentiation, as catalysts, as antioxidants, and as coenzymes. Vitamins are classified as either fat soluble (vitamins A, D, E, K) or water soluble (B group of vitamins and C). Deficiency of most vitamins is rare in Western countries. Certain groups may be prone to vitamin deficiency, and these are discussed here. Vitamin D deficiency is discussed in a separate topic.

SYNONYMS

Hypovitaminosis
Vitamin A: Retinol
Vitamin E: Alpha tocopherol
Vitamin K: Phytonadione or menadiol
Vitamin B_1: Thiamine
Vitamin B_2: Riboflavin
Niacin: Vitamin B_3; nicotinic acid
Vitamin B_5: Pantothenic acid
Vitamin B_6: Pyridoxine; pyridoxal phosphate
Folic acid: Vitamin B_9; folate
Vitamin B_{12}: Cyanocobalamin
Vitamin C: Ascorbic acid

ICD-10CM CODES
E50	Vitamin A deficiency
E51	Thiamine deficiency
E53	Deficiency of other B group vitamins
E55	Vitamin D deficiency
E56	Other vitamin deficiencies
E56.0	Deficiency of vitamin E
E56.1	Deficiency of vitamin K
E53.0	Riboflavin deficiency
E52	Niacin deficiency [pellagra]
E53.1	Pyridoxine deficiency
E53.8	Deficiency of other specified B group vitamins
E54	Ascorbic acid deficiency

EPIDEMIOLOGY & DEMOGRAPHICS

Deficiency can occur in all age groups but is most common in the elderly.
- Vitamin A deficiency: Affects 250 million preschool children worldwide.
- Vitamin E deficiency: Deficiency is rare in humans. Usually occurs in individuals with severe protein-energy malnutrition.
- Vitamin K deficiency: Varies by geographic regions; no race predilection; affects both sexes equally. Encountered often in infants. In normal healthy adults, 8% to 31% have vitamin K deficiency, but it rarely leads to significant bleeding.
- Vitamin B_1 (thiamine) deficiency: Incidence is unknown; no sex, race, or age predilection. Deficiency is usually due to inadequate intake, especially if consuming diet made up of polished rice and grains.
- Vitamin B_2 (riboflavin): More common than previously appreciated. Deficiency is referred to as ariboflavinosis.
- Vitamin B_5 (pantothenic acid) deficiency: Rare, as it is present in all foods.
- Vitamin B_{12} (cobalamin) deficiency: Relatively common. Of patients with anemia, about 1%

to 2% is due to B_{12} deficiency. Among patients with macrocytosis (mean corpuscular volume [MCV] >100) 18% to 20% is due to B_{12} deficiency. Occurs in all age groups but more common in the elderly. B_{12} deficiency due to pernicious anemia is common in Northern Europe.
- Vitamin B_9 (folic acid) deficiency: Mandatory fortification started in 1998. Prevalence before fortification 16% and after 0.5%. Neural tube defect associated with low maternal folate status during pregnancy. Pregnant women and the elderly are at greatest risk of folic acid deficiency.
- Vitamin C (ascorbic acid) deficiency: Smokers and low-income persons are at increased risk. Vitamin C deficiency is associated with access to food and/or socioeconomic status. Prevalence varies worldwide, but the rate is about 7.1% in the U.S.

Fig. 1 shows environmental and nutritional factors in disease.

PHYSICAL FINDINGS & CLINICAL PRESENTATION

- Vitamin A: Xerophthalmia, xerosis of the cornea, keratomalacia, Bitot spots (abnormal squamous cell proliferation and keratinization of the conjunctiva), nyctalopia (poor adaptation to darkness)/night blindness, poor bone growth, dry skin and hair, follicular hyperkeratosis (caused by blockage of hair follicles by keratin), pruritus, broken fingernails
- Vitamin K: Clinical manifestation usually occurs if hypoprothrombinemia is present. Major symptom is bleeding to minor trauma. Also can show easy bruisability, epistaxis, hematoma, gum bleeding, melena, hematuria, or splinter hemorrhage

Vitamin	Function	Consequences of deficiency
A	Retinal function, epithelial growth control	Night blindness, keratomalacia, xerophthalmia
B_1 (thiamine)	Coenzyme	Beriberi, Wernicke's encephalopathy
B_2 (riboflavin)	Coenzyme	Dermatitis, glossitis, keratitis, neuropathy, confusion
B_6 (pyridoxine)	Coenzyme	Neuropathy
B_{12} (cobalamin)	Nucleic acid synthesis	Megaloblastic anemia Subacute combined degeneration of spinal cord
Niacin	Coenzyme NAD, NADP	Pellagra (diarrhea, dermatitis, and dementia)
Folate	Coenzyme in nucleic acid synthesis	Megaloblastic anemia, villous atrophy of gut
Vitamin C	Cofactor in hydroxylation	Scurvy
Vitamin D	Calcium and phosphate absorption	Rickets (childhood) Osteomalacia (adults)
Vitamin E	Antioxidant	Spinocerebellar degeneration
Vitamin K	Cofactor for coagulation factor synthesis	Bleeding due to coagulation defects

FIG. 1 Environmental and nutritional factors in disease. (From Stevens A: *Core pathology,* St Louis, 2009, Elsevier.)

- Vitamin E: Neuromuscular disorders (ataxia; hyporeflexia, peripheral neuropathy); bone weakness, hemolysis
- Vitamin B_1 (thiamine): Beriberi, which has two subtypes (infantile and adult). Adult type is described below:
  1. Dry beriberi (affecting the nervous system): Symmetrical peripheral neuropathy (with sensory and motor impairments), Wernicke encephalopathy (nystagmus, ataxia, ophthalmoplegia, and confusion), Korsakoff syndrome (impaired short-term memory loss and confabulation but normal cognition)
  2. Wet beriberi (affecting the cardiovascular system): Cardiomegaly, cardiomyopathy, heart failure, tachycardia, hypotension, chest pain, peripheral edema
  3. Gastrointestinal (GI): Anorexia; constipation
- Vitamin B_2 (riboflavin):
  1. Cheilosis (chapping and fissure of the lip)
  2. Glossitis (sore red tongue)
  3. Oily, scaly rashes on nasolabial folds, eyelids, scrotum, labia majora
  4. Red itchy eyes
  5. Normocytic or normochromic anemia
  6. Peripheral neuropathy
- Vitamin B_3 (niacin):
  1. Pellagra (4 *D*s—diarrhea, dermatitis, dementia, and ultimately death)
  2. Hyperpigmentation of sun-exposed skin
  3. "Raw beef" swollen and painful tongue
  4. Deficiency can be seen in prolonged use of isoniazid, in carcinoid syndrome, and in Hartnup syndrome
- Vitamin B_5 (pantothenic acid):
  1. Deficiency is rare
  2. Deficiency leads to "burning feet syndrome" (distal paresthesia and dysesthesia)
  3. Anemia
  4. GI symptoms
- Vitamin B_6 (pyridoxine): Rare to see overt deficiency
  1. Mild deficiency: Glossitis, cheilosis, impaired proprioception; sensory ataxia, confusion, depression
  2. Severe deficiency: Seborrheic dermatitis, seizure, microcytic
- Vitamin B_{12} (cyanocobalamin):
  1. Megaloblastic anemia (pernicious anemia)
  2. Neurologic symptoms including peripheral neuropathy, ataxia (shuffling gait), paresthesia; subacute degeneration of the spinal cord (demyelination of the dorsal column), visual disturbances due to optic atrophy
  3. Glossitis and GI symptoms such as nausea, vomiting, and anorexia are also common
  4. Patients may also have dementia/mental sluggishness, depression, and weakness
- Vitamin B_9 (folic acid):
  1. Patchy hyperpigmentation of skin (especially between fingers and toes) and mucous membranes
  2. Moderate fever (temp $<102°F$; $38.9°C$) despite the absence of infection
  3. Neural tube defect
  4. Angular stomatitis
  5. Red, beefy, smooth, and shiny tongue
  6. Megaloblastic anemia

- Vitamin C: Scurvy (bruising, petechiae, follicular hyperkeratosis, perifollicular hemorrhage, corkscrew hairs), poor wound healing, fatigue, gingivitis/bleeding gums, weight loss, bone abnormalities (Fig. E2). Also, loss of teeth, abnormal nail (koilonychia and splint hemorrhages). Vitamin C deficiency may be associated with nonalcoholic fatty liver

ETIOLOGY

- Fat-soluble vitamins (vitamins A, D, E, K):
  1. Decreased ingestion, malnutrition, eating disorders
  2. Diseases that affect fat absorption decrease the absorption of fat-soluble vitamins—for example, cystic fibrosis, celiac sprue, inflammatory bowel disease, cholestasis, hepatobiliary disease, small bowel surgery
  3. Change in vitamin metabolism:
     a. Alcoholism
     b. Drugs such as cholestyramine, warfarin, anticonvulsants, antibiotics (e.g., cephalosporins)
     c. Chronic kidney disease
- Increased risk in:
  1. Vegans
  2. Recent immigrants
  3. Refugees
  4. Toddlers/preschoolers living below the poverty line
- Water-soluble vitamins (the B group of vitamins and vitamin C)—there are several etiologic factors, including:
  1. Inadequate intake
  2. Decreased absorption
  3. Alcoholism
  4. Pregnancy/lactation
  5. Peritoneal dialysis
  6. Medications (e.g., isoniazid, phenothiazines, tricyclic antidepressants, metformin [vitamin B_{12}])
  7. Malabsorption
  8. Low income
  9. Advanced age
- Vitamin B_{12} deficiency—caused by:
  1. Insufficient dietary intake, as in strict vegans
  2. Decreased absorption secondary to intrinsic factor deficiency, decreased intrinsic factor secretion, gastric atrophy, gastrectomy/gastric bypass
  3. Terminal ileum disease such as celiac disease, enteritis, tropical sprue
- Folic acid deficiency:
  1. Increased needs can lead to deficiency (e.g., pregnancy, lactation, malignancy)
  2. Derangement of folate metabolism by:
     a. Medication (e.g., methotrexate)
     b. Disease (e.g., hypothyroidism)
     c. Increased excretion: As seen in alcoholics

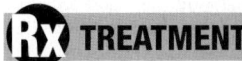 **DIAGNOSIS**

WORKUP

Table 1 summarizes clinical clues in identifying vitamin deficiency.

LABORATORY TESTS

General initial laboratory tests include:
- CBC
- Liver function tests
- Basic metabolic panel
- Albumin
- Measurement of serum levels of the specific vitamin in question

Specific tests may be considered in the following cases:
- Vitamin A:
  1. Serum retinol level (best test, a direct measure, expensive)
  2. Retinol binding protein (easier to perform, less expensive)
  3. Dark-adaptation threshold test
- Vitamin K:
  1. Protein induced by vitamin K absence or antagonism is the current best test available to determine vitamin K status. The level is increased in vitamin K deficiency
  2. Prothrombin time/partial thromboplastin time
  3. Prothrombin
  4. Des-gamma-carboxyprothrombin (most sensitive test)
  5. Niacin: Urine-*N*-methylnicotinamide (level <0.8 mg/day indicates niacin deficiency)
- Vitamin B_1 (thiamine):
  1. Blood thiamine levels
  2. Thiamine pyrophosphate levels in blood
  3. Erythrocyte thiamine transketolase activity
  4. Urinary thiamine excretion
- Vitamin B_3 (niacin): Check urinary N-methylnicotinamide or erythrocyte NAD/NADP ratio (tests are not readily available)
- Vitamin B_2: Check plasma riboflavin concentration
- Vitamin B_{12}:
  1. Serum vitamin B_{12} <190 pg/ml is diagnostic of vitamin B_{12} deficiency
  2. Serum methylmalonic acid, which is elevated in B_{12} deficiency
  3. Antiparietal antibody
  4. Intrinsic factor antibody is decreased
  5. CBC shows increased MCV, anemia with low hemoglobin, and low hematocrit
  6. Blood smear shows macrocytosis and hypersegmentation of megaloblasts
  7. Megaloblastic anemia
- Folic acid:
  1. Check serum folate level.
  2. Additional testing includes checking for serum homocysteine level, which will be elevated.
  3. Red cell folate level shows chronic folate status.

Rx TREATMENT

Most of the vitamins are available over the counter individually or in different multivitamin formulations.
- Vitamin A deficiency: Treat with oral supplementation 10,000 IU daily.
  1. Consume vitamin A–rich foods such as liver, beef, carrots, oranges, mangoes.

TABLE 1 Clinical Clues in Identifying Vitamin Deficiency

Clinical Features	Causes and Diagnosis	Treatment and Notes
Vitamin A deficiency		
Can take years to cause symptoms Xerophthalmia causing night blindness and Bitot spots (conjunctival squamous cell proliferation and keratinization) is the earliest sign Poor bone growth Follicular hyperkeratosis Impaired immune system Conjunctival xerosis Keratomalacia	Low dietary intake (preformed vitamin A is from animals; provitamin A is found in plants) Diagnosis is made by measuring serum retinol levels	Vitamin A supplementation Daily requirement (RDA) for adult males is 3000 IU and for females is 2300 IU Vitamin A toxicity is related to chronic ingestion ($\geq$25,000 IU/day); serum retinol levels are not helpful as vitamin A is stored in the liver
Vitamin B$_{12}$ deficiency		
Can take several years to show symptoms Macrocytic anemia Smooth tongue In severe deficiency—subacute combined degeneration of the spinal cord Peripheral sensory neuropathy affecting large and small fibers Dementia	Low dietary intake Pernicious anemia Terminal ileum disease	Vitamin B$_{12}$ supplementation If both folate and vitamin B$_{12}$ deficiency are present, you must replace vitamin B$_{12}$ first to avoid subacute combined degeneration of the spinal cord
Vitamin B$_6$ (pyridoxine) deficiency		
Can take weeks to become symptomatic Glossitis Cheilosis Vomiting Seizures Scrotal dermatitis	Mainly secondary to drugs (e.g., isoniazid, cycloserine, penicillamine, phenobarbital) Can measure serum levels of pyridoxal-phosphate	Vitamin supplementation Large doses can cause both impaired position and vibratory sense
Vitamin B$_2$ (riboflavin) deficiency		
Can take weeks to become symptomatic Normochromic normocytic anemia Sore throat and magenta tongue Glossitis Cheilosis Seborrheic dermatitis in perianal area, nose	Associated with phenothiazine and tricyclic antidepressants	Vitamin supplementation
Vitamin B$_1$ (thiamine) deficiency		
Can take weeks to become symptomatic Wet beriberi—heart failure secondary to cardiomyopathy Dry beriberi (neuropathy) Wernicke encephalopathy (WE)—nystagmus, ophthalmoplegia, and ataxia Peripheral neuropathy Korsakoff syndrome	Low dietary intake Alcoholic patients, chronic dialysis patients IV glucose can precipitate WE: Give thiamine before glucose Can directly measure thiamine levels in serum	Thiamine supplementation
Vitamin C deficiency (scurvy)		
First symptoms are petechial hemorrhage and ecchymoses Bleeding, swollen gums Hyperkeratotic papules Hemorrhagia into joints, nail beds Loosening of teeth Periosteal hemorrhages Coiled hairs Impaired wound healing Weak bones Sjögren syndrome	Low dietary intake	Vitamin C supplementation Large doses can cause oxalate renal stones and impaired absorption of vitamin B$_{12}$
Iodine deficiency		
Hypothyroidism	Low dietary intake Drug and alcohol abusers	Improve dietary intake
Niacin deficiency (pellagra)		
The 3 Ds: • *D*ermatizis (sun-exposed areas) • *D*iarrhea • *D*epression to dementia to psychosis (altered mental state) Hyperpigmentation Glossitis Stomatitis	Low dietary intake; tryptophan is used in the body to make niacin Carcinoid syndrome (tryptophan is used up) Isoniazid (increased excretion of tryptophan—pyridoxine supplement must be used concurrently to prevent this) Hartnup disease (autosomal recessive, cerebellar ataxia)	Replacement treatment

Continued

TABLE 1 Clinical Clues in Identifying Vitamin Deficiency—cont'd

Clinical Features	Causes and Diagnosis	Treatment and Notes
Zinc deficiency		
Rash (face, body: Pustular, bullous, vesicular, seborrheic, acneiform), skin ulcers, alopecia, dysgeusia Impaired immunity Night blindness Decreased spermatogenesis Diarrhea	Low dietary intake	Zinc supplementation
Vitamin E deficiency		
Peripheral sensory and motor neuropathy Hemolytic anemia Retinal degeneration Dry skin		Vitamin E supplementation Large doses can potentiate the effects of oral anticoagulation
Vitamin K deficiency		
Bleeding tendency Easy bruisability	Low dietary intake Systemic diseases that cause fat-soluble vitamin malabsorption Can detect by checking coagulation profile (INR and PT)	Vitamin K supplementation
Vitamin D deficiency		
The major source of vitamin D is from sun exposure. Secondary sources are from diet or supplementation and intestinal absorption In the liver, vitamin D undergoes hydroxylation by 25-hydroxylase to 25-hydroxyvitamin D, 25 (OH)D. Further hydroxylation takes place in the kidneys to activated vitamin D (1,25-dihydroxyvitamin D). Activated vitamin D is important in bone mineralization Vitamin D deficiency leads to: • Rickets in children • Osteomalacia in adults • Hypocalcemia Secondary hyperparathyroidism which leads to phosphaturia	Decreased exposure to the sun Decreased intestinal absorption from the intestine Renal disease Systemic diseases that cause fat malabsorption Can be directly measured by checking for serum 25(OH)D	Increase casual exposure to sunlight Vitamin D supplementation: • 25(OH)D (Ostelin 1000) • Activated vitamin D (calcitriol; this form should be used in renal disease) The RDA for vitamin D is 600 IU for adults Avoid excessive doses, as toxicity can cause hypercalcemia, confusion, polyuria, polydipsia, anorexia, vomiting, and muscle weakness Long-term toxicity results in bone demineralization and pain

INR, International normalized ratio; *RDA,* recommended dietary allowance; *PT,* prothrombin time.
From Talley NJ et al: *Essentials of internal medicine,* ed 4, Chatswood, NSW, 2021, Elsevier Australia.

2. Five servings of fruit and vegetables give enough carotenoids for a day.
- Vitamin K deficiency: Treatment depends on the severity of bleeding, administered subcutaneously or intramuscularly (IM).
- Vitamin B_1 (thiamine) deficiency: Give IM thiamine 50 mg for several days.
  1. If B_1 deficiency is suspected and patient needs intravenous glucose, give thiamine first before intravenous glucose. This prevents the development of Korsakoff psychosis.
- Vitamin B_{12} deficiency: Give 1000 mcg IM daily for 7 days, then once a wk for 1 mo, then once a mo indefinitely.
  1. A potential option is oral supplementation.

- Folic acid deficiency: Daily requirement is 400 to 1000 mcg (1 mg) daily.
  1. Centers for Disease Control and Prevention recommend that women of childbearing age take 400 mcg of folic acid daily.
  2. The U.S. Preventive Services Task Force (USPSTF) found no benefit and likely harm from use of β-carotene and lack of either benefit or harm from use of vitamin E, leading to a recommendation against use of either one for preventing cardiovascular disease or cancer.[1]

REFERENCE
Available at eBooks.Health.Elsevier.com.

RELATED CONTENT
Anemia, Pernicious (Related Key Topic)
Osteomalacia and Rickets (Related Key Topic)
Vitamin D Deficiency (Related Key Topic)
Wernicke Syndrome (Related Key Topic)
Vitamins and Their Functions (Appendix IIb) (Related Key Topic)

AUTHOR: **FRED F. FERRI, MD**

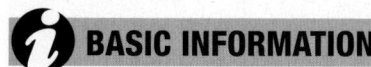 **BASIC INFORMATION**

DEFINITION

von Willebrand disease (vWD) is an inherited disorder of hemostasis characterized by a quantitative or qualitative deficiency in von Willebrand factor (vWF), which results in defective platelet adhesion and aggregation.

SYNONYMS

vWD
Pseudohemophilia

ICD-10CM CODE	
D68.0	von Willebrand disease

EPIDEMIOLOGY & DEMOGRAPHICS

- Most common inherited bleeding disorder.
- Prevalence is 0.6% to 1.3% according to population studies and is consistent across all races and ethnicities.
- Estimates based on referral for symptoms of bleeding suggest a prevalence of 1 case/10,000 persons.[1]

PHYSICAL FINDINGS & CLINICAL PRESENTATION

- Generally normal physical examination.
- Mucosal bleeding (gingival bleeding, epistaxis) and easy bruising occurs.
- GI bleeding may occur because of angiodysplasia in type 2 or type 3 vWD.
- Bleeding after surgery or dental extraction.
- Most women have menorrhagia.
- Rarely, muscle or joint bleeding occurs in type 3 vWD.

ETIOLOGY

- vWD is usually an autosomal-dominant disorder but is rarely recessive or double-heterozygotic.
- vWF is a protein product of a gene located on the short arm of chromosome 12. vWD results from a failure to synthesize or secrete vWF or an accelerated clearance of vWF.
- Binding of vWF multimers to denuded subendothelial collagen or glycosaminoglycans causes platelet adhesion by acting as a ligand for glycoprotein IB on the platelet surface.[2] This latter activity can be measured by the ristocetin cofactor (RCo) assay. In vWD, the RCo level is <30% of normal. Low vWF (mild vWD) exists when the RCo level is between 30% and 60%, with such patients potentially exhibiting a bleeding phenotype.
- There are three broad clinically defined types of vWD:
  1. Type 1 is the most common (80% cases), in which levels of vWF, FVIII:C, and RCo are reduced but concordant. Within type 1, there is type 1 mild, which is common; type 1 severe (T1S), which is rare; and type 1C, in which the low vWF is due to accelerated clearance.
  2. Type 2 has four subtypes: Type 2A, type 2B, type 2N, and type 2M. All of these variants have a qualitative defect in vWF, low

levels of RCo, and show a discordancy between levels of RCo and FVIII:C.
  3. Type 3 is rare and either an autosomal recessive disorder or double heterozygote and has a near-complete quantitative deficiency of vWF and very low FVIII:C.
- Acquired vWD disease presents with mucocutaneous bleeding abnormalities but no family history. It is seen often in association with hematoproliferative or autoimmune disorders or may occur in hypothyroidism. Successful treatment of the underlying illness can reverse the clinical course.

Dx DIAGNOSIS

A definitive diagnosis of vWD may be made if vWF:RCo levels are <30 IU/dl. Typically, a vWD diagnosis requires two criteria: (1) A personal history, family history, or physical evidence of mucocutaneous bleeding and (2) a qualitative or quantitative decrease in functional activity of vWD.

DIFFERENTIAL DIAGNOSIS

Platelet function disorders, clotting factor deficiencies

WORKUP (FIG. 1)

Screening Laboratory Tests:
- Laboratory evaluation (Table 1).
- Initial testing includes prothrombin time (normal), partial thromboplastin time (normal or slightly increased), platelet count (normal),

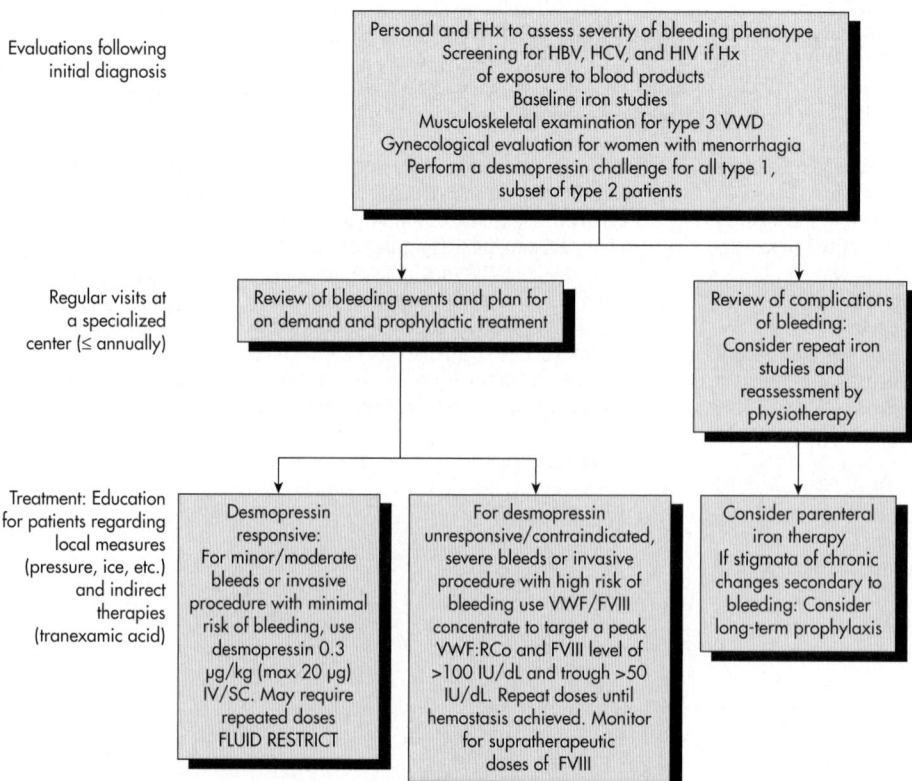

FIG. 1 Approach to the management of von Willebrand disease. *FHx,* Family history; *FVIII,* factor VIII; *HBV,* hepatitis B virus; *HCV,* hepatitis C virus; *HIV,* human immunodeficiency virus; *Hx,* history; *IV,* intravenous; *RCo,* ristocetin cofactor; *SC,* subcutaneous; *vWD,* von Willebrand disease; *vWF,* von Willebrand factor. (From Hoffman R et al: *Hematology, basic principles and practice,* ed 8, Philadelphia, 2023, Elsevier.)

TABLE 1 Table of Investigations

vWD Type	vWF:RCo IU/dl[a]	vWF:Ag IU/dl[a]	RCo/Ag IU/dl[a]	FVIII:C IU/dl[a]	Multimer Pattern[b]	Other
1	Low	Low	Equivalent	~1.5× vWF:Ag	Normal	
2A	Low	Low	vWF:RCo <vWF:Ag	Low or normal	Abnormal↓ HMWM	
2B	Low	Low	vWF:RCo <vWF:Ag	Low or normal	Abnormal↓ HMWM	↑ RIPA[c] (↓ platelet count)
2M	Low	Low	vWF:RCo <vWF:Ag	Low or normal	Normal	
2N	Normal/low	Normal/low	Equivalent	<30	Normal	↓ vWF:FVIIIB[d]
3	Absent	Absent	NA	<10	Absent	

Ag, Antigen; *FVIII:C*, FVIII level; *NA*, not applicable; *RCo*, ristocetin cofactor; *RIPA*, ristocetin-induced platelet aggregation; *vWD*, von Willebrand disease; *vWF:FVIIIB*, FVIII-binding assay.
[a]Relative to the reference range (approximate values); vWF:RCo (50-200 IU/dl); vWF:Ag (50-200 IU/dl); FVIII:C (50-150 IU/dl).
[b]*HMWM*, High-molecular-weight multimers.
[c]Increased agglutination at low concentrations of ristocetin.
[d]The ability of vWF to bind and protect FVIII is reduced. vWF and FVIII levels can look exactly like those in males with mild hemophilia A or in symptomatic hemophilia A carrier females.
From Hoffman R et al: *Hematology, basic principles and practice*, ed 8, Philadelphia, 2023, Elsevier.

TABLE 2 Desmopressin Responsiveness in the Various Subtypes of von Willebrand Disease

vWD Type	vWF:RCo	vWF:Ag	RCo/Ag	FVIII:C IU/dl	vWF:CB	vWF:CB/vWF:Ag
1	Increase	Increase	Remains >0.7	Increase	Increase	Remains >0.7
2A	No/little change	Increase	Remains <0.7	Increase	No/little change	Remains <0.7
2M (GP1B-binding dysfunction)	No/little change	Increase	Remains <0.7	Increase	Increase	Remains >0.7
3	No/little change	No/little change		No/little change	No/little change	

Ag, Antigen; *CB*, collagen assays–binding; *FVIII:C*, factor VIII level; *GP1B*, glycoprotein 1B; *RCo*, ristocetin cofactor; *vWD*, von Willebrand disease; *vWF*, von Willebrand factor.
Modified from Favaloro EJ: Rethinking the diagnosis of von Willebrand disease, *Thromb Res* 127:17, 2011; and Hoffman R et al: *Hematology, basic principles and practice*, ed 8, Philadelphia, 2023, Elsevier.

and PFA-100 (abnormal or may show high normal values in type 1 vWD).

Specific Laboratory Tests:
- Factor VIII coagulant activity (FVIII:C, typically decreased but normal in some type 2 cases).
- vWF antigen, RCo, and collagen binding assay are typically decreased.
- Normal platelet number and morphology.
- Prolonged bleeding time or prolonged PFA-100 closure times.
- von Willebrand propeptide.[3] This measures the N-terminal propeptide of vWF. This vWFpp is secreted in equimolar amounts to the mature vWF. The ratio of vWFpp to vWF assists in identifying vWD due to rapid clearance, as in type 1C.
- Multimeric analysis: Type 2A vWD can be distinguished by absence of medium- and high-molecular-weight multimers.
- Type 2B vWD is distinguished by the absence of high-molecular-weight multimers.
- Type 2N is a defect in the factor VIII:C binding and has normal vWF levels but very low factor VIII:C with a normal multimer pattern.
- Type 2M is a defect in binding to platelets (low RCo, low collagen-binding activity) but normal multimers.
- Response to DDAVP can also be used to diagnose Type 1C or Type 2N

ⓇⓍ TREATMENT

NONPHARMACOLOGIC THERAPY
- Avoidance of aspirin and other NSAIDs.
- Antifibrinolytics such as tranexamic acid (1g PO TID-QID) and aminocaproic acid help, especially for menorrhagia or oral bleeding.
- Topical thrombin soaked in gel foam can be used for controlling oral bleeding.

ACUTE GENERAL Rx
- International Society of Thrombosis and Haemostasis has a Bleeding Assessment Tool (ISTH-BAT) that can be used to quantify the severity of bleeding and the need for treatment.
- Treatment of vWD is based on normalizing factor VIII and vWF levels on spontaneous bleeding or before a planned intervention.
- Desmopressin (DDAVP) (Table 2): This binds to receptors on endothelial cells and causes vWF release and is suitable in milder forms of vWD. DDAVP is administered at a dose of 0.3 mcg/kg in 50 to 100 ml of intravenous normal saline solution infused over 20 to 30 min. It is also available as a nasal spray (150 mcg spray to each nostril) before minor surgery and for the management of minor bleeding episodes.
- The use of therapeutic products to replete vWF levels is required in cases unresponsive to DDAVP or those with severe vWD. Currently available vWF products can be grouped into the following categories: (1) vWF/factor VIII plasma-derived concentrates, (2) plasma-derived vWF-only concentrate, and (3) recombinant-derived vWF-only concentrate.[4]
- Recombinant-derived vWF is a treatment approach that overcomes the limitations associated with plasma-derived vWF concentrates such as variable vWD levels and risk of pathogen transmission.[5] In severe vWD, the prophylactic use of recombinant-derived vWF-only concentrate is superior to on-demand use by reducing rate of bleeding and reduction in bleeding risk.
- In patients with severe vWD undergoing surgery or those who receive repeated therapeutic doses of concentrates, use of a plasma-derived vWF-only concentrate or recombinant-derived vWF-only concentrate need to be administered.
- Platelet transfusions may be given for patients with thrombocytopenia, which occurs in Type 2B vWD.
- Bleeding associated with acquired vWD responds to von Willebrand concentrates. If possible, treat the underlying cause.
- Intravenous immunoglobulin can be used to treat acquired vWD when autoantibodies are present secondary to lymphoproliferative disorder, SLE, and myeloma.[6]

REFERENCES

Available at eBooks.Health.Elsevier.com.

AUTHOR: **JOSEPH EDMUND, MD**

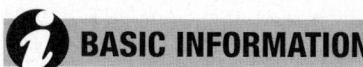
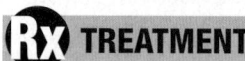 BASIC INFORMATION

DEFINITION
Warts are benign epidermal lesions caused by human papillomavirus (HPV).

SYNONYMS
Verruca vulgaris (common warts)
Verruca plana (flat warts)
Condyloma acuminatum (venereal warts)
Verruca plantaris (plantar warts)
Mosaic warts (cluster of many warts)
HPV infection

ICD-10CM CODES	
B07.9	Viral wart, unspecified
B07.8	Other viral warts
A63.0	Anogenital (venereal) warts
B07.0	Plantar wart

EPIDEMIOLOGY & DEMOGRAPHICS
- HPV infection causes up to 4.5% of all new cancer cases worldwide and represents 29.5% of all infection-related cancers.[1]
- Risk factors include use of communal showers, occupational handling of meat, and immunosuppression. Common warts occur most frequently in children and young adults.
- Anogenital warts are most common in young, sexually active patients. Genital warts are the most common viral sexually transmitted disease in the U.S., with up to 79 million Americans carrying the causative virus and 14 million persons are newly infected each year in the U.S.
- Persistent infection with oncogenic HPV types can cause cervical cancer in women as well as other anogenital and oropharyngeal cancers in women and men. 66% of cervical cancers, 55% of vaginal cancers, 79% of anal cancers, and 62% of oropharyngeal cancers are attributable to HPV types 16 or 18.
- Common warts are longer lasting and more frequent in immunocompromised patients (e.g., lymphoma, AIDS, immunosuppressive drugs).
- Plantar warts occur most frequently at points of maximal pressure (over the heads of the metatarsal bones or on the heels).

PHYSICAL FINDINGS & CLINICAL PRESENTATION (TABLE E1)
- Common warts (Fig. E1) have an initial appearance of a flesh-colored papule with a rough surface; they subsequently develop a hyperkeratotic appearance with black dots on the surface (thrombosed capillaries). They may be single or multiple and are most common on the hands.
- Warts obscure normal skin lines (important diagnostic feature). Cylindrical projections from the wart may become fused, forming a mosaic pattern.
- Flat warts (Fig. E2) generally are pink or light yellow, slightly elevated, and often found on the forehead, back of hands, mouth, and

beard area. They often occur in lines corresponding to trauma (e.g., a scratch), are often misdiagnosed (particularly when present on the face), and are inappropriately treated with topical corticosteroids.
- Filiform warts have a fingerlike appearance with various projections; they are generally found near the mouth, beard, or periorbital and paranasal regions.
- Plantar warts (Fig. E3) are slightly raised and have a roughened surface; they may cause pain when walking; as they involute, small hemorrhages (caused by thrombosed capillaries) may be noted.
- Genital warts (Fig. E4) are generally pale pink with several projections and a broad base. They may coalesce in the perineal area to form masses with a cauliflower-like appearance. Intraanal warts occur predominantly in patients who have had receptive anal intercourse, in contrast with perianal warts, which may occur in men and women without a history of anal sex.
- Genital warts on the cervical epithelium can produce subclinical changes that may be noted on Pap smear or colposcopy.

ETIOLOGY
- HPV infection: >150 types of viral DNA have been identified. Transmission of warts is by direct contact. ~40 different types of HPV are transmitted through sexual contact.
- Genital warts: 90% are caused by HPV types 6 or 11. HPV types 16, 18, 31, 33, and 35 are found occasionally in visible genital warts (usually as coinfections with HPV 6 or 11) and can be associated with foci of high-grade, intraepithelial neoplasia, particularly in persons who are infected with HIV infection. In addition to warts on genital areas, HPV types 6 and 11 have been associated with conjunctival, nasal, oral, and laryngeal warts.

(Dx) DIAGNOSIS

DIFFERENTIAL DIAGNOSIS
- Molluscum contagiosum
- Condyloma latum
- Acrochordon (skin tags) or seborrheic keratosis
- Epidermal nevi
- Hypertrophic actinic keratosis
- Squamous cell carcinomas
- Acquired digital fibrokeratoma
- Varicella-zoster virus in patients with AIDS
- Recurrent infantile digital fibroma
- Plantar corns (may be mistaken for plantar warts)

WORKUP
- Diagnosis is generally based on clinical findings.
- Suspect lesions should be biopsied.
- The application of 3% to 5% acetic acid, which causes skin color to turn white, has been used by some providers to detect HPV-infected genital mucosa. However, acetic acid application is not a specific test for HPV infection. Therefore the routine use of this procedure for screening to detect mucosal

changes attributed to HPV infection is not recommended.

LABORATORY TESTS
- Screening for cervical cancer with cytology, which is performed by either Pap smear or liquid-based cytology. Screening guidelines recommend starting screening at age 21. Annual cytology is recommended until at least three normal cytology results are obtained.
- Colposcopy with biopsy is recommended in patients with cervical squamous cell changes.

(Rx) TREATMENT

NONPHARMACOLOGIC THERAPY
- Importance of use of condoms to reduce transmission of genital warts should be emphasized.
- Watchful waiting is an acceptable option in the treatment of nongenital cutaneous warts because many warts will disappear without intervention over time. However, many patients often request treatment because of social stigma or discomfort.
- Plantar warts that are not painful do not need treatment.
- Factors that influence selection of treatment include wart size, wart number, anatomic site of the wart, wart morphology, patient preference, cost of treatment, convenience, adverse effects, and provider experience. Factors that might affect response to therapy include the presence of immunosuppression and compliance with therapy.

GENERAL Rx
- Common warts:
  1. Application of topical salicylic acid 17%. Soak area for 5 min in warm water and dry. Apply thin layer once or twice daily for up to 12 wk, avoiding normal skin. Bandage.
  2. Liquid nitrogen and electrocautery are also common methods of removal. Cure rates for cryotherapy are 50% to 70% after three or four treatments.
  3. Blunt dissection can be used in large lesions or resistant lesions.
  4. Duct tape occlusion is also effective for treating common warts. It is cut to cover warts and left in place for 6 days. It is removed after 6 days, and the warts are soaked in water and then filed with pumice stones. New tape is applied 12 h later. This treatment can be repeated until warts resolve.
  5. Recalcitrant warts can be treated with injection of *Candida* or mumps skin antigen into the wart every 3 to 4 wk for up to three treatments, photodynamic therapy with aminolevulinic acid, pulsed dye laser, and intralesional bleomycin.
- Filiform warts: Surgical removal is necessary.
- Flat warts: Generally more difficult to treat.
  1. Tretinoin cream applied at bedtime over the involved area for several weeks may be effective.

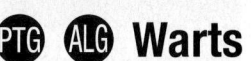
2. Application of liquid nitrogen.
3. Electrocautery.
4. 5-Fluorouracil cream applied once or twice a day for 3 to 5 wk is also effective. Persistent hyperpigmentation may occur after Efudex use.

- Plantar warts:
  1. Salicylic acid therapy (e.g., Occlusal-HP). Soak wart in warm water for 5 min, remove loose tissue, dry. Apply to area, allow to dry, reapply. Use once or twice daily; maximum 12 wk. Use of 40% salicylic acid plasters (Mediplast) is also a safe, nonscarring treatment; it is particularly useful in treating mosaic warts covering a large area.
  2. Blunt dissection is also a fast and effective treatment modality.
  3. Laser therapy can be used for plantar warts and recurrent warts; however, it leaves open wounds that require 4 to 6 wk to fill with granulation tissue.
  4. Interlesional bleomycin is also effective but generally used when all other treatments fail.

- Genital warts:
  1. Can be effectively treated with 20% podophyllin resin in compound tincture of benzoin applied with a cotton tip applicator by the treating physician and allowed to air dry. The treatment can be repeated weekly if necessary.
  2. Podofilox (Condylox 0.5% gel) is available for application by the patient. Local adverse effects include pain, burning, and inflammation at the site.
  3. Cryosurgery with liquid nitrogen delivered with a probe or as a spray is effective for treating smaller genital warts.
  4. Carbon dioxide laser can also be used for treating primary or recurrent genital warts (cure rate >90%).
  5. Imiquimod cream, 5%, is a patient-applied immune response modifier effective in the treatment of external genital and perianal warts (complete clearing of genital warts in >70% of females and >30% of males in 4 to 16 wk). Sexual contact should be avoided while the cream is on the skin. It is applied three times weekly before normal sleeping hours and is left on the skin for 6 to 10 h.
  6. Sinecatechins (Veregen), a botanical drug product, is also effective for treatment of external genital and perianal warts. Formulation is a 15% ointment applied to affected area three times daily for up to 16 wk.

- Application of trichloroacetic acid or bichloroacetic acid 80% to 90% is also effective for external genital warts. A small amount should be applied only to warts and allowed to dry, at which time a white "frosting" develops. This treatment can be repeated weekly if necessary.

DISPOSITION

- Warts can be effectively treated with the previous modalities with complete resolution in the majority of patients; however, the recurrence rate is high.
- Cervical carcinomas and precancerous lesions in women are associated with genital papillomavirus infection.
- Squamous cell anal cancer is also associated with a history of genital warts.

REFERRAL

- Dermatology referral for warts resistant to conservative therapy
- Surgical referral in selected cases
- Sexually transmitted disease counseling for patients with anogenital warts

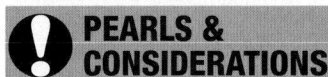

PEARLS & CONSIDERATIONS

COMMENTS

- Subungual and periungual warts are generally more resistant to treatment. Dermatology referral for cryosurgery is recommended in resistant cases.
- Examination of sex partners is not necessary for the management of genital warts because no data indicate that reinfection plays a role.

PREVENTION

- The HPV vaccines (Gardasil, Gardasil-9, Cervarix) have been licensed in the U.S. Advisory Committee on Immunization Practices (ACIP) recommends routine vaccination with HPV4 or HPV2 for females aged 11 to 12 yr and HPV4 for males aged 11 to 12 yr. Vaccination is also recommended for females aged 13 to 26 yr and for males aged 13 through 21 yr who were not vaccinated previously. Delaying vaccination until after first sexual activity is associated with higher prevalence of vaginal human papillomavirus.[2] Males aged 22 through 26 may be vaccinated. ACIP recommends vaccination of men who have sex with men and immunocompromised persons (including those with infection) through age 26 yr if not previously vaccinated. The 9-valent HPV vaccine (Gardasil-9) is approved for use in girls and women 9 to 26 yr old and boys 9 to 15 yr old. It is indicated to prevent diseases associated with HPV infection with types 6, 11, 16, 18, 31, 33, 45, 52, and 58. It appears to be more effective than the other two currently available vaccines. It consists of two doses. The first dose is administered at 11 to 12 yr of age, and the second dose 6 to 12 mo later. However, if the second dose is given <5 mo apart, a third dose will be needed at age 9 to 14. Patients with a weak immune system and in those starting vaccination at age 15 to 26 yr will need three doses. ACIP does not recommend catch-up HPV vaccination for all adults over 26 yr old. Shared decision-making regarding HPV vaccination is recommended for some adults ages 27 through 65 who are unvaccinated.
- Male circumcision decreases heterosexual transmission of HPV.

REFERENCES

Available at eBooks.Health.Elsevier.com.

RELATED CONTENT

Human Papillomavirus Infection (Patient Information)
Warts (Patient Information)
Condyloma Acuminatum (Related Key Topic)
Cervical cancer (Related Key topic)

AUTHOR: **FRED F. FERRI, MD**

ℹ️ BASIC INFORMATION

DEFINITION

Wolff-Parkinson-White (WPW) syndrome is a congenital heart condition in which, in addition to the normal electrical conduction through the atrioventricular (AV) node, there is an accessory pathway (AP) that connects the atria to the ventricles. Consequently, a portion of the ventricular myocardium is depolarized via the AP earlier than the normal AV nodal conduction, resulting in ventricular preexcitation. The terms "WPW syndrome" and "WPW pattern" often are used in describing patients with ventricular preexcitation. Patients with WPW syndrome have ECG findings of preexcitation, including short PR and slurring of the initial segment of the QRS complex known as the delta wave together with symptoms suggestive of arrhythmia or documented arrhythmia, which may be AV reentrant tachycardia, atrial fibrillation (AF), or both. Patients with the WPW pattern have characteristic ECG findings of preexcitation without symptoms or evidence of arrhythmia.

SYNONYMS

WPW
Preexcitation syndrome

ICD-10CM CODE
I45.6   Preexcitation syndrome

EPIDEMIOLOGY & DEMOGRAPHICS[1-5]

- The prevalence of a WPW pattern on the surface ECG is 0.1% to 0.3% in the general population. The prevalence is increased to 0.55% in first-degree relatives of affected patients. It is estimated that ~65% of adolescents and 40% of individuals older than 30 yr with WPW pattern on a resting ECG are asymptomatic.
- The prevalence of WPW is higher among males and decreases with age.
- Most patients with WPW have structurally normal hearts, but it may also occur in patients with congenital heart disease, most notably in patients with Ebstein anomaly, which is associated with right-side AP and often multiple and slowly conducting APs.

PHYSICAL FINDINGS & CLINICAL PRESENTATION

- The physical examination is usually unremarkable.
- Symptoms are typically related to tachyarrhythmias, including the following:
  1. Palpitations, light-headedness, anxiety, dyspnea, or chest pain
  2. Syncope or near syncope
  3. Sudden cardiac death
- The common arrhythmias in WPW syndrome are:
  1. Supraventricular tachycardia (SVT): AV reciprocating tachycardia (AVRT). This is the most common arrhythmia, further classified as orthodromic AVRT (narrow complex tachycardia, with antegrade conduction through the AV node and retrograde conduction via the AP that occurs in 70% of symptomatic patients) or antidromic AVRT (wide complex tachycardia with antegrade conduction via the AP and retrogradely through the AV node, which occurs in 4% to 5% of patients).
  2. AF (~10% to 38%), the second most common tachycardia, can be complicated by a very rapid ventricular response due to conduction over the AP, which can lead to ventricular fibrillation (VF) and sudden death. This risk is dependent on the antegrade refractory period of AP during AF.
  3. The risk of sudden death in symptomatic patients with WPW syndrome is estimated to be ~0.25%/yr or 3% to 4% over a lifetime.
- In a meta-analysis including ~2000 subjects with asymptomatic WPW, children had a sudden death rate of 1.9 compared with 0.9 in adults per 1000 patient-yr of follow-up. This incidence is comparable with the estimated 0.1%/yr risk of death in the general population in Europe, Japan, and the U.S.

ETIOLOGY & PATHOGENESIS[6]

- APs are thought to be an embryologic remnant, as substantiated by reports of SVT in uterus and by a greater prevalence of WPW in newborns and infants.
- Left free wall APs are most common followed by posteroseptal, right free wall, and anteroseptal locations.
- Some patients with WPW syndrome (~5% to 10%) have multiple APs.
- In subjects with WPW, two parallel routes of AV conduction are present: One is subject to delay through the AV node, and the other occurs without delay through the AP and results in preexcitation of the ventricles. The resulting QRS complex is a fusion beat, as a portion of the ventricle is preexcited and activated via the AP giving rise to the delta wave, and the remainder of the ventricle is activated by the normal activation pathway (Fig. 1).
- Reciprocating tachycardias occur when conduction is anterograde in one pathway (usually the AV node, i.e., orthodromic AVRT) and retrograde in the other (usually the AP) as a result of different refractory periods. This is usually initiated by a premature atrial or ventricular depolarization.

Dx DIAGNOSIS

- Three basic features characterize the ECG abnormalities associated with WPW pattern:
  1. PR interval <120 msec.
  2. QRS complex can be >120 msec with a slurred, slowly rising onset of QRS in some leads (delta wave) and a normal terminal QRS portion. The width of the QRS complex depends on the amount of preexcited ventricular tissue.
  3. Secondary ST-T wave changes directed in an opposite direction to the major delta and QRS vectors may be present.

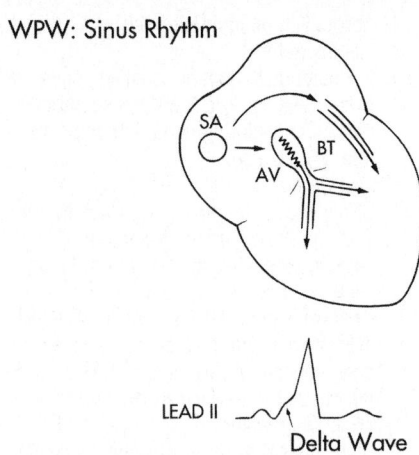

FIG. 1 With Wolff-Parkinson-White *(WPW)* syndrome, an abnormal accessory pathway called a bypass tract connects the atria and the ventricles.

- ECG patterns with abnormal QRS complexes and ST and T changes can mask or mimic myocardial infarction (in particular posteroseptal AP with negative delta waves in the inferior wall, which mimics old inferior wall myocardial infarction), bundle branch block (Fig. 2), or ventricular hypertrophy.
- Most commonly seen tachycardia (orthodromic AVRT) is characterized by a normal QRS with a regular rate of 150 to 250 beats per min. Onset and termination are abrupt.
- Variants of preexcitation:
  1. Lown-Ganong-Levine syndrome is characterized by a short PR interval, a narrow QRS complex without a delta wave, and a clinical syndrome of paroxysmal SVTs. Postulated mechanisms to the short PR interval include a variant of the normal, enhanced sympathetic tone or specialized intranodal fibers with enhanced AV nodal conduction.
  2. Atriofascicular AP: A slowly conducting AP with AV-nodal-like properties that conducts only in antegrade direction and connects the right atrium with the right bundle branch or the apical myocardium. In the baseline state, minimal or no preexcitation may be present. During preexcitation the QRS appears like a typical left bundle branch (LBBB) pattern. The typical arrhythmia in patients with atriofascicular AP is antidromic tachycardia with LBBB morphology.
  3. Nodoventricular or nodofascicular APs (Mahaim fiber): Rare variants that connect the AV node and the ventricle or the bundle branch appropriately.
- An electrophysiology study is the gold standard to confirm the diagnosis, determine the location, and assess the conduction properties of the AP.

RISK STRATIFICATION[7,8]

- Intermittent and abrupt loss of preexcitation on a beat-to-beat basis is usually indicative of lower risk, assessed with Holter monitoring or with an exercise stress test. The loss of

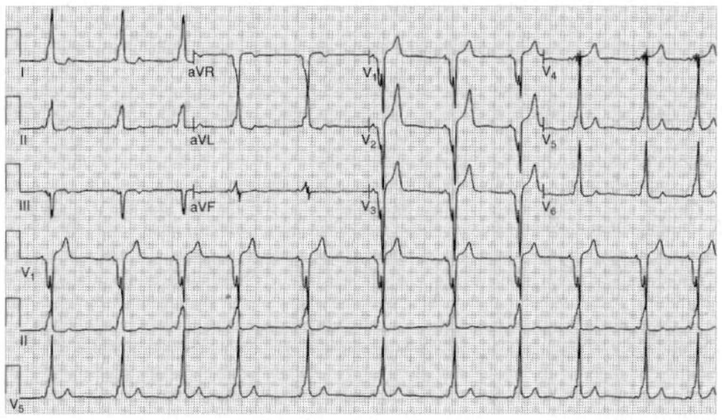

W

Diseases and Disorders

I

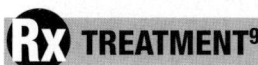

FIG. 2 Wolff-Parkinson-White (WPW) syndrome. This 12-lead electrocardiogram with rhythm strips shows preexcitation with an accessory pathway connecting the right atrium to the right ventricle. This gives rise to a pattern-like left bundle branch block because the ventricles are activated over the right-sided accessory pathway. The tracing shows the typical characteristics of WPW syndrome, including a short PR interval, a wide QRS complex, and a delta wave. From Olshansky B et al: *Arrhythmia essentials,* ed 2, Philadelphia, 2017, Elsevier.

BOX 1 Goals of Electrophysiologic Evaluation in Patients with Wolff-Parkinson-White Syndrome

- Confirmation of the presence of an accessory pathway (AP)
- Evaluation for the presence of multiple APs
- Localization of the AP(s)
- Evaluation of the refractory period of the AP and its implications for life-threatening arrhythmias
- Induction and evaluation of tachycardias
- Demonstration of the AP role in the tachycardia
- Evaluation of other tachycardias not dependent on the presence of the AP
- Ablation of the AP, when indicated.

From Issa Z et al: *Clinical arrhythmology and electrophysiology,* ed 2, Philadelphia, 2012, Saunders.

---

preexcitation after administration of the antiarrhythmic drug procainamide has also been used to indicate a low-risk subgroup. More recent evidence, however, has begun to demonstrate that intermittent preexcitation is not 100% specific for identification of a "low-risk" AP. "High-risk" intracardiac electrophysiology study (EPS) characteristics are found in 5% of patients with intermittent preexcitation and 31% with abrupt loss of preexcitation on exercise test.
- In patients with a persistent preexcitation pattern, electrophysiology study is the procedure of choice for risk stratification.

ⓇⓍ TREATMENT[9]

Goals of electrophysiologic evaluation in patients with WPW syndrome are described in Box 1.

ACUTE MANAGEMENT
- Urgent cardioversion for an acute tachycardia episode with hemodynamic instability.

- Narrow QRS tachycardia (consistent with orthodromic AVRT):
  1. Vagal maneuvers and/or IV adenosine.
  2. IV β-blockers, diltiazem, or verapamil can be administered for regular and **narrow** QRS tachycardia, implying antegrade conduction via the AV node, when the patient is hemodynamically stable and IV adenosine is ineffective.
- Wide QRS complex tachycardias (WCTs):
  1. Most commonly caused by AF with antegrade conduction via the AP and the AV node. AV nodal blocking therapies (i.e., β-blockers, calcium channel blockers, digoxin, and adenosine) are potentially dangerous and should be avoided in these cases because of the risk of causing VF by enhancement of the ventricular response through the AP when the AV node is blocked and the blood pressure is lowered.
  2. Stable patients with preexcited AF can be managed with IV procainamide. Procainamide can decrease ventricular rate by slowing conduction over the AP and

have the additional benefit of possibly terminating AF. Electrical cardioversion should be performed if the patient is hemodynamically unstable.
  3. In a patient with WCT due to antidromic tachycardia, drug treatment may be directed at the AP (IV procainamide) or at the AV node because both are critical components of the tachycardia circuit.

LONG-TERM MANAGEMENT
- Asymptomatic:
  1. In low-risk patients with AP effective refractory period (APERP) >250 msec, or shortest preexcited RR interval (SPERRI) >250 msec, no therapy is required. An electrophysiology study may be considered in asymptomatic patients with intermittent loss of preexcitation for further risk stratification in order to assess the APERP and SPERRI.
  2. In high-risk patients with APERP <250 msec or SPERRI <250 msec, competitive athletes, or high-risk occupation (i.e., pilots), ablation should be considered.
- Symptomatic:
  1. Patients who presented with aborted sudden cardiac death, preexcited tachycardia (i.e., AF, flutter, atrial tachycardia), or syncope suggestive of cardiac origin should undergo an electrophysiology study for further characterization and ablation of the AP accordingly. Patients with symptomatic palpitations or documented AVRT should be offered an electrophysiology study and ablation of the AP to prevent recurrence and to allow the patient to avoid long-term medical therapy. Ongoing management for stable patients with history of orthodromic AVRT who are not candidates for, or prefer not to undergo, catheter ablation:
     a. Class IC antiarrhythmics (flecainide, propafenone), in the absence of structural heart disease.
     b. Class III antiarrhythmics (amiodarone, sotalol, or dofetilide).
     c. Oral β-blockers, diltiazem, or verapamil.

REFERENCES

Available at eBooks.Health.Elsevier.com.

RELATED CONTENT

Wolff-Parkinson-White Syndrome (Patient Information)

AUTHORS: **ROI WESTREICH, MD, PhD** and **YUVAL KONSTANTINO, MD**

SECTION II

Differential Diagnosis

ABDOMINAL DISTENTION

| ICD-10CM # | R14.0 | Abdominal distention (gaseous) |

NONMECHANICAL OBSTRUCTION

Excessive intraluminal gas.
Intraabdominal infection.
Trauma.
Retroperitoneal irritation (renal colic, neoplasms, infections, hemorrhage).
Vascular insufficiency (thrombosis, embolism).
Mechanical ventilation.
Extraabdominal infection (sepsis, pneumonia, empyema, osteomyelitis of spine).
Metabolic/toxic abnormalities (hypokalemia, uremia, lead poisoning).
Chemical irritation (perforated ulcer, bile, pancreatitis).
Peritoneal inflammation.
Severe pain, pain medications.

MECHANICAL OBSTRUCTION

Neoplasm (intraluminal, extraluminal).
Adhesions, endometriosis.
Infection (intraabdominal abscess, diverticulitis).
Gallstones.
Foreign body, bezoars.
Pregnancy.
Hernias.
Volvulus.
Stenosis at surgical anastomosis, radiation stenosis.
Fecaliths.
Inflammatory bowel disease.
Gastric outlet obstruction.
Hematoma.
Other: parasites, superior mesenteric artery (SMA) syndrome, pneumatosis intestinalis, annular pancreas, Hirschsprung disease, intussusception, meconium.

ABDOMINAL PAIN, ADOLESCENCE[1]

| ICD-10CM # | R10.817 | Generalized abdominal tenderness |
| | R10.827 | Generalized rebound abdominal tenderness |

Acute gastroenteritis.
Irritable bowel syndrome.
Anxiety.
Mittelschmerz.
Appendicitis.
Inflammatory bowel disease.
Peptic ulcer disease.
Cholecystitis.
Neoplasm.
Diabetic ketoacidosis.
Functional abdominal pain.
Pelvic inflammatory disease.
Pregnancy.
Pyelonephritis.
Renal stone.
Trauma.

ABDOMINAL PAIN, CHILDHOOD[1]

| ICD-10CM # | R10.817 | Generalized abdominal tenderness |
| | R10.827 | Generalized rebound abdominal tenderness |

Acute gastroenteritis.
Appendicitis.
Constipation.
Cholecystitis, acute.
Intestinal obstruction.
Pancreatitis.
Neoplasm.
Inflammatory bowel disease.
Other:
   Functional abdominal pain.
   Pyelonephritis.
   Pneumonia.
   Diabetic ketoacidosis.
   Heavy metal poisoning.
   Sickle cell crisis.
   Trauma.
   Anxiety.
   Sexual abuse.

ABDOMINAL PAIN, CHRONIC LOWER[2]

ICD-10CM #	R10.814	Left lower quadrant abdominal tenderness
	R10.824	Left lower quadrant rebound abdominal tenderness
	R10.813	Right lower quadrant abdominal tenderness
	R10.823	Right lower quadrant rebound abdominal tenderness
	R10.30	Lower abdominal pain, unspecified

ORGANIC DISORDERS

Common
Gynecologic disease.
Lactase deficiency.
Diverticulitis/diverticulosis.
Crohn disease.
Intestinal obstruction.
Uncommon
Chronic intestinal pseudoobstruction.
Mesenteric ischemia.
Malignancy (e.g., ovarian carcinoma).
Abdominal wall pain.
Spinal disease.
Testicular disease.
Metabolic diseases (e.g., diabetes mellitus, familial Mediterranean fever, C1 esterase deficiency [angioneurotic edema], porphyria, lead poisoning, tabes dorsalis, renal failure).

FUNCTIONAL DISORDERS

Common
Irritable bowel syndrome.

Functional abdominal bloating.
Uncommon
Functional abdominal pain.

ABDOMINAL PAIN, DIFFUSE

| ICD-10CM # | R10.817 | Generalized abdominal tenderness |
| | R10.827 | Generalized rebound abdominal tenderness |

Early appendicitis.
Aortic aneurysm.
Gastroenteritis.
Intestinal obstruction.
Diverticulitis.
Peritonitis.
Mesenteric insufficiency or infarction.
Pancreatitis.
Inflammatory bowel disease.
Irritable bowel.
Mesenteric adenitis.
Metabolic: toxins, lead poisoning, uremia, drug overdose, diabetic ketoacidosis, heavy metal poisoning.
Sickle cell crisis.
Pneumonia (rare).
Trauma.
Urinary tract infection, pelvic inflammatory disease.
Other: anxiety, acute intermittent porphyria, tabes dorsalis, periarteritis nodosa, Henoch-Schönlein purpura, adrenal insufficiency.

ABDOMINAL PAIN, EPIGASTRIC

| ICD-10CM # | R10.816 | Epigastric abdominal tenderness |
| | R10.826 | Epigastric rebound abdominal tenderness |

Gastric: peptic ulcer disease, gastric outlet obstruction, gastric ulcer.
Duodenal: peptic ulcer disease, duodenitis.
Biliary: cholecystitis, cholangitis, biliary dyskinesia.
Hepatic: hepatitis.
Pancreatic: pancreatitis.
Intestinal: high small bowel obstruction, early appendicitis.
Cardiac: angina, myocardial infarction, pericarditis.
Pulmonary: pneumonia, pleurisy, pneumothorax.
Subphrenic abscess.
Vascular: dissecting aneurysm, mesenteric ischemia.
Psychiatric: anxiety.

ABDOMINAL PAIN, EXTRAABDOMINAL AND SYSTEMIC CAUSES[3]

| ICD-10CM # | R10.817 | Generalized abdominal tenderness |

Differential Diagnosis

II

EXTRAABDOMINAL AND SYSTEMIC CAUSES OF ACUTE ABDOMINAL PAIN

Cardiac
Endocarditis.
Heart failure.
Myocardial ischemia and infarction.
Myocarditis.

Thoracic
Empyema.
Esophageal rupture (Boerhaave syndrome).
Esophageal spasm.
Esophagitis.
Pleurodynia (Bornholm disease).
Pneumonitis.
Pneumothorax.
Pulmonary embolism and infarction.

Hematologic
Acute leukemia.
Hemolytic anemia.
Henoch-Schönlein purpura.
Sickle cell disease.

Metabolic
Acute adrenal insufficiency (Addison disease).
Diabetes mellitus (especially with ketoacidosis).
Hyperlipidemia.
Hyperparathyroidism.
Hypersensitivity reactions (e.g., to insect bites, reptile venoms).
Lead poisoning.
Porphyria.
Toxins.
Uremia.

Infections
Herpes zoster.
Osteomyelitis.
Typhoid fever.

Neurologic
Abdominal epilepsy.
Radiculopathy, spinal cord or peripheral nerve tumors, degenerative arthritis of spine, herniated vertebral disk.
Tabes dorsalis.

Miscellaneous
Angioedema.
Familial Mediterranean fever.
Heat stroke.
Muscle contusion, hematoma, tumor.
Narcotic withdrawal.
Psychiatric disorders.

ABDOMINAL PAIN, INFANCY[1]

ICD-10CM #		
	R10.817	Generalized abdominal tenderness
	R10.827	Generalized rebound abdominal tenderness

Acute gastroenteritis.
Appendicitis.
Intussusception.
Volvulus.
Meckel diverticulum.
Other: colic, trauma.

ABDOMINAL PAIN, LEFT LOWER QUADRANT

ICD-10CM #		
	R10.814	Left lower quadrant abdominal tenderness
	R10.824	Left lower quadrant rebound abdominal tenderness

Intestinal: diverticulitis, diverticulosis, intestinal obstruction, perforated ulcer, inflammatory bowel disease, perforated descending colon, inguinal hernia, neoplasm, appendicitis.
Reproductive: ectopic pregnancy, ovarian cyst, torsion of ovarian cyst, tuboovarian abscess, mittelschmerz, endometriosis, seminal vesiculitis.
Renal: renal or ureteral calculi, pyelonephritis, neoplasm.
Vascular: leaking aortic aneurysm.
Psoas abscess.
Trauma.

ABDOMINAL PAIN, LEFT UPPER QUADRANT

ICD-10CM #		
	R19.02	Left upper quadrant abdominal swelling, mass, and lump

Gastric: peptic ulcer disease, gastritis, pyloric stenosis, hiatal hernia.
Pancreatic: pancreatitis, neoplasm, stone in pancreatic duct or ampulla.
Cardiac: myocardial infarction, angina pectoris.
Splenic: splenomegaly, ruptured spleen, splenic abscess, splenic infarction.
Renal: calculi, pyelonephritis, neoplasm.
Pulmonary: pneumonia, empyema, pulmonary infarction.
Vascular: ruptured aortic aneurysm.
Cutaneous: herpes zoster.
Trauma.
Intestinal: high fecal impaction, perforated colon, diverticulitis.

ABDOMINAL PAIN, NONSURGICAL CAUSES

ICD-10CM #		
	R19.8	Other specified symptoms and signs involving the digestive system and abdomen
	R10.817	Generalized abdominal tenderness

Irritable bowel syndrome.
Urinary tract infection, pyelonephritis, salpingitis, pelvic inflammatory disease.
Gastroenteritis, gastritis, peptic ulcer.
Diverticular spasm.
Hepatitis, mononucleosis.
Pancreatitis.
Inferior wall myocardial infarction.
Basilar pneumonia, pulmonary embolism.
Diabetic ketoacidosis.
Strain or hematoma of rectus muscle.
Ruptured Graafian follicle.
Herpes zoster.

Nerve root compression.
Sickle cell crisis.
Acute adrenal insufficiency.
Other: acute porphyria, familial Mediterranean fever, tabes dorsalis, anxiety, sexual abuse.

ABDOMINAL PAIN, PERIUMBILICAL

ICD-10CM #		
	R10.815	Periumbilic abdominal tenderness
	R10.825	Periumbilic rebound abdominal tenderness

Intestinal: small bowel obstruction or gangrene, early appendicitis.
Vascular: mesenteric thrombosis, dissecting aortic aneurysm.
Pancreatic: pancreatitis.
Metabolic: uremia, diabetic ketoacidosis.
Trauma.

ABDOMINAL PAIN, POORLY LOCALIZED[1]

ICD-10CM #		
	R10.819	Abdominal tenderness, unspecified site

EXTRAABDOMINAL

Metabolic
Diabetic ketoacidosis, acute intermittent porphyria, hyperthyroidism, hypothyroidism, hypercalcemia, hypokalemia, uremia, hyperlipidemia, hyperparathyroidism.

Hematologic
Sickle cell crisis, leukemia or lymphoma, Henoch-Schönlein purpura.

Infectious
Infectious mononucleosis, Rocky Mountain spotted fever, acquired immunodeficiency syndrome (AIDS), streptococcal pharyngitis (in children), herpes zoster.

Drugs and Toxins
Heavy metal poisoning, black widow spider bites, withdrawal syndromes, mushroom ingestion.

Referred Pain
Pulmonary: pneumonia, pulmonary embolism, pneumothorax.
Cardiac: angina, myocardial infarction, pericarditis, myocarditis.
Genitourinary: prostatitis, epididymitis, orchitis, testicular torsion.
Musculoskeletal: rectus sheath hematoma.

Functional
Somatization disorder, malingering, hypochondriasis, Munchausen syndrome.

Intraabdominal
Early appendicitis, gastroenteritis, peritonitis, pancreatitis, abdominal aortic aneurysm, mesenteric insufficiency or infarction, intestinal obstruction, volvulus, ulcerative colitis.

ABDOMINAL PAIN, POST-CHOLECYSTECTOMY[3]

ICD-10CM #		
	R10.817	Generalized abdominal tenderness

CAUSES OF ABDOMINAL PAIN AFTER CHOLECYSTECTOMY

Biliary Causes
Biliary stricture.
Biliary tract malignancy.
Choledocholithiasis.
Choledochocele.
Cystic duct remnant.
Sphincter of Oddi dysfunction.

Pancreatic Causes
Pancreatitis.
Pseudocyst.
Malignancy.

Other GI Disorders
Esophageal motor disorders.
Gastroesophageal reflux disease.
Intestinal malignancy.
Intraabdominal adhesions.
IBS.
Mesenteric ischemia.
Peptic ulcer disease.

Extraintestinal Disorders
Coronary artery disease.
Intercostal neuritis.
Neurologic disorders.
Psychiatric disorders.
Wound neuroma.

ABDOMINAL PAIN, PREGNANT PATIENT[4]

ICD-10CM #	R10.817	Generalized abdominal tenderness

COMMON CAUSES OF ABDOMINAL PAIN IN PREGNANT PATIENTS

Right Upper Quadrant
Gastroesophageal reflux.
Peptic ulcer disease.
Acute cholecystitis.
Biliary colic.
Acute pancreatitis.
Hepatitis.
Acute fatty liver of pregnancy.
HELLP syndrome.
Preeclampsia.
Pneumothorax.
Pneumonia.
Acute appendicitis.
Hepatic adenoma.
Hemangioma.

Right Lower Quadrant
Acute appendicitis.
Ectopic pregnancy.
Renal or ureteral colic.
Pelvic inflammatory disease.
Tuboovarian abscess.
Endometriosis.
Adnexal torsion.
Ruptured ovarian cyst.
Ruptured corpus luteum.

Lower Abdomen
Threatened, incomplete, or complete abortion.
Abruptio placentae.
Preterm labor.
Pelvic inflammatory disease.
Tuboovarian abscess.
Inflammatory bowel disease.
Irritable bowel syndrome.
Pyelonephritis.

Flank
Pyelonephritis.
Hydronephrosis of pregnancy.
Acute appendicitis (retrocecal appendix).

Diffuse Abdominal Pain
Early acute appendicitis.
Small bowel obstruction.
Acute intermittent porphyria.
Sickle cell crisis.

HELLP, Hemolysis, elevated liver enzymes, low platelets.

ABDOMINAL PAIN, RIGHT LOWER QUADRANT

ICD-10CM #	R10.813	Right lower quadrant abdominal tenderness
	R10.823	Right lower quadrant rebound abdominal tenderness

Intestinal: acute appendicitis, regional enteritis, incarcerated hernia, cecal diverticulitis, intestinal obstruction, perforated ulcer, perforated cecum, Meckel diverticulitis.
Reproductive: ectopic pregnancy, ovarian cyst, torsion of ovarian cyst, salpingitis, tuboovarian abscess, mittelschmerz, endometriosis, seminal vesiculitis.
Renal: renal and ureteral calculi, neoplasms, pyelonephritis.
Vascular: leaking aortic aneurysm.
Cutaneous: herpes zoster.
Psoas abscess.
Trauma.
Cholecystitis.

ABDOMINAL PAIN, RIGHT UPPER QUADRANT

ICD-10CM #	R10.811	Right upper quadrant abdominal tenderness
	R10.821	Right upper quadrant rebound abdominal tenderness

Biliary: calculi, infection, inflammation, neoplasm.
Hepatic: hepatitis, abscess, hepatic congestion, neoplasm, trauma.
Gastric: peptic ulcer disease, pyloric stenosis, neoplasm, alcoholic gastritis, hiatal hernia.
Pancreatic: pancreatitis, neoplasm, stone in pancreatic duct or ampulla.
Renal: calculi, infection, inflammation, neoplasm, rupture of kidney.
Pulmonary: pneumonia, pulmonary infarction, right-sided pleurisy.
Intestinal: retrocecal appendicitis, intestinal obstruction, high fecal impaction, diverticulitis.

Cardiac: myocardial ischemia (particularly involving the inferior wall), pericarditis.
Cutaneous: herpes zoster.
Trauma.
Fitz-Hugh-Curtis syndrome (perihepatitis).

ABDOMINAL PAIN, SUPRAPUBIC

ICD-10CM #	R10.30	Lower abdominal pain, unspecified

Intestinal: colon obstruction or gangrene, diverticulitis, appendicitis.
Reproductive system: ectopic pregnancy, mittelschmerz, torsion of ovarian cyst, pelvic inflammatory disease, salpingitis, endometriosis, rupture of endometrioma.
Cystitis, rupture of urinary bladder.

ABDOMINAL WALL MASSES[2]

ICD-10CM #	R19.00	Intraabdominal and pelvic swelling, mass and lump, unspecified site

LUMPS ARISING IN THE SKIN AND SUBCUTANEOUS FAT (THAT COULD OCCUR ANYWHERE ON THE BODY)
Lipoma.
Sebaceous cyst.

LUMPS ARISING IN THE SKIN AND SUBCUTANEOUS FAT (SPECIFIC TO THE ANTERIOR ABDOMINAL WALL)
Tumor nodule of the umbilicus (secondary to the intraperitoneal malignancy, also called *Sister Mary Joseph nodule*).

LUMPS ARISING IN THE FASCIA AND MUSCLE
Rectus sheath hematoma (usually painful).
Desmoid tumor (associated with Gardner syndrome).

HERNIA

Incisional: It has an overlying scar. The sac may be very much larger than the neck of the hernia.

Umbilical: The hernia is through the umbilical scar. Those presenting at birth commonly resolve in the first years of life.

Paraumbilical: The neck is just lateral to the umbilical scar. Patients usually present later in life.

Epigastric: It occurs in the midline between the xiphoid process and the umbilicus. They are usually small (<2 cm). They result when a knuckle of extraperitoneal fat extrudes through a small defect in the linea alba. Commonly irreducible and without an expansile cough impulse.

Spigelian: A rare hernia found along the linea semilunaris at the lateral edge of the rectus sheath, most commonly a third of the way between the umbilicus and the pubis.

DIVARICATION OF THE RECTI

Supraumbilical elliptical swelling of the attenuated linea alba (no cough impulse).

ABORTION, RECURRENT

ICD-10CM #	P01.8	Newborn (suspected to be) affected by other maternal complications of pregnancy

Congenital anatomic abnormalities.
Adhesions (uterine synechiae).
Uterine fibroids.
Endometriosis.
Endocrine abnormalities (luteal phase insufficiency, hypothyroidism, uncontrolled diabetes mellitus [DM]).
Parenteral chromosome abnormalities.
Maternal infections (cervical Mycoplasma, Ureaplasma, Chlamydia).
Diethylstilbestrol exposure, heavy metal exposure.
Thrombocytosis.
Allogenic immunity, autoimmunity, lupus anticoagulant.

ACALCULOUS GALLBLADDER DISEASE[5]

ICD-10CM #	K82.9	Other diseases of gallbladder

Biliary tract anomaly (e.g., choledochal cyst).
Bone marrow transplant.
Burns.
Chemotherapy in oncology patients.
Critical illness in intensive care unit patients.
Crohn disease, Henoch-Schönlein purpura, Kawasaki disease, systemic lupus erythematosus.
Infectious agents (atypical microbes).
Microlithiasis.
Postoperative state (e.g., cardiac surgery).
Sepsis.
Sludge.
Systemic inflammatory states.
Total parenteral nutrition.
Traumatic spinal cord injury.

ACHES AND PAINS, DIFFUSE[6]

ICD-10CM #	M25.50	Pain in unspecified joint

Postviral arthralgias/myalgias.
Bilateral soft tissue rheumatism.
Overuse syndromes.
Fibrositis.
Hypothyroidism.
Metabolic bone disease.
Paraneoplastic syndrome.
Myopathy (polymyositis, dermatomyositis).
Rheumatoid arthritis.
Sjögren syndrome.
Polymyalgia rheumatica.

Hypermobility.
Benign arthralgias/myalgias.
Chronic fatigue syndrome.
Hypophosphatemia.

ACIDOSIS, HYPERCHLOREMIC METABOLIC[7]

ICD-10CM #	E87.2	Acidosis

GI BICARBONATE LOSS

Diarrhea.
External pancreatic or small bowel drainage.
Ureterosigmoidostomy, jejunal loop.
Drugs:
  Calcium chloride (acidifying agent).
  Magnesium sulfate (diarrhea).
  Cholestyramine (bile acid diarrhea).

RENAL ACIDOSIS

Hypokalemic
Proximal renal tubular acidosis (RTA) (type 2).
Distal (classic) RTA (type 1).
Drug-induced hypokalemia:
  Acetazolamide (proximal RTA).
  Amphotericin B (distal RTA).

Hyperkalemic
Generalized distal nephron dysfunction (type 4 RTA).
Mineralocorticoid deficiency or resistance (pseudohypoaldosteronism type 1) PHA-I, PHA-II.
$\downarrow Na^+$ delivery to distal nephron.
Tubulointerstitial disease.
Ammonium excretion defect.
Drug-induced hyperkalemia:
  Potassium-sparing diuretics (amiloride, triamterene, spironolactone).
  Trimethoprim.
  Pentamidine.
  ACE inhibitors and angiotensin II receptor blockers.
  NSAIDs.
  Cyclosporine, tacrolimus.

Normokalemic
Early renal insufficiency.

Other
Acid loads (ammonium chloride, hyperalimentation).
Loss of potential bicarbonate: ketosis with ketone excretion.
Dilution acidosis (rapid saline administration).
Hippurate.
Cation-exchange resins.

ACIDOSIS, LACTIC[7]

ICD-10CM #	E87.2	Acidosis

CAUSES OF LACTIC ACIDOSIS

L-Lactic Acidosis
Conditions associated with type A lactic acidosis:
Poor tissue perfusion.
Shock:
  Cardiogenic.
  Hemorrhagic.
  Septic.
Profound hypoxemia:
  Severe asthma.
  Carbon monoxide poisoning.
Conditions associated with type B lactic acidosis:
  Liver disease.

Metformin.
Inborn errors of metabolism.
Pyroglutamic acidosis.
Kombucha tea.

D-Lactic Acidosis
Short bowel syndrome.
Ischemic bowel.
Small bowel obstruction.

ACIDOSIS, METABOLIC

ICD-10CM #	E87.2	Acidosis

METABOLIC ACIDOSIS WITH INCREASED ANION GAP (AG ACIDOSIS)

Lactic acidosis.
Ketoacidosis (diabetes mellitus, alcoholic ketoacidosis).
Uremia (chronic renal failure).
Ingestion of toxins (paraldehyde, methanol, salicylate, ethylene glycol).
High-fat diet (mild acidosis).

METABOLIC ACIDOSIS WITH NORMAL AG (HYPERCHLOREMIC ACIDOSIS)

Renal tubular acidosis (including acidosis of aldosterone deficiency).
Intestinal loss of HCO_3^- (diarrhea, pancreatic fistula).
Carbonic anhydrase inhibitors (e.g., acetazolamide).
Dilutional acidosis (as a result of rapid infusion of bicarbonate-free isotonic saline).
Ingestion of exogenous acids (ammonium chloride, methionine, cystine, calcium chloride).
Ileostomy.
Ureterosigmoidostomy.
Drugs: amiloride, triamterene, spironolactone, β-blockers.

ACIDOSIS, RESPIRATORY

ICD-10CM #	E87.2	Acidosis

Pulmonary disease (chronic obstructive pulmonary disease, severe pneumonia, pulmonary edema, interstitial fibrosis).
Airway obstruction (foreign body, severe bronchospasm, laryngospasm).
Thoracic cage disorders (pneumothorax, flail chest, kyphoscoliosis).
Defects in muscles of respiration (myasthenia gravis, hypokalemia, muscular dystrophy).
Defects in peripheral nervous system (amyotrophic lateral sclerosis, poliomyelitis, Guillain-Barré syndrome, botulism, tetanus, organophosphate poisoning, spinal cord injury).
Depression of respiratory center (anesthesia, narcotics, sedatives, vertebral artery embolism or thrombosis, increased intracranial pressure).
Failure of mechanical ventilator.

ACUTE KIDNEY INJURY AND LIVER DISEASE, CAUSES[8,9]

ICD-10CM #	S37.009A	Unspecified injury of unspecified kidney, initial encounter
	K76.89	Other specified diseases of liver

Prerenal uremia:	Diuretic use, GI loss, peritoneal aspiration, hypoalbuminemia.
Hepatorenal syndrome.	
Acute tubular necrosis:	Hyperbilirubinemia, sepsis, toxic shock syndrome.
Drugs:	Acetaminophen (paracetamol), NSAIDs, tetracycline, rifampicin, isoniazid, anesthetic agents, sulfonamides, allopurinol, methotrexate.
Infections:	Hepatitis C and cryoglobulinemia, hepatitis B and polyarteritis nodosa, leptospirosis, hantavirus, Epstein-Barr virus, gram-negative sepsis, spontaneous bacterial peritonitis.
Other:	Papillary necrosis and obstruction, inhalation of chlorinated hydrocarbons, mushroom poisoning (Amanita phalloides).

ACUTE KIDNEY INJURY DUE TO INTRINSIC RENAL DISEASES[10]

ICD-10CM # Varies with specific diagnosis

INTRINSIC RENAL DISEASES THAT CAUSE ACUTE KIDNEY INJURY

Vascular Diseases
Large-Vessel Diseases
Renal artery thrombosis or stenosis.
Renal vein thrombosis.
Atheroembolic disease.
Small- and Medium-Vessel Diseases
Scleroderma.
Malignant hypertension.
Hemolytic uremic syndrome.
Thrombotic thrombocytopenic purpura.
HIV-associated microangiopathy.

Glomerular Diseases
Systemic Diseases
Systemic lupus erythematosus.
Infective endocarditis.
Systemic vasculitis (e.g., periarteritis nodosa, granulomatosis with polyangiitis).
Henoch-Schönlein purpura.
HIV-associated nephropathy.
Essential mixed cryoglobulinemia.
Goodpasture syndrome.
Primary Renal Diseases
Poststreptococcal glomerulonephritis.
Other postinfectious glomerulonephritis.
Rapidly progressive glomerulonephritis.

Tubulointerstitial Diseases and Conditions
Drugs (many).
Toxins (e.g., heavy metals, ethylene glycol).
Infections.
Multiple myeloma.

Acute Tubular Necrosis
Ischemia
Shock.
Sepsis.
Severe prerenal azotemia.

Nephrotoxins
Antibiotics.
Radiographic contrast agents.
Myoglobinuria.
Hemoglobinuria.
Other Diseases and Conditions
Severe liver disease.
Allergic reactions.
NSAIDs.

ACUTE KIDNEY INJURY, HIV PATIENT, CAUSES[8,9]

ICD-10CM # S37.009A Unspecified injury of unspecified kidney, initial encounter with B20 human immunodeficiency virus (HIV) disease

Prerenal:	Diarrhea, nausea and vomiting, cirrhosis and hepatorenal syndrome, sepsis.
Vascular:	Thrombotic microangiopathy.
Glomerular:	Immune complex glomerulonephritis (MPGN secondary to hepatitis C virus, postinfectious glomerulonephritis), HIVAN.
Acute tubular necrosis:	Sepsis, hypotension, nephrotoxins (aminoglycosides, amphotericin, acyclovir, cidofovir, tenofovir, pentamidine).
Acute interstitial nephritis:	Drug-induced (co-trimoxazole), rifampicin, foscarnet, nevirapine), CMV infection, DILS.
Drug-induced intratubular obstruction:	Sulfadiazine, indinavir, foscarnet, acyclovir.
Postrenal obstruction:	Stones, tuberculosis, fungal ball, tumor.
Associated with IV drug use:	Sepsis, endocarditis, heroin-associated nephropathy (FSGS), rhabdomyolysis.

CMV, Cytomegalovirus; *DILS*, diffusive infiltrative lymphocytosis syndrome; *FSGS*, focal segmental glomerulosclerosis; *HIVAN*, HIV-associated nephropathy; *MPGN*, membranoproliferative glomerulonephritis.

ACUTE KIDNEY INJURY IN SPECIFIC CLINICAL SETTINGS[11]

ICD-10CM # N17.9 Acute kidney failure, unspecified

MAJOR CAUSES OF ACUTE KIDNEY INJURY IN SPECIFIC CLINICAL SETTINGS

AKI in the Cancer Patient
Prerenal azotemia:
Hypovolemia (e.g., poor intake, vomiting, diarrhea).
Intrinsic AKI:
Exogenous nephrotoxins: chemotherapy, antibiotics, contrast media.

Endogenous toxins: hyperuricemia, hypercalcemia, tumor lysis, paraproteins.
Other: radiation, HUS/TTP, glomerulonephritis, amyloid, malignant infiltration.
Postrenal AKI:
Ureteric or bladder neck obstruction.
AKI after Cardiac Surgery
Prerenal azotemia:
Hypovolemia (surgical losses, diuretics), cardiac failure, vasodilators.
Intrinsic AKI:
Ischemic ATN (even in absence of hypotension).
Atheroembolic disease after aortic manipulation/intraaortic balloon pump.
Preoperative or perioperative administration of contrast medium.
Allergic interstitial nephritis induced by perioperative antibiotics.
Postrenal AKI:
Obstructed urinary catheter, exacerbation of voiding dysfunction.
AKI in Pregnancy
Prerenal azotemia:
Acute fatty liver of pregnancy with fulminant hepatic failure.
Intrinsic AKI:
Preeclampsia or eclampsia.
Postpartum HUS/TTP.
HELLP syndrome.
Ischemia: postpartum hemorrhage, abruptio placentae, amniotic fluid embolus.
Direct toxicity of illegal abortifacients.
Postrenal AKI:
Obstruction with pyelonephritis.
AKI after Solid Organ or Bone Marrow Transplantation
Prerenal azotemia:
Intravascular volume depletion (e.g., diuretic therapy).
Vasoactive drugs (e.g., calcineurin inhibitors, amphotericin B).
Hepatorenal syndrome, venoocclusive disease of liver (BMT).
Intrinsic AKI:
Postoperative ischemic ATN (even in absence of hypotension).
Sepsis.
Exogenous nephrotoxins: aminoglycosides, amphotericin B, radiocontrast media.
HUS/TTP (e.g., cyclosporine or myeloablative radiotherapy related).
Allergic tubulointerstitial nephritis.
Postrenal AKI:
Obstructed urinary catheter.
AKI and Pulmonary Disease (Pulmonary Renal Syndrome)
Prerenal azotemia:
Diminished cardiac output complicating pulmonary embolism, severe pulmonary hypertension, or positive-pressure mechanical ventilation.
Intrinsic AKI:
Vasculitis.
Goodpasture syndrome, ANCA-associated vasculitis, SLE, eosinophilic granulomatosis with polyangiitis, polyarteritis nodosa, cryoglobulinemia, right-sided endocarditis, lymphomatoid granulomatosis, sarcoidosis, scleroderma.

Differential Diagnosis

II

Toxins:
  Ingestion of paraquat or diquat.
Infections:
  Legionnaires disease, *Mycoplasma* infection, tuberculosis, disseminated viral or fungal infection.
  AKI from any cause with hypervolemia and pulmonary edema.
  Lung cancer with hypercalcemia, tumor lysis, or glomerulonephritis.

AKI and Liver Disease
Prerenal azotemia:
  Reduced true (GI hemorrhage, GI losses from lactulose, diuretics, large-volume paracentesis) circulatory volume or effective (hypoalbuminemia, splanchnic vasodilation).
  Hepatorenal syndrome type 1 or 2.
  Tense ascites with abdominal compartment syndrome.
Intrinsic AKI:
  Ischemic (severe hypoperfusion—see earlier) or direct nephrotoxicity and hepatotoxicity of drugs or toxins (e.g., carbon tetrachloride, acetaminophen, tetracyclines, methoxyflurane).
  Tubulointerstitial nephritis plus hepatitis caused by drugs (e.g., sulfonamides, rifampin, phenytoin, allopurinol, phenindione), infections (leptospirosis, brucellosis, Epstein-Barr virus infection, cytomegalovirus infection), malignant infiltration (leukemia, lymphoma), or sarcoidosis.
  Glomerulonephritis or vasculitis (e.g., polyarteritis nodosa, ANCA-associated glomerulonephritis, cryoglobulinemia, SLE, postinfectious hepatitis or liver abscess).

AKI and Nephrotic Syndrome
Prerenal azotemia:
  Intravascular volume depletion (diuretic therapy, hypoalbuminemia).
Intrinsic AKI:
  Manifestation of primary glomerular disease.
  Collapsing glomerulopathy (e.g., HIV, pamidronate).
  Associated ATN (older hypertensive males).
  Associated interstitial nephritis (NSAIDs, rifampin, interferon alfa).
Other: amyloid or light-chain deposition disease, renal vein thrombosis, severe interstitial edema.

AKI, Acute kidney injury; *ANCA,* antineutrophil cytoplasmic antibody; *ATN,* acute tubular necrosis; *BMT,* bone marrow transplantation; *HELLP,* hemolysis, elevated liver enzymes, low platelets; *HUS,* hemolytic uremic syndrome; *SLE,* systemic lupus erythematosus; *TTP,* thrombotic thrombocytopenic purpura.

ACUTE KIDNEY INJURY, PIGMENT INDUCED[10]

ICD-10CM # Varies with specific diagnosis

CAUSES OF PIGMENT-INDUCED ACUTE KIDNEY INJURY
Rhabdomyolysis and myoglobinuria.
Vigorous exercise.
Arterial embolization.
Status epilepticus.
Status asthmaticus.

Coma-induced and pressure-induced myonecrosis.
Heat stress.
Diabetic ketoacidosis.
Myopathy.
Alcoholism.
Hypokalemia.
Hypophosphatemia.
Hemoglobinuria.
Transfusion reactions.
Snake envenomation.
Malaria.
Mechanical destruction of RBCs by prosthetic valves.
G6PD deficiency.

G6PD, Glucose-6-phosphate dehydrogenase; *RBCs,* red blood cells.

ACUTE LIVER FAILURE[12]

ICD-10CM # K71.01 Toxic liver disease with hepatic necrosis

DIFFERENTIAL DIAGNOSIS OF ACUTE LIVER FAILURE

Viruses	Hepatitis A and B viruses (typical viruses causing viral hepatitis).
	Hepatitis C virus (rare).
	Hepatitis D virus.
	Hepatitis E virus (often in pregnant women in endemic areas).
	Cytomegalovirus.
	Hemorrhagic fever viruses.
	Herpes simplex virus.
	Paramyxovirus.
	Epstein-Barr virus.
Drugs	Paracetamol hepatotoxicity.
	Idiosyncratic hypersensitivity reactions (e.g., isoniazid, statins, halothane).
	Illicit drugs (e.g., Ecstasy, cocaine).
	Alternative medicines (e.g., chaparral and Teucrium polium), traditional Chinese medicine.
Toxins	Mushroom poisoning (usually *Amanita phalloides*).
	Bacillus cereus toxin.
	Cyanobacteria toxin.
	Organic solvents (e.g., carbon tetrachloride).
	Yellow phosphorus.
Vasculopathy	Ischemic hepatitis.
	Hepatic vein thrombosis (Budd-Chiari syndrome).
	Hepatic venoocclusive disease.
	Portal vein thrombosis.
	Hepatic arterial thrombosis.
Metabolic	Acute fatty liver of pregnancy/hemolysis, elevated liver enzymes, low platelet count (HELLP) syndrome.
	α_1-antitrypsin deficiency.
	Fructose intolerance.
	Galactosemia.
	Lecithin-cholesterol acyltransferase deficiency.
	Reye syndrome.
	Tyrosinemia.
	Wilson disease.

Autoimmune	Autoimmune hepatitis.
Malignancy	Primary liver malignancy (hepatocellular carcinoma or cholangiocarcinoma).
	Secondary (e.g., extensive hepatic metastases or infiltration of adenocarcinoma).
Miscellaneous	Adult-onset Still disease.
	Heat stroke.
	Primary graft nonfunction (in liver transplant recipients).
	Indeterminate etiology (~20% of acute liver failure cases).

ACUTE LUNG INJURY, DISEASE AND DISORDER ASSOCIATIONS[13]

ICD-10CM # S27.3 Injury, lung

CLINICAL DISORDERS ASSOCIATED WITH ACUTE LUNG INJURY

Infectious Causes
Gram-negative or gram-positive sepsis.
Bacterial pneumonia.
Viral pneumonia.
Fungal pneumonia.
Parasitic infections.
Mycobacterial disease.

Aspiration
Gastric acid.
Food and other particulate matter.
Fresh or sea water (near drowning).
Hydrocarbon fluids.

Trauma
Lung contusion.
Fat emboli.
Nonthoracic trauma.
Thermal injury (burns).
Blast injury (explosion, lightning).
Overdistention (mechanical ventilation).
Inhaled gases (phosgene, ammonia).

Hemodynamic Disturbances
Shock of any etiology.
Anaphylaxis.
High-altitude pulmonary edema.
Reperfusion.
Air embolism.
Amniotic fluid embolism.

Drugs
Heroin.
Methadone.
Propoxyphene.
Naloxone.
Cocaine.
Barbiturates.
Colchicine.
Salicylates.
Ethchlorvynol.
Interleukin-2.
Protamine.
Hydrochlorothiazide.

Hematologic Disorders
Disseminated intravascular coagulation.
Incompatible blood transfusion.
Rh incompatibility.
Antileukocyte antibodies.
Leucoagglutinin reactions.
Postcardiopulmonary bypass, pump oxygenator.

Metabolic Disorders
Pancreatitis.
Diabetic ketoacidosis.
Neurologic Disorders
Head trauma.
Grand mal seizures.
Increased intracranial pressure (any cause).
Subarachnoid or intracerebral hemorrhage.
Miscellaneous Disorders
Lung reexpansion.
Upper airway obstruction.

ACUTE RESPIRATORY DISTRESS IN PREGNANCY[14]

ICD-10CM #	J96.00	Acute respiratory failure

Disorder	Distinguishing Features
Pregnancy-Specific	
Amniotic fluid embolism:	Cardiorespiratory collapse, seizures, DIC.
Pulmonary edema secondary to preeclampsia:	Hypertension, proteinuria.
ARDS secondary to obstetric sepsis:	Evidence of obstetric sepsis, shock.
Tocolytic pulmonary edema:	Tocolytic administration, rapid improvement.
Peripartum cardiomyopathy:	Gradual onset, cardiac gallop, cardiomegaly.
Trophoblastic embolism:	Nodular infiltrate, molar pregnancy.
Risk Increased by Pregnancy	
Aspiration pneumonitis:	Vomiting, aspiration.
Venous thromboembolism:	Evidence of DVT, positive V̇/Q̇ scan, leg Doppler, CT angiogram.
Pneumomediastinum:	Occurs during delivery, subcutaneous emphysema.
Valvular heart disease:	Pulmonary edema, cardiac murmur, cardiomegaly.
ARDS secondary to sepsis:	Evidence of sepsis (e.g., pyelonephritis).
Unrelated to Pregnancy	
Asthma:	Features similar to nonpregnant patient.
Pneumonia:	Features similar to nonpregnant patient.

ARDS, Acute respiratory distress syndrome; *CT,* computed tomography; *DIC,* disseminated intravascular coagulopathy; *DVT,* deep venous thrombosis; *V̇/Q̇,* ventilation-perfusion.

ACUTE SCROTUM

ICD-10CM #	R10.2	Pelvic and perineal pain

Testicular torsion.
Epididymitis.
Testicular neoplasm.
Orchitis.
Trauma.

ADNEXAL MASS[1]

ICD-10CM #	R19.00	Intraabdominal and pelvic swelling, mass and lump, unspecified site

Ovary (neoplasm, endometriosis, functional cyst).
Fallopian tube (ectopic pregnancy, neoplasm, tubo-ovarian abscess, hydrosalpinx, paratubal cyst).
Uterus (fibroid, neoplasm).
Retroperitoneum (neoplasm, abdominal wall hematoma or abscess).
Urinary tract (pelvic kidney, distended bladder, urachal cyst).
Inflammatory bowel disease.
GI tract neoplasm.
Diverticular disease.
Appendicitis.
Bowel loop with feces.

ADRENAL CALCIFICATIONS[15]

ICD-10CM #	E27.8	Other specified disorder of adrenal gland

CAUSES OF ADRENAL CALCIFICATION

Infection:
  Tuberculosis.
  Histoplasmosis.
  Echinococcus.
Prior hemorrhage.
Neoplasm:
  Adrenocortical carcinoma.
  Myelolipoma.
  Pheochromocytoma.
Hemangioma (rare).

ADRENAL CYSTIC LESIONS[15]

ICD-10CM #	E27.8	Other specified disorder of adrenal gland

CYSTIC ADRENAL LESIONS

Pseudocyst.
Endothelial cyst.
Epithelial cyst.
Infection (*Echinococcus,* abscess).
Necrotic neoplasm.
Cystic pheochromocytoma.
Lymphangioma.

ADRENAL INSUFFICIENCY, CRITICALLY ILL PATIENT[16]

ICD-10CM #	E27.40	Unspecified adrenocortical insufficiency

CAUSES OF ADRENAL INSUFFICIENCY IN CRITICALLY ILL PATIENTS

Reversible Dysfunction of the HPA Axis
Sepsis/septic shock.
Acute lung injury.
Burns.
Pancreatitis.
Liver failure.
Hypothermia.

Drugs:
  Etomidate (primary AI).
  Corticosteroids (secondary AI).
  Ketoconazole (primary AI).
  Megestrol acetate (secondary AI).
  Rifampin (increased cortisol metabolism).
  Phenytoin (increased cortisol metabolism).
  Metyrapone (primary AI).
  Mitotane (primary AI).
Primary Adrenal Insufficiency (Adrenal Failure)
Autoimmune adrenalitis.
  HIV infection:
    HART therapy.
    HIV virus.
    CMV.
  Metastatic carcinoma:
    Lung.
    Breast.
    Kidney.
  Systemic fungal infection:
    Histoplasmosis.
    Cryptococcus.
    Blastomycosis.
    Tuberculosis.
  Adrenal hemorrhage/infarction:
    DIC.
    Meningococcemia.
    Anticoagulation.
    Antiphospholipid syndrome.
    HIT.
    Trauma.

AI, Adrenal insufficiency; *CMV,* cytomegalovirus; *DIC,* disseminated intravascular coagulation; *HIT,* heparin-induced thrombocytopenia; *HPA,* hypothalamic-pituitary axis.

ADRENAL MASSES[17]

ICD-10CM #	C74.90	Malignant neoplasm of unspecified part of unspecified adrenal gland
	E27.8	Other specified disorders of adrenal gland

UNILATERAL ADRENAL MASSES

Functional Lesions
Adrenal adenoma.
Adrenal carcinoma.
Pheochromocytoma.
Primary aldosteronism, adenomatous type.
Nonfunctional Lesions
Incidentaloma of adrenal.
Ganglioneuroma.
Myelolipoma.
Hematoma.
Adenolipoma.
Metastasis.

BILATERAL ADRENAL MASSES

Functional Lesions
Adrenocorticotropin hormone (ACTH) – dependent Cushing syndrome.
Congenital adrenal hyperplasia.
Pheochromocytoma.
Conn syndrome, hyperplastic variety.
Micronodular adrenal disease.
Idiopathic bilateral adrenal hypertrophy.

Nonfunctional Lesions
Infection (tuberculosis, fungi).
Infiltration (leukemia, lymphoma).
Replacement (amyloidosis).
Hemorrhage.
Bilateral metastases.

ADRENAL PSEUDOMASSES[15]

| ICD-10CM # | E27.8 | Other specified disorder of adrenal gland |

Thickened diaphragmatic crus.
Accessory spleen.
Gastric fundus.
Gastric diverticulum.
Renal vein.
Retrocrural and retroperitoneal adenopathy.
Upper-pole renal cysts and tumors.
Pancreatic tumors.
Hypertrophied caudate lobe of liver.
Fluid-filled colon interposed between stomach and kidney.

ADRENERGIC TOXIDROME[16]

| ICD-10CM # | T44.8X1S | Poisoning by centrally acting and adrenergic-neuron-blocking agents, accidental (unintentional), sequela |

COMMON CAUSES OF THE ADRENERGIC TOXIDROME

Recreational drugs:
 Cocaine.
 Amphetamines and other "designer drugs"; "Ecstasy" (3,4-methylenedioxymethamphetamine [MDMA]); 3,4-methylenedioxyamphetamine (MDA); 3,4-methylenedioxyethylamphetamine (MDEA); paramethoxyamphetamine (PMA); methamphetamine.
β_1-Adrenergic agents:
 Salbutamol.
 Theophylline.
Inotropic agents:
 Norepinephrine.
 Epinephrine.
 Isoproterenol.
Over-the-counter cough and cold preparations and nasal decongestants:
 Phenylpropanolamine.
 Pseudoephedrine.
Amphetamine-like agents prescribed for ADD or weight loss:
 Methylphenidate.
 Dextroamphetamine.
Psychostimulants.

ADD, Attention deficit disorder.

ADRENOCORTICAL HYPERFUNCTION[18]

| ICD-10CM # | E26.9 | Hyperaldosteronism, unspecified |

SYNDROMES OF ADRENOCORTICAL HYPERFUNCTION

States of Glucocorticoid Excess
Physiologic States
Stress.
Strenuous exercise.
Last trimester of pregnancy.
Pathologic States
Psychiatric conditions (pseudo-Cushing disorders):
 Depression.
 Alcoholism.
 Anorexia nervosa.
 Panic disorders.
 Alcohol and drug withdrawal.
ACTH-dependent states:
 Pituitary adenoma (Cushing disease).
 Ectopic ACTH syndrome.
 Bronchial carcinoid.
 Thymic carcinoid.
 Islet cell tumor.
 Small cell lung carcinoma.
 Ectopic CRH secretion.
ACTH-independent states:
 Adrenal adenoma.
 Adrenal carcinoma.
 Micronodular adrenal disease.
Exogenous Sources
Glucocorticoid intake.
ACTH intake.
States of Mineralocorticoid Excess
Primary Aldosteronism
Aldosterone-secreting adenoma.
Bilateral adrenal hyperplasia.
Aldosterone-secreting carcinoma.
Glucocorticoid-suppressible hyperaldosteronism.
Adrenal Enzyme Deficiencies
11b-Hydroxylase deficiency.
17a-Hydroxylase deficiency.
11b-Hydroxysteroid dehydrogenase, type II.
Exogenous Mineralocorticoids
Licorice.
Carbenoxolone.
Fludrocortisone.
Secondary Hyperaldosteronism
Associated with hypertension:
 Accelerated hypertension.
 Renovascular hypertension.
 Estrogen administration.
 Renin-secreting tumors.
Without hypertension:
 Bartter syndrome.
 Sodium-wasting nephropathy.
 Renal tubular acidosis.
 Diuretic and laxative abuse.
 Edematous states (cirrhosis, nephrosis, congestive heart failure).

ACTH, Adrenocorticotropin hormone; CRH, corticotropin-releasing hormone.

ADRENOCORTICAL HYPOFUNCTION

| ICD-10CM # | E27.49 | Other adrenocortical insufficiency |

SYNDROMES OF ADRENOCORTICAL HYPOFUNCTION

Primary Adrenal Disorders
Combined Glucocorticoid and Mineralocorticoid Deficiency
Autoimmune:
 Isolated autoimmune disease (Addison disease).
 Polyglandular autoimmune syndrome, type I.
 Polyglandular autoimmune syndrome, type II.
Infectious:
 Tuberculosis.
 Fungal.
 Cytomegalovirus.
 HIV.
Vascular:
 Bilateral adrenal hemorrhage.
 Sepsis.
 Coagulopathy.
 Thrombosis; embolism.
 Adrenal infarction.
Infiltration:
 Metastatic carcinoma and lymphoma.
 Sarcoidosis.
 Amyloidosis.
 Hemochromatosis.
Congenital:
 Congenital adrenal hyperplasia.
  21-Hydroxylase deficiency.
  3b-o1 Dehydrogenase deficiency.
  20,22-Desmolase deficiency.
 Adrenal unresponsiveness to ACTH.
 Congenital adrenal hypoplasia.
 Adrenoleukodystrophy.
 Adrenomyeloneuropathy.
Iatrogenic
Bilateral adrenalectomy.
Drugs:
 Metyrapone, aminoglutethimide, trilostane, ketoconazole, o,p'-DDD, mifepristone.
Mineralocorticoid Deficiency without Glucocorticoid Deficiency
Corticosterone methyl oxidase deficiency.
Isolated zona glomerulosa defect.
Heparin therapy.
Critical illness.
Converting-enzyme inhibitors.
Secondary Adrenal Disorders
Secondary Adrenal Insufficiency
Hypothalamic-pituitary dysfunction.
Exogenous glucocorticoids.
After removal of an ACTH-secreting tumor.
Hyporeninemic Hypoaldosteronism
Diabetic nephropathy.
Tubulointerstitial diseases.
Obstructive uropathy.
Autonomic neuropathy.
Nonsteroidal antiinflammatory drugs.
β-Adrenergic drugs.

ACTH, Adrenocorticotropic hormone.

ADVERSE FOOD REACTIONS, DIFFERENTIAL DIAGNOSIS[19]

| ICD-10CM # | T78.1XXA | Other adverse food reactions, not elsewhere classified, initial encounter |

GI DISORDERS (WITH VOMITING AND/OR DIARRHEA)

Structural abnormalities (pyloric stenosis, Hirschsprung disease).
Enzyme deficiencies (primary or secondary):
 Disaccharidase deficiency: lactase, fructose, sucrase-isomaltase.
 Galactosemia.
Other: pancreatic insufficiency (cystic fibrosis), peptic disease.

CONTAMINANTS AND ADDITIVES

Flavorings and preservatives—rarely cause symptoms: sodium metabisulfite, monosodium glutamate, nitrites.
Dyes and colorings—very rarely cause symptoms (urticaria, eczema): tartrazine.
Toxins: bacterial, fungal (aflatoxin), fish-related (scombroid, ciguatera).
Infectious organisms:
 Bacteria (Salmonella, Escherichia coli, Shigella).
 Virus (rotavirus, enterovirus).
Parasites (Giardia, Anisakis simplex [in fish]).
Accidental contaminants: heavy metals, pesticides.
Pharmacologic agents: caffeine, glycosidal alkaloid solanine (potato spuds), histamine (fish), serotonin (banana, tomato), tryptamine (tomato), tyramine (cheese).

PSYCHOLOGIC REACTIONS

Food phobias.

ADYNAMIC ILEUS[1]

| ICD-10CM # | K56.0 | Paralytic ileus |
| | K56.7 | Ileus, unspecified |

Abdominal trauma.
Infection (retroperitoneal, pelvic, intrathoracic).
Laparotomy.
Metabolic disease (hypokalemia).
Renal colic.
Skeletal injury (rib fracture, vertebral fracture).
Medications (e.g., narcotics).

AEROPHAGIA (BELCHING, ERUCTATION)

ICD-10CM #	R14.0	Abdominal distention (gaseous)
	R14.1	Gas pain
	R14.2	Eructation
	R14.3	Flatulence

Anxiety disorders.
Rapid food ingestion.
Carbonated beverages.
Nursing infants (especially when nursing in horizontal position).
Eating or drinking in supine position.
Gum chewing.
Poorly fitting dentures, orthodontic appliances.
Hiatal hernia, gastritis, nonnuclear dyspepsia.
Cholelithiasis, cholecystitis.
Ingestion of legumes, onions, peppers.

AGITATION AND CONFUSION[20]

| ICD-10CM # | Varies with specific diagnosis. |

Causes

Epileptic
Absence status.[a]
Complex partial seizure.[a]
Epileptic encephalopathies.[a]
Infectious Disorders
Bacterial infections.
 Cat-scratch disease.[a]
 Meningitis.[a]
Rickettsial infections.
 Lyme disease.[a]
 Rocky Mountain spotted fever.[a]
Viral infections.
 Arboviruses.
 Aseptic meningitis.
 Herpes simplex encephalitis.[a]
 Measles encephalitis.
 Postinfectious encephalomyelitis.
 Reye syndrome.
Metabolic and Systemic Disorders
Disorders of osmolality.
 Hypoglycemia.[a]
 Hyponatremia.[a]
Endocrine disorders.
 Adrenal insufficiency.[a]
 Hypoparathyroidism.[a]
 Thyroid disorders.[a]
Hepatic encephalopathy.
Inborn errors of metabolism.
 Disorders of pyruvate metabolism.
 Medium-chain acyl-CoA dehydrogenase (MCAD) deficiency.
 Respiratory chain disorders.
 Urea cycle disorder, heterozygote.
Renal disease.
 Hypertensive encephalopathy.[a]
 Uremic encephalopathy.[a]
Migraine
Acute confusional.[a]
Aphasic.[a]
Transient global amnesia.[a]
Psychologic
Panic disorder.[a]
Schizophrenia.
Toxic
Immunosuppressive drugs.[a]
Prescription drugs.[a]
Substance abuse.[a]
Toxins.[a]
Vascular
Congestive heart failure.[a]
Embolism.[a]
Hypertensive encephalopathy.[a]
Lupus erythematosus.[a]
Anti-NMDA antibody encephalitis.
Subarachnoid hemorrhage.[a]
 Vasculitis.[a]

[a]Denotes the most common conditions and the ones with disease-modifying treatments.
NMDA, N-methyl-D-aspartate.

AIR-SPACE OPACIFICATION ON X-RAY[21]

| ICD-10CM # | R91.8 | Other nonspecific abnormal finding of lung field |

CAUSES OF AIR-SPACE OPACIFICATION

Edema
Cardiogenic.
Noncardiogenic.
Inflammation/Infection
Granulomatosis with polyangiitis.
Cryptogenic organizing pneumonia.
Blood
Idiopathic pulmonary hemosiderosis.
Antibasement membrane antibody disease.
Systemic lupus erythematosus.
Miscellaneous Causes
Eosinophilic pneumonia.
Alveolar proteinosis.
Alveolar cell carcinoma.
Alveolar microlithiasis.
Lymphoma (MALToma).
Sarcoidosis.

AIRWAY OBSTRUCTION, CENTRAL[22]

| ICD-10CM # | Varies with specific diagnosis |

ETIOLOGY OF CENTRAL AIRWAY OBSTRUCTION

Nonmalignant	Malignant
Vascular sling.	Primary airway tumors.
	Bronchogenic.
	Mucoepidermoid.
	Adenoid cystic.
	Carcinoid.
Lymphadenopathy.	Lymphadenopathy due to malignancy.
Infection (histoplasmosis and tuberculosis).	
Sarcoidosis.	
Relapsing polychondritis.	Metastatic tumor to airway.
	Bronchogenic.
	Renal cell.
	Esophageal carcinoma.
	Breast.
	Thyroid.
	Colon.
	Melanoma.
Granulation tissue associated with:	Mediastinal tumors
Artificial airways.	Lymphoma.
Airway stents.	Thymus.
Aspirated foreign bodies.	Thyroid.
Surgical anastomosis.	
Inflammatory lesions.	
Amyloidosis.	
Papillomatosis.	
Granulomatosis with polyangiitis.	

AIRWAY OBSTRUCTION, PEDIATRIC AGE[23]

ICD-10CM #		
	J44.9	Chronic obstructive pulmonary disease, unspecified
	T17.900A	Unspecified foreign body in respiratory tract, part unspecified causing asphyxiation, initial encounter
	T17.908A	Unspecified foreign body in respiratory tract, part unspecified causing other injury, initial encounter
	T17.910A	Gastric contents in respiratory tract, part unspecified causing asphyxiation, initial encounter
	T17.918A	Gastric contents in respiratory tract, part unspecified causing other injury, initial encounter
	T17.920A	Food in respiratory tract, part unspecified causing asphyxiation, initial encounter
	T17.928A	Food in respiratory tract, part unspecified causing other injury, initial encounter
	T17.990A	Other foreign object in respiratory tract, part unspecified in causing asphyxiation, initial encounter
	T17.998A	Other foreign object in respiratory tract, part unspecified causing other injury, initial encounter
	J38.5	Laryngeal spasm
	J68.9	Unspecified respiratory condition due to chemicals, gases, fumes, and vapors

CONGENITAL CAUSES

Craniofacial dysmorphism.
Hemangioma.
Laryngeal cleft/web.
Laryngoceles, cysts.
Laryngomalacia.
Macroglossia.
Tracheal stenosis.
Vascular ring.
Vocal cord paralysis.

ACQUIRED INFECTIOUS CAUSES

Acute laryngotracheobronchitis.
Epiglottitis.
Laryngeal papillomatosis.
Membranous croup (bacterial tracheitis).
Mononucleosis.
Retropharyngeal abscess.
Spasmodic croup.
Diphtheria.

ACQUIRED NONINFECTIOUS CAUSES

Anaphylaxis.
Foreign body aspiration.
Supraglottic hypotonia.
Thermal/chemical burn.
Trauma.
Vocal cord paralysis.
Angioneurotic edema.

AKINETIC/RIGID SYNDROME[18]

ICD-10CM #	R29.8	Akinesis

Parkinsonism (idiopathic, drug-induced).
Catatonia (psychosis).
Progressive supranuclear palsy.
Multisystem atrophy (Shy-Drager syndrome, olivopontocerebellar atrophy).
Diffuse Lewy-body disease.
Toxins (MPTP, manganese, carbon monoxide).
Huntington disease and other hereditary neurodegenerative disorders.

ALCOHOL-RELATED SEIZURES[10]

ICD-10CM #	F10.232	Alcohol dependence with withdrawal with perceptual disturbance

DIFFERENTIAL DIAGNOSIS OF ALCOHOL-RELATED SEIZURES

Withdrawal (alcohol or drugs).
Exacerbation of idiopathic or posttraumatic seizures.
Acute intoxication (amphetamines, anticholinergics, cocaine, isoniazid, organophosphates, phenothiazines, tricyclic antidepressants, salicylates, lithium).
Metabolic (hypoglycemia, hyponatremia, hypernatremia, hypocalcemia, hepatic failure).
Infectious (meningitis, encephalitis, brain abscess).
Trauma (intracranial hemorrhage).
Cerebrovascular accident.
Sleep deprivation.
Noncompliance with anticonvulsants.

ALKALOSIS, METABOLIC

ICD-10CM #	E87.3	Alkalosis

CAUSES OF METABOLIC ALKALOSIS

Exogenous HCO_3- loads.
Acute alkali administration.
Milk-alkali syndrome.

Effective Extracellular Volume Contraction, Normotension, Hypokalemia, and Secondary Hyperreninemic Hyperaldosteronism
GI origin:
  Vomiting.
  Gastric aspiration.
  Congenital chloridorrhea.
  Villous adenoma.
  Combined administration of sodium polystyrene sulfonate (Kayexalate and aluminum hydroxide).
Renal origin:
  Diuretics (especially thiazides and loop diuretics).
  Acute.
  Chronic.
  Edematous states.
  Posthypercapnic state.
  Hypercalcemia-hypoparathyroidism.
  Recovery from lactic acidosis or ketoacidosis.
  Nonreabsorbable anions such as penicillin, carbenicillin.
  Mg^{++} deficiency.
  K^+ depletion.
  Bartter syndrome (loss-of-function mutation of Cl^- transport in thick ascending limb of Henle loop).
  Gitelman syndrome (loss-of-function mutation in Na^+/Cl^- cotransporter).
  Carbohydrate refeeding after starvation.

Extracellular Volume Expansion, Hypertension, K^+ Deficiency, and Hypermineralocorticoidism
Associated with high renin:
  Renal artery stenosis.
  Accelerated hypertension.
  Renin-secreting tumor.
  Estrogen therapy.
Associated with low renin:
  Primary aldosteronism.
  Adenoma.
  Hyperplasia.
  Carcinoma.
  Glucocorticoid suppressible.
Adrenal enzymatic defects:
  11β-Hydroxylase deficiency.
  17α-Hydroxylase deficiency.
Cushing syndrome or disease:
  Ectopic corticotropin.
  Adrenal carcinoma.
  Adrenal adenoma.
  Primary pituitary.
Other:
  Licorice.
  Carbenoxolone.
  Chewer's tobacco.
  Lydia Pinkham tablets.

Gain-of-Function Mutation of ENaC with Extracellular Fluid Volume Expansion, Hypertension, K⁺ Deficiency, and Hyporeninemic Hypoaldosteronism

Liddle syndrome.

ALKALOSIS, RESPIRATORY

ICD-10CM #	E87.3	Alkalosis

Hypoxemia (pneumonia, pulmonary embolism, atelectasis, high-altitude living).

Drugs (salicylates, xanthenes, progesterone, epinephrine, thyroxine, nicotine).

Central nervous system disorders (tumor, cerebrovascular accident, trauma, infections).

Psychogenic hyperventilation (anxiety, hysteria).

Hepatic encephalopathy.

Gram-negative sepsis.

Hyponatremia.

Sudden recovery from metabolic acidosis.

Assisted ventilation.

ALOPECIA[13,24]

ICD-10CM #	L65.9	Nonscarring hair loss, unspecified
	L63.2	Ophiasis
	L63.8	Other alopecia areata
	Q84.0	Congenital alopecia
	Q84.1	Congenital morphological disturbances of hair, not elsewhere classified
	Q84.2	Other congenital malformations of hair
	F54	Psychological and behavioral factors associated with disorders or diseases classified elsewhere

SCARRING ALOPECIA

Congenital (aplasia cutis).

Tinea capitis with inflammation (kerion).

Bacterial folliculitis.

Discoid lupus erythematosus.

Lichen planopilaris.

Folliculitis decalvans.

Neoplasm.

Trauma.

NONSCARRING ALOPECIA

Cosmetic treatment.

Tinea capitis.

Structural hair shaft disease.

Trichotillomania (hair pulling).

Anagen arrest.

Telogen arrest.

Alopecia areata.

Androgenetic alopecia.

ALOPECIA AND HYPOTRICHOSIS, IN CHILDREN AND ADOLESCENTS

ICD-10CM #	L65.9	Nonscarring hair loss, unspecified
	L63.2	Ophiasis
	L63.8	Other alopecia areata
	Q84.0	Congenital alopecia
	Q84.1	Congenital morphological disturbances of hair, not elsewhere classified
	Q84.2	Other congenital malformations of hair

Congenital total alopecia: atrichia with papules, Moynahan alopecia syndrome.

Congenital localized alopecia: aplasia cutis, triangular alopecia, sebaceous nevus.

Hereditary hypotrichosis: Marie-Unna syndrome, hypotrichosis with juvenile macular dystrophy, hypotrichosis–Mari type, ichthyosis with hypotrichosis, cartilage-hair hypoplasia, Hallermann-Streiff syndrome, trichorhinophalangeal syndrome, ectodermal dysplasia ("pure" hair and nail and other ectodermal dysplasias).

Diffuse alopecia of endocrine origin: hypopituitarism, hypothyroidism, hypoparathyroidism, hyperthyroidism.

Alopecia of nutritional origin: marasmus, kwashiorkor, iron deficiency, zinc deficiency (acrodermatitis enteropathica), gluten-sensitive enteropathy, essential fatty acid deficiency, biotinidase deficiency.

Disturbances of the hair cycle: telogen effluvium.

Toxic alopecia: anagen effluvium.

Autoimmune alopecia: alopecia areata.

Traumatic alopecia: traction alopecia, trichotillomania.

Cicatricial alopecia: lupus erythematosus, lichen planopilaris, pseudopelade, morphea (en coup de saber), dermatomyositis, infection (kerion, favus, tuberculosis, syphilis, folliculitis, leishmaniasis, herpes zoster, varicella), acne keloidalis, follicular mucinosis, sarcoidosis.

Hair shaft abnormalities: monilethrix, pili annulati, pili torti, trichorrhexis invaginata, trichorrhexis nodosa, woolly hair syndrome, Menkes disease, trichothiodystrophy, tricho-dento-osseous syndrome, uncombable hair syndrome (spun-glass hair, pili trianguli et canaliculi).

ALOPECIA, DRUG-INDUCED

ICD-10CM #	L65.9	Nonscarring hair loss, unspecified
	L63.8	Alopecia areata

DRUGS REPORTED TO INDUCE HAIR LOSS

ACE inhibitors (captopril, enalapril, moexipril, ramipril).

Allopurinol.

Amiodarone.

Amphetamines.*,†

Analgesics, antiinflammatories (ibuprofen, indomethacin, naproxen).

Androgens.‡

Anticoagulants (coumarin, dextran, heparin/heparinoids).

Antiepileptics (carbamazepine, hydantoins, lamotrigine, troxidone, valproic acid, vigabatrin).

Antipsychotics (flupentixol decanoate, fluphenazine decanoate).

Antithyroid drugs (carbimazole, iodine, thiouracil).

Appetite suppressants.

Aromatase inhibitors (fadrozole, 4-OHA, vorozole).

Benzimidazoles (albendazole, mebendazole).

β-Blockers (levobunolol, metoprolol, nadolol, propranolol, timolol).

Bromocriptine.

Buspirone.

Butyrophenones.

Cantharidin.

Chloramphenicol.

Cholestyramine.

Cidofovir.

Cimetidine.

Clonazepam.

Clotrimazole.

Colchicine.

Contraceptive (oral).§

Danazol.

Diazoxide.

Diclofenac.

Dixyrazine.

Ethambutol.

Ethionamide.

Fibrates (clofibrate, fenofibrate).

G-CSF (granulocyte-colony stimulating factor).

Gefitinib.¶

Gentamicin.

Glatiramer acetate.

Glibenclamide.

Gold salts.

Haloperidol.

Immunoglobulins.

Indanediones.

Indinavir.

Interferons.

Isonicotinic acid hydrazide.**

Leflunomide.

Levodopa.

Lithium.

Maprotiline.

Mesalazine.

Methyldopa.

Methysergide.

Metyrapone.

Minoxidil.

Nicotinic acid.

Nitrofurantoin.

Octreotide.

*Haidar G, Singh N: Fever of unknown origin, *N Engl J Med* 386(5):463-477, 2022.

†More frequent cause.

‡More frequent cause.

§Genetic transmission.

¶Not listed as a syndrome by ILAE but instead recognized under absence seizures with special features.

**Includes schizophrenia, schizophreniform disorder, brief reactive psychosis.

Differential Diagnosis

II

Olanzapine.
Pentosan polysulfate.
Phenindione.
Potassium thiocyanate.
Pyridostigmine.
Radiation (<700 Gy).
Retinoids (acitretin, etretinate, isotretinoin).
Retinol (vitamin A).
Risperidone.
Salicylates.
Serotonin reuptake inhibitors (fluoxetine, fluvox-
    amine, paroxetine, sertraline).
Sorafenib.
Spironolactone.
Strontium ranelate.
Sulfasalazine.
Tamoxifen.
Terbinafine.
Terfenadine.
Thiamphenicol.
Thyroxine.
Tocopherol (vitamin E).
Trazodone.
Triazoles (fluconazole, itraconazole).
Tricyclic antidepressants (amitriptyline, desipra-
    mine, doxepin, imipramine, maprotiline).
Trimethadione.
Triparanol.
Vasopressin.[††]

[††]Hair loss usually severe.

ALVEOLAR CONSOLIDATION

| ICD-10CM # | J18.2 | Hypostatic pneumonia, unspecified organism |
| | J81.1 | Hypostatic pneumonia, unspecified organism |

Infection.
Neoplasm (bronchoalveolar carcinoma, lym-
    phoma).
Aspiration.
Trauma.
Hemorrhage (granulomatosis with polyangiitis,
    Goodpasture, bleeding diathesis).
Acute respiratory distress syndrome.
Congestive heart failure.
Renal failure.
Eosinophilic pneumonia.
Bronchiolitis obliterans.
Pulmonary alveolar proteinosis.

ALVEOLAR HEMORRHAGE[25]

ICD-10CM #	P26.1	Massive pulmonary hemorrhage originating in the perinatal period
	K08.8	Alveolar hemorrhage
	P26.8	Other pulmonary hemorrhages originating in the perinatal period

Hematologic disorders (coagulopathies, throm-
    bocytopenia).
Goodpasture syndrome (antibasement mem-
    brane antibody disease).
Granulomatosis with polyangiitis.

Immune complex-mediated vasculitis.
Idiopathic pulmonary hemosiderosis.
Drugs (penicillamine).
Lymphangiogram contrast.
Mitral stenosis.

AMENORRHEA

| ICD-10CM # | N91.2 Amenorrhea, unspecified |

PREGNANCY

Early Menopause
Hypothalamic Dysfunction
Defective synthesis or release of LHRH, anorexia
nervosa, stress, exercise.
Pituitary Dysfunction
Neoplasm, postpartum hemorrhage, surgery,
radiotherapy.
Ovarian Dysfunction
Gonadal dysgenesis, 17a-hydroxylase defi-
ciency, premature ovarian failure, polycystic
ovarian disease, gonadal stromal tumors.

UTEROVAGINAL ABNORMALITIES

Congenital: imperforate hymen, imperforate
cervix, imperforate or absent vagina, Müllerian
agenesis.
Acquired: destruction of endometrium with
curettage (Asherman syndrome), closure of
cervix or vagina caused by traumatic injury,
hysterectomy.

OTHER

Metabolic diseases (liver, kidney), malnutrition,
rapid weight loss, exogenous obesity, endocrine
abnormalities (Cushing syndrome, Graves disease, hypothyroidism).

AMNESIA

ICD-10CM #	F19.96	Other psychoactive substance use, unspecified with psychoactive substance-induced persisting amnestic disorder
	F44.0	Dissociative amnesia
	R41.2	Retrograde amnesia
	G45.4	Transient global amnesia

Degenerative diseases (e.g., Alzheimer, Huntington
    disease).
Cerebrovascular accident (especially when
    involving thalamus, basal forebrain, and
    hippocampus).
Head trauma.
Postsurgical (e.g., mammillary body surgery,
    bilateral temporal lobectomy).
Infections (herpes simplex encephalitis, meningitis).
Wernicke-Korsakoff syndrome.
Cerebral hypoxia.
Hypoglycemia.
Central nervous system neoplasms.
Creutzfeldt-Jakob disease.
Medications (e.g., midazolam and other
    benzodiazepines).
Psychosis.
Malingering.

AMNIOTIC FLUID α-FETOPROTEIN ELEVATION[21]

| ICD-10CM # | Z36 | Encounter for antenatal screening of mother |

CAUSES OF ELEVATED AMNIOTIC FLUID α-FETOPROTEIN

Craniospinal defect (open neural tube defect).
Omphalocele.
Gastroschisis.
Duodenal atresia.
Congenital nephrosis.
Cystic hygroma.
Unbalanced dislocation.
Down, Tay-Sachs, Klinefelter, Turner syndromes.
Fetal tumors.
Epidermolysis bullosa.
Pilonidal sinus.
Rhesus disease.
Fetal demise.
Incorrect dates.
Multiple pregnancies.

ANAL ABSCESS AND FISTULA[2]

ICD-10CM #	K61.0	Anal abscess
	K61.1	Rectal abscess
	K61.3	Ischiorectal abscess
	K60.3	Anal fistula

Primary anal gland infection.
Secondary abscess:
    Inflammatory bowel disease:
        Crohn disease.
        Ulcerative colitis.
Infection:
    Tuberculosis.
    Actinomycosis.
    Threadworm.
Trauma.
Leukopenia.
Immunosuppression:
    HIV.
    Drugs.
Rectal cancer.
Diabetes mellitus.

ANAL INCONTINENCE[1]

| ICD-10CM # | R15.9 | Full incontinence of feces |

TRAUMATIC

Nerve injured in surgery.
Spinal cord injury.
Obstetric trauma.
Sphincter injury.

NEUROLOGIC

Spinal cord lesions.
Dementia.
Autonomic neuropathy (e.g., diabetes mellitus).
Obstetrics: pudendal nerve stretched during
    surgery.
Hirschsprung disease.

MASS EFFECT
Carcinoma of anal canal.
Carcinoma of rectum.
Foreign body.
Fecal impaction.
Hemorrhoids.

MEDICAL
Procidentia.
Inflammatory disease.
Diarrhea.
Laxative abuse.

PEDIATRIC
Congenital.
Meningocele.
Myelomeningocele.
Spina bifida.
After corrective surgery for imperforate anus.
Sexual abuse.
Encopresis.

ANAPHYLAXIS[26]

ICD-10CM #	T78.2	Anaphylactic shock, unspecified, initial encounter

PULMONARY
Laryngeal edema.
Epiglottitis.
Foreign body aspiration.
Pulmonary embolus.
Asphyxiation.
Hyperventilation.

CARDIOVASCULAR
Myocardial infarction.
Arrhythmia.
Hypovolemic shock.
Cardiac arrest.

CENTRAL NERVOUS SYSTEM
Vasovagal reaction.
Cerebrovascular accident.
Seizure disorder.
Drug overdose.

ENDOCRINE
Hypoglycemia.
Pheochromocytoma.
Carcinoid syndrome.
Catamenial (progesterone-induced anaphylaxis).

PSYCHIATRIC
Vocal cord dysfunction syndrome.
Munchausen syndrome.
Panic attack/globus hystericus.

OTHER
Hereditary angioedema.
Cord urticaria.
Idiopathic urticaria.
Mastocytosis.
Serum sickness.
Idiopathic capillary leak syndrome.
Sulfite exposure.
Scombroid poisoning (tuna, blue fish, mackerel).

ANAPHYLAXIS MIMICS[27]

ICD-10CM #	Varies with specific diagnosis

CONDITIONS THAT MIMIC ANAPHYLAXIS
Vasovagal episodes.
Acute pulmonary events:
   Acute asthmatic attacks.
   Acute pulmonary edema.
   Pulmonary embolus.
   Spontaneous pneumothorax.
   Foreign body aspiration.
Acute cardiac events:
   Supraventricular tachycardias.
   Acute myocardial infarction/ischemia.
Drug overdoses.
Insulin shock.
Carcinoid attacks.

ANAPHYLAXIS, PATHOPHYSIOLOGIC CLASSIFICATION[28]

ICD-10CM #	T78.2	Anaphylactic shock, unspecified, initial encounter

PATHOPHYSIOLOGIC CLASSIFICATION OF ANAPHYLAXIS
Immunoglobulin E (IgE) Dependent, Immunologic
Foods.
Drugs.
Insect stings and bites.
Exercise (food dependent).
Other causes.
IgE Independent, Immunologic
Immune aggregates.
IgG anti-IgA.
Cytotoxic.
Disturbance of arachidonic acid metabolism:
   Aspirin.
   Other NSAIDs.
Activation of kallikrein-kinin contact system:
   Dialysis membranes.
   Radiocontrast media.
Multimediator recruitment:
   Complement.
   Clotting.
   Clot lysis.
   Kallikrein-kinin contact system.
Other causes.
Nonimmunologic
Direct mediator release from mast cells and basophils:
   Drugs, e.g., opiates.
   Physical factors, e.g., cold and sunlight.
Exercise.
c-kit Mutation (D816V).
Other causes.
Idiopathic.

ANAPHYLACTOID SYNDROME OF PREGNANCY[29]

ICD-10CM #	O88.113

CARDIOVASCULAR COLLAPSE, HYPOTENSION
Acute coronary syndromes, myocardial infarction.
Cardiomyopathy.
Pulmonary embolism.
Anesthesia complications, transfusion reaction.
Sepsis, systemic inflammatory response syndrome.

RESPIRATORY ARREST
Pulmonary embolism, air embolism.
Anesthesia complications, transfusion reaction.
Aspiration.

ALTERED MENTAL STATUS, SEIZURE
Eclampsia.
Cerebrovascular accident.
Hypoglycemia.

COAGULOPATHY
Disseminated intravascular coagulation.
Consumptive coagulopathy from hemorrhage.

ANDROGEN EXCESS, REPRODUCTIVE-AGE WOMAN

ICD-10CM #	E28.1	Androgen excess

Polycystic ovary syndrome.
Idiopathic.
Medications (e.g., anabolizing agents, testosterone, danazol).
Pregnancy (luteoma, hyperreaction luteinalis).
Sertoli-Leydig ovarian neoplasm.
Adrenal adenoma or hyperplasia.
Cushing syndrome.
Glucocorticoid resistance.
Hypothyroidism.
Hyperprolactinemia.

ANDROGEN RESISTANCE[30]

ICD-10CM #	E34.5	Androgen resistance syndrome

CONGENITAL OR DEVELOPMENTAL DISORDERS
Uncommon causes:
   Kennedy disease (spinal and bulbar muscular atrophy).
   Partial androgen insensitivity syndrome (androgen receptor mutations).
   5α-reductase type 2 deficiency.
   Complete androgen insensitivity syndrome (female phenotype).

ACQUIRED DISORDERS
Common causes:
   Androgen receptor antagonists (bicalutamide, nilutamide).
   Drugs (spironolactone, cyproterone acetate, marijuana, histamine 2 receptor antagonists).
Uncommon causes:
   Celiac disease.

ANEMIA, APLASTIC[31]

ICD-10CM #	D61.09	Other constitutional aplastic anemia

ACQUIRED APLASTIC ANEMIA

Secondary aplastic anemia.
Irradiation.
Drugs and chemicals.
Regular effects.
Cytotoxic agents.
Benzene.
Idiosyncratic reactions.
Chloramphenicol.
NSAIDs.
Antiepileptics.
Gold.
Other drugs and chemicals.
Viruses.
Epstein-Barr virus (infectious mononucleosis).
Hepatitis virus (non-A, non-B, non-C, non-G hepatitis).
Parvovirus (transient aplastic crisis, some pure red cell aplasia).
HIV (acquired immunodeficiency syndrome).
Immune diseases.
Eosinophilic fasciitis.
Hyperimmunoglobulinemia.
Thymoma and thymic carcinoma.
Graft-versus-host disease in immunodeficiency.
Paroxysmal nocturnal hemoglobinuria.
Pregnancy.
Idiopathic aplastic anemia.

INHERITED APLASTIC ANEMIA

Fanconi anemia.
Dyskeratosis congenita.
Shwachman-Diamond syndrome.
Reticular dysgenesis.
Amegakaryocytic thrombocytopenia.
Familial aplastic anemias.
Preleukemia (e.g., monosomy 7).
Nonhematologic syndromes (e.g., Down, Dubowitz, Seckel).

ANEMIA, APLASTIC, DUE TO DRUGS AND CHEMICALS[29]

ICD-10CM #	D61.1	Drug-induced aplastic anemia
	D61.2	Aplastic anemia due to other external agents
	D61.89	Other specified aplastic anemias and other bone marrow failure syndromes

Agents that regularly produce marrow depression as a major toxic effect when used in commonly employed doses or normal exposures:
Cytotoxic drugs used in cancer chemotherapy.
Alkylating agents (busulfan, melphalan, cyclophosphamide).
Antimetabolites (antifolic compounds, nucleotide analogs), antimitotics (vincristine, vinblastine, colchicine).
Some antibiotics (daunorubicin, doxorubicin [Adriamycin]).
Benzene (and less often benzene-containing chemicals; kerosene, carbon tetrachloride, Stoddard solvent, chlorophenols).

Agents probably associated with aplastic anemia but with a relatively low probability relative to their use:
Chloramphenicol.
Insecticides.
Antiprotozoals (quinacrine and chloroquine).
NSAIDs (including phenylbutazone, indomethacin, ibuprofen, sulindac, diclofenac, naproxen, piroxicam, fenoprofen, fenbufen, aspirin).
Anticonvulsants (hydantoins, carbamazepine, phenacemide, ethosuximide).
Gold, arsenic, and other heavy metals such as bismuth and mercury.
Sulfonamides as a class.
Antithyroid medications (methimazole, methylthiouracil, propylthiouracil).
Antidiabetes drugs (tolbutamide, carbutamide, chlorpropamide).
Carbonic anhydrase inhibitors (acetazolamide, methazolamide, mesalazine).
D-Penicillamine.
2-Chlorodeoxyadenosine.
Agents more rarely associated with aplastic anemia:
Antibiotics (streptomycin, tetracycline, methicillin, ampicillin, mebendazole and albendazole, sulfonamides, flucytosine, mefloquine, dapsone).
Antihistamines (cimetidine, ranitidine, chlorpheniramine).
Sedatives and tranquilizers (chlorpromazine, prochlorperazine, piperacetazine, chlordiazepoxide, meprobamate, methyprylon, remoxipride).
Antiarrhythmics (tocainide, amiodarone).
Allopurinol (can potentiate marrow suppression by cytotoxic drugs).
Ticlopidine.
Methyldopa.
Quinidine.
Lithium.
Guanidine.
Canthaxanthin.
Thiocyanate.
Carbimazole.
Cyanamide.
Deferoxamine.
Amphetamines.

ANEMIA, CAUSES IN PREGNANCY[32]

ICD-10CM #	D50.8	Other iron deficiency anemias
	D50.9	Iron deficiency anemia, unspecified
	D51.0	Vitamin B_{12} deficiency anemia due to intrinsic factor deficiency
	D51.1	Vitamin B_{12} deficiency anemia due to selective vitamin B_{12} malabsorption with proteinuria
	D51.3	Other dietary vitamin B_{12} deficiency anemia
	D51.8	Other vitamin B_{12} deficiency anemias
	D52.0	Dietary folate deficiency anemia
	D52.1	Drug-induced folate deficiency anemia
	D52.8	Other folate deficiency anemias
	D52.9	Folate deficiency anemia, unspecified
	D53.1	Other megaloblastic anemias, not elsewhere classified
	D53.0	Protein deficiency anemia
	D53.2	Scorbutic anemia
	D53.8	Other specified nutritional anemias
	D53.9	Nutritional anemia, unspecified
	D64.0	Hereditary sideroblastic anemia
	D64.1	Secondary sideroblastic anemia due to disease
	D64.2	Secondary sideroblastic anemia due to drugs and toxins
	D64.3	Other sideroblastic anemias

CAUSES OF ANEMIA DURING PREGNANCY

Common causes—85% of anemia:
Physiologic anemia.
Iron deficiency.
Uncommon causes:
Folic acid deficiency.
Vitamin B_{12} deficiency (due to the rapid increase in bariatric surgery).
Hemoglobinopathies:
Sickle cell disease.
Hemoglobin SC.
β-Thalassemia minor.
Bariatric surgery.
GI bleeding.
Rare causes:
Hemoglobinopathies.
β-Thalassemia major.
α-Thalassemia.
Syndromes of chronic hemolysis:
Hereditary spherocytosis.
Paroxysmal nocturnal hemoglobinuria.
Hematologic malignancy.

ANEMIA, DRUG-INDUCED[33]

ICD-10CM #	D61.1	Drug-induced aplastic anemia

DRUGS THAT MAY INTERFERE WITH RED CELL PRODUCTION BY INDUCING MARROW SUPPRESSION OR APLASIA

Alcohol.
Antineoplastic drugs.
Antithyroid drugs.
Antibiotics.
Oral hypoglycemic agents.
Phenylbutazone.
Azidothymidine (AZT).

DRUGS THAT INTERFERE WITH VITAMIN B$_{12}$, FOLATE, OR IRON ABSORPTION OR UTILIZATION

Nitrous oxide.
Anticonvulsant drugs.
Antineoplastic drugs.
Isoniazid.
Cycloserine A.

DRUGS CAPABLE OF PROMOTING HEMOLYSIS

Immune Mediated

Penicillins.
Quinine.
α-methyldopa.
Procainamide.
Mitomycin C.

Oxidative Stress

Antimalarials.
Sulfonamide drugs.
Nalidixic acid.

DRUGS THAT MAY PRODUCE OR PROMOTE BLOOD LOSS

Aspirin.
Alcohol.
Nonsteroidal antiinflammatory agents.
Corticosteroids.
Anticoagulants.

ANEMIA, HYPOCHROMIC[31]

ICD-10CM #		
D50.8	Other iron deficiency anemias
D50.9	Iron deficiency anemia, unspecified
D64.0	Hereditary sideroblastic anemia
D64.1	Secondary sideroblastic anemia due to disease
D64.2	Secondary sideroblastic anemia due to drugs and toxins
D64.3	Other sideroblastic anemias

DECREASED BODY IRON STORES

Iron deficiency anemia.

NORMAL OR INCREASED BODY IRON STORES

Impaired iron metabolism.
Anemia of chronic disease.
Defective absorption, transport, or use of iron.

Disorders of globin synthesis:
  Thalassemia.
  Other microcytic hemoglobinopathies.
Disorders of heme synthesis: sideroblastic anemias:
  Hereditary.
  Acquired.

ANEMIA, LOW RETICULOCYTE COUNT[18]

ICD-10CM #	D64.9	Anemia, unspecified

MICROCYTIC ANEMIA (MCV <80)

Iron deficiency.
Thalassemia minor.
Sideroblastic anemia.
Lead poisoning.

MACROCYTIC ANEMIA (MCV >100)

Megaloblastic anemias.
Folate deficiency.
Vitamin B$_{12}$ deficiency.
Drug-induced megaloblastic anemia.
Nonmegaloblastic macrocytosis.
Liver disease.
Hypothyroidism.

NORMOCYTIC ANEMIA (MCV 80-100)

Early iron deficiency.
Aplastic anemia.
Myelophthisic disorders.
Endocrinopathies.
Anemia of chronic disease.
Uremia.
Mixed nutritional deficiency.

ANEMIA, MEGALOBLASTIC[17]

ICD-10CM #	D51.0	Vitamin B$_{12}$ deficiency anemia due to intrinsic factor deficiency
	D51.1	Vitamin B$_{12}$ deficiency anemia due to selective vitamin B$_{12}$ malabsorption with proteinuria
	D51.3	Other dietary vitamin B$_{12}$ deficiency anemia
	D51.8	Other vitamin B$_{12}$ deficiency anemias
	D52.0	Dietary folate deficiency anemia
	D52.1	Drug-induced folate deficiency anemia
	D52.8	Other folate deficiency anemias
	D52.9	Folate deficiency anemia, unspecified

	D53.1	Other megaloblastic anemias, not elsewhere classified
	D53.0	Protein deficiency anemia
	D53.2	Scorbutic anemia
	D53.8	Other specified nutritional anemias
	D53.9	Nutritional anemia, unspecified

COBALAMIN (CBL) DEFICIENCY

Nutritional CBL Deficiency (Insufficient CBL Intake)

Vegetarians, vegans, breastfed infants of mothers with pernicious anemia.

Abnormal Intragastric Events (Inadequate Proteolysis of Food CBL)

Atrophic gastritis, partial gastrectomy with hypochlorhydria.

Loss/Atrophy of Gastric Oxyntic Mucosa (Deficient Intrinsic Factor [IF] Molecules)

Total or partial gastrectomy, pernicious anemia (PA), caustic destruction (lye).

Abnormal Events in Small Bowel Lumen

Inadequate pancreatic protease (R-CBL not degraded, CBL not transferred to IF).
  Insufficiency of pancreatic protease—pancreatic insufficiency.
  Inactivation of pancreatic protease—Zollinger-Ellison syndrome.
Usurping of luminal CBL (inadequate CBL binding to IF).
  By bacteria—stasis syndromes (blind loops, pouches of diverticulosis, strictures, fistulas, anastomoses); impaired bowel motility (scleroderma, pseudoobstruction), hypogammaglobulinemia.
  By Diphyllobothrium latum.

Disorders of Ileal Mucosa/IF Receptors (IF-CBL not Bound to IF Receptors)

Diminished or absent IF receptors—ileal bypass/resection/fistula.
Abnormal mucosal architecture/function—tropical/nontropical sprue, Crohn disease, TB ileitis, infiltration by lymphomas, amyloidosis.
IF-/post IF-receptor defects—Imerslund-Gräsbeck syndrome, TC II deficiency.
Drug-induced effects (slow K, biguanides, cholestyramine, colchicine, neomycin, PAS).

DISORDERS OF PLASMA CBL TRANSPORT (TC II-CBL NOT DELIVERED TO TC II RECEPTORS)

Congenital TC II deficiency, defective binding of TC II-CBL to TC II receptors (rare).

METABOLIC DISORDERS (CBL NOT UTILIZED BY CELL)

Inborn enzyme errors (rare).
Acquired disorders: (CBL oxidized to cob[III]alamin)—N$_2$O inhalation.

FOLATE DEFICIENCY

Nutritional Causes
Decreased dietary intake—poverty and famine (associated with kwashiorkor, marasmus), institutionalized individuals (psychiatric/nursing homes), chronic debilitating disease/goats' milk (low in folate), special diets (slimming), cultural/ethnic cooking techniques (food folate destroyed) or habits (folate-rich foods not consumed).

Decreased diet and increased requirements:
- Physiologic: pregnancy and lactation, prematurity, infancy.
- Pathologic: intrinsic hematologic disease (autoimmune hemolytic disease), drugs, malaria; hemoglobinopathies (SS, thalassemia), RBC membrane defects (hereditary spherocytosis, paroxysmal nocturnal hemoglobinopathy); abnormal hematopoiesis (leukemia/lymphoma, myelodysplastic syndrome, agnogenic myeloid metaplasia with myelofibrosis); infiltration with malignant disease; dermatologic (psoriasis).

Folate Malabsorption
With normal intestinal mucosa:
- Some drugs (controversial).
- Congenital folate malabsorption (rare).
- With mucosal abnormalities—tropical and nontropical sprue, regional enteritis.

Defective Cellular Folate Uptake—Familial Aplastic Anemia (Rare), Inadequate Cellular Utilization
Folate antagonists (methotrexate).
Hereditary enzyme deficiencies involving folate.

Drugs (Multiple Effects on Folate Metabolism)
Alcohol, sulfasalazine, triamterene, pyrimethamine, trimethoprim-sulfamethoxazole, diphenylhydantoin, barbiturates.

MISCELLANEOUS MEGALOBLASTIC ANEMIAS (NOT CAUSED BY CBL OR FOLATE DEFICIENCY)

Congenital Disorders of DNA Synthesis (Rare)
Orotic aciduria, Lesch-Nyhan syndrome, congenital dyserythropoietic anemia.

Acquired Disorders of DNA Synthesis
Thiamine-responsive megaloblastosis (rare).
- Malignancy—erythroleukemia—refractory sideroblastic anemias—all antineoplastic drugs that inhibit DNA synthesis.
- Toxins: alcohol.

ANEMIA, MICROCYTIC, HYPOCHROMIC, DIFFERENTIAL DIAGNOSIS[34]

ICD-10CM #		
	D50.8	Other iron deficiency anemias
	D50.9	Iron deficiency anemia, unspecified
	D64.0	Hereditary sideroblastic anemia
	D64.1	Secondary sideroblastic anemia due to disease
	D64.2	Secondary sideroblastic anemia due to drugs and toxins
	D64.3	Other sideroblastic anemias

DIFFERENTIAL DIAGNOSIS OF MICROCYTIC HYPOCHROMIC ANEMIA

Decreased Body Iron Stores
Iron deficiency anemia.

Normal or Increased Body Iron Stores
Anemia of chronic disease.
Defective absorption, transport, or use of iron.
Iron-refractory, iron deficiency anemia after parenteral iron.
Atransferrinemia.
Aceruloplasminemia.
Divalent metal transporter 1 (DMT1 or SLC11A2) deficiency.
Ferroportin-associated hemochromatosis with impaired iron export (type 4A).
Heme oxygenase 1 deficiency.
Disorders of globin synthesis.

Decreased Body Iron Stores
Thalassemia.
- Other microcytic hemoglobinopathies.
- Disorders of heme synthesis.
Sideroblastic anemias.
- Hereditary.
- Acquired.

ANERGY, CUTANEOUS[17]

ICD-10CM #	D89.9	Disorder involving the immune mechanism, unspecified

IMMUNOLOGIC
Acquired (AIDS, acute leukemia, carcinoma, chronic lymphocytic leukemia, Hodgkin lymphoma, non-Hodgkin's lymphoma).
Congenital (ataxia-telangiectasia, Di George syndrome, severe combined immunodeficiency, Wiskott-Aldrich syndrome).

INFECTIONS
Bacterial (bacterial pneumonia, brucellosis).
Disseminated mycotic infections.
Mycobacterial (lepromatous leprosy, TB).
Viral (varicella, hepatitis, influenza, mononucleosis, measles, mumps).

IMMUNOSUPPRESSIVE MEDICATIONS
Systemic corticosteroids.
Methotrexate, cyclophosphamide.
Rifampin.

OTHER
Alcoholic cirrhosis, biliary cirrhosis, sarcoidosis, rheumatic disease.
Diabetes, Crohn disease, uremia.
Anemia, pyridoxine deficiency, sickle cell anemia.
Burns, malnutrition, pregnancy, old age, surgery.

ANEURYSMS, THORACIC AORTA

ICD-10CM #	I71.2	Thoracic aortic aneurysm, without rupture

Trauma.
Infection.
Inflammatory (syphilis, Takayasu disease).
Collagen vascular disease (rheumatoid arthritis, ankylosing spondylitis).
Annuloaortic ectasia (Marfan syndrome, Ehlers-Danlos syndrome).
Congenital.
Coarctation.
Cystic medial necrosis.

ANHIDROSIS

ICD-10CM #	L74.0	Miliaria rubra
	L74.1	Miliaria crystallina
	L74.2	Miliaria profunda

Drugs (anticholinergics).
Dehydration.
Hysteria.
Obstruction of sweat ducts (e.g., inflammation, miliaria).
Local radiant heat or pressure.
Central nervous system lesions (medulla, hypothalamus, pons).
Spinal cord lesions.
Lesions of sympathetic nerves.
Congenital sweat gland disturbances.

ANION GAP ACIDOSIS[7]

ICD-10CM #	E87.2	Acidosis

CLINICAL CAUSES OF HIGH ANION GAP AND NORMAL ANION GAP ACIDOSIS

High Anion Gap
Ketoacidosis:
- Diabetic ketoacidosis (acetoacetate).
- Alcoholic (β-hydroxybutyrate).
- Starvation.
- Lactic acid acidosis:
  - L-Lactic acid acidosis (types A and B).
  - D-Lactic acid acidosis.
- Renal failure: sulfate, phosphate, urate, hippurate.
Ingestions (toxins and their metabolites):
- Ethylene glycol → glycolate, oxalate.
- Methyl alcohol → formate.
- Salicylate → ketones, lactate, salicylate.
- Paraldehyde → organic anions.
- Toluene → hippurate (commonly presents with normal anion gap).
- Propylene glycol → lactate.
- Pyroglutamic acidosis (acetaminophen use) → 5-oxoproline.

Normal Anion Gap
GI loss of HCO_3^- (negative urine anion gap):
- Diarrhea.
- Fistula, external.
Renal loss of HCO_3^- or failure to excrete NH_4^+ (positive urine anion gap):
- Proximal renal tubular acidosis (RTA type 2).
- Acetazolamide.

Classic distal renal tubular acidosis (low serum K^+) RTA type 1.

Generalized distal renal tubular defect (high serum K^+) RTA type 4.

Miscellaneous:

NH₄Cl ingestion.

Sulfur ingestion.

Dilutional acidosis.

Late stages in treatment of diabetic keto-acidosis.

ANION GAP INCREASE

ICD-10CM #	E87.8	Other disorders of electrolyte and fluid balance, not elsewhere classified

Uremia.

Ketoacidosis (diabetic, starvation, alcoholic).

Lactic acidosis.

Ethylene glycol poisoning.

Salicylate overdose.

Methanol poisoning.

ANISOCORIA

ICD-10CM #	H57.02	Anisocoria

Mydriatic or miotic drugs.

Prosthetic eye.

Inflammation (keratitis, iridocyclitis).

Infections (herpes zoster, syphilis, meningitis, encephalitis, TB, diphtheria, botulism).

Subdural hemorrhage.

Cavernous sinus thrombosis.

Intracranial neoplasm.

Cerebral aneurysm.

Glaucoma.

Central nervous system degenerative diseases.

Internal carotid ischemia.

Toxic polyneuritis (alcohol, lead).

Adie syndrome.

Horner syndrome.

Diabetes mellitus.

Trauma.

Congenital.

ANKLE AND FOOT PAIN[35]

ICD-10CM #	M25.579	Pain in unspecified ankle and joint pain in unspecified foot

Anterior ankle:
- Anterior impingement.
- Ankle arthritis or synovitis.
- Osteochondral defect or lesion (cartilage injury).
- Loose body within the joint.
- Talar avascular necrosis.
- Talar stress fracture.
- Tenosynovitis of the extensor hallucis longus, extensor digitorum longus.
- Deep (central) or superficial (anterolateral) peroneal nerve injury.
- Saphenous (anteromedial) nerve injury.

Posterior ankle:
- Os trigonum (accessory ossicle involving the posterior lateral tubercle of the talus).
- Posterior impingement.
- Retrocalcaneal bursitis.
- Achilles tendinopathy.
- Flexor hallucis longus tendinopathy or stenosis.

Posterolateral ankle:
- Peroneal tendinopathy.
- Subfibular impingement caused by flatfoot and impingement.
- Fibular stress fracture.
- Sural nerve injury.
- Lateral ligament injury (sprain).

Posteromedial ankle:
- Posterior tibial tendinopathy.
- Flexor digitorum longus or flexor hallucis longus tendinopathy.
- Tibial stress fracture.
- Medial malleolar stress fracture.
- Tarsal tunnel syndrome.
- Tibial nerve injury.
- Deltoid ligament injury.

Heel:
- Achilles insertional tendinopathy.
- Inflammatory enthesitis.
- Plantar fasciitis.
- Haglund disease (pump bump).
- Calcaneal stress fracture.

Hindfoot:
- Subtalar, talonavicular, or calcaneocuboid arthritis or synovitis.
- Posterior tibial tendon dysfunction or tendinopathy (medial) or peroneal tendon dysfunction (lateral).
- Occult fracture of the talus, calcaneus cuboid, or navicular.
- Accessory navicular.

Midfoot:
- Insertional tendinopathy (peroneal, posterior tibial, tibialis anterior).
- Arthritis or synovitis (navicular–cuneiform, cuneiform–metatarsal, cuboid–metatarsal).
- Navicular stress fracture.
- Spring ligament strain.

Forefoot
First ray, first MTP joint, hallux:
- Arthritis or synovitis MTP (hallux limitus/rigidus) and IP joints.
- Hallux valgus.
- Hallux varus.
- Sesamoiditis.
- Gouty monoarthritis.

Second to fifth rays, MTP joints, lesser toes:
- Arthritis or synovitis (MTP, proximal and distal IP joints).
- Lesser toe deformities (hammer and claw toes).
- Metatarsalgia.
- MTP instability.
- MTP dislocations.
- Morton neuroma (interdigital neuralgia).
- Stress fracture of the metatarsals.
- Bunionette (fifth metatarsal phalangeal deviation).
- Rheumatoid nodules.
- Bursitis (intermetatarsal or adventitious).
- Ulcer.
- Infection.

IP, Interphalangeal; *MTP,* metatarsophalangeal.

ANORECTAL ABSCESS[4]

ICD-10CM #	K61.2	Anorectal abscess

ETIOLOGY OF ANORECTAL ABSCESS

Nonspecific Etiology

Cryptoglandular.

Specific Etiology

Inflammatory condition.

Crohn disease.

Tuberculosis.

Actinomycosis.

Lymphogranuloma venereum.

Traumatic Etiology

Impalement.

Foreign body.

Anal fissure.

Iatrogenic.

Episiotomy.

Hemorrhoidectomy.

Prostatectomy.

Radiation.

Malignancy

Rectal or anal carcinoma.

Leukemia.

Lymphoma.

ANORECTAL DISEASE, AIDS PATIENT[3]

ICD-10CM #	Varies with specific diagnosis

DIFFERENTIAL DIAGNOSIS OF ANORECTAL DISEASE IN PATIENTS WITH AIDS

Infections

Bacteria

*Chlamydia trachomatis.**

Lymphogranuloma venereum.

*Neisseria gonorrhoeae.**

Shigella flexneri.

Mycobacterium tuberculosis.

Protozoa

Entamoeba histolytica.

Leishmania donovani.

Viruses

Herpes simplex virus.*

Cytomegalovirus.*

Differential Diagnosis

II

Fungi
Candida albicans.
Histoplasma capsulatum.
Neoplasms
Lymphoma.*
Kaposi sarcoma.
Squamous cell carcinoma.
Cloacogenic carcinoma.
Condyloma acuminatum.
Other
Idiopathic ulcers.*
Perirectal abscess, fistula.*

*More frequent diagnosis.

ANOREXIA[2]

| ICD-10CM # | R63.0 | Anorexia |

SELECTED CAUSES OF ANOREXIA

Gastrointestinal Tract/Liver
Gastric outlet obstruction or small bowel obstruction.
Gastric cancer.
Hepatic metastases.
Acute viral hepatitis.
Metabolic
Addison disease.
Hypopituitarism.
Hyperparathyroidism.
Functional
Extremely unpleasant sight/smell.
Systemic
Chronic pain.
Renal failure.
Severe congestive heart failure.
Respiratory failure.
Psychiatric
Depression.
Anorexia nervosa.
Medications
Digoxin.
Narcotic analgesics.
Diuretics.
Antihypertensives.
Chemotherapeutic agents.
Amphetamines.
Miscellaneous
Excessive smoking.
Excessive alcohol intake.
Oral cavity disease.
Thiamine deficiency.
Early pregnancy.
Hypogeusia or dysgeusia.

ANOVULATION

| ICD-10CM # | N97.0 | Female infertility associated with anovulation |

Anorexia and bulimia.
Strenuous exercise.
Weight loss/malnutrition.
Empty sella syndrome.
Pituitary disorders (infarction, infection, trauma, irradiation, surgery, microadenomas, macroadenomas).

Idiopathic hypopituitarism.
Drug induced.
Thyroid dysfunction (hypothyroidism, hyperthyroidism).
Systemic diseases (e.g., liver disease).
Adrenal hyperfunction (Cushing syndrome, congenital adrenal hyperplasia).
Polycystic ovarian syndrome.
Isolated gonadotropin deficiency.

ANOVULATION, HYPOTHALAMIC PITUITARY CAUSES[36]

| ICD-10CM # | N97.0 | Female infertility associated with anovulation |

CLASSIFICATION OF ANOVULATION CAUSED BY DISORDERS OF THE HYPOTHALAMIC-PITUITARY UNIT

Functional hypothalamic anovulation (amenorrhea):
Stress (psychogenic or physical).
Dieting.
Vigorous exercise.
Chronic illness (e.g., chronic liver or renal insufficiency, AIDS).
Psychiatric-medical emergencies:
Anorexia nervosa.
Medications:
    Antipsychotics (e.g., olanzapine, risperidone, amisulpride, clozapine).
    Opiates.
    Hypothyroidism.

Anatomically or Genetically Defined Pathologic Conditions of the Hypothalamic-Pituitary Unit
Pituitary tumors.
    Prolactinoma.
    Clinically nonfunctioning adenoma.
    GH-secreting adenoma (acromegaly).
    ACTH-secreting adenoma (Cushing disease).
    Other pituitary tumors (e.g., metastasis, meningioma).
Pituitary stalk section.
Hemorrhagic pituitary destruction, including pituitary apoplexy and Sheehan syndrome.
Pituitary aneurysm.
Infiltrative disease of the pituitary (e.g., lymphocytic hypophysitis, sarcoidosis, histiocytosis X, tuberculosis).
Empty sella syndrome.
Tumors that affect hypothalamic function (e.g., metastasis, craniopharyngioma).
Infiltrative granulomatous disease of the hypothalamus (e.g., sarcoidosis, histiocytosis X, tuberculosis).
Head trauma.
Irradiation to the head.
CNS infection.
Isolated gonadotropin deficiency (including Kallmann syndrome).
Other.

ACTH, Adrenocorticotropic hormone; AIDS, acquired immunodeficiency syndrome; CNS, central nervous system; GH, growth hormone.

AORTIC ARCH SEGMENT ABNORMALITIES[37]

| ICD-10CM # | Q25.49 | Other congenital malformations of aorta |

DIFFERENTIAL DIAGNOSIS OF AORTIC ARCH SEGMENT ABNORMALITIES

Dilated aortic arch:
Aortic aneurysm.
Aortic dissection.
Aortic pseudoaneurysm.
Mass silhouetting aortic arch.
Small or inapparent arch:
    Right-sided aortic arch.
    Coarctation of the aorta.
    Interruption of the aortic arch.
    Double aortic arch.

APPENDICITIS, DIFFERENTIAL DIAGNOSIS IN PREGNANCY[32]

| ICD-10CM # | Varies with specific diagnosis |

DIFFERENTIAL DIAGNOSIS OF APPENDICITIS DURING PREGNANCY

Gynecologic Conditions
Ruptured ovarian cyst.
Adnexal torsion.
Pelvic inflammatory disease or salpingitis.
Endometriosis.
Ovarian cancer.
Obstetrical Causes
Abruptio placentae.
Chorioamnionitis.
Endometritis.
Uterine fibroid degeneration.
Labor (preterm or term).
Viscus perforation after abortion.
Ruptured ectopic pregnancy.
Gastrointestinal Causes
Crohn disease.
Colonic diverticulitis (right side).
Cholecystitis.
Pancreatitis.
Mesenteric lymphadenitis.
Gastroenteritis.
Colon cancer.
Intestinal obstruction.
Hernia (incarcerated inguinal or internal).
Colonic intussusception.
Ruptured Meckel diverticulum.
Colonic perforation.
Acute mesenteric ischemia.
Other Causes
Pyelonephritis.
Urolithiasis.

APPETITE LOSS IN INFANTS AND CHILDREN[23]

ICD-10CM #	R63.0	Anorexia
	F50.8	Other eating disorders
	F98.29	Other feeding disorders of infancy and early childhood

ORGANIC DISEASE

Infection (Acute or Chronic) Neurologic
Congenital degenerative disease.
Hypothalamic lesion.
Increased intracranial pressure (including a brain tumor).
Swallowing disorders (neuromuscular).
GI
Oral lesions (e.g., thrush or herpes simplex).
Gastroesophageal reflux.
Obstruction (especially with gastric or intestinal distention).
Inflammatory bowel disease.
Celiac disease.
Constipation.
Cardiac
Congestive heart failure (especially associated with cyanotic lesions).
Metabolic
Renal failure and/or renal tubule acidosis.
Liver failure.
Congenital metabolic disease.
Lead poisoning.
Nutritional
Marasmus.
Iron deficiency.
Zinc deficiency.
Fever
Rheumatoid arthritis.
Rheumatic fever.
Drugs
Morphine.
Digitalis.
Antimetabolites.
Methylphenidate.
Amphetamines.
Miscellaneous
Prolonged restriction of oral feedings, beginning in the neonatal period.
Systemic lupus erythematosus.
Tumor.

PSYCHOLOGIC FACTORS

Anxiety, fear, depression, mania (limbic influence on the hypothalamus).
Avoidance of symptoms associated with meals (abdominal pain, diarrhea, bloating, urgency, dumping syndrome).
Anorexia nervosa.
Excessive weight loss and food aversion in athletes, simulating anorexia nervosa.

AQUEDUCTAL STENOSIS, CONGENITAL[38]

ICD-10CM #   Varies with specific diagnosis

CAUSES OF CONGENITAL AQUEDUCTAL STENOSIS

Genetic or Presumed Genetic Causes
Holoprosencephaly.
Chiari II malformation.
X-linked hydrocephalus with aqueductal stenosis and pachygyria.
Autosomal recessive hydrocephalus with aqueductal stenosis.
Mutation of dorsalizing gene in vertical axis of neural tube.
Agenesis of mesencephalic and metencephalic neuromeres.

Primary defective ependymal and choroid plexus epithelia.
Acquired Causes in Utero
Intraventricular hemorrhage with thrombus in aqueduct.
Congenital infections (e.g., cytomegalovirus infection, mumps).
Ependymitis/ventriculitis with gliosis around and within aqueduct.
Chronic arachnoiditis.
Hydranencephaly.
Aqueductal membrane across lumen.
Amnion rupture sequence.
Aneurysms, venous angiomas, and other vascular malformations.
Cystic dilation of perivascular Virchow-Robin spaces in midbrain.
Tumors of aqueduct (e.g., ependymoma, astrocytoma, glioneuronal hamartoma, neuroepithelial tumor of subcommissural organ).
Tumors that compress the midbrain tectum from above (e.g., pineal tumors and cysts, arachnoidal cysts, lipomas).

ARTERIAL OCCLUSION[39]

ICD-10CM #	I74.3	Embolism and thrombosis of arteries of the lower extremities
	I74.2	Embolism and thrombosis of arteries of the upper extremities

Thromboembolism (post-myocardial infarction, mitral stenosis, rheumatic valve disease, atrial fibrillation, atrial myxoma, marantic endocarditis, bacterial endocarditis, Libman-Sacks endocarditis).
Atheroembolism (microemboli composed of cholesterol, calcium, and platelets from proximal atherosclerotic plaques).
Arterial thrombosis (endothelial injury, altered arterial blood flow, trauma, severe atherosclerosis, acute vasculitis).
Vasospasm.
Trauma.
Hypercoagulable states.
Miscellaneous (irradiation, drugs, infections, necrotizing).

ARTHRITIS AND ABDOMINAL PAIN

ICD-10CM #	M00.9	Pyogenic arthritis, unspecified
	R10.817	Generalized abdominal tenderness
	M02.9	Reactive arthropathy

Viral syndrome.
Inflammatory bowel disease.
Celiac disease.
Vasculitis.
Systemic lupus erythematosus.
Rheumatoid arthritis.
Scleroderma.
Amyloidosis.
Chronic hepatitis C.

Whipple disease.
Polyarteritis nodosa.
Behçet disease.
Familial Mediterranean fever.
Blind loop syndrome.
Babesiosis.
Lyme disease.
Ehrlichiosis.

ARTHRITIS AND DIARRHEA

ICD-10CM #	M00.9	Pyogenic arthritis, unspecified
	R19.7	Diarrhea, unspecified

Viral syndrome.
Inflammatory bowel disease.
Celiac disease.
Whipple disease.
Enterogenic (bacterial) reactive arthritis.
Collagenous colitis.
Behçet disease.
Hyperthyroidism.
Spondyloarthropathy.
Blind loop syndrome.

ARTHRITIS AND EYE LESIONS[40]

ICD-10CM #	M00.9	Pyogenic arthritis, unspecified
	M02.3	Reiter disease
	M02.9	Reactive arthropathy

Systemic lupus erythematosus.
Sjögren syndrome.
Behçet syndrome.
Sarcoidosis.
Subacute bacterial endocarditis.
Lyme disease.
Granulomatosis with polyangiitis.
Giant cell arteritis.
Takayasu arteritis.
Rheumatoid arthritis, juvenile rheumatoid arthritis.
Scleroderma.
Inflammatory bowel disease.
Whipple disease.
Ankylosing spondylitis.
Reactive arthritis.
Psoriatic arthritis.

ARTHRITIS AND HEART MURMUR[40]

ICD-10CM #	M00.9	Pyogenic arthritis, unspecified
	I01.8	Other acute rheumatic heart disease
	M02.9	Reactive arthropathy

Subacute bacterial endocarditis.
Cardiac myxoma.
Ankylosing spondylitis.
Reactive arthritis.
Acute rheumatic fever.
Rheumatoid arthritis.
Systemic lupus erythematosus with Libman-Sacks endocarditis.
Relapsing polychondritis.

ARTHRITIS AND MUSCLE WEAKNESS[41]

ICD-10CM #	M00.9	Pyogenic arthritis, unspecified
	M62.9	Disorder of muscle, unspecified
	M02.9	Reactive arthropathy

Rheumatoid arthritis.
Ankylosing spondylitis.
Polymyositis.
Dermatomyositis.
Systemic lupus erythematosus, scleroderma, mixed connective tissue disease.
Sarcoidosis.
HIV-associated arthritis.
Whipple disease.

ARTHRITIS AND RASH[40]

ICD-10CM #	M00.9	Pyogenic arthritis, unspecified
	R21	Rash and other nonspecific skin eruption
	M02.9	Reactive arthropathy

Chronic urticaria.
Vasculitic urticaria.
Systemic lupus erythematosus.
Dermatomyositis.
Polymyositis.
Psoriatic arthritis.
Reactive arthritis.
Chronic sarcoidosis.
Serum sickness.
Sweet syndrome.
Leprosy.

ARTHRITIS AND SUBCUTANEOUS NODULES[40]

ICD-10CM #	M00.9	Pyogenic arthritis, unspecified
	A18.4	Tuberculosis of skin and subcutaneous tissue
	M02.9	Reactive arthropathy

Rheumatoid arthritis.
Gout.
Pseudogout (rare).
Sarcoidosis.
Light chain (LA) amyloidosis (primary, multiple myeloma).
Acute rheumatic fever (ARF).
Hemochromatosis.
Whipple disease.
Multicentric reticulohistiocytosis.

ARTHRITIS AND WEIGHT LOSS[40]

ICD-10CM #	M00.9	Pyogenic arthritis, unspecified
	R63.4	Abnormal weight loss
	M02.9	Reactive arthropathy

Severe rheumatoid arthritis.
Rheumatoid arthritis with vasculitis.
Reactive arthritis.
Rheumatoid arthritis or psoriatic arthritis or ankylosing spondylitis with amyloidosis.
Cancer.
Enteropathic arthritis (Crohn, ulcerative colitis).
HIV infection.
Whipple disease.
Blind loop syndrome.
Scleroderma with intestinal bacterial overgrowth.

ARTHRITIS OR EXTREMITY PAIN, IN CHILDREN AND ADOLESCENTS[19]

| ICD-10CM # | M02.9 | Reactive arthropathy |

CAUSES OF ARTHRITIS OR EXTREMITY PAIN IN CHILDREN AND ADOLESCENTS
Rheumatic and Inflammatory Diseases
Juvenile idiopathic arthritis.
Systemic lupus erythematosus.
Juvenile dermatomyositis.
Polyarteritis.
Vasculitis.
Scleroderma.
Sjögren syndrome.
Behçet disease.
Overlap syndromes.
Granulomatosis with polyangiitis (Wegener granulomatosis).
Sarcoidosis.
Kawasaki syndrome.
Henoch-Schönlein purpura.
Chronic recurrent multifocal osteomyelitis.
Seronegative Spondyloarthropathies
Juvenile ankylosing spondylitis.
Inflammatory bowel disease.
Psoriatic arthritis.
Reactive arthritis associated with urethritis, iridocyclitis, and mucocutaneous lesions.
Infectious Illnesses
Bacterial arthritis (septic arthritis, *Staphylococcus aureus*, pneumococcus, gonococcus, *Haemophilus influenzae*).
Lyme disease.
Viral illness (parvovirus, rubella, mumps, Epstein-Barr virus, hepatitis B).
Fungal arthritis.
Mycobacterial infection.
Spirochetal infection.
Endocarditis.
Reactive Arthritis
Acute rheumatic fever.
Reactive arthritis (postinfectious due to *Shigella, Salmonella, Yersinia, Chlamydia*, or meningococcus).
Serum sickness.
Toxic synovitis of the hip.
Postimmunization.
Immunodeficiencies
Hypogammaglobulinemia.
Immunoglobulin A deficiency.
HIV.
Congenital and Metabolic Disorders
Gout.

Pseudogout.
Mucopolysaccharidoses.
Thyroid disease (hypothyroidism, hyperthyroidism).
Hyperparathyroidism.
Vitamin C deficiency (scurvy).
Hereditary connective tissue disease (Marfan syndrome, Ehlers-Danlos syndrome).
Fabry disease.
Farber disease.
Amyloidosis (familial Mediterranean fever).
Bone and Cartilage Disorders
Trauma.
Patellofemoral syndrome.
Hypermobility syndrome.
Osteochondritis dissecans.
Avascular necrosis (including Legg-Calvé-Perthes disease).
Hypertrophic osteoarthropathy.
Slipped capital femoral epiphysis.
Osteolysis.
Benign bone tumors (including osteoid osteoma).
Histiocytosis.
Rickets.
Neuropathic Disorders
Peripheral neuropathies.
Carpal tunnel syndrome.
Charcot joints.
Neoplastic Disorders
Leukemia.
Neuroblastoma.
Lymphoma.
Bone tumors (osteosarcoma, Ewing sarcoma).
Histiocytic syndromes.
Synovial tumors.
Hematologic Disorders
Hemophilia.
Hemoglobinopathies (including sickle cell disease).
Miscellaneous Disorders
Pigmented villonodular synovitis.
Plant-thorn synovitis (foreign body arthritis).
Myositis ossificans.
Eosinophilic fasciitis.
Tendinitis (overuse injury).
Raynaud phenomenon.
Pain Syndromes
Fibromyalgia.
Growing pains.
Depression (with somatization).
Reflex sympathetic dystrophy.
Regional myofascial pain syndromes.

ARTHRITIS, AXIAL SKELETON

ICD-10CM #	M45.9	Ankylosing spondylitis of unspecified sites in spine
	L40.54	Psoriatic juvenile arthropathy
	L40.59	Other psoriatic arthropathy
	M15.9	Polyosteoarthritis, unspecified
	M45.9	Ankylosing spondylitis of unspecified sites in spine

Rheumatoid arthritis.
Psoriatic arthritis.
Reiter syndrome (reactive arthritis).
Ankylosing spondylitis.

Juvenile rheumatoid arthritis.
Degenerative disease of the nucleus pulposus.
Spondylosis deformans.
Diffuse idiopathic skeletal hyperostosis (DISH).
Alkaptonuria.
Infection.

ARTHRITIS, CHRONIC, MONOARTICULAR OR OLIGOARTICULAR, INFECTIOUS CAUSES[42]

ICD-10CM # Varies with specific diagnosis

INFECTIOUS CAUSES OF CHRONIC MONOARTICULAR OR OLIGOARTICULAR ARTHRITIS

Bacterial
Borrelia burgdorferi.
Tropheryma whipplei.
Treponema pallidum.
Nocardia spp.

Fungi
Candida spp.
Cryptococcus neoformans.
Blastomyces dermatitidis.
Coccidioides spp.
Paracoccidioides brasiliensis.
Sporothrix schenckii.
Aspergillus spp. and other molds, including Rhizopus, Scedosporium, and Fusarium.

Mycobacteria
Mycobacterium tuberculosis.
M. kansasii.
M. marinum.
M. avium-intracellulare complex.
M. terrae.
M. fortuitum, M. chelonae, M. abscessus.
M. haemophilum.
M. leprae.

Parasites
Helminths.
Filariae.

ARTHRITIS, FEVER, AND RASH[40]

ICD-10CM #		
	M00.9	Pyogenic arthritis, unspecified
	M02.9	Reactive arthropathy
	R21	Rash and other nonspecific skin eruption
	R50.9	Fever, unspecified

Rubella, parvovirus B19.
Gonococcemia, meningococcemia.
Secondary syphilis, Lyme borreliosis.
Adult acute rheumatic fever, adult Still disease, adult Kawasaki disease.
Vasculitic urticaria.
Acute sarcoidosis.
Familial Mediterranean fever.
Hyperimmunoglobulinemia D and periodic fever syndrome.

ARTHRITIS, MONOARTICULAR AND OLIGOARTICULAR[43]

ICD-10CM #		
	M19.90	Unspecified osteoarthritis, unspecified site
	M01.X0	Direct infection of unspecified joint in infectious and parasitic diseases classified elsewhere
	M13.10	Monoarthritis, not elsewhere classified, unspecified site

Septic arthritis (S. aureus, Neisseria gonorrhoeae, meningococci, streptococci, Streptococcus pneumoniae, enteric gram-negative bacilli).
Crystalline-induced arthritis (gout, pseudogout, calcium oxalate, hydroxyapatite and other basic calcium/phosphate crystals).
Traumatic joint injury.
Hemarthrosis.
Monoarticular or oligoarticular flare of an inflammatory polyarticular rheumatic disease (rheumatoid arthritis, psoriatic arthritis, Reiter syndrome [reactive arthritis], systemic lupus erythematosus).

ARTHRITIS, PEDIATRIC AGE[23]

ICD-10CM #		
	M01.X0	Direct infection of unspecified joint in infectious and parasitic diseases classified elsewhere
	M08.00	Unspecified juvenile rheumatoid arthritis of unspecified site
	M08.3	Juvenile rheumatoid polyarthritis (seronegative)
	M08.40	Pauciarticular juvenile rheumatoid arthritis, unspecified site

RHEUMATIC DISEASES OF CHILDHOOD

Acute rheumatic fever.
Systemic lupus erythematosus.
Juvenile ankylosing spondylitis.
Polymyositis and dermatomyositis.
Vasculitis.
Scleroderma.
Psoriatic arthritis.
Mixed connective tissue disease and overlap syndromes.
Kawasaki disease.
Behçet syndrome.
Familial Mediterranean fever.
Reiter syndrome (reactive arthritis).

Reflex sympathetic dystrophy.
Fibromyalgia (fibrositis).

INFECTIOUS DISEASES
Bacterial arthritis.
Viral or postviral arthritis.
Fungal arthritis.
Osteomyelitis.
Reactive arthritis.

NEOPLASTIC DISEASES
Leukemia.
Lymphoma.
Neuroblastoma.
Primary bone tumors.

NONINFLAMMATORY DISORDERS
Trauma.
Avascular necrosis syndromes.
Osteochondroses.
Slipped capital femoral epiphysis.
Diskitis.
Patellofemoral dysfunction (chondromalacia patellae).
Toxic synovitis of the hip.
Overuse syndromes.

GENETIC OR CONGENITAL SYNDROMES

Hematologic Disorders
Sickle cell disease.
Hemophilia.

INFLAMMATORY BOWEL DISEASE

Miscellaneous
Growing pains.
Psychogenic arthralgias (conversion reactions).
Hypermobility syndrome.
Villonodular synovitis.
Foreign body arthritis.

ARTHRITIS, POLYARTICULAR

ICD-10CM #		
	M15.0	Primary generalized (osteo)arthritis
	M12.89	Other specific arthropathies, not elsewhere classified, multiple sites
	M08.3	Juvenile rheumatoid polyarthritis (seronegative)

Rheumatoid arthritis, juvenile (rheumatoid) polyarthritis.
Systemic lupus erythematosus, other connective tissue diseases, erythema nodosum, palindromic rheumatism, relapsing polychondritis.
Psoriatic arthritis, ankylosing spondylitis.
Sarcoidosis.
Lyme arthritis, bacterial endocarditis, Neisseria gonorrhoeae infection, rheumatic fever, Reiter disease (reactive arthritis).
Crystal deposition disease.
Hypersensitivity to serum or drugs.
Hepatitis B, HIV, rubella, mumps.

Differential Diagnosis

II

Other: serum sickness, leukemias, lymphomas, enteropathic arthropathy, Whipple disease, Behçet syndrome, Henoch-Schönlein purpura, familial Mediterranean fever, hypertrophic pulmonary osteoarthropathy.

ASCENDING AORTA, ABNORMAL SEGMENT[44]

ICD-10CM #	Q25.49	Other congenital malformations of aorta

DIFFERENTIAL DIAGNOSIS OF AN ABNORMAL ASCENDING AORTA SEGMENT

Aortic aneurysm.
Aortic dissection.
Poststenotic dilation in aortic stenosis.
Aortic dilation in aortic insufficiency.

ASCITES

ICD-10CM #	R18.0	Malignant ascites
	C78.6	Secondary malignant neoplasm of retroperitoneum and peritoneum
	I89.8	Other specified noninfective disorders of lymphatic vessels and lymph nodes

Hypoalbuminemia: nephrotic syndrome, protein-losing gastroenteropathy, starvation.
Cirrhosis.
Hepatic congestion: congestive heart failure, constrictive pericarditis, tricuspid insufficiency, hepatic vein obstruction (Budd-Chiari syndrome), inferior vena cava or portal vein obstruction.
Peritoneal infections: TB and other bacterial infections, fungal diseases, parasites.
Neoplasms: primary hepatic neoplasms, metastases to liver or peritoneum, lymphomas, leukemias, myeloid metaplasia.
Lymphatic obstruction: mediastinal tumors, trauma to the thoracic duct, filariasis.
Ovarian disease: Meigs syndrome, struma ovarii.
Chronic pancreatitis or pseudocyst: pancreatic ascites.
Leakage of bile: bile ascites.
Urinary obstruction or trauma: urine ascites.
Myxedema.
Chylous ascites.

ASPIRATION, CHRONIC[22]

ICD-10CM #	Varies with specific diagnosis

CAUSES OF CHRONIC ASPIRATION

Cerebrovascular accidents.
Atherosclerotic thrombosis.
Embolism.
Intracranial hemorrhage.

DEGENERATIVE NEUROLOGIC DISEASES

Parkinson disease.
Amyotrophic lateral sclerosis.

Progressive supranuclear palsy.
Multiple sclerosis.

NEUROMUSCULAR AND MUSCULAR DISORDERS

Poliomyelitis.
Myasthenia gravis.
Muscular dystrophy.
Myopathies.

PERIPHERAL NERVE DISORDERS

Cranial nerves.
Guillain-Barré syndrome.
Intracranial neoplasms.
Primary dysfunction related to neoplasm.
Postsurgical dysfunction.
Trauma.
Closed head injury.
Hematoma.
Anoxic brain injury.
Intracranial infection.

PHARYNGEAL DISORDERS

Neoplasms.
Postsurgical dysfunction.
Postirradiation dysfunction.
Zenker diverticulum.
Cricopharyngeal dysfunction.
Stricture.

ESOPHAGEAL DISORDERS

Reflux.
Achalasia.
Caustic injury.

MISCELLANEOUS

Severe illness.
Multisystem disease.
Drug intoxication.

ASPIRATION LUNG INJURY, CHILDREN[19]

ICD-10CM #	P24.8	Neonatal aspiration syndromes

CONDITIONS PREDISPOSING TO ASPIRATION LUNG INJURY IN CHILDREN

Anatomic and Mechanical
Tracheoesophageal fistula.
Laryngeal cleft.
Vascular ring.
Cleft palate.
Micrognathia.
Macroglossia.
Achalasia.
Esophageal foreign body.
Tracheostomy.
Endotracheal tube.
Nasoenteric tube.
Collagen vascular disease (scleroderma, dermatomyositis).
Gastroesophageal reflux disease.
Obesity.
Neuromuscular
Altered consciousness.
Immaturity of swallowing/prematurity.
Dysautonomia.
Increased intracranial pressure.

Hydrocephalus.
Vocal cord paralysis.
Cerebral palsy.
Muscular dystrophy.
Myasthenia gravis.
Guillain-Barré syndrome.
Werdnig-Hoffmann disease.
Ataxia-telangiectasia.
Cerebral vascular accident.
Miscellaneous
Poor oral hygiene.
Gingivitis.
Prolonged hospitalization.
Gastric outlet or intestinal obstruction.
Poor feeding techniques (bottle propping, overfeeding, inappropriate foods for toddlers).
Bronchopulmonary dysplasia.
Viral infection.

ASTHENIA

ICD-10CM #	G93.3	Postviral fatigue syndrome
	R53.1	Weakness
	R53.81	Other malaise
	R53.83	Other fatigue

Depression.
Chronic fatigue syndrome.
Sleep disorders.
Anemia.
Hypothyroidism.
Sedentary lifestyle.
Medications (e.g., narcotics, sedatives).
Infections.
Dehydration/electrolyte disorders.
Chronic obstructive pulmonary disease and other pulmonary disorders.
Renal failure.
Congestive heart failure.
Diabetes.
Addison disease.
Paraneoplastic syndrome.

ASTHMA, CHILDHOOD[45]

ICD-10CM #	J45.20	Mild intermittent asthma, uncomplicated
	J45.22	Mild intermittent asthma with status asthmaticus

INFECTIONS

Bronchiolitis (respiratory syncytial virus).
Pneumonia.
Croup.
Tuberculosis, histoplasmosis.
Bronchiectasis.
Bronchiolitis obliterans.
Bronchitis.
Sinusitis.

ANATOMIC, CONGENITAL

Cystic fibrosis.
Vascular rings.
Ciliary dyskinesia.
B-lymphocyte immune defect.
Congestive heart failure.
Laryngotracheomalacia.
Tumor, lymphoma.

H-type tracheoesophageal fistula.
Repaired tracheoesophageal fistula.
Gastroesophageal reflux.

VASCULITIS, HYPERSENSITIVITY

Allergic bronchopulmonary aspergillosis.
Allergic alveolitis, hypersensitivity pneumonitis.
Churg-Strauss syndrome.
Periarteritis nodosa.

OTHER

Foreign body aspiration.
Pulmonary thromboembolism.
Psychogenic cough.
Sarcoidosis.
Bronchopulmonary dysplasia.
Vocal cord dysfunction.

ATAXIA

ICD-10CM #		
	R27.0	Ataxia, unspecified
	R27.8	Other lack of coordination
	R27.9	Unspecified lack of coordination
	F10.229	Alcohol dependence with intoxication, unspecified
	F10.20	Alcohol dependence, uncomplicated
	G11.1	Early-onset cerebellar ataxia
	G31.89	Other specified degenerative diseases of nervous system
	F44.4	Conversion disorder with motor symptom or deficit
	F44.6	Conversion disorder with sensory symptom or deficit

Vertebral-basilar artery ischemia.
Diabetic neuropathy.
Tabes dorsalis.
Vitamin B_{12} deficiency.
Multiple sclerosis and other demyelinating diseases.
Meningomyelopathy.
Cerebellar neoplasms, hemorrhage, abscess, infarct.
Nutritional (Wernicke encephalopathy).
Paraneoplastic syndromes.
Parainfectious: Guillain-Barré syndrome, acute ataxia of childhood and young adults.
Toxins: phenytoin, alcohol, sedatives, organophosphates.
Wilson disease (hepatolenticular degeneration).
Hypothyroidism.
Myopathy.
Cerebellar and spinocerebellar degeneration: ataxia/telangiectasia, Friedreich ataxia.
Frontal lobe lesions: tumors, thrombosis of anterior cerebral artery, hydrocephalus.
Labyrinthine destruction: neoplasm, injury, inflammation, compression.
Hysteria.
AIDS.

ATAXIA, ACUTE OR RECURRENT[46]

ICD-10CM #		
	R27.0	Ataxia, unspecified
	R27.8	Other lack of coordination
	R27.9	Unspecified lack of coordination
	F10.229	Alcohol dependence with intoxication, unspecified
	F10.20	Alcohol dependence, uncomplicated
	G11.1	Early-onset cerebellar ataxia
	G31.89	Other specified degenerative diseases of nervous system
	F44.4	Conversion disorder motor symptom or deficit
	F44.6	Conversion disorder with sensory symptom or deficit

Drug ingestion (e.g., phenytoin, carbamazepine, sedatives, hypnotics, and phencyclidine) or intoxication (e.g., alcohol, ethylene glycol, hydrocarbon fumes, lead, mercury, or thallium).
Postinfectious (cerebellitis [e.g., varicella], acute disseminated encephalomyelitis).
Head trauma.
Basilar migraine.
Benign paroxysmal vertigo (migraine equivalent).
Brain tumor or neuroblastoma (if accompanied by opsoclonus or myoclonus [i.e., "dancing eyes, dancing feet"]).
Hydrocephalus.
Infection (e.g., labyrinthitis, abscess).
Seizure (ictal or post-ictal).
Vascular events (e.g., cerebellar hemorrhage or stroke).
Miller-Fisher variant of Guillain-Barré syndrome (ataxia, ophthalmoplegia, and areflexia). Warning: if bulbar signs present, disease is likely progressive; patient may lose ability to protect airway and/or ability to breathe.
Inherited ataxias.
Inborn errors of metabolism (e.g., mitochondrial disorders, amino-acidopathies, urea cycle defects).
Conversion reaction.
Multiple sclerosis.

ATAXIA, CEREBELLAR, ADULT ONSET[47]

ICD-10CM #		
	G11.0	Congenital nonprogressive ataxia
	G11.2	Late-onset cerebellar ataxia

CAUSES OF ADULT-ONSET CEREBELLAR ATAXIA

Inherited
Later onset spinocerebellar ataxia syndromes.
Rarely Friedreich ataxia.

Congenital
Arnold–Chiari malformation (cerebellar ectopia).
Inflammatory
Multiple sclerosis.
Sarcoidosis.
Infections (TB, viral).
Neoplastic
Often metastatic in adults.
Meningioma, neurofibroma.
Hemangioblastoma.
Paraneoplastic
Usually with small cell bronchial carcinoma.
Vascular
Infarction, hemorrhage.
Arteriovenous malformations.
Trauma
Head injury.
Postsurgical.
Toxic
Alcohol, phenytoin, solvent abuse.
Endocrine
Hypothyroidism (very rare).
Degenerative
Multiple system atrophy.

ATAXIA, CEREBELLAR, CHILDREN[47]

ICD-10CM #		
	G11.0	Congenital nonprogressive ataxia
	G11.2	Late-onset cerebellar ataxia

CAUSES OF CEREBELLAR ATAXIA IN CHILDREN

Congenital Malformations
Cerebellar agenesis/hypoplasia.
Dandy–Walker syndrome.
Arnold–Chiari malformation.
Hereditary Ataxias
Friedreich ataxia.
Trauma
Birth trauma.
Head injury in childhood.
Infectious
Secondary to bacterial meningitis.
Secondary to encephalitis.
Hydrocephalus
Tumors
Medulloblastoma.
Astrocytoma.
Hemangioblastoma.

ATAXIA, CHRONIC OR PROGRESSIVE[46]

ICD-10CM #		
	R27.0	Ataxia, unspecified
	R27.8	Other lack of coordination
	R27.9	Unspecified lack of coordination
	G11.1	Early-onset cerebellar ataxia
	G11.0	Congenital nonprogressive ataxia
	G11.2	Late-onset cerebellar ataxia
	G11.3	Cerebellar ataxia with defective DNA repair
	G11.8	Other hereditary ataxia

Differential Diagnosis

II

Hydrocephalus.
Hypothyroidism.
Tumor or paraneoplastic syndrome.
Low vitamin E levels (e.g., cystic fibrosis).
Wilson disease.
Inborn errors of metabolism.
Inherited ataxias (e.g., ataxia-telangiectasia, Friedreich ataxia).

ATAXIA IN CHILDHOOD[48]

ICD-10CM #	G11.1	Early-onset cerebellar ataxia

SELECTED CAUSES OF ATAXIA IN CHILDHOOD

Congenital:
  Agenesis of vermis of the cerebellum.
  Aplasia or dysplasia of the cerebellum.
  Basilar impression.
  Cerebellar dysplasia with microgyria, macrogyria, or agyria.
  Cervical spinal bifida with herniation of the cerebellum (Chiari malformation, type 3).
  Chiari malformation.
  Dandy-Walker syndrome.
  Encephalocele.
  Hydrocephalus (progressive).
  Hypoplasia of the cerebellum.
Degenerative and/or genetic:
  Acute intermittent cerebellar ataxia.
  Ataxia, retinitis pigmentosa, deafness, vestibular abnormality, and intellectual deterioration.
  Ataxia-telangiectasia.
  Biemond posterior column ataxia.
  Cerebellar ataxia with deafness, anosmia, absent caloric responses, nonreactive pupils, and hyporeflexia.
  Cockayne syndrome.
  Dentate cerebellar ataxia (dyssynergia cerebellaris progressiva).
  Familial ataxia with macular degeneration.
  Friedreich ataxia.
  Hereditary cerebellar ataxia, intellectual retardation, choreoathetosis, and eunuchoidism.
  Hereditary cerebellar ataxia with myotonia and cataracts.
  Hypertrophic interstitial neuritis.
  Marie ataxia.
  Marinesco-Sjögren syndrome.
  Pelizaeus-Merzbacher disease.
  Periodic attacks of vertigo, diplopia, and ataxia—autosomal dominant inheritance.
  Posterior and lateral column difficulties, nystagmus, and muscle atrophy.
  Progressive cerebellar ataxia and epilepsy.
  Ramsay Hunt syndrome (myoclonic seizures and ataxia).
  Roussy-Lévy syndrome.
  Spinocerebellar ataxia (SCAs); olivopontocerebellar ataxias.
Endocrinologic:
  Cretinism.
  Hypothyroidism.
Infectious or postinfectious:
  Acute cerebellar ataxia.
  Acute disseminated encephalomyelitis.

Cerebellar abscess.
Coxsackievirus.
Diphtheria.
Echovirus.
Fisher syndrome.
Infectious mononucleosis (Epstein-Barr virus infection).
Infectious polyneuropathy.
Japanese B encephalitis.
Mumps encephalitis.
Mycoplasma pneumoniae.
Pertussis.
Polio.
Postbacterial meningitis.
Rubeola.
Tuberculosis.
Typhoid.
Varicella.
Metabolic:
  Abetalipoproteinemia.
  Argininosuccinic aciduria.
  Ataxia with vitamin E deficiency (AVED).
  GM2 gangliosidosis (late).
  Hartnup disease.
  Hyperalaninemia.
  Hyperammonemia I and II.
  Hypoglycemia.
  Kearns-Sayre syndrome.
  Leigh disease.
  Maple syrup urine disease (intermittent).
  MERRF (myoclonic epilepsy with ragged red fibers).
  Metachromatic leukodystrophy.
  Mitochondrial complex defects (I, III, IV).
  Multiple carboxylase deficiency (biotinidase deficiency).
  Neuronal ceroid-lipofuscinosis.
  Neuropathy, ataxia, retinitis pigmentosa (NARP).
  Niemann-Pick disease (late infantile).
  5-Oxoprolinuria.
  Pyruvate decarboxylase deficiency.
  Refsum disease.
  Sialidosis.
  Triose-phosphate isomerase deficiency.
  Tryptophanuria.
  Wernicke encephalopathy (thiamine or B$_1$ deficiency).
Neoplastic:
  Frontal lobe tumors.
  Hemispheric cerebellar tumors.
  Midline cerebellar tumors.
  Neuroblastoma.
  Pontine tumors (primarily gliomas).
  Spinal cord tumors.
Primary psychogenic:
  Conversion reaction.
Toxic:
  Alcohol.
  Benzodiazepines.
  Carbamazepine.
  Clonazepam.
  Lead encephalopathy.
  Phenobarbital.
  Phenytoin.
  Primidone.
  Tick paralysis poisoning.
Traumatic:
  Acute cerebellar edema.
  Acute frontal lobe edema.

Vascular:
  Angioblastoma of cerebellum.
  Basilar migraine.
  Cerebellar embolism.
  Cerebellar hemorrhage.
  Cerebellar thrombosis.
  Posterior cerebellar artery disease.
  Vasculitis.
  von Hippel-Lindau disease.

ATAXIA, TOXIC CAUSES[49]

ICD-10CM #	R27.0	Early-onset cerebellar ataxia

SELECTED TOXIC CAUSES OF ATAXIA

Medications:
  Acetohexamide.
  Amiodarone.
  Anticholinergic agents.
  Antidepressants, including selective serotonin reuptake inhibitors.
  Antiepileptic drugs.
  Antihistamines.
  Antimicrobials, antifungals.
  Antineoplastics.
  Antiparasitics.
  Baclofen.
  Buspirone.
  Dextromethorphan.
  Disulfiram.
  Ethanol.
  Fenfluramine.
  Lithium.
  Lysergic acid diethylamide (LSD), phencyclidine palmitate (PCP).
  Mexiletine.
  Sedatives, narcotics.
Industrial toxins:
  Aluminum compounds.
  Butyl alcohol.
  Carbon monoxide.
  Carbon tetrachloride.
  Ethylene glycol.
  Formaldehyde.
  Gasoline.
  Manganese.
  Metaldehyde (snail bait, fire starters).
  Paradichlorobenzene (moth repellent, diaper pail deodorant).
  Rodenticides: aluminum phosphide, sodium monofluoroacetate.
  Solvents.
Biologic toxins:
  Belladonna, hyoscyamine.
  Buckeye (*Aesculus* spp.).
  Mayapple (*Podophyllum peltatum*).
  Mescaline, peyote.
  Podophyllum (ingested).
  Poison hemlock (*Conium maculatum*).

ATELECTASIS

ICD-10CM #	J98.11	Atelectasis

Lung neoplasm (primary or metastatic).
Infection (pneumonia, TB, fungal, histoplasmosis).
Postoperative (lower lobes).
Sarcoidosis.

Mucoid impaction.
Foreign body.
Postinflammatory (middle lobe syndrome).
Pneumothorax.
Pleural effusion.
Pneumoconiosis.
Interstitial fibrosis.
Bulla.
Mediastinal or adjacent mass.

ATRIAL ENLARGEMENT, LEFT ATRIUM[21]

ICD-10CM #	I51.7	Cardiomegaly

CAUSES OF LARGE LEFT ATRIUM

Causes Due to Volume Overload

Mitral regurgitation (often with left ventricular failure).
Ventricular septal defect.
Patent ductus arteriosus.
Atrial septal defect with shunt reversal (i.e., pulmonary hypertension).
ASD with tricuspid atresia (obligatory shunt reversal).
Aortopulmonary window.

Causes Due to Pressure Overload

Mitral stenosis.
Noncompliant left ventricle: hypertension, hypertrophic cardiomyopathy, aortic stenosis.
Left ventricular failure (often with secondary mitral regurgitation).
Left atrial myxoma.

Other Causes (Both Rare)

Atrial fibrillation.
Isolated/idiopathic.

ATRIAL ENLARGEMENT, RIGHT ATRIUM

ICD-10CM #	I51.7	Cardiomegaly

Right ventricular failure.
Atrial septal defect.
Tricuspid regurgitation.
Tricuspid stenosis.
Pulmonary hypertension.
Restrictive cardiomyopathy.
Right atrial myxoma.
Ebstein anomaly.
Anomalous pulmonary venous drainage to the right atrium.
Endomyocardial fibrosis.
Sinus of Valsalva fistula.
Arrhythmogenic right ventricular dysplasia.

ATYPICAL LYMPHOCYTOSIS, HETEROPHIL NEGATIVE, INFECTIOUS CAUSES[18]

ICD-10CM #	D72.820	Lymphocytosis (symptomatic)

MOST COMMON INFECTIOUS CAUSES OF HETEROPHIL-NEGATIVE ATYPICAL LYMPHOCYTOSIS

Babesiosis.
Cytomegalovirus.

Epstein-Barr virus (particularly in children).
Human herpesvirus 6.
HIV (especially during acute seroconversion).
Infectious mononucleosis.
Malaria.
Measles.
Toxoplasmosis.
Varicella.
Infectious hepatitis.

AV NODAL BLOCK[39]

ICD-10CM #	I44.30	Unspecified atrioventricular block
	I44.2	Atrioventricular block, complete

Idiopathic fibrosis (Lenègre disease).
Sclerodegenerative processes (e.g., Lev disease with calcification of the mitral and aortic annuli).
AV node radiofrequency ablation procedure.
Medications (e.g., digoxin, β-blockers, calcium channel blockers, class III antiarrhythmics).
Acute inferior wall myocardial infarction.
Myocarditis.
Infections (endocarditis, Lyme disease).
Infiltrative diseases (e.g., hemochromatosis, sarcoidosis, amyloidosis).
Trauma (including cardiac surgical procedures).
Collagen vascular diseases.
Aortic root diseases (e.g., spondylitis).
Electrolyte abnormalities (e.g., hyperkalemia).

BACK PAIN

ICD-10CM #	M54.89	Other dorsalgia
	M54.9	Dorsalgia, unspecified
	M54.5	Low back pain
	F45.42	Pain disorder with related psychological factors
	M54.08	Panniculitis affecting regions of neck and back, sacral and sacrococcygeal region
	S23.9XXA	Sprain of unspecified parts of thorax, initial encounter
	M43.27	Fusion of spine, lumbosacral region
	M43.28	Fusion of spine, sacral and sacrococcygeal region
	M53.2X7	Spinal instabilities, lumbosacral region
	M53.3	Sacrococcygeal disorders, not elsewhere classified

Trauma: injury to bone, joint, or ligament.
Mechanical: pregnancy, obesity, fatigue, scoliosis.
Degenerative: osteoarthritis.

Infections: osteomyelitis, subarachnoid or spinal abscess, TB, meningitis, basilar pneumonia.
Metabolic: osteoporosis, osteomalacia.
Vascular: leaking aortic aneurysm, subarachnoid or spinal hemorrhage/infarction.
Neoplastic: myeloma, Hodgkin disease, carcinoma of pancreas, metastatic neoplasm from breast, prostate, lung.
GI: penetrating ulcer, pancreatitis, cholelithiasis, inflammatory bowel disease.
Renal: hydronephrosis, calculus, neoplasm, renal infarction, pyelonephritis.
Hematologic: sickle cell crisis, acute hemolysis.
Gynecologic: neoplasm of uterus or ovary, dysmenorrhea, salpingitis, uterine prolapse.
Inflammatory: ankylosing spondylitis, psoriatic arthritis, Reiter syndrome (reactive arthritis).
Lumbosacral strain.
Psychogenic: malingering, hysteria, anxiety.
Endocrine: adrenal hemorrhage or infarction.

BACK PAIN, CHILDREN AND ADOLESCENTS[19]

ICD-10CM #	M54.5	Low back pain
	M54.9	Dorsalgia

INFLAMMATORY OR INFECTIOUS

Diskitis.
Vertebral osteomyelitis (pyogenic, tuberculous).
Spinal epidural abscess.
Pyelonephritis.
Pancreatitis.

RHEUMATOLOGIC

Pauciarticular juvenile rheumatoid arthritis.
Reiter syndrome (reactive arthritis).
Ankylosing spondylitis.
Psoriatic arthritis.

DEVELOPMENTAL

Spondylolysis.
Spondylolisthesis.
Scheuermann disease.
Scoliosis.

TRAUMATIC (ACUTE VS. REPETITIVE)

Hip-pelvis anomalies.
Herniated disk.
Overuse syndromes.
Vertebral stress fractures.
Upper cervical spine instability.

NEOPLASTIC

Vertebral Tumors

Benign

Eosinophilic granuloma.
Aneurysmal bone cyst.
Osteoid osteoma.
Osteoblastoma.

Malignant

Osteogenic sarcoma.
Leukemia.
Lymphoma.
Metastatic tumors.

Spinal Cord, Ganglia, and Nerve Roots

Intramedullary spinal cord tumor.

Sympathetic chain.
Ganglioneuroma.
Ganglioneuroblastoma.
Neuroblastoma.

OTHER

Intraabdominal or pelvic pathology.
Following lumbar puncture.
Conversion reaction.
Juvenile osteoporosis.

BACK PAIN, LOW, ACUTE[43]

ICD-10CM #	M54.5	Low back pain

DIFFERENTIAL CONSIDERATIONS IN ACUTE LOW BACK PAIN

Emergent
Aortic dissection.
Cauda equina syndrome.
Epidural abscess or hematoma.
Meningitis.
Ruptured/expanding aortic aneurysm.
Spinal fracture or subluxation with cord or root impingement.
Urgent
Back pain with neurologic deficits.
Disk herniation causing neurologic compromise.
Malignancy.
Sciatica with motor nerve root compression.
Spinal fractures without cord impingement.
Spinal stenosis.
Transverse myelitis.
Vertebral osteomyelitis.
Common or Stable
Acute ligamentous injury.
Acute muscle strain.
Ankylosing spondylitis.
Degenerative joint disease.
Intervertebral disk disease without impingement.
Pathologic fracture without impingement.
Seropositive arthritis.
Spondylolisthesis.
Referred or Visceral
Cholecystitis.
Esophageal disease.
Nephrolithiasis.
Ovarian torsion, mass, or tumor.
Pancreatitis.
Peptic ulcer disease.
Pleural effusion.
Pneumonia.
Pulmonary embolism.
Pyelonephritis.
Retroperitoneal hemorrhage or mass.

BACK PAIN, VISCEROGENIC ORIGIN

ICD-10CM #	F45.41	Pain disorder exclusively related to psychological factors
	M54	Dorsalgia
	M54.5	Low back pain

Urolithiasis.
Aortic aneurysm.
Colorectal carcinoma.

Endometriosis.
Tubal pregnancy.
Prostatitis.
Peptic ulcer.
Pancreatitis.
Diverticular spasm.
Metastatic neoplasm (e.g., bladder, uterus, ovary, kidney).

BACTERIAL OVERGROWTH, SMALL INTESTINE[2]

ICD-10CM #	A04.9	Bacterial intestinal infection, unspecified

Gastric surgery—Billroth II.
Small bowel diverticula.
Small bowel stricture:
  Crohn disease.
  Radiation enteritis.
Impaired small intestinal motility:
  Scleroderma.
  Diabetes mellitus.
  Chronic intestinal pseudoobstruction.
Miscellaneous/multifactorial:
  Elderly.
  Immune deficiency syndromes.
  Chronic pancreatitis.
  Cirrhosis.

BALLISM[43]

ICD-10CM #	G25.4	Drug-induced chorea
	G25.5	Other chorea

Cerebral infarction or hemorrhage.
Medications (e.g., dopamine agonists, phenytoin).
Central nervous system neoplasm (primary or metastatic).
Nonketotic hyperosmolar state.

BENIGN SLEEP MYOCLONUS OF INFANCY (BSMI)[50]

ICD-10CM #	Varies with specific diagnosis

Common Mimics of BSMI

Mimics	Distinguishing Features
Myoclonic seizures.	BSMI occurs only during sleep and stops abruptly and consistently when infants are aroused, whereas seizures can occur during wakefulness. Epileptiform activity on EEG is present during epileptic myoclonus but not with BSMI. BSMI is seen typically in neurologically and developmentally normal infants, whereas myoclonic seizures may be associated with perinatal disorders (i.e., hypoxic-ischemic encephalopathy, infection, or metabolic abnormalities).

Mimics	Distinguishing Features
Infantile spasms (West syndrome).	Often seen after the first month of life. Manifested by sudden head flexion with arm extension and lower extremity flexion. Epileptiform activity on EEG is present; usually associated with an abnormal EEG pattern known as hypsarrhythmia.
Pyridoxine-dependency seizures.	Can occur while infants are awake, whereas BSMI will stop abruptly and consistently when infants are aroused. EEG slowing is supportive of encephalopathy vs. BSMI. Responsive to vitamin B_6 (pyridoxine).
Hyperekplexia (startle disease).	Generalized stiffness while awake. Exaggerated startle reflex. Typical movements occur as an excessive response to stimulation, such as touch or loud noise.
Jitteriness.	Occurs during wakefulness in response to tactile or auditory stimuli, whereas BSMI occurs during sleep.

BSMI, Benign sleep myoclonus of infancy, *EEG*, electroencephalogram.

BILE DUCT, DILATED[2]

ICD-10CM #	K83.1	Obstruction of bile duct

Normal variant.
Postcholecystectomy.
Unsuspected bile duct stone.
Sphincter of Oddi stenosis.
Occult bile duct stricture.
Previous bile duct injury.
Early carcinoma of the pancreas, carcinoma of the bile duct, or carcinoma of the ampulla.
Extrinsic compression of the bile duct by a primary or secondary neoplasm.

BILIARY OBSTRUCTION[15]

ICD-10CM #	Varies with specific diagnosis

CAUSES OF BILIARY OBSTRUCTION

Benign Miscellaneous
Choledocholithiasis.
Hemobilia.
Congenital biliary diseases.
Caroli disease.
Choledochal cysts.
Cholangitis.
Infectious.
Acute pyogenic cholangitis.
Biliary parasites.
Recurrent pyogenic cholangitis.

HIV cholangiopathy.
Sclerosing cholangitis.
Neoplasms
Cholangiocarcinoma.
Gallbladder carcinoma.
Locally invasive tumors (esp. pancreatic adeno-carcinoma).
Ampullary tumors.
Metastases.
Extrinsic Compression
Mirizzi syndrome.
Pancreatitis.
Adenopathy.

BILIARY TREE, REFLUX OF GAS OR BOWEL[48]

ICD-10CM #	Varies with specific diagnosis

CAUSES OF REFLUX OF GAS OR BOWEL CONTRAST INTO THE BILIARY TREE

Iatrogenic.
Sphincterotomy.
Choledochojejunostomy.
Gallstone fistula.
Cholecystoduodenal fistula.
Perforated ulcer.
Choledochoduodenal fistula.
Carcinoma.
Choledochoenteric fistula.

BLADDER (URINARY) WALL THICKENING[15]

ICD-10CM #	Varies with specific diagnosis

CAUSES OF BLADDER WALL THICKENING

Focal
Neoplasm
Transitional cell carcinoma.
Squamous cell carcinoma.
Adenocarcinoma.
Lymphoma.
Metastases.
Infectious/inflammatory.
Tuberculosis (acute).
Schistosomiasis (acute).
Cystitis.
Malakoplakia.
Cystitis cystica.
Cystitis glandularis.
Fistula.
Medical Diseases
Endometriosis.
Amyloidosis.
Trauma
Hematoma.
Diffuse
Neoplasm
Transitional cell carcinoma.
Squamous cell carcinoma.
Adenocarcinoma.
Infectious/Inflammatory
Cystitis.
Tuberculosis (chronic).
Schistosomiasis (chronic).

Medical Diseases
Interstitial cystitis.
Amyloidosis.
Neurogenic Bladder
Detrusor hyperreflexia.
Bladder Outlet Obstruction
With muscular hypertrophy.

BLEEDING, GI IN PATIENTS WITH AIDS[3]

ICD-10CM #	K92.2	Gastrointestinal bleeding, unspecified

(EXCLUDING NON-AIDS-SPECIFIC DIAGNOSES)

Esophagus
Candida spp.
Cytomegalovirus.
Herpes simplex virus.
Idiopathic ulcer.
Stomach
Cytomegalovirus.*
Kaposi sarcoma.*
Cryptosporidiosis.
Lymphoma.
Small Intestine
Kaposi sarcoma.
Lymphoma.
Cytomegalovirus.
Salmonella spp.
Cryptosporidium.
Colon
Cytomegalovirus.*
Kaposi sarcoma.*
Entamoeba histolytica.
Campylobacter jejuni.
Clostridium difficile.
Shigella spp.
Idiopathic ulcerations.
Lymphoma.

*More frequent diagnosis.

BLEEDING, LOWER GI

ICD-10CM #	K92.2	Gastrointestinal hemorrhage, unspecified

(ORIGINATING BELOW THE LIGAMENT OF TREITZ)

Small Intestine
Ischemic bowel disease (mesenteric thrombosis, embolism, vasculitis, trauma).
Small bowel neoplasm: leiomyomas, carcinoids.
Hereditary hemorrhagic telangiectasia (Rendu-Osler-Weber syndrome).
Meckel diverticulum and other small intestine diverticula.
Aortoenteric fistula.
Intestinal hemangiomas: blue rubber-bleb nevi, intestinal hemangiomas, cutaneous vascular nevi.
Hamartomatous polyps: Peutz-Jeghers syndrome (intestinal polyps, mucocutaneous pigmentation).
Infections of small bowel: tuberculous enteritis, enteritis necroticans.

Volvulus.
Intussusception.
Lymphoma of small bowel, sarcoma, Kaposi sarcoma.
Irradiation ileitis.
AV malformation of small intestine.
Inflammatory bowel disease.
Polyarteritis nodosa.
Other: pancreatoenteric fistulas, Henoch-Schönlein purpura, Ehlers-Danlos syndrome, systemic lupus erythematosus, amyloidosis, metastatic melanoma.
Colon
Carcinoma (particularly left colon).
Diverticular disease.
Inflammatory bowel disease.
Ischemic colitis.
Colonic polyps.
Vascular abnormalities: angiodysplasia, vascular ectasia.
Radiation colitis.
Infectious colitis.
Uremic colitis.
Aortoenteric fistula.
Lymphoma of large bowel.
Hemorrhoids.
Anal fissure.
Trauma, foreign body.
Solitary rectal/cecal ulcers.
Long-distance running.

BLEEDING, LOWER GI, PEDIATRIC[43]

ICD-10CM #	K92.2	Gastrointestinal hemorrhage, unspecified

<3 MO
Swallowed maternal blood.
Infectious colitis.
Milk allergy.
Bleeding diathesis.
Intussusception.
Midgut volvulus.
Meckel diverticulum.
Necrotizing enterocolitis.

<2 YR
Anal fissure.
Infectious colitis.
Milk allergy.
Colitis.
Intussusception.
Meckel diverticulum.
Polyp.
Duplication.
Hemolytic-uremic syndrome.
Inflammatory bowel disease.
Pseudomembranous enterocolitis.

<5 YR
Infectious colitis.
Anal fissure.
Polyp.
Intussusception.
Meckel diverticulum.
Henoch-Schönlein purpura.

Hemolytic-uremic syndrome.
Inflammatory bowel disease.
Pseudomembranous enterocolitis.

5 TO 18 YR

Infectious colitis.
Inflammatory bowel disease.
Pseudomembranous enterocolitis.
Polyp.
Hemolytic-uremic syndrome.
Hemorrhoids.

BLEEDING, RECTAL[2]

ICD-10CM #	K92.2	Gastrointestinal hemorrhage, unspecified

IN PATIENTS <40 YR

Very Common
Hemorrhoids.
Anal fissure.
Inflammatory bowel disease (mainly proctitis).
Less Common
Polyps (hamartomatous or adenomatous).
Infective colitis.
Meckel diverticulum.
Intussusception.
Rare
Colorectal cancer.

IN PATIENTS >40 YR

Hemorrhoids.
Anal fissure.
Colorectal cancer.
Colorectal polyps (mostly adenomas).
Angiodysplasia.
Diverticular disease.
Inflammatory bowel disease.
Ischemic colitis.
Infective colitis.

BLEEDING, THIRD TRIMESTER[29]

ICD-10CM #	N93.9	Abnormal uterine and vaginal bleeding, unspecified

Placental abruption.
Placenta previa.
Bloody show (extrusion of cervical mucus).
Vasa previa.
Disseminated intravascular coagulopathy.
Uterine rupture.
Cervicitis, cervical cancer, or other cervical abnormality.
Vaginal laceration.

BLEEDING, UPPER GI

ICD-10CM #	K92.2	Gastrointestinal hemorrhage, unspecified

(ORIGINATING ABOVE THE LIGAMENT OF TREITZ)

Swallowed Hemoptysis
Oral or pharyngeal lesions: swallowed blood from nose or oropharynx.

Esophageal: varices, ulceration, esophagitis, Mallory-Weiss tear, carcinoma, trauma.
Gastric: peptic ulcer (including Cushing and Curling ulcers), gastritis, angiodysplasia, gastric neoplasms, hiatal hernia, gastric diverticulum, pseudoxanthoma elasticum, Rendu-Osler-Weber syndrome.
Duodenal: peptic ulcer, duodenitis, angiodysplasia, aortoduodenal fistula, duodenal diverticulum, duodenal tumors, carcinoma of ampulla of Vater, parasites (e.g., hookworm), Crohn disease.
Biliary: hematobilia (e.g., penetrating injury to liver, hepatobiliary malignancy, endoscopic papillotomy).

BLEEDING, UPPER GI, PEDIATRIC[43]

ICD-10CM #	K92.2	Gastrointestinal hemorrhage, unspecified

<3 MO

Swallowed maternal blood.
Gastritis.
Ulcer, stress.
Bleeding diathesis.
Foreign body (nasogastric tube).
Vascular malformation.
Duplication.

<2 YR

Esophagitis.
Gastritis.
Ulcer.
Pyloric stenosis.
Mallory-Weiss syndrome.
Vascular malformation.
Duplication.

<5 YR

Esophagitis.
Gastritis.
Ulcer.
Esophageal varices.
Foreign body.
Mallory-Weiss syndrome.
Hemophilia.
Vascular malformations.

5 TO 18 YR

Esophagitis.
Gastritis.
Ulcer.
Esophageal varices.
Mallory-Weiss syndrome.
Inflammatory bowel disease.
Hemophilia.
Vascular malformation.

BLEEDING, VAGINAL, NONPREGNANT FEMALE[29]

ICD-10CM #	N93.9	Abnormal uterine and vaginal bleeding, unspecified

TRAUMA

Blunt force.
Penetrating force.
Foreign bodies.

INFECTIOUS

Vaginitis.
Cervicitis.
Endometritis.

DYSFUNCTIONAL UTERINE BLEEDING

Ovulatory.
Anovulatory.
Adenomyosis.

BENIGN GROWTHS

Uterine leiomyomas.
Cervical polyps.

MALIGNANCY

Vulvar.
Cervical.
Uterine.
Ovarian.

SYSTEMIC DISEASE

Medications
Anticoagulation (warfarin [Coumadin], low-molecular-weight heparin, clopidogrel [Plavix]).
Antipsychotics.
Corticosteroids.
Tamoxifen.
Selective serotonin reuptake inhibitors.
Contraceptives (oral, intrauterine devices, intramuscular).

BLINDNESS, GERIATRIC AGE

ICD-10CM #	H54.8	Legal blindness, as defined in USA

Cataracts.
Glaucoma.
Diabetic retinopathy.
Macular degeneration.
Trauma.
Cerebrovascular accident.
Corneal scarring.
Giant cell arteritis.
Ocular herpes zoster.

BLINDNESS, MONOCULAR, TRANSIENT

ICD-10CM #	H54.41	Blindness, right eye, normal vision left eye
	H54.42	Blindness, left eye, normal vision right eye

Migraine (vasospasm).
Embolic cerebrovascular disease.
Intermittent angle-closure glaucoma.
Partial retinal vein occlusion.
Hyphema.
Optic disc edema.
Giant cell arteritis.

Psychogenic.
Hypotension.
Hypercoagulopathy disorders.
Multiple sclerosis.

BLINDNESS, PEDIATRIC AGE[51]

ICD-10CM #	H54.41	Blindness, right eye, normal vision left eye
	H54.42	Blindness, left eye, normal vision right eye

CONGENITAL

Optic nerve hypoplasia or aplasia.
Optic coloboma.
Congenital hydrocephalus.
Hydranencephaly.
Porencephaly.
Microencephaly.
Encephalocele, particularly occipital type.
Morning glory disc.
Aniridia.
Anterior microphthalmia.
Peter anomaly.
Persistent pupillary membrane.
Glaucoma.
Cataracts.
Persistent hyperplastic primary vitreous.

PHAKOMATOSES

Tuberous sclerosis.
Neurofibromatosis (special association with optic glioma).
Sturge-Weber syndrome.
von Hippel–Lindau disease.

TUMORS

Retinoblastoma.
Optic glioma.
Perioptic meningioma.
Craniopharyngioma.
Cerebral glioma.
Posterior and intraventricular tumors when complicated by hydrocephalus.
Pseudotumor cerebri.

NEURODEGENERATIVE DISEASES

Cerebral storage disease.
Gangliosidoses, particularly Tay-Sachs disease (infantile amaurotic familial idiocy), Sandhoff variant, generalized gangliosidosis.
Other lipidoses and ceroid lipofuscinoses, particularly the late-onset amaurotic familial idiocies such as those of Jansky-Bielschowsky and of Batten-Mayou-Spielmeyer-Vogt.
Mucopolysaccharidoses, particularly Hurler syndrome and Hunter syndrome.
Leukodystrophies (dysmyelination disorders), particularly metachromatic leukodystrophy and Canavan disease.
Demyelinating sclerosis (myelinoclastic diseases), especially Schilder disease and Devic neuromyelitis optica.
Special types: Dawson disease, Leigh disease, Bassen-Kornzweig syndrome, Refsum disease.
Retinal degenerations: retinitis pigmentosa and its variants, Leber congenital type.

Optic atrophies: congenital autosomal recessive type, infantile and congenital autosomal dominant types, Leber disease, and atrophies associated with hereditary ataxias—the types of Behr, of Marie, and of Sanger-Brown.

INFECTIOUS PROCESSES

Encephalitis, especially in the prenatal infection syndromes caused by *Toxoplasma gondii,* cytomegalovirus, rubella virus, *Treponema pallidum,* herpes simplex.
Meningitis, arachnoiditis.
Chorioretinitis.
Endophthalmitis.
Keratitis.

HEMATOLOGIC DISORDERS

Leukemia with central nervous system involvement.

VASCULAR AND CIRCULATORY DISORDERS

Collagen vascular diseases.
Arteriovenous malformations: intracerebral hemorrhage, subarachnoid hemorrhage.
Central retinal occlusion.

TRAUMA

Contusion or avulsion of optic nerves, chiasm, globe, cornea.
Cerebral contusion or laceration.
Intracerebral, subarachnoid, or subdural hemorrhage.

DRUGS AND TOXINS OTHER

Retinopathy of prematurity.
Sclerocornea.
Conversion reaction.
Optic neuritis.
Osteopetrosis.

BLISTERS, SUBEPIDERMAL

ICD-10CM #	T07	Unspecified multiple injuries

Burns.
Porphyria cutanea tarda.
Bullous pemphigoid.
Bullous drug reaction.
Arthropod bite reaction.
Toxic epidermal necrosis.
Dermatitis herpetiformis.
Polymorphous light eruption.
Variegate porphyria.
Systemic lupus erythematosus.
Epidermolysis bullosa.
Pseudoporphyria.
Acute graft-versus-host reaction.
Linear IgA disease.
Leukocytoclastic vasculitis.
Pressure necrosis.
Urticaria pigmentosa.
Amyloidosis.

BONE AND/OR SOFT TISSUE HYPERTROPHY[52]

ICD-10CM #	M85.80	Other specified disorders of bone density and structure, unspecified site

DISORDERS ASSOCIATED WITH BONE AND/OR SOFT TISSUE HYPERTROPHY

Conditions Associated with Generalized Overgrowth

Pituitary gigantism and acromegaly.
Other endocrine disorders.
Cerebral gigantism (Sotos).

Conditions Associated with Limb Hemihypertrophy

Lipomatosis.
Idiopathic congenital hemihypertrophy (associated with tumors, e.g., Wilms tumor, adrenocortical tumors, hepatoblastoma).
Proteus syndrome (capillary port-wine hemangiomas, lymphangiomas, lipomas, epidermal nevi, hypertrophy hands and feet, macrocephaly).
Maffucci syndrome (enchondromas, exostosis, lymphangiomas, venous angiomas).
Klippel-Trenaunay syndrome (capillary port-wine hemangiomas, varicosities, lymphangiomas).
Parkes Weber syndrome (capillary port-wine hemangiomas, varicosities, arteriovenous fistula).
Blue rubber bleb nevus syndrome (cavernous hemangiomas of skin, GI tract).
Other angiodysplasias (e.g., Servelle-Martorell syndrome; venous arterial malformations with limb hypertrophy and bony hypoplasia).
Beckwith-Wiedemann syndrome (macroglossia, visceromegaly, omphaloceles, hemihypertrophy, etc.).

Conditions Associated with Macrodactyly

Neurofibromatosis.
Macrodystrophia lipomatosa.
Proteus syndrome.
Bannayan-Zonana syndrome (lipomatosis, angiomatosis, macrocephaly).
Hemangiomatosis and other vascular malformations (Klippel-Trenaunay and Parkes Weber).
Lymphangiomatosis.
Arteriovenous malformation.
Maffucci syndrome, Ollier disease.
Epidermal nevus syndrome.

BONE DENSITY, DECREASED, GENERALIZED[21]

ICD-10CM #	M85.80	Other specified disorders of bone density and structure, unspecified site

DISORDERS ASSOCIATED WITH GENERALIZED LOSS OF BONE DENSITY

Disorders of Multiple or Uncertain Cause

Senile osteoporosis.*
Juvenile osteoporosis.
Osteoporosis imperfecta.†

Secondary Bone Disorders

Endocrine

Adrenal cortex:
    Cushing disease.
    Addison disease.

---

*Patients who cannot synthesize Lewis blood group antigens (~5% of the population) do not produce CA–19–9 antigen.
†Common cause of decrease in bone density in children.

Gonadal disorders:
    Postmenopausal osteoporosis.
    Hypogonadism.
Pituitary:
    Acromegaly.
    Hypopituitarism.
Pancreas:
    Diabetes mellitus.
Thyroid:
    Hyperthyroidism.
    Hypothyroidism.
Parathyroid:
    Hyperparathyroidism.
Marrow Replacement and Expansion
Myeloma.
Leukemia.
Lymphoma.
Metastatic disease.
Gaucher disease.
Anemias (sickle cell, thalassemia, hemophilia).
Drugs and Other Substances
Steroids.
Heparin (osteoporosis).
Anticonvulsants (osteomalacia).
Immunosuppressants.
Alcohol.
Chronic Disease
Chronic renal disease.
Hepatic insufficiency.
GI malabsorption syndromes.
Chronic inflammatory polyarthropathies.
Chronic debility or immobilization.

BONE DENSITY, DECREASED, LOCALIZED[21]

| ICD-10CM # | Z82.62 | Family history of osteoporosis |
| | M85.80 | Other specified disorders of bone density and structure, unspecified site |

DISORDERS ASSOCIATED WITH LOCALIZED LOSS OF BONE DENSITY

Disuse osteoporosis.‡
Reflex sympathetic dystrophy (Sudeck).
Osteolytic syndromes:
    Acroosteolysis, primary and secondary.
    Massive osteolysis of Gorham.
    Carpotarsal osteolysis.
Transient regional osteoporosis.
Neuromuscular disorders.
Infection.
Arthropathies.
Tumors, primary and secondary, myelomatosis.

‡Common causes.

BONE DISEASE, PROLIFERATIVE[53]

ICD-10CM #   Varies with specific diagnosis

CLASSIFICATION CRITERIA FOR SYSTEMIC LUPUS ERYTHEMATOSUS

ACR 1997 Revised Classification Criteria*
Malar rash.
Discoid rash.
Photosensitivity.
Arthritis (nonerosive, affecting two or more joints).
Serositis (pleuritis, pericarditis, or peritonitis).
Seizure or psychosis.
Hematologic manifestations (hemolytic anemia, leukopenia [<4000 leukocytes/mm^3], lymphopenia [<1500 lymphocytes/mm^3], thrombocytopenia [<100,000 platelets/mm^3]).
Immunologic abnormalities (positive anti–double-stranded DNA or anti-Smith antibody).
False-positive RPR, positive lupus anticoagulant test result in elevated anticardiolipin IgG or IgM anticardiolipin antibody.
Antinuclear antibody.

SLICC Classification Criteria†
Clinical Criteria

Acute cutaneous lupus.
Chronic cutaneous lupus.
Oral or nasal ulcers.
Nonscarring alopecia.
Synovitis (two or more joints).
Serositis.
Glomerulonephritis.
Neurologic disorder (seizures, psychosis, mononeuritis multiplex, myelitis, peripheral or cranial neuropathy, acute confusional state).
Hemolytic anemia.
Leukopenia (<4000 leukocytes/mm^3) or lymphopenia (<1000 lymphocytes/mm^3).
Thrombocytopenia (<100,000 platelets/mm^3).

Immunologic Criteria

Antinuclear antibody (ANA).
Anti–double-stranded DNA antibody.
Anti-Smith antibody.
Antiphospholipid antibody (false-positive RPR; medium- or high-titer IgA, IgG, or IgM anticardiolipin antibody; IgG, IgA, or IgM anti–β2 glycoprotein I antibody).
Low complement (C3, C4, CH50).
Positive direct Coombs test in the absence of hemolytic anemia.

ACR, American College of Rheumatology, *Ig,* immunoglobulin, *RPR,* rapid plasma reagin, *SLICC,* Systemic Lupus International Collaborating Clinics.
*For ACR criteria, the presence of 4 or more of 11 criteria is needed.
†For SLICC criteria, the presence of four or more criteria (at least one clinical and one laboratory criterion) is needed or a biopsy demonstrating lupus nephritis with a positive ANA or anti–double-stranded DNA is needed.

BONE LESIONS, PREFERENTIAL SITE OF ORIGIN[54]

ICD-10CM #	C41.0	Malignant neoplasm of bones of skull and face
	C41.1	Malignant neoplasm of mandible
	C41.2	Malignant neoplasm of vertebral column
	C41.3	Malignant neoplasm of ribs, sternum and clavicle
	C40.00	Malignant neoplasm of scapula and long bones of unspecified upper limb
	C40.10	Malignant neoplasm of short bones of unspecified upper limb
	C41.4	Malignant neoplasm of pelvic bones, sacrum and coccyx
	C40.20	Malignant neoplasm of long bones of unspecified lower limb
	C40.30	Malignant neoplasm of short bones of unspecified lower limb
	C41.9	Malignant neoplasm of bone and articular cartilage, unspecified
	C79.51	Secondary malignant neoplasm of bone
	C79.52	Secondary malignant neoplasm of bone marrow

EPIPHYSIS
Chondroblastoma.
Giant cell tumor—after fusion of growth plate.
Langerhans cell histiocytosis.
Clear cell chondrosarcoma.
Osteosarcoma.

METAPHYSIS
Parosteal sarcoma.
Chondrosarcoma.
Fibrosarcoma.
Nonossifying fibroma.
Giant cell tumor—before fusion of growth plate.
Unicameral bone cyst.
Aneurysmal bone cyst.

DIAPHYSIS
Myeloma.
Ewing tumor.
Reticulum cell sarcoma.

METADIAPHYSEAL

Fibrosarcoma.
Fibrous dysplasia.
Enchondroma.
Osteoid osteoma.
Chondromyofibroma.

BONE MARROW FAILURE SYNDROMES, INHERITED[31]

ICD-10CM #	D61.89	Other specified aplastic anemias and other bone marrow failure syndromes

BI-LINEAGE AND TRI-LINEAGE CYTOPENIAS

Fanconi anemia.
Shwachman-Diamond syndrome.
Dyskeratosis congenita.
Amegakaryocytic thrombocytopenia:
    Other inherited thrombocytopenia disorders.
Other genetic syndromes:
    Down syndrome.
    Dubowitz syndrome.
    Seckel syndrome.
    Reticular dysgenesis.
    Schimke immunoosseous dysplasia.
    Noonan syndrome.
    Cartilage-hair hypoplasia.
    Familial marrow failure (non-Fanconi).

UNI-LINEAGE CYTOPENIA

Diamond-Blackfan anemia.
Kostmann syndrome/congenital neutropenia:
    ELA2 mutations.
    HAX1 mutations.
    GFI1 mutations.
    WASP mutations.
    Constitutive cell surface G-CSF-R mutations.
Other inherited neutropenia syndromes:
    Barth syndrome.
    Glycogen storage disease 1b.
    Miscellaneous.
Thrombocytopenia with absent radii.
Congenital dyserythropoietic anemias (CDAs):
    Types I, II, III, IV.
    Variants.
    Nonclassifiable CDAs.
    Groups IV, V, VI, VII.

BONE MARROW FIBROSIS[24]

ICD-10CM #	D75.9	Disease of blood and blood-forming organs, unspecified

MYELOID DISORDERS

Myelofibrosis with myeloid metaplasia.
Metastatic cancer.
Chronic myeloid leukemia.
Myelodysplastic syndrome.
Atypical myeloid disorder.
Acute megakaryocytic leukemia.
Other acute myeloid leukemias.
Gray platelet syndrome.

LYMPHOID DISORDERS

Hairy cell leukemia.
Multiple myeloma.
Lymphoma.

NONHEMATOLOGIC DISORDERS

Connective tissue disorder.
Infections (tuberculosis, kala-azar).
Vitamin D deficiency (rickets).
Renal osteodystrophy.

BONE MASS, LOW[18]

ICD-10CM #	M85.80	Other specified disorders of bone density and structure, unspecified site

SECONDARY CAUSES OF LOW BONE MASS

Endocrine Diseases

Female hypogonadism.
Hyperprolactinemia.
Hypothalamic amenorrhea.
Anorexia nervosa.
Premature and primary ovarian failure.
Female athlete triad.
Male hypogonadism.
Primary gonadal failure (e.g., Klinefelter syndrome).
Secondary gonadal failure (e.g., idiopathic hypo-
    gonadotropic hypogonadism, androgen depri-
    vation therapy for prostate cancer).
Hyperthyroidism.
Hyperparathyroidism.
Hypercortisolism.
Vitamin D insufficiency or deficiency.

GI Diseases

Subtotal gastrectomy.
Gastric bypass surgery.
Malabsorption syndromes.
Chronic obstructive jaundice.
Primary biliary cirrhosis and other cirrhoses.

Bone Marrow Disorders

Multiple myeloma.
Monoclonal gammopathy of unknown signifi-
    cance (MGUS).
Lymphoma.
Leukemia.
Hemolytic anemias.
Systemic mastocytosis.
Disseminated carcinoma.

Connective Tissue Diseases

Osteogenesis imperfecta.
Ehlers-Danlos syndrome.
Marfan syndrome.
Homocystinuria.

Drugs

Alcohol.
Antiseizure medications.
Aromatase inhibitors.
Chemotherapy.
Cyclosporine.
Depo-medroxyprogesterone.
Excess thyroid hormone.
Glucocorticoids.
Gonadotropin-releasing hormone agonists.
Heparin.

Miscellaneous Causes

Immobilization.
Rheumatoid arthritis.
Chronic obstructive pulmonary disease.
Weight loss.

BONE MINERAL DENSITY, INCREASED

ICD-10CM #	M89.30	Hypertrophy of bone, unspecified site
	M89.8X9	Other specified disorders of bone, unspecified site
	M94.8X9	Other specified disorders of cartilage, unspecified sites

Paget disease of bone.
Skeletal metastases.
Diffuse idiopathic skeletal hyperostosis.
Osteonecrosis.
Sarcoidosis.
Hypoparathyroidism, pseudohypoparathyroidism.
Milk-alkali syndrome.
Osteopetrosis.
Hypervitaminosis A or D.
Dysplasias (craniodiaphyseal, craniometaphyseal,
    frontometaphyseal).
Endosteal hyperostosis.
Fluorosis.
Heavy metal poisoning.
Ionizing radiation.
Other: lymphoma, leukemia, mastocytosis, mul-
    tiple myeloma, polycythemia vera.

BONE PAIN

ICD-10CM #	M89.8	Pain, bone

Trauma.
Neoplasm (primary or metastatic).
Osteoporosis with compression fracture.
Paget disease of bone.
Infection (osteomyelitis, septic arthritis).
Osteomalacia.
Viral syndrome.
Sickle cell disease.
Anxiety.

BONE RESORPTION[54]

ICD-10CM #	M89.9	Disorder of bone, unspecified
	M94.9	Disorder of cartilage, unspecified

DISTAL CLAVICLE

Hyperparathyroidism.
Rheumatoid arthritis.
Scleroderma.
Posttraumatic osteolysis.
Progeria.
Pycnodysostosis.
Cleidocranial dysplasia.

INFERIOR ASPECT OF RIBS

Vascular impression associated with but not
    limited to coarctation of the aorta.
Hyperparathyroidism.
Neurofibromatosis.

Differential Diagnosis

II

TERMINAL PHALANGEAL TUFTS

Scleroderma.
Raynaud phenomenon.
Vascular disease.
Frostbite, electrical burns.
Psoriasis.
Tabes dorsalis.
Hyperparathyroidism.

GENERALIZED RESORPTION

Paraplegia.
Myositis ossificans.
Osteoporosis.

BOWEL WALL THICKENING[48]

ICD-10CM # Varies with specific diagnosis

BENIGN VS. MALIGNANT BOWEL WALL THICKENING

Benign
Homogeneous attenuation.
Symmetrical.
Circumferential.
Thickening <1 cm.
Segmental or diffuse involvement.
Double halo sign.
Dark inner ring.
Bright outer ring.
Target sign.
Bright inner ring.
Dark middle ring.
Bright outer ring.
Malignant
Heterogeneous attenuation.
Asymmetrical.
Eccentric.
Thickening >1-2 cm.
Focal mass.
Abrupt transition.
Lobulated contour.
Spiculated contour.
Narrowed bowel lumen.
Enlarged lymph nodes.
Liver metastases.

BOW LEGS (GENU VARUM), CLASSIFICATION[19]

ICD-10CM # E64.3 Genu varum, acquired
Q74.1 Congenital malformation of knee

PHYSIOLOGIC

Asymmetric Growth
Tibia vara (Blount disease):
Infantile.
Juvenile.
Adolescent.
Focal fibrocartilaginous dysplasia.
Physeal injury.
Trauma.
Infection.
Tumor.

METABOLIC DISORDERS

Vitamin D deficiency (nutritional rickets).
Vitamin D–resistant rickets.
Hypophosphatasia.

SKELETAL DYSPLASIA

Metaphyseal dysplasia.
Achondroplasia.
Enchondromatosis.

BRADYCARDIA ICU PATIENT[7]

ICD-10CM # R00.1 Bradycardia, unspecified

COMMON CAUSES OF BRADYCARDIA IN THE ICU

Medications: antiarrhythmics, β-blockers, calcium channel blockers, clonidine, dexmedetomidine, digoxin, lithium, opioids, phenytoin, and propofol.
Age-related degeneration.
Cardiac ischemia.
Electrolyte abnormalities.
Elevated intracranial pressure.
Elevated vagal tone.
Endotracheal intubation.
Hypertension.
Hypothermia.
Hypothyroidism.
Hypoxia.
Inflammatory disease.
Obstructive sleep apnea.
Postcardiac surgery.

BRADYCARDIA, SINUS[39]

ICD-10CM # I49.8 Other specified cardiac arrhythmias
R00.1 Bradycardia, unspecified

Idiopathic.
Degenerative processes (e.g., Lev disease, Lenègre disease).

MEDICATIONS

β-Blockers.
Some calcium channel blockers (diltiazem, verapamil).
Digoxin (when vagal tone is high).
Class I antiarrhythmic agents (e.g., procainamide).
Class III antiarrhythmic agents (amiodarone, sotalol).
Clonidine.
Lithium carbonate.

ACUTE MYOCARDIAL ISCHEMIA AND INFARCTION

Right or left circumflex coronary artery occlusion or spasm.
High vagal tone (e.g., athletes).

BRAIN MASS[29]

ICD-10CM # C71 Malignant neoplasm of brain
D33 Benign neoplasm of brain
I61.9 Intracranial hemorrhage, unspecified

METASTATIC BRAIN TUMOR

Primary Brain Tumor
Meningioma.
Glioma.

Pituitary adenoma.
Vestibular schwannoma.
Primary or secondary central nervous system lymphoma.
Infections
Abscess.
Toxoplasmosis.
Neurocysticercosis.
Tuberculoma.
Progressive multifocal leukoencephalopathy.

VASCULAR DISEASE

Hemorrhage
Anomalies (arteriovenous malformation).
Intratumoral.
Hypertensive.
Infarct
Embolism.
Thrombosis (sinus venous).
Inflammatory
Multiple sclerosis.
Encephalomyelitis.

BRAIN TUMORS, CHILDREN[20]

ICD-10CM # C71 Malignant neoplasm of brain
D33 Benign neoplasm of brain

Brain Tumors in Children

Hemispheric Tumors
Choroid plexus papilloma
Glial tumors:
Astrocytoma.
Ependymoma.
Oligodendroglioma.
Ganglioglioma.
Primitive neuroectodermal tumors.
Pineal region tumors:
Pineal parenchymal tumors.
Pineoblastoma.
Pineocytoma.
Germ cell tumors:
Embryonal cell carcinoma.
Germinoma.
Teratoma.
Other tumors:
Angiomas.
Dysplasia.
Meningioma.
Metastatic tumors.
Middle Fossa Tumors
Optic glioma.
Sellar and parasellar tumors.
Posterior Fossa Tumors
Astrocytoma.
Brain stem glioma.
Ependymoma.
Hemangioblastoma.
Medulloblastoma.

BREAST INFLAMMATORY LESION[55]

ICD-10CM #	N61	Inflammatory disorders of breast
	N60.19	Diffuse cystic mastopathy of unspecified breast
	P39.0	Neonatal infective mastitis
	P83.4	Breast engorgement of newborn

Mastitis (*S. aureus*, β-hemolytic *Streptococcus*).
Trauma.
Foreign body (sutures, breast implants).
Granuloma (TB, fungal).
Fat necrosis post biopsy.
Necrosis or infarction (anticoagulant therapy, pregnancy).
Breast malignancy.

BREAST MASS

ICD-10CM #	N63	Unspecified lump in breast

Fibrocystic breasts.
Benign tumors (fibroadenoma, papilloma).
Mastitis (acute bacterial mastitis, chronic mastitis).
Malignant neoplasm.
Fat necrosis.
Hematoma.
Duct ectasia.
Mammary adenosis.

BREAST MASS, ADOLESCENTS[56]

ICD-10CM #	N63	Unspecified lump in breast

ETIOLOGY OF BREAST MASSES IN ADOLESCENTS

Classic or juvenile fibroadenoma (70%).
Fibrocystic disease.
Breast cyst.
Abscess/mastitis.
Intraductal papilloma.
Fat necrosis/lipoma.
Cystosarcoma phyllodes (low-grade malignancy).
Adenomatous hyperplasia.
Hemangioma, lymphangioma, lymphoma (rare).
Carcinoma (<1%).

BREATH ODOR[57]

ICD-10CM #	R19.6	Halitosis

Sweet, fruity: diabetic ketoacidosis, starvation ketosis.
Fishy, stale: uremia (trimethylamines).
Ammonia-like: uremia (ammonia).
Musty fish, clover: fetor hepaticus (hepatic failure).
Foul, feculent: intestinal obstruction/diverticulum.
Foul, putrid: nasal/sinus pathology (infection, foreign body, cancer), respiratory infections (empyema, lung abscess, bronchiectasis).
Halitosis: tonsillitis, gingivitis, respiratory infections, Vincent angina, gastroesophageal reflux, achalasia, certain foods (garlic, onions, protein drinks, etc.).
Cinnamon: pulmonary TB.

BREATHING DISORDERS, SLEEP RELATED[22]

ICD-10CM #	Varies with specific diagnosis

SLEEP-RELATED BREATHING DISORDERS

Central Sleep Apnea Syndromes
Central sleep apnea with Cheyne-Stokes breathing.
Central sleep apnea due to high-altitude periodic breathing.
Central sleep apnea due to a medical disorder without Cheyne-Stokes breathing.
Central sleep apnea due to a medication or substance.
Primary central sleep apnea.
Primary sleep apnea of infancy.
Primary central sleep apnea of prematurity.
Treatment-emergent central sleep apnea.

OBSTRUCTIVE SLEEP APNEA DISORDERS

Obstructive sleep apnea, adult.
Obstructive sleep apnea, pediatric.

SLEEP-RELATED HYPOVENTILATION/HYPOXEMIC DISORDERS

Obesity hypoventilation syndrome.
Idiopathic central alveolar hypoventilation.

LATE-ONSET CENTRAL HYPOVENTILATION WITH HYPOTHALAMIC DYSFUNCTION

Congenital central alveolar hypoventilation syndrome.
Sleep-related hypoventilation due to a medical disorder.
Sleep-related hypoventilation due to a medication or substance.
Sleep-related hypoxemia.

BREATHING, NOISY[57]

ICD-10CM #	R06.00	Dyspnea, unspecified
	R06.09	Other forms of dyspnea
	R06.3	Periodic breathing
	R06.83	Snoring
	R06.89	Other abnormalities of breathing
	R06.1	Stridor

Infection: upper respiratory infection, peritonsillar abscess, retropharyngeal abscess, epiglottitis, laryngitis, tracheitis, bronchitis, bronchiolitis.
Irritants and allergens: hyperactive airway, asthma (reactive airway disease), rhinitis, angioneurotic edema.
Compression from outside of the airway: esophageal cysts or foreign body, neoplasms, lymphadenopathy.
Congenital malformation and abnormality: vascular rings, laryngeal webs, laryngomalacia, tracheomalacia, hemangiomas within the upper airway, stenoses within the upper airway, cystic fibrosis.
Acquired abnormality (at every level of the airway): nasal polyps, hypertrophied adenoids and/or tonsils, foreign body, intraluminal tumors, bronchiectasis.
Neurogenic disorder: vocal cord paralysis.

BRONCHIAL OBSTRUCTION[21]

ICD-10CM #	J98.0	Tracheobronchial collapse

CAUSES OF BRONCHIAL OBSTRUCTION

Outside the Bronchus
Lymph nodes and other masses.
In the Wall of the Bronchus
Tumors
Lung carcinoma (commonly squamous cell).
Bronchial carcinoid.
Metastasis.
Hamartoma.
Inflammation
Tuberculosis.
Sarcoidosis.
Granulomatosis with polyangiitis.
Inflammatory bowel disease.
Bronchomalacia
Broncholith.
Inside the Bronchus
Mucus plug.
Inhaled foreign body.

BRONCHOPLEURAL FISTULA[21]

ICD-10CM #	J86.0	Bronchopleural fistula

CAUSES OF BRONCHOPLEURAL FISTULA

Trauma
Penetrating.
Iatrogenic (especially postpneumonectomy, postlobectomy, postbiopsy).
Infection
Necrotizing pneumonia.
Empyema.
Tuberculosis.
Septic embolus.
Infected pulmonary infarct.

BROWN URINE

ICD-10CM #	R82	Other abnormal findings in urine

Bile pigments.
Myoglobin.
Concentrated urine.
Use of multivitamin supplements.
Medications (antimalarials, metronidazole, nitrofurantoin, levodopa, methyldopa, phenazopyridine).
Diet rich in fava beans.
Urinary tract infection.

BRUISING

ICD-10CM #	I99.8	Other disorder of circulatory system

Medication-induced (warfarin, aspirin, NSAIDs, prednisone).
Alcohol abuse.
Senile purpura.
Purpura simplex.
Physical abuse.

Differential Diagnosis

II

Vasculitis.
Platelet disorders.
Coagulation factor deficiencies.
Cushing disease.
Vitamin C deficiency.
Marfan syndrome.
Ehlers-Danlos syndrome.
Disseminated intravascular coagulation.
Leukemia.
Hereditary hemorrhagic telangiectasia.

BULLOUS DISEASES

ICD-10CM #	L13.9	Bullous disorder, unspecified
	L12.0	Bullous pemphigoid
	L12.8	Other pemphigoid
	L10.0	Pemphigus vulgaris
	L10.1	Pemphigus vegetans
	L10.2	Pemphigus foliaceous
	L10.4	Pemphigus erythematosus
	L10.9	Pemphigus, unspecified

Bullous pemphigoid.
Pemphigus vulgaris.
Pemphigus foliaceus.
Paraneoplastic pemphigus.
Cicatricial pemphigoid.
Erythema multiforme.
Dermatitis herpetiformis.
Herpes gestationis.
Impetigo.
Erosive lichen planus.
Linear IgA bullous dermatosis.
Epidermolysis bullosa acquisita.

CAFÉ-AU-LAIT SPOTS[19]

| ICD-10CM # | L81.3 | Café au lait spots |

Neurofibromatosis types 1 and 2.
McCune-Albright syndrome.
Russell-Silver syndrome.
Ataxia-telangiectasia.
Fanconi anemia.
Tuberous sclerosis.
Bloom syndrome.
Basal cell nevus syndrome.
Gaucher disease.
Chédiak-Higashi syndrome.
Hunter syndrome.
Maffucci syndrome.
Multiple mucosal neuroma syndrome.
Watson syndrome.
Proteus syndrome.
Turner syndrome.
Ring chromosome syndrome.
Jaffe-Campanacci syndrome.

CALCIFICATION ON CHEST X-RAY

ICD-10CM #	J98.4	Calcification of lung
	M51.84	Other intervertebral disc disorders, thoracic region
	M51.85	Other intervertebral disc disorders, thoracolumbar region

Lung neoplasm (primary or metastatic).
Silicosis.
Idiopathic pulmonary fibrosis.
Tuberculosis.
Histoplasmosis.
Disseminated varicella infection.
Mitral stenosis (end-stage).
Secondary hyperparathyroidism.

CALCIFICATIONS, ABDOMINAL, NONVISCERAL ON X-RAY[21]

| ICD-10CM # | M61.9 | Calcification and ossification of muscle, unspecified |

NONVISCERAL ABDOMINAL CALCIFICATION

Common
Atherosclerosis.
Mesenteric lymph nodes.
Phleboliths.
Aneurysm.
Dermoid cyst.
Differentiate
Rib cartilage.
Injections in the buttocks.
Uncommon
Infestations:
  Armillifer armillatus.
  Cysticercosis.
  Guinea worm.
  Hydatid.
Tumors:
  Lipoma.
  Hemangioma.
  Neuroblastoma.
  Osteo/chondrosarcoma of soft tissues.
  Retroperitoneal sarcoma of soft tissues.
  Peritoneal metastases.
  Pheochromocytoma.
Tuberculosis:
  Peritonitis.
  Psoas abscess.
Meconium peritonitis.
Pseudomyxoma Peritonei
Mesenteric cyst.
Pancreatitis with saponification.
Lithopedion.
Appendices Epiploicae
Ligaments.
Foreign bodies.
Posttraumatic buttock cysts.

CALCIFICATIONS, ADRENAL GLAND ON X-RAY[21]

| ICD-10CM # | E27.4 | Calcification, adrenal gland |

ADRENAL GLAND CALCIFICATION

Common
Idiopathic.
Hemorrhage.
Tuberculosis.
Neuroblastoma/ganglioneuroma.
Pheochromocytoma.

Uncommon
Other tumors:
  Adenoma.
  Carcinoma.
  Dermoid.
Addison disease.
Cyst.
Histoplasmosis.

CALCIFICATIONS, CARDIAC ON X-RAY[21]

| ICD-10CM # | I51.5 | Calcification, myocardium |
| | I25.1 | Calcification, arteriosclerotic |

CAUSES OF VISIBLE CALCIFICATION WITHIN THE HEART

Coronary Artery
Atherosclerosis.
Aortic Root
Atherosclerotic aorta.
Thrombus.
Syphilis.
Ankylosing spondylitis.
Homograft calcification.
Pericardium
Chronic pericarditis, tuberculosis, hemopericardium, pyogenic or viral pericarditis.
Posttraumatic.
Postoperative.
Uremic pericarditis.
Asbestosis (may be pleural calcification applied to pericardium).
Myocardium
Ventricular aneurysm (may mimic pericardial calcification).
Calcified myocardial infarction.
Postmyocarditis.
Endocardium
Endomyocardial fibrosis.
Thrombus.
Valve Cusps
Calcified valves (particularly mitral and aortic valves).
Mitral annulus calcification.
Homograft calcification.
Old vegetation.
Valve Annulus
Submitral.
Mitral.
Aortic.
Left Atrium
Wall.
Thrombus.
Atrial myxoma.
Pulmonary Artery
Pulmonary hypertension.
Postoperative:
  Postoperative serumoma calcified hydatid cyst.

CALCIFICATIONS, CUTANEOUS

| ICD-10CM # | L94.2 | Calcinosis cutis |
| | L98.8 | Other specified disorders of the skin and subcutaneous tissue |

Calcification, Raynaud phenomenon, esophageal dysmotility, sclerodactyly, and telangiectasia (CREST) syndrome.
Trauma.
Pancreatitis or pancreatic cancer.
Chronic renal failure.
Sarcoidosis.
Hyperparathyroidism.
Milk-alkali syndrome.
Hypervitaminosis D.
Panniculitis.
Idiopathic.
Iatrogenic (e.g., application of calcium alginate dressing to skin).
Multiple myeloma.
Dermatomyositis.
Parasitic infections.
Leukemia.
Lymphoma.

CALCIFICATIONS, GENITAL TRACT, FEMALE ON X-RAY[21]

ICD-10CM #	E83.59	Other disorders of calcium metabolism

FEMALE GENITAL TRACT CALCIFICATION

Uterus
Leiomyomas.
Squamous cell carcinoma.
Adenocarcinoma of endometrium.
Leiomyosarcoma.
Lithopedion.
Fallopian Tubes
Ovary.
Dermoid cyst.
Serous cystadenoma/carcinoma.
Tuberculosis.
Cysts.
Autoamputation.

CALCIFICATIONS, LIVER ON X-RAY[21]

ICD-10CM #	K76.89	Other specified diseases of liver
	NEC K75.3	Granuloma, hepatic

LIVER CALCIFICATION

Common
Granuloma (tuberculosis, histoplasmosis, brucellosis).
Multiple scattered round densities.
Hydatid cyst:
Fine curvilinear in wall, or dense and irregular if contracted.
Primary liver tumor (hemangioma, hepatoblastoma, hepatoma, cholangiocarcinoma).
Irregular patterns or multiple nodules.
Metastases (mucinous primary of colon or breast, cystadenocarcinoma of ovary).
Finely stippled, may be extensive.
Uncommon
Hepatic artery aneurysm.
Armillifer armillatus infestation.
Chronic granulomatous disease of childhood.
Cyst (congenital or acquired).

Hematoma.
Intrahepatic gallstones.
Old liver abscess.
Portal vein thrombosis.
Differentiate
Hemochromatosis.
Thorotrast, thallium, iron.

CALCIFICATIONS, PANCREAS ON X-RAY[21]

ICD-10CM #	K86.8	Calcification, pancreas

PANCREATIC CALCIFICATION

Common
Chronic pancreatitis.
Uncommon
Acute pancreatitis (saponification).
Tumors:
Cystadenoma.
Cystadenocarcinoma.
Islet cell tumor.
Metastases.
Hereditary pancreatitis (large clumps).
Hemorrhage.
Hyperparathyroidism.
Pseudocyst.
Cavernous lymphangioma.
Mucoviscidosis.
Kwashiorkor.

CALCIFICATIONS, SPLEEN ON X-RAY[21]

ICD-10CM #	D73.8	Calcification, spleen

SPLENIC CALCIFICATION

Larger than 10 mm
Splenic artery aneurysm.
Splenic artery atheroma.
Cyst:
Posttraumatic.
Dermoid.
Epidermoid.
Hydatid.
Hematoma.
Infarct.
Abscess.
Tuberculosis.
Smaller than 10 mm
Histoplasmosis.
Tuberculosis.
Phleboliths.
Armillifer armillatus infestation.
Brucellosis.
Infarcts.

CALCIFICATIONS, VALVULAR ON X-RAY[21]

ICD-10CM #	I51.5	Calcification, heart

CAUSES OF RADIOGRAPHICALLY VISIBLE VALVE CALCIFICATION

Aortic Valve
Rheumatic aortic valve disease.
Bicuspid aortic valve.
Age/degenerate aortic valve.
Syphilis.

Ankylosing spondylitis.
Homograft calcification.
Mitral Valve
Rheumatic mitral valve disease.
Mitral annulus calcification.
Old vegetation (may only be visible on computed tomography [CT]).
Homograft calcification.
Pulmonary Valve
Congenital pulmonary valve stenosis.
Rheumatic pulmonary valve disease (rare).
Fallot tetralogy (usually after repair).
Pulmonary hypertension.
Homograft calcification.
Tricuspid Valve
Rheumatic tricuspid valve disease.
Old vegetation (may only be visible on ultrafast CT).

CALCIUM STONES

ICD-10CM #	N20.9	Urinary calculus, unspecified

Medications (e.g., antacids, loop diuretics, vitamin D, acetazolamide, glucocorticoids).
Primary hyperparathyroidism.
Hypercalcemia from malignancy.
Sarcoidosis.
Prolonged immobilization.
Hyperoxaluria (e.g., Crohn disease, celiac disease, chronic pancreatitis).
Hyperuricosuria (e.g., hyperuricemia, excessive dietary purine, allopurinol, probenecid).
Renal tubular acidosis.
Milk-alkali syndrome.
Thyrotoxicosis.
Hypocitraturia (e.g., metabolic acidosis, hypomagnesemia, hypokalemia).

CARDIAC ARREST, NONTRAUMATIC[1]

ICD-10CM #	I46.9	Cardiac arrest, cause unspecified

Cardiac (coronary artery disease, cardiomyopathies, structural abnormalities, valve dysfunction, arrhythmias).
Respiratory (upper airway obstruction, hypoventilation, pulmonary embolism, asthma, chronic obstructive pulmonary disease exacerbation, pulmonary edema).
Circulatory (tension pneumothorax, pericardial tamponade, pulmonary embolism, hemorrhage, sepsis).
Electrolyte abnormalities (hypokalemia or hyperkalemia, hypomagnesemia or hypermagnesemia, hypocalcemia).
Medications (tricyclic antidepressants, digoxin, theophylline, calcium channel blockers).
Drug abuse (cocaine, heroin, amphetamines).
Toxins (carbon monoxide, cyanide).
Environmental (drowning/near-drowning, electrocution, lightning, hypothermia or hyperthermia, venomous snakes).

CARDIAC DEATH, SUDDEN[18]

ICD-10CM #	Z86.74	Personal history of sudden cardiac arrest

Differential Diagnosis

II

Ventricular tachycardia.
Bradyarrhythmia, sick sinus syndrome.
Aortic stenosis.
Tetralogy of Fallot.
Pericardial tamponade.
Cardiac tumors.
Complications of infective endocarditis.
Hypertrophic cardiomyopathy (arrhythmia or obstruction).
Myocardial ischemia.
Atherosclerosis.
Prinzmetal angina.
Kawasaki arteritis.

CARDIAC ENLARGEMENT[39]

ICD-10CM #	I51.7	Cardiomegaly
	Q23.8	Other congenital malformations of aortic and mitral valves
	Q24.8	Other specified congenital malformations of heart
	I11.9	Hypertensive heart disease without heart failure

CHAMBER ENLARGEMENT

Chronic Volume Overload
Mitral or aortic regurgitation.
Left-to-right shunt (patent ductus arteriosus, ventricular septal defect, arteriovenous fistula).
Cardiomyopathy
Ischemic.
Nonischemic.
Decompensated Pressure Overload
Aortic stenosis.
Hypertension.
High-Output States
Severe anemia.
Thyrotoxicosis.
Bradycardia
Severe sinus bradycardia.
Complete heart block.
Left Atrium
Left ventricle failure of any cause.
Mitral valve disease.
Myxoma.

RIGHT VENTRICLE

Chronic volume overload.
Tricuspid or pulmonic regurgitation.
Left-to-right shunt (atrial septal defect).
Decompensated pressure overload:
  Pulmonic stenosis.
Pulmonary artery hypertension:
  Primary.
  Secondary (pulmonary embolism, chronic obstructive pulmonary disease).
  Pulmonary venoocclusive disease.

RIGHT ATRIUM

Right ventricle failure of any cause.
Tricuspid valve disease.
Myxoma.
Ebstein anomaly.

MULTICHAMBER ENLARGEMENT

Hypertrophic cardiomyopathy.
Acromegaly.
Severe obesity.

PERICARDIAL DISEASE

Pericardial effusion with or without tamponade.
Effusive constrictive disease.
Pericardial cyst, loculated effusion.

PSEUDOCARDIOMEGALY

Epicardial fat.
Chest wall deformity (pectus excavatum, straight back syndrome).
Low lung volumes.
Anteroposterior chest x-ray examination.
Mediastinal tumor, cyst.

CARDIAC MASSES[58]

ICD-10CM #	C38.0	Malignant neoplasm of heart
	D15.1	Benign neoplasm of heart

Intracardiac thrombus.
Focal myocardial hypertrophy.
Left ventricular noncompaction.
Infectious disease (abscess).
Primary cardiac tumor.
Secondary cardiac tumor (metastasis).
Lipomatous hypertrophy of septum.
Cyst.
Imaging artifact.

CARDIAC MURMURS

ICD-10CM #	R01.0	Benign and innocent cardiac murmurs
	R01.1	Cardiac murmur, unspecified

SYSTOLIC

Mitral regurgitation.
Tricuspid regurgitation.
Ventricular septal defect (VSD).
Aortic stenosis.
Idiopathic hypertrophic subaortic stenosis.
Pulmonic stenosis.
Innocent murmur of childhood.
Coarctation of aorta.
Mitral valve prolapse.

DIASTOLIC

Aortic regurgitation (AR).
Atrial myxoma.
Mitral stenosis.
Pulmonary artery branch stenosis.
Tricuspid stenosis.
Graham Steell murmur (diastolic decrescendo murmur heard in severe pulmonary hypertension).
Pulmonic regurgitation.
Severe MR.
Austin Flint murmur (diastolic rumble heard in severe AR).
Severe VSD and patent ductus arteriosus.

CONTINUOUS

Patent ductus arteriosus.
Pulmonary arteriovenous fistula.

CARDIAC TUMORS[59]

ICD-10CM #	C38.0	Malignant neoplasm of heart
	D15.1	Benign neoplasm of heart

PRIMARY

Benign:
  Myxoma.
  Lipoma.
  Fibroma.
  Rhabdomyoma.
  Fibroelastoma.
Malignant:
  Sarcoma.
  Mesothelioma.
  Lymphoma.

SECONDARY

Direct Extension
Lung cancer.
Breast cancer.
Mediastinal tumors.
Metastatic Tumors
Malignant melanoma.
Leukemia.
Lymphoma.
Venous Extension
Renal cell cancer.
Adrenal cancer.
Liver cancer.

CARDIOEMBOLISM

ICD-10CM #	I21.3 ST	Elevation (STEMI) myocardial infarction of unspecified site
	I21.9	Acute myocardial infarction, unspecified

Acute myocardial infarction.
Atrial fibrillation.
Left ventricular aneurysm.
Valvular heart disease (e.g., rheumatic mitral valve disease, mitral valve prolapse).
Dilated cardiomyopathy.
Atrial septal defect.
Patent foramen ovale.
Cardioversion for atrial fibrillation.
Infective endocarditis.
Atrial septal aneurysm.
Sick sinus syndrome and cardiac arrhythmias.
Nonbacterial thrombotic endocarditis.
Prosthetic heart valves.
Atrial myxoma and other intracardiac tumors.
Cyanotic heart disease.
Balloon angioplasty.
Coronary artery bypass grafting.
Aneurysms of sinus of Valsalva.
Other: VVI pacing, ventricular support devices, heart transplantation, intracardiac defects with paradoxical embolism.

CARDIOGENIC SHOCK

ICD-10CM #	R57.0	Cardiogenic shock

Myocardial infarction.
Arrhythmias.
Pericardial effusion/tamponade.
Chest trauma.
Valvular heart disease.
Myocarditis.
Cardiomyopathy.
Congestive heart failure, end-stage.

CATAPLEXY[38]

ICD-10CM #	G47.4	Narcolepsy and cataplexy

DIFFERENTIAL DIAGNOSIS OF CATAPLEXY

Partial complex seizure.
Absence spell.
Atonic seizure.
Drop attack.
Syncope.
Vertebrobasilar insufficiency.
Basilar migraines.
Pseudocataplexy.

CATARACTS, PEDIATRIC AGE

ICD-10CM #	H26.0	Infantile, juvenile, and presenile cataracts

DEVELOPMENTAL VARIANTS

Prematurity (Y-suture vacuoles) with or without retinopathy of prematurity.

GENETIC DISORDERS

Simple Mendelian Inheritance
Autosomal dominant (most common).
Autosomal recessive.
X-linked.

Major Chromosomal Defects
Trisomy disorders (13, 18, 21).
Turner syndrome (45X).
Deletion syndromes (11p13, 18p, 18q).
Duplication syndromes (3q, 20p, 10q).

Multisystem Genetic Disorders
Alport syndrome (hearing loss, renal disease).
Alström syndrome (nerve deafness, diabetes mellitus).
Apert disease (craniosynostosis, syndactyly).
Cockayne syndrome (premature senility, skin photosensitivity).
Conradi disease (chondrodysplasia punctata).
Crouzon disease (dysostosis craniofacialis).
Hallermann-Streiff syndrome (microphthalmia, small pinched nose, skin atrophy, hypotrichosis).
Hypohidrotic ectodermal dysplasia (anomalous dentition, hypohidrosis, hypotrichosis).
Ichthyosis (keratinizing disorder with thick, scaly skin).
Incontinentia pigmenti (dental anomalies, intellectual disabilities, cutaneous lesions).
Lowe syndrome (oculocerebrorenal syndrome: hypotonia, renal disease).
Marfan syndrome.
Marinesco-Sjögren syndrome (cerebellar ataxia, hypotonia).
Meckel-Gruber syndrome (renal dysplasia, encephalocele).
Myotonic dystrophy.
Nail-patella syndrome (renal dysfunction, dysplastic nails, hypoplastic patella).
Nevoid basal cell carcinoma syndrome (autosomal dominant, basal cell carcinoma erupts in childhood).
Peters anomaly (corneal opacifications with iris-corneal dysgenesis).
Reiger syndrome (iris dysplasia, myotonic dystrophy).

Rothmund-Thomson syndrome (poikiloderma: skin atrophy).
Rubinstein-Taybi syndrome (broad great toe, intellectual disabilities).
Smith-Lemli-Opitz syndrome (toe syndactyly, hypospadias, intellectual disabilities).
Sotos syndrome (cerebral gigantism).
Spondyloepiphyseal dysplasia (dwarfism, short trunk).
Werner syndrome (premature aging in second decade of life).

Inborn Errors of Metabolism
Abetalipoproteinemia (absent chylomicrons, retinal degeneration).
Fabry disease (α-galactosidase A deficiency).
Galactokinase deficiency.
Galactosemia (galactose-1-phosphate uridyl transferase deficiency).
Homocystinemia (subluxation of lens, intellectual disabilities).
Mannosidosis (acid α-mannosidase deficiency).
Niemann-Pick disease (sphingomyelinase deficiency).
Refsum disease (phytanic acid α-hydrolase deficiency).
Wilson disease (accumulation of copper leads to cirrhosis and neurologic symptoms).

ENDOCRINOPATHIES

Hypocalcemia (hypoparathyroidism).
Hypoglycemia.
Diabetes mellitus.

CONGENITAL INFECTIONS

Toxoplasmosis.
Cytomegalovirus infection.
Syphilis.
Rubella.
Perinatal herpes simplex infection.
Measles (rubeola).
Poliomyelitis.
Influenza.
Varicella-zoster.

OCULAR ANOMALIES

Microphthalmia.
Coloboma.
Aniridia.
Mesodermal dysgenesis.
Persistent papillary membrane.
Posterior lenticonus.
Persistent hyperplastic primary vitreous.
Primitive hyaloid vascular system.

MISCELLANEOUS DISORDERS

Atopic dermatitis.
Drugs (corticosteroids).
Radiation.
Trauma.
Idiopathic

CAVITARY LESION ON CHEST X-RAY EXAMINATION[60]

ICD-10CM #	R91.8	Other nonspecific abnormal finding of lung field

NECROTIZING INFECTIONS

Bacteria: anaerobes, *Staphylococcus aureus*, enteric gram-negative bacteria, *Pseudomonas aeruginosa*, *Legionella* spp., *Haemophilus influenzae*, *Streptococcus pyogenes*, *Streptococcus pneumoniae*, *Rhodococcus*, *Actinomyces*.
Mycobacteria: *Mycobacterium tuberculosis*, *Mycobacterium kansasii*, MAI.
Bacteria-like: *Nocardia* spp.
Fungi: Coccidioides *immitis*, *Histoplasma capsulatum*, *Blastomyces hominis*, *Aspergillus* spp., *Mucor* spp.
Parasitic: *Entamoeba histolytica*, *Echinococcus*, *Paragonimus westermani*.

CAVITARY INFARCTION

Bland infarction (with or without superimposed infection).
Lung contusion.

SEPTIC EMBOLISM

S. aureus, anaerobes, others.

VASCULITIS

Granulomatosis with polyangiitis, periarteritis.

NEOPLASMS

Bronchogenic carcinoma, metastatic carcinoma, lymphoma.

MISCELLANEOUS LESIONS

Cysts, blebs, bullae, or pneumatocele with or without fluid collections.
Sequestration.
Empyema with air-fluid level.
Bronchiectasis.

CEREBRAL INFARCTION SECONDARY TO INHERITED DISORDERS

ICD-10CM #	I63.50	Cerebral infarction due to unspecified occlusion or stenosis of unspecified cerebral artery

Homocystinuria.
Marfan syndrome.
Ehlers-Danlos syndrome.
Rendu-Osler-Weber syndrome.
Pseudoxanthoma elasticum.
Fabry disease.

CEREBRAL VASCULITIS, CAUSES[61]

ICD-10CM #	Varies with specific diagnosis

PRIMARY CEREBRAL VASCULITIDES

Takayasu arteritis.
Primary cerebral vasculitis.
Polyarteritis nodosa.

SECONDARY VASCULITIDES

Immune Disorders
Systemic lupus erythematosus.
Wegner granulomatosis.

Differential Diagnosis

II

Kawasaki syndrome.
Sarcoidosis.
Henoch-Schönlein purpura.
Primary Intracranial Infections
Bacterial meningitis (especially *Diplococcus pneumoniae*).
Tuberculous meningitis.
Mycotic infections.
Cat-scratch disease.
HIV/AIDS.
Malaria.
Lyme disease.
Rickettsial infections.
Brucellosis.

CEREBROVASCULAR DISEASE, ISCHEMIC[62]

ICD-10CM #	I67.9	Cerebrovascular disease, unspecified

VASCULAR DISORDERS

Large-vessel atherothrombotic disease.
Lacunar disease.
Arterial-to-arterial embolization.
Carotid or vertebral artery dissection.
Fibromuscular dysplasia.
Migraine.
Venous thrombosis.
Radiation.
Complications of arteriography.
Multiple, progressive intracranial arterial occlusions.

INFLAMMATORY DISORDERS

Giant cell arteritis.
Polyarteritis nodosa.
Systemic lupus erythematosus.
Granulomatous angiitis.
Takayasu disease.
Arteritis associated with amphetamine, cocaine, or phenylpropanolamine.
Syphilis, mucormycosis.
Sjögren syndrome.
Behçet syndrome.

CARDIAC DISORDERS

Rheumatic heart disease.
Mural thrombus.
Arrhythmias.
Mitral valve prolapse.
Prosthetic heart valve.
Endocarditis.
Myxoma.
Paradoxical embolus.

HEMATOLOGIC DISORDERS

Thrombotic thrombocytopenic purpura.
Sickle cell disease.
Hypercoagulable states.
Polycythemia.
Thrombocytosis.
Leukocytosis.
Lupus anticoagulant.

CERVICAL INSTABILITY, PEDIATRIC

ICD-10CM #	M50	Cervical disc disorders

CONGENITAL

Vertebral (Bony Anomalies)
Craniooccipital defects (occipital vertebrae, basilar impression, occipital dysplasias, condylar hypoplasia, occipitalized atlas).
Atlantoaxial defects (aplasia of atlas arch, aplasia of odontoid process).
Subaxial anomalies (failure of segmentation and/or fusion, spina bifida, spondylolisthesis).
Ligamentous or Combined Anomalies
Found at birth as an element of somatogenic aberration.
Syndromic Disorders
Down syndrome.
Klippel-Feil syndrome.
22q11.2 deletion syndrome.
Larsen syndrome.
Marfan syndrome.
Ehlers-Danlos syndrome.

ACQUIRED

Trauma.
Infection (pyogenic, granulomatous).
Tumor (including neurofibromatosis).
Inflammatory conditions (e.g., juvenile rheumatoid arthritis).
Osteochondrodysplasias (e.g., achondroplasia, diastrophic dysplasia, metatropic dysplasia, spondyloepiphyseal dysplasia).
Storage disorders (e.g., mucopolysaccharidoses).
Metabolic disorders (rickets).
Miscellaneous (including osteogenesis imperfecta, sequela of surgery).

CHEST PAIN, CHILDREN[45]

ICD-10CM #	R07.9	Chest pain, unspecified
	R07.82	Intercostal pain
	R07.89	Other chest pain
	R07.1	Chest pain on breathing
	R07.81	Pleurodynia

MUSCULOSKELETAL (COMMON)

Trauma (accidental, abuse).
Exercise, overuse injury (strain, bursitis).
Costochondritis (Tietze syndrome).
Herpes zoster (cutaneous).
Pleurodynia.
Fibrositis.
Slipping rib.
Sickle cell anemia vasoocclusive crisis.
Osteomyelitis (rare).
Primary or metastatic tumor (rare).

PULMONARY (COMMON)

Pneumonia.
Pleurisy.
Asthma.
Chronic cough.
Pneumothorax.
Infarction (sickle cell anemia).
Foreign body.

Embolism (rare).
Pulmonary hypertension (rare).
Tumor (rare).

GI (LESS COMMON)

Esophagitis (gastroesophageal reflux).
Esophageal foreign body.
Esophageal spasm.
Cholecystitis.
Subdiaphragmatic abscess.
Perihepatitis (Fitz-Hugh-Curtis syndrome).
Peptic ulcer disease.

CARDIAC (LESS COMMON)

Pericarditis.
Postpericardiotomy syndrome.
Endocarditis.
Mitral valve prolapse.
Aortic or subaortic stenosis.
Arrhythmias.
Marfan syndrome (dissecting aortic aneurysm).
Anomalous coronary artery.
Kawasaki disease.
Cocaine, sympathomimetic ingestion.
Angina (familial hypercholesterolemia).

IDIOPATHIC (COMMON)

Anxiety, hyperventilation.
Panic disorder.

OTHER (LESS COMMON)

Spinal cord or nerve root compression.
Breast-related pathologic condition.
Castleman disease (lymph node neoplasm).

CHEST PAIN, NONPLEURITIC[63]

ICD-10CM #	R07.9	Chest pain, unspecified
	R07.82	Intercostal pain
	R07.89	Other chest pain

Cardiac: myocardial ischemia/infarction, myocarditis.
Esophageal: spasm, esophagitis, ulceration, neoplasm, achalasia, diverticula, foreign body.
Referred pain from subdiaphragmatic GI structures.
Gastric and duodenal: hiatal hernia, neoplasm, peptic ulcer disease.
Gallbladder and biliary: cholecystitis, cholelithiasis, impacted stone, neoplasm.
Pancreatic: pancreatitis, neoplasm.
Dissecting aortic aneurysm.
Pain originating from skin, breasts, and musculoskeletal structures: herpes zoster, mastitis, cervical spondylosis.
Mediastinal tumors: lymphoma, thymoma.
Pulmonary: neoplasm, pneumonia, pulmonary embolism/infarction.
Psychoneurosis.
Chest pain associated with mitral valve prolapse.

CHEST PAIN, PLEURITIC

ICD-10CM #	R07.1	Chest pain on breathing
	R07.81	Pleurodynia

Cardiac: pericarditis, postpericardiotomy/ Dressler syndrome.

Pulmonary: pneumothorax, hemothorax, embolism/infarction, pneumonia, empyema, neoplasm, bronchiectasis, pneumomediastinum, TB, carcinomatous effusion.

GI: liver abscess, pancreatitis, esophageal rupture, Whipple disease with associated pericarditis or pleuritis.

Subdiaphragmatic abscess.

Pain originating from skin and musculoskeletal tissues: costochondritis, chest wall trauma, fractured rib, interstitial fibrositis, myositis, strain of pectoralis muscle, herpes zoster, soft tissue and bone tumors.

Collagen vascular diseases with pleuritis.

Psychoneurosis.

Familial Mediterranean fever.

CHEST WALL TUMORS, PRIMARY[64]

ICD-10CM #   Varies with specific diagnosis

SOFT TISSUE

Benign
Lipoma.
Hemangioma.
Lymphangioma.
Fibroma.
Rhabdomyoma.
Neurofibroma.
Desmoid tumor.
Malignant
Malignant fibrous histiocytoma.
Rhabdosarcoma.
Liposarcoma.
Neurofibrosarcoma.
Leiomyosarcoma.

BONY AND CARTILAGINOUS

Benign
Fibrous dysplasia.
Osteochondroma.
Chondroma.
Askin tumor.
Plasmacytoma.
Malignant
Chondrosarcoma.
Osteogenic sarcoma.
Ewing sarcoma.

CHIASMAL DISEASE[44]

ICD-10CM #   Varies with specific diagnosis

CAUSES OF CHIASMAL DISEASE

Tumors
Pituitary adenomas.
Craniopharyngioma.
Meningioma.
Glioma.
Chordoma.
Dysgerminoma.
Nasopharyngeal tumors.
Metastases.
Nonneoplastic Masses
Aneurysm.
Rathke pouch cysts.

Fibrous dysplasia.
Sphenoidal sinus mucocele.
Arachnoid cysts.
Miscellaneous
Demyelination.
Inflammation (e.g., sarcoidosis).
Trauma.
Radiation-induced necrosis.
Toxicity (e.g., ethambutol).
Vasculitis.

CHILDHOOD EOSINOPHILIA

| ICD-10CM # | D72.1 | Eosinophilia |

PHYSIOLOGIC

Prematurity.
Infants receiving hyperalimentation.
Familial.

INFECTIOUS

Parasitic (with tissue-invasive helminths, e.g., trichinosis, strongyloidiasis, pneumocystosis, filariasis, cysticercosis, cutaneous and visceral larva migrans, echinococcosis).
Bacterial (brucellosis, tularemia, cat-scratch disease, *Chlamydia*).
Fungal (histoplasmosis, blastomycosis, coccidioidomycosis, allergic bronchopulmonary aspergillosis).
Mycobacterial (tuberculosis, leprosy).
Viral (hepatitis A, hepatitis B, hepatitis C, Epstein-Barr virus).

PULMONARY

Allergic (rhinitis, asthma).
Loeffler syndrome.
Hypersensitivity pneumonitis.
Eosinophilic pneumonia.
Pulmonary interstitial eosinophilia.

DERMATOLOGIC

Atopic dermatitis.
Pemphigus.
Dermatitis herpetiformis.
Infantile eosinophilic pustular folliculitis.
Episodic angioedema and urticaria.
Eosinophilic fasciitis (Shulman syndrome).
Eosinophilic cellulitis (Wells syndrome).
Kimura disease.

ONCOLOGIC

Neoplasm (lung, GI, uterine).
Hodgkin disease.
Leukemia.
Myelofibrosis.

IMMUNOLOGIC

T-cell immunodeficiencies.
Hyperimmunoglobulin E (Job) syndrome.
Wiskott-Aldrich syndrome.
Graft-versus-host disease.
Drug hypersensitivity.
Postirradiation.
Postsplenectomy.

ENDOCRINE

Postadrenalectomy.
Addison disease.
Panhypopituitarism.

CARDIOVASCULAR

Loeffler disease (fibroplastic endocarditis).
Congenital heart disease.
Hypersensitivity vasculitis.

GI

Milk protein allergy.
Inflammatory bowel disease.
Eosinophilic esophagitis.
Eosinophilic gastroenteritis.

CHOLANGITIS, ACUTE[64]

| ICD-10CM # | K83.0 | Cholangitis |

NONIATROGENIC

Benign Conditions
Choledocholithiasis.
  Primary.
  Secondary.
Pancreatitis (chronic/acute), including pancreatic pseudocyst.
Papillary stenosis.
Mirizzi syndrome.
Choledochal cysts (type V, Caroli disease).
Primary sclerosing cholangitis.
Malignancies
Pancreatic cancer.
Cholangiocarcinoma.
Porta hepatis tumor/metastasis.

IATROGENIC

Obstructed biliary endoprosthesis.
Iatrogenic biliary stricture.
Direct surgical trauma.
Ischemia-induced stricture.
Anastomotic stricture (biliobiliary/bilioenteric anastomosis).

CHOLESTASIS[24]

| ICD-10CM # | K80.65 | Calculus of gallbladder and bile duct with chronic cholecystitis with obstruction |

EXTRAHEPATIC

Choledocholithiasis.
Bile duct stricture.
Cholangiocarcinoma.
Pancreatic carcinoma.
Chronic pancreatitis.
Papillary stenosis.
Ampullary cancer.
Primary sclerosing cholangitis.
Choledochal cysts.
Parasites (e.g., ascaris, clonorchis).
AIDS.
Cholangiography.
Biliary atresia.
Portal lymphadenopathy.
Mirizzi syndrome.

INTRAHEPATIC

Viral hepatitis.
Alcoholic hepatitis.
Drug induced.
Ductopenia syndromes.
Primary biliary cirrhosis.
Benign recurrent intrahepatic cholestasis.

Differential Diagnosis

II

Byler disease.
Primary sclerosing cholangitis.
Alagille syndrome.
Sarcoid.
Lymphoma.
Postoperative.
Total parenteral nutrition.
α-1-antitrypsin deficiency.

CHOLESTASIS, NEONATAL AND INFANTILE, DIFFERENTIAL DIAGNOSIS[19]

ICD-10CM # 026.6 Liver disorders in pregnancy, childbirth and the puerperium

INFECTIOUS
Generalized bacterial sepsis.
Viral hepatitis:
  Hepatitis A, B, C, D.
  Cytomegalovirus.
  Rubella virus.
  Herpesvirus: herpes simplex, human herpes-virus 6 and 7.
  Varicella virus.
  Coxsackievirus.
  Echovirus.
  Reovirus type 3.
  Parvovirus B19.
  HIV.
  Adenovirus.
Others:
  Toxoplasmosis.
  Syphilis.
  Tuberculosis.
  Listeriosis.
  Urinary tract infection.

TOXIC
Sepsis.
Parenteral nutrition related.
Drug related.

METABOLIC
Disorders of amino acid metabolism:
  Tyrosinemia.
Disorders of lipid metabolism:
  Wolman disease.
  Niemann-Pick disease (type C).
  Gaucher disease.
Cholesterol ester storage disease.
Disorders of carbohydrate metabolism:
  Galactosemia.
  Fructosemia.
  Glycogenosis IV.
Disorders of bile acid biosynthesis.
Other metabolic defects:
  α1-Antitrypsin deficiency.
  Cystic fibrosis.
  Hypopituitarism.
  Hypothyroidism.
  Zellweger (cerebrohepatorenal) syndrome.
  Neonatal iron storage disease.
  Indian childhood cirrhosis/infantile copper overload.
  Congenital disorders of glycosylation.
  Mitochondrial hepatopathies.
  Citrin deficiency.

GENETIC OR CHROMOSOMAL
Trisomy 17, 18, 21.
Donahue syndrome.

INTRAHEPATIC CHOLESTASIS SYNDROMES
"Idiopathic" neonatal hepatitis.
Alagille syndrome (arteriohepatic dysplasia).
Nonsyndromic bile duct paucity syndrome.
Intrahepatic cholestasis (PFIC):
  FIC-1 deficiency.
  BSEP deficiency.
  MDR3 deficiency.
Familial benign recurrent cholestasis associated with lymphedema (Aagenaes).
Congenital hepatic fibrosis.
Caroli disease (cystic dilation of intrahepatic ducts).

EXTRAHEPATIC DISEASES
Biliary atresia.
Sclerosing cholangitis.
Bile duct stricture/stenosis.
Choledochal-pancreaticoductal junction anomaly.
Spontaneous perforation of the bile duct.
Choledochal cyst.
Mass (neoplasia, stone).
Bile/mucous plug ("inspissated bile").

MISCELLANEOUS
Shock and hypoperfusion.
Associated with enteritis.
Associated with intestinal obstruction.
Neonatal lupus erythematosus.
Myeloproliferative disease (trisomy 21).
Hemophagocytic lymphohistiocytosis.
Arthrogryposis cholestatic pigmentary syndrome.

CHOLESTATIC LIVER ENZYME ELEVATION, EXTRAHEPATIC CAUSES[3]

ICD-10CM # Varies with specific diagnosis

EXTRAHEPATIC CAUSES OF CHOLESTATIC LIVER ENZYMES IN ADULTS
Intrinsic
Choledocholithiasis.
Immune-mediated duct injury:
  Autoimmune pancreatitis.
  PSC.
Malignancy:
  Ampullary cancer.
  Cholangiocarcinoma.
Infections:
  AIDS cholangiopathy:
    Cytomegalovirus.
    Cryptosporidiosis.
    Microsporidiosis.
  Parasitic infections:
    Ascariasis.
Extrinsic
Malignancy:
  Gallbladder cancer.
  Metastases, including portal adenopathy from metastases.
  Pancreatic cancer.
Mirizzi syndrome.
Pancreatitis.
Pancreatic pseudocyst.

CHOLESTATIC LIVER ENZYME ELEVATION, INTRAHEPATIC CAUSES[3]

ICD-10CM # Varies with specific causes

INTRAHEPATIC CAUSES OF CHOLESTATIC LIVER ENZYME ELEVATIONS IN ADULTS
Drugs*
Bland cholestasis:[††]
  Anabolic steroids.
  Estrogens.
Cholestatic hepatitis:
  ACE inhibitors: captopril, enalapril.
  Antimicrobials: amoxicillin-clavulanic acid, ketoconazole.
  Azathioprine.
  Chlorpromazine.
  NSAIDs: sulindac, piroxicam.
Granulomatous hepatitis:
  Allopurinol.
  Antibiotics: sulfonamides.
  Antiepileptics: carbamazepine, phenytoin.
  Cardiovascular agents: hydralazine, procainamide, quinidine.
  Phenylbutazone.
Vanishing bile duct syndrome:
  Amoxicillin-clavulanic acid.
  Chlorpromazine.
  Dicloxacillin.
  Flucloxacillin.
  Macrolides.
Primary biliary cholangitis
PRIMARY SCLEROSING CHOLANGITIS
Granulomatous Liver Disease
Infections:
  Brucellosis.
  Fungal: histoplasmosis, coccidioidomycosis.
  Leprosy.
  Q fever.
  Schistosomiasis.
  TB, *Mycobacterium avium* complex, bacillus Calmette-Guérin.
Sarcoidosis.
Idiopathic granulomatous hepatitis.
Other:
  Crohn disease.
  Heavy metal exposure: beryllium, copper.
  Hodgkin disease.
Viral Hepatitis
Hepatitis A virus and hepatitis E virus.
Hepatitis B virus and hepatitis C virus, including fibrosing cholestatic hepatitis.
Epstein-Barr virus.
Cytomegalovirus.
Idiopathic Adulthood Ductopenia
Genetic Conditions
Progressive familial intrahepatic cholestasis:
  Type 1 (formerly Byler disease).
  Type 2.
  Type 3.

[††]Diffuse, uniform loss, but many hairs left randomly distributed in area of loss.

Benign recurrent intrahepatic cholestasis:
   Type 1.
   Type 2.
Cystic fibrosis.

Malignancy
Hepatocellular carcinoma.
Metastatic disease.
Paraneoplastic syndrome:
   Non-Hodgkin lymphoma.
   Prostate cancer.
   Renal cell cancer.

Infiltrative Liver Disease
Amyloidosis.
Lymphoma.

Intrahepatic Cholestasis of Pregnancy
Total parenteral nutrition:
   Graft-versus-host disease.
   Sepsis.

CHOREA

ICD-10CM #	G25.4	Drug-induced chorea
	G25.5	Other chorea

Medications (e.g., neuroleptics, tricyclics, antiparkinsonian drugs).
Cerebral palsy.
Huntington disease.
Benign hereditary chorea.
Thyroid disorder (hyperthyroidism, hypothyroidism).
Friedreich ataxia.
Ataxia-telangiectasia.
Hypoglycemia, hyperglycemia.
Electrolyte abnormalities (hyponatremia, hypocalcemia, hypomagnesemia, hypernatremia).
Vitamin B_{12} deficiency.
Systemic lupus erythematosus.
Wilson disease.
Alcohol.
Cocaine.
Carbon monoxide poisoning.
Mercury poisoning.

CHOREA, PEDIATRIC PATIENT[49]

ICD-10CM #	G25.5	Other chorea

CAUSES OF CHOREA IN CHILDHOOD

Static Injury/Structural Disorders
Cerebral palsy.
Stroke.
Trauma.
Moyamoya disease.
Vasculitis.
Tumors.
Congenital malformations.
Joubert syndrome.

Hereditary/Degenerative Disorders
Ataxia-telangiectasia (A-T) and ataxia-telangiectasia-like disorder (ATLD).
Ataxia oculomotor apraxia (AOA) (includes AOA-1, AOA-2, and early onset cerebellar ataxia and hypoalbuminemia [EOCA-HA]).
Fahr disease.

Pantothenate kinase-associated neurodegeneration (PKAN, associated with mutations in the pantothenate kinase-2 *[PANK-2]* gene), and other causes of neuronal brain iron accumulation (NBIA).

Metabolic Disorders
Acyl-CoA dehydrogenase deficiencies.
Mitochondrial disorders, including Leigh syndrome.
GM_1 gangliosidosis.
Lesch-Nyhan disease.
Niemann-Pick type C.
Methylmalonic aciduria.
Nonketotic hyperglycemia.
Kernicterus.
Hypoparathyroidism.
Propionic acidemia.
Hypernatremia.
Hypomagnesemia.
Hypocalcemia.
Hypo- or hyperglycemia.
Vitamin E deficiency or malabsorption.
Bassen-Kornzweig disease.
Complications of cardiac bypass.

Infectious/Parainfectious Disease
Encephalitis/postencephalitis.

Immune-Mediated/Demyelinating Disorders
Sydenham chorea.
Lupus erythematosus.
Henoch-Schönlein purpura.
Anticardiolipin or antiphospholipid antibody syndrome.
Anti-NMDA antibody syndrome.

Drugs/Toxins
Neuroleptic medications, and neuroleptic-like antiemetics (haloperidol, chlorpromazine, pimozide, prochlorperazine, metoclopramide).
Calcium channel blockers (flunarizine, cinnarizine).
Antiseizure medications (phenytoin, carbamazepine, valproate, phenobarbital).
Anticholinergic medications (trihexyphenidyl, benztropine).
Antihistamines.
Tricyclic antidepressants.
Clomipramine.
Stimulants (including methylphenidate, dexamphetamine, pemoline, and bronchodilators).
Clonidine.
L-dopa.
Cocaine.
Bismuth.
Lithium.
Manganese.
Ethanol.
Carbon monoxide.
Oral contraceptives.
General anesthesia (including propofol)—during induction or emergence.

Paroxysmal Disorders
Complex migraine.
Alternating hemiplegia of childhood.
Paroxysmal kinesigenic dyskinesia (PKD).
Paroxysmal nonkinesigenic dyskinesia (PNKD).
Paroxysmal exercise-induced dyskinesia (PED).

Endocrine Disorders
Hyperthyroidism.
Pheochromocytoma.

CHOREOATHETOSIS[25]

ICD-10CM #	G25.5	Choreoathetosis

SYSTEMIC DISEASES
Systemic lupus erythematosus.
Polycythemia.
Thyrotoxicosis.
Rheumatic fever.
Cirrhosis of the liver (acquired hepatocerebral degeneration).
Diabetes mellitus.
Wilson disease.

PRIMARY DEGENERATIVE BRAIN DISEASES
Huntington chorea.
Olivopontocerebellar atrophies.
Neuroacanthocytosis.

FOCAL BRAIN DISEASES
Hemichorea.
Stroke.
Tumor.
Arteriovenous malformation.

DRUG-INDUCED CHOREOATHETOSIS
Parkinson Disease Drugs
Levodopa.

EPILEPSY DRUGS
Phenytoin.
Carbamazepine.
Phenobarbital.
Gabapentin.
Valproate.
Psychostimulant Drugs
Cocaine.
Amphetamine.
Methamphetamine.
Dextroamphetamine.
Methylphenidate.
Pemoline.
Psychotropic Drugs
Lithium.
Tricyclic antidepressant drugs.
Oral Contraceptive Drugs
Cimetidine

CHRONIC PNEUMONIA[65]

ICD-10CM #	J17	Pneumonia in diseases classified elsewhere

CAUSES OF CHRONIC PNEUMONIA
Infectious
Bacteria:
   Mixed aerobic and anaerobic bacteria.
   Actinomyces spp.
   Burkholderia pseudomallei.
   Nocardia spp.
   Rhodococcus equi.
Mycobacteria:
   Mycobacterium abscessus.
   Mycobacterium avium complex.
   Mycobacterium kansasii.
   Mycobacterium tuberculosis.

Differential Diagnosis

Parasites:
  Dirofilaria.
  Echinococcus granulosus.
  Filaria.
  Paragonimus westermani.
Fungi:
  Aspergillus spp.
  Blastomyces dermatitidis.
  Coccidioides spp.
  Cryptococcus spp.
  Histoplasma capsulatum.
  Scedosporium spp.
  Sporothrix schenckii.
Noninfectious
Neoplasia.
Cystic fibrosis.
Sarcoidosis.
Amyloidosis.
Vasculitis.
Drugs.
Radiation.
Recurrent pulmonary emboli.
Bronchial obstruction.
Pulmonary infiltration with eosinophilia syndrome.
Pneumoconiosis.

CHYLOTHORAX[4]

ICD-10CM #	I89.8	Other specified noninfective disorders of lymphatic vessels and lymph nodes

Traumatic (Chest and Neck)
Blunt.
Penetrating.
Iatrogenic
Catheterization, particularly subclavian vein.
Postsurgical.
Excision of cervical/supraclavicular lymph nodes.
Radical lymph node dissections of the neck or chest.
Lung, esophageal, or mediastinal resection.
Thoracic aneurysm repair.
Sympathectomy.
Congenital cardiovascular surgery.
Neoplasms
Lymphoma, lung, esophageal, or mediastinal neoplasms.
Metastatic carcinoma.
Infectious
Tuberculous lymphadenosis.
Mediastinitis.
Ascending lymphangitis.
Other
Lymphangioleiomyomatosis.
Venous thrombosis.
Congenital.

CLOUDY URINE

ICD-10CM #	R82	Other abnormal findings in urine

Concentrated urine.
Use of multivitamin supplements.
Diet high in purine-rich foods.
Pyuria.

Phosphaturia.
Urinary tract infection.
Lipiduria.
Chyluria.
Hyperoxaluria.

CLUBBING

ICD-10CM #	R68.3	Clubbing of fingers

Pulmonary neoplasm (lung, pleura).
Other neoplasm (GI, liver, Hodgkin, thymus, osteogenic sarcoma).
Pulmonary infectious process (empyema, abscess, bronchiectasis, TB, chronic pneumonitis).
Extrapulmonary infectious process (subacute bacterial endocarditis, intestinal TB, bacterial or amebic dysentery, arterial graft sepsis).
Pneumoconiosis.
Cystic fibrosis.
Sarcoidosis.
Cyanotic congenital heart disease.
Endocrine (Graves disease, hyperparathyroidism).
Inflammatory bowel disease.
Celiac disease.
Chronic liver disease, cirrhosis (particularly biliary and juvenile).
Pulmonary arteriovenous malformations.
Idiopathic.
Thyroid acropachy.
Hereditary (pachydermoperiostosis).
Chronic trauma (jackhammer operators, machine workers).

COBALAMIN DEFICIENCY[31]

ICD-10CM #	E53.8	Deficiency of other specified B group vitamins

ETIOPATHOPHYSIOLOGIC CLASSIFICATION OF COBALAMIN DEFICIENCY

Nutritional cobalamin deficiency (i.e., insufficient cobalamin intake):
  Vegetarians, poverty-imposed near-vegetarians, breastfed infants of mothers with pernicious anemia.
Abnormal intragastric events (i.e., inadequate proteolysis of food cobalamin):
  Atrophic gastritis, partial gastritis with hypochlorhydria, proton-pump inhibitors, H_2 blockers.
Loss or atrophy of gastric oxyntic mucosa (i.e., deficient intrinsic factor [IF] molecules):
  Total or partial gastrectomy, pernicious anemia, caustic destruction (lye).
Abnormal events in small bowel lumen:
  Inadequate pancreatic protease (e.g., R-cobalamin not degraded, cobalamin not transferred to IF):
    Insufficient pancreatic protease (i.e., pancreatic insufficiency).
    Inactivation of pancreatic protease (i.e., Zollinger-Ellison syndrome).
  Usurping of luminal cobalamin (i.e., inadequate cobalamin binding to IF):
    By bacteria, during stasis syndromes (e.g., blind loops, pouches of diverticulosis, strictures, fistulas, anastomosis), impaired

bowel motility (e.g., scleroderma), hypogammaglobulinemia.
    By Diphyllobothrium latum (fish tapeworm).
Disorders of ileal mucosa/IF–cobalamin receptors (i.e., IF–cobalamin not bound to IF–cobalamin receptors):
  Diminished or absent IF–cobalamin receptors (e.g., ileal bypass, resection, fistula).
  Abnormal mucosal architecture/function (e.g., tropical or nontropical sprue, Crohn disease, tuberculosis ileitis, infiltration by lymphomas, amyloidosis).
  IF-/post-IF–cobalamin receptor defects (e.g., Imerslund-Gräsbeck syndrome, transcobalamin II [TC II] deficiency).
  Drug effects (e.g., slow K, metformin, cholestyramine, colchicine, neomycin).
Disorders of plasma cobalamin transport (i.e., TC II–cobalamin not delivered to TC II receptors):
  Congenital TC II deficiency, defective binding of TC II–cobalamin to TC II receptors (rare).
Metabolic disorders (i.e., cobalamin not used by cells):
  Inborn enzyme errors (rare).
  Acquired disorders (e.g., cobalamin functionally inactivated by irreversible oxidation, N_2O inhalation).

COGNITIVE IMPAIRMENT[66]

ICD-10CM #	G31.84	Mild cognitive impairment, so stated

CAUSES OF COGNITIVE IMPAIRMENT: DIAGNOSES BY CATEGORIES WITH REPRESENTATIVE EXAMPLES

Degenerative
Alzheimer disease.
Frontotemporal dementias.
Dementia with Lewy bodies.
Corticobasal degeneration.
Huntington disease.
Wilson disease.
Parkinson disease.
Multiple system atrophy.
Progressive supranuclear palsy.
Psychiatric
Depression.
Schizophrenia.
Vascular
Vascular dementia.
Binswanger encephalopathy.
Amyloid dementia.
Diffuse hypoxic/ischemic injury.
Obstructive
Normal-pressure hydrocephalus.
Obstructive hydrocephalus.
Traumatic
Chronic subdural hematoma.
Chronic traumatic encephalopathy.
Post Aagenaes concussion syndrome.
Neoplastic
Tumor: malignant, primary and secondary.
Tumor: benign (e.g., frontal meningioma).
Paraneoplastic limbic encephalitis.
Infections
Chronic meningitis.
Postherpes encephalitis.

Focal cerebritis/abscesses.
HIV dementia.
HIV-associated infection.
Syphilis.
Lyme encephalopathy.
Subacute sclerosing panencephalitis.
Creutzfeldt–Jakob disease.
Progressive multifocal leukoencephalopathy.
Parenchymal sarcoidosis.
Chronic systemic infection.

Demyelinating
Multiple sclerosis.
Adrenoleukodystrophy.
Metachromatic leukodystrophy.

Autoimmune
Systemic lupus erythematosus.
Polyarteritis nodosa.

Drugs/Toxins
Medications:
  Anticholinergics.
  Antihistamines.
  Anticonvulsants.
  β-blockers.
  Sedative–hypnotics.

Substance Abuse
Alcohol.
Inhalants.
Phencyclidine (PCP).

Toxins
Arsenic.
Bromide.
Carbon monoxide.
Lead.
Mercury.
Organophosphates.

COLIC, ACUTE ABDOMINAL[2]

ICD-10CM #	R10.0	Acute abdomen

Acute gastroenteritis.
Food poisoning.
Nonspecific causes.
Constipation.
Gastric outlet obstruction:
  Chronic peptic ulceration.
  Gastric cancer.
Small bowel obstruction:
  Adhesions:
    Postsurgical.
    Inflammatory (e.g., diverticular).
    Radiation.
    Meckel diverticulum.
    Metastatic.
  Stricture:
    Ischemic.
    Radiation.
    Inflammatory (e.g., Crohn disease).
  Volvulus intussusception:
    Tumor (e.g., Peutz-Jeghers syndrome).
    Superior mesenteric artery syndrome.
  Intraluminal bolus:
    Gallstone.
    Bezoar.
  Hernia:
    Abdominal wall.
    Internal.
  Neoplasm:
    Benign (e.g., leiomyoma).

Malignant (e.g., carcinoid tumor, adeno-carcinoma).
Large bowel obstruction:
  Colon cancer.
  Diverticular disease.
  Volvulus.
Uterine:
  Missed abortion.
  Parturition.
  Period pain.

COLON ISCHEMIA[3]

ICD-10CM #	Varies with specific diagnosis

CAUSES OF COLON ISCHEMIA

Acute pancreatitis.
Allergy.
Amyloidosis.
Heart failure or cardiac arrhythmias.
Hematologic disorders and coagulopathies:
  Activated protein C resistance.
  Antithrombin deficiency.
  Factor V Leiden mutation.
  Paroxysmal nocturnal hemoglobinuria.
  Polycythemia vera.
  Protein C and S deficiencies.
  Prothrombin G20210A mutation.
  Sickle cell disease.
Infection:
  Bacteria (*Escherichia coli* O157:H7).
  Parasites (*Angiostrongylus costaricensis*).
  Viruses (HBV, HCV, cytomegalovirus).
Inferior mesenteric artery thrombosis.
Long-distance running.
Medications and toxins:
  Alosetron.
  Cocaine.
  Danazol.
  Digitalis compounds.
  Ergots.
  Estrogens.
  Flutamide.
  Glycerin enema.
  Gold salts.
  Immunosuppressive agents.
  Interferon-α.
  Methamphetamine.
  NSAIDs.
  Penicillin.
  Phenylephrine.
  Polyethylene glycol 3350 colon lavage solutions.
  Pit viper toxin.
  Progestins.
  Pseudoephedrine.
  Psychotropic drugs.
  Saline laxatives.
  Sumatriptan.
  Tegaserod.
  Vasopressin.
Pheochromocytoma.
Ruptured ectopic pregnancy.
Shock.
Strangulated hernia.
Surgery/procedures:
  Aortic aneurysmectomy.
  Aortoiliac reconstruction.

Barium enema.
Colectomy with inferior mesenteric artery ligation.
Colon bypass.
Colonoscopy.
Exchange transfusions.
Gynecologic operations.
Lumbar aortography.
Thromboembolism:
  Cholesterol (atheroembolism).
  Myxoma (left atrial).
Trauma (blunt or penetrating).
Vasculitis and vasculopathy:
  Buerger disease.
  Eosinophilic granulomatosis with angiitis.
  Fibromuscular dysplasia.
  Kawasaki disease.
  Polyarteritis nodosa.
  Rheumatoid vasculitis.
  Systemic lupus erythematosus.
  Takayasu arteritis.
Volvulus.

COLOR CHANGES, CUTANEOUS[57]

ICD-10CM #	L81.9	Disorder of pigmentation, unspecified

BROWN

Generalized: pituitary, adrenal, liver disease, adrenocorticotropic hormone–producing tumor (e.g., oat cell lung carcinoma).
Localized: nevi, neurofibromatosis.

WHITE

Generalized: albinism.
Localized: vitiligo, Raynaud phenomenon.

RED (ERYTHEMA)

Generalized: fever, polycythemia, urticaria, viral exanthems.
Localized: inflammation, infection, Raynaud phenomenon.

YELLOW

Generalized: liver disease, chronic renal disease, anemia.
Generalized (except sclera): hypothyroidism, increased intake of vegetables containing carotene.
Localized: resolving hematoma, infection, peripheral vascular insufficiency.

BLUE

Lips, mouth, nail beds: cardiovascular and pulmonary diseases, Raynaud phenomenon.

COMA

ICD-10CM #	R40.20	Unspecified coma

Vascular: hemorrhage, thrombosis, embolism.
Central nervous system infections: meningitis, encephalitis, cerebral abscess.
Cerebral neoplasms with herniation.
Head injury: subdural hematoma, cerebral concussion, cerebral contusion.
Drugs: narcotics, sedatives, hypnotics.

Ingestion or inhalation of toxins: CO, alcohol, lead.
Metabolic disturbances.
Hypoxia.
Acid-base disorders.
Hypoglycemia, hyperglycemia.
Hepatic failure.
Electrolyte disorders.
Uremia.
Hypothyroidism.
Hypothermia, hyperthermia.
Hypotension, malignant hypertension.
Post-ictal.

COMA, NORMAL COMPUTED TOMOGRAPHY[18]

| ICD-10CM # | R40.20 | Unspecified coma |

MENINGEAL DISORDERS

Subarachnoid hemorrhage (uncommon).
Bacterial meningitis.
Encephalitis.
Subdural empyema.

EXOGENOUS TOXINS

Sedative drugs and barbiturates.
Anesthetics and γ hydroxybutyrate.*
Alcohols.
Stimulants:
  Phencyclidines.†
  Cocaine and amphetamines.‡
Psychotropic drugs:
  Cyclic antidepressants.
  Phenothiazines.
  Lithium.
Anticonvulsants.
Opioids.
Clonidine.§
Penicillins.
Salicylates.
Anticholinergics.
Carbon monoxide, cyanide, and methemoglobinemia.

---

*Involvement principally of cancellous bone.
†Involvement of cancellous and cortical bone.
‡Coma after seizures or status (i.e., a prolonged post-ictal state).
§An antihypertensive agent active through the opiate receptor system; frequent overdose when used to treat narcotic withdrawal.

ENDOGENOUS TOXINS/DEFICIENCIES/DERANGEMENTS

Hypoxia and ischemia.
Hypoglycemia.
Hypercalcemia.
Osmolar:
  Hyperglycemia.
  Hyponatremia.
  Hypernatremia.
Organ system failure:
  Hepatic encephalopathy.
  Uremic encephalopathy.
  Pulmonary insufficiency (carbon dioxide narcosis).

SEIZURES

Prolonged post-ictal state.
Spike-wave stupor.

HYPOTHERMIA OR HYPERTHERMIA

Brain stem ischemia.
Basilar artery stroke.
Brain stem or cerebellar hemorrhage.
Conversion or malingering.

COMA, PEDIATRIC POPULATION[67]

| ICD-10CM # | R40.20 | Unspecified coma |

ANOXIA

Birth asphyxia.
Carbon monoxide poisoning.
Croup/epiglottitis.
Meconium aspiration.

INFECTION

Hemolysis.
Blood loss.
Hydrops fetalis.
Infection.
Meningoencephalitis.
Sepsis.
Postimmunization encephalitis.

INCREASED INTRACRANIAL PRESSURE

Anoxia.
Inborn metabolic errors.
Toxic encephalopathy.
Reye syndrome.
Head trauma/intracranial bleed.
Hydrocephalus.
Posterior fossa tumors.

HYPERTENSIVE ENCEPHALOPATHY

Coarctation of aorta.
Nephritis.
Vasculitis.
Pheochromocytoma.

ISCHEMIA

Hypoplastic left heart.
Shunting lesions.
Aortic stenosis.
Cardiovascular collapse (any cause).

PURPURIC CAUSES

Disseminated intravascular coagulation.
Hemolytic-uremic syndrome.
Leukemia.
Thrombotic purpura.

HYPERCAPNIA

Cystic fibrosis.
Bronchopulmonary dysplasia.
Congenital lung anomalies.

NEOPLASM

Medulloblastoma.
Glioma of brain stem.
Posterior fossa tumors.

DRUGS/TOXINS

Maternal sedation.
Alcohol.
Any drug.
Lead.
Salicylism.
Arsenic.
Pesticides.

ELECTROLYTE ABNORMALITIES

Hypernatremia (diarrhea, dehydration, salt poisoning).
Hyponatremia (syndrome of inappropriate antidiuretic hormone secretion, androgenital syndrome, gastroenteritis).
Hyperkalemia (renal failure, salicylism, androgenitalism).
Hypokalemia (diarrhea, hyperaldosteronism, salicylism, diabetic ketoacidosis).
Hypocalcemia (vitamin D deficiency, hyperparathyroidism).
Severe acidosis (sepsis, cold injury, salicylism, diabetic ketoacidosis).

HYPOGLYCEMIA

Birth injury or stress.
Diabetes.
Alcohol.
Salicylism.
Hyperinsulinemia.
Iatrogenic.

POSTSEIZURE

Renal Causes
Nephritis.
Hypoplastic kidneys.
Hepatic Causes
Acute hepatitis.
Fulminant hepatic failure.
Inborn metabolic errors.
Bile duct atresia.

COMPRESSION SYNDROMES, NEUROVASCULAR CAUSES[27]

ICD-10CM #	M47.016	Anterior spinal artery compression syndromes, lumbar region
	M47.019	Anterior spinal artery compression syndromes, site unspecified
	M47.013	Anterior spinal artery compression syndromes, cervicothoracic region
	M47.021	Vertebral artery compression syndromes, occipito-atlanto-axial region
	M47.022	Vertebral artery compression syndromes, cervical region

Anatomic
Potential sites of neurovascular compression:
Interscalene triangle.
Costoclavicular space.
Subcoracoid area.
Congenital
Cervical rib and its fascial remnants.
Rudimentary first thoracic rib.
Scalene muscles:
Anterior.
Middle.
Minimus.
Adventitious fibrous bands.
Bifid clavicle or first rib.
Exostosis of first thoracic rib.
Enlarged transverse process of C7.
Omohyoid muscle.
Anomalous course of transverse cervical artery.
Abnormal lateral insertion of costoclavicular ligament.
Flat clavicle.
Traumatic
Fracture of clavicle.
Dislocation of head of humerus.
Crushing injury to upper thorax.
Sudden, unaccustomed muscular efforts involving shoulder girdle muscles.
Cervical spondylosis and injuries to cervical spine.
Atherosclerosis.

CONGESTIVE HEART FAILURE AND CARDIOMYOPATHY[18]

ICD-10CM #   I50.9   Heart failure, unspecified
         I42.7   Cardiomyopathy due to drug and external agent

CAUSES OF CONGESTIVE HEART FAILURE AND CARDIOMYOPATHY

Coronary Artery Disease
Acute ischemia.
Myocardial infarction.
Ischemic cardiomyopathy with hibernating myocardium.
Idiopathic
Idiopathic dilated cardiomyopathy.
Idiopathic restrictive cardiomyopathy.
Peripartum.
Pressure Overload
Hypertension.
Aortic stenosis.
Volume Overload
Mitral regurgitation.
Aortic insufficiency.
Anemia.
Atrioventricular fistula.
Toxins
Ethanol.
Cocaine.
Doxorubicin (Adriamycin).
Methamphetamine.
Metabolic-Endocrine
Thiamine deficiency.
Diabetes.
Hemochromatosis.
Thyrotoxicosis.

Obesity.
Infiltrative
Amyloidosis.
Inflammatory
Viral myocarditis.
Hereditary
Hypertrophic.
Dilated.

Genetic bases for these cardiomyopathies have been identified in a large number of individual patients and families. Most of the mutations have been found in cardiac contractile or structural proteins.

CONGESTIVE HEART FAILURE, INFANT[29]

ICD-10CM #   I05.9   Heart failure, unspecified

Critical coarctation of the aorta.
Interrupted aortic arch.
Congenital aortic stenosis.
Hypoplastic left heart syndrome.
Large ventricular septal defect.
Truncus arteriosus.
Unrecognized supraventricular tachycardia.
Cardiac tamponade.
Myocarditis.

CONJUNCTIVAL NEOPLASM

ICD-10CM #   Varies with specific diagnosis

MALIGNANT

Squamous cell carcinoma.
Melanoma.
Sebaceous carcinoma.
Kaposi sarcoma.
Metastatic neoplasms.

BENIGN

Melanocytic nevus.
Squamous papilloma.
Hemangioma.
Lymphangioma.
Myxoma.

CONNECTIVE TISSUE DISORDERS, HEREDITARY[38]

ICD-10CM #   Varies with specific diagnosis

CLASSIFICATION OF HEREDITARY DISORDERS OF CONNECTIVE TISSUE

Skeletal (Primarily Type I Collagen)
Osteogenesis imperfecta.
Dermis, Tendons, and Ligaments (Primarily Type I Collagen)
Hypermobile Ehlers-Danlos syndrome (type III).
Classic Ehlers-Danlos syndrome (type I).
Vascular Ehlers-Danlos syndrome.
Cartilage (Primarily Fibrils of Type II Collagen, Proteoglycans)
Chondrodysplasias.
Achondroplasia.
Pseudoachondroplasia.
Stickler syndrome.
Craniosynostosis (syndromic).

Skeletal, Cardiovascular, and Eye (Type I and Type III Collagen, Fibrillin, Elastin)
Marfan syndrome.
MASS phenotype (mitral valve prolapse, aortic dilation, skin, and skeletal features).
Loeys-Dietz syndrome.
Beals syndrome (congenital contractual arachnodactyly).
Dermal/epidermal (keratin, laminin, type VII collagen, plectin, integrin).
Epidermolysis bullosa.
Basal lamina (type IV collagen, laminin, nidogen).
Alport syndrome.

CONSCIOUSNESS IMPAIRMENT, ACUTE, IN CRITICALLY ILL PATIENT

ICD-10CM #   F05.9   Delirium, unspecified

GENERAL CAUSES OF ACUTELY IMPAIRED CONSCIOUSNESS IN THE CRITICALLY ILL

Infection
Sepsis encephalopathy.
Central nervous system infection.
Drugs
Narcotics.
Benzodiazepines.
Anticholinergics.
Anticonvulsants.
Tricyclic antidepressants.
Selective serotonin uptake inhibitors.
Phenothiazines.
Steroids.
Immunosuppressants (cyclosporine, FK-506, OKT3).
Anesthetics.
Electrolyte and Acid-Base Disturbances
Hyponatremia.
Hypernatremia.
Hypercalcemia.
Hypermagnesemia.
Severe acidemia and alkalemia.
Organ System Failure
Shock.
Renal failure.
Hepatic failure.
Pancreatitis.
Respiratory failure (hypoxia, hypercapnia).
Endocrine Disorders
Hypoglycemia.
Hyperglycemia.
Hypothyroidism.
Hyperthyroidism.
Pituitary apoplexy.
Drug Withdrawal
Alcohol.
Opiates.
Barbiturates.
Benzodiazepines.
Vascular Causes
Shock.
Hypotension.
Hypertensive encephalopathy.
Central nervous system vasculitis.
Cerebral venous sinus thrombosis.

Differential Diagnosis

II

Central Nervous System Disorders
Hemorrhage.
Stroke.
Brain edema.
Hydrocephalus.
Increased intracranial pressure.
Meningitis.
Ventriculitis.
Brain abscess.
Subdural empyema.
Seizures.
Vasculitis.
Seizures
Convulsive and nonconvulsive status epilepticus.
Miscellaneous
Fat embolism syndrome.
Neuroleptic malignant syndrome.
Thiamine deficiency (Wernicke encephalopathy).
Psychogenic unresponsiveness.

CONSTIPATION

ICD-10CM #	K59.00	Constipation, unspecified

Intestinal obstruction.
Fecal impaction.
Diverticular disease.
GI neoplasm.
Strangulated femoral hernia.
Gallstone ileus.
Tuberculous stricture.
Adhesions.
Ameboma.
Volvulus.
Intussusception.
Inflammatory bowel disease.
Hematoma of bowel wall, secondary to trauma or anticoagulants.
Poor dietary habits: insufficient bulk in diet, inadequate fluid intake.
Change from daily routine: travel, hospital admission, physical inactivity.
Acute abdominal conditions: renal colic, salpingitis, biliary colic, appendicitis, ischemia.
Hypercalcemia or hypokalemia, uremia.
Irritable bowel syndrome, pregnancy, anorexia nervosa, depression.
Painful anal conditions: hemorrhoids, fissure, stricture.
Decreased intestinal peristalsis: old age, spinal cord injuries, myxedema, diabetes, multiple sclerosis, parkinsonism and other neurologic diseases.
Drugs: codeine, morphine, antacids with aluminum, verapamil, anticonvulsants, anticholinergics, disopyramide, cholestyramine, alosetron, iron supplements.
Hirschsprung disease, meconium ileus, congenital atresia in infants.

CONSTIPATION, ADULT PATIENT[2]

ICD-10CM #	K59.00	Constipation, unspecified

NO GROSS STRUCTURAL ABNORMALITY

Inadequate fiber intake.
Irritable bowel syndrome (associated with abdominal pain) or functional constipation.
Idiopathic slow-transit constipation.
"Obstructed defecation" pelvic floor dysfunction (or dyssynergia).

STRUCTURAL DISORDERS

Anal fissure, infection, or stenosis.
Colon cancer or stricture.
Aganglionosis and/or abnormal myenteric plexus:
 Hirschsprung disease.
 Chagas disease.
 Neuropathic pseudoobstruction.
Abnormal colonic muscle:
 Myopathy.
 Dystrophia myotonica.
 Systemic sclerosis.
Idiopathic megarectum and/or megacolon.
Proximal megacolon.

NEUROLOGIC CAUSES

Diabetic autonomic neuropathy.
Damage to the sacral parasympathetic outflow.
Spinal cord damage or disease (e.g., multiple sclerosis).
Parkinson disease.
Blunting of consciousness, mental retardation, psychosis.
Pain induced by straining (e.g., sciatic nerve compression).

ENDOCRINE OR METABOLIC CAUSES

Hypothyroidism.
Hypercalcemia.
Porphyria.
Pregnancy.

PSYCHOLOGIC DISORDERS

Depression.
Anorexia nervosa.
Denied bowel habit.
Drug side effects.

CONSTIPATION, PEDIATRIC PATIENT[68]

ICD-10CM #	K59.00	Constipation

Nonorganic (Functional)—Retentive
Anatomic
Anal stenosis, atresia with fistula.
Imperforate anus.
Anteriorly displaced anus.
Intestinal stricture (postnecrotizing enterocolitis).
Anal stricture.
Abnormal Musculature
Prune-belly syndrome.
Gastroschisis.
Down syndrome.
Muscular dystrophy.

Nonorganic (Functional)—Retentive
Intestinal Nerve or Muscle Abnormalities
Hirschsprung disease.
Pseudoobstruction (visceral myopathy or neuropathy).
Intestinal neuronal dysplasia.
Spinal cord lesions.
Tethered cord.
Autonomic neuropathy.
Spinal cord trauma.
Spina bifida.
Chagas disease.
Drugs
Anticholinergics.
Narcotics.
Methylphenidate.
Phenytoin.
Antidepressants.
Chemotherapeutic agents (vincristine).
Pancreatic enzymes (fibrosing colonopathy).
Lead, arsenic, mercury.
Vitamin D intoxication.
Calcium channel blocking agents.
Metabolic Disorders
Hypokalemia.
Hypercalcemia.
Hypothyroidism.
Diabetes mellitus, diabetes insipidus.
Porphyria.
Intestinal Disorders
Celiac disease.
Cow's milk protein intolerance.
Cystic fibrosis (meconium ileus equivalent).
Inflammatory bowel disease (stricture).
Tumor.
Connective tissue disorders.
Systemic lupus erythematosus.
Scleroderma.
Psychiatric Diagnosis
Anorexia nervosa.

CHRONIC OBSTRUCTIVE PULMONARY DISEASE DECOMPENSATION[10]

ICD-10CM #	J44.1	Chronic obstructive pulmonary distress with acute exacerbation

CAUSES OF ACUTE DECOMPENSATION IN THE PATIENT WITH CHRONIC OBSTRUCTIVE PULMONARY DISEASE

Acute Exacerbations
Infectious
Viral.
 Rhinovirus, respiratory syncytial virus, coronavirus, influenza virus.
Bacterial.
 Haemophilus influenzae, Streptococcus pneumoniae, Moraxella (Branhamella) catarrhalis, Pseudomonas aeruginosa.
Atypical bacteria.
 Chlamydia pneumoniae, Legionella.

Air Pollution
Nitrogen dioxide.
Ozone.
Particulates, dust.
Other Critical Events
Pneumothorax.
Pulmonary embolism.
Lobar atelectasis.
Congestive heart failure.
Pneumonia.
Pulmonary compression (e.g., obesity, ascites, gastric distention, pleural effusion).
Trauma (e.g., rib fractures, pulmonary contusion).
Neuromuscular and metabolic disorders.
Unrelated treatable chronic pulmonary disease (bronchiectasis, tuberculosis, sarcoidosis).
Noncompliance with prescribed treatment regimens.
Iatrogenic:
    Inadequate therapy.
    Inappropriate therapy (e.g., deleterious drugs).

CORNEAL CLOUDING, PEDIATRIC AGE[20]

ICD-10CM #	Varies with specific diagnosis

Cerebrohepatorenal syndrome (Zellweger syndrome).
Congenital syphilis.[a]
Fabry disease (ceramide trihexosidosis).
Familial high-density lipoprotein deficiency (Tangier Island disease).
Fetal alcohol syndrome.
Glaucoma.[a]
Infantile GM1 gangliosidosis.
Juvenile metachromatic dystrophy.
Marinesco-Sjögren disease.
Mucolipidosis.
Mucopolysaccharidoses.
Multiple sulfatase deficiency.
Pelizaeus-Merzbacher disease.
Trauma (forceps at birth).

[a]Denotes the most common conditions and the ones with disease-modifying treatments.

CORNEAL SENSATION, DECREASED

ICD-10CM #	H18.899	Other specified disorders of cornea, unspecified eye

Herpes (simplex, zoster).
Contact lens wear.
Topical agents (NSAIDs, anesthetics, β-blockers).
Diabetes.
Eye trauma.
Postsurgery.

COUGH

ICD-10CM #	R05	Cough

Infectious process (viral, bacterial).
Postinfectious.

"Smoker's cough."
Rhinitis (allergic, vasomotor, postinfectious).
Asthma.
Exposure to irritants (noxious fumes, smoke, cold air).
Drug-induced (especially ACE inhibitors, β-blockers).
Gastroesophageal reflux disease.
Interstitial lung disease.
Lung neoplasms.
Lymphomas, mediastinal neoplasms.
Bronchiectasis.
Cardiac (congestive heart failure, pulmonary edema, mitral stenosis, pericardial inflammation).
Recurrent aspiration.
Inflammation of larynx, pleura, diaphragm, mediastinum.
Cystic fibrosis.
Anxiety.
Other: pulmonary embolism, foreign body inhalation, aortic aneurysm, Zenker diverticulum, osteophytes, substernal thyroid, thyroiditis, PMR.

COUGH, CHRONIC, ADULT PATIENT[28]

ICD-10CM #	R05	Cough

CAUSES OF CHRONIC COUGH IN ADULTS

Intrathoracic Causes
Lungs and Airways
Asthma.
Nonasthmatic eosinophilic bronchitis.
Chronic bronchitis.
Bronchiectasis.
ACE inhibitors.
Inhaled medications.
Chronic exposure to environmental and occupational irritants.
Bronchogenic and metastatic carcinoma.
Bronchial carcinoid.
Foreign body or endobronchial suture.
Broncholith.
Infectious and noninfectious bronchiolitis.
Chronic infectious pneumonias (e.g., bacterial, tuberculous, fungal, parasitic).
Chronic infectious tracheobronchitis (as in tuberculosis or aspergillosis).
Chronic interstitial lung disease (e.g., sarcoidosis, HSP, IPF, asbestosis).
Pulmonary vasculitis (as in granulomatosis with polyangiitis).
Sjögren syndrome with xerotrachea.
Relapsing polychondritis.
Pleura
Chronic effusion.
Diaphragm
Transvenous pacemaker stimulation.
Mediastinum
Neural tumors.
Thymoma.
Teratoma.
Lymphoma.

Metastatic lymphadenopathy.
Intrathoracic goiter.
Bronchogenic cyst.
Cardiovascular
Mitral stenosis.
Left ventricular failure.
Pulmonary thromboembolism.
Enlarged left atrium.
Vascular ring.
Aberrant innominate artery.
Aortic aneurysm.
Pericardial stimulation by transvenous pacemaker.
Extrathoracic Causes
Head and Neck
Rhinitis and sinusitis.
Nasal polyps.
Rhinolith.
Oropharyngeal dysphagia.
Laryngeal disorders (e.g., vocal fold dysfunction, laryngomalacia).
Postviral vagal neuropathy.
Recurrent aspiration.
Elongated uvula.
Chronically infected tonsils.
Neurilemmoma of vagus nerve.
Neuroma of internal laryngeal nerve.
Ascending palatine artery aneurysm.
Osteophytes of cervical spine.
Mammomanogamus (Syngamus) laryngeus infection.
Thyroiditis.
Upper GI
Gastroesophageal reflux disease.
Esophageal cyst or diverticulum.
Tracheoesophageal fistula.
Central Nervous System
Psychogenic or habit cough.
Tic disorders.
Gilles de la Tourette syndrome.

ACEI, Angiotensin-converting enzyme inhibitor; *HSP*, hypersensitivity pneumonitis; *IPF*, idiopathic pulmonary fibrosis.

COUGH, CHRONIC, PEDIATRIC PATIENT[68]

ICD-10CM #	R05	Cough

DIFFERENTIAL DIAGNOSIS OF RECURRENT AND PERSISTENT COUGH IN CHILDREN

Recurrent Cough

Reactive airway disease (asthma).
Drainage from upper airways.
Aspiration.
Frequently recurring respiratory tract infections in immunocompetent or immunodeficient patients.
Symptomatic Chiari malformation.
Idiopathic pulmonary hemosiderosis.
Hypersensitivity (allergic) pneumonitis.

Persistent Cough

Hypersensitivity of cough receptors after infection.
Reactive airway disease (asthma).
Chronic sinusitis.
Chronic rhinitis (allergic or nonallergic).
Bronchitis or tracheitis caused by infection or smoke exposure.
Bronchiectasis, including cystic fibrosis, primary ciliary dyskinesia, immunodeficiency.
Habit cough.
Foreign-body aspiration.
Recurrent aspiration owing to pharyngeal incompetence, tracheolaryngoesophageal cleft or tracheoesophageal fistula.
Gastroesophageal reflux, with or without aspiration.
Pertussis.
Extrinsic compression of the tracheobronchial tract (vascular ring, neoplasm, lymph node, lung cyst).
Tracheomalacia, bronchomalacia.
Endobronchial or endotracheal tumors.
Endobronchial tuberculosis.
Hypersensitivity pneumonitis.
Fungal infections.
Inhaled irritants, including tobacco smoke.
Irritation of external auditory canal.
ACE inhibitors.

CRAMPS[38]

ICD-10CM #	R25.2	Cramps and spasm

Cramp Syndromes

Ordinary:
   Common in normal individuals, especially gastrocnemius muscle, older age.
   Pregnancy.
Systemic disorders:
   Dehydration: hidrosis, diuretics, hemodialysis.
   Metabolic: low Na^+, $Mg2^+$, $Ca2^+$, glucose, uremia, cirrhosis, Gitelman syndrome.
   Endocrine: thyroid (hyper- or hypothyroid), hypoadrenal, hyperparathyroid.
Ischemia.
Drug-induced.
Denervation, partial: motor neuron disease, spinal stenosis, radiculopathy, neuropathy (including small-fiber neuropathy).
Syndromes: cramp-fasciculation, Satoyoshi syndrome.

Other Contraction Syndromes

Central disorders: stiff person syndrome, spasticity, tetanus, dystonia.
Peripheral nerve disorders: neuromyotonia, tetany, myokymia, partial denervation.
Muscle: contractures, myotonia, myoedema.

Genetic Muscle Contraction Syndromes

Muscular dystrophy: Becker; LGMD 1C.
Myotonia: myotonia congenita, myotonia fluctuans, acetazolamide-responsive myotonia, myotonic dystrophy.
Contractures:
   Brody syndrome: *ATP2A1.*

Glycogen storage disorders: deficiency of myophosphorylase; phosphorylase kinase regulatory subunit $\alpha1$; phosphoglycerate mutase; phosphofructokinase, muscle.
Rippling muscle syndrome: caveolin-3.
Hereditary angiopathy with nephropathy, aneurysms, and muscle cramps (HANAC): *COL4A1.*
Neuropathic.
Cramps: autosomal dominant:
   Schwartz-Jampel: perlecan, *LIFR.*
   Neuromyotonia and myokymia: *KCNQ2; KCNA1.*
   Geniospasm.
   Crisponi: *CRLF1.*
   Myofibrillar myopathy.
Cramps: autosomal recessive:
   Autosomal recessive axonal neuropathy with neuromyotonia *HINT1.*

Possible Treatments for Cramps and Other Muscle Spasms

Normalize metabolic abnormalities.
Quinine sulfate.
Carbamazepine.
Phenytoin.
Gabapentin.
Tocainide.
Verapamil.
Amitriptyline.
Vitamin E.
Riboflavin.
Mexiletine.

CREEPING ERUPTION, TRAVELERS[69]

ICD-10CM #	Varies with specific diagnosis

CAUSES OF CREEPING ERUPTION IN TRAVELERS

Nematode Larvae
Animal hookworms (HrCLM)*, *Pelodera strongyloides*, zoonotic *Strongyloides* spp.
Gnathostomiasis (*Gnathostoma* spp.).
Larva currens (*Strongyloides stercoralis*).
Adult Nematodes
Loiasis (*Loa loa*).
Dracunculiasis (*Dracunculus medinensis*).
Dirofilariasis (*Dirofilaria immitis*).
Trematode Larvae
Fascioliasis (Fasciola gigantica).
Fly Maggots
Migratory myiasis (*Gasterophilus* spp.).
Mites
Scabies (*Sarcoptes scabiei*).*
Pyemotes dermatitis (*Pyemotes ventricosus*).
HrCLM, Hookworm-related cutaneous larva migrans.*

---

*Common cause.

CUTANEOUS CALCIFICATIONS[70]

ICD-10CM #	Varies with specific diagnosis

Disorders of Cutaneous Calcification

Dystrophic

Autoimmune connective tissue diseases, especially dermatomyositis, CREST.
Cutaneous tumors or cysts (e.g., pilomatricomas, pilar cysts).
Infections, especially parasitic.
Trauma, including "heel sticks" in neonates, injection sites, surgical scars.
Panniculitis.
Genetic disorders (e.g., pseudoxanthoma elasticum, Ehlers–Danlos syndrome).

Metastatic

Advanced chronic kidney disease.
Calciphylaxis.*
Benign nodular calcification of renal disease.
Hypervitaminosis D.
Milk-alkali syndrome.
Sarcoidosis.
Tumoral calcinosis (familial).
Hyperparathyroidism.
Neoplasms (e.g., multiple myeloma, adult T-cell leukemia/lymphoma, SCC of the lung or head and neck).

Idiopathic

Idiopathic calcified nodules of the scrotum.
Subepidermal calcified nodule.
Tumoral calcinosis (sporadic).
Milia-like calcinosis.

Iatrogenic

Extravasation of intravenous solutions containing calcium or phosphate.
Application of calcium-containing electrode paste for EMGs and EEGs.
Application of calcium alginate dressings to denuded skin.
Organ transplantation, especially liver.
Gadolinium (nephrogenic systemic fibrosis).

CREST, Calcification, Raynaud phenomenon, esophageal dysmotility, sclerodactyly and telangiectasia; *EEG*, electroencephalogram; *EMG*, electromyography; *SCC*, squamous cell carcinoma.

CUTANEOUS INFECTIONS, ATHLETES

ICD-10CM #	L08.9	Local infection of the skin and subcutaneous tissue, unspecified

Tinea pedis.
Tinea cruris.
Molluscum contagiosum.
Herpes simplex.
Verruca vulgaris.
Folliculitis.
Impetigo.
Furuncles.
Otitis externa.
Erythrasma.

CUTANEOUS ULCERS, TRAVELERS[69]

ICD-10CM #   Varies with specific diagnosis

CAUSES OF CUTANEOUS ULCER IN TRAVELERS

Noninfectious Causes
Spider bite.
Cupping.

Bacterial Infection
Ecthyma.*
Tick eschar* (rickettsiosis).
Anthrax.
Mycobacterial infection *(M. ulcerans)*.
Melioidosis.
Glanders.
Tularemia.
Cutaneous diphtheria.
Plague.

Parasitic Infection
Leishmaniasis.*
Trypanosomal chancre (African trypanosomiasis).
Chagoma (American trypanosomiasis).
Cutaneous amebiasis.

Fungal Infection
Sporotrichosis.
Mycetomas.
West African histoplasmosis.
North American blastomycosis.
Paracoccidioidomycosis.
Chromomycosis.

Viral Infection
Herpes simplex infection.

*Common cause.

CYANOSIS[43]

ICD-10CM #   R23.0   Cyanosis

DIFFERENTIAL DIAGNOSIS OF CYANOSIS

Peripheral Cyanosis
Low Cardiac Output States
Shock.
Left ventricular failure.
Hypovolemia.
Environmental Exposure (Cold)
Air or water.
Arterial Occlusion
Thrombosis.
Embolism.
Vasospasm (Raynaud phenomenon).
Peripheral vascular disease.
Venous Obstruction
Redistribution of blood flow from extremities
Central Cyanosis
Decreased Arterial Oxygen Saturation
High altitude (>8000 ft).
Impaired pulmonary function:
   Hypoventilation.
   Impaired oxygen diffusion.
   Ventilation-perfusion mismatching:
      Pulmonary embolism.
      Acute respiratory distress syndrome.
      Pulmonary hypertension.

Respiratory compromise:
   Upper airway obstruction.
   Pneumonia.
   Diaphragmatic hernia.
   Tension pneumothorax.
   Polycythemia.
Anatomic Shunts
Pulmonary arteriovenous fistulae and intrapulmonary shunts.
Cerebral, hepatic, peripheral arteriovenous fistulae.
Cyanotic congenital heart disease:
   Endocardial cushion defects.
   Ventricular septal defects.
   Coarctation of aorta.
   Tetralogy of Fallot.
   Total anomalous pulmonary venous drainage.
   Hypoplastic left ventricle.
   Pulmonary vein stenosis.
   Tricuspid atresia and anomalies.
   Premature closure of foramen ovale.
   Dextrocardia.
   Pulmonary stenosis of atrial septal defect.
   Patent ductus arteriosus with reversed shunt.
Abnormal Hemoglobin
Methemoglobinemia:
   Hereditary.
   Acquired.
Sulfhemoglobinemia.
Mutant hemoglobin with low oxygen affinity (e.g., hemoglobin Kansas).

CYANOSIS, CENTRAL, SECONDARY TO CARDIAC DEFECT[58]

ICD-10CM #   R23.0   Cyanosis

Note 5 Ts and 2 Es.

Transposition of the great arteries.

Ebstein anomaly.

Tetralogy of Fallot.

Eisenmenger physiology.

Tricuspid atresia.

Critical pulmonary stenosis or atresia.

Truncus arteriosus.

Functionally single ventricle.

Total anomalous pulmonary venous return.

CYANOSIS, NEONATAL[29]

ICD-10CM #   R23.0   Cyanosis

RESPIRATORY

Upper Airway
Choanal atresia.
Macroglossia.
Glossoptosis (secondary to micrognathia).
Laryngomalacia.
Laryngeal web or cyst.
Vascular anomalies (e.g., cystic hygromas, rings).
Subglottic stenosis (commonly secondary to intubation).
Foreign body.
Lower Airway
Pneumonia.
Bronchiolitis.

Pulmonary edema.
Atelectasis.
Bronchopulmonary dysplasia.

SYSTEMIC

Sepsis.
Trauma.
Poisons.

CARDIAC

Cyanotic congenital heart diseases.
Transposition of the great vessels (most common neonatal).
Tetralogy of Fallot.
Truncus arteriosus.
Tricuspid atresia.
Total anomalous pulmonary venous return.
Ebstein anomaly.
GI.
Gastroesophageal reflux.

NEUROLOGIC

Seizures.
Central hypoventilation syndrome (Ondine curse).
Spinal muscular atrophy type I (Werdnig-Hoffmann).
Botulism.
Congenital myopathies.

HEMATOLOGIC

Methemoglobinemia.

CYTOPENIAS, OLDER ADULTS[71]

ICD-10CM #   D46.A   Refractory cytopenia with multilineage dysplasia

Cytopenia of one or more lineages.
Hematologic neoplasm.
Vitamin B_{12} deficiency.
Autoimmune disorder.
Consumptive coagulopathy.
Systemic inflammation.
Alcohol.
Splenomegaly.
Thyroid dysfunction.
HIV.

DAYTIME SLEEPINESS

ICD-10CM #   R53.82   Chronic fatigue, unspecified

Sleep deprivation.
Medication induced (e.g., benzodiazepines, β-blockers, narcotics, sedative antidepressants, gabapentin).
Depression.
Obstructive sleep apnea.
Medical illness (e.g., severe anemia, hypothyroidism, chronic obstructive pulmonary disease, hepatic failure, renal insufficiency, congestive heart failure, electrolyte disturbances).
Circadian rhythm abnormalities (e.g., jet lag, shift work sleep disorder).
Restless legs syndrome.
Posttrauma.
Narcolepsy.

Neurologic disorders (e.g., neurodegenerative disorders; parkinsonism; multiple sclerosis; lesions affecting thalamus, hypothalamus, or brain stem).

DEAFNESS, ACQUIRED

ICD-10CM #	H91.93	Unspecified hearing loss, bilateral
	H91.92	Unspecified hearing loss, left ear
	H91.91	Unspecified hearing loss, right ear
	H91.90	Unspecified hearing loss, unspecified ear
	H91.9	Unspecified hearing loss
	H91	Other and unspecified hearing loss
	H90.5	Unspecified sensorineural hearing loss
	H91.09	Ototoxic hearing loss, unspecified ear
	H90.2	Conductive hearing loss, unspecified
	H91.8X9	Other specified hearing loss, unspecified ear

COMMON CAUSES OF ACQUIRED DEAFNESS

Conductive Hearing Loss
Acute otitis media, otitis media with effusion, chronic otitis media.
Sensorineural Hearing Loss
Severe hypoxia.
Lassa fever.
Sepsis neonatorum.
Bacterial meningitis.
Viral infections (e.g., mumps).
Hyperbilirubinemia.
Noise-induced damage.
Autoimmune sensorineural hearing loss.
Presbycusis.
Head trauma.
Ménière disease.
Scrub typhus.
Sudden idiopathic sensorineural hearing loss.
HIV/AIDS, tuberculosis.
Ototoxicity.
Tumors, hydatid cyst in the cerebellopontine angle.

DELAYED PASSAGE OF MECONIUM[21]

| ICD-10CM # | P76.0 | Meconium plug syndrome |

Ileal atresia.
Meconium ileus.
Functional immaturity of the colon.
Colon atresia.
Anorectal malformations.
Hirschsprung disease.
Megacystis-microcolon-intestinal hypoperistalsis syndrome.

Extrinsic compression of the distal bowel by a mass lesion.
Mesenteric cyst.
Enteric duplication cyst.
Paralytic ileus, sepsis, drugs, and metabolic upset.

DELIRIUM[1]

ICD-10CM #	R40.0	Somnolence
	R40.1	Stupor
	F05	Delirium due to known physiological condition

PHARMACOLOGIC AGENTS

Anxiolytics (benzodiazepines).
Antidepressants (e.g., amitriptyline, doxepin, imipramine).
Cardiovascular agents (e.g., methyldopa, digitalis, reserpine, propranolol, procainamide, captopril, disopyramide).
Antihistamine.
Cimetidine.
Corticosteroids.
Antineoplastics.
Drugs of abuse (alcohol, cannabis, amphetamines, cocaine, hallucinogens, opioids, sedative-hypnotics, phencyclidine).

METABOLIC DISORDERS

Hypercalcemia.
Hypercarbia.
Hypoglycemia.
Hyponatremia.
Hypoxia.

INFLAMMATORY DISORDERS

Sarcoidosis.
Systemic lupus erythematosus.
Giant cell arteritis.

ORGAN FAILURE

Hepatic encephalopathy.
Uremia.

NEUROLOGIC DISORDERS

Alzheimer disease.
Cerebrovascular accident.
Encephalitis (including HIV).
Encephalopathies.
Epilepsy.
Huntington disease.
Multiple sclerosis.
Neoplasms.
Normal-pressure hydrocephalus.
Parkinson disease.
Pick disease.
Wilson disease.

ENDOCRINE DISORDERS

Addison disease.
Cushing syndrome.
Panhypopituitarism.
Parathyroid disease.
Postpartum psychosis.
Recurrent menstrual psychosis.
Sydenham chorea.
Thyroid disease.

DEFICIENCY STATES

Niacin.
Thiamine, vitamin B_{12}, and folate.

DELIRIUM AND AGITATION, DRUG-INDUCED

| ICD-10CM # | F05.9 | Delirium, unspecified |

COMMONLY USED DRUGS ASSOCIATED WITH DELIRIUM AND AGITATION

Benzodiazepines.
Opiates (especially meperidine).
Anticholinergics.
Antihistamines.
H_2 blockers.
Antibiotics.
Corticosteroids.
Metoclopramide.

DELIRIUM, AGITATED[43]

| ICD-10CM # | F05 | Delirium due to known physiological condition |

Metabolic causes:
Electrolyte abnormalities.
Hypoglycemia.
Hypoxia.
Uremia/hyperammonemia.
Structural lesions of the central nervous system:
Trauma.
Stroke.
Hemorrhage.
Mass.
Endocrine disease:
Thyrotoxicosis.
Infections:
Bacterial/viral meningitis/encephalitis.
Toxicologic causes:
Sympathomimetic/stimulants.
Cocaine.
Amphetamines and derivatives.
Caffeine.
Phencyclidine/ketamine.
Anticholinergics.
Serotonin syndrome.
Sedative-hypnotic withdrawal.
Heatstroke.
Post-ictal state.

DELIRIUM, DIALYSIS PATIENT[1]

| ICD-10CM # | F05 | Delirium due to known physiological condition |
| | F06.8 | Other specified mental disorders due to known physiological condition |

STRUCTURAL

Cerebrovascular accident (particularly hemorrhage).
Subdural hematoma.
Intracerebral abscess.
Brain tumor.

METABOLIC

Disequilibrium syndrome.
Uremia.
Drug effects.
Meningitis.
Hypertensive encephalopathy.
Hypotension.
Post-ictal state.
Hypernatremia or hyponatremia.
Hypercalcemia.
Hypermagnesemia.
Hypoglycemia.
Severe hyperglycemia.
Hypoxemia.
Dialysis dementia.

DEMENTIA, ADOLESCENT PATIENT[72]

| ICD-10CM # | F03 | Unspecified dementia |
| | F03.90 | Unspecified dementia without behavioral disturbance |

CAUSES OF DEMENTIA IN ADOLESCENTS

Autoimmune or inflammatory diseases:
  Paraneoplastic syndromes, including NMDA antibody encephalitis.
  Vasculitis.
Cerebral and noncerebral neoplasms:
  Chemotherapy (intrathecal).
  Radiotherapy treatment.
Drug, inhalant, and alcohol abuse, including overdose.
Head trauma, including child abuse.
Infections:
  HIV-associated dementia.
  Variant Creutzfeldt–Jakob disease (vCJD).
  Subacute sclerosing panencephalitis (SSPE).
Metabolic abnormalities:
  Adrenoleukodystrophy.
  Wilson disease.
Neurodegenerative illnesses:
  Huntington disease.
  Metachromatic leukodystrophy.
  Other rare, usually genetically transmitted, illnesses.

DEMENTIAS, NONDEGENERATIVE[38]

| ICD-10CM # | F03 | Unspecified Dementia |

PARTIAL LIST OF NONDEGENERATIVE DEMENTIAS

Vascular

Vasculitis (primary or secondary).
Chronic subdural hematoma.

Infectious Causes

Syphilis.
Chronic meningitis.
CJD and other prion diseases.
Whipple.
PML.
Sequelae of herpes encephalitis.

HIV/AIDS-associated dementia.
Neurobrucellosis.
CNS tuberculosis.
Parasitic infections (e.g., cysticercosis).
Lyme disease.
Subacute sclerosing panencephalitis.

Toxic/Metabolic Causes

Hypothyroidism.
Liver disease.
Kidney disease.
Vitamin B_{12} deficiency.
Thiamine deficiency.
Vitamin E deficiency.
Marchiafava-Bignami disease.
Deficiency of nicotinic acid (pellagra).
Heavy metal toxicity.
Parathyroid hormone dysfunction.
Adrenal and pituitary disorders.
Carbon monoxide poisoning.
Drugs (see prior table for list of drugs that can affect cognition).

Structural Causes

Primary or metastatic neoplasm.
Hydrocephalus.

Immune/Inflammatory

Autoimmune dementia.
Multiple sclerosis.
Sarcoidosis.
Collagen vascular diseases (e.g., systemic lupus erythematosus, Sjögren syndrome).
Behçet.

Neoplastic

Slow-growing neoplasm (e.g., meningioma, pituitary tumors).
Gliomatosis cerebri.
Radiation effect.
Paraneoplastic syndromes.
Lymphoma.

Psychiatric

Depression.

Inherited Disorders

Leukodystrophies (e.g., metachromatic leukodystrophy, adrenoleukodystrophy).
Krabbe disease.
Storage disorders: Gaucher disease, Niemann-Pick disease, cerebrotendinous xanthomatosis, and polysaccharidoses, neuronal ceroid lipofuscinoses.
Wilson disease.

AIDS, acquired immunodeficiency syndrome; *CJD*, Creutzfeldt-Jakob disease; *CNS*, central nervous system; *PML*, progressive multifocal leukoencephalopathy.

DEMYELINATING DISEASES[62]

| ICD-10CM # | G37.9 | Demyelinating disease of central nervous system, unspecified |

MULTIPLE SCLEROSIS

Relapsing and chronic progressive forms.
Acute multiple sclerosis.
Neuromyelitis optica (Devic disease).

DIFFUSE CEREBRAL SCLEROSIS

Schilder encephalitis periaxialis diffusa.
Baló concentric sclerosis.

ACUTE DISSEMINATED ENCEPHALOMYELITIS

After measles, chickenpox, rubella, influenza, mumps.
After rabies or smallpox vaccination.

NECROTIZING HEMORRHAGIC ENCEPHALITIS

Hemorrhagic leukoencephalitis.

LEUKODYSTROPHIES

Krabbe globoid leukodystrophy.
Metachromatic leukodystrophy.
Adrenoleukodystrophy.
Adrenomyeloneuropathy.
Pelizaeus-Merzbacher leukodystrophy.
Canavan disease.
Alexander disease.

DEVELOPMENTAL DELAY, NO REGRESSION[20]

| ICD-10CM # | Varies with specific diagnosis |

Predominant Speech Delay

Bilateral hippocampal sclerosis.
Congenital bilateral perisylvian syndrome.
Hearing impairment.[a]
Autism.

Predominant Motor Delay

Ataxia.
Hemiplegia.
Hypotonia.
Neuromuscular disorders.[a]
Paraplegia.

Global Developmental Delay

Cerebral malformations.
Chromosomal disturbances.
Intrauterine infection.
Perinatal disorders.
Progressive encephalopathies.

[a]Denotes the most common conditions and the ones with disease-modifying treatments.

DEXTROCARDIA[37]

| ICD-10CM # | Q24.0 | Dextrocardia |

TYPES OF DEXTROCARDIA

Primary Dextrocardia

Dextroversion: the left ventricle is to the left of the right ventricle, as it is in the normal heart.
Mirror-image dextrocardia: the left ventricle is to the right of the right ventricle.

Secondary Dextrocardia

Skeletal causes:
  Scoliosis.
  Sternal or rib deformity.

Differential Diagnosis

II

Lung causes:
  Pneumonectomy.
  Collapse.
  Pneumothorax.
  Unilateral airtrapping.
Pleural causes:
  Diaphragmatic hernia with displacement of the gut into left thorax.

DIAPER DERMATITIS[73]

| ICD-10CM # | L22 | Diaper dermatitis |

DIFFERENTIAL DIAGNOSIS OF DIAPER DERMATITIS

Chafing dermatitis.
Irritant contact dermatitis.
Diaper candidiasis.
Seborrheic dermatitis.
Psoriasis.
Intertrigo.
Jacquet dermatitis.
Perianal pseudoverrucous papules and nodules.
Miliaria.
Folliculitis.
Impetigo.
Scabies.
Nutritional deficiency (i.e., acrodermatitis enteropathica, cystic fibrosis, biotin deficiency).
Allergic contact dermatitis.
Atopic dermatitis.
Granuloma gluteale infantum.
Langerhans cell histiocytosis.
Burns.
Child abuse.
Epidermolysis bullosa.
Congenital syphilis.
Varicella/herpes.
Tinea cruris.
Chronic bullous dermatosis of childhood.
Bullous mastocytosis.

DIAPHRAGM ELEVATION, BILATERAL, SYMMETRICAL[21]

| ICD-10CM # | J98.6 | Disorders of diaphragm |

CAUSES OF BILATERAL SYMMETRICAL ELEVATION OF THE DIAPHRAGM

Supine position.
Poor inspiration.
Obesity.
Pregnancy.
Abdominal distention (ascites, intestinal obstruction, abdominal mass).
Diffuse pulmonary fibrosis.
Lymphangitis carcinomatosa.
Disseminated lupus erythematosus.
Bilateral basal pulmonary emboli.
Painful conditions (after abdominal surgery).
Bilateral diaphragmatic paralysis.

DIAPHRAGM ELEVATION, UNILATERAL[21]

| ICD-10CM # | J98.6 | Disorders of diaphragm |

CAUSES OF UNILATERAL ELEVATION OF THE DIAPHRAGM

Posture—lateral decubitus position (dependent side).
Gaseous distention of stomach or colon.
Dorsal scoliosis.
Pulmonary hypoplasia.
Pulmonary collapse.
Phrenic nerve palsy.
Eventration.
Pneumonia or pleurisy.
Pulmonary thromboembolism.
Rib fracture and other painful conditions.
Subphrenic infection.
Subphrenic mass.

DIAPHRAGM WEAKNESS AND PARALYSIS[74]

| ICD-10CM # | J98.6 | Paralysis of diaphragm |

NEUROPATHIC CAUSES

Trauma
Cardiac surgery with cold.
Cardioplegia.
Blunt trauma.
Spinal cord injury.
Radiation injury.
Cervical manipulation.
Scalene and brachial nerve block.
Tumor compression.
Lung cancer.
Metastatic mediastinal tumor.

Metabolic
Diabetes.
Vitamin deficiency (B_6, B_{12}, folate).
Hypothyroidism.

Inflammatory Neuritis
Idiopathic (neuralgic amyotrophy, Parsonage-Turner).
Mononeuritis multiplex.
Vasculitis.
Paraneoplastic.

Miscellaneous
Cervical spondylosis.
Poliomyelitis.
Amyotrophic lateral sclerosis.

MYOPATHIC CAUSES

Muscular Dystrophies
Limb-girdle.
Duchenne and Becker.

Metabolic Myopathies
Hyper- or hypothyroidism.
Acid maltase deficiency.

Rheumatologic
Systemic lupus erythematosus.
Dermatomyositis.
Mixed connective disease.

Miscellaneous
Amyloidosis.
Malnutrition.
Idiopathic.

DIARRHEA, ACUTE WATERY AND BLOODY[2]

ICD-10CM #	K52.2	Allergic and dietetic gastroenteritis and colitis
	K52.89	Other specified noninfective gastroenteritis and colitis
	R19.7	Diarrhea, unspecified

ACUTE WATERY DIARRHEA

GI infections:
  Protozoal (e.g., *Giardia*).
  Bacterial (e.g., enterotoxigenic *Escherichia coli*, cholera).
  Viral (e.g., rotavirus, Norwalk virus).
Drugs.
Toxins.
Dietary constituents (e.g., lactose intolerance).
Onset of chronic diarrheal illness.

ACUTE BLOODY DIARRHEA

Infectious colitis:
  Confluent proctocolitis (e.g., *Shigella*, *Campylobacter*, *Salmonella*, *Entamoeba histolytica*).
  Segmental colitis (e.g., *Campylobacter*, *Salmonella*, enteroinvasive *E. coli*, *Aeromonas*, *E. histolytica*).
  Drug-induced colitis (e.g., NSAIDs).
  Inflammatory bowel disease.
  Ischemic colitis (usually elderly patient with underlying heart disease or arrhythmias).
  Antibiotic-associated colitis.

DIARRHEA, CRITICALLY ILL PATIENT[11]

| ICD-10CM # | R19.7 | Diarrhea, unspecified |

COMMON CAUSES OF DIARRHEA IN CRITICALLY ILL PATIENTS

Medication
Antibiotics.
H_2-receptor antagonists, antacids.
Drugs: significant amounts of sorbitol, magnesium, or hypertonic medications.
Laxative use (unintended).
GI Dysfunction
Gastric or small bowel resection.
Inflammatory bowel disease.
Pancreatic insufficiency.
Radiation enteritis.
Sprue.
Protein-losing gastroenteropathies.
Bowel impaction (paradoxic).
Malnutrition
Hypoproteinemia.
Micronutrient deficiencies.

Enteral Nutrition–Associated
Excessive feeding rate, concentration, volume, or osmolality.
Adaptation in malnourished patients or those whose GI tract has not been used recently.
Intolerance or allergy to feeding formula.
Infection
Clostridium difficile enterocolitis.
Opportunistic GI infection.
Significant amounts of contaminated feeding formula.
Altered GI flora.
Endocrine Dysfunction
Diabetes mellitus.
Hyperthyroidism.
Hypocortisolism.

DIARRHEA, INFECTIOUS[43]

ICD-10CM # A09 Infectious gastroenteritis and colitis, unspecified

ETIOLOGIC AGENTS OF INFECTIOUS DIARRHEA

Viral (60% of Cases)
Astrovirus.
Calicivirus.
Coronavirus.
Cytomegalovirus.*
Enteric adenovirus.
Hepatitis A through G.
Herpes simplex virus.
HIV enteropathy.
Norwalk-like agents.
Pararotavirus.
Norwalk virus.
Picornavirus.
Rotavirus.
Small round viruses.
Bacterial (20% of Cases)
Invasive
Aeromonas spp.
Campylobacter spp.
Clostridium difficile.
Enteroinvasive E. coli.
Mycobacterium spp.
Plesiomonas shigelloides.
Salmonella spp.
Shigella spp.
Vibrio fluvialis.
Vibrio parahaemolyticus.
Vibrio vulnificus.
Yersinia enterocolitica.
Yersinia pseudotuberculosis.
Toxigenic
Food poisoning with preformed toxins:
  Bacillus cereus.
  Clostridium botulinum.
  Staphylococcus aureus.
Toxin formation after colonization:
  Aeromonas hydrophila.
  Clostridium perfringens.
  Enterohemorrhagic E. coli 0157:H7.
  Enterotoxigenic E. coli.
  Klebsiella pneumoniae.
  Shigella spp.

*All of these disorders may cause localized low back pain.

Vibrio cholerae.
  Other bacteria.
Parasitic (5% of Cases)
Protozoa
Balantidium coli.
Blastocystis hominis.
Cryptosporidium.
Cyclospora.
Dientamoeba fragilis.
Entamoeba histolytica.
Entamoeba polecki.
Enteromonas hominis.
Giardia lamblia.
Isospora belli.
Microsporidia.
Sarcocystis hominis.
Helminths
Angiostrongylus costarricense.
Anisakiasis.
Ascaris lumbricoides.
Diphyllobothrium latum.
Enterobius vermicularis.
Hookworms.
Schistosoma spp.
Strongyloides stercoralis.
Taenia spp.
Trichinella spiralis.
Trichuris trichiura.

DIARRHEA, NONINFECTIOUS[43]

ICD-10CM # K59.1 Functional diarrhea

CAUSES OF NONINFECTIOUS DIARRHEA

Toxins
Drugs
ACE inhibitors.
Alprazolam.
Antacids (Mg).
Antibiotics.
Antidepressants.
Antiepileptic drugs.
Antihypertensives.
Antiparkinson drugs.
β-blockers.
Caffeine.
Cardiac antiarrhythmics.
Chemotherapy agents.
Cholesterol-lowering drugs.
Cholinergic agents.
Cholinesterase inhibitors.
Colchicine.
Digitalis.
Diuretics.
Fluorouracil.
Fluoxetine.
Histamine H_2-receptor antagonists.
Hydralazine.
Lactulose.
Laxatives/cathartics.
Levodopa.
Lithium.
NSAIDs.
Neomycin.
Podophyllin.
Procainamide.

Prostaglandins.
Quinidine.
Ricinoleic acid.
Theophylline.
Thyroid hormone.
Valproic acid.
Dietetic Foods
Mannitol.
Sorbitol.
Xylitol.
Fish-Associated Toxins
Amnestic shellfish poisoning.
Ciguatera.
Echinoderms.
Neurotoxic shellfish poisoning.
Paralytic shellfish poisoning.
Scombroid.
Tetroton.
Plant-Associated Toxins
Herbal preparations.
Horse chestnut.
Mushrooms—Amanita spp.
Nicotine.
Other plant toxins:
  Pesticides—organophosphates.
  Pokeweed.
  Rhubarb.
Miscellaneous:
  Allergic reactions.
  Carbon monoxide poisoning.
  Ethanol.
  Heavy metals.
  Monosodium glutamate (MSG).
  Opiate withdrawal.
GI Pathology
Appendicitis.
Autonomic dysfunction.
Bile acid malabsorption.
Blind loop.
Bowel obstruction.
Celiac disease.
Cirrhosis.
Defects in amino acid transport.
Diverticular disease.
Familial dysautonomia.
Fecal impaction.
Fecal incontinence.
GI bleed.
GI cancer.
Hirschsprung disease.
Inflammatory bowel disease (ulcerative colitis, Crohn disease).
Intussusception.
Irritable bowel syndrome.
Ischemic bowel.
Lactose/fructose intolerance.
Malabsorption syndromes.
Malrotation.
Postsurgical.
Postvagotomy.
Radiation therapy.
Short gut syndrome.
Small bowel resection.
Strictures.
Toxic megacolon.
Tropical sprue.
Volvulus.
Whipple disease.

Differential Diagnosis

II

Endocrine Related
Carcinoid syndrome (serotonin).
Hormonal hypersecretion.
Hyperthyroidism (thyroid hormone).
Medullary carcinoma of the thyroid (calcitonin).
Pancreatic cholera (VIP).
Somatostatinoma (somatostatin).
Systemic mastocytosis (histamine).
Zollinger-Ellison syndrome (gastrin).
Endocrine Pathology
Adrenal insufficiency.
Diabetes enteropathy.
Hypoparathyroidism.
Pancreatic insufficiency.
Systemic Illness/Other
Alcoholism.
Amyloidosis.
Connective tissue disease.
Cystic fibrosis.
Ectopic pregnancy.
Hemolytic-uremic syndrome.
Henoch-Schönlein purpura.
Lymphoma.
Otitis media—infants.
Pelvic inflammatory disease.
Pneumonia/sepsis.
Pyelonephritis.
Scleroderma/SLE.
Severe malnutrition.
Stevens-Johnson syndrome.
Toxic shock syndrome.
Wilson disease.
Miscellaneous:
Factitious diarrhea.
Runner's diarrhea.

SLE, Systemic lupus erythematosus; *VIP,* vasoactive intestinal polypeptide.

DIARRHEA IN PATIENTS WITH AIDS[3]

ICD-10CM #   R19.7   Diarrhea, unspecified

PROTOZOA

*Microsporidium.**
Cryptosporidium spp.*
Isospora belli.
Toxoplasma spp.
Giardia lamblia.
Entamoeba histolytica.
Leishmania donovani.
Blastocystis hominis.
Cyclospora spp.
Pneumocystis jirovecii.

BACTERIA

Clostridium difficile.
Salmonella spp.
Shigella spp.
Campylobacter jejuni
Mycobacterium avium complex.
Mycobacterium tuberculosis.
SIBO.
Vibrio spp.

*More frequent cause.

VIRUSES

CMV.
HSV.
Adenoviruses.
Rotavirus spp.
Norovirus.
HIV.

FUNGI

Histoplasmosis.
Coccidioidomycosis.
Cryptococcosis.
Candidiasis.
Penicillium marneffei.

NEOPLASMS

Lymphoma.
Kaposi sarcoma.

IDIOPATHIC

"AIDS enteropathy."

DRUG INDUCED

HIV protease inhibitors.

PANCREATIC DISEASE

Pancreatic insufficiency.
Chronic pancreatitis.
Infectious pancreatitis (CMV, MAC).
Drug-induced pancreatitis (e.g., pentamidine).

CMV, Cytomegalovirus; *HSV,* herpes simplex virus; *MAC,* mycobacterium avium complex.

DIARRHEA, PEDIATRIC PATIENT[68]

ICD-10CM #   R19.7   Diarrhea, unspecified

Acute
Common
Gastroenteritis (viral > bacterial > protozoal).
Systemic infection.
Antibiotic associated.
Overfeeding.
Rare
Primary disaccharidase deficiency.
Hirschsprung toxic colitis.
Adrenogenital syndrome.
Neonatal opiate withdrawal.
Chronic
Common
Postinfectious secondary lactase deficiency.
Cow's milk or soy protein intolerance (allergy).
Chronic nonspecific diarrhea of infancy.
Excessive fruit juice (sorbitol) ingestion.
Celiac disease.
Cystic fibrosis.
AIDS enteropathy.
Rare
Primary immune defects.
Autoimmune enteropathy.
IPEX and IPEX-like syndromes.
Glucose-galactose malabsorption.
Microvillus inclusion disease (microvillus atrophy).
Congenital transport defects (chloride, sodium).
Primary bile acid malabsorption.

Factitious syndrome by proxy.
Hirschsprung disease.
Shwachman syndrome.
Secretory tumors.
Acrodermatitis enteropathica.
Lymphangiectasia.
Abetalipoproteinemia.
Eosinophilic gastroenteritis.
Short bowel syndrome.

CHILD

Acute
Common
Gastroenteritis (viral > bacterial > protozoal).
Food poisoning.
Systemic infection.
Antibiotic associated.
Rare
Toxic ingestion.
Hemolytic uremic syndrome.
Intussusception.
Chronic
Common
Postinfectious secondary.
Lactase deficiency.
Irritable bowel syndrome.
Celiac disease.
Cystic fibrosis.
Lactose intolerance.
Excessive fruit juice (sorbitol) ingestion.
Giardiasis.
Inflammatory bowel disease.
AIDS enteropathy.
Rare
Primary and acquired immune defects.
Secretory tumors.
Pseudoobstruction.
Sucrase-isomaltase deficiency.
Eosinophilic gastroenteritis.
Secretory tumors.

ADOLESCENT

Acute
Common
Gastroenteritis (viral > bacterial > protozoal).
Food poisoning.
Antibiotic associated.
Rare
Hyperthyroidism.
Appendicitis.
Chronic
Common
Irritable bowel syndrome.
Inflammatory bowel disease.
Lactose intolerance.
Giardiasis.
Laxative abuse (anorexia nervosa).
Constipation with encopresis.
Rare
Secretory tumor.
Primary bowel tumor.
Parasitic infections and venereal diseases.
Appendiceal abscess.
Addison disease.

IPEX, Immunodysregulation polyendocrinopathy enteropathy X-linked.

DIARRHEA, TUBE-FED PATIENT[24]

ICD-10CM #   K91.89   Other postprocedural complications and disorders of digestive system

COMMON CAUSES UNRELATED TO TUBE FEEDING

Elixir medications containing sorbitol.
Magnesium-containing antacids.
Antibiotic-induced sterile gut.
Pseudomembranous colitis.

POSSIBLE CAUSES RELATED TO TUBE FEEDING

Inadequate fiber to form stool bulk.
High fat content of formula (in the presence of fat malabsorption syndrome).
Bacterial contamination of enteral products and delivery systems (causal association with diarrhea not documented).
Rapid advancement in rate (after the GI tract is unused for prolonged periods).

UNLIKELY CAUSES RELATED TO TUBE FEEDING

Formula hyperosmolality (proven not to be the cause of diarrhea).
Lactose (absent from nearly all enteral feeding formulas).

DIFFUSE PARENCHYMAL LUNG DISEASE, DRUG-INDUCED[75]

ICD-10CM #   J84.89   Other specified interstitial pulmonary diseases

CYTOTOXIC CHEMOTHERAPY

Bleomycin.
Busulfan.
Cyclophosphamide.
Gemcitabine.
Nitrosoureas.
Taxanes (e.g., paclitaxel, docetaxel).

ANTIMETABOLITES

Methotrexate.

TARGETED BIOLOGIC AGENTS

Tumor necrosis factor (TNF)-α inhibitors or soluble receptors: infliximab.
Adalimumab.
Certolizumab pegol.
Etanercept.
Tyrosine kinase inhibitors:
Afatinib.
Erlotinib.
Gefitinib.
Idelalisib.
Imatinib.
Osimertinib.
Trametinib.

Checkpoint inhibitors (antibodies against PD-1, PD-1 ligand, or CTLA-4):
ipilimumab.
Nivolumab.
Pembrolizumab.
Inhibitors of anaplastic lymphoma kinase (ALK):
Alectinib.
Ceritinib.
Crizotinib.

MISCELLANEOUS

Trastuzumab (monoclonal antibody against HER2).
Rituximab (monoclonal antibody against CD20).
Inhibitors of mechanistic target of rapamycin (mTOR, e.g., everolimus).

MISCELLANEOUS OTHER DRUGS

Nitrofurantoin.
Amiodarone.

DRUG-INDUCED SYNDROMES

Drug-induced lupus (e.g., procainamide, hydralazine).
Drug-induced pulmonary infiltrates with eosinophilia (e.g., sulfa-containing drugs).

DIPLOPIA, BINOCULAR

ICD-10CM #   H53.2   Diplopia

Cranial nerve palsy (third, fourth, sixth).
Thyroid eye disease.
Myasthenia gravis.
Decompensated strabismus.
Orbital trauma with blowout fracture.
Orbital pseudotumor.
Cavernous sinus thrombosis.

DIPLOPIA, MONOCULAR

ICD-10CM #   H53.2   Diplopia

Postoperative corrected long-standing tropia.
Defective contact lenses.
Poorly fitting bifocals.
Trauma to iris.
Corneal disorder (e.g., dry eye, astigmatism).
Cataracts.
Lens subluxation.
Nystagmus.
Eyelid twitching.
Foreign body in aqueous or vitreous media.
Migraine.
Lesions of occipital cortex.
Psychogenic.

DIPLOPIA, VERTICAL[38]

ICD-10CM #   H53.2   Diplopia

COMMON CAUSES

Superior oblique palsy.
Thyroid eye disease (muscle infiltration).
Myasthenia gravis.
Skew deviation (brain stem, cerebellar, hydrocephalus).

LESS COMMON CAUSES

Orbital inflammation (myositis, idiopathic orbital inflammatory syndrome [previously designated "orbital pseudotumor"]).
Orbital infiltration (lymphoma, metastases, amyloid, IgG-4–related disease).
Primary orbital tumor.
Entrapment of the inferior rectus (blowout fracture).
Third nerve palsy with or without aberrant innervation.
Superior division third nerve palsy.

Partial third nuclear lesion (very rare).
Brown syndrome (congenital, acquired).
Congenital extraocular muscle fibrosis or muscle absence.
Double elevator palsy (monocular elevator deficiency); controversial in origin.
Sagging eye syndrome (see discussion in section on sixth nerve mimics).

OTHER CAUSES

Chronic progressive external ophthalmoplegia.
Miller Fisher syndrome.
Botulism.
Monocular supranuclear gaze palsy.
Stiff person syndrome.
Superior oblique myokymia.
Dissociated vertical deviation (divergence).
Wernicke encephalopathy.
Vertical one-and-a-half syndrome.

DIZZINESS

ICD-10CM #   R42   Dizziness and giddiness

Viral syndrome.
Anxiety, hyperventilation.
Benign positional paroxysmal vertigo.
Medications (e.g., sedatives, antihypertensives, analgesics).
Withdrawal from medications (e.g., benzodiazepines, selective serotonin reuptake inhibitors).
Alcohol or drug abuse.
Postural hypotension.
Hypoglycemia, hyperglycemia.
Hematologic disorders (e.g., anemia, polycythemia, leukemia).
Head trauma.
Menière disease.
Vertebrobasilar ischemia.
Cervical osteoarthritis.
Cardiac abnormalities (arrhythmias, cardiomyopathy, congestive heart failure, pericarditis).
Multiple sclerosis.
Peripheral vestibulopathy.
Air or sea travel.
Electrolyte abnormalities.
Eye problems (cornea, lens, retina).
Migraine.
Brain stem infarct.
Autonomic neuropathy.
Chronic otomastoiditis.
Complex partial seizures.
Ramsey Hunt syndrome.
Arteritis.
Syncope and presyncope.
Perilymph fistula.
Cerebellopontine tumor.
Hepatic or renal disease.

DORSAL MIDBRAIN SYNDROME[38]

ICD-10CM #   Code varies with specific diagnosis

Pineal and other tumors.
Stroke.
Trauma (including iatrogenic from surgery).
Hydrocephalus and shunt malfunction.
Multiple sclerosis.

Transtentorial herniation.
Congenital aqueductal stenosis.
Infections:
  Encephalitis.
  Cysticercosis.
  Midbrain arteriovenous malformation.
Metabolic disorders:
  Lipid storage disease.
  Wilson disease.
  Kernicterus.
Wernicke encephalopathy.

DRUG-INDUCED LUPUS[35]

| ICD-10CM # | M32.0 | Drug-induced lupus |

DRY EYE

| ICD-10CM # | H04.129 | Dry eye syndrome of unspecified lacrimal gland |

Contacts.
Medications (antihistamines, clonidine, β-blockers, ibuprofen, scopolamine).
Keratoconjunctivitis sicca.
Trauma.
Environmental causes (air conditioning in patient with contacts).

DYSENTERY AND INFLAMMATORY ENTEROCOLITIS[42]

| ICD-10CM # | Varies with specific diagnosis |

DIFFERENTIAL DIAGNOSIS OF ACUTE BACTERIAL DYSENTERY AND INFLAMMATORY ENTEROCOLITIS

Specific Infectious Processes
Bacillary dysentery (Shigella dysenteriae, Shigella flexneri, Shigella sonnei, Shigella boydii; invasive Escherichia coli).
Campylobacteriosis (Campylobacter jejuni).
Amebic dysentery (Entamoeba histolytica).
Ciliary dysentery (Balantidium coli).
Vibriosis (Vibrio parahaemolyticus).
Salmonellosis (Salmonella typhimurium).
Typhoid fever (Salmonella typhi).
Enteric fever (Salmonella choleraesuis, Salmonella paratyphi).
Yersiniosis (Yersinia enterocolitica).
Proctitis
Gonococcal (Neisseria gonorrhoeae).
Herpetic (herpes simplex virus).
Chlamydial (Chlamydia trachomatis).
Syphilitic (Treponema pallidum).
Other Syndromes
Necrotizing enterocolitis of the newborn.
Enteritis necroticans.
Pseudomembranous enterocolitis or Clostridium difficile colitis without overt pseudomembranes (C. difficile).
Diverticulitis.
Typhlitis.

Chronic Inflammatory Processes
Enteropathogenic and enteroaggregative E. coli.
Syphilis.
GI tuberculosis.
GI mycosis (including Basidiobolus ranarum).
Parasitic enteritis.
Syndromes without Known Infectious Cause
Idiopathic ulcerative colitis.
Crohn disease.
Radiation enteritis.
Ischemic colitis.
Allergic enteritis.
Brainerd diarrhea.

DYSLIPOPROTEINEMIAS, SECONDARY CAUSES[58]

| ICD-10CM # | E78.4 | Other hyperlipidemia |

Cause	Disorder
Metabolic	Diabetes.
	Lipodystrophy.
	Glycogen storage disorders.
Renal	Chronic renal failure.
	Glomerulonephritis with nephritic syndrome.
Hepatic	Cirrhosis.
	Biliary obstruction.
	Porphyria.
	Primary biliary cirrhosis (with secondary LCAT deficiency).
Hormonal	Estrogens.
	Progesterones.
	Growth hormone.
	Thyroid disorders (hypothyroidism).
	Corticosteroids.
Lifestyle	Physical inactivity.
	Obesity.
	Diet rich in fats, saturated fats.
	Alcohol intake.
	Smoking.
Medications	Retinoic acid derivatives.
	Glucocorticoids.
	Exogenous estrogens.
	Thiazide diuretics.
	β-adrenergic blockers (selective).
	Testosterone and other anabolizing steroids.
	Immunosuppressive medications (cyclosporine).
	Antiviral medications (HIV protease inhibitors).
	Antischizophrenic medications.

LCAT, Lecithin-cholesterol acyltransferase.

DYSPAREUNIA[55]

ICD-10CM #	N94.1	Dyspareunia
	N44.8	Other noninflammatory disorders of the testis
	N50.8	Other specified disorders of male genital organs
	N53.12	Painful ejaculation
	F52.6	Dyspareunia not due to a substance or known physiological condition

INTROITAL
Vaginismus.
Intact or rigid hymen.
Clitoral problems.
Vulvovaginitis.
Vaginal atrophy: hypoestrogen.
Vulvar dystrophy.
Bartholin or Skene gland infection.
Inadequate lubrication.
Operative scarring.

MIDVAGINAL
Urethritis.
Trigonitis.
Cystitis.
Short vagina.
Operative scarring.
Inadequate lubrication.

DEEP
Endometriosis.
Pelvic infection.
Uterine retroversion.
Ovarian pathology.
GI.
Orthopedic.
Abnormal penile size or shape.

DYSPEPSIA AND PYROSIS, DIFFERENTIAL DIAGNOSIS DURING PREGNANCY[32]

| ICD-10CM # | K30 | Dyspepsia, atonic |
| | F45.3 | Dyspepsia, psychogenic |

DIFFERENTIAL DIAGNOSIS OF DYSPEPSIA OR PYROSIS DURING PREGNANCY
Gastroesophageal reflux disease.
Peptic ulcer disease.
Nausea and vomiting of pregnancy.
Hyperemesis gravidarum.
Pancreatitis.
Biliary colic.
Acute cholecystitis.
Viral hepatitis.
Appendicitis.
Acute fatty liver of pregnancy (in late pregnancy).
Irritable bowel syndrome/nonulcer dyspepsia.

DYSPHAGIA

ICD-10CM #	R13.10	Dysphagia, unspecified

Esophageal obstruction: neoplasm, foreign body, achalasia, stricture, spasm, esophageal web, diverticulum, Schatzki ring.

Peptic esophagitis with stricture, Barrett stricture.

External esophageal compression: neoplasms (thyroid neoplasm, lymphoma, mediastinal tumors), thyroid enlargement, aortic aneurysm, vertebral spurs, aberrant right subclavian artery (dysphagia lusoria).

Hiatal hernia, gastroesophageal reflux disease.

Oropharyngeal lesions: pharyngitis, glossitis, stomatitis, neoplasms.

Hysteria: globus hystericus.

Neurologic and/or neuromuscular disturbances: bulbar paralysis, myasthenia gravis, amyotrophic lateral sclerosis, multiple sclerosis, parkinsonism, cerebrovascular accident, diabetic neuropathy.

Toxins: poisoning, botulism, tetanus, postdiphtheritic dysphagia.

Systemic diseases: scleroderma, amyloidosis, dermatomyositis.

Candida and herpes esophagitis.

Presbyesophagus.

DYSPHAGIA, ESOPHAGEAL[3]

ICD-10CM #	R13-14	Dysphagia, pharyngoesophageal phase

COMMON CAUSES OF ESOPHAGEAL DYSPHAGIA

Motility (Neuromuscular) Disorders
Primary
Achalasia.
Distal esophageal spasm.
Hypercontractile (jackhammer) esophagus.
Hypertensive LES.
Nutcracker (high-pressure) esophagus.
Other peristaltic abnormalities.*

Secondary
Chagas disease.
Reflux-related dysmotility.
Scleroderma and other rheumatologic disorders.

Structural (Mechanical) Disorders
Intrinsic
Carcinoma and benign tumors.
Diverticula.
Eosinophilic esophagitis.
Esophageal rings and webs (other than Schatzki ring).
Foreign body.
Lower esophageal (Schatzki) ring.
Medication-induced stricture.
Peptic stricture.

Extrinsic
Mediastinal mass.
Spinal osteophytes.
Vascular compression.

---

*Peristaltic abnormalities include absent peristalsis and weak peristalsis, as well as hypertensive peristalsis (nutcracker esophagus).

LES, Lower esophageal sphincter.

DYSPHAGIA, OROPHARYNGEAL[2]

ICD-10CM #	R13.12	Dysphagia, oropharyngeal phase

FUNCTIONAL DISORDERS

Central Nervous System
Stroke.
Head injury.
Parkinson disease.
Motor neuron disease.
Multiple sclerosis.
Tumor.
Drugs (e.g., phenothiazines).
Malformations (e.g., syrinx, Arnold-Chiari).

Neural
Motor neuron disease.
Myasthenia gravis.
Radiotherapy.
Poliomyelitis.
Familial dysautonomia.

Muscle
Autoimmune myopathy (polymyositis, dermatomyositis, systemic lupus erythematosus).
Thyrotoxic myopathy.
Guillain-Barré motor neuropathy.
Muscular dystrophies.

STRUCTURAL DISORDERS

Head/neck surgery.
Stricture.
Radiotherapy.
Tumor.
Pharyngeal pouch.
Web.
Extrinsic (e.g., osteophytes).

MISCELLANEOUS

Xerostomia.

DYSPNEA

ICD-10CM #	R06.9	Unspecified abnormalities of breathing

Upper airway obstruction: trauma, neoplasm, epiglottitis, laryngeal edema, tongue retraction, laryngospasm, abductor paralysis of vocal cords, aspiration of foreign body.

Lower airway obstruction: neoplasm, chronic obstructive pulmonary disease, asthma, aspiration of foreign body.

Pulmonary infection: pneumonia, abscess, empyema, TB, bronchiectasis.

Pulmonary hypertension.

Pulmonary embolism/infarction.

Parenchymal lung disease.

Pulmonary vascular congestion.

Cardiac disease: atherosclerotic heart disease, valvular lesions, cardiac dysrhythmias, cardiomyopathy, pericardial effusion, cardiac shunts.

Space-occupying lesions: neoplasm, large hiatal hernia, pleural effusions.

Disease of chest wall: severe kyphoscoliosis, fractured ribs, sternal compression, morbid obesity.

Neurologic dysfunction: Guillain-Barré syndrome, botulism, polio, spinal cord injury.

Interstitial pulmonary disease: sarcoidosis, collagen vascular diseases, desquamative interstitial pneumonia, Hamman-Rich pneumonitis, etc.

Pneumoconioses: silicosis, berylliosis, etc.

Mesothelioma.

Pneumothorax, hemothorax, pleural effusion.

Inhalation of toxins.

Cholinergic drug intoxication.

Carcinoid syndrome.

Hematologic: anemia, polycythemia, hemoglobinopathies.

Thyrotoxicosis, myxedema.

Diaphragmatic compression caused by abdominal distention, subphrenic abscess, ascites.

Lung resection.

Metabolic abnormalities: uremia, hepatic coma, diabetic ketoacidosis.

Sepsis.

Atelectasis.

Psychoneurosis.

Diaphragmatic paralysis.

Pregnancy.

DYSTONIA, PEDIATRIC PATIENT[49]

ICD-10CM #	G24.9	Dystonia, unspecified
	G24.2	Idiopathic nonfamilial dystonia
	G24.1	Genetic torsion dystonia

CAUSES OF DYSTONIA IN CHILDHOOD

Static Injury/Structural Disorders
Cerebral palsy.
Hypoxic-ischemic injury.
Kernicterus.
Head trauma.
Encephalitis.
Tumors.
Stroke in the basal ganglia (which may be due to vascular abnormalities or varicella).
Congenital malformations affecting basal ganglia.

Hereditary/Degenerative Disorders
DYT1 (autosomal dominant, Torsin A).
DYT2 (autosomal-recessive, hippocalcin).
DYT4 (autosomal dominant, β-tubulin 4a).
DYT5 (autosomal dominant, GTP cyclohydrolase 1).
DYT6 (autosomal dominant, THAP1).
DYT8 (autosomal dominant, myofibrillogenesis regulator 1).
DYT9 (autosomal dominant, GLUT1).
DYT10 (autosomal dominant, PRRT2).
DYT11 (autosomal dominant [maternal imprinting], ε-Sarcoglycan).
DYT12 (autosomal dominant, Na$^+$/K$^+$ATPase α3 subunit).
DYT15 (autosomal dominant, unknown).
DYT16 (autosomal recessive, protein kinase activator PRKRA).
Pantothenate kinase-associated neurodegeneration (PKAN; neuronal brain iron accumulation type 1, due to mutations in *PANK2*).
PLA2G6-associated neurodegeneration (PLAN).
Huntington disease (Westphal variant, IT15–4p16.3).
Spinocerebellar ataxias (SCAs, particularly SCA3/Machado-Joseph disease).
Striatal necrosis.
Leigh syndrome.
Neuroacanthocytosis.

HARP syndrome (hypoprebetalipoproteinemia, acanthocytosis, retinitis pigmentosa, and pallidal degeneration).
Tay-Sachs disease.
Sandhoff disease.
Niemann-Pick type C.
Metabolic Disease
Glutaric aciduria types 1 and 2.
Acyl-CoA dehydrogenase deficiencies.
Neurotransmitter disorders.
Mitochondrial disorders.
GM_1 gangliosidosis.
Lesch-Nyhan disease.
Wilson disease.
Vitamin E deficiency.
Methylmalonic aciduria.
Tyrosinemia.
Drugs/Toxins
Neuroleptic and neuroleptic-like antiemetic medications (haloperidol, chlorpromazine, olanzapine, risperidone, prochlorperazine).
Calcium channel blockers.
Stimulants (amphetamine, cocaine, ergot alkaloids).
Anticonvulsants (carbamazepine, phenytoin).
Thallium.
Manganese.
Carbon monoxide.
Ethylene glycol.
Cyanide.
Methanol.
Paroxysmal Disorders
Paroxysmal kinesigenic dyskinesia (PKD).
Paroxysmal nonkinesigenic dyskinesia (PNKD).
Exercise-induced dyskinesia (PED).

DYSURIA

| ICD-10CM # | R30.0 | Dysuria |
| | R30.9 | Painful micturition, unspecified |

Urinary tract infection.
Estrogen deficiency (in postmenopausal female).
Vaginitis.
Genital infection (e.g., herpes, condyloma).
Interstitial cystitis.
Chemical irritation (e.g., deodorant aerosols, douches).
Meatal stenosis or stricture.
Reiter syndrome.
Bladder neoplasm.
GI etiology (diverticulitis, Crohn disease).
Impaired bladder or sphincter action.
Urethral carbuncle.
Chronic fibrosis posttrauma.
Radiation therapy.
Prostatitis.
Urethritis (gonococcal, *Chlamydia*).
Behçet syndrome.
Stevens-Johnson syndrome.

EARACHE[76]

| ICD-10CM # | H92.09 | Otalgia, unspecified ear |

Otitis media.
Serous otitis media.
Eustachitis.

Otitis externa.
Otitic barotrauma.
Mastoiditis.
Foreign body.
Impacted cerumen.
Referred otalgia, as with TMJ dysfunction, dental problems, and tumors.

ECTOPIC ACTH SECRETION[24]

| ICD-10CM # | E34.2 | Ectopic hormone secretion, not elsewhere classified |

Small cell carcinoma of lung.
Endocrine tumors of foregut origin.
   Thymic carcinoid.
   Islet cell tumor.
   Medullary carcinoid, thyroid.
   Bronchial carcinoid.
Pheochromocytoma.
Ovarian tumors.

EDEMA, CHILDREN[23]

ICD-10CM #	R60.0	Localized edema
	R60.1	Generalized edema
	R60.9	Edema, unspecified

CARDIOVASCULAR
Congestive heart failure.
Acute thrombi or emboli.
Vasculitis of many types.

RENAL
Nephrotic syndrome.
Glomerulonephritis of many types.
End-stage renal failure.

ENDOCRINE OR METABOLIC
Thyroid disease.
Starvation.
Hereditary angioedema.

IATROGENIC
Drugs (diuretics and steroids).
Water or salt overload.

HEMATOLOGIC
Hemolytic disease of the newborn.

GI
Hepatic cirrhosis.
Protein-losing enteritis.
Lymphangiectasis.
Cystic fibrosis.
Celiac disease.
Enteritis of many types.

LYMPHATIC ABNORMALITIES
Congenital (gonadal dysgenesis).
Acquired.

EDEMA, GENERALIZED

ICD-10CM #	R60.0	Localized edema
	R60.1	Generalized edema
	R60.9	Edema, unspecified

Congestive heart failure.
Cirrhosis.
Nephrotic syndrome.
Pregnancy.
Idiopathic.
Acute nephritic syndrome.
Myxedema.
Medications (NSAIDs, estrogens, vasodilators).

EDEMA, LEG, UNILATERAL[1]

| ICD-10CM # | R60.0 | Localized edema |
| | R60.9 | Edema, unspecified |

WITH PAIN
Deep vein thrombosis.
Postphlebitic syndrome.
Popliteal cyst rupture.
Gastrocnemius rupture.
Cellulitis.
Psoas or other abscess.

WITHOUT PAIN
Deep vein thrombosis.
Postphlebitic syndrome.
Other venous insufficiency (after saphenous vein harvest, varicosities).
Lymphatic obstruction/lymphedema (carcinoma, lymphoma, sarcoidosis, filariasis, retroperitoneal fibrosis).

EDEMA OF LOWER EXTREMITIES

| ICD-10CM # | R60.0 | Localized edema |
| | R60.9 | Edema, unspecified |

Congestive heart failure (right-sided).
Hepatic cirrhosis.
Nephrosis.
Myxedema.
Lymphedema.
Pregnancy.
Abdominal mass: neoplasm, cyst.
Venous compression from abdominal aneurysm.
Varicose veins.
Bilateral cellulitis.
Bilateral thrombophlebitis.
Vena cava thrombosis, venous thrombosis.
Retroperitoneal fibrosis.

EJECTION SOUND OR CLICK

| ICD-10CM # | R01.2 | Other cardiac sounds |

Aortic regurgitation.
Aortic root dilation.
Systemic hypertension.
Chronic pulmonary hypertension.
Tetralogy of Fallot.
Atrial septal defect.
Pulmonary valve stenosis.
Aortic aneurysm.

ELBOW PAIN

| ICD-10CM # | M25.529 | Pain in unspecified elbow |

Trauma.
Infection.
Inflammatory arthritis.
Lateral or medial epicondylitis.
Entrapment neuropathy.
Olecranon bursitis.
Osteoarthritis.
Gout.
Cervical disease (referred pain).
Shoulder disease (referred pain).
Partial subluxation.
Synovial osteochondromatosis.
Loose body.

ELEVATED HEMIDIAPHRAGM

ICD-10CM #	J98.6	Disorders of diaphragm
	Q79.0	Congenital diaphrag-matic hernia
	Q79.1	Other congenital malformations of diaphragm

Neoplasm (bronchogenic carcinoma, mediastinal neoplasm, intrahepatic lesion).
Substernal thyroid.
Infectious process (pneumonia, empyema, TB, subphrenic abscess, hepatic abscess).
Atelectasis.
Idiopathic.
Eventration.
Phrenic nerve dysfunction (myelitis, myotonia, herpes zoster).
Trauma to phrenic nerve or diaphragm (e.g., surgery).
Aortic aneurysm.
Intraabdominal mass.
Pulmonary infarction.
Pleurisy.
Radiation therapy.
Rib fracture.

EMBOLI, ARTERIAL[1]

| ICD-10CM # | I74.3 | Embolism and thrombosis of arteries of the lower extremities |
| | I74.2 | Embolism and thrombosis of arteries of the upper extremities |

Myocardial infarction with mural thrombi.
Atrial fibrillation.
Cardiomyopathies.
Prosthetic heart valves.
Congestive heart failure.
Endocarditis.
Left ventricular aneurysm.
Left atrial myxoma.
Sick sinus syndrome.
Paradoxical embolus from venous thrombosis.
Aneurysms of large blood vessels.
Atheromatous ulcers of large blood vessels.

EMESIS, PEDIATRIC AGE[23]

ICD-10CM #	R11.10	Vomiting, unspecified
	R11.11	Vomiting without nausea
	R11.12	Projectile vomiting

INFANCY
GI Tract
Congenital
Regurgitation: chalasia, gastroesophageal reflux.
Atresia: stenosis (tracheoesophageal fistula, prepyloric diaphragm, intestinal atresia).
Duplication.
Volvulus (errors in rotation and fixation, Meckel diverticulum).
Congenital bands.
Hirschsprung disease.
Meconium ileus (cystic fibrosis), meconium plug.
Acquired
Acute infectious gastroenteritis, food poisoning (staphylococcal, clostridial).
Pyloric stenosis.
Gastritis, duodenitis.
Intussusception.
Incarcerated hernia—inguinal, internal secondary to old adhesions.
Cow's milk protein intolerance, food allergy, eosinophilic gastroenteritis.
Disaccharidase deficiency.
Celiac disease—presents after introduction of gluten in diet; inherited risk.
Adynamic ileus—the mediator for many non-GI causes.
Neonatal necrotizing enterocolitis.
Chronic granulomatous disease with gastric outlet obstruction.
Non-GI Tract
Infectious: otitis, urinary tract infection, pneumonia, upper respiratory tract infection, sepsis, meningitis.
Metabolic: aminoaciduria and organic aciduria, galactosemia, fructosemia, adrenogenital syndrome, renal tubular acidosis, diabetic ketoacidosis, Reye syndrome.
Central nervous system: trauma, tumor, infection, diencephalic syndrome, rumination, autonomic responses (pain, shock).
Medications: anticholinergics, aspirin, alcohol, idiosyncratic reaction (e.g., codeine).

CHILDHOOD
GI Tract
Peptic ulcer—vomiting is a common presentation in children younger than 6 yr old.
Trauma: duodenal hematoma, traumatic pancreatitis, perforated bowel.
Pancreatitis: mumps, trauma, cystic fibrosis, hyperparathyroidism, hyperlipidemia, organic acidemias.
Crohn disease.
Idiopathic intestinal pseudoobstruction.
Superior mesenteric artery syndrome.
Non-GI Tract
Central nervous system: cyclic vomiting, migraine, anorexia nervosa, bulimia.

ENCEPHALOMYELITIS, NONVIRAL CAUSES[1]

| ICD-10CM # | G04.81 | Other encephalitis and encephalomyelitis |

Subacute bacterial endocarditis.
Rocky Mountain spotted fever.
Typhus.

Ehrlichia.
Q fever.
Chlamydia.
Mycoplasma.
Legionella.
Brucellosis.
Listeria.
Whipple disease.
Cat-scratch disease.
Syphilis (meningovascular).
Relapsing fever.
Lyme disease.
Leptospirosis.
Nocardia.
Actinomycosis.
Tuberculosis.
Cryptococcus.
Histoplasma.
Toxoplasma.
Plasmodium falciparum.
Trypanosomiasis.
Behçet disease.
Vasculitis.
Carcinoma.
Drug reactions.

ENCEPHALOPATHY, HYPERTENSIVE[7]

| ICD-10CM # | Varies with specific diagnosis |

Cerebral infarction.
Subarachnoid hemorrhage.
Intracerebral hemorrhage.
Subdural or epidural hematoma.
Brain tumor or other mass lesion.
Seizure disorder.
Central nervous system vasculitis.
Encephalitis/meningitis.
Drug ingestion.
Drug withdrawal.

ENCEPHALOPATHY, METABOLIC[17]

ICD-10CM #	F10.27	Alcohol dependence with alcohol-induced persisting dementia
	K72.90	Hepatic failure, unspecified without coma
	K72.91	Hepatic failure, unspecified with coma
	G92	Toxic encephalopathy
	T56.0X1A	Toxic effect of lead and its compounds, accidental (unintentional), initial encounter
	T56.0X2A	Toxic effect of lead and its compounds, intentional self-harm, initial encounter

Differential
Diagnosis

II

Substrate deficiency: hypoxia/ischemia, carbon monoxide poisoning, hypoglycemia.

Cofactor deficiency: thiamine, vitamin B_{12}, pyridoxine (INH administration).

Electrolyte disorders: hyponatremia, hypercalcemia, carbon dioxide narcosis, dialysis, hypermagnesemia, disequilibrium syndrome.

Endocrinopathies: diabetic ketoacidosis, hyperosmolar coma, hypothyroidism, hyperadrenocorticism, hyperparathyroidism.

Endogenous toxins: liver disease, uremia, porphyria.

Exogenous toxins: drug overdose (sedative/hypnotics, ethanol, narcotics, salicylates, tricyclic antidepressants), drug withdrawal, toxicity of therapeutic medications, industrial toxins (e.g., organophosphates, heavy metals), sepsis.

Heat stroke.

Epilepsy (post-ictal).

ENCEPHALOPATHY, PROGRESSIVE, ONSET AFTER AGE 2[20]

ICD-10CM #   Varies with specific diagnosis

DISORDERS OF LYSOSOMAL ENZYMES

Gaucher disease type III (glucosylceramide lipidosis).

Globoid cell leukodystrophy (late-onset Krabbe disease).

Glycoprotein degradation disorders.

Aspartylglycosaminuria.

Mannosidosis type II.

GM2 gangliosidosis (juvenile Tay-Sachs disease).

Metachromatic leukodystrophy (late-onset sulfatide lipidosis).

Mucopolysaccharidoses types II and VII.

Niemann-Pick type C (sphingomyelin lipidosis).

INFECTIOUS DISEASE

Acquired immunodeficiency syndrome encephalopathy.[a]

Congenital syphilis.[a]

Subacute sclerosing panencephalitis.

OTHER DISORDERS OF GRAY MATTER

Ceroid lipofuscinosis.

   Juvenile.

   Late infantile (Bielschowsky-Jansky disease).

Huntington disease.

Mitochondrial disorders.

   Late-onset poliodystrophy.

   Myoclonic epilepsy and ragged-red fibers.

Progressive neuronal degeneration with liver disease.

Xeroderma pigmentosum.

OTHER DISORDERS OF WHITE MATTER

Adrenoleukodystrophy.

Alexander disease.

Cerebrotendinous xanthomatosis.

Progressive cavitating leukoencephalopathy.

---

[a]Denotes the most common conditions and the ones with disease-modifying treatments.

ENCEPHALOPATHY, PROGRESSIVE, ONSET BEFORE AGE 2[20]

ICD-10CM #   Varies with specific diagnosis

Acquired immunodeficiency syndrome encephalopathy.[a]

Disorders of amino acid metabolism.

   Guanidinoacetate methyltransferase deficiency.[a]

   Homocystinuria (21q22).[a]

   Maple syrup urine disease (intermediate and thiamine-response forms).[a]

   Phenylketonuria.

Disorders of lysosomal enzymes.

   Ganglioside storage disorders.

     GM1 gangliosidosis.

     GM2 gangliosidosis (Tay-Sachs disease, Sandhoff disease).

   Gaucher disease type II (glucosylceramide lipidosis).[a]

   Globoid cell leukodystrophy (Krabbe disease).

   Glycoprotein degradation disorders.

   I-cell disease.

     Mucopolysaccharidoses.[a]

     Type I (Hurler syndrome).[a]

     Type III (Sanfilippo disease).

   Niemann-Pick disease type A (sphingomyelin lipidosis).

   Sulfatase deficiency disorders.

     Metachromatic leukodystrophy (sulfatide lipidosis).

     Multiple sulfatase deficiency.

Carbohydrate-deficient glycoprotein syndromes.

Hypothyroidism.[a]

Mitochondrial disorders.

   Alexander disease.

   Mitochondrial myopathy, encephalopathy, lactic acidosis, stroke.

   Progressive infantile poliodystrophy (Alpers disease).

   Subacute necrotizing encephalomyelopathy (Leigh disease).

   Trichopoliodystrophy (Menkes disease).

Neurocutaneous syndromes.

   Chediak-Higashi syndrome.

   Neurofibromatosis.[a]

   Tuberous sclerosis.[a]

Other disorders of gray matter.

   Infantile ceroid lipofuscinosis (Santavuori-Haltia disease).

   Infantile neuroaxonal dystrophy.

   Lesch-Nyhan disease.[a]

   Progressive neuronal degeneration with liver disease.

   Rett syndrome.

Other disorders of white matter.

   Aspartoacylase deficiency (Canavan disease).

   Galactosemia: transferase deficiency.[a]

   Neonatal adrenoleukodystrophy.[a]

   Pelizaeus-Merzbacher disease.

   Progressive cavitating leukoencephalopathy.

Progressive hydrocephalus.[a]

---

[a]Denotes the most common conditions and the ones with disease-modifying treatments.

ENDOMETRIAL THICKENING[15]

ICD-10CM #   Varies with specific diagnosis

CAUSES OF ENDOMETRIAL THICKENING

Early intrauterine pregnancy.

Incomplete abortion.

Ectopic pregnancy.

Retained products of conception.

Trophoblastic disease.

Endometritis.

Adhesions.

Hyperplasia.

Polyps.

Carcinoma.

ENTERIC FEVER[5]

ICD-10CM #	A01.00	Typhoid fever, unspecified
	A01.3	Paratyphoid fever
	R50.9	Fever, unspecified

Epstein-Barr infection.

Dengue.

Tuberculosis.

Brucellosis.

Bartonella henselae.

Leptospirosis.

Tularemia.

Ehrlichiosis.

Plague.

Typhus.

Malaria.

Disseminated histoplasmosis.

ENTHESOPATHY

| **ICD-10CM #** | M46.00 | Spinal enthesopathy, site unspecified |

Viremia or bacteremia.

Ankylosing spondylitis.

Psoriatic arthritis.

Drug-induced (quinolones, etretinate).

Reactive arthritis.

Diffuse idiopathic skeletal hyperostosis.

Reiter syndrome.

EOSINOPHILIA, DISEASE ASSOCIATIONS[77]

| **ICD-10CM #** | D72.1 NEC | Eosinophilia |
| | J82 | Eosinophilia, pulmonary |

DISEASES, SYNDROMES, AND CONDITIONS COMMONLY ASSOCIATED WITH PERIPHERAL BLOOD EOSINOPHILIA AND/OR TISSUE EOSINOPHILIA

Infectious Agents

Parasitic Infections

Tropical eosinophilia.

Visceral larval migrans (VLM, toxocariasis).

Helminth infections.

Filariasis *(Wuchereria bancrofti, Brugia malayi).*

Onchocerciasis.

Schistosomiasis.

Fascioliasis.

Paragonimiasis.
Strongyloidiasis.
Trichinosis.
Hookworm.
Ascariasis.
Echinococcosis/hydatid disease.
Fungal Infections
Coccidioidomycosis.
Cryptococcosis (cerebrospinal fluid eosinophilia) in HIV.
Allergic Diseases
Asthma (atopic and intrinsic, nasal polyps, aspirin intolerance syndromes).
Bronchopulmonary aspergillosis.
Allergic rhinitis.
Urticarias (acute allergic and chronic idiopathic).
Atopic dermatitis.
Acute drug (hypersensitivity) reactions (interstitial nephritis, cholestatic hepatitis, exfoliative dermatitis).
Respiratory Tract Disorders
Hypersensitivity pneumonitis (rare).
Allergic bronchopulmonary aspergillosis.
Eosinophilic pneumonia.
Transient pulmonary infiltrates (Löeffler syndrome).
Prolonged pulmonary infiltrates with eosinophilia (PIE syndrome).
Tropical pulmonary eosinophilia (TPE).
Bronchiectasis.
Cystic fibrosis.
Endocrinologic Disorders
Addison disease.
GI Diseases
Inflammatory bowel disease.
Eosinophilic gastroenteritis, eosinophilic esophagitis (EE).
Allergic gastroenteritis (young children).
Celiac disease (when associated with EE).
Toxic Reactions to Ingested Agents
Eosinophil myalgia syndrome (L-tryptophan).
Toxic oil syndrome.
Reactions to Cytokine Therapies
IL-2 and IL-2 plus lymphokine activated killer (LAK) cells.
GM-CSF therapy.
Cutaneous Disorders
Atopic dermatitis.
Immunologic skin diseases.
Scabies.
Myiasis.
Chlamydial pneumonia of infancy.
Scarlet fever and pneumococcal pneumonia (convalescent phase).
Cat-scratch disease.
Eosinophilic cellulitis (Wells syndrome).
Episodic angioedema with eosinophilia.
Chronic idiopathic urticaria.
Bullous pemphigoid.
Herpes gestationis.
Angioblastic lymphoid hyperplasia (Kimura disease).
Immunodeficiency Syndromes
Wiskott-Aldrich syndrome.
Selective IgA deficiency with atopy.
Hyper-IgE recurrent infection syndrome (Job syndrome).
Swiss-type and sex-linked combined immunodeficiency.
Nezelof syndrome.
Graft-versus-disease (GVHD).

Connective Tissue Diseases
Vasculitis/collagen vascular disorders
  Hypersensitivity vasculitis.
  Allergic granulomatosis with angiitis (Churg-Strauss syndrome).
  Serum sickness.
  Eosinophilic fasciitis.
  Sjögren syndrome.
  Rheumatoid arthritis (severe).
Neoplastic, Myeloproliferative, and Lymphoproliferative Neoplasms and Syndromes
Neoplastic
  Ovarian carcinoma.
  Solid tumors (mucin-secreting, epithelial cell origin).
Chronic eosinophil leukemia.
Idiopathic hypereosinophilic syndromes (HES).
Systemic mastocytosis.
Myeloproliferative
  Chronic myelogenous leukemia (CML), acute myelogenous leukemia (AML), and myelodysplastic syndrome (MDS).
  Myelomonocytic leukemia with bone marrow eosinophilia (M4Eo, inversion 16).
Lymphoproliferative
  T-cell lymphocytic leukemia.
  Lymphomas (T cell, Hodgkin disease).
  Angioimmunoblastic lymphadenopathy.
Rare Causes
Chronic active hepatitis.
Chronic dialysis.
Acute pancreatitis.
Postirradiation.
Hypopituitarism.

EOSINOPHILIA, GI[3]

ICD-10CM #	D72.1	Eosinophilia

CAUSES OF GI EOSINOPHILIA

Gastroesophageal reflux disease.
Eosinophilic GI disorders:
  Eosinophilic esophagitis:
    Connective tissue disease-associated eosinophilic esophagitis.
    Familial eosinophilic esophagitis.
  Eosinophilic gastritis.
  Eosinophilic enteritis.
  Eosinophilic gastroenteritis.
Infections:
  Schistosomiasis.
  Anisakiasis.
  GI basidiobolomycosis.
  Toxocariasis.
Celiac disease.
Hypereosinophilic syndrome.
Drug hypersensitivity response.
Inflammatory bowel disease.
Transplant-associated eosinophilic enteritis.
Eosinophilic granulomatosis with polyangiitis.
Toxic injury.
Graft-versus-host disease.

EOSINOPHILIC LUNG DISEASE[21]

ICD-10CM #	NEC J82	Eosinophilia, pulmonary

IDIOPATHIC
Simple pulmonary eosinophilia (Löffler syndrome).
Acute eosinophilic pneumonia.
Chronic eosinophilic pneumonia.
Hypereosinophilic syndrome.

DRUG-INDUCED
Aminosalicylic acid.
Para-aminosalicylic acid.
NSAIDs.
Captopril.
Cocaine.
Minocycline.
Nitrofurantoin.
Phenytoin.

INFECTION
Parasitic (ascariasis, paragonimiasis. tropical eosinophilia).
Fungal *(Aspergillus).*
Bacterial (TB, atypical mycobacterial infection, brucella).
Viral (respiratory syncytial virus).

IMMUNOLOGIC DISEASES
Granulomatosis with polyangiitis.
Churg-Strauss syndrome.
Rheumatoid disease.
Sarcoidosis.

NEOPLASMS
Bronchogenic carcinoma.
Bronchial carcinoid.
Lymphoma (Hodgkin, non-Hodgkin).

EOSINOPHILIA, PARASITIC CAUSES[42]

ICD-10CM #	Varies with specific diagnosis

PARASITIC CAUSES OF EOSINOPHILIA

Widespread Geographic Distribution
Ascariasis (migratory phase).
Hookworm.[†]
Strongyloidiasis.[*,‡]
Tropical pulmonary eosinophilia.
Lymphatic filariasis.
Schistosomiasis.
Toxocariasis.
Cysticercosis *(Taenia solium).*
Echinococcosis (cyst rupture).
Trichinosis.
Trichuriasis.
Aberrant helminthiasis from animals.
Limited Geographic Distribution
Clonorchiasis.
Paragonimiasis.
Fascioliasis.
Angiostrongyliasis.
Opisthorchiasis.
Onchocerciasis, loiasis, and other nonlymphatic filariases.
Gnathostomiasis.
Capillariasis.
Trichostrongyliasis.

[†]Although these are most common neoplastic lesions of the lumbosacral spine, most occur infrequently.
[*]Most frequent parasitic causes of massive eosinophilia (>5000/mm³).
[‡]Absent in disseminated infection in compromised hosts.

Differential Diagnosis

II

EPIGASTRIC PAIN[2]

ICD-10CM #	R10.816	Epigastric abdominal tenderness
	R10.826	Epigastric rebound abdominal tenderness

Peptic ulceration (uncomplicated).*
Peptic ulceration (perforated).
Biliary colic.
Acute pancreatitis.
Abdominal aortic aneurysm.
Anxiety.
Inferior wall myocardial infarction.

*Conditions that also cause right upper quadrant pain

EPILEPSY

ICD-10CM #	G40.909	Epilepsy, unspecified, not intractable, without status epilepticus

Psychogenic spells.
Transient ischemic attack.
Hypoglycemia.
Syncope.
Narcolepsy.
Migraine.
Paroxysmal vertigo.
Arrhythmias.
Drug reaction.

EPILEPSY MIMICS, PEDIATRIC PATIENT[49]

ICD-10CM #	Varies with specific diagnosis

DISORDERS THAT MAY MIMIC CHILDHOOD EPILEPSY

Confused with Generalized Tonic-Clonic Seizures
Pallid syncope (reflex anoxic seizure).
Vasodepressor syncope (reflex anoxic seizure).
Cyanotic breath-holding attacks.
Collapsing attacks with cardiac dysrhythmias.
Cataplexy.
Confused with Generalized Absence Seizures
Behavioral staring attacks.
Complex partial (dyscognitive) seizures.
Tic disorder.
Confused with Complex Partial (Dyscognitive) Seizures
Self-stimulatory behavior, especially in children with autistic spectrum disorders.
Sleep walking.
Night terrors.
Temper tantrums with amnesia for the rage event.
Benign paroxysmal vertigo.
Migraine-related disorders.
Confused with Epileptic Myoclonus
Physiologic hypnagogic myoclonus.
Benign infantile sleep myoclonus.
Startle disease.

EPILEPSY SYNDROMES, AGE SPECIFIC[5]

ICD-10CM #	G40.90	Epilepsy, unspecified, not intractable
	G40.301	Generalized idiopathic epilepsy and epileptic syndromes, not intractable, with status epilepticus
	G40.40	Other generalized epilepsy and epileptic syndromes, not intractable

EPILEPSY SYNDROMES BY AGE OF ONSET

Neonatal
Benign familial neonatal epilepsy.
Early myoclonic encephalopathy.
Ohtahara syndrome.
Infancy
Epilepsy of infancy with migrating focal seizures.
West syndrome (infantile spasms, hypsarrhythmia; to be distinguished from benign myoclonus of early infancy, a nonepilepsy).
Myoclonic epilepsy in infancy (benign Dravet variant).
Benign infantile epilepsy.
Benign familial infantile epilepsy.
Severe myoclonic epilepsy of infancy (classic Dravet syndrome).
Myoclonic encephalopathy in nonprogressive disorders.
Childhood
Genetic epilepsy with febrile seizures plus (GEFS+; can begin in infancy).
Panayiotopoulos syndrome.
Epilepsy with myoclonic atonic (previously astatic) seizures (Doose syndrome).
Benign epilepsy with centrotemporal spikes (BECTS, or benign rolandic epilepsy).
Autosomal-dominant nocturnal frontal lobe epilepsy (ADNFLE).
Late-onset childhood occipital epilepsy (Gastaut syndrome).
Epilepsy with myoclonic absences (Tassinari syndrome).
Lennox-Gastaut syndrome.
Epileptic encephalopathy with continuous spike-and-wave during sleep (CSWS).
Landau-Kleffner syndrome (LKS).
Childhood absence epilepsy (pyknolepsy).
Generalized epilepsy with eyelid myoclonia (Jeavons syndrome).*
Adolescence–Adult
Juvenile absence epilepsy (JAE).
Juvenile myoclonic epilepsy (JME).
Epilepsy with generalized tonic-clonic seizures alone.
Progressive myoclonus epilepsies (PME).

*Not listed as a syndrome by ILAE but instead recognized under absence seizures with special features.

Autosomal-dominant epilepsy with auditory features.
Other familial temporal lobe epilepsies.
Less Specific Age Relationship
Familial focal epilepsy with variable foci (childhood to adult).
Reflex epilepsies (e.g., photosensitive, audiogenic, or reading-induced seizures; may or may not coexist with spontaneous seizures).

EPISTAXIS

ICD-10CM #	R04.0	Epistaxis

Trauma.
Medications (nasal sprays, NSAIDs, anticoagulants, antiplatelets).
Nasal polyps.
Cocaine use.
Coagulopathy (hemophilia, liver disease, disseminated intravascular coagulation, thrombocytopenia).
Systemic disorders (hypertension, uremia).
Infections.
Anatomic malformations.
Rhinitis.
Nasal polyps.
Local neoplasms (benign and malignant).
Desiccation.
Foreign body.

ERECTILE DYSFUNCTION, ORGANIC[67]

ICD-10CM #	N52.9	Male erectile dysfunction, unspecified

Neurogenic abnormalities: somatic nerve neuropathy, central nervous system abnormalities.
Psychogenic causes: depression, performance anxiety, marital conflict.
Endocrine causes: hyperprolactinemia, hypogonadotropic hypogonadism, testicular failure, estrogen excess.
Trauma: pelvic fracture, prostate surgery, penile fracture.
Systemic disease: diabetes mellitus, renal failure, hepatic cirrhosis.
Medications: diuretics, antidepressants, H_2 blockers, exogenous hormones, alcohol, antihypertensives, nicotine abuse, finasteride, etc.
Structural abnormalities: Peyronie disease.

EROSIONS, GENITALIA

ICD-10CM #	N36.8	Other specified disorders of urethra

Candidiasis.
Intraepithelial neoplasia.
Squamous cell carcinoma.
Lichen planus.
Pemphigus vulgaris.
Erythema multiforme.
Lichen sclerosus.
Bullous pemphigoid.
Extramammary Paget disease.
Impetigo.

ERYTHEMATOUS ANNULAR SKIN LESIONS

ICD-10CM #	L53.8	Other specified erythematous conditions

Tinea corporis.
Warfarin plaques.
Erythema multiforme.
Erythema annulare.
Cutaneous lupus.
Cutaneous sarcoidosis.
Trauma.
Acute febrile neutrophilic dermatosis (Sweet syndrome).

ERYTHROCYTOSIS[31]

ICD-10CM #	D75.0	Familial erythrocytosis

CAUSES OF ERYTHROCYTOSIS

Relative or Spurious Erythrocytosis (Normal Red Cell Mass)
Hemoconcentration secondary to dehydration (diarrhea, diaphoresis, diuretics, water deprivation, emesis, ethanol, hypertension, preeclampsia, pheochromocytoma, carbon monoxide intoxication).

True or Absolute Erythrocytosis
Polycythemia vera.
Primary congenital polycythemia.
Secondary erythrocytosis caused by:
  Congenital causes (e.g., activating mutation of erythropoietin receptor).
  Hypoxia caused by carbon monoxide poisoning, high oxygen affinity hemoglobin, high-altitude residence, chronic pulmonary disease, hypoventilation syndromes such as sleep apnea, right to left cardiac shunt, neurologic defects involving the respiratory center.
Nonhypoxic causes with pathologic erythropoietin production.
Renal disease (cysts, hydronephrosis, renal artery stenosis, focal glomerulonephritis, renal transplantation).
Tumors (renal cell cancer, hepatocellular carcinoma, cerebellar hemangioblastoma, uterine fibromyoma, adrenal tumors, meningioma, pheochromocytoma).
Drug-associated causes:
Androgen therapy.
  Exogenous erythropoietin growth factor therapy.

ERYTHRODERMA

ICD-10CM #	L53.9	Erythematous condition, unspecified

Drug reaction (e.g., allopurinol, ampicillin, phenytoin, vancomycin, dapsone, omeprazole, carbamazepine).
Atopic dermatitis.
Psoriasis.
Contact dermatitis.
Idiopathic.
Pityriasis rubra.
Chronic actinic dermatitis.
Bullous pemphigoid.

Paraneoplastic.
Cutaneous T-cell lymphoma.
Connective tissue disease.
Hypereosinophilia syndrome.

ESOPHAGEAL PERFORATION[1]

ICD-10CM #	K22.3	Perforation of esophagus
	S27.819A	Unspecified injury of esophagus (thoracic part), initial encounter

Trauma.
Caustic burns.
Iatrogenic.
Foreign bodies.
Spontaneous rupture (Boerhaave syndrome).
Postoperative breakdown of anastomosis.

ESOPHAGEAL STRICTURES[78]

ICD-10CM #	Varies with specific diagnosis

BENIGN

Congenital
Esophageal atresia.
Tracheoesophageal fistula.
Web.

ACQUIRED

Peptic:
  Gastroesophageal reflux.
  Scleroderma.
Schatzki ring.
Caustic ingestion.
Drug-induced:
  Anticholinergic medications.
  Aspirin.
  Ferrous sulfate.
  Fosamax.
  Nonsteroidal antiinflammatory.
  Quinidine.
  Potassium supplements.
  Tetracycline.
  Vitamin C.
Eosinophilic esophagitis.
Iatrogenic:
  Variceal ligation/injection.
  Endoscopic mucosal resection.
  Ablation therapy (cryotherapy/radiofrequency).
  Postoperative (anastomotic).
  Radiation.
  Instrumentation.
  Nasogastric tube.
Infections:
  Fungal: moniliasis.
  Bacterial: syphilis.
  Mycobacterial: tuberculosis.
Granulomatous:
  Crohn disease.
Dermatosis:
  Epidermolysis bullosa dystrophica.
  Pemphigoid.
  Behçet syndrome.

MALIGNANT

Primary.
Secondary.

ESOPHAGEAL TUMORS, BENIGN[78]

ICD-10CM #	Varies with specific diagnosis

CLASSIFICATION OF BENIGN ESOPHAGEAL TUMORS

Mucosa (First and Second Esophageal Ultrasound [EUS] Layers)
Squamous papilloma.
Fibrovascular polyp.
Retention cyst.
Submucosa (Third EUS Layer)
Lipoma.
Fibroma.
Neurofibroma.
Granular cell tumor.
Hemangiomas.
Salivary gland–type tumor.
Muscularis Propria (Fourth EUS Layer)
Leiomyoma.
Duplication cyst.
Periesophageal Tissue (Fifth EUS Layer)
Foregut cyst.

ESOPHAGITIS[1]

ICD-10CM #	K20.9	Esophagitis, unspecified

INFECTIOUS

Candidiasis.
Cytomegalovirus.
Herpes simplex virus.
HIV infection, acute.

NONINFECTIOUS

Gastroesophageal reflux.
Mucositis from cancer chemotherapy.
Mucositis from radiation therapy.
Aphthous ulcers.

ESOPHAGUS, SYSTEMIC DISEASES[78]

ICD-10CM #	Varies with specific diagnosis

SYSTEMIC DISEASES OF THE ESOPHAGUS

Connective Tissue Disorders
Scleroderma.
Systemic lupus erythematosus.
Polymyositis.
Dermatomyositis.
Mixed connective tissue disorder.
Raynaud phenomenon.
Allergic Disease
Eosinophilic esophagitis.
Metabolic Diseases
Amyloidosis.
Diabetes mellitus.
Hypothyroidism.
Hyperthyroidism.
Dermatologic Diseases
Epidermolysis bullosa.
Pemphigus vulgaris.
Pemphigoid.
Erythema multiforme.
Lichen planus.

Differential Diagnosis

II

Behçet disease.
Infectious Diseases
Histoplasmosis.
Tuberculosis.
Actinomycosis.
Immunocompromised host:
  Fungal: *Candida* spp.
  Viral: herpes simplex, cytomegalovirus.
  Mycobacterial.
  Bacterial: *Streptococcus viridans, Staphylo-
    coccus,* bacilli, *Treponema pallidum.*
  Protozoal.
Miscellaneous Disorders
Sarcoidosis.
Crohn disease.

ESOTROPIA

ICD-10CM #	H50.00	Unspecified esotropia
	H50.43	Accommodative component in esotropia
	H50.05	Alternating esotropia

Congenital.
Accommodative esotropia.
Myasthenia gravis.
Abducens palsy.
Pseudo-sixth nerve palsy.
Medial rectus entrapment (e.g., blowout fracture).
Posterior internuclear ophthalmoplegia.
Wernicke encephalopathy.
Thyroid myopathy.
Chiari malformation.

EXANTHEMS[25]

| ICD-10CM # | R21 | Rash and other nonspecific skin eruption |

Measles.
Rubella.
Erythema infectiosum (fifth disease).
Roseola exanthema.
Varicella.
Enterovirus.
Adenovirus.
Epstein-Barr virus.
Kawasaki disease.
Staphylococcal scalded skin.
Scarlet fever.
Meningococcemia.
Rocky Mountain spotted fever.

EYELID NEOPLASM

| ICD-10CM # | C44.101 | Unspecified malignant neoplasm of skin of unspecified eyelid, including canthus |

MALIGNANT

Melanoma.
Basal cell carcinoma.
Squamous cell carcinoma.
Bowen disease.
Sebaceous cell carcinoma.
Metastatic lymphoma/leukemia.

BENIGN

Melanocytic nevus.
Pilar, eccrine, or apocrine tumor.

Neurofibroma.
Keratosis.
Squamous papilloma.
Keratoacanthoma.

EYELID RETRACTION

| ICD-10CM # | H02.89 | Other specified disorders of eyelid |

Congenital.
Graves ophthalmopathy.
Myasthenia gravis.
Postsurgical.
Guillain-Barré syndrome.
Cerebellar disease.
Horizontal gaze palsy.
Partial palsy of superior rectus muscle.
Encephalitis.
Closed head injury.
Disseminated sclerosis.
Eye trauma.
Contact lens wear.
Proptosis.
Eyelid neoplasm.
Atopic dermatitis.
Herpes zoster ophthalmicus.
Botulinum toxin injection.
Cyclic oculomotor paralysis.
Spheroid wing meningioma.
Hepatic cirrhosis.
Down syndrome.
Essential hypertension.
Meningitis.
Paget disease of bone.

EYE PAIN

| ICD-10CM # | H57.13 | Ocular pain, bilateral |

Foreign body.
Herpes zoster.
Trauma.
Conjunctivitis.
Iritis.
Iridocyclitis.
Uveitis.
Blepharitis.
Ingrown lashes.
Orbital or periorbital cellulitis/abscess.
Sinusitis.
Headache.
Glaucoma.
Inflammation of lacrimal gland.
Tic douloureux.
Cerebral aneurysm.
Cerebral neoplasm.
Entropion.
Retrobulbar neuritis.
Ultraviolet light.
Dry eyes.
Irritation or inflammation from eye drops, dust, cosmetics, etc.

FACIAL PAIN

| ICD-10CM # | G50.1 | Atypical facial pain |

Infection, abscess.
Postherpetic neuralgia.
Trauma, posttraumatic neuralgia.
Tic douloureux.

Cluster headache, "lower-half headache."
Geniculate neuralgia.
Anxiety, somatization syndrome.
Glossopharyngeal neuralgia.
Carotidynia.

FACIAL PARALYSIS[25]

| ICD-10CM # | G51.0 | Bell palsy |

INFECTION

Bacterial: otitis media, mastoiditis, meningitis, Lyme disease.
Viral: herpes zoster, mononucleosis, varicella, rubella, mumps, Bell palsy.
Mycobacterial: TB, meningitis, leprosy.
Miscellaneous: syphilis, malaria.

TRAUMA

Temporal bone fracture, facial laceration.
Surgery.

NEOPLASM

Malignant: squamous cell carcinoma, basal cell and adenocystic tumors, leukemia, parotid neoplasms, metastatic tumors.
Benign: facial nerve neuroma, vestibular schwannoma, congenital cholesteatoma.

IMMUNOLOGIC

Guillain-Barré syndrome, periarteritis nodosa.
Reaction to tetanus antiserum.

METABOLIC

Pregnancy.
Hypothyroidism.
Diabetes mellitus.

FACIAL WEAKNESS, CONGENITAL[20]

| ICD-10CM # | Varies with specific diagnosis |

CAUSES

Aplasia of facial muscles.
Birth injury.
Congenital myotonic dystrophy.
Congenital bilateral perisylvian syndrome.
Fiber-type disproportion myopathies.
  Myasthenic syndromes.*
  Congenital myasthenia.
  Familial infantile myasthenia.
  Transitory neonatal myasthenia.

*Denotes the most common conditions and the ones with disease-modifying treatments.

FACIAL WEAKNESS, POSTNATAL[20]

| ICD-10CM # | Varies with specific diagnosis |

CAUSES

Autoimmune and postinfectious.
  Bell palsy.[a]
  Idiopathic cranial polyneuropathy.
  Miller Fisher syndrome.[a]
  Myasthenia gravis.[a]

[a]Denotes the most common conditions and the ones with disease-modifying treatments.

Genetic.
  Juvenile progressive bulbar palsy (Fazio-Londe disease).
  Muscular disorders.
  Facioscapulohumeral syndrome.
  Facioscapulohumeral syndrome, infantile form.
  Fiber-type disproportion myopathies.
  Melkersson syndrome.
  Myotonic dystrophy.
  Oculopharyngeal dystrophy.
  Myasthenic syndromes.[a]
  Congenital myasthenia.[a]
  Familial infantile myasthenia.[a]
  Osteopetrosis (Albers-Schönberg disease).
  Recurrent facial palsy.
Hypertension.
Infectious.
  Diphtheria.
  Herpes zoster oticus.[a]
  Infectious mononucleosis.
  Lyme disease.[a]
  Otitis media.[a]
  Sarcoidosis.[a]
  Tuberculosis.[a]
Metabolic disorders.
  Hyperparathyroidism.[a]
  Hypothyroidism.[a]
Multiple sclerosis.
Syringobulbia.[a]
Toxins.
Trauma.
  Delayed.
  Immediate.
Tumor.
  Glioma of brain stem.
  Histiocytosis X.
  Leukemia.
  Meningeal carcinoma.
  Neurofibromatosis.

FAILURE TO THRIVE

ICD-10CM #	R62.50	Unspecified lack of expected normal physiological development in childhood

PSYCHOSOCIAL/BEHAVIORAL

Inadequate diet because of poverty/food insufficiency, errors in food preparation.
Poor parenting skills (lack of knowledge of sufficient diet).
Child/parent interaction problems (autonomy struggles, coercive feeding, maternal depression).
Food refusal.
Rumination.
Parental cognitive or mental health problems.
Child abuse or neglect; emotional deprivation.

NEUROLOGIC

Cerebral palsy.
Hypothalamic and other central nervous system tumors (diencephalic syndrome).
Neuromuscular disorders.
Neurodegenerative disorders.

RENAL

Recurrent urinary tract infection.
Renal tubular acidosis.
Renal failure.

ENDOCRINE

Diabetes mellitus.
Diabetes insipidus.
Hypothyroidism/hyperthyroidism.
Growth hormone deficiency.
Adrenal insufficiency.

GENETIC/METABOLIC/CONGENITAL

Sickle cell disease.
Inborn errors of metabolism (organic acidosis, hyperammonemia, storage disease).
Fetal alcohol syndrome.
Skeletal dysplasias.
Chromosomal disorders.
Multiple congenital anomaly syndromes (VATER [vertebral defects, imperforate anus, tracheoesophageal fistula, radial and renal dysplasia], CHARGE [coloboma, heart disease, atresia choanae, retarded growth and retarded development and/or central nervous system anomalies, genital hypoplasia, ear anomalies and/or deafness]).

GI

Pyloric stenosis.
Gastroesophageal reflux.
Repair of tracheoesophageal fistula.
Malrotation.
Malabsorption syndromes.
Celiac disease.
Milk intolerance: lactose, protein.
Pancreatic insufficiency syndromes (cystic fibrosis).
Chronic cholestasis.
Inflammatory bowel disease.
Chronic congenital diarrhea states.
Short bowel syndrome.
Pseudoobstruction.
Hirschsprung disease.
Food allergy.

CARDIAC

Cyanotic heart lesions.
Congestive heart failure.
Vascular rings.

PULMONARY/RESPIRATORY

Severe asthma.
Cystic fibrosis; bronchiectasis.
Chronic respiratory failure.
Bronchopulmonary dysplasia.
Adenoid/tonsillar hypertrophy.
Obstructive sleep apnea.

MISCELLANEOUS

Collagen vascular disease.
Malignancy.
Primary immunodeficiency.
Transplantation.

INFECTIONS

Perinatal infection (TORCHES [toxoplasma, other, rubella, cytomegalovirus, herpes simplex]).
Occult/chronic infections.
Parasitic infestation.
Tuberculosis.
HIV.

FATIGUE

ICD-10CM #	R53.83	Other fatigue
	F48.0	Neurasthenia

Depression.
Anxiety, emotional stress.
Inadequate sleep.
Chronic fatigue syndrome.
Prolonged physical activity.
Pregnancy and postpartum period.
Anemia.
Hypothyroidism.
Medications (β-blockers, anxiolytics, antidepressants, sedating antihistamines, clonidine, methyldopa).
Viral or bacterial infections.
Sleep apnea syndrome.
Dieting.
Renal failure, congestive heart failure, chronic obstructive pulmonary disease, liver disease.

FATIGUE, CHRONIC

ICD-10CM #	R53.83	Other fatigue
	F48.0	Neurasthenia

CHRONIC INFECTIONS

Hepatitis C.
Lyme disease.
Parasitic and fungal infections.
Tuberculosis.
HIV.
Xenotropic murine leukemia retrovirus.

SLEEP DISORDERS

Obstructive sleep apnea.
Restless leg syndrome.
Circadian rhythm disorder.
Upper airway resistance syndrome.
Narcolepsy/parasomnias.
Alpha-delta sleep disorder.

ENDOCRINE/METABOLIC DISORDERS

Addison disease.
Cushing syndrome.
Poorly controlled diabetes.
Thyroid disorders.
Hemochromatosis.
Hypopituitarism.
Diabetes insipidus.

GENERAL MEDICAL DISORDERS

Anemia (any cause).
Chronic renal/hepatic failure.
Malnutrition.
Medication side effects.
Chronic pain disorders.

PSYCHOLOGIC

Mood disorders (depression, anxiety, bipolar).
Schizophrenia.
Posttraumatic stress disorder.
Anorexia nervosa/bulimia.
Childhood abuse and/or neglect.

Differential Diagnosis

II

CHRONIC INFLAMMATION

Rheumatoid arthritis.
Systemic lupus erythematosus.
Sjögren syndrome.
Polymyositis/dermatomyositis.
Vasculitis.
Sarcoidosis.

CARDIOPULMONARY

Congestive heart failure.
Neurally mediated hypotension.
Postural orthostatic tachycardia syndrome.
Pulmonary hypertension.
Chronic obstructive pulmonary disease.
Mitral valve prolapse.

GASTROINTESTINAL

Celiac disease.
Inflammatory bowel disease.
Autoimmune hepatitis.
Hepatic cirrhosis.

MALIGNANCY

Lymphoma and occult malignancies.
Postchemotherapy syndrome.

NEUROLOGIC DISORDERS

Multiple sclerosis.
Myasthenia gravis.
Muscular dystrophies.
Parkinson disease.
Early dementia.

LIFESTYLE FACTORS

Chronic overwork.
Persistent unresolved stress.
Inadequate exercise.
Morbid obesity (body mass index >40).
Alcoholism/drug abuse.

FATTY LIVER

| ICD-10CM # | K76.0 | Fatty (change of) liver, not elsewhere classified |
| | K76.89 | Other specified diseases of liver |

Obesity.
Alcohol abuse.
Diabetes mellitus.
Acute fatty liver of pregnancy.
Medications (tetracycline, valproic acid, glucocorticoids, amiodarone, estrogen, methotrexate).
Reye syndrome.
Wilson disease.
Nonalcoholic steatosis.

FEVER, ABDOMINAL PAIN, JAUNDICE IN PEDIATRIC PATIENT[5]

| ICD-10CM # | R50.9 | Fever, unspecified |

Cholangitis.
Cholecystitis.
Cholelithiasis.
Sepsis.
Hepatitis.
Choledochal cyst.
Pancreatitis.

Urinary tract infection.
Leptospirosis and other systemic infections with hepatic involvement.
Spontaneous perforation of common bile duct.
Biliary cyst.
Appendicitis.

FEVER AND CARDIOPULMONARY FAILURE[79]

| ICD-10CM # | R50.9 | Fever, unspecified |

DIFFERENTIAL DIAGNOSIS OF FEVER AND RAPIDLY PROGRESSIVE CARDIOPULMONARY FAILURE

Bacterial Infection
Severe community-acquired pneumonia.
Meningitis, endocarditis.
Rickettsial disease (babesiosis, ehrlichiosis, Rocky Mountain spotted fever, scrub typhus, Mediterranean spotted fever).
Q-Fever (Coxiella burnetii).
Brucellosis.
Plague (Yersinia pestis).
Tularemia (Francisella tularensis).
Typhoid fever/salmonellosis.
Leptospirosis (Leptospira interrogans).
Anthrax.
Mycobacterial infections.
Viral Infections
Viral pneumonia (influenza, CMV, EBV, VZV, SARS).
Hantavirus.
Dengue fever and yellow fever.
Hemorrhagic fever (Lassa, Marburg, or Ebola viruses).
Fungal Infections
Coccidiomycosis.
Cryptococcus.
Histoplasmosis.
Blastomycosis.
Parasitic Infections
Malaria.
Leishmaniasis.
Schistosomiasis.
Strongyloides.
Noninfectious Causes
Inflammatory:
   Rapid-onset interstitial pneumonia (acute interstitial pneumonia, acute hypersensitivity pneumonitis).
   Acute eosinophilic pneumonia.
   ARDS due to other causes (inhalation injury, drug overdose, trauma).
Rheumatologic disorders:
   Wegener granulomatosis, Churg-Strauss disease, Goodpasture syndrome.
   Systemic lupus erythematosus, antiphospholipid syndrome.
Other:
   Malignancy, lymphoma, lymphoproliferative disease, leukemia.
   Pulmonary embolism, aortic dissection, acute myocardial infarction.
   Adrenal insufficiency, thyroid storm.

ARDS, Acute respiratory distress syndrome; *CMV,* cytomegalovirus; *EBV,* Epstein-Barr virus; *SARS,* severe acute respiratory syndrome; *VZV,* varicella zoster virus.

FEVER AND JAUNDICE

| ICD-10CM # | R50.9 | Fever, unspecified |
| | R17 | Unspecified jaundice |

Bacterial sepsis.
Cholangitis.
Hepatic abscess.
Leptospirosis.
Malaria.
Viral hepatitis.
Yellow fever.

FEVER AND LYMPHADENOPATHY

| ICD-10CM # | R59.9 | Enlarged lymph nodes, unspecified |
| | R50.9 | Fever, unspecified |

REGIONAL

Cervical
Streptococci.
Tuberculosis.
Viral upper respiratory infection.
Peripheral
Bartonella henselae.
Herpesviruses.
Lymphoma.
Metastatic cancer.
Sporotrichosis.
Streptococci.
Inguinal
Chancroid.
Herpes.
Lymphogranuloma venereum.
Syphilis (primary).

GENERALIZED

Cytomegalovirus.
Epstein-Barr virus.
HIV.
Lymphoma.
Sarcoidosis.
Syphilis (secondary).
Toxoplasmosis.
Viral hepatitis.

FEVER AND RASH

ICD-10CM #	R21	Rash and other nonspecific skin eruption
	R21	Rash and other nonspecific skin eruption
	R50.9	Fever, unspecified

Drug hypersensitivity: penicillin, sulfonamides, thiazides, anticonvulsants, allopurinol.
Viral infection: measles, rubella, varicella, erythema infectiosum, roseola, enterovirus infection, viral hepatitis, infectious mononucleosis, acute HIV.
Other infections: meningococcemia, staphylococcemia, scarlet fever, typhoid fever, *Pseudomonas* bacteremia, Rocky Mountain spotted fever, Lyme disease, secondary syphilis, bacterial endocarditis, babesiosis, brucellosis, listeriosis.

Serum sickness.
Erythema multiforme.
Erythema marginatum.
Erythema nodosum.
Systemic lupus erythematosus.
Dermatomyositis.
Allergic vasculitis.
Pityriasis rosea.
Herpes zoster.

FEVER AND RASH IN ICU[2]

| ICD-10CM # | R21 | Rash and other nonspecific skin eruption |
| | R50.9 | Fever, unspecified |

DIFFERENTIAL DIAGNOSTIC CLINICAL FEATURES OF FEVER AND RASH IN THE ICU

Rash with Shock

Infectious causes: toxic shock syndrome, meningococcemia, postsplenectomy sepsis, overwhelming *Staphylococcus aureus* bacteremia/acute bacterial endocarditis, arboviral hemorrhagic fevers, hemorrhagic smallpox, *Vibrio vulnificus*, gas gangrene, dengue fever.
Noninfectious cause: systemic lupus erythematosus (on steroids).

RASH WITH MENTAL CHANGES

Infectious causes: Rocky Mountain spotted fever, meningococcemia (with meningitis), *S. aureus* acute bacterial endocarditis, Chikungunya fever, typhus.
Noninfectious cause: systemic lupus erythematosus.

RASH WITH CONJUNCTIVAL SUFFUSION

Infectious causes: Rocky Mountain spotted fever, dengue fever, arboviral hemorrhagic fevers, toxic shock syndrome.
Noninfectious cause: adult Kawasaki disease.

RASH WITH RELATIVE BRADYCARDIA

Infectious causes: Rocky Mountain spotted fever, typhus, dengue fever, typhoid, arboviral hemorrhagic fevers.
Noninfectious cause: drug rash.

RASH WITH ABDOMINAL PAIN

Infectious causes: *V. vulnificus*, gas gangrene, *Clostridium sordelli*, scarlet fever.
Noninfectious causes: cholesterol emboli syndrome, systemic lupus erythematosus.

RASH ON PALMS AND SOLES

Infectious causes: Rocky Mountain spotted fever, toxic shock syndrome, chickenpox, smallpox, monkeypox, scarlet fever.
Noninfectious cause: drug rash.

RASH WITH DIARRHEA

Infectious causes: *V. vulnificus*, gas gangrene, toxic shock syndrome, dengue fever, arboviral hemorrhagic fevers.
Noninfectious cause: none.

RASH WITH EDEMA OF DORSUM OF HANDS/FEET

Infectious causes: Rocky Mountain spotted fever, toxic shock syndrome.
Noninfectious cause: adult Kawasaki disease.

RASH WITH BULLAE

Infectious causes: *V. vulnificus*, *S. aureus* complicated skin/skin structure infection, gas gangrene.
Noninfectious cause: none.

RASH WITH HEART MURMUR

Infectious cause: acute bacterial endocarditis.
Noninfectious cause: systemic lupus erythematosus.
Rash with gangrene of nose tip
Infectious cause: *S. aureus* acute bacterial endocarditis.
Noninfectious causes: systemic lupus erythematosus, vasculitis.

RASH WITH CEREBROVASCULAR ACCIDENT

Infectious causes: cholesterol emboli syndrome, *S. aureus* acute bacterial endocarditis.
Noninfectious cause: none.

RASH WITH SPLENOMEGALY

Infectious causes: Rocky Mountain spotted fever, typhus.
Noninfectious causes: systemic lupus erythematosus, adult Kawasaki disease.

RASH WITH DEAFNESS

Infectious causes: Rocky Mountain spotted fever, typhus, meningococcal meningitis.
Noninfectious cause: none.

RASH WITH HEPATOSPLENOMEGALY

Infectious causes: Rocky Mountain spotted fever, typhus.
Noninfectious cause: atypical measles.

RASH WITH HEPATOMEGALY

Infectious cause: typhus.
Noninfectious cause: none.

FEVER, AFTER TRAVEL TO THE TROPICS[18]

| ICD-10CM # | R50.81 | Fever presenting with conditions classified elsewhere |

CAUSES OF FEVER AFTER TRAVEL TO THE TROPICS

80% of Specific Infections Causing Fever (Includes Respiratory and Urinary Tract Infection)
Malaria.
Viral hepatitis.
Febrile illness unrelated to foreign travel.
Dengue fever.
Enteric fever (typhoid and paratyphoid fevers).
Other Causes
Gastroenteritis.

Rickettsia.
Leptospirosis.
Schistosomiasis.
Amebic liver abscess.
Tuberculosis.
Acute HIV infection.
Others.

FEVER, COMMON INFECTIOUS CAUSES[7]

| ICD-10CM # | R50.9 | Fever, unspecified |

CENTRAL NERVOUS SYSTEM

Meningitis:
  Encephalitis.
  Brain abscess.
  Epidural abscess.

HEAD AND NECK

Acute suppurative parotitis:
  Acute sinusitis.
  Parapharyngeal and retropharyngeal space infections.
  Acute suppurative otitis media.

CARDIOVASCULAR

Catheter-related infection:
  Endocarditis.

PULMONARY AND MEDIASTINAL

Pneumonia:
  Empyema.
  Mediastinitis.

HEPATOBILIARY AND GI

Diverticulitis:
  Appendicitis.
  Peritonitis (spontaneous or secondary).
  Intraperitoneal abscess.
  Perirectal abscess.
  Infected pancreatitis.
  Acute cholecystitis.
  Cholangitis.
  Hepatic abscess.
  Acute viral hepatitis.

GENITOURINARY

Bacterial or fungal cystitis:
  Pyelonephritis.
  Perinephric abscess.
  Tuboovarian abscess.
  Endometritis.
  Prostatitis.

BREAST

Mastitis:
  Breast abscess.

CUTANEOUS AND MUSCULAR

Cellulitis:
  Suppurative wound infection.
  Necrotizing fasciitis.
  Bacterial myositis or myonecrosis.
  Herpes zoster.

OSSEOUS

Osteomyelitis.

Differential Diagnosis

II

FEVER, DRUG-INDUCED[59]

ICD-10CM #	R50.2	Drug induced fever

SELECTED AGENTS ASSOCIATED WITH DRUG-INDUCED FEVER

Common

Antimicrobial:
  Amphotericin B.
  β-Lactams.
  Sulfonamides.
Cardiovascular:
  Procainamide.
  Quinidine.
Central nervous system:
  Carbamazepine.
  Phenytoin.
Miscellaneous:
  Bleomycin.
  Interferon-α.
  Interleukin-2.

Less Common

Antimicrobial:
  Clindamycin.
  Fluoroquinolones.
  Rifampin.
Cardiovascular:
  Diltiazem.
  Hydralazine.
Central nervous system:
  Haloperidol.
  Serotonin reuptake inhibitors.
Miscellaneous:
  Allopurinol.
  Cimetidine.
  Tacrolimus.

FEVER, HOSPITAL ASSOCIATED[59]

ICD-10CM #	R50.2	Drug induced fever
	R50.9	Fever, unspecified

SELECTED CAUSES OF HOSPITAL-ASSOCIATED FEVER

Common

Infectious:
  Clostridium difficile enterocolitis.
  Pneumonia.
  Surgical wound.
  Urinary tract.
  Vascular catheter.
Noninfectious:
  Drug-induced fever.
  Hematoma.
  Immediate postoperative state.
  Transfusion reaction.
  Venous thromboembolism.

Less Common

Infectious:
  Biliary tract disease.
  Endometritis.
  Intraabdominal abscess.
  Mediastinitis.
  Sinusitis.

Noninfectious:
  Adrenal insufficiency.
  Gout.
  Myocardial infarction.
  Organ infarction.
  Pancreatitis.

FEVER IN RETURNING TRAVELERS AND IMMIGRANTS[25]

ICD-10CM #	R50.81	Fever presenting with conditions classified elsewhere

COMMON

Acute respiratory tract infection (worldwide).
Gastroenteritis (worldwide) [foodborne, waterborne, fecal-oral].
Enteric fever, including typhoid (worldwide) [food, water].
Urinary tract infection (worldwide) [sexual contact].
Drug reactions [antibiotics, prophylactic agents, other] {rash frequent}.
Malaria (tropics, limited areas of temperate zones) [mosquitoes].
Arboviruses (Africa; tropics) [mosquitoes, ticks, mites].
Dengue (Asia, Caribbean, Africa) [mosquitoes].
Viral hepatitis (worldwide).
Hepatitis A (worldwide) [food, fecal-oral].
Hepatitis B (worldwide, especially Asia, sub-Saharan Africa) [sexual contact] {long incubation period}.
Hepatitis C (worldwide) [blood or sexual contact].
Hepatitis E (Asia, North Africa, Mexico, others) [food, water].
Tuberculosis (worldwide) [airborne, milk] {long period to symptomatic infection}.
Sexually transmitted diseases (worldwide) [sexual contact].

LESS COMMON

Filariasis (Asia, Africa, South America) [biting insects] {long incubation period, eosinophilia}.
Measles (developing world) [airborne] {in susceptible individual}.
Amebic abscess (worldwide) [food].
Brucellosis (worldwide) [milk, cheese, food, animal contact].
Listeriosis (worldwide) [foodborne] {meningitis}.
Leptospirosis (worldwide) [animal contact, open fresh water] {jaundice, meningitis}.
Strongyloidiasis (warm and tropical areas) [soil contact] {eosinophilia}.
Toxoplasmosis (worldwide) [undercooked meat].

RARE

Relapsing fever (western Americas, Asia, northern Africa) [ticks, lice].
Hemorrhagic fevers (worldwide) [arthropod and nonarthropod transmitted].
Yellow fever (tropics) [mosquitoes] {hepatitis}.

Hemorrhagic fever with renal syndrome (Europe, Asia, North America) [rodent urine] {renal impairment}.
Hantavirus pulmonary syndrome (western North America, other) [rodent urine] {respiratory distress syndrome}.
Lassa fever (Africa) [rodent excreta, person to person] {high mortality rate}.
Other: chikungunya, Rift Valley, Ebola-Marburg, etc. (various) [insect bites, rodent excreta, aerosols, person to person] {often severe}.
Rickettsial infections {rashes and eschars}.
Leishmaniasis, visceral (Middle East, Mediterranean, Africa, Asia, South America) [biting flies] {long incubation period}.
Acute schistosomiasis (Africa, Asia, South America, Caribbean) [fresh water].
Chagas disease (South and Central America) [reduviid bug bites] {often asymptomatic}.
African trypanosomiasis (Africa) [tsetse fly bite] {neurologic syndromes, sleeping sickness}.
Bartonellosis (South America) [sandfly bite] {skin nodules}.
HIV infection/AIDS (worldwide) [sexual and blood contact].
Trichinosis (worldwide) [undercooked meat] {eosinophilia}.
Plague (temperate and tropical plains) [animal exposures and fleas].
Tularemia (worldwide) [animal contact, fleas, aerosols] {ulcers, lymph nodes}.
Anthrax (worldwide) [animal, animal product contact] {ulcers}.
Lyme disease (North America, Europe) [tick bites] {arthritis, meningitis, cardiac abnormalities}.

FEVER, NONINFECTIOUS CAUSES[43]

ICD-10CM #	R50.9	Fever, unspecified

DIFFERENTIAL DIAGNOSIS—NONINFECTIOUS CAUSES OF FEVER

Critical Diagnoses

Acute myocardial infarction.
Pulmonary embolism/infarction.
Intracranial hemorrhage.
Cerebrovascular accident.
Neuroleptic-malignant syndrome.
Thyroid storm.
Acute adrenal insufficiency.
Transfusion reaction.
Pulmonary edema.

Emergent Diagnoses

Congestive heart failure.
Dehydration.
Recent seizure.
Sickle cell disease.
Transplant rejection.
Pancreatitis.
Deep vein thrombosis.

Nonemergent Diagnoses

Drug fever.
Malignancy.
Gout.

Sarcoidosis.
Crohn disease.
Postmyocardiotomy syndrome.

FEVER OF UNKNOWN ORIGIN, PEDIATRIC PATIENT[5]

ICD-10CM #   R50.9   Fever, unspecified

INFECTIOUS DISEASES

Bacterial
Bacterial endocarditis.
Brucellosis.
Cat-scratch disease.
Leptospirosis.
Liver abscess.
Mastoiditis (chronic).
Osteomyelitis.
Pelvic abscess.
Perinephric abscess.
Pyelonephritis.
Salmonellosis.
Sinusitis.
Subdiaphragmatic abscess.
Tuberculosis.
Tularemia.
Viral
Adenovirus.
Arboviruses.
Cytomegalovirus.
Epstein-Barr virus (infectious mononucleosis).
Hepatitis viruses.
Chlamydial
Lymphogranuloma venereum.
Psittacosis.
Rickettsial
Q fever.
Rocky Mountain spotted fever.
Fungal
Blastomycosis (nonpulmonary).
Histoplasmosis (disseminated).
Parasitic
Malaria.
Toxoplasmosis.
Visceral larva migrans.
Unclassified
Sarcoidosis.
Collagen Vascular Diseases
Juvenile rheumatoid arthritis.
Polyarteritis nodosa.
Systemic lupus erythematosus.
Malignancies
Hodgkin disease.
Leukemia and lymphoma.
Neuroblastoma.
Miscellaneous
Central diabetes insipidus.
Drug fever.
Ectodermal dysplasia.
Factitious fever.
Familial dysautonomia.
Granulomatous colitis.
Hemophagocytic lymphohistiocytosis.
Infantile cortical hyperostosis.
Kikuchi-Fujimoto disease.
Nephrogenic diabetes insipidus.
Pancreatitis.
Periodic fever.

Serum sickness.
Thyrotoxicosis.
Ulcerative colitis.

FEVER, PEDIATRIC, ACUTE[29]

ICD-10CM #   R50.9   Fever, unspecified

COMMON VIRAL INFECTIONS

Central Nervous System
Meningitis.
Encephalitis.
Tumor.
Brain abscess.
Head, Ears, Eyes, Nose, and Throat
Otitis media.
Pharyngitis.
Retropharyngeal abscess.
Peritonsillar abscess.
Lateral pharyngeal wall abscess.
Stomatitis.
Influenza.
Sinusitis.
Parotitis.
Cervical adenitis.
Periorbital cellulitis.
Orbital cellulitis or abscess.
Respiratory System
Bronchiolitis.
Croup.
Epiglottitis.
Pneumonia.
Upper respiratory infection.
Cardiovascular System
Myocarditis.
Pericarditis.
Endocarditis.
Genitourinary System
Urinary tract infection.
Tuboovarian abscess.
GI Tract
Acute viral gastroenteritis.
Bacterial enteritis.
Appendicitis.
Focal Soft Tissue Infections
Cellulitis.
Musculoskeletal System
Osteomyelitis.
Septic arthritis.
Rheumatologic Disorders
Acute rheumatic fever.
Juvenile rheumatoid arthritis.
Henoch-Schönlein purpura.
Vasculitis
Behçet syndrome.
Malignancy
Leukemia.
Lymphoma.
Sarcoma.
Systemic Illness
Bacteremia.
Viremia.
Sepsis.
Kawasaki disease.
Toxic shock syndrome.
Rocky Mountain spotted fever.
Meningococcemia.

MISCELLANEOUS DISORDERS

Toxicologic
Anticholinergic toxidromes.
Salicylate overdose.
Amphetamine.
Cocaine.
Endocrine
Thyrotoxicosis.

FEVER, PERIODIC[53]

ICD-10CM #   R50.9   Fever, unspecified

DIFFERENTIAL DIAGNOSIS OF PERIODIC FEVER

Hereditary.
Nonhereditary.
  Infectious.
    Hidden infectious focus (e.g., aortoenteric fistula, Caroli disease).
    Recurrent reinfection (e.g., chronic meningococcemia, host defense defect).
    Specific infection (e.g., Whipple disease, malaria).
  Noninfectious inflammatory disorder, e.g.:
    Adult-onset Still disease.
    Juvenile chronic rheumatoid arthritis.
    Periodic fever, aphthous stomatitis, pharyngitis, and adenitis.
    Schnitzler syndrome.
    Behçet disease.
    Crohn disease.
    Sarcoidosis.
    Extrinsic alveolitis.
    Humidifier lung, polymer fume fever.
  Neoplastic
Lymphoma (e.g., Hodgkin disease, angioimmunoblastic lymphoma).
  Solid tumor (e.g., pheochromocytoma, myxoma, colon carcinoma).
Vascular (e.g., recurrent pulmonary embolism).
Hypothalamic.
Psychogenic periodic fever.
Factitious or fraudulent.

FEVER, POSTOPERATIVE[4]

ICD-10CM #   R50.9   Fever, unspecified

Infectious

Abscess.
Acalculous cholecystitis.
Bacteremia.
Decubitus ulcers.
Device-related infections.
Empyema.
Endocarditis.
Fungal sepsis.
Hepatitis.
Meningitis.
Osteomyelitis.
Pseudomembranous colitis.
Parotitis.
Perineal infections.
Peritonitis.
Pharyngitis.
Pneumonia.

Retained foreign body.
Sinusitis.
Soft tissue infection.
Tracheobronchitis.
Urinary tract infection.
Noninfectious
Acute hepatic necrosis.
Adrenal insufficiency.
Allergic reaction.
Atelectasis.
Dehydration.
Drug reaction.
Head injury.
Hepatoma.
Hyperthyroidism.
Lymphoma.
Myocardial infarction.
Pancreatitis.
Pheochromocytoma.
Pulmonary embolus.
Retroperitoneal hematoma.
Solid organ hematoma.
Subarachnoid hemorrhage.
Systemic inflammatory response syndrome.
Thrombophlebitis.
Transfusion reaction.
Withdrawal syndromes.
Wound infection.

FEVER, POSTPARTUM[29]

ICD-10CM #	R50.9	Fever, unspecified

MOST COMMON

Metritis.
Urinary tract infection.
Pneumonia.
Wound infection.
Mastitis.
Superficial or deep vein thrombosis.

MOST THREATENING

Toxic shock syndrome.
Necrotizing fasciitis.
Pelvic phlegmon.
Pelvic abscess.
Peritonitis.
Septic pelvic thrombosis.
Breast abscess.

FEVER, RECURRENT OR PERIODIC, IN CHILDREN[19]

ICD-10CM #	R50.2	Drug induced fever
	R50.9	Fever, unspecified

INFECTIOUS DISEASES

Brucellosis.
Rat-bite fever.
Relapsing fever.

RHEUMATIC DISEASES

Juvenile idiopathic arthritis (systemic onset).
Behçet disease.
Systemic lupus erythematosus.
Relapsing polychondritis.
Crohn disease.

HEREDITARY AUTOINFLAMMATORY SYNDROMES

Familial Mediterranean fever (FMF).
Cryopyrinopathies:
  Familial cold autoinflammatory syndrome (FCAS).
  Muckle-Wells syndrome (MWS).
  Chronic infantile neurologic cutaneous and articular (CINCA) syndrome, also called neonatal-onset multisystem inflammatory disease (NOMID).
Tumor necrosis factor receptor–associated periodic syndrome (TRAPS).
Hyperimmunoglobulinemia D with periodic fever syndrome (HIDS).

CYCLIC HEMATOPOIESIS

Hereditary form.
Acquired form.

IDIOPATHIC CONDITIONS

Periodic fever with aphthous stomatitis, pharyngitis, and adenitis (PFAPA).

FEVER WITH MACULOPAPULAR OR PETECHIAL RASH[27]

ICD-10CM #	R21	Rash and nonspecific skin eruption
ICD-10CM #	R50.9	Fever, unspecified

DIFFERENTIAL DIAGNOSIS OF FEVER WITH MACULOPAPULAR OR PETECHIAL RASH

Rocky Mountain spotted fever.
Meningococcal disease.
Enteroviral infection (echovirus and coxsackievirus).
Human herpesvirus 6 infection (roseola).
Human parvovirus B19 infection (fifth disease).
Epstein-Barr virus infection.
Disseminated gonococcal infection.
Murine typhus.
Ehrlichiosis.
Group A streptococcal pharyngitis.
Mycoplasma pneumoniae infection.
Leptospirosis.
Secondary syphilis.
Kawasaki disease.
Thrombotic thrombocytopenic purpura (TTP).
Drug reactions.
Immune complex–mediated illness.
Toxic shock syndrome.
Erythema multiforme.
Stevens-Johnson syndrome.

FEVERS PRONE TO RELAPSE[35]

ICD-10CM #	R50.9	Fever, unspecified

Infectious Causes

Relapsing fever *(Borrelia recurrentis)*.
Q fever *(Coxiella burnetii)*.
Typhoid fever *(Salmonella typhi)*.
Syphilis *(Treponema pallidum)*.
Tuberculosis.
Histoplasmosis.
Coccidioidomycosis.
Blastomycosis.
Melioidosis *(Pseudomonas pseudomallei)*.
Lymphocytic choriomeningitis (LCM) infection.
Dengue fever.
Yellow fever.
Chronic meningococcemia.
Colorado tick fever.
Leptospirosis.
Brucellosis.
Oroya fever *(Bartonella bacilliformis)*.
Acute rheumatic fever.
Rat-bite fever *(Spirillum minus)*.
Visceral leishmaniasis.
Lyme disease *(Borrelia burgdorferi)*.
Malaria.
Babesiosis.
Noninfluenza respiratory viral infection.
Epstein-Barr virus infection.

Noninfectious Causes

Behçet disease.
Crohn disease.
Weber-Christian disease (panniculitis).
Leukoclastic angiitis syndromes.
Sweet syndrome.
Systemic lupus erythematosus and other autoimmune disorders.

Periodic Fever Syndromes

Familial Mediterranean fever.
Cyclic neutropenia.
Periodic fever, aphthous stomatitis, pharyngitis, and adenopathy (PFAPA).
Hyper–immunoglobulin D syndrome.
Hibernian fever (tumor necrosis factor superfamily immunoglobulin A–associated syndrome [TRAPS]).
Muckle-Wells syndrome.
Others.

FINGER LESIONS, INFLAMMATORY

ICD-10CM #	B08.8	Other specified viral infections characterized by skin and mucous membrane lesions
	L03.0	Cellulitis of finger 6

Paronychia.
Herpes simplex type 1 (herpetic whitlow).
Dyshidrotic eczema (pompholyx).
Herpes zoster.
Bacterial endocarditis (Osler nodes).
Psoriatic arthritis.

FLACCID PARALYSIS, ACUTE, DIFFERENTIAL DIAGNOSIS[19]

ICD-10CM #	G83.9	Paralytic syndrome, unspecified

Brain stem stroke.
Brain stem encephalitis.
Acute anterior poliomyelitis.
   Caused by poliovirus.
   Caused by other neurotropic viruses.
Acute myelopathy.
   Space-occupying lesions.
   Acute transverse myelitis.
Peripheral neuropathy.
   Guillain-Barré syndrome.
   Post-rabies vaccine neuropathy.
   Diphtheritic neuropathy.
   Heavy metals, biologic toxins, or drug intoxication.
   Acute intermittent porphyria.
   Vasculitic neuropathy.
   Critical illness neuropathy.
   Lymphomatous neuropathy.
Disorders of neuromuscular transmission.
   Myasthenia gravis.
   Biologic or industrial toxins.
   Tic paralysis.
Disorders of muscle.
   Hypokalemia.
   Hypophosphatemia.
   Inflammatory myopathy.
   Acute rhabdomyolysis.
   Trichinosis.
   Periodic paralyses.

FLATULENCE AND BLOATING[76]

ICD-10CM #	R14.0	Abdominal distention (gaseous)
	R14.1	Gas pain
	R14.2	Eructation
	R14.3	Flatulence

Ingestion of nonabsorbable carbohydrates.
Ingestion of carbonated beverages.
Malabsorption: pancreatic insufficiency, biliary disease, celiac disease, bacterial overgrowth in small intestine.
Lactase deficiency.
Irritable bowel syndrome.
Anxiety disorders.
Food poisoning, giardiasis.

FLOPPY INFANT[38]

ICD-10CM #	P94.2	Congenital hypotonia

DIFFERENTIAL DIAGNOSIS OF THE FLOPPY INFANT

Cerebral hypotonia.
Chromosomal Disorders
Prader-Willi syndrome.
Chronic nonprogressive encephalopathy.
Chronic progressive encephalopathy.
Benign congenital hypotonia.

Combined Cerebral and Motor Unit Disorders
Acid maltase deficiency.
Congenital myotonic dystrophy.
Syndromic congenital muscular dystrophies.
Congenital disorders of glycosylation.
Lysosomal disorders.
Infantile neuroaxonal dystrophy.
Spinal Cord Disorders
Acquired spinal cord lesions.
Spinal muscular atrophy.
Infantile spinal muscular atrophy with respiratory distress.
X-linked spinal muscular atrophy.
Peripheral Nerve Disorders
Congenital hypomyelinating neuropathy/Dejerine-Sottas disease.
Neuromuscular Junction Disorders
Juvenile myasthenia gravis.
Neonatal myasthenia gravis.
Congenital myasthenic syndromes.
Infant botulism.
Muscle Disorders
Congenital myopathies:
   Centronuclear myopathy.
   Nemaline myopathy.
   Central core disease.
Nonsyndromic congenital muscular dystrophies:
   Merosin-deficient congenital muscular dystrophy.
   Ullrich congenital muscular dystrophy.
Other muscular dystrophies:
   Infantile facioscapulohumeral dystrophy.

FLUSHING[80]

ICD-10CM #	R23.2	Flushing

Physiologic flushing: menopause, ingestion of monosodium glutamate (Chinese restaurant syndrome), ingestion of hot drinks.
Drugs: alcohol (with or without disulfiram, metronidazole, or chlorpropamide), nicotinic acid, diltiazem, nifedipine, levodopa, bromocriptine, vancomycin, amyl nitrate.
Neoplastic disorders: carcinoid syndrome, VIPoma syndrome, medullary carcinoma of thyroid, systemic mastocytosis, basophilic chronic myelocytic leukemia, renal cell carcinoma.
Anxiety.
Agnogenic flushing.

FOLATE DEFICIENCY[31]

ICD-10CM #	D52.0	Dietary folate deficiency anemia
	D52.1	Drug-induced folate deficiency anemia
	D52.8	Other folate deficiency anemias
	D52.9	Folate deficiency anemia, unspecified

ETIOPATHOPHYSIOLOGIC CLASSIFICATION OF FOLATE DEFICIENCY

Nutritional causes:
   Decreased dietary intake:
      Poverty and famine.

   Institutionalized individuals (e.g., psychiatric, nursing homes), chronic debilitating disease.
   Prolonged feeding of infants with goat's milk, special slimming diets or food fads (i.e., folate-rich foods not consumed), cultural or ethnic cooking techniques (i.e., food folate destroyed).
Decreased diet and increased requirements:
   Physiologic (e.g., pregnancy and lactation, prematurity, hyperemesis gravidarum, infancy).
   Pathologic (e.g., intrinsic hematologic diseases involving hemolysis with compensatory erythropoiesis, abnormal hematopoiesis, or bone marrow infiltration with malignant disease and dermatologic disease such as psoriasis).
Folate malabsorption:
   With normal intestinal mucosa:
   Some drugs (controversial).
   Congenital folate malabsorption (rare).
   With mucosal abnormalities (e.g., tropical and nontropical sprue, regional enteritis).
Defective cellular folate uptake:
   Familial aplastic anemia (rare).
   Acute cerebral folate deficiency.
Inadequate cellular use:
   Folate antagonists (e.g., methotrexate).
   Hereditary enzyme deficiencies involving folate.
Drugs:
   Multiple effects on folate metabolism (e.g., alcohol, sulfasalazine, triamterene, pyrimethamine, trimethoprim-sulfamethoxazole, diphenylhydantoin, barbiturates).
Acute folate deficiency:
   Intensive care unit setting.
   Uncertain origin.

FOOT AND ANKLE PAIN[8]

ICD-10CM #	M25.5	Pain in joint
	M25.9	Joint disorder, unspecified

TENDON, LIGAMENT, AND MUSCLE

Gastrocnemius-soleus strain.
Plantaris rupture.
Anterior talofibular ligament tear.
Calcaneofibular ligament tear.
Deltoid ligament tear.
Anterolateral impingement due to complete tear of anterior talofibular ligament and anterior inferior tibiofibular ligament.
Syndesmotic impingement due to tear of syndesmosis.
Sinus tarsi syndrome (lateral hindfoot pain and instability due to injury of contents of the sinus and tarsal tunnel).
Achilles tendinitis.
Achilles rupture.
Plantar fasciitis.
Posterior tibial tendon dysfunction.
Flexor hallucis longus dysfunction.
Tibialis anterior tendon tear.
Peroneus brevis tendon tear.

BONE

Fracture of talus.
Calcaneal fracture.
Navicular fractures.
Lisfranc fracture-dislocation (fracture of the first metatarsal base with dislocation of medial cuneiform).
Metatarsal stress fracture.
Freiberg infraction (sclerosis and flattening of the second metatarsal head due to trauma or microtrauma).
Avascular necrosis of the talus.
Fracture of the phalanges.
Fracture of the sesamoids.
Sesamoiditis.
Metatarsalgia.

JOINT

Osteoarthritis.
Gout.
Rheumatoid arthritis.
Other inflammatory arthritides.
Charcot joint.
Osteochondral lesion of the talus.

PERIARTICULAR STRUCTURES

Shin splint (periosteal avulsion and periostitis at the insertion of the medial soleus due to repetitive overuse, such as in running and hiking).
Hallux rigidus.
Hallux valgus.
Ingrown toenail.
Toe deformities.
Turf toe (sprain of the first metatarsophalangeal joint due to hyperextension forces).
Plantar fasciitis.
Plantar fibromatosis.

NERVES

Anterior tarsal tunnel syndrome (involvement of deep peroneal nerve under the superficial fascia of the ankle).
Morton neuroma.

VESSELS

Atherosclerosis.
Compartment syndrome.

REFERRED PAIN

Complex regional pain syndrome.

FOOT AND ANKLE PAIN, IN DIFFERENT AGE GROUPS[41]

ICD-10CM #	M25.579	Pain in unspecified ankle and joints of unspecified foot

COMMON CAUSES OF FOOT AND ANKLE PAIN IN DIFFERENT AGE GROUPS

Childhood (2 to 10 yr)
Intraarticular
Club foot.
Congenital midfoot and forefoot deformities.
Septic arthritis.

Periarticular
Osteomyelitis.
Adolescence (10 to 18 yr)
Intraarticular
Arch disorders (pes cavus, pes planus).
Periarticular
Osteomyelitis.
Tumors.
Early Adulthood (18 to 30 yr)
Intraarticular
Metatarsalgia.
Hallux valgus.
Hallux rigidus.
Osteochondritis.
Accessory ossicles.
Periarticular
Achilles tendonitis.
Achilles tendon rupture.
Fasciitis.
Referred
Lumbar spine.
Knee.
Adulthood (30 to 50 yr)
Intraarticular
Osteoarthritis.
Inflammatory arthritis.
Gout.
Metatarsalgia.
Hallux valgus.
Hallux rigidus.
Osteochondritis.
Accessory ossicles.
Periarticular
Ischemic foot pain.
Diabetes.
Bursitis.
Tendonitis.
Plantar fasciitis.
Corns.
Referred
Lumbar spine.
Knee.
Old Age (>50 yr)
Intraarticular
Osteoarthritis.
Inflammatory arthritis.
Gout.
Metatarsalgia.
Hallux valgus.
Hallux rigidus.
Periarticular
Ischemic foot pain.
Diabetes.
Bursitis.
Tendonitis.
Plantar fasciitis.
Corns.
Referred
Lumbar spine.
Knee.

FOOT DERMATITIS

ICD-10CM #	B35.3	Tinea pedis
	K25	Unspecified contact dermatitis

Tinea pedis.
Dyshidrotic eczema.
Tylosis (mechanically induced hyperkeratosis, fissuring, and dryness).

Allergic contact dermatitis.
Psoriasis.
Peripheral vascular insufficiency.
Neuropathic foot ulcers (diabetes mellitus, poorly fitting shoes).
Acquired plantar keratoderma.
Sézary syndrome.

FOOTDROP

ICD-10CM #	M21.379	Foot drop, unspecified foot

Peripheral neuropathy.
L5 radiculopathy.
Peroneal nerve compression.
Sciatic nerve palsy.
Scapuloperoneal syndromes.
Spasticity.
Peroneal nerve compression.
Myopathy.
Dystonia.

FOOT LESION, ULCERATING

ICD-10CM #	S90.929A	Unspecified superficial injury of unspecified foot, initial encounter
	S90.933A	Unspecified superficial injury of unspecified great toe, initial encounter
	S90.936A	Unspecified superficial injury of unspecified lesser toe(s), initial encounter
	L08.89	Other specified local infections of the skin and subcutaneous tissue

Cellulitis.
Plantar wart.
Squamous cell carcinoma.
Actinomycosis (Madura foot).
Plantar fibromatosis.
Pseudoepitheliomatous hyperplasia.

FOOT PAIN

ICD-10CM #	M25.579	Pain in unspecified ankle and joints of unspecified foot

Trauma (fractures, musculoskeletal and ligamentous strain).
Inflammation (plantar fasciitis, Achilles tendonitis or bursitis, calcaneal apophysitis).
Arterial insufficiency, Raynaud phenomenon, thromboangitis obliterans.
Gout, pseudogout.
Calcaneal spur.
Infection (cellulitis, abscess, lymphangitis, gangrene).
Decubitus ulcer.

Paronychia, ingrown toenail.
Thrombophlebitis, postphlebitic syndrome.

FOOT PAIN BY AGE[19]

ICD-10CM #	M25.579	Pain in unspecified ankle and joints of unspecified foot

0 TO 6 YEARS

Poorly fitting shoes.
Foreign body.
Fracture.
Osteomyelitis.
Leukemia.
Puncture wound.
Drawing of blood.
Dactylitis.
Juvenile rheumatoid arthritis.

6 TO 12 YEARS

Poorly fitting shoes.
Sever disease.
Enthesopathy (JRA).
Foreign body.
Accessory navicular.
Tarsal coalition.
Ewing sarcoma.
Hypermobile flatfoot.
Trauma (sprains, fractures).
Puncture wound.

12 TO 20 YEARS

Poorly fitting shoes.
Stress fracture.
Foreign body.
Ingrown toenail.
Metatarsalgia.
Plantar fasciitis.
Osteochondroses (avascular necrosis).
Freiberg infarction.
Köhler disease.
Achilles tendinitis.
Trauma (sprains).
Plantar warts.
Tarsal coalition.

FOREARM AND HAND PAIN

ICD-10CM #	S59.809A	Other specified injuries of unspecified elbow, initial encounter
	S59.919A	Unspecified injury of unspecified forearm, initial encounter
	S69.80XA	Other specified injuries of unspecified wrist, hand and finger(s), initial encounter
	S69.90XA	Unspecified injury of unspecified wrist, hand and finger(s), initial encounter

Epicondylitis.
Tenosynovitis.
Osteoarthritis.
Cubital tunnel syndrome.
Carpal tunnel syndrome.
Trauma.
Herpes zoster.
Peripheral vascular insufficiency.
Infection (cellulitis, abscess).

FOREARM FRACTURES[18]

ICD-10CM #	S52	Fracture of forearm

TRAUMATIC

Wrist sprain, elbow sprain.
Ligamentous injuries, forearm contusions, hematomas.
Dislocations of the elbow or wrist (including nursemaid's elbow).

INFECTIOUS

Cellulitis of the forearm, abscesses.
Necrotizing fasciitis.

VASCULAR

Acute arterial occlusion.
Venous thrombosis.

NEUROLOGIC

Neurapraxias, carpal tunnel syndrome.
Systemic neurologic syndromes involving the nerves of the upper extremities.

ARTHRITIS

Septic joint, gonococcal arthritis, rheumatoid arthritis, osteoarthritis.
Pseudogout, gout.
Systemic lupus erythematosus, rheumatic fever, viral syndrome.
Reiter syndrome, Lyme disease, serum sickness.

OTHER

Olecranon bursitis, soft tissue masses.
Normal growth plates, nutrient vessels.

GAIT ABNORMALITY

ICD-10CM #	R26.0	Ataxic gait
	R26.1	Paralytic gait
	R26.89	Other abnormalities of gait and mobility
	R26.9	Unspecified abnormalities of gait and mobility

Parkinsonism.
Degenerative joint disease (hips, back, knees).
Multiple sclerosis.
Trauma, foot pain.
Cerebrovascular accident.
Cerebellar lesions.
Infections (tabes, encephalitis, meningitis).
Sensory ataxia.
Dystonia, cerebral palsy, neuromuscular disorders.
Metabolic abnormalities.

GALACTORRHEA[25]

ICD-10CM #	N64.3	Galactorrhea not associated with childbirth

Prolonged suckling.
Drugs (INH, phenothiazines, reserpine derivatives, amphetamines, spironolactone and tricyclic antidepressants).
Major stressors (surgery, trauma).
Hypothyroidism.
Pituitary tumors.

GALLBLADDER SONOGRAPHIC NONVISUALIZATION[15]

ICD-10CM #	Varies with specific diagnosis

CAUSES OF SONOGRAPHIC NONVISUALIZATION OF GALLBLADDER

Previous cholecystectomy.
Physiologic contraction.
Fibrosed gallbladder duct—chronic cholecystitis.
Air-filled gallbladder or emphysematous cholecystitis.
Tumefactive sludge.
Agenesis of gallbladder.
Ectopic location.

GALLBLADDER WALL THICKENING[15]

ICD-10CM #	Varies with specific diagnosis

CAUSES OF GALLBLADDER WALL THICKENING

Generalized Edematous States
Congestive heart failure.
Renal failure.
End-stage cirrhosis.
Hypoalbuminemia.
Inflammatory Conditions
Primary:
  Acute cholecystitis.
  Cholangitis.
  Chronic cholecystitis.
Secondary:
  Acute hepatitis.
  Perforated duodenal ulcer.
  Pancreatitis.
  Diverticulitis/colitis.
Neoplastic Conditions
Gallbladder adenocarcinoma.
Metastases.
Miscellaneous
Adenomyomatosis.
Mural varicosities.

GALLSTONE DISEASE, PEDIATRIC PATIENT[5]

ICD-10CM #	K80.20	Calculus of gallbladder without cholecystitis without obstruction

Differential Diagnosis

II

Biliary tract anomaly (e.g., choledochal cyst).
Cephalosporin use.
Crohn disease.
Cystic fibrosis.
Genetic predisposition (e.g., ABCB4, UGT1A1 mutations).
Hemolytic disorders (e.g., sickle-cell anemia, hereditary spherocytosis).
Hispanic or Latino ancestry.
Malabsorption.
Metabolic syndrome.
Obesity.
Parasitic disease (Ascaris lumbricoides).
Pregnancy.
Rapid weight loss.
Solid organ and hematologic transplant (e.g., liver, kidney, heart, bone marrow).
Total parenteral nutrition.

GASTRIC DILATION[21]

ICD-10CM #	K31.0	Acute dilation of stomach

CAUSES OF A MASSIVELY DILATED STOMACH

Mechanical Gastric Outlet Obstruction
Duodenal or pyloric canal ulceration.
Carcinoma of pyloric antrum.
Extrinsic compression.
Paralytic Ileus
Surgery.
Trauma.
Peritonitis.
Pancreatitis.
Cholecystitis.
Diabetes mellitus.
Hepatic coma.
Drugs.
Gastric Volvulus
Intubation.
Air swallowing.

GASTRIC EMPTYING, DELAYED[18]

ICD-10CM #	K30	Functional dyspepsia

CAUSES OF DELAYED GASTRIC EMPTYING

Mechanical Causes
Peptic ulcer disease, scarred pylorus.
Malignancy: gastric cancer, gastric lymphoma, pancreatic cancer.
Gastric surgery: vagotomy, gastric resection, Roux-en-Y anastomosis.
Crohn disease.
Endocrine and Metabolic Causes
Diabetes mellitus.
Hypothyroidism.
Hypoadrenal states.
Electrolyte abnormalities.
Chronic renal failure.
Medications.
Anticholinergics.
Opiates.
Dopamine agonists.
Tricyclic antidepressants.

Abnormalities of Gastric Smooth Muscle
Scleroderma.
Polymyositis, dermatomyositis.
Amyloidosis.
Pseudoobstruction.
Myotonic dystrophy.
Neuropathy.
Scleroderma.
Amyloidosis.
Autonomic neuropathy.
Central Nervous System or Psychiatric Disorders
Brain stem tumors.
Spinal cord injury.
Anorexia nervosa.
Stress.
Miscellaneous
Idiopathic gastroparesis.
Gastroesophageal reflux disease.
Nonulcer (functional) dyspepsia.
Cancer cachexia or anorexia.

GASTRIC EMPTYING, RAPID

ICD-10CM #	K30	Functional dyspepsia

Pancreatic insufficiency.
Dumping syndrome.
Peptic ulcer.
Celiac disease.
Promotility agents.
Zollinger-Ellison disease.

GASTROINTESTINAL BLEEDING, PEDIATRIC PATIENT[68]

ICD-10CM #	K92.2	Gastrointestinal hemorrhage, unspecified

INFANT

Common
Bacterial enteritis.
Milk protein allergy intolerance.
Intussusception.
Swallowed maternal blood.
Anal fissure.
Lymphonodular hyperplasia
Rare
Volvulus.
Necrotizing enterocolitis.
Meckel diverticulum.
Stress ulcer, gastritis.
Coagulation disorder (hemorrhagic disease of newborn).
Esophagitis.

CHILD

Common
Bacterial enteritis.
Anal fissure.
Colonic polyps.
Intussusception.
Peptic ulcer/gastritis.
Swallowed epistaxis.
Prolapse (traumatic) gastropathy secondary to emesis.
Mallory-Weiss syndrome.

Rare
Esophageal varices.
Esophagitis.
Meckel diverticulum.
Lymphonodular hyperplasia.
Henoch-Schönlein purpura.
Foreign body.
Hemangioma, arteriovenous malformation.
Sexual abuse.
Hemolytic-uremic syndrome.
Inflammatory bowel disease.
Coagulopathy.
   Duplication cyst:
   Angiodysplasia.
   Angiodysplasia with von Willebrand disease.
   Blue rubber bleb nevus syndrome.

ADOLESCENT

Common
Bacterial enteritis.
Inflammatory bowel disease.
Peptic ulcer/gastritis.
Prolapse (traumatic) gastropathy secondary to emesis.
Mallory-Weiss syndrome.
Colonic polyps.
Anal fissure.
Rare
Hemorrhoids.
Esophageal varices.
Esophagitis.
Pill ulcer.
Telangiectasia-angiodysplasia.
Graft-versus-host disease.
   Duplication cyst:
   Angiodysplasia.
   Angiodysplasia with von Willebrand disease.
   Blue rubber bleb nevus syndrome.

GASTROINTESTINAL OBSTRUCTION, PEDIATRIC PATIENT[68]

ICD-10CM #	K56.2K5.1K56.9 K56.6	Volvulus Intussusception Ileus unspecified Other and unspecified intestinal obstruction

Esophagus
Congenital
Esophageal atresia.
Vascular rings.
Schatzki ring.
Tracheobronchial remnant.
Acquired
Esophageal stricture.
Foreign body.
Achalasia.
Chagas disease.
Collagen vascular disease.
Stomach
Congenital
Antral webs.
Pyloric stenosis.
Acquired

Bezoar, foreign body.
Pyloric stricture (ulcer).
Chronic granulomatous disease of childhood.
Eosinophilic gastroenteritis.
Crohn disease.
Epidermolysis bullosa.

Small Intestine

Congenital

Duodenal atresia.
Annular pancreas.
Malrotation/volvulus.
Malrotation/Ladd bands.
Ileal atresia.
Meconium ileus.
Meckel diverticulum with volvulus or
    intussusception.
Inguinal hernia.
Internal hernia.
Intestinal duplication.
Pseudoobstruction.

Acquired

Postsurgical adhesions.
Crohn disease.
Intussusception.
Distal ileal obstruction syndrome (cystic fibrosis).
Duodenal hematoma.
Superior mesenteric artery syndrome.

Colon

Congenital

Meconium plug.
Hirschsprung disease.
Colonic atresia, stenosis.
Imperforate anus.
Rectal stenosis.
Pseudoobstruction.
Volvulus.
Colonic duplication.

Acquired

Ulcerative colitis (toxic megacolon).
Chagas disease.
Crohn disease.
Fibrosing colonopathy (cystic fibrosis).

GASTROINTESTINAL SYMPTOMS IN CHILDREN, NONDIGESTIVE CAUSES[68]

ICD-10CM # Varies with specific diagnosis

Anorexia

Systemic disease: inflammatory, neoplastic.
Cardiorespiratory compromise.
Iatrogenic: drug therapy, unpalatable therapeutic
    diets.
Depression.
Anorexia nervosa.

Vomiting

Inborn errors of metabolism.
Medications: erythromycin, chemotherapy,
    NSAIDs, marijuana.
Increased intracranial pressure.
Brain tumor.
Infection of the urinary tract.
Labyrinthitis.
Adrenal insufficiency.
Pregnancy.
Psychogenic.
Abdominal migraine.
Poisoning/toxins.
Renal disease.

Diarrhea

Infection: otitis media, urinary tract infection.
Uremia.
Medications: antibiotics, cisapride.
Tumors: neuroblastoma.
Pericarditis.
Adrenal insufficiency.

Constipation

Hypothyroidism.
Spina bifida.
Developmental delay.
Dehydration: diabetes insipidus, renal tubular
    lesions.
Medications: narcotics.
Lead poisoning.
Infant botulism.

Abdominal Pain

Pyelonephritis, hydronephrosis, renal colic.
Pneumonia (lower lobe).
Pelvic inflammatory disease.
Porphyria.
Fabry disease.
Angioedema.
Endocarditis.
Abdominal migraine.
Familial Mediterranean fever.
Sexual or physical abuse.
Systemic lupus erythematosus.
School phobia.
Sickle cell crisis.
Vertebral disk inflammation.
Psoas abscess.
Pelvic osteomyelitis or myositis.
Medications.

Abdominal Distention or Mass

Ascites: nephrotic syndrome, neoplasm, heart
    failure.
Discrete mass: Wilms tumor, hydronephrosis,
    neuroblastoma, mesenteric cyst, hepato-
    blastoma, lymphoma.
Pregnancy.

Jaundice

Hemolytic disease.
Urinary tract infection.
Sepsis.
Hypothyroidism.
Panhypopituitarism.

GAZE PALSIES[20]

ICD-10CM # Varies with specific diagnosis

APRAXIA OF HORIZONTAL GAZE

Ataxia-telangiectasia.
Ataxia-ocular motor apraxia.
Brain stem glioma.
Congenital ocular motor apraxia.
Huntington disease.

INTERNUCLEAR OPHTHALMOPLEGIA

Brain stem stroke.
Brain stem tumor.
Exotropia (pseudo-internuclear ophthalmoplegia
    [INO]).
Multiple sclerosis.
Myasthenia gravis (pseudo-INO).
Toxic-metabolic.

VERTICAL GAZE PALSY

Aqueductal stenosis.
Congenital vertical ocular motor apraxia.
Gaucher disease.
Hydrocephalus.
Miller Fisher syndrome.
Niemann-Pick disease type C.
Tumor:
    Midbrain.
    Pineal region.
    Third ventricle.

HORIZONTAL GAZE PALSY

Adversive seizures.
Brain stem tumors.
Destructive lesions of the frontal lobe.
Familial horizontal gaze palsy.

CONVERGENCE PARALYSIS

Head trauma.
Idiopathic.
Multiple sclerosis.
Pineal region tumors.

GENITAL DISCHARGE, FEMALE[55]

ICD-10CM # N94.9 Unspecified condition
                        associated with
                        female genital organs
                        and menstrual cycle

Physiologic discharge: cervical mucus, vaginal
    transudation, bacteria, squamous epithelial
    cells.
Individual variation.
Pregnancy.
Sexual response.
Menstrual cycle variation.
Infection.
Foreign body: tampon, cervical cap, other.
Neoplasm.
Fistula.
IUD.
Cervical ectropion.
Spermicide.
Nongenital causes: urinary incontinence, urinary
    tract fistula, Crohn disease, rectovaginal fistula.

GENITAL LESIONS, INFECTIOUS CAUSES[42]

ICD-10CM # Varies with specific diagnosis

INFECTIOUS CAUSES OF GENITAL LESIONS

Sexually Transmitted Infections

Syphilis:
    Primary (chancre).
    Secondary (condyloma latum).
Herpes simplex virus types 1 and 2.
Chancroid *(Haemophilus ducreyi)*.
Lymphogranuloma venereum.
Granuloma inguinale (donovanosis).
Human papillomavirus.
Sarcoptes scabiei.
Molluscum contagiosum.

Nonsexually Transmitted Infections

Folliculitis.

Tuberculosis.
Tularemia.
Histoplasmosis.
Candida (balanitis or vaginitis).
Amebiasis.

GENITAL LESIONS, NONINFECTIOUS CAUSES[42]

ICD-10CM #	Varies with specific diagnosis

NONVENEREAL CAUSES OF GENITAL LESIONS

Trauma.
Malignancies (e.g., squamous cell carcinoma).
Behçet syndrome.
Lipschütz vulvar ulcers.
Peyronie disease.
Fixed-drug eruption.
Eczema.
Psoriasis.
Inflammatory bowel disease.
Contact dermatitis.
Lichen planus.
Hidradenitis suppurativa.
Postinflammatory hypopigmentation.
Aphthous ulcers (associated with HIV).

GENITAL SORES[18]

ICD-10CM #	A60.9	Anogenital herpesviral infection, unspecified
	A51.0	Primary genital syphilis
	A63.0	Anogenital (venereal) warts
	A57	Chancroid
	A58	Granuloma inguinale
	A55	Chlamydial lymphogranuloma (venereum)
	N94.89	Other specified conditions associated with female genital organs and menstrual cycle
	N50.8	Other specified disorders of male genital organs

Herpes genitalis.
Syphilis.
Chancroid.
Lymphogranuloma venereum.
Granuloma inguinale.
Condyloma acuminatum.
Neoplastic lesion.
Trauma.

GLOMERULONEPHRITIS ASSOCIATED WITH MALIGNANCY[11]

ICD-10CM #	N00.9	Acute nephritic syndrome with unspecified morphologic changes

Membranous glomerulonephritis:
Breast cancer.
Lung cancer.
Colon cancer.
Prostate cancer.
Graft-versus-host disease.
Minimal change disease:
Hodgkin lymphoma.
Non-Hodgkin lymphoma.
Graft-versus-host disease.
Case reports.
Immunoglobulin A nephritis.
Antineutrophil cytoplasmic antibody vasculitis.
Focal segmental glomerulosclerosis.

GLOMERULONEPHRITIS, RAPIDLY PROGRESSIVE[18]

ICD-10CM #	N05.9	Unspecified nephritic syndrome with unspecified morphologic changes

DIFFERENTIAL DIAGNOSIS OF RAPIDLY PROGRESSIVE GLOMERULONEPHRITIS

Linear Immune Staining
Anti-GBM disease.
Goodpasture syndrome.
Rarely membranous glomerulonephritis.
Granular Immune Staining
Subacute bacterial endocarditis (past infectious).
Lupus nephritis.
Cryoglobulinemia.
Membranoproliferative glomerulonephritis (type II more than type I).
Immunoglobulin A nephropathy, Henoch-Schönlein purpura.
Idiopathic.
No Immune Staining (Pauci-immune)
Antineutrophil cytoplasmic antibody-associated vasculitis (Wegener granulomatosis, microscopic polyangiitis, Churg-Strauss syndrome).
Idiopathic.

GLOMERULOPATHIES, THROMBOTIC, MICROANGIOPATHIC[18]

ICD-10CM #	M31.1	Thrombotic microangiopathy

THROMBOTIC MICROANGIOPATHIC GLOMERULOPATHIES

Thrombotic thrombocytopenic purpura.
Hemolytic-uremic syndrome.
Malignant hypertension.
Scleroderma renal crisis.
Preeclampsia, eclampsia.
HELLP syndrome (hemolysis, elevated liver enzymes, low platelets).
Antiphospholipid antibody syndrome.
Drugs: oral contraceptives, quinine, cyclosporine, tacrolimus, ticlopidine, clopidogrel.

GLOMERULOSCLEROSIS, FOCAL SEGMENTAL[18]

ICD-10CM #	N03.3	Chronic nephritic syndrome with diffuse mesangial proliferative glomerulonephritis

ETIOLOGY OF FOCAL SEGMENTAL GLOMERULOSCLEROSIS (FSGS)

Primary idiopathic FSGS.
Secondary FSGS.
HIV (usually collapsing variant).
Reflux nephropathy.
Heroin abuse.
Sickle cell disease.
Oligomeganephronia.
Renal dysgenesis or agenesis (low nephron mass).
Radiation nephritis.
Familial podocytopathies.
NPHS1 (nephrin) mutation.
NPHS2 (podocin) mutation.
TRPC6 (cation channel) mutation.
ACTN4 (a-actinin 4 mutation).

GLOSSODYNIA[2]

ICD-10CM #	K14.6	Glossodynia

DENTURE-RELATED

Dentures (ill-fitting, monomer from denture base).
Dental plaque.
Oral parafunction.

INFECTIVE/DERMATOLOGIC

Candidiasis.
Lichen planus.

DEFICIENCY STATES

Iron, vitamin B_{12}, folate, B_2 (riboflavin), B_6 (pyridoxine), zinc.

ENDOCRINE

Diabetes.
Myxedema.
Hormonal changes occurring during menopause.

NEUROLOGICALLY MEDIATED

Referred from tonsils, teeth.
Lingual nerve neuropathy.
Glossopharyngeal neuralgia.
Esophageal reflux.

IATROGENIC

Mouthwash.
Xerostomia

GLUCOCORTICOID DEFICIENCY[24]

ICD-10CM #	E27.1	Primary adrenocortical insufficiency
	E27.3	Drug-induced adrenocortical insufficiency

Adrenocorticotropic hormone (ACTH)-independent causes.
TB.
Autoimmune (idiopathic).
Other rare causes:
  Fungal infection.
  Adrenal hemorrhage.
  Metastases.
  Sarcoidosis.
  Amyloidosis.
  Adrenoleukodystrophy.
  Adrenomyeloneuropathy.
  HIV infection.
  Congenital adrenal hyperplasia.
  Medications (e.g., ketoconazole).
ACTH-dependent causes:
  Hypothalamic-pituitary-adrenal suppression.
  Exogenous.
  Glucocorticoid.
  ACTH.
  Endogenous—cure of Cushing syndrome.
Hypothalamic-pituitary lesions.
  Neoplasm:
    Primary pituitary tumor.
    Metastatic tumor.
    Craniopharyngioma.
  Infection:
    Tuberculosis.
    Actinomycosis.
    Nocardiosis.
    Sarcoid.
    Head trauma.
    Isolated ACTH deficiency.

GOITER

ICD-10CM #	E01.2	Iodine-deficiency related (endemic) goiter, unspecified
	E04.9	Nontoxic goiter, unspecified
	E04.9	Nontoxic goiter, unspecified
	E07.1	Dyshormonogenetic goiter
	E01.2	Iodine-deficiency related (endemic) goiter, unspecified
	E04.9	Nontoxic goiter, unspecified
	E04.2	Nontoxic multinodular goiter
	E04.0	Nontoxic diffuse goiter
	E05.10	Thyrotoxicosis with toxic single thyroid nodule without thyrotoxic crisis or storm

Thyroiditis.
Toxic multinodular goiter.
Graves disease.
Medications (PTU, methimazole, sulfonamides, sulfonylureas, ethionamide, amiodarone, lithium, etc.).
Iodine deficiency.
Sarcoidosis, amyloidosis.
Defective thyroid hormone synthesis.
Resistance to thyroid hormone.

GRANULOMATOUS DERMATITIDES

ICD-10CM #	L92.9	Granulomatous disorder of the skin and subcutaneous tissue, unspecified

Granuloma annulare.
Sarcoidosis.
Necrobiosis lipoidica diabeticorum.
Cutaneous Crohn disease.
Rheumatoid nodules.
Annular elastolytic giant cell granuloma (actinic granuloma).
Foreign body granuloma.

GRANULOMATOUS DISORDERS[81]

ICD-10CM #	M31.30	Granulomatosis with polyangiitis without renal involvement
	K75.3	Granulomatous hepatitis
	L92.9	Granulomatous disorder of skin and subcutaneous tissue, unspecified

INFECTIONS
Fungi
Histoplasma.
Coccidioides.
Blastomyces.
Sporothrix.
Aspergillus.
Cryptococcus.
Protozoa
Toxoplasma.
Leishmania.
Metazoa
Toxocara.
Schistosoma.
Spirochetes
Treponema pallidum.
T. pertenue.
T. carateum.
Mycobacteria
M. tuberculosis.
M. leprae.
M. kansasii.
M. marinum.
M. avian.
Bacille Calmette-Guérin (BCG) vaccine.
Bacteria
Brucella.
Yersinia.
Other Infections
Cat-scratch disease.
Lymphogranuloma.

NEOPLASIA
Carcinoma.
Reticulosis.
Pinealoma.
Dysgerminoma.
Seminoma.
Reticulum cell sarcoma.
Malignant nasal granuloma.

CHEMICALS
Beryllium.
Zirconium.
Silica.
Starch.

IMMUNOLOGIC ABERRATIONS
Sarcoidosis.
Crohn disease.
Primary biliary cirrhosis.
Granulomatosis with polyangiitis.
Giant cell arteritis.
Peyronie disease.
Hypogammaglobulinemia.
Systemic lupus erythematosus.
Lymphomatoid granulomatosis.
Histiocytosis X.
Hepatic granulomatous disease.
Immune complex disease.
Rosenthal-Melkersson syndrome.
Churg-Strauss allergic granulomatosis.

LEUKOCYTE OXIDASE DEFECT
Chronic granulomatous disease of childhood.

EXTRINSIC ALLERGIC ALVEOLITIS
Farmer's lung.
Bird fancier's.
Mushroom worker's.
Suberosis (cork dust).
Bagassosis.
Maple bark stripper's.
Paprika splitter's.
Coffee bean.
Spatlese lung.

OTHER DISORDERS
Whipple disease.
Pyrexia of unknown origin.
Radiotherapy.
Cancer chemotherapy.
Panniculitis.
Chalazion.
Sebaceous cyst.
Dermoid.
Sea urchin spine injury.

GRANULOMATOUS LIVER DISEASE

ICD-10CM #	K75.3	Granulomatous hepatitis

Sarcoidosis.
Granulomatosis with polyangiitis.
Vasculitis.
Inflammatory bowel disease.
Allergic granulomatosis.
Erythema nodosum.
Infections (fungal, viral, parasitic).
Primary biliary cirrhosis.
Lymphoma.
Hodgkin disease.
Drugs (e.g., allopurinol, hydralazine, sulfonamides, penicillins).
Toxins (copper sulfate, beryllium).

Differential Diagnosis

II

GREEN OR BLUE URINE

ICD-10CM #   R82   Other abnormal findings
                      in urine

Pseudomonal urinary tract infection
Medications: triamterene, amitriptyline, intravenous cimetidine, intravenous promethazine.
Biliverdin.
Dyes (methylene blue, indigo carmine).

GROIN AND SCROTAL MASSES[4]

ICD-10CM #   Code varies with specific
                diagnosis

DIFFERENTIAL DIAGNOSIS OF GROIN AND SCROTAL MASSES

Inguinal hernia.
Hydrocele.
Varicocele.
Ectopic testis.
Epididymitis.
Testicular torsion.
Lipoma.
Hematoma.
Sebaceous cyst.
Hidradenitis of inguinal apocrine glands.
Inguinal lymphadenopathy.
Lymphoma.
Metastatic neoplasm.
Femoral hernia.
Femoral lymphadenopathy.
Femoral artery aneurysm or pseudoaneurysm.

GROIN LUMP[2]

ICD-10CM #   R19.09   Other intraabdominal
                        and pelvic swelling,
                        mass and lump
             R22.9   Localized swelling,
                        mass and lump,
                        unspecified

COMMON CAUSES

Inguinal hernia.
Femoral hernia.
Lymph node.

OTHER CAUSES

Saphena varix.
Femoral artery aneurysm/pseudoaneurysm.
Psoas abscess.
Lipoma of the cord.
Encysted hydrocele of the cord (male).
Testicular maldescent (male).
Hydrocele of canal of Nuck (female).

GROIN MASSES

ICD-10CM #   R22.9   Localized swelling,
                        mass and lump,
                        unspecified
             S39.848A Other specified
                        injuries of external
                        genitals, initial
                        encounter

Hernia (inguinal, femoral).
Hydrocele.
Varicocele.
Sebaceous cyst.
Hidradenitis of inguinal apocrine glands.
Neoplasm: lymphoma, metastases.
Lipoma.
Hematoma.
Reactive inguinal adenopathy, femoral adenitis.
Folliculitis, psoas abscess.
Epididymitis, testicular torsion, ectopic testes.
Aneurysm or pseudoaneurysm of femoral artery.

GROIN PAIN[64]

ICD-10CM #   R52   Pain, unspecified

DIFFERENTIAL DIAGNOSIS OF GROIN PAIN

Surgery
Workers' compensation.
Hernia.
Recurrent hernia.
Posthernia.
Orthopedic
Hip disorders:
   Acetabular labral tears.
   Avascular necrosis.
   Chondritis dissecans.
   Legg-Calvé-Perthes disease.
   Osteoarthritis.
   Pelvic stress fractures.
   Slipped femoral capital epiphysis.
   Synovitis.
Urology
Cystitis.
Epididymitis.
Nephrolithiasis.
Prostate cancer.
Prostatitis.
Torsion of testes.
Urethral extravasation.
Urinary tract infection.
Vas granuloma/fibrosis.
Dermatology
Lymphadenitis.
Psoriasis/burn.
Sebaceous cyst/hidradenitis.
Thrombophlebitis/cellulitis.
Neurosurgery
Disk disease.
Spinal injuries, inflammation, tumors.
Spondylolisthesis.
Spondylolysis.
Rheumatology
Connective tissue disorders.
Iliopsoas bursitis.
Osteitis pubis.
Systemic lupus erythematosus.
Neurology
Lumbosacral disorders.
Neurofibromatosis.
Infectious Disease
Herpes zoster.
HIV/tuberculosis.
Lyme disease.
Psoas abscess.
Sports Medicine
"Sports hernia" (adductor strains).
Gilmore groin.

Vascular
Abscess hematoma.
Postvein stripping.
Pseudoaneurysm.
Vascular graft.
Gastroenterology
Appendicitis/adhesions.
Diverticulitis.
Inflammatory retroperitoneal phlegmon (pancreatitis).
Meckel diverticulum.
Granulomatous colitis.
Gynecology
Cesarean delivery.
Cervical cancer.
Endometriosis.
Tubal/ovarian disorders.

GROIN PAIN, ACTIVE PATIENT[82]

ICD-10CM #   S39.848A Other specified
                        injuries of
                        external
                        genitals, initial
                        encounter
             R52   Pain, unspecified

MUSCULOSKELETAL

Avascular necrosis of the femoral head.
Avulsion fracture (lesser trochanter, anterior superior iliac spine, anterior inferior iliac spine).
Bursitis (iliopectineal, trochanteric).
Entrapment of the ilioinguinal or iliofemoral nerve.
Gracilis syndrome.
Muscle tear (adductors, iliopsoas, rectus abdominis, gracilis, sartorius, rectus femoris).
Myositis ossificans of the hip muscles.
Osteitis pubis.
Osteoarthritis of the femoral head.
Slipped capital femoral epiphysis.
Stress fracture of the femoral head or neck and pubis.
Synovitis.

HERNIA-RELATED

Avulsion of the internal oblique muscle in the conjoined tendon.
Defect at the insertion of the rectus abdominis muscle.
Direct inguinal hernia.
Femoral ring hernia.
Indirect inguinal hernia.
Inguinal canal weakness.

UROLOGIC

Epididymitis.
Fracture of the testis.
Hydrocele.
Kidney stone.
Posterior urethritis.
Prostatitis.
Testicular cancer.
Torsion of the testis.
Urinary tract infection.
Varicocele.

GYNECOLOGIC

Ectopic pregnancy.
Ovarian cyst.
Pelvic inflammatory disease.
Torsion of the ovary.
Vaginitis.
Lymphatic enlargement in groin.

GROIN PAIN, ATHLETES[83]

ICD-10CM #	R52	Pain, unspecified

DIFFERENTIAL DIAGNOSIS OF GROIN PAIN IN ATHLETES

Hip-Associated Causes
Acetabular labral tear and femoroacetabular impingement.
Osteoarthritis.
Snapping hip syndrome and iliopsoas tendonitis.
Avascular necrosis.
Iliotibial band syndrome.
Visceral Causes
Inguinal hernia.
Other abdominal hernias.
Testicular torsion.
Infectious Causes
Septic arthritis.
Osteomyelitis.
Pelvic inflammatory disease.
Prostatitis.
Epididymitis and orchitis.
Herpes infection.
Inflammatory Causes
Endometriosis.
Inflammatory bowel disease.
Pelvic inflammatory disease.
Primary osteitis pubis.
Traumatic Causes
Stress fracture.
Tendon avulsion.
Muscle contusion.
Baseball pitcher–hockey goalie syndrome.
Developmental Causes
Apophysitis.
Growth plate stress injury or fracture.
Legg-Calvé-Perthes disease.
Developmental dysplasia.
Slipped capital femoral epiphysis.
Neurologic Causes
Nerve entrapment syndromes.
Referred pain.
Sacroiliitis.
Sciatic entrapment (piriformis syndrome).
Hamstring strain.
Knee pain.
Neoplastic Causes
Testicular carcinoma.
Osteoid osteoma.

GYNECOMASTIA

ICD-10CM #	N62	Hypertrophy of breast

Physiologic (puberty, newborns, aging).
Drugs (estrogen and estrogen precursors, 5-a reductase inhibitors, digitalis, testosterone and exogenous androgens, clomiphene, cimetidine, spironolactone, ketoconazole, amiodarone, ACE inhibitors, isoniazid, phenytoin, methyldopa, metoclopramide, phenothiazine).

Increased prolactin level (prolactinoma).
Liver disease.
Adrenal disease.
Thyrotoxicosis.
Increased estrogen production (hCG-producing tumor, testicular tumor, bronchogenic carcinoma).
Secondary hypogonadism.
Primary gonadal failure (trauma, castration, viral orchitis, granulomatous disease).
Defects in androgen synthesis.
Testosterone deficiency.
Klinefelter syndrome.

HAIR LOSS[84]

ICD-10CM #	L63.8	Other alopecia areata
	L63.9	Alopecia areata, unspecified
	L64.0	Drug-induced androgenic alopecia
	L64.8	Other androgenic alopecia

GENERALIZED

Acute blood loss.*
Childbirth.
Crash diets (inadequate protein).
Drugs:
    Coumarin.
    Heparin.
    Propranolol.
    Vitamin A.
    High fever.
Hypothyroidism and hyperthyroidisms.
Physical stress (e.g., surgery).
Physiologic stress (e.g., neonate).
Psychologic stress.
Severe illness (e.g., systemic lupus erythematosus).
Cancer chemotherapeutic agents.
Poisoning:
    Thallium (rat poison).
    Arsenic.
Radiation therapy.
Secondary syphilis: "moth eaten" alopecia.

LOCALIZED

Androgenetic alopecia.†
    Male pattern.
    Female pattern.
Hirsutism.
Alopecia areata.
Trichotillomania.
Traction alopecia.
Scarring alopecia:
    Developmental defects: aplasia cutis.
Physical injury: burns, pressure.
Infection:
    Fungal: kerion.
    Bacterial: folliculitis, furuncle.
    Viral: herpes zoster.
Neoplasms:
    Metastatic carcinoma.
    Sclerosing basal cell carcinoma.
Lupus erythematosus.
Lichen planus.
Cicatricial pemphigoid.
Scleroderma.

*Diffuse, uniform loss, but many hairs left randomly distributed in area of loss.
†Most or all hair missing from involved area.

HALITOSIS

ICD-10CM #	R19.6	Halitosis

Tobacco use.
Alcohol use.
Dry mouth (mouth breathing, inadequate fluid intake).
Foods (onion, garlic, meats, nuts, protein drinks).
Disease of mouth or nose (infections, cancer, inflammation).
Medications (antihistamines, antidepressants).
Systemic disorders (diabetes, uremia).
GI disorders (esophageal diverticula, hiatal hernia, gastroesophageal reflux disease, achalasia).
Sinusitis.
Pulmonary disorders (bronchiectasis, pneumonia, neoplasms, TB).

HALLUCINATIONS, VISUAL, NEUROLOGIC CAUSES[72]

ICD-10CM #	R44.1	Visual hallucinations

Blindness/sensory deprivation—Charles Bonnet syndrome.
Palinopsia.
Dementia-producing diseases:
    Alzheimer.
    Dementia with Lewy bodies.*
    Parkinson.†
Intoxications:
    Alcoholic hallucinosis.
    Delirium tremens (DTs).
Hallucinogens:
    Amphetamines.
    Cocaine.
    Lysergic acid diethylamide (LSD).
    Phencyclidine (PCP).
Medicines:
    Atropine, scopolamine.
    Levodopa and dopamine agonists.
    Steroids.
Migraine with aura (classic migraine).
Narcolepsy: hypnopompic (awakening) and hypnagogic (falling asleep) hallucinations.
Seizures.
Peduncular hallucinations.

*Although visual hallucinations are likely to complicate almost any form of dementia, they are characteristic of dementia with Lewy bodies disease.
†Dopaminergic medications such as levodopa-carbidopa (Sinemet) are more likely than Parkinson disease itself to produce hallucinations.

HAND PAIN AND SWELLING[40]

ICD-10CM #	729.5	Pain in limb

Trauma.
Gout.
Pseudogout.
Cellulitis.
Lymphangitis.
Deep vein thrombosis of upper extremity.
Thrombophlebitis.
Rheumatoid arthritis.
Remitting seronegative symmetrical synovitis with pitting edema (RS3PE).
Polymyalgia rheumatica.

Mixed connective tissue disease.
Scleroderma.
Rupture of the olecranon bursa.
Metzger syndrome (neoplasia).
The puffy hand of drug addiction.
Reflex sympathetic dystrophy.
Eosinophilic fasciitis.
Sickle cell (hand-foot syndrome).
Leprosy.
Factitial (the rubber band syndrome).

HEADACHE[85]

ICD-10CM #	G44.1	Vascular headache, not elsewhere classified
	R51	Headache
	G44.209	Tension-type headache, unspecified, not intractable
	G44.009	Cluster headache syndrome, unspecified, not intractable
	G43.909	Migraine, unspecified, not intractable, without status migrainosus
	G44.1	Vascular headache, not elsewhere classified

Vascular: migraine, cluster headaches, temporal arteritis, hypertension, cavernous sinus thrombosis.
Musculoskeletal: neck and shoulder muscle contraction, strain of extraocular and/or intraocular muscles, cervical spondylosis, temporomandibular arthritis.
Infections: meningitis, encephalitis, brain abscess, sepsis, sinusitis, osteomyelitis, parotitis, mastoiditis.
Cerebral neoplasm.
Subdural hematoma.
Cerebral hemorrhage/infarct.
Pseudotumor cerebri.
Normal-pressure hydrocephalus (NPH).
Postlumbar puncture.
Cerebral aneurysm, arteriovenous malformations.
Posttrauma.
Dental problems: abscess, periodontitis, poorly fitting dentures.
Trigeminal neuralgia, glossopharyngeal neuralgia.
Otitis and other ear diseases.
Glaucoma and other eye diseases.
Metabolic: uremia, carbon monoxide inhalation, hypoxia.
Pheochromocytoma, hypoglycemia, hypothyroidism.
Effort induced: benign exertional headache, cough, headache, coital cephalalgia.
Drugs: alcohol, nitrates, histamine antagonists.
Paget disease of the skull.
Emotional, psychiatric.

HEADACHE, ACUTE[46]

ICD-10CM #	R51	Headache

DIFFERENTIAL DIAGNOSIS OF ACUTE HEADACHE

Evaluation of the first acute headache should exclude pathologic causes listed here before consideration of more common etiologies.
Increased intracranial pressure (ICP): trauma, hemorrhage, tumor, hydrocephalus, pseudotumor cerebri, abscess, arachnoid cyst, cerebral edema.
Decreased ICP: after ventriculoperitoneal shunt, lumbar puncture, cerebrospinal fluid leak from basilar skull fracture.
Meningeal inflammation: meningitis, leukemia, subarachnoid or subdural hemorrhage.
Vascular: vasculitis, arteriovenous malformation, hypertension, cerebrovascular accident.
Bone, soft tissue: referred pain from scalp, eyes, ears, sinuses, nose, teeth, pharynx, cervical spine, temporomandibular joint.
Infection: systemic infection, encephalitis, sinusitis, etc.
First migraine.

HEADACHE AND FACIAL PAIN[17]

ICD-10CM #	R51	Headache
	G44.1	Vascular headache, not elsewhere classified

VASCULAR HEADACHES

Migraine
Migraine with headaches and inconspicuous neurologic features:
　Migraine without aura ("common migraine").
Migraine with headaches and conspicuous neurologic features:
　With transient neurologic symptoms:
　　Migraine with typical aura ("classic migraine").
　　Sensory, basilar, and hemiplegic migraine.
With prolonged or permanent neurologic features ("complicated migraine"):
　Ophthalmoplegic migraine.
　Migrainous infarction.
Migraine without headaches but with conspicuous neurologic features ("migraine equivalents"):
　Abdominal migraine.
　Benign paroxysmal vertigo of childhood.
　Migraine aura without headache ("isolated auras," transient migrainous accompaniments).
Cluster Headaches
Episodic cluster headache ("cyclic cluster headaches").
Chronic cluster headaches.
Chronic paroxysmal hemicrania.
Other Vascular Headaches
Headaches of reactive vasodilation (fever, drug-induced, post-ictal, hypoglycemia, hypoxia, hypercarbia, hyperthyroidism).
Headaches associated with arterial hypertension:
　Chronic severe hypertension (diastolic 120 mm Hg).
　Paroxysmal severe hypertension (pheochromocytoma, some coital headaches).
Headaches caused by cranial arteritis:
　Giant cell arteritis ("temporal arteritis").
　Other vasculitides.

HEADACHES ASSOCIATED WITH DEMONSTRABLE MUSCLE SPASM

Headache caused by posturally induced or perilesional muscle spasm:
　Headaches of sustained or impaired posture (e.g., prolonged close work, driving).
　Headaches associated with cervical spondylosis and other diseases of cervical spine.
　Myofascial pain dysfunction syndrome (headache or facial pain associated with disorders of teeth, jaws, and related structures, or "TMJ syndrome").
Headaches caused by psychophysiologic muscular contraction ("muscle contraction headaches," or tension-type headache associated with disorder of pericranial muscles).

HEADACHES AND FACIAL PAIN WITHOUT DEMONSTRABLE PHYSICAL SUBSTRATE

Headaches of uncertain etiology:
　"Tension headaches" (tension-type headache unassociated with disorder of pericranial muscles).
　Some forms of posttraumatic headache.
Psychogenic headaches (e.g., hypochondriacal, conversional, delusional, malingered).
Facial pain of uncertain etiology ("atypical facial pain").

COMBINED TENSION-MIGRAINE HEADACHES

Episodic migraine superimposed on chronic tension headaches.
Chronic daily headaches:
　Associated with analgesic and/or ergotamine overuse ("rebound headaches").
　Not associated with drug overuse.

HEADACHES AND HEAD PAINS CAUSED BY DISEASES OF EYES, EARS, NOSE, SINUSES, TEETH, OR SKULL

Headaches Caused by Meningeal Inflammation
Subarachnoid hemorrhage.
Meningitis and meningoencephalitis.
Others (e.g., meningeal carcinomatosis).

HEADACHES ASSOCIATED WITH ALTERED INTRACRANIAL PRESSURE ("TRACTION HEADACHES")

Increased Intracranial Pressure
Intracranial mass lesions (neoplasm, hematoma, abscess, etc.).
Hydrocephalus.
Benign intracranial hypertension.
Venous sinus thrombosis.
Decreased Intracranial Pressure
Postlumbar puncture headaches.
Spontaneous hypoliquorrheic headaches.

HEADACHES AND HEAD PAINS CAUSED BY CRANIAL NEURALGIAS

Presumed Irritation of Superficial Nerves
Occipital neuralgia.
Supraorbital neuralgia.

Presumed Irritation of Intracranial Nerves
Trigeminal neuralgia ("tic douloureux").
Glossopharyngeal neuralgia.

HEADACHE, CHRONIC[46]

ICD-10CM #	R51	Headache

DIFFERENTIAL DIAGNOSIS OF RECURRENT OR CHRONIC HEADACHES

Migraine (with or without aura).
Tension.
Analgesic rebound.
Caffeine withdrawal.
Sleep deprivation (e.g., in children with sleep apnea) or chronic hypoxia.
Tumor.
Psychogenic: conversion disorder, malingering.
Cluster headache.

HEAD AND NECK, SOFT TISSUE MASSES

ICD-10CM #	R22.0	Localized swelling, mass and lump, head
	R22.1	Localized swelling, mass and lump, neck

Lipoma.
Pilar cyst.
Epidermal inclusion cyst.
Dermoid cyst.
Bone cyst.
Hemangioma.
Eosinophilic granuloma.
Other: facial nerve neuroma, teratoma, rhabdomyoma, rhabdomyosarcoma, branchial cleft cyst.

HEARING IMPAIRMENT AND DEAFNESS[20]

ICD-10CM #	Varies with specific diagnosis

Congenital.
  Aplasia of inner ear.
  Michel defect.
  Mondini defect.
  Scheibe defect.
Chromosome disorders.
  Trisomy 13.
  Trisomy 18.
  18q syndrome.
Genetic disorders.
  Isolated deafness.
  Pendred syndrome.
  Usher syndrome.
  Waardenburg syndrome.
Intrauterine viral infection.
Maternal drug use.
  Drugs.
  Antibiotics.
  β-Blockers.
  Chemotherapy.
Genetic neurologic disorders.
  Familial spastic paraplegia.
  Hereditary motor sensory neuropathies.

Hereditary sensory autonomic neuropathies.
Infantile Refsum disease.
Neurofibromatosis type 2.
Pontobulbar palsy with deafness.
Mitochondrial disorders.
Spinocerebellar degenerations.
Wolfram syndrome.
Xeroderma pigmentosum.
Infectious diseases.
  Bacterial meningitis.[a]
  Otitis media.[a]
  Sarcoidosis.[a]
  Viral encephalitis.
  Viral exanthemas.
Metabolic disorders.
  Hypothyroidism.[a]
  Ménière disease.
Skeletal disorders.
  Apert acrocephalosyndactyly.
  Cleidocranial dysostosis.
  Craniofacial dysostosis (Crouzon disease).
  Craniometaphyseal dysplasia (Pyle disease).
  Klippel-Feil syndrome.
  Mandibulofacial dysostosis (Treacher-Collins syndrome).
  Osteogenesis imperfecta.
  Osteopetrosis (Albers-Schönberg disease).
Susac syndrome.
Trauma.
Tumor.
  Acoustic neuroma.[a]
  Cholesteatoma.[a]

[a]Denotes the most common conditions and the ones with disease-modifying treatments.

HEARING LOSS, ACUTE[1]

ICD-10CM #	H91.23	Sudden idiopathic hearing loss, bilateral

Infectious: mumps, measles, influenza, herpes simplex, herpes zoster, cytomegalovirus mononucleosis, syphilis.
Vascular: macroglobulinemia, sickle cell disease, Berger disease, leukemia, polycythemia, fat emboli, hypercoagulable states.
Metabolic: diabetes, pregnancy, hyperlipoproteinemia.
Conductive: cerumen impaction, foreign bodies, otitis media, otitis externa, barotrauma, trauma.
Medications: aminoglycosides, loop diuretics, antineoplastics, salicylates, vancomycin.
Neoplasm: acoustic neuroma, metastatic neoplasm.

HEARTBURN AND INDIGESTION[76]

ICD-10CM #	R12	Heartburn
	K30	Functional dyspepsia

Reflux esophagitis.
Gastritis.
Nonulcer dyspepsia.
Functional GI disorder (anxiety disorder, social/environmental stresses).
Excessive intestinal gas (ingestion of flatulogenic foods, GI stasis, constipation).
Gas entrapment (hepatitis or splenic flexure syndrome).

Neoplasm (adenocarcinoma of stomach or esophagus, lymphoma).
Gallbladder disease.

HEART DISEASE, TRAUMATIC CAUSES[86]

ICD-10CM #	S26.020	Mild laceration of heart with hemopericardium
	S26.021	Moderate laceration of heart with hemopericardium
	S26.022	Major laceration of heart with hemopericardium

Penetrating:
  Stab wounds: knives, swords, ice picks, fence posts, wire, sports.
  Projectile wounds: handguns, rifles, nail guns, lawnmower projectiles.
  Shotgun wounds: pellets, close-range vs. distant.
Nonpenetrating (blunt):
  Motor vehicle accident:
    Seat belt.
    Air bag.
    Dashboard/steering wheel.
  Vehicular-pedestrian accident.
  Falls from a height.
  Crushing: industrial accident.
  Blasts: improvised explosive devices, grenades, fragments (combined blunt/penetrating).
  Assault.
  Sternal or rib fractures.
  Recreational: sporting events (e.g., rodeo, baseball).

HEART FAILURE WITH PRESERVED LEFT VENTRICULAR EJECTION FRACTION[59]

ICD-10CM #	I50.9	Heart failure, unspecified

CAUSES OF (AND ALTERNATIVE EXPLANATIONS FOR) HEART FAILURE WITH PRESERVED LEFT VENTRICULAR EJECTION FRACTION (>45% TO 50%)

Inaccurate diagnosis of heart failure (e.g., pulmonary disease, obesity).
Inaccurate measurements of ejection fraction.
Systolic function overestimated by ejection fraction (e.g., mitral regurgitation).
Episodic, unrecognized systolic dysfunction.
Intermittent ischemia.
Arrhythmia.
Severe hypertension.
Alcohol abuse.
Diastolic dysfunction.
Abnormalities of myocardial relaxation:
  Ischemia.
  Hypertrophy.
Abnormalities of myocardial compliance:
  Hypertrophy.
  Aging.
  Fibrosis.

Diabetes mellitus.
Infiltrative disease (amyloidosis, sarcoidosis).
Storage disease (hemochromatosis).
Endomyocardial disease (endomyocardial fibrosis, radiation, anthracyclines).
Pericardial disease (constriction, tamponade).

HEART FAILURE, ACUTE[43]

ICD-10CM #	I50.9	Heart failure, unspecified

COMMON PRECIPITATING CAUSES OF ACUTE HF

Systemic hypertension.
Myocardial infarction or ischemia.
Dysrhythmia.
Systemic infection.
Anemia.
Dietary, physical, environmental, and emotional excesses.
Pregnancy.
Thyrotoxicosis or hypothyroidism.
Acute myocarditis.
Acute valvular dysfunction.
Pulmonary embolus.
Pharmacologic complications.

HEART FAILURE, CHRONIC[87]

ICD-10CM #	I50.9	Heart failure, unspecified

Myocardial disease.
Coronary artery disease:
    Myocardial infarction.*
    Myocardial ischemia.
Chronic pressure overload:
    Hypertension.
    Obstructive valvular disease.
Chronic volume overload:
    Regurgitant valvular disease.
    Intracardiac (left-to-right) shunting.
    Extracardiac shunting.
Nonischemic dilated cardiomyopathy:
    Familial or genetic disorders.
    Infiltrative disorders.
    Toxic or drug-induced damage.
    Metabolic disorder.
    Viral or other infectious agents.
Disorders of rate and rhythm:
    Chronic bradyarrhythmias.
    Chronic tachyarrhythmias.
    Pulmonary heart disease
    Cor pulmonale.
    Pulmonary vascular disorders.
High-output states.
Metabolic disorders:
    Thyrotoxicosis.
    Nutritional disorders (beriberi).
Excessive blood flow requirements:
    Systemic arteriovenous shunting.
    Chronic anemia.

*Indicates conditions that can also lead to heart failure with a preserved ejection fraction.

HEART FAILURE, CONGENITAL HEART DISEASE CAUSES[88]

ICD-10CM #	I50.9	Heart failure, unspecified

CAUSES OF CONGESTIVE HEART FAILURE RESULTING FROM CONGENITAL HEART DISEASE

Age of Onset	Cause
At birth:	HLHS.
	Volume overload lesions: severe tricuspid or pulmonary insufficiency. Large systemic arteriovenous fistula.
First week:	TGA.
	PDA in small premature infants.
	HLHS (with more favorable anatomy).
	TAPVR, particularly those with pulmonary venous obstruction.
	Others.
	Systemic arteriovenous fistula.
	Critical AS or PS.
1 to 4 wk:	COA with associated anomalies.
	Critical AS.
	Large left-to-right shunt lesions (VSD, PDA) in premature infants.
	All other lesions previously listed.
4 to 6 wk:	Some left-to-right shunt lesions such as ECD.
6 wk to 4 mo:	Large VSD.
	Large PDA.
	Others, such as anomalous left coronary artery from the PA.

AS, Aortic stenosis; COA, coarctation of the aorta; ECD, endocardial cushion defect; HLHS, hypoplastic left heart syndrome; PA, pulmonary artery; PDA, patent ductus arteriosus; PS, pulmonary stenosis; TAPVR, total anomalous pulmonary venous return; TGA, transposition of the great arteries; VSD, ventricular septal defect.

HEART FAILURE, PATHOGENIC CAUSES[59]

ICD-10CM #	I50.9	Heart failure, unspecified

IMPAIRED SYSTOLIC (CONTRACTILE) FUNCTION

Ischemic damage or dysfunction:
    Myocardial infarction.
    Persistent or intermittent myocardial ischemia.
    Hypoperfusion (shock).
Chronic pressure overloading:
    Hypertension.
    Obstructive valvular disease.
Chronic volume overload:
    Regurgitant valvular disease.
    Intracardiac left-to-right shunting.
    Extracardiac shunting.

Nonischemic dilated cardiomyopathy:
    Familial/genetic disorders.
    Toxic/drug-induced damage
    Immunologically mediated necrosis.
    Infectious agents.
    Metabolic disorders.
    Infiltrative processes.
    Idiopathic conditions.

IMPAIRED DIASTOLIC FUNCTION (RESTRICTED FILLING, INCREASED STIFFNESS)

Pathologic myocardial hypertrophy:
    Primary (hypertrophic cardiomyopathies).
    Secondary (hypertension).
    Aging.
    Ischemic fibrosis.
    Restrictive cardiomyopathy:
        Infiltrative disorders (amyloidosis, sarcoidosis).
        Storage diseases (hemochromatosis, genetic abnormalities).
Endomyocardial disorders.

MECHANICAL ABNORMALITIES

Intracardiac:
    Obstructive valvular disease.
    Regurgitant valvular disease.
    Intracardiac shunts.
    Other congenital abnormalities.
Extracardiac:
    Obstructive (coarctation, supravalvular aortic stenosis).
    Left-to-right shunting (patent ductus arteriosus).

DISORDERS OF RATE AND RHYTHM

Bradyarrhythmias (sinus node dysfunction, conduction abnormalities).
Tachyarrhythmias (ineffective rhythms, chronic tachycardia).

PULMONARY HEART DISEASE

Cor pulmonale.
Pulmonary vascular disorders.

HIGH-OUTPUT STATES

Metabolic disorders:
    Thyrotoxicosis.
    Nutritional disorders (beriberi).
    Excessive blood flow requirements:
        Chronic anemia.
        Systemic arteriovenous shunting.

HEART FAILURE, PREGNANCY

ICD-10CM #	I50.9	Heart failure, unspecified

Congenital valvular heart disease exacerbated by pregnancy.
Peripartum cardiomyopathy.
Untreated thyrotoxicosis.
Hypothyroidism.
Pulmonary hypertension.
Myocardial infarction.

HEAT STROKE[29]

ICD-10CM #	T67.0	Heatstroke and sunstroke

Sepsis.
Encephalitis.
Meningitis.
Brain abscess.
Malaria (cerebral falciparum).
Typhoid fever.
Tetanus.
Alcohol withdrawal syndrome.
Neuroleptic malignant syndrome.
Anticholinergic toxicity.
Salicylate toxicity.
Phencyclidine hydrochloride (PCP), cocaine, or amphetamine toxicity.
Status epilepticus.
Cerebral hemorrhage.
Diabetic ketoacidosis.
Thyroid storm.

HEEL PAIN

ICD-10CM #	M25.50	Pain in unspecified joint

Achilles tendonitis/tendinopathy (insertional, noninsertional).
Retrocalcaneal bursitis (superficial, deep).
Plantar fasciopathy.
Neuropathy (tarsal tunnel, posterior tibial nerve [medial calcaneal branch], abductor digiti quinti).
Calcaneal stress fracture.
Puncture wound, foreign body.
Cellulitis.
Spondyloarthropathy.
Fat pad atrophy.
Soft tissue tumor.
S1 radiculopathy.
Paget disease of bone.
Haglund deformity.
Primary or metastatic bone tumor.

HEEL PAIN, PLANTAR

ICD-10CM #	M79.609	Pain in unspecified limb

SKIN
Keratoses.
Verruca.
Ulcer.
Fissure.

CONNECTIVE TISSUE
Fat
Atrophy.
Panniculitis.
Dense Connective Tissue
Inflammatory fasciitis.
Fibromatosis.
Enthesopathy.
Bursitis.
Bone (Calcaneus)
Stress fracture.
Paget disease.
Benign bone cyst/tumor.

Malignant bone tumor.
Metabolic bone disease (osteopenia).
Nerve
Tarsal tunnel.
Plantar nerve entrapment.
S1 nerve root radiculopathy.
Painful peripheral neuropathy.

INFECTION
Dermatomycoses.
Acute osteomyelitis.
Plantar abscess.

MISCELLANEOUS
Foreign body.
Nonunion calcaneus fracture.
Psychogenic.
Idiopathic.

HEMARTHROSIS

ICD-10CM #	T14.90	Injury, unspecified

Trauma.
Anticoagulant therapy.
Thrombocytopenia, thrombocytosis.
Bleeding disorders (e.g., von Willebrand disease).
Charcot joint.
Idiopathic.
Other: pigmented villonodular synovitis, hemangioma, synovioma, AV fistula, ruptured aneurysm.

HEMATEMESIS[2]

ICD-10CM #	K92.0	Hematemesis

CAUSES OF HEMATEMESIS
Very Common
Gastric or duodenal ulcer or erosions.
Common
Mallory-Weiss tear (a laceration at the gastroesophageal junction).
Ulcerative esophagitis.
Esophageal varices.
Uncommon
Vascular malformations.
Ulcerated GI stromal tumor.
Carcinoma of esophagus or stomach.
Aortoenteric fistula.

HEMATURIA

ICD-10CM #	R31.9	Hematuria, unspecified

Use the mnemonic TICS:
T (Trauma): blow to kidney, insertion of Foley catheter or foreign body in urethra, prolonged and severe exercise, very rapid emptying of overdistended bladder. (Tumor): hypernephroma, Wilms tumor, papillary carcinoma of the bladder, prostatic and urethral neoplasms. (Toxins): turpentine, phenols, sulfonamides and other antibiotics, cyclophosphamide, NSAIDs.
I (Infections): glomerulonephritis, TB, cystitis, prostatitis, urethritis, *Schistosoma haematobium,* yellow fever, blackwater fever. (Inflammatory processes): Goodpasture syndrome, periarteritis, postirradiation.
C (Calculi): renal, ureteral, bladder, urethra. (Cysts): simple cysts, polycystic disease.

(Congenital anomalies): hemangiomas, aneurysms, arteriovenous malformation.
S (Surgery): invasive procedures, prostatic resection, cystoscopy. (Sickle cell disease and other hematologic disturbances): hemophilia, thrombocytopenia, anticoagulants. (Somewhere else): bleeding genitals, factitious (drug addicts).

HEMATURIA, DIFFERENTIAL BASED ON AGE AND SEX

ICD-10CM #	R31.9	Hematuria, unspecified

0 TO 20 YR
Acute urinary tract infections.
Acute glomerulonephritis.
Congenital urinary tract anomalies with obstruction.
Trauma to genitals.

20 TO 40 YR
Acute urinary tract infection.
Trauma to genitals.
Urolithiasis.
Bladder cancer.

40 TO 60 YR (WOMEN)
Acute urinary tract infection.
Bladder cancer.
Urolithiasis.

40 TO 60 YR (MEN)
Acute urinary tract infection.
Bladder cancer.
Urolithiasis.

60 YR AND OLDER (WOMEN)
Acute urinary tract infection.
Bladder cancer.
Vaginal trauma or irritation.
Urolithiasis.

60 YR AND OLDER (MEN)
Acute urinary tract infection.
Benign prostatic hyperplasia.
Bladder cancer.
Urolithiasis.
Trauma.

HEMATURIA, IN CHILDREN[43]

ICD-10CM #	R31.9	Hematuria, unspecified

EXTRARENAL
Trauma.
Meatal stenosis or posterior urethral valves.
Exercise.
Menstruation or rectal bleeding.
Foreign bodies.
Cystitis, urethritis, or epididymitis.

INTRARENAL
Pyelonephritis.
Renal or bladder stones or tumors.
Poststreptococcal or idiopathic glomerulonephritis.
Acute interstitial nephritis.
Acute tubular necrosis.
Basement membrane glomerular disease.
Renal vein or arterial thrombosis.

Differential Diagnosis

II

Recurrent familial hematuria.
Polycystic kidney disease.

SYSTEMIC
Henoch-Schönlein purpura.
Systemic lupus erythematosus.
Hemolytic-uremic syndrome.
Infectious mononucleosis.
Sickle cell disease or other hemoglobinopathies.
Bacterial endocarditis or artificial cardiac valves.
Bleeding disorders, warfarin, or aspirin.
Medications such as amitriptyline or chlorpromazine, radiocontrast dyes.
Munchausen syndrome or factitious.

HEMIBALLISM[38]

| ICD-10CM # | G25.5 | Other chorea |

ETIOLOGY
Structural Lesions
Cerebrovascular Disease
  Infarction.
  Transient ischemic attack.
  Hemorrhage.
  Arteriovenous malformation.
  Subarachnoid hemorrhage.
  Subclavian steal syndrome.
Infection
Syphilis.
Tuberculoma.
Toxoplasmosis.
Acquired immunodeficiency syndrome.
Influenza A.
Tumor
Pituitary microadenoma.
Metastasis.
Immune-Mediated
Systemic lupus erythematosus.
Sydenham chorea.
Behçet disease.
Scleroderma.
Other
Static encephalopathy.
Head injury.
Demyelinating disease.
Thalamotomy.
Heredodegenerative disease.
Metabolic
Nonketotic hyperosmolar hyperglycemia.
Drug-Induced
Phenytoin and other anticonvulsants.
Oral contraceptives.
Neuroleptics (tardive).

HEMIPLEGIA, ACUTE[20]

| ICD-10CM # | Varies with specific diagnosis |

Alternating hemiplegia.
Asthmatic amyotrophy.
Cerebrovascular disease.[a]
Diabetes mellitus.
Epilepsy.
Hypoglycemia.
Kawasaki disease.
Migraine.[a]

Trauma.
Tumor.[a]

HEMIPLEGIA, PROGRESSIVE[20]

| ICD-10CM # | Varies with specific diagnosis |

Adrenoleukodystrophy.
Arteriovenous malformation.
Brain abscess.
Cerebral hemisphere tumor.
Demyelinating diseases.
Late-onset globoid leukodystrophy.
Multiple sclerosis.
Sturge-Weber syndrome.

HEMIPARESIS/HEMIPLEGIA

| ICD-10CM # | G81.00 | Flaccid hemiplegia affecting unspecified side |
| | G81.10 | Spastic hemiplegia affecting unspecified side |

Cerebrovascular accident.
Transient ischemic attack.
Cerebral neoplasm.
Multiple sclerosis or other demyelinating disorder.
Central nervous system infection.
Migraine.
Hypoglycemia
Subdural hematoma.
Vasculitis.
Todd paralysis.
Epidural hematoma.
Metabolic (hyperosmolar state, electrolyte imbalance).
Psychiatric disorders.
Congenital disorders.
Leukodystrophies.

HEMOLYSIS AND HEMOGLOBINURIA

ICD-10CM #	P55.8	Other hemolytic diseases of newborn
	P55.9	Hemolytic disease of newborn, unspecified
	R82.3	Hemoglobinuria

Erythrocyte trauma (prosthetic cardiac valves, marching and severe trauma, extensive burns).
Infections (malaria, *Bartonella*, *Clostridium welchii*).
Brown recluse spider bite.
Incompatible blood transfusions.
Hemolytic-uremic syndrome.
Thrombotic thrombocytopenic purpura (TTP).
Paroxysmal nocturnal hemoglobinuria (PNH).
Drugs (penicillins, quinidine, methyldopa, sulfonamides, nitrofurantoin).
Erythrocyte enzyme deficiencies (e.g., exposure to fava beans in patients with glucose-6-phosphate dehydrogenase deficiency).

HEMOLYSIS, INTRAVASCULAR

| ICD-10CM # | D59.6 | Hemoglobinuria due to hemolysis from other external causes |
| | D59.8 | Other acquired hemolytic anemias |

Infections.
Exertional hemolysis (e.g., prolonged march).
Valve hemolysis.
Microangiopathic hemolytic anemia.
Osmotic and chemical agents.
Thermal injury.
Cold agglutinins.
Venoms (snakes, spiders).
Paroxysmal nocturnal hemoglobinuria (PNH).

HEMOLYSIS, MECHANICAL

| ICD-10CM # | D59.4 | Other nonautoimmune hemolytic anemias |

Prosthetic heart valves.
Aortic stenosis.
Malignant hypertension.
Metastatic adenocarcinoma.
Traumatic exercise.
Renal transplants.
Renal cortical necrosis.
Glomerulonephritis.
Thrombotic thrombocytopenic purpura (TTP), hemolytic-uremic syndrome (HUS).
Renal vasculitis.
Scleroderma.
Diabetes mellitus.

HEMOLYSIS, OXIDATIVE, DRUG-INDUCED[71]

| ICD-10CM # | D59 | Acquired hemolytic anemia |
| | D59.1 | Other autoimmune hemolytic anemias |

AGENTS THAT CAUSE OXIDATIVE HEMOLYSIS

Therapeutic Agents
Nitrofurantoin (Furadantin).
Sulfasalazine (Azulfidine).
p-Aminosalicylic acid.
Phenazopyridine (Pyridium).
Cotrimoxazole.
Quinolones.
Phenacetin.
Rasburicase.
Dapsone and other sulfones.
Primaquine.
Recreational Drugs
Isobutyl nitrate.
Amyl nitrite.
Miscellaneous Agents
Naphthalene mothballs.
Methylene blue.
Paraquat.
Hydrogen peroxide.

[a]Denotes the most common conditions and the ones with disease-modifying treatments.

HEMOPERITONEUM

ICD-10CM #	K66.1	Hemoperitoneum

Ruptured Graafian follicle.
Ruptured spleen.
Ectopic pregnancy.
Traumatic laceration of liver.
Ruptured aneurysm.
Ruptured bladder.
Traumatic laceration of bowel, pancreas, uterus.

HEMOPTYSIS

ICD-10CM #	R04.2	Hemoptysis

CARDIOVASCULAR

Pulmonary embolism/infarction.
Left ventricular failure.
Mitral stenosis.
AV fistula.
Severe hypertension.
Erosion of aortic aneurysm.

PULMONARY

Neoplasm (primary or metastatic).
Infection.
Pneumonia: *Streptococcus pneumoniae, Klebsiella pneumoniae, Staphylococcus aureus, Legionella pneumophila.*
Bronchiectasis.
Abscess.
TB.
Bronchitis.
Fungal infections (aspergillosis, coccidioidomycosis).
Parasitic infections (amebiasis, ascariasis, paragonimiasis).
Vasculitis: granulomatosis with polyangiitis, Churg-Strauss syndrome, Henoch-Schönlein purpura.
Goodpasture syndrome.
Trauma (needle biopsy, foreign body, right-sided heart catheterization, prolonged and severe cough).
Cystic fibrosis, bullous emphysema.
Pulmonary sequestration.
Pulmonary AV fistula.
Systemic lupus erythematosus.
Idiopathic pulmonary hemosiderosis.
Drugs: aspirin, anticoagulants, penicillamine.
Pulmonary hypertension.
Mediastinal fibrosis.

OTHER

Epistaxis, trauma.
Laryngeal bleeding (laryngitis, laryngeal neoplasm).
Hematologic disorders (clotting abnormalities, disseminated intravascular coagulation, thrombocytopenia).

HEMOPTYSIS/PULMONARY HEMORRHAGE[20]

ICD-10CM #	R04.2	Hemoptysis

CARDIOVASCULAR DISORDERS

Heart failure with pulmonary edema.
Pulmonary hypertension with Eisenmenger syndrome.
Mitral stenosis.
Venoocclusive disease.
Arteriovenous malformation (Osler-Weber-Rendu syndrome).
Pulmonary embolism.
Portal vein obstruction.

PULMONARY DISORDERS

Bronchogenic cyst.
Bronchopulmonary sequestration.
Pneumonia (bacterial, mycobacterial, fungal, parasitic, or viral).
Bronchiectasis (cystic fibrosis, primary ciliary dyskinesia, immunodeficiency, retained foreign body).
Tracheobronchitis.
Lung abscess.
Tumor (adenoma, carcinoid, hemangioma, metastasis).
Trauma (contusion, laceration).

IMMUNE DISORDERS

Henoch-Schönlein purpura.
Pulmonary capillaritis.
Idiopathic pulmonary hemosiderosis.
Anti–glomerular basement membrane disease (Goodpasture disease).
Granulomatosis with polyangiitis (formerly known as Wegener granulomatosis).
Systemic lupus erythematosus.
Polyarteritis nodosa.

OTHER CONDITIONS/FACTORS

Coagulopathy (Von Willebrand factor).
Toxic inhalation (nitrogen dioxide, pesticides, crack cocaine).
Post–bone marrow transplantation.
Catamenial hemoptysis (females).

HEMORRHAGIC CYSTITIS[89]

ICD-10CM #	N39.0	Urinary tract infection

DIFFERENTIAL DIAGNOSIS FOR HEMORRHAGIC CYSTITIS[27]

Infectious.*
  Bacterial.
  Viral (especially BK virus, adenovirus).
  Fungal.
  Parasitic.
Trauma:
  External.
  Postsurgical (e.g., transurethral resection of the bladder).
Malignancy:
  Bladder primary.
  Bladder invasion from local/distant primary.
Vascular malformation.
Chemical exposure:
  Cyclophosphamide.
  Ifosfamide.
  Busulfan.
  Thiotepa.
  Temozolomide.
  Aniline dye.

---

*Bleeding localized to bladder after diagnostic workup for gross hematuria with cystoscopy, urine cytology, and upper tract imaging is without clear cause of alternative bleeding source.

Ether.
Nonoxynol-9 (accidental urethral insertion of vaginal contraceptive).
Radiation therapy history (e.g., prostate cancer, cervical cancer).
Medication induced:
  Penicillin and derivatives (via immune reaction).
  Bleomycin.
  Danazol.
  Tiaprofenic.
  Allopurinol.
  Phensuximide.
  Methenamine mandelate.
  Acetic acid.
Manifestation of systemic disease:
  Amyloidosis.
  Rheumatoid arthritis.
  Crohn disease.

HEPATIC CYSTS[17]

ICD-10CM #	Q44.6	Cystic disease of liver
	B67.8	Echinococcosis, unspecified, of liver

CONGENITAL HEPATIC CYSTS

Parenchymal: solitary cyst, polycystic disease.
Ductal: localized dilation, multiple cystic dilations of intrahepatic ducts (Caroli disease).

ACQUIRED HEPATIC CYSTS

Inflammatory cysts: retention cysts, echinococcal cyst, amebic cyst.
Neoplastic cyst.
Peliosis hepatis.

HEPATIC DYSFUNCTION, POSTOPERATIVE[3]

ICD-10CM #	K91.82	Postprocedural hepatic failure

CAUSES OF POSTOPERATIVE HEPATIC DYSFUNCTION

Hepatocellular Injury (predominant serum ALT elevation, with or without hyperbilirubinemia)
Acute transfusion-associated viral hepatitis.
Hepatic allograft rejection.
Hepatic artery thrombosis.
Inhalational anesthetics: halothane, others.
Ischemic hepatitis (shock liver).
Other drugs: antihypertensives (e.g., labetalol), heparin.
Unrecognized chronic liver disease: NASH, hepatitis C, other disorders.
Cholestatic Jaundice (elevated serum alkaline phosphatase ± ALT; direct hyperbilirubinemia)
Acalculous cholecystitis.
Benign postoperative cholestasis.
Bile duct injury: after cholecystectomy or liver transplantation.
Bile duct obstruction: gallstones, pancreatitis.
Cardiac bypass of prolonged duration.
Cholangitis.
Drugs: amoxicillin-clavulanic acid, chlorpromazine, erythromycin, telithromycin, trimethoprim/sulfamethoxazole, warfarin, others.

Differential Diagnosis

II

Hemobilia.
Microlithiasis (biliary sludge).
Prolonged TPN.
Sepsis.
Indirect Hyperbilirubinemia (serum alkaline phosphatase and ALT often normal)
Gilbert syndrome.
Hemolytic anemia (G6PD deficiency, other causes).
Multiple transfusions.
Resorbing hematoma.

G6PD, Glucose-6-phosphate dehydrogenase; *NASH*, nonalcoholic steatohepatitis.

HEPATIC GRANULOMAS[18]

ICD-10CM #	K75.3	Granulomatous hepatitis

INFECTIONS

Bacterial, spirochetal: TB and atypical mycobacterial infections, tularemia, brucellosis, leprosy, syphilis, Whipple disease, listeriosis.
Viral: mononucleosis, cytomegalovirus.
Rickettsial: Q fever.
Fungal: coccidioidomycosis, histoplasmosis, cryptococcal infections, actinomycosis, aspergillosis, nocardiosis.
Parasitic: schistosomiasis, clonorchiasis, toxocariasis, ascariasis, toxoplasmosis, amebiasis.

HEPATOBILIARY DISORDERS

Primary biliary cirrhosis, granulomatous hepatitis, jejunoileal bypass.

SYSTEMIC DISORDERS

Sarcoidosis, granulomatosis with polyangiitis, inflammatory bowel disease, Hodgkin disease, lymphoma.

DRUGS/TOXINS

Beryllium, parenteral foreign material (starch, talc, silicone, etc.), phenylbutazone, α-methyldopa, procainamide, allopurinol, phenytoin, nitrofurantoin, hydralazine.

HEPATITIS, ACUTE[1]

ICD-10CM #	B17.8	Acute viral hepatitis, unspecified
	B15	Acute hepatitis A
	B16	Acute hepatitis B
	B17.1	Acute hepatitis C
	B17.2	Acute hepatitis E

Infectious:
  Hepatitis A, B, C, D, E.
  Epstein-Barr virus.
  Cytomegalovirus.
  Herpes simplex virus.
  Yellow fever.
  Leptospirosis.
  Q fever.
  HIV.
  Brucellosis.
  Lyme disease.
  Syphilis.

Noninfectious:
  Drug induced.
  Autoimmune.
  Ischemic.
  Acute fatty liver of pregnancy.
  Acute Budd-Chiari syndrome.
  Wilson disease.

HEPATITIS, CHRONIC[1]

ICD-10CM #	K73.9	Chronic hepatitis, unspecified
	B18.0	Chronic viral hepatitis B with δ-agent
	B18.2	Chronic viral hepatitis C

Chronic viral hepatitis:
  Hepatitis B.
  Hepatitis C.
  Hepatitis D.
Autoimmune hepatitis and variant syndromes.
Hereditary hemochromatosis.
Wilson disease.
α_1-Antitrypsin deficiency.
Fatty liver and nonalcoholic steatohepatitis.
Alcoholic liver disease.
Drug-induced liver disease.
Hepatic granulomas:
  Infectious.
  Drug induced.
  Neoplastic.
  Idiopathic.

HEPATITIS, IN CHILDREN[19]

ICD-10CM #	B17.9	Acute viral hepatitis, unspecified
	K73.9	Chronic hepatitis, unspecified

CAUSES AND DIFFERENTIAL DIAGNOSIS OF HEPATITIS IN CHILDREN

Infectious
Hepatotropic viruses:
  Hepatitis A virus.
  Hepatitis B virus.
  Hepatitis C virus.
  Hepatitis D virus.
  Hepatitis E virus.
  Hepatitis non–A-E viruses.
Systemic infection that can include hepatitis:
  Adenovirus.
  Arbovirus.
  Coxsackievirus.
  Cytomegalovirus.
  Enterovirus.
  Epstein-Barr virus.
  "Exotic" viruses (e.g., yellow fever).
  Herpes simplex virus.
  HIV.
  Paramyxovirus.
  Rubella.
  Varicella zoster.
Other.
Nonviral Liver Infections
Abscess.
Amebiasis.

Bacterial sepsis.
Brucellosis.
Fitz-Hugh-Curtis syndrome.
Histoplasmosis.
Leptospirosis.
Tuberculosis.
Other.
Autoimmune
Autoimmune hepatitis.
Sclerosing cholangitis.
Other (e.g., systemic lupus erythematosus, juvenile rheumatoid arthritis).
Metabolic
α_1-Antitrypsin deficiency.
Tyrosinemia.
Wilson disease.
Other.
Toxic
Iatrogenic or drug induced (e.g., acetaminophen).
Environmental (e.g., pesticides).
Anatomic
Choledochal cyst.
Biliary atresia.
Other.
Hemodynamic
Shock.
Congestive heart failure.
Budd-Chiari syndrome.
Other.
Nonalcoholic Fatty Liver Disease
Idiopathic.
Reye syndrome.
Other.

HEPATOMEGALY

ICD-10CM #	R16.0	Hepatomegaly, not elsewhere classified

FREQUENT JAUNDICE

Infectious hepatitis.
Toxic hepatitis.
Carcinoma: liver, pancreas, bile ducts, metastatic neoplasm to liver.
Cirrhosis.
Obstruction of common bile duct.
Alcoholic hepatitis.
Biliary cirrhosis.
Cholangitis.
Hemochromatosis with cirrhosis.

INFREQUENT JAUNDICE

Congestive heart failure.
Amyloidosis.
Liver abscess.
Sarcoidosis.
Infectious mononucleosis.
Alcoholic fatty infiltration.
Nonalcoholic steatohepatitis.
Lymphoma.
Leukemia.
Budd-Chiari syndrome.
Myelofibrosis with myeloid metaplasia.
Familial hyperlipoproteinemia type 1.
Other: amebiasis, hydatid disease of liver, schistosomiasis, kala-azar (*Leishmania donovani*), Hurler syndrome, Gaucher disease, kwashiorkor.

HEPATOMEGALY, BY SHAPE OF LIVER[2]

ICD-10CM #	R16.0	Hepatomegaly, not elsewhere classified

DIFFUSELY ENLARGED AND SMOOTH

Massive
Metastatic disease.
Alcoholic liver disease with fatty infiltration.
Myeloproliferative diseases (e.g., polycythemia rubra vera, myelofibrosis).

Moderate
The above causes.
Hemochromatosis.
Hematologic disease (e.g., chronic myeloid leukemia, lymphoma).
Fatty liver (e.g., diabetes mellitus, obesity).
Infiltrative disorders (e.g., amyloid).

Mild
The above causes.
Hepatitis (viral, drugs).
Cirrhosis.
Biliary obstruction.
Granulomatous disorders (e.g., sarcoid).
HIV infection.

DIFFUSELY ENLARGED AND IRREGULAR

Metastatic disease.
Cirrhosis.
Hydatid disease.
Polycystic liver disease.

LOCALIZED SWELLINGS

Riedel lobe (a normal variant—the lobe may be palpable in the right lumbar region).
Metastasis.
Large simple hepatic cyst.
Hydatid cyst.
Hepatoma.
Liver abscess (e.g., amebic abscess).

HERMAPHRODITISM[45]

ICD-10CM #	Q56.3	Pseudohermaphroditism, unspecified
	Q56.4	Indeterminate sex, unspecified

FEMALE PSEUDOHERMAPHRODITISM

Androgen exposure:
Fetal source:
21-Hydroxylase (P450 c21) deficiency.
11β-Hydroxylase (P450 c11) deficiency.
3β-Hydroxysteroid dehydrogenase II (3β-HSD II) deficiency.
Aromatase (P450arom) deficiency.
Maternal source.
Virilizing ovarian tumor.
Virilizing adrenal tumor.
Androgenic drugs.
Undetermined origin:
Associated with genitourinary and GI tract defects.

MALE PSEUDOHERMAPHRODITISM

Defects in testicular differentiation:
Denys-Drash syndrome (mutation in WT1 gene).
WAGR syndrome (Wilms tumor, aniridia, genitourinary malformation, retardation).
Deletion of 11p13.
Camptomelic syndrome (autosomal gene at 17q24.3-q25.1) and SOX 9 mutation.
XY pure gonadal dysgenesis (Swyer syndrome).
Mutation in SRY gene.
Unknown cause.
XY gonadal agenesis.
Deficiency of testicular hormones:
Leydig cell aplasia.
Mutation in LH receptor.
Lipoid adrenal hyperplasia (P450 scc) deficiency; mutation in StAR (steroidogenic acute regulatory protein).
3α-HSD II deficiency.
17-Hydroxylase/17, 20-lyase (P450 c17) deficiency.
Persistent Müllerian duct syndrome.
Gene mutations, Müllerian-inhibiting substance (MIS).
Receptor defects for MIS.
Defect in androgen action:
5α-Reductase II mutations.
Androgen receptor defects:
Complete androgen insensitivity syndrome.
Partial androgen insensitivity syndrome.
Reifenstein and other syndromes.
Smith-Lemli-Opitz syndrome.
Defect in conversion of 7-dehydrocholesterol to cholesterol.

TRUE HERMAPHRODITISM

XX.
XY.
XX/XY chimeras.

HERNIATION SYNDROMES[20]

ICD-10CM #	Varies with specific diagnosis

UNILATERAL (UNCAL) TRANSTENTORIAL HERNIATION

Declining consciousness.
Increased blood pressure, slow pulse.
Dilated and fixed pupils.
Homonymous hemianopia.
Respiratory irregularity.
Decerebrate rigidity.

BILATERAL (CENTRAL) TRANSTENTORIAL HERNIATION

Decerebrate or decorticate rigidity.
Declining consciousness.
Impaired upward gaze.
Irregular respiration.
Pupillary constriction or dilation.

CEREBELLAR (DOWNWARD) HERNIATION

Declining consciousness.
Impaired upward gaze.
Irregular respirations.
Lower cranial nerve palsies.
Neck stiffness or head tilt.

HICCUPS[26]

ICD-10CM #	R06.6	Hiccough

TRANSIENT HICCUPS

Sudden excitement, emotion.
Gastric distention.
Esophageal obstruction.
Alcohol ingestion.
Sudden change in temperature.

PERSISTENT OR CHRONIC HICCUPS

Toxic/metabolic: uremia, diabetes mellitus, hyperventilation, hypocalcemia, hypokalemia, hyponatremia, gout, fever.
Drugs: benzodiazepines, steroids, α-methyldopa, barbiturates.
Surgery/general anesthesia.
Thoracic/diaphragmatic disorders: pneumonia, lung cancer, asthma, pleuritis, pericarditis, myocardial infarction, aortic aneurysm, esophagitis, esophageal obstruction, diaphragmatic hernia or irritation.
Abdominal disorders: gastric ulcer or cancer, hepatobiliary or pancreatic disease, inflammatory bowel disease, bowel obstruction, intraabdominal or subphrenic abscess, prostatic infection or cancer.
Central nervous system disorders: traumatic, infectious, vascular, structural.
Ear, nose, and throat disorders: pharyngitis, laryngitis, tumor, irritation of auditory canal.
Psychogenic disorders.
Idiopathic disorders.

HILAR AND MEDIASTINAL LYMPH NODE ENLARGEMENT[59]

ICD-10CM #	R59.0	Mediastinal adenopathy

DISORDERS ASSOCIATED WITH HILAR AND MEDIASTINAL LYMPH NODE ENLARGEMENT

Sarcoidosis.
Lymphoma.
Fungal disease.
Tuberculosis.
Metastatic cancer.
Silicosis, coal worker's pneumoconiosis, beryllium lung.

HIP PAIN, CHILDREN[1]

ICD-10CM #	S79.819A	Other specified injuries of unspecified hip, initial encounter
	S79.829A	Other specified injuries of unspecified thigh, initial encounter
	S79.919A	Unspecified injury of unspecified hip, initial encounter

Differential Diagnosis

II

TRAUMA

Hip or pelvis fractures.
Overuse injuries.

INFECTION

Septic arthritis.
Osteomyelitis.

INFLAMMATION

Transient synovitis.
Juvenile rheumatoid arthritis.
Rheumatic fever.

NEOPLASM

Leukemia.
Osteogenic or Ewing sarcoma.
Metastatic disease.

HEMATOLOGIC DISORDERS

Hemophilia.
Sickle cell anemia.

MISCELLANEOUS

Legg-Calvé-Perthes disease.
Slipped capital femoral epiphysis.

HIP PAIN, DIFFERENTIAL DIAGNOSIS[90]

ICD-10CM # M25.559 Pain in unspecified hip

ARTICULAR

Inflammatory Joint Disease
Rheumatoid arthritis.
Spondyloarthropathies.
Polymyalgia rheumatica.
Degenerative Joint Disease
Primary osteoarthritis.
Secondary osteoarthritis.
Metabolic Joint Diseases
Gout.
Pseudogout.
Ochronosis.
Hemochromatosis.
Wilson disease.
Acromegaly.
Femoroacetabular Impingement
Acetabular Labral Tear
Infections.
Tumors.
  Benign:
    Pigmented villonodular sclerosis.
    Osteochondromatosis.
  Malignant:
    Synovial sarcoma.
    Synovial metastasis.
Hemarthrosis in children
Toxic synovitis.
Juvenile chronic arthritis.

REFERRED PAIN

Thoracolumbar spine:
  Intraabdominal structures.
  Retroperitoneal structures.

PERIARTICULAR

Bursitis:
  Trochanteric.
  Iliopsoas.
  Ischiogluteal.

Tendinitis:
  Trochanteric.
  Adductor.
Acute calcific periarthritis.
Heterotropic ossification.

OSSEOUS

Bone lesions.
Fractures.
Neoplasms.
Infection.
Osteonecrosis of the femoral head.
Paget disease.
Metabolic bone disease.
Stress fracture.
Transient osteoporosis.
In children:
  Congenital dislocation of the hip.
  Acetabular dysplasia.
  Coxa vara.
  Slipped capital femoral epiphysis.
  Legg-Calvé-Perthes disease.
  Rickets.

NEUROLOGIC

Entrapment neuropathies.
Lateral femoral cutaneous nerve (meralgia paresthetica).
Lumbar nerve root compression.
L2, L3, and L4.

VASCULAR

Atherosclerosis of aorta, iliac vessels.

HIP PAIN, IN DIFFERENT AGE GROUPS[41]

ICD-10CM # M25.559 Pain in unspecified hip

COMMON CAUSES OF HIP PAIN IN DIFFERENT AGE GROUPS

Childhood (2 to 10 yr)
Intraarticular
Developmental dislocation of the hip.
Perthes disease.
Irritable hip.
Rickets.
Periarticular
Osteomyelitis.
Referred
Abdominal.
Adolescence (10 to 18 yr)
Intraarticular
Slipped upper femoral epiphysis.
Torn labrum.
Periarticular
Trochanteric bursitis.
Snapping hip.
Osteomyelitis.
Tumors.
Referred
Abdominal.
Lumbar spine.
Early Adulthood (18 to 30 yr)
Intraarticular
Inflammatory arthritis.
Torn labrum.
Periarticular
Bursitis.

Referred
Abdominal.
Lumbar spine.
Adulthood (30 to 50 yr)
Intraarticular
Osteoarthritis.
Inflammatory arthritis.
Osteonecrosis.
Transient osteoporosis.
Periarticular
Bursitis.
Referred
Abdominal.
Lumbar spine.
Old Age (50 yr)
Intraarticular
Osteoarthritis.
Inflammatory arthritis.
Referred
Abdominal.
Lumbar spine.

HIP PAIN WITHOUT OBVIOUS FRACTURE[43]

ICD-10CM # R52 Pain, unspecified
  M25.559 Pain in unspecified hip

DIFFERENTIAL DIAGNOSIS OF A PAINFUL HIP WITHOUT OBVIOUS FRACTURE

Referred pain (lumbar spine, hip, or knee).
Avascular necrosis of the femoral head.
Degenerative joint disease or osteoarthritis.
Herniation of a lumbar disk.
Diskitis.
Toxic synovitis of the hip.
Septic arthritis.
Bursitis.
Tendonitis.
Ligamentous injuries of the knee or hip.
Occult fracture.
Slipped capital femoral epiphysis.
Perthes disease.
Tumor (lymphoma).
Deep venous thrombosis.
Arterial insufficiency.
Osteomyelitis.
Iliopsoas abscess.
Retroperitoneal hematoma.
Inguinal hernia.
Inguinal lymphadenopathy.
Genitourinary complaints.
Sports-related hernia.

HIRSUTISM

ICD-10CM # L68.0 Hirsutism

Idiopathic: familial, possibly increased sensitivity to androgens.
Menopause.
Polycystic ovarian syndrome.
Drugs: androgens, anabolic steroids, methyltestosterone, minoxidil, diazoxide, phenytoin, glucocorticoids, cyclosporine.
Congenital adrenal hyperplasia.
Adrenal virilizing tumor.
Ovarian virilizing tumor: arrhenoblastoma, hilus cell tumor.

Pituitary adenoma.
Cushing syndrome.
Hypothyroidism (congenital and juvenile).
Acromegaly.
Testicular feminization.

HIV INFECTION, ANORECTAL LESIONS[1]

| ICD-10CM # | B20 | Human immunodeficiency virus [HIV] disease |
| | Z21 | Asymptomatic human immunodeficiency virus [HIV] infection status |

COMMON CONDITIONS

Anal fissure.
Abscess and fistula.
Hemorrhoids.
Pruritus ani.
Pilonidal disease.

COMMON SEXUALLY TRANSMITTED DISEASES

Gonorrhea.
Chlamydia.
Herpes.
Chancroid.
Syphilis.
Condylomata acuminata.

ATYPICAL CONDITIONS

Infectious: tuberculosis, cytomegalovirus, actinomycosis, *Cryptococcus*.
Neoplastic: lymphoma, Kaposi sarcoma, squamous cell carcinoma.
Other: idiopathic and ulcer.

HIV INFECTION, CHEST RADIOGRAPHIC ABNORMALITIES[1]

| ICD-10CM # | B20 | Human immunodeficiency virus [HIV] disease |
| | Z21 | Asymptomatic human immunodeficiency virus [HIV] infection status |

DIFFUSE INTERSTITIAL INFILTRATION

Pneumocystis jirovecii.
Cytomegalovirus.
Mycobacterium tuberculosis.
Mycobacterium avium complex.
Histoplasmosis.
Coccidioidomycosis.
Lymphoid interstitial pneumonitis.

FOCAL CONSOLIDATION

Bacterial pneumonia.
Mycoplasma pneumoniae.
Pneumocystis jirovecii.
Mycobacterium tuberculosis.
Mycobacterium avium complex.

NODULAR LESIONS

Kaposi sarcoma.
Mycobacterium tuberculosis.
Mycobacterium avium complex.

Fungal lesions.
Toxoplasmosis.

CAVITARY LESIONS

Pneumocystis jirovecii.
Mycobacterium tuberculosis.
Bacterial infection.

PLEURAL EFFUSION

Kaposi sarcoma.
(Small effusion may be associated with any infection).

ADENOPATHY

Kaposi sarcoma.
Lymphoma.
Mycobacterium tuberculosis.
Cryptococcus.

PNEUMOTHORAX

Kaposi sarcoma.

HIV INFECTION, COGNITIVE IMPAIRMENT[1]

| ICD-10CM # | B20 | Human immunodeficiency virus [HIV] disease |

EARLY TO MID-STAGE HIV DISEASE

Depression.
Alcohol and substance abuse.
Medication-induced cognitive impairment.
Metabolic encephalopathies.
HIV-related cognitive impairment.

ADVANCED HIV DISEASE (CD4+ <100/MM[3])

Opportunistic infection of central nervous system.
Neurosyphilis.
Central nervous system lymphoma.
Progressive multifocal leukoencephalopathy.
Depression.
Metabolic encephalopathies.
Medication-induced cognitive impairment.
Stroke.
HIV dementia.

HIV INFECTION, CUTANEOUS MANIFESTATIONS[26]

| ICD-10CM # | B20 | Human immunodeficiency virus [HIV] disease |
| | Z21 | Asymptomatic human immunodeficiency virus [HIV] infection status |

BACTERIAL INFECTION

Bacillary angiomatosis: numerous angiomatous nodules associated with fever, chills, weight loss.
Staphylococcus aureus: folliculitis, ecthyma, impetigo, bullous impetigo, furuncles, carbuncles.
Syphilis: may occur in different forms (primary, secondary, tertiary); chancre may become painful because of secondary infection.

FUNGAL INFECTION

Candidiasis: mucous membranes (oral, vulvovaginal), less commonly candida intertrigo or paronychia.
Cryptococcoses: papules or nodules that strongly resemble molluscum contagiosum; other forms include pustules, purpuric papules, and vegetating plaques.
Seborrheic dermatitis: scaling and erythema in the hair-bearing areas (eyebrows, scalp, chest, and pubic area).

ARTHROPOD INFESTATIONS

Scabies: pruritus with or without rash, usually generalized but can be limited to a single digit.

VIRAL INFECTION

Herpes simplex: vesicular lesion in clusters; perianal, genital, orofacial, or digital; can be disseminated.
Herpes zoster: painful dermatomal vesicles that may ulcerate or disseminate.
HIV: discrete erythematous macules and papules on the upper trunk, palms, and soles are the most characteristic cutaneous finding of acute HIV infection.
Human papillomavirus: genital warts (may become unusually extensive).
Kaposi sarcoma (herpesvirus): erythematous macules or papules; enlarge at varying rates; violaceous nodules or plaques; occasionally painful.
Molluscum contagiosum: discrete umbilicated papules commonly on the face, neck, and intertriginous sites (axilla, groin, or buttocks).

NONINFECTIOUS

Drug reactions: more frequent and severe in HIV patients.
Nutritional deficiencies: mainly seen in children and patients with chronic diarrhea; diffuse skin manifestations, depending upon the deficiency.
Psoriasis: scaly lesions; diffuse or localized; can be associated with arthritis.
Vasculitis: palpable purpuric eruption (can resemble septic emboli).

HIV INFECTION, ESOPHAGEAL DISEASE

| ICD-10CM # | B20 | Human immunodeficiency virus [HIV] disease |
| | K21.9 | Gastro-esophageal reflux disease without esophagitis |

Candida infection.
Cytomegalovirus infection.
Aphthous ulcer.
Herpes simplex.

Differential Diagnosis

II

HIV INFECTION, HEPATIC DISEASE[1]

ICD-10CM # B20 Human immunodeficiency virus [HIV] disease

VIRUSES

Hepatitis A.
Hepatitis B (HBV).
Hepatitis C.
Hepatitis D (with HBV).
Epstein-Barr virus.
Cytomegalovirus.
Herpes simplex virus.
Adenovirus.
Varicella-zoster virus.

MYCOBACTERIA

Mycobacterium avium complex.
Mycobacterium tuberculosis.

FUNGI

Histoplasma capsulatum.
Cryptococcus neoformans.
Coccidioides immitis.
Candida albicans.
Pneumocystis jirovecii.
Penicillium marneffei.

PROTOZOA

Toxoplasma gondii.
Cryptosporidium parvum.
Microsporida.
Schistosoma.

BACTERIA

Bartonella henselae (peliosis hepatis).

MALIGNANCY

Kaposi sarcoma (HHV-8).
Non-Hodgkin lymphoma.
Hepatocellular carcinoma.

MEDICATIONS

Zidovudine.
Didanosine.
Ritonavir.
Other HIV-1 protease inhibitors.
Fluconazole.
Macrolide antibiotics.
Isoniazid.
Rifampin.
Trimethoprim-sulfamethoxazole.

HIV INFECTION, LOWER GI TRACT DISEASE[1]

ICD-10CM # B20 Human immunodeficiency virus [HIV] disease

CAUSES OF ENTEROCOLITIS

Bacteria
Campylobacter jejuni and other spp.
Salmonella spp.
Shigella flexneri.
Aeromonas hydrophila.
Plesiomonas shigelloides.
Yersinia enterocolitica.
Vibrio spp.

Mycobacterium avium complex.
Mycobacterium tuberculosis.
Escherichia coli (enterotoxigenic, enteroadherent).
Bacterial overgrowth.
Clostridium difficile (toxin).
Parasites
Cryptosporidium parvum.
Microsporidia (Enterocytozoon bieneusi, Septata intestinalis).
Isospora belli.
Entamoeba histolytica.
Giardia lamblia.
Cyclospora cayetanensis.
Viruses
Cytomegalovirus.
Adenovirus.
Calicivirus.
Astrovirus.
Picobirnavirus.
HIV.
Fungi
Histoplasma capsulatum.

CAUSES OF PROCTITIS

Bacteria
Chlamydia trachomatis.
Neisseria gonorrhoeae.
Treponema pallidum.
Viruses
Herpes simplex.
Cytomegalovirus.

HIV INFECTION, MUSCULOSKELETAL DISORDERS[52]

ICD-10CM # B20 Human immunodeficiency virus [HIV] disease

MUSCULOSKELETAL DISORDERS ASSOCIATED WITH HIV INFECTION

Joints, Ligaments, and Soft Tissues
Painful articular syndrome.
HIV-associated arthritis.
Reactive arthritis.
Septic arthritis.
Psoriatic arthritis.
Diffuse infiltrative lymphocytosis syndrome.
Systemic lupus erythematosus.
Rheumatoid arthritis.
Vasculitis (polyarteritis nodosa, drug induced).
Immune reconstitution inflammatory syndrome.
Cellulitis and soft tissue abscesses.
Fasciitis (including necrotizing fasciitis).
Bursitis and tenosynovitis.
Muscles
HIV myopathy.
Nucleoside reverse transcriptase inhibitor (NRTI) myopathy.
Muscle infections (pyomyositis, toxoplasmosis).
Other (rhabdomyolysis, non-Hodgkin lymphoma, myasthenia gravis, nemaline [rod] myopathy, and inclusion body myositis).
Bones
Osteomyelitis.
Osteopenia and osteoporosis.
Osteonecrosis.
Hypertrophic osteoarthropathy.

Opportunistic Infections, HIV/AIDS-Defining Neoplastic Disorders, and Other Disorders Affecting Any Part of the Musculoskeletal System in HIV Infection
Neoplasia:
  Kaposi sarcoma.
  Non-Hodgkin lymphoma.
  Hodgkin lymphoma.
  Leiomyosarcoma.
  Ewing sarcoma.
Infection:
  Tuberculosis.
  Disseminated Mycobacterium avium complex infection.
  Coccidioidomycosis.
  Toxoplasmosis.
  Bacillary angiomatosis.
Other:
  HIV-related lipodystrophy.
  HIV wasting syndrome.

HIV INFECTION, OCULAR MANIFESTATIONS[17]

ICD-10CM # B20 Human immunodeficiency virus [HIV] disease
Z21 Asymptomatic human immunodeficiency virus [HIV] infection status

EYELIDS

Molluscum contagiosum.
Kaposi sarcoma.

CORNEA/CONJUNCTIVA

Keratoconjunctivitis sicca.
Bacterial/fungal ulcerative keratitis.
Herpes simplex.
Herpes zoster ophthalmicus.
Conjunctival microvasculopathy.
Kaposi sarcoma.

RETINA, CHOROID, AND VITREOUS

Microvasculopathy.
Endophthalmitis.
Cytomegalovirus retinitis.
Acute retinal necrosis.
Syphilis.
Toxoplasmosis.
Pneumocystis choroidopathy.
Cryptococcosis.
Mycobacterial infection.
Intraocular lymphoma.
Candidiasis.
Histoplasmosis.

DRUGS ASSOCIATED WITH OCULAR TOXICITY

Rifabutin.
Didanosine.

NEUROOPHTHALMIC

Disc edema.
Primary or secondary optic neuropathy.
Cranial nerve palsies.

ORBITAL

Lymphoma.
Infection.
Pseudotumor.

HIV INFECTION, PULMONARY DISEASE[1,42]

ICD-10CM #	B20	Human immunodeficiency virus [HIV] disease
	I28.8	Other diseases of pulmonary vessels

RADIOGRAPHIC APPEARANCE

Diffuse Interstitial Infiltrates
Pneumocystis jirovecii.
Mycobacterium tuberculosis, especially with advanced HIV disease.
Histoplasma capsulatum.
Coccidioides spp.
Cryptococcus neoformans.
Toxoplasma gondii.
Cytomegalovirus.
Influenza.
Lymphocytic interstitial pneumonitis.
Abacavir hypersensitivity.

Focal Consolidation
Pyogenic bacterial pneumonia from Streptococcus pneumoniae, Haemophilus influenzae.
M. tuberculosis.
Legionella spp.
Rhodococcus equi.

Hilar Adenopathy
M. tuberculosis.
H. capsulatum.
Coccidioides spp.
Non-Hodgkin or Hodgkin lymphoma.
Mycobacterium avium complex.

Cavitary Disease
Pyogenic bacterial pneumonia from Pseudomonas aeruginosa, Staphylococcus aureus, Enterobacteriaceae.
M. tuberculosis.
C. neoformans.
R. equi.
Aspergillus spp.
Nocardia spp.
Mycobacterium avium complex.
P. jiroveci.

Nodules or Masses
M. tuberculosis.
C. neoformans.
Aspergillus spp.
H. capsulatum.
Nocardia spp.
Non-Hodgkin lymphoma.
Kaposi sarcoma.
Lung cancer.

Normal Radiograph
P. jiroveci.
M. tuberculosis.

CAUSES

Mycobacterial
M. tuberculosis.
M. kansasii.
M. avium complex.
Other nontuberculous mycobacteria.

Other Bacterial
Streptococcus pneumoniae.
Staphylococcus aureus.
Haemophilus influenzae.
Enterobacteriaceae.

Pseudomonas aeruginosa.
Moraxella catarrhalis.
Group A Streptococcus.
Nocardia spp.
Rhodococcus equi.
Chlamydia pneumoniae.

Fungal
Pneumocystis carinii.
Cryptococcus neoformans.
Histoplasma capsulatum.
Coccidioides immitis.
Aspergillus spp.
Blastomyces dermatitidis.
Penicillium marneffei.

Viral
Cytomegalovirus.
Herpes simplex virus.
Adenovirus.
Respiratory syncytial virus.
Influenza viruses.
Parainfluenza virus.

Other
Toxoplasma gondii.
Strongyloides stercoralis.
Kaposi sarcoma.
Lymphoma.
Lung cancer.
Lymphocytic interstitial pneumonitis.
Nonspecific interstitial pneumonitis.
Bronchiolitis obliterans with organizing pneumonia.
Pulmonary hypertension.
Emphysema-like or bullous disease.
Pneumothorax.
Congestive heart failure.
Diffuse alveolar damage.
Pulmonary embolus.

HOARSENESS

ICD-10CM #	R49.8	Other voice and resonance disorders

Allergic rhinitis.
Infections (laryngitis, epiglottitis, tracheitis, croup).
Vocal cord polyps.
Voice strain.
Irritants (tobacco smoke).
Vocal cord trauma (intubation, surgery).
Neoplastic involvement of vocal cord (primary or metastatic).
Neurologic abnormalities (multiple sclerosis, amyotrophic lateral sclerosis, parkinsonism).
Endocrine abnormalities (puberty, menopause, hypothyroidism).
Other (laryngeal webs or cysts, psychogenic, muscle tension abnormalities).

HYDROCEPHALUS[20]

ICD-10CM #		Varies with specific diagnosis

Head trauma.
Brain neoplasm (primary or metastatic).
Spinal cord tumor.
Cerebellar infarction.
Exudative or granulomatous meningitis.
Cerebellar hemorrhage.
Subarachnoid hemorrhage.
Aqueductal stenosis.
Third ventricle colloid cyst.
Hindbrain malformation.

Viral encephalitis.
Metastases to leptomeninges.
Causes in pediatric age

COMMUNICATING
Achondroplasia.
Basilar impression.
Choroid plexus papilloma.[a]
Meningeal malignancy.
Meningitis.[a]
Posthemorrhagic.

NONCOMMUNICATING
Abscess.[a]
Aqueductal stenosis.[a]
Chiari malformation.
Dandy-Walker malformation.
Hematoma.[a]
Infectious.[a]
Klippel-Feil syndrome.
Mass lesions.[a]
Tumors and neurocutaneous disorders.
Vein of Galen malformation.[a]
Walker-Warburg syndrome.
X-linked.

OTHER CAUSES OF INCREASED INTRACRANIAL CEREBROSPINAL FLUID
Benign enlargement of subarachnoid space.
Holoprosencephaly.
Hydranencephaly.
Porencephaly.

[a]Denotes the most common conditions and the ones with disease-modifying treatments.

HYPERCALCEMIA

ICD-10CM #	E83.52	Hypercalcemia

Malignancy: increased bone resorption via osteoclast-activating factors, secretion of PTH-like substances, prostaglandin E2, direct erosion by tumor cells, transforming growth factors, colony-stimulating activity. Hypercalcemia is common in the following neoplasms:
Solid tumors: breast, lung, pancreas, kidneys, ovary.
Hematologic cancers: myeloma, lymphosarcoma, adult T-cell lymphoma, Burkitt lymphoma.
Hyperparathyroidism: increased bone resorption, GI absorption, and renal absorption; etiology: Parathyroid hyperplasia, adenoma.
Hyperparathyroidism or renal failure with secondary hyperparathyroidism.
Granulomatous disorders: increased GI absorption (e.g., sarcoidosis).
Paget disease: increased bone resorption, seen only during periods of immobilization.
Vitamin D intoxication, milk-alkali syndrome; increased GI absorption.
Thiazides: increased renal absorption.
Other causes: familial hypocalciuric hypercalcemia, thyrotoxicosis, adrenal insufficiency, prolonged immobilization, vitamin A intoxication, recovery from acute renal failure, lithium administration, pheochromocytoma, disseminated systemic lupus erythematosus.

Differential Diagnosis

II

HYPERCALCEMIA, MALIGNANCY-INDUCED

ICD-10CM #	E83.52	Hypercalcemia

Lung carcinoma:	(6% frequency, 35% of hypercalcemic cases)
Breast carcinoma:	(10% frequency, 25% of hypercalcemic cases)
Multiple myeloma:	(33% frequency, 10% of hypercalcemic cases)
Lymphoma:	(4% of hypercalcemic cases)
Genitourinary cancer:	(6% of hypercalcemic cases)

HYPERCAPNIA, PERSISTENT[17]

ICD-10CM #	R06.00	Dyspnea, unspecified
	R06.09	Other forms of dyspnea
	R06.89	Other abnormalities of breathing

Hypercapnia with normal lungs: central nervous system disturbances (cerebrovascular accident, parkinsonism, encephalitis), metabolic alkalosis, myxedema, primary alveolar hypoventilation, spinal cord lesions.

Diseases of the chest wall (e.g., kyphoscoliosis, ankylosing spondylitis).

Neuromuscular disorders (e.g., myasthenia gravis, Guillain-Barré syndrome, amyotrophic lateral sclerosis, muscular dystrophy, poliomyelitis).

Chronic obstructive pulmonary disease.

HYPERCOAGULABLE STATE, ASSOCIATED DISORDERS[31]

ICD-10CM #	D68.69	Other thrombophilia

Systemic lupus erythematosus in association with the presence of a lupus anticoagulant or antiphospholipid antibodies.

MALIGNANCY

Disease-related: includes migratory superficial thrombophlebitis (Trousseau syndrome), nonbacterial thrombotic endocarditis, thrombosis associated with chronic disseminated intravascular coagulation, thrombotic microangiopathy.

Treatment-related: associated with the administration of various chemotherapeutic agents (L-asparaginase, mitomycin, some adjuvant chemotherapeutic agents for treatment of breast cancer, thalidomide or lenalidomide in conjunction with high doses of dexamethasone).

Infusion of prothrombin complex concentrates.

Nephrotic syndrome.

Heparin-induced thrombocytopenia.

Myeloproliferative disorders.

Paroxysmal nocturnal hemoglobinuria.

DIC, Disseminated intravascular coagulopathy.

HYPERGASTRINEMIA

ICD-10CM #	E16.4	Abnormal secretion of gastrin

Decreased gastrin release inhibition from medications (proton pump inhibitors [PPIs], H_2 receptor antagonists), vagotomy.

Chronic renal failure.

Hypochlorhydria due to atrophic gastritis, gastric carcinoma, pernicious anemia.

Gastrinoma (Zollinger-Ellison syndrome).

Pyloric obstruction.

Hyperplasia of antral G cells.

Rheumatoid arthritis.

HYPERHIDROSIS[45]

ICD-10CM #	R61	Generalized hyperhidrosis

CORTICAL

Emotional.

Familial dysautonomia.

Congenital ichthyosiform erythroderma.

Epidermolysis bullosa.

Nail-patella syndrome.

Jadassohn-Lewandowsky syndrome.

Pachyonychia congenita.

Palmoplantar keratoderma.

HYPOTHALAMIC

Drugs

Antipyretics.

Emetics.

Insulin.

Meperidine.

Exercise Infection

Defervescence.

Chronic illness.

Metabolic

Debility.

Diabetes mellitus.

Hyperpituitarism.

Hyperthyroidism.

Hypoglycemia.

Obesity.

Porphyria.

Pregnancy.

Rickets.

Infantile scurvy.

Cardiovascular

Heart failure.

Shock.

Vasomotor

Cold injury.

Raynaud phenomenon.

Rheumatoid arthritis.

Neurologic

Abscess.

Familial dysautonomia.

Postencephalitic.

Tumor.

Miscellaneous

Chédiak-Higashi syndrome.

Compensatory.

Phenylketonuria.

Pheochromocytoma.

Vitiligo.

Medullary

Physiologic gustatory sweating.

Encephalitis.

Granulosis rubra nasi.

Syringomyelia.

Thoracic sympathetic trunk injury.

Spinal

Cord transection.

Syringomyelia.

Changes in Blood Flow

Mallucci syndrome.

Arteriovenous fistula.

Klippel-Trenaunay syndrome.

Glomus tumor.

Blue rubber bleb nevus syndrome.

HYPERKALEMIA

ICD-10CM #	E87.5	Hyperkalemia

Pseudohyperkalemia.

Hemolyzed specimen.

Severe thrombocytosis (platelet count 0.106 ml).

Severe leukocytosis (white blood cell count 0.105 ml).

Fist clenching during phlebotomy.

Excessive potassium intake (often in setting of impaired excretion).

Potassium replacement therapy.

High-potassium diet.

Salt substitutes with potassium.

Potassium salts of antibiotics.

Decreased renal excretion.

Potassium-sparing diuretics (e.g., spironolactone, triamterene, amiloride).

Renal insufficiency.

Mineralocorticoid deficiency.

Hyporeninemic hypoaldosteronism.

Tubular unresponsiveness to aldosterone (e.g., systemic lupus erythematosus, multiple myeloma, sickle cell disease).

Type 4 renal tubular acidosis.

ACE inhibitors.

Heparin administration.

NSAIDs.

Trimethoprim-sulfamethoxazole.

β-blockers.

Pentamidine.

Redistribution (excessive cellular release):

Acidemia (each 0.1 decrease in pH increases the serum potassium by 0.4 to 0.6 mEq/L). Lactic acidosis and ketoacidosis cause minimal redistribution.

Insulin deficiency.

Drugs (e.g., succinylcholine, markedly increased digitalis level, arginine, β-adrenergic blockers).

Hypertonicity.

Hemolysis.

Tissue necrosis, rhabdomyolysis, burns.

Hyperkalemic periodic paralysis.

HYPERKALEMIA, DRUG-INDUCED[7]

ICD-10CM #	E87.5	Hyperkalemia

IMPAIRED RENIN-ALDOSTERONE ELABORATION/FUNCTION

Cyclooxygenase inhibitors (NSAIDs).

β-Adrenergic antagonists.

Spironolactone.

ACE inhibitors and angiotensin II receptor blockers.

Heparin.

INHIBITORS OF RENAL POTASSIUM SECRETION

Potassium-sparing diuretics (amiloride, triamterene).
Trimethoprim.
Pentamidine.
Cyclosporine.
Digitalis overdose.
Lithium.

ALTERED POTASSIUM DISTRIBUTION

Insulin antagonists (somatostatin, diazoxide).
β-Adrenergic antagonists.
α-Adrenergic agonists.
Hypertonic solutions.
Digitalis.
Succinylcholine.
Arginine hydrochloride, lysine hydrochloride.

HYPERKALEMIA IN CHILDREN[11]

ICD-10CM #	E87.5	Hyperkalemia

MOST RELEVANT CAUSES OF HYPERKALEMIA IN PEDIATRIC PATIENTS

Pseudohyperkalemia
Improper collection of blood.
Hematologic disorders: leukocytosis, thrombocytosis, spherocytosis.
Transcellular Shift of Potassium
Acidosis.
Insulin deficiency.
Hyperosmolality.
Exercise with nonselective β-blockers.
Familial hyperkalemic periodic paralysis.
Increased Potassium Load
From exogenous origin: pharmacologic supplements.
From endogenous origin (cellular lysis): burns, trauma, intravascular hemolysis, rhabdomyolysis, tumor mass destruction.
Decreased Urinary Excretion
Renal failure.
Mineralocorticoid deficiency.
Addison disease.
Hypoaldosteronism.
Mineralocorticoid resistance.
Type 1 and type 2 pseudohypoaldosteronism.
Renal tubular acidosis: type 4 and hyperkalemic form of type 1.
"Hyperkalemic" drugs: potassium-sparing diuretics, trimethoprim, calcineurin inhibitors, blockers of the renin angiotensin aldosterone system.

HYPERKINETIC MOVEMENT DISORDERS[91]

ICD-10CM #	F90.8	Attention-deficit hyperactivity disorder, other type
	E83.00	Disorder of copper metabolism, unspecified
	E83.01	Wilson disease
	E83.09	Other disorders of copper metabolism
	G24.02	Drug induced acute dystonia
	G24.1	Genetic torsion dystonia

Chorea, choreoathetosis: drug-induced, Huntington chorea, Sydenham chorea.
Tardive dyskinesia (e.g., phenothiazines).
Hemiballismus (lacunar cerebrovascular accident near subthalamic nuclei in basal ganglia, metastatic lesions, toxoplasmosis [in AIDS]).
Dystonia (idiopathic, familial, drug-induced [prochlorperazine, metoclopramide]), Wilson disease.
Liver failure.
Thyrotoxicosis.
Systemic lupus erythematosus, polycythemia.

HYPERMAGNESEMIA

ICD-10CM #	E83.40	Disorders of magnesium metabolism, unspecified
	E83.41	Hypermagnesemia

Renal failure (decreased glomerular filtration rate).
Decreased renal excretion secondary to salt depletion.
Abuse of antacids and laxatives containing magnesium in patients with renal insufficiency.
Endocrinopathies (deficiency of mineralocorticoid or thyroid hormone).
Increased tissue breakdown (rhabdomyolysis).
Redistribution: acute diabetic ketoacidosis, pheochromocytoma.
Other: lithium, volume depletion, familial hypocalciuric hypercalcemia.

HYPEROSTOSIS, CORTICAL BONE[21]

ICD-10CM #	M48.19	Ankylosing hyperostosis [Forestier], multiple sites in spine

DISORDERS ASSOCIATED WITH HYPEROSTOSIS OF CORTICAL BONE

Progressive diaphyseal dysplasia.
Endosteal hyperostosis.
Pachydermoperiostosis.
Hypertrophic osteoarthropathy.
Thyroid acropachy.
Hypervitaminosis A.
Paget disease.
Infantile cortical hyperostosis.

HYPERPHOSPHATEMIA

ICD-10CM #	E83.30	Disorder of phosphorus metabolism, unspecified

Excessive phosphate administration.
Excessive oral intake or IV administration.
Laxatives containing phosphate (phosphate tablets, phosphate enemas).
Decreased renal phosphate excretion.
Acute or chronic renal failure.
Hypoparathyroidism or pseudohypoparathyroidism.
Acromegaly, thyrotoxicosis.
Bisphosphonate therapy.
Tumor calcinosis.
Sickle cell anemia.
Transcellular shift out of cells.
Chemotherapy of lymphoma or leukemia, tumor lysis syndrome, hemolysis.
Acidosis.
Rhabdomyolysis, malignant hyperthermia.
Artifact: in vitro hemolysis.
Pseudohyperphosphatemia: hyperlipidemia, paraproteinemia, hyperbilirubinemia.

HYPERPHOSPHATEMIA IN CHILDREN[11]

ICD-10CM #	E83.30	Disorder of phosphorus metabolism, unspecified

CAUSES OF HYPERPHOSPHATEMIA

Impaired Renal Excretion of Phosphate
Renal insufficiency.
Hypoparathyroidism, pseudohypoparathyroidism.
Transient parathyroid resistance of infancy.
Acromegaly.
Tumoral calcinosis.
Hyperthyroidism.
Juvenile hypogonadism.
High ambient temperature.
Heparin.
Bisphosphonate etidronate.
Increased Phosphate Intake
Exogenous Loads
Phosphate salts: laxatives and enemas.
Vitamin D intoxication.
Blood transfusion.
White phosphorus burns.
Liposomal amphotericin B.
Fosphenytoin.
Parenteral phosphate.
Endogenous Loads
Crush injury.
Rhabdomyolysis.
Cytotoxic therapy of neoplasms: tumor lysis.
Hemolysis.
Malignant hyperthermia.
Catabolic states.
Lactic acidosis.
Fulminant hepatitis.
Transcellular Shift of Phosphate
Cellular shift in diabetes ketoacidosis.
Metabolic acidosis.
Respiratory acidosis.
Miscellaneous
Hyperostosis.

HYPERPIGMENTATION[92]

ICD-10CM #	L81.4	Other melanin hyperpigmentation

Addison disease.*
Arsenic ingestion.
ACTH- or MSH-producing tumors (e.g., oat cell carcinoma of the lung).
Drug induced (e.g., antimalarials, some cytotoxic agents).
Hemochromatosis ("bronze" diabetes).
Malabsorption syndrome (Whipple disease and celiac sprue).
Melanoma.
Melanotropic hormone injection.
Pheochromocytoma.
Porphyrias (porphyria cutanea tarda and variegate porphyria).
Pregnancy.
Progressive systemic sclerosis and related conditions.
PUVA therapy (psoralen administration) for psoriasis and vitiligo.

---

*Accentuation on sun-exposed surfaces.
ACTH, Adrenocorticotropic hormone; *MSH*, melanocyte-stimulating hormone; *PUVA*, psoralen plus ultraviolet A.

HYPERPROLACTINEMIA[30]

ICD-10CM #	E22.1	Hyperprolactinemia

PHYSIOLOGIC

Pregnancy.
Lactation.
Stress.
Sleep.
Coitus.
Exercise.

PATHOLOGIC

Hypothalamic-Pituitary Stalk Damage
Tumors: craniopharyngioma, suprasellar pituitary mass extension, meningioma, dysgerminoma, hypothalamic metastases.
Granulomas.
Infiltrations.
Rathke cyst.
Irradiation.
Trauma: pituitary stalk section, sellar surgery, head trauma.

Pituitary
Prolactinoma.
Acromegaly.
Macroadenoma (compressive).
Idiopathic.
Plurihormonal adenoma.
Lymphocytic hypophysitis or parasellar mass.
Macroprolactinemia.

Systemic Disorders
Chronic renal failure.
Polycystic ovary syndrome.
Cirrhosis.
Pseudocyesis.
Epileptic seizures.
Cranial irradiation.
Chest: neurogenic chest wall trauma, surgery, herpes zoster.

PHARMACOLOGIC

Neuropeptide
Thyrotropin-releasing hormone.

Drug-Induced Hypersecretion
Dopamine receptor blockers:
    Phenothiazines: chlorpromazine, perphenazine.
    Butyrophenones: haloperidol.
    Thioxanthenes.
    Metoclopramide.
Dopamine synthesis inhibitors:
    α-Methyldopa.
Catecholamine depleters:
    Reserpine.

Cholinergic Agonist
Physostigmine.

Antihypertensives
Labetalol.
Reserpine.
Verapamil.

H_2 Antihistamines
Cimetidine.
Ranitidine.

Estrogens
Oral contraceptives.
Oral contraceptive withdrawal.

Anticonvulsant
Phenytoin.

Anesthetics

Neuroleptics
Chlorpromazine.
Risperidone.
Promazine.
Promethazine.
Trifluoperazine.
Fluphenazine.
Butaperazine.
Perphenazine.
Thiethylperazine.
Thioridazine.
Haloperidol.
Pimozide.
Thiothixene.
Molindone.

Opiates and Opiate Antagonists
Heroin.
Methadone.
Apomorphine.
Morphine.

Antidepressants
Tricyclic antidepressants: clomipramine, amitriptyline.
Selective serotonin reuptake inhibitors: fluoxetine.

HYPERSPLENISM, ASSOCIATED CONDITIONS

ICD-10CM #	D73.1	Hypersplenism

Cirrhosis.
Portal vein thrombosis.
Myeloproliferative diseases.
Lymphomas.
Leukemias.
Splenic vein thrombosis.
Autoimmune disease.
Sickle cell disease.
Thalassemias.
Gaucher disease.
Niemann-Pick disease.

HYPERTENSION, ADRENOCORTICAL CAUSES[30]

ICD-10CM #	I15.8	Other secondary hypertension

LOW RENIN AND HIGH ALDOSTERONE

Primary Aldosteronism

Aldosterone-producing adenoma (APA)	35% of cases
Bilateral idiopathic hyperplasia (IHA)	60% of cases
Primary (unilateral) adrenal hyperplasia	2% of cases
Aldosterone-producing adrenocortical carcinoma	<1% of cases
Familial Hyperaldosteronism (FH)	
Glucocorticoid-remediable aldosteronism (FH type I)	<1% of cases
FH type II (APA or IHA)	<2% of cases
Ectopic aldosterone-producing adenoma or carcinoma	<0.1% of cases

LOW RENIN AND LOW ALDOSTERONE

Hyperdeoxycorticosteronism
Congenital adrenal hyperplasia:
    11β-Hydroxylase deficiency.
    17α-Hydroxylase deficiency.
Deoxycorticosterone-producing tumor.
Primary cortisol resistance.
Apparent mineralocorticoid excess (AME)/11β-HSD* deficiency.
    Genetic: Type 1 AME.
Acquired: licorice or carbenoxolone ingestion (type 1 AME), Cushing syndrome (type 2 AME).

Cushing Syndrome
Exogenous glucocorticoid administration—most common cause.
Endogenous:
    ACH[†]-dependent—85% of cases: pituitary, ectopic.
    ACTH-independent—15% of cases: unilateral adrenal disease (adenoma or carcinoma), bilateral adrenal disease (massive macronodular hyperplasia [rare], primary pigmented nodular adrenal disease [rare]).

---

*Includes alcohol, barbiturates, benzodiazepines.
[†]*ACTH*, corticotropin.

HYPERTENSION, ENDOCRINE CAUSES[30]

ICD-10CM #	I15.8	Other secondary hypertension

ADRENAL-DEPENDENT CAUSES

Pheochromocytoma.
Primary aldosteronism.
Hyperdeoxycorticosteronism:
    Congenital adrenal hyperplasia: 11β-hydroxylase deficiency, 17α-hydroxylase deficiency.

Deoxycorticosterone-producing tumor.
Primary cortisol resistance.
Cushing syndrome.

AME/11β-HSD (HYDROXYSTEROID DEHYDROGENASE) DEFICIENCY

Genetic:
    Type 1 apparent mineralocorticoid excess (AME).
Acquired:
    Licorice or carbenoxolone ingestion (type 1 AME).
    Cushing syndrome (type 2 AME).

THYROID-DEPENDENT CAUSES

Hypothyroidism.
Hyperthyroidism.

PARATHYROID-DEPENDENT CAUSES

Hyperparathyroidism.

PITUITARY-DEPENDENT CAUSES

Acromegaly.
Cushing syndrome.

HYPERTENSION, IN CHILDREN[43]

ICD-10CM #	I10	Essential (primary) hypertension

PRIMARY

Essential hypertension.

SECONDARY

Renal
Glomerulonephritis.
Henoch-Schönlein purpura.
Pyelonephritis.
Obstruction of reflux.
Polycystic kidney disease.
Diabetic nephropathy.
Trauma.
Renal transplant or hemodialysis.
Tuberous sclerosis.
Systemic lupus nephritis.

Endocrine
Pheochromocytoma.
Cushing syndrome.
Congenital adrenal hyperplasia.
Corticosteroid treatment.
Hyperthyroidism.
Neuroblastoma.
Ovarian tumor.

Cardiac
Congestive heart failure.
Coarctation of the aorta.

Vascular
Hemolytic-uremic syndrome.
Kawasaki syndrome.
Renal artery thrombosis or stenosis.

Neurologic
Central nervous system tumor or infection.
Central nervous system trauma or abuse.
Increased intracranial pressure.
Guillain-Barré syndrome.

Neoplastic
Neuroblastoma.
Wilms tumor.
Pheochromocytoma.
Adrenal carcinoma.

Drugs
Corticosteroids.
Cocaine.
Sympathomimetics.
Oral contraceptives.
Phencyclidine.
β-Blocker or clonidine withdrawal.
Lead, mercury.

Others
Iatrogenic fluid overload.
Volume overload from end-stage renal disease.

HYPERTENSION, RESISTANT[11]

ICD-10CM #	I10	Essential (primary) hypertension
ICD-10CM #	I15	Secondary hypertension

CAUSES OF RESISTANT HYPERTENSION

Pseudoresistance:
    White coat hypertension or office elevations.
    Pseudohypertension in older patients.
    Use of small cuff on very obese arm.
Nonadherence to therapeutic regimen.
Volume overload.
Drug-related causes:
    Antihypertensive drug dosage too low.
    Wrong type of diuretic.
    Inappropriate combinations of antihypertensive drugs.
Drug actions and interactions:
    Sympathomimetics.
    Nasal decongestants.
    Appetite suppressants.
    Cocaine.
    Caffeine.
    Oral contraceptives.
    Adrenal steroids.
    Licorice (may be found in chewing tobacco).
    Cyclosporine, tacrolimus.
    Erythropoiesis-stimulating agents (ESAs) and erythropoietin.
    Antidepressants.
    NSAIDs.
Concomitant conditions:
    Obesity.
    Sleep apnea.
    Ethanol intake >1 oz (30 ml)/day.
    Anxiety, hyperventilation.
Secondary causes of hypertension:
    Renovascular hypertension.
    Primary aldosteronism.
    Pheochromocytoma.
    Hypothyroidism.
    Hyperthyroidism.
    Hyperparathyroidism.
    Aortic coarctation.
    Renal disease.

HYPERTENSIVE CRISIS SYNDROMES[7]

ICD-10CM #	I13	Hypertensive heart and renal disease
	I15	Secondary hypertension

Malignant hypertension.
Nonmalignant hypertension with target organ disorders:
    Patient requiring emergency surgery with poorly controlled hypertension.
    Hyperviscosity syndrome.
    Postoperative patient.
    Renal transplant patient: acute rejection, transplant renal artery stenosis.
    Quadriplegic patient with autonomic hyper-reflexia.
    Severe burns.
    Acute aortic dissection.
    Intracranial hemorrhage, ischemic stroke, or subarachnoid hemorrhage.
    Hypertensive encephalopathy.
    Myocardial ischemia/acute left ventricular failure.
    Preeclampsia/eclampsia.
    Antiphospholipid antibody syndrome.
    Acute renal failure:
        Scleroderma renal crisis.
        Chronic glomerulonephritis.
        Reflux nephropathy.
        Analgesic nephropathy.
        Acute glomerulonephritis.
        Radiation nephritis.
        Ask-Upmark kidney.
        Chronic lead intoxication.
Renovascular hypertension:
    Fibromuscular dysplasia.
    Atherosclerosis.
Endocrine hypertension:
    Congenital adrenal hyperplasia.
    Pheochromocytoma.
    Oral contraceptives.
    Aldosteronism.
    Cushing disease.
    Systemic vasculitis.
    Atheroembolic renal crisis.
Drugs:
    Oral contraceptives.
    Nonsteroidal antiinflammatory agents.
    Atropine.
    Corticosteroids.
    Sympathomimetics.
    Cyclosporine.
    Erythropoietin.
Lead intoxication.
Catecholamine excess states:
    Pheochromocytoma.
    MAO/tyramine interaction.
    Antihypertensive withdrawal.
    Cocaine intoxication, sympathomimetic overdose.

HYPERTENSIVE ENCEPHALOPATHY[14]

ICD-10CM #	I67.4	Hypertensive encephalopathy

Differential Diagnosis

II

Ischemic stroke.
Intracerebral hemorrhage.
Subarachnoid hemorrhage.
Subdural hematoma.
Epidural hematoma.
Central nervous vasculitis.
Brain mass.
Seizure disorder.
Central nervous system infection.
Drug toxicity.
Withdrawal syndrome.

HYPERTRICHOSIS[93]

ICD-10CM #	L68.0	Hirsutism
	L68.1	Acquired hypertrichosis lanuginosa
	L68.3	Polytrichia
	L68.9	Hypertrichosis, unspecified
	Q84.1	Congenital morphological disturbances of hair, not elsewhere classified

DRUGS

Dilantin.
Streptomycin.
Hexachlorobenzene.
Penicillamine.
Diazoxide.
Minoxidil.
Cyclosporine.

SYSTEMIC ILLNESS

Hypothyroidism.
Anorexia nervosa.
Malnutrition.
Porphyria.
Dermatomyositis.
Idiopathic

HYPERTRICHOSIS, CONGENITAL, GENERALIZED[73]

ICD-10CM #	L68.9	Hypertrichosis, unspecified

CONGENITAL SYNDROMES ASSOCIATED WITH GENERALIZED HYPERTRICHOSIS

Barber-Say syndrome.
Cantú syndrome (hypertrichosis with osteo-chondrodysplasia).
Coffin-Siris syndrome.
Cornelia de Lange (Brachmann–de Lange) syndrome.
Craniofacial dysostosis.
Hemimaxillofacial dysplasia.
Lipodystrophies:
Berardinelli-Seip syndrome.
Donohue syndrome (leprechaunism).
Mitochondrial encephalopathy, lactic acidosis, and strokelike episodes (MELAS) syndrome.
Mucopolysaccharidoses:
Hunter syndrome.
Hurler syndrome.
Sanfilippo syndrome.

Rubinstein-Taybi syndrome.
Schinzel-Giedion syndrome.
Porphyrias:
Erythropoietic porphyria (Gunther disease).
Familial porphyria cutanea tarda.
Hepatoerythropoietic porphyria.
Stiff skin syndrome.
Toxin exposure:
Fetal alcohol syndrome.
Fetal hydantoin syndrome.
Winchester syndrome.

HYPERTROPHIC OSTEOARTHROPATHY

ICD-10CM #	M89.40	Other hypertrophic osteoarthropathy, unspecified site

Idiopathic.
Pulmonary disease (e.g., pulmonary fibrosis, cystic fibrosis, sarcoidosis).
Bronchogenic carcinoma.
AIDS.
GI neoplasm (e.g., esophagus, colon).
Hepatic neoplasm, cirrhosis.
Cardiovascular diseases, aortic aneurysm, aortic prosthesis.
Congenital cyanotic heart disease, patent ductus arteriosus.
Pulmonary infections, bacterial endocarditis, amebic dysentery.
Inflammatory bowel disease.
Connective tissue diseases.
Lymphomas.
Thyroid acropachy.

HYPERVENTILATION, PERSISTENT[17]

ICD-10CM #	R06.4	Hyperventilation

Fibrotic lung disease.
Metabolic acidosis (e.g., diabetes, uremia).
Central nervous system disorders (midbrain and pontine lesions).
Hepatic coma.
Salicylate intoxication.
Fever.
Sepsis.
Psychogenic (e.g., anxiety).

HYPOCALCEMIA

ICD-10CM #	E83.51	Hypocalcemia

Renal insufficiency: hypocalcemia caused by:
Increased calcium deposits in bone and soft tissue secondary to increased serum phosphate level.
Decreased production of 1,25-dihydroxy-vitamin D.
Excessive loss of 25-OHD (nephrotic syndrome).
Hypoalbuminemia: each decrease in serum albumin (g/L) will decrease serum calcium by 0.8 mg/dl but will not change free (ionized) calcium.
Vitamin D deficiency:
Malabsorption (most common cause).
Inadequate intake.

Decreased production of 1,25-dihydroxy-vitamin D (vitamin D–dependent rickets, renal failure).
Decreased production of 25-OHD (parenchymal liver disease).
Accelerated 25-OHD catabolism (phenytoin, phenobarbital).
End-organ resistance to 1,25-dihydroxy-vitamin D.
Hypomagnesemia: hypocalcemia caused by:
Decreased PTH secretion.
Inhibition of PTH effect on bone.
Pancreatitis, hyperphosphatemia, osteoblastic metastases: hypocalcemia is secondary to increased calcium deposits (bone, abdomen).
Pseudohypoparathyroidism (PHP): autosomal recessive disorder characterized by short stature, shortening of metacarpal bones, obesity, and mental retardation; the hypocalcemia is secondary to congenital end-organ resistance to PTH.
Idiopathic hypoparathyroidism, surgical removal of parathyroids (e.g., neck surgery).
"Hungry bones syndrome": rapid transfer of calcium from plasma into bones after removal of a parathyroid tumor.
Sepsis.
Massive blood transfusion (as a result of EDTA in blood).

HYPOCALCEMIA IN PEDIATRIC PATIENTS[11]

ICD-10CM #	E83.51	Hypocalcemia

CAUSES OF HYPOCALCEMIA

Neonatal Hypocalcemia
Early Neonatal Hypocalcemia (First Few Days of Life)
Maternal hyperparathyroidism.
Maternal diabetes mellitus.
Toxemia of pregnancy.
Sepsis.
Small for gestational age, intrauterine growth restriction, prematurity.
Asphyxia.
Transfusion (citrated blood products).
Congenital rubella.
Hypomagnesemia.
Respiratory or metabolic alkalosis.
Late Neonatal Hypocalcemia (Fourth to Tenth Day of Life)
Vitamin D deficiency: nutritional deficiency; VDR loss-of-function mutation; deficient 1α-hydroxylase activity.
Phosphate overload: excessive intake of evaporated/whole milk.
Nutritional calcium deficiency.
Hypomagnesemia.
Hypoalbuminemia (nephrotic syndrome).
Transfusion (citrated blood products).
Acute/chronic kidney insufficiency.
Diuretics (furosemide).
Organic acidemia.
Primary hypoparathyroidism: DiGeorge syndrome; familial hypoparathyroidism; pseudohypoparathyroidism; Kenny-Caffey syndrome; partial deletion of GCMB; retardation dysmorphism syndrome; Pearson mitochondriopathy;

Kerns-Sayre mitochondriopathy; PTH gene defects; CaSR-activating gene mutation.

Hypocalcemia in Childhood
Parathyroid-Related Hypocalcemia
Primary hypoparathyroidism: DiGeorge syndrome; familial hypoparathyroidism; pseudohypoparathyroidism; Kenny-Caffey syndrome; Sanjad-Sakati syndrome; partial deletion of GCMB; retardation dysmorphism syndrome; Pearson mitochondriopathy; Kerns-Sayre mitochondropathy; PTH gene defects; CaSR-activating gene mutation; Bartter syndrome type 5.

Secondary hypoparathyroidism: radiation; surgery; infiltration (hemochromatosis, thalassemia, Wilson disease).

Autoimmune polyglandular syndrome type 1.

Vitamin D–Related Hypocalcemia
Nutritional vitamin D deficiency.
Defective 1α-hydroxylase activity.
VDR loss-of-function mutation.

Nutritional Calcium Deficiency
Hypomagnesemia
Hyperphosphatemia: kidney failure, rhabdomyolysis, tumor lysis
Hypoalbuminemia (nephrotic syndrome)
Medications: diuretics, chemotherapy, transfusion (citrated blood)
Organic acidemia (IVA, MMA, PPA)

CaSR, Calcium-sensing receptor; *GCMB*, glial cell missing homolog B (a parathyroid-specific transcription factor); *IUGR*, intrauterine growth retardation; *IVA*, isovaleric acidemia; *MMA*, methylmalonic acidemia; *PPA*, propionic acidemia; *PTH*, parathyroid hormone; *SGA*, small for gestational age; *VDR*, vitamin D receptor.

HYPOCAPNIA

ICD-10CM #	R06.8	Hypoventilation

Hyperventilation.
Pneumonia, pneumonitis.
Fever, sepsis.
Medications (salicylates, β-adrenergic agonists, progesterone, methylxanthines).
Pulmonary disease (asthma, interstitial fibrosis).
Pulmonary embolism.
Hepatic failure.
Metabolic acidosis.
High altitude.
Congestive heart failure.
Pregnancy.
Pain.
Central nervous system lesions.

HYPOGLYCEMIA

ICD-10CM #	E16.2	Hypoglycemia, unspecified
	E10.65	Type 1 diabetes mellitus with hyperglycemia
	E15	Nondiabetic hypoglycemic coma
	K91.2	Postsurgical malabsorption, not elsewhere classified
	E16.2	Hypoglycemia, unspecified

Oral hypoglycemics (therapeutic, factitious).
Exogenous insulin (therapeutic, factitious).
Postoperative gastric emptying (alimentary hyperinsulinism).
Severe malnutrition.
Liver disease.
Hypermetabolic state (sepsis).
Ketotic hypoglycemia.
Insulinoma.
Antibodies to endogenous insulin.
Hormone deficiencies (glucagon, growth hormone, hypoadrenalism).
Enzyme disorders in metabolism of glycogen, hexose, glycolysis, and Krebs cycle.
Idiopathic.

HYPOGLYCEMIA, IN INFANTS AND CHILDREN[19]

ICD-10CM #	E16.2	Hypoglycemia, unspecified

CLASSIFICATION OF HYPOGLYCEMIA IN INFANTS AND CHILDREN

Neonatal Transient Hypoglycemia
Associated with Inadequate Substrate or Immature Enzyme Function in Otherwise Normal Neonates
Prematurity.
Small for gestational age.
Normal newborn.

Transient Neonatal Hyperinsulinism Also Present in
Infant of diabetic mother.
Discordant twin.
Birth asphyxia.
Infant of toxemic mother.

NEONATAL, INFANTILE, OR CHILDHOOD PERSISTENT HYPOGLYCEMIAS

Hormonal Disorders
Hyperinsulinism.
Recessive KATP channel HI.
Recessive HADH (hydroxyl acyl CoA dehydrogenase) mutation HI.
Recessive UCP2 (mitochondrial uncoupling protein 2) mutation HI.
Focal KATP channel HI.
Dominant KATP channel HI.
Dominant glucokinase HI.
Dominant glutamate dehydrogenase HI (hyperinsulinism/hyperammonemia syndrome).
Dominant mutation in HNF4A (hepatic nuclear factor 4 alpha) HI with MODY later in life.
Dominant mutation in SLC16A1 (the pyruvate transporter)-exercise-induced hypoglycemia.
Acquired islet adenoma.
Beckwith-Wiedemann syndrome.
Insulin administration (Munchausen syndrome by proxy).
Oral sulfonylurea drugs.
Congenital disorders of glycosylation.

Counter-Regulatory Hormone Deficiency
Panhypopituitarism.
Isolated growth hormone deficiency.

Addison disease.
Epinephrine deficiency.

Glycogenolysis and Gluconeogenesis Disorders
Glucose-6-phosphatase deficiency (GSD 1a).
Glucose-6-phosphate translocase deficiency (GSD 1b).
Amylo-1,6-glucosidase (debranching enzyme) deficiency (GSD 3).
Liver phosphorylase deficiency (GSD 6).
Phosphorylase kinase deficiency (GSD 9).
Glycogen synthetase deficiency (GSD 0).
Fructose-1,6-diphosphatase deficiency.
Pyruvate carboxylase deficiency.
Galactosemia.
Hereditary fructose intolerance.

Lipolysis Disorders
Fatty Acid Oxidation Disorders
Carnitine transporter deficiency (primary carnitine deficiency).
Carnitine palmitoyltransferase-1 deficiency.
Carnitine translocase deficiency.
Carnitine palmitoyltransferase-2 deficiency.
Secondary carnitine deficiencies.
Very long-, long-, medium-, short-chain acyl-CoA dehydrogenase deficiency.

OTHER ETIOLOGIES

Substrate-Limited
Ketotic hypoglycemia.
Poisoning: drugs.
Salicylates.
Alcohol.
Oral hypoglycemic agents.
Insulin.
Propranolol.
Pentamidine.
Quinine.
Disopyramide.
Ackee fruit (unripe): hypoglycin.
Vacor (rat poison).
Trimethoprim-sulfamethoxazole (with renal failure).

Liver Disease
Reye syndrome.
Hepatitis.
Cirrhosis.
Hepatoma.

Amino Acid and Organic Acid Disorders
Maple syrup urine disease.
Propionic acidemia.
Methylmalonic acidemia.
Tyrosinosis.
Glutaric aciduria.
3-Hydroxy-3-methylglutaric aciduria.

Systemic Disorders
Sepsis.
Carcinoma/sarcoma (secreting—insulin-like growth factor II).
Heart failure.
Malnutrition.
Malabsorption.
Antiinsulin receptor antibodies.
Antiinsulin antibodies.
Neonatal hyperviscosity.
Renal failure.
Diarrhea.
Burns.

Differential Diagnosis

II

Shock.
Postsurgical.
Pseudohypoglycemia (leukocytosis, polycythemia).
Excessive insulin therapy of insulin-dependent diabetes mellitus.
Factitious.
Nissen fundoplication (dumping syndrome).
Falciparum malaria.

GSD, Glycogen storage disease; *HI,* hyperinsulinemia; *KATP,* regulated potassium channel.

HYPOGONADISM

ICD-10CM #	E28.310	Symptomatic premature menopause
	E29.1	Testicular hypofunction
	E28.39	Other primary ovarian failure
	E23.6	Other disorders of pituitary gland

HYPERGONADOTROPIC HYPOGONADISM

Hormone resistance (androgen, LH insensitivity).
Gonadal defects (e.g., Klinefelter syndrome, myotonic dystrophy).
Drug-induced (e.g., spironolactone, cytotoxins).
Alcoholism, radiation-induced.
Mumps orchitis.
Anatomic defects, castration.

HYPOGONADOTROPIC HYPOGONADISM

Pituitary lesions (neoplasms, granulomas, infarction, hemochromatosis, vasculitis).
Drug-induced (e.g., glucocorticoids).
Hyperprolactinemia.
Genetic disorders (Laurence-Moon-Biedl syndrome, Prader-Willi).
Delayed puberty.
Other: chronic disease, nutritional deficiency, Kallmann syndrome, idiopathic isolated LH or FSH deficiency.

HYPOKALEMIA

ICD-10CM #	E87.6	Hypokalemia

Cellular shift (redistribution) and undetermined mechanisms.
Alkalosis (each 0.1 increase in pH decreases serum potassium by 0.4 to 0.6 mEq/L).
Insulin administration.
Vitamin B_{12} therapy for megaloblastic anemias, acute leukemias.
Hypokalemic periodic paralysis: rare familial disorder manifested by recurrent attacks of flaccid paralysis and hypokalemia.
β-adrenergic agonists (e.g., terbutaline), decongestants, bronchodilators, theophylline, caffeine.
Barium poisoning, toluene intoxication, verapamil intoxication, chloroquine intoxication.
Correction of digoxin intoxication with digoxin antibody fragments (Digibind).

Increased renal excretion.
Drugs:
  Diuretics, including carbonic anhydrase inhibitors (e.g., acetazolamide).
  Amphotericin B.
  High-dose sodium penicillin, nafcillin, ampicillin, or carbenicillin.
  Cisplatin.
  Aminoglycosides.
  Corticosteroids, mineralocorticoids.
  Foscarnet sodium.
Renal tubular acidosis: distal (type 1) or proximal (type 2).
Diabetic ketoacidosis, ureteroenterostomy.
Magnesium deficiency.
Postobstruction diuresis, diuretic phase of acute tubular necrosis.
Osmotic diuresis (e.g., mannitol).
Bartter syndrome: hyperplasia of juxtaglomerular cells leading to increased renin and aldosterone, metabolic alkalosis, hypokalemia, muscle weakness, and tetany (seen in young adults).
Increased mineralocorticoid activity (primary or secondary aldosteronism), Cushing syndrome.
Chronic metabolic alkalosis from loss of gastric fluid (increased renal potassium secretion).
GI loss:
  Vomiting, nasogastric suction.
  Diarrhea.
  Laxative abuse.
  Villous adenoma.
  Fistulas.
  Inadequate dietary intake (e.g., anorexia nervosa).
  Cutaneous loss (excessive sweating).
  High dietary sodium intake, excessive use of licorice.

HYPOKALEMIA IN PEDIATRIC PATIENTS[11]

ICD-10CM #	E87.6	Hypokalemia

MOST RELEVANT CAUSES OF HYPOKALEMIA IN PEDIATRIC PATIENTS

Acute Redistribution of Potassium to the Intracellular Compartment
Metabolic alkalosis.
Insulin administration.
Hypokalemic periodic paralysis.
Prolonged Lack of Intake
Increased Renal Loss
Drugs: diuretics, antibiotics, aminoglycosides, penicillin, amphotericin B, capreomycin.
Metabolic acidosis and diabetic ketoacidosis.
Increased mineralocorticoid activity.
Cushing syndrome.
Congenital adrenal hyperplasia.
Primary or secondary hyperaldosteronism.
Primary tubulopathies.
Bartter syndrome.
Gitelman syndrome.
Liddle syndrome.
Types 1 and 2 renal tubular acidosis.
Epilepsy, ataxia, sensorineural deafness, and tubulopathy (EAST) syndrome.
Fanconi syndrome.

Increased GI Loss
Vomiting (hypertrophic pyloric stenosis).
Diarrhea.

HYPOMAGNESEMIA

ICD-10CM #	E83.40	Disorders of magnesium metabolism, unspecified
	E83.42	Hypomagnesemia

GI AND NUTRITIONAL

Defective GI absorption (malabsorption).
Inadequate dietary intake (e.g., alcoholics).
Parenteral therapy without magnesium.
Chronic diarrhea, villous adenoma, prolonged nasogastric suction, fistulas (small bowel, biliary).

EXCESSIVE RENAL LOSSES

Diuretics.
Renal tubular acidosis.
Diuretic phase of acute tubular necrosis.
Endocrine disturbances (diabetic ketoacidosis, hyperaldosteronism, hyperthyroidism, hyperparathyroidism), syndrome of inappropriate antidiuretic hormone secretion, Bartter syndrome, hypercalciuria, hypokalemia.
Cisplatin, alcohol, cyclosporine, digoxin, pentamidine, mannitol, amphotericin B, foscarnet, methotrexate.
Antibiotics (gentamicin, ticarcillin, carbenicillin).
Redistribution: hypoalbuminemia, cirrhosis, administration of insulin and glucose, theophylline, epinephrine, acute pancreatitis, cardiopulmonary bypass.
Miscellaneous: sweating, burns, prolonged exercise, lactation, "hungry-bones" syndrome.

HYPOMAGNESEMIA IN PEDIATRIC PATIENTS[11]

ICD-10CM #	E83.42	Hypomagnesemia

MAIN CAUSES OF HYPOMAGNESEMIA IN CHILDREN

Primary Inherited Disorders
Familial hypomagnesemia with hypercalciuria and nephrocalcinosis.
Hypomagnesemia with secondary hypocalcemia.
Autosomal dominant hypomagnesemia.
Isolated autosomal recessive hypomagnesemia with normocalciuria.
Activating mutations of calcium-sensing receptor.
Gitelman syndrome.
Bartter syndrome.
Secondary Disorders
Decreased GI absorption:
  Malabsorptive syndromes.
  Vomiting and diarrhea.
Increased urinary excretion:
  Extracellular volume expansion.
  Polyuric states: obstructive uropathy, kidney transplant.
Drugs:
  Diuretics.
  Calcineurin antagonists.
  Others: cisplatinum, aminoglycosides, amphotericin B.
  Metabolic acidosis.

Miscellaneous: "hungry bone," low-birth-weight newborn, infant of diabetic mother.

HYPONATREMIA

ICD-10CM #	E87.1	Hypo-osmolality and hyponatremia

Renal loss from renal disease, diuretics.
GI loss (diarrhea, vomiting, suction).
Hypertonic hyponatremia (e.g., increased serum osmolality from hyperglycemia).
Transcutaneous loss (extensive burns, excessive sweating).
Fluid sequestration (e.g., ascites).
Osmotic diuresis (e.g., mannitol, glucose).
Dilutional (psychogenic polydipsia, iatrogenic).
Syndrome of inappropriate antidiuretic hormone secretion.
Edema with water and sodium retention.
Artifact (e.g., severe hyperlipidemia).
Laboratory error.
Adrenal insufficiency.

HYPOPHOSPHATEMIA

ICD-10CM #	E83.30	Disorder of phosphorus metabolism, unspecified
	E83.31	Familial hypophosphatemia

Decreased intake (prolonged starvation [alcoholics], hyperalimentation, or IV infusion without phosphate).
Malabsorption.
Phosphate-binding antacids.
Renal loss:
RTA.
Fanconi syndrome, vitamin D–resistant rickets.
ATN (diuretic phase).
Hyperparathyroidism (primary or secondary).
Familial hypophosphatemia.
Hypokalemia, hypomagnesemia.
Acute volume expansion.
Glycosuria, idiopathic hypercalciuria.
Acetazolamide.
Transcellular shift into cells:
Alcohol withdrawal.
Diabetic ketoacidosis (recovery phase).
Glucose-insulin or catecholamine infusion.
Anabolic steroids.
Total parenteral nutrition.
Theophylline overdose.
Severe hyperthermia; recovery from hypothermia.
"Hungry bones" syndrome.

HYPOPHOSPHATEMIA IN PEDIATRIC PATIENTS[11]

ICD-10CM #	E83.30	Disorder of phosphorus metabolism, unspecified

CAUSES OF HYPOPHOSPHATEMIA

Decreased Phosphate Intake

Starvation, inadequate phosphate intake, chronic diarrhea, chronic alcoholism.

Total parenteral nutrition with insufficient phosphate content.

Increased Loss of Phosphate

Increased renal phosphate excretion:
Primary hyperparathyroidism.
Secondary hyperparathyroidism: vitamin D deficiency or resistance (including 1α-hydroxylase deficiency, VDR mutations, VDDR); imatinib.
Excess FGF-23 or phosphatonins: X-linked hypophosphatemia, AD hypophosphatemic rickets, tumor-induced osteomalacia, epidermal nevus, McCune-Albright syndrome.
Fanconi syndrome, cystinosis, Wilson disease Dent disease, Lowe syndrome, multiple myeloma, amyloidosis, heavy-metal toxicity, rewarming of hyperthermia, Na/Pi-IIa and Na/Pi-IIc mutation (HHRH).
PTHrP-dependent hypercalcemia of malignancy.
Hypomagnesemia.
Decreased intestinal absorption:
Vitamin D deficiency or resistance (VDDR I and II).
Malabsorption.
Increased intestinal loss:
Phosphate binding antacids used in treating peptic ulcers.
Increased loss from other routes:
Skin: severe burns.
Vomiting.

Phosphate Shifting from Extracellular Compartment to Cells and Bones

Diabetic ketoacidosis.
Alcohol intoxication.
Acute respiratory alkalosis, salicylate intoxication, gram-negative sepsis, toxic shock syndrome, acute gout.
Refeeding syndromes from starvation, anorexia nervosa, hepatic failure: acute intravenous glucose, fructose, glycerol.
Rapid cellular proliferation: intensive erythropoietin therapy, GM-CSF therapy, leukemic blast crisis.
Recovery from hypothermia.
Heat stroke.
Post parathyroidectomy; "hungry bone" disease: osteoblastic metastases, antiresorptive treatment of severe Paget disease.
Catecholamine (albuterol, dopamine, terbutaline, epinephrine).
Thyrotoxic periodic paralysis.
Hypocalcemic periodic paralysis.

Miscellaneous

Hyperaldosteronism.
Oncogenic hypophosphatemia.
Post kidney transplantation.
Post partial hepatectomy.
High-dose corticosteroids, estrogens.
Medications: ifosfamide, toluene, calcitonin, bisphosphonate, tenofovir, paraquat, cisplatin, acetazolamide, and other diuretics.
Post obstructive diuresis.

AD, Autosomal dominant; *FGF-23,* fibroblast growth factor 23; *GM-CSF,* granulocyte-macrophage colony-stimulating factor; *HHRH,* hereditary hypophosphatemic rickets with hypercalciuria; *Na/Pi-II,* type II sodium-dependent phosphate cotransporter; *PTHrP,* parathyroid hormone–related peptide; *VDR,* vitamin D receptor; *VDDR,* vitamin D–dependent rickets.

HYPOPIGMENTATION

ICD-10CM #	L81.9	Disorder of pigmentation, unspecified

Vitiligo.
Tinea versicolor.
Atopic dermatitis.
Chemical leukoderma.
Idiopathic hypomelanosis.
Sarcoidosis.
Systemic lupus erythematosus.
Scleroderma.
Oculocutaneous albinism.
Phenylketonuria.
Nevoid hypopigmentation.

HYPOTENSION, POSTURAL

ICD-10CM #	I95.89	Other hypotension

Antihypertensive medications (especially α-blockers, diuretics, ACE inhibitors).
Volume depletion (hemorrhage, dehydration).
Impaired cardiac output (constrictive pericarditis, aortic stenosis).
Peripheral autonomic dysfunction (diabetes mellitus, Guillain-Barré).
Idiopathic orthostatic hypotension.
Central autonomic dysfunction (Shy-Drager syndrome).
Peripheral venous disease.
Adrenal insufficiency.

HYPOTHYROIDISM, CONGENITAL[19]

ICD-10CM #	E03.0	Congenital hypothyroidism with diffuse goiter
	E03.1	Congenital hypothyroidism without goiter

ETIOLOGIC CLASSIFICATION OF CONGENITAL HYPOTHYROIDISM

Primary Hypothyroidism

Defect of fetal thyroid development (dysgenesis):
Aplasia.
Hypoplasia.
Ectopia.
Defect in thyroid hormone synthesis (dyshormonogenesis):
Iodide transport defect: mutation in thyroglobulin gene.
Thyroid organification or coupling defect: mutation in thyroid peroxidase gene.
Defects in H_2O_2 generation: mutations in DUOXA2 maturation factor or DUOX2 gene.
Thyroglobulin synthesis defect: mutation in thyroglobulin gene.
Deiodination defect: mutation in *DEHAL1* gene.
TSH unresponsiveness:
$G_s\alpha$ mutation (e.g., type 1A pseudohypothyroidism).
Mutation in TSH receptor.
Defect in thyroid hormone transport: mutation in monocarboxylate transporter 8 (MCT8) gene.

Iodine deficiency (endemic goiter).
Maternal antibodies: thyrotropin receptor–blocking antibody (TRBAb, also termed thyrotropin-binding inhibitor immunoglobulin).
Maternal medications:
Iodides, amiodarone.
Propylthiouracil, methimazole.
Radioiodine.

CENTRAL (HYPOPITUITARY) HYPOTHYROIDISM

PIT-1 mutations:
Deficiency of thyroid-stimulating hormone (TSH).
Deficiency of growth hormone.
Deficiency of prolactin.
PROP-1 mutations:
Deficiency of TSH.
Deficiency of growth hormone.
Deficiency of prolactin.
Deficiency of luteinizing hormone.
Deficiency of follicle-stimulating hormone.
± Deficiency of adrenocorticotropic hormone.
TSH deficiency: mutation in TSH β subunit gene (manifests as primary hypothyroidism with elevated TSH level).
Multiple pituitary deficiencies (e.g., craniopharyngioma).
Thyroid-releasing hormone (TRH) deficiency:
Isolated.
Multiple hypothalamic deficiencies (e.g., septooptic dysplasia).
TRH unresponsiveness.
Mutations in TRH receptor.

HYPOTONIA, INFANTILE, DIFFERENTIAL DIAGNOSIS[19]

ICD-10CM #   H44.40   Unspecified hypotony of eye

Cerebral hypotonia:
Benign congenital hypotonia.
Chromosome disorders.
Prader-Willi syndrome.
Trisomy.
Chronic nonprogressive encephalopathy.
Cerebral malformation.
Perinatal distress.
Postnatal disorders.
Peroxisomal disorders.
Cerebrohepatorenal syndrome (Zellweger syndrome).
Neonatal adrenoleukodystrophy.
Other genetic defects.
Familial dysautonomia.
Oculocerebrorenal syndrome (Lowe syndrome).
Other metabolic defects.
Acid maltase deficiency (see "Metabolic Myopathies").
Infantile GM, gangliosidosis.
Spinal cord disorders.
Spinal muscular atrophies:
Acute infantile.
Autosomal dominant.
Autosomal recessive.
Cytochrome-c oxidase deficiency.
X-linked.

Chronic infantile:
Autosomal dominant.
Autosomal recessive.
Congenital cervical spinal muscular atrophy.
Infantile neuronal degeneration.
Neurogenic arthrogryposis.
Polyneuropathies:
Congenital hypomyelinating neuropathy.
Giant axonal neuropathy.
Hereditary motor-sensory neuropathies.
Disorders of neuromuscular transmission:
Familial infantile myasthenia.
Infantile botulism.
Transitory myasthenia gravis.
Fiber-type disproportion myopathies.
Central core disease.
Congenital fiber-type disproportion myopathy.
Myotubular (centronuclear) myopathy.
Acute.
Chronic.
Nemaline (rod) myopathy.
Autosomal dominant.
Autosomal recessive.
Metabolic myopathies:
Acid maltase deficiency.
Cytochrome-c oxidase deficiency.
Muscular dystrophies:
Bethlem myopathy.
Congenital dystrophinopathy.
Congenital muscular dystrophy.
Merosin deficiency, primary.
Merosin deficiency, secondary.
Merosin positive.
Congenital myotonic dystrophy.

HYPOTONIC POLYURIA[11]

ICD-10CM #   Varies with specific diagnosis

CAUSES OF HYPOTONIC POLYURIA

Central (Neurogenic) Diabetes Insipidus
Congenital (congenital malformations, autosomal dominant, arginine vasopressin [AVP] neurophysin gene mutations).
Drug- or toxin-induced (ethanol, diphenylhydantoin, snake venom).
Granulomatous (histiocytosis, sarcoidosis).
Neoplastic (craniopharyngioma, germinoma, lymphoma, leukemia, meningioma, pituitary tumor; metastases).
Infectious (meningitis, tuberculosis, encephalitis).
Inflammatory, autoimmune (lymphocytic infundibuloneurohypophysitis).
Trauma (neurosurgery, deceleration injury).
Vascular (cerebral hemorrhage or infarction, brain death).
Idiopathic.
Osmoreceptor Dysfunction
Granulomatous (histiocytosis, sarcoidosis).
Neoplastic (craniopharyngioma, pinealoma, meningioma, metastases).
Vascular (anterior communicating artery aneurysm or ligation, intrahypothalamic hemorrhage).
Other (hydrocephalus, ventricular or suprasellar cyst, trauma, degenerative diseases).
Idiopathic.

Increased AVP metabolism.
Pregnancy.
Nephrogenic Diabetes Insipidus
Congenital (X-linked recessive, AVP V2 receptor gene mutations, autosomal recessive or dominant, aquaporin-2 water channel gene mutations).
Drug-induced (demeclocycline, lithium, cisplatin, methoxyflurane).
Hypercalcemia.
Hypokalemia.
Infiltrating lesions (sarcoidosis, amyloidosis).
Vascular (sickle cell anemia).
Mechanical (polycystic kidney disease, bilateral ureteral obstruction).
Solute diuresis (glucose, mannitol, sodium, radiocontrast dyes).
Idiopathic.
Primary Polydipsia
Psychogenic (schizophrenia, obsessive-compulsive behaviors).
Dipsogenic (downward resetting of thirst threshold, idiopathic or similar lesions, as with central DI).

HYPOVOLEMIA[11]

ICD-10CM #   Varies with specific diagnosis

CAUSES OF ABSOLUTE AND RELATIVE HYPOVOLEMIA

Absolute
Extrarenal
GI fluid loss.
Bleeding.
Skin fluid loss.
Respiratory fluid loss.
Extracorporeal ultrafiltration.
Renal
Diuretics.
Obstructive uropathy/postobstructive diuresis.
Hormone deficiency.
Hypoaldosteronism.
Adrenal insufficiency.
Na+ wasting tubulopathies.
Genetic.
Acquired tubulointerstitial disease.
Relative
Extrarenal
Edematous states.
Heart failure.
Cirrhosis.
Generalized vasodilation.
Sepsis.
Drugs.
Pregnancy.
Third-space loss.
Renal
Severe nephrotic syndrome.

HYPOVOLEMIC SHOCK, PEDIATRIC POPULATION[61]

ICD-10CM #   R57.1   Hypovolemic shock
               R57.8   Other shock

ETIOLOGIES OF HYPOVOLEMIC SHOCK

Whole blood loss.
Absolute loss: hemorrhage.
External bleeding.
Internal bleeding:
  GI.
  Intraabdominal (spleen, liver).
  Major vessel injury.
  Intracranial (in infants).
  Fractures.
Relative loss:
  Pharmacologic (barbiturates, vasodilators).
  Positive pressure ventilation.
  Spinal cord injury.
  Sepsis.
  Anaphylaxis.
  Plasma loss.
  Burns.
  Capillary leak syndromes:
  Inflammation, sepsis.
  Anaphylaxis.
Protein-losing syndromes.
Fluid and electrolyte loss.
Vomiting and diarrhea.
Excessive diuretic use.
Endocrine:
  Adrenal insufficiency.
  Diabetes insipidus.
  Diabetes mellitus.

HYPOXEMIA AND HYPERCAPNIC RESPIRATORY FAILURE[27]

ICD-10CM #	Varies with specific diagnosis

COMMON CAUSES OF HYPOXEMIC AND HYPERCAPNIC RESPIRATORY FAILURE

Brain
Bulbar poliomyelitis.
Central alveolar hypoventilation.
Cerebrovascular accident.
Cerebral malignancy.
Drug overdose (e.g., narcotic, sedative/hypnotic).
Elevated intracranial pressure.
Encephalitis and meningitis.
Pontine herniation.
Postoperative anesthetic depression.
Spinal Cord
Amyotrophic lateral sclerosis.
Cervical cordotomy.
Guillain-Barré syndrome.
Poliomyelitis.
Spinal cord trauma.
Neuromuscular System
Acute intermittent porphyria.
Botulism.
Cholinergic crisis.
Curariform drugs.
Electrolyte disorders (e.g., hypophosphatemia, hypomagnesemia).
Hypokalemic periodic paralysis.
Multiple sclerosis.
Myasthenia gravis.
Myxedema.

Neuromuscular blocking antibiotics (e.g., polymyxin, streptomycin).
Organophosphate insecticides.
Peripheral neuritis.
Polymyositis.
Respiratory muscle fatigue—critical illness polyneuropathy/polymyopathy.
Tetanus.
Upper Airway
Epiglottitis and laryngotracheitis.
Large tonsils and adenoids.
Obstructive sleep apnea.
Postintubation laryngeal edema.
Tracheal obstruction.
Vocal cord paralysis.
Thorax and Pleura
Chest wall burn with eschar formation.
Chest wall trauma—flail chest.
Kyphoscoliosis.
Massive abdominal distention.
Massive obesity.
Muscular dystrophy.
Large pleural effusion/pleural fibrosis.
Pneumothorax.
Rheumatoid spondylitis.
Thoracoplasty.
Cardiovascular System
Cardiogenic pulmonary edema.
Left ventricular failure.
Mitral stenosis.
Biventricular failure.
Fat embolism.
Snake bite.
Uremia.
Volume overload.
Pulmonary venoocclusive disease.
Lower Airway and Alveoli
Acute respiratory distress syndrome.
Aspiration.
Asthma.
Atelectasis.
Bronchiectasis.
Bronchiolitis.
Chronic obstructive pulmonary disease.
Cystic fibrosis.
Interstitial lung disease.
Massive bilateral pneumonia.
Near-drowning.
Pancreatitis.
Pulmonary contusion.
Radiation lung injury.
Sepsis.
Smoke inhalation.
Surgical resection of lung parenchyma.

ILIAC FOSSA PAIN, LEFT SIDED[2]

ICD-10CM #	M25.5	Pain in joint

GI CAUSES OF ACUTE LEFT ILIAC FOSSA PAIN

Nonspecific left iliac fossa pain including constipation.
Acute gastroenteritis.
Acute diverticulitis.
Colonic carcinoma.
Colonic ischemia.
Localized small bowel perforation.

ILIAC FOSSA PAIN, RIGHT SIDED[2]

ICD-10CM #	M25.5	Pain in joint

DIFFERENTIAL DIAGNOSIS OF RIGHT ILIAC FOSSA PAIN

GI Causes
Nonspecific right iliac fossa pain.
Acute appendicitis.
Mesenteric adenitis.
Terminal ileitis.
Acute inflammation of Meckel diverticulum.
Crohn disease of the terminal ileum.
Cecal carcinoma.
Inflammatory cecal lesion (e.g., diverticulitis in a solitary cecal diverticulum).
Inflammatory lesion of the terminal ileum (e.g., foreign body perforation).
Non-GI Causes
Ruptured ovarian follicle (mittelschmerz).
Acute salpingitis (pelvic inflammatory disease).
Rupture/torsion or hemorrhage of an ovarian cyst.
Endometriosis.
Ectopic pregnancy.
Urinary tract infection.

IMMUNODEFICIENCY, CONGENITAL (PRIMARY)

ICD-10CM #	D80.0	Hereditary hypogamma-globulinemia
	D80.1	Nonfamilial hypogam-maglobulinemia
	D80.2	Selective deficiency of IgA
	D80.3	Selective deficiency of IgG
	D80.4	Selective deficiency of IgM

CONGENITAL (PRIMARY) CAUSES OF IMMUNODEFICIENCY

T-lymphocyte Deficiencies
DiGeorge syndrome (thymic aplasia with reduced CD4 and CD3 cells).
Purine nucleoside phosphorylase deficiency (marked T-cell depletion).
B-lymphocyte Deficiencies
Bruton X-linked agammaglobulinemia (absence of B cells, plasma cells, and antibody).
Selective immunoglobulin G (IgG) subclass deficiencies.
Selective IgA deficiency.
Hyper-IgM immunodeficiency (elevated IgM but reduced IgG and IgA).
Mixed T- and B-lymphocyte Deficiencies
Common variable immunodeficiency (leads to various B-cell activation or differentiation defects and gradual deterioration of T-cell number and function).
Severe combined immunodeficiency (severe reduction in IgG and absence of T cells).
Wiskott-Aldrich syndrome (decreased T-cell number and function, low IgM, occasionally low IgG).
Ataxia-telangiectasia (decreased T-cell number and function; IgA, IgE, IgG$_2$, and IgG$_4$ deficiency).

Disorders of Complement

C3 deficiency (congenital absence of C3 or consumption of C3 due to deficiency of C3b inactivator).

Phagocyte Defects

Chronic granulomatous disease (defect in nicotinamide adenine dinucleotide phosphate oxidase in phagocytic cells).

Chédiak-Higashi syndrome (impaired microbicidal activity of phagocytes).

Kostmann syndrome, Shwachman-Diamond syndrome, cyclic neutropenia (low neutrophil count).

IMPAIRED CONSCIOUSNESS AND COMA[49]

ICD-10CM #	R40.20	Unspecified coma

INFECTIOUS OR INFLAMMATORY

Infectious

Bacterial meningitis.
Viral encephalitis.
Rickettsial infection.
Protozoan infection.
Helminth infestation.

Inflammatory

Sepsis-associated encephalopathy.
Vasculitis, collagen vascular disorders.
Demyelination.
Acute disseminated encephalomyelitis.
Multiple sclerosis.

STRUCTURAL

Traumatic

Concussion.
Cerebral contusion.
Epidural hematoma or effusion.
Intracerebral hematoma.
Diffuse axonal injury.
Abusive head trauma.

Neoplasms

Vascular Disease

Cerebral infarction:
  Thrombosis.
  Embolism.
  Venous sinus thrombosis.
Cerebral hemorrhage:
  Subarachnoid hemorrhage.
  Arteriovenous malformation.
  Aneurysm.
Congenital abnormality or dysplasia of vascular supply
Trauma to carotid or vertebral arteries in the neck

Focal Infection

Abscess.
Cerebritis.
Hydrocephalus.

METABOLIC, NUTRITIONAL, OR TOXIC

Hypoxic-Ischemic Encephalopathy

Shock.
  Cardiac or pulmonary failure.
  Near-drowning.
  Carbon monoxide poisoning.
  Cyanide poisoning.
  Strangulation.

Metabolic Disorders

Sarcoidosis.
Hypoglycemia.
Fluid and electrolyte imbalance.
Endocrine disorders:
  With acidosis:
  Diabetic ketoacidosis.
  Aminoacidemias.
  Organic acidemias.
With hyperammonemia:
  Hepatic encephalopathy.
  Urea cycle disorders.
  Disorders of fatty acid metabolism.
  Reye syndrome.
  Valproic acid encephalopathy.
  Uremia.
  Porphyria.
  Mitochondrial disorders.
  Leigh syndrome.

Nutritional

Thiamine deficiency.
Niacin or nicotinic acid deficiency.
Pyridoxine dependency.
Folate and vitamin B_{12} deficiency.

Exogenous Toxins and Poisons

Alcohol intoxication.
Over-the-counter medications.
Prescription medications (oral and ophthalmic).
Herbal treatments.
Heavy-metal poisoning.
Mushroom and plant intoxication.
Illegal drugs.
Industrial agents.

Hypertensive Encephalopathy

Burn Encephalopathy

IMPOTENCE[80]

ICD-10CM #	F52.21	Male erectile disorder
	F52.8	Other sexual dysfunction not due to a substance or known physiological condition
	N52.9	Male erectile dysfunction, unspecified

Psychogenic.
Endocrine: hyperprolactinemia, diabetes mellitus, Cushing syndrome, hypothyroidism or hyperthyroidism, abnormality of hypothalamic-pituitary-testicular axis.
Vascular: arterial insufficiency, venous leakage, AV malformation, local trauma.
Medications.
Neurogenic: autonomic or sensory neuropathy, spinal cord trauma or tumor, cerebrovascular accident, multiple sclerosis, temporal lobe epilepsy.
Systemic illness: renal failure, chronic obstructive pulmonary disease, cirrhosis of liver, myotonic dystrophy.
Peyronie disease.
Prostatectomy.

INCONTINENCE, FECAL[2]

ICD-10CM #	R15.9	Full incontinence of feces

NORMAL SPHINCTER

Diarrhea.
Anorectal conditions:
  Rectal carcinoma.
  Inflammatory bowel disease.
  Hemorrhoids.
  Mucosal prolapse.
  Fissure-in-ano.
  Abnormal rectal sensation.

ABNORMAL SPHINCTER

Congenital abnormalities.
Anal sepsis.
Neurologic conditions.
Rectal prolapse.
Sphincter trauma.
Neurogenic (idiopathic) incontinence.

INFECTIOUS DIARRHEA IN TROPICS[3]

ICD-10CM #	R19.7	Diarrhea, unspecified

CAUSES OF INFECTIOUS DIARRHEA IN THE TROPICS

Bacteria

Aeromonas hydrophila.
Arcobacter butzleri.
Bacteroides fragilis, enterotoxigenic.
Campylobacter jejuni.
Escherichia coli: enterotoxigenic, enteroaggregative, enteroinvasive, enterohemorrhagic.
Laribacter hongkongensis.
Plesiomonas shigelloides.
Salmonella, nontyphoidal.
Shigella spp: S. dysenteriae, S. flexneri, S. sonnei, S. boydii.
Vibrio cholerae 01, 0139, non-01 non-0139.
Vibrio parahaemolyticus.
Yersinia enterocolitica.

Helminths

Paracapillaria philippinensis.
Fasciolopsis buski.
Heterophyiasis (Metagonimus yokogawai, Haplorchis taichui).
Schistosoma mansoni.
Strongyloides stercoralis.

Protozoa

Blastocystis hominis.
Cryptosporidium parvum.
Cyclospora cayetanensis.
Encephalitozoon intestinalis.
Enterocytozoon bieneusi.
Giardia lamblia.
Isospora belli.
Leishmania donovani.

Viruses

Astroviruses.
Caliciviruses: norovirus and sapovirus.
Enteric adenoviruses.
HIV.
Picornaviruses.
Rotavirus.

INFERTILITY, FEMALE[24]

ICD-10CM #	N97.9	Female infertility, unspecified

FALLOPIAN TUBE PATHOLOGY

Pelvic inflammatory disease or puerperal infection.
Congenital anomalies.
Endometriosis.
Secondary to past peritonitis of nongenital origin.
Amenorrhea and anovulation.
Minor anovulatory disturbances.

CERVICAL AND UTERINE FACTORS

Leiomyomas and polyps.
Uterine anomalies.
Intrauterine synechiae (Asherman syndrome).
Destroyed endocervical glands (postsurgery or postinfection).

VAGINAL FACTORS

Congenital absence of vagina.
Imperforate hymen.
Vaginismus.
Vaginitis.

IMMUNOLOGIC FACTORS

Sperm-immobilizing antibodies.
Sperm-agglutinating antibodies.

NUTRITIONAL AND METABOLIC FACTORS

Thyroid disorders.
Diabetes mellitus.
Severe nutritional disturbances.

INFERTILITY, MALE[24]

ICD-10CM #	N46.9	Male infertility, unspecified

DECREASED PRODUCTION OF SPERMATOZOA

Varicocele.
Testicular failure.
Endocrine disorders.
Cryptorchidism.
Stress, smoking, caffeine, nicotine, recreational drugs.

DUCTAL OBSTRUCTION

Epididymal (postinfection).
Congenital absence of vas deferens.
Ejaculatory duct (postinfection).
Postvasectomy.

INABILITY TO DELIVER SPERM INTO VAGINA

Ejaculatory disturbances.
Hypospadias.
Sexual problems (i.e., impotence), medical or psychologic.

ABNORMAL SEMEN

Infection.
Abnormal volume.
Abnormal viscosity.
Abnormal sperm motion.

IMMUNOLOGIC FACTORS

Sperm-immobilizing antibodies.
Sperm-agglutinating antibodies.

INSOMNIA[76]

ICD-10CM #	780.51	Insomnia with sleep apnea
	G47.00	Insomnia, unspecified
	F51.01	Primary insomnia
	F51.03	Paradoxical insomnia
	F51.09	Other insomnia not due to a substance or known physiological condition

Anxiety disorder, psychophysiologic insomnia.
Depression.
Drugs (e.g., caffeine, amphetamines, cocaine), hypnotic-dependent sleep disorder.
Pain, fibromyalgia.
Inadequate sleep hygiene.
Restless leg syndrome.
Obstructive sleep apnea.
Sleep bruxism.
Medical illness (e.g., gastroesophageal reflux disease, sleep-related asthma, parkinsonism and movement disorders).
Narcolepsy.
Other: periodic leg movement of sleep, central sleep apnea, rapid eye movement behavioral disorder.

INTESTINAL PSEUDOOBSTRUCTION[17,68]

ICD-10CM #	K56.0	Paralytic ileus
	K56.9	Ileus, unspecified
	K59.9	Functional intestinal disorder, unspecified

"PRIMARY" (IDIOPATHIC INTESTINAL PSEUDOOBSTRUCTION)

Hollow visceral myopathy:
  Familial.
  Sporadic.
Neuropathic:
  Abnormal myenteric plexus.
  Normal myenteric plexus.

SECONDARY

Scleroderma.
Myxedema.
Amyloidosis.
Muscular dystrophy.
Hypokalemia.
Chronic renal failure.
Diabetes mellitus.
Drug toxicity caused by:
  Anticholinergics.
  Opiate narcotics.
Ogilvie syndrome.

CAUSES OF SECONDARY CHRONIC INTESTINAL PSEUDOOBSTRUCTION IN CHILDREN

Causes of Secondary Chronic Intestinal Pseudoobstruction in Children

Autoimmune
Autoimmune myositis.
Autoimmune ganglionitis.
Scleroderma.
Endocrine
Diabetes mellitus.
Hypoparathyroidism.
Hypothyroidism.
Gastrointestinal
Celiac disease.
Eosinophilic gastroenteritis.
Inflammatory bowel disease.
Hematology/Oncology
Multiple myeloma.
Paraneoplastic syndromes.
Pheochromocytoma.
Sickle cell disease.
Infection
Chagas disease.
Cytomegalovirus.
Epstein-Barr virus.
Herpes zoster.
JC virus.
Kawasaki disease.
Postviral neuropathy.
Medications and Toxins
Chemotherapy.
Cyclopentolate and phenylephrine eye drops.
Diltiazem and nifedipine.
Fetal alcohol syndrome.
Jellyfish envenomation.
Opioid medications.
Postanesthesia.
Radiation injury.
Mitochondrial Disorders
Mitochondrial neurogastrointestinal encephalomyopathy.
Musculoskeletal Disorders
Ehlers-Danlos syndrome.
Myotonic dystrophy.
Duchenne muscular dystrophy.
Rheumatology
Amyloidosis.
Dermatomyositis.
Polymyositis.
Systemic lupus erythematous.

From Wyllie R, Hyams JS, Kay M (eds): *Pediatric gastrointestinal and liver disease*, ed 5, Philadelphia, 2016, Elsevier, Box. 44.3, p. 548.

Differential Diagnosis

II

INTRAABDOMINAL MASS LESION, NEONATAL[21]

ICD-10CM #	R19.00	Intraabdominal and pelvic swelling, mass and lump, unspecified site

CAUSES OF A NEONATAL INTRA-ABDOMINAL MASS LESION

Complicated meconium ileus.
Dilated bowel proximal to an obstruction.
Mesenteric or duplication cyst.
Abscess.
Genitourinary causes:
   Hydronephrosis.
   Renal cystic disease.
   Mesoblastic nephroma.
   Wilms tumor.
   Adrenal hemorrhage.
   Neuroblastoma.
   Retroperitoneal teratoma.
   Ovarian cyst.
   Hydrometrocolpos.
Hemangioendothelioma.
Hepatoblastoma.
Choledochal, hepatic, or splenic cysts.

INTRACEREBRAL HEMORRHAGE, NONHYPERTENSIVE CAUSES

ICD-10CM #	I61.9	Nontraumatic intracerebral hemorrhage, unspecified

Trauma.
Anticoagulation.
Intracranial tumors.
Vascular malformations.
Bleeding disorders.
Vasculitides (e.g., polyarteritis nodosa, granulomatous angiitis).
Cocaine and other sympathomimetic agents.
Cerebral amyloid angiopathy.

INTRACRANIAL LESION

ICD-10CM #	G93.89	Other specified disorders of brain

Tumor (primary or metastatic).
Abscess.
Stroke.
Intracranial hemorrhage.
Angioma.
Multiple sclerosis (initial single lesion).
Granuloma.
Herpes encephalitis.
Artifact.

INTRACRANIAL PRESSURE INCREASE[56]

ICD-10CM #	Varies with specific diagnosis

Mass Effect
Hydrocephalus.
Hemorrhage.
Tumor.
Abscess.
Cyst.
Inflammatory mass.
Arterial ischemic stroke with edema.
Cerebral sinovenous thrombosis.

Diffuse Edema
Hypoxic-ischemic injury.
Trauma.
Infection.
Meningitis.
Encephalitis.
Hypertension.
Metabolic derangement or toxin.
Hyponatremia.
Diabetic ketoacidosis.
Dialysis disequilibrium syndrome.
Reye syndrome.
Fulminant hepatic encephalopathy.
Pulmonary insufficiency with hypercarbia.
Lead intoxication.
Idiopathic intracranial hypertension (pseudotumor cerebri).
Drugs.
Withdrawal of long-term steroid administration.
Endocrinologic disturbance.
Obesity.

INTRACRANIAL TUMORS[94]

ICD-10CM #	D33.2	Benign neoplasm of brain, unspecified
	C71.9	Malignant neoplasm of brain, unspecified

DIFFERENTIAL DIAGNOSIS OF INTRACRANIAL TUMORS

Infection.
Brain abscess.
Bacterial.
Fungal.
Parasitic (e.g., cysticercosis).
Herpes encephalitis.
Vascular disease.
Stroke.
Intracranial hemorrhage.
Inflammatory conditions.
Granuloma (sarcoid).
Multiple sclerosis: tumefactive single large lesion.
Vascular malformations.
Cavernous angiomas.
Venous angiomas.
Congenital abnormalities.
Cortical dysplasia.
Heterotopia.

INTRAOCULAR NEOPLASM

ICD-10CM #	C69.9	Malignant disorder of eye, unspecified

MALIGNANT

Retinoblastoma.
Melanoma.
Reticulum cell sarcoma.
Metastatic tumor.

BENIGN

Melanocytic nevus.
Hemangioma.
Reactive lymphoid hyperplasia.

IRON METABOLISM DISORDERS[95]

ICD-10CM #	E83.10	Disorder of iron metabolism, unspecified

IRON DEFICIENCY

Deficient Iron Intake
Diet of low bioavailability.
Increased physiologic requirements due to rapid growth in early childhood and in adolescence.
Blood loss.
Physiologic (e.g., menstruation).
Pathologic (e.g., GI).

Malabsorption of Iron
Reduced or absent gastric acid secretion (e.g., after partial or total gastrectomy or with atrophic gastritis).
Reduced duodenal absorption (e.g., in coeliac disease).
Bypass of stomach and duodenum (bariatric surgery).
Rare, inherited iron-refractory iron deficiency anemia (e.g., deficiency of TMPRSS6 [transmembrane protease, serine 6], also known as matriptase-2).

Redistribution of Iron
Macrophage iron accumulation in reticuloendothelial system in inflammatory, infectious, or malignant diseases (anemia of chronic disease, also known as anemia of inflammation).
Macrophage iron accumulation within the lungs in idiopathic pulmonary hemosiderosis.

IRON OVERLOAD

Due to Increased Iron Absorption
Hereditary hemochromatosis—commonly (among Northern Europeans) homozygosity for *HFE* C282Y but sometimes involving non-C282Y *HFE* or other genes (*HAMP, HFE2* [encoding hemojuvelin], *TFR2, SLC40A1*).
Substantial ineffective erythropoiesis (e.g., β thalassemia intermedia and major, some types of sideroblastic anemia, congenital dyserythropoietic anemia).
Sub-Saharan iron overload ("Bantu siderosis")—only in combination with increased dietary iron.
Other rare inherited disorders (e.g., congenital atransferrinemia, DMT1 deficiency, aceruloplasminemia).
Inappropriate iron therapy (rare).

DUE TO MULTIPLE BLOOD TRANSFUSIONS FOR REFRACTORY ANEMIAS OR FOR OTHER REASONS

Thalassemia major.
Aplastic anemia.
Myelodysplastic syndromes.
Sickle cell disease (when regularly transfused).

IRON OVERLOAD[31]

ICD-10CM #	E83.10	Disorder of iron metabolism, unspecified

HEREDITARY IRON OVERLOAD

Hereditary hemochromatosis:
    HFE-associated (type 1).
    Non–HFE-associated:
        Transferrin receptor 2–associated (type 3).
    Juvenile hemochromatosis (type 2):
        Hemojuvelin-associated (type 2A).
        Hepcidin-associated (type 2B).
    Autosomal dominant hemochromatosis:
        Ferroportin-associated (type 4).
        DMT1-associated hemochromatosis.
        Atransferrinemia.
        Aceruloplasminemia.

ACQUIRED IRON OVERLOAD

Iron-loading anemias (refractory anemias with hypercellular erythroid marrow).
Chronic liver disease.
Porphyria cutanea tarda.
Insulin resistance–associated hepatic iron overload.
African dietary iron overload.*
Medical iron ingestion.
Parenteral iron overload:
    Transfusional iron overload.
    Inadvertent iron overload from therapeutic injections.

PERINATAL IRON OVERLOAD

Neonatal hemochromatosis.
Trichohepatoenteric syndrome.
Cerebrohepatorenal syndrome.
GRACILE (Fellman) syndrome.[†]

FOCAL SEQUESTRATION OF IRON

Idiopathic pulmonary hemosiderosis.
Renal hemosiderosis.
Associated with neurologic abnormalities:
    Pantothenate kinase–associated neurodegeneration (formerly called Hallervorden-Spatz syndrome).
    Neuroferritinopathy.
    Friedreich ataxia.

*May have a genetic component.
[†]GRACILE, Growth retardation, aminoaciduria, cholestasis, iron overload, lactic acidosis, and early death.

ISCHEMIA, UPPER EXTREMITY, CAUSES[60]

ICD-10CM #	S45.809A	Unspecified injury of other specified blood vessels at shoulder and upper arm level, unspecified arm, initial encounter

VASOSPASM

Raynaud disease.
Medication induced: vasopressors, β-blockers.
Ergot poisoning.

INTRINSIC ARTERIAL DISEASE

Atherosclerosis.
Radiation arteritis.
Azotemic arteriopathy.
Spontaneous dissection.
Fibromuscular dysplasia.

INFLAMMATORY DISEASES

Connective tissue disorders.
Buerger disease.
Takayasu arteritis.
Temporal (giant cell) arteritis.
Hypersensitivity angiitis.

NONINFLAMMATORY MEDICAL DISEASE

Thrombophilic states.
Myeloproliferative disorders.
Cold injury.
Hepatitis-associated vasculitis.
Cryoglobulinemia.
Vinyl chloride exposure.

EMBOLISM

Cardiac (most common).
Proximal aneurysm.
Arterial thoracic outlet syndrome.
Atheroembolism.
Paradoxic embolus (with accompanying septal defect).

TRAUMA

Iatrogenic.
Blunt arterial injury.
Penetrating arterial injury.
Hypothenar hammer syndrome.
Vibration.

ISCHEMIC BOWEL DISEASE[29]

ICD-10CM #	K55.1	Vascular disorder of intestine
	I99	Other and unspecified disorders of circulatory system

Abdominal aortic aneurysm: rupture or expansion.
Perforated ulcer or viscus.
Ruptured ectopic pregnancy (woman of childbearing age).
Incarcerated or strangulated hernia.
Septic shock.
Intussusception.
Volvulus.
Salpingitis or tuboovarian abscess.
Torsion of the ovary or testicle.
Appendicitis.
Pelvic mass or torsion.
Pancreatitis.
Diverticulitis.
Ruptured ovarian cyst.
Renal colic.
Biliary colic.
Also consider atypical manifestations of:
    Inferior wall myocardial infarction.
    Pulmonary embolism.
    Pneumonia.
    Diabetic ketoacidosis.
    Acute glaucoma.

Differential diagnoses are listed in order of urgency.

ISCHEMIC COLITIS, NONOCCLUSIVE[26]

ICD-10CM #	K55.1	Chronic vascular disorders of intestine

ACUTE DIMINUTION OF COLONIC INTRAMURAL BLOOD FLOW

Small Vessel Obstruction
Collagen-vascular disease.
Vasculitis, diabetes.
Oral contraceptives.
Nonocclusive Hypoperfusion
Hemorrhage.
Congestive heart failure, myocardial infarction, arrhythmias.
Sepsis.
Vasoconstricting agents: vasopressin, ergot.
Increased viscosity: polycythemia, sickle cell disease, thrombocytosis.

INCREASED DEMAND ON MARGINAL BLOOD FLOW

Increased Motility
Mass lesion, stricture.
Constipation.
Increased Intraluminal Pressure
Bowel obstruction.
Colonoscopy.
Barium enema.

ISCHEMIC NECROSIS OF CARTILAGE AND BONE[24]

ICD-10CM #	M89.9	Disorder of bone, unspecified
	M94.9	Disorder of cartilage, unspecified

ENDOCRINE/METABOLIC

Ethanol abuse.
Glucocorticoid therapy.
Cushing disease.
Diabetes mellitus.
Hyperuricemia.
Osteomalacia.
Hyperlipidemia.

STORAGE DISEASES (E.G., GAUCHER DISEASE)

Hemoglobinopathies (e.g., sickle cell disease).
Trauma (e.g., dislocation, fracture).
HIV infection.
Dysbaric conditions (e.g., caisson disease).
Collagen-vascular disorders.
Irradiation.
Pancreatitis.
Organ transplantation.
Hemodialysis.
Burns.
Intravascular coagulation.
Idiopathic, familial.

JAUNDICE

ICD-10CM #	R17	Unspecified jaundice
	K83.8	Other specified diseases of biliary tract
	E80.7	Disorder of bilirubin metabolism, unspecified

PREDOMINANCE OF DIRECT (CONJUGATED) BILIRUBIN

Extrahepatic obstruction.
Common duct abnormalities: calculi, neoplasm, stricture, cyst, sclerosing cholangitis.
Metastatic carcinoma.
Pancreatic carcinoma, pseudocyst.
Ampullary carcinoma.
Hepatocellular disease: hepatitis, cirrhosis.
Drugs: estrogens, phenothiazines, captopril, methyltestosterone, labetalol.
Cholestatic jaundice of pregnancy.
Hereditary disorders: Dubin-Johnson syndrome, Rotor syndrome.
Recurrent benign intrahepatic cholestasis.

PREDOMINANCE OF INDIRECT (UNCONJUGATED) BILIRUBIN

Hemolysis: hereditary and acquired hemolytic anemias.
Inefficient marrow production.
Impaired hepatic conjugation: chloramphenicol.
Neonatal jaundice.
Hereditary disorders: Gilbert syndrome, Crigler-Najjar syndrome.

JAUNDICE, CLASSIFICATION[18]

ICD-10CM #	R17	Unspecified jaundice

PREHEPATIC (PREDOMINANTLY UNCONJUGATED HYPERBILIRUBINEMIA)

Overproduction

Hemolysis (e.g., spherocytosis, sickle cell disease, hemolysis of the newborn, autoimmune disorders).
Ineffective erythropoiesis (e.g., megaloblastic anemias).
Hematomas.
Pulmonary emboli.

HEPATIC (UNCONJUGATED HYPERBILIRUBINEMIA)

Decreased Hepatic Uptake

Gilbert syndrome.
Drugs (e.g., rifampin, radiographic contrast agents).
Neonatal jaundice.
Posthepatitis.
Decreased systolic binding proteins (e.g., newborn or premature infants).
Portacaval shunt.
Prolonged fasting.

Decreased Conjugation Due to Limited Glucuronyl Transferase Activity

Gilbert disease.
Crigler-Najjar syndrome, types I and II.

Neonatal jaundice.
Breast-milk jaundice.
Chronic persistent hepatitis.
Wilson disease.
Noncirrhotic portal fibrosis.
Drug inhibition (e.g., chloramphenicol).

PREDOMINANTLY CONJUGATED HYPERBILIRUBINEMIA

Impaired Hepatic Excretion

Familial disorders (Dubin-Johnson syndrome, Rotor syndrome, benign recurrent cholestasis, cholestasis of pregnancy).
Hepatocellular infiltrative disorders.
Liver metastasis.
Liver cirrhosis.
Hepatitis (viral, bacterial, parasitic, autoimmune, ethanol, and drug-induced).
Drug-induced cholestasis (especially chlorpromazine, erythromycin estolate, isoniazid, halothane).
Primary biliary cirrhosis.
Primary sclerosing cholangitis.
Pericholangitis.
Congestive heart failure.
Shock.
Toxemia of pregnancy.
Sarcoidosis.
Hepatic trauma.
Amyloidosis.
Autoimmune cholangiopathy.
Vanishing bile duct syndrome.
Sepsis.
Postoperative complications.

EXTRAHEPATIC

Extrahepatic Biliary Obstruction

Gallstones, choledocholithiasis.
Cholecystitis.
Tumors of the head of the pancreas (adenocarcinoma, mucinous duct ectasia, neuroendocrine tumors, metastasis).
Tumors of bile ducts (cholangiocarcinoma, Klatskin tumor: cholangiocarcinoma at the bifurcation).
Gallbladder cancer.
Tumors of the ampulla of Vater (adenoma, adenocarcinoma).
Tumors of the duodenum (adenocarcinoma, lymphoma).
Hemobilia (blood in the biliary tree).
Biliary strictures (postcholecystectomy, post-liver transplantation, primary sclerosing cholangitis).
Congenital disorders (biliary atresia, idiopathic dilation of common bile duct, cystic fibrosis).
Metastasis to the hepatic hilum.
Primary bile duct lymphoma.
Cholangiopathy of acquired immunodeficiency syndrome.
Choledochal cysts.
Infectious cholangiopathy (Clonorchis sinensis, Ascaris lumbricoides, Fasciola hepatica).
Chronic pancreatitis (fibrosis of the head of the pancreas).

JAUNDICE IN PREGNANCY[96]

ICD-10CM #	R17	Unspecified jaundice

DIFFERENTIAL DIAGNOSIS

Drug hepatotoxicity (can be seen with α-methyldopa).
Viral hepatitis.
Autoimmune hepatitis (screen for antimitochondrial antibodies).
Hyperemesis gravidarum (severe).
Cholelithiasis.
Cholangiocarcinoma (extremely rare).
Overlap syndromes:
    Preeclampsia (HELLP syndrome) (liver rupture, and infarction in rare cases).
    Acute fatty liver of pregnancy.

JAUNDICE, NEONATAL[18]

ICD-10CM #	P59.9	Neonatal jaundice, unspecified

PREHEPATIC

Hereditary spherocytosis.
Nonspherocytic hemolytic anemia (glucose-6-phosphate dehydrogenase deficiency, α-thalassemia, vitamin K_3-induced hemolysis, pyruvate kinase deficiency).

HEPATIC

Crigler-Najjar syndrome, types I and II.
α_1-Antitrypsin deficiency.
Sepsis.
Drug-induced.
Hypothyroidism.
Breast-milk jaundice.
Fetomaternal blood group incompatibility (Rhesus, Landsteiner groups ABO).

POSTHEPATIC

Extrahepatic biliary obstruction.
Biliary atresia.
Bile duct paucity.
Alagille syndrome.

JOINT AND PERIARTICULAR PAIN, ACUTE[8]

ICD-10CM #	M25.50	Joint pain

COMMON ACUTE MONOARTHRITIS

Septic arthritis (nongonococcal, gonococcal).
Crystal arthritis (gout, pseudogout).
Reactive arthritides.
Lyme disease.
Plant thorn synovitis.
Other infections (mycobacterial, viral, soft tissue).

TRAUMA OR INTERNAL DERANGEMENT

Loose bodies.
Stress fractures.
Ischemic necrosis.
Hemarthrosis.

ACUTE MONOARTHRITIS OR POLYARTHRITIS

Psoriatic arthritis.
Enteropathic arthritis.
Rheumatoid arthritis/palindromic rheumatism.
Juvenile inflammatory arthritides.

MONOARTHROPATHIES FROM NONINFLAMMATORY DISEASE

Osteoarthritis.
Charcot joints.
Storage diseases (hemochromatosis, ochronosis).

SYNOVIAL DISEASES

Pigmented villonodular synovitis.
Lipoma arborescens.
Synovial osteochondromatosis.
Reflex sympathetic dystrophy.
Sarcoidosis.
Amyloid.

ACUTE MONOARTHRITIS OF SYSTEMIC DISEASE

Systemic lupus erythematosus.
Vasculitides (antineutrophil cytoplasmic antibody positive and negative).
Henoch-Schönlein purpura.
Behçet disease.
Bacterial endocarditis.
Familial Mediterranean fever.
Relapsing polychondritis.

SOFT TISSUE LESIONS

Bone Diseases

Paget disease.
Osteomyelitis (Brodie abscess).
Osteogenic/osteoid tumors.
Metastatic disease.
Pulmonary hypertrophic osteoarthropathy.

JOINT PAIN, ANTERIOR HIP, MEDIAL THIGH, KNEE[25]

ICD-10CM #	M25.50	Pain in unspecified joint
	M25.559	Pain in unspecified hip
	M25.569	Pain in unspecified knee

ACUTE

Acute rheumatic fever.
Adductor muscle strain.
Avascular necrosis.
Crystal arthritis.
Femoral artery (pseudo) aneurysm.
Fracture (femoral neck or intertrochanteric).
Hemarthrosis.
Hernia.
Herpes zoster.
Iliopectineal bursitis.
Iliopsoas tendinitis.
Inguinal lymphadenitis.
Osteomalacia.
Painful transient osteoporosis of hip.
Septic arthritis.

SUBACUTE AND CHRONIC

Adductory muscle strain.
Amyloidosis.
Acute rheumatic fever.
Femoral artery aneurysm.
Hernia (inguinal or femoral).
Iliopectineal bursitis.
Iliopsoas tendinitis.
Inguinal lymphadenopathy.

Osteochondromatosis.
Osteomyelitis.
Osteitis deformans (Paget disease).
Osteomalacia (pseudofracture).
Postherpetic neuralgia.
Sterile synovitis (e.g., rheumatoid arthritis, psoriatic, systemic lupus erythematosus).

JOINT PAIN, HIP, LATERAL THIGH[25]

ICD-10CM #	S79.919A	Unspecified injury of unspecified hip, initial encounter
	S79.929A	Unspecified injury of unspecified thigh, initial encounter
	M25.9	Joint disorder, unspecified

ACUTE

Herpes zoster.
Iliotibial tendinitis.
Impacted fracture of femoral neck.
Lateral femoral cutaneous neuropathy (meralgia paresthetica).
Radiculopathy: L4-5.
Trochanteric avulsion fracture (greater trochanter).
Trochanteric bursitis.
Trochanteric fracture.

SUBACUTE AND CHRONIC

Lateral femoral cutaneous neuropathy (meralgia paresthetica).
Osteomyelitis.
Postherpetic neuralgia.
Radiculopathy: L4-5.
Tumors.

JOINT PAIN, POLYARTICULAR

ICD-10CM #	M25.50	Pain in unspecified joint

Osteoarthritis.
Rheumatoid arthritis.
Fibromyalgia.
Viral syndrome (e.g., human parvovirus B19 infection).
Systemic lupus erythematosus.
Psoriatic arthritis.
Ankylosing spondylitis.

JOINT PAIN, POSTERIOR HIPS, THIGH, BUTTOCKS[25]

ICD-10CM #	M25.50	Pain in unspecified joint
	M25.559	Pain in unspecified hip
	M25.569	Pain in unspecified knee

ACUTE

Gluteal muscle strain.
Herpes zoster.
Ischial bursitis.

Ischial or sacral fracture.
Osteomalacia (pseudofracture).
Sciatic neuropathy.
Radiculopathy: L5-S1.

SUBACUTE AND CHRONIC

Gluteal muscle strain.
Ischial bursitis.
Lumbar spinal stenosis.
Osteoarthritis of hip.
Osteitis deformans (Paget disease).
Osteomyelitis.
Osteochondromatosis.
Osteomalacia (pseudofracture).
Postherpetic neuralgia.
Radiculopathy: L5-S1.
Tumors.

JOINT SWELLING

ICD-10CM #	M25.40	Effusion, unspecified joint

Trauma.
Osteoarthritis.
Gout.
Pyogenic arthritis.
Pseudogout.
Rheumatoid arthritis.
Viral syndrome.

JUGULAR VENOUS DISTENTION

ICD-10CM #	I99.8	Other disorder of circulatory system

Right-sided heart failure.
Cardiac tamponade.
Constrictive pericarditis.
Goiter.
Tension pneumothorax.
Pulmonary hypertension.
Cardiomyopathy (restrictive).
Superior vena cava syndrome.
Valsalva maneuver.
Right atrial myxoma.
Chronic obstructive pulmonary disease.

JUVENILE ARTHRITIS[56]

ICD-10CM #	Varies with specific diagnosis

Connective Tissue Diseases

Juvenile idiopathic arthritis.
Systemic lupus erythematosus.
Juvenile dermatomyositis.
Scleroderma with arthritis.

Infectious Arthritis

Bacterial arthritis.
Viral arthritis.
Fungal arthritis.
Lyme disease.

Reactive Arthritis

Poststreptococcal arthritis.
Rheumatic fever.
Toxic synovitis.
Henoch-Schönlein purpura.
Postinfectious arthritis (formerly Reiter).

Differential
Diagnosis

II

Orthopedic Disorders
Traumatic arthritis.
Legg-Calve-Perthes disease.
Slipped capital femoral epiphysis.
Osteochondritis dissecans.
Chondromalacia patellae.
Musculoskeletal Pain Syndromes
Growing pains.
Hypermobility syndromes.
Myofascial pain syndromes/fibromyalgia.
Complex regional pain syndrome.
Hematologic/Oncologic Disorders
Leukemia.
Lymphoma.
Sickle cell disease.
Thalassemia.
Malignant and benign tumors of bone, carti-
    lage, or synovium.
Metastatic bone disease.
Hemophilia.
Miscellaneous
Rickets/metabolic bone disease.
Lysosomal storage diseases.
Heritable disorders of collagen.

KERATITIS, NONINFECTIOUS

ICD-10CM #	H16.9	Unspecified keratitis

Collagen vascular disease.
Atopic keratoconjunctivitis.
Chemical injury.
Thermal injury.
Ectropion/entropion.
Lid defects.
Exophthalmos.
Keratoconjunctivitis sicca.
Erythema multiforme.
Mucous membrane pemphigoid.
Diabetes mellitus (delayed epithelial healing).
Neuroparalytic (cranial nerve VII).
Neurotrophic (diabetes, cranial nerve V).

KIDNEY CYSTIC DISEASE[89]

ICD-10CM #	Varies with specific diagnosis

CYSTIC DISEASES OF THE KIDNEY

Inheritable
Autosomal recessive (infantile) polycystic kidney
    disease.
Autosomal dominant (adult) polycystic kidney
    disease.
    Juvenile nephronophthisis and medullary
        cystic disease complex.
    Juvenile nephronophthisis (autosomal
        recessive).
Medullary cystic disease (autosomal dominant).
Congenital nephrosis (familial nephrotic syn-
    drome) (autosomal recessive).
Familial hypoplastic glomerulocystic disease
    (autosomal dominant).
Multiple malformation syndromes with renal
    cysts (e.g., tuberous sclerosis, von Hippel-
    Lindau disease).
Nonheritable
Multicystic kidney (multicystic dysplastic
    kidney).

Benign multilocular cyst (cystic nephroma).
Simple cysts.
Medullary sponge kidney.
Sporadic glomerulocystic kidney disease.
Acquired renal cystic disease.
Calyceal diverticulum (pyelogenic cyst).

KIDNEY ENLARGEMENT, UNILATERAL[2]

ICD-10CM #	N13.30	Unspecified hydronephrosis

Hydronephrosis (may be bilateral).
Polycystic kidney (may be bilateral).
Simple cyst of kidney.
Renal cell carcinoma.
Pyonephrosis (may be bilateral).
Acute renal vein thrombosis.

KIDNEY INJURY, CANCER PATIENTS[11]

ICD-10CM #	Varies with specific diagnosis

CAUSES OF ACUTE KIDNEY INJURY IN CANCER PATIENTS

Prerenal
Sepsis
Volume depletion (vomiting, diarrhea, mucositis).
Hepatorenal syndrome (venoocclusive disease
    of the liver).
Capillary leak syndrome (interleukin-2
    administration).
Hypercalcemia.
Intrinsic
Acute tubular necrosis
Ischemia (sepsis/shock).
Nephrotoxic (aminoglycosides, amphotericin B,
    chemotherapy).
Tubulointerstitial Nephritis
    Tumor lysis syndrome (urate and phosphate
        nephropathy).
    Allergic reaction.
    Pyelonephritis.
    Opportunistic infections.
    Infiltration (lymphoma/leukemia).
Vascular
Thrombotic microangiopathy.
Cancer treated.
Drug induced.
Bone marrow transplantation.
Radiation injury.
Amyloidosis
Light-chain deposition disease
Paraneoplastic syndromes (membranous, anti-
    neutrophil cytoplasmic antibody associated,
    focal segmental glomerulosclerosis)
Postrenal
Intrarenal (Urate, Acyclovir, Methotrexate)
Extrarenal (Retroperitoneal Fibrosis,
Lymphadenopathy, Direct Invasion)

KNEE PAIN[25]

ICD-10CM #	S83.419A	Sprain of medial collateral ligament of unspecified knee, initial encounter

	S83.509A	Sprain of unspecified cruciate ligament of unspecified knee, initial encounter
	M23.50	Chronic instability of knee, unspecified knee
	M23.8X9	Other internal derangements of unspecified knee
	S83.289A	Other tear of lateral meniscus, current injury, unspecified knee, initial encounter
	S83.249A	Other tear of medial meniscus, current injury, unspecified knee, initial encounter
	M25.669	Stiffness of unspecified knee, not elsewhere classified

DIFFUSE
Articular.
Anterior.
Prepatellar bursitis.
Patellar tendon enthesopathy.
Chondromalacia patellae.
Patellofemoral osteoarthritis.
Cruciate ligament injury.
Medial plica syndrome.

MEDIAL
Anserine bursitis.
Spontaneous osteonecrosis.
Osteoarthritis.
Medial meniscal tear.
Medial collateral ligament bursitis.
Referred pain from hip and L3.
Fibromyalgia.

LATERAL
Iliotibial band syndrome.
Meniscal cyst.
Lateral meniscal tear.
Collateral ligament.
Peroneal tenosynovitis.

POSTERIOR
Popliteal cyst (Baker cyst).
Tendinitis.
Aneurysms, ganglions, sarcoma.

KNEE PAIN, IN DIFFERENT AGE GROUPS[41]

ICD-10CM #	M25.569	Pain in unspecified knee

COMMON CAUSES OF KNEE PAIN IN DIFFERENT AGE GROUPS

Childhood (2 to 10 yr)
Intraarticular
Juvenile arthritis.
Osteochondritis dissecans.

Infection.
Torn discoid meniscus.
Periarticular
Osteomyelitis.
Referred
Perthes disease.
Irritable hip.
Adolescence (10 to 18 yr)
Intraarticular
Osteochondritis dissecans.
Torn meniscus.
Anterior knee pain syndrome.
Patellar instability.
Periarticular
Osgood-Schlatter disease.
Sinding-Larsen-Johansson syndrome.
Osteomyelitis.
Bone tumors.
Referred
Slipped upper femoral epiphysis.
Early Adulthood (18 to 30 yr)
Intraarticular
Torn meniscus.
Patellar instability.
Anterior knee pain syndrome.
Inflammatory arthritis.
Periarticular
Ligament injuries.
Bursitis.
Adulthood (30 to 50 yr)
Intraarticular
Degenerate meniscal tears.
Osteoarthritis.
Inflammatory arthritis.
Periarticular
Bursitis.
Referred
Osteoarthritis of hip.
Spinal disorders.
Old Age (>50 yr)
Intraarticular
Osteoarthritis.
Inflammatory arthritis.
Periarticular
Bursitis.
Referred
Osteoarthritis of hip.
Spinal disorders.

LARGE BOWEL STRICTURE[21]

ICD-10CM #	S36.5	Injury of colon

CAUSES OF LARGE BOWEL STRICTURES

Physiologic:
  Spasm.
  Distended bladder.
Malignant:
  Annular carcinoma.
  Scirrhous carcinoma.
  Lymphoma.
Diverticular disease:
  Muscle thickening.
  Pericolic abscess.
  Superimposed malignancy.
Ischemia.
Radiation colitis.

Inflammatory bowel disease:
  Ulcerative colitis.
  Crohn disease.
  Tuberculosis.
  Lymphogranuloma venereum.
  Amebiasis.
Extrinsic disease:
  Intraabdominal masses.
  Metastatic carcinoma.
  Endometriosis.
  Pelvic lipomatosis.
  Cholecystitis.
  Pancreatitis.
Miscellaneous:
  Postoperative anastomosis.
  Trauma.
  Hirschsprung disease.

LEFT AXIS DEVIATION[97]

ICD-10CM #	I44.7	Left bundle-branch block, unspecified
	I44.4	Left anterior fascicular block
	I44.5	Left posterior fascicular block
	I44.60	Unspecified fascicular block
	I44.69	Other fascicular block

Normal variation.
  Left anterior fascicular block (hemiblock).
  Left bundle branch block.
  Left ventricular hypertrophy.
  Mechanical shifts causing a horizontal heart, high diaphragm, pregnancy, ascites.
  Some forms of ventricular tachycardia.
  Endocardial cushion defects and other congenital heart disease.

LEFT BUNDLE BRANCH BLOCK

ICD-10CM #	I44.7	Left bundle-branch block, unspecified

Ischemic heart disease.
Electrolyte abnormalities (e.g., hyperkalemia).
Cardiomyopathy.
Idiopathic.
Left ventricular hypertrophy.
Pulmonary embolism.
Cardiac trauma.
Bacterial endocarditis.

LEG CRAMPS, NOCTURNAL

ICD-10CM #	R25.2	Cramp and spasm

Diabetic neuropathy.
Medications.
Electrolyte abnormalities (hypokalemia, hyponatremia, hypocalcemia, hyperkalemia, hypophosphatemia).
Respiratory alkalosis.
Uremia.
Hemodialysis.
Peripheral nerve injury.
Amyotrophic lateral sclerosis.
Alcohol use.

Heat cramps.
Vitamin B_{12} deficiency.
Hyperthyroidism.
Contractures.
DVT.
Hypoglycemia.
Peripheral vascular insufficiency.
Baker cyst.

LEG LENGTH DISCREPANCIES[51]

ICD-10CM #	M21.759	Unequal limb length (acquired), unspecified femur
	M21.769	Unequal limb length (acquired), unspecified tibia and fibula
	Q72.899	Other reduction defects of unspecified lower limb

CONGENITAL

Proximal femoral local deficiency.
Coxa vara.
Hemiatrophy-hemihypertrophy (anisomelia).
Developmental dysplasia of the hip.

DEVELOPMENTAL

Legg-Calvé-Perthes disease.

NEUROMUSCULAR

Polio.
Cerebral palsy (hemiplegia).

INFECTIOUS

Pyogenic osteomyelitis with physeal damage.

TRAUMA

Physeal injury with premature closure.
Overgrowth.
Malunion (shortening).

TUMOR

Physeal destruction.
Radiation-induced physeal injury.
Overgrowth.

LEG MOVEMENT WHEN STANDING, INVOLUNTARY

ICD-10CM #	R25.8	Other abnormal involuntary movements

Benign essential tremor.
Orthostatic tremor.
Spastic ataxia.
Cerebellar truncal tremor.
Postanoxic myoclonus.

LEG PAIN, EXERTIONAL[58]

ICD-10CM #	R25.2	Cramp and spasm

Differential Diagnosis

II

Vascular Causes
Atherosclerosis.
Thrombosis.
Embolism.
Vasculitis:
  Thromboangiitis obliterans.
  Takayasu arteritis.
  Giant cell arteritis.
Aortic coarctation.
Fibromuscular dysplasia.
Irradiation.
Endofibrosis of the external iliac artery.
Extravascular compression:
  Arterial entrapment (e.g., popliteal artery entrapment, thoracic outlet syndrome).
Adventitial cysts.

Nonvascular Causes
Lumbosacral radiculopathy: Degenerative arthritis.
Spinal stenosis.
Herniated disc.
Arthritis:
  Hips, knees.s
  Venous insufficiency.
  Myositis.
  Glycogen storage disease type V (McArdle syndrome).

LEG PAIN WITH EXERCISE

ICD-10CM #	R25.2	Cramp and spasm

Shin splints.
Arteriosclerosis obliterans.
Neurogenic (spinal cord compression or ischemia).
Venous claudication.
Popliteal cyst.
Deep vein thrombosis.
Thromboangiitis obliterans.
Adventitial cysts.
Popliteal artery entrapment syndrome.
McArdle syndrome.

LEG SWELLING[29]

ICD-10CM #	R60.0	Localized edema

Deep vein thrombosis.
Cellulitis.
Baker cyst rupture or inflammation.
Congestive heart failure.
Renal failure.
Liver failure.
Inferior vena cava compression.
Musculoskeletal trauma.
Polyarteritis nodosa.
Erythema nodosum.
Myositis.
Tendinitis.
Lymphedema.
Superficial thrombophlebitis.
Compartment syndrome.

LEG ULCERS[25]

ICD-10CM #	I70.25	Atherosclerosis of native arteries of other extremities with ulceration

	L97.909	Non-pressure chronic ulcer of unspecified part of unspecified lower leg with unspecified severity

VASCULAR

Arterial: arteriosclerosis, thromboangiitis obliterans, arteriovenous malformation, cholesterol emboli.
Venous: superficial varicosities, incompetent perforators, deep vein thrombosis, lymphatic abnormalities.

VASCULITIS HEMATOLOGIC

Sickle cell anemia, thalassemia, polycythemia vera, leukemia, cold agglutinin disease.
Macroglobulinemia, protein C and protein S deficiency, cryoglobulinemia, lupus anticoagulant, antiphospholipid syndrome.

INFECTIOUS

Fungal: blastomycosis, coccidioidomycosis, histoplasmosis, sporotrichosis.
Bacterial: furuncle, ecthyma, septic emboli.
Protozoal: leishmaniasis.

METABOLIC

Necrobiosis lipoidica diabeticorum.
Localized bullous pemphigoid.
Gout, calcinosis cutis, Gaucher disease.

TUMORS

Basal cell carcinoma, squamous cell carcinoma, melanoma.
Mycosis fungoides, Kaposi sarcoma, metastatic neoplasms.

TRAUMA

Burns, cold injury, radiation dermatitis.
Insect bites.
Factitial, excessive pressure.

NEUROPATHIC

Diabetic trophic ulcers.
Tabes dorsalis, syringomyelia.

DRUGS

Warfarin, IV colchicine extravasation, methotrexate, halogens, ergotism, hydroxyurea.

PANNICULITIS

Weber-Christian disease.
Pancreatic fat necrosis, α-antitrypsinase deficiency.

LEPTOMENINGEAL METASTASES[38]

ICD-10CM #		Code varies with specific diagnosis

DIFFERENTIAL DIAGNOSIS

Neoplastic
Parenchymal metastases.
Dural metastases.
Castleman disease.
Infections
Bacterial/viral meningitis.
Fungal infections, including *Cryptococcus*.
Lyme disease.
Neurocysticercosis.
Tuberculosis.
Granulomatous Disorders
Histiocytosis.
Sarcoidosis.
Granulomatosis with polyangiitis.
Inflammatory Disorders
Multiple sclerosis.
Paraneoplastic encephalomyelitis.
Relapsing polychondritis.
Rheumatoid nodules.
Vasculitis (including granulomatous angiitis).
Miscellaneous
Enhancing meningeal blood vessels.
Post–lumbar puncture changes (intracranial hypotension).

LETHARGY AND COMA[20]

ICD-10CM #	Varies with specific diagnosis

EPILEPSY
Epileptic encephalopathies.
Post-ictal state.
Status epilepticus.

HYPOXIA-ISCHEMIA
Cardiac arrest.
Cardiac arrhythmia.
Congestive heart failure.
Hypotension.
  Autonomic dysfunction.
  Dehydration.
  Hemorrhage.
  Pulmonary embolism.
Near-drowning.
Neonatal.

INCREASED INTRACRANIAL PRESSURE
Cerebral abscess.
Cerebral edema.
Cerebral tumor.
Herniation syndromes.
Hydrocephalus.
Intracranial hemorrhage.
  Spontaneous.
  Traumatic.
Infectious Disorders
Bacterial infections.
  Cat-scratch disease.*
  Gram-negative sepsis.*
  Hemorrhagic shock and encephalopathy syndrome.*
  Meningitis.*
  Toxic shock syndrome.
Postimmunization encephalopathy.
Rickettsial infections.
  Lyme disease.*
  Rocky Mountain spotted fever.*
Viral infections.
  Arboviruses.
  Aseptic meningitis.
  Herpes simplex encephalitis.
  Measles encephalitis.

*Denotes the most common conditions and the ones with disease-modifying treatments.

Postinfectious encephalomyelitis.
Reye syndrome.

Metabolic and Systemic Disorders

Disorders of osmolality.
Diabetic ketoacidosis (hyperglycemia).
Hypoglycemia.
Hypernatremia.
Hyponatremia.
Endocrine disorders.
Adrenal insufficiency.
Hypoparathyroidism.
Thyroid disorders.
Hepatic encephalopathy.
Inborn errors of metabolism.
Disorders of pyruvate metabolism.
Glycogen storage disorders.
Medium-chain acyl-CoA dehydrogenase (MCAD) deficiency.
Respiratory chain disorders.
Urea cycle disorder, heterozygote.
Renal disorders.
Acute uremic encephalopathy.
Chronic uremic encephalopathy.
Dialysis encephalopathy.
Hypertensive encephalopathy.
Other metabolic disorders.
Burn encephalopathy.
Hypomagnesemia.
Parenteral hyperalimentation.
Vitamin B complex deficiency.
Migraine coma.
Toxic.
Immunosuppressive drugs.*
Prescription drugs.*
Substance abuse.*
Toxins.*
Trauma.
Concussion.
Contusion.
Intracranial hemorrhage.
Epidural hematoma.
Subdural hematoma.
Intracerebral hemorrhage.
Neonatal.
Vascular.
Hypertensive encephalopathy.*
Intracranial hemorrhage, nontraumatic.*
Lupus erythematosus.*
Neonatal idiopathic cerebral venous thrombosis.
Vasculitis.*

LEUKOCORIA

ICD-10CM #	H57.9	Unspecified disorder of eye and adnexa

Cataract.
Retinal detachment.
Retinoblastoma.
Retinal telangiectasia.
Retrolenticular vascularized membrane.
Familial exudative vitreoretinopathy.

LID RETRACTION, CAUSES[98]

ICD-10CM #	H02.539	Eyelid retraction unspecified eye, unspecified lid

Thyroid eye disease.
Neurogenic:
Contralateral unilateral ptosis.
Unopposed levator action due to facial palsy.
3rd nerve misdirection.
Marcus Gunn jaw-winking syndrome.
Collier sign of the dorsal midbrain (Parinaud syndrome).
Infantile hydrocephalus (setting sun sign).
Parkinsonism.
Sympathomimetic drops.
Mechanical:
Surgical overcorrection of ptosis.
Scarring of upper lid skin.
Congenital:
Isolated.
Duane retraction syndrome.
Down syndrome.
Transient "eye popping" reflex in normal infants.
Miscellaneous:
Prominent globe (pseudo-lid retraction).
Uremia (Summerskill sign).
Idiopathic.

LIGHT-NEAR DISSOCIATION[44]

ICD-10CM #	Varies with specific diagnosis

CAUSES OF LIGHT-NEAR DISSOCIATION

Unilateral

Afferent conduction defect.
Adie pupil.
Herpes zoster ophthalmicus.
Aberrant regeneration of the third cranial nerve.

Bilateral

Neurosyphilis.
Type 1 diabetes mellitus.
Myotonic dystrophy.
Parinaud (dorsal midbrain) syndrome.
Familial amyloidosis.
Encephalitis.
Chronic alcoholism.

LIMB ISCHEMIA, ACUTE, NONTRAUMATIC[64]

ICD-10CM #	I70.2	Atherosclerosis of arteries of extremities

CAUSES OF NONTRAUMATIC ACUTE LIMB ISCHEMIA

Atherosclerotic

In situ thrombosis.
Atheroembolism from thoracic aortic aneurysm/abdominal aortic aneurysm.
Femoral/popliteal aneurysm with or without compression.
Dissection.

Nonatherosclerotic

Embolism from cardiac thrombosis (atrial fibrillation, post–myocardial infarction akinesis).
Graft thrombosis, graft aneurysm.
Mycotic emboli.
Raynaud phenomenon.
Arteritis with thrombosis.
Inherited and acquired hypercoagulable states.

Drug-induced vasospasm.
External compression (Baker cyst, popliteal entrapment).

Mimics

Phlegmasia cerulea dolens.
Acute neuropathy.
Hypovolemia.
Systemic shock.

LIMP

ICD-10CM #	R26.0	Ataxic gait
	R26.1	Paralytic gait
	R26.89	Other abnormalities of gait and mobility
	R26.9	Unspecified abnormalities of gait and mobility
	M25.80	Other specified joint disorders, unspecified joint
	F44.4	Conversion disorder with motor symptom or deficit
	F44.6	Conversion disorder with sensory symptom or deficit

Degenerative joint disease, osteochondritis dissecans, chondromalacia patellae.
Trauma to extremities, vertebral disk, hips.
Poorly fitting shoes, foreign body in shoe, unequal leg length.
Splinter in foot.
Joint infection (septic arthritis, osteomyelitis), viral arthritis.
Abdominal pain (e.g., appendicitis, incarcerated hernia), testicular torsion.
Polio, neuromuscular disorders, Guillain-Barré syndrome, multiple sclerosis.
Osgood-Schlatter disease.
Legg-Calvé-Perthes disease.
Factitious, somatization syndrome.
Neoplasm (local or metastatic).
Other: diskitis, periostitis, sickle cell disease, hemophilia.

LIMPING, PEDIATRIC AGE[51]

ICD-10CM #	R26.0	Ataxic gait
	R26.1	Paralytic gait
	R26.89	Other abnormalities of gait and mobility
	R26.9	Unspecified abnormalities of gait and mobility

TODDLER (1 TO 3 YR)

Infection:
Septic arthritis:
Hip.
Knee.
Osteomyelitis.
Diskitis.
Occult trauma:
Toddler's fracture.
Neoplasia.

CHILDHOOD (4 TO 10 YR)

Infection:
  Septic arthritis:
    Hip.
    Knee.
    Osteomyelitis.
    Diskitis.
Transient synovitis, hip.
LCPD.
Tarsal coalition.
Rheumatologic disorder:
  JRA.
Trauma.
Neoplasia.

ADOLESCENCE (11+ YR)

SCFE.
Rheumatologic disorder:
  JRA.
  Trauma.
  Tarsal coalition.
  Hip dislocation (DDH).
  Neoplasia.

DDH, Developmental dysplasia of the hip; *JRA,* juvenile RA; *LCPD,* Legg-Calvé-Perthes disease; *SCFE,* slipped capital femoral epiphysis.

LIVEDO RETICULARIS

ICD-10CM #	L95.0	Livedoid vasculitis

Emboli (subacute bacterial endocarditis, left atrial myxoma, cholesterol emboli).
Thrombocythemia or polycythemia.
Antiphospholipid antibody syndrome.
Cryoglobulinemia, cryofibrinogenemia.
Leukocytoclastic vasculitis.
Systemic lupus erythematosus, rheumatoid arthritis, dermatomyositis.
Pancreatitis.
Drugs (quinine, quinidine, amantadine, catecholamines).
Physiologic (cutis marmorata).
Congenital.

LIVER DISEASE, PREGNANCY[2]

ICD-10CM #	K75.89	Other specified inflammatory liver diseases

INCIDENTAL TO PREGNANCY

Viral hepatitis.
Alcohol related.
Autoimmune chronic active hepatitis.

RELATED TO PREGNANCY (POSSIBLY INFLUENCED BY HORMONES PRESENT IN PREGNANCY)

Complicated gallstone disease.
Hepatic adenoma.
Focal nodular hyperplasia.
Budd-Chiari syndrome.

SPECIFIC TO PREGNANCY

Severe hyperemesis gravidarum.
Benign intrahepatic cholestasis.
Acute fatty liver of pregnancy.
Preeclampsia (HELLP).

LIVER LESIONS, BENIGN, OFTEN CONFUSED WITH MALIGNANCY

ICD-10CM #	K76.1	Chronic passive congestion of liver
	K76.89	Other specified diseases of liver

Fatty infiltration.
Adenoma.
Hemangioma.
Cysts.
Flow artifacts.
Focal nodular hyperplasia.
Nonenhanced vessels.

LOWER GI ULCERATIVE LESIONS[99]

ICD-10CM #	Varies with specific diagnosis

INFECTIOUS

Epstein-Barr virus.
HIV.
Cytomegalovirus.
Herpes simplex.
Herpes zoster.
Syphilis.
Erosive candidiasis.
Mycobacterial infection.
Chancroid.
Lymphogranuloma venereum.

NOT INFECTIOUS

Behçet disease.
Excoriation.
Aphthous (idiopathic) ulcer.
Erythema multiforme.
Carcinoma.

LOW-VOLTAGE ECG

ICD-10CM #	R94.31	Abnormal electrocardiogram [ECG] [EKG]

Hypothyroidism.
Obesity.
Pericardial effusion.
Anasarca.
Pleural effusion.
Pneumothorax.
Amyloidosis.
Aortic stenosis.

LUMBAR SPINE, VISCEROGENIC PAIN REFERRED TO LUMBAR SPINE[351]*

ICD-10CM #	M54.5	Low back pain

VASCULAR

Expanding aortic aneurysm.

*All of these disorders may cause localized low back pain.

GENITOURINARY

Endometriosis.
Tubal pregnancy.
Kidney stone.
Prostatitis.

GI

Pancreatitis.
Peptic ulcers.
Colon cancer.

LUNG CANCER, OCCUPATIONAL CAUSES[21]

ICD-10CM #	C34.90	Malignant neoplasm of unspecified part of unspecified bronchus or lung

CAUSES OF OCCUPATIONAL LUNG CANCER

Asbestos	Lagging, insulation
Arsenic	Metal smelting, pesticide manufacture
Beryllium	Electronics, dental prosthetic manufacture
Chromium	Coloring pigment production, electroplating
Nickel	Electroplating
Silica	Grinding, quarrying, sandblasting
Radon	Mining
Uranium	Mining

LUNG DISEASE AND GI AND LIVER INVOLVEMENT[13]

ICD-10CM #	Varies with specific diagnosis

ESOPHAGEAL REFLUX

Aspiration pneumonia.
Asthma.
Scleroderma.
Bronchitis.
Bronchiectasis.
Cough.
Pulmonary fibrosis.
Mycobacterial disease.

INFLAMMATORY BOWEL DISEASE

Bronchitis.
Bronchiectasis.
Bronchiolitis.
Colobronchial fistula.
Desquamative interstitial lung disease.
Drug reactions for agents that treat inflammatory bowel disease.
Eosinophilic lung disease.
Interstitial lung disease.
Necrobiotic nodules.
Obstructive lung disease.
Organizing pneumonia.
Reduced diffusing capacity.
Sarcoidosis.
Serositis affecting pleura or pericarditis.
Tracheal stenosis.

LIVER

α1-antitrypsin deficiency.
Chronic active hepatitis.
Hepatopulmonary syndrome.
Portopulmonary hypertension.
Primary biliary cirrhosis.
Hepatosplenomegaly.
  Amyloidosis.
  Collagen vascular disease.
  Eosinophilic granulomatosis.
  Lymphatic interstitial pneumonia.
  Sarcoidosis.

LUNG DISEASE AND RENAL INVOLVEMENT[13]

ICD-10CM #   Varies with specific diagnosis

LUNG DISEASE WITH RENAL INVOLVEMENT

Glomerulonephritis
Systemic vasculitis.
Collagen vascular disease.
Antibasement membrane.
Sarcoidosis.

Nephrotic Syndrome
Amyloidosis.
Disseminated Langerhans cell histiocytosis.
Drug-induced lung disease.
Paraneoplastic syndrome.
Posttransplantation.
Pulmonary hydatid disease.
Systemic lupus erythematosus.
Vasculitis.
Venous thrombosis.
Renal mass
Lymphangioleiomyomatosis.
Metastasis neoplasm.
Renal carcinoid.
Tuberous sclerosis.
Granulomatosis with polyangiitis.

Nephrolithiasis
Alveolar proteinosis.
Cystic fibrosis.
Hypercalcemic syndromes.
Osteolysis from mycobacteria or fungi.
Sarcoidosis.

Systemic Hypertension
Collagen vascular disease.
Diffuse alveolar hemorrhage.
Pulmonary renal syndromes.
Neurofibromatosis.
Sleep apnea.

LUNG DISEASE AND SKIN AND SUBCUTANEOUS LESIONS[13]

ICD-10CM #   Varies with specific diagnosis

SKIN AND SUBCUTANEOUS LESIONS ASSOCIATED WITH LUNG DISEASE

Skin Lesions
Diffuse pigment change:
  Acanthosis nigricans—lung neoplasm.
  Albinism—Hermansky-Pudlak syndrome.
  Bronze pigmentation—hemosiderosis.
  Gray-brown—Whipple disease.

Cutaneous draining sinus:
  Fungal infections (especially histoplasmosis).
  Mycobacterial infections (especially tuberculosis).
  Neoplasms (especially mesothelial tumors).
  Necrotizing vasculitis.
  Other bacterial infections (especially actinomycosis).
Cutaneous ulcers:
  Beryllium disease.
  Chronic venous insufficiency.
  Fungal infections (especially histoplasmosis).
  Mycobacterial disease.
  Necrotizing vasculitis.
  Parasitic disease.
  Polycythemia.
  Sickle cell disease.
  Tularemia.
Cutaneous vasculitis:
  Behçet syndrome.
  Churg-Strauss syndrome.
  Collagen vascular disease.
  Sarcoidosis.
  Granulomatosis with polyangiitis.
Erythema multiforme:
  Drug reactions.
  Fungi (especially coccidiomycosis).
  Mycoplasma and other infectious agents.
  Neoplasms.
  Exfoliative dermatitis.
  Adverse drug reactions.
  Chemotherapy.
  Disseminated malignancy.
  Graft-versus-host disease.
  Radiation therapy.
Flushing:
  Bronchial carcinoid, pheochromocytoma, other neoplasms.
  Carbon dioxide, cyanide, and other toxins.
  Drugs.
  Foods and vasodilatory substances.
  Hormones.
  Mastocytosis.
  Metabolic states (e.g., hyperthyroidism, fever).
Macular rash:
  Antibasement membrane disease.
  Café-au-lait spots (neurofibromatosis).
  Coal miner's scars.
  Collagen vascular disease.
  Idiopathic pulmonary fibrosis.
  Rose spots (psittacosis).
  Sarcoidosis.
  Syphilis.
  Viral pneumonia.
Maculopapular rash:
  Amyloidosis.
  Drug-induced lung disease.
  Collagen vascular disease.
  Gaucher disease.
  Kaposi sarcoma.
  Lung neoplasm.
  Lymphomatoid granulomatosis.
  Lymphoma.
  Parasites.
  Sarcoidosis.
  Syphilis.
  Vasculitis.
  Viral pneumonia
Telangiectasia:
  Arteriovenous malformation.

Ataxia-telangiectasia.
Carcinoid syndrome.
Cushing disease.
Hepatopulmonary syndrome and other chronic liver diseases.
Hereditary hemorrhagic telangiectasia (Osler-Weber-Rendu).
Mastocytosis.
Systemic sclerosis and other collagen vascular diseases.
Urticaria:
  Asthma.
  Drug reactions.
  Cystic fibrosis.
  Exercise-induced urticaria.
  Food allergy.
  Hereditary angioneurotic edema.
  Inhaled antigens.
  Insect bites and stings.
  Infectious agents, such as *Mycoplasma* and *Helicobacter.*
  Mastocytosis.
  Occupational sensitization.
  Parasites.
  Vasculitis.

Nail Changes with Lung Disease
Color changes:
  Cigarette smoking discoloration.
  Splinter hemorrhages.
  Yellow nail syndrome.
Beau lines (any severe illness):
  Dermatomyositis.
  Sarcoidosis.
  Seronegative arthropathies.
  Systemic sclerosis.

Lung Disease with Subcutaneous Involvement
Adenopathy:
  Environmental mycobacteria.
  Fungal infections.
  HIV infections.
  Metastatic neoplasm.
  Leukemia.
  Lymphoma.
  Sarcoidosis.
  Tuberculosis.
Calcinosis:
  Dermatomyositis.
  Metastatic osteosarcoma.
  Mixed connective tissue disease.
  Scleroderma.
  Tuberculosis.
  Uremic metastatic calcification.
Erythema induratum (Bazin disease):
  Aortic stenosis.
  Cryoglobulinemia.
  Nodular vasculitis.
  Panniculitis.
  Peripheral neuropathy.
  Takayasu disease.
  Streptococcus infection.
  Tuberculosis and other mycobacterial disease.
  Weber-Christian disease.
Erythema nodosum:
  Neoplasm.
  Other infectious and inflammatory diseases.
  Primary coccidiomycosis, histoplasmosis.
  Primary tuberculosis.
  Psittacosis.
  Sarcoidosis.

Subcutaneous nodules:
  Amyloidosis.
  Neoplasm.
  Neurofibromatosis.
  Rheumatoid arthritis.
  Tuberous sclerosis (angiofibromas).
  von Recklinghausen.
  Weber-Christian disease.
Lung Disease with Salivary Gland Enlargement
Bulimia and aspiration.
Gaucher disease.
Lymphoid interstitial pneumonitis.
Lymphatic carcinoma.
Lymphoma.
Other causes of lymphadenopathy.
Sarcoidosis.
Sjögren disease.

LUNG DISEASE WITH BONE, JOINT, NERVE, AND MUSCLE INVOLVEMENT[13]

ICD-10CM #	Varies with specific diagnosis

ARTHRITIS
Ankylosing spondylitis.
Collagen vascular diseases.
Reactive arthritis.
Sarcoidosis.
Systemic vasculitis.
Tuberculosis.

BONE LESIONS
Ankylosing spondylitis.
Blastomycosis and other fungal disease.
Collagen vascular diseases.
Eosinophilic granulomatosis.
Fibrous histiocytoma.
Gaucher disease.
Neoplasm.
Sarcoidosis.
Tuberculosis.

MUSCLE DISEASE
Collagen vascular disease.
l-Tryptophan.
Diabetes insipidus.
Eosinophilic granulomatosis.
Polymyositis.
Sarcoidosis.

NEUROLOGIC DISEASE
Acute inflammatory polyneuropathy.
Amyotrophic lateral sclerosis.
Aspiration.
Botulism.
Lambert-Eaton syndrome.
Myasthenia gravis.
Organophosphate poisoning.
Polio and postpolio syndrome.
Sarcoidosis.
Churg-Strauss syndrome.
Granulomatosis with polyangiitis.

LUNG TUMORS, BENIGN[78]

ICD-10CM #	Varies with specific disorder

COMMON BENIGN TUMORS OF THE LUNG BASED ON CELLS OF ORIGIN

Tumors of Epithelial Origin
Mucous gland adenoma.
Clara cell adenoma.
Mucous cystadenoma.
Pleomorphic adenoma.
Tumors of Mesenchymal Origin
Hamartoma.
Inflammatory pseudotumor.
Chondroma.
Fibroma.
Benign endobronchial fibrous histiocytoma.
Leiomyoma.
Lipoma.
Lymphatic lesions.
Tumors of Miscellaneous Origin
Nodular pulmonary amyloidosis.
Clear cell tumor (sugar tumor).
Thymoma.
Granular cell tumor.
Teratoma.
Pulmonary paraganglioma.

LUNG VOLUMES IN DIFFUSE LUNG DISEASE[59]

ICD-10CM #	Varies with specific disorder

LARGE LUNG VOLUMES
Emphysema.
Chronic asthma.
Diffuse bronchiolitis obliterans.
Highly trained athletes.
Lymphangioleiomyomatosis.

SMALL LUNG VOLUMES
End-stage lung fibrosis.
Bilateral diaphragmatic paralysis.
Massive ascites.

NORMAL LUNG VOLUMES
Sarcoidosis.
Langerhans cell histiocytosis.
Neurofibromatosis.
Emphysema with pulmonary fibrosis.

LYMPHADENOPATHY[24]

ICD-10CM #	R59.9	Enlarged lymph nodes, unspecified

GENERALIZED
AIDS.
Lymphoma: Hodgkin disease, non-Hodgkin lymphoma.
Leukemias, reticuloendotheliosis.
Infectious mononucleosis, cytomegalovirus, and other viral infections.
Diffuse skin infection: generalized furunculosis, multiple tick bites.
Parasitic infections: toxoplasmosis, filariasis, leishmaniasis, Chagas disease.
Serum sickness.
Collagen vascular diseases (rheumatoid arthritis, systemic lupus erythematosus).
Dengue (arbovirus infection).
Sarcoidosis and other granulomatous diseases.

Drugs: INH, hydantoin derivatives, antithyroid and antileprosy drugs.
Secondary syphilis.
Hyperthyroidism, lipid-storage diseases.

LOCALIZED
Cervical Nodes
Infections of the head, neck, ears, sinuses, scalp, pharynx.
Mononucleosis.
Lymphoma.
TB.
Malignancy of head and neck.
Rubella.
Scalene/Supraclavicular Nodes
Lymphoma.
Lung neoplasm.
Bacterial or fungal infection of thorax or retroperitoneum.
GI malignancy.
Axillary Nodes
Infections of hands and arms.
Cat-scratch disease.
Neoplasm (lymphoma, melanoma, breast carcinoma).
Brucellosis.
Epitrochlear Nodes
Infections of the hand.
Lymphoma.
Tularemia.
Sarcoidosis, secondary syphilis (usually bilateral).
Inguinal Nodes
Infections of leg or foot, folliculitis (pubic hair).
LGV, syphilis.
Lymphoma.
Pelvic malignancy.
Pasteurella pestis.
Hilar Nodes
Sarcoidosis.
TB.
Lung carcinoma.
Fungal infections, systemic.
Mediastinal Nodes
Sarcoidosis.
Lymphoma.
Lung neoplasm.
TB.
Mononucleosis.
Histoplasmosis.
Abdominal/Retroperitoneal Nodes
Lymphoma.
TB.
Neoplasm (ovary, testes, prostate, and other malignancies).

LYMPHANGITIS[1]

ICD-10CM #	I89.1	Lymphangitis

Acute:
  Group A streptococci.
  Staphylococcus aureus.
  Pasteurella multocida.
Chronic:
  Sporothrix schenckii (sporotrichosis).
  Mycobacterium marinum (swimming pool granuloma).
  Mycobacterium kansasii.
  Nocardia brasiliensis.
  Wuchereria bancrofti.

LYMPHEDEMA[100]

ICD-10CM #	i89.0	Lymphedema, not elsewhere classified
	I97.2	Postmastectomy lymphedema syndrome
	Q82.0	Hereditary lymphedema

CLASSIFICATION OF LYMPHEDEMA

Primary Lymphedema
Congenital lymphedema (Milroy disease).
Lymphedema praecox.
Lymphedema tarda.
Syndromes Associated with Primary Lymphedema
Yellow nail syndrome.
Turner syndrome.
Noonan syndrome.
Pes cavus.
Phakomatosis pigmentovascularis.
Distichiasis-lymphedema.
Emberger syndrome.
WILD syndrome.
Hypotrichosis-telangiectasia-lymphedema syndrome.
Cutaneous Disorders Sometimes Associated with Primary Lymphedema
Yellow nails.
Hemangiomas.
Xanthomatosis and chylous lymphedema.
Congenital absence of nails.
Secondary Lymphedema
Postmastectomy lymphedema.
Melphalan isolated limb perfusion.
Malignant occlusion with obstruction.
Extrinsic pressure.
Factitial lymphedema.
Postradiation therapy.
Following recurrent lymphangitis/cellulitis.
Lymphedema of upper limb in recurrent eczema.
Granulomatous disease.
Rosaceous lymphedema.
Primary amyloidosis.
Complications of Lymphedema
Cellulitis of lymphedema.
Elephantiasis nostras verrucosa.
Ulceration.
Lymphangiosarcoma.

LYMPHOCYTOSIS, ATYPICAL[1]

ICD-10CM #	D72.89	Other specified disorders of white blood cells

Epstein-Barr virus primary infection (infectious mononucleosis).
Cytomegalovirus primary infection (heterophile-negative mono).
Human herpesvirus 6 primary infection (roseola).
Primary HIV infection.
Toxoplasmosis.
Acute viral hepatitis.
Rubella, mumps.
Drug reactions (e.g., phenytoin, sulfa).

MACROCEPHALY[101]

ICD-10CM #	Varies with specific diagnosis

CAUSES

Hydrocephalus.
Obstructive hydrocephalus from aqueductal stenosis.
Communicating hydrocephalus from meningitis.
Mass lesions.
Subdural hematoma.
Tumors.
Neurocutaneous disorders.
Neurofibromatosis (NF1).
Tuberous sclerosis.
Metabolic storage diseases.
Hurler syndrome.
Leukodystrophies.
Tay-Sachs disease.
Genetic mutations.
47,XYY.
PTEN mutation.
Trisomy 13.
Trisomy 18.
Abnormal skull growth.
Achondroplasia.
Benign familial trait.

MACROTHROMBOCYTOPENIA, INHERITED[31]

ICD-10CM #	Varies with specific disorder

Bernard-Soulier syndrome.
MHY9-related disorders:
    May-Hegglin anomaly.
    Sebastian syndrome.
    Fechtner syndrome.
    Epstein syndrome.
Gray platelet syndrome.
Montreal platelet syndrome.
Mediterranean macrothrombocytopenia.
Mediterranean stomatocytosis/macrothrombocytemia.
GATA1 mutations.
Sialyl-Lewis-S antigen deficiency.
Paris-Trousseau syndrome.
Platelet-type von Willebrand disease.

MACULAR CRYSTALS[44]

ICD-10CM #	Varies with specific diagnosis

OTHER CAUSES OF MACULAR CRYSTALS

Primary hyperoxaluria.
Bietti corneoretinal crystalline dystrophy.
Cystinosis.
Sjögren–Larsson syndrome.
Gyrate atrophy.
Acquired parafoveal telangiectasis.
Talc-corn starch emboli.
West African crystalline maculopathy.

MADAROSIS[44]

ICD-10CM #	H02.729	Madarosis of unspecified eye, unspecified eyelid and periocular area

CAUSES OF MADAROSIS

Local
Chronic anterior lid margin disease.
Infiltrating lid tumors.
Burns.
Radiotherapy or cryotherapy of lid tumors.
Skin Disorders
Generalized alopecia.
Psoriasis.
Systemic diseases.
Myxedema.
Systemic lupus erythematosus.
Acquired syphilis.
Lepromatous leprosy.
Following Removal
Procedures for trichiasis.
Trichotillomania (psychiatric disorder of hair removal).

MALABSORPTION[2]

ICD-10CM #	K90.89	Other intestinal malabsorption

CAUSES OF MALABSORPTION

More Common
Celiac disease.
Chronic pancreatitis.
Post gastrectomy.
Crohn disease.
Small bowel resection.
Small intestinal bacterial overgrowth.
Lactase deficiency.
Less Common
AIDS (Mycobacterium avium intracellulare, AIDS enteropathy).
Whipple disease.
Intestinal lymphoma.
Immunoproliferative small intestinal disease (alpha heavy chain disease).
Radiation enteritis.
Collagenous sprue.
Tropical sprue.
Nongranulomatous ulcerative jejunoileitis.
Eosinophilic gastroenteritis.
Amyloidosis.
Zollinger-Ellison syndrome.
Intestinal lymphangiectasia.
Systemic mastocytosis.
Chronic mesenteric ischemia.
Abetalipoproteinemia (autosomal recessive).

MALABSORPTION SYNDROME IN TROPICS[3]

ICD-10CM #	K90.89	Other intestinal malabsorption

CAUSES OF MALABSORPTION SYNDROME IN THE TROPICS

SIBO
Following ulcer surgery.
Secondary to intestinal TB and Crohn disease.
Infections
Bacteria
Mycobacterium avium intracellulare complex.
Mycobacterium tuberculosis.
Helminths
Paracapillaria philippinensis.
Strongyloides stercoralis.

Protozoa
Cryptosporidium parvum.
Cyclospora cayetanensis.
Encephalitozoon intestinalis.
Enterocytozoon bieneusi.
Giardia lamblia.
Isospora belli.
Leishmania donovani.
Lymphatic Obstruction
Intestinal lymphangiectasia.
Mucosal Diseases
Autoimmune enteropathy.
Celiac disease.
Eosinophilic gastroenteritis.
HIV enteropathy.
Immunoproliferative small intestinal disease.
Intestinal lymphoma.
Primary immunodeficiencies.
Tropical sprue.
Neonatal Diseases
Microvillus inclusion disease.
Tufting enteropathy.
Pancreatic Insufficiency
Alcoholic pancreatitis.
CF.
Tropical pancreatitis.
Specific Transport Disorders
Abetalipoproteinemia.
Fructose malabsorption.
Glucose-galactose malabsorption.
Hypolactasia.
Sucrose intolerance.

MALNUTRITION, CAUSES IN EARLY LIFE[19]

ICD-10CM #	E46	Unspecified protein-energy malnutrition

0 TO 6 MO

Breastfeeding difficulties.
Improper formula preparation.
Impaired parent/child interaction.
Congenital syndromes.
Prenatal infections or teratogenic exposures.
Poor feeding (sucking, swallowing) or feeding refusal (aversion).
Maternal psychologic disorder (depression or attachment disorder).
Congenital heart disease.
Cystic fibrosis.
Neurologic abnormalities.
Child neglect.
Recurrent infections.

6 TO 12 MO

Celiac disease.
Food intolerance.
Child neglect.
Delayed introduction of age-appropriate foods or poor transition to food.
Recurrent infections.
Food allergy.

AFTER INFANCY

Acquired chronic diseases.
Highly distractible child.
Inappropriate mealtime environment.

Inappropriate diet (e.g., excessive juice consumption, avoidance of high-calorie foods).
Recurrent infections.

MASTALGIA, MEDICATION INDUCED[102]

ICD-10CM #	N64.4	Mastodynia

MEDICATIONS ASSOCIATED WITH MASTALGIA

Antihypertensives.
Atenolol and other beta-blockers.
Hydrochlorothiazide.
Methyldopa.
Minoxidil.
Spironolactone.
Antidepressants and antipsychotic agents.
Amitriptyline and other tricyclic antidepressants.
Chlorpromazine/promethazine.
Fluoxetine.
Haloperidol.
Hormonal agents.
Estrogens.
Progestins.
Androgens.
Ginseng.
Clomiphene citrate.
Digoxin.
Chlorpropamide.

MEDIASTINAL COMPARTMENTS, ANATOMY AND PATHOLOGY[103]

ICD-10CM #	Varies with specific disorder

ANTERIOR

Normal Structures
Lymph nodes.
Connective tissue.
Thymus (remnant in adults).
Masses
Thymoma.
Germ cell neoplasm.
Lymphoma.
Thyroid enlargement (intrathoracic goiter).
Other tumors.

MIDDLE

Normal Structures
Pericardium.
Heart.
Vessels: ascending aorta, venae cavae, main pulmonary arteries.
Trachea.
Lymph nodes.
Nerves: phrenic, upper vagus.
Masses
Carcinoma.
Lymphoma.
Pericardial cyst.
Bronchogenic cyst.
Benign lymph node enlargement (granulomatous disease).

POSTERIOR

Normal Structures
Vessels: descending aorta.

Esophagus.
Vertebral column.
Nerves: sympathetic chain, lower vagus.
Lymph nodes.
Connective tissue.
Masses
Neurogenic tumor.
Diaphragmatic hernia.

MEDIASTINAL MASSES OR WIDENING ON CHEST X-RAY

ICD-10CM #	R59.9	Enlarged lymph nodes, unspecified
	J98.5	Diseases of mediastinum, not elsewhere classified

Lymphoma: Hodgkin disease and non-Hodgkin lymphoma.
Sarcoidosis.
Vascular: aortic aneurysm, ectasia, or tortuosity of aorta or bronchocephalic vessels.
Carcinoma: lungs, esophagus.
Esophageal diverticula.
Hiatal hernia.
Achalasia.
Prominent pulmonary outflow tract: pulmonary hypertension, pulmonary embolism, right-to-left shunts.
Trauma: mediastinal hemorrhage.
Pneumomediastinum.
Lymphadenopathy caused by silicosis and other pneumoconioses.
Leukemias.
Infections: TB, viral (rare), *Mycoplasma* (rare), fungal, tularemia.
Substernal thyroid.
Thymoma.
Teratoma.
Bronchogenic cyst.
Pericardial cyst.
Neurofibroma, neurosarcoma, ganglioneuroma.

MEDIASTINAL MASSES, SITES OF ORIGIN[48]

ICD-10CM #	Varies with specific diagnosis

DIFFERENTIAL DIAGNOSIS OF MEDIASTINAL MASSES BASED ON COMMON SITES OF ORIGIN

Prevascular Space (Anterior Mediastinum)
Thymic masses.
Thymoma.
Thymic carcinoma.
Thymic neuroendocrine tumor.
Thymolipoma.
Thymic cyst.
Thymic hyperplasia.
Thymic lymphoma.
Germ cell tumors.
Teratoma and dermoid cyst.
Seminoma.
Nonseminomatous germ cell tumors.
Thyroid abnormalities (goiter and neoplasm).
Parathyroid tumor or hyperplasia.
Lymph node masses (particularly Hodgkin lymphoma).

Vascular abnormalities (aorta and great vessels).
Mesenchymal abnormalities (e.g., lipomatosis, lipoma).
Foregut cyst.
Lymphangioma.
Hemangioma.

Retrosternal Space (Anterior Mediastinum)
Lymph node masses.

Pretracheal Space (Middle Mediastinum)
Lymph node masses.
Lung carcinoma.
Sarcoidosis.
Lymphoma (particularly Hodgkin disease).
Metastases.
Infections (e.g., tuberculosis).
Foregut cyst.
Tracheal tumor.
Mesenchymal masses (e.g., lipomatosis, lipoma).
Thyroid abnormalities.
Vascular abnormalities (aorta and great vessels).
Lymphangioma and hemangioma.

Aortopulmonary Window (Middle Mediastinum)
Lymph node masses.
Lung carcinoma.
Sarcoidosis.
Lymphoma.
Metastases.
Infections (e.g., tuberculosis).
Mesenchymal masses (e.g., lipomatosis, lipoma).
Vascular abnormalities (aorta or pulmonary artery).
Chemodectoma.
Foregut cyst.

Subcarinal Space and Azygoesophageal Recess (Middle Mediastinum)
Lymph node masses.
Lung carcinoma.
Sarcoidosis.
Lymphoma.
Metastases.
Infections (e.g., tuberculosis).
Foregut cyst.
Dilated azygos vein.
Esophageal masses.
Varices.
Hernia.

Paravertebral Masses (Posterior Mediastinum)
Neurogenic tumor.
Nerve sheath tumors.
Sympathetic ganglia tumors.
Paraganglioma.
Meningocele.
Foregut cyst.
Neurenteric cyst.
Thoracic spine abnormalities.
Extramedullary hematopoiesis.
Fluid collections and pseudocyst.
Vascular abnormalities.
Hernias.
Esophageal masses.
Varices.
Mesenchymal masses (e.g., lipomatosis, lipoma).
Lymph node masses.
Lymphoma (particularly non-Hodgkin).
Metastases.
Dilated azygos or hemiazygos vein.
Hernia.

Lymphangioma and hemangioma.
Thymic mass or germ cell tumor.
Anterior cardiophrenic angle masses.
Lymph node masses (particularly lymphoma and metastases).
Pericardial cyst.
Fat pad.
Morgagni hernia.
Thymic masses.
Germ cell tumors.

MEDIASTINITIS, ACUTE[1]

ICD-10CM #   J98.5   Diseases of mediastinum, not elsewhere classified

Esophageal perforation.
Iatrogenic.
EGD, esophageal dilation, esophageal variceal sclerotherapy, nasogastric tube, Sengstaken-Blackmore tube, endotracheal intubation, esophageal surgery, paraesophageal surgery, transesophageal echocardiography, anterior stabilization of cervical vertebral bodies.
Swallowed foreign bodies.
Trauma.
Spontaneous perforation (e.g., emesis, carcinoma).
Head and neck infections (e.g., tonsillitis, pharyngitis, parotitis, epiglottitis, odontogenic).
Infections originating at another site (e.g., TB, pneumonia, pancreatitis, osteomyelitis of sternum, clavicle, ribs).
Cardiothoracic surgery (median sternotomy) (e.g., CABG, valve replacement, other types of cardiothoracic surgery).

MELANONYCHIA

ICD-10CM #   NEC L81.4   Melanin hyperpigmentation

Pregnancy.
Trauma.
Medications (e.g., AZT, 5-fluorouracil, doxorubicin, psoralens).
Nail matrix nevus.
HIV infection.
Onychomycosis.
Melanocyte hyperplasia.
Verrucae.
Pustular psoriasis.
Lichen planus.
Basal cell carcinoma.
Nail matrix melanoma.
Subungual keratosis.
Addison disease.
Bowen disease.

MEMORY LOSS SYMPTOMS, ELDERLY PATIENTS

ICD-10CM #   R41.2   Retrograde amnesia

Age-related mild cognitive impairment.
Depression (pseudodementia).
Medications (e.g., anticholinergics, sedatives).
Hypothyroidism.
Chronic hypoxia.
Cerebrovascular infarcts.
Alzheimer disease.

Hepatic disease.
Chronic renal failure.
Hyperthyroidism.
Frontotemporal dementia.
Lewy body dementia.

MENINGITIS, CHRONIC[1]

ICD-10CM #   G03.1   Chronic meningitis

TB.
Fungal central nervous system infection.
Tertiary syphilis.
Central nervous system neoplasm.
Metabolic encephalopathies.
Multiple sclerosis.
Chronic subdural hematoma.
Systemic lupus erythematosus cerebritis.
Encephalitides.
Sarcoidosis.
NSAIDs.
Behçet syndrome.
Anatomic defects (traumatic, congenital, postoperative).
Granulomatous angiitis.

MENINGITIS, RECURRENT[1]

ICD-10CM #   G03.2   Benign recurrent meningitis [Mollaret]

Drug induced (with rechallenge).
Parameningeal focus.
    Infection (sinusitis, mastoiditis, osteomyelitis, brain abscess).
    Tumor (epidermoid cyst, craniopharyngioma).
Posttraumatic (bacterial).
Mollaret meningitis.
Systemic lupus erythematosus.
Herpes simplex virus.

MENTAL STATUS CHANGES AND COMA[43]

ICD-10CM #   R41.82   Altered mental status, unspecified

METABOLIC/SYSTEMIC ETIOLOGY OF ALTERED MENTAL STATUS AND COMA

Hypoxia
Severe pulmonary disease (hypoventilation).
Severe anemia.
Environmental/toxin:
Methemoglobinemia:
    Cyanide.
    Carbon monoxide.
    Decreased atmospheric oxygen (high altitude).
    Near-drowning.

Disorders of Glucose
Hypoglycemia:
    Chronic alcohol abuse and liver disease.
    Excessive use of insulin or other hypoglycemic agents.
    Insulinoma.
Hyperglycemia:
    Diabetic ketoacidosis.
    Nonketotic hyperosmolar coma.

Decreased Cerebral Blood Flow
Hypovolemic shock.
Cardiac:

Vasovagal syncope.
Arrhythmias.
Myocardial infarction.
Valvular disorders.
Congestive heart failure.
Pericardial effusion/tamponade.
Myocarditis.
Infectious:
Septic shock.
Bacterial meningitis.
Vascular/hematologic:
Hypertensive encephalopathy.
Pseudotumor cerebri.
Hyperviscosity (sickle cell, polycythemia).
Hyperventilation.
Cerebral lupus vasculitis.
Thrombotic thrombocytopenic purpura.
Disseminated intravascular coagulation.
Metabolic Cofactor Deficiency
Thiamine (Wernicke-Korsakoff syndrome).
Pyridoxine (isoniazid overdose).
Folic acid (chronic alcohol abuse).
Cyanocobalamin.
Niacin.
Electrolyte/pH Disturbances
Acidosis/alkalosis.
Hypernatremia/hyponatremia.*
Hypercalcemia/hypocalcemia.
Hypophosphatemia.
Hypermagnesemia/hypomagnesemia.
Endocrine Disorders
Myxedema coma, thyrotoxicosis.
Hypopituitarism.
Addison disease (primary or secondary).
Cushing disease.
Pheochromocytoma.
Hyperparathyroidism/hypoparathyroidism.
Endogenous Toxins
Hyperammonemia (liver failure).
Uremia (renal disease).
Carbon dioxide narcosis (pulmonary disease).
Porphyria.
Exogenous Toxins
Alcohols:
Ethanol, isopropyl alcohol, methanol, ethylene glycol.
Acid poisons:
Salicylates.
Paraldehyde.
Ammonium chloride.
Antidepressant medications:
Lithium.
Tricyclic antidepressants (TCAs).
Selective serotonin reuptake inhibitors (SSRIs).
Monoamine oxidase inhibitors (MAOIs).
Stimulants:
Amphetamines/methamphetamines.
Cocaine.
Over-the-counter sympathomimetics.
Narcotics/opiates:
Morphine.
Heroin.
Codeine, oxycodone, meperidine, hydrocodone.
Methadone.
Fentanyl.
Propoxyphene.

*Can be associated with dilution of formula in infant feeding.

Sedative-hypnotics:
Benzodiazepines.
Barbiturates.
Rohypnol.
Bromide.
Hallucinogens:
Lysergic acid diethylamide (LSD).
Marijuana.
Mescaline, peyote.
Mushrooms.
Phencyclidine (PCP).
Herbs/plants:
Aconite.
Jimson weed.
Morning glory.
Volatile substances:
Hydrocarbons (gasoline, butane, toluene, benzene, chloroform).
Nitrites.
Anesthetic agents (nitrous oxide, ether).
Other:
γ-Hydroxybutyrate (GHB).
Ketamine.
Penicillin.
Cardiac glycosides.
Anticonvulsants.
Steroids.
Heavy metals.
Cimetidine.
Organophosphates.
Disorders of Temperature Regulation/ Environmental
Hypothermia.
Heat stroke.
Malignant hyperthermia.
Neuroleptic malignant syndrome.
High-altitude cerebral edema (HACE).
Dysbarism.
Primary Glial or Neuronal Disorders
Adrenoleukodystrophy.
Creutzfeldt-Jakob disease.
Progressive multifocal leukoencephalopathy.
Marchiafava-Bignami disease.
Gliomatosis cerebri.
Central pontine myelinolysis.
Other Disorders of Unknown Etiology
Seizures.
Post-ictal states.
Reye syndrome.[†]
Intussusception.

[†]Prominent in the pediatric population.

MENTAL STATUS CHANGES AND COMA, STRUCTURAL CAUSES[29]

ICD-10CM #	R40.1	Stupor

COMMON AGE-RELATED CAUSES OF ALTERED MENTAL STATUS AND COMA

Infant
Infection.
Trauma, abuse.
Metabolic.
Child
Toxic ingestion.

Adolescent, Young Adult
Toxic ingestion.
Recreational drug use.
Trauma.
Elderly
Medication changes.
Over-the-counter medications.
Infection.
Alterations in living environment.
Stroke.
Trauma.

MENTAL STATUS CHANGES AND COMA, METABOLIC AND SYSTEMIC CAUSES

ICD-10CM #	F05.9	Delirium, unspecified

METABOLIC AND SYSTEMIC CAUSES OF ALTERED MENTAL STATUS AND COMA

Hypoxia, Hypercapnia
Severe pulmonary disease (hypoventilation).
Severe anemia.
Environmental, toxic.
Methemoglobinemia.
Cyanide.
Carbon monoxide.
Decreased atmospheric oxygen (high altitude).
Near-drowning.
Glucose Disorders
Hypoglycemia:
Chronic alcohol abuse and liver disease.
Excessive dosage of insulin or other hypogly-cemic agents.
Insulinoma.
Hyperglycemia:
Diabetic ketoacidosis.
Nonketotic hyperosmolar coma.
Decreased Cerebral Blood Flow
Hypovolemic shock.
Cardiac:
Vasovagal syncope.
Arrhythmias.
Myocardial infarction.
Valvular disorders.
Congestive heart failure.
Pericardial effusion, tamponade.
Myocarditis.
Infectious:
Septic shock.
Bacterial meningitis.
Vascular, hematologic:
Hypertensive encephalopathy.
Pseudotumor cerebri.
Hyperviscosity (sickle cell, polycythemia).
Hyperventilation.
Cerebral vasculitis as a manifestation of sys-temic lupus erythematosus.
Thrombotic thrombocytopenic purpura.
Disseminated intravascular coagulation.
Metabolic Cofactor Deficiency
Thiamine (Wernicke-Korsakoff syndrome).
Pyridoxine (isoniazid overdose).
Folic acid (chronic alcohol abuse).
Cyanocobalamin.
Niacin.
Electrolyte, pH Disturbances
Acidosis, alkalosis.

Hypernatremia, hyponatremia.*
Hypercalcemia, hypocalcemia.
Hypophosphatemia.
Hypermagnesemia, hypomagnesemia.
Endocrine Disorders
Myxedema coma, thyrotoxicosis.
Hypopituitarism.
Addison disease (primary or secondary).
Cushing disease.
Pheochromocytoma.
Hyperparathyroidism, hypoparathyroidism.
Endogenous Toxins
Hyperammonemia (liver failure).
Uremia (renal disease).
Carbon dioxide narcosis (pulmonary disease).
Porphyria.
Exogenous Toxins
Alcohols:
  Ethanol, isopropyl alcohol, methanol, ethylene glycol.
Acid poisons:
  Salicylates.
  Paraldehyde.
  Ammonium chloride.
Antidepressant medications:
  Lithium.
  Tricyclic antidepressants.
  Selective serotonin reuptake inhibitors.
  Monoamine oxidase inhibitors.
Stimulants:
  Amphetamines, methamphetamines.
  Cocaine.
  Over-the-counter sympathomimetics.
Narcotics, opiates:
  Morphine.
  Heroin.
  Codeine, oxycodone, meperidine, hydrocodone.
  Methadone.
  Fentanyl.
  Propoxyphene.
Sedative-hypnotics:
  Benzodiazepines.
  Barbiturates.
  Rohypnol.
  Bromide.
Hallucinogens:
  Lysergic acid diethylamide.
  Marijuana.
  Mescaline, peyote.
  Mushrooms.
  Phencyclidine.
Herbs, plants:
  Aconite.
  Jimsonweed.
  Morning glory.
Volatile substances:
  Hydrocarbons (gasoline, butane, toluene, benzene, chloroform).
  Nitrites.
  Anesthetic agents (nitrous oxide, ether).
Other:
  γ-Hydroxybutyrate.
  Ketamine.
  Penicillin.
  Cardiac glycosides.
  Anticonvulsants.

*Can be associated with dilution of formula in infant feeding.

Steroids.
Heavy metals.
Cimetidine.
Organophosphates.
Disorders of Temperature Regulation, Environmental
Hypothermia.
Heat stroke.
Malignant hyperthermia.
Neuroleptic malignant syndrome.
High-altitude cerebral edema.
Dysbarism.
Primary Glial or Neuronal Disorders
Adrenoleukodystrophy.
Creutzfeldt-Jakob disease.
Progressive multifocal leukoencephalopathy.
Marchiafava-Bignami disease.
Gliomatosis cerebri.
Central pontine myelinolysis.
Other Disorders with Unknown Etiology
Seizures.
Post-ictal states.
Reye syndrome.
Intussusception.

MESENTERIC ARTERIAL EMBOLISM, ASSOCIATED FACTORS[43]

ICD-10CM #	I74.09	Other arterial embolism and thrombosis of abdominal aorta

FACTORS ASSOCIATED WITH MESENTERIC ARTERIAL EMBOLISM

Coronary artery disease:
  Postmyocardial infarction mural thrombi.
  Congestive heart failure.
Valvular heart disease:
  Rheumatic mitral valve disease.
  Nonbacterial endocarditis.
Arrhythmias:
  Chronic atrial fibrillation.
  Aortic aneurysms or dissections.
  Coronary angiography.

MESENTERIC ISCHEMIA, NONOCCLUSIVE[1]

ICD-10CM #	K55.0	Acute vascular disorders of intestine
	K55.1	Chronic vascular disorders of intestine
	S35.8X9A	Unspecified injury of other blood vessels at abdomen, lower back and pelvis level, initial encounter

Cardiovascular disease resulting in low-flow states (congestive heart failure, cardiogenic shock, post cardiopulmonary bypass, dysrhythmias).

Septic shock.
Drug induced (cocaine, vasopressors, ergot alkaloid poisoning).

MESENTERIC VENOUS THROMBOSIS[1]

ICD-10CM #	I82.91	Chronic embolism and thrombosis of unspecified vein

Hypercoagulable states (protein C or S deficiency, antithrombin III deficiency, Factor V Leyden, malignancy, polycythemia vera, sickle cell disease, homocystinemia, lupus anticoagulant, cardiolipin antibody).
Trauma (operative venous injury, abdominal trauma, postsplenectomy).
Inflammatory conditions (pancreatitis, diverticulitis, appendicitis, cholangitis).
Other: Congestive heart failure, renal failure, portal hypertension, decompression sickness.

METASTATIC NEOPLASMS

ICD-10CM #	C79.51	Secondary malignant neoplasm of bone
	C79.52	Secondary malignant neoplasm of bone marrow
	C79.31	Secondary malignant neoplasm of brain
	C78.7	Secondary malignant neoplasm of liver and intrahepatic bile duct
	C78.00	Secondary malignant neoplasm of unspecified lung

To Bone
Breast.
Lung.
Prostate.
Thyroid.
Kidney.
Bladder.
Endometrium.
Cervix.
Melanoma.

To Liver
Colon.
Stomach.
Pancreas.
Breast.
Lymphomas.
Bronchus.
Lung.
Sarcoma.
Choriocarcinoma.
Kidney.

To Brain
Lung.
Breast.
Melanoma.
GU tract.
Colon.
Sinuses.
Sarcoma.
Skin.
Thyroid.

To Lung
Breast.
Colon.
Kidney.
Testis.
Stomach.
Thyroid.
Melanoma.

METHEMOGLOBINEMIA, DRUG-INDUCED[34]

ICD-10CM #	D74	Methemoglobinemia

Differential Diagnosis

II

SUBSTANCES ASSOCIATED WITH METHEMOGLOBINEMIA

Acetaminophen (nitrobenzene derivative).
Acetanilide.
Local anesthetics:
   Benzocaine.
   Lidocaine.
   Prilocaine.
Aniline dyes.
Celecoxib.
Dapsone.
Flutamide.
Ifosfamide.
Metoclopramide.
Nitric oxide.
Nitrites:
   Amyl nitrite.
   Isobutyl nitrite.
   Sodium nitrite.
   Nitrates (bacterial conversion to nitrites).
Nitrobenzenes/nitrobenzoates.
Nitroethane (nail polish remover).
Nitrofurans.
Nitroglycerin.
Paraquat/monolinuron.
Phenacetin.
Phenazopyridine (pyridium).
Primaquine.
Rasburicase.
Sulfamethoxazole.

MICROCEPHALY[45,101]

ICD-10CM #	Varies with specific diagnosis

PRIMARY (GENETIC)

Familial (autosomal recessive).
Autosomal dominant.
Syndromes:
   Down (21-trisomy).
   Edward (18-trisomy).
   Cri-du-chat (5 p-).
   Cornelia de Lange.
   Rubinstein-Taybi.
   Smith-Lemli-Opitz.

SECONDARY (NONGENETIC)

Radiation.
   Congenital infections:
      Cytomegalovirus.
      Rubella.
      Toxoplasmosis.
Drugs:
Fetal alcohol.
Fetal hydantoin.
Meningitis/encephalitis.
Malnutrition.
Metabolic.
Hyperthermia.
Hypoxic-ischemic encephalopathy.

COMMONLY CITED CAUSES

In utero infections.
   Zika, HIV, toxoplasmosis, rubella, cytomegalovirus, herpes.[a]

---

[a]Often neurologists apply the mnemonic "TORCHES" to Toxoplasmosis, Rubella, Cytomegalovirus, Herpes.

In utero and neonatal cerebral insults.
   Hypoxia, stroke.
Congenital malformations.
   Neural tube defects, anencephaly.
Genetic mutation syndromes.
   Angelman, Rett, velocardiofacial (VCF).
Toxic exposures.
   Fetal alcohol syndrome.
   Cocaine exposure.

MICROPENIS[80]

ICD-10CM #	N48.89	Other specified disorders of penis
	Q55.62	Hypoplasia of penis

HYPOGONADOTROPIC HYPOGONADISM (HYPOTHALAMIC OR PITUITARY DEFICIENCIES)

Kallmann syndrome: autosomal dominant; associated with hyposmia.
Prader-Willi syndrome: hypotonia, mental retardation, obesity, small hands and feet.
Rud syndrome: hyposomia, ichthyosis, mental retardation.
De Morsier syndrome (septooptic dysplasia): hypopituitarism, hypoplastic optic discs, absent septum pellucidum.

HYPERGONADOTROPIC HYPOGONADISM

Primary testicular defect: disorders of testicular differentiation or inborn errors of testosterone synthesis.
Klinefelter syndrome.
Other X polysomies (i.e., XXXXY, XXXY).
Robinow syndrome: brachymesomelic dwarfism, dysmorphic facies.

PARTIAL ANDROGEN INSENSITIVITY

Idiopathic
Defective morphogenesis of the penis.

MIOSIS

ICD-10CM #	H57.03	Miosis

Medications (e.g., morphine, pilocarpine).
Neurosyphilis.
Congenital.
Iritis.
Central nervous system pontine lesion.
Central nervous system infections.
Cavernous sinus thrombosis.
Inflammation/irritation of cornea or conjunctiva.

MONOARTHRITIS, ACUTE

ICD-10CM #	M13.10	Monoarthritis, not elsewhere classified, unspecified site

Overuse.
Trauma.
Gout.
Pseudogout.
Osteoarthritis.

Infectious arthritis (e.g., gonococcal, Lyme disease, viral, mycobacteria, fungi).
Osteomyelitis.
Avascular necrosis of bone.
Hemarthrosis.
Bowel disease–associated arthritis.
Bone malignancy.
Psoriatic arthritis.
Juvenile rheumatoid arthritis.
Sarcoidosis.
Hemoglobinopathies.
Vasculitic syndromes.
Behçet syndrome.
Foreign body synovitis.
Hypertrophic pulmonary osteoarthropathy.
Amyloidosis, familial Mediterranean fever.

MONOCYTOSIS[31]

ICD-10CM #	D72.821	Monocytosis (symptomatic)

Inflammatory diseases:
   Autoimmune/granulomatous.
   Systemic lupus erythematosus.
   Rheumatoid arthritis.
   Giant cell arteritis.
   Myositis.
   Polyarteritis.
   Ulcerative colitis.
   Regional enteritis.
   Sarcoidosis.
Infectious diseases:
   Tuberculosis.
   Syphilis.
   Subacute bacterial endocarditis.
Malignant disorders:
   Preleukemia.
   Nonlymphocytic leukemia.
   Histiocytoses.
   Hodgkin disease.
   Non-Hodgkin lymphoma.
   Carcinomas.
Miscellaneous:
   Chronic neutropenia.
   Post splenectomy.

MONONEUROPATHY

ICD-10CM #	G58.9	Mononeuropathy, unspecified

Herpes zoster.
Herpes simplex.
Vasculitis.
Trauma, compression.
Diabetes.
Postinfectious or inflammatory.

MONONEUROPATHY, ISOLATED[43]

ICD-10CM #	G56.90	Unspecified mononeuropathy of unspecified upper limb

UPPER EXTREMITY

Radial nerve:
   Axilla.
   Humerus.

Elbow (posterior interosseous neuropathy).
Wrist (superficial cutaneous radial neuropathy).
Ulnar nerve:
  Axilla.
  Humerus.
  Elbow.
  Condylar groove.
  Cubital tunnel.
Wrist (Guyon canal):
Hand:
  Superficial terminal ulnar neuropathy.
  Deep terminal ulnar neuropathy:
    Proximal hypothenar.
    Distal hypothenar.
Median nerve.
Axilla.
Humerus (musculocutaneous mononeuropathy).
Forearm:
  Anterior interosseus.
  Pronator syndrome.
Wrist (carpal tunnel).
Hand (recurrent motor branch).
Suprascapular mononeuropathy:
  Axillary mononeuropathy.

LOWER EXTREMITY

Sciatic nerve.
Femoral nerve:
  Iliacus compartment (proximal).
  Saphenous mononeuropathy (distal).
Lateral femoral cutaneous (meralgia paresthetica).
Peroneal nerve:
  Common peroneal mononeuropathy (fibular head, popliteal fossa).
  Deep peroneal mononeuropathy (anterior compartment).
Tibial nerve:
  Popliteal fossa (proximal).
  Tarsal tunnel (distal).
Sural nerve:
  Popliteal fossa, calf (proximal).
  Fifth metatarsal base (distal).
Plantar nerve:
  Distal to tarsal tunnel.
  Interdigital neuropathies (Morton neuroma).
Obturator mononeuropathy.

MONONEUROPATHY MULTIPLEX[10]

ICD-10CM #	G58.9	Mononeuropathy, unspecified

MONONEUROPATHY MULTIPLEX

Vasculitis
Systemic vasculitis:
  Polyarteritis nodosa.
  Rheumatoid arthritis.
  Systemic lupus erythematosus.
  Sjögren syndrome (keratoconjunctivitis sicca).
Nonsystemic vasculitis
Diabetes Mellitus
Neoplastic
Paraneoplastic.
Direct infiltration.
Infectious
Lyme disease.
HIV infection.

Sarcoid
Toxic (lead)
Transient (polycythemia vera)
Cryoglobulinemia (hepatitis C)

MONONUCLEOSIS, MONOSPOT NEGATIVE[18]

ICD-10CM #	B27.90	Infectious mononucleosis, unspecified without complication

DIFFERENTIAL DIAGNOSIS OF MONOSPOT-NEGATIVE MONONUCLEOSIS

Acute HIV infection.
Epstein-Barr virus mononucleosis (particularly in children).
Cytomegalovirus.
Acute toxoplasmosis.
Streptococcal pharyngitis.
Acute hepatitis B infection.

MONOPLEGIA, ACUTE[20]

ICD-10CM #	Varies with specific diagnosis

Complicated migraine.[a]
Dislocation of the radial head.
Hemiparetic seizures.[a]
Monomelic spinal muscular atrophy.
Plexopathy and neuropathy.
  Acute neuritis.
    Asthmatic plexitis.
    Idiopathic plexitis.[a]
    Osteomyelitis plexitis.
    Poliomyelitis.
    Tetanus toxoid plexitis.
  Hereditary.
    Hereditary brachial neuritis.
    Hereditary neuropathy with liability to pressure palsy.
  Injury.
    Lacerations.
    Pressure injuries.
    Traction injuries.[a]
Stroke.

---

[a]Denotes the most common conditions and the ones with disease-modifying treatments.

MOVEMENT DISORDER, HYPERKINETIC[94]

ICD-10CM #	G25.9	Extrapyramidal and movement disorder, unspecified

HYPERKINETIC MOVEMENT DISORDERS

Tremor.
Chorea.
Ballism.
Dystonia.
Athetosis.
Tics.
Myoclonus.

Startle.
Stereotypies.
Miscellaneous.

MOVEMENT DISORDER, PEDIATRIC PATIENT[72]

ICD-10CM #	G25.9	Extrapyramidal and movement disorder, unspecified

COMMONLY CITED MOVEMENT DISORDERS THAT MAY BEGIN IN CHILDHOOD OR ADOLESCENCE

Early Childhood
Athetosis or choreoathetosis.
Lesch-Nyhan syndrome.
Childhood
Dopa-responsive dystonia.
Dystonia associated with DYT1 gene.
Myoclonus from subacute sclerosing panencephalitis (SSPE).
Parkinson disease.
Sydenham chorea.
Tourette disorder.
Withdrawal-emergent dyskinesia.
Adolescence
Essential tremor.*
Huntington disease (juvenile Huntington disease).*
Medication- and drug-induced movements.
Tardive dyskinesias.
Wilson disease.*

---

*Despite incapacitating movements, many choreoathetosis patients have no mental retardation.

MOVEMENT DISORDERS AND COGNITIVE IMPAIRMENT[72]

ICD-10CM #	G25.9	Extrapyramidal and movement disorder, unspecified

MOVEMENT DISORDERS ASSOCIATED WITH COGNITIVE IMPAIRMENT

Young Children
Athetosis or choreoathetosis.*
Lesch-Nyhan syndrome.
Rett syndrome.
Older Children and Adolescents
Huntington disease.
Subacute sclerosing panencephalitis.
Wilson disease.
Adults
Creutzfeldt-Jakob disease.[†]
Huntington disease.
Parkinson disease.

---

*Genetic transmission.
[†]Myoclonus.

MOVEMENT DISORDERS, NEUROLEPTIC-INDUCED[72]

ICD-10CM #	G25.70	Drug-induced movement disorder, unspecified

II

Differential Diagnosis

Acute dyskinesias:
  Akathisia.
  Neuroleptic-malignant syndrome.
  Oculogyric crisis and other dystonias.
Tardive dyskinesias:
  Akathisia.
  Dystonia.
  Oral-buccal-lingual dyskinesia.*
  Tics.
  Tremor.
  Stereotypies.
  Dose-dependent dyskinesia:
    Parkinsonism.
Withdrawal-emergent dyskinesias.

*Commonly referred to as "tardive dyskinesia."

MULTIVALVULAR HEART DISEASE[58]

ICD-10CM #   Varies with specific diagnosis

Acquired
Systemic diseases:
  Infective endocarditis.
  Carcinoid heart disease.
  Systemic lupus erythematosus.
Cardiac diseases:
  Infective endocarditis.
  Rheumatic heart disease.
Degenerative:
  Calcific diseases, increased with age, prior
    radiation, chronic kidney disease.
Iatrogenic:
  Adverse drug effects: ergot-related antagonists.
  Radiation therapy.
Functional (annulus dilation), caused by:
  Ischemic heart disease.
  Hypertensive heart disease.
  Chronic arrhythmia.
  Pulmonary hypertension.
  Cardiomyopathy.

Congenital
Connective tissue disorders:
  Marfan syndrome.
  Ehlers-Danlos syndrome.
Other:
  Trisomy 18, 13, and 15.
  Shone syndrome.
  Ochronosis.

Mixed
Multiple conditions may contribute to valve
  dysfunction, such as: Degenerative diseases
  may lead to associated functional disease.
  Congenital heart disease may predispose to
  infective endocarditis or degenerative disease.

MUSCLE DISCOMFORT DUE TO DRUGS AND TOXINS[38]

ICD-10CM #   Varies with specific diagnosis

INFLAMMATORY MYOPATHY
Definite:
  Hydralazine.
  Penicillamine.
  Procainamide.
  1,1'-Ethylidenebis (tryptophan).

Immune checkpoint inhibitors (ipilimumab,
  nivolumab, more so anti-PD-1 agents).
Statin (HMG-CoA reductase antibody
  myopathy).
Toxic oil syndrome.
Possible:
  Cimetidine.
  Imatinib mesylate.
  Interferon-α.
  Ipecac.
  Lansoprazole.
  Leuprolide.
  Levodopa.
  Penicillin.
  Phenytoin.
  Propylthiouracil.
  Proton pump inhibitors.
  Sulfonamide.

RHABDOMYOLYSIS ± CHRONIC MYOPATHY
Alcohol.
ε-Amino caproic acid.
Amphetamines.
Cocaine.
Cyclosporine.
Daptomycin.
Hypokalemia.
Isoniazid.
Lipid-lowering agents:*
  Bezafibrate.
  Clofibrate.
  Fenofibrate.
  Gemfibrozil.
  Lovastatin.
  Simvastatin.
  Pravastatin.
  Fluvastatin.
  Atorvastatin.
  Cerivastatin.
  Nicotinic acid.
  Red yeast rice.
Labetalol.
Lithium.
Organophosphates.
Propofol.
Snake venom.
Tacrolimus.
Zidovudine.

PAINFUL MYOPATHY ± RHABDOMYOLYSIS
Colchicine.
Emetine.
Fenoverine.
Germanium.
Hypervitaminosis E.
Taxenes.
Zidovudine.

MYALGIA ± MYOPATHY
Amiodarone.
Amphotericin.
Aromatase inhibitors.
Azathioprine.
Beta-blockers (rare).

*Especially with concurrent cyclosporine A, danazol, erythro-
  mycin, gemfibrozil, niacin, or colchicine.

Bevacizumab.
Bisphosphonates.
Bortezomib.
Brentuximab.
Bumetanide.
Calcium channel blockers.
Cholesterol-lowering agents.
Corticosteroid withdrawal.
Danazol.
Denosumab.
Eculizumab.
Estrogen.
Evolocumab.
Fluoroquinolones.
HER2 antibodies (trastuzumab, pertuzumab).
Inotersen.
Interferon-α: 2a and 2b.
Ivosidenib.
Lanadelumab (anti-kallikrein monoclonal antibody).
Mercury (organic).
Methotrexate.[†]
Metolazone.
Mushrooms (orellanine/*Psilocybe*).
Opioids.
Oral contraceptives.
Paclitaxel.
Retinoids (all-*trans*-retinoic acid, isotretinoin).
Rifampin.
  Serotonin reuptake inhibitor treatment and
    withdrawal.[‡]
  Succinylcholine.
  Tyrosine kinase inhibitors (alectinib, acala-
    brutinib, dasatinib, imatinib, larotrectinib,
    lenvatinib, lorlatinib, nilotinib, pazopanib,
    sunitinib, trametinib, as well as BRAF in-
    hibitors [dabrafenib, vemurafenib]).
  Vaccines.
  Vinca alkaloids.

CRAMPS
Albuterol.
Anticholinesterase.
Bergamot (bergapten).
Caffeine.
Clofibrate.
Cyclosporine.
Diuretics (chronic, excessive use).
Lithium.
Nifedipine.
Terbutaline.
Tetanus.
Theophylline.
Vitamin A.

†With concurrent pantoprazole.
‡Especially with withdrawal of medications with a short half-
  life (paroxetine, venlafaxine).

MUSCLE DISEASE[47]

ICD-10CM #   M60.009   Infective myositis,
                          unspecified site

CLASSIFICATION OF MUSCLE DISEASE

Muscular Dystrophies
Duchenne.
Becker.
Limb girdle.

Childhood.
Facioscapulohumeral.

Myotonic Disorders

Dystrophia myotonica.
Myotonica congenita.

Inflammatory

Infective: bacterial, viral, parasitic.
  Unknown cause: polymyositis, dermatomyositis, sarcoidosis.

Endocrine

Thyroid disease—hyper- and hypothyroidism.
Cushing disease.
Addison disease.
Hyperparathyroidism.

Metabolic

Glycogen storage diseases.
Periodic paralyses.
Mitochondrial diseases.

Drug-Induced

Corticosteroids.
Chloroquine.
Amiodarone.
Penicillamine.
Alcohol.
Zidovudine.
Clofibrate.

Other

Inclusion body myositis.

MUSCLE WEAKNESS

ICD-10CM #	M62.9	Disorder of muscle, unspecified

Physical deconditioning.
Impaired cardiac output (e.g., mitral stenosis, mitral regurgitation).
Uremia, liver failure.
Electrolyte abnormalities (hypokalemia, hyperkalemia, hypophosphatemia, hypercalcemia), hypoglycemia.
Drug induced (e.g., statin myopathy).
Muscular dystrophies.
Steroid myopathy.
Alcoholic myopathy.
Myasthenia gravis, Lambert-Eaton syndrome.
Infections (polio, botulism, HIV, hepatitis, diphtheria, tick paralysis, neurosyphilis, brucellosis, TB, trichinosis).
Pernicious anemia, other anemias, beriberi.
Psychiatric illness (depression, somatization syndrome).
Organophosphate or arsenic poisoning.
Inflammatory myopathies (e.g., collagen vascular disease, rheumatoid arthritis, sarcoidosis).
Endocrinopathies (e.g., adrenal insufficiency, hypothyroidism), diabetic neuropathy.
Other: motor neuron disease, mitochondrial myopathy, L-tryptophan (eosinophilia-myalgia), rhabdomyolysis, glycogen storage disease, lipid storage disease.

MUSCLE WEAKNESS, LOWER MOTOR NEURON VS. UPPER MOTOR NEURON

ICD-10CM #	M62.9	Disorder of muscle, unspecified

LOWER MOTOR NEURON

Weakness, usually severe.
Marked muscle atrophy.
Fasciculations.
Decreased muscle stretch reflexes.
Clonus not present.
Flaccidity.
No Babinski sign.
Asymmetric and may involve one limb only in the beginning to become generalized as the disease progresses.

UPPER MOTOR NEURON

Weakness, usually less severe.
Minimal disuse muscle atrophy.
No fasciculations.
Increased muscle stretch reflexes.
Clonus may be present.
Spasticity.
Babinski sign.
Often initial impairment of only skilled movements.
In the limbs the following muscles may be the only ones weak or weaker than the others: triceps; wrist and finger extensors; interossei; iliopsoas; hamstrings; and foot dorsiflexors, inverters, and extroverters.

MUSCULOSKELETAL BENIGN TUMORS AND TUMORLIKE LESIONS[52]

ICD-10CM #	Varies with specific diagnosis

Fibrous dysplasia.
Enchondromatosis.
Osteochondromatosis.
Synovial cysts.
Brown tumors in hyperparathyroidism.
Langerhans cell histiocytosis (eosinophilic granuloma).
Hemangiomatosis.
Bone islands, osteoma (Gardner syndrome).
Fibrous cortical defect, nonossifying fibroma.
Giant cell tumor.
Neurofibromatosis.
Amyloidosis.
Mastocytosis.
SAPHO, chronic multifocal osteomyelitis.

SAPHO, Synovitis, acne, pustulosis, hyperostosis, osteitis.

MUSCULOSKELETAL MALIGNANT TUMORS AND TUMORLIKE LESIONS[52]

ICD-10CM #	Varies with specific diagnosis

Metastases.
Myeloma.
Angiosarcoma.
Leukemia.
Neuroblastoma.
Ewing sarcoma.
Osteosarcomatosis.
Lymphoma.

MYDRIASIS

ICD-10CM #	H57.04	Mydriasis

Coma.
Medications (cocaine, atropine, epinephrine, etc.).
Glaucoma.
Cerebral aneurysm.
Ocular trauma.
Head trauma.
Optic atrophy.
Cerebral neoplasm.
Iridocyclitis.

MYELIN DISEASES[38]

ICD-10CM #	Varies with specific diagnosis

AUTOIMMUNE

Acute disseminated encephalomyelitis.
Acute hemorrhagic leukoencephalopathy.
Multiple sclerosis.

INFECTIOUS

Progressive multifocal leukoencephalopathy.

TOXIC/METABOLIC

Carbon monoxide poisoning.
Vitamin B_{12} deficiency.
Mercury intoxication (Minamata disease).
Alcohol/tobacco amblyopia.
Central pontine myelinolysis.
Marchiafava-Bignami syndrome.
Hypoxia.
Radiation.

VASCULAR

Binswanger disease.

HEREDITARY DISORDERS OF MYELIN METABOLISM

Adrenoleukodystrophy.
Metachromatic leukodystrophy.
Krabbe disease.
Alexander disease.
Canavan-van Bogaert-Bertrand disease.
Pelizaeus-Merzbacher disease.
Phenylketonuria.

MYELITIS[7]

ICD-10CM #	G04.91	Myelitis, unspecified
	G04.89	Other myelitis

VIRAL

HIV.
Herpes simplex virus (HSV)-1 and HSV-2.
Varicella-zoster virus.
Cytomegalovirus.
Epstein-Barr virus.
West Nile virus.
Human T-lymphotropic virus.

BACTERIAL

Mycoplasma pneumoniae.
Borrelia burgdorferi.
Treponema pallidum.
Pyogenic bacteria.
Mycobacterium tuberculosis.

FUNGAL

Coccidioides immitis.
Actinomyces.
Aspergillus.
Blastomyces dermatitidis.
Histoplasmosis.

IMMUNE-MEDIATED

Multiple sclerosis.
Neuromyelitis optica.
Connective tissue disorders (neuro-lupus, neuro-Sjögren).
Neurosarcoidosis.
Paraneoplastic.

NONINFLAMMATORY MYELOPATHIES

Vitamin B_{12} deficiency.
Folic acid deficiency.
Copper deficiency.
Vitamin E deficiency.
Nitrous oxide toxicity.
Heroin.
Radiation myelopathy.
Traumatic/compressive myelopathy.
Vascular myelopathy.

MYELOPATHY AND MYELITIS[17]

ICD-10CM #	M51.9	Unspecified thoracic, thoracolumbar and lumbosacral intervertebral disc disorder
	G95.9	Disease of spinal cord, unspecified

INFLAMMATORY

Infectious: spirochetal TB, zoster, rabies, HIV, polio, rickettsial, fungal, parasitic.
Noninfectious: idiopathic transverse myelitis, multiple sclerosis.

TOXIC/METABOLIC

Diabetes mellitus, pernicious anemia, chronic liver disease, pellagra, arsenic.

TRAUMA COMPRESSION

Spinal neoplasm, cervical spondylosis, epidural abscess, epidural hematoma.

VASCULAR

AV malformation, systemic lupus erythematosus, periarteritis nodosa, dissecting aortic aneurysm.

PHYSICAL AGENTS

Electrical injury, irradiation.

NEOPLASTIC

Spinal cord tumors, paraneoplastic myelopathy.

MYOCARDIAL ISCHEMIA[17]

ICD-10CM #	I25.5	Ischemic cardiomyopathy
	I25.89	Other forms of chronic ischemic heart disease
	I25.9	Chronic ischemic heart disease, unspecified
	I24.8	Other forms of acute ischemic heart disease

Atherosclerotic obstructive coronary artery disease.
Nonatherosclerotic coronary artery disease:
Coronary artery spasm.
Congenital coronary artery anomalies:
Anomalous origin of coronary artery from pulmonary artery.
Aberrant origin of coronary artery from aorta or another coronary artery.
Coronary arteriovenous fistula.
Coronary artery aneurysm.
Acquired disorders of coronary arteries:
Coronary artery embolism.
Dissection:
Surgical.
During percutaneous coronary angioplasty.
Aortic dissection.
Spontaneous (e.g., during pregnancy).
Extrinsic compression:
Tumors.
Granulomas.
Amyloidosis.
Collagen-vascular disease:
Polyarteritis nodosa.
Temporal arteritis.
Rheumatoid arthritis.
Systemic lupus erythematosus.
Scleroderma.
Miscellaneous disorders:
Irradiation.
Trauma.
Kawasaki disease.
Syphilis.
Hereditary disorders:
Pseudoxanthoma elasticum.
Gargoylism.
Progeria.
Homocystinuria.
Primary oxaluria.
"Functional" causes of myocardial ischemia in absence of anatomic coronary artery disease:
Syndrome X.
Hypertrophic cardiomyopathy.
Dilated cardiomyopathy.
Muscle bridge.
Hypertensive heart disease.
Pulmonary hypertension.
Valvular heart disease; aortic stenosis, aortic regurgitation.

MYOCLONUS

ICD-10CM #	G25.3	Myoclonus

Physiologic (e.g., exercise or anxiety induced).
Renal failure.
Hepatic failure.
Hyponatremia.
Hypoglycemia or severe hyperglycemia.
Postdialysis.
Epileptic myoclonus.
Postencephalitis.
Central nervous system lesion (stroke, neoplasm).
Central nervous system trauma.
Parkinson disease.
Medications (e.g., tricyclics, L-dopa).
Friedreich ataxia.
Ataxia-telangiectasia.
Wilson disease.
Huntington disease.
Progressive supranuclear palsy.
Heavy metal poisoning.
Benign familial.

MYOCLONUS, DRUG-INDUCED[49]

ICD-10CM #	G25.79	Other drug-induced movement disorders

SELECTED AGENTS ASSOCIATED WITH MYOCLONUS

Medications

Antibiotics (β-lactams).
Antidepressants.
Antineoplastics: busulfan, chlorambucil.
Carbamazepine, vigabatrin.
Clozapine.
L-dopa.
Lidocaine.
Lithium.
Lorazepam (preterm infants).
Methaqualone.
Morphine.
Nitroprusside.
Piperazine.

Industrial Toxins

Camphor.
Chlorophenoxy herbicides.
Gasoline.

Biologic Toxins

Buckeye (Aesculus spp.).
Lupine.
Shellfish (domoic acid poisoning).

MYOCLONUS, PEDIATRIC PATIENT[68]

ICD-10CM #	G25.3	Myoclonus

SELECTED CAUSES OF MYOCLONUS IN CHILDREN

Physiologic Causes

Hiccups.
Hypnic jerks (sleep starts).
Nocturnal (sleep) myoclonus.

Developmental Causes

Benign neonatal sleep myoclonus.
Benign myoclonus of early infancy.
Myoclonus with fever.

Storage Diseases

Juvenile Gaucher disease (type III).
Sialidosis type 1 (cherry-red spot–myoclonus).
GM_1 gangliosidosis.
Neuronal ceroid-lipofuscinosis (late infantile).

Inherited Degenerative Diseases

Dentatorubral-pallidoluysian atrophy (DRPLA).
Huntington disease.
Progressive myoclonus ataxia.
Ramsay Hunt syndrome.
Early myoclonic encephalopathy.
Rasmussen encephalitis.

Infectious and Postinfectious Diseases

Meningitis (viral or bacterial).
Encephalitis.
Epstein-Barr virus (EBV).
Coxsackievirus.
Influenza.
HIV.
Acute disseminated encephalomyelitis (ADEM).

Metabolic Causes

Uremia.
Hepatic failure.
Electrolyte disturbances.
Hypoglycemia or hyperglycemia.
Aminoacidurias.
Organic acidurias.
Urea cycle disorders.
POLG1 mutations.
Myoclonic epilepsy with ragged red fibers (MERRF).
Mitochondrial encephalomyopathy, lactic acidosis, and stroke-like episodes (MELAS).
Biotinidase deficiency (usually epileptic).
Cobalamin deficiency (infantile).
Leigh syndrome.

Toxic Causes

Psychotropic medications (tricyclic antidepressants, lithium, selective serotonin reuptake inhibitors, monoamine oxidase inhibitors, neuroleptics).
Antibiotics (penicillin, cephalosporins, quinolones).
Antiepileptics (phenytoin, carbamazepine, lamotrigine, gabapentin, benzodiazepines [in infants], vigabatrin).
Opioids.
General anesthetics.
Antineoplastic drugs.
Strychnine, toluene, lead, carbon monoxide, mercury.

Hypoxia

Lance-Adams syndrome.

Functional (Psychogenic) Causes

MYOPATHIC PAIN SYNDROMES[38]

ICD-10CM #	Code varies with specific diagnosis

INFLAMMATORY

Inflammatory and immune myopathies:
  Systemic connective tissue disease.
  Perimysial pathology: tRNA synthetase antibodies.
  Fasciitis.
  Childhood dermatomyositis.
Muscle infections:
Viral myositis (including hepatitis C [possibly], enterovirus, dengue virus).
Pyomyositis.
Toxoplasmosis.
Trichinosis.
Spirochete (*Borrelia burgdorferi*/Lyme disease).

RHABDOMYOLYSIS ± METABOLIC DISORDER

Glycogen storage disease type V (myophosphorylase deficiency): McArdle disease.
Glycogen storage disease type VII (phosphofructokinase deficiency).
Carnitine palmitoyltransferase II.
Mitochondrial myopathies.
Malignant hyperthermia syndromes.
Familial recurrent rhabdomyolysis (myoglobinuria) in childhood (LPIN1 mutations).

OTHER MYOPATHIES WITH PAIN OR DISCOMFORT

Myopathy with tubular aggregates ± cylindrical spirals.
Adult-onset nemaline rod myopathy.
Multicore disease.
Fiber-type disproportion myopathy.
Myopathy with deficiency of iron-sulfur clusters.
Myopathy with tubulin-reactive crystalline inclusions.
Myopathy with hexagonally cross-linked crystalloid inclusions.
Myoadenylate deaminase deficiency.
Neuromyopathy with internalized capillaries.
Myotonias: myotonic dystrophy 2; dominant myotonia congenita (occasional).
Muscular dystrophies (occasional): Duchenne, Becker, limb-girdle dystrophy types 1A, 1C, 2C, 2D, 2E, 2H, 2I, 2L; ANO5-deficient myopathy.
Selenium deficiency.
Vitamin D deficiency.
Toxic myopathy: eosinophilia myalgia, rhabdomyolysis.
Hypothyroid myopathy.
Mitochondrial disorders (fatigue or myalgias with exercise).
Camurati-Engelmann syndrome (bone pain).
Drugs and toxins

MYOPATHIC SYNDROMES, DRUG-INDUCED[90]

ICD-10CM #	G72.9 Myopathy, unspecified

TYPE OF MYOPATHY

Necrotizing myopathy.
Inflammatory myopathy.
Mitochondrial myopathy.
Hypokalemic myopathy.
Antimicrotubular myopathy.
Lysosomal storage myopathy.
Corticosteroid myopathy.
Others.

DRUGS

HMG-CoA reductase inhibitors (statins), fibrates, alcohol.
Penicillamine, interferon-a, procainamide.
Zidovudine.
Diuretics, laxatives, licorice, amphotericin B, alcohol.
Colchicine, vincristine.
Chloroquine, hydroxychloroquine, quinacrine, amiodarone, perhexiline.
Corticosteroids, especially fluorinated.
Ipecac syrup, emetine.

MYOPATHIES ASSOCIATED WITH REST PAIN[90]

ICD-10CM #	G72.9 Myopathy, unspecified

Childhood dermatomyositis.
Hypothyroid myopathy.
Acute alcoholic myopathy.
Drug-induced myopathies.
Infectious myopathies.
Myopathies associated with metabolic bone disease.
Carnitine palmitoyl transferase deficiency.
Rhabdomyolysis from any cause.

MYOPATHIES, HIV-ASSOCIATED[8]

ICD-10CM #	G72.9	Myopathy, unspecified

HIV-Associated Myopathies	Myopathies Secondary to Antiretrovirals	Others
HIV polymyositis.	Zidovudine myopathy.	Opportunistic infections involving muscle (toxoplasmosis).
Inclusion body myositis.	Toxic Mitochondrial myopathies related to other NRTIs.	
Nemaline myopathy.		Tumor infiltrations of skeletal muscle.
Diffuse infiltrative lymphocytosis syndrome.	HIV-associated lipodystrophy syndrome.	Rhabdomyolysis.
HIV wasting syndrome.	Immune Reconstitution syndrome related to ART.	
Vasculitic processes.		
Myasthenia gravis and other myasthenic syndromes.		
Chronic fatigue and fibromyalgia.		

ART, Antiretroviral therapy; *NRTIs,* nucleoside reverse transcriptase inhibitors.

MYOPATHIES, INFECTIOUS

ICD-10CM #	G72.9	Myopathy, unspecified

HIV.
Viral myositis.
Trichinosis.
Toxoplasmosis.
Cysticercosis.

MYOPATHIES, INFLAMMATORY

ICD-10CM # G72.9 Myopathy, unspecified

Systemic lupus erythematosus, rheumatoid arthritis.
Sarcoidosis.
Paraneoplastic syndrome.
Polymyositis, dermatomyositis.
Polyarteritis nodosa.
Mixed connective tissue disease.
Scleroderma.
Inclusion body myositis.
Sjögren syndrome.
Cimetidine, D-penicillamine.

MYOPATHIES, METABOLIC[90]

ICD-10CM # G72.9 Myopathy, unspecified

DISORDERED GLYCOGEN METABOLISM

Myophosphorylase deficiency (McArdle disease).
Phosphorylase b kinase deficiency.
Phosphofructokinase deficiency.
Debrancher enzyme deficiency.
Brancher enzyme deficiency.
Phosphoglycerate kinase deficiency.
Phosphoglycerate mutase deficiency.
Lactate dehydrogenase deficiency.
Acid maltase deficiency.
Aldolase deficiency.
β-Enolase deficiency.

DISORDERED LIPID METABOLISM

Carnitine deficiencies.
Carnitine palmitoyltransferase deficiency.
Fatty acid acyl-CoA dehydrogenase deficiencies.

MITOCHONDRIAL MYOPATHIES

Coenzyme Q10 deficiency.
Respiratory chain complex deficiencies.

ENDOCRINE

Acromegaly.
Hypothyroidism.
Hyperthyroidism.
Hyperparathyroidism.
Cushing disease.
Addison disease.
Hyperaldosteronism.

METABOLIC-NUTRITIONAL

Uremia.
Hepatic failure.
Malabsorption.
Periodic paralysis.
Vitamin D deficiency.
Vitamin E deficiency.

ELECTROLYTE DISORDERS

Sodium: hypernatremia and hyponatremia.
Potassium: hyperkalemia and hypokalemia.
Calcium: hypercalcemia and hypocalcemia.
Phosphate: hypophosphatemia.
Magnesium: hypomagnesemia.

MYOPATHIES, TOXIC[18]

ICD-10CM # G72.2 Myopathy due to other toxic agents

Inflammatory: cimetidine, D-penicillamine.
Noninflammatory necrotizing or vacuolar: cholesterol-lowering agents, chloroquine, colchicine.
Acute muscle necrosis and myoglobinuria: cholesterol-lowering drugs, alcohol, cocaine.
Malignant hyperthermia: halothane, ethylene, others; succinylcholine.
Mitochondrial: zidovudine.
Myosin loss: nondepolarizing neuromuscular blocking agents; glucocorticoids.

MYOPATHY, DRUG-INDUCED[35]

ICD-10CM # G72.9 Myopathy, unspecified

DRUGS AND TOXINS THAT MAY INDUCE MYOPATHY

Example	Comments
Cimetidine.	
Chloroquine.	Vacuolar myopathy.
Colchicine.	Vacuolar myopathy.
Emetine.	
Ethanol.	Acute rhabdomyolysis and chronic myopathy.
Glucocorticoids.	Type II fiber atrophy.
Heroin.	
IFN-α.	Dermatomyositis and polymyositis reported.
Penicillamine.	Typical polymyositis. Mitochondrial myopathy.
Statins and fibrates.	Cases of autoimmune necrotizing myopathy, polymyositis, rhabdomyolysis, and noninflammatory myopathies reported.
Anti-TNF.	In RA patients existing reports of polymyositis, dermatomyositis and anti–Jo-1–positive myositis during TNF blockade.
Zidovudine (AZT). (Many others reported at the case level.)	

AZT, Zidovudine; *IFN,* interferon; *RA,* rheumatoid arthritis; *TNF,* tumor necrosis factor.

MYOSITIS, INFECTIOUS CAUSES[90]

ICD-10CM # M60.009 Infective myositis, unspecified site

VIRAL

Influenza A and B viruses.
Enteroviruses (coxsackieviruses, echoviruses).
HIV.
Human T-cell lymphotrophic virus type 1.
Hepatitis B and C viruses.
Cytomegalovirus.
Epstein-Barr virus.
Adenovirus.
Varicella-zoster virus.
Parainfluenza.

PARASITIC

Trichinella spp.
Echinococcus spp.
Schistosoma spp.
Toxoplasma gondii.
Trypanosoma cruzi.
Sarcocystis spp.

BACTERIAL

Staphylococcus aureus.
Streptococcus, groups A and B.
Aeromonas hydrophila.
Borrelia burgdorferi.
Clostridium perfringens.
Anaerobic streptococci.
Mycobacterium spp.
Rickettsia spp.

FUNGAL

Candida spp.
Cryptococcus neoformans.
Microsporida.

MYOSITIS, INFLAMMATORY[18]

ICD-10CM #	M60.009	Infective myositis, unspecified site
	M60.9	Myositis, unspecified
	M60.10	Interstitial myositis of unspecified site

INFECTIOUS

Viral myositis:
  Retroviruses (HIV, human T-lymphotropic virus type 1).
  Enteroviruses (echovirus, coxsackievirus).
  Other viruses (influenza, hepatitis A and B, Epstein-Barr virus).
Bacterial: pyomyositis.
  Parasites: trichinosis, cysticercosis.
  Fungi: candidiasis.

IDIOPATHIC

Granulomatous myositis (sarcoid, giant cell).
Eosinophilic myositis.
Eosinophilia-myalgia syndrome.

ENDOCRINE/METABOLIC DISORDERS

Hypothyroidism.
Hyperthyroidism.
Hypercortisolism.
Hyperparathyroidism.
Hypoparathyroidism.
Hypocalcemia.
Hypokalemia.

METABOLIC MYOPATHIES

Myophosphorylase deficiency (McArdle disease).
Phosphofructokinase deficiency.
Myoadenylate deaminase deficiency.
Acid maltase deficiency.

Lipid storage diseases.
Acute rhabdomyolysis.

DRUG-INDUCED MYOPATHIES

Alcohol.
D-Penicillamine.
Zidovudine.
Colchicine.
Chloroquine, hydroxychloroquine.
Lipid-lowering agents.
Cyclosporine.
Cocaine, heroin, barbiturates.
Corticosteroids.

NEUROLOGIC DISORDERS

Muscular dystrophies.
Congenital myopathies.
Motor neuron disease.
Guillain-Barré syndrome.
Myasthenia gravis.

NAIL CLUBBING

ICD-10CM #	R68.3	Clubbing of nails

Chronic obstructive pulmonary disease.
Pulmonary malignancy.
Cirrhosis.
Inflammatory bowel disease.
Chronic bronchitis.
Congenital heart disease.
Endocarditis.
AV malformations.
Asbestosis.
Trauma.
Idiopathic.

NAIL, HORIZONTAL WHITE LINES (BEAU LINES)

ICD-10CM #	L60.4	Beau lines

Malnutrition.
Idiopathic.
Trauma.
Prolonged systemic illnesses.
Pemphigus.
Raynaud phenomenon.

NAIL KOILONYCHIA

ICD-10CM #	L60.8	Other nail disorders

Trauma.
Iron deficiency.
Systemic lupus erythematosus.
Hemochromatosis.
Raynaud phenomenon.
Nail-patella syndrome.
Idiopathic.

NAIL ONYCHOLYSIS

ICD-10CM #	L60.1	Onycholysis

Infection.
Trauma.
Psoriasis.
Connective tissue disorders.
Sarcoidosis.
Hyperthyroidism.
Amyloidosis.
Nutritional deficiencies.

NAIL PITTING

ICD-10CM #	L60.8	Other nail disorders

Psoriasis.
Alopecia areata.
Reiter syndrome.
Trauma.
Idiopathic.

NAIL SPLINTER HEMORRHAGE

ICD-10CM #	L60.8	Other nail disorders

SBE.
Trauma.
Malignancies.
Oral contraceptives.
Pregnancy.
Systemic lupus erythematosus.
Antiphospholipid syndrome.
Psoriasis.
Rheumatoid arthritis.
Peptic ulcer disease.

NAIL STRIATIONS

ICD-10CM #	L60.8	Other nail disorders

Psoriasis.
Alopecia areata.
Trauma.
Atopic dermatitis.
Vitiligo.

NAIL TELANGIECTASIA

ICD-10CM #	L60.8	Other nail disorders

Rheumatoid arthritis.
Scleroderma.
Trauma.
Systemic lupus erythematosus.
Dermatomyositis.

NAIL WHITENING (TERRY NAILS)

ICD-10CM #	L60.8	Other nail disorders

Malnutrition.
Trauma.
Liver disease (cirrhosis, hepatic failure).
Diabetes mellitus.
Hyperthyroidism.
Idiopathic.

NAIL YELLOWING

ICD-10CM #	L60.8	Other nail disorders

Tobacco abuse.
Nephrotic syndrome.
Chronic infections (TB, sinusitis).
Bronchiectasis.
Lymphedema.
Raynaud phenomenon.
Rheumatoid arthritis.
Pleural effusions.
Thyroiditis.
Immunodeficiency.

NASAL AND PARANASAL SINUS TUMORS[21]

ICD-10CM #	C30.0	Malignant neoplasm of nasal cavity

BENIGN AND MALIGNANT NASAL AND PARANASAL SINUS TUMORS

Epithelial tumors

BENIGN

Papilloma.
Adenoma.
Inverting papilloma.

MALIGNANT

Squamous carcinoma.
Adenocarcinoma.
Melanoma.
Adenoid cystic carcinoma.
Malignant salivary tumors.

MESENCHYMAL TUMORS

Benign
Osteoma.
Ossifying fibroma complex.
Angiofibroma.
Chondroma.
Malignant
Osteogenic sarcoma.
Fibrosarcoma.
Angiosarcoma.
Chondrosarcoma.
Lymphoma.
Rhabdomyosarcoma.

NASAL BLOCKAGE[96]

ICD-10CM #	Code varies with specific diagnosis

CAUSES

Nasal mucosal conditions:
   Allergic rhinitis.
   Nonallergic rhinitis.
   Infective rhinitis.
   Chronic rhinosinusitis (with or without nasal polyps).
Adenoidal hypertrophy.
Vasculitic conditions:
   ANCA-positive vasculitis.
Granulomatous disorders:
   Sarcoidosis.
Mass lesions:
   Tumors of the nasal cavity, paranasal sinuses, or nasopharynx.
Anatomical obstruction:
   Nasal septal deviation.
   Trauma.
   Foreign bodies.

NASAL MASSES, CONGENITAL[21]

ICD-10CM #	J34.1	Cyst and mucocele of nose and nasal sinus
	J34.89	Other specified disorders of nose and nasal sinuses

Differential Diagnosis

II

Dermoid.
Nasal cerebral heterotopia (glioma).
Frontal meningoencephalocele.
Nasolacrimal duct mucocele.
Nasal hamartoma.
Nasal hemangioma.

NASOPHARYNGEAL TUMORS[22]

ICD-10CM #	C10.6	Benign neoplasm of nasopharynx
ICD-10CM #	C11.3	Malignant neoplasm of nasopharynx

BENIGN TUMORS

Developmental
Thornwaldt cyst.
Hairy polyp.
Teratomas (varied origin).

ECTODERMAL

Papilloma.
Adenomatous polyps.

MESODERMAL

Juvenile angiofibroma.
Fibromyxomatous polyps.
Choanal polyps.
Osteomas.
Fibrous dysplasia.
Craniopharyngioma.
Solitary fibrous tumor.
Desmoid fibromatosis.
Schwannoma.

BENIGN SALIVARY GLAND TUMORS

Pleomorphic adenoma.
Monomorphic adenoma.

MALIGNANT TUMORS

Epithelial
Nasopharyngeal cancer.
Undifferentiated carcinoma.
Squamous cell carcinoma.

EMBRYONAL

Chordoma.

LYMPHOID

Lymphoma.

MESODERMAL

Hemangiopericytoma.
Malignant fibrous histiocytoma.
Rhabdomyosarcoma.

MALIGNANT SALIVARY GLAND TUMORS

Adenoid cystic carcinoma.
Mucoepidermoid carcinoma.
Acinic cell carcinoma.
Adenocarcinoma.

METASTATIC TUMORS

Adenocarcinoma.
Papillary carcinoma.

NAUSEA AND VOMITING

ICD-10CM #	R11.2	Nausea with vomiting, unspecified

Infections (viral, bacterial).
Intestinal obstruction.
Metabolic (uremia, electrolyte abnormalities, diabetic ketoacidosis, acidosis, etc.).
Severe pain.
Anxiety, fear.
Psychiatric disorders (bulimia, anorexia nervosa).
Pregnancy.
Medications (NSAIDs, erythromycin, morphine, codeine, aminophylline, chemotherapeutic agents, etc.).
Withdrawal from substance abuse (drugs, alcohol).
Head trauma.
Vestibular or middle ear disease.
Migraine headache.
Central nervous system neoplasms.
Radiation sickness.
Peptic ulcer disease.
Carcinoma of GI tract.
Reye syndrome.
Eye disorders.
Abdominal trauma.

NAUSEA AND VOMITING, CAUSES DURING PREGNANCY[32]

ICD-10CM #	R11.2	Nausea with vomiting, unspecified

DIFFERENTIAL DIAGNOSIS OF NAUSEA AND VOMITING DURING PREGNANCY

Nausea and vomiting of pregnancy.
Hyperemesis gravidarum.
Pancreatitis.
Symptomatic cholelithiasis.
Viral hepatitis.
Peptic ulcer disease.
Gastric cancer.
Intestinal obstruction.
Intestinal pseudoobstruction.
Gastroparesis diabeticorum.
Gastritis.
Gastroesophageal reflux disease.
Acute pyelonephritis.
Drug toxicity.
Vagotomy.
Preeclampsia/eclampsia.
Acute fatty liver of pregnancy.
Hemolysis, elevated liver enzymes, and low platelets (HELLP) syndrome.
Anorexia nervosa/bulimia.
Other neuropsychiatric disorders.

NAUSEA AND VOMITING, CHRONIC[3]

ICD-10CM #	R11.2	Nausea with vomiting, unspecified

DIFFERENTIAL DIAGNOSIS OF CHRONIC NAUSEA AND VOMITING

Mechanical GI tract obstruction (pylorus, bile duct, small intestine, colon).
Mucosal inflammation.
Peritoneal irritation.
Carcinomas (e.g., gastric, ovarian, renal, bronchogenic).
Metabolic/endocrine disorders (diabetic mellitus, hypothyroidism, hyperthyroidism, adrenal insufficiency, uremia).
Medications (anticholinergics, narcotics, L-dopa, progesterone, calcium channel blockers, digitalis, NSAIDs, antidysrhythmic agents, lubiprostone, cannabis, metformin, amylin analogs).
Gastroparesis.
Gastric dysrhythmias (tachygastria, bradygastria, mixed).
Central nervous system disorders (tumors, migraine, seizures, stroke, orthostatic intolerance).
Psychogenic disorders (anorexia nervosa, bulimia nervosa).

NECK AND ARM PAIN

ICD-10CM #	M54.2	Cervicalgia
	S46.919A	Strain of unspecified muscle, fascia and tendon at shoulder and upper arm level, unspecified arm, initial encounter

Cervical disk syndrome.
Trauma, musculoskeletal strain.
Rotator cuff syndrome.
Bicipital tendonitis.
Glenohumeral arthritis.
Acromioclavicular arthritis.
Thoracic outlet syndrome.
Pancoast tumor.
Infection (cellulitis, abscess).
Angina pectoris.

NECK MASS[25]

ICD-10CM #	R22.1	Localized swelling, mass and lump, neck

CONGENITAL ANOMALIES

Thyroglossal duct cyst.
Bronchial apparatus anomalies.
Teratomas.
Ranula.
Dermoid cysts.
Hemangioma.
Laryngoceles.
Cystic hygroma.

NONNEOPLASTIC INFLAMMATORY ETIOLOGIES

Folliculitis.
Adenopathy secondary to peritonsillar abscess.
Retropharyngeal or parapharyngeal abscess.

Salivary gland infections.
Viral infections (mononucleosis, HIV, cytomegalovirus).
TB.
Cat-scratch disease.
Toxoplasmosis.
Actinomyces.
Atypical *Mycobacterium.*
Jugular vein thrombus.

NEOPLASM (PRIMARY OR METASTATIC)

Lipoma

NECK PAIN[25]

ICD-10CM #	M54.2	Cervicalgia

INFLAMMATORY DISEASES

Rheumatoid arthritis.
Spondyloarthropathies.
Juvenile rheumatoid arthritis.

NONINFLAMMATORY DISEASE

Cervical osteoarthritis.
Diskogenic neck pain.
Diffuse idiopathic skeletal hyperostosis.
Fibromyalgia or myofascial pain.

INFECTIOUS CAUSES

Meningitis.
Osteomyelitis.
Infectious diskitis.

NEOPLASMS

Primary.
Metastatic.

REFERRED PAIN

Temporomandibular joint pain.
Cardiac pain.
Diaphragmatic irritation.
GI sources (gastric ulcer, gallbladder, pancreas).

NECK PAIN FROM RHEUMATOLOGIC DISORDERS[8]

ICD-10CM #	M54.2	Cervicalgia

Rheumatoid arthritis:
    Without disease of the C1-C2 joint.
    With structural cervical abnormalities: C1-C2 subluxation, C1-C2 facet involvement.
Spondyloarthropathies.
Reactive arthritis.
Psoriatic arthritis.
Enteropathic arthritis.
Polymyalgia rheumatica.
Osteoarthritis.
Fibromyalgia.
Nonspecific musculoskeletal pain.
Miscellaneous spondyloarthropathies.
    Whipple disease.
    Behçet disease.
    Paget disease.
    Acromegaly.
    Ossification of the posterior longitudinal ligament.
    Diffuse idiopathic skeletal hyperostosis.

NECK PAIN, NONMUSCULAR CAUSES[35]

ICD-10CM #	M54.2	Cervicalgia

Structure	Condition
Pharynx.	Pharyngitis.
Larynx.	Laryngitis.
	Carcinoma.
Trachea.	Tracheitis.
Thyroid.	Thyroiditis.
Lymph nodes.	Lymphadenitis.
Carotid arteries.	Carotidynia.
	Dissection.
	Inflammation.
Aorta.	Aneurysm.
	Dissection.
Heart.	Angina.
	Infarction.
Pericardium.	Pericarditis.
Diaphragm.	Inflammation by blood, infection.

NECROTIZING PNEUMONIAS[18]

ICD-10CM #	J15.8	Pneumonia due to other specified bacteria

COMMON

Tuberculosis.
Staphylococcus.
Gram-negative bacilli.
Anaerobes.
Fungi.
Pneumocystis jirovecii.

RARE

Streptococcus pneumoniae.
Legionella.
Viruses.
Mycoplasma pneumoniae.

NEONATAL SEIZURES MIMICS[20]

ICD-10CM #	Varies with specific diagnosis

Benign nocturnal myoclonus.[a]
Jitteriness.*
Nonconvulsive apnea.
Normal movement.
Opisthotonos.
Pathologic myoclonus.

[a]Denotes the most common conditions and the ones with disease-modifying treatments.

NEOPLASTIC LESIONS, LUMBOSACRAL SPINE[35]

ICD-10CM #	M54.5	Low back pain

BENIGN

Osteoid osteoma.
Osteoblastoma.
Osteochondroma.

Giant cell tumor.
Aneurysmal bone cyst.
Hemangioma.
Eosinophilic granuloma.
Sacroiliac lipoma.

MALIGNANT

Multiple myeloma.
Chondrosarcoma.
Chordoma.
Lymphoma.
Skeletal metastases.

SPINAL CORD TUMORS

Extradural metastases.
Intradural–extramedullary:
    Neurofibroma.
    Meningioma.
Intramedullary:
    Ependymoma.
    Astrocytoma.

NEPHRITIC SYNDROME, ACUTE[18]

ICD-10CM #	N00.8	Acute nephritic syndrome with other morphologic changes

LOW SERUM COMPLEMENT LEVEL

Acute postinfectious glomerulonephritis.
Membranoproliferative glomerulonephritis.
Systemic lupus erythematosus.
Subacute bacterial endocarditis.
Visceral abscess "shunt" nephritis.
Cryoglobulinemia.

NORMAL SERUM COMPLEMENT LEVEL

IgA nephropathy.
Antiglomerular basement membrane disease.
Polyarteritis nodosa.
Granulomatosis with polyangiitis.
Henoch-Schönlein purpura.
Goodpasture syndrome.

NEPHROCALCINOSIS

ICD-10CM #	E83.59	Other disorders of calcium metabolism

Sarcoidosis.
Hyperparathyroidism.
Chronic glomerulonephritis.
Milk-alkali syndrome.
Distal renal tubular acidosis.
Medullary sponge kidney.
Bartter syndrome.
Hypervitaminosis D.
Idiopathic hypercalciuria.
Hyperoxaluria.
Cortical necrosis.
Tuberculosis.
Idiopathic hypercalciuria.
Rapidly progressive osteoporosis.

NEPHROPATHY, OBSTRUCTIVE[89]

ICD-10CM #   Varies with specific diagnosis

POSSIBLE CAUSES OF OBSTRUCTIVE NEPHROPATHY

Renal
Congenital
Polycystic kidney.
Renal cyst.
Peripelvic cyst.
Ureteropelvic junction obstruction.
Neoplastic
Wilms tumor.
Renal cell carcinoma.
Transitional cell carcinoma of the collecting system.
Multiple myeloma.
Inflammatory
Tuberculosis.
Echinococcus infection.
Metabolic
Calculi.
Miscellaneous
Sloughed papillae.
Trauma.
Renal artery aneurysm.
Ureter
Congenital
Stricture.
Ureterocele.
Obstructing megaureter.
Retrocaval ureter.
Prune belly syndrome.
Neoplastic
Primary carcinoma of ureter.
Metastatic carcinoma.
Inflammatory
Tuberculosis.
Amyloidosis.
Schistosomiasis.
Abscess.
Ureteritis cystica.
Endometriosis.
Miscellaneous
Retroperitoneal fibrosis.
Pelvic lipomatosis.
Aortic aneurysm.
Radiation therapy.
Lymphocele.
Trauma.
Urinoma.
Pregnancy.
Radiofrequency ablation.
Bladder and Urethra
Congenital
Posterior urethral valve.
Phimosis.
Hydrocolpos.
Neoplastic
Bladder carcinoma.
Prostate carcinoma.
Carcinoma of urethra.
Carcinoma of penis.
Inflammatory
Prostatitis.
Paraurethral abscess.

Miscellaneous
Benign prostatic hypertrophy.
Neurogenic bladder.
Urethral stricture.

NEUROGENIC BLADDER[104]

ICD-10CM #   N31.9   Neuromuscular dysfunction of bladder, unspecified

SUPRATENTORIAL

Cerebrovascular accident.
Parkinson disease.
Alzheimer disease.
Cerebral palsy.

SPINAL CORD

Spinal cord injury.
Spinal stenosis.
Central cord syndrome.
Amyotrophic lateral sclerosis.
Multiple sclerosis.
Myelodysplasia.

PERIPHERAL NEUROPATHY

Diabetes.
Alcohol.
Shingles.
Syphilis.

NEUROLOGIC DEFICIT, FOCAL[1]

ICD-10CM #   G45.9   Transient cerebral ischemic attack, unspecified
                I67.848 Other cerebrovascular vasospasm and vasoconstriction

TRAUMATIC: INTRACRANIAL, INTRASPINAL

Subdural hematoma.
Intraparenchymal hemorrhage.
Epidural hematoma.
Traumatic hemorrhagic necrosis.

INFECTIOUS

Brain abscess.
Epidural and subdural abscesses.
Meningitis.

NEOPLASTIC

Primary central nervous system tumors.
Metastatic tumors.
Syringomyelia.
Vascular.
Thrombosis.
Embolism.
Spontaneous hemorrhage: arteriovenous malformation, aneurysm, hypertensive.

METABOLIC

Hypoglycemia.
Vitamin B$_{12}$ deficiency.
Postseizure.
Hyperosmolar nonketotic.

OTHER

Migraine.
Bell palsy.
Psychogenic.

NEUROLOGIC DEFICIT, MULTIFOCAL[1]

ICD-10CM #   I67.89 Other cerebrovascular disease
                G45.9   Transient cerebral ischemic attack, unspecified
                I67.848 Other cerebrovascular vasospasm and vasoconstriction

Acute disseminated encephalomyelitis: postviral or postimmunization.
Infectious encephalomyelitis: poliovirus, enteroviruses, arbovirus, herpes zoster, Epstein-Barr virus.
Granulomatous encephalomyelitis: sarcoid.
Autoimmune: systemic lupus erythematosus.
Other: familial spinocerebellar degenerations.

NEUROMUSCULAR JUNCTION DYSFUNCTION[18]

ICD-10CM #   N31.9   Neuromuscular dysfunction of bladder, unspecified

DISORDERS OF THE NEUROMUSCULAR JUNCTION

Autoimmune
Myasthenia gravis.
Lambert-Eaton myasthenic syndrome.
Congenital
Presynaptic defects in ACh resynthesis, packaging, or release.
Synaptic defect: congenital end plate AChE deficiency.
Postsynaptic defects: slow-channel syndromes.
Postsynaptic defects: decreased response to ACh.
  Fast-channel syndromes.
  AChR deficiency without kinetic abnormality.
Familial limb-girdle myasthenia.
Toxic
Botulism.
Drug-induced disorders.
Organophosphate intoxication.

Ach, Acetylcholine; *AChE,* acetylcholinesterase; *AChR,* acetylcholine receptor.

NEURONOPATHIES, SENSORY (GANGLIONOPATHIES)[43]

ICD-10CM #   G60.0   Hereditary motor and sensory neuropathy

Herpes:
  Herpes simplex I and II.
  Varicella zoster (shingles).
Inflammatory sensory polyganglionopathy (ISP).
Paraneoplastic.
Primary biliary cirrhosis.
Sjögren syndrome (keratoconjunctivitis sicca).

Toxin-induced:
Pyridoxine (vitamin B$_6$) overdose.
Metals:
Platinum (cisplatin).
Methyl mercury.
Vitamin E deficiency.

NEUROPATHIC BLADDER (HEAD) NEUROPATHIES, AUTONOMIC[19]

ICD-10CM #	G63	Polyneuropathy in diseases classified elsewhere

GUILLAIN-BARRÉ SYNDROME

Non–Guillain-Barré syndrome autoimmunity.
Paraneoplastic (type I antineuronal nuclear antibody).
Lambert-Eaton syndrome.
Antibodies to neuronal nicotinic acetylcholine receptors.
Antibodies to P/Q type calcium channels.
Other autoantibodies.
Systemic lupus erythematosus.

HEREDITARY

Type I autosomal dominant.
Type II autosomal recessive (Morvan disease).
Type III autosomal recessive (Riley-Day).
Type IV autosomal recessive (congenital insensitivity to pain with anhidrosis).
Type V absence of pain.

METABOLIC

Fabry disease.
Diabetes mellitus.
Tangier disease.
Porphyria.

INFECTIOUS

HIV.
Chagas disease.
Botulism.
Leprosy.
Diphtheria.
Toxins.

OTHER

Triple A (Allgrove) syndrome.
Navajo Indian neuropathy.
Multiple endocrine neoplasia type 2b.

NEUROPATHIES, AUTONOMIC, PERIPHERAL, CAUSES[59]

ICD-10CM #	G90.09	Other idiopathic peripheral autonomic neuropathy

METABOLIC

Diabetes mellitus.
Alcohol.
Acute intermittent porphyria.
Uremia.

AUTOIMMUNE

Autoimmune autonomic ganglionopathy.
Guillain-Barré syndrome.
Morvan syndrome.
Lambert-Eaton myasthenic syndrome.
Chronic inflammatory demyelinating polyradiculoneuropathy.
Sjögren syndrome.
Systemic lupus erythematosus.
Mixed connective tissue diseases.

PARAPROTEINEMIC

Amyloidosis.

NUTRITIONAL

Cyanocobalamin deficiency.
Thiamine deficiency.
Gluten-sensitive neuropathy.

TOXIC

Heavy metals.
Organic solvents.
Organophosphates.
Vacor.
Acrylamide.

DRUG INDUCED

Cisplatin.
Vincristine.
Amiodarone.
Metronidazole.
Perhexiline.
Paclitaxel.

INFECTIOUS

HIV.
Leprosy.
Chagas disease.
Botulism.
Diphtheria.
Lyme disease.

GENETIC

Hereditary sensory and autonomic neuropathies:
Types I and II.
Type III (familial dysautonomia).
Type IV (congenital insensitivity to pain).
Type V.
Fabry disease.

IDIOPATHIC

Adie syndrome.
Ross syndrome.
Acute cholinergic neuropathy.
Chronic idiopathic anhidrosis.
Amyotrophic lateral sclerosis.

NEUROPATHIES, PAINFUL[62]

ICD-10CM #	G58.9	Mononeuropathy, unspecified
	G62.1	Alcoholic polyneuropathy
	G61.89	Other inflammatory polyneuropathies
	G60.0	Hereditary motor and sensory neuropathy

	G60.0	Hereditary motor and sensory neuropathy
	E11.42	Type 2 diabetes mellitus with diabetic polyneuropathy
	E10.42	Type 1 diabetes mellitus with diabetic polyneuropathy

MONONEUROPATHIES

Compressive neuropathy (carpal tunnel, meralgia paresthetica).
Trigeminal neuralgia.
Ischemic neuropathy.
Polyarteritis nodosa.
Diabetic mononeuropathy.
Herpes zoster.
Idiopathic and familial brachial plexopathy.

POLYNEUROPATHIES

Diabetes mellitus.
Paraneoplastic sensory neuropathy.
Nutritional neuropathy.
Multiple myeloma.
Amyloid.
Dominantly inherited sensory neuropathy.
Toxic (arsenic, thallium, metronidazole).
AIDS-associated neuropathy.
Tangier disease.
Fabry disease.

NEUROPATHIES, PERIPHERAL, ASYMMETRICAL PROXIMAL/ DISTAL[43]

ICD-10CM #	G99.0	Autonomic neuropathy in diseases classified elsewhere

BRACHIAL PLEXOPATHY

Open
Direct plexus injury (knife or gunshot wound).
Neurovascular (plexus ischemia).
Iatrogenic (central line insertion).
Closed
Traction injuries:
"Stingers."
Traction neurapraxia.
Partial or complete nerve root avulsion.
Radiation.
Neoplastic.
Idiopathic brachial plexitis.
Thoracic outlet.

LUMBOSACRAL PLEXOPATHIES

Open
Closed
Traction injuries:
Pelvic double vertical shearing fracture.
Posterior hip dislocation.
Retroperitoneal hemorrhage.
Vasospastic (deep buttock injection).
Neoplastic.

Radiation.
Idiopathic lumbosacral plexitis.
Infectious:
    Herpesvirus (sacrococcygeal).
    Herpes simplex II.
    Herpes zoster.
Cytomegalovirus (CMV) polyradiculopathy (HIV).

NEUROPATHIES, SENSORY ATAXIC[38]

ICD-10CM #	Code varies with specific diagnosis

Sensory neuronopathies (polyganglionopathies):
    Paraneoplastic sensory neuronopathy (malignant inflammatory sensory polyganglionopathy):
    Sjögren syndrome.
    Idiopathic.
    Toxic (cisplatin and analogs, vitamin B_6 excess).
Chronic immune sensory polyradiculopathy.
Demyelinating polyradiculoneuropathies:
    Guillain-Barré syndrome (Miller-Fisher variant).
    Immunoglobulin M monoclonal gammopathy MAG** antibody.
Canomad.*
Tabes dorsalis.

**Myelin-associated glycoprotein.
*Chronic ataxic neuropathy with ophthalmoplegia, IgM paraprotein, cold agglutinins, and anti-GD1b disialosyl antibodies.

NEUROPATHIES, SMALL FIBER[38]

ICD-10CM #	Code varies with specific diagnosis

Diabetes mellitus and impaired glucose tolerance.
Sjögren (sicca) syndrome.
Celiac disease.
Amyloid neuropathy (early familial and primary).
HIV–associated sensory neuropathy.
Hereditary sensory and autonomic neuropathies.
Fabry disease.
Tangier disease.
Cryptogenic small-fiber neuropathy.

NEUROPATHIES, TOXIC AND METABOLIC[19]

ICD-10CM #	NEC G62.2	Toxic neuropathy

METALS

Arsenic (insecticide, herbicide).
Lead (paint, batteries, pottery).
Mercury (metallic, vapor).
Thallium (rodenticides).
Gold.

OCCUPATIONAL OR INDUSTRIAL CHEMICALS

Acrylamide (grouting, flocculation).
Carbon disulfide (solvent).
Cyanide.
Dichlorophenoxyacetate.
Dimethylaminopropionitrite.

Ethylene oxide (gas sterilization).
Hexacarbons (glue, solvents).
Organophosphates (insecticides, petroleum additive).
Polychlorinated biphenyls.
Tetrachlorbiphenyl.
Trichloroethylene.

DRUGS

Amiodarone.
Chloramphenicol.
Chloroquine.
Cisplatin.
Colchicine.
Dapsone.
Ethambutol.
Ethanol.
Gold.
Hydralazine.
Isoniazid.
Metronidazole.
Nitrofurantoin.
Nitrous oxide.
Nucleosides (antiretroviral agents ddC, ddl, d4T, others).
Penicillamine.
Pentamidine.
Phenytoin.
Pyridoxine (excessive).
Statins.
Stilbamidine.
Suramin.
Taxanes (paclitaxel, docetaxel).
Thalidomide.
Tryptophan (eosinophilia-myalgia syndrome).
Vincristine.

METABOLIC DISORDER

Fabry disease.
Krabbe disease.
Leukodystrophies.
Porphyria.
Tangier disease.
Tyrosinemia.
Uremia.

NEUROPATHIES WITH AUTONOMIC NERVOUS SYSTEM INVOLVEMENT[38]

ICD-10CM #	Code varies with specific diagnosis

ACUTE

Acute pandysautonomic neuropathy (autoimmune, paraneoplastic).
Guillain-Barré syndrome.
Porphyria.
Toxic: vincristine, Vacor (rodenticide).

CHRONIC

Diabetes mellitus.
Amyloid neuropathy (familial and primary).
Paraneoplastic sensory neuronopathy (malignant inflammatory sensory polyganglionopathy).
HIV–related autonomic neuropathy.
Hereditary sensory and autonomic neuropathy.

NEUROPATHIES WITH FACIAL NERVE INVOLVEMENT

ICD-10CM #	G51.8	Other disorders of facial nerve

Sarcoidosis.
HIV.
Lyme disease.
Guillain-Barré.
Others: chronic inflammatory polyneuropathy, Tangier disease, amyloidosis.

NEUTROPENIA, DRUG-INDUCED[34]

ICD-10CM #	D70.9	Other neutropenia

DRUGS COMMONLY ASSOCIATED WITH NEUTROPENIA

Antibiotics:
    Vancomycin.
    Semisynthetic penicillins.
    Chloramphenicol.
    Sulfa.
    Linezolid.
Antithyroid drugs:
    Methimazole.
    Propylthiouracil.
Cardiovascular:
    Ticlopidine.
    Procainamide.
Antipsychotics:
    Clozapine.
    Olanzapine.
    Chlorpromazine.
Anticonvulsants:
    Phenytoin.
    Carbamazepine
    Valproic acid.
Antiinflammatory agents:
    Indomethacin.
    Sulfasalazine.
    Phenylbutazone.
H_2 blockers:
    Cimetidine.
    Ranitidine.
Analgesics:
    Dipyrone.
Antineoplastic:
    Rituximab.
Anthelminthic:
    Levamisole.

NEUTROPENIA WITH DECREASED MARROW RESERVE[31]

ICD-10CM #	D70.8	Other neutropenia

PRIMARY

Severe congenital neutropenia.
Shwachman-Diamond syndrome.
Cyclic neutropenia.

SECONDARY

Lymphoproliferative disorder of granular lymphocytes.
Chemotherapy.

Drug induced (nonimmune).
Nutritional.
Viral infection (varicella, EBV, measles, CMV, hepatitis, HIV).

NEUTROPENIA WITH NORMAL MARROW RESERVE[31]

ICD-10CM #	D70.9	Neutropenia, unspecified

Chronic benign neutropenia of infancy and childhood.
Ethnic or benign familial neutropenia.
Autoimmune neutropenia.
Alloimmune neutropenia.
Drug-induced neutropenia.
Infection-related neutropenia.
Hypersplenism.

NEUTROPENIA, IN CHILDHOOD[105]

ICD-10CM #	D70.8	Other neutropenia
	D70.9	Neutropenia unspecified

ACQUIRED

Infection.
Immune mediated.
Hypersplenism.
Vitamin B_{12}, folate, copper deficiency.
Drugs or toxic substances.
Aplastic anemia.
Malignancies or preleukemic disorders.
Ionizing radiation.

CONGENITAL

Cyclic neutropenia.
Severe congenital neutropenia (Kostmann syndrome).
Chronic benign neutropenia of childhood.
Shwachman-Diamond syndrome.
Fanconi anemia.
Metabolic disorders (amino acidopathies, Barth syndrome, glycogen storage disorders).
Osteopetrosis.
Neutropenia with pigmentation abnormalities, e.g., Chédiak-Higashi.

NEUTROPHILIA[31]

ICD-10CM #	D72.0	Neutrophilia, hereditary giant
	D71	Functional disorders of polymorphonuclear neutrophils

CLASSIFICATION OF NEUTROPHILIA

Primary (No Other Evident Associated Disease)
Hereditary neutrophilia.
Chronic idiopathic neutrophilia.
Chronic myelogenous leukemia (CML) and other myeloproliferative diseases.
Familial myeloproliferative disease.

Congenital anomalies and leukemoid reaction.
Leukocyte adhesion factor deficiency (LAD).
Familial cold urticaria and leukocytosis.
Secondary
Infection.
Stress neutrophilia.
Chronic inflammation.
Drug induced.
Nonhematologic malignancy.
Generalized marrow stimulation as in hemolysis.
Asplenia and hyposplenism.

NIPPLE DISCHARGE[68]

ICD-10CM #	Varies with specific diagnosis

Pregnancy.
Hormones (oral contraceptives, estrogen, progesterone).
Blood pressure drugs (methyldopa, verapamil).
Tricyclic antidepressants.
Tranquilizers (antipsychotics).
Antinausea drugs (metoclopramide).
Herbs (nettle, fennel, blessed thistle, anise, fenugreek seed).
Illicit drugs (marijuana, opiates).
Stimulation of the breast (sexual or from exercise).
Thyroid abnormalities.
Chronic emotional stress.
Hypothalamic tumors.
Chest wall conditions.
Herpes zoster.
Trauma.
Burns.
Tumors.
Breast conditions:
Mammary duct ectasia.
Chronic cystic mastitis.
Intraductal cysts.
Intraductal papillomas.

NIPPLE LESIONS

ICD-10CM #	Varies with specific diagnosis

Contact dermatitis.
Trauma.
Paget disease.
Sebaceous hyperplasia.
Neurofibroma.
Accessory nipple.
Papillary adenoma.
Nevoid hyperkeratosis.
Cellulitis.

NODULAR LESIONS, SKIN

ICD-10CM #	R22.9	Localized swelling, mass and lump, unspecified

Lipoma.
Cherry angioma.
Angiokeratoma.
Hemangioma.
Classic Kaposi sarcoma.
Nodular melanoma.
Pyogenic granuloma.

Angiosarcoma.
Eccrine poroma.

NODULES, PAINFUL

ICD-10CM #	R22.9	Localized swelling, mass and lump, unspecified

Arthropod bite or sting.
Erythema nodosum.
Glomus tumor.
Neuroma.
Leiomyoma.
Angiolipoma.
Dermatofibroma.
Osler node.
Blue rubber bleb nevus.
Vasculitis.
Sweet syndrome.

NYSTAGMUS

ICD-10CM #	H55.00	Unspecified nystagmus
	H55.89	Other irregular eye movements

Medications (meperidine, barbiturates, phenytoin, phenothiazines, etc.).
Multiple sclerosis.
Congenital.
Neoplasm (cerebellar, brain stem, cerebral).
Labyrinthine or vestibular lesions.
Central nervous system infections.
Optic atrophy.
Other: Arnold-Chiari malformation, syringobulbia, chorioretinitis, meningeal cysts.

NYSTAGMUS, DOWNBEAT[38]

ICD-10CM #	H55.09	Other forms of nystagmus

CAUSES

Congenital (rare).
Transiently in normal neonates.
Idiopathic (common).
Craniocervical junction abnormalities:
Basilar invagination (e.g., Paget disease).
Chiari malformations.
Dolichoectasia of the vertebrobasilar arterial system.
Foramen magnum tumors.
Syringobulbia.
Cerebellar disorders:
Alcoholic cerebellar degeneration (chronic usage).
Anoxic cerebellar degeneration.
Antiglutamic acid decarboxylase antibodies (anti-GAD65 antibodies).
Cerebellar degeneration following human T-lymphotropic virus types I and II.
Episodic ataxia.
Familial spinocerebellar degeneration, particularly SCA-6, and with multiple system atrophy.
Heat stroke–induced cerebellar degeneration.
Paraneoplastic cerebellar degeneration.

Differential Diagnosis

II

Metabolic disorders (drugs, toxins, and deficiencies):
  Alcohol intoxication.
  Amiodarone.
  Anticonvulsants.
  Lithium.
  Magnesium depletion.
  Opioids.
  Toluene abuse.
  Vitamin B_{12} deficiency.
  Wernicke encephalopathy (as a chronic, persistent late-stage finding).
Other:
  Benign paroxysmal positional vertigo: positional downbeat nystagmus with an anterior canal lesion.
  Brain stem encephalitis.
  Cardiogenic vertigo.
  Cephalic tetanus.
  Finger extensor weakness and downbeat nystagmus motor neuron disease (FEWDON-MND).
  Hydrocephalus.
  Leukodystrophy.
  Multiple sclerosis.
  Small-amplitude downbeat nystagmus in carriers of blue-cone monochromatism.
  Syncope.
  Vertebrobasilar ischemia.

NYSTAGMUS, MONOCULAR

| ICD-10CM # | H55.09 | Other forms of nystagmus |
| | H55.00 | Unspecified nystagmus |

Amblyopia.
Strabismus.
Multiple sclerosis.
Monocular blindness.
Internuclear ophthalmoplegia.
Lid fasciculations.
Brain stem infarct.

OCULAR MOTOR APRAXIA, ASSOCIATED DISORDERS[38]

| ICD-10CM # | Varies with specific diagnosis |

ASSOCIATED DISORDERS

Aicardi syndrome.
Aplasia or hypoplasia of the corpus callosum.
Aplasia or hypoplasia of the cerebellar vermis (up to 53% of patients).
Ataxia with "ocular motor" apraxia type I syndrome.
Ataxia telangiectasia.
Autosomal recessive AOA associated with axonal peripheral neuropathy, areflexia, and pes cavus (may be the same as EOAH).
Bardet-Biedl syndrome.
Bilateral cerebral cortical lesions.
Birth injuries (see perinatal/postnatal disorders).
Carbohydrate-deficient glycoprotein syndrome type Ia.
Carotid fibromuscular hypoplasia.
Cockayne syndrome.

COMA (occasionally may be familial).
Congenital vertical ocular motor apraxia (rare).
Cornelia de Lange syndrome.
Dandy-Walker malformation.
EOAH (may be the same disorder as AOA).
GM1 gangliosidosis.
Hydrocephalus.
Infantile Gaucher disease.
Infantile Refsum disease.
Joubert syndrome.
Krabbe leukodystrophy.
Leber congenital amaurosis.
Megalocephaly.
Microcephaly.
Microphthalmos.
Neurovisceral lipidosis (e.g., Niemann-Pick type C).
Occipital porencephalic cysts.
Pelizaeus-Merzbacher disease.
Perinatal and postnatal disorders (hypoxia, meningitis, PV leukomalacia, athetoid cerebral palsy, perinatal septicemia and anemia, herpes encephalitis, epilepsy).
Propionic acidemia.
Succinic semialdehyde dehydrogenase deficiency.
Wieacker syndrome.

ODYNOPHAGIA[2]

| ICD-10CM # | Varies with specific diagnosis |

CAUSES OF ODYNOPHAGIA

Infections
Herpes simplex virus.
Cytomegalovirus.
Candidiasis.
Chemical, Inflammatory
Gastroesophageal reflux.
Drug induced (slow-K, tetracyclines, quinidine).
Radiation.
Graft-versus-host disease.
Crohn disease.
Dermatologic diseases (pemphigus and pemphigoid).

OLFACTORY FUNCTION IMPAIRMENT[38]

| ICD-10CM # | G52.0 | Disorders of olfactory nerve |

ASSOCIATED DISORDERS AND CONDITIONS, AS MEASURED BY OLFACTORY TESTING

22q11 deletion syndrome.
AIDS/HIV infection.
Adenoid hypertrophy.
Adrenal cortical insufficiency.
Age.
Alcoholism.
Allergies.
Alzheimer disease.
Amyotrophic lateral sclerosis.
Anorexia nervosa.
Asperger syndrome.
Ataxias.

Attention deficit hyperactivity disorder.
Bardet-Biedl syndrome.
Chemical exposure.
Chronic obstructive pulmonary disease.
Congenital COVID-19 infection.
Creutzfeldt-Jakob disease.
Cushing syndrome.
Cystic fibrosis.
Degenerative ataxias.
Diabetes.
Down syndrome.
Epilepsy.
Facial paralysis.
Frontotemporal lobe degeneration.
Gonadal dysgenesis (Turner syndrome).
Guamanian ALS/PD/dementia syndrome.
Head trauma.
Herpes simplex encephalitis.
Hypothyroidism.
Huntington disease.
Iatrogenesis.
Kallmann syndrome.
Korsakoff psychosis.
Leprosy.
Liver disease.
Lubag.
Medications.
Migraine.
Multiple sclerosis.
Multiple system atrophy.
Multiinfarct dementia.
Narcolepsy with cataplexy.
Neoplasms, cranial/nasal.
Nutritional deficiencies.
Obesity.
Obsessive compulsive disorder.
Obstructive pulmonary disease.
Orthostatic tremor.
Panic disorder.
Parkinson dementia complex of Guam.
Parkinson disease.
Pick disease.
Posttraumatic stress disorder.
Pregnancy.
Pseudohypoparathyroidism.
Psychopathy.
Radiation (therapeutic, cranial).
REM behavior disorder.
Refsum disease.
Renal failure/end-stage kidney disease.
Restless leg syndrome.
Rhinosinusitis/polyposis.
Schizophrenia.
Seasonal affective disorder.
Sjögren syndrome.
Stroke.
Tobacco smoking.
Toxic chemical exposure.
Upper respiratory infections.
Usher syndrome.
Vascular disorders (e.g., aneurysms, hemorrhages).
Vitamin B_{12} deficiency.

AIDS, Acquired immunodeficiency syndrome; *ALS*, advanced life support; *PD*, Parkinson disease; *REM*, rapid eye movement.

OPACIFICATION OF HEMIDIAPHRAGM ON X-RAY[21]

ICD-10CM #   Varies with specific diagnosis

CAUSES OF OPACIFICATION OF A HEMITHORAX

Pleural effusion.
Consolidation.
Collapse.
Massive tumor.
Fibrothorax.
Combination of above lesions.
Pneumonectomy.
Lung agenesis.

OPHTHALMOPLEGIA[18]

ICD-10CM #	H51.9	Unspecified disorder of binocular movement
	H49.00	Third [oculomotor] nerve palsy, unspecified eye

BILATERAL

Botulism.
Myasthenia gravis.
Wernicke encephalopathy.
Acute cranial polyneuropathy.
Brain stem stroke.

UNILATERAL

Carotid-posterior (third cranial nerve, pupil involved communicating aneurysm).
Diabetic-idiopathic (third or sixth cranial nerve, pupil spared).
Myasthenia gravis.
Brain stem stroke.[‡]

[‡]Spontaneous, multivector, chaotic eye movement.

OPHTHALMOPLEGIA, ACUTE, BILATERAL[38]

ICD-10CM #   Varies with specific diagnosis

Basilar meningitis, hypertrophic cranial pachymeningitis, or neoplastic infiltration.[†]
Botulism.
Brain stem encephalitis.[†]
Brain stem stroke.[†]
Carotid-cavernous or dural shunt fistula.[†]
Cavernous sinus thrombosis (febrile, ill patient).[†]
Central herniation syndrome.
Ciguatera poisoning.
Diphtheria.
Fisher syndrome (Miller Fisher syndrome) with or without ataxia.
Intoxication (sedatives, tricyclics, organophosphates, anticonvulsants—consciousness impaired).
Leigh disease (subacute necrotizing encephalomyelitis).
Multiple sclerosis.
Myasthenia.

[†]Pain may be present.

Neuroleptic malignant syndrome (personal observation).
Orbital pseudotumor.[†]
Paraneoplastic encephalomyelitis.
Pituitary apoplexy.[†]
Progressive encephalomyelitis with rigidity and myoclonus, a variant of stiff person syndrome.
Psychogenic.
Stiff person syndrome.
Thallium poisoning.
Tick paralysis.
Tolosa-Hunt syndrome.[†]
Trauma (impaired consciousness, signs of injury).[†]
Wernicke encephalopathy.

*All may be unilateral.

OPHTHALMOPLEGIA, ACUTE, UNILATERAL[20]

ICD-10CM #   Varies with specific diagnosis

Aneurysm.[a,b]
Brain tumors.
   Brain stem glioma.
   Parasellar tumors.
   Tumors of pineal region.
Brain stem stroke.[a]
Cavernous sinus fistula.
Cavernous sinus thrombosis.
Gradenigo syndrome.
Idiopathic ocular motor nerve palsy.[a]
Increased intracranial pressure.
Multiple sclerosis.[a]
Myasthenia gravis.[a]
Ophthalmoplegic migraine.[a,b]
Orbital inflammatory disease.[a,b]
Orbital tumor.[b]
Recurrent familial.[a]
Trauma.
   Head.
   Orbital.

[a]May be recurrent.
[b]May be associated with pain.

OPHTHALMOPLEGIA AND GAZE PALSIES[38]

ICD-10CM #   Varies with specific diagnosis

CAUSES OF OPHTHALMOPLEGIA AND GAZE PALSIES

Site	Disorder
Muscle:	Ocular myopathies: Congenital myopathies:
	Central core.
	Centronuclear (myotubular).
	Fiber-type disproportion.
	Multicore (ptosis, spares EOM).
	Nemaline.
	Neurocristopathy (EOM fibrosis).
	Oculopharyngodistal myopathy (Satoyoshi myopathy).
	Autosomal dominant. Autosomal recessive.
	Reducing body myopathy (ptosis, spares EOM).
	Dystrophies:
	Myotonic dystrophy (ptosis, usually spares EOM).
	Oculopharyngeal dystrophy.
	Inflammatory myopathies:
	Dermatomyositis.
	Giant cell arteritis (typically by muscle ischemia).
	Idiopathic orbital inflammatory syndrome (orbital pseudotumor).
	Metabolic and toxic myopathies (act at multiple sites, e.g., anticonvulsants).
	Mitochondrial cytopathy:
	Chronic progressive external ophthalmoplegia (CPEO).
	CPEO-like syndrome: mitochondrial toxicity in long-standing AIDS and long exposure to HAART.
	Kearns-Sayre syndrome.
	Pearson syndrome.
	POLIP syndrome (polyneuropathy, ophthalmoplegia, leukoencephalopathy, intestinal pseudoobstruction).
	Infiltrative disorders (thyroid, amyloid, metastases, congenital familial fibrosis, cystinosis).
	High myopia (large globes cause mechanical restriction).
	Trauma (orbital entrapment).
Neuromuscular junction:	Myasthenia gravis.
	Toxins (e.g., botulism, cosmetic botulinum toxin, organophosphates).
	Lambert-Eaton syndrome (rarely affects EOM, mainly causes ptosis).
Ocular motor nerves:	
Gaze palsies:	Nuclear and paranuclear:
	Brain stem injury (vascular, multiple sclerosis, neuromyelitis optica, encephalitis, paraneoplastic, toxins, tumor).
	Familial congenital gaze palsy.
	Glycine encephalopathy (nonketotic hyperglycinemia: hiccups, seizures, apneic spells).

II

Site	Disorder
	Internuclear ophthalmoplegia.
	Leigh disease.
	Machado-Joseph disease (SCA3).
	Maple syrup urine disease.
	Möbius and Duane syndromes (agenesis of cranial nerve nuclei).
	One-and-a-half syndrome.
	Progressive encephalitis with rigidity and myoclonus (PERM), a variant of the stiff person syndrome.
	Spinocerebellar degeneration.
	Tangier disease.
	Vitamin E deficiency.
	Prenuclear:
	Monocular "supranuclear" elevator palsy.
	Ocular tilt reaction.
	Skew deviation.
	Vertical one-and-a-half syndrome.
	Supranuclear (predominantly horizontal).
	Acutely, after hemispheric stroke:
	Congenital ocular motor apraxia or congenital saccadic palsy.
	Ipsiversive or contraversive (wrong-way eyes).
	Gaucher disease (types 2 and 3).
	Ictal (transient, adversive).
	Juvenile-onset GM2 gangliosidosis (mimics juvenile SMA).
	Post-ictal (transient, ipsiversive).
	Paraneoplastic disorders.
	Supranuclear (predominantly vertical): Adult-onset GM2 gangliosidosis (mimics multisystem atrophy or spinocerebellar degeneration) (V>H).
	Amyotrophic lateral sclerosis (rare, V>H).
	Autosomal dominant parkinsonian-dementia complex with pallidopontonigral degeneration (dementia, dystonia, frontal and pyramidal signs, urinary incontinence).
	Cerebral amyloid angiopathy with leukoencephalopathy.

Site	Disorder
	Congenital vertical ocular motor apraxia (rare).
	Dentatorubral-pallidoluysian atrophy (autosomal dominant, dementia, ataxia, myoclonus, choreoathetosis).
	Diffuse Lewy body disease (ophthalmoplegia may be global).
	Dorsal midbrain syndrome.
	Familial Creutzfeldt-Jakob disease (U>D).
	Familial paralysis of vertical gaze.
	Gerstmann-Sträussler-Scheinker disease (U>D, dysmetria, nystagmus).
	Guamanian Parkinson disease-dementia complex (Lytico-Bodig disease).
	HARP syndrome (hypoprebetalipoproteinemia, acanthocytosis, retinitis pigmentosa, pallidal degeneration).
	Hydrocephalus (untreated, decompensated shunt).
	Joseph disease.
	Kernicterus (U>D).
	Late-onset cerebellopontomesencephalic degeneration (D>U).
	Neurovisceral lipidosis; synonyms: DAF syndrome (downgaze palsy-ataxia-foamy macrophages); dystonic lipidosis; Niemann-Pick disease type C (initially loss of downgaze, which may become global, and be associated with ataxia, cognitive changes, sensory neuropathy, and pyramidal findings).
	Pallidoluysian atrophy (dysarthria, dystonia, bradykinesia).
	Paraneoplastic disorders.
	Progressive supranuclear palsy (PSP).
	Stiff person syndrome.
	Subcortical gliosis (U>D).
	Variant Creutzfeldt-Jakob disease (U>D).
	Vitamin B_{12} deficiency (U>D).
	AIDS encephalopathy.

Site	Disorder
	Alzheimer disease (pursuit). Cerebral adrenoleukodystrophy.
	Corticobasal ganglionic degeneration.
	Fahr disease (idiopathic striatopallidodentate calcification).
	Gaucher disease.
	Hexosaminidase A deficiency.
	Huntington disease.
	Joubert syndrome.
	Leigh disease (infantile striatonigral degeneration).
	Malignant neuroleptic syndrome (personal observation). Methylmalonomocystinuria.
	Neurosyphilis.
	Opportunistic infections.
	Paraneoplastic disorders.
	Pelizaeus-Merzbacher disease (H>V).
	Pick disease (impaired saccades).
	Progressive multifocal leukoencephalopathy.
	Pseudo-PSP, a selective saccadic palsy, associated with progressive ataxia, dysarthria, and dysphagia over several months following aortic/cardiac surgery under hypothermic circulatory arrest.
	Stiff person syndrome—late.
	Tay-Sachs disease (infantile GM2 gangliosidosis) (V>H).
	Wernicke encephalopathy.
	Whipple disease (V>H).
	X-linked dystonia-parkinsonism (Lubag disease).

AIDS, Acquired immunodeficiency syndrome; *D,* loss of downgaze; *EOM,* extraocular muscles; *global,* loss of horizontal and vertical gaze; *H,* loss of horizontal gaze; *HAART,* highly active antiretroviral therapy; *SMA,* spinal muscular atrophy; *U,* loss of upgaze; *V,* loss of vertical gaze.

OPHTHALMOPLEGIA, CHRONIC[38]

ICD-10CM # Varies with specific diagnosis

Brain stem neoplasm.
Chronic ataxic neuropathy, ophthalmoplegia, monoclonal protein, cold agglutinins, and di-sialosyl antibodies (CANOMAD).
Chronic basal meningitis (infection, sarcoid, or carcinoma).
Chronic ophthalmoplegia with anti-GQ1b antibody.
Congenital extraocular muscle fibrosis.
Dysthyroidism.
Leigh disease.
Multiple sclerosis.
Myasthenia gravis.

Myopathies (e.g., mitochondrial, fiber-type disproportion).

Nuclear, paranuclear, and supranuclear gaze palsies.

OPHTHALMOPLEGIA, COMBINED VERTICAL GAZE[38]

ICD-10CM # Varies with specific diagnosis

DIFFERENTIAL DIAGNOSIS

Stroke.
Progressive supranuclear palsy.
Cortical-basal ganglionic degeneration.
Arteriovenous malformation.
Multiple sclerosis.
Tumor (thalamic, mesencephalic, pineal).
Hydrocephalus.
Whipple disease.
Syphilis.
Metabolic disorders:
  Lipid and lysosomal storage diseases (e.g., Niemann-Pick type C).
  Wilson disease.
  Kernicterus.
  Wernicke encephalopathy.
Bulbar-onset amyotrophic lateral sclerosis (associated with TDP-43–positive inclusions).
Paraneoplastic brain stem encephalitis (e.g., with Ma-2 antibodies).
Creutzfeldt-Jakob disease.

OPHTHALMOPLEGIA, INTERNUCLEAR[38]

ICD-10CM # Varies with specific diagnosis

Brain stem (pontine) stroke—unilateral.
Multiple sclerosis—unilateral or bilateral.
Intrinsic tumor—primary or metastatic.
Meningitis (especially tuberculosis, also acquired immunodeficiency syndrome, brucellosis, cysticercosis, syphilis).
Brain stem encephalitis (infective, inflammatory, lupus, paraneoplastic, sarcoid).
Chemotherapy with radiation therapy.
Drug intoxication:
Comatose—anticonvulsants, phenothiazines, tricyclics.
Awake—lithium.
Spinocerebellar degeneration.
Fabry disease (vascular).
Herniation (epidural and acute and chronic subdural hemorrhage, cerebral hematoma).
Vascular malformations.
Vasculitis.
Wernicke encephalopathy.
Progressive supranuclear palsy.
Syringobulbia associated with a Chiari malformation.
Trauma (closed head injury, neck/vertebral artery injury).
Hexosaminidase A deficiency.
Kennedy disease (X-linked recessive progressive spinomuscular atrophy).
Maple syrup urine disease.

Cerebral air embolism.
Vitamin B_{12} deficiency.
Pseudointernuclear ophthalmoplegia.
  Long-standing exotropia.
  Myasthenia.
  Myotonic dystrophy.
  Neuromyotonia of the lateral rectus muscle.
  Partial palsy of cranial nerve III.
  Previous extraocular muscle surgery.
  Thyroid orbitopathy (lateral rectus restriction).
  Orbital pseudotumor.
  Other infiltrative disorders of extraocular muscle (neoplasm, amyloid, etc.).
  Miller Fisher syndrome (sometimes may be a true internuclear ophthalmoplegia).

OPHTHALMOPLEGIA, TOTAL[38]

ICD-10CM # Varies with specific diagnosis

ACUTE

Miller Fisher syndrome.
Guillain-Barré syndrome.
Bilateral pontine or midbrain-thalamic stroke.
Myasthenia gravis.
Pituitary apoplexy.
Botulism.
Anticonvulsant intoxication.
Multiple cranial neuropathies from infection or neoplasm.
Wernicke encephalopathy.

CHRONIC/PROGRESSIVE

Chronic progressive external ophthalmoplegia syndromes.
Oculopharyngeal muscular dystrophy.
Myotonic dystrophy and other congenital myopathies.
Congenital cranial dysinnervation syndromes.
Neurodegenerative diseases (e.g., progressive supranuclear palsy, late spinocerebellar ataxia type 2).
Myasthenia gravis.
Thyroid eye disease (especially in combination with myasthenia gravis).

OPSOCLONUS[61]

ICD-10CM # H55.89 Other irregular eye movements

Multiple sclerosis.
Encephalitis.
Central nervous system lymphoma.
Hydrocephalus.
Pontine hemorrhage.
Thalamic disorder (glioma, hemorrhage).
Hyperosmolar coma.
Carcinoma, paraneoplastic.
Cocaine.
Medications (e.g., phenytoin, haloperidol, amitriptyline, diazepam, vidarabine).

OPTIC ATROPHY[47]

ICD-10CM # H47.20 Unspecified optic atrophy

CAUSES OF OPTIC ATROPHY

Optic Nerve Compression
Pituitary tumor.
Carotid aneurysm.
Glaucoma.
Optic nerve tumor.
Sphenoid meningioma.
Olfactory groove meningioma.
Optic Neuritis Following Long-Standing Papilledema Central Retinal Artery Occlusion Toxic/Metabolic
Diabetes.
Methyl alcohol.
Tobacco.
Quinine.
Ethambutol.
Lead and arsenic.
Anemia.
Secondary to Retinal Disease
Senile macular degeneration.
Retinitis pigmentosa.
Severe chorioretinitis.
Secondary to Trauma
Orbital fracture.
Hereditary
Leber optic atrophy.
Hereditary ataxias.
Spinocerebellar degeneration.

OPTIC DISC ELEVATION[44]

ICD-10CM # Varies with specific diagnosis

CAUSES OF OPTIC DISC ELEVATION

Papilledema.
Accelerated hypertension.
Anterior optic neuropathy.
Ischemic.
Inflammatory.
Infiltrative.
Compressive, including orbital disease.
Pseudopapilledema.
Disc drusen.
Tilted optic disc.
Peripapillary myelinated nerve fibers.
Crowded disc in hypermetropia.
Mitochondrial optic neuropathies.
Leber hereditary optic neuropathy.
Methanol poisoning.
Intraocular disease.
Central retinal vein occlusion.
Uveitis.
Posterior scleritis.
Hypotony.

OPTIC DISC SWELLING[20]

ICD-10CM # Varies with specific diagnosis

Congenital disk elevation.
Increased intracranial pressure.
Ischemic neuropathy.
Optic glioma.
Optic nerve drusen.
Papillitis.
Retrobulbar mass.

Differential Diagnosis

II

ORAL MUCOSA, ERYTHEMATOUS LESIONS[63]

ICD-10CM #	K12.2	Cellulitis and abscess of mouth
	K13.70	Unspecified lesions of oral mucosa
	K13.79	Other lesions of oral mucosa

Allergy.
Erythroplakia.
Candidiasis.
Geographic tongue.
Stomatitis areata migrans.
Plasma cell gingivitis.
Pemphigus vulgaris.

ORAL MUCOSA, PIGMENTED LESIONS[63]

ICD-10CM #	K12.2	Cellulitis and abscess of mouth
	K13.70	Unspecified lesions of oral mucosa
	K13.79	Other lesions of oral mucosa
	K13.5	Oral submucous fibrosis

Racial pigmentation.
Oral melanotic macule.
Peutz-Jeghers syndrome.
Neurofibromatosis.
Albright syndrome.
Addison disease.
Chloasma.
Drug reaction: quinacrine, Minocin, chlorpromazine, Myleran.
Amalgam tattoo.
Lead line.
Smoker's melanosis.
Nevi.
Melanoma.

ORAL MUCOSA, PUNCTATE EROSIVE LESIONS[63]

ICD-10CM #	K12.2	Cellulitis and abscess of mouth
	K13.70	Unspecified lesions of oral mucosa
	K13.79	Other lesions of oral mucosa

Viral lesion: herpes simplex, coxsackievirus (A, B, A16), herpes zoster.
Aphthous stomatitis.
Sutton disease (giant aphthae).
Behçet syndrome.
Reiter syndrome.
Neutropenia.
Acute necrotizing ulcerative gingivostomatitis (ANUG).
Drug reaction.
Inflammatory bowel disease.
Contact allergy.

ORAL MUCOSA, WHITE LESIONS[63]

ICD-10CM #	K12.2	Cellulitis and abscess of mouth
	K13.70	Unspecified lesions of oral mucosa
	K13.79	Other lesions of oral mucosa
	K13.5	Oral submucous fibrosis

Leukoplakia.
White, hairy leukoplakia.
Squamous cell carcinoma.
Lichen planus.
Stomatitis nicotinica.
Benign intraepithelial dyskeratosis.
White spongy nevus.
Leukoedema.
Darier-White disease.
Pachyonychia congenital.
Candidiasis.
Allergy.
Systemic lupus erythematosus.

ORAL SOFT TISSUE TUMORS[94]

ICD-10CM #	Varies with specific diagnosis

Connective Tissue Hyperplasia (Normal-Appearing Overlying Mucosa)
Irritation fibroma.
Denture-associated hyperplasia.
Palatal papillomatosis (papillary hyperplasia).
Generalized gingival hyperplasias.
Drug-induced (phenytoin, nifedipine, cyclosporine).
Hereditary.
Reactive Hyperplasia (Erythematous Overlying Mucosa)
Pyogenic granuloma/pregnancy tumor.
Peripheral giant cell granuloma.
Inflammatory gingival hyperplasia.
Hyperplastic lingual tonsil.
Epithelial Masses (Usually Irregular White Surface)
Papilloma/oral wart.
Squamous cell carcinoma.
Verrucous carcinoma.
Focal epithelial hyperplasia (Heck disease).
Condyloma acuminatum (venereal wart).
Keratoacanthoma (on lips).
Salivary Duct Obstruction (Minor Salivary Glands)
Mucocele/ranula (usually fluctuant).
Salivary stone (sialolith).
Subepithelial Neoplasms
Primary connective tissue or salivary gland tumors.
Metastatic Lesions (Especially in the Mandible).
Lymphoma (especially in the palate or posterior mandible).
Focal or generalized leukemic infiltrates in the gingiva (especially with acute monocytic leukemia).

ORAL ULCERS, ACUTE

ICD-10CM #	K13.70	Unspecified lesions of oral mucosa
	K13.79	Other lesions of oral mucosa

Trauma (including thermal trauma).
Aphthous stomatitis.
Syphilis.
Herpes simplex infection.
Herpes zoster.

ORAL VESICLES AND ULCERS[18]

ICD-10CM #	K13.70	Unspecified lesions of oral mucosa
	K13.79	Other lesions of oral mucosa

Aphthous stomatitis.
Primary herpes simplex infection.
Vincent stomatitis.
Syphilis.
Coxsackievirus A (herpangina).
Fungi (histoplasmosis).
Behçet syndrome.
Systemic lupus erythematosus.
Reiter syndrome.
Crohn disease.
Erythema multiforme.
Pemphigus.
Pemphigoid.

ORBITAL INFLAMMATION[44]

ICD-10CM #	H05.019	Cellulitis of unspecified orbit
	C69.10	Malignant neoplasm of unspecified orbit
	D31.60	Benign neoplasm of unspecified orbit
	H05.029	Osteomyelitis of unspecified orbit
	H05.049	Tendonitis of unspecified orbit
	H05.229	Edema of unspecified orbit
	H05.239	Hemorrhage of unspecified orbit

DIFFERENTIAL DIAGNOSIS OF AN ACUTELY INFLAMED ORBIT

Infection
Bacterial orbital cellulitis.
Fungal orbital infection.
Dacryocystitis.
Infective dacryoadenitis.
Vascular lesions
Acute orbital hemorrhage,
Cavernous sinus thrombosis.
Carotid–cavernous fistula.
Neoplasia
Rapidly progressive retinoblastoma.
Lacrimal gland tumor.
Other neoplasms (e.g., metastatic lesion with inflammation, lymphoma, Waldenström macroglobulinemia).

Rhabdomyosarcoma, leukemia, lymphangioma, or neuroblastoma in children

Endocrine
Thyroid eye disease of rapid onset.

Nonneoplastic inflammation
Idiopathic orbital inflammatory disease.
Tolosa-Hunt syndrome.
Orbital myositis.
Acute allergic conjunctivitis with lid swelling.
Herpes zoster ophthalmicus.
Herpes simplex skin rash.
Sarcoidosis.
Vasculitides: Wegener granulomatosis, polyarteritis nodosa.
Scleritis, including posterior scleritis.
Ruptured dermoid cyst.

ORBITAL LESIONS, CALCIFIED

ICD-10CM #	H05.89	Other disorders of orbit

Chronic inflammation.
Phlebolith.
Dermoid cyst.
Mucocele walls.
Tumors (lacrimal gland, fibroosseous).
Meningioma (optic sheath).
Lymphangioma.
Orbital varix.

ORBITAL LESIONS, CYSTIC

ICD-10CM #	H05.9	Unspecified disorder of orbit

Sweat gland cyst.
Dermoid cyst.
Lacrimal gland cyst.
Abscess.
Conjunctival cyst.
Lymphangioma.
Schwannoma.

ORBITAL NEOPLASMS, MALIGNANT[106]

ICD-10CM #	C69.10	Malignant neoplasm of unspecified orbit

LESIONS WITH CLINICALLY MALIGNANT BEHAVIOR

Langerhans cell tumors.*
Non-Langerhans cell tumors.
Atypical lymphoid hyperplasia.
Meningioma of optic nerve.

PRIMARY MALIGNANT TUMORS OF ORBIT

Lymphoma.
Lacrimal gland carcinomas.
Rhabdomyosarcoma.
Primitive neuroectodermal tumors.
Malignant peripheral nerve sheath tumor.
Alveolar soft part sarcoma.
Melanoma.
Osteosarcoma.

*Relatively common tumor.

Fibrosarcoma.
Leiomyosarcoma.
Chondrosarcoma.
Liposarcoma.
Glioma of optic nerve.

SECONDARY MALIGNANT TUMORS OF ORBIT

Eyelid malignancies.
Conjunctival malignancies.
Uveal melanoma.
Retinoblastoma.
Lacrimal drainage system malignancies.
Paranasal sinus and nasal carcinoma.
Brain tumors.

METASTATIC TUMORS OF ORBIT

Distant carcinomas (e.g., breast, lung, GI tract).
Neuroblastoma.
Leukemia (granulocytic sarcoma).
Carcinoid tumor.
Metastatic melanoma.

ORGASM DYSFUNCTION[55]

ICD-10CM #	F52.31	Female orgasmic disorder
	F52.32	Male orgasmic disorder

Anorgasmia: inadequate stimulation or learning.
Spinal cord lesion or injury.
Multiple sclerosis.
Alcoholic neuropathy.
Amyotrophic lateral sclerosis.
Spinal cord accident.
Spinal cord trauma.
Peripheral nerve damage.
Radical pelvic surgery.
Herniated lumbar disk.
Hypothyroidism.
Addison disease.
Cushing disease.
Acromegaly.
Hypopituitarism.
Pharmacologic agents (e.g., selective serotonin reuptake inhibitors, β-blockers).
Psychogenic.

OROFACIAL PAIN

ICD-10CM #	R51	Facial pain

Dental abscess.
Sinusitis.
Otitis media.
Otitis externa.
Wisdom tooth eruption.
Sialoadenitis.
Herpes zoster.
Trigeminal neuralgia.
Parotitis.
Anxiety disorder.
Malingering.

OSTEOLYTIC BENIGN BONE LESIONS, MULTIPLE[52]

ICD-10CM #	Varies with specific diagnosis

COMMON MULTIPLE OSTEOLYTIC BENIGN LESIONS

Cystic lesions in joint disease.
Amyloidosis.
Brown tumors in hyperparathyroidism.
Enchondromatosis.
Fibrous dysplasia.
Osteomyelitis (including tuberculosis, hydatid, sarcoid, etc.).
Massive osteolysis (Gorham disease).
Mastocytosis.
Neurofibromatosis.
Langerhans cell histiocytosis (histiocytosis X).

OSTEOMYELITIS, PEDIATRIC PATIENT[5]

ICD-10CM #	M86	Osteomyelitis

Fractures.
Thrombophlebitis.
Scurvy.
Septicemia.
Cellulitis.
Septic bursitis.
Myositis.
Pyomyositis.
Rheumatic fever.
Toxic synovitis.
Reactive arthritis.
Complex regional pain syndrome.
Chronic recurrent multifocal osteomyelitis.
Osteoid osteoma.
Langerhans cell histiocytosis.
Leukemia.
Ewing sarcoma.
Malignant primary bone tumors.
Bone infarction (sickle-cell or Gaucher disease).

OSTEOPOROSIS IN CHILDREN[52]

ICD-10CM #	M81.8	Other osteoporosis without current pathological fracture

CAUSES OF OSTEOPOROSIS IN CHILDREN

Systemic long-term oral glucocorticoid therapy.
Chronic inflammatory disease (e.g., juvenile inflammatory arthritis).
Hypogonadism—primary or secondary.
Prolonged immobilization.
Osteogenesis imperfecta.
Idiopathic juvenile osteoporosis.

OSTEOPOROSIS, SECONDARY CAUSES

ICD-10CM #	M81.0	Age-related osteoporosis without current pathological fracture

Medication induced (e.g., glucocorticoids, anticonvulsants, heparin, LHRH agonists or antagonists).

Differential Diagnosis

II

Hyperparathyroidism.
Hyperthyroidism.
Prolonged immobilization.
Chronic renal failure.
Sickle cell disease.
Multiple myeloma.
Myeloproliferative diseases.
Leukemias and lymphomas.
Acromegaly.
Prolactinoma.
Diabetes mellitus.
Total parenteral nutrition.
Malabsorption.
Chronic hypophosphatemia.
Connective tissue disorders (e.g., osteogenesis imperfecta, Marfan syndrome, Ehlers-Danlos).
Hepatobiliary disease.
Postgastrectomy.
Aluminum-containing antacids.
Systemic mastocytosis.
Homocystinuria.*

*Involvement principally of cancellous bone.

OSTEOSCLEROSIS, DIFFUSE[21]

ICD-10CM #	Q77.4	Congenital osteosclerosis

DISORDERS ASSOCIATED WITH DIFFUSE OSTEOSCLEROSIS

Neoplastic Causes*
Prostate carcinoma, breast carcinoma, GI adenocarcinoma, carcinoid tumors, transitional cell carcinoma of the bladder, myeloma, lymphoma, leukemia.

Hematologic Causes
Sickle cell disorders, mastocytosis, myelofibrosis, polycythemia vera.

Metabolic Causes
Renal osteodystrophy, primary hyperparathyroidism, familial hypophosphatemic osteomalacia, hypervitaminosis D, fluorosis, hypoparathyroidism, pseudohypoparathyroidism.[†]

Primary Osseous Disorders[†]
Osteoporosis.
Pyknodysostosis.
Paget disease.

[†]Involvement of cancellous and cortical bone.

OSTEOSCLEROTIC BENIGN BONE LESIONS, MULTIPLE[52]

ICD-10CM #	Q78.2	Osteosclerosis

COMMON MULTIPLE OSTEOSCLEROTIC BENIGN LESIONS

Bone infarcts.
Bone islands.
Callus.
Osteomyelitis (chronic, multifocal).
Paget disease.
Fibrous dysplasia.
Enchondromatosis.
Mastocytosis.
Matured benign lesions (e.g., nonossifying fibromas).
Osteomas (Gardner syndrome).

Osteopathia striata.
Osteopoikilosis.

OVARIAN ENLARGEMENT, NONNEOPLASTIC[99]

ICD-10CM #	N83.209	Unspecified ovarian cyst, unspecified side
	N83.29	Other ovarian cysts
	N80.1	Endometriosis of ovary
	O00.209	Unspecified ovarian pregnancy without intrauterine pregnancy

NONNEOPLASTIC CAUSES OF OVARIAN ENLARGEMENT IN THE NONPREGNANT PATIENT

Functional
Hemorrhagic corpus luteum.
Follicle cyst.
Cortical stromal hyperplasia (hyperthecosis).
Polycystic ovarian syndrome (PCOS).
Mesothelial/Müllerian.
Endometriotic cyst.
Xanthomatous pseudotumor.
Cystic adhesions/cystic mesothelioma.
Simple cyst.

Vascular
Ovarian torsion/infarction.
Massive ovarian edema.

OVULATORY DYSFUNCTION[26]

ICD-10CM #	N97.0	Female infertility associated with anovulation
	N92.3	Ovulation bleeding

HYPERANDROGENIC ANOVULATION

Polycystic ovarian syndrome.
Late-onset congenital adrenal hyperplasias.
Ovarian hyperthecosis.
Androgen-producing ovarian tumors.
Androgen-producing adrenal tumors.
Cushing syndrome.

HYPOESTROGENIC ANOVULATION (HYPOTHALAMIC OR PITUITARY ETIOLOGY)

Hypogonadotropic Hypoestrogenic States
Reversible:
    Functional hypothalamic amenorrheas:
        Eating disorders (anorexia nervosa, excessive weight loss).
        Excessive athletic training.
Neoplastic:
    Craniopharyngioma.
    Pituitary stalk compression.
Infiltrative diseases:
    Histiocytosis-X.
    Sarcoidosis.
Hypophysitis.
Pituitary adenomas:
    Hyperprolactinemia.
    Euprolactinemic galactorrhea.

Endocrinopathies:
    Hypothyroidism/hyperthyroidism.
    Cushing disease.
Irreversible:
    Kallmann syndrome.
    Isolated gonadotropin deficiency (hypothalamic or pituitary origin).
    Panhypopituitarism/pituitary insufficiency:
        Sheehan syndrome, pituitary apoplexy.
        Pituitary irradiation or ablation.

Hypergonadotropic Hypoestrogenic States
Physiologic states:
    Menopause.
    Perimenopause.
Premature ovarian failure.
Immune-related:
    Radiation/chemotherapy-induced.
Ovarian dysgenesis.
Turner syndrome.
46XX with mutations of X.
Androgen insensitivity syndrome.

Miscellaneous
Endometriosis.
Luteal phase defect.

PAIN, MIDFOOT

ICD-10CM #	M25.579	Pain in unspecified ankle and joints of unspecified foot

MEDIAL ASPECT

Tendonitis of posterior tibialis.
Tendonitis of flexor digitorum longus.
Tendonitis of flexor hallucis longus.
Infection (osteomyelitis, septic arthritis, cellulitis) of foot.
Peripheral vascular insufficiency.
Fracture.
Osteoarthritis.
Gout, pseudogout.
Neuropathy.
Tumor.

LATERAL ASPECT

Peroneus longus tendonitis.
Peroneus brevis tendonitis.
Infection (osteomyelitis, septic arthritis, cellulitis) of foot.
Peripheral vascular insufficiency.
Fracture.
Osteoarthritis.
Gout, pseudogout.
Neuropathy.
Tumor.

PAIN, PLANTAR ASPECT, HEEL

ICD-10CM #	M25.579	Pain in unspecified ankle and joints of unspecified foot

Plantar fasciitis.
Tarsal tunnel syndrome.
Neuroma.
Infection (osteomyelitis, septic arthritis, cellulitis) of foot.
Peripheral vascular insufficiency.

Fracture.
Bone cyst.
Osteoarthritis.
Gout, pseudogout.
Neuropathy.
Tumor.
Heel pad atrophy.
Plantar fascia rupture.

PAIN, POSTERIOR HEEL

ICD-10CM #	M79.609	Pain in unspecified limb

Achilles tendonitis.
Retrocalcaneal bursitis.
Retroachilles bursitis.
Infection (osteomyelitis, septic arthritis, cellulitis) of foot.
Peripheral vascular insufficiency.
Fracture.
Osteoarthritis.
Gout, pseudogout.
Neuropathy.
Tumor.

PAIN SYNDROMES WITHOUT CHRONIC MYOPATHY[38]

ICD-10CM #	Code varies with specific diagnosis

PAIN OF UNCERTAIN ORIGIN

Polymyalgia rheumatica.
Infections:
    Viral and postviral syndromes.
    Brucellosis.

ENDOCRINE

Thyroid: decreased (mainly) or increased.
Parathyroid: increased or decreased.
Adrenal insufficiency.
    Familial Mediterranean fever.

PAIN WITH DEFINED ORIGIN

Connective tissue disorders:
    Systemic.
    Fasciitis.
Joint disease.
Bone: osteomalacia, fracture, neoplasm.
Vascular: ischemia, thrombophlebitis.
Polyneuropathy:
    Small-fiber polyneuropathies.
    Guillain-Barré syndrome.
Radiculoneuropathy.
Central nervous system: restless legs syndrome, dystonias (focal).

PAIN OF MUSCLE FROM CENTRAL SENSITIZATION

Fibromyalgia.
Chronic fatigue syndrome/systemic exertion intolerance disease.
Myofascial pain syndrome.
Joint hypermobility syndrome/Ehlers-Danlos syndrome.

PAIN OF MUSCLE ORIGIN WITHOUT CHRONIC MYOPATHY

Muscle ischemia: atherosclerosis, calciphylaxis.

Muscle overuse syndromes:
    Delayed-onset muscle soreness (DOMS).
    Cramps.
Drugs, toxins.
Muscle injury (strain).
Usual features: muscle pain; may interfere with effort but no true weakness; present at rest, may increase with movement; muscle morphology and serum creatine kinase normal.

PALINDROMIC RHEUMATISM[40]

ICD-10CM #	M12.30	Palindromic rheumatism, unspecified site
	M12.319	Palindromic rheumatism, unspecified shoulder
	M12.329	Palindromic rheumatism, unspecified elbow
	M12.339	Palindromic rheumatism, unspecified wrist
	M12.349	Palindromic rheumatism, unspecified hand
	M12.359	Palindromic rheumatism, unspecified hip
	M12.369	Palindromic rheumatism, unspecified knee
	M12.379	Palindromic rheumatism, unspecified ankle and foot
	M12.38	Palindromic rheumatism, vertebrae
	M12.39	Palindromic rheumatism, multiple sites

Palindromic rheumatoid arthritis.
Essential palindromic rheumatism.
Crystal synovitis (gout, CPPD, pseudogout, calcific periarthritis).
Lyme borreliosis, stages 2 and 3.
Sarcoidosis.
Whipple disease.
Acute rheumatic fever.
Reactive arthritis (rare).

PALMOPLANTAR HYPERKERATOSIS

ICD-10CM #	L85.1	Acquired keratosis [keratoderma] palmaris et plantaris
	L85.2	Keratosis punctata (palmaris et plantaris)
	L87.0	Keratosis follicularis et parafollicularis in cutem penetrans

Superficial skin infection.
Chronic eczema.
Repeated trauma.
Psoriasis.
Reiter syndrome.
Paraneoplastic acrokeratosis.

PALPABLE GALLBLADDER[96]

ICD-10CM #	Varies with specific diagnosis

CAUSES

With Jaundice
Carcinoma of the head of the pancreas.
Carcinoma of the ampulla of Vater.
Mucocele of the gallbladder due to a stone in Hartmann pouch and a stone in the common bile duct (rare).
Without Jaundice
Mucocele of the gallbladder.
Carcinoma of the gallbladder.

PALPITATIONS[76]

ICD-10CM #	R00.2	Palpitations

Anxiety.
Electrolyte abnormalities (hypokalemia, hypomagnesemia).
Exercise.
Hyperthyroidism.
Ischemic heart disease.
Ingestion of stimulant drugs (cocaine, amphetamines, caffeine).
Medications (digoxin, β-blockers, calcium channel antagonists, hydralazines, diuretics, minoxidil).
Hypoglycemia in type 1 diabetes mellitus.
Mitral valve prolapse.
Wolff-Parkinson-White (WPW) syndrome.
Sick sinus syndrome.

PANCOAST SYNDROME[14]

ICD-10CM #	Varies with specific diagnosis

CAUSES OF PANCOAST SYNDROME

Neoplasms
Primary bronchogenic carcinomas.
Other primary thoracic neoplasms: adenoid cystic carcinomas.
Hemangiopericytoma.
Mesothelioma.
Metastatic neoplasms: carcinoma of the larynx, cervix, urinary bladder, and thyroid gland.
Hematologic neoplasms: plasmacytoma, lymphoid granulomatosis, lymphoma.
Infectious Processes
Bacterial: staphylococcal and pseudomonal pneumonia, thoracic actinomycosis.
Fungal: aspergillosis, allescheriasis, cryptococcosis.
Tuberculosis.
Parasitic: echinococcosis (hydatid cyst).

PANCREATIC CALCIFICATIONS

ICD-10CM #	K86.1	Other chronic pancreatitis
	K86.8	Other specified diseases of pancreas

Chronic pancreatitis.
Hyperparathyroidism.
Metastatic neoplasm.
Pseudocyst.
Hereditary pancreatitis.
Cystoadenoma.
Cystoadenocarcinoma.
Cavernous lymphangioma.
Hemorrhage.
Acute pancreatitis (saponification).

PANCREATIC CYSTIC LESIONS[48]

ICD-10CM #	K86.2	Cyst of pancreas
	K86.3	Pseudocyst of pancreas

Pseudocyst.
Serous cystadenoma.
Mucinous cystic neoplasm.
Intraductal papillary mucinous neoplasm.
Solid and papillary epithelial neoplasm.
True epithelial cyst.
Duodenal diverticulum.
Cystic neuroendocrine tumors.
Ductal adenocarcinoma with cystic degeneration.
Cystic metastases.
Cystic degeneration in sarcoma, hemangioma, and paraganglioma.

PANCREATIC SOLID LESIONS[48]

ICD-10CM #	C25.9	Malignant neoplasm of pancreas, unspecified
	D13.6	Benign neoplasm of pancreas

Neoplastic solid tumors.
Ductal adenocarcinoma.
Pancreatic neuroendocrine tumor.
Pancreatic lymphoma.
Metastases to the pancreas.
Solid pseudopapillary tumor.
Pancreaticoblastoma.
Acinar cell carcinoma.
Mesenchymal tumors (sarcoma, fibrous histio-cytoma, etc.).
Nonneoplastic solid lesions.
Focal chronic pancreatitis.
Autoimmune pancreatitis.
Groove pancreatitis.
Focal sparing of diffuse pancreatic fatty infiltration.
Intrapancreatic accessory spleen.
Developmental pancreas lobulation.
Sarcoidosis of the pancreas.

PANCREATITIS, ACUTE, IN CHILDREN[19]

ICD-10CM #	K85	Acute pancreatitis

CAUSES OF ACUTE PANCREATITIS IN CHILDREN

Drugs and Toxins
Acetaminophen overdose.
Alcohol.

L-Asparaginase.
Azathioprine.
Carbamazepine.
Cimetidine.
Corticosteroids.
Enalapril.
Erythromycin.
Estrogen.
Furosemide.
Isoniazid.
Lisinopril.
6-Mercaptopurine.
Methyldopa.
Metronidazole.
Organophosphate poisoning.
Pentamidine.
Retrovirals: DDC, DDI, tenofovir.
Sulfonamides: mesalamine, 5-aminosalicylates, sulfasalazine, trimethoprim/sulfamethoxazole.
Sulindac.
Tetracycline.
Thiazides.
Valproic acid.
Venom (spider, scorpion, Gila monster lizard).
Vincristine.
Genetic
Cationic trypsinogen gene (PRSS1).
Chymotrypsin C gene (CTRC).
Cystic fibrosis gene (CFTR).
Trypsin inhibitor gene (SPINK1).
Infectious
Ascariasis.
Coxsackie B virus.
Epstein-Barr virus.
Hepatitis A, B.
Influenza A, B.
Leptospirosis.
Malaria.
Measles.
Mumps.
Mycoplasma.
Reye syndrome: varicella, influenza B.
Rubella.
Rubeola.
Septic shock.
Obstructive
Ampullary disease.
Ascariasis.
Biliary tract malformations.
Choledochal cyst.
Choledochocele.
Cholelithiasis, microlithiasis, and choledocholi-thiasis (stones or sludge).
Duplication cyst.
Endoscopic retrograde cholangiopancreatogra-phy (ERCP) complication.
Pancreas divisum.
Pancreatic ductal abnormalities.
Postoperative.
Sphincter of Oddi dysfunction.
Tumor.
Systemic Disease
Autoimmune pancreatitis.
Brain tumor.
Collagen vascular diseases.
Crohn disease.
Diabetes mellitus.
Head trauma.
Hemochromatosis.

Hemolytic-uremic syndrome.
Hyperlipidemia: type I, IV, V.
Hyperparathyroidism/hypercalcemia.
Kawasaki disease.
Malnutrition.
Organic acidemia.
Peptic ulcer.
Periarteritis nodosa.
Renal failure.
Systemic lupus erythematosus.
Transplantation: bone marrow, heart, liver, kidney, pancreas.
Vasculitis.
Traumatic
Blunt injury.
Burns.
Child abuse.
Hypothermia.
Surgical trauma.
Total body cast.

PANCREATITIS, DRUG-INDUCED[43]

ICD-10CM #	K85.3	Drug induced acute pancreatitis

DEFINITE
Acetaminophen.
Azathioprine.
Cimetidine.
Cisplatin.
Corticosteroids.
Didanosine.
Erythromycin.
Estrogens.
Ethyl alcohol.
Furosemide.
L-Asparaginase.
Mercaptopurine.
Metronidazole.
Methyldopa.
Nitrofurantoin.
Octreotide.
Organophosphates.
Pentamidine.
Ranitidine.
Tetracycline.
Salicylates.
Sulfonamides, trimethoprim-sulfamethoxazole, sulfasalazine.
Sulindac.
Valproic acid.

POSSIBLE
Bumetanide.
Carbamazepine.
Chlorthalidone.
Clonidine.
Colchicine.
Cyclosporine.
Cytarabine.
Diazoxide.
Enalapril.
Ergotamine.
Ethacrynic acid.
Indomethacin.
Isoniazid.
Isotretinoin.

Mefenamic acid.
Opiates.
Phenformin.
Piroxicam.
Procainamide.
Rifampin.
Thiazides.

PANCYTOPENIA[31]

ICD-10CM #   D61.818   Other pancytopenia

PANCYTOPENIA WITH HYPOCELLULAR BONE MARROW

Acquired aplastic anemia.
Inherited aplastic anemia (Fanconi anemia and others).
Some myelodysplasia syndromes.
Rare aleukemic leukemia (acute myelogenous leukemia).
Some acute lymphoblastic leukemias.
Some lymphomas of bone marrow.

PANCYTOPENIA WITH CELLULAR BONE MARROW

Primary bone marrow diseases.
Myelodysplasia syndromes.
Paroxysmal nocturnal hemoglobinuria.
Myelofibrosis.
Some aleukemic leukemias.
Myelophthisis.
Bone marrow lymphoma.
Hairy cell leukemia.
Secondary to systemic diseases.
Systemic lupus erythematosus, Sjögren syndrome.
Hypersplenism.
Vitamin B$_{12}$, folate deficiency (familial defect).
Overwhelming infection.
Alcohol.
Brucellosis.
Ehrlichiosis.
Sarcoidosis.
Tuberculosis and atypical mycobacteria.

HYPOCELLULAR BONE MARROW ± CYTOPENIA

Q fever.
Legionnaires disease.
Mycobacteria.
Tuberculosis.*
Anorexia nervosa, starvation.
Hypothyroidism.

---

*Pancytopenia in tuberculosis only rarely is associated with a hypocellular bone marrow at biopsy or autopsy. Marrow failure in the setting of tuberculosis is almost always fatal; exceptional patients probably had underlying myelodysplasia or acute leukemia.

PANCYTOPENIA SYNDROME, INHERITED[19]

ICD-10CM #   D61.818   Other pancytopenia

Fanconi anemia.
Shwachman-Diamond syndrome.
Dyskeratosis congenita.
Congenital amegakaryocytic thrombocytopenia.
Unclassified inherited bone marrow failure syndromes.

Other genetic syndromes:
   Down syndrome.
   Dubowitz syndrome.
   Seckel syndrome.
   Reticular dysgenesis.
   Schimke immunoosseous dysplasia.
   Familial aplastic anemia (non-Fanconi).
   Cartilage-hair hypoplasia.
   Noonan syndrome.

PAPILLEDEMA

ICD-10CM #   H47.10   Unspecified papilledema

Central nervous system infections (viral, bacterial, fungal).
Medications (lithium, cisplatin, corticosteroids, tetracycline, etc.).
Head trauma.
Central nervous system neoplasm (primary or metastatic).
Pseudotumor cerebri.
Cavernous sinus thrombosis.
Systemic lupus erythematosus.
Sarcoidosis.
Subarachnoid hemorrhage.
Carbon dioxide retention.
Arnold-Chiari malformation and other developmental or congenital malformations.
Orbital lesions.
Central retinal vein occlusion.
Hypertensive encephalopathy.
Metabolic abnormalities.

PAPULOSQUAMOUS DISEASES[24]

ICD-10CM #   L98.8   Other specified disorders of the skin and subcutaneous tissue

Psoriasis.
Pityriasis rubra pilaris.
Pityriasis rosea.
Lichen planus.
Lichen nitidus.
Secondary syphilis.
Pityriasis lichenoides.
Parapsoriasis.
Mycosis fungoides.
Dermatophytosis.
Tinea versicolor.

PARALYSIS AND MUSCULAR RIGIDITY, DRUG-INDUCED[49]

ICD-10CM #   G83   Other paralytic syndromes
               R29.818   Other symptoms and signs involving the nervous system

SELECTED AGENTS ASSOCIATED WITH PARALYSIS AND MUSCULAR RIGIDITY

Paralysis
Medications and Industrial Toxins
Aminoglycoside antibiotics.
β-blockers.

Chloroquine (with color vision shift).
Cholinesterase inhibitors: neostigmine, pyridostigmine.
D-Penicillamine.
Pesticides: organophosphates, carbamates.
Pyrithioxine.
Trimethadione.
Biologic Toxins
Cobra venom.
Poison hemlock (Conium maculatum).
Scorpion fish (Scorpaenidae).
Snake venom, ticks, botulinum toxin.
Star of Bethlehem (Hippobroma longiflora).
Sweet pea (Lathyrus odoratus).
Tetrodotoxin (puffer fish, blue-ringed octopus, others).
Muscular Rigidity
Black widow spider venom (Latrodectus mactans).
Strychnine (Strychnos nux vomica, "slang nut").
Tetanus toxin.

PARALYTIC ILEUS[107]

ICD-10CM #   K56   Paralytic ileus and intestinal obstruction

CAUSES OF A PARALYTIC ILEUS

Peritonitis.
Surgery.
Trauma:
   Spine.
   Ribs.
   Hip.
Retroperitoneum.
Inflammation:
   Appendicitis.
   Pancreatitis.
   Cholecystitis.
   Salpingitis.
Congestive heart failure.
Pneumonia.
Renal colic.
Renal failure.
Leaking abdominal aortic aneurysm.
Low serum potassium.
Drugs (e.g., morphine).
Spinal lesions.
General debility or infection.
Vascular occlusion.

PARANASAL SINUS MALIGNANCIES[22]

ICD-10CM #   Code varies with specific diagnosis

EPITHELIAL MALIGNANCIES

Squamous cell carcinoma:
Verrucous carcinoma.
Papillary squamous cell carcinoma.
Basaloid squamous cell carcinoma.
Spindle cell carcinoma.
Adenosquamous carcinoma.
Acantholytic squamous cell carcinoma.
Lymphoepithelial carcinoma.
Sinonasal undifferentiated carcinoma.
Adenocarcinoma:
Intestinal-type adenocarcinoma.
Nonintestinal-type adenocarcinoma.
Salivary gland–type carcinomas:
Adenoid cystic carcinoma.
Acinic cell carcinoma.
Mucoepidermoid carcinoma.
Epithelial-myoepithelial carcinoma.
Clear cell carcinoma not otherwise specified.
Myoepithelial carcinoma.
Carcinoma ex pleomorphic adenoma.
Polymorphous low-grade adenocarcinoma.

Neuroendocrine tumors:
Typical carcinoid.
Atypical carcinoid.
Small cell carcinoma, neuroendocrine type.

SOFT TISSUE MALIGNANCIES

Fibrosarcoma.
Malignant fibrous histiocytoma.
Leiomyosarcoma.
Rhabdomyosarcoma.
Angiosarcoma.
Malignant peripheral nerve sheath tumor.

BONE AND CARTILAGE MALIGNANCIES

Chondrosarcoma.
Mesenchymal chondrosarcoma.
Osteosarcoma.
Chordoma.

HEMATOLYMPHOID MALIGNANCIES

Extranodal natural killer/T-cell lymphoma.
Diffuse large B-cell lymphoma.
Extramedullary plasmacytoma.
Extramedullary myeloid sarcoma.
Histiocytic sarcoma.
Langerhans cell histiocytosis.

NEUROECTODERMAL MALIGNANCIES

Ewing sarcoma.
Primitive neuroectodermal tumor.
Olfactory neuroblastoma.
Melanotic neuroectodermal tumor of infancy.
Mucosal malignant melanoma.

GERM CELL MALIGNANCIES

Teratoma with malignant transformation.
Sinonasal teratocarcinosarcoma.

PARANEOPLASTIC NEUROLOGIC SYNDROMES

ICD-10CM #	G13.0	Paraneoplastic neuromyopathy and neuropathy

Lambert-Eaton myasthenic syndrome.
Myasthenia gravis.
Guillain-Barré syndrome.
Amyotrophic lateral sclerosis.
Dermatomyositis.
Carcinoid myopathy.
Cerebellar degeneration.
Encephalomyelitis.
Optic neuritis, uveitis, retinopathy.
Stiff-man syndrome.
Autonomic neuropathy.
Brachial neuritis.
Sensory neuropathy.
Progressive multifocal leukoencephalopathy.

PARANEOPLASTIC SYNDROMES, ENDOCRINE[17]

ICD-10CM #	G13.0	Paraneoplastic neuromyopathy and neuropathy

Hypercalcemia.
Syndrome of inappropriate secretion of antidiuretic hormone.
Hypoglycemia.
Zollinger-Ellison syndrome.
Ectopic secretion of human chorionic gonadotropin.
Cushing syndrome.

PARANEOPLASTIC SYNDROMES, NONENDOCRINE[17]

ICD-10CM #	G13.0	Paraneoplastic neuromyopathy and neuropathy

CUTANEOUS

Dermatomyositis.
Acanthosis nigricans.
Sweet syndrome.
Erythema gyratum repens.
Systemic nodular panniculitis (Weber-Christian disease).

RENAL

Nephrotic syndrome.
Nephrogenic diabetes insipidus.

NEUROLOGIC

Subacute cerebellar degeneration.
Progressive multifocal leukoencephalopathy.
Subacute motor neuropathy.
Sensory neuropathy.
Ascending acute polyneuropathy (Guillain-Barré syndrome).
Myasthenic syndrome (Eaton-Lambert syndrome).

HEMATOLOGIC

Microangiopathic hemolytic anemia.
Migratory thrombophlebitis (Trousseau syndrome).
Anemia of chronic disease.

RHEUMATOLOGIC

Polymyalgia rheumatica.
Hypertrophic pulmonary osteoarthropathy.

PARAPARESIS[101]

ICD-10CM #	Varies with specific diagnosis

CAUSES

Inflammatory central nervous system diseases.
Multiple sclerosis.
Neuromyelitis optica.
Genetic disorders.
Spinal cerebellar ataxias.
Hereditary spastic paraparesis.
Infectious illnesses.
Human T-lymphotropic virus type 1 myelopathy.
Compressive lesions.
Cervical spondylosis.
Spinal meningiomas.
Metastatic tumors.

Neurodegenerative illnesses.
Amyotrophic lateral sclerosis.
Nutritional deficiencies.
Copper deficiency.
Vitamin B_{12} deficiency (combined system disease).

PARAPARESIS, ACUTE OR SUBACUTE[47]

ICD-10CM #	G82.2	Paraparesis

CAUSES OF ACUTE OR SUBACUTE PARAPARESIS

Trauma to a Previously Normal Spine
Vertebral Disease
Metastatic carcinoma.
Cervical spondylosis.
Dorsal disk prolapse.
Paget disease.
Rheumatoid arthritis.
Pott disease of spine.
Tumors
Extradural or intradural carcinoma, lymphoma, myeloma, leukemia.
Dorsal meningioma.
Neurofibroma.
Hematologic Disease
Any cause of thrombocytopenia.
Other clotting disorders.
Leukemia.
Anticoagulant treatment.
Epidural or intramedullary hemorrhage.
Infection
Epidural abscess.
TB abscess.
Syphilitic myelitis.
HIV infection.
Vascular myelopathy.
Vascular
Anterior spinal artery occlusion.
Infarction secondary to hypotension.
Embolic infarction.
Infarction secondary to aortic dissection.
Arteriovenous malformation: infarction or hemorrhage.
Primary intramedullary hemorrhage.
Vasculitis—polyarteritis nodosa (PAN).
Inflammatory
Myelitis of unknown cause.
Multiple sclerosis.
Systemic lupus erythematosus.
Sarcoidosis.
Metabolic
Subacute degeneration of the cord.

PARAPARESIS, CHRONIC PROGRESSIVE[47]

ICD-10CM #	G82.2	Paraparesis

CAUSES OF CHRONIC PROGRESSIVE PARAPARESIS

Vertebral Disease
Cervical spondylosis.
Dorsal disk prolapse.
Rheumatoid arthritis.
Pott disease of spine.
Ankylosing spondylitis.

Tumors
Meningioma.
Neurofibroma.
Glioma.
Ependymoma.
Chordoma.
Lipoma.
Syringomyelia
With Arnold-Chiari malformation.
With tumor.
Posttraumatic.
Infection
Tropical spastic paraparesis (HTLV-1 infection).
Syphilitic myelitis.
Vascular
Arteriovenous malformation.
Inflammatory
Multiple sclerosis.
Sarcoidosis.
Radiation myelopathy.
Arachnoiditis.
Metabolic
Subacute combined degeneration of the cord.
Paget disease.
Degenerative
Motor neuron disease.
Hereditary
Hereditary spastic paraplegia.

PARAPARESIS, PAINLESS[72]

ICD-10CM #	G82	Paraplegia (paraparesis) and quadriplegia (quadriparesis)

FREQUENTLY OCCURRING CAUSES OF PAINLESS PARAPARESIS

Inflammatory central nervous system diseases:
  Multiple sclerosis.
  Neuromyelitis optica.
Genetic disorders:
  Spinal cerebellar ataxias.
  Hereditary spastic paraparesis
Infectious illnesses:
  Human T-lymphotropic virus type 1 myelopathy.
Compressive lesions:*
  Cervical spondylosis.
  Spinal meningiomas.
  Metastatic tumors.
Neurodegenerative illnesses:
  amyotrophic lateral sclerosis.
Nutritional deficiencies:
  Copper deficiency.
  Vitamin B_{12} deficiency (combined system disease).

*Frequently presents with wrist drop.

PARAPLEGIA

ICD-10CM #	G82.20	Paraplegia, unspecified
	G80.1	Spastic diplegic cerebral palsy

I69.969	Other paralytic syndrome following unspecified cerebrovascular disease affecting unspecified side

Trauma: penetrating wounds to motor cortex, fracture-dislocation of vertebral column with compression of spinal cord or cauda equina, prolapsed disk, electrical injuries.
Neoplasm: parasagittal region, vertebrae, meninges, spinal cord, cauda equina, Hodgkin disease, NHL, leukemic deposits, pelvic neoplasms.
Multiple sclerosis and other demyelinating disorders.
Mechanical compression of spinal cord, cauda equina, or lumbosacral plexus: Paget disease, kyphoscoliosis, herniation of intervertebral disk, spondylosis, ankylosing spondylitis, rheumatoid arthritis, aortic aneurysm.
Infections: spinal abscess, syphilis, TB, poliomyelitis, leprosy.
Thrombosis of superior sagittal sinus.
Polyneuritis: Guillain-Barré syndrome, diabetes, alcohol, beriberi, heavy metals.
Heredofamilial muscular dystrophies.
Amyotrophic lateral sclerosis.
Congenital and familial conditions: syringomyelia, myelomeningocele, myelodysplasia.
Hysteria.

PARASELLAR MASSES[30]

ICD-10CM #	Varies with specific diagnosis

GENETIC
Transcription factor mutations (e.g., PROP1*).

CYSTS
Rathke.
Arachnoid.
Epidermoid.
Dermoid.

TUMORS
Hormone-secreting or nonfunctional pituitary adenoma.
Granular cell tumor.
Craniopharyngioma (cystic components).
Chordoma.
Meningioma.
Sarcoma.
Glioma.
Schwannoma.
Germ cell tumor.
Vascular tumor.
Solid or hematologic metastasis.

MALFORMATION AND HAMARTOMAS
Ectopic pituitary, neurohypophyseal, or salivary tissue.

*PROP1, prophet of Pit1 (pairedlike homeodomain transcription factor).

Hypothalamic hamartoma.
Gangliocytoma.

MISCELLANEOUS LESIONS
Aneurysms.
Hypophysitis.
Infections.
Sarcoidosis.
Giant cell granuloma.
Histiocytosis X.

PARESTHESIAS

ICD-10CM #	R20.2	Paresthesia of skin
	G54.8	Other nerve root and plexus disorders

Multiple sclerosis.
Nutritional deficiencies (thiamin, vitamin B_{12}, folic acid).
Compression of spinal cord or peripheral nerves.
Medications (e.g., INH, lithium, nitrofurantoin, gold, cisplatin, hydralazine, amitriptyline, sulfonamides, amiodarone, metronidazole, dapsone, disulfiram, chloramphenicol).
Toxic chemicals (e.g., lead, arsenic, cyanide, mercury, organophosphates).
Diabetes mellitus.
Myxedema.
Alcohol.
Sarcoidosis.
Neoplasms.
Infections (HIV, Lyme disease, herpes zoster, leprosy, diphtheria).
Charcot-Marie-Tooth syndrome and other hereditary neuropathies.
Guillain-Barré neuropathy.

PARKINSONISM[49]

ICD-10CM #	G20	Parkinson disease
	G21	Secondary parkinsonism
	G21.9	Secondary parkinsonism, unspecified
	G21.19	Other drug-induced Secondary parkinsonism
	G21.4	Vascular parkinsonism
	G21.2	Secondary parkinsonism due to other external agents

CAUSES OF PARKINSONISM
Static Injury/Structural Disorders
Basal ganglia infarcts.
Brain tumor.
Hydrocephalus.
Hereditary/Degenerative Disorders
Juvenile Parkinson disease.
Spinocerebellar ataxia.
Huntington disease (Westphal variant).
Pallidal-pyramidal disorder.
Neurodegeneration with brain iron accumulation (NBIA).

Pantothenate kinase-associated neurodegeneration (PKAN).

Rett syndrome.

Pelizaeus-Merzbacher disease.

Machado-Joseph disease (spinocerebellar ataxia type 3).

Neuronal ceroid lipofuscinoses.

Neuronal intranuclear inclusion body disease.

Metabolic Disorders

Dopa-responsive dystonia.

Tyrosine hydroxylase deficiency and other abnormalities of bioamine metabolism.

Abnormalities of folate metabolism.

Wilson disease.

Basal ganglia calcification (Fahr syndrome, hypoparathyroidism).

Infectious/Parainfectious Disorders

Encephalitis lethargica (Von Economo disease).

Autoimmune encephalitides, including anti-NMDA receptor associated encephalitis.

Viral encephalitis.

Acute demyelinating encephalomyelitis.

Drugs/Toxins

1-methyl-4-phenyl-1,2,3,6-tetrahydropyridine (MPTP) poisoning.

Rotenone.

Tetrabenazine.

Reserpine.

Methyldopa.

Sedatives.

Neuroleptics.

Antiemetics.

Calcium channel blockers.

Isoniazid.

Serotonin reuptake inhibitors (sertraline, fluoxetine).

Meperidine.

Disorders That Mimic Parkinsonism

Catatonia.

Spasticity.

Hypothyroidism.

Depression (with psychomotor retardation).

PARKINSONISM AND OTHER ACUTE EXTRAPYRAMIDAL REACTIONS, DRUG-INDUCED[49]

ICD-10CM #	G21.19	Other drug-induced secondary parkinsonism

SELECTED AGENTS ASSOCIATED WITH PARKINSONISM AND OTHER ACUTE EXTRAPYRAMIDAL REACTIONS

Medications

Amiodarone.

Anticholinergic agents: benztropine.

Antidepressants (including selective serotonin reuptake inhibitors).

Antiepileptic drugs.

Antifungal agents.

Antihistamines.

Antipsychotics and related drugs (including "novel" agents).

Bethanechol.

Bupropion (acute).

Buspirone.

Captopril (acute).

Clonazepam.

Diazoxide.

Digoxin (chorea).

Estrogen (chorea).

Heroin.

Ketamine.

L-dopa.

Lithium (chorea).

l-Methyl-4-phenyl-1,2,3,6,-tetrahydropyridine (MPTP).

Metronidazole (oculogyric crisis).

Ofloxacin (Tourette-like syndrome).

Opiates/opioids.

Reserpine.

Stimulants.

Sulfasalazine (chorea).

Vinblastine.

Industrial Toxins

Carbon monoxide.

Metals: manganese, thallium, aluminum.

Methanol.

Trichloroethylene.

Biologic Toxins

Arthrinium mycotoxin.

PARKINSONISM-PLUS SYNDROMES

ICD-10CM #	G21.8	Other secondary parkinsonism

Parkinson disease.

Shy-Drager syndrome.

Corticobasal degeneration.

Olivo-ponto-cerebellar atrophy.

Dementia with Lewy bodies.

Progressive supranuclear palsy.

Striatonigral degeneration.

PAROTID SWELLING[108]

ICD-10CM #	K11.20	Sialoadenitis, unspecified
	B26.9	Mumps without complication
	K11.8	Other diseases of salivary glands
	K11.5	Sialolithiasis
	K11.3	Abscess of salivary gland

INFECTIOUS

Mumps.

Parainfluenza.

Influenza.

Cytomegalovirus infection.

Coxsackievirus infection.

Lymphocytic choriomeningitis.

Echovirus infection.

Suppuration (bacterial).

Actinomyces infection.

Mycobacterial infection.

Cat-scratch disease.

NONINFECTIOUS

Drug hypersensitivity (thiouracil, phenothiazines, thiocyanate, iodides, copper, isoprenaline, lead, mercury, phenylbutazone).

Sarcoidosis.

Tumors, mixed.

Hemangioma, lymphangioma.

Sialectasis.

Sjögren syndrome.

Mikulicz syndrome (scleroderma, mixed connective tissue disease, systemic lupus erythematosus).

Recurrent idiopathic parotitis.

Pneumoparotitis.

Trauma.

Sialolithiasis.

Foreign body.

Cystic fibrosis.

Malnutrition (marasmus, alcohol cirrhosis).

Dehydration.

Diabetes mellitus.

Waldenström macroglobulinemia.

Reiter syndrome (reactive arthritis).

Amyloidosis.

NONPAROTID SWELLING

Hypertrophy of masseter muscle.

Lymphadenopathy.

Rheumatoid mandibular joint swelling.

Tumors of jaw.

Infantile cortical hyperostosis.

PELVIC AVULSION FRACTURES[52]

ICD-10CM #	M84.350A	Stress fracture pelvis, initial encounter
	M84.454A	Pathological fracture pelvis, initial encounter

ACUTE AVULSION FRACTURE

Nontraumatic avulsion fracture:	Bone metastasis, prior graft harvesting.
Soft tissue injury:	Tendon tear, muscle strain.
Aggressive-looking appearance:	Osteomyelitis, tumor.
Incidental normal variant:	Accessory bone.

CHRONIC AVULSION FRACTURE

Apophyseal avulsion injury:	Apophysitis, traction periostitis.
Soft tissue injury:	Bursitis, degenerative tendinopathy, calcific tendinitis.

PELVIC MASS

ICD-10CM #	R19.09	Other intraabdominal and pelvic swelling, mass and lump

Hemorrhagic ovarian cyst.

Simple ovarian cyst (follicle or corpus luteum).

Ovarian carcinoma, carcinoma of fallopian tube, colorectal carcinoma, metastatic carcinoma, prostate carcinoma, bladder carcinoma, lymphoma, Hodgkin disease.

Cystadenoma, teratoma, endometrioma.

Leiomyoma.

Leiomyosarcoma.

Diverticulitis, diverticular abscess.
Appendiceal abscess, tuboovarian abscess.
Ectopic pregnancy, intrauterine pregnancy.
Paraovarian cyst.
Hydrosalpinx.

PELVIC PAIN, CAUSES IN WOMEN[43]

ICD-10CM #	N94	Pain and other conditions associated with female genital organs and menstrual cycle
	G10.2	Pelvic and perineal pain
	G89.4	Chronic pain syndrome

POTENTIAL CAUSES OF PELVIC PAIN IN WOMEN

Reproductive Tract
Ovarian torsion.
Ovarian cyst.
Salpingitis/tuboovarian abscess.
Septic pelvic thrombophlebitis.
Endometritis.
Endometriosis.
Uterine perforation.
Uterine fibroids.
Dysmenorrhea.

Pregnancy-related
First Trimester
Ectopic pregnancy.
Threatened abortion.
Nonviable pregnancy.
Ovarian hyperstimulation syndrome.

Second and Third Trimesters
Placenta previa.
Placental abruption.
Round ligament pain.

Intestinal Tract
Appendicitis.
Diverticulitis.
Ischemic bowel.
Perforated viscus.
Bowel obstruction.
Incarcerated/strangulated hernia.
Inflammatory bowel disease.
Gastroenteritis.

Urinary Tract
Pyelonephritis.
Cystitis.
Ureteral stone.

PELVIC PAIN, CHRONIC[93]

ICD-10CM #	N94.89	Other specified conditions associated with female genital organs and menstrual cycle
	R10.2	Pelvic and perineal pain
	R10.10	Upper abdominal pain, unspecified
	R10.2	Pelvic and perineal pain
	R10.30	Lower abdominal pain, unspecified

GYNECOLOGIC DISORDERS

Primary dysmenorrhea.
Endometriosis.
Adenomyosis.
Adhesions.
Fibroids.
Retained ovary syndrome after hysterectomy.
Previous tubal ligation.
Chronic pelvic infection.

MUSCULOSKELETAL DISORDERS

Myofascial pain syndrome.

GI DISORDERS

Irritable bowel syndrome.
Inflammatory bowel disease.

URINARY TRACT DISORDERS

Interstitial cystitis.
Nonbacterial urethritis.

PELVIC PAIN, CYCLIC AND ACYCLIC[12]

ICD-10CM #	R10.10	Abdominal and pelvic pain

CAUSES OF CYCLIC AND ACYCLIC PELVIC PAIN

Cyclic
Mittelschmerz.
Endometriosis.*
Adenomyosis.
Cervical stenosis.*
Leiomyoma (fibroid).
Primary dysmenorrhea.

Acyclic
Chronic PID.
Pelvic adhesions.
Uterine prolapse.
Chronic urethritis.
Diverticulitis.
Irritable bowel syndrome.
Levator syndrome.
Detrusor instability.
Interstitial cystitis.
Abdominal hernia.
Abdominal wall myofascial pain.
Abuse syndromes: physical and sexual.
Depression.

*May become acyclic.
PID, Pelvic inflammatory disease.

PELVIC PAIN, GENITAL ORIGIN[1]

ICD-10CM #	N94.89	Other specified conditions associated with female genital organs and menstrual cycle
	R10.2	Pelvic and perineal pain
	R10.10	Upper abdominal pain, unspecified
	R10.2	Pelvic and perineal pain
	R10.30	Lower abdominal pain, unspecified

PERITONEAL IRRITATION

Ruptured ectopic pregnancy.
Ovarian cyst rupture.
Ruptured tuboovarian abscess.
Uterine perforation.

TORSION

Ovarian cyst or tumor.
Pedunculated fibroid.

INTRATUMOR HEMORRHAGE OR INFARCTION

Ovarian cyst.
Solid ovarian tumor.
Uterine leiomyoma.

INFECTION

Endometritis.
Pelvic inflammatory disease.
Trichomonas cervicitis or vaginitis.
Tuboovarian abscess.

PREGNANCY-RELATED

First Trimester
Ectopic pregnancy.
Abortion.
Corpus luteum hematoma.
Late Pregnancy
Placental problems.
Preeclampsia.
Premature labor.

MISCELLANEOUS

Endometriosis.
Foreign objects.
Pelvic adhesions.
Pelvic neoplasm.
Primary dysmenorrhea.

PELVIC PAIN, NONPREGNANT FEMALE[29]

ICD-10CM #	N94.89	Other specified conditions associated with female genital organs and menstrual cycle
	R10.2	Pelvic and perineal pain
	R10.10	Upper abdominal pain, unspecified
	R10.30	Lower abdominal pain, unspecified

DIFFERENTIAL DIAGNOSIS OF PELVIC PAIN IN NONPREGNANT FEMALES

Gynecologic Diagnoses
Infectious:
    Vaginitis.
    Cervicitis.
    Endometritis.
    Tuboovarian abscess.
    Pelvic inflammatory disease.
Ovarian:
    Ovarian torsion.
    Ruptured ovarian cyst.
    Ovarian tumor.

Degenerating ovarian tumor.
Mittelschmerz.
Cervical:
Cervical polyps.
Cervical stenosis.
Cervical cancer.
Uterine:
Uterine fibroids.
Degenerating uterine fibroids.
Adenomyosis.
Endometrial carcinoma.
Extrauterine:
Endometriosis.
Adhesions.
Residual accessory ovary.
Nongynecologic Diagnoses
GI:
Acute appendicitis.
Mesenteric lymphadenitis.
Diverticulitis.
Inflammatory bowel disease.
Irritable bowel syndrome.
Bowel obstruction.
Intraabdominal abscess.
Colorectal carcinoma.
Urinary:
Cystitis.
Renal colic.
Bladder cancer.
Musculoskeletal:
Abdominal wall pain.
Lumbar back pain.
Fibromyalgia.
Muscular strain.
Piriformis syndrome.
Neurologic:
Lumbar radiculopathy.
Shingles.
Spondylosis.
Psychologic:
Personality disorders.
Major depressive disorder.

PENILE RASH

ICD-10CM #	R21	Rash and other nonspecific skin eruption

Herpes simplex 2.
Balanitis (*Candida*).
Condyloma acuminatum.
Molluscum contagiosum.
Scabies.
Pediculosis pubis.
Pearly penile papules.
Lichen nitidus.
Fox-Fordyce disease (follicular papules).
Trauma.

PERIANAL PAIN[2]

ICD-10CM #	K62.89	Other specified diseases of anus and rectum

Fissure-in-ano.
Anal sepsis:
Anal abscess.
Anal fistula.

Hemorrhoids:
Internal hemorrhoids.
External hemorrhoids.
Pruritus ani.
Proctalgia fugax.
Chronic perianal pain syndromes:
Coccygodynia.
Descending perineum syndrome.
Levator ani syndrome.
Idiopathic perineal pain.

PERICARDIAL EFFUSION

ICD-10CM #	I30.9	Acute pericarditis, unspecified
	I31.3	Pericardial effusion

Pericarditis.
Uremia.
Myxedema.
Neoplasm (leukemia, lymphoma, metastatic).
Hemorrhage (trauma, leakage of thoracic aneurysm).
Systemic lupus erythematosus, rheumatoid disease.
Myocardial infarction.

PERIPHERAL ARTERIAL DISEASE, NONATHEROSCLEROTIC CAUSES[71]

ICD-10CM #	I73.9	Peripheral vascular disease, unspecified
	I73.8	Other specified peripheral vascular diseases
	I79.8	Other disorders of arteries, arterioles, and capillaries in diseases classified elsewhere

NONATHEROSCLEROTIC CAUSES OF PERIPHERAL ARTERY DISEASE

Thromboembolism.
Atheroembolism.
Vasculitides:
Large vessel vasculitides, such as giant cell arteritis and Takayasu arteritis.
Small vessel vasculitides, such as thromboangiitis obliterans (Buerger disease).
Trauma.
Popliteal artery entrapment.
Cystic adventitial disease.
Fibromuscular dysplasia.
Iliac artery endofibrosis.

PERIPHERAL INFLAMMATORY ARTHRITIS[53]

ICD-10CM #		Code varies with specific diagnosis

DIFFERENTIAL DIAGNOSIS FOR PATIENTS WITH A NEW ONSET OF PERIPHERAL INFLAMMATORY ARTHRITIS

Crystal arthritis (e.g., gout, pseudogout).
Inflammatory osteoarthritis.
Rheumatoid arthritis.
Psoriatic arthritis.
Other spondyloarthropathy.
Systemic lupus erythematosus.
Other connective tissue diseases/vasculitis.
Postinfective arthritis (e.g., reactive arthritis, postviral arthritis).
Sarcoidosis.
Malignancy-associated arthritis.
RS3PE.
Septic arthritis.
Other.

RS3PE, Remitting seronegative symmetrical synovitis with pitting edema.

PERIODIC PARALYSIS, HYPERKALEMIC

ICD-10CM #	G83.9	Paralytic syndrome, unspecified

Chronic renal failure.
Renal insufficiency with excessive potassium supplementation.
Potassium-sparing diuretics.
Endocrinopathies (hypoaldosteronism, adrenal insufficiency).

PERIODIC PARALYSIS, HYPOKALEMIC

ICD-10CM #	G83.9	Paralytic syndrome, unspecified

Chronic diarrhea (laxative abuse, sprue, villous adenoma).
Potassium-depleting diuretics.
Medications (amphotericin B, corticosteroids).
Chronic licorice ingestion.
Thyrotoxicosis.
Renal tubular acidosis.
Conn syndrome.
Bartter syndrome.
Barium intoxication.

PERITONEAL CARCINOMATOSIS[24]

ICD-10CM #	C78.6	Secondary malignant neoplasm of retroperitoneum and peritoneum

PRIMARY DISORDERS OF THE PERITONEUM: MESOTHELIOMA

Metastatic spread from:
Stomach.
Colon.
Pancreas.
Carcinoid.
Other Intraabdominal Organs
Ovary.
Pseudomyxoma peritonei.

Differential Diagnosis

II

Extraabdominal Primary Tumors
Breast.
Lung.
Hematologic Malignancy
Lymphoma.

PERITONEAL EFFUSION[109]

ICD-10CM #	R18	Ascites
	R85.9	Unspecified abnormal finding in specimens from digestive organs and abdominal cavity
	R88.8	Abnormal findings in other body fluids and substances

TRANSUDATES

Increased hydrostatic pressure or decreased plasma oncotic pressure.
Congestive heart failure.
Hepatic cirrhosis.
Hypoproteinemia.

EXUDATES

Increased capillary permeability or decreased lymphatic resorption.
Infections (TB, spontaneous bacterial peritonitis, secondary bacterial peritonitis).
Neoplasms (hepatoma, metastatic carcinoma, lymphoma, mesothelioma).
Trauma.
Pancreatitis.
Bile peritonitis (e.g., ruptured gallbladder).

CHYLOUS EFFUSION

Damage or obstruction to thoracic duct.
Trauma.
Lymphoma.
Carcinoma.
Tuberculosis.
Parasitic infection.

PERIUMBILICAL SWELLING

ICD-10CM #	R19.00	Intraabdominal and pelvic swelling, mass and lump, unspecified site

Umbilical hernia.
Lipoma.
Epigastric hernia.
Umbilical granuloma.
Omphalocele.
Gastroschisis.
Caput medusae.

PHARYNGEAL OBSTRUCTION, CAUSES[13]

ICD-10CM #	Varies with specific diagnosis

CAUSES OF PHARYNGEAL OBSTRUCTION

Malignant or benign tumors (e.g., papillomas, polyps).
Infection (e.g., croup, epiglottitis, tonsillar abscess).

Edema or hypertrophy (e.g., angioneurotic edema, anaphylactic reactions, postradiation therapy, obstructive sleep apnea).
Trauma (e.g., cricoid fracture, cervical subluxation, precervical hematoma).
Burn injury.
Extrinsic compression (e.g., goiter or pregnancy-related thyroid enlargement).
Foreign body.
Congenital web (infants).
Sarcoidosis and other granulomatous diseases.
Amyloid.

PHEOCHROMOCYTOMA-TYPE SPELLS[30]

ICD-10CM #	I15.2	Hypertension due to pheochromocytoma

DIFFERENTIAL DIAGNOSIS OF PHEOCHROMOCYTOMA-TYPE SPELLS

Endocrine Causes
Carbohydrate intolerance.
Hyperadrenergic spells.
Hypoglycemia.
Pancreatic tumors (e.g., insulinoma).
Pheochromocytoma.
Primary hypogonadism (menopausal syndrome).
Thyrotoxicosis.
Cardiovascular Causes
Angina.
Cardiovascular deconditioning.
Labile essential hypertension.
Orthostatic hypotension.
Paroxysmal cardiac arrhythmia.
Pulmonary edema.
Renovascular disease.
Syncope (e.g., vasovagal reaction).
Psychologic Causes
Factitious (e.g., drugs, Valsalva).
Hyperventilation.
Severe anxiety and panic disorders.
Somatization disorder.
Pharmacologic Causes
Chlorpropamide-alcohol flush.
Combination of a monoamine oxidase inhibitor and a decongestant.
Illegal drug ingestion (cocaine, phencyclidine, lysergic acid diethylamide).
Sympathomimetic drug ingestion.
Vancomycin ("red man syndrome").
Withdrawal of adrenergic-inhibitor.
Neurologic Causes
Autonomic neuropathy.
Cerebrovascular insufficiency.
Diencephalic epilepsy (autonomic seizures).
Migraine headache.
Postural orthostatic tachycardia syndrome.
Stroke.
Other Causes
Carcinoid syndrome:
  Mast cell disease.
  Recurrent idiopathic anaphylaxis.
  Unexplained flushing spells.

PHOTODERMATOSES[24]

ICD-10CM #	L56.0	Drug phototoxic response
	L56.1	Drug photoallergic response
	L56.2	Photocontact dermatitis [berloque dermatitis]

Polymorphous light eruption.
Chronic actinic dermatitis.
Solar urticaria.
Phototoxicity and photoallergy.
Porphyrias.

PHOTOSENSITIVITY

ICD-10CM #	L56.0	Drug phototoxic response
	L56.1	Drug photoallergic response
	L56.2	Photocontact dermatitis [berloque dermatitis]

Solar urticaria.
Photoallergic reaction.
Phototoxic reaction.
Polymorphous light eruption.
Porphyria cutanea tarda.
Systemic lupus erythematosus.
Drug induced (e.g., tetracyclines).

PIGMENTURIA[43]

ICD-10CM #	R82	Other abnormal findings in urine

HEMOGLOBINURIA

Hemolysis.

HEMATURIA

Renal causes.
Trauma.

ACUTE INTERMITTENT PORPHYRIA

Bilirubinuria
Food
Beets.
Drugs
Vitamin B_{12}.
Rifampin.
Phenytoin.
Laxatives.

PITUITARY INSUFFICIENCY, ACQUIRED[36]

ICD-10CM #	E23.0	Hypopituitarism
	E89.3	Postprocedural hypopituitarism
	E23.1	Drug-induced hypopituitarism

CAUSES OF ACQUIRED PITUITARY INSUFFICIENCY

Traumatic
Surgical resection.
Radiation damage.
Traumatic brain injury.

Infiltrative/Inflammatory
Primary Hypophysitis
Lymphocytic.
Granulomatous.
Xanthomatous.
Secondary Hypophysitis
Sarcoidosis.
Histiocytosis X.
Infections.
Wegener granulomatosis.
Takayasu disease.
Hemochromatosis.

Infections
Tuberculosis.
Pneumocystis jirovecii infection.
Fungal (histoplasmosis, aspergillosis).
Parasites (toxoplasmosis).
Viral (cytomegalovirus).

Vascular
Pregnancy related.
Aneurysm.
Apoplexy.
Diabetes.
Hypotension.
Arteritis.
Sickle cell disease.

Neoplastic
Pituitary adenoma.
Parasellar mass:
Rathke cyst.
Dermoid cyst.
Meningioma.
Germinoma.
Ependymoma.
Glioma.
Craniopharyngioma.
Hypothalamic hamartoma, gangliocytoma.
Pituitary metastatic deposits.
Hematologic malignancy:
Leukemia.
Lymphoma.

PITUITARY REGION TUMORS[21]

ICD-10CM #	Varies with specific diagnosis

PRIMARY TUMORS IN THE SELLAR AND PARASELLAR REGION
Pituitary macroadenoma.
Meningioma.
Schwannoma (e.g., of fifth nerve).
Chordoma.
Chondrosarcoma.
Craniopharyngioma.
Rathke cleft cyst.
Dermoid.
Epidermoid.
Tuber cinereum hamartoma.
Optic glioma.
Germ cell tumors.

PLATELET DYSFUNCTION, DRUG-INDUCED[71]

ICD-10CM #	D69.1	Qualitative platelet defects

Antiplatelet Drugs
COX inhibitors: aspirin.
ADP receptor antagonists:
Thienopyridines: clopidogrel, ticlopidine, prasugrel.
Nonthienopyridines: ticagrelor, cangrelor.
$\alpha_{IIb}\beta_3$ inhibitors: abciximab, eptifibatide, tirofiban.
PDE inhibitors:
Nonselective PDE inhibitors: pentoxifylline, caffeine, theophylline.
PDE3 inhibitors: cilostazol, milrinone, anagrelide.
PDE5 inhibitors: dipyridamole, sildenafil.
Adenyl cyclase stimulators: epoprostenol, iloprost, beraprost.
Drugs that adversely affect platelet function.
NSAIDs: ibuprofen, naproxen, indomethacin.
Cardiovascular agents:
Calcium channel blockers: nifedipine, diltiazem, verapamil.
β-Blockers: propranolol.
Vasodilators: nitrates, nitroprusside.
Diuretics: furosemide.
Angiotensin II receptor antagonist: losartan, valsartan, and olmesartan.
Antibiotics: β-lactams, amphotericin, hydroxychloroquine, nitrofurantoin.
Antifungal drugs: Miconazole, amphotericin B:
Psychiatric drugs: TCAs, fluoxetine, chlorpromazine, promethazine, trifluoperazine.
Oncologic drugs: mithramycin, daunorubicin, BCNU, asparaginase, vincristine, dasatinib, ibrutinib.
Anesthetics: dibucaine, procaine, halothane, sevoflurane, propofol.
Plasma expanders: dextran, hydroxyl ethyl starch.
Heparins and thrombolytic agents.
Miscellaneous: clofibrate, statins, cocaine, ketanserin, radiographic contrast agents, antihistamines, immunosuppressive drugs.

ADP, Adenosine diphosphate; *BCNU*, carmustine; *COX*, cyclooxygenase; *NSAID*, nonsteroidal antiinflammatory drug; *PDE*, phosphodiesterase; *TCA*, tricyclic antidepressant.

PLEURAL EFFUSIONS

ICD-10CM #	J91.8	Pleural effusion in other conditions classified elsewhere

EXUDATIVE
Neoplasm: bronchogenic carcinoma, breast carcinoma, mesothelioma, lymphoma, ovarian carcinoma, multiple myeloma, leukemia, Meigs syndrome.
Infections: viral pneumonia, bacterial pneumonia, *Mycoplasma*, TB, fungal and parasitic diseases, extension from subphrenic abscess.
Trauma.
Collagen vascular diseases: systemic lupus erythematosus, rheumatoid arthritis, scleroderma, polyarteritis, granulomatosis with polyangiitis.
Pulmonary infarction.
Pancreatitis.
Postcardiotomy/Dressler syndrome.
Drug-induced systemic lupus erythematosus (hydralazine, procainamide).
Postabdominal surgery.
Ruptured esophagus.
Chronic effusion secondary to congestive failure.

TRANSUDATIVE
Congestive heart failure.
Hepatic cirrhosis.
Nephrotic syndrome.
Hypoproteinemia from any cause.
Meigs syndrome.

PLEURAL EFFUSIONS, MALIGNANCY-ASSOCIATED

ICD-10CM #	C78.2	Secondary malignant neoplasm of pleura

Lung cancer	(30%-40%)
Breast cancer	(20%-25%)
Lymphoma	(10%-15%)
Leukemia	(5%-10%)
GI tract	(5%)
GU tract	(5%)
Reproductive	(3%)

PLEURAL HYPERPLASIA[78]

ICD-10CM #	Varies with specific diagnosis

BENIGN CAUSES OF PLEURAL HYPERPLASIA
Pleural infections.
Radiation.
Surgery.
Trauma.
Intracavitary treatments (chemotherapy or sclerosing agents).
Collagen vascular diseases.
Systemic immune diseases (systemic lupus erythematosus, rheumatoid arthritis, Sjögren syndrome, Wegener granulomatosis).
Subpleural pulmonary abnormalities (infarction, infection, neoplasia).
Pneumothorax.
Drug reactions (nitrofurantoin, bromocriptine, methysergide, procarbazine).
Pancreatitis, uremia.
Pneumoconiosis (asbestosis).

PLEURAL MASSES[78]

ICD-10CM #	Varies with specific diagnosis

CAUSES OF PLEURAL MASSES
Inflammatory pleural reactions:
Reactive mesothelial hyperplasia or organizing pleuritis vs. atypical mesothelial hyperplasia.
Nodular pleural plaques.

Pulmonary tumors that may resemble pleural tumors:
  Inflammatory pseudotumor of the lung.
Benign pleural tumors:
  Solitary fibrous tumor.
  Lipomas and lipoblastomas.
  Adenomatous tumors.
  Calcifying fibrous tumors.
  Mesothelial cysts.
  Multicystic mesothelioma.
  Schwannoma.
Pleural tumors with low malignant potential:
  Desmoid tumors.
  Well-differentiated papillary mesothelioma.
  Pleural thymoma.
Primary malignant pleural tumors that may look like benign tumors:
  Malignant solitary fibrous tumor.
  Pleuropulmonary blastoma.
  Localized malignant mesothelioma.
  Vascular sarcoma.
  Liposarcoma.
  Pleuropulmonary synovial sarcoma.
  Askin tumor or primitive neuroectodermal tumor (PNET).
  Desmoplastic small round cell tumor.
Malignant pleural tumors:
  Metastatic malignancies to the pleura.
  Malignant mesothelioma.

PNEUMATOSIS INTESTINALIS IN NEONATE AND OLDER CHILD[21]

ICD-10CM #   Varies with specific diagnosis

CAUSES OF PNEUMATOSIS INTESTINALIS IN THE NEONATE AND THE OLDER CHILD

Necrotizing enterocolitis.
Bowel ischemia, inflammation, and obstruction.
Cyanotic congenital heart disease.
Hirschsprung disease.
Gastroschisis.
Anorectal atresia.
Inflammatory bowel disease.
Lymphoma.
Leukemia.
CMV and rotavirus gastroenteritis.
Colonoscopy.
Caustic ingestion.
Short bowel syndrome.
Congenital immune deficiency states.
Clostridium infection.
Chronic steroid use.
Posthepatic, renal, or bone marrow transplant.
Collagen vascular disease.
Graft-versus-host disease.
AIDS.

PNEUMONIA, CHRONIC[42]

ICD-10CM #	J15.9	Unspecified bacterial pneumonia
	J12.9	Viral pneumonia, unspecified
	B25.0	Cytomegaloviral pneumonitis
	J18.0	Bronchopneumonia, unspecified organism

INFECTIOUS AGENTS THAT TYPICALLY CAUSE CHRONIC PNEUMONIA

Bacteria
Mixed aerobic and anaerobic bacteria.
Actinomyces spp.
Nocardia spp.
Rhodococcus equi.
Burkholderia pseudomallei.
Mycobacteria
Mycobacterium tuberculosis.
Mycobacterium kansasii.
Mycobacterium avium complex.
Mycobacterium abscessus.
Mycobacterium terrae.
Fungi
Aspergillus spp.
Blastomyces dermatitidis.
Coccidioides spp.
Cryptococcus neoformans.
Cryptococcus gattii.
Dark-walled molds.
Emmonsia parvum var. crescens.
Histoplasma capsulatum.
Sporothrix schenckii complex.
Paracoccidioides brasiliensis.
Penicillium marneffei.
Scedosporium apiospermum.
Parasites
Dirofilaria:
  Echinococcus granulosus.
  Filaria (tropical pulmonary eosinophilia).
  Paragonimus westermani.

NONINFECTIOUS CAUSES OF CHRONIC PNEUMONIA

Neoplasia
Carcinoma (primary or metastatic).
Hodgkin disease and non-Hodgkin lymphoma.
Other lymphoproliferative disorders.
Cystic Fibrosis
Sarcoidosis
Amyloidosis
Vasculitis (autoimmune diseases)
Systemic lupus erythematosus.
Polyarteritis nodosa.
Granulomatosis with polyangiitis.
Allergic angiitis and granulomatosis (Churg-Strauss syndrome).
Goodpasture syndrome.
Microscopic polyangiitis.
Lymphomatoid granulomatosis.
Progressive systemic sclerosis.
Rheumatoid arthritis.
Mixed connective tissue syndrome (overlap syndrome).
Chemicals, Drugs
Radiation
Recurrent pulmonary emboli
Bronchial obstruction with atelectasis (e.g., tumor, foreign body)
Pulmonary sequestration
Pulmonary infiltration with eosinophilia syndrome (Löffler syndrome—usually transient.)
Pneumonia plus asthma (e.g., allergic bronchopulmonary aspergillosis).
Bronchocentric granulomatosis.
Chronic eosinophilic pneumonia.

Pneumoconiosis
Asbestosis.
Berylliosis.
Silicosis.
Anthracosilicosis.

OTHER LUNG DISEASES: CAUSE UNKNOWN

Chronic Organizing Pneumonia
Chronic Interstitial Pneumonia (Fibrosing Alveolitis, Idiopathic Pulmonary Fibrosis)
Usual interstitial pneumonia (UIP).
Desquamative interstitial pneumonia (DIP).
Lymphocytic interstitial pneumonia (LIP).
Giant cell interstitial pneumonia (GIP).
Eosinophilic granuloma (histiocytosis X).
Lymphangioleiomyomatosis.
Pulmonary alveolar proteinosis.
Pulmonary alveolar microlithiasis.
Idiopathic pulmonary hemosiderosis.
Angiocentric immunoproliferative lesions.

PNEUMONIA MIMICS[110]

ICD-10CM #   Varies with specific diagnosis

NONINFECTIOUS CAUSES THAT MAY PRESENT AS PNEUMONIA

Radiologic Technique
Inadequate inspiration.
Breast shadow.
Thymus.
Uneven grid on film.
Underpenetrated film.
Primary Pulmonary
Asthma.
Bronchiectasis.
Atelectasis.
Bronchopulmonary dysplasia.
Cystic fibrosis.
Pulmonary sequestration.
Congenital cystic adenomatoid malformation.
α_1-Antitrypsin deficiency.
Aspiration
Foreign body.
Chemical.
Recurrent caused by anatomic or physiologic disorders.
Primary Cardiac
Congenital heart disease.
Congestive heart failure.
Pulmonary Infarction
Sickle cell vasoocclusive crisis.
Pulmonary embolism.
Collagen Vascular Disorders
Acute Respiratory Distress Syndrome
Pleural effusion
Neoplasm.

PNEUMONIA, NONRESPONDING, CAUSES[13]

ICD-10CM #	J15.9	Unspecified bacterial pneumonia
	J12.9	Viral pneumonia, unspecified
	B25.0	Cytomegaloviral pneumonitis
	J18.0	Bronchopneumonia, unspecified organism

CAUSES OF NONRESPONDING PNEUMONIA

Infectious Pneumonia

Resistant microorganisms:

Community-acquired pneumonia (e.g., Streptococcus pneumoniae, Staphylococcus aureus).

Nosocomial pneumonia (e.g., Acinetobacter, methicillin-resistant Staphylococcus aureus (MRSA), Pseudomonas aeruginosa).

Uncommon microorganisms (e.g., *Mycobacterium tuberculosis, Nocardia* spp., fungi, *Pneumocystis jirovecii*).

Complications of pneumonia:

Empyema.

Abscess or necrotizing pneumonia.

Metastatic infection.

Noninfectious Pneumonia

Neoplasms.

Pulmonary hemorrhage.

Pulmonary embolism.

Sarcoidosis.

Eosinophilic pneumonia.

Pulmonary edema.

Acute respiratory distress syndrome.

Bronchiolitis obliterans with organizing pneumonia.

Drug-induced pulmonary disease.

Pulmonary vasculitis.

PNEUMONIA, RECURRENT

ICD-10CM #	J15.9	Unspecified bacterial pneumonia
	J12.9	Viral pneumonia, unspecified
	B25.0	Cytomegaloviral pneumonitis
	J18.0	Bronchopneumonia, unspecified organism

Mechanical obstruction from neoplasm.

Chronic aspiration (tube feeding, alcoholism, cerebrovascular accident, neuromuscular disorders, seizure disorder, inability to cough).

Bronchiectasis.

Kyphoscoliosis.

Chronic obstructive pulmonary disease, congestive heart failure, asthma, silicosis, pulmonary fibrosis, cystic fibrosis.

Pulmonary TB, chronic sinusitis.

Immunosuppression (HIV, corticosteroids, leukemia, chemotherapy, splenectomy).

PNEUMOPERITONEUM, NEONATAL[21]

| ICD-10CM # | Varies with specific diagnosis |

CAUSES OF NEONATAL PNEUMOPERITONEUM

Necrotizing enterocolitis.

Spontaneous perforation of a hollow viscus:

Stomach.

Duodenum.

Ileum.

Colon.

Malrotation and volvulus.

Distal obstruction.

Perforation of Meckel diverticulum.

Anterior abdominal wall defects:

Pentalogy of Cantrell.

Omphalocele.

Gastroschisis.

Cloacal exstrophy.

Stress and peptic ulcers.

Mechanical ventilation (air leak) or resuscitation ("bagging").

Postlaparotomy.

Iatrogenic gastric perforation with an orogastric tube.

Iatrogenic colon perforation:

Thermometer.

During an enema.

Indomethacin.

Dexamethasone treatment.

PNEUMOTHORAX, IN CHILDREN[19]

ICD-10CM #	J93.0	Spontaneous tension pneumothorax
	J93	Pneumothorax
	J93.9	Pneumothorax unspecified

SPONTANEOUS

Primary idiopathic—usually resulting from ruptured subpleural blebs.

Secondary blebs.

Congenital lung disease:

Congenital cystic adenomatoid malformation.

Bronchogenic cysts.

Pulmonary hypoplasia.

Conditions associated with increased intrathoracic pressure:

Asthma.

Bronchiolitis.

Air-block syndrome in neonates.

Cystic fibrosis.

Airway foreign body.

Infection:

Pneumatocele.

Lung abscess.

Bronchopleural fistula.

Diffuse lung disease:

Langerhans cell histiocytosis.

Tuberous sclerosis.

Marfan syndrome.

Ehlers-Danlos syndrome.

Metastatic neoplasm—usually osteosarcoma (rare).

TRAUMATIC

Noniatrogenic:

Penetrating trauma.

Blunt trauma.

Loud music (air pressure).

Iatrogenic:

Thoracotomy.

Thoracoscopy, thoracentesis.

Tracheostomy.

Tube or needle puncture.

Mechanical ventilation.

POLIOSIS[44]

| ICD-10CM # | Varies with specific diagnosis |

CAUSES OF POLIOSIS

Ocular

Chronic anterior blepharitis.

Sympathetic ophthalmitis.

Idiopathic uveitis.

Systemic

Vogt-Koyanagi-Harada syndrome.

Waardenburg syndrome.

Vitiligo.

Marfan syndrome.

Tuberous sclerosis.

POLYCYTHEMIA

| ICD-10CM # | D45 | Polycythemia primary |
| | D75.1 | Polycythemia secondary |

Tobacco abuse.

Chronic lung disease.

High altitude.

Sleep apnea.

Right-to-left cardiac shunts.

Erythropoietin administration.

Androgens/anabolic steroids.

Polycystic kidney disease.

Renal cell carcinoma.

Hepatocellular carcinoma.

Polycythemia vera.

Carbon monoxide exposure.

Primary familial and congenital polycythemia.

High-oxygen–affinity hemoglobins.

Uterine leiomyoma, meningioma, pheochromocytoma, parathyroid carcinoma.

Cobalt exposure.

POLYCYTHEMIAS, DIFFERENTIAL DIAGNOSIS[34]

| ICD-10CM # | D45 | Polycythemia primary |
| | D75.1 | Polycythemia secondary |

DIFFERENTIAL DIAGNOSIS OF THE POLYCYTHEMIAS

Relative or Spurious Polycythemia

Decreased plasma volume—reduced fluid intake, marked loss of body fluids (diaphoresis, vomiting, diarrhea, "third spacing").

Gaisböck syndrome.

Overfilling of blood in collection vacuum tubes.

Absolute polycythemia

Secondary polycythemia.

Acquired.

Hypoxia:

Pulmonary disease.

Cyanotic congenital heart disease.

Hypoventilation syndromes:

Sleep apnea.

Pickwickian syndrome.

High altitude.

Smokers' polycythemia, hookah polycythemia, carbon monoxide intoxication caused by industrial exposure.

Postrenal transplantation erythrocytosis.

Aberrant erythropoietin production.

Tumors:

Renal cell carcinoma.

Wilms tumor.

Hepatic carcinoma.

Uterine leiomyomata.

Virilizing ovarian tumors.

Vascular cerebellar tumors.
Miscellaneous renal and hepatic disorders:
    Solitary renal cysts.
    Polycystic kidney disease.
    Renal artery stenosis hydronephrosis.
    Viral hepatitis.
    Endocrine disorders:
    Cushing syndrome.
    Primary aldosteronism.
    Androgen use.
    Erythropoietin use.
    Congenital polycythemias:
        Abnormal high-affinity hemoglobin variants.
        Bisphosphoglycerate deficiency.
        Congenital methemoglobinemia.
        Chuvash polycythemia (von Hippel Lindau mutations).
        Prolyl hydroxylase mutations.
        Hypoxia-inducible factor gene mutations.
Primary polycythemias:
    Primary congenital and familial polycythemia.
    Polycythemia vera.

POLYCYTHEMIA, RELATIVE VS. ABSOLUTE[31]

ICD-10CM #   D75.1   Secondary polycythemia

RELATIVE OR SPURIOUS POLYCYTHEMIA

Decreased plasma volume—reduced fluid intake, marked loss of body fluids (diaphoresis, vomiting, diarrhea, "third-spacing").
Gaisböck syndrome.
Overfilling of blood in collection vacuum tubes.

ABSOLUTE POLYCYTHEMIA

Primary Congenital and Familial Polycythemia
Secondary Polycythemia Acquired
Hypoxia:
    Pulmonary disease.
    Cyanotic congenital heart disease.
    Hypoventilation syndromes: sleep apnea, Pickwickian syndrome.
High altitude.
Smokers' polycythemia, carbon monoxide intoxication due to industrial exposure.
Postrenal transplantation erythrocytosis.
Aberrant erythropoietin production.
Tumors: renal cell carcinoma, Wilms tumor, hepatic carcinoma, uterine leiomyomata, virilizing ovarian tumors, vascular cerebellar tumors.
Miscellaneous renal and hepatic disorders: solitary renal cysts, polycystic kidney disease, renal artery stenosis, hydronephrosis, viral hepatitis.
Endocrine disorders: Cushing syndrome, primary aldosteronism.
Androgen use.
Erythropoietin use.
Congenital:
    Abnormal high-affinity hemoglobin variants.
    Bisphosphoglycerate deficiency.
    Congenital methemoglobinemia.
    Chuvash polycythemia (von Hippel-Lindau mutations).
    Prolyl hydroxylase mutations.
Polycythemia vera.

POLYMYALGIAS[90]

ICD-10CM #   M35.3   Polymyalgia rheumatica

DISEASE ENTITIES WITH POLYMYALGIAS

Rheumatoid arthritis.
Rotator cuff syndrome.
Osteoarthritis of shoulder and hip joints.
Fibromyalgia.
Polymyositis/dermatomyositis.
Spondyloarthritis.
Systemic lupus erythematosus.
Vasculitides.
Paraneoplastic myalgias.
Infection-associated myalgias.
Statin therapy.
RS3PE (remitting seronegative symmetric synovitis and pitting edema).
Parkinson disease.
Hypothyroidism.

POLYNEUROPATHIES WITH PREDOMINANTLY UPPER LIMB MOTOR INVOLVEMENT[38]

ICD-10CM #   Code varies with specific diagnosis

Multifocal motor neuropathy.
Multifocal acquired demyelinating sensory and motor neuropathy (MADSAM, Lewis-Sumner syndrome).
Lead neuropathy.*
Porphyria.
Tangier disease.
Familial amyloid neuropathy type 2.
Hereditary motor neuropathy (uncommon forms).

---

*May be associated with spine pain.

POLYNEUROPATHY[62]

ICD-10CM #   G61.9   Inflammatory polyneuropathy, unspecified

PREDOMINANTLY MOTOR

Guillain-Barré syndrome.
Porphyria.
Diphtheria.
Lead.
Hereditary sensorimotor neuropathy, types I and II.
Paraneoplastic neuropathy.

PREDOMINANTLY SENSORY

Diabetes.
Amyloidosis.
Leprosy.
Lyme disease.
Paraneoplastic neuropathy.
Vitamin B_{12} deficiency.
Hereditary sensory neuropathy, types I-IV.

PREDOMINANTLY AUTONOMIC

Diabetes.
Amyloidosis.
Alcoholic neuropathy.
Familial dysautonomias.

MIXED SENSORIMOTOR

Systemic diseases: renal failure, hypothyroidism, acromegaly, rheumatoid arthritis, periarteritis nodosa, systemic lupus erythematosus, multiple myeloma, macroglobulinemia, remote effect of malignancy.
Medications: isoniazid, nitrofurantoin, ethambutol, chloramphenicol, chloroquine, vincristine, vinblastine, dapsone, disulfiram, diphenylhydantoin, cisplatin, 1-tryptophan.
Environmental toxins: *N*-hexane, methyl *N*-butyl ketone, acrylamide, carbon disulfide, carbon monoxide, hexachlorophene, organophosphates.
Deficiency disorders: malabsorption, alcoholism, vitamin B_1 deficiency, Refsum disease, metachromatic leukodystrophy.

POLYNEUROPATHY, DEMYELINATING[43]

ICD-10CM #   G37.9   Demyelinating disease of central nervous system, unspecified

Guillain-Barré syndrome:
    Acute inflammatory demyelinating polyradiculoneuropathy (AIDP).
    Acute motor axonal neuropathy (AMAN).
    Acute motor and sensory axonal neuropathy (AMSAN).
    Miller Fisher syndrome.
Chronic inflammatory demyelinating polyradiculoplexo-neuropathy.
    Malignancy.
    HIV.
    Hepatitis B.
    Buckthorn.
    Diphtheria.

POLYNEUROPATHY, DISTAL SENSORIMOTOR[43]

ICD-10CM #   G63   Polyneuropathy in diseases classified elsewhere

Diabetes mellitus.
Alcoholism.
Neoplastic or paraneoplastic.
Hereditary motor and sensory neuropathies (Charcot-Marie-Tooth).
Cryptogenic sensorimotor polyneuropathies (CSPN).
HIV.
Toxins:
    Organic or industrial agents:
        Acrylamide.
        Allyl chloride.
        Carbon disulfide.
        Ethylene oxide.
        Hexacarbons.
        Methyl bromide.
        Organophosphate-induced delayed polyneuropathy (OPIDP).
        Polychlorinated biphenyls (PCBs).
        Trichloroethylene.
        Vacor.
Metals:
    Arsenic.
    Gold.

Mercury (inorganic).
Thallium.
Therapeutic agents:
  Amiodarone.
  Antiretrovirals.
  Dapsone.
  Disulfiram.
  Isoniazid.
  Metronidazole.
  Nitrofurantoin.
  Paclitaxel (Taxol).
  Phenytoin.
  Statins (HMG-CoA reductase inhibitors).
  Thalidomide.
  Vinca alkaloids (vincristine, vinblastine).
Nutritional:
  Beriberi (thiamine or vitamin B_1).
  Pellagra (niacin, B vitamins).
  Pernicious anemia (vitamin B_{12}).
  Pyridoxine deficiency (vitamin B_6).
End-organ dysfunction
  Acromegaly.
  Chronic pulmonary disease.
  Hypothyroidism.
  Renal failure (uremic neuropathy).
Paraproteinemias:
  Amyloidosis.
  Monoclonal gammopathy of unknown significance (MGUS).
  Multiple myeloma.
  Waldenström macroglobulinemia.
Porphyria

HMG-CoA, Hydroxymethylglutaryl coenzyme A.

POLYNEUROPATHY, DRUG-INDUCED[62]

ICD-10CM #	G62.0	Drug-induced polyneuropathy

DRUGS IN ONCOLOGY

Vincristine.
Procarbazine.
Cisplatin.
Misonidazole.
Metronidazole
Taxol.

DRUGS IN INFECTIOUS DISEASES

Isoniazid.
Nitrofurantoin.
Dapsone.
ddC (dideoxycytidine).
ddI (dideoxyinosine).

DRUGS IN CARDIOLOGY

Hydralazine.
Perhexiline maleate.
Procainamide.
Disopyramide.

DRUGS IN RHEUMATOLOGY

Gold salts.
Chloroquine.

DRUGS IN NEUROLOGY AND PSYCHIATRY

Diphenylhydantoin.
Glutethimide.
Methaqualone.

MISCELLANEOUS

Disulfiram (Antabuse).
Vitamin: (pyridoxine in megadoses).

POLYNEUROPATHY, SYMMETRIC[62]

ICD-10CM #	G61.9	Inflammatory polyneuropathy, unspecified

ACQUIRED NEUROPATHIES

Toxic:
  Drugs.
  Industrial toxins.
  Heavy metals.
  Abused substances.
Metabolic/endocrine:
  Diabetes.
  Chronic renal failure.
  Hypothyroidism.
  Polyneuropathy of critical illness.
Nutritional deficiency:
  Vitamin B_{12} deficiency.
  Alcoholism.
  Vitamin E deficiency.
Paraneoplastic:
  Carcinoma.
  Lymphoma.
Plasma cell dyscrasia:
  Myeloma, typical, atypical, and solitary forms.
  Primary systemic amyloidosis.
Idiopathic chronic inflammatory demyelinating polyneuropathies.
Polyneuropathies associated with peripheral nerve autoantibodies.
AIDS.

INHERITED NEUROPATHIES

Neuropathies with Biochemical Markers
Refsum disease.
Bassen-Kornzweig disease.
Tangier disease.
Metachromatic leukodystrophy.
Krabbe disease.
Adrenomyeloneuropathy.
Fabry disease.
Neuropathies without Biochemical Markers or Systemic Involvement
Hereditary motor neuropathy.
Hereditary sensory neuropathy.
Hereditary sensorimotor neuropathy.

POLYURIA

ICD-10CM #	R35.8	Other polyuria

Diabetes mellitus.
Diabetes insipidus.
Primary polydipsia (compulsive water drinking).
Hypercalcemia.
Hypokalemia.
Postobstructive uropathy.
Diuretic phase of renal failure.

Drugs: diuretics, caffeine, alcohol, lithium.
Sickle cell trait or disease, chronic pyelonephritis (failure to concentrate urine).
Anxiety, cold weather.

POPLITEAL SWELLING

ICD-10CM #	I87.1	Compression of vein
	I72.4	Aneurysm of artery of lower extremity
	S85.009A	Unspecified injury of popliteal artery, unspecified leg, initial encounter
	I77.3	Arterial fibromuscular dysplasia
	M71.20	Synovial cyst of popliteal space [Baker], unspecified knee
	I80.3	Phlebitis and thrombophlebitis of lower extremities, unspecified
	M66.369	Spontaneous rupture of flexor tendons, unspecified lower leg

Phlebitis (superficial).
Lymphadenitis.
Trauma: fractured tibia or fibula, contusion, traumatic neuroma.
DVT.
Ruptured varicose vein.
Baker cyst.
Popliteal abscess.
Osteomyelitis.
Ruptured tendon.
Aneurysm of popliteal artery.
Neoplasm: lipoma, osteogenic sarcoma, neurofibroma, fibrosarcoma.

PORTAL HYPERTENSION[18]

ICD-10CM #	K76.6	Portal hypertension

INCREASED RESISTANCE TO FLOW

Presinusoidal
Portal or splenic vein occlusion (thrombosis, tumor).
Schistosomiasis.
Congenital hepatic fibrosis.
Sarcoidosis.
Sinusoidal
Cirrhosis (all causes).
Alcoholic hepatitis.
Postsinusoidal
Venoocclusive disease.
Budd-Chiari syndrome.
Constrictive pericarditis.

INCREASED PORTAL BLOOD FLOW

Splenomegaly not caused by liver disease.
Arterioportal fistula.

POSTMENOPAUSAL BLEEDING

ICD-10CM #	N95.0	Postmenopausal bleeding

Hormone replacement therapy.
Neoplasm (uterine, ovarian, cervical, vaginal, vulvar).
Atrophic vaginitis.
Vaginal infection.
Polyp.
Extragenital (GI, urinary).
Tamoxifen.
Trauma.

POSTURAL HYPOTENSION, NONNEUROLOGIC CAUSES

ICD-10CM #	I95.1	Orthostatic hypotension

Diuretics and hypertensive agents.
GI hemorrhage.
Alcohol.
Excessive heat.
Rapid volume loss from diarrhea, vomiting.
Hemodialysis.
Extensive burns.
Pyrexia.
Aortic stenosis (impaired output).
Constrictive pericarditis, atrial myxoma (impaired cardiac filling).
Adrenal insufficiency.
Diabetes insipidus.
Vasodilatory agents (e.g., nitrates).

POSTURING ABNORMALITY[20]

ICD-10CM #	Varies with specific diagnosis

Dystonia.[a]
Conversion disorder.
Muscular dystrophy.
Myotonia.
Neuromyotonia.
Rigidity.
Spasticity.[a]
Stiff person syndrome (stiff man syndrome).

[a]Denotes the most common conditions and the ones with disease-modifying treatments.

PREMATURE GRAYING, SCALP HAIR

ICD-10CM #	Varies with specific diagnosis

Chemical exposure (e.g., phenol/catechol derivatives, sulfhydryls, arsenic).
Physical agents (e.g., ionizing radiation, lasers).
Hyperthyroidism.
Vitamin B_{12} deficiency.
Down syndrome.
Chronic and severe protein deficiency.
Vitiligo.
Idiopathic.
Myotonic dystrophy.
Ataxia-telangiectasia.
Progeria.
Werner syndrome.

PREMATURE VENTRICULAR CONTRACTIONS AND VENTRICULAR TACHYCARDIA[43]

ICD-10CM #	I49.40	Unspecified premature depolarization
	I47.2	Ventricular tachycardia

CAUSES OF PREMATURE VENTRICULAR CONTRACTIONS AND VENTRICULAR TACHYCARDIA

Acute or previous myocardial infarction/ischemia.
Hypokalemia.
Hypoxemia.
Ischemic heart disease.
Valvular disease.
Catecholamine excess.*
Other drug intoxications (especially cyclic antidepressants).
Idiopathic causes.†
Digitalis toxicity.
Hypomagnesemia.
Hypercapnia.
Class I antidysrhythymic agents.
Ethanol.
Myocardial contusion.
Cardiomyopathy.
Acidosis.
Alkalosis.
Methylxanthine toxicity.

*Relative increase in sympathetic tone from drugs (direct or indirect) or conditions that augment catecholamine release or decrease parasympathetic tone.
†Isolated premature ventricular contractions (PVCs) can occur in up to 50% of young subjects without obvious cardiac or noncardiac disease; however, multiform and repetitive PVCs and ventricular tachycardia are rarely seen in this population.

PREPUBERTAL BLEEDING WITHOUT BREAST DEVELOPMENT[102]

ICD-10CM #	Varies with specific diagnosis

Foreign object.
Genital trauma.
Sexual abuse.
Lichen sclerosus.
Infectious vaginitis (especially from *Shigella*).
Urethral prolapse.
Breakdown of labial adhesions.
Friable genital warts or vulvar lesions.
Vaginal tumor.
Rare presentation of McCune-Albright syndrome (typically have breast development).
Isolated menarche (controversial).
Dermatologic conditions with secondary excoriation.
Nongenital bleeding; mistaken as genital: rectal and urinary.

PRESACRAL MASSES IN CHILDREN[15]

ICD-10CM #	Varies with specific diagnosis

PRESACRAL MASSES IN CHILDREN

Solid
Sacrococcygeal teratoma.
Neuroblastoma.
Rhabdomyosarcoma.
Fibroma.
Lipoma.
Leiomyoma.
Lymphoma.
Hemangioendothelioma.
Sacral bone tumors.
Cystic
Abscess.
Rectal duplication.
Hematoma.
Lymphocele.
Neurenteric cyst.
Sacral osteomyelitis.
Ulcerative colitis.
Anterior meningocele.

PRIMARY ANGIITIS OF CENTRAL NERVOUS SYSTEM[111]

ICD-10CM #	Varies with specific diagnosis

Differential Diagnosis of Primary Angiitis of the CNS

Secondary Cerebral Vasculitis
Primary Systemic Vasculitides
Granulomatosis with polyangiitis.
Microscopic polyangiitis.
Eosinophilic granulomatosis with polyangiitis.
Polyarteritis nodosa.
Behçet disease.
Systemic Autoimmune Disease
Systemic lupus erythematosus.
Sjögren syndrome.
Inflammatory myositis.
Rheumatoid arthritis.
Mixed connective tissue disease.
Other Multisystem Inflammatory Disorders
Sarcoidosis.
Susac syndrome.
Infection
Bacterial.
Mycobacterial.
Fungal.
Viral.
Protozoal.
Malignancy
Central nervous system lymphoma.
Glioma.
Angiocentric lymphoma.
Lymphomatoid granulomatosis.
Metastatic malignancy.
Vasospastic Disorders
Reversible cerebral vasoconstrictive syndrome.
Drug exposures.

Differential Diagnosis

II

Secondary Cerebral Vasculitis

Other Arterial Diseases

Atherosclerosis.
Fibromuscular dysplasia.
Moyamoya disease.
Dissection.

Hypercoagulable States

Antiphospholipid antibody syndrome.
Thrombotic thrombocytopenic purpura.

Stroke-like Syndromes

CADASIL.
Mitochondrial diseases.
Sickle cell disease.
Fabry disease.
Sneddon syndrome.

Leukoencephalopathies

Progressive multifocal leukoencephalopathy.
Reversible posterior leukoencephalopathy
　syndrome.

Cerebral Hemorrhage

Hypertensive.
Aneurysmal.
Amyloid angiopathy.
Arteriovenous malformation.

Embolic Disease

Thrombus.
Cholesterol emboli.
Myxoma.
Endocarditis.
Air emboli.

CADASIL, Cerebral autosomal dominant arteriopathy with subcortical infarcts and leukoencephalopathy.
From *Firestein & Kelley's textbook of rheumatology*, ed 11, Philadelphia, 2021, Elsevier.

PROLONGED QT SYNDROMES[10]

ICD-10CM #	I45.81	Long QT syndrome

CLASSIFICATION AND CAUSES OF PROLONGED QT SYNDROMES THAT PRODUCE TORSADES DE POINTES

Pause Dependent (Acquired)

Drug induced: class IA and IC antidysrhythmics; many phenothiazines and butyrophenones (notably haloperidol and droperidol), cyclic antidepressants, antibiotics (especially macrolides), organophosphates, antihistamines, antifungals, antiseizure and antiemetic agents.
Electrolyte abnormalities: hypokalemia, hypomagnesemia, hypocalcemia (rarely).
Diet related: starvation, low protein.
Severe bradycardia or atrioventricular block.
Hypothyroidism.
Contrast injection.
Cerebrovascular accident (especially intraparenchymal).
Myocardial ischemia.

Adrenergic Dependent (Tachycardia Prompted)

Congenital:
　Jervell and Lange-Nielsen syndrome (deafness, autosomal recessive).

Romano-Ward syndrome (normal hearing, autosomal dominant).
Sporadic (normal hearing, no familial tendency).
Mitral valve prolapse.
Acquired (rare):
　Cerebrovascular disease (especially subarachnoid hemorrhage).
　Autonomic surgery: radical neck dissection, carotid endarterectomy, truncal vagotomy.

PROPTOSIS[22]

ICD-10CM #	H05.2	Ocular proptosis

Endocrine:
　Graves ophthalmopathy.
　Cushing syndrome.
Orbital neoplasms:
　Primary neoplasms.
　Hemangioma.
　Lymphoma (may be systemic).
　Optic nerve glioma.
　Choroidal melanoma.
　Lacrimal gland tumors.
　Meningioma.
　Rhabdomyosarcoma.
Extension of paranasal sinus tumors.
Metastatic disease:
　Malignant melanoma.
　Breast carcinoma.
　Lung carcinoma.
　Kidney.
　Prostate.
Inflammatory:
　Orbital pseudotumor.
　Orbital myositis.
Granulomatous:
　Sarcoidosis.
　Wegener granulomatosis.
Infectious:
　Orbital cellulitis.
　Syphilis.
　Mucormycosis.
　Parasitic (trypanosomiasis, schistosomiasis, cysticercosis, echinococcal disease).
Vascular/miscellaneous:
　Carotid-cavernous fistula.
　Lithium therapy.
　Cirrhosis.
　Obesity.
　Amyloidosis.
　Dermoid and epidermoid cysts.
Foreign body.

PROPTOSIS AND PALATAL NECROTIC ULCERS

ICD-10CM #	K13.70	Unspecified lesions of oral mucosa
	K13.79	Other lesions of oral mucosa
	H05.20	Unspecified exophthalmos

Cavernous sinus thrombosis.
Bacterial orbital cellulitis.
Metastatic neoplasm.
Rhinocerebral mucormycosis.
Ecthyma gangrenosum.
Central nervous system aspergillosis.

PROTEIN-LOSING ENTEROPATHY, PEDIATRIC AGE[19]

ICD-10CM #	E44.0	Moderate protein-energy malnutrition

CAUSES OF PROTEIN-LOSING ENTEROPATHY

Mucosal inflammation:
Infection:
　Cytomegalovirus.
　Bacterial overgrowth.
　Invasive bacterial infection.
Gastric inflammation:
　Ménétrier disease.
　Eosinophilic gastroenteropathy.
Intestinal inflammation:
　Celiac disease.
　Crohn disease.
Eosinophilic gastroenteropathy:
　Tropical sprue.
　Radiation enteritis.
Primary intestinal lymphangiectasia.
Secondary intestinal lymphangiectasia:
Constrictive pericarditis.
Congestive heart failure.
Post–Fontan procedure.
Malrotation.
Lymphoma.
Sarcoidosis.
Radiation therapy.
Colonic inflammation:
　Inflammatory bowel diseases.
　Necrotizing enterocolitis.
Congenital disorders of glycosylation.

PROTEINURIA

ICD-10CM #	R80.9	Proteinuria, unspecified

Nephrotic syndrome as a result of primary renal diseases.
Malignant hypertension.
Malignancies: multiple myeloma, leukemias, Hodgkin disease.
Congestive heart failure.
Diabetes mellitus.
Systemic lupus erythematosus, rheumatoid arthritis.
Sickle cell disease.
Goodpasture syndrome.
Malaria.
Amyloidosis, sarcoidosis.
Tubular lesions: cystinosis.
Functional (after heavy exercise).
Pyelonephritis.
Pregnancy.
Constrictive pericarditis.
Renal vein thrombosis.
Toxic nephropathies: heavy metals, drugs.
Radiation nephritis.
Orthostatic (postural) proteinuria.
Benign proteinuria: fever, heat, or cold exposure.

PRURITUS

ICD-10CM #	L29.9	Pruritus, unspecified
	L29.3	Anogenital pruritus, unspecified

Dry skin.
Drug-induced eruption, fiberglass exposure.
Scabies.
Skin diseases.
Myeloproliferative disorders: mycosis fungoides, Hodgkin lymphoma, multiple myeloma, polycythemia vera.
Cholestatic liver disease.
Endocrine disorders: diabetes mellitus, thyroid disease, carcinoid, pregnancy.
Carcinoma: breast, lung, gastric.
Chronic renal failure.
Iron deficiency.
AIDS.
Neurosis.
Sjögren syndrome.

PRURITUS ANI[10]

| ICD-10CM # | L29.0 | Pruritus ani |

FECAL IRRITATION

Poor hygiene.
Anorectal conditions (fissure, fistula, hemorrhoids, skin tags, perianal clefts).
Spicy foods, citrus foods, caffeine, colchicine, quinidine.

CONTACT DERMATITIS

Anesthetic agents, topical corticosteroids, perfumed soap.

DERMATOLOGIC DISORDERS

Psoriasis, seborrhea, lichen simplex, or sclerosus.

SYSTEMIC DISORDERS

Chronic renal failure, myxedema, diabetes mellitus, thyrotoxicosis, polycythemia vera, Hodgkin disease.

SEXUALLY TRANSMITTED DISEASES

Syphilis, herpes simplex virus, human papillomavirus.

OTHER INFECTIOUS AGENTS

Pinworms.
Scabies.
Bacterial infection, viral infection.

PRURITUS VULVAE[47]

| ICD-10CM # | L29.3 | Anogenital pruritus, unspecified |

CAUSES OF PRURITUS VULVAE

Diseases Special to Vulval Skin
Lichen sclerosus et atrophicus.
Leukoplakia.
Carcinoma.
Skin Disease
Psoriasis.
Atopic dermatitis.
Irritant and allergic contact dermatitis (especially medicaments).
Infection
Candidiasis.
Trichomonas.
Infestation
Pediculosis.

Psychogenic
Anxiety.
Depression.
Unknown.

PSEUDOCELLULITIS[70]

| ICD-10CM # | Varies with specific diagnosis |

CAUSES OF PSEUDOCELLULITIS

Infections and Bites
Arthropod bite reactions (e.g., insect, spider).
Erythema migrans.
Herpes zoster.
Toxin-mediated erythema (e.g., recurrent toxin-mediated perineal erythema).
Neutrophilic Dermatoses
Sweet syndrome, neutrophilic panniculitis.
Familial Mediterranean fever, other autoinflammatory syndromes.
Drug Reactions
Fixed drug eruptions (especially nonpigmenting).
Vaccine/injection site reactions.
Toxic erythema of chemotherapy (e.g., due to gemcitabine), neutrophilic eccrine hidradenitis.*
Other Inflammatory Disorders
Allergic contact dermatitis (including airborne and dermal), stasis dermatitis.
Phytophotodermatitis.
Well syndrome.
Panniculitis (e.g., lipodermatosclerosis, erythema nodosum).
Thrombophlebitis.
Angioedema.
Interstitial granulomatous dermatitis, patch type granuloma annulare.
Inflammatory morphea.
Acute inflammatory edema of the ICU.
Metabolic Disorders
Gout.
Malignancy
Erysipeloid skin metastases (especially breast carcinoma).

*ICU, Intensive care unit. Occasionally develops before onset of leukemia or due to infection.

PSEUDOCYANOSIS, ETIOLOGY

| ICD-10CM # | Varies with etiology |

Medications: amiodarone, minocycline, chlorpromazine.
Heavy metals:
Gold (systemic absorption).
Silver (systemic absorption).
Local contact with color dyes, gold, silver.

PSEUDOHERMAPHRODITISM, FEMALE

ICD-10CM #	E25.0	Congenital adrenogenital disorders associated with enzyme deficiency
	E25.8	Other adrenogenital disorders
	E25.9	Adrenogenital disorder, unspecified
	Q56.3	Pseudohermaphroditism, unspecified
	Q56.4	Indeterminate sex, unspecified

Congenital adrenal hyperplasia.
Maternal use of testosterone or related steroids.
Virilizing ovarian or adrenal tumor.
Virilizing luteoma of pregnancy.
Disturbances in differentiation of urogenital structures, nonandrogen related.
Maternal virilizing adrenal hyperplasia.
Fetal P450 aromatase deficiency.

PSEUDOHERMAPHRODITISM, MALE

ICD-10CM #	E25.0	Congenital adrenogenital disorders associated with enzyme deficiency
	E25.8	Other adrenogenital disorders
	E25.9	Adrenogenital disorder, unspecified
	Q56.3	Pseudohermaphroditism, unspecified
	Q56.4	Indeterminate sex, unspecified

Maternal ingestion of progestogens.
End-organ resistance to androgenic hormones.
5-α-reductase-2 deficiency.
XY gonadal dysgenesis.
Testicular regression syndrome.
Defects in testosterone metabolism by peripheral tissues.
Testosterone biosynthesis defects.

PSEUDOINFARCTION[97]

| ICD-10CM # | Varies with specific diagnosis |

Cardiac tumors, primary and secondary.
Cardiomyopathy (particularly hypertrophic and dilated).
Chagas disease.
Chest deformity.
Chronic obstructive pulmonary disease (particularly emphysema).
HIV infection.
Hyperkalemia.
Left anterior fascicular block.
Left bundle branch block.
Left ventricular hypertrophy.
Myocarditis and pericarditis.
Normal variant.
Pneumothorax.
Poor R wave progression, rotational changes, and lead placement.
Pulmonary embolism.
Trauma to chest (nonpenetrating).
Wolff-Parkinson-White syndrome.
Rare causes: pancreatitis, amyloidosis, sarcoidosis, scleroderma.

Differential Diagnosis

II

PSYCHOSIS[25]

ICD-10CM #	F29	Unspecified psychosis not due to a substance or known physiological condition
	F29	Unspecified psychosis not due to a substance or known physiological condition
	F10.231	Alcohol dependence with withdrawal delirium
	F01.51	Vascular dementia with behavioral disturbance

PRIMARY

Schizophrenia-related.*
Major depression.
Dementia.
Bipolar disorder.

SECONDARY

Drug use.[†]
Drug withdrawal.[‡]
Drug toxicity.[§]
Charles Bonnet syndrome.
Infections (pneumonia).
Electrolyte imbalance.
Syphilis.
Congestive heart failure.
Parkinson disease.
Trauma to temporal lobe.
Postpartum psychosis.
Hypothyroidism/hyperthyroidism.
Hypomagnesemia.
Epilepsy.
Meningitis.
Encephalitis.
Brain abscess.
Herpes encephalopathy.
Hypoxia.
Hypercarbia.
Hypoglycemia.
Thiamine deficiency.
Postoperative states.

---

*Includes schizophrenia, schizophreniform disorder, brief reactive psychosis.
[†]Includes hypnotics, glucocorticoids, marijuana, phencyclidine, atropine, dopaminergic agents (e.g., amantadine, bromocriptine, L-dopa), immunosuppressants.
[‡]Includes alcohol, barbiturates, benzodiazepines.
[§]Includes digitalis, theophylline, cimetidine, anticholinergics, glucocorticoids, catecholaminergic agents.

PSYCHOSIS, MEDICAL DISORDERS-INDUCED[10]

ICD-10CM #	F29	Unspecified psychosis not due to a substance or known physiological condition
	F53	Puerperal psychosis

MEDICAL DISORDERS THAT MAY CAUSE ACUTE PSYCHOSIS

Metabolic Disorders
Hypercalcemia.
Hypercarbia.
Hypoglycemia.
Hyponatremia.
Hypoxia.

Inflammatory Disorders
Sarcoidosis.
Systemic lupus erythematosus.
Temporal (giant cell) arteritis.

Organ Failure
Hepatic encephalopathy.
Uremia.

Neurologic Disorders
Alzheimer disease.
Cerebrovascular disease.
Encephalitis (including HIV infection).
Encephalopathies.
Epilepsy.
Huntington disease.
Multiple sclerosis.
Neoplasms.
Normal-pressure hydrocephalus.
Parkinson disease.
Pick disease.
Wilson disease.

Endocrine Disorders
Addison disease.
Cushing disease.
Panhypopituitarism.
Parathyroid disease.
Postpartum psychosis.
Recurrent menstrual psychosis.
Sydenham chorea.
Thyroid disease.

Deficiency States
Niacin.
Thiamine.
Vitamin B_{12} and folate.

PSYCHOSIS, MEDICATION-INDUCED[10]

ICD-10CM #	F10.5	Psychotic disorder due to psychoactive substance use

PHARMACOLOGIC AGENTS THAT MAY CAUSE ACUTE PSYCHOSIS

Antianxiety Agents
Alprazolam.
Chlordiazepoxide.
Clonazepam.
Clorazepate.
Diazepam.
Ethchlorvynol.

Antibiotics
Isoniazid.
Rifampin.

Anticonvulsants
Ethosuximide.
Phenobarbital.
Phenytoin.
Primidone.

Antidepressants
Amitriptyline.
Doxepin.
Imipramine.
Protriptyline.
Trimipramine.

Cardiovascular Drugs
Captopril.
Digitalis.
Disopyramide.
Methyldopa.
Procainamide.
Propranolol.
Reserpine.

Drugs of Abuse
Alcohol.
Amphetamines.
Cannabis.
Cocaine.
Hallucinogens.
Opioids.
Phencyclidine.
Sedative-hypnotics.

Miscellaneous Drugs
Antihistamines.
Antineoplastics.
Bromides.
Cimetidine.
Corticosteroids.
Disulfiram.
Heavy metals.

PTOSIS[20]

ICD-10CM #	Varies with specific diagnosis

CONGENITAL

Congenital fibrosis of extraocular muscles.
Horner syndrome.[a]
Myasthenia.[a]
Oculomotor nerve palsy.[a]

ACQUIRED

Horner syndrome.[a]
Lid inflammation.
Mitochondrial myopathies.
Myasthenia gravis.[a]
Oculomotor nerve palsy.[a]
Oculopharyngeal dystrophy.
Ophthalmoplegic migraine.
Orbital cellulitis.
Trauma.

---

[a]Denotes the most common conditions and the ones with disease-modifying treatments.

PUBERTY, DELAYED[80]

ICD-10CM #	E30.0	Delayed puberty

NORMAL OR LOW SERUM GONADOTROPIN LEVELS

Constitutional delay in growth and development.
Hypothalamic and/or pituitary disorders:
    Isolated deficiency of growth hormone.
    Isolated deficiency of GnRH.
    Isolated deficiency of LH and/or FSH.
    Multiple anterior pituitary hormone deficiencies.
    Associated with congenital anomalies: Kallmann syndrome; Prader-Willi syndrome; Laurence-Moon-Biedl syndrome; Friedreich ataxia.
    Trauma.
    Postinfection.
    Hyperprolactinemia.
    Postirradiation.
    Infiltrative disease (histiocytosis).

Tumor.
Autoimmune hypophysitis.
Idiopathic.
Functional:
Chronic endocrinologic or systemic disorders.
Emotional disorders.
Drugs: cannabis.

INCREASED SERUM GONADOTROPIN LEVELS

Gonadal abnormalities:
Congenital:
Gonadal dysgenesis.
Klinefelter syndrome.
Bilateral anorchism.
Resistant ovary syndrome.
Myotonic dystrophy in males.
17-Hydroxylase deficiency in females.
Galactosemia.
Acquired:
Bilateral gonadal failure resulting from trauma or infection or after surgery, irradiation, or chemotherapy.
Oophoritis: isolated or with other autoimmune disorders.
Uterine or vaginal disorders:
Absence of uterus and/or vagina.
Testicular feminization: complete or incomplete androgen insensitivity.

PUBERTY, PRECOCIOUS

ICD-10CM #	E25.0	Congenital adrenogenital disorders associated with enzyme deficiency
	E25.8	Other adrenogenital disorders
	E25.9	Adrenogenital disorder, unspecified

Idiopathic.
Congenital virilizing adrenal hyperplasia.
Hypothalamic tumors.
Head trauma.
Hydrocephalus.
Degenerative central nervous system disease.
Arachnoid cyst.
Sex chromosome abnormalities (e.g., 47, XXY, 48, XXXY).
Perinatal asphyxia.
Central nervous system infection (e.g., meningitis, encephalitis).

PULMONARY ARTERY SEGMENT ABNORMALITIES[37]

ICD-10CM #	Q25.72	Congenital pulmonary arteriovenous malformation

DIFFERENTIAL DIAGNOSIS OF THE MAIN PULMONARY ARTERY SEGMENT

DILATED MPA SEGMENT

Increased pulmonary artery volume (shunt):
VSD.
ASD.
PDA.

Increased pulmonary artery pressure (pulmonary hypertension):
Mitral stenosis.
COPD/emphysema.
Interstitial pulmonary fibrosis.
Cystic fibrosis.
Chronic thromboembolism.
Primary PH.
Increased pulmonary artery volume and pressure:
ASD with PH.
Normal pulmonary artery pressure and flow:
Valvular pulmonic stenosis.

FLAT OR CONCAVE MPA SEGMENT

Tetralogy of Fallot.
Tetralogy variants.
Tetralogy with pulmonary atresia.
Pulmonary atresia with VSD.
Double-chamber RV.
Double-outlet RV.
Tricuspid atresia.
Ebstein malformation.

NO MPA SEGMENT PRESENT

Persistent truncus arteriosus.
D-transposition of the great arteries.

ASD, Atrial septal defect; *COPD*, chronic obstructive pulmonary disease; *MPA*, main pulmonary artery; *PDA*, patent ductus arteriosus; *PH*, pulmonary hypertension; *RV*, right ventricle; *VSD*, ventricular septal defect.

PULMONARY CRACKLES

ICD-10CM #	R09.8	Friction sounds, chest

Pneumonia.
Left ventricular failure.
Asbestosis, silicosis, interstitial lung disease.
Chronic bronchitis.
Alveolitis (allergic, fibrosing).
Neoplasm.

PULMONARY CYSTS ON X-RAY[21]

ICD-10CM #	Q33.0	Polycystic lungs, congenital
	J98.4	Pulmonary manifestations

CAUSES OF CYSTS IN THE LUNG ON CHEST RADIOGRAPH

Cystic fibrosis.
Cystic bronchiectasis.
Bronchopulmonary dysplasia (neonate and older).
Tuberculosis (apical thick walled).
Pulmonary abscess (thick wall, fluid level).
Empyema.
Streptococcal pneumatocele (thin wall, postinfective).
Cavitating pneumonia.
Mycetoma (apical cyst with contents).
Cystic congenital adenomatoid malformation (basal cysts of varying size).
Diaphragmatic hernia (cysts of similar size).
Hiatal hernia (posterior).
Morgagni hernia (midline anterior).
Bronchopulmonary sequestration (basal).

Congenital lobar emphysema.
Hydatid disease (in endemic areas).
Kerosene inhalation (pneumatocele).
Histiocytosis and other causes of interstitial disease.

PULMONARY EDEMA, NONCARDIOGENIC[21]

ICD-10CM #	J81.0	Acute pulmonary edema

CAUSES OF NONCARDIOGENIC PULMONARY EDEMA

Adult respiratory distress syndrome.
Drowning.
Asphyxia.
Upper airway obstruction (usually with cardiomegaly).
High altitude.
Increased intracranial pressure.
Post-ictal.
Noxious gases:
Smoke.
Nitrous dioxide (silo filler's disease).
Sulfur dioxide.
Nitrogen mustard.
Drugs:
Aspirin.
Diazepam, chlordiazepoxide, barbiturates.
Narcotics (heroin, methadone, morphine).
β-adrenergic drugs (terbutaline).
Contrast media.
Colchicine.
Fluorescein.
Hydrochlorothiazide.
Nitrofurantoin.
Propoxyphene.
Poisons:
Parathion.
Transfusion reactions.
Renal failure: transplantation.
Bone marrow transplantation.
Fat embolism.
Pancreatitis.

PULMONARY EOSINOPHILIA[28]

ICD-10CM #	NEC J82	Eosinophilia, pulmonary

TYPES AND CAUSES OF PULMONARY EOSINOPHILIA

Drug- and toxin-induced eosinophilic lung diseases.
Helminth and fungal infection-related eosinophilic lung diseases:
Transpulmonary passage of larvae (i.e., Löffler syndrome): *Ascaris*, hookworm, *Strongyloides*.
Pulmonary parenchymal invasion: mostly helminths, paragonimiasis.
Heavy hematogenous seeding with helminths: trichinellosis, disseminated strongyloidiasis, cutaneous and visceral larva migrans, schistosomiasis.
Tropical pulmonary eosinophilia: filaria.
Allergic bronchopulmonary aspergillosis.
Chronic eosinophilic pneumonia.
Acute eosinophilic pneumonia.

Churg-Strauss syndrome (vasculitis).
Other: neoplasia, idiopathic hypereosinophilic syndrome, bronchocentric granulomatosis.

PULMONARY HEMORRHAGE, DIFFUSE, ALVEOLAR[14]

ICD-10CM #	R04.8	Pulmonary hemorrhage

IMMUNOLOGIC DISEASES

Antiglomerular basement membrane antibody disease (Goodpasture syndrome).
Vasculitides associated with circulating or in situ immune complexes:
  Systemic lupus erythematosus.
  Mixed connective tissue disease.
  Schönlein-Henoch purpura.
  Essential mixed cryoglobulinemia.
  Tumor-related vasculitis.
  Endocarditis-related vasculitis.
  Polyarteritis nodosa.
  Systemic necrotizing vasculitis.
  Vasculitides associated with antineutrophil cytoplasmic antibodies:
    Wegener granulomatosis.
    Microscopic polyangiitis.
    Idiopathic necrotizing crescentic glomerulonephritis.
Rapidly progressive glomerulonephritis.
Associated with other connective tissue diseases, pathophysiology unknown:
  Rheumatoid arthritis.
  Progressive systemic sclerosis.
  Behçet disease.
  Associated with other renal diseases.
  Immunoglobulin A nephropathy.
  Diabetic nephropathy.
  Associated with precipitating antibodies to milk (Heiner syndrome).
  Idiopathic pulmonary hemosiderosis.
  Primary antiphospholipid antibody syndrome.

CHEMICAL OR DRUG-RELATED CAUSES

Amiodarone.
D-Penicillamine.
Isocyanates.
Nitrofurantoin.
Retinoic acid.
Trimellitic anhydride.
"Crack" cocaine.
Sirolimus.
Everolimus.
Propylthiouracil-induced vasculitis.
Erlotinib.
Bevacizumab.
Gemcitabine.
Infliximab.

TRANSPLANT-RELATED CAUSES

Bone marrow transplant.
Renal transplant.
Lung transplant.

BLEEDING DIATHESIS

Thrombocytopenia.
Leukemia with diffuse alveolar damage.
Viral pneumonia.

Bacterial or fungal sepsis.
Radiation.
Chemotherapy toxic to lung.
Blast counts >80,000/μL.
Extrinsic anticoagulants/thrombolytics.
Warfarin overdose.
Tissue plasminogen activator.
Platelet glycoprotein IIb/IIIa inhibitors.
Coagulopathies.
Cirrhosis.
Disseminated intravascular coagulation.

INFECTIONS

Adenovirus.
Aspergillosis (invasive).
Cytomegalovirus.
Dengue.
Hantavirus.
Influenza.
Legionella.
Leptospirosis.
Malaria.
Mycoplasma.
Staphylococcus aureus.

PULMONARY VENOUS HYPERTENSION

Mitral stenosis.
Mitral regurgitation.
Pulmonary capillary hemangiomatosis.
Pulmonary venoocclusive disease.
Fibrosing mediastinitis.
Congenital heart disease.

DIFFUSE LUNG INJURY

Negative-pressure pulmonary hemorrhage.
Breath-hold diving.
Post-ictal neurogenic pulmonary edema.

PULMONARY HEMORRHAGE, FOCAL[27]

ICD-10CM #	R04.8	Pulmonary hemorrhage

CAUSES OF FOCAL PULMONARY HEMORRHAGE

Iatrogenic Disorders
Bronchoscopy.
Lung biopsy.
Pulmonary artery catheterization.
Transtracheal aspiration.
Radiofrequency ablation.
Brachytherapy.

Infectious Disorders
Lung abscess.
Mycetoma.
Necrotizing pneumonia (*Staphylococcus aureus*, gram-negative aerobes, *Legionella*, *Actinomyces* spp., *Stenotrophomonas*, *Kytococcus sedentarius*, *Leptospira* spp., *Yersinia pestis*, *Francisella tularensis*).
Parasitic infection (paragonimiasis, amebiasis, ascariasis, clonorchiasis, echinococcosis, hookworm infestation, strongyloidiasis, trichinosis, schistosomiasis).
Parenchymal fungal infection (aspergillosis, mucormycosis, coccidioidomycosis, histoplasmosis, maduromycosis, botryomycosis).

Tuberculosis (active or inactive).
Viral tracheitis.
Herpetic tracheobronchitis.
Interstitial Lung Diseases
Lymphangioleiomyomatosis.
Sarcoidosis.
Tuberous sclerosis.
Pneumoconiosis.
Langerhans cell granulomatosis.
Miscellaneous Disorders
Amyloidosis.
Bronchogenic cyst.
Broncholithiasis.
Bronchopleural fistula.
Thoracic endometriosis.
Foreign body.
Tracheopathia osteoplastica.
Lipoid pneumonia.
Organophosphate aspiration.
Chronic pancreatitis.
Neoplastic Disorders
Bronchial adenoma.
Lung cancer.
Tracheal tumors (mucoepidermoid, squamous cell, adenoid cystic, glomus).
Pulmonary blastoma.
Pleuropulmonary angiosarcoma.
Sarcoma (synovial, myofibroblastic).
Clear cell tumor.
Metastatic disease (prostate, renal, breast, ovarian).
Tracheobronchial schwannoma.
Pulmonary Airway Diseases
Bronchiectasis.
Bronchitis.
Granulomatous tracheobronchitis (ulcerative colitis, Crohn disease, granulomatosis with polyangiitis).
Cystic fibrosis.
Bullous emphysema.
Traumatic Injury
Blunt chest trauma.
Penetrating injury.
Ruptured bronchus.
Lightning injury.
Thoracic splenosis.
Vascular Disorders
Pulmonary embolism, infarction.
Systemic cholesterol emboli.
Intralobar sequestration.
Pulmonary artery aneurysms.
Behçet disease, Hughes-Stovin syndrome, traumatic pseudoaneurysms.
Acquired arteriovenous malformations.
Osler-Weber-Rendu syndrome (hereditary hemorrhagic telangiectasia).
Takayasu arteritis.
Aortic aneurysms.
Trachea–innominate artery fistulas.
Scimitar syndrome.
Vena cava-bronchial.
Dieulafoy disease of bronchus.
Ventriculopulmonary fistulas.
Hemangioma (sclerosing, cavernous, tracheal).

PULMONARY HEMORRHAGE, PEDIATRIC AGE

ICD-10CM #	P26.9	Pulmonary hemorrhage newborn

CAUSES OF PULMONARY HEMORRHAGE (HEMOPTYSIS)

Focal Hemorrhage

Bronchitis and bronchiectasis (especially cystic fibrosis related).
Infection (acute or chronic), pneumonia, abscess.
Tuberculosis.
Trauma.
Pulmonary arteriovenous malformation.
Foreign body (chronic).
Neoplasm including hemangioma.
Pulmonary embolus with or without infarction.
Bronchogenic cysts.
Diffuse hemorrhage
Idiopathic of infancy.
Congenital heart disease (including pulmonary hypertension, venoocclusive disease, congestive heart failure).
Prematurity.
Cow's milk hyperreactivity (Heiner syndrome).
Goodpasture syndrome.
Collagen vascular diseases (systemic lupus erythematosus, rheumatoid arthritis).
Henoch-Schönlein purpura and vasculitic disorders.
Granulomatous disease (Wegener granulomatosis).
Celiac disease.
Coagulopathy (congenital or acquired).
Malignancy.
Immunodeficiency.
Exogenous toxins.
Hyperammonemia.
Pulmonary hypertension.
Pulmonary alveolar hemosiderosis.
Tuberous sclerosis.
Lymphangiomyomatosis or lymphangioleiomyomatosis.
Physical injury or abuse.

PULMONARY HEMORRHAGIC SYNDROMES, DIFFUSE[21]

| ICD-10CM # | P26.1 | Massive pulmonary hemorrhage originating in the perinatal period |
| | R04.8 | Pulmonary hemorrhage |

CLASSIFICATION OF DIFFUSE PULMONARY HEMORRHAGE SYNDROMES

Nonimmunocompromised Patients

Antibasement membrane antibody disease/Goodpasture syndrome.
Diseases of presumed immune etiology, with or without nephropathy:
Systemic lupus erythematosus.
Rheumatoid arthritis.
Systemic sclerosis.
Systemic necrotizing vasculitis.
Granulomatosis with polyangiitis.
Microscopic polyarteritis.
Diseases with no known immune etiology:
Idiopathic pulmonary hemosiderosis.
Rapidly progressive glomerulonephritis without immune complexes.
Fibrillary glomerulonephritis.

Drug-induced (anticoagulants, trimellitic anhydride, cocaine, lymphangiography).
Valvular heart disease.
Disseminated intravascular coagulation.
Acute lung injury.
Tumors.

Immunocompromised Patients

Blood dyscrasias.
Infection.
Tumors.

PULMONARY INFILTRATES ASSOCIATIONS[106]

| ICD-10CM # | Varies with specific diagnosis |

PULMONARY INFILTRATES AND THEIR ASSOCIATION WITH SPECIFIC INFECTIOUS AND NONINFECTIOUS DISORDERS

Radiologic Sign	Potential Etiologic Disorder(s)
Interstitial infiltrates:	Pulmonary edema.
Diffuse alveolar damage:	Idiopathic pneumonia syndrome. Respiratory virus infection: RSV, parainfluenza virus, influenza virus, adenovirus, enterovirus. Herpesvirus infection: CMV, HSV, VZV, HHV-6. *Pneumocystis* pneumonia.
Focal airspace disease:	Bacterial pneumonia. Fungal pneumonia.
Nodules:	Fungal pneumonia (aspergillosis). *Nocardia* infection. *Legionella* infection. Septic bacterial emboli. Mycobacterial infection (with cavitation). EBV lymphoproliferative disorder. Relapsed malignancy. Pulmonary embolism (pleura based).
Halo sign or air-crescent sign:	Aspergillosis.

CMV, Cytomegalovirus; *EBV*, Epstein-Barr virus; *HHV*, human herpesvirus; *HSV*, herpes simplex virus; *RSV*, respiratory syncytial virus; *VZV*, varicella-zoster virus.

PULMONARY INFILTRATES, IMMUNOCOMPROMISED HOST[103]

| ICD-10CM # | J82 | Pulmonary eosinophilia, not elsewhere classified |
| | J98.4 | Other disorders of lung |

CAUSES OF PULMONARY INFILTRATES IN THE IMMUNOCOMPROMISED HOST

Infections:
Bacteria:
Gram-positive cocci, especially *Staphylococcus.*
Gram-negative bacilli.
Mycobacterium tuberculosis.
Nontuberculous mycobacteria.
Nocardia.
Viruses:
Cytomegalovirus.
Herpesvirus.
Fungi:
Aspergillus.
Cryptococcus.
Candida.
Mucor.
Pneumocystis jirovecii.
Protozoa:
Toxoplasma gondii (rare).
Pulmonary effects of therapy:
Chemotherapeutic agents.
Radiation therapy.
Pulmonary hemorrhage.
Congestive heart failure.
Disseminated malignancy.
Nonspecified interstitial pneumonitis (no defined etiology).

PULMONARY LESIONS

ICD-10CM #	J98.4	Other disorders of lung
	J70.9	Respiratory conditions due to unspecified external agent
	S27.309A	Unspecified injury of lung, unspecified, initial encounter

TB.
Legionella pneumonia.
Mycoplasma pneumonia.
Viral pneumonia.
Pneumocystis carinii.
Hypersensitivity pneumonitis.
Aspiration pneumonia.
Fungal disease (aspergillosis, histoplasmosis).
Acute respiratory distress syndrome associated with pneumonia.
Psittacosis.
Sarcoidosis.
Septic emboli.
Metastatic cancer.
Multiple pulmonary emboli.
Rheumatoid nodules.

PULMONARY MASS, SOLITARY, CAUSES[21]

| ICD-10CM # | R91.1 | Solitary pulmonary nodule |

CAUSES OF A SOLITARY PULMONARY MASS

Bronchial carcinoma.
Bronchial carcinoid.

Differential Diagnosis

II

Granuloma.
Hamartoma.
Metastasis.
Chronic pneumonia or abscess.
Hydatid cyst.
Pulmonary hematoma.
Bronchocele.
Fungus ball.
Massive fibrosis in coal workers.
Bronchogenic cyst.
Sequestration.
Arteriovenous malformation.
Pulmonary infarct.
Round atelectasis.

PULMONARY MASS, SOLITARY, MIMICS[21]

ICD-10CM #   Varies with specific diagnosis

SIMULANTS OF A SOLITARY PULMONARY MASS

Extrathoracic artifacts.
Cutaneous masses.
Bony lesions.
Pleural tumors or plaques.
Encysted pleural fluid.
Pulmonary vessels.

PULMONARY NODULE, SOLITARY

ICD-10CM #   J98.4 Other disorders of lung

Bronchogenic carcinoma.
Granuloma from histoplasmosis.
TB granuloma.
Granuloma from coccidioidomycosis.
Metastatic carcinoma.
Bronchial adenoma.
Bronchogenic cyst.
Hamartoma.
Arteriovenous malformation.
Other: fibroma, intrapulmonary lymph node, sclerosing hemangioma, bronchopulmonary sequestration.

PULMONARY NODULES, MULTIPLE IN PATIENT WITH PRIOR CANCER[74]

ICD-10CM #   Varies with specific diagnosis

Malignant.
Metastasis.
Primary lung cancer.
Benign.
Infectious
Fungal infection.
Mycobacterial infection.
Nocardiosis.
Septic emboli.
Noninfectious
Rheumatoid nodules.
Hamartoma.
Carcinoid.
Sarcoidosis.
Cryptogenic organizing pneumonia.
Vasculitis (granulomatosis with polyangiitis).

PULMONARY OPACITIES[94]

ICD-10CM #   Varies with specific diagnosis

CLASSIFICATION OF LARGE PULMONARY OPACITIES

Diffuse homogeneous.
Multifocal patchy.
Lobar without atelectasis.
Lobar with atelectasis.
Perihilar.
Peripheral.

PULMONARY–RENAL SYNDROMES, CAUSES[9]

ICD-10CM #   Varies with specific diagnosis

Systemic vasculitis: ANCA associated:	Anti-GBM disease (Goodpasture). Granulomatosis with polyangiitis. Microscopic polyarteritis. Churg-Strauss syndrome. Drugs (penicillamine, hydralazine, propylthiouracil). Immune complex disease. Lupus erythematosus. Henoch-Schönlein purpura. Mixed cryoglobulinemia. Rheumatoid vasculitis.
Infection:	Severe bacterial pneumonia, postinfectious glomerulonephritis, *Legionella,* hantavirus, opportunistic infection in immunocompromised patients, infective endocarditis.
Pulmonary edema and AKI:	Volume overload, severe left ventricular failure.
Multiorgan failure:	Acute respiratory distress syndrome and AKI.
Other:	Paraquat poisoning, renal vein or IVC thrombosis with pulmonary emboli.

AKI, Acute kidney injury; *ANCA,* antineutrophil cytoplasmic antibody; *GBM,* glomerular basement membrane; *IVC,* inferior vena cava.

PULSATILE TINNITUS[22]

ICD-10CM #	H93.A9	Pulsatile tinnitus, unspecified ear
	H93.A1	Pulsatile tinnitus right ear
	H93.A2	Pulsatile tinnitus left ear
	H93.A3	Pulsatile tinnitus bilateral

Synchronous with Pulse
Arterial Etiologies

Cardiovascular:	Hypertension. Valvular heart disease.
Intraosseous:	Paget disease, otosclerosis.
Neoplasm:	Paraganglioma (glomus tympanicum or jugulare). Vestibular schwannoma, endolymphatic sac tumor, hemangiopericytoma, temporal bone hemangioma, meningioma, and vascular metastases to the skull base.
Vascular stenosis:	Carotid artery atherosclerosis and subsequent stenosis. Other atherosclerotic disease (subclavian, external carotid). Fibromuscular dysplasia of the carotid artery.
Skull base variant:	Persistent stapedial artery. Aberrant or dehiscent internal carotid artery (intratympanic). Arteriovenous fistula or malformation, aneurysm. Arterial dissection (carotid, vertebral). Vascular compression of cranial nerve VIII. Hyperdynamic states with increased cardiac output (anemia, thyrotoxicosis, pregnancy).
Venous etiologies:	Sigmoid sinus and jugular bulb anomalies. Idiopathic intracranial hypertension. Dilated mastoid or condylar emissary veins. Dural sinus stenosis (transverse or sigmoid sinus). Idiopathic tinnitus, essential tinnitus, or venous hum.*

Asynchronous with Pulse

Muscular myoclonus:	Palatal, tensor tympani, or stapedial muscle myoclonus.
Otologic— middle ear:	Patulous eustachian tube. Ossicular or tympanic membrane abnormality. Otosclerosis. Semicircular canal dehiscence. Middle ear effusion.
Joints:	Temporomandibular joint disease.

*Venous hum, also known as idiopathic or essential tinnitus, is a subtype of pulsatile tinnitus whose existence is controversial. Historical cases of venous hum are thought to be secondary to undiagnosed idiopathic intracranial hypertension.

PULSELESS ELECTRICAL ACTIVITY

ICD-10CM #	I46.9	Cardiac arrest, cause unspecified

Hypovolemia.
Hypoxia.
Hyperkalemia.
Acidosis.
Cardiac tamponade.
Tension pneumothorax.
Pulmonary embolus.
Drug overdose.
Hypothermia.

PUPILLARY DILATATION, POOR RESPONSE TO DARKNESS

ICD-10CM #	H21.569	Pupillary abnormality, unspecified eye

Drugs (narcotics, general anesthetics, cholinergics).
Acute trauma (spasm from prostaglandin release).
Inflammation, infection (interruption of inhibitory fibers to the Edinger-Westphal nucleus).
Old age (loss of inhibition at midbrain from reticular activating formation).
Horner syndrome (sympathetic neuron interruption).
Adie syndrome tonic pupil.
Lymphoma.
Congenital miosis.

PURPURA

ICD-10CM #	D69.2	Other nonthrombocytopenic purpura
	D69.0	Allergic purpura
	D69.49	Other primary thrombocytopenia
	M31.1	Thrombotic microangiopathy

THROMBOTIC

Trauma.
Septic emboli, atheromatous emboli.
Disseminated intravascular coagulation.
Thrombocytopenia.
Meningococcemia.
Rocky Mountain spotted fever.
Hemolytic-uremic syndrome.
Viral infection: echo, coxsackie.
Scurvy.
Other: left atrial myxoma, cryoglobulinemia, vasculitis, hyperglobulinemic purpura.

PURPURA, NONPALPABLE[31]

ICD-10CM #	D69.2	Other nonthrombocytopenic purpura

INCREASED TRANSMURAL PRESSURE GRADIENT

Acute (Valsalva, coughing, vomiting, high altitude, weight lifting).
Chronic—venous stasis.

DECREASED MECHANICAL INTEGRITY OF MICROCIRCULATION AND SUPPORTING TISSUES

Age related (infancy and actinic purpura).
Glucocorticoid excess—Cushing syndrome and glucocorticoid therapy.
Vitamin C deficiency (scurvy).
Abnormal connective tissue—Ehlers-Danlos syndrome.
Amyloid infiltration of blood vessels.
Colloid milium.
Hormonal—female easy bruising syndrome (purpura simplex).
Lorenzo oil.
MELAS syndrome.

TRAUMA TO BLOOD VESSELS

Physical:
   Injuries.
   Child abuse.
   Factitial purpura.
Ultraviolet purpura:
   Purpuric sunburn.
   Solar purpura.
Infectious:
   Bacterial.
   Rickettsial.
   Fungal.
   Viral.
   Parasitic.
Embolic:
   Infectious organisms.
   Atheroemboli (cholesterol crystal emboli).
   Fat emboli.
Allergic and/or inflammatory:
   Serum sickness.
   Pigmented purpuric eruptions.
   Pyoderma gangrenosum.
   Contact dermatitis.
   Familial Mediterranean fever.
Neoplastic.
Metabolic:
   Erythropoietic porphyria.
   Calciphylaxis.
Immunoglobulin related (hyperglobulinemic purpura of Waldenström and light-chain vasculitis).
Drug related.
Thrombotic:
   Disseminated intravascular coagulation.
   Warfarin (Coumadin)-induced skin necrosis.
   Protein C or protein S deficiency, factor V Leiden, prothrombin G20201A.
   Purpura fulminans.
   Paroxysmal nocturnal hemoglobinuria.
   Antiphospholipid antibody syndrome.
Hemangioma with thrombocytopenia and consumptive coagulopathy (Kasabach-Merritt syndrome).
Unknown cause—psychogenic purpura.

PURPURA, NONPURPURIC DISORDERS SIMULATING PURPURA[18]

ICD-10CM #	Varies with specific diagnosis

Disorders with telangiectasias:
   Cherry angiomas.
   Hereditary hemorrhagic telangiectasia.
   Chronic actinic telangiectasia.
   Scleroderma.
   CREST syndrome.
   Ataxia-telangiectasia.
   Chronic liver disease.
   Pregnancy-related telangiectasia.
Kaposi sarcoma and other vascular sarcomas.
Fabry disease.
Neonatal extramedullary hematopoiesis.
Angioma serpiginosum.

PURPURA, PALPABLE[31]

ICD-10CM #	D69.2	Other nonthrombocytopenic purpura

Cutaneous vasculitis:
   Systemic vasculitides.
   Paraneoplastic vasculitis.
   Henoch-Schönlein purpura.
   Acute hemorrhagic edema of infancy.
   Livedoid vasculitis.
   Idiopathic.
   Urticarial.
   Cryoglobulinemia.
   Cryofibrinogenemia.
   Primary cutaneous diseases

QT INTERVAL PROLONGATION[97]

ICD-10CM #	R94.31	Abnormal electrocardiogram [ECG] [EKG]
	I45.81	Long QT syndrome

Drugs:
   Class I antiarrhythmics (e.g., disopyramide, procainamide, quinidine).
   Class III antiarrhythmics.
   Tricyclic antidepressants.
   Phenothiazines.
   Astemizole.
   Terfenadine.
   Adenosine.
   Antibiotics (e.g., erythromycin and other macrolides):
      Antifungal agents.
      Pentamidine, chloroquine.
Ischemic heart disease.
Cerebrovascular disease.
Rheumatic fever.
Myocarditis.
Mitral valve prolapse.
Electrolyte abnormalities.
Hypocalcemia.
Hypothyroidism.
Liquid protein diets.
Organophosphate insecticides.
Congenital prolonged QT syndrome.

RADIATION-INDUCED NEOPLASMS[54]

ICD-10CM #	Varies with specific diagnosis

RADIATION-INDUCED NEOPLASMS

Osteochondroma
Benign.
Exclusively with childhood irradiation.

Differential Diagnosis

II

Histologically identical to spontaneous osteochondroma.

Sarcoma

Malignant.

Latent period of 4 years or more.

Histologically identical to spontaneous sarcoma.

Commonly malignant fibrous histiocytoma or osteosarcoma.

Occurs in either bone or soft tissue.

Tumors in Other Organ Systems

Squamous cell cancer of the skin.

Breast cancer.

Leukemia, with shorter latent period than sarcoma.

RECTAL MASS, PALPABLE[2]

ICD-10CM #	R22.9	Localized swelling, mass and lump, unspecified

Rectal carcinoma.

Rectal polyp.

Hypertrophied anal papilla.

Diverticular phlegmon (prolapsing into the pouch of Douglas).

Sigmoid colon carcinoma (prolapsing into the pouch of Douglas).

Metastatic deposits at the pelvic reflection (Blumer shelf).

Primary pelvic malignancy (uterine, ovarian, prostatic, or cervical).

Mesorectal lymph nodes.

Endometriosis.

Solitary rectal ulcer syndrome.

Foreign body.

Feces.

Presacral cyst.

Amebic granuloma.

Vaginal tampon and even the pubic bone may be mistaken for a rectal mass.

RECTAL PAIN

ICD-10CM #	K62.89	Other specified diseases of anus and rectum

Anal fissure.

Thrombosed hemorrhoid.

Anorectal abscess.

Foreign bodies.

Fecal impaction.

Endometriosis.

Neoplasms (primary or metastatic).

Pelvic inflammatory disease.

Inflammation of sacral nerves.

Compression of sacral nerves.

Prostatitis.

Other: proctalgia fugax, uterine abnormalities, myopathies, coccygodynia.

RED BLOOD CELL APLASIA, ACQUIRED, ETIOLOGY

ICD-10CM #	D61.01	Constitutional (pure) red blood cell aplasia

Idiopathic (>50% of cases).

Medications (most frequent with phenytoin).

Non-Hodgkin lymphoma.

Viral infections (parvovirus B19, EB virus, mumps, hepatitis).

Myelodysplastic syndromes.

Thymoma.

Autoimmune diseases.

Allogenic bone marrow transplant from ABO incompatible donor.

Pregnancy.

RED BLOOD CELL FRAGMENTATION HEMOLYSIS, CAUSES[34]

ICD-10CM #	Varies with specific disorder

CAUSES OF RED BLOOD CELL FRAGMENTATION HEMOLYSIS

Damaged microvasculature.

Thrombotic thrombocytopenic purpura–hemolytic uremic syndrome (TTP–HUS).

Associated with pregnancy: preeclampsia or eclampsia; hemolysis plus elevated liver enzymes plus low platelets (HELLP syndrome).

Associated with malignancy, with or without mitomycin C treatment.

Vasculitis: polyarteritis, Wegener granulomatosis, acute glomerulonephritis, or Rickettsia-like infections.

Systemic lupus erythematosus.

Abnormalities of renal vasculature: malignant hypertension, acute glomerulonephritis, scleroderma, or allograft rejection with or without cyclosporine treatment.

Disseminated intravascular coagulation.

Malignant hypertension.

Catastrophic antiphospholipid antibody syndrome.

Atrioventricular malformations.

Kasabach-Merritt syndrome.

Hemangioendotheliomas.

Atrioventricular shunts for congenital and acquired conditions (e.g., stents, coils, transjugular intrahepatic portosystemic shunt, Levine shunts).

Cardiac abnormalities:

Replaced valve, prosthesis, graft, or patch.

Aortic stenosis or regurgitant jets (e.g., in ruptured sinus of Valsalva).

Drugs:

Cyclosporine.

Mitomycin.

Ticlopidine.

Clopidogrel.

Tacrolimus.

Cocaine.

Systemic infection:

Bacterial endocarditis.

Brucellosis.

Cytomegalovirus.

HIV.

Ehrlichiosis.

Rocky Mountain spotted fever

RED EYE

ICD-10CM #	H57.8	Other specified disorders of eye and adnexa

Infectious conjunctivitis (bacterial, viral).

Allergic conjunctivitis.

Acute glaucoma.

Keratitis (bacterial, viral).

Iritis.

Trauma.

RED EYE, ACUTE[112]

ICD-10CM #	H57.8	Other specified disorders of eye and adnexa

Obvious open globe.

Corneal abrasion.

Corneal ulcer.

Subconjunctival hemorrhage.

Hyphema.

Occult open globe.

Herpes simplex virus glaucoma.

Iritis, traumatic iritis.

Scleritis.

Conjunctivitis.

Blepharitis.

Ultraviolet keratitis.

Episcleritis.

Conjunctival foreign body.

Dry eye.

Contact lens overwear syndrome.

RED HOT JOINT

ICD-10CM #	Varies with specific diagnosis

Trauma.

Gout.

Infection (septic joint).

Pseudogout (calcium pyrophosphate dehydrate crystal deposition).

Psoriatic arthropathy.

Reactive arthritis.

Palindromic rheumatism.

RED URINE

ICD-10CM #	R39.19	Other difficulties with micturition

Hematuria.

Porphyrins.

Hemoglobinuria.

Myoglobinuria.

Medications (phenazopyridine, aminosalicylic acid, deferoxamine, phenazopyridine, phenolphthalein, NSAIDs, rifampin, phenytoin, methyldopa, doxorubicin, phenacetin).

Foods (beets, berries, maize).

Urate crystalluria.

RENAL ALLOGRAFT DYSFUNCTION[59]

ICD-10CM #	T86.1	Complications of renal allograft

IMMEDIATE/DELAYED GRAFT FUNCTION (1 TO 3 DAYS)

Acute tubular necrosis.

Hyperacute humoral rejection.

Urinary leak or obstruction.

Renal artery or vein thrombosis.

Recurrence of disease (e.g., focal segmental glomerulosclerosis).

EARLY POSTTRANSPLANTATION PERIOD (FIRST MONTH)

Acute cellular rejection.
Acute humoral rejection.
Calcineurin inhibitor toxicity.
Urinary tract obstruction.
Volume depletion.
Recurrence of disease.

Late Acute Dysfunction

Acute rejection.
Cyclosporine or tacrolimus toxicity.
Recurrence of primary disease.
Tubulointerstitial nephritis, drug-induced.
Renal artery stenosis.
Infection (bacterial urinary tract infection [UTI], cytomegalovirus, BK virus).
Hemodynamic (volume; use of angiotensin-converting enzyme inhibitor, angiotensin II receptor blocker).

Chronic Dysfunction

Chronic rejection.
Cyclosporine or tacrolimus toxicity.
Recurrent renal disease.
De novo renal disease.
Urinary tract obstruction.
Bacterial UTI.
Hypertensive nephrosclerosis.

RENAL ARTERY OCCLUSION, CAUSES

ICD-10CM # N28.0 Ischemia and infarction of kidney

Atrial fibrillation.
Angiography or stent placement.
Abdominal aortic surgery.
Trauma.
Renal artery aneurysm/dissection.
Vasculitis.
Thrombosis in patient with fibromuscular dysplasia.
Atherosclerosis.
Septic embolism.
Mural thrombus thromboembolism.
Atrial myxoma thromboembolism.
Mitral stenosis thromboembolism.
Prosthetic valve thromboembolism.
Renal cell carcinoma.

RENAL COLIC[112]

ICD-10CM # N23 Unspecified renal colic

Vascular:
    Abdominal aortic aneurysm.
    Aortic dissection.
    Renal artery dissection.
    Renal artery stenosis.
    Renal vein thrombosis.
    Renal infarct.
    Mesenteric ischemia.
    Retroperitoneal hemorrhage.
GI:
    Incarcerated hernia.
    Appendicitis.
    Cholecystitis.
    Biliary colic.
    Pancreatitis.
    Bowel obstruction.
    Diverticulitis.

Gynecologic:
    Ectopic pregnancy.
    Ovarian torsion.
    Tuboovarian abscess.
    Pelvic inflammatory disease.
    Endometriosis.
Genitourinary:
    Testicular torsion.
    Pyelonephritis.
    Perinephric abscess.
    Urinary tract tumor.
    Renal papillary necrosis.
    Upper urinary tract hemorrhage.
Musculoskeletal:
    Lumbar strain.
    Radiculopathy.
    Disk herniation.
    Vertebral compression fracture.
Dermatologic:
    Herpes zoster.
Miscellaneous:
    Factitious.

RENAL CYSTIC DISORDERS

ICD-10CM # Q61.01 Congenital single renal cyst

Simple cysts.
Acquired cystic kidney disease.
Autosomal dominant polycystic kidney disease.
Autosomal recessive polycystic kidney disease.
Medullary cystic disease.
Medullary sponge kidney.

RENAL DISEASE, SKIN MANIFESTATIONS[11]

ICD-10CM # Varies with specific diagnosis

SKIN MANIFESTATIONS SECONDARY TO RENAL DISEASE

Nonspecific

Pruritus.
Xerosis.
Acquired ichthyosis.
Pigmentary alteration:
    Pallor (secondary to anemia).
    Hyperpigmentation.
    Dyspigmentation (yellow tint).
Infections (fungal, bacterial, viral).
Purpura.

Somewhat Specific

Acquired perforating dermatosis.
Calciphylaxis.
Metastatic calcification.
Blistering disorders:
    Porphyria cutanea tarda.
    Pseudoporphyria.
Eruptive xanthomas.
Pseudo–Kaposi sarcoma.

Specific

Nephrogenic systemic fibrosis.
Dialysis-associated steal syndrome.
Metastatic renal cell carcinoma.
Dialysis-related amyloidosis.
Arteriovenous shunt dermatitis.
Uremic frost.

RENAL FAILURE, ACUTE, PIGMENT-INDUCED[43]

ICD-10CM # N19 Unspecified kidney failure

CAUSES OF PIGMENT-INDUCED ACUTE RENAL FAILURE

Rhabdomyolysis and myoglobinuria.
Vigorous exercise.
Arterial embolization.
Status epilepticus.
Status asthmaticus.
Coma-induced and pressure-induced myonecrosis.
Heat stress.
Diabetic ketoacidosis.
Myopathy.
Alcoholism.
Hypokalemia.
Hypophosphatemia.
Hemoglobinuria.
Transfusion reactions.
Snake envenomation.
Malaria.
Mechanical destruction of RBCs by prosthetic valves.
G6PD deficiency.

G6PD, Glucose-6-phosphate dehydrogenase; *RBCs*, red blood cells.

RENAL FAILURE, CHRONIC[59]

ICD-10CM # N18.9 Chronic kidney disease, unspecified

CAUSES OF CHRONIC RENAL FAILURE

Diabetic glomerulosclerosis (systemic disease involving the kidney).
Hypertensive nephrosclerosis.
Glomerular disease:
    Glomerulonephritis.
    Amyloidosis, light chain disease (systemic disease involving the kidney).
    Systemic lupus erythematosus, Wegener granulomatosis (systemic disease involving the kidney).
Tubulointerstitial disease:
    Reflux nephropathy (chronic pyelonephritis).
    Analgesic nephropathy.
    Obstructive nephropathy (stones, benign prostatic hypertrophy).
    Myeloma kidney (systemic disease involving the kidney).
Vascular disease:
    Scleroderma (systemic disease involving the kidney).
    Vasculitis (systemic disease involving the kidney).
    Renovascular renal failure (ischemic nephropathy).
    Atheroembolic renal disease (systemic disease involving the kidney).
Cystic disease:
    Autosomal dominant polycystic kidney disease.
    Medullary cystic kidney disease.

RENAL FAILURE, INTRINSIC OR PARENCHYMAL CAUSES[17]

ICD-10CM #	N17.0	Acute kidney failure with tubular necrosis
	N17.1	Acute kidney failure with acute cortical necrosis
	N17.2	Acute kidney failure with medullary necrosis
	N17.8	Other acute kidney failure
	N17.9	Acute kidney failure, unspecified
	N18.9	Chronic kidney disease, unspecified

ABNORMALITIES OF THE VASCULATURE

Renal arteries: atherosclerosis, thromboembolism, arteritis.
Renal veins: thrombosis.
Microvasculature: vasculitis, thrombotic microangiopathy.

ABNORMALITIES OF GLOMERULI (ACUTE GLOMERULONEPHRITIS)

Antiglomerular membrane disease (Goodpasture syndrome).
Immune complex glomerulonephritis: systemic lupus erythematosus, postinfectious, idiopathic, membranoproliferative.

ABNORMALITIES OF INTERSTITIUM (ACUTE INTERSTITIAL NEPHRITIS)

Drugs (e.g., antibiotics, NSAIDs, diuretics, anticonvulsants, allopurinol).
Infectious pyelonephritis.
Infiltrative: lymphoma, leukemia, sarcoidosis.

ABNORMALITIES OF TUBULES

Physical obstruction (uric acid, oxalate, light chains).
Acute tubular necrosis:
  Ischemic.
  Toxic (antibiotics, chemotherapy, immunosuppressives, radiocontrast dyes, heavy metals, myoglobin, hemolyzed RBCs).

RENAL FAILURE, POSTRENAL CAUSES[17]

ICD-10CM #	N17.0	Acute kidney failure with tubular necrosis
	N17.1	Acute kidney failure with acute cortical necrosis
	N17.2	Acute kidney failure with medullary necrosis
	N17.8	Other acute kidney failure
	N17.9	Acute kidney failure, unspecified
	N18.9	Chronic kidney disease, unspecified

URETER AND RENAL PELVIS

Intrinsic obstruction:
  Blood clots.
  Stones.
  Sloughed papillae: diabetes, sickle cell disease, analgesic nephropathy.
  Inflammatory: fungus ball.
Extrinsic obstruction:
  Malignancy.
  Retroperitoneal fibrosis.
  Iatrogenic: inadvertent ligation of ureters.

BLADDER

Prostatic hypertrophy or malignancy.
Neuropathic bladder.
Blood clots.
Bladder cancer.
Stones.

URETHRAL

Strictures.
Congenital valves.

RENAL FAILURE, PRERENAL CAUSES[17]

ICD-10CM #	N17.0	Acute kidney failure with tubular necrosis
	N17.1	Acute kidney failure with acute cortical necrosis
	N17.2	Acute kidney failure with medullary necrosis
	N17.8	Other acute kidney failure
	N17.9	Acute kidney failure, unspecified
	N18.9	Chronic kidney disease, unspecified

DECREASED CARDIAC OUTPUT

Congestive heart failure.
Arrhythmias.
Pericardial constriction or tamponade.
Pulmonary embolism.

HYPOVOLEMIA

GI tract loss (vomiting, diarrhea, nasogastric suction).
Blood losses (trauma, GI tract surgery).
Renal losses (diuretics, mineralocorticoid deficiency, postobstructive diuresis).
Skin losses (burns).

VOLUME REDISTRIBUTION (DECREASE IN EFFECTIVE BLOOD VOLUME)

Hypoalbuminemic states (cirrhosis, nephrosis).
Sequestration of fluid in "third" space (ischemic bowel, peritonitis, pancreatitis).
Peripheral vasodilation (sepsis, vasodilators, anaphylaxis).

ALTERED RENAL VASCULAR RESISTANCE

Increase in afferent vascular resistance (NSAIDs, liver disease, sepsis, hypercalcemia, cyclosporine).
Decrease in efferent arteriolar tone (ACE inhibitors).

RENAL INFARCTION[9]

ICD-10CM #	N28.0	Ischemia and infarction of kidney

CAUSES OF RENAL INFARCTION

Thrombosis: Spontaneous
Atherosclerotic disease of aorta and renal artery.
Fibromuscular dysplasia of renal artery.
Aneurysms of aorta or renal artery.
Dissection of aorta or renal artery:
  Marfan syndrome.
  Ehlers-Danlos syndrome.
Vasculitis involving renal artery:
  Polyarteritis nodosa.
  Takayasu arteritis.
  Kawasaki disease.
  Thromboangiitis obliterans.
  Other necrotizing vasculitides.
Inflammatory disease of the aorta or renal artery:
  Syphilis.
  Tuberculosis.
  Mycoses.
Hypercoagulable states:
  Nephrotic syndrome.
  Antiphospholipid syndrome.
  Antithrombin III deficiency.
  Homocystinuria.
Thrombotic microangiopathies:
  Hemolytic-uremic syndrome.
  Thrombotic thrombocytopenic purpura.
  Antiphospholipid syndrome.
  Malignant hypertension.
  Scleroderma.
  Sickle cell nephropathy.
  Polycythemia vera.
  Postpartum hemolytic-uremic syndrome.
  Hyperacute vascular allograft rejection.
Thrombosis: Induced
Traumatic.
Following endovascular intervention.
Postrenal transplantation.
Embolism
Cardiac source:
  Atrial fibrillation or other arrhythmias.
  Native and prosthetic valvular heart disease.
  Infective endocarditis.
  Marantic endocarditis.
Myocardial infarction with mural thrombi.
Left atrial myxoma or other tumor.
Noncardiac sources:
  Atheromatous embolic disease.
  Paradoxical emboli.
  Fat emboli.
  Tumor emboli.
Therapeutic renal embolization.
Segmental renal infarction of childhood.
Cisplatinum and gemcitabine.
Sickle cell disease or sickle cell trait.

RENAL PARENCHYMAL DISEASE, CHRONIC[21]

ICD-10CM #	N28.9	Disorder of kidney and ureter, unspecified

DIFFERENTIAL DIAGNOSIS OF CHRONIC RENAL PARENCHYMAL DISEASE

No Papillary/Caliceal Abnormality
Diffuse Parenchymal Loss
Bilateral:
   Chronic glomerulonephritis.
   Diffuse small-vessel disease.
   Hereditary nephropathies.
Unilateral:
   Renal artery stenosis.
   Postirradiation.
   Rare:
      Hypoplastic kidney.
      Postobstructive atrophy.

FOCAL PARENCHYMAL LOSS

Infarct.
Previous trauma.
Papillary/Caliceal Abnormality
Diffuse Parenchymal Loss
Obstructive nephropathy.
Generalized reflux nephropathy.
No Parenchymal Loss
Papillary necrosis.
TB.
Medullary sponge kidney.
Megacalices.
Pelvicaliceal cyst.
Focal Parenchymal Loss
Focal reflux nephropathy (chronic atrophic pyelonephritis).
TB.
Calculus disease.

RENAL VEIN THROMBOSIS, CAUSES

ICD-10CM #	I82.3	Embolism and thrombosis of renal vein

Nephrotic syndrome.
Renal cell carcinoma.
Aortic aneurysm causing compression.
Lymphadenopathy.
Retroperitoneal fibrosis.
Estrogen therapy.
Pregnancy.
Renal cell carcinoma with vein invasion.
Severe dehydration.

RESPIRATORY DISTRESS IN THE NEWBORN, CAUSES[32]

ICD-10CM #	J96.00	Acute respiratory failure

RESPIRATORY DISTRESS IN THE NEWBORN

Noncardiopulmonary
Hypothermia or hyperthermia.
Hypoglycemia.
Metabolic acidosis.
Drug intoxications; withdrawal.
Polycythemia.
Central nervous system insult.
Asphyxia.
Hemorrhage.

Neuromuscular disease.
Werdnig-Hoffman disease.
Myopathies.
Phrenic nerve injury.
Skeletal abnormalities.
Asphyxiating thoracic dystrophy.
Cardiovascular
Left-sided outflow obstruction.
Hypoplastic left heart.
Aortic stenosis.
Coarctation of the aorta.
Cyanotic lesions.
Transposition of the great vessels.
Total anomalous pulmonary venous return.
Tricuspid atresia.
Right-sided outflow obstruction.
Pulmonary
Upper airway obstruction.
Choanal atresia.
Vocal cord paralysis.
Meconium aspiration.
Clear fluid aspiration.
Transient tachypnea.
Pneumonia.
Pulmonary hypoplasia.
Primary.
Secondary.
Hyaline membrane disease.
Pneumothorax.
Pleural effusions.
Mass lesions.
Lobar emphysema.
Cystic adenomatoid malformation.

RESPIRATORY DYSFUNCTION ASSOCIATED WITH CENTRAL NERVOUS SYSTEM[74]

ICD-10CM #	Code varies with specific diagnosis

CEREBRAL CORTEX

Stroke.
Neoplasm.
Cerebral degeneration.
Seizures.

BRAIN STEM/BASAL GANGLIA

Stroke.
Neoplasm.
Poliomyelitis.
Central alveolar hypoventilation.
Progressive bulbar palsy.
Multiple system atrophy.
Anoxic encephalopathy.
Encephalitis.
Multiple sclerosis.
Parkinson disease.
Chorea.
Dyskinesias.

SPINAL CORD

Trauma.
Infarction or hemorrhage.
Demyelinating disease.
Disc compression.
Syringomyelia.
Tumor.
Epidural abscess.

RESPIRATORY DYSFUNCTION ASSOCIATED WITH PERIPHERAL NERVOUS SYSTEM[74]

ICD-10CM #	Code varies with specific diagnosis

MOTOR NERVES/ANTERIOR HORN CELL

Acute idiopathic polyneuropathy (Guillain-Barré syndrome).
Motor neuron disease.
Amyotrophic lateral sclerosis.
Spinal muscular atrophy.
Primary lateral sclerosis.
Critical illness neuropathy.
Vasculitides.
Toxins (e.g., lithium, arsenic, gold).
Metabolic.
Diabetes.
Porphyria.
Uremia.
Diphtheria.

NEUROMUSCULAR JUNCTION

Myasthenia gravis.
Lambert-Eaton myasthenic syndrome.
Toxins.
Botulism.
Snake venoms.
Scorpion bites.
Shellfish.
Crab poisoning.
Drugs.
Antibiotics.
Neuromuscular junction blockers.
Anticholinesterase inhibitors.
Corticosteroids.
Lidocaine.
Quinidine.
Lithium.
Antirheumatics.

MYOPATHIES

Muscular dystrophies.
Myotonic dystrophy.
Dermatomyositis.
Polymyositis.
Inclusion body myositis.
Glycogen storage diseases.
Pompe disease.
Forbes-Cori disease.
Thick filament myopathy.
Mitochondrial myopathy.
Nemaline body myopathy.
Severe hypokalemia.
Hypophosphatemia.

RESPIRATORY FAILURE, HYPOVENTILATORY[25]

ICD-10CM #	J96.00	Acute respiratory failure, unspecified whether with hypoxia or hypercapnia
	J96.90	Respiratory failure, unspecified, unspecified whether with hypoxia or hypercapnia

Differential Diagnosis

II

ABNORMAL RESPIRATORY CAPACITY (NORMAL RESPIRATORY WORKLOADS)

Acute depression of central nervous system:
Various causes.
Chronic central hypoventilation syndromes:
Obesity-hypoventilation syndrome.
Sleep apnea syndrome.
Hypothyroidism.
Shy-Drager syndrome (multisystem atrophy syndrome).
Acute toxic paralysis syndromes:
Botulism.
Tetanus.
Toxic ingestion or bites.
Organophosphate poisoning.
Neuromuscular disorders (acute and chronic):
Myasthenia gravis.
Guillain-Barré syndrome.
Drugs.
Amyotrophic lateral sclerosis.
Muscular dystrophies.
Polymyositis.
Spinal cord injury.
Traumatic phrenic nerve paralysis.

ABNORMAL PULMONARY WORKLOADS

Chronic obstructive pulmonary disease:
Chronic bronchitis.
Asthmatic bronchitis.
Emphysema.
Asthma and acute bronchial hyperreactivity syndromes.
Upper airway obstruction.
Interstitial lung diseases.

ABNORMAL EXTRAPULMONARY WORKLOADS

Chronic thoracic cage disorders:
Severe kyphoscoliosis.
After thoracoplasty.
After thoracic cage injury.
Acute thoracic cage trauma and burns.
Pneumothorax.
Pleural fibrosis and effusions.
Abdominal processes.

RESPIRATORY MUSCLE WEAKNESS[27]

ICD-10CM #   Varies with specific diagnosis

CAUSES OF DECREASED RESPIRATORY MUSCLE STRENGTH OR ENDURANCE

Disorders of the phrenic nerve:
Guillain-Barré syndrome.
Poliomyelitis.
Respiratory muscle atrophy.
Disorders of neuromuscular transmission:
Myasthenia gravis.
Ventilator dependence.
Malnutrition.
Myopathy.
Critical illness polyneuropathy/myopathy.
Altered diaphragmatic force-length relationship:
Dynamic hyperinflation and diaphragmatic flattening.

RETINOPATHY, HYPERTENSIVE

ICD-10CM #	H35.039	Hypertensive retinopathy, unspecified eye

Retinal venous obstruction.
Diabetic retinopathy.
Ocular ischemic syndrome.
Hyperviscosity.
Tortuosity of retinal artery.

RHINITIS

ICD-10CM #	J31.0	Chronic rhinitis
	J30.0	Vasomotor rhinitis
	J30.1	Allergic rhinitis due to pollen
	J30.2	Other seasonal allergic rhinitis
	J30.5	Allergic rhinitis due to food
	J30.89	Other allergic rhinitis
	J30.9	Allergic rhinitis, unspecified

Allergic rhinitis.
Infectious rhinitis.
Vasomotor rhinitis.
Exercise-induced rhinitis.
Emotional rhinitis.
Rhinitis medicamentosa.
Hormone-mediated rhinitis (menses, pregnancy, oral contraceptives, hypothyroidism).
GERD.
Chemical- or irritant-induced rhinitis.
Rhinitis mimics:
Deviated septum.
Enlarged adenoids.
Nasal polyps/tumors.
Foreign bodies.
Cerebrospinal fluid rhinorrhea.
Sarcoidosis.
Midline granuloma.
Granulomatosis with polyangiitis.
Systemic lupus erythematosus.
Sjögren syndrome.

RHINITIS, CHRONIC[28]

ICD-10CM #	J31.0	Chronic rhinitis

CLASSIFICATION OF CHRONIC RHINITIS

Allergic
Systemic.
Local (entopy).
Work-Related
Irritant.
Corrosive.
Immunologic.
Infectious (Rhinosinusitis)
Allergic.
Nonallergic.
Nonallergic
Idiopathic.
Nonallergic with eosinophilia.
Atrophic.

Primary.
Secondary.
Medication-related.
Topical vasoconstrictors (rhinitis medicamentosa).
Oral medications.
Exercise-induced.
Cold air-induced.
Gustatory.
Hormonal.
Aging.
Systemic diseases.

RHINOSINUSITIS, DIFFERENTIAL DIAGNOSIS[13]

ICD-10CM #	Varies with specific diagnosis

DIFFERENTIAL DIAGNOSIS OF RHINOSINUSITIS

Allergic Rhinitis
Seasonal.
Perennial.
Combined seasonal and perennial.
Allergic fungal rhinosinusitis.
Nonallergic Rhinitis
Nonallergic, noninflammatory idiopathic rhinopathy (vasomotor rhinitis).
Nonallergic rhinitis with eosinophilia syndrome (NARES).
Cold dry air-induced rhinitis.
Gustatory rhinitis.
Infectious Rhinosinusitis
Bacterial.
Viral.
Fungal.
Granulomatous.
Drug-Induced Rhinitis
Oral contraceptives.
Various antihypertensives and ocular β-blockers.
Topical decongestants (rhinitis medicamentosa).
Phosphodiesterase-5 antagonists.
Mechanical Causes of Rhinosinusitis
Septal deviation.
Nasal foreign body.
Choanal atresia or stenosis.
Adenoid hypertrophy.
Encephalocele.
Glioma.
Dermoid.
Innate and Acquired Immunity Disorders
Congenital or acquired immunodeficiencies.
Cystic fibrosis.
Immotile cilia syndrome.
Systemic Inflammatory Disorders
Sarcoidosis.
Granulomatosis with polyangiitis.
Vasculitis.
Neoplastic Causes
Benign:
Polyps.
Nasopharyngeal angiofibroma.
Inverting papilloma.
Malignant:
Adenocarcinoma.
Squamous cell carcinoma.
Esthesioneuroblastoma.
Lymphoma.
Rhabdomyosarcoma.

RIB DEFECTS ON X-RAY[21]

ICD-10CM #   Varies with specific diagnosis

CAUSES OF SUPERIOR MARGINAL RIB DEFECTS

Normal
Isolated defects.
Projectional artifacts (due to lordosis).
Neurologic
Paralytic poliomyelitis.
Quadriparesis.
Collagen Vascular Disease
Rheumatoid arthritis.
Systemic lupus erythematosus.
Systemic sclerosis.
Local Pressure
Chest drainage tube.
Osteochondroma.
Neural tumor.
Coarctation of aorta.
Hyperparathyroidism Miscellaneous
Osteogenesis imperfecta.
Marfan syndrome.

RIB NOTCHING ON X-RAY[21]

ICD-10CM #   Varies with specific diagnosis

CAUSES OF INFERIOR RIB NOTCHING
ARTERIAL

Aortic Obstruction
Aortic coarctation.
Aortic thrombosis.
Aortitis.

SUBCLAVIAN ARTERY OBSTRUCTION

Blalock-Taussig operation.
Arteritis.
Atherosclerotic occlusion.

PULMONARY OLIGEMIA

Pulmonary atresia.
Tetralogy of Fallot.
Multiple pulmonary arterial stenoses.

VENOUS
CHRONIC SUPERIOR VENA CAVAL OBSTRUCTION

Arteriovenous
Arteriovenous Malformation
Pulmonary.
Chest wall.

NEURAL

Neurofibromas.

RIGHT AXIS DEVIATION[97]

ICD-10CM #   Varies with specific diagnosis

Normal variation.
Right ventricular hypertrophy.
Left posterior fascicular block.
Lateral myocardial infarction.
Pulmonary embolism.
Dextrocardia.

Mechanical shifts or emphysema causing a vertical heart.

SACCADIC INTRUSIONS AND OSCILLATIONS[38]

ICD-10CM #   H55.81   Deficient saccadic eye movements

Square-wave jerks and square-wave oscillations.
Flutter (voluntary, involuntary).
Flutter dysmetria.
Microsaccadic flutter (variant of voluntary flutter?).
Opsoclonus.
Macro–square wave jerks (now designated square-wave pulses).
Ocular bobbing, reverse and inverse bobbing, dipping, and reverse dipping.
Superior oblique myokymia.
Convergence-retraction nystagmus.
Abduction nystagmus with internuclear ophthalmoplegia.
Ticlike ocular myoclonic jerks (eye tics).

SALIVARY GLAND ENLARGEMENT

ICD-10CM #   K11.1   Hypertrophy of salivary gland

Neoplasm.
Sialolithiasis.
Infection (mumps, bacterial infection, HIV, TB).
Sarcoidosis.
Idiopathic.
Acromegaly.
Anorexia/bulimia.
Chronic pancreatitis.
Medications (e.g., phenylbutazone).
Cirrhosis.
Diabetes mellitus.

SALIVARY GLAND SECRETION, DECREASED

ICD-10CM #   K11.7   Disturbances of salivary secretion
          R68.2   Dry mouth, unspecified

Medications (antihistamines, antidepressants, neuroleptics, antihypertensives).
Dehydration.
Anxiety.
Sjögren syndrome.
Sarcoidosis.
Mumps.
Amyloidosis.
Central nervous system disorders.
Head and neck radiation.

SCLERODERMA-LIKE SYNDROMES[18]

ICD-10CM #   Varies with specific diagnosis

OTHER DISEASES

Morphea.
Eosinophilic fasciitis.

Scleredema (of Buschke).
Scleromyxedema.
Graft-versus-host disease.
Nephrogenic-fibrosing dermopathy.

ENVIRONMENTAL AGENTS AND DRUGS

Bleomycin.
L-Tryptophan.
Organic solvents.
Pentazocine.
Toxic oil syndrome.
Vinyl chloride disease.
Gadolinium.

SCLERODERMA-LIKE SYNDROMES, DRUG-INDUCED[53]

ICD-10CM #   M34.2   Systemic sclerosis induced by drug or chemical

CHEMICALS

Silica.
Heavy metals.
Mercury.

ORGANIC CHEMICALS

Vinyl chloride.
Benzene.
Toluene.
Trichloroethylene.

DRUGS

Bleomycin.
Pentazocine.
Taxol.
Cocaine.

DIETARY SUPPLEMENT/ APPETITE SUPPRESSANTS

L-tryptophan (or contaminant).
Mazindol.
Fenfluramine.
Diethylpropion.

SCROTAL CALCIFICATIONS[15]

ICD-10CM #   Varies with specific diagnosis

SCROTAL CALCIFICATIONS

Testicular
Solitary, postinflammatory granulomatous, vascular.
Microlithiasis.
"Burned-out" germ cell tumor.
Large-cell calcifying Sertoli cell tumor.
Teratoma.
Mixed germ cell tumor.
Sarcoid.
TB.
Chronic infarct.
Extratesticular
Tunica vaginalis "scrotal pearls."
Chronic epididymitis.
Schistosomiasis.

Differential Diagnosis

II

SCROTAL MASSES, BOYS AND ADOLESCENTS[19]

ICD-10CM #	R22.9	Localized swelling, mass and lump, unspecified

PAINFUL

Testicular torsion.
Torsion of appendix testis.
Epididymitis.
Trauma: ruptured testis, hematocele.
Inguinal hernia (incarcerated).
Mumps orchitis.

PAINLESS

Hydrocele.
Inguinal hernia.*
Varicocele.
Spermatocele.
Testicular tumor.
Henoch-Schönlein purpura.
Idiopathic scrotal edema.

*May be associated with discomfort.

SCROTAL PAIN[25]

ICD-10CM #	S31.30XA	Unspecified open wound of scrotum and testes, initial encounter
	N50.9	Disorder of male genital organs, unspecified
	R10.2	Pelvic and perineal pain
	N49.9	Inflammatory disorder of unspecified male genital organ
	N50.1	Vascular disorders of male genital organs
	N49.9	Inflammatory disorder of unspecified male genital organ

Torsion:
    Appendages.
    Spermatic cord.
Infection:
    Orchitis.
    Abscess.
    Epididymitis.
Neoplasia:
    Benign.
    Malignant.
    Incarcerated hernia.
    Trauma.
    Hydrocele.
    Spermatocele.
    Varicocele.

SCROTAL PAIN, ADOLESCENT OR PEDIATRIC PATIENT[89]

ICD-10CM #	Varies with specific diagnosis

DIFFERENTIAL DIAGNOSIS OF PEDIATRIC ADOLESCENT ACUTE SCROTAL PAIN

Appendage torsion:
    Appendix testis.
    Other appendage (epididymis, paradidymis, vas aberrans).
Spermatic cord torsion:
    Intravaginal, acute or intermittent.
    Extravaginal.
Epididymitis:
    Infectious:
        Urinary tract infection.
        Sexually transmitted disease.
        Viral.
    Sterile or traumatic.
Scrotal edema or erythema:
    Diaper dermatitis, insect bite, or other skin lesions.
    Idiopathic scrotal edema.
Orchitis:
    Associated with epididymitis with or without abscess.
    Vasculitis (e.g., Henoch-Schönlein purpura).
    Viral illness (mumps).
Trauma:
    Hematocele or scrotal contusion or testis rupture.
Hernia or hydrocele:
    Inguinal hernia with or without incarceration.
    Communicating hydrocele.
    Encysted hydrocele with or without torsion.
    Associated with acute abdominal pathology (e.g., appendicitis, peritonitis).
    Varicocele.
    Intrascrotal mass:
    Cystic dysplasia or tumor of testis.
    Epididymal cyst, spermatocele or tumor.
    Other paratesticular tumors.
Musculoskeletal pain from inguinal tendonitis or muscle strain.
Referred pain (e.g., ureteral calculus or anomaly).

SCROTAL SWELLING

ICD-10CM #	N50.8	Other specified disorders of male genital organs

Hydrocele.
Varicocele.
Neoplasm.
Acute epididymitis.
Orchitis.
Trauma.
Hernia.
Torsion of spermatic cord.
Torsion of epididymis.
Torsion of testis.
Insect bite.
Folliculitis.
Sebaceous cyst.
Thrombosis of spermatic vein.

Other: lymphedema, dermatitis, fat necrosis, Henoch-Schönlein purpura, idiopathic scrotal edema.

SEIZURE

ICD-10CM #	R56.9	Unspecified convulsions

Syncope.
Alcohol abuse/withdrawal.
TIA.
Hemiparetic migraine.
Psychiatric disorders.
Carotid sinus hypersensitivity.
Hyperventilation, prolonged breath holding.
Hypoglycemia.
Narcolepsy.
Movement disorders (tics, hemiballismus).
Hyponatremia.
Brain tumor (primary or metastatic).
Tetanus.
Strychnine, phencyclidine poisoning.

SEIZURE, PEDIATRIC[43]

ICD-10CM #	R56.9	Unspecified convulsions
	P90	Convulsions of newborn

FIRST MONTH OF LIFE

First Day
Hypoxia.
Drugs.
Trauma.
Infection.
Hyperglycemia.
Hypoglycemia.
Pyridoxine deficiency.
Day 2 to 3
Infection.
Drug withdrawal.
Hypoglycemia.
Hypocalcemia.
Developmental malformation.
Intracranial hemorrhage.
Inborn error of metabolism.
Hyponatremia or hypernatremia.
Day >4
Infection.
Hypocalcemia.
Hyperphosphatemia.
Hyponatremia.
Developmental malformation.
Drug withdrawal.
Inborn error of metabolism.

1 TO 6 MO

As above.

6 MO TO 3 YR

Febrile seizures.
Birth injury.
Infection.
Toxin.
Trauma.
Metabolic disorder.
Cerebral degenerative disease.

>3 YR

Idiopathic.
Infection.
Trauma.
Cerebral degenerative disease.

SEIZURE MIMICS[18]

ICD-10CM #   Varies with specific diagnosis

NONEPILEPTIC EPISODIC DISORDERS THAT MAY RESEMBLE SEIZURES

Movement disorders: myoclonus, paroxysmal choreoathetosis, episodic ataxias, hyperexplexia (startle disease).
Migraine: confusional, vertebrobasilar, visual auras.
Syncope.
Behavioral and psychiatric: psychogenic nonepileptic attacks (pseudoseizures), hyperventilation syndrome, panic or anxiety disorder, dissociative states.
Cataplexy (usually associated with narcolepsy).
Transient ischemic attack.
Alcoholic blackouts.
Hypoglycemia.

SEIZURES, NEONATAL, DUE TO NEUROCUTANEOUS DISORDERS[20]

ICD-10CM #   Varies with specific diagnosis

INCONTINENTIA PIGMENTI

Seizure type.
    Neonatal seizures.
Generalized tonic-clonic.
Cutaneous manifestations.
Erythematous bullae (newborn).
Pigmentary whorls (infancy).
Depigmented areas (childhood).

LINEAR NEVUS SEBACEOUS SYNDROME

Seizure type.
    Infantile spasms.
    Lennox-Gastaut syndrome.
    Generalized tonic-clonic.
Cutaneous manifestation.
    Linear facial sebaceous nevus.

NEUROFIBROMATOSIS

Seizure type.
    Generalized tonic-clonic.
    Partial complex.
    Partial simple motor.
Cutaneous manifestations.
    Cafe au lait spots.
    Axillary freckles.
    Neural tumors.

STURGE-WEBER SYNDROME

Seizure type.
    Epilepsia partialis continua.
    Partial simple motor.
    Status epilepticus.

Cutaneous manifestation.
    Hemifacial hemangioma.

TUBEROUS SCLEROSIS

Seizure type.
    Neonatal seizures.
    Infantile spasms.
    Lennox-Gastaut syndrome.
    Generalized tonic-clonic.
    Partial simple motor.
    Partial complex.

CUTANEOUS MANIFESTATIONS

Abnormal hair pigmentation.
Adenoma sebaceum.
Café-au-lait spots.
Depigmented areas.
Shagreen patch.

SEIZURES, NEONATAL PEAK TIME OF ONSET[20]

ICD-10CM #   Varies with specific diagnosis

24 H

Bacterial meningitis and sepsis.[a]
Direct drug effect.
Hypoxic-ischemic encephalopathy.[a]
Intrauterine infection.
Intraventricular hemorrhage at term.[a]
Laceration of tentorium or falx.
Pyridoxine dependency.[a]
Subarachnoid hemorrhage.*

24 TO 72 H

Bacterial meningitis and sepsis.[a]
Cerebral contusion with subdural hemorrhage.
Cerebral dysgenesis.[a]
Cerebral infarction.[a]
Drug withdrawal.
Glycine encephalopathy.
Glycogen synthase deficiency.
Hypoparathyroidism-hypocalcemia.
Idiopathic cerebral venous thrombosis.
Incontinentia pigmenti.
Intracerebral hemorrhage.
Intraventricular hemorrhage in premature newborns.[a]
Pyridoxine dependency.[a]
Subarachnoid hemorrhage.
Tuberous sclerosis.
Urea cycle disturbances.

72 H TO 1 WK

Cerebral dysgenesis.
Cerebral infarction.[a]
Familial neonatal seizures.
Hypoparathyroidism.
Idiopathic cerebral venous thrombosis.[a]
Intracerebral hemorrhage.
Kernicterus.
Methylmalonic acidemia.
Nutritional hypocalcemia.[a]
Propionic acidemia.
Tuberous sclerosis.
Urea cycle disturbances.

1 TO 4 WK

Adrenoleukodystrophy, neonatal.
Cerebral dysgenesis.
Fructose dysmetabolism.
Gaucher disease type 2.
GM1 gangliosidosis type 1.
Herpes simplex encephalitis.[a]
Idiopathic cerebral venous thrombosis.[a]
Ketotic hyperglycinemias.
Maple syrup urine disease, neonatal.[a]
Tuberous sclerosis.
Urea cycle disturbances.

---

[a]Denotes the most common conditions and the ones with disease-modifying treatments.

SEXUAL DIFFERENTIATION ABNORMALITIES[89]

ICD-10CM #   Varies with specific diagnosis

ABNORMAL SEXUAL DIFFERENTIATION

Disorders of gonadal differentiation.
    Seminiferous tubule dysgenesis.
    Klinefelter syndrome.
    46,XX male.
    Syndromes of gonadal dysgenesis:
       Turner syndrome.
       Pure gonadal dysgenesis.
       Mixed gonadal dysgenesis.
       Partial gonadal dysgenesis (dysgenetic male pseudohermaphroditism).
       Bilateral vanishing testis, testicular regression syndromes.
Ovotesticular DSD (true hermaphroditism).
46,XX DSD (masculinized female):
    Congenital adrenal hyperplasia (21-hydroxylase, 11β-hydroxylase, 3β-hydroxysteroid dehydrogenase deficiencies).
Maternal androgens.
46,XY DSD (undermasculinized male).
    Leydig cell agenesis, unresponsiveness.
    Disorders of testosterone biosynthesis.
    Variants of congenital adrenal hyperplasia affecting corticosteroid and testosterone synthesis:
       StAR deficiency (congenital lipoid adrenal hyperplasia).
       Cytochrome P450 oxidoreductase (POR) deficiency.
       3β-Hydroxysteroid dehydrogenase deficiency.
       17β-Hydroxylase deficiency.
Disorders of testosterone biosynthesis:
    17, 20-Lyase deficiency.
    17β-Hydroxysteroid oxidoreductase deficiency.
Disorders of androgen-dependent target tissue:
    Androgen receptor and postreceptor defects.
    Syndrome of complete (severe) androgen insensitivity.
    Syndrome of partial androgen insensitivity.
    Mild androgen insensitivity syndrome (MAIS).
Disorders of testosterone metabolism by peripheral tissues:
    5α-Reductase deficiency.
    Disorders of synthesis, secretion, or response to Müllerian-inhibiting substance.

Persistent Müllerian duct syndrome.
Unclassified forms:
    In females: Mayer-Rokitansky-Küster-Hauser
        syndrome.
    Disorder of sex development (DSD).

SEXUAL DYSFUNCTION, FEMALE[18]

ICD-10CM #	R37	Sexual dysfunction, unspecified

FACTORS THAT MAY INFLUENCE SEXUAL FUNCTIONING IN WOMEN

Biologic
Medications (e.g., antidepressants, antihypertensives).
Vaginal atrophy, pain with intercourse.
Low testosterone levels (e.g., bilateral oophorectomy).
Illness (e.g., diabetes, hypothyroidism, cerebrovascular accident).
Sleep disturbances, fatigue.
Disability or pain from illness (e.g., arthritis).
Incontinence.
Psychologic
Depression.
Body image.
Interpersonal
Marital issues.
Poor communication.
Partner's sexual problems (e.g., erectile dysfunction).
Partner's health problems (e.g., myocardial infarction).
Sociocultural
Ageism ("too old" to want sex).
Multiple other obligations and commitments.
Lack of partner.

SEXUALLY TRANSMITTED DISEASES, ANORECTAL REGION[10]

ICD-10CM #	K62.89	Other specified diseases of anus and rectum

ULCERATIVE
Lymphogranuloma venereum.
Herpes simplex virus.
Early (primary) syphilis.
Chancroid (*Haemophilus ducreyi*).
Cytomegalovirus.
Idiopathic (usually HIV positive).

NONULCERATIVE
Condyloma acuminatum.
Gonorrhea.
Chlamydia (*Chlamydia trachomatis*).
Syphilis.

SEXUAL PRECOCITY[113]

ICD-10CM #	E30.1	Precocious puberty
	E30.8	Other disorders of puberty

TRUE PRECOCIOUS PUBERTY
Premature reactivation of LHRH pulse generator.

INCOMPLETE SEXUAL PRECOCITY
(Pituitary gonadotropin independent).
Males
Chorionic gonadotropin-secreting tumor.
Leydig cell tumor.
Familial testotoxicosis.
Virilizing congenital adrenal hyperplasia.
Virilizing adrenal tumor.
Premature adrenarche.
Females
Granulosa cell tumor (follicular cysts may be manifested similarly).
Follicular cyst.
Feminizing adrenal tumor.
Premature thelarche.
Premature adrenarche.
Late-onset virilizing congenital adrenal hyperplasia.
In Both Sexes
McCune-Albright syndrome.
Primary hypothyroidism.

SHOULDER PAIN

ICD-10CM #	M24.819	Other specific joint derangements of unspecified shoulder, not elsewhere classified
	M75.80	Other shoulder lesions, unspecified shoulder
	S43.409A	Unspecified sprain of unspecified shoulder joint, initial encounter
	S46.919A	Strain of unspecified muscle, fascia and tendon at shoulder and upper arm level, unspecified arm, initial encounter

WITH LOCAL FINDINGS IN SHOULDER
Trauma: contusion, fracture, muscle strain, trauma to spinal cord.
Arthrosis, arthritis, rheumatoid arthritis, ankylosing spondylitis.
Bursitis, synovitis, tendinitis, tenosynovitis.
Aseptic (avascular) necrosis.
Local infection: septic arthritis, osteomyelitis, abscess, herpes zoster, TB.

WITHOUT LOCAL FINDINGS IN SHOULDER
Cardiovascular disorders: ischemic heart disease, pericarditis, aortic aneurysm.
Subdiaphragmatic abscess, liver abscess.
Cholelithiasis, cholecystitis.

Pulmonary lesions: apical bronchial carcinoma, pleurisy, pneumothorax, pneumonia.
GI lesions: peptic ulcer disease, gastric neoplasm, peptic esophagitis.
Pancreatic lesions: carcinoma, calculi, pancreatitis.
Central nervous system abnormalities: neoplasm, vascular abnormalities.
Multiple sclerosis.
Syringomyelia.
Polymyositis/dermatomyositis.
Psychogenic.
Polymyalgia rheumatica.
Ectopic pregnancy.

SHOULDER PAIN BY LOCATION

ICD-10CM #	M75.80	Other shoulder lesions, unspecified shoulder
	S43.499A	Other sprain of unspecified shoulder joint, initial encounter
	S46.019A	Strain of muscle(s) and tendon(s) of the rotator cuff of unspecified shoulder, initial encounter
	S46.819A	Strain of other muscles, fascia and tendons at shoulder and upper arm level, unspecified arm, initial encounter

TOP OF SHOULDER (C4)
Cervical source.
Acromioclavicular.
Sternoclavicular.
Diaphragmatic.

SUPEROLATERAL (C5)
Rotator cuff tendinitis.
Impingement.
Adhesive capsulitis.
Glenohumeral arthritis.

ANTERIOR
Bicipital tendinitis and rupture.
Glenoid labral tear.
Adhesive capsulitis.
Glenohumeral arthritis.
Osteonecrosis.

AXILLARY
Neoplasm (Pancoast, mediastinal).
Herpes zoster.

SHOULDER PAIN, IN DIFFERENT AGE GROUPS[41]

ICD-10CM #	M25.519	Pain in unspecified shoulder

COMMON CAUSES OF SHOULDER PAIN IN DIFFERENT AGE GROUPS

Childhood (2 to 10 yr)
Intraarticular
Instability.
Periarticular
Osteochondromas.
Adolescence (10 to 18 yr)
Intraarticular
Instability.
Early Adulthood (18 to 30 yr)
Intraarticular
Instability.
Acromioclavicular joint sprain.
Periarticular
Calcific tendonitis.
Impingement.
Referred
Cervical.
Adulthood (30 to 60 yr)
Intraarticular
Osteochondritis.
Osteoarthritis.
Frozen shoulder.
Inflammatory arthritis.
Periarticular
Calcific tendonitis.
Impingement.
Rotator cuff tear.
Bicipital tendonitis.
Referred
Cervical.
Old Age (>60 yr)
Intraarticular
Osteochondritis.
Osteoarthritis.
Frozen shoulder.
Inflammatory arthritis.
Periarticular
Impingement.
Rotator cuff tear.
Referred
Cervical.

SINOVENOUS OCCLUSIVE DISEASE, INTRACRANIAL[38]

ICD-10CM #   Varies with specific diagnosis

Facial/orbital/paranasal sinuses/middle ear infections.
Trichinosis.
Syphilis.
Varicella-zoster virus infections.
HIV infections.
Sepsis.
Pregnancy and puerperium.
Carcinoma.
Dehydration.
Marasmus.
L-Asparaginase therapy.
Androgen therapy.
Cisplatin and etoposide therapy.
Epsilon-aminocaproic acid therapy.
Medroxyprogesterone therapy.
Cis-diamminedichloroplatinum (CDDP) and etoposide (VP-16) therapy.
catheters, cardiac pacemakers.

Polyarteritis nodosa.
Systemic lupus erythematosus.
Granulomatosis with polyangiitis.
Behçet disease.
Kohlmeier-Degos disease (malignant atrophic papulosis).
Osteopetrosis.
Inflammatory bowel disease.
Sarcoidosis.
Osteoporosis.
Congestive heart failure.
Nephrotic syndrome.
Budd-Chiari syndrome.
Chronic lung disease.
Diabetes mellitus.
Cerebral arterial occlusions.
Homocystinuria.
Head injury.
Paroxysmal nocturnal hemoglobinuria.
Sickle cell disease and trait.
Polycythemia vera.
Essential thrombocythemia.
Iron-deficiency anemia.
Hypoplasminogenemia.
Afibrinogenemia.
Cryofibrinogenemia.
Antiphospholipid antibody syndrome (APAS).
Disseminated intravascular coagulation.
Antithrombin deficiency.
Protein S deficiency.
Protein C deficiency.
Combined deficiencies (protein C, protein S, and antithrombin III).
Activated protein C resistance.
Factor V Leiden mutation.
Prothrombin G20210 mutation.
Elevated factor VIII plasma levels.
Heparin-induced thrombocytopenia.
Maternal coagulopathy (twin transfusion reaction).
Familial histidine-rich glycoprotein deficiency.
Arteriovenous malformations.
Sturge-Weber syndrome.
Neoplasm (meningioma, metastasis, glomus tumors).
Idiopathic.

SINUS NODE DYSFUNCTION[59]

ICD-10CM #   Varies with specific diagnosis

CAUSES OF SINUS NODE DYSFUNCTION

Intrinsic
Hypothyroidism.
Fibrocalcific degeneration.
Increased vagal tone, especially in sleep apnea.
Congenital mutations.
Scleroderma.
Amyloidosis.
Chagas disease.
Extrinsic
Trauma, including cardiac surgery.
Drugs:
  Calcium-channel blockers.
  β-Blockers.
  Digoxin.
  Antiarrhythmic medications (amiodarone, dronedarone, sotalol, flecainide, propafenone).
  Lithium.

SINUS OF VALSALVA ANEURYSMS[37]

ICD-10CM #   Varies with specific diagnosis

Congenital: single cusp involved with normal aorta.
  Localized deficiency of the tissue in the aortic annulus.
  Retraction of a cusp into a closing ventricular septal defect.
Inherited: all cusps involved with annuloaortic ectasia.
  Marfan syndrome.
  Ehlers-Danlos syndrome.
Acquired: saccular false aneurysms.
  Aortic root abscess with endocarditis.
  Luetic aortitis.
  Aortic dissection.

SINUS OSTIAL OBSTRUCTION[42]

ICD-10CM #   Varies with specific diagnosis

FACTORS THAT PREDISPOSE TO SINUS OSTIAL OBSTRUCTION

Mucosal Swelling
Systemic factors:
  Viral upper respiratory infection.
  Allergic inflammation.
  Cystic fibrosis.
  Immune disorders.
  Ciliary dyskinesia.
  Tobacco smoke.
Local insult:
  Facial trauma.
  Swimming, diving.
  Rhinitis medicamentosa.
  Nasal intubation.
Mechanical Obstruction
Choanal atresia.
Deviated septum.
Nasal polyps.
Foreign body.
Tumor.
Ethmoid bullae.

SINUS TACHYCARDIA[27]

ICD-10CM # R00.0 Tachycardia, unspecified

DIFFERENTIAL DIAGNOSIS OF SINUS TACHYCARDIA

Etiologic Category
Specific Disorders
Hemodynamic:
  Heart failure: systolic and diastolic heart failure caused by ischemic, valvular, or nonischemic myopathy.
  Loss of circulating blood volume: GI bleeding, anemia, shifts of intravascular fluid due to changes in colloidal osmotic pressure or inflammation.
  Septic shock: dehydration.
  Vascular shunts: intracardiac as well as aortovenous malformations, fistulas.
  Pulmonary embolism.
Metabolic and neurohumoral:

Differential Diagnosis

II

Sepsis: infections and inflammatory conditions.
Hyperthyroidism.
Paget disease of the bone.
Pheochromocytoma.
Carcinoid syndrome.
Beriberi heart disease.
Carcinoma.
Hyperpyrexia.
Acidosis.
Exercise.
Pharmacologic:
Sympathomimetic agents: isoproterenol, epinephrine, or dopamine.
Vagolytic agents, atropine, scopolamine.
Vasodilators: nitrates, ACE inhibitors, angiotensin receptor blockers, hydrazine, as well as centrally acting vasodilators.
Thyroid preparations, caffeine and nicotine.
Bronchodilators, including theophylline and terbutaline.
Anesthetic agents, including spinal anesthetics, causing peripheral vasodilation.
Drugs of abuse: amphetamines, cocaine, "ecstasy," cannabis.
Neurologic/psychologic:
Pain.
Fear, anxiety, and hysteria.
Hyper-β adrenergic phase of neurocardiogenic syncope.
Autonomic dysfunction such as with diabetes.

SKIN AND RENAL[11]

| ICD-10CM # | Varies with specific diagnosis |

SELECTED CONDITIONS WITH CONCURRENT SKIN AND RENAL INVOLVEMENT

More Common
Lupus erythematosus.
Leukocytoclastic vasculitis.
Henoch-Schönlein purpura.
Mixed cryoglobulinemia.
Diabetes mellitus.
Systemic vasculitis.

Less Common
Nail-patella syndrome.
Hemolytic-uremic syndrome.
Toxic shock syndrome.
Mixed connective tissue disease.
Dermatomyositis.
Rheumatoid arthritis.
Sjögren syndrome.
Dermatitis herpetiformis.
Sarcoidosis.
Systemic sclerosis.
Ulcerative colitis.
Amyloidosis.
Toxic epidermolysis.
Hypothyroidism.
Graves disease.
Fabry disease.
Neurofibromatosis.
Hurler syndrome.
Castleman disease.
Infectious endocarditis.
Staphylococcal scalded skin syndrome (in adults).

SKIN INDURATION, CHRONIC[90]

| ICD-10CM # | Varies with specific diagnosis |

CONDITIONS ASSOCIATED WITH CHRONIC SKIN INDURATION

Systemic sclerosis.
Localized scleroderma.
Scleroderma variants.
Scleredema:
Scleredema adultorum of Buschke.
Scleredema diabeticorum.
Scleredema neonatorum.
Scleromyxedema.
Nephrogenic fibrosing dermopathy.
Eosinophilic syndromes:
Eosinophilic fasciitis (diffuse fasciitis with eosinophilia, Shulman disease).
Eosinophilia-myalgia syndrome.
Toxic oil syndrome.
Chronic graft-versus-host disease.
Pseudoscleroderma (local injection of vitamin K, bleomycin, pentazocine).
Metabolic diseases:
Porphyria cutanea tarda.
Phenylketonuria.
Werner syndrome.
Acromegaly.
Pachydermoperiostosis.
Polyneuropathy, organomegaly, endocrinopathy, monoclonal gammopathy (POEMS).
Stiff skin syndrome.
Reflex sympathetic dystrophy.
Hemiplegia.

SKIN, THICKENED AND TETHERED[96]

| ICD-10CM # | Varies with specific diagnosis |

CREST syndrome, scleroderma, or mixed connective tissue disease.
Eosinophilic fasciitis.
Localized morphea—small areas of sclerosis.
Chemicals—vinyl chloride, pentazocine, bleomycin, toxic oil syndrome.
Pseudoscleroderma—secondary to porphyria cutanea tarda, acromegaly, carcinoid syndrome.
Scleredema—people with diabetes develop thick skin over the shoulders and upper back.
Graft-versus-host disease.
Silicosis.

SLEEP-RELATED HALLUCINATIONS[50]

| ICD-10CM # | Varies with specific diagnosis |

HYPNAGOGIC AND HYPNOPOMPIC HALLUCINATIONS

Sleep deprivation.[‡]
Narcolepsy.[§¶]

[‡]American Academy of Sleep Medicine: *International classification of sleep disorders,* ed 3, Darien, 2014, American Academy of Sleep Medicine.
[§]Leu-Semenescu S et al: Hallucinations in narcolepsy with and without cataplexy: contrasts with Parkinson disease, *Sleep Med* 12:497-504, 2011.
[¶]Szucs A et al: Misleading hallucinations in unrecognized narcolepsy, *Acta Psychiatr Scand* 108:314-317, 2003.

COMPLEX NOCTURNAL VISUAL HALLUCINATIONS

Parkinson disease.[*,†,‡,§]
Dementia with Lewy bodies.[¶,**]
Peduncular hallucinosis.[††,‡‡,§§]
Charles Bonnet syndrome.[*,¶¶]
Schizophrenia.[¶¶]
Metabolic encephalopathy.[*]
Posterior cerebral artery infarction.[*]
Delirium tremens.[*]
Migraine.[*]
Focal epilepsy.[*]
Guillain-Barré syndrome.[***]
Sleepwalking.[†††,‡‡‡]
Night terrors.[†††]
Idiopathic hypersomnia.[§§§]
Anxiety disorder.[§§§]
Acute alcohol withdrawal.[¶¶¶]
Acute barbiturate withdrawal.[§§§]
Acute benzodiazepine withdrawal.[§§§]
Lipophilic beta-blockers.[†††]
Dopaminergic agents.[†††]
Substances with hallucinogenic properties, such as mescaline, LSD, amphetamine, and cocaine.[†††]

---

[*]Manford M, Andermann F: Complex visual hallucinations, *Brain* 121:1819-1840, 1998.
[†]Kulisevsky J, Roldan E: Hallucinations and sleep disturbances in Parkinson's disease, *Neurology* 63(Suppl 3): S28-S30, 2004.
[‡]Arnulf I et al: Hallucinations, REM sleep, Parkinson's disease, *Neurology* 55:281-288, 2000.
[§]Arnulf I et al: Parkinson's disease and sleepiness. An integral part of PD, *Neurology* 58:1019-1024, 2002.
[¶]McKeith IG et al: Diagnosis and management of dementia with Lewy bodies: fourth consensus report of the DLB Consortium, *Neurology* 89:88-100, 2017.
[**]Tiraboschi P et al: Absence of rapid eye movement sleep with hypnopompic visual hallucinations; a possible harbinger of dementia with Lewy bodies, *Sleep Med* 14:377-379, 2013.
[††]Benke T: Peduncular hallucinosis, *J Neurol* 253:1561-1571, 2006.
[‡‡]Cervera A et al: Sleep studies in two patients with pontine haematomas and "peduncular" hallucinosis, *J Neurol* 246(Suppl 1):139, 1999.
[§§]Vetrugno R et al: Peduncullar hallucinosis: a polysomnographic and SPECT study of a patient and efficacy of serotonergic therapy, *Sleep Med* 90:1158-1160, 2009.
[¶¶]Lerario A et al: Charles Bonnet syndrome: two case reports and review of the literature, *J Neurol* 260:1180-1186, 2013.
[***]De Cock VC et al: Vivid dreams, hallucinations, psychosis and REM sleep in Guillain-Barré syndrome, *Brain* 128:2535-2545, 2005.
[†††]Rao SC, Silber MH: Sleep-related hallucinations and exploding head syndrome. In Thorpy MJ, Plazzi G (eds): *The parasomnias and other related sleep-related movement disorders,* Cambridge, United Kingdom, 2010, Cambridge University Press, 194-201.
[‡‡‡]Mantoan L et al: Adult-onset NREM parasomnia with hypnopompic hallucinatory pain: a case report, *Sleep* 36: 287-290, 2013.
[§§§]Silber MH et al: Complex nocturnal visual hallucinations, *Sleep Med* 6:363-366, 2005.
[¶¶¶]The US Xyrem Multicenter Study Group: A randomized, double blind, placebo-controlled multicenter trial comparing the effects of three doses of orally administered sodium oxybate with placebo for the treatment of narcolepsy, *Sleep* 25:42-49, 2002.

SLEEPTALKING[50]

ICD-10CM #   Varies with specific diagnosis

Confusional arousals.*
Night terrors.*
Sleepwalking.*
Sleep-related eating syndrome.[†]
Sexsomnia.[‡]
REM sleep behavior disorder.[§,¶,**,††]
Status dissociatus.[‡‡]
Parasomnia overlap disorder.[§§]
Agrypnia excitata.[¶¶]
Anti-IgLON5 disease.[***]
Sleep-related hypermotor epilepsy.[†††]
Periodic limb movement disorder.[‡‡‡]
Obstructive sleep apnea.[§§§]
Nocturnal panic attacks.[†††]
Sleep-related dissociative disorder.[†††]

---

*Oudiette D et al: Dreamlike mentations during sleepwalking and sleep terrors in adults, *Sleep* 32:1621-1627, 2009.

[†]Vinai P et al: Defining the borders between sleep-related eating disorder and night eating syndrome, *Sleep Med* 13:686-690, 2012.

[‡]Schenck CH et al: Sleep and sex: what can go wrong? A review of the literature on sleep related disorders and abnormal sexual behaviors and experiences, *Sleep* 30:683-702, 2007.

[§]Iranzo A et al: The clinical and pathophysiological relevance of REM sleep behavior disorder in neurodegenerative diseases, *Sleep Med Rev* 13:385-401, 2009.

[¶]Santamaria J et al: Relation between dream content and movement intensity in REM behavior disorder, *Sleep* 27(Suppl):A289, 2003.

**De Cock VC et al: Restoration of normal control in Parkinson's disease during REM sleep, *Brain* 130:450-456, 2007.

[††]De Cock VC et al: The improvement of movement and speech during rapid eye movement sleep behavior disorder in multiple system atrophy, *Brain* 134:856-862, 2011.

[‡‡]Mahowald MW, Schenck CH: Dissociated states of wakefulness and sleep, *Neurology* 42(Suppl 6):44-52, 1992.

[§§]Schenck CH et al: A parasomnia overlap disorder involving sleepwalking, sleep terrors, and REM sleep behavior disorder in 33 polysomnographic confirmed cases, *Sleep* 20:972-981, 1997.

[¶¶]Provini F: Agrypnia excitata, *Curr Neurol Neurosci Rep* 13:341, 2013.

[***]Sabater L et al: A novel non-rapid-eye movement and rapid-eye-movement parasomnia with sleep breathing disorder associated with antibodies to IgLON5: an observational study: a case series, characterisation of the antigen, and postmortem study, *Lancet Neurol* 13:575-586, 2014.

[†††]American Academy of Sleep Medicine: *International classification of sleep disorders*, ed 3, Darien, 2014, American Academy of Sleep Medicine.

[‡‡‡]Gaig C et al: Periodic limb movements during sleep mimicking REM sleep behavior disorder: a new form of periodic limb movement disorder, *Sleep* 40(3), 2017, http://dx.doi.org/10.1093/sleep/zsw063.

[§§§]Iranzo A, Santamaria J: Severe obstructive sleep apnea/hypopnea syndrome mimicking REM sleep behavior disorder, *Sleep* 28:203-206, 2005.

SMALL BOWEL MASSES[2]

ICD-10CM #   Varies with specific diagnosis

Cyst:
  Mesenteric cyst.
Tumor:
  Benign.
  Malignant.
Intussusception.
Inflammation:
  Crohn disease.

SMALL BOWEL OBSTRUCTION[10]

| ICD-10CM # | K56.5 | Intestinal adhesions [bands] with obstruction (postprocedural) (postinfection) |
| | Q41.9 | Congenital absence, atresia and stenosis of small intestine, part unspecified |

INTRINSIC

Congenital (atresia, stenosis).
Inflammatory (Crohn, radiation enteritis).
Neoplasms (metastatic or primary).
Intussusception.
Traumatic (hematoma).

EXTRINSIC

Hernias (internal and external).
Adhesions.
Volvulus.
Compressing masses (tumors, abscesses, hematomas).

INTRALUMINAL

Foreign body.
Gallstones.
Bezoars.
Barium.
Ascaris infestation.

SMALL INTESTINE ULCERATION

| ICD-10CM # | K63.3 | Ulcer of intestine |

Inflammatory bowel disease.
Celiac disease.
Vasculitis, systemic lupus erythematosus, Behçet syndrome.
Uremia.
Infections (*Campylobacter*, TB, *Yersinia*, parasites, typhoid, cytomegalovirus, *Clostridium*).
Mesenteric insufficiency.
Neoplasms.
Radiation.
Drugs (salicylates, potassium, indomethacin, antimetabolites).
Meckel diverticulum.
Zollinger-Ellison syndrome.
Lymphocytic enterocolitis.
Stomal ulceration.

SMELL DISTURBANCE

| ICD-10CM # | R43.8 | Other disturbances of smell and taste |

Upper respiratory tract infection.
Nasal or paranasal sinus disease.
Exposure to noxious vapors.
Head trauma.
Idiopathic.
Dental caries, periodontal disease.
Medications.

SODIUM RETENTION, RENAL CAUSES[11]

ICD-10CM #   Varies with specific diagnosis

CAUSES OF RENAL SODIUM RETENTION

Primary
Oliguric acute kidney injury.
Chronic kidney disease.
Glomerular disease.
Severe bilateral renal artery stenosis.
Na^+-retaining tubulopathies (genetic).
Mineralocorticoid excess.
Secondary
Heart failure.
Cirrhosis.
Idiopathic edema.

SOFT TISSUE MASS MIMICKING MALIGNANCY[52]

ICD-10CM #   Varies with specific diagnosis

OVERVIEW OF DISEASES THAT CAN PRESENT AS A SOFT TISSUE MASS MIMICKING MALIGNANCY

Etiology	Disease Entity
Trauma:	Muscle contusion.
	Hematoma.
	Muscle herniation.
	Calcific myonecrosis.
	Hypothenar hammer syndrome.
	Myositis ossificans.
Metabolic:	Diabetic myopathy.
	Gout.
	Pseudogout.
	Calcific tendinosis.
Congenital:	Accessory muscle.
Infectious:	Necrotizing fasciitis.
	Abscess.
	Pyomyositis.
	Hydatid cystic disease.
	Cat-scratch disease.
	Actinomycosis.
Inflammation:	Bursitis.
	Sarcoidosis.
	Foreign body reaction.
	Injection granuloma.
	Granuloma annulare.
	Epidermal inclusion cyst.
Vascular:	Adventitial cystic disease.
	Pseudoaneurysm.
	Thrombosed vein.
	Arteriovenous vascular malformation.
Miscellaneous:	Focal myositis.
	Amyloid tumor of soft tissue.

SOFT TISSUE TUMORS, PEDIATRIC PATIENTS[52]

ICD-10CM # Varies with specific diagnosis

PEDIATRIC SOFT TISSUE TUMORS

Vascular lesions:
  Hemangioma of infancy.*
  Congenital hemangioma.
  Hemangioendothelioma (Kasabach-Merritt syndrome).
  Arteriovenous malformation.
  Venous malformations.
  Lymphatic malformation (lymphangioma, cystic hygroma).
  Capillary malformation.
Adipocytic tumors:
  Lipoma.
  Lipoblastoma.
  Liposarcoma.
Fibrohistiocytic tumors:
  Pigmented villonodular synovitis.
  Giant cell tumor of tendon sheath.
Fibroblastic and myofibroblastic tumors:
  Nodular fasciitis.
  Fibrous hamartoma of infancy.
  Myofibroma, myofibromatosis.
  Infantile fibrosarcoma.
  Fibromatosis colli.
Neurogenic tumors:
  Schwannoma.
  Neurofibroma.
  Malignant nerve sheath tumor.
Leiomyoma.
Rhabdomyosarcoma.
Tumors of uncertain differentiation:
  Synovial cell sarcoma.
  Primitive neuroectodermal tumor (Ewing sarcoma).
Pilomatricoma.

*Lesions with MR-specific features.

SORE THROAT[43]

ICD-10CM # J02 Acute pharyngitis

DIFFERENTIAL DIAGNOSIS FOR SORE THROAT

Infectious Causes
Aerobes
Common:
  Streptococcus pyogenes (GABHS).
  Peptostreptococcus spp.
  Nongroup A *Streptococcus*.
  Neisseria gonorrhoeae.
  Neisseria meningitides.
  Mycoplasma pneumoniae.
  Arcanobacterium hemolyticum.
  Chlamydia trachomatis.
  Staphylococcus aureus.
Uncommon:
  Haemophilus influenzae.
  Haemophilus parainfluenzae.
  Coccidioides spp.
  Corynebacterium diphtheriae.
  Streptococcus pneumoniae.

Yersinia enterocolitica.
Treponema pallidum.
Francisella tularensis.
Legionella pneumophila.
Mycobacterium spp.

ANAEROBES

Bacteroides spp.
Peptococcus spp.
Clostridium spp.
Fusobacterium spp.
Prevotella spp.

OTHER

Candida spp.

VIRAL

Rhinovirus.
Adenovirus.
Coronavirus.
Herpes simplex 1, 2.
Influenza A, B.
Parainfluenza.
Cytomegalovirus.
Epstein-Barr.
Varicella-zoster.
Hepatitis virus.

NONINFECTIOUS CAUSES SYSTEMIC

Kawasaki disease.
Stevens-Johnson syndrome.
Cyclic neutropenia.
Thyroiditis.
Connective tissue disease.

TRAUMA, MISCELLANEOUS

Penetrating injury.
Angioneurotic edema.
Retained foreign body.
Anomalous aortic arch.
Laryngeal fracture.
Calcific retropharyngeal tendinitis.
Retropharyngeal hematoma.
Caustic exposure.

TUMOR

Tongue.
Larynx.
Thyroid.
Leukemia.

SPASTIC PARAPLEGIAS

ICD-10CM # G82.20 Paraplegia, unspecified

Cervical spondylosis.
Friedreich ataxia.
Multiple sclerosis.
Spinal cord tumor.
HIV.
Tertiary syphilis.
Vitamin B_{12} deficiency.
Spinocerebellar ataxias.
Syringomyelia.
Spinal cord AV malformations.
Adrenoleukodystrophy.

SPINAL CORD COMPRESSION, EPIDURAL

ICD-10CM # Varies with specific diagnosis

Osteoarthritis.
Meningioma.
Spinal epidural abscess.
Spinal epidural hematoma.
Spinal epidural vascular malformations.
Rheumatoid arthritis.
Metastatic cancer (vertebral, intramedullary, leptomeninges).
Radiation myelopathy.
Neurofibroma.
Sarcoidosis.
Paraneoplastic myelopathy.
Histiocytosis.

SPINAL CORD DYSFUNCTION

ICD-10CM #		
	G95.9	Disease of spinal cord, unspecified
	Q07.9	Congenital malformation of nervous system, unspecified
	D51.1	Vitamin B_{12} deficiency anemia due to selective vitamin B_{12} malabsorption with proteinuria
	D51.3	Other dietary vitamin B_{12} deficiency anemia
	D51.8	Other vitamin B_{12} deficiency anemias
	G95.89	Other specified diseases of spinal cord
	G95.19	Other vascular myelopathies

Trauma.
Multiple sclerosis.
Transverse myelitis.
Neoplasm (primary, metastatic).
Syringomyelia.
Spinal epidural abscess.
HIV myelopathy.
Diskitis.
Spinal epidural hematoma.
Spinal cord infarction.
Spinal AV malformation.
Subarachnoid hemorrhage.

SPINAL CORD DYSFUNCTION, NONTRAUMATIC[43]

ICD-10CM #	Q07.9	Congenital malformation of nervous system, unspecified

NONTRAUMATIC ETIOLOGIES OF SPINAL CORD DYSFUNCTION

Processes Affecting the Spinal Cord or Blood Supply Directly

Multiple sclerosis.
Transverse myelitis.
Spinal arteriovenous malformation/subarachnoid hemorrhage.
Syringomyelia.
HIV myelopathy.
Other myelopathies.
Spinal cord infarction.

Compressive Lesions Affecting the Spinal Cord

Spinal epidural abscess.
Spinal epidural hematoma.
Diskitis.
Neoplasm.
Metastatic.
Primary central nervous system.

SPINAL CORD ISCHEMIC SYNDROMES[38]

ICD-10CM #	G95.9	Acute infarction of spinal cord

Local mechanical vascular compression.
Regional hemodynamic compromise.
Systemic hypotension.
Occlusive vascular disease.
Thromboembolism.
Endovascular procedures.
Fibrocartilaginous (intervertebral disk) embolism.
Vasculitis.
Arterial dissection.
Thrombosis.
Venous occlusion.

SPINAL TUMORS[24]

ICD-10CM #	Varies with specific diagnosis

EXTRADURAL

Metastases.
Primary bone tumors arising in spine.

INTRADURAL EXTRAMEDULLARY

Meningiomas.
Neurofibromas.
Schwannomas.
Lipomas.
Arachnoid cysts.
Epidermoid cysts.
Metastasis.

INTRAMEDULLARY

Ependymoma.
Glioma.
Hemangioblastoma.
Lipoma.
Metastases.

SPINAL PARAPLEGIA[20]

ICD-10CM #	Varies with specific diagnosis

Congenital malformations.
    Arachnoid cyst.
    Arteriovenous malformations.

Atlantoaxial dislocation.
Caudal regression syndrome.
Dysraphic states.
Chiari malformation.
Myelomeningocele.
Tethered spinal cord.
Syringomyelia.
Familial spastic paraplegia.
    Autosomal dominant.
    Autosomal recessive.
    X-linked recessive.
Infections.
    Asthmatic amyotrophy.
    Diskitis.
    Epidural abscess.
    Herpes zoster myelitis.
    Polyradiculoneuropathy.
    Tuberculous osteomyelitis.
Lupus myelopathy.
Metabolic disorders.
    Adrenomyeloneuropathy (adrenoleukodystrophy).
    Argininemia.
    Krabbe disease.
Neonatal cord infarction.
Transverse myelitis.
    Devic disease.
    Encephalomyelitis.
    Idiopathic.
    Trauma.
Concussion.
    Epidural hematoma.
    Fracture dislocation.
Neonatal cord trauma.
Tumors.
    Astrocytoma.
    Ependymoma.
    Ewing sarcoma.
    Neuroblastoma.

SPLENIC CYSTS, CLASSIFICATION[64]

ICD-10CM #	D73.4	Cyst of spleen

Primary (true).
Parasitic.
Nonparasitic.
Congenital.
Epidermoid.
Dermoid.
Mesothelial (serous).
Transitional.
Neoplastic.
Secondary (false): pseudocysts.
Traumatic.
Degenerative.
Inflammatory.
Hemorrhagic.

SPLENIC MASSES, FOCAL SOLID[15]

ICD-10CM #	Varies with specific diagnosis

FOCAL SOLID SPLENIC MASSES

Benign
Hemangioma.
Hamartoma.
Littoral cell angioma.

Lymphangioma.
Sclerosing angiomatoid nodular transformation (SANT).
Inflammatory pseudotumor.
Malignant
Lymphoma.
Metastases.
Angiosarcoma.
Hemangiopericytoma.
Other
Infarct.

SPLENIC NODULES[15]

ICD-10CM #	Varies with specific diagnosis

CAUSES OF SPLENIC NODULES

Infectious
Tuberculosis/Mycobacterium avium-intracellulare complex.
Pyogenic abscesses.
Histoplasmosis.
Candida abscesses.
Cat-scratch disease.
Pneumocystis jirovecii (formerly P. carinii pneumonia).
Inflammatory
Sarcoidosis.
Malignant
Lymphoma.
Metastases.
Other
Gamna-Gandy bodies.
Gaucher disease.

SPLENIC TUMORS, CLASSIFICATION[64]

ICD-10CM #	C26.1	Malignant neoplasm of spleen

Malignant.
Lymphoproliferative disease.
Non-Hodgkin lymphoma.
Hodgkin disease.
Hairy cell leukemia.
Chronic lymphocytic leukemia.
Myeloproliferative disease.
Chronic myelogenous leukemia.
Myelofibrosis.
Primary tumors.
Angiosarcoma.
Metastatic tumors.
Benign.
Hemangiomas.
Hamartomas.
Lymphangiomas.
Sclerosing angiomatoid nodular transformation (SANT).

SPLENOMEGALY

ICD-10CM #	R16.1	Splenomegaly, not elsewhere classified
	D73.2	Chronic congestive splenomegaly
	R16.1	Splenomegaly, not elsewhere classified

Hepatic cirrhosis.

Neoplastic involvement: CML, CLL, lymphoma, multiple myeloma.

Bacterial infections: TB, infectious endocarditis, typhoid fever, splenic abscess.

Viral infections: infectious mononucleosis, viral hepatitis, HIV.

Gaucher disease and other lipid storage diseases.

Sarcoidosis.

Parasitic infections (malaria, kala-azar, histoplasmosis).

Hereditary and acquired hemolytic anemias.

Idiopathic thrombocytopenic purpura (ITP).

Collagen vascular disorders: systemic lupus erythematosus, rheumatoid arthritis (Felty syndrome), polyarteritis nodosa.

Serum sickness, drug hypersensitivity reaction.

Splenic cysts and benign tumors: hemangioma, lymphangioma.

Thrombosis of splenic or portal vein.

Polycythemia vera, myeloid metaplasia.

SPLENOMEGALY AND HEPATOMEGALY[2]

| ICD-10CM # | R16.1 | Splenomegaly, not elsewhere classified |
| | R16.0 | Hepatomegaly, not elsewhere classified |

CAUSES OF SPLENOMEGALY AND HEPATOSPLENOMEGALY

Massive Splenomegaly

Hematologic disease (e.g., chronic myeloid leukemia, myelofibrosis).

Moderate Splenomegaly

The above causes.

Portal hypertension.

Hematologic disease (e.g., lymphoma, leukemia, thalassemia).

Storage disease (e.g., Gaucher disease).

Small Splenomegaly

The above causes.

Infective (hepatitis, leptospirosis, malaria, bacterial endocarditis).

Hematologic disease (e.g., hemolytic anemias, essential thrombocythemia, polycythemia rubra vera).

Connective tissue diseases or vasculitis (e.g., rheumatoid arthritis, systemic lupus erythematosus, polyarteritis nodosa).

Solitary cyst, polycystic syndrome, hydatid cyst.

Infiltration (amyloid, sarcoid).

Hepatosplenomegaly

Chronic liver disease with portal hypertension.

Hematologic disease (e.g., myeloproliferative disease, lymphoma).

Infection (e.g., amyloid, sarcoid).

Connective tissue disease (e.g., systemic lupus erythematosus).

SPLENOMEGALY AND HYPERSPLENISM[71]

ICD-10CM #	R16.1	Splenomegaly, not elsewhere classified
	D73.1	Hypersplenism
	D73.81	Neutropenic splenomegaly

DIFFERENTIAL DIAGNOSIS OF SPLENOMEGALY AND HYPERSPLENISM

Infections

Acute

Viral (viral hepatitis, infectious mononucleosis, CMV infection).

Bacterial (septicemia, salmonellosis, brucellosis, splenic abscess).

Parasite (toxoplasmosis).

Subacute and Chronic

Subacute bacterial endocarditis.

Tuberculosis.

Malaria.

Kala-azar.

Fungal disease.

Inflammation

Felty syndrome.

SLE.

Serum sickness.

Rheumatic fever.

Sarcoidosis.

ALPS.

Congestive Splenomegaly

Intrahepatic

Cirrhosis.

Extrahepatic

Portal vein obstruction.

Splenic vein obstruction.

Hepatic vein occlusion (Budd-Chiari syndrome).

Chronic Passive Congestion

Heart failure.

Hematologic Disorders

RBC disorders: hemolytic anemias, thalassemia, sickle cell disorders.

Neoplasia

Malignant

MPDs.

Myeloid metaplasia.

Polycythemia rubra vera.

Essential thrombocythemia.

Chronic leukemia.

Chronic myeloid leukemia.

Chronic lymphocytic leukemia.

Hairy cell leukemia.

Lymphoma.

Acute leukemia.

Malignant histiocytosis.

Benign

Hamartoma.

Hemangioma.

Lymphangioma.

Fibroma.

Storage Diseases

Gaucher disease.

Niemann-Pick disease.

Miscellaneous

Amyloidosis.

Cysts.

ALPS, Autoimmune lymphoproliferative syndrome; *CMV*, cytomegalovirus; *MPD*, myeloproliferative disorder; *RBC*, red blood cell; *SLE*, systemic lupus erythematosus.

SPLENOMEGALY, CHILDREN[31]

| ICD-10CM # | R16.1 | Splenomegaly, not elsewhere classified |

DISORDERS OF THE BLOOD

Hemolytic anemia: congenital/acquired.

Thalassemia.

Sickle cell disease.

Leukemia.

Osteopetrosis.

Myelofibrosis/myeloid metaplasia/thrombocythemia.

INFECTIONS: ACUTE AND CHRONIC

Viral:

Congenital (e.g., TORCH association).

Mononucleosis (e.g., EBV, CMV infection).

Virus-associated hemophagocytic syndrome.

HIV.

Bacterial:

Sepsis/abscess.

Brucellosis.

Salmonellosis.

Tularemia.

Tuberculosis.

Subacute bacterial endocarditis.

Syphilis.

Lyme disease.

Fungal:

Histoplasmosis (disseminated).

Rickettsial:

Rocky Mountain spotted fever.

Cat-scratch disease.

Parasitic:

Toxoplasmosis.

Malaria.

Leishmaniasis (kala-azar).

Schistosomiasis.

Echinococcosis.

HEPATIC/PORTAL SYSTEM DISORDERS

Acute/chronic active hepatitis.

Cirrhosis/hepatic fibrosis/biliary atresia.

Portal or splenic venous obstruction (Banti syndrome).

AUTOIMMUNE DISEASE

Juvenile rheumatoid arthritis.

Systemic lupus erythematosus.

Autoimmune lymphoproliferative syndrome (Canale-Smith syndrome).

NEOPLASMS/CYSTS

Lymphomas (Hodgkin and non-Hodgkin).

Hemangiomas/lymphangiomas.

Hamartomas.

Congenital or acquired (posttraumatic) cysts.

STORAGE DISEASES/INBORN ERRORS OF METABOLISM

Lipidoses: Gaucher disease, Niemann–Pick disease, others.

Mucopolysaccharidoses.

Defects in carbohydrate metabolism: galactosemia, fructose intolerance.

Sea-blue histiocyte syndrome.

MISCELLANEOUS DISORDERS

Histiocytoses:

Reactive.

Langerhans cell.

Malignant.

Sarcoidosis.

Congestive heart failure.
Familial Mediterranean fever.

CMV, Cytomegalovirus; *EBV,* Epstein-Barr virus; *TORCH,* toxoplasmosis, other infections, rubella, cytomegalovirus infection, herpes simplex.

SPONTANEOUS PNEUMOTHORAX[10]

ICD-10CM #	J93.0	Spontaneous tension pneumothorax
	J93.11	Primary spontaneous pneumothorax
	J93.12	Secondary spontaneous pneumothorax

CAUSES OF SECONDARY SPONTANEOUS PNEUMOTHORAX

Airway Disease
Chronic obstructive pulmonary disease.
Asthma.
Cystic fibrosis.
Infections
Necrotizing bacterial pneumonia, lung abscess.
Pneumocystis jirovecii pneumonia.
Tuberculosis.
Interstitial Lung Disease
Sarcoidosis.
Idiopathic pulmonary fibrosis.
Lymphangiomyomatosis.
Tuberous sclerosis.
Pneumoconioses.
Neoplasms
Primary lung cancers.
Pulmonary or pleural metastases.
Miscellaneous
Connective tissue diseases.
Pulmonary infarction.
Endometriosis, catamenial pneumothorax.

STATURAL OVERGROWTH[30]

| ICD-10CM # | E34.4 | Constitutional tall stature |

FETAL OVERGROWTH

Maternal diabetes mellitus.
Cerebral gigantism (Sotos syndrome).
Weaver syndrome.
Beckwith-Wiedemann syndrome.
Other insulin-like growth factor 2 (IGF2) excess syndromes.

POSTNATAL OVERGROWTH LEADING TO CHILDHOOD TALL STATURE

Familial (constitutional) tall stature.
Cerebral gigantism.
Beckwith-Wiedemann syndrome.
Exogenous obesity.
Excess growth hormone (GH) secretion (pituitary gigantism).
McCune-Albright syndrome or multiple endocrine neoplasia (MEN) associated with excess GH secretion.
Precocious puberty.
Marfan syndrome.
Klinefelter syndrome (XXY).
Weaver syndrome.
Fragile X syndrome.
Homocystinuria.

XYY.
Hyperthyroidism.

POSTNATAL OVERGROWTH LEADING TO ADULT TALL STATURE

Familial (constitutional) tall stature.
Androgen or estrogen deficiency/estrogen resistance (in males).
Testicular feminization.
Excess GH secretion.
Marfan syndrome.
Klinefelter syndrome (XXY).
XYY.

STEATOHEPATITIS

| ICD-10CM # | K76.0 | Fatty (change of) liver, not elsewhere classified |
| | K76.89 | Other specified diseases of liver |

Alcohol abuse.
Obesity.
Diabetes mellitus.
Parenteral nutrition.
Medications (high-dose estrogen, amiodarone, corticosteroids, methotrexate, nifedipine).
Jejunoileal bypass.
Abetalipoproteinemia.
Wilson disease, Weber-Christian disease.

STEATOSIS, MACROVESICULAR AND MICROVESICULAR[94]

| ICD-10CM # | K75.81 | Nonalcoholic steatohepatitis (NASH) |
| | K70.9 | Alcoholic liver disease, unspecified |

Common Causes of Macrovesicular and Microvesicular Steatosis

Macrovesicular Steatosis	Microvesicular Steatosis
Obesity, type 2 diabetes, metabolic syndrome, and dyslipidemia (nonalcoholic fatty liver disease).	Reye syndrome.
	Medications (valproate, antiretroviral medicines, intravenous tetracycline).
Excessive alcohol consumption.	Heat stroke.
Hepatitis C (genotype 3).	Acute fatty liver of pregnancy.
Wilson disease.	HELLP syndrome.
Lipodystrophy starvation.	Inborn errors of metabolism (lecithin–cholesterol acyltransferase deficiency, cholesterol ester storage disease, Wolman disease).
Jejunoileal bypass.	
Parenteral nutrition.	
Medications (amiodarone, methotrexate, tamoxifen, corticosteroids, antipsychotics).	

HELLP, Hemolysis, elevated liver enzymes, and low platelets.

STERILE PYURIA[12]

| ICD-10CM # | R82.998 | Other abnormal findings in urine |

Common causes of sterile pyuria:
Nonspecific urethritis in males.
Prostatitis.
Renal tract neoplasm.
Renal calculi.
Catheterization.
Renal tuberculosis.
Previous antibiotic treatment.

STOMATITIS, BULLOUS

| ICD-10CM # | K12.30 | Oral mucositis (ulcerative), unspecified |

Erythema multiforme.
Erosive lichen planus.
Bullous pemphigoid.
Systemic lupus erythematosus.
Pemphigus vulgaris.
Mucous membrane pemphigoid.

STRIDOR IN NEONATES[29]

| ICD-10CM # | R06.1 | Stridor |

INTRINSIC LESIONS

Larynx
Laryngomalacia.
Infection (laryngitis).
Vocal cord paralysis.
Laryngeal web.
Laryngocele or laryngeal cyst.
Laryngotracheal esophageal cleft.
Foreign body.
Trachea
Tracheomalacia.
Tracheal stenosis.
Tracheoesophageal fistula.
Subglottic hemangioma.
Tracheal web.
Extrinsic Compression
Vascular ring.
Anomalous innominate artery.
Mediastinal mass.
Esophageal foreign body.
Other
Macroglossia.
Gastroesophageal reflux.

STRIDOR, PEDIATRIC AGE[45]

| ICD-10CM # | R06.1 | Stridor |

RECURRENT

Allergic (spasmodic) croup.
Respiratory infections in a child with otherwise asymptomatic anatomic narrowing of the large airways.
Laryngomalacia.

PERSISTENT

Laryngeal obstruction:
Laryngomalacia.
Papillomas, other tumors.
Cysts and laryngoceles.

Laryngeal webs.
Bilateral abductor paralysis of the cords.
Foreign body.
Tracheobronchial disease:
  Tracheomalacia.
  Subglottic tracheal webs.
Endotracheal, endobronchial tumors.
Subglottic tracheal stenosis.
Congenital.
Acquired.
Extrinsic masses.
Mediastinal masses.
Vascular ring.
Lobar emphysema.
Bronchogenic cysts.
Thyroid enlargement.
Esophageal foreign body.
Tracheoesophageal fistulas.
Other.
Gastroesophageal reflux.
Macroglossia, Pierre Robin syndrome.
Cri-du-chat syndrome.
Hysterical stridor.
Hypocalcemia.

STROKE[17]

ICD-10CM #	Varies with specific diagnosis

STROKE "MIMICS"

Hypoglycemia.
Drug overdose or intoxication.
Hysterical conversion reaction.
Hyperventilation.
Metabolic encephalopathy.
Migraine.
Syncope.
Transient global amnesia.
Seizures.
Vestibular vertigo.

STROKE, PEDIATRIC AGE[97]

ICD-10CM #	I67.89	Other cerebrovascular disease

CARDIAC DISEASE

Congenital:
  Aortic stenosis.
  Mitral stenosis; mitral prolapse.
  Ventricular septal defects.
  Patent ductus arteriosus.
  Cyanotic congenital heart disease involving right-to-left shunt.
Acquired:
  Endocarditis (bacterial, systemic lupus erythematosus).
  Kawasaki disease.
  Cardiomyopathy.
  Atrial myxoma.
  Arrhythmia.
  Paradoxical emboli through patent foramen ovale.
  Rheumatic fever.
  Prosthetic heart valve.

HEMATOLOGIC ABNORMALITIES

Hemoglobinopathies:
  Sickle cell (SS) disease.
  Sickle (SC) disease.

Polycythemia.
Leukemia/lymphoma.
Thrombocytopenia.
Thrombocytosis.
Disorders of coagulation:
  Protein C deficiency.
  Protein S deficiency.
  Factor V Leiden.
  Antithrombin III deficiency.
  Lupus anticoagulant.
Oral contraceptive pill use.
Pregnancy and the postpartum state.
Disseminated intravascular coagulation.
Paroxysmal nocturnal hemoglobinuria.
Inflammatory bowel disease (thrombosis).

INFLAMMATORY DISORDERS

Meningitis:
  Viral.
  Bacterial.
  Tuberculosis.
Systemic infection:
  Viremia.
  Bacteremia.
  Local head and neck infections.
Drug-induced inflammation:
  Amphetamine.
  Cocaine.
Autoimmune disease:
  Systemic lupus erythematosus.
  Juvenile rheumatoid arthritis.
  Takayasu arteritis.
  Mixed connective tissue disease.
  Polyarteritis nodosum.
  Primary CNS vasculitis.
  Sarcoidosis.
  Behçet syndrome.
  Granulomatosis with polyangiitis.

METABOLIC DISEASE ASSOCIATED WITH STROKE

Homocystinuria.
Pseudoxanthoma elasticum.
Fabry disease.
Sulfite oxidase deficiency.
Mitochondrial disorders:
  MELAS.
  Leigh syndrome.
Ornithine transcarbamylase deficiency.

INTRACEREBRAL VASCULAR PROCESSES

Ruptured aneurysm.
Arteriovenous malformation.
Fibromuscular dysplasia.
Moyamoya disease.
Migraine headache.
Postsubarachnoid hemorrhage vasospasm.
Hereditary hemorrhagic telangiectasia.
Sturge-Weber syndrome.
Carotid artery dissection.
Postvaricella.

TRAUMA AND OTHER EXTERNAL CAUSES

Child abuse.
Head trauma/neck trauma.
Oral trauma.

Placental embolism.
ECMO therapy.

CNS, Central nervous system; *ECMO*, extracorporeal membrane oxygenation; *MELAS*, mitochondrial encephalomyopathy, lactic acidosis, and stroke.

STROKE, YOUNG ADULT, CAUSES[18]

ICD-10CM #	I64	Stroke
	I67.89	Other cerebrovascular disease

Cardiac factors (ASD, MVP, patent foramen ovale).
Inflammatory factors (systemic lupus erythematosus, polyarteritis nodosa).
Infections (endocarditis, neurosyphilis).
Drugs (cocaine, heroin, oral contraceptives, decongestants).
Arterial dissection.
Hematologic factors (disseminated intravascular coagulation, TTP, deficiency of protein S, protein C, antithrombin III).
Migraine.
Postpartum angiopathy.
Other: premature atherosclerosis, fibromuscular dysplasia.

ST-SEGMENT DEPRESSION, NONCORONARY CAUSES[87]

ICD-10CM #	R94.31	Abnormal electrocardiogram

NONCORONARY CAUSES OF ST-SEGMENT DEPRESSION

Anemia.
Cardiomyopathy.
Digitalis use.
Glucose load.
Hyperventilation.
Hypokalemia.
Intraventricular conduction disturbance.
Left ventricular hypertrophy.
Mitral valve prolapse.
Preexcitation syndrome.
Severe aortic stenosis.
Severe hypertension.
Severe hypoxia.
Severe volume overload (aortic, mitral regurgitation).
Sudden excessive exercise.
Supraventricular tachyarrhythmias.

ST-SEGMENT ELEVATION[29]

ICD-10CM #	R94.31	Abnormal electrocardiogram [ECG] [EKG]

DIFFERENTIAL DIAGNOSIS OF ST-SEGMENT ELEVATION ON ELECTROCARDIOGRAPHY

ST-segment elevation myocardial infarction.
Pericarditis.
Benign early repolarization.
Left bundle branch block.
Left ventricular hypertrophy.
Left ventricular aneurysm.
Paced ventricular rhythms.
Prinzmetal angina.

Hyperkalemia.
Hypothermia with Osborne waves.
Intracranial hemorrhage.
Brugada syndrome.
Normal variant.

ST-SEGMENT ELEVATIONS, NONISCHEMIC

ICD-10CM #	R94.31	Abnormal electrocardiogram [ECG] [EKG]

Early repolarization.
Acute pericarditis.
LVH.
Normal pattern variant.
LBBB.
Pulmonary embolism.
Hyperkalemia.
Postcardioversion.

SUDDEN CARDIAC DEATH[86]

ICD-10CM #	Z86.74	Personal history of sudden cardiac arrest
	Z82.41	Family history of sudden cardiac death

CAUSES OF AND CONTRIBUTING FACTORS IN SUDDEN CARDIAC DEATH

Coronary Artery Abnormalities
Coronary atherosclerosis:
Chronic coronary atherosclerosis with acute or transient myocardial ischemia—thrombosis, spasm, physical stress.
Acute myocardial infarction, onset and early phase.
Chronic atherosclerosis with a change in myocardial substrate, including previous myocardial infarction.
Congenital abnormalities of coronary arteries:
Anomalous origin from the pulmonary artery.
Other coronary arteriovenous fistula.
Origin of a left coronary branch from the right or noncoronary sinus of Valsalva.
Origin of the right coronary artery from the left sinus of Valsalva.
Hypoplastic or aplastic coronary arteries.
Coronary-intracardiac shunt.
Coronary artery embolism:
Aortic or mitral endocarditis.
Prosthetic aortic or mitral valves.
Abnormal native valves or left ventricular mural thrombus.
Platelet embolism.
Coronary arteritis:
Polyarteritis nodosa, progressive systemic sclerosis, giant cell arteritis.
Mucocutaneous lymph node syndrome (Kawasaki disease).
Syphilitic coronary ostial stenosis.
Miscellaneous mechanical obstruction of the coronary arteries:
Coronary artery dissection in Marfan syndrome.
Coronary artery dissection in pregnancy.
Prolapse of aortic valve myxomatous polyps into the coronary ostia.
Dissection or rupture of the sinus of Valsalva.

Functional obstruction of the coronary arteries:
Coronary artery spasm with or without atherosclerosis.
Myocardial bridges.

Hypertrophy of the Ventricular Myocardium
Left ventricular hypertrophy associated with coronary heart disease.
Hypertensive heart disease without significant coronary atherosclerosis.
Hypertrophic myocardium secondary to valvular heart disease.
Hypertrophic cardiomyopathy:
Obstructive.
Nonobstructive.
Primary or secondary pulmonary hypertension:
Advanced chronic right ventricular overload.
Pulmonary hypertension in pregnancy (highest risk peripartum).

Myocardial Diseases and Dysfunction, with or without Heart Failure
Chronic congestive heart failure:
Ischemic cardiomyopathy.
Idiopathic dilated cardiomyopathy, acquired.
Hereditary dilated cardiomyopathy.
Alcoholic cardiomyopathy.
Hypertensive cardiomyopathy.
Postmyocarditis cardiomyopathy.
Peripartum cardiomyopathy.
Idiopathic fibrosis.
Acute and subacute cardiac failure:
Massive acute myocardial infarction.
Myocarditis, acute or fulminant.
Acute alcoholic cardiac dysfunction.
Takotsubo syndrome (uncertain risk for sudden death).
Ball valve embolism in aortic stenosis or prosthesis.
Mechanical disruptions of cardiac structures:
Rupture of the ventricular free wall.
Disruption of the mitral apparatus:
Papillary muscle.
Chordae tendineae.
Leaflet.
Rupture of the interventricular septum.
Acute pulmonary edema in noncompliant ventricles.

Inflammatory, Infiltrative, Neoplastic, and Degenerative Processes
Viral myocarditis, with or without ventricular dysfunction:
Acute phase.
Postmyocarditis interstitial fibrosis.
Myocarditis associated with the vasculitides.
Sarcoidosis.
Progressive systemic sclerosis.
Amyloidosis.
Hemochromatosis.
Idiopathic giant cell myocarditis.
Chagas disease.
Cardiac ganglionitis.
Arrhythmogenic right ventricular dysplasia, right ventricular cardiomyopathy.
Neuromuscular diseases (e.g., muscular dystrophy, Friedreich ataxia, myotonic dystrophy).
Intramural tumors:
Primary.
Metastatic.
Obstructive intracavitary tumors:
Neoplastic.
Thrombotic.

Diseases of the Cardiac Valves
Valvular aortic stenosis/insufficiency.
Mitral valve disruption.
Mitral valve prolapse.
Endocarditis.
Prosthetic valve dysfunction.

Congenital Heart Disease
Congenital aortic (potentially high risk) or pulmonic (low risk) valve stenosis.
Congenital septal defects with Eisenmenger physiology:
Advanced disease.
During labor and delivery.
Late after surgical repair of congenital lesions (e.g., tetralogy of Fallot).

Electrophysiologic Abnormalities
Abnormalities of the conducting system:
Fibrosis of the His-Purkinje system:
Primary degeneration (Lenègre disease).
Secondary to fibrosis and calcification of the "cardiac skeleton" (Lev disease).
Postviral conducting system fibrosis.
Hereditary conducting system disease.
Anomalous pathways of conduction (Wolff-Parkinson-White syndrome, short refractory period bypass).
Abnormalities of repolarization:
Congenital abnormalities in duration of the QT interval:
Congenital long–QT interval syndromes:
Romano-Ward syndrome (without deafness).
Jervell and Lange-Nielsen syndrome (with deafness).
Congenital short–QT interval syndrome.
Acquired (or provoked) long–QT interval syndromes:
Drug effect (with genetic predisposition?):
Cardiac, antiarrhythmic.
Noncardiac.
Drug interactions.
Electrolyte abnormality (response modified by genetic predisposition?).
Toxic substances.
Hypothermia.
Central nervous system injury, subarachnoid hemorrhage.
Brugada syndrome—right bundle branch block and ST-segment elevations in the absence of ischemia:
Early repolarization syndrome.
Ventricular fibrillation of unknown or uncertain cause:
Absence of identifiable structural or functional causes:
"Idiopathic" ventricular fibrillation.
Short-coupled torsades de pointes, polymorphic ventricular tachycardia.
Nonspecific fibrofatty infiltration in a previously healthy victim (variation of right ventricular dysplasia?).
Sleep-death in Southeast Asians (see VIIB3, Brugada syndrome):
Bangungut.
Pokkuri.
Lai-tai.

Electrical Instability Related to Neurohumoral and Central Nervous System Influences
Catecholaminergic polymorphic ventricular tachycardia.

Other catecholamine-dependent arrhythmias.
Central nervous system related:
  Psychic stress, emotional extremes (Takotsubo syndrome).
Auditory related:
  "Voodoo death" in primitive cultures.
  Diseases of the cardiac nerves.
  Arrhythmia expression in congenital long–QT interval syndrome.

Sudden Infant Death Syndrome and Sudden Death in Children

Sudden infant death syndrome:
  Immature respiratory control function.
  Long–QT interval syndrome.
  Congenital heart disease.
  Myocarditis.
Sudden death in children:
  Eisenmenger syndrome, aortic stenosis, hypertrophic cardiomyopathy, pulmonary atresia.
  After corrective surgery for congenital heart disease.
  Myocarditis.
  Genetic disorders of electrical function (e.g., long–QT interval syndrome).
  No identified structural or functional cause.

Miscellaneous

Sudden death during extreme physical activity (seek predisposing causes).
Commotio cordis—blunt chest trauma.
Mechanical interference with venous return:
  Acute cardiac tamponade.
  Massive pulmonary embolism.
  Acute intracardiac thrombosis.
Dissecting aneurysm of the aorta.
Toxic and metabolic disturbances (other than the QT interval effects listed above):
  Electrolyte disturbances.
  Metabolic disturbances.
  Proarrhythmic effects of antiarrhythmic drugs.
  Proarrhythmic effects of noncardiac drugs.
Mimics sudden cardiac death:
  "Café coronary."
  Acute alcoholic states ("holiday heart").
  Acute asthmatic attacks.
  Air or amniotic fluid embolism.

SUDDEN DEATH, PEDIATRIC AGE[45]

ICD-10CM #	R99	Ill-defined and unknown cause of mortality

SIDS AND SIDS "MIMICS"

SIDS.
Long QT syndromes.
Inborn errors of metabolism.
Child abuse.
Myocarditis.
Duct-dependent congenital heart disease.

CORRECTED OR UNOPERATED CONGENITAL HEART DISEASE

Aortic stenosis.
Tetralogy of Fallot.
Transposition of great vessels (postoperative atrial switch).
Mitral valve prolapse.
Hematologic left heart syndrome.
Eisenmenger syndrome.

CORONARY ARTERIAL DISEASE

Anomalous origin.
Anomalous tract.
Kawasaki disease.
Periarteritis.
Arterial dissection.
Marfan syndrome.
Myocardial infarction.

MYOCARDIAL DISEASE

Myocarditis.
Hypertrophic cardiomyopathy.
Dilated cardiomyopathy.
Arrhythmogenic right ventricular dysplasia.

CONDUCTION SYSTEM ABNORMALITY/ARRHYTHMIA

Long QT syndromes.
Proarrhythmic drugs.
Preexcitation syndromes.
Heart block.
Commotio cordis.
Idiopathic ventricular fibrillation.
Heart tumor.

MISCELLANEOUS

Pulmonary hypertension.
Pulmonary embolism.
Heat stroke.
Cocaine.
Anorexia nervosa.
Electrolyte disturbances.

SIDS, Sudden infant death syndrome.

SUDDEN DEATH, YOUNG ATHLETE

ICD-10CM #	R99	Ill-defined and unknown cause of mortality

Hypertrophic cardiomyopathy.
Coronary artery anomalies.
Myocarditis.
Ruptured aortic aneurysm (Marfan syndrome).
Arrhythmias.
Aortic valve stenosis.
Asthma.
Trauma (cerebral, cardiac).
Drug and alcohol abuse.
Heat stroke.
Cardiac sarcoidosis.
Atherosclerotic coronary artery disease.
Dilated cardiomyopathy.

SUPERIOR VENA CAVA SEGMENT ABNORMALITIES[37]

ICD-10CM #	Q26.8	Other congenital malformations of great veins

DIFFERENTIAL DIAGNOSIS OF AN ABNORMAL SUPERIOR VENA CAVA SEGMENT

Increased SVC Pressure
SVC obstruction:
  Lung cancer.
  Stricture resulting from long-term cannulation.
  Right-sided heart failure.

Increased SVC Volume
Vein of Galen aneurysm.
Upper extremity AVM.
Partial anomalous pulmonary venous connection.
Interruption of the IVC with azygos continuation.

AVM, Arteriovenous malformation; *IVC*, inferior vena cava; *SVC*, superior vena cava.

SWOLLEN LIMB

ICD-10CM #	M79.89	Other specified soft tissue disorders

Trauma.
Insect bite.
Abscess.
Lymphedema.
Thrombophlebitis.
Lipoma.
Neurofibroma.
Postphlebitic syndrome.
Myositis ossificans.
Nephrosis, cirrhosis, congestive heart failure.
Hypoalbuminemia.
Varicose veins.

SYMPATHOMIMETIC TOXICITY[12]

ICD-10CM #	Varies with specific diagnosis

SUBSTANCES THAT CAN CAUSE SYMPATHOMIMETIC TOXICITY

Methamphetamines (ice [crystals]); speed (powder), pills, base (oily powder).
3, 4-methylenedioxymethamphetamine (MDMA or Ecstasy).
Phenylethylamines (bath salts).
Cocaine.
Ma huang (herbal ecstasy).
Paramethoxyamphetamine (PMA or "death").
Mephedrone (4-MMC).
Pseudoephedrine.
Methylphenidate.
Imidazolines: decongestants (naphazoline, oxymetazoline, tetrahydrozoline).
Clonidine withdrawal.*
Dexamphetamine.
Caffeine.
Yohimbe-containing supplements (used in combinations with stimulants).

*Clonidine is a central α_2 agonist; it does not cause acute sympathomimetic syndrome except in abrupt withdrawals.

TALL STATURE[80]

ICD-10CM #	E22.0	Acromegaly and pituitary gigantism

CONSTITUTIONAL (FAMILIAL OR GENETIC)—MOST COMMON CAUSE

Endocrine Causes

Growth hormone excess—gigantism.
Sexual precocity (tall as children, short as adults):
  True sexual precocity.
  Pseudosexual precocity.

Androgen deficiency:
  Klinefelter syndrome.
  Bilateral anorchism.

GENETIC CAUSES

Klinefelter syndrome.
Syndromes of XYY, XXYY.

MISCELLANEOUS SYNDROMES AND DISORDERS

Cerebral gigantism or Sotos syndrome: prominent forehead, hypertelorism, high arched palate, dolichocephaly, mental retardation, large hands and feet, and premature eruption of teeth. Large at birth, with most rapid growth in first 4 yr of life.

Marfan syndrome: disorder of mesodermal tissues, subluxation of the lenses, arachnodactyly, and aortic aneurysm.

Homocystinuria: same phenotype as Marfan syndrome.

Obesity: tall as infants, children, and adolescents.

Total lipodystrophy: large hands and feet, generalized loss of subcutaneous fat, insulin-resistant diabetes mellitus, and hepatomegaly.

Beckwith-Wiedemann syndrome: neonatal tallness, omphalocele, macroglossia, and neonatal hypoglycemia.

Weaver-Smith syndrome: excessive intrauterine growth, mental retardation, megalocephaly, widened bifrontal diameter, hypertelorism, large ears, micrognathia, camptodactyly, broad thumbs, and limited extension of elbows and knees.

Marshall-Smith syndrome: excessive intrauterine growth, mental retardation, blue sclerae, failure to thrive, and early death.

TARDIVE DYSKINESIA[85]

ICD-10CM #		
	R27.9	Unspecified lack of coordination
	F44.4	Conversion disorder with motor symptom or deficit
	F44.6	Conversion disorder with sensory symptom or deficit
	G24.4	Idiopathic orofacial dystonia

DIFFERENTIAL DIAGNOSIS

Medications (antidepressants, anticholinergics, amphetamines, lithium, L-dopa, phenytoin).
Brain neoplasms.
Ill-fitting dentures.
Huntington disease.
Idiopathic dystonias (tics, blepharospasm, aging).
Wilson disease.
Extrapyramidal syndrome (postanoxic or postencephalitic).
Torsion dystonia.

TASTE AND SMELL LOSS[18]

ICD-10CM #		
	R43.0	Anosmia
	R43.1	Parosmia
	R43.2	Parageusia

TASTE

Local: radiation therapy.
Systemic: cancer, renal failure, hepatic failure, nutritional deficiency (vitamin B_{12}, zinc), Cushing syndrome, hypothyroidism, diabetes mellitus, infection (influenza), drugs (antirheumatic and antiproliferative).
Neurologic: Bell palsy, familial dysautonomia, multiple sclerosis.

SMELL

Local: allergic rhinitis, sinusitis, nasal polyposis, bronchial asthma.
Systemic: renal failure, hepatic failure, nutritional deficiency (vitamin B_{12}), Cushing syndrome, hypothyroidism, diabetes mellitus, infection (viral hepatitis, influenza), drugs (nasal sprays, antibiotics).
Neurologic: head trauma, multiple sclerosis, Parkinson disease, frontal brain tumor.

TELANGIECTASIA

ICD-10CM #		
	I78.8	Other diseases of capillaries
	I78.9	Disease of capillaries, unspecified

Oral contraceptive agents.
Pregnancy.
Rosacea.
Varicose veins.
Trauma.
Drug induced (corticosteroids, systemic or topical).
Spider telangiectases.
Hepatic cirrhosis.
Mastocytosis.
Systemic lupus erythematosus, dermatomyositis, systemic sclerosis.

TENDINOPATHY[10]

ICD-10CM #		
	M67.90	Unspecified disorder of synovium and tendon, unspecified site
	M71.9	Bursopathy, unspecified

INTRINSIC FACTORS

Anatomic Factors
Malalignment.
Muscle weakness or imbalance.
Muscle inflexibility.
Decreased vascularity.
Systemic Factors
Inflammatory conditions (e.g., systemic lupus erythematosus).
Pregnancy.
Quinolone-induced tendinopathy.
Age-Related Factors
Tendon degeneration.
Increased tendon stiffness.
Tendon calcification.
Decreased vascularity.

EXTRINSIC FACTORS

Repetitive Mechanical Load
Excessive duration.
Excessive frequency.

Excessive intensity.
Poor technique.
Workplace factors.
Equipment Problems
Footwear.
Athletic field surface.
Equipment factors (e.g., racquet size).
Protective gear.

TESTICULAR CYSTIC LESIONS[15]

ICD-10CM #	Varies with specific diagnosis

BENIGN

Tunica albuginea cysts.
Tunica vaginalis cysts.
Intratesticular cysts.
Tubular ectasia of rete testis.
Cystic dysplasia.
Epidermoid cysts.
Abscess.

MALIGNANT

Nonseminomatous germ cell tumor.
Necrosis or hemorrhage in tumor.
Tubular obstruction by tumor.
Lymphoma.

TESTICULAR FAILURE[114]

ICD-10CM #	E29	Testicular dysfunction

PRIMARY

Klinefelter syndrome (XXY).
XYY.
Vanishing testes syndrome (in utero or early postnatal torsion).
Noonan syndrome.
Varicocele.
Myotonic dystrophy.
Orchitis (mumps, gonorrhea).
Cryptorchidism.
Chemical exposure.
Irradiation to testes.
Spinal cord injury.
Polyglandular failure.
Idiopathic oligospermia or azoospermia.
Germinal cell aplasia (Sertoli cell-only syndrome).
Idiopathic testicular failure.
Testicular torsion.
Testicular trauma.
Diethylstilbestrol (maternal use during pregnancy leading to in utero estrogen exposure).
Testicular tumor with subsequent irradiation therapy, chemotherapy, or surgery (retroperitoneal lymph node dissection or orchiectomy).

SECONDARY

Delayed puberty.
Kallmann syndrome.
Isolated gonadotropin deficiency.
Prader-Labhart-Willi syndrome.
Lawrence-Moon-Biedl syndrome.
Central nervous system irradiation.
Prepubertal panhypopituitarism.
Postpubertal panhypopituitarism.

Differential Diagnosis

II

Hypogonadism secondary to hyperprolactinemia.
Adrenogenital syndrome.
Chronic liver disease.
Chronic renal failure/uremia.
Hemochromatosis.
Cushing syndrome.
Malnutrition.
Massive obesity.
Sickle cell anemia.
Hyper/hypothyroidism.
Anabolic steroid use.

TESTICULAR PAIN

| ICD-10CM # | N50.9 | Disorder of male genital organs, unspecified |
| | R10.2 | Pelvic and perineal pain |

Testicular torsion.
Trauma.
Epididymitis.
Orchitis.
Neoplasm.
Urolithiasis.
Inguinal hernia.
Infection (cellulitis, abscess, folliculitis).
Anxiety.

TESTICULAR SIZE VARIATIONS[114]

ICD-10CM #	N50.0	Atrophy of testis
	N44.2	Benign cyst of testis
	N44.8	Other noninflammatory disorders of the testis
	N50.3	Cyst of epididymis
	N50.8	Other specified disorders of male genital organs
	N53.12	Painful ejaculation
	E29.1	Testicular hypofunction

SMALL TESTES
Hypothalamic-pituitary dysfunction.
Gonadotropin deficiency.
Growth hormone deficiency.
Normal variant.
Primary hypogonadism.
Autoimmune destruction.
Chemotherapy.
Cryptorchidism.
Irradiation.
Klinefelter syndrome.
Orchiditis.
Testicular regression syndrome.
Torsion.
Trauma.

LARGE TESTES
Adrenal rest tissue.
Compensatory.
Fragile X syndrome.
Idiopathic.
Tumor.

TETANUS[10]

| ICD-10CM # | A35 | Other tetanus |

TETANUS "MIMICS"
Acute abdomen.
Black widow spider bite.
Dental abscess.
Dislocated mandible.
Dystonic reaction.
Encephalitis.
Head trauma.
Hyperventilation syndrome.
Hypocalcemia.
Meningitis.
Peritonsillar abscess.
Progressive fluctuating muscular rigidity (stiff-man syndrome).
Psychogenic.
Rabies.
Sepsis.
Subarachnoid hemorrhage.
Status epilepticus.
Strychnine poisoning.
Temporomandibular joint syndrome.

THORACIC AORTIC ANEURYSMS[37]

| ICD-10CM # | I71.2 | Thoracic aortic aneurysm, without rupture |

ANEURYSMS OF THE THORACIC AORTA
By Location
Sinuses of Valsalva:
  Infected.
  Congenital.
  Trauma.
  Annuloaortic ectasia.
Ascending aorta:
  Aortitis.
  Takayasu disease.
  Syphilis.
  Trauma.
  Annuloaortic ectasia.
  Marfan syndrome.
  Ehlers-Danlos syndrome.
Aortic arch:
  Trauma.
  Infected.
  Syphilis.
  Of patent ductus arteriosus.
  Coarctation.
  Takayasu disease.
  Duct of Kommerell from aberrant right subclavian artery.
Descending aorta:
  Atherosclerosis.
  Infected.
  Inflammatory.
  Syphilis.
  Takayasu disease.
By Shape
Saccular:
  Trauma.
  Infected.
  Of ductus arteriosus.
  Syphilis.
  Penetrating ulcer.
Fusiform:
  Cystic medial necrosis.
  Atherosclerosis.
By Integrity of the Aortic Wall
True:
  Cystic medial necrosis.
  Atherosclerosis.
  Collagen vascular disease.
  Rheumatoid arthritis.
  Ankylosing spondylitis.
  Aortitis.
False:
  Trauma.
  Infected.
  Penetrating ulcer.
  Rupture.
  After aortotomy.

THROMBOCYTOPENIA

ICD-10CM #	D47.3	Essential (hemorrhagic) thrombocythemia
	D69.59	Other secondary thrombocytopenia
	D69.6	Thrombocytopenia, unspecified

INCREASED DESTRUCTION
Immunologic
Drugs: quinine, quinidine, digitalis, procainamide, thiazide diuretics, sulfonamides, phenytoin, aspirin, penicillin, heparin, gold, meprobamate, sulfa drugs, phenylbutazone, NSAIDs, methyldopa, cimetidine, furosemide, INH, cephalosporins, chlorpropamide, organic arsenicals, chloroquine, platelet glycoprotein IIb/IIIa receptor inhibitors, ranitidine, indomethacin, carboplatin, ticlopidine, clopidogrel.
Idiopathic thrombocytopenic purpura (ITP).
Transfusion reaction: transfusion of platelets with plasminogen activator (PLA) in recipients without PLA-1.
Fetal/maternal incompatibility.
Collagen vascular diseases (e.g., systemic lupus erythematosus).
Autoimmune hemolytic anemia.
Lymphoreticular disorders (e.g., CLL).
Nonimmunologic
Prosthetic heart valves.
Thrombotic thrombocytopenic purpura.
Sepsis.
disseminated intravascular coagulation.
Hemolytic-uremic syndrome.
Giant cavernous hemangioma.

DECREASED PRODUCTION
Abnormal marrow.
Marrow infiltration (e.g., leukemia, lymphoma, fibrosis).
Marrow suppression (e.g., chemotherapy, alcohol, radiation).
Hereditary disorders.
Wiskott-Aldrich syndrome: X-linked disorder characterized by thrombocytopenia, eczema, and repeated infections.

May-Hegglin anomaly: increased megakaryocytes but ineffective thrombopoiesis.

Vitamin deficiencies (e.g., vitamin B_{12}, folic acid).

SPLENIC SEQUESTRATION, HYPERSPLENISM

Dilutional, as a result of massive transfusion.

THROMBOCYTOPENIA, IN PREGNANCY[31]

ICD-10CM #	D69.59	Other secondary thrombocytopenia

Incidental thrombocytopenia of pregnancy (gestational thrombocytopenia).

Preeclampsia/eclampsia.
  Peripartum/postpartum thrombotic microangiopathy.

Disseminated intravascular coagulation secondary to:
  Abruptio placentae.
  Endometritis.
  Amniotic fluid embolism.
  Retained fetus.

Thrombotic thrombocytopenic purpura.

Hemolytic-uremic syndrome.

THROMBOCYTOPENIA, INHERITED DISORDERS[18]

ICD-10CM #	D47.3	Essential (hemorrhagic) thrombocythemia

Amegakaryocytic thrombocytopenia.

Thrombocytopenia–absent radii.

MYH9-related thrombocytopenia:

May-Hegglin anomaly.

Fechtner syndrome.

Epstein syndrome.

Sebastian syndrome.

X-linked macrothrombocytopenia.

Wiskott-Aldrich syndrome.

X-linked thrombocytopenia.

Thrombocytopenia and radioulnar synostosis.

Familial platelet disorder—AML.

Familial dominant thrombocytopenia.

Paris-Trousseau thrombocytopenia.

Bernard-Soulier syndrome.

Bernard-Soulier carrier/Mediterranean macrothrombocytopenia.

THROMBOCYTOPENIA IN NEWBORNS, DIFFERENTIAL DIAGNOSIS[34]

ICD-10CM #	D47.3	Essential (hemorrhagic) thrombocythemia
	D69.59	Other secondary thrombocytopenia
	D69.6	Thrombocytopenia, unspecified

DIFFERENTIAL DIAGNOSIS OF THROMBOCYTOPENIA IN NEWBORNS

Perinatal hypoxemia.

Placental insufficiency.

Congenital infection.
  Sepsis.
  Toxoplasmosis.
  Rubella.
  Cytomegalovirus.

Autoimmune:
  Maternal immune thrombocytopenia.
  Maternal systemic lupus erythematosus.

Disseminated intravascular coagulation.

Maternal drug exposure.

Congenital heart disease.

Hereditary thrombocytopenia.
  MYH9 macrothrombocytopenia (including May-Hegglin anomaly).
  Thrombocytopenia absent radii syndrome.
  Amegakaryocytic thrombocytopenia.
  Wiskott-Aldrich syndrome.
  Fanconi anemia.

Hemangioma with thrombocytopenia.
  Kasabach-Merritt syndrome.

Bone marrow infiltration.
  Congenital leukemia.

THROMBOCYTOSIS

ICD-10CM #	D75.9	Disease of blood and blood-forming organs, unspecified

Iron deficiency.

Posthemorrhage.

Neoplasms (GI tract).

CML.

Polycythemia vera.

Myelofibrosis with myeloid metaplasia.

Infections.

After splenectomy.

Postpartum.

Hemophilia.

Pancreatitis.

Cirrhosis.

Idiopathic.

THROMBOSIS OR THROMBOTIC DIATHESIS[18]

ICD-10CM #	I74.09	Other arterial embolism and thrombosis of abdominal aorta

DIFFERENTIAL DIAGNOSIS OF THE PATIENT PRESENTING WITH THROMBOSIS OR THROMBOTIC DIATHESIS

Inherited (Primary) Hypercoagulable States

Activated protein C resistance caused by factor V Leiden mutation.

Prothrombin gene mutation (G to A transition at position 20210 in the 3-untranslated region).

Antithrombin III deficiency.

Protein C deficiency.

Protein S deficiency.

Dysfibrinogenemias (rare).

Acquired (Secondary) Hypercoagulable States

In association physiologic or thrombogenic stimuli:
  Pregnancy (especially the postpartum period).
  Estrogen use (oral contraceptives, hormone replacement therapy).

Immobilization.

Trauma.

Postoperative state.

Advancing age.

Obesity.

Prolonged air travel.

Lupus anticoagulant or antiphospholipid antibody syndrome.

In association with other clinical disorders.

Mixed/Unknown

Activated protein C resistance in the absence of factor V Leiden.

Elevated factor VIII level.

Elevated factor XI level.

Elevated factor IX level.

Elevated thrombin activatable fibrinolysis inhibitor (TAFI) level.

Decreased free tissue factor pathway inhibitor (TFPI) level.

Decreased plasma fibrinolytic activity.

THYMIC MASSES[78]

ICD-10CM #	Varies with specific diagnosis

THYMIC MASSES

Thymic hyperplasia.

Thymoma.

Thymic carcinoma.

Thymic neuroendocrine tumors.
  Carcinoid.
  Small-cell carcinoma.

Thymic cysts (not rhizomatous).

Thymolipoma.

Metastases to the thymus.

THYMOMA, DISEASES ASSOCIATIONS[78]

ICD-10CM #	Varies with specific diagnosis

SYSTEMIC DISEASES MOST COMMONLY ASSOCIATED WITH THYMOMA

Myasthenia gravis.

Cytopenias (most commonly red cell hypoplasia).

Nonthymic malignancies.

Hypogammaglobulinemia.

Systemic lupus erythematosus.

Polymyositis.

Rheumatoid arthritis.

Thyroiditis.

Sjögren syndrome.

Ulcerative colitis.

THYROMEGALY

ICD-10CM #	Varies with specific diagnosis

Goiter.

Graves disease.

Thyroiditis (lymphocytic, granulomatous, suppurative).

Toxic adenoma.

Neoplasm (primary, metastatic).

THYROTOXICOSIS[30]

ICD-10CM #	E05.80

Differential Diagnosis

II

CAUSES OF THYROTOXICOSIS

Sustained Hormone Overproduction (Hyperthyroidism)

Low TSH, high RAIU:
Graves disease (von Basedow disease).
Toxic multinodular goiter.
Toxic adenoma.
Chorionic gonadotropin-induced:
Gestational hyperthyroidism: physiologic hyperthyroidism of pregnancy, familial gestational hyperthyroidism due to TSH receptor mutations.
Trophoblastic tumors.
Inherited nonimmune hyperthyroidism associated with TSH receptor or G protein mutations.
Low TSH, low RAIU:
Iodide-induced hyperthyroidism (Jod-Basedow effect).
Amiodarone-associated hyperthyroidism due to iodide release.
Struma ovarii:
Metastatic functioning thyroid carcinoma.
Normal or elevated TSH:
TSH-secreting pituitary tumors.
Thyroid hormone resistance with pituitary predominance.

TRANSIENT HORMONE EXCESS (THYROTOXICOSIS)

Low TSH, low RAIU
Thyroiditis:
Autoimmune: lymphocytic thyroiditis (silent thyroiditis, painless thyroiditis, postpartum thyroiditis), acute exacerbation of Hashimoto disease.
Viral or postviral:
Subacute (granulomatous, painful, postviral) thyroiditis.
Drug-induced or associated thyroiditis:
Amiodarone.
Lithium, interferon-α, interleukin-2, GM-CSF.
Infectious thyroiditis.
Exogenous thyroid hormone:
Iatrogenic overreplacement.
Thyrotoxicosis factitia.
Ingestion of natural products containing thyroid hormone:
"Hamburger" thyrotoxicosis.
Natural foodstuffs.
Thyromimetic compounds (e.g., tiratricol PLB).
Occupational exposure to thyroid hormone (e.g., pill manufacturing, veterinary occupations).

GM-CSF, granulocyte-macrophage colony-stimulating factor; *RAIU,* radioactive iodine uptake; *TSH,* thyroid-stimulating hormone.

TICK-RELATED INFECTIONS

ICD-10CM #	A77.0	Spotted fever due to *Rickettsia rickettsii*
	A93.2	Colorado tick fever
	B60.0	Babesiosis
	A77.8	Other spotted fevers
	A69.20	Lyme disease, unspecified

Lyme disease.
Rocky Mountain spotted fever.
Babesiosis.
Tularemia.
Q fever.
Colorado tick fever.
Ehrlichiosis.
Relapsing fever.

TICS

| ICD-10CM # | F95.9 | Tic disorder, unspecified |

Tourette syndrome.
Physiologic tic.
Anxiety disorder.
Huntington disease.
Medications (e.g., antipsychotics, carbamazepine, phenytoin, phenobarbital).
Encephalitis.
Head trauma.
Schizophrenia.
Carbon monoxide poisoning.
Stroke.
Sydenham chorea.
Creutzfeldt-Jakob disease.

TORSADES DE POINTES[97]

| ICD-10CM # | I47.2 | Ventricular tachycardia |

Antiarrhythmics known to increase the QT interval (e.g., quinidine, procainamide, amiodarone, disopyramide, sotalol).
Tricyclic antidepressants and phenothiazines.
Histamine (H_1) antagonists (e.g., astemizole, terfenadine).
Antiviral and antifungal agents and antibiotics.
Hypokinemia.
Hypomagnesemia.
Insecticide poisoning.
Bradyarrhythmias.
Congenital long QT syndrome.
Subarachnoid hemorrhage.
Chloroquine, pentamidine.
Cocaine abuse.

TOXIC MEGACOLON, CAUSES[64]

| ICD-10CM # | K59.3 | Megacolon, not elsewhere classified |

INFLAMMATORY

Ulcerative colitis.
Crohn disease.

INFECTIOUS

Bacterial:
Clostridium difficile pseudomembranous colitis.
Salmonella (typhoid and nontyphoid).
Shigella.
Campylobacter.
Yersinia.
Parasitic:
Entamoeba histolytica.
Cryptosporidium.

Viral:
Cytomegalovirus colitis.

OTHER

Ischemia.
Kaposi sarcoma.

TRACHEOBRONCHIAL NARROWING ON X-RAY[21]

| ICD-10CM # | Varies with specific diagnosis |

CAUSES OF TRACHEOBRONCHIAL NARROWING

Long-Segment/Diffuse Narrowing
Sarcoidosis.
Amyloidosis.
Granulomatosis with polyangiitis.
Relapsing polychondritis.
Tracheobronchopathia osteochondroplastica.
Pemphigoid.
Short-Segment Narrowing
Previous intubation or tracheostomy.
Congenital stenosis or web.
Extrinsic compression (from thyroid).
Adenoid cystic carcinoma.
Squamous carcinoma.

TRANSIENT AMNESIA[101]

| ICD-10CM # | Varies with specific diagnosis |

Alcohol abuse.
Wernickea-Korsakoff syndrome.
Alcoholic blackouts.
Electroconvulsive therapy (ECT).
Head trauma.
Medications.
Benzodiazepines.
Fentanyl.
Gamma hydroxybutyrate (GHB).[a]
Scopolamine, other anticholinergic medications.
Sildenafil (Viagra), tadalafil (Cialis).
Zolpidem (Ambien).

[a]When used illicitly, people call GHB the "date-rape drug." Under carefully controlled conditions, neurologists prescribe GHB as oxybate (Xyrem) to treat cataplexy.

TREMOR

ICD-10CM #	R25.0	Abnormal head movements
	R25.1	Tremor, unspecified
	R25.2	Cramp and spasm
	R25.3	Fasciculation
	R25.9	Unspecified abnormal involuntary movements
	G25.0	Essential tremor
	G25.1	Drug-induced tremor
	G25.2	Other specified forms of tremor

REST TREMORS

Parkinson disease.
Other parkinsonian syndromes (less commonly).
Midbrain (rubral) tremor: rest <postural <kinetic.

Wilson disease (also acquired hepatocerebral degeneration).

Essential tremor—only if severe: rest <postural and action.

POSTURAL AND ACTION (TERMINAL) TREMORS

Physiologic tremor.

Exaggerated physiologic tremor (these factors can also aggravate other forms of tremor).

Stress, fatigue, anxiety, emotion.

Endocrine: hypoglycemia, thyrotoxicosis, pheochromocytoma, adrenocorticosteroids.

Drugs and toxins: β-agonists, dopamine agonists, amphetamines, lithium, tricyclic antidepressants, neuroleptics, theophylline, caffeine, valproic acid, alcohol withdrawal, mercury (Hatter shakes), lead, arsenic, others.

Essential tremor (familial or sporadic):

Primary writing tremor.

With other central nervous system disorders:

Parkinson disease.

Other akinetic-rigid syndromes.

Idiopathic dystonia, including focal dystonias.

With peripheral neuropathy:

Charcot-Marie-Tooth syndrome (controversial whether to call this the Roussy-Levy syndrome).

Variety of other peripheral neuropathies (especially dysgammaglobulinemia).

Cerebellar tremor.

KINETIC (INTENTION) TREMOR

Disease of cerebellar outflow (dentate nucleus and superior cerebellar peduncle): multiple sclerosis, trauma, tumor, vascular disease, Wilson acquired hepatocerebral degeneration, drugs, toxins (e.g., mercury), others.

MISCELLANEOUS RHYTHMICAL MOVEMENT DISORDERS

Psychogenic tremor.

Orthostatic tremor.

Rhythmical movements in dystonia (dystonic tremor).

Rhythmical myoclonus (segmental myoclonus—e.g., palatal or branchial myoclonus, spinal myoclonus, limb myorhythmia).

Oscillatory myoclonus.

Asterixis.

Clonus.

Epilepsia partialis continua.

Hereditary chin quivering.

Spasmus nutans.

Head bobbing with third ventricular cysts.

Nystagmus.

TREMOR, IN CHILDREN, CAUSES[19]

ICD-10CM #	R25.0	Abnormal head movements
	R25.1	Tremor, unspecified
	R25.2	Cramp and spasm
	R25.3	Fasciculation
	R25.9	Unspecified abnormal involuntary movements

BENIGN

Enhanced physiologic tremor.

Shuddering attacks.

Jitteriness.

Spasmus nutans.

STATIC INJURY/STRUCTURAL

Cerebellar malformation.

Stroke (particularly in the midbrain or cerebellum).

Multiple sclerosis.

HEREDITARY/DEGENERATIVE

Familial essential tremor.

Fragile X premutation.

Wilson disease.

Huntington disease.

Juvenile parkinsonism (tremor is rare).

Pallidonigral degeneration.

METABOLIC

Hyperthyroidism.

Hyperadrenergic state (including pheochromocytoma and neuroblastoma).

Hypomagnesemia.

Hypocalcemia.

Hypoglycemia.

Hepatic encephalopathy.

Vitamin B_{12} deficiency.

Inborn errors of metabolism.

Mitochondrial disorders.

DRUGS/TOXINS

Valproate, phenytoin, carbamazepine, lamotrigine, gabapentin, lithium, tricyclic antidepressants, stimulants (cocaine, amphetamine, caffeine, thyroxine, bronchodilators), neuroleptics, cyclosporin, toluene, mercury, thallium, amiodarone, nicotine, lead, manganese, arsenic, cyanide, naphthalene, ethanol, lindane, serotonin reuptake inhibitors.

PERIPHERAL NEUROPATHIES

Psychogenic.

TRICHOMEGALY[44]

| ICD-10CM # | | Not available |

CAUSES OF TRICHOMEGALY

Drug-induced: topical prostaglandin analogues, phenytoin and cyclosporine.

Malnutrition.

AIDS.

Porphyria.

Hypothyroidism.

Familial.

Congenital: Oliver-McFarlane, Cornelia de Lange, Goldstein-Hutt, Hermansky-Pudlak syndromes.

TUBULOINTERSTITIAL DISEASE, ACUTE[24]

| ICD-10CM # | N17.0 | Acute kidney failure with tubular necrosis |

DRUGS

Antibiotics, penicillins, cephalosporins, rifampin.

Sulfonamides: cotrimoxazole, sulfamethoxazole.

NSAIDs: propionic acid derivatives.

Miscellaneous: phenytoin, thiazides, allopurinol, cimetidine, ifosfamide.

INFECTIONS

Invasion of renal parenchyma.

Reaction to systemic infections: streptococcal, diphtheria, hantavirus.

SYSTEMIC DISEASES

Immune mediated: systemic lupus erythematosus, transplanted kidney, cryoglobulinemias.

Metabolic: urate, oxalate.

Neoplastic: lymphoproliferative diseases.

IDIOPATHIC

TUBULOINTERSTITIAL KIDNEY DISEASE[24]

| ICD-10CM # | N17.0 | Acute kidney failure with tubular necrosis |

Ischemic and toxic acute tubular necrosis.

Allergic interstitial nephritis.

Interstitial nephritis secondary to immune complex-related collagen vascular disease (e.g., systemic lupus erythematosus, Sjögren).

Granulomatous diseases (sarcoidosis, uveitis).

Pigment-related tubular injury (myoglobinuria, hemoglobinuria).

Hypercalcemia with nephrocalcinosis.

Tubular obstruction (drugs such as indinavir, uric acid in tumor lysis syndrome).

Myeloma kidney or cast nephropathy.

Infection-related interstitial nephritis: *Legionella*, *Leptospira*.

Infiltrative diseases (e.g., lymphoma).

TUMOR MARKERS ELEVATION[2]

| ICD-10CM # | R97.8 | Other abnormal tumor markers |

CAUSES OF ELEVATED LEVELS OF TUMOR MARKERS

Carcinoembryonic Antigen (CEA)

Colonic cancer (higher levels if the tumor is more differentiated or is extensive or has spread to the liver).

Lung or breast cancer; seminoma.

Cigarette smokers.

Cirrhosis, inflammatory bowel disease, rectal polyps, pancreatitis.

Advanced age.

α-Fetoprotein

Hepatocellular cancer: very high titers or a rising titer is strongly suggestive, but >10% of patients do not have an elevated level.

Hepatic regeneration (e.g., cirrhosis, alcoholic or viral hepatitis).

Cancer of the stomach, colon, pancreas, or lung.

Teratocarcinoma or embryonal cell carcinoma (testis, ovary, extragonadal).

Pregnancy.

Ataxia-telangiectasia.

Normal variant.

Prostate-Specific Antigen
Prostate carcinoma (localized disease).
Prostatic hyperplasia.
Prostatitis.
Prostatic infarction.

Cancer-Associated Antigen (CA-19-9)
Pancreatic carcinoma (80% with advanced, well-differentiated cancer have an elevated level).
Other GI cancers: colon, stomach, bile duct.
Acute or chronic pancreatitis.
Chronic liver disease.
Biliary tract disease.

UPPER AIRWAY OBSTRUCTION[12]

ICD-10CM # Varies with specific diagnosis

CAUSES OF UPPER AIRWAY OBSTRUCTION
Altered conscious state:
  Head injury.
  Cerebrovascular accident.
  Drugs and toxins.
  Metabolic—hypoglycemia, hyponatremia.
Foreign bodies.
Infections:
  Tonsillitis.
  Peritonsillar abscess (quinsy).
  Epiglottitis.
  Ludwig angina.
  Other abscesses and infections.
Trauma:
  Blunt or penetrating trauma resulting in edema or hematoma formation.
  Uncontrolled hemorrhage.
  Thermal injuries.
  Inhalation burns.
Neoplasms:
  Larynx, trachea, thyroid.
Allergic reactions:
  Anaphylaxis.
  Angioedema.
Anatomic:
  Tracheomalacia—congenital or acquired (secondary to prolonged intubation).
  Other congenital malformations.
Functional upper airway obstruction syndrome.
Acute-on-chronic causes.
Patients with chronic narrowing of the airway (e.g., due to tracheomalacia) may present with worsening obstruction from an acute upper respiratory tract illness or injury.

UREMIC ENCEPHALOPATHY, DIFFERENTIAL DIAGNOSIS[9]

ICD-10CM # G93.40 Encephalopathy, unspecified

Differential Diagnosis	Comment
Hypertensive encephalopathy	
Systemic inflammatory response syndrome (SIRS):	Observed in septic patients.
Systemic vasculitis:	Vasculitis or lupus with cerebral involvement.

Differential Diagnosis	Comment
Drug-induced neurotoxicity	
Analgesics:	Meperidine, codeine, morphine, gabapentin.
Antibiotics:	High-dose penicillins (may cause seizures), acyclovir, ethambutol (optic nerve damage), erythromycin and aminoglycosides (may cause ototoxicity), nitrofurantoin and isoniazid (peripheral neuropathy).
Psychotropics:	Lithium, haloperidol, clonazepam, diazepam, chlorpromazine.
Immunosuppressants:	Cyclosporine, tacrolimus.
Chemotherapeutics:	Cisplatinum, ifosfamide.
Others:	High doses of loop diuretics (ototoxic), ephedrine, methyldopa, aluminum.
Cerebral atheroembolic disease:	Follows recent aortic or cardiac angiography; associated with peripheral manifestations, including lower extremity cyanosis, livedo reticularis, and eosinophilia.
Subdural hematoma	
Posterior leukoencephalopathy:	Observed particularly following renal transplantation due to reversible, abnormal permeability of the blood-brain barrier. Often manifests as headache followed by mental depression, visual loss, and seizures in the context of volume expansion, acute hypertension, and often treatment with corticosteroids or calcineurin inhibitors. Lesions in the parietal, temporal, and occipital lobes may be seen on imaging studies.

URETERAL COLIC[115]

ICD-10CM # R33.8 Other retention of urine
N13.8 Other obstructive and reflux uropathy

DIAGNOSTIC DIFFERENTIALS OF RENAL OR URETERAL COLIC
Acute cholecystitis, acute cholelithiasis.
Acute appendicitis.
Pelvic inflammatory disease.
Diverticulosis and/or diverticulitis.
Intestinal obstruction.
Leaking abdominal aortic aneurysm.
Musculoskeletal sprains.
Herniated disk.
Herpes zoster (shingles).
GI dysfunction with ileus and/or toxic colonic dilatation.

URETERAL STRICTURE[89]

ICD-10CM # Varies with specific diagnosis

ETIOLOGY OF URETERAL STRICTURE
Malignancy (e.g., transitional cell carcinoma, cervical cancer).
Ureteral calculus.
Radiation.
Ischemia or trauma caused by surgical dissection.
Periureteral fibrosis caused by abdominal aortic aneurysm or endometriosis.
Endoscopic instrumentation.
Renal ablation injury.
Infection (tuberculosis).
Idiopathic condition.

URETERIC OBSTRUCTION, CONGENITAL[21]

ICD-10CM # N13.8 Other obstructive and reflux uropathy
N20.9 Urolithiasis

CONGENITAL CAUSES OF URETERIC OBSTRUCTION
Primary megaureter.
Ureterocele (ectopic and orthotopic).
Ureteric valve.
Distal ureteric stenosis.
Ureteric atresia.
Circumcaval ureter and variants.
Bladder diverticulum.

URETHRAL BLEEDING[89]

ICD-10CM # Varies with specific diagnosis

DIFFERENTIAL DIAGNOSIS FOR URETHRAL BLEEDING
Male
Trauma:
  Blunt (straddle injury, kick to perineum).
  Penetrating (foreign body insertion, failed urethral catheterization).
  Intercourse related (penile fracture, masturbation).

Urethritis:
  Bacterial (gonococcal, nongonococcal).
  Viral.
  Chemical.
  Autoimmune (Reiter syndrome).
Malignancy:
  Urothelial carcinoma.
  Squamous cell carcinoma (meatus/glans).
Condyloma.
Calculus disease.
Female
Trauma:
  Blunt (pelvic fracture).
  Penetrating (foreign body).
Urethral diverticulum.
Urethral caruncle.
Urethritis.
Malignancy.
Calculus disease.

URETHRAL DISCHARGE AND DYSURIA

ICD-10CM #		
R36.0	Urethral discharge without blood
R36.9	Urethral discharge, unspecified
N36.9	Urethral disorder, unspecified
N39.9	Disorder of urinary system, unspecified
R30.0	Dysuria
R30.9	Painful micturition, unspecified

Urethritis (gonococcal, chlamydial, trichomonal).
Cystitis.
Prostatitis.
Vaginitis (candidiasis, chemical).
Meatal stenosis.
Interstitial cystitis.
Trauma (foreign body, masturbation, horseback or bike riding).

URETHRAL OBSTRUCTION, CHILDREN[21]

ICD-10CM #	N13.8	Other obstructive and reflux uropathy

CAUSES OF URETHRAL OBSTRUCTION IN CHILDREN

Intrinsic Lesions
Valve (posterior, anterior, saccular diverticulum).
Stenosis, atresia.
Inflammatory stricture.
Traumatic stricture:
  External trauma (saddle injury, and so on).
  Iatrogenic trauma (catheter, cystoscopy, surgery).
Urethral "tumors":
  Girls: leiomyoma.
  Boys: polyp, rhabdomyosarcoma.
Miscellaneous (epidermolysis bullosa).
Extrinsic Lesions
Presacral mass dissecting inferiorly (tumor, cyst).
Fecal impaction (Hirschsprung, postrepair anal atresia, habitual constipation, neuropathy).

Mass originating in genital organs:
  Boys: utricle cyst, prostate rhabdomyosarcoma, seminal vesicle cyst, Cowper duct cyst.
  Girls: hydrometrocolpos, hydrocolpos, fused labia.

URETHRITIS, PEDIATRIC PATIENT[5]

ICD-10CM #	N34.1	Nonspecific urethritis
	N34.2	Other urethritis

ETIOLOGY OF URETHRITIS

Infectious	Noninfectious
Sexually Transmitted Infections	*Vasculitides*
Neisseria gonorrhoeae.	Reiter syndrome.
Chlamydia trachomatis.	Erythema multiforme.
Trichomonas vaginalis.	Kawasaki disease.
Herpes simplex virus type 2.	Mechanical.
Mycoplasma spp.	Masturbation.
Nonsexually Transmitted Infections	Foreign body.
	Trauma.
Staphylococcus saprophyticus.	Dysfunctional elimination.
Enterobacteriaceae.	Chemical
Gardnerella vaginalis.	Soaps.
Streptococcus spp.	Detergents.
Enterobius vermicularis.	Drugs.

URIC ACID STONES

ICD-10CM #	N20.9	Urolithiasis

Hyperuricemia.
Excessive dietary purine.
Medications (salicylates, allopurinol, probenecid).
Urine pH <5.5 (e.g., diarrhea, high animal protein diet).
Decreased urine output (dehydration, malabsorption, diarrhea, inadequate fluid intake).
Tumor lysis.
Hemolytic anemia.
Myeloproliferative disorders.

URINARY INCONTINENCE, CHILDREN[19]

ICD-10CM #	R32	Unspecified urinary incontinence

CAUSES OF URINARY INCONTINENCE IN CHILDHOOD

Overactive bladder.
Infrequent voiding.
Detrusor-sphincter dyssynergia.
Nonneurogenic neurogenic bladder (Hinman syndrome).
Vaginal voiding.
Giggle incontinence.
Cystitis.
Bladder outlet obstruction (posterior urethral valves).
Ectopic ureter and fistula.

Sphincter abnormality (epispadias, exstrophy; urogenital sinus abnormality).
Neuropathic.
Overflow incontinence.
Traumatic.
Iatrogenic.
Behavioral.
Combination.

URINARY RETENTION[115]

ICD-10CM #	R33.9	Retention of urine, unspecified

COMMON CAUSES OF URINARY RETENTION

Obstructive Cause
Urethral stricture.
Enlarged prostate.
Lower genitourinary tract malignancy.
Pelvic malignancy.
Bladder stones.
Foreign body.
Blood clot.
Posterior urethral valves.
Ureterocele.
Primary Detrusor Insufficiency
Detrusor areflexia.
Multiple sclerosis.
Iatrogenic injury during abdominal or back surgery.
Spinal cord injury.
Myelomeningocele.

URINARY RETENTION, ACUTE

ICD-10CM #	R33.9	Retention of urine, unspecified

Mechanical obstruction: urethral stone, foreign body, urethral stricture, BPH, prostate carcinoma, prostatitis, trauma with hematoma formation.
Neurogenic bladder.
Neurologic disease (MS, parkinsonism, tabes dorsalis, cerebrovascular accident).
Spinal cord injury.
Central nervous system neoplasm (primary or metastatic).
Spinal anesthesia.
Lower urinary tract instrumentation.
Medications (antihistamines, antidepressants, narcotics, anticholinergics).
Abdominal or pelvic surgery.
Alcohol toxicity.
Pregnancy.
Anxiety.
Encephalitis.
Postoperative pain.
Spina bifida occulta.

URINARY TRACT BLEEDING, UPPER[89]

ICD-10CM #	Varies with specific diagnosis

DIFFERENTIAL DIAGNOSIS FOR UPPER URINARY TRACT BLEEDING

Renal glomerular diseases:
  IgA nephropathy (Berger disease).
  Thin basement membrane disease.

Acute glomerulonephritis (e.g., poststrepto-coccal).

Lupus nephritis.

Hereditary nephritis (e.g., Alport syndrome).

Renal tubulointerstitial diseases:

Papillary necrosis.

Sickle cell nephropathy.

Analgesic nephropathy.

Polycystic kidney disease.

Medullary sponge kidney.

Vasculitis:

Henoch-Schönlein purpura.

Wegener granulomatosis.

Infection:

Pyelonephritis.

Xanthogranulomatous pyelonephritis.

Renal tuberculosis.

Fungal infection.

Obstruction:

Ureteropelvic junction obstruction.

Ureteral stricture.

Nephrolithiasis.

Malignancy:

Renal cortical tumors (renal cell carcinoma, benign tumors).

Upper tract urothelial carcinoma.

Fibroepithelial polyp.

Vascular diseases:

Renal arteriovenous malformations (congenital, acquired).

Iliac arterio-ureteral fistula.

Renal artery aneurysm (especially ruptured).

Renal artery pseudoaneurysm.

Renal artery and/or vein thrombosis.

Hemangioma.

Atheroembolic disease.

Nutcracker syndrome.

Loin-pain hematuria syndrome.

Trauma:

Blunt.

Penetrating.

Lateralizing essential hematuria.

URINARY TRACT OBSTRUCTION[59]

| ICD-10CM # | N21.8 | Other lower urinary tract calculus |
| | N20.9 | Urolithiasis |

INTRARENAL

Uric acid nephropathy.

Sulfonamide precipitates.

Acyclovir, indinavir precipitates.

Multiple myeloma.

URETERAL

Intrinsic

Intraluminal:

Nephrolithiasis.

Papillary necrosis.

Blood clots.

Fungus balls.

Intramural:

Ureteropelvic junction dysfunction.

Ureterovesical junction dysfunction.

Ureteral valve, polyp, or tumor.

Ureteral stricture.

Schistosomiasis.

Tuberculosis.

Scarring from instrumentation.

Drugs (e.g., NSAIDs).

Extrinsic

Vascular system:

Aneurysm: abdominal aorta or iliac vessels.

Aberrant vessels: ureteropelvic junction.

Venous: retrocaval ureter.

GI tract:

Crohn disease.

Diverticulitis.

Appendiceal abscess.

Colon cancer.

Pancreatic tumor, abscess, or cyst.

Reproductive system:

Uterus: pregnancy, prolapse, tumor, endometriosis.

Ovary: abscess, tumor, ovarian remnants.

Gartner duct cyst, tuboovarian abscess.

Retroperitoneal disease:

Retroperitoneal fibrosis: radiation, drugs, idiopathic.

Inflammatory: tuberculosis, sarcoidosis.

Hematoma.

Primary tumor (e.g., lymphoma, sarcoma).

Metastatic tumor (e.g., cervix, ovarian, bladder, colon).

Lymphocele.

Pelvic lipomatosis.

BLADDER

Neurogenic bladder:

Diabetes mellitus.

Spinal cord defect.

Trauma.

Multiple sclerosis.

Stroke.

Parkinson disease.

Spinal anesthesia.

Anticholinergics.

Bladder neck dysfunction.

Bladder calculus.

Bladder cancer.

URETHRA

Urethral stricture.

Prostate hypertrophy or cancer.

Obstruction from instrumentation.

URINARY TRACT OBSTRUCTION, CONGENITAL CAUSES[11]

| ICD-10CM # | Varies with specific diagnosis |

CONGENITAL CAUSES OF URINARY TRACT OBSTRUCTION

Ureteropelvic Junction

Ureteropelvic junction obstruction.

Proximal and Middle Ureter

Ureteral folds.

Ureteral valves.

Strictures.

Benign fibroepithelial polyps.

Retrocaval ureter.

Distal Ureter

Ureterovesical junction obstruction.

Vesicoureteral reflux.

Prune-belly syndrome.

Ureteroceles.

Bladder

Bladder diverticula.

Neurologic conditions (e.g., spina bifida).

Urethra

Posterior urethral valves.

Urethral diverticula.

Anterior urethral valves.

Urethral atresia.

Labial fusion.

URINE CASTS

| ICD-10CM # | R82.99 | Other abnormal findings in urine |

Normal finding.

Pyelonephritis.

Chronic renal disease.

Nephrotic syndrome.

Acute tubular necrosis.

Interstitial nephritis.

Nephritic syndrome.

Glomerulonephritis.

Eclampsia.

Heavy metal ingestion.

Allograft rejection.

Hypothyroidism.

URINE COLOR ABNORMALITIES[115]

| ICD-10CM # | R82.5 | Elevated urine levels of drugs, medicaments and biological substances |
| | R82.99 | Other abnormal findings in urine |

COMMON CAUSES OF ABNORMAL URINE COLOR

Colorless.

DISEASE

Diabetes mellitus.

Diabetes insipidus.

DRUG

Ethyl alcohol.

Diuretics.

MISCELLANEOUS

Overhydration.

Yellow-orange

DRUG

Tetracycline.

Flutamide.

Pyridium.

Azo Gantrisin (Roche Labs, Nutley, NJ).

Sulfasalazine.

Vitamin B.

MISCELLANEOUS

Dehydration.

Milky white

DISEASE

Urinary tract infection/pyuria.

Blue-green

DISEASE

Pseudomonas urinary tract infection.

DRUG

Methylene blue.
Urised (Polymedica Pharmaceuticals, Woburn, MA).
Indigo carmine.
Doan's pills (Novartis Consumer Health, Parsippany, NJ).
Clorets (Cadbury Adams, Parsippany, NJ).
Amitriptyline.
    Red-brown

DISEASE

Hematuria.
Hemolytic anemia.
Hemoglobinuria.
Lead poisoning.
Mercury poisoning.
Porphyria.

DRUG

Rifampin.
Ex-Lax (Novartis Consumer Health, Parsippany, NJ).
Phenolphthalein.
Phenothiazines.
Nitrofurantoin.
Doxorubicin.

MISCELLANEOUS

Beets.
Blackberries.
Rhubarb.
    Brown-black

DISEASE

Fecaluria.
Methemoglobinuria.
Melaninuria.

DRUG

Metronidazole.
Methyldopa.
Methocarbamol.

MISCELLANEOUS

Fava beans.
Aloe.

URINE, RED[104]

ICD-10CM #	Varies with specific diagnosis

WITH A POSITIVE DIPSTICK

Hematuria.
Hemoglobinuria: negative urinalysis.
Myoglobinuria: negative urinalysis.

WITH A NEGATIVE DIPSTICK

Drugs
Aminosalicylic acid.
Deferoxamine mesylate.
Ibuprofen.
Phenacetin.
Phenolphthalein.
Phensuximide.
Rifampin.
Anthraquinone laxatives.

Doxorubicin.
Methyldopa.
Phenazopyridine.
Phenothiazine.
Phenytoin.
Dyes
Azo dyes.
Eosin.
Foods
Beets, berries, maize.
Rhodamine B.
Metabolic
Porphyrins.
Serratia marcescens (red diaper syndrome).
Urate crystalluria.

UROLITHIASIS-LIKE PAIN[11]

ICD-10CM #	Varies with specific diagnosis

DIFFERENTIAL DIAGNOSIS OF UROLITHIASIS-LIKE PAIN

Category
Disorders
Renal:
    Pyelonephritis.
    Blood clot.
    Renal infarction.
    Tumor (kidney or pelvis).
    Papillary necrosis.
Ureteral:
    Tumor.
    Blood clot.
    Stricture.
Bladder:
    Tumor.
    Blood clot.
    Urinary retention.
Intraabdominal:
    Peritonitis.
    Appendicitis.
    Biliary disease.
    Bowel obstruction.
    Vascular disorder.
    Aortic aneurysm.
    Mesenteric insufficiency.
Retroperitoneal:
    Lymphadenopathy.
    Fibrosis.
    Tumor.
Gynecologic:
    Ectopic or tubal pregnancy.
    Ovarian torsion, cyst rupture.
    Pelvic inflammatory disease.
    Cervical cancer.
    Endometriosis.
    Ovarian vein syndrome.
Neuromuscular:
    Muscle pain.
    Rib fracture.
    Radiculitis.
Infectious:
    Herpes zoster.
    Pleuritis, pneumonia.
    Fungal bezoar.

UROPATHY, OBSTRUCTIVE[17]

ICD-10CM #	N13.9	Obstructive and reflux uropathy, unspecified
	N20.9	Urolithiasis

INTRINSIC CAUSES

Intraluminal
Intratubular deposition of crystals (uric acid, sulfas).
Stones.
Papillary tissue.
Blood clots.
Intramural
Functional.
Ureter (ureteropelvic or ureterovesical dysfunction).
Bladder (neurogenic): spinal cord defect or trauma, diabetes, multiple sclerosis, Parkinson disease, cerebrovascular accidents.
Bladder neck dysfunction.
Anatomic
Tumors.
Infection, granuloma.
Strictures.

EXTRINSIC CAUSES

Originating in the Reproductive System
Prostate: benign hypertrophy or cancer.
Uterus: pregnancy, tumors, prolapse, endometriosis.
Ovary: abscess, tumor, cysts.
Originating in the Vascular System
Aneurysms (aorta, iliac vessels).
Aberrant arteries (ureteropelvic junction).
Venous (ovarian veins, retrocaval ureter).
Originating in the GI Tract
Crohn disease.
Pancreatitis.
Appendicitis.
Tumors.
Originating in the Retroperitoneal Space
Inflammations.
Fibrosis.
Tumor, hematomas.

UROSEPSIS[115]

ICD-10CM #	A41.9	Sepsis, unspecified organism

COMMON CAUSES OF UROSEPSIS

Obstructing ureteral stone with pyonephrosis.
Staghorn calculus with urinary tract infection.
Ureteral obstruction with proximal urinary tract infection.
Urinary retention with urinary tract infection.
Acute prostatitis with prostatic abscess.
Perinephric abscess or renal carbuncle.
Urethral stricture with periurethral abscess.
Fournier gangrene.
Foreign body within urinary tract (e.g., Foley catheter).

URTICARIA IN TRAVELERS[69]

ICD-10CM #	L50.9	Urticaria, unspecified

II

Differential Diagnosis

CAUSES OF URTICARIA IN TRAVELERS

Noninfectious causes: adverse drug reaction.*
Viral infection: hepatitis A infection.
Parasitic infection: invasive phase of helminthic diseases (ascariasis, hookworm, strongyloidiasis, anisakiasis, gnathostomiasis, schistosomiasis,* fascioliasis), chronic helminthic infections where humans are dead-end host (trichinellosis, toxocariasis), and rupture of cyst during hydatid disease.

*Common cause.

UTERINE BLEEDING, ABNORMAL[55]

| ICD-10CM # | N92.6 | Irregular menstruation, unspecified |
| | N93.9 | Abnormal uterine and vaginal bleeding, unspecified |

PREGNANCY

Threatened abortion.
Incomplete abortion.
Complete abortion.
Molar pregnancy.
Ectopic pregnancy.
Retained products of conception.

OVULATORY

Vulva: infection, laceration, tumor.
Vagina: infection, laceration, tumor, foreign body.
Cervix: polyps, cervical erosion, cervicitis, carcinoma.
Uterus: fibroids (submucous fibroids most likely to cause abnormal bleeding), polyps, adenomyosis, endometritis, intrauterine device, atrophic endometrium.
Pregnancy complications: ectopic pregnancy; threatened, incomplete, complete abortion; retained products of conception.
Abnormality of clotting system.
Midcycle bleeding.
Halban disease (persistent corpus luteum).
Menorrhagia.
Pelvic inflammatory disease.

ANOVULATORY

Physiologic causes:
Puberty.
Perimenopausal.
    Pathologic causes:
    Ovarian failure (FSH over 40 IU/ml).
    Hyperandrogenism.
    Hyperprolactinemia.
    Obesity.
    Hypothalamic dysfunction (polycystic ovaries); LH/FSH ratio greater than 2:1.
    Hyperplasia.
    Endometrial carcinoma.
    Estrogen-producing tumors.
    Hypothyroidism.

UVEITIS, PEDIATRIC AGE

| ICD-10CM # | H20.9 | Anterior uveitis |

ANTERIOR UVEITIS

Juvenile rheumatoid arthritis (pauciarticular).
Sarcoidosis.
Trauma.
Tuberculosis.
Kawasaki disease.
Ulcerative colitis.
Postinfectious (enteric or genital) with arthritis and rash.
Spirochetal (syphilis, leptospiral).
Heterochromic iridocyclitis (Fuchs).
Viral (herpes simplex, herpes zoster).
Ankylosing spondylitis.
Stevens-Johnson syndrome.
Idiopathic.
Drugs.

POSTERIOR UVEITIS (CHOROIDITIS—MAY INVOLVE RETINA)

Toxoplasmosis.
Parasites (toxocariasis).
Sarcoidosis.
Tuberculosis.
Viral (rubella, herpes simplex, HIV, cytomegalovirus).
Subacute sclerosing panencephalitis.
Idiopathic.

ANTERIOR AND/OR POSTERIOR UVEITIS

Sympathetic ophthalmia (trauma to other eye).
Vogt-Koyanagi-Harada syndrome (uveo-otocutaneous syndrome: poliosis, vitiligo, deafness, tinnitus, uveitis, aseptic meningitis, retinitis).
Behçet syndrome.
Lyme disease.

VAGINAL BLEEDING, ABNORMAL

| ICD-10CM # | N93.9 | Abnormal uterine and vaginal bleeding, unspecified |

DIFFERENTIAL DIAGNOSIS OF ABNORMAL VAGINAL BLEEDING

Ovulatory Bleeding—Menorrhagia
Anovulatory bleeding—sometimes known as dysfunctional uterine bleeding (DUB).
Uterine and Ovarian Pathology
Uterine fibroids (pelvic pain, dysmenorrhea).
Endometriosis; adenomyosis (dysmenorrhea, dyspareunia, pelvic pain, infertility).
Pelvic inflammatory disease and pelvic infection (fever, vaginal discharge, pelvic pain, intermenstrual and postcoital bleeding).
Endometrial polyps (intermenstrual bleeding).
Endometrial hyperplasia; endometrial carcinoma (pelvic pain, abnormal bleeding, postcoital bleeding).
Polycystic ovary syndrome (irregular bleeding, infertility, and hirsutism).

Systemic Disease

Coagulation disorder; bleeding diathesis such as von Willebrand disease.
Liver or renal disease.
Hypothyroidism (fatigue, constipation, coarse features, alopecia).

IATROGENIC CAUSE

Anticoagulation.
Intrauterine device.
Chemotherapy.
Sex steroids.

VAGINAL BLEEDING, PREGNANCY[93]

| ICD-10CM # | N93.9 | Abnormal uterine and vaginal bleeding, unspecified |

FIRST TRIMESTER

Implantation bleeding.
Abortion:
    Threatened.
    Complete.
    Incomplete.
    Missed.
Ectopic pregnancy.
Neoplasia.
Hydatidiform mole.
Cervix.

THIRD TRIMESTER

Placenta previa.
Placental abruption.
Premature labor.
Choriocarcinoma.

VAGINAL DISCHARGE, PREPUBERTAL GIRLS[23]

| ICD-10CM # | N89.8 | Other specified noninflammatory disorders of vagina |

Irritative (bubble baths, sand):
    Poor perineal hygiene.
    Foreign body.
    Associated systemic illness (group A streptococci, chickenpox).
Infections:
    Escherichia coli with foreign body.
    Shigella organisms.
    Yersinia organisms.
    Infections (consider sexual abuse):
        Chlamydia trachomatis.
        Neisseria gonorrhoeae.
        Trichomonas vaginalis.
Tumor (rare).

VALVULAR HEART DISEASE[18]

| ICD-10CM # | Varies with specific diagnosis |

MAJOR CAUSES OF VALVULAR HEART DISEASE IN ADULTS

Aortic Stenosis
Bicuspid aortic valve.
Rheumatic fever.

Degenerative stenosis.
Aortic Regurgitation
Bicuspid aortic valve.
Aortic dissection.
Endocarditis.
Rheumatic fever.
Aortic root dilation.
Mitral Stenosis
Rheumatic fever.
Mitral Regurgitation

CHRONIC

Mitral valve prolapse.
Left ventricular dilation.
Posterior wall myocardial infarction.
Rheumatic fever.
Endocarditis.

ACUTE

Posterior wall or papillary muscle ischemia.
Papillary muscle or chordal rupture.
Endocarditis.
Prosthetic valve dysfunction.
Systolic anterior motion of mitral valve.

TRICUSPID REGURGITATION

Functional (annular) dilation.
Tricuspid valve prolapse.
Endocarditis.
Carcinoid heart disease.

VASCULAR LESIONS OF GI TRACT[3]

ICD-10CM #   Varies with specific diagnosis

PRIMARY VASCULAR LESIONS

Aneurysms of the aorta and its branches.
Angioectasia (angiodysplasia, vascular ectasia).
Arteriovenous malformation.
Blue rubber bleb nevus.
Capillary phlebectasia.
Dieulafoy lesion.
Glomus tumor.
Hemangioma.
Hemangiomatosis.
Hemangioendothelioma.
Hemangiopericytoma.
Hemangiosarcoma.
Hemorrhoids.
Kaposi sarcoma.

DISEASES AND SYNDROMES WITH VASCULAR LESIONS

Blue rubber bleb nevus syndrome.
Ehlers-Danlos syndrome.
Hereditary hemorrhagic telangiectasia (Osler-Weber-Rendu disease).
Klippel-Trenaunay or Parkes Weber syndrome.
Kohlmeier-Degos syndrome.
Marfan syndrome.
Pseudoxanthoma elasticum.
PSS (scleroderma, CREST).
Scurvy.
Turner syndrome.
von Willebrand disease.

SYSTEMIC DISORDERS ASSOCIATED WITH VASCULAR LESIONS

Portal hypertension:
  Congestive gastropathy and colopathy.
  GAVE (watermelon stomach).
  Spider telangiectasias.
  Varices.
Renal failure:
  GI telangiectasias.
  GAVE (watermelon stomach).
Vasculitis (e.g., polyarteritis nodosa).
Iatrogenic lesions:
  Radiation telangiectasia.

CREST, Calcinosis, Raynaud phenomenon, esophageal dysmotility, sclerodactyly, telangiectasia; *GAVE*, gastric antral vascular ectasia

VASCULITIS, CLASSIFICATION

ICD-10CM #   I77.6   Arteritis, unspecified

LARGE VESSEL DISEASE

Arteritis
Giant cell arteritis.
Takayasu arteritis.
Arteritis associated with Reiter syndrome (reactive arthritis), ankylosing spondylitis.

MEDIUM AND SMALL VESSEL DISEASE

Polyarteritis Nodosa
Primary (idiopathic).
Associated with viruses (hepatitis B or C, CMV, HIV, herpes zoster).
Associated with malignancy (hairy cell leukemia).
Familial Mediterranean fever.
Granulomatous Vasculitis
Granulomatosis with polyangiitis.
Lymphomatoid granulomatosis.
Behçet Disease
Kawasaki disease (mucocutaneous lymph node syndrome)

PREDOMINANTLY SMALL VESSEL DISEASE

Hypersensitivity Vasculitis (Leukocytoclastic Vasculitis)
Henoch-Schönlein purpura.
Mixed cryoglobulinemia.
Serum sickness.
Vasculitis associated with connective tissue diseases (systemic lupus erythematosus, Sjögren syndrome).
Vasculitis associated with specific syndromes:
  Primary biliary cirrhosis.
  Lyme disease.
  Chronic active hepatitis.
  Drug-induced vasculitis.
Churg-Strauss Syndrome
Goodpasture syndrome.
Erythema nodosum.
Panniculitis.
Buerger disease (thrombophlebitis obliterans).

VASCULITIS (DISEASES THAT MIMIC VASCULITIS)[25]

ICD-10CM #   Varies with specific diagnosis

EMBOLIC DISEASE

Infectious or marantic endocarditis.
Cardiac mural thrombus.
Atrial myxoma.
Cholesterol embolization syndrome.

NONINFLAMMATORY VESSEL WALL DISRUPTION

Atherosclerosis.
Arterial fibromuscular dysplasia.
Drug effects (vasoconstrictors, anticoagulants).
Radiation.
Genetic disease (neurofibromatosis, Ehlers-Danlos syndrome).
Amyloidosis.
Intravascular malignant lymphoma.

DIFFUSE COAGULATION

Disseminated intravascular coagulation.
Thrombotic thrombocytopenic purpura.
Hemolytic-uremic syndrome.
Protein C and S deficiencies, factor V/Leiden mutation.
Antiphospholipid syndrome.

VEGETATIVE STATE, PERSISTENT[18]

ICD-10CM #   R40.3   Persistent vegetative state

PERSISTENT VEGETATIVE STATE: COMMON CAUSES*

Trauma (diffuse axonal injury).
Cardiac arrest and hypoperfusion (laminar necrosis of cortical mantle and/or thalamic necrosis).
Bihemispheric infarctions.
Purulent meningitis or encephalitis (cortical injury).
Carbon monoxide.
Prolonged hypoglycemic coma.

VENTILATION DISORDERS[96]

ICD-10CM #   Varies with specific diagnosis

UPPER AIRWAY PATHOLOGY

Obstructive sleep apnea.
Upper airway mechanical dysfunction (e.g., tracheal stenosis, vocal cord dysfunction).
Foreign body inhalation.
Oropharyngeal disorders (e.g., tonsillar hypertrophy, epiglottitis, malignancies).

LOWER AIRWAY OBSTRUCTIVE PATHOLOGY

Reversible airway disease: asthma.
Chronic obstructive pulmonary disease: emphysema, chronic bronchitis.
Bronchiectasis.
Lobar collapse (foreign body, neoplasm, mucus plug).

Differential Diagnosis

II

LOWER AIRWAY PARENCHYMAL PATHOLOGY

Infection: pneumonia.
Interstitial disease: idiopathic, pneumoconiosis, autoimmune, granulomatous, drug-induced, hypersensitivity.
Neoplasm.

CHEST WALL AND PLEURAL ABNORMALITIES

Pleural effusion.
Empyema.
Skeletal deformity (e.g., kyphoscoliosis, fractured ribs).
Malignancy—mesothelioma.
Pneumothorax.
Primary or secondary muscle disease (e.g., polymyositis, muscular dystrophy, drug-induced myopathy).

CENTRAL CONTROL PROBLEMS

Central sleep apnea.
Sedation (e.g., due to drugs, primary cerebral disease).

VENTILATION–PERFUSION MISMATCH ON LUNG SCAN

ICD-10CM #   Varies with specific diagnosis

Pulmonary embolism.
Emphysema.
Irradiation.
Pulmonary hypertension.
AV malformations.
Pulmonary thrombosis.
External compression of pulmonary artery (neoplasm, cysts, fibrosing mediastinitis).
Vasculitis.
Tuberculosis.
Pulmonary thrombosis.
Congenital (pulmonary artery hypoplasia, congenital heart disease with upper lobe diversion).
Sequestered segment.
Parasitic lung disease.
Intraluminal obstruction from catheter fragments.

VENTRICULAR FAILURE

ICD-10CM #   I51.9   Heart disease, unspecified

LEFT VENTRICULAR FAILURE

Systemic hypertension.
Valvular heart disease (AS, AR, MR).
Cardiomyopathy, myocarditis.
Bacterial endocarditis.
Myocardial infarction.
Idiopathic hypertrophic subaortic stenosis.

RIGHT VENTRICULAR FAILURE

Valvular heart disease (mitral stenosis).
Pulmonary hypertension.
Bacterial endocarditis (right-sided).
Right ventricular infarction.

BIVENTRICULAR FAILURE

Left ventricular failure.
Cardiomyopathy.

Myocarditis.
Arrhythmias.
Anemia.
Thyrotoxicosis.
Arteriovenous fistula.
Paget disease.
Beriberi.

VERRUCOUS LESIONS

ICD-10CM #   Varies with specific diagnosis

Warts.
Seborrheic keratosis.
Lichen simplex.
Acanthosis nigricans.
Scabies (Norwegian, crusted).
Verrucous carcinoma.
Nevus sebaceous.
Deep fungal infection.

VERTEBRAL LESIONS[106]

ICD-10CM #   Varies with specific diagnosis

Anatomic Distribution Of Vertebral Lesions

Anterior Elements of the Spine	Posterior Elements of the Spine	Both Anterior and Posterior Elements of the Spine
Multiple myeloma.	Osteoid osteoma.	Metastasis (spares disc end plates).
Hemangioma.	Osteoblastoma.	Infection (involves disc end plates).
Paget disease of bone.	Aneurysmal bone cyst.	Classic osteosarcoma.
Histiocytosis X (vertebra plana).		Postradiation sarcoma.
Giant cell tumor of bone.		Malignant histiocytoid variety.
Reparative granuloma.		Osteosarcoma.
Ewing sarcoma (primitive neuroectodermal tumor).		Osteochondroma.
Lymphoma of bone.		Primary chondrosarcoma.
Malignant fibrous histiocytoma.		Secondary chondrosarcoma.
Chordoma.		

VERTIGO

| ICD-10CM # | R42 | Dizziness and giddiness |
| | H81.13 | Benign paroxysmal vertigo, bilateral |

	H81.49	Vertigo of central origin, unspecified ear
	H81.399	Other peripheral vertigo, unspecified ear
	H81.23	Vestibular neuronitis, bilateral

PERIPHERAL

Otitis media.
Acute labyrinthitis.
Vestibular neuronitis.
Benign positional vertigo.
Ménière disease.
Ototoxic drugs: streptomycin, gentamicin.
Lesions of the eighth nerve: acoustic neuroma, meningioma, mononeuropathy, metastatic carcinoma.
Mastoiditis.

CENTRAL NERVOUS SYSTEM OR SYSTEMIC

Vertebrobasilar artery insufficiency.
Posterior fossa tumor or other brain tumors.
Infarction/hemorrhage of cerebral cortex, cerebellum, or brain stem.
Basilar migraine.
Metabolic: drugs, hypoxia, anemia, fever.
Hypotension/severe hypertension.
Multiple sclerosis.
Central nervous system infections: viral, bacterial.
Temporal lobe epilepsy.
Arnold-Chiari malformation, syringobulbia.
Psychogenic: ventilation, hysteria.

VERTIGO, CENTRAL[29]

ICD-10CM #   R42

MAJOR CAUSES OF CENTRAL VERTIGO

Demyelination:
  Acquired.
  Leukodystrophies.
  Multiple sclerosis.
Familial disorders:
  Friedreich ataxia.
  Spinocerebellar ataxia.
  Familial episodic ataxia (type 1 and type 2).
  Olivopontocerebellar atrophy.
Central nervous system infections:
  Lyme neuroborreliosis.
  Meningitis.
  Tuberculosis.
Intrinsic brain stem lesion:
  Tumor.
  Arteriovenous malformation.
  Trauma.
Migraine:
  Basilar.
  Benign paroxysmal positional vertigo of childhood.
Toxins:
  Drugs, alcohol.
  Analgesics.
  Anticonvulsants.
  Antihypertensives.

Hypnotics.
Tranquilizers.
Metabolic and endocrine disorders:
  Hyperinsulinism.
  Impaired glucose tolerance.
  Diabetes mellitus.
  Hypertriglyceridemia.
  Hypothyroidism.
Systemic conditions:
  Paget disease.
Stroke/ischemia:
  Vertebrobasilar.
  Cerebellar.
  Posterior inferior cerebellar artery syndrome.
  Lateral medullary syndrome.
  Medial medullary infarct.
  Basilar artery syndrome.
  Anterior inferior cerebellar artery.
Other causes of posterior ischemia:
  Subclavian steal syndrome.
  Rotational vertebral artery occlusion syndrome.
  Vertebral artery dissection.
  Vertebral or basilar artery dolichoectasia.
  Neoplasm of the fourth ventricle.
  Chiari malformation.
  Superficial siderosis of the central nervous system.
  Vestibular epilepsy.

VESICULAR OR BULLOUS SKIN RASH[12]

ICD-10CM #	R21	Rash and other nonspecific skin eruption

CAUSES OF A VESICULAR OR BULLOUS SKIN RASH

Most Common

Viral:
  Herpes zoster.
  Herpes simplex.
Impetigo.
Scabies.
Insect bites and papular urticaria.
Bullous eczema and pompholyx.
Drugs:
  Sulfonamides.
  Penicillin.
  Barbiturates.

Less Common

Erythema multiforme major ("target lesions" rash, plus one mucous membrane involved) or erythema multiforme minor (1 to 2 cm "target lesions" only):
  Mycoplasma pneumonia.
  Herpes simplex.
  Drugs such as sulfur, penicillins.
  Idiopathic (50%).
SJS and TEN with epidermal detachment and mucosal erosions:
  Drugs such as anticonvulsants, sulfonamides, NSAIDs, and penicillins.
Staphylococcal scalded-skin syndrome (children).
Dermatitis herpetiformis (gluten sensitivity).
Pemphigus and pemphigoid.

Rare

Porphyria cutanea tarda.
Epidermolysis bullosa.

NSAIDs, Nonsteroidal antiinflammatory drugs; *SJS,* Stevens-Johnson syndrome; *TEN,* toxic epidermal necrolysis.

VESICULOBULLOUS DISEASES[24]

ICD-10CM #	L94.2	Calcinosis cutis
	L98.8	Other specified disorders of the skin and subcutaneous tissue

IMMUNOLOGICALLY MEDIATED DISEASES

Bullous pemphigoid.
Herpes gestationis.
Mucous membrane pemphigoid.
Epidermolysis bullosa acquisita.
Dermatitis herpetiformis.
Pemphigus (vulgaris, foliaceus, paraneoplastic).

HYPERSENSITIVITY DISEASES

Erythema multiforme minor.
Erythema multiforme major (Stevens-Johnson syndrome).
Toxic epidermal necrolysis.

METABOLIC DISEASES

Porphyria cutanea tarda.
Pseudoporphyria.
Diabetic blisters.

INHERITED GENETIC DISORDERS

Epidermolysis bullosa:
Simplex.
Junctional.
Dystrophic.

INFECTIOUS DISEASES

Impetigo.
Staphylococcal scalded skin syndrome.
Herpes simplex.
Varicella.
Herpes zoster.

VIRAL ENCEPHALITIS, COMMON CAUSES[94]

ICD-10CM #	A86	Unspecified viral encephalitis
	A85.2	Arthropod-borne viral encephalitis, unspecified
	A84.9	Tick-borne viral encephalitis, unspecified
	A83.9	Mosquito-borne viral encephalitis, unspecified
	A85.8	Other specified viral encephalitis
	A85	Other viral encephalitis, not elsewhere classified

COMMON CAUSES OF VIRAL ENCEPHALITIS

Causes of Viral Encephalitis

Nonseasonal:
  Herpes simplex virus type 1 (herpes simplex encephalitis).
  Herpes simplex virus type 2 (neonatal encephalitis or adult meningoencephalitis).
Seasonal—summer and fall—arboviruses (arthropod borne):
  West Nile virus.
  St. Louis encephalitis virus.
  Eastern equine encephalitis virus.
  Western equine encephalitis virus.
  La Crosse/California encephalitis virus.
  Powassan encephalitis virus.
  Chikungunya virus.
Seasonal—nonarthropod borne:
  Summer and fall: enteroviruses (including coxsackieviruses, echoviruses, polioviruses, and enterovirus 71).
  Winter: influenza virus.
Immunosuppressed patients:
  HIV (chronic HIV encephalitis).
  Varicella-zoster virus (subacute encephalitis).
  JC virus (progressive multifocal leukoencephalopathy).
  Cytomegalovirus (ventriculitis or encephalitis).
  Human herpesvirus 6 (subacute encephalitis).
  Epstein-Barr virus (subacute encephalitis).

Uncommon Causes in the U.S.

Powassan encephalitis virus.
Zika virus.
Chikungunya virus.
Variegated squirrel bornavirus.
Lymphotropic choriomeningitis virus.
Rabies.
Measles (subacute sclerosing panencephalitis).
Mumps.
Adenovirus.
Herpes B virus (of monkeys).
Rubella (progressive rubella panencephalitis).

Causes Outside the United States

Zika virus (Africa, Asia, Caribbean, Central America, Pacific Islands, South America).
Chikungunya virus (Africa, Asia, Central America, Pacific Islands, South America, Western Europe).
Tick-borne encephalitis virus (Russia, Asia).
Japanese encephalitis virus (Japan, Southeast Asia, Malaysia).
Venezuelan equine encephalitis virus (Central and South America).
Dengue virus (Southern Asia, Africa, South America).
Rift Valley fever virus (east central Africa).
Murray Valley encephalitis virus (Australia).
Powassan encephalitis virus (Canada).
Nipah virus (Malaysia and Bangladesh).

VISION LOSS, ACUTE, PAINFUL

ICD-10CM #	H53.139	Sudden visual loss, unspecified eye

Differential Diagnosis

II

Acute angle-closure glaucoma.
Corneal ulcer.
Uveitis.
Endophthalmitis.
Factitious.
Somatization syndrome.
Trauma.

VISION LOSS, ACUTE, PAINLESS

ICD-10CM # H53.139 Sudden visual loss, unspecified eye

Retinal artery occlusion.
Optic neuritis.
Retinal vein occlusion.
Vitreous hemorrhage.
Retinal detachment.
Exudative macular degeneration.
Cerebrovascular accident.
Ischemic optic neuropathy.
Factitious.
Somatization syndrome, anxiety reaction.

VISION LOSS, ACUTE, PEDIATRIC AGE[20]

ICD-10CM # Varies with specific diagnosis

Carotid dissection.[a]
Cortical blindness.
  Anoxic encephalopathy.
  Benign occipital epilepsy.[a]
  Hydrocephalus.[a]
  Hypoglycemia.[a]
  Hypertension[a] (malignant or accelerated).
  Hyperviscosity.
  Hypotension.
  Migraine.[a]
  Occipital metastatic disease.
  Posttraumatic transient cerebral blindness.
  Systemic lupus erythematosus.
  Toxic[a] (e.g., cyclosporine).
  Trauma.
  Disorders affecting the optic nerves.
  Optic neuropathy.[a]
    Demyelinating.
    Idiopathic optic neuritis.
    Multiple sclerosis.
    Neuromyelitis optica.
  Ischemic.
  Toxic.
  Traumatic.
  Pituitary apoplexy.
  Pseudotumor cerebri.[a]
Retinal disease.
  Central retinal artery occlusion.
  Migraine.
  Trauma.

[a]Denotes the most common conditions and the ones with disease-modifying treatments.

VISION LOSS AFTER DIVING[112]

ICD-10CM # H53.139 Sudden visual loss, unspecified eye

DIFFERENTIAL DIAGNOSIS OF DECREASED VISION AFTER DIVING

Decompression sickness.
Arterial gas embolism.
Bubbles under contact lenses.
Displaced contact lens.
Antifog agent keratopathy.
Contact lens adherence syndrome.
Transdermal scopolamine
Hyperoxic myopia.
Oxymetazoline optic neuropathy.
Diving-induced migraine phenomena.
Eye disorders not related to diving.

VISION LOSS, CHILDREN

ICD-10CM # H53.9 Unspecified visual disturbance

Craniopharyngioma.
Hereditary optic atrophy.
Optic nerve glioma.
Glioma of chiasm.
Albinism.
Optic nerve hypoplasia.

VISION LOSS, CHRONIC, PROGRESSIVE

ICD-10CM # H54.7 Unspecified visual loss

Cataract.
Macular degeneration.
Cerebral neoplasm.
Refractive error.
Open-angle glaucoma.

VISION LOSS, MONOCULAR, TRANSIENT

ICD-10CM # H54.7 Unspecified visual loss

Thromboembolism.
Vasculitis.
Migraine (vasospasm).
Anxiety reaction.
Central nervous system tumor.
Temporal arteritis.
Multiple sclerosis.

VISION LOSS, PROGRESSIVE, PEDIATRIC AGE[20]

ICD-10CM # Varies with specific diagnosis

Compressive optic neuropathies.
  Aneurysm.[a]
  Arteriovenous malformations.[a]
  Craniopharyngioma.[a]
  Hypothalamic and optic tumors.[a]
  Pituitary adenoma.[a]
  Pseudotumor cerebri.[a]
Disorders of the lens.
  Cataract.
  Dislocation of the lens.

[a]Denotes the most common conditions and the ones with disease-modifying treatments.

Hereditary optic atrophy.
  Leber hereditary optic neuropathy.
  Wolfram syndrome.
Intraocular tumors.
Tapetoretinal degenerations.
  Abnormal carbohydrate metabolism.
    Mucopolysaccharidosis.
    Primary hyperoxaluria.
Abnormal lipid metabolism.
  Abetalipoproteinemia.
  Hypobetalipoproteinemia.
  Multiple sulfatase deficiency.
  Neuronal ceroid lipofuscinosis.
  Niemann-Pick disease.
  Refsum disease.
Other syndromes of unknown etiology.
  Bardet-Biedl syndrome.
  Cockayne syndrome.
  Laurence-Moon syndrome.
  Refsum disease.
  Usher syndrome.

VISUAL HALLUCINATIONS[101]

ICD-10CM # Varies with specific diagnosis

Blindness/sensory deprivation—Charles Bonnet syndrome.
Palinopsia.
Dementia-producing diseases.
Alzheimer disease.
Dementia with Lewy bodies.[a]
Parkinson disease.[b]
Intoxications.
Alcoholic hallucinosis.
Delirium tremens (DTs).
Hallucinogens.
Amphetamines.
Cocaine.
Lysergic acid diethylamide (LSD).
Phencyclidine (PCP).
Medicines.
Atropine, scopolamine.
Levodopa and dopamine agonists.
Steroids.
Migraine with aura (classic migraine).
Narcolepsy: hypnopompic (awakening) and hypnagogic (falling asleep) hallucinations.
Seizures.
Peduncular hallucinations.

[a]Although visual hallucinations are likely to complicate almost any form of dementia, they are characteristic of dementia with Lewy bodies.
[b]Dopaminergic medications such as levodopa-carbidopa (Sinemet) are more likely than Parkinson disease itself to produce hallucinations.

VISUAL IMPAIRMENT, ELDERLY PATIENT[101]

ICD-10CM # Varies with specific diagnosis

Cataracts.
Diabetic retinopathy.
Macular degeneration.
Glaucoma.
Presbyopia and other accommodation problems.
Temporal (giant cell) arteritis.
Visual agnosia and cortical blindness from multiple strokes or Alzheimer disease.

VITREOUS HEMORRHAGE[98]

ICD-10CM #	H43.13	Vitreous hemorrhage, bilateral

CAUSES OF VITREOUS HEMORRHAGE

Acute posterior vitreous detachment associated either with a retinal tear or avulsion of a peripheral vessel.
Proliferative retinopathies:
  Diabetic.
  Following retinal vein occlusion.
  Sickle cell disease.
  Eales disease.
  Vasculitis.
Miscellaneous retinal disorders:
  Macroaneurysm.
  Telangiectasis.
  Capillary hemangioma.
Trauma:
  Blunt.
  Penetrating.
  Iatrogenic.
Systemic:
  Bleeding disorders.
  Terson syndrome.

VOCAL CORD PARALYSIS

ICD-10CM #	J38.00	Paralysis of vocal cords and larynx, unspecified
	J38.01	Paralysis of vocal cords and larynx, unilateral
	J38.02	Paralysis of vocal cords and larynx, bilateral

Neoplasm: primary or metastatic (e.g., lung, thyroid, parathyroid, mediastinum).
Neck surgery (parathyroid, thyroid, carotid endarterectomy, cervical spine).
Idiopathic.
Viral, bacterial, or fungal infection.
Trauma (intubation, penetrating neck injury).
Cardiac surgery.
Rheumatoid arthritis.
Multiple sclerosis.
Parkinsonism.
Toxic neuropathy.
Cerebrovascular accident.
Central nervous system abnormalities: hydrocephalus, Arnold–Chiari malformation, meningomyelocele.

VOLUME DEPLETION[18]

ICD-10CM #	E86.9	Volume depletion, unspecified

GI losses:
  Upper: bleeding, nasogastric suction, vomiting.
  Lower: bleeding, diarrhea, enteric or pancreatic fistula, tube drainage.
Renal losses:
  Salt and water: diuretics, osmotic diuresis, postobstructive diuresis, acute tubular necrosis (recovery phase), salt-losing nephropathy, adrenal insufficiency, renal tubular acidosis.
Water loss: diabetes insipidus.
Skin and respiratory losses:
  Sweat, burns, insensible losses.
Sequestration without external fluid loss:
  Intestinal obstruction, peritonitis, pancreatitis, rhabdomyolysis, internal bleeding.

VOLUME EXCESS[18]

ICD-10CM #		Varies with specific diagnosis

PRIMARY RENAL SODIUM RETENTION (INCREASED EFFECTIVE CIRCULATING VOLUME)

Renal failure, nephritic syndrome, acute glomerulonephritis.
Primary hyperaldosteronism.
Cushing syndrome.
Liver disease.

SECONDARY RENAL SODIUM RETENTION (DECREASED EFFECTIVE CIRCULATING VOLUME)

Heart failure.
Liver disease.
Nephrotic syndrome (minimal change disease).
Pregnancy.

VOMITING

ICD-10CM #	R11.10	Vomiting, unspecified
	R11.11	Vomiting without nausea
	R11.12	Projectile vomiting

GI disturbances:
  Obstruction: esophageal, pyloric, intestinal.
  Infections: viral or bacterial enteritis, viral hepatitis, food poisoning, gastroenteritis.
  Pancreatitis.
  Appendicitis.
  Biliary colic.
  Peritonitis.
  Perforated bowel.
  Diabetic gastroparesis.
Other: gastritis, peptic ulcer disease, inflammatory bowel disease, GI tract neoplasms.
Drugs: morphine, digitalis, cytotoxic agents, bromocriptine.
Severe pain: myocardial infarction, renal colic.
Metabolic disorders: uremia, acidosis/alkalosis, hyperglycemia, diabetic ketoacidosis, thyrotoxicosis.
Trauma: blows to the testicles, epigastrium.
Vertigo.
Reye syndrome.
Increased intracranial pressure.
Central nervous system disturbances: trauma, hemorrhage, infarction, neoplasm, infection, hypertensive encephalopathy, migraine.
Radiation sickness.
Nausea and vomiting of pregnancy, hyperemesis gravidarum.
Motion sickness.
Bulimia, anorexia nervosa.
Psychogenic: emotional disturbances, offensive sights or smells.
Severe coughing.
Pyelonephritis.
Boerhaave syndrome.
Carbon monoxide poisoning.

VOMITING, NEONATAL[29]

ICD-10CM #	R11.10	Vomiting, unspecified

CAUSES OF NEONATAL VOMITING

Anatomic Causes
Esophagus, trachea, great vessels:
  Stricture.
  Web.
  Tracheoesophageal fistula.
  Laryngeal cleft.
  Double aortic arch.
Stomach and duodenum:
  Pyloric stenosis.
  Duodenal atresia (usually noted on the first day of life).
Small and large intestine:
  Volvulus secondary to malrotation.
  Incarcerated hernia.
  Hirschsprung disease (secondary to obstipation).
  Necrotizing enterocolitis.
Genitourinary:
  Testicular torsion.
Nonanatomic Causes
Infection:
  Septicemia.
  Meningitis.
  Urinary tract infection.
  Gastroenteritis.
  Otitis media.
Increased intracranial pressure:
  Cerebral edema.
  Subdural hematoma.
  Hydrocephalus.
  Brain tumor.
Congenital adrenal hyperplasia (salt-losing variety).
Inborn errors of metabolism.
Renal disease.

VULVAR LESIONS[55]

ICD-10CM #	N77.0	Ulceration of vulva in diseases classified elsewhere
	N90.7	Vulvar cyst
	N90.89	Other specified noninflammatory disorders of vulva and perineum
	D07.1	Carcinoma in situ of vulva
	N90.89	Other specified noninflammatory disorders of vulva and perineum
	N90.5	Atrophy of vulva

RED LESION

Infection/Infestation
Fungal infection:
  Candida.
  Tinea cruris.
  Intertrigo.
  Pityriasis versicolor.

Differential Diagnosis

II

Sarcoptes scabiei.
   Erythrasma: *Corynebacterium minutissimum.*
   Granuloma inguinale: *Calymmatobacterium granulomatis.*
   Folliculitis: *Staphylococcus aureus.*
   Hidradenitis suppurativa.
   Behçet syndrome.

Inflammation
Reactive vulvitis.
Chemical irritation:
   Detergent.
   Dyes.
   Perfume.
   Spermicide.
   Lubricants.
   Hygiene sprays.
   Podophyllum.
   Topical 5-FU.
   Saliva.
   Gentian violet.
   Semen.
Mechanical trauma: scratching.
Vestibular adenitis.
Essential vulvodynia.
Psoriasis.
Seborrheic dermatitis.

Neoplasm
Vulvar intraepithelial neoplasia (VIN):
   Mild dysplasia.
   Moderate dysplasia.
   Severe dysplasia.
   Carcinoma-in-situ.
   Vulvar dystrophy.
   Bowen disease.
Invasive cancer:
   Squamous cell carcinoma.
   Malignant melanoma.
   Sarcoma.
   Basal cell carcinoma.
   Adenocarcinoma.
   Paget disease.
   Undifferentiated.

WHITE LESION
Vulvar dystrophy:
   Lichen sclerosus.
   Vulvar dystrophy.
   Vulvar hyperplasia.
   Mixed dystrophy.
VIN.
Vitiligo.
Partial albinism.
Intertrigo.
Radiation treatment.

DARK LESION
Lentigo.
Nevi (mole).
Neoplasm (see "Neoplasm, Vulvar," below).
Reactive hyperpigmentation.
Seborrheic keratosis.
Pubic lice.

ULCERATIVE LESION
Infection
Herpes simplex.
Vaccinia.
Treponema pallidum.

Granuloma inguinale.
Pyoderma.
Tuberculosis.
Noninfectious
Behçet disease.
Crohn disease.
Pemphigus.
Pemphigoid.
Hidradenitis suppurativa (see "Neoplasm, Vulvar," below).
Neoplasm
Basal cell carcinoma.
Squamous cell carcinoma.
Vulvar tumor <1 cm:
   Condyloma acuminatum.
   Molluscum contagiosum.
   Epidermal inclusion.
   Vestibular cyst.
   Mesonephric duct.
   VIN.
   Hemangioma.
   Hidradenoma.
   Neurofibroma.
   Syringoma.
   Accessory breast tissue.
   Acrochordon.
   Endometriosis.
   Fox-Fordyce disease.
   Pilonidal sinus.
Vulvar tumor >1 cm:
   Bartholin cyst or abscess.
   Lymphogranuloma venereum.
   Fibroma.
   Lipoma.
   Verrucous carcinoma.
   Squamous cell carcinoma.
   Hernia.
   Edema.
   Hematoma.
   Acrochordon.
   Epidermal cysts.
   Neurofibromatosis.
   Accessory breast tissue.

VULVAR PAIN[99]

ICD-10CM #	N94.81	Vulvodynia
	R10.2	Pelvic and perineal pain

DISEASES ASSOCIATED WITH VULVAR PAIN, NOT QUALIFYING FOR THE DIAGNOSIS OF VULVODYNIA
Podophyllin overdose.
Condylox (podofilox) overdose.
Behçet disease.
Aphthous ulcers.
Herpes (simplex and zoster).
Candidiasis.
Trichomonas.
Chancroid.
Sjögren disease.
Contact dermatitis.
Endometriosis.
Pemphigus.
Pemphigoid.
Atrophy.

Lichen sclerosus.
Lichen planus.
Crohn disease.
Bartholin abscess.
Trauma.
Imperforate hymen.
Prolapsed urethra.
Vulvar intraepithelial neoplasia.
Carcinoma.

VULVITIS, GRANULOMATOUS

ICD-10CM #	N76.2	Acute vulvitis
	N76.3	Subacute and chronic vulvitis

Differential diagnosis of granulomatous vulvitis
Syphilis.
Lymphogranuloma venereum.
Mycobacteria.
Fungus.
Bacillary angiomatosis.
Folliculitis.
Ruptured pilosebaceous unit.
Ruptured cyst.
Crohn disease.
Vulvitis granulomatosa.
Hydradenitis suppurativa.

WEAKNESS, ACUTE, EMERGENT[10]

ICD-10CM #	M62.81	Muscle weakness (generalized)

Demyelinating disorders (Guillain-Barré, chronic inflammatory demyelinating polyneuropathy [CIDP]).
Myasthenia gravis.
Infectious (poliomyelitis, diphtheria).
Toxic (botulism, tick paralysis, paralytic shellfish toxin, puffer fish, newts).
Metabolic (acquired or familial hypokalemia, hypophosphatemia, hypermagnesemia).
Metal poisoning (arsenic, thallium).
Porphyria.

WEAKNESS, GRADUAL ONSET

ICD-10CM #	M62.81	Muscle weakness (generalized)

Depression.
Malingering.
Anemia.
Hypothyroidism.
Medications (e.g., sedatives, antidepressants, narcotics).
Congestive heart failure.
Renal failure.
Liver failure.
Respiratory insufficiency.
Alcoholism.
Nutritional deficiencies.
Disorders of motor unit.
Basal ganglia disorders.
Upper motor neuron lesions.

WEAKNESS, NONNEUROMUSCULAR CAUSES

ICD-10CM #	G93.3	Postviral fatigue syndrome
	R53.1	Weakness
	R53.81	Other malaise
	R53.83	Other fatigue

Anxiety disorder.
Infectious process.
Anemia.
Renal insufficiency.
Hyperventilation.
Malignancy.
Hypothyroidism.
Hypotension.
Hypercapnia.
Hypoglycemia.
Cardiac arrhythmias.
Hepatic insufficiency.
Electrolyte imbalance.
Malnutrition.
Cerebrovascular insufficiency.

WEIGHT GAIN

ICD-10CM #	R63.5	Abnormal weight gain
	E66.9	Obesity, unspecified

Sedentary lifestyle.
Fluid overload.
Discontinuation of tobacco abuse.
Endocrine disorders (hypothyroidism, hyperin-sulinism associated with maturity-onset diabetes mellitus, Cushing syndrome, hypogonadism, insulinoma, hyperprolactinemia, acromegaly).
Medications (nutritional supplements, oral contraceptives, glucocorticoids, etc.).
Anxiety disorders with compulsive eating.
Laurence-Moon-Biedl syndrome, Prader-Willi syndrome, other congenital diseases.
Hypothalamic injury (rare; <100 cases reported in medical literature).

WEIGHT LOSS

ICD-10CM #	R63.4	Abnormal weight loss

Malignancy.
Psychiatric disorders (depression, anorexia nervosa).
New-onset diabetes mellitus.
Malabsorption.
Chronic obstructive pulmonary disease.
AIDS.
Uremia, liver disease.
Thyrotoxicosis, pheochromocytoma, carcinoid syndrome.
Addison disease.
Intestinal parasites.
Peptic ulcer disease.
Inflammatory bowel disease.
Food faddism.
Postgastrectomy syndrome.

WHEEZING

ICD-10CM #	R06.2	Wheezing

Asthma.
Chronic obstructive pulmonary disease.
Interstitial lung disease.
Infections (pneumonia, bronchitis, bronchiolitis, epiglottitis).
Cardiac asthma.
GERD with aspiration.
Foreign body aspiration.
Pulmonary embolism.
Anaphylaxis.
Obstruction of airway (neoplasm, goiter, edema or hemorrhage from trauma, aneurysm, congenital abnormalities, strictures, spasm).
Carcinoid syndrome.

WHEEZING, PEDIATRIC AGE[45]

ICD-10CM #	R06.2	Wheezing

Reactive airways disease.
Atopic asthma.
Infection-associated airway reactivity.
Exercise-induced asthma.
Salicylate-induced asthma and nasal polyposis.
Asthmatic bronchitis.
Other hypersensitivity reactions:
  Hypersensitivity pneumonitis.
  Tropical eosinophilia.
  Visceral larva migrans.
  Allergic bronchopulmonary aspergillosis.
Aspiration:
  Foreign body.
  Food, saliva, gastric contents.
  Laryngotracheoesophageal cleft.
  Tracheoesophageal fistula, H-type.
  Pharyngeal incoordination or neuromuscular weakness.
Cystic fibrosis.
Primary ciliary dyskinesia.
Cardiac failure.
Bronchiolitis obliterans.
Extrinsic compression of airways:
  Vascular ring.
  Enlarged lymph node.
  Mediastinal tumor.
  Lung cysts.
Tracheobronchomalacia.
Endobronchial masses.
Gastroesophageal reflux.
Pulmonary hemosiderosis.
Sequelae of bronchopulmonary dysplasia.
"Hysterical" glottic closure.
Cigarette smoke, other environmental insults.

WRIST AND HAND PAIN[35]

ICD-10CM #	S69.90XA	Unspecified injury of unspecified wrist, hand, and finger(s), initial encounter

Articular

Arthritis of the wrist, MCP, PIP, or DIP as a result of:	Trauma, hypermobility, sprain. RA (wrist, MCP, PIP joints). Osteoarthritis (first CMC, PIP, and DIP joints). Other forms of arthritis: gout, psoriatic arthritis, infection. Joint neoplasm.

Periarticular

Subcutaneous.	RA nodules, gouty tophi, painful subcutaneous calcific nodules in scleroderma, glomus tumor of the nail bed.
Palmar fascia.	Dupuytren contracture.
Tendon sheath.	Wrist extensor tenosynovitis, including de Quervain tenosynovitis and extensor carpi radialis tenosynovitis. Wrist volar flexor tenosynovitis (including carpal tunnel syndrome). Thumb flexor tenosynovitis (trigger or snapping thumb). Finger flexor tenosynovitis (trigger finger). Pigmented villonodular tenosynovitis (giant cell tumor of the tendon sheath).
Acute calcific periarthritis ganglion.	Wrist, MCP, and rarely the PIP and DIP joints.

Osseous

Bone lesions.	Fractures; neoplasm; infection; osteonecrosis, including Kienböck disease (lunate) and Preiser disease (scaphoid).

Neurologic

Nerve entrapment syndromes

Median nerve.	Carpal tunnel syndrome (at the wrist). Pronator teres syndrome (at the pronator teres). Anterior interosseous nerve syndrome.
Ulnar nerve.	Cubital tunnel syndrome (at the elbow). Guyon canal (at the wrist).
Posterior interosseous nerve syndrome.	Radial nerve palsy (spiral groove syndrome).
Lower brachial plexus.	Thoracic outlet syndrome, Pancoast tumor.
Cervical nerve roots.	Herniated cervical disk, tumors.

Differential Diagnosis

II

Spinal Cord Lesion

Spinal tumors, syringomyelia.

Vascular

Vasoplastic disorders with Raynaud phenomenon.	Scleroderma, occupational vibration syndrome.
Small- or large-vessel vasculitis.	With digital ischemia, ischemic ulcers (e.g., SLE, RA, and Takayasu arthritis).

Referred Pain

Cervical spine disorders.	Shoulder–hand syndrome and causalgia.
Reflex sympathetic dystrophy syndrome.	
Cardiac.	Angina pectoris.

CMC, Carpometacarpal; *DIP*, distal interphalangeal; *MCP*, metacarpophalangeal; *PIP*, proximal interphalangeal; *RA*, rheumatoid arthritis; *SLE*, systemic lupus erythematosus.

WRIST AND HAND PAIN, IN DIFFERENT AGE GROUPS[41]

ICD-10CM #	S69.80XA	Other specified injuries of unspecified wrist, hand and finger(s), initial encounter
	S69.90XA	Unspecified injury of unspecified wrist, hand and finger(s), initial encounter

COMMON CAUSES OF WRIST AND HAND PAIN IN DIFFERENT AGE GROUPS

Childhood (2 to 10 yr)
Intraarticular
Infection.
Periarticular
Fracture.
Osteomyelitis.
Adolescence (10 to 18 yr)
Intraarticular
Infection.
Periarticular
  Trauma.
  Osteomyelitis.
  Tumors.
  Ganglion.
  Idiopathic wrist pain.
Early Adulthood (18 to 30 yr)
Intraarticular
Inflammatory arthritis.
Infection.
Osteoarthritis.
Periarticular
Peripheral nerve entrapment.
Tendonitis.

Referred
Cervical.
Adulthood (30 to 50 yr)
Intraarticular
Inflammatory arthritis.
Infection.
Osteoarthritis.
Periarticular
Peripheral nerve entrapment.
Tendonitis.
Referred
Cervical.
Chest.
Cardiac.
Old Age (>50 yr)
Intraarticular
Inflammatory arthritis.
Osteoarthritis.
Periarticular
Peripheral nerve entrapment.
Tendonitis.
Referred
Cervical.
Chest.
Cardiac.

WRIST PAIN

ICD-10CM #	S69.80XA	Other specified injuries of unspecified wrist, hand and finger(s), initial encounter
	S69.90XA	Unspecified injury of unspecified wrist, hand and finger(s), initial encounter

MECHANICAL

Osteoarthritis.
Ligament tear.
Fracture.
Ganglion.
De Quervain tenosynovitis.
Avascular necrosis (scaphoid, lunate).
Nonunion of scaphoid or lunate.
Neoplasm.

METABOLIC

Pregnancy.
Diabetes.
Gout.
Pseudogout.
Paget disease.
Acromegaly.
Hypothyroidism.
Hyperparathyroidism.

INFECTIOUS

Osteomyelitis.
Septic arthritis.
Cat-scratch disease.
Tick bite (Lyme disease, babesiosis).
Tuberculosis.

NEUROLOGIC

Peripheral neuropathy.
Nerve injury (median, ulnar, radial nerve).
Thoracic outlet compression syndrome.
Distal posterior interosseous nerve syndrome.

RHEUMATOLOGIC

Psoriasis.
Rheumatoid arthritis.
Systemic lupus erythematosus, mixed connective tissue disorder (MCTD).
Scleroderma.

MISCELLANEOUS

Granulomatous (sarcoidosis).
Amyloidosis.
Multiple myeloma.
Leukemia.

XANTHOMAS[70]

ICD-10CM #	L99	Other disorders of skin and subcutaneous tissue in diseases classified elsewhere

Differential Diagnosis of Xanthomas

Eruptive xanthomas:
  Non-Langerhans cell histiocytosis.
Xanthoma disseminatum.
Papular xanthoma.
Generalized eruptive histiocytomas.
Indeterminate cell histiocytosis.
Rosai-Dorfman disease.
Juvenile xanthogranuloma (micronodular form).
Xanthomatous lesions of Langerhans cell histiocytosis.
Disseminated granuloma annulare.
Tuberous xanthomas:
  Erythema elevatum diutinum.
  Multicentric reticulohistiocytosis.
Tendinous xanthomas:
  Giant cell tumor of the tendon sheath.
  Rheumatoid nodule.
  Subcutaneous granuloma annulare.
  Erythema elevatum diutinum.
Xanthelasma:
  Syringomas.
  Necrobiotic xanthogranuloma.
  Adult-onset asthma and periocular xanthogranuloma (AAPOX).
  Sebaceous hyperplasia.
  Palpebral sarcoidosis.

XEROPHTHALMIA[25]

ICD-10CM #	H11.149	Conjunctival xerosis, unspecified, unspecified eye

MEDICATIONS

Tricyclic antidepressants: amitriptyline, doxepin.
Antihistamines: diphenhydramine, chlorpheniramine, promethazine, and many cold and decongestant preparations.
Anticholinergic agents: antiemetics such as scopolamine, antispasmodic agents such as oxybutynin chloride.

ABNORMALITIES OF EYELID FUNCTION

Neuromuscular disorders.
Aging.
Thyrotoxicosis.

ABNORMALITIES OF TEAR PRODUCTION

Hypovitaminosis A.
Stevens-Johnson syndrome.
Familial diseases affecting sebaceous secretions.

ABNORMALITIES OF CORNEAL SURFACES

Scarring from past injuries and herpes simplex infection.

XEROSTOMIA[25]

| ICD-10CM # | K11.7 | Disturbances of salivary secretion |
| | R68.2 | Dry mouth, unspecified |

MEDICATIONS

Tricyclic antidepressants: amitriptyline, doxepin.
Antihistamines: diphenhydramine, chlorpheniramine, promethazine, and many cold and decongestant preparations.
Anticholinergic agents: antiemetics such as scopolamine, antispasmodic agents such as oxybutynin chloride.

DEHYDRATION

Debility.
Fever.

POLYURIA

Alcohol intake.
Arrhythmia.
Diabetes.

PREVIOUS HEAD AND NECK IRRADIATION SYSTEMIC DISEASES

Sjögren syndrome.
Sarcoidosis.
Amyloidosis.
HIV infection.
Graft-versus-host disease.

YELLOW URINE

| ICD-10CM # | R82 | Other abnormal findings in urine |

Normal coloration.
Concentrated urine.
Use of multivitamin supplements.
Diet rich in carrots.
Use of Cascara.
Urinary tract infection.

REFERENCES

1. Mandell GL et al: *Mandell, Douglas, and Bennett's principles and practice of infectious diseases,* ed 6, New York, 2009, Churchill Livingstone.
2. Talley NJ, Martin CJ: *Clinical gastroenterology,* ed 2, Sydney, 2006, Churchill Livingstone.
3. Feldman M et al: *Sleisenger and Fordtran's gastrointestinal and liver disease,* ed 10, Philadelphia, 2016, Elsevier.
4. Townsend CM: *Sabiston textbook of surgery,* ed 21, Philadelphia, 2021, Elsevier.
5. Cherry JD: *Feigin and Cherry's pediatric infectious diseases,* ed 8, Philadelphia, 2017, Elsevier.
6. Hochberg M et al: *Practical rheumatology,* ed 3, London, 2004, Mosby.
7. Vincent JL et al: *Textbook of critical care,* ed 6, Philadelphia, 2011, Saunders.
8. Firestein GS et al: *Kelly's textbook of rheumatology,* ed 9, Philadelphia, 2013, Saunders.
9. Floege J et al: *Comprehensive clinical nephrology,* ed 4, Philadelphia, 2010, Saunders.
10. Marx JA: *Rosen's emergency medicine,* ed 8, Philadelphia, 2014, Saunders.
11. Skorecki K et al: *Brenner & Rector's the kidney,* ed 10, Philadelphia, 2016, Elsevier.
12. Cameron P et al: *Textbook of adult emergency medicine,* ed 5, Philadelphia, 2020, Elsevier.
13. Mason RJ et al: *Murray & Nadel's textbook of respiratory medicine,* ed 5, Philadelphia, 2010, Saunders.
14. Parrillo JE, Dellinger RP: *Critical care medicine, principles of diagnosis and management in the adult,* ed 5, Philadelphia, 2019, Elsevier.
15. Rumack CM: *Diagnostic ultrasound,* ed 4, Philadelphia, 2011, Elsevier.
16. Ronco C: *Critical care nephrology,* ed 3, Philadelphia, 2019, Elsevier.
17. Stein JH et al: *Internal medicine,* ed 5, St Louis, 1998, Mosby.
18. Andreoli TE et al: *Cecil essentials of medicine,* ed 5, Philadelphia, 200 Saunders.
19. Kliegman RM et al: *Nelson textbook of pediatrics,* ed 19, Philadelphia, 2011, Saunders.
20. Pina-Garza J, James KC: *Fenichel's clinical pediatric neurology,* ed 8, Philadelphia, 2019, Elsevier.
21. Grainger RG, Allison D: *Grainger & Allison's diagnostic radiology, a textbook of medical imaging,* ed 4, London, 2001, Churchill Livingstone.
22. Flint PW et al: *Cummings otolaryngology,* ed 7, Philadelphia, 2021, Elsevier.
23. Hoekelman R et al: *Primary pediatric care,* ed 3, St Louis, 1997, Mosby.
24. Goldman L, Ausiello D: *Cecil textbook of medicine,* ed 21, Philadelphia, 1999, Saunders.
25. Noble J: *Primary care medicine,* ed 3, St Louis, 2001, Mosby.
26. Kassirer J: *Current therapy in adult medicine,* ed 4, St Louis, 1997, Mosby.
27. Parrillo JE, Dellinger RP: *Critical care medicine, principles of diagnosis and management in the adult,* ed 4, Philadelphia, 2014, Elsevier.
28. Adkinson NF et al: *Middleton's allergy principles and practice,* ed 8, Philadelphia, 2014, Saunders.
29. Adams JG et al: *Emergency medicine, clinical essentials,* ed 2, Philadelphia, 2013, Elsevier.
30. Melmed S et al: *Williams textbook of endocrinology,* ed 12, Philadelphia, 2011, Saunders.
31. Hoffmann R et al: *Hematology: basic principles and practice,* ed 5, 2008, Churchill Livingstone.
32. Gabbe SG et al: *Gabbe's Obstetrics,* ed 6, Philadelphia, 2012, Saunders.
33. Harrington J: *Consultation in internal medicine,* ed 2, St Louis, 1997, Mosby.
34. Hoffman R et al: *Hematology: basic principles and practice,* ed 6, Philadelphia, 2013, Saunders.
35. Hochberg MC: *Rheumatology,* ed 7, Philadelphia, 2019, Elsevier.
36. Melmed S et al: *Williams textbook of endocrinology,* ed 14, Philadelphia, 2020, Elsevier.
37. Boxt LM, Abbara S: *Cardiac imaging: the requisites,* ed 4, Philadelphia, 2016, Elsevier.
38. Jankovic J et al: *Bradley and Daroff's neurology in clinical practice,* ed 8, Philadelphia, 2022, Elsevier.
39. Goldman L, Braunwald E: *Braunwauld primary cardiology,* ed 2, Philadelphia, 2003, Saunders.
40. Canoso J: *Rheumatology in primary care,* Philadelphia, 1997, Saunders.
41. Carr A, Hamilton W: *Orthopedics in primary care,* ed 2, Philadelphia, 2005, Saunders.
42. Bennett JE et al: *Mandell, Douglas, and Bennett's principles and practice of infectious diseases,* ed 8, Philadelphia, 2015, Saunders.
43. Barkin RM, Rosen P: *Emergency pediatrics: a guide to ambulatory care,* ed 5, St Louis, 2003, Mosby.
44. Bowling B: *Kanski's clinical ophthalmology,* ed 8, Philadelphia, 2016, Elsevier.
45. Behrman RE et al: *Nelson textbook of pediatrics,* ed 16, Philadelphia, 2000, Saunders.
46. Custer JW, Rau RE: *The Harriet Lane handbook,* ed 18, St Louis, 2008, Mosby.
47. Souhami RL, Moxham J: *Textbook of medicine,* ed 4, London, 2002, Churchill Livingstone.
48. Webb WR et al: *Fundamentals of body CT,* ed 4, Philadelphia, 2015, Saunders.
49. Swaiman KF et al: *Swaiman's pediatric neurology, principles and practice,* ed 6, Philadelphia, 2017, Elsevier.
50. Kryger M et al: *Principles and practice of sleep medicine,* ed 7, Philadelphia, 2023, Elsevier.
51. Kliegman R: *Practical strategies in pediatric diagnosis and therapy,* ed 2, Philadelphia, 2004, Saunders.
52. Pope TL et al: *Musculoskeletal imaging,* ed 2, Philadelphia, 2014, Saunders.
53. Firestein GS et al: *Firestein & Kelley's textbook of rheumatology,* ed 11, Philadelphia, 2021, Elsevier.
54. Specht N: *Practical guide to diagnostic imaging,* St Louis, 1997, Mosby.
55. Danakas G: *Practical guide to the care of the gynecologic/obstetric patient,* ed 2, St Louis, 2008, Mosby.
56. Marcdante KJ et al: *Nelson essentials of pediatrics,* ed 9, 2023, Elsevier.
57. Siedel HM et al: *Mosby's guide to physical examination,* ed 4, St Louis, 1998, Mosby.
58. Zipes DP: *Braunwald's heart disease, a textbook of cardiovascular medicine,* ed 11, Philadelphia, 2019, Elsevier.
59. Goldman L, Schafer AI: *Goldman's Cecil medicine,* ed 24, Philadelphia, 2011, Saunders.
60. Gorbach SL et al (eds): *Infectious diseases,* ed 2, Philadelphia, 1998, Saunders.
61. Fuhrman BP et al: *Pediatric critical care,* ed 4, Philadelphia, 2011, Saunders.
62. Wiederholt WC: *Neurology for non-neurologists,* ed 4, Philadelphia, 2000, Saunders.
63. Conn R: *Current diagnosis,* ed 9, Philadelphia, 1997, Saunders.
64. Cameron JL, Cameron AM: *Current surgical therapy,* ed 10, Philadelphia, 1994, Saunders.

65. Spec A et al: *Comprehensive review of infectious diseases,* Elsevier, 2020.

66. Stern TA: *Massachusetts General Hospital handbook of general hospital psychiatry,* ed 7, Philadelphia, 2018, Elsevier.

67. Rakel RE: *Principles of family practice,* ed 6, Philadelphia, 2001, Saunders.

68. Kliegman RM: *Nelson textbook of pediatrics,* ed 21, Philadelphia, 2020, Elsevier.

69. Ryan ET et al: *Hunter's tropical medicine and emerging infectious diseases,* ed 10, Philadelphia, 2020, Elsevier.

70. Bolognia JL et al: *Dermatology,* ed 4, Philadelphia, 2018, Elsevier.

71. Hoffman R: *Hematology, basic principles and practice,* ed 7, Philadelphia, 2018, Elsevier.

72. Kaufman DM et al: *Kaufman's clinical neurology for psychiatrists,* ed 8, Philadelphia, 2017, Elsevier.

73. Paller AS, Mancini AU: *Hurwitz clinical pediatric dermatology,* ed 5, Philadelphia, 2016, Elsevier.

74. Broaddus VC et al: *Murray & Nadel's textbook of respiratory medicine,* ed 7, Philadelphia, 2022, Elsevier.

75. Weinberger SE et al: *Principles of pulmonary medicine,* ed 7, Philadelphia, 2019, Elsevier.

76. Seller RH: *Differential diagnosis of common complaints,* ed 4, Philadelphia, 2000, Saunders.

77. Mahanty S, Nutman TB: Eosinophilia and eosinophil-related disorders. In Middleton EJ et al (eds): *Allergy: principles and practice,* ed 4, St Louis, 1993, Mosby-Year Book, p. 1077.

78. Sellke FW et al: *Sabiston & Spencer surgery of the chest,* ed 9, Philadelphia, 2016, Elsevier.

79. Eberlein M: *A fall in Ghana,* Am J Med 122:1091, 2009.

80. Moore WT, Eastman RC: *Diagnostic endocrinology,* ed 2, St Louis, 1990, Mosby.

81. Schwarz MI: *Interstitial lung disease,* ed 2, St Louis, 2003, Mosby.

82. Swain R, Snodgrass JG: Managing groin pain, *Phys Sportsmed* 23(56), 1995.

83. Cameron JL, Cameron AM: *Current surgical therapy,* ed 12, Philadelphia, 2017, Elsevier.

84. Habif TP: *Clinical dermatology,* ed 6, Philadelphia, 2016, Elsevier.

85. Goldberg RJ: *Practical guide to the care of the psychiatric patient,* ed 3, St Louis, 2007, Mosby.

86. Mann DL et al: *Braunwald's heart disease,* ed 10, Philadelphia, 2015, Elsevier.

87. Bonow RO et al: *Braunwauld's heart disease,* ed 9, Philadelphia, 2011, Elsevier.

88. Park MK: *Park's pediatric cardiology for practitioners,* ed 6, Philadelphia, 2014, Saunders.

89. Wein AU: *Campbell-Walsh urology,* ed 11, Philadelphia, 2016, Elsevier.

90. Hochberg MC et al: *Rheumatology,* ed 5, St Louis, 2010, Mosby.

91. Palay D: *Ophthalmology for the primary care physician,* St Louis, 1997, Mosby.

92. Callen JP: *Color atlas of dermatology,* ed 2, Philadelphia, 2000, WB Saunders.

93. Carlson KJ: *Primary care of women,* ed 2, St Louis, 2002, Mosby.

94. Goldman L, Schafer AI: *Goldman-Cecil medicine,* ed 26, Philadelphia, 2020, Elsevier.

95. Bain BJ et al: *Dacie and Lewis practical haematology,* ed 12, Philadelphia, 2017, Elsevier.

96. Talley NJ et al: *Essentials of internal medicine,* ed 4, Chatswood, 2021, Elsevier Australia.

97. Khan MG: *Rapid ECG interpretation,* ed 4, Philadelphia, 2019, Jaypee Brothers Medical Publishers Pvt. Ltd.

98. Kanski JJ, Bowlng B: *Clinical ophthalmology,* a systematic approach, ed 7, Philadelphia, 2011, Saunders.

99. Crum CP: *Diagnostic gynecologic and obstetric pathology,* ed 3, Philadelphia, 2018, Elsevier.

100. James WD: *Andrews' diseases of the skin,* ed 12, Philadelphia, 2016, Saunders.

101. Kaufman DM et al: *Kaufman's clinical neurology for psychiatrists,* ed 9, Philadelphia, 2023, Elsevier.

102. Gershenson DM et al: *Comprehensive Gynecology,* ed 8, Philadelphia, 2022, Elsevier.

103. Weinberger SE et al: *Principles of pulmonary medicine,* ed 5, Philadelphia, 2008, Saunders.

104. Nseyo UO: *Urology for primary care physicians,* Philadelphia, 1999, Saunders.

105. Tschudy MM, Arcara KM: *The Harriet Lane handbook,* ed 19, Philadelphia, 2011, Mosby.

106. Niederhuber JE et al: *Abeloff's clinical oncology,* ed 6, Philadelphia, 2020, Elsevier.

107. Grant LA, Griffin N: *Grainger & Allison's diagnostic radiology essentials,* ed 2, Philadelphia, 2019, Elsevier.

108. Baude AI: *Infectious diseases and medical microbiology,* ed 2, Philadelphia, 1985, Saunders.

109. Henry JB: *Clinical diagnosis and management by laboratory methods,* ed 20, Philadelphia, 2001, Saunders.

110. Boyer KM: Nonbacterial pneumonia. In Feigin RD, Cherry JD, (eds): *Textbook of pediatric infectious diseases,* ed 4, Philadelphia, 1998, WB Saunders, pp 260-273.

111. Hull KM et al: The expanding spectrum of systemic autoinflammatory disorders and their rheumatic manifestations, *Curr Opin Rheumatol* 15:61-69, 2003.

112. Auerbach P: *Wilderness medicine,* ed 7, Philadelphia, 2016, Saunders.

113. Wilson JD: *Williams textbook of endocrinology,* ed 9, Philadelphia, 1998, Saunders.

114. Copeland LJ: *Textbook of gynecology,* ed 2, Philadelphia, 1999, Saunders.

115. Lipshultz LI et al: *Urology and the primary care practitioner,* ed 3, Philadelphia, 2008, Elsevier.

SECTION III

Clinical Algorithms

INTRODUCTION

PLEASE NOTE: These algorithms are designed to assist clinicians in the evaluation and treatment of patients. They may not apply to all patients with a particular disorder and are not intended to replace the clinician's individual judgment.

Additional Algorithms Content Is Available at Elsevier Ebooks+ (eBooks.Health.Elsevier.com).

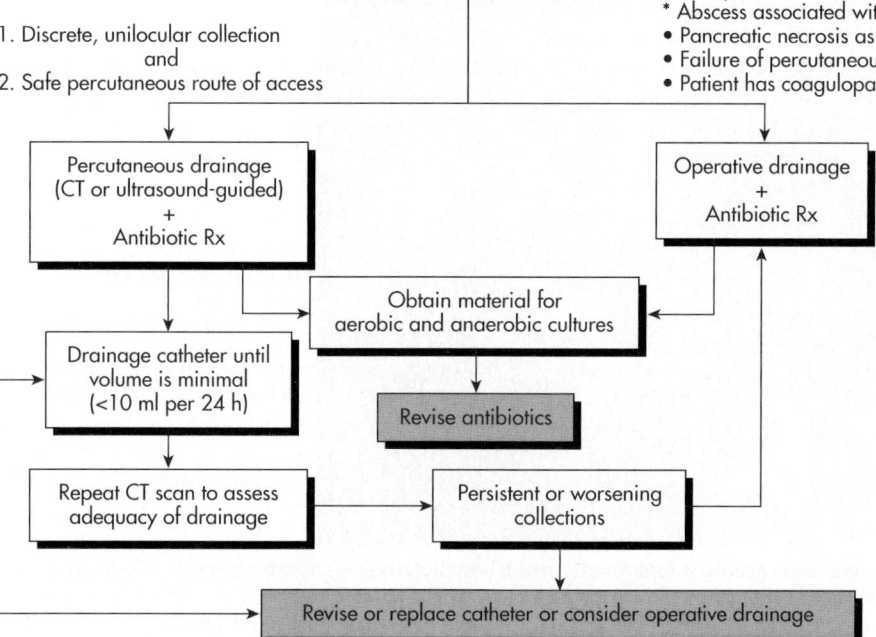

FIG. 1 Approach to management of intraabdominal abscesses including indications for consideration of percutaneous versus operative drainage. *CT,* Computed tomography; *Rx,* treatment. (From Parrillo JE, Dellinger RP: *Critical care medicine, principles of diagnosis and management in the adult,* ed 5, Philadelphia, 2019, Elsevier.)

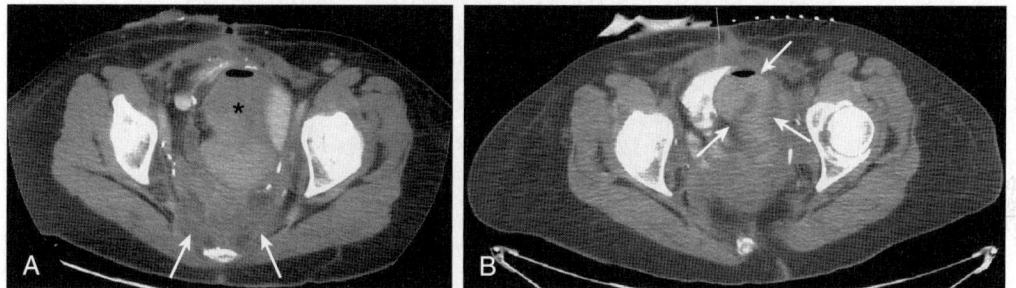

FIG. 2 **A,** Axial computed tomography (CT) image shows an apparently rim-enhancing structure containing gas *(asterisk)* in the deep pelvis adjacent to tethered bowel loops in a patient with prior pelvic irradiation. The structure could represent an abscess or a dilated loop of small bowel. The presacral inflammation *(arrows)* is related to radiation change. **B,** CT image obtained 2 h later shows ingested oral contrast in this structure *(arrows)* confirming that this is a bowel loop rather than an abscess. (From Feldman M et al: *Sleisenger and Fortran's gastrointestinal and liver disease,* ed 10, Philadelphia, 2016, Elsevier.)

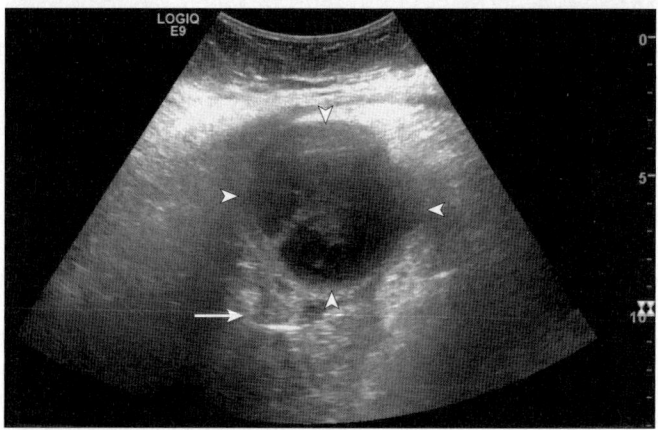

FIG. 3 Abdominal ultrasound of a typical abscess *(arrowheads)* demonstrating central decreased echogenicity, thickened wall, and debris arising anterior to the descending colon *(arrow)* in a patient with diverticulosis compatible with a diverticular abscess. (From Feldman M et al: *Sleisenger and Fortran's gastrointestinal and liver disease,* ed 10, Philadelphia, 2016, Elsevier.)

Clinical Algorithms

III

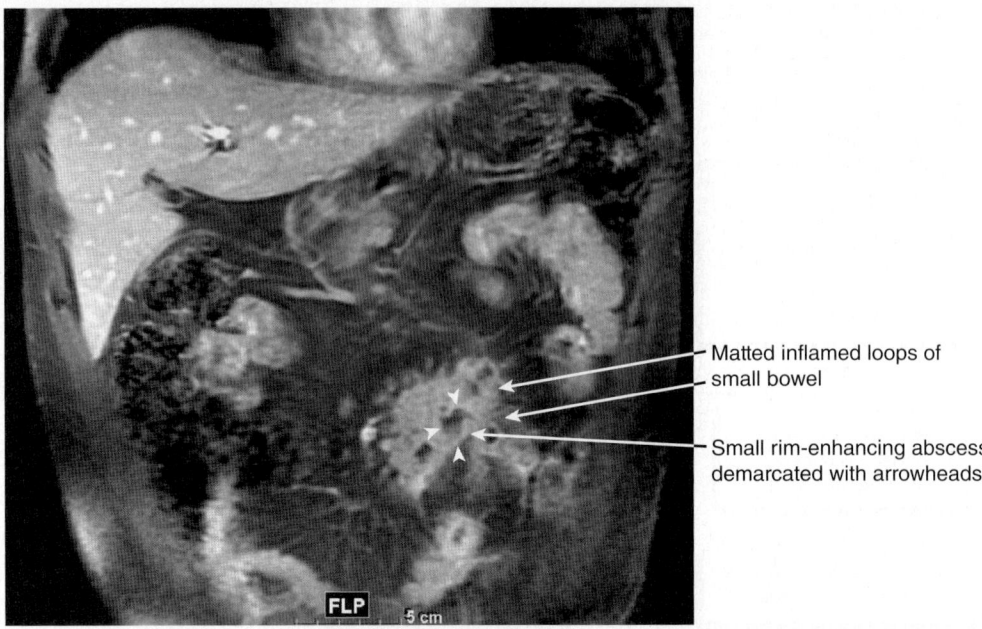

Matted inflamed loops of
small bowel

Small rim-enhancing abscess
demarcated with arrowheads

FIG. 4 Coronal magnetic resonance image with gadolinium contrast of a patient with Crohn disease showing a small rim-enhancing collection *(arrowheads)* **interposed between several loops of inflamed bowel** *(arrows)* **compatible with an interloop abscess.** Interloop abscesses are not amenable to percutaneous drain placement. (From Feldman M et al: *Sleisenger and Fortran's gastrointestinal and liver disease,* ed 10, Philadelphia, 2016, Elsevier.)

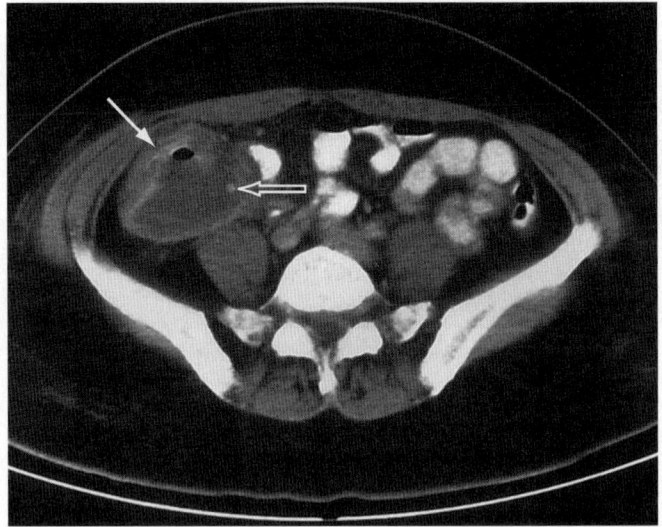

FIG. 5 Axial computed tomography demonstrating a right lower quadrant abscess *(closed arrow)* **with an appendicolith** *(open arrow).* Such extraluminal appendicoliths may predict clinical failure with percutaneous drainage. (From Feldman M et al: *Sleisenger and Fortran's gastrointestinal and liver disease,* ed 10, Philadelphia, 2016, Elsevier.)

BOX 1   Causes of Intraabdominal Abscesses

Abdominal trauma
Appendicitis
Cholecystectomy and other operations or invasive procedures
Crohn disease
Diverticulitis
Neoplastic disease
Pancreatitis
Perforated hollow viscus (e.g., duodenal or gastric ulcer)

From Feldman M et al: *Sleisenger and Fortran's gastrointestinal and liver disease,* ed 10, Philadelphia, 2016, Elsevier.

BOX 2   Clinical Risk Factors for Intraabdominal Abscess

Chronic glucocorticoid use
Increasing age
Malnutrition
Preexisting organ dysfunction
Transfusion
Underlying malignancy

From Feldman M et al: *Sleisenger and Fortran's gastrointestinal and liver disease,* ed 10, Philadelphia, 2016, Elsevier.

BOX 3   Antibiotic Choices in the Treatment of Intraabdominal Infections

Single-Agent Therapy
Second-Generation Cephalosporins
Cefoxitin
Carbapenems
Imipenem-cilastatin
Meropenem
Doripenem
Ertapenem (no *Pseudomonas* coverage)

Extended-Spectrum Penicillin–β-Lactamase Inhibitor Combinations
Piperacillin sodium-tazobactam
Ticarcillin disodium-clavulanate

Glycylcyclines
Tigecycline

Combination Therapy (Antiaerobe[a] + Antianaerobe)
Third- or Fourth-Generation Cephalosporins
Ceftriaxone + metronidazole
Cefotaxime + metronidazole
Ceftazidime (*Pseudomonas* coverage) + metronidazole
Cefepime (*Pseudomonas* coverage) + metronidazole

Fluoroquinolones
Ciprofloxacin + metronidazole
Levofloxacin + metronidazole
Moxifloxacin[b]

[a]Aminoglycoside therapy as an antiaerobic drug should not be used in routine practice owing to an increase in nephrotoxicity and possible worsened patient outcomes with its use.
[b]Moxifloxacin has adequate anaerobic coverage, making metronidazole unnecessary.
From Feldman M et al: *Sleisenger and Fortran's gastrointestinal and liver disease,* ed 10, Philadelphia, 2016, Elsevier.

Clinical Algorithms

III

TABLE 1 Comparison of Common Causes of Acute Abdominal Pain

Cause	Onset	Location	Character	Descriptor	Radiation	Intensity
Appendicitis	Gradual	Periumbilical area early; RLQ late	Diffuse early; localized later	Aching	None	++
Cholecystitis	Acute	RUQ	Localized	Constricting	Scapula	++
Pancreatitis	Acute	Epigastrium, back	Localized	Boring	Midback	++ to +++
Diverticulitis	Gradual	LLQ	Localized	Aching	None	++ to +++
Perforated peptic ulcer	Sudden	Epigastrium	Localized early, diffuse later	Burning	None	+++
Small bowel obstruction	Gradual	Periumbilical area	Diffuse	Cramping	None	++
Mesenteric ischemia, infarction	Sudden	Periumbilical area	Diffuse	Agonizing	None	+++
Ruptured abdominal aortic aneurysm	Sudden	Abdomen, back, flank	Diffuse	Tearing	None	+++
Gastroenteritis	Gradual	Periumbilical area	Diffuse	Spasmodic	None	+ to ++
Pelvic inflammatory disease	Gradual	Either LQ, pelvis	Localized	Aching	Upper thigh	++
Ruptured ectopic pregnancy	Sudden	Either LQ, pelvis	Localized	Sharp	None	++

+, Mild; ++, moderate; +++, severe; *LLQ,* left lower quadrant; *LQ,* lower quadrant; *RLQ,* right lower quadrant; *RUQ,* right upper quadrant.
From Feldman M et al: *Sleisenger and Fordtran's gastrointestinal and liver disease,* ed 10, Philadelphia, 2016, Elsevier.

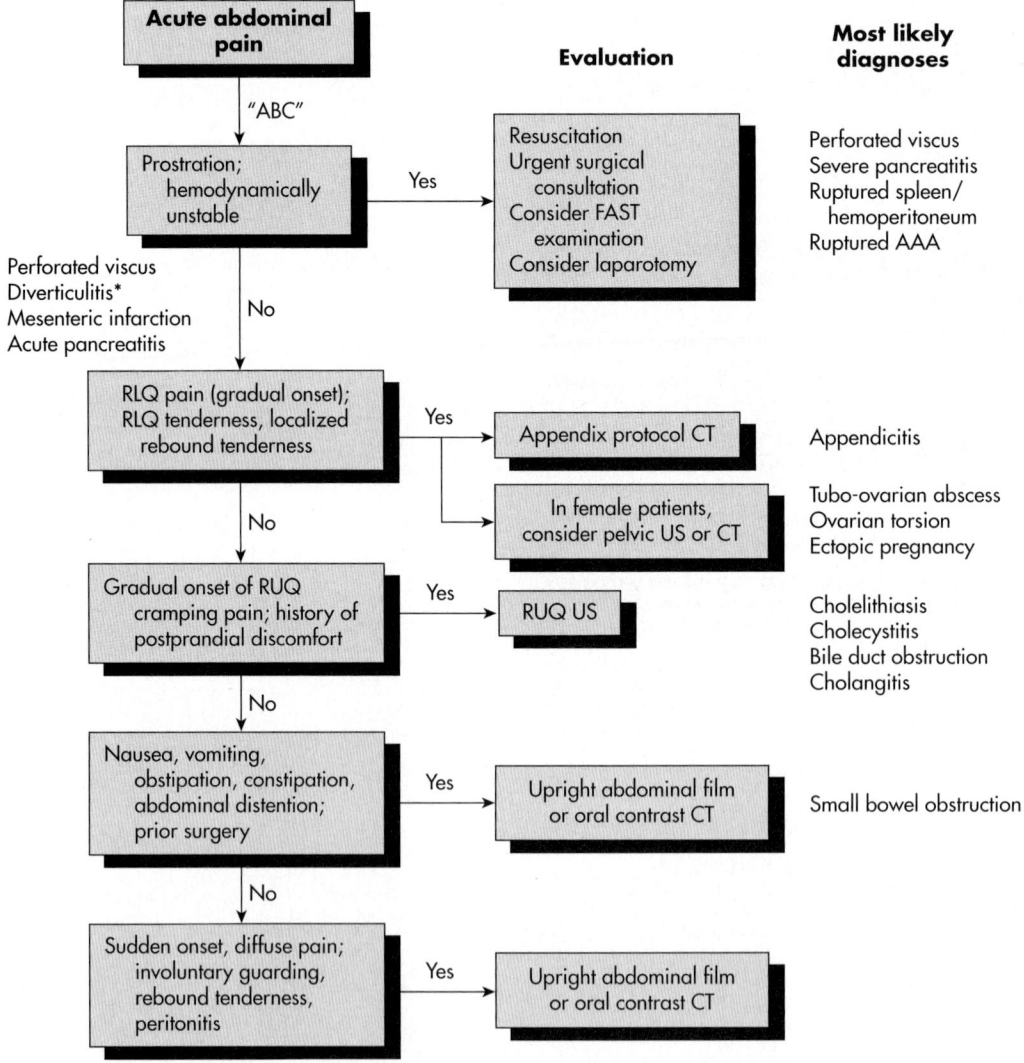

FIG. 6 An approach to the urgent evaluation of abdominal pain. Specific complaints and physical examination findings are coupled with appropriate radiologic imaging. *For left lower quadrant pain, the most likely diagnosis is diverticulitis. *AAA,* Abdominal aortic aneurysm; *ABC,* airway, breathing, circulation; *CT,* computed tomography; *FAST,* focused abdominal sonogram for trauma; *RLQ,* right lower quadrant; *RUQ,* right upper quadrant; *US,* ultrasound. (From Feldman M et al: *Sleisenger and Fordtran's gastrointestinal and liver disease,* ed 10, Philadelphia, 2016, Elsevier.)

BOX 4   Nonsurgical Causes of the Acute Abdomen

Endocrine and Metabolic Causes
Acute intermittent porphyria
Addisonian crisis
Diabetic crisis

Hereditary Mediterranean Fever
Uremia

Hematologic Causes
Acute leukemia
Sickle cell crisis

Toxins and Drugs
Black widow spider poisoning
Lead poisoning
Other heavy metal poisoning
Narcotic withdrawal

From Townsend CM et al: *Sabiston textbook of surgery,* ed 21, St Louis, 2022, Elsevier.

BOX 5   Surgical Acute Abdominal Conditions

Hemorrhage
Aortoduodenal fistula after aortic vascular graft
Arteriovenous malformation of the gastrointestinal tract
Bleeding gastrointestinal diverticulum
Hemorrhagic pancreatitis

Intestinal ulceration
Leaking or ruptured arterial aneurysm
Mallory-Weiss syndrome
Ruptured ectopic pregnancy
Solid organ trauma
Spontaneous splenic rupture

Infection
Appendicitis
Cholecystitis
Diverticulitis
Hepatic abscess
Meckel diverticulitis
Psoas abscess

Ischemia
Buerger disease
Ischemic colitis
Mesenteric thrombosis or embolism
Ovarian torsion
Strangulated hernia
Testicular torsion

Obstruction
Cecal volvulus
Gastrointestinal malignancy
Incarcerated hernias
Inflammatory bowel disease
Intussusception
Sigmoid volvulus
Small bowel obstruction

Perforation
Boerhaave syndrome
Perforated diverticulum
Perforated gastrointestinal cancer
Perforated gastrointestinal ulcer

From Townsend CM et al: *Sabiston textbook of surgery,* ed 21, St Louis, 2022, Elsevier.

BOX 6   Laboratory Tests for Abdominal Pain

- White blood cell count with differential
- Hemoglobin
- Platelets
- Electrolytes
- Creatinine and blood urea nitrogen
- Amylase and lipase
- Total and fractionated serum bilirubin
- Serum lactate levels
- Viral hepatitis panel
- Urinalysis
- Urine human chorionic gonadotropin
- *Clostridium difficile* culture and toxin assay

From Townsend CM et al: *Sabiston textbook of surgery,* ed 21, St Louis, 2022, Elsevier.

Clinical
Algorithms

TABLE 2 Abdominal Examination Signs

History	Physical Exam	Likely Diagnosis
Danforth sign	Shoulder pain on inspiration	Hemoperitoneum
Inspection		
Cruveilhier sign	Varicose veins at umbilicus	
Cullen sign	Periumbilical bruising	
Grey Turner sign	Local areas of discoloration near umbilicus and flanks	
Ransohoff sign	Yellow discoloration of umbilical region	
Palpation		
Aaron sign	Pain or pressure in epigastrium or anterior chest with persistent firm pressure applied to McBurney point	Acute appendicitis
Bassler sign	Sharp pain created by compressing appendix between abdominal wall and iliacus	Chronic appendicitis
Blumberg sign	Transient abdominal wall rebound tenderness	Peritoneal inflammation
Carnett sign	Loss of abdominal tenderness when abdominal wall muscles contracted	Intraabdominal source of abdominal pain
Chandelier sign	Extreme pelvic pain with movement of the cervix	Pelvic inflammatory disease
Courvoisier sign	Palpable gallbladder when jaundice is present	Periampullary mass
Fothergill sign	Abdominal wall mass that does not cross midline and is palpable when rectus is contracted	Rectus muscle hematoma
Iliopsoas sign	Elevation of extended leg against resistance is painful	Retrocecal acute appendicitis
Murphy sign	Pain caused by inspiration while applying pressure to right upper abdomen	Acute cholecystitis
Obturator sign	Flexion and external rotation of right thigh creates hypogastric pain	Pelvic abscess or inflammatory mass (appendicitis)
Rovsing sign	Pain at McBurney point when palpating the left lower quadrant	Acute appendicitis
Ten Horn sign	Pain caused by gentle traction of right testicle	Acute appendicitis

From Townsend CM et al: *Sabiston textbook of surgery,* ed 21, St Louis, 2022, Elsevier.

TABLE 3 Differential Diagnosis of Pain by Location (List Is Not Exhaustive)

Right upper quadrant	Epigastrium	Left upper quadrant
Hepatobiliary pathology	Gastritis, peptic ulcer	Gastritis, peptic ulcer
Duodenal ulcer, duodenitis	Hepatobiliary pathology	Renal colic, pyelonephritis
Renal colic, pyelonephritis	Pancreatitis	Splenic pathology
Retrocecal appendicitis	Aortic aneurysm	Pancreatitis
Pneumonia, pulmonary embolism	Early appendicitis	Pneumonia
	Myocardial infarction	

Right lumbar or flank	Midline or periumbilical	Left lumbar or flank
Renal colic, pyelonephritis	Visceral pain from midgut structures	Renal colic, pyelonephritis
Aortic aneurysm	Early appendicitis	Aortic aneurysm
Psoas abscess	Aortic aneurysm	Psoas abscess
Appendicitis		

Right lower quadrant	Suprapubic	Left lower quadrant
Appendicitis	Cystitis, bladder pathology	Similar to causes for right lower quadrant pain except for appendicitis (very rarely left-sided)
Ectopic pregnancy, tuboovarian pathology, endometriosis, pelvic inflammatory disease	Urinary tract infection	
Urinary tract infection, ureteric colic	Prostatitis	
Diverticulitis	Ectopic pregnancy, tuboovarian pathology, endometriosis, pelvic inflammatory disease	
Hernia		
Aortic aneurysm		
Testicular torsion, epididymoorchitis		

Pain radiating to the back

Perforated peptic ulcer
Acute pancreatitis
Abdominal aortic aneurysm, aortic dissection

NOTE: Pain from inflammatory bowel disease, diverticulitis, colitis, gastroenteritis, volvulus, intestinal obstruction, adhesions, ischemic colitis, and constipation may localize to any part of the abdomen.
From Cameron P et al: *Textbook of adult emergency medicine,* ed 5, Philadelphia, 2019, Elsevier.

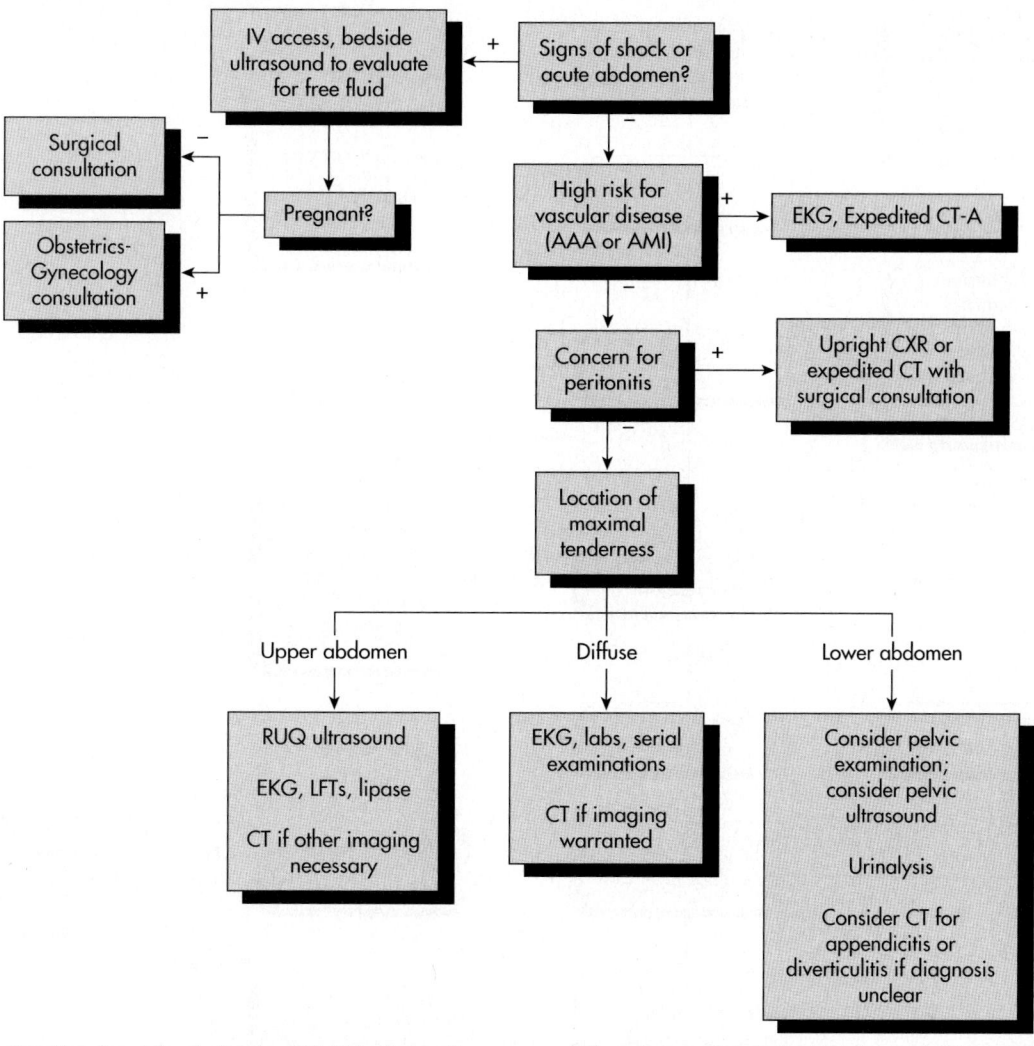

FIG. 7 Diagnostic algorithm for abdominal pain. *AAA,* Abdominal aortic aneurysm; *AMI,* acute mesenteric ischemia; *CT,* computed tomography; *CT-A,* Computed tomography angiography; *CXR,* chest x-ray; *EKG,* electrocardiogram; *IV,* intravenous; *LFTs,* liver function tests; *RUQ,* right upper quadrant. (From Walls RM et al: *Rosen's emergency medicine, concepts and clinical practice,* ed 10, Philadelphia, 2023, Elsevier.)

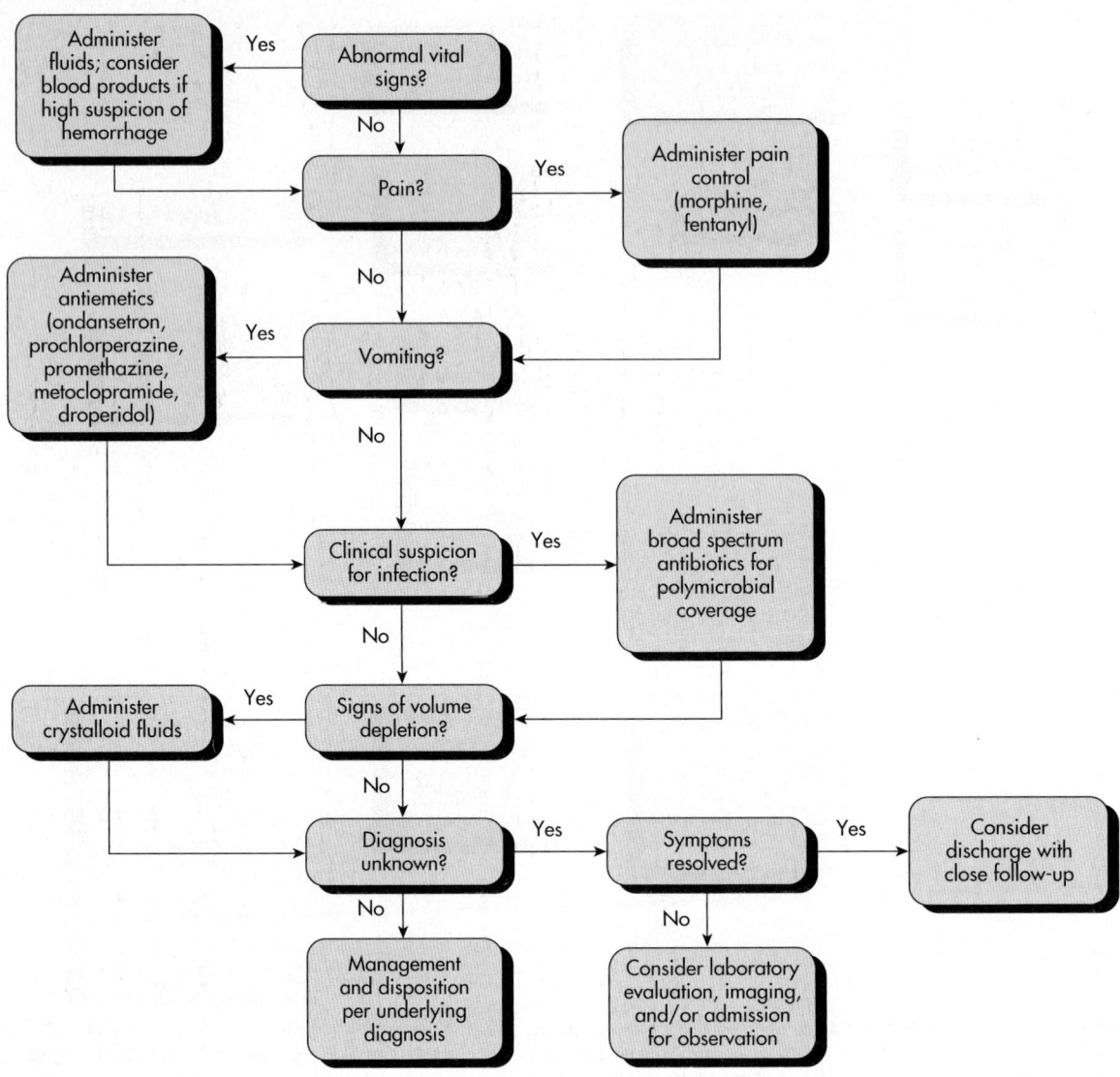

FIG. 8 Management algorithm for abdominal pain. (From Walls RM et al: *Rosen's emergency medicine, concepts and clinical practice,* ed 10, Philadelphia, 2023, Elsevier.)

TABLE 4   Critical Causes of Abdominal Pain

Cause	Epidemiology	Etiology	Presentation	Physical Examination	Useful Tool(s)	Pearls/Pitfalls
Ruptured ectopic pregnancy	Occurs in females of childbearing age. No method of contraception prevents ectopic pregnancy. Approximately 1 in every 100 pregnancies. Heterotopic pregnancy seen increasingly with ART.	Risk factors include nonwhite race, older gestational age, prior history of STD or PID, infertility treatment (ART), IUD placed within the past year, tubal sterilization, or previous ectopic pregnancy.	Severe, sharp, constant pain often localized to the affected side. More diffuse abdominal pain with intraperitoneal hemorrhage. Signs of shock may be present.	Shock or evidence of peritonitis may be present. Lateralized abdominal tenderness. Localized adnexal tenderness or cervical motion tenderness increases the likelihood of ectopic pregnancy. Vaginal bleeding does not have to be present.	β-hCG testing should be considered in all females of childbearing age or reproductive capacity (10-55 yr old); Pelvic ultrasonography is a critical diagnostic tool in evaluation. FAST examination is useful in evaluating for free fluid in patients with shock or peritonitis.	ART patients should not be considered to have an ectopic pregnancy ruled-out when intrauterine pregnancy is found given incidence of multiple gestations with ART.
Ruptured abdominal aortic aneurysm	Incidence increases with advancing age. More frequent in men. Risk factors include HTN, DM, smoking, COPD, and CAD.	Exact cause is undetermined. Contributing factors include atherosclerosis, genetic predisposition, HTN, connective tissue disease, trauma, or infection.	Patient is often asymptomatic until rupture. Acute epigastric and back pain is often associated with, or followed by, syncope or signs of shock. Pain may radiate to back, groin, or testes.	Vital signs may be normal (in 70%) to severely abnormal. Palpation of a pulsatile mass is possible in aneurysms 5 cm or greater. The physical examination may be nonspecific. Bruits or inequality of femoral pulses may be evident.	Abdominal plain films are abnormal in 80% of cases. Ultrasound can define diameter and length but can be limited by obesity or bowel gas. FAST examination can be helpful in evaluating for leak by looking for free fluid. CT-A test of choice in stable patients.	Endovascular repair possible, even in some complex cases. Permissive hypotension allowable.
Acute mesenteric ischemia	Occurs most commonly in elders with CV disease, CHF, cardiac dysrhythmias, DM, sepsis, dialysis, or dehydration. Mortality is 70%. MVT is associated with hypercoagulable states, hematologic inflammation, or trauma. MVT often presents less acute and in younger patients.	20%-30% of lesions are nonocclusive. The causes of ischemia are multifactorial, including transient hypotension in the presence of preexisting atherosclerotic lesion. The arterial occlusive causes (65%) are secondary to emboli (75%) or acute arterial thrombosis (25%).	Pain can be severe and colicky starting in the periumbilical region and then becomes diffuse. Often associated with vomiting and diarrhea. May be preceded by months of postprandial pain or "intestinal angina."	Early examination results can be remarkably benign in the presence of severe ischemia. Bowel sounds are often still present.	Often a pronounced leukocytosis is present. Metabolic acidosis caused by lactic acidemia is often seen with infarction. CT-A is now test of choice, but traditional angiography allows for therapy as well.	Needs multidisciplinary approach in most cases (general surgery, vascular surgery, interventional radiology, critical care). Interventional approaches can usually be pursued first, unless frank peritonitis.
Perforated viscus	Incidence increases with advancing age. History of peptic ulcer disease or diverticular disease common.	More often a duodenal ulcer that erodes through the serosa. Colonic diverticula, large bowel, and gallbladder perforations are rare. Spillage of bowel contents causes peritonitis.	Acute onset of epigastric pain is common. Vomiting in 50%. Fever may develop later. Pain may localize with omental walling off of peritonitis. Shock may be present with bleeding or sepsis.	Fever, usually of low grade, is common; worsens over time. Tachycardia is common. Abdominal examination reveals diffuse guarding and rebound. "Boardlike" abdomen in later stages. Bowel sounds are decreased.	WBC count is usually elevated owing to peritonitis. Amylase may be elevated; LFT results are variable. The upright radiographic view reveals free air in 70%-80% of cases with perforated ulcers.	Elderly rarely have rigidity (absent in almost 90% of cases).
Massive gastrointestinal bleeding	More common in adults ages 40-70.	History of peptic ulcer disease, gastritis, or liver disease; prior GI bleeding history.	Nausea and vomiting typically occur with upper GI bleeding with hallmark coffee-ground or hematemesis; slow transit can lead to melena; lower GI bleeds associated with poorly localized discomfort and bright red blood per rectum.	Nonfocal abdominal tenderness; large bleeds may result in tachycardia or hypotension with significant blood loss. Hemoglobin/hematocrit may be falsely reassuring in acute, massive bleeding.	Stool guaiac if there is a question of bleeding; massive bleeds may require emergent consultation by gastroenterology, interventional radiology, or surgery to intervene.	Stigmata of liver disease should prompt consideration of esophageal varices.
Acute myocardial infarction	Elderly women in particular may present with GI symptoms.	Plaque rupture leads to coronary vessel occlusion.	Nausea, vomiting, or epigastric discomfort may be the sole presenting symptoms, particularly in inferior events or in elderly females.	Nonspecific. Bradycardia often seen with inferior myocardial infarction.	Rapid electrocardiogram in evaluation of abdominal pain if possibility of coronary ischemia is suspected.	Mortality increases with delays in care.

ART, Assisted reproductive technologies; β-hCG, beta-human chorionic gonadotropin; CAD, coronary artery disease; CHF, congestive heart failure; COPD, chronic obstructive pulmonary disease; CV, cardiovascular; DM, diabetes mellitus; FAST, focused assessment by sonography in trauma; GI, gastrointestinal; HTN, hypertension; IUD, intrauterine contraceptive device; LFT, liver function test; MVT, mesenteric venous thrombosis; PID, pelvic inflammatory disease; STD, sexually transmitted disease; WBC, white blood cell.
From Walls RM et al: Rosen's emergency medicine, concepts and clinical practice, ed 10, Philadelphia, 2023, Elsevier.

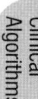

Clinical Algorithms

III

TABLE 5 Emergent Causes of Abdominal Pain

Causative Disorder or Condition	Epidemiology	Etiology	Presentation	Physical Examination	Useful Test(s)
Gastric, esophageal, or duodenal inflammation	Occurs in all age groups.	Caused by imbalance between digestive enzymes and mucoprotective barriers, infection, or exogenous sources.	Pain is epigastric, radiating or localized, associated with certain foods. Pain may be burning. In some cases, exacerbation in supine position.	Epigastric tenderness without rebound or guarding. Perforation or bleeding leads to more profound clinical findings.	Uncomplicated cases are treated with antacids or histamine H_2 blockers before invasive studies are contemplated. Gastroduodenoscopy is valuable in diagnosis and biopsy. Testing for *Helicobacter pylori* with blood or biopsy specimens. If perforation is suspected, an upright chest radiograph is obtained early to rule out free air. CT may be beneficial.
Acute appendicitis	Peak age in adolescence and young adulthood; less common in children and elders. Higher perforation rate in women, children, and elders, or in pregnancy. Mortality rate is 0.1% but increases to approximately 2% with perforation.[11]	Appendiceal lumen obstruction leads to swelling, ischemia, infection, and perforation.	Epigastric or periumbilical pain migrates (+LR 1.8 child/3.2 adult) to RLQ over 8-12 h. RLQ pain common (+LR 1.4 in child/7.3-8.5 in adult).[12] Later presentations associated with higher perforation rates. Pain, low-grade fever (+LR 1.2 in child/1.9 in adult), and anorexia (80%) common; vomiting less common (50%-70%).	Mean temperature 38°C (100.5°F). Higher temperature associated with perforation. RLQ tenderness (90%-95%) with rebound (40%-70%) in majority of cases. Rectal tenderness in 30%.	Leukocyte count is nonspecific and may be normal or elevated. If elevated, may or may not show left shift. Urinalysis may show sterile pyuria. CT is sensitive and specific. US may have use in those with nonobese body habitus, women, pregnancy, and children with RLQ pain. MRI has excellent diagnostic accuracy in pregnant women.
Biliary tract disease	Peak age 35-60 yr old; unlikely in patients younger than 20. Female-to-male ratio of 3:1. Risk factors include multiparity, obesity, alcohol intake, and use of birth control pills.	Presence of gallstones may cause biliary colic. Impaction of a stone in cystic duct or common duct may lead to cholecystitis or cholangitis, respectively.	Crampy RUQ pain radiates to right subscapular area. Prior history of pain is common. May have nausea or postprandial pain. Longer duration of pain favors diagnosis of cholecystitis or cholangitis.	Temperature is normal in biliary colic, may be elevated in cholecystitis or cholangitis. RUQ tenderness, rebound, or jaundice (less common) may be present.	WBC may be elevated in cholecystitis and cholangitis. US may demonstrate wall thickening, pericholecystic fluid, stones, or duct dilation. Hepatobiliary scintigraphy (HIDA scan) evaluates gallbladder function.
Ureteral colic	Average age for first episode is 30-40 yr, primarily in men. Prior history or family history of kidney stones is common.	Family history, gout, *Proteus* infection. Renal tubular acidosis or cystinuria lead to stone formation.	Acute onset of flank pain radiating to groin. Nausea, vomiting, and pallor are common. Patients are usually restless and unable to find position of comfort.	Vital signs are usually normal. Tenderness on CVA percussion with benign abdominal examination.	Urinalysis usually shows hematuria. Non-contrast CT is sensitive and specific. Ultrasound to evaluate for hydronephrosis may be sufficient if diagnosis previously established.
Diverticulitis	Incidence increases with advancing age, affects males more often than females. Recurrences are common.	Colonic diverticula may become infected, perforate, or cause local colitis. Obstruction, peritonitis, abscesses, fistulae result from infection or swelling.	Change in stool frequency or consistency commonly reported. LLQ pain is common. Associated with fever, nausea, and vomiting; rectal bleeding may be seen.	Fever usually low grade. LLQ pain without rebound is common. Stool may be heme positive.	Results on most tests usually normal. Plain radiographs not indicated. CT is diagnostic, but diagnosis can also be made clinically, without imaging, in selected lower-risk patients.
Acute gastroenteritis	Seasonal. Most common misdiagnosis of appendicitis and of acute mesenteric ischemia. May be seen in multiple family members. History of travel or immunocompromise. Most common GI disease in the United States.	Usually viral. Consider invasive bacterial or parasitic cause in prolonged cases, in travelers, or immunocompromised patients.	Pain usually poorly localized, intermittent, crampy, and diffuse. Diarrhea is key element in diagnosis; usually large volume, watery. Nausea and vomiting usually begin before pain.	Abdominal examination usually nonspecific without peritoneal signs. Watery diarrhea or no stool noted or rectal examination. Fever may be present.	Usually symptomatic care with antiemetics and volume repletion. Heme-positive stools may be a clue to invasive pathogens. Also consider more serious causes prior to concluding on diagnosis of acute gastroenteritis.

Causative Disorder or Condition	Epidemiology	Etiology	Presentation	Physical Examination	Useful Test(s)
Constipation and obstipation	More common in females, elders, the very young, and patients on narcotics.	Idiopathic, or bowel hypokinesis secondary to disease states (low motility) or exogenous sources (diet, medications).	Abdominal pain; change in bowel habits.	Variable, nonspecific without peritoneal signs. Rectal examination may reveal hard stool or impaction.	Radiographs may show large amounts of stool. Constipation or obstipation are diagnoses of exclusion.
Intestinal obstruction	Peaks in infancy and in the elderly. More common with history of previous abdominal surgery.	Adhesions, carcinoma, hernias, abscesses, volvulus, or infarction. Obstruction leads to vomiting, extravascular fluid accumulation; strangulation and necrosis of bowel may occur.	Crampy diffuse abdominal pain associated with vomiting.	Vital signs are usually normal unless dehydration or bowel strangulation has occurred. Abdominal distention, hyperactive bowel sounds, and diffuse tenderness. Local peritoneal signs may indicate strangulation.	Elevated WBC count may suggest advanced disease or strangulation. Volume depletion may be severe. Electrolytes may be abnormal if associated with vomiting or prolonged symptoms. Abdominal radiographs, CT, and ultrasound are useful in diagnosis.
Acute pancreatitis	Peak age is adulthood; rare in children. Male preponderance. Alcohol abuse and biliary tract disease are risk factors.	Alcohol, gallstones, hyperlipidemia, hypercalcemia, or endoscopic retrograde pancreatography causing pancreatic damage, saponification, or necrosis. ARDS, sepsis, hemorrhage, or renal failure may be secondary complications.	Acute onset of epigastric pain radiating to the mid-back. Nausea and vomiting are common. Pain disproportionate to physical findings. Adequate volume repletion is important in the initial therapy.	Low-grade fever is common. Patient may be hypotensive or tachypneic. Some epigastric tenderness is usually present. Because the pancreas is a retroperitoneal organ, guarding or rebound not present unless condition is severe. Flank or periumbilical ecchymosis may be seen with hemorrhagic pancreatitis.	Serum lipase is the test of choice. Ultrasound examination may show edema, pseudocyst, or biliary tract disease. CT scan may show abscesses, necrosis, hemorrhage, or pseudocysts. Ultrasound is recommended to assess for gallstones while CT is recommended if severe acute pancreatitis is suspected.

ARDS, Acute respiratory distress syndrome; *CT*, computed tomography; *CVA*, costovertebral angle; *HIDA*, hepatobiliary scintigraphy; *LLQ*, left lower quadrant; *LR*, likelihood ratio; *RLQ*, right lower quadrant; *RUQ*, right upper quadrant; *US*, ultrasound; *WBC*, white blood cell.
From Walls RM et al: *Rosen's emergency medicine, concepts and clinical practice*, ed 10, Philadelphia, 2023, Elsevier.

Clinical Algorithms

III

BOX 7 Extra-abdominal and Systemic Causes of Acute Abdominal Pain

Cardiac
- Endocarditis
- Heart failure
- Myocardial ischemia and infarction
- Myocarditis

Thoracic
- Empyema
- Esophageal rupture (Boerhaave syndrome)
- Esophageal spasm
- Esophagitis
- Pleurodynia (Bornholm disease)
- Pneumonitis
- Pneumothorax
- Pulmonary embolism and infarction

Hematologic
- Acute leukemia
- Hemolytic anemia
- Henoch-Schönlein purpura
- Sickle cell disease

Metabolic
- Acute adrenal insufficiency (Addison disease)
- Diabetes mellitus (especially with ketoacidosis)
- Hyperlipidemia
- Hyperparathyroidism

- Hypersensitivity reactions (e.g., to insect bites, reptile venoms)
- Lead poisoning
- Porphyria
- Toxins
- Uremia

Infections
- Herpes zoster
- Osteomyelitis
- Syphilis
- Typhoid fever

Neurologic
- Abdominal epilepsy
- Radiculopathy, spinal cord or peripheral nerve tumors, degenerative arthritis of the spine, herniated vertebral disk
- Tabes dorsalis

Miscellaneous
- Angioedema
- Familial Mediterranean fever
- Heat stroke
- Muscle contusion, hematoma, tumor
- Narcotic withdrawal
- Psychiatric disorders

From Feldman M et al: *Sleisenger and Fordtran's gastrointestinal and liver disease,* ed 11, Philadelphia, 2021, Elsevier.

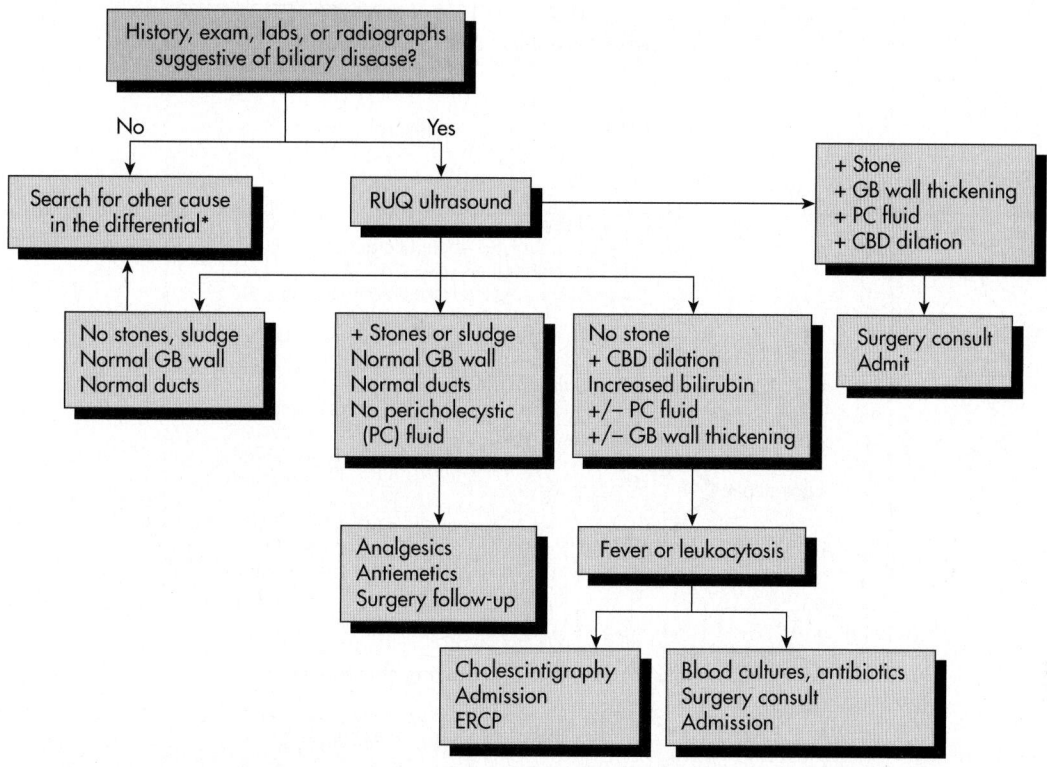

FIG. 9 Treatment algorithm for right upper quadrant *(RUQ)* pain. *Refer to Section II, Differential Diagnosis: Abdominal Pain, Right Upper Quadrant. *CBD,* Common bile duct; *ERCP,* endoscopic retrograde cholangiopancreatography; *GB,* gallbladder; *RUQ,* right upper quadrant; +, with; −, without; ±, with or without. (From Adams JG et al: *Emergency medicine, clinical essentials,* ed 2, Philadelphia, 2013, Elsevier.)

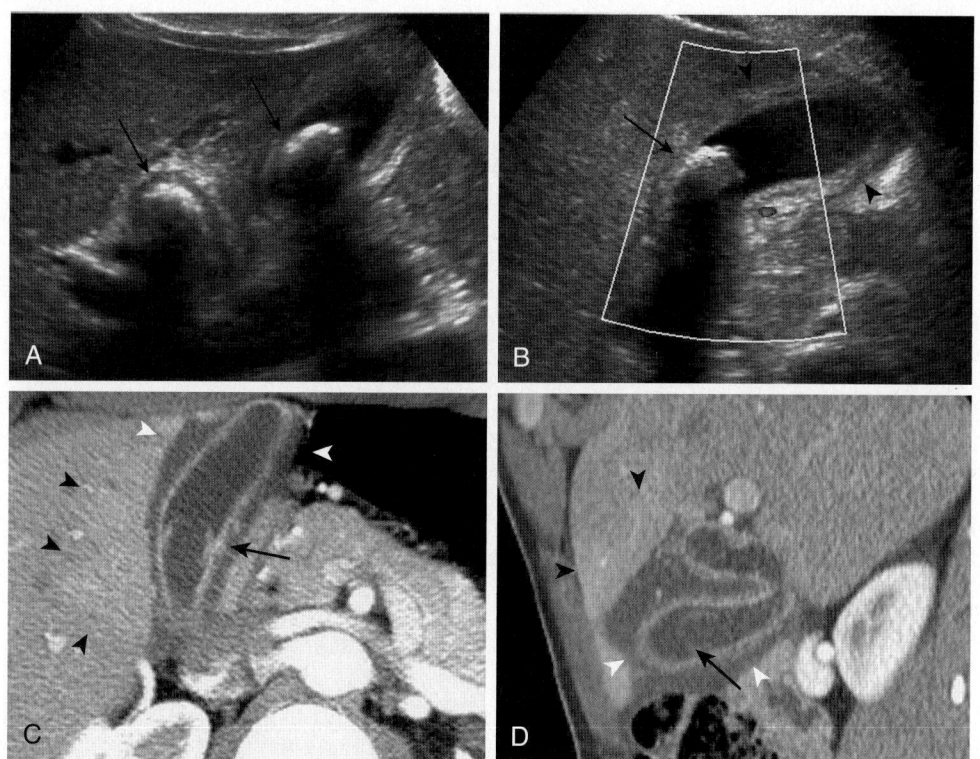

FIG. 10 A 43-yr-old man with acute cholecystitis. Ultrasound images (**A** and **B**) demonstrate echogenic, shadowing gallstones *(arrows)* with gallbladder wall thickening *(arrowheads)* in a patient in whom a sonographic Murphy sign was elicited. Axial (**C**) and sagittal (**D**) portal venous phase computed tomography images reveal a gallstone *(arrows)*, as well as a thickened gallbladder wall *(white arrowheads)*. Although not acquired in the arterial phase of contrast, hepatic hyperenhancement consistent with secondary inflammation is nevertheless seen *(black arrowheads)*. These findings are specific for this life-threatening complication and should be recognized and treated urgently. (From Soto JA, Lucey BC: *Emergency radiology, the requisites,* ed 2, Philadelphia, 2017, Elsevier.)

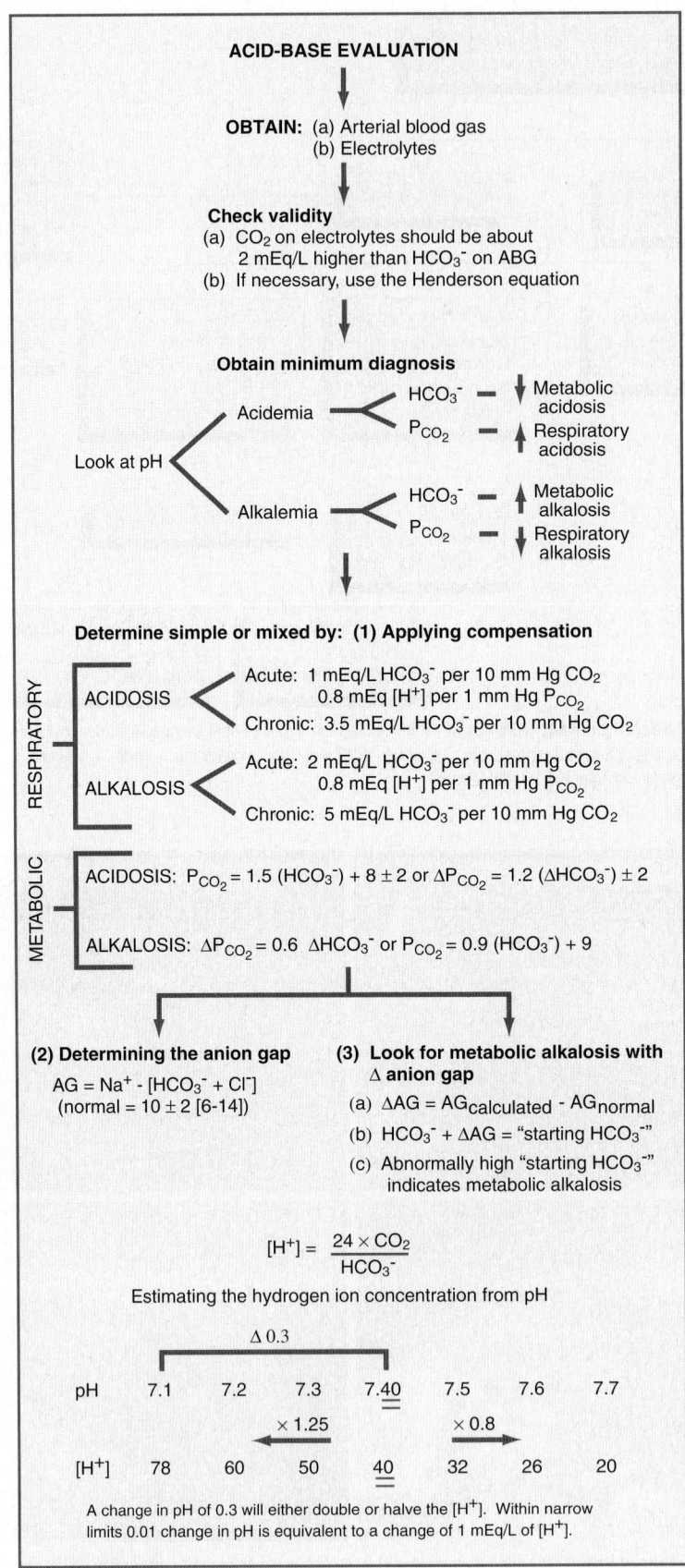

FIG. 11 Scheme for assessing acid-base homeostasis. *ABG,* Arterial blood gases; *AG,* anion gap; *PCO2,* partial pressure of carbon dioxide. (Modified from Andreoli TE [ed]: *Cecil essentials of medicine,* ed 7, Philadelphia, 2008, Saunders.)

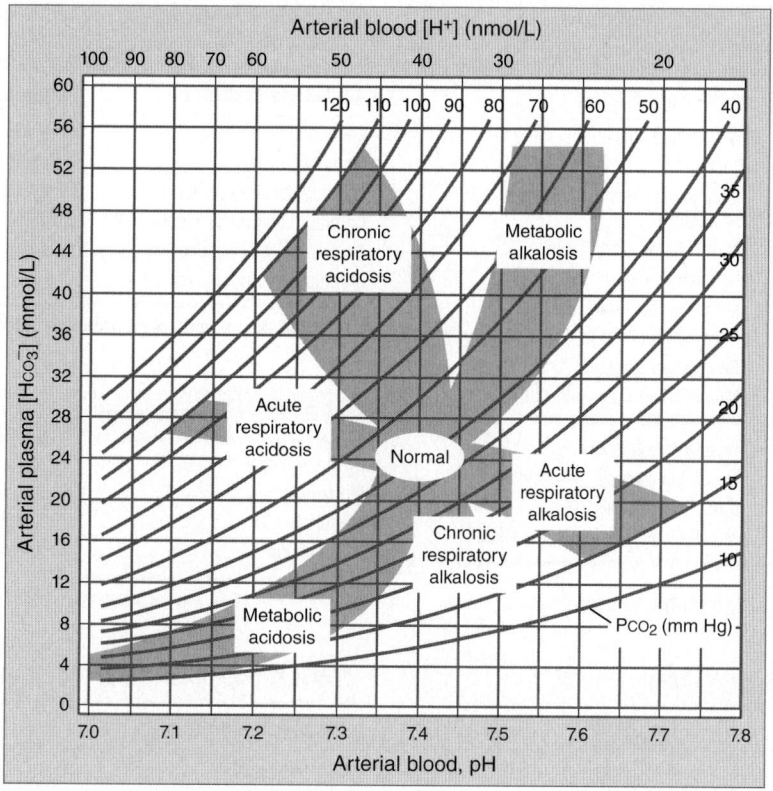

FIG. 12 Acid base normogram. Shaded areas represent 95% confidence limits of normal respiratory and metabolic compensations for primary disturbances. Points outside shaded areas represent a mixed disorder, assuming absence of laboratory error. (From Vincent JL et al: *Textbook of critical care*, ed 6, Philadelphia, 2011, Saunders.)

TABLE 6   Rules of Chronic Compensation

Primary Disorder	Secondary Compensation	EXAMPLES	
		Primary Change	Compensation
↑ Pco_2	↑ HCO_3^- : 4 mEq/L for each 10 mm Hg increase in Pco_2 (±3 mEq/L)	Pco_2: 40 → 80	HCO_3^-: 24 → 40 pH: 7.1 → 7.32
↓ Pco_2	↓ HCO_3^-: 2.5 mEq/L for each 10 mm Hg decrease in Pco_2 (±3 mEq/L)*	Pco_2: 40 → 20	HCO_3^-: 24 → 19 pH: 7.70 → 7.60
↓ HCO_3^-	↓ Pco_2: 1-1.5 mm Hg for each mEq/L decrease in HCO_3^-	HCO_3^-: 24 → 9	Pco_2: 40 → 25 pH: 7.00 → 7.20
↑ HCO_3^-	↑ Pco_2: 0.5-1.0 mm Hg for each mEq/L increase in HCO_3^-	HCO_3^-: 24 → 34	Pco_2: 40 → 50 pH: 7.56 → 7.46

*HCO_3^- seldom falls below 18 mEq/L in acute and 16 mEq/L in chronic respiratory alkalosis.
From Broaddus VC et al: *Murray & Nadel's textbook of respiratory medicine*, ed 7, Philadelphia 2022, Elsevier.

Clinical
Algorithms

III

TABLE 7 Common Clinical Presentations and Associated Acid-Base Disorders

Phenotype	Acid-Base Status
Pulmonary embolism	Respiratory alkalosis
Shock	Lactic acidosis (metabolic)
Sepsis	Metabolic acidosis and respiratory alkalosis
Vomiting	Metabolic alkalosis
Diarrhea	Metabolic acidosis
Acute kidney injury	Metabolic acidosis
Cirrhosis	Respiratory alkalosis
Pregnancy	Respiratory alkalosis
Diuretics	Metabolic alkalosis unless thiazides are used
COPD	Respiratory acidosis
Diabetic ketosis	Metabolic acidosis (ketoacidosis)
Ethylene glycol poisoning (antifreeze)	Metabolic acidosis
Excessive 0.9% saline use	Metabolic nonanion gap acidosis

COPD, Chronic obstructive pulmonary disease.
From Vincent JL et al: *Textbook of critical care,* ed 8, Philadelphia, 2024, Elsevier.

TABLE 8 Normal Acid-Base Values

	Mean	1 ± SD	2 ± SD
$PaCO_2$ (mm Hg)	40	38-42	35-45
pH	7.4	7.38-7.42	7.35-7.45
HCO_3-	24	23-25	22-26

SD, standard deviation.
From Vincent JL et al: *Textbook of critical care,* ed 8, Philadelphia, 2024, Elsevier.

TABLE 9 Acid-Base Disorders

Phenotype	Diagnostic Criteria
Respiratory acidosis	$PaCO_2$ >45 mm Hg
Respiratory alkalosis	$PaCO_2$ <35 mm Hg
Acute respiratory acidosis	$PaCO_2$ >45 mm Hg and pH <7.35
Chronic respiratory acidosis	$PaCO_2$ >45 mm Hg and pH = 7.36-7.44
Acute respiratory alkalosis	$PaCO_2$ <35 mm Hg and pH >7.45
Chronic respiratory alkalosis	$PaCO_2$ <35 mm Hg and pH = 7.36-7.44
Acidemia	pH <7.35
Alkalemia	pH >7.45
Acidosis	HCO_3- < 22 mEq/L
Alkalosis	HCO_3- >26 mEq/L

From Vincent JL et al: *Textbook of critical care,* ed 8, Philadelphia, 2024, Elsevier.

TABLE 10 Compensation Formulas for Simple Acid-Base Disorders

Acid-Base Disorder	Compensation
Metabolic acidosis	Change in $PaCO_2$ = 1.2 × change in HCO_3-
Metabolic alkalosis	Change in $PaCO_2$ = 0.6 × change in HCO_3-
Acute respiratory acidosis	Change in HCO_3- = 0.1 × change in $PaCO_2$
Chronic respiratory acidosis	Change in HCO_3- = 0.35 × change in $PaCO_2$
Acute respiratory alkalosis	Change in HCO_3- = 0.2 × change in $PaCO_2$
Chronic respiratory alkalosis	Change in HCO_3- = 0.5 × change in $PaCO_2$

From Vincent JL et al: *Textbook of critical care,* ed 8, Philadelphia, 2024, Elsevier.

TABLE 11 Causes of an Increased Osmolal Gap

Ethylene glycol	Alcohol
Methanol	Isopropyl alcohol (nongap)
Mannitol	Sorbitol
Paraldehyde	Acetone

From Vincent JL et al: *Textbook of critical care,* ed 8, Philadelphia, 2024, Elsevier.

TABLE 12 Causes of Metabolic Acidosis

Increased Anion Gap	Normal Anion Gap
Acute kidney injury	Hypokalemic acidosis
Rhabdomyolysis	Hyperkalemic acidosis
Ketoacidosis	
Lactic acidosis	
Toxins: 5-oxoproline	
Beriberi	

From Vincent JL et al: *Textbook of critical care,* ed 8, Philadelphia, 2024, Elsevier.

TABLE 13 Causes of Metabolic Alkalosis

Low Urine Chloride (Volume or Saline Responsive)	High Urine Chloride With Hypertension
Gastric volume loss	Primary and secondary hyperaldosteronism
Diuretics	Apparent mineralocorticoid excess
Posthypercapnia	Liddle syndrome (autosomal dominant, pseudoaldosteronism)
Villous adenoma (rare)	Conn syndrome
Cystic fibrosis (if there has been excessive sweating)	Cushing disease

High Urine Chloride Without Hypertension

Bartter syndrome

Gitelman syndrome (autosomal recessive hypokalemic metabolic alkalosis)

Excess bicarbonate administration

From Vincent JL et al: *Textbook of critical care,* ed 8, Philadelphia, 2024, Elsevier.

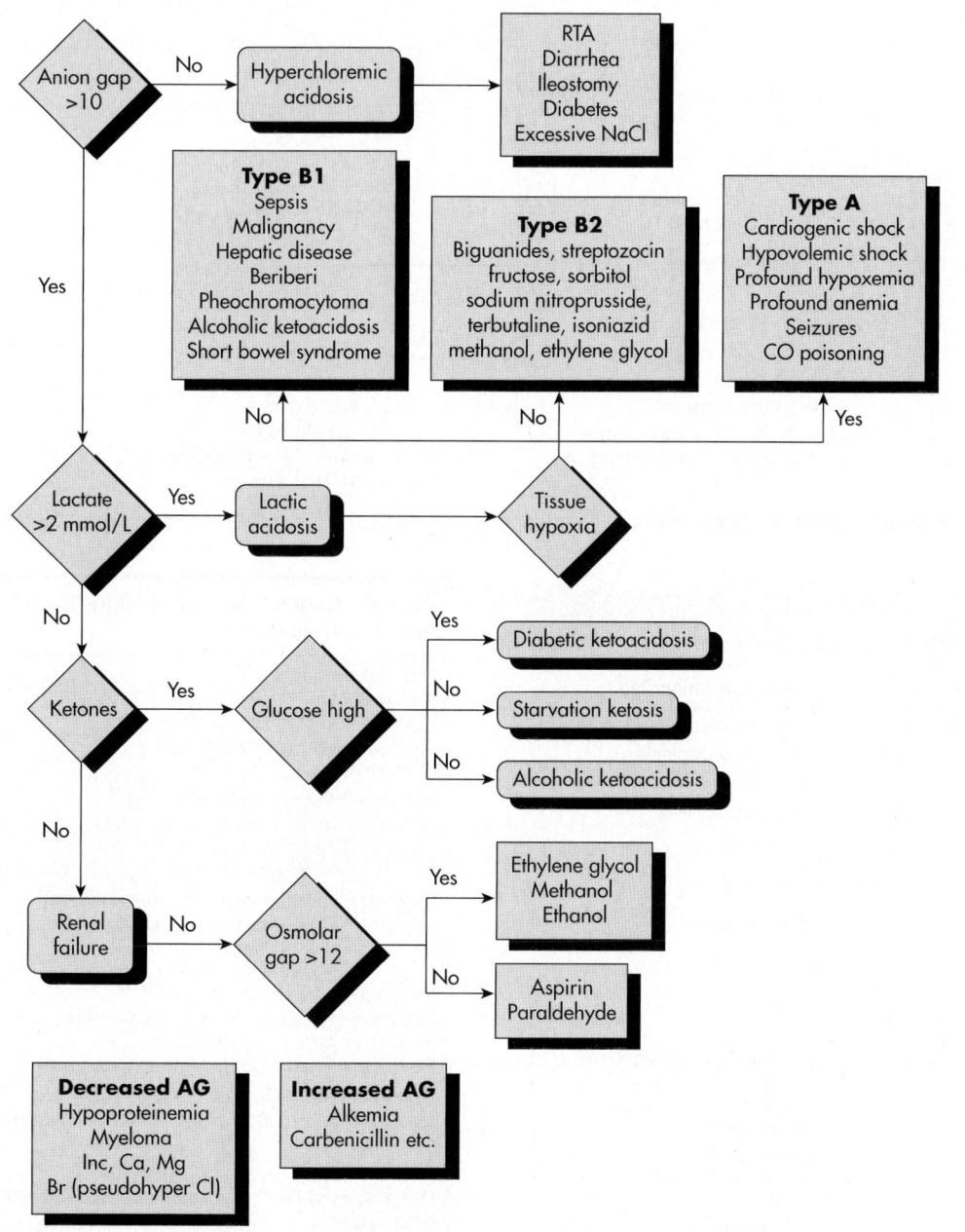

FIG. 13 Diagnostic approach to metabolic acidosis. *AG,* Anion gap; *CO,* carbon monoxide; *RTA,* renal tubular acidosis. (From Vincent JL et al: *Textbook of critical care,* ed 7, Philadelphia, 2017, Elsevier.)

Clinical
Algorithms

III

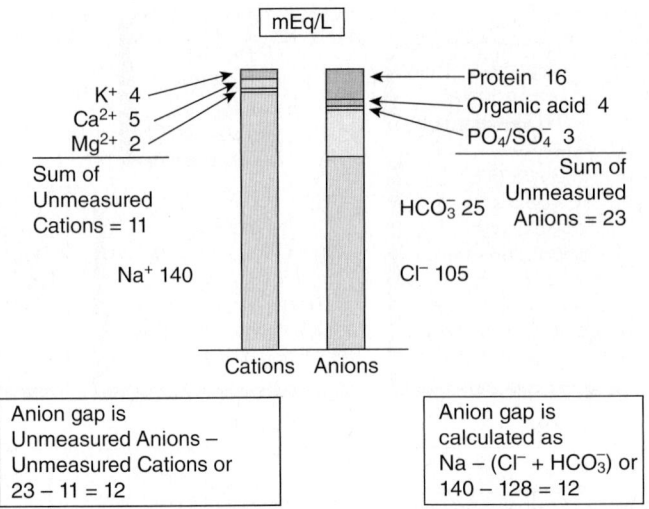

FIG. 14 Components of the serum anion gap. (From Vincent JL et al: *Textbook of critical care,* ed 8, Philadelphia, 2024, Elsevier.)

TABLE 14 Anion Gap in the Diagnosis of Metabolic Acidosis Anion Gap=Na$^+$ – (Cl$^-$+ HCO$_3^-$)=9 + 3 mEq/L

Decreased Anion Gap	Increased Anion Gap
Increased cations (not Na$^+$)	Increased anions (not Cl$^-$ or HCO$_3^-$)
↑Ca^{2+}, Mg^{2+}	↑Albumin concentration
↑Li$^+$	Alkalosis
↑IgG	↑Inorganic anions
Decreased anions:	Phosphate
(not Cl$^-$ or HCO$_3^-$)	Sulfate
Hypoalbuminemia*	
Acidosis	↑Organic anions
Laboratory error	L-Lactate
	D-Lactate
Hyperviscosity	Ketones
Bromism	Uremic
	↑Exogenously supplied anions
	Toxins
	Salicylate
	Paraldehyde
	Ethylene glycol
	Methanol
	Toluene
	Pyroglutamic acid
	↑Unidentified anions
	Uremic
	Hyperosmolar, nonketotic states
	Myoglobinuric acute renal failure
	Decreased cations (not Na$^+$)
	↑Ca^{2+}, Mg^{2+}

*Albumin is the major unmeasured anion. A decline in serum albumin of 1.0 g/dl from the normal value of 4.5 g/dl decreases the anion gap by 2.3-2.5 mEq/L. Correction is very important to diagnose anion gap acidosis in the setting of hypoalbuminemia.

Adapted from Emmett M, Narins RG: Clinical use of the anion gap, *Medicine* 56:38–54, 1997; Oh MS, Carroll HJ: The anion gap, *N Engl J med* 297:814-817, 1977; Kraut JA, Madisa NE, Serum anion gap: its uses and limitations in clinical medicine, *Clin J Am Soc Nephrol* 2: 162-174, 2007.

BOX 8 Clinical Causes of High Anion Gap and Normal Anion Gap Acidosis

High anion gap
Ketoacidosis
Diabetic ketoacidosis (acetoacetate)
Alcoholic (beta-hydroxybutyrate)
Starvation

Lactic acid acidosis (see Box 9)
L-Lactic acid acidosis (types A and B)
D-Lactic acid acidosis
Renal failure: Sulfate, phosphate, urate, hippurate

Ingestions (toxins and their metabolites)
Ethylene glycol → glycolate, oxalate
Methyl alcohol → formate
Salicylate → ketones, lactate, salicylate
Paraldehyde → organic anions
Toluene → hippurate (commonly presents with normal anion gap)
Propylene glycol → lactate
Pyroglutamic acidosis (acetaminophen use) → 5-oxoproline

Normal anion gap
Gastrointestinal loss of HCO$_3^-$ (negative urine anion gap)
Diarrhea
Fistula, external

Renal loss of HCO$_3^-$ or failure to excrete NH$_4^+$ (positive urine anion gap)
Proximal renal tubular acidosis (RTA type 2)
Acetazolamide
Classic distal renal tubular acidosis (low serum K+) RTA type 1
Generalized distal renal tubular defect (high serum K+) RTA type 4

Miscellaneous
NH4Cl ingestion
Sulfur ingestion
Dilutional acidosis
Late stages in treatment of diabetic ketoacidosis

Adapted in part from DuBose TD Jr: Acid-base disorders. In Brenner BM (ed): *Brenner and Rector's the kidney,* ed 8, Philadelphia, 2008, Saunders, pp. 513-546.

BOX 9   Differential Diagnosis of Hyperchloremic Metabolic Acidosis

Gastrointestinal bicarbonate loss
Diarrhea
External pancreatic or small bowel drainage
Ureterosigmoidostomy, jejunal loop

Drugs
Calcium chloride (acidifying agent)
Magnesium sulfate (diarrhea)
Cholestyramine (bile acid diarrhea)

Renal acidosis
Hypokalemic
Proximal renal tubular acidosis (RTA) (type 2) (see Box 10)
Distal (classic) RTA (type 1)

Drug-induced hypokalemia
Acetazolamide (proximal RTA)
Amphotericin B (distal RTA)

Hyperkalemic
Generalized distal nephron dysfunction (type 4 RTA) (see Box 10)
Mineralocorticoid deficiency or resistance (pseudohypoaldosteronism type 1) PHA-I, PHA-II

↓Na^+ delivery to distal nephron
Tubulointerstitial disease
Ammonium excretion defect

Drug-induced hyperkalemia
Potassium-sparing diuretics (amiloride, triamterene, spironolactone)
Trimethoprim
Pentamidine
Angiotensin-converting enzyme inhibitors and angiotensin II receptor blockers
Nonsteroidal antiinflammatory drugs
Cyclosporine, tacrolimus

Normocalcemic
Early renal insufficiency

Other
Acid loads (ammonium chloride, hyperalimentation)
Loss of potential bicarbonate: Ketosis with ketone excretion
Dilution acidosis (rapid saline administration)
Hippurate
Cation-exchange resins

Adapted in part from DuBose TD Jr: Acid-base disorders. In Brenner BM (ed): *Brenner and Rector's the kidney,* ed 8, Philadelphia, 2008, Saunders, pp. 513-546.

BOX 10   List of Select Disorders Associated with Renal Tubular Acidosis*

Renal defect in net acid excretion, classic distal renal tubular acidosis (type 1 RTA)
Systemic or tubulointerstitial disease
Medullary sponge kidney
Cryoglobulinemia
Balkan nephropathy
Nephrocalcinosis
Chronic pyelonephritis
HIV nephropathy
Renal transplant
Sjögren syndrome
Thyroiditis
Hyperparathyroidism

Drug or toxin induced
Ifosfamide
Amphotericin B
Foscarnet
Toluene
Mercury
Classic analgesic nephropathy

Renal defect in HCO_3^- reclamation, proximal renal tubular acidosis (type 2 RTA)
Selective (unassociated with Fanconi syndrome)
Idiopathic
Carbonic anhydrase deficiency or inhibition
Drugs such as acetazolamide
Carbonic anhydrase II deficiency with osteopetrosis (Sly syndrome)

Generalized (associated with Fanconi syndrome)
Primary: Inherited or sporadic
Genetically transmitted systemic diseases: Cystinosis, Lowe syndrome, Wilson syndrome

Dysproteinemic states
Multiple myeloma
Monoclonal gammopathy

Secondary hyperparathyroidism with chronic hypocalcemia
Vitamin D deficiency or resistance
Vitamin D dependency

Drugs or toxins
Ifosfamide
Lead
Outdated tetracycline
Streptozotocin
Mercury
Amphotericin B (historic)

Tubulointerstitial diseases
Sjögren syndrome
Medullary cystic disease
Renal transplantation

Generalized defect of the distal nephron with hyperkalemia (type 4 RTA)
Mineralocorticoid deficiency
Primary aldosterone deficiency
Adrenal disease (hemorrhage, destruction, infarction)
Heparin (low-molecular-weight or unfractionated)
Persistent hypotension in critically ill patient
Renin–angiotensin system modulating agents (ACEI, ARB)

Secondary aldosterone deficiency (hyporeninemic hypoaldosteronism)
Diabetic nephropathy
HIV disease
Tubulointerstitial nephropathy
NSAID use

Renal tubular dysfunction (voltage defect)
Drugs that interfere with sodium channel or NA^+/K^+-ATPase
Amiloride
Pentamidine
Triamterene
Trimethoprim
Cyclosporine
Tacrolimus

Disorders associated with tubulointerstitial disease
Renal failure
Lupus nephritis
Obstructive uropathy
Renal transplant rejection
Sickle cell disease

*See source for complete list of disorders.
ACEI, angiotensin-converting enzyme inhibitor; *ARB,* angiotensin receptor blocker; *HIV,* human immunodeficiency virus; *NSAID,* nonsteroidal antiinflammatory drugs; *RTA,* renal tubular acidosis.
Adapted in part from DuBose TD Jr: Acid-base disorders. In Brenner BM (ed): *Brenner and Rector's the kidney,* ed 8, Philadelphia, 2008, Saunders, pp. 513-546.

Clinical Algorithms

III

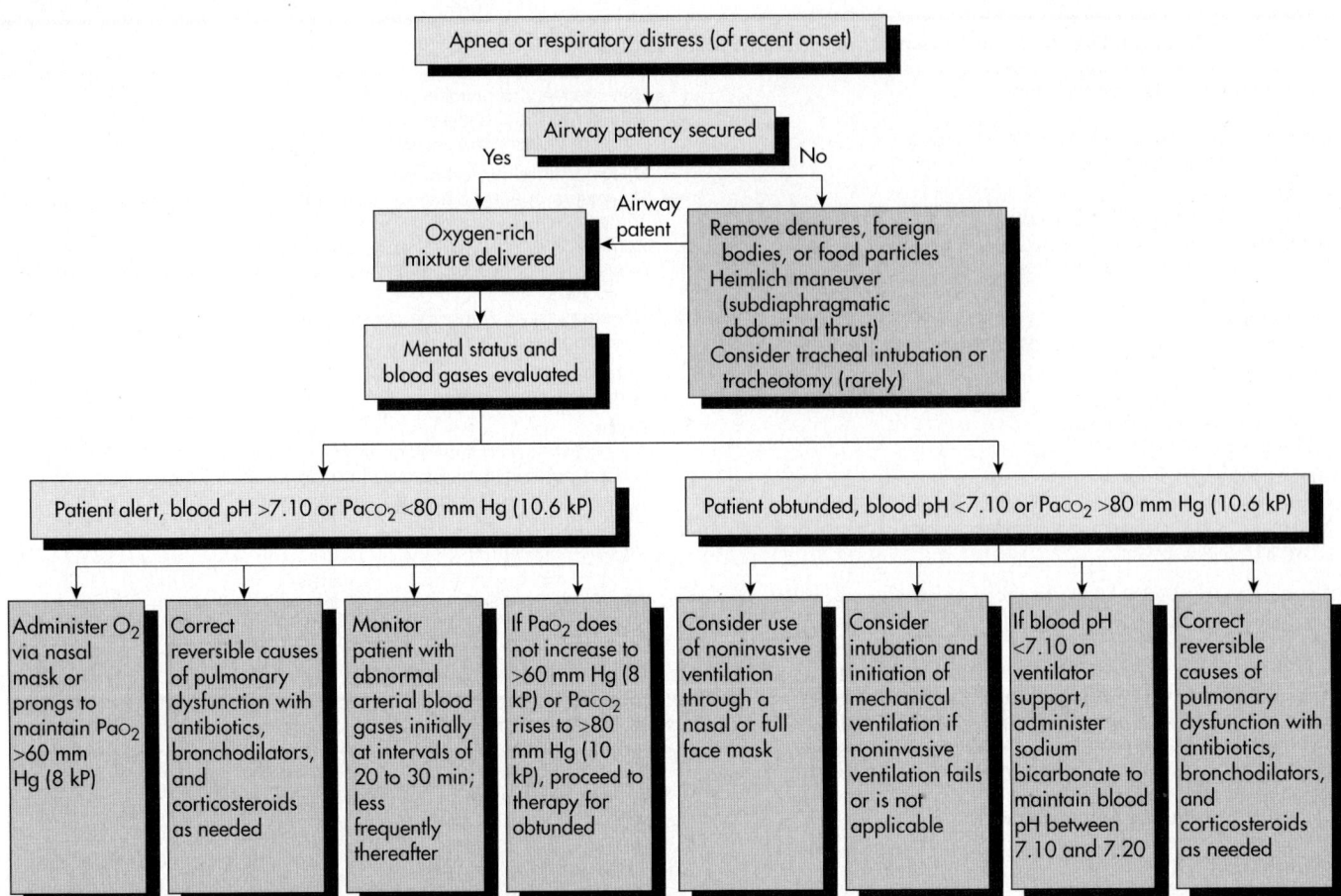

FIG. 15 Algorithm for management of acute respiratory acidosis. *PCO₂*, Partial pressure of carbon dioxide. (From Johnson R et al: *Comprehensive clinical nephrology,* ed 5, Philadelphia, 2015, Saunders.)

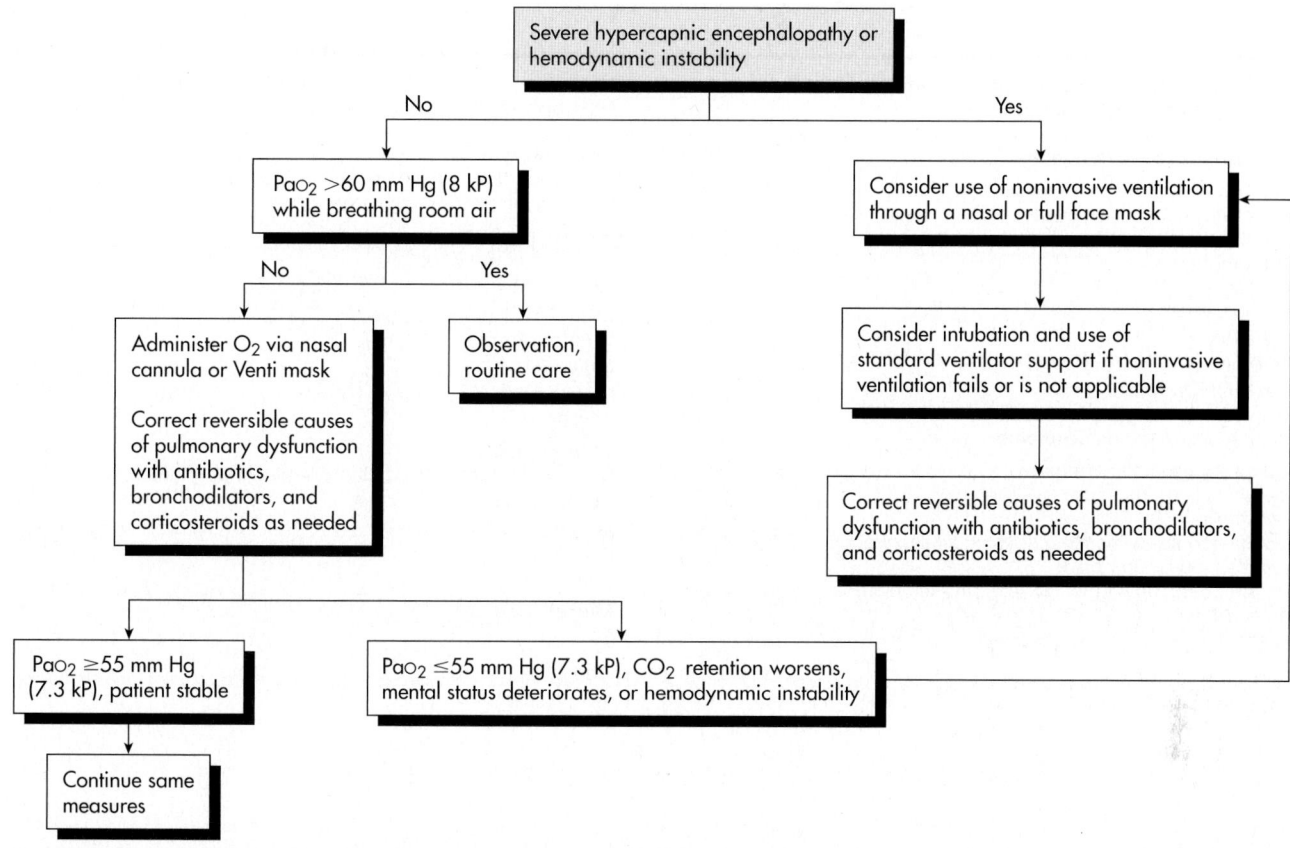

FIG. 16 Algorithm for management of chronic respiratory acidosis. *PaO₂*, Partial pressure of oxygen. (From Johnson R et al: *Comprehensive clinical nephrology,* ed 5, Philadelphia, 2015, Saunders.)

TABLE 15 Causes of Chronic Alveolar Hypoventilation/Respiratory Acidosis

	Site of Defect	Condition
Defects in respiratory drive	Central and peripheral chemoreceptors	Brainstem lesions Primary alveolar hypoventilation syndrome (Ondine curse), extreme obesity (Pickwickian syndrome) Spinal cord lesions
Neuromuscular defects	*Neuromuscular*	*Motor neuron disease:* Critical illness polyneuropathy, multiple sclerosis, amyotrophic lateral sclerosis
	Muscular disease	Myasthenia gravis, critical illness myopathy
Defects in respiratory mechanics and gas exchange	*Lung*	*Increased dead space:* Chronic obstructive pulmonary disease, chronic pulmonary embolism *Increased lung elastance:* Pulmonary fibrosis *Increased chest wall elastance:* Extreme obesity, fibrothorax, kyphoscoliosis *Increased respiratory resistance:* Airway stenosis, chronic obstructive pulmonary disease

From Ronco C: *Critical care nephrology,* ed 3, Philadelphia, 2019, Elsevier.

Clinical Algorithms

III

BOX 11 Causes of Respiratory Acidosis Based on Pathophysiologic Mechanism

Respiratory disease (lungs and airways)

Airway obstruction

Obstructive pulmonary diseases (e.g., chronic obstructive pulmonary disease)

Pneumothorax

Pulmonary effusion

Pulmonary edema

Pneumonia

Mechanical ventilation (iatrogenic hypoventilation)

Chest wall disease

Chest wall trauma (e.g., flail chest)

Obesity hypoventilation syndrome

Respiratory muscle weakness

Myopathies (e.g., muscular dystrophy)

Neuropathies (e.g., Guillain-Barré)

Electrolyte abnormalities (e.g., hypokalemia, hypophosphatemia)

Decreased respiratory drive

Brain space-occupying lesion (e.g., intracranial mass, intracranial hemorrhage)

Drugs/toxins (e.g., sedative-hypnotics, narcotics)

From Walls RM et al: *Rosen's emergency medicine, concepts and clinical practice,* ed 10, Philadelphia, 2023, Elsevier.

BOX 12 Causes of Respiratory Alkalosis Based on Pathophysiologic Mechanism

Respiratory

Conditions that cause hypoxemia (e.g., pulmonary embolus)

Mechanical ventilation (iatrogenic hyperventilation)

Gastrointestinal

Hepatic encephalopathy

Neurologic

Brain lesion

Genitourinary

Pregnancy

Psychiatric

Anxiety

Toxic-metabolic

Drugs (e.g., salicylates, catecholamines, progesterone)

Hyperthyroidism

Infectious

Fever

Sepsis

Miscellaneous

Pain

From Walls RM et al: *Rosen's emergency medicine, concepts and clinical practice,* ed 10, Philadelphia, 2023, Elsevier.

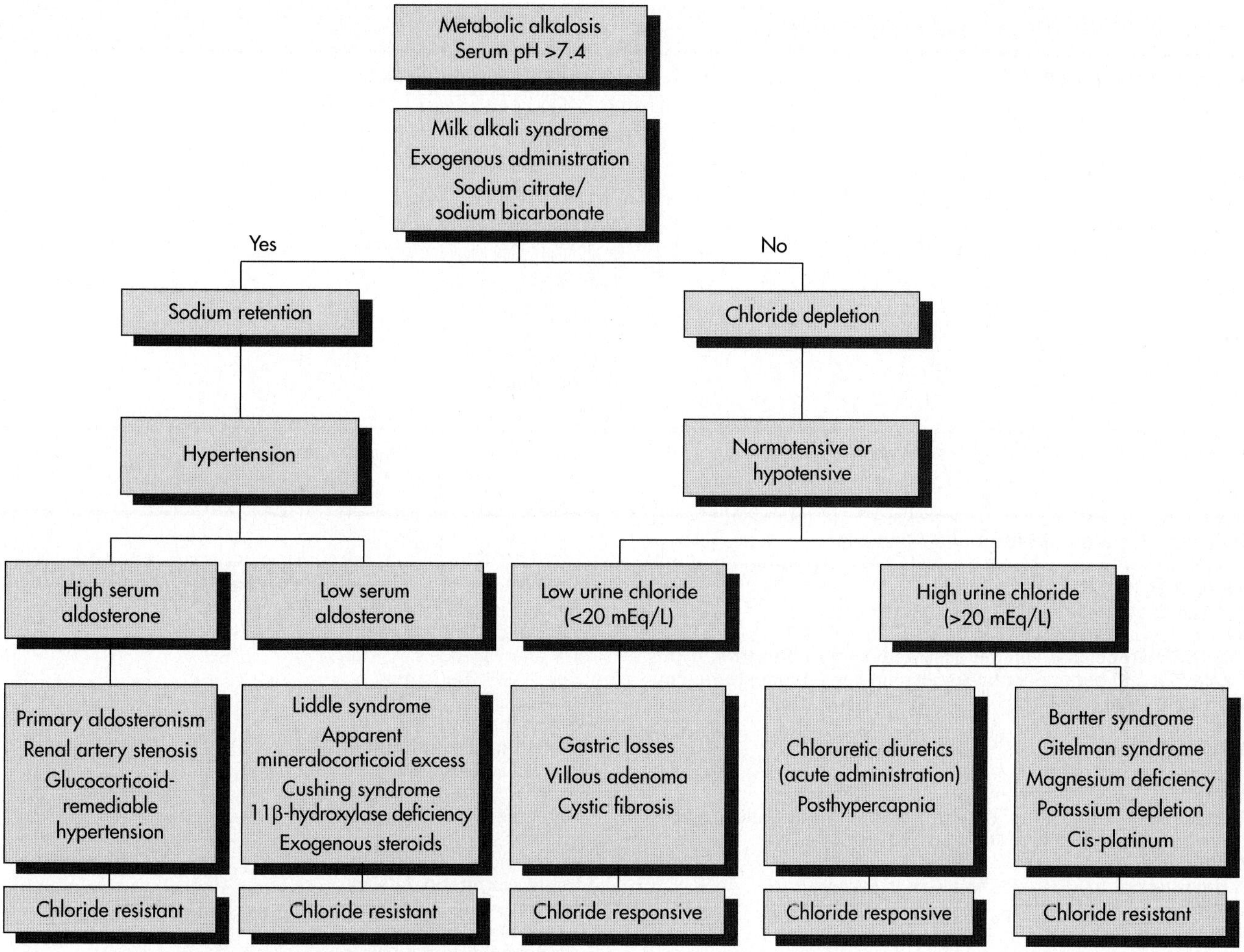

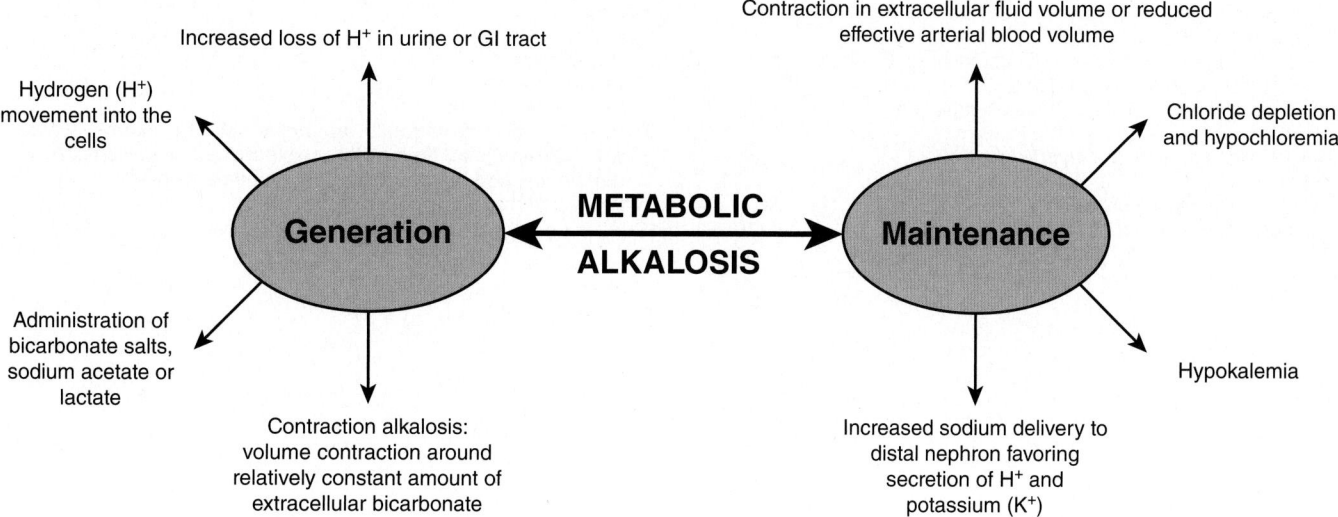

FIG. 19 Differential diagnosis of metabolic alkalosis. (From Ronco C: *Critical care nephrology,* ed 3, Philadelphia, 2019, Elsevier.)

FIG. 20 Pathogenesis and maintenance of metabolic alkalosis. (From Vincent JL et al: *Textbook of critical care,* ed 8, Philadelphia, 2024, Elsevier.)

TABLE 16 Diagnosis of Metabolic Alkalosis

Saline-Responsive Alkalosis	Saline-Unresponsive Alkalosis
Low urinary [Cl⁻]	High or normal urinary [Cl⁻]
Normotensive	Hypertensive
Vomiting, nasogastric aspiration	Primary aldosteronism
Diuretics	Cushing syndrome
Posthypercapnia	Renal artery stenosis
Bicarbonate therapy of organic acidosis	Renal failure plus alkali therapy
K⁺ deficiency	Normotensive
Hypertensive	Mg²⁺ deficiency
Liddle syndrome	Severe K⁺ deficiency
	Bartter syndrome
	Gitelman syndrome
	Diuretics

From Vincent JL et al: *Textbook of critical care,* ed 8, Philadelphia, 2024, Elsevier.

BOX 13 Causes of Metabolic Alkalosis

Exogenous HCO_3^- loads
Acute alkali administration
Milk-alkali syndrome
Effective extracellular volume contraction, normotension, hypokalemia, and secondary hyperreninemic hyperaldosteronism
Gastrointestinal origin
Vomiting
Gastric aspiration
Congenital chloridorrhea
Villous adenoma
Combined administration of sodium polystyrene sulfonate (Kayexalate and aluminum hydroxide)
Renal origin
Diuretics (especially thiazides and loop diuretics)
Acute
Chronic
Edematous states
Posthypercapnic state
Hypercalcemia-hypoparathyroidism
Recovery from lactic acidosis or ketoacidosis
Nonreabsorbable anions such as penicillin, carbenicillin
Mg^{2+} deficiency
K^+ depletion
Bartter syndrome (loss-of-function mutation of Cl⁻ transport in thick ascending limb of loop of Henle)
Gitelman syndrome (loss-of-function mutation in Na⁺/Cl⁻ cotransporter)
Carbohydrate refeeding after starvation
Other
Sweat loss in cystic fibrosis
Loss of fluid in third space

Extracellular volume expansion, hypertension, K^+ deficiency, and hypermineralocorticoidism
Associated with high renin
Renal artery stenosis
Accelerated hypertension
Renin-secreting tumor
Estrogen therapy
Associated with low renin
Primary aldosteronism
Adenoma
Hyperplasia
Carcinoma
Glucocorticoid suppressible
Adrenal enzymatic defects
11β-Hydroxylase deficiency
17α-Hydroxylase deficiency
Cushing syndrome or disease
Ectopic corticotropin
Adrenal carcinoma
Adrenal adenoma
Primary pituitary
Other
Licorice
Carbenoxolone
Chewing tobacco
Lydia Pinkham tablets
Gain-of-function mutation of epithelial sodium channel (ENaC) with extracellular fluid volume expansion, hypertension, K^+ deficiency, and hyporeninemic hypoaldosteronism
Liddle syndrome

From Vincent JL et al: *Textbook of critical care,* ed 8, Philadelphia, 2024, Elsevier.

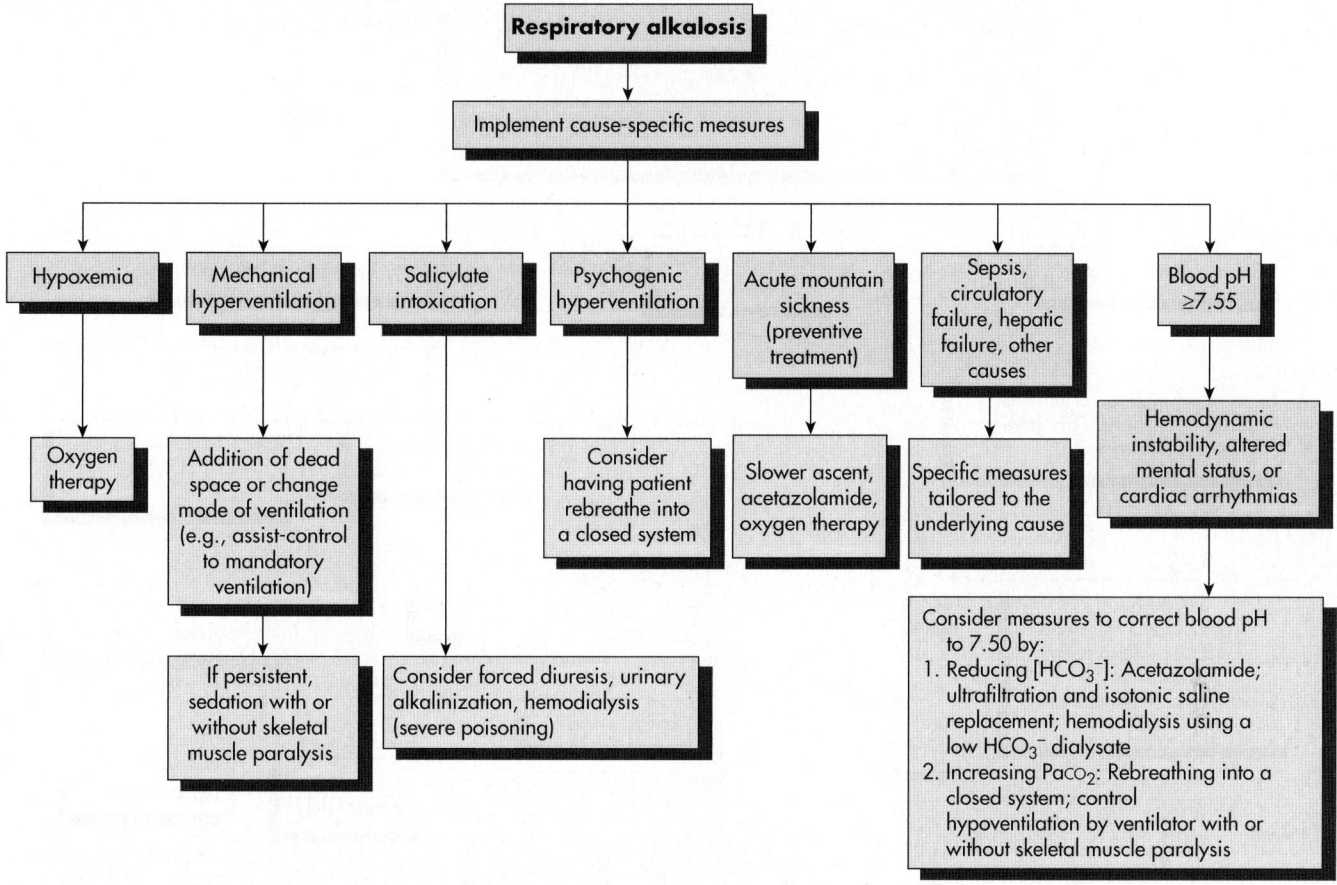

FIG. 21 Recommended treatment of respiratory alkalosis. *PCO₂*, Partial pressure of carbon dioxide. (From Johnson R et al: *Comprehensive clinical nephrology,* ed 5, Philadelphia, 2015, Saunders.)

TABLE 17　Causes of Alveolar Hyperventilation/Respiratory Alkalosis

	Site of Defect	Condition
Defects in respiratory drive	*Central chemoreceptors*	*Voluntary hyperventilation psychogenic:* Pain, panic attack
		Central neurogenic hyperventilation: Brainstem injuries, brain tumors
		Hormonal: Increased progesterone levels in pregnancy and liver cirrhosis
		Infectious: Meningitis, encephalitis
		Thermal hyperpnea: Fever, hyperthermia
		Intoxication: Salicylate, topiramate
		Therapeutic: Doxapram
	Peripheral chemoreceptors	*Increased activity of peripheral chemoreceptors:* Hypoxic pulmonary disease, high altitude
		Increased activity of lung receptors, e.g., pulmonary edema, pneumonia, pulmonary embolism, interstitial fibrosis
Iatrogenic		*Mechanical ventilation:* Excessive mechanical ventilation (accidental, or therapeutic for traumatic brain injury)
		Extracorporeal gas exchange: Excessive extracorporeal CO₂ removal

From Ronco C: *Critical care nephrology,* ed 3, Philadelphia, 2019, Elsevier.

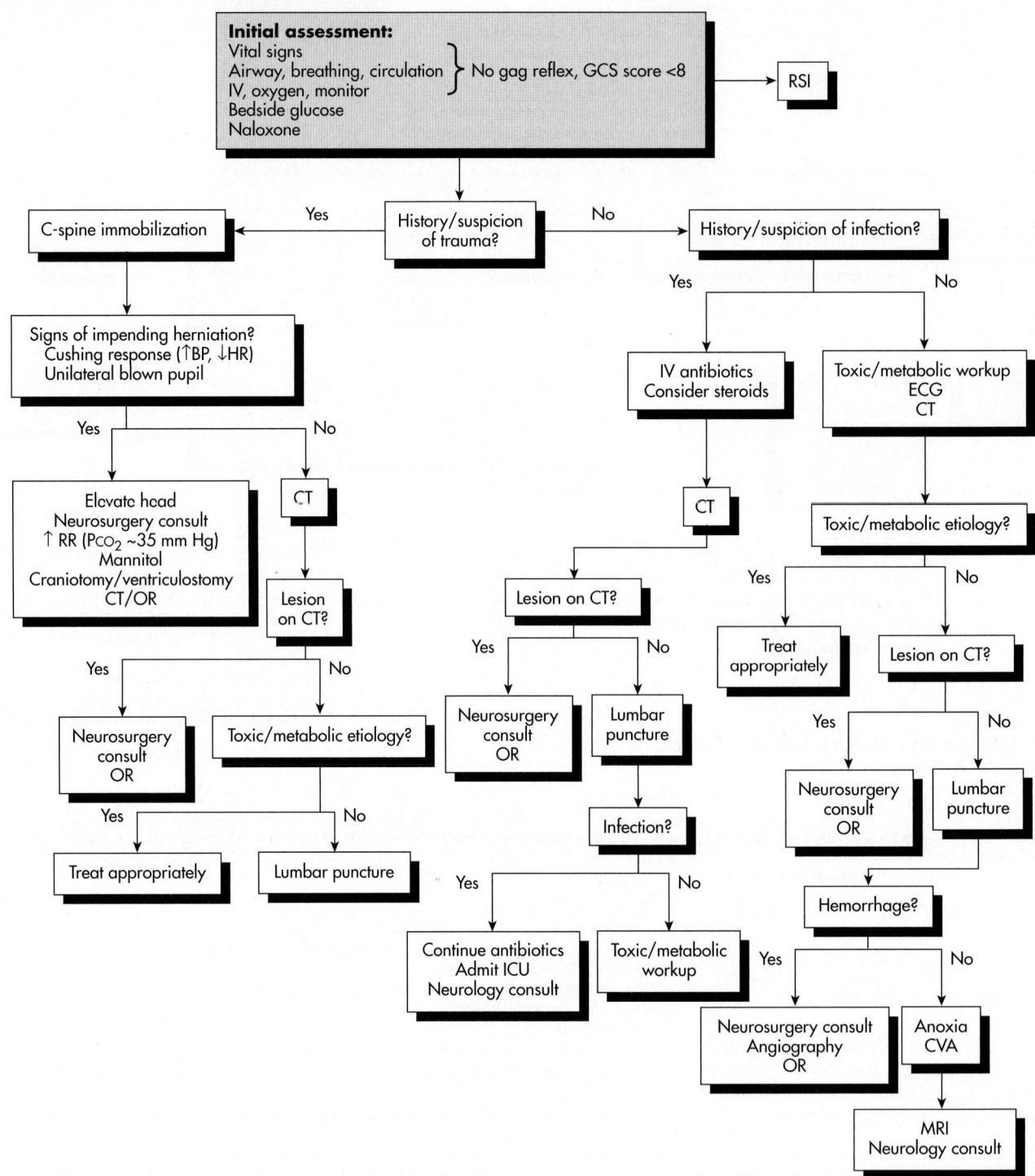

FIG. 23 Diagnostic approach to altered mental status and coma. *BP,* Blood pressure; *C-spine,* cervical spine; *CT,* computed tomography; *CVA,* cerebrovascular accident; *ECG,* electrocardiography; *GCS,* Glasgow Coma Scale; *HR,* heart rate; *ICU,* intensive care unit; *IV,* intravenous; *MRI,* magnetic resonance imaging; *OR,* operating room; *PCO₂,* Partial pressure of carbon dioxide; *RR,* respiratory rate; *RSI,* rapid-sequence intubation. (From Adams JG et al: *Emergency medicine, clinical essentials,* ed 2, Philadelphia, 2013, Elsevier.)

Hb below expected and/or falling over time
- Female: Black Hb <11.5g/dl, white <12.2 g/dl
- Males: Black Hb <12.7g/dl, white <13.2g/dl

Review patient history
- Signs and symptoms and risk factors, attention to iron deficiency (blood thinners or bleeding)

Review prior hematologic laboratories
- Assess available past hemoglobin values

Routine laboratory tests
- Complete blood count, white blood cell differential, RBC indices
- Iron studies: Serum ferritin, serum iron, total iron binding capacity, transferrin saturation
- Vitamin B_{12}
- Serum creatinine for estimated GFR
- C-reactive protein
- Reticulocyte count
- Thyroid stimulating hormone
- RBC or serum folate (only when specific risk factors)

Diagnostic considerations of common anemias in older adults   **Treatment considerations**

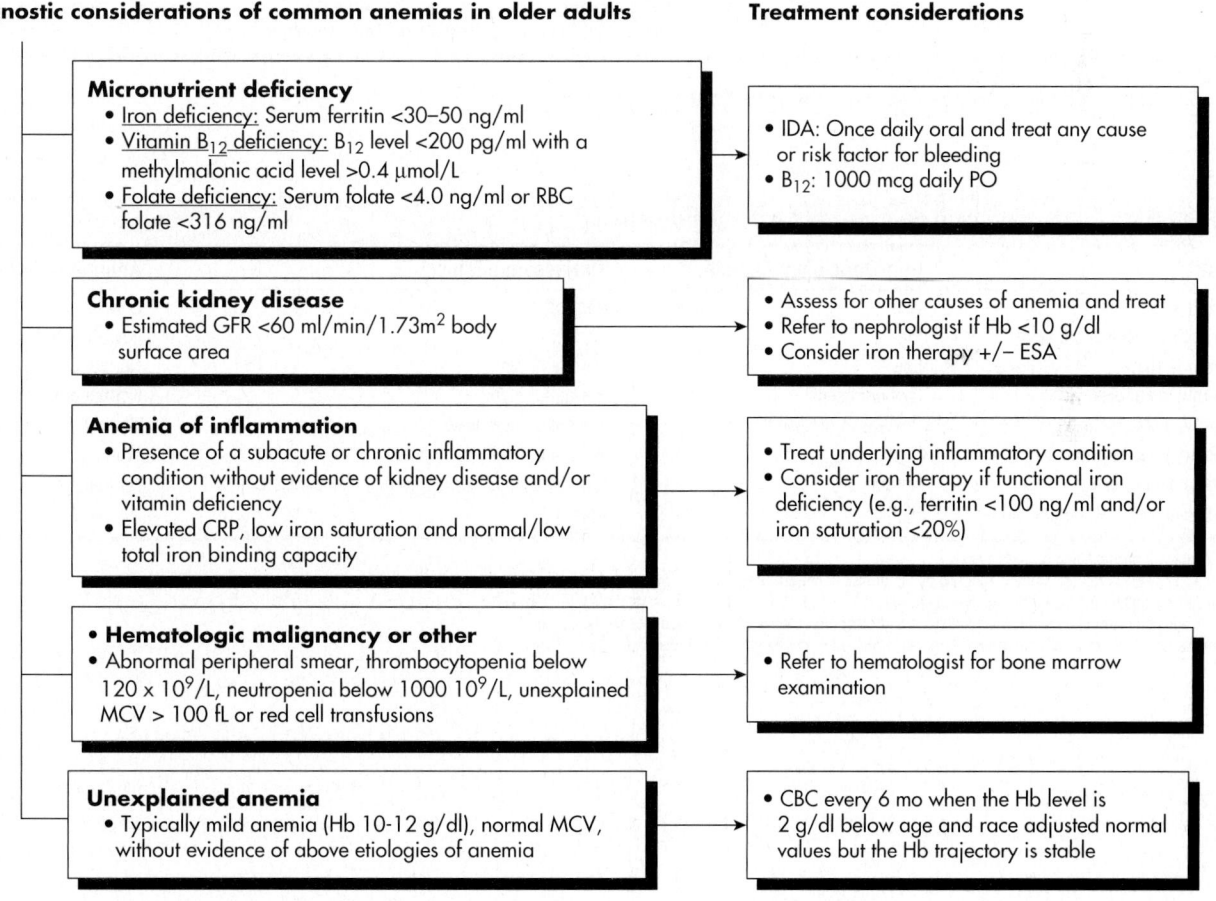

Micronutrient deficiency
- Iron deficiency: Serum ferritin <30–50 ng/ml
- Vitamin B_{12} deficiency: B_{12} level <200 pg/ml with a methylmalonic acid level >0.4 μmol/L
- Folate deficiency: Serum folate <4.0 ng/ml or RBC folate <316 ng/ml

- IDA: Once daily oral and treat any cause or risk factor for bleeding
- B_{12}: 1000 mcg daily PO

Chronic kidney disease
- Estimated GFR <60 ml/min/1.73m² body surface area

- Assess for other causes of anemia and treat
- Refer to nephrologist if Hb <10 g/dl
- Consider iron therapy +/− ESA

Anemia of inflammation
- Presence of a subacute or chronic inflammatory condition without evidence of kidney disease and/or vitamin deficiency
- Elevated CRP, low iron saturation and normal/low total iron binding capacity

- Treat underlying inflammatory condition
- Consider iron therapy if functional iron deficiency (e.g., ferritin <100 ng/ml and/or iron saturation <20%)

- **Hematologic malignancy or other**
- Abnormal peripheral smear, thrombocytopenia below 120 x 10⁹/L, neutropenia below 1000 10⁹/L, unexplained MCV > 100 fL or red cell transfusions

- Refer to hematologist for bone marrow examination

Unexplained anemia
- Typically mild anemia (Hb 10-12 g/dl), normal MCV, without evidence of above etiologies of anemia

- CBC every 6 mo when the Hb level is 2 g/dl below age and race adjusted normal values but the Hb trajectory is stable

FIG. 29 Workup of older adult presenting with anemia. *CRP,* C-Reactive protein; *ESA,* erythropoietin stimulating agents; *GFR,* glomerular filtration rate; *Hb,* hemoglobin; *IDA,* iron deficiency anemia; *MCV,* mean corpuscular volume; *PO,* by mouth (per os); *RBC,* red blood cell count. (From Warshaw G et al: *Ham's primary care geriatrics,* ed 7, Philadelphia, 2022, Elsevier.)

Clinical
Algorithms

III

TABLE 19 Anemia Workup

	Parameters	Interpretation
History	Diet (meat and green vegetables)	Risk of malnutrition if lacking: Suggests susceptibility to iron and folic acid deficiency
	Blood loss	Obvious gastrointestinal bleeding
		Chronic subclinical blood loss (e.g., NSAIDs, colon polyps, hereditary telangiectasias, menorrhagia)
	Gastrointestinal surgery	Gastrectomy or ileal resection: Vitamin B_{12} deficiency
		Small bowel resections: Iron, folate deficiency
	Comorbidity	Chronic infections and inflammatory disorders suggest risk of anemia of chronic disease
Examination	Pallor	Severity of anemia
	Icterus	May suggest hemolysis
	Lymphadenopathy, hepatomegaly, splenomegaly, bone tenderness	Coexistence of another primary hematologic disorder
	Evidence of portal hypertension	Hypersplenism and potential for variceal bleed
Red cell size and hemoglobinization	Microcytic hypochromic	Iron deficiency
		Thalassemia
		Anemia of chronic disease
		Sideroblastic anemia
	Normocytic	Acute bleeding
		Bone marrow infiltration
		Aplastic anemia
		Renal failure
	Macrocytic	Vitamin B_{12}/folate deficiencies
		Myelodysplasia
		Medication effects
		Other medical conditions: Hypothyroidism, liver impairment

NSAIDs, Nonsteroidal antiinflammatory drugs.
From Talley NJ et al: *Essentials of internal medicine,* ed 4, Chatswood, NSW, 2021, Elsevier Australia.

TABLE 20 Differentiating Features of Microcytic Anemias*

Test	Iron-Deficiency Anemia	Thalassemia Minor[†]	Anemia of Inflammation[‡]
Serum iron	Low	Normal	Low
Serum iron-binding capacity	High	Normal	Low or normal
Serum ferritin	Low	Normal or high	Normal or high
Marrow iron stores	Low or absent	Normal or high	Normal or high
Marrow sideroblasts	Decreased or absent	Normal or increased	Normal or increased
Free erythrocyte protoporphyrin	High	Normal or slightly increased	High
Hemoglobin A_2 or F	Normal	High beta-thalassemia; normal alpha-thalassemia	Normal
Red blood cell distribution width[§]	High	Normal	Normal/↑

*See Table 22 for definition of microcytosis.
[†]Alpha-thalassemia minor can be diagnosed by the presence of Bart hemoglobin on newborn screening.
[‡]Usually normochromic; 25% of cases are microcytic.
[§]Red blood cell distribution width quantitates the degree of anisocytosis (different sizes) of red blood cells.
From Marcdante KJ et al: *Nelson essentials of pediatrics,* ed 9, Philadelphia, 2023, Elsevier.

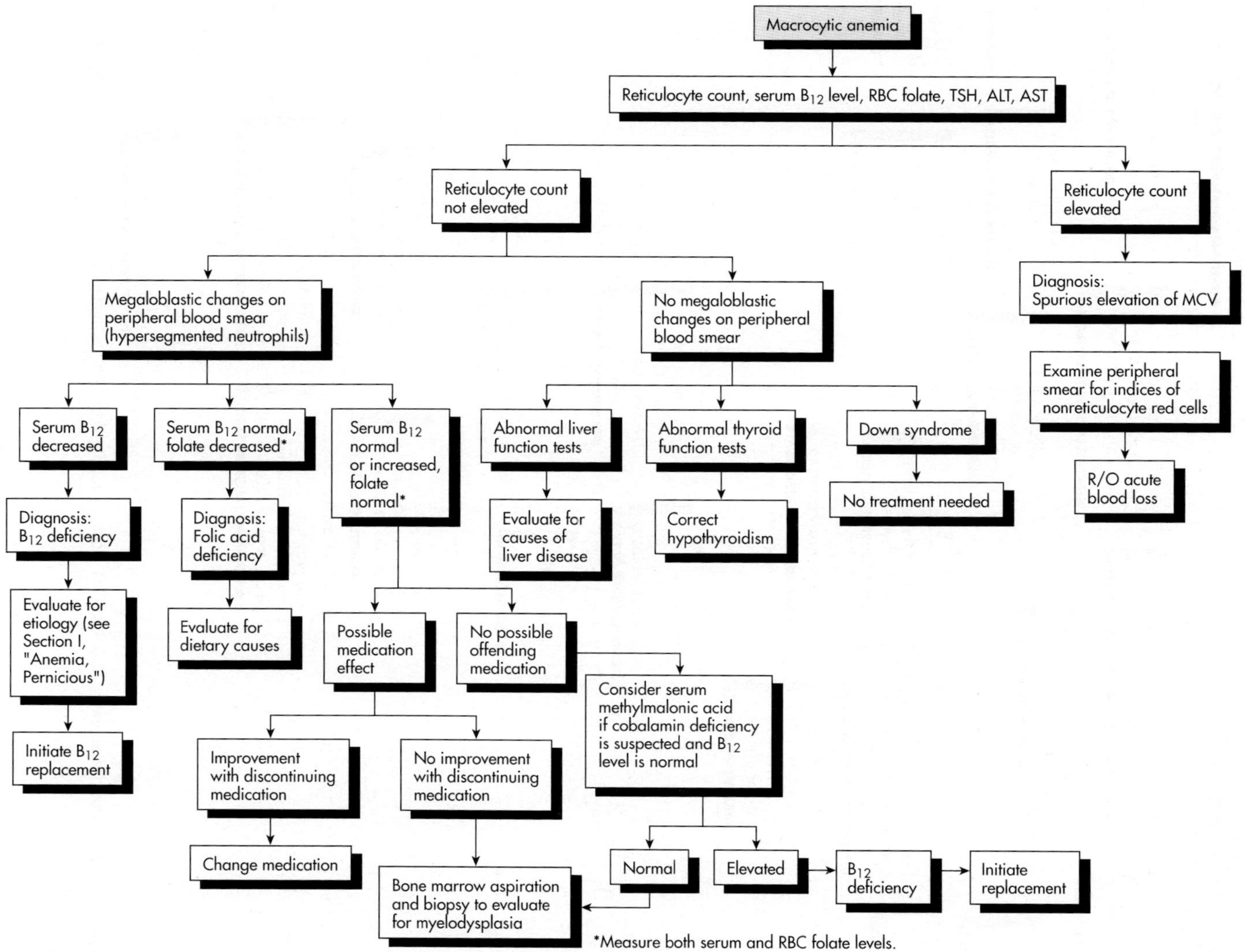

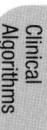

FIG. 30 Differential diagnosis of macrocytic anemia. *ALT,* Alanine transaminase; *AST,* aspartate aminotransferase; *MCV,* mean corpuscular volume; *RBC,* red blood cell; *R/O,* rule out; *TSH,* thyroid-stimulating hormone. (Modified and updated from Rakel RE [ed]: *Principles of family practice,* ed 7, Philadelphia, 2007, Saunders.)

Clinical
Algorithms

III

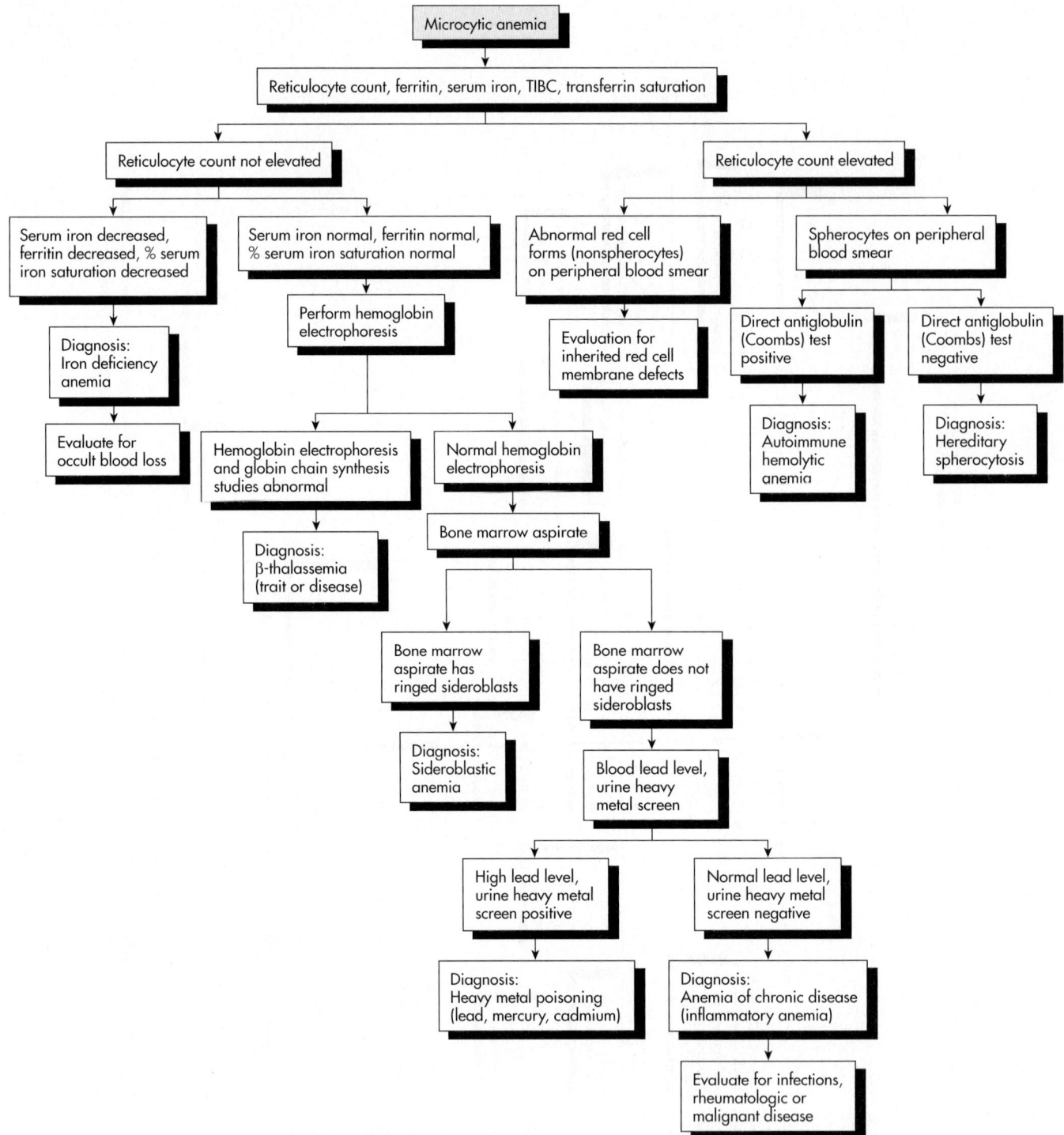

FIG. 31 Differential diagnosis of microcytic anemia. *TIBC*, Total iron binding capacity. (Modified and updated from Rakel RE [ed]: *Principles of family practice,* ed 7, Philadelphia, 2007, Saunders.)

TABLE 21   Differential Diagnosis of Microcytic Hypochromic Anemia

Parameter	Iron-Deficiency Anemia	Anemia of Chronic Disease (Anemia of Inflammation)	Thalassemias	Sideroblastic Anemia
MCV	↓	↓ / N	↓	↓ / N
Serum iron	↓	↓	N	↑
Transferrin saturation	↓	↓ / N	N	↑
TIBC	↓	↓ / N	N	N
Serum transferrin receptor	↑	↓	N	N / ↑
Serum ferritin	↓	↑/ N	N	↑
Serum hepcidin	↓	↑	N / ↓	↓
Bone marrow iron stores	↓	↑/ N	↑/ N	↑/ N Ring sideroblasts

MCV, Mean corpuscular volume; *N,* normal; *TIBC,* total iron-binding capacity.
Talley NJ et al: *Essentials of internal medicine,* ed 4, Chatswood, NSW, 2021, Elsevier Australia.

TABLE 22   Stages in the Development of Iron Deficiency Anemia

Hemoglobin (g/dL)	Peripheral Smear	Serum Iron (μg/dl)	Bone Marrow Iron	Serum Ferritin (ng/ml)
13+ (normal)	nc/nc	50-150	Fe^{2+}	*Male:* 40-340 *Female:* 40-150
10-12	nc/nc	↓	Fe^{2+} absent, erythroid hyperplasia	<12
8-10	hypo/nc	↓	Fe^{2+} absent, erythroid hyperplasia	<12
<8	hypo/micro*	↓	Fe^{2+} absent, erythroid hyperplasia	<12

Hypo/micro, Hypochromic, microcytic; *hypo/nc,* hypochromic, normocytic; *nc/nc,* normochromic, normocytic.
*Microcytosis, determined by a mean corpuscular volume (in fL) <2 standard deviations (SD) below the mean, must be adjusted for age (e.g., −2 SD at 3-6 mo = 74; at 0.5-2 yr = 70; at 2-6 yr = 75; at 6-12 yr = 77; and at 12-18 yr = 78).
From Andreoli TE et al: *Cecil essentials of medicine,* ed 4, Philadelphia, 1997, Saunders.

BOX 16   Causes of Iron Deficiency

Inadequate Intake
- Veganism, dietary choices

Inadequate Absorption
- High gastric pH or antacid therapy
- Excess tannins and phytates in diet
- Bowel resection
- Celiac disease
- Inflammatory bowel disease

Increased Physiologic Requirement
- Pregnancy and breastfeeding
- Infancy, puberty

Increased Loss
- Gastrointestinal blood loss
- Genitourinary blood loss
- Menorrhagia
- Operative blood loss
- Parasitosis
- Trauma
- Excessive phlebotomy

From Talley NJ et al: *Essentials of internal medicine,* ed 4, Chatswood, NSW, 2021, Elsevier Australia.

Clinical
Algorithms

III

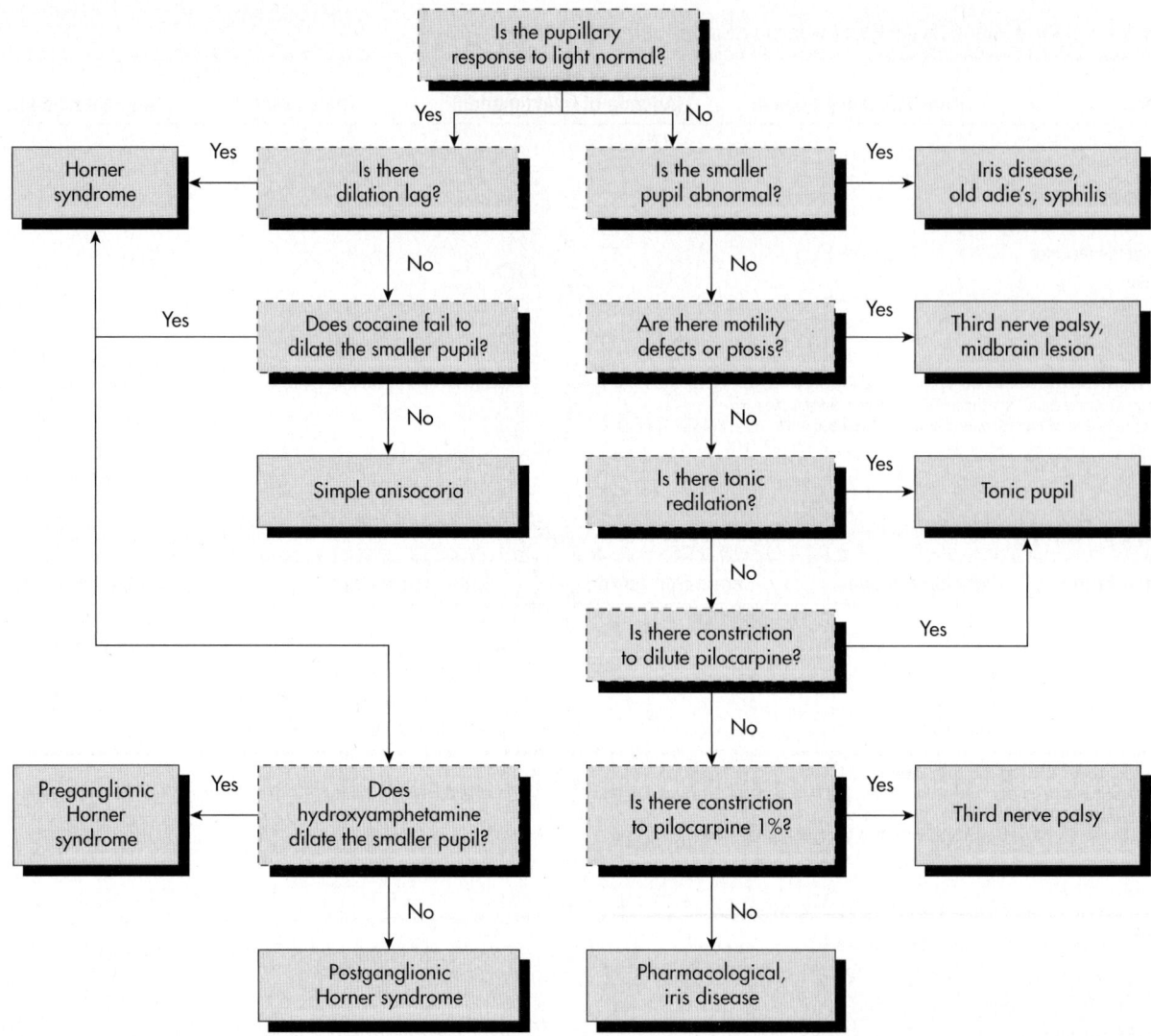

FIG. 32 Flowchart with systematic guidelines for evaluation of anisocoria. (From Jankovic J et al: *Bradley and Daroff's neurology in clinical practice,* ed 8, Philadelphia, 2022, Elsevier.)

TABLE 23 Diagnostic Pupillary Eyedrop Testing

Testing	Mechanism of Action	Diagnostic Utility and Expected Response
Anisocoria Greater in the Light (Abnormal Larger Pupil)		
Dilute pilocarpine (0.0625% or 0.1%)	Parasympathomimetic; direct sphincter stimulation	Tonic pupil will constrict and pupil affected by oculomotor palsy may constrict (denervation supersensitivity)
		Normal pupil and pupil affected by pharmacologic blockade will not respond
Pilocarpine (1%)	Parasympathomimetic; direct sphincter stimulation	Normal pupil and pupil affected by oculomotor palsy will constrict fully
		Pupil affected by pharmacologic blockade will not or only partially respond
Anisocoria Greater in the Dark (Abnormal Smaller Pupil)		
Cocaine (2%-10%)	Inhibits norepinephrine reuptake at the sympathetic terminus	Horner pupil will not dilate
		Normal pupil will dilate
Hydroxyamphetamine (1%)	Induces third-order sympathetic neuron to release any stored norepinephrine	Preganglionic (first- or second-order neuron) Horner pupil will dilate
		Postganglionic (third-order neuron) Horner pupil will not dilate
Apraclonidine (0.5%)	Weak sympathetic agonist	Horner pupil will dilate (denervation supersensitivity)
		Normal pupil will not change or will constrict slightly

From Jankovic J et al: *Bradley and Daroff's neurology in clinical practice,* ed 8, Philadelphia, 2022, Elsevier.

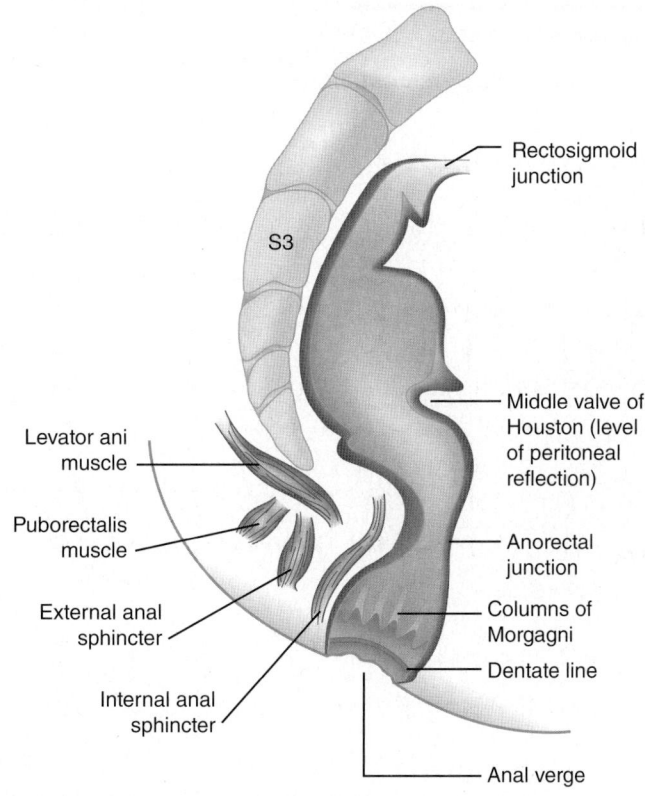

FIG. 34 Anorectal anatomy. (From Walls RM et al: *Rosen's emergency medicine, concepts and clinical practice,* ed 10, Philadelphia, 2023, Elsevier.)

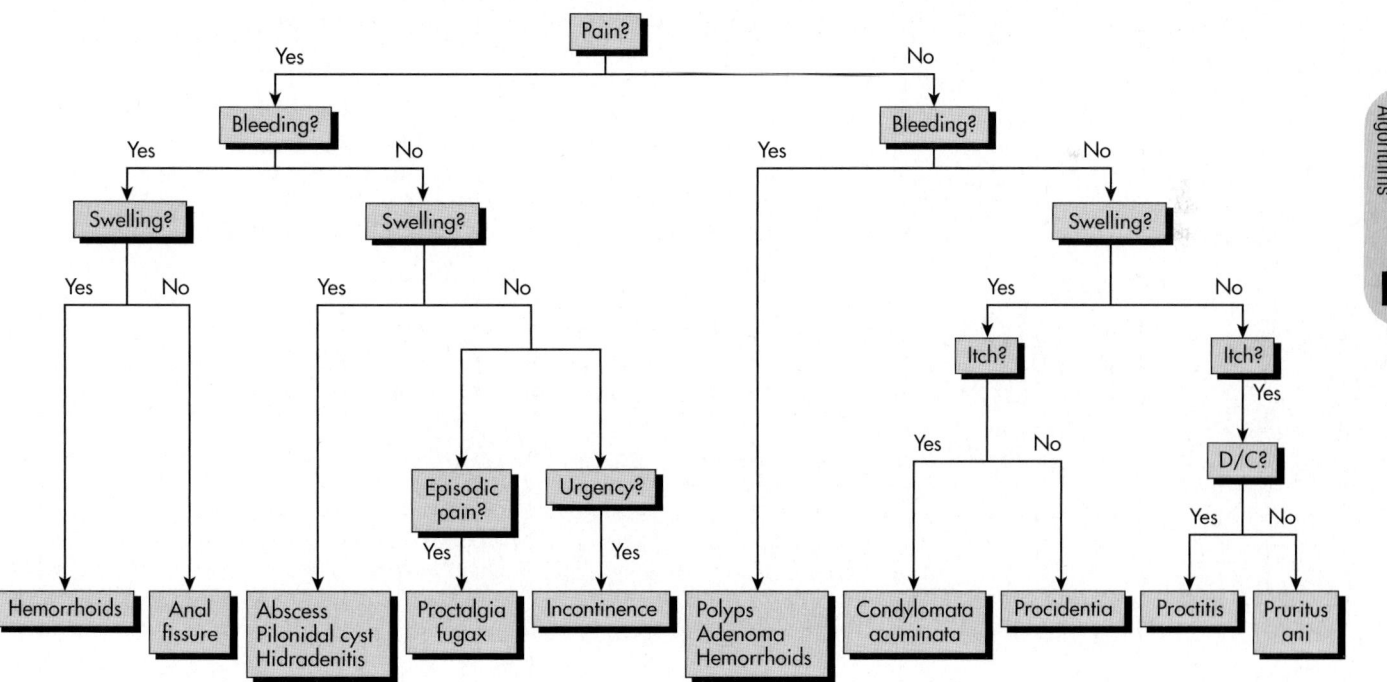

FIG. 35 Algorithm for anorectal complaints. *D/C,* Discharge. (From Walls RM et al: *Rosen's emergency medicine, concepts and clinical practice,* ed 10, Philadelphia, 2023, Elsevier.)

Clinical
Algorithms

III

BOX 17   Medical History in Diagnosis of Anorectal Disorders

Anorectal History
Pain
Bleeding
Swelling
Itching
Discharge
Urgency

Gastrointestinal History
Change in bowel habits (straining, flatus, color, consistency, frequency)
Nausea or vomiting
Incontinence of stool
Underlying GI disease (Crohn disease, cancer, polyps)

Systemic Disease History
Diabetes mellitus
Coagulopathy
Cancer
HIV infection

Sexual History of the Anus
Penetration
Known STDs
Assault

GI, Gastrointestinal; *HIV,* human immunodeficiency virus; *STD,* sexually transmitted disease.
From Walls RM et al: *Rosen's emergency medicine, concepts and clinical practice,* ed 10, Philadelphia, 2023, Elsevier.

ICD-10CM # M54.5   Low back pain
            L29   Pruritus
            M54.89   Other dorsalgia
            M54.9   Dorsalgia, unspecified
            F45.42   Pain disorder with related psychological factors
            M54.08   Panniculitis affecting regions of neck and back, sacral
                     and sacrococcygeal region
            S23.9XXA Sprain of unspecified parts of thorax, initial encounter
            M43.27   Fusion of spine, lumbosacral region
            M43.28   Fusion of spine, sacral and sacrococcygeal region
            M53.2X7 Spinal instabilities, lumbosacral region
            M53.3   Sacrococcygeal disorders, not elsewhere classified

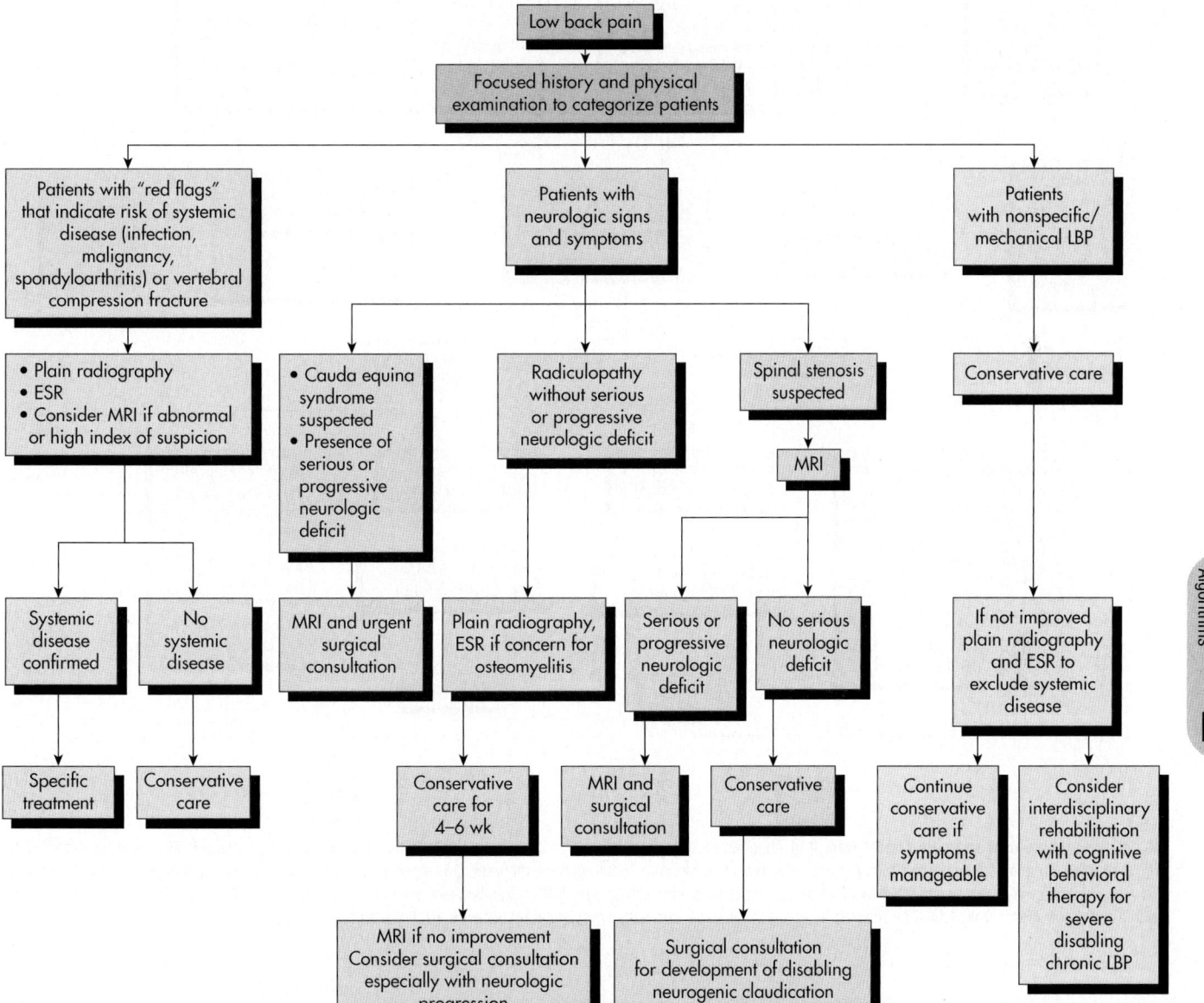

FIG. 38 Algorithm for the differential diagnosis and treatment of low back pain. *ESR,* Erythrocyte sedimentation rate; *LBP,* low back pain; *MRI,* magnetic resonance imaging. (From Firestein GS et al: *Firestein & Kelley's textbook of rheumatology,* ed 11, Philadelphia, 2021, Elsevier.)

Clinical Algorithms

III

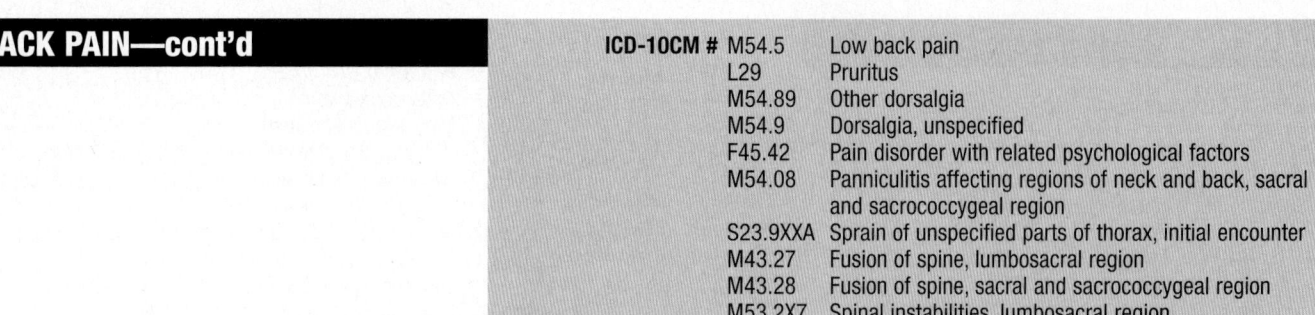

ICD-10CM #	M54.5	Low back pain
	L29	Pruritus
	M54.89	Other dorsalgia
	M54.9	Dorsalgia, unspecified
	F45.42	Pain disorder with related psychological factors
	M54.08	Panniculitis affecting regions of neck and back, sacral and sacrococcygeal region
	S23.9XXA	Sprain of unspecified parts of thorax, initial encounter
	M43.27	Fusion of spine, lumbosacral region
	M43.28	Fusion of spine, sacral and sacrococcygeal region
	M53.2X7	Spinal instabilities, lumbosacral region
	M53.3	Sacrococcygeal disorders, not elsewhere classified

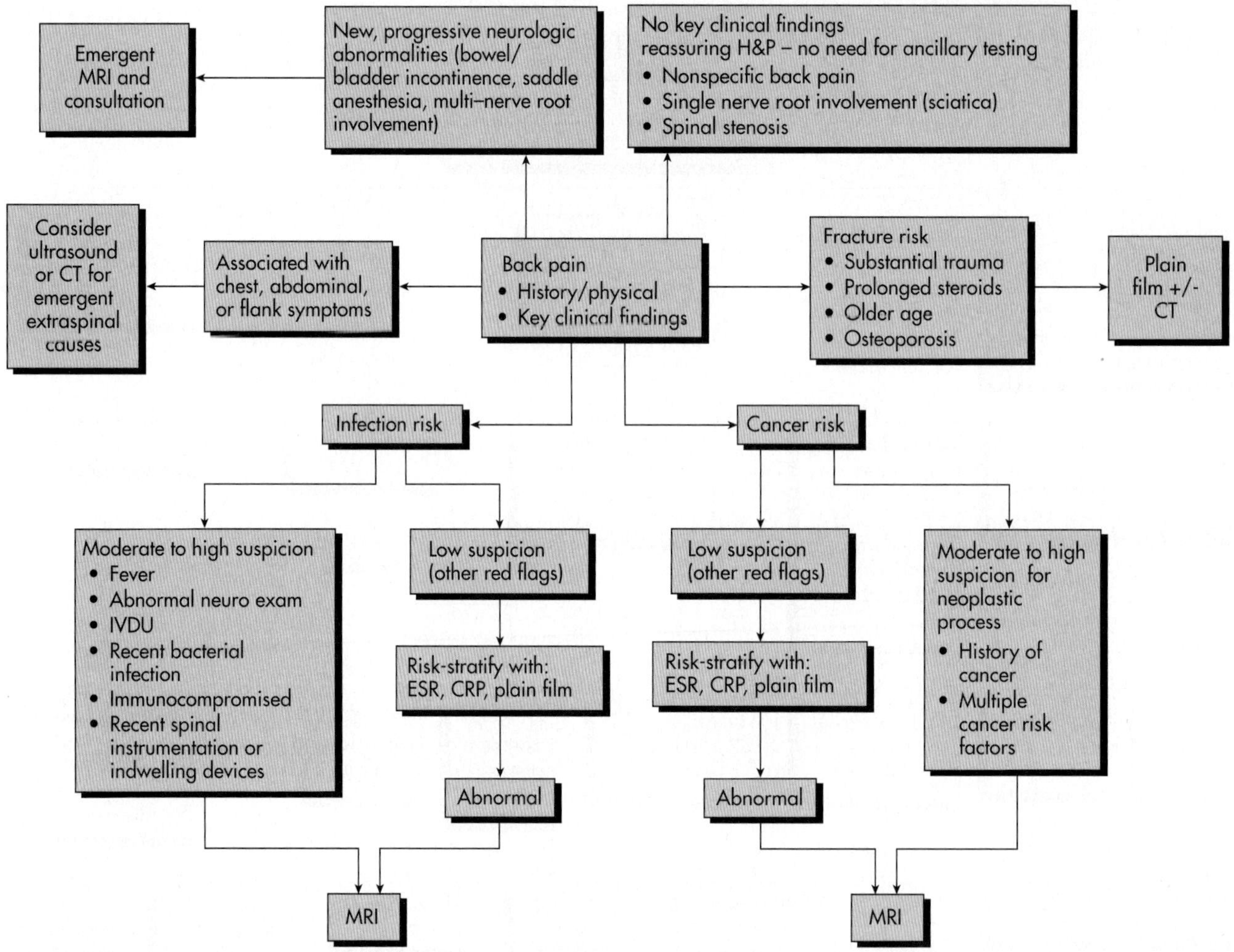

FIG. 39 Management of acute low back pain. *AAA,* Abdominal aortic aneurysm; *ADLs,* activities of daily living; *ASAP,* as soon as possible; *CBC,* complete blood count; *CRP,* C-reactive protein; *CT,* computed tomography; *ECG,* electrocardiogram; *echo,* echocardiogram; *ED,* emergency department; *ESR,* erythrocyte sedimentation rate; *exam,* examination; *H&P,* history and physical examination; *IVDU,* intravenous drug use; *MRI,* magnetic resonance imaging; *neuro,* neurologic; *NSAIDs,* nonsteroidal antiin-flammatory drugs. (From Walls RM et al: *Rosen's emergency medicine, concepts and clinical practice,* ed 10, Philadelphia, 2023, Elsevier.)

TABLE 24 Red Flags for Potentially Serious Conditions

Possible Fracture	Possible Tumor or Infection	Possible Cauda Equina Syndrome
From Medical History		
Major trauma, such as vehicle accident or fall from height	Age over 50 or under 20 yr	Saddle anesthesia
	History of cancer	Recent onset of bladder dysfunction, such as urinary retention, increased frequency, or overflow incontinence
Minor trauma or even strenuous lifting (in older or potentially osteoporotic patient)	Constitutional symptoms, such as recent fever or chills or unexplained weight loss	Severe or progressive neurologic deficit in the lower extremity
	Risk factors for spinal infection: Recent bacterial infection (e.g., urinary tract infection), intravenous drug abuse, or immune suppression (from steroids, transplant, or human immunodeficiency virus)	
	Pain that worsens when supine; severe nighttime pain	

ICD-10CM #	M54.5	Low back pain
	L29	Pruritus
	M54.89	Other dorsalgia
	M54.9	Dorsalgia, unspecified
	F45.42	Pain disorder with related psychological factors
	M54.08	Panniculitis affecting regions of neck and back, sacral and sacrococcygeal region
	S23.9XXA	Sprain of unspecified parts of thorax, initial encounter
	M43.27	Fusion of spine, lumbosacral region
	M43.28	Fusion of spine, sacral and sacrococcygeal region
	M53.2X7	Spinal instabilities, lumbosacral region
	M53.3	Sacrococcygeal disorders, not elsewhere classified

TABLE 25 Motor and Sensory Function of Lumbosacral Nerves

Nerve	Origin	Motor Function	Sensory Function
Femoral	Lumbar plexus, L2-L4	Extension of knee, flexion of thigh	Anterior thigh
Saphenous	Distal sensory branch of femoral nerve	None	Inside aspect of lower leg
Lateral femoral cutaneous	Branch of lumbar plexus, L2-L3	None	Lateral thigh
Obturator	Lumbar plexus, L2-L4	Adduction of thigh	Medial aspect of upper thigh
Sciatic	Combined roots from lumbosacral plexus, partially separated into tibial and peroneal divisions	Foot plantar (tibial division) and dorsiflexion (peroneal division), foot inversion (tibial) and eversion (peroneal)	Lateral, anterior, and posterior aspects of lower leg and foot
Tibial	Lumbosacral plexus, L4-S3	Plantar flexion and inversion of foot	Posterior lower leg and sole of foot
Peroneal	Lumbosacral plexus, L5-S2	Dorsiflexion and eversion of foot	Dorsum of foot and lateral lower leg
Superficial peroneal	Distal sensory branch of peroneal nerve	None	Dorsum of foot
Sural	Cutaneous branches of peroneal and tibial nerves	None	Lateral foot to sole

From Jankovic J et al: *Bradley and Daroff's neurology in clinical practice,* ed 8, Philadelphia, 2022, Elsevier.

TABLE 26 Classification of Lower Back and Lower Limb Pain

Type	Examples
Mechanical pain	Facet pain
	Bony destruction
	Sacroiliac joint inflammation
	Osteomyelitis
	Diskitis
	Lumbar spondylosis
Neuropathic pain	Polyneuropathy
	Radiculopathy from disk disease, zoster, and diabetes
	Mononeuropathy including sciatic, femoral, lateral femoral cutaneous, and peroneal neuropathies
	Plexopathy from cancer, abscess, hematoma, and autoimmune processes
Nonneurologic pain	Urolithiasis
	Retroperitoneal mass
	Ovarian cyst or carcinoma
	Endometriosis

From Jankovic J et al: *Bradley and Daroff's neurology in clinical practice,* ed 8, Philadelphia, 2022, Elsevier.

TABLE 27 Differential Diagnosis of Lower Back and Leg Pain

Disorder	Clinical Features	Diagnostic Findings
Radiculopathy	Back pain radiating into leg in a dermatomal distribution. Sensory loss and motor loss are in a root distribution. Increased pain with coughing or straining.	Suspected when neuropathic pain radiates from back down into leg in a single root distribution. Disk or mass can be seen on MRI or CT. Zoster and diabetes can cause radiculopathy without abnormal studies.
Plexopathy	Back and leg pain with a neuropathic character, dysesthesias, burning, or electric sensation. Back pain can develop when cause is mass lesion in region of plexus.	Suspected when patient has leg pain in more than one peripheral nerve or root distribution. MRI of plexus or CT of abdomen and pelvis can show mass or hematoma.
Spinal stenosis	Pain in lower back, buttocks, and legs, especially with standing, walking, and lumbar spine extension.	MRI or CT shows obliteration of subarachnoid space.

CT, Computed tomography; *MRI,* magnetic resonance imaging.
From Jankovic J et al: *Bradley and Daroff's neurology in clinical practice,* ed 8, Philadelphia, 2022, Elsevier.

Clinical
Algorithms

III

ICD-10CM #	
M54.5	Low back pain
L29	Pruritus
M54.89	Other dorsalgia
M54.9	Dorsalgia, unspecified
F45.42	Pain disorder with related psychological factors
M54.08	Panniculitis affecting regions of neck and back, sacral and sacrococcygeal region
S23.9XXA	Sprain of unspecified parts of thorax, initial encounter
M43.27	Fusion of spine, lumbosacral region
M43.28	Fusion of spine, sacral and sacrococcygeal region
M53.2X7	Spinal instabilities, lumbosacral region
M53.3	Sacrococcygeal disorders, not elsewhere classified

TABLE 28 Differential Diagnosis of Isolated Lower Back Pain

Disorder	Clinical Features	Diagnostic Findings
Sacroiliac joint inflammation	Pain lateral to spine where sacrum inserts into top of iliac bone. Pain is exacerbated by movement and pressure but does not radiate down leg.	Clinical diagnosis. Radiographs can show degenerative changes in joint. Bone scan shows increased uptake in region.
Facet pain	Unilateral or bilateral paraspinal pain without radiation. Pain is increased by spine motion, especially extension.	Clinical diagnosis. Radiographs can show facet degeneration.
Ovarian cyst or cancer	Pain in hip and lower back, often but not always extending into lower quadrant. Bowel disturbance may develop with advanced disease.	Abdominal and pelvic CT shows mass lesion in ovary.
Endometriosis	Usually pelvic pain but occasionally pain in back and legs. Pain is often timed to menses.	Diagnosis suspected during pelvic examination. Vaginal ultrasound is supportive. Laparoscopy is diagnostic.
Retroperitoneal mass, abdominal aortic aneurysm, abscess, hematoma	Pain in back. May be bilateral to spine. May be associated with superimposed neuropathic pain in cases with plexus or proximal nerve involvement.	CT or MRI shows hematoma, aneurysm, eroding vertebral bodies, or abdominal mass.
Urolithiasis	Pain in upper to mid-back laterally that may radiate to groin. No radiation into leg.	Radiographs may show stones. Intravenous pyelography typically shows obstruction of flow. Contrasted abdominal CT usually shows the stone and obstruction.
Diskitis	Pain in lower back exacerbated by movement. Some patients may have radiation of pain to abdomen, hip, or leg.	MRI shows characteristic changes in disk and surrounding tissues.

CT, Computed tomography; *MRI,* magnetic resonance imaging.
From Jankovic J et al: *Bradley and Daroff's neurology in clinical practice,* ed 8, Philadelphia, 2022, Elsevier.

TABLE 29 Diagnostic Studies for Lower Back and Lower Limb Pain

Diagnostic Test	Advantages	Disadvantages
Magnetic resonance imaging	Sensitive for identification of lumbar disk herniation, spinal stenosis, paravertebral mass in region of plexus, perineural tumors, and diskitis.	May overemphasize structural lesions. May miss vascular lesions of spinal cord. Paravertebral disorders may be overlooked if they are not the focus of interest. Cannot be performed on patients with some implanted metallic and electrical devices.
Noncontrast CT	Shows osteophytes and lateral disk herniations best. Can show bone fractures and extension of fragments into regions that may contain neural elements.	Cannot identify neural elements without intrathecal contrast. Disk herniations without bone involvement may be missed.
Myelography with postmyelographic CT	Many neurosurgeons consider this the definitive test for identification of lumbar disk herniation, osteophytes, and intervertebral foraminal stenosis. Postmyelographic CT should be routinely performed.	May miss far-lateral herniations. Is invasive with a small risk of serious adverse effects.
Nerve conduction studies and EMG	Sensitive for identification of specific nerve root or peripheral neuropathic involvement.	Patients may have clinically significant radiculopathy without EMG evidence of denervation (or vice versa if radiculopathy is old).
Diskogram	Can identify disk anatomy in comparison with bony and neural anatomy. May confirm disk level if it produces pain that reproduces patient's complaints.	Invasive test, but risk of serious complications is low. Seldom performed in routine practice.

CT, Computed tomography; *EMG,* electromyography.
From Jankovic J et al: *Bradley and Daroff's neurology in clinical practice,* ed 8, Philadelphia, 2022, Elsevier.

ICD-10CM # M54.5   Low back pain
            L29   Pruritus
            M54.89   Other dorsalgia
            M54.9   Dorsalgia, unspecified
            F45.42   Pain disorder with related psychological factors
            M54.08   Panniculitis affecting regions of neck and back, sacral
                       and sacrococcygeal region
            S23.9XXA   Sprain of unspecified parts of thorax, initial encounter
            M43.27   Fusion of spine, lumbosacral region
            M43.28   Fusion of spine, sacral and sacrococcygeal region
            M53.2X7   Spinal instabilities, lumbosacral region
            M53.3   Sacrococcygeal disorders, not elsewhere classified

TABLE 30 Classical Findings in Selected Serious Causes of Acute Back Pain

Findings	Diagnoses	History	Important Physical Examination Findings	Ancillary Testing	Comments
Critical					
Vascular	Aortic dissection	Often sudden-onset, tearing, severe chest and/or back pain; associated nausea, vomiting, acute anxiety common; syncope can occur.	Associated diaphoresis, unstable vital signs; hypertension common; unequal upper extremity blood pressure; new-onset aortic insufficiency murmur; central and peripheral neurologic deficits secondary to ischemia	Choice of CT, transesophageal ECHO, MRI; depends on patient stability and availability of equipment	More common as cause of thoracic back pain.
	AAA, Abdominal aortic aneurysm (ruptured, expanding)	Pain typically noted in the abdomen, but back, flank, or pelvic pain, or radiation to groin may occur; syncope may be present.	Pulsatile abdominal mass, abdominal bruits; hypoperfusion	Bedside US; if stable, abdominal CT with contrast; plain films may show calcified, enlarged, aortic contour	Can also mimic renal colic, GI bleeding, diverticulitis, myocardial infarction; 30% of signs are misdiagnosed.
Infectious	Spinal epidural abscess	At-risk population with diabetes, chronic renal failure, dialysis, IV drug use, HIV/AIDS, immunosuppression, steroid use, alcoholism, cancer, recent spinal surgery, trauma, recent bacterial infection, bacteremia	Fever (50%), back pain (75%); focal neurologic deficits are late findings (<50% of patients); all three (classic triad) present in 15%; localized body tenderness along spine; rare cauda equina–like syndrome	Elevated WBC (66%), ESR/CRP (80%-100%) sensitive but nonspecific; MRI with contrast is modality of choice; CT if MRI contraindicated; search for source of infection; obtain blood cultures; *Staphylococcus aureus* most common cause (>50%)	Manifests as mass-occupying lesion compressing spinal cord; may be mistaken for hematoma, malignancy, herniated disc; abscess drainage may be necessary; start IV antibiotics immediately as 5% will die from sepsis.
Mechanical	Epidural compression syndrome (e.g., cauda equina syndrome, neoplastic cord compression)	Usually history of back pain, cancer; symptoms may develop over hours; sciatica (96%), urinary dysfunction (89%), bowel dysfunction (47%)	Urinary retention, fecal incontinence; saddle anesthesia (81%), bilateral leg pain; lower extremity weakness with hyporeflexia	Evaluate postvoid residual; MRI makes the diagnosis, consider performing with contrast if infection or cancer highly suspected; if contra-indicated, then obtain CT	Emergent condition caused by compression of lumbosacral nerve roots; functional status at diagnosis highly predictive of longer term outcomes.
	Spinal fracture with cord impingement, or unstable fracture	Acute onset, localized pain; usually trauma history; older adults; chronic steroid use; osteoporosis	Bone tenderness, radiculopathy or myelopathy symptoms	Plain films initially, then CT or MRI	Symptoms, signs depend on level.
	Epidural hematoma	Usually seen in patients with coagulation disorder, hereditary or acquired (e.g., anticoagulants); may occur after epidural anesthesia	Radiculopathy or myelopathy symptoms	MRI or CT	Can also occur in AV malformations
Emergent					
Infectious	Vertebral osteomyelitis	At-risk group similar to that for epidural abscess; onset may be insidious; back pain, tenderness, and stiffness may precede neurologic findings by significant time period.	May have fever (poorly sensitive or specific), other constitutional symptoms; localized tenderness of two adjacent vertebrae	CBC, blood cultures, generally low yield; ESR/CRP usually elevated but nonspecific; diagnose using MRI with contrast	Biopsy may be necessary for diagnosis; *S. aureus* most common, ideally hold antibiotics until bacteria isolated unless unstable patient; if cultures positive for GPC, consider endocarditis; can lead to pathologic fracture

Continued

Clinical
Algorithms

III

ICD-10CM #	
M54.5	Low back pain
L29	Pruritus
M54.89	Other dorsalgia
M54.9	Dorsalgia, unspecified
F45.42	Pain disorder with related psychological factors
M54.08	Panniculitis affecting regions of neck and back, sacral and sacrococcygeal region
S23.9XXA	Sprain of unspecified parts of thorax, initial encounter
M43.27	Fusion of spine, lumbosacral region
M43.28	Fusion of spine, sacral and sacrococcygeal region
M53.2X7	Spinal instabilities, lumbosacral region
M53.3	Sacrococcygeal disorders, not elsewhere classified

TABLE 30 Classical Findings in Selected Serious Causes of Acute Back Pain—cont'd

Findings	Diagnoses	History	Important Physical Examination Findings	Ancillary Testing	Comments
Immune	Transverse myelitis	Back pain, neurologic deficits; Almost 50% of patients worsen maximally in 24 h	Presentation similar to other causes of myelopathy, including motor and sensory abnormalities, risk of progressive paralysis; bladder, bowel, sexual dysfunction; most common thoracic followed by lumbosacral; likely bilateral	Goal is to rule out mass lesion compressing the cord; thought to be autoimmune origin; MRI imaging modality of choice; contrast CT if MRI contra-indicated.	May be associated with multiple sclerosis, SLE, sarcoidosis; also associated with Lyme disease, Epstein-Barr virus, other viral (e.g., herpes, enterovirus) or bacterial (e.g., tuberculosis, syphilis) infections
Mechanical	Back pain with neurologic deficits; central disc herniation; spinal stenosis; spinal fractures without cord impingement; malignancy; sciatica with potential for nerve root compression	Search for key clinical findings to rule out serious underlying disease.	Positive straight leg raise test; muscular weakness; sensory deficits; absent or diminished deep tendon reflexes	Plain films not indicated; Perform MRI or CT for complete assessment if infection, mass, cord hematoma, or cord compression is suspected	Perform complete neurologic examination including motor, sensory, reflex, and gait testing.

AV, Arteriovenous; *CBC*, complete blood count; *CRP*, C-reactive protein; *CT*, computed tomography; *ECHO*, echocardiogram; *ESR*, erythrocyte sedimentation rate; *GI*, gastrointestinal; *GPC*, gram positive cocci; *MRI*, magnetic resonance imaging; *SLE*, systemic lupus erythematous; *US*, ultrasound; *WBC*, white blood cell.

From Walls RM et al: *Rosen's emergency medicine, concepts and clinical practice,* ed 10, Philadelphia, 2023, Elsevier.

Assess reason for referral, previous diagnosis/investigations, and patient's concerns about bleeding.

↓

Evaluate the history for unprovoked, unexpected, significant, and recurrent bleeding (current and previous). Assess for symptoms of bruising, prolonged bleeding with cuts, nosebleeds, gum and oral bleeding, gastrointestinal bleeding, joint or muscle bleeds, urinary tract bleeding, and other bleeding (e.g., intracranial, umbilical stump). Evaluate the drug history and family history of bleeding problems. Evaluate other medical problems. Determine the nature and timing of any abnormal bleeding with challenges (right away, within hours or days after) and the severity (e.g., required transfusion, longer hospital stay, developed large hematomas).

↓

If symptoms suggest an underlying bleeding problem, evaluate whether the cause could be an acquired or congenital problem (e.g., symptoms from childhood, positive family history).

↓

If bleeding problems are new, consider potential reasons and triggers (e.g., a first major hemostatic challenge could be the first presentation of a mild bleeding disorder; trigger could be drugs, development of an immune disorder, or blood, endocrine, liver, or renal disease).

↓

Formulate a differential diagnosis for the potential inherited and acquired causes that should be investigated.

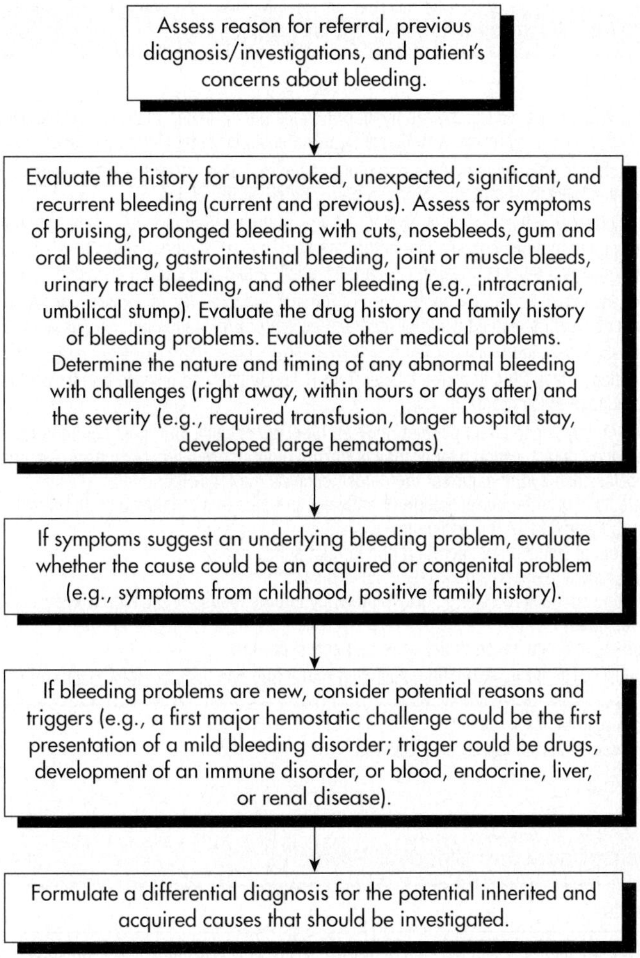

FIG. 40 Steps to evaluate bleeding and bruising problems. (From Hoffman R: *Hematology, basic principles and practice*, ed 7, Philadelphia, 2018, Elsevier.)

Clinical Algorithms

III

TABLE 31   Differential Diagnosis of Bleeding Problems

Major Categories	Comments
No bleeding disorder	Symptoms do not reflect a bleeding disorder and have another explanation (e.g., a surgical bleed, not caused by a bleeding disorder).
Possible bleeding disorder	The laboratory findings are nondiagnostic, and the bleeding history is considered equivocal (e.g., unexplained serious bleed with one surgical procedure; unexplained menorrhagia without other bleeding problems).
Definite bleeding disorder, undefined or indeterminate type	The bleeding history is consistent with a bleeding disorder; however, the laboratory findings are nondiagnostic. Commonly the bleeding history resembles mild to moderate defects in platelet function or von Willebrand factor. The diagnosis should only be made once an adequate evaluation for common bleeding disorders (e.g., for von Willebrand disease and platelet aggregation and release defects) is completed. If testing is not complete, the classification should indicate the types of conditions excluded or not excluded, for example, mild mucocutaneous bleeding problem, von Willebrand disease excluded, mild mucocutaneous bleeding problem, platelet release defects not yet excluded.
Definite bleeding disorder with cause	The symptoms and laboratory findings are considered diagnostic of a bleeding disorder.

From Hoffman R: *Hematology, basic principles and practice*, ed 7, Philadelphia, 2018, Elsevier.

TABLE 32 Differential Diagnosis of Congenital Bleeding Disorders

Disorder	Comments
Fibrinogen deficiency or dysfunction	Deficiencies can be mild-moderate hypofibrinogenemia or severe afibrinogenemia. Fibrinogen function is abnormal in dysfibrinogenemias, which can present with bleeding, thrombosis, or both. Fibrinogen levels can be reduced in some dysfibrinogenemias.
X-linked coagulation factor deficiencies—hemophilia	Presentation is influenced by the degree of deficiency. Factor VIII deficiency is more common than factor IX deficiency. If factor VIII is low, von Willebrand disease needs to be excluded as the cause.
Rarer, coagulation factor deficiencies	Deficiencies can affect factors XI, V, II, VII, or X, and the presentation is dependent on the severity of the deficiency. Hereditary deficiencies of multiple coagulation factors are rare (e.g., of factors V and VIII, or multiple vitamin K-dependent coagulation factors for congenital defects impairing γ-carboxylation) and can easily be excluded by measuring multiple factors.
Fibrinolytic defects	Causes include disorders caused by loss of function, such as α2-antiplasmin or PAI-1 deficiency, and by gain-of-function defects, such as Quebec platelet disorder (overexpression of urokinase plasminogen activator in megakaryocytes).
von Willebrand disease	Causes include quantitative (partial type 1 to severe type 3) and qualitative defects (loss of function in type 2M and 2A, gain of function in type 2B and platelet-type). Type 1 von Willebrand disease can be confused with low von Willebrand factor levels (e.g., because of blood group O).
Platelet disorders	These conditions can affect platelet number, function, or both. The most common type of platelet function disorder is a platelet secretion defect, which may or may not also impair aggregation responses. Disorders of platelet function are commonly subclassified by the nature of the defect, such as the following: Defects of membrane receptors for adhesive proteins (e.g., Glanzmann thrombasthenia and Bernard-Soulier syndrome) or agonists (e.g., P2Y$_{12}$ deficiency) Defects of signaling or secretion (the largest subcategory) Cytoskeletal defects (e.g., MYH9-related disorders) Storage pool disorders (e.g., gray platelet syndrome, dense granule deficiency, $\alpha\gamma$-storage pool deficiency, Quebec platelet disorder) Defects of procoagulant function (e.g., Scott syndrome)
Vascular disorders	Congenital vascular malformation, including hereditary hemorrhagic telangiectasia, Ehlers-Danlos syndrome

MYH9, Myosin heavy polypeptide 9; *PAI-1,* plasminogen activator inhibitor 1.
From Hoffman R: *Hematology, basic principles and practice,* ed 7, Philadelphia, 2018, Elsevier.

TABLE 33 Differential Diagnosis of Acquired Bleeding Problems

Disorder	Comments
Drug induced	Aspirin, NSAIDs, other platelet function inhibitors (e.g., P2Y$_{12}\alpha_{IIb}\beta_3$ inhibitors), anticoagulants, fibrinolytic drugs, and antidepressants are common causes.
Acquired factor deficiencies	The causes can be immune (e.g., acquired factor VIII deficiency, acquired factor V deficiency) or nonimmune. Reductions in multiple factors can result from vitamin K deficiency, treatment with vitamin K antagonists, liver disease, hemodilution, and rarely snakebites. Severe acquired hypofibrinogenemia is commonly caused by a postpartum coagulopathy or severe liver disease. Prothrombin deficiency occurs with some lupus anticoagulants. Amyloidosis can cause an acquired factor X deficiency, which may be associated with reductions in other coagulation factors synthesized in the liver if the liver is involved.
Disseminated intravascular coagulation	The manifestations can include thrombocytopenia, consumption of coagulation factors, including fibrinogen, and impairment of hemostatic mechanisms from the fibrin/fibrinogen degradation products. Causes are wide ranging and include postpartum consumptive states, prostate and other cancers, and snakebites.
Acquired von Willebrand disease	The cause can be immune (often in association with an IgG paraprotein) or nonimmune (e.g., increased proteolysis of von Willebrand factor with stenotic aortic valvular disease).
Immune thrombocytopenia	Bleeding is usually influenced by the extent of the thrombocytopenia. Some autoantibodies interfere with platelet membrane receptor function, causing bleeding disproportionate to the thrombocytopenia.
Nondrug-induced, acquired platelet function disorders	The cause can be immune (see earlier) or nonimmune, typically from bone marrow disorders, although secretion defects can be secondary to Cushing syndrome or hypothyroidism.
Liver disease	Liver disease can cause thrombocytopenia, deficiencies of coagulation factors, hypofibrinogenemia and dysfibrinogenemia, and increased fibrinolysis. In mild liver disease, factor VII and sometimes factors XI and XII are low. Fibrinogen is often increased in early liver disease, and if low, the finding suggests severe liver disease.
Renal disease	Anemia is an important predictor of uremic bleeding. Uremic bleeding is typically associated with severe renal impairment.
Hypothyroidism	Hypothyroidism can cause an acquired von Willebrand disease and acquired defects in platelet function.
Cushing syndrome	This syndrome should be suspected when there are symptoms and findings suggestive of Cushing syndrome or treatment with systemic or topical glucocorticoids.
Surgical bleeding	This is often a diagnosis of exclusion, although the procedural notes sometimes document that a technical problem was encountered that led to abnormal bleeding.
Vitamin K deficiency	Newborns are at risk, as are individuals with malabsorption and/or receiving broad-spectrum antibiotics that reduce vitamin K production by reducing gut bacteria. Older adults are also at greater risk for developing vitamin K deficiency because of reduced stores from poorer intake of vitamin K. If the patient does not respond to parenteral vitamin K, other causes should be considered.
Vitamin C deficiency (scurvy)	This diagnosis should be considered when there is lethargy with skin and gum bleeding (perifollicular hemorrhages, gum bleeding with swelling). The condition is rare in developed countries. The cause is usually a very poor diet or malabsorption.

IgG, Immunoglobulin G; *NSAID,* nonsteroidal antiinflammatory drug.
From Hoffman R: *Hematology, basic principles and practice,* ed 7, Philadelphia, 2018, Elsevier.

TABLE 34 The Effect of Anticoagulants on Commonly Ordered Coagulation Tests

Test	Warfarin	UFH	LMWH	Direct Thrombin Inhibitors (e.g., Dabigatran)	Factor Xa Inhibitors (e.g., Rivaroxaban, Apixaban, Edoxaban)
PT/INR (clot based)	Increases	No effect or increases	No effect	No effect or increases	No effect or increases
APTT (clot based)	Increases	Increases	No effect or increases	No effect or increases	No effect or increases
Thrombin time (clot based)	No effect	Increases	No effect or increases	Increases	No effect
Clauss fibrinogen (clot based)	No effect	No effect	No effect	Minimal effect to falsely decrease (if direct thrombin inhibitor level very high)	No effect
Antithrombin (chromogenic anti-Xa based)	No effect	Decreases	No effect to decreases	No effect	Falsely increases
Antithrombin (chromogenic anti-IIa based)	No effect	Decreases	No effect to decreases	Falsely increases	No effect
Protein C—functional (clot based)	Decreases	No effect (neutralizer in reagent)	No effect	Falsely increases	Falsely increases
Protein C—functional (chromogenic)	Decreases	No effect (neutralizer in reagent)	No effect	No effect	No effect
Protein S—free (latex immunoassay)	Decreases	No effect	No effect	No effect	No effect
Activated protein C (APC) resistance (clot based)	Unknown	Unknown	Unknown	Unknown, may be falsely normal	Unknown, may be falsely normal
Lupus anticoagulant—lupus sensitive APTT (clot based)	Falsely increases, may correct on mixing	Falsely increases, generally does not correct on mixing	Possibly falsely increases, generally does not correct on mixing	Falsely increases, generally does not correct on mixing	Falsely increases, generally does not correct on mixing
Lupus anticoagulant—DRVVT (dilute Russell viper venom time) (clot based)	Falsely increases, does not correct on mixing	No effect	No effect	Falsely increases, does not correct on mixing	Falsely increases, does not correct on mixing

APTT, Activated partial thromboplastin time; *INR,* international normalized ratio; *PT,* prothrombin time.
From Hoffman R et al: *Hematology, basic principles and practice,* ed 8, Philadelphia, 2023, Elsevier.

BOX 18 The Laboratory Manifestations of Bleeding Disorders

- The laboratory manifestations of bleeding disorders can include abnormalities from the following:
  The underlying hemostatic defect
  Bleeding complications (e.g., anemia, iron deficiency, coagulopathy secondary to hemodilution after resuscitation for a massive bleed, development of red cell antibodies after transfusion)
  False-positive abnormalities (e.g., prolonged aPTT caused by incidental mild factor XII deficiency, which is found in about 1 of 200 patients, or a lupus anticoagulant, which can be a transient finding in about 5% of hospitalized patients)
  Extremes of normal variation (e.g., mildly low von Willebrand factor levels in an individual who is blood group O, absent secondary aggregation with epinephrine in adjusted platelet-rich plasma aggregation studies)

From Hoffman R: *Hematology, basic principles and practice,* ed 7, Philadelphia, 2018, Elsevier.

BOX 19 Influences on Presenting Problems

When evaluating a bleeding history, it is important to recognize that the presenting problems are influenced by the following factors:
  The nature and severity of the defect, and the presence of single or multiple risk factors for bleeding
  Whether the bleeding problem is congenital or acquired
  Antecedent exposure to hemostatic challenges (such as surgery, dental extraction, menses, and childbirth) and the risk for bleeding with each of these challenges
  The presence of other medical problems (e.g., renal, hepatic, or thyroid disease), including anemia
  Variability in the bleeding symptoms experienced by individuals without bleeding disorders (e.g., nosebleeds, bruising) and by individuals with known bleeding disorders, even within families with the same defect
  Local factors (e.g., sun-damage to the skin, vascular lesions, diverticular disease, or cancerous lesions in the gastrointestinal tract) and the possibility of nonaccidental trauma
  Treatments that increase the risk for bleeding (e.g., antiplatelet drugs, such as aspirin and nonsteroidal antiinflammatory drugs used for pain control, anticoagulant therapy, etc.)
  Whether treatments were used to prevent or control bleeding
  Whether treatments prescribed for other reasons may have reduced bleeding (e.g., reduced menstrual bleeding while on oral contraceptives to prevent pregnancy)

From Hoffman R: *Hematology, basic principles and practice,* ed 7, Philadelphia, 2018, Elsevier.

BOX 20   Case 1: Illustration of a Mild, Inherited Bleeding Problem

A 77-yr-old man who is starting treatment for multiple myeloma was discovered to have a prolonged activated partial thromboplastin time. Review of his records indicated that the abnormality was present on a previous admission for spinal cord compression, which was treated with surgery. He required 4 units of packed red blood cells several days after this surgery because of delayed postoperative bleeding. There was no other bleeding history. He was found to have mild factor IX deficiency, unrelated to the myeloma, and his daughter proved to be a carrier of this defect.

From Hoffman R: *Hematology, basic principles and practice,* ed 7, Philadelphia, 2018, Elsevier.

BOX 21   Case 2: Illustration of the Importance of Assessing Both Personal and Familial Bleeding Problems

A 22-yr-old woman was referred for evaluation of a possible platelet disorder. She had a history of menorrhagia (4 days out of 7 days of menstrual flow were heavy when not on treatment), prolonged nosebleeds in childhood, and hematuria with urinary tract infections. She did not have thrombocytopenia, and she had no exposure to major hemostatic challenges. Her father, uncle, and grandfather had a striking bleeding history, and two of them had thrombocytopenia. The bleeding in her relatives included joint bleeds with trauma and severe, delayed-onset bleeding after trauma and surgery (usually more than a day later), which continued for weeks despite platelet transfusions. One of these relatives reported no bleeding when he had a tooth extracted while receiving fibrinolytic inhibitor therapy. Although menorrhagia is not specific to any one type of bleeding disorder, the delayed bleeding in affected relatives suggests a possible autosomal dominant disorder and either a fibrinolytic defect of a factor defect or deficiency (e.g., affected relatives). Because of the family history of thrombocytopenia, joint bleeds, and delayed bleeding, which did not respond well to platelet transfusions, testing was done for the Quebec platelet disorder. Genetic testing for duplication mutation of the urokinase plasminogen activator gene confirmed this diagnosis in the patient and her relatives. The case illustrates the importance of evaluating both the personal and family bleeding history and highlights the fact that bleeding-symptom severity can vary among affected family members, in part because of their different exposures to challenges and treatments.

From Hoffman R: *Hematology, basic principles and practice,* ed 7, Philadelphia, 2018, Elsevier.

BOX 22   Case 3: Illustration of the Importance of Assessing Bleeding Problems Over Time

A 72-yr-old man was referred for evaluation of a severe bleed after receiving a single dose of low–molecular-weight heparin for unconfirmed deep vein thrombosis. He had a history of a similar bleeding episode several years previously while on warfarin treatment for atrial fibrillation. There was no other bleeding history, and the patient subsequently developed a spontaneous iliopsoas bleed. He had undergone numerous surgeries earlier in life without any bleeding problems, and there was no family history of bleeding. The bleeding history suggested the possibility of an acquired bleeding problem, possibly acquired von Willebrand disease or an acquired factor XIII deficiency. Diagnostic testing indicated that he had acquired factor XIII deficiency. This case illustrates the fact that there may be more than one risk factor for bleeding: In this case, several exposures to anticoagulants triggered bleeding in a patient with an acquired factor deficiency. On initial treatment of his iliopsoas bleed with factor XIII concentrate, there was partial neutralization of the infused factor followed by accelerated clearance, consistent with acquired factor XIII deficiency secondary to an autoantibody.

From Hoffman R: *Hematology, basic principles and practice,* ed 7, Philadelphia, 2018, Elsevier.

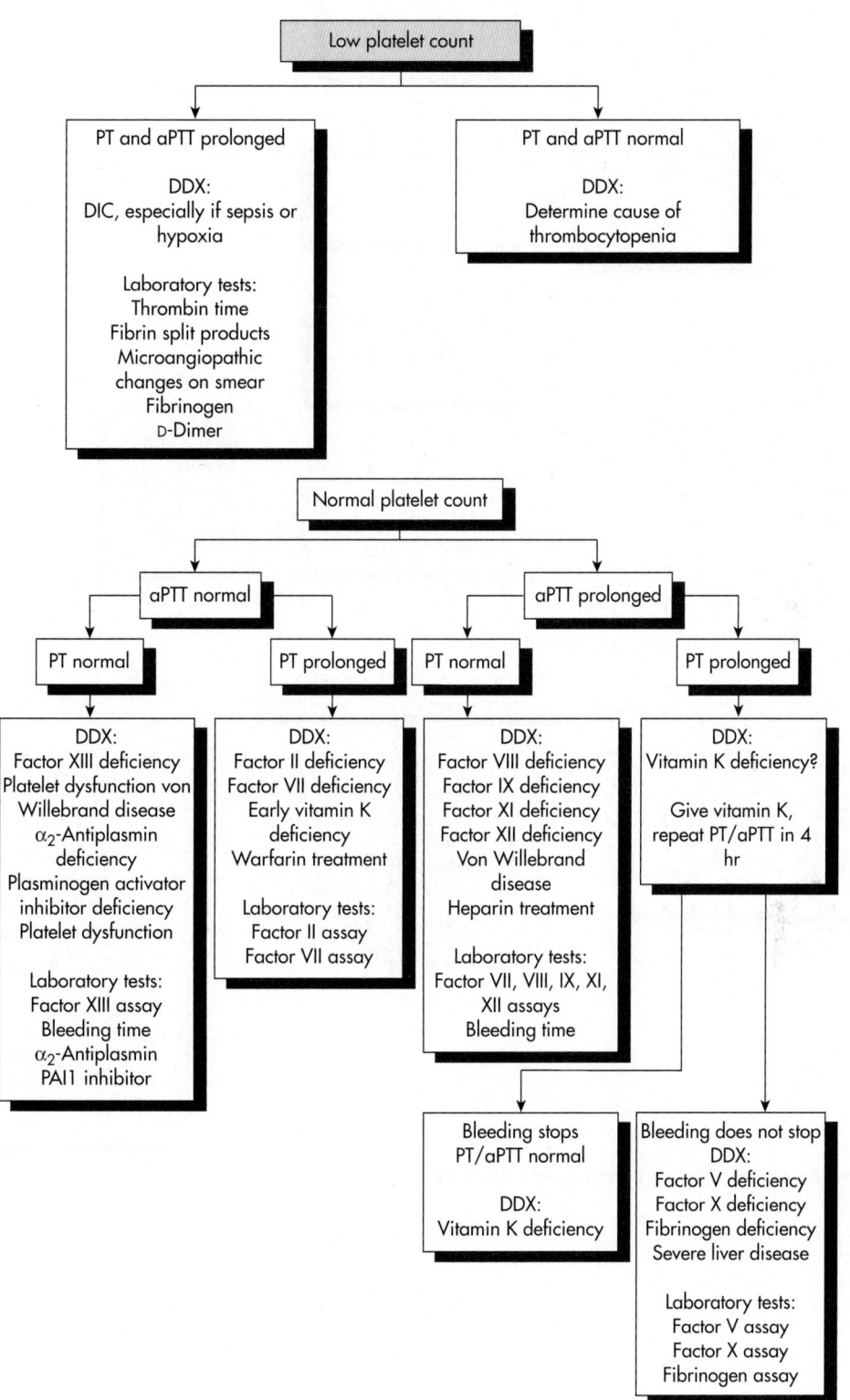

FIG. 41 Differential diagnosis *(DDx)* of bleeding disorders. *aPTT,* Activated partial thromboplastin time; *DDX,* differential diagnosis; *DIC,* disseminated intravascular coagulation; *PT,* prothrombin time. (From Hughes HK, Kahl LK: *The Harriet Lane handbook,* ed 21, St Louis, 2018, Mosby.)

Clinical
Algorithms

III

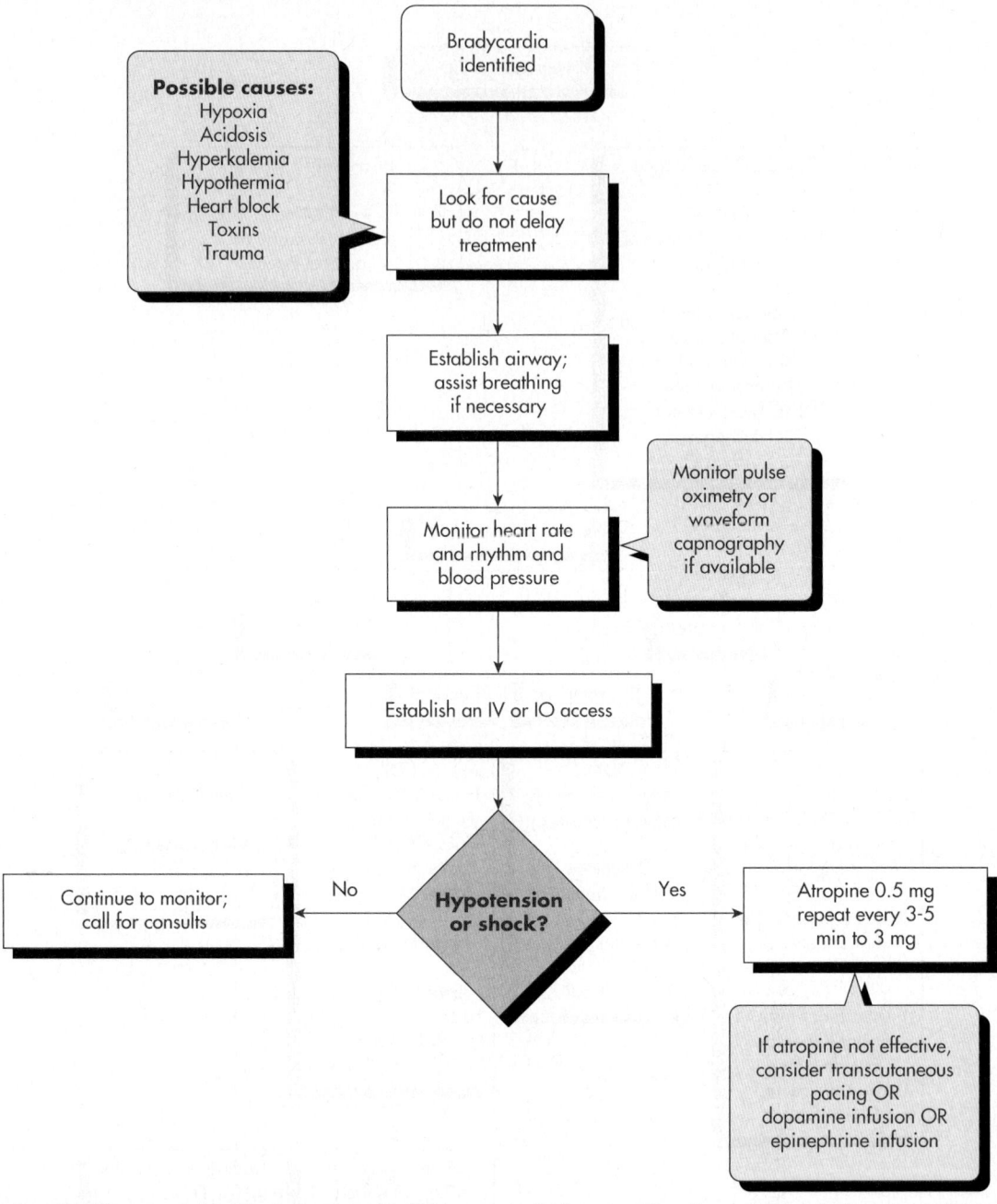

FIG. 46 Advanced cardiac life support algorithm for bradycardia. *IO,* Intraosseous; *IV,* intravenous. (From Newman M et al: *Perioperative medicine,* ed 2, Philadelphia, 2022, Elsevier.)

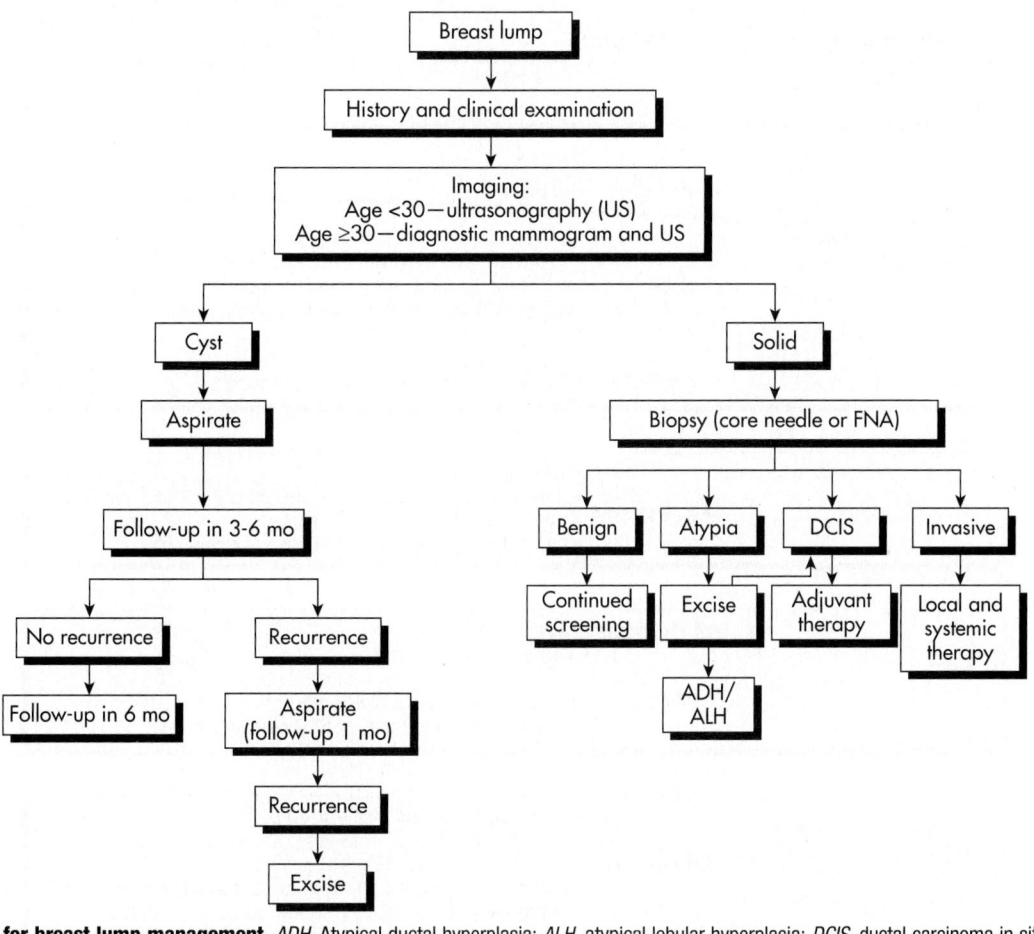

FIG. 47 Algorithm for breast lump management. *ADH,* Atypical ductal hyperplasia; *ALH,* atypical lobular hyperplasia; *DCIS,* ductal carcinoma in situ; *FNA,* fine-needle aspiration. (From Niederhuber JE: *Abeloff's clinical oncology,* ed 6, Philadelphia, 2020, Elsevier.)

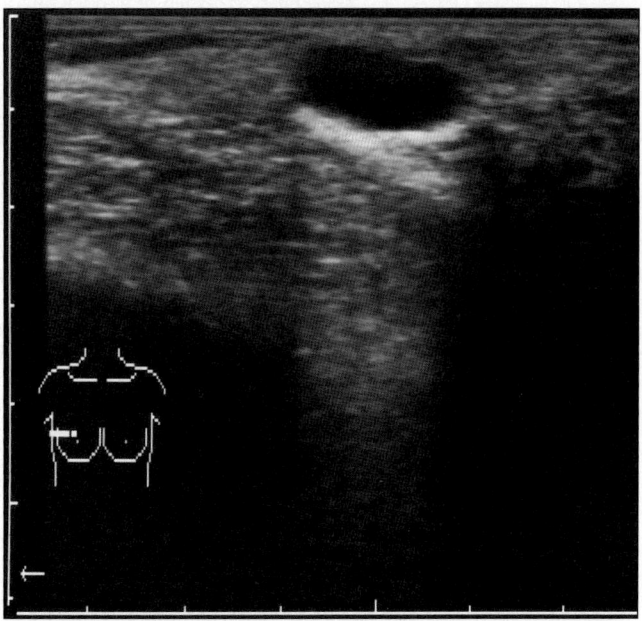

FIG. 48 Ultrasound image of the breast showing the palpable lump to be cystic. Cystic lesions have a characteristic hypoechoic pattern, with prominent acoustic shadowing. (From Niederhuber JE: *Abeloff's clinical oncology,* ed 6, Philadelphia, 2020, Elsevier.)

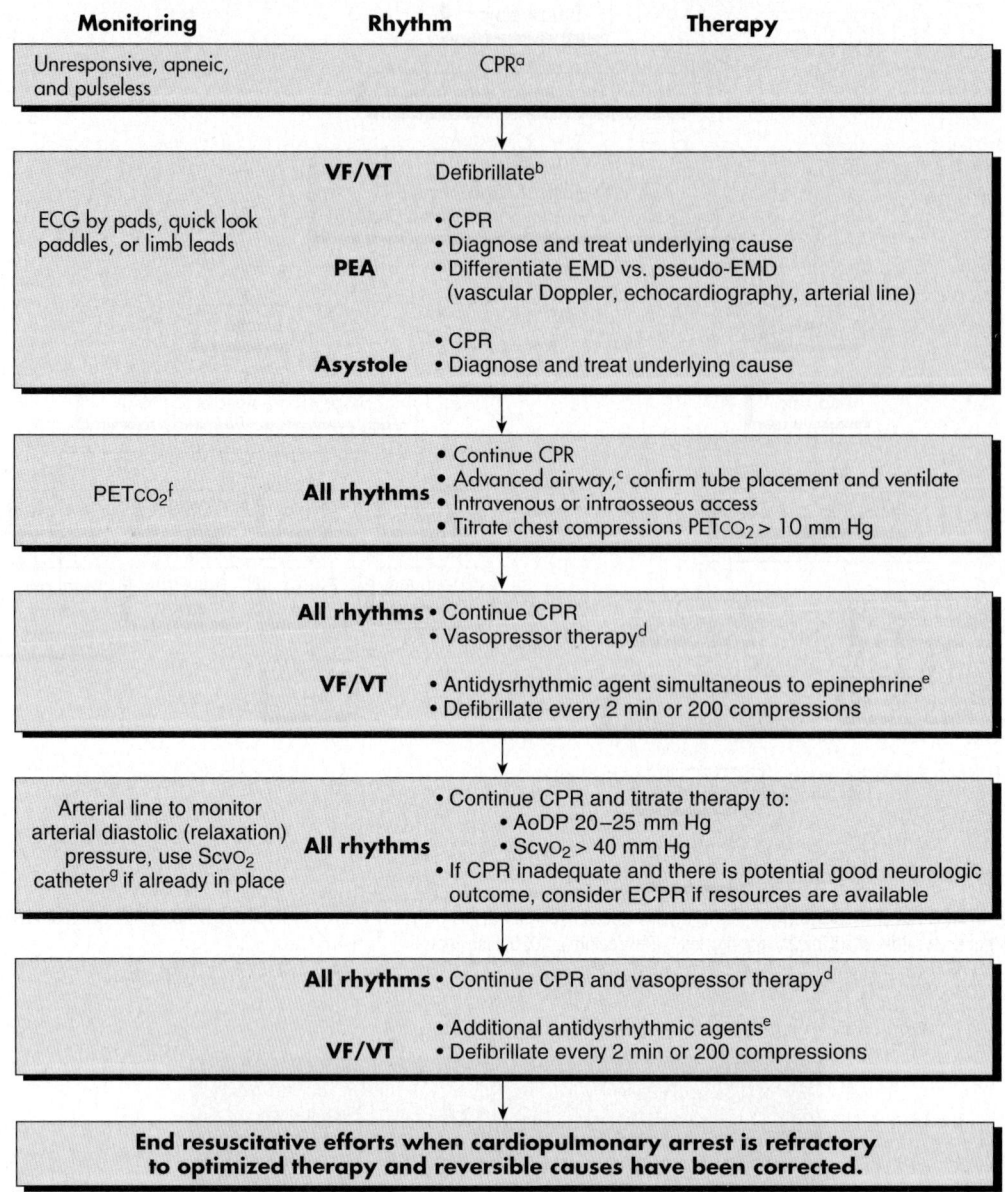

FIG. 52 Emergency treatment algorithm for treatment of cardiac arrest. [a]If arrest is witnessed and known to be of short duration, immediate rhythm assessment and defibrillation of ventricular fibrillation/ventricular tachycardia *(VF/VT)* precede cardiopulmonary resuscitation *(CPR)*. [b]Biphasic defibrillation should use manufacturer-recommended energy versus monophasic defibrillation (360 J). [c]Endotracheal intubation or supraglottic airway, when feasible, with minimal interruption in chest compressions. [d]Epinephrine, initial dose of 1 mg IV or IO. Repeat every 3 to 5 minutes. [e]Amiodarone, 300 mg via IV push, followed by 150 mg. Lidocaine is an alternative antidysrhythmic if amiodarone is not available. Magnesium sulfate may be given in torsades de pointes or hypomagnesemia. [f]Changes in the partial pressure of end-tidal carbon dioxide (PETco2) may not be predictive of myocardial blood flow in the setting of high-dose vasopressor therapy. [g]Invasive monitoring should be performed only if adequate personnel are available and if it would not delay therapeutic interventions. *AoDP,* Aortic diastolic pressure; *ECG,* electrocardiogram; *EMD,* electromechanical dissociation; *PEA,* pulseless electrical activity; *Scvo2,* central venous oxygen saturation. (From Walls RM et al: *Rosen's emergency medicine, concepts and clinical practice,* ed 10, Philadelphia, 2023, Elsevier.)

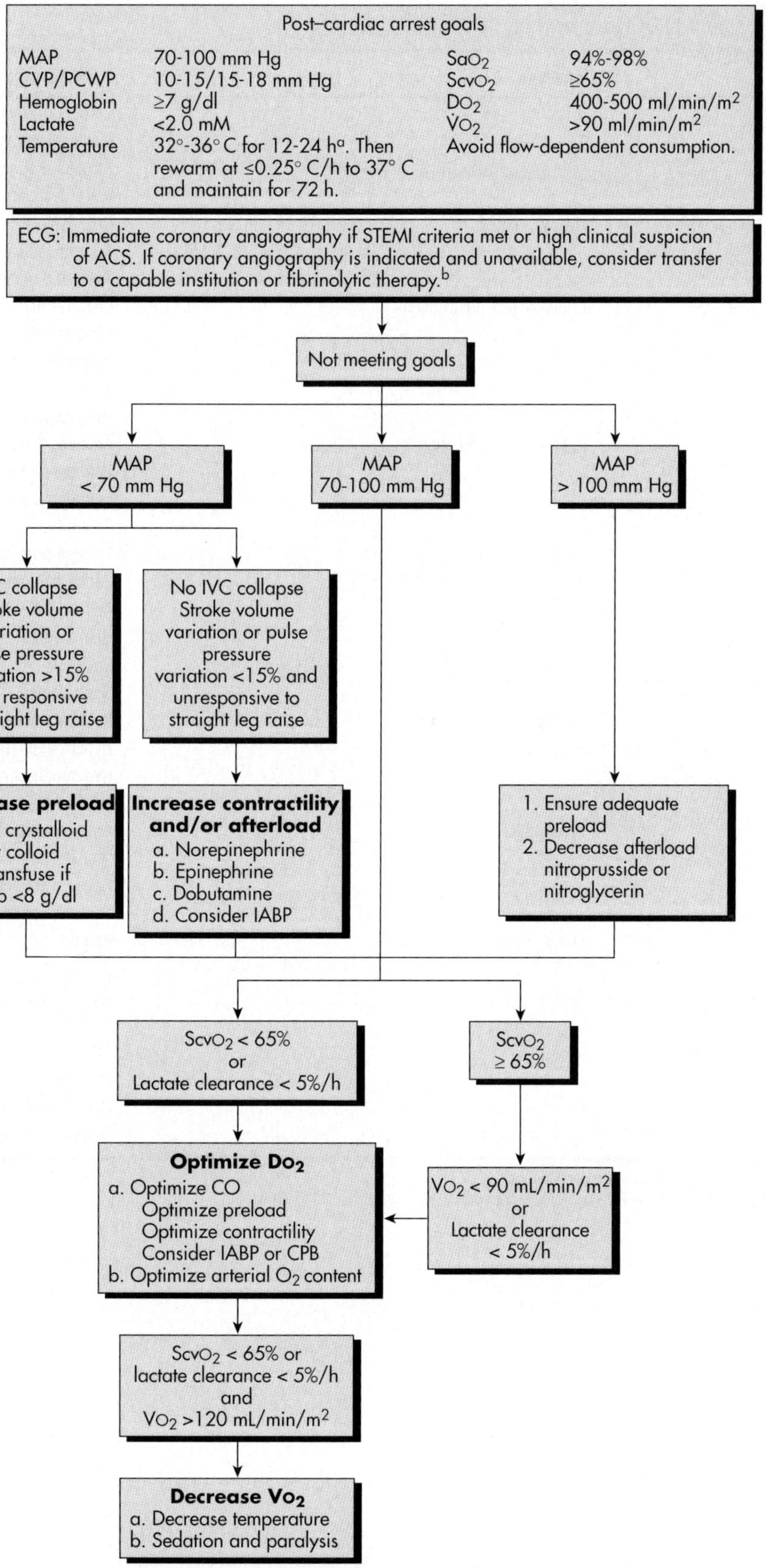

Post–cardiac arrest goals

MAP	70-100 mm Hg	SaO_2	94%-98%
CVP/PCWP	10-15/15-18 mm Hg	$ScvO_2$	≥65%
Hemoglobin	≥7 g/dl	DO_2	400-500 ml/min/m^2
Lactate	<2.0 mM	VO_2	>90 ml/min/m^2
Temperature	32°-36° C for 12-24 h[a]. Then rewarm at ≤0.25° C/h to 37° C and maintain for 72 h.	Avoid flow-dependent consumption.	

ECG: Immediate coronary angiography if STEMI criteria met or high clinical suspicion of ACS. If coronary angiography is indicated and unavailable, consider transfer to a capable institution or fibrinolytic therapy.[b]

Not meeting goals

MAP < 70 mm Hg

MAP 70-100 mm Hg

MAP > 100 mm Hg

IVC collapse
Stroke volume variation or Pulse pressure variation >15% and responsive to straight leg raise

No IVC collapse
Stroke volume variation or pulse pressure variation <15% and unresponsive to straight leg raise

Increase preload
a. IV crystalloid or colloid
b. transfuse if Hb <8 g/dl

Increase contractility and/or afterload
a. Norepinephrine
b. Epinephrine
c. Dobutamine
d. Consider IABP

1. Ensure adequate preload
2. Decrease afterload nitroprusside or nitroglycerin

$ScvO_2$ < 65% or Lactate clearance < 5%/h

$ScvO_2$ ≥ 65%

Optimize Do_2
a. Optimize CO
   Optimize preload
   Optimize contractility
   Consider IABP or CPB
b. Optimize arterial O_2 content

VO_2 < 90 mL/min/m^2 or Lactate clearance < 5%/h

$ScvO_2$ < 65% or lactate clearance < 5%/h and VO_2 >120 mL/min/m^2

Decrease Vo_2
a. Decrease temperature
b. Sedation and paralysis

Clinical Algorithms

FIG. 53   Goal-directed post-arrest treatment algorithm. [a]Hypothermic targeted temperature management (HTTM) is indicated in comatose survivors of cardiac arrest. Relative contraindications include uncontrolled bleeding, preexisting coagulopathy, another obvious reason for coma (e.g., drug overdose, status epilepticus), known end-stage terminal illness, and a preexisting do-not-resuscitate status. [b]Initiation of HTTM is not a contraindication to thrombolytic therapy. *CPB,* cardiopulmonary bypass; *CVP,* central venous pressure; *Do₂,* oxygen delivery; *ECG,* electrocardiogram; *Hb,* hemoglobin; *IABP,* intra-aortic balloon pump; *MAP,* mean arterial pressure; *MI,* myocardial infarction; *NTG,* nitroglycerin; *PCWP,* pulmonary capillary wedge pressure; *Sao₂,* arterial oxygen saturation; *Scvo₂,* central venous oxygen saturation; *VO₂,* oxygen consumption. (From Walls RM et al: *Rosen's emergency medicine, concepts and clinical practice,* ed 10, Philadelphia, 2023, Elsevier.)

TABLE 37   Common Causes of Nontraumatic Cardiac Arrest

General	Specific	Disease or Agent
Cardiac		Coronary artery disease
		Cardiomyopathies
		Structural abnormalities
		Valve dysfunction
Respiratory	Hypoventilation	CNS dysfunction
		Neuromuscular disease
		Toxic and metabolic encephalopathies
	Upper airway obstruction	CNS dysfunction
		Foreign body
		Infection
		Trauma
		Neoplasm
	Pulmonary dysfunction	Asthma, COPD
		Pulmonary edema
		Pulmonary embolus
		Pneumonia
Circulatory	Mechanical obstruction	Tension pneumothorax
		Pericardial tamponade
		Pulmonary embolus
	Hypovolemia	Hemorrhage
	Vascular tone	Sepsis
		Neurogenic
Metabolic	Electrolyte abnormalities	Hypokalemia or hyperkalemia
		Hypermagnesemia
		Hypomagnesemia
		Hypocalcemia
Toxic	Prescription medications	Antidysrhythmics
		Digoxin, beta blockers
		Calcium channel blockers
		Tricyclic antidepressants
	Drugs of abuse	Cocaine
		Heroin
	Toxins	Carbon monoxide
		Cyanide
Environmental		Lightning
		Electrocution
		Hypothermia or hyperthermia
		Drowning or near-drowning

CNS, Central nervous system; *COPD,* chronic obstructive pulmonary disease.
From Walls RM et al: *Rosen's emergency medicine, concepts and clinical practice,* ed 10, Philadelphia, 2023, Elsevier.

TABLE 38   Physical Examination Findings Indicating Potential Cause of Cardiac Arrest and Complications of Therapy

Physical Examination	Abnormalities	Potential Causes
General	Pallor	Hemorrhage
	Cold	Hypothermia
Airway	Secretions, vomitus, or blood	Aspiration
		Airway obstruction
	Resistance to positive-pressure ventilation	Tension pneumothorax
		Airway obstruction
		Bronchospasm
Neck	Jugular venous distention	Tension pneumothorax
		Cardiac tamponade
		Pulmonary embolus
	Tracheal deviation	Tension pneumothorax
Chest	Median sternotomy scar	Underlying cardiac disease
Lungs	Unilateral breath sounds	Tension pneumothorax
		Right mainstem intubation
		Aspiration
	Distant or no breath sounds or no chest expansion	Esophageal intubation
		Airway obstruction
		Severe bronchospasm
	Wheezing	Aspiration
		Bronchospasm
		Pulmonary edema
	Rales	Aspiration
		Pulmonary edema
		Pneumonia
Heart	Diminished heart tones	Hypovolemia
		Cardiac tamponade
		Tension pneumothorax
		Pulmonary embolus
Abdomen	Distended and dull	Ruptured abdominal aortic aneurysm or ruptured ectopic pregnancy
	Distended, tympanitic	Esophageal intubation
	Gastric insufflation	
Rectal	Blood, melena	Gastrointestinal hemorrhage
Extremities	Asymmetrical pulses	Aortic dissection
	Arteriovenous shunt or fistula	Hyperkalemia
Skin	Needle tracks or abscesses	Intravenous drug abuse
	Burns	Smoke inhalation
		Electrocution

From Walls RM et al: *Rosen's emergency medicine, concepts and clinical practice*, ed 10, Philadelphia, 2023, Elsevier.

Clinical Algorithms

III

ICD-10CM # I51.7   Cardiomegaly
Q24.8   Other specified congenital malformations of heart
I11.9   Hypertensive heart disease without heart failure
I11.0   Hypertensive heart disease with heart failure
Q23.8   Other congenital malformations of aortic and mitral valves

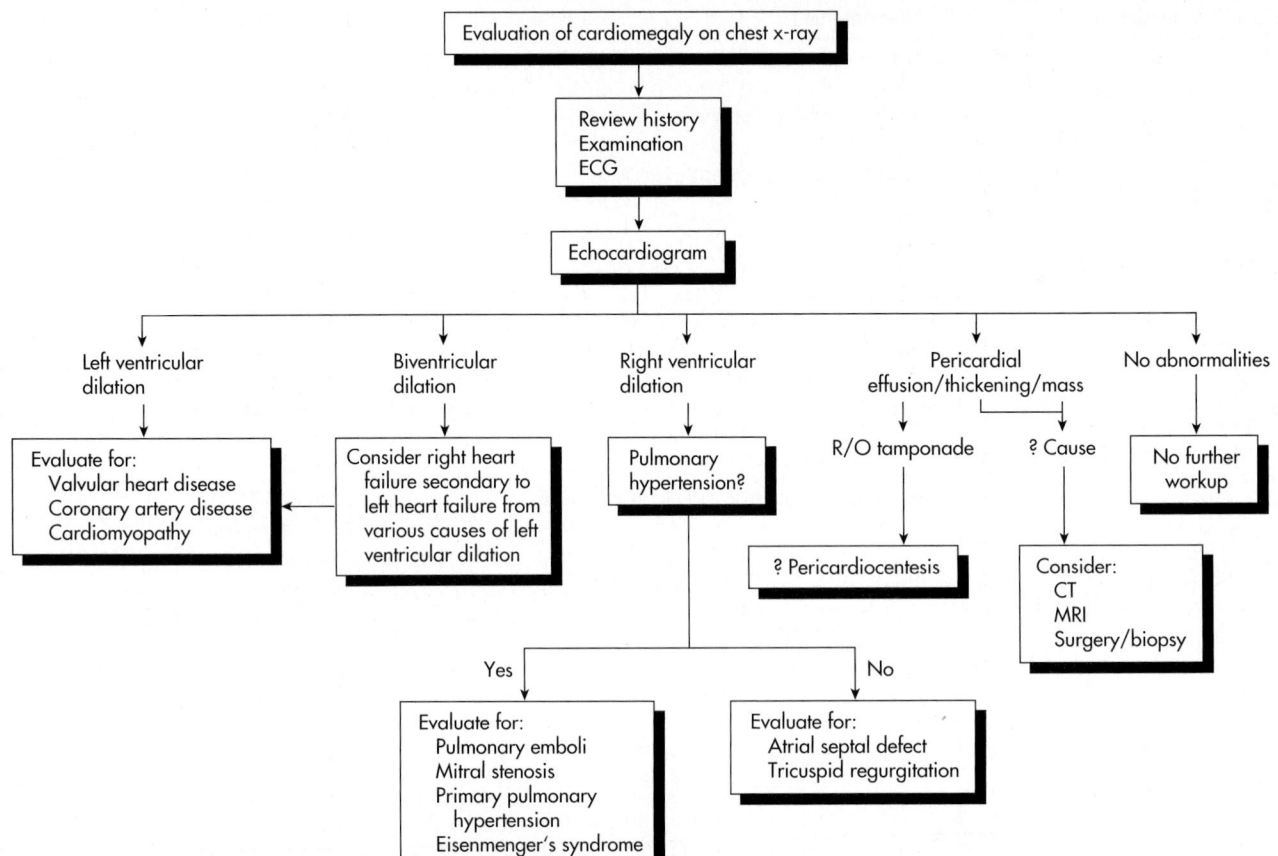

FIG. 55 Approach to the patient with cardiomegaly. When cardiomegaly is found on the chest radiograph, the history and physical examination should be reviewed and an electrocardiogram *(ECG)* performed before obtaining a two-dimensional Doppler echocardiographic study. Cardiomegaly may be explained by left ventricular dilation, biventricular dilation, right ventricular dilation, or pericardial abnormalities, or it may be found to be spurious on the echocardiogram. Rarely, isolated abnormalities of the atrium, particularly the left atrium, may cause abnormalities on the chest radiograph but will not cause true cardiomegaly. Depending on the echocardiographic findings, further tests can help elucidate the cause of echocardiographically confirmed cardiomegaly. *CT,* Computed tomography; *MRI,* magnetic resonance imaging; *R/O,* rule out. (From Goldman L, Braunwald E [eds]: *Primary cardiology,* ed 2, Philadelphia, 2003, Saunders.)

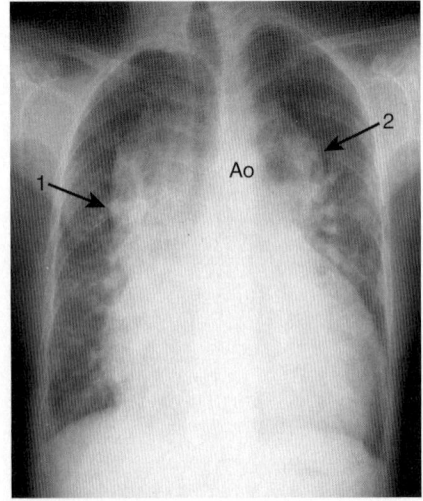

FIG. 56 "Snowman" heart in a 36-yr-old man with increasing shortness of breath. Posteroanterior chest film examination shows cardiomegaly and increased pulmonary blood flow. The superior mediastinum is widened, the result of dilation of the left vertical vein *(arrow 2)* and the right-sided superior vena cava *(arrow 1).* The trachea is displaced by a normal left-sided aortic arch *(Ao).* (From Boxt LM, Abbara S: *Cardiac imaging: the requisites,* ed 4, Philadelphia, 2016, Elsevier.)

CARDIOMEGALY ON CHEST X-RAY—cont'd

ICD-10CM #	I51.7	Cardiomegaly
	Q24.8	Other specified congenital malformations of heart
	I11.9	Hypertensive heart disease without heart failure
	I11.0	Hypertensive heart disease with heart failure
	Q23.8	Other congenital malformations of aortic and mitral valves

1397

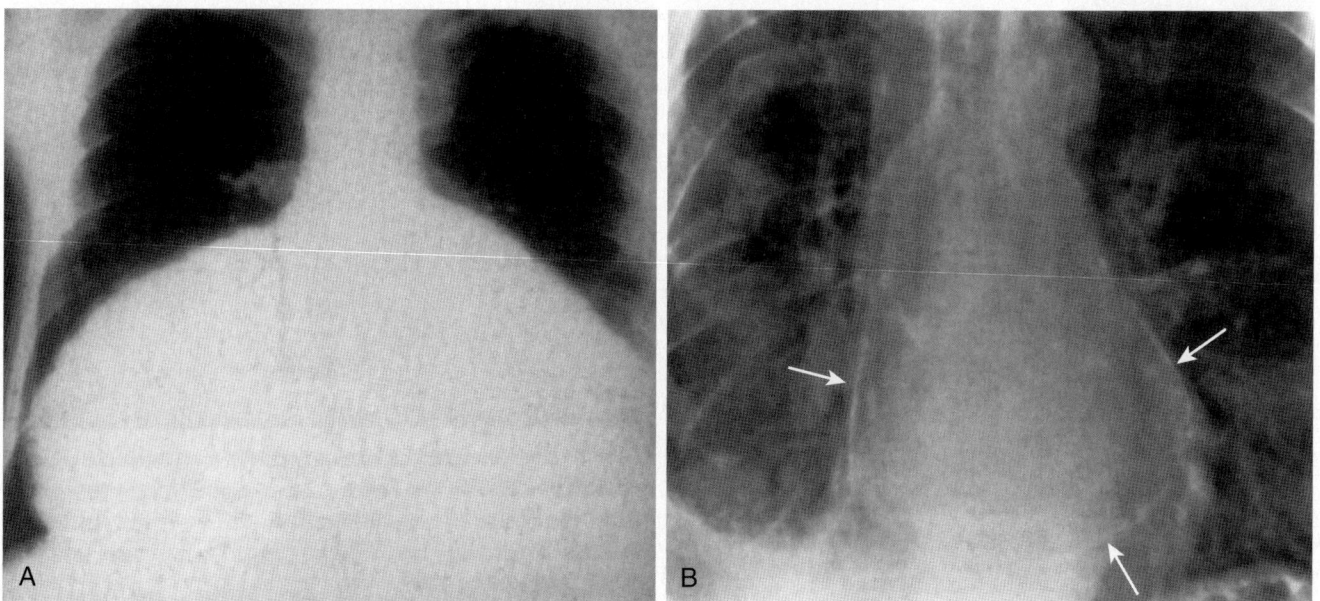

FIG. 57 Chest radiographs in a patient with a very large pericardial effusion. A, "Water bottle" sign. **B,** A patient with constrictive pericarditis and pericardial calcifications *(white arrows)*. (From Vincent JL et al: *Textbook of critical care,* ed 7, Philadelphia, 2017, Elsevier.)

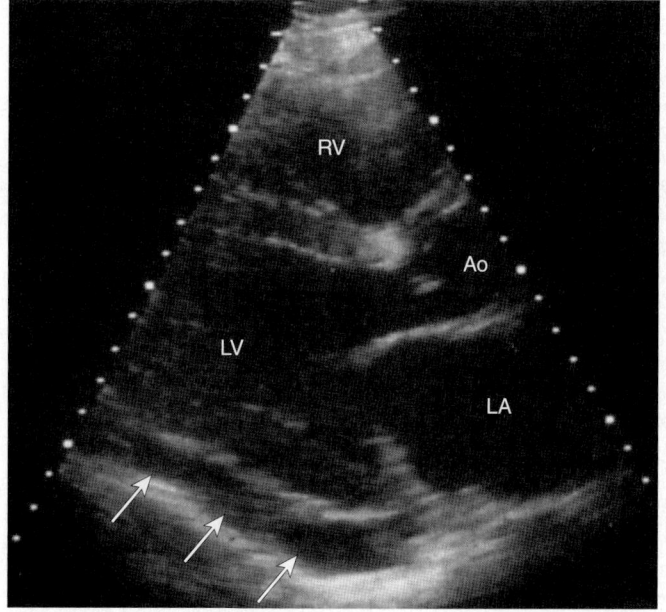

FIG. 58 Echocardiographic findings in a small to moderate pericardial effusion *(white arrows)*. *Ao,* Aortic root; *LA,* left atrium; *LV,* left ventricle; *RV,* right ventricle. (From Vincent JL et al: *Textbook of critical care,* ed 7, Philadelphia, 2017, Elsevier.)

Clinical Algorithms

III

ICD-10CM # I51.7   Cardiomegaly
Q24.8   Other specified congenital malformations of heart
I11.9   Hypertensive heart disease without heart failure
I11.0   Hypertensive heart disease with heart failure
Q23.8   Other congenital malformations of aortic and mitral valves

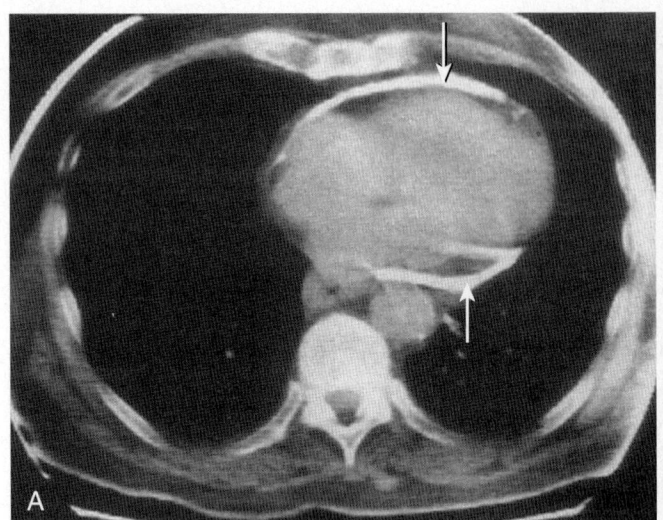 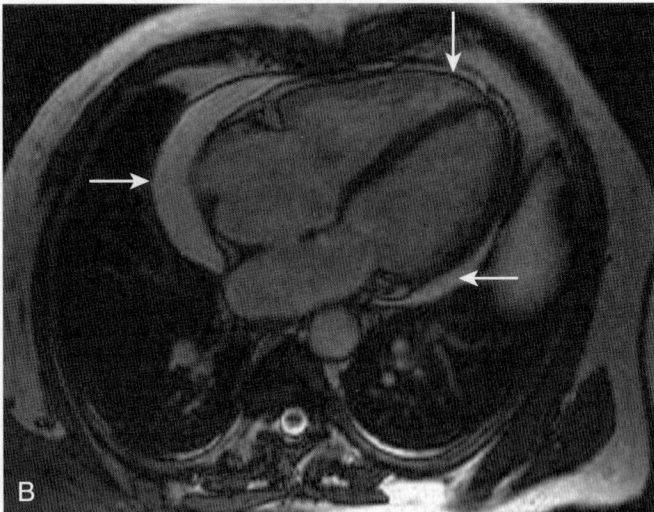

FIG. 59 A, Computed tomography findings in constrictive pericarditis. *White vertical arrows* are depicting thickened pericardium and pericardial calcification. **B,** The magnetic resonance imaging results of a patient with effusive-constrictive pericarditis are shown in the right image. *Horizontal arrows* show a loculated pericardial effusion, and the *vertical arrow* shows thickened pericardium. (From Vincent JL et al: *Textbook of critical care,* ed 7, Philadelphia, 2017, Elsevier.)

TABLE 39   Diagnosis of Cardiac Tamponade

Clinical presentation	Elevated systemic venous pressure,* hypotension,† pulsus paradoxus,‡ tachycardia,§ dyspnea, or tachypnea with clear lungs
Precipitating factors	Drugs (cyclosporine, anticoagulants, thrombolytics), recent cardiac surgery, indwelling instrumentation, blunt chest trauma, malignancies, connective tissue disease, renal failure, septicemia‖
ECG	Can be normal or nonspecifically changed (ST-T wave), electrical alternans (QRS, rarely T), bradycardia (end stage), electromechanical dissociation (agonal phase)
Chest radiograph	Enlarged cardiac silhouette with clear lungs
M-mode/two-dimensional echocardiogram	Diastolic collapse of the anterior RV free wall,¶ RA collapse, LA and rarely LV collapse, increased LV diastolic wall thickness "pseudohypertrophy," IVC dilation (no collapse in inspiration), "swinging heart"
Doppler	Tricuspid flow increases and mitral flow decreases during inspiration (reverse in expiration)
	Systolic and diastolic flows are reduced in systemic veins in expiration and reverse flow with atrial contraction is increased
M-mode color Doppler	Large respiratory fluctuations in mitral/tricuspid flows
Cardiac catheterization	Confirmation of the diagnosis and quantification of the hemodynamic compromise
	RA pressure is elevated (preserved systolic × descent and absent or diminished diastolic y descent)
	Intrapericardial pressure is also elevated and virtually identical to RA pressure (both pressures fall in inspiration)
	RV mid-diastolic pressure is elevated and equal to the RA and pericardial pressures (no dip-and-plateau configuration)
	Pulmonary artery diastolic pressure is slightly elevated and may correspond to the RV pressure
	Pulmonary capillary wedge pressure is also elevated and nearly equal to intrapericardial and right atrial pressure
	LV systolic and aortic pressures may be normal or reduced
	Documenting that pericardial aspiration is followed by hemodynamic improvement**
	Detection of coexisting hemodynamic abnormalities (LV failure, constriction, pulmonary hypertension)
	Detection of associated cardiovascular diseases (cardiomyopathy, coronary artery disease)
RV/LV angiography	Atrial collapse and small hyperactive ventricular chambers
Coronary angiography	Coronary compression in diastole

ECG, Electrocardiogram; *IVC,* inferior vena cava; *LA,* left atrium; *LV,* left ventricle; *QRS,* Q wave, R wave, S wave; *RA,* right atrium; *RV,* right ventricle.

*Jugular venous distention is less notable in hypovolemic patients or in "surgical tamponade." An inspiratory increase or lack of fall of pressure in the neck veins (Kussmaul sign), when verified by tamponade or after pericardial drainage, indicates effusive-constrictive disease.

†Heart rate is usually greater than 100 beats per min but may be lower in patients with hypothyroidism or uremia.

‡Pulsus paradoxus is defined as a drop in systolic blood pressure greater than 10 mm Hg during inspiration, while diastolic blood pressure remains unchanged. It is easily detected by simply feeling the pulse, which diminishes significantly during inspiration. Clinically significant pulsus paradoxus is apparent when the patient is breathing normally. When this sign is present only in deep inspiration, it should be interpreted with caution. The magnitude of pulsus paradoxus is evaluated by sphygmomanometry. If pulsus paradoxus is present, the first Korotkoff sound is not heard equally well throughout the respiratory cycle but only during expiration at a given blood pressure. The blood pressure cuff is therefore inflated above the patient's systolic pressure. Then it is slowly deflated, while the clinician observes the phase of respiration. During deflation, the first Korotkoff sound is intermittent. Correlation with the patient's respiratory cycle identifies a point at which the sound is audible during expiration but disappears when the patient breathes in. As the cuff pressure drops further, another point is reached when the first blood pressure sound is audible throughout the respiratory cycle. The difference in systolic pressure between these two points is the clinical measure of pulsus paradoxus. Pulsus paradoxus is absent in tamponade complicating an atrial septal defect and in patients with significant aortic regurgitation.

§Occasional patients are hypertensive, especially if they have preexisting hypertension.

‖Febrile tamponade may be misdiagnosed as septic shock.

¶Right ventricular collapse can be absent in elevated right ventricular pressure and right ventricular hypertrophy or in right ventricular infarction.

**If after drainage of the pericardial effusion, the intrapericardial pressure does not fall below atrial pressure, effusive-constrictive disease should be considered.

From Vincent JL et al: *Textbook of critical care,* ed 7, Philadelphia, 2017, Elsevier.

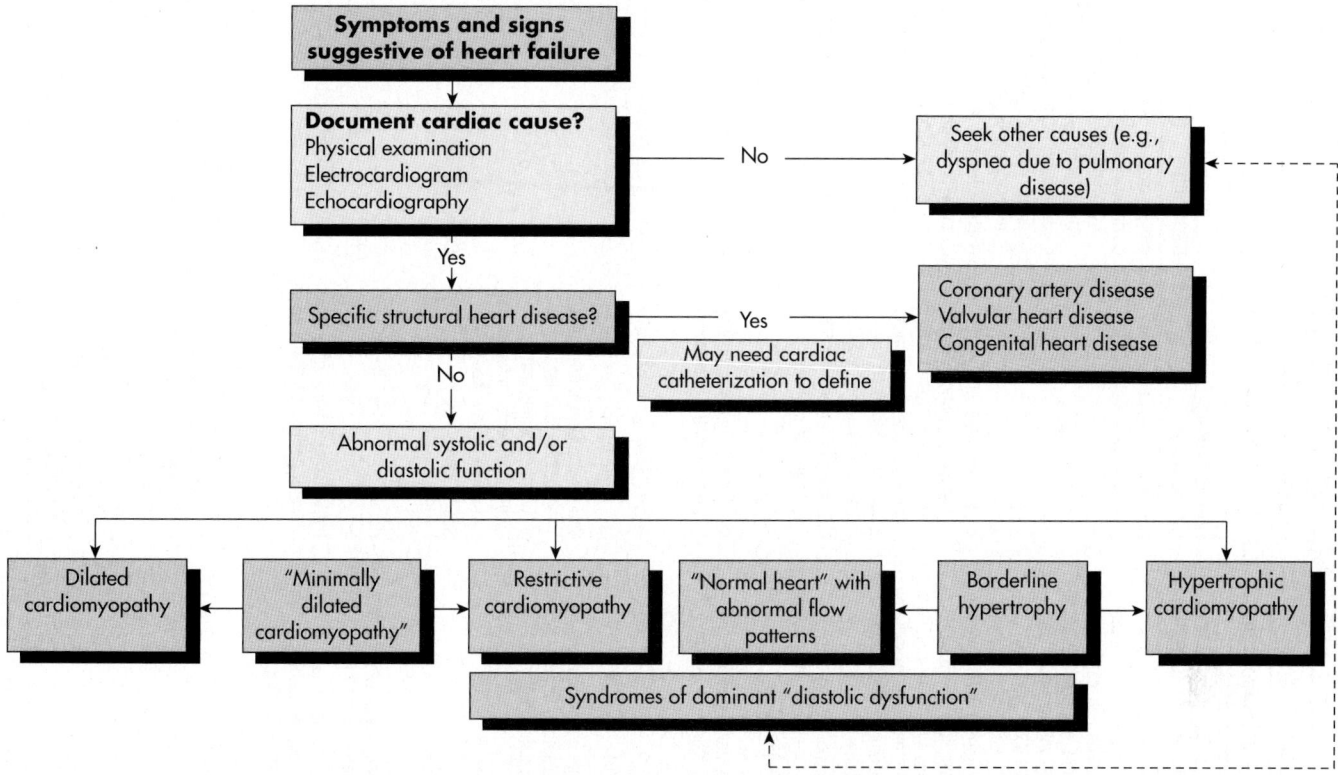

FIG. 60 Initial approach to classification of cardiomyopathy. The evaluation of symptoms or signs consistent with heart failure first includes confirmation that they can be attributed to a cardiac cause. Although this conclusion is often apparent from routine physical examination and electrocardiography, echocardiography serves to confirm cardiac disease and provides clues to the presence of other cardiac diseases, such as focal abnormalities suggesting primary valve disease or congenital heart disease. Having excluded these conditions, cardiomyopathy is generally considered to be dilated, restrictive, or hypertrophic, as shown in the figure. Patients with apparently normal cardiac structure and contraction are occasionally found to demonstrate abnormal intracardiac flow patterns consistent with diastolic dysfunction but should also be evaluated carefully for other causes of their symptoms. Most patients with so-called diastolic dysfunction also demonstrate at least borderline criteria for left ventricular hypertrophy, frequently in the setting of chronic hypertension and diabetes. A moderately decreased ejection fraction without marked dilation or a pattern of restrictive cardiomyopathy is sometimes referred to as minimally dilated cardiomyopathy, which may represent either a distinct entity or a transition between acute and chronic disease. (From Goldman L, Schafer AI: *Goldman Cecil medicine,* ed 25, Philadelphia, 2016, Saunders.)

Clinical Algorithms

III

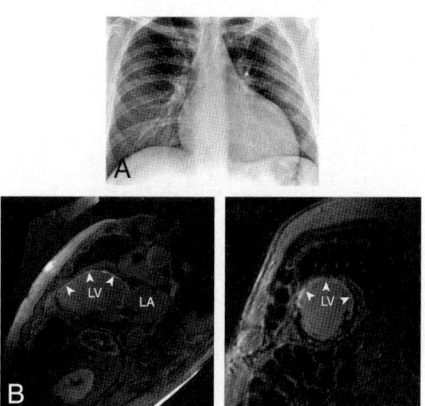

FIG. 61 Dilated cardiomyopathy. A, The heart shows enlargement of all four chambers. The azygos vein and superior vena cava are slightly dilated, reflecting high central venous pressure. **B,** Delayed enhanced magnetic resonance images demonstrate ischemic dilated cardiomyopathy. Extensive subendocardial delayed hyperenhancement *(arrowheads)* demonstrates features of old myocardial infarction—it follows a vascular territory (the left anterior descending), it is based on the subendocardium, and there is thinning of the affected myocardium. *LA,* Left atrium; *LV,* left ventricle. (From Boxt LM, Abbara S: *Cardiac imaging: the requisites,* ed 4, Philadelphia, 2016, Elsevier.)

TABLE 40 Classification of the Cardiomyopathies by Phenome and Genome

Type	PHENOME			Systemic Conditions or Diseases, Clinically Relevant Features, Classic Risk Factors, Associations	GENOME	
	Morphology	Physiology	Pathology		Nonsyndromic, Usually Single Gene	Syndromic
Dilated (DCM)	LV/RV dilation with minimal or no wall thickening	Reduced contractility is the primary defect; variable degree of diastolic dysfunction	Myocyte hypertrophy; scattered fibrosis	Hypertension; alcohol use; thyrotoxicosis, myxedema; persistent tachycardia; toxins, e.g., chemotherapy, especially anthracyclines; radiation; pregnancy	Diverse gene ontology with >30 genes implicated	Diverse array of associated conditions, especially muscular dystrophies (MDs): Emery-Dreifuss MD, limb-girdle MD, Duchenne/Becker MD; Laing distal myopathy; Barth syndrome; Kearns-Sayre; others
Restrictive (RCM)	Usually normal chamber sizes; minimal wall thickening	Contractility normal or near-normal with a marked increase in end-diastolic filling pressure	Specific to type, diagnosis: Amyloid, iron, glycogen storage disease, others	Endomyocardial fibrosis, amyloid, sarcoid, scleroderma, Churg-Strauss syndrome, cystinosis, lymphoma, pseudoxanthoma elasticum, hypereosinophilic syndrome, carcinoid	If not associated with a systemic genetic disease (e.g., hemochromatosis), genetic cause found most commonly to result from sarcomeric gene mutations	Gaucher disease, hemochromatosis, Fabry disease, familial amyloidosis. Mucopolysaccharidoses, Noonan syndrome
Hypertrophic (HCM)	Usually normal or reduced internal chamber dimension; wall thickening pronounced, especially septal hypertrophy	Systolic function increased or normal	Myocyte hypertrophy, classically with disarray	Severe hypertension can onfound clinical, morphologic diagnosis	Mutations of genes encoding sarcomeric proteins	Noonan/Leopard, Danon, Fabry, WPW, Friedrich ataxia, MERRF, MELAS
Arrhythmogenic cardiomyopathy (ACM)	Scattered fibrofatty infiltration, classically of the right ventricle but also commonly involving the left ventricle; RV dilation, LV dilation, or both are common although not universal	Ventricular arrhythmias (VT, VF) early or late; reduced contractility with progressive disease; can mimic DCM	Islands of fatty replacement; fibrosis	Palmoplantar keratoderma, wooly hair in Naxos syndrome	Mutations of genes encoding proteins of the desmosome	Naxos syndrome
Left ventricular noncompaction (LVNC)	Ratio of noncompacted to compacted myocardium increased; normal chamber dimensions varying to a DCM phenotype	Normal to reduced systolic function	Myocardium normal and ranging to findings consistent with other coexisting cardiomyopathy	Phenotype has been observed in the setting of other types of cardiomyopathy	Various cardiomyopathy genes associated but uncertain whether genetic cause or developmental defect during organogenesis; see text	See "RCM" above
Infiltrative	Usually thickened walls; occasional dilation	Restrictive physiology; systolic function usually mildly reduced	Specific to type, diagnosis: Amyloid, iron, glycogen storage disease, others		See "RCM" above	
Inflammatory	Normal or dilated without hypertrophy	Reduced systolic function	Inflammatory infiltrates	Hypereosinophilic syndrome (see text); acute myocarditis		
Ischemic	Normal or dilated without hypertrophy	Reduced systolic function	Areas of infarcted myocardium	Hypercholesterolemia, hypertension, diabetes, cigarette smoking, family history	Familial hypercholesterolemia; other heritable lipid disorders	Familial hypercholesterolemia
Infectious	Normal or dilated without hypertrophy	Reduced systolic function		Specific to infection	Viral (especially acute myocarditis); protozoal (e.g., Chagas); bacterial; direct infection (e.g., Lyme disease), or from acute cellular toxicity as a result of systemic toxins (Streptococcus, gram-negatives, etc.)	Genetic predisposition to infection and/or variable response to infective agent

LV, Left ventricle; MELAS, mitochondrial encephalopathy, lactic acidosis, and strokelike symptoms; MERRF, myoclonic epilepsy associated with ragged red fibers; RV, right ventricle; VF, ventricular fibrillation; VT, ventricular tachycardia; WPW, Wolff-Parkinson-White syndrome.

From Mann DL et al: Braunwald's heart disease, ed 10, Philadelphia, 2015, Elsevier.

CHEST PAIN

ICD-10CM # R07.4 Pain(s) chest
R07.2 Pain(s) heart
R07.3 Pain(s) chest anterior wall

1401

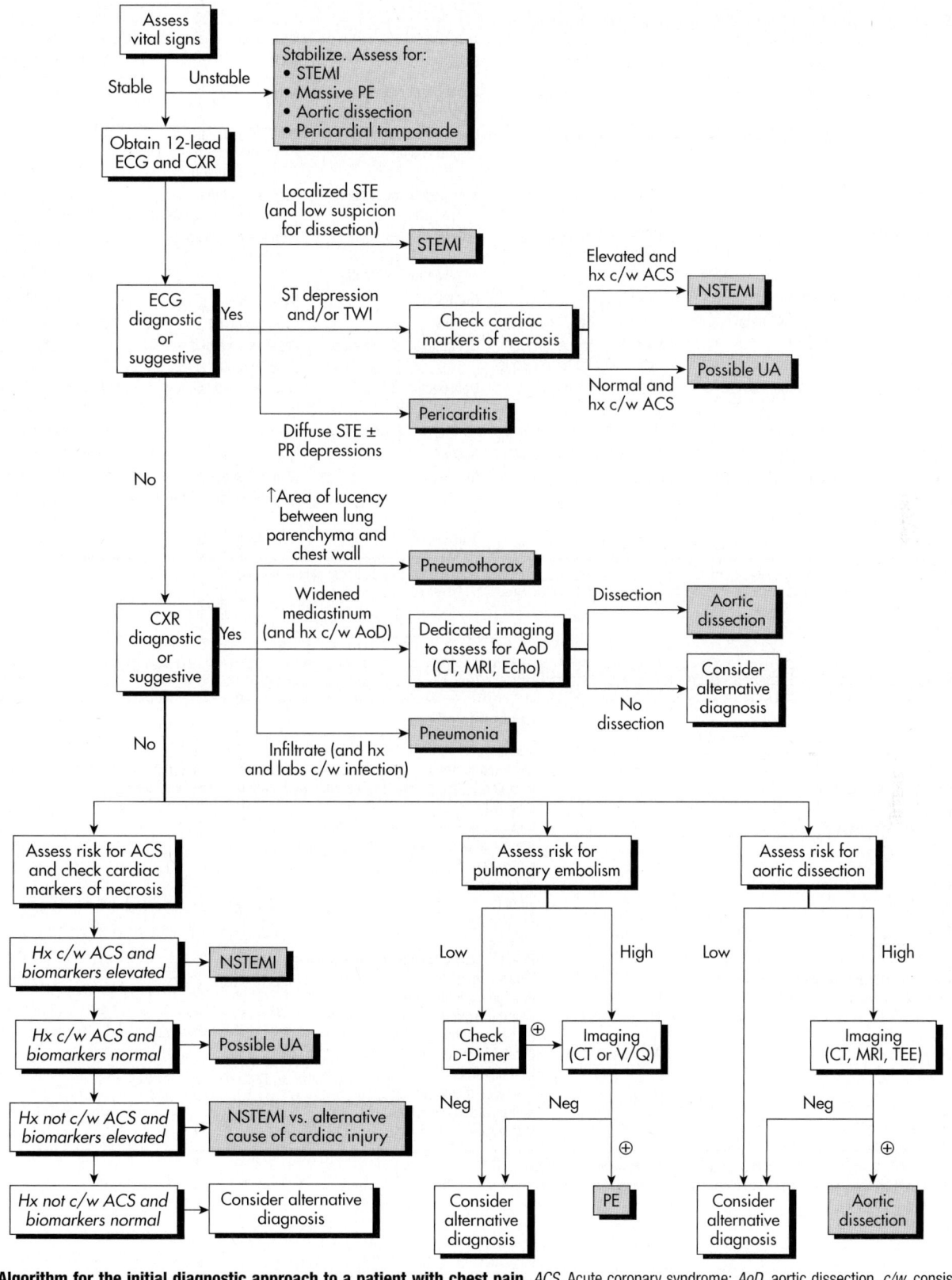

FIG. 63 Algorithm for the initial diagnostic approach to a patient with chest pain. *ACS,* Acute coronary syndrome; *AoD,* aortic dissection, *c/w,* consistent with; *CT,* computed tomography; *CXR,* chest x-ray; *ECG,* electrocardiogram; *Hx,* history; *NSTEMI,* non-ST-elevation myocardial infarction; *PE,* pulmonary embolism; *PR, STE,* ST elevation; *STEMI,* ST elevation myocardial infarction; *TEE,* transesophageal echocardiography; *TWI,* T wave inversion; *UA,* unstable angina; *V/Q,* ventilation-perfusion scan. (From Libby P et al: *Braunwald's heart disease, a textbook of cardiovascular medicine,* ed 12, Philadelphia, 2022, Elsevier.)

Clinical
Algorithms

ICD-10CM # R07.4 Pain(s) chest
R07.2 Pain(s) heart
R07.3 Pain(s) chest anterior wall

TABLE 41   Differential Diagnosis of Chest Pain in Adults

Diagnosis	Pain	Characteristics	ECG	CXR	Associated Features
Angina pectoris	Substernal, constricting	Transient, effort-related	Local ST depression; occasional elevation	Normal	Relief with NTG
MI	Substernal, crushing	Persistent, severe	Local ST elevation or depression	Possible vascular congestion or cardiomegaly	Relief with opiates; possible hypotension; ↑ troponin
Pulmonary embolism	Pleuritic	Sudden onset with dyspnea	Nonspecific; occasional RV strain	Normal or opacities ± small pleural effusion	Risk factor(s) for venous thrombosis
Pulmonary hypertension	Gradual onset	Associated with dyspnea, fatigue, and edema	Tall right precordial R waves, right axis deviation, RV strain	Prominent pulmonary arteries	Exclude pulmonary thromboembolism and interstitial lung disease
Bacterial pneumonia	Pleuritic	Onset in minutes to hours	Normal	Consolidation	Fever, productive cough
Pneumothorax	Sharp, unilateral	Sudden onset with dyspnea	Normal	Collapsed lung	Asthenic habitus, recurrence
Pericarditis	Pleuritic	Either side; gradual onset; pain referred to trapezius	Generalized ST elevation	Possible enlarged silhouette	Friction rub
Aortic dissection	Substernal, severe	Radiation to the back	Nonspecific; LVH or inferior MI	Widened mediastinum	Prostration, loss of pulse, aortic insufficiency
Esophageal spasm/reflux	Substernal	May mimic angina; burning	Normal or ST-T changes	Normal	Relief with NTG or antacids
Costochondritis	Dull-achy, localized	↑ by cough or deep breath	Normal	Normal	Localized tenderness
Mediastinitis	Interscapular, upper back, can be pleuritic	Severe	Normal	Widened mediastinum, mediastinal emphysema	Associated with fever, odynophagia
Herpes zoster	Sharp, unilateral	Dysesthesia	Normal	Normal	Vesicular rash

CXR, Chest x-ray; *ECG,* electrocardiography; *LVH,* left ventricular hypertrophy; *MI,* myocardial infarction; *NTG,* nitroglycerin; *RV,* right ventricular.
From Broaddus VC et al: *Murray & Nadel's textbook of respiratory medicine,* ed 7, Philadelphia, 2022, Elsevier.

TABLE 42   Differential Diagnosis of Pediatric Chest Pain

Common	Uncommon/Rare
Musculoskeletal	Cardiac
Costochondritis	Ischemia (coronary artery abnormalities, severe AS or PS, HOCM, cocaine)
Trauma or muscle overuse/strain	Infection/inflammation (myocarditis, pericarditis, Kawasaki disease)
Pulmonary	Dysrhythmia
Asthma (often exercise induced)	Musculoskeletal
Severe cough	Abnormalities of rib cage/thoracic spine
Pneumonia	Tietze syndrome
Gastrointestinal	Slipping rib
Reflux esophagitis	Tumor
Psychogenic	Pulmonary
Anxiety, hyperventilation	Pleurisy
Miscellaneous	Pneumothorax, pneumomediastinum
Precordial catch syndrome (Texidor twinge)	Pleural effusion
Sickle cell vasoocclusive crisis	Pulmonary embolism
Idiopathic	Gastrointestinal
	Esophageal foreign body
	Esophageal spasm
	Psychogenic
	Conversion symptoms
	Somatization disorders
	Depression

AS, Aortic stenosis; *HOCM,* hypertrophic obstructive cardiomyopathy; *PS,* pulmonary stenosis.
From Marcdante KJ et al: *Nelson essentials of pediatrics,* ed 9, Philadelphia, 2023, Elsevier.

CHEST PAIN—cont'd

ICD-10CM # R07.4 Pain(s) chest
R07.2 Pain(s) heart
R07.3 Pain(s) chest anterior wall

1403

TABLE 43 Pivotal Findings in Physical Examination

Sign	Finding	Diagnoses
Appearance	Acute respiratory distress	PE, tension pneumothorax, acute MI, pneumothorax
	Diaphoresis	Acute MI, aortic dissection, coronary ischemia, PE, esophageal rupture, unstable angina, cholecystitis, perforated peptic ulcer
Vital signs	Hypotension	Tension pneumothorax, PE, acute MI, aortic dissection (late), coronary ischemia, esophageal rupture, pericarditis, myocarditis
	Tachycardia	Acute MI, PE, aortic dissection, coronary ischemia, tension pneumothorax, esophageal rupture, coronary spasm, pericarditis, myocarditis, mediastinitis, cholecystitis, esophageal tear (Mallory-Weiss)
	Bradycardia	Acute MI, coronary ischemia, unstable angina
	Hypertension	Acute MI, coronary ischemia, aortic dissection (early)
	Fever	PE, esophageal rupture, pericarditis, myocarditis, mediastinitis, cholecystitis
	Hypoxemia	PE, tension pneumothorax, pneumothorax
Cardiovascular examination	Significant difference in upper extremity blood pressures	Aortic dissection
	Narrow pulse pressure	Pericarditis (with effusion)
	New murmur	Acute MI, aortic dissection, coronary ischemia
	S3-S4 gallop	Acute MI, coronary ischemia
	Pericardial rub	Pericarditis
	Audible systolic "crunch" on cardiac auscultation (Hamman sign)	Esophageal rupture, mediastinitis
	JVD	Acute MI, coronary ischemia, tension pneumothorax, PE, pericarditis
Pulmonary examination	Unilateral diminished or absent breath sounds	Tension pneumothorax, pneumothorax
	Pleural rub	PE
	Subcutaneous emphysema	Tension pneumothorax, esophageal rupture, pneumothorax, mediastinitis
	Rales	Acute MI, coronary ischemia, table angina
Abdominal examination	Epigastric tenderness	Esophageal rupture, esophageal tear, cholecystitis, pancreatitis
	Left upper quadrant tenderness	Pancreatitis
	Right upper quadrant tenderness	Cholecystitis
Extremity examination	Unilateral leg swelling, warmth, pain, tenderness, or erythema	PE
Neurologic examination	Focal findings	Aortic dissection
	Stroke	Acute MI
	Coronary ischemia	Aortic dissection, coronary spasm

JVD, Jugular venous distention; *MI,* myocardial infarction; *PE,* pulmonary embolism.
From Walls RM et al: *Rosen's emergency medicine, concepts and clinical practice,* ed 10, Philadelphia, 2023, Elsevier.

Clinical
Algorithms

TABLE 44 Electrocardiographic Findings in Ischemic Chest Pain

	Findings
Classic myocardial infarction	ST segment elevation (>1 mm) in contiguous leads; new LBBB
	Q waves > 0.04-s duration
Subendocardial infarction	T wave inversion or ST segment depression in concordant leads
Unstable angina	Most often normal or nonspecific changes; may see T wave inversion
Pericarditis	Diffuse ST segment elevation; PR segment depression

LBBB, Left bundle branch block.
From Walls RM et al: *Rosen's emergency medicine, concepts and clinical practice,* ed 10, Philadelphia, 2023, Elsevier.

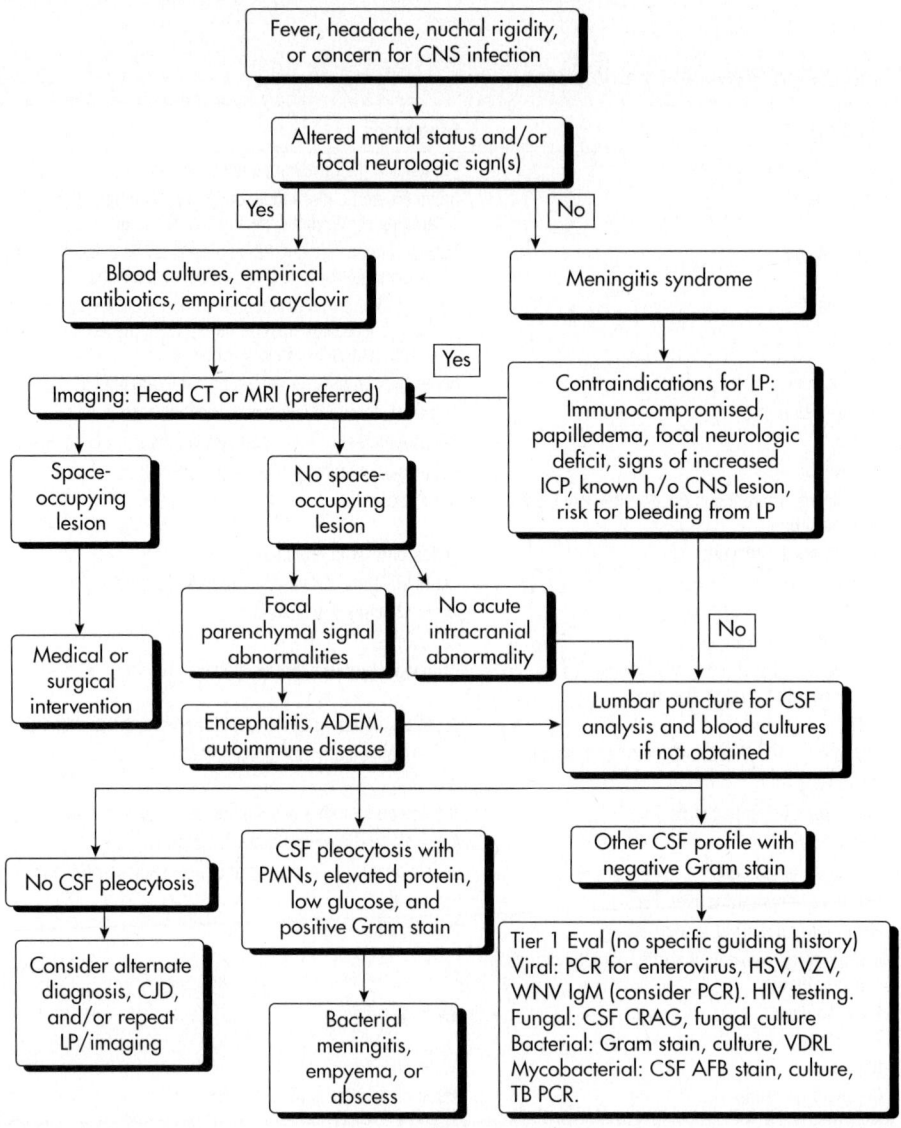

FIG. 64 **Approach to the patient with possible central nervous system** *(CNS)* **infection.** *ADEM,* Acute disseminated encephalomyelitis; *AFB,* acid-fast bacilli; *CJD,* Creutzfeldt-Jakob disease; *CSF,* cerebrospinal fluid; *CRAG,* cryptococcal antigen; *CT,* computed tomography; *HIV,* human immunodeficiency virus; *HSV,* herpes simplex virus; *ICP,* intracranial pressure; *IgM,* immunoglobulin M; *LP,* lumbar puncture; *MRI,* magnetic resonance imaging; *PCR,* polymerase chain reaction; *PMN,* polymorphonuclear leukocyte; *TB,* tuberculosis; *VDRL,* Venereal Disease Research Laboratory; *VZV,* varicella zoster virus; *WNV,* West Nile virus. Tier 1 evaluation described. See text for subsequent evaluation based on exposures. (From Bennett JE et al: *Mandell, Douglas, and Bennett's principles and practice of infectious diseases,* ed 9, Philadelphia, 2020, Elsevier.)

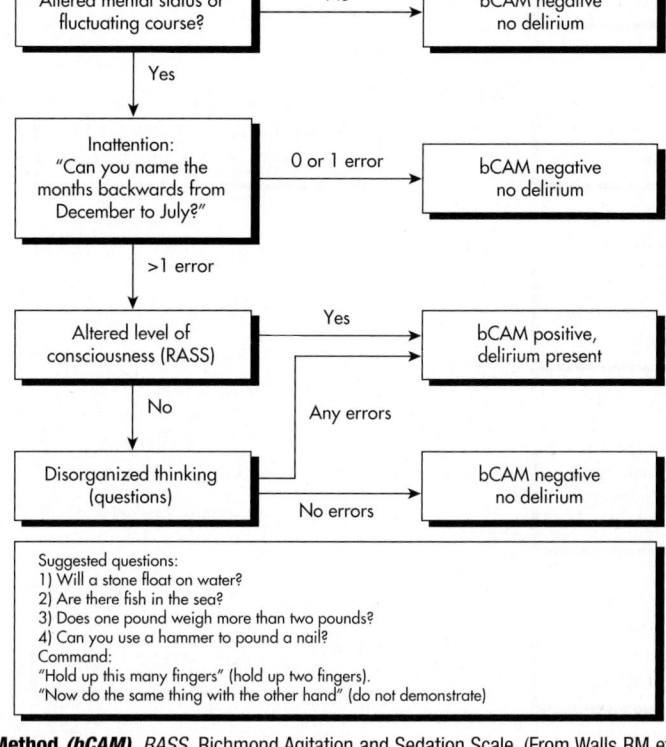

FIG. 65 Brief Confusion Assessment Method *(bCAM)*. *RASS,* Richmond Agitation and Sedation Scale. (From Walls RM et al: *Rosen's emergency medicine, concepts and clinical practice,* ed 10, Philadelphia, 2023, Elsevier.)

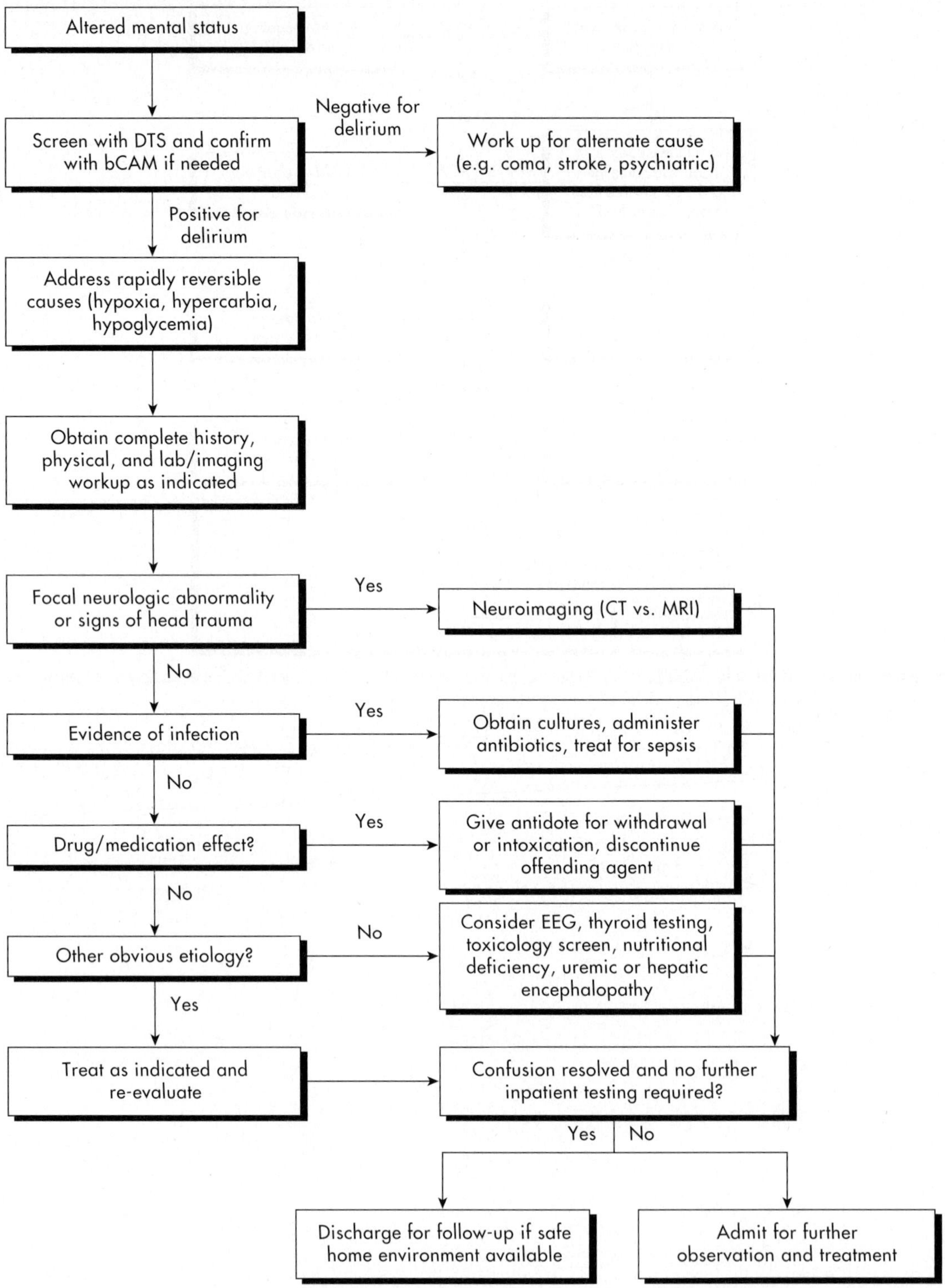

FIG. 66 Diagnostic algorithm for confusion. *bCAM,* Brief Confusion Assessment Method; *CT,* computed tomography; *DTS,* Delirium Triage Screen; *EEG,* electroencephalography; *MRI,* magnetic resonance imaging. (From Walls RM et al: *Rosen's emergency medicine, concepts and clinical practice,* ed 10, Philadelphia, 2023, Elsevier.)

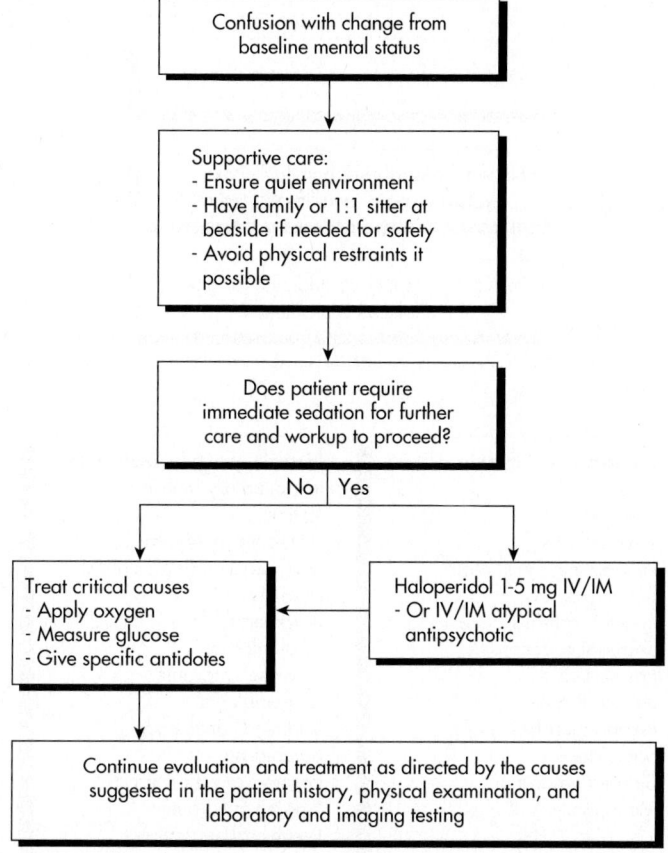

FIG. 67 **Management algorithm for confusion.** *IM,* Intramuscular; *IV,* intravenous. (From Walls RM et al: *Rosen's emergency medicine, concepts and clinical practice,* ed 10, Philadelphia, 2023, Elsevier.)

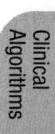

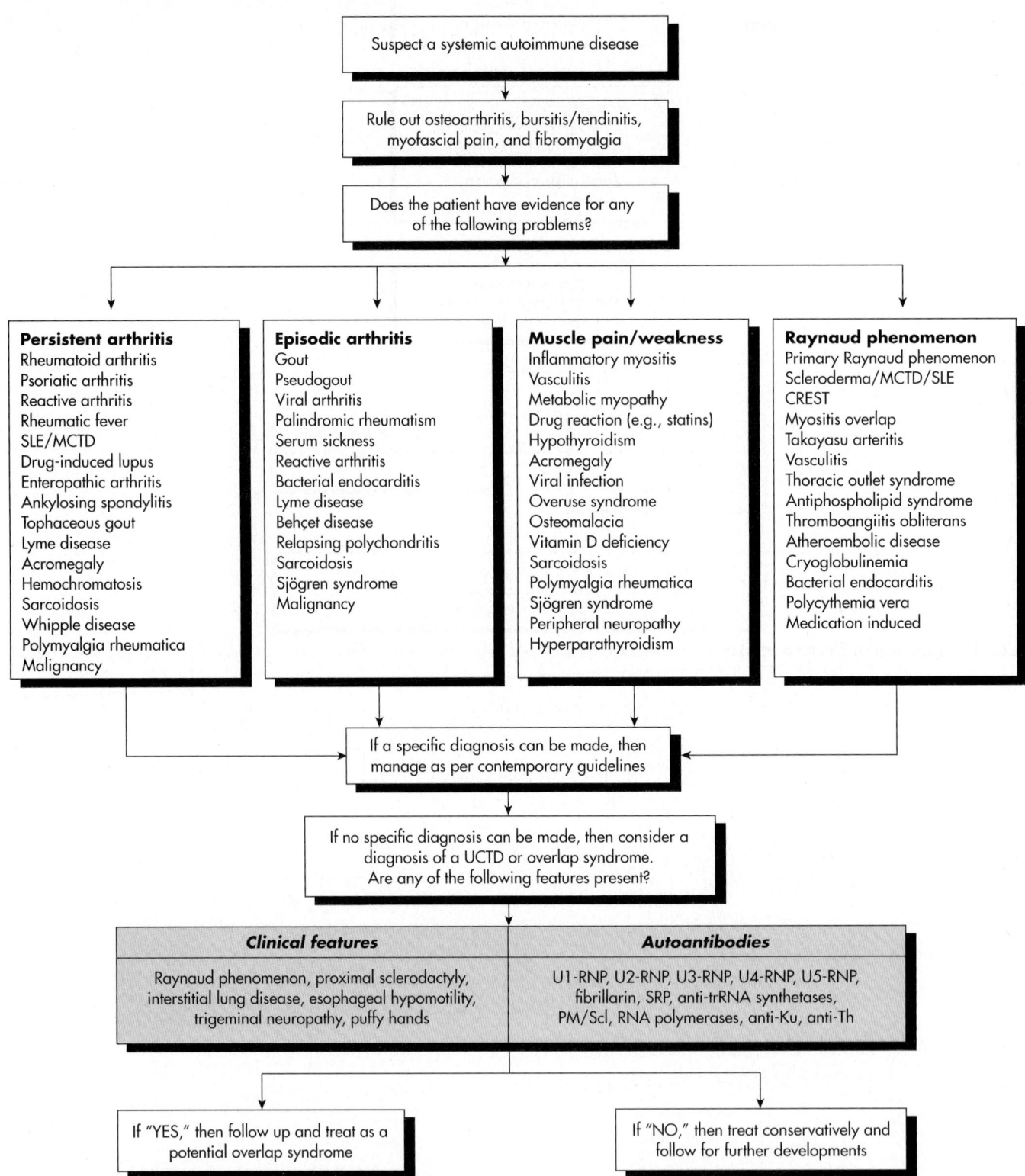

FIG. 68 Algorithm for evaluating patients with undifferentiated connective tissue disease (UCTD). *CREST,* Calcinosis, Raynaud phenomenon, esophageal dysmotility, sclerodactyly, and telangiectasia; *MCTD,* mixed connective tissue disease; *PM/Scl,* polymyositis/scleroderma; *RNA,* ribonucleic acid; *SLE,* systemic lupus erythematosus; *SRP,* signal recognition particle; *trRNA,* transfer ribonucleic acid; *UCTD,* undifferentiated connective tissue disease. (From Firestein GS et al: *Kelley and Firestein's textbook of rheumatology,* ed 10, Philadelphia, 2017, Elsevier.)

CONNECTIVE TISSUE LABORATORY SCREENING TESTS

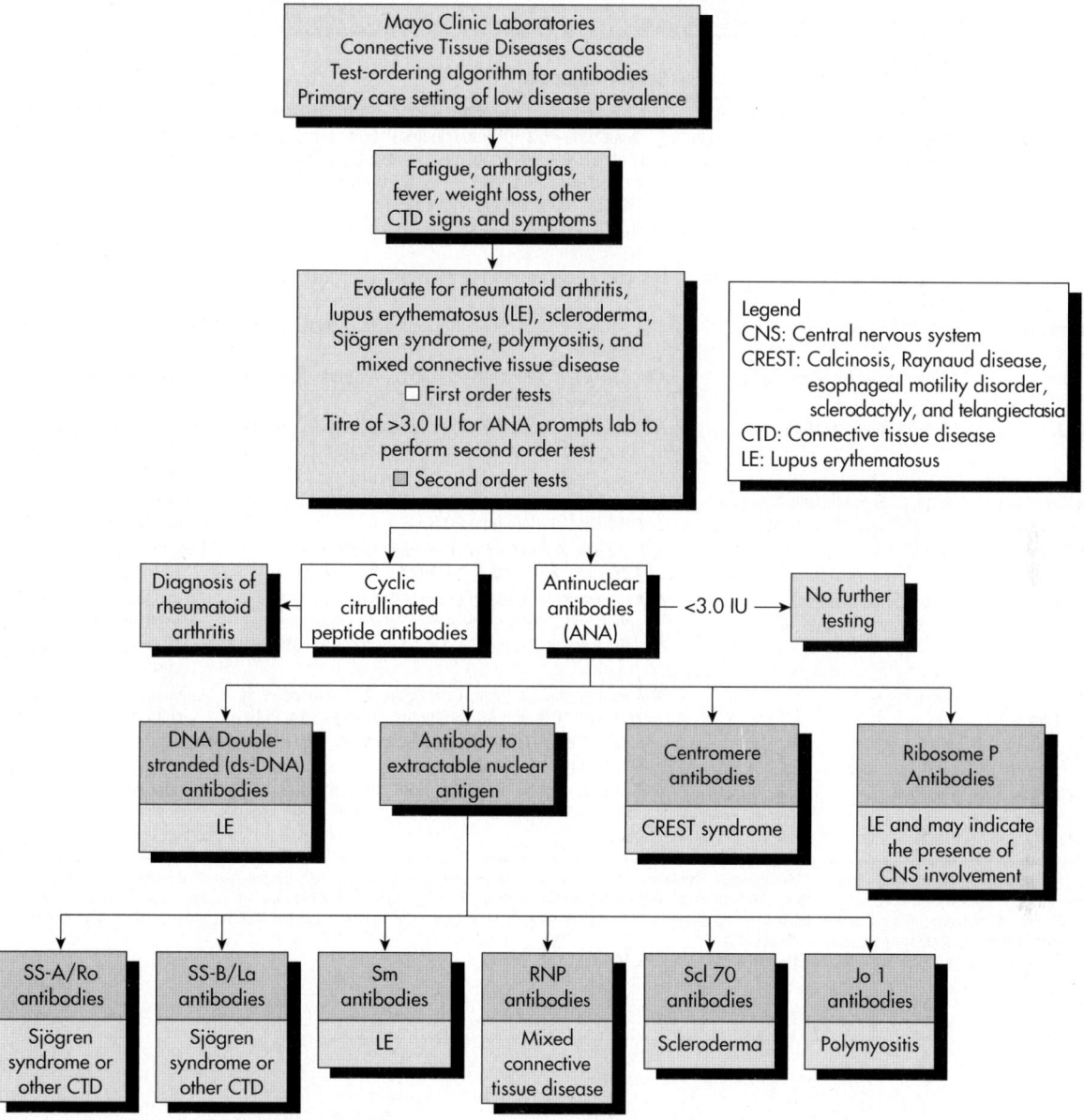

FIG. 69 Algorithm for connective tissue laboratory screening tests. (From Habif TP: *Clinical dermatology, a color guide to diagnosis and therapy,* ed 6, Philadelphia, 2016, Elsevier.)

TABLE 45 Autoantibody Tests for Connective Tissue Diseases

Antibody	Clinical Significance
Antinuclear antibodies	Screening for SLE and PSS
Centromere antibodies	Marker for CREST
Histone antibodies	To exclude drug-induced LE
ENA: Sm antibodies	Marker for SLE
RNP antibodies	SLE, MCTD, scleroderma
SS-A (Ro)/SS-B (La) antibodies	SLE, Sjögren syndrome, SCLE, and others
Scl-70 antibodies	Marker for scleroderma
Jo-1 antibodies	Marker for polymyositis
Ku (Ki) antibodies	Polymyositis/scleroderma overlap, SLE
Phospholipid antibodies (lupus anticoagulant)	Marker for SLE subset with thrombosis: Frequent aborters

CREST, Calcinosis, Raynaud phenomenon, esophageal dysmotility, sclerodactyly, and telangiectasia; *ENA,* extractable nuclear antigen; *LE,* lupus erythematosus; *MCTD,* mixed connective tissue disease; *PSS,* progressive systemic sclerosis; *RNP,* ribonucleoprotein; *SCLE,* subacute cutaneous lupus erythematosus; *SLE,* systemic lupus erythematosus.
From Habif TP: *Clinical dermatology, a color guide to diagnosis and therapy,* ed 6, Philadelphia, 2016, Elsevier.

TABLE 46 Diagnostic Significance of Immunologic Findings in Serum and Skin Biopsies in Connective Tissue Diseases

Disease	Biopsy Findings: Direct Immunofluorescence	Serum Findings	Relevance
Systemic LE	LE band (granular immune deposits, IgG, and/or IgM) IgA, C3 at DEJ in lesional and/or normal skin (over 90% in sun-exposed skin)	ANA elevated titers (about 95%-99%); nDNA antibodies about 50%-75%; DNP antibodies <50%; Sm antibodies in about 20%; RNP antibodies in about 5%-30%; SS-A antibodies in about 30%-40%; SS-B antibodies in about 1%-15%; phospholipid antibodies in about 30%-50%; PCNA antibodies in about 2%-10%; Ku(Ki) antibodies in about 10%	DIF, ANA, and ENA usually diagnostic; nDNA and Sm antibodies are diagnostic markers
Discoid LE	LE band, mostly IgG and C in lesion ONLY	Essentially negative; ANA titers usually in normal range	LE band highly characteristic
Subacute, cutaneous LE	LE band in lesion	ANA positive in 70%; SS-A (Ro) antibodies positive in more than 60%	DIF and anti–SS-A (Ro) highly characteristic
Neonatal LE	LE band in lesion (about 50%)	ANA positive in 30%; antibodies to SS-A (Ro) in 100%; antibodies to SS-B (La) in about 60%	DIF and anti–SS-A (Ro) highly characteristic
Drug-induced LE	LE band in lesion (rare)	ANA positive in more than 90%; histone positive about 90%; other antibodies to nDNA and ENA negative	DIF and histone antibodies in absence of other nuclear antibodies highly characteristic
Mixed connective tissue disease	Nuclear IgG or LE band in normal and/or lesional epidermis	Speckled ANA antibodies in more than 95% and RNP antibodies in more than 90%	Serology and/or DIF of nuclei diagnostic for MCTD, SLE, or PSS
Sjögren syndrome	Negative	ANA positive in about 55%; antibodies to SS-A (Ro) in 43%-88%; SS-B (La) in 14%-60%; RF positive	Positive serum results support diagnosis
Progressive systemic sclerosis (scleroderma)	Nucleolar IgG in epidermis in few cases; most negative	ANA (about 85%) speckled or nucleolar; centromere antibody in CREST (70%-90%); Scl-70 antibodies in diffuse sclerosis (45%) and in acrosclerosis (15%-20%)	DIF limited value; centromere antibodies are diagnostic marker in CREST; Scl-70 antibodies are diagnostic marker in scleroderma
Polymyositis/dermatomyositis	Negative	ANA usually positive (more than 80%); Jo-1 antibodies in 30% PM, 10% DM; SS-A (Ro) antibodies in 55% PM/scleroderma overlap; Ku (Ki) antibodies in 10% PM/scleroderma overlap	Limited value, but positive serum results support diagnosis
Rheumatoid arthritis	Negative	ANA usually negative or low titer; RF positive in about 90%; RNA positive in about 70%-90% and 95% of RF-negative cases	Positive serum results support diagnosis

ANA, Antinuclear antibodies; *CREST,* calcinosis, Raynaud phenomenon, esophageal dysmotility, sclerodactyly, and telangiectasia; *DEJ,* dermal-epidermal junction; *DIF,* direct immunofluorescence; *DM,* dermatomyositis; *DNP,* deoxyribonucleoprotein protein; *ENA,* extractable nuclear antigen; *Ig,* immunoglobulin; *LE,* lupus erythematosus; *MCTD,* mixed connective tissue disease; *nDNA,* nuclear deoxyribonucleic acid; *PCNA,* proliferating cell nuclear antigen; *PM,* polymyositis; *PSS,* progressive systemic sclerosis; *RF,* rheumatoid factor; *RNA,* antibodies to rheumatoid arthritis-associated nuclear antigen; *RNP,* ribonucleoprotein; *SLE,* systemic lupus erythematosus.

From Habif TP: *Clinical dermatology, a color guide to diagnosis and therapy,* ed 6, Philadelphia, 2016, Elsevier.

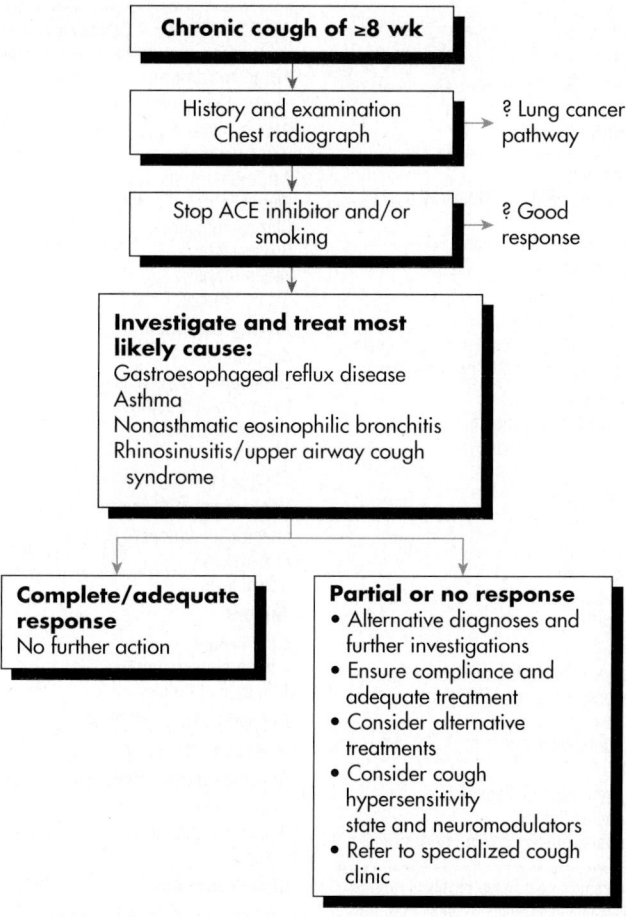

FIG. 71 Algorithm for the management of chronic cough in adult patients. For a chronic cough lasting for >8 wk, the evaluation and management should be methodical. After a thorough history and physical examination and chest imaging to exclude lung cancer or other intrathoracic pathology, and after stopping angiotensin-converting enzyme (ACE) inhibitor and/or smoking, the workup proceeds through the most common likely entities. These are listed as gastroesophageal reflux disease, asthma, nonasthmatic eosinophilic bronchitis and rhinosinusitis, or upper airway cough syndrome. Exclusion can be determined either by investigations or trial of therapy or both. Ultimately, patients with persistent chronic cough can be referred to specialized cough clinics for alternative diagnosis and treatment. (From Broaddus VC et al: *Murray & Nadel's textbook of respiratory medicine,* ed 7, Philadelphia, 2022, Elsevier.)

TABLE 47   Testing Characteristics of Diagnostic Protocol for Evaluation of Chronic Cough

Tests	Diagnosis	Positive Predictive Value (%)	Negative Predictive Value (%)
Sinus radiograph	Sinusitis	57-81	95-100
Methacholine inhalation challenge	Asthma	60-82	100
Modified barium esophagography	GERD, esophageal stricture	38-63	63-93
Esophageal pH*	GERD	89-100	>100
Bronchoscopy	Endobronchial mass/lesion	50-89	100

GERD, Gastroesophageal reflux disease.
*24-h esophageal pH monitoring.
From Goldman L, Schafer AI (eds): *Goldman's Cecil medicine,* ed 24, Philadelphia, 2012, Saunders.

TABLE 48 Definitions and Common Causes of Cough in Adults and Children

Age Group	Type of Cough	Duration (wk)	Common Causes
Adults	Acute	<3	Common cold Exacerbation of lung disease (e.g., asthma) Acute environmental exposure Acute cardiopulmonary disease
	Subacute	3-8	Postinfectious cough Pertussis infection Exacerbation of underlying lung disease (e.g., asthma, COPD, bronchiectasis)
	Chronic	>8	ACEI therapy Smoking/chronic bronchitis Underlying lung disease UACS Asthma NAEB GERD
Children	Acute	<4	Common cold Exacerbation of underlying lung disease Acute cardiopulmonary disease
	Chronic	>4	Asthma Protracted bacterial bronchitis Tracheobronchomalacia Chronic rhinosinusitis Recurrent aspiration GERD Underlying lung disease (e.g., bronchiectasis) Pulmonary infections (e.g., pertussis)

ACEI, Angiotensin-converting enzyme inhibitor; *COPD,* chronic obstructive pulmonary disease; *GERD,* gastroesophageal reflux disease; *NAEB,* nonasthmatic eosinophilic bronchitis; *UACS,* upper airway cough syndrome.
From Adkinson NF et al: *Middleton's allergy principles and practice,* ed 8, Philadelphia, 2014, Saunders.

TABLE 49 Common Causes of Cough

Acute Infections
Tracheobronchitis
Bronchopneumonia
Viral pneumonia
Acute-on-chronic bronchitis
Pertussis
Chronic infections
Bronchiectasis
Tuberculosis
Cystic fibrosis

Airway Diseases
Asthma
Eosinophilic bronchitis
Cough-variant asthma
Chronic bronchitis
COPD
Chronic postnasal drip

Parenchymal Diseases
Interstitial pulmonary fibrosis
Emphysema
Sarcoidosis

Tumors
Lung cancer
Benign airway tumors
Mediastinal tumors

Aspirated Foreign Bodies
Middle ear pathology

Cardiovascular Diseases
Left ventricular failure
Pulmonary infarction
Aortic aneurysm

Other Diseases
Gastroesophageal reflux disease
Laryngopharyngeal reflux
Recurrent microaspiration
Endobronchial sutures
Obstructive sleep apnea
Laryngeal dysfunction
Drugs
Angiotensin-converting enzyme inhibitors

From Broaddus VC et al: *Murray & Nadel's textbook of respiratory medicine,* ed 7, Philadelphia, 2022, Elsevier.

TABLE 50 Diagnostic Evaluation of Chronic Cough

- History and physical examination.
- Chest radiograph, particularly in smokers.
- Initial evaluation may lead to diagnosis of chronic bronchitis in cigarette smokers and of angiotensin-converting enzyme inhibitor cough. Discontinue cigarette smoking and offending drug.
- Further diagnostic evaluation on basis of initial evaluation:
  If suggestive of postnasal drip, order a computed tomography (CT) scan of sinuses, and allergy tests.
  If suggestive of asthma, request a record of peak expiratory flow measurements at home for 2 wk and a bronchoprovocation test with histamine or methacholine, and/or a trial of antiasthma treatment.
  If suggestive of gastroesophageal reflux disease, request 24-h pH monitoring and, if necessary, an endoscopic examination of the esophagus or a barium swallow series.
  If the chest radiograph is abnormal, consider examination of sputum and a fiberoptic bronchoscopy. A high-resolution CT scan of the thorax and further lung function evaluation may be necessary.
- Treat specifically for associated conditions. The cause(s) of cough is (are) determined when specific therapies eliminate or improve the cough. There may be more than one associated cause for the cough.

From Broaddus VC et al: *Murray & Nadel's textbook of respiratory medicine,* ed 7, Philadelphia, 2022, Elsevier.

TABLE 51   Potential Complications from Excessive Cough

Respiratory

Pneumothorax
Subcutaneous emphysema
Pneumomediastinum
Pneumoperitoneum
Laryngeal damage

Cardiovascular

Cardiac dysrhythmias
Loss of consciousness

Central Nervous System

Syncope
Headaches
Cerebral air embolism

Musculoskeletal

Intercostal muscle pain
Rupture of rectus abdominis muscle
Increase in serum creatine phosphokinase
Cervical disc prolapse

Gastrointestinal

Esophageal perforation

Other

Social embarrassment
Depression
Sleep disruption

Urinary incontinence

Disruption of surgical wounds
Subconjunctival hemorrhage
Petechiae
Purpura

From Broaddus VC et al: *Murray & Nadel's textbook of respiratory medicine,* ed 7, Philadelphia 2022, Elsevier.

TABLE 52   Treatments for Chronic Cough

Treating the Specific Underlying Cause(s)

Asthma, cough-variant asthma	Bronchodilators and inhaled corticosteroids
Eosinophilic bronchitis	Inhaled corticosteroids; leukotriene inhibitors
Allergic rhinitis and postnasal drip	Topical nasal steroids and antihistamines
	Topical nasal anticholinergics (with antibiotics, if indicated)
Gastroesophageal reflux	Conservative measures
	Histamine H_2-antagonist or proton pump inhibitor
Angiotensin-converting enzyme inhibitor	Discontinue and replace with alternative drug such as angiotensin II receptor antagonist
Chronic bronchitis/COPD	Smoking cessation
	Treat for COPD
Bronchiectasis	Postural drainage
	Treat infective exacerbation and airflow obstruction
Infective tracheobronchitis	Appropriate antibiotic therapy
	Treat any postnasal drip

Symptomatic Antitussive Treatment: Neuromodulators (Only after Consideration of Cause of Cough)

Chronic cough (all)	Speech and language therapy
Chronic cough affecting quality of life	Amitriptyline
	Gabapentin
Chronic refractory cough	Slow-release morphine

From Broaddus VC et al: *Murray & Nadel's textbook of respiratory medicine,* ed 7, Philadelphia, 2022, Elsevier.

BOX 23 Pitfalls and Errors in the Diagnosis and Management of Chronic Cough in Adults

General Considerations
Failing to consider that UACS, asthma/NAEB, and/or GERD are likely when the chest radiograph is normal or near-normal in appearance and the patient is a nonsmoker and is not taking an ACEI
Failing to include UACS, asthma/NAEB, and/or GERD in the differential diagnosis because clinical or radiographic evidence confirms the presence of an "obvious" cause of the patient's cough (e.g., solitary pulmonary nodule, idiopathic pulmonary fibrosis)
Not recognizing multiple simultaneous causes of cough
Failing to continue treatment trials long enough to accurately assess their effectiveness
Prematurely diagnosing "unexplained" cough before a bronchoscopy has been performed to assess for unsuspected airway disease
Mistakenly diagnosing "unexplained" cough or diagnosing psychogenic cough before a complete evaluation for cough has been performed

Upper Airway Cough Syndrome
Failing to realize that UACS can manifest as cough productive of phlegm
Not recognizing that chronic cough can be the sole manifestation of UACS in at least 20% of the cases
Failing to consider sinusitis as a cause of UACS
Mistakenly assuming that selective histamine H_1 receptor antagonists are effective in treating nonallergic causes of UACS
Missing allergic rhinitis because symptoms are perennial
Missing aspirin-exacerbated disease in a patient with nasal polyps

Asthma/NAEB
Failing to realize that these conditions can sometimes manifest as cough productive of phlegm
Not recognizing that chronic cough can sometimes be the sole manifestation of asthma (so-called cough variant asthma)
Mistakenly assuming that a positive result on bronchial challenge (e.g., methacholine challenge) is diagnostic of asthma when it is merely consistent with the diagnosis
Failing to consider NAEB when the bronchial challenge test yields a negative result
Not recognizing that inhaled medications can sometimes provoke cough
Failing to consider occupational and environmental causes of asthma/NAEB

Gastroesophageal Reflux Disease
Failing to realize that GERD can sometimes manifest as cough productive of phlegm
Not recognizing that chronic cough can sometimes be the sole manifestation of GERD (so-called silent GERD)
Mistakenly concluding that cough cannot be due to GERD simply because cough does not resolve with relief of gastrointestinal symptoms
Not considering nonacid reflux and mistakenly assuming that cough will always respond to acid suppression
Failing to assess the adequacy of GERD treatment by using 24-h monitoring of esophageal pH and impedance
Not recognizing coexisting diseases (e.g., sleep apnea) and medications (e.g., nitrates, progesterone) that may impair the effectiveness of GERD treatment
Failing to recognize that surgery may help when intensive medical therapy has failed

Angiotensin-Converting Enzyme Inhibitor
Failing to consider ACEI therapy as a cause of chronic cough simply because the cough predated initiation of the ACEI
Mistakenly concluding that ACEI therapy is not the cause of chronic cough because the cough did not resolve within 1-3 wk of stopping the ACEI

ACEI, Angiotensin-converting enzyme inhibitor; *GERD*, gastroesophageal reflux disease; *NAEB*, thematicmatic eosinophilic bronchitis; *UACS*, upper airway cough syndrome.
From Adkinson NF et al: *Middleton's allergy principles and practice,* ed 8, Philadelphia, 2014, Saunders.

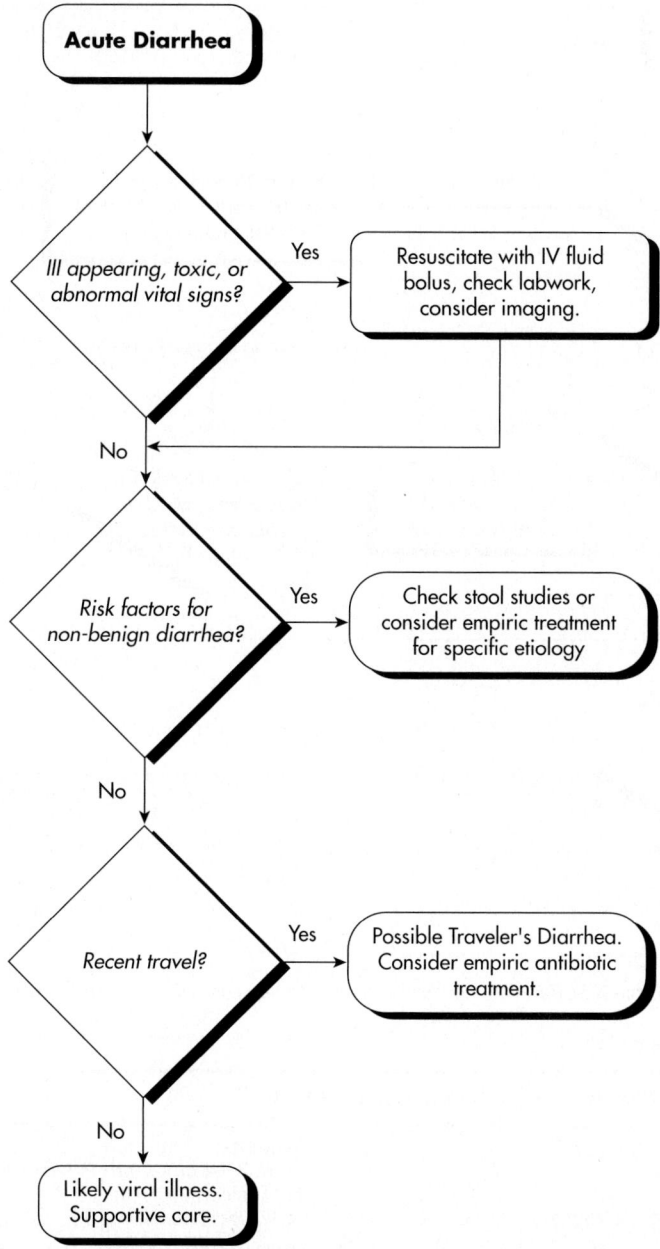

FIG. 76 Diagnostic algorithm. *IV,* Intravenous. (From Walls RM et al: *Rosen's emergency medicine, concepts and clinical practice,* ed 10, Philadelphia, 2023, Elsevier.)

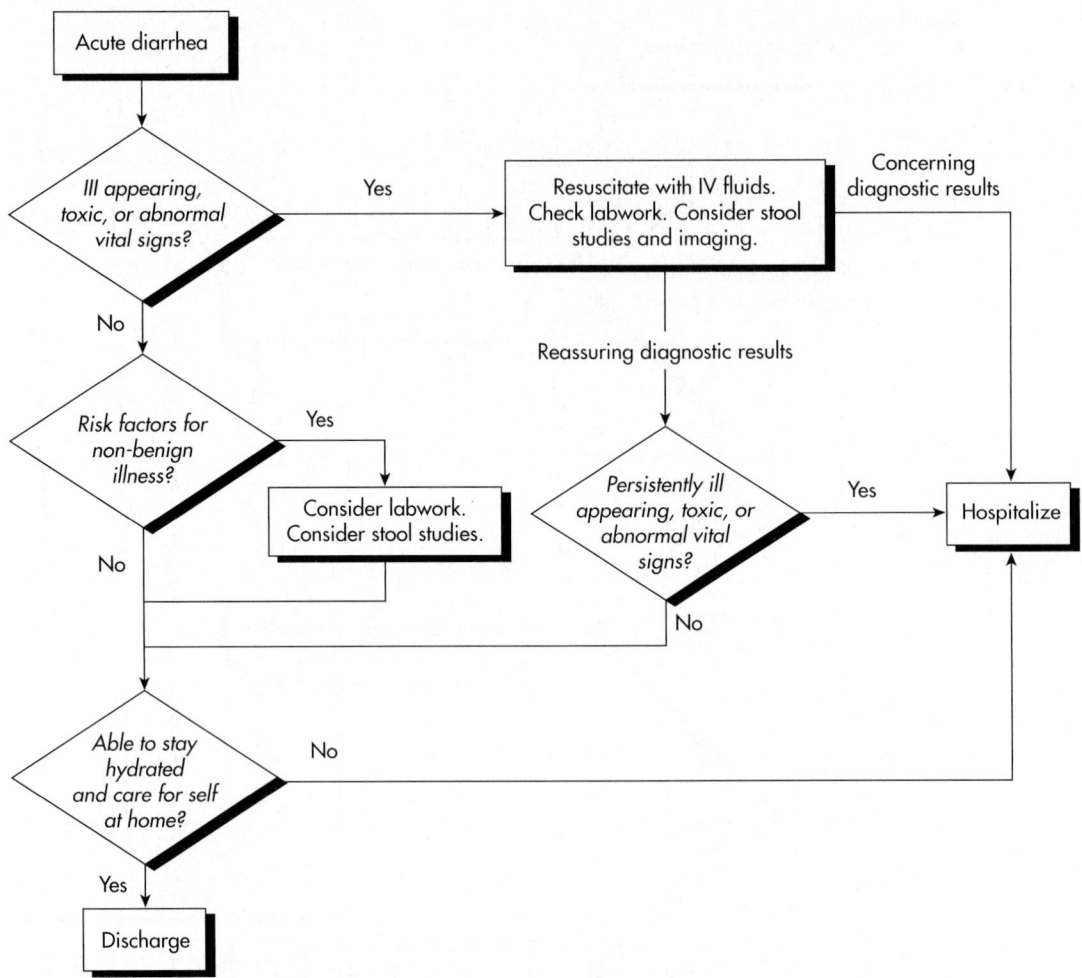

FIG. 77 Approach to disposition. (From Walls RM et al: *Rosen's emergency medicine, concepts and clinical practice,* ed 10, Philadelphia, 2023, Elsevier.)

BOX 24 Common Causative Agents of Acute Infectious Diarrhea

Viral
Cytomegalovirus
Enteric adenovirus
Human immunodeficiency virus (HIV) enteropathy
Norovirus
Rotavirus

Bacterial
Invasive
Campylobacter species
Clostridioides difficile
Enteroinvasive *Escherichia coli*
Salmonella species
Shigella species
Vibrio vulnificus
Yersinia enterocolitica

Toxigenic
Food Poisoning with Preformed Toxins
Bacillus cereus
Staphylococcus aureus

Toxin Formation after Colonization
Shiga toxin–producing *E. coli* 0157:H7 (STEC) [also known as enterohemorrhagic *E. coli* (EHEC) or verocytotoxin-producing *E. coli* (VTEC)]
Enterotoxigenic *E. coli*
Shigella species
Vibrio cholerae

Protozoa
Cryptosporidium
Cyclospora
Entamoeba histolytica
Giardia

From Walls RM et al: *Rosen's emergency medicine, concepts and clinical practice,* ed 10, Philadelphia, 2023, Elsevier.

BOX 25 Selected Causes of Noninfectious Diarrhea

Pharmaceuticals
Antacids (magnesium)
Antimicrobials
Antiretrovirals
Chemotherapeutic agents
Cholinergic agents
Cholinesterase inhibitors
Colchicine
Lactulose
Laxatives/cathartics
Prostaglandins

Dietetic Supplements
Caffeine
Sorbitol
Xylitol

Seafood-Associated Toxins
Ciguatera
Paralytic shellfish poisoning
Scombroid

Plant and Herbal Preparations
Aloe vera juice
Senna
Pokeweed
Turmeric

Miscellaneous
Pesticides—organophosphates
Opiate withdrawal

Gastrointestinal Pathology
Celiac disease
Irritable bowel syndrome with diarrhea
Lactose intolerance
Malabsorption syndromes
Post vagotomy
Radiation enteritis
Short gut syndrome

Endocrine-Related Conditions
Carcinoid syndrome
Adrenal insufficiency
Diabetic enteropathy
Pancreatic insufficiency

Systemic Illness and Other Causes
Alcoholism
Connective tissue disease/scleroderma
Cystic fibrosis
Runners diarrhea

From Walls RM et al: *Rosen's emergency medicine, concepts and clinical practice*, ed 10, Philadelphia, 2023, Elsevier.

TABLE 54 Epidemiology, Clinical Syndrome, Characteristic Virulence Factors, and Treatment Considerations for Diarrheagenic *Escherichia coli* Pathotypes

Pathotype	Epidemiology	Clinical Syndrome	Characteristic Virulence Factors	Treatment Considerations[a]
ETEC	Pediatric diarrhea, particularly in the developing world Traveler's diarrhea Foodborne outbreaks	Acute nonbloody diarrhea	Heat-labile (LT) and/or heat-stable toxin (ST) Heterogeneous adhesins; also called colonization factors (CFs)	Traveler's diarrhea[b]
EPEC	Pediatric diarrhea, particularly in the developing world Atypical EPEC (aEPEC) increasingly recognized to cause diarrhea regardless of age Traveler's diarrhea Nosocomial and child care center outbreaks	Acute nonbloody diarrhea Associated with vomiting and sometimes protracted disease	Attaching and effacing lesions (A/E) Typical EPEC (tEPEC) defined by type IV bundle-forming pili (BFP)	Traveler's diarrhea[b] Antimicrobial therapy for severe endemic disease, including nosocomial outbreaks
STEC (including EHEC)	Foodborne outbreaks; person-to-person and animal contact transmission	Acute, often bloody diarrhea Can progress to hemolytic-uremic syndrome (HUS)	Shiga toxin EHEC produces attaching and effacing lesions (A/E) like EPEC	Antimicrobial and antimotility agents associated with increased risk of HUS
EAEC	Increasingly recognized to cause diarrhea in all ages, including developed countries Associated with growth impairment in children from developing countries Traveler's diarrhea Foodborne outbreaks	Acute nonbloody diarrhea Chronic diarrhea in some children and HIV patients	Aggregative adherence fimbriae (AAF) Enteroaggregative heat-stable toxin 1 (EAST-1) and several SPATE proteins	Traveler's diarrhea[b] Case reports support antimicrobial therapy for chronic disease in HIV patients
EIEC	Pediatric diarrhea, particularly in the developing world Foodborne outbreaks; person-to-person transmission	Acute, sometimes bloody diarrhea Clinically indistinguishable from shigellosis, although typically less severe	Cellular invasion then cell-to-cell spread orchestrated by *pInv* plasmid	Antimicrobial therapy recommended for severe cases, but must first exclude STEC
DAEC	Pediatric diarrhea in somewhat older children Not an established cause of diarrhea in adults	Acute nonbloody diarrhea	Afa/Dr family adhesins	
AIEC	Associated with Crohn disease pathogenesis, although not with diarrhea per se		Adherence to M cells of Peyer patches by type I and long polar fimbriae Cell invasion facilitated by membrane-bound protein OmpA	

AIEC, Adherent-invasive *E. coli*; *DAEC*, diffuse-adhering *E. coli*; *EAEC*, enteroaggregative *E. coli*; *EHEC*, enterohemorrhagic *E. coli*; *EIEC*, enteroinvasive *E. coli*; *EPEC*, enteropathogenic *E. coli*; *ETEC*, enterotoxigenic *E. coli*; *HIV*, human immunodeficiency virus; *SPATE*, serine protease autotransporters of the *Enterobacteriaceae*; *STEC*, Shiga toxin–producing *E. coli*.
[a]Volume resuscitation is the most important treatment for diarrhea regardless of etiology. Most diarrheagenic *E. coli* infections are self-limiting with supportive care.
[b]Data support the use of antimicrobial therapy for shortening the duration of traveler's diarrhea with loperamide in combination with single-dose azithromycin, levofloxacin, or rifaximin.
From Bennett JE et al: *Mandell, Douglas, and Bennett's principles and practice of infectious diseases*, ed 9, Philadelphia, 2020, Elsevier.

Clinical Algorithms

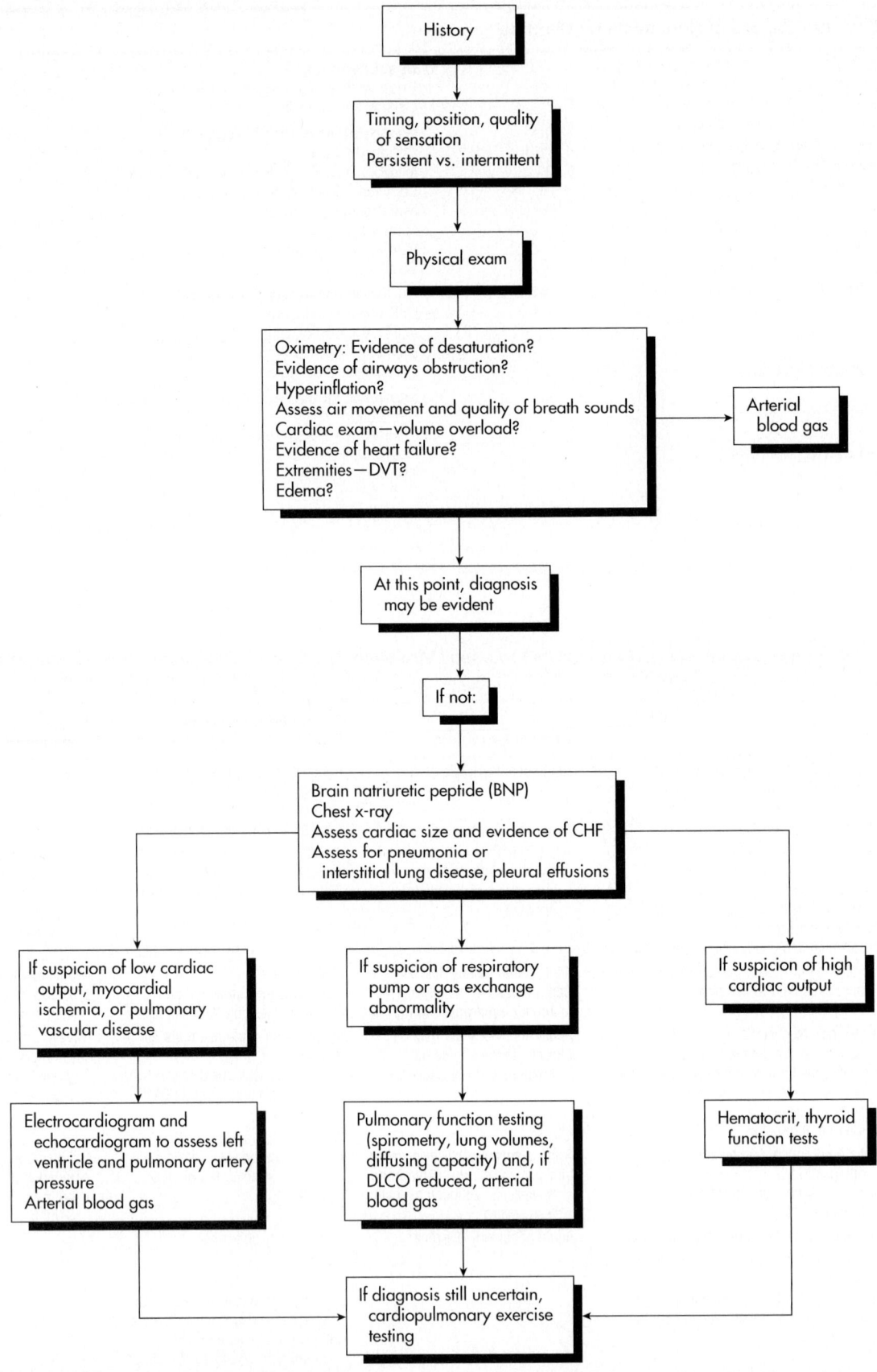

FIG. 80 Algorithm for the evaluation of the patient with dyspnea. The pace and completeness with which one approaches this framework depends on the intensity and acuity of the patient's symptoms. In a patient with severe, acute dyspnea, for example, an arterial blood gas measurement may be one of the first laboratory evaluations, whereas this measurement might not be obtained until much later in the workup in a patient with chronic breathlessness of unclear cause. A therapeutic trial of a medication, for example, a bronchodilator, may be instituted at any point if one is fairly confident of the diagnosis based on the data available at that time. *CHF,* Congestive heart failure; *DLCO,* diffusing capacity of the lung for carbon monoxide; *DVT,* deep venous thrombosis. (Modified from Schwartzstein RM, Feller-Kopman D: Approach to the patient with dyspnea. In Braunwald E, Goldman L [eds]: *Primary cardiology,* ed 2, Philadelphia, 2003, Saunders.)

TABLE 55 Differential Diagnoses for Acute Dyspnea

Organ System	Critical Diagnoses	Emergent Diagnoses	Nonemergent Diagnoses
Pulmonary	Airway obstruction	Spontaneous pneumothorax	Pleural effusion
	Pulmonary embolus	Asthma	Neoplasm
	Noncardiogenic edema	Cor pulmonale	Pneumonia (CAP score ≤70)
	Anaphylaxis	Aspiration	COPD
	Ventilatory failure	Pneumonia (CAP score >70)	
Cardiac	Pulmonary edema	Pericarditis	Congenital heart disease
	Myocardial infarction		Valvular heart disease
	Cardiac tamponade		Cardiomyopathy
Primarily Associated with Normal or Increased Respiratory Effort			
Abdominal		Mechanical interference	Pregnancy
		Hypotension, sepsis from ruptured viscus, bowel obstruction, inflammatory or infectious process	Ascites obesity
Psychogenic			Hyperventilation syndrome
			Somatization disorder
			Panic attack
Metabolic or endocrine	Toxic ingestion	Renal failure	Fever
	DKA	Electrolyte abnormalities	Thyroid disease
		Metabolic acidosis	
Infectious	Epiglottitis	Pneumonia (CAP score >70)	Pneumonia (CAP score ≤70)
Traumatic	Tension pneumothorax	Simple pneumothorax, hemothorax	Rib fractures
	Cardiac tamponade	Diaphragmatic rupture	
	Flail chest		
Hematologic	Carbon monoxide poisoning	Anemia	
	Acute chest syndrome		
Primarily Associated with Decreased Respiratory Effort			
Neuromuscular	CVA, intracranial insult	Multiple sclerosis	ALS
	Organophosphate poisoning	Guillain-Barré syndrome	Polymyositis
		Tick paralysis	Porphyria

ALS, Amyotrophic lateral sclerosis; *CAP*, community-acquired pneumonia; *COPD*, chronic obstructive pulmonary disease; *CVA*, cerebrovascular accident; *DKA*, diabetic ketoacidosis.
From Marx JA et al: *Rosen's emergency medicine*, ed 8, Philadelphia, 2014, Saunders.

Clinical
Algorithms

III

TABLE 56 Pivotal Findings in Physical Examination

Sign	Physical Finding	Diagnoses to Consider
Vital signs	Tachypnea	Pneumonia, pneumothorax
	Hypopnea	Intracranial insult, drug or toxin ingestion
	Tachycardia	PE, traumatic chest injury
	Hypotension	Tension pneumothorax
	Fever	Pneumonia, PE
General appearance	Cachexia, weight loss	Malignancy, acquired immune disorder, mycobacterial infection
	Obesity	Hypoventilation, sleep apnea, PE
	Pregnancy	PE
	Barrel chest	COPD
	"Sniffing" position	Epiglottitis
	"Tripoding" position	COPD or asthma with severe distress
	Traumatic injury	Pneumothorax (simple, tension), rib fractures, flail chest, hemothorax, pulmonary contusion
Skin and nails	Tobacco stains or odor	COPD, malignancy, infection
	Clubbing	Chronic hypoxia, intracardiac shunts, or pulmonary vascular anomalies
	Pallid skin or conjunctivae	Anemia
	Muscle wasting	Neuromuscular disease
	Bruising	Chest wall: Rib fractures, pneumothorax
		Diffuse: Thrombocytopenia, chronic steroid use, anticoagulation
	Subcutaneous emphysema	Rib fractures, pneumothorax, tracheobronchial disruption
	Hives, rash	Allergic reaction, infection, tick-borne illness
Neck	Stridor	Upper airway edema or infection, foreign body, traumatic injury, anaphylaxis
	JVD	Tension pneumothorax, COPD or asthma exacerbation, fluid overload or CHF, PE
Lung examination	Wheezes	CHF, anaphylaxis
		Bronchospasm
	Rales	CHF, pneumonia, PE
	Unilateral decrease	Pneumothorax, pleural effusion, consolidation, rib fractures or contusion, pulmonary contusion
	Hemoptysis	Malignancy, infection, bleeding disorder, CHF
	Sputum production	Infection (viral, bacterial)
	Friction rub	Pleurisy
	Abnormal respiratory pattern (e.g., Cheyne-Stokes)	Intracranial insult
Chest examination	Crepitance or pain on palpation	Rib or sternal fractures
	Subcutaneous emphysema	Pneumothorax, tracheobronchial rupture
	Thoracoabdominal desynchrony	Diaphragmatic injury with herniation; cervical spinal cord trauma
	Flail segment	Flail chest, pulmonary contusion
Cardiac examination	Murmur	PE
	S₃ or S₄ gallop	PE
	S₂ accentuation	PE
	Muffled heart sounds	Cardiac tamponade
Extremities	Calf tenderness, Homans sign	PE
	Edema	CHF
Neurologic examination	Focal deficits (motor, sensory, cognitive)	Stroke, intracranial hemorrhage causing central abnormal respiratory drive; if long-standing, risk of aspiration pneumonia
	Symmetric deficits	Neuromuscular disease
	Diffuse weakness	Metabolic or electrolyte abnormality (hypocalcemia, hypomagnesemia, hypophosphatemia), anemia
	Hyporeflexia	Hypermagnesemia
	Ascending weakness	Guillain-Barré syndrome

CHF, Congestive heart failure; *COPD,* chronic obstructive pulmonary disease; *JVD,* jugular venous distention; *PE,* pulmonary embolism.
From Marx JA et al: *Rosen's emergency medicine,* ed 8, Philadelphia, 2014, Saunders.

TABLE 57 Diagnostic Table: Patterns of Diseases Often Resulting in Dyspnea

Disease	History (Dyspnea)	Associated Symptoms	Signs and Physical Findings	Tests
Pulmonary embolism	HPI: Abrupt onset, pleuritic pain, immobility (travel, recent surgery) PMH: Malignancy, DVT, PE, hypercoagulability, oral contraception, obesity	Diaphoresis, exertional dyspnea	Tachycardia, tachypnea, low-grade fever	Pulse oximetry, ABG (A-a gradient), D-dimer ECG (dysrhythmia, right-sided heart strain) CXR (Westermark sign, Hampton hump), spiral CT, MRV Pulmonary angiogram Ultrasound positive for DVT
Pneumonia	Fever, productive cough, chest pain	Anorexia, chills, nausea, vomiting, exertional dyspnea, cough	Fever, tachycardia, tachypnea, rales, or decreased breath sounds	CXR, CBC, sputum and blood cultures
Bacterial	SH: Tobacco use			Pulse oximetry Waveform capnography if altered mental status, ABG if capnography unavailable and acid-base derangement or hypercarbia suspected
Viral	Exposure (e.g., influenza, varicella)			
Opportunistic	Immune disorder, chemotherapy			
Fungal or parasitic	Exposure (e.g., birds), indolent onset	Episodic fever, nonproductive cough		
Pneumothorax	Abrupt onset: Trauma, chest pain, thin males more likely to have spontaneous pneumothorax	Localized chest pain	Decreased breath sounds, subcutaneous emphysema, chest wall wounds or instability	CXR: Pneumothorax, rib fractures, hemothorax Ultrasound: Pneumothorax, pleural effusion
Simple				Ultrasound positive for pneumothorax
Tension	Decompensation of simple pneumothorax	Diaphoresis	JVD, tracheal deviation, muffled heart sounds, cardiovascular collapse	Clinical diagnosis: Requires immediate decompression. May verify via bedside ultrasound
COPD or asthma	Tobacco use, medication noncompliance, URI symptoms, sudden weather change PMH: Environmental allergies FH: Asthma	Air hunger, diaphoresis	Retractions, accessory muscle use, tripoding, cyanosis "Shark fin" capnograph	CXR: Rule out infiltrate, pneumothorax, atelectasis (mucus plug) Ultrasound: Distinguish from heart failure Waveform capnography
Malignancy	Weight loss, tobacco, or other occupational exposure	Dysphagia	Hemoptysis	CXR, chest CT: Mass, hilar adenopathy, focal atelectasis
Fluid overload	Gradual onset, dietary indiscretion or medication noncompliance, chest pain PMH: Recent MI, diabetes, CHF	Worsening orthopnea, PND	JVD, peripheral edema, S_3 or S_4 gallop, new cardiac dysrhythmia, hepatojugular reflux	CXR and/or ultrasound: Pleural effusion, interstitial edema, Kerley B lines, cardiomegaly ECG: Ischemia, dysrhythmia NT-proBNP
Anaphylaxis	Abrupt onset, exposure to allergen	Dysphagia	Oral swelling, stridor, wheezing, hives	

A-a, Alveolar-arterial; *ABG,* arterial blood gas; *CBC,* complete blood count; *CHF,* congestive heart failure; *COPD,* chronic obstructive pulmonary disease; *CT,* computed tomography; *CXR,* chest x-ray examination; *DVT,* deep vein thrombosis; *ECG,* electrocardiogram; *FH,* family history; *HPI,* history of present illness; *JVD,* jugular venous distention; *MI,* myocardial infarction; *MRV,* magnetic resonance venography; *NT-proBNP,* amino-terminal pro–B-type natriuretic peptide; *PE,* pulmonary embolism; *PMH,* past medical history; *PND,* paroxysmal nocturnal dyspnea; *SH,* social history; *URI,* upper respiratory infection.

From Marx JA et al: *Rosen's emergency medicine,* ed 8, Philadelphia, 2014, Saunders.

TABLE 58 Relationships among Qualities of Dyspnea, Physiology, and Symptomatic Treatment

Quality of Dyspnea	Physiology	Symptomatic Treatment
Air hunger, urge to breathe, need more air	Stimulation of respiratory controller via chemoreceptors, pulmonary receptors, vascular receptors	Supplemental oxygen; nasal flow of gas; cool air on the face; chest wall vibration; inhaled furosemide; opiates
Chest tightness	Stimulation of airway receptors	Inhaled bronchodilators (beta agonists, anticholinergics, steroids)
Cannot get a deep breath	Stimulation of respiratory controller; dynamic hyperinflation	Breathing retraining (slower breathing); pursed lips breathing
Increased work or effort to breathe	Mechanical load on the respiratory system; neuromuscular weakness	Inspiratory muscle training; noninvasive ventilation/BPAP
Breathing more	Increased ventilation; stimulation of metaboreceptors in muscles	Exercise training
All qualities	Altered perception/processing of information centrally	Desensitization treatment in pulmonary rehabilitation; morphine

BPAP, Bilevel positive airway pressure.

From Broaddus VC et al: *Murray & Nadel's textbook of respiratory medicine,* ed 7, Philadelphia, 2022, Elsevier.

Clinical Algorithms

III

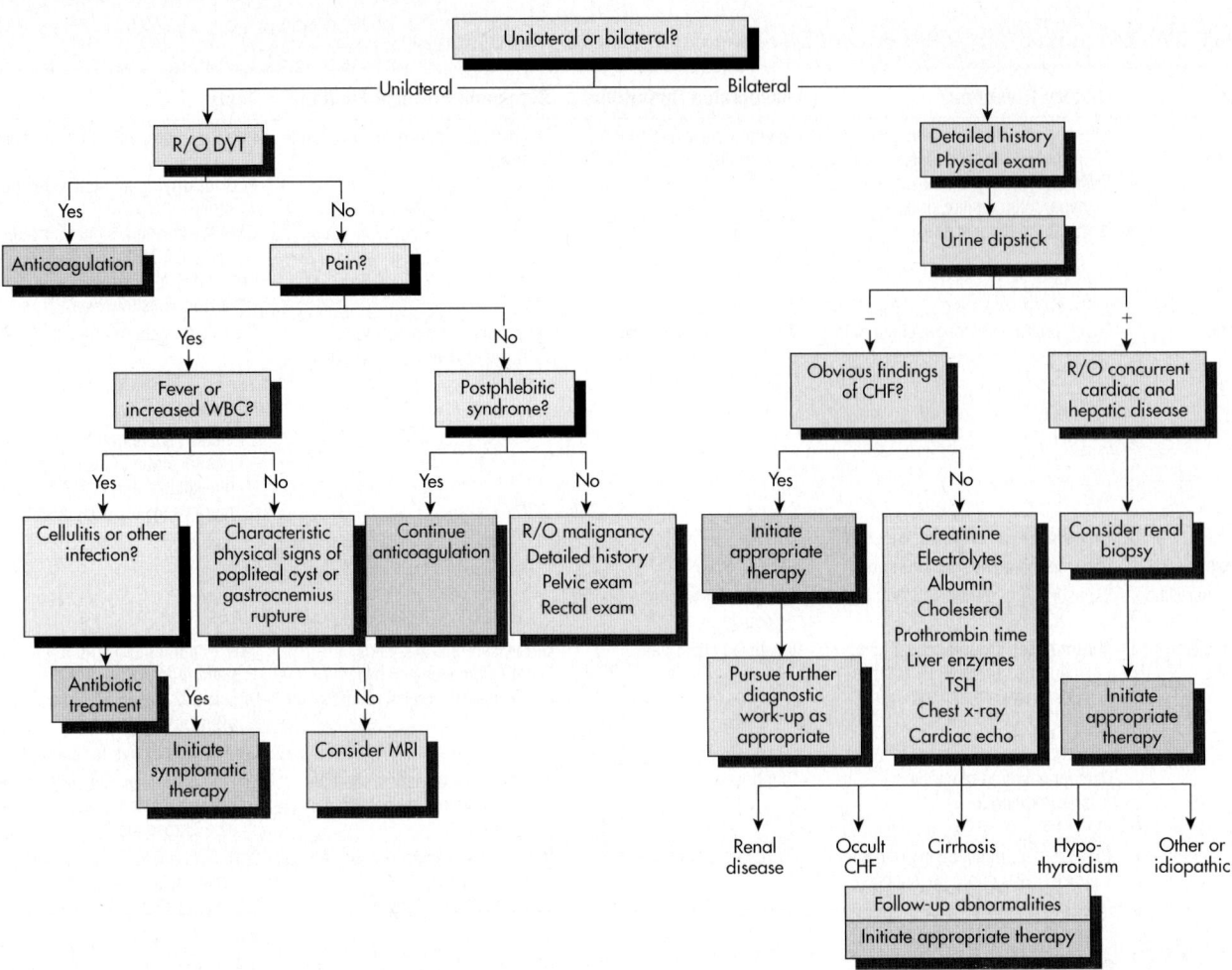

FIG. 81 Diagnostic approach to patients with edema. *CHF,* Congestive heart failure; *DVT,* deep vein thrombosis; *MRI,* magnetic resonance imaging; *R/O,* rule out; *TSH,* thyroid-stimulating hormone; *WBC,* white blood cell count. (From Chertow G: Approach to the patient with edema. In: Braunwald E, Goldman L [eds]: *Primary cardiology,* ed 2, Philadelphia, 2003, Saunders.)

ERYTHROCYTOSIS, ACQUIRED

ICD-10CM # D75.0 Familial erythrocytosis
D75.1 Secondary polycythemia
D45 Polycythemia vera
P61.1 Polycythemia neonatorum

1423

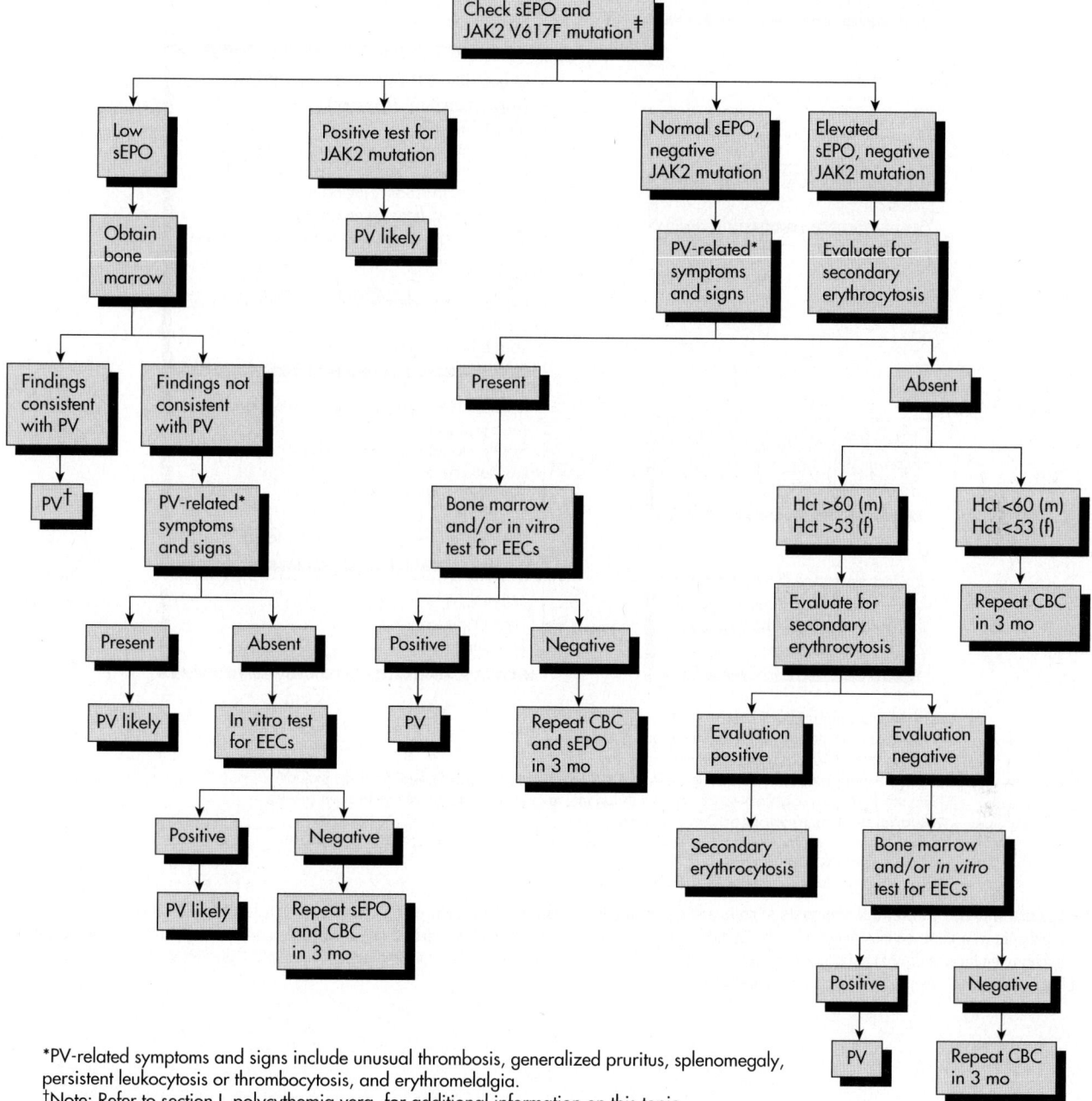

*PV-related symptoms and signs include unusual thrombosis, generalized pruritus, splenomegaly, persistent leukocytosis or thrombocytosis, and erythromelalgia.
†Note: Refer to section I, polycythemia vera, for additional information on this topic.
‡The JAK2 mutation is found in >95% of patients with PV and can be used for diagnostic purposes.

FIG. 84 A diagnostic approach to acquired erythrocytosis. *CBC*, Complete blood cell count; *EEC*, endogenous (spontaneous) erythroid colonies; *f*, female; *Hct*, hematocrit; *m*, male; *PV*, polycythemia vera; *sEPO*, serum erythropoietin level. (Modified from Goldman L, Schafer AL [eds]: *Cecil textbook of medicine*, ed 24, Philadelphia, 2012, Saunders.)

Clinical
Algorithms

III

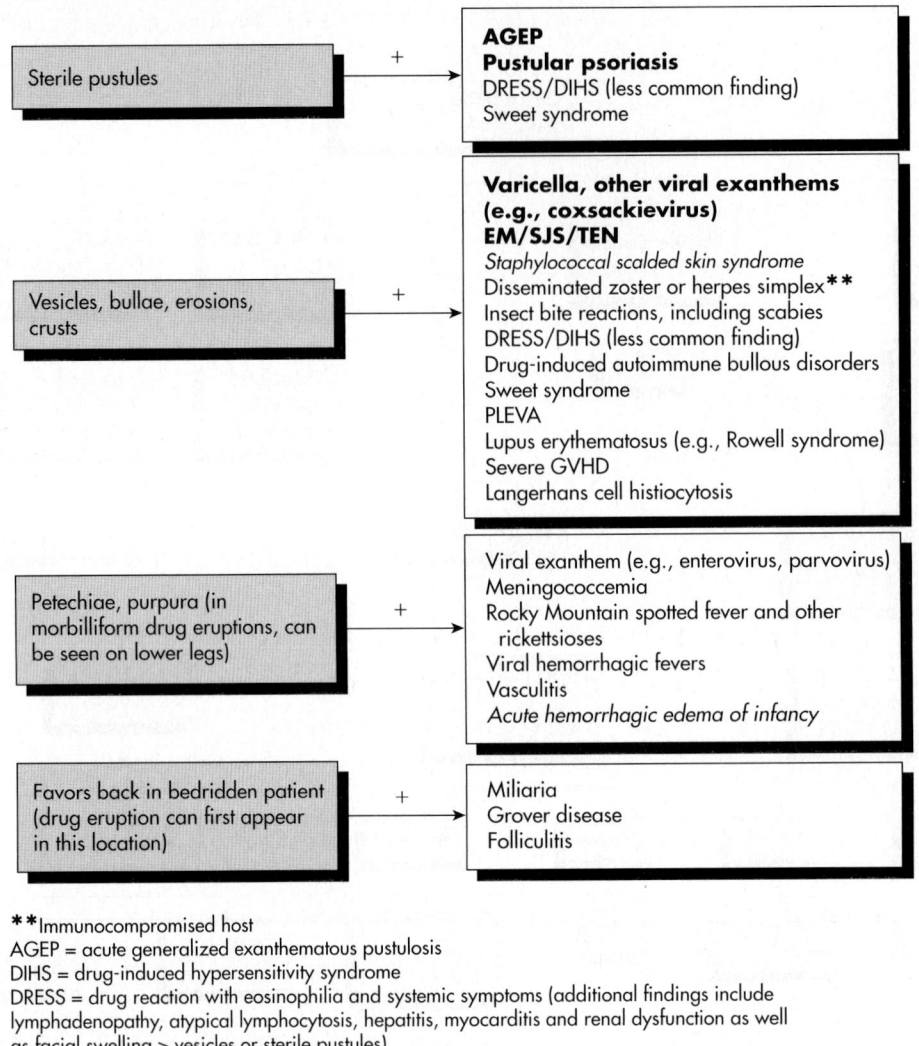

FIG. 91 Approach to the differential diagnosis of an exanthematous drug reaction. With a few exceptions (e.g., pityriasis rosea, drug-induced autoimmune bullous disorders), patients with these entities may be febrile. Entities in italics occur primarily in children. Toxic shock syndrome can be staphylococcal or streptococcal. Drug-induced autoimmune bullous disorders: Bullous pemphigoid or linear IgA bullous dermatosis > drug-induced pemphigus. *CMV,* Cytomegalovirus; *EBV,* Epstein-Barr virus. (From Bolognia JL: *Dermatology,* ed 4, Philadelphia, 2018, Elsevier.)

Continued

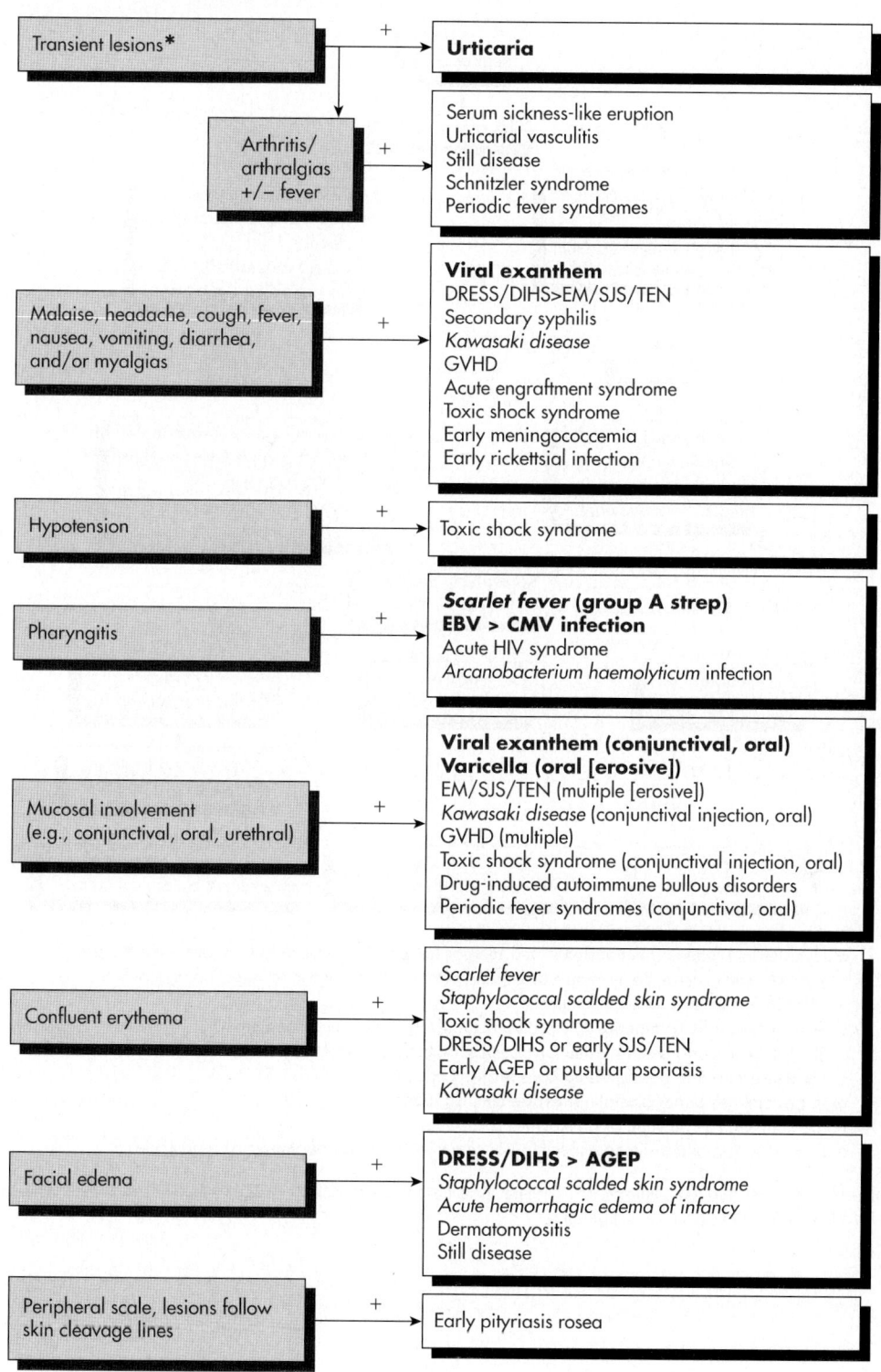

| Transient lesions* | + | **Urticaria** |

| Arthritis/ arthralgias +/– fever | + | Serum sickness-like eruption
Urticarial vasculitis
Still disease
Schnitzler syndrome
Periodic fever syndromes |

| Malaise, headache, cough, fever, nausea, vomiting, diarrhea, and/or myalgias | + | **Viral exanthem**
DRESS/DIHS>EM/SJS/TEN
Secondary syphilis
Kawasaki disease
GVHD
Acute engraftment syndrome
Toxic shock syndrome
Early meningococcemia
Early rickettsial infection |

| Hypotension | + | Toxic shock syndrome |

| Pharyngitis | + | ***Scarlet fever* (group A strep)**
EBV > CMV infection
Acute HIV syndrome
Arcanobacterium haemolyticum infection |

| Mucosal involvement (e.g., conjunctival, oral, urethral) | + | **Viral exanthem (conjunctival, oral)**
Varicella (oral [erosive])
EM/SJS/TEN (multiple [erosive])
Kawasaki disease (conjunctival injection, oral)
GVHD (multiple)
Toxic shock syndrome (conjunctival injection, oral)
Drug-induced autoimmune bullous disorders
Periodic fever syndromes (conjunctival, oral) |

| Confluent erythema | + | *Scarlet fever*
Staphylococcal scalded skin syndrome
Toxic shock syndrome
DRESS/DIHS or early SJS/TEN
Early AGEP or pustular psoriasis
Kawasaki disease |

| Facial edema | + | **DRESS/DIHS > AGEP**
Staphylococcal scalded skin syndrome
Acute hemorrhagic edema of infancy
Dermatomyositis
Still disease |

| Peripheral scale, lesions follow skin cleavage lines | + | Early pityriasis rosea |

*Individual lesions last <24 h, which can be documented by outlining them with ink; exceptions include urticarial vasculitis and, occasionally, Schnitzler or periodic fever syndromes

FIG. 91, cont'd

Clinical Algorithms

III

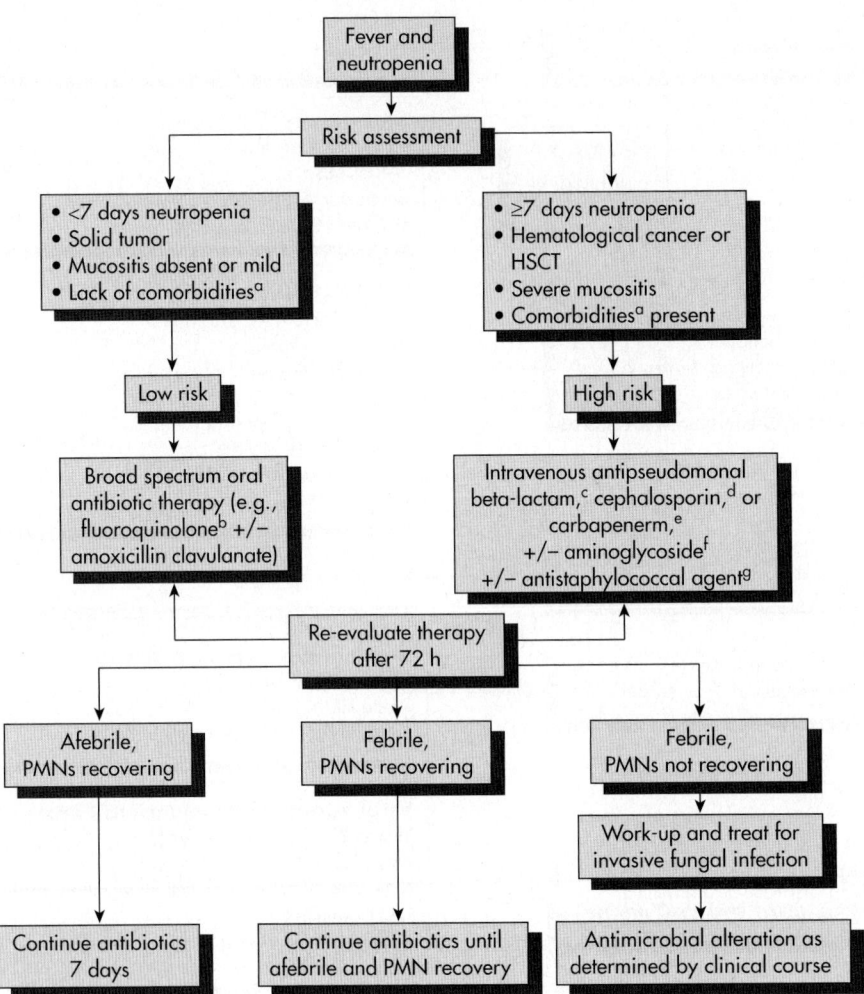

a Hypotension, altered mental status, neurologic changes, respiratory failure, abdominal pain, hemorrhage, cardiac compromise or new arrhythmia, catheter tunnel infection, extensive cellulitis, acute renal or liver failure
b Institution sensitivity dependent, ciprofloxacin, levofloxacin, moxifloxacin
c Drug selection and dosing institution-specific: Piperacillin tazobactam, ticarcillin/clavulanate
d Drug selection and dosing institution-specific: Ceftazidime
e Imipenem, cefepime/cilastatin, meropenem, doripenem
f Gentamicin, tobramycin, or amikacin
g Drug selection and institution-specific: Vancomycin, linezolid, daptomycin, ceftaroline

FIG. 93 Approach to patient with fever and neutropenia. *HSCT,* Hematopoietic stem cell transplant; *PMN,* polymorphonuclear neutrophil. (From Hoffman R: *Hematology: basic principles and practice,* ed 7, Philadelphia, 2018, Elsevier.)

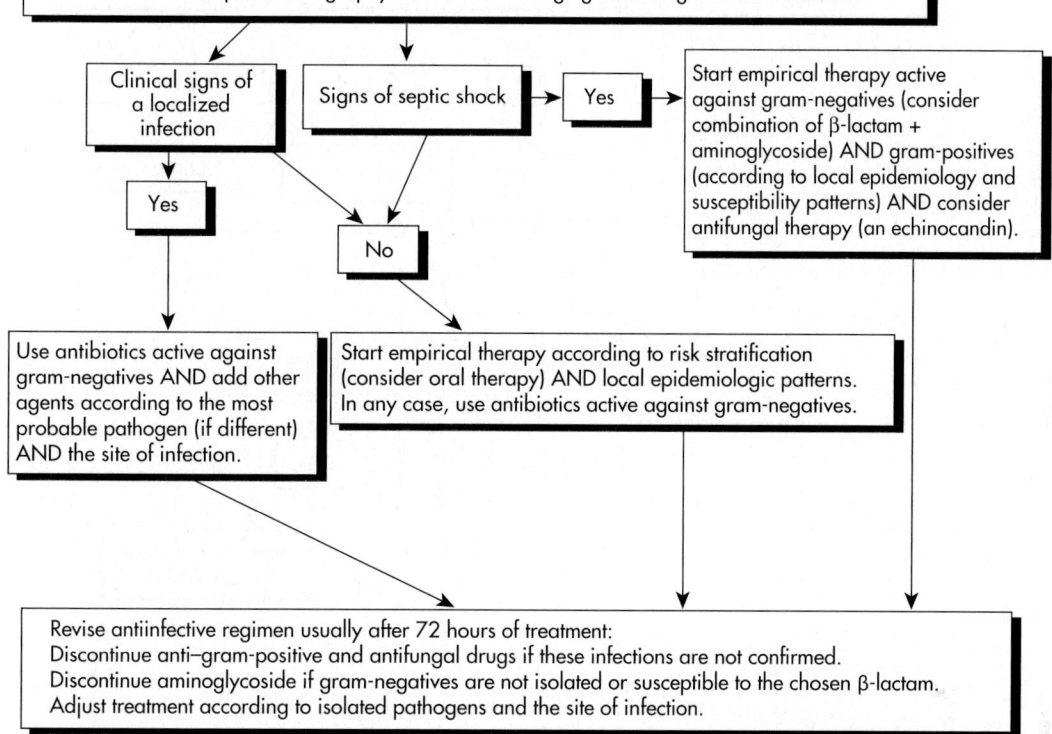

At onset of febrile neutropenia consider:
1. Type of patient: underlying disease, time from chemotherapy, and previous history of prophylactic antimicrobials and infectious complications, particularly if caused by resistant pathogens.
2. Type of center: knowledge of epidemiology of infections and susceptibility patterns.
If available, use a risk stratification system.
For antibiotic choice, consider the local resistance patterns.
Perform blood cultures (at least three) and other cultures from sites of suspected infection.
Consider chest computed tomography scan or other imaging according to clinical features.

Clinical signs of a localized infection

Signs of septic shock → Yes →

Start empirical therapy active against gram-negatives (consider combination of β-lactam + aminoglycoside) AND gram-positives (according to local epidemiology and susceptibility patterns) AND consider antifungal therapy (an echinocandin).

Yes

No

Use antibiotics active against gram-negatives AND add other agents according to the most probable pathogen (if different) AND the site of infection.

Start empirical therapy according to risk stratification (consider oral therapy) AND local epidemiologic patterns. In any case, use antibiotics active against gram-negatives.

Revise antiinfective regimen usually after 72 hours of treatment:
Discontinue anti–gram-positive and antifungal drugs if these infections are not confirmed.
Discontinue aminoglycoside if gram-negatives are not isolated or susceptible to the chosen β-lactam.
Adjust treatment according to isolated pathogens and the site of infection.

FIG. 94 Possible initial approach to a patient with febrile neutropenia. (From Bennett JE et al: *Mandell, Douglas, and Bennett's principles and practice of infectious diseases,* ed 9, Philadelphia, 2020, Elsevier.)

Clinical
Algorithms

III

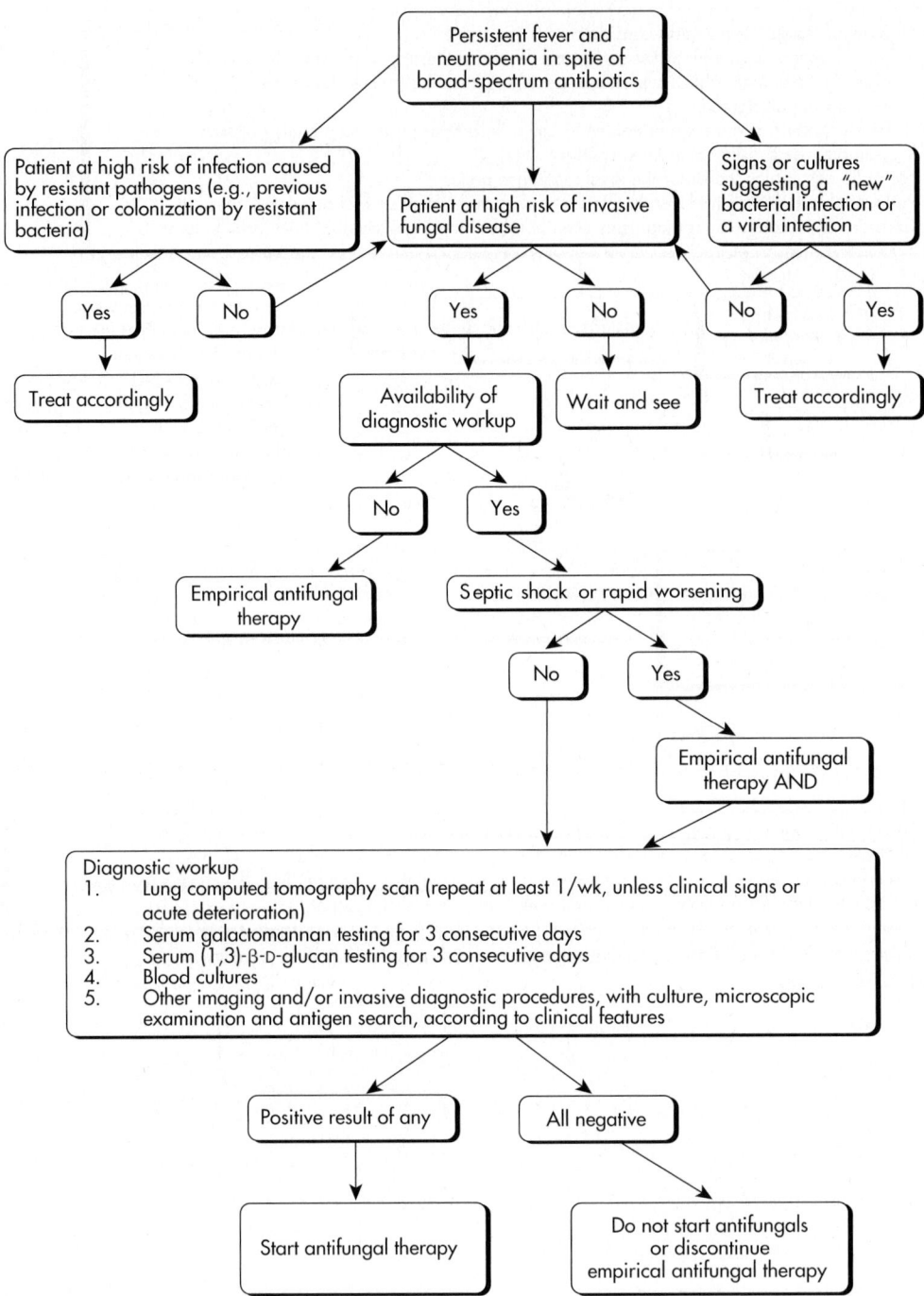

FIG. 95 Management of a persistently febrile neutropenic patient. (From Bennett JE et al: *Mandell, Douglas, and Bennett's principles and practice of infectious diseases,* ed 9, Philadelphia, 2020, Elsevier.)

TABLE 62   What Should a Clinician Wonder about and Look for When Approaching a Cancer Patient with a Suspected Infection?

Questions	Rationale for the Question

The underlying disease:
  1. Acute leukemia? Solid tumor? Lymphoma? Other?
  2. Active disease? In remission? Not evaluable?
	The incidence of infectious complications is different according to the underlying disease and consequent intensity of chemotherapy.
	The stage of disease may influence type, risk, and outcome of infection.

Recent treatments:
  1. Did the patient recently (within 1 mo) receive chemotherapy?
  2. Which drugs and which schedule? How long ago?
  3. Did the patient receive autologous or allogeneic HSCT?
  4. If allogeneic HSCT, what donor type?
  5. Did the patient receive monoclonal antibodies (anti-CD20, anti-CD52, etc.) in the past 6 months?
	Different drugs may give different types of immunosuppression and favor different infectious complications.
	Previous transplantation might result in long-term immunodeficiency, particularly if immunosuppressive treatment is continued.
	
	Immune reconstitution depends on the type of donor and conditioning regimens used in allogeneic HSCT.

White blood cell count:
  1. Is the patient neutropenic (PMNs <500/mm³ or <1000/mm³ but rapidly decreasing)?
  2. Was the patient neutropenic in the previous 30 days?
	The presence of neutropenia increases significantly the risk of infection. The knowledge of local epidemiologic data on antimicrobial susceptibility is mandatory for a correct choice of empirical therapy.

Risk of infection caused by resistant bacteria:
  1. Is the patient colonized with resistant bacteria, particularly gram-negatives?
  2. Is the hospital or the country endemic for resistant organisms?
  3. Any previous infections caused by resistant pathogens?
	In patients colonized by resistant bacteria, particularly if neutropenic, initial empirical therapy should cover these pathogens.
	If not colonized, but cared for in a setting where resistance is an issue, then consider the possibility of deescalation strategy.

Central venous catheter:
  1. Yes or no?
  2. Has the catheter been manipulated (including infusions) within a few hours before the onset of fever?
	The central venous access may be an important source of infection.

Past history of infections (both before and after the diagnosis of cancer)	It may suggest the etiology and drive the therapeutic choice (e.g., tuberculosis, toxoplasmosis, multidrug-resistant bacteria, or opportunistic fungal infections).
Country of origin	Specific endemic infections can reactivate (Chagas disease, strongyloidiasis, tuberculosis, endemic mycoses). Epidemiology of antibacterial resistance varies worldwide; thus patients coming from areas endemic for resistant bacteria should be treated accordingly.

The clinical picture:
  1. Presence of (severe) mucositis?
  2. New onset of pain (perianal, chest, everywhere)?
	It may suggest the etiology and drive the therapeutic choice.
	The presence of mucositis is suggestive of infection with pathogens from oral flora or gastrointestinal tract.
	The pain may help to locate formation of abscesses or indicate presence of a locally invasive process, such as pulmonary aspergillosis.

Administration of prophylaxis (no, yes, which drugs):
  1. Antibacterial?
  2. Antifungal, including *Pneumocystis jirovecii*?
  3. Antiviral?
  4. Was the patient compliant?
  5. Is there the possibility of inadequate blood levels due to lack of absorption or PK/PD problems?
	Breakthrough infections are possible, and fever during prophylaxis should be considered as failure of prophylaxis, unless proven otherwise.
	The occurrence of a bacterial/fungal/viral infection during specific prophylaxis may influence the choice of empirical therapy, depending on the drug used for prophylaxis. A resistant pathogen should be suspected in every case, unless the patient was clearly noncompliant or there is the possibility of low drug levels caused by poor absorption, increased metabolism, or drug interaction (e.g., azoles such as itraconazole, voriconazole, or posaconazole), or both. Knowledge of local epidemiology, including susceptibility pattern, is mandatory for correct diagnostic and therapeutic management.

HSCT, Hematopoietic stem cell transplantation; *PK/PD*, pharmacokinetic/pharmacodynamic; *PMNs*, polymorphonuclear neutrophils.
From Bennett JE et al: *Mandell, Douglas, and Bennett's principles and practice of infectious diseases*, ed 9, Philadelphia, 2020, Elsevier.

Clinical
Algorithms

III

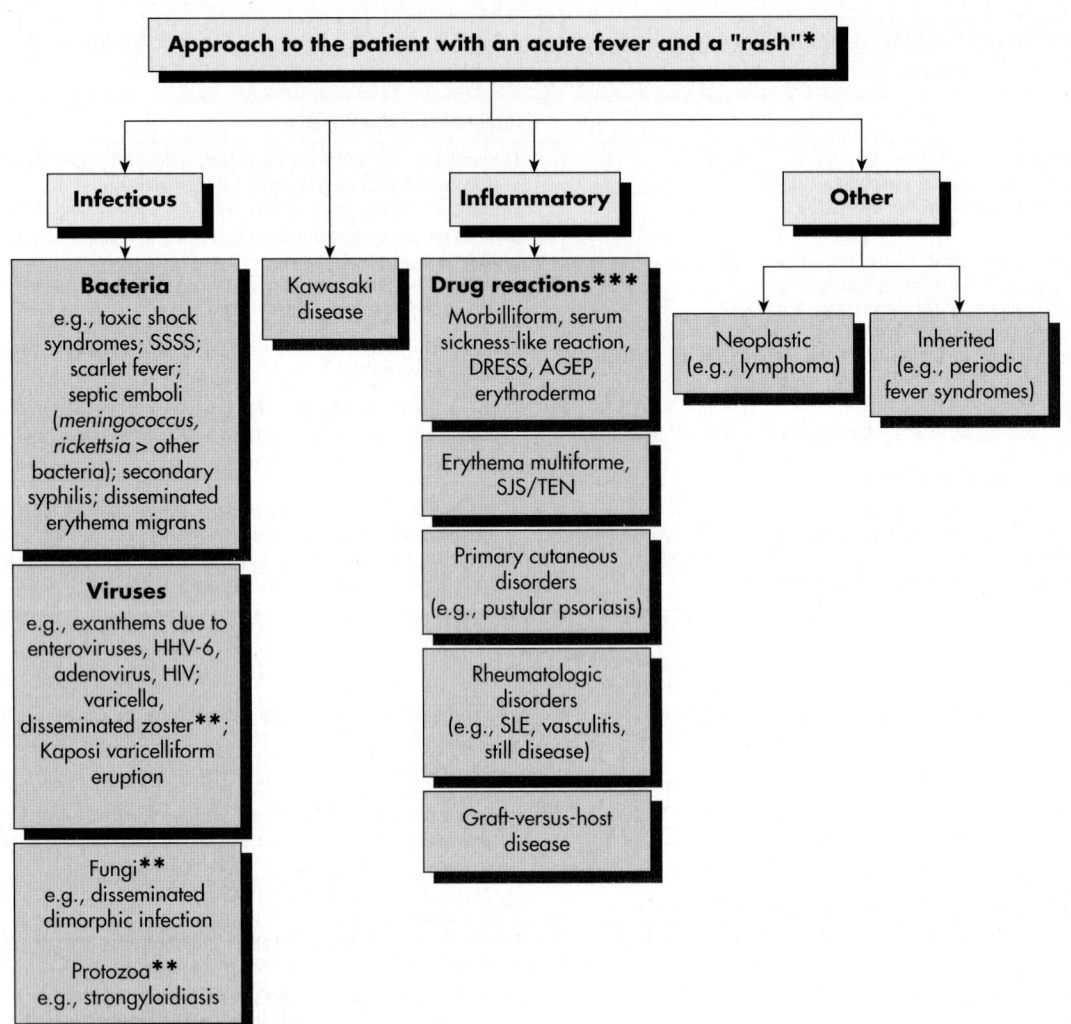

* Not a single site as in cellulitis, necrotizing fasciitis
** More likely in immunocompromised patient
*** Early on, more serious drug reactions, e.g., DRESS, may resemble a morbilliform eruption

FIG. 97 Approach to the patient with an acute fever and a "rash." *AGEP,* Acute generalized exanthematous pustulosis; *DRESS,* drug reaction with eosinophilia and systemic symptoms (also referred to as drug-induced hypersensitivity syndrome [DIHS]); *HHV,* human herpes virus; *HIV,* human immunodeficiency virus; *SJS,* Stevens-Johnson syndrome; *SLE,* systemic lupus erythematosus; *SSSS,* staphylococcal scalded skin syndrome; *TEN,* toxic epidermal necrolysis. (From Bolognia J: *Dermatology,* ed 4, Philadelphia, 2018, Elsevier.)

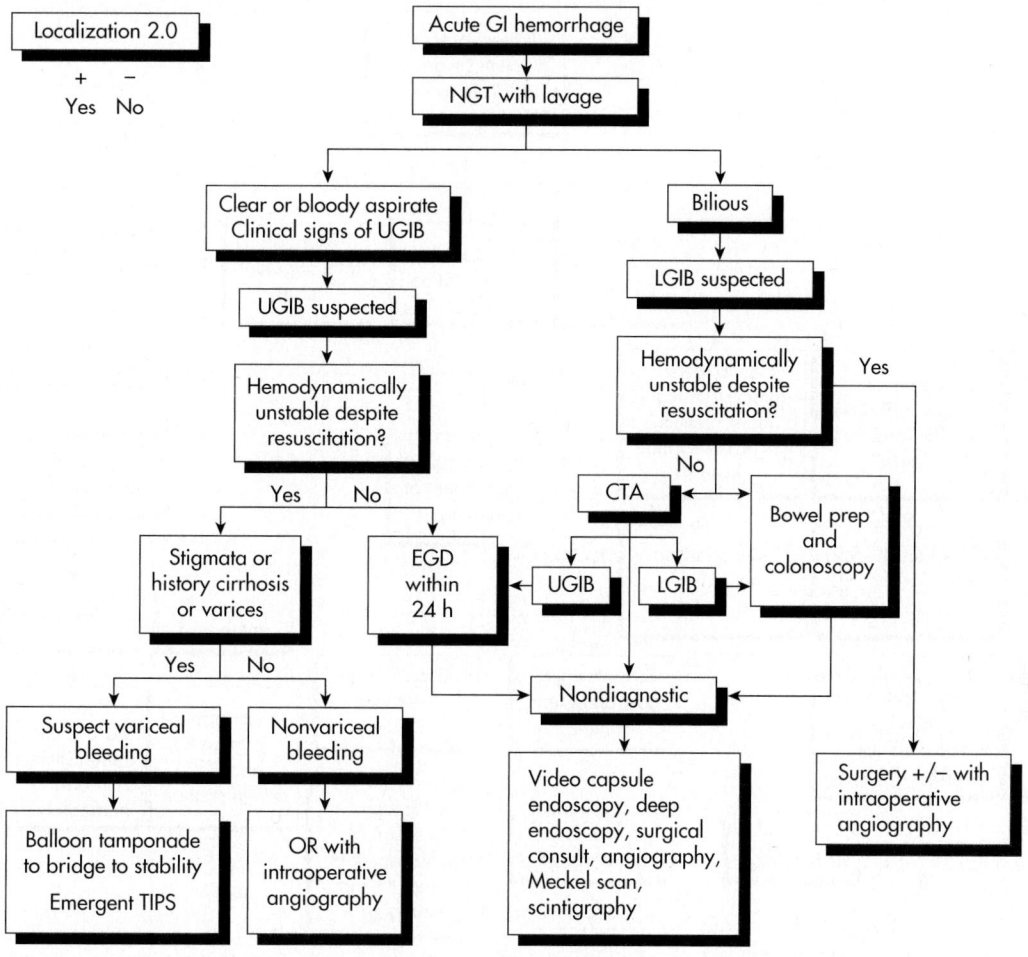

FIG. 98 Algorithm for the diagnosis of acute gastrointestinal *(GI)* hemorrhage. *CTA*, Computed tomography angiogram; *EGD*, esophagogastroduodenoscopy; *GI*, gastrointestinal; *LGIB*, lower GI bleed; *NGT*, nasogastric tube; *TIPS*, transjugular intrahepatic portosystemic shunt; *UGIB*, upper GI bleed. (From Townsend CM et al: *Sabiston textbook of surgery*, ed 21, St Louis, 2022, Elsevier.)

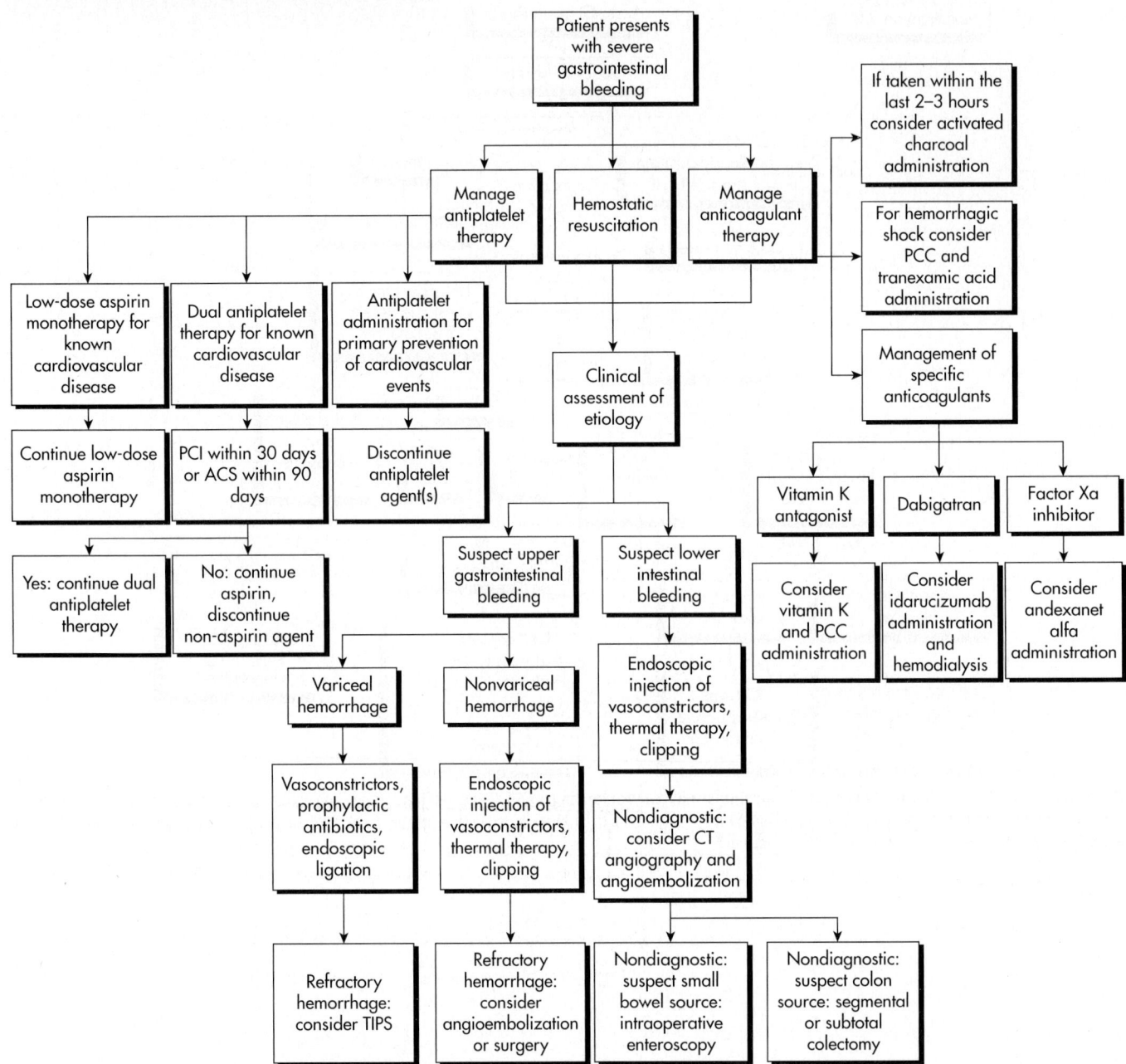

FIG. 99 Severe gastrointestinal bleeding management algorithm. *ACS,* Acute coronary syndrome; *CT,* computed tomography; *PCI,* percutaneous coronary intervention; *PCC,* prothrombin complex concentrate; *TIPS,* transjugular intrahepatic portosystemic shunt. (From Vincent JL et al: *Textbook of critical care,* ed 8, Philadelphia, 2024, Elsevier.)

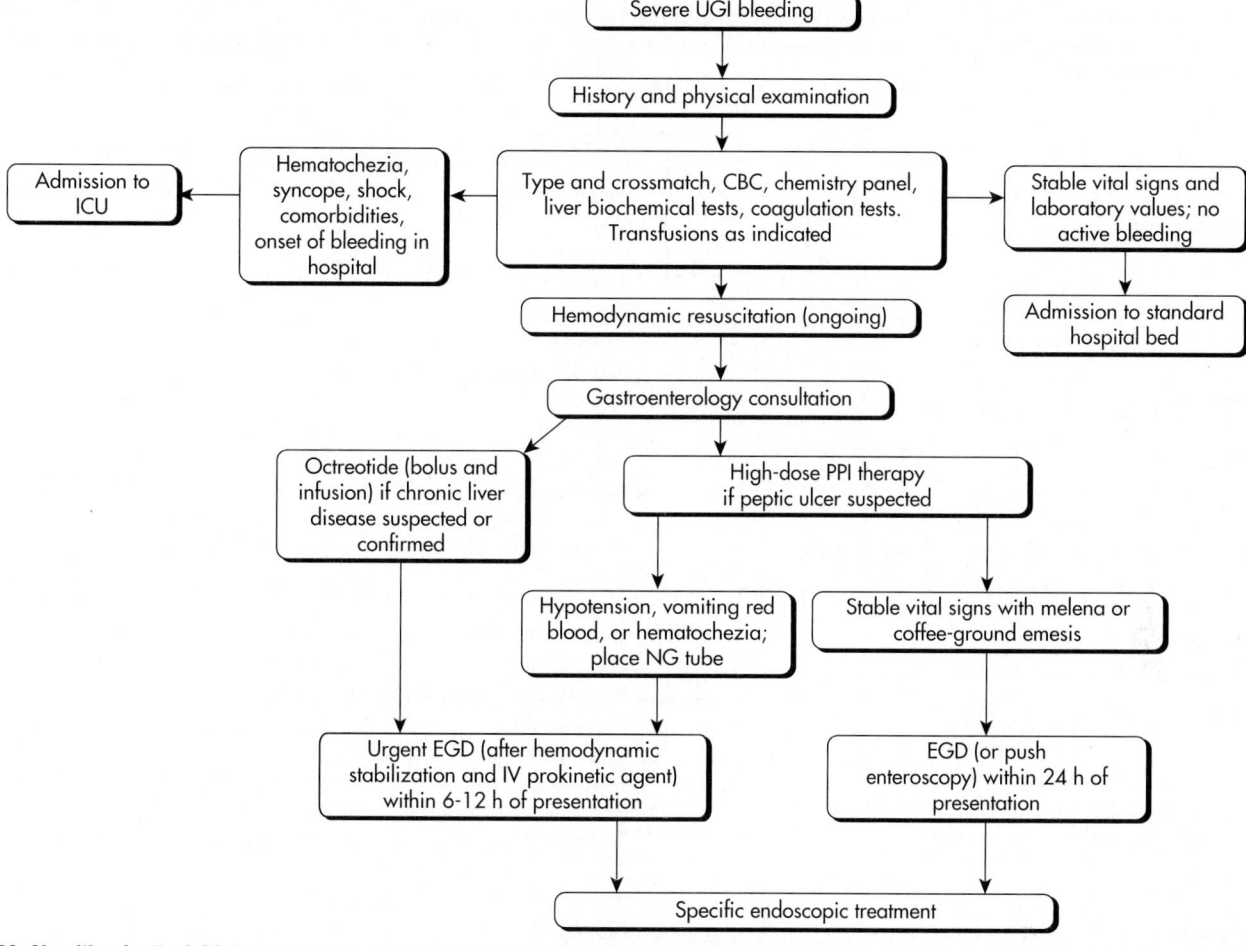

FIG. 100 Algorithm for the initial management of severe upper gastrointestinal *(UGI)* bleeding. Some steps may take place simultaneously or in varying order and in the emergency department, depending on the clinical situation. *CBC,* Complete blood cell count; *EGD,* esophagogastroduodenoscopy; *ICU,* intensive care unit; *IV,* intravenous; *NG,* nasogastric; *PPI,* proton pump inhibitors. (From Feldman M et al: *Sleisenger and Fordtran's gastrointestinal and liver disease,* ed 11, Philadelphia, 2021, Elsevier.)

TABLE 63 Rockall Scoring System for UGI Bleeding

Variable	POINTS			
	0	**1**	**2**	**3**
Age (yr)	<60	60-79	≥80	—
Pulse rate (beats/min)	<100	≥100	—	—
Systolic blood pressure (mm Hg)	Normal	≥100	<100	—
Comorbidity	None	—	Ischemic heart disease, cardiac failure, other major illness	Renal failure, hepatic failure, metastatic cancer
Diagnosis	Mallory-Weiss tear or no lesion observed	All other benign diagnoses	Malignant lesion	—
Endoscopic stigmata of recent hemorrhage	No stigmata or dark spot in ulcer base	—	Blood in UGI tract, adherent clot, visible vessel, active bleeding	—

Total Score	Frequency (% of Total)	Rebleeding Rate (%)	Mortality Rate (%)
0	4.9	4.9	0
1	9.5	3.4	0
2	11.4	5.3	0.2
3	15.0	11.2	2.9
4	17.9	14.1	5.3
5	15.3	24.1	10.8
6	10.6	32.9	17.3
7	9.0	43.8	27.0
≥8	6.4	41.8	41.1

Modified from Rockall TA, Logan RF (eds): Selection of patients for early discharge or outpatient care after acute upper gastrointestinal haemorrhage. National Audit of Acute Upper Gastrointestinal Haemorrhage, *Lancet* 347:1138-40, 1996.

Clinical Algorithms

III

TABLE 64   Suspected Source of GI Bleeding as Suggested by a Patient's History

Suspected Source of Bleeding	Patient History
Nasopharynx	History of nasopharyngeal radiation
	Recurrent epistaxis
	Prior nasopharyngeal malignancy
Lungs	Hemoptysis
Esophageal ulceration	GERD
	Heartburn
	Heavy alcohol use
	Odynophagia
	Pill ingestion
	Traumatic nasogastric tube placement
Esophageal cancer	Dysphagia
	Weight loss
Mallory-Weiss tear	Alcohol binge
	Vomiting
Cameron lesions	Large hiatal hernia
Esophageal or gastric varices or portal hypertensive gastropathy	Chronic liver disease
	Cirrhosis
	Heavy alcohol use
Gastric angiodysplasia	Chronic kidney disease
Peptic ulcer	Epigastric discomfort
	Frequent aspirin or other NSAID use
	History of PUD
Gastric cancer	Early satiation
	Weight loss
Primary aortoenteric fistula	Prior severe acute unexplained bleeding
Secondary aortoenteric fistula	Prior surgical repair of an abdominal aortic aneurysm with synthetic graft
Ampulla of Vater	Recent endoscopic sphincterotomy
Bile ducts	Recent liver biopsy or cholangiography
Pancreatic ducts	Pancreatitis
	Pseudocyst
	Recent pancreatography
Small intestinal malignancy	Hereditary nonpolyposis colorectal cancer
	History of intraabdominal metastatic cancer
	Intermittent small intestinal obstruction
	Recurrent unexplained GI bleeding
	Weight loss
Meckel diverticulum	Unexplained GI bleeding since childhood
Small intestinal or colonic ulcerations	Use of aspirin or other NSAID
Small intestinal telangiectasias	Frequent nosebleeds
	Hereditary hemorrhagic telangiectasia (Osler-Weber-Rendu disease)
Small intestinal angiodysplasia	Age >60 yr
Colonic diverticulosis	Hematochezia without abdominal pain
	History of diverticulosis
Colonic neoplasia	Change in bowel habits
	Personal or family history colon neoplasia
	Subacute bleeding
	Weight loss
Ischemic colitis	Cardiovascular disease
	Hematochezia with abdominal pain or discomfort
UC	Bloody diarrhea
	Family history of IBD
	History of UC
Crohn disease	Chronic abdominal discomfort
	Family history of IBD
	History of Crohn disease
Anal fissure	Hematochezia with anal pain
Hemorrhoids	Dripping blood with bowel movements
	Hematochezia with normal bowel movements

TABLE 64   Suspected Source of GI Bleeding as Suggested by a Patient's History—cont'd

Suspected Source of Bleeding	Patient History
Postpolypectomy ulcer	Recent colonoscopy with polypectomy
	Use of anticoagulants or antiplatelet drugs
Colonic or small intestinal angioectasias	Age >70 yr
	Cardiovascular disease
	Recurrent bleeding of variable severity
Anastomotic ulceration	Prior intestinal surgical anastomosis
Radiation enteritis or proctitis	History of abdominal radiation therapy

GERD, Gastroesophageal reflux disease; *GI*, gastrointestinal; *IBD*, inflammatory bowel disease; *NSAID*, nonsteroidal antiinflammatory drug; *PUD*, peptic ulcer disease; *UC*, ulcerative colitis.
From Feldman M et al: *Sleisenger and Fordtran's gastrointestinal and liver disease*, ed 10, Philadelphia, 2016, Elsevier.

TABLE 65   Evaluation of Gastrointestinal Bleeding, Pediatric Patient

Laboratory Investigation
All Patients
CBC and platelet count
Coagulation tests: prothrombin time, partial thromboplastin time
Tests of liver dysfunction: AST, ALT, GGT, bilirubin
Occult blood test of stool or vomitus
Blood type and crossmatch
Evaluation of Bloody Diarrhea
Stool culture or PCR, *Clostridium difficile* toxin
Sigmoidoscopy or colonoscopy
CT or MRI enteroscopy
Evaluation of Rectal Bleeding with Formed Stools
External and digital rectal examination
Sigmoidoscopy or colonoscopy
Meckel scan
Mesenteric arteriogram
Video capsule endoscopy
Initial Radiologic Evaluation
All Patients
Abdominal x-ray series
Evaluation of Hematemesis
Barium upper GI series if endoscopy not available
Evaluation of Bleeding with Pain and Vomiting (Bowel Obstruction)
Abdominal x-ray series
Pneumatic or contrast enema
Upper GI series

ALT, Alanine aminotransferase; *AST*, aspartate aminotransferase; *CBC*, complete blood count; *CT*, computed tomography; *GGT*, γ-glutamyltransferase; *GI*, gastrointestinal.
From Marcdante KJ et al: *Nelson essentials of pediatrics*, ed 9, Philadelphia, 2023, Elsevier.

Clinical
Algorithms

III

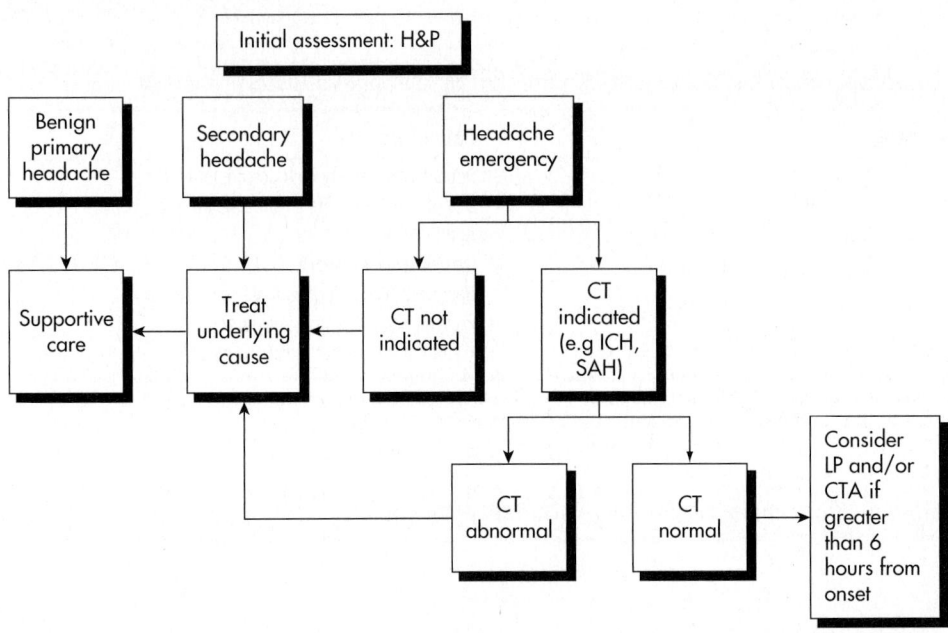

FIG. 104 Evaluation algorithm for presentation of headache. *CO,* Carbon monoxide; *CT,* computed tomography; *CTA,* computed tomography angiography; *HA,* headache; *H&P,* history and physical examination; *ICH,* intracranial hemorrhage; *LP,* lumbar puncture; *SAH,* subarachnoid hemorrhage. (From Walls RM et al: *Rosen's emergency medicine, concepts and clinical practice,* ed 10, Philadelphia, 2023, Elsevier.)

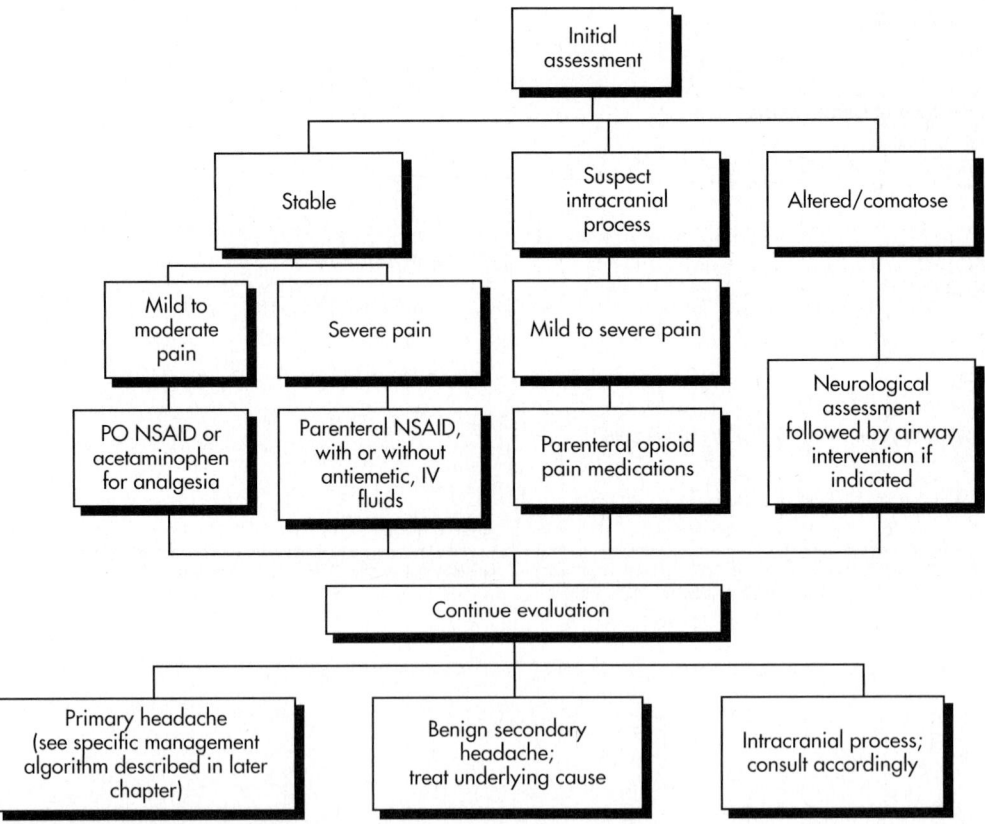

FIG. 105 Management algorithm. *IV,* Intravenous; *NSAID,* nonsteroidal antiinflammatory drug; *PO, per os* (by mouth). (From Walls RM et al: *Rosen's emergency medicine, concepts and clinical practice,* ed 10, Philadelphia, 2023, Elsevier.)

BOX 26   Emergent Causes of Headache and Associated Risk Factors

1. Carbon monoxide poisoning
   a. Breathing in enclosed or confined spaces with engine exhaust or ventilation of heating equipment
   b. Multiple household members with the same symptoms
   c. Wintertime and working around machinery or equipment producing carbon monoxide (e.g., furnaces, heaters)
2. Meningitis, encephalitis, abscess
   a. History of sinus or ear infection or recent surgical procedure
   b. Immunocompromised state
   c. General debilitation with decreased immunologic system function
   d. Acute febrile illness—any type
   e. Extremes of age
   f. Impacted living conditions (e.g., military barracks, college dormitories)
   g. Lack of primary immunization
3. Temporal arteritis
   a. Age >50
   b. Females more often than males (4:1)
   c. History of other collagen vascular diseases (e.g., systemic lupus)
   d. Previous chronic meningitis
   e. Previous chronic illness, such as tuberculosis, parasitic or fungal infection
4. Glaucoma—acute angle closure
   a. Not associated with any usual or customary headache patterns
   b. History of previous glaucoma
   c. Age >30
   d. History of pain increasing in a dark environment
5. Increased intracranial pressure
   a. History of previous benign intracranial hypertension
   b. Presence of cerebrospinal fluid (CSF) shunt
   c. History of congenital brain or skull abnormalities
   d. Female gender
   e. Obesity
6. Cerebral venous sinus thrombosis
   a. Female gender
   b. Pregnancy, peripartum, hormone replacement therapy or oral contraceptive use
   c. Prothrombotic conditions
7. Reversible cerebral vasoconstriction syndrome
   a. Episodic sudden severe pain, with or without focal neurological findings or seizure
   b. Recurrent episodes over a period up to several weeks
   c. Exposure to adrenergic or serotonergic drugs
   d. Postpartum state
8. Intracranial hemorrhage (ICH)
   a. Subarachnoid hemorrhage (SAH)
      i. Sudden and severe pain; "worst headache of life"
      ii. Acute severe pain after sexual intercourse or exertion
      iii. History of SAH or cerebral aneurysm
      iv. History of polycystic kidney disease
      v. Family history of SAH
      vi. Hypertension—severe
      vii. Previous vascular lesions in other areas of the body
      viii. Young and middle-aged
   b. Subdural hematoma
      i. History of alcohol dependency with or without trauma
      ii. Current use of anticoagulation
   c. Epidural hematoma
      i. Traumatic injury
      ii. Lucid mentation followed by acute altered mentation or somnolence
      iii. Anisocoria

From Walls RM et al: *Rosen's emergency medicine, concepts and clinical practice,* ed 10, Philadelphia, 2023, Elsevier.

Clinical
Algorithms

III

TABLE 67　Headache Etiologies and Associated Spectrum of Severity of Disease by System

Organ System	Critical	Emergent	Nonemergent
CNS, neurologic, vessels	SAH Carotid dissection Venous sinus thrombosis	Shunt failure Traction headaches Tumor or mass Subdural hematoma Reversible cerebral vasoconstriction syndrome	Migraine, various types Vascular headache, various types Trigeminal neuralgia Post-traumatic (concussion) Post LP headache
Toxic/metabolic, environmental	Carbon monoxide poisoning	Mountain sickness	
Collagen vascular disease	Temporal arteritis		
Ocular/ENT		Glaucoma	Sinusitis Dental problems TMJ disease
Musculoskeletal			Tension headache Cervical strain
Allergy			Cluster or histamine headaches
Infectious disease	Bacterial meningitis Encephalitis	Brain abscess	Febrile headaches, non-neurologic source
Pulmonary or oxygen		Anoxic headache	
Cardiovascular		Hypertensive crisis	Hypertension (rare)
Unspecified		Preeclampsia IIH	Effort-dependent or coital headaches Medication overuse/rebound

CNS, Central nervous system; *ENT,* ear, nose, and throat; *IIH,* idiopathic intracranial hypertension; *LP,* lumbar puncture; *SAH,* subarachnoid hemorrhage; *TMJ,* temporomandibular joint.
From Walls RM et al: *Rosen's emergency medicine, concepts and clinical practice,* ed 10, Philadelphia, 2023, Elsevier.

TABLE 68　Signs and Symptoms of Various Headache Etiologies

Symptom	Finding	Possible Diagnosis
Sudden onset of pain	"Thunderclap" with any decreased mentation, any positive focal finding, meningismus or intractable pain	SAH, cervical artery dissection, cerebral venous thrombosis, acute angle closure glaucoma
Sudden onset of pain	Recurrent thunderclap episodes, may be associated with strokelike symptoms	Reversible cerebral vasoconstriction syndrome
"Worst headache of my life"	Associated with sudden onset	SAH, cervical artery dissection, cerebral venous thrombosis
Near syncope or syncope	Associated with sudden onset	SAH, cervical artery dissection, cerebral venous thrombosis
Increased with jaw movement	Clicking or snapping; pain with jaw movement	TMJ disease
Facial pain	Fulminant pain of the forehead and area of maxillary sinus; nasal congestion	Sinus pressure or dental infection
Jaw, forehead and/or temporal area pain	Tender temporal arteries	Temporal arteritis
Periorbital or retro-orbital pain	Sudden onset with tearing	Temporal arteritis or acute angle closure glaucoma

SAH, Subarachnoid hemorrhage; *TMJ,* temporomandibular joint.
From Walls RM et al: *Rosen's emergency medicine, concepts and clinical practice,* ed 10, Philadelphia, 2023, Elsevier.

TABLE 69   Signs and Symptoms Associated with Different Headache Etiologies

Sign	Finding	Possible Diagnoses
General appearance	Nonfocal mental status changes	Meningitis, encephalitis, SAH, subdural hematoma, anoxia, increased intracranial pressure, carbon monoxide poisoning
	Mental status changes with focal findings	Intraparenchymal bleed, tentorial herniation, stroke
	Severe nausea, vomiting	Increased intracranial pressure, acute-angle closure glaucoma, SAH, carbon monoxide poisoning
Vital signs	Hypertension with normal heart rate or bradycardia	Increased intracranial pressure, SAH, tentorial herniation, intraparenchymal bleed, preeclampsia, reversible cerebral vasoconstriction syndrome
	Tachycardia	Anoxia, anemia, febrile headache, exertional or coital headache
	Fever	Febrile headache, meningitis, encephalitis
HEENT	Tender temporal arteries	Temporal arteritis
	Increased intraocular pressure	Acute angle closure glaucoma
	Loss of venous pulsations on fundoscopy or papilledema	Increased intracranial pressure, mass lesions, subhyaloid hemorrhage, SAH, cerebral venous thrombosis
	Acute red eye (severe ciliary flushing) and poorly reactive pupils	Acute angle closure glaucoma
Neurologic	Enlarged pupil with third nerve palsy	Tentorial pressure cone, mass effect (aneurysm, bleed, abscess, or tumor)
	Lateralized motor or sensory deficit	Stroke, subdural hematoma, epidural hematoma, hemiplegic or anesthetic migraine (rare), reversible cerebral vasoconstriction syndrome, central venous thrombosis
	Balance and coordination deficits	Cervical artery dissection, acute cerebellar hemorrhage, acute cerebellitis (mostly children),[9] chemical intoxication of various types
	Extraocular movement deficits (CN III, IV, and VI)	Mass lesion, neurapraxia (post-traumatic headache), IIH

CN, Cranial nerve; *HEENT,* head, eyes, ears, nose, and throat; *IIH,* idiopathic intracranial hypertension; *SAH,* subarachnoid hemorrhage.
From Walls RM et al: *Rosen's emergency medicine, concepts and clinical practice,* ed 10, Philadelphia, 2023, Elsevier.

TABLE 70   Diagnostic Findings in Emergent Causes of Headache

Diagnosis	Test	Finding
Temporal arteritis	Erythrocyte sedimentation rate (ESR) or C-reactive protein (CRP)	ESR greater than 50 mm/H Elevated CRP
SAH Increased intracranial pressure	Electrocardiogram (ECG)	Nonspecific ST/T wave changes
Anoxia	Complete blood count (CBC)	Severe anemia
Increased intracranial pressure	Computed tomography (CT) scan: Head	Increased ventricular size
SAH		Blood in subarachnoid space
Epidural or subdural hematoma		Blood in epidural or subdural space
Intraparenchymal hemorrhage		Bleeding into parenchyma of brain
Pale infarct		Areas of poor vascular flow
Traction headache secondary to mass effect		Structural, mass lesion
IIH	Lumbar puncture (LP) and cerebrospinal fluid (CSF) analysis	Increased opening pressure
Mass lesion		
Shunt failure		
Cryptococcal meningitis		
Tumor or other structural lesions, infection		Increased protein
SAH		Increased RBCs
Infection		Increased WBCs
Infection		Positive Gram stain
Infection		Decreased glucose

IIH, Idiopathic intracranial hypertension; *RBC,* red blood cell; *SAH,* subarachnoid hemorrhage; *WBC,* white blood cell.
From Walls RM et al: *Rosen's emergency medicine, concepts and clinical practice,* ed 10, Philadelphia, 2023, Elsevier.

Clinical Algorithms

III

TABLE 71 Causes and Differentiation of Potentially Catastrophic Illness Manifesting with Nontraumatic Headache

Disease Entities	Pain History	Associated Symptoms	Support History	Prevalence
Carbon monoxide poisoning	Usually gradual, subtle, dull, nonfocal throbbing pain	May wax and wane as individual leaves and enters the involved area of carbon monoxide; throbbing may vary considerably	Exposure to engine exhaust, old or defective heating systems, most common in winter months	Rare
Subarachnoid hemorrhage (SAH)	Sudden onset, "thunderclap," severe throbbing	Symptoms variable; may present from relatively asymptomatic to altered mental status or focal neurological deficit	History of polycystic kidney disease; history of HTN	Uncommon
Meningitis, encephalitis, abscess	Gradual; as general symptoms increase, headache increases. Nonfocal pain	Decreased mentation prominent, irritability prominent. With abscess, focal neurologic findings may be present	Recent infection, recent facial or dental surgery or other ENT surgery, unimmunized state	Uncommon
Temporal arteritis	Pain often develops over a few hours from mild to severe, almost always localized to temporal area(s)	Decreased vision, nausea, vomiting may be intense and confound diagnosis	Age over 50; other collagen vascular diseases or inflammatory diseases	Uncommon
Acute angle closure glaucoma	Sudden in onset	Nausea, vomiting, decreased vision	History of glaucoma; history of pain increasing in dark areas	Rare
Increased intracranial pressure syndromes	Gradual, dull, nonfocal	Vomiting, decreased mentation	History of CSF shunt or congenital brain or skull abnormality	Uncommon

CSF, Cerebrospinal fluid; *ENT,* ear, nose, and throat; *HTN,* hypertension.
From Walls RM et al: *Rosen's emergency medicine, concepts and clinical practice,* ed 10, Philadelphia, 2023, Elsevier.

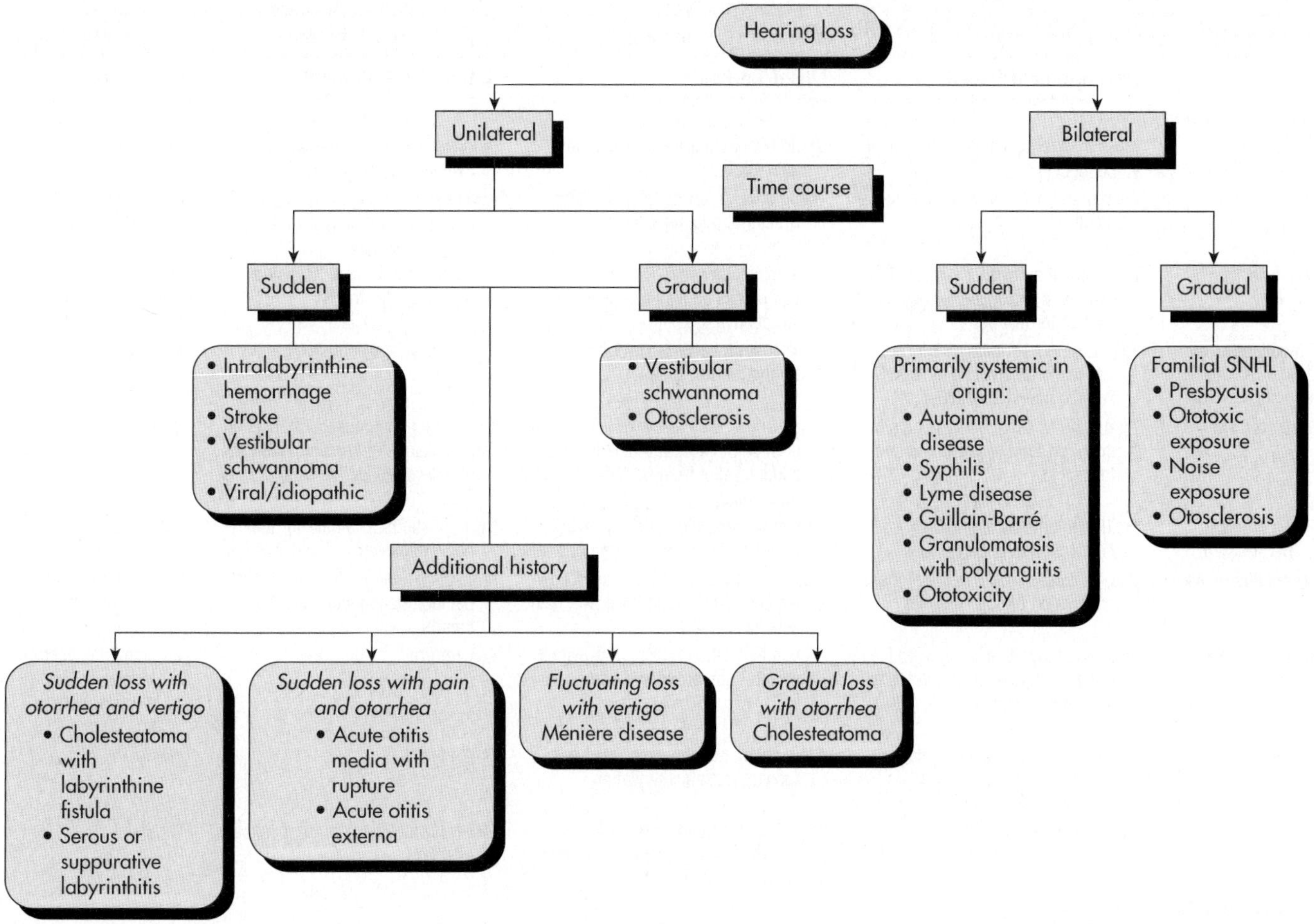

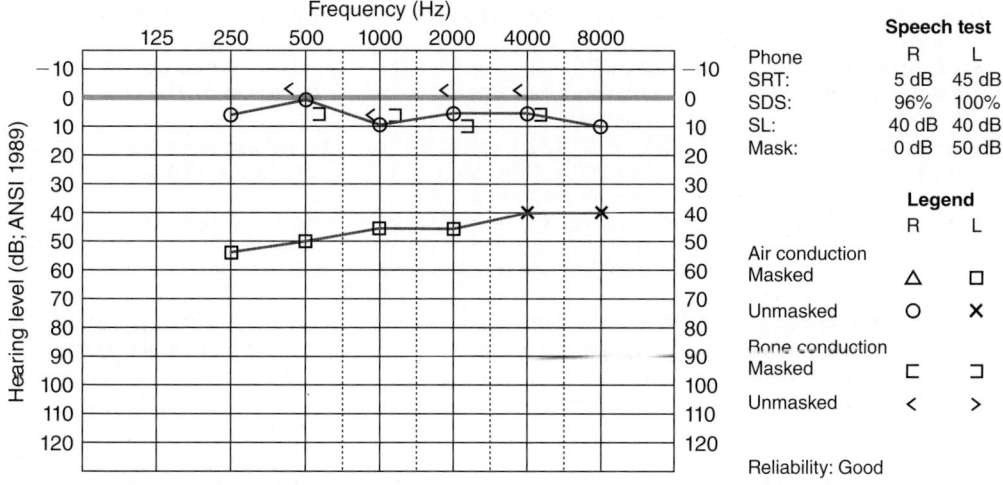

FIG. 106 Establishing a differential diagnosis with a chief complaint of hearing loss. This algorithm encourages the clinician to consider the patient complaint in categorical differential diagnosis families. It is not exhaustive. *SNHL,* Sensorineural hearing loss. (From Flint PW et al: *Cummings otolaryngology, head and neck surgery,* ed 7, Philadelphia, 2021, Elsevier.)

Clinical
Algorithms

FIG. 107 An audiogram showing a clinically significant left-sided conductive hearing loss. Note the air-bone gap, normal speech discrimination, and normal masked bone conduction in the left ear. *SDS,* Speech discrimination score; *SL,* sensory level; *SRT,* speech reception threshold. (From Flint PW et al: *Cummings otolaryngology, head and neck surgery,* ed 7, Philadelphia, 2021, Elsevier.)

TABLE 72 Lesions That Cause Hearing Loss

	Description of Pathology	Onset/Course	Actions or Treatment	Prognosis
Conductive Lesion				
Foreign body	Mass in external canal blocks sound conduction	Acute onset associated or not with pain, drainage, or odor	Removal. Evaluate for infection. Evaluate for TM perforation	Excellent
Otitis externa	Edema and detritus obstruct external canal	Rapid onset. Pain, edema, swelling. Drainage, odor often present	Aural toilet to remove debris. Topical (±oral) antibiotics. Evaluate for necrotizing otitis	Excellent if treated appropriately
Exostosis	Bony growths obstruct canal. Often seen with prolonged exposure to cold water (divers)	Slow insidious onset. No pain or drainage unless causes complete obstruction	Evaluate for infection. Reassure patient. Refer to ENT	Good
Tympanosclerosis	TM scarring from perforations or infections. Decreased mobility impairs sound conduction	Slow onset following perforations, trauma, or infections	ENT referral. Reassurance	Variable
Perforated TM	Disruption of TM integrity results in impaired transmission of sound to ossicle	Acute onset. May follow direct trauma or sudden barotrauma. May have sudden relief from pain if caused by otitis media	Treat infectious causes. Counsel on importance of keeping water out of ear canal. ENT referral	Good
Sterile effusion (barotrauma)	Fluid in middle ear dampens conduction through ossicles	Often following flight, diving, or URI. Bubbles can cause intermittent pain	Decongestants. Evaluate for infection. Follow-up	Excellent
Acute otitis media	Pus (or fluid) in middle ear dampens conduction through ossicles	Acute to subacute onset, often following URI. Often associated with pain ± fever	Antibiotics (unless viral cause suspected), decongestants, pain control	Excellent if treated appropriately
Cholesteatoma	Trapped stratified squamous epithelial mass in middle ear. Interferes with ossicle conduction	Slow onset. Often history of previous perforations or chronic infections	ENT referral	Variable. May destroy ossicles or erode into surrounding structures
Glomus tumor	Vascular tumor occupies middle ear space. Interferes with ossicle conduction	Slow onset. May be associated with rushing pulsatile sensation	ENT referral	Variable
Cancer	Squamous cell most common. Obstructs external canal	Slow onset. Often noticed first by others. Painless unless occlusion causes otitis externa	ENT referral. Evaluate for secondary infection	Variable
Sensorineural Lesion				
Perilymph fistula (inner ear barotrauma)	Disruption of round or oval window allows leakage of perilymph into middle ear	Sudden onset of hearing loss often with tinnitus and vertigo. Frequently follows straining or abrupt change in pressure. Turning in direction of fistula exacerbates symptoms	Complete bed rest. Elevate head of bed and avoid increases in CSF pressure. Severe symptoms or noncompliance may require hospitalization. ENT consultation for possible oval or round window patch	Variable
Viral cochleitis	Cochlear inflammation. Often following URI	Rapid onset. Often following URI	Steroids often used (no good data)	Variable
Presbycusis	Age-related hearing loss. May be related to previous chronic noise exposure	Slow onset. Usually symmetric. High frequencies most affected. Tinnitus may occur	Hearing aid may help with both hearing loss and tinnitus	Variable
Acoustic neuroma	Benign schwannoma of 8th cranial nerve	Slow onset. Usually unilateral. May exhibit tinnitus, vertigo. May exhibit facial hyperesthesias or twitching	May require surgical excision if symptoms debilitating	Variable
Ototoxic agents	Direct toxicity to inner ear structures	Variable onset. High frequency most affected. Exposure to ototoxic drugs. May have associated tinnitus	Stop use of offending agent	Variable. Hearing loss at time of stopping offending agent is usually permanent
Multiple sclerosis	Multiple demyelinating lesions interfere with nerve conduction	Often other associated neurologic findings. May wax and wane	Standard multiple sclerosis treatment (steroids, cytotoxic agents)	Variable
Stroke/CVA	Focal ischemic lesion of auditory nerve or auditory cortex	Sudden onset. Often associated with other neurologic deficits	Treat CVA risk factors (ASA, anticoagulants, glycemic control, BP control)	Variable
Meningitis	Infection enters inner ear through CNS-perilymph connection. Damages organ of Corti	Follows clinical picture of meningitis	Treat infection. Steroids may limit inflammation and damage	Variable
Ménière disease (endolymphatic hydrops)	Abnormal homeostasis of inner ear fluids (clinical diagnosis; definitive diagnosis made histologically)	Episodic spells of vertigo. Associated sensation of fullness, tinnitus, and SNHL or auditory distortion. Low-frequency ranges most affected	Reduce salt, caffeine, nicotine (vasoconstrictors) intake. Consider diuretics, antihistamines, anticholinergics. ENT referral	Variable
Chronic noise exposure	Direct mechanical damage to cochlear structures and hair cells	Slow onset. Usually high frequency most affected	Prevention measures (earplugs). Stop exposure	Usually permanent

Continued

TABLE 72 Lesions That Cause Hearing Loss—cont'd

	Description of Pathology	Onset/Course	Actions or Treatment	Prognosis
Skull trauma	Interruption of cranial nerve VIII, ossicle disruption, or shearing effects on organ of Corti	Sudden onset after trauma	ENT consultation for possible surgical repair	Variable: Ossicle disruption has better prognosis than nerve or organ of Corti damage
Autoimmune causes	Vascular or neuronal inflammatory changes	Bilateral asymmetric SNHL. May be fluctuating or progressive. Often other systemic autoimmune findings	Outpatient autoimmune evaluation. Steroids and cytotoxic agents may slow progression	Variable

ASA, Acetylsalicylic acid; *BP,* blood pressure; *CNS,* central nervous system; *CSF,* cerebrospinal fluid; *CVA,* cerebrovascular accident; *ENT,* ear, nose, and throat; *SNHL,* sensorineural hearing loss; *TM,* tympanic membrane; *URI,* upper respiratory infection.
From Adams JG et al: *Emergency medicine, clinical essentials,* ed 2, Philadelphia, 2013, Elsevier.

TABLE 73 A Summary of Diagnostic Audiology Tests and Applications

Audiologic Test Battery	Hearing acuity	*Air conduction thresholds*	Measures function of the external, middle, and inner ear.
		Bone conduction thresholds	Measures function of the inner ear, bypassing external and middle ear structures.
	Speech testing	*Speech detection threshold (SDT)*	The speech (spondee word) level where an individual can discern the presence of a speech signal 50% of the time.
		Speech reception threshold (SRT)	The intensity level where an individual can correctly repeat spondee words 50% of the time.
		Speech recognition	Measures an individual's ability to recognize speech—typically monosyllabic words presented at supra-threshold levels, under well-controlled conditions. Testing may be open or closed set.
		Subjective report scales	Questionnaires or inventories related to everyday listening situations for adults or that use parental reporting to evaluate a child's listening skills in his or her daily environment.
Evaluating Middle Ear Function	Tympanometry		Measures the acoustic immittance of the tympanic membrane and middle ear ossicular chain as a function of air pressure variations in the ear canal. Estimates intratympanic pressure, eustachian tube function, tympanic membrane integrity and mobility, and continuity of the ossicular chain.
	Stapedial reflexes		Determines the softest level of sound that will elicit stapedial muscle contraction. Typically occurs at 70-100 dB HL for a normal-hearing ear.
	Acoustic reflex decay		Measures the ability of the stapedius muscle to maintain sustained contraction. A response is abnormal if its amplitude decreases to half or less of its original measurement over 5 sec.
Objective Tests for Differential Diagnostic Applications	Otoacoustic emissions	*Transient-evoked otoacoustic emissions*	Audiofrequency signals generated by outer hair cells measured in the ear canal elicited by a transient, brief stimulus such as a click or tone burst. Presence indicates cochlear outer hair cell integrity.
		Distortion-product otoacoustic emissions	Audiofrequency signals generated by outer hair cells measured in the ear canal elicited by a pair of pure tones separated by a specific frequency difference. Presence indicates cochlear outer hair cell integrity.
	ECochG		Measurement of neuroelectric events at the tympanic membrane or promontory generated by cochlear structures and the auditory nerve in response to acoustic stimulation. Response may consist of the cochlear microphonic, summating potential, and/or action potential.
	Sonomotor responses	*C-VEMP and O-VEMP*	Vestibular evoked myogenic potentials elicited from the sternocleidomastoid muscle (inferior vestibular nerve) or inferior rectus/inferior oblique of contralateral eye (superior vestibular nerve) that are useful to evaluate the function of the superior versus inferior vestibular nerve.
	Auditory brainstem response	*Threshold estimation ABR*	Surface-recorded averaged responses to click or tone burst stimuli that represent activity of the distal portion of the auditory pathway. Wave V threshold may be used to estimate behavioral auditory thresholds.
		Neurodiagnostic ABR	Surface-recorded averaged response to click stimuli that represents activity of the distal portion of the auditory pathway. Responses are typically assessed for amplitude, morphology, and absolute and inter-peak latencies of waves I-V.
	Auditory steady-state response		Far-field recording of EEG activity evoked using a continuous sinusoidal acoustic stimulus that is amplitude and frequency modulated at slow rates. Response presence/absence is analyzed automatically using statistical procedures.
	Electrically evoked auditory potentials	*Electrically evoked ABR*	Surface-recorded averaged responses to electrical stimuli delivered to promontory or via a cochlear implant that represents activity of the distal portion of the auditory pathway.
		Electrically evoked compound action potential	Recording of the synchronized discharge of a large number of electrically stimulated auditory nerve fibers. The primary response is a single negative peak (N1) occurring at 0.3-0.5 ms with amplitude up to 2-3 mV.
		Electrically evoked middle-latency response	A series of electrically evoked vertex-positive peaks that occur within a time window of 10-50 ms after stimulation and is thought to be generated by neurons in the auditory midbrain and primary cortex.
		Cortical auditory evoked potentials	Most frequently refers to the long-latency, obligatory P1-N1-P2 complex. Components have latencies between 70 and 300 ms and arise from cortical or precortical levels of the auditory system.

Clinical Algorithms

III

Continued

TABLE 73 A Summary of Diagnostic Audiology Tests and Applications—cont'd

Evaluating Functional HL	PTA/SRT agreement	The average of the air conduction thresholds at 500, 1000, and 2000 Hz should agree with the speech reception threshold within 5 dB.
	Stenger test	A tone is presented to the better ear at 10 dB above its threshold simultaneously with an identical tone to the poorer ear at 10 dB below its voluntary threshold. The individual will respond if the hearing loss is genuine. A nonresponse is a positive Stenger test and indicates pseudohypacusis.

ABR, Auditory brainstem responses; *C-VEMP,* cervical vestibular evoked myogenic potential; *ECochG,* electrocochleography; *HL,* hearing level; *O-VEMP,* ocular vestibular-evoked myogenic potential; *PTA,* pure-tone average; *SDT,* speech detection threshold; *SRT,* speech reception threshold.
From Flint PW et al: *Cummings otolaryngology, head and neck surgery,* ed 7, Philadelphia, 2021, Elsevier.

TABLE 74 History Taking for a Chief Complaint of Hearing Loss

Duration	What difficulty is this causing the individual?
Progression	Prior ear infection/trauma/surgery
Slow versus rapid	Noise exposure
Sudden	Family history of hearing loss
Fluctuating	Ototoxic medication exposure
Symmetric or asymmetric?	Prior amplification experience
Associated ear symptoms	
Tinnitus	
Vertigo	
Otalgia	
Otorrhea	

From Flint PW et al: *Cummings otolaryngology, head and neck surgery,* ed 7, Philadelphia, 2021, Elsevier.

TABLE 75 Red Flags for Hearing Loss History

Unilateral	Otalgia
Sudden onset	Accompanying cranial nerve signs
Fluctuation	Numbness
Rapidly progressive	Diplopia
Vertigo or ataxia	Facial paresis
Otorrhea	Voice/swallowing changes

From Flint PW et al: *Cummings otolaryngology, head and neck surgery,* ed 7, Philadelphia, 2021, Elsevier.

TABLE 76 History Taking for a Chief Complaint of Tinnitus

Duration	Associated ear symptoms
Progression	Vertigo
Slow versus rapid	Hearing loss
Sudden	Otalgia
Fluctuating	Otorrhea
Symmetric or asymmetric?	Prior ear infection/trauma/surgery
Pulsatile or nonpulsatile?	Noise exposure
How does it sound?	Family history of hearing loss
Mitigating factors	Caffeine or other stimulant consumption
Prior therapies	

From Flint PW et al: *Cummings otolaryngology, head and neck surgery,* ed 7, Philadelphia, 2021, Elsevier.

TABLE 77 Interpreting the Weber and Rinne Tuning Fork Tests

	Weber to Left	Weber to Right
Rinne + AU	SNHL AD (or mild CHL AS)	SNHL AS (or mild CHL AD)
Rinne − AS	CHL AS	Mixed HL AS[a]
Rinne − AD	Mixed HL AD[a]	CHL AD
Rinne − AU	CHL AS, Mixed HL AD	CHL AD, Mixed HL AS

AD, Right ear; *AS,* left ear; *AU,* bilateral; *CHL,* conductive HL; *HL,* hearing loss; *SNHL,* sensorineural hearing loss.
[a]It is also possible that the Rinne could be heard in the normal-hearing contralateral ear in cases of profound SNHL in the test ear due to inability to mask.
From Flint PW et al: *Cummings otolaryngology, head and neck surgery,* ed 7, Philadelphia, 2021, Elsevier.

TABLE 78 Hearing Loss Classification and Features

Criteria	Classification	Comment
Causality	Genetic	Hereditary
	Environmental	Nonhereditary
	Multifactorial	
Time of onset	Congenital	At birth
	Acquired	Develops any time after birth
Age of onset	Prelingual	Before speech development
	Postlingual	After speech development
Clinical presentation	Nonsyndromic	Hearing loss only symptom
	Syndromic	Hearing loss and other symptoms
Anatomic defect	Conductive	Dysfunction of outer or middle ear
	Sensorineural	Dysfunction of inner ear or auditory
	Mixed	nerve
Severity	Slight	16-25 dB
	Mild	26-40 dB
	Moderate	41-55 dB
	Moderately severe	56-70 dB
	Severe	71-90 dB
	Profound	>90 dB
Frequency loss	Low frequency	<500 Hz
	Mid frequency	501-2000 Hz
	High frequency	>2000 Hz
Ears affected	Unilateral	One ear affected
	Bilateral	Both ears affected
	Symmetric	Both ears affected equally
	Asymmetric	Both ears not affected equally
Prognosis	Stable	Severity remains unchanged
	Progressive	Severity increases over time

From Flint PW et al: *Cummings otolaryngology, head and neck surgery,* ed 7, Philadelphia 2021, Elsevier.

TABLE 79 Quantification of Hearing Impairment

Impairment (%)	Pure Tone Average (dB)[a]	Residual Hearing (%)
100	91	0
80	78	20
60	65	40
30	45	70

[a]Pure tone average of 500, 1000, 2000, and 3000 Hz.
From Flint PW et al: *Cummings otolaryngology, head and neck surgery,* ed 7, Philadelphia 2021, Elsevier.

TABLE 80 Differential Diagnosis of Sudden Sensorineural Hearing Loss

Category	Etiology
Infectious	Serous or suppurative labyrinthitis
	Viral (e.g., mumps, rubella, rubeola, varicella zoster, herpes simplex, HIV/AIDS, mononucleosis, Lassa fever, Zika, West Nile virus)
	Bacterial (e.g., streptococcal meningitis, syphilis, Lyme, mycoplasma, cryptococcal meningitis)
Neoplastic	Acoustic neuroma/vestibular schwannoma
	Meningioma
	Epidermoid
	Hemangioma
	Arachnoid cyst
	Temporal bone metastasis, meningeal carcinomatosis
	Lymphoma, leukemia, myeloma
Traumatic	Acoustic trauma
	Temporal bone fracture, penetrating trauma
	Inner ear concussion
	Perilymphatic fistula
	Barotrauma
Ototoxic	Ototoxic medications (e.g., aminoglycosides, chemotherapeutics)
	Medication overuse or abuse (e.g., acetaminophen/opiate combinations, heroin, methadone, cocaine)
Immunologic	Autoimmune inner ear disease
	Autoimmune disease (e.g., Cogan syndrome, systemic lupus erythematosus, granulomatosis with polyangiitis, polyarteritis nodosa, relapsing polychondritis, sarcoidosis)
	Multiple sclerosis
Vascular	Cerebrovascular accident
	Vertebrobasilar insufficiency
	Migraine
	Sickle cell disease
	Macroglobulinemia
	Cardiopulmonary bypass
Developmental	Large vestibular aqueduct
Idiopathic	Idiopathic sudden sensorineural hearing loss
	Ménière disease
	Nonorganic hearing loss (factitious, malingering, or conversion disorder)

From Flint PW et al: *Cummings otolaryngology, head and neck surgery,* ed 7, Philadelphia 2021, Elsevier.

Clinical Algorithms

III

ICD-10CM # H90.2 Conductive hearing loss, unspecified
H90.5 Unspecified sensorineural hearing loss

TABLE 81 Comparison of Conventional Hearing Aids and Implantable Hearing Devices

Device	Sensor	Actuator	Regulatory Approval	Totally/Partially Implanted	Surgical Placement	Audiologic Indications	MRI	Special Advantages/Disadvantages	EAC Occlusion
Conventional digital BTE device	External BTE microphone	Acoustic, to TM	Yes	NA	NA	Mild to severe CHL or SNHL	NA	No surgery required; visible; EAC occlusion	Yes, unless open fit
Conventional digital CIC device	External microphone at lateral end of CIC device	Acoustic, to TM	Yes	NA	NA	Mild to moderate CHL or SNHL	NA	No surgery required, low visibility; EAC occlusion	Yes
Esteem (Envoy Medical)	Piezoelectric, coupled to malleus/TM	Piezoelectric, to stapes	FDA CE mark	Total	Transmastoid, mandatory partial incus removal		No	Very high power; requires partial incus removal	No
Carina (Cochlear)	Subcutaneous microphone	Piezoelectric, to incus	CE mark, FDA Phase II clinical trials	Total	Transmastoid	Moderate to severe	No	High-powered output, fully implantable; ossicles remain intact; adjustable for ossicular abnormalities	No
Vibrant Soundbridge (Med-El)	External BTE microphone	Electromagnetic, clipped to incus	FDA CE mark	Partial	Transmastoid and endaural		No	First FDA approved; largest install base	No
Baha (Cochlear)	External microphone	Electromagnetic vibrator, coupled to titanium screw in skull	FDA CE mark	Partial	Cortical skull bone screw	CHL, inability to tolerate conventional HA, SSD	Yes	Simple placement, nothing in ear or mastoid	No
Ponto (Oticon Medical)	External microphone	Electromagnetic vibrator, coupled to titanium screw in skull	FDA CE mark	Partial	Cortical skull bone screw	CHL, inability to tolerate conventional HA, SSD	Yes	Simple placement, nothing in ear or mastoid	No
Alpha 2 (Sophono)	External microphone	Electromagnetic vibrator, transcutaneously coupled to osseointegrated implant	FDA CE mark	Partial	Cortical skull bone well and screws	CHL unable to tolerate conventional HA, SSD	No	No percutaneous abutment	No
Bonebridge (Med-El)	External microphone	Electromagnetic vibrator, transcutaneously coupled to osseointegrated implant	CE mark	Partial	Cortical skull bone well and screws	CHL, inability to tolerate conventional HA, SSD	No	No percutaneous abutment	No
SoundBite (Sonitus Medical)	External BTE microphone	Piezoelectric, to maxillary molars	FDA CE mark	NA	NA	CHL, inability to tolerate conventional HA, SSD	NA	No surgery required; visible; EAC occlusion	No

BTE, Behind the ear; CE, Communauté Européenne; CHL, conductive hearing loss; CIC, completely in canal; EAC, external auditory canal; FDA, U.S. Food and Drug Administration; HA, hearing aid; MRI, magnetic resonance imaging; NA, not applicable; SNHL, sensorineural hearing loss; SSD, single-sided deafness; TM, tympanic membrane.
From Flint PW et al: Cummings otolaryngology, head and neck surgery, ed 7, Philadelphia, 2021, Elsevier.

BOX 27 History and Physical Examination for Hearing Loss

Onset
Age at onset
Abrupt versus gradual
Progressive, intermittent, or continuous
Antecedent illness
Duration of symptoms

Associated Symptoms
Tinnitus
Dizziness or vertigo
Aural fullness
Pain
Allergy symptoms
Actions that change intensity of symptoms
Distorted auditory perception
Worsening with pregnancy or oral contraceptive use

Further History
Family history of hearing loss
Occupational noise exposure
Recreational noise exposure
Trauma
Surgical history
Previous or current drainage from ear
Quality of drainage
Systemic infections and treatments
Meningitis
Syphilis
Previous use of a hearing aid
Ototoxic medications
Cancer chemotherapy
Antibiotics
Recent air travel
Recent underwater diving

Examination
Complete head and neck examination
Cranial nerve examination
Otoscopy with microscope as needed
Otoneurologic examination as indicated
Tuning fork testing (256 Hz, 512 Hz, 1024 Hz)
Weber test
Rinne test

Radiographic and Laboratory Evaluation
Computed tomography as indicated
Magnetic resonance imaging as indicated
Erythrocyte sedimentation rate; fluorescent treponemal antibody, absorbed; Lyme titers; complete blood count; thyroid function tests; electrolytes; urinalysis (additional studies are indicated to work up suspected systemic diseases)

Audiometric Evaluation
Pure tone audiometry
Air conduction
Bone conduction
Speech testing
Speech reception threshold
Speech discrimination testing
Immittance testing
Static compliance
Tympanometry
Acoustic reflexes

Additional Audiometric Testing
Auditory brain stem response
Electrocochleography
Otoacoustic emissions

From Flint PW et al: *Cummings otolaryngology, head and neck surgery,* ed 7, Philadelphia, 2021, Elsevier.

Clinical
Algorithms

III

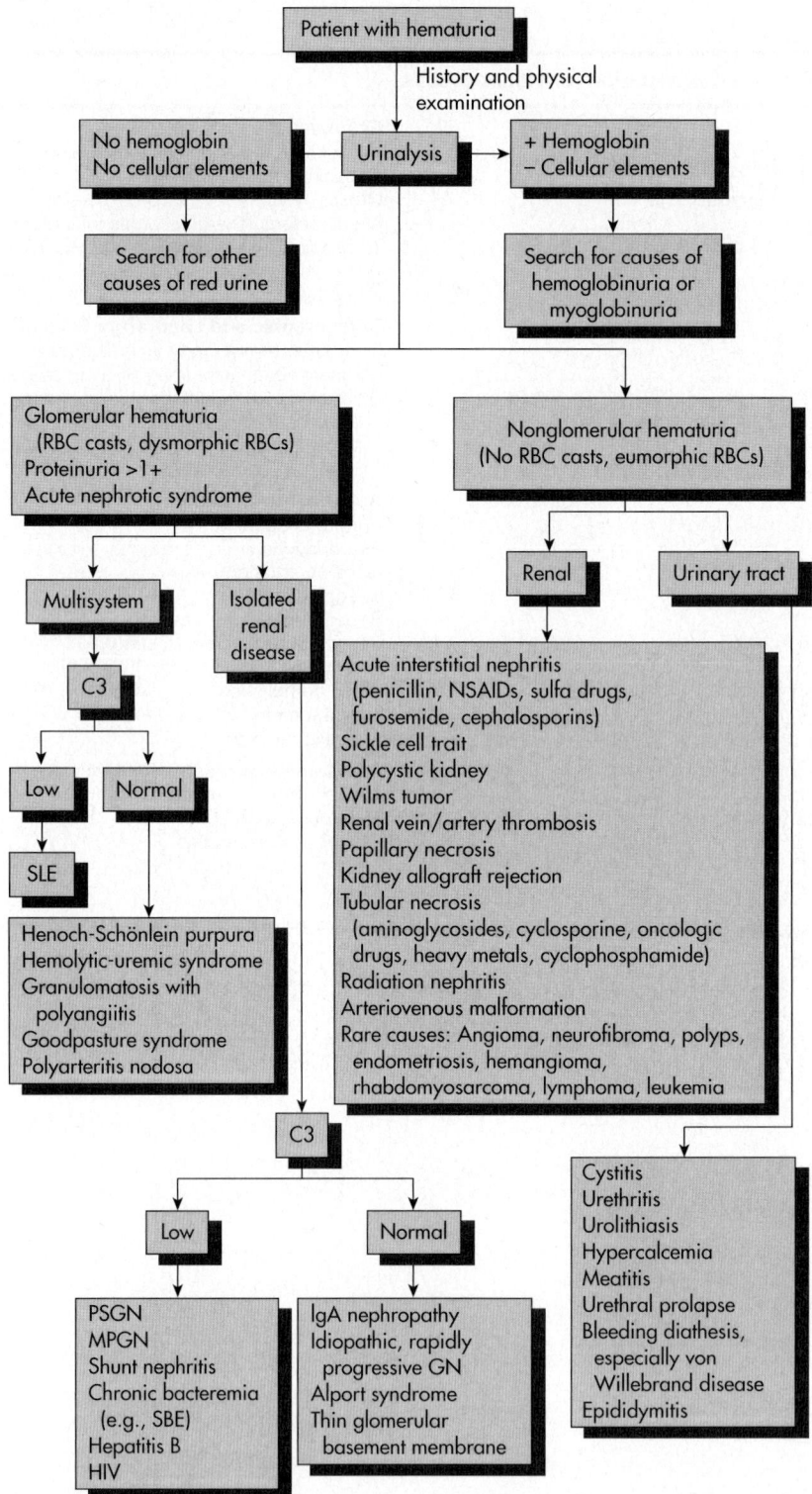

FIG. 109 Diagnostic strategy for hematuria. *GN,* Glomerulonephritis; *HIV,* human immunodeficiency virus; *Ig,* immunoglobulin; *MPGN,* membranoproliferative glomerulonephritis; *NSAIDs,* nonsteroidal antiinflammatory drugs; *PSGN,* poststreptococcal glomerulonephritis; *RBC,* red blood cell; *SBE,* subacute bacterial endocarditis; *SLE,* systemic lupus erythematosus. (From The Johns Hopkins Hospital et al [eds]: *The Harriet Lane handbook,* ed 21, St Louis, 2018, Elsevier.)

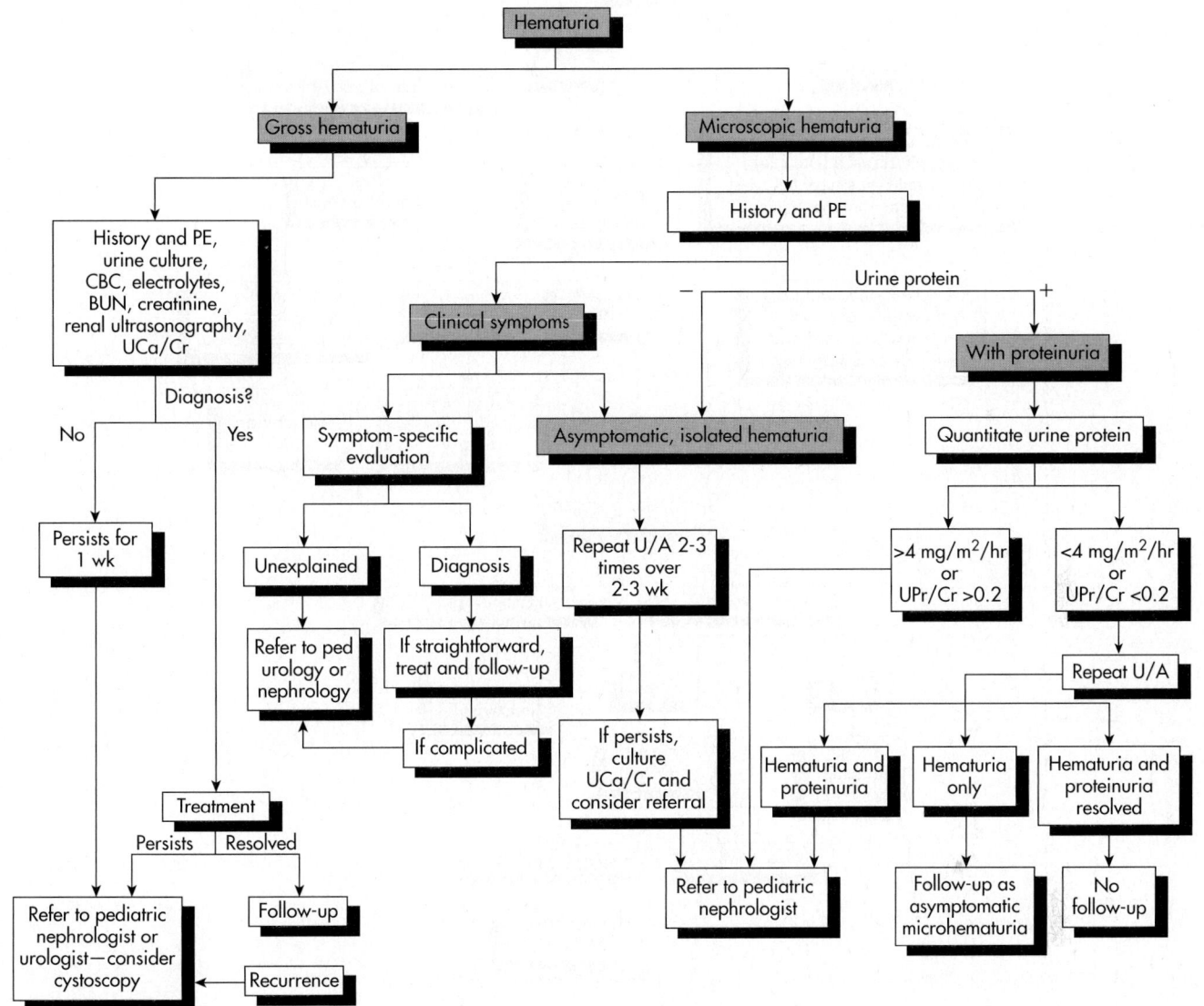

FIG. 110 Algorithm for the treatment of hematuria. *BUN,* Blood urea nitrogen; *CBC,* complete blood cell count; *PE,* physical examination; *U/A,* urinalysis; *UCa/Cr,* urinary calcium/creatinine ratio; *UPr/Cr,* urinary protein/creatinine ratio. (From Wein AJ et al: *Campbell-Walsh urology,* ed 11, Philadelphia, 2016, Elsevier.)

Clinical Algorithms

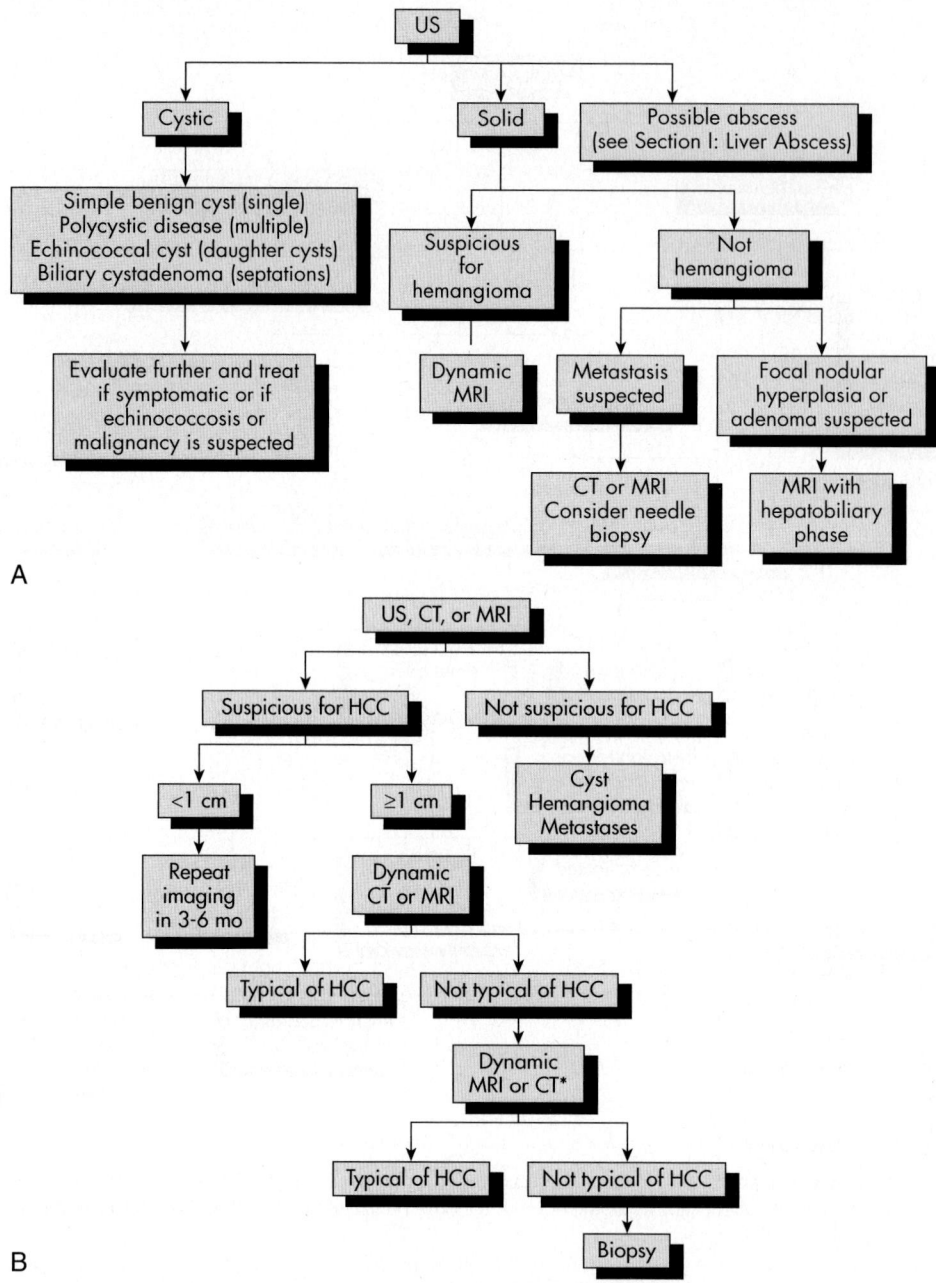

FIG. 111 A, Algorithm for the approach to the management of a patient, not known to have cirrhosis, with a hepatic mass (often incidental, possibly symptomatic). **B,** Algorithm for the approach to the management of a patient with known or suspected cirrhosis and a hepatic mass (found on routine surveillance, because of symptoms, or because of an increasing alpha-fetoprotein level). *Perform imaging modality not previously performed. *CT,* Computed tomography; *HCC,* hepatocellular carcinoma; *MRI,* magnetic resonance imaging; *US,* ultrasound. (From Feldman M et al: *Sleisenger and Fordtran's gastrointestinal and liver disease,* ed 10, Philadelphia, 2016, Elsevier.)

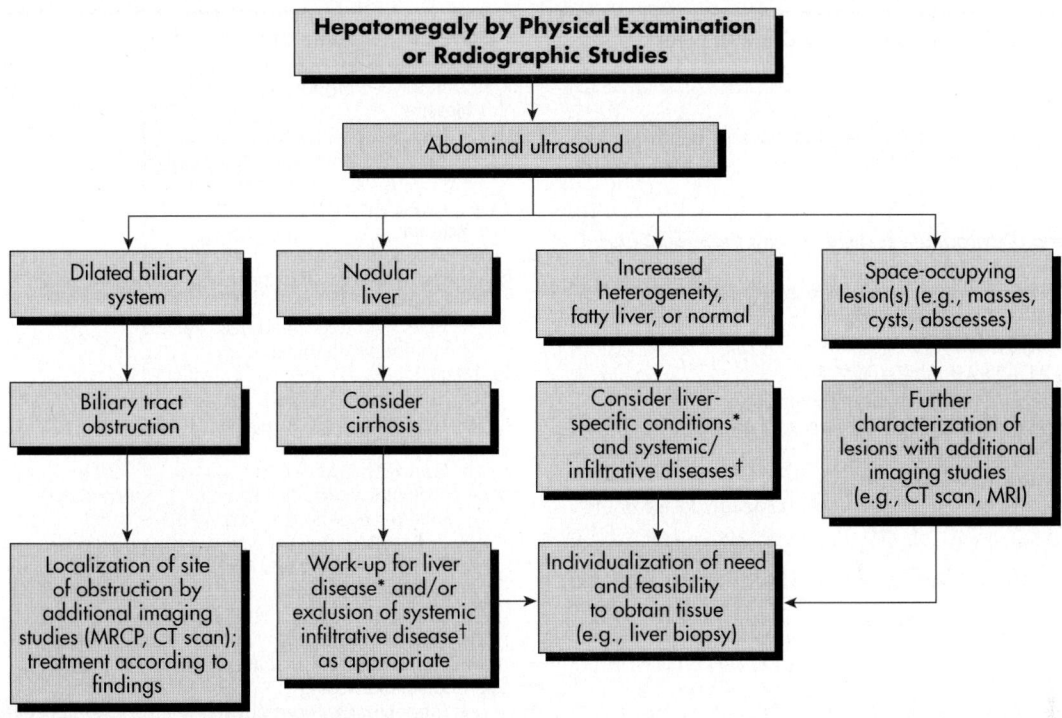

FIG. 112 Diagnostic approach to hepatomegaly. *Conditions to be excluded include viral hepatitis; alcohol- and drug-induced liver disease; steatohepatitis; autoimmune liver diseases; and metabolic disorders, including hemochromatosis, Wilson disease, and α1-antitrypsin deficiency. †Systemic and infiltrative diseases include amyloidosis, lymphoma, sarcoidosis, and infectious processes such as disseminated tuberculosis and fungemia. *CT,* Computed tomography; *MRCP,* magnetic resonance cholangiopancreatography; *MRI,* magnetic resonance imaging. (From Goldman L, Shafer AI: *Goldman-Cecil medicine,* ed 26, Elsevier, 2020.)

TABLE 82 Approach to Common Hepatic Complaints

Presentation	Common Symptoms	Common Physical Signs	Diagnostic Studies	Common Diagnoses
Ascites	Abdominal distention and pain, ankle edema	Flank dullness Shifting dullness Fluid wave	Ultrasound with Doppler Diagnostic paracentesis Urinalysis	Cirrhosis Budd-Chiari syndrome Heart failure Nephrotic syndrome
Hepatic encephalopathy	Sleep disorientation, confusion, coma	Asterixis Altered mentation Fetor hepaticus	Serum ammonia Blood cultures Stool hemoccult Serum creatinine and electrolytes	Decompensated cirrhosis Acute liver failure Other metabolic encephalopathies (renal, respiratory)
Hepatic mass	None or abdominal pain	Hepatic bruit or rub	α-Fetoprotein Ultrasound CT scan MRI Biopsy	Benign lesions: Hemangioma, adenoma, focal nodular hyperplasia Malignant lesions: Hepatocellular carcinoma, cholangiocarcinoma, metastases
Abdominal pain	Nausea, vomiting, fever	Right upper quadrant tenderness Palpable gallbladder Murphy sign	Ultrasound HIDA scan Paracentesis for ascites if present	Biliary colic Acute cholecystitis Hepatic congestion Hepatic metastases

CT, Computed tomography; *HIDA,* hepatobiliary iminodiacetic acid; *MRI,* magnetic resonance imaging.
From Goldman L, Shafer AI: *Goldman-Cecil medicine,* ed 26, Philadelphia, 2020, Elsevier.

Clinical Algorithms

III

BOX 28 Clinical Clues Suggesting Chronic Liver Disease

Symptoms

Fatigue, pruritus, bleeding, abdominal pain, nausea, anorexia, myalgia, jaundice, dark urine, pale stools, fever, weight loss; may be no symptoms

Signs

Peripheral signs of chronic liver disease with hepatocellular dysfunction:

Spider nevi, palmar erythema, white nails, gynecomastia, body hair loss, testicular atrophy, hepatomegaly

Signs of portal hypertension:

Splenomegaly, ascites, peripheral edema

Signs of poor hepatocellular synthetic function:

Bruising, peripheral edema (reflecting depleted coagulation factors and albumin levels)

Signs of end-stage liver disease:

Wasting, progressive severe fatigue, encephalopathy (asterixis, fetor, coma)

From Talley NJ et al: *Essentials of internal medicine,* ed 4, Chatswood, NSW, 2021, Elsevier Australia.

BOX 29 Causes of Hepatomegaly

1. Diffusely enlarged and smooth
   Massive
   - Metastatic disease
   - Alcoholic liver disease with fatty infiltration
   - Myeloproliferative diseases (e.g., polycythemia rubra vera, myelofibrosis)
   Moderate
   - The above causes
   - Hematologic disease (e.g., chronic myeloid leukemia, lymphoma)
   - Fatty liver (e.g., diabetes mellitus)
   - Hemochromatosis
   Mild
   - The above causes
   - Hepatitis (viral, drugs)
   - Cirrhosis
   - Biliary obstruction
   - Granulomatous disorders (e.g., sarcoidosis)
   - Infiltrative disorders (e.g., amyloidosis)
   - Human immunodeficiency virus infection
2. Diffusely enlarged and irregular
   - Metastatic disease
   - Cirrhosis
   - Hydatid disease
   - Polycystic liver disease
3. Localized swelling
   - Riedel lobe (a normal variant—the lobe may even be palpable in the right lumbar region)
   - Metastasis
   - Large simple hepatic cyst
   - Hydatid cyst
   - Hepatoma
   - Liver abscess (e.g., amebic abscess)
4. Hepatosplenomegaly
   - Chronic liver disease with portal hypertension
   - Hematologic disease (e.g., myeloproliferative disease, lymphoma)
   - Infection (e.g., acute viral hepatitis, infectious mononucleosis)
   - Infiltration (e.g., amyloidosis, sarcoidosis)
   - Connective tissue disease (e.g., systemic lupus erythematosus)

From Talley NJ et al: *Essentials of internal medicine,* ed 4, Chatswood, NSW, 2021, Elsevier Australia.

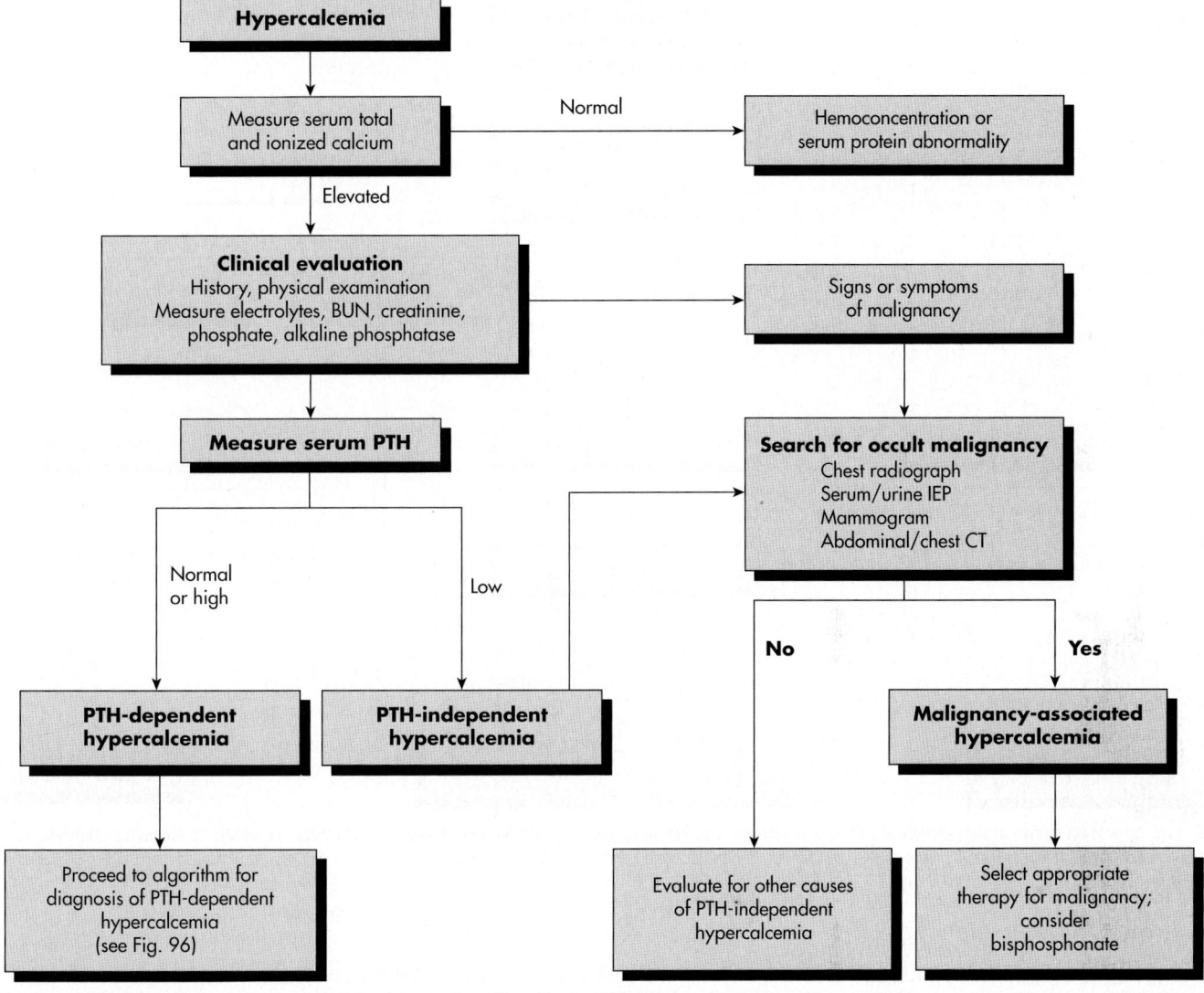

FIG. 113 Approach to the management of the hypercalcemic patient. *BUN,* Blood urea nitrogen; *CT,* computed tomography; *IEP,* immunoelectrophoresis; *PTH,* parathyroid hormone. (From Melmed S et al. *Williams textbook of endocrinology,* ed 14, Philadelphia, 2019, Elsevier.)

Clinical
Algorithms

III

PTH-dependent hypercalcemia
24-h urine calcium and creatinine
Urine calcium <100 mg/day, or Cl_{Ca}/Cl_{Cr} <0.01
Yes
No
PTH normal
PTH high
Primary hyperparathyroidism
Li therapy
Age <40, or Fam. Hx.
Perform bone densitometry
Consider stopping Li therapy
Yes
No
Review criteria for surgery
Calcium high
Calcium normal
No
Yes
Presumptive FHH; consider family screening
Medical observation
Parathyroidectomy
Li-induced hyperparathyroidism

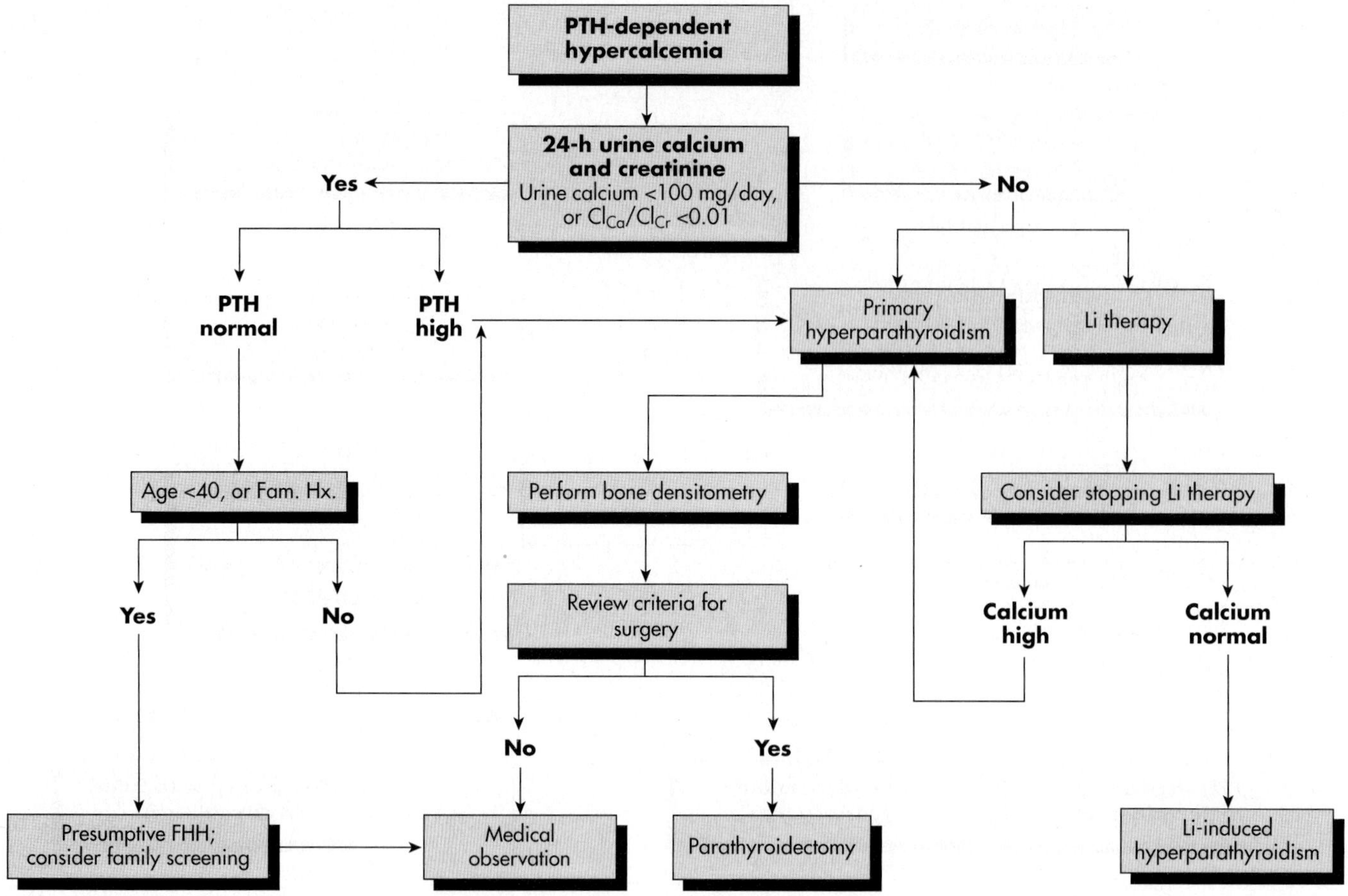

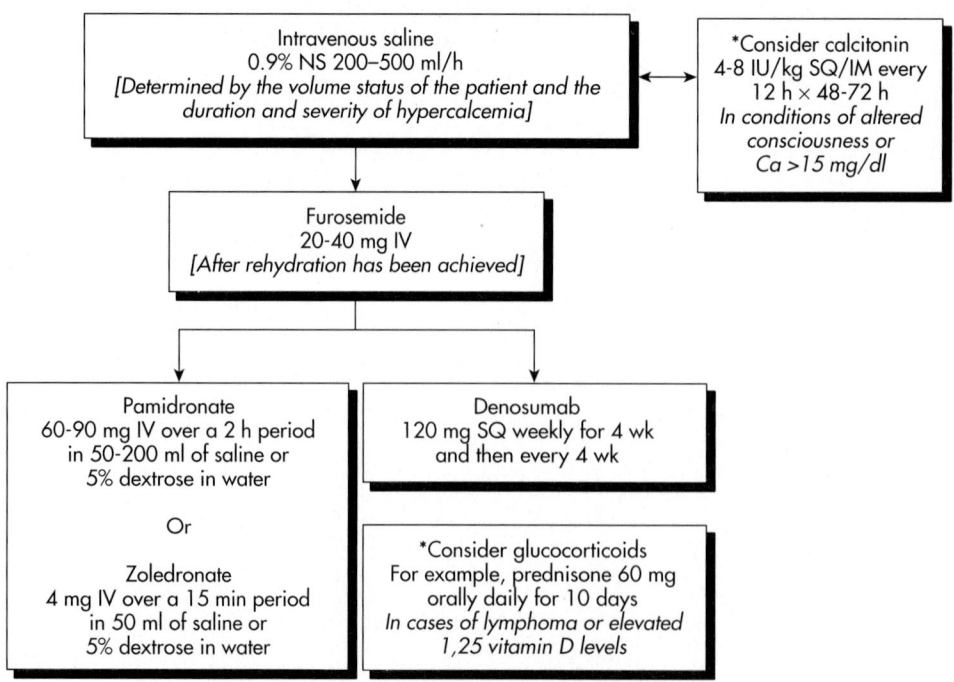

FIG. 114 Approach to the management of the hypercalcemic patient with parathyroid hormone–dependent hypercalcemia. *Cl,* Clearance; *Fam. Hx.,* family history; *FHH,* familial hypocalciuric hypercalcemia; *Li,* lithium; *PTH,* parathyroid hormone. (From Melmed S et al. *Williams textbook of endocrinology,* ed 14, Philadelphia, 2019, Elsevier.)

SUGGESTED TREATMENT OF MALIGNANCY ASSOCIATED HYPERCALCEMIA
Intravenous saline
0.9% NS 200–500 ml/h
[Determined by the volume status of the patient and the duration and severity of hypercalcemia]
*Consider calcitonin
4-8 IU/kg SQ/IM every 12 h × 48-72 h
In conditions of altered consciousness or Ca >15 mg/dl
Furosemide
20-40 mg IV
[After rehydration has been achieved]
Pamidronate
60-90 mg IV over a 2 h period in 50-200 ml of saline or 5% dextrose in water
Or
Zoledronate
4 mg IV over a 15 min period in 50 ml of saline or 5% dextrose in water
Denosumab
120 mg SQ weekly for 4 wk and then every 4 wk
*Consider glucocorticoids
For example, prednisone 60 mg orally daily for 10 days
In cases of lymphoma or elevated 1,25 vitamin D levels

FIG. 115 Suggested treatment for malignancy-associated hypercalcemia. *IM,* Intramuscular; *IV,* Intravenous; *NS,* Normal saline; *SQ,* Subcutaneous. (From Robertson RP et al: *DeGroot's endocrinology, basic science and clinical practice,* ed 8, Philadelphia, 2023, Elsevier.)

DIAGNOSTIC IMAGING

- Radiograph of painful bones (r/o bone neoplasm, multiple myeloma)
- Tc-99m parathyroid scan (r/o parathyroid adenoma)
- Ultrasound of parathyroid glands
- Ultrasound of kidneys (r/o renal cell carcinoma)

LAB EVALUATION

- Serum calcium level
- Parathyroid hormone level
- Serum phosphate, magnesium, alkaline phosphatase, albumin
- Electrolytes, blood urea nitrogen creatinine
- 24-h urine collection for calcium
- Urinary cyclic adenosine monophosphate
- Prostate-specific antigen (if prostate carcinoma is suspected)
- Serum and urine protein immunoelectrophoresis (if multiple myeloma suspected)

TABLE 83 Important Physiologic Changes in Bone and Mineral Diseases

Condition	Calcium	Phosphate	Parathyroid Hormone	25(OH)D
Primary hypoparathyroidism	↓	↑	↓	NI
Pseudohypoparathyroidism	↓	↑	↑	NI
Vitamin D deficiency	NI(↓)	↓	↑	↓
Familial hypophosphatemic rickets	NI	↓	NI (sl↑)	NI
Hyperparathyroidism	↑	↓	↑	NI
Immobilization	↑	↑	↓	NI

25(OH)D, 25-hydroxyvitamin D; *NI*, normal; *sl*, slight; ↑, high; ↓, low.
From Marcdante KJ et al: *Nelson essentials of pediatrics*, ed 9, Philadelphia, 2023, Elsevier.

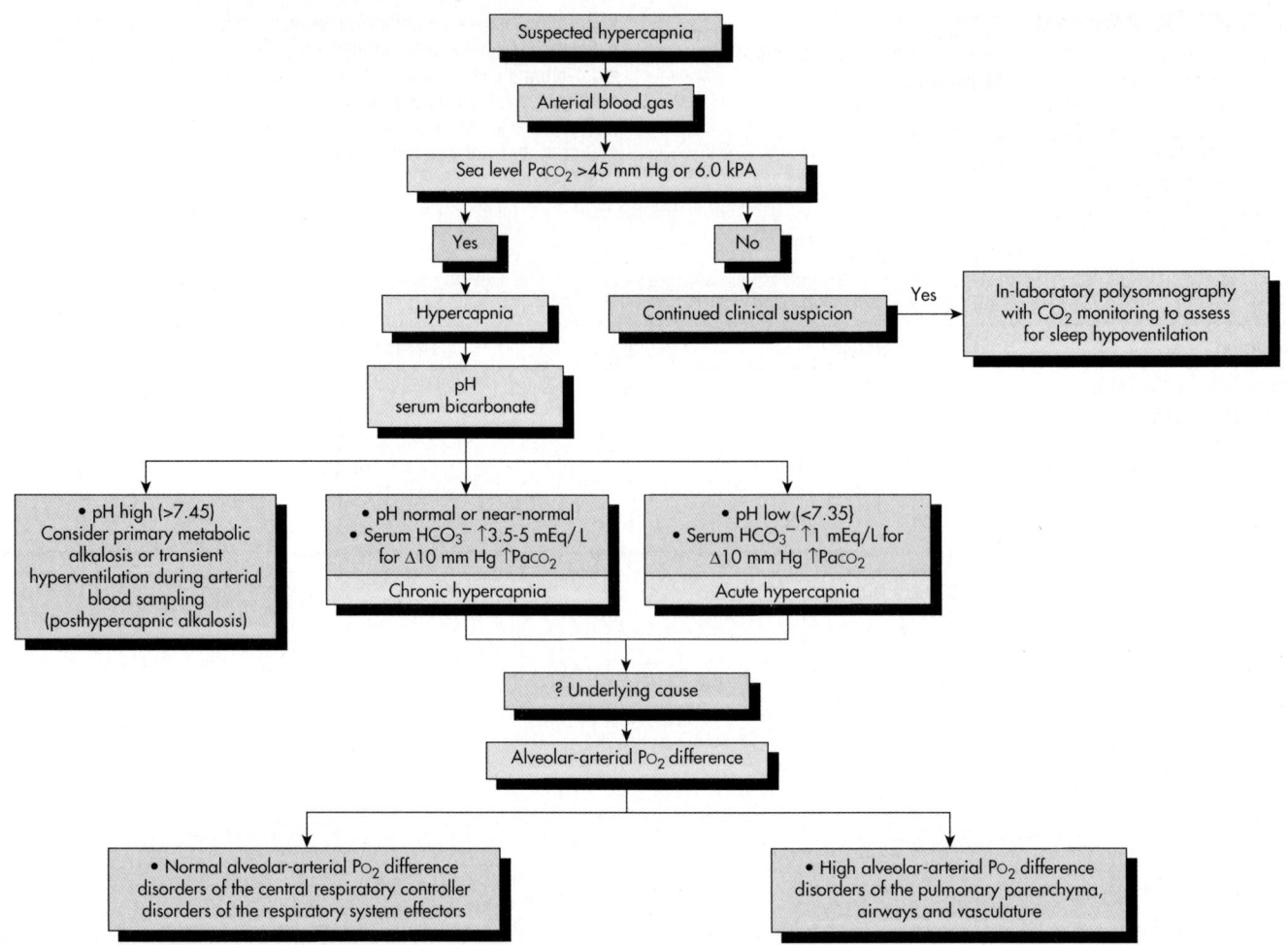

FIG. 116 Algorithm demonstrating a diagnostic approach to a patient with suspected hypercapnia. *Paco₂*, Partial pressure of carbon dioxide; *Pc₂*, partial pressure of oxygen. (From Broaddus VC et al: *Murray & Nadel's textbook of respiratory medicine*, ed 7, Philadelphia, 2022, Elsevier.)

TABLE 84   Classification of Hypercapnic Diseases

	Mechanism	Diagnosis	Treatment
Acquired Disease			
Narcotic overdose	Reduced central drive	History, narcotized pupils, toxicology	Supportive care, naloxone
Acute severe asthma	Severe airflow obstruction, high dead space	Typical history, wheezing on examination, low FEV₁/FVC	Bronchodilators, antiinflammatories, mechanical ventilation (usually invasive)
Acute exacerbation of COPD	Airflow obstruction, high dead space	History, cigarette smoking, low FEV₁/FVC, infectious etiology	Bronchodilators, antiinflammatories, noninvasive ventilation
Obesity-hypoventilation syndrome	Low respiratory system compliance, high upper airway resistance, low central drive	High BMI, lack of other diagnoses; blunted carbon dioxide response	Weight loss, nocturnal bilevel positive airway pressure
Neuromuscular disease (e.g., myasthenia gravis, ALS, polymyositis, GBS/AIDP)	Lack of respiratory muscle force	Immediate orthopnea, low VC, low MIPs/ MEPs	Underlying cause, nocturnal noninvasive ventilation, supportive care
Severe parenchymal lung disease, e.g., COPD	Lack of alveolar surface area; high pulmonary dead space and work of breathing	Typical history, smoking, low FEV₁ and FEV₁/FVC	Bronchodilator, antiinflammatory therapy, possible nocturnal noninvasive ventilation, smoking cessation
Kyphoscoliosis	Low respiratory system compliance	Physical examination	Supportive care, noninvasive ventilation
Congenital Disease			
Central congenital hypoventilation syndrome	*PHOX2B* mutation, lack of central drive	Genetic testing	Supportive care, mechanical ventilation (usually noninvasive)

AIDP, Acute inflammatory demyelinating polyneuropathy; *ALS,* amyotrophic lateral sclerosis; *BMI,* body mass index; *COPD,* chronic obstructive pulmonary disease; *FEV₁,* forced expiratory volume in 1 second; *FVC,* forced vital capacity; *GBS,* Guillain-Barré syndrome; *MEPs,* maximal expiratory pressures; *MIPs,* maximal inspiratory pressures; *VC,* vital capacity.
From Goldman L, Shafer AI: *Goldman-Cecil medicine,* ed 26, Philadelphia, 2019, Elsevier.

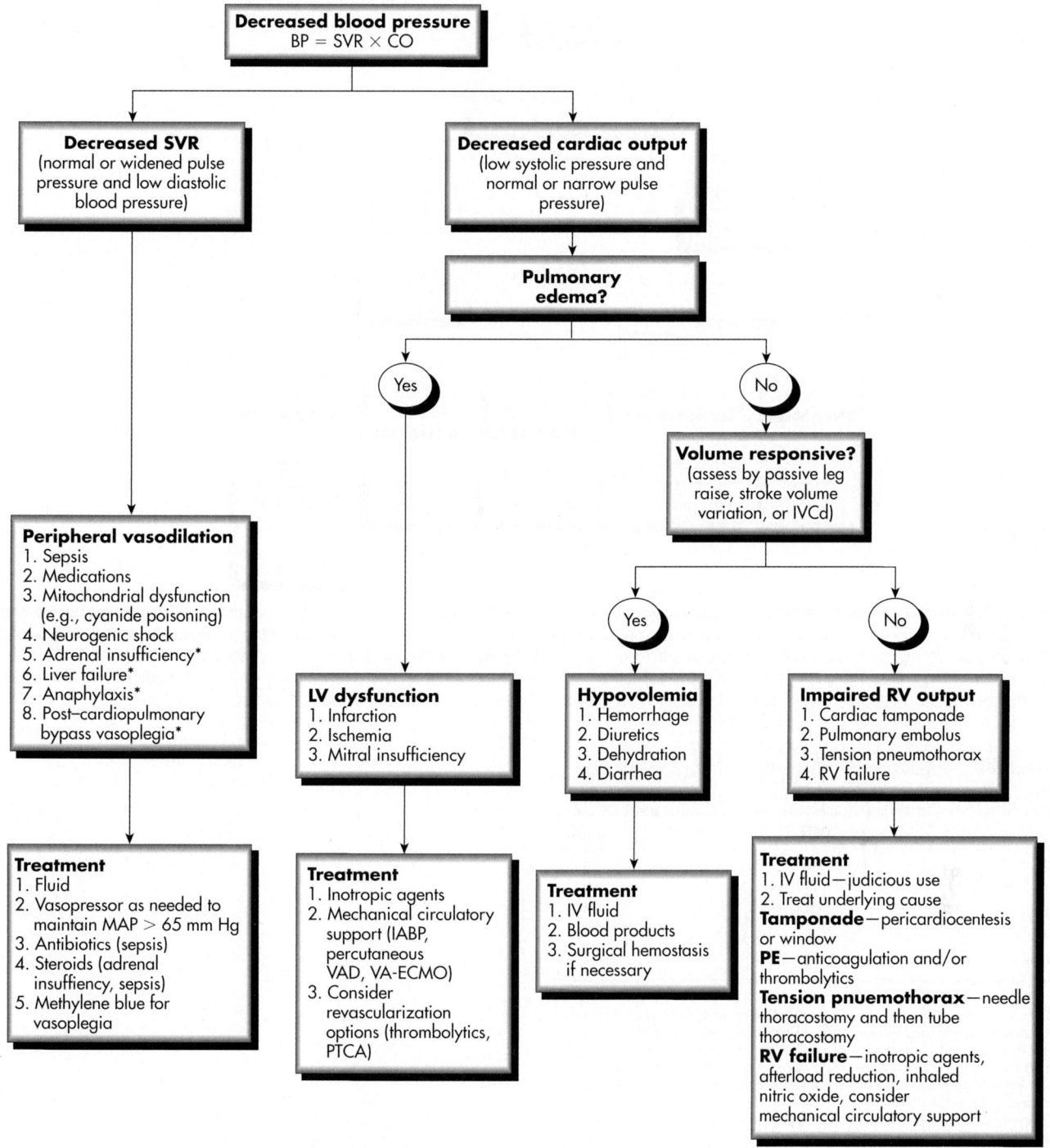

FIG. 120 Initial approach to a patient with low systemic arterial blood pressure. *Adrenal insufficiency, liver failure, post–cardiopulmonary bypass vasoplegia, and anaphylaxis are commonly listed as vasodilatory shock; however, data are inconclusive, and components of other types of shock (hypovolemic, cardiogenic) may also be present. *BP,* Blood pressure; *CO,* cardiac output; *IABP,* intraaortic balloon pump; *IV,* intravenous; *IVCd,* inferior vena cava diameter; *LV,* left ventricle; *MAP,* mean arterial pressure; *PE,* pulmonary embolism; *PTCA,* percutaneous transluminal coronary angioplasty; *RV,* right ventricle; *SVR,* systemic vascular resistance; *VAD,* ventricular assist device; *VA-ECMO,* venovenous extracorporeal membrane oxygenation. (From Vincent JL et al: *Textbook of critical care,* ed 8, Philadelphia, 2024, Elsevier.)

Clinical
Algorithms

III

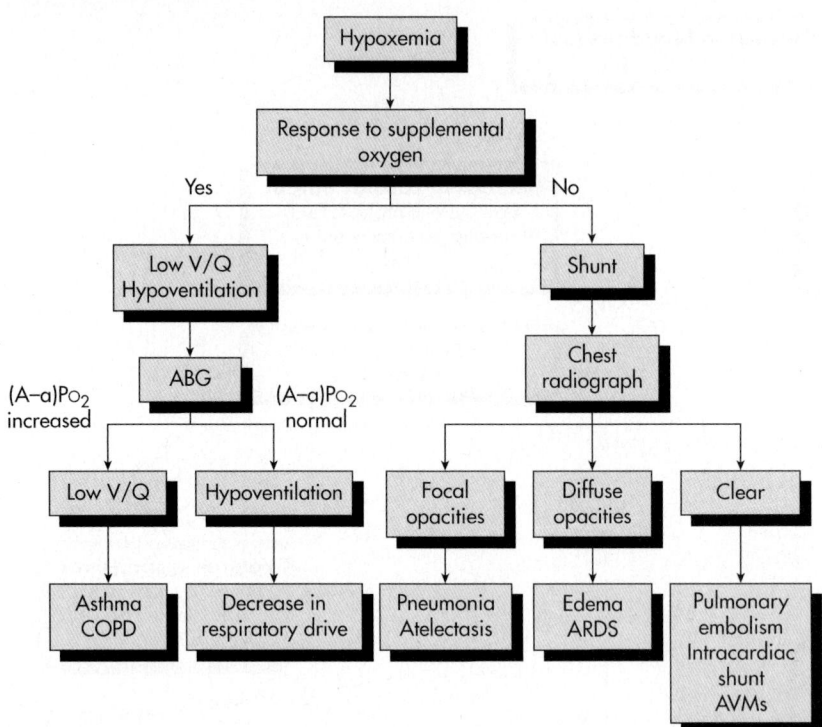

FIG. 123 A simplified algorithm for distinguishing the major clinical causes of hypoxemia. Clinically, the most important first step is in knowing whether the patient responds well to supplemental oxygen. If the response is good, the likely mechanisms are low ventilation-perfusion (V/Q) or hypoventilation; if so, an arterial blood gas (ABG) determination will be the next step. If the response to oxygen is poor, one is likely dealing with a shunt. Imaging with chest radiography will help determine the likely cause and next steps, recognizing that the chest radiograph is not as sensitive as chest computed tomography. *ARDS,* Acute respiratory distress syndrome; *AVMs,* arteriovenous malformations. (From Broaddus VC et al: *Murray & Nadel's textbook of respiratory medicine,* ed 7, Philadelphia, 2022, Elsevier.)

TABLE 87 The Danger of Undetected Hypoventilation When a Patient Is Receiving Supplemental Oxygen*

	paO$_2$	paCO$_2$
Room air	55	50
2 L/min	110	50
2 L/min	97.5	60
2 L/min	85	70
Room air	**30**	70

*In this patient receiving supplemental oxygen, the arterial pCO$_2$ starts to rise. With each 10 mm Hg rise, the arterial pO$_2$ falls 12.5 mm Hg (see text), although the arterial pO$_2$ (and oxygen saturation, not shown) never falls into a range to trigger the pulse oximeter. At the higher arterial pCO$_2$, supplemental oxygen becomes a lifeline. The supplemental oxygen in effect allows the arterial pCO$_2$ to rise without detection of a drop in oxygen saturation by the pulse oximeter. Removing the oxygen when the paCO$_2$ has risen can lead to a precipitous fall in arterial pO$_2$ (the calculated value of 30).

paCO$_2$, Arterial partial pressure of carbon dioxide; *paO$_2$,* arterial partial pressure of oxygen. All values in mm Hg.

INFECTIONS OF SOFT TISSUE, JOINTS, AND BONE

ICD-10CM # T84.3 Infection and inflammatory reaction
M00.9 Pyogenic arthritis, unspecified
M86.9 Osteomyelitis unspecified
M79.9 Soft tissue disorder, unspecified

1459

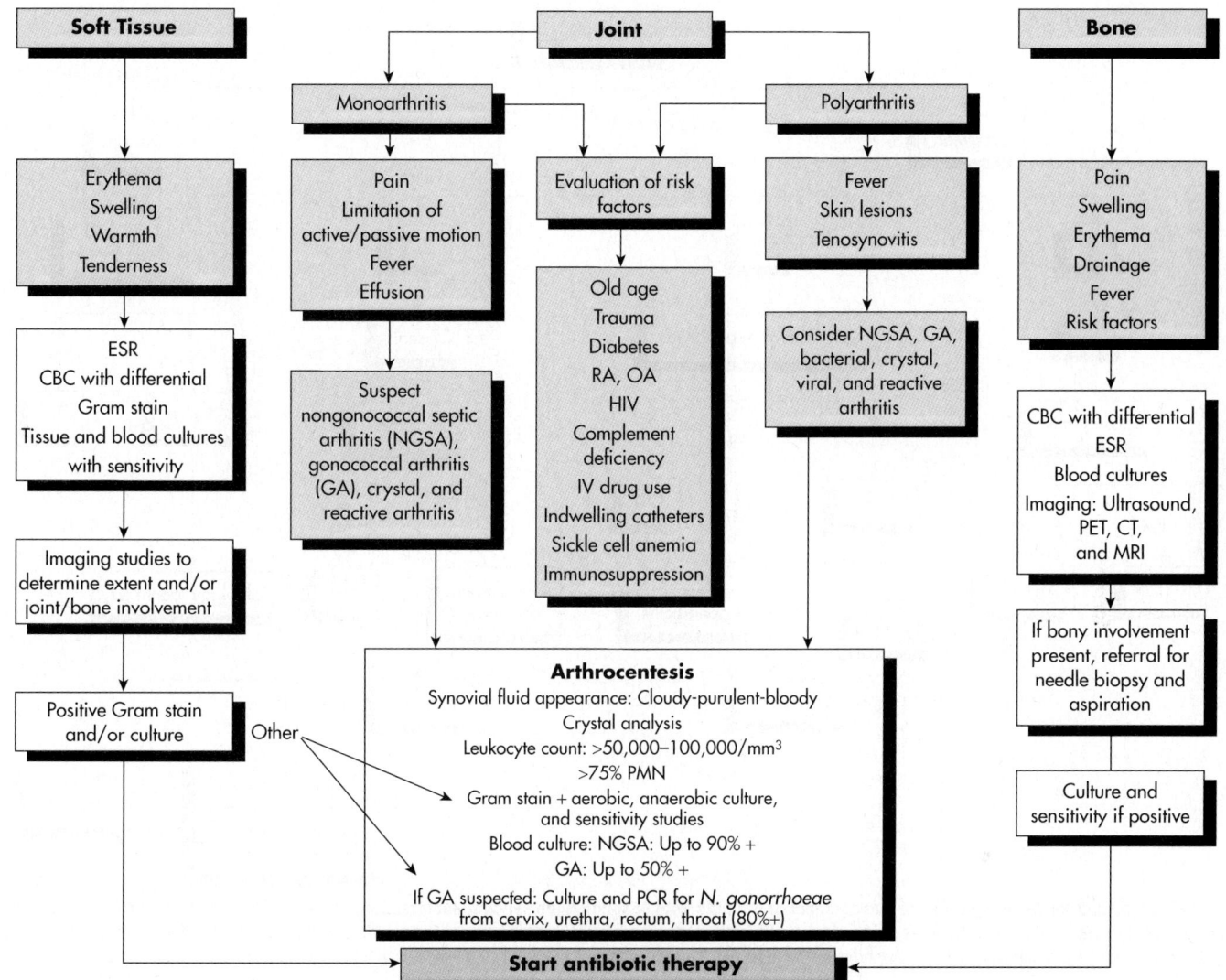

FIG. 125 Clinical evaluation of infections of soft tissues, joints, and bone. *CBC,* Complete blood count; *CT,* computed tomography; *ESR,* erythrocyte sedimentation rate; *HIV,* human immunodeficiency virus; *IV,* intravenous; *MRI,* magnetic resonance imaging; *OA,* osteoarthritis; *PCR,* polymerase chain reaction; *PET,* positron emission tomography; *PMN,* polymorphonuclear leukocyte; *RA,* rheumatoid arthritis. (From Goldman L, Schafer AI: *Goldman Cecil medicine,* ed 25, Philadelphia, 2016, Saunders.)

Clinical Algorithms

III

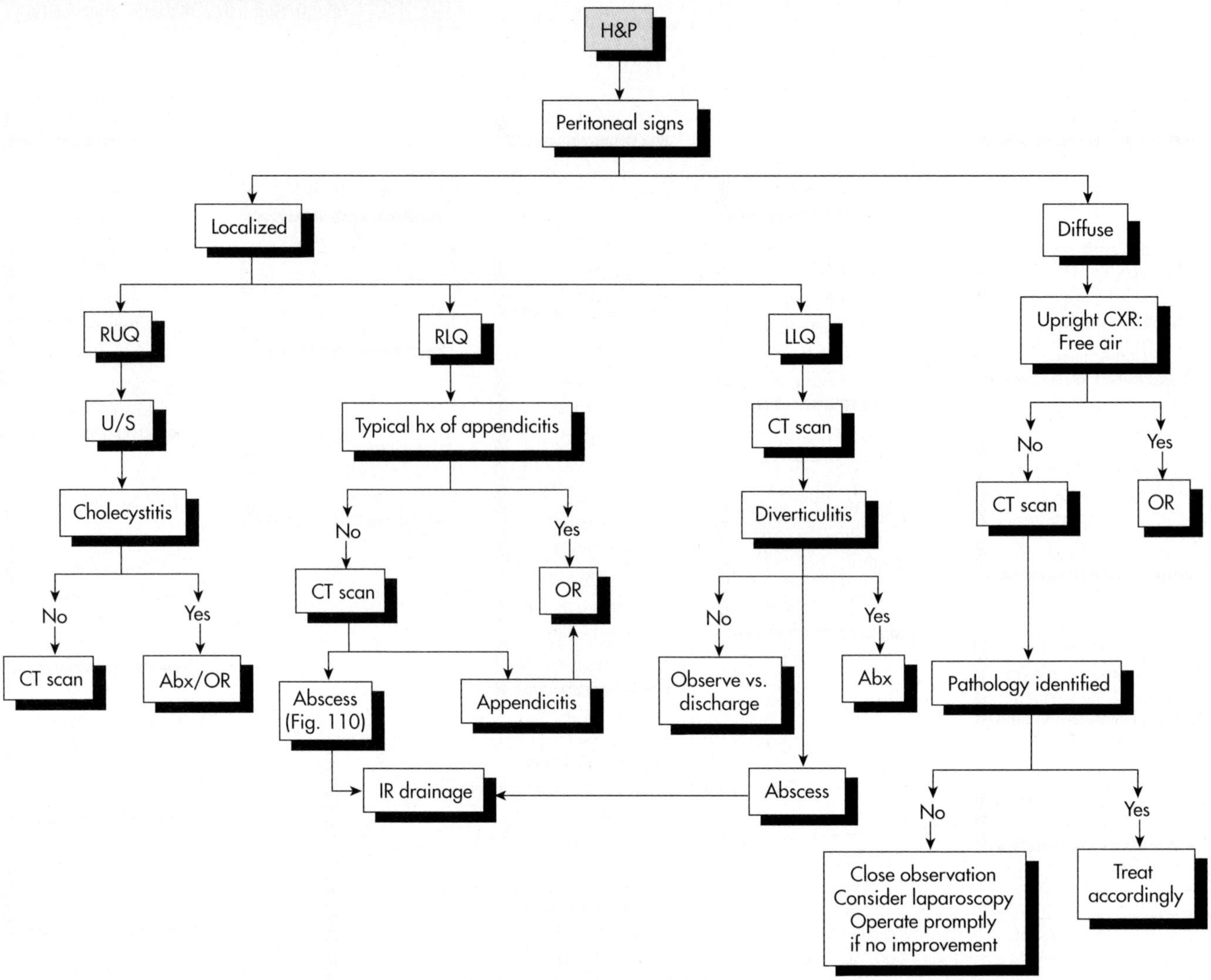

H&P

↓

Peritoneal signs

Localized | Diffuse

Localized:

RUQ | RLQ | LLQ

RUQ → U/S → Cholecystitis
- No → CT scan
- Yes → Abx/OR

RLQ → Typical hx of appendicitis
- No → CT scan → Abscess (Fig. 110) → IR drainage
- Yes → OR → Appendicitis

LLQ → CT scan → Diverticulitis
- No → Observe vs. discharge
- Yes → Abx
- → Abscess → IR drainage

Diffuse:

Upright CXR: Free air
- No → CT scan → Pathology identified
  - No → Close observation / Consider laparoscopy / Operate promptly if no improvement
  - Yes → Treat accordingly
- Yes → OR

FIG. 126 Algorithm for the diagnosis and management of patients with suspected intraabdominal infection. *Abx,* Antibiotics; *CT,* computed tomography; *CXR,* chest radiograph; *H&P,* history and physical exam; *hx,* history; *IR,* interventional radiology; *LLQ,* left lower quadrant; *OR,* operating room; *RLQ,* right lower quadrant; *RUQ,* right upper quadrant; *U/S,* ultrasound. (From Cameron JL, Cameron AM: *Current surgical therapy,* ed 10, Philadelphia, 2011, Saunders.)

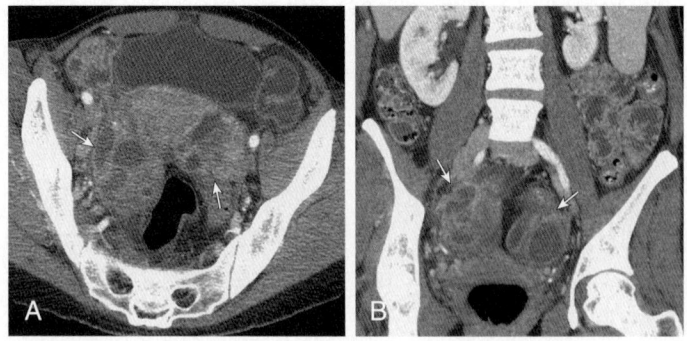

FIG. 127 Axial **(A)** and coronal **(B)** postcontrast computed tomographic images showing bilateral tuboovarian abscesses *(arrows).* (From Fielding JR et al: *Gynecologic imaging,* Philadelphia, 2011, Saunders.)

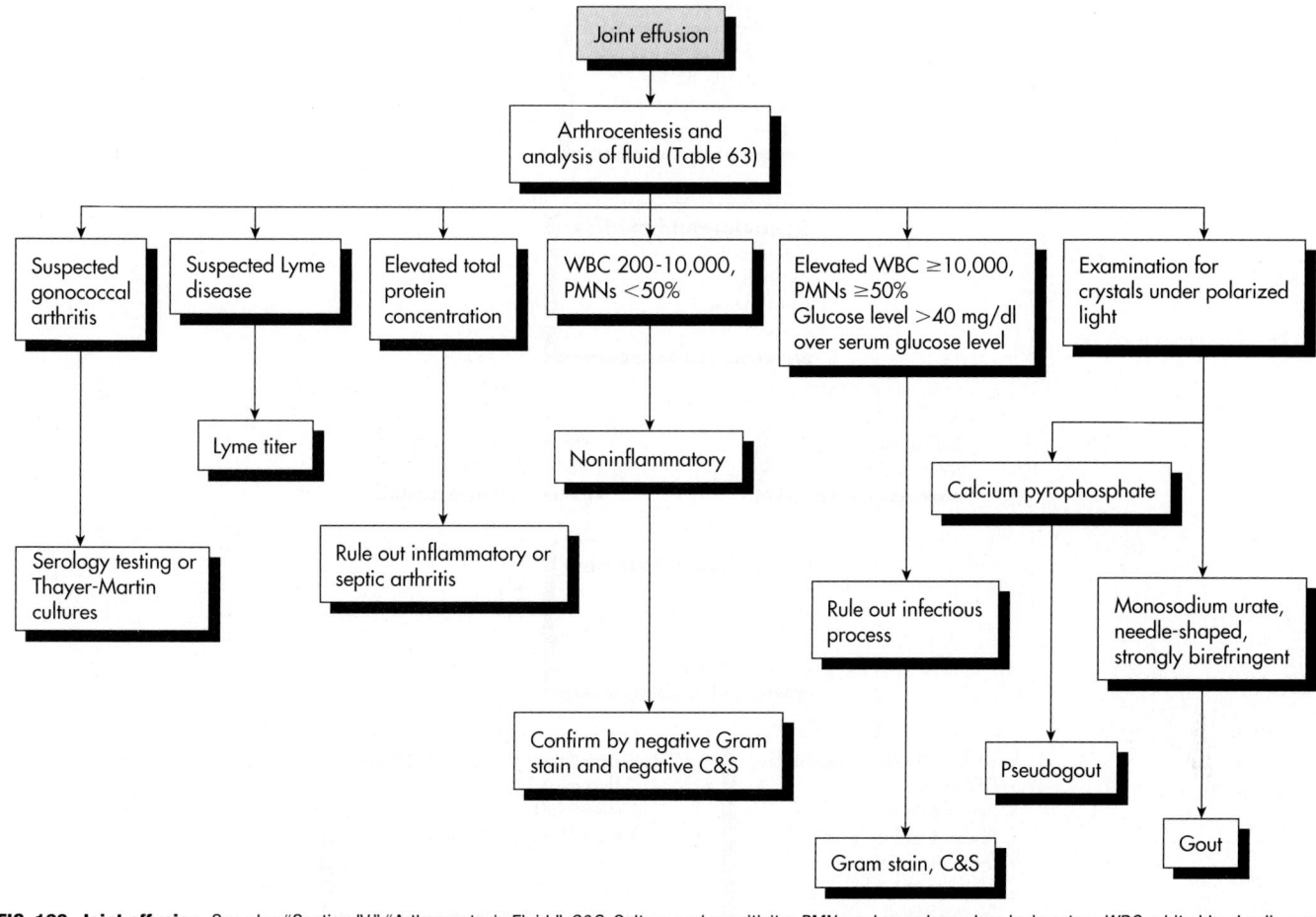

FIG. 128 Joint effusion. See also "Section IV," "Arthrocentesis Fluid." *C&S,* Culture and sensitivity; *PMNs,* polymorphonuclear leukocytes; *WBC,* white blood cell count.

TABLE 88   Indications for Arthrocentesis

Undiagnosed Arthritis with Effusion

Characterize type of arthritis
- Noninflammatory (WBC <2000/mm^3)
- Inflammatory (WBC >2000/mm^3)
- Septic (WBC >50,000/mm^3)
- Definitive diagnosis
- Gout (urate crystals)
- Pseudogout (calcium pyrophosphate dihydrate crystals)
- Septic arthritis (Gram stain [rare] or culture)

Undiagnosed Arthritis without Effusion

May be definitive in gout (knee, first metatarsophalangeal joint)

Patient with Known Diagnosis

Septic arthritis (repeated taps for adequate drainage)
Other types of arthritis for symptomatic relief (with or without injection)*

WBC, White blood cells.
*Most studies show improved effect if fluid is aspirated before injection.
From Firestein GS et al: *Kelley's textbook of rheumatology,* ed 9, Philadelphia, 2013, Saunders.

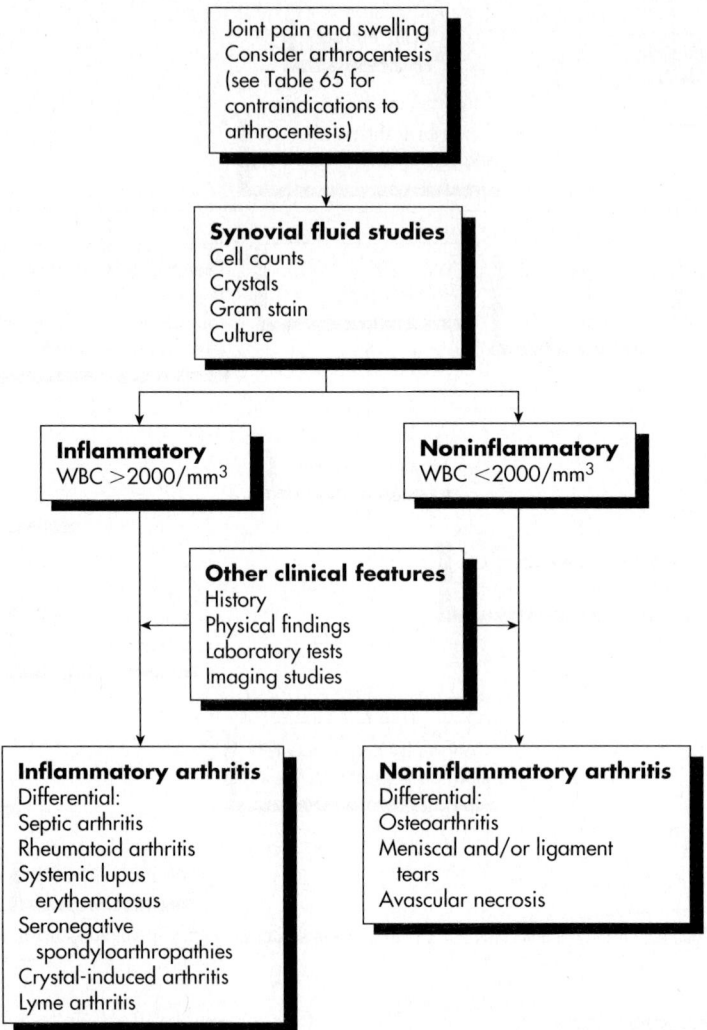

FIG. 129 Diagnostic approach for swollen joints. *WBC,* White blood cell count. (From Goldman L, Schafer AL [eds]: *Cecil textbook of medicine,* ed 24, Philadelphia, 2012, Saunders.)

TABLE 89 Clinical and Radiologic Findings in Joint Disease

Condition	Site of Involvement	Discriminatory Findings
Primary osteoarthritis (F>M • >45 yr)	Hands	PIP and DIP joint involvement (Heberden and Bouchard nodes) No osteopenia
	Large joints (e.g., hip, knee)	Joint space narrowing Subchondral sclerosis Subchondral cysts Marginal osteophytes
	Spine	Degenerative disc disease Spondylosis deformans Apophyseal joint involvement Spinal stenosis Foraminal stenosis
Erosive osteoarthritis (affects middle-aged females)	Hands	PIP and DIP joint involvement Joint ankylosis "Gull-wing" deformities (central erosions and marginal osteophytes)
Rheumatoid arthritis (F>M • Rh factor positive)	Hand and wrist	Symmetric arthritis MCP and PIP joint involvement Periarticular (early) and diffuse (late) osteopenia Marginal erosions Subluxation (swan neck and boutonnière deformities) Periostitis is uncommon

Continued

TABLE 89 Clinical and Radiologic Findings in Joint Disease—cont'd

Condition	Site of Involvement	Discriminatory Findings
	Large joints	Joint space narrowing Marginal erosions Synovial cysts Protrusio acetabulae
	Spine	Atlantoaxial subluxation
Juvenile idiopathic arthritis (M = F • affects children)	Hands	Joint ankylosis Florid periosteal reaction Osteopenia
	Large joints (e.g., knee)	Abnormalities of growth and maturation Epiphyseal overgrowth and premature closure of the physis Widened intercondylar notch
	Cervical spine	Apophyseal joint fusion Atlantoaxial subluxation
Psoriatic arthritis (M>F •nail changes • HLA-B27 +ve)	Upper extremities (e.g., hands)	"Sausage" digit DIP joint involvement Terminal tuft erosion Pencil-in-cup deformity Joint ankylosis Arthritis mutilans Periosteal reaction No osteopenia
	SI joints	Asymmetric or unilateral sacroiliitis
	Spine	Coarse syndesmophytes
Reites syndrome (affects young male adults)	Lower extremities (e.g., foot)	Hallux involvement Periosteal reaction Calcaneal erosions Osteopenia not prominent
	Spine	Coarse syndesmophytes
	SI joints	Asymmetric or unilateral sacroiliitis
Ankylosing spondylitis (M>F • affects young adults • HLA-B27 +ve in 95%)	SI joints	Bilateral symmetric sacroiliitis Ankylosis
	Spine	Anterior vertebral body squaring • Syndesmophytes • Paravertebral ossification • Bamboo spine
	Pelvis	"Whiskering" of the iliac crests and ischial tuberosities
Enteropathic arthropathies	SI joints	Symmetric sacroiliitis
Gout (M>F)	Hands and feet (especially the great toe)	MTP joint of the great toe Juxta-articular erosions Punched-out lesions with an overhanging margin No periarticular osteopenia Tophi
CPPD crystal deposition disease (M = F)	Any peripheral joint Predilection for the knee	Degenerative changes Chondrocalcinosis Paucity of subchondral sclerosis
HA crystal deposition disease (M = F)	Predilection for the shoulder (supraspinatus tendon)	Periarticular calcification
Hemochromatosis (M>F)	Hands	2nd and 3rd MCP joint involvement ("squared" metacarpal heads) Joint space narrowing "Hooklike" osteophytes Numerous subchondral cysts
Alkaptonuria (ochronosis) (M = F)	Intervertebral discs • SI joints • Large joints	Degenerative changes: Disc calcification • Joint space narrowing • Periarticular sclerosis
Systemic lupus erythematosus (F>M • affects young adults)	Hands	Reversible MCP joint subluxation
Scleroderma (F>M • affects adults)	Hands	IP joint arthritis • Acroosteolysis • Soft tissue calcifications
Mixed connective tissue disease (overlap syndrome)	Hands	PIP joint, MCP joint, mid-carpal involvement • Soft tissue swelling, calcifications, or atrophy
Multicentric reticulohistiocytosis (F>M)	Hands and feet	DIP joint and carpal involvement Soft tissue swelling Articular erosions No osteopenia
Polymyositis/dermatomyositis	Proximal extremities	Soft tissue calcification
	Hands	DIP joint erosions

Continued

TABLE 89 Clinical and Radiologic Findings in Joint Disease—cont'd

Condition	Site of Involvement	Discriminatory Findings
Sarcoidosis	Distal and middle phalanges of the hands and feet	Punched-out cystlike lesions • "Lacelike" appearance
Hemophilic arthropathy (affecting males—but with female carriers)	Predilection for large joints (e.g., knee)	Epiphyseal overgrowth • Juxtaarticular osteopenia • Erosion and cartilage destruction • Widened intercondylar and trochlear notches • Squared patella
Neuropathic arthropathy	Any joint	5 "Ds": Normal bone Density • Joint Distension • Bony Debris • Joint Disorganization • Dislocation
Hypertrophic osteoarthropathy	Tubular bones (radius and ulna > tibia and fibula)	Diaphyseal and metaphyseal painful periostitis

CPPD, Calcium pyrophosphate deposition disease; *DIP,* distal interphalangeal; *F,* female; *HA,* hydroxyapatite; *HLA,* human leukocyte antigen; *IP,* interphalangeal; *M,* male; *MCP,* metacarpophalangeal; *MTP,* metatarsophalangeal; *PIP,* proximal interphalangeal; *Rh,* Rhesus; *SI,* sacroiliac.
From Grant LA, Griffin N: *Grainger & Allison's diagnostic radiology essentials,* ed 2, Philadelphia, 2019, Elsevier.

TABLE 90 Contraindications to Arthrocentesis and Joint Injection

Contraindication	Comment
Established infection in nearby structures (e.g., cellulitis, septic bursitis)	Sometimes gout mimics cellulitis, creating a confusing picture
Septicemia (theoretic risk of introducing organism into joint)	Need to tap suspected septic joints in septic patients
Disrupted skin barrier (e.g., psoriasis)	Do not tap through lesions
Bleeding disorder (not absolute, but use more care)	Risk of bleeding very low, even in patients taking warfarin
Septic joint	Steroid injection contraindicated
Prior lack of response	Relative contraindication
Difficult-to-access joint	Relative contraindication without imaging aid

From Firestein GS et al: *Kelley's textbook of rheumatology,* ed 9, Philadelphia, 2013, Saunders.

TABLE 91 Synovial Fluid Characteristics in Clinical Situations, with Imaging and Investigation Techniques to Identify the Cause

Diagnosis	Cells	Microorganisms	Appearance	Imaging Modality	Comments
Bacterial arthritis	Neutrophils, 10,000->100,000	Gram stain usually positive	Turbid/pus	May need ultrasound to aspirate dryness	Systemic symptoms, Gram stain, blood and synovial fluid culture
Gonococcal arthritis	Neutrophils, 10,000-100,000	Gram stain usually positive	Turbid/pus	May need ultrasound to aspirate dryness	Systemic symptoms, Gram stain, blood and synovial fluid culture
Crystal arthritis	Neutrophils, 10,000->100,000	—	Turbid/pus	Radiographs, CPPD	Presence of appropriate crystals Acute serum urate unreliable
Tuberculous arthritis	Mononuclear 5000-50,000	Acid-fast stain often negative, may need to culture synovial tissue	Turbid/pus		At-risk population; Ziehl-Neelsen stain biopsy may be necessary
Inflammatory monoarthropathies	Neutrophils 5000-50,000	—	Slightly turbid	Ultrasound/MRI for early synovitis and erosions	Serum autoantibodies such as RF, ACPA, ANA
Osteoarthritis	Mononuclear 0-2000	—	Clear	Radiographic changes	Usually noninflammatory CPPD may be present
Internal derangement	Red blood cells	—	Clear/turbid	MRI	Arthroscopy may be necessary
Trauma	Red blood cells	—	Clear/turbid	Radiographs	Tc bone scan may aid diagnosis if radiograph normal
Ischemic necrosis		—		MRI in early disease	XR abnormal only in advanced cases
Uncommon Causes					
Sarcoidosis	Mononuclear, 5000-20,000	—		CXR	
PVNS	Red blood cells	—	Turbid	Ultrasound and MRI	Synovial biopsy essential
Charcot disease	Mononuclear, 0-2000	—		Radiographs	CPPD may be present
Lyme disease	Neutrophils, 0-5000	—	Clear/turbid		SF eosinophilia may be found Serology for *Borrelia*
Amyloid	Mononuclear, 2000-10,000	—	Turbid		Synovial biopsy for Congo red stain

ACPA, Anticitrullinated protein antibody; *ANA,* antinuclear antibody; *CPPD,* calcium pyrophosphate dehydrate deposition; *CXR,* chest radiograph; *PVNS,* pigmented villonodular synovitis; *RF,* rheumatoid factor; *SF,* synovial fluid; *Tc,* technetium; *XR,* radiograph.
From Firestein GS et al: *Firestein & Kelley's textbook of rheumatology,* ed 11, Philadelphia, 2021, Elsevier.

TABLE 92 The Differential Diagnosis of Polyarthritis

Disease Category	Specific Disease	Mono-, Oligo-, or Polyarthritis (Most Common Presentation)
Infections		
Viral	Parvovirus B19	Poly
	Rubella virus	Poly
	Hepatitis A, B, C	Poly
	HIV	Oligo, poly
	Alphaviruses, including chikungunya infection	Poly
Bacterial	Gram-positive and gram-negative infections	Mono, occasionally oligo/poly
	Initial phase of gonorrhea	Poly
	Later phase of gonorrhea	Mono
	Early phase of Lyme arthritis	Poly
	Later phase of Lyme arthritis	Oligo, mono
Diseases Triggered by Infection but Presumed to Be Autoimmune		
Reactive arthritis	After urogenital infections (*Chlamydia* and *Ureaplasma*); after gastrointestinal infections (*Yersinia*, *Shigella*, *Campylobacter*, and *Salmonella*)	Mono, oligo, poly
Acute rheumatic fever	After infection with group A streptococcus	Oligo
Autoimmune Diseases		
Primary arthritides	Rheumatoid arthritis	Poly
	Psoriatic arthritis	Oligo, poly
	Spondyloarthropathies	Oligo, poly
	Juvenile inflammatory arthritis	Mono, oligo, poly
Transient and recurring polyarthritides	Palindromic rheumatism	Poly
	Recurrent symmetric seronegative synovitis with pitting edema (RS3PE syndrome)	Poly
Systemic autoimmune disease	Systemic lupus erythematosus	Poly
	Mixed connective tissue disease	Poly
	Primary Sjögren syndrome	Poly
	Progressive systemic sclerosis and limited scleroderma	Poly
	Behçet disease	Oligo, poly
	Sarcoidosis	Oligo, poly
	Vasculitis	Poly
Autoinflammatory diseases	Adult-onset Still disease	Oligo, poly
	Familial Mediterranean fever and other cryopyrin-associated fever syndromes	Poly
	Various genetic autoinflammatory conditions usually manifested first in childhood	Poly
Degenerative diseases Osteoarthritis	Includes erosive inflammatory osteoarthritis	Poly
Hypertrophic osteoarthropathy		Poly
Osteonecrosis		Mono, oligo
Metabolic Diseases		
Thyroid diseases	Hypothyroidism	Mono, oligo
Hemochromatosis	Hyperthyroidism (Graves disease; early phase of Hashimoto disease)	Oligo, poly
Hemoglobinopathies	Sickle cell anemia	Oligo, poly
Hemochromatosis	Thalassemia	Oligo, poly
Crystal diseases	Gout	Mono (initial), oligo, poly (late stage)
	Pseudogout	Mono, oligo, poly
Deposition diseases	Glycogen storage diseases; amyloid deposition in primary amyloidosis; mucopolysaccharidoses; light- and heavy-chain deposition diseases; others	Oligo, poly
Drug-Induced Diseases		
Vasculitic drug reactions, serum sickness		Poly

From Firestein GS et al: *Firestein & Kelley's textbook of rheumatology,* ed 11, Philadelphia, 2021, Elsevier.

Clinical Algorithms

III

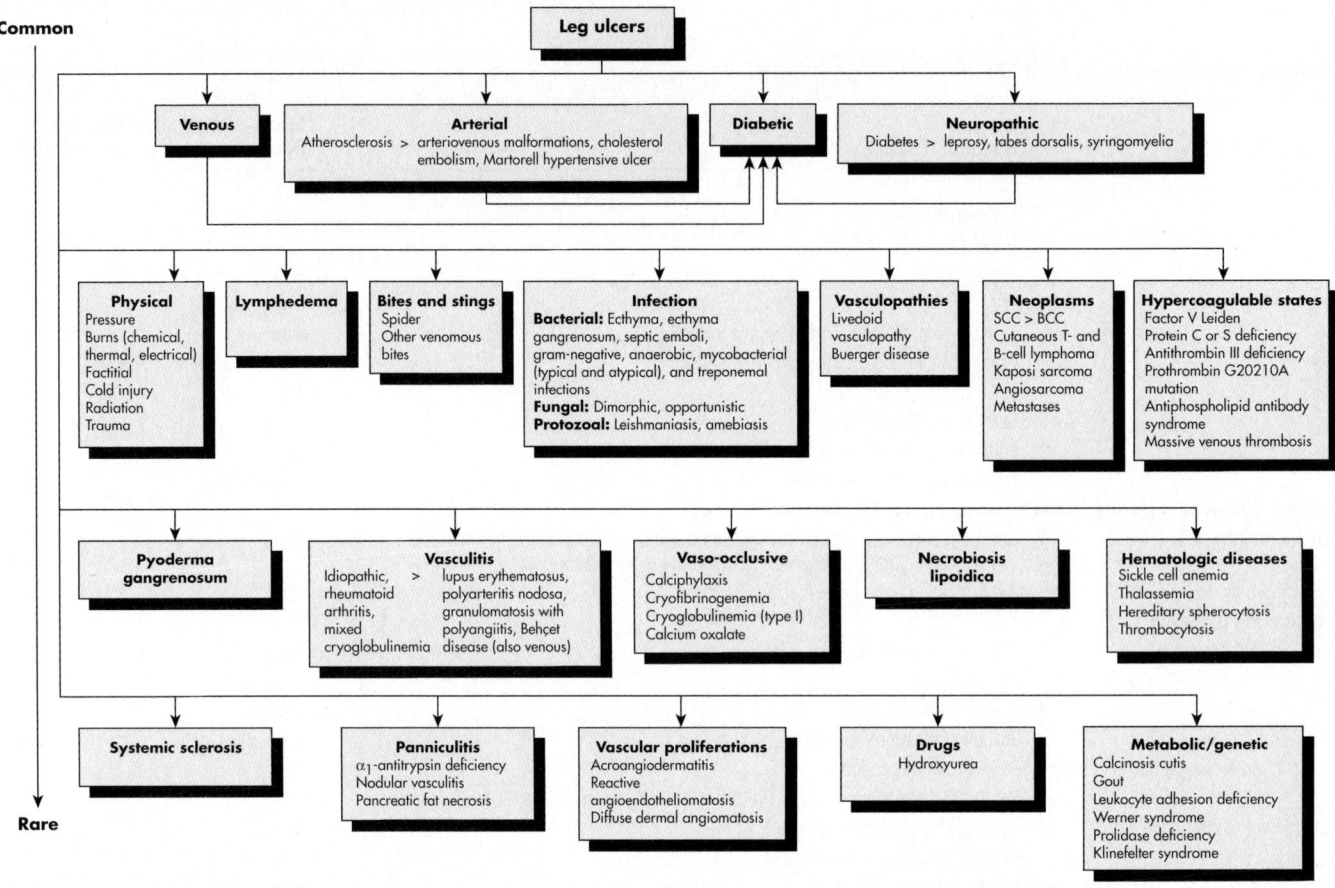

FIG. 130 Causes of leg ulcers. Patients with Behçet disease also develop lower extremity ulcers due to vasculitis and/or venous insufficiency related to deep vein thromboses, and, occasionally, erosive pustular dermatosis is a cause of leg ulcers. Hydroxyurea-induced leg ulcers are often on the malleolus or tibial crest, exceedingly painful, and surrounded by atrophic skin. (From Bolognia J: *Dermatology,* ed 4, Philadelphia, 2018, Elsevier.)

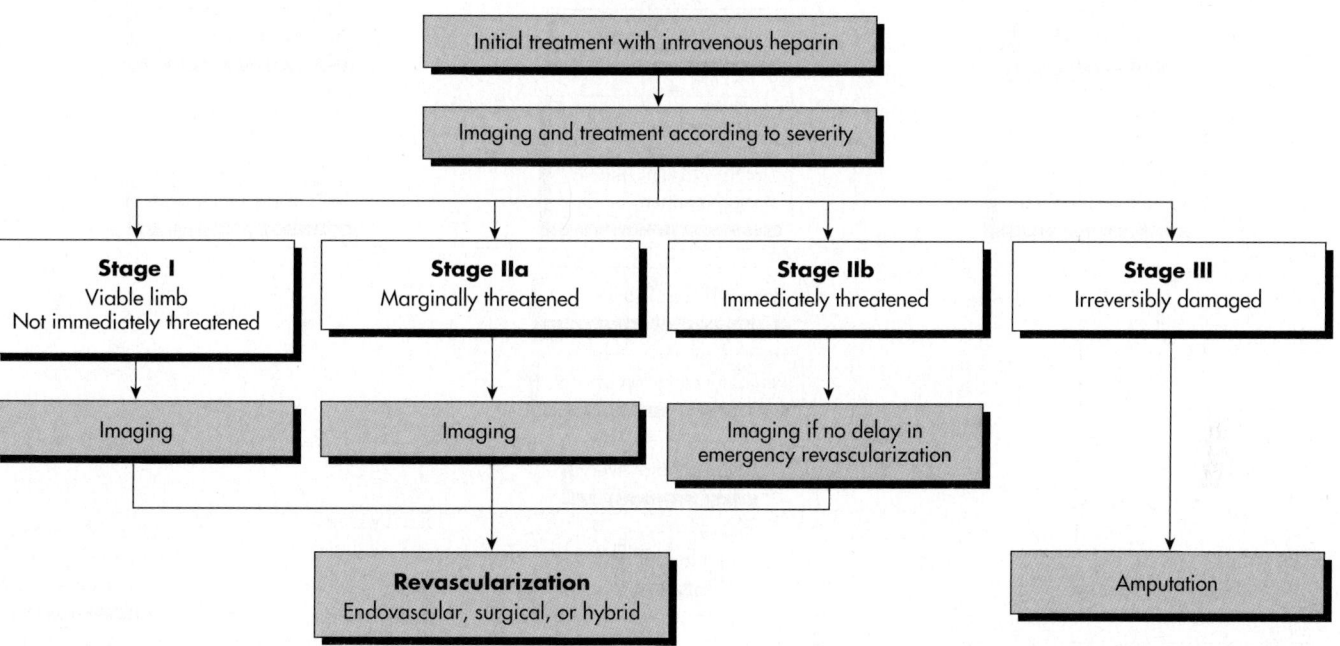

Diagnosis

Symptoms Pain
Paresthesia
Weakness or paralysis

Signs Absent pulses
Pallor
Cool skin
Decreased sensation
Decreased strength
Limb blood pressure <50 mm Hg

Potential causes Thrombosis of artery
or bypass graft
Embolism from heart
or proximal vessel
Dissection
Trauma

Management

Initial treatment with intravenous heparin

Imaging and treatment according to severity

Stage I
Viable limb
Not immediately threatened

Stage IIa
Marginally threatened

Stage IIb
Immediately threatened

Stage III
Irreversibly damaged

Imaging

Imaging

Imaging if no delay in
emergency revascularization

Revascularization
Endovascular, surgical, or hybrid

Amputation

FIG. 131 Diagnostic and treatment approach for patients presenting with acute limb ischemia. (From Zipes DP: *Braunwald's heart disease, a textbook of cardiovascular medicine,* ed 11, Philadelphia, 2019, Elsevier.)

TABLE 93 Rutherford Classification of Acute Limb Ischemia

Category	Description/Prognosis	CLINICAL EXAMINATION		DOPPLER SIGNAL	
		Sensory Loss	Muscle Weakness	Arterial	Venous
I. Viable	Not immediately threatened	None	None	Audible	Audible
II. Threatened					
IIa. Marginally	Salvageable if promptly treated	Minimal (toes) or none	None	(Often) audible	Audible
IIb. Immediately	Salvageable with immediate revascularization	More than toes, associated with rest pain	Mild, moderate	(Usually) audible	Audible
III. Irreversible	Major tissue loss or permanent damage inevitable	Profound, anesthetic	Profound, paralysis (rigor)	Inaudible	Inaudible

From Hoffman R: *Hematology, basic principles and practice,* ed 7, Philadelphia, 2018, Elsevier.

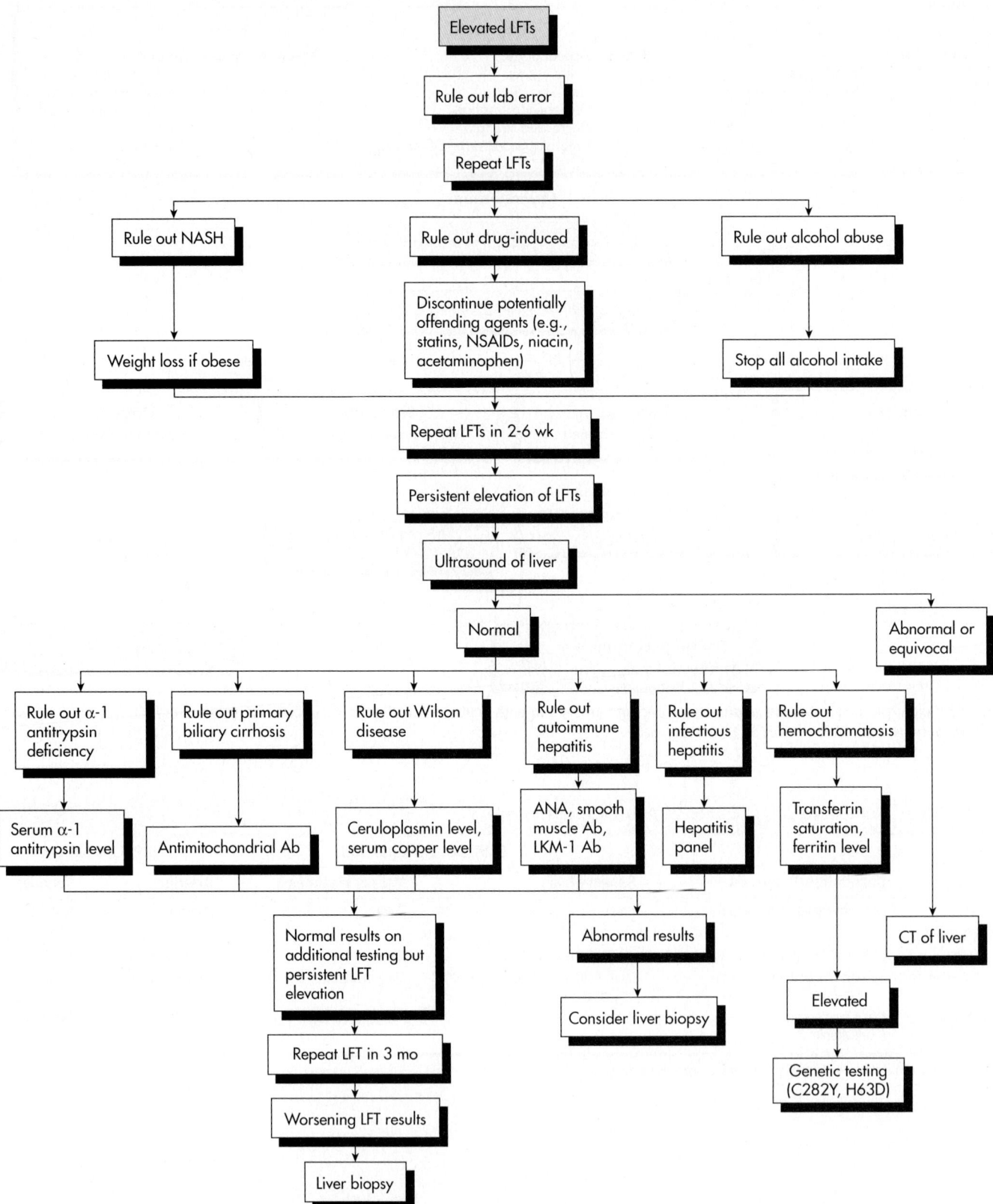

FIG. 132 Liver function test elevations. *Ab,* Antibody; *ANA,* antibody to nuclear antigens; *CT,* computed tomography; *LFTs,* liver function tests; *LKM,* liver-kidney microsome; *NASH,* nonalcoholic steatohepatitis; *NSAIDs,* nonsteroidal antiinflammatory drugs.

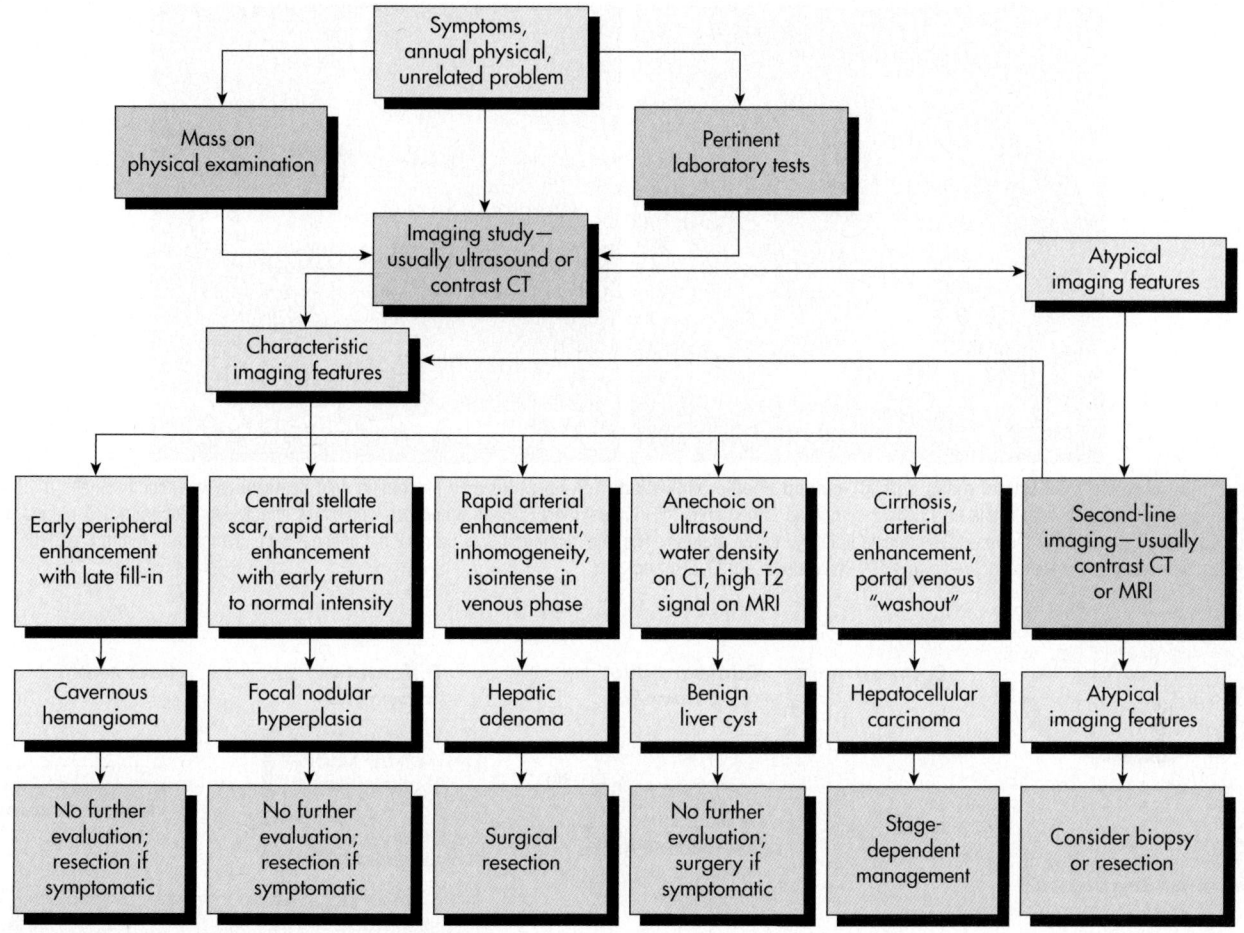

FIG. 133 Approach to evaluating the patient with a mass lesion in the liver. This flow chart shows an algorithm for evaluating and managing common liver mass lesions. *CT,* Computed tomography; *MRI,* magnetic resonance imaging. (From Roberts LR: Liver and biliary tract tumors. In Goldman L, Schafer AI [eds]: *Goldman's Cecil medicine,* ed 24, Philadelphia, 2012, Saunders.)

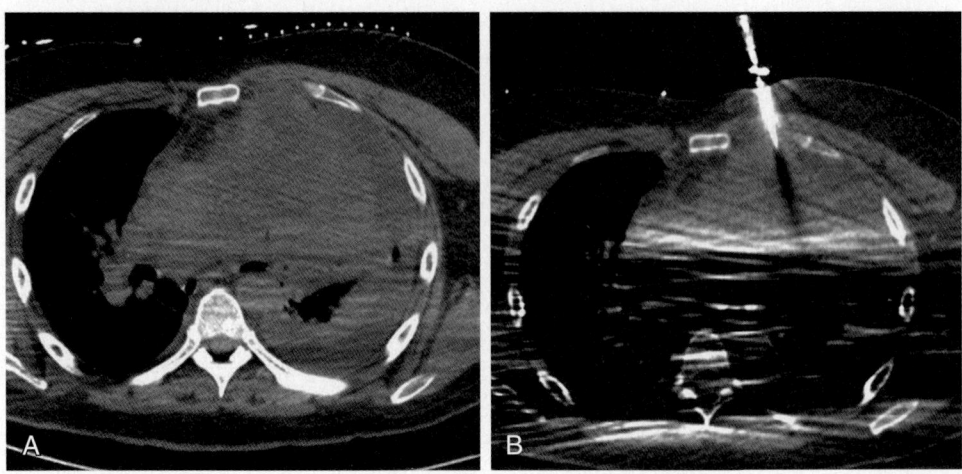

FIG. 134 Bulky anterior mediastinal mass with CT-guided needle aspiration. A, A 45-yr-old man presenting with hoarseness was found to have a 12 × 10 × 11 cm anterior mediastinal mass. On this noncontrast computed tomography (CT) image, there is central necrosis and mass effect with concurrent left pleural effusion. **B,** CT-guided needle aspiration of the mass. The needle is lateral to the sternum. The final diagnosis was primary mediastinal B-cell lymphoma. (From Broaddus VC et al: *Murray & Nadel's textbook of respiratory medicine,* ed 7, Philadelphia, 2022, Elsevier.)

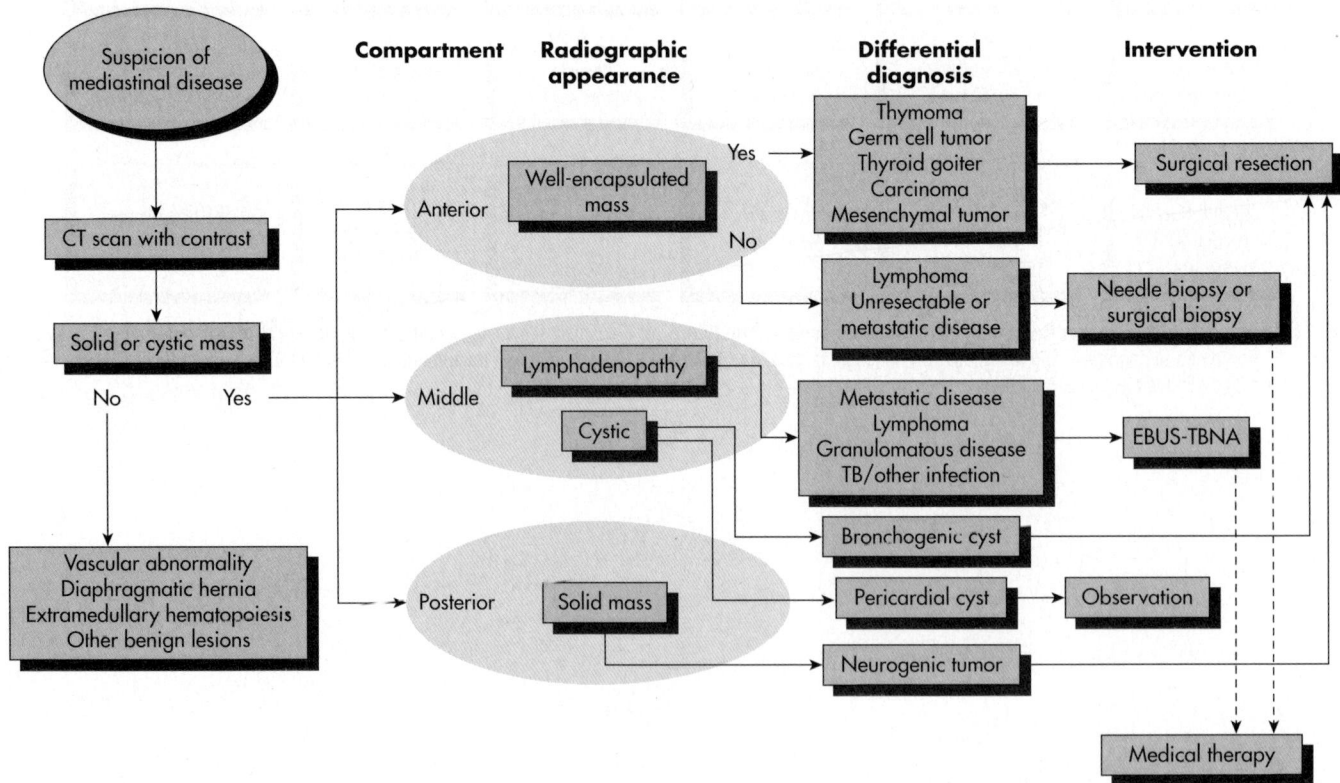

FIG. 135 Suggested algorithm for the diagnostic approach to mediastinal masses. *CT,* Computed tomography; *EBUS-TBNA,* endobronchial ultrasound-guided transbronchial needle aspiration; *TB,* tuberculosis. (From Broaddus VC et al: *Murray & Nadel's textbook of respiratory medicine,* ed 7, Philadelphia, 2022, Elsevier.)

TABLE 94   Disorders Presenting as a Mass in the Mediastinum

Anterior/Prevascular Mediastinum	Middle/Visceral Mediastinum	Posterior/Paravertebral Mediastinum
Thymic neoplasms	Lymphadenopathy	Neurogenic tumors
Germ cell tumors	Reactive and granulomatous inflammation	Meningocele
Teratoma	Metastasis	Diaphragmatic hernia (Bochdalek)
Seminoma	Angiofollicular lymphoid hyperplasia (Castleman disease)	Extramedullary hematopoiesis
Nonseminomatous germ cell tumors	Lymphoma	Lymphadenopathy
Embryonal cell carcinoma	Developmental cysts	Lesions arising from posterior spine
Choriocarcinoma	Pericardial cyst	Metastases
Lymphoma	Foregut duplication cysts	Discitis/osteomyelitis
Hodgkin lymphoma	Bronchogenic cyst	Thoracic duct cyst
Non-Hodgkin lymphoma	Enteric cyst	
Thyroid neoplasms/goiter	Others	
Parathyroid neoplasms	Vascular enlargements (i.e., descending aortic aneurysm)	
Mesenchymal tumors	Diaphragmatic hernia (hiatal)	
Lipoma	Esophageal lesions	
Fibroma	Carcinoma	
Lymphangioma	Diverticula	
Hemangioma	Varices	
Mesothelioma		
Sarcoma		
Diaphragmatic hernia (Morgagni)		
NUT midline carcinoma		
Lymphadenopathy		
Vascular lesions		

NUT, Nuclear protein in testis.
From Broaddus VC et al: *Murray & Nadel's textbook of respiratory medicine,* ed 7, Philadelphia, 2022, Elsevier.

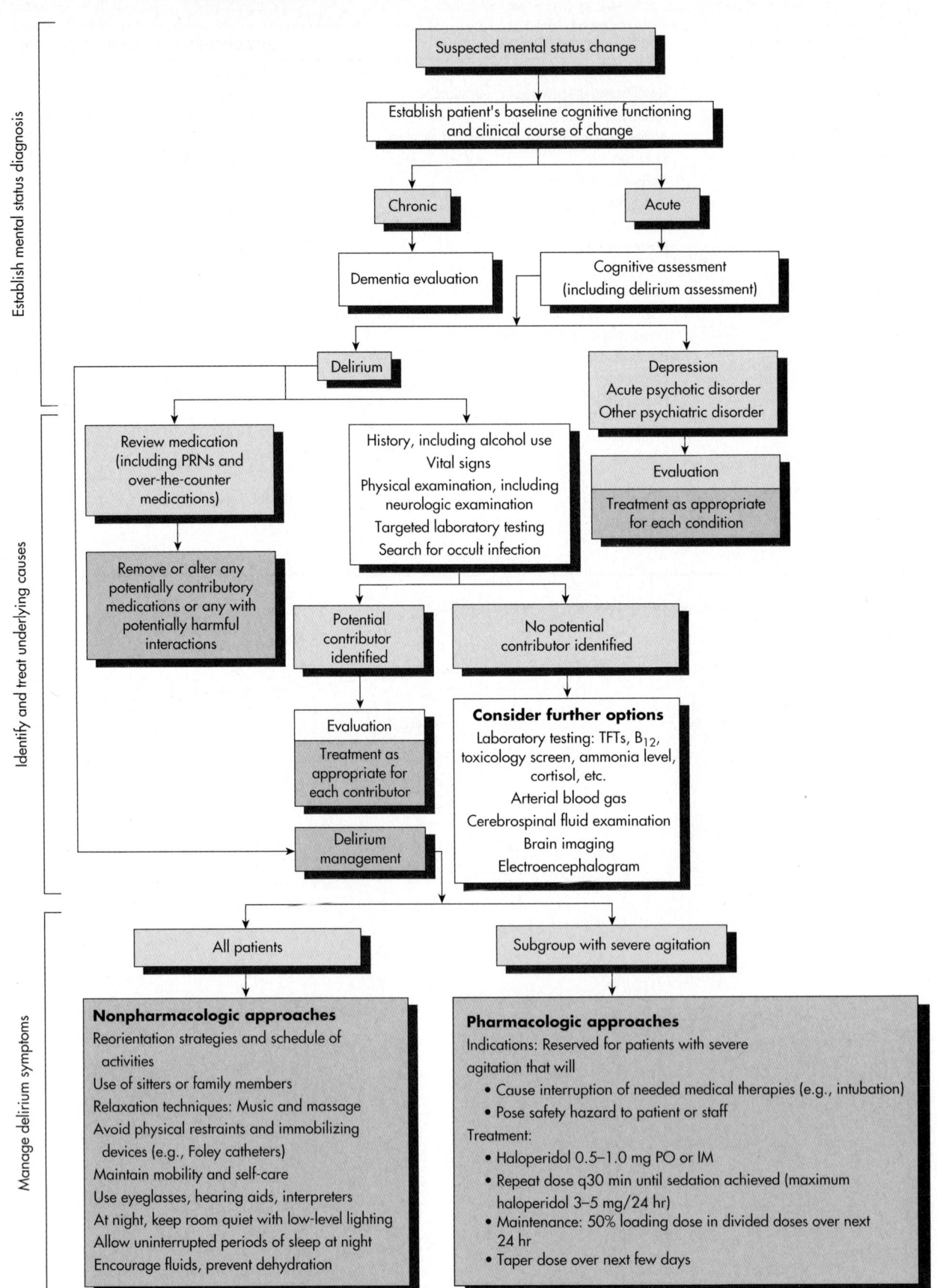

FIG. 136 Algorithm for the evaluation of suspected mental status change in older patients. *IM,* Intramuscular; *PO,* by mouth; *PRN,* as needed; *TFTs,* thyroid function tests. (From Goldman L, Schafer AI: *Goldman Cecil medicine,* ed 25, Philadelphia, 2016, Saunders.)

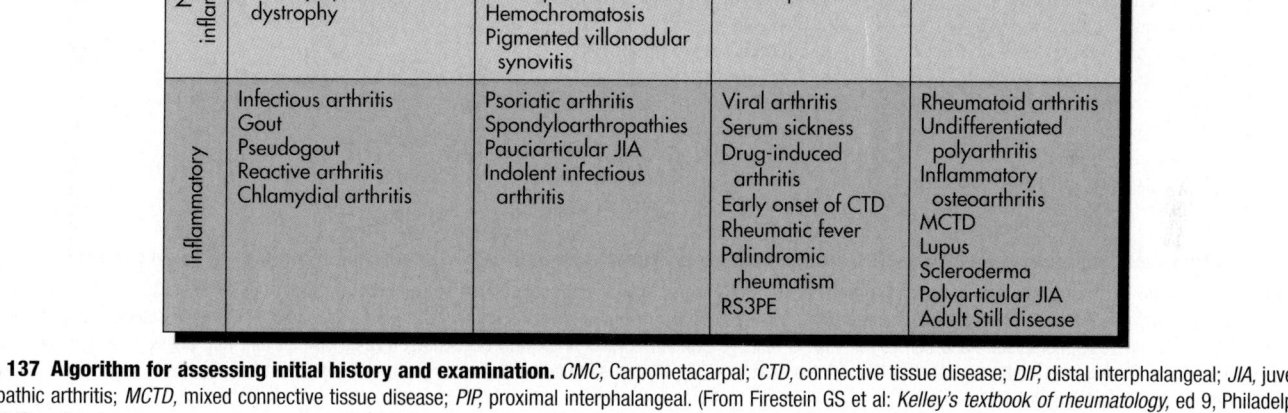

FIG. 137 Algorithm for assessing initial history and examination. *CMC,* Carpometacarpal; *CTD,* connective tissue disease; *DIP,* distal interphalangeal; *JIA,* juvenile idiopathic arthritis; *MCTD,* mixed connective tissue disease; *PIP,* proximal interphalangeal. (From Firestein GS et al: *Kelley's textbook of rheumatology,* ed 9, Philadelphia, 2013, Saunders.)

Clinical
Algorithms

III

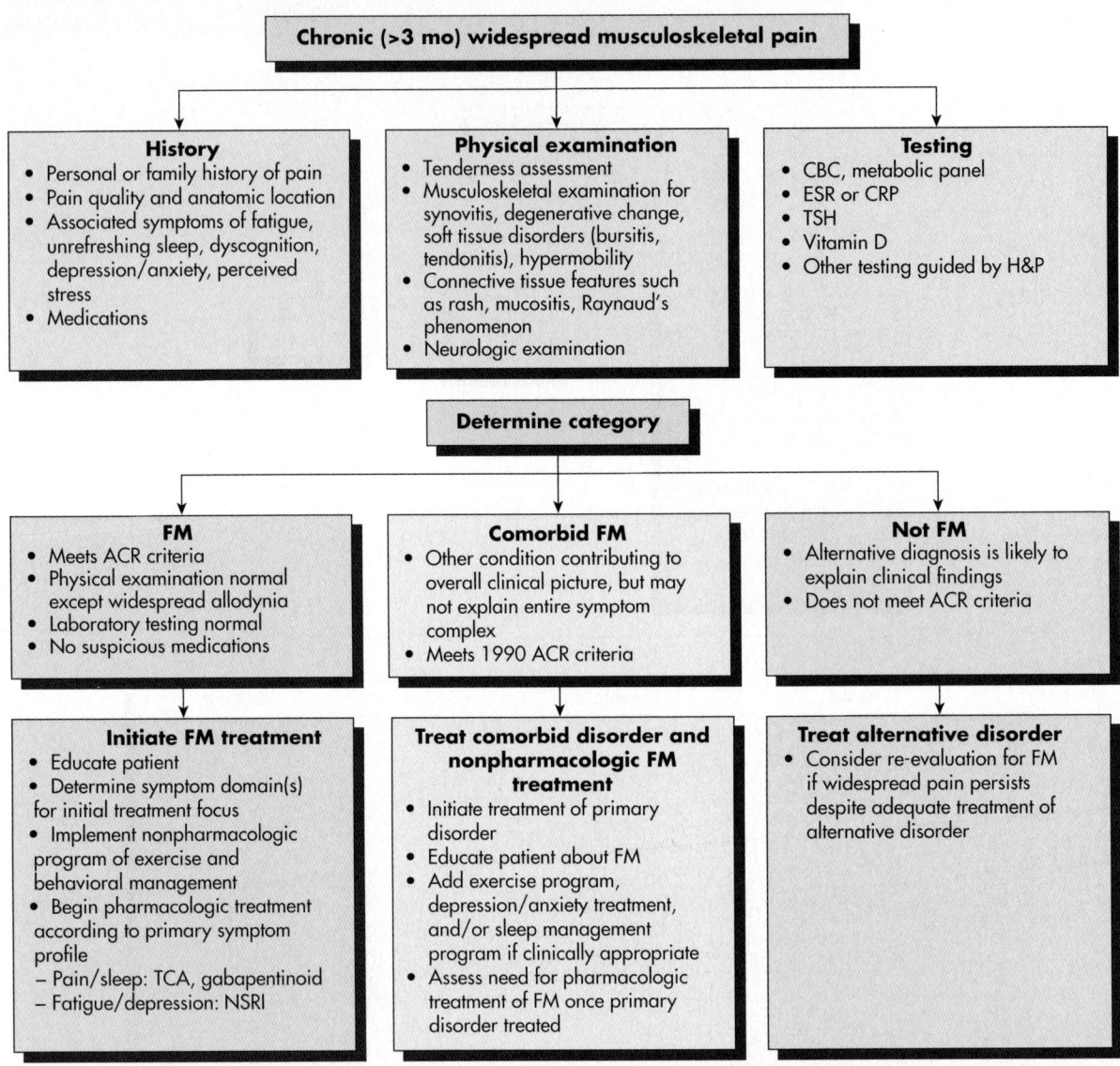

FIG. 138 Strategy for evaluation and initial management of patients with chronic widespread musculoskeletal pain. After initial evaluation, patients may be diagnosed with fibromyalgia (FM), FM comorbid with another diagnosis, or not FM. The figure presents strategies for initial management of each category. *ACR,* American College of Rheumatology; *CBC,* complete blood cell count; *CRP,* C-reactive protein; *ESR,* erythrocyte sedimentation rate; *H&P,* history and physical examination; *NSRI,* norepinephrine serotonin reuptake inhibitor; *TCA,* tricyclic antidepressants; *TSH,* thyroid-stimulating hormone. (From Firestein GS et al: *Firestein & Kelley's textbook of rheumatology,* ed 11, Philadelphia, 2021, Elsevier.)

TABLE 95   Differential Diagnosis of Diffuse Myalgias

Diagnosis	Findings[a]
Inflammatory	
Polymyalgia rheumatica	Elevated ESR and/or CRP
Seronegative spondyloarthropathies	Abnormal imaging
Connective tissue diseases	Positive serologies
Systemic vasculitis	Systemic inflammation, end-organ damage
Infectious	
Hepatitis C	Positive antibodies
HIV	Positive antibodies
Lyme disease	Positive antibodies
Parvovirus B19	Positive antibodies
Epstein-Barr virus	Positive antibodies
Noninflammatory	
Degenerative joint/spine disease	Abnormal imaging
Fibromyalgia	Widespread allodynia/hyperalgesia
Myofascial pain	Localized allodynia/hyperalgesia
Joint hypermobility	Joint hypermobility
Metabolic myopathies	Abnormal muscle biopsy
Endocrine	
Hypo- or hyperthyroidism	Abnormal thyroid function tests
Hyperparathyroidism	Elevated serum calcium
Addison disease	Abnormal serum cortisol
Vitamin D deficiency	Low serum vitamin D
Neurologic Diseases	
Multiple sclerosis	Abnormal neurologic examination and imaging
Neuropathic pain	Reasonable cause or abnormal imaging
Psychiatric Diseases	
Major depressive disorder	Positive depression screening
Drugs	
Statins	History of exposure
Aromatase inhibitors	History of exposure

CRP, C-reactive protein; *ESR,* erythrocyte sedimentation rate.

[a]Recommended routine testing includes ESR or CRP and thyroid-stimulating hormone. Other diagnostic testing should be guided by risk profile and history and physical examination. Repeated diagnostic testing is discouraged.

From Firestein GS et al: *Firestein & Kelley's textbook of rheumatology,* ed 11, Philadelphia, 2021, Elsevier.

TABLE 96   Patterns of Arthritis

	PATTERN				
	Monoarthritis	**Inflammatory Spinal Disease Sacroiliitis**	**Asymmetrical Large Joint Arthritis**	**Symmetrical Small Joint Arthritis (MCP, PIP, MTP)**	**DIP Hands**
Differential diagnosis	Trauma Hemophilia Septic Gout Pseudogout	Ankylosing spondylitis Psoriatic arthritis IBD	Psoriatic arthritis Reactive arthritis IBD	RA SLE Psoriatic arthritis	Inflammatory OA (if involves PIP and first CMC) Psoriatic arthritis
Further investigations	X-ray Aspirate for crystals and culture	Review personal and family history HLA- B27 X- ray lumbar spine and SI joints MRI sacroiliac joints	Review personal and family history Examine scalp and buttocks for psoriasis Examine for conjunctivitis and urethritis Infection screen	Examine for rheumatoid nodules, skin rashes, serositis or mucositis Urinalysis RF, CCP antibodies, ANA X-ray hands and feet	X-ray hands

ANA, Antinuclear antibodies; *CCP,* cyclic citrullinated peptides; *CMC,* carpometacarpophalangeal; *DIP,* distal interphalangeal; *HLA,* human leukocyte antigen; *IBD,* inflammatory bowel disease; *MCP,* metacarpophalangeal; *MTP,* metatarsophalangeal; *OA,* osteoarthritis; *PIP,* proximal interphalangeal; *RA,* rheumatoid arthritis; *RF,* rheumatoid factor; *SI,* sacroiliac; *SLE,* systemic lupus erythematosus.

From Talley NJ et al: *Essentials of internal medicine,* ed 4, Chatswood, 2021, Elsevier Australia.

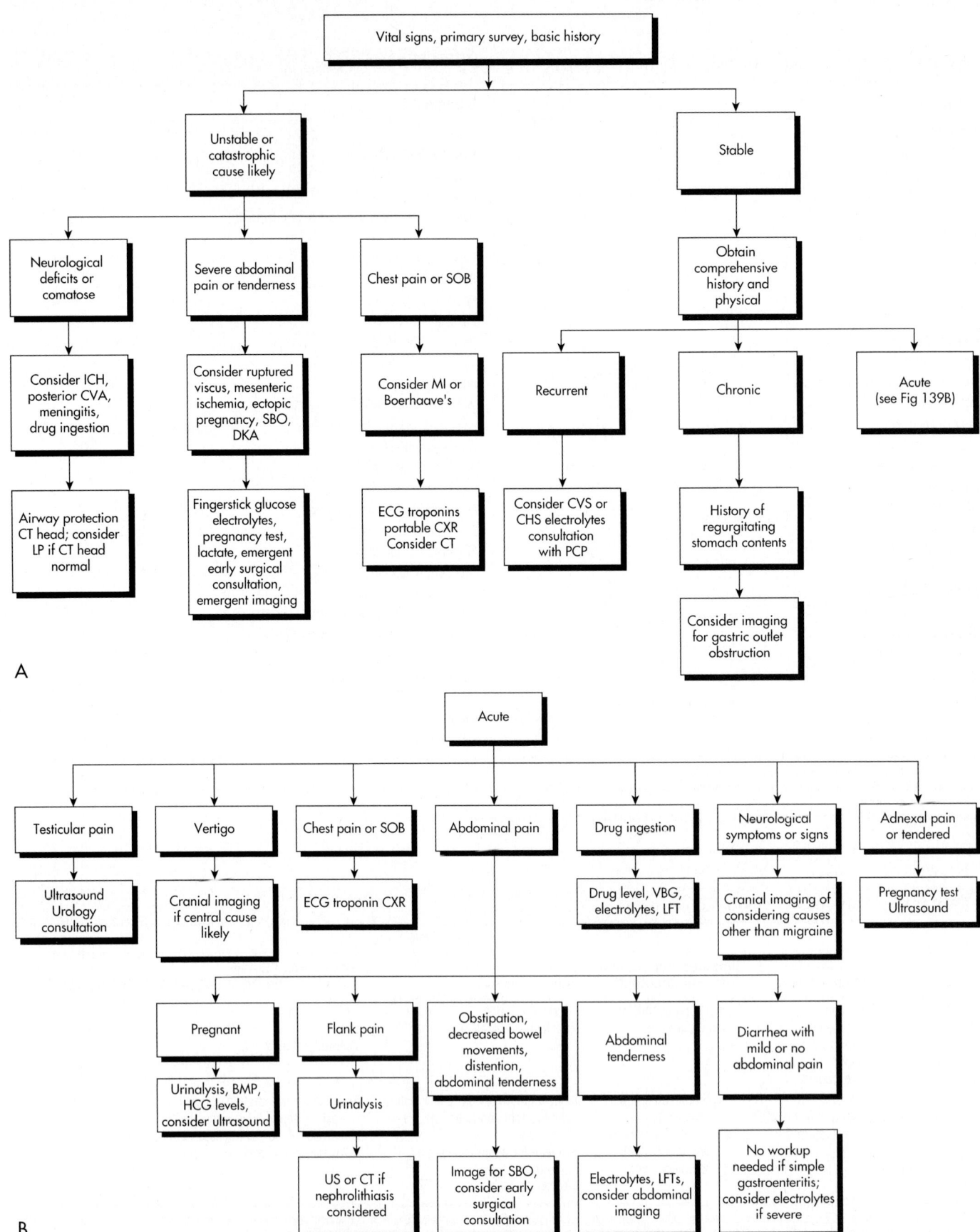

FIG. 139 (A and B) Approach to the patient with nausea and vomiting. *BMP,* Basic metabolic panel; *CT,* computed tomography; *CVA,* Cerebrovascular accident; *CVS,* cyclical vomiting syndrome; *CXR,* chest x-ray; *DKA,* diabetic ketoacidosis; *ECG,* electrocardiogram; *ICH,* intracranial hemorrhage; *LFT,* liver function test; *LP,* lumbar puncture; *MI,* myocardial infarction; *PCP,* phencyclidine; *SBO,* small bowel obstruction; *SOB,* shortness of breath; *US,* ultrasound; *VBG,* venous blood gas. (From Walls RM et al: *Rosen's emergency medicine, concepts and clinical practice,* ed 10, Philadelphia, 2023, Elsevier.)

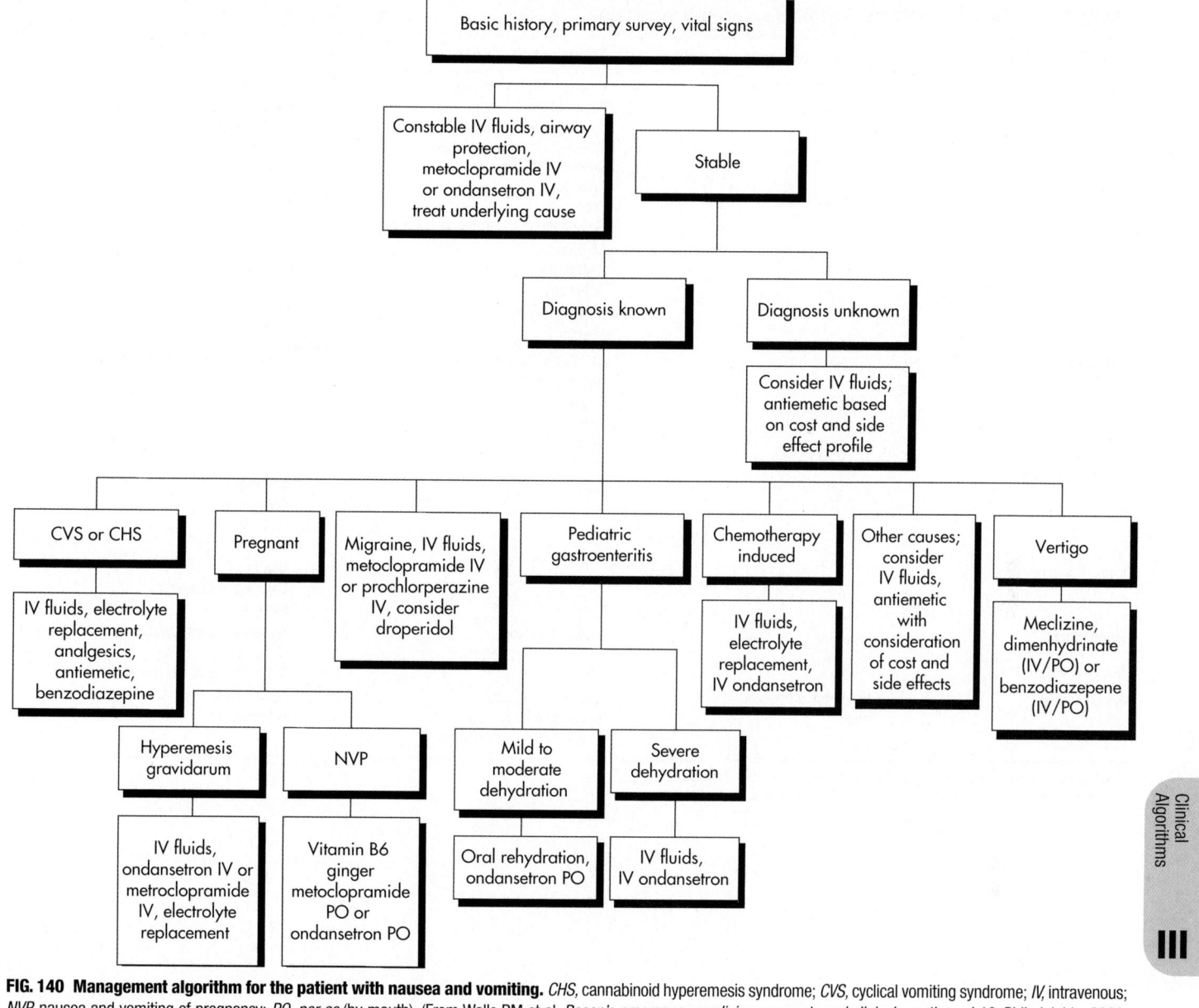

FIG. 140 Management algorithm for the patient with nausea and vomiting. *CHS,* cannabinoid hyperemesis syndrome; *CVS,* cyclical vomiting syndrome; *IV,* intravenous; *NVP,* nausea and vomiting of pregnancy; *PO, per os* (by mouth). (From Walls RM et al: *Rosen's emergency medicine, concepts and clinical practice,* ed 10, Philadelphia, 2023, Elsevier.)

Clinical
Algorithms

III

TABLE 97 Differential Diagnosis of Nausea and Vomiting

Etiologic Category	Critical Diagnoses	Emergent Diagnoses	Nonemergent Diagnoses
Gastrointestinal (GI)	Boerhaave syndrome Ischemic bowel GI bleeding	Gastric outlet obstruction Pancreatitis Cholecystitis or cholangitis Bowel obstruction or ileus Ruptured viscus Appendicitis Peritonitis Spontaneous bacterial peritonitis	Gastritis Gastroparesis Peptic ulcer disease Inflammatory bowel disease Biliary colic Hepatitis Gastroenteritis
Neurologic	Intracerebral bleed Meningitis	Migraine CNS tumor Raised ICP	
Endocrine	DKA	Adrenal insufficiency Uremia	Thyroid
Pregnancy		Hyperemesis gravidarum	Nausea and vomiting of pregnancy
Drug toxicity		Acetaminophen Digoxin Aspirin Theophylline	
Therapeutic drug use			Aspirin Antibiotics Erythromycin Ibuprofen Chemotherapy
Drugs of abuse			Narcotics Narcotic withdrawal Alcohol
Genitourinary		Gonadal torsion	Urinary tract infection Poisoning Nephrolithiasis
Miscellaneous	Myocardial infarction Sepsis	Carbon monoxide Electrolyte disorders Organophosphate poisoning	Motion sickness Labyrinthitis

CNS, Central nervous system; *DKA*, diabetic ketoacidosis; *ICP*, intracranial pressure.
From Marx JA et al: *Rosen's emergency medicine*, ed 8, Philadelphia, 2014, Saunders.

TABLE 98   Disorders Commonly Associated with Vomiting

Disorder	History	Prevalence	Physical Examination	Useful Tests	Comments
Nausea and vomiting of pregnancy (NVP)	Vomiting occurs predominantly in the morning. Associated breast tenderness. NVP typically starts in wk 4-7, peaks in wk 10-16, and disappears by wk 20. Vomiting that begins after wk 12 or continues past wk 20 should prompt a search for another cause.	Very common Affects 75% of all pregnancies	Benign abdomen	Urine pregnancy test Serum electrolytes, urine ketones to exclude hyperemesis gravidarum	Consider NVP in all females of childbearing age. Prognosis for mother and infant is excellent. NVP is associated with a decreased risk of miscarriage, fetal growth retardation, and fetal mortality.
Hyperemesis gravidarum	Severe, protracted form of NVP. No universally accepted definition of the disease. Generally accepted hallmarks include 5% weight loss, ketonuria, and electrolyte disturbance. Hyperemesis is associated with multiple gestation, molar pregnancy, and nulliparity.	Uncommon Affects <1% of pregnancies	Signs of dehydration Benign abdomen	β-hCG Urinalysis for ketones Serum electrolytes Ultrasound examination to exclude molar pregnancy or multiple gestation	Most studies have found no adverse outcomes for the fetus. A few studies, however, have shown a correlation with fetal growth retardation.
Gastroenteritis	Fever, diarrhea, and crampy abdominal pain. Vomiting and pain occur early, usually followed by diarrhea within 24 h.	Very common	Benign abdomen	Usually not necessary	Early gastroenteritis, when only vomiting and periumbilical pain are present, may be confused with early appendicitis. Diarrhea is usually in the diagnosis of gastroenteritis.
Gastritis	Epigastric pain, belching, bloating, fullness, heartburn, and food intolerance. Use of NSAIDs or ETOH common.	Very common	Mild epigastric tenderness may be present.	Lipase and pregnancy test may be necessary to exclude other diagnoses.	Removal of inciting agent along with antacid therapy will resolve symptoms in most patients.
Peptic ulcer disease (PUD)	Epigastric pain present in 90% of cases. Classically, duodenal ulcer pain is relieved by food whereas gastric ulcer pain is made worse. Presence of severe pain should raise suspicion of perforation.	Very common	Mild epigastric tenderness	Hemoglobin if bleeding is suspected Heme-positive stool Upright abdominal film if perforation is suspected	Three major causes of PUD are NSAIDs, *Helicobacter pylori* infection, and hypersecretory states.
Biliary disease	Abdominal pain may be midepigastric or right upper quadrant (RUQ). Onset frequently after a fatty meal. May have history of similar episodes in the past.	Very common	RUQ tenderness present in most cases. If instructed to breathe deeply during palpation in the RUQ, the patient experiences heightened tenderness and inspiratory arrest (Murphy sign).	WBCs Lipase Serum bilirubin Alkaline phosphatase RUQ ultrasound examination ERCP	Normal temperature, WBCs, and spontaneous resolution of symptoms suggest biliary colic. Fever, Murphy sign, elevated WBCs, and suggestive ultrasound indicate cholecystitis.
Myocardial infarction (MI)	Patients typically have substernal chest pain that may radiate to left arm or jaw. Often associated with dyspnea, diaphoresis, or dizziness.	Common	Patients often are anxious and in distress from pain. No diagnostic examination findings.	ECG (new Q waves, ST segment changes, or T wave inversions) troponin	Not all patients have chest pain. A subset of patients, particularly diabetics and elders, may have only nausea, vomiting, and epigastric discomfort.
Diabetic ketoacidosis (DKA)	Polydipsia and polyuria occur early Without treatment, altered mental status and coma may develop. In patients with long-standing diabetes, DKA may be triggered by infection, trauma, MI, or surgery.	Common	"Fruity" breath odor results from serum acetone. Tachypnea occurs with attempts to "blow off" carbon dioxide to compensate for metabolic acidosis. Signs of dehydration may be present. Severe cases often manifest with altered mental status or coma.	Serum glucose, urine ketones, ABGs	DKA may be the first manifestation of diabetes in some patients. These patients often do not recognize the importance of polydipsia and polyuria. They often report only nausea, vomiting, and epigastric pain.
Pancreatitis	Presenting symptom is epigastric pain, which often radiates to the back. Most cases are caused by gallstones or alcoholism. Other causes include hypercalcemia, hyperlipidemia, drugs (sulfas and thiazides), ERCP.	Common	Epigastric tenderness is present. Associated paralytic ileus may cause abdominal distention and decreased bowel sounds. Frank shock may be present in severe cases.	Lipase WBCs, serum glucose, LDH, AST Hematocrit, BUN, calcium, ABGs	Criteria correlating with higher mortality: *At admission*—age >55 yr, WBCs >16,000/mm³, glucose >200 dl, base deficit >4, LDH >350 IU/L, AST >250 U/L *Within 48 hr*—Hct drop of 10%, BUN >2 mg/dl, pO₂ <60 mm Hg, calcium <8 mg, fluid sequestration >4 L *Continued*

Clinical Algorithms

III

TABLE 98 Disorders Commonly Associated with Vomiting—cont'd

Disorder	History	Prevalence	Physical Examination	Useful Tests	Comments
Appendicitis	Abdominal pain classically begins in periumbilical region and later moves to right lower quadrant. Anorexia is common.	Common	Localized tenderness over right lower quadrant. Low-grade fever may be present.	WBCs Ultrasound Abdominal CT	Early appendicitis can be a difficult diagnosis to make. It is still frequently missed on the first physician encounter.
Bowel obstruction	Classically, abdominal pain consists of intermittent cramps occurring at regular intervals. The frequency of the cramps varies with the level of the obstruction; the higher the level, the more frequent the cramps. The location of the pain also varies with the level of the obstruction; high obstruction causes epigastric pain, midlevel obstruction causes periumbilical pain, colonic obstruction causes hypogastric pain.	Common	Abdominal distention, mild diffuse tenderness, and high-pitched "tinkling" bowel sounds may be present. Thorough search for hernias should be performed.	Supine and upright plain abdominal films Abdominal CT	Adhesions, hernias, and tumors account for 90% of bowel obstructions. Other causes include intussusception, volvulus, foreign bodies, gallstone ileus, inflammatory bowel disease, stricture, cystic fibrosis, and hematoma.
Carbon monoxide (CO) poisoning	Headache is usually present. CO poisoning often occurs during winter months when furnaces are turned on. Family members may have similar symptoms if they also have been exposed.	Uncommon	No reliable signs of early CO poisoning	CO level	Because CO is a tasteless, odorless gas, patients may not realize they have been exposed. It is important to keep a high index of suspicion during the cold months.
Boerhaave syndrome	Patients may have neck, chest, or epigastric pain. Forceful, protracted vomiting usually causes the tear. Most cases follow a bout of heavy eating and drinking. Other reported causes include childbirth, defecation, seizures, and heavy lifting.	Uncommon	Tachypnea, tachycardia, and hypotension may be present. Escaped air from the esophagus may produce subcutaneous emphysema. Air in the mediastinum produces a "crunching" sound as the heart beats (Hamman sign).	CXR may show pleural effusion, widened mediastinum, pneumothorax, or pneumomediastinum. Esophagogram with water-soluble contrast is definitive.	The classic presentation includes forceful vomiting, severe chest pain, subcutaneous emphysema, and multiple CXR findings. There is a growing body of evidence that most cases do not have this "classic" picture. In more subtle presentations, the diagnosis can be difficult to make.

ABGs, Arterial blood gases; *AST,* aspartate aminotransferase; β-*hCG,* β-human chorionic gonadotropin; *BUN,* blood urea nitrogen; *CT,* computed tomography; *CXR,* chest radiography; *ECG,* electrocardiogram; *ERCP,* endoscopic retrograde cholangiopancreatography; *ETOH,* ethyl alcohol; *Hct,* hematocrit; *LDH,* lactate dehydrogenase; *NSAID,* nonsteroidal antiinflammatory drug; *pO2,* partial pressure of oxygen; *RUQ,* right upper quadrant; *WBC,* white blood cell.

From Marx JA et al: *Rosen's emergency medicine,* ed 8, Philadelphia, 2014, Saunders.

TABLE 99 Etiology of Nausea and Vomiting in Pediatric Age Groups

Etiologic Category	Newborn	Infant	Child	Adolescent
Infectious	Sepsis, meningitis, UTI, thrush	Pneumonia, otitis media, thrush	Gastroenteritis	Gastroenteritis, URI
Anatomic	Atresia and webs, malrotation, stenosis, meconium ileus, Hirschsprung disease	Pyloric stenosis, intussusception, Hirschsprung disease	Bezoars, chronic granulomatous disease	PUD, superior mesenteric syndrome
Gastrointestinal	Reflux, overfeeding, gastric outlet obstruction, volvulus	Reflux, gastritis, milk intolerance	Appendicitis, pancreatic, hepatitis, other food intolerance	Achalasia, hepatitis
Neurologic	Subdural hematoma, hydrocephalus	Subdural hematoma	Neoplasia, migraine, Reye syndrome, motion sickness, hypertension	Neoplasia, migraine, motion sickness, hypertension
Metabolic	Organic or amino acidemias, urea cycle defects, galactosemia, hypercalcemia, phenylketonuria, kernicterus	Hereditary fructose intolerance, disorders of fatty acid metabolism, uremia, adrenal hyperplasia, kernicterus	Diabetes, vitamin A excess	Diabetes, pregnancy, acute intermittent porphyria
Other	Idiopathic, cardiac failure	Rumination, cardiac failure	Cyclic vomiting syndrome, toxins, food poisoning, Munchausen syndrome by proxy	Psychogenic, anorexia

PUD, Peptic ulcer disease; *URI*, upper respiratory infection; *UTI*, urinary tract infection.
Adapted from Li HK, Sunku BK: Vomiting and nausea. In Wyllie R, Hyams JS (eds): *Pediatric gastrointestinal and liver disease: pathophysiology, diagnosis, management*, Philadelphia, 2005, Saunders, pp. 127-149. From Marx JA et al: *Rosen's emergency medicine*, ed 8, Philadelphia, 2014, Saunders.

TABLE 100 Commonly Used Medications for the Treatment of Nausea and Vomiting

Medication	Dose	Comments
Promethazine (Phenergan)	*Adult:* 12.5-25 mg IV, IM, PO, or by rectum *Pediatric:* 0.25-1 mg/kg/dose q4-6h prn IV, IM, PO, or by rectum; max 25 mg/dose	May be repeated every 4-6 h until cessation of vomiting. May cause dry mouth, dizziness, blurred vision. Boxed warning for use under 2 yr old.
Prochlorperazine (Compazine)	*Adult:* 5-10 mg IM or PO; 2.5-10 mg IV; 25 mg by rectum *Pediatric:* 0.4 mg/kg/24 h tid-qid PO or by rectum; 0.1-0.15 mg/kg/dose tid-qid IM; max 40 mg/24 h	May be repeated every 4 h IV or IM or every 12 h by rectum until cessation of vomiting. May cause lethargy, hypotension, extrapyramidal effects.
Metoclopramide (Reglan)	*Adult:* 10 mg IM or IV, may repeat q6h *Pediatric:* 1-2 mg/kg/dose q2-6h IV q2-3h	May cause dystonic reactions, tardive dyskinesia, neuroleptic malignant syndrome.
Ondansetron (Zofran)	*Adult:* 4 mg IV single dose *Pediatric:* Up to 40 kg: 0.1 mg/kg; >40 kg: 4 mg/dose IV single dose	May cause headache, dizziness, and musculoskeletal pain.

IM, Intramuscularly; *IV,* intravenously; *PO,* orally; *prn,* as needed; *q,* every.
From Marx JA et al: *Rosen's emergency medicine*, ed 8, Philadelphia, 2014, Saunders.

Clinical Algorithms

III

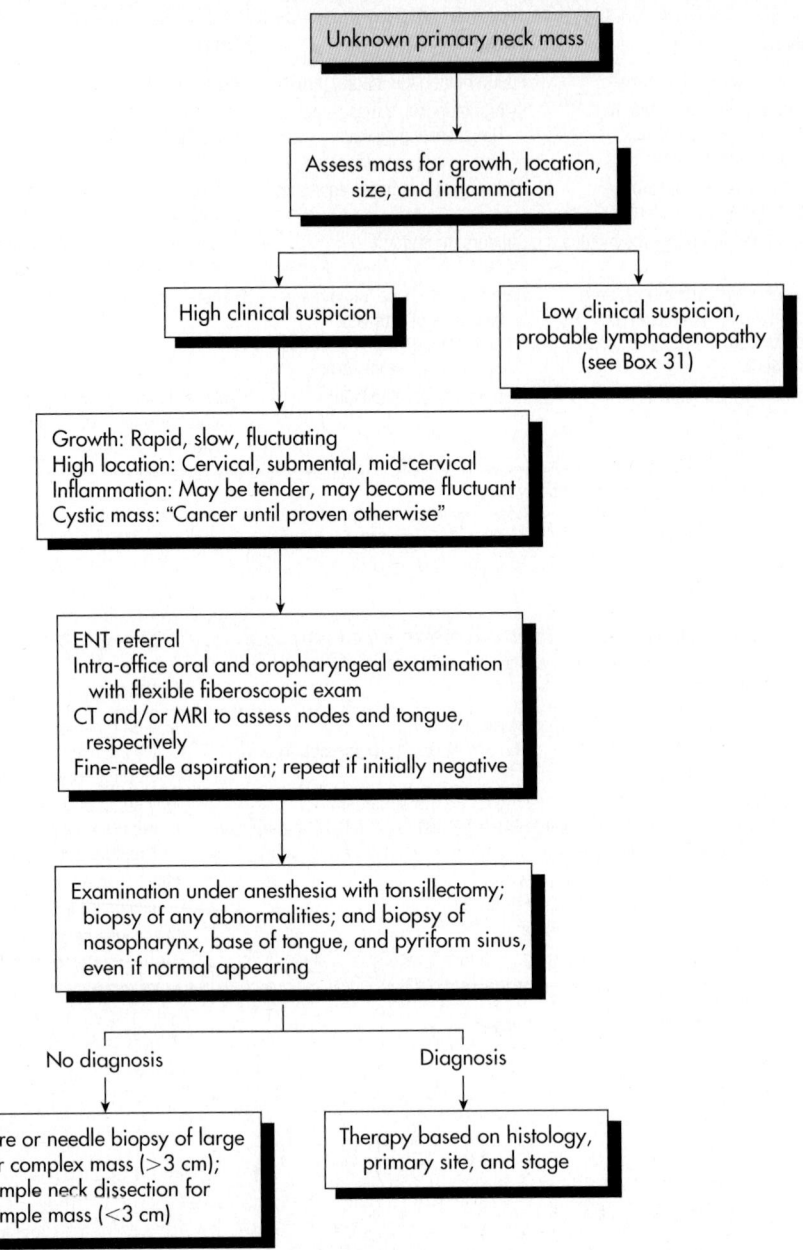

FIG. 141 Evaluation of an unknown primary neck mass. *CT,* Computed tomography; *ENT,* ear, nose, and throat; *MRI,* magnetic resonance imaging. (From Goldman L, Schafer AL [eds]: *Cecil textbook of medicine,* ed 24, Philadelphia, 2012, Saunders.)

BOX 31   An Approach to the Patient with Lymphadenopathy

- Does the patient have a known illness that causes lymphadenopathy? Treat and monitor for resolution.
- Is there an obvious infection to explain the lymphadenopathy (e.g., infectious mononucleosis)? Treat and monitor for resolution.
- Are the nodes very large and/or very firm and thus suggestive of malignancy? Perform a biopsy.
- Is the patient very concerned about malignancy and unable to be reassured that malignancy is unlikely? Perform a biopsy.
- If none of the preceding are true, perform a complete blood cell count, and if it is unrevealing, monitor for a predetermined period (usually 2-6 wk). If the nodes do not regress or if they increase in size, perform a biopsy.

From Goldman L, Ausiello D (eds): *Cecil textbook of medicine,* ed 23, Philadelphia, 2008, Saunders.

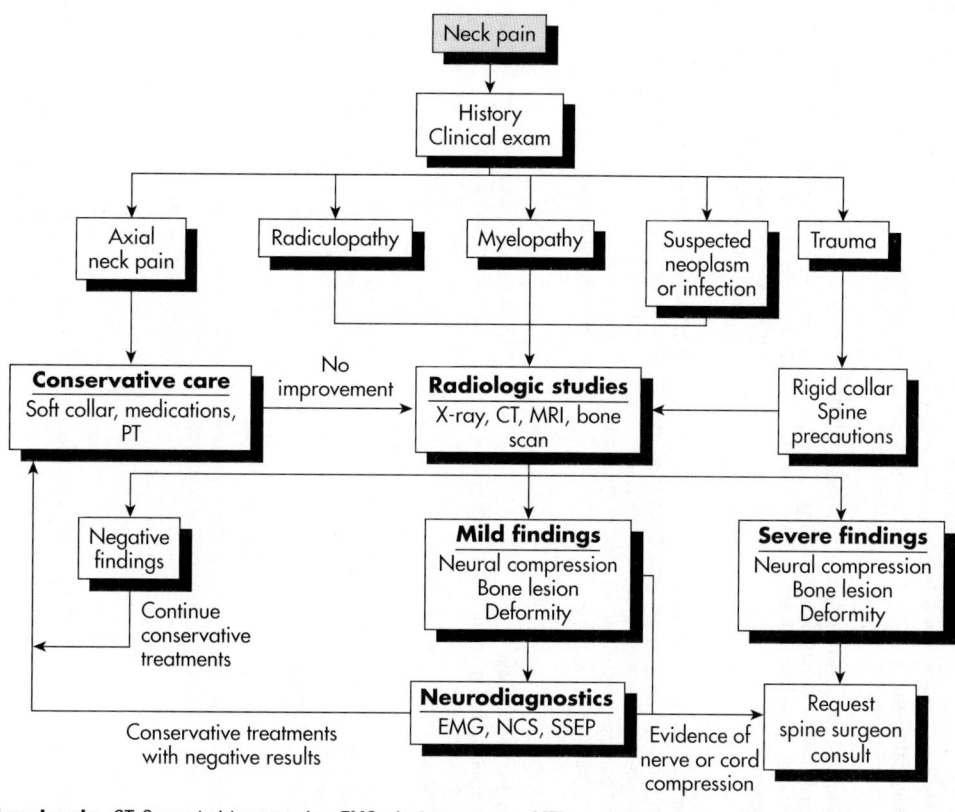

FIG. 142 Algorithm of neck pain. *CT,* Computed tomography; *EMG,* electromyogram; *MRI,* magnetic resonance imaging; *NCS,* nerve conduction study; *PT,* physical therapy; *SSEP,* somatosensory evoked potentials. (From Firestein GS et al: *Kelley's textbook of rheumatology,* ed 9, Philadelphia, 2013, Saunders.)

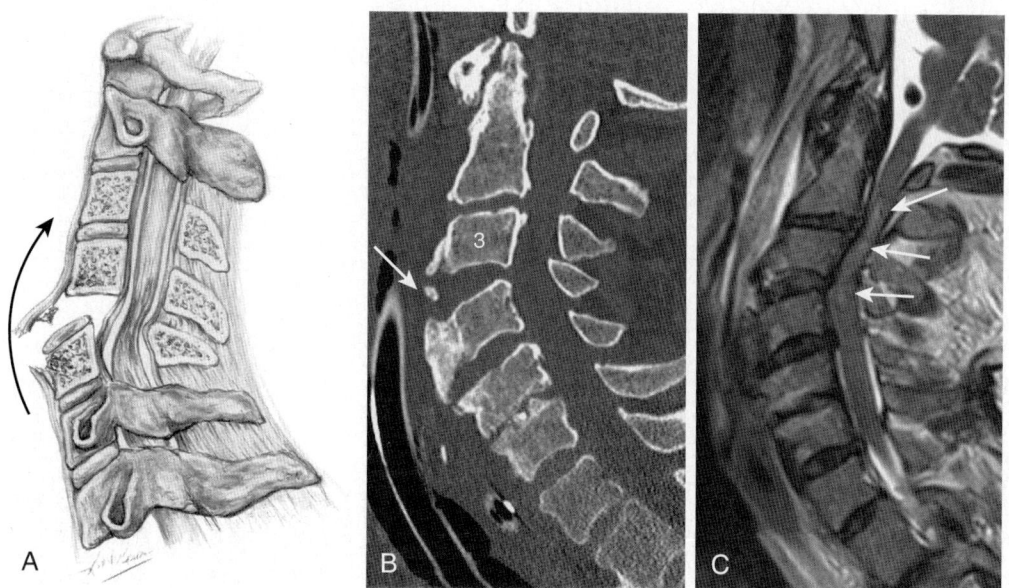

FIG. 143 Extension injury. A, Drawing shows mechanism and injury. There is a small avulsion from the anterosuperior margin of the vertebra immediately below the affected level. Note the wide disk space and retrolisthesis, hallmarks of this injury. The spinal cord is frequently injured in this setting. **B,** Sagittal reconstructed computed tomography image shows widening of the C3 disk space with an avulsed fragment of bone *(arrow)* and retrolisthesis. **C,** T2-weighted magnetic resonance image shows cord hemorrhage *(arrows).* The patient is quadriplegic. (From Pope TL et al: *Musculoskeletal imaging,* ed 2, Philadelphia, 2015, Elsevier.)

TABLE 101 Differential Diagnosis of Common Causes of Axial Neck Pain

Etiology	Cause	Characteristics	Physical Exam	Treatment
Trauma	Irritation of muscles, facets, intervertebral discs, and ligaments (i.e., "whiplash") Bony fractures	History of trauma Neck stiffness Pain worsens with movement May have accompanying neurologic deficits	Guarding of the neck muscles leading to reduced ROM Severe midline tenderness with fractures Moderate tenderness with whiplash type injuries Neurologic deficit	Physical therapy and antiinflammatories may be beneficial in the case of whiplash Bracing may be necessary for minor fractures Surgical intervention may be necessary for instability or neurologic compression
Degenerative Changes (Nonneuropathic)	Irritation of zygapophyseal (facet) joints Irritation of cervical discs	Often chronic in nature Pain radiates to shoulders Suboccipital headaches Facet pain improves with injections targeting the joint capsule or block of dorsal primary ramus	Limited neck range of motion Facet pain worsened by palpation of paraspinal region Discogenic pain worsened by midline palpation Discogenic pain worsened with neck extension and rotation	Physical therapy, antiinflammatories Medial branch blocks or radiofrequency ablation for facet pain Surgical intervention may be considered if instability or deformity is present
Cervical Radiculopathy	Herniated cervical disc Spondylosis Noncompressive pathologies (diabetes, herpes zoster, etc.)	Sharp, shooting pain Radiation into the associated dermatome	Positive Spurling sign Numbness, tingling, and/or pain in associated dermatomes Weakness in associated myotomes	Physical therapy, antiinflammatories, oral steroids, and epidural steroid injections Surgery for failure of conservative therapy or if weakness is present
Cervical Stenosis	Spondylosis Congenitally narrow canal Postsurgical Traumatic Rheumatologic	Often accompanied by myelopathy (deterioration in fine motor skills, gait and balance disturbances, incontinence, etc.)	Broad-based, spastic gait Hyperreflexia Weakness Positive Hoffman sign	Symptomatic treatment may be beneficial in the absence of a neurologic deficit Surgical intervention warranted in the presence of neurologic deficits or hyperreflexia
Myofascial Pain	Chronic irritation of neck muscles May be due to postural or biomechanical imbalance, trauma, emotional stress, and endocrine or hormone abnormalities	Dull and persistent pain without clear exacerbating or alleviating factors Sometimes worsened with neck flexion May be associated with fibromyalgia	Patient may have trigger points, or palpable muscle bands that refer pain when pressure is applied	Physical therapy and antiinflammatories Psychotherapy Trigger point injections
Rheumatologic Disease Rheumatoid arthritis (RA) Ankylosing spondylitis (AS) Others	Joint inflammation Cervical stenosis Musculoskeletal strain from cervicothoracic kyphotic deformity in AS	Morning stiffness and rigidity RA may lead to atlanto-axial instability AS may lead to cervicothoracic kyphosis	Additional symptoms related to systemic disorder	Physical therapy and antiinflammatories may be considered to alleviate symptoms Surgery may be necessary to address instability or deformity

Continued

TABLE 101   Differential Diagnosis of Common Causes of Axial Neck Pain—cont'd

Etiology	Cause	Characteristics	Physical Exam	Treatment
Infection				
Osteomyelitis	Bone destruction	Severe neck pain that is present at rest and worsened with movement	Severe pain that is worsened with movement	IV antibiotics
Diskitis	Irritation of periosteal nerves	Signs/symptoms of infection	Neurologic deficits may be due to epidural abscess	Surgery may be necessary in the presence of an epidural abscess
Epidural abscess	Instability	Patients with history of IVDU or immunocompromise	Stigmata of bacteremia	Bracing may offer symptomatic relief
	Altered biomechanics			
Neoplasm				
Metastatic tumors	Bone destruction	Neck pain worsens with movement	Severe neck tenderness	Symptomatic treatment with antiinflammatories and pain medications
Multiple myeloma/plasmacytoma	Irritation of periosteal nerves	Pain awakens patient from sleep	Neck pain worsens with movement	Radiation
Primary bone tumors	Mechanical instability	Systemic symptoms such as unexplained weight loss, anorexia, malaise, etc.	Neurologic deficits present from epidural tumor	Surgical intervention may be warranted for decompression and/or stabilization
Vascular				
Cervical carotid dissection	Traumatic or spontaneous tear in the tunica intima	Sudden onset	Horner syndrome	Antiplatelet agents, anticoagulants, stenting
	Blood enters the space between the inner and outer wall	Tearing sensation	Carotid bruit	
		Headache	Expanding hematoma	
		Facial or eye pain	Neurologic deficit	
		Pulsatile tinnitus		
		Ischemic events		
Postsurgical				
Pseudoarthrosis (failed fusion)	Hardware loosening	Improvement in neck pain after surgery ("honeymoon period") with worsening neck and interscapular pain	Painful range of motion in the neck	Revision surgical procedure
Postsurgical iatrogenic instability	Instability due to disruption of disc and joints		History of cervical surgery	

From Firestein GS et al: *Firestein & Kelley's textbook of rheumatology*, ed 11, Philadelphia, 2021, Elsevier.

Clinical
Algorithms

III

TABLE 102   Rheumatologic Disorders Causing Neck Pain

- Rheumatoid arthritis
  - Without disease of the C1-C2 joint
  - With structural cervical abnormalities
  - C1-C2 subluxation
  - C1-C2 facet involvement
- Spondyloarthropathies
  - Ankylosing spondylitis
  - Reactive arthritis
  - Psoriatic arthritis
  - Enteropathic arthritis
- Polymyalgia rheumatica
- Osteoarthritis
- Fibromyalgia
- Nonspecific musculoskeletal pain
- Miscellaneous spondyloarthropathies
  - Whipple disease
  - Behçet disease
  - Paget disease
  - Acromegaly
  - Ossification of the posterior longitudinal ligament
  - Diffuse idiopathic skeletal hyperostosis

From Firestein GS et al: *Firestein & Kelley's textbook of rheumatology,* ed 11, Philadelphia, 2021, Elsevier.

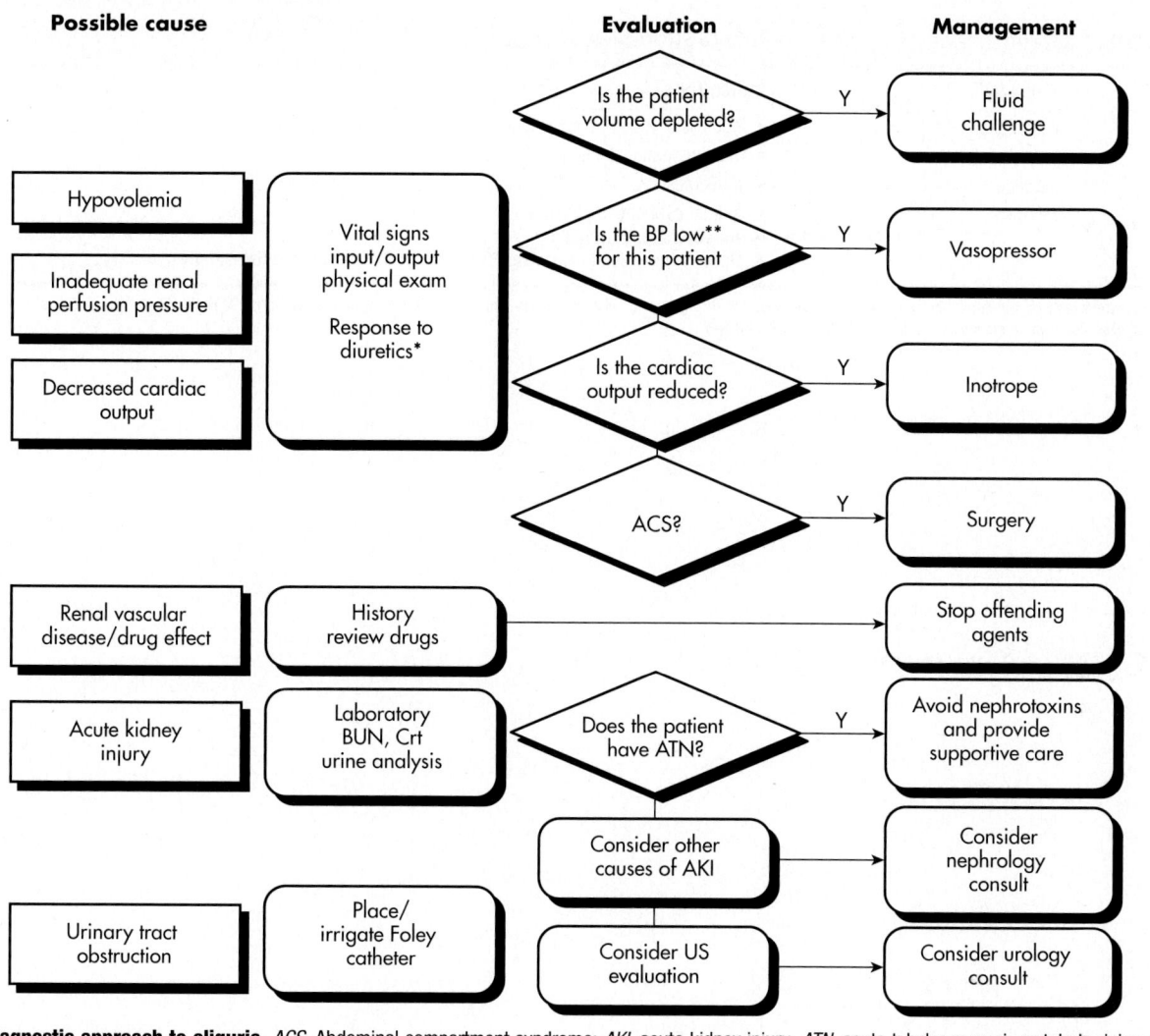

FIG. 144 Diagnostic approach to oliguria. *ACS*, Abdominal compartment syndrome; *AKI*, acute kidney injury; *ATN*, acute tubular necrosis or tubular injury; *BP*, blood pressure; *BUN*, blood urea nitrogen; *Crt*, creatinine; *US*, ultrasound. (From Vincent JL et al: *Textbook of critical care*, ed 8, Philadelphia, 2024, Elsevier.)

TABLE 103   Diagnostic Tests and Their Utility in an Oliguric Patient

S. No.	Diagnostic Test	Comments
1	Urine microscopy	• Often noncontributory • RBC casts, when present, indicate glomerular pathology
2	Urine indices	• Very low utility in the ICU • Not recommended in the evaluation of oliguria
3	Renal ultrasound	• Should be routinely performed to rule out obstruction • Provides information on existence of chronic kidney disease
4	Biomarkers (NGAL, TIMP-2, and IGFBP-7)	• Consider when available • Elevation indicates structural kidney damage
5	Hemodynamic evaluation	• Mandatory to ensure fluid responsiveness and fluid tolerance
6	Measurement of intraabdominal pressure	• Suggested in patients with high risk for ACS

ACS, Abdominal compartment syndrome; *ICU*, intensive care unit; *IGFBP-7*, insulin-like growth factor binding protein-7; *NGAL*, neutrophil gelatinase–associated lipocalcin; *RBC*, red blood cell; *TIMP-2*, tissue inhibitor of metalloproteinases.
From Vincent JL et al: *Textbook of critical care*, ed 8, Philadelphia, 2024, Elsevier

TABLE 104	Effectiveness of Various Treatment Strategies in Oliguria	

S. No.	Therapy	Indications
1	Fluid bolus	• Administer if overt hypovolemia and if fluid responsive and tolerant
2	Vasopressors	• In septic patients with MAP ≤65 mm Hg1
3	Inotropes	• If decreased LV and/or RV function with cardiorenal syndrome
4	Diuretics	• In fluid-overloaded patients
		• To prevent fluid overload
		• Once volume replete, consider FST2 to assess response and risk stratify

FST, Furosemide stress test; *LV*, left ventricular; *MAP*, mean arterial pressure; *RV*, right ventricular. In patients with known chronic hypertension, target MAP 70-75 mm Hg; *S. No.*, strategy number.
From Vincent JL et al: *Textbook of critical care*, ed 8, Philadelphia, 2024, Elsevier

ICD-10CM #
H92.0	Otalgia
H92.01	Otalgia, right ear
H92.02	Otalgia, left ear
H92.03	Bilateral otalgia
H92.09	Unspecified otalgia
H92.1	Otorrhea
H92. 13	Bilateral otorrhea
H92.11	Otorrhea, right ear
H92.12	Otorrhea, left ear
H92.10	Otorrhea, unspecified ear

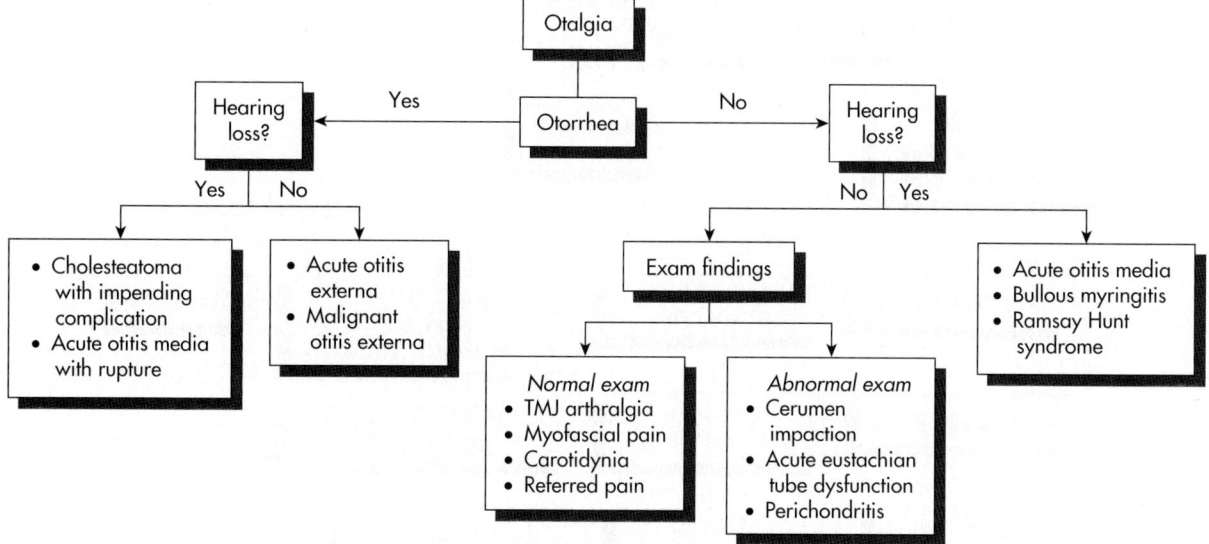

FIG. 145 Establishing a differential diagnosis with a chief complaint of otalgia. This algorithm encourages the clinician to consider the patient complaint in categoric differential diagnosis families. It is not exhaustive. (From Flint PW et al: *Cummings otolaryngology, head and neck surgery,* ed 7, Philadelphia, 2021, Elsevier.)

Clinical Algorithms

III

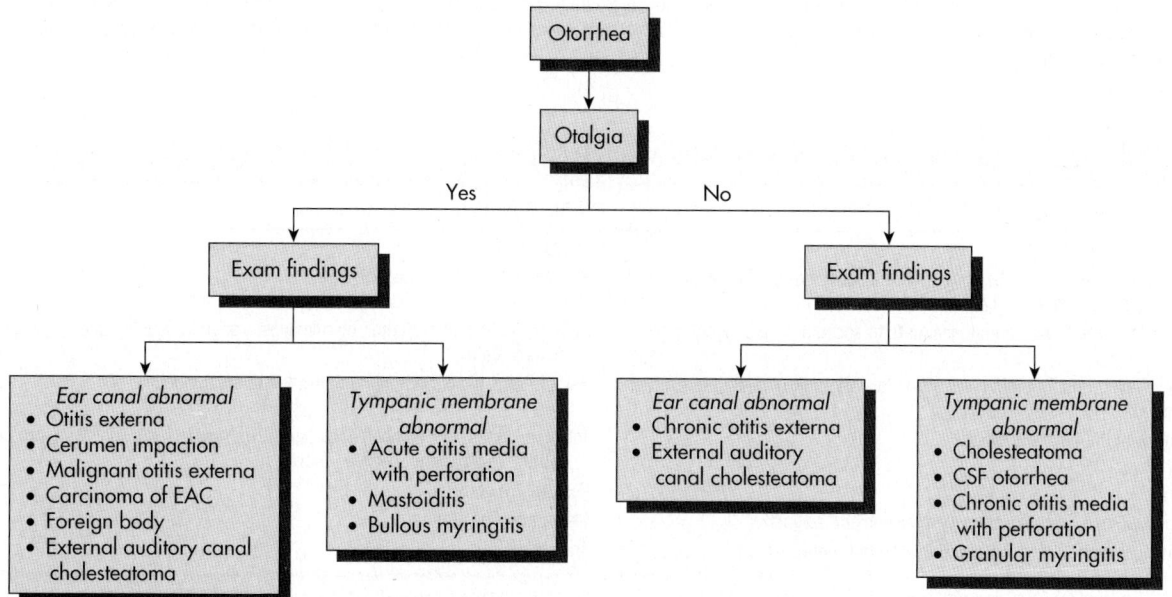

FIG. 146 Establishing a differential diagnosis with a chief complaint of otorrhea. This algorithm encourages the clinician to consider the patient complaint in categoric differential diagnosis families. It is not exhaustive. *CSF,* Cerebrospinal fluid; *EAC,* external auditory canal. (From Flint PW et al: *Cummings otolaryngology, head and neck surgery,* ed 7, Philadelphia, 2021, Elsevier.)

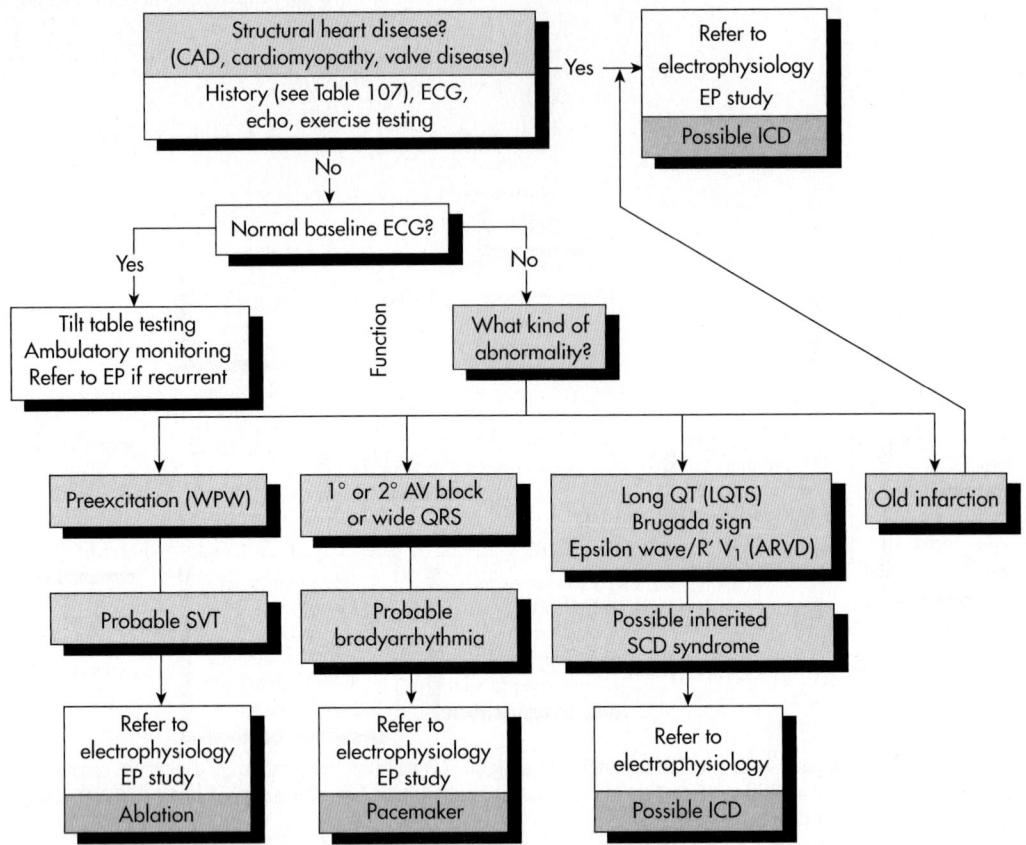

FIG. 147 Algorithm for evaluating patients with symptoms of palpitation, dizziness, or syncope. *ARVD,* Arrhythmogenic right ventricular dysplasia; *AV,* atrioventricular; *CAD,* coronary artery disease; *ECG,* electrocardiogram; *echo,* echocardiogram; *EP,* electrophysiology; *ICD,* implantable cardioverter-defibrillator; *LQTS,* long QT syndrome; *SCD,* sudden cardiac death; *SVT,* supraventricular tachycardia; *WPW,* Wolff-Parkinson-White syndrome. (From Goldman L, Schafer AI: *Goldman Cecil medicine,* ed 25, Philadelphia, 2016, Saunders.)

TABLE 105 Items to Be Covered in History of Patient with Palpitation

Does the Palpitation Occur:	If So, Suspect:
As isolated "jumps" or "skips"?	Extrasystoles
In attacks known to be of abrupt beginning, with a heart rate of 120 beats/min or over, with regular or irregular rhythm?	Paroxysmal rapid heart action
Independent of exercise or excitement adequate to account for the symptom?	Atrial fibrillation, atrial flutter, thyrotoxicosis, anemia, febrile states, hypoglycemia, anxiety state
In attacks developing rapidly, though not absolutely abruptly, unrelated to exertion or excitement?	Hemorrhage, hypoglycemia, tumor of the adrenal medulla
In conjunction with the taking of drugs?	Tobacco, coffee, tea, alcohol, epinephrine, ephedrine, aminophylline, atropine, thyroid extract, monoamine oxidase inhibitors
On standing?	Postural hypotension
In middle-aged women, in conjunction with flushes and sweats?	Menopausal syndrome
When the rate is known to be normal and the rhythm regular?	Anxiety state

From Goldman L, Braunwald E: Chest discomfort and palpitation. In Isselbacher KJ et al (eds): *Harrison's principles of internal medicine,* ed 13, New York, 1994, McGraw-Hill.

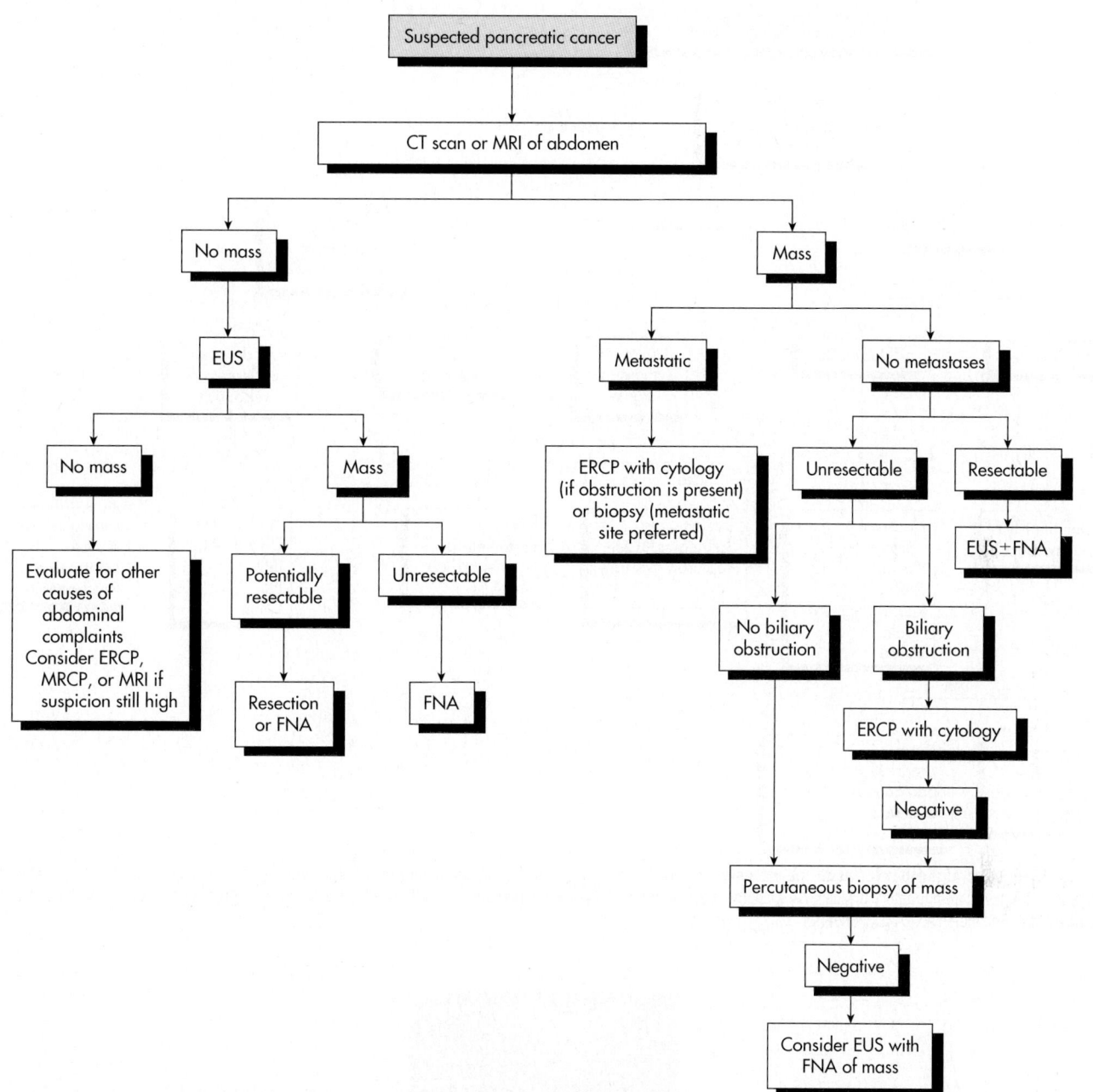

FIG. 150 Diagnostic algorithm for pancreatic cancer. Intraoperative fine-needle aspiration *(FNA)* if found inoperable during surgery. *CT,* Computed tomography; *ERCP,* endoscopic retrograde cholangiopancreatography; *EUS,* endoscopic ultrasonography; *MRCP,* magnetic resonance cholangiopancreatography; *MRI,* magnetic resonance imaging. (From Goldman L, Schafer AL [eds]: *Cecil textbook of medicine,* ed 24, Philadelphia, 2012, Saunders.)

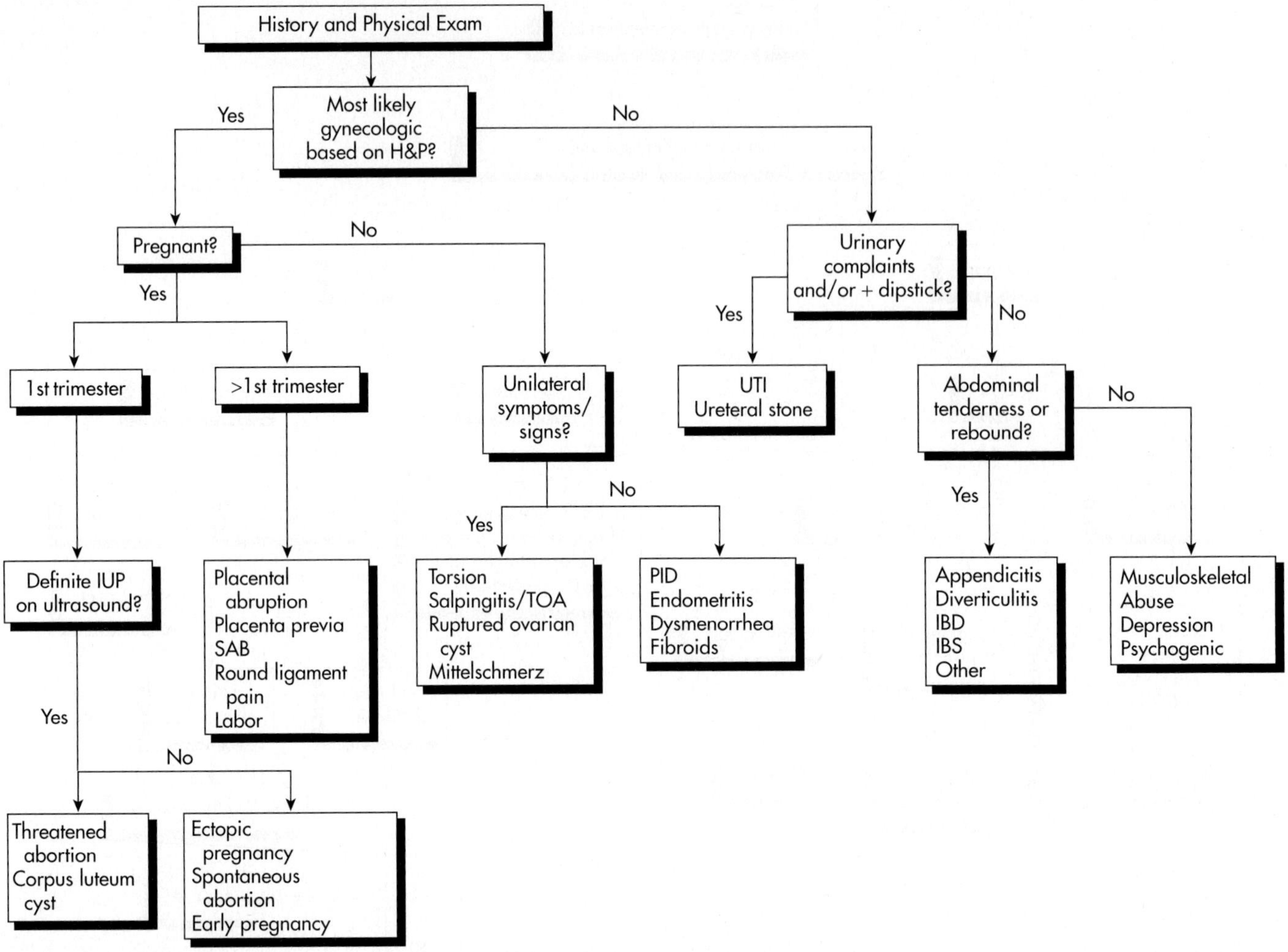

History and Physical Exam

Most likely gynecologic based on H&P?

Yes → Pregnant?

No →

Pregnant?
- Yes
- No →

Urinary complaints and/or + dipstick?
- Yes
- No

1st trimester

>1st trimester

Unilateral symptoms/signs?
- Yes
- No

UTI
Ureteral stone

Abdominal tenderness or rebound?
- Yes
- No

Definite IUP on ultrasound?
- Yes
- No

Placental abruption
Placenta previa
SAB
Round ligament pain
Labor

Torsion
Salpingitis/TOA
Ruptured ovarian cyst
Mittelschmerz

PID
Endometritis
Dysmenorrhea
Fibroids

Appendicitis
Diverticulitis
IBD
IBS
Other

Musculoskeletal
Abuse
Depression
Psychogenic

Threatened abortion
Corpus luteum cyst

Ectopic pregnancy
Spontaneous abortion
Early pregnancy

FIG. 151 Diagnostic algorithm for acute pelvic pain. *H&P,* History and physical; *IBD,* inflammatory bowel disease; *IBS,* irritable bowel syndrome; *IUP,* intrauterine pregnancy; *PID,* pelvic inflammatory disease; *SAB,* spontaneous abortion; *TOA,* tuboovarian abscess; *UTI,* urinary tract infection. (From Marx JA et al: *Rosen's emergency medicine,* ed 8, Philadelphia, 2014, Saunders.)

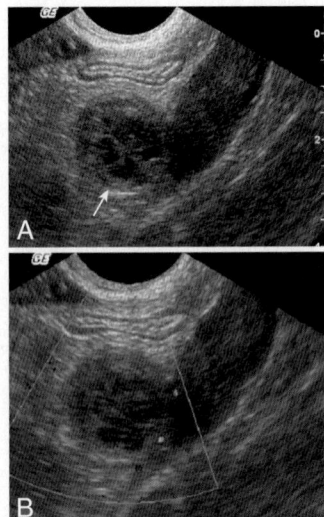

FIG. 152 Ectopic pregnancy seen as mixed-echogenicity mass. A 30-yr-old woman presented with left lower quadrant pain at 7 wk gestation and β-hCG of 500 mIU/ml and falling over a 3-day period. **A,** In the left adnexa, medial to the left ovary, there was a 2-cm mass *(arrow)* with mixed echogenicity, and **B,** only minimal peripheral vascularity. A left ectopic pregnancy was confirmed and, based on a falling β-hCG, was treated expectantly and resolved without complication. (From Rumack CM et al: *Diagnostic ultrasound,* ed 4, Philadelphia, 2011, Elsevier.)

ICD-10CM # G60.9   Hereditary and idiopathic neuropathy, unspecified
G57.10   Meralgia paresthetica, unspecified lower limb
G90.09   Other idiopathic peripheral autonomic neuropathy

APPROACH TO EVALUATION OF PERIPHERAL NEUROPATHIES

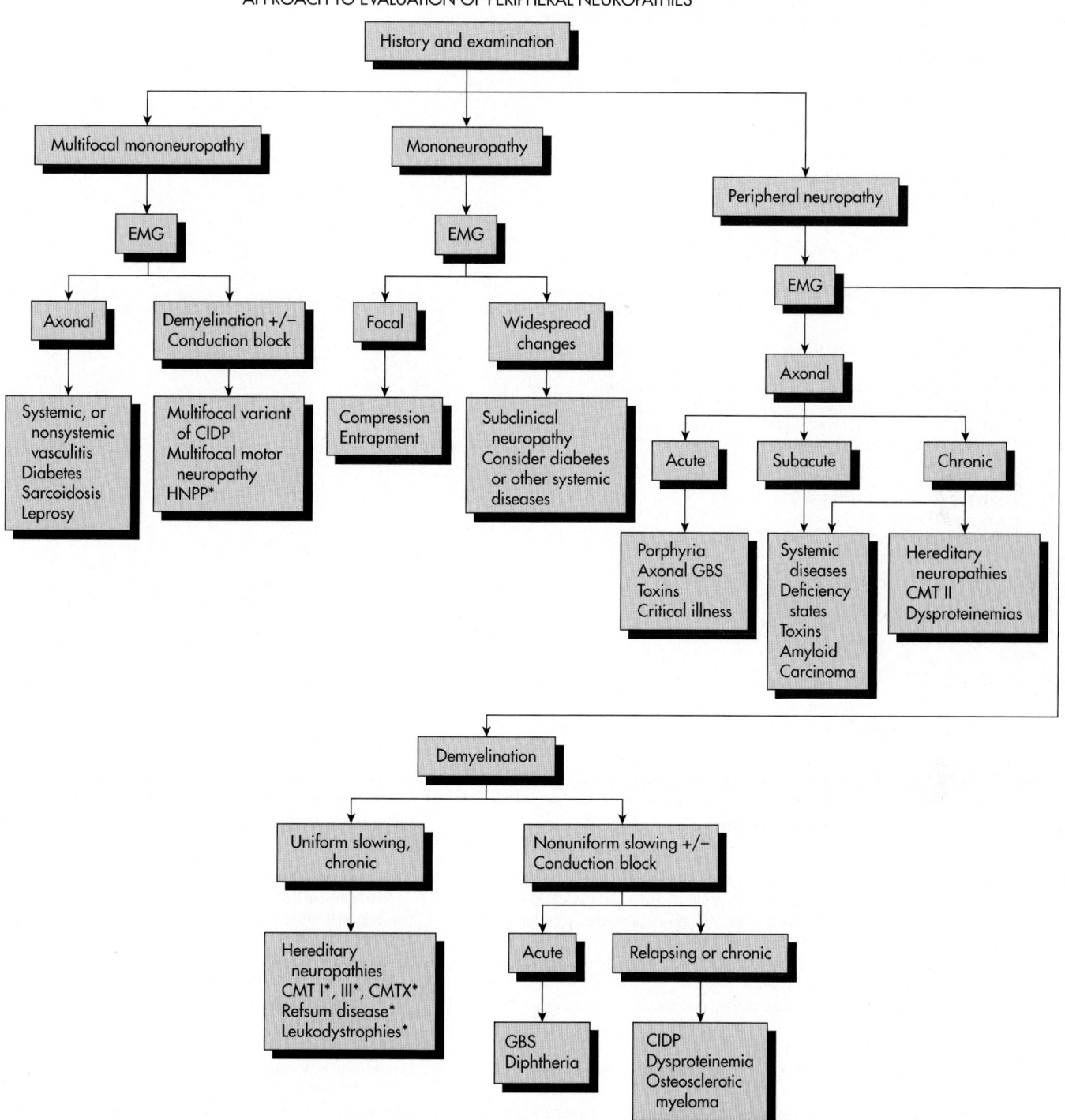

FIG. 154 Diagnostic approach to evaluation of a patient with peripheral neuropathy. Electromyography *(EMG)* denotes electrodiagnostic studies including nerve conduction studies and needle EMG. DNA diagnostic testing or specific biochemical tests are available for conditions marked with asterisks. *CIDP,* Chronic inflammatory demyelinating polyradiculoneuropathy; *CMT,* Charcot-Marie-Tooth disease; *CMTX,* Charcot-Marie-Tooth disease X-linked; *GBS,* Guillain-Barré syndrome; *HNPP,* hereditary liability to pressure palsies. (From Jankovic J et al: *Bradley and Daroff's neurology in clinical practice,* ed 8, Philadelphia, 2022, Elsevier.)

Clinical
Algorithms

III

ICD-10CM # G60.9 Hereditary and idiopathic neuropathy, unspecified
G57.10 Meralgia paresthetica, unspecified lower limb
G90.09 Other idiopathic peripheral autonomic neuropathy

BOX 32 Ancillary Diagnostic Testing in Suspected Peripheral Neuropathy

Obtained in Most Patients
Complete blood count
Erythrocyte sedimentation rate
Glucose
Creatine kinase
Creatinine

Obtained in Some Patients Based on History
Human chorionic gonadotropin
Magnesium
Phosphate
Vitamin B_{12}
Hemoglobin A_{1c}
Serum protein electrophoresis with immune fixation electrophoresis
Venereal Disease Research Laboratory (VDRL) or rapid plasma reagin screen with fluorescent treponemal antibody absorption test, as appropriate
Thyroid function
Human immunodeficiency virus (HIV) titer
Lyme enzyme-linked immunosorbent assay and Western blot
Rheumatoid factor and antinuclear antibody
Blood, urine, hair, or nails for metal, depending on suspected chronicity of exposure
Specific serum antibodies to components of peripheral nervous system (PNS)
Cerebrospinal fluid (CSF) for cells, protein, Lyme titer
Electrodiagnostic testing
Nerve conduction studies (NCS)
Electromyography (EMG)
Neurodiagnostic imaging
Magnetic resonance imaging (MRI)
Computed tomography (CT)
Sonography
Quantitative sensory testing
Nerve biopsy
Sural
Intraepidermal nerve fiber density

From Walls RM et al: *Rosen's emergency medicine, concepts and clinical practice,* ed 10, Philadelphia, 2023, Elsevier.

TABLE 107 Peripheral Nerve Lesions of the Arm

Lesion	Clinical Findings	Electromyography Findings
Median Neuropathy		
Carpal tunnel syndrome	Weakness and wasting of abductor pollicis brevis if severe; sensory loss on palmar aspect of first through third digits	Slow median motor and sensory NCV through the carpal tunnel; denervation of abductor pollicis brevis if severe
Anterior interosseous syndrome	Weakness of flexor digitorum profundus, pronator quadratus, flexor pollicis longus	Denervation in flexor digitorum profundus, flexor pollicis longus, pronator quadratus
Pronator teres syndrome	Weakness of distal median-innervated muscles; tenderness of pronator teres	Slow median motor NCV through proximal forearm denervation of distal median-innervated muscles
Compression at the ligament of Struthers	Weakness of distal median-innervated muscles	As for pronator teres syndrome, with the addition of denervation of pronator teres
Ulnar Neuropathy		
Palmar branch damage	Weakness of dorsal interossei; no sensory loss	Normal ulnar NCV; denervation of first dorsal interosseus but not abductor digiti minimi
Entrapment at Guyon canal	Weakness of ulnar intrinsic muscles; numbness over fourth and fifth digits	Slow ulnar motor and sensory NCV through wrist
Entrapment at or near the elbow	Weakness of ulnar intrinsic muscles; numbness over fourth and fifth digits	Slow ulnar motor NCV across elbow, denervation in first dorsal interosseus, abductor digiti minimi, and ulnar half of flexor digitorum profundus
Radial Neuropathy		
Posterior interosseus syndrome	Weakness of finger and wrist extensors; no sensory loss	Denervation in wrist and finger extensors; sparing of the supinator and extensor carpi radialis
Compression at the spiral groove	Weakness of finger and wrist extensors; triceps usually spared; sensory loss on dorsal aspects of first digit	Slow radial motor NCV across spiral groove; denervation in distal radial-innervated muscles; triceps may be affected with proximal lesions

NCV, Nerve conduction velocity.
From Jankovic J et al: *Bradley and Daroff's neurology in clinical practice,* ed 8, Philadelphia, 2022, Elsevier.

PERIPHERAL NEUROPATHY—cont'd

ICD-10CM # G60.9 Hereditary and idiopathic neuropathy, unspecified
G57.10 Meralgia paresthetica, unspecified lower limb
G90.09 Other idiopathic peripheral autonomic neuropathy

1497

TABLE 108 Peripheral Nerve Lesions of the Leg

Lesion	Clinical Findings	Electromyography Findings
Sciatic neuropathy	Weakness of tibial- and peroneal-innervated muscles, with sensory loss on posterior leg and foot	Denervation distally in tibial- and peroneal-innervated muscles
Peroneal neuropathy	Weakness of foot extension and eversion and toe extension	Denervation in tibialis anterior; NCV across fibular neck may be slowed
Tibial neuropathy	Weakness of foot plantar flexion	Denervation of gastrocnemius
Femoral neuropathy	Weakness of knee extension; weakness of hip flexion if psoas involved	Denervation in quadriceps, sometimes psoas

NCV, Nerve conduction velocity.
From Jankovic J et al: *Bradley and Daroff's neurology in clinical practice,* ed 8, Philadelphia, 2022, Elsevier.

TABLE 109 Radiculopathies

Level	Motor Deficit	Sensory Deficit
Cervical Radiculopathy		
C5	Deltoid, biceps	Lateral upper arm
C6	Biceps, brachioradialis	Radial forearm and first and second digits
C7	Wrist extensors, triceps	Third and fourth digits
C8	Intrinsic hand muscles	Fifth digit and ulnar forearm
T1	Intrinsic muscles of the hand, especially APB	Axilla
Lumbar Radiculopathy		
L2	Psoas, quadriceps	Lateral and anterior thigh
L3	Psoas, quadriceps	Lower medial thigh
L4	Tibialis anterior, quadriceps	Medial lower leg
L5	Peroneus longus, gluteus medius, tibialis anterior, extensor hallucis longus	Lateral lower leg
S1	Gastrocnemius, gluteus maximus	Lateral foot and fourth and fifth digits

APB, Abductor pollicis brevis.
From Jankovic J et al: *Bradley and Daroff's neurology in clinical practice,* ed 8, Philadelphia, 2022, Elsevier.

TABLE 110 Some of the More Common Causes of Peripheral Neuropathy

Disease	Sensory	Motor	Autonomic	Fiber Size	Common Clinical Presentation
Diabetes	+++	±	++	S > L	Burning starting in feet; 'glove and stocking'
Alcohol	+++	±	++	S > L	Burning in feet Often cerebellar, ocular or cognitive features
Critical illness	++	++	++	Mixed	Weakness, difficulty weaning from ventilator
Vitamin B$_{12}$	+++	−	−	L > S	Sensory ataxia; often dorsal column signs
Uremia	+++	±	+	S > L	Glove and stocking
Malignancy	+++	++	±	Variable	Variable; may have other neurologic features; may have cachexia and muscle weakness
Liver failure	+++	+	±	Often S > L	Glove and stocking
Paraprotein	++	++	−	Both	Slowly progressive glove and stocking
Anti-MAG	++	++	+	S > L	Glove and stocking
MGUS	++	++	+	Both	Progressive sensorimotor involvement with other features of myeloma
POEMS Amyloidosis	++	±	+++	S >> L	Painful neuropathy with autonomic dysfunction
Chemotherapy (platinum, taxanes, etc.)	+++	+	±	L > S	Glove and stocking pattern—may be rapidly progressive with repeat exposure
HIV	+++	+	±	Both	Progressive glove and stocking
Hereditary (multiple disorders)	Variable	Variable	Variable	Variable	Typically do not have dysesthesia or pain (may be present late)

HIV, Human immunodeficiency virus; *L,* large; *MAG,* myelin-associated glycoproteins; *MGUS,* monoclonal gammopathy of uncertain significance; *POEMS,* polyneuropathy, organomegaly, endocrinopathy, M-spike, skin changes; *S,* small.
L > S indicates that large fibers are affected more than small fibers.
From Talley NJ et al: *Essentials of internal medicine,* ed 4, Chatswood, NSW, 2021, Elsevier Australia.

Clinical Algorithms

III

ICD-10CM # G60.9   Hereditary and idiopathic neuropathy, unspecified
G57.10   Meralgia paresthetica, unspecified lower limb
G90.09   Other idiopathic peripheral autonomic neuropathy

BOX 33   Indications for Nerve Biopsy

Nerve Biopsy Is Diagnostic and Essential for Diagnosis
- Vasculitis*
- Amyloidosis*
- Sarcoidosis*
- Hansen disease (leprosy)
- Giant axonal neuropathy
- Tumor infiltration
- Polyglucosan body disease

Nerve Biopsy Is Suggestive and Only Supportive of Diagnosis
- Charcot-Marie-Tooth disease types 1 and 3
- Chronic inflammatory demyelinating polyradiculoneuropathy
- Paraproteinemic neuropathy (immunoglobulin M monoclonal gammopathy with antimyelin-associated glycoprotein antibody)

*Consider combined distal nerve and muscle biopsies.
From Jankovic J et al: *Bradley and Daroff's neurology in clinical practice,* ed 8, Philadelphia, 2022, Elsevier.

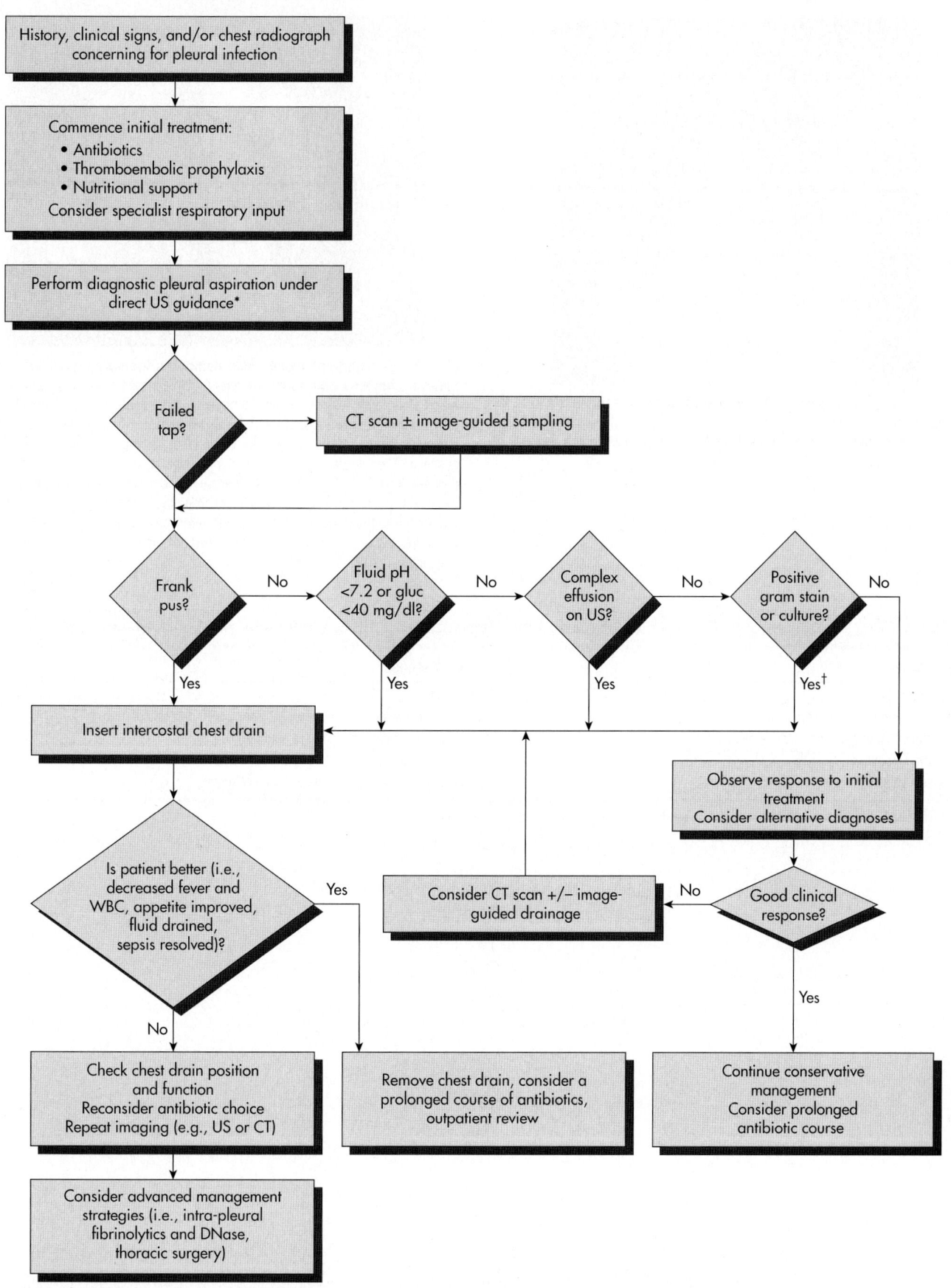

FIG. 156 Algorithm demonstrating the investigation and management of suspected pleural infection. *Ideally this should be performed before administration of antibiotics; however, treatment should not be delayed if aspiration cannot be performed immediately. †A positive pleural culture or Gram stain result usually means that a chest drain is required; however, the patient's clinical course should be considered when making this decision. *CT*, Computed tomography; *US*, ultrasound; *WBC*, white blood cells. (From Broaddus VC et al: *Murray & Nadel's textbook of respiratory medicine,* ed 7, Philadelphia, 2022, Elsevier.)

Clinical
Algorithms

III

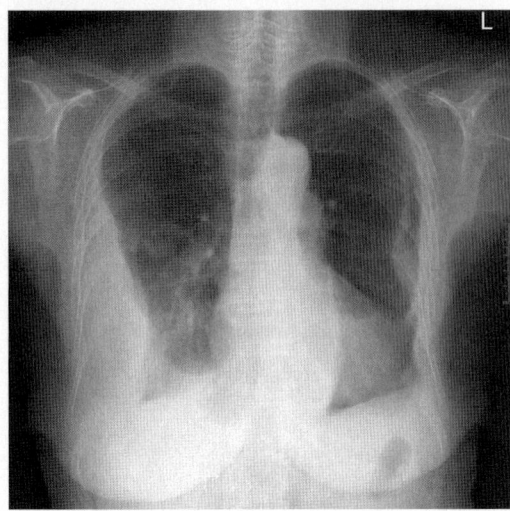

FIG. 157 Pleural empyema seen on a frontal chest radiograph. The D-shaped opacity, suggesting an extraparenchymal process, is commonly seen in cases of pleural infection. (From Broaddus VC et al: *Murray & Nadel's textbook of respiratory medicine,* ed 7, Philadelphia, 2022, Elsevier.)

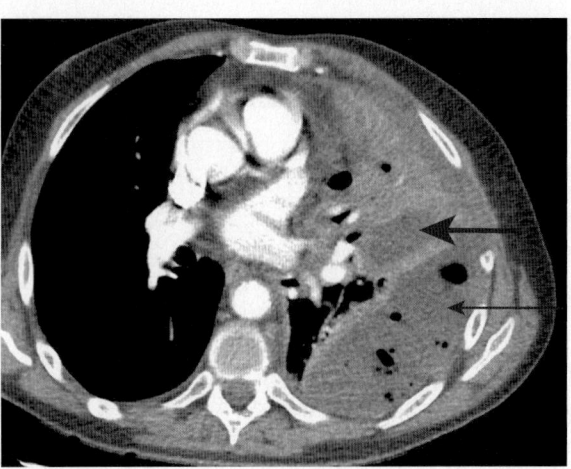

FIG. 158 Contrast-enhanced chest computed tomography showing both pleural empyema and a lung abscess. With contrast-enhanced computed tomography, pleural lesions can be discriminated from parenchymal lesions. The *thin arrow* shows empyema, and the *thick arrow* indicates a lung abscess. Note the lenticular shape of the empyema in contrast to the rounded shape of the abscess. The pleural collection does not have a visible "wall," whereas the abscess wall is thick and irregular. Within the empyema are multiple separate locules of gas, suggesting that the pleural collection is septated. Also see Table 111 for features that differentiate between empyema and lung abscess. (From Broaddus VC et al: *Murray & Nadel's textbook of respiratory medicine,* ed 7, Philadelphia, 2022, Elsevier.)

TABLE 111 Key Differences Between the Radiographic Appearance of Pleural Infection and Lung Abscesses

Empyema	Lung Abscess
Lenticular shape	Rounded
Surrounding lung often compressed	Boundary between lung and fluid indistinct, with necrosis of lung
Margins of collection creating obtuse angles with chest wall	Contact with chest wall made at acute angle
Thick smooth wall	Thick irregular wall
No vessels close by	Vessels seen passing through or near collection

From Broaddus VC et al: *Murray & Nadel's textbook of respiratory medicine,* ed 7, Philadelphia, 2022, Elsevier.

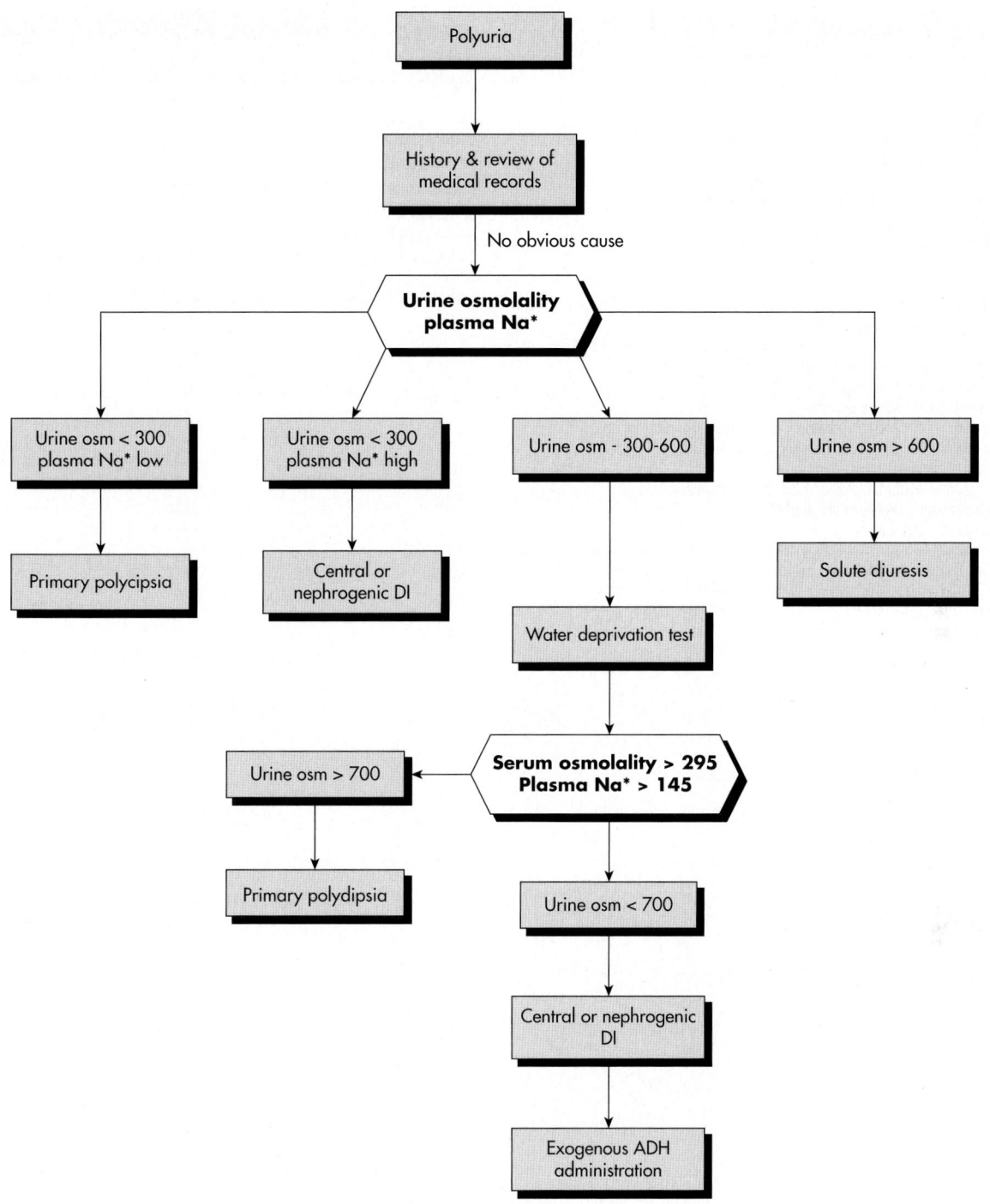

FIG. 161 Approach to polyuria. *ADH,* Antidiuretic hormone; *DI,* diabetes insipidus; osm, osmolality. (From Vincent JL et al: *Textbook of critical care*, ed 8, Philadelphia, 2024, Elsevier.)

TABLE 112 Cause of Polyuria

1. Polyuria secondary to water diuresis
   a. Excessive intake of water
      i. Psychogenic polydipsia
      ii. Drugs—anticholinergic drugs, thioridazin
      iii. Hypothalamic diseases—trauma, sarcoidosis
   b. Defective water reabsorption by the kidney
      i. Central diabetes insipidus (vasopressin deficiency)
      ii. Renal tubular resistance to AVP
2. Congenital nephrogenic diabetes insipidus
3. Acquired nephrogenic diabetes insipidus
   a. Hypercalcemia
   b. Hypokalemia
   c. Drugs—lithium, demeclocycline
   d. Chronic renal diseases—postobstructive diuresis, polyuric phase of ATN
   e. Other systemic diseases—amyloidosis, sickle cell anemia
4. Polyuria secondary to solute diuresis
   a. Electrolyte-induced solute diuresis
      i. Iatrogenic—excessive sodium chloride load, loop diuretic use
      ii. Salt-wasting nephropathy (rarely causes polyuria)
   b. Nonelectrolyte solute–induced diuresis
      i. Glucosuria—diabetic ketoacidosis, hyperosmolar coma
      ii. Urea diuresis—high-protein diet, ATN
      iii. Iatrogenic—mannito

ATN, Acute tubular necrosis; *AVP,* arginine vasopressin.
From Vincent JL et al: *Textbook of critical care,* ed 8, Philadelphia, 2024, Elsevier.

TABLE 113 Differentiation of Cerebral Salt Wasting vs. Central DI

	Cerebral Salt Wasting	**Central DI**
Urine osmolality	High (>300 mOsm)	Low (<300 mOsm)
Serum osmolality	Low	High
Urine sodium	High (>40 mEq/L)	Low (<20 mEq/L)
Serum sodium	Low	High
Intravascular volume	Low	Low

DI, Diabetes insipidus.
From Vincent JL et al: *Textbook of critical care,* ed 8, Philadelphia, 2024, Elsevier.

SOLID & PART-SOLID NODULES

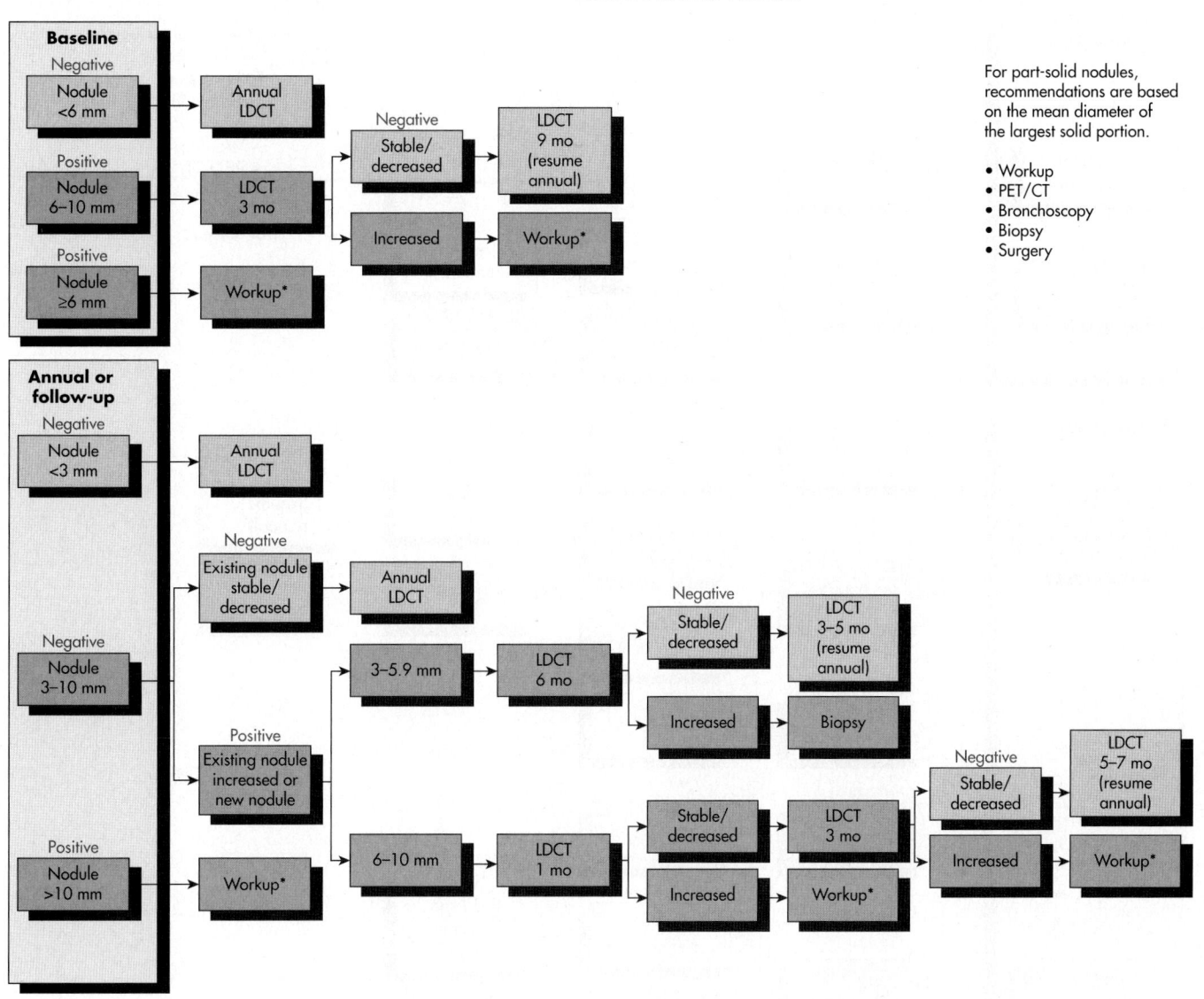

For part-solid nodules, recommendations are based on the mean diameter of the largest solid portion.

- Workup
- PET/CT
- Bronchoscopy
- Biopsy
- Surgery

A

FIG. 165 The diagnostic algorithm for (A) solid or part-solid nodules and (B) nonsolid nodules. This algorithm was created through discussion by a multidisciplinary group composed of thoracic surgeons, radiologists, pulmonologists, oncologists, and pathologists. *Workup is at the discretion of the treating physicians but typically consists of a PET/CT and tissue diagnosis, either by bronchoscopy, CT-guided biopsy, or for highly suspicious nodules, minimally invasive surgery. *CT,* Computed tomography; *LDCT,* low-dose computed tomography; *PET,* positron emission tomography. (From Sellke FW: *Sabiston & Spencer surgery of the chest,* ed 9, Philadelphia, 2016, Elsevier.) The Fleischner Society recommendations for computed tomography follow-up of pulmonary nodules are summarized in Tables 114-116.

NONSOLID NODULES

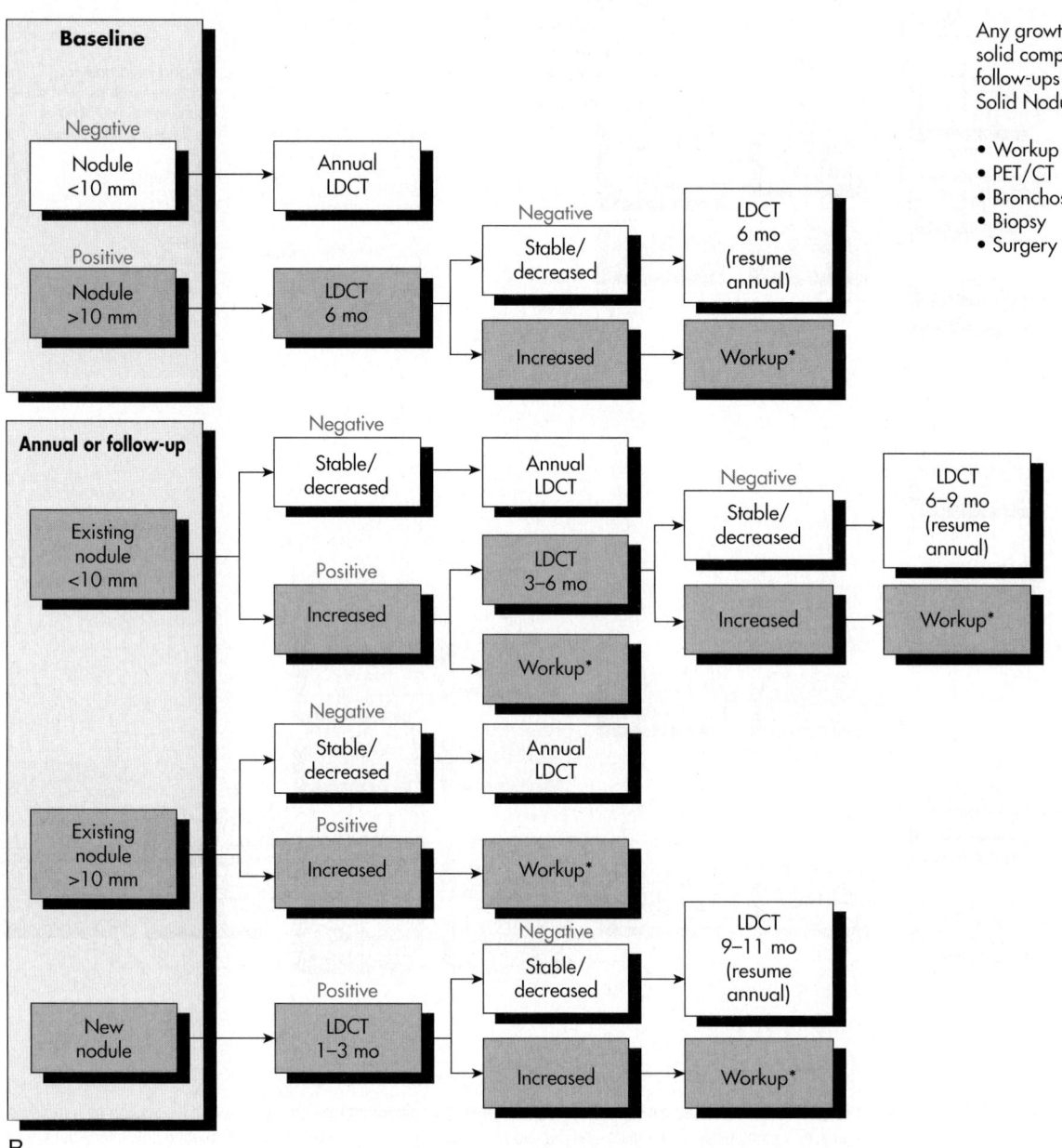

Any growth or development of solid components prompts follow-ups as per Solid & Part-Solid Nodule algorithm.

• Workup
• PET/CT
• Bronchoscopy
• Biopsy
• Surgery

B

FIG. 165, cont'd

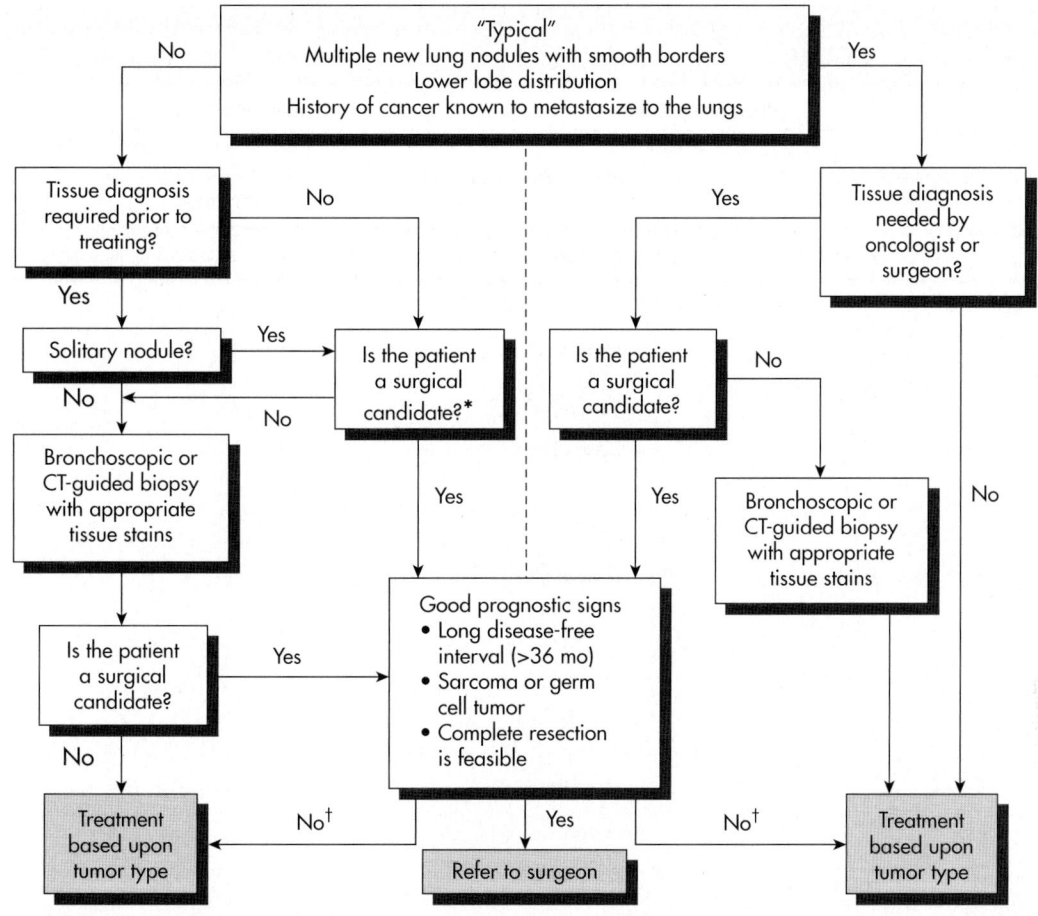

FIG. 166 Suggested management algorithm for patients with known prior cancer and new lung nodule or nodules. Decisions take into account the typical or atypical appearance of a lung nodule in a patient with prior known cancer, the utility of a tissue diagnosis to the treating physicians, the physiologic fitness of the patient for surgery, and the known prognostic indicators for a favorable outcome after metastectomy. Each patient should be managed individually, within the context of the skills and experience of local providers with the varied diagnostic and therapeutic options. *Patients at high risk for primary lung cancer may be considered for diagnostic lobectomy, when appropriate. †These are suggested criteria for surgical resection of lung metastases, and multidisciplinary teams should make this decision. Radiofrequency ablation or stereotactic ablative body radiotherapy may also be an excellent choice for these patients. *CT,* Computed tomography. (From Broaddus VC et al: *Murray & Nadel's textbook of respiratory medicine,* ed 7, Philadelphia, 2022, Elsevier.)

TABLE 114 Fleischner Society Recommendations for Computed Tomography (CT) Follow-Up (FU) of Solid Nodules*

Nodule Size	Low-Risk Patient	High-Risk Patient
≤4 mm	No FU CT needed (FU is optional)	FU CT at 12 mo; if unchanged, no further FU
>4-6 mm	FU CT at 12 mo; if unchanged, no further FU	FU CT at 6-12 mo, then at 18-24 mo if no change
>6-8 mm	FU CT at 6-12 mo, then at 18-24 mo if no change	FU CT at 3-6 mo, then at 9-12 and 24 mo if no change
>8 mm	Options: FU CT at 3, 9, and 24 mo; positron emission tomography; biopsy; video-assisted thoracic surgery	

*Nodule size is average of length and width. Low-risk patient, minimal or absent history of smoking or other known risk factors; high-risk patient, history of smoking or other known risk factors.
From Webb WR et al: *Fundamentals of body CT,* ed 4, Philadelphia, 2015, Saunders.

TABLE 115 Fleischner Society Recommendations for Computed Tomography (CT) Follow-Up (FU) of Solitary Ground-Glass Opacity (GGO) or Part-GGO Nodules

Nodule Type	Recommendation	Additional Remarks
Solitary pure GGO ≤5 mm	No FU CT required	Use 1-mm slices to confirm nodule is pure GGO
Solitary pure GGO >5 mm	FU CT at 3 mo; if persistent, yearly FU for at least 3 yr	Positron emission tomography of limited value and not recommended
Solitary part-solid nodules	FU CT at 3 mo; if persistent and solid component <5 mm, yearly FU for at least 3 yr; if persistent and solid component ≥5 mm, then biopsy or resection	Consider positron emission tomography if nodule >1 cm

From Webb WR et al: *Fundamentals of body CT,* ed 4, Philadelphia, 2015, Saunders.

TABLE 116 Fleischner Society Recommendations for Computed Tomography (CT) Follow-Up (FU) of Multiple Ground-Glass Opacity (GGO) or Part-GGO Nodules

Nodule Type	Recommendation	Additional Remarks
Multiple pure GGO ≤5 mm	FU CT at 2 and 4 yr	Consider alternate cause for GGO nodules
Multiple pure GGO >5 mm; no dominant lesion	FU CT at 3 mo; if persistent, yearly FU for at least 3 yr	Positron emission tomography of limited value and not recommended
Dominant part-solid nodule(s)	FU CT at 3 mo; if persistent, then biopsy or resection, particularly if solid component ≥ 5 mm	Consider lung-sparing surgery in patients with a dominant lesion suspicious for lung cancer

From Webb WR et al: *Fundamentals of body CT,* ed 4, Philadelphia, 2015, Saunders.

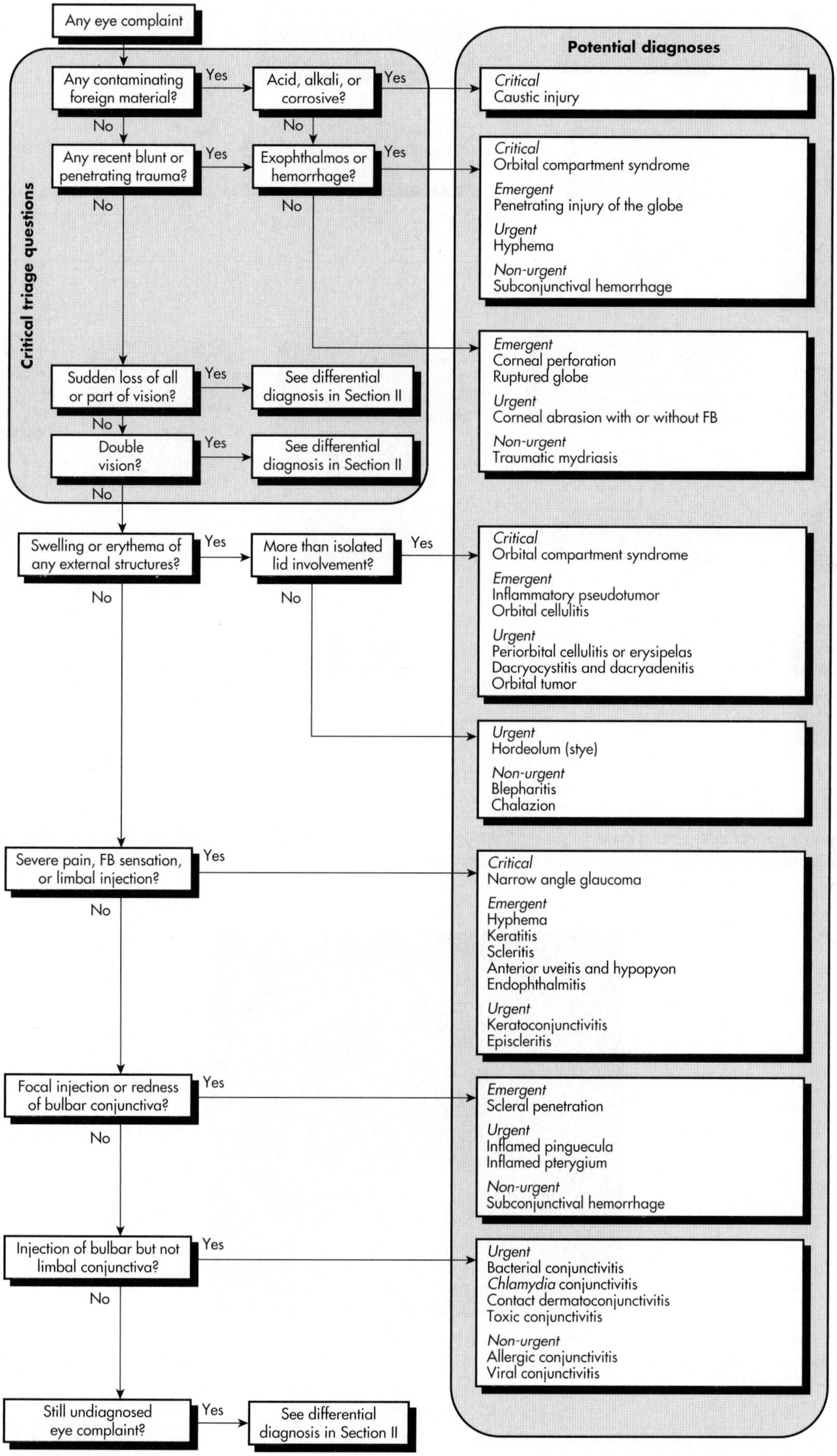

Critical triage questions

Any eye complaint

Any contaminating foreign material? — Yes → Acid, alkali, or corrosive? — Yes →
No ↓   No ↓

Any recent blunt or penetrating trauma? — Yes → Exophthalmos or hemorrhage? — Yes →
No ↓   No ↓

Sudden loss of all or part of vision? — Yes → See differential diagnosis in Section II
No ↓

Double vision? — Yes → See differential diagnosis in Section II
No ↓

Swelling or erythema of any external structures? — Yes → More than isolated lid involvement? — Yes →
No ↓   No ↓

Severe pain, FB sensation, or limbal injection? — Yes →
No ↓

Focal injection or redness of bulbar conjunctiva? — Yes →
No ↓

Injection of bulbar but not limbal conjunctiva? — Yes →
No ↓

Still undiagnosed eye complaint? — Yes → See differential diagnosis in Section II

Potential diagnoses

Critical
Caustic injury

Critical
Orbital compartment syndrome
Emergent
Penetrating injury of the globe
Urgent
Hyphema
Non-urgent
Subconjunctival hemorrhage

Emergent
Corneal perforation
Ruptured globe
Urgent
Corneal abrasion with or without FB
Non-urgent
Traumatic mydriasis

Critical
Orbital compartment syndrome
Emergent
Inflammatory pseudotumor
Orbital cellulitis
Urgent
Periorbital cellulitis or erysipelas
Dacryocystitis and dacryadenitis
Orbital tumor

Urgent
Hordeolum (stye)
Non-urgent
Blepharitis
Chalazion

Critical
Narrow angle glaucoma
Emergent
Hyphema
Keratitis
Scleritis
Anterior uveitis and hypopyon
Endophthalmitis
Urgent
Keratoconjunctivitis
Episcleritis

Emergent
Scleral penetration
Urgent
Inflamed pinguecula
Inflamed pterygium
Non-urgent
Subconjunctival hemorrhage

Urgent
Bacterial conjunctivitis
Chlamydia conjunctivitis
Contact dermatoconjunctivitis
Toxic conjunctivitis
Non-urgent
Allergic conjunctivitis
Viral conjunctivitis

Clinical
Algorithms

FIG. 170 Diagnostic algorithm for red and painful eyes. *FB,* Foreign body. (From Walls RM et al: *Rosen's emergency medicine, concepts and clinical practice,* ed 10, Philadelphia, 2023, Elsevier.)

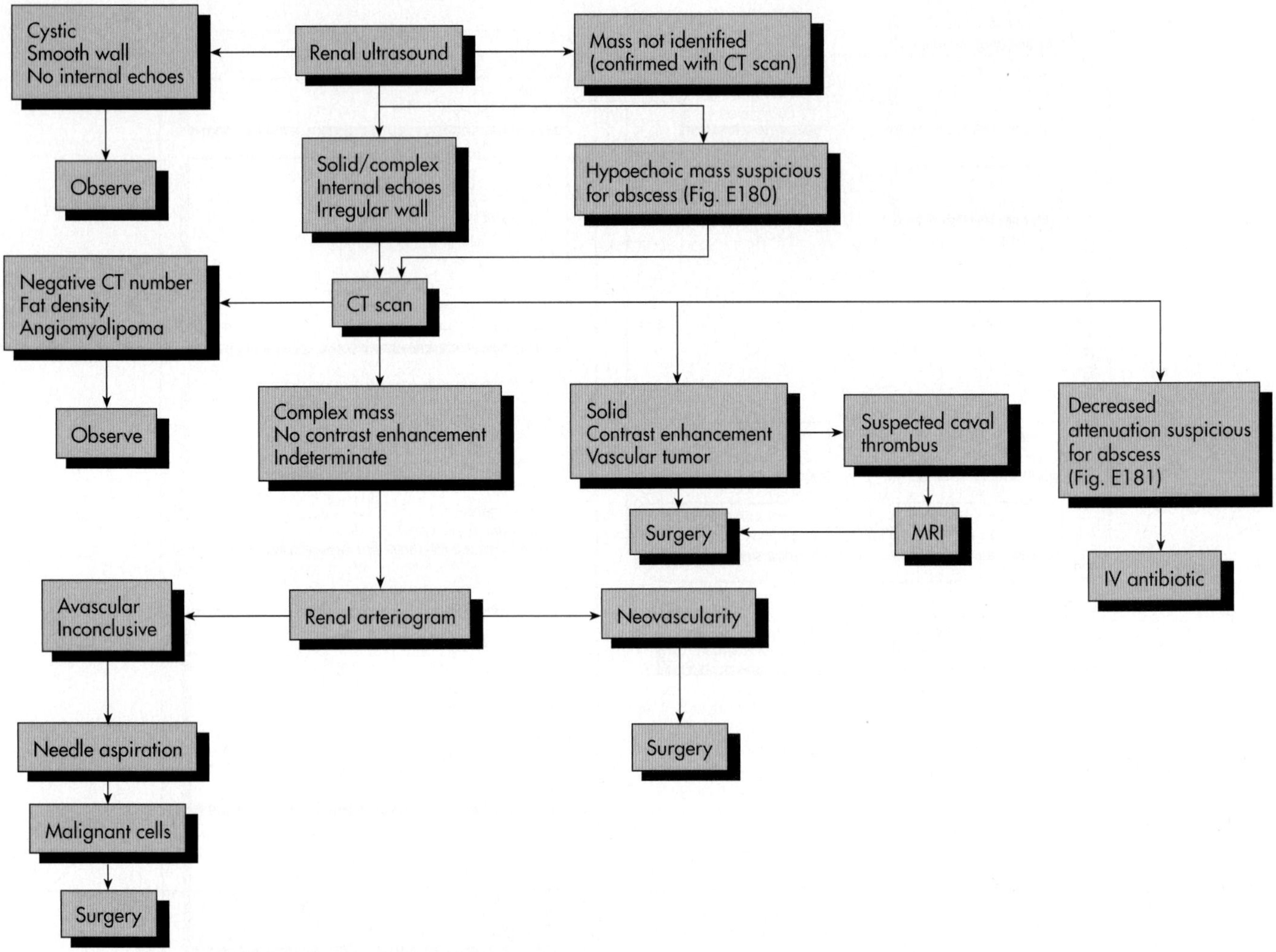

Cystic
Smooth wall
No internal echoes → Renal ultrasound → Mass not identified (confirmed with CT scan)

Observe

Solid/complex
Internal echoes
Irregular wall

Hypoechoic mass suspicious for abscess (Fig. E180)

Negative CT number
Fat density
Angiomyolipoma ← CT scan

Observe

Complex mass
No contrast enhancement
Indeterminate

Solid
Contrast enhancement
Vascular tumor → Suspected caval thrombus

Decreased attenuation suspicious for abscess (Fig. E181)

Surgery ← MRI

IV antibiotic

Avascular
Inconclusive ← Renal arteriogram → Neovascularity

Needle aspiration

Surgery

Malignant cells

Surgery

FIG. 177 Evaluation of a patient with a renal mass on renal ultrasound. *CT,* Computed tomography; *MRI,* magnetic resonance imaging. (Modified from Williams RD: Tumors of the kidney, ureter, and bladder. In Goldman L, Schafer AL [eds]: *Cecil textbook of medicine,* ed 23, Philadelphia, 2008, Saunders.)

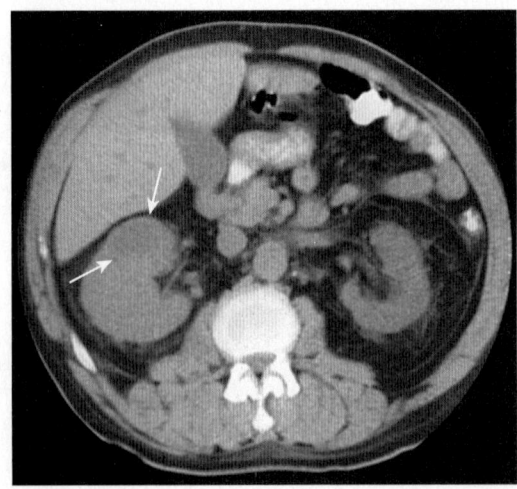

FIG. 179 Acute renal abscess. Nonenhanced computed tomography scan through the mid-pole of the right kidney demonstrates right renal enlargement and an area of decreased attenuation *(arrows).* After antimicrobial therapy, a follow-up scan showed complete regression of these findings. (From Wein AJ et al: *Campbell-Walsh urology,* ed 11, Philadelphia, 2016, Elsevier.)

ICD-10CM # N44.2 Benign cyst of testis
N44.8 Other noninflammatory disorders of the testis
N50.3 Cyst of epididymis
N50.8 Other specified disorders of male genital organs

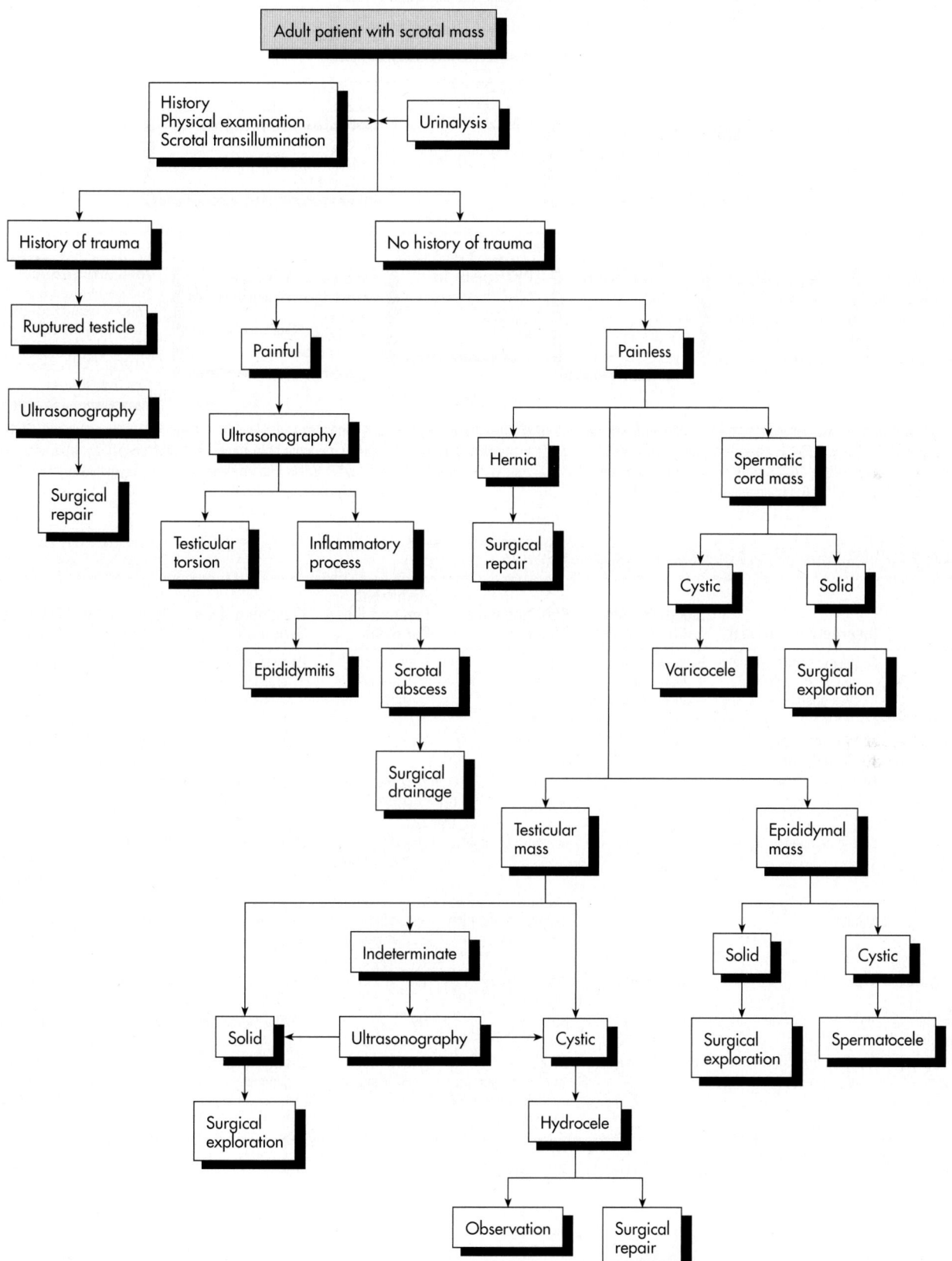

FIG. 182 Evaluation of scrotal mass. (Modified from Greene HL et al [eds]: *Decision making in medicine,* ed 2, St Louis, 1998, Mosby.)

Clinical
Algorithms

III

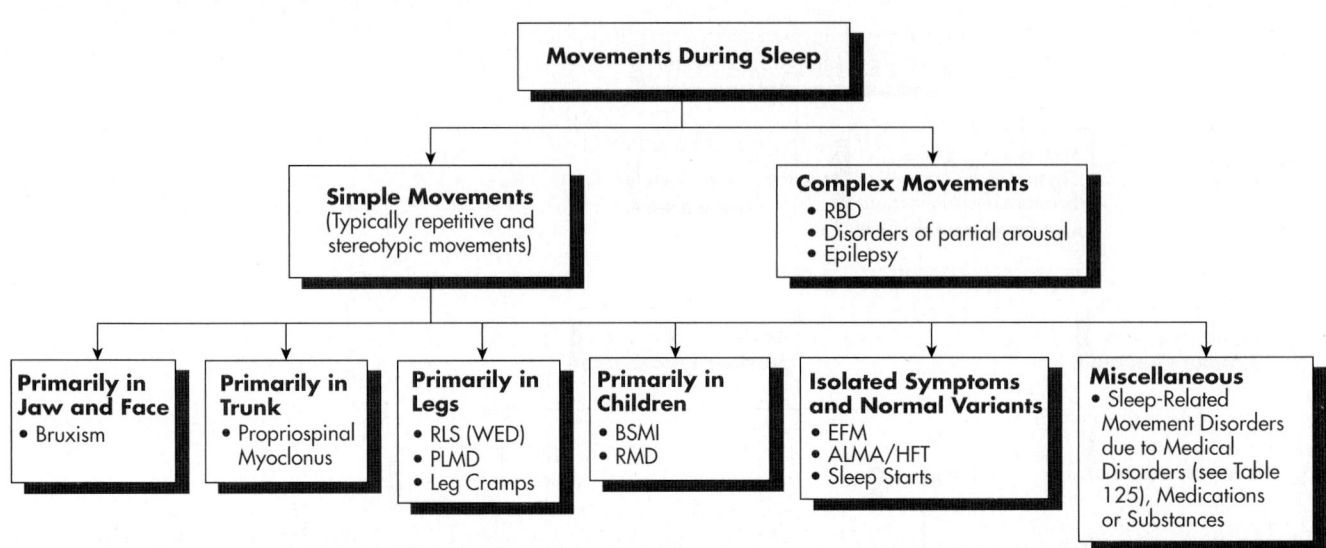

FIG. 194 Flow chart for the approach to the differential diagnosis of sleep-related movement disorders. *ALMA,* Alternating leg muscle activation; *BSMI,* benign sleep myoclonus of infancy; *EFM,* excessive fragmentary myoclonus; *HFT,* hypnagogic foot tremor; *PLMD,* periodic limb movement disorder; *RBD,* rapid eye movement *(REM)* sleep behavior disorder; *RLS (WED),* restless legs syndrome; *RMD,* rhythmic movement disorder; *WED,* Willis-Ekbom disease. (From Kryger M et al: *Principles and practice of sleep medicine,* ed 6, Philadelphia, 2017, Elsevier.)

TABLE 125 Distinguishing Features of Nocturnal Events

Feature	Disorders of Arousal	Sleep-Related Eating Disorder	REM Behavior Disorder	Recurrent Isolated Sleep Paralysis	Exploding Head Syndrome	Psychogenic Events	Nocturnal Seizures
Behavior	Confused; semipurposeful movement with eyes open	Eating typically high-calorie foods; eyes open	Sometimes combative with eyes closed	Episodes of inability to move	Painless sensation of explosion inside the head	Variable	Dependent on the portion of brain involved
Age of onset	Childhood and adolescence	Variable	Older adult	Variable	Adult	Adolescence to adulthood	Variable
Time of occurrence	First third of night	First half of night	During REM	Typically on awakening	Usually near sleep onset but can be variable	Anytime	Anytime
Frequency of events	Less than one per night	Variable	Multiple per night	Variable less than weekly	Rare	Variable	Frontal seizures—multiple per night
Duration	Minutes	Minutes	Seconds to minutes	Seconds to minutes	Seconds	Variable minutes or longer	Usually under 3 min
Memory of event	Usually none	Usually none or limited	Dream recall	Yes	Yes	None	Usually none
Stereotypical movements	No	No	No	No	Similar sensation	No	Yes
Polysomnogram findings	Arousals from slow wave sleep	Arousal from NREM sleep	Excessive electromyogram tone during REM sleep	Arousal from REM sleep	Usually occurs in light sleep	Occur from awake state	Potentially epileptiform activity

NREM, Nonrapid eye movement; *REM,* rapid eye movement.
From Kryger M et al: *Principles and practice of sleep medicine,* ed 6, Philadelphia, 2017, Elsevier.

DIAGNOSTIC ALGORITHM

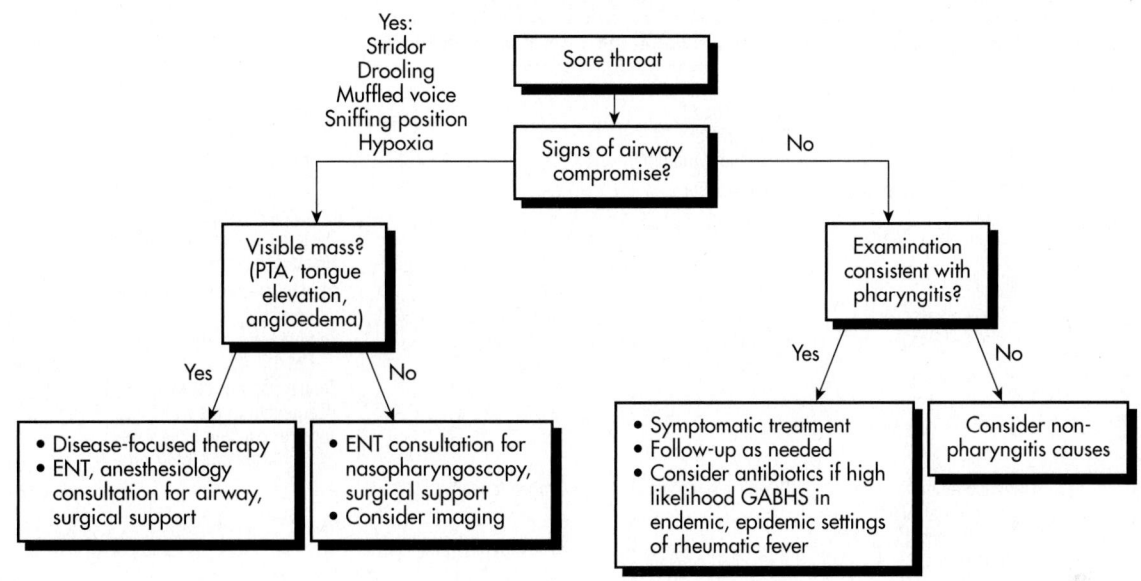

A

MANAGEMENT ALGORITHM

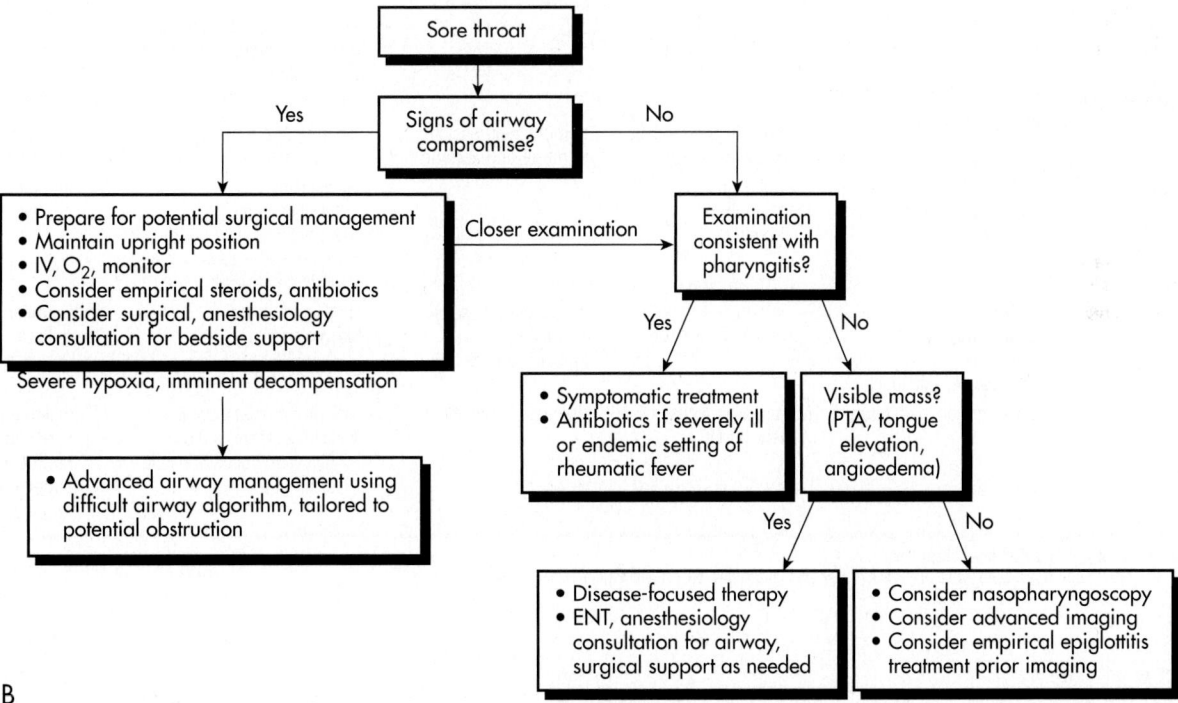

B

FIG. 195 Approach to the patient with sore throat, diagnostic and management algorithms. *ENT,* Ear-nose-throat; *GABHS,* group A beta-hemolytic streptococci; *IV,* intravenous; *PTA,* peritonsillar abscess. (From Walls RM et al: *Rosen's emergency medicine, concepts and clinical practice,* ed 10, Philadelphia, 2023, Elsevier.)

TABLE 126 Differential Diagnosis of Sore Throat

Type of Pharyngitis	Nature of Patient	Nature of Symptoms	Predisposing Factors	Physical Findings	Diagnostic Studies
Without Pharyngeal Ulcers					
Viral	All ages	Pain in throat Rapid onset Systemic symptoms	—	Exudate less likely than with streptococcal infections	—
Infectious mononucleosis	Adolescents and young adults Uncommon in elderly	Gradual onset	—	Low-grade temperature Occasional exudate Posterior cervical adenopathy Hepatosplenomegaly	Monospot test
Streptococcal pharyngitis	Patients younger than 25 yr, especially age 6-12 yr	Pain in throat Rapid onset Few systemic symptoms	Fall and winter Streptococcal infection in family Diabetes	Marked erythema and throat swelling Temperature >101° F (38.33° C) Tender anterior cervical nodes Scarlatiniform rash Tonsillar exudate more likely than with viral infection	Culture Rapid streptococcal antigen screening Increased antistreptol-ysin O titer
Gonococcal pharyngitis	Most common in male homosexuals and people with anogenital gonorrhea	Often no symptoms	Orogenital sex	—	Culture
Sinusitis with postnasal drip	Adults	Mild throat soreness Symptoms often worse with recumbency	—	Evidence of sinusitis Postnasal drip	CT/flexible rhinoscopy (in recalcitrant cases)
Allergic pharyngitis	—	—	Seasonal allergies	No fever Intermittent postnasal drip Swollen pharynx with minimal injection	Allergy testing
With Pharyngeal Ulcers					
Herpangina	More common in children	Painful ulcers on tonsils, pillars, or uvula	Immunosuppression Summer and autumn	Vesicles 1-2-mm ulcers	Serologic tests
Fusospirochetal infection (Vincent angina)	Children and people with poor oral hygiene	Painful ulcers Bleeding gums Foul breath	—	No vesicles Ulcerative gingivitis Gray, necrotic ulcers 2-30-mm ulcers Pseudomembrane	Gram stain: Spiro-chetes
Candidiasis	Children Immunosuppressed patients Those taking antibiotics	—	Immunosuppression Antibiotics Inhaled steroids	3-11-mm ulcers No vesicles	KOH smear: *Candida* culture
Herpes simplex	Most common in children	Not usually a cause of sore throat	Immunosuppression	1-2-mm painful ulcers Vesicles present on lips, gingivae, buccal mucosa, or tongue	Tzanck smear (not very sensitive) viral culture, PCR, herpes simplex virus antibody assay

CT, Computed tomography; *PCR,* polymerase chain reaction.
Modified from Seller RH, Symons AB: *Differential diagnosis of common complaints,* ed 7, Philadelphia, 2018, Elsevier.

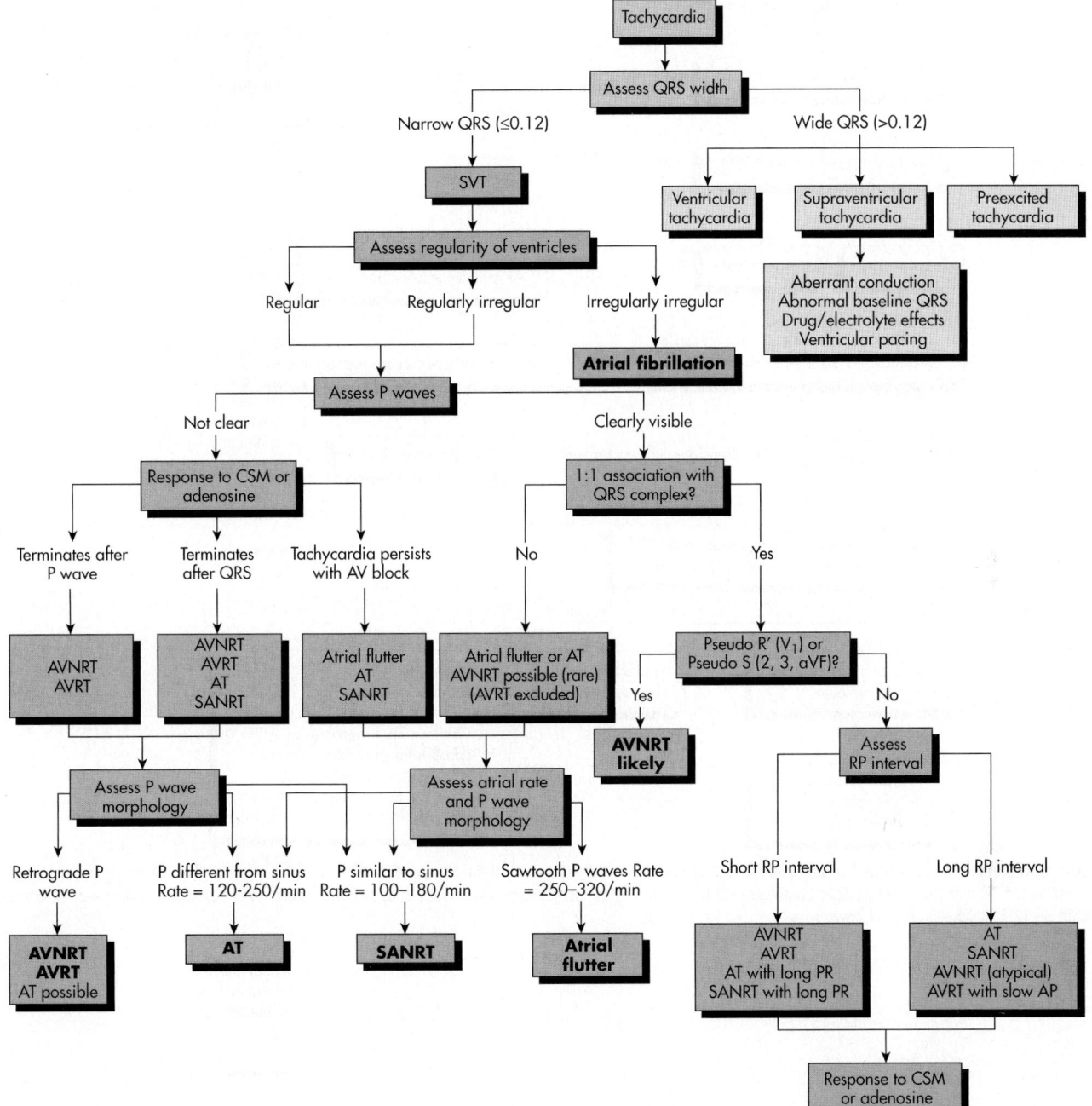

FIG. 201 Stepwise approach to diagnosis of the type of tachycardia based on a 12-lead electrocardiogram during the episode. The initial step is to determine whether the tachycardia has a wide or narrow QRS complex. For wide-complex tachycardia, see Table 129; the remainder of the algorithm is helpful in diagnosis of the type of narrow-complex tachycardia. *AP,* Accessory pathway; *AT,* atrial tachycardia; *AVNRT,* atrioventricular nodal reentrant tachycardia; *AVRT,* atrioventricular reciprocating tachycardia; *CSM,* carotid sinus massage; *SANRT,* sinoatrial nodal reentry tachycardia. (From Libby P et al: *Braunwald's heart disease, a textbook of cardiovascular medicine,* ed 12, Philadelphia, 2022, Elsevier.)

Clinical Algorithms

III

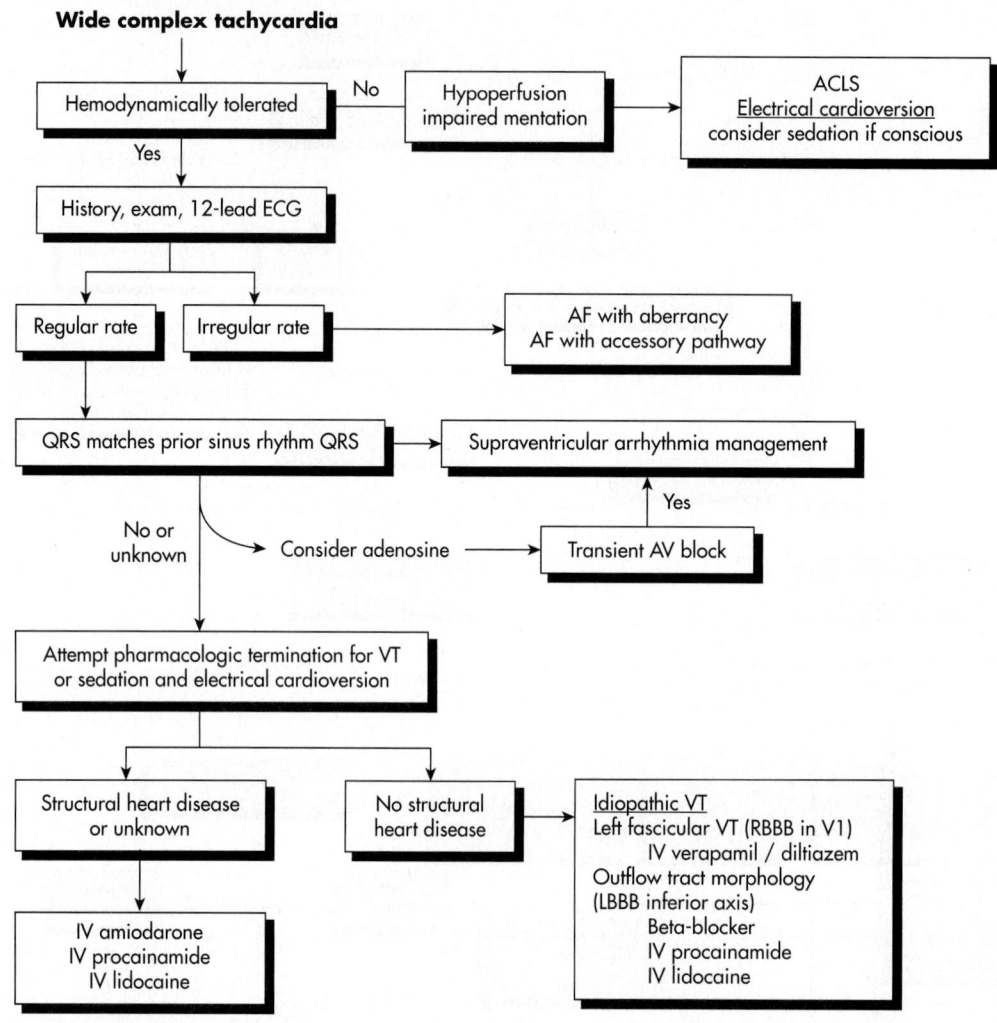

FIG. 202 Management of the patient with a wide QRS tachycardia. *ACLS,* Advanced cardiac life support; *AF,* atrial fibrillation; *ECG,* electrocardiogram; *IV,* intravenous; *LBBB,* left bundle branch block; *RBBB,* right bundle branch block; *VT,* ventral tachycardia. (From Libby P et al: *Braunwald's heart disease, a textbook of cardiovascular medicine,* ed 12, Philadelphia, 2022, Elsevier.)

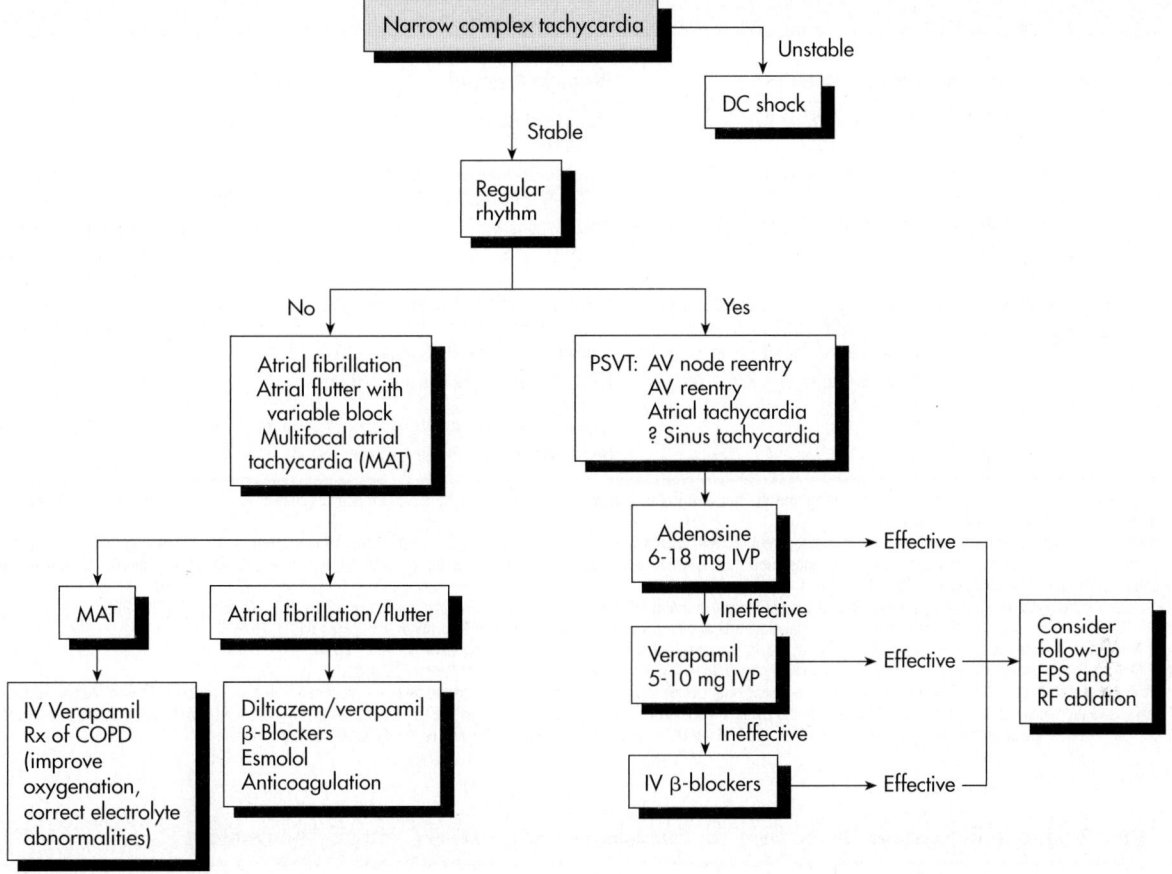

FIG. 203 Evaluation and management of narrow complex tachycardia. *AV,* Atrioventricular; *COPD,* chronic obstructive pulmonary disease; *DC,* direct current; *EPS,* electrophysiologic studies; *IV,* intravenous; *IVP,* intravenous push; *PSVT,* paroxysmal supraventricular tachycardia; *RF,* radiofrequency; *Rx,* treatment.

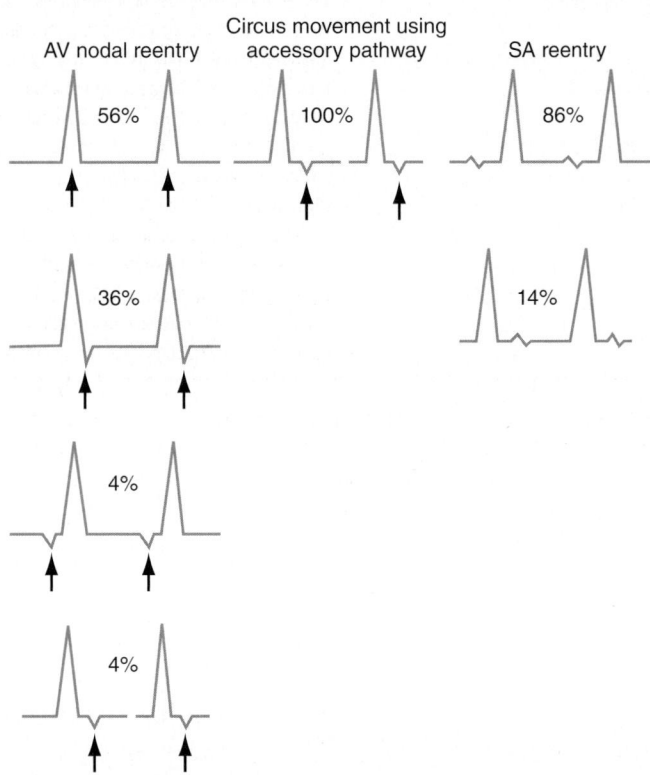

FIG. 204 Location of P waves in common causes of regular narrow-complex tachycardia. *AV,* Atrioventricular; *SA,* sinoatrial. (From Marriott HJL, Conover MB: *Advanced concepts in dysrhythmias,* ed 2, St Louis, 1989, Mosby. In Marx JA et al: *Rosen's emergency medicine,* ed 8, Philadelphia, 2014, Saunders.)

TABLE 128 Stepwise Criteria Favoring Ventricular Tachycardia Patients with Wide-Complex Tachycardias Using Different Algorithms

ACC/AHA/ESC Algorithm*	Kindwall Criteria[†]	Wellens Criteria[‡]	Brugada Criteria[§]	Miller criteria[§]
See FIG. 206	R >30 ms in V_1 or $V_2 \rightarrow$ VT	AV dissociation $\rightarrow$ VT	Absence of RS complex in all precordial leads $\rightarrow$ VT	Initial R wave in aVR $\rightarrow$ VT
	Any Q in $V_6 \rightarrow$ VT	QRS width >140 ms $\rightarrow$ VT	Longest R/S interval >100 ms in any precordial lead $\rightarrow$ VT	aVR with initial r or q >40 sec in duration $\rightarrow$ VT
	>60 ms to S wave nadir in V_1 or $V_2 \rightarrow$ VT	Left axis deviation >$-30° \rightarrow$ VT	AV dissociation $\rightarrow$ VT	aVR with a notch on the descending limb of a negative-onset and predominantly negative QRS in aVR $\rightarrow$ VT
	Notched downstroke S wave in V_1 or $V_2 \rightarrow$ VT	If RBBB morphology, monophasic or biphasic QRS in $V_1 \rightarrow$ SVT or R-to-S ratio of <1 in $V_6 \rightarrow$ VT	If RBBB morphology, monophasic R or qR in $V_1 \rightarrow$ VT R taller than R' $\rightarrow$ VT rS in $V_6 \rightarrow$ VT	In aVR, mV of initial 40 msec divided by terminal 40 msec ($v/v_t \le 1$) $\rightarrow$ VT
		If LBBB morphology, S in V_1-$V_2 \rightarrow$ VT	If LBBB morphology, initial R >40 ms in duration $\rightarrow$ VT Slurred or notched S in V_1 or $V_2 \rightarrow$ VT Beginning Q or QS in $V_6 \rightarrow$ VT	

ACC, American College of Cardiology; AHA, American Heart Association; AV, atrioventricular; aVR, augmented vector right; ESC, European Society of Cardiology; LBBB, left bundle branch block; RBBB, right bundle branch block; VT, ventricular tachycardia.

*Blomström-Lundqvist C et al: ACC/AHA/ESC guidelines for the management of patients with supraventricular arrhythmias—executive summary: a report of the American College of Cardiology/American Heart Association Task Force on Practice Guidelines and the European Society of Cardiology Committee for Practice Guidelines (Writing Committee to Develop Guidelines for the Management of Patients with Supraventricular Arrhythmias), Circulation 108:1871, 2003.
[†]Kindwall KE et al: Electrocardiographic criteria for ventricular tachycardia in wide complex left bundle branch block morphology tachycardias, Am J Cardiol 61:1279, 1988.
[‡]Wellens HJ et al: The value of the electrocardiogram in the differential diagnosis of a tachycardia with a widened QRS complex, Am J Med 64:27, 1978.
[§]Brugada P et al: A new approach to the differential diagnosis of a regular tachycardia with a wide QRS complex, Circulation 83:1649, 1991.
[‖]Vereckei A et al: New algorithm using only lead aVR for differential diagnosis of wide QRS complex tachycardia, Heart Rhythm 5:89, 2008.
From Bloomstrom-Lundqvist C et al: ACC/AHA/ESC guidelines for the management of patients with supraventricular arrhythmias—executive summary: a report of the American College of Cardiology/ American Heart Association Task Force on Practice Guidelines and the European Society of Cardiology Committee for Practice Guidelines (Writing Committee to Develop Guidelines for the Management of Patients with Supraventricular Arrhythmias), Circulation 108:1871, 2003; Mann DL et al: Braunwald's heart disease, ed 10, Philadelphia, 2015, Elsevier.

TABLE 129 Electrocardiographic Distinctions for Diagnosis of Wide–QRS Complex Tachycardia

Favor Supraventricular Tachycardia	Favor Ventricular Tachycardia
Initiation with a premature P wave	Initiation with a premature QRS complex
Tachycardia complexes identical to those in resting rhythm	Tachycardia beats identical to PVCs during sinus rhythm
"Long-short" sequence preceding initiation	"Short-long" sequence preceding initiation
Changes in the P-P interval preceding changes in the R-R interval	Changes in the R-R interval preceding changes in the P-P interval
QRS contours consistent with aberrant conduction (V_1, V_6)	QRS contours inconsistent with aberrant conduction (V_1, V_6)
Slowing or termination with vagal maneuvers	AV dissociation or other non-1:1 AV relationship
Onset of the QRS to its peak (positive or negative) <50 msec	Onset of the QRS to its peak (positive or negative) ≥50 msec
	Fusion beats, capture beats
QRS duration ≤0.14 sec	QRS duration >0.14 sec
Normal QRS axis (0−+90 degrees)	Left-axis deviation (especially −90-180 degrees)
	Concordant R-wave progression pattern
	Contralateral bundle branch block pattern from the resting rhythm
	Initial R, q, or r >40 msec or notched Q in aVR
	Absence of an "rS" complex in any precordial lead

AV, Atrioventricular; PVC, premature ventricular complexes.
From Libby P et al: Braunwald's heart disease, a textbook of cardiovascular medicine, ed 12, Philadelphia, 2022, Elsevier.

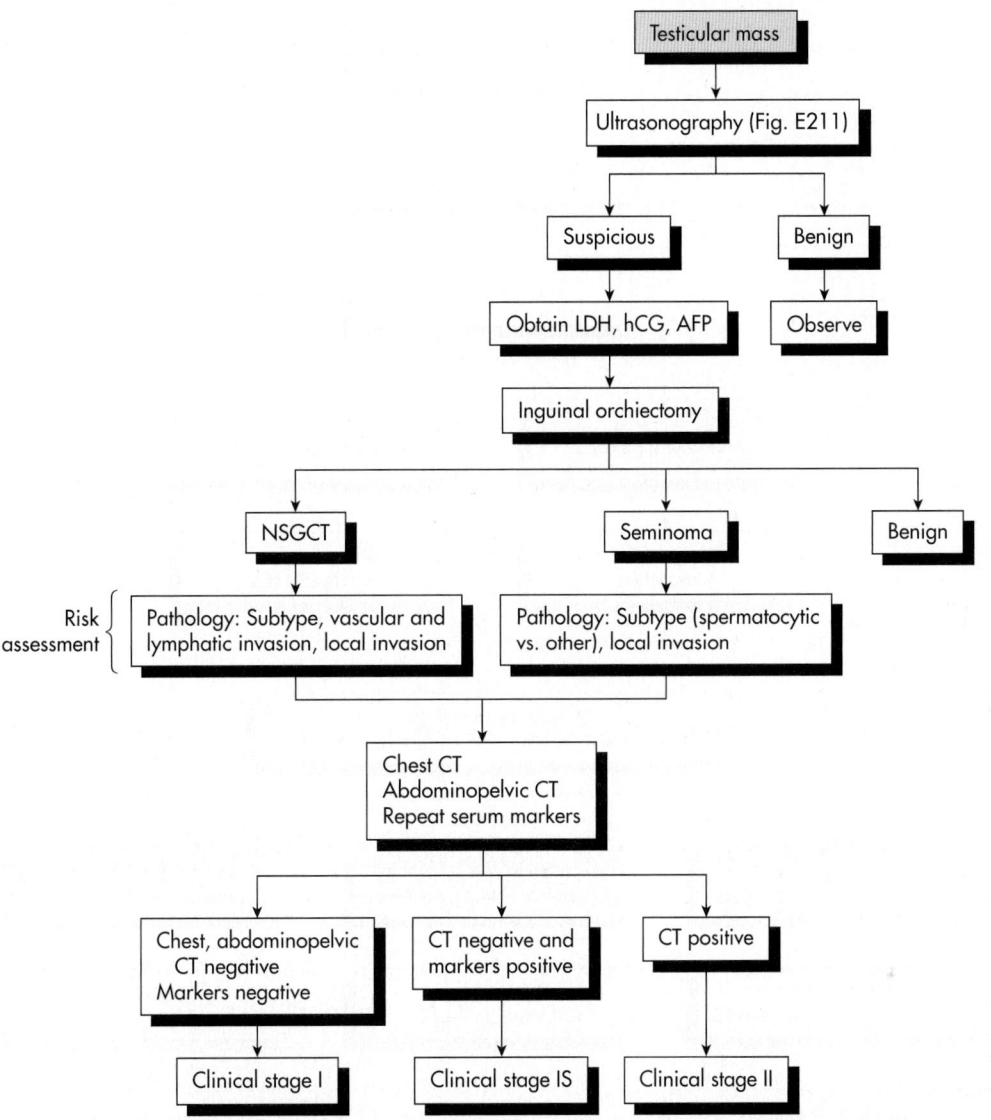

FIG. 206 Diagnosis, staging, and risk assessment of patients with testicular germ cell tumor. See "Section I Topic Testicular Cancer" for additional information. *AFP*, α-Fetoprotein; *CT*, computed tomography; *hCG*, human chorionic gonadotropin; *LDH*, lactic dehydrogenase; *NSGCT*, nonseminoma germ cell tumor. (From Abeloff MD: *Clinical oncology*, ed 4, New York, 2007, Churchill Livingstone.)

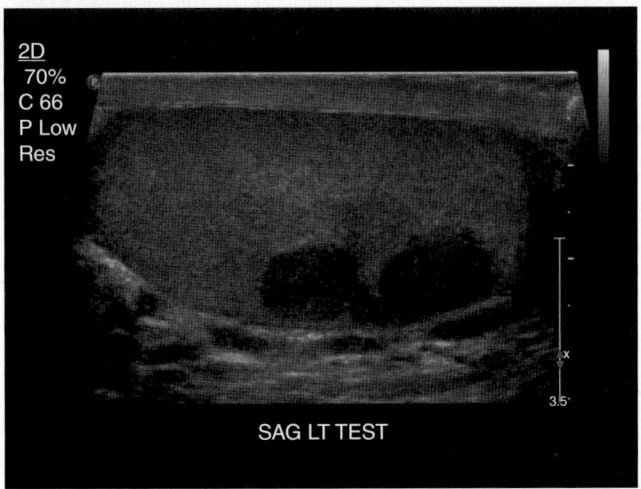

FIG. 207 Sagittal view of ultrasound of left testis showing multinodular hypoechoic intratesticular lesion confirmed to be pure seminoma at orchiectomy. (From Wein AJ et al: *Campbell-Walsh urology*, ed 11, Philadelphia, 2016, Elsevier.)

ICD-10CM # R36   Urethral discharge
R36.9 Urethral discharge, unspecified
R36.0 Urethral discharge without blood

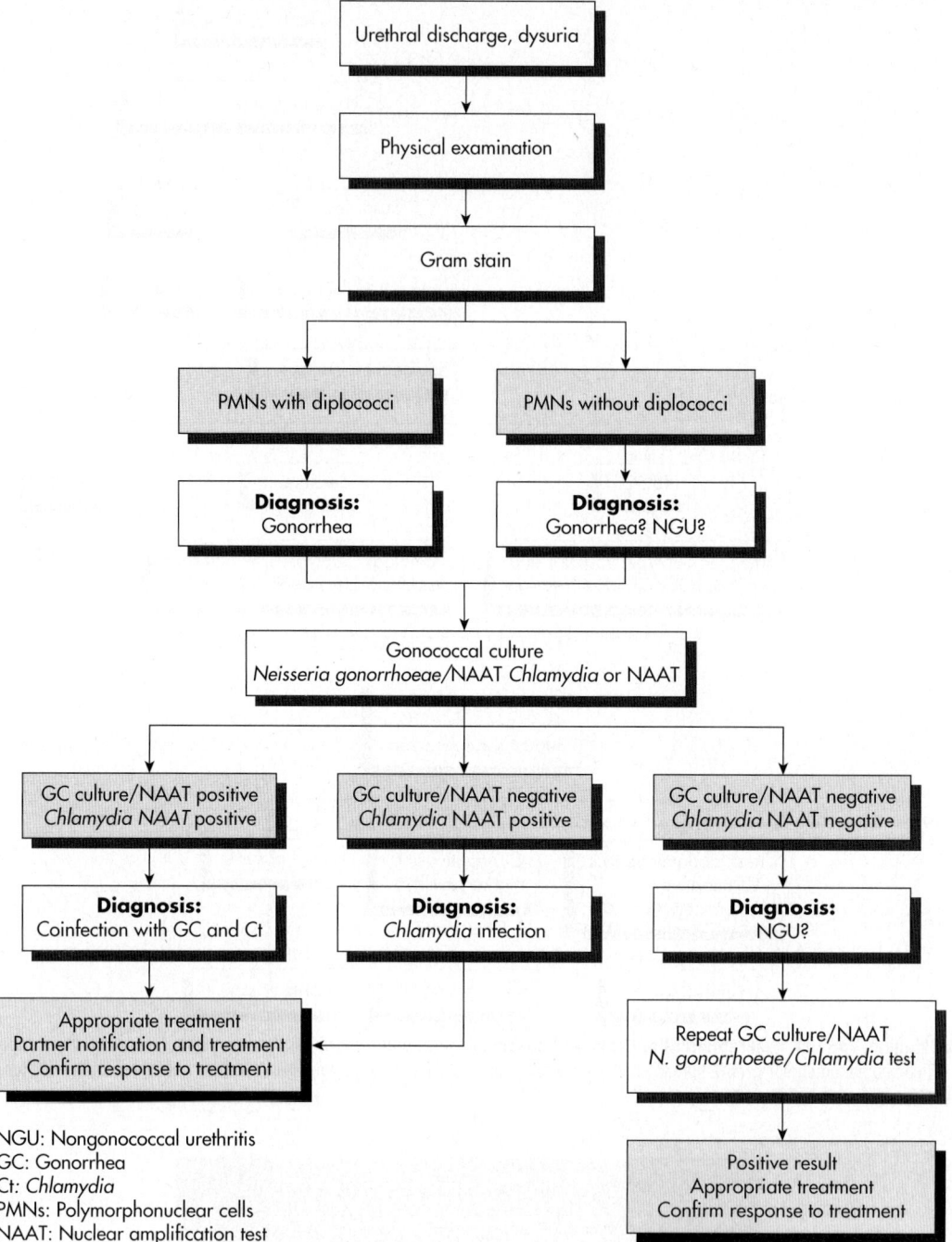

NGU: Nongonococcal urethritis
GC: Gonorrhea
Ct: *Chlamydia*
PMNs: Polymorphonuclear cells
NAAT: Nuclear amplification test

FIG. 211 Diagnostic algorithm for evaluation of urethral discharge or dysuria. (From Bolognia J: *Dermatology,* ed 4, Philadelphia, 2018, Elsevier.)

URINARY SYMPTOMS, LOWER URINARY TRACT

ICD-10CM # R33.9 Retention of urine, unspecified
N21.8 Other lower urinary tract calculus
R32 Unspecified urinary incontinence

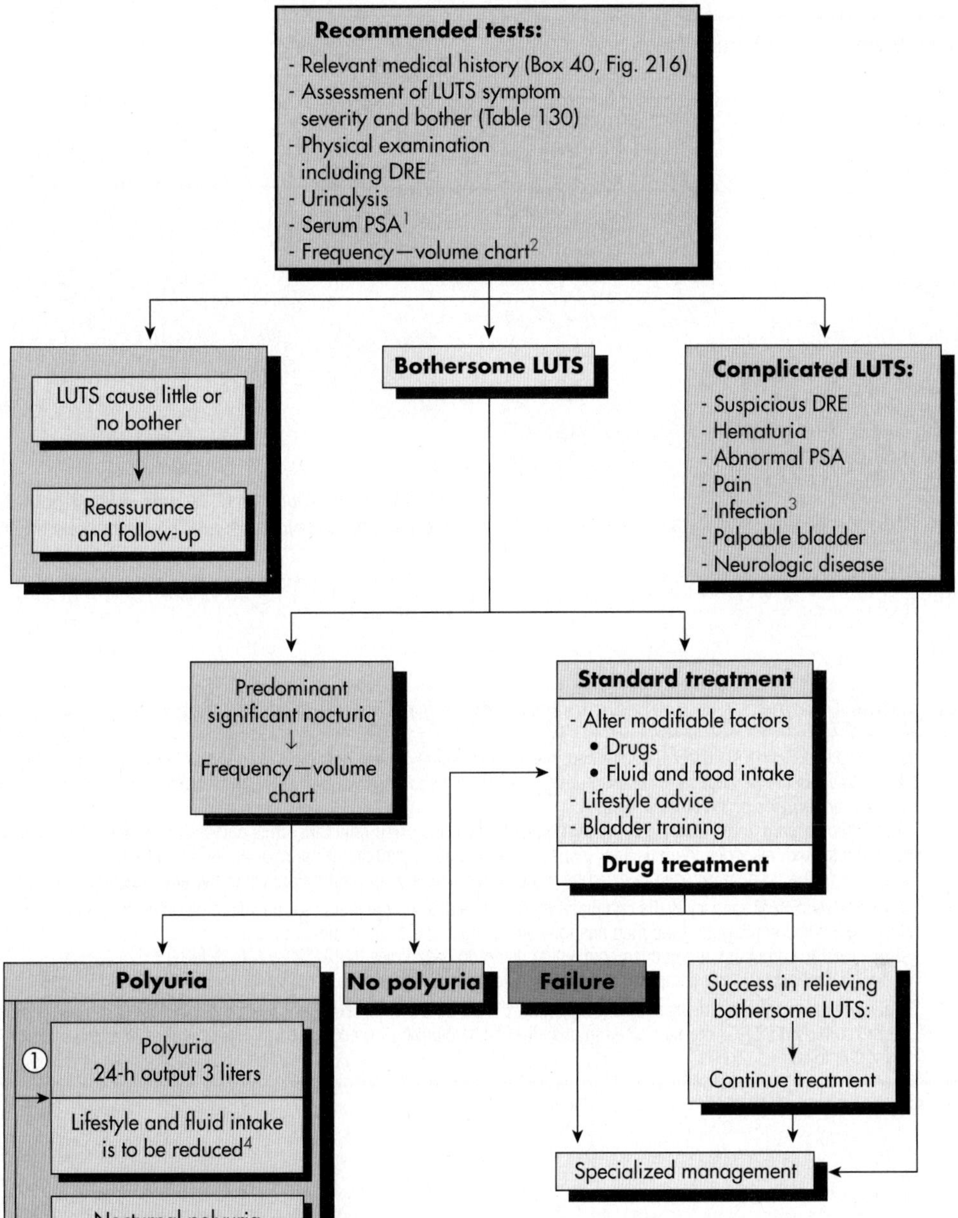

1519

Recommended tests:
- Relevant medical history (Box 40, Fig. 216)
- Assessment of LUTS symptom severity and bother (Table 130)
- Physical examination including DRE
- Urinalysis
- Serum PSA[1]
- Frequency—volume chart[2]

LUTS cause little or no bother

→

Reassurance and follow-up

Bothersome LUTS

Complicated LUTS:
- Suspicious DRE
- Hematuria
- Abnormal PSA
- Pain
- Infection[3]
- Palpable bladder
- Neurologic disease

Predominant significant nocturia
↓
Frequency—volume chart

Standard treatment
- Alter modifiable factors
  - Drugs
  - Fluid and food intake
- Lifestyle advice
- Bladder training

Drug treatment

Polyuria

① Polyuria 24-h output 3 liters

Lifestyle and fluid intake is to be reduced[4]

② Nocturnal polyuria 33% output at night

Fluid intake to be reduced; consider desmopressin

No polyuria

Failure

Success in relieving bothersome LUTS:
↓
Continue treatment

Specialized management

[1]When life expectancy is >10 yr and if the diagnosis of prostate cancer can modify the management
[2]When significant nocturia is a predominant symptom
[3]Assess and start treatment before referral
[4]In practice, advise patients with symptoms to aim for a urine output of about 1 L/24 h

FIG. 212 Basic management of lower urinary tract symptoms *(LUTS)* in men. *DRE,* Digital rectal examination; *PSA,* prostate-specific antigen. (From Fillit HM: *Brocklehurst's textbook of geriatric medicine and gerontology,* ed 8, Philadelphia, 2017, Elsevier.)

Clinical Algorithms

III

1520 **URINARY SYMPTOMS, LOWER URINARY TRACT—cont'd**

ICD-10CM # R33.9 Retention of urine, unspecified
N21.8 Other lower urinary tract calculus
R32 Unspecified urinary incontinence

BOX 40   Causes of Male Lower Urinary Tract Symptoms

Benign prostatic enlargement (secondary to benign prostatic hyperplasia)
Urinary tract infection
Prostatitis
Overactive bladder
Neurogenic bladder dysfunction
Urethral stricture
Bladder neck contracture
Phimosis
Urinary tract stones
Bladder tumor
Advanced prostate cancer
Foreign body in the bladder
Medications, illicit drugs, and dietary factors (including caffeine, alcohol, ketamine, and decongestants)
Diabetes mellitus

From Fillit HM: *Brocklehurst's textbook of geriatric medicine and gerontology,* ed 8, Philadelphia, 2017, Elsevier.

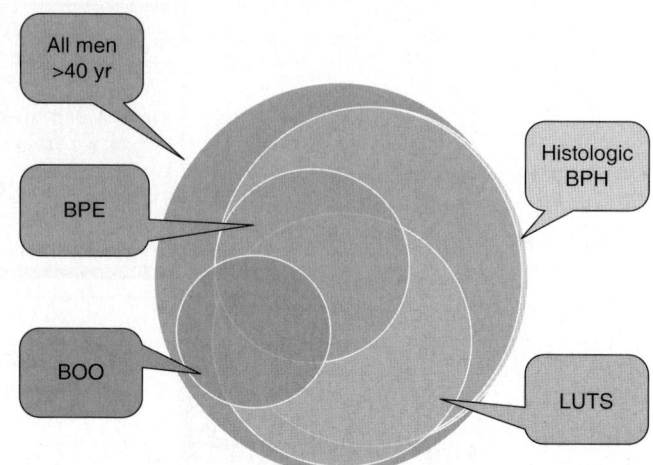

FIG. 213 Occurrence of LUTS with and without BOO, BPE, or BPH. *BOO,* Bladder outflow obstruction; *BPH,* benign prostate hyperplasia; *BPE,* benign prostate enlargement; *LUTS,* lower urinary tract symptoms. (From Fillit HM: *Brocklehurst's textbook of geriatric medicine and gerontology,* ed 8, Philadelphia, 2017, Elsevier.)

TABLE 130   International Continence Society Definitions of Lower Urinary Tract Symptoms

Voiding symptoms	*Hesitancy* is difficulty in initiating micturition, resulting in a delay in the onset of voiding after being ready to pass urine.
	Slow stream is the perception of reduced urine flow, usually compared to previous performance or in comparison to others.
	Splitting or spraying of the urine stream.
	Intermittent stream (intermittency) is the term used to describe urine flow that stops and starts, on one or more occasions, during micturition.
	Straining to void describes the muscular effort used to initiate, maintain, or improve the urinary stream.
	Terminal dribble is the term used to describe a prolonged final part of micturition, when the flow has slowed to a trickle or dribble.
Storage symptoms	*Increased daytime frequency* is the complaint by the patient who considers that he voids too often during the day.
	Nocturia is the complaint that the man has to wake at night one or more times to void.
	Urgency is the complaint of a sudden compelling desire to pass urine that is difficult to defer.
	Urinary incontinence is the complaint of any involuntary leakage of urine.
Postmicturition symptoms	*Feeling of incomplete emptying* is a self-explanatory term for a feeling experienced by the individual after passing urine.
	Postmicturition dribble is the term used to describe the involuntary loss of urine immediately after finishing passing urine, usually after leaving the toilet.

From Fillit HM: *Brocklehurst's textbook of geriatric medicine and gerontology,* ed 8, Philadelphia, 2017, Elsevier.

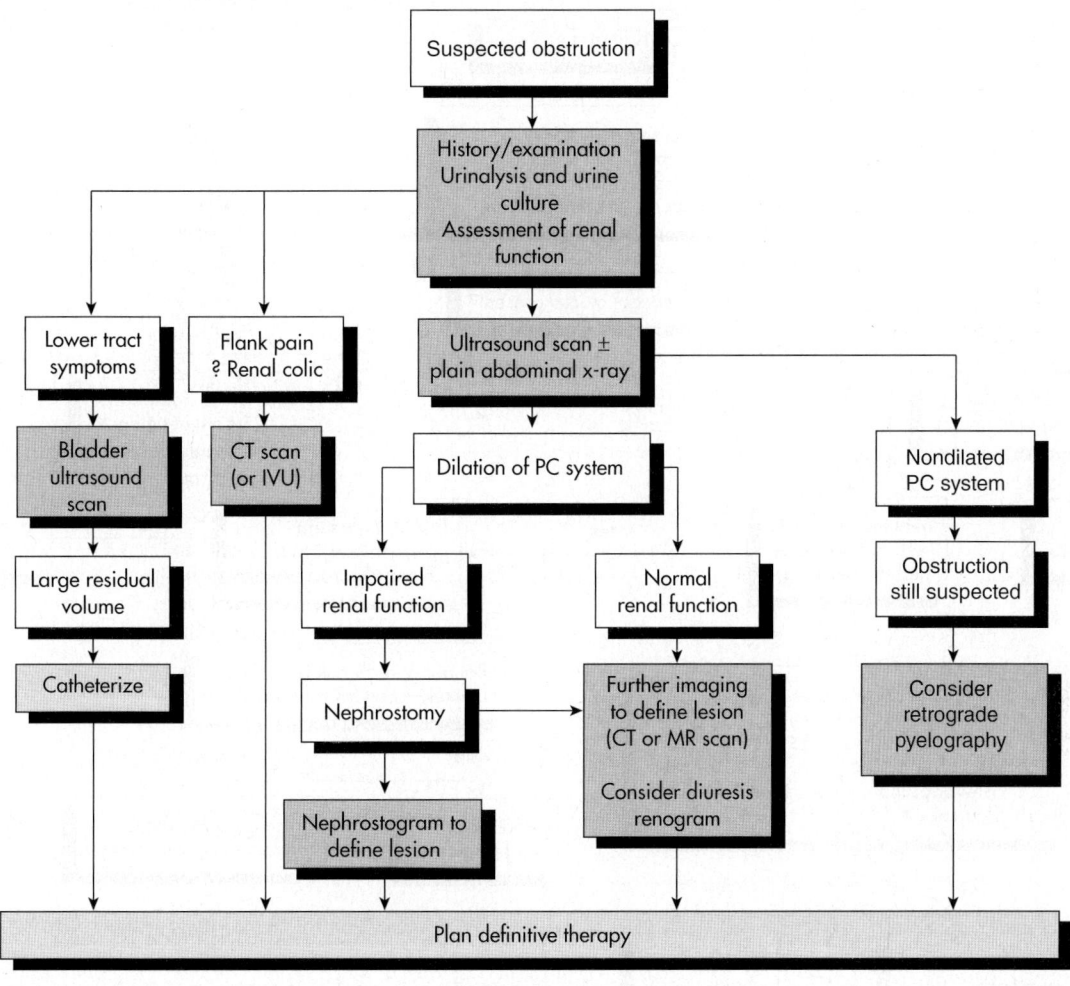

FIG. 214 Investigation and management of suspected urinary tract obstruction. A full history should be taken and a thorough examination performed, together with urinalysis, urine microscopy and culture, and measurement of renal function and serum electrolytes. Ultrasound is a useful first-line investigation for any patient with suspected urinary tract obstruction. Computed tomography *(CT)* is now the preferred imaging technique when renal calculi are suspected. Either CT or magnetic resonance *(MR)* urography can accurately diagnose both the site and cause of obstruction in most cases. If there is renal impairment, a nephrostomy allows the effective relief of the obstruction and time for renal function to recover while definitive therapy is planned. *IVU,* Intravenous urography; *PC,* pelvicalyceal. (From Johnson R et al: *Comprehensive clinical nephrology,* ed 5, Philadelphia, 2015, Saunders.)

Clinical Algorithms

III

BOX 41 Diagnostic Tests Used in Obstructive Uropathy

Upper Urinary Tract Obstruction
Sonography (ultrasound)
Plain films of the abdomen (KUB)
Excretory or intravenous pyelography (very rarely needed)
Retrograde pyelography
Isotopic renography
Computed tomography (helical CT)
Magnetic resonance imaging
Pressure flow studies (the Whitaker test)

Lower Urinary Tract Obstruction
Some of the tests listed above
Cystoscopy
Voiding cystourethrogram
Retrograde urethrography
Urodynamic tests
Debimetry
Cystometrography
Electromyography
Urethral pressure profile

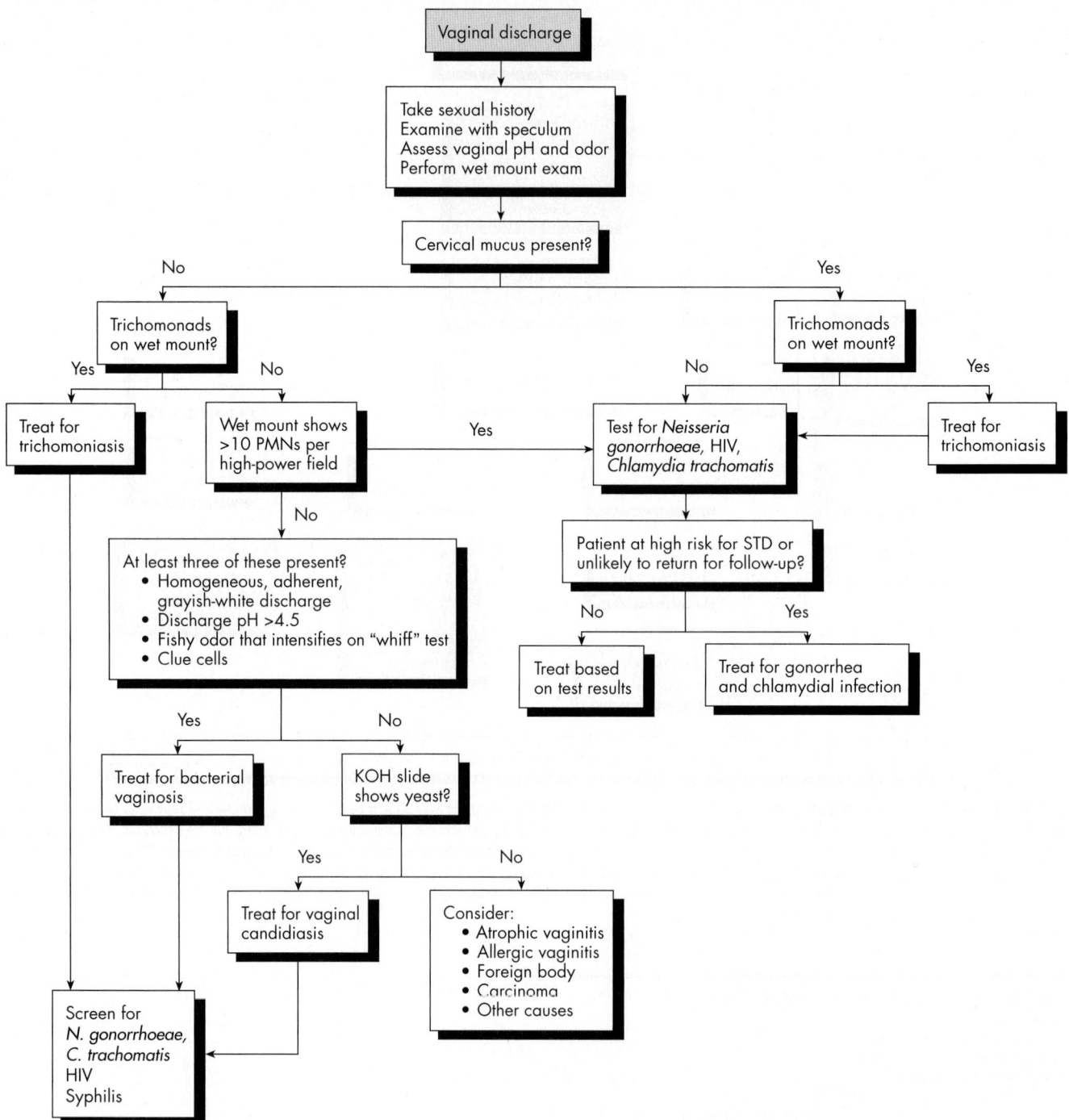

FIG. 215 Evaluation of vaginal discharge. See "Section I" topics "Vaginal Trichomoniasis," "Vulvovaginal Candidiasis," "Vaginosis, Bacterial" for additional information. *HIV,* Human immunodeficiency virus; *KOH,* potassium hydroxide; *PMN,* polymorphonuclear leukocyte; *STD,* sexually transmitted disease.

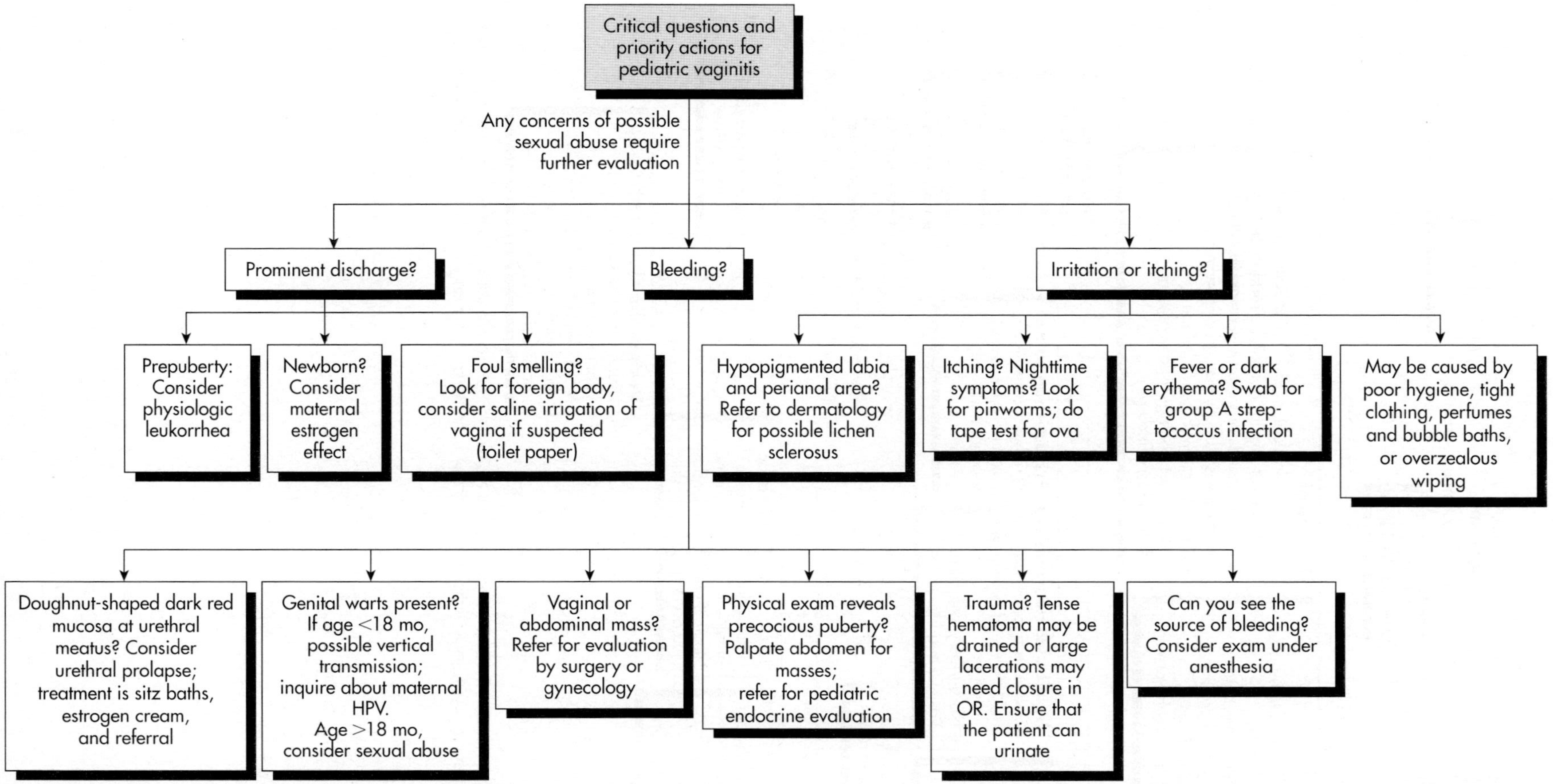

Critical questions and priority actions for pediatric vaginitis

Any concerns of possible sexual abuse require further evaluation

Prominent discharge?

Prepuberty: Consider physiologic leukorrhea

Newborn? Consider maternal estrogen effect

Foul smelling? Look for foreign body, consider saline irrigation of vagina if suspected (toilet paper)

Doughnut-shaped dark red mucosa at urethral meatus? Consider urethral prolapse; treatment is sitz baths, estrogen cream, and referral

Genital warts present? If age <18 mo, possible vertical transmission; inquire about maternal HPV. Age >18 mo, consider sexual abuse

Vaginal or abdominal mass? Refer for evaluation by surgery or gynecology

Bleeding?

Hypopigmented labia and perianal area? Refer to dermatology for possible lichen sclerosus

Physical exam reveals precocious puberty? Palpate abdomen for masses; refer for pediatric endocrine evaluation

Trauma? Tense hematoma may be drained or large lacerations may need closure in OR. Ensure that the patient can urinate

Can you see the source of bleeding? Consider exam under anesthesia

Irritation or itching?

Itching? Nighttime symptoms? Look for pinworms; do tape test for ova

Fever or dark erythema? Swab for group A streptococcus infection

May be caused by poor hygiene, tight clothing, perfumes and bubble baths, or overzealous wiping

FIG. 216 Algorithm showing critical questions and priority actions for pediatric vaginitis. Additional information available in "Section I" topic "Vaginitis, Prepubescent." *HPV,* Human papillomavirus; *OR,* operating room. (From Adams JG et al: *Emergency medicine: clinical essentials,* ed 2, Philadelphia, 2013, Elsevier.)

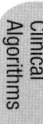

Clinical Algorithms

III

ICD-10CM # H81.13 Benign paroxysmal vertigo, bilateral
R42 Dizziness and giddiness
H81.49 Vertigo of central origin, unspecified ear
H81.399 Other peripheral vertigo, unspecified ear
H81.23 Vestibular neuronitis, bilateral

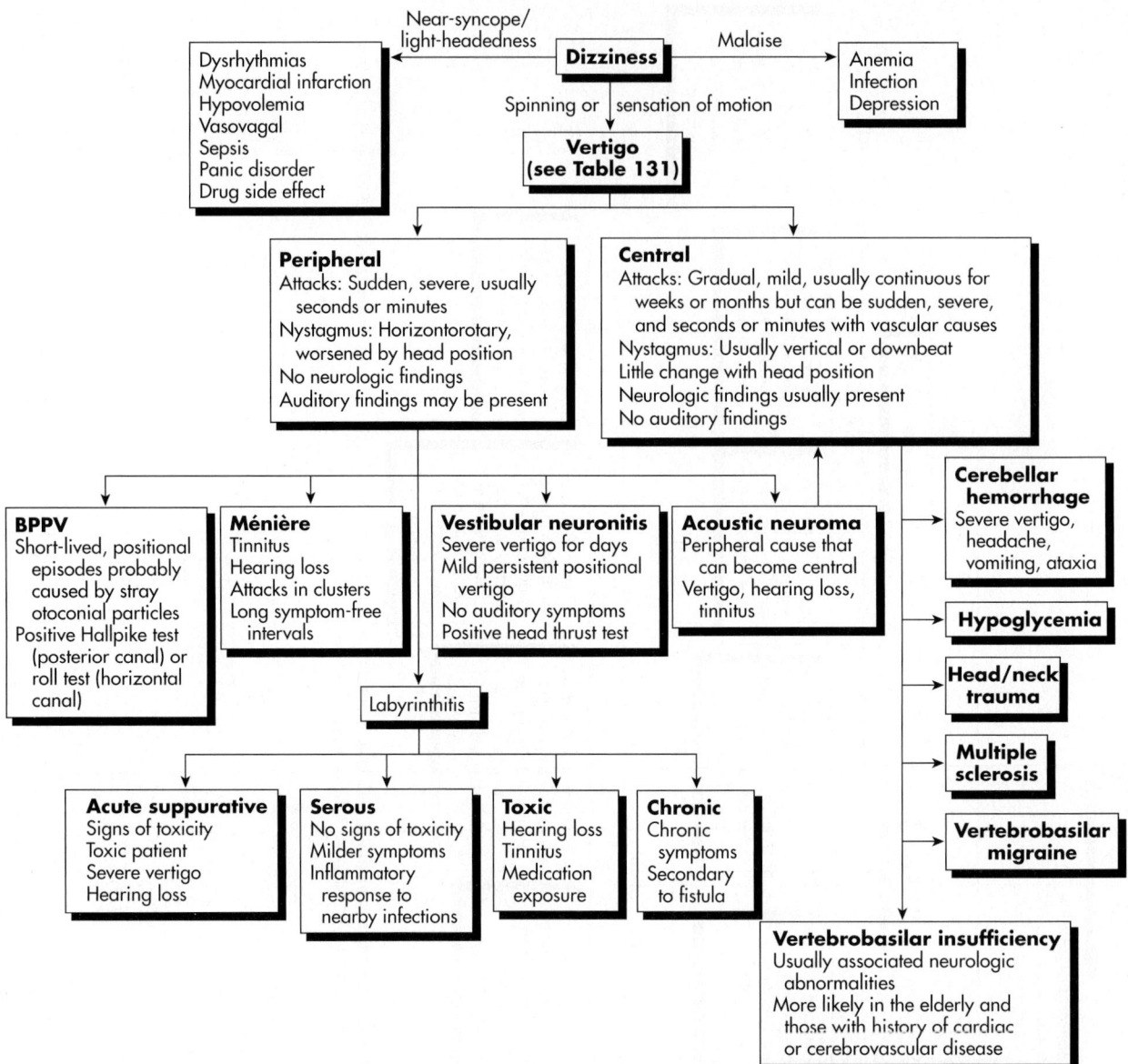

FIG. 219 Diagnostic algorithm for dizziness and vertigo. Also see "Section I" topics "Vestibular Neuronitis," "Acoustic Neuroma," "Labyrinthitis," "Ménière Disease," and "Benign Paroxysmal Positional Vertigo." *BPPV,* Benign paroxysmal positional vertigo. (From Marx JA et al: *Rosen's emergency medicine,* ed 8, Philadelphia, 2014, Saunders.)

ICD-10CM #	H81.13	Benign paroxysmal vertigo, bilateral
	R42	Dizziness and giddiness
	H81.49	Vertigo of central origin, unspecified ear
	H81.399	Other peripheral vertigo, unspecified ear
	H81.23	Vestibular neuronitis, bilateral

1525

TABLE 131 Differential Diagnosis of Patients with True Vertigo

Cause	History	Associated Symptoms	Physical
Peripheral			
Benign paroxysmal positional vertigo	Short-lived, positional, fatigable episodes.	Nausea, vomiting	Single position can precipitate vertigo. Positive result on Hallpike test (posterior semicircular canal) or Roll test (horizontal canal).
Serous	Mild to severe positional symptoms. Usually coexisting or antecedent infection of ear, nose, throat, or meninges.	Mild to severe hearing loss can occur	Usually nontoxic patient with minimal fever elevation.
Acute suppurative	Coexisting acute exudative infection of the inner ear. Severe symptoms.	Usually severe hearing loss, nausea, vomiting	Febrile patient showing signs of toxicity. Acute otitis media.
Toxic	Gradually progressive symptoms: Patients on medication causing toxicity.	Hearing loss that may become rapid and severe, nausea and vomiting	Hearing loss. Ataxia common feature in chronic phase.
Ménière disease	Recurrent episodes of severe rotational vertigo usually lasting hours. Onset usually abrupt. Attacks may occur in clusters. Long symptom-free remissions.	Nausea, vomiting, tinnitus, hearing loss	Positional nystagmus not present.
Vestibular neuritis	Sudden onset of severe vertigo, increasing in intensity for hours, then gradually subsiding over several days but can last weeks to months. Can be worsened with positional change. Sometimes history of infection or toxic exposure that precedes initial attack. Highest incidence is found in third and fifth decades.	Nausea, vomiting. Auditory symptoms do not occur.	Spontaneous nystagmus toward the involved ear may be present.
Acoustic neuroma	Gradual onset and increase in symptoms. Neurologic signs in later stages. Most occur in women aged 30-60.	Hearing loss, tinnitus. True ataxia and neurologic signs as tumor enlarges.	Unilateral decreased hearing. True truncal ataxia and other neurologic signs when tumor enlarges. May have diminution or absence of corneal reflex. Eighth cranial nerve deficit may be present.
Central			
Vertebrobasilar insufficiency	Should be considered in any patient of advanced age with isolated new-onset vertigo without an obvious cause. More likely with history of atherosclerosis. Can occur with neck trauma. Initial episode usually lasts seconds to minutes.	Often headache. Usually neurologic symptoms including dysarthria, ataxia, weakness, numbness, double vision. Tinnitus and deafness uncommon.	Neurologic deficits usually present, but initially neurologic examination can be normal.
Cerebellar hemorrhage	Sudden onset of severe symptoms.	Headache, vomiting, ataxia	Signs of toxicity. Dysmetria, true ataxia. Ipsilateral sixth cranial nerve palsy may be present.
Occlusion of posterior inferior cerebellar artery (Wallenberg syndrome)	Vertigo associated with significant neurologic complaints.	Nausea, vomiting, loss of pain and temperature sensation, ataxia, hoarseness	Loss of pain and temperature sensation on the side of the face ipsilateral to the lesion and on the opposite side of the body, paralysis of the palate, pharynx, and larynx. Horner syndrome (ipsilateral ptosis, miosis, and decreased facial sweating).
Head trauma	Symptoms begin with or shortly after head trauma. Positional symptoms most common type after trauma. Self-limited symptoms that can persist weeks to months.	Usually mild nausea	Occasionally, basilar skull fracture.
Vertebrobasilar migraine	Vertigo almost always followed by headache. Patient has usually had similar episodes in past. Most patients have a family history of migraine. Syndrome usually begins in adolescence.	Dysarthria, ataxia, visual disturbances, or paresthesias usually precede headache	No residual neurologic or otologic signs are present after attack.
Multiple sclerosis	Vertigo presenting symptom in 7%-10% and appears in the course of the disease in a third. Onset may be severe and suggest labyrinth disease. Disease onset usually between ages 20 and 40. Often history of other attacks with varying neurologic signs or symptoms.	Nausea and vomiting, which may be severe	May have horizontal, rotary, or vertical nystagmus. Nystagmus may persist after the vertiginous symptoms have subsided. Bilateral internuclear ophthalmoplegia and ataxic eye movements suggest multiple sclerosis.
Temporal lobe epilepsy	Can be initial or prominent symptom in some patients with the disorder.	Memory impairment, hallucinations, trancelike states, seizures	May have aphasia or convulsions.
Hypoglycemia	Should be considered in diabetics and any other patient with unexplained symptoms.	Sweating, anxiety	Tachycardia, mental status change may be present.

From Marx JA et al: *Rosen's emergency medicine*, ed 8, Philadelphia, 2014, Saunders.

ICD-10CM #	H81.13	Benign paroxysmal vertigo, bilateral
	R42	Dizziness and giddiness
	H81.49	Vertigo of central origin, unspecified ear
	H81.399	Other peripheral vertigo, unspecified ear
	H81.23	Vestibular neuronitis, bilateral

TABLE 132 Distinguishing Among Common Peripheral and Central Vertigo Syndromes

Cause	History of Vertigo	Duration of Vertigo	Associated Symptoms	Physical Examination
Peripheral				
Vestibular neuritis	Single prolonged episode	Days to weeks	Nausea, imbalance	"Peripheral" nystagmus, positive head-thrust test, imbalance
BPPV	Positionally triggered episodes	<1 min	Nausea	Characteristic positionally triggered burst of nystagmus
Ménière disease	May be triggered by salty foods	Hours	Unilateral ear fullness, tinnitus, hearing loss, nausea	Unilateral low-frequency hearing loss
Vestibular paroxysmia	Abrupt onset; spontaneous or positionally triggered	Seconds	Tinnitus, hearing loss	Usually normal
Perilymph fistula	Triggered by sound or pressure changes	Seconds	Hearing loss, hyperacusis	Nystagmus triggered by loud sounds or pressure changes
Central				
Stroke/TIA	Abrupt onset; spontaneous	Stroke, >24 h; TIA, <24 h	Brainstem, cerebellar	Spontaneous "central" nystagmus; gaze-evoked nystagmus; focal neurologic signs; negative head-thrust test; skew deviation
MS	Subacute onset	Minutes to weeks	Unilateral visual loss, diplopia, incoordination, ataxia	"Central" types or rarely "peripheral" types of spontaneous or positional nystagmus; usually other focal neurologic signs
Neurodegenerative disorders	May be spontaneous or positionally triggered	Minutes to hours	Ataxia	"Central" types of spontaneous or positional nystagmus; gaze-evoked nystagmus; impaired smooth pursuit; cerebellar, extrapyramidal and frontal signs
Migraine	Onset usually associated with typical migraine triggers	Seconds to days	Headache, visual aura, photo-/phonophobia	Normal interictal examination; ictal examination may show "peripheral" or "central" types of spontaneous or positional nystagmus
Familial ataxia syndromes	Acute-subacute onset; usually triggered by stress, exercise, or excitement	Hours	Ataxia	"Central" types of spontaneous or positional nystagmus Ictal, or even interictal, gaze-evoked nystagmus; ataxia; gait disorders

BPPV, Benign paroxysmal positional vertigo; *MS,* multiple sclerosis; *TIA,* transient ischemic attack.
From Jankovic J et al: *Bradley and Daroff's neurology in clinical practice,* ed 8, Philadelphia, 2022, Elsevier.

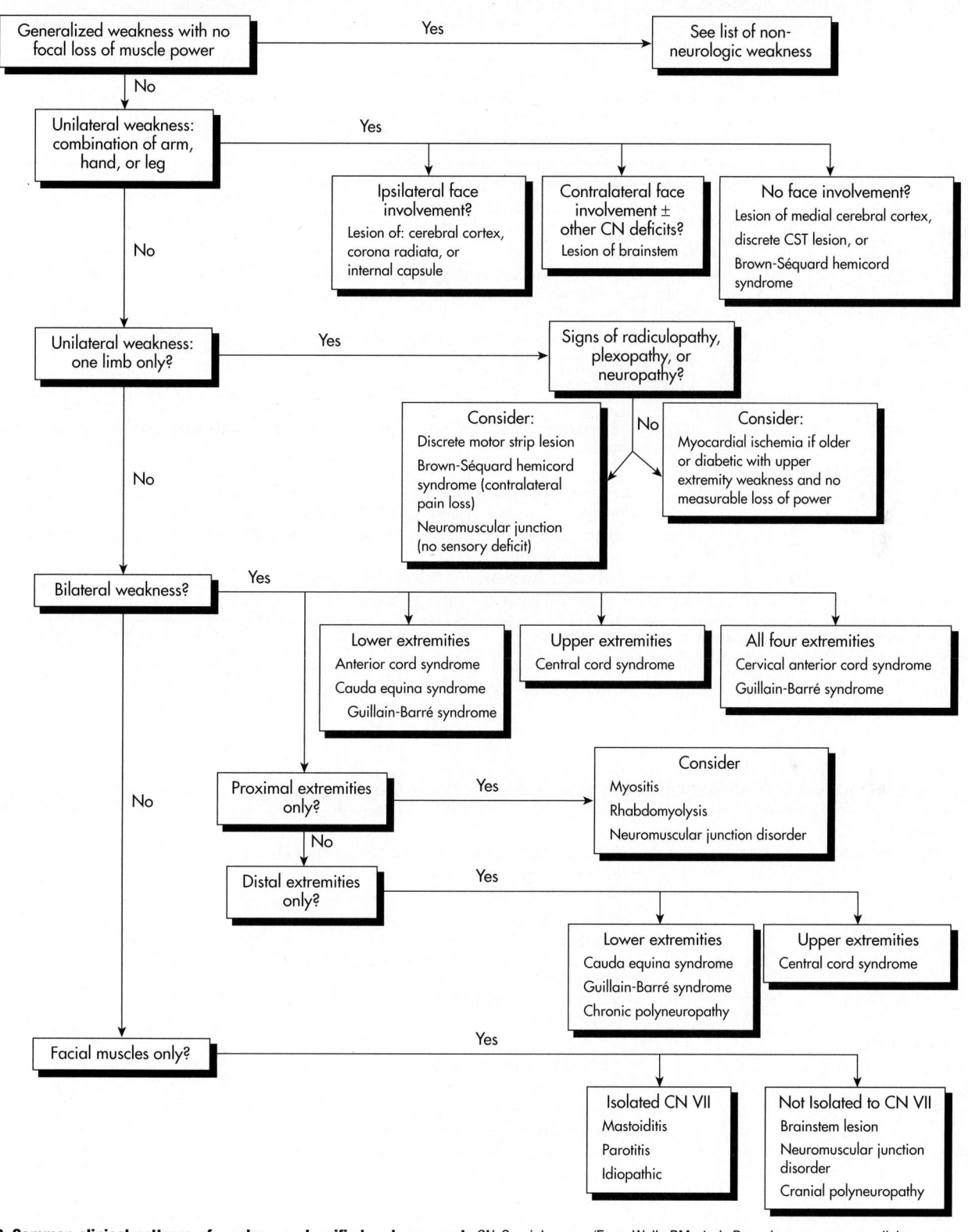

FIG. 222 Common clinical patterns of weakness, classified and assessed. *CN*, Cranial nerve. (From Walls RM et al: *Rosen's emergency medicine, concepts and clinical practice,* ed 10, Philadelphia, 2023, Elsevier.)

Clinical
Algorithms

TABLE 134 Differential Diagnosis of Muscle Weakness

General Type	Subtypes/Examples
Denervating conditions	Spinal muscular atrophy,[a] amyotrophic lateral sclerosis[a]
Neuromuscular junction disorders	Eaton-Lambert syndrome,[a] myasthenia gravis[a]
Genetic muscular dystrophies	Duchenne, facioscapulohumeral, limb-girdle,[a] Becker, Emery-Dreifuss types,[a] distal, ocular
Myotonic diseases	Dystrophia myotonica,[a] myotonia congenita
Congenital myopathies	Nemaline, mitochondrial, centronuclear, central core
Glycogen storage diseases	Adult-onset acid maltase deficiency (Pompe),[a] McArdle disease
Lipid storage myopathies	Carnitine deficiency,[a] carnitine palmitoyltransferase deficiency[a]
Periodic paralyses	
Myositis ossificans[a]	Generalized and local
Endocrine myopathies[a]	Hypothyroidism, hyperthyroidism, acromegaly, Cushing disease, Addison disease, hyperparathyroidism, hypoparathyroidism, vitamin D deficiency myopathy, hypokalemia, hypocalcemia
Metabolic myopathies[a]	Uremia, hepatic failure
Toxic myopathies[a]	Acute and chronic alcoholism; drugs, including penicillamine,[a] clofibrate,[a] chloroquine, emetine
Nutritional myopathies	Vitamin E deficiency,[a] malabsorption[a]
Carcinomatous neuromyopathy[a]	Carcinomatous cachexia
Acute rhabdomyolysis[a]	
Proximal neuropathies	Guillain-Barré syndrome,[a] acute intermittent porphyria,[a] diabetic lower limb chronic plexopathies,[a] chronic autoimmune polyneuropathy
Microembolization by atheroma or carcinoma	
Polymyalgia rheumatica[a]	
Other collagen vascular diseases	Rheumatoid arthritis, scleroderma, systemic lupus erythematosus, polyarteritis nodosa
Infections	Acute viral, including influenza, mononucleosis, coxsackievirus, and rubella and rubella vaccination; *Rickettsia*; acute bacterial, including typhoid
Parasites	*Toxoplasma, Trichinella, Schistosoma, Cysticercus,* Sarcosporidia
Septic myositis	*Staphylococcus, Streptococcus, Clostridium perfringens (welchii)*, and leprosy

[a]Conditions most commonly confused with muscle weakness.
From Hochberg MC et al: *Rheumatology,* ed 8, Philadelphia, 2023, Elsevier.

TABLE 135 Critical and Emergent Causes of Neuromuscular Weakness

Critical Diagnoses

Cerebral cortex or subcortical	Ischemic or hemorrhagic cerebrovascular accident (CVA)
Brainstem	Ischemic or hemorrhagic CVA
Spinal cord	Ischemia, compression (disc, abscess, or hematoma)
Peripheral nerve	Acute demyelination (Guillain-Barré syndrome)
Neuromuscular junction	Myasthenic or cholinergic crisis
	Botulism
	Tick paralysis
	Organophosphate poisoning
Muscle	Rhabdomyolysis

Emergent Diagnoses

Cerebral cortex or subcortical	Tumor, abscess, demyelination
Brainstem	Demyelination
Spinal cord	Demyelination (transverse myelitis)
	Compression (disk, spondylosis)
Peripheral nerve	Compressive plexopathy (hematoma, aneurysm)
	Paraneoplastic vasculitis uremia
Muscle	Inflammatory myositis

From Marx JA et al: *Rosen's emergency medicine,* ed 8, Philadelphia, 2014, Saunders.

TABLE 136   Clinical Signs That Point to the Origin of Neuromuscular Weakness

Sign	UMNs	LMNs	NMJ	Myopathy
Atrophy	None	Severe	Mild	Mild
Fasciculation	None	Common	None	None
Deep tendon reflexes	Hyperreflexic	Areflexic/hyporeflexic	Normal/hyporeflexic	Normal/hyporeflexic
Distribution of weakness	Pyramidal/regional	Distal/segmental	Variable/fatigable weakness	Proximal > distal
Tone	Spastic	Decreased/flaccid	Decreased/flaccid	Normal/decreased
Plantar response	Upgoing	Downgoing or absent	Downgoing or absent	Downgoing or absent

LMNs, Lower motor neurons; *NMJ,* neuromuscular junction; *UMNs,* upper motor neurons.
From Cameron P et al: *Textbook of adult emergency medicine,* ed 5, Edinburgh, 2019, Elsevier.

TABLE 137   Nonneuromuscular Conditions Associated with Weakness

Condition	Manifestations
Anemia	Breathlessness and fatigue usually worse with acute-onset anemia
Cardiac failure	Fatigue and weakness are common symptoms of heart failure in elderly patients, especially weakness in females over 50 yr
Malignancy	Paraneoplastic syndromes (e.g., generalized wasting)
Psychologic disorders	Depression/anxiety, psychosis, medication side effects, malingering
Malnutrition	Institutionalized patients, impoverished elderly, anorexia nervosa
Chronic fatigue syndrome	Possibly postviral syndrome
Rheumatologic disorders	Rheumatoid arthritis, systemic lupus erythematosus, fibromyalgia
Medications	Many medications have been associated with weakness; the commonly encountered ones include glucocorticoids, statins, antiretrovirals, alcohol, colchicine, and polypharmacy, especially in the elderly
Acute electrolyte derangement (e.g., hypokalemia and hyperkalemia, hypocalcemia)	Acute-onset weakness and/or tetany with hypocalcemia
Sepsis	Acidosis, deranged metabolic state
Dehydration	Lethargy/fatigue
Hypothyroidism	Lethargy, cold intolerance, weight gain, weakness
Chronic disease	Respiratory, renal, hepatic failure

From Cameron P et al: *Textbook of adult emergency medicine,* ed 5, Edinburgh, 2019, Elsevier.

Clinical
Algorithms

III

TABLE 138   Key Features of Conditions Associated with the Symptom of Weakness

Disease	Pathophysiology	Assessment	ED Management
Primary Neurologic			
Guillain-Barré syndrome, most common cause of acute symmetric weakness	Immune-mediated polyradiculopathy Postinfective (15%-40%), esp. due to *Campylobacter* or viral infection; >50% are idiopathic	Suggestive history (e.g., diarrhea) Symmetric ascending flaccid weakness; loss of DTRs; early facial palsy common; ± autonomic dysfunction Serial assessment of respiratory function crucial to predict need for intubation/ ventilation CSF high protein with normal glucose and cell count	Supportive care; early intubation for respiratory failure Early neurology and ICU consultation Early administration of IVIG ± plasmapheresis beneficial Corticosteroids *not* indicated
Myasthenia gravis, localized variant more common Myasthenic crises/respiratory decompensation (rare) are main ED issues	Immune-mediated Ach receptor dysfunction; may be precipitated by thymic disorders	Fluctuating, fatigable weakness of voluntary muscles, especially ocular muscles or proximal limbs. Cranial nerve involvement with ptosis in >25% cases; ± dysphagia, weakness of masticatory muscles; normal sensation; normal reflexes Improves with rest Serial respiratory assessment if severe Ice-pack test if there is ptosis	Supportive care Avoid potential precipitants including corticosteroids Anticholinesterase treatment as directed by neurologist

Continued

TABLE 138 Key Features of Conditions Associated with the Symptom of Weakness—cont'd

Disease	Pathophysiology	Assessment	ED Management
Multiple sclerosis, relapsing/remitting course most common	Immune-mediated scattered neuron demyelination; affects motor, sensory, visual, and cerebellar function Classically ≥2 separate episodes of neurologic dysfunction indicating white matter or spinal cord lesions at distinct locations	Acute exacerbations, acute worsening of clinical signs; variable weakness, hypertonicity, spasticity, clonus, altered pain/temp/vibration and proprioceptive senses Lhermitte sign Optic neuritis in up to 30% with acute central vision loss, afferent papillary defect, red desaturation lung puncture, MRI, evoked potentials in consultation with neurologist	Pulse methylprednisolone therapy for exacerbations Supportive care for generalized weakness Neurology consultation Long-term disease modification and lifestyle strategies (e.g., vitamin D)
Cord compression	Spinal stenosis ± malignancy or infection	Thorough neurologic examination Red flags (e.g., fever, malignancy, IVDU warrant MRI)	Neurosurgical consultation Decompression, antibiotics, targeted radiotherapy as indicated
Myopathies			
Congenital Dystrophin disorders, Duchenne muscular dystrophy (DMD); Becker muscular dystrophy (BMB) DMD/BMD, mitochondrial disorders	X-linked dystrophin gene dysfunction Males affected more severely by DMD; life expectancy to early 20s; BMD of later onset less severe	Generalized weakness Usual ED presentation is acute deterioration with respiratory compromise Spirometry/respiratory assessment Mitochondrial disorders—variable episodic weakness and fluctuating consciousness	Supportive care Discussion with patient, advocates, neurologists regarding appropriateness of intensive intervention Consider advance care directives Ventilatory support as appropriate
Acquired Metabolic/electrolyte disorders Hypokalemic periodic paralysis Endocrine Cushing disease Addison disease Thyrotoxicosis Toxic Statins, corticosteroids	Variable weakness; may be acute episodic weakness with hypokalemia ± thyrotoxicosis Drug-induced or history of endocrine myopathies suggestive	Periodic paralysis; may be preceded by vomiting/diarrheal illness; may have family history Check electrolytes, especially K⁺ ECG if K⁺ deranged Endocrine—assess for other stigmata of endocrinopathy (e.g., cushingoid, addisonian)	Electrolyte (K⁺) reconstitution Supportive care Correct endocrine abnormalities Discontinue offending medications
Intoxications			
Botulism due to *Clostridium botulinum* toxin	Deranged neurotransmission Ingested botulinum toxin prevents Ach release at NMJ	History of ingestion GI symptoms in 50% Descending flaccid paralysis Postural hypotension, diplopia, blurred vision, ptosis, dysphagia, respiratory compromise, progressing to limb weakness Ileus common	Supportive care ICU admission for ventilatory support as needed Specific antiserum in consultation with toxicology/neurology
Tetanus due to *Clostridium tetani* tetanospasmin toxin Endemic in developing countries	Impaired inhibitory neurotransmission causing skeletal muscle spasm and rigidity Classically infected deep wounds in nonimmunized patients	Suggestive history—recent wound, vulnerable patient (e.g., elderly, nonimmune) Trismus/dysphagia common early; progressive to painful skeletal muscle spasms; exacerbated by minor stimuli (e.g., touch) May be a localized form Clinical diagnosis	Supportive care, ICU for ventilatory support and sedation Tetanus antitoxin Tetanus immunization is protective Antibiotics (penicillin) to treat clostridial infection
Tick paralysis due to tick toxin, ascending flaccid paralysis mimics Guillain-Barré syndrome	Impaired neurotransmission *Ixodes holocyclus* (Australian paralysis tick) Death from respiratory paralysis	Mostly children in tick-endemic area ± tick found on patient; ataxia, weakness ± extraocular palsy/dysphagia May progress after tick removal to generalized/respiratory paralysis	Tick removal/observation sufficient in most cases If severe, ventilatory support Antiserum administration as directed by toxicology/neurology
Marine intoxications Ciguatera Puffer fish Blue-ringed octopus	Ciguatera toxin (from reef fish) Tetrodotoxin (puffer fish, blue-ringed octopus) block sodium channels and impair neurotransmission Tetrodotoxin also acts on CTZ and impairs ventilation	History of tropical fish ingestion; onset of symptoms within a few hours Ciguatera—paresthesias, electrical sensations in response to hot/cold Tetrodotoxin—progressive flaccid weakness with respiratory compromise	Supportive treatment esp. ventilatory support

CSF, Cerebrospinal fluid; *CTZ*, chemoreceptor trigger zone; *DTRs*, deep tendon reflexes; *ECG*, electrocardiogram; *ED*, emergency department; *GI*, gastrointestinal; *ICU*, intensive care unit; *IVDU*, intravenous drug user; *IVIG*, intravenous immunoglobulin; *MRI*, magnetic resonance imaging; *NMJ*, neuromuscular junction.
From Cameron P et al: *Textbook of adult emergency medicine*, ed 5, Edinburgh, 2019, Elsevier.

BOX 42   Progressive Proximal Weakness

Spinal cord disorders
Juvenile spinal muscular atrophies
- Autosomal dominant
- Autosomal recessive
- GM$_2$ gangliosidosis (hexosaminidase A deficiency)
- Myasthenic syndromes

Acquired limb-girdle myasthenia
Slow-channel syndrome
Muscular dystrophies
Bethlem myopathy
Dystrophinopathies
Facioscapulohumeral syndrome
Severe childhood autosomal recessive muscular
Dystrophy
Inflammatory myopathies
Dermatomyositis[a]
Polymyositis[a]
Metabolic myopathies
Acid maltase deficiency[a]
Carnitine deficiency[a]
Debrancher enzyme deficiency[a]
Lipid storage myopathies
Mitochondrial myopathies
Myophosphorylase deficiency
Endocrine myopathies
Adrenal cortex[a]
Parathyroid[a]
Thyroid[a]

[a]Denotes the most common conditions and the ones with disease-modifying treatments.
From Pina-Garza J, James KC: *Fenichel's clinical pediatric neurology,* ed 8, Philadelphia, 2019, Elsevier.

BOX 44   Acute Generalized Weakness

Infectious Disorders
Acute infectious myositis
Acute inflammatory polyradiculoneuropathy[a] (Guillain-Barré syndrome)
Acute axonal neuropathies
Chronic inflammatory polyradiculoneuropathy[a] (CIDP)
Enterovirus infections

Metabolic Disorders
Acute intermittent porphyria
Hereditary tyrosinemia

Neuromuscular Blockade
Botulism[a]
Corticosteroid-induced quadriplegia[a]
Intensive care unit weakness
Tick paralysis[a]

Periodic Paralysis
Andersen-Tawil syndrome
Familial hypokalemic[a] (FPPI)
Familial hyperkalemic[a] (FPPII)
Familial normokalemic (FPPIII)

[a]Denotes the most common conditions and the ones with disease-modifying treatments.
From Pina-Garza J, James KC: *Fenichel's clinical pediatric neurology,* ed 8, Philadelphia, 2019, Elsevier.

BOX 43   Progressive Distal Weakness

Spinal cord disorders
Motor neuron diseases
Juvenile amyotrophic lateral sclerosis
Monomelic
Spinal muscular atrophies
Autosomal dominant forms
Autosomal recessive forms
Neuropathies
Hereditary motor sensory neuropathies
Charcot-Marie-Tooth disease
Familial amyloid neuropathy
Giant axonal neuropathy (16q24)
Other genetic neuropathies
Other lipid neuropathies
Pyruvate dehydrogenase deficiency
Refsum disease
Sulfatide lipidosis: metachromatic leukodystrophy
Neuropathies with systemic diseases
Drug-induced[a]
Systemic vasculitis[a]
Toxins[a]
Uremia[a]
Idiopathic neuropathy
Chronic axonal neuropathy[a]
Chronic demyelinating neuropathy[a]
Myopathies
Autosomal dominant childhood myopathy
Autosomal dominant infantile myopathy
Autosomal recessive distal (Miyoshi) myopathy
Inclusion body myopathies
Myotonic dystrophy
Scapulo (humeral) peroneal syndrome
- Emery-Dreifuss muscular dystrophy type 1
- Emery-Dreifuss muscular dystrophy type 2
- Scapuloperoneal myopathy
- Scapuloperoneal neuronopathy

[a]Denotes the most common conditions and the ones with disease-modifying treatments.
From Pina-Garza J, James KC: *Fenichel's clinical pediatric neurology,* ed 8, Philadelphia, 2019, Elsevier.

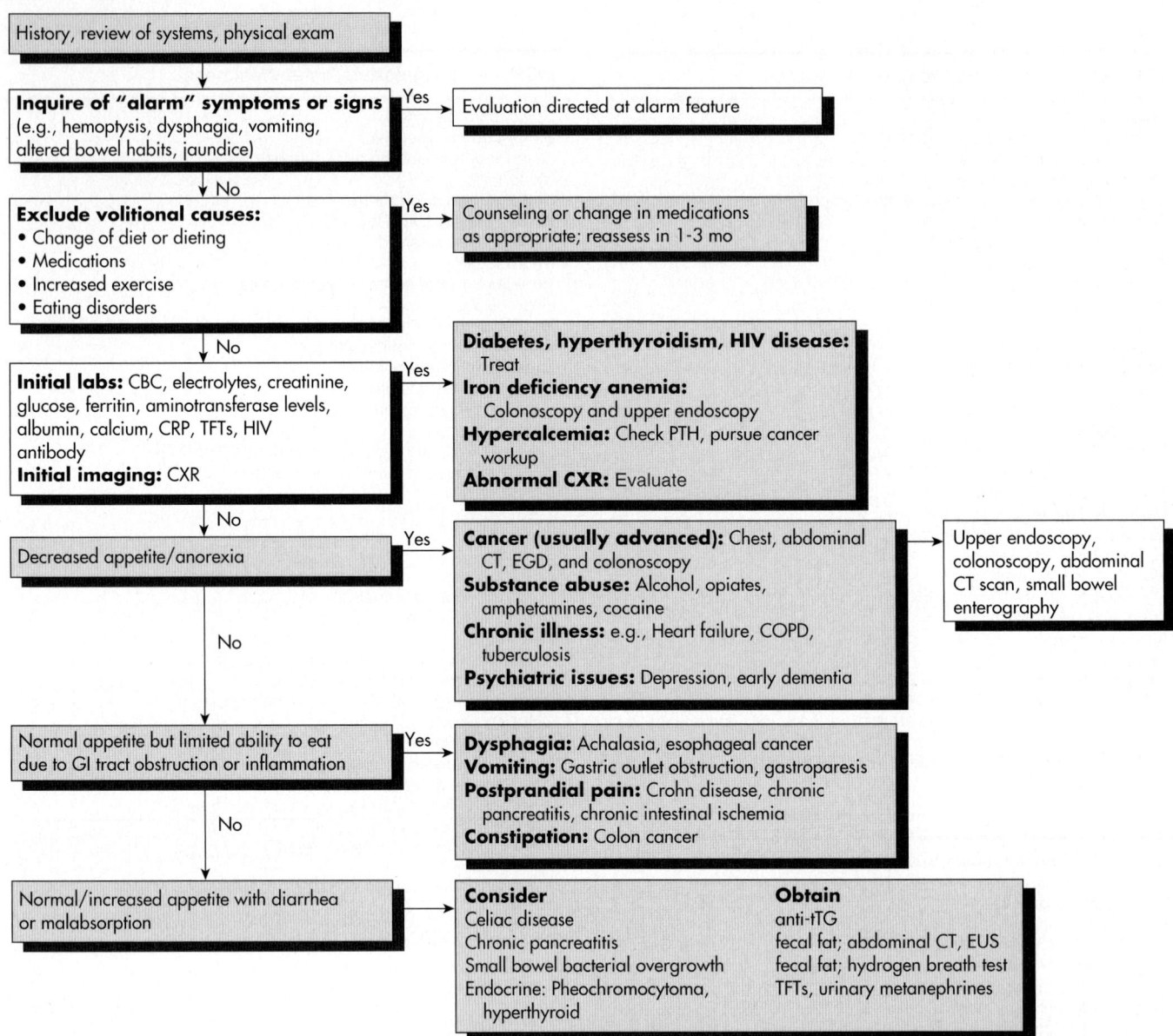

FIG. 224 Approach to the patient with unintentional weight loss of more than 5%. *CBC,* Complete blood count; *COPD,* chronic obstructive pulmonary disease; *CRP,* C-reactive protein; *CT,* computed tomography; *CXR,* chest radiograph; *EGD,* esophagogastroduodenoscopy; *EUS,* endoscopic ultrasound; *GI,* gastrointestinal; *HIV,* human immunodeficiency virus; *PTH,* parathyroid hormone; *TFTs,* thyroid function tests; *tTG,* tissue transglutaminase. (From Goldman L, Schafer AI: *Goldman Cecil medicine,* ed 25, Philadelphia, 2016, Saunders.)

TABLE 139 Causes of Involuntary Weight Loss

Condition	Quality	Duration	Aggravating or Relieving Factors	Associated Symptoms or Signs	Diagnostic Studies
Weight Loss Secondary to Gastrointestinal Causes					
GI, pancreatic, or hepatobiliary malignant disease	Progressive, fast	Months	Better with cancer therapy (e.g., surgery, XRT, chemotherapy)	Dysphagia (esophageal); anorexia, nausea, vomiting (gastric, small or large bowel obstruction); visible or occult blood in stool; altered bowel habits; jaundice or hepatomegaly (biliary obstruction, hepatic tumor, metastatic disease); iron deficiency anemia	CBC, FOBT, ferritin, CEA, CA19-9, AFP, EGD, colonoscopy, abdominal CT, PET
Malabsorption (poor absorption of nutrients due to pancreatic insufficiency, small intestinal mucosal disorders, or bacterial overgrowth)	Progressive, slow	Months to years	Diarrhea or steatorrhea, excessive flatulence; worse with eating and resolves with NPO status	Usually associated with increased appetite; may have anemia (iron, B_{12}, folate); osteoporosis, or osteomalacia (vitamin D, calcium, phosphorus); easy bruising (vitamin K), night blindness (vitamin A)	72-h stool for fecal fat; fecal elastase; vitamins A and D and INR; calcium, ferritin, B_{12}, albumin; celiac disease antibodies (e.g., anti-tTG, anti-endomysial antibodies); EGD with small bowel biopsy; breath test for bacterial overgrowth
Inflammatory bowel disease (especially Crohn disease)	Progressive, slow	Months	Eating causes pain, cramps, increased diarrhea and urgency; improved by low-residue diet or NPO status	Bloody stools, abdominal cramps and pain, perianal disease, extraintestinal manifestations (e.g., oral ulcers, uveitis, erythema nodosum, arthralgias)	CBC, albumin, ESR, CRP, colonoscopy with biopsies, CT or MR enterography, wireless capsule study
GI motility disorders	Intermittent, slow	Years	Worse with eating	Nausea, vomiting, distention, diarrhea, or constipation may be present	EGD and colonoscopy, gastric emptying study, CT or MR enterography, surgical full-thickness intestinal biopsies
Cirrhosis	Muscle wasting with edema, so weight may increase	Months to years	Worse with salt or fluid intake	Ascites, peripheral edema	Liver biopsy
Chronic intestinal ischemia	Progressive	Months to years	Worse with eating	Afraid to eat; postprandial abdominal pain, nausea; associated atherosclerotic disease	CT or MR angiography
Weight Loss Secondary to Nongastrointestinal Causes					
Poor or inadequate calorie intake due to social factors	Intermittent or progressive, acute (hospitalized) or chronic	Days to months to years	Common in elderly, teenagers; exacerbated by poor dentition or poorly fitting dentures	Will eat if food is made available	Review dietary log and how food is obtained and prepared
Medications	Intermittent or progressive	Months	Worse with medication; resolves with discontinuation of offending drug	Anorexia, nausea, vomiting	Review drug profile
Non-GI malignant disease	Progressive	Months	Better with cancer therapy (e.g., surgery, XRT, chemotherapy)	Anorexia, nausea, vomiting; pain; metastatic disease	Calcium, cortisol; CT for underlying disease, PET
Endocrine disorders: DM, hyperthyroidism, adrenal insufficiency	DM—appetite increased or decreased, early satiety; hyperthyroidism—increased appetite	Months to years	Worse with disease chronicity	DM: Gastroparesis, neuropathy, retinopathy, nephropathy; Adrenal insufficiency: Nausea, vomiting, diarrhea, abdominal pain	Serum glucose, TFT, cortisol
Chronic infections, including HIV and TB	Progressive, fast	Months	Better with directed therapy, megestrol acetate (Megace)	Nausea, anorexia, other infections	HIV test, PPD, cultures, biopsies if necessary
Systemic inflammatory disorders	Progressive, moderate	Months to years	Better with directed therapy, megestrol acetate (Megace)	Arthritis, rash, vasculitis	ANA, RF, ESR, CRP
Chronic renal failure	Progressive, slow; edema may increase weight	Months to years	Better with dialysis, megestrol acetate (Megace)	Nausea, anorexia, weight gain	BUN, Cr, 24-h creatinine clearance
Advanced COPD or heart failure	Progressive, slow	Months to years	Better with oxygen and specific treatment	Fatigue, dyspnea, edema, wasting	Pulmonary function testing or two-dimensional echocardiography
Psychiatric illness: Depression, manic-depressive illness	Progressive, slow	Months to years	Depression common in elderly; flat affect; manic phase associated with hyperactivity and decreased intake	Psychologic testing	Psychiatric testing
Psychogenic eating disorders—anorexia nervosa, bulimia	Intermittent or progressive	Months to years	Worse with stressors	Refusal to eat, loss of tooth enamel, calluses and healing ulcerations of hand	Psychiatric testing
Substance abuse (alcohol, opiates, CNS stimulants)	Intermittent or progressive	Months	Resolves with discontinuation	Anorexia, nausea, vomiting	Careful interview; patients may deny or minimize

AFP, α-Fetoprotein; *ANA,* antinuclear antibody; *BUN,* blood urea nitrogen; *CBC,* complete blood count; *CEA,* carcinoembryonic antigen; *CNS,* central nervous system; *COPD,* chronic obstructive pulmonary disease; *Cr,* creatinine; *CRP,* C-reactive protein; *CT,* computed tomography; *DM,* diabetes mellitus; *EGD,* esophagogastroduodenoscopy; *ESR,* erythrocyte sedimentation rate; *FOBT,* fecal occult blood test; *GI,* gastrointestinal; *HIV,* human immunodeficiency virus; *INR,* international normalized ratio; *MR,* magnetic resonance; *NPO,* nothing orally; *PET,* positron emission tomography; *PPD,* purified protein derivative; *RF,* rheumatoid factor; *TB,* tuberculosis; *TFT,* thyroid function test; *tTG,* tissue transglutaminase; *XRT,* x-ray therapy.
From Goldman L, Shafer AI: *Goldman-Cecil medicine,* ed 26, Philadelphia, 2020, Elsevier.

Clinical Algorithms

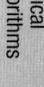

SECTION IV

Laboratory Tests and Interpretation of Results

INTRODUCTION

This section contains over 300 commonly performed laboratory tests. In general, the tests are discussed in the following format:

1. Laboratory test.
2. Normal range in adult patients. Normal values are given using the present (traditional) reference interval, followed by the Système Internationale (SI) reference interval, the conversion factor (CF), and the suggested minimum increment (SMI).
3. Common abnormalities, such as a positive test or increased or decreased value.
4. Causes of abnormal result.
5. The normal ranges may differ slightly, depending on the laboratory. The reader should be aware of the "normal range" of the particular laboratory performing the test. Every attempt has been made to present current laboratory test data, with an emphasis on practical considerations.

ACE LEVEL
See "ANGIOTENSIN-CONVERTING ENZYME"

ACETONE (SERUM OR PLASMA)
Normal: Negative
Elevated in: Diabetic ketoacidosis (DKA), starvation, isopropanol ingestion

ACETYLCHOLINE RECEPTOR (AChR) ANTIBODY
Normal: <0.03 nmol/L
Elevated in: Myasthenia gravis. Changes in AChR concentration correlate with the clinical severity of myasthenia gravis after therapy and during therapy with prednisone and immunosuppressants. False-positive AChR antibody results may be found in patients with Eaton-Lambert syndrome.

ACID-BASE REFERENCE VALUES
See Tables 1, 2, and 3. Fig. 1 illustrates the relationship between bicarbonate and pCO$_2$ in a variety of clinical disorders.

ACID PHOSPHATASE (SERUM)
Normal range: 0 to 5.5 U/L (0 to 90 nkat/L [CF: 16.67; SMI: 2 nkat/L])
Elevated in: Carcinoma of the prostate, other neoplasms (breast, bone), Paget disease, osteogenesis imperfecta, malignant invasion of bone, Gaucher disease, multiple myeloma, myeloproliferative disorders, benign prostatic hypertrophy, prostatic palpation or surgery, hyperparathyroidism, liver disease, chronic renal failure, idiopathic thrombocytopenic purpura, bronchitis

ACID SERUM TEST
See "HAM TEST"

ACTIVATED CLOTTING TIME (ACT)
Normal: This test is used to determine the dose of protamine sulfate to reverse the effect of heparin as an anticoagulant during angioplasty, cardiac surgery, and hemodialysis. The accepted goal during cardiopulmonary bypass surgery is usually 400 to 500 sec.

ACTIVATED PARTIAL THROMBOPLASTIN TIME (APTT, aPTT)
See "PARTIAL THROMBOPLASTIN TIME"

ADRENOCORTICOTROPIC HORMONE (ACTH)
Normal: 9 to 52 pg/ml. Table E4 describes patterns of serum levels of ACTH and cortisol in different adrenal gland disorders.
Elevated in: Addison disease, ectopic ACTH-producing tumors, congenital adrenal hyperplasia, Nelson syndrome, pituitary-dependent Cushing disease
Decreased in: Secondary adrenocortical insufficiency, hypopituitarism, adrenal adenoma or adrenal carcinoma

ALANINE AMINOPEPTIDASE
Normal:
Male: 1.11 to 1.71 mcg/ml
Female: 0.96 to 1.52 mcg/ml
Elevated in: Liver or pancreatic disease, ethanol use, oral contraceptive use, malignancy, tobacco use, pregnancy
Decreased in: Abortion

ALANINE AMINOTRANSFERASE (ALT, SGPT)
See Fig. E2 for an algorithm for the evaluation of elevated ALT. Table E5 describes patterns of liver function tests in liver disorders.
Normal range: 0 to 35 U/L (0.058 μkat/L [CF: 0.02 μkat/L])
Elevated in: Liver disease (hepatitis, cirrhosis, Reye syndrome), hepatic congestion, infectious mononucleosis, myocardial infarction, myocarditis, severe muscle trauma, dermatomyositis/polymyositis, muscular dystrophy, drugs (antibiotics, narcotics, antihypertensive agents, heparin, labetalol, statins, NSAIDs, amiodarone, chlorpromazine, phenytoin), malignancy, renal and pulmonary infarction, seizures, eclampsia, shock liver

TABLE 1 Commonly Used Acid-Base Reference Values for Arterial and Venous Plasma or Serum (Averaged from Various Sources)

	ARTERIAL		VENOUS	
	Conventional Units	SI Units[a]	Conventional Units	SI Units[a]
pH	7.40 (7.35-7.45)	7.40 (7.35-7.45)	7.37 (7.32-7.42)	7.37 (7.32-7.42)
Pco$_2$	40 mm Hg (35-45)	5.33 kPa (4.67-6.10)	45 mm Hg (45-50)	6.10 kPa (5.33-6.67)
Po$_2$	80-100 mm Hg	10.66-13.33 kPa	40 mm Hg (37-43)	5.33 kPa (4.93-5.73)
HCO$_3^-$ (CO$_2$ combining power)	24 mEq/L (20-28)	24 mmol/L (20-28)	26 mEq/L (22-30)	26 mmol/L (22-30)
CO$_2$ content	25 mEq/L (22-28)	25 mmol/L (22-28)	27 mEq/L (24-30)	27 mmol/L (24-30)

[a]International system.
From Ravel R: *Clinical laboratory medicine,* ed 6, St Louis, 1995, Mosby.

TABLE 2 Summary of Laboratory Findings in Primary Uncomplicated Respiratory and Metabolic Acid-Base Disorders[a]

Disorder	Pco$_2$	pH	Base Excess
Acute primary respiratory hypoactivity (respiratory acidosis)	Increase	Decrease	Normal/positive
Acute primary respiratory hyperactivity (respiratory alkalosis)	Decrease	Increase	Normal/negative
Uncompensated metabolic acidosis	Normal	Decrease	Negative
Uncompensated metabolic alkalosis	Normal	Increase	Positive
Partially compensated metabolic acidosis	Decrease	Decrease	Negative
Partially compensated metabolic alkalosis	Increase	Increase	Positive
Chronic primary respiratory hypoactivity (compensated respiratory acidosis)	Increase	Normal	Positive
Fully compensated metabolic alkalosis	Increase	Normal	Positive
Chronic primary respiratory hyperactivity (compensated respiratory alkalosis)	Decrease	Normal	Negative
Fully compensated metabolic acidosis	Decrease	Normal	Negative

[a]Base excess results refer to negative (−) values more than 22 and positive (+) values more than 12.
From Vincent JL et al: *Textbook of critical care,* ed 7, Philadelphia, 2017, Elsevier. Adapted and updated from Bidani A et al: Regulation of whole body acid-base balance. In DuBose TD, Hamm LL (eds): *Acid base and electrolytes disorders: a companion to Brenner and Rector's the kidney,* Philadelphia, 2002, Saunders, p. 1-21.

Laboratory Tests

IV

TABLE 3 Acid-Base Abnormalities and Appropriate Compensatory Responses for Simple Disorders

Primary Acid-Base Disorders	Primary Defect	Effect on pH	Compensatory Response	Expected Range of Compensation	Limits of Compensation
Respiratory acidosis	Alveolar hypoventilation ($\uparrow$ P_{CO_2})	$\downarrow$	$\uparrow$ Renal HCO_3^- reabsorption ($HCO_3^-\uparrow$)	Acute: $\Delta[HCO_3^-] = +1$ mEq/L for each $\uparrow\Delta P_{CO_2}$ of 10 mm Hg	$[HCO_3^-] = 38$ mEq/L
				Chronic: $\Delta[HCO_3^-] = +4$ mEq/L for each $\uparrow\Delta P_{CO_2}$ of 10 mm Hg	$[HCO_3^-] = 45$ mEq/L
Respiratory alkalosis	Alveolar hyperventilation ($\downarrow$ P_{CO_2})	$\uparrow$	$\downarrow$ Renal HCO_3^- reabsorption ($HCO_3^-\downarrow$)	Acute: $\Delta[HCO_3^-] = -2$ mEq/L for each $\downarrow\Delta P_{CO_2}$ of 10 mm Hg	$[HCO_3^-] = 18$ mEq/L
				Chronic: $\Delta[HCO_3^-] = -5$ mEq/L for each $\downarrow\Delta P_{CO_2}$ of 10 mm Hg	$[HCO_3^-] = 15$ mEq/L
Metabolic acidosis	Loss of HCO_3^- or gain of H^+ ($\downarrow$ HCO_3^-)	$\downarrow$	Alveolar hyperventilation to $\uparrow$ pulmonary CO_2 excretion ($\downarrow$ P_{CO_2})	$P_{CO_2} = 1.5[HCO_3^-] + 8 \pm 2$ P_{CO_2} = last 2 digits of pH $\times$ 100 P_{CO_2} = 15 + $[HCO_3^-]$	$P_{CO_2} = 15$ mm Hg
Metabolic alkalosis	Gain of HCO_3^- or loss of H^+ ($\uparrow$ HCO_3^-)	$\uparrow$	Alveolar hypoventilation to $\downarrow$ pulmonary CO_2 excretion ($\uparrow$ P_{CO_2})	$P_{CO_2} = +0.6$ mm Hg for $\Delta[HCO_3^-]$ of 1 mEq/L. $P_{CO_2} = 15 + [HCO_3^-]$	$P_{CO_2} = 55$ mm Hg

From Vincent JL et al: *Textbook of critical care,* ed 7, Philadelphia, 2017, Elsevier. Adapted and updated from Bidani A et al: Regulation of whole body acid-base balance. In DuBose TD, Hamm LL (eds): *Acid base and electrolytes disorders: a companion to Brenner and Rector's the kidney,* Philadelphia, 2002, Saunders, p. 1-21.

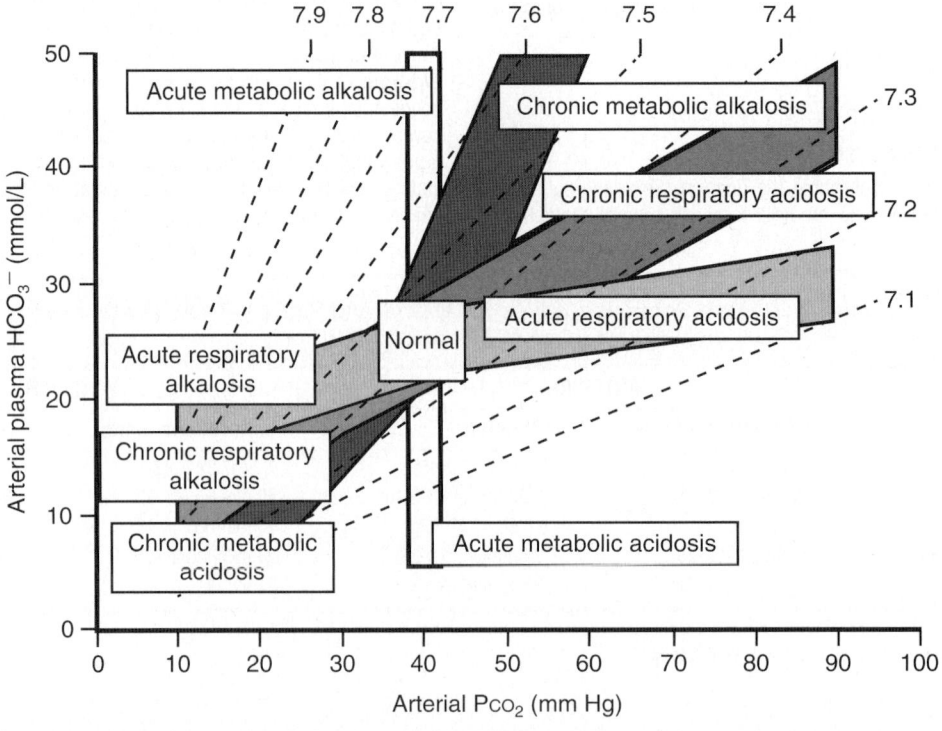

FIG. 1 The relation between bicarbonate (HCO_3^-) and pCO$_2$ in a variety of clinical disorders. The 95% confidence levels for acute and chronic respiratory and metabolic abnormalities are denoted by the colored boxes. The vertical transparent bar indicates the absence of any change in arterial pCO$_2$ with acute changes in HCO_3^-. However, the respiratory response to the onset of metabolic acidosis and alkalosis is rapid, and the metabolic band rotates clockwise toward the chronic metabolic position within a matter of minutes to hours. Compensatory metabolic responses to respiratory changes in arterial pCO$_2$ are much slower, making it easier to observe the acute respiratory bands before metabolic compensation. (From Broaddus VC et al: *Murray & Nadel's textbook of respiratory medicine,* ed 7, Philadelphia, 2022, Elsevier.)

ALBUMIN (SERUM)

Normal range: 4 to 6 g/dl (40 to 60 g/L [CF:10; SMI: 1 g/L])
Elevated in: Dehydration (relative increase)
Decreased in: Liver disease, nephrotic syndrome, poor nutritional status, rapid intravenous (IV) hydration, protein-losing enteropathies (e.g., inflammatory bowel disease), severe burns, neoplasia, chronic inflammatory diseases, pregnancy, oral contraceptives, prolonged immobilization, lymphomas, hypervitaminosis A, chronic glomerulonephritis

ALCOHOL DEHYDROGENASE

Normal: 0 to 7 U/L
Elevated in: Drug-induced hepatocellular damage, obstructive jaundice, malignancy, inflammation, infection

ALDOLASE (SERUM)

Normal range: 0 to 6 U/L (0 to 100 nkat/L [CF: 16.67; SMI: 20 nkat/L])
Elevated in: Muscular dystrophy, rhabdomyolysis, dermatomyositis/polymyositis, trichinosis, acute hepatitis and other liver diseases, myocardial infarction, prostatic carcinoma, hemorrhagic pancreatitis, gangrene, delirium tremens, burns
Decreased in: Loss of muscle mass, late stages of muscular dystrophy

ALDOSTERONE

Normal range:
Recumbent: 50 to 150 ng/L
Upright: 150 to 300 ng/L
(Highest levels in neonates, decreasing over time to adult levels.) The normal renin-angiotensin-aldosterone axis is illustrated in Fig. E3.
Elevated in: Primary aldosteronism, secondary aldosteronism, pseudoprimary aldosteronism. Table E6 differentiates the various causes of hyperaldosteronism.
Decreased in:
Patients with hypertension: Diabetes mellitus; Turner syndrome; acute alcohol intoxication; excess secretion of deoxycorticosterone, corticosterone, and 18-hydroxycorticosterone
Patients without hypertension: Addison disease, hypoaldosteronism resulting from renin deficiency, isolated aldosterone deficiency. Table E7 differentiates the various causes of hypoaldosteronism.

ALKALINE PHOSPHATASE (ALP) (SERUM)

See Fig. E4 for investigating a raised ALP in general practice.
    See Fig. E5 for an approach to elevated ALP.
Normal range: 30 to 120 U/L (0.5 to 2 μkat/L [CF:0.01667; SMI: 0.1 μkat/L])
Elevated in: LIVER AND BILIARY TRACT ORIGIN
Extrahepatic bile duct obstruction
Intrahepatic biliary obstruction
Liver cell acute injury
Liver passive congestion
Drug-induced liver cell dysfunction
Space-occupying lesions
Primary biliary cirrhosis
Sepsis
BONE ORIGIN (OSTEOBLAST HYPERACTIVITY)
Physiologic (rapid) bone growth (childhood and adolescence)
Metastatic tumor with osteoblastic reaction
Fracture healing
Paget disease of bone
CAPILLARY ENDOTHELIAL ORIGIN
Granulation tissue formation (active)
PLACENTAL ORIGIN
Pregnancy
Some parenteral albumin preparations
OTHER
Thyrotoxicosis
Benign transient hyperphosphatasemia
Primary hyperparathyroidism
Decreased in: Hypothyroidism, pernicious anemia, hypophosphatemia, hypervitaminosis D, malnutrition

ALPHA-1-ANTITRYPSIN (SERUM)

Normal range: 110 to 140 mg/dl
Decreased in: Homozygous or heterozygous deficiency

ALPHA-1-FETOPROTEIN (SERUM)

See "α-1 FETOPROTEIN"

ALT

See "ALANINE AMINOTRANSFERASE"

ALUMINUM (SERUM)

Normal range: 0 to 6 ng/ml
Elevated in: Chronic renal failure on dialysis, parenteral nutrition, industrial exposure

AMA

See "ANTIMITOCHONDRIAL ANTIBODY"

AMEBIASIS SEROLOGIC TEST

Test description: Test is used to support the diagnosis of amebiasis caused by *Entamoeba histolytica*. Serum acute and convalescent titers are drawn 1 to 3 wk apart. A fourfold increase in titer is the most indicative result.

AMINOLEVULINIC ACID (δ-ALA) (24-H URINE COLLECTION)

Normal: 1.5 to 7.5 mg/day
Elevated in: Acute porphyrias, lead poisoning, DKA, pregnancy, anticonvulsant drugs, hereditary tyrosinemia
Decreased in: Alcoholic liver disease

AMMONIA (SERUM)

See Box E1 for the differential diagnosis of hyperammonemia.
    See Fig. E6 for an approach to hyperammonemia in pediatric patients.
Normal range: 10 to 80 μg/dl (5 to 50 μmol/L [CF: 0.5872; SMI: 5 μmol/L])
Elevated in: Hepatic failure, hepatic encephalopathy, Reye syndrome, portacaval shunt, drugs (diuretics, polymyxin B, methicillin)
Decreased in: Drugs (neomycin, lactulose, tetracycline), renal failure

AMYLASE (SERUM)

Normal range: 0 to 130 U/L (0 to 2.17 μkat/L [CF: 0.01667; SMI: 0.01 μkat/L])
Elevated in: Acute pancreatitis, pancreatic neoplasm, abscess, pseudocyst, ascites, macroamylasemia, perforated peptic ulcer, intestinal obstruction, intestinal infarction, acute cholecystitis, appendicitis, ruptured ectopic pregnancy, salivary gland inflammation, peritonitis, burns, diabetic ketoacidosis, renal insufficiency, drugs (morphine), carcinomatosis (of lung, esophagus, ovary), acute ethanol ingestion, mumps, prostate tumors, postendoscopic retrograde cholangiopancreatography, bulimia, anorexia nervosa (Table E8)
Decreased in: Advanced chronic pancreatitis, hepatic necrosis, cystic fibrosis

AMYLASE, URINE

See "URINE AMYLASE"

AMYLOID A PROTEIN (SERUM)

Normal: <10 mcg/ml
Elevated in: Inflammatory disorders (acute phase-reacting protein), infections, acute coronary syndrome, malignancies

ANA

See "ANTINUCLEAR ANTIBODY"

ANCA

See "ANTINEUTROPHIL CYTOPLASMIC ANTIBODY"

ANDROSTENEDIONE (SERUM)

Normal:
Male: 75 to 205 ng/dl
Female: 85 to 275 ng/dl
Elevated in: Congenital adrenal hyperplasia, polycystic ovary syndrome, ectopic ACTH-producing tumor, Cushing syndrome, hirsutism, hyperplasia of ovarian stroma, ovarian neoplasm
Decreased in: Ovarian failure, adrenal failure, sickle cell anemia

ANGIOTENSIN II

Normal: 10 to 60 pg/ml
Elevated in: Hypertension, congestive heart failure (CHF), cirrhosis, renin-secreting renal tumor, volume depletion
Decreased in: ACE inhibitor drugs, angiotensin-converting enzyme inhibitor (ARB) drugs, primary aldosteronism, Cushing syndrome

Laboratory Tests

IV

ANGIOTENSIN-CONVERTING ENZYME (ACE LEVEL)

Normal range: <40 nmol/ml/min (<670 nkat/L [CF: 16.67; SMI: 10 nkat/L])
Elevated in: Sarcoidosis, primary biliary cirrhosis, alcoholic liver disease, hyperthyroidism, hyperparathyroidism, diabetes mellitus, amyloidosis, multiple myeloma, lung disease (asbestosis, silicosis, berylliosis, allergic alveolitis, coccidioidomycosis), Gaucher disease, leprosy

ANH

See "ATRIAL NATRIURETIC HORMONE"

ANION GAP (AG)

The AG is the net change difference between the cations Na^+, K^+, and the anions Cl^- and HCO_3^-.
    See Fig. E7 for charge balance in blood plasma.
    See Tables E9, E10, and E11.
Normal range: 9 to 14 mEq/L
Elevated in: Lactic acidosis, ketoacidosis (diabetes, alcoholic starvation), uremia (chronic renal failure), ingestion of toxins (paraldehyde, methanol, salicylates, ethylene glycol), hyperosmolar nonketotic coma, antibiotics (carbenicillin)
Decreased in: Hypoalbuminemia, severe hypermagnesemia, IgG myeloma, lithium toxicity, laboratory error (falsely decreased sodium or overestimation of bicarbonate or chloride), hypercalcemia of parathyroid origin, antibiotics (e.g., polymyxin)

ANTICARDIOLIPIN ANTIBODY (ACA)

Normal range: Negative. Test includes detection of IgG, IgM, and IgA antibodies to phospholipid, cardiolipin
Present in: Antiphospholipid antibody syndrome, chronic hepatitis C

ANTICOAGULANT

See "CIRCULATING ANTICOAGULANT"

ANTIDIURETIC HORMONE

Normal range: mOsm/kg 295 to 300 (4 to 12 pg/ml)
Elevated in: SIADH, antipsychotic medications, ectopic ADH from systemic neoplasm, Guillain-Barré syndrome, central nervous system (CNS) infections, brain tumors, nephrogenic diabetes insipidus
Decreased in: Central diabetes insipidus, nephritic syndrome, psychogenic polydipsias, demeclocycline, lithium, phenytoin, alcohol. Table E12 describes the water deprivation test used for diagnosing and classifying diabetes insipidus. Table E13 summarizes tests in the differential diagnosis of water homeostasis. Causes of polyuria due to water diuresis are described in Box E2.

ANTI-DNA

Normal range: Absent
Present in: Systemic lupus erythematosus, chronic active hepatitis, infectious mononucleosis, biliary cirrhosis

ANTI-DS DNA

Normal: <25 U
Elevated in: Systemic lupus erythematosus

ANTIGLOBULIN TEST

See "DIRECT ANTIGLOBULIN (COOMBS DIRECT)"
See "INDIRECT ANTIGLOBULIN (COOMBS INDIRECT)"

ANTIGLOMERULAR BASEMENT ANTIBODY

See "GLOMERULAR BASEMENT MEMBRANE ANTIBODY"

ANTIHISTONE

Normal: <1 U
Elevated in: Drug-induced lupus erythematosus

ANTIMITOCHONDRIAL ANTIBODY (AMA, MITOCHONDRIAL ANTIBODY)

Normal range: <1:20 titer
Elevated in: Primary biliary cirrhosis (85% to 95%), chronic active hepatitis (25% to 30%), cryptogenic cirrhosis (25% to 30%)

ANTINEUTROPHIL CYTOPLASMIC ANTIBODY (ANCA)

Positive test: Cytoplasmic pattern (c-ANCA): Positive in granulomatosis with polyangiitis (see Fig. E8 and Table E14 for approach to patient with positive c-ANCA)
Perinuclear pattern (p-ANCA): Positive in inflammatory bowel disease, primary biliary cirrhosis, primary sclerosing cholangitis, autoimmune chronic active hepatitis, crescentic glomerulonephritis (see Table E14 for approach to patient with positive p-ANCA)

ANTINUCLEAR ANTIBODY (ANA)

Fig. E9 describes an algorithm for the use of antinuclear antibodies in the diagnosis of connective tissue disorders. See Fig. E10 for approach to positive ANA pattern. Table E15 shows the frequency of antinuclear antibodies in autoimmune and nonrheumatic diseases.
Normal range: <1:20 titer
Positive test: Systemic lupus erythematosus (more significant if titer >1:160), drugs (phenytoin, ethosuximide, primidone, methyldopa, hydralazine, carbamazepine, penicillin, procainamide, chlorpromazine, griseofulvin, thiazides), chronic active hepatitis, autoimmune thyroid disease (positive ANA is found in up to 45% of patients), idiopathic thrombocytopenic purpura, multiple sclerosis, rheumatoid arthritis, scleroderma, mixed connective tissue disease, necrotizing vasculitis, Sjögren syndrome, tuberculosis, pulmonary interstitial fibrosis. Positive ANA results are nonspecific and can be found in healthy individuals (13.8% of the adult general population). Table E16 describes diseases associated with ANA subtypes. Fig. 11 illustrates various fluorescent ANA test patterns.

ANTI-RNP ANTIBODY

See "EXTRACTABLE NUCLEAR ANTIGEN"

ANTI-SCL-70

Normal: Absent
Elevated in: Scleroderma

ANTI-SM (ANTI-SMITH) ANTIBODY

See "EXTRACTABLE NUCLEAR ANTIGEN"

ANTI-SMOOTH MUSCLE ANTIBODY

See "SMOOTH MUSCLE ANTIBODY"

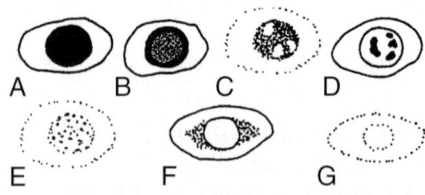

FIG. 11 Fluorescent antinuclear antibody test patterns (HEP-2 cells). A, Solid (homogeneous). **B,** Peripheral (rim). **C,** Speckled. **D,** Nucleolar. **E,** Anticentromere. **F,** Antimitochondrial. **G,** Normal (nonreactive).

ANTISTREPTOLYSIN O TITER (STREPTOZYME, ASLO TITER)

Normal range for adults: <160 Todd units
Elevated in: Streptococcal upper airway infection, acute rheumatic fever, acute glomerulonephritis, increased levels of β-lipoprotein

NOTE: A fourfold increase in titer between acute and convalescent specimens is diagnostic of streptococcal upper airway infection regardless of the initial titer.

ANTITHROMBIN III

See Table E17.
Normal range: 81% to 120% of normal activity; 17 to 30 mg/dl
Decreased in: Hereditary deficiency of antithrombin III, disseminated intravascular coagulation, pulmonary embolism, cirrhosis, thrombolytic therapy, chronic liver failure, postsurgery, third trimester of pregnancy, oral contraceptives, nephrotic syndrome, IV heparin >3 days, sepsis, acute leukemia, carcinoma, thrombophlebitis
Elevated in: Warfarin drugs, postmyocardial infarction

APOLIPOPROTEIN A-1 (APO A-1)

Normal: Desirable >120 mg/dl
Elevated in: Familial hyperalphalipoproteinemia, statins, niacin, estrogens, weight loss, familial cholesteryl ester transfer protein (CETP) deficiency
Decreased in: Familial hypoalphalipoproteinemia, Tangier disease, diuretics, androgens, cigarette smoking, hepatocellular disorders, chronic renal failure, nephritic syndrome, coronary heart disease, cholestasis

APOLIPOPROTEIN B (APO B)

Normal: Desirable <100 mg/dl; high risk >120 mg/dl
Elevated in: High saturated fat diet, high-cholesterol diet, hyperapobetalipoproteinemia, familial combined hyperlipidemia, anabolic steroids, diuretics, β-blockers, corticosteroids, progestins, diabetes, hypothyroidism, chronic renal failure, liver disease, Cushing syndrome, coronary heart disease
Decreased in: Statins, niacin, low-cholesterol diet, malnutrition, abetalipoproteinemia, hypobetalipoproteinemia, hyperthyroidism

ARTERIAL BLOOD GASES

Normal range:
Po_2: 75 to 100 mm Hg
Pco_2: 35 to 45 mm Hg
HCO_3^-: 24 to 28 mEq/L
pH: 7.35 to 7.45
Abnormal values: Acid-base disturbances (see the following)
METABOLIC ACIDOSIS
Causes of metabolic acidosis by net acid excretion are summarized in Box E3.
RESPIRATORY ACIDOSIS
Pulmonary disease (chronic obstructive pulmonary disease [COPD], severe pneumonia, pulmonary edema, interstitial fibrosis)
Airway obstruction (foreign body, severe bronchospasm, laryngospasm)
Thoracic cage disorders (pneumothorax, flail chest, kyphoscoliosis)
Defects in muscles of respiration (myasthenia gravis, hypokalemia, muscular dystrophy)
Defects in peripheral nervous system (amyotrophic lateral sclerosis, poliomyelitis, Guillain-Barré syndrome, botulism, tetanus, organophosphate poisoning, spinal cord injury)
Depression of respiratory center (anesthesia, narcotics, sedatives, vertebral artery embolism or thrombosis, increased intracranial pressure)
Failure of mechanical ventilator
METABOLIC ALKALOSIS
Divided into chloride-responsive (urinary chloride <15 mEq/L) and chloride-resistant forms (urinary chloride level >15 mEq/L)
CHLORIDE-RESPONSIVE
Vomiting
Nasogastric (NG) suction
Diuretics
Posthypercapnic alkalosis
Stool losses (laxative abuse, cystic fibrosis, villous adenoma)
Massive blood transfusion
Exogenous alkali administration

CHLORIDE-RESISTANT
Hyperadrenocorticoid states (Cushing syndrome, primary hyperaldosteronism, secondary mineralocorticoidism [licorice, chewing tobacco])
Hypomagnesemia
Hypokalemia
Bartter syndrome
RESPIRATORY ALKALOSIS
Hypoxemia (pneumonia, pulmonary embolism, atelectasis, high-altitude living)
Drugs (salicylates, xanthines, progesterone, epinephrine, thyroxine, nicotine)
CNS disorders (tumor, cerebrovascular accident [CVA], trauma, infections)
Psychogenic hyperventilation (anxiety, hysteria)
Hepatic encephalopathy
Gram-negative sepsis
Hyponatremia
Sudden recovery from metabolic acidosis
Assisted ventilation

ARTHROCENTESIS FLUID

Reference intervals for synovial fluid constituents are described in Table 18. Also see Fig. E12.
Interpretation of results:
1. **Color:** Normally it is clear or pale yellow; cloudiness indicates inflammatory process or presence of crystals, cell debris, fibrin, or triglycerides.
2. **Viscosity:** Normally it has a high viscosity because of hyaluronate; when fluid is placed on a slide, it can be stretched to a string >2 cm in length before separating (low viscosity indicates breakdown of hyaluronate [lysosomal enzymes from leukocytes] or the presence of edema fluid).
3. **Mucin clot:** Add 1 ml of fluid to 5 ml of a 5% acetic acid solution and allow 1 min for the clot to form; a firm clot (does not fragment on shaking) is normal and indicates the presence of large molecules of hyaluronic acid (this test is nonspecific and infrequently done).
4. **Glucose:** Normally it approximately equals serum glucose level; a difference of more than 40 mg/dl is suggestive of infection.
5. **Protein:** Total protein concentration is <2.5 g/dl in the normal synovial fluid; it is elevated in inflammatory and septic arthritis.
6. Microscopic examination for crystals.
   a. **Gout:** Monosodium urate crystals
   b. **Pseudogout:** Calcium pyrophosphate dihydrate crystals

ASO TITER

See "ANTISTREPTOLYSIN O TITER"

ASPARTATE AMINOTRANSFERASE (AST, SGOT)

Normal range: 0 to 35 U/L (0 to 0.58 µkat/L [CF: 0.01667, SMI: 0.01µkat/L])
Elevated in: *HEART*
Acute myocardial infarction
Pericarditis (active—some cases)
LIVER
Hepatitis virus, Epstein-Barr, or cytomegalovirus infection
Active cirrhosis
Liver passive congestion or hypoxia
Alcohol- or drug-induced liver dysfunction
Space-occupying lesions (active)
Fatty liver (severe)
Extrahepatic biliary obstruction (early)
Drug-induced
SKELETAL MUSCLE
Acute skeletal muscle injury
Muscle inflammation (infectious or noninfectious)
Muscular dystrophy (active)
Recent surgery
Delirium tremens
KIDNEY
Acute injury or damage
Renal infarct

IV

Laboratory Tests

TABLE 18 Reference Intervals for Synovial Fluid Constituents

Constituent	Synovial Fluid	Plasma
Total protein	1-3 g/dl	6-8 g/dl
Albumin	55%-70%	50%-65%
α1-Globulin	6%-8%	3%-5%
α2-Globulin	5%-7%	7%-13%
β-Globulin	8%-10%	8%-14%
γ-Globulin	10%-14%	12%-22%
Hyaluronic acid	0.3-0.4 g/dl	
Glucose	70-110 mg/dl	70-110 mg/dl
Uric acid	2-8 mg/dl	2-8 mg/dl
Lactate	9-29 mg/dl	9-29 mg/dl

From McPherson RA, Pincus MR (eds): *Henry's clinical diagnosis and management by laboratory methods,* ed 23, Philadelphia, 2017, Elsevier.

OTHER
Intestinal infarction
Shock
Cholecystitis
Acute pancreatitis
Hypothyroidism
Heparin therapy (60% to 80% of cases)
Fig. E2 describes an approach to the evaluation of AST elevation.
Box E5 describes causes of elevated serum aminotransferase levels.

ATRIAL NATRIURETIC HORMONE (ANH)
Normal: 20 to 77 pg/ml
Elevated in: CHF, volume overload, cardiovascular disease with high filling pressure
Decreased with: Prazosin and other alpha blockers

B-TYPE NATRIURETIC PEPTIDE (BNP)
Normal range: Up to 100 mcg/L. Natriuretic peptides are secreted to regulate fluid volume, blood pressure, and electrolyte balance. They have activity in both the central and peripheral nervous systems. In humans the main source of circulatory BNP is the heart ventricles.
Elevated in: Heart failure. This test is useful to differentiate heart failure patients from those with chronic obstructive pulmonary disease presenting with dyspnea. Levels are also increased in asymptomatic left ventricular dysfunction, arterial and pulmonary hypertension, cardiac hypertrophy, valvular heart disease, arrhythmia, and acute coronary syndrome. See Fig. 13.

BASOPHIL COUNT
Key causes of basophilia are summarized in Box 6.
Normal range: 0.4% to 1% of total white blood cells (WBCs); 40 to 100/mm^3
Elevated in: Leukemia, inflammatory processes, polycythemia vera, Hodgkin lymphoma, hemolytic anemia, after splenectomy, myeloid metaplasia, myxedema
Decreased in: Stress, hypersensitivity reaction, steroids, pregnancy, hyperthyroidism, postirradiation

BICARBONATE
Normal:
Arterial: 21 to 28 mEq/L
Venous: 22 to 29 mEq/L
Elevated in: Metabolic alkalosis, compensated respiratory acidosis, diuretics, corticosteroids, laxative abuse
Decreased in: Metabolic acidosis, compensated respiratory alkalosis, acetazolamide, cyclosporine, cholestyramine, methanol or ethylene glycol poisoning

BILE, URINE
See "URINE BILE"

BILIRUBIN, DIRECT (CONJUGATED BILIRUBIN)
Normal range: 0 to 0.2 mg/dl (0 to 4 µmol/L [CF: 17.10; SMI: 2 µmol/L])
Elevated in: Hepatocellular disease, biliary obstruction, drug-induced cholestasis, hereditary disorders (Dubin-Johnson syndrome, Rotor syndrome)

BILIRUBIN, INDIRECT (UNCONJUGATED BILIRUBIN)
Normal range: 0 to 1.0 mg/dl (2 to 18 µmol/L [CF: 17.10; SMI: 2 µmol/L])
Elevated in: Increased bilirubin production (if normal liver, serum unconjugated bilirubin is usually <4 mg/100 ml)
1. Hemolytic anemia
   a. Acquired
   b. Congenital
2. Resorption from extravascular sources
   a. Hematomas
   b. Pulmonary infarcts
3. Excessive ineffective erythropoiesis
   a. Congenital (congenital dyserythropoietic anemias)
   b. Acquired (pernicious anemia, severe lead poisoning; if present, bilirubinemia is usually mild)
4. Defective hepatic unconjugated bilirubin clearance (defective uptake or conjugation)
   a. Severe liver disease
   b. Gilbert syndrome
   c. Crigler-Najjar type I or II
   d. Drug-induced inhibition
   e. Portacaval shunt
   f. Congestive heart failure
   g. Hyperthyroidism (uncommon)

BILIRUBIN, TOTAL
See Fig. E14, Table E19, and Table E20 for evaluation of hyperbilirubinemia and liver disease.
Normal range: 0 to 1.0 mg/dl (2 to 18 µmol/L [CF: 17.10, SMI: 2 µmol/L])
Elevated in: Liver disease (hepatitis, cirrhosis, cholangitis, neoplasm, biliary obstruction, infectious mononucleosis), hereditary disorders (Gilbert disease, Dubin-Johnson syndrome), drugs (steroids, statins, niacin, acetaminophen, diphenylhydantoin, phenothiazines, penicillin, erythromycin, clindamycin, captopril, amphotericin B, sulfonamides, azathioprine, isoniazid, 5-aminosalicylic acid, allopurinol, methyldopa, indomethacin, halothane, oral contraceptives, procainamide, tolbutamide, labetalol), hemolysis, pulmonary embolism or infarct, hepatic congestion secondary to congestive heart failure

BILIRUBIN, URINE
See "URINE BILE"

BLADDER TUMOR ASSOCIATED ANTIGEN
Normal: ≤14 U/ml. Test is used to detect bladder cancer recurrence. Sensitivity 57% to 83% and specificity 68% to 72%.
Elevated in: Bladder cancer, renal stones, nephritis, UTI, hematuria, renal cancer, cystitis, recent bladder or urinary tract trauma

BLEEDING TIME (MODIFIED IVY METHOD)
See Fig. E15 for evaluation of patients with prolonged bleeding time.
Normal range: 2 to 9.5 min
Elevated in: Thrombocytopenia, capillary wall abnormalities, platelet abnormalities (Bernard-Soulier disease, Glanzmann disease), drugs (aspirin, warfarin, antiinflammatory medications, streptokinase, urokinase, dextran, β-lactam antibiotics, moxalactam), disseminated intravascular coagulation, cirrhosis, uremia, myeloproliferative disorders, von Willebrand disease
Bleeding time tests are no longer performed at many hospitals and have been replaced by the platelet function analyzer (PFA-100) assay.

BLOOD TYPE
Blood components must be serologically compatible with the recipient. ABO compatibility is the primary consideration. Transfused red cells must be compatible with recipient antibodies, and transfused plasma must be compatible with recipient red cells. Therefore, whole blood must be of identical ABO type to the recipient. Red blood cells contain a limited

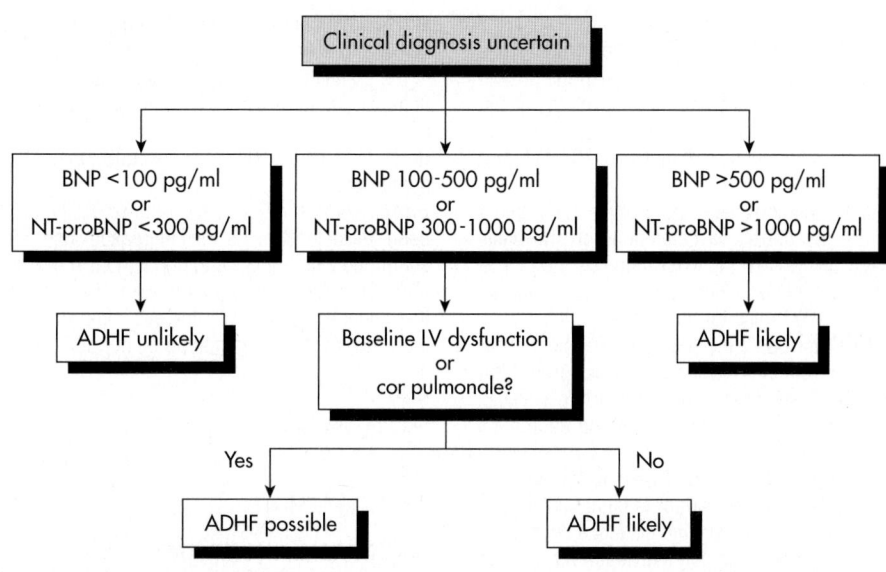

FIG. 13 Interpretation of natriuretic peptide levels. *ADHF,* Acute decompensated heart failure; *BNP,* B-type natriuretic peptide; *LV,* left ventricle; *NT-proBNP,* inactive N-terminal fragment of BNP. (From Adams JG et al: *Emergency medicine: clinical essentials,* ed 2, Philadelphia, 2013, Elsevier.)

BOX 6   Key Causes of Basophilia

Myeloproliferative disease
Allergic—food, drugs, foreign proteins
Infectious—variola, varicella
Chronic hemolytic anemia—especially postsplenectomy
Inflammatory—collagen vascular disease, ulcerative colitis

From McPherson RA, Pincus MR: *Henry's clinical diagnosis and management by laboratory methods,* ed 23, St Louis, 2017, Elsevier.

TABLE 21   ABO Compatibility

Donor Type	RECIPIENT TYPE			
	O	A	B	AB
O	R	R	R	R
	P			
A		R		R
	P	P		
B			R	R
			P	
AB				R
	P	P	P	P

P, Plasma-containing components (platelets, fresh frozen plasma) are compatible; *R,* red cells are compatible.

From McPherson RA, Pincus MR: *Henry's clinical diagnosis and management by laboratory methods,* ed 23, St Louis, 2017, Elsevier.

---

amount of plasma and need to be compatible but not necessarily identical to the ABO type of the recipient. Similarly, plasma and platelet concentrates contain few, if any, red cells. ABO-compatible blood component selection is summarized in Table 21. Red blood cells must also be negative for clinically significant antigens when transfused to alloimmunized recipients. It is highly desirable to transfuse only Rh-negative red cells to Rh-negative recipients because there is approximately a 30% risk for immunization to Rh(D). This is particularly important for women of childbearing potential because of the risk for hemolytic disease of the newborn in subsequent pregnancies. Special considerations apply to recipients of ABO-incompatible hematopoietic progenitor cell transplants. During the course of transplantation, such individuals will change their blood type.

Transfused red cells should be compatible with both donor and recipient isohemagglutinins, and transfused plasma–containing components should be compatible with both donor and recipient red cells. Thus, the optimal choice for such a patient will depend on current and expected future typing results.

BLOOD VOLUME, TOTAL

Normal range: 60 to 80 ml/kg
Elevated in: Polycythemia vera, pulmonary disease, CHF, renal insufficiency, pregnancy, acidosis, thyrotoxicosis
Decreased in: Anemia, hemorrhage, vomiting, diarrhea, dehydration, burns, starvation

BNP

See "B-TYPE NATRIURETIC PEPTIDE"

BORDETELLA PERTUSSIS SEROLOGY

Test description: Polymerase chain reaction (PCR) of nasopharyngeal aspirates or secretions is used to identify *Bordetella pertussis,* the organism responsible for whooping cough.

BRCA ANALYSIS
DESCRIPTION OF ANALYSIS
Comprehensive BRCA analysis:
BRCA1: Full sequence determination in both forward and reverse directions of approximately 5500 base pairs comprising 22 coding exons and one noncoding exon (exon 4) and approximately 800 adjacent base pairs in the noncoding intervening sequence (intron). Exon 1, which is noncoding, is not analyzed. The wild-type *BRCA1* gene encodes a protein comprising 1863 amino acids.
BRCA2: Full sequence determination in both forward and reverse directions of approximately 10,200 base pairs comprising 26 coding exons and approximately 900 adjacent base pairs in the noncoding intervening sequence (intron). Exon 1, which is noncoding, is not analyzed. The wild-type *BRCA2* gene encodes a protein comprising 3418 amino acids.
The noncoding intronic regions of *BRCA1* and *BRCA2* that are analyzed do not extend more than 20 base pairs proximal to the 5′ end and 10 base pairs distal to the 3′ end of each exon.
Single-site *BRCA* analysis: DNA sequence analysis for a specified mutation in *BRCA1* and/or *BRCA2.*
Multisite 3 *BRCA* analysis: DNA sequence analysis of specific portions of *BRCA1* exon 2, *BRCA1* exon 20, and *BRCA2* exon 11 designed to detect only mutations 187delAG and 5385insC in *BRCA1* and 6174delT in *BRCA2.*

Interpretive criteria:

"Positive for a deleterious mutation": Includes all mutations (nonsense, insertions, deletions) that prematurely terminate ("truncate") the protein product of *BRCA1* at least 10 amino acids from the C-terminus, or the protein product of *BRCA2* at least 110 amino acids from the C-terminus (based on documentation of deleterious mutations in *BRCA1* and *BRCA2*).

In addition, specific missense mutations and noncoding intervening sequence (IVS) mutations are recognized as deleterious on the basis of data derived from linkage analysis of high-risk families, functional assays, biochemical evidence, and/or demonstration of abnormal messenger ribonucleic acid (mRNA) transcript processing.

"Genetic variant, suspected deleterious": Includes genetic variants for which the available evidence indicates a likelihood, but not proof, that the mutation is deleterious. The specific evidence supporting such an interpretation will be summarized for individual variants on each such report.

"Genetic variant, favor polymorphism": Includes genetic variants for which available evidence indicates that the variant is highly unlikely to contribute substantially to cancer risk. The specific evidence supporting such an interpretation will be summarized for individual variants on each such report.

"Genetic variant of uncertain significance": Includes missense mutations and mutations that occur in analyzed intronic regions whose clinical significance has not yet been determined, as well as chain-terminating mutations that truncate *BRCA1* and *BRCA2* distal to amino acid positions 1853 and 3308, respectively.

"No deleterious mutation detected": Includes nontruncating genetic variants observed at an allele frequency of approximately 1% of a suitable control population (providing that no data suggest clinical significance), as well as all genetic variants for which published data demonstrate absence of substantial clinical significance. Also includes mutations in the protein-coding region that neither alter the amino acid sequence nor are predicted to significantly affect exon splicing, and base pair alterations in noncoding portions of the gene that have been demonstrated to have no deleterious effect on the length or stability of the mRNA transcript.

There may be uncommon genetic abnormalities in *BRCA1* and *BRCA2* that will not be detected by *BRCA* analysis. This analysis, however, is believed to rule out the majority of abnormalities in these genes, which are believed responsible for most hereditary susceptibility to breast and ovarian cancer.

"Specific variant/mutation not identified": Specific and designated deleterious mutations or variants of uncertain clinical significance are not present in the individual being tested. If one (or rarely two) specific deleterious mutations have been identified in a family member, a negative analysis for the specific mutation(s) indicates that the tested individual is at the general population risk of developing breast or ovarian cancer.

BREATH HYDROGEN TEST (HYDROGEN BREATH TEST)

Normal: This test is for bacterial overgrowth. H_2 excretion fasting: 4.6 ± 5.1, after lactulose, early increase <12. Lactulose usually results in a colonic response >30 min after ingestion.

Elevated in: A high fasting breath H_2 level and an increase of at least 12 ppm within 30 min after lactulose challenge are indicative of bacterial overgrowth in the small intestine. The increase must precede the colonic response.

False positives in: Accelerated gastric emptying, laxative use

False negatives in: Use of antibiotics and patients who are nonhydrogen producers

BUN

See "UREA NITROGEN, BLOOD"

C282Y AND H63D MUTATION ANALYSIS

Procedure: Detection of the C282Y and H63D mutations is accomplished by amplification of exons 2 and 4 of the *HFE* gene on chromosome 6 by polymerase chain reaction (PCR) followed by allele-specific hybridization

and chemiluminescent detection of hybridized probes. H63D is viewed by some as a polymorphism rather than a mutation because of its prevalence in the population, because 15% of the individuals affected with hereditary hemochromatosis (HH) are compound heterozygotes for C282Y and H63D and about 1% of patients are H63D homozygotes, which suggests that H63D may be causative in the development of the disorder at reduced penetrance.

Interpretation of results: Homozygosity for the C282Y mutation has been associated with an increased risk of being affected with HH compared with the general population. The genotype is observed in 60% to 90% of individuals affected with HH and occurs in less than 1% of the general population. However, approximately 25% of asymptomatic individuals with this genotype do not develop the disorder.

C3

See "COMPLEMENT"

C4

See "COMPLEMENT"

CALCITONIN (SERUM)

Normal range: <100 pg/ml (<100 ng/L [CF: 1; SMI: 10 ng/L])

Elevated in: Medullary carcinoma of the thyroid (particularly if level >1500 pg/ml), carcinoma of the breast, apudomas, carcinoids, renal failure, thyroiditis

CALCIUM (SERUM)

Laboratory values in various altered states of calcium metabolism are summarized in Table E22.

See Figs. E16 and E17.

Normal range: 8.8 to 10.3 mg/dl (2.2 to 2.58 µmol/L [CF: 0.2495; SMI: 0.02 µmol/L])

ELEVATED

Relatively common:

1. Neoplasia
2. Bone primary
3. Myeloma
4. Acute leukemia
5. Nonbone solid tumors
6. Breast
7. Lung
8. Squamous nonpulmonary
9. Kidney
10. Neoplasm secretion of parathyroid hormone-related protein (PTHrP, "ectopic PTH")
11. Primary hyperparathyroidism
12. Thiazide diuretics
13. Tertiary (renal) hyperparathyroidism
14. Idiopathic
15. Spurious (artifactual) hypercalcemia
16. Dehydration
17. Serum protein elevation
18. Laboratory technical problem (lab error)
19. Relatively uncommon
20. Sarcoidosis
21. Hyperthyroidism
22. Immobilization (mostly seen in children and adolescents)
23. Diuretic phase of acute renal tubular necrosis
24. Vitamin D intoxication
25. Milk-alkali syndrome
26. Addison disease
27. Lithium therapy
28. Idiopathic hypercalcemia of infancy
29. Acromegaly
30. Theophylline toxicity

Table E23 describes the laboratory differential diagnosis of hypercalcemia.

Box E7 describes the differential diagnosis of hypercalcemia in older adults.

Table E24 describes the laboratory differential diagnosis of hypocalcemia.

CALCIUM, URINE
See "URINE CALCIUM"

CANCER ANTIGEN 15-3 (CA 15-3)
Normal: <30 U/ml
Elevated in: Approximately 80% of women with metastatic breast cancer. Clinical sensitivity is 0.60, specificity 0.87, positive predictive value 0.91. This test is generally used to predict recurrence of breast cancer and evaluate response to therapy. May also be elevated in liver cancer, pancreatic cancer, ovarian cancer, colorectal cancer. Elevations can also occur with benign breast and liver disease.

CANCER ANTIGEN 27-29 (CA 27-29)
Normal: <38 U/ml
Elevated in: Approximately 75% of women with metastatic breast cancer. Clinical sensitivity is 0.57, specificity 0.97, positive predictive value 0.83, negative predictive value 0.92. This test is generally used to predict recurrence of breast cancer and evaluate response to therapy. May also be elevated in liver cancer, pancreatic cancer, ovarian cancer, colorectal cancer. Elevations can also occur with benign breast and liver disease.

CANCER ANTIGEN 72-4 (CA 72-4)
Normal: <4.0 ng/ml
Elevated in: Gastric cancer (elevated in >50% of patients). Often used in combination with CA 72-4, CA 19-9, and CEA to monitor gastric cancer after treatment.

CANCER ANTIGEN 125 (CA 125)
Normal range: <1.4%
This test uses an antibody against antigen from tissue culture of an ovarian tumor cell line. Various published evaluations report sensitivity of about 75% to 80% in patients with ovarian carcinoma. There is also an appreciable incidence of elevated values in nonovarian malignancies and in certain benign conditions (see "BENIGN" below). Test values may transiently increase during chemotherapy.

MALIGNANT
1. Epithelial ovarian carcinoma, 75% to 80% (range, 25% to 92%; better in serous than mucinous cystadenocarcinoma)
2. Endometrial carcinoma, 25% to 48% (2% to 90%)
3. Pancreatic carcinoma, 59%
4. Colorectal carcinoma, 20% (15% to 56%)
5. Endocervical adenocarcinoma, 83%
6. Squamous cervical or vaginal carcinoma, 7% to 14%
7. Lung carcinoma, 32%
8. Breast carcinoma, 12% to 40%
9. Lymphoma, 35%

BENIGN
1. Cirrhosis, 40% to 80%
2. Acute pancreatitis, 38%
3. Acute peritonitis, 75%
4. Endometriosis, 88%
5. Acute pelvic inflammatory disease, 33%
6. Pregnancy first trimester, 2% to 24%
7. During menstruation (occasionally)
8. Renal failure (?frequency)
9. Normal persons, 0.6% to 1.4%

CAPTOPRIL STIMULATION TEST
Normal: Test performed by giving 25 mg captopril orally after overnight fast. Patient should be seated during test. After captopril, aldosterone <15 ng/dl, renin >2 ng angiotensin L/ml/h.
Interpretation of results: In patients with primary aldosteronism, plasma aldosterone remains high and plasma renin activity remains low after captopril.

CARBAMAZEPINE (TEGRETOL)
Normal therapeutic range: 4 to 12 mcg/ml

TABLE 25 Carbamazepine (Tegretol)

Purpose	Treatment of Generalized Tonic-Clonic Seizures, Simple Partial Seizures, Complex Partial Seizures, Trigeminal Neuralgia, and Glossopharyngeal Neuralgia
General adult dose	Oral: 0.8-1.2 g/day maintenance for seizure control; 0.2-1.2 g/day for neuralgia
Usual bioavailability	70%
Half-life	Initially approximately 35 h; approximately 8-20 h after 3-4 wk of administration
General therapeutic range	4-12 mcg/ml
General toxic level	>12 mcg/ml
Transport	60%-70% plasma protein bound
Metabolism	Hepatic: Carbamazepine-10,11-epoxide (active); carbamazepine-10,11-transdihydrodiol (inactive)
Elimination	1%-2% unchanged in urine
Steady state	3-7 days
Mechanism of action	Decreases sodium and calcium ion influx into repeatedly depolarizing CNS neurons; reduces excitatory synaptic transmission in the spinal trigeminal nucleus
Toxic effects	Drowsiness, ataxia, dizziness, nausea, vomiting, involuntary movements, abnormal reflexes, irregular pulse

CNS, Central nervous system.
From McPherson RA, Pincus MR: *Henry's clinical diagnosis and management by laboratory methods*, ed 23, St Louis, 2017, Elsevier.

CARBAMAZEPINE LEVEL
Therapeutic range and general information are summarized in Table 25.

CARBOHYDRATE ANTIGEN 19-9
Normal: <37.0 U/ml
Elevated in: GI cancer, most frequently pancreatic cancer. Amount of elevation has no relation to tumor mass. Elevations can also occur with cirrhosis, cholangitis, and chronic or acute pancreatitis.

CARBON DIOXIDE, PARTIAL PRESSURE
Normal:
Male: 35 to 48 mm Hg
Female: 32 to 45 mm Hg
Elevated in: Respiratory acidosis
Decreased in: Respiratory alkalosis

CARBON MONOXIDE
See "CARBOXYHEMOGLOBIN"

CARBOXYHEMOGLOBIN
Normal range: Saturation of hemoglobin <2%; smokers <9%
Elevated in: Smoking, exposure to smoking, exposure to automobile exhaust fumes, malfunctioning gas-burning appliances

CARCINOEMBRYONIC ANTIGEN (CEA)
Normal range:
Nonsmokers: 0 to 2.5 ng/ml (0 to 2.5 µg/L [CF: 1; SMI: 0.1 µg/L])
Smokers: 0 to 5 ng/ml (0 to 5 µg/L [CF: 1; SMI: 0.1 µg/L])
Elevated in:
Colorectal carcinomas,* pancreatic carcinomas, and metastatic disease (usually produce higher elevations: >20 ng/ml)
Carcinomas of the esophagus, stomach, small intestine, liver, breast, ovary, lung, and thyroid (usually produce lesser elevations)

*To detect colorectal cancer, the sensitivity of CEA ranges from 68% for a threshold of 10 mcg/L to 82% for a threshold of 2.5 mcg/L, and the specificity ranges from 97% for a threshold of 10 mcg/L to 80% for a threshold of 2.6 mcg/L.

Laboratory Tests

IV

Benign conditions (smoking, inflammatory bowel disease, hypothyroidism, cirrhosis, pancreatitis, infections) (usually produce levels <10 ng/ml)

CAROTENE (SERUM)

Normal range: 50 to 250 µg/dl (0.9 to 4.6 µmol/L [CF: 0.01863; SMI: 0.1 µmol/L])
Elevated in: Carotenemia, chronic nephritis, diabetes mellitus, hypothyroidism, nephrotic syndrome, hyperlipidemia
Decreased in: Fat malabsorption, steatorrhea, pancreatic insufficiency, lack of carotenoids in diet, high fever, liver disease

CATECHOLAMINES, URINE

See "URINE CATECHOLAMINES"

CBC

See "COMPLETE BLOOD COUNT"

CD40 LIGAND

Normal: <5 mcg/L. CD40 ligand is a soluble protein that is shed from activated leukocytes and platelets and used in risk stratification for acute coronary syndrome.
Elevated in: Acute coronary syndrome. Increased CD40 ligand is associated with higher incidence of death or nonfatal myocardial infarction (MI).

CD4+ T-LYMPHOCYTE COUNT (CD4+ T CELLS)

Calculated as total WBC × % lymphocytes × % lymphocytes stained with CD4.

This test is used primarily to evaluate immune dysfunction in HIV infection. It is useful as a prognostic indicator and as a criterion for initiating prophylaxis for several opportunistic infections that are sequelae of HIV infection. Progressive depletion of CD4+ T lymphocytes is associated with an increased likelihood of clinical complications (Table E26).

CEA

See "CARCINOEMBRYONIC ANTIGEN"

CEREBROSPINAL FLUID (CSF)

Adult lumbar CSF reference values are summarized in Table 27. CSF proteins in various central nervous system diseases are described in Table E28.

Interpretation of results:
1. Appearance of the fluid.
2. Clear: Normal.
3. Yellow color (xanthochromia) in the supernatant of centrifuged CSF within ≤1 h after collection is usually the result of previous bleeding (subarachnoid hemorrhage); it may also be caused by increased CSF protein, melanin from meningeal melanosarcomas, or carotenoids.
4. Pinkish color is usually the result of a bloody tap; the color generally clears progressively from tubes 1 to 4 (the supernatant is usually crystal clear in traumatic taps).
5. Turbidity usually indicates the presence of leukocytes (bleeding introduces approximately 1 WBC/500 RBCs into the CSF).
6. CSF pressure: Elevated pressure can be seen with meningitis, meningoencephalitis, pseudotumor cerebri, mass lesions, and intracerebral bleeding.
7. Cell count: In the adult the CSF is normally free of cells (although up to five mononuclear cells/mm^3 is considered normal); the presence of granulocytes is never normal.
   Neutrophils: Seen in bacterial meningitis, early viral meningoencephalitis, and early tuberculosis (TB) meningitis. Box 8 summarizes causes of increased CSF neutrophils.
   Increased lymphocytes: TB meningitis, viral meningoencephalitis, syphilitic meningoencephalitis, fungal meningitis. Causes of CSF lymphocytosis are summarized in Box 9.
   CSF plasmacytosis: Box 10 describes inflammatory and infectious causes of CSF plasmacytosis.
   CSF eosinophilia: Causes of CSF eosinophilic pleocytosis are summarized in Box 11.
   Protein: Serum proteins are generally too large to cross the normal blood-CSF barrier; however, increased CSF protein is seen with meningeal inflammation, traumatic tap, increased CNS synthesis,

---

TABLE 27   Adult Lumbar CSF Reference Values

Analyte	Conventional Units	SI Units
Protein	15-60 mg/dl	0.15-0.60 g/L
Prealbumin	2%-7%	
Albumin	56%-76%	
α_1-Globulin	2%-7%	
α_2-Globulin	4%-12%	
β-Globulin	8%-18%	
γ-Globulin	3%-12%	
Electrolytes		
Osmolality	280-300 mOsm/L	280-300 mmol/L
Sodium	135-150 mEq/L	135-150 mmol/L
Potassium	2.6-3.0 mEq/L	2.6-3.0 mmol/L
Chloride	115-130 mEq/L	115-130 mmol/L
Carbon dioxide	20-25 mEq/L	20-25 mmol/L
Calcium	2.0-2.8 mEq/L	1.0-1.4 mmol/L
Magnesium	2.4-3.0 mEq/L	1.2-1.5 mmol/L
Lactate	10-22 mg/dl	1.1-2.4 mmol/L
pH		
Lumbar fluid	7.28-7.32	
Cisternal fluid	7.32-7.34	
pCO$_2$		
Lumbar fluid	44-50 mm Hg	
Cisternal fluid	40-46 mm Hg	
pO$_2$	40-44 mm Hg	
Other Constituents		
Ammonia	10-35 µg/dl	6-20 µmol/L
Glutamine	5-20 mg/dl	0.3-1.4 mmol/L
Creatinine	0.6-1.2 mg/dl	45-92 µmol/L
Glucose	50-80 mg/dl	2.8-4.4 mmol/L
Iron	1-2 µg/dl	0.2-0.4 µmol/L
Phosphorus	1.2-2.0 mg/dl	0.4-0.7 mmol/L
Total lipid	1-2 mg/dl	0.01-0.02 g/L
Urea	6-16 mg/dl	2.0-5.7 mmol/L
Urate	0.5-3.0 mg/dl	30-180 µmol/L
Zinc	2-6 µg/dl	0.3-0.9 µmol/L

CSF, Cerebrospinal fluid; *pCO$_2$,* partial pressure of carbon dioxide; *pO$_2$,* partial pressure of oxygen.
From McPherson RA, Pincus MR: *Henry's clinical diagnosis and management by laboratory methods,* ed 23, St Louis, 2017, Elsevier.

BOX 8   Causes of Increased CSF Neutrophils

Meningitis
  Bacterial meningitis
  Early viral meningoencephalitis
  Early tuberculous meningitis
  Early mycotic meningitis
  Amebic encephalomyelitis
Other infections
  Cerebral abscess
  Subdural empyema
  AIDS-related CMV radiculopathy
Following seizures
Following CNS hemorrhage
  Subarachnoid
  Intracerebral
Following CNS infarct
Reaction to repeated lumbar punctures
Injection of foreign material in subarachnoid space (e.g., methotrexate, contrast media)
Metastatic tumor in contact with CSF

AIDS, Acquired immunodeficiency virus; *CMV,* cytomegalovirus; *CNS,* central nervous system; *CSF,* cerebrospinal fluid.
From McPherson RA, Pincus MR: *Henry's clinical diagnosis and management by laboratory methods,* ed 23, St Louis, 2017, Elsevier.

BOX 9   Causes of CSF Lymphocytosis

Meningitis
Viral meningitis
Tuberculous meningitis
Fungal meningitis
Syphilitic meningoencephalitis
Leptospiral meningitis
Bacterial due to uncommon organisms
Early bacterial meningitis where leukocyte counts are relatively low
Parasitic infestations (e.g., cysticercosis, trichinosis, toxoplasmosis)
Aseptic meningitis due to septic focus adjacent to meninges

Degenerative Disorders
Subacute sclerosing panencephalitis
Multiple sclerosis
Drug abuse encephalopathy
Guillain-Barré syndrome
Acute disseminated encephalomyelitis

Other Inflammatory Disorders
HaNDL syndrome (headache with neurologic deficits and CSF lymphocytosis)
Sarcoidosis
Polyneuritis
CNS periarteritis

CNS, Central nervous system; *CSF,* cerebrospinal fluid.
From McPherson RA, Pincus MR: *Henry's clinical diagnosis and management by laboratory methods,* ed 23, St Louis, 2017, Elsevier.

BOX 10   Inflammatory and Infectious Causes of CSF Plasmacytosis

Guillain-Barré syndrome
Multiple sclerosis
Parasitic CNS infestations
Sarcoidosis
Subacute sclerosing panencephalitis
Syphilitic meningoencephalitis
Tuberculous meningitis
Acute viral infections

CNS, Central nervous system; *CSF,* cerebrospinal fluid.
From McPherson RA, Pincus MR: *Henry's clinical diagnosis and management by laboratory methods,* ed 23, St Louis, 2017, Elsevier.

BOX 11   Causes of CSF Eosinophilic Pleocytosis

Commonly Associated With
Acute polyneuritis
CNS reaction to foreign material (drugs, shunts)
Fungal infections
Idiopathic eosinophilic meningitis
Idiopathic hypereosinophilic syndrome
Parasitic infections

Infrequently Associated With
Bacterial meningitis
Leukemia/lymphoma
Myeloproliferative disorders
Neurosarcoidosis
Primary brain tumors
Tuberculous meningoencephalitis
Viral meningitis

CNS, Central nervous system; *CSF,* cerebrospinal fluid.
Modified from Kjeldsberg CR, Knight JA: *Body fluids: laboratory examination of amniotic, cerebrospinal, seminal, serous and synovial fluids,* ed 3, Chicago, 1993, American Society for Clinical Pathology, with permission. In McPherson RA, Pincus MR: *Henry's clinical diagnosis and management by laboratory methods,* ed 23, St Louis, 2017, Elsevier.

---

tissue degeneration, obstruction to CSF circulation, and Guillain-Barré syndrome. Mean concentrations of plasma and CSF proteins are summarized in Table E29. Conditions associated with increased CSF total protein are summarized in Box 12.

Glucose: Decreased glucose is seen with bacterial meningitis, TB meningitis, fungal meningitis, subarachnoid hemorrhage, and some cases of viral meningitis.

A mild increase in CSF glucose can be seen in patients with very elevated serum glucose levels.

Table E30 describes CSF findings in infectious and inflammatory diseases of the central nervous system and meninges.

Causes of xanthochromia are summarized in Table E31.

CERULOPLASMIN (SERUM)

Normal range: 20 to 35 mg/dl (200 to 350 mg/L [CF: 10; SMI: 10 mg/L])
Elevated in: Pregnancy, estrogens, oral contraceptives, neoplastic diseases (leukemias, Hodgkin lymphoma, carcinomas), inflammatory states, systemic lupus erythematosus, primary biliary cirrhosis, rheumatoid arthritis
Decreased in: Wilson disease (values often <10 mg/dl), nephrotic syndrome, advanced liver disease, malabsorption, total parenteral nutrition, Menkes syndrome

CHLAMYDIA GROUP ANTIBODY SEROLOGIC TEST

Test description: Acute and convalescent sera is drawn 2 to 4 wk apart. A fourfold increase in titer between acute and convalescent sera is necessary for confirmation. A single titer ≥1:64 is considered indicative of psittacosis or lymphogranuloma venereum (LGV).

CHLAMYDIA TRACHOMATIS PCR

Test description: Test is performed on endocervical swab, urine, and intraurethral swab (Table E32).
Normal: Negative

BOX 12   Conditions Associated With Increased CSF Total Protein

Traumatic Spinal Puncture
Increased blood-CSF permeability
Arachnoiditis (e.g., following methotrexate therapy)
Meningitis (bacterial, viral, fungal, tuberculous)
Hemorrhage (subarachnoid, intracerebral)
Endocrine/metabolic disorders
    Milk-alkali syndrome with hypercalcemia
    Diabetic neuropathy
    Hereditary neuropathies and myelopathies
    Decreased endocrine function (thyroid, parathyroid)
    Other disorders (uremia, dehydration)

Drug Toxicity
Ethanol, phenothiazines, phenytoin

CSF Circulation Defects
Mechanical obstruction (tumor, abscess, herniated disk)
Loculated CSF effusion

Increased Immunoglobulin (Ig)G Synthesis
Multiple sclerosis

Neurosyphilis
Subacute sclerosing panencephalitis

Increased IgG Synthesis and Blood-CSF Permeability
Guillain-Barré syndrome
Collagen vascular diseases (e.g., lupus, periarteritis)
Chronic inflammatory demyelinating polyradiculopathy

CNS, Central nervous system; *CSF,* cerebrospinal fluid.
From McPherson RA, Pincus MR: *Henry's clinical diagnosis and management by laboratory methods,* ed 23, St Louis, 2017, Elsevier.

Laboratory Tests

IV

CHLORIDE (SERUM)

Normal range: 95 to 105 mEq/L (95 to 105 mmol/L [CF: 1; SMI: 1 mmol/L])

Elevated in: Dehydration, excessive infusion of normal saline solution, cystic fibrosis (sweat test), hyperparathyroidism, renal tubular disease, metabolic acidosis, prolonged diarrhea, drugs (ammonium chloride administration, acetazolamide, boric acid, triamterene)

Decreased in: Congestive heart failure, syndrome of inappropriate antidiuretic hormone secretion, Addison disease, vomiting, gastric suction, salt-losing nephritis, continuous infusion of D_5W, thiazide diuretic administration, diaphoresis, diarrhea, burns, diabetic ketoacidosis

CHLORIDE (SWEAT)

Normal: 0 to 40 mmol/L

Borderline/indeterminate: 41 to 60 mmol/L

Consistent with cystic fibrosis: >60 mmol/L

False low results can occur with edema, excessive sweating, and hypoproteinemia.

CHLORIDE, URINE

See "URINE CHLORIDE"

CHOLECYSTOKININ-PANCREOZYMIN (CCK, CCK-PZ)

Normal: <80 pg/ml

Elevated in: Pancreatic disease, celiac disease, gastric ulcer, postgastrectomy, irritable bowel syndrome (IBS), fatty food intolerance

CHOLESTEROL, HIGH-DENSITY LIPOPROTEIN

See "HIGH-DENSITY LIPOPROTEIN CHOLESTEROL"

CHOLESTEROL, LOW-DENSITY LIPOPROTEIN

See "LOW-DENSITY LIPOPROTEIN CHOLESTEROL"

CHOLESTEROL, TOTAL

Normal range:

Varies with age

Generally <200 mg/dl (<5.20 mmol/L [CF: 0.02586; SMI: 0.05 mmol/L])

Elevated in: Primary hypercholesterolemia, biliary obstruction, diabetes mellitus, nephrotic syndrome, hypothyroidism, primary biliary cirrhosis, high-cholesterol diet, pregnancy third trimester, myocardial infarction, drugs (steroids, phenothiazines, oral contraceptives). Classic hyperlipidemia phenotypes are summarized in Table E33.

Decreased in: Medications (statins, niacin), starvation, malabsorption, sideroblastic anemia, thalassemia, abetalipoproteinemia, hyperthyroidism, Cushing syndrome, hepatic failure, multiple myeloma, polycythemia vera, chronic myelocytic leukemia, myeloid metaplasia, Waldenström macroglobulinemia, myelofibrosis

CHORIONIC GONADOTROPINS, HUMAN (SERUM) (hCG)

Normal range, serum:

Female, premenopausal: <0.8 IU/L; postmenopausal <3.3 IU/L

Male: <0.7 IU/L

Elevated in:

Pregnancy, choriocarcinoma, gestational trophoblastic neoplasia (including molar gestations), placental site trophoblastic tumors; human antimouse antibodies (HAMA) can produce false serum assay for hCG.

The principal use of this test is to diagnose pregnancy. The concentration of hCG increases significantly during the initial 6 wk of pregnancy.

Normal range: Varies with gestational stage:

1 wk: 5 to 50 mU/ml

1 to 2 wk: 50 to 550 mU/ml

2 to 3 wk: Up to 5000 mU/ml

3 to 4 wk: Up to 10,000 mU/ml

4 to 5 wk: Up to 50,000 mU/ml

2 to 3 mo: 10,000 to 100,000 mU/ml

Peak values approaching 100,000 IU/L occur 60 to 70 days following implantation.

hCG levels generally double every 1 to 3 days. In patients with concentration <2000 IU/L, an increase of serum hCG <66% after 2 days is suggestive of spontaneous abortion or ruptured ectopic gestation.

CHYMOTRYPSIN

Normal: <10 mcg/L

Elevated in: Acute pancreatitis, chronic renal failure, oral enzyme preparations, gastric cancer, pancreatic cancer

Decreased in: Chronic pancreatitis, late cystic fibrosis

CIRCULATING ANTICOAGULANT (LUPUS ANTICOAGULANT)

Normal: Negative

Detected in: Systemic lupus erythematosus, drug-induced lupus, long-term phenothiazine therapy, multiple myeloma, ulcerative colitis, rheumatoid arthritis, postpartum, hemophilia, neoplasms, chronic inflammatory states, AIDS, nephrotic syndrome

NOTE: The name is a misnomer because these patients are prone to hypercoagulability and thrombosis.

CK

See "CREATINE KINASE"

CLONIDINE SUPPRESSION TEST

Interpretation of results

Clonidine inhibits neurogenic catecholamine release and will cause a decrease in plasma norepinephrine into the reference interval in hypertensive subjects without pheochromocytoma. Test is performed by giving 4.3 mcg clonidine/kg orally after overnight fast. Norepinephrine is measured at 3 h. Result should be within established reference range and decrease to <50% of baseline concentration. Lack of decrease in norepinephrine is suggestive of pheochromocytoma.

CLOSTRIDIUM DIFFICILE TOXIN ASSAY (STOOL)

Normal: Negative

Detected in: Antibiotic-associated diarrhea and pseudomembranous colitis

CO

See "CARBOXYHEMOGLOBIN"

COAGULATION FACTORS

A differential diagnosis of abnormal coagulation screening tests is described in Table 34.

See Table E35 for characteristics of coagulation factors.

See Table E36 for differential diagnosis of low factor VIII.

TABLE 34 Differential Diagnosis of Abnormal Coagulation Screening Tests

Abnormal Activated Partial Thromboplastin Time (APTT) Alone

Associated with bleeding: VIII, IX, and XI defects

Not associated with bleeding: XII, prekallikrein (PK), high molecular weight kininogen, lupus anticoagulants

Abnormal Prothrombin Time (PT) Alone

Factor VII defects

Combined Abnormal APTT and PT

Medical conditions: Anticoagulants, disseminated intravascular coagulation (DIC), liver disease, vitamin K deficiency, massive transfusion

Rarely dysfibrinogenemia; factor X, V, and II defects

From McPherson RA, Pincus MR: *Henry's clinical diagnosis and management by laboratory methods*, ed 23, St Louis, 2017, Elsevier.

Factor reference ranges:

V: >10%
VII: >10%
VIII: 50% to 170%
IX: 60% to 136%
X: >10%
XI: 50% to 150%
XII: >30%

Table E37 describes screening laboratory results in coagulation factor deficiencies. Characterization of coagulation factors and their deficiencies is summarized in Table E38.

COBALAMIN, SERUM

See "VITAMIN B12"

COLD AGGLUTININS TITER

Normal range: <1:32
Elevated in:

1. Primary atypical pneumonia (*Mycoplasma* pneumonia), infectious mononucleosis, CMV infection
2. Others: Hepatic cirrhosis, acquired hemolytic anemia, frostbite, multiple myeloma, lymphoma, malaria

COMPLEMENT

Inherited deficiencies in complement and complement-related proteins are summarized in Table E39.
Normal range:
C3: 70 to 160 mg/dl (0.7 to 1.6 g/L [CF: 0.01; SMI: 0.1 g/L])
C4: 20 to 40 mg/dl (0.2 to 0.4 g/L [CF: 0.01; SMI: 0.1 g/L])
Abnormal values:
Decreased C3: Active SLE, immune complex disease, acute glomerulonephritis, inborn C3 deficiency, membranoproliferative glomerulonephritis, infective endocarditis, serum sickness, autoimmune/chronic active hepatitis
Decreased C4: Immune complex disease, active SLE, infective endocarditis, inborn C4 deficiency, hereditary angioedema, hypergammaglobulinemic states, cryoglobulinemic vasculitis
NOTE: The complement system has daunting nomenclature; accordingly, some basic definitions are given in Box 13.

COMPLETE BLOOD COUNT (CBC)

Common types of anemias and their diagnostic workups are summarized in Table 40.
See Fig. E18, which describes an algorithm for the evaluation of patients with neutropenia.

BOX 13   Definitions

Classical pathway: C1, C4, C2, C3, and the terminal components.
Alternative pathway: Factor B, factor D, properdin, and the terminal components.
Lectin activation pathway: MBL, MASP1, MASP2, C3, and the terminal components.
Anaphylatoxins: C3a, C4a, C5a. These are mediators of smooth muscle contraction, degranulation of mast cells, enhanced neutrophil aggregation, increased vascular permeability.
Opsonization: Renders a particle more easily phagocytosed.
C3 tickover: This term occasionally is used to describe spontaneous C3 hydrolysis.
Membrane attack complex (terminal components): C5, C6, C7, C8, C9.
CH50: Used to define the dilution of serum capable of lysing 50% of sensitized sheep red cells. This assay measures the intactness of the classical pathway through the terminal components.
AH50: Used to define the dilution of serum capable of lysing 50% of nonsensitized rabbit red cells. This assay measures the intactness of the alternative pathway through the terminal components.

From Adkinson NF et al: *Middleton's allergy principles and practice*, ed 8, Philadelphia, 2014, Saunders.

White blood cells 3200 to 9800/mm³ (3.2 to 9.8 × 10⁹/L [CF: 0.001; SMI: 0.1 × 10⁹/L])
Red blood cells
- Male: 4.3 to 5.9 × 10⁶/mm³ (4.3 to 5.9 × 10¹²/L [CF: 0.001; SMI: 0.1 × 10¹²/L])
- Female: 3.5 to 5 × 10⁶/mm³ (3.5 to 5 × 10¹²/L [CF: 0.001; SMI: 0.1 × 10¹²/L])

Hemoglobin
- Male: 13.6 to 17.7 g/dl (136 to 172 g/L [CF: 10; SMI: 1 g/L])
- Female: 12 to 15 g/dl (120 to 150 g/L [CF: 10; SMI: 1 g/L])

Hematocrit
- Male: 39% to 49% (0.39 to 0.49 [CF: 0.01; SMI: 0.01])
- Female: 33% to 43% (0.33 to 0.43 [CF: 0.01; SMI: 0.01])

Mean corpuscular volume (MCV): 76 to 100 μm³ (76 to 100 fL [CF: 1; SMI: 1 fL])
Mean corpuscular hemoglobin (MCH): 27 to 33 pg (27 to 33 pg [CF: 1; SMI: 1 pg])
Mean corpuscular hemoglobin concentration (MCHC): 33 to 37 g/dl (330 to 370 g/L [CF: 10; SMI: 10 g/L])
Red blood cell distribution width index (RDW): 11.5% to 14.5%
Platelet count: 130 to 400 × 10³/mm³ (130-400 × 10⁹/L [CF: 1; SMI: 5 × 10⁹/L])

TABLE 40   Common Types of Anemias and Their Diagnostic Workups[a]

Anemia	Cause	Common Laboratory Abnormality
Hypoproliferative, microcytic	Iron deficiency	Low ferritin Increased IBC Decreased serum iron Reduced Fe/TIBC ratio Generally increased RDW
Hypoproliferative, microcytic	Anemia of chronic disease	Generally high ferritin Normal IBC Decreased serum iron Normal Fe/TIBC ratio Generally normal RDW
Hyperproliferative, normocytic	Hemolytic anemia	Schistocytosis Increased reticulocytes Low haptoglobin Elevated carboxyhemoglobin Elevated LD and potassium Elevated indirect bilirubin Generally increased RDW
Hypoproliferative, normocytic	Aplastic anemia	Leukopenia Thrombocytopenia Hypocellular bone marrow Generally normal RDW
Hypoproliferative, normocytic	Renal failure	Elevated BUN and creatinine Low erythropoietin Burr cells may be present Generally normal RDW
Hypoproliferative, macrocytic		
Megaloblastic	Vitamin B₁₂ and/or folate deficiency	Low vitamin B₁₂ and/or folate Hyperlobulated polymorphonuclear leukocytes Macro-ovalocytes Increased RDW
Nonmegaloblastic	Hypothyroidism	Elevated TSH Normal RDW

BUN, Blood urea nitrogen; *Fe*, iron; *IBC*, iron-binding capacity; *LD*, lactate dehydrogenase; *RDW*, red cell distribution width; *TIBC*, total IBC; *TSH*, thyroid-stimulating hormone.
[a]Low is equivalent to depressed, and high is equivalent to elevated. Ferritin, haptoglobin, LD, bilirubin, BUN, creatinine, erythropoietin, TSH, and T4 are all expressed as concentrations. All of these analytes are measured in serum.

From McPherson RA, Pincus MR: *Henry's clinical diagnosis and management by laboratory methods*, ed 23, St Louis, 2017, Elsevier.

Differential:
- 2 to 6 stabs (bands, early mature neutrophils)
- 60 to 70 segs (mature neutrophils)
- 1 to 4 eosinophils
- 0 to 1 basophils
- 2 to 8 monocytes
- 25 to 40 lymphocytes

CONJUGATED BILIRUBIN

See "BILIRUBIN, DIRECT"

COPPER (SERUM)

Normal range: 70 to 140 µg/dl (11 to 22 µmol/L [CF: 0.1574, SMI: 0.2 µmol/L])

Decreased in: Wilson disease, Menkes syndrome, malabsorption, malnutrition, nephrosis, total parenteral nutrition, acute leukemia in remission

Elevated in: Aplastic anemia, biliary cirrhosis, systemic lupus erythematosus, hemochromatosis, hyperthyroidism, hypothyroidism, infection, iron deficiency anemia, leukemia, lymphoma, oral contraceptives, pernicious anemia, rheumatoid arthritis

COPPER, URINE

See "URINE COPPER"

CORTICOTROPIN RELEASING HORMONE (CRH) STIMULATION TEST

Normal: A dose of 0.5 mg of dexamethasone is given every 6 h for 2 days; 2 h after last dose 1 mcg/kg CRH is given IV. Samples are drawn after 15 min. Normally there is a twofold to fourfold increase in mean baseline concentration of ACTH or cortisol. Cortisol >1.4 mcg/L is virtually 100% specific and 100% diagnostic.

Interpretation of results:

Normal or exaggerated response: Pituitary Cushing disease

No response: Ectopic ACTH-secreting tumor

A positive response to CRH or a suppressed response to high-dose dexamethasone has a 97% positive predictive value for Cushing disease. However, a lack of response to either test excludes Cushing disease in only 64% to 78% of patients. When the tests are considered together, negative responses from both have a 100% predictive value for ectopic ACTH secretion.

CORTISOL, PLASMA

Normal range: Varies with time of collection (circadian variation):

8 A.M.: 4 to 19 µg/dl (110 to 520 nmol/L [CF: 27.59; SMI: 10 nmol/L])

4 P.M.: 2 to 15 µg/dl (50 to 410 nmol/L [CF: 27.59; SMI: 10 nmol/L])

Elevated in: Ectopic adrenocorticotropic hormone production (i.e., oat cell carcinoma of lung), loss of normal diurnal variation, pregnancy, chronic renal failure, iatrogenic, stress, adrenal or pituitary hyperplasia, or adenomas

Decreased in: Primary adrenocortical insufficiency, anterior pituitary hypofunction, secondary adrenocortical insufficiency, adrenogenital syndromes

COOMBS DIRECT

See "DIRECT ANTIGLOBULIN"

COOMBS INDIRECT

See "INDIRECT ANTIGLOBULIN"

COVID-19

Name: Coronavirus

Value: Not detected

Reference range: Not detected

A Not Detected (negative) test result for this test means that SARS-CoV-2 RNA was not present in the specimen above the limit of detection. A negative test does not rule out the possibility of COVID-19 and should not be used as the sole basis for treatment or patient management decisions. If COVID-19 is still suspected, based on exposure history together with other clinical findings, re-testing should be considered in consultation with public health authorities.

Laboratory test results should always be considered in the context of clinical observations and epidemiologic data in making a final diagnosis and patient management decisions.

C-PEPTIDE

Elevated in: Insulinoma, sulfonylurea administration

Decreased in: Insulin-dependent diabetes mellitus, factitious insulin administration

CPK

See "CREATINE KINASE"

C-REACTIVE PROTEIN

Normal range: 6.8 to 820 µg/dl (68 to 8200 µg/L [CF: 10; SMI: 10 µg/L])

Elevated in: Rheumatoid arthritis, rheumatic fever, inflammatory bowel disease, bacterial infections, myocardial infarction, oral contraceptives, third trimester of pregnancy (acute phase reactant), inflammatory and neoplastic diseases. Table 41 shows a comparison of erythrocyte sedimentation rate and C-reactive protein, and Table 42 shows conditions associated with elevated C-reactive protein levels.

C-REACTIVE PROTEIN, HIGH SENSITIVITY (hs-CRP, CARDIO-CRP)

This is a cardiac risk marker. It is increased in patients with silent atherosclerosis years before a cardiovascular event and is independent of cholesterol level and other lipoproteins. It can be used to help stratify cardiac risk.

Interpretation of Results:

Cardio-CRP result (mg/L)	Risk
0.6	Lowest risk
0.7-1.1	Low risk
1.2-1.9	Moderate risk
2.0-3.8	High risk
3.9-4.9	Highest risk
≥5.0	Results may be confounded by acute inflammatory disease. If clinically indicated, a repeat test should be performed in 2 or more wk

TABLE 41 Comparison of Erythrocyte Sedimentation Rate and C-Reactive Protein

	Erythrocyte Sedimentation Rate	C-Reactive Protein
Advantages	Much clinical information in the literature. May reflect overall health status	Rapid response to inflammatory stimuli. Wide range of clinically relevant values are detectable Unaffected by age and sex Reflects value of a single acute phase protein Can be measured on stored sera Quantitation is precise and reproducible
Disadvantages	Affected by age and sex Affected by red blood cell morphology Affected by anemia and polycythemia Reflects levels of many plasma proteins, not all of which are acute phase proteins Responds slowly to inflammatory stimuli Requires fresh sample May be affected by drugs	None

From Firestein GS et al: *Kelley's textbook of rheumatology*, ed 9, Philadelphia, 2013, Saunders.

TABLE 42 Conditions Associated With Elevated C-Reactive Protein Levels

Normal or Minor Elevation (<1 mg/dl)	Moderate Elevation (1-10 mg/dl)	Marked Elevation (>10 mg/dl)
Vigorous exercise	Myocardial infarction	Acute bacterial infection (80%-85%)
Common cold	Malignancies	
Pregnancy	Pancreatitis	Major trauma
Gingivitis	Mucosal infection (bronchitis, cystitis)	Systemic vasculitis
Seizures		
Depression	Most connective tissue diseases	
Insulin resistance and diabetes	Rheumatoid arthritis	
Several genetic polymorphisms		
Obesity		

From Firestein GS et al: *Kelley's textbook of rheumatology,* ed 9, Philadelphia, 2013, Saunders.

CREATINE KINASE (CK, CPK)
Fig. E19 describes a diagnostic approach to creatine kinase elevation.
Normal range: 0 to 130 U/L (0 to 2.16 µkat/L [CF: 0.01667; SMI: 0.01 µkat/L])
Elevated in: Myocardial infarction, myocarditis, rhabdomyolysis, myositis, crush injury/trauma, polymyositis, dermatomyositis, vigorous exercise, muscular dystrophy, myxedema, seizures, malignant hyperthermia syndrome, intramuscular (IM) injections, cerebrovascular accident, pulmonary embolism and infarction, acute dissection of aorta
Decreased in: Corticosteroid use, decreased muscle mass, connective tissue disorders, alcoholic liver disease, metastatic neoplasms

CREATINE KINASE ISOENZYMES
CK-BB
Elevated in: Cerebrovascular accident, subarachnoid hemorrhage, neoplasms (prostate, gastrointestinal tract, brain, ovary, breast, lung), severe shock, bowel infarction, hypothermia, meningitis
CK-MB
Elevated in: Myocardial infarction (MI), myocarditis, pericarditis, muscular dystrophy, cardiac defibrillation, cardiac surgery, extensive rhabdomyolysis, strenuous exercise (marathon runners), mixed connective tissue disease, cardiomyopathy, hypothermia
NOTE: CK-MB exists in the blood in two subforms. MB_2 is released from cardiac cells and converted in the blood to MB_1. Rapid assay of CK-MB subforms can detect MI (CK-$MB_2 \geq$ 1.0 U/L, with a ratio of CK-MB_2/CK-$MB_1 \geq$ 1.5) within 6 h of onset of symptoms.
Fig. E20 illustrates the time course of CK, AST, troponins, and lactate dehydrogenase (LDH) activity after acute MI.
CK-MM
Elevated in: Crush injury, seizures, malignant hyperthermia syndrome, rhabdomyolysis, myositis, polymyositis, dermatomyositis, vigorous exercise, muscular dystrophy, IM injections, acute dissection of aorta

CREATININE (SERUM)
Normal range: 0.6 to 1.2 mg/dl (50 to 110 µmol/L [CF: 88.4; SMI: 10 µmol/L]). Fig. E21 illustrates the relationship between creatinine clearance and serum creatinine. Factors that may alter serum creatinine level are described in Box 14.
Elevated in: Renal insufficiency (acute and chronic), decreased renal perfusion (hypotension, dehydration, congestive heart failure), urinary tract infection, rhabdomyolysis, ketonemia
Drugs (antibiotics [aminoglycosides, cephalosporins], hydantoin, diuretics, methyldopa)
The RIFLE criteria for acute kidney injury is summarized in Table E43. A classification of acute kidney injury (AKI) is described in Table E44.
Falsely elevated in: Diabetic ketoacidosis, administration of some cephalosporins (e.g., cefoxitin, cephalothin)
Decreased in: Decreased muscle mass (including amputees and older persons), pregnancy, prolonged debilitation

BOX 14 Factors That May Alter Serum Creatinine (Cr) Level

Endogenous
Reduced muscle mass: ↓
Hyperbilirubinemia: ↓
Exogenous
Medications inhibiting tubular secretion (trimethoprim, cimetidine): ↑
Medications Interfering with Laboratory Assays*
Flucytosine and cefoxitin: ↑
Catecholamines: ↓

BOX 15 Cockcroft-Gault Formula to Calculate Creatinine Clearance (C_{cr})

$$C_{cr} = \frac{(140 - \text{age in ear}) \times (\text{lean body weight in kg})}{S_{cr} \text{ in mg/dl} - 72}$$

CREATININE CLEARANCE
Normal range: 75 to 124 ml/min (1.24 to 2.08 ml/sec [CF: 0.01667; SMI: 0.02 ml/sec])
Table E45 shows equations commonly used to estimate renal clearance.
The Cockcroft-Gault formula to calculate creatinine clearance is described in Box 15.
Elevated in: Pregnancy, exercise
Decreased in: Renal insufficiency, drugs (cimetidine, procainamide, antibiotics, quinidine)

CREATININE, URINE
See "URINE CREATININE"

CRYOGLOBULINS (SERUM)
Normal range: Not detectable
Present in: Collagen vascular diseases, chronic lymphocytic leukemia, hemolytic anemias, multiple myeloma, Waldenström macroglobulinemia, chronic active hepatitis, Hodgkin disease

CRYPTOSPORIDIUM ANTIGEN BY EIA (STOOL)
Normal range: Not detected
Present in: Cryptosporidiosis

CSF
See "CEREBROSPINAL FLUID"

CYSTATIN C
Normal: Cystatin C is a cysteine protease inhibitor that is produced at a constant rate by all nucleated cells. It is freely filtered by the glomerulus and reabsorbed (but not secreted) by the renal tubules with no extrarenal excretion. Its concentration is not affected by diet, muscle mass, or acute inflammation. Normal range when measured by particle-enhanced nephelometric immunoassay (PENIA) is <0.28 mg/L.
Elevated in: Renal disorders. Good predictor of the severity of acute tubular necrosis. Cystatin C increases more rapidly than creatinine in the early stages of GFR impairment. The cystatin C concentration is an independent risk factor for heart failure in older adults and appears to provide a better measure of risk assessment than the serum creatinine concentration.

CYSTIC FIBROSIS PCR
Test description: Test can be performed on whole blood or tissue. Common mutations in the cystic fibrosis transmembrane regulator (CFTR) gene can be used to detect 75% to 80% of mutant alleles.

CYTOMEGALOVIRUS BY PCR
Test description: Test can be performed on whole blood, plasma, or tissue. Qualitative PCR is highly sensitive but may not be able to differentiate between latent and active infection.

IV

Laboratory Tests

D-DIMER

Normal range: <0.5 mcg/ml
Elevated in:
1. DVT, pulmonary embolism, high levels of rheumatoid factor, activation of coagulation and fibrolytic system from any cause
2. D-dimer assay by enzyme-linked immunosorbent assay (ELISA) assists in the diagnosis of DVT and pulmonary embolism. This test has significant limitations because it can be elevated whenever the coagulation and fibrinolytic systems are activated and can also be falsely elevated with high rheumatoid factor levels.
3. A positive D-dimer is suggestive but not diagnostic for pulmonary embolism (PE). Patients with positive D-dimer and clinical suspicion for PE need additional tests such as chest CT to confirm diagnosis.
4. PE might be ruled out in patients with negative D-dimer and low pretest probability for PE.

DEHYDROEPIANDROSTERONE SULFATE

Normal:

Males

Ages 19-30:	125-619 mcg/dl
31-50:	59-452 mcg/dl
51-60:	20-413 mcg/dl
61-83:	10-285 mcg/dl

Females

Ages 19-30:	29-781 mcg/dl
31-50:	12-379 mcg/dl
Postmenopausal:	30-260 mcg/dl

Elevated in: Hirsutism, congenital adrenal hyperplasia, adrenal carcinomas, adrenal adenomas, polycystic ovary syndrome, ectopic ACTH-producing tumors, Cushing disease, spironolactone

DEOXYCORTICOSTERONE (11-DEOXYCORTICOSTERONE, DOC) (SERUM)

Normal: 2 to 19 ng/dl. Normal secretion depends on ACTH and is suppressible by dexamethasone.
Elevated in: Adrenogenital syndromes due to 17- and 11-hydroxylase deficiencies, pregnancy
Decreased in: Preeclampsia

DEXAMETHASONE SUPPRESSION TEST, OVERNIGHT

Normal: Test is performed by giving 1 mg dexamethasone orally at 11 P.M. and measuring serum cortisol at 8 A.M. the following morning. Normal response is cortisol suppression to <3 mcg/dl; if dose of 4 mg dexamethasone is given, cortisol suppression will be to <50% of baseline.
Interpretation of results: Cushing syndrome (<10 mcg/dl), endogenous depression (half of patients suppress test values <5 mcg/dl). Most patients with pituitary Cushing disease demonstrate suppression, whereas patients with adrenal adenoma, carcinoma, and ectopic ACTH-producing tumors do not.

DIGOXIN

Normal therapeutic range: 0.5 to 2 ng/ml
Elevated in: Impaired renal function, excessive dosing, concomitant use of quinidine, amiodarone, verapamil, fluoxetine, nifedipine. Toxicity may occur at a lower blood concentration in the presence of hypokalemia, hypomagnesemia, and hypercalcemia. See Table E46.

DIGOXIN LEVEL

Therapeutic range and general information are summarized in Table 47.

DIHYDROTESTOSTERONE (SERUM, URINE)

Normal:
Serum: Males: 30 to 85 ng/dl; females: 4 to 22 ng/dl
Urine, 24 h: Males: 20 to 50 mcg/day; females: <8 mcg/day
Elevated in: Hirsutism
Decreased in: 5-α-reductase deficiency, hypogonadism

TABLE 47 Digoxin

Purpose	Treatment of Congestive Heart Failure and Atrial Fibrillation-Flutter
General adult dose	Oral: 0.75-1.5 mg for digitalization, 0.125-0.5 mg/day for maintenance
Usual bioavailability	Approximately 60%-85% for tablet or elixir; 90%-100% for liquid-filled capsules
Half-life	Approximately 35-40 h; however, prolonged in patients with decreased renal function
General therapeutic range	0.5-2 ng/ml
General toxic level	>2 ng/ml, but somewhat variable
Transport	Approximately 20%-25% plasma protein bound
Metabolism	Generally, only small amounts are metabolized (liver, lumen of large intestine)
Elimination	Approximately 50%-75% unchanged in urine
Steady state	Approximately 7 days in undigitalized patients with normal renal function
Mechanism of action	Causes release of calcium ions in T-system of myocardium; slows AV node conduction
Toxic effects	Gastric disturbances, nausea, vomiting, atrial and ventricular arrhythmias, irregular pulse

AV, Atrioventricular.
From McPherson RA, Pincus MR: *Henry's clinical diagnosis and management by laboratory methods,* ed 23, St Louis, 2017, Elsevier.

DILANTIN

See "PHENYTOIN"

DIRECT ANTIGLOBULIN (COOMBS DIRECT)

Normal: Negative
Positive: Autoimmune hemolytic anemia, erythroblastosis fetalis, transfusion reactions, drugs (α-methyldopa, penicillins, tetracycline, sulfonamides, levodopa, cephalosporins, quinidine, insulin)
False positive: May be seen with cold agglutinins

DISACCHARIDE ABSORPTION TESTS

Normal: Test is used to diagnose malabsorption due to disaccharide deficiency. It is performed by giving disaccharide orally 1 g/kg body weight to a total of 25 g. Blood is drawn at 0, 30, 60, 90, and 120 min. Normal response is a change in glucose from fasting value >30 mg/dl, inconclusive when increase is 20 to 30 mg/dl, abnormal when increase is >20 mg/dl. Test can also be performed by measuring air at 0, 30, 60, 90, and 120 min. Normal is H_2>20 ppm above baseline level before a colonic response.
Decreased in: Disaccharide deficiency (lactose, fructose, sorbitol), celiac disease, sprue, acute gastroenteritis

DOC

See "DEOXYCORTICOSTERONE"

DONATH-LANDSTEINER (D-L) TEST FOR PAROXYSMAL COLD HEMOGLOBINURIA

Normal: No hemolysis
Interpretation of result: Hemolysis indicates presence of bithermic cold hemolysins or Donath-Landsteiner antibodies (D-L Ab)

DOPAMINE

Normal range: 175 pg/ml
Elevated in: Pheochromocytomas, neuroblastomas, stress, vigorous exercise, certain foods (bananas, chocolate, coffee, tea, vanilla)

D-XYLOSE ABSORPTION

Normal range: 21% to 31% excreted in 5 h
Decreased in: Malabsorption syndrome

D-XYLOSE ABSORPTION TEST

Normal range:
URINE: ≥4 g/5 h (5-h urine collection in adults >12 y [25-g dose])
SERUM: ≥25 mg/dl (adult, 1 h, 25-g dose, normal renal function)
Normal results: In patients with malabsorption, normal results suggest pancreatic disease as an etiology of the malabsorption.
Abnormal results: Celiac disease, Crohn disease, tropical sprue, surgical bowel resection, AIDS. False positives can occur with decreased renal function, dehydration/hypovolemia, surgical blind loops, decreased gastric emptying, vomiting.

ELECTROPHORESIS, HEMOGLOBIN

See "HEMOGLOBIN ELECTROPHORESIS"

ELECTROPHORESIS, PROTEIN

See "PROTEIN ELECTROPHORESIS"

ENA COMPLEX

See "EXTRACTABLE NUCLEAR ANTIGEN"

ENDOMYSIAL ANTIBODIES

Normal: Not detected
Present in: Celiac disease, dermatitis herpetiformis

EOSINOPHIL COUNT

Normal range: 1% to 4% eosinophils (0 to 440/mm³)
Elevated in: HELMINTHIC PARASITE
Ascaris lumbricoides (invasive larval stage)
Hookworms (invasive larval stage)
Strongyloides stercoralis (initial infection and autoinfection)
Trichinosis
Filariasis
Echinococcus granulosus and *E. multilocularis*
Toxocara species
Animal hookworms
Angiostrongylus cantonensis and *A. costaricensis*
Schistosomiasis
Liver flukes
Fasciolopsis buski
Anisakiasis
Capillaria philippinensis
Paragonimus westermani
"Tropical eosinophilia" (unidentified microfilariae)
  NOTE: Table E48 describes an approach to investigation of eosinophilia in returning travelers.
OTHER INFECTIONS/INFESTATIONS
Pulmonary aspergillosis
Severe scabies
ALLERGIES
Asthma
Hay fever
Drug reactions
Atopic dermatitis
AUTOIMMUNE AND RELATED DISORDERS
Polyarteritis nodosa
Necrotizing vasculitis
Eosinophilic fasciitis
Pemphigus
NEOPLASTIC DISEASES
Hodgkin disease
Mycosis fungoides
Chronic myelocytic leukemia
Eosinophilic leukemia
Polycythemia vera
Mucin-secreting adenocarcinomas
IMMUNODEFICIENCY STATES
Hyperimmunoglobulin E with recurrent infection
Wiskott-Aldrich syndrome

OTHER
Addison disease
Inflammatory bowel disease
Dermatitis herpetiformis
Toxic/chemical syndrome
Eosinophilic myalgia syndrome, tryptophan, toxic oil syndrome
Hypereosinophilic syndrome (unknown etiology)
  Fig. E22 describes an algorithm for patients with eosinophil disorders.
  Table E49 describes hematopoietic neoplasms accompanied by eosinophilia.
  Table E50 describes the differential diagnosis of childhood eosinophilia.

EPINEPHRINE, PLASMA

Normal range: 0 to 90 pg/ml
Elevated in: Pheochromocytomas, neuroblastomas, stress, vigorous exercise, certain foods (bananas, chocolate, coffee, tea, vanilla), hypoglycemia (Box E16)

EPSTEIN-BARR VIRUS SEROLOGY

Normal range: IgG antiviral capsid antigen (VCA) <1:10 or negative
Abnormal:
IgG anti-VCA >1:10 or positive indicates either current or previous infection.
IgM anti-VCA >1:10 or positive indicates current or recent infection.
Anti-Epstein-Barr virus nuclear antigen (EBNA) ≥1.5 or positive indicates previous infection.
  Table E51 and Fig. 23 describe test interpretation.

ERYTHROCYTE SEDIMENTATION RATE (ESR, SED RATE, SEDIMENTATION RATE)

See Table E52 for erythrocyte sedimentation rate ranges in health.
Normal range:
Male: 0 to 15 mm/h
Female: 0 to 20 mm/h
Elevated in: Collagen vascular diseases, infections, myocardial infarction, neoplasms, inflammatory states (acute phase reactant), hyperthyroidism, hypothyroidism, rouleaux formation
Decreased in: Sickle cell disease, polycythemia, corticosteroids, spherocytosis, anisocytosis, hypofibrinogenemia, increased serum viscosity

ERYTHROPOIETIN (EP)

Normal: 3.7 to 16.0 IU/L by radioimmunoassay
  Erythropoietin is a glycoprotein secreted by the kidneys that stimulates RBC production by acting on erythroid-committed stem cells.
Increased in:
1. **Extremely high:** Generally seen in patients with severe anemia (Hct, <25; Hb<7) such as in cases of aplastic anemia, severe hemolytic anemia, hematologic cancers
2. **Very high:** Patients with mild to moderate anemia (Hct, 25 to 35; Hb, 7 to 10)
3. **High:** Patients with mild anemia (e.g., AIDS, myelodysplasia)
  Erythropoietin can be inappropriately elevated in patients with malignant neoplasms, renal cysts, postrenal transplant, meningioma, hemangioblastoma, and leiomyoma.
Decreased in: Renal failure, polycythemia vera, autonomic neuropathy

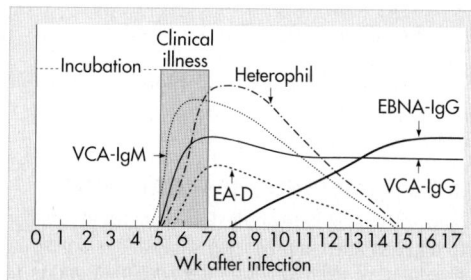

FIG. 23 Tests in Epstein-Barr viral infection. See Table E51 for abbreviations.

IV

Laboratory Tests

ESTRADIOL (SERUM)

Normal range:
Female, premenopausal: 30 to 400 pg/ml, depending on phase of menstrual cycle
Female, postmenopausal: 0 to 30 pg/ml
Male, adult: 10 to 50 pg/ml
Decreased in: Ovarian failure
Elevated in: Tumors of ovary, testis, adrenal, or nonendocrine sites (rare)

ESTROGEN

Normal range (serum):

Males:	20-80 pg/ml
Females:	
Follicular:	60-200 pg/ml
Luteal:	160-400 pg/ml
Postmenopausal:	<130 pg/ml

Normal range (urine):

Males:	4-23 µg/g creatinine
Females:	
Follicular:	7-65 µg/g creatinine
Midcycle:	32-104 µg/g creatinine
Luteal:	8-135 µg/g creatinine

Elevated in: Hyperplasia of adrenal cortex, ovarian tumors producing estrogen, granulosa and thecal cell tumors, testicular tumors
Decreased in: Menopause, hypopituitarism, primary ovarian malfunction, anorexia nervosa, hypofunction of adrenal cortex, ovarian agenesis, psychogenic stress, gonadotropin-releasing hormone deficiency

ETHANOL (BLOOD)

Normal range: Negative (values <10 mg/dl are considered negative)
Ethanol is metabolized at 10 to 25 mg/dl/h. Levels ≥80 mg/dl are considered evidence of impairment for driving. Fatal blood concentration is considered to be >400 mg/dl. Table E53 summarizes the influence of acute ethanol ingestion on ethanol levels and behavior.

EXTRACTABLE NUCLEAR ANTIGEN (ENA COMPLEX, ANTI-RNP ANTIBODY, ANTI-SM, ANTI-SMITH)

Normal: Negative
Present in: Systemic lupus erythematosus, rheumatoid arthritis, Sjögren syndrome, mixed connective tissue disease

FACTOR V LEIDEN

Test description: PCR test performed on whole blood or tissue. This single mutation, found in 2% to 8% of the general White population, is the single most common cause of hereditary thrombophilia.

FASTING BLOOD SUGAR

See "GLUCOSE, FASTING"

FBS

See "GLUCOSE, FASTING"

FDP

See "FIBRIN DEGRADATION PRODUCT"

FECAL FAT, QUANTITATIVE (72-H COLLECTION)

Normal range: 2 to 6 g/24 h (7 to 21 mmol/dl [CF: 3.515; SMI: 1 mmol/dl])
Elevated in: Malabsorption syndrome

FECAL GLOBIN IMMUNOCHEMICAL TEST

Normal: Negative. This test is performed by immunochromatography on a cellulose strip that has been impregnated with various antibodies. The test uses a small amount of toilet water as the specimen and is placed onto absorbent pads of card similar to traditional occult blood (OB) card. There is no direct handling of stool. This test is specific for the globin portion of the hemoglobin molecule, which confers lower GI bleeding specificity. It specifically detects blood from the lower GI tract; guaiac tests are not lower GI specific. It is more sensitive than typical Hemoccult test (detection limit 50 mcg Hb/g feces versus >500 mcg Hb/g feces for Hemoccult). It has no dietary restrictions and gives no false positives due to plant peroxidases and red meats. It has no medication restrictions. Iron supplements and NSAIDs do not cause false positives. Vitamin C does not cause false negatives.
Positive in: Lower GI bleeding

FERRITIN (SERUM)

Normal range: 18 to 300 ng/ml (18 to 300 µg/L [CF: 1; SMI: 10 µg/L])
Elevated in: Hyperthyroidism, inflammatory states, liver disease (ferritin elevated from necrotic hepatocytes), neoplasms (neuroblastomas, lymphomas, leukemia, breast carcinoma), iron replacement therapy, hemochromatosis, hemosiderosis. Table E54 summarizes hereditary iron overload disorders.
Decreased in: Iron deficiency anemia

α-1 FETOPROTEIN

Normal range: 0 to 20 ng/ml (0 to 20 µg/L [CF: 1; SMI: 1 µg/L])
Elevated in: Hepatocellular carcinoma (usually values >1000 ng/ml), germinal neoplasms (testis, ovary, mediastinum, retroperitoneum), liver disease (alcoholic cirrhosis, acute hepatitis, chronic active hepatitis), fetal anencephaly, spina bifida, basal cell carcinoma, breast carcinoma, pancreatic carcinoma, gastric carcinoma, retinoblastoma, esophageal atresia

FIBRIN DEGRADATION PRODUCT (FDP)

Normal range
<10 µg/ml
Elevated in: Disseminated intravascular coagulation, primary fibrinolysis, pulmonary embolism, severe liver disease
NOTE: The presence of rheumatoid factor may cause falsely elevated FDP.

FIBRINOGEN

Normal range: 200 to 400 mg/dl (2 to 4 g/L [CF: 0.01; SMI: 0.1 g/L])
Elevated in: Tissue inflammation or damage (acute phase protein reactant), oral contraceptives, pregnancy, acute infection, myocardial infarction
Decreased in: Disseminated intravascular coagulation, hereditary afibrinogenemia, liver disease, primary or secondary fibrinolysis, cachexia

FOLATE (FOLIC ACID)

Normal range:
Plasma: 2 to 10 ng/ml (4 to 22 nmol/L [CF: 2.266; SMI: 2 nmol/L])
Red blood cells: 140 to 960 ng/ml (550 to 2200 nmol/L [CF: 2.266; SMI: 10 nmol/L])
Decreased in: Folic acid deficiency (inadequate intake, malabsorption), alcoholism, drugs (methotrexate, trimethoprim, phenytoin, oral contraceptives, Azulfidine), vitamin B_{12} deficiency (defective red cell folate absorption), hemolytic anemia. Box E17 summarizes an etiophysiologic classification of folate deficiency.
Elevated in: Folic acid therapy

FOLLICLE-STIMULATING HORMONE (FSH)

Normal range: 5 to 20 mIU/ml
Elevated in: Menopause, primary gonadal failure, alcoholism, castration, Klinefelter syndrome, gonadotropin-secreting pituitary hormones
Decreased in: Pregnancy, polycystic ovary disease, anorexia nervosa, anterior pituitary hypofunction

FREE T₄

See "T₄, FREE"

FREE THYROXINE INDEX

Normal range: 1.1 to 4.3
INCREASED THYROXINE OR FREE THYROXINE VALUES
- Laboratory error
- Primary hyperthyroidism (T₄/T₃ type)
- Severe thyroxine-binding globulin elevation
- Excess therapy of hypothyroidism

- Excessive dose of levothyroxine
- Active thyroiditis (subacute, painless, early active Hashimoto disease)
- Familial dysalbuminemic hyperthyroxinemia (some FT_4 kits, especially analog types)
- Peripheral resistance to T_4 syndrome
- Amiodarone or propranolol
- Postpartum transient toxicosis
- Factitious hyperthyroidism
- Jod-Basedow (iodine-induced) hyperthyroidism
- Severe nonthyroid illness
- Acute psychosis (especially paranoid schizophrenia)
- T_4 sample drawn 2 to 4 h after levothyroxine dose
- Struma ovarii
- Pituitary thyroid-stimulating hormone-secreting tumor
- Certain x-ray contrast media (Telepaque and Oragrafin)
- Acute porphyria
- Heparin effect (some T_4 and FT_4 kits)
- Amphetamine, heroin, methadone, and phencyclidine abuse
- Perphenazine or 5-fluorouracil
- Antithyroid or anti-IgG heterophil (HAMA) autoantibodies
- "T_4" hyperthyroidism
- Hyperemesis gravidarum; about 50% of patients
- High altitudes

DECREASED THYROXINE OR FREE THYROXINE VALUES
- Laboratory error
- Primary hypothyroidism
- Severe nonthyroid illness
- Lithium therapy
- Severe thyroxine-binding globulin decrease (congenital, disease, or drug-induced) or severe albumin decrease
- Dilantin, Depakene, or high-dose salicylate drugs
- Pituitary insufficiency
- Large doses of inorganic iodide (e.g., saturated solution of potassium iodide)
- Moderate or severe iodine deficiency
- Cushing syndrome
- High-dose glucocorticoid drugs
- Pregnancy, third trimester (low normal or small decrease)
- Addison disease; some patients (30%)
- Heparin effect (a few FT_4 kits)
- Desipramine or amiodarone drugs
- Acute psychiatric illness

FTA-ABS (SERUM)

Normal: Nonreactive

Reactive in: Syphilis, other treponemal diseases (yaws, pinta, bejel), SLE, pregnancy

FUROSEMIDE STIMULATION TEST

Normal: Test is performed by giving 60 mg furosemide orally after overnight fast. Patient should be on a normal diet without medications the week before the test. Normal results: Renin 1 to 6 ng angiotensin L/ml/h.

Elevated in: Renovascular hypertension, Bartter syndrome, high-renin essential hypertension, pheochromocytoma

No response in: Primary aldosteronism, low-renin essential hypertension, hyporeninemic hypoaldosteronism

GAMMA-GLUTAMYL TRANSFERASE (GGT)

See "γ-GLUTAMYL TRANSFERASE"

GASTRIN (SERUM)

Normal range: 0 to 180 pg/ml (0 to 180 ng/L [CF: 1; SMI: 10 ng/L])

Elevated in: Zollinger-Ellison syndrome (gastrinoma), pernicious anemia, hyperparathyroidism, retained gastric antrum, chronic renal failure, gastric ulcer, chronic atrophic gastritis, pyloric obstruction, malignant neoplasms of the stomach, H_2-blockers, omeprazole, calcium therapy, ulcerative colitis, rheumatoid arthritis

GASTRIN STIMULATION TEST

Normal: Gastrin stimulation test after calcium infusion is performed by giving a calcium infusion (15 mg/kg in 500 ml normal saline over 4 h). Serum is drawn in fasting state before infusion and at 1, 2, 3, and 4 h. Normal response is little or no increase over baseline gastrin level.

Elevated in: Gastrinoma (gastrin >400 pg/ml), duodenal ulcer (gastrin level increase <400 ng/L)

Decreased in: Pernicious anemia, atrophic gastritis

GLIADIN ANTIBODIES, IGA AND IGG

Normal: <25 U, equivocal 20 to 25 U, positive >25 U. Test is useful to monitor compliance with gluten-free diet in patients with celiac disease.

Elevated in: Celiac disease with dietary noncompliance

GLOMERULAR BASEMENT MEMBRANE (GBM) ANTIBODY

Normal: Negative

Present in: Goodpasture syndrome

GLOMERULAR FILTRATION RATE

See Box E18 for a summary of common equations for calculating GFR or creatinine clearance. Chronic kidney disease stages based on GFR are summarized in Table 55.

Normal:

Ages 20-29	116 ml/min/1.73 m^2
Ages 30-39	107 ml/min/1.73 m^2
Ages 40-49	99 ml/min/1.73 m^2
Ages 50-59	93 ml/min/1.73 m^2
Ages 60-69	85 ml/min/1.73 m^2
Ages >75	75 ml/min/1.73 m^2

Decreased in: Renal insufficiency, decreased renal blood flow

GLUCAGON

Normal: 20 to 100 pg/ml

Elevated in: Glucagonoma (900 to 7800 pg/ml), chronic renal failure, diabetes mellitus, glucocorticoids, insulin, nifedipine, danazol, sympathomimetic amines

Decreased in: Hyperlipoproteinemia (types III, IV), β-blockers, secretin

GLUCOSE, FASTING (FBS, FASTING BLOOD SUGAR)

Fig. E24 describes the approach to hypoglycemia. An algorithm for evaluation of hypoglycemia in children is described in Fig. E25.

Normal range: 60 to 99 mg/dl (3.8 to 6.0 mmol/L [CF: 0.05551; SMI: 0.1 mmol/L])

Elevated in: Diabetes mellitus, stress, infections, myocardial infarction, cerebrovascular accident, Cushing syndrome, acromegaly, acute pancreatitis, glucagonoma, hemochromatosis, drugs (glucocorticoids, diuretics [thiazides, loop diuretics]), glucose intolerance, impaired fasting glucose

TABLE 55   Chronic Kidney Disease Stages

Stage	eGFR (ml/min/1.73 m^2)	Urinalysis Findings
1	≥90	Hematuria, proteinuria, or imaging abnormalities at >3 mo
2	60-89	Hematuria, proteinuria, or imaging abnormalities at >3 mo
3	30-59	↑ or normal
4	15-29	↑ or normal
5	0-14	↑ or normal

eGFR, Estimated glomerular filtration rate.
From Parrillo JE, Dellinger RP: *Critical care medicine, principles of diagnosis and management in the adult*, ed 4, Philadelphia, 2014, Elsevier.

Decreased in: Sulfonylurea therapy, insulin therapy, reactive hypoglycemia (e.g., subtotal gastrectomy), starvation, insulinoma, glycogen storage disorders, severe liver disease or renal disease, ethanol-induced hypoglycemia, mesenchymal tumors that secrete insulin-like hormones

GLUCOSE, POSTPRANDIAL

Normal range: <140 mg/dl (<7.8 mmol/L [CF: 0.05551; SMI: 0.1 mmol/L])
Elevated in: Diabetes mellitus, glucose intolerance
Decreased in: Post-gastrointestinal resection, reactive hypoglycemia, hereditary fructose intolerance, galactosemia, leucine sensitivity

GLUCOSE TOLERANCE TEST

Normal values above fasting:
30 min: 30 to 60 mg/dl (1.65 to 3.3 mmol/L [CF: 0.05551; SMI: 0.1 mmol/L])
60 min: 20 to 50 mg/dl (1.1 to 2.75 mmol/L [CF: 0.05551; SMI: 0.1 mmol/L])
120 min: 5 to 15 mg/dl (0.28 to 0.83 mmol/L [CF: 0.05551; SMI: 0.1 mmol/L])
180 min: Fasting level or below
Abnormal in: Glucose intolerance, diabetes mellitus, Cushing syndrome, acromegaly, pheochromocytoma, gestational diabetes

GLUCOSE-6-PHOSPHATE DEHYDROGENASE (G6PD) SCREEN (BLOOD)

Normal: G6PD enzyme activity detected
Abnormal: If a deficiency is detected, quantitation of G6PD is necessary; a G6PD screen may be falsely interpreted as "normal" after an episode of hemolysis because most G6PD-deficient cells have been destroyed.

γ-GLUTAMYL TRANSFERASE (GGT)

Normal range: 0 to 30 U/L (0.050 µkat/L [CF: 0.01667; SMI: 0.01 µkat/L])
Elevated in: Chronic alcoholic liver disease, neoplasms (hepatoma, metastatic disease to the liver, carcinoma of the pancreas), systemic lupus erythematosus, congestive heart failure, trauma, nephrotic syndrome, sepsis, cholestasis, drugs (phenytoin, barbiturates)

GLYCOHEMOGLOBIN (GLYCATED GLYCOSYLATED HEMOGLOBIN), (HBA$_{1C}$)

Normal range: 4.0% to 5.9%. Glycemic goals in adults are summarized in Table E56.
Elevated in: Uncontrolled diabetes mellitus (glycated hemoglobin levels reflect the level of glucose control over the preceding 120 days), lead toxicity, alcoholism, iron deficiency anemia, hypertriglyceridemia
Decreased in: Hemolytic anemias, decreased red blood cell survival, pregnancy, acute or chronic blood loss, chronic renal failure, insulinoma, congenital spherocytosis, hemoglobin S, C, and D diseases

GROWTH HORMONE

Normal: Male: 1 to 9 ng/ml; female: 1 to 16 ng/ml
Elevated in: Pituitary gigantism, acromegaly, ectopic GH secretion, cirrhosis, renal failure, anorexia nervosa, stress, exercise, prolonged fasting, amphetamines, β-blockers, insulin, levodopa, metoclopramide, clonidine, vasopressin, human growth hormone (HGH) supplementation
Decreased in: Hypopituitarism, pituitary dwarfism, adrenocortical hyperfunction, bromocriptine, corticosteroids, glucose

GROWTH HORMONE–RELEASING HORMONE (GHRH)

Normal: <50 pg/ml
Elevated in: Acromegaly caused by GHRH secretion by neoplasms

GROWTH HORMONE SUPPRESSION TEST (AFTER GLUCOSE)

Normal: Test is done by giving 1.75 g glucose/kg orally after overnight fast. Blood is drawn at baseline, after 60 min, and after 120 min of glucose load. Normal response is growth hormone suppression to <2 ng/ml or undetectable levels.
Abnormal: There is no or incomplete suppression from the high basal level in gigantism or acromegaly.

HAM TEST (ACID SERUM TEST)

Normal: Negative
Positive in: Paroxysmal nocturnal hemoglobinuria
False-positive in: Hereditary or acquired spherocytosis, recent transfusion with aged red blood cells, aplastic anemia, myeloproliferative syndromes, leukemia, hereditary dyserythropoietic anemia type II

HAPTOGLOBIN (SERUM)

Normal range: 50 to 220 mg/dl (0.50 to 2.2 g/L [CF: 0.01; SMI: 0.01 g/L])
Elevated in: Inflammation (acute phase reactant), collagen vascular diseases, infections (acute phase reactant), drugs (androgens), obstructive liver disease
Decreased in: Hemolysis (intravascular more than extravascular), megaloblastic anemia, severe liver disease, large tissue hematomas, infectious mononucleosis, drugs (oral contraceptives)

HBA$_{1C}$

See "GLYCOHEMOGLOBIN"

HDL

See "HIGH-DENSITY LIPOPROTEIN CHOLESTEROL"

HELICOBACTER PYLORI (SEROLOGY, STOOL ANTIGEN)

Normal range: Not detected
Detected in: *H. pylori* infection. Positive serology can indicate current or past infection. Positive stool antigen test indicates acute infection (sensitivity and specificity >90%). Stool testing should be delayed at least 4 wk after eradication therapy.

HEMATOCRIT

Normal range:
Male: 39% to 49% (0.39 to 0.49 [CF: 0.01; SMI: 0.01])
Female: 33% to 43% (0.33 to 0.43 [CF: 0.01; SMI: 0.01])
Elevated in: Polycythemia vera, smoking, chronic obstructive pulmonary disease, high altitudes, dehydration, hypovolemia
Decreased in: Blood loss (gastrointestinal, genitourinary) anemia

HEMOGLOBIN

Normal range:
Male: 13.6 to 17.7 g/dl (136 to 172 g/L [CF: 10; SMI: 1 g/L])
Female: 12.0 to 15.0 g/dl (120 to 150 g/L [CF: 10; SMI: 1 g/L])
Elevated in: Hemoconcentration, dehydration, polycythemia vera, chronic obstructive pulmonary disease, high altitudes, false elevations (hyperlipemic plasma, white blood cells >50,000/mm³), stress
Decreased in: Hemorrhagic (gastrointestinal, genitourinary) anemia

HEMOGLOBIN A$_{1C}$

See "GLYCOHEMOGLOBIN"

HEMOGLOBIN ELECTROPHORESIS

Table E57 describes neonatal hemoglobin electrophoresis patterns, Table 58 summarizes types of hemoglobin, and Table E59 describes classifications of hemoglobinopathies.
Normal range:
HbA$_1$: 95% to 98%
HbA$_2$: 1.5% to 3.5%
HbF: <2%
HbC: Absent
HbS: Absent

HEMOGLOBIN, GLYCATED

See "GLYCOHEMOGLOBIN"

HEMOGLOBIN, GLYCOSYLATED

See "GLYCOHEMOGLOBIN"

HEMOGLOBIN H

See Table 58.

TABLE 58   Types of Hemoglobin

	Hemoglobin	Structure	Comment
Normal	A	$\alpha 2\beta 2$	97% of adult hemoglobin
	A2	$\alpha 2\delta 2$	2% of adult Hb; elevated in β-thalassemia
	F	$\alpha 2\gamma 2$	Normal Hb in fetus from 3rd-9th mo; increased in β-thalassemia
Abnormal chain production	H	$\beta 4$	Found in α-thalassemia, biologically useless
	Barts	$\gamma 4$	Found in α-thalassemia, biologically useless
Abnormal chain structure	S	$\alpha 2\beta 2$	Substitution of valine for glutamic acid in position 6 of β chain
	C	$\alpha 2\beta 2$	Substitution of lysine for glutamic acid in position 6 of β chain

From Ballinger A: *Kumar & Clark's essentials of clinical medicine,* ed 6, Edinburgh, 2012, Saunders.

Normal: Negative
Present in
Hemoglobin H disease, α-thalassemia trait, unstable hemoglobin disorders

HEMOGLOBIN, URINE
See "URINE HEMOGLOBIN, FREE"

HEMOSIDERIN, URINE
See "URINE HEMOGLOBIN, FREE"

HEPARIN-INDUCED THROMBOCYTOPENIA ANTIBODIES
Normal: Antigen assay: Negative, <0.45; weak, 0.45-1.0; strong, >1.0
Elevated in: Heparin-induced thrombocytopenia

HEPATITIS A ANTIBODY
Normal: Negative
Present in: Viral hepatitis A; can be IgM or IgG (if IgM, acute hepatitis A; if IgG, previous infection with hepatitis A)
   See Fig. 26 for serologic tests in HAV infection.
   See Table E60 for serologic and virologic tests for hepatitis viruses.

Hepatitis A viral infection:
Best all-purpose test(s) to diagnose acute HAV infection = HAV-Ab (IgM)
Best all-purpose test(s) to demonstrate past HAV infection/immunity = HAV-Ab (total)

HEPATITIS A VIRUS-IGM ANTIBODY
Appearance: About the same time as clinical symptoms (3 to 4 wk after exposure; range, 14 to 60 days), or just before beginning of AST/ALT elevation (range, 10 days before to 7 days after)
Peak: About 3 to 4 wk after onset of symptoms (1 to 6 wk)
Becomes nondetectable: 3 to 4 mo after onset of symptoms (1 to 6 mo)
In a few cases, HAV-IgM antibody can persist as long as 12 to 14 mo.

HEPATITIS A VIRUS TOTAL ANTIBODY
Appearance: About 3 wk after IgM becomes detectable (therefore about the middle of clinical symptom period to early convalescence)
Peak: About 1 to 2 mo after onset
Becomes nondetectable: Remains elevated for life but can somewhat slowly fall

HEPATITIS B SURFACE ANTIGEN (HBSAG)
Normal: Not detected
Detected in: Acute viral hepatitis type B, chronic hepatitis B
Appearance: 2 to 6 wk after exposure (range, 6 days to 6 mo); 5% to 15% of patients are negative at onset of jaundice
Peak: 1 to 2 wk before to 1 to 2 wk after onset of symptoms
Becomes nondetectable: 1 to 3 mo after peak (range, 1 wk to 5 mo)

HEPATITIS B VIRAL INFECTION
See Table 61
   Figs. 27, 28, and 29 illustrate antigens and antibodies in hepatitis B infection.
HB$_S$
-Ag:
HB$_S$Ag: Shows current active hepatitis B virus (HBV) infection
Persistence over 6 mo indicates carrier/chronic HBV infection
HBV nucleic acid probe: Present before and longer than HB$_S$Ag
More reliable marker for increased infectivity than HB$_S$Ag and/or HB$_e$Ag
-Ab: HB$_S$Ab-total: Shows previous healed HBV infection and evidence of immunity
HB$_C$
-Ab:
HB$_C$Ab-IgM: Shows either acute or very recent infection by HBV
In convalescent phase of acute HBV, may be elevated when HB$_S$Ag has disappeared (core window)

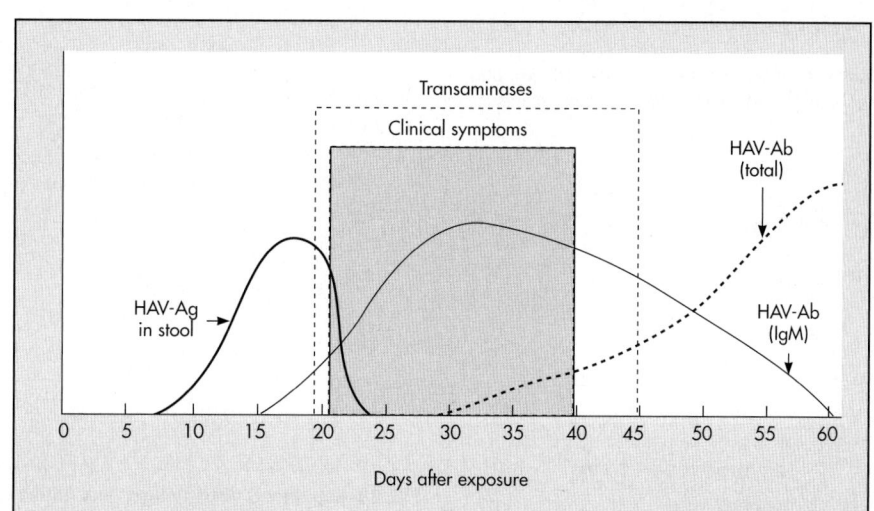

FIG. 26 Serologic tests in hepatitis A viral infection. *HAV,* Hepatitis A virus; *HAV-Ab,* hepatitis A virus antibodies test; *HAV-Ag,* hepatitis A virus antigen test; *Ig,* immunoglobulin.

TABLE 61 Serologic Markers of Hepatitis B Infection

	HBsAg	anti-HBc	anti-HBs	IgM anti-HBc
Susceptible to infection	Negative	Negative	Negative	Negative
Immune due to natural infection	Negative	Positive	Positive	Negative
Immune due to hepatitis B vaccination	Negative	Negative	Positive	Negative
Acutely infected	Positive	Positive	Negative	Positive
Chronically infected	Positive	Positive	Negative	Negative

HBsAg, Hepatitis B surface antigen; *Ig*, immunoglobulin.

From Ballinger A: *Kumar & Clark's essentials of clinical medicine*, ed 6, Edinburgh, 2012, Saunders.

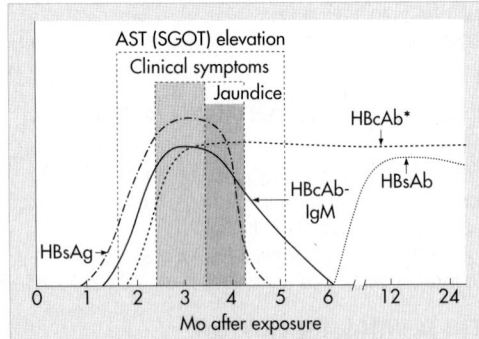

FIG. 27 Hepatitis B virus surface antigen-antibody and core antibodies. Note "core window." *$HB_CAb = HB_CAb\text{-}IgM + HBCAb\text{-}IgG$ (combined). *AST,* Aspartate aminotransferase; *HBcAb,* hepatitis B core antibody; *HBsAb,* hepatitis B surface antibody; *HBsAg,* hepatitis B surface antigen; *Ig,* immunoglobulin; *SGOT,* serum glutamic-oxaloacetic transaminase.

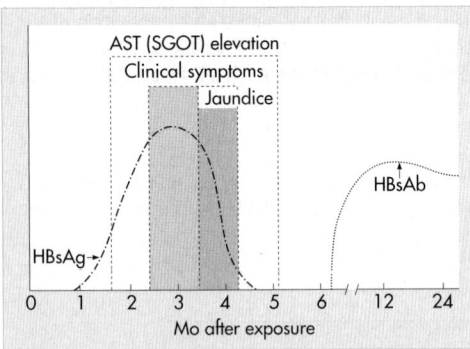

FIG. 28 Hepatitis B virus surface antigen and antibody (HB$_S$Ag and HB$_S$Ab-total). *AST,* Aspartate aminotransferase; *SGOT,* serum glutamic-oxaloacetic transaminase.

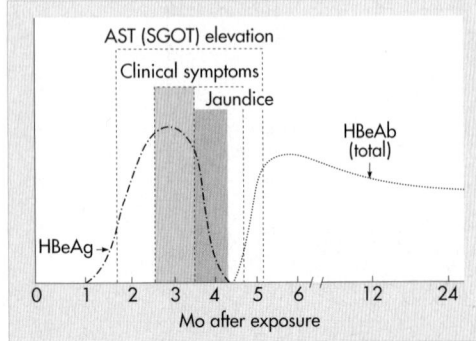

FIG. 29 HBVe antigen and antibody. *AST,* Aspartate aminotransferase; *HBeAb,* hepatitis B e-antibody; *SGOT,* serum glutamic-oxaloacetic transaminase.

Negative $HB_CAb\text{-}IgM$ with positive HB_SAg suggests either very early acute HBV or carrier/chronic HBV

HB_CAb-total: Only useful to show past HBV infection if HB_SAg and HB_CAb-IgM are both negative

HB$_e$-Ag:

HB_e-AbAg: When present, especially without HB_eAb, suggests increased patient infectivity

HB_eAb-total: When present, suggests less patient infectivity

1. HB_SAg positive, HB_CAb negative
   a. About 5% (range, 0% to 17%) of patients with early-stage HBV acute infection (HB_CAb rises later)
2. HB_SAg positive, HB_CAb positive, HB_SAb negative
   a. Most of the clinical symptom stage
   b. Chronic HBV carriers without evidence of liver disease ("asymptomatic carriers")
   c. Chronic HBV hepatitis (chronic persistent type or chronic active type)
3. HB_SAg negative, HB_CAb positive, HB_SAb negative
   a. Late clinical symptom stage or early convalescence stage (core window)
   b. Chronic HBV infection with HB_SAg below detection levels with current tests
   c. Old previous HBV infection
4. HB_SAg negative, HB_CAb positive, HB_SAb positive
   a. Late convalescence to complete recovery
   b. Old infection

HEPATITIS C RNA

Normal: Negative

Elevated in: Hepatitis C. Detection of hepatitis C-RNA is used to confirm current infection and to monitor treatment. Quantitative assays (viral load) are needed before treatment to assess response (<2 log decrease after 12-wk treatment indicates lack of response).

HCV

-Ag: HCV nucleic acid probe: Shows current infection by HCV (especially with PCR amplification).

-Ab: HCV-Ab (IgG): Current, convalescent, or old HCV infection.

HAV

-Ag: HAV-Ag by EM: Shows presence of virus in stool early in infection.

-Ab:

HAV-Ab (IgM): Current or recent HAV infection.

HAV-Ab (total): Convalescent or old HAV infection.

HEPATITIS C VIRAL INFECTION

Fig. 30 illustrates antigens and antibodies in hepatitis C infection. Table 62 summarizes interpretation of patterns of HCV markers.

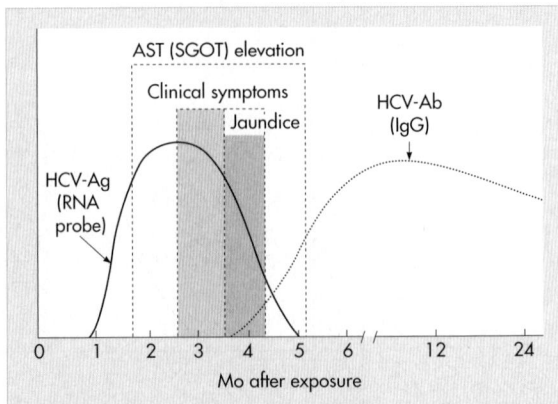

FIG. 30 Hepatitis C virus antigen and antibody. *AST,* Aspartate aminotransferase; *HCV-Ab,* hepatitis C virus antibody; *HCV-Ag,* hepatitis C virus core antigen; *Ig,* immunoglobulin; *RNA,* ribonucleic acid; *SGOT,* serum glutamic-oxaloacetic transaminase.

TABLE 62 Interpretation of Patterns of HCV Markers

Interpretation	Anti-HCV	RIBA	HCV RNA
Acute HCV infection	−	−	+
Active HCV infection	+	+	+
Possible HCV clearance	+	+	−
False-positive HCV test	+	−	−
Requires further study	+	Indeterminate[a]	−

HCV, Hepatitis C; *RIBA*, recombinant immunoassay; *RNA*, ribonucleic acid.
[a]Indeterminate result: Only one band positive, or more than one band and nonspecific reactivity.
From McPherson RA, Pincus MR: *Henry's clinical diagnosis and management by laboratory methods*, ed 23, St Louis, 2017, Elsevier.

HEPATITIS D VIRAL INFECTION

Fig. 31 illustrates antigens and antibodies in hepatitis D infection.
Best current all-purpose screening test = HDV-Ab (total)
Best test to differentiate acute from chronic infection = HDV-Ab (IgM)

HEPATITIS DELTA COINFECTION (ACUTE HDV1 ACUTE HBV) OR SUPERINFECTION (ACUTE HDV1 CHRONIC HBV)

HDV
-Ag:
HDV-Ag: Shows current infection (acute or chronic) by HDV
HDV nucleic acid probe: Detects antigen before and longer than HDV-Ag by EIA
-Ab:
HDV-Ab (IgM): High elevation in acute HDV; does not persist
Low or moderate elevation in convalescent HDV; does not persist
Low to high persistent elevation in chronic HDV (depends on degree of cell injury and sensitivity of the assay)
HDV-Ab (total): High elevation in acute HDV; does not persist
High persistent elevation in chronic HDV

HEPATITIS D VIRUS-AB (IGM)

Appearance: About 10 days after symptoms begin (range, 1 to 28 days)
Peak: About 2 wk after first detection
Becomes nondetectable: About 35 days (range, 10 to 80 days) after first detection (most other IgM antibodies take 3 to 6 mo to become nondetectable)

HEPATITIS D VIRUS-AG

Detected by DNA probe, less often by immunoassay
Appearance: Prodromal stage (before symptoms); just at or after initial rise in ALT (about a week after appearance of HB$_S$Ag and about the time HB$_C$Ab-IgM level begins to rise)
Peak: 2 to 3 days after onset
Becomes nondetectable: 1 to 4 days (may persist until shortly after symptoms appear)

HEPATITIS D VIRUS-AB (TOTAL)

Appearance: About 50 days after symptoms begin (range, 14 to 80 days); about 5 wk after HDV-Ag (range, 3 to 11 wk)
Peak: About 2 wk after first detection
Becomes nondetectable: About 7 mo after first detection (range, 4 to 14 mo)

HER-2/*NEU*

Normal: Negative
Present in: 25% to 30% of primary breast cancers. It can also be found in other epithelial tumors, including lung, hepatocellular, pancreatic, colon, stomach, ovarian, cervical, and bladder cancer. Trastuzumab (Herceptin) is a humanized monoclonal antibody against Her-2/*neu*. This test is useful to identify patients with metastatic; recurrent; and/or treatment-refractory, unresectable, locally advanced breast cancer for trastuzumab treatment.

HERPES SIMPLEX VIRUS (HSV)

Test description: The PCR test can be performed on serum biopsy samples, CSF, vitreous humor.

HETEROPHIL ANTIBODY

Normal: Negative
Positive in: Infectious mononucleosis

HFE SCREEN FOR HEREDITARY HEMOCHROMATOSIS

Test description: PCR test can be performed on whole blood or tissue. One mutation (C282Y) and two polymorphisms (H63D, S65C) account for the majority of alleles associated with this disease.

HIGH-DENSITY LIPOPROTEIN (HDL) CHOLESTEROL

Normal range:
Male: 40 to 70 mg/dl (0.8 to 1.8 mmol/L [CF: 0.02586; SMI: 0.05 mmol/L])
Female: 50 to 90 mg/dl (1.1 to 2.35 mmol/L [CF: 0.02586; SMI: 0.05 mmol/L])

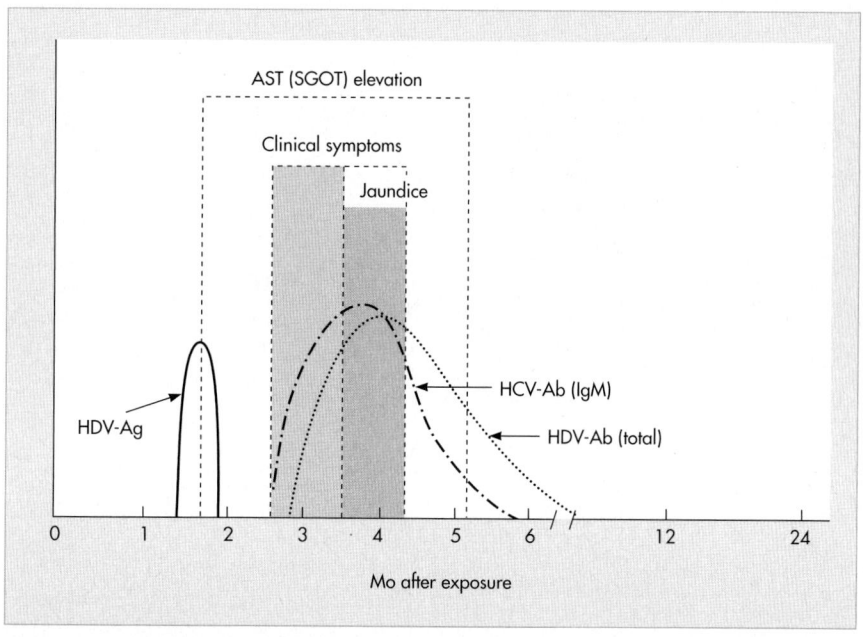

FIG. 31 Hepatitis D virus antigen and antibodies. *AST,* Aspartate aminotransferase; *HCV-Ab,* hepatitis C virus antibody; *HDV-Ab,* hepatitis D virus antibody; *HDV-Ag,* hepatitis D virus antigen; *Ig,* immunoglobulin; *SGOT,* serum glutamic-oxaloacetic transaminase.

Laboratory Tests

IV

Increased in: Use of gemfibrozil, statins, fenofibrate, nicotinic acid, estrogens, regular aerobic exercise, small (1 oz) daily alcohol intake

Decreased in: Deficiency of apoproteins, liver disease, probucol ingestion, Tangier disease

NOTE: A cholesterol/HDL ratio >4.0 is associated with increased risk of coronary artery disease. Table E63 summarizes significant human apolipoproteins.

HLA ANTIGENS

Associated disorders: See Table 64.

HOMOCYSTEINE (PLASMA)

Normal range:

0-30 yr:	4.6-8.1 µmol/L
30-59 yr:	6.3-11.2 µmol/L (males), 4.5-7.9 µmol/L (females)
>59 yr:	5.8-11.9 µmol/L

Increased: Thrombophilic states, B_6, B_{12}, folic acid, riboflavin deficiency, pregnancy, homocystinuria

NOTE: An increased homocysteine level is an independent risk factor for atherosclerosis.

TABLE 64 HLA Antigens Associated With Specific Diseases

Antigen	Condition	Antigen	Condition
HLA-B27	Ankylosing spondylitis	HLA-B8, Dw3	Celiac disease
	Reiter syndrome	HLA-B8, Dw3	Dermatitis herpetiformis
	Psoriatic arthritis	HLA-B8	Myasthenia gravis
HLA-A10, B18, Dw2	C2 deficiency	HLA-B8	Chronic active hepatitis in children
HLA-A2, B40, Cw3	C4 deficiency	HLA-Drw4	Active chronic hepatitis in adults
HLA-B7, Dw2	Multiple sclerosis	HLA-B13, Bw17	Psoriasis
HLA-A3	Hemochromatosis		

HLA, Human leukocyte antigen.
From Cerra FB: *Manual of critical care,* St Louis, 1987, Mosby.

HUMAN CHORIONIC GONADOTROPIN (HCG)

Normal range: Varies with gestational stage:

1 wk:	5-50 mU/ml
1-2 wk:	50-550 mU/ml
2-3 wk:	up to 5000 mU/ml
3-4 wk:	up to 10,000 mU/ml
4-5 wk:	up to 50,000 mU/ml
2-3 mo:	10,000-100,000 mU/ml

Elevated in: Normal pregnancy, hydatidiform mole, choriocarcinoma, germ cell tumors of testicle, some nontrophoblastic neoplasms (e.g., neoplasms of cervix, gastrointestinal tract, ovary, lung, breast)

HUMAN HERPES VIRUS 8 (HHV8)

Test description: PCR test can be performed on whole blood, tissue, bone marrow, and urine. HHV8 is found in all forms of Kaposi sarcoma.

HUMAN IMMUNODEFICIENCY VIRUS ANTIBODY, TYPE 1 (HIV-1)

Normal range: Not detected.

Abnormal result: HIV antibodies usually appear in the blood 1 to 4 mo after infection.

Testing sequence: ELISA is the recommended initial screening test. Sensitivity and specificity are >99%. False-positive ELISA may occur with autoimmune disorders, administration of immune globulin manufactured before 1985, within 6 wk of testing, in the presence of rheumatoid factor, in the presence of DLA-DR antibodies in multigravida female, with administration of influenza vaccine within 3 mo of testing, with hemodialysis, with positive plasma reagin test, and with certain medical disorders (hemophilia, hypergammaglobulinemia, alcoholic hepatitis).

A positive ELISA is confirmed with western blot (Fig. E32). False-positive western blot may result from connective tissue disorders, human leukocyte antigen antibodies, polyclonal gammopathies, hyperbilirubinemia, presence of antibody to another human retrovirus, or cross-reaction with other nonvirus-derived proteins in healthy persons. Undetermined western blot may occur in AIDS patients with advanced immunodeficiency (caused by loss of antibodies) and in recent HIV infections.

PCR is used to confirm indeterminate western blot results or negative results in persons with suspected HIV infection.

Fig. 33 describes tests in HIV infection; indications for plasma HIV RNA testing are described in Table E65.

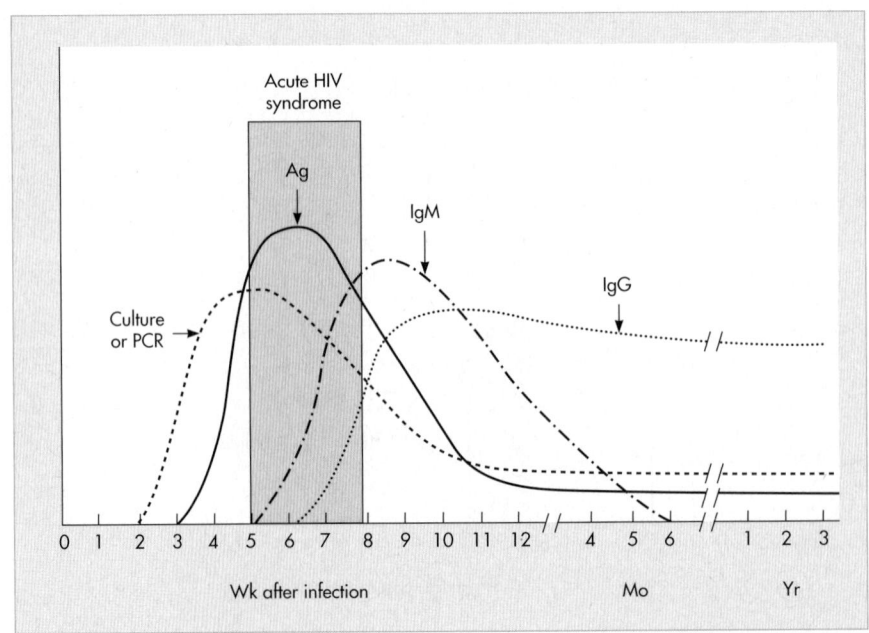

FIG. 33 Tests in human immunodeficiency virus (HIV)-1 infection. *Ag,* Antigen; *Ig,* immunoglobulin; *PCR,* polymerase chain reaction. (From Ravel R [ed]: *Clinical laboratory medicine,* ed 6, St Louis, 1995, Mosby.)

HUMAN IMMUNODEFICIENCY VIRUS TYPE 1 (HIV-1) ANTIGEN (P24), QUALITATIVE (P24 ANTIGEN)

Normal range: Negative. This test detects uncomplexed HIV-1 p24 antigen. The core protein p24 is the first detectable protein encoded by the group-specific antigen *(gag)* gene. This protein is a marker for viremia. This test should not be used in place of HIV-1 antibody testing as a screen for HIV-1 infection. HIV-1 p24 may be detectable in the first mo of acute HIV-1 infection and generally falls to undetectable levels during the asymptomatic stage of HIV-1 infection. A negative result does not exclude the possibility of infection or exposure to HIV-1. It is recommended that a negative result be followed with repeat testing at least 8 wk after the original test. This test is used primarily for screening of donated blood and plasma and as an aid for the prognosis of HIV-1 infection.

HUMAN IMMUNODEFICIENCY VIRUS TYPE 1 (HIV-1) VIRAL LOAD

Normal range: HIV-1 RNA, quant. bDNA 3: <50 copies/ml or <1.7 log copies/ml

This test should be used only in individuals with documented HIV-1 infection for monitoring the progression of infection, response to antiretroviral therapy, and disease prognosis. It is not indicated for diagnosis of HIV infection.

HUMAN PAPILLOMAVIRUS (HPV)

Test description: PCR test can be performed on cervical smears, biopsies, scrapings, liquid cytology specimen, and anogenital tissues.

HUNTINGTON DISEASE PCR

Test description: PCR can be performed on whole blood. Huntington disease is caused by the expansion of the trinucleotide repeat cytosine-adenine-guanine (CAG) within IT 15 (huntingtin). Pretest and posttest counseling should be performed when ordering this test.

HYDROGEN BREATH TEST

See "BREATH HYDROGEN TEST"

5-HYDROXYINDOLE-ACETIC ACID, URINE

See "URINE 5-HYDROXYINDOLE-ACETIC ACID"

IMMUNE COMPLEX ASSAY

Normal: Negative
Detected in: Collagen vascular disorders, glomerulonephritis, neoplastic diseases, malaria, primary biliary cirrhosis, chronic acute hepatitis, bacterial endocarditis, vasculitis

IMMUNOGLOBULINS

Normal range:

IgA:	50-350 mg/dl (0.5-3.5 g/L [CF: 0.01; SMI: 0.01 g/L])
IgD:	<6 mg/dl (<60 mg/L [CF: 0.01; SMI: 0.01 g/L])
IgE:	<25 µg/dl (<0.00025 g/L [CF: 0.01; SMI: 0.01 g/L])
IgG:	800-1500 mg/dl (8-15 g/L [CF: 0.01; SMI: 0.01 g/L])
IgM:	45-150 mg/dl (0.45-1.5 g/L [CF: 0.01; SMI: 0.01 g/L])

Table E66 summarizes biologic properties of human immunoglobulin isotopes. Box 19 summarizes selected conditions associated with monoclonal immunoglobulins. Disease states associated with polyclonal hyperimmunoglobulinemia are described in Table E67.
Elevated in:
1. **IgA:** Lymphoproliferative disorders, Berger nephropathy, chronic infections, autoimmune disorders, liver disease
2. **IgE:** Allergic disorders, parasitic infections, immunologic disorders, IgE myeloma (see Box E20 for summary of nonallergic diseases associated with high levels of IgE. Box 21
3. **IgG:** Chronic granulomatous infections, infectious diseases, inflammation, myeloma, liver disease
4. 4.**IgM:** Primary biliary cirrhosis, infectious diseases (brucellosis, malaria), Waldenström macroglobulinemia, liver disease

---

BOX 19   Selected Conditions Associated with Monoclonal Immunoglobulins

Multiple myeloma
Macroglobulinemia of Waldenström
Chronic lymphocytic leukemia
Other leukemias
Lymphomas
"Benign" monoclonal gammopathy
Systemic capillary leak syndrome
Amyloidosis
Chronic liver disease such as chronic active hepatitis, primary biliary cirrhosis
Autoimmune disorders, including rheumatoid arthritis, systemic lupus erythematosus, thyroiditis, pernicious anemia, polyarteritis nodosa, Sjögren syndrome
Gaucher disease
Malignancies of various types
Hereditary spherocytosis
HIV infection, including AIDS

From McPherson RA, Pincus MR: *Henry's clinical diagnosis and management by laboratory methods,* ed 23, St Louis, 2017, Elsevier.

BOX 21   Conditions Associated With Unusually High Serum Immunoglobulin E Concentrations (≥500 IU/ml)

Allergic bronchopulmonary mycosis
Allergic fungal sinusitis
Atopic dermatitis
Human immunodeficiency virus (HIV) infection
Hyperimmunoglobulin E (hyper-IgE) syndrome
Immunoglobulin E myeloma
Kimura disease
Lymphoma
Netherton syndrome
Systemic helminthic parasitosis
Tuberculosis

From Adkinson NF et al: *Middleton's allergy principles and practice,* ed 8, Philadelphia, 2014, Saunders.

Decreased in:
IgA: Nephrotic syndrome, protein-losing enteropathy, congenital deficiency, lymphocytic leukemia, ataxia-telangiectasia, chronic sinopulmonary disease
IgE: Hypogammaglobulinemia, neoplasms (breast, bronchial, cervical), ataxia-telangiectasia, primary biliary cirrhosis (see Box E20)
IgG: Congenital or acquired deficiency, lymphocytic leukemia, phenytoin, methylprednisolone, nephrotic syndrome, protein-losing enteropathy
IgM: Congenital deficiency, lymphocytic leukemia, nephrotic syndrome

INDIRECT ANTIGLOBULIN (COOMBS INDIRECT)

Normal: Negative
Positive: Acquired hemolytic anemia, incompatible cross-matched blood, anti-Rh antibodies, drugs (methyldopa, mefenamic acid, levodopa)
Fig. E34 illustrates the mechanism of Coombs test.

INFLUENZA A AND B TESTS

Test description: PCR can be performed on nasopharyngeal swab, wash, or aspirate.
Normal: Negative

INSULIN AUTOANTIBODIES

Normal: Negative
Present in: Exogenous insulin from insulin therapy. The presence of islet cell antibodies indicates ongoing beta cell destruction. This test is useful in the early diagnosis of type 1a diabetes mellitus and in the identification of patients at high risk for type 1a diabetes.

INSULIN, FREE

Normal: <17 mcU/ml
Elevated in: Insulin overdose, insulin resistance syndromes, endogenous hyperinsulinemia
Decreased in: Inadequately treated type 1 diabetes mellitus

INSULIN-LIKE GROWTH FACTOR-1 (IGF-1) (SERUM)

Normal range:

Ages 16-24:	182-780 ng/ml
Ages 25-39:	114-492 ng/ml
Ages 40-54:	90-360 ng/ml
Ages >55:	71-290 ng/ml

Elevated in: Adolescence, acromegaly, pregnancy, precocious puberty, obesity
Decreased in: Malnutrition, delayed puberty, diabetes mellitus, hypopituitarism, cirrhosis, old age

INSULIN-LIKE GROWTH FACTOR-II

Normal range: 288 to 736 ng/ml
Elevated in: Hypoglycemia associated with nonislet cell tumors, hepatoma, and Wilms tumor
Decreased in: Growth hormone deficiency

INTERNATIONAL NORMALIZED RATIO (INR)

The INR is a comparative rating of prothrombin time (PT) ratios. The INR represents the observed PT ratio adjusted by the International Reference Thromboplastin. It provides a universal result indicative of what the patient's PT result would have been if measured using the primary World Health Organization International Reference reagent. For proper interpretation of INR values, the patient should be on stable anticoagulant therapy.

RECOMMENDED INR RANGES

Proximal deep vein thrombosis:	2-3
Pulmonary embolism:	2-3
Transient ischemic attacks:	2-3
Atrial fibrillation:	2-3
Mechanical prosthetic valves:	2.5-3.5
Recurrent venous thromboembolic disease:	2.5-3.5

INTRINSIC FACTOR ANTIBODIES

Normal: Negative
Present in: Pernicious anemia (>50% of patients). Cyanocobalamin may give false-positive results.

IRON (SERUM)

Normal: Male: 65 to 175 mcg/dl; female: 50 to 1170 mcg/dl
Elevated in: Hemochromatosis, excessive iron therapy, repeated transfusions, lead poisoning, hemolytic anemia, aplastic anemia, pernicious anemia
Decreased in: Iron deficiency anemia, hypothyroidism, chronic infection

IRON-BINDING CAPACITY, TOTAL (TIBC)

Normal range: 250 to 460 µg/dl (45 to 82 µmol/L [CF: 0.1791; SMI: 1 µmol/L])
Elevated in: Iron deficiency anemia, pregnancy, polycythemia, hepatitis, weight loss
Decreased in: Anemia of chronic disease, hemochromatosis, chronic liver disease, hemolytic anemias, malnutrition (protein depletion)
Table 68 describes TIBC and serum iron abnormalities.

IRON SATURATION (% TRANSFERRIN SATURATION)

Normal:
Male: 20% to 50%
Female: 15% to 50%

TABLE 68 Serum Iron and Total Iron-Binding Capacity Patterns

SI↓	TIBC↓	Chronic diseases; uremia
SI↓	TIBC↑	Chronic iron deficiency anemia; pregnancy in third trimester
SI↑	TIBC↓	Hemochromatosis iron therapy overload (TIBC may be normal); hemolytic anemia; thalassemia; lead poisoning; megaloblastic anemia; aplastic, pyridoxine deficiency, or other sideroblastic anemias
SI↑	TIBC↑	Oral contraceptives; acute hepatitis (some report TIBC is low normal); chronic hepatitis (some patients)
SI↑	TIBCNL	B₁₂ or folate deficiency
SI↓	TIBCNL	Chronic iron deficiency (some patients); acute infection, surgery, tissue damage
SI NL	TIBC↑	B₁₂/folate deficiency plus iron deficiency

NL, Normal; *SI*, serum iron; *TIBC*, total iron-binding capacity.

Elevated in: Hemochromatosis, excessive iron intake, aplastic anemia, thalassemia, vitamin B₆ deficiency
Decreased in: Hypochromic anemias, GI malignancy

LACTATE (BLOOD)

Normal range: 0.5 to 2.0 mEq/L
Elevated in: Tissue hypoxia (shock, respiratory failure, severe CHF, severe anemia, carbon monoxide or cyanide poisoning), systemic disorders (liver or renal failure, seizures), abnormal intestinal flora (D-lactic acidosis), drugs or toxins (salicylates, ethanol, methanol, ethylene glycol), G6PD deficiency

LACTATE DEHYDROGENASE (LDH)

Normal range: 50 to 150 U/L (0.82 to 2.66 µkat/L [CF: 0.01667; SMI: 0.02 µkat/L])
Elevated in:
1. Infarction of myocardium, lung, kidney
2. Diseases of cardiopulmonary system, liver, collagen, central nervous system
3. Hemolytic anemias, megaloblastic anemias, transfusions, seizures, muscle trauma, muscular dystrophy, acute pancreatitis, hypotension, shock, infectious mononucleosis, inflammation, neoplasia, intestinal obstruction, hypothyroidism

LACTATE DEHYDROGENASE ISOENZYMES

Normal range:

LDH₁:	22%-36% (cardiac, red blood cell) (0.22-0.36 [CF: 0.01, SMI: 0.01])
LDH₂:	35%-46% (cardiac, red blood cell) (0.35-0.46)
LDH₃:	13%-26% (pulmonary) (0.15-0.26)
LDH₄:	3%-10% (striated muscle, liver) (0.03-0.1)
LDH₅:	2%-9% (striated muscle, liver) (0.02-0.09)

Normal ratios:
$LDH_1 < LDH_2$
$LDH_5 < LDH_4$
Abnormal values:
$LDH_1 > LDH_2$: Myocardial infarction (can also be seen with hemolytic anemias, pernicious anemia, folate deficiency, renal infarct)
$LDH_5 > LDH_4$: Liver disease (cirrhosis, hepatitis, hepatic congestion)

LACTOSE TOLERANCE TEST (SERUM)

Normal: Test is performed by giving 2 g/kg body weight lactose orally and drawing glucose level at 0, 30, 45, 60, and 90 min. Normal response is change in glucose from fasting value to >30 mg/dl. Inconclusive response is increase of 20 to 30 mg/dl, abnormal response is increase <20 mg/dl. Table E69 summarizes laboratory tests in the differential diagnosis of diarrhea.
Abnormal in: Lactase deficiency

LAP SCORE
See "LEUKOCYTE ALKALINE PHOSPHATASE"

LEAD
Normal: Child, <10 mcg/dl; adult, <25 mcg/dl; acceptable for industrial exposure, <50 mcg/dl
Elevated in: Lead exposure, lead poisoning

LDH
See "LACTATE DEHYDROGENASE"

LDL
See "LOW-DENSITY LIPOPROTEIN CHOLESTEROL"

LEGIONELLA PNEUMOPHILA PCR
Test description: PCR can be performed on lung tissue, water sputum, bronchoalveolar lavage, and other respiratory fluids.

LEGIONELLA TITER
Normal: Negative
Positive in: Legionnaires disease (presumptive: ≥1:256 titer; definitive: fourfold titer increase to ≥1:128)

LEUKOCYTE ALKALINE PHOSPHATASE (LAP)
Normal range: 13 to 100 (33 to 188 U)
Elevated in: Leukemoid reactions, neutrophilia secondary to infections (except in sickle cell crisis—no significant increase in LAP score), Hodgkin disease, polycythemia vera, hairy cell leukemia, aplastic anemia, Down syndrome, myelofibrosis
Decreased in: Acute and chronic granulocytic leukemia, thrombocytopenic purpura, paroxysmal nocturnal hemoglobinuria, hypophosphatemia, collagen disorders

LEUKOCYTE COUNT
See "COMPLETE BLOOD COUNT"

LIPASE
Normal range: 0 to 160 U/L (0 to 2.66 μkat/L [CF: 0.01667; SMI: 0.02 μkat/L])
Elevated in: Acute pancreatitis, perforated peptic ulcer, carcinoma of pancreas (early stage), pancreatic duct obstruction, bowel infarction, intestinal obstruction

LIPOPROTEIN(A)
Normal: Male: 1.35 to 19.6 mg/dl; female: 1.24 to 20.1 mg/dl. Fig. E35 illustrates lipoprotein structure. Table E70 summarizes the major classes of human plasma lipoproteins. The chemical composition of major classes of plasma lipoproteins is described in Table E71.
Elevated in: Coronary artery disease, uncontrolled diabetes, hypothyroidism, chronic renal failure, pregnancy, tobacco use, infections, nephritic syndrome
Decreased in: Niacin, omega-3 fatty acids, estrogens, tamoxifen, statins

LIPOPROTEIN CHOLESTEROL, HIGH-DENSITY
See "HIGH-DENSITY LIPOPROTEIN CHOLESTEROL"

LIPOPROTEIN CHOLESTEROL, LOW-DENSITY
See "LOW-DENSITY LIPOPROTEIN CHOLESTEROL"

LIVER KIDNEY MICROSOME TYPE 1 ANTIBODIES (LKM1)
Normal: <20 U
Elevated in: Autoimmune hepatitis type 2

LKM1
See "LIVER KIDNEY MICROSOME TYPE 1 ANTIBODIES"

LOW-DENSITY LIPOPROTEIN (LDL) CHOLESTEROL
Normal range: 50 to 130 mg/dl (1.30 to 1.68 mmol/L [CF: 0.02586; SMI: 0.05 mmol/L]). Fig. E36 illustrates the LDL receptor pathway and regulation of cholesterol metabolism.

<70	Optimal in diabetics, prior MI, and patients with cardiac risk factors
100-129	Near or above optimal
130-159	Borderline high
160-189	High
≥190	Very high

LUPUS ANTICOAGULANT
See "CIRCULATING ANTICOAGULANT"

LUTEINIZING HORMONE
Luteinizing hormone (LH) changes during the menstrual cycle are illustrated in Fig. E37. LH changes in different disease states are summarized in Table E72.
Normal range: 5 to 25 mIU/ml
Elevated in: Postmenopause, pituitary adenoma, primary gonadal dysfunction, polycystic ovary syndrome
Decreased in: Severe illness, anorexia nervosa, malnutrition, pituitary or hypothalamic impairment, severe stress

LYME DISEASE ANTIBODY TITER
Normal range: Negative
Positive result: Fig. E38 illustrates the usual serologic response in Lyme disease.

LYMPHOCYTES
Normal range:
15% to 40%
Total lymphocyte count = 800 to 2600/mm³
Total T lymphocyte = 800 to 2200/mm³
CD4 lymphocytes = ≥400/mm³
CD8 lymphocytes = 200 to 800/mm³
Normal CD4/CD8 ratio is 2.0.
Elevated in: Chronic infections, infectious mononucleosis and other viral infections, chronic lymphocytic leukemia, Hodgkin disease, ulcerative colitis, hypoadrenalism, idiopathic thrombocytopenia
Decreased in: AIDS, bone marrow suppression from chemotherapeutic agents or chemotherapy, aplastic anemia, neoplasms, steroids, adrenocortical hyperfunction, neurologic disorders (multiple sclerosis, myasthenia gravis, Guillain-Barré syndrome)

CD4 lymphocytes are calculated as total white blood cells × % lymphocytes × % lymphocytes stained with CD4. They are decreased in AIDS and other immune dysfunction.

Table E73 describes various lymphocyte abnormalities in peripheral blood.

Box E22 summarizes key causes of lymphocytopenia.

MAGNESIUM (SERUM)
See Figs. E39 and E40.
Normal range: 1.8 to 3.0 mg/dl (0.80 to 1.20 mmol/L [CF: 0.4114; SMI: 0.02 mmol/L])
CAUSES OF HYPERMAGNESEMIA
1. Decreased renal excretion
2. Renal failure—glomerular filtration rate less than 30 ml/min
3. Hyperparathyroidism
4. Hypothyroidism
5. Addison disease
6. Lithium intoxication
7. Familial hypocalciuric hypercalcemia
8. Other causes: Usually in association with decrease in glomerular filtration rate

9. Endogenous loads
10. Diabetic ketoacidosis
11. Severe tissue injury: Burns
12. Exogenous loads
13. Gastrointestinal
14. Magnesium-containing laxatives and antacids
15. High-dose vitamin D analogs
16. Parenteral: Management of toxemia of pregnancy

CAUSES OF HYPOMAGNESEMIA

1. Alcohol abuse
2. Diuretic use
3. Renal losses
4. Acute and chronic renal failure
5. Postobstructive diuresis
6. Acute tubular necrosis
7. Chronic glomerulonephritis
8. Chronic pyelonephritis
9. Interstitial nephropathy
10. Renal transplantation
11. Gastrointestinal losses
12. Chronic diarrhea
13. Nasogastric suctioning
14. Short bowel syndrome
15. Protein-calorie malnutrition
16. Bowel fistula
17. Total parenteral nutrition
18. Acute pancreatitis
19. Endocrine
20. Diabetes mellitus
21. Hyperaldosteronism
22. Hyperthyroidism
23. Hyperparathyroidism
24. Acute intermittent porphyria
25. Pregnancy
26. Drugs
27. Aminoglycosides
28. Amphotericin
29. β-agonists
30. Cisplatin
31. Cyclosporine
32. Diuretics
33. Foscarnet
34. Pentamidine
35. Theophylline
36. Congenital disorders
37. Familial hypomagnesemia
38. Maternal diabetes
39. Maternal hypothyroidism
40. Maternal hyperparathyroidism

MEAN CORPUSCULAR VOLUME (MCV)

Laboratory features in microcytic hypochromic anemias are summarized in Table E74.

Normal range: 76 to 100 μm^3 (76 to 100 fL [CF: 1; SMI: 1 fL])

Table E75 summarizes clinical conditions not to be confused with megaloblastosis. See Tables E76 and E77 for descriptions of MCV abnormalities. Table E78 describes the usefulness of the MCV and RBC distribution width in the diagnosis of anemia. Table E79 describes peripheral blood film evaluation in a patient with red cell membrane disorder.

METANEPHRINES, URINE

See "URINE METANEPHRINES"

METHYLMALONIC ACID (SERUM)

Normal: <0.2 μmol/L
Elevated in: Vitamin B_{12} deficiency, pregnancy, methylmalonic acidemia

MITOCHONDRIAL ANTIBODY (AMA)

Normal: Negative
Present in: Primary biliary cirrhosis (>90% of patients)

MONOCYTE COUNT

Normal range: 2% to 8%
Elevated in: Viral diseases, parasites, infections, neoplasms, inflammatory bowel disease, monocytic leukemia, lymphomas, myeloma, sarcoidosis
Decreased in: Aplastic anemia, lymphocytic leukemia, glucocorticoid administration
See Table E80 for changes in monocyte number.

MYCOPLASMA PNEUMONIAE PCR

Test description: PCR can be performed on sputum, bronchoalveolar lavage, nasopharyngeal and throat swabs, other respiratory fluids, and lung tissue.

MYELIN BASIC PROTEIN, CEREBROSPINAL FLUID

Normal: <2.5 ng/ml
Elevated in: Multiple sclerosis, CNS trauma, stroke, encephalitis

MYOGLOBIN, URINE

See "URINE MYOGLOBIN"

NEISSERIA GONORRHOEAE PCR

Test description: Test can be performed on endocervical swab, urine, and intraurethral swab
Normal: Negative

NEUTROPHIL COUNT

Normal range: 50% to 70%
Subsets
Stabs (bands, early mature neutrophils): 2% to 6%
Segs (mature neutrophils): 60% to 70%
Elevated in: Acute bacterial infections, acute myocardial infarction, stress, neoplasms, myelocytic leukemia
Decreased in: Viral infections, aplastic anemias, immunosuppressive drugs, radiation therapy to bone marrow, agranulocytosis, drugs (antibiotics, antithyroidals, clopidogrel), lymphocytic and monocytic leukemias

Box 23 describes various drugs that can cause neutropenia. Table E81 describes miscellaneous inherited neutropenia disorders. Classification of neutropenia is covered in Table E82. Table E83 lists drugs associated with agranulocytosis. Table E84 describes causes of neutrophilia.

NOREPINEPHRINE

Normal range: 0 to 600 pg/ml
Elevated in: Pheochromocytomas, neuroblastomas, stress, vigorous exercise, certain foods (bananas, chocolate, coffee, tea, vanilla)

5′-NUCLEOTIDASE

Normal range: 2 to 16 IU/L (3-27 × 10^8 kat/L [CF: 1.67 × 10^8; SMI: 1 × 10^8 kat/L])

BOX 23 Drugs That Cause Neutropenia

Antiarrhythmics: Tocainide, procainamide, propranolol, quinidine
Antibiotics: Chloramphenicol, penicillins, sulfonamides, *p*-aminosalicylic acid (PAS), rifampin, vancomycin, isoniazid, nitrofurantoin
Antimalarials: Dapsone, quinine, pyrimethamine
Anticonvulsants: Phenytoin, mephenytoin, trimethadione, ethosuximide, carbamazepine
Hypoglycemic agents: Tolbutamide, chlorpropamide
Antihistamines: Cimetidine, brompheniramine, tripelennamine
Antihypertensives: Methyldopa, captopril
Antiinflammatory agents: Aminopyrine, phenylbutazone, gold salts, ibuprofen, indomethacin
Antithyroid agents: Propylthiouracil, methimazole, thiouracil
Diuretics: Acetazolamide, hydrochlorothiazide, chlorthalidone
Phenothiazines: Chlorpromazine, promazine, prochlorperazine
Immunosuppressive agents: Antimetabolites
Cytotoxic agents: Alkylating agents, antimetabolites, anthracyclines, *Vinca* alkaloids, cisplatin, hydroxyurea, dactinomycin
Other agents: Recombinant interferons, allopurinol, ethanol, levamisole, penicillamine, zidovudine, streptokinase, carbamazepine, clopidogrel, ticlopidine

Elevated in: Biliary obstruction, metastatic neoplasms to liver, primary biliary cirrhosis, renal failure, pancreatic carcinoma, chronic active hepatitis

OSMOLALITY (SERUM)

Normal range:
280 to 300 mOsm/kg (280 to 300 mmol/kg [CF: 1; SMI: 1 mmol/kg])
It can also be estimated by the following formula: 2([Na]+[K]+glucose/18+BUN/2.8)

The relationship between plasma osmolality and plasma arginine vasopressin is illustrated in Fig. E41.

The relationships between plasma and urine osmolality are illustrated in Fig. E42.

Elevated in: Dehydration, hypernatremia, diabetes insipidus, uremia, hyperglycemia, mannitol therapy, ingestion of toxins (ethylene glycol, methanol, ethanol), hypercalcemia, diuretics

Decreased in: Syndrome of inappropriate diuretic hormone secretion, hyponatremia, overhydration, Addison disease, hypothyroidism

OSMOLALITY, URINE

Normal range: 50 to 1200 mOsm/kg (50 to 1200 mmol/kg [CF: 1; SMI: 1 mmol/kg])

Elevated in: Syndrome of inappropriate antidiuretic hormone secretion, dehydration, glycosuria, adrenal insufficiency, high-protein diet

Decreased in: Diabetes insipidus, excessive water intake, IV hydration with D_5W, acute renal insufficiency, glomerulonephritis

The relationship between plasma urine osmolality and plasma arginine vasopressin in patients with polyuria is illustrated in Fig. E43. Box E24 describes urine osmolality variances in common clinical situations.

OSMOTIC FRAGILITY TEST

Normal: Hemolysis begins at 0.50, w/v [5.0 g/L] and is complete at 0.30, w/v [3.0 g/L] NaCl.

Elevated in: Hereditary spherocytosis, hereditary stomatocytosis, spherocytosis associated with acquired immune hemolytic anemia

Decreased in: Iron deficiency anemia, thalassemias, liver disease, leptocytosis associated with asplenia

PARACENTESIS FLUID

Testing and evaluation of results: Process the fluid as follows:
- Tube 1: LDH, glucose, albumin.
- Tube 2: Protein, specific gravity.
- Tube 3: Cell count and differential.
- Tube 4: Save until further notice.
- Draw serum LDH, protein, albumin.
- Gram stain, acid-fast bacilli stain, bacterial and fungal cultures, amylase, and triglycerides should be ordered only when clearly indicated; bedside inoculation of blood-culture bottles with ascitic fluid improves sensitivity in detecting bacterial growth.
- If malignant ascites is suspected, consider a carcinoembryonic antigen level on the paracentesis fluid and cytologic evaluation.
- In suspected spontaneous bacterial peritonitis (SBP) the incidence of positive cultures can be increased by injecting 10 to 20 ml of ascitic fluid into blood culture bottles.
- Peritoneal effusion can be subdivided as exudative or transudative based on its characteristics (see "Section II").
- The serum-ascites albumin gradient (serum albumin level-ascitic fluid albumin level [SAAG]) correlates directly with portal pressure and can also be used to classify ascites. Patients with gradients ≥1.1 g/dl have portal hypertension, and those with gradients ≤1.1 g/dl do not; the accuracy of this method is >95%.
- For the differential diagnosis of ascites, refer to Section II.
- An ascitic fluid polymorphonuclear leukocyte count >500/μL is suggestive of SBP.
- A blood-ascitic fluid albumin gradient. Box E25 summarizes causes of peritoneal effusions. Useful criteria for evaluation of peritoneal lavage is summarized in Box E26. Recommended tests in peritoneal effusions are summarized in Box E27.

PARATHYROID HORMONE (PTH)

Table E85 describes serum PTH and calcium patterns in various disorders.

Normal:
Serum, intact molecule 10 to 65 pg/ml
Plasma 1.0 to 5.0 pmol/L

Elevated in: Hyperparathyroidism (primary or secondary), pseudohypoparathyroidism, anticonvulsants, corticosteroids, lithium, isoniazid (INH), rifampin, phosphates, Zollinger-Ellison syndrome, hereditary vitamin D deficiency

Decreased in: Hypoparathyroidism, sarcoidosis, cimetidine, β-blockers, hyperthyroidism, hypomagnesemia

PARIETAL CELL ANTIBODIES

Normal: Negative
Present in: Pernicious anemia (>90%), atrophic gastritis (up to 50%), thyroiditis (30%), Addison disease, myasthenia gravis, Sjögren syndrome, type 1 DM

PARTIAL THROMBOPLASTIN TIME (PTT), ACTIVATED PARTIAL THROMBOPLASTIN TIME (APTT)

See Table E86 for interpretation of coagulation protein screening tests.
Normal range: 25 to 41 sec
Elevated in: Heparin therapy, coagulation factor deficiency (I, II, V, VIII, IX, X, XI, XII), liver disease, vitamin K deficiency, disseminated intravascular coagulation, circulating anticoagulant, warfarin therapy, specific factor inhibition (penicillin [PCN] reaction, rheumatoid arthritis), thrombolytic therapy, nephrotic syndrome

NOTE: Useful to evaluate the intrinsic coagulation system.

PEPSINOGEN I

Normal: 124 to 142 ng/ml
Elevated in: Zollinger-Ellison (ZE) syndrome, duodenal ulcer, acute gastritis
Decreased in: Atrophic gastritis, gastric carcinoma, myxedema, pernicious anemia, Addison disease

PH, BLOOD

Normal values:
Arterial: 7.35 to 7.45
Venous: 7.32 to 7.42
For abnormal values, refer to "ARTERIAL BLOOD GASES."

PH, URINE

See "URINE pH"

PHENOBARBITAL

Therapeutic range and general information are summarized in Table 87.
Normal therapeutic range: 15 to 30 mcg/ml for epilepsy control

TABLE 87	Phenobarbital
Purpose	**Treatment of Generalized Tonic-Clonic Seizures, Simple Partial Seizures, Anxiety, Insomnia**
General adult dose	Oral: 100-200 mg/day for seizure control; 30-120 mg/day for anxiety; 100-320 mg for sleep induction
Usual bioavailability	Approximately 90%-100%
Half-life	Approximately 5-6 days in adults; approximately 3-4 days in children
General therapeutic range	15-30 mcg/ml for epilepsy control
General toxic level	>40 mcg/ml, although tolerance may develop
Transport	Approximately 40%-60% plasma protein bound
Metabolism	Approximately 75% hepatic:*p*-hydroxyphenobarbital, inactive
Elimination	Approximately 25% unchanged in urine
Steady state	Approximately 14-21 days
Mechanism of action	Stabilizes damaged membranes and raises threshold for neuronal membrane depolarization
Toxic effects	Drowsiness, depression, respiratory depression, coma, sedation, hypotension. Respiratory depression may be caused by rapid intravenous administration

From McPherson RA, Pincus MR: *Henry's clinical diagnosis and management by laboratory methods,* ed 23, St Louis, 2017, Elsevier.

	Treatment of Generalized Tonic-Clonic Seizures, Simple Partial Seizures, Complex
Purpose	**Partial Seizures**
General adult dose	Oral: 300-400 mg/day maintenance dose
Usual bioavailability	Variable: 30%-95%
Half-life	24 ± 12 h, and dose dependent
General therapeutic range	10-20 mcg/ml
General toxic level	>20 mcg/ml
Transport	Approximately 90%-95% plasma protein bound
Metabolism	Hepatic: 5-(p-hydroxyphenyl)5-phenylhydantoin, inactive
Elimination	Approximately 5% unchanged in urine
Steady state	Approximately 7-8 days
Mechanism of action	Appears to block sodium and calcium ion influxes into repeatedly depolarizing CNS neurons
Toxic effects	Nystagmus, ataxia, diplopia, drowsiness, coma; rapid intravenous administration may produce cardiovascular collapse and/or CNS depression

TABLE 88 Phenytoin (Dilantin)

CNS, Central nervous system.
From McPherson RA, Pincus MR: *Henry's clinical diagnosis and management by laboratory methods,* ed 23, St Louis, 2017, Elsevier.

PHENYTOIN (DILANTIN)

Therapeutic range and general information are summarized in Table 88.
Normal therapeutic range: 10 to 20 mcg/ml

PHOSPHATASE, ACID

See "ACID PHOSPHATASE"

PHOSPHATASE, ALKALINE

See "ALKALINE PHOSPHATASE"

PHOSPHATE (SERUM)

Phosphate levels in various disorders are summarized in Table E89.
Normal range: 2.5 to 5 mg/dl (0.8 to 1.6 mmol/L [CF: 0.3229; SMI: 0.05 mmol/L])
DECREASED
Parenteral hyperalimentation
Diabetic acidosis
Alcohol withdrawal
Severe metabolic or respiratory alkalosis
Antacids that bind phosphorus
Malnutrition with refeeding using low-phosphorus nutrients
Renal tubule failure to reabsorb phosphate (Fanconi syndrome; congenital disorder; vitamin D deficiency)
Glucose administration
Nasogastric suction
Malabsorption
Gram-negative sepsis
Primary hyperthyroidism
Chlorothiazide diuretics
Therapy of acute severe asthma
Acute respiratory failure with mechanical ventilation
INCREASED
Renal failure
Severe muscle injury
Phosphate-containing antacids
Hypoparathyroidism
Tumor lysis syndrome

PLASMA CELLS

Plasma cells are not normally present in circulating blood. They are increased in a variety of chronic infections, in allergic states, in the presence of neoplasms, and in other conditions in which the serum γ-globulin concentration is elevated. Plasma cells have also been recorded in the blood of patients with viral disorders, including rubella, measles, chickenpox, and mumps. They are moderately increased in cutaneous exanthemas, infectious mononucleosis, syphilis, subacute bacterial endocarditis, sarcoidosis, and collagen disease. Rarely, bacterial sepsis may show a peripheral plasmacytosis mimicking plasma cell leukemia. Their increase is usually linked with increases in lymphocytes, monocytes, and eosinophils. Causes and conditions associated with plasmacytosis include those listed in Box E28.

PLASMINOGEN

Normal: Immunoassay (antigen): <20 mg/dl
Elevated in
Infection, trauma, neoplasm, myocardial infarction (acute phase reactant), pregnancy, bilirubinemia
Decreased in: Disseminated intravascular coagulation (DIC), severe liver disease, thrombolytic therapy with streptokinase or urokinase, alteplase

PLATELET AGGREGATION

Normal: Full aggregation (generally >60%) in response to epinephrine, thrombin, ristocetin, adenosine diphosphate (ADP), collagen
Elevated in: Heparin, hemolysis, lipemia, nicotine, hereditary and acquired disorders of platelet adhesion, activation, and aggregation
Decreased in: Aspirin, some penicillins, chloroquine, chlorpromazine, clofibrate, captopril, Glanzmann thrombasthenia, Bernard-Soulier syndrome, Wiskott-Aldrich syndrome, cyclooxygenase deficiency. In von Willebrand disease there is normal aggregation with ADP, collagen, and epinephrine but abnormal agglutination with ristocetin.

PLATELET ANTIBODIES

Normal: Absent
Present in: Idiopathic thrombocytopenic purpura (ITP) (>90% of patients with chronic ITP). Patients with nonimmune thrombocytopenias may have false-positive results.

PLATELET COUNT

A classification of inherited thrombocytopenias by platelet size is described in Table E90.
See Fig. E44 for evaluation of thrombocytosis. Box E29 describes testing for thrombocytopenia. See Table E91 for differential diagnosis. Table E92 describes antibody-mediated thrombocytopenic disorders caused by autoantibodies, alloantibodies, or potentially both. Tables E93 and E94 indicate differential diagnosis of thrombocytopenia in newborns and differential diagnosis of thrombocytopenia in pregnancy, respectively. Table E95 describes laboratory tests used to investigate a patient with thrombocytopenia.
Normal range: 130 to 400 × 10³/mm³ (130 to 400 × 10⁹/L [CF: 1; SMI: 5 × 10⁹/L])
Elevated in: *REACTIVE THROMBOCYTOSIS*
Infections or inflammatory states: Vasculitis, allergic reactions, etc.
Surgery and tissue damage: Myocardial infarction, pancreatitis, etc.
Postsplenectomy state
Malignancy: Solid tumors, lymphoma
Iron deficiency anemia, hemolytic anemia, acute blood loss
Uncertain etiology
Rebound effect after chemotherapy or immune thrombocytopenia
Renal disorders: Renal failure, nephrotic syndrome
MYELOPROLIFERATIVE DISORDERS
Chronic myeloid leukemia
Primary thrombocythemia
Polycythemia vera
Idiopathic myelofibrosis
Decreased: Increased destruction (see Table E96)
Immunologic
Drugs: Quinine, quinidine, digitalis, procainamide, thiazide diuretics, sulfonamides, phenytoin, aspirin, penicillin, heparin, gold, meprobamate, sulfa drugs, phenylbutazone, NSAIDs, methyldopa, cimetidine, furosemide, INH, cephalosporins, chlorpropamide, organic arsenicals, chloroquine
Idiopathic thrombocytopenic purpura

Transfusion reaction: Transfusion of platelets with platelet antigen HPA-1a (PL^{A1}) in recipients without PL^{A1}

Fetal/maternal incompatibility

Vasculitis (e.g., systemic lupus erythematosus)

Autoimmune hemolytic anemia

Lymphoreticular disorders (e.g., chronic lymphocytic leukemia)

Nonimmunologic

    Prosthetic heart valves

    Thrombotic thrombocytopenic purpura

    Sepsis

    Disseminated intravascular coagulation

    Hemolytic-uremic syndrome

    Giant cavernous hemangioma

Decreased production

    Abnormal marrow

        Marrow infiltration (e.g., leukemia, lymphoma, fibrosis)

        Marrow suppression (e.g., chemotherapy, alcohol, radiation)

    Hereditary disorders (see Table E97)

    Wiskott-Aldrich syndrome: X-linked disorder characterized by thrombocytopenia, eczema, and repeated infections

    May-Hegglin anomaly: Increased megakaryocytes but ineffective thrombopoiesis

    Vitamin deficiencies (e.g., vitamin B$_{12}$, folic acid)

    Splenic sequestration, hypersplenism

    Dilutional, secondary to massive transfusion

PLATELET FUNCTION ANALYSIS 100 ASSAY (PFA)

Normal: This test is a two-component assay where blood is aspirated through two capillary tubes, one of which is coated with collagen and ADP (COL/ADP) and the other with collagen and epinephrine (COL/EPI). The test measures the ability of platelets to occlude an aperture in a biologically active membrane treated with COL/ADP and COL/EPI. During the test, the platelets adhere to the surface of the tube and cause blood flow to cease. The closing time refers to the cessation of blood flow and is reported in conjunction with the hematocrit and platelet count. Hematocrit count must be >25% and platelet count >50 K/microliter for the test to be performed.

    COL/ADP: 70 to 120 sec

    COL/EPI: 75 to 120 sec

Elevated in: Acquired platelet dysfunction, von Willebrand disease, anemia, thrombocytopenia, use of aspirin and NSAIDs

PLEURAL FLUID

Testing and evaluation of results:

Pleural effusion fluid should be differentiated in exudate or transudate.

The initial laboratory studies should be aimed only at distinguishing an exudate from a transudate.

Tube 1: Protein, LDH, albumin.

Tubes 2, 3, 4: Save the fluid until further notice. In selected patients with suspected empyema, a pH level may be useful (generally ≤7.0). See following for proper procedure to obtain a pH level from pleural fluid.

A serum/effusion albumin gradient of ≤1.2 g/dl is indicative of exudative effusions, especially in patients with congestive heart failure (CHF) treated with diuretics.

Note the appearance of the fluid:

    A grossly hemorrhagic effusion can be a result of a traumatic tap, neoplasm, or an embolus with infarction.

    A milky appearance indicates either of the following:

        Chylous effusion: Caused by trauma or tumor invasion of the thoracic duct; lipoprotein electrophoresis of the effusion reveals chylomicrons and triglyceride levels >115 mg/dl.

        Pseudochylous effusion: Often seen with chronic inflammation of the pleural space (e.g., TB, connective tissue diseases).

If transudate, consider CHF, cirrhosis, chronic renal failure, and other hypoproteinemic states and perform subsequent workup accordingly.

If exudate, consider ordering these tests on the pleural fluid:

    Cytologic examination for malignant cells (for suspected neoplasm).

    Gram stain, cultures (aerobic and anaerobic), and sensitivities (for suspected infectious process).

    AFB stain and cultures (for suspected TB).

    pH: A value <7.0 suggests parapneumonic effusion or empyema; a pleural fluid pH must be drawn anaerobically and iced immediately; the syringe should be prerinsed with 0.2 ml of 1:1000 heparin.

    Glucose: A low glucose level suggests parapneumonic effusions and rheumatoid arthritis.

    Amylase: A high amylase level suggests pancreatitis or ruptured esophagus.

Perplexing pleural effusions are often a result of malignancy (e.g., lymphoma, malignant mesothelioma, ovarian carcinoma), TB, subdiaphragmatic processes, prior asbestos exposure, and postcardiac injury syndrome.

Box E30 describes a cellular differential of pleural effusions. Features differentiating exudative from transudative pleural effusion are summarized in Table E98.

POTASSIUM (SERUM)

Normal range: 3.5 to 5 mEq/L (3.5 to 5 mmol/L [CF: 1; SMI: 0.1 mmol/L])

CAUSES OF HYPERKALEMIA

See Fig. E45 for evaluation and treatment of hyperkalemia, and Fig. E46 for electrocardiographic changes in hyperkalemia.

Pseudohyperkalemia

    Hemolysis of sample

    Thrombocytosis

    Leukocytosis

    Laboratory error

Increased potassium intake and absorption

    Potassium supplements (oral and parenteral)

    Dietary: Salt substitutes

    Stored blood

    Potassium-containing medications

Impaired renal excretion

    Acute renal failure

    Chronic renal failure

    Tubular defect in potassium secretion

        Renal allograft

        Analgesic nephropathy

        Sickle cell disease

        Obstructive uropathy

    Hypoaldosteronism

        Primary (Addison disease)

        Secondary

            Hyporeninemic hypoaldosteronism (type IV renal tubular acidosis [RTA])

            Congenital adrenal hyperplasia

            Drug-induced

            NSAIDs

            ACE inhibitors

            Heparin

            Cyclosporine

    Transcellular shifts

        Acidosis

        Hypertonicity

        Insulin deficiency

        Drugs

            β-Blockers

            Digitalis toxicity

            Succinylcholine

Exercise

Hyperkalemic periodic paralysis

Cellular injury

    Rhabdomyolysis

    Severe intravascular hemolysis

    Acute tumor lysis syndrome

    Burns and crush injuries

CAUSES OF HYPOKALEMIA

For the clinical approach to hypokalemia, see Fig. 47.

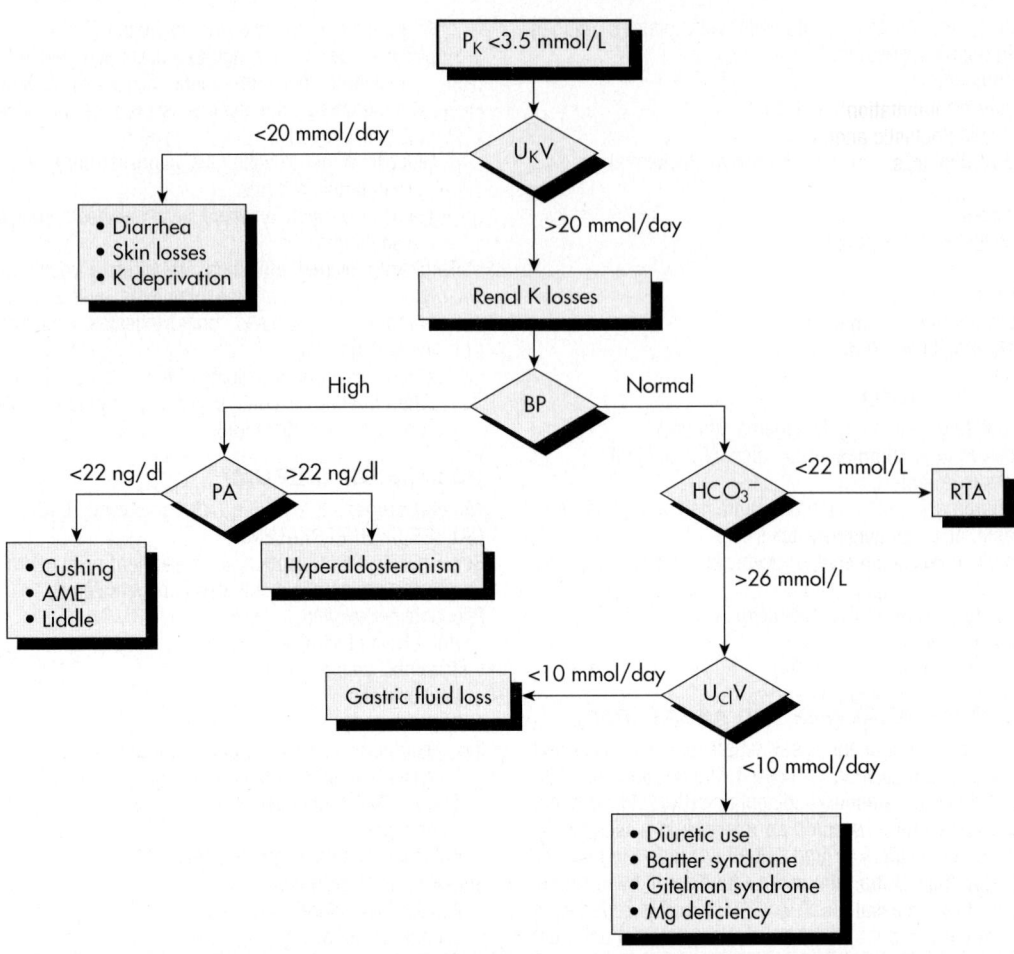

FIG. 47 Diagnostic evaluation of chronic hypokalemia. *AME,* Syndrome of apparent mineralocorticoid excess; *BP,* blood pressure; *HCO₃⁻,* bicarbonate; *PA,* stimulated plasma aldosterone (see text); *RTA,* renal tubular acidosis; *U_Cl V,* urinary chloride excretion; *U_k V,* urinary potassium excretion. (From Parrillo JE, Dellinger RP: *Critical care medicine, principles of diagnosis and management in the adult,* ed 5, Philadelphia, 2019, Elsevier.)

Decreased intake
  Decreased dietary potassium
  Impaired absorption of potassium
  Clay ingestion
  Kayexalate
Increased loss
  Renal
  Hyperaldosteronism
    Primary
      Conn syndrome
      Adrenal hyperplasia
    Secondary
      Congestive heart failure
      Cirrhosis
      Nephrotic syndrome
      Dehydration
      Bartter syndrome
  Glycyrrhizic acid (licorice, chewing tobacco)
  Excessive adrenal corticosteroids
    Cushing syndrome
    Steroid therapy
    Adrenogenital syndrome
  Renal tubular defects
    Renal tubular acidosis
    Obstructive uropathy
    Salt-wasting nephropathy
  Drugs
    Diuretics

    Aminoglycosides
    Mannitol
    Amphotericin
    Cisplatin
    Carbenicillin
  Gastrointestinal
    Vomiting
    Nasogastric suction
    Diarrhea
    Malabsorption
    Ileostomy
    Villous adenoma
    Laxative abuse
  Increased losses from the skin
    Excessive sweating
    Burns
Transcellular shifts
  Alkalosis
    Vomiting
    Diuretics
    Hyperventilation
    Bicarbonate therapy
  Insulin
    Exogenous
    Endogenous response to glucose
  β₂-Agonists (albuterol, terbutaline, epinephrine)
  Hypokalemia periodic paralysis
  Familial

Throtoxic
Miscellaneous
    Anabolic state
    Intravenous hyperalimentation
    Treatment of megaloblastic anemia
    Acute mountain sickness

POTASSIUM, URINE

See "URINE POTASSIUM"

PROCAINAMIDE

Therapeutic range and general information are summarized in Table 99.
Normal therapeutic range: 4 to 10 mcg/ml

PROGESTERONE (SERUM)

Normal:
Female: Follicular phase: 15 to 70 ng/dl
Luteal phase: 200 to 2500 ng/dl
Male: 15 to 70 ng/dl
Elevated in: Congenital adrenal hyperplasia, clomiphene, corticosterone, 11-deoxycortisol, dihydroprogesterone, molar pregnancy, lipoid ovarian tumor
Decreased in: Primary or secondary hypogonadism, oral contraceptives, ampicillin, threatened abortion

PROLACTIN

See Fig. E48 for the evaluation of hyperprolactinemia.
Normal range: <20 ng/ml (<20 µg/L [CF: 1; SMI: 1 µg/L])
Elevated in: Prolactinomas (level >200 mcg/L highly suggestive), drugs (phenothiazines, cimetidine, tricyclic antidepressants, metoclopramide, estrogens, antihypertensives [methyldopa], verapamil, haloperidol), postpartum, stress, hypoglycemia, hypothyroidism, chronic liver disease, end-stage renal disease, brain radiation therapy, polycystic ovary syndrome, seizures, exercise, coitus, lactation. Mild hyperprolactinemia (<100 mcg/L) can also be caused by large sellar masses, including nonfunctioning pituitary adenoma.

PROSTATE-SPECIFIC ANTIGEN (PSA)

Normal range: 0 to 4 ng/ml
Table E100 describes age-specific reference ranges for PSA.
Elevated in: Benign prostatic hypertrophy, carcinoma of prostate, prostatitis, postrectal examination, prostate trauma
Factors affecting serum PSA are described in Table E101.
NOTE: Measurement of free PSA is useful to assess the probability of prostate cancer in patients with normal digital rectal examination and total PSA between 4 and 10 ng/ml. In these patients, the global risk of prostate cancer is 25%; however, if the free PSA is >25%, the risk of prostate cancer decreases to 8%, whereas if the free PSA is <10%, the risk of cancer increases to 56%. Free PSA is also useful to evaluate the aggressiveness of prostate cancer. A low free PSA percentage generally indicates a high-grade cancer, whereas a high free PSA percentage is generally associated with a slower-growing tumor.
Decreased in: 5-α reductase inhibitors (finasteride, dutasteride), saw palmetto use, antiandrogens

PROSTATIC ACID PHOSPHATASE

Normal: 0 to 0.8 U/L
Elevated in: Prostate cancer (especially in metastatic prostate cancer), BPH, prostatitis, post–prostate surgery or manipulation, hemolysis, androgens, clofibrate
Decreased in: Ketoconazole

PROTEIN (SERUM)

Normal range: 6 to 8 g/dl (60 to 80 g/L [CF: 10; SMI: 1 g/L])
Elevated in: Dehydration, multiple myeloma, Waldenström macroglobulinemia, sarcoidosis, collagen vascular diseases
Decreased in: Malnutrition, low-protein diet, overhydration, malabsorption, pregnancy, severe burns, neoplasms, chronic diseases, cirrhosis, nephrosis

PROTEIN C ASSAY

See Table E102 and Fig. E49.
Normal: 70% to 140%
Elevated in: Oral contraceptives, stanozolol
Decreased in: Congenital protein C deficiency, warfarin therapy, vitamin K deficiency, renal insufficiency, consumptive coagulopathies

PROTEIN ELECTROPHORESIS (SERUM)

Normal range:
Albumin: 60% to 75% (0.6 to 0.75 [CF: 0.01; SMI: 0.01])
    α-1: 1.7% to 5% (0.02 to 0.05)
    α-2: 6.7% to 12.5% (0.07 to 0.13)
    β: 8.3% to 16.3% (0.08 to 0.16)
    γ: 10.7% to 20% (0.11 to 0.2)
Albumin: 3.6 to 5.2 g/dl (36 to 52 g/L [CF: 0.01; SMI: 1 g/L])
    α-1: 0.1 to 0.4 g/dl (1 to 4 g/L)
    α-2: 0.4 to 1 g/dl (4 to 10 g/L)
    β: 0.5 to 1.2 g/dl (5 to 12 g/L)
    γ: 0.6 to 1.6 g/dl (6 to 16 g/L)
Elevated in:
Albumin: Dehydration
    α-1: Neoplastic diseases, inflammation
    α-2: Neoplasms, inflammation, infection, nephrotic syndrome
    β: Hypothyroidism, biliary cirrhosis, diabetes mellitus
    γ: See "IMMUNOGLOBULINS"
Decreased in:
Albumin: Malnutrition, chronic liver disease, malabsorption, nephrotic syndrome, burns, systemic lupus erythematosus
    α-1: Emphysema (α-1 antitrypsin deficiency), nephrosis
    α-2: Hemolytic anemias (decreased haptoglobin), severe hepatocellular damage
    β: Hypocholesterolemia, nephrosis
    γ: See "IMMUNOGLOBULINS"
Fig. E50 describes serum protein electrophoretic patterns.

PROTEIN S ASSAY

See Table E103.
Normal: 65% to 140%
Elevated in: Presence of lupus anticoagulant
Decreased in: Hereditary deficiency, acute thrombotic events, DIC, surgery, oral contraceptives, pregnancy, hormone replacement therapy, l-asparaginase treatment

PROTHROMBIN TIME (PT)

See Table E104.

TABLE 99	Procainamide

Purpose	Treatment of Supraventricular or Ventricular Arrhythmias
General adult dose	Oral: 4 g/day, in divided doses, for maintenance therapy
Usual bioavailability	75%-95%
Half-life	Approximately 3.5 h in patients with normal renal function
General therapeutic range	4-10 mcg/ml
General toxic level	>12 mcg/ml
Transport	Approximately 15% plasma protein bound
Metabolism	Hepatic: *N*-acetylprocainamide (active), with approximately 7 h in patients with normal renal function
Elimination	Approximately 50%-60% unchanged in urine
Steady state	Minimum of 12 h
Mechanism of action	Prolongation of atrial refractory period and decreased myocardial excitability
Toxic effects	Reversible lupus erythematosus-like syndrome, irregular pulse, hypotension, rash, agranulocytosis

From McPherson RA, Pincus MR: *Henry's clinical diagnosis and management by laboratory methods*, ed 23, St Louis, 2017, Elsevier.

Normal range: 10 to 12 sec

Elevated in: Liver disease, oral anticoagulants (warfarin), heparin, factor deficiency (I, II, V, VII, X), disseminated intravascular coagulation, vitamin K deficiency, afibrinogenemia, dysfibrinogenemia, drugs (salicylate, chloral hydrate, diphenylhydantoin, estrogens, antacids, phenylbutazone, quinidine, antibiotics, allopurinol, anabolic steroids). Table E105 describes a differential diagnosis of abnormal coagulation screening tests

Decreased in: Vitamin K supplementation, thrombophlebitis, drugs (glutethimide, estrogens, griseofulvin, diphenhydramine)

PROTOPORPHYRIN (FREE ERYTHROCYTE)

Normal range: 16 to 36 µg/dl of red blood cells (0.28 to 0.64 µmol/L [CF: 0.0177; SMI: 0.02 µmol/L])

Elevated in: Iron deficiency, lead poisoning, sideroblastic anemias, anemia of chronic disease, hemolytic anemias, erythropoietic protoporphyria

PSA

See "PROSTATE-SPECIFIC ANTIGEN"

PT

See "PROTHROMBIN TIME"

PTH

See "PARATHYROID HORMONE"

PTT

See "PARTIAL THROMBOPLASTIN TIME"

RAPID PLASMA REAGIN (RPR)

Description: Nontreponemal test traditionally used as a screening test for syphilis. It is a quantitative test, and antibody titers can be monitored to assess treatment response.

Normal: Negative

Positive: Syphilis. False-positive results may occur with pregnancy, autoimmune diseases, tuberculosis, and other inflammatory conditions. Positive results should be confirmed with treponemal serologic tests (e.g., T-pallidum enzyme immunoassay [TP-EIA]).

RDW

See "RED BLOOD CELL DISTRIBUTION WIDTH"

RED BLOOD CELL (RBC) COUNT

Normal range:

Male: 4.3 to $5.9 \times 10^6/mm^3$ (4.3 to $5.9 \times 10^{12}/L$ [CF: 1; SMI: $0.1 \times 10^{12}/L$])
Female: 3.5 to $5 \times 10^6/mm^3$ (3.5 to $5 \times 10^{12}/L$ [CF: 1; SMI: $0.1 \times 10^{12}/L$])

Elevated in

Polycythemia vera, smokers, high altitude, cardiovascular disease, renal cell carcinoma and other erythropoietin-producing neoplasms, stress, hemoconcentration/dehydration

Decreased in: Anemias, hemolysis, chronic renal failure, hemorrhage, failure of marrow production

RED BLOOD CELL DISTRIBUTION WIDTH (RDW)

Measures variability of red cell size (anisocytosis)

Normal range: 11.5 to 14.5

Normal RDW and elevated mean corpuscular volume (MCV):

Aplastic anemia, preleukemia

Normal MCV: Normal, anemia of chronic disease, acute blood loss or hemolysis, chronic lymphocytic leukemia (CLL), chronic myelocytic leukemia, nonanemic enzymopathy or hemoglobinopathy

Decreased MCV: Anemia of chronic disease, heterozygous thalassemia

Elevated RDW and elevated MCV: Vitamin B$_{12}$ deficiency, folate deficiency, immune hemolytic anemia, cold agglutinins, CLL with high count, liver disease

Normal MCV: Early iron deficiency, early vitamin B$_{12}$ deficiency, early folate deficiency, anemic globinopathy

Decreased MCV: Iron deficiency, red blood cell fragmentation, HbH disease, thalassemia intermedia

See Table E106 for combining the reticulocyte count and RBC parameters for diagnosis.

RED BLOOD CELL FOLATE

See "FOLATE"

RED BLOOD CELL MASS (VOLUME)

Normal range:

Male: 20 to 36 ml/kg body weight (1.15 to 1.21 L/m^2 body surface area)
Female: 19 to 31 ml/kg body weight (0.95 to 1.00 L/m^2 body surface area)

Elevated in: Polycythemia vera, hypoxia (smokers, high altitude, cardiovascular disease), hemoglobinopathies with high oxygen affinity, erythropoietin-producing tumors (renal cell carcinoma)

Decreased in: Hemorrhage, chronic disease, failure of marrow production, anemias, hemolysis

RED BLOOD CELL MORPHOLOGY

Table E107 describes features of the peripheral blood smear. Table E108 summarizes peripheral blood film evaluation in a patient with red cell membrane disorder. See Fig. E51 for useful peripheral blood and RBC features in the evaluation of anemia.

RENIN (SERUM)

Blood causes of hypertension associated with high levels of plasma renin are summarized in Box E31. Low levels of renin and hypertension are listed in Box E32.

Elevated in: Drugs (thiazides, estrogen, minoxidil), chronic renal failure, Bartter syndrome, pregnancy (normal), pheochromocytoma, renal hypertension, reduced plasma volume, secondary aldosteronism.

Decreased in: Adrenocortical hypertension, increased plasma volume, primary aldosteronism, drugs (propranolol, reserpine, clonidine).

Table 109 describes typical renin-aldosterone patterns in various conditions.

RESPIRATORY SYNCYTIAL VIRUS (RSV) SCREEN

Test description: PCR test can be performed on nasopharyngeal swab, wash, or aspirate

RETICULOCYTE COUNT

See Fig. E52, Fig. E53, and Table E110.

TABLE 109 Typical Renin-Aldosterone Patterns in Various Conditions

	Plasma Renin	Aldosterone
Primary aldosteronism	Low	High
"Low-renin" essential hypertension	Low	Normal
Cushing syndrome	Low	Low-normal
Licorice ingestion syndrome	Low	Low
High-salt diet	Low	Low
Oral contraceptives	High	Normal
Cirrhosis	High	High
Malignant hypertension	High	High
Unilateral renal disease	High	High
"High-renin" essential hypertension	High	High
Pregnancy	High	High
Diuretic overuse	High	High
Juxtaglomerular tumor (Bartter syndrome)	High	High
Low-salt diet	High	High
Addison disease	High	Low
Hypokalemia	High	Low

Normal range: 0.5% to 1.5%

Elevated in: Hemolytic anemia (sickle cell crisis, thalassemia major, autoimmune hemolysis), hemorrhage, postanemia therapy (folic acid, ferrous sulfate, vitamin B_{12}), chronic renal failure

Decreased in: Aplastic anemia, marrow suppression (sepsis, chemotherapeutic agents, radiation), hepatic cirrhosis, blood transfusion, anemias of disordered maturation (iron deficiency anemia, megaloblastic anemia, sideroblastic anemia, anemia of chronic disease)

RHEUMATOID FACTOR

Normal: Negative. Present in titer >1:20
RHEUMATIC DISEASES
Rheumatoid arthritis
Sjögren syndrome
Systemic lupus erythematosus
Polymyositis/dermatomyositis
Mixed connective tissue disease
Scleroderma
INFECTIOUS DISEASES
Subacute bacterial endocarditis
Tuberculosis
Infectious mononucleosis
Hepatitis
Syphilis
Leprosy
Influenza
MALIGNANCIES
Lymphoma
Multiple myeloma
Waldenström macroglobulinemia
Postradiation or postchemotherapy
MISCELLANEOUS
Normal adults, especially the elderly
Sarcoidosis
Chronic pulmonary disease (interstitial fibrosis)
Chronic liver disease (chronic active hepatitis, cirrhosis)
Mixed essential cryoglobulinemia
Hypergammaglobulinemic purpura
RNP
See "EXTRACTABLE NUCLEAR ANTIGEN"

RPR

See "RAPID PLASMA REAGIN"

ROTAVIRUS SEROLOGY

Test description: PCR test is performed on stool specimen
Normal: Negative

SARS-COV-2 ANTIBODIES

Name	Value	Reference Range
SARS-COV-2 ABS Interp.	Negative	Negative
SARS-COV-2 ABS INDEX	0.09	<1.0 (Index)

Index (COI) Value	Interpretation
<1.0	Negative for ANTI-SARS COV 2 antibodies
≥1.0	Positive for ANTI-SARS COV 2 antibodies

The ANTI-SARS-COV-2 assay is intended for the qualitative detection of antibodies to SARS-COV-2 in human serum and as an aid in identifying individuals with an adaptive immune response to SARS-COV-2, indicating recent or prior infection. At the time of this publication, it is unknown for how long antibodies persist following infection and to what degree the presence of antibodies confers protective immunity. This assay should not be used to diagnose acute SARS-COV-2 infection.

Negative results do not preclude acute SARS-COV-2 infection. If acute infection is suspected, direct PCR testing is recommended. False-positive results may occur due to cross-reactivity from preexisting antibodies or other possible causes. This assay has overall sensitivity of 100% and specificity of 99.8% in patients ≥14 days post-PCR confirmation.

SED RATE

See "ERYTHROCYTE SEDIMENTATION RATE"

SEDIMENTATION RATE

See "ERYTHROCYTE SEDIMENTATION RATE"

SEMEN ANALYSIS

Table 111 describes semen analysis reference ranges.

SGOT

See "ASPARTATE AMINOTRANSFERASE"

SGPT

See "ASPARTATE AMINOTRANSFERASE"

SICKLE CELL TEST

Normal: Negative
Positive in: Sickle cell anemia, sickle cell trait, combination of *Hb S* gene with other disorders such as alpha-thalassemia, beta-thalassemia

SMOOTH MUSCLE ANTIBODY

Normal: Negative
Present in: Chronic acute hepatitis, primary sclerosing cholangitis, primary biliary cirrhosis, autoimmune hepatitis, infectious mononucleosis

SODIUM (SERUM)

Normal range: 135 to 147 mEq/L (135 to 147 mmol/L [CF: 1; SMI: 1 mmol/L]). Electrolyte concentrations in extracellular and intracellular fluid are summarized in Table E112.
HYPONATREMIA
See Fig. E54.
1. Common causes of hyponatremia and electrolyte patterns in serum and urine with normal renal function are described in Table E113. Table E114 describes drugs associated with hyponatremia.

TABLE 111	Semen Analysis Reference Ranges
Color	Grayish White
pH	7.3-7.8 (literature range, 7.0-7.8)
Volume	2.0-5.0 ml (literature range, 1.5-6.0 ml)
Sperm count	20-250 million/ml (literature range for upper limit varies from 100-250 million/ml)
Motility	>60% motile <3 h after specimen is obtained (literature range, >40% to >70%)
% Normal sperm	>60% (literature range, >60% to >70%)
Viscosity	Can be poured from a pipet in droplets rather than a thick strand

2. Sodium and water depletion (deficit hyponatremia)
   Loss of gastrointestinal secretions with replacement of fluid but not electrolytes
      Vomiting
      Diarrhea
      Tube drainage
   Loss from skin with replacement of fluids but not electrolytes
      Excessive sweating
      Extensive burns
   Loss from kidney
      Diuretics
      Chronic renal insufficiency (uremia) with acidosis
   Metabolic loss
      Starvation with acidosis
      Diabetic acidosis
   Endocrine loss
      Addison disease
      Sudden withdrawal of long-term steroid therapy
   Iatrogenic loss from serous cavities
      Paracentesis or thoracentesis
   Excessive water (dilution hyponatremia)
      Excessive water administration
      Congestive heart failure
      Cirrhosis
      Nephrotic syndrome
      Hypoalbuminemia (severe)
      Acute renal failure with oliguria
   Inappropriate antidiuretic hormone (IADH) syndrome
   Intracellular loss (reset osmostat syndrome)
   False hyponatremia (actually a dilutional effect)
      Marked hypertriglyceridemia
      Marked hyperproteinemia
      Severe hyperglycemia

HYPERNATREMIA

See Fig. E55.
   Common causes of hypernatremia and electrolyte patterns in serum and urine with normal renal function are summarized in Table E115
Dehydration is the most frequent overall clinical finding in hypernatremia
Deficient water intake (either orally or intravenously)
Excess kidney water output (diabetes insipidus, osmotic diuresis)
Excess skin water output (excess sweating, loss from burns)
Excess gastrointestinal tract output (severe protracted vomiting or diarrhea without fluid therapy)
Accidental sodium overdose
High-protein tube feedings

STREPTOZYME

See "ANTISTREPTOLYSIN O TITER"

SUCROSE HEMOLYSIS TEST (SUGAR WATER TEST)

Normal: Absence of hemolysis
Positive in:
Paroxysmal nocturnal hemoglobinuria
False positive: Autoimmune hemolytic anemia, megaloblastic anemias
False negative: May occur with use of heparin or EDTA

SUDAN III STAIN (QUALITATIVE SCREENING FOR FECAL FAT)

Normal: Negative. Test should be preceded by diet containing 100 to 150 g of dietary fat/day for 1 wk, avoidance of high-fiber diet, and avoidance of suppositories or oily material before specimen collection.
Positive in: Steatorrhea, use of castor oil or mineral oil droplets

SYNOVIAL FLUID ANALYSIS

Table E116 describes the classification and interpretation of synovial fluid analysis. An algorithm for analysis of joint fluid is illustrated in Fig. E56.

T₃ (TRIIODOTHYRONINE)

See Table 117 for T_3 abnormalities.

TABLE 117   Findings in Thyroid Function Tests in Various Clinical Conditions

Condition	T_4	FT_4I	T_3	FT_3I	TSH	TSI	TRH Stimulation
Hyperthyroidism							
Graves disease	↑	↑	↑	↑	↓	+	↓
Toxic nodular goiter	↑	↑	↑	↑	↓	−	↓
Pituitary TSH-secreting tumors	↑	↑	↑	↑	↑	−	↓
T_3 thyrotoxicosis	N	N	↑	↑	↓	+,−	↓
T_4 thyrotoxicosis	↑	↑	N	N	↓	+,−	↓
Hypothyroidism							
Primary	↓	↓	↓	↓	↑	+,−	↑
Secondary	↓	↓	↓	↓	↓ N	−	↓
Tertiary	↓	↓	↓	↓	↓, N	−	N
Peripheral unresponsiveness	↑, N	↑, N	↑, N	↑	↑, N	−	N, ↑

↑, Increased; ↓, decreased; +, − variable; *FTI*, free thyroid index; *N*, normal; *T_3*, triiodothyronine; *T_4*, thyroxine; *TRH*, thyrotropin-releasing hormone; *TSH*, thyroid-stimulating hormone; *TSI*, thyroid stimulating immunoglobulin.

Normal range: 75 to 220 ng/dl (1.2 to 3.4 nmol/L [CF: 0.01536; SMI: 0.1 nmol/L])
Abnormal values:
1. Elevated in hyperthyroidism (usually earlier and to a greater extent than serum T_4)
2. Useful in diagnosing:
   T_3 hyperthyroidism (thyrotoxicosis): Increased T_3, normal free thyroxine index (FTI)
   Toxic nodular goiter: Increased T_3, normal or increased T_4
   Iodine deficiency: Normal T_3, possibly decreased T_4
   Thyroid replacement therapy with liothyronine (Cytomel): Normal T_4, increased T_3 if patient is symptomatically hyperthyroid
   Not ordered routinely but indicated when hyperthyroidism is suspected and serum-free T_4 or FTI inconclusive

T₃ RESIN UPTAKE (T₃RU)

Normal range: 25% to 35%
Abnormal values: Increased in hyperthyroidism. T_3 resin uptake (T_3RU or RT_3U) measures the percentage of free T_4 (not bound to protein); it does not measure serum T_3 concentration; T_3RU and other tests that reflect thyroid hormone binding to plasma protein are also known as *thyroid hormone-binding ratios* (THBR).

T₄, FREE (FREE THYROXINE)

Normal range: 0.8 to 2.8 ng/dl
Elevated in:
Graves disease, toxic multinodular goiter, toxic adenoma, iatrogenic and factitious causes, transient hyperthyroidism.
Serum-free T_4 directly measures unbound thyroxine. Free T_4 can be measured by equilibrium dialysis (gold standard of free T_4 assays) or by immunometric techniques (influenced by serum levels of lipids, proteins, and certain drugs). The FTI can also be easily calculated by multiplying T_4 times T_3RU and dividing the result by 100; the FTI corrects for any abnormal T_4 values secondary to protein binding: FTI = $T_4 \times T_3RU/100$. Normal values equal 1.1 to 4.3.

T₄, SERUM T₄

Normal range: 0.8 to 2.8 ng/dl (10 to 36 pmol/L [CF: 12.87; SMI: 1 pmol/L])
Abnormal values: Serum thyroxine (T_4)
Elevated in:
Graves disease
Toxic multinodular goiter

Toxic adenoma
latrogenic and factitious
Transient hyperthyroidism
    Subacute thyroiditis
    Hashimoto thyroiditis
    Silent thyroiditis
- Rare causes: Hypersecretion of TSH (e.g., pituitary neoplasms), struma ovarii, ingestion of large amounts of iodine in a patient with preexisting thyroid hyperplasia or adenoma (Jod-Basedow phenomenon), hydatidiform mole, carcinoma of thyroid, amiodarone therapy of arrhythmias
- Serum thyroxine test measures both circulating thyroxine bound to protein (represents >99% of circulating T_4) and unbound (free) thyroxine. Values vary with protein binding; changes in the concentration of T_4 secondary to changes in thyroxine-binding globulin (TBG) can be caused by the following:

Increased TBG ($\uparrow T_4$)	Decreased TBG ($\downarrow T_4$)
Pregnancy	Androgens, glucocorticoids
Estrogens	Nephrotic syndrome, cirrhosis
Acute infectious hepatitis	Acromegaly
Oral contraceptives	Hypoproteinemia
Familial	Familial
Fluorouracil, clofibrate	Phenytoin, acetylsalicylic acid (ASA) and other NSAIDs, heroin, methadone, high-dose penicillin, asparaginase, chronic debilitating illness

To eliminate the suspected influence of protein binding on thyroxine values, two additional tests are available: T_3 resin uptake and serum free thyroxine. Table E118 summarizes the effects of pregnancy on thyroid physiology, and Table E119 describes changes in thyroid hormone levels during illness.

TEGRETOL
See "CARBAMAZEPINE"

TESTOSTERONE (TOTAL TESTOSTERONE)

Normal range: Variable with age and sex. Testosterone circulates in plasma mostly bound to plasma proteins and sex hormone–binding globulin (SHBG). Approximately 2% of testosterone circulates in free form (biologically active form). Low testosterone levels in obese patients may be due to reduced levels of SHBG; therefore, it is essential to measure free testosterone when evaluating androgen deficiency in obese patients.

Serum/Plasma
Males: 280-1100 ng/dl   Females: 15-70 ng/dl
Urine
Males: 50-135 µg/day   Females: 2-12 µg/day

Elevated in: Testicular tumors, ovarian masculinizing tumors, testosterone replacement therapy
Decreased in: Hypogonadism, obesity, insulin resistance, sleep apnea. Fig. E57 illustrates testosterone level changes with age. The diagnosis of androgen deficiency should be based on at least two morning testosterone measurements (collected on separate days) in a symptomatic patient.

THEOPHYLLINE
Normal therapeutic range: 10 to 20 mcg/ml

THORACENTESIS FLUID
See "PLEURAL FLUID"

THROMBIN TIME (TT), THROMBIN CLOTTING TIME (TCT)
Normal range: 11.3 to 18.5 sec
Elevated in: Thrombolytic and heparin therapy, disseminated intravascular coagulation, hypofibrinogenemia, dysfibrinogenemia
   See Table E120 for synthesizing results of PT, APTT, and TCT. Also see Fig. E58.

THYROGLOBULIN
Normal: 3 to 40 ng/ml. Thyroglobulin is a tumor marker for monitoring the status of patients with papillary or follicular thyroid cancer following resection.
Elevated in: Papillary or follicular thyroid cancer, Hashimoto thyroiditis, Graves disease, subacute thyroiditis

THYROID MICROSOMAL ANTIBODIES
Normal: Undetectable. Low titers may be present in 5% to 10% of normal individuals.
Elevated in: Hashimoto disease, thyroid carcinoma, early hypothyroidism, pernicious anemia

THYROID-STIMULATING HORMONE (TSH)
Changes in TSH levels during illness are summarized in Table E121.
   See Fig. E59 for an algorithmic approach to thyroid testing.
Normal range: 2 to 11 µU/ml (2 to 11 mU/L [CF: 1; SMI: 1 mU/L])
CONDITIONS THAT INCREASE SERUM THYROID-STIMULATING HORMONE VALUES
1. Laboratory error
2. Primary hypothyroidism
3. Synthroid therapy with insufficient dose
4. Lithium or amiodarone; some patients
5. Hashimoto thyroiditis in later stage
6. Large doses of inorganic iodide (e.g., potassium iodide [SSKI])
7. Severe nonthyroid illness in recovery phase
8. Iodine deficiency (moderate or severe)
9. Addison disease
10. TSH specimen drawn in evening (peak of diurnal variation)
11. Pituitary TSH-secreting tumor
12. Therapy of hypothyroidism (3 to 6 wk after beginning therapy [range, 1 to 8 wk]; sometimes longer when pretherapy TSH is over 100 µU/ml)
13. Acute psychiatric illness
14. Peripheral resistance to T_4 syndrome
15. Antibodies (e.g., human antimouse antibody [HAMA]) interfering with monoclonal sandwich method of TSH assay
16. Telepaque (iopanoic acid) and Oragrafin (ipodate) x-ray contrast media
17. Amphetamines
18. High altitudes
CONDITIONS THAT DECREASE SERUM THYROID-STIMULATING HORMONE VALUES
1. Laboratory error
2. T_4/T_3 toxicosis (diffuse or nodular etiology)
3. Excessive therapy for hypothyroidism
4. Active thyroiditis (subacute, painless, or early active Hashimoto disease)
5. Multinodular goiter containing areas of autonomy
6. Severe nonthyroid illness (especially acute trauma, dopamine, or glucocorticoid)
7. T_3 toxicosis
8. Pituitary insufficiency
9. Cushing syndrome (and some patients on high-dose glucocorticoid)
10. Jod-Basedow (iodine-induced) hyperthyroidism
11. Thyroid-stimulating hormone drawn 2 to 4 h after levothyroxine dose
12. Postpartum transient toxicosis

13. Factitious hyperthyroidism
14. Struma ovarii
15. Radioimmunoassay, surgery, or antithyroid drug therapy for hyperthyroidism 4 to 6 wk (range, 2 wk to 2 yr) after the treatment
16. Interleukin-2 drugs (3% to 6% of cases) or α-interferon therapy (1% of cases)
17. Hyperemesis gravidarum
18. Amiodarone therapy
   See Table E119 for changes in thyroid hormone levels during illness.

THYROTROPIN (TSH) RECEPTOR ANTIBODIES

Normal: <130% of basal activity
Elevated in: Values between 1.3 and 2.0 are found in 10% of patients with thyroid disease other than Graves disease. Values >2.8 have been found only in patients with Graves disease.

THYROTROPIN-RELEASING HORMONE (TRH) STIMULATION TEST

Normal: Baseline TSH <11 microU/ml; stimulated TSH: More than double the baseline

In primary hypothyroidism the TSH increase is 2 to 3× the normal result. In secondary hypothyroidism no TSH response occurs. In tertiary hypothyroidism (hypothalamic failure) there is a delayed rise in the TSH level.

THYROXINE (T₄)

Patterns in T_4 levels in different thyroid gland conditions are summarized in Table 122.
Normal range: 4 to 11 µg/dl (51 to 142 nmol/L [CF: 12.87; SMI: 1 nmol/L])
Elevated: Hyperthyroidism (see Fig. E59)

TIBC

See "IRON-BINDING CAPACITY, TOTAL"

TISSUE TRANSGLUTAMINASE ANTIBODY

Normal: Negative
Present in: Celiac disease (specificity; 94% to 97%, sensitivity, 90% to 98%), dermatitis herpetiformis

TRANSFERRIN

Normal range: 170 to 370 mg/dl (1.7 to 3.7 g/L [CF: 0.01; SMI: 0.01 g/L])
Elevated in: Iron deficiency anemia, oral contraceptive administration, viral hepatitis, late pregnancy
Decreased in: Nephrotic syndrome, liver disease, hereditary deficiency, protein malnutrition, neoplasms, chronic inflammatory states, chronic illness, thalassemia, hemochromatosis, hemolytic anemia

TRIGLYCERIDES

Normal range: <150 mg/dl (<1.80 mmol/L [CF: 0.01129; SMI: 0.02 mmol/L])
Elevated in: Hyperlipoproteinemias (types I, IIb, III, IV, V), hypothyroidism, pregnancy, estrogens, acute myocardial infarction, pancreatitis, alcohol intake, nephrotic syndrome, diabetes mellitus, glycogen storage disease
Decreased in: Malnutrition, congenital abetalipoproteinemias, drugs (e.g., gemfibrozil, fenofibrate, nicotinic acid, clofibrate)

TRIIODOTHYRONINE

See "T₃"

TROPONINS (SERUM)

Box E33 summarizes the differential diagnosis of elevated troponin other than acute coronary syndrome.
Normal range: 0 to 0.4 ng/ml (negative). If there is clinical suspicion of evolving acute MI or ischemic episode, repeat testing in 5 to 6 h is recommended.
Indeterminate: 0.05 to 0.49 ng/ml. Suggest further tests. In a patient with unstable angina and this troponin I level, there is an increased risk of a cardiac event in the near future.
Strong probability of acute MI: ≥0.05 ng/ml
Cardiac troponin T (cTnT) is a highly sensitive marker for myocardial injury for the first 48 h after MI and for up to 5 to 7 days (see Fig. E21, under "Creatine Kinase Isoenzymes"). It may also be elevated in renal failure, chronic muscle disease, and trauma.
Cardiac troponin I (cTnI) is highly sensitive and specific for myocardial injury (≥CK-MB) in the initial 8 h, peaks within 24 h, and lasts up to 7 days. With progressively higher levels of cTnI, the risk of mortality increases because the amount of necrosis increases.

TSH

See "THYROID-STIMULATING HORMONE"

TT

See "THROMBIN TIME"

TUBERCULIN TEST (PPD)

Abnormal results: See Box 34. Box E35 describes factors associated with false-negative tuberculin tests.

BOX 34 PPD Reaction Size Considered "Positive" (Intracutaneous 5 TU Mantoux Test at 48 H)

5 mm or More
HIV infection or risk factors for HIV
Close recent contact with active TB case
Persons with chest x-ray examination consistent with healed TB

10 mm or More
Foreign-born persons from countries with high TB prevalence in Asia, Africa, and Latin America
IV drug users
Medically underserved low-income population groups (including Native Americans, Hispanics, and Blacks)
Residents of long-term care facilities (nursing homes, mental institutions)
Medical conditions that increase risk for TB (silicosis, gastrectomy, undernourishment, diabetes mellitus, high-dose corticosteroids or immunosuppression Rx, leukemia or lymphoma, other malignancies)
Employees of long-term care facilities, schools, child care facilities, health care facilities

15 mm or More
All others not already listed

TABLE 122 Patterns of Serum Levels of TSH and T₄ in Different Thyroid Gland Conditions

Condition	T₄ (Most Accurate, Free T₄)	TSH	Site of Disease
Euthyroid	Normal	Normal	None
Primary hypothyroidism	Low	High	Thyroid gland
Secondary hypothyroidism	Low	Low to normal	Pituitary
Primary hyperthyroidism	High	Low	Thyroid
Secondary hyperthyroidism	High	High	Pituitary

TSH, Thyroid-stimulating hormone.
From McPherson RA, Pincus MR: *Henry's clinical diagnosis and management by laboratory methods,* ed 23, St Louis, 2017, Elsevier.

HIV, Human immunodeficiency virus; *IV,* intravenous; *PPD,* purified protein derivative; *Rx,* prescription; *TB,* tuberculosis; *TU,* tuberculin units.

UNCONJUGATED BILIRUBIN

See "BILIRUBIN, DIRECT"

UREA NITROGEN, BLOOD (BUN)

Normal range: 8 to 18 mg/dl (3 to 6.5 mmol/L [CF: 0.357; SMI: 0.5 mmol/L])

Box E36 describes factors affecting BUN level independent of renal function.

Elevated in: Dehydration, drugs (aminoglycosides and other antibiotics, diuretics, lithium, corticosteroids), gastrointestinal bleeding, decreased renal blood flow (shock, congestive heart failure, myocardial infarction), renal disease (glomerulonephritis, pyelonephritis, diabetic nephropathy), urinary tract obstruction (prostatic hypertrophy)

Decreased in: Liver disease, malnutrition, third trimester of pregnancy, overhydration, acromegaly, celiac disease

URIC ACID (SERUM)

Normal range: 2 to 7 mg/dl

Elevated in: Renal failure, gout, excessive cell lysis (chemotherapeutic agents, radiation therapy, leukemia, lymphoma, hemolytic anemia), hereditary enzyme deficiency (hypoxanthine-guanine-phosphoribosyl transferase), acidosis, myeloproliferative disorders, diet high in purines or protein, drugs (diuretics, low doses of ASA, ethambutol, nicotinic acid), lead poisoning, hypothyroidism, Addison disease, nephrogenic diabetes insipidus, active psoriasis, polycystic kidneys

Decreased in: Drugs (allopurinol, febuxostat, high doses of ASA, probenecid, warfarin, corticosteroid), deficiency of xanthine oxidase, syndrome of inappropriate antidiuretic hormone secretion, renal tubular deficits (Fanconi syndrome), alcoholism, liver disease, diet deficient in protein or purines, Wilson disease, hemochromatosis

URINALYSIS

Blood urinalysis abnormalities in various urinary system diseases are summarized in Table E123.

Normal range:
Color: Light straw
Appearance: Clear
Ketones: Absent
pH: 4.5 to 8 (average, 6)
Protein: Absent
Glucose: Absent
Specific gravity: 1.005 to 1.030
Occult blood absent
Microscopic examination:
Red blood cells: 0 to 5 (high-power field)
White blood cells: 0 to 5 (high-power field)
Bacteria (spun specimen): Absent
Casts: 0 to 4 hyaline (low-power field)

Abnormalities in the microscopic examination of urine are described in Table E124. Causes of abnormal appearance and color of urine are described in Table E125. Urine color changes with commonly used drugs are summarized in Table E126.

URINE AMYLASE

Normal range: 35 to 260 U Somogyi/h (6.5 to 48.1 U/h [CF: 0.185; SMI: 1 U/h])
Elevated in: Pancreatitis, carcinoma of the pancreas

URINE BILE

Normal: Absent
Abnormal:
Urine bilirubin: Hepatitis (viral, toxic, drug-induced), biliary obstruction
Urine urobilinogen: Hepatitis (viral, toxic, drug-induced), hemolytic jaundice, liver cell dysfunction (cirrhosis, infection, metastases)

URINE CALCIUM

Normal range: <250 mg/24 h (<6.2 mmol/dl [CF: 0.02495; SMI: 0.1 mmol/dl])
Elevated in: Primary hyperparathyroidism, hypervitaminosis D, bone metastases, multiple myeloma, increased calcium intake, steroids, prolonged immobilization, sarcoidosis, Paget disease, idiopathic hypercalciuria, renal tubular acidosis

Decreased in: Hypoparathyroidism, pseudohypoparathyroidism, vitamin D deficiency, vitamin D–resistant rickets, diet low in calcium, drugs (thiazide diuretics, oral contraceptives), familial hypocalciuric hypercalcemia, renal osteodystrophy, potassium citrate therapy

URINE CAMP

Elevated in: Hypercalciuria, familial hypocalciuric hypercalcemia, primary hyperparathyroidism, pseudohypoparathyroidism, rickets
Decreased in: Vitamin D intoxication, sarcoidosis

URINE CATECHOLAMINES

Normal range
Norepinephrine: <100 μg/24 h (<590 nmol/day [CF: 5.911; SMI: 10 nmol/day])
Epinephrine: <10 μg/24 h (55 nmol/day [CF: 5.458; SMI: 5 nmol/day])
Elevated in: Pheochromocytoma, neuroblastoma, severe stress

URINE CHLORIDE

Normal range: 110 to 250 mEq/day (110 to 250 mmol/day [CF: 1; SMI: 1 mmol/day])
Elevated in: Corticosteroids, Bartter syndrome, diuretics, metabolic acidosis, severe hypokalemia
Decreased in: Chloride depletion (vomiting), colonic villous adenoma, chronic renal failure, renal tubular acidosis

URINE COPPER

Normal range: <40 μg/24 h (<0.6 μmol/day [CF: 0.01574; SMI: 0.2 μmol/day])

URINE CORTISOL, FREE

Normal range: 10 to 110 μg/24 h (30 to 300 nmol/day [CF: 2.759; SMI: 10 nmol/day])
Elevated: See "CORTISOL, PLASMA"

URINE CREATININE (24 H)

Normal range:
Male: 0.8 to 1.8 g/day (7 to 16 mmol/day [CF: 8.840; SMI: 0.1 mmol/day])
Female: 0.6 to 1.6 g/day (5.3 to 14 mmol/day)
NOTE: Useful test as an indicator of completeness of 24-h urine collection.

URINE CRYSTALS

Uric acid: Acid urine, hyperuricosuria, uric acid nephropathy
Sulfur: Antibiotics containing sulfa
Calcium oxalate: Ethylene glycol poisoning, acid urine, hyperoxaluria
Calcium phosphate: Alkaline urine
Cystine: Cystinuria

URINE EOSINOPHILS

Normal: Absent
Present in: Interstitial nephritis, acute tubular necrosis, urinary tract infection, kidney transplant rejection, hepatorenal syndrome

URINE GLUCOSE (QUALITATIVE)

Normal: Absent
Present in: Diabetes mellitus, renal glycosuria (decreased renal threshold for glucose), glucose intolerance

URINE HEMOGLOBIN, FREE

Normal: Absent
Present in: Hemolysis (with saturation of serum haptoglobin binding capacity and renal threshold for tubular absorption of hemoglobin)

URINE HEMOSIDERIN

Normal: Absent
Present in: Paroxysmal nocturnal hemoglobinuria, chronic hemolytic anemia, hemochromatosis, blood transfusion, thalassemias

URINE 5-HYDROXYINDOLE-ACETIC ACID (URINE 5-HIAA)

Normal range: 2 to 8 mg/24 h (10 to 40 µmol/day [CF: 5.23; SMI: 5 µmol/day])
Elevated in: Carcinoid tumors, after ingestion of certain foods (bananas, plums, tomatoes, avocados, pineapples, eggplant, walnuts), drugs (monoamine oxidase inhibitors, phenacetin, methyldopa, glycerol guaiacolate, acetaminophen, salicylates, phenothiazines, imipramine, methocarbamol, reserpine, methamphetamine). See Table E127.

URINE INDICAN

Normal: Absent
Present in: Malabsorption secondary to intestinal bacterial overgrowth

URINE KETONES (SEMIQUANTITATIVE)

Normal: Absent
Present in: Diabetic ketoacidosis, alcoholic ketoacidosis, starvation, isopropanol ingestion

URINE METANEPHRINES

Normal range: 0 to 2.0 mg/24 h (0 to 11.0 µmol/day [CF: 5.458; SMI: 0.5 µmol/day])
Elevated in: Pheochromocytoma, neuroblastoma, drugs (caffeine, phenothiazines, monoamine oxidase inhibitors), stress. Table E128 summarizes medications that may increase metanephrine levels.

URINE MYOGLOBIN

Normal: Absent
Present in: Severe trauma, hyperthermia, polymyositis/dermatomyositis, carbon monoxide poisoning, drugs (narcotic and amphetamine toxicity), hypothyroidism, muscle ischemia
   Table 129 differentiates hematuria and hemoglobinuria from myoglobinuria.

URINE NITRITE

Normal: Absent
Present in: Urinary tract infections

URINE OCCULT BLOOD

Normal: Negative
Positive in: Trauma to urinary tract, renal disease (glomerulonephritis, pyelonephritis), renal or ureteral calculi, bladder lesions (carcinoma, cystitis), prostatitis, prostatic carcinoma, menstrual contamination, hematopoietic disorders (hemophilia, thrombocytopenia), anticoagulants, ASA

URINE OSMOLALITY

See "OSMOLALITY, URINE"

URINE PH

Normal range: 4.6 to 8 (average, 6)
Elevated in: Bacteriuria, vegetarian diet, renal failure with inability to form ammonia, drugs (antibiotics, sodium bicarbonate, acetazolamide)
Decreased in: Acidosis (metabolic, respiratory), drugs (ammonium chloride, methenamine mandelate), diabetes mellitus, starvation, diarrhea

URINE PHOSPHATE

Normal range: 0.8 to 2.0 g/24 h
Elevated in: Acute tubular necrosis (diuretic phase), chronic renal disease, uncontrolled diabetes mellitus, hyperparathyroidism, hypomagnesemia, metabolic acidosis, metabolic alkalosis, neurofibromatosis, adult-onset vitamin D-resistant hypophosphatemic osteomalacia
Decreased in: Acromegaly, acute renal failure, decreased dietary intake, hypoparathyroidism, respiratory acidosis

URINE POTASSIUM

Normal range: 25 to 100 mEq/24 h (25 to 100 mmol/day [CF: 1; SMI: 1 mmol/day])
Elevated in: Aldosteronism (primary, secondary), glucocorticoids, alkalosis, renal tubular acidosis, excessive dietary potassium intake
Decreased in: Acute renal failure, potassium-sparing diuretics, diarrhea, hypokalemia
   Box E37 describes urine potassium in hypokalemia.

URINE PROTEIN (QUANTITATIVE)

Normal range: <150 mg/24 h (<0.15 g/day [CF: 0.001; SMI: 0.01 g/day])
Elevated in:
1. Nephrotic syndrome as a result of primary renal diseases
2. Malignant hypertension
3. Malignancies: Multiple myeloma, leukemias, Hodgkin disease
4. Congestive heart failure
5. Diabetes mellitus
6. Systemic lupus erythematosus, rheumatoid arthritis
7. Sickle cell disease
8. Goodpasture syndrome
9. Malaria
10. Amyloidosis, sarcoidosis
11. Tubular lesions: Cystinosis
12. Functional (after heavy exercise)
13. Pyelonephritis
14. Pregnancy
15. Constrictive pericarditis
16. Renal vein thrombosis
17. Toxic nephropathies: Heavy metals, drugs
18. Radiation nephritis
19. Orthostatic (postural) proteinuria
20. Benign proteinuria: Fever, heat or cold exposure

URINE SEDIMENT

See Fig. E60 for visual evaluation of common abnormalities. Table E130 summarizes characteristics of amorphous and crystalline urinary sediments.

URINE SODIUM (QUANTITATIVE)

See Table E131 for use of urine electrolytes in the differential diagnosis of hypokalemia. Table E132 describes urine sodium findings in acute kidney injury (AKI).
Normal range: 40 to 220 mEq/day (40 to 220 mmol/day [CF: 1; SMI: 1 mmol/day])

TABLE 129 Differentiation of Hematuria, Hemoglobinuria, and Myoglobinuria

Condition	Plasma Findings	Urine Findings
Hematuria	Color—normal	Color—normal, smoky, pink, red, brown
		Erythrocytes—many
		Renal—red blood cell casts
		Protein—marked increase
		Lower urinary tract—no casts
		Protein—present or absent
Hemoglobinuria	Color—pink (early)	Color—pink, red, brown
	Haptoglobin—low	Erythrocytes—occasional
		Pigment casts—occasional
		Protein—present or absent
		Hemosiderin—late
Myoglobinuria	Color—normal	Color—red, brown
	Haptoglobin—normal	Erythrocytes—occasional
	Creatine kinase—marked increase	Dense brown casts—occasional
	Aldolase—increased	Protein—present or absent

From McPherson RA, Pincus MR: *Henry's clinical diagnosis and management by laboratory methods*, ed 23, St Louis, 2017, Elsevier.

Elevated in: Diuretic administration, high sodium intake, salt-losing nephritis, acute tubular necrosis, vomiting, Addison disease, syndrome of inappropriate antidiuretic hormone secretion, hypothyroidism, congestive heart failure, hepatic failure, chronic renal failure, Bartter syndrome, glucocorticoid deficiency, interstitial nephritis caused by analgesic abuse, mannitol, dextran, or glycerol therapy, milk-alkali syndrome, decreased renin secretion, postobstructive diuresis

Decreased in: Increased aldosterone, glucocorticoid excess, hyponatremia, prerenal azotemia, decreased salt intake

URINE SPECIFIC GRAVITY

Normal range: 1.005 to 1.030

Elevated in: Dehydration, excessive fluid losses (vomiting, diarrhea, fever), x-ray contrast media, diabetes mellitus, congestive heart failure, syndrome of inappropriate antidiuretic hormone secretion, adrenal insufficiency, decreased fluid intake

Decreased in: Diabetes insipidus, renal disease (glomerulonephritis, pyelonephritis), excessive fluid intake or IV hydration

URINE VANILLYLMANDELIC ACID (VMA)

Normal range: <6.8 mg/24 h (<35 µmol/day [CF: 5.046; SMI: 1 µmol/day])

Elevated in: Pheochromocytoma, neuroblastoma, ganglioblastoma, drugs (isoproterenol, methocarbamol, levodopa, sulfonamides, chlorpromazine), severe stress; after ingestion of bananas, chocolate, vanilla, tea, coffee

Decreased in: Drugs (monoamine oxidase inhibitors, reserpine, guanethidine, methyldopa)

VARICELLA-ZOSTER VIRUS (VZV) SEROLOGY

Test description: Test can be performed on whole blood, tissue, skin lesions, and CSF.

VASOACTIVE INTESTINAL PEPTIDE (VIP)

Normal: <50 pg/ml

Elevated in: Pancreatic VIP-omas, neuroblastoma, pancreatic islet cell hyperplasia, liver disease, multiple endocrine neoplasia (MEN) I, ganglioneuroma, ganglioneuroblastoma

VDRL

Normal range: Negative

Positive test: Syphilis, other treponemal diseases (yaws, pinta, bejel)

NOTE: A false-positive test may be seen in patients with systemic lupus erythematosus and other autoimmune diseases, infectious mononucleosis, HIV, atypical pneumonia, malaria, leprosy, typhus fever, rat-bite fever, relapsing fever.

NOTE: See Table E133 for interpretation of serologic tests for syphilis.

VISCOSITY (SERUM)

Normal range: 1.4 to 1.8 relative to water (1.10 to 1.22 centipoise)

Elevated in: Monoclonal gammopathies (Waldenström macroglobulinemia, multiple myeloma), hyperfibrinogenemia, systemic lupus erythematosus, rheumatoid arthritis, polycythemia, leukemia

VITAMIN B₁₂ (COBALAMIN)

See Box E38 for etiopathophysiologic classification of cobalamin deficiency. Causes of false-positive and false-negative serum cobalamin levels are summarized in Table E134. Table E135 describes causes of megaloblastosis not responding to therapy with cobalamin or folate. Table E136 summarizes indications for prophylaxis with cobalamin or folate.

Normal:

190 to 900 ng/ml

Causes of vitamin B₁₂ deficiency:
1. Pernicious anemia (antibodies against intrinsic factor and gastric parietal cells)
2. Dietary (strict lacto-ovo vegetarians, food faddists)
3. Malabsorption (achlorhydria, gastrectomy, ileal resection, pancreatic insufficiency, drugs [omeprazole, cholestyramine])

Falsely low levels occur in patients with severe folate deficiency, in patients using high doses of ascorbic acid, and when cobalamin levels are measured after nuclear medicine studies (radioactivity interferes with cobalamin radioimmunoassay).

Falsely high or normal levels in patients with cobalamin deficiency can occur in severe liver disease and chronic granulocytic leukemia.

The absence of anemia or macrocytosis does not exclude the diagnosis of cobalamin deficiency.

VITAMIN D, 1,25 DIHYDROXY CALCIFEROL

Normal: 16 to 65 pg/ml

Elevated in: Tumor calcinosis, primary hyperparathyroidism, sarcoidosis, tuberculosis, idiopathic hypercalciuria

Decreased in: Nutritional deficiency, postmenopausal osteoporosis, chronic renal failure, hypoparathyroidism, tumor-induced osteomalacia, rickets, elevated blood lead levels. Table E137 compares vitamin D levels in various disorders. Fig. E61 illustrates vitamin D physiology.

VITAMIN K

Normal: 0.10 to 2.20 ng/ml

Decreased in: Primary biliary cirrhosis, anticoagulants, antibiotics, cholestyramine, GI disease, pancreatic disease, cystic fibrosis, obstructive jaundice, hypoprothrombinemia, hemorrhagic disease of the newborn

VON WILLEBRAND FACTOR

Normal: Levels vary according to blood type; blood type O: 50 to 150 U/dl; blood type non-O: 90 to 200 U/dl

Decreased in: von Willebrand disease (however, in type II von Willebrand disease the antigen may be normal but the function is impaired)

SECTION V

Clinical Practice Guidelines

INTRODUCTION

Childhood and Adolescent Immunizations

Recommended Child and Adolescent Immunization Schedule
for ages 18 years or younger

UNITED STATES 2024

Vaccines and Other Immunizing Agents in the Child and Adolescent Immunization Schedule*

Monoclonal antibody	Abbreviation(s)	Trade name(s)
Respiratory syncytial virus monoclonal antibody (Nirsevimab)	RSV-mAb	Beyfortus™
Vaccine	**Abbreviation(s)**	**Trade name(s)**
COVID-19	1vCOV-mRNA	Comirnaty®/Pfizer-BioNTech COVID-19 Vaccine
		Spikevax®/Moderna COVID-19 Vaccine
	1vCOV-aPS	Novavax COVID-19 Vaccine
Dengue vaccine	DEN4CYD	Dengvaxia®
Diphtheria, tetanus, and acellular pertussis vaccine	DTaP	Daptacel® Infanrix®
Haemophilus influenzae type b vaccine	Hib (PRP-T)	ActHIB® Hiberix®
	Hib (PRP-OMP)	PedvaxHIB®
Hepatitis A vaccine	HepA	Havrix® Vaqta®
Hepatitis B vaccine	HepB	Engerix-B® Recombivax HB®
Human papillomavirus vaccine	HPV	Gardasil 9®
Influenza vaccine (inactivated)	IIV4	Multiple
Influenza vaccine (live, attenuated)	LAIV4	FluMist® Quadrivalent
Measles, mumps, and rubella vaccine	MMR	M-M-R II® Priorix®
Meningococcal serogroups A, C, W, Y vaccine	MenACWY-CRM	Menveo®
	MenACWY-TT	MenQuadfi®
Meningococcal serogroup B vaccine	MenB-4C	Bexsero®
	MenB-FHbp	Trumenba®
Meningococcal serogroup A, B, C, W, Y vaccine	MenACWY-TT/ MenB-FHbp	Penbraya™
Mpox vaccine	Mpox	Jynneos®
Pneumococcal conjugate vaccine	PCV15	Vaxneuvance™
	PCV20	Prevnar 20®
Pneumococcal polysaccharide vaccine	PPSV23	Pneumovax 23®
Poliovirus vaccine (inactivated)	IPV	Ipol®
Respiratory syncytial virus vaccine	RSV	Abrysvo™
Rotavirus vaccine	RV1	Rotarix®
	RV5	RotaTeq®
Tetanus, diphtheria, and acellular pertussis vaccine	Tdap	Adacel® Boostrix®
Tetanus and diphtheria vaccine	Td	Tenivac® Tdvax™
Varicella vaccine	VAR	Varivax®
Combination vaccines *(use combination vaccines instead of separate injections when appropriate)*		
DTaP, hepatitis B, and inactivated poliovirus vaccine	DTaP-HepB-IPV	Pediarix®
DTaP, inactivated poliovirus, and *Haemophilus influenzae* type b vaccine	DTaP-IPV/Hib	Pentacel®
DTaP and inactivated poliovirus vaccine	DTaP-IPV	Kinrix® Quadracel®
DTaP, inactivated poliovirus, *Haemophilus influenzae* type b, and hepatitis B vaccine	DTaP-IPV-Hib-HepB	Vaxelis®
Measles, mumps, rubella, and varicella vaccine	MMRV	ProQuad®

*Administer recommended vaccines if immunization history is incomplete or unknown. Do not restart or add doses to vaccine series for extended intervals between doses. When a vaccine is not administered at the recommended age, administer at a subsequent visit. The use of trade names is for identification purposes only and does not imply endorsement by the ACIP or CDC.

11/16/2023

How to use the child and adolescent immunization schedule

1 Determine recommended vaccine by age **(Table 1)**

2 Determine recommended interval for catch-up vaccination **(Table 2)**

3 Assess need for additional recommended vaccines by medical condition or other indication **(Table 3)**

4 Review vaccine types, frequencies, intervals, and considerations for special situations **(Notes)**

5 Review contraindications and precautions for vaccine types **(Appendix)**

6 Review new or updated ACIP guidance **(Addendum)**

Recommended by the Advisory Committee on Immunization Practices (www.cdc.gov/vaccines/acip) and approved by the Centers for Disease Control and Prevention (www.cdc.gov), American Academy of Pediatrics (www.aap.org), American Academy of Family Physicians (www.aafp.org), American College of Obstetricians and Gynecologists (www.acog.org), American College of Nurse-Midwives (www.midwife.org), American Academy of Physician Associates (www.aapa.org), and National Association of Pediatric Nurse Practitioners (www.napnap.org).

Report
* Suspected cases of reportable vaccine-preventable diseases or outbreaks to your state or local health department
* Clinically significant adverse events to the Vaccine Adverse Event Reporting System (VAERS) at www.vaers.hhs.gov or 800-822-7967

Questions or comments
Contact www.cdc.gov/cdc-info or 800-CDC-INFO (800-232-4636), in English or Spanish, 8 a.m.–8 p.m. ET, Monday through Friday, excluding holidays

 Download the CDC Vaccine Schedules app for providers at www.cdc.gov/vaccines/schedules/hcp/schedule-app.html

Helpful information
* Complete Advisory Committee on Immunization Practices (ACIP) recommendations: www.cdc.gov/vaccines/hcp/acip-recs/index.html
* ACIP Shared Clinical Decision-Making Recommendations: www.cdc.gov/vaccines/acip/acip-scdm-faqs.html
* *General Best Practice Guidelines for Immunization* (including contraindications and precautions): www.cdc.gov/vaccines/hcp/acip-recs/general-recs/index.html
* Vaccine information statements: www.cdc.gov/vaccines/hcp/vis/index.html
* Manual for the Surveillance of Vaccine-Preventable Diseases (including case identification and outbreak response): www.cdc.gov/vaccines/pubs/surv-manual

Scan QR code for access to online schedule

CDC

U.S. Department of Health and Human Services
Centers for Disease Control and Prevention

CS310020-D

TABLE 1 Recommended Child and Adolescent Immunization Schedule for Ages 18 Years or Younger, United States, 2024. (For those who fall behind or start late, see the catch-up schedule [Table 2])

These recommendations must be read with the notes that follow. For those who fall behind or start late, provide catch-up vaccination at the earliest opportunity as indicated by the green bars.
To determine minimum intervals between doses, see the catch-up schedule (Table 2).
From Centers for Disease Control and Prevention.

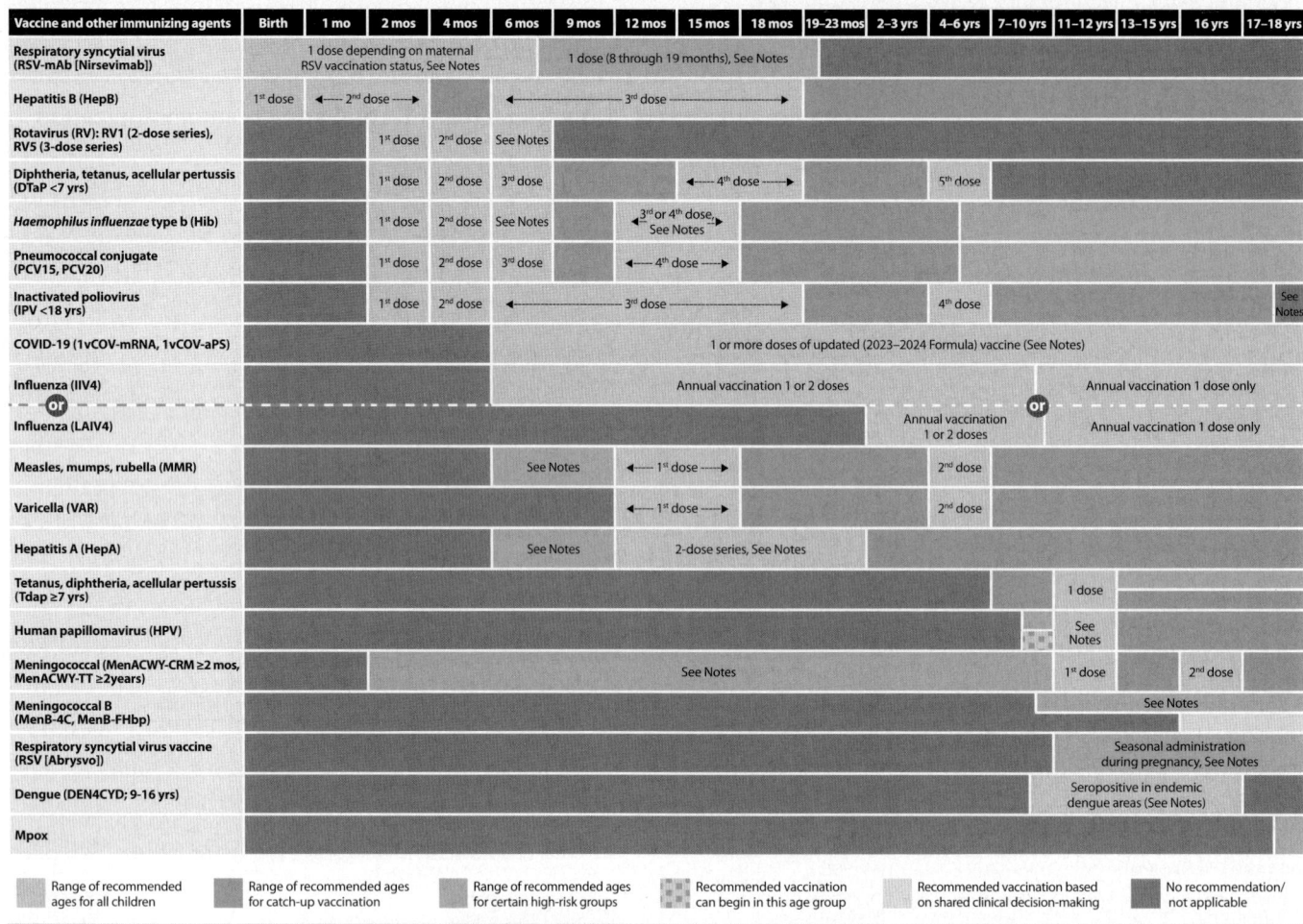

Vaccine and other immunizing agents	Birth	1 mo	2 mos	4 mos	6 mos	9 mos	12 mos	15 mos	18 mos	19–23 mos	2–3 yrs	4–6 yrs	7–10 yrs	11–12 yrs	13–15 yrs	16 yrs	17–18 yrs
Respiratory syncytial virus (RSV-mAb [Nirsevimab])		1 dose depending on maternal RSV vaccination status, See Notes			1 dose (8 through 19 months), See Notes												
Hepatitis B (HepB)	1st dose	←— 2nd dose —→			←————————— 3rd dose —————————→												
Rotavirus (RV): RV1 (2-dose series), RV5 (3-dose series)			1st dose	2nd dose	See Notes												
Diphtheria, tetanus, acellular pertussis (DTaP <7 yrs)			1st dose	2nd dose	3rd dose			←—— 4th dose ——→				5th dose					
Haemophilus influenzae type b (Hib)			1st dose	2nd dose	See Notes		3rd or 4th dose, See Notes										
Pneumococcal conjugate (PCV15, PCV20)			1st dose	2nd dose	3rd dose		←—— 4th dose ——→										
Inactivated poliovirus (IPV <18 yrs)			1st dose	2nd dose	←————————— 3rd dose —————————→							4th dose					See Notes
COVID-19 (1vCOV-mRNA, 1vCOV-aPS)					1 or more doses of updated (2023–2024 Formula) vaccine (See Notes)												
Influenza (IIV4)					Annual vaccination 1 or 2 doses									Annual vaccination 1 dose only			
or																	
Influenza (LAIV4)											Annual vaccination 1 or 2 doses			Annual vaccination 1 dose only			
Measles, mumps, rubella (MMR)					See Notes		←—— 1st dose ——→					2nd dose					
Varicella (VAR)							←—— 1st dose ——→					2nd dose					
Hepatitis A (HepA)					See Notes		2-dose series, See Notes										
Tetanus, diphtheria, acellular pertussis (Tdap ≥7 yrs)														1 dose			
Human papillomavirus (HPV)														See Notes			
Meningococcal (MenACWY-CRM ≥2 mos, MenACWY-TT ≥2years)						See Notes								1st dose		2nd dose	
Meningococcal B (MenB-4C, MenB-FHbp)															See Notes		
Respiratory syncytial virus vaccine (RSV [Abrysvo])														Seasonal administration during pregnancy, See Notes			
Dengue (DEN4CYD; 9-16 yrs)														Seropositive in endemic dengue areas (See Notes)			
Mpox																	See Notes

Range of recommended ages for all children		Range of recommended ages for catch-up vaccination		Range of recommended ages for certain high-risk groups	Recommended vaccination can begin in this age group	Recommended vaccination based on shared clinical decision-making	No recommendation/ not applicable

TABLE 2 Recommended Catch-up Immunization Schedule for Children and Adolescents Who Start Late or Who Are More than 1 Month Behind, United States, 2024

The table below provides catch-up schedules and minimum intervals between doses for children whose vaccinations have been delayed. A vaccine series does not need to be restarted, regardless of the time that has elapsed between doses. Use the section appropriate for the child's age. Always use this table in conjunction with Table 1 and the footnotes that follow.
From Centers for Disease Control and Prevention.

Vaccine	Minimum Age for Dose 1	Minimum Interval Between Doses			
		Dose 1 to Dose 2	**Dose 2 to Dose 3**	**Dose 3 to Dose 4**	**Dose 4 to Dose 5**
Children age 4 months through 6 years					
Hepatitis B	Birth	**4 weeks**	**8 weeks *and* at least 16 weeks after first dose** minimum age for the final dose is 24 weeks		
Rotavirus	6 weeks Maximum age for first dose is 14 weeks, 6 days.	**4 weeks**	**4 weeks** maximum age for final dose is 8 months, 0 days		
Diphtheria, tetanus, and acellular pertussis	6 weeks	**4 weeks**	**4 weeks**	**6 months**	**6 months** A fifth dose is not necessary if the fourth dose was administered at age 4 years or older *and* at least 6 months after dose 3
Haemophilus influenzae type b	6 weeks	**No further doses needed** if first dose was administered at age 15 months or older. **4 weeks** if first dose was administered before the 1st birthday. **8 weeks (as final dose)** if first dose was administered at age 12 through 14 months.	**No further doses needed** if previous dose was administered at age 15 months or older **4 weeks** if current age is younger than 12 months *and* first dose was administered at younger than age 7 months *and* at least 1 previous dose was PRP-T (ActHib®, Pentacel®, Hiberix®), Vaxelis® or unknown **8 weeks *and* age 12 through 59 months (as final dose)** if current age is younger than 12 months *and* first dose was administered at age 7 through 11 months; OR if current age is 12 through 59 months *and* first dose was administered before the 1st birthday *and* second dose was administered at younger than 15 months; OR if both doses were PedvaxHIB® and were administered before the 1st birthday	**8 weeks (as final dose)** This dose only necessary for children age 12 through 59 months who received 3 doses before the 1st birthday.	
Pneumococcal conjugate	6 weeks	**No further doses needed** for healthy children if first dose was administered at age 24 months or older **4 weeks** if first dose was administered before the 1st birthday **8 weeks (as final dose for healthy children)** if first dose was administered at the 1st birthday or after	**No further doses needed** for healthy children if previous dose was administered at age 24 months or older **4 weeks** if current age is younger than 12 months *and* previous dose was administered at <7 months old **8 weeks (as final dose for healthy children)** if previous dose was administered between 7–11 months (wait until at least 12 months old); OR if current age is 12 months or older *and* at least 1 dose was administered before age 12 months	**8 weeks (as final dose)** This dose is only necessary for children age 12 through 59 months regardless of risk, or age 60 through 71 months with any risk, who received 3 doses before age 12 months.	
Inactivated poliovirus	6 weeks	**4 weeks**	**4 weeks** if current age is <4 years **6 months (as final dose)** if current age is 4 years or older	**6 months (minimum age 4 years for final dose)**	
Measles, mumps, rubella	12 months	**4 weeks**			
Varicella	12 months	**3 months**			
Hepatitis A	12 months	**6 months**			
Meningococcal ACWY	2 months MenACWY-CRM 2 years MenACWY-TT	**8 weeks**	See Notes	See Notes	
Children and adolescents age 7 through 18 years					
Meningococcal ACWY	Not applicable (N/A)	**8 weeks**			
Tetanus, diphtheria; tetanus, diphtheria, and acellular pertussis	7 years	**4 weeks**	**4 weeks** if first dose of DTaP/DT was administered before the 1st birthday **6 months (as final dose)** if first dose of DTaP/DT or Tdap/Td was administered at or after the 1st birthday	**6 months** if first dose of DTaP/DT was administered before the 1st birthday	
Human papillomavirus	9 years	**Routine dosing intervals are recommended.**			
Hepatitis A	N/A	**6 months**			
Hepatitis B	N/A	**4 weeks**	**8 weeks *and* at least 16 weeks after first dose**		
Inactivated poliovirus	N/A	**4 weeks**	**6 months** A fourth dose is not necessary if the third dose was administered at age 4 years or older *and* at least 6 months after the previous dose.	A fourth dose of IPV is indicated if all previous doses were administered at <4 years OR if the third dose was administered <6 months after the second dose.	
Measles, mumps, rubella	N/A	**4 weeks**			
Varicella	N/A	**3 months** if younger than age 13 years. **4 weeks** if age 13 years or older			
Dengue	9 years	**6 months**	6 months		

TABLE 3 Recommended Child and Adolescent Immunization Schedule by Medical Indication, United States, 2024

Always use this table in conjunction with Table 1 and the notes that follow.
From Centers for Disease Control and Prevention.

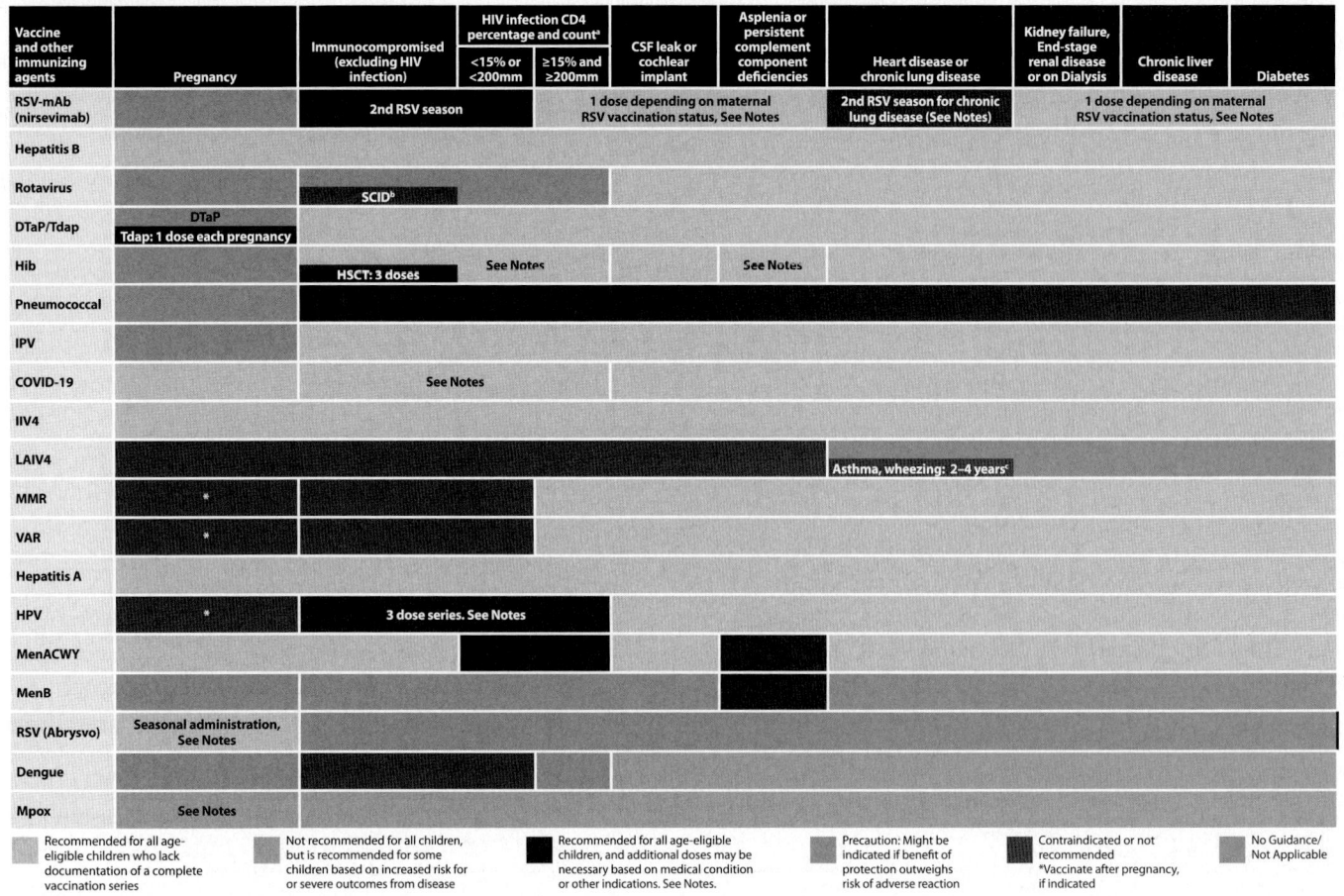

Vaccine and other immunizing agents	Pregnancy	Immunocompromised (excluding HIV infection)	HIV infection CD4 percentage and count[a]		CSF leak or cochlear implant	Asplenia or persistent complement component deficiencies	Heart disease or chronic lung disease	Kidney failure, End-stage renal disease or on Dialysis	Chronic liver disease	Diabetes
			<15% or <200mm	≥15% and ≥200mm						
RSV-mAb (nirsevimab)		2nd RSV season	1 dose depending on maternal RSV vaccination status, See Notes				2nd RSV season for chronic lung disease (See Notes)	1 dose depending on maternal RSV vaccination status, See Notes		
Hepatitis B										
Rotavirus		SCID[b]								
DTaP/Tdap	DTaP / Tdap: 1 dose each pregnancy									
Hib		HSCT: 3 doses	See Notes			See Notes				
Pneumococcal										
IPV										
COVID-19		See Notes								
IIV4										
LAIV4							Asthma, wheezing: 2–4 years[c]			
MMR	*									
VAR	*									
Hepatitis A										
HPV	*	3 dose series. See Notes								
MenACWY										
MenB										
RSV (Abrysvo)	Seasonal administration, See Notes									
Dengue										
Mpox	See Notes									

Legend:
- Recommended for all age-eligible children who lack documentation of a complete vaccination series
- Not recommended for all children, but is recommended for some children based on increased risk for or severe outcomes from disease
- Recommended for all age-eligible children, and additional doses may be necessary based on medical condition or other indications. See Notes.
- Precaution: Might be indicated if benefit of protection outweighs risk of adverse reaction
- Contraindicated or not recommended *Vaccinate after pregnancy, if indicated
- No Guidance/ Not Applicable

a. For additional information regarding HIV laboratory parameters and use of live vaccines, see the General Best Practice Guidelines for Immunization, "Altered Immunocompetence," at www.cdc.gov/vaccines/hcp/acip-recs/general-recs/immunocompetence.html and Table 4-1 (footnote J) at www.cdc.gov/vaccines/hcp/acip-recs/general-recs/contraindications.html.

b. Severe Combined Immunodeficiency

c. LAIV4 contraindicated for children 2–4 years of age with asthma or wheezing during the preceding 12 months

For vaccination recommendations for persons ages 19 years or older, see the Recommended Adult Immunization Schedule, 2024.

Additional information

- For calculating intervals between doses, 4 weeks = 28 days. Intervals of ≥4 months are determined by calendar months.

- Within a number range (e.g., 12–18), a dash (–) should be read as "through."

- Vaccine doses administered ≤4 days before the minimum age or interval are considered valid. Doses of any vaccine administered ≥5 days earlier than the minimum age or minimum interval should not be counted as valid and should be repeated as age appropriate. **The repeat dose should be spaced after the invalid dose by the recommended minimum interval.** For further details, see Table 3-2, Recommended and minimum ages and intervals between vaccine doses, in *General Best Practice Guidelines for Immunization* at www.cdc.gov/vaccines/hcp/acip-recs/general-recs/timing.html.

- Information on travel vaccination requirements and recommendations is available at www.cdc.gov/travel/.

- For vaccination of persons with immunodeficiencies, see Table 8-1, Vaccination of persons with primary and secondary immunodeficiencies, in *General Best Practice Guidelines for Immunization* at www.cdc.gov/vaccines/hcp/acip-recs/general-recs/immunocompetence.html, and Immunization in Special Clinical Circumstances (In: Kimberlin DW, Barnett ED, Lynfield Ruth, Sawyer MH, eds. *Red Book: 2021–2024 Report of the Committee on Infectious Diseases*. 32nd ed. Itasca, IL: American Academy of Pediatrics; 2021:72–86).

- For information about vaccination in the setting of a vaccine-preventable disease outbreak, contact your state or local health department.

- The National Vaccine Injury Compensation Program (VICP) is a no-fault alternative to the traditional legal system for resolving vaccine injury claims. All vaccines included in the child and adolescent vaccine schedule are covered by VICP except dengue, PPSV23, RSV, Mpox and COVID-19 vaccines. Mpox and COVID-19 vaccines are covered by the Countermeasures Injury Compensation Program (CICP). For more information, see www.hrsa.gov/vaccinecompensation or www.hrsa.gov/cicp.

COVID-19 vaccination
(minimum age: 6 months [Moderna and Pfizer-BioNTech COVID-19 vaccines], 12 years [Novavax COVID-19 Vaccine])

Routine vaccination

Age 6 months–4 years

- **Unvaccinated:**
  - 2-dose series of updated (2023–2024 Formula) Moderna at 0, 4-8 weeks
  - 3-dose series of updated (2023–2024 Formula) Pfizer-BioNTech at 0, 3-8, 11-16 weeks

- **Previously vaccinated* with 1 dose of any Moderna:** 1 dose of updated (2023–2024 Formula) Moderna 4-8 weeks after the most recent dose.

- **Previously vaccinated* with 2 or more doses of any Moderna:** 1 dose of updated (2023–2024 Formula) Moderna at least 8 weeks after the most recent dose.

- **Previously vaccinated* with 1 dose of any Pfizer-BioNTech:** 2-dose series of updated (2023–2024 Formula) Pfizer-BioNTech at 0, 8 weeks (minimum interval between previous Pfizer-BioNTech and dose 1: 3-8 weeks).

- **Previously vaccinated* with 2 or more doses of any Pfizer-BioNTech:** 1 dose of updated (2023–2024 Formula) Pfizer-BioNTech at least 8 weeks after the most recent dose.

Age 5–11 years

- **Unvaccinated:** 1 dose of updated (2023–2024 Formula) Moderna or Pfizer-BioNTech vaccine.

- **Previously vaccinated* with 1 or more doses of Moderna or Pfizer-BioNTech:** 1 dose of updated (2023–2024 Formula) Moderna or Pfizer-BioNTech at least 8 weeks after the most recent dose.

Age 12–18 years

- **Unvaccinated:**
  - 1 dose of updated (2023–2024 Formula) Moderna or Pfizer-BioNTech vaccine
  - 2-dose series of updated (2023–2024 Formula) Novavax at 0, 3-8 weeks

- **Previously vaccinated* with any COVID-19 vaccine(s):** 1 dose of any updated (2023–2024 Formula) COVID-19 vaccine at least 8 weeks after the most recent dose.

Special situations
Persons who are moderately or severely immunocompromised**

Age 6 months–4 years

- **Unvaccinated:**
  - 3-dose series of updated (2023–2024 Formula) Moderna at 0, 4, 8 weeks
  - 3-dose series of updated (2023–2024 Formula) Pfizer-BioNTech at 0, 3, 11 weeks.

- **Previously vaccinated* with 1 dose of any Moderna:** 2-dose series of updated (2023–2024 Formula) Moderna at 0, 4 weeks (minimum interval between previous Moderna and dose 1: 4 weeks).

- **Previously vaccinated* with 2 doses of any Moderna:** 1 dose of updated (2023–2024 Formula) Moderna at least 4 weeks after the most recent dose.

- **Previously vaccinated* with 3 or more doses of any Moderna:** 1 dose of updated (2023–2024 Formula) Moderna at least 8 weeks after the most recent dose.

- **Previously vaccinated* with 1 dose of any Pfizer-BioNTech:** 2-dose series of updated (2023–2024 Formula) Pfizer-BioNTech at 0, 8 weeks (minimum interval between previous Pfizer-BioNTech and dose 1: 3 weeks).

- **Previously vaccinated* with 2 or more doses of any Pfizer-BioNTech:** 1 dose of updated (2023–2024 Formula) Pfizer-BioNTech at least 8 weeks after the most recent dose.

Age 5–11 years

- **Unvaccinated:**
  - 3-dose series of updated (2023–2024 Formula) Moderna at 0, 4, 8 weeks
  - 3-dose series updated (2023–2024 Formula) Pfizer-BioNTech at 0, 3, 7 weeks.

- **Previously vaccinated* with 1 dose of any Moderna:** 2-dose series of updated (2023–2024 Formula) Moderna at 0, 4 weeks (minimum interval between previous Moderna and dose 1: 4 weeks).

- **Previously vaccinated* with 2 doses of any Moderna:** 1 dose of updated (2023–2024 Formula) Moderna at least 4 weeks after the most recent dose.

- **Previously vaccinated* with 1 dose of any Pfizer-BioNTech:** 2-dose series of updated (2023–2024 Formula) Pfizer-BioNTech at 0, 4 weeks (minimum interval between previous Pfizer-BioNTech and dose 1: 3 weeks)

- **Previously vaccinated* with 2 doses of any Pfizer-BioNTech:** 1 dose of 2023–2024 Pfizer-BioNTech at least 4 weeks after the most recent dose.

Notes Recommended Child and Adolescent Immunization Schedule for Ages 18 Years or Younger, United States, 2024

- **Previously vaccinated* with 3 or more doses of any Moderna or Pfizer-BioNTech:** 1 dose of updated (2023–2024 Formula) Moderna or Pfizer-BioNTech at least 8 weeks after the most recent dose.

Age 12–18 years

- **Unvaccinated:**
  - 3-dose series of updated (2023–2024 Formula) Moderna at 0, 4, 8 weeks
  - 3-dose series of updated (2023–2024 Formula) Pfizer-BioNTech at 0, 3, 7 weeks
  - 2-dose series of updated (2023–2024 Formula) Novavax at 0, 3 weeks

- **Previously vaccinated* with 1 dose of any Moderna:** 2-dose series of updated (2023–2024 Formula) Moderna at 0, 4 weeks (minimum interval between previous Moderna dose and dose 1: 4 weeks).

- **Previously vaccinated* with 2 doses of any Moderna:** 1 dose of updated (2023–2024 Formula) Moderna at least 4 weeks after the most recent dose.

- **Previously vaccinated* with 1 dose of any Pfizer-BioNTech:** 2-dose series of updated (2023–2024 Formula) Pfizer-BioNTech at 0, 4 weeks (minimum interval between previous Pfizer-BioNTech dose and dose 1: 3 weeks).

- **Previously vaccinated* with 2 doses of any Pfizer-BioNTech:** 1 dose of updated (2023–2024 Formula) Pfizer-BioNTech at least 4 weeks after the most recent dose.

- **Previously vaccinated* with 3 or more doses of any Moderna or Pfizer-BioNTech:** 1 dose of any updated (2023–2024 Formula) COVID-19 vaccine at least 8 weeks after the most recent dose.

- **Previously vaccinated* with 1 or more doses of Janssen or Novavax or with or without dose(s) of any Original monovalent or bivalent COVID-19 vaccine:** 1 dose of any updated (2023–2024 Formula) COVID-19 vaccine at least 8 weeks after the most recent dose.

There is no preferential recommendation for the use of one COVID-19 vaccine over another when more than one recommended age-appropriate vaccine is available.

Administer an age-appropriate COVID-19 vaccine product for each dose. For information about transition from age 4 years to age 5 years or age 11 years to age 12 years during COVID-19 vaccination series, see Tables 1 and 2 at www.cdc.gov/vaccines/covid-19/clinical-considerations/interim-considerations-us.html#covid-vaccines.

Current COVID-19 schedule and dosage formulation available at www.cdc.gov/covidschedule. For more information on Emergency Use Authorization (EUA) indications for COVID-19 vaccines, see www.fda.gov/emergency-preparedness-and-response/coronavirus-disease-2019-covid-19/covid-19-vaccines

*Note: Previously vaccinated is defined as having received any Original monovalent or bivalent COVID-19 vaccine (Janssen, Moderna, Novavax, Pfizer-BioNTech) prior to the updated 2023–2024 formulation.

**Note: Persons who are moderately or severely immunocompromised have the option to receive one additional dose of updated (2023–2024 Formula) COVID-19 vaccine at least 2 months following the last recommended updated (2023–2024 Formula) COVID-19 vaccine dose. Further additional updated (2023–2024 Formula) COVID-19 vaccine dose(s) may be administered, informed by the clinical judgement of a healthcare provider and personal preference and circumstances. Any further additional doses should be administered at least 2 months after the last updated (2023–2024 Formula) COVID-19 vaccine dose. Moderately or severely immunocompromised children 6 months–4 years of age should receive homologous updated (2023–2024 Formula) mRNA vaccine dose(s) if they receive additional doses.

Dengue vaccination
(minimum age: 9 years)

Routine vaccination

- Age 9–16 years living in areas with endemic dengue **AND** have laboratory confirmation of previous dengue infection
  - 3-dose series administered at 0, 6, and 12 months

- Endemic areas include Puerto Rico, American Samoa, US Virgin Islands, Federated States of Micronesia, Republic of Marshall Islands, and the Republic of Palau. For updated guidance on dengue endemic areas and pre-vaccination laboratory testing see www.cdc.gov/mmwr/volumes/70/rr/rr7006a1.htm?s_cid=rr7006a1_w and www.cdc.gov/dengue/vaccine/hcp/index.html

- Dengue vaccine should not be administered to children traveling to or visiting endemic dengue areas.

Diphtheria, tetanus, and pertussis (DTaP) vaccination (minimum age: 6 weeks [4 years for Kinrix® or Quadracel®])

Routine vaccination

- 5-dose series (3-dose primary series at age 2, 4, and 6 months, followed by a booster doses at ages 15–18 months and 4–6 years

- **Prospectively:** Dose 4 may be administered as early as age 12 months if at least 6 months have elapsed since dose 3.
- **Retrospectively:** A 4th dose that was inadvertently administered as early as age 12 months may be counted if at least 4 months have elapsed since dose 3.

Catch-up vaccination

- Dose 5 is not necessary if dose 4 was administered at age 4 years or older and at least 6 months after dose 3.
- For other catch-up guidance, see Table 2.

Special situations

- **Wound management** in children less than age 7 years with history of 3 or more doses of tetanus-toxoid-containing vaccine: For all wounds except clean and minor wounds, administer DTaP if more than 5 years since last dose of tetanus-toxoid-containing vaccine. For detailed information, see www.cdc.gov/mmwr/volumes/67/rr/rr6702a1.htm.

Haemophilus influenzae type b vaccination (minimum age: 6 weeks)

Routine vaccination

- **ActHIB®, Hiberix®, Pentacel®, or Vaxelis®:** 4-dose series (3-dose primary series at age 2, 4, and 6 months, followed by a booster dose* at age 12–15 months)
  - *Vaxelis® is not recommended for use as a booster dose. A different Hib-containing vaccine should be used for the booster dose.
- **PedvaxHIB®:** 3-dose series (2-dose primary series at age 2 and 4 months, followed by a booster dose at age 12–15 months)

Catch-up vaccination

- **Dose 1 at age 7–11 months:** Administer dose 2 at least 4 weeks later and dose 3 (final dose) at age 12–15 months or 8 weeks after dose 2 (whichever is later).
- **Dose 1 at age 12–14 months:** Administer dose 2 (final dose) at least 8 weeks after dose 1.
- **Dose 1 before age 12 months and dose 2 before age 15 months:** Administer dose 3 (final dose) at least 8 weeks after dose 2.
- **2 doses of PedvaxHIB® before age 12 months:** Administer dose 3 (final dose) at age 12–59 months and at least 8 weeks after dose 2.
- **1 dose administered at age 15 months or older:** No further doses needed
- **Unvaccinated at age 15–59 months:** Administer 1 dose.

Notes Recommended Child and Adolescent Immunization Schedule for Ages 18 Years or Younger, United States, 2024

- **Previously unvaccinated children age 60 months or older who are not considered high risk:** Do not require catch-up vaccination

For other catch-up guidance, see Table 2. Vaxelis® can be used for catch-up vaccination in children less than age 5 years. Follow the catch-up schedule even if Vaxelis® is used for one or more doses. For detailed information on use of Vaxelis® see www.cdc.gov/mmwr/volumes/69/wr/mm6905a5.htm.

Special situations
- **Chemotherapy or radiation treatment:**
  Age 12–59 months
  - Unvaccinated or only 1 dose before age 12 months: 2 doses, 8 weeks apart
  - 2 or more doses before age 12 months: 1 dose at least 8 weeks after previous dose

  Doses administered within 14 days of starting therapy or during therapy should be repeated at least 3 months after therapy completion.
- **Hematopoietic stem cell transplant (HSCT):**
  - 3-dose series 4 weeks apart starting 6 to 12 months after successful transplant, regardless of Hib vaccination history
- **Anatomic or functional asplenia (including sickle cell disease):**
  Age 12–59 months
  - Unvaccinated or only 1 dose before age 12 months: 2 doses, 8 weeks apart
  - 2 or more doses before age 12 months: 1 dose at least 8 weeks after previous dose

  Unvaccinated* persons age 5 years or older
  - 1 dose
- **Elective splenectomy:**
  Unvaccinated* persons age 15 months or older
  - 1 dose (preferably at least 14 days before procedure)
- **HIV infection:**
  Age 12–59 months
  - Unvaccinated or only 1 dose before age 12 months: 2 doses, 8 weeks apart
  - 2 or more doses before age 12 months: 1 dose at least 8 weeks after previous dose

  Unvaccinated* persons age 5–18 years
  - 1 dose
- **Immunoglobulin deficiency, early component complement deficiency:**
  Age 12–59 months
  - Unvaccinated or only 1 dose before age 12 months: 2 doses, 8 weeks apart

- 2 or more doses before age 12 months:
  1 dose at least 8 weeks after previous dose

Unvaccinated = Less than routine series (through age 14 months) **OR no doses (age 15 months or older)*

Hepatitis A vaccination
(minimum age: 12 months for routine vaccination)

Routine vaccination
- 2-dose series (minimum interval: 6 months) at age 12–23 months

Catch-up vaccination
- Unvaccinated persons through age 18 years should complete a 2-dose series (minimum interval: 6 months).
- Persons who previously received 1 dose at age 12 months or older should receive dose 2 at least 6 months after dose 1.
- Adolescents age 18 years or older may receive the combined HepA and HepB vaccine, **Twinrix®**, as a 3-dose series (0, 1, and 6 months) or 4-dose series (3 doses at 0, 7, and 21–30 days, followed by a booster dose at 12 months).

International travel
- Persons traveling to or working in countries with high or intermediate endemic hepatitis A (www.cdc.gov/travel/):
  - **Infants age 6–11 months:** 1 dose before departure; revaccinate with 2 doses (separated by at least 6 months) between age 12–23 months.
  - **Unvaccinated age 12 months or older:** Administer dose 1 as soon as travel is considered.

Hepatitis B vaccination
(minimum age: birth)

Routine vaccination
- 3-dose series at age 0, 1–2, 6–18 months **(use monovalent HepB vaccine for doses administered before age 6 weeks)**
  - Birth weight ≥2,000 grams: 1 dose within 24 hours of birth if medically stable
  - Birth weight <2,000 grams: 1 dose at chronological age 1 month or hospital discharge (whichever is earlier and even if weight is still <2,000 grams).
- Infants who did not receive a birth dose should begin the series as soon as possible (see Table 2 for minimum intervals).
- Administration of 4 doses is permitted when a combination vaccine containing HepB is used after the birth dose.
- **Minimum intervals (see Table 2):** when 4 doses are administered, substitute "dose 4" for "dose 3" in these calculations

- **Final (3rd or 4th) dose:** age 6–18 months **(minimum age 24 weeks)**
- **Mother is HBsAg-positive**
  - **Birth dose (monovalent HepB vaccine only):** administer **HepB vaccine** and **hepatitis B immune globulin (HBIG)** (in separate limbs) within 12 hours of birth, regardless of birth weight.
  - **Birth weight <2000 grams:** administer 3 additional doses of HepB vaccine beginning at age 1 month (total of 4 doses)
  - **Final (3rd or 4th) dose:** administer at age 6 months **(minimum age 24 weeks)**
  - Test for HBsAg and anti-HBs at age 9–12 months. If HepB series is delayed, test 1–2 months after final dose. Do not test before age 9 months.
- **Mother is HBsAg-unknown**

  If other evidence suggestive of maternal hepatitis B infection exists (e.g., presence of HBV DNA, HBeAg-positive, or mother known to have chronic hepatitis B infection), manage infant as if mother is HBsAg-positive.
  - **Birth dose (monovalent HepB vaccine only):**
    - Birth weight ≥2,000 grams: administer **HepB vaccine** within 12 hours of birth. Determine mother's HBsAg status as soon as possible. If mother is determined to be HBsAg-positive, administer **HBIG** as soon as possible (in separate limb), but no later than 7 days of age.
    - Birth weight <2,000 grams: administer **HepB vaccine** and **HBIG** (in separate limbs) within 12 hours of birth. Administer 3 additional doses of **HepB vaccine** beginning at age 1 month (total of 4 doses)
  - **Final (3rd or 4th) dose:** administer at age 6 months **(minimum age 24 weeks)**
  - If mother is determined to be HBsAg-positive or if status remains unknown, test for HBsAg and anti-HBs at age 9–12 months. If HepB series is delayed, test 1–2 months after final dose. Do not test before age 9 months.

Catch-up vaccination
- Unvaccinated persons should complete a 3-dose series at 0, 1–2, 6 months. See Table 2 for minimum intervals
- Adolescents age 11–15 years may use an alternative 2-dose schedule with at least 4 months between doses (adult formulation **Recombivax HB®** only).
- Adolescents age 18 years may receive:
  - **Heplisav-B®:** 2-dose series at least 4 weeks apart
  - **PreHevbrio®:** 3-dose series at 0, 1, and 6 months
  - Combined HepA and HepB vaccine, **Twinrix®:** 3-dose series (0, 1, and 6 months) or 4-dose series (3 doses at 0, 7, and 21–30 days, followed by a booster dose at 12 months).

Notes Recommended Child and Adolescent Immunization Schedule for Ages 18 Years or Younger, United States, 2024

Special situations

- Revaccination is not generally recommended for persons with a normal immune status who were vaccinated as infants, children, adolescents, or adults.

- **Post-vaccination serology testing and revaccination** (if anti-HBs <10mIU/mL) is recommended for certain populations, including:
  - Infants born to HBsAg-positive mothers
  - Persons who are predialysis or on maintenance dialysis
  - Other immunocompromised persons
  - For detailed revaccination recommendations, see www.cdc. gov/vaccines/hcp/acip-recs/vacc-specific/hepb.html.

Note: Heplisav-B and PreHevbrio are not recommended in pregnancy due to lack of safety data in pregnant persons

Human papillomavirus vaccination
(minimum age: 9 years)

Routine and catch-up vaccination

- HPV vaccination routinely recommended at **age 11–12 years (can start at age 9 years)** and catch-up HPV vaccination recommended for all persons through age 18 years if not adequately vaccinated

- 2- or 3-dose series depending on age at initial vaccination:
  - **Age 9–14 years at initial vaccination:** 2-dose series at 0, 6–12 months (minimum interval: 5 months; repeat dose if administered too soon)
  - **Age 15 years or older at initial vaccination:** 3-dose series at 0, 1–2 months, 6 months (minimum intervals: dose 1 to dose 2: 4 weeks / dose 2 to dose 3: 12 weeks / dose 1 to dose 3: 5 months; repeat dose if administered too soon)

- No additional dose recommended when any HPV vaccine series **of any valency** has been completed using recommended dosing intervals.

Special situations

- **Immunocompromising conditions, including HIV infection:** 3-dose series, even for those who initiate vaccination at age 9 through 14 years.

- **History of sexual abuse or assault:** Start at age 9 years

- **Pregnancy:** Pregnancy testing not needed before vaccination; HPV vaccination not recommended until after pregnancy; no intervention needed if vaccinated while pregnant

Influenza vaccination
(minimum age: 6 months [IIV], 2 years [LAIV4], 18 years [recombinant influenza vaccine, RIV4])

Routine vaccination

- Use any influenza vaccine appropriate for age and health status annually:
  - **Age 6 months–8 years** who have received **fewer** than 2 influenza vaccine doses before July 1, 2023, or whose influenza vaccination history is unknown: 2 doses, separated by at least 4 weeks. Administer dose 2 even if the child turns 9 years between receipt of dose 1 and dose 2.
  - **Age 6 months–8 years** who have received **at least** 2 influenza vaccine doses before July 1, 2023: 1 dose
  - **Age 9 years or older:** 1 dose

- For the 2023-2024 season, see www.cdc.gov/mmwr/volumes/72/rr/rr7202a1.htm.

- For the 2024–25 season, see the 2024–25 ACIP influenza vaccine recommendations.

Special situations

- **Close contacts (e.g., household contacts) of severely immunosuppressed persons who require a protected environment:** should not receive LAIV4. If LAIV4 is given, they should avoid contact with for such immunosuppressed persons for 7 days after vaccination.

Note: Persons with an egg allergy can receive any influenza vaccine (egg-based and non-egg-based) appropriate for age and health status.

Measles, mumps, and rubella vaccination
(minimum age: 12 months for routine vaccination)

Routine vaccination

- 2-dose series at age 12–15 months, age 4–6 years

- MMR or MMRV* may be administered

Note: For dose 1 in children age 12–47 months, it is recommended to administer MMR and varicella vaccines separately. MMRV* may be used if parents or caregivers express a preference.

Catch-up vaccination

- Unvaccinated children and adolescents: 2-dose series at least 4 weeks apart*

- The maximum age for use of MMRV* is 12 years.

Special situations

- **International travel**
  - **Infants age 6–11 months:** 1 dose before departure; revaccinate with 2-dose series at age 12–15 months (12 months for children in high-risk areas) and dose 2 as early as 4 weeks later.*
  - **Unvaccinated children age 12 months or older:** 2-dose series at least 4 weeks apart before departure*

- In mumps outbreak settings, for information about additional doses of MMR (including 3rd dose of MMR), see www.cdc.gov/mmwr/volumes/67/wr/mm6701a7.htm

*Note: If MMRV is used, the minimum interval between MMRV doses is 3 months

Meningococcal serogroup A,C,W,Y vaccination
(minimum age: 2 months [MenACWY-CRM, Menveo], 2 years [MenACWY-TT, MenQuadfi]), 10 years [MenACWY-TT/MenB-FHbp, Penbraya])

Routine vaccination

- 2-dose series at age 11–12 years; 16 years

Catch-up vaccination

- Age 13–15 years: 1 dose now and booster at age 16–18 years (minimum interval: 8 weeks)

- Age 16–18 years: 1 dose

Special situations

Anatomic or functional asplenia (including sickle cell disease), HIV infection, persistent complement component deficiency, complement inhibitor (e.g., eculizumab, ravulizumab) use:

- **Menveo®***
  - Dose 1 at age 2 months: 4-dose series (additional 3 doses at age 4, 6, and 12 months)
  - Dose 1 at age 3–6 months: 3- or 4-dose series (dose 2 [and dose 3 if applicable] at least 8 weeks after previous dose until a dose is received at age 7 months or older, followed by an additional dose at least 12 weeks later and after age 12 months)
  - Dose 1 at age 7–23 months: 2-dose series (dose 2 at least 12 weeks after dose 1 and after age 12 months)
  - Dose 1 at age 24 months or older: 2-dose series at least 8 weeks apart

- **MenQuadfi®**
  - Dose 1 at age 24 months or older: 2-dose series at least 8 weeks apart

Notes Recommended Child and Adolescent Immunization Schedule for Ages 18 Years or Younger, United States, 2024

Travel to countries with hyperendemic or epidemic meningococcal disease, including countries in the African meningitis belt or during the Hajj (www.cdc.gov/travel/):

- Children less than age 24 months:
  - **Menveo®® (age 2–23 months)**
    - Dose 1 at age 2 months: 4-dose series (additional 3 doses at age 4, 6, and 12 months)
    - Dose 1 at age 3–6 months: 3- or 4-dose series (dose 2 [and dose 3 if applicable] at least 8 weeks after previous dose until a dose is received at age 7 months or older, followed by an additional dose at least 12 weeks later and after age 12 months)
    - Dose 1 at age 7–23 months: 2-dose series (dose 2 at least 12 weeks after dose 1 and after age 12 months)
- Children age 2 years or older: 1 dose Menveo®® or MenQuadfi®

First-year college students who live in residential housing (if not previously vaccinated at age 16 years or older) or military recruits:

- 1 dose **Menveo®®** or **MenQuadfi®**

Adolescent vaccination of children who received MenACWY prior to age 10 years:

- **Children for whom boosters are recommended** because of an ongoing increased risk of meningococcal disease (e.g., those with complement component deficiency, HIV, or asplenia): Follow the booster schedule for persons at increased risk.
- **Children for whom boosters are not recommended** (e.g., a healthy child who received a single dose for travel to a country where meningococcal disease is endemic): Administer MenACWY according to the recommended adolescent schedule with dose 1 at age 11–12 years and dose 2 at age 16 years.

Menveo has two formulations: lyophilized and liquid. The liquid formulation should not be used before age 10 years. See www.cdc.gov/vaccines/vpd/mening/downloads/menveo-single-vial-presentation.pdf.

Note: For MenACWY **booster dose recommendations** for groups listed under "Special situations" and in an outbreak setting and additional meningococcal vaccination information, see www.cdc.gov/mmwr/volumes/69/rr/rr6909a1.htm.

Children age 10 years or older may receive a single dose of Penbraya™ as an alternative to separate administration of MenACWY and MenB when both vaccines would be given on the same clinic day (see "Meningococcal serogroup B vaccination" section below for more information).

Meningococcal serogroup B vaccination
(minimum age: 10 years [MenB-4C, Bexsero®; MenB-FHbp, Trumenba®; MenACWY-TT/MenB-FHbp, Penbraya™])

Shared clinical decision-making

- **Adolescents not at increased risk** age 16–23 years (preferred age 16–18 years) based on shared clinical decision-making:
  - **Bexsero®:** 2-dose series at least 1 month apart
  - **Trumenba®:** 2-dose series at least 6 months apart (if dose 2 is administered earlier than 6 months, administer a 3rd dose at least 4 months after dose 2)

For additional information on shared clinical decision-making for MenB, see www.cdc.gov/vaccines/hcp/admin/downloads/isd-job-aid-scdm-mening-b-shared-clinical-decision-making.pdf

Special situations

Anatomic or functional asplenia (including sickle cell disease), persistent complement component deficiency, complement inhibitor (e.g., eculizumab, ravulizumab) use:

- **Bexsero®:** 2-dose series at least 1 month apart
- **Trumenba®:** 3-dose series at 0, 1–2, 6 months (if dose 2 was administered at least 6 months after dose 1, dose 3 not needed; if dose 3 is administered earlier than 4 months after dose 2, a 4th dose should be administered at least 4 months after dose 3)

Note: Bexsero® and **Trumenba®** are not interchangeable; the same product should be used for all doses in a series.

For MenB **booster dose recommendations** for groups listed under "Special situations" and in an outbreak setting and additional meningococcal vaccination information, see www.cdc.gov/mmwr/volumes/69/rr/rr6909a1.htm.

Children age 10 years or older may receive a dose of Penbraya™ as an alternative to separate administration of MenACWY and MenB when both vaccines would be given on the same clinic day. For age-eligible children not at increased risk, if Penbraya™ is used for dose 1 MenB, MenB-FHbp (Trumenba) should be administered for dose 2 MenB. For age-eligible children at increased risk of meningococcal disease, Penbraya™ may be used for additional MenACWY and MenB doses (including booster doses) if both would be given on the same clinic day **and** at least 6 months have elapsed since most recent Penbraya™ dose.

Mpox vaccination
(minimum age: 18 years [Jynneos®])

Special situations

- **Age 18 years and at risk for Mpox infection:** 2-dose series, 28 days apart.

  Risk factors for Mpox infection include:
  - Persons who are gay, bisexual, and other MSM, transgender or nonbinary people who in the past 6 months have had:
    - A new diagnosis of at least 1 sexually transmitted disease
    - More than 1 sex partner
    - Sex at a commercial sex venue
    - Sex in association with a large public event in a geographic area where Mpox transmission is occurring
  - Persons who are sexual partners of the persons described above
  - Persons who anticipate experiencing any of the situations described above
- **Pregnancy:** There is currently no ACIP recommendation for Jynneos use in pregnancy due to lack of safety data in pregnant persons. Pregnant persons with any risk factor described above may receive Jynneos.

For detailed information, see: www.cdc.gov/vaccines/acip/meetings/downloads/slides-2023-10-25-26/04-MPOX-Rao-508.pdf

Pneumococcal vaccination
(minimum age: 6 weeks [PCV15], [PCV 20]; 2 years [PPSV23])

Routine vaccination with PCV

- 4-dose series at 2, 4, 6, 12–15 months

Catch-up vaccination with PCV

- Healthy children ages 2–4 years with any incomplete* PCV series: 1 dose PCV
- For other catch-up guidance, see Table 2.

Note: For children **without** risk conditions, PCV20 is not indicated if they have received 4 doses of PCV13 or PCV15 or another age appropriate complete PCV series.

Notes Recommended Child and Adolescent Immunization Schedule for Ages 18 Years or Younger, United States, 2024

Special situations

Children and adolescents with cerebrospinal fluid leak; chronic heart disease; chronic kidney disease (excluding maintenance dialysis and nephrotic syndrome); chronic liver disease; chronic lung disease (including moderate persistent or severe persistent asthma); cochlear implant; or diabetes mellitus:

Age 2–5 years

- Any incomplete* PCV series with:
  - 3 PCV doses: 1 dose PCV (at least 8 weeks after the most recent PCV dose)
  - Less than 3 PCV doses: 2 doses PCV (at least 8 weeks after the most recent dose and administered at least 8 weeks apart)
- Completed recommended PCV series but have not received PPSV23
  - Previously received at least 1 dose of PCV20: no further PCV or PPSV23 doses needed
  - Not previously received PCV20: administer 1 dose PCV20 OR 1 dose PPSV23 administer at least 8 weeks after the most recent PCV dose.

Age 6–18 years

- Not previously received any dose of PCV13, PCV15, or PCV20: administer 1 dose of PCV15 or PCV20. If PCV15 is used and no previous receipt of PPSV23, administer 1 dose of PPSV23 at least 8 weeks after the PCV15 dose.**
- Received PCV before age 6 years but have not received PPSV23
  - Previously received at least 1 dose of PCV20: no further PCV or PPSV23 doses needed
  - Not previously received PCV20: 1 dose PCV20 OR 1 dose PPSV23 administer at least 8 weeks after the most recent PCV dose.
- Received PCV13 only at or after age 6 years: administer 1 dose PCV20 OR 1 dose PPSV23 at least 8 weeks after the most recent PCV13 dose.
- Received 1 dose PCV13 and 1 dose PPSV23 at or after age 6 years: no further doses of any PCV or PPSV23 indicated.

Children and adolescents on maintenance dialysis, or with immunocompromising conditions such as nephrotic syndrome; congenital or acquired asplenia or splenic dysfunction; congenital or acquired immunodeficiencies; diseases and conditions treated with immunosuppressive drugs or radiation therapy, including malignant neoplasms, leukemias, lymphomas, Hodgkin disease, and solid organ transplant; HIV infection; or sickle cell disease or other hemoglobinopathies:

Age 2–5 years

- Any incomplete* PCV series:
  - 3 PCV doses: 1 dose PCV (at least 8 weeks after the most recent PCV dose)
  - Less than 3 PCV doses: 2 doses PCV (at least 8 weeks after the most recent dose and administered at least 8 weeks apart)
- Completed recommended PCV series but have not received PPSV23
  - Previously received at least 1 dose of PCV20: no further PCV or PPSV23 doses needed
  - Not previously received PCV20: administer 1 dose PCV20 OR 1 dose PPSV23 at least 8 weeks after the most recent PCV dose. If PPSV23 is used, administer 1 dose of PCV20 or dose 2 PPSV23 at least 5 years after dose 1 PPSV23.

Age 6–18 years

- Not previously received any dose of PCV13, PCV15, or PCV20: administer 1 dose of PCV15 or 1 dose of PCV20. If PCV15 is used and no previous receipt of PPSV23, administer 1 dose of PPSV23 at least 8 weeks after the PCV15 dose.**
- Received PCV before age 6 years but have not received PPSV23
  - Previously received at least 1 dose of PCV20: no additional dose of PCV or PPSV23
  - Not previously received PCV20: administer 1 dose PCV20 OR 1 dose PPSV23 at least 8 weeks after the most recent PCV dose. If PPSV23 is used, administer either PCV20 or dose 2 PPSV23 at least 5 years after dose 1 PPSV23.
- Received PCV13 only at or after age 6 years: administer 1 dose PCV20 OR 1 dose PPSV23 at least 8 weeks after the most recent PCV13 dose. If PPSV23 is used, administer 1 dose of PCV20 or dose 2 PPSV23 at least 5 years after dose 1 PPSV23.
- Received 1 dose PCV13 and 1 dose PPSV23 at or after age 6 years: administer 1 dose PCV20 OR 1 dose PPSV23 at least 8 weeks after the most recent PCV13 dose and at least 5 years after dose 1 PPSV23.

Incomplete series = Not having received all doses in either the recommended series or an age-appropriate catch-up series. See Table 2 in ACIP pneumococcal recommendations at stacks.cdc.gov/view/cdc/133252

**When both PCV15 and PPSV23 are indicated, administer all doses of PCV15 first. PCV15 and PPSV23 should not be administered during the same visit.*

For guidance on determining which pneumococcal vaccines a patient needs and when, please refer to the mobile app, which can be downloaded here:
www.cdc.gov/vaccines/vpd/pneumo/hcp/pneumoapp.html

Poliovirus vaccination
(minimum age: 6 weeks)

Routine vaccination

- 4-dose series at ages 2, 4, 6–18 months, 4–6 years; administer the final dose on or after age 4 years and at least 6 months after the previous dose.
- 4 or more doses of IPV can be administered before age 4 years when a combination vaccine containing IPV is used. However, a dose is still recommended on or after age 4 years and at least 6 months after the previous dose.

Catch-up vaccination

- In the first 6 months of life, use minimum ages and intervals only for travel to a polio-endemic region or during an outbreak.
- **Adolescents age 18 years known or suspected to be unvaccinated or incompletely vaccinated:** administer remaining doses (1, 2, or 3 IPV doses) to complete a 3-dose primary series.* Unless there are specific reasons to believe they were not vaccinated, most persons aged 18 years or older born and raised in the United States can assume they were vaccinated against polio as children.

Series containing oral poliovirus vaccine (OPV), either mixed OPV-IPV or OPV-only series:

- Total number of doses needed to complete the series is the same as that recommended for the U.S. IPV schedule. See www.cdc.gov/mmwr/volumes/66/wr/mm6601a6.htm?s_%20 cid=mm6601a6_w.
- Only trivalent OPV (tOPV) counts toward the U.S. vaccination requirements.
  - Doses of OPV administered before April 1, 2016, should be counted (unless specifically noted as administered during a campaign).
  - Doses of OPV administered on or after April 1, 2016, should not be counted.
  - For guidance to assess doses documented as "OPV," see www.cdc.gov/mmwr/volumes/66/wr/mm6606a7.htm?s_ cid=mm6606a7_w.
- For other catch-up guidance, see Table 2.

Notes   Recommended Child and Adolescent Immunization Schedule for Ages 18 Years or Younger, United States, 2024

Special situations

- **Adolescents aged 18 years at increased risk of exposure to poliovirus and completed primary series*:** may administer one lifetime IPV booster

*Note: Complete primary series consist of at least 3 doses of IPV or trivalent oral poliovirus vaccine (tOPV) in any combination.

For detailed information, see: www.cdc.gov/vaccines/vpd/polio/hcp/recommendations.html

Respiratory syncytial virus immunization (minimum age: birth [Nirsevimab, RSV-mAb (Beyfortus™)])

Routine immunization

- **Infants born October – March in most of the continental United States***
  - Mother did not receive RSV vaccine OR mother's RSV vaccination status is unknown: administer 1 dose nirsevimab within 1 week of birth in hospital or outpatient setting
  - Mother received RSV vaccine **less than 14 days** prior to delivery: administer 1 dose nirsevimab within 1 week of birth in hospital or outpatient setting
  - Mother received RSV vaccine **at least 14 days** prior to delivery: nirsevimab not needed but can be considered in rare circumstances at the discretion of healthcare providers (see special populations and situations at www.cdc.gov/vaccines/vpd/rsv/hcp/child-faqs.html)
- **Infants born April–September in most of the continental United States***
  - Mother did not receive RSV vaccine OR mother's RSV vaccination status is unknown: administer 1 dose nirsevimab shortly before start of RSV season*
  - Mother received RSV vaccine **less than 14 days** prior to delivery: administer 1 dose nirsevimab shortly before start of RSV season*
  - Mother received RSV vaccine **at least 14 days** prior to delivery: nirsevimab not needed but can be considered in rare circumstances at the discretion of healthcare providers(see special populations and situations at www.cdc.gov/vaccines/vpd/rsv/hcp/child-faqs.html)

Infants with prolonged birth hospitalization** (e.g., for prematurity) discharged October through March should be immunized shortly before or promptly after discharge.

Special situations

- **Ages 8–19 months with chronic lung disease of prematurity requiring medical support (e.g., chronic corticosteroid therapy, diuretic therapy, or supplemental oxygen) any time during the 6-month period before the start of the second RSV season; severe immunocompromise; cystic fibrosis with either weight for length <10th percentile or manifestation of severe lung disease (e.g., previous hospitalization for pulmonary exacerbation in the first year of life or abnormalities on chest imaging that persist when stable)**:**
  - 1 dose nirsevimab shortly before start of second RSV season*
- **Ages 8–19 months who are American Indian or Alaska Native:**
  - 1 dose nirsevimab shortly before start of second RSV season*
- **Age-eligible and undergoing cardiac surgery with cardiopulmonary bypass**:** 1 additional dose of nirsevimab after surgery. For additional details see special populations and situations at www.cdc.gov/vaccines/vpd/rsv/hcp/child-faqs.html

*Note: While the timing of the onset and duration of RSV season may vary, nirsevimab may be administered October through March in most of the continental United States. Providers in jurisdictions with RSV seasonality that differs from most of the continental United States (e.g., Alaska, jurisdiction with tropical climate) should follow guidance from public health authorities (e.g., CDC, health departments) or regional medical centers on timing of administration based on local RSV seasonality. Although optimal timing of administration is just before the start of the RSV season, nirsevimab may also be administered during the RSV season to infants and children who are age-eligible.

**Note: Nirsevimab can be administered to children who are eligible to receive palivizumab. Children who have received nirsevimab should not receive palivizumab for the same RSV season.

For further guidance, see www.cdc.gov/mmwr/volumes/72/wr/mm7234a4.htm and www.cdc.gov/vaccines/vpd/rsv/hcp/child-faqs.html

Respiratory syncytial virus vaccination (RSV [Abrysvo™])

Routine vaccination

- **Pregnant at 32 weeks 0 days through 36 weeks and 6 days gestation from September through January in most of the continental United States*:** 1 dose RSV vaccine (Abrysvo™). Administer RSV vaccine regardless of previous RSV infection.
  - Either maternal RSV vaccination or infant immunization with nirsevimab (RSV monoclonal antibody) is recommended to prevent respiratory syncytial virus lower respiratory tract infection in infants.
- **All other pregnant persons:** RSV vaccine not recommended.

There is currently no ACIP recommendation for RSV vaccination in subsequent pregnancies. No data are available to inform whether additional doses are needed in later pregnancies.

*Note: Providers in jurisdictions with RSV seasonality that differs from most of the continental United States (e.g., Alaska, jurisdiction with tropical climate) should follow guidance from public health authorities (e.g., CDC, health departments) or regional medical centers on timing of administration based on local RSV seasonality.

Rotavirus vaccination (minimum age: 6 weeks)

Routine vaccination

- **Rotarix®:** 2-dose series at age 2 and 4 months
- **RotaTeq®:** 3-dose series at age 2, 4, and 6 months
- If any dose in the series is either **RotaTeq®** or unknown, default to 3-dose series.

Catch-up vaccination

- Do not start the series on or after age 15 weeks, 0 days.
- The maximum age for the final dose is 8 months, 0 days.
- For other catch-up guidance, see Table 2.

Tetanus, diphtheria, and pertussis (Tdap) vaccination
(minimum age: 11 years for routine vaccination, 7 years for catch-up vaccination)

Routine vaccination

- **Age 11–12 years:** 1 dose Tdap (adolescent booster)
- **Pregnancy:** 1 dose Tdap during each pregnancy, preferably in early part of gestational weeks 27–36.

Note: Tdap may be administered regardless of the interval since the last tetanus- and diphtheria-toxoid-containing vaccine.

Catch-up vaccination

- **Age 13–18 years who have not received Tdap:** 1 dose Tdap (adolescent booster)
- **Age 7–18 years not fully vaccinated* with DTaP:** 1 dose Tdap as part of the catch-up series (preferably the first dose); if additional doses are needed, use Td or Tdap.
- **Tdap administered at age 7–10 years:**
  - **Age 7–9 years** who receive Tdap should receive the adolescent Tdap booster dose at age 11–12 years.
  - **Age 10 years** who receive Tdap do not need the adolescent Tdap booster dose at age 11–12 years.
- **DTaP inadvertently administered on or after age 7 years:**
  - **Age 7–9 years:** DTaP may count as part of catch-up series. Administer adolescent Tdap booster dose at age 11–12 years.
  - **Age 10–18 years:** Count dose of DTaP as the adolescent Tdap booster dose.
- For other catch-up guidance, see Table 2.

Special situations

- **Wound management** in persons age 7 years or older with history of 3 or more doses of tetanus-toxoid-containing vaccine: For clean and minor wounds, administer Tdap or Td if more than 10 years since last dose of tetanus-toxoid-containing vaccine; for all other wounds, administer Tdap or Td if more than 5 years since last dose of tetanus-toxoid-containing vaccine. Tdap is preferred for persons age 11 years or older who have not previously received Tdap or whose Tdap history is unknown. If a tetanus-toxoid-containing vaccine is indicated for a pregnant adolescent, use Tdap.
- For detailed information, see www.cdc.gov/mmwr/volumes/69/wr/mm6903a5.htm.

*Fully vaccinated = 5 valid doses of DTaP OR 4 valid doses of DTaP if dose 4 was administered at age 4 years or older

Varicella vaccination
(minimum age: 12 months)

Routine vaccination

- 2-dose series at age 12–15 months, 4–6 years
- VAR or MMRV may be administered*
- Dose 2 may be administered as early as 3 months after dose 1 (a dose inadvertently administered after at least 4 weeks may be counted as valid)

***Note**: For dose 1 in children age 12–47 months, it is recommended to administer MMR and varicella vaccines separately. MMRV may be used if parents or caregivers express a preference.

Catch-up vaccination

- Ensure persons age 7–18 years without evidence of immunity (see *MMWR* at www.cdc.gov/mmwr/pdf/rr/rr5604.pdf) have a 2-dose series:
  - **Age 7–12 years:** Routine interval: 3 months (a dose inadvertently administered after at least 4 weeks may be counted as valid)
  - **Age 13 years and older:** Routine interval: 4–8 weeks (minimum interval: 4 weeks)
  - The maximum age for use of *MMRV* is 12 years.

11/16/2023

Centers for Disease Control and Prevention | Recommended Child and Adolescent Immunization Schedule, United States, 2024

Appendix Recommended Child and Adolescent Immunization Schedule for Ages 18 Years or Younger, United States, 2024

Guide to Contraindications and Precautions to Commonly Used Vaccines

Adapted from Table 4-1 in Advisory Committee on Immunization Practices (ACIP) General Best Practice Guidelines for Immunization: Contraindication and Precautions, Prevention and Control of Seasonal Influenza with Vaccines: Recommendations of the Advisory Committee on Immunization Practices—United States, 2023–24 Influenza Season | MMWR (cdc.gov), Contraindications and Precautions for COVID-19 Vaccination, and Contraindications and Precautions for JYNNEOS Vaccination

Vaccines and other Immunizing Agents	Contraindicated or Not Recommended[1]	Precautions[2]
COVID-19 mRNA vaccines [Pfizer-BioNTech, Moderna]	• Severe allergic reaction (e.g., anaphylaxis) after a previous dose or to a component of an mRNA COVID-19 vaccine[4]	• Diagnosed non-severe allergy (e.g., urticaria beyond the injection site) to a component of an mRNA COVID-19 vaccine[4]; or non-severe, immediate (onset less than 4 hours) allergic reaction after administration of a previous dose of an mRNA COVID-19 vaccine • Myocarditis or pericarditis within 3 weeks after a dose of any COVID-19 vaccine • Multisystem inflammatory syndrome in children (MIS-C) or multisystem inflammatory syndrome in adults (MIS-A) • Moderate or severe acute illness, with or without fever
COVID-19 protein subunit vaccine [Novavax]	• Severe allergic reaction (e.g., anaphylaxis) after a previous dose or to a component of a Novavax COVID-19 vaccine[4]	• Diagnosed non-severe allergy (e.g., urticaria beyond the injection site) to a component of Novavax COVID-19 vaccine[4]; or non-severe, immediate (onset less than 4 hours) allergic reaction after administration of a previous dose of a Novavax COVID-19 vaccine • Myocarditis or pericarditis within 3 weeks after a dose of any COVID-19 vaccine • Multisystem inflammatory syndrome in children (MIS-C) or multisystem inflammatory syndrome in adults (MIS-A) • Moderate or severe acute illness, with or without fever
Influenza, egg-based, inactivated injectable (IIV4)	• Severe allergic reaction (e.g., anaphylaxis) after previous dose of any influenza vaccine (i.e., any egg-based IIV, ccIIV, RIV, or LAIV of any valency) • Severe allergic reaction (e.g., anaphylaxis) to any vaccine component[3] (excluding egg)	• Guillain-Barré syndrome (GBS) within 6 weeks after a previous dose of any type of influenza vaccine • Moderate or severe acute illness with or without fever
Influenza, cell culture-based inactivated injectable (ccIIV4) [Flucelvax Quadrivalent]	• Severe allergic reaction (e.g., anaphylaxis) to any ccIIV of any valency, or to any component[3] of ccIIV4	• Guillain-Barré syndrome (GBS) within 6 weeks after a previous dose of any type of influenza vaccine • Persons with a history of severe allergic reaction (e.g., anaphylaxis) after a previous dose of any egg-based IIV, RIV, or LAIV of any valency. If using ccIIV4, administer in medical setting under supervision of health care provider who can recognize and manage severe allergic reactions. May consult an allergist. • Moderate or severe acute illness with or without fever
Influenza, recombinant injectable (RIV4) [Flublok Quadrivalent]	• Severe allergic reaction (e.g., anaphylaxis) to any RIV of any valency, or to any component[3] of RIV4	• Guillain-Barré syndrome (GBS) within 6 weeks after a previous dose of any type of influenza vaccine • Persons with a history of severe allergic reaction (e.g., anaphylaxis) after a previous dose of any egg-based IIV, ccIIV, or LAIV of any valency. If using RIV4, administer in medical setting under supervision of health care provider who can recognize and manage severe allergic reactions. May consult an allergist. • Moderate or severe acute illness with or without fever
Influenza, live attenuated (LAIV4) [Flumist Quadrivalent]	• Severe allergic reaction (e.g., anaphylaxis) after previous dose of any influenza vaccine (i.e., any egg-based IIV, ccIIV, RIV, or LAIV of any valency) • Severe allergic reaction (e.g., anaphylaxis) to any vaccine component[3] (excluding egg) • Children age 2–4 years with a history of asthma or wheezing • Anatomic or functional asplenia • Immunocompromised due to any cause including, but not limited to, medications and HIV infection • Close contacts or caregivers of severely immunosuppressed persons who require a protected environment • Pregnancy • Cochlear implant • Active communication between the cerebrospinal fluid (CSF) and the oropharynx, nasopharynx, nose, ear or any other cranial CSF leak • Children and adolescents receiving aspirin or salicylate-containing medications • Received influenza antiviral medications oseltamivir or zanamivir within the previous 48 hours, peramivir within the previous 5 days, or baloxavir within the previous 17 days	• Guillain-Barré syndrome (GBS) within 6 weeks after a previous dose of any type of influenza vaccine • Asthma in persons age 5 years old or older • Persons with underlying medical conditions other than those listed under contraindications that might predispose to complications after wild-type influenza virus infection, e.g., chronic pulmonary, cardiovascular (except isolated hypertension), renal, hepatic, neurologic, hematologic, or metabolic disorders (including diabetes mellitus) • Moderate or severe acute illness with or without fever

1. When a contraindication is present, a vaccine should **NOT** be administered. Kroger A, Bahta L, Hunter P. ACIP General Best Practice Guidelines for Immunization.
2. When a precaution is present, vaccination should generally be deferred but might be indicated if the benefit of protection from the vaccine outweighs the risk for an adverse reaction. Kroger A, Bahta L, Hunter P. ACIP General Best Practice Guidelines for Immunization.
3. Vaccination providers should check FDA-approved prescribing information for the most complete and updated information, including contraindications, warnings, and precautions. See Package inserts for U.S.-licensed vaccines.
4. See package inserts and FDA EUA fact sheets for a full list of vaccine ingredients. mRNA COVID-19 vaccines contain polyethylene glycol (PEG).

Appendix	Recommended Child and Adolescent Immunization Schedule for Ages 18 Years or Younger, United States, 2024

Vaccines and other Immunizing Agents	Contraindicated or Not Recommended[1]	Precautions[2]
Dengue (DEN4CYD)	• Severe allergic reaction (e.g., anaphylaxis) after a previous dose or to a vaccine component[3] • Severe immunodeficiency (e.g., hematologic and solid tumors, receipt of chemotherapy, congenital immunodeficiency, long-term immunosuppressive therapy or patients with HIV infection who are severely immunocompromised) • Lack of laboratory confirmation of a previous Dengue infection	• Pregnancy • HIV infection without evidence of severe immunosuppression • Moderate or severe acute illness with or without fever
Diphtheria, tetanus, pertussis (DTaP)	• Severe allergic reaction (e.g., anaphylaxis) after a previous dose or to a vaccine component[3] • For DTaP only: Encephalopathy (e.g., coma, decreased level of consciousness, prolonged seizures) not attributable to another identifiable cause within 7 days of administration of previous dose of DTP or DTaP	• Guillain-Barré syndrome (GBS) within 6 weeks after previous dose of tetanus-toxoid–containing vaccine • History of Arthus-type hypersensitivity reactions after a previous dose of diphtheria-toxoid–containing or tetanus-toxoid–containing vaccine; defer vaccination until at least 10 years have elapsed since the last tetanus-toxoid-containing vaccine • For DTaP only: Progressive neurologic disorder, including infantile spasms, uncontrolled epilepsy, progressive encephalopathy; defer DTaP until neurologic status clarified and stabilized • Moderate or severe acute illness with or without fever
Haemophilus influenzae type b (Hib)	• Severe allergic reaction (e.g., anaphylaxis) after a previous dose or to a vaccine component[3] • Less than age 6 weeks	• Moderate or severe acute illness with or without fever
Hepatitis A (HepA)	• Severe allergic reaction (e.g., anaphylaxis) after a previous dose or to a vaccine component[3] including neomycin	• Moderate or severe acute illness with or without fever
Hepatitis B (HepB)	• Severe allergic reaction (e.g., anaphylaxis) after a previous dose or to a vaccine component[3] including yeast • Pregnancy: Heplisav-B and PreHevbrio are not recommended due to lack of safety data in pregnant persons. Use other hepatitis B vaccines if HepB is indicated[4].	• Moderate or severe acute illness with or without fever
Hepatitis A-Hepatitis B vaccine (HepA-HepB) [Twinrix]	• Severe allergic reaction (e.g., anaphylaxis) after a previous dose or to a vaccine component[3] including neomycin and yeast	• Moderate or severe acute illness with or without fever
Human papillomavirus (HPV)	• Severe allergic reaction (e.g., anaphylaxis) after a previous dose or to a vaccine component[3] • Pregnancy: HPV vaccination not recommended.	• Moderate or severe acute illness with or without fever
Measles, mumps, rubella (MMR) Measles, mumps, rubella, and varicella (MMRV)	• Severe allergic reaction (e.g., anaphylaxis) after a previous dose or to a vaccine component[3] • Severe immunodeficiency (e.g., hematologic and solid tumors, receipt of chemotherapy, congenital immunodeficiency, long-term immunosuppressive therapy or patients with HIV infection who are severely immunocompromised) • Pregnancy • Family history of altered immunocompetence, unless verified clinically or by laboratory testing as immunocompetent	• Recent (≤11 months) receipt of antibody-containing blood product (specific interval depends on product) • History of thrombocytopenia or thrombocytopenic purpura • Need for tuberculin skin testing or interferon-gamma release assay (IGRA) testing • Moderate or severe acute illness with or without fever • For MMRV only: Personal or family (i.e., sibling or parent) history of seizures of any etiology
Meningococcal ACWY (MenACWY) MenACWY-CRM [Menveo] MenACWY-TT [MenQuadfi]	• Severe allergic reaction (e.g., anaphylaxis) after a previous dose or to a vaccine component[3] • For Men ACWY-CRM only: severe allergic reaction to any diphtheria toxoid—or CRM197—containing vaccine • For MenACWY-TT only: severe allergic reaction to a tetanus toxoid-containing vaccine	• For MenACWY-CRM only: Preterm birth if less than age 9 months • Moderate or severe acute illness with or without fever
Meningococcal B (MenB) MenB-4C [Bexsero] MenB-FHbp [Trumenba]	• Severe allergic reaction (e.g., anaphylaxis) after a previous dose or to a vaccine component[3]	• Pregnancy • For MenB-4C only: Latex sensitivity • Moderate or severe acute illness with or without fever
Meningococcal ABCWY (MenACWY-TT/MenB-FHbp) [Penbraya]	• Severe allergic reaction (e.g., anaphylaxis) after a previous dose or to a vaccine component[3] • Severe allergic reaction to a tetanus toxoid-containing vaccine	• Moderate or severe acute illness, with or without fever
Mpox [Jynneos]	• Severe allergic reaction (e.g., anaphylaxis) after a previous dose or to a vaccine component[3]	• Moderate or severe acute illness, with or without fever
Pneumococcal conjugate (PCV)	• Severe allergic reaction (e.g., anaphylaxis) after a previous dose or to a vaccine component[3] • Severe allergic reaction (e.g., anaphylaxis) to any diphtheria-toxoid-containing vaccine or its component[3]	• Moderate or severe acute illness with or without fever
Pneumococcal polysaccharide (PPSV23)	• Severe allergic reaction (e.g., anaphylaxis) after a previous dose or to a vaccine component[3]	• Moderate or severe acute illness with or without fever
Poliovirus vaccine, inactivated (IPV)	• Severe allergic reaction (e.g., anaphylaxis) after a previous dose or to a vaccine component[3]	• Pregnancy • Moderate or severe acute illness with or without fever
RSV monoclonal antibody (RSV-mAb)	• Severe allergic reaction (e.g., anaphylaxis) after a previous dose or to a vaccine component[3]	• Moderate or severe acute illness with or without fever
Respiratory syncytial virus vaccine (RSV)	• Severe allergic reaction (e.g., anaphylaxis) after a previous dose or to a vaccine component[3]	• Moderate or severe acute illness with or without fever
Rotavirus (RV) RV1 [Rotarix] RV5 [RotaTeq]	• Severe allergic reaction (e.g., anaphylaxis) after a previous dose or to a vaccine component[3] • Severe combined immunodeficiency (SCID) • History of intussusception	• Altered immunocompetence other than SCID • Chronic gastrointestinal disease • RV1 only: Spina bifida or bladder exstrophy • Moderate or severe acute illness with or without fever
Tetanus, diphtheria, and acellular pertussis (Tdap) Tetanus, diphtheria (Td)	• Severe allergic reaction (e.g., anaphylaxis) after a previous dose or to a vaccine component[3] • For Tdap only: Encephalopathy (e.g., coma, decreased level of consciousness, prolonged seizures) not attributable to another identifiable cause within 7 days of administration of previous dose of DTP, DTaP, or Tdap	• Guillain-Barré syndrome (GBS) within 6 weeks after a previous dose of tetanus-toxoid–containing vaccine • History of Arthus-type hypersensitivity reactions after a previous dose of diphtheria-toxoid–containing or tetanus-toxoid–containing vaccine; defer vaccination until at least 10 years have elapsed since the last tetanus-toxoid–containing vaccine • For Tdap only: Progressive or unstable neurological disorder, uncontrolled seizures, or progressive encephalopathy until a treatment regimen has been established and the condition has stabilized • Moderate or severe acute illness with or without fever
Varicella (VAR)	• Severe allergic reaction (e.g., anaphylaxis) after a previous dose or to a vaccine component[3] • Severe immunodeficiency (e.g., hematologic and solid tumors, receipt of chemotherapy, congenital immunodeficiency, long-term immunosuppressive therapy or patients with HIV infection who are severely immunocompromised) • Pregnancy • Family history of altered immunocompetence, unless verified clinically or by laboratory testing as immunocompetent	• Recent (≤11 months) receipt of antibody-containing blood product (specific interval depends on product) • Receipt of specific antiviral drugs (acyclovir, famciclovir, or valacyclovir) 24 hours before vaccination (avoid use of these antiviral drugs for 14 days after vaccination) • Use of aspirin or aspirin-containing products • Moderate or severe acute illness with or without fever • If using MMRV, see MMR/MMRV for additional precautions

1. When a contraindication is present, a vaccine should NOT be administered. Kroger A, Bahta L, Hunter P. ACIP General Best Practice Guidelines for Immunization. www.cdc.gov/vaccines/hcp/acip-recs/general-recs/contraindications.html
2. When a precaution is present, vaccination should generally be deferred but might be indicated if the benefit of protection from the vaccine outweighs the risk for an adverse reaction. Kroger A, Bahta L, Hunter P. ACIP General Best Practice Guidelines for Immunization. www.cdc.gov/vaccines/hcp/acip-recs/general-recs/contraindications.html
3. Vaccination providers should check FDA-approved prescribing information for the most complete and updated information, including contraindications, warnings, and precautions. Package inserts for U.S.-licensed vaccines are available at www.fda.gov/vaccines-blood-biologics/approved-products/vaccines-licensed-use-united-states.
4. For information on the pregnancy exposure registries for persons who were inadvertently vaccinated with Heplisav-B or PreHevbrio while pregnant, please visit heplisavbpregnancyregistry.com or www.prehevbrio.com/#safety.
5. Full prescribing information for BEYFORTUS (nirsevimab-alip) www.accessdata.fda.gov/drugsatfda_docs/label/2023/761328s000lbl.pdf

Addendum Recommended Child and Adolescent Immunization Schedule for Ages 18 Years or Younger, United States, 2024

In addition to the recommendations presented in the previous sections of this immunization schedule, ACIP has approved the following recommendations by majority vote since October 26, 2023. The following recommendations have been adopted by the CDC Director and are now official. Links are provided if these recommendations have been published in *Morbidity and Mortality Weekly Report (MMWR)*.

Vaccines	Recommendations	Effective Date of Recommendation*
No new vaccines or vaccine recommendations to report		

*The effective date is the date when the CDC director adopted the recommendation and when the ACIP recommendation became official.

VACCINE ADMINISTRATION*

INFECTION CONTROL AND STERILE TECHNIQUE

Persons administering vaccines should follow appropriate precautions to minimize risk for spread of disease. Hands should be cleansed with an alcohol-based, waterless antiseptic hand rub or washed with soap and water between each patient contact. Occupational Safety and Health Administration (OSHA) regulations do not require that gloves be worn when administering vaccinations unless persons administering vaccinations are likely to come into contact with potentially infectious body fluids or have open lesions on their hands. Needles used for injections must be sterile and disposable to minimize the risk for contamination. A separate needle and syringe should be used for each injection. Changing needles between drawing vaccine from a vial and injecting it into a recipient is not necessary. Different vaccines should never be mixed in the same syringe unless specifically licensed for such use, and no attempt should be made to transfer between syringes.

For all intramuscular injections, the needle should be long enough to reach the muscle mass and prevent vaccine from seeping into subcutaneous tissue, but not so long as to involve underlying nerves, blood vessels, or bone. Vaccinators should be familiar with the anatomy of the area where they are injecting vaccine. Intramuscular injections are administered at a 90-degree angle to the skin, preferably into the anterolateral aspect of the thigh or the deltoid muscle of the upper arm depending on the age of the patient.

Decision on needle size and site of injection must be made for each person on the basis of the size of the muscle, the thickness of adipose tissue at the injection site, the volume of the material to be administered, injection technique, and the depth below the muscle surface into which the material is to be injected. Aspiration before injection of vaccines or toxoids (i.e., pulling back on the syringe plunger after needle insertion before injection) is not required because no large blood vessel exists at the recommended injection sites.

INFANTS (AGED <12 MO)

For the majority of infants, the anterolateral aspect of the thigh is the recommended site for injection because it provides a large muscle mass. The muscles of the buttock have not been used for administration of vaccines in infants and children because of concern about potential injury to the sciatic nerve, which is well documented after injection of antimicrobial agents into the buttock. If the gluteal muscle must be used, care should be taken to define the anatomic landmarks. Injection technique is the most important parameter to ensure efficient intramuscular vaccine delivery. If the subcutaneous and muscle tissue are bunched to minimize the chance of striking bone, a 1-inch needle is required to ensure intramuscular administration in infants. For the majority of infants, a 1-inch, 22- to 25-gauge needle is sufficient to penetrate muscle in an infant's thigh. For newborn (first 28 days of life) and premature infants, a ⅝-inch-long needle usually is adequate if the skin is stretched flat between thumb and forefinger and the needle inserted at a 90-degree angle to the skin.

TODDLERS AND OLDER CHILDREN (AGED 12 MO TO 10 YR)

The deltoid muscle should be used if the muscle mass is adequate. The needle size for deltoid site injections can range from 22 to 25 gauge and from ⅝ to 1 inch on the basis of the size of the muscle and the thickness of adipose tissue at the injection site. A ⅝-inch needle is adequate only for the deltoid muscle and only if the skin is stretched flat between the thumb and forefinger and the needle inserted at a 90-degree angle to the skin. For toddlers, the anterolateral thigh can be used, but the needle should be at least 1 inch in length.

ADOLESCENTS AND ADULTS (AGED >11 YR)

For adults and adolescents, the deltoid muscle is recommended for routine intramuscular vaccinations. The anterolateral thigh also can be used. For men and women weighing <130 lb (<60 kg) a ⅝- to 1-inch needle is sufficient to ensure intramuscular injection. For women weighing 130 to 200 lb (60 to 90 kg) and men 130 to 260 lb (60 to 118 kg), a 1- to 1½-inch needle is needed. For women weighing >200 lb (>90 kg) or men weighing >260 lb (>118 kg), a 1½-inch needle is required.

SUBCUTANEOUS INJECTIONS

Subcutaneous injections are administered at a 45-degree angle, usually into the thigh for infants younger than 12 mo and in the upper-outer triceps area of persons aged 12 mo and older. Subcutaneous injections can be administered into the upper-outer triceps area of an infant if necessary. A ⅝-inch, 23- to 25-gauge needle should be inserted into the subcutaneous tissue.

IMMUNIZATIONS FOR ADULTS

RECOMMENDED ADULT IMMUNIZATION SCHEDULE BY AGE GROUP, UNITED STATES, 2024

The *Recommended Adult Immunization Schedule by Age Group, United States* became effective, as recommended by the Advisory Committee on Immunization Practices (ACIP) and approved by the Centers for Disease Control and Prevention (CDC). The adult immunization schedule was also reviewed and approved by the following professional medical organizations:
American College of Physicians (http://www.acponline.org/)
American Academy of Family Physicians (http://www.aafp.org/)
American College of Obstetricians and Gynecologists (http://www.acog.org/)
American College of Nurse-Midwives (http://www.midwife.org/)

CDC announced the availability of the 2024 adult immunization schedule at https://www.cdc.gov/vaccines/schedules/easy-to-read/adult.html.

The adult immunization schedule describes the age groups and medical conditions and other indications for which licensed vaccines are recommended. The 2024 adult immunization schedule consists of:

Table 13. Recommended immunization schedule for adults by age group

Table 14. Recommended immunization schedule for adults by medical condition and other indications

Footnotes that accompany each vaccine containing important general information and considerations for special populations

Consider the following information when reviewing the adult immunization schedule:

The tables in the adult immunization schedule should be read with the footnotes that contain important general information and information about vaccination of special populations.

When indicated, administer recommended vaccines to adults whose vaccination history is incomplete or unknown.

Increased interval between doses of a multi-dose vaccine does not diminish vaccine effectiveness; therefore, it is not necessary to restart the vaccine series or add doses to the series because of an extended interval between doses.

Adults with immunocompromising conditions should generally avoid live vaccines, e.g., measles, mumps, and rubella vaccine. Inactivated vaccines, e.g., pneumococcal or inactivated influenza vaccines, are generally acceptable.

Combination vaccines may be used when any component of the combination is indicated and when the other components of the combination vaccine are not contraindicated.

The use of trade names in the adult immunization schedule is for identification purposes only and does not imply endorsement by the ACIP or CDC.

Details on vaccines recommended for adults and complete ACIP statements are available at https://www.cdc.gov/vaccines/hcp/acip-recs/index.html. Additional CDC resources include:

A summary of information on vaccination recommendations, vaccination of persons with immunodeficiencies, preventing and managing adverse reactions, vaccination contraindications and precautions, and other information can be found in *General Recommendations on Immunization* at https://www.cdc.gov/mmwr/preview/mmwrhtml/rr6002a1.htm.

Vaccine Information Statements that explain benefits and risks of vaccines are available at https://www.cdc.gov/vaccinesafety/Concerns/Index.html.

Information and resources regarding vaccination of pregnant women are available at http://www.cdc.gov/vaccines/pregnancy/pregnant-women/index.html.

Information on travel vaccine requirements and recommendations is available at https://www.cdc.gov/travel/destinations/list.

CDC Vaccine Schedules App for clinicians and other immunization service providers to download is available at https://www.cdc.gov/vaccines/schedules/.

Recommended Immunization Schedule for Children and Adolescents Aged 18 Years or Younger is available at https://www.cdc.gov/vaccines/schedules/hcp/child-adolescent.html.

Report suspected cases of reportable vaccine-preventable diseases to the local or state health department.

Report all clinically significant postvaccination reactions to the Vaccine Adverse Event Reporting System at http://www.vaers.hhs.gov/ or by telephone, 800-822-7967. All vaccines included in the 2024 adult immunization schedule except herpes zoster and 23-valent pneumococcal polysaccharide vaccines are covered by the Vaccine Injury Compensation Program. Information on how to file a vaccine injury claim is available at https://www.hrsa.gov/vaccinecompensation or by telephone, 800-338-2382.

The following acronyms are used for vaccines recommended for adults:

HepA	hepatitis A vaccine
HepA-HepB	hepatitis A and hepatitis B vaccines
HepB	hepatitis B vaccine
Hib	*Haemophilus influenzae* type b conjugate vaccine
HPV vaccine	human papillomavirus vaccine
HZV	herpes zoster vaccine
IIV	inactivated influenza vaccine
LAIV	live attenuated influenza vaccine
MenACWY	serogroups A, C, W, and Y meningococcal conjugate vaccine
MenB	serogroup B meningococcal vaccine
MMR	measles, mumps, and rubella vaccine
MPSV4	serogroups A, C, W, and Y meningococcal polysaccharide vaccine
PCV13	13-valent pneumococcal conjugate vaccine
PPSV23	23-valent pneumococcal polysaccharide vaccine
RIV	recombinant influenza vaccine
Td	tetanus and diphtheria toxoids
Tdap	tetanus toxoid, reduced diphtheria toxoid, and acellular pertussis vaccine
VAR	varicella vaccine

Recommended Adult Immunization Schedule
for ages 19 years or older

UNITED STATES
2024

Vaccines in the Adult Immunization Schedule*

Vaccine	Abbreviation(s)	Trade name(s)
COVID-19 vaccine	1vCOV-mRNA	Comirnaty®/Pfizer-BioNTech COVID-19 Vaccine Spikevax®/Moderna COVID-19 Vaccine
	1vCOV-aPS	Novavax COVID-19 Vaccine
Haemophilus influenzae type b vaccine	Hib	ActHIB® Hiberix® PedvaxHIB®
Hepatitis A vaccine	HepA	Havrix® Vaqta®
Hepatitis A and hepatitis B vaccine	HepA-HepB	Twinrix®
Hepatitis B vaccine	HepB	Engerix-B® Heplisav-B® PreHevbrio® Recombivax HB®
Human papillomavirus vaccine	HPV	Gardasil 9®
Influenza vaccine (inactivated)	IIV4	Many brands
Influenza vaccine (live, attenuated)	LAIV4	FluMist® Quadrivalent
Influenza vaccine (recombinant)	RIV4	Flublok® Quadrivalent
Measles, mumps, and rubella vaccine	MMR	M-M-R II® Priorix®
Meningococcal serogroups A, C, W, Y vaccine	MenACWY-CRM MenACWY-TT	Menveo® MenQuadfi®
Meningococcal serogroup B vaccine	MenB-4C MenB-FHbp	Bexsero® Trumenba®
Meningococcal serogroup A, B, C, W, Y vaccine	MenACWY-TT/ MenB-FHbp	Penbraya™
Mpox vaccine	Mpox	Jynneos®
Pneumococcal conjugate vaccine	PCV15 PCV20	Vaxneuvance™ Prevnar 20™
Pneumococcal polysaccharide vaccine	PPSV23	Pneumovax 23®
Poliovirus vaccine	IPV	Ipol®
Respiratory syncytial virus vaccine	RSV	Arexvy® Abrysvo™
Tetanus and diphtheria toxoids	Td	Tenivac® Tdvax™
Tetanus and diphtheria toxoids and acellular pertussis vaccine	Tdap	Adacel® Boostrix®
Varicella vaccine	VAR	Varivax®
Zoster vaccine, recombinant	RZV	Shingrix

*Administer recommended vaccines if vaccination history is incomplete or unknown. Do not restart or add doses to vaccine series if there are extended intervals between doses. The use of trade names is for identification purposes only and does not imply endorsement by the ACIP or CDC.

12/28/2023

How to use the adult immunization schedule

1 Determine recommended vaccinations by age **(Table 1)**

2 Assess need for additional recommended vaccinations by medical condition or other indication **(Table 2)**

3 Review vaccine types, dosing frequencies and intervals, and considerations for special situations **(Notes)**

4 Review contraindications and precautions for vaccine types **(Appendix)**

5 Review new or updated ACIP guidance **(Addendum)**

Recommended by the Advisory Committee on Immunization Practices (www.cdc.gov/vaccines/acip) and approved by the Centers for Disease Control and Prevention (www.cdc.gov), American College of Physicians (www.acponline.org), American Academy of Family Physicians (www.aafp.org), American College of Obstetricians and Gynecologists (www.acog.org), American College of Nurse-Midwives (www.midwife.org), American Academy of Physician Associates (www.aapa.org), American Pharmacists Association (www.pharmacist.com), and Society for Healthcare Epidemiology of America (www.shea-online.org).

Report
- Suspected cases of reportable vaccine-preventable diseases or outbreaks to the local or state health department
- Clinically significant adverse events to the Vaccine Adverse Event Reporting System at www.vaers.hhs.gov or 800-822-7967

Questions or comments
Contact www.cdc.gov/cdc-info or 800-CDC-INFO (800-232-4636), in English or Spanish, 8 a.m.–8 p.m. ET, Monday through Friday, excluding holidays.

 Download the CDC Vaccine Schedules app for providers at www.cdc.gov/vaccines/schedules/hcp/schedule-app.html.

Helpful information
- Complete Advisory Committee on Immunization Practices (ACIP) recommendations: www.cdc.gov/vaccines/hcp/acip-recs/index.html
- ACIP Shared Clinical Decision-Making Recommendations: www.cdc.gov/vaccines/acip/acip-scdm-faqs.html
- *General Best Practice Guidelines for Immunization* www.cdc.gov/vaccines/hcp/acip-recs/general-recs/index.html
- Vaccine information statements: www.cdc.gov/vaccines/hcp/vis/index.html
- Manual for the Surveillance of Vaccine-Preventable Diseases (including case identification and outbreak response): www.cdc.gov/vaccines/pubs/surv-manual

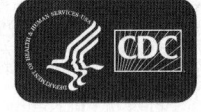 **U.S. Department of Health and Human Services** Centers for Disease Control and Prevention

 Scan QR code for access to online schedule

CS310021-D

TABLE 13 Recommended Adult Immunization Schedule by Age Group, United States, 2024

These recommendations must be read with the footnotes that follow.
From Centers for Disease Control and Prevention.

Vaccine	19–26 years	27–49 years	50–64 years	≥65 years
COVID-19	\multicolumn — 1 or more doses of updated (2023–2024 Formula) vaccine (See Notes)			
Influenza inactivated (IIV4) or **Influenza recombinant** (RIV4)	**or**	1 dose annually **or**		
Influenza live, attenuated (LAIV4)	1 dose annually			
Respiratory Syncytial Virus (RSV)	Seasonal administration during pregnancy. See Notes.			≥60 years
Tetanus, diphtheria, pertussis (Tdap or Td)	1 dose Tdap each pregnancy; 1 dose Td/Tdap for wound management (see notes)			
	1 dose Tdap, then Td or Tdap booster every 10 years			
Measles, mumps, rubella (MMR)	1 or 2 doses depending on indication (if born in 1957 or later)			For healthcare personnel, see notes
Varicella (VAR)	2 doses (if born in 1980 or later)		2 doses	
Zoster recombinant (RZV)	2 doses for immunocompromising conditions (see notes)		2 doses	
Human papillomavirus (HPV)	2 or 3 doses depending on age at initial vaccination or condition	27 through 45 years		
Pneumococcal (PCV15, PCV20, PPSV23)				See Notes
				See Notes
Hepatitis A (HepA)	2, 3, or 4 doses depending on vaccine			
Hepatitis B (HepB)	2, 3, or 4 doses depending on vaccine or condition			
Meningococcal A, C, W, Y (MenACWY)	1 or 2 doses depending on indication, see notes for booster recommendations			
Meningococcal B (MenB)	19 through 23 years	2 or 3 doses depending on vaccine and indication, see notes for booster recommendations		
Haemophilus influenzae type b (Hib)	1 or 3 doses depending on indication			
Mpox				

Recommended vaccination for adults who meet age requirement, lack documentation of vaccination, or lack evidence of immunity

Recommended vaccination for adults with an additional risk factor or another indication

Recommended vaccination based on shared clinical decision-making

No recommendation/ Not applicable

TABLE 14 Recommended Adult Immunization Schedule by Medical Condition or Other Indication, United States, 2024

These recommendations must be read with the footnotes that follow.
From Centers for Disease Control and Prevention.

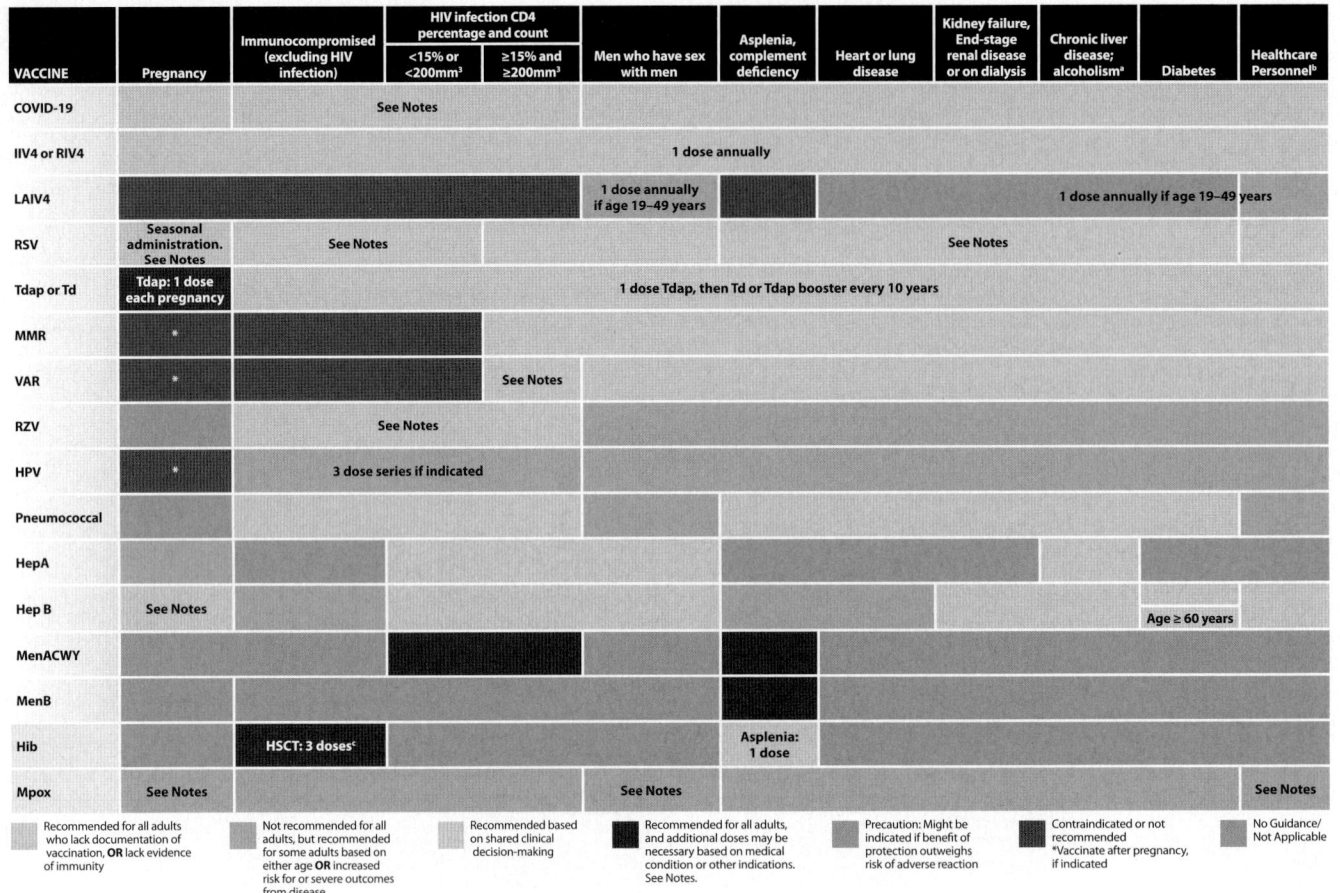

VACCINE	Pregnancy	Immunocompromised (excluding HIV infection)	HIV infection CD4 percentage and count		Men who have sex with men	Asplenia, complement deficiency	Heart or lung disease	Kidney failure, End-stage renal disease or on dialysis	Chronic liver disease; alcoholism[a]	Diabetes	Healthcare Personnel[b]
			<15% or <200mm³	≥15% and ≥200mm³							
COVID-19			See Notes								
IIV4 or RIV4					1 dose annually						
LAIV4					1 dose annually if age 19–49 years				1 dose annually if age 19–49 years		
RSV	Seasonal administration. See Notes		See Notes					See Notes			
Tdap or Td	Tdap: 1 dose each pregnancy				1 dose Tdap, then Td or Tdap booster every 10 years						
MMR	*										
VAR	*			See Notes							
RZV			See Notes								
HPV	*		3 dose series if indicated								
Pneumococcal											
HepA											
Hep B	See Notes									Age ≥ 60 years	
MenACWY											
MenB											
Hib		HSCT: 3 doses[c]				Asplenia: 1 dose					
Mpox	See Notes				See Notes						See Notes

Recommended for all adults who lack documentation of vaccination, **OR** lack evidence of immunity

Not recommended for all adults, but recommended for some adults based on either age **OR** increased risk for or severe outcomes from disease

Recommended based on shared clinical decision-making

Recommended for all adults, and additional doses may be necessary based on medical condition or other indications. See Notes.

Precaution: Might be indicated if benefit of protection outweighs risk of adverse reaction

Contraindicated or not recommended *Vaccinate after pregnancy, if indicated

No Guidance/ Not Applicable

a. Precaution for LAIV4 does not apply to alcoholism.
b. See notes for influenza; hepatitis B; measles, mumps, and rubella; and varicella vaccinations.
c. Hematopoietic stem cell transplant.

Notes Recommended Adult Immunization Schedule for Ages 19 Years or Older, United States, 2024

For vaccination recommendations for persons ages 18 years or younger, see the Recommended Child and Adolescent Immunization Schedule, 2024: www.cdc.gov/vaccines/schedules/hcp/child-adolescent.html

Additional Information

- For calculating intervals between doses, 4 weeks = 28 days. Intervals of ≥4 months are determined by calendar months.
- Within a number range (e.g., 12–18), a dash (–) should be read as "through."
- Vaccine doses administered ≤4 days before the minimum age or interval are considered valid. Doses of any vaccine administered ≥5 days earlier than the minimum age or minimum interval should not be counted as valid and should be repeated. **The repeat dose should be spaced after the invalid dose by the recommended minimum interval.** For further details, see Table 3-2, Recommended and minimum ages and intervals between vaccine doses, in *General Best Practice Guidelines for Immunization* at www.cdc.gov/vaccines/hcp/acip-recs/general-recs/timing.html.
- Information on travel vaccination requirements and recommendations is available at www.cdc.gov/travel/.
- For vaccination of persons with immunodeficiencies, see Table 8-1, Vaccination of persons with primary and secondary immunodeficiencies, in *General Best Practice Guidelines for Immunization* at www.cdc.gov/vaccines/hcp/acip-recs/general-recs/immunocompetence.html.
- For information about vaccination in the setting of a vaccine-preventable disease outbreak, contact your state or local health department.
- The National Vaccine Injury Compensation Program (VICP) is a no-fault alternative to the traditional legal system for resolving vaccine injury claims. All vaccines included in the adult immunization schedule except PPSV23, RSV, RZV, Mpox, and COVID-19 vaccines are covered by the National Vaccine Injury Compensation Program (VICP). Mpox and COVID-19 vaccines are covered by the Countermeasures Injury Compensation Program (CICP). For more information, see www.hrsa.gov/vaccinecompensation or www.hrsa.gov/cicp.

COVID-19 vaccination

Routine vaccination

Age 19 years or older

- **Unvaccinated:**
  - 1 dose of updated (2023–2024 Formula) Moderna or Pfizer-BioNTech vaccine
  - 2-dose series of updated (2023–2024 Formula) Novavax at 0, 3–8 weeks
- **Previously vaccinated* with 1 or more doses of any COVID-19 vaccine:** 1 dose of any updated (2023–2024 Formula) COVID-19 vaccine administered at least 8 weeks after the most recent COVID-19 vaccine dose.

Special situations

Persons who are moderately or severely immunocompromised**

- **Unvaccinated:**
  - 3-dose series of updated (2023–2024 Formula) Moderna at 0, 4, 8 weeks
  - 3-dose series of updated (2023–2024 Formula) Pfizer-BioNTech at 0, 3, 7 weeks
  - 2-dose series of updated (2023–2024 Formula) Novavax at 0, 3 weeks
- **Previously vaccinated* with 1 dose of any Moderna:** 2-dose series of updated (2023–2024 Formula) Moderna at 0, 4 weeks (minimum interval between previous Moderna dose and dose 1: 4 weeks)
- **Previously vaccinated* with 2 doses of any Moderna:** 1 dose of updated (2023–2024 Formula) Moderna at least 4 weeks after most recent dose.
- **Previously vaccinated* with 1 dose of any Pfizer-BioNTech:** 2-dose series of updated (2023–2024 Formula) Pfizer-BioNTech at 0, 4 weeks (minimum interval between previous Pfizer-BioNTech dose and dose 1: 3 weeks).
- **Previously vaccinated* with 2 doses of any Pfizer-BioNTech:** 1 dose of updated (2023–2024 Formula) Pfizer-BioNTech at least 4 weeks after most recent dose.

- **Previously vaccinated* with 3 or more doses of any Moderna or Pfizer-BioNTech:** 1 dose of any updated (2023–2024 Formula) COVID-19 vaccine at least 8 weeks after the most recent dose.
- **Previously vaccinated* with 1 or more doses of Janssen or Novavax with or without dose(s) of any Original monovalent or bivalent COVID-19 vaccine:** 1 dose of any updated (2023–2024 Formula) of COVID-19 vaccine at least 8 weeks after the most recent dose.

There is no preferential recommendation for the use of one COVID-19 vaccine over another when more than one recommended age-appropriate vaccine is available.

Current COVID-19 vaccine information available at www.cdc.gov/covidschedule. For information on Emergency Use Authorization (EUA) indications for COVID-19 vaccines, see www.fda.gov/emergency-preparedness-and-response/coronavirus-disease-2019-covid-19/covid-19-vaccines.

*Note: Previously vaccinated is defined as having received any Original monovalent or bivalent COVID-19 vaccine (Janssen, Moderna, Novavax, Pfizer-BioNTech) prior to the updated 2023–2024 formulation.

**Note: Persons who are moderately or severely immunocompromised have the option to receive one additional dose of updated (2023–2024 Formula) COVID-19 vaccine at least 2 months following the last recommended updated (2023–2024 Formula) COVID-19 vaccine dose. Further additional updated (2023–2024 Formula) COVID-19 vaccine dose(s) may be administered, informed by the clinical judgement of a healthcare provider and personal preference and circumstances. Any further additional doses should be administered at least 2 months after the last updated (2023–2024 Formula) COVID-19 vaccine dose.

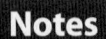 **Notes** Recommended Adult Immunization Schedule for Ages 19 Years or Older, United States, 2024

Haemophilus influenzae type b vaccination

Special situations

- **Anatomical or functional asplenia (including sickle cell disease):** 1 dose if previously did not receive Hib vaccine; if elective splenectomy, 1 dose preferably at least 14 days before splenectomy.

- **Hematopoietic stem cell transplant (HSCT):** 3-dose series 4 weeks apart starting 6–12 months after successful transplant, regardless of Hib vaccination history.

Hepatitis A vaccination

Routine vaccination

- **Any person who is not fully vaccinated and requests vaccination** (identification of risk factor not required): 2-dose series HepA (Havrix 6–12 months apart or Vaqta 6–18 months apart [minimum interval: 6 months]) or 3-dose series HepA-HepB (Twinrix at 0, 1, 6 months [minimum intervals: dose 1 to dose 2: 4 weeks / dose 2 to dose 3: 5 months])

Special situations

- **Any person who is not fully vaccinated and who is at risk for hepatitis A virus infection:** 2-dose series HepA or 3-dose series HepA-HepB as above. Risk factors for hepatitis A virus infection include:
  - **Chronic liver disease** (e.g., persons with hepatitis B, hepatitis C, cirrhosis, fatty liver disease, alcoholic liver disease, autoimmune hepatitis, alanine aminotransferase [ALT] or aspartate aminotransferase [AST] level greater than twice the upper limit of normal)
  - **HIV infection**
  - **Men who have sex with men**
  - **Injection or noninjection drug use**
  - **Persons experiencing homelessness**
  - **Work with hepatitis A virus** in research laboratory or with nonhuman primates with hepatitis A virus infection

- **Travel in countries with high or intermediate endemic hepatitis A** (HepA-HepB [Twinrix] may be administered on an accelerated schedule of 3 doses at 0, 7, and 21–30 days, followed by a booster dose at 12 months)
- **Close, personal contact with international adoptee** (e.g., household or regular babysitting) in first 60 days after arrival from country with high or intermediate endemic hepatitis A (administer dose 1 as soon as adoption is planned, at least 2 weeks before adoptee's arrival)
- **Pregnancy** if at risk for infection or severe outcome from infection during pregnancy
- **Settings for exposure,** including health care settings targeting services to injection or noninjection drug users or group homes and nonresidential day care facilities for developmentally disabled persons (individual risk factor screening not required)

Hepatitis B vaccination

Routine vaccination

- **Age 19 through 59 years:** complete a 2- or 3- or 4-dose series
  - 2-dose series only applies when 2 doses of Heplisav-B* are used at least 4 weeks apart
  - 3-dose series Engerix-B, PreHevbrio*, or Recombivax HB at 0, 1, 6 months [minimum intervals: dose 1 to dose 2: 4 weeks / dose 2 to dose 3: 8 weeks / dose 1 to dose 3: 16 weeks])
  - 3-dose series HepA-HepB (Twinrix at 0, 1, 6 months [minimum intervals: dose 1 to dose 2: 4 weeks / dose 2 to dose 3: 5 months])
  - 4-dose series HepA-HepB (Twinrix) accelerated schedule of 3 doses at 0, 7, and 21–30 days, followed by a booster dose at 12 months

*__Note:__ Heplisav-B and PreHevbrio are not recommended in pregnancy due to lack of safety data in pregnant persons.

- **Age 60 years or older without** known risk factors for hepatitis B virus infection **may** receive a HepB vaccine series.
- **Age 60 years or older with** known risk factors for hepatitis B virus infection **should** receive a HepB vaccine series.
- **Any adult age 60 years of age or older** who requests HepB vaccination should receive a HepB vaccine series.
  - **Risk factors for hepatitis B virus infection include:**
    - **Chronic liver disease** e.g., persons with hepatitis C, cirrhosis, fatty liver disease, alcoholic liver disease, autoimmune hepatitis, alanine aminotransferase (ALT) or aspartate aminotransferase (AST) level greater than twice the upper limit of normal
    - **HIV infection**
    - **Sexual exposure risk** e.g., sex partners of hepatitis B surface antigen (HBsAg)-positive persons, sexually active persons not in mutually monogamous relationships, persons seeking evaluation or treatment for a sexually transmitted infection, men who have sex with men
    - **Current or recent injection drug use**
    - **Percutaneous or mucosal risk for exposure to blood** e.g., household contacts of HBsAg-positive persons, residents and staff of facilities for developmentally disabled persons, health care and public safety personnel with reasonably anticipated risk for exposure to blood or blood-contaminated body fluids; persons on maintenance dialysis (including in-center or home hemodialysis and peritoneal dialysis), persons who are predialysis, and patients with diabetes*
    - **Incarceration**
    - **Travel in countries with high or intermediate endemic hepatitis B**

*__Age 60 years or older with diabetes:__ Based on shared clinical decision making, 2-, 3-, or 4-dose series as above.

Notes Recommended Adult Immunization Schedule for Ages 19 Years or Older, United States, 2024

Special situations

- **Patients on dialysis:** complete a 3- or 4-dose series
  - 3-dose series Recombivax HB at 0, 1, 6 months (Note: Use Dialysis Formulation 1 mL = 40 mcg)
  - 4-dose series Engerix-B at 0, 1, 2, and 6 months (Note: Use 2 mL dose instead of the normal adult dose of 1 mL)

Human papillomavirus vaccination

Routine vaccination

- **All persons up through age 26 years:** 2- or 3-dose series depending on age at initial vaccination or condition
  - **Age 9–14 years at initial vaccination and received 1 dose or 2 doses less than 5 months apart:** 1 additional dose
  - **Age 9–14 years at initial vaccination and received 2 doses at least 5 months apart:** HPV vaccination series complete, no additional dose needed
  - **Age 15 years or older at initial vaccination:** 3-dose series at 0, 1–2 months, 6 months (minimum intervals: dose 1 to dose 2: 4 weeks / dose 2 to dose 3: 12 weeks / dose 1 to dose 3: 5 months; repeat dose if administered too soon)
- No additional dose recommended when any HPV vaccine series of any valency has been completed using the recommended dosing intervals.

Shared clinical decision-making

- **Adults age 27–45 years:** Based on shared clinical decision-making, complete a 2-dose series (if initiated age 9-14 years) or 3-dose series (if initiated ≥15 years)

For additional information on shared clinical decision-making for HPV; see www.cdc.gov/vaccines/hcp/admin/downloads/isd-job-aid-scdm-hpv-shared-clinical-decision-making-hpv.pdf

Special situations

- **Age ranges recommended above for routine and catch-up vaccination or shared clinical decision-making also apply in special situations**
  - **Immunocompromising conditions, including HIV infection:** 3-dose series, even for those who initiate vaccination at age 9 through 14 years.
  - **Pregnancy:** Pregnancy testing is not needed before vaccination. HPV vaccination is not recommended until after pregnancy. No intervention needed if inadvertently vaccinated while pregnant.

Influenza vaccination

Routine vaccination

- **Age 19 years or older:** 1 dose any influenza vaccine appropriate for age and health status annually.
  - **Age 65 years or older:** Any one of quadrivalent high-dose inactivated influenza vaccine (HD-IIV4), quadrivalent recombinant influenza vaccine (RIV4), or quadrivalent adjuvanted inactivated influenza vaccine (aIIV4) is preferred. If none of these three vaccines are available, then any other age-appropriate influenza vaccine should be used.
- For the 2023–2024 season, see www.cdc.gov/mmwr/volumes/72/rr/rr7202a1.htm
- For the 2024–2025 season, see the 2024–2025 ACIP influenza vaccine recommendations.

Special situations

- **Close contacts (e.g., caregivers, healthcare workers) of severely immunosuppressed persons who require a protected environment:** should not receive LAIV4. If LAIV4 is given, they should avoid contact with/caring for such immunosuppressed persons for 7 days after vaccination.

Note: Persons with an egg allergy can receive any influenza vaccine (egg-based and non-egg based) appropriate for age and health status.

Measles, mumps, and rubella vaccination

Routine vaccination

- **No evidence of immunity to measles, mumps, or rubella:** 1 dose
  - **Evidence of immunity:** Born before 1957 (except for health care personnel, see below), documentation of receipt of MMR vaccine, laboratory evidence of immunity or disease (diagnosis of disease without laboratory confirmation is not evidence of immunity)

Special situations

- **Pregnancy with no evidence of immunity to rubella:** MMR contraindicated during pregnancy; after pregnancy (before discharge from health care facility), 1 dose
- **Nonpregnant persons of childbearing age with no evidence of immunity to rubella:** 1 dose
- **HIV infection with CD4 percentages ≥15% and CD4 count ≥200 cells/mm³ for at least 6 months and no evidence of immunity to measles, mumps, or rubella:** 2-dose series at least 4 weeks apart; MMR contraindicated for HIV infection with CD4 percentage <15% or CD4 count <200 cells/mm³
- **Severe immunocompromising conditions:** MMR contraindicated
- **Students in postsecondary educational institutions, international travelers, and household or close, personal contacts of immunocompromised persons with no evidence of immunity to measles, mumps, or rubella:** 2-dose series at least 4 weeks apart if previously did not receive any doses of MMR or 1 dose if previously received 1 dose MMR
- **In mumps outbreak settings,** for information about additional doses of MMR (including 3rd dose of MMR), see www.cdc.gov/mmwr/volumes/67/wr/mm6701a7.htm

Notes Recommended Adult Immunization Schedule for Ages 19 Years or Older, United States, 2024

- **Health care personnel:**
  - **Born before 1957 with no evidence of immunity to measles, mumps, or rubella:** Consider 2-dose series at least 4 weeks apart for protection against measles or mumps or 1 dose for protection against rubella
  - **Born in 1957 or later with no evidence of immunity to measles, mumps, or rubella:** 2-dose series at least 4 weeks apart for protection against measles or mumps or at least 1 dose for protection against rubella

Meningococcal vaccination

Special situations for MenACWY

- **Anatomical or functional asplenia (including sickle cell disease), HIV infection, persistent complement component deficiency, complement inhibitor (e.g., eculizumab, ravulizumab) use:** 2-dose series MenACWY (Menveo or MenQuadfi) at least 8 weeks apart and revaccinate every 5 years if risk remains

- **Travel in countries with hyperendemic or epidemic meningococcal disease, or microbiologists routinely exposed to *Neisseria meningitidis*:** 1 dose MenACWY (Menveo or MenQuadfi) and revaccinate every 5 years if risk remains

- **First-year college students who live in residential housing (if not previously vaccinated at age 16 years or older) or military recruits:** 1 dose MenACWY (Menveo or MenQuadfi)

- For MenACWY **booster dose recommendations** for groups listed under "Special situations" and in an outbreak setting (e.g., in community or organizational settings, or among men who have sex with men) and additional meningococcal vaccination information, see www.cdc.gov/mmwr/volumes/69/rr/rr6909a1.htm

Shared clinical decision-making for MenB

- **Adolescents and young adults age 16–23 years (age 16–18 years preferred) not at increased risk for meningococcal disease:** Based on shared clinical decision-making, 2-dose series MenB-4C (Bexsero) at least 1 month apart or 2-dose series MenB-FHbp (Trumenba) at 0, 6 months (if dose 2 was administered less than 6 months after dose 1, administer dose 3 at least 4 months after dose 2); MenB-4C and MenB-FHbp are not interchangeable (use same product for all doses in series).

For additional information on shared clinical decision-making for MenB, see www.cdc.gov/vaccines/hcp/admin/downloads/isd-job-aid-scdm-mening-b-shared-clinical-decision-making.pdf

Special situations for MenB

- **Anatomical or functional asplenia (including sickle cell disease), persistent complement component deficiency, complement inhibitor (e.g., eculizumab, ravulizumab) use, or microbiologists routinely exposed to *Neisseria meningitidis*:**
2-dose primary series MenB-4C (Bexsero) at least 1 month apart or 3-dose primary series MenB-FHbp (Trumenba) at 0, 1–2, 6 months (if dose 2 was administered at least 6 months after dose 1, dose 3 not needed; if dose 3 is administered earlier than 4 months after dose 2, a fourth dose should be administered at least 4 months after dose 3); MenB-4C and MenB-FHbp are not interchangeable (use same product for all doses in series); 1 dose MenB booster 1 year after primary series and revaccinate every 2–3 years if risk remains.

- **Pregnancy:** Delay MenB until after pregnancy unless at increased risk and vaccination benefits outweigh potential risks.

- For MenB **booster dose recommendations** for groups listed under "Special situations" and in an outbreak setting (e.g., in community or organizational settings and among men who have sex with men) and additional meningococcal vaccination information, see www.cdc.gov/mmwr/volumes/69/rr/rr6909a1.htm

Note: MenB vaccines may be administered simultaneously with MenACWY vaccines if indicated, but at a different anatomic site, if feasible.

Adults may receive a single dose of Penbraya as an alternative to separate administration of MenACWY and MenB when both vaccines would be given on the same clinic day. For adults not at increased risk, if Penbraya is used for dose 1 MenB, MenB-FHbp (Trumenba) should be administered for dose 2 MenB. For adults at increased risk of meningococcal disease, Penbraya may be used for additional MenACWY and MenB doses (including booster doses) if both would be given on the same clinic day **and** at least 6 months have elapsed since most recent Penbraya dose.

Mpox vaccination

Special situations

- **Any person at risk for Mpox infection:** 2-dose series, 28 days apart.

  Risk factors for Mpox infection include:
  - Persons who are gay, bisexual, and other MSM, transgender or nonbinary people who in the past 6 months have had:
    - A new diagnosis of at least 1 sexually transmitted disease
    - More than 1 sex partner
    - Sex at a commercial sex venue
    - Sex in association with a large public event in a geographic area where Mpox transmission is occurring
  - Persons who are sexual partners of the persons described above
  - Persons who anticipate experiencing any of the situations described above

Notes — Recommended Adult Immunization Schedule for Ages 19 Years or Older, United States, 2024

- **Pregnancy:** There is currently no ACIP recommendation for Jynneos use in pregnancy due to lack of safety data in pregnant persons. Pregnant persons with any risk factor described above may receive Jynneos.

- **Healthcare personnel:** Except in rare circumstances (e.g. no available personal protective equipment), healthcare personnel who do not have any of the sexual risk factors described above should not receive Jynneos.

  For detailed information, see: www.cdc.gov/vaccines/acip/meetings/downloads/slides-2023-10-25-26/04-MPOX-Rao-508.pdf

Pneumococcal vaccination

Routine vaccination

- **Age 65 years or older who have:**
  - **Not previously received a dose of PCV13, PCV15, or PCV20 or whose previous vaccination history is unknown:** 1 dose PCV15 OR 1 dose PCV20.
    - If PCV15 is used, administer 1 dose PPSV23 at least 1 year after the PCV15 dose (may use minimum interval of 8 weeks for adults with an immunocompromising condition,* cochlear implant, or cerebrospinal fluid leak).
  - **Previously received only PCV7:** follow the recommendation above.
  - **Previously received only PCV13:** 1 dose PCV20 OR 1 dose PPSV23.
    - If PCV20 is selected, administer at least 1 year after the last PCV13 dose.
    - If PPSV23 is selected, administer at least 1 year after the last PCV13 dose (may use minimum interval of 8 weeks for adults with an immunocompromising condition,* cochlear implant, or cerebrospinal fluid leak).
  - **Previously received only PPSV23:** 1 dose PCV15 OR 1 dose PCV20. Administer either PCV15 or PCV20 at least 1 year after the last PPSV23 dose.
    - If PCV15 is used, no additional PPSV23 doses are recommended.

- **Previously received both PCV13 and PPSV23 but NO PPSV23 was received at age 65 years or older:** 1 dose PCV20 OR 1 dose PPSV23.
  - If PCV20 is selected, administer at least 5 years after the last pneumococcal vaccine dose.
  - If PPSV23 is selected, see dosing schedule at www.cdc.gov/vaccines/vpd/pneumo/downloads/pneumo-vaccine-timing.pdf.

- **Previously received both PCV13 and PPSV23, AND PPSV23 was received at age 65 years or older:** Based on shared clinical decision-making, 1 dose of PCV20 at least 5 years after the last pneumococcal vaccine dose.

- For guidance on determining which pneumococcal vaccines a patient needs and when, please refer to the mobile app, which can be downloaded here: www.cdc.gov/vaccines/vpd/pneumo/hcp/pneumoapp.html.

Special situations

- **Age 19–64 years with certain underlying medical conditions or other risk factors** who have:
  - **Not previously received a PCV13, PCV15, or PCV20 or whose previous vaccination history is unknown:** 1 dose PCV15 OR 1 dose PCV20.
    - If PCV15 is used, administer 1 dose PPSV23 at least 1 year after the PCV15 dose (may use minimum interval of 8 weeks for adults with an immunocompromising condition,* cochlear implant, or cerebrospinal fluid leak).
  - **Previously received only PCV7:** follow the recommendation above.
  - **Previously received only PCV13:** 1 dose PCV20 OR 1 dose PPSV23.
    - If PCV20 is selected, administer at least 1 year after the PCV13 dose.
    - If PPSV23 is selected, see dosing schedule at www.cdc.gov/vaccines/vpd/pneumo/downloads/pneumo-vaccine-timing.pdf
  - **Previously received only PPSV23:** 1 dose PCV15 OR 1 dose PCV20. Administer either PCV15 or PCV20 at least 1 year after the last PPSV23 dose.

  - If PCV15 is used, no additional PPSV23 doses are recommended.
- **Previously received PCV13 and 1 dose of PPSV23:** 1 dose PCV20 OR 1 dose PPSV23.
  - If PCV20 is selected, administer at least 5 years after the last pneumococcal vaccine dose.
  - If PPSV23 is selected, see dosing schedule at www.cdc.gov/vaccines/vpd/pneumo/downloads/pneumo-vaccine-timing.pdf

- For guidance on determining which pneumococcal vaccines a patient needs and when, please refer to the mobile app which can be downloaded here: www.cdc.gov/vaccines/vpd/pneumo/hcp/pneumoapp.html

*Note: Immunocompromising conditions include chronic renal failure, nephrotic syndrome, immunodeficiencies, iatrogenic immunosuppression, generalized malignancy, HIV infection, Hodgkin disease, leukemia, lymphoma, multiple myeloma, solid organ transplant, congenital or acquired asplenia, or sickle cell disease or other hemoglobinopathies.

**Note: Underlying medical conditions or other risk factors include alcoholism, chronic heart/liver/lung disease, chronic renal failure, cigarette smoking, cochlear implant, congenital or acquired asplenia, CSF leak, diabetes mellitus, generalized malignancy, HIV infection, Hodgkin disease, immunodeficiencies, iatrogenic immunosuppression, leukemia, lymphoma, multiple myeloma, nephrotic syndrome, solid organ transplant, or sickle cell disease or other hemoglobinopathies.

Poliovirus vaccination

Routine vaccination

- **Adults known or suspected to be unvaccinated or incompletely vaccinated:** administer remaining doses (1, 2, or 3 IPV doses) to complete a 3-dose primary series.* Unless there are specific reasons to believe they were not vaccinated, most adults who were born and raised in the United States can assume they were vaccinated against polio as children.

Notes Recommended Adult Immunization Schedule for Ages 19 Years or Older, United States, 2024

Special situations

- **Adults at increased risk of exposure to poliovirus who completed primary series*:** may administer one lifetime IPV booster

*Note: Complete primary series consists of at least 3 doses of IPV or trivalent oral poliovirus vaccine (tOPV) in any combination.

For detailed information, see: www.cdc.gov/vaccines/vpd/polio/hcp/recommendations.html

Respiratory syncytial virus vaccination

Routine vaccination

- **Pregnant at 32 weeks 0 days through 36 weeks and 6 days gestation from September through January in most of the continental United States*:** 1 dose RSV vaccine (Abrysvo™). Administer RSV vaccine regardless of previous RSV infection.
  - Either maternal RSV vaccination or infant immunization with nirsevimab (RSV monoclonal antibody) is recommended to prevent respiratory syncytial virus lower respiratory tract infection in infants.

- **All other pregnant persons:** RSV vaccine not recommended

There is currently no ACIP recommendation for RSV vaccination in subsequent pregnancies. No data are available to inform whether additional doses are needed in later pregnancies.

Special situations

- **Age 60 years or older:** Based on shared clinical decision-making, 1 dose RSV vaccine (Arexvy® or Abrysvo™). Persons most likely to benefit from vaccination are those considered to be at increased risk for severe RSV disease.** For additional information on shared clinical decision-making for RSV in older adults, see www.cdc.gov/vaccines/vpd/rsv/downloads/provider-job-aid-for-older-adults-508.pdf

For further guidance, see www.cdc.gov/mmwr/volumes/72/wr/mm7229a4.htm

*Note: Providers in jurisdictions with RSV seasonality that differs from most of the continental United States (e.g., Alaska, jurisdiction with tropical climate) should follow guidance from public health authorities (e.g., CDC, health departments) or regional medical centers on timing of administration based on local RSV seasonality. Refer to the 2024 Child and Adolescent Immunization Schedule for considerations regarding nirsevimab administration to infants.

**Note: Adults age 60 years or older who are at increased risk for severe RSV disease include those with chronic medical conditions such as lung diseases (e.g., chronic obstructive pulmonary disease, asthma), cardiovascular diseases (e.g., congestive heart failure, coronary artery disease), neurologic or neuromuscular conditions, kidney disorders, liver disorders, hematologic disorders, diabetes mellitus, and moderate or severe immune compromise (either attributable to a medical condition or receipt of immunosuppressive medications or treatment); those who are considered to be frail; those of advanced age; those who reside in nursing homes or other long-term care facilities; and those with other underlying medical conditions or factors that a health care provider determines might increase the risk of severe respiratory disease.

Tetanus, diphtheria, and pertussis vaccination

Routine vaccination

- **Previously did not receive Tdap at or after age 11 years*:** 1 dose Tdap, then Td or Tdap every 10 years

Special situations

- **Previously did not receive primary vaccination series for tetanus, diphtheria, or pertussis:** 1 dose Tdap followed by 1 dose Td or Tdap at least 4 weeks later, and a third dose of Td or Tdap 6–12 months later (Tdap is preferred as first dose and can be substituted for any Td dose), Td or Tdap every 10 years thereafter.
- **Pregnancy:** 1 dose Tdap during each pregnancy, preferably in early part of gestational weeks 27–36.

- **Wound management:** Persons with 3 or more doses of tetanus-toxoid-containing vaccine: For clean and minor wounds, administer Tdap or Td if more than 10 years since last dose of tetanus-toxoid-containing vaccine; for all other wounds, administer Tdap or Td if more than 5 years since last dose of tetanus-toxoid-containing vaccine. Tdap is preferred for persons who have not previously received Tdap or whose Tdap history is unknown. If a tetanus-toxoid-containing vaccine is indicated for a pregnant woman, use Tdap. For detailed information, see www.cdc.gov/mmwr/volumes/69/wr/mm6903a5.htm

*Note: Tdap administered at age 10 years may be counted as the adolescent dose recommended at age 11–12 years

Varicella vaccination

Routine vaccination

- **No evidence of immunity to varicella:** 2-dose series 4–8 weeks apart if previously did not receive varicella-containing vaccine (VAR or MMRV [measles-mumps-rubella-varicella vaccine] for children); if previously received 1 dose varicella-containing vaccine, 1 dose at least 4 weeks after first dose.
  - **Evidence of immunity:** U.S.-born before 1980 (except for pregnant persons and health care personnel [see below]), documentation of 2 doses varicella-containing vaccine at least 4 weeks apart, diagnosis or verification of history of varicella or herpes zoster by a health care provider, laboratory evidence of immunity or disease.

Special situations

- **Pregnancy with no evidence of immunity to varicella:** VAR contraindicated during pregnancy; after pregnancy (before discharge from health care facility), 1 dose if previously received 1 dose varicella-containing vaccine or dose 1 of 2-dose series (dose 2: 4–8 weeks later) if previously did not receive any varicella-containing vaccine, regardless of whether U.S.-born before 1980.

Notes   Recommended Adult Immunization Schedule for Ages 19 Years or Older, United States, 2024

- **Health care personnel with no evidence of immunity to varicella:** 1 dose if previously received 1 dose varicella-containing vaccine; 2-dose series 4–8 weeks apart if previously did not receive any varicella-containing vaccine, regardless of whether U.S.-born before 1980.

- **HIV infection with CD4 percentages ≥15% and CD4 count ≥200 cells/mm³ with no evidence of immunity:** Vaccination may be considered (2 doses 3 months apart); VAR contraindicated for HIV infection with CD4 percentage <15% or CD4 count <200 cells/mm³

- **Severe immunocompromising conditions:** VAR contraindicated.

Zoster vaccination

Routine vaccination

- **Age 50 years or older*:** 2-dose series recombinant zoster vaccine (RZV, Shingrix) 2–6 months apart (minimum interval: 4 weeks; repeat dose if administered too soon), regardless of previous herpes zoster or history of zoster vaccine live (ZVL, Zostavax) vaccination.

*Note: Serologic evidence of prior varicella is not necessary for zoster vaccination. However, if serologic evidence of varicella susceptibility becomes available, providers should follow ACIP guidelines for varicella vaccination first. RZV is not indicated for the prevention of varicella, and there are limited data on the use of RZV in persons without a history of varicella or varicella vaccination.

Special situations

- **Pregnancy:** There is currently no ACIP recommendation for RZV use in pregnancy. Consider delaying RZV until after pregnancy.

- **Immunocompromising conditions (including persons with HIV regardless of CD4 count)**:** 2-dose series recombinant zoster vaccine (RZV, Shingrix) 2–6 months apart (minimum interval: 4 weeks; repeat dose if administered too soon). For detailed information, see www.cdc.gov/shingles/vaccination/immunocompromised-adults.html

**Note: If there is no documented history of varicella, varicella vaccination, or herpes zoster, providers should refer to the clinical considerations for use of RZV in immunocompromised adults aged ≥19 years and the ACIP varicella vaccine recommendations for further guidance: www.cdc.gov/mmwr/volumes/71/wr/mm7103a2.htm

Appendix — Recommended Adult Immunization Schedule for Ages 19 Years or Older, United States, 2024

Contraindications and Precautions to Commonly Used Vaccines

Adapted from Table 4-1 in Advisory Committee on Immunization Practices (ACIP) General Best Practice Guidelines for Immunization: Contraindication and Precautions, Prevention and Control of Seasonal Influenza with Vaccines: Recommendations of the Advisory Committee on Immunization Practices—United States, 2023–24 Influenza Season | MMWR (cdc.gov), Contraindications and Precautions for COVID-19 Vaccination, **and** Contraindications and Precautions for Jynneos Vaccination

Vaccines and Other Immunizing Agents	Contraindicated or Not Recommended[1]	Precautions[2]
COVID-19 mRNA vaccines [Pfizer-BioNTech, Moderna]	• Severe allergic reaction (e.g., anaphylaxis) after a previous dose or to a component of an mRNA COVID-19 vaccine[4]	• Diagnosed non-severe allergy (e.g., urticaria beyond the injection site) to a component of an mRNA COVID-19 vaccine[4]; or non-severe, immediate (onset less than 4 hours) allergic reaction after administration of a previous dose of an mRNA COVID-19 vaccine • Myocarditis or pericarditis within 3 weeks after a dose of any COVID-19 vaccine • Multisystem inflammatory syndrome in children (MIS-C) or multisystem inflammatory syndrome in adults (MIS-A) • Moderate or severe acute illness, with or without fever
COVID-19 protein subunit vaccine [Novavax]	• Severe allergic reaction (e.g., anaphylaxis) after a previous dose or to a component of a Novavax COVID-19 vaccine[4]	• Diagnosed non-severe allergy (e.g., urticaria beyond the injection site) to a component of Novavax COVID-19 vaccine[4]; or non-severe, immediate (onset less than 4 hours) allergic reaction after administration of a previous dose of a Novavax COVID-19 vaccine • Myocarditis or pericarditis within 3 weeks after a dose of any COVID-19 vaccine • Multisystem inflammatory syndrome in children (MIS-C) or multisystem inflammatory syndrome in adults (MIS-A) • Moderate or severe acute illness, with or without fever
Influenza, egg-based, inactivated injectable (IIV4)	• Severe allergic reaction (e.g., anaphylaxis) after previous dose of any influenza vaccine (i.e., any egg-based IIV, ccIIV, RIV, or LAIV of any valency) • Severe allergic reaction (e.g., anaphylaxis) to any vaccine component[3] (excluding egg)	• Guillain-Barré syndrome (GBS) within 6 weeks after a previous dose of any type of influenza vaccine • Moderate or severe acute illness with or without fever
Influenza, cell culture-based inactivated injectable (ccIIV4) [Flucelvax Quadrivalent]	• Severe allergic reaction (e.g., anaphylaxis) to any ccIIV of any valency, or to any component[3] of ccIIV4	• Guillain-Barré syndrome (GBS) within 6 weeks after a previous dose of any type of influenza vaccine • Persons with a history of severe allergic reaction (e.g., anaphylaxis) after a previous dose of any egg-based IIV, RIV, or LAIV of any valency. If using ccIIV4, administer in medical setting under supervision of health care provider who can recognize and manage severe allergic reactions. May consult an allergist. • Moderate or severe acute illness with or without fever
Influenza, recombinant injectable (RIV4) [Flublok Quadrivalent]	• Severe allergic reaction (e.g., anaphylaxis) to any RIV of any valency, or to any component[3] of RIV4	• Guillain-Barré syndrome (GBS) within 6 weeks after a previous dose of any type of influenza vaccine • Persons with a history of severe allergic reaction (e.g., anaphylaxis) after a previous dose of any egg-based IIV, ccIIV, or LAIV of any valency. If using RIV4, administer in medical setting under supervision of health care provider who can recognize and manage severe allergic reactions. May consult an allergist. • Moderate or severe acute illness with or without fever
Influenza, live attenuated (LAIV4) [Flumist Quadrivalent]	• Severe allergic reaction (e.g., anaphylaxis) after previous dose of any influenza vaccine (i.e., any egg-based IIV, ccIIV, RIV, or LAIV of any valency) • Severe allergic reaction (e.g., anaphylaxis) to any vaccine component[3] (excluding egg) • Anatomic or functional asplenia • Immunocompromised due to any cause including, but not limited to, medications and HIV infection • Close contacts or caregivers of severely immunosuppressed persons who require a protected environment • Pregnancy • Cochlear implant • Active communication between the cerebrospinal fluid (CSF) and the oropharynx, nasopharynx, nose, ear, or any other cranial CSF leak • Received influenza antiviral medications oseltamivir or zanamivir within the previous 48 hours, peramivir within the previous 5 days, or baloxavir within the previous 17 days.	• Guillain-Barré syndrome (GBS) within 6 weeks after a previous dose of any type of influenza vaccine • Asthma in persons aged 5 years or older • Persons with underlying medical conditions (other than those listed under contraindications) that might predispose to complications after wild-type influenza virus infection [e.g., chronic pulmonary, cardiovascular (except isolated hypertension), renal, hepatic, neurologic, hematologic, or metabolic disorders (including diabetes mellitus)] • Moderate or severe acute illness with or without fever

1. When a contraindication is present, a vaccine should NOT be administered. Kroger A, Bahta L, Hunter P. ACIP General Best Practice Guidelines for Immunization.
2. When a precaution is present, vaccination should generally be deferred but might be indicated if the benefit of protection from the vaccine outweighs the risk for an adverse reaction. Kroger A, Bahta L, Hunter P. ACIP General Best Practice Guidelines for Immunization.
3. Vaccination providers should check FDA-approved prescribing information for the most complete and updated information, including contraindications, warnings, and precautions. See Package inserts for U.S.-licensed vaccines.
4. See package inserts and FDA EUA fact sheets for a full list of vaccine ingredients. mRNA COVID-19 vaccines contain polyethylene glycol (PEG).

Appendix — Recommended Adult Immunization Schedule for Ages 19 Years or Older, United States, 2024

Vaccine	Contraindicated or Not Recommended[1]	Precautions[2]
Haemophilus influenzae type b (Hib)	• Severe allergic reaction (e.g., anaphylaxis) after a previous dose or to a vaccine component[3]	• Moderate or severe acute illness with or without fever
Hepatitis A (HepA)	• Severe allergic reaction (e.g., anaphylaxis) after a previous dose or to a vaccine component[3] including neomycin	• Moderate or severe acute illness with or without fever
Hepatitis B (HepB)	• Severe allergic reaction (e.g., anaphylaxis) after a previous dose or to a vaccine component[3] including yeast • *Pregnancy: Heplisav-B and PreHevbrio are not recommended due to lack of safety data in pregnant persons. Use other hepatitis B vaccines if HepB is indicated[4]*	• Moderate or severe acute illness with or without fever
Hepatitis A-Hepatitis B vaccine (HepA-HepB) [Twinrix]	• Severe allergic reaction (e.g., anaphylaxis) after a previous dose or to a vaccine component[3] including neomycin and yeast	• Moderate or severe acute illness with or without fever
Human papillomavirus (HPV)	• Severe allergic reaction (e.g., anaphylaxis) after a previous dose or to a vaccine component[3] • *Pregnancy: HPV vaccination not recommended*	• Moderate or severe acute illness with or without fever
Measles, mumps, rubella (MMR)	• Severe allergic reaction (e.g., anaphylaxis) after a previous dose or to a vaccine component[3] • Severe immunodeficiency (e.g., hematologic and solid tumors, receipt of chemotherapy, congenital immunodeficiency, long-term immunosuppressive therapy or patients with HIV infection who are severely immunocompromised) • Pregnancy • Family history of altered immunocompetence, unless verified clinically or by laboratory testing as immunocompetent	• Recent (≤11 months) receipt of antibody-containing blood product (specific interval depends on product) • History of thrombocytopenia or thrombocytopenic purpura • Need for tuberculin skin testing or interferon-gamma release assay (IGRA) testing • Moderate or severe acute illness with or without fever
Meningococcal ACWY (MenACWY) (MenACWY-CRM) [Menveo] (MenACWY-TT) [MenQuadfi]	• Severe allergic reaction (e.g., anaphylaxis) after a previous dose or to a vaccine component[3] • For MenACWY-CRM only: severe allergic reaction to any diphtheria toxoid–or CRM197–containing vaccine • For MenACWY-TT only: severe allergic reaction to a tetanus toxoid-containing vaccine	• Moderate or severe acute illness with or without fever
Meningococcal B (MenB) MenB-4C [Bexsero] MenB-FHbp [Trumenba]	• Severe allergic reaction (e.g., anaphylaxis) after a previous dose or to a vaccine component[3]	• Pregnancy • For MenB-4C only: Latex sensitivity • Moderate or severe acute illness with or without fever
Meningococcal ABCWY (MenACWY-TT/MenB-FHbp) [Penbraya]	• Severe allergic reaction (e.g., anaphylaxis) after a previous dose or to a vaccine component[3] • Severe allergic reaction to a tetanus toxoid-containing vaccine	• Moderate or severe acute illness, with or without fever
Mpox [Jynneos]	• Severe allergic reaction (e.g., anaphylaxis) after a previous dose or to a vaccine component[3]	• Moderate or severe acute illness, with or without fever
Pneumococcal conjugate (PCV15, PCV20)	• Severe allergic reaction (e.g., anaphylaxis) after a previous dose or to a vaccine component[3] • Severe allergic reaction (e.g., anaphylaxis) to any diphtheria-toxoid–containing vaccine or to its vaccine component[3]	• Moderate or severe acute illness with or without fever
Pneumococcal polysaccharide (PPSV23)	• Severe allergic reaction (e.g., anaphylaxis) after a previous dose or to a vaccine component[3]	• Moderate or severe acute illness with or without fever
Poliovirus vaccine, inactivated (IPV)	• Severe allergic reaction (e.g., anaphylaxis) after a previous dose or to a vaccine component[3]	• Pregnancy • Moderate or severe acute illness with or without fever
Respiratory syncytial virus vaccine (RSV)	• Severe allergic reaction (e.g., anaphylaxis) to a vaccine component	• Moderate or severe acute illness with or without fever
Tetanus, diphtheria, and acellular pertussis (Tdap) Tetanus, diphtheria (Td)	• Severe allergic reaction (e.g., anaphylaxis) after a previous dose or to a vaccine component[3] • For Tdap only: Encephalopathy (e.g., coma, decreased level of consciousness, prolonged seizures), not attributable to another identifiable cause, within 7 days of administration of previous dose of DTP, DTaP, or Tdap	• Guillain-Barré syndrome (GBS) within 6 weeks after a previous dose of tetanus-toxoid–containing vaccine • History of Arthus-type hypersensitivity reactions after a previous dose of diphtheria-toxoid– containing or tetanus-toxoid–containing vaccine; defer vaccination until at least 10 years have elapsed since the last tetanus-toxoid–containing vaccine • Moderate or severe acute illness with or without fever • For Tdap only: Progressive or unstable neurological disorder, uncontrolled seizures, or progressive encephalopathy until a treatment regimen has been established and the condition has stabilized
Varicella (VAR)	• Severe allergic reaction (e.g., anaphylaxis) after a previous dose or to a vaccine component[3] • Severe immunodeficiency (e.g., hematologic and solid tumors, receipt of chemotherapy, congenital immunodeficiency, long-term immunosuppressive therapy or patients with HIV infection who are severely immunocompromised) • Pregnancy • Family history of altered immunocompetence, unless verified clinically or by laboratory testing as immunocompetent	• Recent (≤11 months) receipt of antibody-containing blood product (specific interval depends on product) • Receipt of specific antiviral drugs (acyclovir, famciclovir, or valacyclovir) 24 hours before vaccination (avoid use of these antiviral drugs for 14 days after vaccination) • Use of aspirin or aspirin-containing products • Moderate or severe acute illness with or without fever
Zoster recombinant vaccine (RZV)	• Severe allergic reaction (e.g., anaphylaxis) after a previous dose or to a vaccine component[3]	• Moderate or severe acute illness with or without fever • Current herpes zoster infection

1. When a contraindication is present, a vaccine should NOT be administered. Kroger A, Bahta L, Hunter P. ACIP General Best Practice Guidelines for Immunization. www.cdc.gov/vaccines/hcp/acip-recs/general-recs/contraindications.html
2. When a precaution is present, vaccination should generally be deferred but might be indicated if the benefit of protection from the vaccine outweighs the risk for an adverse reaction. Kroger A, Bahta L, Hunter P. ACIP General Best Practice Guidelines for Immunization. www.cdc.gov/vaccines/hcp/acip-recs/general-recs/contraindications.html
3. Vaccination providers should check FDA-approved prescribing information for the most complete and updated information, including contraindications, warnings, and precautions. Package inserts for U.S.-licensed vaccines are available at www.fda.gov/vaccines-blood-biologics/approved-products/vaccines-licensed-use-united-states.
4. For information on the pregnancy exposure registries for persons who were inadvertently vaccinated with Heplisav-B or PreHevbrio while pregnant, please visit heplisavbpregnancyregistry.com/ or www.prehevbrio.com/#safety.

Addendum — Recommended Adult Immunization Schedule for Ages 19 Years or Older, United States, 2024

In addition to the recommendations presented in the previous sections of this immunization schedule, ACIP has approved the following recommendations by majority vote since October 26, 2023. The following recommendations have been adopted by the CDC Director and are now official. Links are provided if these recommendations have been published in *Morbidity and Mortality Weekly Report (MMWR)*.

Vaccines	Recommendations	Effective Date of Recommendation*
No new vaccines or vaccine recommendations to report		

*The effective date is the date when the CDC director adopted the recommendation and when the ACIP recommendation became official.

The Advisory Committee on Immunization Practices (ACIP) recommendations and package inserts for vaccines provide information on contraindications and precautions related to vaccines. Contraindications are conditions that increase chances of a serious adverse reaction in vaccine recipients, and the vaccine should not be administered when a contraindication is present. Precautions should be reviewed for potential risks and benefits for vaccine recipient. For a person with a severe allergy to latex, e.g., anaphylaxis, vaccines supplied in vials or syringes that contain natural rubber latex should not be administered unless the benefit of vaccination clearly outweighs the risk for a potential allergic reaction. For latex allergies other than anaphylaxis, vaccines supplied in vials or syringes that contain dry, natural rubber or natural rubber latex may be administered.

TABLE 15 Immunization and Pregnancy

Vaccine	Before Pregnancy	During Pregnancy	After Pregnancy	Type of Vaccine	Route
Hepatitis A	If at high risk for disease	If at high risk for disease	If at high risk for disease	Inactivated	IM
Hepatitis B	Yes, if at risk	Yes, if at risk	Yes, if at risk	Inactivated	IM
Human papillomavirus (HPV)	Yes, if 9-26 yr of age	No, under study	Yes, if 9-26 yr of age	Inactivated	IM
Influenza TIV	Yes	Yes	Yes	Inactivated	IM
Influenza LAIV	Yes, if <50 yr and healthy; avoid conception for 4 wk	No	Yes, if <50 yr and healthy; avoid conception for 4 wk	Live	Nasal spray
MMR	Yes, avoid conception for 4 wk	No	Yes, give immediately postpartum if susceptible to rubella	Live	SC
Meningococcal	If indicated	If indicated	If indicated		
Polysaccharide				Inactivated	SCIM
Conjugate				Inactivated	
Pneumococcal polysaccharide	If indicated	If indicated	If indicated	Inactivated	IM or SC
Tetanus/diphtheria Td	Yes, Tdap preferred	If indicated	Yes, Tdap preferred	Toxoid	IM
Tdap, one dose only	Yes, preferred	If high risk of pertussis; otherwise, Td preferred	Yes, preferred	Toxoid/inactivated	IM
Varicella	Yes, avoid conception for 4 wk	No	Yes, give immediately postpartum if susceptible	Live	SC

IM, Intramuscular; *LAIV,* live, attenuated influenza vaccine; *SC,* subcutaneous; *Tdap,* tetanus and diphtheria toxoids and acellular pertussis; *TIV,* trivalent inactivated influenza vaccine.

TABLE 16 Immunizing Agents and Immunization Schedules for Health Care Workers (HCWs)*

Generic Name	Primary Schedule and Booster(s)	Indications	Major Precautions and Contraindications	Special Considerations
Immunizing Agents Strongly Recommended for Health Care Workers				
Hepatitis B (HB) recombinant vaccine	Two doses IM 4 wk apart; third dose 5 mo after second; booster doses not necessary	**Preexposure:** HCWs at risk for exposure to blood or body fluids	Based on limited data no risk of adverse effects to developing fetuses is apparent. Pregnancy should *not* be considered a contraindication to vaccination of women. Previous anaphylactic reaction to common baker's yeast is a contraindication to vaccination	The vaccine produces neither therapeutic nor adverse effects on HB-infected persons. Prevaccination serologic screening is not indicated for persons being vaccinated because of occupational risk. HCWs who have contact with patients or blood should be tested 1-2 mo after vaccination to determine serologic response
Hepatitis B immune globulin (HBIG)	0.06 ml/kg IM as soon as possible after exposure. A second dose of HBIG should be administered 1 mo later if the HB vaccine series has not been started	**Postexposure prophylaxis:** For persons exposed to blood or body fluids containing HBsAg and who are not immune to HBV infection— 0.06 ml/kg IM as soon as possible (but no later than 7 days after exposure)		
Influenza vaccine (inactivated whole-virus and split-virus vaccines)	Annual vaccination with current vaccine Administered IM	HCWs who have contact with patients at high risk for influenza or its complications; HCWs who work in long-term care facilities; HCWs with high-risk medical conditions or who are aged ≥65 yr	History of anaphylactic hypersensitivity to egg ingestion	No evidence exists of risk to mother or fetus when the vaccine is administered to a pregnant woman with an underlying high-risk condition. Influenza vaccination is recommended during second and third trimesters of pregnancy because of increased risk for hospitalization
Measles live-virus vaccine	One dose SC; second dose at least 1 mo later	HCWs† born during or after 1957 who do not have documentation of having received two doses of live vaccine on or after the first birthday **or** a history of physician-diagnosed measles or serologic evidence of immunity. Vaccination should be considered for all HCWs who lack proof of immunity, including those born before 1957	Pregnancy; immunocompromised persons,‡ including HIV-infected persons who have evidence of severe immunosuppression; anaphylaxis after gelatin ingestion or administration of neomycin; recent administration of immune globulin	MMR is the vaccine of choice if recipients are likely to be susceptible to rubella and/or mumps as well as measles. Persons vaccinated between 1963 and 1967 with a killed measles vaccine alone, killed vaccine followed by live vaccine, or with a vaccine of unknown type should be revaccinated with two doses of live measles virus vaccine
Mumps live-virus vaccine	One dose SC; second dose at least 1 mo later	HCWs† believed to be susceptible can be vaccinated. Adults born before 1957 can be considered immune	Pregnancy; immunocompromised persons,‡ history of anaphylactic reaction after gelatin ingestion or administration of neomycin	MMR is the vaccine of choice if recipients are likely to be susceptible to measles and rubella, as well as mumps
Hepatitis A virus (HAV) vaccine	Two doses of vaccine either 6-12 mo apart (HAVRIX), or 6 mo apart (VAQTA)	Not routinely indicated for HCWs in the United States. Persons who work with HAV-infected primates or with HAV in a research laboratory setting should be vaccinated	History of anaphylactic hypersensitivity to alum or, for HAVRIX, the preservative 2-phenoxyethanol. The safety of the vaccine in pregnant women has not been determined; the risk associated with vaccination should be weighed against the risk for hepatitis A in women who may be at high risk for exposure to HAV	
Meningococcal vaccine	One dose in volume and by route specified by manufacturer; single booster for adults 19-21 yr of age if the first dose was given before age 16	Laboratory personnel and others with exposure risk	The safety of the vaccine in pregnant women has not been evaluated; it should not be administered during pregnancy unless the risk for infection is high	
Typhoid vaccine, IM, SC, and oral	IM vaccine: One 0.5-ml/dose, booster 0.5 ml every 2 yr SC vaccine: Two 0.5-ml doses, ≥4 wk apart, booster 0.5 ml SC or 0.1 ID every 3 yr if exposure continues Oral vaccine: Four doses on alternate days. The manufacturer recommends revaccination with the entire 4-dose series every 5 yr	Workers in microbiology laboratories who frequently work with *Salmonella typhi*	Severe local or systemic reaction to a previous dose. Ty21a (oral) vaccine should not be administered to immunocompromised persons† or to persons receiving antimicrobial agents	Vaccination should not be considered an alternative to the use of proper procedures when handling specimens and cultures in the laboratory

Continued

TABLE 16 Immunizing Agents and Immunization Schedules for Health Care Workers (HCWs)*—cont'd

Generic Name	Primary Schedule and Booster(s)	Indications	Major Precautions and Contraindications	Special Considerations
Vaccinia vaccine (smallpox)	One dose administered with a bifurcated needle; boosters administered every 10 yr	Laboratory workers who directly handle cultures with vaccinia, recombinant vaccinia viruses, or orthopox viruses that infect human beings	The vaccine is contraindicated in pregnancy, in persons with eczema or a history of eczema, and in immunocompromised persons[†] and their household contacts	Vaccination may be considered for HCWs who have direct contact with contaminated dressings or other infectious material from volunteers in clinical studies involving recombinant vaccinia virus
COVID-19	A person is fully vaccinated 2 wk after receiving all recommended doses in the primary series of their COVID-19 vaccination. A person is up to date with their COVID-19 vaccination if they have received all recommended doses in the primary series and boosters when eligible.			

Other Vaccine-Preventable Diseases

Generic Name	Primary Schedule and Booster(s)	Indications	Major Precautions and Contraindications	Special Considerations
Tetanus and diphtheria and pertussis (Tdap)	Two IM doses 4 wk apart or tetanus and diphtheria toxoid for adults with uncertain or incomplete primary vaccination; third dose 6-12 mo after second dose; booster every 10 yr. Substitute a one-time dose of Tdap for one of the doses of Td, either in the primary series or for the routine booster, whichever comes first	All adults	Except in the first trimester, pregnancy is not a precaution. History of a neurologic reaction or immediate hypersensitivity reaction after a previous dose. History of severe local (Arthus-type) reaction after a previous dose. Such persons should not receive further routine or emergency doses of Td for 10 yr	Tetanus prophylaxis in wound management[‡]
Pneumococcal polysaccharide vaccine (23 valent)	One dose, 0.5 ml, IM or SC; revaccination recommended for those at highest risk ≥5 yr after the first dose	Adults who are at increased risk of pneumococcal disease and its complications because of underlying health conditions; older adults, especially those age ≥65 who are healthy	The safety of vaccine in pregnant women has not been evaluated; it should not be administered during pregnancy unless the risk for infection is high. Previous recipients of any type of pneumococcal polysaccharide vaccine who are at highest risk for fatal infection or antibody loss may be revaccinated ≥5 yr after the first dose	
Rubella live-virus vaccine	One dose SC; second dose at least 1 mo later	Indicated for HCWs,[†] both men and women, who do not have documentation of having received live vaccine on or after their first birthday **or** laboratory evidence of immunity. Adults born before 1957, **except women who can become pregnant,** can be considered immune	Pregnancy; immunocompromised persons[†]; history of anaphylactic reaction after administration of neomycin	The risk for rubella vaccine-associated malformations in the offspring of women pregnant when vaccinated or who become pregnant within 3 mo after vaccination is negligible. Such women should be counseled regarding the theoretic basis of concern for the fetus. MMR is the vaccine of choice if recipients are likely to be susceptible to measles or mumps as well as rubella
Varicella-zoster live-virus vaccine	Two 0.5-ml doses SC 4-8 wk apart if ≥13 yr	Indicated for HCWs[†] who do not have either a reliable history of varicella or serologic evidence of immunity	Pregnancy, immunocompromised persons,[‡] history of anaphylactic reaction after receipt of neomycin or gelatin. Avoid salicylate use for 6 wk after vaccination	Vaccine is available from the manufacturer for certain patients with acute lymphocytic leukemia in remission. Because 71%-93% of persons without a history of varicella are immune, serologic testing before vaccination is likely to be cost effective
Varicella-zoster immune globulin (VZIG)	Persons <50 kg: 125 μg/10 kg IM; persons ≥50 kg: 625 μg[§]	Persons known or likely to be susceptible (particularly those at high risk for complications, e.g., pregnant women) who have close and prolonged exposure to a contact case or to an infectious hospital staff worker or patient		Serologic testing may help in assessing whether to administer VZIG. If use of VZIG prevents varicella disease, patient should be vaccinated subsequently

Continued

TABLE 16 Immunizing Agents and Immunization Schedules for Health Care Workers (HCWs)*—cont'd

Generic Name	Primary Schedule and Booster(s)	Indications	Major Precautions and Contraindications	Special Considerations
BCG Vaccination				
Bacille Calmette-Guérin (BCG) vaccine (TB)	One percutaneous dose of 0.3 ml; no booster dose recommended	Should be considered only for HCWs in areas where multidrug TB is prevalent, a strong likelihood of infection exists, and where comprehensive infection control precautions have failed to prevent TB transmission to HCWs	Should not be administered to immunocompromised persons,‡ pregnant women	In the United States, TB-control efforts are directed toward early identification, treatment of cases, and preventive therapy with isoniazid
Other Immunobiologics that Are or May Be Indicated for HCWs				
Immune globulin (hepatitis A)	**Postexposure**—One IM dose of 0.02 ml/kg administered ≤2 wk after exposure	Indicated for HCWs exposed to feces of infectious patients	Contraindicated in persons with IgA deficiency; do not administer within 2 wk after MMR vaccine or 3 wk after varicella vaccine. Delay administration of MMR vaccine for ≥3 mo and varicella vaccine ≥5 mo after administration of immune globulin	Administer in large muscle mass (deltoid, gluteal)

HBsAg, Hepatitis B surface antigen; *HBV,* hepatitis B virus; *HIV,* human immunodeficiency virus; *IM,* intramuscular; *MMR,* measles, mumps, rubella vaccine; *SC,* subcutaneous; *TB,* tuberculosis.

*Persons who provide health care to patients or work in institutions that provide patient care (e.g., physicians, nurses, emergency medical personnel, dental professionals and students, medical and nursing students, laboratory technicians, hospital volunteers, and administrative and support staff in health care institutions).

†All HCWs (i.e., medical or nonmedical, paid or volunteer, full time or part time, student or nonstudent, with or without patient-care responsibilities) who work in health care institutions (e.g., inpatient and outpatient, public and private) should be immune to measles, rubella, and varicella.

‡Persons immunocompromised because of immune deficiency diseases, HIV infection, leukemia, lymphoma or generalized malignancy, or immunosuppressed as a result of therapy with corticosteroids, alkylating drugs, antimetabolites, or radiation.

§Some experts recommend 125 μg/10 kg regardless of total body weight.

Modified from Centers for Disease Control and Prevention: Immunization of health-care workers: recommendations of the Advisory Committee on Immunization Practices (ACIP) and the Hospital Infection Control Practices Advisory Committee (HICPAC), *MMWR Recomm Rep* 46(RR-18):1-42, 1997.

Recommendations for Providing Sexually Transmitted Diseases Clinical Services

BOX 1 Recommendations for Obtaining a Sexual History and Conducting a Physical Examination as Part of Sexually Transmitted Diseases Care in Primary Care and Sexually Transmitted Diseases Specialty Care Settings*

STD care in primary care settings

A sexual history and risk assessment **should** be available as part of basic STD care services at the following patient visits:

Initial comprehensive or annual visit

Each visit concerning reproductive, genital, or urologic issues

A physical examination **should** be available as a basic STD care service for male and female patients with STD-related symptoms, STD-related concerns, or those at high behavioral risk for incident STDs.

A pelvic examination **should** be available as a basic STD care service.

A sexual history and risk assessment **could** be available as basic STD care services at each visit unrelated to reproductive, genital, or urologic concerns.

Anoscopy **could** be available as a basic STD care service.

STD care in STD specialty care settings

- A sexual history and risk assessment **should** be part of specialized STD care services at every visit for patients with STD-related symptoms, STD-related concerns, or concerns about preventing or achieving pregnancy.
- A physical examination **should** be available as a specialized STD care service for male and female patients with STD-related symptoms, STD-related concerns, or high behavioral risk for incident STDs.
- A pelvic examination **should** be available as a specialized STD care service.
- Colposcopy **should** be available as a specialized STD care service for female patients with abnormal Pap smears.
- Anoscopy **should** be available as a specialized STD care service.
- A high-resolution anoscopy **could** be available as a specialized STD care service for patients with abnormal anal Pap smears.

*Primary care setting is defined as a place where patients are evaluated for various health conditions. An STD specialty care setting is defined as a place where the focus is on providing patients with timely, comprehensive, confidential, and culturally sensitive STD care. STD care delivered in STD specialty care settings includes all care delivered in primary care settings.

STD, Sexually transmitted disease.

Barrow RY, Ahmed F, Bolan GA, Workowski KA: Recommendations for providing quality sexually transmitted diseases clinical services, 2020, *MMWR Recomm Rep* 68(No. RR-5):1-20, 2020. https://doi.org/10.15585/mmwr.rr6805a1.

BOX 2 Prevention Recommendations for Sexually Transmitted Diseases Care in Primary Care and Sexually Transmitted Diseases Specialty Care Settings*

STD care in primary care settings
- The following prevention services should be available as basic STD care services:
  1. On-site hepatitis B vaccination or referral
  2. On-site HPV vaccination or referral
  3. Brief single STD/HIV prevention counseling session (up to 30 min)[†]
  4. PrEP for HIV prevention and nPEP of HIV risk assessment, education, and referral or link to HIV care[†]
  5. Emergency contraceptive pills[§]
  6. Brief contraceptive counseling or referral
  7. Referral or link to HIV care, family planning services, and behavioral health services, if indicated
- The following prevention services could be available as basic STD care services:
  1. On-site condom provision[¶]
  2. On-site hepatitis A vaccination
  3. Provision of PrEP for HIV prevention[**]
  4. Provision of nPEP of HIV[††]
  5. Moderate-intensity STD behavioral counseling (≥30 min)[†]

STD care in STD specialty care settings
- The following prevention services should be available as specialized STD care services:
  1. On-site condom provision
  2. On-site hepatitis A vaccination
  3. On-site hepatitis B vaccination
  4. On-site HPV vaccination
  5. Brief single STD/HIV prevention counseling session (up to 30 min)[†]
  6. PrEP for HIV prevention and nPEP of HIV risk assessment, education, counseling, and referral or link to HIV care[†]
  7. Provision of PrEP for HIV prevention[§§]
  8. Provision of nPEP of HIV[¶¶]
  9. Brief contraceptive counseling or referral
  10. Emergency contraceptive pills[§]
  11. Referral or link to HIV care, family planning services, and behavioral health services, if indicated
- The following prevention services could be available as specialized STD care services:
  1. Moderate-intensity STD behavioral counseling (≥30 min)[†]
  2. High-intensity STD behavioral counseling (≥2 h)[†]

*Primary care setting is defined as a place where patients are evaluated for various health conditions. STD specialty care setting is defined as a place where the focus is on providing patients with timely, comprehensive, confidential, and culturally sensitive STD care. STD care delivered in STD specialty care settings includes all care delivered in primary care settings.

[†]Provided by a clinician or other appropriately trained staff.

[§]If emergency contraceptive pills are not available on site or by prescription, patients can be advised that levonorgestrel emergency contraceptive pills are available over the counter and ulipristal acetate emergency contraceptive pills are only available by prescription. Emergency contraceptive pills should be taken as soon as possible within 5 days of unprotected sex.

[¶]Providers can partner with local organizations, such as the local health department and community-based organizations, to procure condoms. In some states, prescriptions can be written for condoms. For certain settings, such as family planning clinics, condoms should be available on site.

[**]PrEP could be available by starter packs or prescription with on-site follow-up care for basic STD care. If PrEP is not provided, navigator-assisted referral for PrEP should be provided with first appointment made while the patient is on site.

[††]nPEP starter pack (3-7 days of medication) could be available on site, with either on-site follow-up care or referral for basic STD care. nPEP starter pack or complete 28-day course could be available by prescription, with either on-site follow-up care or referral, with first appointment made while the patient is on site. Provision of the complete 28-day nPEP medication supply at the initial visit rather than a starter pack of 3-7 days has been reported to increase likelihood of adherence, especially when patients find returning for multiple follow-up visits difficult. Routinely providing starter packs or the complete 28-day course requires that health care providers stock nPEP drugs in their practice setting or have an established agreement with a pharmacy to stock, package, and urgently dispense nPEP drugs with required administration instructions (https://www.cdc.gov/hiv/pdf/programresources/cdc-hiv-npep-guidelines.pdf).

[§§]PrEP should be available in starter packs or by prescription with on-site follow-up care for specialized STD care. If PrEP is not provided, navigator-assisted referral for PrEP should be provided with first appointment made while the patient is on site.

[¶¶]nPEP starter pack (3-7 days of medication) should be available on site, with either on-site follow-up care or referral to specialized STD care. nPEP complete 28-day course should be available by prescription, with either on-site follow-up care or referral, with first appointment made while the patient is on site. Provision of the complete 28-day nPEP medication supply at the initial visit rather than a starter pack of 3-7 days has been reported to increase likelihood of adherence, especially when patients find returning for multiple follow-up visits difficult.

Barrow RY et al: Recommendations for providing quality sexually transmitted diseases clinical services, 2020, *MMWR Recomm Rep* 68(No. RR-5):1-20, 2020. https://doi.org/10.15585/mmwr.rr6805a1.

BOX 3 Screening Recommendations for Sexually Transmitted Diseases Care in Primary Care and Sexually Transmitted Diseases Specialty Care Settings*

STD care in primary care settings
- Screening and assessment for the following STDs **should** be available as basic STD care services:
    1. Gonorrhea
    2. Chlamydia
    3. Syphilis
    4. Hepatitis B
    5. Hepatitis C
    6. HIV
    7. Cervical cancer
- Screening and assessment for the following STD **could** be available as a basic STD care service:
    1. Trichomoniasis

STD care in STD specialty care settings
- Screening and assessment for the following STDs **should** be available as specialized STD care services:
    1. Gonorrhea
    2. Chlamydia
    3. Syphilis
    4. Hepatitis B
    5. Hepatitis C
    6. HIV
    7. Cervical cancer
    8. Trichomoniasis
- Screening and assessment for the following STD could be available as a specialized STD care service:
    1. Anal cancer

*Primary care setting is defined as a place where patients are evaluated for various health conditions. STD specialty care setting is defined as a place where the focus is on providing patients with timely, comprehensive, confidential, and culturally sensitive STD care. STD care delivered in STD specialty care settings includes all care delivered in primary care settings.
Barrow RY et al: Recommendations for providing quality sexually transmitted diseases clinical services, 2020, *MMWR Recomm Rep* 68(No. RR-5):1-20, 2020. https://doi.org/10.15585/mmwr.rr6805a1.

BOX 4 Partner Services Recommendations for Sexually Transmitted Diseases Care in Primary Care and Sexually Transmitted Diseases Specialty Care Settings*

STD care in primary care settings
- The following partner services **should** be available as basic STD care services:
    1. Guidance regarding notification and care of sex partners
    2. EPT (where legal and where local or state jurisdictions do not prohibit by regulation)[†]
- The following partner services **could** be available as a basic STD care service:
    1. Interactive counseling for partner notification

STD care in STD specialty care settings
- The following partner services **should** be available as specialized STD care services:
    1. Guidance regarding notification and care of sex partners
    2. Interactive counseling for partner notification
    3. EPT (where legal and where local or state jurisdictions do not prohibit by regulation)[†]
    4. Health department DIS elicitation of sex partner information to identify those who might have been exposed and to identify patient follow-up needs[§]

*Primary care setting is defined as a place where patients are evaluated for various health conditions. STD specialty care setting is defined as a place where the focus is on providing patients with timely, comprehensive, confidential, and culturally sensitive STD care. STD care delivered in STD specialty care settings includes all care delivered in primary care settings.
[†]Information on legal status of EPT for each state is available at https://www.cdc.gov/std/ept/legal/default.htm.
[§]Partner services can be provided on site or by referral.
Barrow RY et al: Recommendations for providing quality sexually transmitted diseases clinical services, 2020, *MMWR Recomm Rep* 68(No. RR-5):1-20, 2020. https://doi.org/10.15585/mmwr.rr6805a1.

BOX 5 Evaluation of Sexually Transmitted Disease–Related Conditions Recommendations in Primary Care and Sexually Transmitted Diseases Specialty Care Settings*

STD care in primary care settings
- Evaluation (history and examination) for the following STD-related conditions **should** be available as basic STD care services:
    1. Genital ulcer disease
    2. Male urethritis syndrome
    3. Vaginal discharge
    4. PID
    5. Genital warts
    6. Proctitis[†]
    7. Ectoparasitic infections
    8. Pharyngitis
    9. Epididymitis
    10. Systemic or dermatologic conditions compatible with or suggestive of an STD etiology

STD care in STD specialty care settings
- Evaluation (history and examination) for the following STD-related conditions **should** be available as specialized STD care services:
    1. Genital ulcer disease
    2. Male urethritis syndrome
    3. Vaginal discharge
    4. PID
    5. Genital warts
    6. Proctitis[†]
    7. Ectoparasitic infections
    8. Pharyngitis
    9. Epididymitis
    10. Systemic or dermatologic conditions compatible with or suggestive of an STD etiology

PID, Pelvic inflammatory disease; *STD*, sexually transmitted disease.
*Primary care setting is defined as a place where patients are evaluated for various health conditions. STD specialty care setting is defined as a place where the focus is on providing patients with timely, comprehensive, confidential, and culturally sensitive STD care. STD care delivered in STD specialty care settings includes all care delivered in primary care settings.
[†]Evaluation for proctitis might include visual examination of the anus, anorectal examination with a rectal swab, digital anorectal examination, or anoscopy. For specialized STD care, high-resolution anoscopy might be included.
Barrow RY et al: Recommendations for providing quality sexually transmitted diseases clinical services, 2020, *MMWR Recomm Rep* 68(No. RR-5):1-20, 2020. https://doi.org/10.15585/mmwr.rr6805a1.

BOX 6 Laboratory Recommendations for Sexually Transmitted Diseases Care in Primary Care and Sexually Transmitted Diseases Specialty Care Settings*

STD care in primary care settings
At the time of the patient visit
- The following general services, equipment, or tests **should** be available as basic STD care services at the time of the patient visit:
  1. Thermometer
  2. pH paper
- The following general services, equipment, or tests **could** be available as basic STD services with test results available during the patient visit:
  1. Phlebotomy
  2. Test for trichomoniasis[†]
  3. Test for bacterial vaginosis[§]
  4. Test for vulvovaginal candidiasis[¶]
  5. Urine dipstick
  6. Urinalysis with microscopy
  7. Test for pregnancy
  8. Test for HIV

Clinical laboratory
- The following tests should be available through clinical laboratory as basic STD care services:
  1. Urogenital NAAT for gonorrhea and chlamydia
  2. Extragenital (pharynx and rectum) NAAT for gonorrhea and chlamydia
  3. Quantitative nontreponemal serologic test for syphilis
  4. Treponemal serologic test for syphilis
  5. HSV viral culture or PCR
  6. HSV serology
  7. Fourth-generation antigen/antibody HIV test
  8. Oncogenic HPV NAATs with Pap smear
  9. nPEP and PrEP
  10. Serologic tests for hepatitis A, B, and C
  11. Test for pregnancy
- The following tests **could** be available through clinical laboratory as basic STD care services:
  1. Gram stain, methylene blue, or gentian violet stain for urethritis
  2. Gonorrhea culture
  3. Gonorrhea antimicrobial susceptibility testing**
  4. NAAT for trichomoniasis

STD care in STD specialty care settings
At the time of the patient visit
- The following general services, equipment, or tests **should** be available as specialized STD care services at the time of the patient visit:
  1. Thermometer
  2. pH paper
  3. Phlebotomy
  4. Test for trichomoniasis[†]
  5. Test for bacterial vaginosis[§]
  6. Test for vulvovaginal candidiasis[¶]
  7. Urine dipstick
  8. Urinalysis with microscopy
  9. Test for pregnancy
  10. Gram stain, methylene blue, or gentian violet stain for urethritis
  11. On-site qualitative nontreponemal serologic test for syphilis
- The following general services, equipment, or tests **could** be available as specialized STD care services with test results available during the patient visit:
  1. Dark-field microscopy for syphilis
  2. Test for HIV

Clinical laboratory
- The following tests **should** be available through a clinical laboratory as specialized STD care services:
  1. Urogenital NAAT for gonorrhea and chlamydia
  2. Extragenital (pharynx and rectum) NAAT for gonorrhea and chlamydia
  3. Quantitative nontreponemal serologic test for syphilis
  4. Treponemal serologic test for syphilis
  5. HSV viral culture or PCR
  6. HSV serology
  7. Fourth-generation antigen/antibody HIV test
  8. Oncogenic HPV NAATs with Pap smear
  9. nPEP and PrEP
  10. Serologic tests for hepatitis A, B, and C
  11. Gonorrhea culture
  12. Gonorrhea antimicrobial susceptibility testing**
  13. NAAT for trichomoniasis

*Primary care setting is defined as a place where patients are evaluated for various health conditions. STD specialty care setting is defined as a place where the focus is on providing patients with timely, comprehensive, confidential, and culturally sensitive STD care. STD care delivered in STD specialty care settings includes all care delivered in primary care settings.

[†]On-site test for trichomoniasis can include wet mount microscopy and OSOM Trichomonas.

[§]On-site test for bacterial vaginosis can include wet mount microscopy, OSOM BVBlue, and Affirm.

[¶]On-site test for vulvovaginal candidiasis can include wet mount microscopy.

**Access needs to be established for transport medium that adequately maintains the viability of *Neisseria gonorrhoeae* until the specimen reaches a laboratory (e.g., transport medium in transport container, transport system, or transport swab). Providers should contact their state or local health department if they have concerns about resistant *N. gonorrhoeae* infection or if assistance is required for culture and antimicrobial susceptibility testing.

Barrow RY et al: Recommendations for providing quality sexually transmitted diseases clinical services, 2020, *MMWR Recomm Rep* 68(No. RR-5):1-20, 2020. https://doi.org/10.15585/mmwr.rr6805a1.

BOX 7 Persons Recommended to Receive Hepatitis B Vaccination

- All infants
- Unvaccinated children aged <19 yr
- Persons at risk for infection by sexual exposure
  1. Sex partners of hepatitis B surface antigen (HBsAg)-positive persons
  2. Sexually active persons who are not in a long-term, mutually monogamous relationship (e.g., persons with more than one sex partner during the previous 6 mo)
  3. Persons seeking evaluation or treatment for a sexually transmitted infection
  4. Men who have sex with men
- Persons at risk for infection by percutaneous or mucosal exposure to blood
  1. Current or recent injection-drug users
  2. Household contacts of HBsAg-positive persons
  3. Residents and staff of facilities for developmentally disabled persons
  4. Health care and public safety personnel with reasonably anticipated risk for exposure to blood or blood-contaminated body fluids
  5. Hemodialysis patients and predialysis, peritoneal dialysis, and home dialysis patients
  6. Persons with diabetes aged 19-59 yr; persons with diabetes aged ≥60 yr at the discretion of the treating clinician
- Others
  1. International travelers to countries with high or intermediate levels of endemic hepatitis B virus (HBV) infection (HBsAg prevalence of ≥2%)
  2. Persons with hepatitis C virus infection
  3. Persons with chronic liver disease (including persons with cirrhosis, fatty liver disease, alcoholic liver disease, autoimmune hepatitis, and an alanine aminotransferase [ALT] or aspartate aminotransferase [AST] level greater than twice the upper limit of normal)
  4. Persons with human immunodeficiency virus infection
  5. Incarcerated persons
- All other persons seeking protection from HBV infection

From Schillie S et al: Prevention of hepatitis B virus infection in the United States: recommendations of the Advisory Committee on Immunization Practices, *MMWR Recomm Rep* 67(No. RR-1):1-31, 2018.

BOX 8 Testing Anti-Hbs for Health Care Personnel (HCP) Vaccinated in the Past

The issue: An increasing number of HCP have received routine hepatitis B (HepB) vaccination during childhood. No postvaccination serologic testing is recommended after routine infant or adolescent HepB vaccination. Because vaccine-induced antibody to hepatitis B surface antigen (anti-HBs) wanes over time, testing HCP for anti-HBs years after vaccination might not distinguish vaccine nonresponders from responders.

Guidance for health care institutions: Health care institutions may measure anti-HBs upon hire or matriculation for HCP who have documentation of a complete HepB vaccine series in the past (e.g., as part of routine infant or adolescent vaccination). HCP with anti-HBs <10 mIU/ml should receive one or more additional doses of HepB vaccine and retesting (see Fig. 1). Institutions that decide to not measure anti-HBs upon hire or matriculation for HCP who have documentation of a complete HepB vaccine series in the past should ensure timely assessment and postexposure prophylaxis following an exposure (see Table E26).

Considerations: The risk for occupational HBV infection for vaccinated HCP might be low enough in certain settings so that assessment of anti-HBs status and appropriate follow-up should be done at the time of exposure to potentially infectious blood or body fluids. This approach relies on HCP recognizing and reporting blood and body fluid exposures and therefore may be applied on the basis of documented low risk, implementation, and cost considerations. Certain HCP occupations have lower risk for occupational blood and body fluid exposures (e.g., occupations involving counseling versus performing procedures), and nontrainees have lower risks for blood and body fluid exposures than trainees. Some settings also will have a lower prevalence of HBV infection in the patient population served than in other settings, which will influence the risk for HCP exposure to HBsAg-positive blood and body fluids.

From Schillie S et al: Prevention of hepatitis B virus infection in the United States: recommendations of the Advisory Committee on Immunization Practices, *MMWR Recomm Rep* 67(No. RR-1):1-31, 2018.

BOX 9 Persons Recommended to Receive Serologic Testing Before Vaccination*

- Human immunodeficiency virus-positive persons[†]
- Persons with elevated alanine aminotransferase/aspartate aminotransferase of unknown etiology[†]
- Hemodialysis patients[†]
- Men who have sex with men[†]
- Past or current persons who inject drugs[†]
- Persons born in countries of high and intermediate hepatitis B virus (HBV) endemicity (HBsAg prevalence ≥2%)
- U.S.-born persons not vaccinated as infants whose parents were born in countries with high HBV endemicity (≥8%)
- Persons needing immunosuppressive therapy, including chemotherapy, immunosuppression related to organ transplantation, and immunosuppression for rheumatologic or gastroenterologic disorders
- Donors of blood, plasma, organs, tissues, or semen

*Serologic testing comprises testing for hepatitis B surface antigen (HBsAg), antibody to HBsAg, and antibody to hepatitis B core antigen.
[†]Denotes persons also recommended for hepatitis B vaccination. Serologic testing should occur before vaccination. Serologic testing should not be a barrier to vaccination of susceptible persons. The first dose of vaccine should typically be administered immediately after collection of the blood for serologic testing.
From Schillie S et al: Prevention of hepatitis B virus infection in the United States: recommendations of the Advisory Committee on Immunization Practices, *MMWR Recomm Rep* 67(No. RR-1):1-31, 2018.

BOX 10 Persons Recommended to Receive Postvaccination Serologic Testing* After a Complete Series of Hepatitis B Vaccination

- Infants born to hepatitis B surface antigen (HBsAg)-positive mothers or mothers whose HBsAg status remains unknown (e.g., when a parent or person with lawful custody safely surrenders an infant confidentially shortly after birth)†
- Health care personnel and public safety workers
- Hemodialysis patients and others who might require outpatient hemodialysis (e.g., predialysis, peritoneal dialysis, and home dialysis)
- HIV-infected persons
- Other immunocompromised persons (e.g., hematopoietic stem-cell transplant recipients or persons receiving chemotherapy)
- Sex partners of HBsAg-positive persons

*Postvaccination serologic testing for persons other than infants born to HBsAg-positive (or HBsAg-unknown) mothers consists of anti-HBs.
†Postvaccination serologic testing for infants born to HBsAg-positive (or HBsAg-unknown) mothers consists of anti-HBs and HBsAg. Persons with anti-HBs <10 mIU/ml after the primary vaccine series should be revaccinated. Infants born to HBsAg-positive mothers or mothers with an unknown HBsAg status should be revaccinated with a single dose of HepB vaccine and receive postvaccination serologic testing 1-2 mo later. Infants whose anti-HBs remains <10 mIU/ml after single dose revaccination should receive two additional doses of HepB vaccine, followed by postvaccination serologic testing 1-2 mo after the final dose. Based on clinical circumstances or family preference, HBsAg-negative infants with anti-HBs <10 mIU/ml may instead be revaccinated with a mo complete 3-dose series, followed by postvaccination serologic testing performed 1-2 mo after the final dose of vaccine. For others with anti-HBs <10 mIU/ml after the primary series, administration of 3 additional HepB vaccine doses on an appropriate schedule, followed by anti-HBs testing 1-2 mo after the final dose, is usually more practical than serologic testing after ≥1 dose of vaccine.
From Schillie S et al: Prevention of hepatitis B virus infection in the United States: recommendations of the Advisory Committee on Immunization Practices, *MMWR Recomm Rep* 67(No. RR-1):1-31, 2018.

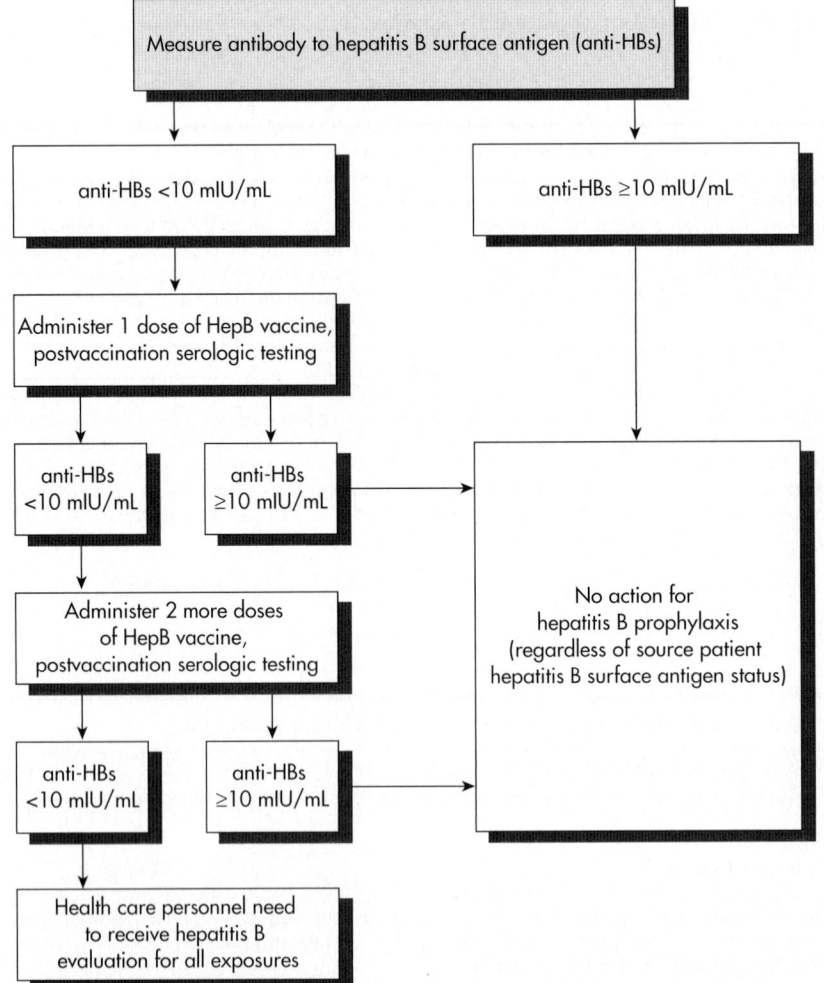

FIG. 1 Preexposure evaluation for health care personnel previously vaccinated with complete ≥3-dose HepB vaccine series who have not had postvaccination serologic testing.*
*Should be performed 1-2 mo after the last dose of vaccine using a quantitative method that allows detection of the protective concentration of anti-HBs (≥10 mIU/ml) (e.g., enzyme-linked immunosorbent assay [ELISA]).
(From Schillie S et al: Prevention of hepatitis B virus infection in the United States: recommendations of the Advisory Committee on Immunization Practices, *MMWR Recomm Rep* 67[No. RR-1]:1-31, 2018.) (Source: Adapted from CDC: a comprehensive immunization strategy to eliminate transmission of hepatitis B virus infection in the United States: recommendations of the Advisory Committee on Immunization Practices [ACIP]. Part II: immunization of adults, *MMWR* 55 [No. RR-16], 2006.)

Influenza Treatment and Prophylaxis

BOX 11 Summary of Seasonal Influenza Vaccination Recommendations

Children

All children aged 6 mo to 18 yr should be vaccinated annually. Children and adolescents at higher risk for influenza complications should continue to be a focus for vaccination efforts as providers and programs transition to routinely vaccinating all children and adolescents, including those who:

- Are aged 6 mo to 4 yr (59 mo)
- Have chronic pulmonary (including asthma), cardiovascular (except hypertension), renal, hepatic, cognitive, neurologic/neuromuscular, hematologic, or metabolic disorders (including diabetes mellitus)
- Are immunosuppressed (including immunosuppression caused by medications or by human immunodeficiency virus)
- Are receiving long-term aspirin therapy and therefore might be at risk for experiencing Reye syndrome after influenza virus infection
- Are residents of long-term care facilities
- Will be pregnant during the influenza season
- NOTE: Children aged <6 mo cannot receive influenza vaccination. Household and other close contacts (e.g., day-care providers) of children aged <6 mo, including older children and adolescents, should be vaccinated.

Adults

Annual vaccination against influenza is recommended for any adult who wants to reduce the risk of becoming ill with influenza or of transmitting it to others. Vaccination is recommended for all adults without contraindications in the following groups, because these persons either are at higher risk for influenza complications, or are close contacts of the persons at higher risk:

- Persons aged ≥50 yr
- Women who will be pregnant during the influenza season
- Persons who have chronic pulmonary (including asthma), cardiovascular (except hypertension), renal, hepatic, cognitive, neurologic/neuromuscular, hematologic, or metabolic disorders (including diabetes mellitus)
- Persons who have immunosuppression (including immunosuppression caused by medications or by human immunodeficiency virus)
- Residents of nursing homes and other long-term care facilities
- Health care personnel
- Household contacts and caregivers of children aged <5 yr and adults aged ≥50 yr, with particular emphasis on vaccinating contacts of children aged <6 mo
- Household contacts and caregivers of persons with medical conditions that put them at higher risk for severe complications from influenza

Centers for Disease Control and Prevention: Prevention and control of seasonal influenza with vaccines: recommendations of the Advisory Committee on Immunization Practices (ACIP), 2009, *MMWR Recomm Rep* 58(RR-8):1-52, 2009.

INDICATIONS FOR USE OF ANTIVIRALS

PERSONS FOR WHOM ANTIVIRAL TREATMENT SHOULD BE CONSIDERED

If possible, antiviral treatment should be started within 48 h of influenza illness onset. The effectiveness of initiating antiviral treatment more than 48 h after illness onset has not been established. Persons for whom antiviral treatment should be considered include:

- Persons hospitalized with laboratory-confirmed influenza (limited data suggest benefit even for persons whose antiviral treatment is initiated more than 48 h after illness onset)
- Persons with laboratory-confirmed influenza pneumonia
- Persons with laboratory-confirmed influenza and bacterial coinfection
- Persons with laboratory-confirmed influenza infection who are at higher risk for influenza complications
- Persons presenting to medical care with laboratory-confirmed influenza within 48 h of influenza illness onset who want to decrease the duration or severity of their symptoms and transmission of influenza to others at higher risk for complications

PERSONS FOR WHOM ANTIVIRAL CHEMOPROPHYLAXIS SHOULD BE CONSIDERED DURING PERIODS OF INCREASED INFLUENZA ACTIVITY IN THE COMMUNITY

- Persons at high risk during the 2 wk after influenza vaccination (after the second dose for children younger than 9 yr who have not previously been vaccinated) if influenza viruses are circulating in the community

- Persons at high risk for whom influenza vaccine is contraindicated
- Family members or health care providers who are unvaccinated and are likely to have ongoing, close exposure to persons at high risk or unvaccinated persons or infants younger than 6 mo
- Persons and their family members and close contacts and health care workers when circulating strains of influenza virus in the community are not matched with vaccine strains
- Persons with immune deficiencies or those who might not respond to vaccination (e.g., persons infected with HIV or other immunosuppressed conditions or who are receiving immunosuppressive medications)
- Unvaccinated staff and persons during response to an outbreak in a closed institutional setting with residents at high risk (e.g., extended-care facilities)

Centers for Disease Control and Prevention: Prevention and control of influenza: recommendations of the Advisory Committee on Immunization Practices (ACIP), 2008, *MMWR Recomm Rep* 57(RR-7):1-60, 2008.

NOTE: Recommended antiviral medications (neuraminidase inhibitors) are not licensed for chemoprophylaxis of children younger than 1 yr (oseltamivir) or younger than 5 yr (zanamivir). Updates or supplements to these recommendations (e.g., expanded age or risk group indications for licensed vaccines) might be required. Health care providers should be alert to announcements of recommendation updates and should check the Centers for Disease Control and Prevention influenza website periodically for additional information (https://www.cdc.gov/flu).

TESTING AND CLINICAL MANAGEMENT OF HEALTH CARE PERSONNEL POTENTIALLY EXPOSED TO HEPATITIS C VIRUS

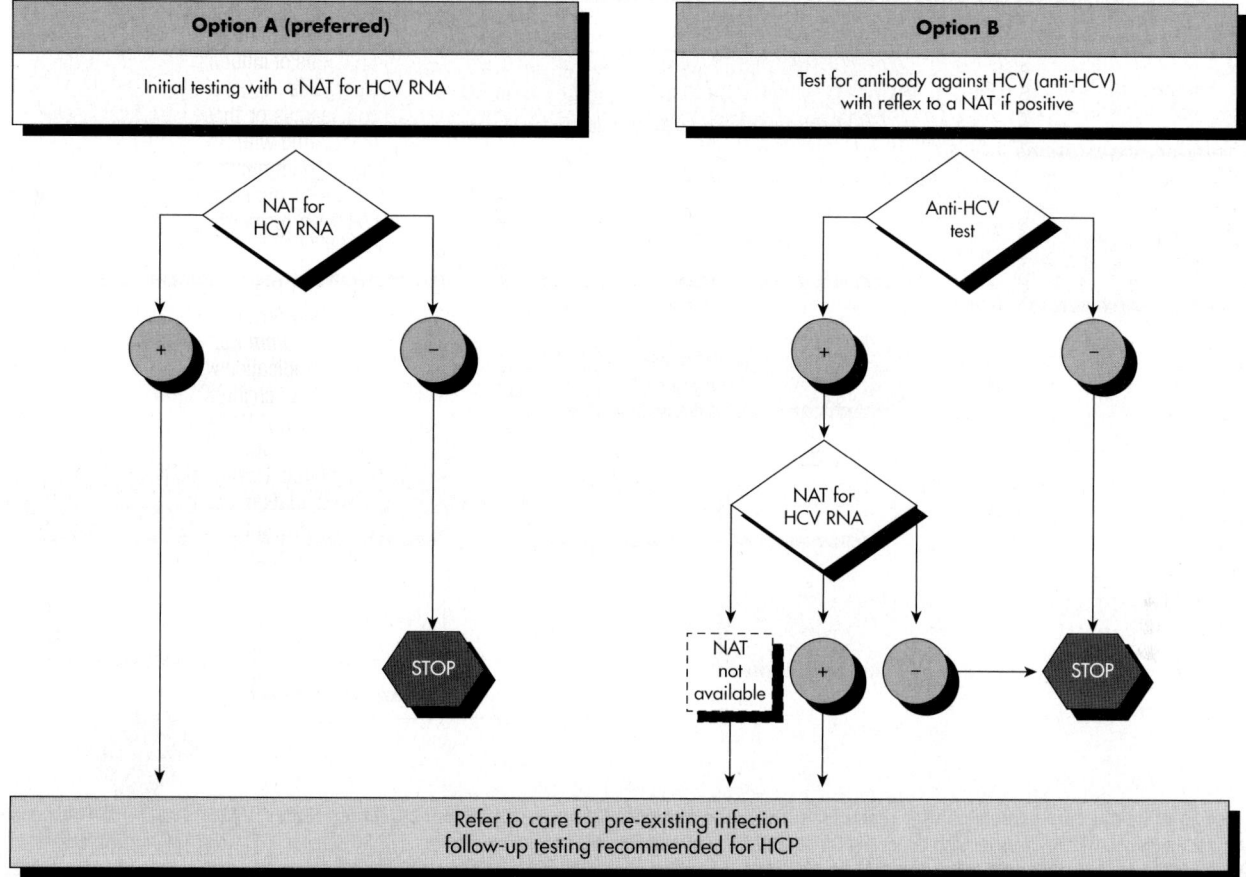

FIG. 2 Testing of source patients after potential exposure of health care personnel to hepatitis C virus—CDC guidance, United States, 2020.* *AASLD-IDSA,* American Association for the Study of Liver Diseases and the Infectious Diseases Society of America; *HCP,* health care personnel; *HCV,* hepatitis C virus; *NAT,* nucleic acid test. **Testing of the source patient should be performed as soon as possible (preferably within 48 h) after exposure.* Testing may follow option A (preferred), which is testing with a NAT for HCV RNA, or option B, which is testing for anti-HCV with reflex to a NAT for HCV RNA if positive. If the source patient is known or suspected to have recent behaviors that increase risk for HCV acquisition (e.g., injection drug use within the previous 4 mo) or if risk cannot be reliably assessed, initial testing of the source patient should include an NAT for HCV RNA. A source patient found to be positive for HCV RNA should be referred to care. Follow-up testing of HCP is recommended if the source patient is HCV RNA positive, is anti-HCV positive with HCV RNA status unknown, or cannot be tested. *Persons with detectable HCV RNA at any point* should be referred to care consistent with current AASLD-IDSA guidelines for evaluation and treatment of all persons with acute or chronic HCV infection. Guidance for hepatitis C treatment (https://www.hcvguidelines.org/) is evolving with emerging data on treatment with direct-acting antivirals.
(From Moorman AC et al: Testing and clinical management of health care personnel potentially exposed to hepatitis C virus—CDC Guidance, United States, 2020, *MMWR Recomm Rep* 69(No. RR-6):1-8, 2020.)

BOX 12 Testing of Source Patients and Health Care Personnel Potentially Exposed to Hepatitis C Virus—CDC Guidance, United States, 2020

Source-patient testing
- Testing of the source patient may follow option A (preferred), which is testing with a nucleic acid test (NAT) for hepatitis C virus (HCV) RNA, **or** option B, which is testing for anti-HCV with reflex to a NAT if positive.
- If a source patient is known or suspected to have recent behaviors that increase risk for HCV acquisition (e.g., injection drug use within the previous 4 mo) or if risk cannot be reliably assessed, initial testing should include a NAT.
- Follow-up testing of health care personnel (HCP) is recommended if the source patient is HCV RNA positive, is anti-HCV positive with RNA status unknown, or cannot be tested.

HCP testing*
- Baseline testing of HCP for anti-HCV with reflex to a NAT if positive should be conducted as soon as possible (preferably within 48 h) after the exposure and may be simultaneous with source-patient testing.
- If follow-up testing of HCP is recommended based on the source-patient's status, test with an NAT at 3-6 wk postexposure.
- If the HCP is NAT negative at 3-6 wk postexposure, a final test for anti-HCV at 4-6 mo postexposure is recommended.
- A source patient or HCP who is positive for HCV RNA should be referred to care.

CDC, Centers for Disease Control and Prevention.
*Follow-up testing of HCP is also warranted when concerns exist about specimen integrity, including handling and storage conditions that might have compromised source-patient test results, or if they exhibit any clinical signs of HCV infection.
From Moorman AC et al: Testing and clinical management of health care personnel potentially exposed to hepatitis C virus—CDC guidance, United States, 2020, *MMWR Recomm Rep* 69(No. RR-6):1-8, 2020.

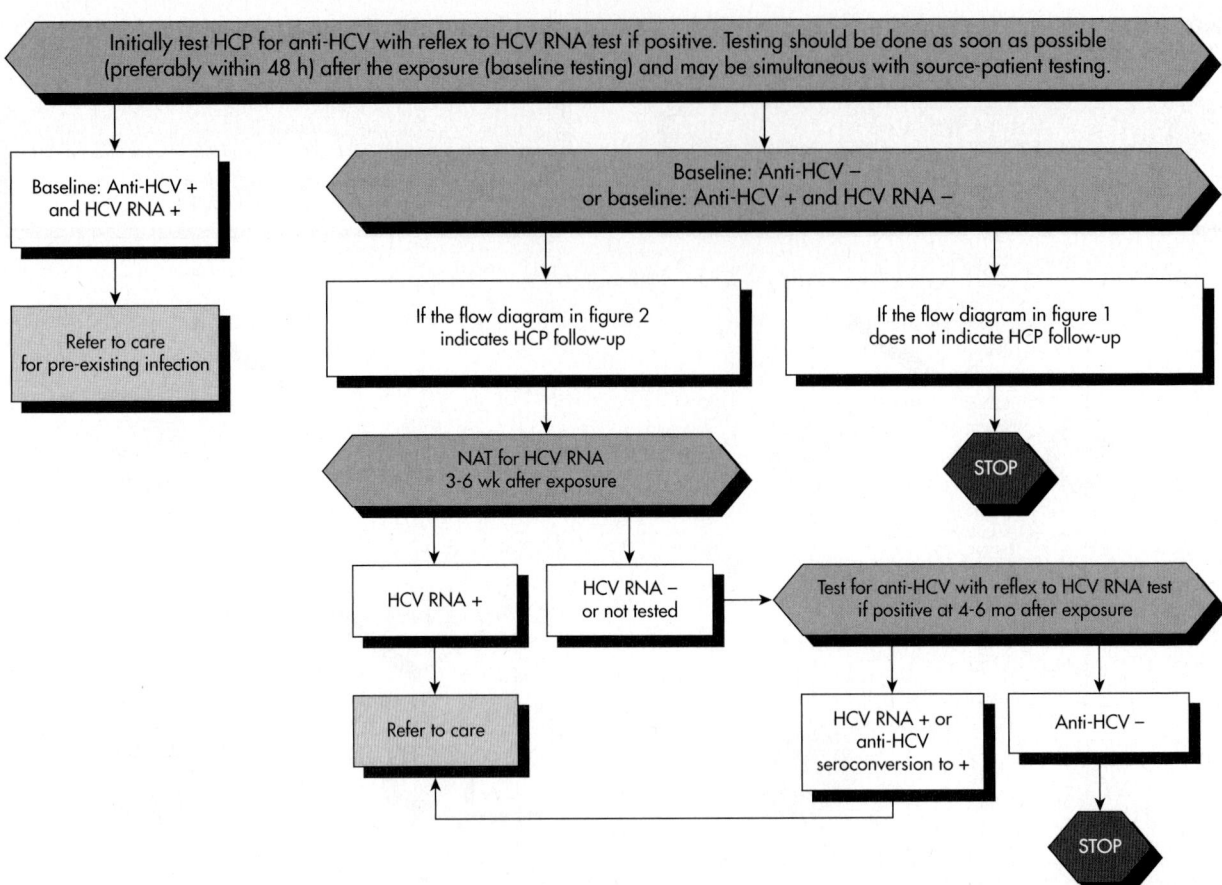

FIG. 3 Testing of health care personnel after potential exposure to hepatitis C virus—CDC guidance, United States, 2020. *AASLD-IDSA,* American Association for the Study of Liver Diseases and the Infectious Diseases Society of America; *HCP,* health care personnel; *HCV,* hepatitis C virus; *NAT,* nucleic acid test. *Baseline testing of HCP for anti-HCV with reflex to a NAT for HCV RNA if positive should be done as soon as possible* (preferably within 48 h) after the exposure and may be simultaneous with source-patient testing. *If follow-up testing is recommended based on the source-patient's status, test for HCV RNA at 3-6 wk postexposure.* Testing for HCV RNA performed at 6 wk postexposure has the advantage of coinciding with human immunodeficiency virus (HIV) postexposure testing schedules if HIV surveillance is recommended. *If HCV RNA is negative at 3-6 wk postexposure, a final test for anti-HCV at 4-6 mo postexposure is recommended* due to the possibility of intermittent periods of aviremia in acute HCV infection. *If the HCP was anti-HCV positive and HCV RNA negative at baseline, testing at this time should be conducted for HCV RNA detection, as persons successfully treated for HCV infection will remain anti-HCV positive and HCV RNA negative unless reinfected.* Testing performed at 6 mo postexposure has the advantage of coinciding with hepatitis B virus (HBV) postexposure testing schedules if HBV testing is recommended. *HCP with anti-HCV seroconversion and negative HCV RNA should be referred for further evaluation.* False-positive anti-HCV results are known to occur among low-risk populations. Anti-HCV seroconversion occurs on average 8-11 wk after exposure, although cases of delayed seroconversion have been documented among persons with immunosuppression such as in HIV infection. *For persons who had a negative anti-HCV result and are immunocompromised, testing for HCV RNA can be considered.* Also, for persons with a positive anti-HCV and negative HCV RNA result, HCV RNA testing should be repeated if an additional potential HCV exposure occurred within the past 6 mo, clinical evidence of HCV infection is present, or concerns exist about specimen integrity, including handling and storage conditions that might have compromised test results. *Exposed persons who develop viral syndromes suggestive of acute HCV infection at any point* should be retested for HCV RNA. *Persons with detectable HCV RNA at any point* should be referred to care consistent with current AASLD-IDSA guidelines for evaluation and treatment of all persons with acute or chronic HCV infection. Those persons with acute infection should be treated on initial diagnosis without awaiting spontaneous resolution. Guidance for hepatitis C treatment (https://www.hcvguidelines.org/) is evolving with emerging data on treatment with direct-acting antivirals. (From Moorman AC et al: Testing and clinical management of health care personnel potentially exposed to hepatitis C virus—CDC guidance, United States, 2020, *MMWR Recomm Rep* 69[No. RR-6]:1-8, 2020.)

HIV Testing and Postexposure Prophylaxis

RECOMMENDATIONS FOR HIV TESTING OF ADULTS, ADOLESCENTS, AND PREGNANT WOMEN

RECOMMENDATIONS FOR ADULTS AND ADOLESCENTS

The CDC recommends that diagnostic human immunodeficiency virus (HIV) testing and opt-out HIV screening be a part of routine clinical care in all health care settings while also preserving the patient's option to decline HIV testing and ensuring a provider-patient relationship conducive to optimal clinical and preventive care. The recommendations are intended for providers in all health care settings, including hospital emergency departments, urgent-care clinics, inpatient services, sexually transmitted disease (STD) clinics or other venues offering clinical STD services, tuberculosis (TB) clinics, substance abuse treatment clinics, other public health clinics, community clinics, correctional health care facilities, and primary care settings. The guidelines address HIV testing in health care settings only; they do not modify existing guidelines concerning HIV counseling, testing, and referral for persons at high risk for HIV who seek or receive HIV testing in nonclinical settings (e.g., community-based organizations, outreach settings, or mobile vans).[3]

SCREENING FOR HIV INFECTION

- In all health care settings, screening for HIV infection should be performed routinely for all patients aged 13 to 64 yr. Health care providers should initiate screening unless prevalence of undiagnosed HIV infection in their patients has been documented to be less than 0.1%. In the absence of existing data for HIV prevalence, health care providers should initiate voluntary HIV screening until they establish that the diagnostic yield is less than 1 per 1000 patients screened, at which point such screening is no longer warranted.
- All patients initiating treatment for TB should be screened routinely for HIV infection.
- All patients seeking treatment for STDs, including all patients visiting STD clinics, should be screened routinely for HIV during each visit for a new complaint, regardless of whether the patient is known or suspected to have specific behavior risks for HIV infection.

REPEAT SCREENING

- Health care providers should subsequently test all persons likely to be at high risk for HIV at least annually. Persons likely to be at high risk include users of injection drugs and their sex partners, persons who exchange sex for money or drugs, sex partners of persons who are HIV infected, and men who have sex with men (MSM) or heterosexual persons who themselves or whose sex partners have had more than one sex partner since their most recent HIV test.
- Health care providers should encourage patients and their prospective sex partners to be tested before initiating a new sexual relationship.
- Repeat screening of persons not likely to be at high risk for HIV should be performed on the basis of clinical judgment.
- Unless recent HIV test results are immediately available, any person whose blood or body fluid is the source of an occupational exposure for a health care provider should be informed of the incident and tested for HIV infection at the time the exposure occurs.

CONSENT AND PRETEST INFORMATION

- Screening should be voluntary and undertaken only with the patient's knowledge and understanding that HIV testing is planned.
- Patients should be informed orally or in writing that HIV testing will be performed unless they decline (opt-out screening). Oral or written information should include an explanation of HIV infection and the meanings

of positive and negative test results, and the patient should be offered an opportunity to ask questions and decline testing. With such notification, consent for HIV screening should be incorporated into the patient's general informed consent for medical care on the same basis as are other screening or diagnostic tests; a separate consent form for HIV testing is not recommended.
- Easily understood informational materials should be made available in the languages of the commonly encountered populations within the service area. The competence of interpreters and bilingual staff to provide language assistance to patients with limited English proficiency must be ensured.
- If a patient declines an HIV test, this decision should be documented in the medical record.

DIAGNOSTIC TESTING FOR HIV INFECTION

- All patients with signs or symptoms consistent with HIV infection or an opportunistic illness characteristic of acquired immunodeficiency syndrome (AIDS) should be tested for HIV.
- Clinicians should maintain a high level of suspicion for acute HIV infection in all patients who have a compatible clinical syndrome and who report recent high-risk behavior. When acute retroviral syndrome is a possibility, a plasma RNA test should be used in conjunction with an HIV antibody test to diagnose acute HIV infection.
- Patients or persons responsible for the patient's care should be notified orally that testing is planned, advised of the indication for testing and the implications of positive and negative test results, and offered an opportunity to ask questions and decline testing. With such notification, the patient's general consent for medical care is considered sufficient for diagnostic HIV testing.

HIV SCREENING FOR PREGNANT WOMEN AND THEIR INFANTS

Universal Opt-Out Screening
- All pregnant women in the United States should be screened for HIV infection.
- Screening should occur after a woman is notified that HIV screening is recommended for all pregnant patients and that she will receive an HIV test as part of the routine panel of prenatal tests unless she declines (opt-out screening).
- HIV testing must be voluntary and free from coercion. No woman should be tested without her knowledge.
- Pregnant women should receive oral or written information that includes an explanation of HIV infection, a description of interventions that can reduce HIV transmission from mother to infant, and the meanings of positive and negative test results. They should be offered an opportunity to ask questions and decline testing.
- No additional process or written documentation of informed consent beyond what is required for other routine prenatal tests should be required for HIV testing.
- If a patient declines an HIV test, this decision should be documented in the medical record.

ADDRESSING REASONS FOR DECLINING TESTING

- Providers should discuss and address reasons for declining an HIV test (e.g., lack of perceived risk, fear of the disease, and concerns regarding partner violence or potential stigma or discrimination).
- Women who decline an HIV test because they have had a previous negative test result should be informed of the importance of retesting during each pregnancy.
- Logistical reasons for not testing (e.g., scheduling) should be resolved.
- Certain women who initially decline an HIV test might accept at a later date, especially if their concerns are discussed. Certain women will continue to decline testing, and their decisions should be respected and documented in the medical record.

Timing of HIV Testing
- To promote informed and timely therapeutic decisions, health care providers should test women for HIV as early as possible during each pregnancy. Women who decline the test early in prenatal care should be encouraged to be tested at a subsequent visit.

---

[3]Data from Centers for Disease Control and Prevention: Revised surveillance case definitions for HIV infection among adults, adolescents, and children aged <18 months and for HIV infection and AIDS among children aged 18 months to <13 years—United States, 2008, *MMWR Recomm Rep* 57(10):1-12, 2008.

- A second HIV test during the third trimester, preferably less than 36 wk of gestation, is cost effective even in areas of low HIV prevalence and may be considered for all pregnant women. A second HIV test during the third trimester is recommended for women who meet one or more of the following criteria:
  1. Women who receive health care in jurisdictions with elevated incidence of HIV or AIDS among women aged 15 to 45 yr. In 2004, these jurisdictions included Alabama, Connecticut, Delaware, the District of Columbia, Florida, Georgia, Illinois, Louisiana, Maryland, Massachusetts, Mississippi, Nevada, New Jersey, New York, North Carolina, Pennsylvania, Puerto Rico, Rhode Island, South Carolina, Tennessee, Texas, and Virginia.[4]
  2. Women who receive health care in facilities in which prenatal screening identifies at least one pregnant woman who is infected with HIV per 1000 women screened.
  3. Women who are known to be at high risk for acquiring HIV (e.g., users of injection drugs and their sex partners, women who exchange sex for money or drugs, women who are sex partners of persons who are infected with HIV, and women who have had a new or more than one sex partner during this pregnancy).
  4. Women who have signs or symptoms consistent with acute HIV infection. When acute retroviral syndrome is a possibility, a plasma RNA test should be used in conjunction with an HIV antibody test to diagnose acute HIV infection.

Rapid Testing During Labor

- Any woman with undocumented HIV status at the time of labor should be screened with a rapid HIV test unless she declines (opt-out screening).
- Reasons for declining a rapid test should be explored (see "Addressing Reasons for Declining Testing").

---

[4]A second HIV test in the third trimester is as cost effective as other common health interventions when HIV incidence among women of childbearing age is =17 HIV cases per 100,000 person-yr. In 2004, in jurisdictions with available data on HIV case rates, a rate of 17 new HIV diagnoses per yr per 100,000 women aged 15 to 45 yr was associated with an AIDS case rate of at least nine AIDS diagnoses per yr per 100,000 women aged 15 to 45 yr (CDC, unpublished data, 2005). As of 2004, the jurisdictions listed above exceeded these thresholds. The list of specific jurisdictions where a second test in the third trimester is recommended will be updated periodically based on surveillance data.

- Immediate initiation of appropriate antiretroviral prophylaxis should be recommended to women on the basis of a reactive rapid test result without waiting for the result of a confirmatory test.

Postpartum/Newborn Testing

- When a woman's HIV status is still unknown at the time of delivery, she should be screened immediately postpartum with a rapid HIV test unless she declines (opt-out screening).
- When the mother's HIV status is unknown postpartum, rapid testing of the newborn as soon as possible after birth is recommended so that antiretroviral prophylaxis can be offered to infants exposed to HIV. Women should be informed that identifying HIV antibodies in the newborn indicates that the mother is infected.
- For infants whose HIV exposure status is unknown and who are in foster care, the person legally authorized to provide consent should be informed that rapid HIV testing is recommended for infants whose biologic mothers have not been tested.
- The benefits of neonatal antiretroviral prophylaxis are best realized when it is initiated within 12 h after birth.

Confirmatory Testing

- Whenever possible, uncertainties regarding laboratory test results indicating HIV infection status should be resolved before final decisions are made regarding reproductive options, antiretroviral therapy, cesarean delivery, or other interventions.
- If the confirmatory test result is not available before delivery, immediate initiation of appropriate antiretroviral prophylaxis should be recommended to any pregnant patient whose HIV screening test result is reactive to reduce the risk for perinatal transmission.

BOX 13   Situations for Which Expert Consultation for HIV Postexposure Prophylaxis Is Advised*

- Delayed (i.e., later than 24-36 h) exposure report
  1. The interval after which there is no benefit from postexposure prophylaxis (PEP) is undefined
- Unknown source (e.g., needle in sharps disposal container or laundry)
  1. Decide use of PEP on a case-by-case basis
  2. Consider the severity of the exposure and the epidemiologic likelihood of human immunodeficiency virus (HIV) exposure
  3. Do not test needles or other sharp instruments for HIV
- Known or suspected pregnancy in the exposed person
  1. Does not preclude the use of optimal PEP regimens
  2. Do not deny PEP solely on the basis of pregnancy
- Resistance of the source virus to antiretroviral agents
  1. Influence of drug resistance on transmission risk is unknown
  2. Selection of drugs to which the source person's virus is unlikely to be resistant is recommended if the source person's virus is known or suspected to be resistant to one or more of the drugs considered for the PEP regimen
  3. Resistance testing of the source person's virus at the time of the exposure is not recommended
- Toxicity of the initial PEP regimen
  1. Adverse symptoms such as nausea and diarrhea are common with PEP
  2. Symptoms often can be managed without changing the PEP regimen by prescribing antimotility and/or antiemetic agents
  3. Modification of dose intervals (i.e., administering a lower dose of drug more frequently throughout the day, as recommended by the manufacturer) in other situations might help alleviate symptoms

*Local experts and/or the National Clinicians' Postexposure Prophylaxis Hotline (PEPline [888-448-4911]).

BOX 14   Occupational Exposure Management Resources

National Clinicians' Postexposure Prophylaxis Hotline (PEPline) Run by University of California–San Francisco/San Francisco General Hospital staff; supported by the Health Resources and Services Administration, Ryan White CARE Act, HIV/AIDS Bureau, AIDS Education and Training Centers, and CDC	Phone: 888-448-4911 Internet: https://nccc.ucsf.edu/clinician-consultation;/pep-post-exposure-prophy-laxis/
Hepatitis Hotline	Phone: 888-443-7232 Internet: https://www.cdc.gov/ncidod/diseases/hepatitis/index.htm
Reporting to CDC: Occupationally acquired HIV infections and failures of PEP	Phone: 800-893-0485
HIV Antiretroviral Pregnancy Registry	Phone: 800-258-4263 Fax: 800-800-1052 Address: 1410 Commonwealth Dr., Suite 215, Wilmington, NC 28405 Internet: https://www.apregistry.com/
Food and Drug Administration Report unusual or severe toxicity to antiretroviral agents	Phone: 800-332-1088 Address: MedWatch, HF-2, FDA, 5600 Fishers Lane, Rockville, MD 20857 Internet: https://www.fda.gov/medwatch
HIV/AIDS Treatment Information Service	Internet: http://www.hivatis.org/

BOX 15 Management of Occupational Blood Exposures

Provide Immediate Care to the Exposure Site
- Wash wounds and skin with soap and water
- Flush mucous membranes with water

Determine Risk Associated With Exposure
- Type of fluid (e.g., blood, visibly bloody fluid, other potentially infectious fluid or tissue, and concentrated virus)
- Type of exposure (e.g., percutaneous injury, mucous membrane or nonintact skin exposure, and bites resulting in blood exposure)

Evaluate Exposure Source
- Assess the risk of infection using available information
- Test known sources for HBsAg, anti-HCV, and HIV antibodies (consider using rapid testing)
- For unknown sources, assess risk of exposure to HBV, HCV, or HIV infection
- Do not test discarded needles or syringes for virus contamination

Evaluate the Exposed Person
- Assess immune status for HBV infection (i.e., by history of hepatitis B vaccination and vaccine response)

Give PEP for Exposures Posing Risk of Infection Transmission
- HBV: See Table E6
- HCV: PEP not recommended
- HIV: See Tables E34, E35, and E36
  1. Initiate PEP as soon as possible, preferably within hours of exposure
  2. Offer pregnancy testing to all women of childbearing age not known to be pregnant
  3. Seek expert consultation if viral resistance is suspected
  4. Administer PEP for 4 wk if tolerated

Perform Follow-up Testing and Provide Counseling
- Advise exposed persons to seek medical evaluation for any acute illness occurring during follow-up

HBV Exposures
- Perform follow-up anti-HBs testing in persons who receive hepatitis B vaccine
  1. Test for anti-HBs 1-2 mo after last dose of vaccine
  2. Anti-HBs response to vaccine cannot be ascertained if HBIG was received in the previous 3-4 mo

HCV Exposures
- Perform baseline and follow-up testing for anti-HCV and alanine aminotransferase 4-6 mo after exposure
- Perform HCV RNA at 4-6 wk if earlier diagnosis of HCV infection desired
- Confirm repeatedly reactive anti-HCV enzyme immunoassays with supplemental tests

HIV Exposures
- Perform HIV-antibody testing for at least 6 mo after exposure (e.g., at baseline, 6 wk, 3 mo, and 6 mo)
- Perform HIV-antibody testing if illness compatible with an acute retroviral syndrome occurs
- Advise exposed persons to use precautions to prevent secondary transmission during the follow-up period
- Evaluate exposed persons taking PEP within 72 h after exposure and monitor for drug toxicity for at least 2 wk

HBIG, Hepatitis B immune globulin; *HBsAg,* hepatitis B surface antigen; *HBV,* hepatitis B virus; *HCV,* hepatitis C virus; *HIV,* human immunodeficiency virus; *PEP,* postexposure prophylaxis.

Recommendations for Meningococcal Vaccination

BOX 16 Meningococcal Vaccination Recommendations—Advisory Committee on Immunization Practices, United States, 2020

ACIP recommends MenACWY vaccination for the following groups:
- Routine vaccination for adolescents aged 11 or 12 yr, with a booster dose at age 16 yr.
- Routine vaccination of persons aged ≥2 mo at increased risk for meningococcal disease (dosing schedule varies by age and indication, and interval for booster dose varies by age at time of previous vaccination):
  - Persons with certain medical conditions including anatomic or functional asplenia, complement component deficiencies (e.g., C3, C5-C9, properdin, factor H, or factor D), complement inhibitor (e.g., eculizumab [Soliris] or ravulizumab [Ultomiris]) use, or human immunodeficiency virus infection.
  - Microbiologists with routine exposure to *Neisseria meningitidis* isolates.
  - Persons at increased risk during an outbreak (e.g., in community or organizational settings, and among men who have sex with men [MSM]).
  - Persons who travel to or live in countries in which meningococcal disease is hyperendemic or epidemic.
  - Unvaccinated or undervaccinated first-year college students living in residence halls.
  - Military recruits.
  - Booster doses for previously vaccinated persons who become or remain at increased risk.

ACIP recommends MenB vaccination for the following groups:
- Routine vaccination of persons aged ≥10 yr at increased risk for meningococcal disease (dosing schedule varies by vaccine brand; boosters should be administered at 1 yr after primary series completion, then every 2-3 yr thereafter):
  - Persons with certain medical conditions, such as anatomic or functional asplenia, complement component deficiencies, or complement inhibitor use.
  - Microbiologists with routine exposure to *N. meningitidis* isolates.
  - Persons at increased risk during an outbreak (e.g., in community or organizational settings, and among MSM).
  - Vaccination of adolescents and young adults aged 16-23 yr with a 2-dose MenB series on the basis of shared clinical decision-making. The preferred age for MenB vaccination is 16-18 yr. Booster doses are not recommended unless the person becomes at increased risk for meningococcal disease.
  - Booster doses for previously vaccinated persons who become or remain at increased risk.

ACIP, Advisory Committee on Immunization Practices; *MenACWY,* quadrivalent (serogroups A, C, W, Y) meningococcal conjugate vaccine; *MenB,* serogroup B meningococcal vaccine.
From Mbaeyi SA et al: Meningococcal vaccination: recommendations of the Advisory Committee on Immunization Practices, United States, 2020, *MMWR Recomm Rep* 69(No. RR-9):1-41, 2020.

Vaccine Websites and Resources

TABLE 46 Vaccine Websites and Resources	
Organization	**Website**
Health Professional Associations	
American Academy of Family Physicians (AAFP)	https://www.familydoctor.org/online/famdocen/home.html
American Academy of Pediatrics (AAP)	https://www.aap.org/
AAP Childhood Immunization Support Program	https://www.aap.org/immunization/
American Association of Occupational Health Nurses (AAOHN)	https://www.aaohn.org/
American College Health Association (ACHA)	https://www.acha.org/
American College of Obstetricians and Gynecologists (ACOG)–Immunization for Women	https://www.immunizationforwomen.org/
American Medical Association (AMA)	https://www.ama-assn.org/
American Nurses Association (ANA)	https://www.nursingworld.org/
American Pharmacists Association (APhA)	https://www.pharmacist.com/
American School Health Association (ASHA)	https://www.ashaweb.org/
American Travel Health Nurses Association (ATHNA)	https://www.athna.org/
Association for Professionals in Infection Control and Epidemiology (APIC)	https://www.apic.org/
Association of State and Territorial Health Officials (ASTHO)	https://www.astho.org/
Association of Teachers of Preventive Medicine (ATPM)	https://www.atpm.org/
National Medical Association (NMA)	https://www.nmanet.org/
Society of Teachers of Family Medicine—Group on Immunization Education	https://www.immunizationed.org/
Nonprofit Groups and Universities	
Albert B. Sabin Vaccine Institute	https://www.sabin.org/
Brighton Collaboration	
Center for Vaccine Awareness and Research—Texas Children's Center	https://www.texaschildrens.org/departments/immunization-project
Children's Vaccine Program	
Every Child by Two (ECBT)	https://www.ecbt.org/
Families Fighting Flu	https://www.familiesfightingflu.org/
GAVI, the Vaccine Alliance	
Health on the Net Foundation (HON)	https://www.hon.ch/
Immunization Action Coalition (IAC)	https://www.immunize.org/
Infectious Diseases Society of America (IDSA)	https://www.idsociety.org/Index.aspx
Institute for Vaccine Safety (IVS), Johns Hopkins Bloomberg School of Public Health	https://www.vaccinesafety.edu/
National Academies: Health and Medicine Division	https://www.nationalacademies.org/hmd/
National Alliance for Hispanic Health	https://www.hispanichealth.org/
National Foundation for Infectious Diseases (NFID)	http://www.nfid.org/
National Foundation for Infectious Diseases (NFID)—Childhood Influenza Immunization Coalition (CIIC)	
National Network for Immunization Information (NNii)	
Parents of Kids with Infectious Diseases (PKIDS)	https://www.pkids.org/
PATH Vaccine Resource Library	
Vaccine Education Center at the Children's Hospital of Philadelphia	https://www.chop.edu/service/vaccine-education-center/home.html
Vaccinate Your Baby	https://www.vaccinateyourbaby.org/
Government Organizations	
Centers for Disease Control and Prevention (CDC)	
Advisory Committee on Immunization Practices (ACIP)	https://www.cdc.gov/vaccines/acip/index.html
ACIP Vaccine Recommendations	https://www.cdc.gov/vaccines/hcp/acip-recs/index.html
Current Vaccine Delays and Shortages	https://www.cdc.gov/vaccines/vac-gen/shortages/
Epidemiology and Prevention of Vaccine-Preventable Diseases (also known as the Pink Book)	https://www.cdc.gov/vaccines/pubs/pinkbook/index.html
Manual for the Surveillance of Vaccine-Preventable Diseases	https://www.cdc.gov/vaccines/pubs/surv-manual/index.html
Public Health Image Library	http://www.phil.cdc.gov/phil/home.asp
Travelers' Health	https://www.cdc.gov/travel/
CDC Health Information for International Travel (also known as the Yellow Book)	https://www.c.cdc.gov/travel/yellowbook/2016/table-of-contents
Vaccine Adverse Events Reporting System (VAERS)	
Vaccine Administration: Recommendations and Guidelines	
Vaccines and Immunizations	https://www.cdc.gov/vaccines/
Vaccines for Children Program	https://www.cdc.gov/vaccines/programs/vfc/index.html
Vaccines for Children—Vaccine Price List	https://www.cdc.gov/vaccines/programs/vfc/awardees/vaccine-management/price-list/index.html

Continued

TABLE 46 Vaccine Websites and Resources—cont'd

Organization	Website
Vaccine Information Statements	https://www.cdc.gov/vaccines/hcp/vis/index.html
Vaccine Safety	https://www.cdc.gov/vaccinesafety/index.html
Vaccine Storage and Handling	https://www.cdc.gov/vaccines/recs/storage/default.htm
Department of Health and Human Services (HHS)	
National Vaccine Program Office (NVPO)	https://www.hhs.gov/nvpo/
Health Resources and Services Administration	
National Vaccine Injury Compensation Program	https://www.hrsa.gov/vaccinecompensation/
National Institute of Allergy and Infectious Diseases (NIAID)	
Vaccines	https://www.niaid.nih.gov/about/vrc
World Health Organization (WHO)	
Immunization, Vaccines, and Biologicals	https://www.who.int/immunization/en/

From Kliegman RM: *Nelson textbook of pediatrics,* ed 21, Philadelphia, 2020, Elsevier.

Index

Note: Page numbers followed by *f* indicate figures, *b* indicate boxes, *t* indicate tables, and *e* and **bold** indicate online content.

Note: Page numbers followed by *f* indicate figures, *b* indicate boxes, *t* indicate tables, and *e* and **bold** indicate online content.

Note: Page numbers followed by *f* indicate figures, *b* indicate boxes, *t* indicate tables, and *e* and **bold** indicate online content.

Note: Page numbers followed by *f* indicate figures, *b* indicate boxes, *t* indicate tables, and *e* and **bold** indicate online content.

Note: Page numbers followed by *f* indicate figures, *b* indicate boxes, *t* indicate tables, and *e* and **bold** indicate online content.

Note: Page numbers followed by *f* indicate figures, *b* indicate boxes, *t* indicate tables, and *e* and **bold** indicate online content.

Note: Page numbers followed by *f* indicate figures, *b* indicate boxes, *t* indicate tables, and *e* and **bold** indicate online content.

Note: Page numbers followed by *f* indicate figures, *b* indicate boxes, *t* indicate tables, and *e* and **bold** indicate online content.

Note: Page numbers followed by *f* indicate figures, *b* indicate boxes, *t* indicate tables, and *e* and **bold** indicate online content.

Note: Page numbers followed by *f* indicate figures, *b* indicate boxes, *t* indicate tables, and *e* and **bold** indicate online content.

Note: Page numbers followed by *f* indicate figures, *b* indicate boxes, *t* indicate tables, and *e* and **bold** indicate online content.

Note: Page numbers followed by *f* indicate figures, *b* indicate boxes, *t* indicate tables, and *e* and **bold** indicate online content.

Note: Page numbers followed by *f* indicate figures, *b* indicate boxes, *t* indicate tables, and *e* and **bold** indicate online content.

Note: Page numbers followed by *f* indicate figures, *b* indicate boxes, *t* indicate tables, and *e* and **bold** indicate online content.

Note: Page numbers followed by *f* indicate figures, *b* indicate boxes, *t* indicate tables, and *e* and **bold** indicate online content.

Note: Page numbers followed by *f* indicate figures, *b* indicate boxes, *t* indicate tables, and *e* and **bold** indicate online content.

Note: Page numbers followed by *f* indicate figures, *b* indicate boxes, *t* indicate tables, and *e* and **bold** indicate online content.

Note: Page numbers followed by *f* indicate figures, *b* indicate boxes, *t* indicate tables, and *e* and **bold** indicate online content.

Note: Page numbers followed by *f* indicate figures, *b* indicate boxes, *t* indicate tables, and *e* and **bold** indicate online content.

Note: Page numbers followed by *f* indicate figures, *b* indicate boxes, *t* indicate tables, and *e* and **bold** indicate online content.

Note: Page numbers followed by *f* indicate figures, *b* indicate boxes, *t* indicate tables, and *e* and **bold** indicate online content.

Note: Page numbers followed by *f* indicate figures, *b* indicate boxes, *t* indicate tables, and *e* and **bold** indicate online content.

Note: Page numbers followed by *f* indicate figures, *b* indicate boxes, *t* indicate tables, and *e* and **bold** indicate online content.

Note: Page numbers followed by *f* indicate figures, *b* indicate boxes, *t* indicate tables, and *e* and **bold** indicate online content.

Note: Page numbers followed by *f* indicate figures, *b* indicate boxes, *t* indicate tables, and *e* and **bold** indicate online content.

Note: Page numbers followed by *f* indicate figures, *b* indicate boxes, *t* indicate tables, and *e* and **bold** indicate online content.

Spur cells, **292.e1f, 1570.e1t**
SQTS. *See* Short QT syndrome
Squamous cell carcinoma
  in actinic keratosis, 21.e9
  bladder, 185
  characteristics of, 438,
    **1007.e68–1007.e70,
    1007.e68f, 1007.e69f,
    1007.e70f, 1007.e70t**
  head and neck, 483–485, **483.e1f,
    483.e2f, 484.e1f,** 484t
  keratinizing, **767.e1f**
  lip, 1007.e69f
  lung, 675
  oral, **483.e1f,** 793–795, **794.e1f**
  oropharyngeal, 793t
  penile, 845.e17
  of trachea, **1366.e1f**
  vaginal, 1108.e19
  vulvar, 1133.e2, 1133.e3f
Squamous cell hyperplasia, 926.e2
Squint, 1012.e10
SS. *See* Serotonin syndrome; Sjögren
    syndrome
SSc. *See* Systemic sclerosis
SSM. *See* Smoldering systemic
    mastocytosis
SSRIs. *See* Selective serotonin
    reuptake inhibitors
SSS. *See* Sick sinus syndrome
SSSIs. *See* Skin and skin structure
    infections
St. Anthony's fire, 434.e47
St. John's wort, for major depression,
    352
St. Louis encephalitis virus,
    410.e2–410.e5t
St. Louis University Mental Status, 716
Stable ischemic heart disease, 85,
    320, **322.e1f**
Staging. *See also* TNM staging
  of amyloidosis, 80.e19b
  of breast cancer, 200t, 201t
  of cervical cancer, 251t
  of chronic lymphocytic leukemia,
    270
  of colon cancer, 308
  of hepatocellular carcinoma, 533
  of Hodgkin lymphoma, 546, 548b
  of lymphomas, 779
  of melanoma, 695
  of multiple myeloma, 741.e6t
  **of mycosis fungoides,
    751.e2–751.e3, 751.e4**
  of neuroblastoma, 770.e2t
  of pancreatic cancer, 820
  of prostate cancer, 920t
  of renal cell carcinoma, 951t
  of thymoma, 1063.e7t
Stalevo, for Parkinson disease, 836
**Stanford classification, of acute
    aortic syndromes, 21.e13,
    21.e14t**
Stapedectomy, 813.e4
Stapedotomy, 813.e4
**Staphylococcal toxic shock
    syndrome, 1080.e7–1080.e10,
    1080.e8t**
Staphylococcus aureus
  **cardiac implantable electronic
    device infection caused by,
    227.e11**

Staphylococcus aureus (Continued)
  **chronic rhinosinusitis caused by,
    291.e4**
  food poisoning, 457
  glomerulonephritis associated with,
    34t
  **impetigo caused by,
    633.e2–633.e3**
  methicillin-resistant, **485.e3,** 691,
    712.e9–712.e10
  **toxic shock syndrome caused by,
    1080.e7–1080.e10**
Stapled hemorrhoidopexy, 515.e26
STARI. *See* Southern tick-associated
    rash illness
Stasis dermatitis, 1118
Stasis ulcers, 1120, **1120.e1f**
Statin(s), 89
  for atherosclerotic cardiovascular
    disease, 564f, 565t
  for coronary artery disease, 323
  for hypercholesterolemia, 563–565,
    564t, 565t
  for hyperlipidemia, 584t
  for IgA nephropathy, 631.e4
  lipoprotein metabolism affected by,
    566f
  for myocardial infarction, 760
  for peripheral artery disease, 862t
Statin-associated autoimmune
    myopathy, 1008
Statin-induced muscle syndromes,
    1008–1009, **1009.e1b**
Statin-induced myalgias, 1008
Statin-induced myopathies,
    643.e2–643.e3t, 1008
Statin-induced myositis, 1008
Statin-induced rhabdomyolysis, 959,
    1008
Statural overgrowth, 1319
Stature
  short
    differential diagnosis of, **1509.e8f**
    **in Turner syndrome, 1092.e42,
      1092.e43f**
  tall, 1322–1323
Status asthmaticus, 115
Status epilepticus, **798.e5t,**
    1010–1012, 1010t, 1011f, 1012t
Stavudine, for human
    immunodeficiency virus,
    1628.e2t
Staxyn. *See* Vardenafil
STDs. *See* Sexually transmitted
    diseases
Steatohepatitis, 1319
Steatorrhea, 290, **390.e6**
Steatosis, 1319
**Steele-Richardson-Olszewski
    syndrome, 918.e4**
Steinberg test, 689.e24f
Stein-Leventhal syndrome, 890.e8
ST-elevation myocardial infarction, 31t
**Stem cell transplantation
  for amyloidosis, 80.e17**
  for aplastic anemia, 104.e11
  **for multiple myeloma, 741.e4,
    741.e6**
STEMI. *See* ST-segment elevation
    myocardial infarction
Stemmer sign, 684
Stenosing cholangitis, 915

**Stenosing flexor tenosynovitis,
    1092.e14**
Stenosing tendovaginitis, 1092.e14
**Stenosing tenosynovitis of the
    radial styloid process, 331.e55**
**Stenosing tenovaginitis of the first
    dorsal compartment, 331.e55**
Stenosis
  aortic, 100–104, 100f, 102f, 103f,
    1332–1333
  carotid artery, 240–242
Stenosis of the pylorus, 467
Stenotrophomonas maltophilia,
    737.e5–737.e6
Stents/stenting
  for abdominal aortic aneurysm, 5f
  for angina pectoris, 90, **91.e2**
  **for aortic coarctation,
    94.e56–94.e58**
  **for Budd-Chiari syndrome,
    212.e15**
  **for superior vena cava syndrome,
    1029.e13**
Steppage gait, 669.e29
Stereotactic biopsy
  for astrocytoma, 132
  for breast cancer, 203b
**Stereotactic body radiosurgery,
    946.e21**
**Stereotactic radiosurgery
  for acromegaly, 21.e3**
  for brain metastases, 192.e3
  for prolactinoma, 918.e9
Sterile pyuria, 1319
Sterility, **639.e8–639.e9.** *See also*
    Infertility
Sterilization, for contraception, 318
Stevens-Johnson syndrome, 9,
    **1012.e2–1012.e4, 1012.e2f,
    1012.e3b, 1012.e3f, 1080.e2,
    1391.e1t**
Stickler syndrome, 1012.e5
Stiff person syndrome, 243.e11
Still's disease, 1044.e5
  adult-onset, 62.e21–62.e22
Stimulant use disorder, 80.e12
Stimulants
  for attention-deficit/hyperactivity
    disorder, 153
  for Tourette syndrome, 1079–1080
Stings
  **insect, 645.e11–645.e14,
    645.e11f, 645.e12f, 645.e13f**
  scorpion, 183
Stomach cancer, 464, 465t
Stomatitis, **1012.e6–1012.e9,
    1012.e7f, 1012.e8f**
  bullous, 1319
  **recurrent aphthous, 104.e7–104.e9,
    104.e7f, 104.e9t**
Stomatocytes, **1564.e2t, 1570.e2t**
Stomatodynia, 217.e4
Stones, kidney, 1105
Stool antigen test
  description of, 468.e6
  for *Helicobacter pylori*, 511, 847
Stool/fecal incontinence, 447.e1
STOP-BANG questionnaire, 1001f
Storage diseases, 1318–1319
Strabismic amblyopia, 80.e2
**Strabismus, 1012.e10, 1012.e11f,
    1012.e12f**

Strangulated bowel obstruction, 1005
Strangulated inguinal hernia, 645.e8
Strattera. *See* Atomoxetine
Strawberry tongue, 971.e2f
Streptococcal myonecrosis, 767.e5t
Streptococcal pharyngitis, **960.e2,
    971.e2,** 1512t
Streptococcal tonsillitis, 869, 871b
**Streptococcal toxic shock
    syndrome, 1080.e7, 1080.e7b,
    1080.e8t**
Streptococcus spp.
  **impetigo caused by,
    633.e2–633.e3**
  S. pneumoniae, 885f
Streptokinase
  for deep vein thrombosis, 335
  for myocardial infarction, 758t
Streptomycin, 1092.e36
Streptozyme. *See* Antistreptolysin O titer
**Stress cardiomyopathy, 1052.e9,
    1052.e9f, 1052.e10f**
Stress disorder, acute, 59.e2–59.e3
Stress echocardiography, for angina
    pectoris, 87–88
Stress incontinence, 634, 634t,
    634.e1f, 639.e2f, 845.e3f
Stress test algorithm, 87
Stress ulcer, 53
Striatonigral degeneration, 747.e2
**Stricture, anorectal, 94.e23b,
    94.e23–94.e24, 94.e23t**
Stridor
  causes of, 1173
  in neonates, 1319
  in pediatric age, 1319–1320
Stroke, 1013, **1024.e2.** *See also*
    Brainstem ischemic stroke
    syndromes
  acute ischemic, **197.e5b, 197.e6t,**
    1013–1020, 1013b, 1014b,
    1015f, 1015t, 1016t, 1017t,
    1018b, 1018t, 1019f
  **aphasia syndromes caused by,
    104.e5t**
  bilateral, 197.e3
  cardioembolic, 1024.e2–1024.e3
  cigarette smoking and, 1024.e3
  differential diagnosis of, 1320
  hemorrhagic, 1021–1024, 1022t,
    1023b, **1023.e1f,** 1024t
  imaging of, 197.e5t
  lateral pontine, 197.e2–197.e3
  **long-term complications of,
    1024.e3**
  medial pontine, 197.e3
  medullary, 197.e4t
  midbrain, 197.e3t
  **obstructive sleep apnea and,
    1024.e3**
  in pediatric patients, 1320
  pontine, 197.e2–197.e3, 197.e4t
  prevention of, **142.e1f**
  risk factors for, 1024.e3
  **secondary prevention of,
    1024.e2–1024.e4**
  thromboembolism as cause of, 136
  in young adults, 1320
Strongyloides stercoralis, **106.e3t**
**Structured Clinical Interview for
    Dissociative Disorders, 392.e2**
Struvite stones, 1105

Note: Page numbers followed by *f* indicate figures, *b* indicate boxes, *t* indicate tables, and *e* and **bold** indicate online content.

Note: Page numbers followed by *f* indicate figures, *b* indicate boxes, *t* indicate tables, and *e* and **bold** indicate online content.

Note: Page numbers followed by *f* indicate figures, *b* indicate boxes, *t* indicate tables, and *e* and **bold** indicate online content.

Note: Page numbers followed by *f* indicate figures, *b* indicate boxes, *t* indicate tables, and *e* and **bold** indicate online content.

Note: Page numbers followed by *f* indicate figures, *b* indicate boxes, *t* indicate tables, and *e* and **bold** indicate online content.

Note: Page numbers followed by *f* indicate figures, *b* indicate boxes, *t* indicate tables, and *e* and **bold** indicate online content.